Brief Contents of Volume 2

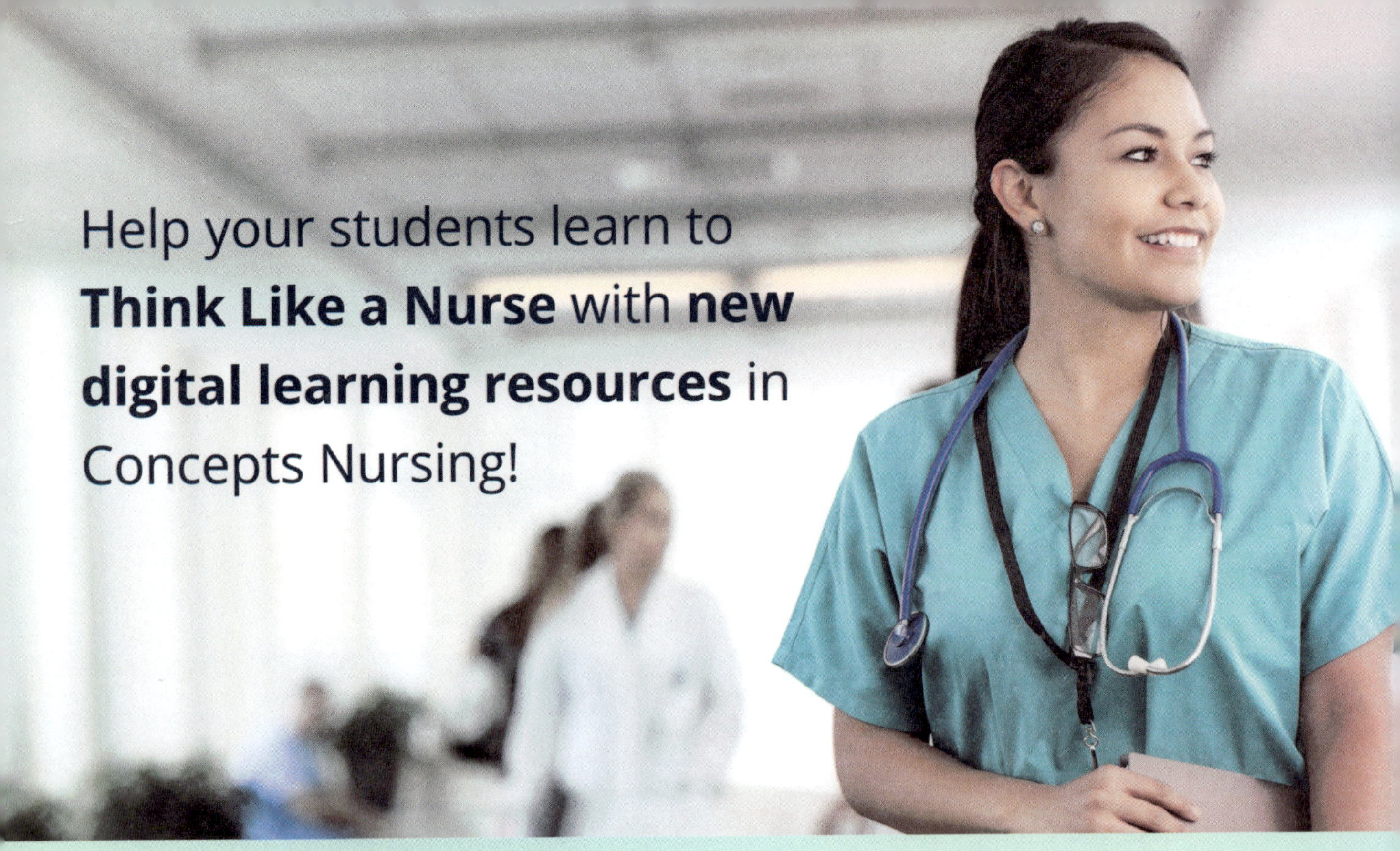

Help your students learn to **Think Like a Nurse** with **new digital learning resources** in Concepts Nursing!

MyLab® Nursing

MyLab Nursing helps students master key concepts, prepare for success on the NCLEX-RN® exam, and develop clinical reasoning skills.

NEW! Adaptive, mobile-enabled Dynamic Study Modules with personalized learning and remediation help students focus their studies and retain information over the long term.

Learn more at pearson.com/mylab/nursing

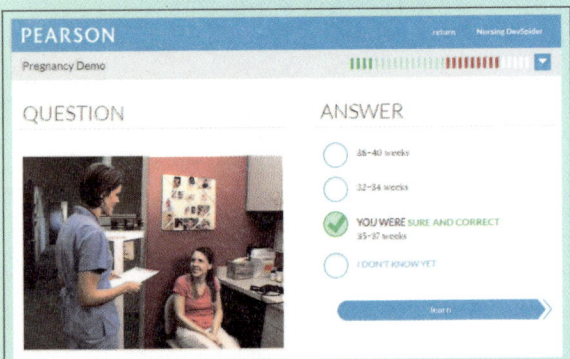

NEW! Concepts Connection in Nursing App

The Concepts Connections in Nursing app helps students make important connections between concepts in nursing and exemplars or alterations. Understanding these key concepts and the connectio between them enables students to focus on the critic thinking and decision-making skills necessary for successful clinical practice. Now available on both the Apple App Store and Google Play.

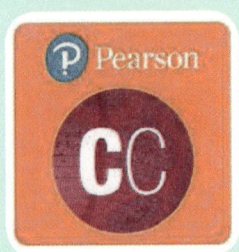

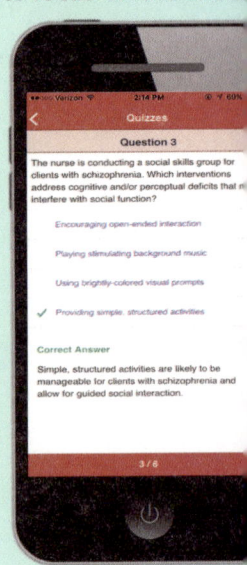

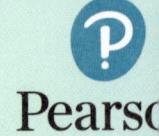

Pearso

VOLUME 1

NURSING
A Concept-Based Approach to Learning

Third Edition

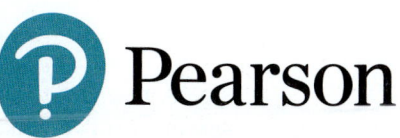

330 Hudson Street, NY, NY 10013

Vice President, Health Science and TED: Julie Levin Alexander
Director of Portfolio Management and Portfolio Manager: Katrin Beacom
Development Editors: Laura S. Horowitz and Adelaide R. McCulloch
Portfolio Management Assistant: Erin Sullivan
Vice President, Content Production and Digital Studio: Paul DeLuca
Managing Producer, Health Science: Melissa Bashe
Content Producer: Bianca Sepulveda
Diversity & Inclusion Specialists: Kendra R. Thomas, JD, and Chuin Phang
Operations Specialist: Maura Zaldivar-Garcia
Creative Director: Blair Brown
Creative Digital Lead: Mary Siener
Director of Digital Production, Digital Studio, Health Science: Amy Peltier
Digital Studio Producer, REVEL and eText 2.0: Jeff Henn
Digital Content Team Lead: Brian Prybella
Digital Content Project Lead: William Johnson
Vice President, Field Marketing: David Gesell
Executive Product Marketing Manager: Christopher Barry
Sr. Field Marketing Manager: Brittany Hammond
Full-Service Project Management and Composition: iEnergizer Aptara®, Ltd.
Project Manager: Kelly Ricci
Inventory Manager: Vatche Demirdjian
Interior Design: Studio Montage
Cover Design: Mary Siener
Cover Art: Studio Montage
Printer/Binder: LSC Communications, Inc.
Cover Printer: Phoenix Color/Hagerstown

Library of Congress Cataloging-in-Publication Data

Title: Nursing: a concept-based approach to learning.
Other titles: Nursing (Pearson)
Description: Third edition. | Boston : Pearson, [2019] | Includes bibliographical references and index.
Identifiers: LCCN 2017043040 | ISBN 9780134616803 (v. 1) | ISBN 0134616804 (v. 1) |
ISBN 9780134616810 (v. 2) | ISBN 0134616812 (v. 2)
Subjects: | MESH: Nursing Care Classification: LCC RT40 | NLM WY 100.1 | DDC 610.73--dc23 LC
record available at https://lccn.loc.gov/2017043040

1 18

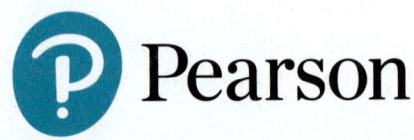

ISBN 13: 978-0-13-461680-3

ISBN 10:   0-13-461680-4

Pearson's Concepts Solution

Nursing: A Concept-Based Approach to Learning is the number one choice for schools of nursing that use a concept-based curriculum. It is the *only* true concept-based learning solution and the *only* concepts curriculum developed from the ground up as a cohesive, comprehensive learning system. The three-volume series, along with MyLab Nursing, provides everything you need to deliver an effective concept-based program that teaches students to think like a nurse and develops practice-ready nurses.

Nursing: A Concept-Based Approach to Learning, Third Edition, represents the cutting edge in nursing education. This uniquely integrated solution provides students with a

consistent design of content and assessment that specifically supports a concept-based curriculum. Available as a fully integrated digital experience or in print format, this solution meets the needs of today's nursing student.

Starting with the cover, our goal for the Third Edition is to help students learn the essential knowledge they will need for patient care. The cover, a Möbius strip, represents the relationships among the concepts and how they are all interconnected. By understanding important connections of concepts, students are able to relate topics to broader contexts.

What Makes Pearson's S[...]

As demonstrated with the previous two editions of *Nu[...] ing: A Concept-Based Approach to Learning,* Pearson's p[...] gram has successfully met the needs of tens of thousan[...] of students and instructors in concept-based educati[...] programs. The Third Edition builds on our commitment [...] excellence: Every page, every word, every feature has be[...] examined—all to help enhance the learning and teach[...] process. The result is an integration of content and f[...] tures that *you*, our customer, have asked for and that [...] will not find anywhere else.

[...] in one package: [...] tools. [...]ers for concep-[...]enabling objec-[...]rable outcomes [...] pregnancy and [...]ence, and into [...]e.

Why Teach Concept-based Lea[...]

University and college nursing programs across the United States have begun evaluating how their programs can meet the needs of today's nursing students. The vast array of new knowledge in the "information age" has left nursing students feeling overwhelmed by the quantity of knowledge and skills they must gain in order to become practicing nurses. In light of this, many programs are moving to the model of concept-based learning in an effort to meet the challenges facing nursing students and new nurses today. Aside from creating a streamlined approach in response to content overload/saturation in nursing education, there are a multitude of reasons for nursing programs to consider a concept-based program.

This model provides the impetus for educators to transition away from traditional methods of faculty-centered teaching and passive learning toward active, focused,

participative, and collaborative teaching and learning. Pearson's *Nursing: A Concept-Based Approach to Learning,* Third Edition, is designed to assist nursing faculty in providing students with a broader perspective while promoting a deeper understanding of content across the lifespan in a focused, participative, and collaborative learning environment.

What are the benefits of conceptual learning? Some of the often-referenced benefits of conceptual learning in nursing programs are that it:

- Focuses on problems
- Fosters systematic observations
- Fosters understanding of relationships
- Focuses on nursing actions and interprofessional efforts
- Challenges students to be excellent learners.

Organization and Structure of the Third Edition

The basic structure of the Second Edition was retained for the Third Edition. There are:

- Five parts:
  - I: The Biophysical Modules (in the Individual Domain)
  - II: The Psychosocial Modules (in the Individual Domain)
  - III: Reproduction (in the Individual Domain)
  - IV: The Nursing Domain
  - V: The Healthcare Domain
- Fifty-one concepts
- One hundred fifty-eight exemplars

The Concepts were chosen after surveying numerous concept-based curricula and finding the common elements. Some Concepts were added or revised in response to requests by users. The result is a comprehensive set of Concepts that cover the essentials of nursing education.

The Exemplars were chosen based on selected national models and initiatives such as those of the Institute of Medicine, *Healthy People 2020,* The Centers for Disease Control and Prevention, The Joint Commission, the National Institutes of Health, the National Institute of Mental Health, the NCLEX Test Plan, The Centers for Medicare and Medicaid, the Occupational Safety and Health Administration, and Quality and Safety Education for Nurses, among others. Prevalence rates were considered for the biophysical and psychosocial exemplars, with more common disorders prioritized over less common ones. Certain Exemplars were chosen because they lend themselves to teaching across concepts or across the lifespan. In the Third Edition, some Exemplars that focused on a particular stage of the lifespan, such as Diabetes in Children, have been folded into the Lifespan Considerations of another exemplar. Now there are two separate Exemplars on diabetes: one focusing on type 1 diabetes mellitus and the other focusing on type 2 diabetes mellitus. In the Third Edition, nine new/expanded Exemplars have been added:

- Cystic Fibrosis
- Delirium
- Environmental Quality
- Nurse Safety
- Patient Safety
- Sexual Dysfunction
- Traumatic Brain Injury
- Type 1 Diabetes Mellitus
- Type 2 Diabetes Mellitus

For the Third Edition, as shown in the Module Outline and Learning Outcomes listed at the beginning of each module, each main section has a dedicated learning outcome. Our editorial and instructional design teams worked to create consistent, accurate, challenging, achievable, and measurable objective statements based on objective-driven design practices to better engage students, improve performance, increase student gains, and promote deep learning.

Module Outline and Learning Outcomes

The Concept of Acid–Base Balance

Normal Acid–Base Balance

1.1 Analyze the physiology of normal acid–base balance.

Alterations to Acid–Base Balance

1.2 Differentiate alterations in acid–base balance.

Concepts Related to Acid–Base Balance

1.3 Outline the relationship between acid–base balance and other concepts.

Health Promotion

1.4 Explain the promotion of healthy acid–base balance.

Nursing Assessment

1.5 Differentiate common assessment procedures and tests used to examine acid–base balance.

Independent Interventions

1.6 Analyze independent interventions nurses can implement for patients with alterations in acid–base balance.

Collaborative Therapies

1.7 Summarize collaborative therapies used by interprofessional teams for patients with alterations in acid–base balance.

Acid–Base Balance Exemplars

Exemplar 1.A Metabolic Acidosis

1.A Analyze metabolic acidosis as it relates to acid–base balance.

Exemplar 1.B Metabolic Alkalosis

1.B Analyze metabolic alkalosis as it relates to acid–base balance.

Exemplar 1.C Respiratory Acidosis

1.C Analyze respiratory acidosis as it relates to acid–base balance.

Exemplar 1.D Respiratory Alkalosis

1.D Analyze respiratory alkalosis as it relates to acid–base balance.

Structure and Features of the Concepts

The Concepts feature a consistent design throughout the program. This allows students to anticipate the learning they will experience. Special features, which students can use for learning and review, recur in each Concept. The basic structure of the Concepts is shown below with visuals and annotations describing the content. Note that each **red heading** has a corresponding learning outcome.

Normal Presentation ... Each Concept starts with a review of normal, healthy function, including subsections on Physiology Review and Genetic Considerations where appropriate.

Physiology Review

Genetic Considerations

Alterations ... The second section of each Concept focuses on alterations, including subheads on Alterations and Manifestations, Prevalence, and Genetic Considerations and Risk Factors. A standard feature in this section is the Alterations and Therapies table.

Alterations and Manifestations

Prevalence

Genetic Considerations and Risk Factors

Alterations and Therapies
Oxygenation

ALTERATION	DESCRIPTION	MANIFESTATIONS	INTERVENTIONS AND THERAPIES
Hypoxemia	Decreased level of oxygen	▪ Chest wall in-drawing (early manifestation) ▪ Cyanosis (late manifestation)	▪ Identify and treat the underlying cause. ▪ Administer oxygen if O_2 saturation level falls below 90%.
Dyspnea	Labored breathing or shortness of breath	▪ Clearly audible, labored breathing; anxiety ▪ Distressed facial expression ▪ Nasal flaring	▪ Identify and treat the underlying cause. ▪ Administer oxygen if O_2 saturation level falls below 90%.
Apnea	Absence of breathing	▪ Lack of respiratory effort that can lead to respiratory arrest	▪ Identify and treat the underlying cause. ▪ Administer respiratory stimulants, as appropriate.
Tachypnea	A respiratory rate greater than 20 breaths per minute for children and adults, 60 breaths per minute for an infant	▪ Excessive rapid breathing ▪ Rapid breathing at rest ▪ Shallow breathing	▪ Identify and treat the underlying cause.
Orthopnea	Difficulty breathing when lying down	▪ Dyspnea while lying down	▪ Identify and treat the underlying cause. ▪ Elevate the head, neck, and chest while sleeping.
Pneumothorax	Lung collapse caused by the collection of free air within the pleural space	▪ Chest pain ▪ Shortness of breath	▪ Identify and treat the underlying cause. ▪ Observe the patient. ▪ Use needle decompression or chest tube insertion. ▪ Surgery

Case Studies

Each Concept contains a three-part unfolding case study to help students apply what they are learning to a sample patient.

Case Study » Part 1

Dennis Welborn is a 52-year-old Caucasian man who visits his primary care physician with complaints of severe pain in his back and abdomen and painful urination with hematuria. As the nurse working at the clinic, you take Mr. Welborn's medical history and make a preliminary assessment. Mr. Welborn is 6'2" tall and weighs 265 pounds. His vital signs include temperature 100.8°F oral, pulse 95 bpm, respirations 22/min, and BP 140/92 mmHg. Mr. Welborn rates his back and abdominal pain as 9 on a scale of 0–10, and his midline abdominal pain level is a 7 when he is urinating. When asked about his diet, Mr. Welborn admits that as a widower, he often eats out with coworkers for lunch and picks up fast food on the way home for his evening meal. He usually drinks three cups of coffee in the morning and diet soda throughout the afternoon and evening. When he gets heartburn, he chews several antacid tablets for relief. An abdominal assessment reveals a distended bladder. Mr. Welborn states he delays urination as long as possible because of the pain. When he does urinate, he has noticed that he has a weak stream and continues to feel the urge to urinate when he has finished. The medical care provider orders lab tests, so a

blood and urine sample are obtained for analysis. Mr. Welborn is transferred to the radiology department to have an abdominal x-ray. The x-ray reveals a large stone (1.2 cm) in Mr. Welborn's proximal right ureter, and the urinalysis indicates the presence of small calcium crystals, RBCs, and bacteria. The blood test also detects high blood calcium levels.

Clinical Reasoning Questions Level I

1. What risk factors does Mr. Welborn have for developing urinary calculi?
2. Other than a distended bladder, what findings might you discover...
3. How...nary...

Clinical Reas...

4. What...
5. What...Mr. W...
6. *Refer*...ment...

Case Study » Part 3

After 3 days in the hospital, Mr. Welborn is discharged to home. His urinary catheter has been removed, and he states that he can urinate without pain. However, the nephrostomy tube remains in place. In addition, his IV morphine has been discontinued, and he now receives acetaminophen (1000 mg q6h). With consistent ambulation and discontinuation of morphine, Mr. Welborn had two bowel movements before discharge.

Clinical Reasoning Questions Level I

1. What methods can you teach Mr. Welborn to help prevent future renal calculi?
2. Describe the patient teaching you will provide Mr. Welborn about caring for his nephrostomy tube.
3. What assessment should be performed on Mr. Welborn before discharge?

Clinical Reasoning Questions Level II

4. What medications might the healthcare provider prescribe for Mr. Welborn upon discharge?
5. What follow-up appointments should you schedule for Mr. Welborn? Why?
6. How would a referral to a nutritionist benefit Mr. Welborn?

Case Study » Part 2

Mr. Welborn's physician consults with a urologist, who suggests that Mr. Welborn be admitted to the hospital for a percutaneous nephrolithotomy. The urologist prescribes intravenous (IV) morphine for pain and schedules the surgery for 8:00 the next morning. The procedure is successful, without complications, and a urinary catheter and nephrostomy tube are put in place during surgery to drain urine. Postoperative pain is again managed with IV morphine, and Mr. Welborn states that his pain is manageable. He is confined to bed until 1 day postsurgery. The day after surgery, Mr. Welborn reports that he did not have his normal morning bowel movement. When he sat on the toilet, he was unable to defecate, and he was afraid to push too hard because of his surgery. He was also unable to have a bowel movement the previous morning because of anxiety about the surgery, and his abdomen is feeling full. Abdominal assessment reveals diminished bowel sounds and dullness to percussion.

Clinical Reasoning Questions Level I

1. What factors may have contributed to Mr. Welborn's constipation?
2. What independent nursing interventions can you implement to help Mr. Welborn eliminate feces?
3. What patient teaching can you provide to help Mr. Welborn prevent constipation in the future?

Clinical Reasoning Questions Level II

4. What effects might Mr. Welborn's constipation have on his urinary problems?
5. What complications may develop as a result of Mr. Welborn's constipation? What assessments should you perform to detect these complications?
6. What side effects of the percutaneous nephrolithotomy may Mr. Welborn experience related to his urinary system?

Concepts Related to
Immunity

CONCEPT	RELATIONSHIP TO IMMUNITY	NURSING IMPLICATIONS
Comfort	Painful conditions, such as swelling and skin reactions, often occur during immune response.	■ Assess related symptoms, such as edema, rash, malaise, loss of appetite, and trouble sleeping. ■ Be alert to topical and latex allergies that could worsen symptoms. ■ *Anticipate:* Additional assessments, comfort measures
Infection	Patients with alterations in immunity can experience acute or chronic infections.	■ Assess area of suspected infection (see Infection Assessment section in the module on Infection). ■ Educate patients regarding the importance of immunizations and encourage their use. ■ Educate patients regarding the importance of avoiding situations that could increase exposure to infection. ■ Practice standard precautions, proper hand hygiene, and aseptic/sterile technique with all procedures. ■ Assess complete blood count (CBC) results; be alert for elevated WBC count.
Inflammation	Movement of fluid and cells to the site of injury or infection causes inflammation during an immune response.	■ Assess for fever, skin warmth and redness, edema, and generalized pain. ■ Be alert for abscess formation, purulent exudate, and increased WBC count. ■ *Anticipate:* Aspirin, antipyretics, cold packs
Managing Care	Patients with alterations in their immune system can greatly benefit from participating in managed care and have more positive health outcomes.	■ Assess the needs of patients to identify actual or potential problems related to care. ■ Advocate for patients in relation to their care needs.

Concepts Related to ... Enhanced for the Third Edition, the Concepts Related to section and feature are designed to help students make linkages between and among different Concepts.

Health Promotion ... New to the Third Edition is a focus on health promotion, one of the foundations of nursing. Many Health Promotion sections include a Patient Teaching feature. Examples of subsections include:

Modifiable Risk Factors

Care in the Community

Patient Teaching
Health Promotion for Cancer Prevention: Modifiable Risk Factors

■ *Discourage smoking or use of other tobacco products.* Emphasize the importance of patients protecting children and themselves from exposure to tobacco smoke. This is one of the most important health decisions an individual can make.

■ *Encourage patients, especially children, to consume a healthy diet.* This should include a minimum of five servings of fruits and vegetables daily as well as whole grains, iron-rich foods, and foods that are rich in vitamin B_{12}. Teach patients to limit their consumption of processed meats; drink alcohol in moderation; and choose fewer high-calorie foods.

■ *Explain the importance of maintaining a healthy weight and being physically active.* Physical activity helps to control weight. Together, these factors may lower the risk for various types of cancer.

■ *Teach patients effective ways to protect themselves from ultraviolet radiation.* Early excessive exposure to sun and one or more severe sunburns during childhood increase the chances of skin cancers developing in adulthood. Patients who work outdoors, athletes, coaches, and others who spend time outside regularly should use sunscreen daily (SPF 15 or greater), regardless of the climate in which they live. Emphasize the importance of avoiding midday sun, when the sun's rays are strongest. Instruct patients to cover exposed skin and wear a hat with a wide brim. They should avoid tanning beds and sunlamps.

■ *Explain the importance of avoiding risky behaviors.* Practicing risky behaviors such as needle sharing or unsafe sexual contact can increase the risk of developing certain cancers.

■ *Suggest that patients have their homes tested for radon and explore their exposure to harmful chemicals.* Patients may be exposed to hazardous substances in the home or in the workplace.

■ *Stress the importance of getting immunizations, receiving regular medical care, and doing self-examinations.* By protecting against certain viral infections, immunizations can decrease the risk of some cancers. Regular screenings and self-examinations increase the chances of early detection of cancer, allowing for a better chance of successful treatment (Mayo Clinic, 2015a).

Oxygenation Assessment

ASSESSMENT/ METHOD	NORMAL FINDINGS	ABNORMAL FINDINGS	LIFESPAN OR DEVELOPMENTAL CONSIDERATIONS
Nasal Assessment			
Inspect the nose symmetry.	The nose should be midline and symmetrical.	■ Asymmetry indicates trauma or surgery.	■ Nasal flaring in the neonate may be indicative of respiratory compromise.
Inspect nasal cavity using a flashlight.	The septum should fall midline and be intact. The mucosa of the nares should be pink and moist without drainage. Both nares should be patent.	■ Redness and/or swelling is observed. ■ Deviated septum narrows or occludes one naris. ■ Foreign bodies may be found in the nares, especially of infants, toddlers, and preschoolers. ■ Purulent or watery nasal drainage is present. ■ Pale turbinates are seen.	■ Nasal passages of neonates and small children are smaller than those of adults. Ensuring a clear nasal cavity may decrease the risk for respiratory compromise, as neonates and infants are nasal breathers.
Respiratory Rate Assessment			
Count respiratory rate for one full minute, counting one inspiration and one expiration as one breath.	Normal respiratory rate is eupnea (see Table 15–1 for developmental impact on rate).	■ Bradypnea ■ Tachypnea ■ Apnea ■ Cheyne-Stokes respirations	■ A child's respiratory rate is higher than that of an adult's. Rely on both sight and touch to obtain an accurate respiratory rate. Neonates are sporadic breathers so short periods of apnea (less than 15 seconds) are expected.
Assess quality of breathing: determine regularity in timing. Assess depth of inspiration. Observe effort to breathe.	The I:E ratio is normally 1:2. The cycle of inspiration and expiration should be followed by a resting period in which the sensors of the respiratory system will initiate the next cycle. Normal breathing is referred to as eupnea.	■ Shortness of breath ■ Dyspnea ■ Orthopnea	■ Infants and children have softer chest walls and depend more heavily on the diaphragm to breathe. Therefore, they exhibit what is known as "seesaw" breathing, an indicator of severe distress. ■ In older adults, lifestyle choices such as smoking can affect the quality of breathing, as can the development of respiratory diseases.
Inspection of Thoracic Cavity			
Anteroposterior diameter is half the transverse diameter.	Normal ratio is 1:2. (See **Figures 15–5 >>** and **15–6 >>**.)	■ Anteroposterior equals transverse thoracic diameter measurements, called a barrel chest.	■ Rapid growth early in life, the plateau in young adulthood, and decline in later life can affect normal ratios.

Nursing Assessment ... Restructured for the Third Edition, this section covers everything the new nurse needs to know about assessing patients. It includes information on:

Observation and Patient Interview

Physical Examination

Diagnostic Tests

Independent Interventions ... Emphasizes interventions that nurses can perform on their own, without an order from the healthcare provider. Examples of subsections include:

Prevent Infection

Promote Safety

Sleep Hygiene

Medications
Antimicrobial Agents

CLASSIFICATION AND DRUG EXAMPLES	MECHANISMS OF ACTION	NURSING CONSIDERATIONS
Antibiotics • Amino-glycosides • Macrolides • Tetracyclines • Cephalosporins • Penicillins • Sulfonamides • Fluoroquinolones *Drug examples:* Cefaclor, erythromycin, penicillin, tobramycin, trimethoprim-sulfamethoxazole	Antibiotics may be used prophylactically to prevent infection or used to treat existing bacterial infection. A specific antibiotic is chosen on the basis of the pathogen causing the infection.	• Teach patients the importance of taking the entire prescribed amount. • Encourage adequate fluid intake. • Monitor for signs of allergic reaction. • Assess renal and hepatic function and vital signs.
Antifungal *Drug examples:* Amphotericin B, anidulafungin, caspofungin acetate, flucytosine, micafungin, fluconazole, nystatin	These drugs are selective for fungal plasma membranes. They inhibit ergosterol synthesis.	• Carefully monitor the patient's condition. • Use cautiously in patients with renal impairment and severe bone marrow suppression as well as patients who are pregnant. • Closely monitor kidney function (intake and output, BUN, creatinine, daily weights). • Monitor serum electrolytes.
Antipyretic, Analgesic *Drug example:* Acetaminophen	These drugs relieve pain and reduce fever.	• Monitor temperature. • Assess pain level. • Teach proper administration.
Antipyretic, Analgesic, Anti-inflammatory *Drug examples:* Aspirin, ibuprofen	These drugs reduce fever and inflammation, in addition to relieving pain.	• Monitor temperature. • Assess pain level. • Teach proper administration.

Collaborative Therapies ... Each Concept includes an overview of relevant therapies that require collaboration with the interprofessional team. A Medications feature covers the most common drugs used to treat alterations. Examples of subsections include:

Surgery

Pharmacologic Therapy

Nonpharmacologic Therapy

Complementary Health Approaches

REVIEW The Concept of ... As in the Second Edition, each Concept ends with a review that includes linking questions, a list of relevant skills from Volume 3, and a short case study with questions so students can apply their knowledge.

REVIEW The Concept of Elimination

RELATE Link the Concepts

Linking the concept of elimination with the concept of infection:
1. What changes in urinary elimination indicate the presence of a UTI?
2. List the effects viral gastroenteritis has on bowel elimination.

Linking the concept of elimination with the concept of communication:
3. How can therapeutic communication be beneficial when assessing patients with urinary or bowel elimination problems?
4. Describe the importance of accurate documentation when caring for a hospitalized patient with urinary or bowel elimination problems.

READY Go to Volume 3: Clinical Nursing Skills

▪ SKILL 1.10	Abdomen: Assessing
▪ SKILL 2.25	Rectal Medication: Administering
▪ SKILLS 4.1–4.5	Elimination: Assessment—Collecting Specimens
▪ SKILLS 4.6–4.16	Elimination: Bladder Interventions
▪ SKILLS 4.17–4.23	Elimination: Bowel Interventions
▪ SKILLS 4.24–4.27	Elimination: Dialysis
▪ SKILL 6.1	Hand Hygiene: Performing

REFER Go to Pearson MyLab Nursing and eText
▪ Additional review materials
▪ MiniModule: Anatomy and Physiology of Urinary Elimination

REFLECT Apply Your Knowledge
Tony Norwinski is a 7-year-old boy in the second grade. He and his 4-year-old sister, Nyla, live at home with their mother, Diane Norwinski.

Ms. Norwinski is a single parent who works in the cafeteria at the high school. Tony has a problem with wetting the bed occasionally and is too embarrassed to discuss it with anyone. Ms. Norwinski thinks Tony wets the bed because of emotional problems caused by his father leaving them when he was so young. Ms. Norwinski does not want to try anything new to help with the bedwetting because she is afraid it will cause Tony more embarrassment and emotional upset. They try not to talk about the bedwetting because Ms. Norwinski thinks it will make matters worse for Tony and prolong the problem.

Today, both children have an appointment for an annual physical examination with the nurse practitioner prior to starting the new school year. Tony is soft spoken and reserved when questioned about his general heath. Ms. Norwinski is a good historian and offers complete answers about Tony's health history. The nurse notices the odor of urine on Tony's undergarments during the initial assessment. When questioned, Tony looks at his mother and does not answer. Ms. Norwinski looks away and does not answer right away. The nurse remains silent, waiting for a response to the questions.

After a period of silence, Ms. Norwinski reassures Tony and answers the nurse's questions about the odor. Though embarrassed, Tony appears to trust the nurse because he helps his mother explain about the bedwetting.

1. What therapeutic communication techniques could the nurse use to facilitate a full disclosure of the problem?
2. What are some questions the nurse could ask Tony and his mother to obtain the most pertinent information about Tony's situation? What nursing diagnosis would best describe the priority problem?
3. List four other possible nursing diagnoses the nurse may want to incorporate in the plan of care.

Structure and Features of the Exemplars

The structure of the Exemplars is picked up from the Second Edition. Note that each Exemplar has one main learning outcome with multiple enabling objectives.

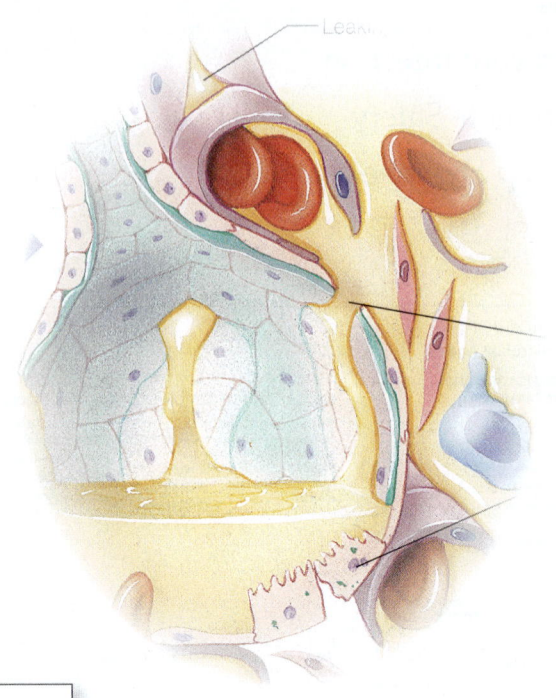

Overview ... Sets the stage for the Exemplar and often includes information on the prevalence of the disorder.

Pathophysiology and Etiology ... Describes not only the pathophysiology and etiology of the disorder, but also risk factors and prevention methods.

Pathophysiology

Etiology

Risk Factors

Prevention

Clinical Manifestations and Therapies
Chronic Obstructive Pulmonary Disease

ETIOLOGY	CLINICAL MANIFESTATIONS	CLINICAL THERAPIES
Bronchitis	■ Chronic cough with mucus production ■ Dyspnea ■ Tachycardia ■ Narrowed airway passages ■ Wheezing ■ Air trapping	■ Smoking cessation ■ Bronchodilators ■ Corticosteroids ■ Fluids to thin secretions ■ Elevating the head of the bed ■ Low-flow oxygen ■ Monitoring of ABGs and oxygen ■ Mechanical ventilation if patient cannot meet oxygen demands
Emphysema	■ Air trapping ■ Possible wheezing ■ Dyspnea ■ Barrel chest ■ Pursed-lip breathing ■ Posturing	■ Oxygen administration as needed ■ Pursed-lip breathing technique ■ Patient education of posture changes to improve ventilation ■ Low-flow oxygen ■ Monitoring of ABGs and oxygen ■ Mechanical ventilation if patient cannot meet oxygen demands ■ Nutritional assessment and increased calorie intake

Cardiac dysfunction	■ Chest pain
	■ Poor perfusion
	■ Arrhythmias, particularly premature ventricular contractions
	■ Hypertension
	■ Cardiac hypertrophy
	■ Congestive heart failure
		■ Medications:
		  a. Positive inotropics
		  b. Calcium blockers
		  c. Antiarrhythmic medications
		  d. Diuretics
		  e. Nitrites
		  f. Antihypertensives
		■ Monitoring of exercise tolerance
		■ Holter monitoring
		■ Antiembolism stockings to improve venous return
		■ Fluid restrictions if cardiac dysfunction not medically managed

Clinical Manifestations ... Includes information on clinical manifestations the nurse might see in a patient with the disorder. The Clinical Manifestations and Therapies feature is an excellent tool for review.

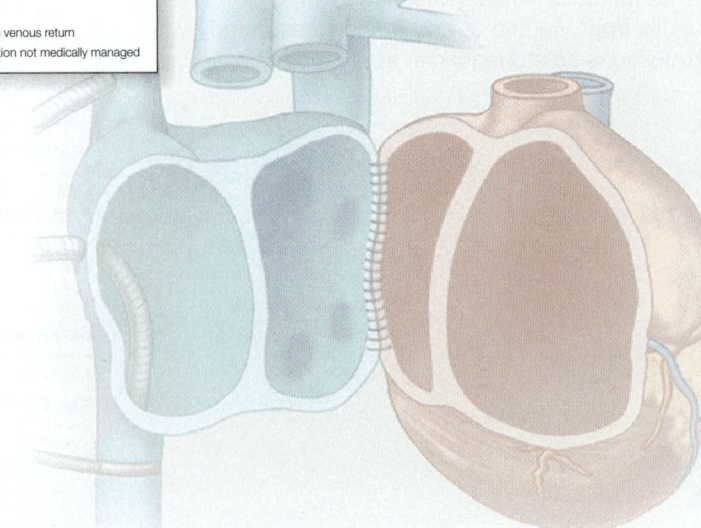

Collaboration ... Outlines interprofessional interventions and therapies appropriate for patients with the disorder.

Diagnostic Tests

Surgery

Pharmacologic Therapy

Nonpharmacologic Therapy

Complementary Health Approaches

Lifespan Considerations ... New to the Third Edition, all specifics relevant to the lifespan are gathered in one section. Lifespan Considerations are provided as appropriate for both Concepts and Exemplars. Examples of subsections include:

Considerations for Infants

Considerations for Children and Adolescents

Considerations for Pregnant Women

Considerations for Older Adults

Nursing Process ... A detailed look at the nursing process helps students put together all of the content in the exemplar and learn the essentials of providing care to patients with the disorder.

Assessment

Diagnosis

Planning

Implementation

Evaluation

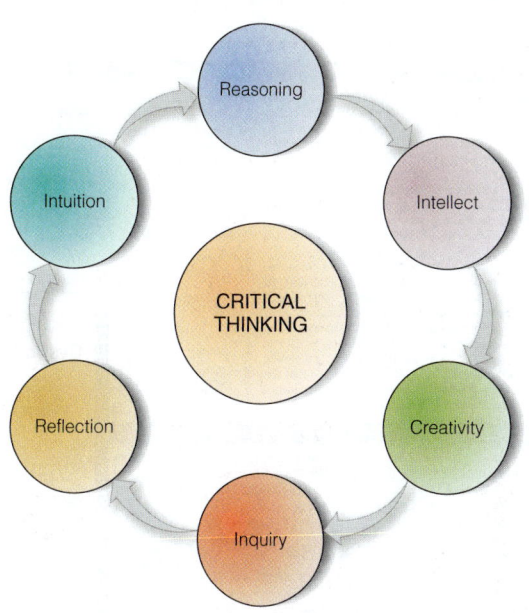

REVIEW Exemplar ... As in the Second Edition, each exemplar ends with a Review that includes linking questions and a short case study with questions to help students apply their knowledge.

REVIEW Benign Prostatic Hyperplasia

RELATE Link the Concepts and Exemplars

Linking the exemplar of BPH with the concept of sexuality:

1. What communication strategies would the nurse use to discuss the impact BPH will have on sexuality without making an older man feel uncomfortable?

2. How can you assess his concerns, fears, and knowledge regarding the impact of BPH on his sexuality?

Linking the exemplar of BPH with the concept of infection:

3. What pathophysiology of BPH could increase the risk of UTIs?

4. What nursing interventions will reduce the risk of UTIs?

READY Go to Volume 3: Clinical Nursing Skills

REFER Go to Pearson MyLab Nursing and eText

■ Additional review materials

REFLECT Apply Your Knowledge

Clifford Allen is a middle manager for a small manufacturing company where he has worked for the last 20 years. Overall, Mr. Allen is in good health, although he has been undergoing treatment recently for BPH. He has a history of depression, for which he does not seek treatment because he fears the social stigma connected to the diagnosis. Mr. Allen has been considering retiring within the next few years so he and his wife can travel, but mostly to escape his stressful work environment. He enjoys bowling and is involved in activities at church. He and his wife go for a walk each evening after supper.

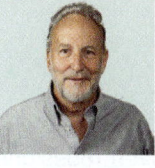

One evening while bowling, he notices that his bladder feels somewhat full. Mr. Allen calls to make an appointment to see his urologist for a follow-up examination. He has been taking finasteride (Proscar) for the last 6 months but does not believe it has been particularly effective. He still has trouble urinating and believes that his symptoms are worse than before he started taking the drug. When he sees the urologist 2 weeks later, he reports that he often feels his bladder is full after voiding, he has difficulty starting his stream of urine, and his stream is weak once started. He gets up frequently at night to void. His score on the AUASI is 28, which has increased from his score of 18 six months ago. The urologist confirms that the medication has not been effective and schedules further tests, including uroflowmetry, check postvoid residual, a PSA blood test, and a urinalysis. Results from the uroflowmetry and postvoid residual test show a significant obstruction of urinary flow. The serum PSA is negative, and the urinalysis is consistent with bladder inflammation. A TURP is recommended in the upcoming weeks.

1. To determine Mr. Allen's understanding of the procedure, what will the nurse want to ask him upon admission to the surgical center?

2. What teaching will the nurse prepare regarding postoperative self-care?

3. Design a nursing plan of care for this patient postoperatively.

Additional Features

Additional features found throughout the program include numbered tables, figures, and boxes that contain content presented in visual formats, and the following highlighted features: Safety Alert, Stay Current, Evidence-Based Practice, Nursing Care Plan, Focus on Diversity and Culture, and Focus on Integrative Health.

Nursing Care Plan
A Patient with Asthma

Sarah Mitchell is a 35-year-old working mother with moderate persistent asthma. Her known triggers are allergies to dust mites, cockroach feces, grass and tree pollens, and some molds. She takes immunotherapy once a week and takes maintenance medications daily. She works as a full-time preschool teacher.

Ms. Mitchell calls her allergist's office asking to be seen because she is having a bad asthma flare. She reports having to use her rescue inhaler every 3–4 hours, that her chest is very tight, and that she is having trouble breathing. She has used her home peak flow meter three times since late yesterday and has been in the yellow zone each time. She did not sleep last night because of her asthma symptoms.

ASSESSMENT	DIAGNOSES	PLANNING
The nurse, Clancy O'Hara, admits Ms. Mitchell when she arrives at the allergist's office. During the health history Ms. Mitchell confirms she is compliant with her medication regimen. She takes a LABA in combination with a low-dose corticosteroid, a daily antihistamine, and montelukast. In checking Ms. Mitchell's medical record, Nurse O'Hara notes that the patient is maintaining her scheduled immunotherapy appointments. Ms. Mitchell reports that she is not aware of any unusual allergy exposure but says that several of her students have a cold this week. On physical examination, Nurse O'Hara notes that Ms. Mitchell's vital signs are as follows: T 37°C (98.6°F); P 96 bpm; R 36/min; BP 128/86 mmHg. Other assessment data include needing to pause frequently while speaking, use of accessory muscles for respirations, and scattered wheezes audible over both lung fields with stethoscope. ABG results are pH 7.32, PaO_2 88 mmHg, $PaCO_2$ 47 mmHg, and HCO_3 38 mEq/L. Pulses are strong and equal bilaterally, and the patient expectorates a small amount of white mucus into a tissue.	■ *Ineffective Breathing Pattern* related to exacerbation of asthma ■ *Impaired Gas Exchange* related to bronchoconstriction and mucus in airways ■ *Fatigue* related to ineffective sleep pattern ■ *Activity Intolerance* related to inadequate oxygenation (NANDA-I © 2014)	Together Nurse O'Hare and Ms. Mitchell agree on the following outcomes: ■ The patient's breathing will return to the green zone within 24 hours. ■ The patient's need for her rescue inhaler will decline within 3 days and return to baseline within 1 week. ■ The patient will maintain baseline respiratory rate and pattern sufficient to meet her ADLs within

IMPLEMENTATION

Ms. Mitchell's provider prescribes a higher-dose inhaled steroid to use 10–15 minutes after she uses her LABA. The provider also gives Ms. Mitchell a short, tapered course of prednisone. Ms. O'Hare initiates the following implementations:

■ Teaches Ms. Mitchell how to properly self-administer medications and about possible side effects associated with steroid use, including those that should be reported immediately

■ Explains the importance of taking the steroid as ordered and not stopping the medication suddenly

■ Provides strategies for managing fatigue, including a handout with written instructions

■ Teaches Ms. [...] hydration in a [...]
■ Observes Ms. [...]
■ Reviews sig[...] and instructs [...]
■ Schedules M[...] evaluation bu[...] or if she sees [...]

Many exemplars contain **Nursing Care Plans**, and additional ones can be found in the Pearson eText in MyLab Nursing. The Nursing Care Plans follow the nursing process with sections on assessment, diagnosis, planning, implementation, and evaluation. They end with a series of Critical Thinking questions.

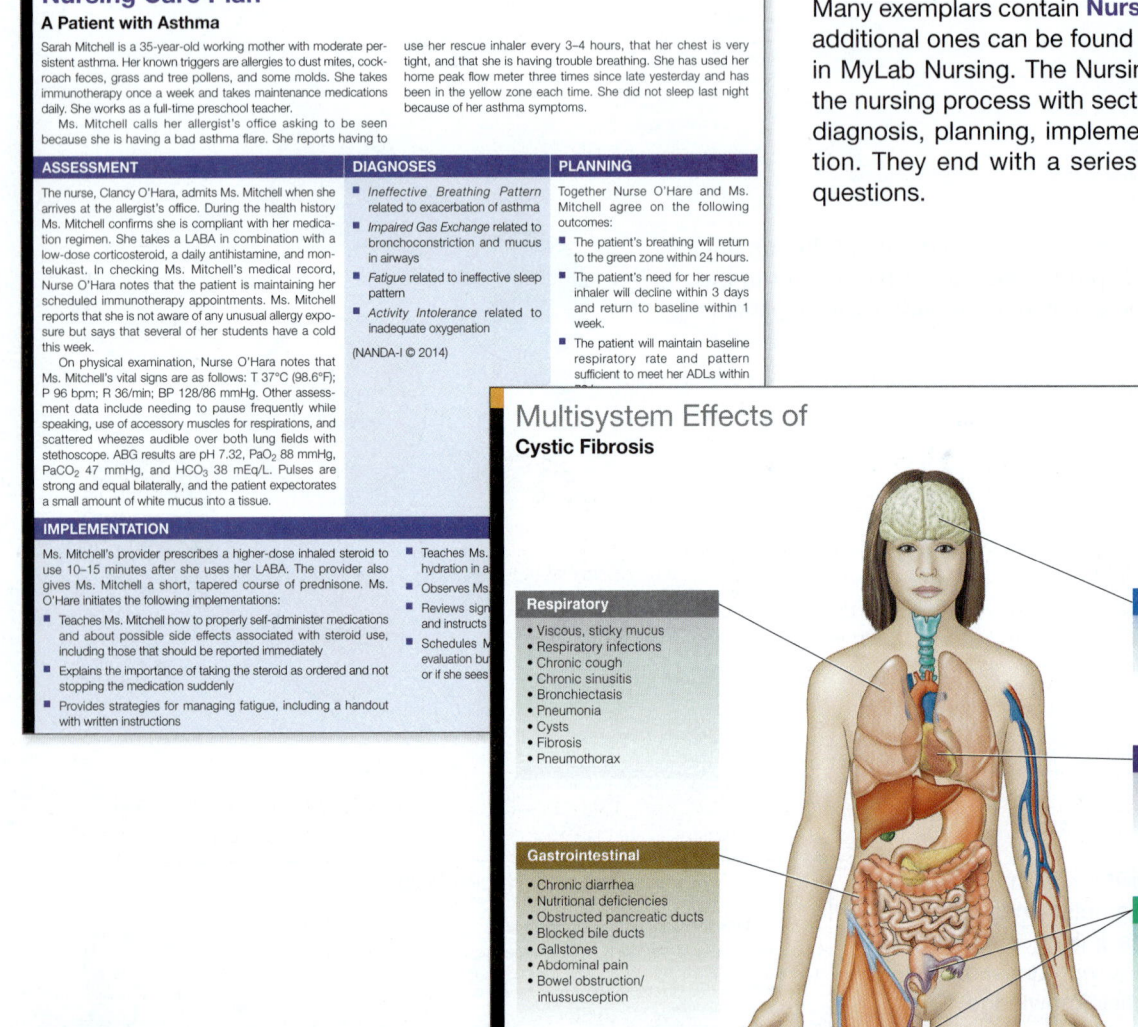

Multisystem Effects of
Cystic Fibrosis

Respiratory
- Viscous, sticky mucus
- Respiratory infections
- Chronic cough
- Chronic sinusitis
- Bronchiectasis
- Pneumonia
- Cysts
- Fibrosis
- Pneumothorax

Gastrointestinal
- Chronic diarrhea
- Nutritional deficiencies
- Obstructed pancreatic ducts
- Blocked bile ducts
- Gallstones
- Abdominal pain
- Bowel obstruction/intussusception

Musculoskeletal
- Delayed growth and development
- Osteopenia
- Osteoporosis
- Fractures

Neurologic
- Depression
- Anxiety

Cardiovascular
- Clubbing of fingers and toes
- Cyanosis

Reproductive
- Delayed puberty
- Blockage or absence of vas deferens
- Decreased fertility (men and women)
- Pregnancy complications

Integumentary
- Salty skin

Metabolic Processes
- Diabetes

The **Multisystem Effects** features have been redesigned for the Third Edition. Each one highlights the effects that a disorder has on various systems of the body.

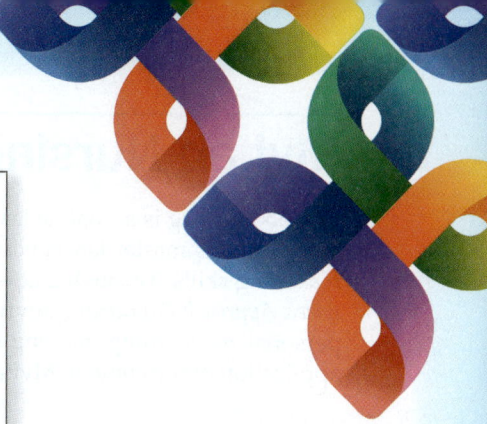

Focus on Integrative Health
Chronic Obstructive Pulmonary Disease

Complementary health approaches may be useful to help manage symptoms of COPD. Dietary measures, such as minimizing intake of dairy products and salt, may help reduce mucus
production and keep mucus more liquefied. Be sure to recommend measures to replace the protein and calcium in dairy
products to help maintain nutritional balance. Hot herbal teas
made with peppermint may act as expectorants to help relieve
chest congestion.

Patients may be interested in trying complementary health
approaches to assist them in quitting smoking. While additional
studies are needed to evaluate the effectiveness of complementary health approaches for use in quitting smoking, current
research suggests that acupuncture and hypnotherapy may be
effective in promoting smoking cessation (Tahiri et al., 2012).
Likewise, Hasan et al. (2014) found that hypnotherapy may be
more effective than NRT for promotion of smoking cessation.

Focus on Diversity and Culture
Assessing for Cyanosis

When assessing for cyanosis, normal assessment findings vary
depending on the individual's normal skin tones. For example,
in a white or light-skinned individual, cyanosis due to hypoxemia most often manifests as a bluish discoloration of the lips,
oral mucosa, and nail beds. Among dark-skinned individuals,
cyanosis may be difficult to detect and may actually cause the
skin to appear darker. Typical manifestations of cyanosis in
dark-skinned individuals include pallor or an ash-gray discoloration of the skin surrounding the mouth. Conjunctivae appear
gray or blue-tinged among dark-skinned individuals. Among
patients whose normal skin tone is yellowish, cyanosis may
manifest as a gray–green skin discoloration (Sommers, 2011).

For the most part, care of patients from different cultures is covered in the basal text. **Focus
on Diversity and Culture** features are used only for unique situations of which the nurse
should be aware.

Focus on Integrative Health boxes highlight the use of complementary health approaches
in addition to traditional nursing practice.

SAFETY ALERT Chronic cough and sputum are not normal
occurrences. An individual experiencing chronic cough and sputum
beyond 3–4 days should consult with a healthcare professional. Individuals with a smoking history as well as chronic cough and sputum
production should have PFTs to determine lung function.

Each **Safety Alert** provides critical information the
nurse needs to know to keep patients and staff safe.

>> **Stay Current:** Visit the Safe to Sleep website at https://
www.nichd.nih.gov/sts/Pages/default.aspxto learn more about
SIDS prevention.

The **Stay Current** feature provides a weblink (which
is a hot link in the eText) to a website that will keep
students informed on the most recent updates.

The goal of the **Evidence-Based Practice**
features is to show students the necessity of
evidence driving practice. Each starts with a
problem, delves into the research, presents implications for the nurse, and ends with critical thinking questions for the student.

Evidence-Based Practice
Compliance with Safe to Sleep Recommendations

Problem

Compared to previous recommendations for preventing SIDS, current recommendations are more complex. For example, the Safe to
Sleep guidelines address not only infant positioning but also maintaining a safe sleep environment and abstaining from co-sleeping
(bed sharing). The increased complexity of the recommendations
may lead to decreased parental compliance with current guidelines
for the prevention of SIDS (Goodstein, Bell, & Krugman, 2015).

Evidence

The Safe to Sleep recommendations include supine positioning during sleep, using a firm sleep surface, breastfeeding, room sharing
without co-sleeping, routine immunizations, and the use of a pacifier.
Items that should be avoided include soft bedding, toys, layered
clothing, and crib bumpers (USDHHS, 2015). Research suggests
that parental adherence to current recommendations for the prevention of SIDS is significantly increased when nurses model the behaviors that are reflective of all current guidelines for preventing SIDS and
obtain parental signatures on a document acknowledging receipt of
education related to current guidelines (Goodstein et al., 2015).

Implications

Nurses should demonstrate endorsement of all current recommendations for reducing SIDS-related deaths, including modeling and
implementing all recommendations as soon as the infant is clinically stable and up to discharge. Nurses working with parents of
newborns must provide additional patient teaching and follow-up,
as well as ensuring that parents understand the teaching. All parents should receive documented education on safe infant sleep
practices, including voluntary acknowledgement forms indicating
that education has been provided with regard to the specific current guidelines (Goodstein et al., 2015).

Critical Thinking Application

1. Identify barriers to educating parents and caregivers about
   current recommendations for preventing sleep-associated
   deaths.
2. Describe methods for evaluating parental understanding of
   the current guidelines for prevention of SIDS.

MyLab Nursing

MyLab Nursing is an online learning and practice environment that works with the text to help students master key concepts, prepare for the NCLEX-RN exam, and develop clinical reasoning skills. Through a new mobile experience, students can study *Nursing: A Concept-Based Approach to Learning* anytime, anywhere. New adaptive technology with remediation personalizes learning, moving students beyond memorization to true understanding and application of the content. MyLab Nursing contains the following features:

Dynamic Study Modules ... New adaptive learning modules with remediation that personalize the learning experience by allowing students to increase both their confidence and their performance while being assessed in real time.

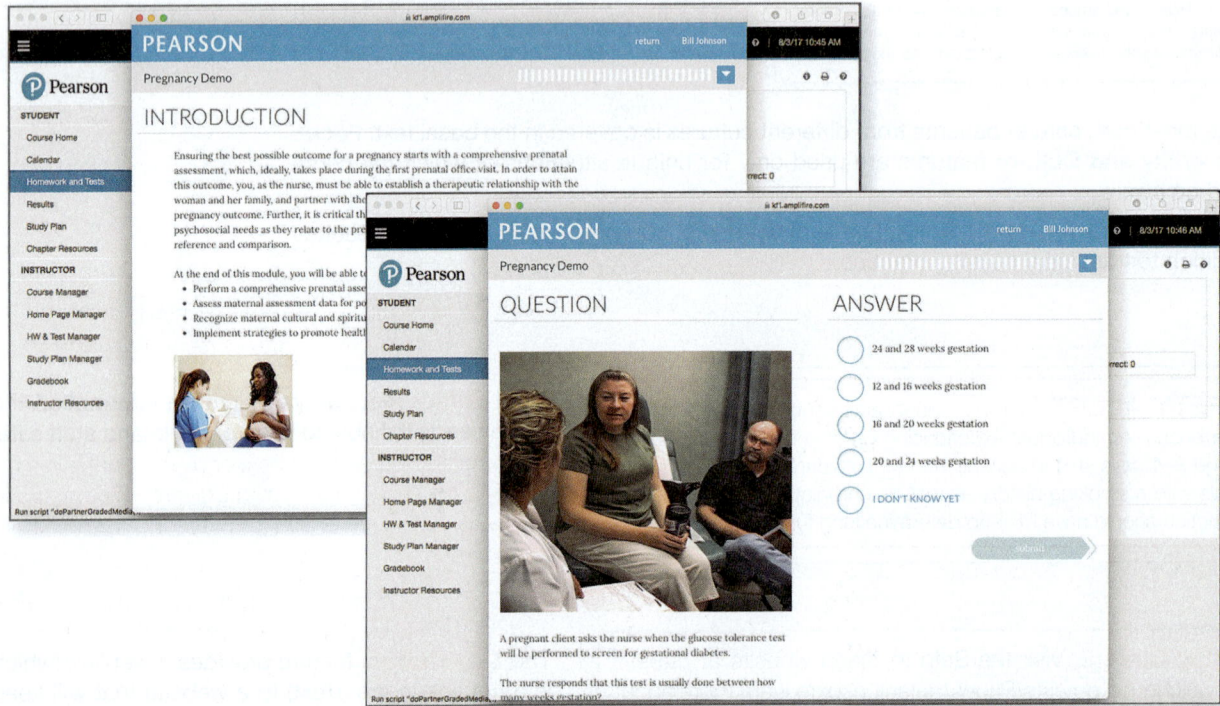

NCLEX-Style Questions ... Practice tests with more than 3000 NCLEX-style questions of various types build student confidence and prepare them for success on the NCLEX-RN exam. Questions are organized by Concept and Exemplar.

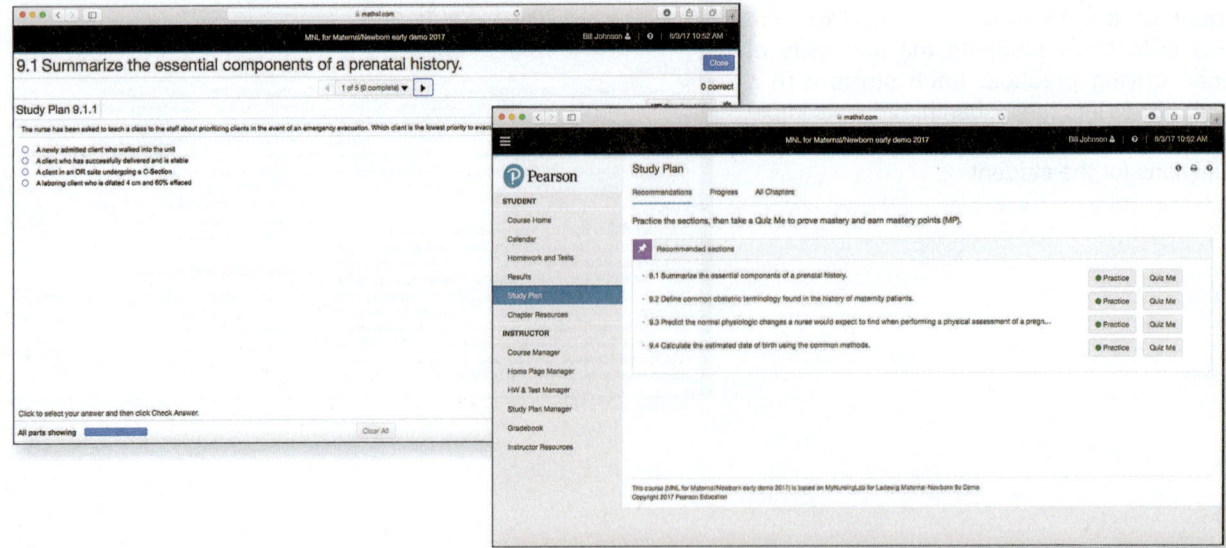

Decision Making Cases ... Clinical case studies that provide opportunities for students to practice analyzing information and making important decisions at key moments in patient care scenarios. These case studies are designed to help prepare students for clinical practice.

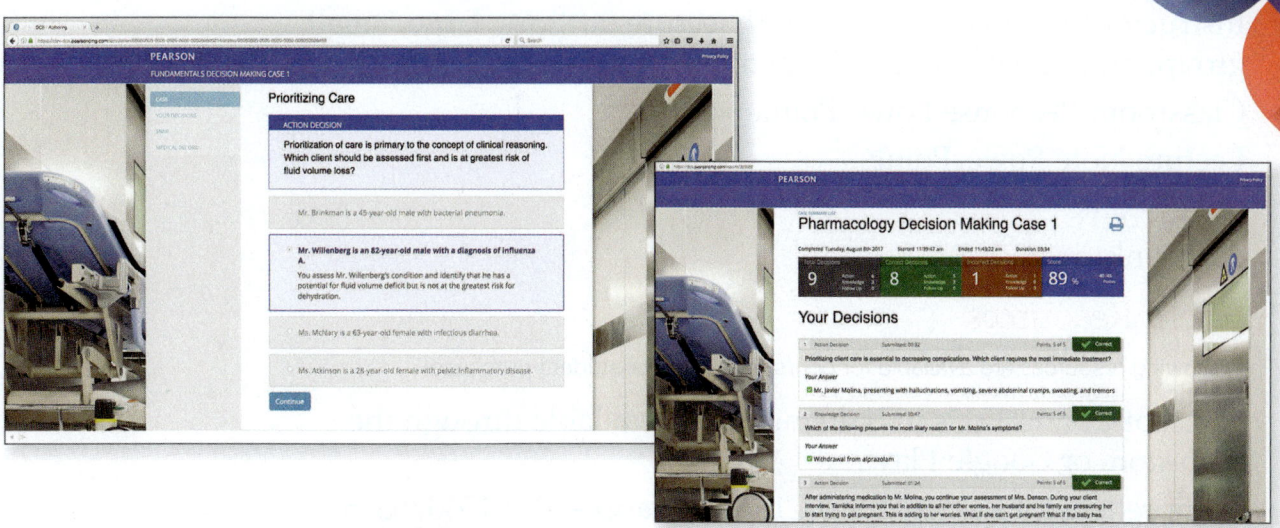

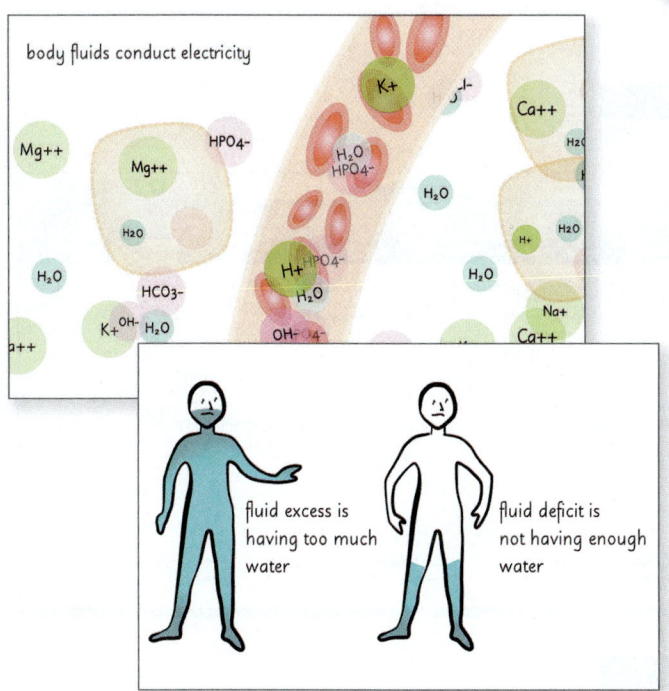

Pearson eText ... Enhances student learning both in and outside the classroom. Students can take notes, highlight, and bookmark important content, or engage with interactive and rich media to achieve greater conceptual understanding of the Concepts and their Exemplars. Interactive features include audio clips, pop-up definitions, figures, questions and answers, the nursing process, hotspots, and video animations. Some examples of video animations include:

- **Fluid and Electrolyte Animations** provide students with the necessary information about the balance and imbalance of fluids and electrolytes to think, reason, and make clinical judgments.

- **Congenital Heart Defect Animations** illustrate the many congenital heart defects that may occur in newborns and provide students the opportunity to see, hear, and understand how congenital heart defects impair the correct functioning of the heart and how they may be corrected.

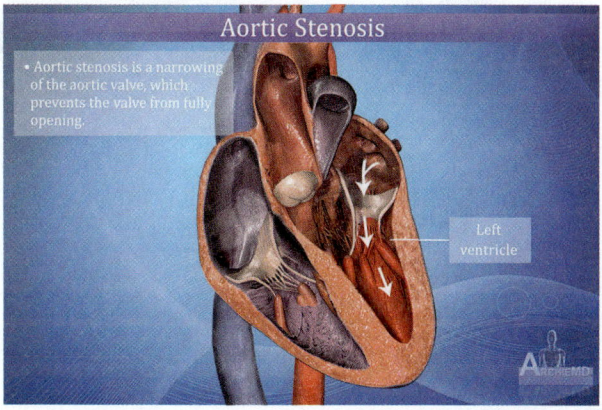

Resources

Instructor Resources

Instructor Resource Manual—with lecture outlines, large/small group, individual, and clinical activities

Classroom Response PowerPoints

Lecture Note PowerPoints

Image bank

Test bank

Student Resources

The following resources are available for course adoption or student purchase:

Concept Connections in Nursing app—available through the App store or Google Play

Comprehensive Review for NCLEX-RN app—9780134376325

RealEHRprep with iCare

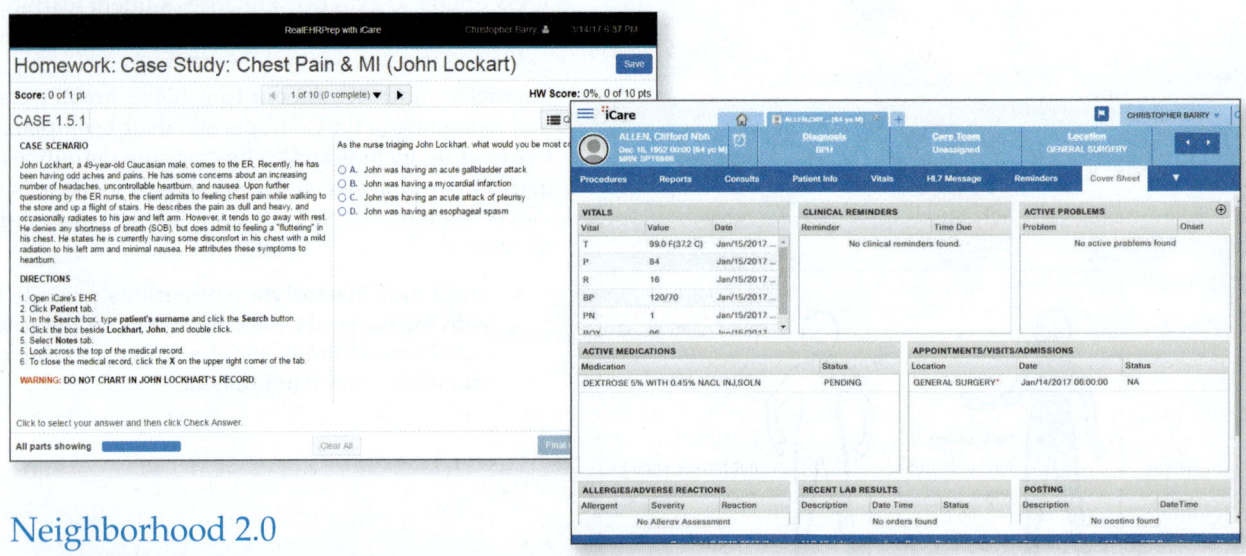

Neighborhood 2.0

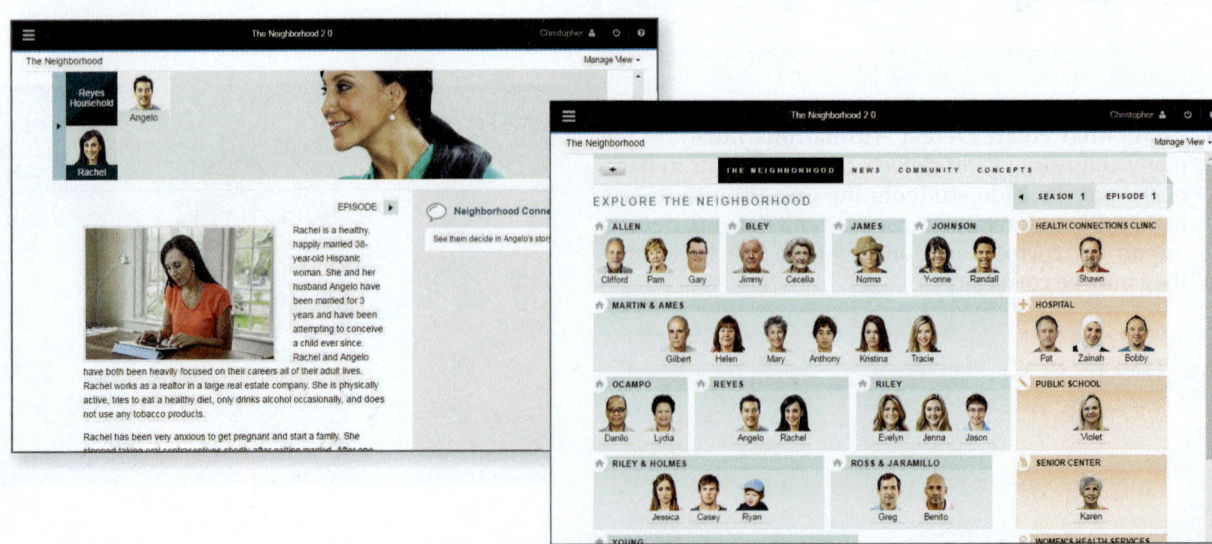

Acknowledgments

We would like to extend our heartfelt thanks to more than 80 instructors from schools of nursing across the country who have given their time generously during the past few years to help us create this concept-based learning package. The talented faculty on our Concepts Editorial Board and all of the Contributors and Reviewers helped us to develop this Third Edition through a variety of contributions and by answering myriad questions right up to the time of publication. *Nursing: A Concept-Based Approach to Learning,* Third Edition, has benefited immeasurably from their efforts, insights, suggestions, objections, encouragement, and inspiration, as well as from their vast experience as faculty and practicing nurses.

We would like to thank the editorial team, especially Julie Alexander, Publisher, for her continuous support throughout this process; Katrin Beacom, Director of Portfolio Management for championing this project; Erin Sullivan, the editorial assistant for helping to keep all the balls in the air; Bianca Sepulveda and Melissa Bashe for keeping us organized and putting together all of the components of the concepts program; and most of all, Laura Horowitz and Addy McCulloch, development editors, for their dedication and attention to detail that promoted an excellent outcome once again. Special thanks to the design team, led by Mary Siener, and Studio Montage for the thoughtful and integrated design of our concepts solution. Many thanks to Kelly Ricci and the Aptara team for producing this book with precision.

Concepts Editorial Board

Barbara Arnoldussen, MBA, BSN, RN, CPHQ
International Technological University
San Jose, CA

Barbara Callahan, MEd, RN, NCC, CHSE
Lenoir Community College
Kinston, NC

Linda K. Daley, PhD, RN, ANEF
The Ohio State University
Columbus, OH

Mark C. Hand, PhD, RN, MSN, CNE
East Carolina University
Greenville, NC

Pamela Phillips, PhD, RN
University of South Carolina Beaufort
Beaufort, SC

T. Kim Rodehorst, PhD, RN
University of Nebraska Medical Center
Scottsbluff, NE

Contributors

Michelle Aebersold, PhD, RN, CHSE, FAAN
University of Michigan
Ann Arbor, MI

Eleisa Bennett, RN, MSN
James Sprunt Community College
Kenansville, NC

Marlena Bushway, PhD, MSNEd, RN, CNE
New Mexico Junior College
Hobbs, NM

Barbara Callahan, MEd, RN, NCC, CHSE
Lenoir Community College
Kinston, NC

Linda Daley, PhD, RN
The Ohio State University
Columbus, OH

Christi Emerson, EdD, MSN, RN
University of Mary Hardin-Baylor
Belton, TX

Michele G. Hackney, EdD, MSN, RN, CNE
University of Mary Hardin-Baylor
Belton, TX

Elizabeth Johnston Taylor, PhD, RN
Loma Linda University
Loma Linda, CA

Amy Mitchell Kennedy, MSN, RN
Nursing Content Manager
Newport News, VA

Christine Kleckner, MA, MAN, RN
Minneapolis Community and Technical College
Minneapolis, MN

Juleann H. Miller, RN, PhD
St. Ambrose University
Davenport, IA

Jeanne Papa, MSN, MBE, ACNP
Neumann University
Aston, PA

Cynthia Parkman, PhD, RN
National University
San Diego, CA

Pamela Phillips, PhD, RN
University of South Carolina Beaufort
Beaufort, SC

T. Kim Rodehorst, PhD, RN
University of Nebraska Medical Center
Scottsbluff, NE

Judith Rolph, MSN, RN
MassBay Community College
Framingham, MA

Sharon Souter, RN, PhD, CNE
University of Mary Hardin-Baylor
Belton, TX

Patricia Vasquez, MSN, RN
Trinity Valley Community College
Kaufman, TX

Jacqueline M. Loversidge, PhD, RNC-AWHC, CNS
The Ohio State University
Columbus, OH

Reviewers

Folake Elizabeth Adelakun, RN, MSN, MBA-HC, DNP
Minneapolis Community and Technical College
Minneapolis, MN

Carol S. Amis, MSN, RN, CCRN
Minneapolis Community and Technical College
Minneapolis, MN

Barbara Arnoldussen, MBA, BSN, RN, CPHQ
International Technological University
San Jose, CA

Jacqueline Bencker, BSN, RN, CNOR
St. Mary Medical Center
Langhorne, PA

Eleisa Bennett, RN, MSN
James Sprunt Community College
Kenansville, NC

Shelley Layne Blackwood, EdS, MSN, RN-BC, PCCN
University of Mary Hardin-Baylor
Belton, TX

Karen Bledsoe, MSN, RN-C
University of Mary Hardin-Baylor
Belton, TX

Tracy Booth, MSEd, BSN, RN
University of Mary Hardin-Baylor
Belton, TX

Wendy Buchanan, RN, MSN-E
Southwestern Community College
Sylva, NC

Becky Bunn, MSN, RN
University of Mary Hardin-Baylor
Belton, TX

Regina Burgin, MSN, RN-BC
Sampson Community College
Clinton, NC

Marlena Bushway, PhD, MSNEd, RN, CNE
New Mexico Junior College
Hobbs, NM

Marcy Caplin, PhD, RN, CNE
Kent State University
Kent, OH

Kristine Carey, MSN, RN
Normandale Community College
Bloomington, MN

Diane Cohen, MSN, RN
MassBay Community College
Framingham, MA

Barbara E. Connell, RN, MSN
Southwestern Community College
Sylva, NC

Ann Crawford, RN, PhD, CNS, CEN, CPEN
University of Mary Hardin-Baylor
Belton, TX

Diane Daddario, MSN, ANP-C, ACNS-BC, RN, BC, CMSRN
Pennsylvania State University
University Park, PA

Linda Daley, PhD, RN
The Ohio State University
Columbus, OH

Carrie Dickson, MS, APRN, CNM, CNE
Normandale Community College
Bloomington, MN

Barbara Dixon, MSN, RN
University of Mary Hardin-Baylor
Belton, TX

Patricia Ann Durham-Taylor, RN, PhD
Truckee Meadows Community College
Reno, NV

Mary Ervi, MSN, RN, CNE
University of Mary Hardin-Baylor
Belton, TX

Vicki Evans, MSN, RN, CEN, CNE
University of Mary Hardin-Baylor
Belton, TX

Abimbola Farinde, PhD
Columbia Southern University
Orange Beach, AL

Pamela Fauskee, MN, RN, CNE
Anoka-Ramsey Community College
Cambridge, MN

James R. Fell, MSN, MBA, RN
The Breen School of Nursing, Ursuline University
Pepper Pike, OH

Judy Flowers, MSN, MS, RN
Catawba Valley Community College
Hickory, NC

Tobi Fuller, MSN, MS, RN
El Centro College
Dallas, TX

Frederick Gunzel
Independent Contractor
Farmingville, NY

Michele G. Hackney, EdD, MSN, RN, CNE
University of Mary Hardin-Baylor
Belton, TX

Mark C. Hand, PhD, RN, MSN, CNE
Durham Technical Community College
Durham, NC

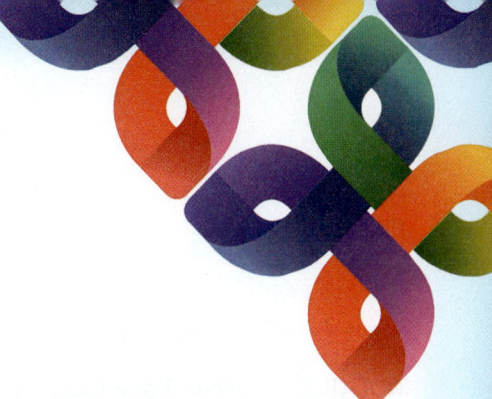

Lori Kelty, MSNEd, RN, CCRN, CEN, NE
Mercer County Community College
Windsor Township, NJ

Amy Mitchell Kennedy, MSN, RN
Nursing Content Manager
Newport News, VA

Christine Kleckner, MA, MAN, RN
Minneapolis Community and Technical
College
Minneapolis, MN

Dawna Martich, MSN, RN
Nursing Education Consultant
Pittsburgh, PA

Belle McGinty, MEd, RN, BSN
Brunswick Community College
Bolivia, NC

Kimi C. McMahan, RN, MSNEd
Southwestern Community College
Sylva, NC

Amy Mersiovsky, MSN, RN, BC
University of Mary Hardin-Baylor
Belton, TX

Juleann H. Miller, RN, PhD
St. Ambrose University
Davenport, IA

Michelle Natrop, RN, BAN, MSN
Normandale Community College
Bloomington, MN

Lynn Perkins, PhD, MSN, RN
Minneapolis Community and Technical
College
Minneapolis, MN

Margaret Prydun, PhD, RN, CNE
University of Mary Hardin-Baylor
Belton, TX

Judith Rolph, MSN, RN
MassBay Community College
Framingham, MA

John E. Scarbrough, PhD, PT,
RN, CNE
New Mexico State University
Las Cruces, NM

Cynthia K. Schweizer, MSN, RN
Brunswick Community College
Bolivia, NC

Amber J. Seidel, PhD
Pennsylvania State University
University Park, PA

Brenda L. Shostrom, RN, PhD
St. Ambrose University
Davenport, IA

Amy B. Sneed
Brunswick Community College
Bolivia, NC

Ami Stone, RN, MSN
University of Mary Hardin-Baylor
Belton, TX

Betsy Swinny, MSN, RN, CCRN
Baptist Health System
San Antonio, TX

Lori L. Thompson, APRN, MSN, NP-C
Vance–Granville Community College
Henderson, NC

Carolina Partners in Mental HealthCare
Wake Forest, NC

Patricia Vasquez, MSN, RN
Trinity Valley Community College
Kaufman, TX

Paulette Whitfield, PhD, RN, ANP-BC
University of Mary Hardin-Baylor
Belton, TX

Joanne Woods, BS, MSN
University of Mary Hardin-Baylor
Belton, TX

Contents

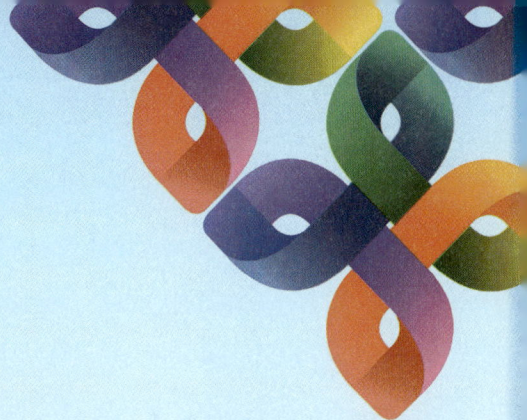

Part I
Biophysical Modules

Part I consists of the biophysical modules within the individual domain. Each module presents a biophysical concept—such as oxygenation or perfusion—and selected alterations of that concept are presented as exemplars. For example, in the module on Oxygenation, exemplars include asthma and chronic obstructive pulmonary disease. Each module addresses the impact of that concept and selected alterations on individuals across the life span, inclusive of cultural, gender, and developmental considerations.

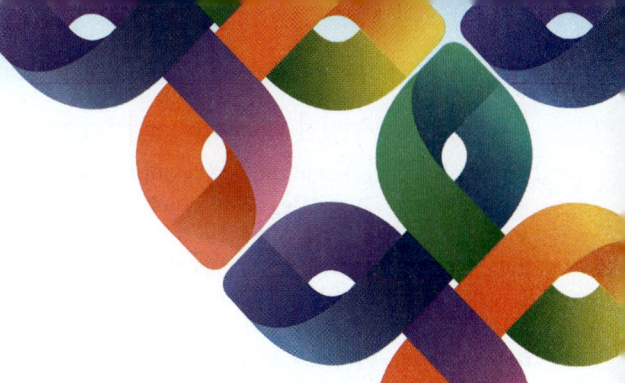

Module 1
Acid–Base Balance

Module Outline and Learning Outcomes

The Concept of Acid–Base Balance

Normal Acid–Base Balance

1.1 Analyze the physiology of normal acid–base balance.

Alterations to Acid–Base Balance

1.2 Differentiate alterations in acid–base balance.

Concepts Related to Acid–Base Balance

1.3 Outline the relationship between acid–base balance and other concepts.

Health Promotion

1.4 Explain the promotion of healthy acid–base balance.

Nursing Assessment

1.5 Differentiate common assessment procedures and tests used to examine acid–base balance.

Independent Interventions

1.6 Analyze independent interventions nurses can implement for patients with alterations in acid–base balance.

Collaborative Therapies

1.7 Summarize collaborative therapies used by interprofessional teams for patients with alterations in acid–base balance.

Acid–Base Balance Exemplars

Exemplar 1.A Metabolic Acidosis

1.A Analyze metabolic acidosis as it relates to acid–base balance.

Exemplar 1.B Metabolic Alkalosis

1.B Analyze metabolic alkalosis as it relates to acid–base balance.

Exemplar 1.C Respiratory Acidosis

1.C Analyze respiratory acidosis as it relates to acid–base balance.

Exemplar 1.D Respiratory Alkalosis

1.D Analyze respiratory alkalosis as it relates to acid–base balance.

The Concept of Acid–Base Balance

Concept Key Terms

Acidosis, **4**	Allen test, **9**	Bases, **3**	Hypoxemia, **10**	Serum bicarbonate, **4**
Acids, **3**	Arterial blood gases (ABGs), **9**	Buffers, **4**	$PaCO_2$, **5**	Serum carbonic acid, **4**
Alkalis, **3**	Base excess (BE), **10**	Hypercapnia, **10**	PaO_2, **10**	Volatile acid, **4**
Alkalosis, **4**		Hypocapnia, **10**	pH, **3**	

Acid–base balance is critical to homeostasis and optimal cellular function. To maintain acid–base balance, the hydrogen ion (H+) concentration of body fluids must be kept within a relatively narrow range. Hydrogen ions determine the relative acidity of body fluids. **Acids** release hydrogen ions in solution; **bases** (or **alkalis**) accept hydrogen ions in solution. The hydrogen ion concentration of a solution is measured as its **pH**. The relationship between hydrogen ion concentration and pH is inverse: As hydrogen ion concentration increases, the pH falls, and the solution becomes more acidic; as hydrogen ion concentration falls, the pH

rises, and the solution becomes more alkaline or basic. The normal pH of body fluids is slightly basic, ranging from 7.35 to 7.45. (A pH of 7 is neutral.) Normal pH indicates acid–base balance.

Acid–base imbalance results from any one of several underlying causes and can be an important clue in diagnosing illness or disease. Failure to restore acid–base balance can lead to impairment of organs and critical bodily functions. The body's tolerance for alterations in acid–base levels is very narrow; a pH below 7 or above 7.6 for even a short time can result in death.

Normal Acid–Base Balance

Metabolic processes in the body continuously produce acids, which fall into two categories: volatile acids and nonvolatile acids. A **volatile acid** can be eliminated from the body as a gas. Carbonic acid (H_2CO_3) is the only volatile acid produced in the body. It dissociates (separates) into carbon dioxide (CO_2) and water (H_2O); the lungs eliminate the carbon dioxide. All other acids produced in the body are nonvolatile acids that must be metabolized or excreted in fluid. Examples are lactic acid (resulting from cellular destruction), hydrochloric acid (found in stomach secretions), phosphoric acid (from the oxidation of phospholipids and phosphoproteins), and sulfuric acid (formed by oxidation of sulfur-containing amino acids). Most acids and bases in the body are weak; that is, they neither release nor accept a significant number of hydrogen ions.

Despite the body's continuous acid production, three systems work together to maintain pH within a normal range: buffer systems, the respiratory system, and the renal system.

Physiology Review

Buffer Systems

Buffers are substances that prevent major changes in pH by releasing hydrogen ions. When excess acid is present in body fluid, buffers bind with hydrogen ions to minimize the change in pH. If body fluids become too basic or too alkaline, buffers release hydrogen ions, restoring the pH. Although buffers act within a fraction of a second, their capacity to maintain pH is limited. The body's major buffer systems are the bicarbonate–carbonic acid buffer system, the phosphate buffer system, and protein buffers.

The normal **serum bicarbonate** level is 24–28 mEq/L, and the normal **serum carbonic acid** level is 1.2 mEq/L. Thus, the ratio of bicarbonate (HCO_3) to carbonic acid (H_2CO_3) is 20:1. Although the amounts of bicarbonate and carbonic acid in the body vary somewhat, as long as this ratio is maintained, the pH remains within the 7.35–7.45 range (**Figure 1–1 》**).

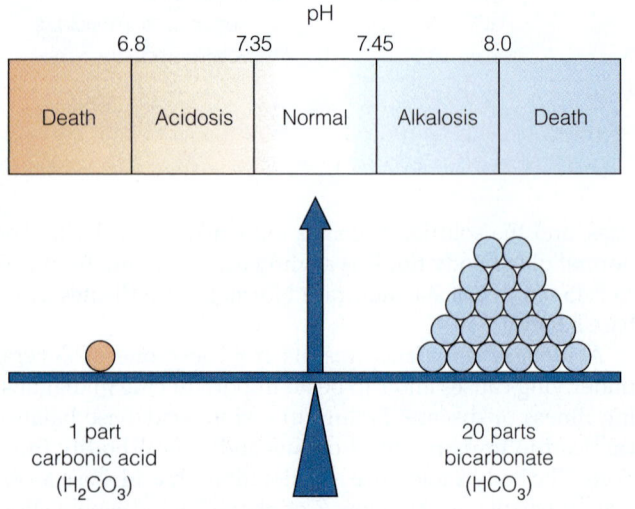

Figure 1–1 》 The normal ratio of bicarbonate to carbonic acid is 20:1. As long as this ratio is maintained, the pH remains within the normal range of 7.35–7.45.

Bicarbonate (HCO_3) is a weak base. When an acid is added to the system, the hydrogen ion in the acid combines with bicarbonate, and the pH changes only slightly. Carbonic acid is a weak acid produced when carbon dioxide dissolves in water. When a base is added to the system, it combines with carbonic acid, and the pH remains within the normal range.

Adding a strong acid to extracellular fluid (ECF) depletes bicarbonate, changing the 20:1 ratio and causing the pH to drop below 7.35. This is known as **acidosis**. Adding a strong base depletes carbonic acid, as it combines with the base, again disrupting the 20:1 ratio. The pH rises above 7.45, a condition known as **alkalosis**.

Respiratory System

The respiratory system (and the brain's respiratory center) regulates carbonic acid by eliminating or retaining carbon dioxide. Carbon dioxide is a potential acid; when combined with water, it forms carbonic acid, a volatile acid. Acute increases in carbon dioxide or hydrogen ions in the blood stimulate the brain's respiratory center, increasing both the rate and depth of respiration. As a result, carbon dioxide is eliminated and carbonic acid levels fall, bringing the pH to a more normal range. Although this compensation for increased hydrogen ion concentration occurs within minutes, it becomes less effective over time. For example, patients with chronic lung disease (such as chronic obstructive pulmonary disease, COPD) may have consistently high carbon dioxide levels in their blood.

Alkalosis, by contrast, depresses the respiratory center, decreasing both the rate and depth of respiration and causing carbon dioxide retention. The retained carbon dioxide then combines with water to restore carbonic acid levels and bring the pH back within the normal range.

Renal System

The renal system is responsible for the long-term regulation of acid–base balance. The kidneys normally eliminate the excess nonvolatile acids produced during metabolism. The kidneys also regulate bicarbonate levels in ECF by regenerating or reabsorbing bicarbonate ions in the renal tubules. Although the kidneys respond more slowly to changes in pH (over hours to days), they can generate bicarbonate and selectively excrete or retain hydrogen ions as needed. In acidosis, when excess hydrogen ions are present and the pH falls, the kidneys excrete hydrogen ions and retain bicarbonate. In alkalosis, the kidneys retain hydrogen ions and excrete bicarbonate to restore acid–base balance.

Alterations to Acid–Base Balance

Acid–base imbalances fall into two major categories: acidosis and alkalosis. As noted previously, acidosis occurs when the hydrogen ion concentration increases above normal (pH below 7.35). Alkalosis occurs when the hydrogen ion concentration falls below normal (pH above 7.45).

Alterations and Manifestations

Acid–base imbalances are further classified as *metabolic* or *respiratory* disorders. In metabolic disorders, the primary change is in the concentration of bicarbonate. In *metabolic acidosis*, the

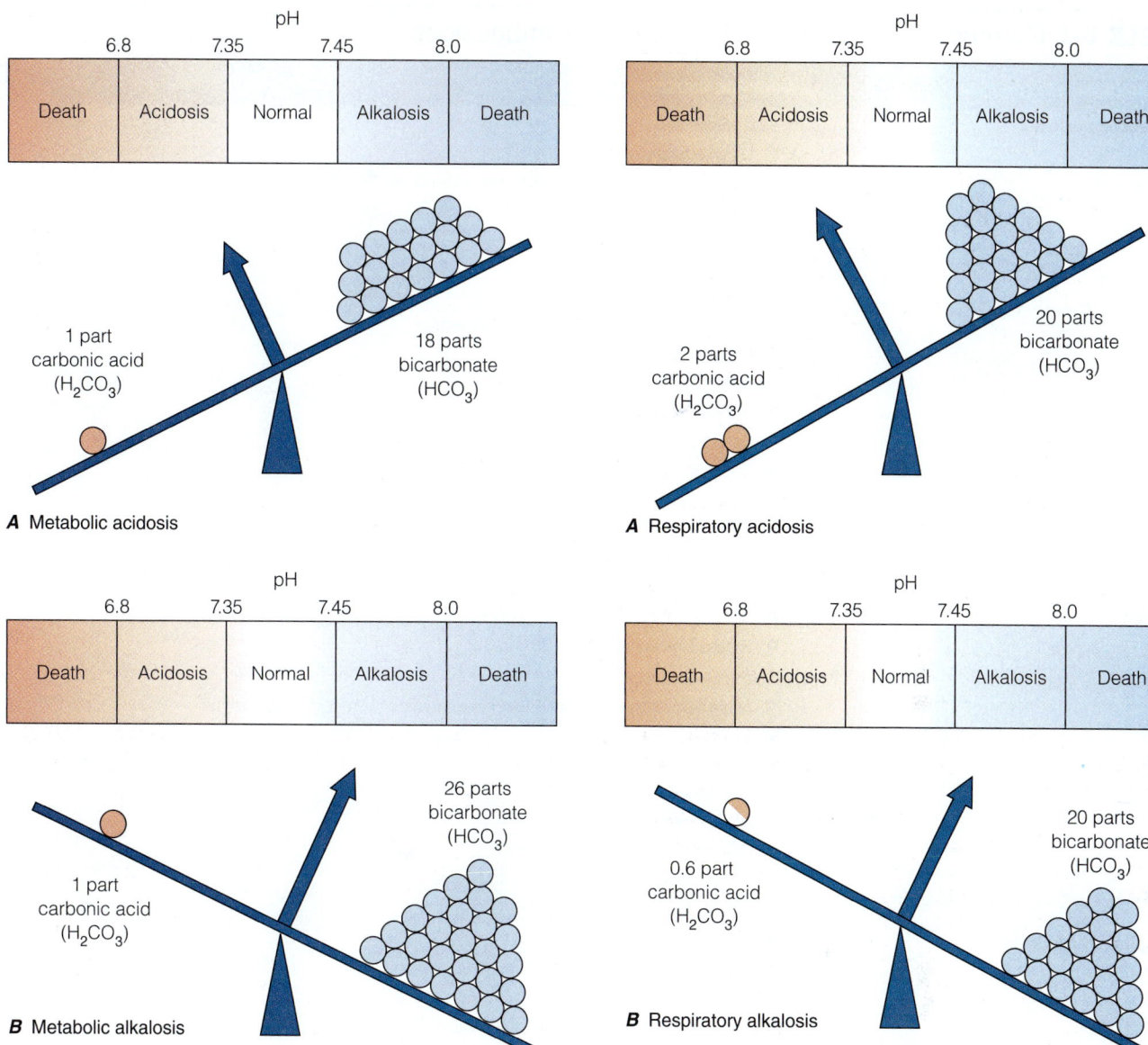

Figure 1–2 》 Metabolic acid–base imbalances. **A,** Metabolic acidosis. **B,** Metabolic alkalosis.

Figure 1–3 》 Respiratory acid–base imbalances. **A,** Respiratory acidosis. **B,** Respiratory alkalosis.

amount of bicarbonate decreases in relation to the amount of acid in the body (**Figure 1–2A 》**). This condition can develop from abnormal bicarbonate losses or from excess nonvolatile acids in the body. The pH falls below 7.35, and the bicarbonate concentration is less than 24 mEq/L. *Metabolic alkalosis,* by contrast, occurs when there is an excess of bicarbonate in relation to the amount of hydrogen ion (Figure 1–2B). The pH is above 7.45, and the bicarbonate concentration is greater than 28 mEq/L.

In respiratory disorders, the primary change is in the concentration of carbonic acid. *Respiratory acidosis* occurs when carbon dioxide is retained, increasing the amount of carbonic acid in the body (**Figure 1–3A 》**). As a result, the pH falls to less than 7.35, and the **PaCO$_2$** (pressure exerted by dissolved carbon dioxide in the blood) is greater than 45 mmHg. When too much carbon dioxide is lost, carbonic acid levels fall and *respiratory alkalosis* develops (Figure 1–3B). The pH rises to above 7.45, and the PaCO$_2$ is less

than 35 mmHg. Any condition that causes hypoventilation may result in respiratory acidosis and hypoxemia, while any condition that causes hyperventilation often results in respiratory alkalosis.

Acid–base disorders are further defined as *primary* (simple) and *mixed.* Primary disorders usually have one cause. For example, respiratory failure often causes respiratory acidosis due to retained carbon dioxide; renal failure usually causes metabolic acidosis due to retained hydrogen ion and impaired bicarbonate production. **Table 1–1 》** summarizes primary acid–base imbalances with the common causes of each. Mixed disorders occur from combinations of respiratory and metabolic disturbances. For example, a patient in cardiac arrest develops a mixed respiratory and metabolic acidosis due to lack of ventilation (and retained CO$_2$) and hypoxia of body tissues that leads to anaerobic metabolism and acid by-products (excess nonvolatile acids).

TABLE 1–1 Common Causes of Primary Acid–Base Imbalances

Imbalance	Common Causes

Metabolic acidosis
pH < 7.35
HCO_3 < 24 mEq/L
Critical values
pH < 7.20
HCO_3 < 10 mEq/L
	↑ Acid production
	  ■ Lactic acidosis
	  ■ Ketoacidosis related to diabetes, starvation, or alcoholism
	  ■ Salicylate toxicity
	↓ Acid excretion
	  ■ Renal failure
	↑ Bicarbonate loss
	  ■ Diarrhea, ileostomy drainage, intestinal fistula
	  ■ Biliary or pancreatic fistulas
	↑ Chloride
	  ■ Sodium chloride intravenous (IV) solutions
	  ■ Renal tubular acidosis
	  ■ Carbonic anhydrase inhibitors

Metabolic alkalosis
pH > 7.45
HCO_3 > 28 mEq/L
Critical values
pH > 7.60
HCO_3 > 40 mEq/L
	↑ Acid loss or excretion
	  ■ Vomiting, gastric suction
	  ■ Hypokalemia
	↑ Bicarbonate
	  ■ Alkali ingestion (bicarbonate of soda)
	  ■ Excess bicarbonate administration

Respiratory acidosis
pH < 7.35
$PaCO_2$ > 45 mmHg
Critical values
pH < 7.20
$PaCO_2$ > 77 mmHg
	Acute respiratory acidosis
	  ■ Acute respiratory conditions (pulmonary edema, pneumonia, acute asthma)
	  ■ Opiate overdose
	  ■ Foreign body aspiration
	  ■ Chest trauma
	Chronic respiratory acidosis
	  ■ Chronic respiratory conditions (COPD, cystic fibrosis)
	  ■ Multiple sclerosis, other neuromuscular diseases
	  ■ Stroke

Respiratory alkalosis
pH > 7.45
$PaCO_2$ < 35 mmHg
Critical values
pH > 7.60
$PaCO_2$ < 20 mmHg
	■ Anxiety-induced hyperventilation
	  ■ Fever
	  ■ Early salicylate intoxication
	  ■ Hyperventilation with mechanical ventilator

Compensation

With primary acid–base disorders, compensatory changes in other parts of the regulatory system occur to restore a normal pH and homeostasis. In metabolic acid–base disorders, the change in pH affects the rate and depth of respirations, which, in turn, affects carbon dioxide elimination and the $PaCO_2$ and helps restore the ratio of carbonic acid to bicarbonate. The kidneys compensate for simple respiratory imbalances. The change in pH affects both bicarbonate conservation and hydrogen ion elimination (**Table 1–2** »).

Compensatory changes in respirations occur within minutes of a change in pH. These changes, however, become less effective over time. The renal response takes longer to restore the pH, but it is a more effective long-term mechanism. If the pH is restored to normal limits, the disorder is *fully compensated*. When these changes are reflected in arterial blood gas

(ABG) values but the pH remains outside normal limits, the disorder is *partially compensated*.

Risk Factors

Acid–base imbalances occur in critically ill patients. There are many underlying causes of these disturbances. Each acid–base disorder is treated separately, with the underlying cause considered in the critically ill patients.

Clinical Example A

Jay James is a 24-year-old man who was rock climbing with his friends at a national park 25 miles from the nearest hospital when he suddenly lost his footing and slid 20 feet to the ground. Mr. James was alert and oriented when his friends reached him, and he could move all extremities quite easily. He had multiple scrapes over his anterior chest and a large gash over his left thigh (near the groin),

TABLE 1–2 Compensation for Simple Acid–Base Imbalances

Primary Disorder	Cause	Compensation	Effect on ABGs
Metabolic acidosis	Excess nonvolatile acids; bicarbonate deficiency	Rate and depth of respirations increase, eliminating additional CO_2.	$\downarrow$ pH $\downarrow$ HCO_3 $\downarrow$ $PaCO_2$
Metabolic alkalosis	Bicarbonate excess	Rate and depth of respirations decrease; CO_2 is retained.	$\uparrow$ pH $\uparrow$ HCO_3 $\uparrow$ $PaCO_2$
Respiratory acidosis	Retained CO_2 and excess carbonic acid	Kidneys conserve bicarbonate to restore carbonic acid: bicarbonate ratio of 1:20.	$\downarrow$ pH $\uparrow$ $PaCO_2$ $\uparrow$ HCO_3
Respiratory alkalosis	Loss of CO_2 and deficient carbonic acid	Kidneys excrete bicarbonate and conserve H^+ to restore carbonic acid: bicarbonate ratio.	$\uparrow$ pH $\downarrow$ $PaCO_2$ $\downarrow$ HCO_3

which was bleeding profusely. His friends made a makeshift tourniquet, which slowed the bleeding. They immediately contacted the park ranger, who secured a helicopter to evacuate Mr. James to the nearest hospital.

Two large-bore IVs were placed in each arm in-flight, and normal saline was administered. The flight medic placed a 100% nonrebreathing mask on Mr. James. Mr. James became disoriented and confused during the flight. Mr. James arrived in the emergency department (ED) in 45 minutes after the fall.

On arrival in the ED, Mr. James is lethargic but responsive to painful stimuli. He has multiple abrasions over his chin and neck. His pulse oximetry is 99% on the nonrebreather mask, so the ED team replaces the mask with a nasal cannula at 4 L/min. A repeat pulse oximeter reads 95% saturation.

Vital signs are as follows: T_O 99.1°F; HR 130 bpm; R 30/min; BP 100/60 mmHg. Skin is cool and clammy, nail beds are pale, and mucous membranes are dry. All pulses are palpable but weak and thready. Lungs are clear, heart sounds regular. Output via urinary catheter for the past hour is 20 mL.

Clinical Reasoning Questions Level I

1. What is the most likely cause of Mr. James's high heart rate and low blood pressure?
2. If you were the nurse assigned to Mr. James, what would be your primary concerns at this time?

Clinical Reasoning Questions Level II

3. What is the priority nursing diagnosis for Mr. James at this time?
4. Why is Mr. James exhibiting confusion and disorientation?
5. What diagnostic tests would you expect to be ordered for Mr. James?

Concepts Related to Acid–Base Balance

Although the human body is made up of numerous systems that can be studied individually, no system is truly isolated. Instead, the function of one body system can greatly affect the function of one or more other body systems. For example, changes in acid–base balance can result in decreased tissue perfusion, leading to cardiac arrest. Acidosis or alkalosis may result in a decreasing level of consciousness (LOC), and

patients with acute respiratory acidosis may also experience irritability and altered mental status. Chronic respiratory acidosis can manifest in impaired memory and/or personality changes. Metabolic acidosis resulting from fluid or electrolyte imbalance can be particularly dangerous, especially in the case of diabetic ketoacidosis (DKA). The Concepts Related to Acid-Base Balance feature links some, but not all, of the concepts related to acid–base balance. They are presented in alphabetical order.

Health Promotion

Health promotion focuses on maintaining fluid balance. Both overhydration and dehydration can result in acid–base imbalances. Chronic conditions that can easily cause a change in fluid status and subsequent acid–base imbalances include diabetes, Crohn disease, chronic kidney disease, and chronic lung diseases such as COPD. Electrolyte imbalances, particularly sodium and potassium, may be caused by certain medications, supplements, or changes in diet. Nurses focus on patient teaching regarding adequate nutrition, taking medications as prescribed, and following treatment regimens for chronic illnesses.

Nursing Assessment

Focused assessment related to acid–base imbalances includes the following: You should begin by identifying patients at risk for acid–base disturbances, including those who have a risk for significant electrolyte imbalances, net gain or loss of acids, net gain or loss of bases, ventilation abnormalities, abnormal kidney function, and metabolic malfunction. Consider what the patient's vital signs are telling you. Count the patient's respirations for a full minute. Consider the rate and depth of respirations in your assessment. Do you see any reasons why the patient should have impending or underlying respiratory or metabolic problems? What is the patient's LOC? Decreased LOC can be a sign of an acid–base disturbance. What are the fluid balance and kidney function of the patient? Do your findings correlate with the patient's diagnosis?

Alterations and Therapies
Acid–Base Imbalances

ALTERATION	DESCRIPTION/ DEFINITION	MANIFESTATIONS	INTERVENTIONS AND THERAPIES
Metabolic acidosis	Metabolic acidosis (bicarbonate deficit) may be caused by excess acid in the body or loss of bicarbonate from the body.	▪ Nausea and vomiting ▪ Weakness ▪ Fatigue ▪ Headache ▪ ↓ Level of consciousness (LOC) ▪ Hyperventilation *Laboratory findings:* ▪ Arterial blood pH below 7.35 ▪ Serum bicarbonate less than 24 mEq/L ▪ $PaCO_2$ less than 38 mmHg with respiratory compensation	▪ Monitor ABG values, intake and output, and LOC. ▪ Administer IV sodium bicarbonate carefully as ordered. ▪ Treat underlying problem as ordered.
Metabolic alkalosis	Metabolic alkalosis (bicarbonate excess) may be caused by loss of acid or excess bicarbonate in the body.	▪ Confusion ▪ ↓ LOC ▪ Hypotension ▪ Tetany ▪ Seizures ▪ Respiratory failure *Laboratory findings:* ▪ Arterial blood pH above 7.45 ▪ Serum bicarbonate greater than 28 mEq/L ▪ $PaCO_2$ higher than 45 mmHg with respiratory compensation	▪ Monitor intake and output closely. ▪ Monitor vital signs, especially respirations, and LOC. ▪ Administer ordered IV fluids carefully. ▪ Treat underlying problem as ordered.
Respiratory acidosis	Respiratory acidosis is caused by an excess of dissolved carbon dioxide, or carbonic acid; it can be acute or chronic.	*Acute:* ▪ Headache ▪ Irritability, altered mental status ▪ ↓ LOC ▪ Cardiac arrest *Chronic:* ▪ Dull headache ▪ Impaired memory ▪ Personality changes ▪ Weakness *Laboratory findings:* ▪ Arterial blood pH less than 7.35 ▪ $PaCO_2$ above 45 mmHg ▪ HCO_3 normal or slightly elevated çin acute; above 28 mEq/L in chronic	▪ Frequently assess respiratory status and lung sounds. ▪ Monitor airway and ventilation; assist with insertion of artificial airway and prepare for mechanical ventilation as necessary. ▪ Administer pulmonary therapy measures such as inhalation therapy, percussion and postural drainage, bronchodilators, and antibiotics as ordered. ▪ Monitor fluid intake and output, vital signs, and ABGs. ▪ Administer narcotic antagonists as indicated. ▪ Maintain adequate hydration (2–3 L of fluid per day unless contraindicated by other health conditions).
Respiratory alkalosis	Respiratory alkalosis is caused by hyperventilation, leading to a carbon dioxide deficit.	▪ Hyperventilation ▪ Dizziness ▪ Palpitations ▪ Anxiety–panic ▪ Tetany ▪ ↓ LOC *Laboratory findings (in uncompensated respiratory alkalosis):* ▪ Arterial blood pH above 7.45 ▪ $PaCO_2$ less than 35 mmHg *Laboratory findings (in chronic hyperventilation):* ▪ Serum bicarbonate less than 24 mEq/L ▪ Arterial blood pH near normal	▪ Monitor vital signs and ABGs. ▪ Teach patient to breathe more slowly. ▪ Reduce stimuli in environment and speak in calm, quiet voice.

Concepts Related to
Acid–Base Balance

CONCEPT	RELATIONSHIP TO ACID–BASE BALANCE	NURSING IMPLICATIONS
Cognition	$\downarrow O_2$ can cause changes in cognition, leading to impaired communication.	■ Maintain adequate oxygenation. ■ Monitor closely for change in LOC. ■ LOC changes can lead to stupor and coma. ■ Ask yes/no questions. ■ Observe for nonverbal cues.
Fluids and Electrolytes	Another primary disorder causes metabolic results.	■ Focus treatment on primary disorder, reduce the effects of acidosis on cardiac function, and restore fluid levels in the body. ■ Administer IV bicarbonate as ordered. ■ Administer IV fluids with insulin to correct acidosis in patients with DKA. ■ Rapid administration of sodium bicarbonate leads to metabolic alkalosis and hypokalemia. ■ Monitor ABG values.
Oxygenation	**Hypoventilation:** $\downarrow$ Respiratory rate causes increased PCO_2. **Hyperventilation:** $\uparrow$ Respiratory rate causes decreased PCO_2.	■ Monitor respiration in all patients. ■ Monitor vital signs and pulse oximetry. ■ Give special attention when respirations are 12 breaths per minute or less. ■ Determine course of treatment based on underlying cause. ■ Severe hypoventilation requires opioid antagonist (e.g., naloxone). Monitor respiration in all patients. ■ Calm patient if cause is panic. ■ Offer stress reduction counseling if cause is anxiety. ■ Speak in a slow, calm voice.
Perfusion	$\downarrow$ Tissue perfusion results from shock or cardiac arrest.	■ Administer oxygen therapy as ordered. ■ Correct underlying problem to improve tissue perfusion.
Stress and Coping	Anxiety can lead to difficulty breathing, dizziness, and central nervous system (CNS) symptoms.	■ Reassure patient. ■ Provide distractions. ■ Teach guided imagery and relaxation therapy.

Observation and Patient Interview

Acid–base balance is a function of the chemical and physiologic components of the body. A complete health history is necessary to determine the underlying acid–base imbalance. Each specific disorder has different symptoms. It is important to identify any prescribed and over-the-counter medications that the patient is currently taking, as well as any complementary health approaches, such as vitamins and herbal supplements.

Physical Examination

Assess the patient's vital signs, including pulse oximetry. Assess mentation. Use fall precautions for patients with decreased LOC. Skin color and temperature, rate of respirations, lung sounds, bowel sounds, and urine output may be among the indicators of a change in acid–base balance. See the exemplars for more specific details on manifestations and assessment considerations.

Diagnostic Tests

Acid–base balance is assessed primarily by measuring **arterial blood gases (ABGs)**. Arterial blood is most often used because it reflects acid–base balance throughout the entire body better than venous or capillary blood that has dispersed oxygen into the tissues and has collected carbon dioxide. However, venous blood gases are occasionally ordered when frequent ABGs have resulted in damage to normal arterial gas sampling sites. Arterial blood also provides information about the effectiveness of the lungs in oxygenating blood. However, when a patient has chronic retention of serum carbon dioxide (CO_2), it is reflected in a metabolic panel. If the history of long-standing chronic lung disease is unknown, it is often helpful to look at serum CO_2 to see a trend.

The examiner must perform a modified **Allen test** before drawing arterial blood gases. A modified Allen test is a measurement of ulnar patency. The patient elevates the hand and repeatedly makes a fist while the examiner places digital occlusive pressure over the radial and ulnar arteries of the wrist. The hand will lose its normal color. Digital pressure is released from one artery while the other remains compressed. The return of color indicates that the hand has good collateral supply of blood and that arterial puncture can safely be performed (Venes, 2013). Blood gases may be

Box 1–1
Interpreting ABGs

1. **Look at the pH.**
   - pH < 7.35 = acidosis
   - pH > 7.45 = alkalosis
2. **Look at the PaCO$_2$.**
   - PaCO$_2$ < 35 mmHg = hypocapnia; more carbon dioxide is being exhaled than normal.
   - PaCO$_2$ > 45 mmHg = hypercapnia; carbon dioxide is being retained.
3. **Evaluate the pH–PaCO$_2$ relationship for a possible respiratory problem.**
   - If the pH is < 7.35 (acidosis) and the PaCO$_2$ is > 45 mmHg (hypercapnia), retained carbon dioxide is causing increased H$^+$ concentration and respiratory acidosis.
   - If the pH is > 7.45 (alkalosis) and the PaCO$_2$ is < 35 mmHg (hypocapnia), low carbon dioxide levels and decreased H$^+$ concentration are causing respiratory alkalosis.
4. **Look at the bicarbonate.**
   - If the HCO$_3$ is < 24 mEq/L, bicarbonate levels are lower than normal.
   - If the HCO$_3$ is > 28 mEq/L, bicarbonate levels are higher than normal.
5. **Evaluate the pH, HCO$_3$, and BE for a possible metabolic problem.**
   - If the pH is < 7.35, the HCO$_3$ is < 24 mEq/L, and the BE is < –3 mEq/L, then low bicarbonate levels and high H$^+$ concentrations are causing metabolic acidosis.
   - If the pH is > 7.45, the HCO$_3$ is > 28 MEq/L, and the BE is > +3 mEq/L, then high bicarbonate levels are causing metabolic alkalosis.
6. **Look for compensation.**
   - Renal compensation
     a. In respiratory acidosis (pH < 7.35, PaCO$_2$ > 45 mmHg), the kidneys retain HCO$_3$ to buffer the excess acid, so the HCO$_3$ is > 28 mEq/L.
     b. In respiratory alkalosis (pH > 7.45, PaCO$_2$ < 35 mmHg), the kidneys excrete HCO$_3$ to minimize the alkalosis, so the HCO$_3$ is < 24 mEq/L.
   - Respiratory compensation
     a. In metabolic acidosis (pH < 7.35, HCO$_3$ < 24 mEq/L), the rate and depth of respirations increase, increasing carbon dioxide elimination, so the PaCO$_2$ is < 35 mmHg.
     b. In metabolic alkalosis (pH > 7.45, HCO$_3$ > 28 mEq/L), respirations slow and carbon dioxide is retained, so the PaCO$_2$ is > 45 mmHg.
7. **Evaluate oxygenation.**
   - PaO$_2$ < 80 mmHg = hypoxemia; possible hypoventilation.
   - PaO$_2$ > 100 mmHg = hyperventilation.

drawn by respiratory therapists, healthcare providers, or nurses with specialized skills (intensive care-trained). Because blood is drawn from a high-pressure artery, it is important to apply pressure to the puncture site for 10 minutes (more than 10–15 minutes if the patient is receiving anticoagulant therapy) after the procedure to reduce the risk of bleeding or bruising. A systematic approach is important in the analysis of ABG results. First, evaluate each individual measurement; then, analyze the interrelationships to determine the patient's acid–base status (**Box 1–1 »**).

The PaCO$_2$ measures the pressure exerted by dissolved carbon dioxide in the arterial blood and reflects the respiratory component of acid–base regulation and balance because it is regulated by the lungs. The normal value is 35–45 mmHg. PaCO$_2$ less than 35 mmHg is known as **hypocapnia**; PaCO$_2$ greater than 45 mmHg is known as **hypercapnia**. Healthcare providers often look at venous CO$_2$ when chronic CO$_2$ retention occurs.

PaCO$_2$ and PaO$_2$ can be abbreviated further as pCO$_2$ and pO$_2$. The *P* stands for partial pressure, or the pressure exerted by the gas dissolved in the blood. The *a* indicates that the sample is arterial blood. Because these measurements are rarely done on venous or capillary blood, the *a* is often deleted from the abbreviation.

The **PaO$_2$** is a measure of the pressure exerted by oxygen that is dissolved in the plasma. Only about 3% of oxygen in the blood is transported in solution; most is combined with hemoglobin. However, only dissolved oxygen is available to the cells for metabolism. As dissolved oxygen diffuses out of plasma into the tissues, more is released from hemoglobin. The normal value for PaO$_2$ is 75–100 mmHg. PaO$_2$ less than

80 mmHg indicates **hypoxemia**. The PaO$_2$ is valuable for evaluating respiratory function, but it is not used as a primary measurement in determining acid–base status. The serum bicarbonate (HCO$_3$) reflects the renal regulation of acid–base balance. The normal HCO$_3$ value is 24–28 mEq/L.

The **base excess (BE)** is a calculated value also known as *buffer base capacity*. The BE measures substances that can accept or combine with hydrogen ions. It reflects the degree of acid–base imbalance by indicating the status of the body's total buffering capacity. It represents the amount of acid or base that must be added to a blood sample to achieve a pH of 7.4 and is essentially a measure of increased or decreased bicarbonate. The normal BE value for arterial blood is –3 to +3.

It is important to correlate the results of the pulse oximeter with ABG results. When pulse oximetry is reading a low percentage, it may not correlate to the accurate number in the arterial sample. For example when perfusion is low, your pulse oximetry reading does not correlate to arterial oxygenation. Therefore, it may be necessary to record the pulse oximetry reading and perform an arterial blood gas at the same time to correlate differences. The oxygen saturation of 90% corresponds to about PaO$_2$ of 60 mmHg.

Other reasons for false readings may include anemia, carbon monoxide poisoning, hypothermia, hypotension, peripheral vasoconstriction, and poor peripheral perfusion caused by disease. Remember that arterial blood is the gold standard and most accurate reading for the patient.

*» Go to **Pearson MyLab Nursing and eText** to see Appendix B for information on normal and abnormal values and on how to evaluate ABG measurements.*

Clinical Example B

Anna Zemakis is a 49-year-old woman admitted to the hospital with severe vomiting and muscle weakness. She fell 2 weeks ago and reports not feeling well since. Four days ago, she developed abdominal discomfort with vomiting. The vomiting has been severe, and she has not been able to eat or drink very much. She says she has lost a significant amount of weight. She has felt very weak, anorexic, and lethargic. She has not had diarrhea or urinary symptoms. There is no significant past medical history, and she reports she is not on any prescribed medications or taking anything over-the-counter. Ms. Zemakis's vital signs are as follows: T_O 98.9°F; HR 84 bpm; R 18/min; BP 90/58 mmHg (sitting); BP 110/60 mmHg (lying); pulse oximetry 98% on room air. Her lungs are clear, and her heart sounds normal. You observe she has dry mucous membranes. Initial examination reveals slight abdominal tenderness.

Clinical Reasoning Questions Level I
1. What is Ms. Zemakis's primary health problem?
2. As the nurse assigned to Ms. Zemakis, what are your concerns at this time?

Clinical Reasoning Questions Level II
3. What nursing diagnoses are appropriate for Ms. Zemakis at this time? Which takes priority?
4. What therapies would assist Ms. Zemakis in returning to homeostasis?
5. Referring to the module on Perfusion, what is the significance of the different blood pressure readings in different positions?

Independent Interventions

The nurse approaches acid–base imbalances by taking vital signs and obtaining a thorough patient history, which includes risk factors; cardiac, renal, pulmonary symptoms; current medications; medical conditions; and other symptoms. For patients in severe distress, family members may need to be consulted for critical information, including recent eating habits and history of vomiting. When taking the patient's health history, the nurse should consider conditions potentially related to culture and developmental stages.

Independent interventions related to acid–base management may include the following:

- Taking weight daily
- Monitoring intake and output
- Assessing respiratory and renal function
- Maintaining a patent airway
- Monitoring oxygen saturation
- Taking vital signs
- Assessing LOC and neurologic function
- Prompt reporting of changes in patient condition.

Collaborative Therapies

Untreated, severe metabolic acidosis can lead to myocardial depression, seizures, shock, and multi-organ failure. The goal of treatment is to restore or maintain normal body balance. Treatment of acid–base imbalance depends on identification and treatment of the underlying cause; collaborative care for an acid–base imbalance also depends on identification of the underlying cause. There is ongoing collaboration with the healthcare team for all patients.

Pharmacologic Therapy

Specific pharmacologic therapies are available to treat acidosis and alkalosis. Careful monitoring of ABG levels prevents overtreatment that causes pH to alter in the opposite direction, changing alkalosis to acidosis or acidosis to alkalosis.

In patients with acidosis, the therapeutic goal is to reverse the effects of excess acids in the blood and return the patient to normal pH levels as quickly as possible. The pharmacologic treatment of choice for acute acidosis is sodium bicarbonate infusions, provided that the patient's bicarbonate level is low. The bicarbonate ion acts quickly as a base to neutralize acids in the blood and other body fluids. Carefully monitor the patient's ABGs during infusions and watch for signs of alkalosis; sodium bicarbonate can "overcorrect" the acidosis, causing blood pH to turn alkaline. Symptoms of alkalosis include irritability, confusion, cyanosis, slow respirations, irregular pulse, and muscle weakness. If these symptoms occur, withhold the medication and notify the healthcare provider.

The nurse's role in sodium bicarbonate therapy involves carefully monitoring a patient's condition and educating the patient and family about the prescribed treatment. Sodium bicarbonate is given to neutralize acidotic states, so first analyze the ABG reports of pH, carbon dioxide levels ($PaCO_2$), bicarbonate levels (HCO_3), and oxygenation status (PaO_2 and O_2 saturation). Assess the patient for symptoms associated with acidosis, such as sleepiness, coma, disorientation, dizziness, headache, seizures, and hypoventilation. Also assess the patient for causative factors that could produce acidosis, such as diabetes mellitus, shock, and diarrhea. Successful management of the underlying disease condition frequently corrects acidosis.

Sodium bicarbonate is used only in patients with a pH less than 7.2 (Wiederkehr & Emmett, 2016). Several contraindications and precautions are related to the administration of sodium bicarbonate. It should be used judiciously in patients with cardiac disease and renal impairment because of the sodium content.

Sodium bicarbonate is also used to alkalinize the urine and speed the excretion of acidic substances. This process is useful in treating overdoses of certain acidic medications such as aspirin and phenobarbital and is useful as adjunctive therapy for certain chemotherapeutic drugs such as methotrexate.

Sodium bicarbonate is also used in chronic renal failure to neutralize the metabolic acidosis that occurs when the kidneys cannot excrete hydrogen ion. Intravenous (IV) sodium bicarbonate causes the urine to become more alkaline. Less acid is reabsorbed in the renal tubules, so more acid and acidic medicine is excreted. This process is known as *ion trapping*. During ion trapping, monitor the patient's acid–base status closely and report symptoms of imbalance. Provide care directed toward supporting critical body functions such as cardiovascular, respiratory, and neurologic status, which may be impaired secondary to the drug overdose.

Sodium bicarbonate (baking soda) is used as a home remedy to neutralize gastric acid, relieving heartburn and sour stomach. Although occasional use is acceptable, nurses should be aware that patients may misinterpret cardiac symptoms as heartburn, and overuse of sodium bicarbonate may lead to systemic alkalosis.

Patient Teaching

Sodium Bicarbonate

Include the following points when teaching patients and their families about sodium bicarbonate:

- Immediately contact the primary healthcare provider if gastric discomfort continues or is accompanied by chest pain, dyspnea, or diaphoresis.
- Use nonsodium antacids to prevent the absorption of excess sodium or bicarbonate into the systemic circulation.
- Do not use any antacid, including sodium bicarbonate, for longer than 2 weeks without consulting your healthcare provider.

Patient education as it relates to sodium bicarbonate should include the goals of therapy, the reasons for obtaining baseline data such as vital signs and electrolyte levels, and possible drug side effects.

Airway Management

Patients experiencing respiratory distress may require intubation. Although there is no specific rule for when to intubate, generally intubation is indicated if the patient has a $PaCO_2$ greater than 77 mmHg, a PaO_2 less than 60 mmHg, and a pH less than 7.20. Patients with chronic hypercarbia require care to correct their status slowly, as correcting $PaCO_2$ too quickly may result in metabolic alkalosis due to excessive retention of bicarbonate. Patients with hypoxemia may also require supplemental oxygen, which has been shown to improve outcomes and reduce mortality rates (Feller-Kopman & Schwartzstein, 2015). Mechanical ventilation and oxygen administration are discussed in detail in the module on Oxygenation.

Bilevel positive airway pressure (bipap) may be an option for certain patients who are not in immediate need of intubation and who meet certain criteria that include severe respiratory distress and acute respiratory acidosis, especially if intubation is contraindicated. Monitor patients receiving bipap therapy for pneumothorax and hypotension secondary to decreased venous return (Melanson, 2015).

Clinical Example C

John Quinland is a 60-year-old man with a 45-year history of smoking two packs of cigarettes a day. Over the past year, he has become increasingly short of breath. At first, he noticed this only when exercising, but now he is short of breath even at rest. Over the past year, he has had several infections of the lower respiratory tract that were treated successfully with antibiotics at the local ED. His shortness of breath has not subsided, and he uses his accessory muscles of respiration to assist him in breathing. Mr. Quinland does not have a primary care provider and does not get physical examinations. He had his last physical over 20 years ago to meet a work requirement. Mr. Quinland goes to the nearest hospital when he has a respiratory infection. The ED physician advises Mr. Quinland to find a healthcare provider because he needs routine checkups, but Mr. Quinland does not take the advice.

Clinical Reasoning Questions Level I

1. If you were the nurse taking Mr. Quinland's health history during his latest trip to the ED, what would be your primary concerns?
2. What nursing diagnoses are appropriate for Mr. Quinland at this time?
3. Is Mr. Quinland's smoking the priority consideration at this time? Why or why not?

Clinical Reasoning Questions Level II

4. Refer to the exemplar on COPD in the module on Oxygenation. What signs/symptoms of COPD does Mr. Quinland exhibit? What risk factors does he have?
5. Refer to the exemplar on Nicotine Use in the module on Addiction. Why/how does smoking result in alterations such as chronic hypercapnia and COPD?
6. What patient teaching would you attempt to provide Mr. Quinland prior to discharge?

REVIEW　The Concept of Acid–Base Balance

RELATE Link the Concepts

Linking the concept of acid–base balance with the concept of oxygenation:

1. What oxygenation changes are seen in patients with acidosis and alkalosis?
2. Why does hypoventilation decrease oxygenation? Why does hyperventilation increase oxygenation?

Linking the concept of acid–base balance with the concept of communication:

3. How might an acid–base imbalance impair a patient's ability to communicate?
4. Give some examples of therapeutic communication techniques to use when addressing concerns of patients whose communication is limited due to severity of illness?

Linking the concept of acid–base balance with the concept of safety:

5. Why would it be particularly important to guard against medication errors for a patient with acid–base imbalance?
6. In what situations or for what patients might it be necessary to arrange for a home safety assessment prior to discharge?

READY Go to Volume 3: Clinical Nursing Skills

- SKILL 1.5 　Blood Pressure: Newborn, Infant, Child, Adult, Obtaining
- SKILL 1.7 　Pulse Oximeter: Using
- SKILL 1.8 　Respirations: Newborn, Infant, Child, Adult, Obtaining
- SKILL 1.22 　Neurologic Status: Assessing
- SKILL 11.8 　Oxygen Delivery Systems: Using
- SKILL 11.14 Suctioning, Oropharyngeal and Nasopharyngeal: Newborn, Infant, Child, Adult

REFER Go to Pearson MyLab Nursing and eText

- Additional review materials

REFLECT Apply Your Knowledge

Maria Hernandez is an 80-year-old woman (weight 40 kg) who is admitted to the intensive care unit following a motor vehicle collision. She was driving and wearing her seat belt when she ran her car off the road and hit a tree. She remembers the collision and did not lose consciousness. Her injuries include a left anterior flail segment of the rib, a fractured left shoulder, and facial bruising. She is hemodynamically stable but has respiratory distress with paradoxical movement of her left anterior chest wall. She has no head or neck injury. She has recently had several unexplained blackouts. She takes a beta-blocker daily for hypertension.

She was intubated and ventilated in the ED because of respiratory distress. Initial ventilation was tidal volume 700 mL at a rate of 12 breaths with 100% oxygen. Peripheral perfusion was good. An intravenous infusion of lactated Ringer solution was started at 100 mL per hour. Arterial blood gases were obtained half an hour later.

At this time, Ms. Hernandez's vital signs are T_O 98.8°F; HR 110 bpm; R 16/min; BP 120/60 mmHg; pulse oximeter 99% on 100% oxygen. Her ABG values are pH 7.32; pCO_2 48 mmHg; pO_2 86 mmHg; HCO_3 21 mEq/L.

Clinical Reasoning Questions Level I

1. What is Ms. Hernandez's primary problem?
2. What is the cause of her respiratory distress?
3. What do her ABG results indicate?

Clinical Reasoning Questions Level II

4. Refer to the module on Oxygenation. What will you need to monitor Ms. Hernandez while she is intubated?
5. Refer to the module on Oxygenation. How will you help Ms. Hernandez communicate while she is intubated?
6. Refer to the module on Legal Issues. Ms. Hernandez's nephew calls to inquire about her condition. What regulations or policies apply when an individual calls seeking information about a patient? How do you respond to the nephew?

Exemplar 1.A
Metabolic Acidosis

Exemplar Learning Outcomes

1.A Analyze metabolic acidosis as it relates to acid–base balance.

- Describe the pathophysiology of metabolic acidosis.
- Describe the etiology of metabolic acidosis.
- Compare the risk factors and prevention of metabolic acidosis.
- Identify the clinical manifestations of metabolic acidosis.
- Summarize diagnostic tests and therapies used by interprofessional teams in the collaborative care of an individual with metabolic acidosis.

- Differentiate care of patients with metabolic acidosis across the lifespan.
- Apply the nursing process in providing culturally competent care to an individual with metabolic acidosis.

Exemplar Key Terms

Kussmaul respirations, *15*
Metabolic acidosis, *13*

Overview

Metabolic acidosis (bicarbonate deficit) is characterized by a low pH (less than 7.35) and a low bicarbonate (less than 24 mEq/L). It may be caused by excess acid in the body or loss of bicarbonate from the body. When metabolic acidosis develops, the respiratory system attempts to return the pH to normal by increasing the rate and depth of respirations. Carbon dioxide elimination increases, and the $PaCO_2$ falls (to less than 35 mmHg).

Pathophysiology and Etiology
Pathophysiology

Four basic mechanisms can cause metabolic acidosis:

1. Accumulation of metabolic acids
2. Excess loss of bicarbonate
3. An increase in chloride levels
4. Fluid imbalance.

An accumulation of metabolic acids can result from excess acid production or impaired renal elimination of metabolic acids. Lactic acidosis develops due to tissue hypoxia and a shift to anaerobic metabolism by the cells. Lactate and hydrogen ions are produced, forming lactic acid. Both oxygen and glucose are necessary for normal cell metabolism. When intracellular glucose is inadequate because of starvation or a lack of insulin to move it into cells, the body breaks down fatty tissue to meet its metabolic needs. In this process, fatty acids are released and converted to ketones; ketoacidosis results. Aspirin (acetylsalicylic acid) breaks down into salicylic acid in the body. Substances such as aspirin, methanol (wood alcohol), and ethylene (contained in antifreeze and solvents) cause a toxic increase in body acids by either breaking down into acid products (salicylic acid) or stimulating metabolic acid production (Porth & Gross, 2014). Hypovolemia from dehydration will cause metabolic acidosis, contributing to other conditions such as bicarbonate lost in stool, ketones produced with starvation (as seen in eating disorders), ketoacidosis from decreased tissue perfusion, and decreased renal perfusion. Renal failure impairs the body's ability to excrete excess hydrogen ions and form bicarbonate.

Excess metabolic acids increase the hydrogen ion concentration of body fluids. The buffering of excess acid by bicarbonate leads to what is known as a *high anion gap acidosis*.

The pancreas secretes bicarbonate-rich fluid into the small intestine. Intestinal suction, severe diarrhea, ileostomy drainage, or fistulas can lead to excess losses of bicarbonate. Hyperchloremic acidosis can develop when excess of a chloride solution (e.g., NaCl) is infused, causing a rise in chloride concentrations. It also may be related to renal disease or administration of carbonic anhydrate inhibitor diuretics. The anion gap remains normal in metabolic acidosis because of bicarbonate loss or excess chloride.

Acidosis depresses cell membrane excitability, affecting neuromuscular function. It also increases the amount of free calcium in ECF by interfering with protein binding. Severe acidosis (pH of 7 or less) depresses myocardial contractility, leading to decreased cardiac output. If kidney function is normal, acid excretion and ammonia production increase to eliminate excess hydrogen ions.

Acid–base imbalances also affect electrolyte balance. In acidosis, potassium is retained as the kidney excretes excess hydrogen ions. Excess hydrogen ions also enter the cells, displacing potassium from the intracellular space to maintain the balance of cations and anions within the cells. The effect of both processes is to increase serum potassium levels. Also in acidosis, calcium is released from its bonds with plasma proteins, increasing the amount of ionized (free) calcium in the blood. Magnesium levels may fall in acidosis.

Etiology

Metabolic acidosis is rarely a primary disorder; it usually develops during the course of another disease, as follows:

- Acute lactic acidosis usually results from tissue hypoxia due to shock or cardiac arrest.
- Patients with type 1 diabetes mellitus are at risk for developing DKA.
- Acute or chronic renal failure impairs the excretion of metabolic acids.
- Diarrhea, intestinal suction, or abdominal fistulas increase the risk for excess bicarbonate loss.
- Ingestion of an acidic substance or a substance that can be metabolized to an acid.

Risk Factors

Risk factors for metabolic acidosis include DKA, renal failure, severe sepsis, liver failure, and salicylate intoxication. Metabolic acidosis from severe diarrhea can occur at any age. Young women with eating disorders who abuse laxatives or engage in severe diet restriction to the point of cachexia (wasting with acute weight loss and muscle loss) are at an increased risk of metabolic acidosis due to the resulting decrease in bicarbonate. Other common causes of metabolic acidosis are listed in Table 1–1.

Clinical Manifestations

Metabolic acidosis affects the function of many body systems. Its general manifestations include weakness and fatigue, headache, and general malaise. The effects on gastrointestinal function cause diminished appetite, nausea, vomiting, and abdominal pain. The LOC may decline into stupor and coma.

Clinical Manifestations and Therapies
Metabolic Acidosis

ETIOLOGY	CLINICAL MANIFESTATIONS	CLINICAL THERAPIES
Conditions that increase nonvolatile acids in the blood (e.g., renal impairment, diabetes mellitus, starvation)	■ Diminished appetite ■ Nausea and vomiting ■ Abdominal pain	■ Monitor ABG values, intake and output, and LOC. ■ Position patient to facilitate chest expansion.
Conditions that decrease bicarbonate (e.g., prolonged diarrhea, excessive use of laxatives)	■ Weakness ■ Fatigue	■ Provide oral care for dry mouth. ■ Administer IV sodium bicarbonate carefully if ordered.
Excessive infusion of chloride-containing IV fluids (e.g., NaCl)	■ Headache ■ General malaise	■ Treat underlying problem as ordered.
Excessive ingestion of acids (e.g., salicylates)	■ Decreasing LOC ■ Dysrhythmia	
Cardiac arrest	■ Bradycardia ■ Warm, flushed skin ■ Skeletal problems ■ Hyperventilation (Kussmaul respirations) ■ Dyspnea	

Cardiac dysrhythmias develop, and cardiac arrest may occur. The skin is often warm and flushed. Skeletal problems may develop in chronic acidosis, as calcium and phosphate are released from the bones. Manifestations of compensatory mechanisms are seen. The deep and rapid respirations that may occur are known as **Kussmaul respirations**. The patient may complain of shortness of breath, or dyspnea.

Collaboration

As stated earlier, metabolic acidosis normally results from another primary disorder. Therefore the focus is on treating the primary disorder, reducing the effects of acidosis on cardiac function, and ensuring adequate oxygenation. Refer to the patient's history for listing of predisposing/contributing factors. Monitor serum electrolytes, especially potassium. Replace fluids as needed. Modify diet as indicated.

Diagnostic Tests

Diagnostic tests include ABGs, serum electrolytes, and tests as indicated by the underlying primary disorder.

Pharmacologic Therapy

To reduce the effects of acidosis on cardiac function, an alkalinizing solution such as bicarbonate may be given if the pH is less than 7.1. Sodium bicarbonate is the most commonly used alkalinizing solution; others include lactate, citrate, and acetate solutions (which are metabolized to bicarbonate). Give alkalinizing solutions intravenously for severe acute metabolic acidosis. Use the oral route for chronic metabolic acidosis.

Carefully monitor patients treated with bicarbonate. Rapid correction of the acidosis may lead to metabolic alkalosis and hypokalemia. Hypernatremia and hyperosmolality may develop as well, leading to water retention and fluid overload.

SAFETY ALERT As metabolic acidosis is corrected, potassium shifts back into the intracellular space. This shift can lead to hypokalemia and cardiac dysrhythmias. Carefully monitor serum potassium levels during treatment.

Treatment for DKA includes intravenous insulin and fluid replacement. Alcoholic ketoacidosis is treated with saline solutions and glucose. Treatment for lactic acidosis from decreased tissue perfusion (e.g., shock, cardiac arrest, rhabdomyolysis due to crush injuries) focuses on correcting the underlying problem and improving tissue perfusion. Patients with chronic renal failure and mild or moderate metabolic acidosis may or may not require treatment, depending on their pH and bicarbonate levels. When metabolic acidosis is due to diarrhea, treatment includes correcting the underlying cause and providing fluid and electrolyte replacement.

Lifespan Considerations
Metabolic Acidosis in Infants and Children

Metabolic acidosis can occur in any age group. Metabolic acidosis is an acid–base disorder characterized by a decrease in serum pH that results from either a primary decrease in plasma bicarbonate concentration or an increase in hydrogen ion concentration. Infants are more likely to develop metabolic acidosis from significant losses of bicarbonate in diarrhea. Children with congenital or acquired renal tubular acidosis can lose large amounts of bicarbonate, with or without potassium depletion. Children with metabolic disease, such as type 1 diabetes, need lifelong insulin administration and good nutritional education and support (Huang, 2015).

Metabolic Acidosis in Older Adults

Many older adults can maintain acid–base balance under normal conditions. However, metabolic acidosis in an older adult who presents to the ED may be a consequence of diabetes, renal failure, or ketoacidosis. Accidental overdose of salicylic acid (aspirin) may also cause metabolic acidosis. Older adults experience a higher concentration of hydrogen ion in metabolic acidosis, which inversely correlates with serum bicarbonate and $PaCO_2$ (Lewis et al., 2014). Older adults may take more medications because of the increased incidence of disease. Diuretics, certain antidepressants, antiseizure medications, and angiotensin-converting enzyme (ACE) inhibitors may affect acid–base balance in older adults. Outcome depends on the nature of the illness and early diagnosis and treatment.

NURSING PROCESS

Nurses frequently provide care for patients with metabolic acidosis, although the focus of care is usually the underlying disorder (e.g., diabetes mellitus, renal failure) rather than the acidosis itself. For this reason, nurses must know the effects of acidosis and its implications for nursing care.

To promote health in patients at risk for metabolic acidosis, discuss management of the underlying disease process (e.g., type 1 diabetes, renal failure) to help patients prevent complications such as DKA and metabolic acidosis. Because early manifestations of metabolic acidosis (e.g., fatigue, general malaise, diminished appetite, nausea, abdominal pain) resemble those of common viral disorders such as influenza, stress the importance of promptly seeking treatment if these symptoms develop.

Assessment

- *Observation and patient interview.* Ask the patient about current manifestations, including diminished appetite, nausea, vomiting, abdominal discomfort, fatigue, lethargy, and other symptoms; duration of symptoms and any precipitating factors such as diarrhea and ingestion of a toxin such as aspirin, methanol, or ethylene; chronic diseases such as diabetes or renal failure, cirrhosis of the liver, or endocrine disorders; and current medications.
- *Physical examination.* Examine mental status and LOC, vital signs including respiratory rate and depth, apical and peripheral pulses, skin color and temperature, abdominal contour and distention, bowel sounds, and urine output.

Diagnosis

Although the focus of nursing management is on the primary disorder, the acidosis itself has effects that require care.

Possible nursing diagnoses for the patient with metabolic acidosis are the following:

- *Cardiac Output, Decreased, Risk for*
- *Electrolyte Imbalance, Risk for*
- *Fluid Volume: Deficient*
- *Fluid Volume: Excess*
- *Falls, Risk for.*

(NANDA-I © 2014)

Planning

Planning for the patient with metabolic acidosis involves identification and treatment of the underlying cause and restoration and maintenance of acid–base balance. (Refer to other modules for a discussion of interventions specific to the underlying disorder.) Potential goals for the patient with metabolic acidosis may be the following:

- Patient will describe and demonstrate preventive measures related to chronic disease process.
- pH will remain within normal range.
- Disease process causing acid–base imbalance will be controlled to reduce acid production or alkaline loss.
- Patient will maintain vital signs within normal range for age and condition.
- Patient will maintain baseline cardiac rhythm.

Implementation

Metabolic acidosis affects cardiac output by decreasing myocardial contractility, slowing the heart rate, and increasing the risk for dysrhythmias. The accompanying hyperkalemia increases the risk for decreased cardiac output as well. (See the module on Fluids and Electrolytes for discussion about hyperkalemia.) In the acute care setting:

- Monitor vital signs, including peripheral pulses and capillary refill. Hypotension, diminished pulse strength, and slowed capillary refill may indicate decreased cardiac output and impaired tissue perfusion. Poor tissue perfusion can increase the risk for lactic acidosis.
- Monitor intake and output. In particular, patients with eating disorders may attempt to continue self-imposed dietary restrictions. These patients can be resistant to treatment and may try to conceal the true nature of their disorders.
- Monitor the ECG pattern for dysrhythmias and changes characteristic of hyperkalemia, such as peaked T waves. Notify the physician of changes. Progressive ECG changes such as widening of the QRS complex indicate an increasing risk of dysrhythmias and cardiac arrest. Dysrhythmias further decrease cardiac output, possibly intensifying the degree of acidosis.
- Monitor laboratory values, including ABGs, serum electrolytes, and renal function studies (serum creatinine and blood urea nitrogen [BUN]). Frequent monitoring of laboratory values allows evaluation of the effectiveness of treatment as well as early identification of potential problems.

SAFETY ALERT Administering bicarbonate to correct acidosis increases the risk for hypernatremia, hyperosmolality, and fluid volume excess. Sodium bicarbonate is only administered when pH is less than 7.1.

Monitor Potential for Excess Fluid Volume

- Monitor and maintain fluid replacement as ordered. Monitor serum sodium levels and osmolality.
- Monitor heart and lung sounds, central venous pressure (CVP), and respiratory status. Increasing dyspnea, adventitious lung sounds, a third heart sound (S_3) due to the volume of blood flow through the heart, and high CVP readings indicate hypervolemia and should be reported to the healthcare provider.
- Assess for edema, particularly in the back, sacral, and periorbital areas. Edema initially affects dependent tissues—the back and sacrum in patients who are bedridden. Periorbital edema indicates more generalized edema.
- Assess urine output hourly. Maintain accurate intake and output records. Note urine output less than 30 mL/hour or a positive fluid balance on 24-hour total intake and output calculations. Heart failure and inadequate renal perfusion may lead to decreased urine output.
- Obtain daily weights using consistent conditions (same time of day, clothing, and scale). Daily weights are an accurate indicator of fluid balance.
- Administer prescribed diuretics as ordered, monitoring the patient's response to therapy. Loop or high-ceiling diuretics such as furosemide can lead to further electrolyte imbalances, especially hypokalemia. This is a significant risk, like that seen during correction of metabolic acidosis.

Reduce Risk for Injury

Mental status and brain function are affected by acidosis, increasing the risk for injury. Nurses working with patients who exhibit altered mental status related to acidosis should:

- Monitor neurologic function, including mental status, LOC, and muscle strength. As the pH falls, the resulting decline in mental functioning leads to confusion, stupor, and a decreasing LOC.
- Institute safety precautions as necessary: Keep the bed in its lowest position, make sure the call light can be reached, and assign a sitter if necessary. These measures help protect the patient from injury resulting from confusion or disorientation.
- Keep clocks, calendars, and familiar objects at bedside. Orient to time, place, and circumstances as needed. Allow significant others to remain with the patient as much as possible. An unfamiliar environment and altered thought processes can further increase the risk for injury. Significant others provide a sense of security and reduce anxiety.

Plan for Discharge

When preparing the patient with metabolic acidosis for discharge, consider the cause of the acidosis and any underlying factors. Patients who have developed ketoacidosis as a result of diabetes mellitus, starvation, or alcoholism need interventions and teaching to prevent future episodes of acidosis. Diet, medication management, and alcohol dependency treatment are vital teaching areas. When metabolic acidosis is related to renal failure, the patient should be referred for management of the renal failure itself. Patients who have experienced diarrhea or excess ileostomy drainage leading to bicarbonate loss need information about appropriate diarrhea treatment strategies and need to know when to call their primary care provider. Provide teaching to patients and their families about the following:

- Using appropriate resources to get medical assistance.
- Contacting the primary care provider immediately if the patient experiences dizziness, nausea, vomiting, and fatigue.

Evaluation

Expected outcomes of nursing care relate to prevention of acidosis and restoration of normal body balance during disease processes. During the recovery period, frequently monitor pH levels and vital signs, and reassess the patient's condition to revise care plans as necessary. Expected outcomes include the following:

- Patient maintains pH within normal range.
- Patient's vital signs remain within normal range based on age and condition.
- Patient maintains adequate oxygenation of tissues.
- Patient is able to describe or demonstrate measures to control the disease process to prevent future complications of pH imbalance.

Nursing Care Plan
A Patient with Metabolic Acidosis

Mary Groverman, a 29-year-old patient, is admitted with generalized weakness, nausea, and diarrhea. The patient was a poor historian. Her electronic records reveal a long history of laxative abuse and one hospital admission for diuretic abuse. There was difficulty in obtaining records from outside hospitals because of incorrect address and phone numbers.

ASSESSMENT	DIAGNOSES	PLANNING
Ms. Groverman states that she has been tired and weak but does not admit to an eating disorder or to any behaviors that may have caused symptoms. Physical examination findings include weight 40 kg; temperature 97.8°F oral; pulse 105 bpm; respirations 16/min; and BP 85/55 mmHg. The nurse observes poor skin turgor and dry mucous membranes. Bilateral breath sounds are clear. Her abdominal assessment is essentially normal with hyperactive bowel sounds. Ms. Groverman's urine is dark, amber, and concentrated. Electrolytes reveal: - Sodium—132 mEq/L - Chloride—105 mEq/L - Potassium—2.9 mEq/L - Sodium bicarbonate—14.0 mmol/L - Serum glucose—87 mm/dL Complete blood count (CBC) results are as follows: - Hemoglobin—8.2 g/dL - Hematocrit—38% - BUN—35 mg/dL - Creatinine—2.8 mg/dL ABGs: - pH—7.29 - pCO_2—33 mmHg - PO_2—119 mmHg - HCO_3—18 mmol/L	- *Activity Intolerance* related to fluid volume deficiency, weakness, and fatigue - *Electrolyte Imbalance, Risk for* related dehydration and acidosis - *Gas Exchange, Impaired* related to acidotic state - *Fluid Volume: Deficient* related to abuse of laxatives - *Imbalanced Nutrition: Less than Body Requirements* related to malnutrition - *Self-Esteem, Situational Low* related to eating disorder - *Urinary Elimination, Impaired* related to dehydration and acidosis (NANDA-I © 2014)	- The patient will have normal physiologic balance. - The patient will have normal electrolytes and acid–base status. - The patient will have normal cardiac function. - The patient will maintain daily weights. - The patient will demonstrate normal extracellular fluid volume by gaining weight and maintaining normal urine output. - The patient will discuss proper use of laxatives. - The patient will follow up with psychologic counseling for evaluation and treatment of an eating disorder (bulimia).

IMPLEMENTATION	
- Provide hydration initially by IV and then by oral intake when patient is able. - Provide fluids and encourage good nutrition when patient is able. - Weigh daily before breakfast; monitor vital signs and heart rate every 4 hours.	- Document intake and output every 4 hours. - Monitor food intake, noting percentage and types of food consumed. - Add supplemental vitamins and minerals. - Arrange nutrition and mental health consults.

(continued on next page)

Nursing Care Plan *(continued)*

EVALUATION

Ms. Groverman was hospitalized for 4 days, during which her appetite improved and she gave no evidence of laxative abuse or purging. Ms. Groverman remains slightly nauseated but is eating most of her prescribed diet and snacks. She has gained 3 pounds over the course of 4 days. Ms. Groverman has agreed to be treated as an outpatient in the nearby center for eating disorders.

CRITICAL THINKING

1. How does a history of laxative and diuretic abuse in the setting of an eating disorder cause metabolic acidosis?
2. How do electrolyte and renal dysfunction cause changes in cognition and mental status?
3. Normal hematocrit is 3 times the hemoglobin. Why is the hematocrit elevated?

REVIEW   Metabolic Acidosis

RELATE Link the Concepts and Exemplars

The ambulance arrives with a patient who presents with Kussmaul respirations and a history of diabetes mellitus.

Linking the exemplar of metabolic acidosis with the concept of metabolism:

1. Based on the patient's history, what impact does the nurse expect to find on acid–base balance?
2. When the nurse is assessing this patient, what symptoms of acidosis would be directly related to alterations in pH?

Linking the exemplar of metabolic acidosis with the concept of fluids and electrolytes:

3. When assessing the patient, what electrolyte imbalances should the nurse monitor in acidosis?
4. What signs of dehydration will the nurse observe in a patient in acute metabolic acidosis?

Linking the exemplar of metabolic acidosis with the concept of safety:

5. What precautions should the nurse implement for the patient with metabolic acidosis to prevent potential injury?
6. The patient with metabolic acidosis becomes confused and disoriented. What nursing care should the nurse provide to this patient to maintain safety?

READY Go to Volume 3: Clinical Nursing Skills

REFER Go to Pearson MyLab Nursing and eText

- Additional review materials

REFLECT Apply Your Knowledge

Reread Clinical Example A. Mr. James's arterial blood gas values were pH 7.28; $PaCO_2$ 31 mmHg; PaO_2 95 mmHg; and HCO_3 15 mEq/L. CVP or right atrial pressure (RAP) ranged from 1 to 3 cm H_2O pressure. ECG revealed sinus tachycardia with ST depression in most leads. Two units of packed red blood cells were ordered and rapidly transfused into the patient. His hemoglobin was 10 g/dL and his hematocrit was 40% before the transfusion.

1. What is the priority nursing diagnosis for Mr. James at this time? Why?
2. What is the interpretation of the ABG results?
3. How is the patient compensating for the acidosis?
4. Refer to the module on Perfusion. Why was the CVP catheter placed in this patient? What are normal CVP values?
5. Why is the hematocrit falsely elevated?
6. What safety precautions should be implemented for Mr. James at this time?

›› Exemplar 1.B
Metabolic Alkalosis

Exemplar Learning Outcomes

1.B Analyze metabolic alkalosis as it relates to acid–base balance.

- Describe the pathophysiology of metabolic alkalosis.
- Describe the etiology of metabolic alkalosis.
- Compare the risk factors and prevention of metabolic alkalosis.
- Identify the clinical manifestations of metabolic alkalosis.
- Summarize diagnostic tests and therapies used by interprofessional teams in the collaborative care of an individual with metabolic alkalosis.
- Differentiate care of patients with metabolic alkalosis across the lifespan.
- Apply the nursing process in providing culturally competent care to an individual with metabolic alkalosis.

Exemplar Key Term

Metabolic alkalosis, *19*

Overview

Metabolic alkalosis (bicarbonate excess) is characterized by a high pH (greater than 7.45) and a high bicarbonate (greater than 28 mEq/L). It may be caused by loss of acid or excess bicarbonate in the body. When metabolic alkalosis develops, the respiratory system attempts to return the pH to normal by slowing the respiratory rate. Carbon dioxide is retained, and the $PaCO_2$ increases (to greater than 45 mmHg).

Pathophysiology and Etiology

Pathophysiology

Hydrogen ions may be lost through the kidneys or via gastric secretions or because of a shift of hydrogen ions into the cells. Metabolic alkalosis due to loss of hydrogen ions usually occurs because of vomiting or gastric suction. Gastric secretions are highly acidic (pH 1–3). When these are lost through vomiting or gastric suction, the alkalinity of body fluids increases. This increased alkalinity results from the loss of acid and from selective retention of bicarbonate by the kidneys as chloride is depleted. (Chloride is the major anion in ECF; when it is lost, bicarbonate is retained as a replacement anion.)

Increased renal excretion of hydrogen ions can be prompted by hypokalemia as the kidneys try to conserve potassium, excreting hydrogen ions instead. Hypokalemia contributes to metabolic alkalosis in another way as well. When potassium shifts out of cells to maintain extracellular potassium levels, hydrogen ions shift into the cells to maintain the balance between cations and anions within the cells.

Excess bicarbonate usually occurs as a result of ingesting antacids that contain bicarbonate (e.g., soda bicarbonate, Alka-Seltzer) or overzealous administration of bicarbonate to treat metabolic acidosis. Common causes of metabolic alkalosis are summarized in Table 1–1.

In alkalosis, more calcium combines with serum proteins, reducing the amount of ionized (physiologically active) calcium in the blood. This reduction in ionized calcium accounts for many of the common manifestations of metabolic alkalosis. Alkalosis also affects potassium balance: Hypokalemia not only can cause metabolic alkalosis (see earlier), but also can result from metabolic alkalosis. Hydrogen ions shift out of the intracellular space to help restore the pH, prompting

more potassium to enter the cells and depleting ECF potassium. The high pH depresses the respiratory system as the body retains carbon dioxide to restore the ratio of carbonic acid to bicarbonate.

Etiology

Metabolic alkalosis is a primary problem seen in excessive ingestion of antacids, excessive use of bicarbonate, and lactate administration in hemodialysis. Metabolic alkalosis may also develop from hyperaldosteronism, hypokalemia, hypochloremia, nasogastric suctioning, use of loop diuretics, and vomiting.

Risk Factors

Like other acid–base imbalances, metabolic alkalosis rarely occurs as a primary disorder. Risk factors include hospitalization, hypokalemia, and treatment with alkalinizing solutions (e.g., bicarbonate). Metabolic alkalosis can occur in patients of any age, but older adults are at risk because of their delicate fluid and electrolyte status, and treatment focuses on the underlying cause. Young women who practice self-induced vomiting are also at risk for developing metabolic alkalosis. Finally, men and women with chronic hypercapnia respiratory failure are at risk for metabolic alkalosis if their $PaCO_2$ levels are rapidly reduced in mechanical ventilation.

Clinical Manifestations

Manifestations of metabolic alkalosis result from decreased calcium ionization and are similar to those of hypocalcemia. They include numbness and tingling around the mouth, fingers, and toes; dizziness; Trousseau sign (spasmodic contraction of hand/fingers in response to occlusion of the blood supply); and muscle spasm. As the respiratory system compensates for metabolic alkalosis, respirations are depressed and respiratory failure with hypoxemia and respiratory acidosis may develop.

Collaboration

Metabolic alkalosis typically arises as a consequence of an underlying primary disorder. The plan of care and therapeutic regimen are aimed at controlling alkalosis while treating the underlying cause.

Clinical Manifestations and Therapies
Metabolic Alkalosis

ETIOLOGY	CLINICAL MANIFESTATIONS	CLINICAL THERAPIES
Excessive acid losses due to vomiting or gastric suction	▪ Confusion	▪ Monitor intake and output closely.
Excessive use of potassium-losing diuretics	▪ Decreasing LOC	▪ Monitor vital signs, especially respirations and LOC.
Excessive adrenal corticoid hormones due to:	▪ Hyperreflexia	▪ Administer ordered IV fluids carefully.
▪ Cushing syndrome	▪ Tetany	▪ Administer oxygen as ordered.
▪ Hyperaldosteronism	▪ Dysrhythmias	▪ Treat underlying problem.
▪ Excessive bicarbonate intake from antacids	▪ Hypotension	
▪ Parenteral sodium bicarbonate infusion	▪ Seizures	
	▪ Respiratory failure	

Laboratory and Diagnostic Tests

The following laboratory and diagnostic tests may be ordered:

- **ABGs** show a pH greater than 7.45 and bicarbonate level greater than 28 mEq/L. With compensatory hypoventilation, carbon dioxide is retained and the $PaCO_2$ is greater than 45 mmHg.
- **Serum electrolytes** often demonstrate decreased serum potassium (less than 3.5 mEq/L) and decreased chloride (less than 95 mEq/L) levels. The serum bicarbonate level is high. Although the total serum calcium may be normal, the ionized fraction of calcium is low.
- **Urine pH** may be low (pH 1–3) if metabolic acidosis is caused by hypokalemia. The kidneys selectively retain potassium and excrete hydrogen ion to restore ECF potassium levels. Urinary chloride levels may be normal or greater than 250 mEq/24 hours.
- **The ECG pattern** shows changes similar to those seen with hypokalemia. (See the module on Fluids and Electrolytes for more information related to symptoms of hypokalemia.) These changes may be due to hypokalemia or to the alkalosis.

Pharmacologic Therapy

Treatment of metabolic alkalosis includes restoring normal fluid volume and administering potassium chloride and sodium chloride solution. The potassium restores serum and intracellular potassium levels, allowing the kidneys to conserve hydrogen ions more effectively. Chloride promotes renal excretion of bicarbonate. Sodium chloride solutions restore fluid volume deficits that can contribute to metabolic alkalosis. In severe alkalosis, an acidifying solution such as dilute hydrochloric acid or ammonium chloride may be administered. In addition, drugs may be used to treat the underlying cause of the alkalosis.

Lifespan Considerations
Metabolic Alkalosis in Infants and Children

Metabolic alkalosis is an acid–base disturbance caused by an elevation in the plasma bicarbonate concentration. It refers to a loss of acid or a gain of base in the extracellular fluid. Although metabolic alkalosis can occur at any age, a higher incidence is seen in younger children post cardiac surgery (Huang, 2013). Other causes of metabolic alkalosis in children include prolonged vomiting (as seen in pyloric stenosis), nasogastric suctioning, cystic fibrosis, use of diuretics, and hypokalemia. Nursing management for infants and children experiencing metabolic alkalosis includes (Ball et al., 2017):

- Ongoing monitoring of LOC and neuromuscular irritability
- Monitoring for nausea and vomiting
- Careful assessment of respiration rate and depth
- Obtaining ABGs as ordered
- Positioning to facilitate ease of respirations and to prevent aspiration of vomitus.

Metabolic Alkalosis in Older Adults

Many older adults can maintain acid–base balance under normal conditions. Metabolic alkalosis may be a consequence of a disorder in older adults. Vomiting may lead to dehydration. Because older adults have a diminished sense of thirst, they can become volume depleted and dehydrated much quicker than younger adults. Metabolic alkalosis results when loss of fluids and volume contraction lower serum potassium (Lewis et al. 2014). Outcome depends on the nature of the illness and early diagnosis/treatment.

NURSING PROCESS

Health promotion activities focus on teaching patients the risks of using sodium bicarbonate as an antacid to relieve heartburn or gastric distress. Stress the availability of other effective antacid preparations and the need to seek medical evaluation for persistent gastric symptoms.

In the hospital setting, carefully monitor laboratory values for patients at risk for developing metabolic alkalosis, particularly patients undergoing continuous gastric suction.

Assessment

Focused assessment data related to metabolic alkalosis are gathered from the patient interview, physical examination, and diagnostic tests.

- **Observation and patient interview.** Ask the patient about current manifestations such as numbness and tingling, muscle spasms, dizziness, or other symptoms; duration of symptoms and any precipitating factors such as bicarbonate ingestion, vomiting, diuretic therapy, or endocrine disorders; and current medications.
- **Physical examination.** Examine vital signs, including apical pulse and rate and depth of respirations; muscle strength; and deep tendon reflexes.
- **Diagnostic tests.** Examine test results of ABGs and serum electrolytes.

Diagnosis

Nursing care of the patient with metabolic alkalosis, as with metabolic acidosis, often focuses on intervention for the primary problem rather than the alkalosis itself. However, the risk for impaired gas exchange is a priority problem, especially with severe metabolic alkalosis. Possible nursing diagnoses for the patient with metabolic alkalosis include the following:

- *Breathing Pattern, Ineffective*
- *Cardiovascular Function, Impaired, Risk for*
- *Fluid Volume: Deficient, Risk for*
- *Injury, Risk for.*

(NANDA-I © 2014)

Planning

Planning for the patient with metabolic alkalosis depends on identification and treatment of the underlying cause.

Restoring and maintaining normal acid–base balance is the desired outcome. Nursing care will also include measures to treat the underlying disorder, such as hypokalemia. (Refer to other modules for a discussion of interventions specific to the underlying disorder.) Appropriate outcomes will include resolution of the underlying cause and the patient's return to:

- Oxygen saturation level of 95% or greater.
- Normal or near normal fluid and electrolyte volumes.

Implementation

Nursing care of the patient with metabolic alkalosis is focused on controlling pH while treating the underlying causative disorder and preventing complications.

Monitor for Impaired Gas Exchange

Respiratory compensation for metabolic alkalosis depresses the respiratory rate and reduces the depth of breathing to promote carbon dioxide retention. As a result, the patient is at risk for impaired gas exchange, especially in the presence of underlying lung disease.

- Monitor respiratory rate, depth, and effort. Monitor oxygen saturation continuously, reporting an oxygen saturation level of less than 95% (or as ordered). The depressed respiratory drive associated with metabolic alkalosis can lead to hypoxemia and impaired oxygenation of tissues. Oxygen saturation levels of less than 90% indicate significant oxygenation problems.
- Assess skin color; note and report cyanosis around the mouth. Central cyanosis, seen around the mouth and oral mucous membranes, indicates significant hypoxia and is a late sign.
- Monitor mental status and LOC. Report decreasing LOC or behavior changes such as restlessness, agitation, or confusion. Changes in mental status or behavior may be early signs of hypoxia.
- Place in semi-Fowler or Fowler position as tolerated. Elevating the head of the bed facilitates alveolar ventilation and gas exchange.
- Administer oxygen as ordered or as necessary to maintain oxygen saturation levels. Supplemental oxygen can help maintain blood and tissue oxygenation despite depressed respirations.
- Schedule nursing care activities to allow rest periods. The patient with hypoxemia has limited energy reserves, necessitating frequent rest and limited activities.

Monitor for Fluid Volume Deficit

Patients with metabolic alkalosis often have an accompanying fluid volume deficit.

- Assess intake and output accurately, monitoring fluid balance. In acute situations, hourly intake and output assessment may be indicated. Urine output of less than 30 mL/hr indicates inadequate tissue perfusion, inadequate renal perfusion, and an increased risk for acute renal failure.

- Assess vital signs, CVP, and peripheral pulse volume at least every 4 hours. Hypotension, tachycardia, low CVP, and weak, easily obliterated peripheral pulses indicate hypovolemia.
- Weigh daily under standard conditions (time of day, clothing, and scale). Rapid weight changes accurately reflect fluid balance.
- Administer IV fluids as prescribed using an electronic infusion pump. If rapid fluid replacement is ordered, monitor for the following indicators of fluid overload: dyspnea, tachypnea, tachycardia, increased CVP, jugular vein distention, and edema. Rapid fluid replacement may lead to hypervolemia, resulting in pulmonary edema and cardiac failure, particularly in patients with compromised cardiac and renal function.
- Monitor serum electrolytes, osmolality, and ABG values. Rehydration and administration of potassium chloride affect both acid–base and fluid and electrolyte balance. Careful monitoring is important to identify changes.

Plan for Discharge

When preparing the patient with metabolic alkalosis for discharge, consider the cause of the alkalosis and any underlying factors. For example, provide teaching to the patient and family about the following:

- Using appropriate antacids for heartburn and gastric distress
- Using potassium supplements as ordered or eating high-potassium foods to prevent hypokalemia if taking a potassium-wasting diuretic or if aldosterone production is impaired
- Contacting the primary care provider if uncontrolled or extended vomiting develops.

Evaluation

Expected outcomes of nursing care relate to restoration of normal body balance. Revisions in the care plan may need to be made if patients do not respond to some aspect of the plan. Nurses may need to follow up with patients released from hospital care to determine whether they are continuing to follow instructions for self-monitoring and self-care. Possible outcomes for patients with metabolic alkalosis include the following:

- Patient reports use of antacids that are acceptable for use and that reduce risk of recurrence of metabolic alkalosis.
- Patient describes proper self-administration procedure for oral potassium supplements.
- Patient describes when to notify provider about changes in daily weight.
- Patient's arterial pH returns to normal range.
- Patient's serum electrolyte values are within normal range.

REVIEW   Metabolic Alkalosis

RELATE Link the Concepts and Exemplars

Linking the exemplar of metabolic alkalosis with the concept of fluids and electrolytes:

1. What pathophysiologic process is involved with metabolic alkalosis that leads to a decrease in mental function?

2. What changes in serum electrolyte levels could indicate a risk for metabolic alkalosis?

Linking the exemplar of metabolic alkalosis with the concept of tissue integrity:

3. What caring interventions might be implemented (independently by the nurse or collaboratively by the healthcare team) to prevent metabolic alkalosis?

Linking the exemplar of metabolic alkalosis with the concept of communication:

4. What information about the patient with metabolic alkalosis should the nurse include in the end-of-shift report?

5. The patient with metabolic alkalosis becomes confused and disoriented. What strategies will help promote communication with this patient?

READY Go to Volume 3: Clinical Nursing Skills

REFER Go to Pearson MyLab Nursing and eText

- Additional review questions

Chart 1: Nursing Care Plan: A Patient with Metabolic Alkalosis

REFLECT Apply Your Knowledge

Reread Clinical Example B. Ms. Zemakis's initial labs reveal Na 130; K 2.0; Cl 103; Mg 1.4; BUN 10; creatinine 1.2 mmol/l. ABG values are pH 7.47; $PaCO_2$ 26 mmHg; PaO_2 88 mmHg; HCO_3 29 mEq/L.

Ms. Zemakis is transferred to the intensive care step-down unit for fluid and electrolyte replacement with ECG monitoring.

1. What are the priority nursing interventions for Ms. Zemakis at this time?

2. What is the interpretation of the ABG results?

3. What is the cause of her muscle weakness?

4. Why is ECG monitoring necessary?

5. Why does this patient need closer monitoring in the intensive care step-down unit?

» Exemplar 1.C Respiratory Acidosis

Exemplar Learning Outcomes

1.C Analyze respiratory acidosis as it relates to acid–base balance.

- Describe the pathophysiology of respiratory acidosis.
- Describe the etiology of respiratory acidosis.
- Compare the risk factors and prevention of respiratory acidosis.
- Identify the clinical manifestations of respiratory acidosis.
- Summarize diagnostic tests and therapies used by interprofessional teams in the collaborative care of an individual with respiratory acidosis.

- Differentiate care of patients with respiratory acidosis across the lifespan.
- Apply the nursing process in providing culturally competent care to an individual with respiratory acidosis.

Exemplar Key Terms

Hypercapnia, *22*
Hypoxemia, *22*
Respiratory acidosis, *22*
Ventilation, *22*

Overview

Respiratory acidosis is caused by an excess of dissolved carbon dioxide, or carbonic acid. It is characterized by a pH less than 7.35 and a $PaCO_2$ greater than 45 mmHg. Respiratory acidosis may be acute or chronic. In chronic respiratory acidosis, the bicarbonate level is higher than 28 mEq/L, as the kidneys compensate by retaining bicarbonate.

Pathophysiology and Etiology

Both acute and chronic respiratory acidosis result from carbon dioxide retention caused by alveolar hypoventilation. **Hypoxemia** (decreased oxygen) frequently accompanies respiratory acidosis.

Acute Respiratory Acidosis

Acute respiratory acidosis results from a sudden failure of **ventilation** (the exchange of oxygen and carbon dioxide). Chest trauma, aspiration of a foreign body, acute pneumonia, and overdoses of narcotic or sedative medications can lead to this condition. Because acute respiratory acidosis occurs with the sudden onset of hypoventilation—for example, with cardiac arrest—the $PaCO_2$ rises rapidly and the pH falls markedly. A pH of 7 or lower can occur within minutes, resulting in death if not corrected (Metheny, 2012). The serum bicarbonate level is unchanged initially because the compensatory response of the kidneys continues over hours to days.

Hypercapnia (increased carbon dioxide levels) affects neurologic function and the cardiovascular system. Carbon dioxide rapidly crosses the blood–brain barrier. Cerebral blood vessels dilate, and if the condition continues, intracranial pressure increases and papilledema (swelling and inflammation of the optic nerve where it enters the retina) develops (Porth & Gross, 2014). Peripheral vasodilation also occurs, and the pulse rate increases to maintain cardiac output.

The primary problem is alveolar hypoventilation with increased $PaCO_2$. Respiratory acidosis can be caused by acute pulmonary edema, central nervous system depression, chest wall disorders, trauma, oversedation, asthma, obstructive sleep apnea, obesity, and pulmonary infections.

Chronic Respiratory Acidosis

Chronic respiratory acidosis is associated with chronic respiratory or neuromuscular conditions such as COPD, asthma, cystic fibrosis, and multiple sclerosis. These conditions affect alveolar ventilation because of airway obstruction, structural changes in the lung, and limited chest wall expansion. Most patients with chronic respiratory acidosis have COPD with chronic bronchitis and emphysema. In chronic respiratory acidosis, the $PaCO_2$ increases over time and remains elevated. The kidneys retain bicarbonate, increasing bicarbonate levels, and the pH often remains close to the normal range because of adequate metabolic compensation.

The acute effects of hypercapnia may not develop when carbon dioxide levels rise gradually, allowing compensatory changes to occur. When carbon dioxide levels are chronically elevated, the respiratory center becomes less sensitive to the gas as a stimulant of the respiratory drive. The PaO_2 provides the primary stimulus for respirations. Patients with chronic respiratory acidosis are at risk for developing carbon dioxide narcosis (with manifestations of acute respiratory acidosis) if the respiratory center is suppressed by the administration of excess supplemental oxygen. Manifestations include confusion, tremors, and convulsions; coma can

occur if blood levels of $PaCO_2$ reach 70 mmHg or higher. Patients with chronic respiratory acidosis can tolerate $PaCO_2$ levels that are much higher than normal.

SAFETY ALERT Carefully monitor neurologic and respiratory status in patients with chronic respiratory acidosis who are receiving oxygen therapy. Immediately report a decreasing LOC or depressed respirations.

Risk Factors

Acute or chronic lung disease (e.g., pneumonia, COPD) or trauma is the primary risk factor for respiratory acidosis. Other conditions that depress or interfere with ventilation, such as excess narcotic analgesics, airway obstruction, and neuromuscular disease, also are risk factors for respiratory acidosis. Selected causes of respiratory acidosis are listed in Table 1–1.

Clinical Manifestations

The manifestations of acute and chronic respiratory acidosis differ. In acute respiratory acidosis, the rapid rise in $PaCO_2$ levels causes manifestations of hypercapnia. Cerebral vasodilation causes manifestations such as headache, blurred vision, irritability, and mental cloudiness. If the condition continues, the LOC progressively decreases. Rapid and dramatic changes in ABGs can lead to unconsciousness and ventricular fibrillation, a potentially lethal cardiac dysrhythmia. The skin of the patient with acute respiratory acidosis may be warm and flushed, and the pulse rate is elevated.

The manifestations of chronic respiratory acidosis include weakness and a dull headache. Sleep disturbances, daytime sleepiness, impaired memory, and personality changes also may be manifestations of chronic respiratory acidosis. Patients with acute respiratory failure require treatment in

Clinical Manifestations and Therapies
Respiratory Acidosis

ETIOLOGY	CLINICAL MANIFESTATIONS	CLINICAL THERAPIES
Diseases of the airways, such as asthma, chronic obstructive lung disease Disease of the chest Drugs that suppress breathing, such as opioids, or alcohol Obstructive sleep apnea	*Acute respiratory acidosis:* ■ Headache ■ Warm, flushed skin ■ Elevated pulse ■ Blurred vision ■ Irritability or altered mental status ■ Decreasing LOC ■ Cardiac dysrhythmias ■ Cardiac arrest *Chronic respiratory acidosis:* ■ Weakness ■ Dull headache ■ Sleep disturbances with daytime sleepiness ■ Impaired memory ■ Personality changes	■ Assist with identification/treatment of underlying cause. ■ Observe for altered respiratory excursion, rate, and depth. Auscultate breath sounds. ■ Assess LOC and progressive changes. ■ Place in semi-Fowler position or Fowler position as tolerated. ■ Encourage the patient with chronic respiratory acidosis to use pursed-lip breathing. ■ Administer oxygen as indicated by mask, cannula, or mechanical ventilation. Increase or decrease respiratory rate on ventilator. Modify respiratory settings as needed. ■ Administer medications as indicated; for example, naloxone hydrochloride (Narcan). ■ Use continuous positive airway pressure (CPAP).

the ED or intensive care unit. The focus is on restoring adequate ventilation and gas exchange.

Acute respiratory acidosis is often the result of inadequate breathing patterns resulting in retained carbon dioxide and inadequate intake of oxygen. As a result, hypoxemia often accompanies hypercapnia, requiring administration of supplemental oxygen. The administration of oxygen to the patient with chronic hypercapnia, such as the patient with COPD, must be done cautiously to prevent removing the respiratory drive in those who breathe as a result of minor hypoxia. See the exemplar on COPD in the module on Oxygenation, for more information about the administration of oxygen to those with chronic hypercapnia.

Collaboration

Care of the patient experiencing respiratory acidosis involves the efforts of the entire healthcare team. A respiratory therapist may provide breathing treatments and related therapies as ordered. Consultation with the pharmacist and the patient's primary care provider prevents administration of medications that may be contraindicated. Patients who are using accessory muscles to breathe may require increased caloric intake and the participation of a dietitian.

Diagnostic Tests

The following diagnostic tests may be ordered:

- **ABGs** show a pH of less than 7.35 and a $PaCO_2$ of more than 45 mmHg. In acute respiratory acidosis, the bicarbonate level is initially within the normal range but increases to greater than 28 mEq/L if the condition persists. In chronic respiratory acidosis, both the $PaCO_2$ and the HCO_3 may be significantly elevated.
- **Serum electrolytes** may show hypochloremia (chloride level below normal) in chronic respiratory acidosis.
- **Pulmonary function studies** may be done to determine whether chronic lung disease is the cause of the respiratory acidosis. However, these studies are not done during the acute period.

Additional diagnostic tests may be done to identify the underlying cause of the respiratory acidosis. Chest x-ray and sputum studies (cytology and culture) may be ordered to identify an acute or chronic lung disorder. If drug overdose is suspected, serum levels of the drug may be obtained.

Pharmacologic Therapy

A bronchodilator may be administered to open the airways. Antibiotics are prescribed to treat respiratory infections. If excess narcotics or anesthetic caused the acute respiratory acidosis, narcotic antagonists such as naloxone may be given to reverse the effects.

Respiratory Support

Treatment of respiratory acidosis, either acute or chronic, focuses on improving alveolar ventilation and gas exchange. Patients with severe respiratory acidosis and hypoxemia may require intubation and mechanical ventilation. The $PaCO_2$ level is lowered slowly to prevent complications

such as cardiac dysrhythmias and decreased cerebral perfusion. In patients with chronic respiratory acidosis, oxygen is administered cautiously to prevent carbon dioxide narcosis.

Pulmonary hygiene measures may be instituted, such as deep breathing and coughing exercises, breathing treatments, and percussion and drainage. Adequate hydration is important to promote removal of respiratory secretions.

Lifespan Considerations

Respiratory Acidosis in Infants and Children

Respiratory acidosis is an acid–base disturbance caused by an elevation of $PaCO_2$ with resultant excess of carbonic acid owing to primary defects in lung function or changes in the respiratory pattern. Children with asthma, pneumonia, airway obstruction, acute pulmonary edema, acute respiratory distress syndrome (ARDS), head trauma, and poisoning are at high risk for respiratory acidosis (Doenges, Moorhouse, & Murr, 2014). In children, the critical ABG result is increased $PaCO_2$, indicating increased carbonic acid; serum pH can be normal or decreased.

Clinical manifestations of respiratory acidosis in children of all ages are similar to those in adults: decreased LOC, increased intracranial pressure, and eventually coma. Acute respiratory acidosis may result in tachycardia and arrhythmias. Nursing management includes ongoing assessment of mental and respiratory status, positioning, suctioning as needed, and encouraging deep breathing (Ball et al., 2017).

Respiratory Acidosis in Older Adults

Many illnesses common to older adults may result in acid–base imbalance if not properly treated. COPD, chest wall abnormalities, pneumonia, and respiratory muscle weakness are some of the common causes of respiratory acidosis in older adults. CO_2 retention from hypoventilation occurs, and the compensatory response is HCO_3 retention by the kidneys (Lewis et al., 2014). Older adults are more prone to have COPD. Outcome depends on the nature of the illness and early diagnosis/treatment. Nursing interventions are as described in the Nursing Process section.

Patient Teaching

Instructions for Parents of Children with Airway Disorders or Lung Infection

Children with asthma, airway obstruction, influenza, and pneumonia are at risk for respiratory acidosis. Patient teaching includes teaching parents prevention methods such as (Ball et al., 2017):

- Deep breathing (several times a day)
- Signs of infection
- Positioning to facilitate chest expansion
- Medication administration (as appropriate)
- Use of any ordered devices such as home respirators and nebulizers.

NURSING PROCESS

Nursing care of patients with respiratory acidosis is focused on improving breathing patterns and maintaining a patent airway. Because of the link between smoking and chronic pulmonary diseases, nursing care may include teaching patients how to make healthier lifestyle choices.

Assessment

- ■ *Observation and patient interview.* Ask the patient about current manifestations, including headache, irritability, lethargy, difficulty thinking, blurred vision, and other symptoms; duration of symptoms and any precipitating factors such as drug use or respiratory infection; chronic diseases such as cystic fibrosis or COPD; and current medications.
- ■ *Physical examination.* Examine mental status and LOC; vital signs, skin color and temperature; and rate and depth of respirations, pulmonary excursion, and lung sounds.

Diagnosis

Restoring effective alveolar ventilation and gas exchange is the priority of interprofessional and nursing care for patients with respiratory acidosis. Possible nursing diagnoses for the patient with respiratory acidosis include the following:

- ■ *Airway Clearance, Ineffective*
- ■ *Anxiety*
- ■ *Breathing Pattern, Ineffective*
- ■ *Cardiac Output, Decreased*
- ■ *Gas Exchange, Impaired.*

(NANDA-I © 2014)

Planning

Planning for the patient with respiratory acidosis involves both restoration of acid–base balance and appropriate treatment for any underlying disease or cause. Expected outcomes include resolution of the underlying illness and the patient's maintaining

- ■ Adequate fluid intake
- ■ Oxygenation saturation greater than 90%
- ■ Normal $PaCO_2$ levels
- ■ pH balance.

Implementation

Frequently assess respiratory status, including rate, depth, effort, and oxygen saturation levels. Decreasing respiratory rate and effort along with decreasing oxygen saturation levels may signal worsening respiratory failure and respiratory acidosis.

SAFETY ALERT Frequently assess LOC. A decline in LOC may indicate increasing hypercapnia and the need for increasing ventilatory support (e.g., intubation, mechanical ventilation).

Promote Gas Exchange

- ■ Promptly evaluate and report ABG results to the physician and respiratory therapist. Rapid changes in carbon dioxide or oxygen levels may necessitate modification of the treatment plan to prevent complications of overcorrection of respiratory acidosis.
- ■ Place in semi-Fowler to Fowler position as tolerated. Elevating the head of the bed promotes lung expansion and gas exchange.
- ■ Administer oxygen as ordered. Carefully monitor response. Reduce the oxygen flow rate or percentage and immediately report increasing somnolence. Supplemental oxygen can suppress the respiratory drive in patients with chronic respiratory acidosis.

Promote Effective Airway Clearance

- ■ Frequently auscultate lung sounds (whether the patient is on or off a mechanical ventilator). Increasing adventitious sounds or decreasing breath sounds (faint or absent) may indicate worsening airway clearance due to obstruction or fatigue.
- ■ Encourage the patient with chronic respiratory acidosis to use pursed-lip breathing. Pursed-lip breathing helps maintain open airways throughout exhalation, promoting carbon dioxide elimination. See the Patient Teaching feature on Effective Coughing in the module on Oxygenation for detailed instructions on purse-lipped breathing.
- ■ Frequently reposition and encourage ambulation as tolerated. Repositioning, sitting at the bedside, and ambulation promote airway clearance and lung expansion.
- ■ Encourage fluid intake. Fluids help liquefy secretions and hydrate respiratory mucous membranes, promoting airway clearance.
- ■ Administer medications such as inhaled bronchodilators as ordered. Inhaled bronchodilators help relieve bronchial spasm, dilating airways.
- ■ Provide percussion, vibration, and postural drainage as ordered. Pulmonary hygiene measures such as these help loosen respiratory secretions.

Reduce Anxiety Levels

Anxiety is a common result of both hypoxia and hypercapnia triggered by insufficient oxygen supply to neurons. Patients with respiratory disorders commonly experience anxiety that is eliminated by improved ventilation and oxygenation. The nurse can help the patient reduce anxiety levels through the following interventions:

- ■ Remain with the patient and monitor for changes in condition.
- ■ Explain procedures and treatments using short, simple sentences. Providing clearly understood information reduces fear of the unknown.
- ■ Reduce environmental stimuli, and use a calm, reassuring manner. These measures help reduce anxiety.
- ■ Allow supportive family members to remain with the patient as much as possible to provide further reassurance.

Reduce Risk for Injury

Patients with respiratory acidosis may experience blurred vision and an altered LOC, putting them at risk for injuries. Nurses working with these patients should:

- Assess LOC, mental status, orientation frequently.
- Place call alarm controls within reach.
- Manage rest and activity patterns to improve gas exchange and reduce oxygen demands.
- Administer supplemental oxygen as needed to prevent cellular hypoxia and tissue damage.

Plan for Discharge

Planning and teaching for home care focus on the problem that caused the respiratory acidosis.

- Teach the patient and family about preventive measures and equipment that may be used in the home. The patient who developed acute respiratory acidosis as a result of acute pneumonia or chest trauma may require only teaching to prevent future problems.
- If acute respiratory acidosis occurred secondarily to a narcotic overdose, determine whether the drug was prescribed for pain or whether it was an illicit street drug. Provide teaching to the patient who requires continuous narcotic medication. Refer the patient using illicit drugs to a substance abuse counselor, treatment center, or Narcotics Anonymous, as appropriate; refer the family to support groups as well.
- For patients with chronic lung disease and their families, discuss ways to avoid future episodes of acute

respiratory failure. Encourage the patient to receive immunization against pneumococcal pneumonia and influenza. Discuss with the patient and family ways to avoid acute respiratory infections, such as good hand hygiene, crowd avoidance, and respiratory cough etiquette.

- Provide instructions regarding measures to take when respiratory status is further compromised. The patient and family should be alerted that symptoms such as headache accompanied by blurred vision or weakness, irritability and confusion, or sleep disturbances and memory impairments warrant immediate medical attention. Shortness of breath or activity intolerance are often the earliest symptoms of worsening respiratory status. Wheezing, grunting, use of accessory muscles, and cyanosis are often late signs.

Evaluation

The evaluation of nursing care is based on the patient's progress in meeting goals, and the nurse revises the plan of care as indicated by outcomes. Expected outcomes of nursing care for a patient with respiratory acidosis include the following:

- Patient maintains patent airway.
- Patient maintains appropriate breathing patterns to meet oxygen demands.
- Patient remains conscious and does not display anxiety indicating potential hypoxia.
- ABG reflects pH and $PaCO_2$ within an acceptable range for the patient.

REVIEW Respiratory Acidosis

RELATE Link the Concepts and Exemplars

Linking the exemplar of respiratory acidosis with the concept of perfusion:

1. Describe the pathophysiologic process that leads from cardiac arrest to respiratory acidosis.
2. Describe how pulmonary embolism might affect the patient's pH.

Linking the exemplar of respiratory acidosis with the concept of mobility:

3. An older adult experienced a hip fracture that was repaired in surgery earlier today. How might the patient's reduced mobility increase the risk of respiratory acidosis?
4. What independent and collaborative nursing interventions might be initiated to prevent respiratory acidosis in this patient?

Linking the exemplar of respiratory acidosis with the concept of safety:

5. What precautions would the nurse implement for the patient with respiratory acidosis to prevent potential injury?
6. The patient with respiratory acidosis becomes confused and disoriented. What is the first intervention needed?

READY Go to Volume 3: Clinical Nursing Skills

REFER Go to Pearson MyLab Nursing and eText

- Additional review materials

Chart 2: Nursing Care Plan: A Patient with Respiratory Acidosis

REFLECT Apply Your Knowledge

Reread Clinical Example C. Mr. Quinland's vitals were as follows: T_O 101.1°F; HR 125 bpm; R 32/min; BP 150/90 mmHg. ABGs were immediately drawn by the respiratory therapist. ABG values were pH 7.32; $PaCO_2$ 50 mmHg; PaO_2 78 mmHg; HCO_3 45 mEq/L. The nurse auscultated decreased breath sounds with scattered rhonchi in the right upper and middle lobes. The patient was placed on a 2L nasal cannula, and pulse oximetry was 90%. The respiratory therapist administered a nebulizer treatment, and a chest x-ray was performed.

The hospital admitted Mr. Quinland overnight. The chest x-ray revealed hyperinflation with flattened diaphragm and right lobular bacterial pneumonia. He was started on antibiotics and remained on low-flow oxygen. A pulmonologist consult was ordered, and Mr. Quinland was discharged after seeing the pulmonary physician. He was scheduled for pulmonary function studies after the pneumonia cleared. The discharge medications were antibiotics, respiratory inhalers, and oxygen. Discharge teaching included information on smoking cessation. Unfortunately Mr. Quinland was not able to wean to room air, and he was discharged on a 2L nasal cannula with oximetry of 91%. Home care services have been arranged for Mr. Quinland.

1. What is the interpretation of the ABG results?

2. How is the patient compensating for the acidosis?

3. How can you determine if this is a chronic problem?

4. Mr. Quinland's pO_2 is clearly below the normal range. An instinct might be to give 100% oxygen. Why would this be dangerous for him?

5. Why is it important for the patient to follow up with the pulmonologist?

» Exemplar 1.D
Respiratory Alkalosis

Exemplar Learning Outcomes

1.D Analyze respiratory alkalosis as it relates to acid–base balance.

- Describe the pathophysiology of respiratory alkalosis.
- Describe the etiology of respiratory alkalosis.
- Compare the risk factors and prevention of respiratory alkalosis.
- Identify the clinical manifestations of respiratory alkalosis.
- Summarize diagnostic tests and therapies used by interprofessional teams in the collaborative care of an individual with respiratory alkalosis.

- Differentiate care of patients with respiratory alkalosis across the lifespan.
- Apply the nursing process in providing culturally competent care to an individual with respiratory alkalosis.

Exemplar Key Terms

Hyperventilation, *27*
Respiratory alkalosis, *27*

Overview

Respiratory alkalosis is characterized by a pH greater than 7.45 and a $PaCO_2$ of less than 35 mmHg. It is always caused by **hyperventilation** (unusually fast respirations, or overbreathing), leading to a carbon dioxide deficit.

Pathophysiology and Etiology

Pathophysiology

In acute respiratory alkalosis, the pH rises rapidly as the $PaCO_2$ falls. Because the kidneys are unable to adapt rapidly to the change in pH, the bicarbonate level remains within normal limits.

Etiology

Anxiety-based hyperventilation is the most common cause of acute respiratory alkalosis. Other physiologic causes of hyperventilation include high fever, hypoxia, gram-negative bacteremia, and thyrotoxicosis (excessive amounts of thyroid hormones). Early salicylate intoxication (aspirin overdose), encephalitis, and high progesterone levels in pregnancy directly stimulate the respiratory center, potentially leading to hyperventilation and respiratory alkalosis. Hyperventilation also can occur during anesthesia and mechanical ventilation if the rate and tidal volume (depth) of ventilation are excessive.

If hyperventilation continues, the kidneys compensate by eliminating bicarbonate to restore the ratio of bicarbonate to carbonic acid. The bicarbonate level is lower than normal in chronic respiratory alkalosis, and the pH may be close to the normal range.

Alkalosis increases binding of extracellular calcium to albumin, reducing ionized calcium levels. As a result, neuromuscular excitability increases, and manifestations similar to hypocalcemia develop. Low carbon dioxide levels in the blood cause vasoconstriction of cerebral vessels, increasing the neurologic manifestations of the disorder.

Risk Factors

Anxiety with hyperventilation is the most common cause of respiratory alkalosis; therefore anxiety disorders increase the risk for this acid–base imbalance. In the patient who is critically ill, mechanical ventilation is a risk factor for respiratory alkalosis if breaths per minute or peak pressures are set too high for the patient's needs.

Clinical Manifestations

The manifestations of respiratory alkalosis include light-headedness, a feeling of panic and difficulty concentrating, circumoral and distal extremity paresthesias (numbness or tingling), tremors, and positive Chvostek sign (a type of facial spasm, usually indicative of hypocalcemia) and Trousseau sign (a spasm of the hand and forearm). The patient also may experience tinnitus, a sensation of chest tightness, and palpitations (cardiac dysrhythmias). Seizures and loss of consciousness may occur.

ABGs generally show a pH greater than 7.45 and a $PaCO_2$ of less than 35 mmHg. In chronic hyperventilation, there is a compensatory decrease in serum bicarbonate to less than 24 mEq/L, and the pH may be near normal.

Collaboration

Management of respiratory alkalosis focuses on correcting the imbalance and treating the underlying cause. It is important to create a calm, quiet, low-stimulation environment to reduce the patient's anxiety or panic. ABGs must be ordered prior to administration of medications or oxygen therapy.

Pharmacologic Therapy

A sedative or antianxiety agent may be necessary to relieve anxiety and restore a normal breathing pattern. Additional

Clinical Manifestations and Therapies
Respiratory Alkalosis

ETIOLOGY	CLINICAL MANIFESTATIONS	CLINICAL THERAPIES
Hyperventilation due to: ■ Brainstem injury ■ Elevated body temperature or fever ■ Extreme anxiety ■ Hypoxia ■ Increased basal metabolic rate ■ Overventilation with a mechanical ventilator ■ Salicylate overdose	■ Dizziness ■ Numbness and tingling around mouth, hands, and feet ■ Palpitations ■ Dyspnea ■ Chest tightness ■ Anxiety/panic ■ Tremors ■ Tetany ■ Seizures or loss of consciousness	■ Monitor vital signs, LOC, and ABGs. ■ Encourage patient to breathe more slowly; teach breathing and stress reduction techniques. ■ Administer sedative or antianxiety agent as ordered. ■ Monitor ventilator settings. ■ Administer oxygen as ordered. ■ Maintain fluid status.

drugs may be ordered to correct underlying problems other than anxiety-induced hyperventilation.

Respiratory Therapy

Use of paper bags has historically been a recommended treatment for hyperventilation. While use of paper bags helps to raise carbon dioxide levels in patients with true hyperventilation syndrome, it can also cause hypoxia. Other diseases can mimic hyperventilation, such as myocardial infarction, pneumothorax, and pulmonary embolism (PE), and rebreathing into a paper bag is not always recommended (Kern, 2014). Elevated carbon dioxide levels have been found to trigger panic attacks, which can further exacerbate hyperventilation. The best treatment for suspected hyperventilation is to teach breathing exercises, encouraging the patient to take slow, regular breaths and breathe into cupped hands. Stress reduction should be strongly encouraged.

Lifespan Considerations
Respiratory Alkalosis in Infants and Children

In respiratory alkalosis there is a decrease in $PaCO_2$ with a deficit of carbonic acid, owing to a marked increase in the rate of respirations. This disorder can be seen in children with hypoxia, sepsis (gram-negative organism), pneumonia, meningitis, brain trauma/lesions, and salicylate poisoning (Doenges et al., 2014). Symptoms and treatment are similar to those seen in adults. Paresthesias can be particularly troublesome for children (and parents). Infants may be comforted by swaddling, calming touch, and/or speaking with a quiet voice. Toddlers and preschoolers may benefit from holding a stuffed animal, singing familiar songs with a parent or caregiver, and talking quietly about their feelings with a supportive adult. Younger school-age children may be comforted by talking about something they enjoy, reading a familiar book aloud with a caregiver, and supportive listening and reassurance that the pain will go away. For older children and adolescents experiencing parathesias, inquire about typical coping mechanisms, reassure them the pain will go away, and offer distraction via music or videos on an iPad or other electronic device (Ball et al., 2017).

Respiratory Alkalosis in Older Adults

Many older adults can maintain acid–base balance under normal conditions. Respiratory distress and chest pain are commonly seen in older adults with respiratory alkalosis. Increased $PaCO_2$ excretion from hyperventilation occurs with compensatory response of HCO_3 excretion of the kidneys. Hyperventilation in older adults may originate from hypoxia, pulmonary emboli, or anxiety (Lewis et al., 2014). Inpatient care is usually not required with hyperventilation related to an anxiety disorder. Pharmacotherapy is often helpful but should be used with caution in older adults who take multiple medications. Regardless, it is important to rule out any serious problems, such as encephalitis and septicemia, before discharging older adults. Outcome depends on the nature of the illness and early diagnosis/treatment.

NURSING PROCESS

Nursing care is focused on reducing anxiety through manipulation of the environment to reduce stimuli and to create a sense of peace. This restful environment will help the patient breathe more slowly and effectively.

Assessment

■ *Observation and patient interview.* Observe the patient for signs of anxiety. Discuss the triggering event for the onset of hyperventilation. Ask the patient about mental health disorders, coping mechanisms, and available support systems.

■ *Physical examination.* Examine breath sounds, neurologic function, respiratory and cardiac status, and any changes in LOC.

Diagnosis

Possible nursing diagnoses for the patient with respiratory alkalosis include the following:

- *Breathing Pattern, Ineffective*
- *Anxiety*
- *Injury, Risk for.*

(NANDA-I © 2014)

Planning

Planning for the patient with respiratory alkalosis involves identification and treatment of its underlying cause and the restoration of acid–base balance. Appropriate outcomes include resolution of the underlying cause and that the patient will manifest normal respiratory rate and rhythm, maintain safety, and maintain appropriate fluid status.

Implementation

It is important not only to address the hyperventilation but also to identify the underlying cause. The usual cause of hyperventilation and respiratory alkalosis is psychologic, although physiologic disorders also can lead to hyperventilation.

- Assess respiratory rate, depth, and ease. Monitor vital signs (including temperature) and skin color. Assessment data can help identify the underlying cause, such as a fever or hypoxia.

- Obtain subjective assessment data such as the circumstances leading up to the current situation, current health and recent illnesses or medication use, and current manifestations. Subjective data provide clues to the cause and circumstances of the hyperventilation response.

- Reassure the patient that the symptoms do not indicate a heart attack and will resolve when breathing returns to normal. Manifestations of hyperventilation and respiratory alkalosis such as dyspnea, chest tightness or pain, and palpitations can mimic those of a heart attack.

- Instruct the patient to maintain eye contact and breathe with you to slow the respiratory rate. These measures help make the patient aware of respirations and provide a sense of support and control (Ackley & Ladwig, 2014). Be aware that some patients are uncomfortable making eye contact for cultural reasons.

- Protect the patient from injury. If hyperventilation continues to the point where the patient loses consciousness, respirations will return to normal, as will acid–base balance.

- Refer for counseling a patient who has experienced repeated episodes of hyperventilation or who has a chronic anxiety disorder. Counseling can help the patient develop alternative strategies for dealing with anxiety.

Planning and teaching for home care is directed toward the underlying cause of hyperventilation. If anxiety precipitated the episode, discuss anxiety and stress management strategies with the patient. Teach the patient how to identify a hyperventilation reaction and provide self-care, and when to seek medical intervention.

Evaluation

The evaluation of care is based on the patient's ability to meet goals set during the planning stage and the outcomes achieved. Nursing care is reformulated as needed if outcomes are not met. Expected outcomes for the patient with respiratory alkalosis include the following:

- Patient experiences no subsequent episodes of hyperventilation.

- Patient describes strategies for coping with anxiety in the future.

- Family displays ability to contribute to calming patient during times of anxiety.

- Patient and/or family participate in support groups that will help the patient cope with an anxiety disorder.

REVIEW Respiratory Alkalosis

RELATE Link the Concepts and Exemplars

Linking the exemplar of respiratory alkalosis with the concept of oxygenation:

1. Why is oxygenation often a concern when dealing with a patient with respiratory alkalosis?

2. What ventilator settings need to be adjusted if the ABGs of a patient using mechanical ventilation demonstrate respiratory alkalosis?

Linking the exemplar of respiratory alkalosis with the concept of anxiety:

3. What would be an expected outcome for a patient with hyperventilation syndrome?

4. What occurs if the patient loses consciousness from hyperventilation related to anxiety?

Linking the exemplar of respiratory alkalosis with the concept of safety:

5. What would be the nurse's specific concerns regarding safety for a patient with respiratory alkalosis?

6. What safety precautions might the nurse employ to prevent injury to the patient with respiratory alkalosis related to hyperventilation caused by anxiety?

READY Go to Volume 3: Clinical Nursing Skills

REFER Go to Pearson MyLab Nursing and eText

- Additional review questions
- Chart 3: Nursing Care Plan: A Patient with Respiratory Alkalosis

REFLECT Apply Your Knowledge

Reread Clinical Example D. The respiratory therapist made changes to Ms. Hernandez's ventilator. A half hour after the ventilator changes were made, the ABG values were pH 7.42; $PaCO_2$ 35 mmHg; PaO_2 100 mmHg; and HCO_3 24 mEq/L.

1. What is the interpretation of the ABG results?

2. Why is it important to wait 20–30 minutes after making ventilator changes to draw ABGs?

3. Refer to the module on Oxygenation. What are some signs that Ms. Hernandez is ready to be weaned from the ventilator?

References

Ackley, B. J., & Ladwig, G. B. (2014). *Nursing diagnosis handbook: A guide to planning care* (10th ed.). St. Louis, MO: Mosby.

Ball, J. W., Bindler, R. C., Cowen, K., & Shaw, M. (2017). *Principles of pediatric nursing: Caring for children* (7th ed.). Hoboken, NJ: Pearson Education.

Doenges, M., Moorhouse, M., & Murr, A. (2014). *Nursing care plans: Guidelines for individualizing client care across the life span* (9th ed.). Philadelphia, PA: F.A. Davis.

Feller-Kopman, D. J., & Schwartzstein, R. M. (2015). *The evaluation, diagnosis and treatment of adult patients with acute hypercarbia.* Retrieved from UpToDate website: http://www.uptodate.com/contents/the-evaluation-diagnosis-and-treatment-of-the-adult-patient-with-acute-hypercapnic

Herdman, T. H. & Kamitsuru, S. (Eds.). *Nursing Diagnoses—Definitions and Classification 2015–2017.*

Copyright © 2014, 1994–2014 NANDA International. Used by arrangement with John Wiley & Sons, Inc. Companion website: www.wiley.com/go/nursingdiagnoses

Huang, L. (2013). Pediatric metabolic alkalosis. *Medscape.* Retrieved from http://emedicine.medscape.com/article/906819-overview

Huang, L. (2015). Pediatric metabolic acidosis. *Medscape.* Retrieved from http://emedicine.medscape.com/article/906440-overview

Kern, B. (2014). Hyperventilation syndrome treatment and management. *Medscape.* Retrieved from http://emedicine.medscape.com/article/807277-treatment

Lewis, S., Dirksen, S., Heitkemper, M., & Bucher, L. (2014). *Medical surgery nursing assessment and management of clinical problems* (9th ed., pp. 304–306). St. Louis, MO: Elsevier-Mosby.

Melanson, P. (2015). *Preventing intubation in acute respiratory failure: Use of CPAP and bipap.* Retrieved from McGill Critical Care Medicine website: https://www.mcgill.ca/criticalcare/teaching/files/intubation

Metheny, N. M. (2012). *Fluid and electrolyte balance: Nursing considerations* (5th ed.) Philadelphia, PA: Lippincott Williams & Wilkins.

Porth, C. M., & Gross, S. (2014). *Pathophysiology: Concepts of altered health states* (9th ed.). Philadelphia, PA: Lippincott Williams & Wilkins.

Venes, D. (Ed.). (2013). *Taber's cyclopedic medical dictionary* (22nd ed.) Philadelphia, PA: F. A. Davis.

Wiedkerkehr, M., & Emmett, M. (2016). *Bicarbonate therapy in lactic acidosis.* Retrieved from UpToDate website: http://www.uptodate.com/contents/bicarbonate-therapy-in-lactic-acidosis

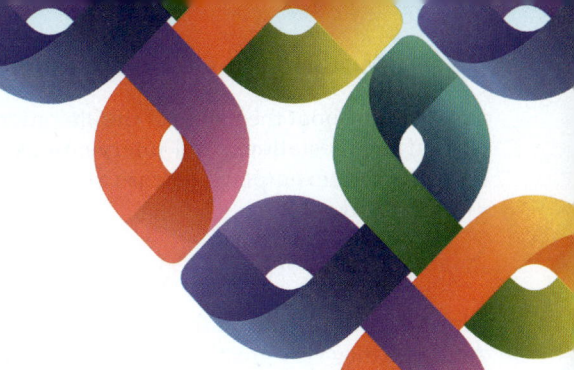

Module 2
Cellular Regulation

Module Outline and Learning Outcomes

The Concept of Cellular Regulation

Normal Cellular Regulation

2.1 Analyze the physiology of cellular regulation in the body.

Alterations to Cellular Regulation

2.2 Differentiate alterations in cellular regulation.

Concepts Related to Cellular Regulation

2.3 Outline the relationship between cellular regulation and other concepts.

Health Promotion

2.4 Explain the promotion of healthy cellular regulation.

Nursing Assessment

2.5 Differentiate common assessment procedures and tests used to examine cellular regulation.

Independent Interventions

2.6 Analyze independent interventions nurses can implement for patients with alterations in cellular regulation.

Collaborative Therapies

2.7 Summarize collaborative therapies used by interprofessional teams for patients with alterations in cellular regulation.

Lifespan Considerations

2.8 Differentiate considerations related to the care of patients with alterations in cellular regulation throughout the lifespan.

Cellular Regulation Exemplars

Exemplar 2.A Cancer

2.A Analyze cancer as it relates to cellular regulation.

Exemplar 2.B Anemia

2.B Analyze anemia as it relates to cellular regulation.

Exemplar 2.C Breast Cancer

2.C Analyze breast cancer as it relates to cellular regulation.

Exemplar 2.D Colorectal Cancer

2.D Analyze colorectal cancer as it relates to cellular regulation.

Exemplar 2.E Leukemia

2.E Analyze leukemia as it relates to cellular regulation.

Exemplar 2.F Lung Cancer

2.F Analyze lung cancer as it relates to cellular regulation.

Exemplar 2.G Prostate Cancer

2.G Analyze prostate cancer as it relates to cellular regulation.

Exemplar 2.H Sickle Cell Disease

2.H Analyze sickle cell disease as it relates to cellular regulation.

Exemplar 2.I Skin Cancer

2.I Analyze skin cancer as it relates to cellular regulation.

 ## The Concept of Cellular Regulation

Concept Key Terms

Anaplasia, **34**
Autosomes, **33**
Cell cycle, **33**
Chromosomes, **33**

Deoxyribonucleic acid (DNA), **32**
Differentiation, **34**
Dysplasia, **34**

Genome, **33**
Homologous chromosomes, **33**
Hyperplasia, **34**

Meiosis, **33**
Metaplasia, **34**
Mitosis, **33**
Ribonucleic acid (RNA), **32**

Sex chromosomes, **33**
Somatic cells, **33**

The cell is the basic unit of all living systems. Although each human life begins with just a single cell, by adulthood nearly 75 trillion cells combine to form the body (Roberts, 2016). The many types of specialized cells in the body function differently depending on their location. For example, pancreatic cells have a very different function from that of nerve cells. However, all cells have common features, such as a nucleus and mitochondria.

Cell reproduction, proliferation, and growth are regulated by the body. Alterations in cellular regulation can have devastating consequences for body tissues and functions. This concept and its exemplars provide essential information about the nature of the alterations, risk factors, clinical manifestations, and interventions and treatment options. The exemplars discuss selected alterations in greater detail.

Normal Cellular Regulation

Almost all of the cells in the human body are microscopic. Although they vary greatly in size, shape, and function, they all share certain features. Any change in or disturbance to one or more of these features can result in abnormal cell development or replication. To understand alterations in cellular function, nurses must first understand the common characteristics of cells.

Physiology Review

A discussion of cellular regulation begins with an exploration of the cell, which is the site of numerous metabolic and regulatory processes.

Cell Membrane

Every cell, regardless of its shape or function, must have a cell membrane to maintain its integrity and survive. The membrane is a defined boundary that possesses a definite shape and holds the cell contents together. The cell membrane acts as a protective covering and is responsible for allowing materials into and out of the cell. It is called a selectively permeable (or semipermeable) membrane because it allows only certain things to move into or out of the cell. Substances are transported across the cell membrane in various ways (see **Table 2–1 »**).

The cell membrane also has identification markers, which signal that it is the cell of a specific individual. If a foreign cell shows up (e.g., in a transplanted organ), the body signals an attack on that cell or group of cells.

Cytoplasm

Inside the cell is a watery soup of proteins, nucleic acids, gases, salts, and other substances that are essential for life. This internal environment of the cell, known as the cytoplasm, must be maintained in balance for the cell to survive.

Nucleus and Nucleolus

The nucleus is sometimes described as the brain of the cell. Within the nucleus is the biological "software" that regulates and directs the activities of the organelles in the cell. The nucleus of a cell is surrounded by a double-walled nuclear membrane that has large pores that allow certain materials to pass in and out.

Chromatin is tightly wound into bundles called chromosomes and is the material found in the nucleus that contains **deoxyribonucleic acid (DNA)**. Coded into DNA are instructions that determine the individual's inherited characteristics, such as hair and eye color, as well as the production of every protein needed by the body. These instructions are called *genes*.

The nucleolus, a spherical body made up of dense fibers, is found within the cell nucleus. Its major function is to synthesize the **ribonucleic acid (RNA)** that forms ribosomes.

Centrosomes are tubular structures usually found in pairs in the nucleus. They contain centrioles, which are involved in cell division.

Ribosomes

Ribosomes are organelles found on the endoplasmic reticulum or floating around in the cytoplasm. Ribosomes are made of RNA and assist in the production of enzymes and other proteins needed for cell repair and reproduction.

Endoplasmic Reticulum

The endoplasmic reticulum is a series of channels, formed from folded membranes, set up in the cytoplasm. The endoplasmic reticulum has two distinct forms. The rough endoplasmic reticulum, which has a sandpaper-like appearance due to the ribosomes on its surface, is responsible for the synthesis of protein. Once the protein has been synthesized, it is sent to the Golgi apparatus for processing. The smooth endoplasmic reticulum has no ribosomes on its surface, making it appear smooth. It synthesizes lipids (fats) and steroids.

Mitochondria

Mitochondria are tiny, bean-shaped organelles that act as the cell's power plant, providing up to 95% of the energy that

TABLE 2–1 Methods of Cellular Transportation

Cellular Transportation Methods	Description
Passive Transportation (no energy required)	
Diffusion	Movement of a substance from an area of high concentration to an area of low concentration
Facilitated diffusion	Movement of a substance that is assisted via certain transmembrane proteins in the direction it was already traveling, from an area of high concentration to an area of low concentration
Osmosis	Movement of water across a membrane from an area that has a low concentration of a solute to an area that has a higher concentration until the concentration is the same on both sides of the membrane
Filtration	Application of pressure to force water and dissolved materials across a membrane
Active Transport (energy required)	
Active transport pumps	A method that requires additional energy (in the form of adenosine triphosphate) to move substances against the concentration gradient (from low concentration to high concentration)
Endocytosis	Ingestion of substances that are too large to diffuse across the cell membrane
Phagocytosis	Form of endocytosis in which solid particles are brought into the cell via vesicles
Pinocytosis	Form of endocytosis in which liquid is brought into the cell via vesicles
Exocytosis	Transportation of material outside of the cell

the body needs for cellular repair, movement, and reproduction. Special enzymes in the mitochondria help to take in oxygen and turn it into energy.

Golgi Apparatus

The Golgi apparatus looks like a bunch of flattened, membranous sacs. When a protein is received from the endoplasmic reticulum, a portion of the Golgi apparatus envelops the protein, which is pinched off and moved to the cell membrane to be released or secreted. For example, organs and glands with a high level of secretion or storage, such as the digestive system, salivary glands, and pancreatic glands, are made of cells containing a large Golgi apparatus.

Lysosomes

Lysosomes are vesicles containing powerful enzymes that clean up intercellular debris and other waste. They also aid in maintaining health by destroying unwanted bacteria through phagocytosis (the process by which microorganisms and cellular debris are engulfed and destroyed).

Genetic Considerations

Certain factors predispose an individual for the development of alterations in cellular regulation. Even before birth, genetic processes are at work in determining whether any number of alterations will be present.

DNA and Genes

Every human cell except mature red blood cells (RBCs) contains a complete set of DNA molecules. These molecules consist of long sequences of nucleotides, or bases, represented by the letters A, T, C, and G. The order of the bases dictates the exact instructions for the functioning of that particular cell. All of the DNA in a human cell is referred to as the human **genome**, or the complete set of inheritance for an individual. The genome includes the DNA in the cell nucleus as well as the DNA in the mitochondria (see **Figure 2–1 》**). Each individual's genome is unique.

The cell nucleus contains about 2 meters of DNA that is tightly wound and packaged into 23 pairs of **chromosomes** (threadlike strands of DNA in the cell that carry the genes), making a complete set of 46 chromosomes. One member of each pair of chromosomes is inherited from the mother, and the other is inherited from the father. These pairs of inherited chromosomes are called **homologous chromosomes**.

Chromosomes are numbered according to size, chromosome 1 being the largest and chromosome 22 being the smallest. The first 22 pairs of chromosomes, known as **autosomes**, are alike in men and women. The 23rd pair, the **sex chromosomes**, determines an individual's gender. A daughter has two copies of the X chromosomes (one copy inherited from each parent), and a son has one X chromosome (inherited from his mother) and a Y chromosome (inherited from his father).

The Cell Cycle

The **cell cycle** comprises the four phases of cell growth and development. Human cells divide in two ways: mitosis and meiosis. **Mitosis**, the process of making new cells, takes place in the **somatic cells** (tissue) of the body. Cell division through mitosis results in two cells, called daughter cells, that are genetically identical to the original cell, or mother

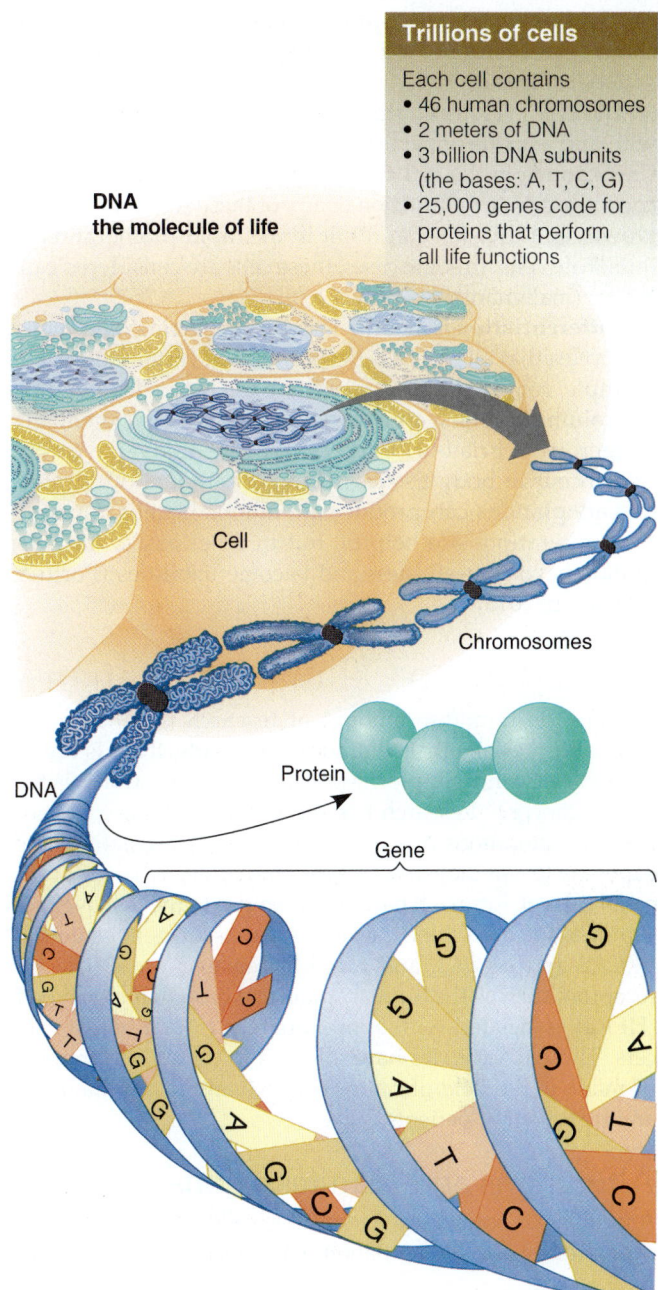

Trillions of cells

Each cell contains
- 46 human chromosomes
- 2 meters of DNA
- 3 billion DNA subunits (the bases: A, T, C, G)
- 25,000 genes code for proteins that perform all life functions

DNA
the molecule of life

Cell

Chromosomes

Protein

DNA

Gene

Figure 2–1 》 Each cell nucleus throughout the body contains the genes, DNA, and chromosomes that make up the majority of an individual's genome. The remaining portion of the human genome is in the mitochondria.

cell, and to each other. Cell division through mitosis heals wounds and replaces the cells lost daily on skin surfaces and in the lining of gastrointestinal and respiratory tracts. In addition, the mitotic activity of the zygote and its daughter cells is the foundation for human growth and development. The zygote undergoes mitosis to form a multicellular embryo, which develops into a fetus and then an infant.

Meiosis is a type of cell division that takes place in the sex cells of the testes and ovaries and results in formation of the sperm and oocytes (gametes). Through a series of complex mechanisms, the amount of genetic material is reduced by half (23 chromosomes). Thus, when the two sex cells combine during fertilization, the necessary number of chromosomes

(46) is present in the offspring's cells. This combination of chromosomes from two different cells with different genetic material allows diversity in the human population.

The cell cycle is controlled by cyclins, which combine with and activate enzymes called cyclin-dependent kinases. Checkpoints in the cell cycle ensure that it proceeds in the correct order. A malfunction of any of these regulators of cell growth and division can result in the rapid proliferation of immature cells. In some cases, these cells are considered cancerous (malignant).

Differentiation is a normal process occurring over many cell cycles that allows cells to specialize in certain tasks. For example, some epithelial cells lining the lungs develop into tall columnar cells with cilia. These cells sweep potentially dangerous debris out of the lungs. When adverse conditions occur in body tissues during differentiation, protective adaptations can produce alterations in cells. Some of these alterations are helpful, but in other cases, the cells mutate beyond usefulness and become liabilities (Porth & Grossman, 2013).

Alterations to Cellular Regulation

Despite the immense amount of research that has taken place and progress that continues to be made, there is unfortunately still no simple response to the question "What causes cancer?" Research has shown that there is a genetic basis for alterations that occur with cellular regulation, and exposure to carcinogens can cause mutations to occur at the cellular level. Research has also given rise to the discovery of tumor-associated genes, tumor suppressor genes such as *BRCA1* and *BRCA2*, and tumor-associated growth factor receptors such as the human epidermal growth factor type 2 (HER2) associated with approximately 25% of breast cancers. These discoveries have allowed for many advances to be made in the field of cancer research and in the diagnosis and treatment of patients.

Alterations and Manifestations

A number of potentially undesirable cellular alterations can occur during cell differentiation. These include the following:

- **Hyperplasia** is an increase in the number or density of normal cells. Hyperplasia occurs in response to stress, increased metabolic demands, or elevated levels of hormones. Examples include the hyperplasia of myocardial cells in response to a prolonged increase in the body's demand for oxygen and hyperplasia of uterine cells in response to rising levels of estrogen during pregnancy. Hyperplastic cells are under normal DNA control.

- **Metaplasia** is a change in the normal pattern of differentiation such that dividing cells differentiate into cell types not normally found at that location in the body. The metaplastic cell is normal for its particular type but is not in its normal location. Some metaplastic cells are less functional than the cells they replace. Metaplasia is a protective response to adverse conditions, often the result of inflammation. Metaplastic cells are under normal DNA control, and the metaplasia is reversible when the stressor or other disruptive condition ceases. Metaplasia often

occurs in the lungs of smokers, where normal ciliated epithelium may be replaced by a squamous stratified epithelium known as squamous metaplasia (Herfs et al., 2012).

- **Dysplasia** represents a loss of DNA control over differentiation in response to adverse conditions. Dysplastic cells show abnormal variations in size, shape, and appearance and a disturbance in their usual arrangement. Examples of dysplasia include changes in the cervix in response to continued irritation, such as from the human papillomavirus, and leukoplakia on oral mucous membranes in response to chronic irritation from smoking.

- **Anaplasia** is the regression of a cell to an immature or undifferentiated cell type. Anaplastic cell division is no longer under DNA control. Anaplasia usually occurs when a damaging or transforming event takes place inside the dividing, still undifferentiated cell, leading to loss of useful function. Anaplasia may occur in response to overwhelmingly destructive conditions inside the cell or in surrounding tissue (Porth & Grossman, 2013). It is often associated with malignancies and is one of the criteria used to grade the aggressiveness of cancer cells.

Although hyperplasia, metaplasia, and dysplasia often reverse after the irritating factor is eliminated, they can lead to malignancy under certain conditions. This is especially true of dysplasia, which represents a loss of DNA control. Anaplasia is not reversible, and the degree of anaplasia determines the potential risk for cancer.

Any one of these alterations in cellular regulation has the potential to become cancerous or cause disorders that can compromise a patient's health. The most common of these are cancer, anemia, sickle cell disease (SCD), leukemia, and polycythemia (see the Alterations and Manifestations feature and the exemplars in this module). Others, such as endometriosis and HIV, are discussed in other modules.

Although the human body's numerous systems can be studied individually, no system is truly isolated. The function of one body system can greatly affect the function of one or more other systems. Likewise, psychosocial factors can affect a number of body systems and physiologic processes.

Prevalence

Although disorders of cellular regulation affect millions of people throughout the world, certain populations tend to be more susceptible to certain disorders.

Cancer

According to the ACS's Cancer Facts and Figures 2016, the United States was home to more than 1.6 million people living with some form of cancer (ACS, 2016b). Although the age at onset varies for different forms of cancer, of the men and woman born today, an estimated 39.0% will be diagnosed with cancer at some point in their lives (Surveillance, Epidemiology, and End Results Program [SEER], 2017).

>> **Stay Current:** For current statistics related to the prevalence of cancer, visit the website of the National Cancer Institute (NCI) at http://seer.cancer.gov/statfacts and the ACS's Cancer Facts & Figures 2016 report at http://www.cancer.org/acs/groups/content/@research/documents/document/acspc-047079.pdf.

Alterations and Manifestations
Cellular Regulation

ALTERATION	DESCRIPTION	MANIFESTATIONS	INTERVENTIONS AND THERAPIES
Cancer (e.g., breast, colon, lung, ovarian, prostate, and testicular)	Abnormal and rapid growth of body cells that may invade surrounding body tissues and spread (metastasize) to other sites	■ Manifestations are variable, depending on the location and size of the growth, as well as on whether other tissues and organs are affected. ■ Surrounding blood vessels and organs may also be affected, producing varying effects. ■ General signs and symptoms may include lethargy, fever, and weight loss (American Cancer Society [ACS], 2014a).	■ Identify and treat the affected organ(s) and/or tissue(s). Conventional treatments may include chemotherapy, radiation, and surgical removal of the affected organ/tissue. Alternative treatments may include relaxation therapy, guided imagery, and certain homeopathic supplements.
Anemia (e.g., aplastic, hemolytic, and iron deficiency)	Deficiency of hemoglobin or reduction of number of RBCs that leads to inadequate delivery of oxygenation to cells, tissues, and organs; may also be caused by blood loss, impaired RBC production, or excessive RBC destruction	■ Manifestations are variable, depending on the underlying cause. ■ General signs and symptoms may include lethargy, pallor, dyspnea, dizziness, and confusion.	■ Identify and treat the underlying cause. Medical interventions may include blood transfusions and surgical measures to stop internal bleeding. Nutritional supplements may include iron (for treatment of iron deficiency anemia) and folate or vitamin B_{12} (for treatment of anemia due to vitamin deficiency). ■ When possible, aplastic anemia is treated through elimination of the known cause. Pharmacologic treatments may include medications that induce RBC production, such as erythropoietin and colony-stimulating factors. Other treatments include blood and marrow stem cell transplants (National Heart, Lung, and Blood Institute [NHLBI], 2012a).
Leukemia	Form of cancer in which abnormal and rapid formation of white blood cells (WBCs) leads to circulation of increased numbers of abnormal, immature WBCs	■ Manifestations include fatigue, pallor, weight loss, bruising, unusual bleeding, recurrent infections, joint or bone pain, and weakness.	■ Intervention varies depending on type of leukemia, patient age, and other factors. Conventional treatments may include chemotherapy, radiation, biological therapy, bone marrow transplantation, and surgical removal of the spleen (splenectomy) (Mayo Clinic, 2016a). Alternative treatments may include relaxation therapy, guided imagery, and certain homeopathic supplements.
Sickle cell disease	Inherited alteration of hemoglobin S that results in deformed (sickle-shaped) RBCs	■ Trapping of misshapen RBCs in blood vessels may cause vascular occlusion, leading to reduced or blocked blood flow to organs and tissues. ■ Symptoms may include anemia, pain, recurrent infections, or growth retardation. In infants, hand-foot syndrome (swollen hands and feet due to blockage of blood flow) may be the first sign of this disorder (Mayo Clinic, 2014a).	■ Supplemental oxygen, intravenous (IV) fluids (for hydration), and analgesics may be administered during an acute crisis. Long-term management may include RBC transfusion therapy. General pharmacologic management may include antibiotics and immunizations for infection prevention (Maakaron, 2015). Hydroxyurea may be administered to stimulate production of fetal hemoglobin (which appears to help prevent the formation of sickled cells) (Mayo Clinic, 2014a).
Polycythemia	Abnormal increase in the production of erythrocytes (RBCs) leading to increased blood viscosity	■ Increased coagulability of blood leads to increased risks for injury, including myocardial infarction, cerebrovascular accident, and heart failure (Mayo Clinic, 2014b).	■ Intervention includes phlebotomy (to reduce RBC count). ■ Treatment also includes hydration with IV fluids. Hydroxyurea may be administered to decrease RBC and platelet production. Aspirin may be administered for analgesia and to reduce blood coagulability (Mayo Clinic, 2014c).

Anemia

Rather than being a primary disease, anemia is the result of an underlying pathologic process; the prevalence of anemia depends on its cause. Anemia is most often linked to blood loss, impaired production of RBCs, or increased destruction of RBCs (Osborn et al., 2013), all of which will be discussed in greater detail in Exemplar 2.B on Anemia.

Sickle Cell Disease

An estimated 100,000 people in the United States are affected by SCD. Although its prevalence is greater among African Americans, the disorder is not limited to that population. Throughout the world, SCD affects millions of people from a variety of cultural backgrounds. However, this condition is more prevalent among those whose ancestry includes African, southern European, Hispanic, Middle Eastern, or Asian Indian origins (NHLBI, 2016).

Genetic Considerations and Risk Factors

Cancer

According to the NCI (2016a), certain forms of cancer may have a genetic component. For example, skin cancer (melanoma), ovarian cancer, breast cancer, and cancers of the prostate and colon tend to occur more commonly in some families. Regardless of genetics, socioeconomic factors have a major impact for all forms of cancer. In general, a low socioeconomic status and lack of healthcare coverage are associated with an increased risk for developing cancer (U.S. Department of Health and Human Services, 2014).

Anemia

Genetic considerations and nonmodifiable risk factors for anemia depend on the underlying cause of the disorder. For example, between menarche and menopause, women are at greater risk for development of anemia that results from blood loss. Considerations related to some of the more common forms of anemia are discussed in Exemplar 2.B on Anemia.

Sickle Cell Disease

The development of SCD depends entirely on genetics. People with this disease are born with two hemoglobin S genes, one from each parent. If only one hemoglobin S gene is inherited, the individual has a condition called sickle cell trait. Although people with sickle cell trait do not have SCD, they may pass the hemoglobin S gene to their offspring (NHLBI, 2016).

Case Study >> Part 1

Andrew Ladeaux, an 8-year-old boy, is brought to the emergency department by his mother. On arrival, Andrew is pressing a bloody towel against his nose. As the triage nurse, you direct the boy and his mother to the assessment station. Andrew's mother explains that Andrew's nose began bleeding "about an hour ago" during a baseball tournament. Andrew denies any traumatic injury, and his mother reports that her son's game had not yet begun when the bleeding started. Andrew appears to be in no acute distress. His respiratory rate is 28/min, and his respirations are regular and not labored.

Andrew's pulse rate is 136 bpm, which is elevated. As you apply a blood pressure cuff to Andrew's arm, you notice light, scattered bruising along his forearm. His blood pressure is 118/71 mmHg, which is slightly elevated. Although Andrew denies any additional complaints, during further exploration of his health status, his mother reports that her son has seemed "really tired lately" and that he "seems like he's been bruising very easily."

Clinical Reasoning Questions Level I

1. Considering your assessment of Andrew, which findings might suggest an alteration in cellular regulation?
2. Why might Andrew's blood pressure and pulse rate be elevated?
3. What is the relationship between bleeding and bruising?

Clinical Reasoning Questions Level II

4. At this time, presuming that Andrew has lost a significant amount of blood, what is the priority nursing diagnosis for this patient?
5. *Refer to Exemplar 2.E on Leukemia.* Which blood test do you expect to be ordered for further assessment of Andrew's condition?

Concepts Related to Cellular Regulation

The human body is composed of trillions of cells, all working together through various systems to maintain homeostasis. Homeostatic balance can be disrupted by both internal and external factors such as genetic influences, lifestyle choices, or environmental exposure. When there is a prolonged disruption in this homeostatic balance, cellular malfunction and disease may result.

Consider the impact of the body's inflammatory response on the activity of WBCs. In a healthy individual, any type of trauma can trigger the inflammatory process, causing a number of responses at the cellular level. (For a detailed discussion of the inflammatory process, see the module on Inflammation.) One response to trauma involves the recruitment of WBCs to the site of the injury. At the injury site, WBCs fight infection, increase blood flow to the injured area, and summon additional WBCs to the site.

To further explore the relationships between concepts, consider the effects of oxidative stress (OS), which is the body's physiologic response to both external and internal stress factors. OS occurs when the body cannot adequately manage or neutralize molecules called *free radicals* (Osborn et al., 2013). These may be end products of food breakdown or may be produced when the body is exposed to certain environmental toxins, such as radiation and tobacco smoke (MedlinePlus, 2013). Research suggests that OS may play a role in psychiatric disorders, such as depression, bipolar disorder, and certain anxiety disorders (Salim, 2014). Research has also suggested that there is a close relationship between OS and inflammation and that the cellular damage caused by OS is linked to a number of disorders and diseases, including cancer, diabetes, and Alzheimer disease (Biswas, 2015; NCCIH, 2016). The Concepts Related to Cellular Regulation feature links some, but not all, of the concepts integral to cellular regulation. They are presented in alphabetical order.

Concepts Related to
Cellular Regulation

CONCEPT	RELATIONSHIP TO CELLULAR REGULATION	NURSING IMPLICATIONS
Advocacy	The nurse should ensure that patients receive sufficient information on which to base their consent for care and related treatment. The nurse provides an environment favorable for patients to make their own care decisions, as appropriate.	■ Assess the patient's level of understanding related to care and treatment options. ■ Discuss the plan of care with the patient and allow for self-determination such as which treatment may be the best option, as appropriate. ■ Assess your own values and beliefs related to refusal of treatment/procedures. ■ Recognize the patient's right to refuse treatment/procedures.
Infection	Introduction of bacteria, viruses, fungi, or foreign substances → activation of immune response → increased production of WBCs	■ Assess for signs and symptoms of infection, including redness, swelling, and draining from the injured site. Be aware that fever often accompanies infectious processes. ■ Anticipate potential need for blood and/or wound cultures and administration of antibiotics. ■ Antipyretics may be indicated. ■ Be aware that increased WBC count may indicate an inflammatory process, infection, or a combination of both.
Inflammation	Trauma → activation of inflammatory response → recruitment of WBCs to site of injury and increased WBC production	■ Assess for signs and symptoms of inflammation, including redness and swelling. Be aware that fever may accompany inflammatory processes even in the absence of infection. ■ Anticipate administration of anti-inflammatory medications, possible application of ice to inflamed area, and, if possible, elevation of injured site. ■ Be aware that an increased WBC count may indicate an inflammatory process, infection, or a combination of both.
Managing Care	Patients with alterations in cellular regulation can greatly benefit from participating in managed care and have more positive health outcomes.	■ Assess the needs of the patient to identify actual or potential problems related to care. ■ Advocate for the patient in relation to their care needs. ■ Participate in coordination of care to secure the patient's well-being.
Stress and Coping	Physical and/or emotional stress → OS → production of free radicals → increased risk for development of diseases and disorders	■ Assess psychosocial factors that affect the patient. ■ Recognize the potential health effects of physical and emotional stressors. ■ Anticipate the need for patient teaching related to coping and relaxation. When indicated, referral to other healthcare professionals may be appropriate for both disease prevention and health promotion.

Health Promotion

Although genetic factors play a part in the development of some illnesses caused by impaired cellular regulation, an individual's health is also affected by many personal choices. Wellness promotion and simple health practices can significantly affect the risk for developing disorders of cellular regulation.

Modifiable Risk Factors

Risk of cellular regulation disorders is increased by the following factors, among others:

- Smoking, use of other tobacco products, and exposure to secondhand tobacco smoke
- Poor diet, including consumption of processed meat and other processed foods, excessive consumption of sugar and fatty foods, and excessive consumption of alcohol
- Lack of physical activity
- Infection with hepatitis B, hepatitis C, HIV, or *Helicobacter pylori*
- Exposure to ultraviolet radiation
- Exposure to certain cancer treatments
- Hormone replacement therapy
- Exposure to some chemicals, including those found in the workplaces of chemical, metal, and textile workers; hairdressers; and printers as well as some herbicides and insecticides
- Living in areas with high levels of air pollution
- Exposure to radon.

The Patient Teaching feature provides guidance for helping patients manage their risk of developing alterations in cellular regulation.

Patient Teaching
Health Promotion for Cancer Prevention: Modifiable Risk Factors

- *Discourage smoking or use of other tobacco products.* Emphasize the importance of patients protecting children and themselves from exposure to tobacco smoke. This is one of the most important health decisions an individual can make.

- *Encourage patients, especially children, to consume a healthy diet.* This should include a minimum of five servings of fruits and vegetables daily as well as whole grains, iron-rich foods, and foods that are rich in vitamin B_{12}. Teach patients to limit their consumption of processed meats; drink alcohol in moderation; and choose fewer high-calorie foods.

- *Explain the importance of maintaining a healthy weight and being physically active.* Physical activity helps to control weight. Together, these factors may lower the risk for various types of cancer.

- *Teach patients effective ways to protect themselves from ultraviolet radiation.* Early excessive exposure to sun and one or more severe sunburns during childhood increase the chances of skin cancers developing in adulthood. Patients who work outdoors, athletes, coaches, and others who spend time outside

regularly should use sunscreen daily (SPF 15 or greater), regardless of the climate in which they live. Emphasize the importance of avoiding midday sun, when the sun's rays are strongest. Instruct patients to cover exposed skin and wear a hat with a wide brim. They should avoid tanning beds and sunlamps.

- *Explain the importance of avoiding risky behaviors.* Practicing risky behaviors such as needle sharing or unsafe sexual contact can increase the risk of developing certain cancers.

- *Suggest that patients have their homes tested for radon and explore their exposure to harmful chemicals.* Patients may be exposed to hazardous substances in the home or in the workplace.

- *Stress the importance of getting immunizations, receiving regular medical care, and doing self-examinations.* By protecting against certain viral infections, immunizations can decrease the risk of some cancers. Regular screenings and self-examinations increase the chances of early detection of cancer, allowing for a better chance of successful treatment (Mayo Clinic, 2015a).

Screenings

When there is a familial history of cancer, anemia, SCD, other disorders of cellular regulation, nurses should encourage families to learn more about the disorder and teach children to receive regular surveillance as they enter young adulthood. Nurses should inform adolescent and adult patients in all families about screenings, such as the Papanicolaou (Pap) test, breast self-examination, and testicular examination, that can lead to early detection.

>> **Stay Current:** Visit http://www.cancer.org/healthy/findcancerearly/cancerscreeningguidelines/american-cancer-society-guidelines-for-the-early-detection-of-cancer to see the ACS's screening guidelines for early detection of cancer.

Nursing Assessment

The assessment of the patient with alterations in cellular regulation is highly dependent on the specific alteration and the organ systems involved. For example, when the alteration involves cells directly related to the transport of oxygen, the nurse should assess oxygenation and breathing patterns.

Observation and Patient Interview

Observation is a vital part of the assessment process and should be done at every patient encounter. Patient observation should include level of consciousness, state of health, mood, facial expressions, affect, probable nutritional status, and signs of discomfort. Ongoing observation and assessment of all patients with alterations in cellular regulation should include assessment of stress and coping abilities and psychosocial supports. Grief is a normal response when receiving a diagnosis of cancer, SCD, or another cellular regulation disorder, and the nurse should observe patients during each visit for clues to their progression through the

stages of grief and to determine how the patients are coping with actual or potential alterations in body image. The patients' ability to discuss the diagnosis and prognosis with family members should also be assessed. The assessment should also include noting the stress levels and coping abilities of spouses, parents, and/or caregivers and how these individuals are gaining access to support groups, financial resources, and spiritual aid.

Because early intervention and treatment of cancer improve patient outcomes, nurses should use observation and the patient interview to assess for early warning signs of cancer and teach patients the signs to watch for and report. The early warning signs include change in bowel or bladder habits, a sore that does not heal, unusual bleeding or discharge, thickening or lump in the breast or elsewhere, indigestion or difficulty swallowing, obvious change in wart or mole, or a nagging cough or hoarseness (ACS, 2014b).

Physical Examination

When assessing patients with an alteration in cellular regulation, the nurse should begin with a general survey, including the cardiovascular, respiratory, integumentary, and digestive systems. See the modules on Assessment, Digestion, Oxygenation, Perfusion, and Tissue Integrity for more detailed information related to the assessment process and the assessment of each individual system. Other specific physical assessment recommendations are listed in the exemplars.

Patients with alterations in cellular function may display activity intolerance, which can result in reduced activity, risk for injury, and alterations in skin integrity. Assessing activity tolerance, promoting safety, and helping patients remain as active as possible all play roles in the patients' eventual outcomes.

Diagnostic Tests

Patients with disorders of cellular regulation may need diagnostic tests or procedures to assist in decision making and treatment. Useful tests may include the following:

- Biopsy
- Bone marrow aspiration
- CT or computed axial tomography
- MRI
- Positron-emission tomography
- Radiography (x-ray)
- Scans
- Ultrasonography
- Complete blood count (CBC)
- Red blood indices
- Serum chemistry panel
- Tumor markers
- Urinalysis
- Lumbar puncture.

Case Study >> Part 2

Andrew Ladeaux is admitted to the emergency department. During the emergency department physician's assessment, Andrew tells the physician he feels "a little short of breath," especially when he runs. Andrew's mother reports that he has been treated for strep throat three times and has had several ear infections within the past 6 months. The physician orders a CBC with differential for Andrew. After the phlebotomist draws Andrew's blood, she has to apply pressure to the puncture site for nearly 2 minutes before the site stops bleeding. You return to check on Andrew's status. The physician tells you he suspects that Andrew may have developed leukemia.

Clinical Reasoning Questions Level I

1. Which two components of the CBC will be most useful for evaluation of Andrew's shortness of breath with physical activity?
2. On the basis of Andrew's recurrent nosebleeds and his delayed clotting response after venipuncture, which particular blood component would you expect to be impaired?
3. Describe methods by which you could explain venipuncture to Andrew. How could you involve his mother when explaining the procedure?

Clinical Reasoning Questions Level II

Refer to Exemplar 2.E on Leukemia.

4. If Andrew has developed leukemia, what results would you expect the CBC to reveal?
5. For which invasive diagnostic test might Andrew be scheduled to further evaluate for leukemia?
6. Explain the relationship between frequent or recurrent infections and leukemia.

Independent Interventions

For patients with alterations in cellular regulation, nursing interventions focus on reducing complications and maintaining optimal homeostasis. Common interventions for patients with cellular alterations are directed at nutrition, hydration, activity, breathing, fatigue, and comfort. Nurses also provide interventions and patient teaching to help patients manage side effects and provide patients and their families with psychosocial support. These interventions are critical to the patients' successful recovery.

For patients with impaired cellular regulation, independent nursing interventions include providing education about the disease and offering emotional support to the patients and family members. In many cases, patients can greatly improve their health status by recognizing and avoiding situations that exacerbate their condition. In addition to teaching about the patients' condition and treatments, the nurse should focus on helping the patients and family members understand how to prevent complications.

Providing Psychosocial Support

A diagnosis of cancer, leukemia, or SCD can create a whirlwind of emotions. Patients and family members may initially experience shock and anger. They need basic information about the disease and the purposes of the tests that will be performed. Because of increased stress levels, they may not process information well the first time it is presented and may need instructions to be repeated. For pediatric patients, nurses should assist the parents to plan how and when to tell the child the diagnosis. What the child needs to know is based on his or her developmental level and understanding.

After progressing from the initial state of shock about the diagnosis, the family needs to learn more about the disease, including the pathophysiology, treatment, and expected outcome or the prognosis. Knowing what to expect can help to decrease anxiety. Nurses should clarify the family's understanding of these areas and be ready to answer questions. They should provide both verbal explanations and written material. Patients and family members may talk with friends, purchase books, or search the internet for information. Nurses should find out where they are getting information and provide additional resources when appropriate. Nurses may also need to correct misconceptions and misinformation.

As a patient experiences remissions, exacerbations, or complications, the family will feel alternately hopeful and discouraged. Nurses should help the family to identify support systems and intervene as needed to enhance these systems. They should facilitate contact with extended family members who might be of help, faith-based or spiritual connections, social service agencies, and other resources such as the internet and parent and caregiver support groups. Nurses can assist patients and caregivers who are worried about job obligations and financial concerns.

Nurses should provide opportunities for patients to express thoughts and feelings. They may simply listen, educate, or dispel fears that stem from lack of understanding. Nurses can suggest that patients make use of area support groups and provide referrals as appropriate. Sharing with others who have had similar experiences can reduce anxiety and provide much-needed support.

Promoting Healthy Coping

Early in the disease continuum, threats to or changes in health status, physical comfort, role functioning, or even socioeconomic status can cause anxiety in patients. Later, anxiety may result from the anticipation of pain, disfigurement, or the threat of death. Patients whose coping skills have been poor in the past may find themselves at a loss to manage the current crisis. They may manifest overt signs of anxiety: trembling, restlessness, irritability, hyperactivity, stimulation of the sympathetic nervous system (e.g., increased blood pressure, pulse, respiration, excessive perspiration, pallor), withdrawal, worried facial expressions, and poor eye contact. Patients may report insomnia and feelings of tension and apprehension or express concerns regarding perceived changes brought about by the disease and fear of future events.

Nurses should carefully assess the patient's level of anxiety and the reality of the threats represented in the patient's current situation. These will influence the type of intervention that is appropriate. A patient in panic may need medical intervention with appropriate medications, whereas a patient with moderate or severe anxiety may be managed by the nurse through counseling and teaching new coping skills.

Nurses should establish a therapeutic relationship by conveying warmth and empathy and by listening nonjudgmentally. A patient who feels safe in the relationship with the nurse more easily expresses feelings and thoughts. The nurse should encourage the patient to acknowledge and express feelings, no matter how inappropriate they may seem to the patient. Just by expressing his or her feelings, the patient often can significantly diminish anxiety. Expressing feelings also allows the patient to direct energy toward healing and thus has a positive therapeutic effect. Moreover, acknowledging feelings, especially those the patient considers unacceptable, can lay the groundwork for new coping behaviors.

The nurse should review the coping strategies the patient has used in the past, and build on past successful behaviors, introducing new strategies as appropriate. The nurse should explain why inappropriate strategies, such as repressing anger or turning to alcohol, are not helpful. The patient will be more willing to make changes that build on what has already worked in the past. The patient will also be more willing to reject inappropriate strategies if given a persuasive reason why they have not had the desired effect in managing previous crises.

Collaborative Therapies

Nurses will provide appropriate pain management interventions, both pharmacologic and nonpharmacologic, to patients experiencing discomfort as rapid cellular reproduction in patients with cancer places pressure on healthy cells or alterations in cellular function result in inadequate oxygenation of tissues (anemias). Patients with disorders of cellular regulation who need surgery or radiation will require careful management related to these interventions. Patients with alterations in cellular regulation will require some assistance from members of the healthcare team in managing nutrition and hydration and managing treatment side effects.

Surgery

Surgery to treat cancer works best for solid tumors that are contained in one area. Surgery is not used to treat cancer that has metastasized, leukemia, or anemia if the underlying cause does not require surgery. The rationale for using surgery as treatment depends on the type of cancer being treated and the current stage of the cancer.

Surgery can be used to remove the entire tumor; to debulk a tumor, removing part of a tumor that could be threatening to damage an organ or to allow treatment to be more effective; or to ease symptoms when tumors are causing blockages, pain, or pressure (NCI, 2015a).

Management of patients who require surgery is discussed in the respective cancer exemplars and in the module on Perioperative Care.

Radiation

Radiation therapy is the application of high-energy x-rays or particles for the purpose of damaging or killing cancer cells. It has multiple applications in the treatment of cancer. In this type of therapy, high doses of radiation are used to:

- Treat cancer by preventing cancer from returning through stopping or slowing cancer growth.
- Ease cancer symptoms by shrinking tumors to treat pain or other problems caused by the tumor or decrease problems caused by a growing tumor such as difficulty breathing or loss of bowel and bladder control (NCI, 2015b).

Management of patients who require radiation is discussed in the respective cancer exemplars.

Management of Nutrition and Hydration

Cells cannot function properly if the body is not provided with all of the essential nutrients. Assessment of nutritional status and promotion of good nutrition play important roles in supporting the patient's recovery as well as reducing the likelihood of cellular alterations.

The goals of nutrition therapy during treatment for cellular regulation disorders are to prevent or reverse any nutritional deficiencies, preserve the patient's lean body mass, minimize any side effects that influence nutritional state, allow for the growth needs of pediatric patients, and improve overall quality of life. The nurse should offer frequent, small meals and administer antiemetic drugs to lessen nausea from chemotherapy. It may be helpful to offer the patient's favorite foods at times when nausea and vomiting are less. The nurse should perform 24-hour dietary recalls to assess the patient's intake, and evaluate height and weight regularly. When the patient's nutritional status is deteriorating or parenteral nutrition is used, the nurse should perform weekly studies of serum electrolytes, liver chemistry, glucose, and triglycerides. The nurse can partner with both the oncologist and the dietitian to plan interventions appropriate for meeting the needs of the patient.

Hydration management can be challenging, because the patient may not be thirsty but is excreting large numbers of cell fragments and other substances as a result of treatment. Children in particular are at risk for dehydration due to a higher concentration of fluid within the body. The nurse should offer small amounts of fluid frequently. Frozen ice pops or other fluid-containing foods such as Jell-O, fruit, or soups should be included, avoiding citrus fruits. The nurse should measure intake and output.

Management of Treatment Side Effects

All cancer treatments affect some normal body cells along with cancer cells, causing a wide variety of side effects. Nurses should teach patients and their caregivers that some side effects may not develop until after therapy is completed. They should emphasize the importance of all follow-up visits for monitoring of late effects.

A frequent occurrence is *myelosuppression,* or suppression of blood cell production in the bone marrow. Suppression of the immune response may lead to increased susceptibility to infection. *Neutropenia* is present when the absolute neutrophil count (ANC) is less than 500 cells/mm^3 or when it is between 500 and 1000 cells/mm^3 while the patient is receiving chemotherapy and falling levels are anticipated. At these levels, the patient will be given a broad-spectrum antibiotic and possibly granulocyte colony-stimulating factor (G-CSF). The nurse should take the patient's temperature, isolate the patient from others with infections, and perform serum laboratory studies as ordered.

The nurse should protect the patient from bruises and be alert for hemorrhage or signs of bleeding such as petechiae, nosebleeds, dark-colored or bloody stools, and the presence of blood in vomit and urine, which may occur due to thrombocytopenia. The patient may need to receive infusions of platelets if thrombocytopenia is severe. If thrombocytopenia develops, the nurse should minimize needlesticks and other intrusive procedures and should report any bleeding episodes to the oncologist. Patients, family members, and caregivers need to know that the patient should avoid contact sports and other rough activities and that any healthcare provider, such as a dentist, should be informed of the patient's treatment and condition.

Pharmacologic Therapy

Pharmacologic therapy, in the form of chemotherapy, plays an important role in treating alterations in cellular regulation (see the Medications feature). The three typical goals of chemotherapy are cure, control, and palliation (ACS, 2015b). Cure is the primary goal for most patients with a cancer diagnosis (**Figure 2–2 》**). However, sometimes cancer has progressed, and cure is not possible. Then, the goal of chemotherapy is to control or manage the disease by preventing tumor growth and spread, which may extend the patient's life. In the advanced stages of cancer, chemotherapy may be used for palliation by reducing tumor size to decrease pain and tumor-related symptoms, thus improving a patient's quality of life. In some patients, chemotherapy may be used as adjuvant therapy after surgery or radiation to aid in the removal of any remaining cancerous cells or to treat microscopic metastases (Adams, Holland, & Urban, 2017).

Individuals who handle chemotherapeutic drugs are at constant risk of exposure because of the toxicity of antineoplastic medications. This includes nurses who administer chemotherapy and requires them to obtain advanced training. This risk of exposure can be minimized through the use of personal protective equipment (PPE) (i.e., gowns, gloves, eye and face shields, and respirator protection), a needle-less system, and ventilation cabinets (Oncology Nursing Society [ONS], 2016a). The handling of chemotherapy drugs by pregnant nurses may be especially risky; unfortunately, information related to the level of toxicity during pregnancy is limited. Pregnant healthcare professionals should use an additional level of protection when handling chemotherapeutic agents. However, the risks cannot be completely eliminated for anyone who handles these medications, even with adherence to all precautions (Gilani & Giridharan, 2014).

Biological Therapy

Biological therapies, also called biotherapies, enhance the ability of the body to use its natural defenses to fight cancer, i.e., the immune system is stimulated to stop the growth of the cancer, increase the immune system cells so they can destroy the cancer cells, and keep the cancer from spreading to other sites. Bacillus Calmette-Guérin (BCG) was the first biologic therapy to be approved by the FDA for use in patients with bladder cancer. BCG is a weakened form of a live tuberculosis bacterium that does not cause disease in humans. It is inserted directly into the bladder with a catheter and stimulates a general immune response that is directed against the foreign bacterium itself and against bladder cancer cells. Approximately 70 percent of patients with early-stage bladder cancer experience a remission after BCG therapy (Steinberg, 2017).

Targeted therapy for cancer has moved the focus of treatment from an "empiric guess to a predictive choice" (Vanneman & Dranoff, 2012). These agents, also termed personalized medicine, target the hallmarks of cancer growth with less toxicity than conventional chemotherapy. Currently there are FDA approved medications that target tumor angiogenesis, growth signals and signaling pathways, plus cell cycle apoptosis.

The experimental procedure of gene therapy focuses on the use of genes to treat or prevent disease. Most commonly a normal gene is inserted, using a variety of placement techniques, to replace an abnormal gene. Other possibilities include repairing an abnormal gene or altering the amount a gene can be turned "on" or "off." Currently, research directions include killing cancer cells by replacing or knocking out the gene, incorporating genes that will boost the immune system that will in turn destroy the cancer, utilization of viruses that occur naturally (like retroviruses that cause the common cold) to selectively infect cancer cells and then cause them to be destroyed, or inject viruses that will replicate selectively in the cancer cells and then destroy the cancer cells or perhaps not even allow replication and just induce cell death. Gene therapy is currently available only through clinical trials (NIH U.S. National Library of Medicine, 2017).

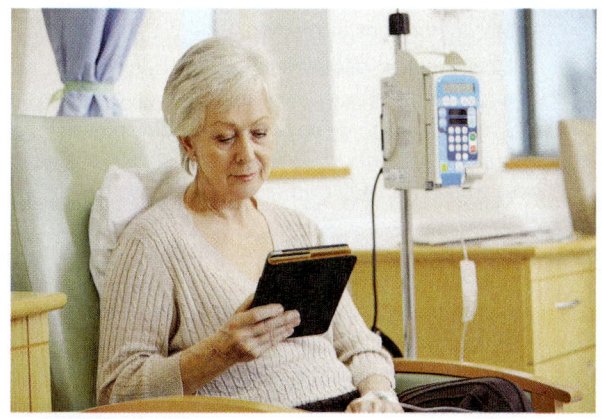

Source: Stockbroker/MBI/Alamy Stock Photo.

Figure 2–2 》 Chemotherapy is often administered in a comfortable outpatient setting.

Complementary Health Approaches

An increasing number of patients are using complementary health approaches to address their concerns related to

Medications
Cellular Regulation

CLASSIFICATION AND DRUG EXAMPLES	MECHANISMS OF ACTION	NURSING CONSIDERATIONS
Antineoplastics: Alkylating Agents *Drug examples:* Busulfan, carboplatin, carmustine, cisplatin, chlorambucil, cyclophosphamide, ifosfamide, lomustine, melphalan	These drugs interfere with DNA production, causing cellular death. They are not cell specific, so both cancerous and noncancerous cells are destroyed.	▪ Monitor CBC with differential, platelet count, uric acid levels, and kidney and liver function studies. ▪ Monitor temperature; avoid rectal temperature assessment. ▪ Assess mentation and neurologic status. ▪ Monitor nutritional and fluid intake. ▪ Monitor respiratory status, cardiovascular status, and skin. ▪ Concurrent administration with drugs that are toxic to kidneys or liver is contraindicated. ▪ Use in patients with liver, kidney, or gastrointestinal disorders is contraindicated.
Antineoplastics: Antitumor Antibiotics *Drug examples:* Bleomycin, dactinomycin, daunorubicin, doxorubicin, epirubicin, idarubicin, mitomycin	These drugs interfere with production and action of nucleic acids to inhibit DNA and RNA replication.	▪ Monitor CBC with differential and electrolytes. ▪ Monitor cardiovascular, respiratory, and neurologic status. ▪ Monitor for bleeding and protect the patient from traumatic injury. ▪ Monitor for signs of infection. ▪ Monitor nutritional and fluid intake. ▪ Use in patients with liver, kidney, cardiac, pulmonary, gastrointestinal, or lung disease is contraindicated.
Antineoplastics: Antimetabolites *Drug examples:* Capecitabine, cytarabine, fluorouracil, methotrexate, pemetrexed, pralatrexate	These drugs interfere with either the use of folate by the cell, which is essential for cell maintenance, or with pyrimidine and purine synthesis, which is essential for DNA production.	▪ Monitor CBC with differential, electrolytes, and kidney and liver function studies. ▪ Monitor for bleeding and protect the patient from traumatic injury. ▪ Monitor for signs of infection. ▪ Monitor nutritional and fluid intake. ▪ Monitor for dyspnea and cough.
Hormones and Hormone Agonists *Drug examples:* *Hormones:* dexamethasone, diethylstilbestrol, ethinyl estradiol, medroxyprogesterone, prednisone *Hormone antagonists:* abiraterone, anastrozole, bicalutamide, exemestane, goserelin, leuprolide, tamoxifen	These drugs help block cancerous cells from utilizing the hormones that promote their growth and inhibit the body's natural production of hormones that promote growth of the cancerous cells.	▪ Monitor CBC with differential and serum calcium (tamoxifen). ▪ Monitor blood pressure. ▪ Monitor for signs of bleeding and protect the patient from traumatic injury. ▪ Monitor for signs of infection. ▪ Monitor cardiovascular status. ▪ Advise the patient to discontinue this medication only when advised to do so by the healthcare provider.
Biological Response Modifiers and Targeted Therapy *Drug examples:* *Biological response modifiers:* interferon alfa-2b, interferon alfacon-1, peginterferon alfa-2a *Targeted therapy:* axitinib, bilnatumomab, brentuximab, ibritumomab, rituximab, trastuzumab	These drugs stimulate immune function or block tumor growth. They block cellular replication or attack specific tumor cells.	▪ Monitor electrolytes and assess for signs of dehydration. ▪ Monitor for signs of infection. ▪ Monitor nutritional and fluid intake. ▪ Monitor for capillary leak syndrome (hypotension, generalized edema, decreased urine output). ▪ Monitor respiratory status.

Medications *(continued)*

CLASSIFICATION AND DRUG EXAMPLES	MECHANISMS OF ACTION	NURSING CONSIDERATIONS
Natural Products: Vinca Alkaloids, Taxanes and Topisomerase Inhibitors *Drug examples:* Paclitaxel, teniposide, vinblastine, vincristine, vinorelbine	These drugs cause immediate cellular death by inhibition of mitosis or by inhibiting topoisomerase I, causing permanent damage to tumor cell DNA.	▪ Monitor CBC with differential and liver function studies. ▪ Monitor for bleeding and protect the patient from traumatic injury. ▪ Monitor for signs of infection. ▪ Monitor nutritional and fluid intake. ▪ Monitor neurologic and cardiovascular status.
Antianemic Agents: Iron Supplements *Drug examples:* Ferrous fumarate, ferrous gluconate, ferrous sulfate	These drugs provide additional iron intake for the purpose of correcting RBC abnormalities caused by iron deficiency. They do not stimulate RBC production (erythropoiesis).	▪ Monitor hemoglobin and reticulocyte counts. ▪ To avoid staining teeth, thoroughly dilute liquid preparations and administer by using a straw or a dropper to apply medication to the back of the tongue. ▪ Advise the patient of potential side effects, including black or dark green stools and constipation.
Antianemic Agents *Drug examples:* Folic acid (vitamin B_9 or folate) and vitamin B_{12} (cyanocobalamin)	Folic acid stimulates production of RBCs, WBCs, and platelets in patients with megaloblastic anemia. Vitamin B_{12} (cyanocobalamin) is necessary for the production of RBCs and is used to treat vitamin B_{12} deficiency and pernicious anemia.	▪ Monitor CBC with reticulocyte count, vitamin B_{12}, and serum folate levels. ▪ Monitor serum potassium for 48 hours following initiation of cyanocobalamin treatment. ▪ Especially in patients with cardiovascular disease, monitor for signs and symptoms of pulmonary edema.

Source: Data from Adams, M. P., Holland, L. N., & Urban, C. (2017). *Pharmacology for nurses: A pathophysiologic approach* (5th ed.). Hoboken, NJ: Pearson Education.

alterations in cellular regulation and the pharmacologic therapies used to treat them (pain, nausea, vomiting, fatigue, insomnia, depression, and anxiety) in an attempt to improve their quality of life. When such an approach is used as an adjunct to other cancer treatment, it is referred to as complementary therapy, and the use of conventional and complementary treatments together is called integrative therapy. If it is used alone or instead of conventional treatment, it is referred to as alternative therapy. These health approaches include herbal and dietary supplements, meditation, spinal manipulation, acupuncture, biofeedback, exercise, meditation, music, visualization/guided imagery, yoga, kinesiology, massage, reflexology, healing touch, Qigong, Reiki, and transcutaneous electrical nerve stimulation. Healthcare providers often integrate these therapies into conventional treatment plans to provide a more holistic approach to patient care. Because the safety and efficacy of many of these therapies have not been scientifically proven, patients should consult with their healthcare provider before beginning any type of complementary health approach (Kravits, 2013; Leukemia and Lymphoma Society [LLS], 2015a; National Center for Complementary and Integrative Health [NCCIH], 2014a).

There is substantial evidence that acupuncture is beneficial in the management of treatment-related nausea and vomiting (see the Focus on Integrative Therapy feature). Ginger has also been shown to aid in the reduction of chemotherapy-related nausea. Massage therapy is another approach that has proven to be beneficial in relieving pain, nausea, anxiety, and depression.

Meditation training has been shown to assist patients in relieving anxiety, stress, fatigue, and general mood, thereby improving overall quality of life. Evidence has shown meditation to be most effective with patients in the early stages of the disease process. Other studies have examined the possible benefits of yoga, hypnosis, relaxation therapies, and biofeedback to help patients manage their symptoms and treatment side effects (NCCIH, 2014b).

Patients should consult with their healthcare provider before taking any herbal supplements because of the risk of potential negative interactions with conventional cancer treatments (NCCIH, 2014a).

Lifespan Considerations

Cellular Regulation Disorders in Infants, Children, and Adolescents

The diagnosis of a cellular regulation disorder can be devastating at any age; however, the blow seems to be more difficult when it involves a child or adolescent. The age, developmental level, and personality of the child or adolescent have an effect on their response to the diagnosis. Although every child is different, there are some common themes among age groups. Each age group also has a multitude of different developmental milestones that must continue to be assessed for regularly while they are undergoing treatment. Cellular regulation disorders can influence each age group in different psychologic ways as well.

Focus on Integrative Health
Acupuncture

Acupuncture is an alternative health approach that involves the placement of special needles at certain points in the skin. Needle placement can be followed by manual manipulation or the application of heat or electrical impulses that stimulate nervous system activity. Clinical trials have indicated that acupuncture is both safe and effective in relieving numerous symptoms experienced by patients with cancer. The scientific evidence provides the most support for the use of acupuncture in reducing chemotherapy-induced nausea and vomiting. It has also been proven beneficial in reducing certain types of pain and radiation-induced xerostomia (excessive dryness of the mucous membranes), relieving anxiety, treating insomnia, and decreasing lymphedema in breast cancer patients. The practice of acupuncture is generally safe when performed by qualified practitioners. The most common adverse effects include minor bleeding or bruising and pain at the acupuncture sites. Acupuncture should not be used in patients with cancer who have severe neutropenia or thrombocytopenia because of an increased risk for infection or bleeding. Acupuncture should not be used as first-line treatment for symptom relief but may be considered for inclusion in the treatment plan when conventional treatment is unsuccessful or not well tolerated by the patient (Deng & Cassileth, 2013; NCI, 2016b).

Nurses caring for these patients must be aware of the ways these disorders can affect individuals across the lifespan (NCI, 2015c, 2016c).

Children and adolescents who survive any type of cellular regulation disorder diagnosis are at risk of being affected later in life as a result of treatments received. The risks are related to the type of disorder and its location in the body, the type of treatment received, and multiple patient factors, including gender, age and developmental stage. Areas affected may include organs and other tissues, body function, growth and development, thinking, learning and memory, and social and psychologic adjustment (NCI, 2016d).

Infants, toddlers, and young children are unable to understand what the diagnosis of a cellular regulation disorder actually means. If they are hospitalized, familiar items from home such as toys or a blanket can help them feel more secure. The use of skin to skin contact by the parent, singing, or talking to the infant can also be soothing. The nurse should try to maintain feeding and bedtime routines as much as possible.

Toddlers understand things they can see and touch. They fear being separated from their parents and may cling to them when they are afraid or overly anxious. Toddlers need to be prepared ahead of time for painful medical procedures to decrease their level of fear and anxiety. This age group likes to start making choices. The nurse can allow a toddler to choose a flavor of medicine if appropriate or choose a sticker. The older toddler may regress to behaviors such as thumb sucking or bedwetting if potty trained (NCI, 2015d).

School-age children are able to understand that the treatments and medicines are to help them get better. They are more cooperative but want to know what to expect. This age group often asks many questions related to treatment and how it works (NCI, 2015d). School-age children may show

anger and sadness over the losses they are experiencing (health, school, normal life). They look for more emotional and social support from family and friends. Therefore, children this age should return to school as soon as possible after diagnosis. Teachers should be informed of the child's condition before the return to school so they can assist with plans to prepare classmates for the child's return. Arrangements can also be made for tutors to assist the child with schoolwork during hospitalization and home care if needed.

Assessment of children's physical and neurologic development helps in determining the progress made during treatment and provides a baseline for evaluating the long-term effects of treatment. Developmental assessment of children should be performed regularly during treatment for cellular regulation disorders, at times when the child feels well so that the results are accurate (see the module on Development). The nurse should observe developmental milestones at each contact with the child and refer for further assessment if regression is observed. Performance in school and social activities with friends provides important information about expected developmental milestones in older children.

A major developmental task of adolescence is to attain independence and control, but a cellular regulation diagnosis often interferes with adolescents' ability to achieve this task. They may be upset by the disruption of school and their activities with friends. Friendships are very important for this age group. Helping the adolescent maintain connections with friends through texting, video chats, e-mails, social media, and visits can be beneficial. Adolescents may feel the need to protect others who are close to them by withholding their feelings; they may confide in a friend or member of the healthcare team instead (NCI, 2015d). Planning nursing strategies that empower adolescents such as asking them whether they prefer morning or afternoon appointments and encouraging parents to allow them to make choices about issues at home can be beneficial.

Cellular Regulation Disorders in Pregnant Women

During pregnancy, cellular regulation disorders can pose problems to both the mother and the fetus. Maternal issues can arise from underlying organ dysfunction such as renal disease or pulmonary hypertension, caused by the cellular regulation disorder. These women are also more likely to experience preeclampsia and eclampsia. The fetus can also be affected by cellular regulation disorders. Concerns for the fetus include alloimmunization, consequences of utero-placental insufficiency, and opioid exposure. Specific treatments involved with cellular regulation disorder diagnoses can also have an impact on the fetus. Women who have a diagnosis of a cellular regulation disorder should receive preconception counseling and be made aware of the health risks involved, not only for herself, but for her unborn child (James, 2014).

Cellular Regulation Disorders in Older Adults

Cellular regulation disorders can affect the older adult population, and certain disorders tend to be more prevalent in this age group. Older adults experiencing cellular regulation disorders are more likely to have comorbidities such as lung, kidney, or heart disease, which can increase their risk of treatment complications. These individuals are also less likely to tolerate the necessary treatment or its adverse reactions. Older adults with cellular regulation disorders who have a lower functional status are generally predisposed to poorer outcomes (Phillips, 2012).

Case Study » Part 3

Andrew Ladeaux's laboratory results are available. His CBC results include the following:

WBC: 37.8 (normal = 4.5–10 K/μL)

RBC: 3.2 (normal = 4.6–6 M/μL)

PLT (platelets): 90 (normal = 150–400 K/μL)

Lymphocytes: 70 (normal = 25–35%)

At the emergency department physician's request, the pediatric oncologist arrives to examine Andrew and review his laboratory test results. Her conclusion is that Andrew's signs and symptoms may be caused by acute lymphoblastic leukemia (ALL). Andrew is admitted to the hospital for further evaluation and treatment.

Clinical Reasoning Questions Level I

1. What diagnostic test will likely be included in Andrew's plan of care to confirm the suspected diagnosis of ALL?
2. Which component of Andrew's CBC suggests thrombocytopenia?
3. In reacting to the potential diagnosis of cancer, what response(s) might you anticipate from Andrew and his family members?

Clinical Reasoning Questions Level II
Refer to the Exemplar 2.E Leukemia.

4. What does Andrew's lymphocyte measurement suggest about his body's ability to fight infection?
5. As you prepare to transfer Andrew to the pediatric oncology unit, he asks you why he has to stay in the hospital. How should you respond?
6. Formulate three nursing diagnoses that are appropriate for inclusion in the nursing plan of care for Andrew and his family.

REVIEW The Concept of Cellular Regulation

RELATE Link the Concepts

Linking the concept of cellular regulation with the concept of infection:

1. How does impaired cellular regulation influence a patient's susceptibility to infection?
2. What can the nurse do to help reduce the likelihood of infection in patients with disorders related to impaired cellular regulation?

Linking the concept of cellular regulation with the concept of stress and coping:

3. What is the relationship between poor coping abilities and disorders of cellular regulation?
4. Which personality types are most often correlated with a risk for ineffective coping?
5. Is there a relationship between personality and impaired cellular regulation? Explain your answer.

Linking the concept of cellular regulation with the concept of safety:

6. Identify three safety concerns specific to the patient with a disorder related to impaired cellular regulation.
7. Based on QSEN competencies, how can the nurse promote safety for the patient with a disorder of cellular regulation?

READY Go to Volume 3: Clinical Nursing Skills

- SKILLS 1.5–1.9   Vital Signs
- SKILL 2.10   Automated Dispensing System: Using
- SKILL 3.1   Pain in Newborn, Infant, Child, or Adult: Assessing
- SKILL 5.9   Infusion: Initiating
- SKILL 5.10   Infusion: Maintaining
- SKILL 6.1   Hand Hygiene: Performing
- SKILL 6.7   Isolation, Transporting Patient Outside Room
- SKILL 6.8   PPE, Clean Gloves: Donning and Doffing
- SKILL 6.9   PPE, Face Masks: Donning and Doffing
- SKILL 10.5   Nutrition: Assessing
- SKILL 11.8   Oxygen Delivery Systems: Using
- SKILL 13.1   Perioperative Patient Teaching
- SKILL 15.5   Environmental Safety: Healthcare Facility, Community, Home
- SKILL 15.9   Immobilizer, Mummy: Applying

REFER Go to Pearson MyLab Nursing and eText

- Additional review materials
- Chart 1: Case Study

REFLECT Apply Your Knowledge

Jason Marchetti is a 25-year-old man who has been regularly going to the gym daily after work for the past 8 months. Approximately 4 months ago, he noticed a small nodule on the left side of his chest. Now the nodule is somewhat larger, and the nipple had an odd shape. The area is not painful, but Mr. Marchetti is worried that he may have injured a muscle at the gym and decides to go to his primary healthcare provider to have the area evaluated. Upon examination, the provider finds a 2.5 cm, nontender, movable nodule in Mr. Marchetti's left breast area. There are no risk factors for breast cancer in Mr. Marchetti's previous medical or family history. The provider tells Mr. Marchetti that he is concerned about the nodule and a biopsy is needed to determine whether it is benign or cancer. The biopsy is performed, and Mr. Marchetti returns the next week to get the results. The provider informs Mr. Marchetti that he has invasive ductal carcinoma of the breast and that they should discuss options for treatment. Mr. Marchetti sits in the examination room in disbelief. "I don't understand how I can have breast cancer. I thought only women got that," he says to the nurse.

1. What treatment options are available for Mr. Marchetti and could be recommended by the provider?
2. What nursing diagnoses might the nurse use when writing out the plan of care?
3. What would be appropriate primary nursing interventions for the nurse to implement for Mr. Marchetti at this time?

» Exemplar 2.A
Cancer

Exemplar Learning Outcomes

2.A Analyze cancer as it relates to cellular regulation.

- Describe the pathophysiology of cancer.
- Describe the etiology of cancer.
- Compare the risk factors for and prevention of cancer.
- Identify the clinical manifestations of cancer.
- Summarize diagnostic tests and therapies used by interprofessional teams in the collaborative care of an individual with cancer.
- Differentiate considerations for care of patients with cancer across the lifespan.
- Apply the nursing process in providing culturally competent care to an individual with cancer.

Exemplar Key Terms

Benign, *46*
Cachexia, *52*

Overview

Cancer refers to a group of complex diseases whose manifestations depend on the affected body system and the type of cells involved. It is marked by uncontrolled growth and the spread of abnormal cells. Cancer can affect people of any age, gender, ethnicity, or geographic region. Although the incidence and mortality rates of cancer have continued to decline since 1990, it remains one of the most feared diseases. Even the suggestion of a cancer diagnosis often evokes feelings of hopelessness and helplessness. African Americans are more likely to develop cancer than any other ethnic or racial group in the United States (Centers for Disease Control and Prevention [CDC], 2015a). Asians and Native Americans have the lowest incidence of prostate cancer. Cancer incidence and mortality are lower in Native American men and women than in any other ethnic or racial group, but mortality rates are lowest among the Asian/Pacific Islander population.

Cancer results when normal cells mutate into abnormal, deviant cells that then perpetuate within the body. It can affect any body tissue. Nursing care of the patient with cancer is holistic and comprehensive, focusing on cancer not as one disease but as a constellation of many diseases. The nurse recognizes that cancer is a disruptive and life-threatening process that affects the whole individual and the patient's significant others. Nursing interventions are based on the understanding that cancer is a chronic disease with acute episodes, that the patient is often treated in the home, and that the patient is usually treated with a combination of therapeutic modalities. Equally important, the nurse recognizes that caring for the patient with cancer involves prevention, early detection, treatment, supportive care, long-term follow-up, and, for some patients, end-of-life care (ONS, 2016b).

Oncology is the study of cancer. The term is derived from the Greek word *oncoma* ("bulk"). Oncologists specialize in caring for patients with cancer and may be medical doctors, surgeons, radiologists, immunologists, or researchers. The oncology nurse has received specialized training in cancer care and treatment and is an important and significant member of the oncology team. Oncology nurses have special skills in assisting the patient and family with the psychosocial issues associated with cancer and terminal illness. Collaboration among healthcare professionals (e.g., surgeons, oncologists, nurses, social workers) ensures the most effective care and treatment for the patient with cancer.

Pathophysiology and Etiology

A **neoplasm** is a mass of new tissue (a collection of cells) that grows independently of its surrounding structures and has no physiologic purpose. The term *neoplasm* is often used interchangeably with *tumor* (from the Latin word meaning "swelling"). Neoplasms are said to be autonomous for these reasons:

- They grow at a rate uncoordinated with the needs of the body.
- They share some of the properties of the parent cells but with altered size and shape.
- They do not benefit the host and, in some cases, are actively harmful.

Neoplasms are not completely autonomous, however, because they require a blood supply with nutrients and oxygen to sustain their growth. Neoplasms typically are classified as benign or malignant on the basis of their potential to damage the body and their growth characteristics. A **benign** growth is one that does not endanger life or health; it tends not to recur after treatment. A **malignant** growth is one that, if not treated, will recur, continue to grow, and spread to other sites in the body, ending in death.

Benign Neoplasms

Benign neoplasms are localized growths. They form a solid mass, have well-defined borders, and are frequently encapsulated. Benign neoplasms tend to respond to the body's homeostatic controls. Thus, they often stop growing when they reach the boundaries of another tissue (a process called contact inhibition). They grow slowly and often remain stable in size. Because they are usually encapsulated, benign neoplasms often are easily removed and tend not to recur.

Although typically harmless, benign neoplasms can be destructive if they crowd surrounding tissue and obstruct the function of organs. For example, a benign meningioma (from the meninges of the brain and spinal cord) can cause severely increased intracranial pressure, which progressively impairs the individual's cerebral function. Unless the meningioma can be successfully removed, the steadily rising intracranial pressure will eventually lead to coma and death.

Malignant Neoplasms

Malignant neoplasms grow aggressively and do not respond to the body's homeostatic controls. Malignant neoplasms are not cohesive, and they present with an irregular shape. Instead of slowly crowding other tissues aside, malignant neoplasms cut through surrounding tissues (a process known as **invasion**), causing bleeding, inflammation, and necrosis (tissue death) as they grow. This invasive quality of malignant neoplasms is reflected in the origin of the word *cancer* (from the Greek *karkinos*, meaning "crab"). Healthcare professionals are referring to a malignant neoplasm when they use the term *cancer.*

Malignant cells from the primary tumor may travel through the blood or lymph to invade other tissues and organs of the body and form a secondary tumor. The spreading of malignant neoplasms to other areas of the body—perhaps their most destructive trait—is called **metastasis**. Malignant neoplasms can recur after surgical removal of the primary and secondary tumors and after other treatments. **Table 2–2 »** compares benign and malignant neoplasms.

Malignant neoplasms vary in their degree of differentiation from the parent tissue. Highly differentiated cancer cells try to mimic the specialized function of the parent tissue, but undifferentiated cancers, consisting of immature cells, have almost no resemblance to the parent tissue and perform no useful function. Furthermore, undifferentiated cancers rob the body of its energy and nutrition as they grow. Undifferentiated anaplastic cells, which have little structural or functional relationship to the parent cells, are the basis of many malignant neoplasms. The degree of differentiation of anaplastic cells is a consideration in the classification and staging of neoplasms.

Characteristics of Malignant Cells

Malignant neoplasms may be identified by the following predictable cellular characteristics:

- ***Loss of regulation of the rate of mitosis.*** This results in rapid cell division and growth of the neoplasm.

- ***Loss of specialization and differentiation.*** Malignant cells do not perform typical cellular functions. Many produce hormones and enzymes similar to those of the parent tissue, but usually in excessive amounts, possibly revealing their presence.

- ***Loss of contact inhibition.*** Malignant cells do not respect other cellular boundaries. They easily invade and destroy other tissues.

- ***Progressive acquisition of a cancerous phenotype.*** Cellular mutation seems to be a sequential process involving successive generations of cells, with each generation becoming more deviant than the previous one. In addition, malignant cells seem to be "immortal"—that is, they do not stop growing and die, as do normal cells, which have a genetically determined lifespan.

- ***Irreversibility.*** The transformation into a malignant cell is irreversible. Rarely does a malignant neoplasm revert to a benign state.

- ***Altered cell structure.*** Cytologic examination of malignant cells reveals distinct differences in the cell nucleus and cytoplasm as well as an overall cell shape that differs from that of normal cells of the particular tissue type.

- ***Simplified metabolic activities.*** The work of malignant cells is simpler than that of normal cells; they show an increased synthesis of substances needed for cell division, and they have no need to create proteins for the specialized functions of the tissues they invade.

- ***Transplantability.*** Malignant cells often break away from the primary tissue site and travel to other locations in the body, where they establish new growths.

- ***Ability to promote their own survival.*** Malignant cells may create ectopic sites to produce the hormones they need for their growth. By their very presence and their ability to initiate vascular permeability, malignant cells promote the development of nonneoplastic stroma, a connective tissue framework consisting of collagen and other components, which then supports the neoplasm. Malignant cells may also create their own blood supply. Through a process called angiogenesis, tumor cells secrete a polypeptide angiogenic growth factor that stimulates blood vessels from surrounding normal tissue to grow into the tumor. Finally, malignant cells divert nutrition from the host to meet their own needs, by diffusion when the tumor is less than 1 mm and by means of the newly formed blood vessels thereafter. If unchecked, malignant cells eventually destroy their host.

TABLE 2–2 Comparison of Benign and Malignant Neoplasms

Benign	Malignant
Local	Invasive
Cohesive	Noncohesive
Well-defined borders	Does not stop at tissue border
Pushes other tissues out of the way	Invades and destroys surrounding tissues
Slow growth	Rapid growth
Encapsulated	Metastasizes to distant sites
Easily removed	Not always easy to remove
Does not recur	Can recur

Tumor Invasion and Metastasis

Cancer cells may overtake adjacent tissues (invasion) and spread from their primary site to distant organs (metastasis). Aggressive tumors possess several qualities that facilitate invasion:

- *Ability to cause pressure atrophy.* The pressure of a growing tumor can cause atrophy and necrosis of adjacent tissues. The malignancy then moves into the vacated space.

- *Ability to disrupt the basement membrane of normal cells.* Many cancer cells can bind to elements of the basement membrane and secrete enzymes that degrade that physical barrier, thus facilitating their movement into normal tissues, lymph, and blood circulation.

- *Motility.* Because malignant cells are less tightly bound to each other than normal cells (reduced adhesiveness), they easily separate from the neoplasm and move into surrounding body fluids and tissues.

- *Response to chemical signals from adjacent tissues.* **Chemotaxis** (the movement of cells in response to a chemical stimulus) draws the tumor cells into the normal tissues, possibly as a result of the degrading of the basement membranes of the normal cells. This breakdown of normal cellular membranes releases the chemical stimulus that is physiologically designed to draw normal phagocytic cells to clean up the debris. Malignant cells are also known to respond chemotactically to the end product of cellular metabolism. Some cancer cells even produce a substance called autocrine motility factor, which calls other malignant cells to a normal tissue. The first invading cells produce this substance, which then actively draws other malignant cells from the primary tumor into the invaded normal tissue.

The factors that favor invasion also contribute to the process of metastasis. Metastasis can occur by means of one or more mechanisms, including embolism in the blood or lymph or spread by way of body cavities.

A blood- or lymph-borne metastasis allows a new tumor to be established in a distant organ. **Figure 2–3** ❯❯ shows metastasis through the bloodstream. A tumor's ability to metastasize in this manner requires the following steps:

1. Intravasation of malignant cells through blood or lymphatic vessel walls and into the circulation
2. Survival of the malignant cells in the blood (to survive, the cells must escape the notice of the body's immune surveillance; only about 1 in 1000 cells does so)
3. Extravasation from the circulation and implantation in a new tissue.

The tumor cells tend to clump together, forming an embolus, and continue growing until their size prevents further travel in the vessel or lymph channel. The growing neoplastic mass then uses its invasive abilities (secreting enzymes and motility factor) to move into the nearest organ.

Approximately 60% of metastatic lesions tend to occur in a pattern reflective of blood or lymph circulation. Some malignant cells, however, defy a bloodborne pattern and target specific organs to which they prefer to metastasize. For example, lung cancer frequently metastasizes to the adrenal glands, and breast cancer frequently metastasizes to bone.

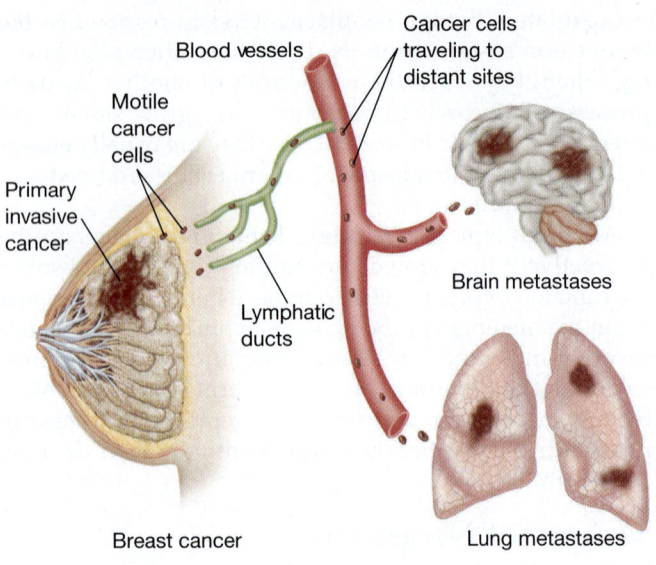

Figure 2–3 ❯❯ Metastasis through the bloodstream. Cancer cells secrete enzymes and a motility factor that disrupt the basement membrane in the blood vessel. In this way, the cancer cells gain access to the circulation. Once cancer cells are in the blood, only about 1 in 1000 escapes immune detection, but that can be enough. Undetected cells move out of the blood, again secreting enzymes and cutting through the vessel wall into new tissue. The tissue in which a new tumor is established may be downstream from the original tumor, or a chemical attraction may cause the malignant cells to target a specific site. Once in the new site, the malignant cells multiply and establish a metastatic tumor.

Malignant cells that gain access to the lymph channels may travel to a preferred organ and then move into it the same way they migrate through blood vessels. The malignant cells may alternatively become trapped in the lymph node and continue to grow. The malignant cells eventually replace the node's tissues. At this point, emboli from the cancerous node disseminate to other nodes, creating a cascade reaction. The malignant cascade causes widespread transfer of the tumor to uncharacteristic sites.

A malignant tumor may break through the walls of the organ in which it is primarily housed, in the process shedding cells into the nearby body cavity. Those cells are then free to establish new tumors in a distant area of that cavity. For example, malignant cells from a colon cancer may be seeded into the peritoneal cavity, establishing a new tumor in the mesenteric epithelium.

Metastatic lesions are differentiated from primary neoplasms by cell morphology: Metastatic cells do not resemble the tissue in which they reside. The most common sites of metastasis are the lymph nodes, liver, lungs, bones, and brain.

For metastasis to occur, the cancerous cells must avoid detection by the immune system. Thus, impairment of the immune system is a major factor in the establishment of metastatic lesions. Cells may escape detection in several different ways:

- Aggressive cancer cells may compile a large mass (greater than 1 cm) so rapidly that the immune system is unable to overcome the tumor before it takes hold in a new tissue.

- For tumor cells to be recognized as foreign by the immune system, they must display on their surface a special antigen called *tumor-associated antigen* (TAA). TAA marks tumor cells for destruction by the lymphocytes. Some oncogenic viruses depress the expression of TAA on infected cells. Also, some tumors in advanced stages of growth no longer display TAA. Thus, such tumor cells escape detection as they travel through the blood or lymph.

- If the individual's immune response is weakened or altered, then a metastatic tumor may take hold with little opposition.

An estimated 50–60% of all cancers have already metastasized by the time the primary tumor is identified. Cancer accounts for nearly 1 in 4 deaths in the United States (ACS, 2016b), which certainly supports the need for patient education to facilitate early diagnosis. The time it takes for metastasis to occur is extremely variable and often difficult to predict. Some cancers, such as basal cell carcinomas, do not metastasize. The aggressiveness and location of the tumor and the state of the individual's immune system determine whether and how rapidly metastasis takes place.

Immune System Response

When the immune system discovers a neoplasm, it tries to destroy it using the resources of the body. The body mounts an all-out assault on the foreign invader, calling on many resources, including chemical mediators, hormones and enzymes, blood cells, antibodies, proteins, and inflammatory and immune responses.

These protective responses also mobilize the fluid, electrolyte, and nutritional systems. This massive effort requires tremendous energy. If the neoplasm is small enough (i.e., microscopic), the immune system can destroy it, and a tumor will never manifest. A neoplasm of 1 cm is large enough to overwhelm most immune systems; however, the body will continue trying to fight until it reaches the stage of exhaustion and is no longer capable (Selye, 1984). Thus, many patients with cancer present with fatigue, weight loss, anemia, dehydration, and electrolyte imbalances.

Etiology

Theories of **carcinogenesis** (the production or origin of cancer) include the involvement of cellular mutation, oncogenes, and tumor suppressor genes. Central to these theories are two important concepts about the etiology of cancer. First, damaged DNA, whether inherited or from external sources, sets up the necessary initial step for cancer to occur. Second, impairment of the human immune system, from whatever cause, lessens its ability to destroy abnormal cells.

Cellular Mutation

The theory of cellular mutation suggests that **carcinogens** (cancer-causing substances) cause mutations in cellular DNA. According to this theory, the carcinogenic process has three stages: (1) initiation, (2) promotion, and (3) progression. The initiation stage involves permanent damage in the cellular DNA as a result of exposure to a carcinogen (e.g., radiation, chemicals) that was not repaired or that had a defective repair. Promotion may last for years and includes conditions such as smoking or alcohol use that act repeatedly on the already affected cells. In the progression stage, further inherited changes acquired during cell replication develop into a cancer.

Oncogenes

Oncogenes are genes that promote cell proliferation and are capable of triggering cancerous characteristics. Oncogenes can be classified according to their overall function. Several oncogenes and their relationship to human cancers have been identified. For example, *BRCA1* and *BRCA2* are associated with breast cancer (NCI, 2015e).

A decrease in the body's immune surveillance may allow the expression of oncogenes; this can occur during times of stress or in response to certain carcinogens. For example, cytomegaloviruses (CMVs), which frequently occur in patients who are HIV positive, are associated with a higher incidence of Kaposi sarcoma (Osborn et al., 2013).

Tumor Suppressor Genes

Tumor suppressor genes normally slow cell division or repair errors in DNA replication. Thus, they tend to work against the growth of cancerous cells. Tumor suppressor genes can become inactive by deletion or mutation. Inherited cancers have been associated with inactivation of tumor suppressor genes. For example, abnormalities in *Tp53*, a suppressor gene, have been associated with over half of human cancers (ACS, 2014c).

Causative Agents

A number of agents are known to cause cancer or at least are strongly linked to certain kinds of cancers. These carcinogens may be external (e.g., chemicals, radiation, viruses) or internal (e.g., hormones, immune conditions, inherited mutations). Causal factors may act together or in sequence to initiate or promote carcinogenesis. Ten or more years often pass between exposures or mutations and detectable cancer.

Carcinogens can be categorized in two groups: genotoxic carcinogens, which directly alter DNA and cause mutations, and promoter substances, which cause other adverse biological effects, such as cytotoxicity, hormonal imbalances, altered immunity, or chronic tissue damage. Promoter substances do not cause cancer in the absence of previous cell damage (initiation), and they often require high-level and long-term contact with the altered cells.

Although everyone comes into contact with a vast number of substances that are considered carcinogenic, not everyone develops cancer. Other factors, such as genetic predisposition, impairment of the immune response, and repeated exposure to the carcinogen, are necessary for a cancer to develop.

Several viruses have been associated with the development of cancer. These viruses damage cells and induce hyperplastic cell growth. Viral infection may play a role in cell mutation that can progress to malignant cells. Normal aging and immune system dysfunction increase an individual's susceptibility to viral carcinogens (Osborn et al., 2013). **Box 2–1 »** identifies these viruses and the cancers with which they are associated.

In addition, viruses play a significant role in weakening immunologic defenses against neoplasms. For example,

Box 2–1
Cancers Associated with Viral Etiology

Herpes Simplex Virus Types 1 and 2 (HSV-1 and HSV-2)
- Carcinoma of the lip
- Cervical carcinoma
- Kaposi sarcoma

Human Cytomegalovirus (HCMV)
- Kaposi sarcoma
- Prostate cancer

Epstein-Barr Virus (EBV)
- Burkitt lymphoma

Human Herpesvirus 6 (HHV-6)
- Lymphoma

Hepatitis B Virus (HBV)
- Primary hepatocellular cancer

Papillomavirus
- Malignant melanoma
- Cervical, penile, and laryngeal cancers

Human T-lymphotropic Viruses (HTLV)
- Adult T-cell leukemia and lymphoma
- T-cell variant of hairy-cell leukemia
- Kaposi sarcoma

HIV, which infects helper T lymphocytes and monocytes, impairs an individual's protection against certain cancers, such as lymphoma and Kaposi sarcoma.

Risk Factors

Risk factors make an individual or a population vulnerable to a specific disease or other unhealthy outcome. Risk factors can be divided into those that are modifiable and those that are nonmodifiable. Knowledge and assessment of risk factors are especially important in counseling patients and families about measures to prevent cancer.

Heredity

It is estimated that 5–10% of cancers may have a hereditary component (ACS, 2014a). The familial pattern of some breast and colon cancers has been well documented. Lung, ovarian, and prostate cancers have also shown some familial relationships. For most cancers, however, research has yet to distinguish true genetic transfer from environmental causes. Although further research is needed to identify cancers that are caused by the inheritance of defective genes, familial predisposition to malignancies should be counted among risk factors. This allows people at risk to reduce behaviors that promote cancer. For example, a nurse should counsel a patient with a family history of lung cancer to avoid smoking, to avoid areas where smoking is allowed, and to avoid working in an occupation that may expose the patient to inhaled carcinogens.

Age

Cancer is a disease associated with aging; approximately 86% of cancer diagnoses occur after age 50 (ACS, 2016b). A number of factors are associated with this increased risk in older adults. One possible factor is that at least five cycles of genetic mutations seem necessary to cause permanent damage to the afflicted cells. In addition, long-term exposure to high doses of promotional agents is usually necessary to allow the cancer to take hold. Another factor may be the immune system's decline with aging (Osborn et al., 2013). Another problem is that free radicals (molecules resulting from the body's metabolic and oxidative processes) tend to accumulate in the cells over time, causing damage and mutation.

Hormonal changes that occur with aging can be associated with cancer. Postmenopausal women receiving exogenous estrogen have an increased risk for breast and uterine cancers. Older men are at risk for prostate cancer, possibly as a result of the breakdown of testosterone into carcinogenic forms.

Gender

Gender is a risk factor for certain types of cancer. Breast cancer is the most frequently diagnosed cancer in women; prostate cancer is the most frequently diagnosed cancer in men. The incidence of bladder cancer is approximately 3 times higher in men than in women, whereas thyroid cancer occurs more commonly among women (ACS, 2016b).

Poverty

Individuals living in poverty are at higher risk for cancer than the population in general. Inadequate access to healthcare, especially preventive screening and counseling, may be a major factor. Although other factors that may be involved, such as diet and stress, usually come under the category of modifiable risks, these risks are frequently nonmodifiable in this population.

Stress

Although some studies suggest a direct link between stress and cancer development, other studies are unable to establish such a link. Perhaps more easily supported is a link between cancer risks and unhealthy coping mechanisms that may emerge under stressful conditions. Unhealthy coping behaviors such as overeating, smoking, and alcohol abuse may lead to physical conditions that are associated with higher risks for developing cancer (NCI, 2012a).

Diet

Examination of human populations has not yet indicated that any specific dietary component causes or protects against cancer. The results indicate only that there is association between the dietary component and change in cancer risk (NCI, 2015f). Some foods are considered genotoxic, such as the nitrosamines found in preserved meats and pickled, salted foods. Other foods, such as high-fat, low-fiber foods—the mainstay of many American diets—promote colon, breast, and sex hormone–dependent tumors. When fish and meat are excessively fried or broiled, potent carcinogenic compounds can form that may cause tumors in the mammary glands, colon, liver, pancreas, and bladder. Also, repeatedly using fat to fry foods at high temperatures produces high levels of polycyclic hydrocarbons, which increase the risk for cancer considerably. Other food-related substances believed to increase cancer risk include sodium, saccharine, red food dyes, and both regular and decaffeinated coffee.

Occupation

Occupational risk might be considered either modifiable or nonmodifiable. For many people, both education and ability limit their choice of occupation; moreover, during times of high unemployment, changing occupations because the job poses risk factors may not be a viable option. Federal standards are designed to protect workers from hazardous substances, but many observers believe that these standards are not strict enough and that inspections are not frequent enough to prevent violations.

Specific risks vary according to the occupation. For example, individuals who work outdoors, such as farmers and construction workers, are exposed to solar radiation. Healthcare workers, such as x-ray technicians and biomedical researchers, are exposed to ionizing radiation and carcinogenic substances.

Infection

Because a number of viruses have been linked to some cancers, avoiding those specific infections will decrease risk. Some infections may be unavoidable, but others, such as genital herpes and papillomavirus-induced genital warts, can be avoided by following safer sex practices (e.g., the use of condoms).

Tobacco Use

Lung cancer is considered highly preventable because of its relationship to smoking. The genotoxic carcinogenic substances in tobacco are considered weak; therefore, stopping smoking can reverse the damage it causes. However, many other substances in tobacco are highly promotional, so the larger the dose and the longer the use, the higher the risk for developing cancer. Research has shown a significantly lower risk for death from lung cancer among former smokers compared to current smokers. For smokers who quit before 40 years of age, the risk of death due to conditions associated with continued smoking is reduced by approximately 90% (Jha et al., 2013).

Smokers also face an increased risk for oropharyngeal, esophageal, laryngeal, gastric, pancreatic, and bladder cancers. Pipe and cigar smokers are especially susceptible to oropharyngeal and laryngeal cancers. Oral and esophageal cancers are more common among those who chew tobacco or use snuff. Smokers who have a genetic decrease in α_1-antitrypsin (an enzyme that protects lung tissue) that results in emphysema face an even higher risk for cancer than smokers without this defect.

Secondhand tobacco smoke has also been identified as a cause of cancer. According to some researchers, among adults, secondhand smoke may increase the risk of developing breast, stomach, and bladder cancer as well as nasal sinus cavity and nasopharyngeal cancer. In children, secondhand smoke is believed to increase the risk of developing brain tumors, lymphoma, and leukemia (ACS, 2015a).

Alcohol Use

Alcohol promotes cancer by enhancing the contact between carcinogens, such as those in tobacco, and the stem cells that line the oral cavity, larynx, and esophagus (Porth & Grossman, 2013). People who both smoke and drink a considerable amount of alcohol daily have an increased risk for oral, esophageal, and laryngeal cancers.

Recreational Drug Use

Recreational drug use often promotes an unhealthy lifestyle that increases an individual's general risk for cancer; for example, habitual drug users often do not maintain adequate nutrition. Furthermore, recreational drugs are implicated as promoters because of their suppressive effect on the immune system. Research findings suggest that marijuana use is linked to the development of testicular cancer. Men who had testicular germ cell tumors were twice as likely to report having used marijuana than men without these types of tumors (Simon, 2012a). Although some studies suggest smoking marijuana may increase the risk for developing lung cancer, the results of these studies are often affected by the subjects' concurrent cigarette smoking. What is known is that marijuana smoke and tobacco smoke contain many of the same carcinogens, some of which are found in higher concentrations in marijuana smoke. A strong dose–response relationship has also appeared during these studies (Callaghan, Allebeck, & Sidorchuk, 2013; Volkow et al., 2014).

Obesity

Excessive body fat has been linked to an increased risk for hormone-dependent cancers. Because sex hormones are synthesized from fat, people who are obese often have excessive amounts of the hormones that feed hormone-dependent malignancies of the breast, bowel, ovary, endometrium, and prostate.

Sun Exposure

As the protective ozone layer thins, more of the sun's damaging ultraviolet (UV) radiation reaches the earth. As a consequence, the rate of skin cancers has increased. Sun-related skin cancers are now considered a problem for all people, regardless of skin color, but people of northern European extraction with very fair skin, blue or green eyes, and light-colored hair are most vulnerable. Older adults with decreased pigment, even those with darker skin, are also more at risk.

Prevention

Cancer prevention centers on making healthy lifestyle choices, such as avoiding smoking and limiting alcohol consumption, as well as eating a balanced diet. A healthy diet combined with regular exercise is an effective means of avoiding obesity, which is a risk factor for several types of cancer. Good physical health also allows for optimal immune function, reducing the risk of infection and thereby reducing the risk for developing certain types of cancer. Wearing sunscreen and avoiding prolonged sun exposure are simple but effective preventive steps for avoiding skin cancer. In the occupational setting, it is especially important to follow safety protocols, including those designed to prevent exposure to carcinogens.

Clinical Manifestations

Much of the nursing care for patients with cancer is related to the generalized effects of cancer on the body and to the side effects of the treatments used to remove or destroy the cancer. Although the pathophysiologic effects of a cancer vary with the type and location of the cancer, the effects detailed in this section are common among many types of cancer.

Disruption of Function

Physiologic functioning can be upset by obstruction or pressure. For example, a large tumor in the bowel can stop intestinal motility, resulting in a bowel obstruction. Prostatic tumors can obstruct the bladder neck or urethra, resulting in urine retention. Intracranial pressure can be dangerously increased by a glioma.

Obstruction or pressure can cause anoxia and necrosis of surrounding tissues, which in turn cause a loss of function of the involved organ or tissue. For example, a kidney tumor may progress to renal failure. Pressure against the superior vena cava from an adjacent lung tumor or tumor-infiltrated lymph nodes can interrupt the blood flow to the heart.

In the liver, either a primary hepatocellular cancer or a metastatic lesion can have several significant effects:

- In liver parenchymal tissue, it can impair the multiple life-sustaining functions of the liver, such as carbohydrate metabolism, synthesis of plasma proteins, detoxification, and immunologic functions. These functional impairments result in severe nutritional, hormonal, hematologic, and immunologic problems.
- Because more than 1 L of blood per minute passes through the liver via the portal vein, obstruction to this flow by a tumor can cause portal hypertension. This results in backup of fluid and increased pressure in the splanchnic circulation. The end result is ascites (third-spaced fluid in the peritoneal cavity) and varices (friable, overdistended blood vessels) of the esophageal, gastric, mesenteric, and hemorrhoidal vessels.

Hematologic Alterations

Hematologic alterations can impair the normal function of blood cells. For example, in leukemia, a malignant proliferative disease of the hematopoietic (blood cell–producing) system, the immature leukocytes cannot perform the normal protective phagocytic functions, and immunity is compromised. In addition, the excessive numbers of immature leukocytes in the bone marrow impair production of erythrocytes (RBCs) and thrombocytes (platelets), resulting in secondary anemia and clotting disorders (American Society of Hematology, 2016).

Other examples of hematologic alteration include the following:

- Gastrointestinal tumors disrupt the absorption of vitamin B_{12} and iron.
- Growing tumors need purines and folate and have a unique ability to accumulate and store these substances. Thus, the tumor deprives the bone marrow of these substances, which are needed for erythropoiesis (RBC production).
- Renal cell carcinoma produces its own erythropoietin hormone, which causes an excessively large number of RBCs to be produced and dumped into the bloodstream. The resulting polycythemia causes viscous blood, which impairs circulation, plugs small capillaries, and promotes thrombus formation.

Infection

If the tumor invades and connects two incompatible organs, such as the bowel and the bladder, and thus creates a fistula, infection becomes a serious problem. As they destroy viable tissue and thus their own source of nutrition, tumors may become necrotic; septicemia may result. Some tumors are less efficient in creating capillaries; as a consequence, the center of the tumor may become necrotic and infected. When a tumor grows near the surface of the body, it may erode through to the surface, thus breaking down the natural defenses of intact skin and mucous membranes and providing a site for the entry of microorganisms. Any malignant involvement of the organs or tissues of immunity—such as the liver, bone marrow, Peyer patches in the small intestine, spleen, or lymph nodes—can seriously impair the immune response, allowing infections to develop in vulnerable tissues.

Hemorrhage

Tumor erosion through blood vessels can cause extensive bleeding, giving rise to severe anemia. Hemorrhage can be serious enough to cause life-threatening hypovolemic shock.

Anorexia-Cachexia Syndrome

A characteristic feature of cancer is the wasting syndrome called **cachexia**, which includes malnutrition and unexplained loss of weight and muscle mass. In many cases, unexplained rapid weight loss in a short period of time is the first symptom that brings the patient to a healthcare provider. Weight loss can result from a variety of problems associated with cancer, such as pain, infection, depression, or the side effects of chemotherapy and radiation. However, the emaciation, malnutrition, and loss of energy are usually attributed to anorexia-cachexia syndrome. These patients can also have anthropometric measurements below 85% of standard for fat and muscle tissue, decreases in serum proteins, and negative responses to antigen testing.

Cancer cachexia is caused by the effect of cancer cells on the host's metabolism. The neoplastic cells divert nutrition to their own use while causing changes that reduce the patient's appetite. Early in the disease, glucose metabolism is altered, causing an increase in serum glucose levels. Through the process of negative feedback, anorexia (loss of appetite) results. In addition, the tumor secretes substances that decrease appetite by altering taste and smell and producing early satiety. Some types of cancers cause specific food aversions, such as to red meat, coffee, or chocolate.

A starvation state typically reduces the body's basal metabolic rate. However, in many people with cancer, the metabolic rate is increased, probably because of the hyperactive metabolic and reproductive activities of the malignant cells. Cancers of the gastrointestinal system further promote anorexia-cachexia by decreasing absorption and use of nutrients; the side effects of some treatment modalities enhance this effect. **Figure 2–4 》** shows the characteristic appearance of an individual with cachexia.

Paraneoplastic Syndromes

Paraneoplastic syndromes are rare disorders triggered by an altered immune system response. When a tumor develops,

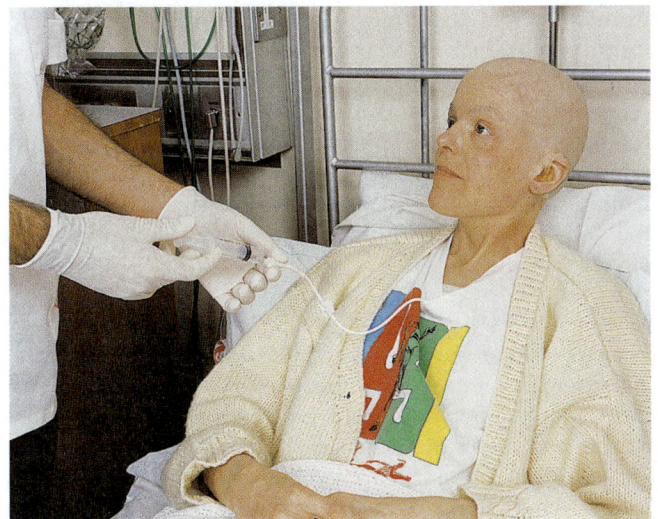

Source: Simon Fraser/RVI, Newcastle upon Tyne/Science Source.

Figure 2–4 ›› Individual with cachexia. Cancer robs its host of nutrients and increases body catabolism of fat and muscle to meet its metabolic needs.

this response may cause the body to produce antibodies to attack and destroy tumor cells. Paraneoplastic syndromes may also result from the production and release of physiologically active substances (e.g., hormones) by the tumor, known as tumor markers. The symptoms of these syndromes occur away from the site of the tumor itself and may be early warning signs of cancer, indicate complications, or suggest the return of a malignancy (Santacroce, 2015). For example, breast, ovarian, and renal cancers may set up ectopic parathyroid hormone sites, causing severe hypercalcemia. Paraneoplastic syndromes can affect practically any body system.

Pain

Pain is one of the most serious concerns of patients, families, and oncology healthcare professionals. Because pain management for people with cancer has a reputation as being ineffective, the anticipation of pain may engender fear in even the most stoic people. Most individuals fear pain and suffering even more than possible death. Although pain management strategies have improved tremendously, undertreatment and inadequate pain management are still significant issues for patients with cancer (Rozzi, Lanzetta, & Salerno, 2014).

Types of Cancer Pain

Cancer pain can be divided into two main categories, acute and chronic, with subgroupings. Acute pain has a well-defined pattern of onset, exhibits common signs and symptoms, and is often identified with hyperactivity of the autonomic system. Chronic pain, which lasts more than 6 months, frequently lacks the objective manifestations of acute pain, primarily because the autonomic nervous system adapts to this chronic stress. Chronic pain unfortunately often results in personality changes, alterations in functional abilities, and lifestyle disruptions that can seriously affect compliance with treatment and the quality of life.

Most patients with cancer who cite acute pain as the primary symptom that led to the diagnosis tend to associate pain with the introduction to their disease. If these patients experience pain during the illness or after therapy, they often perceive the pain as the introduction to another cancer or as a recurrence of the original cancer. Other patients report experiencing pain as a component of cancer therapy. These patients often are able to endure the pain in anticipation of a successful outcome of treatment.

Chronic pain may be related to treatment or may indicate progression of the disease. Determining whether the pain is treatment related or tumor related is extremely important. For the patient whose pain is caused by advancement of the disease, psychologic factors play an even more important role. Hopelessness and fear of impending death intensify physiologic pain and contribute to overall suffering.

Three other categories are used for patients with cancer pain: patients with preexisting pain, those with a history of drug abuse, and dying patients with cancer-related pain. The first two groups may have altered perceptions of pain and may not have the anticipated response to pain medication. For the dying patient, pain is strongly associated with both the patient's and family's confrontation of issues of hopelessness and death. Confronting these issues can intensify the perception of pain.

Causes of Cancer Pain

Direct tumor involvement is the primary cause of the pain experienced by people with cancer. This pain may result from metastatic bone disease, nerve compression, or involvement of visceral organs. The pain from tumor involvement is believed to be mechanical, resulting from stretching of tissues and compression. Chemicals from ischemia or tumor metabolites and toxins that activate and sensitize nociceptors and mechanoreceptors also cause tumor pain.

Side effects or toxic effects of cancer therapies (e.g., surgery, radiation, chemotherapy) may also cause cancer pain. These are usually the result of traumatized tissue; one example is the oropharyngeal ulcerations that occur with some types of chemotherapy. However, these therapies may also be used to manage pain, such as radiation to decrease pain associated with bone metastasis.

Psychologic Stress

People confronted with a cancer diagnosis exhibit a variety of psychologic and emotional responses. Some see cancer as a death sentence and experience overwhelming grief, often giving up. Others may feel guilt, considering the cancer a punishment for past behaviors, such as smoking, unhealthy eating habits, or delaying diagnosis or treatment. The patient may experience anger, especially if the individual believes that he or she had been practicing a healthful lifestyle; beneath that anger may reside feelings of powerlessness. Fear is common: fear of the outcome of the illness, fear of the effects of treatment, fear of pain, and fear of death. Some people feel isolated because of the stigma of cancer and old beliefs about contagion. Body image concerns and sexual dysfunction may be present but are often unexpressed, especially if the cancer is of the breast or sexual organs or causes visible body changes.

Oncologic Emergencies

Patients may experience oncologic emergencies resulting from the cancer itself or as a side effect of treatment. Oncologic emergencies can be organized into three groups: metabolic, hematologic, and those involving space-occupying lesions. Overall, the most common oncologic emergencies are tumor lysis syndrome, septic shock, brain herniation, spinal cord compression, and superior vena cava compression from a superior mediastinal mass.

Metabolic Emergencies

Metabolic emergencies result from the lysis (dissolving or decomposing) of tumor cells, a process called **tumor lysis syndrome (TLS)**. In TLS, cellular lysis leads to the release of intracellular contents into the circulation, causing hyperkalemia, hyperuricemia, and hyperphosphatemia. Consequences of this syndrome may include cardiac arrhythmias, renal failure, and death. Although usually associated with rapid cell lysis due to chemotherapy, TLS may also occur without any apparent cause. TLS is most often seen in cancers with high growth rates, acute leukemias, and high-grade non-Hodgkin lymphomas (Ikeda, 2016; Osborn et al., 2013).

A second type of metabolic emergency is septic shock. During periods of immune suppression, the patient is vulnerable to overwhelming infection. Systemic infection that progresses to septic shock may lead to circulatory failure and death. For these patients, prompt, aggressive treatment is critical to survival. (See the exemplar on Sepsis in the module on Infection for a full description of septicemia and septic shock.)

A third type of metabolic emergency involves the development of cancer-related hypercalcemia (elevated calcium in the serum). When cancer causes bone to break down, the calcium that is released into the circulation may lead to hypercalcemia. There are also other potential causes of hypercalcemia. For example, certain types of tumors release proteins that mimic parathyroid hormone, causing bones to release calcium. Treatment depends on the cause of the hypercalcemia and may include administration of medications such as bisphosphonates, which stop bone breakdown (American Society of Clinical Oncology [ASCO], 2015a).

Hematologic Emergencies

Hematologic emergencies result from bone marrow suppression or infiltration of brain and respiratory tissue with high numbers of leukemic blast cells (hyperleukocytosis). Bone marrow suppression results in anemia and *thrombocytopenia* (decreased platelets) with resultant coagulation disturbance. Idiopathic bleeding (bleeding with no known cause) may be a sign of thrombocytopenia. Examples of external idiopathic bleeding include bleeding from the nose that is not due to trauma and bleeding from the gums after brushing the teeth. Thrombocytopenia may also lead to bruising easily or bruising that is not related to injury. Disseminated intravascular coagulation (DIC), which occurs when the body's intricate clotting mechanisms are impaired, occurs in some cases. DIC may lead to rapid, profuse blood loss and is a life-threatening complication. Gastrointestinal and central nervous system bleeding (strokes) are common. Disruption of normal WBC production and resulting hyperleukocytosis can lead to obstruction of small blood vessels throughout the body.

Treatment of DIC may include infusion of packed RBCs for anemia, platelet transfusion, and administration of vitamin K and fresh frozen plasma for thrombocytopenia and hemorrhage. Management of hyperleukocytosis may include transfusion of platelets, hemodialysis, administration of hydroxyurea and urate oxidase, and leukapheresis if needed (Sung et al., 2012).

Space-Occupying Lesions

Extensive tumor growth may result in spinal cord compression, increased intracranial pressure, brain herniation, seizures, massive hepatomegaly, gastrointestinal obstruction, cardiac and respiratory complications, and superior vena cava syndrome (obstruction of the superior vena cava by tumor). After biopsy of the mass, treatment involves radiation therapy, antineoplastic agents (chemotherapy), and corticosteroids.

Collaboration

A team approach is essential to the care of patients diagnosed with cancer. For some forms of cancer, including breast and colorectal cancer, early diagnosis is associated with treatment that is both more successful and less extensive in nature (ACS, 2016b). Diagnosis, treatment, and aftercare of patients with cancer are complex processes that require all members of the healthcare team to combine knowledge with compassion throughout each phase of care.

Diagnostic Tests

Several procedures are used to diagnose cancer. X-ray imaging, CT, ultrasonography, and MRI can locate abnormal tissues or tumors. However, only microscopic histologic examination of the tissue reveals the type of cell and its structural difference from the parent tissue. Tissue samples are acquired through biopsy, shed cells (e.g., Pap smear), or collections of secretions (e.g., sputum). Lymph nodes are also biopsied to determine whether metastasis has begun. Simple screening procedures can be used to pick up substances secreted by the tumor, such as the prostate-specific antigen (PSA) blood test.

Increases in enzymes or hormones that are released by normal tissues when they are damaged can also contribute to the diagnosis. For example, increased alkaline phosphatase is noted in patients with bone metastases and osteosarcoma.

Some investigators studying chemical mediators of the immune system have noted that communication seems to occur between the chemical mediators and the emotional centers of the brain (Newman, 2016). Healthcare providers should listen carefully to patients who feel that they have cancer and should investigate thoroughly.

To help standardize diagnosis and treatment protocols, an elaborate identification system has been developed. This consists of naming the tumor (classification) and describing its aggressiveness (grading) and spread within or beyond the tissue of origin (staging).

Tumors are classified and named by the tissue or cell of origin. Tumor nomenclature often incorporates the Latin stem identifying the tissue from which the tumor arises. For

Clinical Manifestations and Therapies
Cancer

ETIOLOGY	CLINICAL MANIFESTATIONS	CLINICAL THERAPIES
Direct tumor involvement with the tissues often results in pain.	■ The patient experiences pain, often severe in nature and described as any type, depending on the tissue involved.	■ Pain management usually requires narcotic analgesics with escalating dosages as tolerance develops.
Anorexia-cachexia syndrome often results from rapid growth and reproduction of cancer cells and their need for increased nutrients.	■ The patient experiences muscle wasting, weight loss, and emaciated appearance, with resulting weakness and fatigue.	■ Offer nutritional counseling. ■ Increase caloric intake. ■ Reduce activity level. ■ Provide vitamin and mineral supplementation. ■ Dietary supplements, such as liquid formulas, may help provide extra calories between meals.
Risk for infection may increase as a result of bone marrow suppression secondary to both the tumor growth and treatments.	■ Manifestations include fever, malaise, and fatigue with minor infections ranging to septicemia with systemic infection.	■ Teach infection prevention techniques, including hand hygiene, cough etiquette, and crowd avoidance. ■ Antimicrobial medications are used to treat existing infections. ■ Monitor and maintain hydration.
Paraneoplastic syndrome often results from tumor growth that usually involves the endocrine system but may also involve the renal, integumentary, neurologic, or other systems.	■ Manifestations depend on the system involved. Increased hormone production from ectopic tumor sites will produce symptoms similar to those seen in hypersecretion of hormone.	■ Treatment includes surgery to remove the tumor. ■ Provide palliative treatment of symptoms until tumor reduction therapies diminish the impact of the tumor. ■ Offer supportive treatment.

example, a carcinoma arises from epithelial tissue; adjectives are added to further specify the location. A glandular malignancy arising from epithelial tissue is classified as an adenocarcinoma. A tumor arising from supportive tissues is called a sarcoma; the specific type of tissue is added as a prefix. For example, a cancer of fibrous connective tissue is called a fibrosarcoma, and a smooth muscle cancer is a leiomyosarcoma. A tumor from seminal or germ tissue is called a seminoma. **Table 2–3 》** compares the nomenclature of benign and malignant neoplasms.

Other names for tumors incorporate the name of the discoverer of that particular cancer, such as Burkitt lymphoma or Hodgkin disease. Hematopoietic malignancies (also known as liquid tumors) are usually named by the type of immature blood cell that dominates. For example, myelocytic leukemia is named for the immature form of the granulocyte that is predominant in this malignancy.

Grading and Staging

Grading evaluates the amount of differentiation (level of functional maturity) of the cell and estimates the rate of growth based on the mitotic rate. Cells that are the most differentiated—that is, cells that are most like the parent tissue and therefore the least malignant—are classified as grade 1 and are associated with a better prognosis. Grade 4 is reserved for the least differentiated and most aggressively malignant cells. Because of the differences inherent in tumor appearance and biological behavior, grading criteria may vary with different locations and types of tumors.

Staging is a system of classifying cancer according to the size of the tumor, involvement of lymph nodes, and the presence or absence of distant metastasis The TNM staging system is internationally recognized: The T stands for the relative tumor size, depth of invasion, and surface spread; N indicates the presence and extent of lymph node involvement; and M denotes the presence or absence of distant metastases. **Table 2–4 》** shows the basic outline of the TNM system; however, other systems are also used to differentiate types and locations of tumors (e.g., melanomas, cervical cancer, Hodgkin disease).

Cytologic Examination

For malignant tissues to be identified by name, grade, and stage, they must first be subjected to histologic and cytologic examination by light microscopy or electron microscopy. Specimens are collected by three basic methods:

1. **Exfoliation from an epithelial surface.** Examples include scraping cells from the cervix (Pap smear) or bronchial washings.
2. **Aspiration of fluid from body cavities or blood.** Examples include WBCs for evaluation of hematopoietic cancers, pleural fluid, and cerebrospinal fluid.
3. **Needle aspiration of solid tumors.** This could include the breast, lung, or prostate.

Cytologic examination is also carried out on specimens from biopsied tissues or tumors and on collected body secretions, such as sputum or urine.

TABLE 2–3 Nomenclature for Benign and Malignant Neoplasms

Tissue of Origin	Benign	Malignant
Ectoderm/Endoderm		
Epithelium	Papilloma	Carcinoma
Gland	Adenoma	Adenocarcinoma
Liver cells	Hepatocellular adenoma	Hepatocellular carcinoma
Neuroglia	Glioma	Glioma
Melanocytes	Melanoma	Malignant melanoma
Basal cells	Basal cell carcinoma	Basal cell carcinoma
Germ cells	Tetroma	Seminoma
Mesoderm: Connective Tissue		
Adipose tissue	Lipoma	Liposarcoma
Fibrous tissue	Fibroma	Fibrosarcoma
Bone tissue	Osteoma	Osteosarcoma
Cartilage	Chondroma	Chondrosarcoma
Mesoderm: Muscle		
Smooth muscle	Leiomyoma	Leiomyosarcoma
Striated muscle	Rhabdomyoma	Rhabdomyosarcoma
Mesoderm: Neural Tissue		
Nerve cells	Ganglioneuroma	Neuroblastoma
Mesoderm: Endothelial Tissues		
Blood vessels	Hemangioma	Angiosarcoma
		Kaposi sarcoma
Meninges	Meningioma	Malignant meningioma
Hematopoietic Tissues		
Granulocytes	Granulocytosis	Leukemia
Plasma cells		Multiple myeloma
Lymphocytes		Lymphomas

TABLE 2–4 The TNM Staging System

	Stage	Manifestations
Tumor	T0	No evidence of primary tumor
	Tis	Tumor in situ
	T1, T2, T3, T4	Ascending degrees of tumor size and involvement
Nodes	N0	No abnormal regional nodes
	N1a, N2a	Regional nodes—no metastasis
	N1b, N2b, N3b	Regional lymph nodes—metastasis suspected
	Nx	Regional nodes cannot be assessed clinically
Metastasis	M0	No evidence of distant metastasis
	M1, M2, M3	Ascending degrees of metastatic involvement of the host, including distant nodes

After collection, specimens are spread on a glass slide, fixed, and stained if necessary. The morphologic features of the cells are examined, with special attention to the nucleus and cytoplasm. Other special pathologic procedures can be carried out on the specimen, but they must be ordered ahead of time if special preparations of the specimen are necessary.

Tumor Markers

A **tumor marker** is a protein molecule detectable in serum or other body fluids. This marker is used as a biochemical indicator for the presence of a malignancy. Small amounts of tumor marker proteins are found in normal body tissues or benign tumors and are not specific for malignancy. However, high levels are suspicious and mandate follow-up diagnostic studies. Some of the cancers identified using tumor marker testing include breast, ovarian, colon, lung, and liver cancers (American Association for Clinical Chemistry, 2016).

TABLE 2–5 Selected Tumor-Derived Markers Associated with Specific Neoplasms

Type of Tumor Marker	Tumor Marker	Associated Neoplasm
Oncofetal antigens	CEA	Adenocarcinomas of the colon, lung, breast, ovary, stomach, and pancreas
	AFP	Primary liver cell cancer, ovarian cancer, gonadal germ cell tumors
Hormones	HCG	Gonadal germ cell tumors
	Calcitonin	Medullary cancer of the thyroid
	Catecholamines/metabolites	Pheochromocytoma
Enzymes	Lactate dehydrogenase	Leukemia, lymphoma, gonadal germ cell tumors, melanoma, neuroblastoma
Isoenzymes	PAP	Adenocarcinoma of prostate
	NSE	Small-cell lung carcinoma, neuroblastoma
Specific proteins	PSA	Adenocarcinoma of the prostate
	Immunoglobin	Multiple myeloma
	CA 125	Epithelial ovarian cancer
	CA 19-9	Adenocarcinoma of the pancreas or colon
	CA 15-3	Breast cancer
	CA 27-29	Breast cancer
	Bladder tumor antigen (BTA)	Bladder cancer
	Epidermal growth factor receptor (EGFR)	Non-small-cell, lung, head and neck, colon, pancreas, and breast cancers
	HER1	Breast cancer
	HER2	Breast cancer

Source: Based on American Cancer Society (ACS). (2014d). *Advanced cancer: Tests to find advanced cancer.* Retrieved from http://www.cancer.org/treatment/understandingyourdiagnosis/advancedcancer/advanced-cancer-diagnosis; American Society of Clinical Oncology (ASCO). (2013). *What to know: ASCO's guideline on tumor markers for testicular cancer and extragonadal germ cell tumors in teenage boys and men.* Retrieved from http://www.cancer.net/publications-and-resources/what-know-ascos-guidelines/what-know-ascos-guideline-tumor-markers-testicular-cancer-and-extragonadal-germ-cell-tumors-teenage; Medline Plus. (2014a). *Lactate dehydrogenase test.* Retrieved from http://www.nlm.nih.gov/medlineplus/ency/article/003471.htm.

Tumor marker tests are useful in guiding treatment decisions, monitoring the patient's response to therapy, detecting residual disease, and predicting the chance of recovery. However, this testing does have limitations. Not all cancers produce detectable tumor marker levels, and other testing is required for a definitive diagnosis to be made (ASCO, 2016a).

Tumor markers fall into two general categories: those derived from the tumor itself and those associated with host (immune) response to the tumor. Examples of tumor markers include the following:

- **Antigens.** These are present in fetal tissue but normally are suppressed after birth. Thus, their presence in large amounts may reflect an anaplastic process in tumor cells. Alpha-fetoprotein (AFP) and carcinoembryonic antigen (CEA) are oncofetal antigens.
- **Hormones.** Hormones are, of course, present in human blood and tissues in considerable amounts, but very high levels not related to other conditions may signify the presence of a hormone-secreting malignancy. Some common hormones seen as tumor markers include human chorionic gonadotropin (HCG), antidiuretic hormone, parathyroid hormone, calcitonin, and catecholamines.
- **Proteins.** These narrow down the type of tissue that may be malignant, although they can also be increased in hyperplastic disorders. Examples of tissue-specific proteins include serum immunoglobin and beta$_2$-microglobulin.

- **Enzymes.** Rapid, excessive growth of a tissue may cause some of the enzymes and isoenzymes normally present in that particular tissue to spill into the bloodstream. Elevated levels can point to either hyperplasia of the tissue or cancer. Prostatic acid phosphatase (PAP) and neuron-specific enolase (NSE) are examples. **Table 2–5** compares selected tumor-derived markers with their presence in neoplasms and other conditions.

Oncologic Imaging

Because physical assessment usually cannot detect cancer until the tumor has reached a size that poses a major risk for metastasis, radiologic examination is extremely important in early diagnosis. This diagnostic process may involve routine x-ray imaging (usually for screening only), CT, MRI, ultrasonography, nuclear imaging, angiography, and positron-emission tomography.

X-ray imaging is considered the least expensive and least invasive diagnostic procedure and is the method of choice for screening such body areas as the breast (mammography), lung, and bone to identify changes in tissue density that may indicate malignancies. X-ray studies are limited in that they do not easily distinguish among calcifications, benign cystic growths, and true malignancies. However, as a screening tool, x-ray imaging can usually reassure the patient if findings are negative or encourage follow-up studies if findings are suspicious. X-ray imaging is still the method of choice for lung cancer. However, it does not usually reveal tumors until they have reached about 1 cm in size, which is late in their development.

By applying computers and mathematics to diagnostic imaging, CT allows for visualization of cross sections of the anatomy. Because CT scans reveal subtle differences in tissue densities, they provide much greater accuracy in tumor diagnosis than traditional x-rays. CT is useful in screening for some cancers such as renal cell and most gastrointestinal tumors and in evaluating possible lymph node involvement.

Like CT, MRI involves computerized mathematical technology. The patient is placed within a strong magnetic field, pulsed radio waves are directed at the patient, and transmitted signals based on tissue characteristics are analyzed by a computer. Related diagnostic imaging procedures—positron-emission tomography and single-photon-emission computed tomography—create visible images by measuring electrical impulses from different body structures. Despite its expense, MRI is the diagnostic tool of choice for both screening and follow-up of cranial as well as head and neck tumors.

Ultrasonography is relatively safe and noninvasive. It measures sound waves as they bounce off various body structures, giving an image of normal anatomy as well as revealing abnormalities that indicate tumors. Ultrasonography has been adapted for diagnosing some specific tumors. For example, transrectal ultrasonography has provided excellent imaging of early prostate cancers and is used to guide needle biopsy. Ultrasound imaging is also more useful for detecting masses in the denser breast tissue of young women.

Nuclear imaging involves the use of a special scintillation scanner in conjunction with the ingestion or injection of specific radioactive isotopes. The principle underlying the technology is that certain isotopes have an affinity for specific tissues; for example, radioactive iodine (I-131) has an affinity for the thyroid gland. Malignancies in these tissues sequester an abnormally large amount of the isotope, which then can be traced and measured by the scintillation scanner. This procedure is considered safe, because the amount of isotope used is small enough not to damage normal cells.

For the patient with a newly diagnosed cancer, nuclear imaging is often used to check for possible bone or other organ metastases. This evaluation helps the healthcare provider determine appropriate treatment. Though invasive, the procedure is usually only minimally distressing for patients. Drinking the isotope solution is not pleasant but is tolerable; some anxious patients may have difficulty lying still during the scan. Antianxiety medication may help. Some patients may experience nausea from drinking the isotope and require antiemetic drugs to complete the procedure. Patient preparation may include complete restriction of fluids and food by mouth or allowing only clear fluids after midnight.

Angiography, an expensive and invasive procedure, is used infrequently for tumor diagnosis. Angiography is performed when the precise location of the tumor cannot be identified or the tumor's extent needs to be visualized before surgery. The procedure involves injecting a radiopaque dye into a major blood vessel proximal to the organ or tissue to be examined. The movement of the dye through the vasculature of the organ or tissue is then traced by means of x-ray, MRI, or CT scan. In some cases, small catheters are threaded through the vein under fluoroscopy to ensure the specific placement of the dye. Blockage to the flow of the dye indicates the tumor's location. Dye may also be used to identify blood vessels supplying a tumor, allowing the surgeon to know where to safely ligate vessels.

Angiography requires preparation similar to that for minor surgery. The nurse should inform the patient that injection of the dye used to enhance imaging may cause a hot, flushing sensation or nausea and vomiting. Although angiography is usually done on an outpatient basis, the patient will be kept in a short-stay unit for several hours and monitored for such complications as bleeding at the catheter insertion site.

Direct Visualization

Procedures for direct visualization are invasive but do not require the use of radiography. Examples include sigmoidoscopy (viewing the sigmoid colon with a fiberoptic flexible sigmoidoscope), cystoscopy (viewing the urethra and bladder), endoscopy (viewing the upper gastrointestinal tract), and bronchoscopy (inspecting the tracheobronchial tree).

These methods allow visual identification of the organs within the limits of the scope and usually permit biopsy of suspicious lesions or masses. Flexible fiberoptic scopes may be more useful, because they allow deeper penetration than traditional scopes. These procedures all require some patient preparation, cause moderate to considerable discomfort, and may require sedation or even anesthesia, as in the case of bronchoscopy. Some procedures, such as sigmoidoscopy and cystoscopy, may be performed in the physician's office rather than a hospital and therefore cost less, making these screening procedures more accessible.

Patient preparation includes a thorough bowel cleansing before the sigmoidoscopy and cystoscopy; the patient may ingest only liquids the morning of the procedure. Because anesthesia may be required, patients undergoing bronchoscopy and endoscopy may be instructed to have nothing by mouth from midnight until the procedure.

A more radical method of direct visualization for suspected malignancies is exploratory surgery with biopsy. In this method, the patient undergoes the usual preoperative preparation for the type of surgery anticipated. When the tumor is exposed, a sample of tissue (biopsy) is sent to the pathology laboratory for a "frozen-section" histologic examination. This can be done rapidly while the patient remains on the operating table under anesthesia. If the initial report is negative, the benign mass is usually removed to prevent further symptoms. If the report is positive for cancer, the tumor and often the adjacent lymph nodes are resected, along with any other suspicious tissue. The tumor, nodes, and any other specimens are sent to the pathology laboratory for more in-depth analysis. The patient then receives the usual postoperative care.

Laboratory Tests

Most laboratory tests of blood, urine, and other body fluids are used to rule out nutritional disorders and other noncancerous conditions that may be causing the patient's symptoms. When combined with other diagnostic tests, routine laboratory tests can also be used to form a differential diagnosis and, in certain forms of cancer, can also give clues about disease progression. These tests include evaluating levels of enzymes such as alanine aminotransferase, aspartate aminotransferase, and lactic dehydrogenase for liver metastases and protein tumor markers such as PSA for prostate cancer and CEA for colon cancer.

>> Go to **Pearson MyLab Nursing and eText** to see Chart 2, a table listing common laboratory tests, their normal values, and their possible indications.

Surgery

In many cases, the primary treatment is surgical removal of the cancerous lesion along with a portion of the normal surrounding tissue. The nature of the surgery depends on the location of the cancer and on whether or not the cancer has metastasized. Surgery may also be used for diagnostic confirmation (e.g., a biopsy) and to relieve secondary effects of the cancer, including pain and obstruction of other organs or impairment of physiologic processes.

Pharmacologic Therapy

Pharmacologic treatment of cancer, commonly referred to as **chemotherapy**, is the administration of chemicals that destroy cancer cells. Chemotherapeutic medications attack growing cells. Compared to normal cells, cancer cells usually replicate at a faster rate; as a result, cancerous cells are particularly susceptible to these medications. However, the attack on cancer cells is accompanied by unavoidable damage to normal, healthy cells. Chemotherapy medications may be administered via numerous routes, including oral, IV, subcutaneous, intramuscular (IM), topical, arterial, and intrathecal. Certain chemotherapeutic agents may be administered intraperitoneally (directly into the abdominal cavity) (ASCO, 2015b).

Total pharmacologic eradication of cancer cells is nearly impossible. Rather, the goal of chemotherapy is to kill the greatest possible number of cancer cells and then to allow the patient's immune system to complete the process (Osborn et al., 2013). In addition to being used as a primary treatment in certain cases, chemotherapy may be administered prior to surgery or radiation therapy to cause tumor shrinkage. Following surgery or radiation therapy, chemotherapeutic agents may be administered to help kill remaining cancer cells (ASCO, 2015b).

A simple method of classifying this complex group of drugs includes the following six categories:

1. Alkylating agents
2. Antitumor antibiotics
3. Antimetabolites
4. Hormones and hormone agonists
5. Biological response modifiers and targeted therapies
6. Natural products.

For an overview of select chemotherapeutic medications, including their mechanism of action and important nursing considerations for each drug category, see the Medications feature in the Concept of Cellular Regulation section.

SAFETY ALERT Workplace exposure to antineoplastic agents is believed to be linked to the development of cancer, as well as potentially causing adverse reproductive effects, including infertility, spontaneous abortion, and birth defects. Pharmacists who prepare chemotherapy agents and the nurses who administer the drugs are included among the individuals at greatest risk for exposure to antineoplastic agents (CDC, 2015b). Adherence to safety regulations regarding the preparation and handling of antineoplastic agents remains voluntary; however, nurses and other individuals who are exposed to antineoplastic agents are urged to follow all established safety guidelines and standards (CDC, 2016a).

Radiation Therapy

More than half of all patients diagnosed with cancer will be treated with radiation therapy (Osborn et al., 2013). Rather than being systemic in nature, like many forms of chemotherapy, radiation therapy is a localized treatment intended to affect only one body region. Goals of therapy include tumor shrinkage prior to surgery, prevention of postoperative tumor recurrence, and eradication of cancer cells in other parts of the body (ASCO, 2015b). Radiation therapy may also be used for **palliation**, which aims not to cure the disease but to relieve disease-related symptoms and enhance the patient's quality of life (Osborn et al., 2013).

The most common type of radiation therapy is external-beam radiation therapy, during which radiation is administered from a source outside the body. In addition to using x-rays, external-beam radiation therapy may incorporate the use of high-energy protons, which can kill cancer cells. Internal radiation therapy delivered by way of implants is called brachytherapy (ASCO, 2015b).

Lifespan Considerations

A diagnosis of cancer can be devastating to children and their family members or to women who are pregnant. These patients face specific challenges related to psychosocial needs and treatment considerations. Older adults are more likely to get cancer, and the presence of chronic conditions can affect the cancer and treatment choices.

Children and Adolescents with Cancer

Nurses caring for the child or adolescent with cancer provide care for the entire family. This care ranges from assessing the child's physiologic and psychologic status at the bedside or during an office visit to assessing the parent's need for respite care or additional resources and the sibling's need for a more predictable schedule. In particular, nurses need to be knowledgeable about the patient's and family's psychosocial needs and issues related to survival and treatment of children with cancer (see **Figure 2–5 >>**).

Psychosocial Needs

The diagnosis of cancer is overwhelming for families. While attempting to cope with the diagnosis, parents must simultaneously gather resources to support the child, make treatment decisions, and adjust family life to integrate the needs of the child with cancer. Some families need to travel a great distance for the child's treatments, and others may have financial constraints that make healthcare costs a major concern. Parental

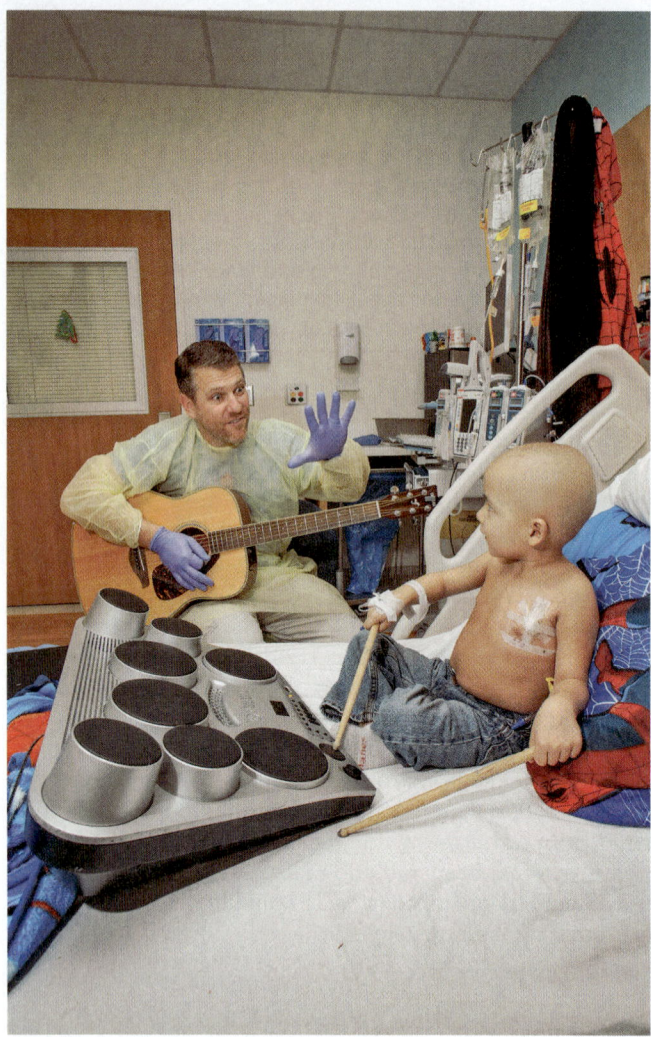

Source: Spencer Grant/Alamy Stock Photo.

Figure 2–5 ⟫ A music therapist with a guitar and portable drum kit engages a young child with cancer at a children's hospital.

work schedules and arrangements for other children will have to be adjusted. Both parents should be included in plans of care; extended family members may also be important sources of help. Most cancer treatments last for a minimum of several months and may last several years, necessitating nearly constant adaptation by the child and family.

A child's developmental stage significantly affects the child's reaction to the illness:

- Infants and toddlers are unaware of the severity of the disease but deal with issues such as pain and separation from parents.
- Preschoolers are beginning to understand illness. However, they may think they caused their illness and may be confused about why the parent cannot make the illness go away.
- School-age children can understand a diagnosis of cancer and benefit from opportunities to talk about the experience.
- Adolescents find contact with others who have gone through their experience reassuring and supportive.

Nearly all children with cancer are hospitalized after diagnosis. Care should include being in proximity to parents, involvement in self-care appropriate for age, positive relationships with staff, and emotional care (Hockenberry & Wilson, 2014). Programs such as group therapy sessions, computer programs about cancer and treatment, and school reintegration can assist children and adolescents who are adjusting to cancer (see Figure 2–5).

Treatment of Cancer in Children

Although children under the age of 18 are not legally entitled to make their own decisions regarding treatment,

Patient Teaching
Parents of Children with Cancer

The diagnosis and treatment of a child with cancer causes great anxiety for the parents. Patient teaching can help alleviate some of the anxiety parents experience by providing information about key aspects of treatment. Depending on the stage and type of treatment, the following suggestions may be helpful for parents:

- Children being treated with radiation and chemotherapy experience fatigue. Parents should provide extra rest periods with shorter activity periods between them.
- Children should have an overnight bag ready in case they develop a complication and need to stay in the hospital for a few days. Several hospital stays of a few days are normal during treatment.
- When parents are concerned about a symptom in their child, they should ask the healthcare provider. Parents are often key in identifying problems early.
- Because poor appetite can interfere with nutrition intake, children with cancer need to eat when they express hunger.
- The loss of the child's hair during treatment can be devastating for many parents. The nurse should ask parents how they plan to cope. They need to be prepared for the fact that hair loss can be rapid or slow. The nurse can offer resources for wigs, hats, or other ideas. Children with hair loss need to cover the head, wear sunscreen when outside, and avoid the sun as much as possible to minimize chance of burn to the head, which is prone to burning because of its usual lack of sun exposure.
- Parents should remember that the child is still at the normal developmental age. They should treat the child as a reflection of his or her age, not as if the child is older or younger.
- Parents should try to maintain contact with the child's peer group and extended family members.
- Parents should seek information from other parents and resources on cancer care.
- Siblings of a child with cancer need attention too. They may feel scared about what is happening; worried that this will happen to them too; mad that this is happening to their family; guilty about being healthy; jealous of the attention received by the other sibling; or alone, neglected, ignored, and left out. Their behavior may change, and their school progress may be slowed.
- Parents need time for relaxation so that their own energy remains sufficient to deal with the child's therapy and the strains on the family.

they should be allowed to take part in decision-making processes whenever possible and appropriate and to actively participate in their plan of care (NCI, 2015g). This provides them with a sense of control and promotes effective coping.

Treatment for cancer in children may have long-lasting effects. According to the ACS, radiation can impair the growth of bones and teeth, leading to conditions such as leg length discrepancy, osteoporosis, or poor dental health. Chronic pain can result from skeletal toxicity. Hypothyroidism can be observed in those who have had head and neck radiation. Cardiotoxicity and pulmonary toxicity can result from mediastinal radiation, and delayed puberty and sterility can result from radiation effects to the cranium and spinal regions. Impaired neurocognitive performance may occur with long-term effects of treatment, especially with higher doses of radiation (ACS, 2014e). Some studies have found lower behavioral and social competence in treated children and higher rates of posttraumatic stress disorder (Hockenberry & Wilson, 2014).

Cardiomyopathy can occur with some chemotherapy drugs, especially the anthracyclines. Temporary or permanent pulmonary toxicity and renal complications can develop. Certain chemotherapy drugs and antibiotics, as well as radiation to the ear or brain, can lead to hearing loss. Radiation to the eye and certain chemotherapy medications can cause cataracts and other eye problems. Learning disabilities and change in IQ occur in some children. Infertility may also result (ACS, 2014e).

Cancer treatment during childhood may predispose the patient to developing secondary cancers, also called secondary malignant neoplasms (SMNs), of a different histologic type from the original or primary cancer. For example, survivors of childhood cancer tend to have a higher risk for developing cancer in areas that were previously treated with radiation. Although radiation is responsible for most secondary tumors, some chemotherapy drugs have also been implicated. Survivors of childhood cancer are also at higher risk for developing cancers commonly seen in adults, such as colon, breast, or prostate cancer (ACS, 2014e).

Research suggests that survivors of childhood cancer may demonstrate higher rates of depression and recurrent suicidal ideation (Brinkman et al., 2014). On the other hand, hopefulness and the sense of having an added purpose in life can be positive outcomes for many cancer survivors. The highest risk for long-term emotional and psychologic distress in adult survivors of childhood cancer occurs in those with poor health status, low income, low education, and unemployment (Oancea et al., 2014).

Pregnant Women with Cancer

Approximately 1 out of 1000 pregnant women will be diagnosed with cancer. While some cancers are capable of spreading to the placenta, most are unable to spread to the fetus. Nevertheless, recognition and treatment of cancer remains a critical concern for both mother and baby (ASCO, 2015c).

Because cancer-related symptoms may be similar to those that normally accompany pregnancy, delayed diagnosis may be an issue. For example, frequent headaches and abdominal bloating, which are commonly associated with pregnancy, may be overlooked or accepted as being normal pregnancy-related manifestations. However, the converse is also true: Pregnancy can lead to detection of cancerous conditions that otherwise may not have been recognized. For example, a prenatal ultrasound may reveal ovarian cancer (ASCO, 2015c).

When a pregnancy is involved, the approach to treating cancer becomes even more complex. Although surgery is considered to be the safest treatment option for pregnant women with cancer, certain types of chemotherapy may be administered during the second and third trimester. Treatment with radiation generally is avoided because of the potential for harm to the fetus (ASCO, 2015c). Nursing considerations include acknowledging the immense physical and psychosocial stress these patients face, as well as being aware of the latest treatment approaches for the specific form of cancer involved.

>> **Stay Current:** To learn more about the management of breast cancer in pregnant women, visit the NCI's website at http://www.cancer.gov/types/breast/hp/pregnancy-breast-treatment-pdq. For an overview of the treatment of other forms of cancer in pregnant women, visit the National Institutes of Health website at https://medlineplus.gov/tumorsandpregnancy.html.

Older Adults with Cancer

Approximately 60% of cancers occur in adults age 65 and older, with the cancer mortality rate averaging 70%. The number of older adults is expected to double by the year 2030, which will give rise to a 67% increase in cancer diagnoses in this age group. Members of this age group unfortunately have not been allowed access to clinical research trials regarding treatment, so much about their behavioral responses to cancer treatment remains unknown (ASCO, 2016b; Dennis, 2015). The ASCO has recommended including this patient population in current clinical trials to ensure the development of evidence-based practice to guarantee that patients of all ages are receiving high-quality, evidence-based cancer care (Dennis, 2015). Older adults do not respond to cancer treatment in the same way younger adults respond because of their age-associated physiologic changes, higher incidence of comorbidities, and use of associated medications. Older adults' functional age correlates more accurately with their overall health status than does their chronologic age, which is another consideration when treatment options are being explored (Hurria et al., 2015).

Recent studies have examined cancer screening for older adults. These studies examined the risks and benefits of cancer screening for this population and recommended that screenings for specific cancers, such as colorectal and breast, target older adults who have a life expectancy greater than 10 years. The risk-to-benefit ratio in screening for these cancers was greater for older adults with a life expectancy of less than 5 years. Screenings in this age group should be performed on an individualized basis to enhance informed decision making regarding care (Nelson, 2014).

Older adults experience many of the same symptoms caused by cancer as younger adults. However, the presence of chronic conditions in the older adult, such as heart, lung, or kidney disease or diabetes, can affect cancer treatment.

Risks involved with chronic health conditions and cancer treatments can include the following:

- Reactions between medications for cancer treatment and other medications
- Interruption of or change in cancer treatment due to the chronic health condition
- Delayed recovery from cancer treatment.

Cancer treatment may worsen chronic health conditions. Therefore, older adults should continue to visit their regular healthcare provider for management of any comorbidities (ASCO, 2016b).

NURSING PROCESS

Nursing care is vitally important to the recovery of patients with cancer. Patients, family members, and loved ones are often very frightened by the diagnosis and require emotional as well as physical support. Patients may become very sick during treatment as a result of side effects or complications or if the neoplasm does not respond to treatment. Nursing care focuses on teaching patients about self-care to avoid complications and minimize side effects of treatment as well as on providing emotional, spiritual, and psychologic support.

Assessment

Assessment of the patient who is suspected of having cancer begins with a focused assessment of the organ system involved, then broadens to include a full assessment to determine sites of possible metastasis. For example, the patient who presents with a lump in the breast will have a focused assessment looking for changes in the breast that may indicate the cause of the lump. Then, if the patient is diagnosed with cancer, a more thorough assessment will be required that looks for any abnormality that could indicate metastasis, side effects of treatment, or complications of therapy.

- ***Observation and patient interview.*** Observation provides information related to the overall state of the patient and should begin at the time of initial contact and continue throughout the assessment process. Observation of the patient during the initial interview and at subsequent assessments should include level of consciousness; facial expressions, affect, mood, and manner; state of health; signs of discomfort; and nutritional status.

    The patient interview generally progresses from exploration of the patient's current complaint to a broader health history and physical status. In addition, for patients who are diagnosed with cancer, the nurse should discuss functional limitations, psychosocial considerations, and the patient's understanding of the treatment plan. The following are appropriate questions to ask the patient during the initial interview and at subsequent assessments:

    a. *"What brought you in today?"* Asking open-ended, introductory questions may elicit more information than asking specific questions. For patients who offer insufficient information in response to this open-ended question, more specific questions may be necessary, such as "Did you have pain or any specific physical problems that caused you to seek healthcare?"

    b. *"Do you have any history of other medical conditions or health problems? If so, can you tell me about them?"* Thorough knowledge of the patient's health history is essential to the patient's overall care and can also help the nurse anticipate problems and formulate potential nursing diagnoses related to other diseases that may interact with the cancer.

    c. *"What kinds of physical problems are you having? Do you have pain? Are you nauseated? Have you lost weight? Are you having difficulty carrying out your daily activities? Are you feeling sad or discouraged because of your illness?"* For each positive response, the nurse should ask follow-up questions to narrow down or define the exact nature of the problem.

    d. *"What options has your physician suggested for treating your cancer?"* The answer will indicate the patient's knowledge about the treatment and, possibly, the patient's communication with the physician. Often, under the stress of a cancer diagnosis, patients do not hear or understand what the physician is saying and are afraid to ask questions. Lack of knowledge indicates a need to collaborate with the physician to explain the information to the patient so that the patient can absorb and understand it.

    e. *"What do you expect to happen as a result of this treatment?"* The patient's answer may be used to gauge his or her expectations, as well as to determine education needs regarding the goals and effects of the treatment.

    f. *"What effect is the disease and/or treatment having on your ability to carry on with your usual daily activities?"* The response to this question should provide information regarding the patient's functional status. Additional questions may be needed to pinpoint the types of limitations.

    g. *"Who is available to help you at home and run errands for you? Who can provide transportation for you to get to your appointments or treatments? Who can you rely on to be a good listener when you're sad or need companionship? Is there someone you would like to make healthcare decisions for you if there is a time when you are unable to make them for yourself?"* This information can identify how much support and help the patient has or needs. The last question introduces the concept of advance directives and durable power of attorney regarding healthcare (see the module on Legal Issues).

    h. *"How do you manage your stress or your feelings of discomfort? What helps you feel better? Do you think these measures work well for you?"* The responses to these questions provide information about the patient's coping strategies and may identify maladaptive strategies, such as alcohol or drug use. Lack of appropriate coping methods can interfere with the patient's response to treatment and decrease overall quality of life.

Other assessment questions may be useful at different stages of the patient's illness. For example, if the patient is not expected to survive the cancer, the nurse should ask whether the patient has made decisions about last wishes (e.g., for a funeral and burial), whether these wishes have been discussed with significant others, and whether the patient has made out a will.

■ ***Physical examination.*** As soon as the patient is admitted to the healthcare service or agency, the nurse should conduct a complete physical assessment to establish a baseline against which to evaluate changes. The nurse should document the nutritional status of the patient using anthropomorphic measurements (i.e., frame size, height, weight, body fat, and muscle mass), evaluate laboratory results, and note any specific signs and symptoms. For discussion of assessment of nutritional status, refer to the module on Nutrition.

The nurse should assess the patient's hydration status, especially if the patient is not taking oral food and fluids well or is having bouts of vomiting. (See the module on Fluids and Electrolytes for information on assessment of fluid status.)

When screening for cancer, nurses should keep in mind the ACS's guidelines for early detection (see **Box 2–2** ≫). Cancer-related screening should include assessment for cancers of the thyroid, testicles, ovaries, lymph nodes, oral region, and skin.

Diagnosis

Relevant nursing diagnoses vary depending on the individual patient, as well as the patient's stage of care. Examples of nursing diagnoses that may be appropriate for inclusion in the plan of care for the patient with cancer include the following:

■ *Infection, Risk for*
■ *Injury, Risk for*
■ *Imbalanced Nutrition: Less Than Body Requirements*
■ *Tissue Integrity, Impaired*
■ *Pain, Acute*

■ *Anxiety*
■ *Body Image, Disturbed*
■ *Grieving, Risk for Complicated.*

(NANDA-I © 2014)

Planning

Nursing goals focus on supporting the whole individual and managing specific problems, such as pain, poor nutrition, dehydration, fatigue, adverse emotional responses, altered individual and family coping, and the side effects of medical treatment. Nursing goals may include the following:

■ The patient will demonstrate no signs or symptoms of infection.
■ The patient will sustain no injuries.
■ Using a predetermined pain rating scale of 0–10 in which 10 represents "the worst possible pain," the patient will consistently rate pain at a level of 3 or less.
■ The patient will maintain weight within the normal range based on height and body type.
■ The patient will remain hydrated, as evidenced by assessment of skin turgor and mucous membranes.
■ The patient and family will vocalize feelings related to the cancer diagnosis and seek support from others to improve coping.
■ The patient will relate potential side effects of chosen therapies and list strategies for minimizing or coping with symptoms.

Box 2–2
Selected Cancer Screening Guidelines for Asymptomatic Individuals of Average Risk

Colorectal Cancer (Men and Women)
■ Fecal occult blood test (FOBT) or immunochemical FOBT annually beginning at age 50 *or*
■ Stool DNA test every 3 years *or*
■ As alternatives to fecal testing, beginning at age 50, either a flexible sigmoidoscopy every 5 years, *or* double contrast barium enema every 5 years *or*
■ Colonoscopy every 10 years, *or* CT colonography every 5 years.

Breast Cancer (Women)
■ There are no clear benefits currently indicated by physical breast examinations performed by either the patients themselves or by a healthcare professional. Education should emphasize benefits and limitations of breast self-examination, as well as the importance of immediately reporting any changes or symptoms to a healthcare provider.
■ Choice of mammogram annually beginning at age 40.
■ Mammogram annually beginning at age 45.
■ Mammogram annually or biannually at age 55 and older (good overall health; life expectancy 10 years or more).

Cervical and Uterine Cancer (Women)
■ Pap test and HPV test every 3 years for women ages 21–29.
■ For women ages 30–65, screening with both HPV testing and Pap test (preferred) every 3–5 years *or* every 3 years with Pap test alone (acceptable).
■ Screening may be discontinued in women ages 66 or older who demonstrate three or more consecutive negative Pap tests and no positive Pap test in the last 10 years.
■ Cervical cancer screening may be discontinued following total hysterectomy.

Prostate Cancer (Men)
■ Men ages 50 years or older who have at least a 10-year life expectancy should be educated as to the benefits and limitations of PSA testing and digital rectal examination. Screening should be completed only in conjunction with an informed decision-making process.

Sources: Based on American Cancer Society (ACS). (2015c). *American Cancer Society recommendations for early breast cancer detection in women without breast symptoms: Clinical breast exam and breast self-exam.* Retrieved from http://www.cancer.org/cancer/breastcancer/moreinformation/breastcancerearlydetection/breast-cancer-early-detection-acs-recs; American Cancer Society (ACS). (2016b). *Cancer facts and figures 2016.* Retrieved from http://www.cancer.org/acs/groups/content/@research/documents/acspc-047079.pdf; National Cancer Institute (NCI). (2016e). *PDQ cancer information summaries: Screening/detection (testing for cancer).* Retrieved from http://www.cancer.gov/publications/pdq/information-summaries/screening; University of Texas MD Anderson Cancer Center. (2016a). *Cancer screening guidelines.* Retrieved from https://www.mdanderson.org/prevention-screening/get-screened.html.

Implementation

Nursing interventions are evidence-based strategies geared toward helping the patient meet the measurable goals associated with each nursing diagnosis. As with all elements of the care plan, the selection and implementation of nursing interventions must be tailored to reflect the individual patient's needs. For the patient diagnosed with cancer, nursing interventions also vary significantly depending on the type and location of the cancer cells.

In addition to physical care, patients diagnosed with cancer have critical comfort-related and psychosocial needs that must be addressed to promote recovery. While management of life-threatening physiologic conditions always takes priority over pain management, treatment of pain remains a priority concern in the stable patient. Analgesics should be administered as ordered; collaboration with the prescribing provider may be needed to achieve a pain management regimen that affords the patient consistently acceptable pain relief. (For a detailed discussion of the nurse's role in pain management, see the module on Comfort.)

Prevent Infection

The patient with cancer faces multiple risks for infection as a result of malnutrition, tumor necrosis, suppression of WBCs from chemotherapy or radiation, and anorexia resulting from nausea and other treatment side effects. The patient may exhibit the classic signs of infection: lethargy, fever, anorexia, pain in the affected area, and physical evidence of infection, such as a purulent, draining lesion or wound. Bone marrow depression resulting from certain types of cancer and chemotherapy undermines the body's ability to respond to infection. If the bone marrow is compromised, the usual signs and symptoms of infection may be absent or reduced.

- Protect skin and mucous membranes from injury. Explain that the patient may experience scaling, flaking, dryness, itching, rash, or dry desquamation of the skin, particularly after radiation therapy. Teach appropriate skin care measures, such as good hygiene, use of a moisturizing lotion to prevent dryness and cracking, frequent changes of position for individuals who are bedbound, and immediate attention to skin breaks or lesions. Ensuring intact skin strengthens the first line of defense against infection.

- Encourage the patient to consume a diet high in protein, minerals, and vitamins, especially vitamin C. Improving nutrition decreases the risk of infection. Vitamin C has been shown to help prevent certain types of infection, such as colds.

- Teach the patient to avoid crowds, small children, and people with infections when the patient's WBC count is at nadir (lowest point during chemotherapy) and to practice scrupulous personal hygiene. During periods of leukopenia, patients may lose immunity to their own natural flora. Careful attention to hygiene reduces the risk of infection. Small children should be avoided because they often have microbes to which most people are usually immune but that the patient may not be able to resist.

- Monitor vital signs. Fever and sympathetic nervous system responses, such as increased pulse and respiration, are the usual early signs of infection. However, patients with severe immunosuppression may be unable to mount a fever; therefore, the absence of fever cannot rule out infection.

- Monitor WBC counts frequently, especially if the patient is receiving chemotherapy that is known to cause bone marrow suppression. Notify the physician at the first sign of diminishing WBC counts so that corrective action can be taken.

- Avoid invasive procedures when possible, including injections, IV catheters, catheterizations, and rectal and vaginal procedures. When necessary, use strict aseptic technique for all invasive procedures and monitor carefully for infection.

Prevent Injury

In addition to infection, cancer can pose a risk for injury from, for example, obstruction by a large tumor or one located in a limited body space (e.g., in the brain, bowel, or bronchial airways). If the cancer is one that creates ectopic sites of hormones, elevated levels of hormones that are not under the control of the pituitary gland can injure the patient in a variety of ways. Signs of obstruction depend on the organ involved: Bowel obstruction presents with pain, distention, and cessation of bowel activities; obstruction in the brain gives signs of increased intracranial pressure or personality/behavioral change; bronchial obstruction manifests as respiratory distress, cyanosis, and altered arterial blood gases. Ectopic production of parathyroid hormone manifests as high serum calcium levels as well as signs of hypercalcemia; ectopic production of antidiuretic hormone causes fluid retention and manifests as hypertension and peripheral and pulmonary edema.

- Teach the patient to differentiate minor problems from those of a serious nature. Encourage the patient to consult with the nurse or physician if in doubt or to call 9-1-1 if he or she becomes very ill. The Patient Teaching feature provides guidelines to help patients identify serious problems. Having guidelines for when to call the physician provides an anxiety-reducing safety net for the patient and family and promotes early detection of complications.

- Assess frequently for signs and symptoms indicating problems with organ obstruction. Early detection of major problems allows the nurse to seek medical help before the problem evolves into a physiologic crisis.

- Monitor laboratory values that may indicate the presence of ectopic functioning, and report abnormal findings to the physician immediately. **Table 2–6 》** provides laboratory indicators of ectopic functioning. Refer to the respective modules for specific signs and symptoms of alterations in acid–base, electrolytes, and endocrine function. Early detection promotes early medical intervention and prevents serious consequences from the ectopic secretion.

Manage Pain Effectively

The patient with cancer may experience pain related to preparatory procedures, diagnostic examinations, and surgery. Also, the primary tumor itself and, potentially, metastatic tumors may impinge on nerves and other organs, causing pain. In the patient with terminal cancer, chronic and acute pain must be managed effectively to allow a peaceful death.

Patient Teaching

When Patients with Cancer Should Call for Help

Instruct the patient or family member to call the nurse or physician if any of the following signs or symptoms occur:

- Oral temperature greater than 38.6°C (101.5°F)
- Severe headache
- Significant increase in pain at the usual site, especially if the pain is not relieved by the medication regimen, or severe pain at a new site
- Difficulty breathing
- New bleeding from any site, such as rectal or vaginal bleeding
- Confusion, irritability, or restlessness
- Withdrawal, greatly decreased activity level, or frequent crying
- Verbalizations of deep sadness or a desire to end life
- Changes in body functioning, such as the inability to void or severe diarrhea or constipation
- Changes in eating patterns, such as refusal to eat, extreme hunger, or a significant increase in nausea and vomiting
- Appearance of edema in the extremities or significant increase in edema already present.

Instruct the patient or family member to call 9-1-1 if the patient:

- Is having much difficulty breathing or if the lips or face has a bluish tinge
- Becomes unconscious or has a convulsion
- Exhibits unmanageable behavior, such as being physically abusive, hurting self, or engaging in uncontrollable activity.

A cardinal rule of successful pain management is the importance of reducing or eliminating the cause of pain. Appropriate interventions are based on a careful assessment of the patient's pain. The nurse can assist the patient in managing pain effectively by doing the following:

- Assess the intensity, location, and quality of the pain. Be alert for nonverbal signs, such as grimacing, muscle tension, apparent dozing, changes in pulse or blood pressure, and rapid, shallow respirations. The patient may assume that pain is to be expected or tolerated or may fear becoming addicted to analgesic medications.

TABLE 2–6 Laboratory Indicators of Ectopic Functioning

Hormone	Specific Laboratory Test
Antidiuretic hormone	Serum and urine osmolality
Adrenocorticotropic hormone (ACTH)	Plasma ACTH, ACTH suppression test, ACTH stimulation test, urine catecholamines
Calcitonin	Serum calcitonin
Insulin	Serum glucose, glucose tolerance test
Parathyroid hormone	Serum parathyroid hormone, serum calcium
Thyroxine (T_4)	Serum thyroid-stimulating hormone, triiodothyronine, T_4

- Provide analgesics as needed. Postoperative recovery and restoration of function is facilitated by adequate pain management.
- Monitor analgesic effectiveness 30 minutes after administration. Monitor for pain relief and adverse effects. The method of delivery, dosage, or medication itself may need to be adjusted to provide adequate pain relief.
- In the early postoperative period, an epidural infusion or patient-controlled analgesia often is used to manage pain. Patient-controlled analgesia, routine administration of ordered analgesics, or a continuous analgesia delivery system may be used for pain management when the tumor is far enough advanced to preclude surgical resection.
- For cancer pain, maintain an around-the-clock medication schedule using narcotics, nonsteroidal anti-inflammatory drugs, and other medications as ordered. In the patient with terminal cancer, addiction is not a concern. Providing adequate pain relief that does not allow "breakthrough" pain is important.
- Teach the patient and family noninvasive methods of pain control. Various modalities can be successful in alleviating pain or reducing its perception, thus enhancing the comfort of the patient. For example, some research suggests massage therapy and touch therapy may be useful in reducing cancer-related pain. Patients should always confer with their healthcare provider before using any complementary health approaches. Any treatment that requires applying pressure to a tumor is discouraged (NCCIH, 2014c).
- Provide or assist with comfort measures, such as massage, positioning, distraction, and relaxation techniques. These techniques promote relaxation and enhance pain relief.
- Assist the patient and family to plan and engage in activities that distract from pain, such as reading, watching television, and engaging in social interactions. Distraction helps the patient focus away from the pain.
- Spend as much time with the patient as possible, and allow family members to remain with the patient. The physical presence of the nurse and family provides emotional support for the patient.

Pain management is discussed further in the exemplar on Acute and Chronic Pain in the module on Comfort. Care for the patient at the end of life is discussed in the exemplar on End-of-Life Care in the module on Comfort.

Promote Balanced Nutrition

The high metabolic rate of cancer growth depletes the patient's nutritional stores, so many patients have lost weight and muscle mass at the time of diagnosis. In addition, the catabolic effect of chemotherapy and radiation on normal cells necessitates further cellular replacement. Loss of appetite, food aversion, taste changes, nausea and vomiting, and painful oral lesions from chemotherapy or radiation may contribute to impaired nutrition. The nurse should do the following:

- Assess current eating patterns, including usual likes and dislikes, and identify factors that impair food intake. This allows for a more individualized plan based on needs and preferences.

- Weigh the patient daily. Weight fluctuation may indicate adequate or inadequate dietary intake.

- Teach the principles of maintaining good nutrition by using the federal government's MyPlate recommendations and adapting the diet to medical restrictions and current preferences. This tailors the food plan to the patient's needs and thereby promotes compliance.

- Evaluate degree of malnutrition:
  a. Check laboratory values for total serum protein, serum albumin and globins, total lymphocyte count, serum transferrin, hemoglobin, and hematocrit. These values represent the laboratory values that are most likely to decrease with malnutrition.
  b. Calculate nitrogen balance and creatinine-height index. Calculate skeletal muscle mass, and compare findings to normal ranges. Urinary creatinine is an index of lean body mass and decreases in malnutrition. Lean muscle mass is catabolized for energy in patients with cancer.
  c. Take anthropometric measurements, and compare them to standards: height, weight, elbow breadth, arm circumference, triceps skinfold thickness, and arm muscle mass. This estimates the degree of wasting; findings below 85% of standard are considered malnutrition.

- Manage nausea and vomiting by administering anti-emetic drugs (around-the-clock medication may be an effective preventive measure). Encourage the patient to eat small, frequent, low-fat meals with dry foods (e.g., crackers and toast), to avoid liquids with meals, and to sit upright for an hour after meals. Remove emesis basins, and encourage oral hygiene before eating. Dry, low-fat foods are more readily tolerated when the patient is nauseated.

- Administer parenteral nutrition via central line or other venous access device (VAD). For these patients, teach safety measures, care of the VAD, and explain how the pump delivering solution works. Provide an emergency phone number for help with administration problems.

- Assess readiness for resumption of oral intake after surgery or procedures using data such as statements of hunger, presence of bowel sounds, passage of flatus, and minimal abdominal distention. Manipulation of the bowel interrupts peristalsis of the gastrointestinal tract. Ensure that peristalsis has resumed before oral intake begins.

The nurse can teach the patient ways to help manage nutrition and problems interfering with nutrition. Refer to the Patient Teaching feature.

》Stay Current: For more information on nutrition in cancer care, go to the NCI's website at http://www.cancer.gov/about-cancer/treatment/side-effects/appetite-loss/nutrition-pdq.

Protect Tissue Integrity

The most common impairment of tissue integrity in patients with cancer occurs in the oral-pharyngeal-esophageal mucous membranes. It is secondary to the effects of some chemotherapeutic drugs and radiation treatment to the head and neck. The oral-pharyngeal-esophageal tissues are lined with cells that have a high mitotic turnover rate and are therefore vulnerable to many chemotherapeutic drugs. Leukemias, bone marrow transplants, and herpes viral infections also disrupt oral-pharyngeal-esophageal tissue. Manifestations of this problem include small ulcers that occur on the tongue and mucous membranes in the mouth and throat; herpes simplex type 1 lesions or vesicles that evolve into ulcerations; fungal infections, such as thrush (resulting from *Candida* infections), that manifest as a white, yellow, or tan coating with dry, red, fissured tissue underneath; red, swollen, friable gums that bleed with minimal or no trauma; and **xerostomia**, which is excessive dryness of the mucous membranes caused by chemotherapy or radiation.

To promote the integrity of oral-pharyngeal-esophageal tissues, the nurse should do the following:

- Carefully assess and evaluate the type of tissue impairment present. Identify possible sources, such as chemotherapy or radiation therapy to the head and neck, and implement corrective measures appropriate to the type of problem.

- Implement and teach measures for preventing oropharyngeal infection:
  a. Culture any oral lesions, and report the problem to the physician. Herpes lesions may not follow a typical

Patient Teaching
Nutrition Management

Following are some teaching points for helping patients with cancer who have difficulty maintaining good nutrition:

- Eat whatever is appealing, and consider adding nutritional supplements, such as Ensure Plus or Isocal, to the diet. Increase calorie intake by adding ice cream or frozen yogurt to liquid supplements and commercial protein powders to milk or juice. It is better to eat something, even if it is not nutritionally balanced.

- Eat small, frequent meals. These are more easily digested and absorbed and are usually better tolerated by the patient with anorexia.

- Try icy-cold foods (e.g., ice cream) or those that are more highly seasoned if food has no taste. Chemotherapy and radiation therapy may harm taste buds and prevent distinguishing the taste of foods. Strong seasonings and coldness can make food more enjoyable to the patient with diminished taste. However, if painful oropharyngeal ulcers are present, spicy foods are not recommended.

- If the patient has oropharyngeal ulcers, cold and bland, semisoft and liquid foods are less irritating to sensitive mucous membranes. Use an anesthetic, alcohol-free mouthwash before eating because deadening the pain can make chewing and swallowing easier.

- Removing vomiting cues, such as odor and supplies associated with vomiting, can reduce nausea. Take prescribed antinausea medication on a schedule to help prevent nausea.

- Keep a food diary to document food intake. By seeing how little is being consumed, the patient may eat more.

pattern in patients who are immunosuppressed. Identifying the cause of the infection, whether viral, fungal, or bacterial, allows the physician to prescribe the appropriate treatment.

b. Encourage cleaning teeth gently and using a nonalcohol mouthwash several times a day. Reducing the oral flora by performing frequent hygiene decreases the risk of infection. Review the contents of each mouthwash, and assist in patient teaching to prevent hypersensitivity reactions to ingredients (e.g., lidocaine).

■ Implement and teach measures for reducing trauma to delicate tissues:

a. Avoid putting sharp instruments in the mouth. Use smooth plastic spoons and forks for eating, especially when a bleeding disorder is present. Dental work should be done by dental oncologists.

b. Counteract dry mouth and lips with lubricating and moisturizing agents, such as Gatorade, sugarless gum, and lip balm. This protects mucous membranes from infection and trauma.

c. Brush teeth with a very soft toothbrush, and obtain a new toothbrush monthly. If gums are friable and bleeding, clean teeth with a soft cloth placed over a finger or with toothpaste on the finger. Chlorhexidine mouthwash (Peridex) may be used. This protects gums from trauma and decreases the risk of hemorrhage.

Promote Healthy Body Image

Cancer and cancer treatments frequently result in major physiologic and psychologic changes in body image. Loss of a body part (e.g., through amputation, prostatectomy, or mastectomy), skin changes and hair loss due to treatment, disfigurement (e.g., lymphedema in the affected extremities), or creation of unnatural openings on the body for elimination (e.g., colostomy, ileostomy) may drastically affect the individual's self-image. Body image can also be significantly affected by the development of anorexia-cachexia syndrome or the appearance of draining, malodorous lesions that result when cancer breaks through the skin. Visible changes or disfigurement may also give rise to fear of rejection, which can play a major role in sexual dysfunction. Typical patient responses include verbalizing negative feelings about the body and/or fear of rejection by others, refusing to look at the affected site, and depersonalizing the body change or lost part (e.g., calling the colostomy "that thing"). The nurse should do the following:

■ Observe and evaluate the patient's interaction with significant others. People who are important to the patient may unintentionally reinforce negative feelings about body image; on the other hand, the patient may perceive rejection where none exists.

■ Allow denial, but do not participate in it. For example, if the patient does not want to look at the wound, the nurse may say, "I am going to change the dressing on your breast incision now." During the initial stage of shock at the loss of a body part, denial is a protective mechanism and should not be challenged, nor should

it be promoted. A matter-of-fact approach and an empathetic attitude will go far to facilitate the eventual acceptance of the change.

■ Teach the patient or significant others to participate in the care of the afflicted body area. Active involvement in providing care empowers the patient and/or significant others and can desensitize feelings about disfigurement and promote acceptance. Supporting and validating their efforts will promote continued participation.

■ Teach strategies for minimizing physical changes, such as providing skin care during radiation therapy and dressing to enhance appearance and minimize the change in the body part. Early intervention can limit the negative side effects of treatment and promote recovery. Involving the patient provides additional ways for the patient to maintain control of a difficult situation.

■ Hair loss can be devastating for patients. Interventions to reduce that loss can have a significant impact on body image concerns. Teach ways to reduce the hair loss that results from chemotherapy and to enhance appearance until the hair grows back:

a. Discuss the pattern and timing of hair loss. This allows the patient to cope with changes and incorporate them into daily activities.

b. Encourage wearing cheerful, brightly colored head coverings; assist in color coordinating them with usual clothing. Attractive head coverings protect the bald head while allowing the patient to feel stylish and well dressed.

c. Refer the patient to a good wig shop before hair loss is experienced. Hair color and texture can be matched to minimize obvious changes in appearance.

d. Refer the patient to support programs such as "Look Good . . . Feel Better," which is sponsored by the ACS and the Cosmetic, Toilet, and Fragrance Association Foundation. A support group can diminish feelings of isolation and provide practical tips for managing problems.

e. Reassure the patient that hair will grow back after chemotherapy is discontinued, though the color and texture of the new hair may be different. Knowing what to expect may decrease anxiety and distress.

Promote Healthy Grieving

Although 50% of people with cancer fully recover, many do not, and certain types of cancer have a much higher death rate than others. Thus, the patient with cancer is often confronted with facing death and making preparations for it. This can be a healthy response that allows the patient and family to work through the dying process and achieve growth in the final stage of life. Perceived changes in body image and lifestyle also can prompt anticipatory grieving. The patient or significant others may show sorrow, anger, depression, or withdrawal, expressing distress at the potential loss or verbalizing concern about unfinished life business.

■ Spend time with the patient and family. Time is necessary to develop a trusting, therapeutic relationship.

- Use the therapeutic communication skills of active listening, silence, and nonverbal support to provide an open environment for the patient and significant others to discuss their feelings realistically and to express anger or other negative feelings appropriately.

- Answer questions about illness and prognosis honestly, but always encourage hope. This allows for realistic appraisal of the situation and planning while helping to combat feelings of hopelessness and depression.

- Discuss advance directives, such as do-not-resuscitate orders, and powers of attorney for healthcare with the patient and family. These documents give the patient and family a sense of control over medical care provided if the patient is no longer able to express his or her own wishes.

- Encourage the patient who is dying to make funeral and burial plans ahead of time and to be sure his or her will is in order. Make sure the necessary phone numbers can be easily located. This gives a sense of control and relieves family members of these concerns.

- Demonstrate respect for cultural, spiritual, and religious values and beliefs; encourage use of these resources to cope with losses.

- Encourage the patient to continue taking part in activities he or she enjoys, including maintaining employment as long as possible. This gives a sense of continuity of life even in the face of severe losses.

- If the patient wishes you to do so, involve the partner in helping the patient cope with the loss. Remember that the partner may also be grieving. Not all patients want to share their grief, and not all partners are interested and supportive.

Evaluation

When evaluating the patient's response to therapy, the nurse should remember that while hopeful outcomes should always include patient recovery and absence of complications, this is not realistic for every individual diagnosed with cancer. In some cases, outcomes may include the patient's acceptance of and preparedness for death. Other expected outcomes may include the following:

- The patient demonstrates no evidence of infection.

- Using a predetermined pain rating scale of 0–10, the patient reports a pain level of 3 or less, allowing for adequate rest and performance of activities of daily living (ADLs).

- The patient reports reduction in side effects of the treatment regimen.

- The patient demonstrates appropriate dietary choices to increase caloric intake.

Even if evaluation shows no current evidence of infection, the patient and family need to be educated about the continued risk for infection due to the myelosuppression. Constipation or diarrhea may also be an issue for the patient due to treatment, nutritional intake, disease process, or use of pain medications. Ascertaining the patient's usual elimination habits will provide a baseline by which to evaluate therapeutic interventions. Educating the patient on the adjustment of fluid and fiber intake as appropriate can assist in prevention of constipation; low-fiber foods can decrease irritability and provide bowel rest if diarrhea is present.

REVIEW Cancer

RELATE Link the Concepts and Exemplars

Linking the exemplar of cancer with the concept of evidence-based practice:

1. How does evidence-based practice affect cancer screening guidelines?

2. In what ways can the nurse ensure that he or she is adhering to current principles of evidenced-based practice?

Linking the exemplar of cancer with the concept of comfort.

3. Describe pharmacologic and nonpharmacologic comfort measures that can be used by a patient with a cancer diagnosis.

4. Describe barriers related to adequate pain relief that patients with a cancer diagnosis may encounter.

Linking the exemplar of cancer with the concept of development.

5. Using Erikson's Eight Stages of Development, describe how the development of a school-age child might be affected by a cancer diagnosis.

6. Describe how the normal developmental tasks of an adolescent could be affected by a diagnosis of cancer.

READY Go to Volume 3: Clinical Nursing Skills

REFER Go to Pearson MyLab Nursing and eText

- Additional review materials
- Chart 2: Laboratory Tests Used for Cancer Diagnosis
- Nursing Care Plan: A Patient with Cancer

REFLECT Apply Your Knowledge

Mandy Leno, 63 years old, has lived with bipolar disorder since young adulthood. She has recently been diagnosed with pancreatic cancer. Following her diagnosis of cancer, Ms. Leno experiences an acute manic episode and is admitted to an inpatient psychiatric unit for evaluation and treatment. She is currently pacing up and down the hall, stating that she will conquer her cancer without drugs or surgery. She is refusing all medications. She has barely slept and has deep circles under her eyes. She has eaten very little in the past few days. Her urine output is low, she is disheveled, and her clothes are dirty. Ms. Leno is divorced and has no family nearby. Her only daughter lives across the country and has three small children.

1. What are the priorities of care for Ms. Leno?

2. Is Ms. Leno capable of giving consent for surgery? Is surgical consent needed? Why or why not?

3. Should Ms. Leno's daughter be contacted? Explain your answer.

» Exemplar 2.B
Anemia

Exemplar Learning Outcomes

2.B Analyze anemia as it relates to cellular regulation.

- Describe the pathophysiology of anemia.
- Describe the etiology of anemia.
- Compare the risk factors for and prevention of anemia.
- Identify the clinical manifestations of anemia.
- Summarize diagnostic tests and therapies used by interprofessional teams in the collaborative care of an individual with anemia.
- Differentiate considerations for care of patients with anemia across the lifespan.
- Apply the nursing process in providing culturally competent care to an individual with anemia.

Exemplar Key Terms

Anemia, *69*
Aplastic anemia, *74*
Hemolytic anemias, *73*
Iron deficiency anemia, *72*
Neonatal anemia, *77*
Pernicious anemia, *72*
Physiologic anemia of the newborn, *77*
Thalassemia, *73*

Overview

The erythrocyte, or RBC, carries oxygen throughout the body. Oxygen binds to hemoglobin, which is the main component of the RBC. **Anemia** occurs when oxygen delivery is inadequate as a result of a deficient hematocrit (the volume percentage of healthy RBCs) or a decreased amount of normal hemoglobin. In some cases, even though the number of RBCs is adequate, a defect in the structure and function of the RBC prevents adequate oxygen transport, which causes anemia. Symptoms of anemia can be very vague; in many cases, fatigue is the first symptom of this disorder.

Anemia that occurs because of a decreased hematocrit may be caused by blood loss, inadequate RBC production, or increased RBC destruction. Insufficient or defective hemoglobin may occur because of nutritional deficiencies and physiologic disorders.

Pathophysiology and Etiology

Pathophysiology

Because RBCs are needed to carry oxygen throughout the body, all types of anemia, regardless of their cause, reduce the oxygen-carrying capacity of the blood. Therefore, anemia results in less oxygen reaching cells and tissues, which can lead to tissue hypoxia.

When the onset of anemia is slow, compensatory mechanisms may prevent or mask the appearance of symptoms. When oxygen demands increase, such as during exercise or with infection, the symptoms of anemia may become more apparent. During these times, as blood is redistributed to the vital organs, the skin, mucous membranes, conjunctiva, and nail beds may develop pallor (see **Figure 2–6** »). Tissue hypoxia triggers a compensatory increase in heart rate and respiratory rate. Increased heart rate promotes an increase in cardiac output, while increased respiratory rate allows for greater delivery of oxygen to the lungs and, subsequently, to the blood. Tissue hypoxia may cause angina, fatigue, dyspnea on exertion, and night cramps. It also stimulates erythropoietin release; in turn, increased erythropoietin activity stimulates RBC production in the bone marrow and may lead to bone pain. Cerebral hypoxia can lead to headache, dizziness, and visual disturbances. Severe anemia may cause heart failure.

Etiology

Although a number of different pathologic mechanisms can lead to anemia, iron deficiency is the most common cause (see **Box 2–3** »). Iron deficiency anemia occurs when there is an insufficient amount of mineral iron present in the body to produce the necessary hemoglobin to make RBCs. Insufficient iron supply will first cause iron stores in the bone marrow to be depleted. As iron deficiencies develop, hemoglobin production will be affected, and blood tests will indicate a decrease in hemoglobin and hematocrit levels. Anemia develops as hemoglobin production continues to decline. Iron deficiency can result from several conditions, including nutritional iron deficiency, conditions causing internal blood loss, and impaired iron absorption. Nutritional iron deficiency

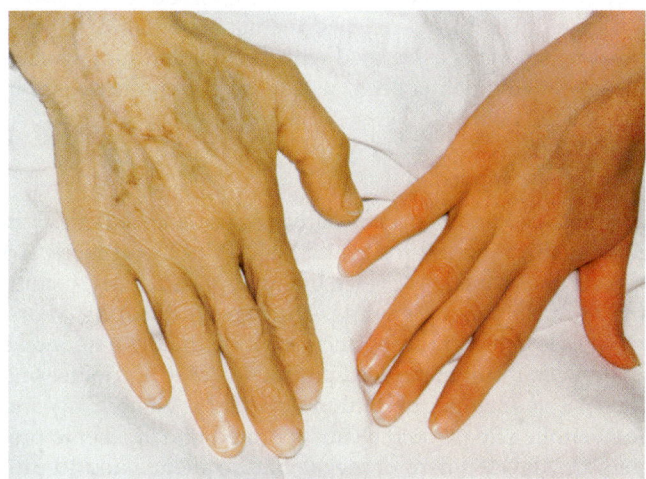

Source: Westminster Hospital/Science Source.

Figure 2–6 » The skin of the patient with anemia appears pale beside that of an individual with a normal hemoglobin and hematocrit.

Box 2–3
Pathophysiologic Mechanisms of Anemia

Decreased RBC Production	Increased RBC Loss or Destruction

■ Altered hemoglobin synthesis:
  a. Iron deficiency
  b. Thalassemia
  c. Chronic inflammation
■ Altered DNA synthesis:
  a. Vitamin B_{12} malabsorption or deficiency
  b. Folic acid malabsorption or deficiency
■ Bone marrow failure:
  a. Aplastic anemia (stem cell dysfunction)
  b. Red cell aplasia
  c. Myeloproliferative leukemias
  d. Cancer metastasis, lymphoma
  e. Chronic infection or inflammation, physical and emotional fatigue
	■ Acute or chronic blood loss:
	  a. Hemorrhage or trauma
	  b. Chronic gastrointestinal bleeding, menorrhagia
	■ Increased hemolysis:
	  a. Hereditary cell membrane disorders
	  b. Defective hemoglobin—SCD or trait
	  c. Pyruvate kinase or glucose-6-phosphate dehydrogenase (G6PD) deficiency affecting glycolysis or cell oxidation
	  d. Immune mechanisms and disorders (e.g., blood reaction, hypersensitivity responses, autoimmune disorders)
	  e. Splenomegaly and hypersplenism
	  f. Infection
	  g. Erythrocyte trauma (e.g., caused by cardiopulmonary bypass, hemolytic uremic syndrome)

affects approximately 2 billion individuals worldwide, and although the majority of American adults consume an adequate amount of iron in their diet, iron deficiency is the most prevalent nutritional deficiency in the United States. This is attributed to the consumption of diets high in processed foods or strict vegetarian diets (University of Maryland Medical Center [UMMC], 2013a). See the Clinical Manifestations and Therapies feature for a summary of common causes of iron deficiency anemia.

Iron deficiency anemia is particularly common in older adults and in women of childbearing age. Iron deficiency anemia can result from chronic, occult (hidden) blood loss caused by slowly bleeding peptic ulcers, gastrointestinal inflammation, hemorrhoids, and cancer. Depending on its severity, anemia may affect all major organ systems.

Iron deficiency is one of the most common nutritional deficiencies seen in children (Hockenberry & Wilson, 2014). Pica (consumption of or cravings for nonfood items) also is associated with iron deficiency anemia in pediatric patients. Lead poisoning is associated with anemia and may worsen in those with anemia because lead absorption increases in the anemic state.

Risk Factors

Patients who do not eat a healthy, well-balanced diet rich in meat, fish, and fresh fruits and vegetables are at increased risk for those anemias caused by nutrient deficiency, including iron deficiency anemia. During childbearing years, women lose blood during menstruation. Inadequate intake of iron can result in reduced production of RBCs, increasing the risk of anemia due to iron deficiency. Vitamin B_{12} and folate (folic acid) should be incorporated into the diet to prevent the development of megaloblastic anemia and to promote overall good health (UMMC, 2013a).

Prevention

Several forms of anemia are genetic in origin and cannot be prevented. However, for cases of anemia that are caused by iron deficiency, adequate nutrition is a major factor. General guidelines include a balanced diet that combines iron-rich foods with vegetables, fruits, whole grains, low-fat milk products, eggs, lean meat, and fish. Meals ideally should combine nonheme iron sources with foods that are rich in vitamin C, which promotes the absorption of nonheme iron (Lichtin, 2013). Likewise, anemia that is due primarily to insufficient intake of vitamin B_{12} can be prevented through dietary modifications.

Clinical Manifestations

Anemia is categorized by cause: blood loss, nutritional, hemolytic, and bone marrow suppression (aplastic). A neonatal anemia also is recognized. Each type has its own specific pathophysiology and manifestations; see the Multisystem Effects of Anemia feature.

Blood Loss Anemia

All bleeding involves the loss of RBCs and other blood components. However, the effects and manifestations related to this process depend on the volume and rate of blood loss and on whether the bleeding is acute or chronic.

Acute loss of a significant volume of blood triggers compensatory mechanisms (including an increase in heart rate and constriction of peripheral blood vessels) that help maintain cardiac output. Vessels in the liver, a blood storage organ, also constrict, increasing circulating volume. Fluid shifts from the interstitial spaces into the vascular compartment to maintain blood volume, diluting the cellular components of the blood and reducing its viscosity. If hemorrhage continues, compensatory mechanisms become less effective, increasing the risk for hypovolemic shock and circulatory failure. Initial manifestations of hypovolemic shock include tachycardia and tachypnea; the skin may be pale, cool, and clammy as peripheral vessels constrict to maintain blood flow to the heart and brain. With continued blood loss, hypotension, increased tachycardia, decreased level of consciousness, and oliguria develop.

Multisystem Effects of
Anemia

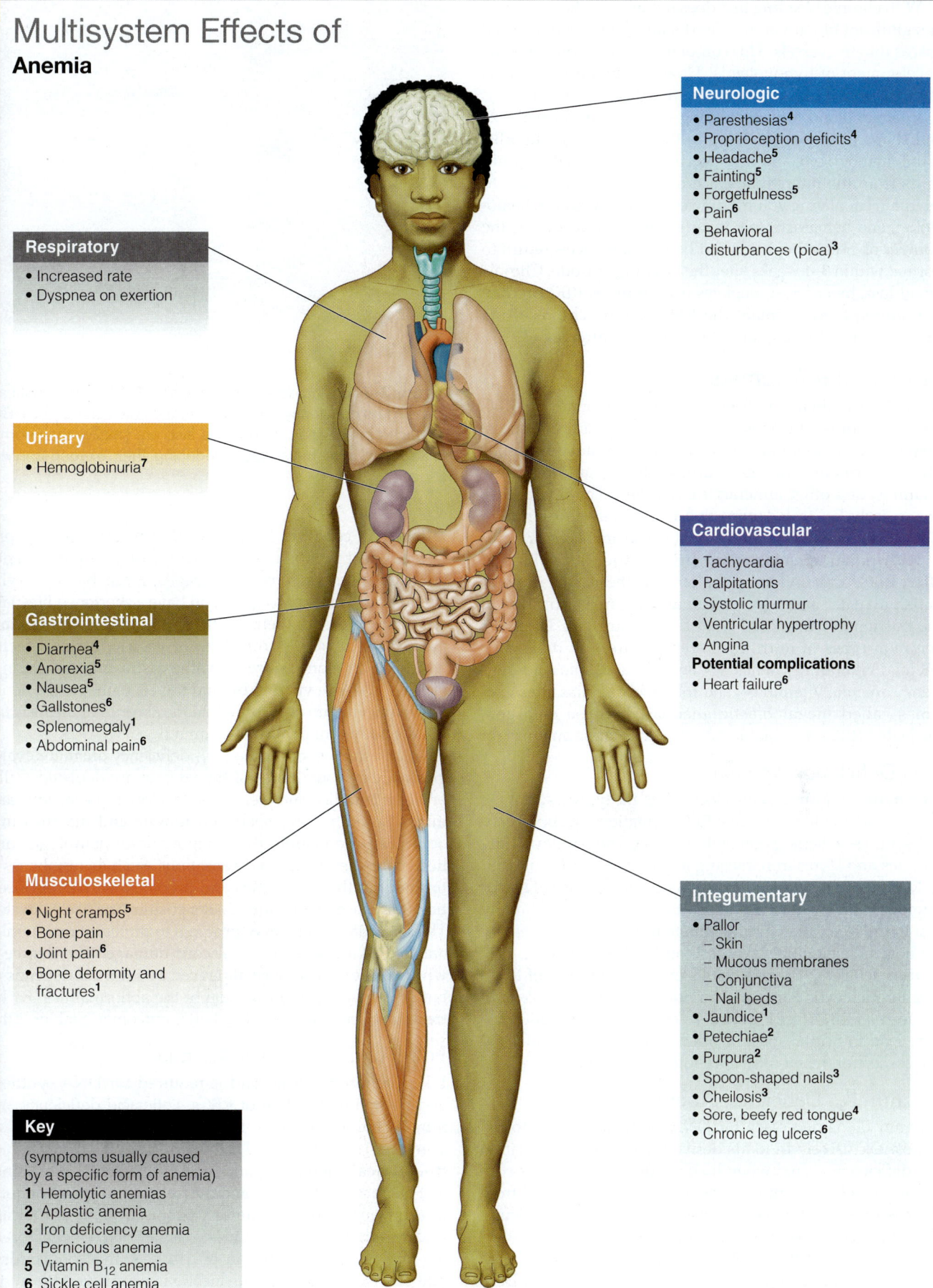

Neurologic
- Paresthesias[4]
- Proprioception deficits[4]
- Headache[5]
- Fainting[5]
- Forgetfulness[5]
- Pain[6]
- Behavioral
  disturbances (pica)[3]

Respiratory
- Increased rate
- Dyspnea on exertion

Urinary
- Hemoglobinuria[7]

Gastrointestinal
- Diarrhea[4]
- Anorexia[5]
- Nausea[5]
- Gallstones[6]
- Splenomegaly[1]
- Abdominal pain[6]

Cardiovascular
- Tachycardia
- Palpitations
- Systolic murmur
- Ventricular hypertrophy
- Angina
Potential complications
- Heart failure[6]

Musculoskeletal
- Night cramps[5]
- Bone pain
- Joint pain[6]
- Bone deformity and
  fractures[1]

Integumentary
- Pallor
  - Skin
  - Mucous membranes
  - Conjunctiva
  - Nail beds
- Jaundice[1]
- Petechiae[2]
- Purpura[2]
- Spoon-shaped nails[3]
- Cheilosis[3]
- Sore, beefy red tongue[4]
- Chronic leg ulcers[6]

Key

(symptoms usually caused
by a specific form of anemia)
1 Hemolytic anemias
2 Aplastic anemia
3 Iron deficiency anemia
4 Pernicious anemia
5 Vitamin B_{12} anemia
6 Sickle cell anemia
7 G6PD anemia

With chronic bleeding that does not involve the acute loss of significant blood volume, fluid shifts from the interstitial spaces into the vessels. This compensatory shift prevents the development of hypovolemia. However, blood viscosity is reduced, which may result in a systolic heart murmur.

In acute blood loss, circulating RBCs are of normal size and shape (normocytic). Early in the hemorrhage, the RBC count, hemoglobin, and hematocrit may be normal. As fluid shifts from the interstitial space into the vascular space to maintain circulating volume, however, the RBC count, hemoglobin, and hematocrit fall. If sufficient iron is available, the number of circulating RBCs and hemoglobin levels return to normal within 3–4 weeks after the bleeding episode. Chronic blood loss, by contrast, depletes iron stores as RBC production attempts to maintain the RBC supply. The resulting RBCs are small (microcytic) and pale (hypochromic).

Nutritional Anemias

A number of different nutrients are required for normal RBC development (erythropoiesis). Iron is a key nutrient necessary for hemoglobin synthesis. In addition, adequate supplies of protein (and its building blocks, amino acids), vitamins, and other minerals are required. The B vitamins, particularly B_{12} (cobalamin) and folate, play a key role in RBC development. Vitamins C and E also are necessary.

Nutritional anemias result from nutrient deficits that affect RBC formation or hemoglobin synthesis. The nutrient deficit may be caused by inadequate diet, malabsorption of the nutrient, or increased need for the nutrient. The most common types of nutritional anemias are iron deficiency anemia, vitamin B_{12} deficiency anemia, and folic acid deficiency anemia. Vitamin B_{12} and folic acid anemias are sometimes called megaloblastic anemias, because enlarged, nucleated RBCs (megaloblasts) are seen in these anemias.

Iron Deficiency Anemia

Iron deficiency anemia develops when the body's supply of iron is inadequate for optimal RBC formation. The body cannot synthesize hemoglobin without iron. The body typically recycles and stores iron, reusing much of the iron contained in RBCs that are removed from circulation because of age or damage. However, small amounts of iron are continually lost in the feces; therefore, adequate iron intake is necessary for normal hemoglobin synthesis and RBC production.

Iron deficiency anemia results in fewer numbers of RBCs and in microcytic (smaller than normal), hypochromic, and malformed RBCs (see **Figure 2–7 »**). Chronic iron deficiency may lead to brittle, spoon-shaped nails; cheilosis (cracks at the corners of the mouth); a smooth, sore tongue; and pica.

Vitamin B_{12} Deficiency Anemia

Vitamin B_{12} is necessary for DNA synthesis and is found almost exclusively in foods derived from animals. Vitamin B_{12} deficiency occurs when inadequate vitamin B_{12} is consumed or, more commonly, when it is poorly absorbed from the gastrointestinal tract. Resection of the stomach or ileum, loss of pancreatic secretions, and chronic gastritis can affect vitamin B_{12} absorption. Dietary deficiencies of vitamin B_{12} are rare, usually occurring only among strict vegetarians. Deficiency of this vitamin impairs cell division and maturation of the cell nucleus, especially in rapidly proliferating RBCs. As a result, macrocytic (larger than normal), misshapen (oval

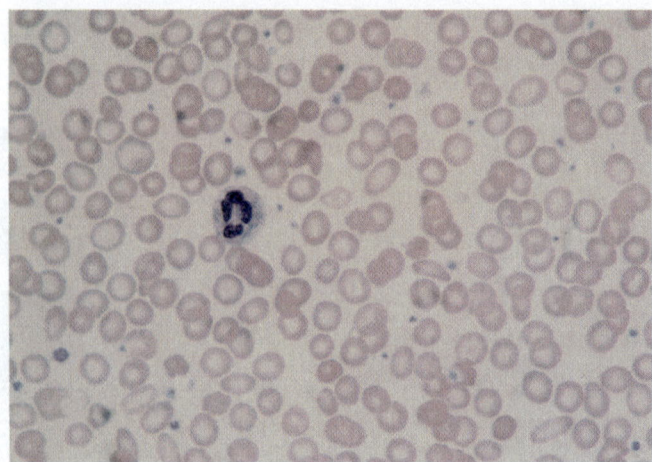

Source: Dr. E. Walker/Science Source.

Figure 2–7 » A blood smear showing RBCs characteristically seen in iron deficiency anemia. Note the pale color of the RBCs (hypochromic). Many of the cells also are smaller than normal (microcytic) and misshapen, reducing their oxygen-carrying capacity.

rather than concave) RBCs with thin membranes are produced. Great numbers of these large, immature RBCs enter the circulation. These cells are fragile, incapable of carrying adequate amounts of oxygen, and have a shortened lifespan.

Failure to absorb dietary vitamin B_{12} produces **pernicious anemia**. It develops from lack of gastric intrinsic factor, which is a substance secreted by the gastric mucosa. Intrinsic factor binds with vitamin B_{12} and travels with it to the ileum, where the vitamin is absorbed. In the absence of intrinsic factor, the body cannot absorb vitamin B_{12}.

Manifestations of vitamin B_{12} deficiency anemia develop gradually as body stores of the vitamin are depleted. Pallor or slight jaundice and weakness develop. In pernicious anemia, a smooth, sore, beefy red tongue and diarrhea may occur. Because vitamin B_{12} is important for neurologic function, paresthesias (altered sensations, such as numbness or tingling) in the extremities and problems with proprioception (the sense of the individual's position in space) develop. These manifestations may progress to difficulty maintaining balance as a result of spinal cord damage. The degree to which neurologic abnormalities can be reversed depends on both the severity and duration of the abnormalities. Earlier treatment generally produces better outcomes (Stabler, 2013).

Folic Acid Deficiency Anemia

Like vitamin B_{12}, folic acid is required for DNA synthesis and normal maturation of RBCs. Folic acid deficiency anemia is characterized by fragile, megaloblastic (large and immature) cells. Folic acid is found in green leafy vegetables, fruits, cereals, and meats and is absorbed from the intestines.

Folic acid deficiency anemia as a result of inadequate intake is more common among people who are chronically undernourished. This includes older adults, patients receiving total parenteral nutrition, and those with alcohol or drug addictions. Individuals with alcoholism are especially at risk because alcohol suppresses folate metabolism, which forms folic acid; their diets are usually also lacking in the vitamin. Because increased folic acid levels also may lead to anemia, pregnant women are at greater risk for anemia due to increased intake of folic acid to promote fetal development. Infants and teenagers can develop temporary folic acid deficiencies during periods of rapid growth. Impaired folic acid absorption and metabolism can cause folic acid deficiency anemia. Malabsorption disorders, such as celiac sprue (a hereditary gastrointestinal disorder characterized by the inability to metabolize amino acids found in gluten), and certain medications, such as methotrexate and some chemotherapeutic agents, may be implicated.

The manifestations of folic acid deficiency anemia develop gradually as folic acid stores are depleted. Signs and symptoms may include pallor, progressive weakness and fatigue, shortness of breath, and heart palpitations. Manifestations similar to those associated with vitamin B_{12} anemia, such as glossitis, cheilosis, and diarrhea, are common. No neurologic symptoms occur with folic acid deficiency anemia; this helps clinicians to differentiate it from vitamin B_{12} deficiency anemia. However, these two nutritional anemias do sometimes coexist.

Maternal folic acid deficiency is strongly associated with neural tube defects, such as meningomyelocele. The neural tube develops early in the process of fetal development, often before pregnancy is recognized.

Hemolytic Anemias

Hemolytic anemias are characterized by premature destruction (lysis) of RBCs. When RBCs break down, iron and other by-products of their destruction remain in the plasma. RBC lysis (hemolysis) may occur within the circulatory system or as a result of phagocytosis by WBCs, such as circulating monocytes and macrophages in the spleen. In response to hemolysis, the hematopoietic activity of bone marrow increases, leading to increased reticulocytes (immature RBCs) in circulating blood. Most types of hemolytic anemia are characterized by normocytic and normochromic RBCs.

There are multiple causes of hemolytic anemias, which may be either *intrinsic*, arising from disorders within the RBC itself, or *extrinsic*, originating outside the RBC. Intrinsic disorders include cell membrane defects, defects in hemoglobin structure and function (e.g., SCD, thalassemia), and inherited enzyme deficiencies (e.g., G6PD deficiency). Extrinsic causes of hemolytic anemia include drugs, chemicals, toxins, venoms, trauma, burns, and bacterial or other infections. This section discusses thalassemia, acquired hemolytic anemia, and G6PD anemia. (For details regarding sickle cell anemia, see Exemplar 2.H on Sickle Cell Disease.)

Thalassemia

Thalassemia refers to inherited disorders of hemoglobin synthesis in which either the alpha or beta chains of the hemoglobin molecule are missing or defective. This leads to deficient hemoglobin production and fragile hypochromic, microcytic RBCs called target cells because of their distinctive bull's-eye appearance (NHLBI, 2012b).

Thalassemia is more prevalent among certain populations. People of Mediterranean, African, and South Asian descent are more likely to have beta-defect thalassemia. People of Southeast Asian descent more commonly have alpha-defect thalassemia, with up to 30% of the population having the trait. There are high numbers of carriers of alpha-defect

thalassemia in Sub-Saharan Africa and the Western Pacific Regions. There is a higher prevalence of both alpha- and beta-defect thalassemias in the tropical and subtropical regions of the world (India and Thailand). In Europe, the southern regions of Italy and Greece are more commonly affected, while countries north of the African continent also have a higher prevalence of thalassemia (Smith, 2015a).

Treatment for thalassemia can vary depending on the patient's situation and presenting symptoms. Individuals who have thalassemia minor (having inherited a mutated gene from one parent) often experience no symptoms and require no treatment. Those with mild cases of the disease may be required only to make small lifestyle and dietary modifications to aid in the management of the condition. Others with more severe cases of the disease will require regular or frequent blood transfusions throughout their lives. However, lifelong blood transfusions create additional health risks, including the potential for iron overload. Many patients who require regular blood transfusions also need iron chelation therapy to prevent iron-related damage to the heart, liver, and other organs. An individual who has a severe case of thalassemia may benefit from stem cell or bone marrow transplantation. However, this treatment is reserved as last-line therapy, because the side effects can be serious and sometimes fatal (Smith, 2015b).

Individuals with thalassemia minor often are asymptomatic. Individuals who have thalassemia major (a mutated gene inherited from each parent) may experience mild to moderate anemia, mild splenomegaly, bronze skin coloring, and bone marrow hyperplasia. The major form of the disease causes severe anemia, heart failure, and liver and spleen enlargement from increased RBC destruction. Fractures of the long bones, ribs, and vertebrae may result from bone marrow expansion and thinning as a result of increased hematopoiesis. Jaundice, hepatomegaly, and splenomegaly may develop because of hemolysis.

Acquired Hemolytic Anemia

Acquired hemolytic anemia is caused by hemolysis resulting from factors outside of the RBCs. Causes of acquired hemolytic anemias include the following:

- Mechanical trauma to RBCs produced by prosthetic heart valves, severe burns, hemodialysis, or radiation
- Autoimmune disorders
- Bacterial or protozoal infection
- Immune system–mediated responses, such as transfusion reactions
- Drugs, toxins, chemical agents, or venoms.

The manifestations of acquired hemolytic anemia depend on the extent of hemolysis and the body's ability to replace destroyed RBCs. The anemia itself often is mild to moderate as erythropoiesis increases to replace the destroyed RBCs. The spleen enlarges as it removes damaged or destroyed RBCs. If the breakdown of heme units exceeds the liver's ability to conjugate and excrete bilirubin, jaundice develops. When the condition is severe, bone marrow expands, and bones may be deformed or may develop pathologic fractures. The severity of generalized manifestations of anemia (e.g., tachycardia, pallor) depends on the degree of anemia and deficiency of tissue oxygenation.

Glucose-6-Phosphate Dehydrogenase Anemia

Glucose-6-phosphate dehydrogenase (G6PD) anemia is caused by a hereditary defect in RBC metabolism. It is relatively common in people of African and Mediterranean descent. The defective gene is located on the X chromosome and therefore affects more men than women. There are many variations of this genetic defect.

G6PD is an enzyme that catalyzes glycolysis, the process in which an RBC derives cellular energy. A defect in G6PD action causes direct oxidation of hemoglobin, damaging the RBC. Hemolysis usually occurs only when the affected individual is exposed to stressors (e.g., drugs such as aspirin, sulfonamides, or vitamin K derivatives) that increase the metabolic demands on RBCs. The G6PD deficiency impairs the necessary compensatory increase in glucose metabolism and causes cellular damage. Damaged RBCs are destroyed over a period of 7–12 days.

When the patient is exposed to a stressor that triggers G6PD anemia, symptoms develop within several days. These may include pallor, jaundice, hemoglobinuria (hemoglobin in the urine), and an elevated reticulocyte count. As new RBCs develop, counts return to normal.

Aplastic Anemia

In **aplastic anemia**, the bone marrow fails to produce all three types of blood cells, leading to pancytopenia, a deficiency in both red and white blood cells. Normal bone marrow is replaced by fat. Aplastic anemia fortunately is rare.

A rare form of aplastic anemia, Fanconi anemia, is caused by defects of DNA repair. For approximately 50% of acquired aplastic anemias, however, the underlying cause is unknown (idiopathic aplastic anemia). Other cases of aplastic anemia follow stem cell damage caused by exposure to radiation or certain chemical substances, such as benzene, arsenic, pesticides, certain antibiotics (especially chloramphenicol), and chemotherapeutic drugs (NHLBI, 2012c). Aplastic anemia also may occur with viral infections, such as mononucleosis, hepatitis C, and HIV (Porth & Grossman, 2013).

In aplastic anemia, the number of stem cells in the bone marrow is significantly reduced. The stem cell pool may be less than 1% of normal when the disease is recognized. Anemia develops as the bone marrow fails to replace RBCs that have reached the end of their life span. Remaining RBCs may be normochromic and normocytic, or they may be large, with increased mean corpuscular volume.

Manifestations of aplastic anemia vary with the severity of the pancytopenia. Its onset usually is insidious but may be sudden. Manifestations include fatigue, pallor, progressive weakness, exertional dyspnea, headache, and ultimately tachycardia and heart failure. Platelet deficiency leads to bleeding problems; bleeding gums, excessive bruising, and nosebleeds may be the initial symptoms. A deficiency in the number of WBCs increases the risk of infection, causing manifestations such as sore throat and fever.

Collaboration

Ensuring adequate tissue oxygenation is the priority of care in treating anemia. The specific therapy is determined by the underlying cause of the disorder. Anemia that results from nutritional deficiencies is addressed through dietary counseling. Some cases of anemia may be treated with drugs. In severe cases, the patient with anemia may need a blood transfusion. (For an overview of treatments used in the management of various types of anemia, see the Clinical Manifestations and Therapies feature.) Members of the interprofessional healthcare team may include pharmacists and nutritionists or dietitians in addition to nurses, physicians, and other healthcare professionals.

Diagnostic Tests

The diagnosis of anemia is based on laboratory studies. The CBC, which is a routine diagnostic test, measures both RBCs and hemoglobin and is useful in identification of anemia related to inadequate RBC count or hemoglobin. However, additional analysis is needed to confirm adequate RBC structure and function. A diet history and analysis can provide information related to food intake. Tests that may be ordered include the following:

- CBC
- Hemoglobin and hematocrit
- Hemoglobin electrophoresis
- Serum iron
- Serum ferritin
- Iron-binding capacity
- Microscopic analysis
- Schilling test
- Bone marrow examination
- Quantitative assay of G6PD.

Surgery

For the patient diagnosed with anemia that is due to blood loss, treatment focuses on identifying the source of the bleeding and, if possible, surgically repairing the damaged organ or tissues. Treatment of aplastic anemia resulting from damaged bone marrow may include a stem cell transplantation (also referred to as a bone marrow transplantation). The patient with pernicious anemia may require surgical exploration to assess for disorders such as celiac disease, Crohn disease, and diverticuli, which are conditions known to decrease the production of gastric intrinsic factor (Osborn et al., 2013). Splenectomy may be indicated in treatment of the patient with thalassemia major.

Pharmacologic Therapy

Medications used to treat anemia depend on the underlying cause. Pharmacologic agents used to treat and manage anemia include vitamin B_{12}, ferrous sulfate (or other iron sources), and folic acid.

For treatment of symptomatic iron deficiency anemia that does not respond to dietary modifications alone, supplemental iron may be administered orally or parenterally. IV and IM administration of iron are becoming more common, particularly in patients with an acute deficiency or an anemia associated with chronic gastrointestinal blood loss, chronic renal failure, and other chronic conditions that increase the need for blood cell production (e.g., cancers). Hypersensitivity reactions to parenterally administered iron preparations are rare and range from a mild hypersensitivity reaction to anaphylaxis. Although rare, theses reactions are potentially life-threatening (Rampton et al., 2014). For this reason, patients who receive IV iron supplementation must be closely observed for signs and symptoms of an adverse reaction. For oral preparations, common side effects include constipation, nausea, and heartburn.

Parenteral vitamin B_{12} is given when malabsorption or lack of intrinsic factor leads to vitamin B_{12} deficiency anemia. Folic acid is ordered for women of childbearing age, pregnant women, and patients with folic acid deficiency or SCD to meet the increased demands of the bone marrow. Hydroxyurea, a drug that promotes fetal hemoglobin production, may be prescribed for patients with SCD, particularly those with frequent crises or severe disease. Resulting increased levels of fetal hemoglobin interfere with the sickling process and reduce the incidence of painful crises (UMMC, 2013b).

Erythropoietin may be ordered for patients with low erythropoietin levels (e.g., patients with chronic renal failure) and for people who have anemia associated with other chronic diseases. Erythropoietin is given subcutaneously, and it may be given as often as three times a week in chronic renal failure. Because erythropoietin stimulates RBC production, adequate iron must be present; patients receiving erythropoietin may require regular IV iron therapy as well.

Immunosuppressive therapy with antithymocyte globulin, corticosteroids, and cyclosporine may be used to treat aplastic anemia. Androgens may stimulate blood cell production in some patients with aplastic anemia.

SAFETY ALERT In rare cases, parenteral iron administration may cause anaphylaxis. Should signs and symptoms of anaphylaxis develop, discontinue the infusion, remain with the patient, closely monitor for signs and symptoms of airway compromise and other complications, and notify the primary care provider immediately.

Nonpharmacologic Therapy

Good nutrition and awareness of the signs and symptoms related to exacerbations of anemia are essential to health promotion for patients diagnosed with this disorder. Because of the inherent relationship between anemia and impaired oxygenation, activity tolerance is a primary consideration for these patients, and a healthy balance between rest and activity is also essential.

Nutrition

Dietary modifications are recommended for nutritional deficiency anemias, such as iron deficiency anemia, vitamin B_{12} deficiency anemia, or folic acid deficiency anemia. **Box 2–4 »** identifies good sources of dietary iron, folic acid, and vitamin B_{12}. For individuals whose condition cannot be managed or reversed strictly through diet, good nutrition is still extremely important for optimizing energy levels and promoting general wellness.

Blood Transfusion

Blood transfusions may be indicated to treat anemias resulting from major blood loss, such as from trauma or major surgery, and severe anemia regardless of cause. In acute hemorrhage, whole blood may be given to replace both blood cells and volume. A unit of packed RBCs may be given when anemia is severe and the patient demonstrates cardiovascular instability or compromise. Treatment of aplastic anemia may also incorporate blood transfusions. For individuals diagnosed with thalassemia, blood transfusions will be required throughout their lifespan.

Lifespan Considerations

There are specific groups at higher risk for developing anemia than others. Neonates can develop anemia because of

---

Box 2–4
Dietary Sources of Iron, Folic Acid, and Vitamin B_{12}

Iron

Iron in the diet comes from two sources. The first, heme iron, makes up about one half of the iron from animal sources. The second, nonheme iron, includes the remaining iron from animal sources and all the iron from plants, legumes, and nuts. Heme iron promotes absorption of nonheme iron from other foods when both forms are consumed at the same time. Absorption of nonheme iron is enhanced by vitamin C and is inhibited by tea and coffee.

Sources of Heme Iron

- Beef
- Chicken
- Egg yolk
- Clams, oysters
- Pork loin
- Turkey
- Veal

Sources of Nonheme Iron

- Bran flakes
- Brown rice
- Whole-grain breads
- Dried beans
- Dried fruits
- Greens
- Oatmeal

Sources of Folic Acid

- Green leafy vegetables
- Broccoli
- Organ meats
- Eggs
- Wheat germ
- Asparagus
- Milk
- Yeast
- Kidney beans

Sources of Vitamin B_{12}

- Liver
- Fresh shrimp and oysters
- Eggs
- Milk
- Kidney
- Meats (muscle)
- Cheese

Clinical Manifestations and Therapies
Anemia

ETIOLOGY	CLINICAL MANIFESTATIONS	CLINICAL THERAPIES
Iron deficiency anemia ■ Dietary deficiencies: Vegetarian diet Inadequate protein intake ■ Decreased absorption: Partial or total gastrectomy Chronic diarrhea Malabsorption syndromes ■ Increased metabolic requirements: Pregnancy Lactation ■ Blood loss: Gastrointestinal bleeding (especially caused by ulcers or chronic aspirin use) Menorrhagia ■ Chronic hemoglobinuria	■ Onset is usually insidious (manifested slowly over a period of time); early signs and symptoms may include headache, pallor, lethargy, fatigue, shortness of breath, and intolerance of cold temperatures. ■ Late manifestations may include pica, glossitis (inflamed tongue), stomach irritation, and cheilosis (cracks at the corners of the mouth).	■ Increased dietary intake of iron-rich foods ■ Oral or parenteral iron supplements
Vitamin B_{12} deficiency	■ Onset is usually insidious; signs and symptoms include nausea; anorexia; swollen, sore tongue; and skin discoloration (hyperpigmentation) of the hands and knuckles. ■ Neurologic symptoms may include diminished reflexes, confusion, memory loss, gait disturbances, and peripheral neuropathy.	■ Increased dietary intake of foods containing vitamin B_{12} (e.g., meats, eggs, dairy products) ■ Oral or parenteral vitamin B_{12} supplements ■ Parenteral vitamin B_{12} for deficiency caused by malabsorption or lack of intrinsic factor
Folic acid deficiency	■ Onset is usually insidious; signs and symptoms include pallor, progressive weakness and fatigue, shortness of breath, and heart palpitations, as well as manifestations similar to those associated with vitamin B_{12} anemia, such as glossitis and cheilosis.	■ Increased dietary intake of foods rich in folic acid (folate) ■ Oral folic acid supplements ■ Folic acid supplements recommended for women who are pregnant or may become pregnant in order to prevent neural tube defects
Sickle cell disease	■ General symptoms include moderate to severe lethargy and pain (due to vascular occlusion). ■ Reduced tissue oxygenation and blood stagnation can lead to altered levels of consciousness. ■ Sickle cell crisis is marked by trapping of sickled RBCs in the spleen and subsequent splenomegaly; reduced or absent RBC production by bone marrow leading to severe decrease in hemoglobin; and rarely, hyperhemolytic crisis, which manifests as an extreme increase in RBC destruction. ■ Acute chest syndrome leads to an increase in hemoglobin sickling, which exacerbates hypoxia and can be life-threatening.	■ Primarily supportive treatment ■ Hydroxyurea ■ *Sickle cell crisis:* Rest Oxygen therapy Narcotic analgesia Vigorous hydration Treatment of precipitating factors ■ *Acute chest syndrome:* Careful hydration; hemodynamic monitoring Oxygen therapy Transfusion Folic acid supplements ■ Blood transfusions during surgery or pregnancy as necessary ■ Genetic counseling recommended

Clinical Manifestations and Therapies (continued)

ETIOLOGY	CLINICAL MANIFESTATIONS	CLINICAL THERAPIES
Thalassemia	▪ General symptoms include mild to moderate anemia, mild splenomegaly, bronze skin coloring, and bone marrow hyperplasia. ▪ Thalassemia major produces severe anemia, heart failure, and liver and spleen enlargement from increased RBC destruction. ▪ Fractures of the long bones, ribs, and vertebrae may occur. ▪ Accumulation of iron in the heart, liver, and pancreas following repeated transfusions for treatment may eventually cause failure of these organs.	▪ Regular blood transfusions ▪ Folic acid supplements ▪ Possible splenectomy ▪ Genetic counseling
Aplastic anemia	▪ Onset of manifestations may be insidious or sudden and include fatigue, pallor, progressive weakness, exertional dyspnea, headache, and ultimately tachycardia and heart failure. ▪ Initial symptoms may include bleeding gums, excessive bruising, and nosebleeds. ▪ Deficiency of WBCs increases the risk of infection, causing manifestations such as sore throat and fever.	▪ Withdrawal of the causative agent, if known ▪ Blood transfusions ▪ Bone marrow transplantation as indicated

issues related to the blood itself, while infants, children, adolescents, and pregnant women have the highest risk for developing anemia related to nutritional deficiency (Abbaspour, Hurrell, & Kelishadi, 2014). Older adults are also at risk for the development of anemia; however, it is caused by multiple factors.

Anemia in Neonates

Neonatal anemia may be caused by blood loss, hemolysis/erythrocyte destruction, and impaired RBC production (Paul, 2013). Blood loss (hypovolemia) occurs in utero from placental bleeding (placenta previa or abruptio placentae). Intrapartum blood loss may be feto-maternal, feto-fetal, or the result of umbilical cord bleeding. Birth trauma to abdominal organs (adrenal hemorrhage) or the cranium (sublegal bleed) may produce significant blood loss, and cerebral bleeding may occur because of hypoxia.

Excessive hemolysis of RBCs is usually a result of blood group incompatibilities, but it may be caused by infections. The most common cause of impaired RBC production is a genetically transmitted deficiency in G6PD.

Physiologic anemia of the newborn occurs as a result of the normal, gradual drop in hemoglobin for the first 6–12 weeks of life. When the amount of hemoglobin decreases in term infants, the bone marrow begins production of RBCs again, and the anemia disappears.

Anemia in Infants and Children

In infancy, the body's iron requirements markedly increase between 4 and 6 months after birth. Between the ages of 1 and 6 years, the amount of iron required by the body increases again. These increases in the amount of iron required during these periods are attributed to rapid growth. If there is inadequate access to foods rich in absorbable iron during these periods of increased demand, deficiency can result (Abbaspour et al., 2014). The primary etiology of anemia in young children is nutritional deficiency due to excessive intake of milk and/or prolonged breastfeeding without adequate iron supplementation. Parents should be educated on the importance of limiting the intake of cow's milk (20 ounces/24 hours) and providing a well-balanced diet that includes iron-rich foods. Iron deficiency anemia in young children has been associated with deficits in mental and motor development, some of which are long lasting (Powers & Buchanan, 2014).

Anemia in Adolescents

Adolescents have very high requirements for iron because of their increased metabolic needs, expansion of blood volume, and increases in muscle mass (Abrams, 2016). Adolescent girls are also at risk for the development of anemia related to heavy menstrual bleeding, and regulation with hormone therapy may be necessary to control excessive blood loss (Powers & Buchanan, 2014). Both boys and girls who are underweight, malnourished, overweight, or obese appear to be at increased risk as well, with obese girls having a higher risk than obese boys (Abrams, 2016). Adolescents should be educated about the importance of including iron-rich foods in their diet.

Anemia in Pregnant Women and Women of Reproductive Age

Iron deficiency anemia represents 75% of all cases of anemia experienced in pregnancy. During pregnancy, a gain in plasma volume dilutes the RBCs and may be reflected as anemia. (Refer to the module on Reproduction for a discussion on physiologic anemia of pregnancy.) There is also a significant increase in the amount of iron required by the body due to rapid placental and fetal growth. Adverse outcomes for both mother and fetus associated with anemia during pregnancy include an increased risk of sepsis, maternal and perinatal mortality, and low birth weight. In women of reproductive age, heavy menstruation, high parity, use of an intrauterine device, and vegetarian diets are risk factors for iron deficiency anemia (Abbaspour et al., 2014). Nutritional counseling and education related to the inclusion of iron-rich foods are beneficial.

Anemia in Older Adults

Anemia can be a significant problem in older adults, and identifying the cause is essential. The most common causes of anemia in older adults include iron deficiency, chronic disease or inflammation, and chronic kidney disease (Artz, 2015). The normal effects of aging, such as the decreasing ability of the bone marrow to respond to the body's signals to increase blood cell production, can also play a role in the development of anemia. Medications can have a myelosuppressive effect on the bone marrow, another factor that can result in the development of anemia.

The bodies of older adults who develop anemia cannot adapt as well as those of younger individuals, and older adults can display symptoms of fatigue, dyspnea, and confusion more easily. In addition, the prevalence of anemia in older adults who have chronic disease is even greater, and those with existing renal or cardiac disease have an increased mortality risk if they are anemic. Anemia is more common in older Black adults than in other races and ethnicities. Older adults with anemia have been found to have increased mortality, increased difficulty with mobility, increased hospitalizations, and a decrease in their ADLs (Artz, 2015). Education regarding the importance of including iron-rich foods in their diet can benefit older adults, as can referral to community services such as Meals on Wheels.

NURSING PROCESS

Nursing care includes screening patients at risk for anemia to promote early intervention and to prevent complications. Acute exacerbations and crises related to anemia warrant emergent care, such as oxygen administration and administration of IV fluid, as described earlier in this exemplar.

Long-term care for patients with anemia centers on prevention of complications and optimization of health and wellness. Patient teaching is directed toward self-care and will often include dietary counseling.

Assessment

Assessment data to collect for patients with suspected anemia include the following:

- **Observation and patient interview.** Observe the patient for pallor of the skin and mucous membranes, cheilosis, obvious bruising or bleeding, loss of balance, or dyspnea on exertion. Ask whether the patient has experienced any shortness of breath with activity, fatigue, weakness, dizziness or fainting, or palpitations. Ask about the patient's history of anemia or bleeding episodes, menstrual history (if appropriate), medications, chronic diseases, usual diet, and patterns of alcohol intake or cigarette smoking.

- **Physical examination.** The physical assessment should include general appearance; vital signs, including temperature; skin color; mucous membranes; heart and lung sounds; peripheral pulses; capillary refill; abdominal tenderness; and signs of obvious bleeding or bruising.

Diagnosis

Anemia affects circulating oxygen levels and tissue oxygenation. Priority nursing diagnoses include the following:

- *Gas Exchange, Impaired*
- *Decreased Cardiac Output, Risk for*
- *Ineffective Cerebral Tissue Perfusion, Risk for*
- *Pain, Acute*
- *Fatigue*
- *Activity Intolerance*
- *Self-Neglect.*

(NANDA-I © 2014)

Planning

Treatment goals may include the following:

- The patient will report an absence of dyspnea.

- The patient will verbalize awareness of signs and symptoms associated with exacerbations of conditions related to anemia.

- The patient will describe a plan for balancing activity with rest.

- The patient will make appropriate dietary choices to increase iron intake.

- The patient will demonstrate appropriate self-administration of supplements.

- The patient's RBC count (or hemoglobin) will be maintained within a specified acceptable range.

Implementation

Nursing implementation for the patient with anemia is directed toward minimizing the impact of the symptoms while promoting resolution of the condition. While management of life-threatening physiologic needs always takes priority over pain management, treatment of pain remains a priority concern. Analgesics should be administered as ordered, preferably using a routine schedule of administration in order to maintain a consistent level of pain control. Patient preferences, culture, and specific symptoms must all be considered before implementing care.

Promote Optimal Cardiorespiratory Function

Cardiac output may be affected by acute bleeding and volume loss or by heart failure resulting from severe anemia. Impaired tissue oxygenation leads to an increased respiratory rate and dyspnea. Weakness, fatigue, and/or vertigo may occur even during ADLs, including those associated with self-care, home life, job performance, and social roles. See the Patient Teaching feature for strategies to help the patient conserve energy and improve performance of necessary or desired activities.

- Monitor vital signs, breath sounds, and apical pulse. Increased cardiac workload can affect the blood pressure, heart, and respiratory rates. Increased blood flow can lead to heart murmur or abnormal heart sounds, such as S_3 or S_4. Tachypnea and dyspnea may affect the depth of respirations, alveolar ventilation, and blood and tissue oxygenation.

- Assess the patient for pallor, cyanosis, and dependent edema. Blood is shunted to the vital organs, causing vasoconstriction of skin vessels. This, in addition to lower levels of hemoglobin, causes pallor. Cyanosis, especially of the lips and nail beds, indicates inadequate oxygenation of blood. Dependent edema occurs in response to right ventricular failure.

- Closely monitor the patient for manifestations of anaphylaxis (e.g., urticaria, erythema or flushing, edema, wheezing, dyspnea, nausea and vomiting, anxiety) when administering parenteral iron preparations. Anaphylaxis, a systemic type I hypersensitivity (allergic) reaction, can lead to severe cardiopulmonary compromise, necessitating emergency measures to preserve life. Should signs and symptoms of anaphylaxis develop, discontinue administration of the iron and immediately notify the physician. Continuously monitor the patient and prepare to administer medications such as diphenhydramine (Benadryl) or epinephrine, as ordered. Institute cardiopulmonary resuscitation measures as necessary.

Facilitate Enhanced Self-Care

Glossitis (inflammation of the tongue that may cause the tongue and lips to turn red) and cheilosis (fissures or cracks at the corners of the mouth) may occur with nutritional deficiencies of iron, folate, and vitamin B_{12}. Patient education should include the following recommendations:

- Monitor the condition of the lips and tongue daily. Glossitis and cheilosis increase the risk for bleeding and infection and may require medical treatment. Pain and discomfort may interfere with oral intake, further worsening the nutritional deficiency.

- Use a mouthwash of saline, saltwater, or half-strength peroxide and water to rinse the mouth every 2–4 hours.

Patient Teaching
Energy Supply and Demand

- Work with the patient and family to identify alternative ways of performing tasks. For example, sitting when performing hygiene care and kitchen tasks may reduce oxygen demands. Assistance from others may be necessary to conserve energy and reduce symptoms.

- Help the patient and family establish priorities for tasks and activities. Because family members may need to assume responsibility for additional tasks, the plan's success depends on mutually established goals.

- Assist the patient to develop a schedule of alternating periods of activity and rest throughout the day. Rest periods decrease oxygen needs, reducing strain on the heart and lungs and allowing restoration of homeostasis before further activities.

- Encourage 8–10 hours of sleep at night. Rest decreases oxygen demands and increases available energy for morning activities.

- Instruct the patient not to smoke. Smoking causes vasoconstriction and increases carbon monoxide levels in the blood, interfering with tissue oxygenation.

- Teach the patient or family members to monitor vital signs before and after activity. These provide a measure of activity tolerance. Increased heart and respiratory rates or a change in blood pressure may indicate intolerance of the activity.

- Ensure that the patient understands that chest pain, breathlessness, or vertigo; palpitations or tachycardia that does not return to normal within 4 minutes of resting; bradycardia; tachypnea or dyspnea; and/or decreased systolic blood pressure changes may signify cardiac decompensation resulting from insufficient oxygenation. The patient should discontinue the activity and reduce the intensity, duration, or frequency of the activity.

This cleanses and soothes oral mucous membranes. Alcohol-based mouthwashes further irritate and dry oral tissues and should be avoided.

- Provide frequent oral hygiene (after each meal and at bedtime) with a soft bristle toothbrush or sponge. A soft toothbrush reduces irritation or bleeding of oral mucosa. Keeping the oral cavity clean also reduces the risk of infection.

- Apply a petroleum-based lubricating jelly or ointment to the lips after oral care to help retain moisture and protect the lips from other drying agents.

- Encourage soft, cool, bland foods to promote comfort and help maintain adequate food and fluid intake. Instruct the patient to avoid hot, spicy, or acidic foods. Such foods may further irritate and dry mucous membranes.

- Encourage the patient to eat four to six small meals with high protein and vitamin content each day. Small, frequent meals may be better tolerated, increasing intake. Nutrient-rich meals promote healing of the mucous membranes.

SAFETY ALERT Report signs and symptoms of decreased cardiac output to the physician. Severe anemia can lead to heart failure and may be fatal.

Evaluation

Expected outcomes of nursing care include the following:

- The patient's RBC count and hemoglobin level are within normal limits.
- The patient and/or family verbalizes understanding of the treatment regimen.
- The patient consumes the recommended dietary intake of iron.
- The patient is free of side effects of iron therapy.
- The patient is active and able to maintain normal activity levels.

- The pediatric patient achieves appropriate growth and development milestones.

The nurse should educate the patient on the importance of increasing intake of iron-rich foods and taking prescribed supplements as directed. The nurse should also instruct the patient on self-monitoring for signs and symptoms associated with exacerbations of anemia such as increased fatigue, dyspnea on exertion, weakness, or dizziness. The nurse should evaluate the patient's understanding of the importance of follow-up with the healthcare provider.

Nursing Care Plan
A Patient with Folic Acid Deficiency Anemia

Sheri Matthews is a 76-year-old widow who lives alone. Mrs. Matthews visits her primary care physician for evaluation of her decreased energy level. In particular, Mrs. Matthews complains that she does not have "enough energy to clean the house anymore." She also reports shortness of breath when she vacuums. When asked about her current diet, Mrs. Matthews tells Lisa Apana, RN, the nurse in her care provider's office, that she liked to cook when her husband was alive, but preparing an entire meal just for herself seems senseless. She relates that her typical day's menu includes coffee for breakfast; a bologna sandwich and coffee for lunch; and a hot dog or two, a few cookies, and a glass of milk for dinner.

ASSESSMENT

Mrs. Matthews's nursing history includes a 9-kg (20-lb) weight loss since her husband died 8 months ago. She states that she sometimes has heart palpitations and always feels weak. Physical assessment reveals the following: T 98.8°F; P 110 bpm; R 22/min; BP 90/52 mmHg. Her skin is warm, pale, and dry. Diagnostic tests indicate folic acid deficiency anemia. Mrs. Matthews is started on an oral folic acid supplement and instructed about foods containing folic acid.

DIAGNOSES

- *Activity Intolerance* related to weakness secondary to decreased tissue oxygenation
- *Imbalanced Nutrition: Less Than Body Requirements* related to lack of motivation to cook and understanding of nutritional needs, as manifested by weight loss of 20 lb and folic acid deficiency
- *Deficient Knowledge* related to lack of information about a well-balanced diet and foods containing folic acid

(NANDA-I © 2014)

PLANNING

- The patient will verbalize the importance of taking folic acid supplements and eating a balanced diet.
- The patient will gain at least 1 lb (0.45 kg) per week.
- The patient will return to her previous level of physical energy.
- The patient will consume a balanced diet, including foods containing folic acid.

IMPLEMENTATION

- Discuss foods required for a well-balanced diet as well as dietary sources of folic acid.
- Develop a dietary plan with Mrs. Matthews that includes food preferences and foods that are easy and quick to prepare.

- Discuss the importance of taking the folic acid supplement. Advise Mrs. Matthews to continue taking it even after she begins to feel better.
- Help Mrs. Matthews develop a schedule of activities that provides adequate rest and energy for cooking.

EVALUATION

Mrs. Matthews gained 1 lb (0.45 kg) during the first week of treatment. She has met with a nutritionist and has a better understanding of her nutritional needs. She states that she can prepare hot meals when she schedules a rest period before and after lunch. Ms. Apana has provided written and verbal information about the folic acid supplement and diet. Mrs. Matthews verbalizes understanding, stating, "I will continue to take the folic acid until the doctor tells me to stop. I'm beginning to enjoy cooking again, now that I have a reason to cook!" Ms. Apana contacts the local senior services representative to determine whether Mrs. Matthews is eligible to participate in the local Meals on Wheels program.

CRITICAL THINKING

1. What is the pathophysiologic basis for Mrs. Matthews's abnormal vital signs during her initial assessment?
2. Design a week's menu that includes foods high in folic acid.
3. Why was Mrs. Matthews placed on a folic acid supplement in addition to dietary modifications?
4. Why is the older adult at increased risk for developing folic acid deficiency anemia? Consider physiologic, economic, and social factors.

REVIEW Anemia

RELATE Link the Concepts and Exemplars

Linking the exemplar of anemia with the concept of development:

1. What effects will anemia have on the development of the school-age child?

2. A young woman in her fifth month of pregnancy develops severe anemia. What independent nursing interventions might you initiate to resolve this problem?

Linking the exemplar of anemia with the concept of family:

3. What nursing diagnoses does the nurse create for the mother of three who has anemia?

4. What effect will anemia have on family processes?

Linking the exemplar of anemia with the concept of perfusion:

5. How does chronic anemia eventually cause progressive cardiac enlargement and left ventricular hypertrophy?

6. Describe the relationship between anemia and tissue perfusion.

READY Go to Volume 3: Clinical Nursing Skills

REFER Go to Pearson MyLab Nursing and eText

- Additional review materials

REFLECT Apply Your Knowledge

Jessica Riley, 17 years old, is 6 months pregnant with her first child. The father of the baby has ended their relationship. Jessica tried living with her mother, but they fought constantly. Jessica has moved into her own apartment. She is working as a waitress to try to support herself and has plans to attend cosmetology school.

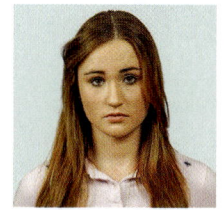

1. What preventive interventions would you plan for Jessica to reduce her risk of developing anemia?

2. How could the development of anemia affect Jessica and her fetus?

3. What nutrition counseling would you provide Jessica to reduce the risk of anemia

---

» Exemplar 2.C
Breast Cancer

Exemplar Learning Outcomes

2.C Analyze breast cancer as it relates to cellular regulation.

- Describe the pathophysiology of breast cancer.
- Describe the etiology of breast cancer.
- Compare the risk factors for and prevention of breast cancer.
- Identify the clinical manifestations of breast cancer.
- Summarize diagnostic tests and therapies used by interprofessional teams in the collaborative care of an individual with breast cancer.
- Differentiate considerations for care of patients with breast cancer across the lifespan.
- Apply the nursing process in providing culturally competent care to an individual with breast cancer.

Exemplar Key Terms

Breast cancer, *81*
Hormone therapy, *84*
Lumpectomy, *84*
Lymphedema, *84*
Metastasis, *81*
Modified radical mastectomy, *84*
Radical mastectomy, *83*
Segmental mastectomy, *84*
Simple mastectomy, *84*

Overview

Breast cancer is the unregulated growth of abnormal cells in breast tissue. It is the second most commonly occurring cancer in women (skin cancer being first) and the second leading cause of cancer-related death in women in the United States (lung cancer being first). The ACS (2016b) estimated that in the United States, more than 249,000 individuals would be diagnosed with breast cancer in 2016; approximately 246,600 would be women, and approximately 2600 would be men. More women (40,450) than men (440) were expected to die from breast cancer in 2016. In the United States, breast cancer is more prevalent among Caucasian/White women than women of African American/Black, Hispanic/Latina, American Indian/Alaska Native, or Asian/Pacific Islander heritage (CDC, 2015c; NCI, 2012b).

Pathophysiology and Etiology
Pathophysiology

Cancer of the breast begins as a single, transformed cell and is often hormone dependent. These cancers are classified as noninvasive (in situ) or invasive, depending on the penetration of the tumor into surrounding tissue. Breast cancer may remain a noninvasive disease or an invasive disease without **metastasis** (spreading to other organs) for long periods of time.

Breast cancer may be categorized as carcinoma of the mammary ducts, carcinoma of mammary lobules, or sarcoma of the breast. Most breast cancers are adenocarcinomas and appear to arise in the terminal section of the breast ductal tissue. There are many histologic types of breast cancer;

TABLE 2–7 Staging of Breast Cancer

Stage	Tumor	Node	Metastasis
Stage 0	Tis—Carcinoma in situ or Paget disease of the nipple	N0—No regional lymph node metastasis	M0—No evidence of distant metastasis
Stage I	T1—Tumor no larger than 2 cm	N0	M0
Stage IIA	T0–T1—No evidence of primary tumor	N1—Metastasis to movable ipsilateral axillary nodes	M0
	T2—Tumor no larger than 5 cm	N0	M0
Stage IIB	T2	N1	M0
	T3—Tumor larger than 5 cm	N0	M0
Stage IIIA	T0, T1, T2	N2—Metastasis to ipsilateral fixed axillary nodes	M0
	T3	N1–N2	M0
Stage IIIB	T4—Tumor of any size with direct extension to chest wall or skin	N0–N2	M0
	Any T	N3—Metastasis to ipsilateral internal mammary lymph nodes	M0
Stage IV	Any T	Any N	M1—Distant metastasis

only some examples are described here. The most common type is infiltrating ductal carcinoma. Two atypical types of breast cancer are inflammatory carcinoma and Paget disease. Inflammatory carcinoma of the breast, a systemic disease, is the most malignant form of breast cancer. Edema with skin dimpling that resembles an orange peel (peau d'orange) is usually present. Paget disease is a rare type of breast cancer involving infiltration of the nipple epithelium.

Breast cancer can metastasize to other sites through the bloodstream or lymphatic system. The common sites of metastasis of breast cancer are bone, brain, lung, liver, skin, and lymph nodes. The staging of the breast cancer provides important information for making decisions about treatment options and is also used as a basis for prognosis (see **Table 2–7 》》**).

Etiology

Possible causes of breast cancer include environmental, hormonal, reproductive, and hereditary factors. Two breast cancer susceptibility genes have been identified: *BRCA1* on chromosome 17 and *BRCA2* on chromosome 13. Both belong to a group of genes known as tumor suppressors (NCI, 2015e). These genes may be responsible for approximately 20–25% of cases of hereditary breast cancer, and approximately 5–10% of all breast cancer in women. Research also suggests that there are undiscovered breast cancer genes that may be unique to African Americans (Donovan, 2015).

Risk Factors

Some risk factors for breast cancer can be changed, and some cannot. Nonmodifiable risk factors are as follows:

- *Age and gender.* Women are much more likely to have breast cancer than men, and the risk increases with age.
- *Genetic risk factors.* Compared to a woman who does not have an undesirable genetic mutation, a woman with

identified harmful mutations in *BRCA1* or *BRCA2* suppression is 5 times more likely to develop breast cancer and also has an increased risk for ovarian cancer (NCI, 2015e). These mutations may also cause breast cancer in men.

- *Family history of breast cancer.* Having a first-degree relative (parent, sibling, or child) with breast cancer increases an individual's risk for development of breast cancer. Having a male family member with breast cancer also poses an increased risk.
- *Personal history of breast cancer.* A woman with cancer in one breast has an increased risk for developing a new cancer in the other breast or in a different part of the same breast.
- *Previous chest irradiation.* Radiation of the chest as a child or young woman for other cancer (e.g., Hodgkin disease) significantly increases the risk of breast cancer.
- *Menstrual history.* Women who begin menstruating before the age of 12 or who have menopause after the age of 55 may be at a higher risk (ACS, 2016b; NCI, 2012b).

Modifiable factors that are associated with risk for breast cancer include using oral contraceptives, not having children or having them after the age of 30, using hormone replacement therapy for more than 5 years, not breastfeeding, drinking alcohol, obesity, high-fat diets, physical inactivity, and (possibly) environmental pollution. Breastfeeding, moderate or vigorous physical activity, and maintaining a healthy body weight lower an individual's risk for breast cancer.

Prevention

Prevention of breast cancer essentially involves actively limiting exposure to risk factors linked to its development. For example, because alcohol use is a known risk factor, recommendations include limiting alcohol intake to a maximum of one drink per day. Maintaining body weight within normal limits and engaging in physical activity can also reduce the risk for developing breast cancer. Recommendations also include refraining from smoking, avoiding exposure to environmental pollution and radiation, and limiting hormone therapy in terms of both duration and dose (Mayo Clinic, 2016b).

Although early detection cannot prevent breast cancer, it is essential to reducing the patient's risk for mortality and promoting positive patient outcomes. Early detection begins with monthly breast self-examinations, which women should do 3–5 days after their period starts. Postmenopausal women should conduct self-examinations on the same day each month (MedlinePlus, 2015). The nurse's role in patient self-examinations is to assess and encourage patients to do them and to provide instructions as necessary.

>> **Stay Current:** For information on breast self-examinations, go to the National Institute of Health's website at http://www.nlm.nih.gov/medlineplus/ency/article/001993.htm.

Clinical Manifestations

The manifestations of breast cancer may include a nontender lump in the breast (most often in the upper outer quadrant, the area with the most glandular tissue), abnormal nipple discharge, a rash around the nipple area, nipple retraction, dimpling of the skin, or a change in the position of the nipple. There may also be nipple pain, scaliness, ulceration, skin irritation, or discharge. Breast cancer is usually painless, but some women report a burning or stinging sensation. Many patients with breast cancer have no manifestations, and their tumors are detected by mammography. However, most breast cancers are found by the women themselves during breast self-examination or by their partners during sexual activity.

>> Go to **Pearson MyLab Nursing and eText** to Appendix B for details about mammography.

Collaboration

Palpation of a mass on self-examination or appearance of a mass on mammography may be the first indicator of breast cancer. Any palpable mass requires evaluation. Clinical examination and mammography begin the process of diagnosis. Once the diagnosis is made, a number of treatment options are available. The choice of treatment depends on several factors, such as the stage of the cancer, the age of the patient, and the patient's preferences.

Diagnostic Tests

Although clinical examination and mammography both are valuable screening tools, mammography can buy the patient precious time. Tumors may be present as many as 8–10 years before they can be detected by palpation, and mammography can detect a tumor up to 2 years before it reaches palpable size.

Although some research has cast doubt on the ability of screening mammography to improve mortality rates for women under the age of 60 (Miller et al., 2014), the ACS recommends annual mammograms beginning at age 45 and either annually or biannually beginning at age 55 (ACS, 2015c).

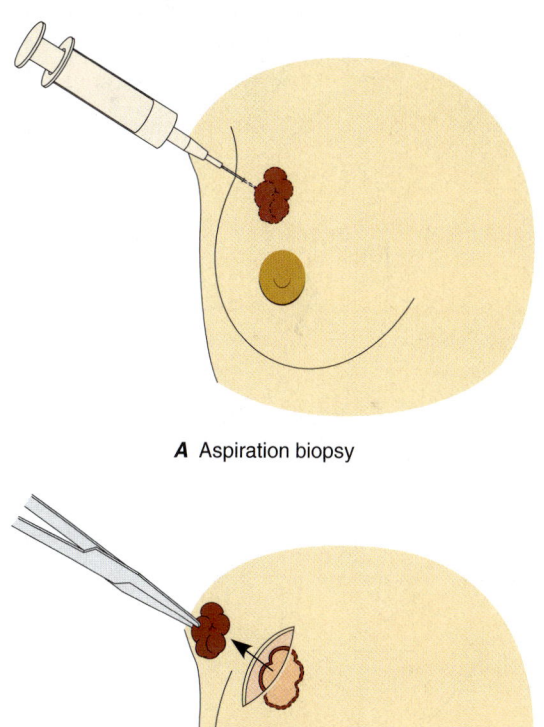

A Aspiration biopsy

B Excisional biopsy

Figure 2–8 >> Types of breast biopsy. **A,** In an aspiration biopsy, a needle is used to aspirate fluid or tissue from the breast. **B,** In an excisional biopsy, tissue from the breast lesion is removed surgically.

Education should emphasize the benefits and limitations of breast self-examination as well as the importance of immediately reporting any changes of symptoms to the healthcare provider.

Other diagnostic tests include a percutaneous needle biopsy (to define a cystic mass or fibrocystic changes and provide specimens for cytologic examination) and a breast biopsy once a suspicious lump is identified. In aspiration biopsy or fine-needle aspiration biopsy, a needle is used to remove cells or fluid from the breast lesion (see **Figure 2–8** >>). In many facilities, fine-needle aspiration biopsies are performed using a stereotactic biopsy device; mammography and a computer are used to guide the needle.

Surgery

Until recently, the treatment of choice for breast cancer was a radical mastectomy. The trend now is toward more conservative surgery combined with chemotherapy, hormone therapy, or radiation, depending on the stage of the tumor and the age of the patient.

Mastectomy

Various types of mastectomy surgeries are used to treat breast cancer (**Figure 2–9** >>). **Radical mastectomy** is the

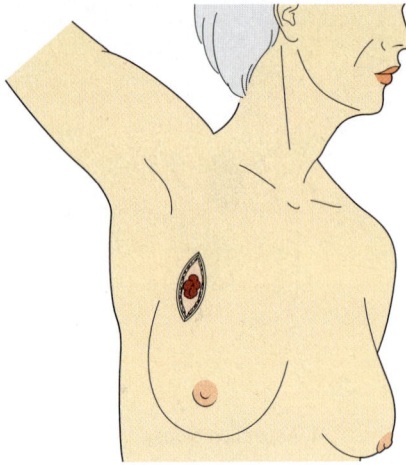

A Lumpectomy

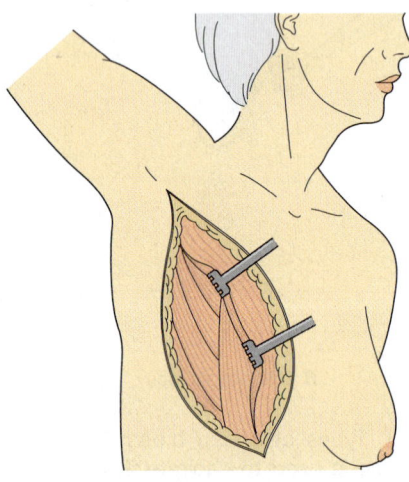

B Modified radical mastectomy

Figure 2–9 ›› Types of mastectomy. *A,* In a lumpectomy, only the tumor and a small margin of surrounding tissue are removed. *B,* In a modified radical mastectomy, all breast tissue and the underarm lymph nodes are removed, but the underlying muscles remain.

removal of the entire affected breast, the underlying chest muscles, and the lymph nodes under the arms. **Simple mastectomy** is the removal of the complete breast only. **Segmental mastectomy** (also referred to as breast conservation surgery or lumpectomy) is the removal of the tumor and the surrounding margin of breast tissues (see Figure 2–9*A*). **Modified radical mastectomy** is the removal of the breast tissue and lymph nodes under the arm (axillary node dissection), leaving the chest wall muscles intact (see Figure 2–9*B*).

Axillary node dissection is generally performed during surgery for all invasive breast carcinoma to stage the tumor. Because this surgery can cause **lymphedema** (accumulation of fluid in the soft tissues of the arm caused by removal of lymph channels), nerve damage, and adhesions, and because of the role the lymph nodes play in immune system function, nonsurgical methods of detecting lymph node involvement now are being used. A sentinel node biopsy is performed before a node dissection by injecting a radioactive substance or dye into the region of the tumor. The dye is carried to the first (sentinel) lymph node, which is the first node to receive lymph from the tumor and is therefore the most likely to contain cancer cells (if the cancer has metastasized). If the sentinel node is positive, more nodes are removed. If the sentinel node is negative, further node evaluation is usually not indicated.

Lumpectomy

Breast conservation surgery (**lumpectomy**) may be defined as excision of the primary tumor and adjacent breast tissue followed by radiation therapy. Many women are candidates for this procedure; however, some women, such as those who have multicentric breast neoplasms and those who have large tumors in relation to their breast size, are unsuitable candidates. Selection of patients for lumpectomy is guided by the need for local control of the lesion, cosmetic results, and personal preference. In men with breast cancer, lumpectomy may be an option, but because men have a relatively small amount of breast tissue, the whole breast is usually removed (ACS, 2014f).

Breast Reconstruction

After a mastectomy, some women may choose to have their breast reconstructed. They report that surgical reconstruction of the breast simplifies their lives and restores a sense of body integrity. Other women choose to use a removable breast prosthesis, and some women are comfortable without reconstruction or a prosthesis.

Breast reconstruction may be performed at the time of the mastectomy or at any time thereafter, depending on the woman's preference. A number of procedures may be used to reconstruct a breast (see **Figure 2–10** ››). These include placement of a submuscular implant, use of a tissue expander followed by an implant, transposition of muscle and blood supply from the abdomen or back, or (most often) use of a transverse rectus abdominis myocutaneous (TRAM) free-tissue flap.

›› **Stay Current:** Learn about the latest techniques for breast reconstruction at the NCI's website: http://www.cancer.gov/types/breast/reconstruction-fact-sheet.

Pharmacologic Therapy

Hormone therapy is often used in the treatment of individuals with breast cancer. One of the most commonly used hormone therapy drugs is tamoxifen citrate (Nolvadex). Tamoxifen is a selective estrogen receptor modulator (SERM). It works by preventing estrogen from attaching to estrogen receptors on the cancer cells, which inhibits tumor growth and ultimately kills tumor cells (Mayo Clinic, 2015b). It is used to treat advanced breast cancer, as an adjuvant for early-stage breast cancer, and as a preventive treatment in women at high risk for developing breast cancer. Aromatase inhibitors are another type of hormone therapy used to treat breast cancer. They block the action of an enzyme that converts androgens into estrogen. Anastrozole (Arimidex) is the aromatase inhibitor used as first line treatment in postmenopausal women (Breastcancer.org, 2016b; Mayo Clinic, 2015b). Hormone therapy may be used in treating breast cancer in men, but there is little research on its effectiveness. The best-studied drug in men is tamoxifen (ACS, 2014g).

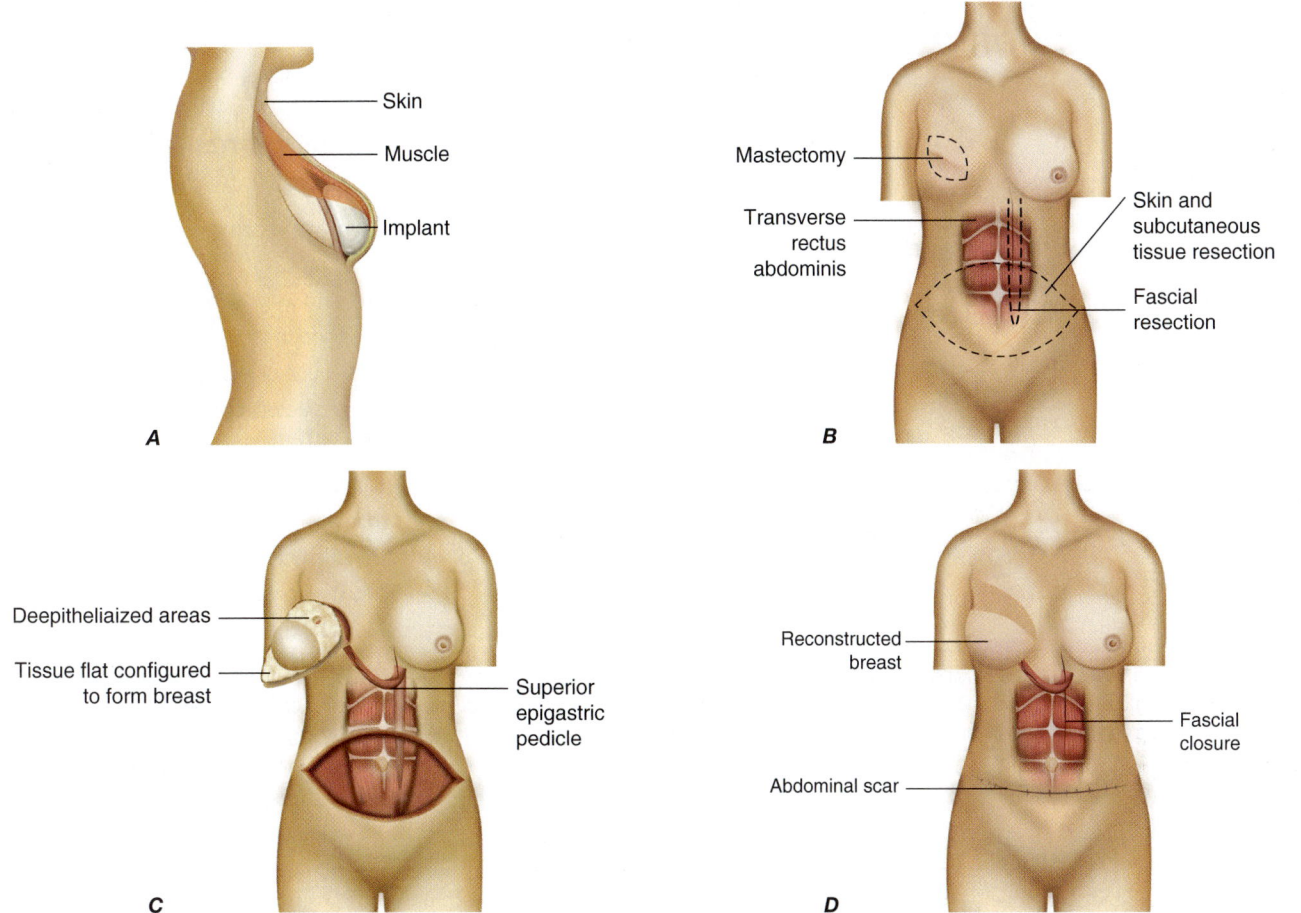

Skin
Muscle
Implant

A

Mastectomy
Transverse rectus abdominis
Skin and subcutaneous tissue resection
Fascial resection

B

Deepitheliaized areas
Tissue flat configured to form breast
Superior epigastric pedicle

C

Reconstructed breast
Fascial closure
Abdominal scar

D

Figure 2–10 ⟫ Types of breast reconstruction surgeries. **A,** A breast implant is inserted under the pectoris muscle. **B,** In an autogenous procedure, a flap of skin, muscle, and fat from the donor site on the woman's body is transferred to the mastectomy site (**C** and **D**). The most frequently used donor muscle sites are the latissimus dorsi and the rectus abdominis (the TRAM flap).

Targeted drugs may be used to counteract specific genetic mutations that promote cancer growth. For example, trastuzumab (Herceptin) is used to stop the growth of breast tumors that express the HER2/neu receptor (which binds an EGFR that contributes to cancer cell growth) on their cell surface. This drug is a recombinant DNA-derived monoclonal antibody that binds to the receptor, inhibiting tumor cell proliferation.

Chemotherapy has become the standard of care for the majority of breast cancer cases with axillary node involvement. In late metastatic disease, chemotherapy becomes the primary treatment to prolong the patient's life. Adjuvant (additional) systemic therapy following primary treatment for early-stage breast cancer refers to the administration of chemotherapy and other pharmacologic agents. This type of therapy has been widely studied; its use reduces both the rate of recurrence and the rate of death from breast cancer. For example, the drug bevacizumab, when combined with chemotherapy to treat metastatic breast cancer, has extended cancer-free survival; letrozole (an aromatase inhibitor) has reduced the risk of recurrence after surgery (in some cases more effectively than tamoxifen).

Radiation Therapy

Radiation therapy typically follows breast cancer surgery to destroy any remaining cancer cells that could cause recurrence or metastasis. If a tumor is unusually large, radiation may be used to shrink the tumor before surgery. Radiation therapy is most commonly used in combination with lumpectomy for early-stage (stage I or II) breast cancer. Palliative radiation therapy is also used to treat chest wall recurrences and some bone metastases to help control pain and prevent fractures. Radiation therapy is administered by means of an external beam or tissue implants.

Lifespan Considerations

Breast Cancer in Young Women

Approximately 11% of all new breast cancer cases affect women younger than age 45. Diagnosis and treatment can be devastating at any age; however, younger women may find it overwhelming. Breast cancer in younger women has a tendency to be more aggressive, and the survival rates are lower than those for older women. Some younger women have a higher risk for developing breast cancer than others in this same age group. These risk factors include having a close relative such as a parent, sibling, or child diagnosed with breast or ovarian cancer prior to age 45 or a male relative who has had breast cancer; having been treated with radiation therapy to the breast or chest during childhood or early adulthood; having changes in the *BRCA1* or *BRCA2* gene or close relatives with these changes; having other

Clinical Manifestations and Therapies
Breast Cancer

ETIOLOGY	CLINICAL MANIFESTATIONS	CLINICAL THERAPIES
Lymphedema (accumulation of fluid in the soft tissues of the arm) may occur following radical mastectomy secondary to removal of axillary lymph nodes.	▪ Swelling of the arm and hand on the side of the mastectomy ▪ May be acute, temporary, and mild if occurring immediately postoperative; acute and painful if occurring 4–6 weeks postoperative; or more commonly, chronic and painless if occurring 18–24 months after surgery	▪ Exercise ▪ Customized compression sleeve ▪ Arm pump ▪ Diet and weight control ▪ Elevation of the arm ▪ Prevention of infection ▪ Avoidance of invasive procedures on affected arm
Cachexia occurs in most patients with advanced cancer.	▪ Weight loss, fatigue, weakness, loss of strength, activity intolerance, and constipation	▪ Nutritional counseling ▪ Increased caloric intake ▪ Periods of rest and activity ▪ Monitoring weight ▪ Monitoring intake and output
Memory loss and difficulty concentrating may follow treatment with chemotherapy (sometimes referred to as chemo-brain).	▪ Memory loss, difficulty focusing on tasks, changes in mood and affect, as well as fatigue ▪ Generally lasts for 1–2 years after completing treatment	▪ Warning patients in advance of possible occurrence, because it can be very frightening to patients ▪ Recommending use of memory aids (e.g., making notes) ▪ Providing emotional support to patients

breast health problems (atypical ductal or lobular hyperplasia); and having the presence of dense breast tissue appear in a mammogram (CDC, 2015d).

Breast Cancer in Older Women

The incidence of breast cancer in the United States is greatest in women ages 75–79. This population requires a multifaceted treatment approach, as there are many factors to consider. Upon diagnosis, the functional level and overall health status of the patient must be assessed as well as knowledge of the disease, resources, and level of support. The impact that the treatment will have on the patient's quality of life should also be a consideration.

For too long, mastectomy was perceived as the only treatment option open to most older women with breast cancer, even those with early-stage disease. That perception is slowly changing as breast-conservation treatment gains greater acceptance. The choice of surgical treatment, particularly for older women, is highly individual. Many older women wish to preserve their breasts.

Although older women with breast cancer may experience coexisting chronic illnesses and impaired physical function, research suggests that they show lower levels of emotional distress compared to younger women. The need for services such as personal care, shopping, housekeeping, and transportation increases as the ages of both the patient and the caregiver increase.

It can be challenging for healthcare providers not to overtreat or undertreat the older adult patient. Comorbidities and life expectancy are also factors that can affect treatment options for breast cancer. There is a need for the inclusion of older adults in cancer research trials based on the aging population and lack of evidence related to the effects of cancer treatment on the older adult (Schapira & Muss, 2013).

NURSING PROCESS

The patient diagnosed with breast cancer requires holistic care that addresses physical, psychologic, social, and spiritual needs. Careful assessment of the patient's response to therapy will improve the care planning process.

Assessment

Collect the following data through the health history and physical examination:

▪ *Observation and patient interview.* Observe the patient's overall health status and general appearance for evidence of discomfort such as facial grimacing or guarding of the affected breast. Ask whether the patient has noticed any breast changes or nipple discharge. Obtain information about family history of breast cancer, use of hormone replacement therapy, personal history of breast cancer, previous diagnostic tests and treatment for cancer, menstrual history, pregnancies, alcohol intake, physical activity, and dietary history.

▪ *Physical examination.* Assess general appearance, height, and weight. Assess the patient's heart and lung sounds, breasts, and lymph glands.

Further focused assessments are described in the Implementation section that follows.

Diagnosis

Although each patient has individual needs, nursing diagnoses relevant to the plan of care for the individual with breast cancer may include the following:

- *Infection, Risk for*
- *Injury, Risk for*
- *Pain, Acute*
- *Anxiety*
- *Decisional Conflict*
- *Grieving*
- *Body Image, Disturbed.*

(NANDA-I © 2014)

Planning

Goals for treatment may include the following:

- The patient will maintain a WBC count less than 10,000 and a normal body temperature.
- The patient will make informed treatment decisions.
- The patient will express feelings regarding diagnosis, treatment, and prognosis.
- The family and significant others will provide appropriate support for the patient.

Implementation

Nursing interventions are evidence-based strategies geared toward helping the patient meet the goals outlined in the nursing plan of care. As with all elements of the care plan, the selection and implementation of nursing interventions must be individualized and tailored to meet the individual patient's needs. Examples of nursing interventions that may be appropriate for inclusion in the plan of care for the patient with breast cancer follow.

Prevent Infection

Like any surgical patient, the patient who has breast surgery is at risk for infection. Removal of lymph nodes and the presence of a draining wound increase the risk. See Exemplar 2.A on Cancer for more information about infection prevention. To assist the patient with breast cancer in preventing infection, the nurse can implement the following interventions:

- Tell the patient to avoid deodorants and talcum powder on the affected side until the incision is completely healed. These substances may irritate the skin and impede healing.
- Assess the surgical dressings for bleeding, drainage, color, and odor every 4 hours for 24 hours, and document your findings. Circle any visible bleeding and drainage on the dressing as a baseline for subsequent assessment. Excessive bleeding or drainage signals postoperative complications that may require emergency attention.
- Observe the incision and IV sites for pain, redness, swelling, and drainage. Assess the drainage system for patency and adequate suction; note the color and amount of drainage. Careful observation for any signs of infection is essential, because the patient's immune system is

compromised. IV catheters should be placed on the uninvolved side only.

- Change dressings and IV tubing using aseptic technique. Moist dressings and IV tubing provide sites for bacterial growth. Routine dressing and IV tubing changes using aseptic technique reduce the risk for infection.
- Teach the patient how to care for the drainage system, if present (i.e., clean the site; empty the device; and record the amount, color, and type of drainage). The patient is often discharged before removal of the drainage system and dressings and needs instruction to provide self-care.
- At discharge, teach the patient to watch for and report to the healthcare provider the manifestations of infection: fever, redness or hardness at the surgical site, or purulent drainage. Any of these manifestations should be reported to the physician or surgeon.

Promote Optimal Circulation

Removal of the lymph nodes puts the patient at risk for injury and long-term complications, such as lymphedema and infection.

- Encourage range-of-motion exercises in the affected arm. Exercise helps develop collateral drainage.
- Explain that lymphedema massage and an elastic compression bandage may help control the swelling after the patient has recovered from surgery.
- When obtaining blood pressure and starting IVs, use the nonsurgical side. Compression of the arm on the surgical side may cause lymphedema.
- Elevate the affected arm higher than the shoulder on a pillow, but do not abduct it. The hand should be higher than the elbow. Elevating the arm permits drainage, prevents swelling, and promotes circulation.

Promote a Healthy Body Image

Breast surgery can change the patient's body image. The surgical changes may be compounded by weight gain and other side effects of chemotherapy or hormone therapy. Self-esteem also affects adjustment to a changed body image.

- Assess the patient's current body image. Self-image is related to self-esteem. Discuss whether her self-image has changed.
- Explain that redness and swelling in the scar will fade with time. Knowledge that the scar will fade may give the woman a more realistic view of the changes.
- Encourage the patient to look at the incision when she or he feels ready; often, the reality is not as frightening as what the patient had imagined. Explain that it is normal to be afraid to look. Reassurance that the patient's behavior is normal decreases anxiety.
- Breast reconstruction options are available for women and men (NCI, 2016f). If the patient is interested in breast reconstruction, provide written material and encourage discussion with a plastic surgeon and with others who have had reconstruction. It is important for the patient to be fully knowledgeable about available options to make an informed decision. **Box 2–5** » discusses the various types of breast reconstructive surgery.

Box 2–5
Reconstructive Surgery After Breast Cancer

Breast reconstruction surgery is performed by plastic surgeons. Breast reconstruction may be performed immediately after a mastectomy (immediate reconstruction), at a later time (delayed reconstruction), or in stages (delayed-immediate reconstruction) (ACS, 2016c; Breastcancer.org, 2016a).

There are two types of breast reconstruction: those that use breast implants (saline or silicone inserts) and those that use the body's tissue (called *flap procedures*). Surgeons occasionally use both procedures to get a good result. A third type of procedure is nipple and areola reconstruction, which is performed to make the reconstructed breast look more realistic.

It is important for patients to understand that reconstructed breasts, nipples, and areolas have little to no sensation. In some patients, nipple-sparing mastectomy is possible, which preserves some sensation.

Implant reconstruction requires less surgery than flap reconstruction, but it still may require more than one procedure, and the implants will need to be replaced every 10–20 years (Breastcancer.org, 2016a). The implants are placed under the pectoral chest muscle.

Flap reconstruction (autologous reconstruction) uses tissue from another place on the patient's body to form a new breast. The skin, fat, and sometimes muscle (together called the *flap*) may come from the back, belly, buttocks, or inner thighs. The tissue may be completely separated from its original blood vessels and moved to the chest (called a *free flap*), or it may remain attached to its original blood vessels, which are moved under the skin up to the chest (called a *pedicle flap*). Flap procedures are named for the area from which the flap is taken. For example, flap procedures using tissue from the belly include DIEP (deep inferior epigastric perforator artery), TRAM (transverse rectus abdominus), and SIEA (superficial inferior epigastric artery); flaps from the back are called latissimus dorsi flaps.

Flap reconstruction surgery is more difficult to perform than implant reconstruction, is a longer surgery, and requires a longer recovery period. Flap surgery usually requires two procedures—the main procedure and a follow-up procedure to make adjustments—but flaps will usually last a lifetime.

» Stay Current: Breast reconstruction techniques are always being refined. Visit http://www.breastcancer.org to learn about all current techniques.

Evaluation

Patients are evaluated for expected outcomes based on specific patient needs and care planning. Potential outcomes may include the following:

- The patient experiences no complications resulting from treatment.
- Side effects from medications are minimized.
- Pain is managed to allow the patient to rest and perform essential ADLs.

If the patient appears to be having difficulty reaching these outcomes, the nurse can assist the patient by administering antinausea medication and ensuring that the patient is well hydrated prior to treatment, monitoring the infusion site closely for extravasation if vesicant agents are used, and administering pain medication as prescribed.

Nursing Care Plan
A Patient with Breast Cancer

Rachel Clemments is a 42-year-old mother of two: Sarah, age 12, and Jennifer, age 18. Because of a family history of breast cancer, she has been closely monitored (annual mammograms and clinical breast examination, monthly breast self-examination, a needle aspiration biopsy with negative findings) for 4 years before her diagnosis. Mrs. Clemments discovers a lump in her left breast during her monthly breast self-examination. An incisional biopsy reveals invasive lobular carcinoma in the left breast. Mrs. Clemments is debating whether to have reconstructive breast surgery. One of her greatest concerns is how her illness will affect her ability to support and care for her daughters. The breast cancer diagnosis seems part of the family legacy. She wonders, "When will it happen to Jennifer? To Sarah?"

ASSESSMENT	DIAGNOSES	PLANNING
During the history, Laura Nelson, RN, the nurse admitting Mrs. Clemments, learns that her mother, two of her aunts, and one sister were diagnosed with breast cancer. Her mother and one of the aunts died before age 45. Physical assessment findings include temperature 98.5°F oral; pulse 65 bpm; respirations 14/min; and BP 110/62 mmHg. Her weight is 54 kg (120 lb); she is 168 cm (66 in.) tall. Modified radical mastectomy is performed. Histologic examination shows a 3-cm tumor; axillary node dissection shows that 4 of 16 lymph nodes are positive.	• *Infection, Risk for*, related to surgical incision • *Pain, Acute*, related to surgery • *Body Image, Disturbed* • *Decisional Conflict* related to concerns about risks and benefits • *Fear* related to disease process/prognosis (NANDA-I © 2014)	• The patient will remain free of infection. • The patient will experience minimal pain or discomfort during her recovery. • The patient will maintain a positive body image, regardless of her decision about reconstruction. • The patient will evaluate the treatment options in relation to personal values and decide on a course of action. • The patient will identify the sources of her fear and demonstrate behaviors that may reduce fears.

Nursing Care Plan *(continued)*

IMPLEMENTATION

- Teach the patient about hand hygiene and wound care.
- Assess the patient's pain tolerance, and administer analgesics as prescribed.
- Teach the patient to use caution when moving the affected arm, to avoid lifting heavy objects, and to wear gloves when gardening.
- Encourage the patient to express thoughts and feelings. Refer to appropriate support groups if the patient is amenable.

- Assess the patient's interest in spiritual or religious support, and refer if appropriate.
- Encourage the patient to verbalize fears about her own prognosis and about her daughters' future risks for breast cancer; assess the need or interest for referral to psychologic counseling.

EVALUATION

At discharge, Mrs. Clemments has no signs of physical complications and is looking forward to being at home with her daughters as temporary caregivers. Mrs. Clemments met with a Reach to Recovery volunteer, who brought her a temporary prosthesis and booklets about postmastectomy exercises, chemotherapy, and breast reconstruction.

The volunteer also referred her to a local cancer support group. Mrs. Clemments has talked about her concerns related to breast reconstruction. "I want to avoid anything that would increase the risk of complications. The possibility of recurrence and my fear for my daughters' future health are more than enough to worry about."

CRITICAL THINKING

1. What role could genetic counseling play in helping Mrs. Clemments and her daughters better understand the daughters' risks for breast cancer?
2. Describe the types of mastectomies and their implications for nursing care.
3. What medications might help minimize the side effects of chemotherapy?
4. Develop a plan of care for Mrs. Clemments for the nursing diagnosis Disturbed Sleep Pattern.

REVIEW Breast Cancer

RELATE Link the Concepts and Exemplars

Linking the exemplar of breast cancer with the concept of advocacy:

1. How might the nurse advocate for the prevention of breast cancer or its early detection?
2. What role can the nurse play in advocating to make men more aware of the role they can play in breast cancer prevention and early detection?

Linking the exemplar of breast cancer with the concept of sexuality:

3. A patient who is preparing for a radical mastectomy says, "My husband says if I only have one breast I am only half a woman." How can you help this patient adapt to the perceived change in her femininity?
4. Is the impact on a patient's sexuality completely reversed if the patient has plastic surgery to repair the appearance of the breast? Is plastic surgery always an option? Explain your answer.

READY Go to Volume 3: Clinical Nursing Skills

REFER Go to Pearson MyLab Nursing and eText

- Additional review materials

REFLECT Apply Your Knowledge

Judy Franklin, 22 years old, has just graduated from college and is about to start a job as a graphic arts designer in a large marketing company. She is also planning her wedding, which is to take place 6 months from now. She found a lump in her left breast during self-exam and has come to the physician for an initial consultation. During the assessment, the nurse learns that Ms. Franklin has not told her fiancé about her findings. She will not make eye contact with the nurse and appears distracted during the interview.

1. What nursing diagnoses would be appropriate for Ms. Franklin?
2. How might you assist Ms. Franklin to inform her fiancé if the lump is determined to be a malignant tumor?
3. What support interventions would you initiate to help Ms. Franklin as she waits for the results of diagnostic testing to determine the cause of the lump?

≫ Exemplar 2.D Colorectal Cancer

Exemplar Learning Outcomes

2.D Analyze colorectal cancer as it relates to cellular regulation.

- Describe the pathophysiology of colorectal cancer.
- Describe the etiology of colorectal cancer.
- Compare the risk factors for and prevention of colorectal cancer.
- Identify the clinical manifestations of colorectal cancer.
- Summarize diagnostic tests and therapies used by interprofessional teams in the collaborative care of an individual with colorectal cancer.

- Differentiate considerations for care of patients with colorectal cancer across the lifespan.
- Apply the nursing process in providing culturally competent care to an individual with colorectal cancer.

Overview

Colon cancer is cancer of the third segment of the large bowel and may or may not include the anus. **Colorectal cancer** involves both the colon and the rectum. Although the terms are often used interchangeably, they differ in terms of whether the rectum is involved.

Regular colonoscopies can greatly reduce the risk for colorectal cancer by allowing removal of polyps before they become malignant tumors that invade the bowel and metastasize to other areas of the body. The nurse's role focuses on promoting the need for regular screening as well as reporting the early warning signs of the disease in order to reduce occurrence and improve outcomes.

Pathophysiology and Etiology

Pathophysiology

Nearly all colorectal cancers are adenocarcinomas that begin as adenomatous **polyps** (small vascular growths on the surface of any mucous membrane, referring in this exemplar to growths on the internal surface of the bowel). Most tumors develop in the rectum and sigmoid colon, although any portion of the colon may be affected (see **Figure 2–11 》**).

The tumor typically grows undetected, producing few manifestations. By the time manifestations occur, the disease may have spread into deeper layers of the bowel tissue and adjacent organs. Colorectal cancer spreads by direct extension to involve the entire bowel circumference, the submucosa, and outer bowel wall layers. Neighboring structures, such as the liver, greater curvature of the stomach, duodenum, small intestine, pancreas, spleen, genitourinary tract, and abdominal wall, also may be involved by direct extension.

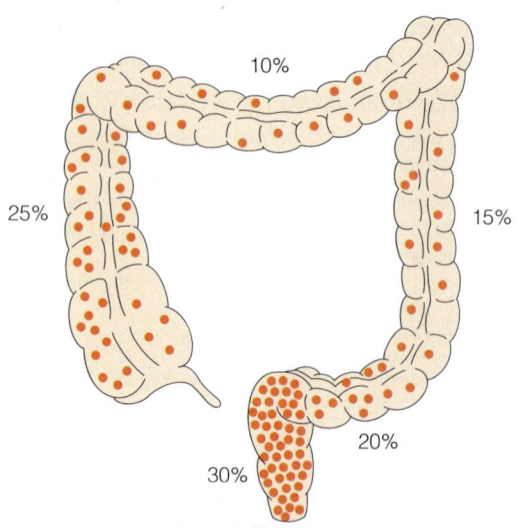

Figure 2–11 》 The distribution and frequency of cancer of the colon and rectum.

Exemplar Key Terms

Colon cancer, *90*
Colorectal cancer, *90*
Colostomy, *92*
Fulguration, *92*
Polyps, *90*

Metastasis to regional lymph nodes is the most common form of tumor spread. This is not always an orderly process; distal nodes may contain cancer cells while regional nodes remain normal. Cancerous cells from the primary tumor may also spread by way of the lymphatic system or circulatory system to secondary sites, such as the liver, lungs, brain, bones, and kidneys. In addition, "seeding" of the tumor to other areas of the peritoneal cavity can occur when the tumor extends through the serosa or during surgical resection.

Current staging methods primarily use the TNM system, as outlined in **Table 2–8 》**.

Etiology

Colorectal cancer (cancer of the colon or rectum) is the third most common cancer diagnosed in the United States. The ACS (2016b) estimated that in 2016, more than 95,000 new cases of colon cancer and more than 39,000 new cases of rectal cancer were diagnosed in the United States.

The incidence of colorectal cancer, which is slightly higher among men than among women (ACS, 2016b), has been declining in the United States for the past several decades (Welch & Robertson, 2016). Earlier diagnosis and improved treatment are credited with increasing the survival rate. Colorectal cancer occurs most frequently after age 50. The incidence continues to rise with increasing age. With early diagnosis and treatment, the 5-year survival rate for colorectal cancer is 90%; however, only 39% of colorectal cancers are diagnosed at this early stage (ACS, 2016b).

Risk Factors

Genetic factors are strongly linked to the risk for colorectal cancer. Family history of the disease increases an individual's risk for its development (ACS, 2016b). Individuals with familial adenomatous polyposis inevitably will develop colon cancer unless the colon is removed. Hereditary nonpolyposis colorectal cancer (also known as Lynch syndrome) is an autosomal dominant disorder that significantly increases the risk for developing colorectal and other cancers. Tumors associated with Lynch syndrome often affect the ascending colon and tend to occur at an earlier age. Inflammatory bowel diseases also increase the risk of colorectal cancer. Additional risk factors include being over age 50 and previous exposure to radiation.

Diet plays a role in the development of colorectal cancer. The disease is prevalent in economically prosperous countries where people consume diets high in calories, meat proteins, and fats. This dietary pattern, common in the United States, is thought to increase the population of anaerobic bacteria in the gut. These anaerobes convert bile acids into carcinogens. Diets high in fruits and vegetables, folic acid, and calcium appear to reduce the risk of colorectal cancer. Cereal fiber, once thought to reduce colorectal cancer risk, now does not appear to play a role either way in its development. Other factors that may reduce the risk of colorectal cancer include

TABLE 2–8 The TNM Staging System for Colorectal Cancer

Stage	Primary Tumor (T)	Regional Lymph Nodes (N)	Distant Metastasis (M)
	TX—Primary tumor cannot be assessed T0—No evidence of primary tumor	NX—Regional lymph node cannot be assessed	MX—Presence of distant metastasis cannot be assessed
Stage 0	Tis—Carcinoma in situ	N0—No regional lymph node metastasis	M0—No distant metastasis
Stage I	T1—Tumor invades submucosa	N0	M0
	T2—Tumor invades muscularis propria	N0	M0
Stage IIA	T3—Tumor invades through muscularis propria into subserosa or into nonperitonealized pericolic or perirectal tissues	N0	M0
Stage IIB	T4a—Tumor perforates visceral peritoneum or directly invades other organs or structures	N0	M0
Stage IIC	T4b	N0	M0
Stage IIIA	T1–T2	N1—Metastasis in one to three pericolic or perirectal lymph nodes	M0
Stage IIIB	T3–T4a	N1–N2—Metastasis in four or more pericolic or perirectal lymph nodes	M0
Stage IIIC	T3–T4b	N1–N2b—Metastasis in any lymph node along course of a major named vascular trunk	M0
Stage IV	Any T	Any N	M1—Distant metastasis

regular exercise, taking a daily multivitamin, and the use of aspirin and other nonsteroidal anti-inflammatory drugs.

Prevention

The ACS (2016b) recommends one of the following testing schedules for early detection of colorectal cancer, beginning at age 50. These options are acceptable choices for average-risk adults:

- Yearly fecal occult blood test or fecal immunochemical test (For fecal occult blood test, the take-home, multiple-sample method should be used.)
- Stool DNA test every 3 years
- Flexible sigmoidoscopy every 5 years
- Double-contrast barium enema every 5 years

- Colonoscopy every 10 years
- CT colonography every 5 years.

Clinical Manifestations

Bowel cancer often produces no manifestations until it is advanced. Because it grows slowly, 5–15 years of growth may occur before manifestations develop. The manifestations depend on its location, type and extent, and complications.

Rectal bleeding is often the initial manifestation that prompts patients to seek medical care. Other common early manifestations include a change in bowel habits, either diarrhea or constipation. Pain, anorexia, and weight loss are characteristic in advanced disease. A palpable abdominal or rectal mass may be present. On occasion, the patient presents with anemia from occult bleeding.

Clinical Manifestations and Therapies
Colorectal Cancer

ETIOLOGY	CLINICAL MANIFESTATIONS	CLINICAL THERAPIES
Rectal bleeding may occur as the cancer cells invade or irritate the bowel mucosa.	■ Symptoms include dark color to stool, blood may or may not be visible without guaiac testing, classic alteration in smell of stools with frank blood, anemia, decreasing hemoglobin and hematocrit, and decreased RBCs. Patient is often asymptomatic unless guaiac is tested.	■ Treatment may include surgical removal of the tumor and involved segment of bowel. ■ Blood transfusions and hydration may be needed if blood loss is significant.
Change in bowel habits may occur as cancer cells grow.	■ Stools may be pencil thin as the bowel lumen diminishes. ■ Diarrhea or constipation may occur.	■ Treatment may include surgical resection of the involved bowel. ■ Antidiarrheals may be indicated if diarrhea results. ■ Monitor for signs of complete obstruction of bowel, including emesis, acute abdominal pain, or abdominal distention, accompanied by absence of stool for several days.

Collaboration

The patient with a diagnosis of colorectal cancer needs a collaborative approach, often requiring intervention from surgeons, nurses specializing in care of ostomies, dietary counselors, radiation therapists, as well as the nurse providing primary care. A holistic approach to the patient's care improves both patient outcomes and chances for survival.

Diagnostic Tests

Diagnostic and laboratory tests are used for screening, diagnosis, and monitoring purposes. Diagnostic tests include a sigmoidoscopy or colonoscopy as the primary means used to detect and visualize tumors. While flexible sigmoidoscopy can detect 50–65% of colorectal cancers, many clinicians recommend colonoscopy. Tissue for biopsy is obtained at the time of endoscopy to evaluate for cancerous tissue and cell differentiation. Current staging methods primarily use the TNM system, as outlined in Table 2–8. Radiologic examinations may include a chest x-ray to detect tumor metastasis to the lung; and CT, MRI, or ultrasonic examination may be used to assess tumor depth and involvement of other organs by direct extension or metastasis.

Laboratory tests include a fecal occult blood test (by guaiac or Hemoccult testing) to detect blood in the feces, a CBC to detect anemia resulting from chronic blood loss and tumor growth, and a CEA level, which is a tumor marker that can be detected in the blood of patients with colorectal cancer. CEA levels are used to estimate prognosis, monitor treatment, and detect cancer recurrence.

Surgery

Surgical resection of the tumor, adjacent colon, and regional lymph nodes is the treatment of choice for colorectal cancer. Options for surgical treatment vary from destruction of the tumor by laser photocoagulation performed during endoscopy to abdominoperineal resection with permanent colostomy. When possible, the anal sphincter is preserved and colostomy avoided.

Other surgical treatment options for small, localized tumors include local excision and fulguration. These procedures also may be performed during endoscopy, eliminating the need for abdominal surgery. Local excision may be used to remove a disk of rectum containing a tumor in patients with a small, well-differentiated, mobile polypoid lesion. **Fulguration**, also known as electrocoagulation, is a procedure used to reduce the size of some large tumors for patients who are poor surgical risks. Fulguration requires general anesthesia and may need to be repeated at intervals.

Most patients with colorectal cancer undergo surgical resection of the colon with anastomosis of the remaining bowel as a curative procedure. The distribution of regional lymph nodes determines the extent of resection, because they may contain metastatic lesions. Most tumors of the ascending, transverse, descending, and sigmoid colon can be resected.

Tumors of the rectum usually are treated with an abdominoperineal resection, in which the sigmoid colon, rectum, and anus are removed through both abdominal and perineal incisions. A permanent sigmoid colostomy is performed to provide for elimination of feces.

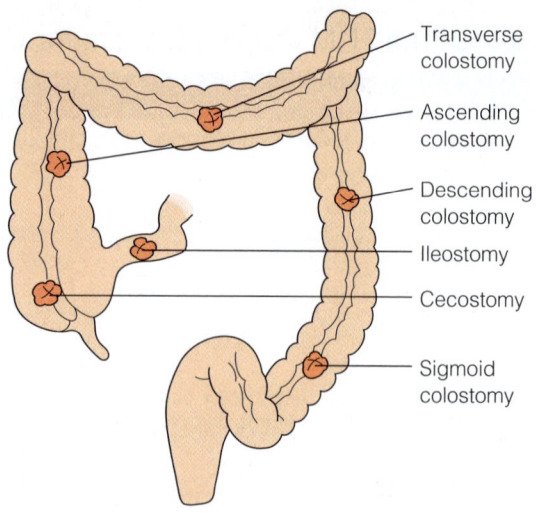

Figure 2–12 » Various ostomy levels and sites.

Colostomy

Surgical resection of the bowel may be accompanied by a colostomy for diversion of fecal contents. A **colostomy** is an ostomy made in the colon. It may be created if the bowel is obstructed by the tumor, as a temporary measure to promote healing of anastomoses, or as a permanent means of fecal evacuation when the distal colon and rectum are removed. Colostomies take the name of the portion of the colon from which they are formed: ascending colostomy, transverse colostomy, descending colostomy, and sigmoid colostomy (see **Figure 2–12 »**).

A sigmoid colostomy is the most common permanent colostomy, particularly for cancer of the rectum. It is usually created during an abdominoperineal resection. The anal canal is closed, and a stoma is formed from the proximal sigmoid colon. The stoma usually is located on the lower left quadrant of the abdomen.

When a double-barrel colostomy is performed, two separate stomas are created (see **Figure 2–13 »**). The distal colon

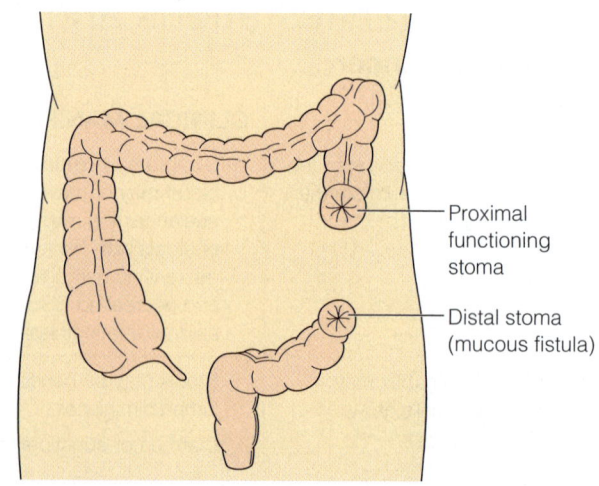

Figure 2–13 » A double-barrel colostomy. The proximal stoma is the functioning stoma; the distal stoma expels mucus from the distal colon.

is not removed, but bypassed. The proximal stoma, which is functional, diverts feces to the abdominal wall. The distal stoma, also called the mucous fistula, expels mucus from the distal colon. It may be pouched or dressed with a 4-in. × 4-in. gauze dressing. A double-barrel colostomy may be created for cases of trauma, tumor, or inflammation; it may be temporary or permanent.

An emergency procedure used to relieve an intestinal obstruction or perforation is called a transverse loop colostomy. During this procedure, a loop of the transverse colon is brought out from the abdominal wall and suspended over a plastic rod or bridge, which prevents the loop from slipping back into the abdominal cavity. The loop stoma may be opened at the time of surgery or a few days later at the patient's bedside. The bridge may be removed in 1–2 weeks. Transverse loop colostomies are typically temporary.

In a Hartmann procedure, a common temporary colostomy procedure, the distal portion of the colon is left in place and is oversewn for closure. A temporary colostomy may be done to allow bowel rest or healing, such as following tumor resection or inflammation of the bowel. It also may be created following traumatic injury to the colon, such as a gunshot wound. Anastomosis of the severed portions of the colon is delayed, because bacterial colonization of the colon would prevent proper healing of the anastomosis. Approximately 3–6 months following a temporary colostomy, the colostomy is closed, and the colon is reconnected. Patients with temporary colostomies require the same care as patients with permanent colostomies.

Laser Photocoagulation

Laser photocoagulation uses a very small, intense beam of light to generate heat in tissues toward which it is directed. The heat generated by the laser beam can be used to destroy small tumors. It is also used for palliative surgery of advanced tumors to remove obstruction. Laser photocoagulation can be performed endoscopically and is useful for patients who cannot tolerate major surgery.

Pharmacologic Therapy

Chemotherapeutic agents, such as IV fluorouracil (5-FU) and folinic acid (leucovorin), are used postoperatively as adjunctive therapy for colorectal cancer. When combined with radiation therapy, chemotherapy reduces the rate of tumor recurrence and prolongs survival for patients with stage II and stage III rectal tumors. The benefit for patients with colon cancer is less clear, but chemotherapy may be used to reduce its spread to the liver and prevent recurrence. Irinotecan (CPT-11) or oxaliplatin also may be used in chemotherapy regimens for colorectal cancer.

Radiation Therapy

Although radiation therapy is not used as a primary treatment for colon cancer, it is used with surgical resection for treating rectal tumors. Small rectal cancers may be treated with intracavitary, external, or implantation radiation. Rectal cancer has a high rate of regional recurrence following complete surgical resection, particularly when the tumor has invaded tissues outside the bowel wall or regional lymph nodes. Pre- or postoperative radiation therapy reduces the recurrence of pelvic tumors, although the effect of radiation therapy on long-term survival is less clear. Radiation therapy also is used preoperatively to shrink large rectal tumors enough to permit surgical removal of the tumor.

Lifespan Considerations

Colorectal Cancer in Children and Adolescents

Polyps can occur in children and adolescents, isolated juvenile polyps being the most common type (80%). These polyps lack malignant potential, but they are the most frequent cause of lower gastrointestinal bleeding in this population. The development of isolated juvenile polyps is highest in children 3–5 years of age, and these polyps are rarely seen after adolescence. Juvenile polyposis is a group of syndromes with varying degrees of severity. Diffuse juvenile polyposis of infancy is almost always fatal. Juvenile polyposis and juvenile polyposis coli can increase the risk of developing colorectal cancer in adulthood by as much as 50%. Adenomas are quite unusual in this population (less than 3%) and represent a genetic alteration in the mucosa placing the child or adolescent at risk for the development of malignancy as adults. If a child or adolescent is diagnosed as having any of the polyposis syndromes, annual screenings are recommended to detect the development of other cancers (Shalkow, 2014).

Colorectal Cancer in Pregnant Women

Colorectal cancer is among the eight most common cancers in pregnancy, and although its occurrence is rare, diagnosis and treatment options are challenging for healthcare providers. The common manifestations of the disease (nausea, vomiting, abdominal pain, and altered bowel elimination) mimic manifestations associated with normal pregnancy. This can cause the malignancy to initially be missed, leading to later diagnosis and poorer prognosis. Other manifestations include anemia and rectal bleeding, which may also be attributed to pregnancy. Diagnostic imaging and other procedures are limited during pregnancy, as are the use of chemotherapeutic agents. The gestational age of the fetus and tumor stage must also be considered. In some cases, the choice must be made to save the life of the mother over the life of the fetus (Khodaverdi, Valeshabad, & Khodaverdi, 2013).

Colorectal Cancer in Older Adults

The majority (approximately 60%) of patients with colorectal cancer are older than 70 years of age, and 43% are older than age 75. A major challenge providers face in treating this population is the frequent discrepancy between physiologic and chronologic age together with coexisting medical conditions and the potential psychologic and social care issues that may be involved. Thus, care of the older adult with colorectal cancer requires a multidisciplinary approach. Studies have recommended the use of a geriatric assessment to evaluate a patient's functional status, physical performance, comorbidities, polypharmacy, nutritional status, cognitive function, emotional function (anxiety and depression), and social support to assist in treatment decisions. The individualization of treatment for older adults and the inclusion of members of this age group in clinical trials are absolute necessities for improving care management for these patients (Papamichael et al., 2015).

NURSING PROCESS

In planning and implementing care, consider both physical care needs and the patient's emotional response to the diagnosis. Because colorectal cancer is often advanced at the time of diagnosis, the prognosis, even with treatment, may be poor. Denial and anger are common. Extensive abdominal surgery and a colostomy may be necessary, and the effects of chemotherapy and radiation therapy can leave the patient fatigued and discouraged.

Assessment

Collect the following data through the health history and physical examination:

- *Observation and patient interview.* Observe the patient's general appearance and state of health, and be alert for signs of discomfort. Ask the patient about any unusual bowel patterns and any recent changes, weight loss, fatigue, or decreased activity tolerance; presence of blood in the stool; and pain with defecation, abdominal discomfort, or perineal pain. Ask the patient questions related to usual diet, whether there is a family history of colorectal cancer, and other specific risk factors, such as inflammatory bowel disease or colon polyps.
- *Physical examination.* The physical assessment should include general appearance, weight, abdominal shape and contour, bowel sounds, presence of abdominal tenderness, and stool Hemoccult or guaiac test.

Diagnosis

Nursing diagnoses for the patient with colorectal cancer are individualized to each patient's needs and may include the following:

- *Infection, Risk for*
- *Pain, Acute*
- *Imbalanced Nutrition: Less Than Body Requirements*
- *Anticipatory Grieving*
- *Sexuality Pattern, Ineffective.*

(NANDA-I © 2014)

Planning

The goals for the patient are determined by the patient's condition and prognosis, the amount of tissue involved, and staging of the tumor. Potential goals may include the following:

- The patient will not demonstrate evidence of infection.
- Using a predetermined pain rating scale of 0–10, with 10 representing "the worst imaginable pain," the patient will consistently rate pain at 3 or less.

- The patient will demonstrate proper ostomy care and management.
- The patient will verbalize feelings related to diagnosis and prognosis.
- The family or significant others will provide adequate emotional and physical support for the patient upon discharge.
- The patient will make an informed choice related to treatment options.

Implementation

Nursing care for the patient with colorectal cancer includes providing emotional support, teaching, and direct care before and after diagnostic procedures and surgery as well as during adjunctive treatments. The risk for sexual dysfunction should be addressed as a nursing diagnosis if a colostomy has been created.

Patients with colorectal cancer are at risk for infection, and nursing care aimed at reducing this is essential. Guidance regarding good hygiene, promoting skin integrity, and avoiding circumstances that elevate risk (e.g., crowds, exposure to individuals who are ill) is part of the nurse's focus. See Exemplar 2.A on Cancer for a full discussion of nursing interventions to prevent infection in patients with cancer.

Manage Pain Effectively

Besides pain from diagnostic procedures and surgery, the patient with colorectal cancer may experience "phantom" rectal pain after an abdominoperineal resection related to the severing of nerves during the wide excision of the rectum. See Exemplar 2.A on Cancer for detailed information on managing the patient's pain effectively.

Reduce Risk for Sexual Dysfunction

Colorectal cancer and ostomy surgery increase the risk for sexual dysfunction. Physical factors that can lead to sexual dysfunction include disruption of nerves and blood vessels that supply the genitals, radiation therapy, chemotherapy, and other medications prescribed after surgery.

Psychologically, a patient with an ostomy experiences an altered body image and may develop low self-esteem. The patient may feel undesirable and fear rejection. If the patient is concerned about odors or pouch leakage during sexual activity, this emotional stress can contribute to sexual dysfunction. The nurse should do the following:

- Encourage the patient to express sexual concerns. Sexuality is a very private concern to most people. The patient and family are not likely to express their concerns openly unless trust has been established.
- Reassure the patient and significant other that the effect of physical illness and prescribed interventions on sexuality usually is temporary. The patient and partner may misinterpret an initial decrease in libido as evidence that sexual activity will not be possible or will not resume following recovery.
- Refer the patient and partner to social services or a family counselor for further interventions. Patients are often discharged from acute care settings well before concerns about sexual activity surface. Ongoing counseling provides a continuing resource.

- Arrange for a visit from a member of the United Ostomy Association. People who are living and coping with an ostomy can provide information and support, helping the patient with a new ostomy overcome feelings of isolation and rejection.

Evaluation

Patient outcomes are evaluated based on goals of care. Expected outcomes may include the following:

- The patient does not demonstrate any signs or symptoms of infection.

- The patient maintains adequate hydration, as evidenced by urinary output of at least 0.5 mL/kg/hr.

- Using a predetermined pain rating scale of 0–10 in which 10 represents "the worst possible pain," the patient consistently rates his or her pain at a level of 3 or less.

- The patient is able to perform essential daily ADLs.

The patient ideally will show no signs or symptoms of infection. However, if infection is present, early identification of stomal necrosis, ischemia, or skin irritation can prevent serious complications.

Nursing Care Plan
A Patient with Colorectal Cancer

William Cunningham is a 65-year-old retired railroad employee, husband, and father of three grown children. For the past 3 months, Mr. Cunningham has noticed small amounts of blood and occasional mucus in his stools. He has a sensation of pressure in the rectum, and he notices that his stools are smaller in diameter, about the size of pencil. After palpating a mass on digital examination of the rectum, the physician orders a colonoscopy. A large sessile lesion is found in the rectum and biopsied. The pathology report shows the lesion to be adenocarcinoma. Mr. Cunningham is scheduled for an abdominoperineal resection and sigmoid colostomy.

ASSESSMENT	DIAGNOSES	PLANNING
Madonna Hart, RN, completes the admission assessment. Mr. Cunningham states that his bowel habits have recently changed, but he denies pain or other symptoms. Physical assessment findings include temperature 36.9°C (98.4°F) oral; pulse 82 bpm; respirations 18/min; and BP 118/78 mmHg. He is 178 cm (70 in.) tall and weighs 84 kg (185 lb). Laboratory findings are normal except for the previous pathology report of adenocarcinoma of rectal lesion. Mr. Cunningham states, "I really don't want a colostomy, but if that is what it takes to get rid of this, I'm ready to get it over with."	• *Pain, Acute,* related to surgical intervention • *Skin Integrity, Risk for Impaired* (peristomal) related to fecal drainage and pouch adhesive • *Gastrointestinal Motility, Risk for Dysfunctional,* related to effects of surgery on bowel function • *Body Image, Disturbed,* related to colostomy • *Sexuality Pattern, Ineffective,* related to wide rectal incision, radiation therapy, and colostomy (NANDA-I © 2014)	• The patient will report pain within an acceptable range that allows ease of movement and ambulation. • The patient will perform colostomy care using correct technique. • The patient will demonstrate willingness to discuss changes in sexual function. • The patient will wear clothing to enhance physical and emotional self-esteem.

IMPLEMENTATION

- Provide analgesia as ordered, evaluating its effectiveness.
- Discuss foods that cause odor and gas.
- Teach colostomy care.
- Teach the patient to avoid the use of rectal suppositories and rectal enemas and to not take temperatures rectally.

- Refer to the local United Ostomy Association.
- Provide a list of local medical supply companies that carry ostomy supplies.
- Provide for privacy when teaching and discussing concerns about ostomy.

EVALUATION

On discharge, Mr. Cunningham is able to empty and rinse out his colostomy pouch. He is changing the pouch and caring for surrounding skin appropriately. Ms. Hart has given him verbal and written instructions on colostomy care. He verbalizes understanding of phantom rectal pain and the importance of avoiding rectal suppositories.

He expresses an understanding of the need to avoid heavy lifting and the importance of follow-up care. Ms. Hart has referred Mr. Cunningham to a home health agency in his community for further questions and follow-up care.

CRITICAL THINKING

1. What is the cause of phantom rectal pain?
2. Why is it important to discuss dietary concerns with a patient with a colostomy, especially odor- and gas-forming foods?
3. Outline a plan to teach Mr. Cunningham how to irrigate a colostomy.
4. Develop a care plan for Mr. Cunningham for the nursing diagnosis of Disturbed Body Image.

REVIEW Colorectal Cancer

RELATE Link the Concepts and Exemplars

Linking the exemplar of colorectal cancer with the concept of elimination:

1. What alterations in bowel elimination increase the patient's risk for colorectal cancer?

2. What preventive teaching can you provide the patient with altered bowel elimination to reduce the risk of colorectal cancer?

Linking the exemplar of colorectal cancer with the concept of self:

3. How might a patient's self-concept be altered as the result of treatment for colorectal cancer resulting in a colostomy?

4. You are caring for a patient with end-stage colorectal cancer who appears emaciated, has cachexia, and has lost most of her hair as a result of treatment. She refuses visitors because she does not want friends and loved ones to see her looking like this. What nursing interventions can you implement to help her cope with her altered body image and self-concept while promoting socialization?

READY Go to Volume 3: Clinical Nursing Skills

REFER Go to Pearson MyLab Nursing and eText

- Additional review materials

REFLECT Apply Your Knowledge

Pamela Allen is a 65-year-old woman who has been married to Clifford for 40 years. Their only child, 24-year-old Gary, has Down syndrome and lives with them. In the past, Mrs. Allen worked as an administrative assistant in a law firm. After Gary was born, Mrs. Allen gave up her career to care for him.

Mrs. Allen frequently experiences constipation, which she treats with over-the-counter agents. She considers the constipation more of

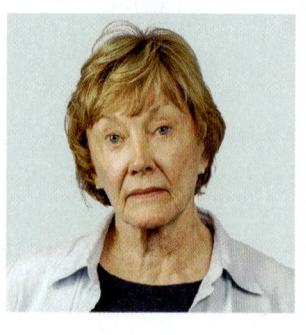

an annoyance than anything else. The only medical condition she has ever had requiring treatment was endometrial cancer at age 50. The cancer was diagnosed at a very early stage, and she underwent a total hysterectomy and bilateral salpingo-oophorectomy. Because there was no evidence of lymph node involvement, she was considered cured and has been cancer free ever since. Her last examination was 14 months ago.

One day Mrs. Allen experiences diarrhea with odor and an odd reddish-brown color. The next day, she is again constipated. She has been straining to have a bowel movement and notes that her stools are thinner than usual. A few weeks later, while still experiencing constipation and odd-shaped stools, she begins to feel a sense of fullness in her rectum and pelvic area, even after defecation. The appearance of the reddish-brown color in her stools has been more regular. She has often been feeling tired lately. On Friday afternoon, she finally makes a decision to call for an appointment with her physician about the symptoms. She is told to come to the office on the following Monday morning. She has a feeling of dread and becomes worried that something serious may be wrong.

1. What specific symptoms described by Mrs. Allen would cause you to suspect colorectal cancer?

2. What diagnostic test would you anticipate will be performed in the physician's office on her first visit?

3. Develop a plan of care for Mrs. Allen addressing both her physical and psychosocial needs.

≫ Exemplar 2.E Leukemia

Exemplar Learning Outcomes

2.E Analyze leukemia as it relates to cellular regulation.

- Describe the pathophysiology of leukemia.
- Describe the etiology of leukemia.
- Compare the risk factors for and prevention of leukemia.
- Identify the clinical manifestations of leukemia.
- Summarize diagnostic tests and therapies used by interprofessional teams in the collaborative care of an individual with leukemia.
- Differentiate considerations for care of patients with leukemia across the lifespan.
- Apply the nursing process in providing culturally competent care to an individual with leukemia.

Exemplar Key Terms

Acute lymphocytic leukemia (ALL), *98*
Acute myeloid leukemia (AML), *98*
Allogeneic bone marrow transplant, *100*
Autologous bone marrow transplant, *102*
Bone marrow transplant (BMT), *100*
Chronic lymphocytic leukemia (CLL), *99*
Chronic myeloid leukemia (CML), *98*
Leukemia, *96*
Philadelphia chromosome, *98*
Remission, *100*
Stem cell transplant (SCT), *102*

Overview

Leukemia (literally, "white blood") is a group of chronic malignant disorders of WBCs and WBC precursors. In leukemia, the usual ratio of RBCs to WBCs is reversed. Leukemias are characterized by replacement of bone marrow by malignant immature WBCs; abnormal immature circulating WBCs; and infiltration of these cells into the liver, spleen, and lymph nodes throughout the body.

Pathophysiology and Etiology

Leukemia occurs when the stem cells in the bone marrow produce immature WBCs that cannot function normally. These cells proliferate rapidly by cloning instead of through normal mitosis, causing the bone marrow to fill with abnormal WBCs. The abnormal cells then spill out into the circulatory system, where they steadily replace the normally functioning WBCs. As this occurs, the protective lymphocytic functions, such as cellular and humoral immunity, are reduced, leaving the body vulnerable to infections.

The malignant WBCs rapidly fill the bone marrow, replacing stem cells that produce erythrocytes (RBCs) and other blood products, such as platelets, thereby decreasing the amount of these products in circulation. The stem cells are replaced by leukemic clones, eventually resulting in anemia. Patients with leukemia commonly experience abnormal bleeding because of the reduced platelet amounts.

Leukemias are classified by their acuity and by the predominant cell type involved. The *acute* leukemias are characterized by an acute onset, rapid disease progression, and immature or undifferentiated blast cells. *Chronic* leukemias, by contrast, have a gradual onset, prolonged course, and abnormal mature-appearing cells. Lymphocytic (or lymphoblastic) leukemias involve immature lymphocytes and their precursor cells in the bone marrow. Lymphocytic leukemias infiltrate the spleen, lymph nodes, central nervous system, and other tissues. Myeloid (also called myelogenous, myelocytic, or myeloblastic) leukemias involve myeloid stem cells in the bone marrow, interfering with the maturation of all types of blood cells, including granulocytes, RBCs, and thrombocytes (Porth & Grossman, 2013). Acute lymphocytic (lymphoblastic) leukemia is the most common type of leukemia in children (see **Figure 2–14** 》). In adults, acute myeloid

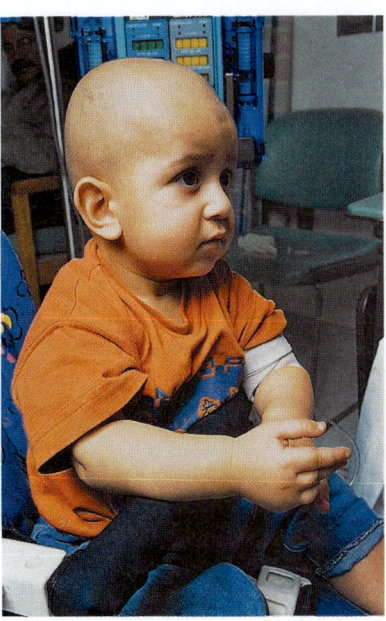

Figure 2–14 》 Acute lymphoblastic leukemia is the most common type of leukemia in children and the most common cancer affecting children under 5 years of age.

leukemia and chronic lymphocytic leukemia are the most common types (ACS, 2016b).

The major types of leukemia are summarized in **Table 2–9** 》. However, this general system of classifying leukemias does not differentiate subtypes of acute leukemias. In the 1970s, the French–American–British (FAB) system for classifying acute leukemias was introduced, which further differentiated acute leukemias by the predominant cell

TABLE 2–9 Primary Forms of Leukemia

Type and Description	Clinical Manifestations	Curative Treatment

Acute lymphoblastic leukemia (ALL)
 	
 Abnormal growth of marrow cells that form lymphocytes
   Primarily affects children and young adults; rapid onset and disease progression
	Weakness, decreased energy, recurrent infections, bleeding; pallor, bone pain, weight loss, sore throat, night sweats	Potential central nervous system manifestations if brain and/or spinal cord is infiltrated include headaches, vomiting, visual disturbances, and seizures
		   Chemotherapy, bone marrow transplant (BMT), or stem cell transplant (SCT)

Chronic lymphocytic leukemia (CLL) Abnormal growth of marrow cells that form lymphocytes Primarily affects older adults; insidious onset and slow, chronic course	Fatigue; exercise intolerance; lymphadenopathy and splenomegaly; recurrent infections, pallor, edema, and thrombophlebitis	Often requires no treatment, depending on rate of progression; chemotherapy, BMT
Acute myeloid leukemia (AML) Abnormal growth of marrow cells that form RBCs, WBCs (other than lymphocytes), and platelets Common in older adults, rarely seen in children and young adults	Fatigue, weakness, fever; anemia; headache; bone and joint pain; abnormal bleeding and bruising; recurrent infection; lymphadenopathy, splenomegaly, and hepatomegaly	Chemotherapy; SCT
Chronic myeloid leukemia (CML) Abnormal growth of marrow cells that form RBCs, WBCs (other than lymphocytes), and platelets Primarily affects adults; usually associated with Philadelphia chromosome	Early course slow and stable, progressing to aggressive phase in 3–4 years *Chronic phase:* asymptomatic or very mild, vague symptoms *Accelerated phase:* decreased appetite, weight loss, and fever *Acute phase* (*blast crisis* or *blast phase*): progression includes splenomegaly, bone damage, abnormal platelet count	Interferon alfa; chemotherapy with imatinib mesylate (Gleevec), SCT

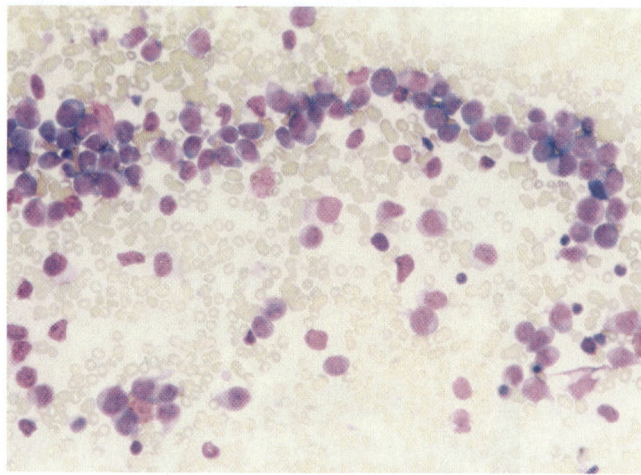

Source: Dr. Gopal Murti/Science Source.

Figure 2–15 ⟫ A blood smear from the bone marrow of a patient with acute myeloid leukemia. Note the abnormally large number of myelocyte WBCs (stained purple) among the small RBCs.

involved and the degree of cell differentiation. Later, the World Health Organization (WHO) designed a similar system of classification; the WHO system takes into account factors that affect prognosis, such as genetic mutations and previous exposures to radiation (ACS, 2016d).

Acute Myeloid Leukemia

Acute myeloid leukemia (AML) is characterized by uncontrolled proliferation of myeloblasts (the precursors of granulocytes) and hyperplasia of the bone marrow and spleen (see **Figure 2–15** ⟫). Between 45,000 and 50,000 new cases of all forms of leukemia occur annually. Nearly 90% of leukemia cases involve adults ages 20 years or older. Among adults, AML accounts for 31% of newly diagnosed leukemia cases (ACS, 2016b). However, AML is uncommon in individuals younger than 40 years of age. On average, the individual diagnosed with AML is approximately 67 years old (ACS, 2016d). For these individuals, the 5-year relative survival rate is approximately 25% (ACS, 2016b).

The manifestations of AML result from neutropenia and thrombocytopenia. Decreased neutrophils lead to recurrent severe infections, such as pneumonia, septicemia, abscesses, and mucous membrane ulceration. The manifestations of thrombocytopenia include petechiae (red or purple spots that looks like a spider caused by a broken capillary), purpura (small areas of subcutaneous bleeding), ecchymoses (bruising), epistaxis (nosebleeds), hematomas, hematuria, and gastrointestinal bleeding. Bone infarctions or subperiosteal infiltrates of leukemic cells may cause bone pain. Anemia is a late manifestation, causing fatigue, headaches, pallor, and dyspnea on exertion. Death usually results from infection or hemorrhage.

Bone marrow aspiration shows a proliferation of immature WBCs. The CBC shows thrombocytopenia and normocytic, normochromic anemia.

Chronic Myeloid Leukemia

Chronic myeloid leukemia (CML) is characterized by abnormal proliferation of all bone marrow elements. This

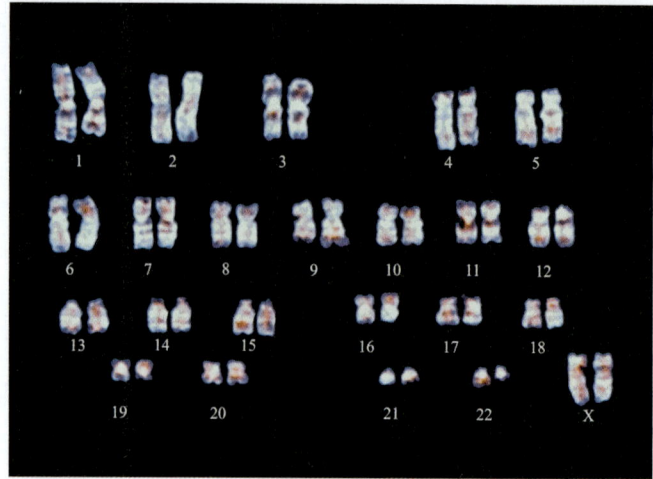

Source: Addenbrookes Hospital/Science Source.

Figure 2–16 ⟫ The Philadelphia chromosome. Note the chromosomes of pairs 9 and 22. In each instance, the left-hand chromosome of the pair is normal, whereas an exchange of material between chromosomes has made the right-hand chromosome 9 larger and the right-hand chromosome 22 smaller. In stem cells within the bone marrow, the chromosome 22 defect leads to chronic myeloid leukemia.

type of leukemia constitutes approximately 15% of adult leukemias. It affects women slightly more frequently than men. The average age of the individual with CML is approximately 65 years. This form of leukemia is very rarely seen in children (ACS, 2015d).

CML usually is associated with a chromosome abnormality called the **Philadelphia chromosome**, a balanced translocation of chromosome 22 to chromosome 9 (see **Figure 2–16** ⟫). The fusion gene produced by this translocation, known as *bcr/abl*, is an oncogene capable of initiating malignancy. Very large doses of ionizing radiation also may induce CML in some patients (ACS, 2015d).

In the early or *chronic phase* of CML, the patient often is either asymptomatic or demonstrates very mild, vague symptoms. In fact, CML is often diagnosed when a routine blood test reveals abnormal cell counts. In the *accelerated phase*, common symptoms include decreased appetite, weight loss, and fever. During the *acute phase*, also called the *blast crisis* or *blast phase*, blast cells have proliferated and spread beyond the bone marrow, infiltrating tissues and organs. In addition to decreased appetite, weight loss, and fever, manifestations of the acute phase may include splenomegaly, bone damage, and an extremely high or low platelet count (ACS, 2015d).

Acute Lymphocytic Leukemia

Acute lymphocytic leukemia (ALL) is the most common type of leukemia in children and adolescents. The incidence of ALL decreases after the mid-20s and then gradually increases after about age 50. Genetic factors may play a role in its development, particularly the *bcr/abl* translocation also implicated in CML (ACS, 2014h).

Most cases of ALL (80%) result from malignant transformation of B cells, with the remaining 20% arising from T cells. The malignant cells resemble immature lymphocytes

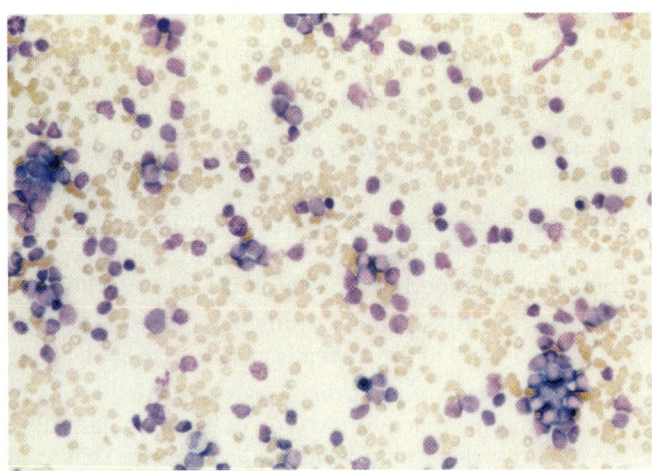

Source: Dr. Gopal Murti/Science Source.

Figure 2–17 » A blood smear from the bone marrow of a patient with acute lymphocytic leukemia. Note the abnormally large number of lymphocytes (stained purple) crowding the bone marrow. As a result, normal production of RBCs, functional WBCs, and platelets is suppressed.

(lymphoblasts); however, they do not mature or function effectively to maintain immunity. These lymphoblasts accumulate in the bone marrow, lymph nodes, and spleen as well as in circulating blood. Some types of lymphoma are thought to represent a later stage of the same disease.

The onset of ALL is usually rapid. Lymphoblasts proliferating in bone marrow and peripheral tissues crowd the growth of normal cells (see **Figure 2–17 »**). Normal hematopoiesis is suppressed, leading to thrombocytopenia, leukopenia, and anemia. Manifestations of infections, bleeding, and anemia develop. Lymphadenopathy, liver enlargement, and bone pain resulting from rapid generation of marrow elements are also common. Infiltration of the central nervous system causes headaches, visual disturbances, vomiting, and seizures.

The CBC shows an elevated WBC count with increased lymphocytes on the differential. The RBC and platelet counts are decreased. Bone marrow studies reveal a hypercellular marrow with growth of lymphoblasts. Combination chemotherapy produces complete remission in 80–90% of adults with ALL. However, because relapse is common among adults, the rate of cure for this population is closer to 40% (ACS, 2014h). With treatment, the survival rate among children with ALL is estimated to be more than 85% (ACS, 2016e).

Chronic Lymphocytic Leukemia

Chronic lymphocytic leukemia (CLL) is characterized by proliferation and accumulation of small, abnormal, mature lymphocytes in the bone marrow, peripheral blood, and body tissues. The abnormal cells are usually B lymphocytes that are unable to produce adequate antibodies to maintain normal immune function. CLL statistically is the most common form of leukemia diagnosed in adults 20 years of age and older (ACS, 2016b). However, it is rarely seen in children or in adults under the age of 40 years. The average age at the time of diagnosis is 72 years (ACS, 2015e).

Chronic lymphocytic leukemia has a slow onset and is often diagnosed during a routine physical examination. If symptoms are present, they usually include vague complaints of weakness or malaise. Possible clinical findings include anemia; infection; and enlarged lymph nodes, spleen, and liver. As in other leukemias, bone marrow hyperplasia is present. Erythrocyte and platelet counts are reduced. Leukocyte counts may be either elevated or reduced, but abnormal cells are always present. In CLL, years may elapse before treatment is required. The 5-year survival rate for individuals diagnosed with CLL is 82% (ACS, 2016b).

Etiology

Although leukemia is often thought of as a childhood disease, adults ages 20 years or older account for approximately 90% of new diagnoses. In 2016, an estimated 60,140 individuals were newly diagnosed with leukemia, while approximately 24,400 individuals died from leukemia-related complications that same year (ACS, 2016b).

The causes of leukemia are not well understood. Some investigators theorize that exposure to infectious agents can predispose people to leukemia. Genetic factors are also believed to play a role in some types of the disease.

Risk Factors

While the cause of most leukemias is unknown, certain risk factors have been identified. Men are affected more frequently than women. Children with immunodeficiency states, such as ataxia-telangiectasia, congenital hypogammaglobulinemia, and Wiskott-Aldrich syndrome, have an increased risk of ALL. Patients who have undergone treatment for cancer may also have an increased risk. The human T-cell leukemia/lymphoma virus 1, a retrovirus, is known to cause certain leukemias and lymphomas (ACS, 2014i).

People with certain genetic disorders have a higher incidence of leukemia. Children with chromosomal defects, such as Down syndrome, Klinefelter syndrome, Bloom syndrome, and Fanconi anemia, have an increased incidence of ALL. While chromosomal abnormalities are present in many patients with ALL, these mutations are generally believed to have transpired during the individual's lifetime, rather than being inherited (ACS, 2014h). In addition, several chromosomal and genetic abnormalities are associated with AML; however, these abnormalities are rarely due to inherited DNA mutations.

Environmental risk factors play a role as well. Risk factors for AML include cigarette smoking and exposure to chemicals such as benzene (present in cigarette smoke and gasoline). Exposure to high-dose ionizing radiation, such as from a nuclear reactor or atomic blast, increases the risk for both AML and ALL.

There are very few known environmental or lifestyle-related causes of childhood or other leukemias; therefore, there is no sure way to prevent them from developing (ACS, 2016a). Exposure to high-dose radiation is the only proven modifiable risk factor for CML (ACS, 2015d). CLL has no known modifiable risk factors; diet, radiation exposure, smoking, and infection do not appear to be linked to its development (ACS, 2015e).

Clinical Manifestations

The general manifestations of leukemia (regardless of type) result from anemia, infection, and bleeding. These include pallor, fatigue, tachycardia, malaise, lethargy, and dyspnea on exertion. Infection may cause fever, night sweats, oral ulcerations, and frequent or recurrent respiratory, urinary, integumentary, or other infections. Increased bleeding as a result of thrombocytopenia leads to bruising, petechiae, bleeding gums, and bleeding within specific organs and tissues.

Other manifestations result from leukemic cell infiltration, increased metabolism, and increased leukocyte destruction (see the Multisystem Effects of Leukemia feature). Infiltration of the liver, spleen, lymph nodes, and bone marrow causes pain and tissue swelling in the involved areas. Meningeal infiltration may cause manifestations of increased intracranial pressure, such as headache, altered level of consciousness, cranial nerve impairment, and nausea and vomiting. Infiltration of the kidneys may affect renal function, with decreased urine output and increased blood urea nitrogen and creatinine. Increased metabolism causes heat intolerance, weight loss, dyspnea on exertion, and tachycardia. Destruction of large numbers of WBCs releases substantial amounts of uric acid into the circulation; uric acid crystals may obstruct renal tubules, causing renal insufficiency.

Collaboration

Treatment for leukemia focuses on achieving remission or cure and relieving symptoms. The methods of treatment may include chemotherapy, radiation therapy, and bone marrow or stem cell transplantation. Cure is more often achieved in children with acute leukemia than in adults, although long-term **remission** (a disease-free period with no signs or symptoms) often can be achieved. The nurse's role

as a member of the interprofessional healthcare team is outlined in the Nursing Process section that follows this section.

Diagnostic Tests

The following diagnostic tests are useful in the diagnosis of leukemia:

- **CBC with differential** is done to evaluate cell counts; hemoglobin and hematocrit levels; and the number, distribution, and morphology (size and shape) of WBCs.
- **Platelets** are measured to identify possible thrombocytopenia secondary to the leukemia and the risk of bleeding.
- **Bone marrow examination** provides information about cells within the marrow, the type of erythropoiesis, and the maturity of erythropoietic and leukopoietic cells.

Table 2–10 » outlines usual diagnostic test results in the various forms of leukemia.

Surgery

Surgical procedures include transplantation of bone marrow or stem cells. Cells may be obtained either from a donor or from the recipient, depending on the procedure.

Bone Marrow Transplant

Bone marrow transplant (BMT) is the treatment of choice for some types of leukemia (see Table 2–9). BMT often is used in conjunction with or following chemotherapy or radiation. There are two major categories of BMT: In allogeneic BMT, the bone marrow of a healthy donor is infused into the patient with the illness; in autologous BMT, the patient is infused with his or her own bone marrow.

Allogeneic Bone Marrow Transplant

Allogeneic bone marrow transplant uses bone marrow cells from a donor. The donor is often a sibling with closely matched tissue antigens; a closely matched unrelated

Clinical Manifestations and Therapies
Leukemia

ETIOLOGY	CLINICAL MANIFESTATIONS	CLINICAL THERAPIES
Anemia may result because the bone marrow is so busy producing WBCs that it produces inadequate numbers of RBCs.	▪ Pallor, fatigue, tachycardia, malaise, lethargy, and dyspnea on exertion	▪ Improve nutritional status. ▪ Stimulate RBC production with medications (e.g., epoetin). ▪ Perform blood transfusions. ▪ Promote rest. ▪ Monitor vital signs and CBC.
Infection risk increases because of immature WBCs that are ineffective in responding to pathogens.	▪ Fever, night sweats, oral ulcerations, and frequent or recurrent respiratory, urinary, integumentary, or other infections	▪ Teach infection prevention strategies (e.g., hand hygiene, cough etiquette, crowd avoidance). ▪ Teach symptoms to report. ▪ Give antimicrobials as indicated to treat infections. ▪ Monitor vital signs and CBC.
Bleeding may result from reduced coagulation factors, increased fibrinolytic activity, and accelerated intravascular coagulation.	▪ Petechiae, bruising, bleeding from gums, hematuria, hematemesis, and rectal bleeding	▪ Monitor coagulation studies. ▪ Provide patient teaching to reduce injury risk. ▪ Administer platelets and clotting factors. ▪ Replace blood if bleeding occurs.

Multisystem Effects of
Leukemia

Neurologic
- Headache
- Altered LOC
- Cranial nerve impairment

Potential complications
- Subarachnoid hemorrhage
- Retinal hemorrhage
- Seizures, coma

Respiratory
- Dyspnea on exertion
- Pharyngitis, sore throat
- Frequent respiratory infections

Potential complication
- Pulmonary bleeding

Gastrointestinal
- Anorexia, nausea
- Oral ulcerations, infection
- Bleeding gums
- Gingival hyperplasia (gum overgrowth)
- Abdominal pain
- Hepatomegaly
- Occult GI bleeding

Urinary
- Urinary tract infection
- Hematuria

Potential complication
- Renal insufficiency or failure

Musculoskeletal
- Weakness
- Bone tenderness, pain
- Joint pain

Metabolic Processes
- Malaise, lethargy
- Heat intolerance
- Diaphoresis
- Chills, fever
- Night sweats
- Weight loss

Cardiovascular
- Tachycardia, palpitations
- Orthostatic hypotension
- Heart murmurs
- Hematomas
- Edema

Potential complications
- Hemorrhage
- Thrombophlebitis

Hematologic
- Anemia
- Thrombocytopenia
- Leukopenia
- Bleeding (epistaxis)
- Splenomegaly

Potential complication
- DIC

Immunologic
- Frequent or recurrent infections
- Lymphadenopathy

Potential complications
- Abscesses
- Septicemia

Integumentary
- Skin and mucous membrane pallor
- Petechiae
- Bruising, purpura
- Ulcerations
- Chloromas (skin infiltrations near bony prominences)

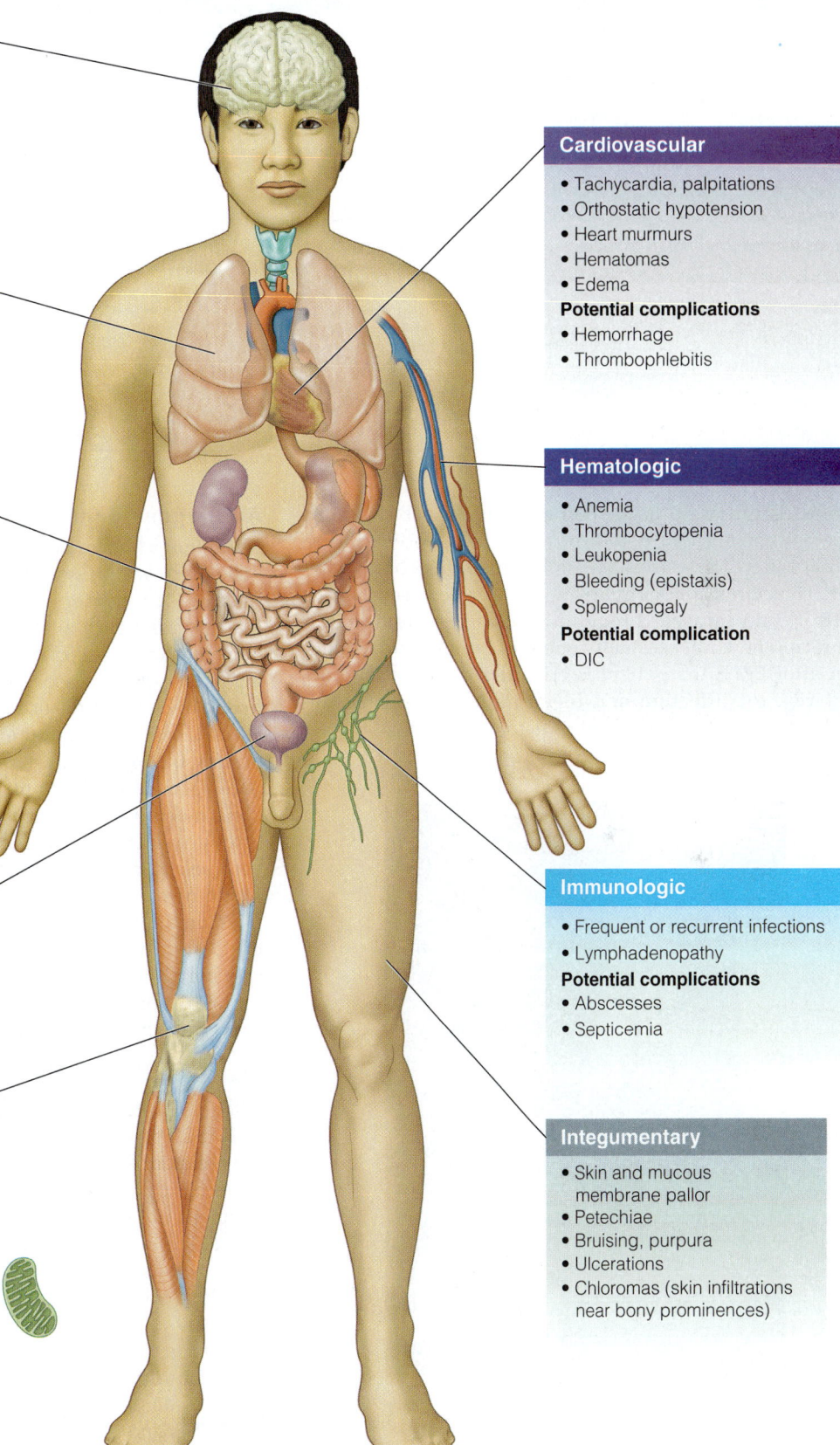

TABLE 2–10 Diagnostic Findings by Type of Leukemia

Test	Acute Myeloid Leukemia	Chronic Myeloid Leukemia	Acute Lymphocytic Leukemia	Chronic Lymphocytic Leukemia
RBC count	Low	Low	Low	Low
Hemoglobin	Low	Low	Low	Low
Hematocrit	Low	Low	Low	Low
Platelet count	Very low	High early, low late	Low	Low
WBC count	Varies	Increased	Varies	Increased
Myeloblasts	Present			
Neutrophils	Decreased	Increased	Decreased	Normal
Lymphocytes		Normal		Increased
Monocytes		Normal/low		
Blasts	Present	Present (crisis)	Present	
Bone marrow	Hypercellular		Hypercellular	
Myeloblasts	Present			
Lymphoblasts			Present	
Lymphocytes				Present

donor also may be used. Before allogeneic BMT, high doses of chemotherapy and possibly total body irradiation are used to destroy leukemic cells in the bone marrow. The donor's bone marrow is aspirated (see **Figure 2–18** 》) and infused through a central venous line into the recipient. Until reestablishment of bone marrow function after BMT, the patient is critically ill and at significant risk for infection and bleeding as a result of the depletion of WBCs and platelets.

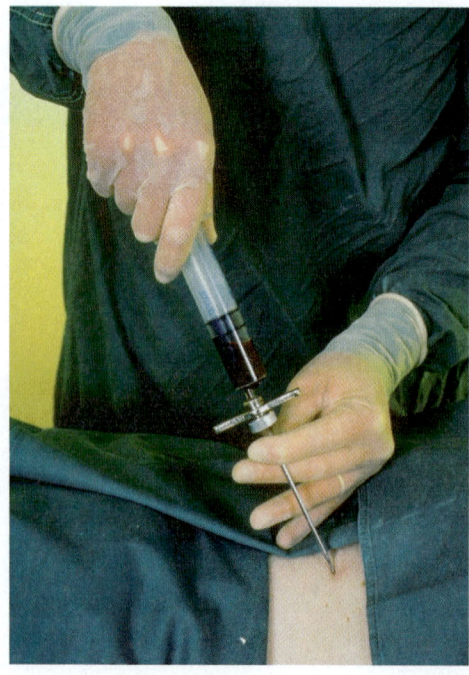

Source: Simon Fraser/Science Source.

Figure 2–18 》 Allogeneic bone marrow transplant. Bone marrow from the donor is aspirated, then filtered and infused into the recipient.

Autologous Bone Marrow Transplant

Autologous bone marrow transplant uses the patient's own bone marrow to restore bone marrow function after chemotherapy or radiation; this procedure is often called bone marrow rescue. In autologous BMT, approximately 1 L of bone marrow is aspirated (usually from the iliac crests) during a period of disease remission. The bone marrow is then frozen and stored for use after treatment. If relapse occurs, lethal doses of chemotherapy or radiation are given to destroy the immune system and malignant cells and to prepare space in the bone marrow for new cells. The filtered bone marrow is then thawed and infused intravenously through a central line. The infused marrow cells slowly become a part of the patient's bone marrow, the neutrophil count increases, and normal hematopoiesis takes place.

As in allogeneic BMT, the patient is critically ill during the period of bone marrow destruction and immunosuppression. The patient is hospitalized in a private room for 6–8 weeks or more. Potential complications include malnutrition, infection, and bleeding.

Stem Cell Transplant

Allogeneic **stem cell transplant (SCT)** is an alternative to BMT. SCT results in complete and sustained replacement of the recipient's blood cell lines (WBCs, RBCs, and platelets) with cells derived from the donor stem cells. Before SCT, the recipient undergoes treatment similar to that before BMT. The risks for infection and other complications, as well as graft-versus-host disease (GVHD), which occurs when immune cells of the donated bone marrow identify the recipient's body tissue as foreign, are similar as well.

Donors for SCT must have tissue that is closely matched with that of the recipient. Before harvesting, hematopoietic growth factors, including granulocyte-macrophage CSF (GM-CSF) and granulocyte CSF (G-CSF), are administered to the donor for 4–5 days. This increases the concentration of stem cells in peripheral blood, allowing it to be used for the transplant instead of bone marrow. Peripheral blood is removed, and WBCs are separated from the plasma, then administered via a large central venous catheter. Large concentrations of stem cells also are present in umbilical cord blood. This may be stored and used in some cases (Osborn et al., 2013).

Allogeneic BMT or SCT may precipitate GVHD. During GVHD, T lymphocytes in the donated marrow attack the liver, skin, and gastrointestinal tract. Acute GVHD develops within the first 3 months following a transplant and is usually marked by a pruritic, maculopapular rash that begins on the palms and soles of the feet and may extend over the entire body. Additional manifestations of acute GVHD may include jaundice, nausea, vomiting, diarrhea, and dry eyes. Chronic GVHD develops more than 3 months after a transplant procedure. Chronic GVHD may be accompanied by chronic pain, fatigue, weakness, and shortness of breath (MedlinePlus, 2014b). In some cases, chronic GVHD may follow acute GVHD; however, it may also develop in patients with no previous symptoms. GVHD is treated with antibiotics and steroids; immunosuppressant drugs, such as thalidomide and immunotoxin (XomaZyme), may be used if necessary.

Pharmacologic Therapy

Treatment for leukemia, as well as for other forms of cancer, often incorporates two main approaches: killing the cancerous cells and changing the way the body responds to the cancerous cells. Chemotherapy medications have cytotoxic effects. Biological therapies, which alter the body's response to cancer cells, may also be cytotoxic.

Chemotherapy

Single-agent or combination chemotherapy is the treatment of choice for most types of leukemia, with the goal of eradicating leukemic cells and producing remission. **Table 2–11** outlines typical chemotherapeutic regimens for different types of leukemia. Combination chemotherapy reduces drug resistance and toxicity and interrupts cell growth at various stages of the cell cycle, producing a complementary effect of the drugs used.

Chemotherapy for leukemia generally is divided into the induction phase and postremission therapy. During induction, drug doses are high to eradicate leukemic cells from the bone marrow. Often, however, these high doses also damage stem cells and interfere with production of normal blood cells. Circulating mature blood cells are not affected, because they are no longer dividing. The degree of bone marrow suppression is influenced by a number of factors, including age, nutritional status, concurrent chronic diseases (e.g., impaired liver or renal function), the drug and drug dose, and previous treatment.

Tumor lysis syndrome (TLS) also is a risk in patients with leukemia who are undergoing their initial treatment with chemotherapy. TLS develops when a large number of malignant cells are destroyed by treatment with chemotherapy or radiation. With cellular lysis, intracellular contents are released into the circulation, causing hyperkalemia, hyperuricemia, and hyperphosphatemia. As a result, the patient may experience cardiac arrhythmias, renal failure, and even death. Acute leukemia is among the conditions most commonly associated with TLS (Ikeda, 2016; Osborn et al., 2013).

Once remission has been achieved, postremission chemotherapy is continued to eradicate any additional leukemic cells, prevent relapse, and prolong survival. A single chemotherapeutic agent, combination therapy, or BMT may be used for postremission treatment.

Biological Therapy

Cytokines, such as interferons and interleukins, are biological agents that may be used to treat some leukemias. These agents modify the body's response to cancer cells; in some cases, the agents are cytotoxic as well. Interferons are a complex group of messenger proteins normally produced in response to antigens such as viruses. They have multiple effects, including moderating immune function and inhibiting abnormal cell proliferation and growth. Interferon alfa may be used to treat some leukemias, particularly CML. Side effects commonly associated with interferon therapy include flulike symptoms, persistent fatigue and lethargy, weight loss, and muscle and joint pain.

Biological response modifiers such as colony-stimulating factors (CSFs), also called hematopoietic growth factors, may be administered to "rescue" the bone marrow following induction chemotherapy. CSFs are cytokines that regulate the growth and differentiation of blood cells. Factors that support neutrophil maturation, GM-CSF, and G-CSF are included among these medications. Bone pain is a common side effect of therapy with these agents. Patients also may experience fevers, chills, anorexia, muscle aches, and lethargy (Wilson, Shannon, & Shields, 2016).

Radiation Therapy

Radiation therapy uses high doses of x-rays or other forms of energy to damage cellular DNA. Although the cell continues to function, it cannot divide and multiply. Cells that divide rapidly, such as bone marrow and cancer cells (radiosensitive cells), respond quickly to radiation therapy. Although normal cells are affected, they are better able than cancer cells to recover from the damage caused by the radiation.

TABLE 2–11 Chemotherapeutic Regimens Used to Treat Leukemia

Type of Leukemia	Chemotherapeutic Regimen
Acute myeloid leukemia (AML)	■ Cytarabine (Cytoxan, an alkylating agent) *with* daunorubicin (Cerubidine, an antitumor antibiotic) *or* idarubicin (Idamycin, an antitumor antibiotic) ■ All-*trans* retinoic acid (ATRA) added for patients with promyelocytic leukemia
Chronic myeloid leukemia (CML)	■ Imatinib mesylate (Gleevec), a *bcr/abl* tyrosine kinase (enzyme) inhibitor ■ Hydroxyurea (a DNA inhibitor) *or* homoharringtonine (HHT, a plant alkaloid) if imatinib is not tolerated
Acute lymphocytic leukemia (ALL)	■ Daunorubicin (Cerubidine, an antitumor antibiotic) *with* vincristine (Oncovin, a plant alkaloid) *with* prednisone *with* asparaginase (Elspar)
Chronic lymphocytic leukemia (CLL)	■ Fludarabine (Fludara, an antimetabolite) *or* chlorambucil (Chloromycetin, an antitumor antibiotic) ■ Cyclophosphamide (Cytoxan, an alkylating agent), vincristine, and prednisone ■ Cyclophosphamide, doxorubicin (Adriamycin, an antitumor antibiotic), vincristine, and prednisone

Lifespan Considerations

Leukemia in Children

Leukemia accounts for almost one out of every three cancers diagnosed in children. Most cases are ALL; the remaining cases are usually AML. The incidence of ALL peaks between the ages of 2 and 4 years but is slightly more common during the first 2 years of life and during the teenage years. ALL is also more common among Hispanic and Caucasian children than African American and Asian children; boys appear to have a higher incidence than girls. AML occurs equally among both sexes of all races. Juvenile myelomonocytic leukemia (JMML), a rare form of leukemia in which too many immature WBCs are made in the bone marrow, occurs most often in children under the age of 4 years.

There are currently no screening procedures or blood tests to identify the disease before it begins to cause symptoms, which are normally what prompt the parent or caregiver to seek medical care for the child. Children known to have increased risk for leukemia (see the Risk Factors section) should have regular medical checkups and other testing as recommended by their healthcare provider. The majority of symptoms of leukemia such as weakness, fatigue, dizziness, headache, and pallor may also be associated with other causes. These symptoms are related to a decrease in RBCs. Other symptoms such as infection, fever, and easy bruising and bleeding result from a decrease in WBCs and platelets. Depending on the type of leukemia, the child may also present with bone or joint pain, weight loss, anorexia, swollen lymph nodes, or swelling of the face and arms. Symptoms of JMML differ slightly from those of the other childhood leukemias and can include cough, difficulty breathing from too many WBCs in the lungs, and enlarged spleen and lymph nodes.

The type of leukemia a child has plays a major role in both treatment options and the child's prognosis. Leukemia is not staged in the same manner as other cancers. However, it is still important to know whether leukemia cells have begun collecting in other organs, lymph nodes, testicles, or the central nervous system. Age at diagnosis and the initial WBC count are thought to be the two most important prognostic factors for children with ALL. Children between the ages of 1 and 9 years with B-cell ALL tend to have better cure rates than others. Children diagnosed with AML who are younger than age 2 years appear to have a better prognosis than others, especially teenagers. Disease response to the initial treatment for both ALL and AML affects long-term prognosis.

The main treatment for childhood leukemia is chemotherapy and involves a multidisciplinary team approach. This treatment is very intensive, and the type of leukemia being treated affects the number of phases of treatment the child must endure. ALL is treated in three phases, which can last a total of 2–3 years: induction, to achieve remission; consolidation, to reduce the number of remaining leukemia cells; and maintenance, which begins if the leukemia remains in remission. The treatment plan for ALL can change if the disease does not go into or remain in remission. Treatment of AML involves two phases (induction and consolidation), and higher doses of chemotherapy are used for a shorter period of time. These children must be treated in facilities that are experienced in disease treatment because of the risk

of serious complications from the intensive treatment. Children with higher-risk leukemias may also be treated with SCT. This is the treatment of choice for children with JMML. Other therapies, such as targeted therapy or radiation, may be used in special circumstances. The 5-year survival rates for children with ALL are now greater than 85% with rates for ALL survival ranging from 60 to 70%.

Research related to the causes, diagnosis, and treatment of leukemia is ongoing. Progress continues to be made in understanding the relationship between DNA changes in stem cells and the development of leukemia and how this can affect the intensity of treatment received. It has already led to the development of immensely improved, very sensitive tests for the detection of leukemia cells in both blood and bone marrow samples. Children with leukemia are often involved in clinical trials, which allow them to receive the most current treatments. The use of chimeric antigen receptor (CAR) T-cell therapy and monoclonal antibody therapy are two areas of immunotherapy treatment that have shown promise in treating ALL (ACS, 2016e).

Children who are successfully treated for leukemia during childhood have an increased risk for various health problems in their adult years. Nurses caring for children with leukemia should help them prepare for the challenges they may face in the future (see the Evidence-Based Practice feature).

Leukemia in Pregnant Women

Acute leukemia is one of the most common types of hematologic cancers diagnosed in pregnant women, although its occurrence is rare. It is also one of the most challenging cancers to treat during pregnancy. Diagnosis during pregnancy can result in a complicated situation because the chemotherapy and/or targeted therapies used for treatment are teratogenic to the fetus. Delaying treatment may be too risky for the mother, and termination of the pregnancy may be necessary to save her life. Providing the mother with information related to the possible risks and benefits will allow her to make an informed decision about treatment. Researchers have noted that it may be possible to treat the mother if the initial leukemia diagnosis is made later in the pregnancy; however, additional studies are needed to determine its safety (Simon, 2012b).

Leukemia in Older Adults

CLL is considered to be a disease of the older adult, the median age of onset being approximately 70 years of age. Because this age group has been poorly represented in clinical trials, there is uncertainty about optimal treatment. The majority of patients with CLL are diagnosed in the early stages of the disease process and can remain asymptomatic for several years, requiring no treatment (Shanafelt, 2013). One of the most important prognostic factors is the presence of comorbidities, which can also affect treatment options. As with other cancers, age and functional status are also considerations. Treatment for CLL should be given only to patients who exhibit symptoms of active disease; there is no evidence to support improved clinical outcomes with earlier treatment. Chlorambucil remains the current standard of treatment for the older adult patient with CLL. However, other therapies with reduced toxic effects are being investigated in clinical trials and will eventually replace chemotherapy (Molica et al., 2013).

Evidence-Based Practice
Preparing Childhood ALL Survivors for Challenges in Adulthood

Problem

In addition to the emotional and psychosocial challenges faced by children with ALL, treatment also requires an immense physical battle. Because of the major advances in leukemia treatment, most children with the disease are now living into adulthood. This victory over leukemia can unfortunately set the stage for future battles that may be equally intense. Childhood survivors are at an increased risk for numerous potential late effects of their treatment, including chronic conditions and premature death. These effects are related to multiple factors, such as type of leukemia, type and dose of treatment, and age of the child when treatment was received (ACS, 2016e).

Evidence

Patients who overcome lymphoma and ALL during childhood demonstrate a much higher incidence of chronic fatigue in adulthood. For long-term survivors, research suggests that 20 years after diagnosis, the incidence of chronic fatigue among childhood leukemia/lymphoma survivors is roughly 3 times higher than that in the general population (Hamre et al., 2013). In the past, some researchers linked the development of chronic fatigue to many potential causes, including previous exposure to viruses associated with specific forms of leukemia. However, current researchers have found that this is not the case (Alter et al., 2012).

Adult survivors of ALL also face other chronic health challenges. The medications and therapies used in treatment of ALL are associated with lasting effects, including myocardial impairment, growth hormone deficiency, infertility, osteoporosis, and the development of secondary cancers. Adult survivors of ALL also have a higher incidence of obesity and hypertension, which can add to the heart and lung problems caused by therapy (ACS, 2016e).

Implications

While providing the highest quality care to pediatric patients diagnosed with ALL, nurses should also consider the future ramifications of treatment. Remission is the immediate goal. However, promotion of healthy habits and lifestyle choices, such as balanced nutrition and regular exercise, may have far-reaching effects on the quality of life these patients experience in adulthood. It is also important that young patients and their caregivers receive factual information about the risks the patients may face in the future.

Critical Thinking Application

1. How might emotion-based care of pediatric patients with ALL unintentionally lead to promotion of unhealthy habits by caregivers and family members?

2. Considering the physiologic effects of treatments for ALL and the pediatric patient's need for rest, in what ways can the nurse still promote physical exercise?

3. Explain how the long-term effects of medications used in the treatment of ALL could influence the activity tolerance, exercise habits, and overall level of fitness of an adult survivor of childhood ALL.

AML is the second most common type of leukemia diagnosed in adults, the median age at diagnosis being 67 years of age; 60% of newly diagnosed patients are older than age 60. These individuals account for more than 75% of all annual AML-related deaths. Treatment for AML in the older adult is highly individualized. Recent studies have indicated that 50–60% of newly diagnosed patients with AML do not receive any form of treatment after diagnosis, and age has been indicated as having a major role in treatment protocols, which are usually intensive. Clinical trials indicate promising results for the future (Medeiros, 2015).

NURSING PROCESS

When caring for the patient with leukemia, the nurse considers the chronic and life-threatening nature of the disease as well as the effects of treatment in planning care.

Assessment

Focused assessment data related to leukemia include the following:

- **Observation and patient interview.** During the initial interview, observe the general appearance of the patient. The patient may be pale and have visible bruising on the skin. Ask whether the patient has any complaints of fatigue, weakness, dyspnea on exertion, frequent infections, sore throat, night sweats, bleeding gums, or nose bleeds. Ask about recent weight loss, exposure to ionizing radiation (multiple x-rays, residence near a site of radiation or atomic testing) or chemicals (occupational), previous treatment for cancer, and history of immune disorders.

- **Physical examination.** The physical assessment should include the skin and mucous membranes for color, bruising, purpura, petechiae, ulcers, or lesions; pallor; vital signs, including orthostatic vitals; heart and lung sounds; abdominal examination; and stool for occult blood.

Diagnosis

Nursing diagnoses for the patient with leukemia include the following:

- *Infection, Risk for*
- *Bleeding, Risk for*
- *Imbalanced Nutrition: Less Than Body Requirements*
- *Mucous Membrane: Oral, Impaired*
- *Grieving.*

  (NANDA-I © 2014)

Planning

Goals for patient care include the following:

- The patient and family members/significant others will describe strategies to reduce risk of infection.

- The patient will demonstrate no signs or symptoms of infection.

- The pediatric patient will meet developmental milestones.

- The patient will express emotions related to the diagnosis.

- The patient will receive adequate dietary intake that is sufficient for meeting nutritional needs.
- The patient will promptly report symptoms of complications.

Implementation

Nurses play a key role in the long-term multidisciplinary treatment of patients with leukemia. The impact of a diagnosis of leukemia and the long-term nature of treatment can severely stress the coping abilities of both the patient and the family. Ongoing psychosocial assessment and emotional support are essential. Referral to support groups and social services may be beneficial. Assist the family in exploration of complementary health approaches, such as relaxation, imagery, and nutritional support. Be alert for any interactions that could occur between complementary health approaches and the medical regimen. Many patients are treated in an oncology clinic, staying in the hospital only on the day of IV drug administration, and receive oral medications at home. The time at the hospital is used to assess how the family is managing issues such as nutrition, sleep, medication administration, and obtaining psychosocial support. Careful teaching for the family is needed to ensure safe drug administration and identification of issues requiring further care.

Prevent and Manage Adverse Medication Effects

The nurse should carefully monitor the patient with leukemia receiving treatment to prevent or manage any adverse medication effects. The nurse should check drug references carefully for recommendations specific to each drug. Other nursing interventions regarding medications include the following:

- Obtain daily weight measurements. Daily weight measurements are important to assist in planning adequate hydration during chemotherapy as well as to measure nutritional status.
- Evaluate the infusion site before and frequently during infusion. Although extravasation is not as common with central lines used in cancer treatment as in peripheral lines, it still can occur. Many chemotherapeutic agents are extremely toxic to tissues. In addition, lysis of the cancer cells can produce toxic side effects.
- Monitor the patient's intake and output. Careful monitoring of intake and output is required to record the IV fluids, assess kidney functioning, and monitor excretion of by-products. Monitor specific gravity every 8 hours as well as before and during administration of the drug and when the IV fluids are reduced to maintenance volume levels.
- Renal function must be carefully monitored in patients receiving cyclophosphamide. Gross hematuria is a side effect of this drug. Hydration with IV fluids to attain a specific gravity of less than 1.010 prevents or reduces the severity of hematuria. It also prepares the kidneys to manage products of tumor cell breakdown. To achieve this desired specific gravity, the patient receives IV fluids at 1.5 times maintenance volume for at least 6–8 hours

before and at least 1.5 hours after administration of the drug. Other chemotherapeutic drugs have different infusion times, while some do not require hydration before infusion.

- Administer prescribed medications, such as allopurinol and diuretics, as ordered. Allopurinol reduces the risk of uric acid crystallization in the kidneys and other tissues (Wilson et al., 2016).

Prevent Infection

Infection is the major cause of death in patients with leukemia. Mucous membranes are especially susceptible to breakdown and infection as a result of tissue damage from chemotherapy or radiation. Changes in WBC function impair the immune and inflammatory responses in the patient with leukemia, increasing the risk for infection. WBCs may be immature and ineffective or, in some cases, deficient. Chemotherapy or radiation therapy further depresses bone marrow function and increases the risk for infection. See Exemplar 2.A on Cancer for more on infection prevention.

Protect from Injury Related to Bleeding

Bleeding is the second most common cause of leukemia deaths. As the platelet counts decrease, the risk of bleeding increases. Internal hemorrhage may lead to tachycardia, hypotension, pallor, and diaphoresis. Bleeding into the lungs may cause dyspnea; bleeding into the abdomen causes increased girth, pain, and guarding. Intracranial bleeding affects mental status and level of consciousness. Early identification of bleeding helps to prevent significant blood loss and potential shock. The nurse can perform the following interventions to reduce the patient's risk of bleeding:

- Instruct the patient to avoid forceful blowing or picking of the nose, forceful coughing or sneezing, and straining to have a bowel movement. These activities can damage mucous membranes, increasing the risk for bleeding.
- Monitor and promptly report abnormal blood levels of electrolytes, uric acid, urea nitrogen, and creatinine or manifestations of TLS. Significant alterations in electrolyte levels can lead to complications, such as cardiac dysrhythmias, muscle weakness or tetany, paresthesias, and mental status changes. Excess uric acid can compromise renal function and lead to metabolic acidosis and gout.
- Assess vital signs every 4 hours and body systems every shift for bleeding:
  a. Skin and mucous membranes for petechiae, ecchymoses, and purpura
  b. Gums, nasal membranes, and conjunctiva for bleeding
  c. Vomitus, stool, and urine for visible or occult blood
  d. Vaginal bleeding
  e. Prolonged bleeding from puncture sites
  f. Neurologic changes, such as headache, visual changes, altered mentation, decreased level of consciousness, and seizures
  g. Abdomen for complaints of epigastric pain, diminished bowel sounds, increasing abdominal girth, rigidity, or guarding.

- Avoid invasive procedures, such as taking the temperatures rectally and the use of suppositories, vaginal douches and suppositories, tampons, urinary catheterization, and parenteral injections, if possible. Invasive diagnostic procedures, such as biopsy or lumbar puncture, should not be done if the platelet count is less than 50,000. Invasive procedures can cause tissue trauma and bleeding. Procedures that use large-bore needles should be delayed until the platelet count is increased.

- Apply pressure to injection sites for 3–5 minutes and to arterial punctures for 15–20 minutes. Pressure prevents prolonged bleeding by prompting hemostasis and clot formation.

Evaluation

Expected outcomes for nursing care of the patient with leukemia include the following:

- The patient remains free from signs and symptoms of infection.

- The patient maintains urinary output of at least 0.5 mL/kg/hr.

- The patient is adequately hydrated to allow elimination of drugs and cell components.

- The patient's electrolyte values are maintained within normal limits.

- The patient rates pain as absent or at a level that is tolerable.

- The patient demonstrates adequate knowledge related to the disease process and treatment regimens.

If one or more of the expected outcomes are not met, further nursing interventions may be needed. These might include further patient teaching regarding the disease process, the importance of hydration, and the connection between good nutrition and minimizing the risk of infection. If infection is present, the nurse should report to the healthcare provider and determine whether further infection protection measures are needed.

Nursing Care Plan
A Patient with AML

Catherine Cole is a 37-year-old secretary who lives with her husband, Ray, and teenage daughter, Amy, in an apartment in a large metropolitan area. Approximately 2 months ago, Ms. Cole began to tire easily and experience night sweats several times a week. She also noted that she was pale, bruised easily, and was having heavier than normal menstrual periods. Blood tests ordered by her primary care provider had abnormal results. She has been admitted for a bone marrow biopsy.

ASSESSMENT	DIAGNOSES	PLANNING
Mary Losapio, RN, obtains a nursing history and physical assessment for Ms. Cole. Ms. Cole tells her, "I'm so tired, and I have these bruises all over me. I'm so afraid of the results of the bone marrow examination. I don't know what we will do if I have cancer." Ms. Cole clutches her husband's hand and then begins to cry. Physical assessment data include the following: height, 156 cm (64 in.); weight, 48.1 kg (106 lb); and temperature 37.8°C (100°F) oral, pulse 102 bpm, respirations 22/min, and BP 130/82 mmHg. Numerous petechiae are scattered over the trunk and arms; ecchymoses are noted on lower right arm and right calf. Oral mucosa is red, with several small ulcerations in buccal areas. Blood count shows reduced RBCs, hemoglobin, and hematocrit levels. The WBC count is high, with myeloblasts seen on differential. The platelet count is very low. A tentative diagnosis of AML is made.	■ *Infection, Risk for* related to altered WBC production and immune function ■ *Bleeding, Risk for* ■ *Impaired Oral Mucous Membrane* secondary to anemia and reduced platelets ■ *Fatigue* related to anemia ■ *Anxiety* related to fear of leukemia diagnosis (NANDA-I © 2014)	■ The patient will remain free of infection. ■ The patient will experience no significant bleeding. ■ The patient will have intact oral mucous membranes. ■ The patient will manage self-care activities despite fatigue. ■ The patient will verbalize decreased anxiety.

IMPLEMENTATION

- Place the patient in a private room, and limit visitors to immediate family for the present.
- Instruct all staff, the family, and the patient to perform careful hand hygiene. Post a sign over the washbasin in the room as a reminder.
- Record vital signs every 4 hours.
- Avoid invasive procedures unless absolutely necessary.
- Monitor for bleeding every 4 hours, including skin, oral mucosa, abdominal assessment, body fluids, and menstrual pad count.
- Instruct to perform oral hygiene every 2–4 hours, using a soft-bristle toothbrush.

- Ask the dietitian to work with the patient to identify preferred foods. Instruct the patient to avoid foods that may damage oral mucosa, such as very hot, very cold, or highly acidic or spicy foods.
- Provide for periods of rest alternating with activity.
- Teach about the bone marrow biopsy. Allow time for questions and for the patient to verbalize fears.
- Refer to the oncology nurse specialist for further teaching and support.

(continued on next page)

Nursing Care Plan (continued)

EVALUATION

The bone marrow biopsy confirms the diagnosis of AML. Ms. Cole is very upset, but she calms as the physician and the oncology nurse discuss treatment plans and the possibility of remission. She decides to have outpatient chemotherapy. During her hospital stay, Ms. Cole remained free of infection or further bleeding.

She tells Nurse Losapio that her mouth feels better, although it is still painful. During routine assessment, Ms. Cole remarks, "You know, I was so scared when I came here, but I think I am a little less so now. Sometimes not knowing what is wrong is worse than knowing."

CRITICAL THINKING

1. Describe how alterations in WBCs can increase an individual's susceptibility to infection.

2. List sources of potential infection for the patient who is hospitalized.

3. What is the rationale for having the patient do her own oral and physical hygiene?

4. Outline a teaching plan for this patient and her family for home care to prevent infection.

5. Develop a care plan for Ms. Cole for the nursing diagnosis of Activity Intolerance.

REVIEW Leukemia

RELATE Link the Concepts and Exemplars

Linking the exemplar of leukemia with the concept of comfort:

1. When caring for a patient diagnosed with leukemia, what nursing diagnoses would you implement to address comfort?

2. What interventions would be appropriate for the patient receiving chemotherapy who reports fatigue and difficulty meeting self-care needs?

Linking the exemplar of leukemia with the concept of culture:

3. How will you meet the cultural needs of the patient who recently moved from Mexico, does not speak English, and has been diagnosed with leukemia?

4. What assessment data will you collect to prioritize nursing diagnoses for a patient from India who has been diagnosed with leukemia?

READY Go to Volume 3: Clinical Nursing Skills

REFER Go to Pearson MyLab Nursing and eText

- Additional review materials

REFLECT Apply Your Knowledge

Johnny O'Malley is 4 years old and was brought to the clinic by his mother, who reports that she cannot put her finger on what is wrong but he has not looked well lately. He is pale, has dark circles under his eyes, and has bruising on his arms and legs. His mother states that he does not seem to have any energy lately. Johnny tells you that he is very tired all the time.

1. What is your priority when assessing Johnny during this visit?

2. What patient teaching will you provide to maintain Johnny's safety?

3. What interventions will you initiate to support Johnny and his family through a new diagnosis of leukemia?

›› Exemplar 2.F Lung Cancer

Exemplar Learning Outcomes

2.F Analyze lung cancer as it relates to cellular regulation.

- Describe the pathophysiology of lung cancer.
- Describe the etiology of lung cancer.
- Compare the risk factors for and prevention of lung cancer.
- Identify the clinical manifestations of lung cancer.
- Summarize diagnostic tests and therapies used by interprofessional teams in the collaborative care of an individual with lung cancer.

- Differentiate considerations for care of patients with lung cancer across the lifespan.
- Apply the nursing process in providing culturally competent care to an individual with lung cancer.

Exemplar Key Terms

Brachytherapy, *113*
Bronchogenic carcinomas, *109*
Hemoptysis, *110*
Non-small-cell carcinomas, *109*
Small-cell carcinomas, *109*

Overview

Of all forms of cancer in men and women, lung cancer accounts for the greatest number of deaths. In 2016, an estimated 158,080 deaths (26% of all cancer-related deaths) were due to lung cancer, while an estimated 224,390 individuals were expected to be newly diagnosed with lung cancer that same year (ACS, 2016b). Despite advances in surgical techniques and therapeutic treatments, lung cancer remains a significant health threat with dire consequences.

Pathophysiology and Etiology

Pathophysiology

The vast majority of primary lung lesions are **bronchogenic carcinomas** (tumors of the airway epithelium). These tumors are further differentiated by cell type: small-cell carcinoma, adenocarcinoma, squamous cell carcinoma, and large-cell carcinoma. For clinical purposes, the latter three cell types frequently are classified together as non-small-cell carcinomas. **Small-cell carcinomas**, which account for approximately 13% of lung cancers, grow rapidly and spread early (ACS, 2016b). These tumors have paraneoplastic properties; that is, they produce manifestations at sites that are not directly affected by the tumor. Small-cell lung carcinomas can synthesize bioactive products and hormones, such as adrenocorticotropic hormones, antidiuretic hormone, a parathormone-like hormone, and gastrin-releasing peptide. **Non-small-cell carcinomas** account for approximately 83% of lung cancers (ACS, 2016b). Each cell type differs in its incidence, presentation, and manner of spread. **Table 2–12** » outlines the incidence and unique characteristics of each type of small-cell and non-small-cell carcinomas.

TABLE 2–12 Comparison of Lung Cancer Cell Types

	Cell Type	Presentation and Associated Manifestations	Spread
	Small-cell (oat cell) carcinoma	Central lesion with hilar mass common, early mediastinal involvement, no cavitation; syndrome of inappropriate antidiuretic hormone (SIADH), Cushing syndrome, thrombophlebitis	Aggressive tumor; more than 40% of patients have distant metastasis at time of presentation
	Adenocarcinoma	Peripheral mass involving bronchi; few local symptoms; hypertrophic pulmonary osteoarthropathy	Early metastasis to central nervous system, skeleton, and adrenal glands
	Squamous cell carcinoma	Central lesion located in large bronchi; patient presents with cough, dyspnea, atelectasis, and wheezing; hypercalcemia common	Spreads by local invasion
	Large-cell carcinoma	Usually peripheral lesion that is larger than associated with adenocarcinoma and tends to cavitate; gynecomastia, thrombophlebitis	Early metastasis

Bronchogenic cancer, regardless of cell type, tends to be aggressive, locally invasive, and have widespread metastatic lesions. Tumors begin as mucosal lesions that grow to form masses that obstruct the bronchi or invade adjacent lung tissue. All types frequently spread via the lymph system to nodes and other organs, such as the brain, bones, and liver.

Etiology

Tobacco smoking is the leading cause of lung cancer (ACS, 2016f). Cigarette smoke contains more than 7000 chemicals, more than 70 of which are known carcinogens. Although not everyone who gets lung cancer is a smoker, approximately 90% of diagnosed cases are linked to smoking (CDC, 2015e). Lung cancer develops as damaged bronchial epithelial cells mutate over time to become neoplastic. Genetic changes are also linked to the development of lung cancer. Some of these genetic changes are inherited; others are acquired. The inherited genetic abnormality commonly seen is on chromosome 6, with loss of genetic material, and individuals with this mutation are more likely to develop lung cancer regardless of their smoking history. Acquired genetic changes develop over the lifetime of an individual; most of them result from exposure to cancer-causing chemicals in the environment, such as those in tobacco smoke, though some may be random changes without an external cause (ACS, 2016g). Alterations in specific tumor suppressor genes are thought to be important in the development of non-small-cell lung cancer (ACS, 2016f). The incidence of lung cancer varies from state to state and among nations. The incidence increases with age, occurring most commonly in patients over age 50.

Risk Factors and Prevention

Smoking is the strongest risk factor related to the development of lung cancer; however, it often interacts with other factors (ACS, 2016f). There is a dose–response relationship between smoking and lung cancer: The more the individual smokes and the longer the individual smokes, the greater the risk. Even former smokers who have abstained for a number of years have a higher risk for developing lung cancer compared with individuals who have never smoked. Exposure to ionizing radiation and inhaled irritants, asbestos in particular, is also recognized as a risk factor for lung cancer. Exposure to radon, a radioactive gas, is another lung cancer risk factor (CDC, 2015e). Radon forms as radium, an element in the earth's crust, disintegrates. Radon tends to accumulate in closed spaces where air circulation is poor, such as caves, mines, and energy-efficient houses.

Given the link between lung cancer and smoking, prevention of lung cancer is highly dependent on refraining from or stopping smoking. Despite the increased risk for lung cancer demonstrated among former smokers, there is still good reason to quit. Among smokers who quit before 40 years of age, the risk of death due to conditions associated with continued smoking decreases by approximately 90% (Jha et al., 2013). Aside from avoidance or cessation of smoking, prevention of lung cancer includes preventing environmental and occupational exposure to known carcinogens, such as radon and asbestos.

Clinical Manifestations

The manifestations of lung cancer are related to the location and spread of the tumor. Patients may present with symptoms related to the primary tumor, manifestations of metastatic disease, or systemic symptoms. Initial symptoms often are attributed to smoking or chronic bronchitis. Chronic cough is common, as is hemoptysis. Wheezing and shortness of breath occur as a result of airway obstruction. Dull, aching chest pain occurs as the tumor spreads to the mediastinum; pleuritic pain occurs when the pleura is invaded. Hoarseness and/or dysphagia indicates pressure of the tumor on the trachea or esophagus.

Systemic and paraneoplastic manifestations of lung cancer include weight loss, anorexia, fatigue, and weakness; bone pain, tenderness, and swelling; clubbing of the fingers and toes; and various endocrine, neuromuscular, cardiovascular, and hematologic symptoms. See the Multisystem Effects feature for more information.

Confusion, impaired gait and balance, headache, and personality changes may indicate brain metastasis. Bone metastases cause bone pain, pathologic fractures, and possible spinal cord compression, as well as thrombocytopenia and anemia if bone marrow is invaded. When the liver is affected, symptoms of liver dysfunction and biliary obstruction, including jaundice, anorexia, and upper right quadrant pain, are evident.

Lung cancer has both local and systemic effects. Local effects include cough, excess mucus production, shortness of breath or dyspnea, **hemoptysis** (bloody sputum), and chest pain. Systemic effects may include fever, anorexia and malaise, cyanosis, and other manifestations of impaired gas exchange.

Collaboration

Because lung cancer typically is advanced when diagnosed and the prognosis generally is poor, prevention of the disease must be a primary goal for all healthcare providers. With 90% of lung cancers related to cigarette smoking, reducing tobacco use can have a significant impact on the death rate from lung cancer—a far greater impact than advances in treatment.

Establishing an accurate diagnosis is the first step in treating lung cancer. Treatment decisions are based on the tumor location, the type of cancer cell, the staging of the tumor, and the patient's ability to tolerate treatment. Lung cancer is staged by the tumor size, location, degree of invasion of the primary tumor, and the presence of metastatic disease. Lung cancer staging is summarized in **Table 2–13 ≫**. Surgery is the treatment of choice for most forms of lung cancer.

Diagnostic Tests

Diagnostic tests for lung cancer are based on location and size of the tumor along with the patient's condition. Once lung cancer has been diagnosed, additional tests may be ordered to rule out possible metastasis. Common diagnostic tests include the following:

- ***Chest x-ray*** usually provides the first evidence of lung cancer. It is particularly reliable as a diagnostic tool when

Multisystem Effects of
Lung Cancer

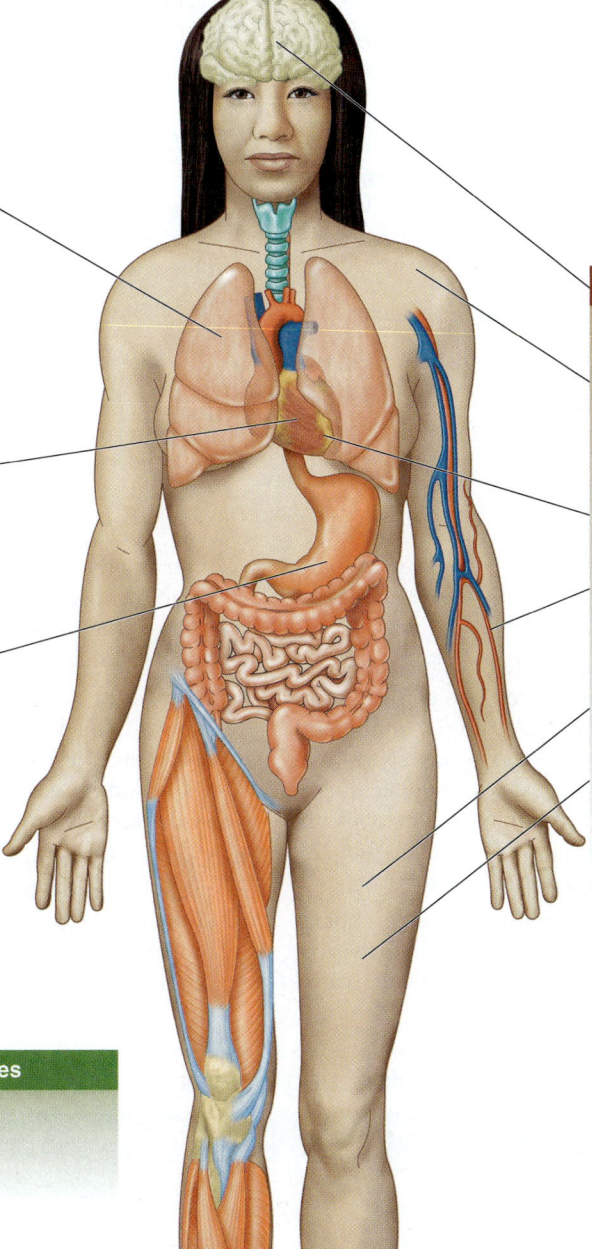

Respiratory

- Cough
- Hemoptysis
- Wheezing and dyspnea
- Chest pain, dull or pleuritic
- Hoarseness and dysphagia
- Pleural effusion

Cardiovascular

- Compression of the superior vena cava

Gastrointestinal

- Anorexia

Metabolic processes

- Weight loss
- Fever

Paraneoplastic syndromes

Endocrine system
- Hypercalcemia
- Hyperphosphatemia
- Cushing syndrome
- Syndrome of inappropriate antidiuretic hormone (SIADH) with water retention and hyponatremia

Cardiovascular system
- Thrombophlebitis
- Endocarditis

Hematologic effects
- Anemia
- Disseminated intravascular coagulation (DIC)
- Eosinophillia

Connective tissue
- Osteoarthropathy with clubbing and periosteal inflammation

Neuromuscular effects
- Peripheral neuropathy
- Cerebellar degeneration
- Myasthenia-like muscle weakness

Clinical Manifestations and Therapies
Lung Cancer

ETIOLOGY	CLINICAL MANIFESTATIONS	CLINICAL THERAPIES
Hypoxia	▪ Shortness of breath, chest pain, reduced oxygen saturation, tachypnea, chronic cough, dyspnea, and cyanosis	▪ Administer oxygen. ▪ Reduce activity level. ▪ Position in Fowler's or tripod position.
Paraneoplastic syndrome resulting from growth and metastasis of the tumor	▪ Weight loss, anorexia, fatigue, and weakness; bone pain, tenderness, and swelling; clubbing of the fingers and toes; and various endocrine, neuromuscular, cardiovascular, and hematologic symptoms	▪ Treatment may include surgical removal of the tumor. ▪ Chemotherapy or radiation therapy may be used to reduce metastasis and tumor size. ▪ Use palliative treatments to reduce symptoms. ▪ Use pain management as indicated.
Metastasis to brain	▪ Confusion, impaired gait and balance, headache, and personality changes	▪ Maintain familiar items in the room to promote orientation. ▪ Protect from falls and reduce the risk for injury. ▪ Explain the impact of brain metastasis to the family in order to prepare them for personality changes.

it can be compared with a previous chest x-ray. In high-risk populations, the chest x-ray may be used as a screening tool for lung cancer.

- **Sputum specimen** is sent for cytologic examination to establish the diagnosis of lung cancer. The sputum sample is collected on arising in the morning. If malignant cells are found in the sputum, more expensive and invasive examinations may be unnecessary. However, a sputum sample that is negative for malignant cells does not rule out lung cancer; it may simply indicate that the tumor is not shedding cells into mucous secretions.
- **Bronchoscopy** is frequently done to visualize and obtain a biopsy specimen from the tumor. When a tumor mass or suspicious tissue is identified visually, a cable-activated instrument is used to obtain a tissue specimen. If the tumor cannot be seen, the airways may be flushed with a saline solution (bronchial washing) to obtain cells for cytologic examination.
- **CT** is used to evaluate and localize tumors, particularly tumors in the lung parenchyma and pleura. It also is done before needle biopsy to localize the tumor. In addition, CT scanning can detect distant tumor metastasis and evaluate tumor response to treatment.
- **Cytologic examination and biopsy** involve cells or tissue obtained by aspirating fluid from a pleural effusion, percutaneous needle biopsy, and lymph node biopsy. These procedures may be done in an outpatient or surgical setting.

TABLE 2–13 The TNM Staging System for Lung Cancer

	Primary Tumor (T)	Regional Lymph Nodes (N)	Distant Metastasis (M)
Stage 0	TX—Malignant cells in bronchopulmonary secretions, but no tumor visualized		MX—Presence of distant metastasis cannot be assessed
Stage IA	T1a,b—Tumor of 3 cm or less in diameter, with no evidence of invasion	N0—No regional lymph node metastasis	M0—No distant metastasis
Stage IB	T2a	N0	M0
Stage IIA	T1a,b–T2ab—Tumor greater than 3 cm in diameter, or invades visceral pleura, or has associated atelectasis or pneumonitis	N1—Metastasis or direct extension to peribronchial or ipsilateral hilar nodes	M0
Stage IIB	T2b–T3—Tumor with direct extension into an adjacent structure, or any tumor with associated pleural effusion or atelectasis or pneumonitis of entire lung	N1	M0
Stage IIIA	T3–T4	N1–N2—Metastasis to ipsilateral mediastinal or subcarinal nodes	M0
Stage IIIB	T4—Tumor that invades mediastinum or involves the heart, great vessels, trachea, esophagus, vertebral body, or carina; presence of malignant pleural effusion	N3—Metastasis to contralateral mediastinal, scalene, or supraclavicular nodes	M0
Stage IV	Any T	Any N	M1—Distant metastasis present

- **CBC, liver function studies, and serum electrolytes,** including calcium are obtained to evaluate for evidence of metastatic disease or paraneoplastic syndromes.
- **Tuberculin test** is performed to rule out tuberculosis as the cause of symptoms and abnormalities seen on chest x-ray.
- **Pulmonary function tests and arterial blood gases** may be performed before the initiation of treatment if the patient has manifestations of respiratory insufficiency (e.g., dyspnea, activity intolerance, low oxygen saturation levels).

These tests are described in greater detail in Appendix B available online at Pearson MyLab Nursing and eText.

Surgery

Surgery offers the only real chance for a cure in patients with non-small-cell lung cancer. Most tumors unfortunately are inoperable or only partially resectable at the time of diagnosis. The type of surgery that is performed depends on the location and size of the tumor as well as on the patient's pulmonary and general health. The goal of surgery is to remove all involved tissue while preserving as much functional lung as possible. **Table 2–14** ›› outlines various surgical procedures used to diagnose and treat lung cancer.

Pharmacologic Therapy

Combination chemotherapy (often combined with radiation therapy and/or surgery) is the treatment of choice for small-cell lung cancer because of the rapid growth, dissemination, and sensitivity to cytotoxic drugs of this type of cancer. Used in combination, chemotherapeutic drugs allow tumor cells to be attacked at different parts of the cell cycle and in different ways, increasing the effectiveness of therapy. Fifty percent of patients with tumors at early stages achieve complete tumor remission with combination chemotherapy. When a complete tumor response is achieved in the first few cycles of chemotherapy, the chances for long-term survival are much greater.

Combination chemotherapy also is used as an adjunct to surgery or radiation therapy for other types of lung cancer. It may be used to reduce the size of advanced local tumors before surgery and to lengthen survival when distant metastases are present.

Bronchodilators may be prescribed to reduce airway obstruction. Analgesics and pain management strategies are vital when the cancer is advanced. See the module on Comfort for more information about postoperative and cancer pain management.

Radiation Therapy

Radiation therapy is used alone or in combination with surgery or chemotherapy for lung cancer. The goal of treatment may be either cure or symptom relief (palliation). Before surgery, radiation therapy is used to debulk tumors. When cancer has spread by direct extension to other thoracic structures and surgery is not feasible, radiation therapy may be the treatment of choice. It also may be used to relieve manifestations such as cough, hemoptysis, pain resulting from bone metastasis, and dyspnea from bronchial obstruction. Complications of lung cancer, such as superior vena cava syndrome, may be treated with radiation. Radiation therapy may be delivered by external beam to the primary tumor site or by **brachytherapy**, in which a radioactive source is implanted in the body near the tumor, providing a high dose of radiation to the tumor and allowing the surrounding healthy tissues to be exposed to less radiation than they would be with external beam therapy.

Lifespan Considerations

Lung Cancer in Children

Lung cancer is a rare occurrence in children. However, when lung tumors occur in children, they are most often malignant. Treatment generally involves surgery to remove the tumor. The type of tumor and amount of metastasis dictate additional treatment (NCI, 2015g).

Lung Cancer in Pregnant Women

Lung cancer during pregnancy is uncommon, but when it does occur, it typically has poor maternal and fetal outcomes. This is generally due to the presence of metastasis at diagnosis and effects of treatment on the pregnancy (Boussios et al., 2013). However, most infants who survive to term in mothers with lung cancer are healthy at birth (Mitou et al., 2016).

TABLE 2–14 Types of Surgery for Lung Cancer

Procedure	Description	Used for
Laser bronchoscopy	Bronchoscopy-guided laser used to resect tumor	Tumors localized in a main bronchus
Mediastinoscopy	Visualization of the mediastinum using an endoscope passed through a suprasternal incision	Evaluation and biopsy of a mediastinal tumor and lymph nodes
Thoracotomy	Incision into the chest wall	Access to the lung and thoracic cavity for surgery
Wedge resection	Removal of a small section (wedge) of peripheral lung tissue	Small, peripheral lung tumors
Segmental resection	Removal of an individual bronchovascular segment of a lobe	Peripheral lung tumor with no evidence of extension to the chest wall or metastasis
Sleeve resection (bronchoplastic reconstruction)	Resection of a section of a major bronchus with reconstruction of remaining normal bronchus	Small lesion of a major bronchus
Lobectomy	Removal of a single lung lobe	Tumors confined to a single lobe
Pneumonectomy	Removal of an entire lung	Tumor widespread throughout the lung, involving the main bronchus, or fixed to the hilum

Lung Cancer in Older Adults

Lung cancer is the most common cause of cancer death in the older adult population. Approximately 81% of individuals diagnosed with lung cancer are over the age of 65, the median age at diagnosis being approximately 70 years of age (Karve et al., 2014; Nadpara, Madhavan, & Tworek, 2015; News Medical, 2016). This number is expected to increase as the estimated number of older adults in the United States doubles to approximately 70 million by 2030. The majority of new lung cancer diagnoses are classified as non-small-cell lung cancer (85%); the remaining cases are classified as small-cell lung cancer. A higher percentage of these cancers have metastasized to other organs at the time of initial diagnosis, which is a contributing factor to the low overall 5-year survival rate of 16.6% for this age group (Caprario & Strauss, 2014; Nadpara et al., 2015).

Combination chemotherapy has been used as the main treatment for older adult patients with lung cancer for decades; however, this has not been shown to improve overall survival rates in older adults. Older adult patients may also be less tolerant to chemotherapy treatment as a result of comorbidities and the development of toxicity (Caprario & Strauss, 2014). Recent research has revealed important information related to the long-term survival of these patients, which will improve treatment decision making. It also revealed a greater than expected survival rate for older adults undergoing surgery for lung cancer (News Medical, 2016).

Another important factor in the quality of care received by older adult patients with cancer is the timeliness in which the care is received. Studies by the Institute of Medicine (IOM) have indicated that delays in time from diagnosis to initiation of treatment may affect the patient's prognosis. This delay can be minimized through the use of a multidisciplinary team approach. These studies also indicated that patients who were diagnosed in the earlier stages of the disease process were less likely to receive care in a timely manner than were those diagnosed in the later stages. Results of the IOM studies show that delays in diagnosis and treatment should be avoided to prevent the risk of disease progression and increased psychologic stress in the patient. Improvement in the coordination of care for the older adult with lung cancer is still needed among healthcare providers to reduce delays in diagnosis and treatment (Nadpara et al., 2015).

NURSING PROCESS

The patient with lung cancer is facing invasive treatments with undesirable side effects, possibly surgery, and typically a poor prognosis for long-term survival. Nursing care components are diverse, related to respiratory status, the cancer itself and possible metastases, and the treatment plan.

Assessment

Nursing assessment related to lung cancer focuses on identifying risk factors for the disease, early manifestations of lung cancer, and respiratory function in the patient undergoing treatment. The nurse should collect the following data through the health history and physical examination:

- **Observation and patient interview.** Observe the patient for dyspnea with exertion, signs of discomfort, presence of cough, and visible signs of alterations in nutritional status. Ask about current symptoms, including chronic cough, shortness of breath, and blood-tinged sputum; systemic manifestations such as recent weight loss, fatigue, anorexia, and bone pain; smoking history; occupational exposure to carcinogens; and chronic diseases such as chronic obstructive pulmonary disease.
- **Physical examination.** Assess respiratory function, including respiratory rate, depth, breath sounds, and chest excursion. Assess oxygenation using pulse oximetry, arterial blood gas results, and pulmonary function studies.

Diagnosis

Priority nursing diagnoses related to respiratory function for the patient with lung cancer include the following:

- *Gas Exchange, Impaired*
- *Breathing Pattern, Ineffective*
- *Decreased Cardiac Tissue Perfusion, Risk for*
- *Activity Intolerance*
- *Pain*
- *Grieving.*

(NANDA-I © 2014)

Planning

Goals and identified outcomes for the patient with lung cancer depend on the specific nursing diagnoses included in the patient's plan of care, as well as the individual patient. The wide range of possible outcomes relevant to the plan of care for the patient with lung cancer may include the following:

- The patient will maintain an oxygen saturation of greater than 90%.
- The patient's respiratory rate will range between 12 and 20 breaths per minute.
- The patient will deny dyspnea.
- The patient's heart rate will be maintained within normal limits.
- The patient will demonstrate the ability to make informed decisions regarding all treatments.
- Using a predetermined pain rating scale, the patient will report that pain is maintained at a level deemed by the patient to be tolerable.
- The patient will verbalize emotions and concerns related to diagnosis and treatment.

Implementation

Nurses take a holistic approach to providing care for the patient with lung cancer, meeting both the physical and psychosocial needs of the patient. Airway and breathing are always the greatest priority, followed by circulation. The patient who has hypoxia will be anxious, so reducing anxiety is a priority intervention for that patient.

Promote Effective Cardiorespiratory Function

Breathing pattern and ventilation of the patient with lung cancer may be affected by the tumor itself or by treatment of the tumor. Thoracic surgery increases the risk caused by the incision and disruption of the muscles of respiration. Maintaining effective lung ventilation is particularly important postoperatively to re-expand remaining lung tissue and prevent surgical complications. The nurse should do the following:

- Assess and document respiratory rate, depth, and lung sounds at least every 4 hours; evaluate more frequently in the immediate postoperative period or as indicated by condition. Early detection of signs of respiratory compromise or adventitious lung sounds is vital for effective intervention.

- Suction the airway as needed. Suctioning may be required to remove secretions that the patient is unable to cough up and expectorate.

- Provide chest physiotherapy with percussion and postural drainage as needed or ordered. Percussion and postural drainage help maintain airway patency and effective respirations.

- Administer supplemental oxygen as ordered and as needed per protocols.

- Impaired oxygenation can lead to inadequate perfusion of cardiac tissue, which can cause cardiac complications, including tachycardia and dysrhythmias. For some patients, especially those with compromised respiratory function, continuous electrocardiogram (ECG) monitoring is indicated.

- Elevate the head of the bed to 60 degrees. Elevating the head of the bed reduces pressure on the diaphragm and permits optimal lung expansion.

- Assist the patient to turn, cough, and deep-breathe and to use incentive spirometry. Help splint the chest with a pillow or blanket when coughing. These measures promote airway clearance.

- If mechanical ventilation is instituted, work with respiratory therapy and use analgesia or sedation as needed to synchronize respirations with the ventilator. Coordination of the patient's respiratory effort with ventilator-delivered breaths is important for fully effective mechanical ventilation.

Manage Fatigue and Activity Intolerance

Both resectional lung surgery and inoperable lung cancer reduce the amount of functional lung tissue and surface area for gas diffusion. This can lead to activity intolerance if the oxygen supply is insufficient to meet the body's oxygen demand. The nurse should do the following:

- Keep frequently used objects within easy reach. This helps to conserve energy.

- Plan rest periods between activities and procedures. Rest periods reduce oxygen demands and fatigue.

- Teach measures to conserve energy while performing ADLs, such as sitting while showering and dressing and wearing slip-on shoes. These energy-conserving measures

reduce oxygen demand and help the patient to remain independent.

- Encourage maintenance of physical activity to tolerance. Maintaining activity levels to the degree possible improves physical and emotional well-being.

- Allow family members to provide assistance as needed. This helps the patient conserve energy and allows the family to retain a sense of usefulness.

- Provide reassurance and emotional support. These measures help to relieve anxiety and promote an effective breathing pattern.

- Administer oxygen as prescribed. Teach the patient and family about home oxygen use if appropriate. Supplemental oxygen can help improve activity and exercise tolerance.

- Assist the postoperative patient to increase activities gradually, which improves exercise tolerance.

Evaluation

The patient's response to care is evaluated according to how well the goals of care have been met. Desired outcomes may include the following:

- The patient maintains an oxygen saturation of greater that 90% at rest and with activity.

- The patient's respiratory rate ranges between 12 and 24 breaths per minute.

- The patient denies dyspnea at rest and during appropriate levels of activity.

- The patient's heart rate is maintained within 10% of the upper and lower limits of this patient's normal range.

- The patient makes informed decisions regarding all treatments.

- Using a predetermined pain rating scale, the patient reports maintenance of pain at a level deemed by the patient to be tolerable.

- The patient verbalizes grief and fears related to the diagnosis and treatment.

Secondary interventions for the patient with lung cancer may include education related to adequate nutrition. Patients receiving cancer treatment will need to increase their intake of high-calorie nutrient-rich foods and take in adequate fluid. The use of supplements may be necessary to achieve this increase. Eating small, more frequent meals can also help patients increase their intake. Increased metabolic needs related to treatment and healing processes require these dietary changes. The nurse should instruct patients to avoid spicy, overly sweet, fatty foods and to use antinausea medications as prescribed if chemotherapy-related nausea is an issue. Referral to a dietitian may also be beneficial. The nurse should also instruct patients about prevention of infection because of myelosuppression related to treatment. Proper hand cleansing and personal hygiene, as well as limiting exposure to crowds and those who are ill, will limit potential sources of infection. Radiation and chemotherapy treatments can damage the skin; therefore, education related to proper skin care will prevent breakdown and allow for early recognition of delayed wound healing.

Nursing Care Plan
A Patient with Lung Cancer

After coughing up bloody sputum one morning, James Mueller, a 68-year-old retired mill worker, sees his physician. A chest x-ray shows a suspicious density in the central portion of his right lung. Mr. Mueller is admitted to the hospital the following Monday for diagnostic tests.

ASSESSMENT

Anita Sarros, RN, admits Mr. Mueller to the oncology unit and obtains a nursing history. Mr. Mueller is married and has three grown children. He worked in a local paper mill for 35 years before retiring at age 62. He describes himself as "pretty healthy" except for a chronic smoker's cough. He started smoking as a young man in the army. He has a 50-year smoking history, having smoked a pack a day since age 18. Mr. Mueller says that he briefly quit smoking after a small heart attack 3 years ago but started again 4 months later. On further questioning, Mr. Mueller says that his cough has been productive for the past few months, especially in the morning, and that he is shorter of breath than usual with activity.

Mr. Mueller's vital signs include temperature 98.4°F oral; pulse 78 bpm; respirations 20/min; and BP 162/86 mmHg. His color is good, and his skin is warm and dry. Inspiratory and expiratory wheezes are noted in right chest, but good breath sounds are heard throughout. No other abnormal findings are noted on examination. The physician orders early-morning sputum specimens times 3 days for cytologic examination and schedules a CT scan of the chest the morning after admission.

Mr. Mueller's CBC shows mild anemia, but remaining routine laboratory tests are essentially normal. Sputum cytology is positive for small-cell bronchogenic cancer. The CT scan shows a central mass approximately 4 cm in diameter with involved mediastinal and subclavicular lymph nodes. A small mass is also noted on the lumbar spine. After conferring with his physician and an oncologist, Mr. Mueller decides to undergo a trial course of chemotherapy.

DIAGNOSES

- *Airway Clearance, Ineffective,* related to tumor mass
- *Imbalanced Nutrition: Less Than Body Requirements, Risk for,* related to effects of chemotherapy
- *Family Coping, Compromised,* related to new diagnosis of lung cancer
- *Deficient Knowledge* about lung cancer and aids to smoking cessation

(NANDA-I © 2014)

PLANNING

- The patient will maintain a patent airway.
- The patient will maintain current weight.
- The patient will express feelings and concerns about the effect of cancer on the family.
- The patient will participate in care.
- The patient will contact appropriate support groups.
- The patient will verbalize an understanding of the disease, its treatment, and its prognosis.
- The patient will develop a plan to stop smoking.

IMPLEMENTATION

- Teach Mr. Mueller coughing, deep breathing, and hydration measures to facilitate airway clearance.
- Discuss symptoms to report to the physician: increased dyspnea or hemoptysis, severe stridor or wheezing, and chest pain.
- Discuss measures to relieve nausea associated with chemotherapy, including premedication with a prescribed antiemetic.
- Have a dietitian consult with Mr. Mueller and his wife to develop a diet plan for maintaining ideal weight.
- Discuss possible effects of lung cancer with Mr. and Mrs. Mueller.
- Encourage Mr. and Mrs. Mueller to call a family conference to discuss the disease with their children and grandchildren.
- Evaluate family members' knowledge and understanding of lung cancer, correcting misinformation and teaching as needed.
- Have an American Cancer Society volunteer contact the family.
- Refer the Muellers to a local cancer support group.
- Refer the Muellers to a home health service for follow-up and further teaching.
- Work with Mr. Mueller to develop a plan to stop smoking.
- Ask the physician for a prescription for nicotine patches or gum for Mr. Mueller.

EVALUATION

Mr. Mueller had his first chemotherapy treatment in the hospital and was discharged 4 days after admission. After 3 months of chemotherapy, his tumor shows little regression, and a liver scan reveals further metastasis. He and his wife decide to stop chemotherapy, a decision with which the children reluctantly agree. Mr. and Mrs. Mueller are referred to hospice services. With the help of hospice nurses and volunteers, Mr. Mueller is able to remain at home. His pain is managed initially with oral MS Contin, a sustained-release form of morphine sulfate, and later with an IV morphine infusion. Mr. Mueller dies at home with his family at his side, 9 months after his diagnosis of lung cancer.

CRITICAL THINKING

1. The oncologist prescribed a chemotherapy regimen of cyclophosphamide, doxorubicin, and vincristine. Describe how each of these drugs works against cancer cells, and discuss the rationale for using this combination.

2. Develop a care plan to deal with the specific side effects for the above treatment regimen.

3. Mr. Mueller had small-cell cancer. How would his presentation and treatment differ if the diagnosis had been non-small-cell adenocarcinoma, stage T2N2M0?

REVIEW Lung Cancer

RELATE Link the Concepts and Exemplars

Linking the exemplar of lung cancer with the concept of acid–base balance:

1. What effect might lung cancer have on the patient's acid–base balance?
2. What patient teaching will you provide to assist with normalizing acid–base balance?

Linking the exemplar of lung cancer with the concept of infection:

3. What priority patient teaching can you provide to reduce the risk of infection in the patient diagnosed with lung cancer?
4. When caring for the patient with lung cancer, what interventions will you initiate to reduce the risk of infection?

READY Go to Volume 3: Clinical Nursing Skills

REFER Go to Pearson MyLab Nursing and eText

■ Additional review materials

REFLECT Apply Your Knowledge

Michael Harris, 66 years old, has abused alcohol for many years and has smoked two packs of cigarettes a day since age 19. He has been diagnosed with lung cancer. Mr. Harris is divorced and lives alone in a fourth-floor apartment. He has two children who are grown and live out of town. Mr. Harris has a girlfriend who also smokes and abuses alcohol. The physician in charge of Mr. Harris's care has told him that he will need a lobectomy of the left lung, radiation therapy, and chemotherapy. Mr. Harris thanks the doctor and says he will get back to him. The nurse remains with Mr. Harris after the doctor leaves the room and overhears him say under his breath, "Fat chance I'm going to do all that. I'd rather die in peace."

1. How would you respond to this statement?
2. What are the priorities for Mr. Harris's care at this time?
3. What interventions can you initiate to help Mr. Harris make the best healthcare and lifestyle decisions?
4. What would your personal feelings and thoughts be if you were caring for Mr. Harris and he decided not to pursue treatment? How might your biases affect your approach to caring for him?

≫ Exemplar 2.G
Prostate Cancer

Exemplar Learning Outcomes

2.G Analyze prostate cancer as it relates to cellular regulation.

■ Describe the pathophysiology of prostate cancer.
■ Describe the etiology of prostate cancer.
■ Compare the risk factors for and prevention of prostate cancer.
■ Identify the clinical manifestations of prostate cancer.
■ Summarize diagnostic tests and therapies used by interprofessional teams in the collaborative care of an individual with prostate cancer.

■ Differentiate considerations for care of patients with prostate cancer across the lifespan.
■ Apply the nursing process in providing culturally competent care to an individual with prostate cancer.

Exemplar Key Terms

Androgens, *117*
Orchiectomy, *120*
Prostatectomy, *119*

Overview

Cancer of the prostate is the most common type of cancer and the second leading cause of death among men in North America. It is primarily a disease of older men, increasing in incidence with age. The majority of diagnosed cases are in men older than 65 years. Researchers anticipated diagnosis of more than 180,890 new cases of prostate cancer in 2016, and more than 26,120 men were expected to die from this disease that same year (ACS, 2016b). Prostate cancer is a major health problem for older men, but the death rate is decreasing as a result of advances in diagnosis and treatment.

Abnormal growth of prostate tissue may be related to benign prostatic hyperplasia (covered in more detail in the module on Elimination), or it may be an indication of prostate cancer. The diagnosis of prostate cancer is very frightening for most men, who fear death, disfigurement, and loss of sexual function.

When diagnosed early, prostate cancer is curable. When the cancer is confined to the prostate at diagnosis, the

5-year survival rate is 100%. Even when the cancer has spread regionally, approximately 99% of patients are alive after 5 years. More than 92% of prostate cancer diagnoses are made at one of these stages (ACS, 2016b). Many men are found to have prostate cancer on autopsy. The cancer usually has produced no manifestations or complications, and these men may have died with no knowledge of the developing disease.

Pathophysiology and Etiology
Pathophysiology

The prostate gland consists primarily of glandular epithelial cells. The exact etiology of prostate cancer is unknown, although **androgens** (hormones synthesized in the testes, ovaries, and adrenal cortex that promote expression of male sex characteristics) are believed to have a role in its development. Almost all primary prostate cancers are adenocarcinomas, and they develop in the peripheral zones of the prostate gland. This location increases the risk of local spread to the prostatic capsule. Despite its proximity to the rectum, metastasis to the bowel is uncommon, because a tough sheet of tissue, Denonvilliers fascia, acts as an effective physical barrier.

As the tumor enlarges, it may compress the urethra, obstructing urinary flow. The tumor may metastasize and involve the seminal vesicles or bladder by direct extension. Metastasis by lymph and venous channels is common.

Etiology

The exact cause of prostate cancer is unknown, but researchers believe it to be linked to changes in the DNA of the normal prostate cell. Inherited genetic mutations have been linked to hereditary prostate cancer. These mutated genes include *RNASFL, BRCA 1, BRCA2, MSN2, MLH1,* and *HOXB13.* Men with these mutations have an increased risk for developing prostate cancer. Some studies have found a relationship between acquired genetic mutations caused by increased hormone levels and inflammation and the development of prostate cancer, while others have not. Additional research is needed in this area (ACS, 2016h).

Risk Factors

The greatest risk factor for prostate cancer is age. Approximately one in eight men age 70 years and older will be diagnosed with prostate cancer (ACS, 2016b). Race is also a significant risk factor for prostate cancer; African American men are at particularly high risk. According to recent studies, a diet high in dairy foods or processed meat may increase the risk for developing prostate cancer, and obesity may increase the risk for developing an aggressive form of this disease. Some research suggests that firefighters may be at increased risk for prostate cancer (ACS, 2016b). Other risk factors being investigated include the following:

- Genetic and hereditary factors, with increased risk in men who have a family history of the disease
- Having a vasectomy, which is believed to increase the levels of circulating free testosterone
- Dietary factors, including a diet high in animal fat and excessive supplemental vitamin A.

Prevention

Prevention of prostate cancer through use of medications is a prominent area of research. The drugs dutasteride and finasteride, which reduce the amount of certain male hormones, are already being used in the management of symptoms related to benign prostate enlargement. Although neither drug is approved for the prevention of prostate cancer, owing to lack of evidence to support improvement of overall prostate cancer survival, they do appear to reduce cancer risk. However, side effects such as risk of erectile dysfunction and diminished libido make these drugs less than ideal for use as prophylactic treatments (ACS, 2016b).

Screening recommendations center on the optimal timing for discussing the benefits and limitations associated with available tests for early prostate cancer detection. Following this discussion between the patient and his healthcare provider, the patient should be encouraged to consider testing and to make an informed decision that incorporates

his individual preferences and values. Guidelines include the following (ACS, 2016b):

- For men at average risk of prostate cancer and whose life expectancy is at least 10 years, this discussion and informed decision should be initiated at 50 years of age.
- For men at high risk for developing prostate cancer, including those whose close relative was diagnosed with prostate cancer before age 65 and African Americans, this discussion and informed decision should begin at 45 years of age.
- For men at even higher risk, including those for whom several close relatives have been diagnosed with prostate cancer at an early age, this discussion and informed decision about testing should commence at age 40 years.

Clinical Manifestations

Men with early-stage prostate cancer are often asymptomatic. Pain from metastasis to bones is frequently the initial manifestation noted. Urinary manifestations depend on the size and location of the tumor and on the stage of the malignancy. They are often much like manifestations of benign prostatic hyperplasia: urgency, frequency, hesitancy, dysuria, and nocturia. The man may also notice hematuria or blood in the ejaculate (Porth & Grossman, 2013). For an overview of manifestations associated with prostate cancer, see the Clinical Manifestations and Therapies feature.

Collaboration

Care of the patient with prostate cancer focuses on diagnosis, elimination, or containment of the cancer and prevention or treatment of complications. There are currently no clinical strategies to prevent the development of prostate cancer. Therefore, early detection remains the major emphasis for control of this disease.

The treatment of prostate cancer is complex and depends on the grade and stage of the cancer as well as on the age, general health, and preference of the patient. In some cases, for example, when the patient with a slow-growing tumor is older or has a limited life expectancy, *watchful waiting* is the treatment of choice. Treatments for prostate cancer include surgery, radiation therapy, and hormone manipulation.

Diagnostic Tests

Although many patients with prostate cancer have either locally advanced cancer or distant metastasis at the time of diagnosis, an increasing number of patients are being diagnosed with asymptomatic prostate cancer. The definitive diagnosis can be made only by biopsy; however, other tests may suggest the presence of prostate cancer.

DRE will find the prostate gland nodular and fixed in the patient with prostate cancer. Levels of *prostate-specific antigen (PSA)* are used to screen for prostate cancer and to monitor initial responses to treatment. In addition, the PSA test is used to monitor effects of treatment. Until recently, the National Cancer Institute guidelines included considering a PSA level of 4.0 ng/mL or lower to be normal. However, current research suggests that men with normal PSA levels may nevertheless have prostate cancer. Likewise, an elevated or fluctuating PSA level, which previously was considered to be

Clinical Manifestations and Therapies
Prostate Cancer

ETIOLOGY	CLINICAL MANIFESTATIONS	CLINICAL THERAPIES
Enlarged prostate	▪ Dysuria ▪ Frequency of urination ▪ Reduction in urinary stream ▪ Nocturia ▪ Hematuria ▪ Abnormal prostate on digital rectal examination (DRE)	Treatment may include the following: ▪ Surgery ▪ Radiation ▪ Chemotherapy ▪ Hormone therapy
Metastasis of cancer to bones	▪ Bone or joint pain ▪ Migratory bone pain ▪ Back pain	▪ Administer analgesics as ordered. ▪ Promote balance between rest and activity. ▪ Massage the patient.
Nerve impingement due to mechanical compression by enlarged prostate	▪ Nerve pain ▪ Bilateral lower extremity weakness ▪ Bowel or bladder dysfunction ▪ Muscle spasms	▪ Administer analgesics as ordered. ▪ Administer muscle relaxants as ordered. ▪ Assist with ambulation, and institute safety protocols. ▪ Provide teaching to optimize patterns of urinary elimination (including instructions for Kegel exercises, if appropriate). ▪ As ordered, implement interventions to promote urinary elimination (e.g., insertion of indwelling urinary catheter).
Increased metabolic demands	▪ Weight loss ▪ Fatigue	▪ Encourage balanced nutrition. ▪ Offer foods that appeal to the patient. ▪ Promote balance between activity and rest.

a relative indication for prostate biopsy, has been known to occur also in conditions such as prostatitis and urinary tract infection. Therefore, PSA levels are now interpreted in conjunction with the patient's health history. Prior to prostate biopsy, additional testing (e.g., x-rays, cystoscopy) may be warranted to rule out other causative factors (NCI, 2012c).

Transrectal ultrasonography may be used when the DRE is abnormal or when the PSA is elevated without otherwise apparent cause. In this test, a small probe is inserted in the rectum. The probe gives off sound waves that create a picture of the prostate on a video screen. Guided by this picture, the physician inserts a narrow needle through the rectal wall into the prostate gland, and the needle removes a sample of tissue for examination. Other tests that may be ordered include a urinalysis or cystoscopy. Bone scan, MRI, or CT may be performed to determine the presence of tumor metastasis.

Grade and stage help determine prognosis and guide treatment decisions. Grade (cancer cell differentiation) is determined by the pathologist. Prostate cancer is staged with a variety of tests. **Table 2–15 》** outlines treatment options according to the stage of the cancer.

Surgery

Surgery for prostate cancer generally involves **prostatectomy**, or removal of all or part of the prostate. Types of prostatectomies include the following:

■ ***Transurethral resection of the prostate (TURP)*** involves removal of parts of the prostate gland by a surgical instrument that is inserted into the end of the penis and through the urethra. For very early disease in older men, TURP may achieve cure of prostate cancer.

■ ***Radical prostatectomy*** involves removal of the prostate, prostate capsule, seminal vesicles, and a portion of the bladder neck. Many patients experience varying degrees of urinary incontinence and erectile dysfunction (see **Table 2–16 》**). A fairly new treatment is laparoscopic radical prostatectomy, in which small incisions are made in the abdomen and a laparoscope is inserted and used to remove the prostate. Some surgeons do this from an area other than the operating room by using a robotic interface.

■ ***Retropubic prostatectomy*** may be performed because it allows adequate control of bleeding, visualization of the prostate bed and bladder neck, and access to pelvic lymph nodes.

■ ***Perineal prostatectomy*** is often preferred for older men or those who are poor surgical risks. This approach requires less time and involves less bleeding.

■ ***Suprapubic prostatectomy*** is rarely used; it may be done when problems with the bladder are expected. Control of bleeding is more difficult because the surgical approach is through the bladder.

For patients with stage III prostate cancer that is locally advanced (beyond the prostatic capsule), surgery is controversial because of the likelihood of hidden lymph node metastasis and relapse. TURP is not performed as curative therapy for patients with advanced disease (stage III or IV), but it may be used to relieve urinary obstruction.

TABLE 2–15 Prostate Cancer Staging and Treatment

Stage	Description	Treatment
Stage I	Confined to prostate; nonpalpable, focal involvement; well differentiated	▪ Observation and follow-up ▪ Interstitial or external-beam radiation therapy ▪ Prostatectomy
Stage II	Confined to prostate; palpable, involves one or both lobes; poorly differentiated	▪ Careful observation in selected patients ▪ Prostatectomy ▪ Interstitial or external-beam radiation therapy ▪ Ultrasound-guided percutaneous cryosurgery
Stage III	Extension of the tumor outside the prostate capsule; possible seminal vesicle involvement	▪ External-beam radiation therapy ▪ Interstitial radiation ▪ Radical prostatectomy ▪ Adjunctive hormone therapy ▪ Palliative surgery (transurethral prostatectomy or transurethral resection of the prostate (TURP)—removal of the prostate through the urethra)
Stage IV	Extension of the tumor into surrounding tissues; lymph node involvement or distant metastasis	▪ Hormone therapy ▪ External-beam radiation therapy ▪ Palliative treatment with radiation therapy and/or TURP ▪ Radical prostatectomy with orchiectomy ▪ Chemotherapy

Surgical intervention is now available for men with urinary sphincter insufficiency, which is the major cause of incontinence after prostatectomy. An artificial urinary sphincter is surgically implanted (see **Figure 2–19** »). To be eligible, the man must be able to manipulate the pump placed in the scrotum and have adequate cognitive function to be able to recognize when a problem with the appliance occurs.

Pharmacologic Therapy

Androgen deprivation therapy is used to treat advanced prostate cancer. Many cells in the growing tumor are androgen dependent and either die or cease to grow if deprived of androgens. Other cancer cells unfortunately thrive without androgen and are unaffected by therapy to reduce circulating androgens. Therefore, the effects of hormone manipulations vary from complete but temporary regression of the tumor to no response at all.

TABLE 2–16 Potential Complications Related to Radical Prostatectomy and Radiation Therapy

Radical Prostatectomy	Radiation Therapy
Erectile dysfunction	Erectile dysfunction[a]
Urethral stricture	Urethral stricture
Fistula/rectal injury	Rectal/anal stricture[a]
Urinary incontinence	Cystitis
Surgical/anesthetic risk	Diarrhea
	Proctitis
	Rectal ulcer
	Bowel obstruction[a]
	Urinary incontinence

[a]Delayed complications; may appear months or years after completion of therapy.

Strategies to induce androgen deprivation vary from **orchiectomy** (surgical removal of one or both testicles) to oral administration of hormonal agents. **Table 2–17** » compares surgical and hormone therapies and the advantages and disadvantages of each. In addition, new drugs are being

TABLE 2–17 Surgical and Hormone Therapy in the Management of Advanced Prostate Cancer

Treatment	Advantages	Disadvantages
Orchiectomy	Inexpensive Immediate effect; men report diminished pain from metastasis in the recovery room	Body image problems resulting from loss of testicles
Estrogen compounds (diethylstilbestrol)	Inexpensive Effects reversible	Increased risk of cardiovascular problems More likely to cause gynecomastia, hypertrophy of breast tissue
Luteinizing hormone-releasing hormone agonist (LHRH) (leuprolide)	Effects reversible No cardiovascular risk Monthly administration	Very expensive Subcutaneous injection route Slow onset: up to 4 weeks
Steroidal antiandrogens (megestrol [Megace])	Effects reversible No cardiovascular risk Inexpensive	May not drop testosterone levels sufficiently Weight gain
Nonsteroidal antiandrogens (flutamide; often used in conjunction with LHRH)	Does not alter circulating androgens Blocks some side effects of LHRH May be effective if other methods fail	Very expensive

Note: All hormonal manipulations have the potential disadvantage of loss of libido, erectile dysfunction, hot flashes, and gynecomastia (enlarged breasts).

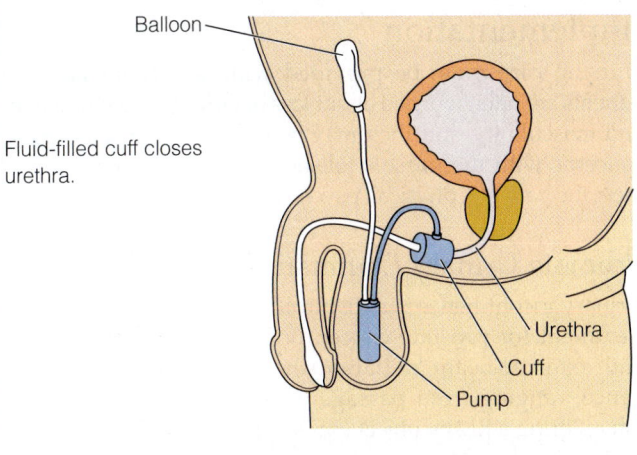

Balloon

Fluid-filled cuff closes urethra.

Urethra

Cuff

Pump

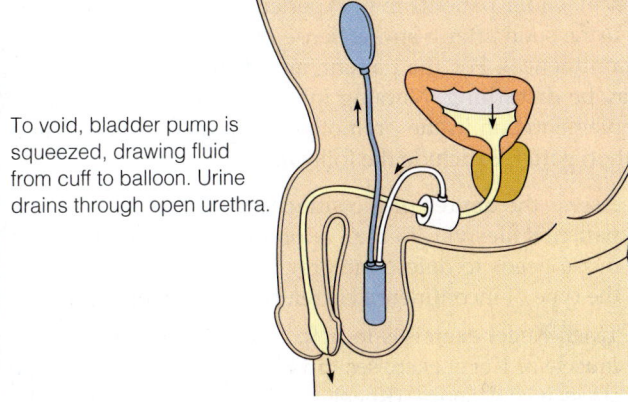

To void, bladder pump is squeezed, drawing fluid from cuff to balloon. Urine drains through open urethra.

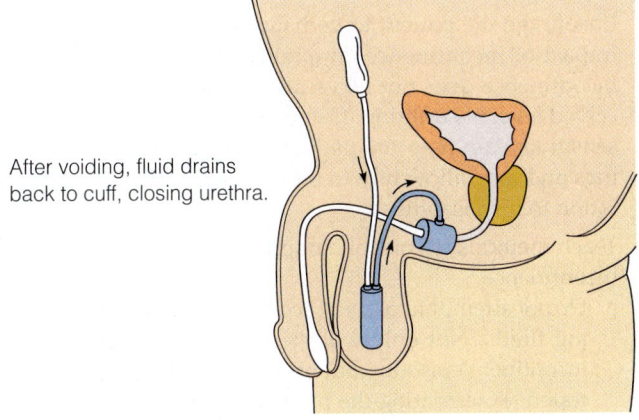

After voiding, fluid drains back to cuff, closing urethra.

Figure 2–19 》 Operation of an artificial urinary sphincter.

developed that block the effects of male hormones, and research is being conducted to determine which mix of hormones is best and at what time in the perioperative period they are most effective.

Radiation Therapy

Radiation therapy may be used as a primary treatment for prostate cancer because it reduces the risk of long-term problems of impotence and urinary incontinence associated with surgery. Radiation may be delivered either by external beam or interstitial implants of radioactive seeds of iodine, gold, palladium, or iridium (brachytherapy). Interstitial radiation has a lower risk of impotence and

Focus on Integrative Health
Vitamin Supplements

As a component of wellness promotion, the nurse should emphasize disease prevention, including avoidance of unintentional harm. Natural and over-the-counter therapies and supplements should not be presumed to be safe. For example, according to the NCCIH (2015), recent studies demonstrate an increased risk of prostate cancer among men who take vitamin E supplements. Nursing assessment should include interviewing the patient as to his use of nutritional supplements and nonprescription therapies. Likewise, patients should be urged to consult their healthcare provider regarding the safety and efficacy of complementary health approaches before starting to use them.

rectal damage than external-beam radiation. Radiation therapy also has a palliative role for patients with metastatic prostate cancer; it can reduce the size of bone metastasis, assist in controlling pain, and restore function, such as continence or the ability to ambulate for patients with spinal cord compression.

Nonpharmacologic Therapy

One risk factor that can be easily addressed is diet. Men should know that they may lower their risk of prostate cancer by consuming a diet that limits dairy products and processed meats. The nurse should advise patients to follow the recommended balanced nutrition of fruits and vegetables as outlined in the federal government's MyPlate guidelines.

Lifespan Considerations

Although prostate cancer typically occurs most frequently in older men, the number of younger men being diagnosed with prostate cancer has significantly increased over the past 20 years. According to the ACS (2016i), prostate cancer is rarely diagnosed prior to age 40, with 4 out of 10 cases being diagnosed in men younger than age 65. Prostate cancer is generally slow-growing, and patients who develop this type of cancer usually die from causes other than the cancer. Research has found that prostate cancers that are diagnosed at a younger age tend to be more aggressive, and metastasis may have already occurred, given the advanced disease state at time of diagnosis. Studies are continuing to examine the link between genetic variants and early-onset prostate cancer. Individuals who are at increased risk of developing early-onset prostate cancer have been found to have a family history of prostate cancer before age 50, and recommendations have been made for those at higher risk to have genetic counseling and increased screening (University of Michigan Cancer Center, 2014).

NURSING PROCESS

Nurses plan and implement interventions to help prevent prostate cancer and to facilitate a return to functional health status once prostate cancer is diagnosed. Nurses are in a unique position to increase public awareness about early detection of prostate cancer. Every encounter with men and their families—in clinics, hospital units, or in the home—is an opportunity to provide information about early detection and to identify needs. Several studies have shown a positive correlation between increased awareness of and participation in prostate cancer screening procedures.

>> **Stay Current:** The National Cancer Institute has free pamphlets about prostate cancer that are useful for educating the public. Download a pamphlet at http://www.cancer.gov/publications/patient-education/wyntk-prostate-cancer.

Assessment

Collect the following data through the health history and physical examination:

- **Observation and patient interview.** Observe the patient for signs of discomfort or pain in the spine, hips, or other bones and for signs of weakness or numbness in the legs or feet, which may suggest that a tumor is pressing on the spinal cord. Ask the patient about risk factors, urinary elimination patterns and manifestations, hematuria, and pain.
- **Physical examination.** The physical assessment should include DRE to assess prostate size, symmetry, firmness, and nodules; assess for bladder distention, urinary flow, and urine retention.

Note that a DRE is an advanced nursing assessment.

Diagnosis

Potential nursing diagnoses appropriate for inclusion in the nursing care plan for a patient with prostate cancer will vary, depending on the individual patient and the medical interventions used. Although not intended to be all inclusive, nursing diagnoses relevant to the care of a patient with prostate cancer may include the following:

- *Urinary Elimination, Impaired*
- *Urinary Retention*
- *Stress Urinary Incontinence*
- *Sexual Dysfunction*
- *Comfort, Impaired.*

(NANDA-I © 2014)

Planning

Goals of nursing care may include the following:

- The patient will express concerns and emotions related to his diagnosis and the potential effects of treatment.
- The patient will demonstrate optimal urinary function, including urine elimination of at least 0.5 mL/kg/hr.
- The patient will verbalize awareness of strategies for promoting urinary continence.
- The patient will demonstrate the ability to make informed decisions regarding all treatments.
- Using a predetermined pain rating scale, the patient will report his pain is maintained at a level deemed by him to be tolerable.

Implementation

Nursing care must be provided with sensitivity because patients are often worried about loss of virility, sexual function, and masculinity, and they may be reluctant to discuss these concerns with the nurse. Holistic care must be provided to meet the patient's physical, psychosocial, and spiritual needs.

Promote Urinary Elimination

Urinary incontinence is a disturbing complication following treatment for prostate cancer. Both radical prostatectomy and external-beam radiation therapy can cause incontinence, ranging from passage of a small amount of urine when lifting a heavy object (stress incontinence) to complete and unpredictable loss of urinary control (total incontinence). Older patients may experience involuntary passage of urine soon after a strong sense of urgency to void (urge incontinence). For the patient, any degree of incontinence may be disturbing. Nursing interventions appropriate for implementation in the promotion of optimal urinary elimination patterns include the following:

- Assess the degree of incontinence and its effects on the patient's lifestyle. To plan appropriate interventions, the nurse needs to determine previous urinary patterns and the type of incontinence currently being experienced.
- Teach Kegel exercises to help restore continence. Pelvic muscle or Kegel exercises can often improve or eliminate stress incontinence. (Kegel exercises are discussed in the module on Elimination.)
- Encourage the patient to verbalize his feelings about the impact of incontinence on quality of life. The degree of incontinence does not necessarily correlate with the perceived level of suffering. Listening to these concerns with sensitivity can help the patient work through these feelings and may allow him to move toward a healthy adaptation to his disability.
- Teach methods to control dampness and odor from stress incontinence:
  a. Do not attempt to prevent accidental voiding by restricting fluids. Not only will the patient continue to have incontinent episodes, but his urine will become concentrated, exacerbating the problem with odor. Restricting fluids may also lead to insufficient hydration, which can have negative effects on several body systems.
  b. Manage occasional episodes (one to three small-volume accidents per day) with absorbent pads worn inside the underwear and changed as needed. Most pads are made with a polymer gel that controls odor. Appropriate measures help promote good hygiene, decrease anxiety, and increase comfort.
- Refer to physical therapy or a continence specialist for additional measures to promote continence. Special exercises, restricting some types of fluids, and other measures (e.g., bladder training) can help the patient deal with incontinence.
- Explore options such as an external collection device (external catheter or Texas catheter) for the patient with total incontinence. This device may improve his self-esteem and allow resumption of social activities.

Patient Teaching

Home Care for the Patient with Prostate Cancer

Depending on the type of treatment, the following topics should be addressed in preparing the patient and his family for home care:

- For the patient having a surgical procedure: manifestations of infection and excessive bleeding, catheter care, and wound care pain management
- For the patient receiving radiation therapy:
  a. Danger of radiation damage to others (sleep in a room alone for a week; avoid close contact with pregnant women, infants, and children)
  b. Condom use during sexual contact (ejaculate may be discolored, distressing the patient's sexual partner)
- The importance of keeping appointments with healthcare providers and having yearly PSA and rectal examinations
- If appropriate, community services, such as support groups, home health nurses, and hospice
- Helpful resources, such as the American Cancer Society (http://www.cancer.org), the American Urological Association (http://www.auanet.org), and the National Cancer Institute (http://www.cancer.gov).

Promote Communication Related to Sexual Function

Surgical treatment for prostate cancer may cause erectile dysfunction and changes in ejaculatory function. Hormone therapy for advanced prostate cancer lowers libido and may cause erectile dysfunction. The diagnosis of cancer and the body image changes caused by hormone therapy may lower self-esteem, which in turn can diminish sexual desire and willingness to interact sexually with a partner. Most older men are sexually active and fully capable of sustaining an erection. They are likely to fear the effect of treatment on their sexual health. They may allow this concern to guide their decision about the course of treatment, or they may refuse all therapy because of this fear. Reactions vary greatly, and the nurse must maintain a sensitive, nonjudgmental approach to education and support.

- Interview the patient about his pretreatment level of sexual function. Knowledge of previous sexual function is necessary to plan appropriate interventions.

- Teach the patient about the actual or potential effects of therapy on sexual function. The incidence of erectile dysfunction varies with different therapies for prostate cancer.
- Provide an opportunity for the patient and his partner to discuss implications of and concerns about the diagnosis and treatment of sexual function. The treatments for prostate cancer often affect the physiology of erection. The patient and his partner need support and counseling during the period of adjustment.
- Refer for sexual counseling as appropriate. The patient and his partner may benefit from therapy beyond that provided by nurses.
- Discuss medical and surgical treatments for erectile dysfunction. Many men are as devastated by the loss of erectile function as they are by the diagnosis of cancer. Information about achieving erection and maintaining sexual intimacy is essential to a good quality of life.

Evaluation

Expected outcomes to evaluate patient care are based on goals set during the planning stage and may include the following:

- Using a predetermined pain rating scale, the patient reports managing pain at a tolerable level.
- The patient is able to discuss sexual function with his partner.
- The patient lists strategies for managing urinary incontinence.
- The patient maintains adequate urine output without complications related to altered urinary elimination.

In evaluating the patient who is being treated for prostate cancer, the nurse will need to provide an open, nonjudgmental environment and use therapeutic communication skills to encourage truthful discussion about the patient's experiences and concerns. The patient may be unwilling to reveal that he is finding it difficult to maintain urinary continence or is having sexual difficulties. Further treatment might be necessary, or the patient might be open to referral to the appropriate counseling; the process will begin with the nurse's ability to communicate compassionately with the patient.

Nursing Care Plan

A Patient with Prostate Cancer

William Turner, a 71-year-old African American man, lives with his wife in a small retirement community in Florida. His wife had a stroke 2 years ago, and Mr. Turner does all the cooking and housework. He has been in good health for most of his life, having only "a small touch" of osteoarthritis in his knees and hands. He has noticed a gradual onset of urinary urgency and frequency during the past 2 years but has never had incontinence.

During a routine checkup, the nurse practitioner at the local health clinic performs a DRE and palpates a hard nodule on the surface of Mr. Turner's prostate. After his PSA is found to be elevated, he is

referred to a urologist, who diagnoses prostate cancer. Mr. Turner chooses to have surgery, and a radical retropubic prostatectomy and lymph node dissection are performed. The lymph nodes are negative for metastasis. Following surgery, his recovery is uncomplicated. However, the nurse caring for Mr. Turner is concerned about his ability to care for his indwelling catheter because of his arthritis and his wife's physical disabilities from the stroke. The nurse makes a referral to a home health agency to ensure that Mr. Turner can manage his care at home. An initial home health assessment is scheduled for the day after Mr. Turner is discharged from the hospital.

(continued on next page)

Nursing Care Plan (continued)

ASSESSMENT	DIAGNOSES	PLANNING
The home health nurse notes that the house is clean and neat. Mr. Turner is dressed but still wearing his night urinary drainage bag, although it is well past noon. Mr. Turner tells the nurse that his main problem is going to get groceries, because he is embarrassed to be seen with the drainage bag. He says that he has not been able to remove the drainage bag and attach the leg bag because of his arthritis. Physical assessment findings include healing of the pelvic incision without signs of infection. There is no tenderness in his calves, no chest pain, and no shortness of breath. The urine is yellow, without odor. Mr. Turner states that he sees no need for the pelvic exercises, since he is no longer in the hospital. He also expresses the belief that he is cured of cancer and questions the need for follow-up care.	■ *Stress Urinary Incontinence* related to surgical procedure ■ *Health Maintenance, Ineffective* related to inability to care for the urinary drainage system, not understanding need for postoperative exercises, and questions about follow-up care (NANDA-I © 2014)	■ The patient will regain urinary continence after catheter removal. ■ The patient will change the urinary drainage bag with the appropriate assistance. ■ The patient will verbalize the rationale for performing postoperative exercises. ■ The patient will verbalize the need for continued follow-up care.

IMPLEMENTATION

- Discuss the possibility of stress incontinence after the catheter is removed.
- Reinforce the need for Kegel exercises while the catheter is still in place.

- Explore Mr. Turner's support system to identify people who could assist him with catheter care, and arrange a teaching session with them.
- Teach Mr. Turner the importance of follow-up care, relating the care to the history of the disease.

EVALUATION

Good friends from Mr. Turner's church have assisted him with care of his drainage bag and have reminded him to do his Kegel exercises several times a day while the catheter is in place. When the catheter is removed, Mr. Turner has only a small amount of urine leakage after voiding. He understands that it may take several weeks for this to resolve. Efforts to help him understand the need for continued medical care have been less successful. Mr. Turner continues to state that he is cured, his wife needs him, and he sees no need to go back to the doctor.

CRITICAL THINKING

1. Outline a teaching plan for Mr. Turner for the nursing diagnosis Risk for Impaired Skin Integrity related to urinary incontinence.
2. As a result of Mr. Turner's refusal to get ongoing medical care, he might be labeled as noncompliant. Would you make the nursing diagnosis of Noncompliance? Why, or why not?
3. If you were the home health nurse making a home visit and found that Mr. Turner had had no urinary drainage for 16 hours, what assessments would you make? How would you handle this problem?

REVIEW Prostate Cancer

RELATE Link the Concepts and Exemplars

Linking the exemplar of prostate cancer with the concept of elimination:

1. What effect might prostate cancer have on the patient's ability to urinate if he chooses to treat the cancer by medical, rather than surgical, therapies?
2. How can you promote adequate urinary elimination for this patient?

Linking the exemplar of prostate cancer with the concept of tissue integrity:

3. What nursing interventions can promote tissue integrity in the patient who recently had surgical removal of the prostate?
4. Write a teaching plan for the patient preparing for discharge to home following prostatectomy.

READY Go to Volume 3: Clinical Nursing Skills

REFER Go to Pearson MyLab Nursing and eText

■ Additional review materials

REFLECT Apply Your Knowledge

Maury Blarden is a 45-year-old patient who has been diagnosed with prostate cancer. He is married and has a 3-year-old daughter. Mr. Blarden and his wife own a company that offers home renovation and decoration services. Mr. and Ms. Blarden have been told that surgery is necessary, along with radiation and chemotherapy. Mr. Blarden tells the nurse that he and his wife are trying to have another child. He is not sure that he can take the time away from the business for surgery and therapy. The couple has minimal healthcare coverage and is worried about the costs of care because they barely make enough to get by.

1. What expected outcomes would be appropriate for this patient?
2. Ms. Blarden asks you, while her husband is out of the room, whether the procedure will result in impotence. How will you respond to this question?
3. Will the Blardens be able to have children if he decides to undergo surgery? Explain your answer.

» Exemplar 2.H
Sickle Cell Disease

Exemplar Learning Outcomes

2.H Analyze sickle cell disease (SCD) as it relates to cellular regulation.

- Describe the pathophysiology of SCD.
- Describe the etiology of SCD.
- Compare the risk factors for and prevention of SCD.
- Identify the clinical manifestations of SCD.
- Summarize diagnostic tests and therapies used by interprofessional teams in the collaborative care of an individual with SCD.
- Differentiate considerations for care of patients with SCD across the lifespan.
- Apply the nursing process in providing culturally competent care to an individual with SCD.

Exemplar Key Terms

Alloimmunization, *128*
Hemoglobinopathy, *125*
Hemosiderosis, *128*
Priapism, *126*
Sickle cell anemia, *125*
Sickle cell crisis, *125*
Sickle cell disease (SCD), *125*
Sickle cell trait, *126*
Sickling, *125*
Vaso-occlusive crisis, *125*

Overview

Sickle cell disease (SCD) is a hereditary **hemoglobinopathy**, a type of disorder characterized by replacement of normal hemoglobin with abnormal hemoglobin S (HbS) in RBCs. **Sickle cell anemia**, a chronic hemolytic anemia, is the most common type of SCD. (See Exemplar 2.B on Anemia and **Table 2–18 »**.)

Pathophysiology and Etiology

Pathophysiology

When RBCs that contain HbS pass through blood vessels, deoxygenation of HbS causes the RBCs to become rigid and deformed. As a result of this distortion, the RBCs take on a crescent or sickle shape. Because of the characteristic shape of malformed RBCs associated with this disorder, the process is called **sickling**. Unlike healthy RBCs, sickled RBCs are more rigid and inflexible, and they can occlude small blood vessels, especially capillaries. Vascular occlusion can cause tissue ischemia and organ damage.

Repeated or prolonged ischemia resulting from sickle cell–induced occlusions causes damage to tissues and organs. For example, children with SCD can experience life-threatening splenic sequestration due to trapping of blood in the spleen. Many children must undergo splenectomy in early childhood, leading to severely compromised immunity. Their infection rate is subsequently high because of impaired immunity, and bacterial infections are the leading cause of death in young children with SCD. Repeated sickling episodes weaken RBC cell membranes and shorten the lifespan of affected RBCs. Early destruction of RBCs can lead to anemia.

Sickling may be triggered by any condition that increases the body's need for oxygen, including fever, emotional or physical stress, high altitudes, poorly pressurized airplanes, hypoventilation, and vasoconstriction due to cold temperatures. **Sickle cell crisis** (also called **vaso-occlusive crisis**) is the term used to describe painful periods resulting from ischemia due to vascular occlusion. Any condition that increases the body's need for oxygen or alters the transport of oxygen, such as infection or trauma, may result in sickle cell crisis. Although potential causes include those known to trigger sickling, in more than 50% of cases, the exact cause of sickle cell crisis is not identifiable (UMMC, 2013b). Dehydration increases blood viscosity, which can predispose an individual to sickle cell crisis.

Sickled cells can resume a normal shape when they are rehydrated and reoxygenated. The membranes of these cells

TABLE 2–18 Forms of Sickle Cell Disease

Sickle Cell Disease	Description
Sickle cell trait HbAS	This is the most common form of SCD in the United States.
	This is a heterozygous condition in which the child inherits one sickle cell (HbS) gene and one normal hemoglobin (HbA) gene.
	The child is a carrier of SCD and rarely has symptoms of the disease.
Sickle cell anemia HbSS	This is a homozygous condition. (The child inherits two HbS genes.)
	The child is subject to sickle cell crises.
Sickle cell syndromes HbSC	In this variation, the child inherits a sickle cell gene (HbS) from one parent and an abnormal hemoglobin gene from the other parent (HbC). Most often, this produces a less severe form of SCD.
Hb S beta thalassemia	The child inherits a sickle cell gene (HbS) from one parent and one of two types of genes for beta thalassemia from the other parent.
	Manifestations of SCD can range from mild to severe.

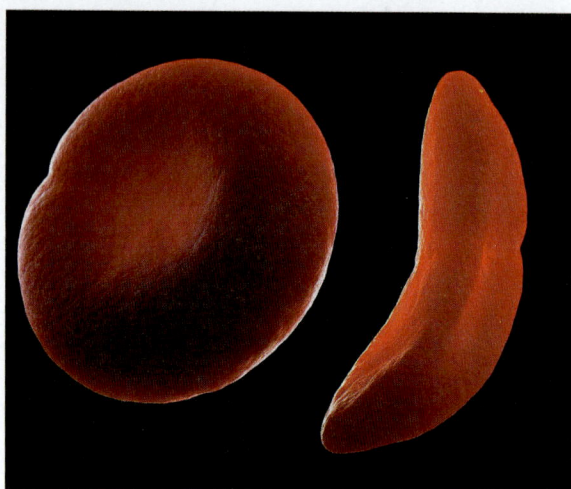

Source: SCIEPRO/Science Photo Library/Getty Images.

Figure 2–20 》 Blood smear containing normal red blood cells and sickle cells.

become more fragile, however, and cell life is shortened to 10–20 days rather than the usual 120 days. In response, bone marrow spaces enlarge to produce more RBCs. In some individuals with SCD, bone marrow ceases to produce new RBCs, leading to aplastic crisis (CDC, 2016b).

Etiology

SCD is transmitted as an autosomal recessive genetic defect. If both parents have the trait, then with each pregnancy, the risk of having a child with the disease is 25%. The HbS gene changes the structure of the beta chain of the hemoglobin molecule. When hypoxemia develops and HbS is deoxygenated, it crystallizes into rodlike structures. Clusters of these rods form long chains that deform the erythrocyte into a crescent or sickle shape (see **Figure 2–20 》**). The sickled cells tend to clump together and obstruct capillary blood flow, causing ischemia and possible infarction of surrounding tissue.

Risk Factors and Prevention

The risk of inheriting SCD is related to genetics. The disease is most common among people of African descent. An estimated 1 in 13 African Americans carries one abnormal hemoglobin (HbS) gene and thus has **sickle cell trait**. These carriers are likely to remain asymptomatic unless stressed by severe hypoxemia. SCD, which requires inheritance of two HbS genes (one from each parent), occurs in approximately 1 in 365 African American newborns. Individuals with SCD are at risk for sickle cell crisis. Those who are uncertain whether they are carriers of abnormal hemoglobin can have their blood tested for the HbS gene. If a couple is planning to have children and know that there is a risk of having a child with SCD, referral to a genetics counselor can assist with their understanding of the risks and the choices available (NHLBI, 2016).

Clinical Manifestations

The acute and chronic manifestations of SCD arise from episodes of RBC sickling. Sickling causes general manifestations

of hemolytic anemia, including pallor, fatigue, jaundice, and irritability. Repeated infarcts associated with sickling can affect the structure and function of nearly every organ system. Patients with SCD may develop an enlarged spleen and liver, renal insufficiency, gallstones, and other manifestations of organ dysfunction. **Priapism** (painful, prolonged penile erection) may develop. Abdominal pain may signal infarction of abdominal organs and structures. Skin ulcers may develop as the result of occluded vessels supplying the dermis.

Pain intensity and duration vary depending on the individual and the location. Pain may be transient in a localized area, such as the wrist, to severe, generalized pain that lasts for several days or weeks and may require hospitalization. The pain is often severe enough to require opioid analgesics and the use of a patient-controlled analgesic pump.

Stroke is a significant risk for all patients diagnosed with SCD. Other complications of SCD include aplastic crisis or temporary cessation of bone marrow blood cell production (UMMC, 2013b). Extensive sickling can precipitate a crisis as a result of occluded circulation, impaired erythropoiesis, or sequestration of large amounts of blood in the liver or spleen (see **Table 2–19 》**).

Sickle cell crisis occurs when sickled cells obstruct vascular blood flow, which can lead to tissue ischemia and infarction. These excruciating vaso-occlusive crises last an average of 4–6 days. (For a basis of comparison, vaso-occlusion occurs on a much smaller scale when an individual wraps a rubber band around a finger so tightly that blood flow is obstructed.) For the individual experiencing the intense vaso-occlusion associated with sickle cell crisis, infarction of small vessels in the extremities causes painful swelling of the hands and feet; the large joints also may be affected. Infarction also may affect bone marrow or lead to aseptic necrosis of affected bones, resulting in pain from avascular necrosis of the bone marrow, and is typically experienced in the back, abdomen, chest, and joints. Acute chest syndrome, a symptom complex that includes fever, chest pain, an increasing WBC count, and pulmonary infiltrates, may develop, as well as other complications, such as pneumonia, pulmonary infarction, pulmonary embolism, and even death (CDC, 2016b; Porth & Grossman, 2013).

TABLE 2–19 Overview of Sickle Cell Crisis

Etiology	Clinical Manifestations
Vaso-occlusion (thrombotic)	■ Vaso-occlusion is the most common type of crisis. It may last for days or weeks. ■ It is precipitated by dehydration, exposure to cold, acidosis, or localized hypoxia. ■ It is caused by stasis of blood with clumping of cells in the microcirculation, ischemia, and infarction. ■ Thrombosis and infarction of local tissue may occur if the crisis is not reversed. ■ Cerebral occlusion can result in stroke, manifested by paralysis or other central nervous system complications. ■ It is extremely painful; symptoms include fever, tissue engorgement, painful swelling of joints in hands and feet, priapism, and severe abdominal pain.
Splenic sequestration	■ Splenic sequestration is a life-threatening crisis; death can occur within hours. ■ It is caused by pooling of blood in the spleen; because the spleen can hold much of the body's blood supply, cardiovascular collapse can result. It is most commonly seen in children and adolescents and may be seen in young adults. ■ Clinical manifestations include profound anemia, hypovolemia, and shock.
Aplastic crisis	■ Aplastic crisis is caused by diminished production and increased destruction of RBCs. ■ It is often triggered by human parvovirus B19 viral infection. ■ Signs include profound anemia, pallor, and fatigue.
Acute chest syndrome	■ Acute chest syndrome is a common cause of hospitalization for patients with SCD. ■ It is associated with a pediatric mortality rate of 2% and an adult mortality rate of 4%. ■ Pulmonary infiltrate of abnormal blood cells leads to lower respiratory tract symptoms. ■ Clinical manifestations include fever, cough, chest and back pain, dyspnea, and hypoxemia. ■ Pulmonary infection, infarction, and fat embolism may occur and can lead to pulmonary failure and death.

Sources: Data from Centers for Disease Control and Prevention (CDC). (2016c). *Sickle cell disease (SDC)—Data & statistics.* Retrieved from http://www.cdc.gov/ncbddd/sicklecell/data.html. University of Maryland Medical Center (UMMC). (2013b). *Sickle cell disease.* Retrieved from http://www.umm.edu/health/medical/reports/articles/sickle-cell-disease.

Collaboration

Optimal care for the patient with SCD involves coordinated efforts by members of a healthcare team. Neonatal screening, early intervention, prophylactic antibiotics, and parent education have allowed children with SCD to live into adulthood. A nurse with a specialty in genetics or a genetics counselor may be involved in sickle cell gene testing and counseling to identify and inform carriers and children who have the disease.

Diagnostic Tests

In the United States, newborn screening for SCD is mandatory. While prenatal diagnosis of SCD is possible using amniocentesis, the initial diagnosis of SCD in newborns is most often made by testing a few drops of blood obtained by way of a heelstick. For adults, a venous blood sample is usually obtained from the arm. Blood samples are evaluated for the presence of HbS. Positive samples are further evaluated to identify the number of sickle cell genes present. The presence of two HbS genes, which correlates with a diagnosis of SCD, warrants further testing (including RBC count) to assess for anemia (Mayo Clinic, 2014d).

For the pediatric patient with SCD, additional diagnostic testing may be indicated for prevention of stroke. Beginning at age 2 years, children with SCD should undergo routine ultrasound scanning of the head to assess cerebral blood flow (NHLBI, 2016).

Surgery

Bone marrow or hematopoietic stem cell transplantation may be considered. However, the disease recurs in approximately 10% of transplant recipients. For patients experiencing splenic sequestration of RBCs, blood transfusion is the most common treatment. In life-threatening instances of splenic RBC sequestration, splenectomy may be necessary (CDC, 2016b).

Pharmacologic Therapy

For the patient experiencing complications related to SCD, mainstays of treatment include oxygenation, hydration, and analgesic administration. Oxygen is usually administered to reduce the risk of hypoxemia and associated complications and to promote comfort and minimize dyspnea. Oral and IV fluid replacement also promotes pain relief, since dehydration is often a cause of crisis. Fluids reduce the viscosity of the blood, so adequate hydration is essential. Parenteral analgesics, such as morphine, are generally administered around the clock or via patient-controlled analgesia. Particularly in children, pain medications should not be ordered on an "as needed" basis, because this increases the child's anxiety and delays medication administration.

Treatment with hydroxyurea has been helpful in adults and is now being used more frequently in children. This cytotoxic medication decreases production of abnormal blood cells and leads to a lesser amount of pain being experienced. In addition, hydroxyurea increases fetal hemoglobin production and red cell mean corpuscular volume (NHLBI, 2016). Side effects of hydroxyurea include bone marrow suppression, headaches, dizziness, nausea, and vomiting.

For children between 2 months and 5 years of age who are diagnosed with SCD, treatment often includes daily administration of prophylactic penicillin (NHLBI, 2016). Children who are functionally asplenic or have had a splenectomy have a resultant decreased capability to fight infection. For this reason, infection is a serious condition requiring immediate attention. When an infection is suspected, cultures (blood, urine, and throat) are obtained to identify the

Clinical Manifestations and Therapies
Sickle Cell Disease

ETIOLOGY	CLINICAL MANIFESTATIONS	CLINICAL THERAPIES
Dyspnea ■ Due to inadequate delivery of oxygen to cells, tissues, and organs	■ Hypoxia, lethargy, fatigue, shortness of breath, tachypnea, and decreased oxygen saturation level	■ Provide supplemental oxygen. ■ Elevate head of bed to the point of patient comfort. ■ Provide blood transfusions. ■ Monitor oxygen saturation level. ■ Auscultate lungs at least every 4 hours and as needed.
Anemia ■ May be due to increased RBC destruction, impaired RBC production, or both	■ Hypoxia, lethargy, fatigue, pallor, shortness of breath, complaints of dyspnea, tachycardia, and decreased RBC and Hb measurements	■ Provide blood transfusions. ■ BMT or SCT may be used.
Impaired circulation ■ Due to impaired flow of sickled RBCs	■ Impaired oxygenation, tachypnea, tachycardia, edema, and splenic sequestration of RBCs ■ In pediatric patients (usually in those younger than 4 years old), sickle cells can obstruct small blood vessels in the hands and feet, causing hand-foot syndrome, which manifests as pain, fever, and swelling	■ Provide blood transfusions. ■ Offer IV and oral hydration. ■ Prevent physical exacerbation and exposure to environments or circumstances that increase oxygen demand. ■ Splenectomy may be needed.
Risk for infection ■ Due to inadequate circulation	■ Fever, tachypnea, tachycardia, increased WBC count, localized symptoms of infection (e.g., redness, drainage, and swelling at a specific site) ■ Blood cultures positive for infectious organism	■ Administer antibiotics as ordered for prophylactic and acute treatment. ■ Encourage the patient to adhere to current vaccination recommendations, as well as to receive annual influenza and pneumococcal vaccinations. ■ Adhere to standard precautions and organizational protocols for infection prevention.
Pain ■ Due to vascular occlusion by RBCs	■ Complaints of pain or discomfort ■ Increased blood pressure, pulse, and respiratory rate due to sympathetic nervous system stimulation (may or may not be present) ■ Objective indicators of pain, including crying, grimacing, and guarding affected sites	■ Promote oxygenation and vascular flow of blood through hydration and, if indicated, transfusion of RBCs. ■ Administer analgesics as ordered. ■ Administer hydroxyurea as ordered. ■ Massage the patient.

source of infection and the offending organism. Aggressive antibiotic therapy is implemented immediately.

Nonpharmacologic Therapy

Blood transfusions are also a core component of treatment for the patient with SCD. Benefits of transfusions include improved blood and tissue oxygenation, a reduction in sickling, and a temporary suppression of the production of RBCs containing HbS. Several types of blood transfusion are used.

A complication associated with frequent transfusions is an overload of iron in the body. The iron is stored in tissues and organs (**hemosiderosis**) because the body has no way of excreting it. For this reason, an iron-chelating drug, such as deferoxamine, may be given with vitamin C to promote iron excretion. Another complication of multiple transfusions is the development of alloimmunization to red cell and platelet antigens (Osborn et al., 2013). **Alloimmunization** occurs

when the child's immune system reacts against antigens on the donated tissues (e.g., blood and stem cells).

Periodic transfusions have proven to be an effective treatment for stroke complications related to SCD. In children who have had strokes from the disease, transfusions approximately every 3–4 weeks can reduce the incidence of strokes (UMMC, 2013b). If administered early in the crisis, blood transfusions may relieve the ischemia caused by vaso-occlusion in major organs and body parts, such as the spleen, lung, kidney, brain, and penis. Exchange transfusion is preferred to reduce the potential of fluid volume excess.

Lifespan Considerations
Sickle Cell Disease in Children

Children affected with SCD are usually asymptomatic until 4–6 months of age because sickling is inhibited by

Patient Teaching

The Child with Sickle Cell Disease

- Provide parents with information about SCD and the child's treatment. Even parents of a child previously diagnosed with the disorder may benefit from information about the disease process and its management. Explain the basic effect of tissue hypoxia and the effects of sickling on circulation.

- Teach parents to look for signs of dehydration, such as dry mucous membranes, weight loss, and sunken fontanelles in infants. Give specific instructions about how many ounces of liquid the child needs to drink each day. Emphasize that increased fluid intake is needed to replace the fluids lost from overheating or exposure to hot weather.

- Make sure both the child and the family understand the triggers and precipitating factors for sickle cell crises. Encourage them to avoid situations that cause crises. Instruct the child and parents about signs and symptoms of crises that should be reported to the healthcare provider.

- Provide the family with careful instructions about infusion therapy. When regular blood infusions are used, the resulting iron overload is damaging to body organs. Children treated with transfusions need infusion of deferoxamine (Desferal) for iron overload. The medication is usually given by subcutaneous or IV routes over 8–10 hours. Prompt recognition of side effects and careful management of the lengthy infusion process are important. The child needs to be monitored for skin reactions and allergic responses. Have parents demonstrate the infusion technique and state what to do in case of reactions. Pain management is needed during infusion because the site may be tender and uncomfortable.

- Instruct parents that it is important to inform all treating physicians and dentists of the child's medical condition. Special precautions are necessary when the child undergoes surgery of any kind, because hypoxemia resulting from anesthesia is a major surgical risk. The child should also wear a medical identification tag or bracelet.

- Because infection is especially dangerous for the patient with SCD, recommendations for patients of all ages include keeping current with vaccinations, plus receiving annual influenza and pneumococcal vaccinations (NHLBI, 2016). The Haemophilus influenzae type b (Hib) vaccine series should be started at 2 months of age and continued at recommended ages.

- Family members need ongoing support to deal with the stress of having a child with a chronic condition. Provide resources, respite care for parents, and information as needed for siblings.

- Encourage older children with SCD to participate in activities with other children between crises but to avoid strenuous physical exertion and contact sports. Play and social interactions that promote learning and development are important.

high levels of fetal hemoglobin. Children with SCD can experience chest tightness and shortness of breath, which are diagnostic for acute chest syndrome and medical crisis. Among children with SCD, 10% will experience a stroke, which can result in permanent disabilities, learning impairment, and other neurologic outcomes (CDC, 2016b). Research has investigated two new areas of disease management in children. The use of hydroxyurea and screening with transcranial doppler for primary stroke prevention in children with SCD appears to be a viable alternative to treating with periodic blood transfusions. The second area of investigation is the use of an anti-sickling hemoglobin modifier (GBT440) that works by increasing hemoglobin's affinity for oxygen and can potentially prevent sickling of RBCs. The results of the study indicated that GBT440 rapidly reduced the rate of RBC destruction, improved oxygen delivery to tissues, and decreased the number of sickled cells circulating in the blood stream. These results support the need for further investigation of GBT440 as potential disease-modifying therapy (American Society of Hematology, 2015).

Children with sickle cell trait rarely experience sickle cell crisis. However, because they have some abnormal hemoglobin, they may develop symptoms of the disease under conditions of abnormally low oxygen, such as flying in an unpressurized airplane over 7000 feet or when anesthesia is administered. The most common symptoms experienced by those with sickle cell trait are splenic infarction and hematuria. However, most individuals who carry the trait never have symptoms, even with low oxygen concentrations.

Sickle Cell Disease in Pregnant Women

Pregnant women diagnosed with SCD often experience more frequent pain crises, along with more intense symptoms. In addition, they are at higher risk for complications, including miscarriage, premature birth, and low birth weight. With vigilant prenatal care and monitoring, the majority of pregnant women with SCD can expect positive outcomes (CDC, 2016c).

Sickle Cell Disease in Older Adults

The estimated mean life expectancy for patients with SCD is 39 years of age, and it is rare for patients with this disorder to live past the age of 50. However, some are living to become older adults. This improvement in overall patient survival has been attributed to the increase in prophylactic penicillin use and standard newborn screening. SCD is now becoming a chronic condition because of the increasing age of these patients. Another issue that has surfaced in relation to the increasing age of patients with SCD is the lack of available healthcare providers to care for these individuals, causing them to often rely on emergency department physicians and inpatient treatment for their care. This is an area for improvement in continuity of care for these patients (Kanter & Kruse-Jarres, 2013).

NURSING PROCESS

For the patient diagnosed with SCD, a comprehensive physical assessment is essential because any body system can be affected. The nurse focuses on providing care to the patient as well as teaching both the patient and family how to reduce sickling, how to provide home care, and what symptoms to report to the provider immediately.

Assessment

Collect the following data through the health history and physical examination:

- **Observation and patient interview.** Observe overall appearance and nonverbal pain cues such as gait disturbances, positioning, guarding, or facial grimacing. In patients who are known to have SCD, obtain a detailed history from the patient or caregivers about past crises, precipitating events, medical treatment, and home management. Ask adult patients to rate chronic or acute pain using a pain rating scale. For pediatric patients, use age-appropriate pain rating scales and objective (visual) assessment for indicators of pain. (See the module on Comfort for discussion of pain assessment across the lifespan.) Pain may occur in nearly any body part but most commonly manifests as headache, extremity pain, or abdominal discomfort. Assess the methods of pain management protocols used, and ask which interventions have been most effective. Because failure to thrive is common among children with SCD, obtain a height and weight for pediatric patients for comparison with previous measurements or to serve as a baseline for future comparison.

- **Physical examination.** Assess the patient for fever, neurologic changes (e.g., decreased alertness or behavioral changes), and respiratory symptoms, which are emergency conditions that necessitate prompt treatment. For the patient experiencing sickle cell crisis, in addition to assessing for indicators of inflammation or infection, be aware that a crisis can deteriorate into a life-threatening situation. Carefully monitor the patient for signs of shock (hypotension, changes in level of consciousness, dizziness or light-headedness, increased capillary refill time).

SCD is a chronic illness that can interfere with self-concept, level of independent function, and ADLs. Depending on the patient's age and developmental stage, disturbed self-concept and body image, guilt about upsetting the family's routines, depression, and isolation can occur.

The family of a child with SCD requires ongoing, thorough psychosocial assessment. If the child is newly diagnosed with the disorder, the family will need assistance to deal with feelings related to the disease's serious, life-threatening nature. Assess parents' understanding of the disease transmission, and ask whether genetic counseling has been obtained. Determine whether the family has adequate healthcare coverage to pay for the child's medical expenses. Ask older children about their knowledge of the disease, and explore their feelings related to the management of a chronic condition. When siblings or other family members are carriers, they should receive periodic counseling during the lifespan so that they understand the implications for dating, marriage, and having children.

Diagnosis

Using the assessment data, nurses choose diagnoses to reflect the needs of the specific patient and family members. Examples of nursing diagnoses that may be appropriate for inclusion in the plan of care for a patient with SCD include the following:

- *Gas Exchange, Impaired*
- *Breathing Pattern, Ineffective*
- *Decreased Cardiac Tissue Perfusion, Risk for*
- *Imbalanced Fluid Volume, Risk for*
- *Ineffective Cerebral Tissue Perfusion, Risk for*
- *Infection, Risk for*
- *Pain, Acute*
- *Caregiver Role Strain*
- *Family Processes, Interrupted*
- *Disproportionate Growth, Risk for*
- *Physical Mobility, Impaired.*

    (NANDA-I © 2014)

Planning

Identified outcomes are specific to the nursing diagnoses included in the patient's plan of care. Identified outcomes and goals appropriate for the patient with SCD may include the following:

- The patient's oxygen saturation will be maintained at greater than 90%.

- The patient's respiratory rate will range between 12 and 20 breaths per minute at rest and with appropriate activity.

- The patient will deny shortness of breath and dyspnea at rest and with appropriate activity.

- The patient will deny manifestations of acute cardiac syndrome, including chest pain, adventitious breath sounds, pulmonary infiltrates, and increased WBC count.

- The patient will demonstrate no signs or symptoms of stroke.

- The patient will demonstrate urine output of at least 0.5 mL/kg/hr.

- The patient will demonstrate no signs or symptoms of infection.

- Using a predetermined pain rating scale of 0–10 in which 10 represents "the worst possible pain," the adult patient will consistently rate pain at a level of 3 or less.

- Using a predetermined, developmentally appropriate pain rating scale, the pediatric patient will consistently rate pain as being tolerable or absent.

- The patient will meet criteria (e.g., height and weight) for normal growth and development.

Implementation

Nursing management for the patient in crisis focuses on optimizing tissue perfusion, promoting hydration, controlling pain, preventing infection, ensuring adequate nutrition, preventing complications, and providing emotional support to the child and family.

Promote Optimal Oxygenation and Circulation

Good tissue perfusion is extremely important in patients with SCD. The nurse can assist by doing the following:

- Encourage the patient to balance activity and rest.
- Work with the patient and family to identify healthy methods of coping with emotional stress, and plan with the family for the trips to the healthcare facility. Any activities that increase cellular metabolism also increase oxygen demands, so the patient or family may need assistance with planning daily activities. For pediatric patients, schedule play as well as caregiving activities during hospitalizations and clinic visits to allow for optimal rest.
- Administer oxygen, IV fluids, and blood transfusions as ordered.
- Because children with SCD receive treatment every 3 weeks, nurses commonly insert the IV access devices and maintain the lines and infusions used. To prevent hemolysis, the IV fluid administered with a blood transfusion must be normal saline (0.9% NS) rather than D_5W.
- In small children, the blood is usually infused without saline, because the child cannot tolerate the additional fluid volume. Monitor for transfusion reactions.

Maintain Fluid Volume Balance

Proper fluid balance is vital for patients with SCD. The nurse's interventions may include the following:

- Teach patients and parents how to monitor intake and output, and provide patient teaching regarding fluid management.
- Adjust oral intake as necessary to keep the child well hydrated. Calculate the patient's fluid maintenance requirements (minimum daily fluid intake), and monitor oral and IV fluid intake.
- For the patient with SCD, dehydration can lead to life-threatening consequences. Administer IV fluids as ordered.

Manage Pain

Pain management is important for comfort, healing, and for promoting physical mobility in patients with SCD. Nursing implementations to manage the patient's pain include the following:

- Reposition the infant or young child carefully, supporting joints and extremities on pillows or special mattresses. Assist the child to assume a comfortable position. Avoid putting stress on painful joints or other body parts.
- Administer prescribed analgesics around the clock during crises. If patient-controlled analgesia is used, be sure that the constant infusions run as ordered and that the parent and child understand the use of bolus infusions when needed.

SAFETY ALERT Neither hot nor cold compresses should be used for pain management in the child with SCD. Ischemic tissue is fragile and has reduced sensation, increasing the risk of burn injury from hot compresses. Cold compresses promote sickling.

Prevent and Manage Infection

Infection is especially dangerous for the patient with SCD. Infection makes the patient more susceptible to a crisis, and the crisis in turn increases susceptibility to infection.

- Teach the patient or parents how to administer antibiotics for prophylaxis or treatment of infection. Be sure the family has the finances and other resources to obtain and give daily antibiotics.
- Because infections can be particularly virulent and can cause death in these children, instruct parents to obtain immediate care when the child is ill.

Reduce Risk for Caregiver Role Strain

SCD is a chronic disease accompanied by life-threatening episodic crises. Family members often need support to deal with their feelings about the diagnosis and its implications.

- Explore resources in the home and community to determine whether parents will be able to administer medications and fluids and to provide adequate nutrition.
- Assess parents' knowledge of signs of infection and of sickle cell crisis and when to seek medical care for the child.
- Refer the parents for genetic counseling, particularly if they plan to have more children. Encourage adolescents and young adults in the family to receive genetic counseling and testing as well.
- Referrals to support groups and contact with others with the disease can be helpful.
- Collaborate with family members, and provide them with ongoing support to deal with the stress of having a child with a chronic condition.
- Provide resources, including information about respite care for parents and information as needed for siblings.

>> **Stay Current:** Visit the website of the Sickle Cell Disease Association of America at http://www.sicklecelldisease.org to find resources for families.

Evaluation

Expected outcomes of nursing care for the patient with SCD include the following:

- The patient demonstrates no signs or symptoms of hypoxia or dyspnea.
- The patient experiences no complications of SCD, including stroke or acute chest syndrome.
- The patient demonstrates indicators of adequate hydration, including urine output of at least 0.5 mL/kg/hr and moist mucous membranes.

- The patient demonstrates no signs or symptoms of infection.
- The patient is up to date with all recommended vaccinations.
- The patient reports absence of pain or pain at a level the patient finds tolerable.
- The pediatric patient meets normal growth and developmental milestones.
- The family demonstrates adequate knowledge of the disease and treatment regimens.

If the patient reports pain that is not at a tolerable level, the nurse can educate the patient and family in the use of alternative or complementary pain relief measures, including relaxation techniques, biofeedback, yoga, meditation, distraction techniques, guided imagery, and breathing techniques. Cognitive–behavioral pain management may reduce reliance on pharmacologic means of pain control and enhance the patient's sense of control.

Nursing Care Plan

A Patient with Sickle Cell Disease

Mark Gotham is 10 years old. He was diagnosed with SCD shortly after birth. Both his mother and father carry the trait, but neither has the disease. Mark started fifth grade at a new school last week and was worried that the kids would make fun of him because of his small stature and occasional limp. Instead of going to lunch with his classmates, he stayed in the classroom so that no one would see how he limps when he walks. He became dehydrated and started to feel severe pain in his right leg. His mother brought him to the emergency department.

ASSESSMENT	DIAGNOSES	PLANNING
Mark is crying in pain and holding his right upper thigh. His vital signs include: temperature 98.4°F oral; pulse 112 bpm; respirations 24/min; and BP 118/65 mmHg. Popliteal, dorsalis pedis, and posterior tibial pulses are palpable in both legs.	■ *Peripheral Tissue Perfusion, Ineffective* related to alteration in hemoglobin ■ *Deficient Fluid Volume, Risk for* related to inadequate fluid intake and dehydration ■ *Chronic Pain* related to chronic physical disability and clustering of sickled cells ■ *Infection, Risk for* related to chronic disease and splenic malfunction ■ *Deficient Knowledge* (child and parents) related to lack of exposure about cause and treatment of SCD (NANDA-I © 2014)	■ The child will show no signs and symptoms of acute tissue hypoxia. ■ The child will maintain or be restored to adequate hydration. ■ The child will verbalize that pain is controlled. ■ The child will not develop infection. ■ The child and family will verbalize understanding of risk factors for sickle cell crises and how to minimize them.

IMPLEMENTATION

- Assess oxygenation status and efficacy of breathing.
- Position the patient to minimize the work of breathing and promote comfort.
- Give oxygen as ordered.
- Administer IV fluids and blood transfusions as ordered.
- Calculate the patient's daily fluid requirements and ensure appropriate fluid intake.
- Monitor and record fluid intake and output.
- Assess for signs and symptoms of dehydration.
- Administer analgesics, such as morphine or hydromorphone (Dilaudid), as ordered.
- Isolate the child from possible sources of infection. Instruct the parents about signs of infection, and encourage them to seek prompt healthcare.

- Instruct the child to avoid physical exertion, emotional stress, low-oxygen environments (e.g., airplanes and high altitudes), and known sources of infection.
- Instruct the family to report fever, vomiting, diarrhea, or other signs of fluid imbalance immediately.
- Ask the family what pain relief measures are helpful, and integrate these into the child's care.
- Ensure adequate nutrition through a high-calorie, high-protein diet. Ensure that the child's immunizations are up to date. Report any signs of infection to the physician immediately.
- Review the basics of SCD. Teach the child and family about signs and symptoms of crises.
- Arrange for genetic counseling and testing for sickle cell trait for family members if desired.

EVALUATION

- The child demonstrates no shortness of breath and shows no signs of hypoxia.
- The child demonstrates no signs or symptoms of stroke.
- The child shows indicators of adequate hydration, including sufficient urine production.

- Using a predetermined, developmentally appropriate pain rating scale, the patient consistently rates his pain as being tolerable or absent.
- The child demonstrates no signs or symptoms of infection.
- The child and parent can verbalize precipitating events of crises.

Nursing Care Plan (continued)

CRITICAL THINKING

1. What factors in Mark's history may have precipitated sickling?
2. When you admit Mark to the emergency department, what is your priority of care? Explain your answer.
3. What teaching will you provide to reduce the risk of future recurrence of sickling?

REVIEW Sickle Cell Disease

RELATE Link the Concepts and Exemplars

Linking the exemplar of SCD with the concept of oxygenation:

1. You admit a child in sickle cell crisis. How will you assess oxygenation?
2. How will you promote oxygenation for the patient in sickle cell crisis?

Linking the exemplar of SCD with the concept of infection:

3. What teaching priorities will you provide the parents of a young child who has SCD to reduce the risk of infection?
4. What interventions will you implement during hospitalization for a 9-year-old admitted in sickle cell crisis to reduce the risk of infection?

READY Go to Volume 3: Clinical Nursing Skills

REFER Go to Pearson MyLab Nursing and eText

- Additional review materials

REFLECT Apply Your Knowledge

Wendell Kozier is a 7-year-old boy with SCD. Wendell has had many absences during sickle cell crises and is now in first grade. Wendell is very bright and inquisitive. He tells the nurse he wants to play hockey when he grows up. Wendell's father is African American, and his mother is Caucasian and African American. Wendell is in the physician's office today for a checkup and immunizations. He was discharged from the hospital following sickle cell crisis 1 month ago.

1. What nursing diagnoses are appropriate for Wendell?
2. How will you respond to Wendell's desire to play hockey? What will you teach his parents about sports and sickle cell crisis?
3. What teaching will you provide to Wendell and his family to help reduce the frequency of sickle cell crisis?

» Exemplar 2.I
Skin Cancer

Exemplar Learning Outcomes

2.I Analyze skin cancer as it relates to cellular regulation.

- Describe the pathophysiology of skin cancer.
- Describe the etiology of skin cancer.
- Compare the risk factors for and prevention of skin cancer.
- Identify the clinical manifestations of skin cancer.
- Summarize diagnostic tests and therapies used by interprofessional teams in the collaborative care of an individual with skin cancer.
- Differentiate considerations for care of patients with skin cancer across the lifespan.
- Apply the nursing process in providing culturally competent care to an individual with skin cancer.

Exemplar Key Terms

Actinic keratosis, *136*
Basal cell cancer, *135*
Keratotic basal cell carcinoma, *136*
Melanomas, *133*
Microstaging, *138*
Morpheaform basal cell carcinoma, *136*
Nevi, *134*
Nodular basal cell carcinoma, *135*
Pigmented basal cell carcinoma, *136*
Squamous cell cancer, *136*
Superficial basal cell carcinoma, *135*

Overview

The skin, despite its ability to protect the internal body from external damage, is a fragile organ and is subject to damage from UV radiation and chemicals. Over time, this damage may result in alterations in cellular structure and function, leading to malignancies of the skin.

The skin is a common site for malignant lesions. Many of these lesions are found on skin surfaces that have undergone long-term exposure to the sun or the environment. Malignant skin tumors (**melanomas**) are the most common of all cancers. The nonmelanoma skin cancers are basal cell cancer and squamous cell cancer.

Pathophysiology and Etiology

Skin cancer can be classified as melanoma or nonmelanoma in type. Each classification will be considered independently.

Melanoma

Malignant melanomas arise from melanocytes, cells located at or near the basal layer (the deepest epidermal layer).

These cells produce melanin, the dark skin pigment. Melanin is made in granules and transferred to keratinocytes (primary cell of the epidermis), where it accumulates on the superficial side of each keratinocyte and forms a shield of pigment over the nucleus as protection against UV rays. Malignant melanomas can develop wherever there is pigment, but about one third of them originate in existing **nevi** (moles).

Almost all malignant melanomas are more than 6 mm in diameter, are asymmetric, and initially develop within the epidermis over a long period. While they are still confined to the epidermis, the lesions (called malignant melanoma in situ) are flat and relatively benign. However, when they penetrate the dermis, they mingle with blood and lymph vessels and are capable of metastasizing. At this latter stage, the tumors develop a raised or nodular appearance and often have smaller nodules, called satellite lesions, around the periphery.

The prognosis for survival among people diagnosed with malignant melanoma is determined by several variables, including tumor thickness, ulceration, metastasis, site, and the patient's age and gender. Younger patients and women have a somewhat better chance of survival. Tumors on the hands, feet, and scalp have a poorer prognosis; tumors of the feet and scalp are less visible and may not be diagnosed until they grow into the dermis.

Precursor Lesions

The three specific precursor lesions for the development of malignant melanoma are congenital nevi, dysplastic nevi, and lentigo maligna. A precursor lesion is also called a premalignant lesion, a name that indicates that the lesion's risk of becoming malignant is greater than normal.

- *Congenital nevi.* Congenital nevi are present at birth. Some lesions are small; others are large enough to cover an entire body area. Their color can range from brown to black. They are often slightly raised, with an irregular surface and a fairly regular border.

- *Dysplastic nevi.* Dysplastic nevi are also called atypical moles. Although dysplastic nevi are not present at birth, they appear as normal nevi during childhood and become dysplastic (having abnormal development) after puberty. A patient with classic dysplastic nevi has more than 100 nevi, at least one of which is larger than 8 mm in diameter and at least one of which has the characteristics of malignant melanoma (asymmetry, irregular border, color variegation, and a diameter greater than 6 mm). A familial tendency to dysplastic nevi increases the risk for development of malignant melanoma. However, it is not known whether people with dysplastic nevi and no family history of melanoma face a higher risk for melanoma.

  Dysplastic nevi most often appear on the face, trunk, and arms but also are seen on the scalp, female breast, groin, and buttocks. The pigmentation of the nevi is irregular, with mixtures of tan, brown, black, red, and pink. An area of lighter pigmentation is surrounded by a papular area of deeper pigmentation (described as a "fried egg appearance"). The borders of the nevi are irregular.

- *Lentigo maligna.* Lentigo maligna, also called Hutchinson freckle, is a tan or black patch on the skin that looks like a freckle. It grows slowly, becoming mottled, dark, thick, and nodular. It is usually seen on one side of the face of an older adult who has had a large amount of sun exposure.

Classifications of Malignant Melanomas

Malignant melanomas are classified into different types. The major types are superficial spreading melanoma, lentigo maligna melanoma, nodular melanoma, and acral lentiginous melanoma. Each is characterized by a radial and/or vertical growth phase. During the initial radial phase, which may last from 1 to 25 years (depending on the type), the melanoma grows parallel to the skin surface. During this phase, the tumor rarely metastasizes and is often curable by surgical excision. However, during the vertical growth phase, atypical melanocytes rapidly penetrate into the dermis and subcutaneous tissue, greatly increasing the risk for metastasis and death.

- *Superficial spreading melanoma.* Superficial spreading melanoma is the most common type, comprising approximately 50% of all melanomas (Osborn et al., 2013). The lesions are usually flat and scaly or crusty and are approximately 2 cm in diameter. They often arise from a preexisting nevus. This type of melanoma is found on the trunk and back of men and on the legs of women. Superficial spreading melanomas occur more often in women than in men. The median age of occurrence is the 50s.

  The radial growth phase lasts from 1 to 5 or more years. When the lesion enters the vertical growth phase, it grows rapidly, and its color changes from a mixture of tan, brown, and black to a characteristic red, white, and blue. The lesion also develops irregular borders and often has raised nodules and ulcerations (see **Figure 2–21 »**).

- *Lentigo maligna melanoma.* Lentigo maligna melanoma often arises from the precursor lesion, lentigo maligna. The lesions are large and tan, with different shades of brown. This type of melanoma makes up 15% of malignant melanomas and is the least serious form (Osborn et al., 2013). It occurs on skin that has had long-term sun exposure, such as the face, neck, and sometimes the dorsal surface of the hands and lower extremities. Lentigo maligna melanoma affects women more than men. It is typically diagnosed in people in their 60s and 70s.

- Lentigo maligna melanoma is characterized by a proliferation of atypical melanocytes parallel to the basal layer of the epidermis. The radial growth phase may last from 10 to 25 years, with the lesion growing to as large as 10 cm. The lesion becomes malignant as soon as the melanocytes invade the dermis. In the vertical growth phase, raised nodules may appear on the surface of the lesion. The lesion tends to acquire a freckled or mottled appearance.

- *Nodular melanoma.* Nodular melanoma lesions are raised, dome-shaped, blue-black or red nodules on areas of the head, neck, and trunk that may or may not have been exposed to the sun. The lesions may look like a blood blister, or they may ulcerate and bleed. The lesions arise from unaffected skin rather than from a preexisting lesion. This type makes up 20–25% of malignant

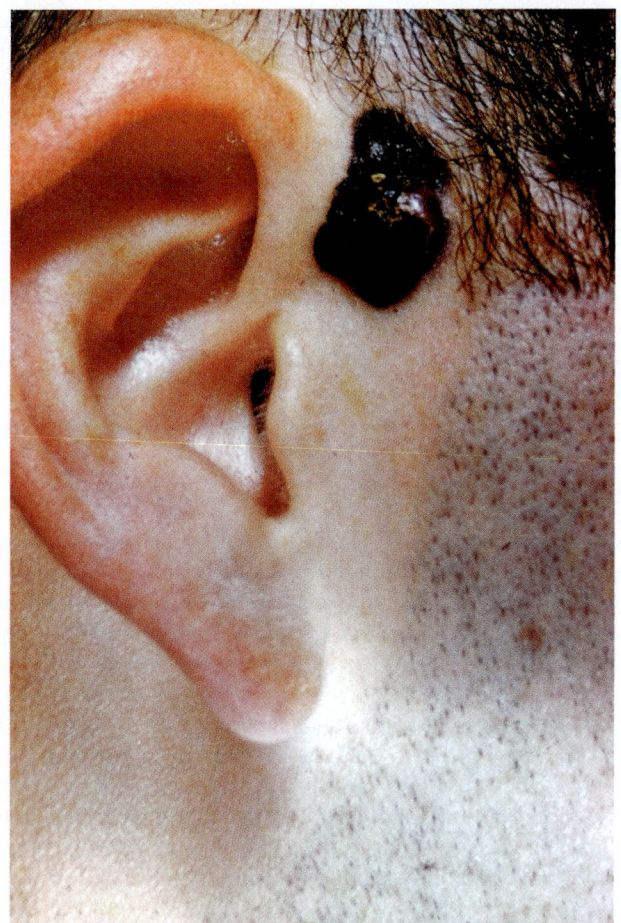

Source: Custom Medical Stock Photo/Alamy Stock Photo.

Figure 2–21 》 Malignant melanoma is a serious skin cancer that arises from melanocytes.

melanomas and is often diagnosed in people in their 50s (Osborn et al., 2013).

- Nodular melanoma has only a vertical growth phase, but it grows aggressively during that phase. However, the absence of a radial growth phase makes this type of melanoma more difficult to diagnose before it metastasizes.

- *Acral lentiginous melanoma.* Acral lentiginous melanoma is the least common form of melanoma, comprising less than 10% of all new cases (Osborn et al., 2013). Also called mucocutaneous melanoma, this condition is less common in people with fair skin and more common in people with dark skin. The lesions progress from tan, brown, or black flat lesions to elevated nodules and are approximately 3 cm in diameter. The radial phase lasts from 2 to 5 years. The nodules are found on the palms of the hands, the soles of the feet, the mucous membranes, and the nail beds. Acral lentiginous melanoma affects men and women equally and is most often diagnosed in people in their 50s and 60s.

Nonmelanoma Skin Cancer

Basal cell cancer and squamous cell cancer arise from epithelial tissue but have different pathophysiologies, classifications, and manifestations.

Basal Cell Cancer

Basal cell cancer is an epithelial tumor that is believed to originate either from the basal layer of the epidermis or from cells in the surrounding dermal structures. These tumors are characterized by an impaired ability of the basal cells of the epidermis to mature into keratinocytes, with mitotic division beyond the basal layer. This results in a bulky neoplasm that grows by direct extension and destroys surrounding tissue, including healthy skin, nerves, blood vessels, lymphatic tissue, cartilage, and bone. Basal cell cancer is the most common but least aggressive type of skin cancer, rarely metastasizing.

Basal cell cancers tend to recur. Tumors greater than 2 cm in diameter have a high recurrence rate. Predisposing factors for metastasis are the size of the tumor and the patient's resistance to treatment with surgery or chemotherapy. Although they rarely metastasize, untreated basal cell cancers invade surrounding tissue and may destroy body parts, such as the nose or eyelid.

Basal cell cancer is classified into different types: nodular, superficial, pigmented, morpheaform, and keratotic. These types are described below and are summarized in **Table 2–20 》**.

- **Nodular basal cell carcinoma**, the most common type of basal cell cancer, most often appears on the face, neck, and head. The tumor is made up of masses of cells that resemble epidermal basal cells and grow in a bulky, nodular form from lack of keratinization. In early stages, the tumor is a papule that looks like a smooth pimple. It is often pruritic and continues to grow at a steady rate, doubling in size every 6–12 months. As the tumor grows, the epidermis thins but remains intact. The skin over the tumor is shiny and pearly white, pink, or flesh colored. Telangiectasis (red, purple, or blue discoloration under the skin caused by abnormal dilation of a vessel) may be visible over the area of the tumor. As the tumor continues to increase in size, the center or periphery may ulcerate, and the tumor develops well-circumscribed borders. It bleeds easily from mild injury.

- **Superficial basal cell carcinoma**, found most often on the trunk and extremities, is the second most common type of

TABLE 2–20 Types and Characteristics of Basal Cell Cancers

Type	Common Location	Manifestation
Nodular	Face, neck, head	Small, firm papule; pearly, white, pink, or flesh colored; telangiectasis; enlarges; may ulcerate
Superficial	Trunk, extremities	Papules or plaque that is flat, erythematous, or scaling; pink color; well-defined borders; may have shallow erosions and surface crusting
Pigmented	Head, neck, face	Dark brown, blue, or black color; border is shiny and well defined
Morpheaform	Head, neck	Looks like a flat scar; ivory or flesh colored
Keratotic	Ear	Small, firm papule; pearly, white, pink, or flesh colored; may ulcerate

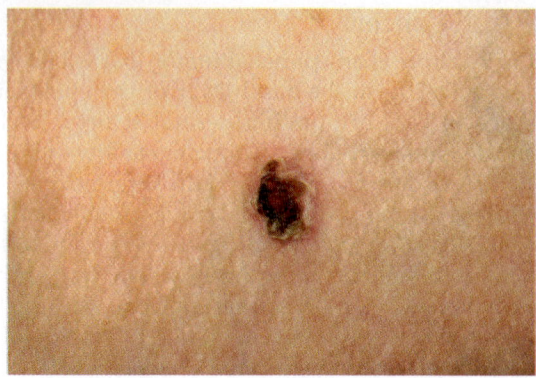

Source: Girand/BSIP SA/Alamy Stock Photo.

Figure 2–22 》 A superficial basal cell cancer is characterized by erythema, ulcerations, and well-defined borders.

basal cell cancer. This tumor is a proliferating tissue that attaches to the undersurface of the epithelium. The tumor is a flat papule or plaque, often erythematous, with well-defined borders. The tumor may ulcerate and be covered with crusts or shallow erosions (see **Figure 2–22** 》).

■ **Pigmented basal cell carcinoma**, found on the head, neck, and face, is less common. This tumor concentrates melanin pigment in the center of the basal cancer cells, giving it a dark brown, blue, or black appearance. The border of the tumor is shiny and well defined.

■ **Morpheaform basal cell carcinoma**, the rarest form of basal cell cancer, usually develops on the head and neck. The tumor forms finger-like projections that extend in any direction along dermal tissue planes. The tumor resembles a flat ivory or flesh-colored scar. This form is more likely to extend into and destroy adjacent tissue, especially muscle, nerve, and bone. It is often more difficult to diagnose because of its appearance.

■ **Keratotic basal cell carcinoma** (basosquamous) is found on the preauricular and postauricular groove. It contains both basal cells and squamoid-appearing cells that keratinize. Its appearance is much like that of nodular basal cell cancer. This type of basal cell cancer tends to recur locally and also is the type most likely to metastasize.

Squamous Cell Cancer

Squamous cell cancer is a malignant tumor of the squamous epithelium of the skin or mucous membranes. It occurs most often on areas of skin exposed to UV rays and weather, such as the forehead, helix of the ear, top of the nose, lower lip, and back of the hands. Squamous cell cancer may also arise on skin that has been burned or has chronic inflammation. This is a much more aggressive cancer than basal cell cancer, with a faster growth rate and a much greater potential for metastasis if untreated.

The tumors arise when the keratinizing cells of the squamous epithelium proliferate, producing a growth that eventually fills the epidermis and invades the dermal tissue planes. Keratinization of some cells is present, and the formation of keratin "pearls" is common. The keratin formation diminishes as the tumor grows. As the tumor grows, the tumor cells increase in number and rate of mitosis, forming odd shapes.

Squamous cell cancer begins as a small, firm, red nodule. The tumor may be crusted with keratin products. As it grows, it may ulcerate, bleed, and become painful. As the tumor extends into the surrounding tissue and becomes a nodule, the area around the nodule becomes indurated (hardened) (see **Figure 2–23** 》).

Recurrent squamous cell cancer can be invasive, increasing the risk of metastasis. Invasive squamous cell cancer may arise from preexisting skin lesions, such as scars and actinic keratosis, and extend into the dermis (called intraepidermal squamous cell cancer). This form appears as a slightly raised erythematous plaque with well-defined borders. Metastasis occurs most often via the lymphatics. The degree of risk for metastasis depends on the size and depth of penetration of the tumor.

Actinic Keratosis

Actinic keratosis, also called senile or solar keratosis, is an epidermal skin lesion directly related to chronic sun exposure and photo damage. Actinic keratosis may progress to squamous cell carcinoma. Because of this tendency, the lesions are classified as premalignant.

Actinic keratosis lesions are erythematous, rough macules a few millimeters in diameter. They are often shiny but may be scaly; if the scales are removed, the underlying skin bleeds. They occur in multiple patches, primarily on the face, dorsa of the hands, the forearms, and sometimes, on the upper trunk (see **Figure 2–24** 》). Enlargement or ulceration of the lesions suggests transformation to malignancy.

Etiology

UV rays can actually change the DNA in cells; this is believed to be the cause of most skin cancers. Although UV rays account for only a small part of the sun's radiation, exposure to UV radiation from sunlight is a major cause of skin cancer. Tanning beds are another dangerous form of UV exposure. Other etiologic factors are age, skin type, skin color, and genetic predisposition.

Risk Factors

Risk factors vary according to type of lesion. Melanoma, nonmelanoma, and actinic keratosis each have specific considerations related to risk.

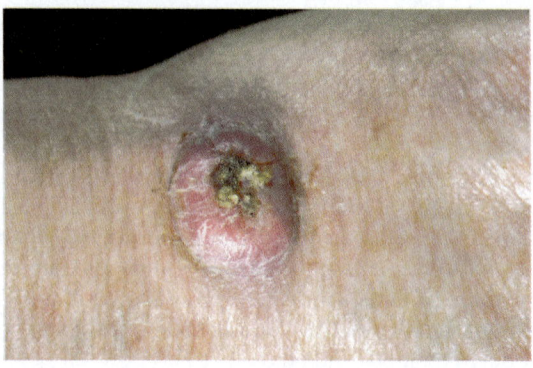

Source: Mediscan/Alamy Stock Photo.

Figure 2–23 》 As a squamous cell cancer grows, it tends to invade surrounding tissue. It also ulcerates, may bleed, and is painful.

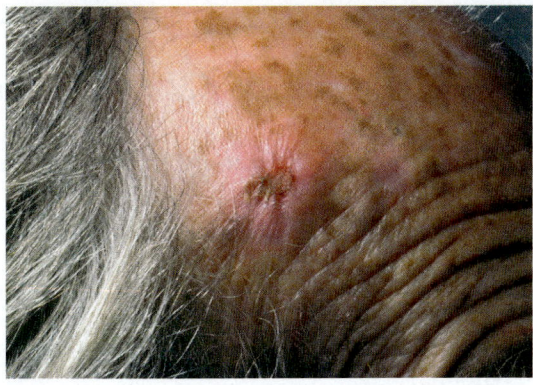

Source: Mediscan/Alamy Stock Photo.

Figure 2–24 >> The effects of long-term sun exposure are illustrated in this epidermal skin lesion, called actinic keratosis.

Melanoma Skin Cancer

Although the exact cause of melanoma is unknown, certain risk factors are associated with the disease. Even a single blistering sunburn during childhood or adolescence more than doubles a child's risk for developing melanoma in later years (Skin Cancer Foundation, n.d.a). The risk factors for melanoma are listed in **Box 2–6** >>.

Nonmelanoma Skin Cancer

Multiple etiologic factors are involved in the development of nonmelanoma skin cancer, including environmental factors and host factors. Unknown factors may also play a role.

The environmental factors implicated in the nonmelanoma skin cancers are UV radiation, pollutants, chemicals, ionizing radiation, viruses, and physical trauma.

Ultraviolet radiation from the sun is believed to be the cause of most nonmelanoma skin cancers. Sunlight contains both short-length rays (UVB) and long-length rays (UVA). UVB rays are absorbed by the top layer of skin and cause sunburn. UVA rays penetrate deeper into the skin layers, causing tissue damage. Both types of rays are believed to cause DNA alterations and also suppress T-cell and B-cell immunity. The amount of UV radiation reaching the earth is increasing, most likely from depletion of the ozone layer surrounding the planet. The U.S.

Box 2–6
Risk Factors for Melanoma Skin Cancer

- A high number of moles or large moles
- Fair skin, freckling, blond hair, or blue eyes
- Close relative with the disease
- Men with gene changes from a family history of breast or ovarian cancer
- Treatment with medications that suppress the immune system
- Too much exposure to UV radiation from sunlight, tanning lamps, or tanning booths
- Age older than 50 years
- Xeroderma pigmentosus, a rare, inherited disease in which people are less able to repair damage caused by sunlight
- Past history of melanoma

Environmental Protection Agency predicts that for every 1% decrease in the ozone layer, a corresponding 1–3% increase in cases of nonmelanoma skin cancer per year will occur.

Geographic, environmental, and lifestyle factors affect the amount of exposure to the sun and the risk for nonmelanoma skin cancer. People who live in latitudes close to the equator and those who live at higher altitudes receive greater UV radiation exposure. The amount of clothing worn, the time of day, and the amount of time in the sun also determine the amount of exposure. Exposure to UV radiation in tanning booths has also been implicated in the development of nonmelanoma skin cancer.

Certain chemicals have long been associated with nonmelanoma skin cancer. Polycyclic aromatic hydrocarbons, found in mixtures of coal, tar, asphalt, soot, and mineral oils, have been linked with skin cancers. Psoralens, used in conjunction with UVA for treatment of psoriasis and cutaneous T-cell lymphoma, increase the risk of squamous cell cancer.

Other factors associated with nonmelanoma skin cancer are the use of ionizing radiation, viruses, and physical trauma. X-ray therapy for tinea capitis and the use of radium to treat other malignancies are risk factors. Human papillomavirus is implicated in the development of squamous cell cancer, as is damage to the skin from burns.

Certain host factors increase the risk for nonmelanoma skin cancer. These include skin pigmentation as well as the presence of premalignant lesions.

Skin pigmentation is an important factor in the development of nonmelanoma skin cancer. The amount of melanin pigment produced by the melanocytes determines an individual's skin color. The more melanin, the more the skin is protected from the damage produced by UV rays. Thus, some darker-skinned African Americans, Asian Americans, and people of Mediterranean descent have a much lower incidence of nonmelanoma skin cancer than do people who have fair complexions and tend to freckle or sunburn easily, such as some people of Irish, Scandinavian, or English ancestry.

Although most people have numerous pigmented lesions on their body, almost all of these are normal. However, a major risk factor in the development of nonmelanoma skin cancer is a change in an existing lesion or the presence of a premalignant lesion, such as actinic keratosis. Organ transplant recipients who undergo immunosuppression to prevent rejection are also at risk for the development of squamous cell cancer.

Actinic Keratosis

The prevalence of actinic keratosis is highest in people with light-colored skin. These lesions are rare in people with dark skin.

Prevention

Primary prevention includes avoiding prolonged sun exposure and refraining from the use of artificial tanning machines. Recommendations for protection from the sun's harmful rays include daily application of sunscreen that provides a sun protection factor (SPF) of 15 or higher. Before extended periods of sun exposure, sunscreen that provides an SPF of 30 or higher should be applied. Sunscreen should be applied 30 minutes before anticipated sun exposure and reapplied every 2 hours, with reapplication immediately after swimming or following periods of excessive perspiration. Broad-brimmed hats and sunglasses that block UV rays should be worn. Patients should be encouraged to perform head-to-toe skin exams and to seek an annual skin exam from their healthcare provider. Newborns should not be exposed to direct sunlight. For infants 6 months or older, sunscreen should be applied (Skin Cancer Foundation, n.d.b).

SAFETY ALERT In the prevention of skin cancer, wellness promotion includes educating patients about the risks associated with indoor tanning devices. With just one indoor tanning session, an individual's risk for developing melanoma increases by 20%. With each additional tanning session during the same year, the individual's risk for melanoma increases by nearly an additional 2% (Boniol et al., 2012). Tanning beds are so dangerous, especially for younger individuals, that several states in the United States have banned the use of tanning beds by anyone under age 18 (Simon, 2015c).

Clinical Manifestations

The clinical manifestations of the various types of skin cancer differ. It is often possible to determine the likelihood of a specific classification based on appearance, although further testing is generally done to confirm the diagnosis. Manifestations of skin cancers are summarized in the Clinical Manifestations and Therapies feature.

Collaboration

Care of the patient with skin cancer requires a collaborative team of healthcare providers to promote early detection and prompt intervention and to improve patient outcomes. Numerous treatment options may be offered, and the nurse's role is to help the patient make an informed decision about the treatment option that is best for his or her needs and circumstances.

Treatment of nonmelanoma skin cancer focuses on removal of all malignant tissue using such methods as surgery, curettage and electrodessication, cryotherapy, or radiotherapy. These modalities offer a greater than 90% cure rate. Other methods of treatment are chemotherapy, immunotherapy, and radiation therapy. Biological therapies with interleukin-2 and interferon and therapeutic vaccines containing melanoma antigens are sometimes used. After the malignant tissue is removed, the patient should have regular examinations for recurrence.

The management of the patient with malignant melanoma begins with identification, diagnosis, and tumor staging. If treatable, the tumor is removed through surgical excision. Malignant melanoma is also treated with chemotherapy, immunotherapy, and radiation therapy.

Diagnostic Tests

Malignant melanoma is most often found on the trunk of men and on the lower extremities of women. Nevertheless, it is important for the patient to have a complete physical examination and total skin assessment. A change in the color or size of a nevus is reported in 70% of people diagnosed with a malignant melanoma. The **ABCD** rule is used to assess suspicious lesions:

Asymmetry (one half of the nevus does not match the other half)

Border irregularity (edges are ragged, blurred, or notched)

Color variation or dark black color

Diameter greater than 6 mm (size of a pencil eraser).

Along with visual examination of all skin surfaces, palpation of regional lymph nodes, the liver, and the spleen is essential to assess for metastasis when a melanoma is suspected or found.

In addition to biopsy of any suspicious lesion, diagnostic tests are conducted to determine whether the tumor has metastasized. Because malignant melanoma may metastasize to any organ or tissue of the body, a variety of tests may be conducted, including microscopic examination, biopsy, and tests for metastasis. These test may include liver function tests, CT of the liver, CBC, serum blood chemistry profile, chest x-ray, bone scan, and CT or MRI of the brain.

Microstaging

Microstaging describes the assessment of the level of invasion of a malignant melanoma and the maximum tumor thickness. In the Clark system of microstaging, the vertical growth of the lesion is measured from the epidermis to the subcutaneous tissue to determine the level of invasion (see **Figure 2–25 »**). However, variations in individual skin thicknesses and different anatomical sites can affect the accuracy of the measurement. In the Breslow system, an adaptation of the Clark system of assessment, the vertical thickness is measured from the granular level of the epidermis to the deepest level of tumor invasion. This determination is important, because as the thickness of the melanoma increases, survival rate decreases.

After the thickness and depth of the tumor have been determined, a clinical stage is assigned. The traditional three-stage system is still used, although it does not include tumor thickness. The American Joint Committee on Cancer has adopted a four-stage system that includes tumor thickness, level of invasion, lymph node involvement, and evidence of metastasis.

Surgery

Surgical excision is the preferred treatment for malignant melanoma. If a biopsy identifies the lesion as a melanoma, a

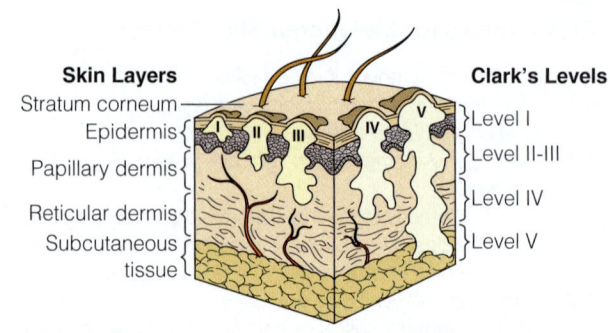

Figure 2–25 » The Clark system for staging the invasion of a melanoma from the epidermis to the subcutaneous tissue.

Clinical Manifestations and Therapies
Skin Cancer

ETIOLOGY	CLINICAL MANIFESTATIONS	CLINICAL THERAPIES
Melanomas		
Congenital nevi, precursor to melanoma	▪ Range in color from brown to black ▪ Often slightly raised, with an irregular surface and fairly regular border ▪ Can range in size from small to covering entire body	▪ Surgical excision ▪ Chemotherapy ▪ Immunotherapy ▪ Radiation therapy ▪ Regular examinations to assess for recurrence
Dysplastic nevi, precursor to melanoma	▪ Have irregular pigmentation with mixtures of tan, brown, black, red, and pink ▪ May have an area of lighter pigmentation surrounded by an area of deeper pigmentation ▪ Irregular borders ▪ Often appear on the face, trunk, and arms but can be seen on the scalp, female breast, groin, and buttocks	
Lentigo maligna, precursor to melanoma	▪ Tan or black patch on the skin that looks like a freckle ▪ Grows slowly, becoming mottled, dark, thick, and nodular ▪ Usually seen on one side of the face in an older adult who has had a large amount of sun exposure	
Malignant melanoma	▪ Asymmetrical, with an irregular border ▪ Color variegation ▪ Diameter greater than 6 mm (the size of a pencil eraser)	
Nonmelanomas		
Nodular basal cell carcinoma	▪ Papule that looks like a smooth pimple that grows at a steady rate ▪ Skin over the tumor that is shiny and may be pearly white, pink, or flesh colored ▪ Chance of visible telangiectasis ▪ Tumor that may ulcerate at the center or periphery and bleed easily from mild injury	▪ Surgical excision ▪ Curettage and electrodesiccation ▪ Cryotherapy ▪ Radiotherapy ▪ Chemotherapy ▪ Immunotherapy ▪ Radiation therapy ▪ Biological therapy ▪ Vaccines ▪ Regular examinations to assess for recurrence
Superficial basal cell carcinoma	▪ Appears as a flat papule or plaque, often erythematous, with well-defined borders ▪ Tumor that may ulcerate and be covered with crusts or shallow erosions ▪ Most common on the trunk and extremities	
Pigmented basal cell carcinoma	▪ Dark brown, blue, or black, with a shiny surface and well-defined borders ▪ Typically found on the head, face, and neck	
Morpheaform basal cell carcinoma	▪ Resembles a flat ivory or flesh-colored scar that forms finger-like projections that extend along dermal tissue planes ▪ Usually develops on the head and neck	
Keratotic basal cell carcinoma	▪ Appears similar to nodular basal cell carcinoma	
Squamous cell cancer	▪ Begins as a small, firm, red nodule that may be crusted with keratin products ▪ Tumors that ulcerate, bleed, and become painful as they grow ▪ Causes the area around the nodule to harden as the tumor extends into the surrounding tissue and becomes a nodule ▪ Most common on areas of skin exposed to UV rays and weather, such as the forehead, helix of the ear, top of the nose, lower lip, and back of the hands	
Other types of lesions		
Actinic keratosis	▪ Erythematous, rough macules a few millimeters in diameter ▪ Often shiny but may be scaly; if scales are removed, underlying skin bleeds ▪ Occur in multiple patches, primarily on the face, dorsa of the hands, the forearms, and sometimes, on the upper trunk ▪ Enlargement or ulceration of the lesions suggests transformation to malignancy	▪ Cryosurgery ▪ Topical creams or gels ▪ Shave excision ▪ Curettage and electrodesiccation ▪ Photodynamic therapy ▪ Chemical peels ▪ Laser surgery ▪ Monitoring for changes or abnormalities in lesion(s)

wide excision is performed that includes the full thickness of the skin and subcutaneous tissue. Because the risk of local recurrence for thin melanomas (those smaller than 0.76 mm) is quite low, margins of 0.5–1.0 cm of normal skin are excised around the tumor. Thick tumors require a 1- to 3-cm margin excision because they are at risk for local recurrence or satellite lesions.

Regional lymph nodes are the most common sites for metastasis of malignant melanoma. Standard surgical treatment for clinically suspicious lymph node involvement includes excision of the primary lesions as well as surgical dissection of the involved lymph nodes. Elective lymph node dissection (ELND) in the treatment of localized malignant melanoma remains controversial. Advocates of ELND believe that the procedure benefits patients with intermediate-thickness tumors, because approximately 20% of people whose lymph nodes were clinically negative at diagnosis show some metastasis on removal of the nodes. Those opposed to ELND believe the risks associated with the procedure are too high for the 80% of people who have no evidence of metastasis after removal of the nodes (McNeil, 2013).

Surgery also is indicated for palliative management of isolated metastasis. Removal of metastatic tumors in the brain, liver, lung, gastrointestinal tract, or subcutaneous tissue may relieve symptoms and prolong life.

Pharmacologic Therapy

In addition to surgical procedures, treatment of the patient with melanoma may include immunotherapy. Very sensitive new tests can better detect the spread of melanoma to lymph nodes and can possibly better identify people who could be helped by a treatment such as immunotherapy after surgery.

Immunotherapy is an emerging treatment modality for malignant melanoma. The role of the immunologic response initially was recognized because of the numerous spontaneous remissions seen in patients with melanoma—a higher occurrence than with any other adult tumor. In addition, researchers have recently identified tumor-specific antigen-antibodies in patients with melanoma. This also has stimulated an interest in immunotherapeutic interventions for the treatment of malignant melanoma.

Agents such as interferons, interleukins, monoclonal antibodies, bacille Calmette-Guérin, levamisole, transfer factors, and tumor vaccines have been used to treat melanoma, with varying response rates. The effectiveness of these agents, used either alone, in combination with chemotherapy, or in combination with each other, is under investigation.

>> **Stay Current:** Visit the website of the National Cancer Institute to stay abreast of current treatment options for melanoma: http://www.cancer.gov/types/skin/patient/melanoma-treatment-pdq.

Radiation Therapy

Melanoma responds to higher-dose radiation, especially if the tumor is small. Response rates to radiation therapy depend on the site of the tumor, the thickness of the tumor, the type of melanoma, and the patient's general health, but may range from 0 to 71%. Radiation frequently is used for palliation of symptoms resulting from metastasis to the brain, bone, lymph nodes, gastrointestinal tract, skin, or

subcutaneous tissue. Liver and lung metastases are not treated with radiation therapy, because a loss of organ function may result.

Knowledge of how UV light harms DNA is increasing, providing support for referral to genetic counseling for people with a strong family history of melanoma.

Lifespan Considerations

Skin Cancer in Children

Melanoma, although rare in children, is the most common type of pediatric skin cancer. Approximately 500 children are diagnosed each year, and melanoma accounts for about 2% of all childhood cancers. Melanoma occurs more commonly as children get older, with 8% of teenagers, especially girls, developing this type of cancer. Research has indicated that sun exposure and tanning beds increase the risk for melanoma in this population (University of Texas MD Anderson Cancer Center, 2016b).

Skin Cancer in Older Adults

The incidence of malignant lesions is increasing among older adults, with the majority of basal cell and squamous cell carcinomas occurring in this age group. The incidence of malignant melanoma is also 10 times higher. Symptom presentation of these lesions differs from that in younger adults, and prognosis tends to be poorer because of the advanced disease state when the patient seeks treatment. Melanoma is frequently asymptomatic, and the subtypes of this skin cancer are more aggressive. Older adults are at greater risk for developing skin cancer because of immunoescence (a decrease in immune function with aging), which physiologically makes them more susceptible, and cumulative risk factors such as exposure to carcinogens and UV radiation. This population can also have greater difficulty identifying new or changing skin lesions.

As with all suspected cases of skin cancer, a biopsy should be performed. However, sentinel node biopsies are less frequently positive in the older adult population. Treatment for the older adult with skin cancer is similar to that for the younger adult. However, not all older adults are candidates for surgery, owing to comorbidities such as diabetes; cardiac, vascular, or coagulation conditions; and arthritis. Radiotherapy may be appropriate treatment for squamous cell carcinoma or basal cell carcinoma if the older adult is not a candidate for surgery; it offers a 90% 5-year cure rate. The use of topical treatments may also be an option, but the presence and levels of arthritis and dementia need to be considered prior to prescribing this treatment. Comorbidities should also be considered when prescribing adjuvant therapies. Complete lymph node dissection may be needed if malignant melanoma has spread and the sentinel lymph node is positive; however, the morbidity of the procedure is significant for the older adult. Systemic therapies are generally not well tolerated by older adults and may complicate other coexisting diseases. Healthcare providers need to take significant action in the prevention of skin cancer for the older adult population by performing proper skin assessments and providing education related to risk reduction and available treatment options (Johnson & Taylor, 2012).

NURSING PROCESS

Nursing care of patients diagnosed with any form of skin cancer requires careful assessment and documentation of lesions, monitoring for any change in appearance, and support of the patient's physical and emotional needs. Fear of death, altered body image, and painful treatments often result from the diagnosis, and the nurse must provide holistic care that addresses both the physical and emotional needs of the patient.

Assessment

- **Observation and patient interview.** Patients with skin cancer should undergo a skin assessment. Specific health history questions include the following:
  a. Have any members of your family ever been treated for skin cancer?
  b. Have you had a skin cancer removed from any part of your body?
  c. Have you noticed any change in the size, shape, or color of a mole, wart, birthmark, or scar?
  d. Do you have any moles, warts, birthmarks, or scars that itch, are painful, have crusting, or bleed?
  e. In what parts of the country or world have you lived?
  f. Have you ever been badly sunburned?
  g. Do you visit tanning salons?
  h. Are you exposed to any hazardous chemicals in your job?
  i. Have you been taught how to examine your skin? If so, how do you do this examination? How often?

- **Physical examination.** The physical assessment should include the following:
  1. Ask the patient to remove all clothing and put on an examination gown. Ensure good light; natural, bright light is best for inspection of lesions. The patient may sit, stand, or lie down.
  2. Inspect and palpate the skin. Stretching the skin tightly during assessment facilitates assessment of nodular and scaly lesions and lesions in the dermis. Assess for the following:
     a. Obvious lesions
     b. Visible swellings
     c. Alterations in normal contour and borders of nevi
     d. Enlarged lymph glands
     e. Skin or mucosal discolorations
     f. Areas of ulceration, scaling, crusting, or erosion.
  3. The order of assessment is as follows:
     a. Head and neck: entire scalp, eyelids, external ear, auditory canals, external surface of the nose, internal surface of the nose, the oral cavity, facial skin, and the facial glands (parotid, submaxillary, sublingual)
     b. Thyroid and neck, including lymph glands
     c. Chest and abdomen, with special attention under pendulous breasts, in skinfolds, and in areas covered with hair
     d. Back and buttocks, with special attention to the area between the buttocks
     e. Extremities, with special attention to the axillae, nail beds, webs between the fingers and toes, and soles of the feet
     f. External genitals, with special attention to skinfolds, mucous membranes, and areas covered with hair.

  4. Measure and record a description of all skin lesions on an anatomical chart. Take photographs (if possible) of any suspicious lesion, and include them in the patient's record for future reference.

Diagnosis

Although many different nursing diagnoses may be appropriate for the patient with a malignant melanoma, common responses are the following:

- *Skin Integrity, Impaired*
- *Knowledge, Deficient*
- *Infection, Risk for*
- *Hopelessness*
- *Anxiety.*

(NANDA-I © 2014)

Planning

Planning care for the patient diagnosed with skin cancer is highly individualized. It depends on where the cells are located, the presence of metastasis, the treatment indicated, and the age of the patient. Suggested goals for care may include the following:

- The patient will describe different treatment options available and the pros and cons of each in order to make an informed decision about treatment.
- The patient will demonstrate no signs or symptoms of infection postoperatively.
- The patient will conduct skin self-examinations at least once monthly and will report any abnormalities or changes in skin.
- The patient will verbalize awareness of measures to prevent skin cancer recurrence, including proper use of sunscreen and clothing and avoidance of artificial tanning machines.
- The patient will verbalize emotions and concerns related to diagnosis of skin cancer and the available treatments.

Implementation

In addition to providing patient care, nurses play an important role in promoting awareness of skin cancer prevention. Teaching the need for sun protection and avoidance of tanning beds is an important role for the nurse advocate. Additional nursing interventions target preventing infection and facilitating open communication, as well as promoting psychosocial well-being.

Address Feelings of Hopelessness

The diagnosis of malignant melanoma threatens the quality and quantity of life as the patient faces the possibility or reality of metastasis; the possibility that the cancer may recur and cause death; and alterations in self-concept, roles, and relationships. Patients with this diagnosis may lose hope, becoming withdrawn, passive, and apathetic. Verbalizing feelings, concerns, and goals allows others to validate or correct them, promotes a therapeutic nurse–patient relationship, and fosters feelings of self-worth. Expressing positive emotions and calling on support systems and sources of

Patient Teaching
The Patient with Malignant Melanoma

Health education for the patient and family experiencing the diagnosis and treatment of malignant melanoma involves self-care and ongoing self-monitoring. Education for the patient and family is specific to the type of treatment. In addition to wound care, patients who have had a lymph node dissection need instructions on how to protect against bleeding, trauma, and infection. Address the following topics:

- The importance of regular medical checkups every 3 months for the first 2 years, every 6 months for the next 5 years, and yearly thereafter
- How proper self-care combined with regular medical care can help the patient lead a fairly normal life
- If assistance for home care is necessary, referrals to a community health agency or a home care agency, as well as referral to a local cancer support group if desired. Other resources in this area include the American Cancer Society (http://www.cancer.org) and the Skin Cancer Foundation (http://www.skincancer.org).

strength that were effective in coping with past crises help the individual resolve the crisis and develop hope. The nurse should do the following:

- Provide an environment that encourages the patient to identify and express feelings, concerns, and goals. Using active listening, ask open-ended questions and reflect on the patient's statements. Acknowledge and respect feelings of apathy and/or anger as expressions of distress, and convey an empathetic understanding of fears and concerns. Also provide opportunities to express positive emotions, such as hope, faith, a sense of purpose, and the will to live. Explore the patient's perceptions, and modify or clarify them if necessary by providing information and correcting misconceptions. Encourage the patient to identify support systems and sources of strength and coping in the past.
- Encourage active participation in self-care as well as in mutual decision making and goal setting. Meeting self-care needs and making decisions about care increase the patient's personal confidence in his or her capacity for coping.
- Encourage a focus not only on the present but also on the future: Review past occasions for hope, discuss the patient's personal meaning of hope, establish and evaluate short-term goals with the patient and family, and encourage them to express hope for the future. The nurse mobilizes the patient's resources to strengthen motivation, hope, and the will to live.

Reduce Anxiety

Anxiety is one of the most common psychosocial responses in patients with cancer. The intensity of the anxiety depends on the severity of the present situation and on the patient's ability to handle the threat. Anxiety increases at the time of diagnosis and remains a constant emotion throughout the course of treatment, regardless of treatment type or setting. Interventions focus on helping the patient recognize the manifestations of anxiety, determining whether the patient wishes to do anything about the anxiety, and facilitating coping strategies. Although the prognosis and treatment of melanoma depend on various factors, the prognosis of complete cure is decreased with metastasis. Surgical incisions include excision with wide margins, which may cause disfigurement. Active participation in care gives the patient some control over the future and is often an effective means of coping with anxiety. The nurse should do the following:

- Provide reassurance and comfort by setting aside time to sit quietly with the patient, speak slowly and calmly, and conveying empathetic understanding by touch and supporting coping mechanisms, such as crying and talking. Do not make demands or expect the patient to make decisions.
- Decrease sensory stimuli by using short, simple sentences; focusing on the here and now; and providing concise information. Higher levels of anxiety result in a focus on the present, inability to concentrate, and difficulty in understanding verbal communications.
- Provide accurate information about the illness, treatment, and expected length of recovery. Encourage the patient's and family's participation in care. Encourage discussion of expected physical changes and ways to minimize disfigurement through cosmetics and clothing.

Evaluation

The efficacy of the nursing care plan is evaluated based on the patient's progress in meeting goals of care. Possible expected outcomes used to evaluate care include the following:

- The patient demonstrates no signs or symptoms of infection.
- The patient's postoperative wound demonstrates signs of adequate healing, including well-approximated wound edges and granulation of tissue.
- Using a predetermined pain rating scale, the patient consistently rates pain at a level he or she considers to be tolerable or denies pain.
- The patient verbalizes awareness of the need to examine all skin lesions for changes or unusual appearance.
- The patient describes indications for reporting integumentary changes to the healthcare provider.
- The patient makes informed decisions regarding treatment options.
- The patient avoids unprotected sun exposure and use of tanning beds.
- The patient demonstrates healthy methods of coping with alterations in body image.

If the patient does not yet understand the importance of continuing to be vigilant for changes in the skin, the nurse should provide further education. The nurse should teach the patient to inspect moles for changes using the ABCD guidelines. Suspicious moles, actinic dermatoses, and other precancerous lesions found on evaluation should be removed.

REVIEW Skin Cancer

RELATE Link the Concepts and Exemplars

Linking the exemplar of skin dancer with the concept of development:

1. What teaching points will you include when teaching a group of teens about skin cancer prevention?

2. How will you respond to an adolescent girl who tells you she has to use the tanning bed or she looks too pale and ugly?

Linking the exemplar of skin cancer with the concept of advocacy:

3. How can you, as a student nurse, advocate for patients to reduce the rate of skin cancer as the result of tanning bed usage?

4. What is the role of the nurse advocate in reducing the rate of skin cancer diagnoses?

READY Go to Volume 3: Clinical Nursing Skills

REFER Go to Pearson MyLab Nursing and eText

- Additional review materials
- Chart 1: Case Study
- Nursing Care Plan: A Patient with Malignant Melanoma

REFLECT Apply Your Knowledge

Roe Jefferson is a nurse on vacation in Hampton Bays, Long Island. Ms. Jefferson has worked in pediatrics for 4 years now and really enjoys her work with parents and children. As she walks along the beach, she sees families with kids swimming and sunning themselves. She notices that there are no umbrellas and that, when not in the water, the children are not wearing hats or shirts. Several families have infants in car seats sitting in the sun.

1. What interventions would you implement to advocate for the children on the beach if you were Ms. Jefferson?

2. What is the teaching priority for families regarding the use of sunscreen?

3. What safety strategies would you teach families when they plan a day at the beach?

References

Abbaspour, N., Hurrell, R., & Kelishadi, R. (2014). Review on iron and its importance for human health. *Journal of Research in Medical Sciences, 19*(2), 164–174. Retrieved from http://www.ncbi.nlm.nih.gov/pmc/articles/PMC3999603/?report=printable

Abrams, S.A. (2016). Iron requirements and iron deficiency in adolescents. *UpToDate.* Retrieved from http://www.uptodate.com/contents/iron-requirements-and-iron-deficiency-in-adolescents

Adams, M. P., Holland, L. N., & Urban, C. (2017). *Pharmacology for nurses: A pathophysiologic approach* (5th ed.). Hoboken, NJ: Pearson Education.

Alter, H. J., Mikovits, J. A., Switzer, W. M., Ruscetti, F. W., Lo, S., Klimas, N. … Lipkin, W. I. (2012). A multicenter blinded analysis indicates no association between chronic fatigue syndrome/myalgic encephalomyelitis and either xenotropic murine leukemia virus-related virus or polytropic murine leukemia virus. *mBio, 3*(5), e00266–e00212.

American Association for Clinical Chemistry. (2016). *Tumor markers: What are tumors markers?* Retrieved from https://labtestsonline.org/understanding/analytes/tumor-markers

American Cancer Society (ACS). (2014a). *Genetics and cancer: Family cancer syndromes.* Retrieved from http://www.cancer.org/cancer/cancercauses/geneticsandcancer/heredity-and-cancer

American Cancer Society (ACS). (2014b). *Signs and symptoms of cancer: What are signs and symptoms?* Retrieved from http://www.cancer.org/cancer/cancerbasics/signs-and-symptoms-of-cancer

American Cancer Society (ACS). (2014c). *Genes and cancer: Oncogenes and tumor suppressor genes.* Retrieved from http://www.cancer.org/cancer/cancercauses/geneticsandcancer/genesandcancer/genes-and-cancer-oncogenes-tumor-suppressor-genes

American Cancer Society (ACS). (2014d). *Advanced cancer: Tests to find advanced cancer.* Retrieved

from http://www.cancer.org/treatment/understandingyourdiagnosis/advancedcancer/advanced-cancer-diagnosis

American Cancer Society (ACS). (2014e). *Children diagnosed with cancer: Late effects of cancer treatment.* Retrieved from http://www.cancer.org/treatment/childrenandcancer/whenyourchildhascancer/children-diagnosed-with-cancer-late-effects-of-cancer-treatment

American Cancer Society (ACS). (2014f). *Surgery for breast cancer in men.* Retrieved from http://www.cancer.org/cancer/breastcancerinmen/detailedguide/breast-cancer-in-men-treating-surgery

American Cancer Society (ACS). (2014g). *Hormone therapy for breast cancer in men.* Retrieved from http://www.cancer.org/cancer/breastcancerinmen/detailedguide/breast-cancer-in-men-treating-hormone-therapy

American Cancer Society (ACS). (2014h). *Leukemia—Acute lymphocytic (adults).* Retrieved from http://www.cancer.org/acs/groups/cid/documents/webcontent/003109-pdf.pdf

American Cancer Society (ACS). (2014i). *Infections that can lead to cancer.* Retrieved from http://www.cancer.org/acs/groups/cid/documents/webcontent/002782-pdf.pdf

American Cancer Society (ACS). (2015a). *Health risks of secondhand smoke: What is secondhand smoke?* Retrieved from http://www.cancer.org/cancer/cancercauses/tobaccocancer/secondhand-smoke

American Cancer Society (ACS). (2015b). *Chemotherapy drugs: How they work.* Retrieved from http://www.cancer.org/acs/groups/cid/documents/webcontent/002995-pdf.pdf

American Cancer Society (ACS). (2015c). *American Cancer Society recommendation for early breast cancer detection in women without breast symptoms: Clinical breast exam and breast self-exam.* Retrieved from http://www.cancer.org/cancer/breastcancer/

moreinformation/breastcancerearlydetection/breast-cancer-early-detection-acs-recs

American Cancer Society (ACS). (2015d). *Leukemia—Chronic myeloid leukemia (CML).* Retrieved from http://www.cancer.org/acs/groups/cid/documents/webcontent/003112-pdf.pdf

American Cancer Society (ACS). (2015e). *Leukemia—Chronic lymphocytic leukemia (CLL).* Retrieved from http://www.cancer.org/acs/groups/cid/documents/webcontent/003111-pdf.pdf

American Cancer Society (ACS). (2016a). *Can childhood leukemia be prevented?* Retrieved from http://www.cancer.org/leukemiainchildren/detailedguide/childhood-leukemia-prevention

American Cancer Society (ACS). (2016b). *Cancer facts & figures 2016.* Retrieved from http://www.cancer.org/acs/groups/content/@research/documents/acspc-047079.pdf

American Cancer Society (ACS). (2016c). *Breast reconstruction.* Retrieved from http://www.cancer.org/cancer/breastcancer/moreinformation/breastreconstructionaftermastectomy/breast-reconstruction-after-mastectomy-toc

American Cancer Society (ACS). (2016d). *Leukemia—Acute myeloid leukemia (AML).* Retrieved from http://www.cancer.org/acs/groups/cid/documents/webcontent/003110-pdf.pdf

American Cancer Society (ACS). (2016e). *Leukemia in children.* Retrieved from http://www.cancer.org/acs/groups/cid/documents/webcontent/003095-pdf.pdf

American Cancer Society (ACS). (2016f). *What causes non-small cell lung cancer.* Retrieved from http://www.cancer.org/cancer/lungcancer-non-smallcell/detailedguide/non-small-cell-lung-cancer-what-causes

American Cancer Society (ACS). (2016g). *What causes small cell lung cancer?* Retrieved from http://www.cancer.org/cancer/lungcancer-smallcell/detailedguide/small-cell-lung-cancer-what-causes

American Cancer Society (ACS). (2016h). *Prostate cancer*. Retrieved from http://www.cancer.org/acs/groups/cid/documents/webcontent/003134-pdf.pdf

American Cancer Society (ACS). (2016i). *Treating actinic keratosis and Bowen disease*. Retrieved from http://www.cancer.org/cancer/skincancer-basalandsquamouscell/detailedguide/skin-cancer-basal-and-squamous-cell-treating-actinic-keratosis

American Society of Clinical Oncology (ASCO). (2013). *What to know: ASCO's guideline on tumor markers for testicular cancer and extragonadal germ cell tumors in teenage boys and men*. Retrieved from http://www.cancer.net/publications-and-resources/what-know-ascos-guidelines/what-know-ascos-guideline-tumor-markers-testicular-cancer-and-extragonadal-germ-cell-tumors-teenage

American Society of Clinical Oncology (ASCO). (2015a). *Hypercalcemia*. Retrieved from http://www.cancer.net/navigating-cancer-care/side-effects/hypercalcemia

American Society of Clinical Oncology (ASCO). (2015b). *Understanding radiation therapy*. Retrieved from http://www.cancer.net/navigating-cancer-care/how-cancer-treated/radiation-therapy/understanding-radiation-therapy

American Society of Clinical Oncology (ASCO). (2015c). *Cancer during pregnancy*. Retrieved from http://www.cancer.net/navigating-cancer-care/dating-sex-and-reproduction/cancer-during-pregnancy

American Society of Clinical Oncology (ASCO). (2016a). *Tumor marker tests*. Retrieved from http://www.cancer.net/navigating-cancer-care/diagnosing-cancer/tests-and-procedures/tumor-marker-tests

American Society of Clinical Oncology (ASCO). (2016b). *Navigating cancer care—for older adults*. Retrieved from http://www.cancer.net/navigating-cancer-care/older-adults/multiple-health-concerns-older-adults

American Society of Hematology. (2015). *New sickle cell disease research shows improved patient outcomes*. Retrieved from http://www.hematology.org/Newsroom/Press-Releases/2015/4746.aspx

American Society of Hematology. (2016). *Leukemia*. Retrieved from http://www.hematology.org/Patients/Cancers/Leukemia.aspx

Artz, A. S. (2015). Anemia in elderly persons. *Medscape*. Retrieved from http://emedicine.medscape.com/article/1339998-overview#a1

Biswas, S. K. (2015). Does the interdependence between oxidative stress and inflammation explain the antioxidant paradox? *Oxidative Medicine and Cellular Longevity, 2016*, 1–9. http://dx.doi.org/10.1155/2016/5698931

Boniol, M., Autier, P., Boyle, P., & Gandini, S. (2012). Cutaneous melanoma attributable to sun-bed use: Systematic review and meta-analysis. *BMJ, 345*, e4757.

Boussios, S., Han, S. N., Fruscio, R., Halaska, M. J., Ottevanger, P. B., Peccatori, F. A., ... Amant, F. (2013). Lung cancer in pregnancy: Report of nine cased from an international collaborative study [Abstract]. *Lung Cancer, 82*(3), 499–505. http://dx.doi.org/10.1016/j.lungcan.2013.09.002

Breastcancer.org. (2016a). *Breast reconstruction*. Retrieved from http://www.breastcancer.org/treatment/surgery/reconstruction

Breastcancer.org. (2016b). *Aromatase inhibitors*. Retrieved from http://www.breastcancer.org/treatment/hormonal/aromatase_inhibitors

Brinkman, T. M., Zhang, N., Recklitis, C. J., Kimberg, C., Zeltzer, L. K., Muriel, A. C., ... Krull, K. R. (2014). Suicide ideation and associated mortality in adult survivors of childhood cancer. *Cancer, 120*(2), 271–277. doi:10.1002/cncr.28385

Callaghan, R. C., Allebeck, P., & Sidorchuck, A. (2013). Marijuana use and risk of lung cancer: A 40-year cohort study. *Cancer Causes & Control, 24*(10), 1811–1820. doi:10.1007/s10552-013-0259-0

Caprario, L. C., & Strauss, G. M. (2014). The benefit of chemotherapy in elderly patients with small cell lung cancer. *Expert Review of Anticancer Therapy, 14*(6), 645–647. Retrieved from http://search.proquest.com.proxy092.nclive.org/central/docview/1527340983/fulltextPDF/D9A2282E72FC4D1DPQ/17?accountid=14003

Centers for Disease Control and Prevention (CDC). (2015a). *Cancer rates by race/ethnicity and sex*. Retrieved from http://www.cdc.gov/cancer/dcpc/data/race.htm

Centers for Disease Control and Prevention (CDC). (2015b). *Occupational exposure to antineoplastic agents and other hazardous drugs*. Retrieved from http://www.cdc.gov/niosh/topics/antineoplastic/default.html

Centers for Disease Control and Prevention (CDC). (2015c). *Breast cancer rates by race and ethnicity*. Retrieved from http://www.cdc.gov/cancer/breast/statistics/race.htm

Centers for Disease Control and Prevention (CDC). (2015d). *Breast cancer in young women*. Retrieved from http://www.cdc.gov/cancer/breast/young_women/bringyourbrave/breast_cancer_young_women/index.htm

Centers for Disease Control and Prevention (CDC). (2015e). *Lung cancer—What are the risk factors of lung cancer?* Retrieved from http://www.cdc.gov/cancer/lung/basic_info/risk_factors.htm

Centers for Disease Control and Prevention (CDC). (2016a). *Workplace safety & health topics: Hazardous drug exposures in health care*. Retrieved from http://www.cdc.gov/niosh/topics/hazdrug/

Centers for Disease Control and Prevention (CDC). (2016b). *Sickle cell disease (SCD)—Complications and treatments*. Retrieved from http://www.cdc.gov/ncbddd/sicklecell/treatments.html

Centers for Disease Control and Prevention (CDC). (2016c). *Sickle cell disease (SDC)—Data & statistics*. Retrieved from http://www.cdc.gov/ncbddd/sicklecell/data.html

Deng, G., & Cassileth, B. (2013). Complementary or alternative medicine in cancer care—myths and realities. *Nature Reviews Clinical Oncology, 10*, 656–664. doi:10.1038/nrclinonc.2013.125

Dennis, T. (2015). *Clinical trials need older adults, ASCO says. City of Hope's Arti Hurria explains*. Retrieved from http://www.cityofhope.org/blog/clinical-trials-older-adults

Donovan, P. (2015). Study links new genetic anomalies to breast cancer in African American families. *University at Buffalo News Center*. Retrieved from http://www.buffalo.edu/news/releases/2015/02/006.html

Gilani, S., & Giridharan, S. (2014). Is it safe for pregnant health-care professionals to handle cytotoxic drugs? A review of the literature and recommendations. *Ecancermedicalscience, 8*(418). http://doi.org/10.3332/ecancer.2014.418

Hamre, H., Zeller, B., Kanellopoulos, A., Kiserud, C. E., Aakhus, S., Lund, M. B., ...Rudd, E. (2013). High prevalence of chronic fatigue in adult long-term survivors of acute lymphoblastic leukemia and lymphoma during childhood and adolescence. *Journal of Adolescent and Young Adult Oncology, 2*(1), 2–9. doi:10.1089/jayao.2012.0015

Herdman, T. H. & Kamitsuru, S. (Eds.) *Nursing Diagnoses—Definitions and Classification 2015–2017.* Copyright © 2014, 1994–2014 NANDA International. Used by arrangement with John Wiley & Sons, Inc. Companion website: www.wiley.com/go/nursingdiagnoses

Herfs, M., Hubert, P., Poirrier, A., Vandevenne, P., Renoux, V., Habraken, Y., ... Delvenne, P. (2012). Proinflammatory cytokines induce bronchial hyperplasia and squamous metaplasia in smokers. *American Journal of Respiratory Cell and Molecular Biology, 47*(1), 67–79. doi:10.1165/rcmb.2011-0353OC

Hockenberry, M. J., & Wilson, D. (2014). Family centered care of the child with chronic illness or disability and family centered palliative care. In *Wong's Nursing Care of Infants and Children* (10th ed.). St. Louis, MO: Mosby.

Hurria, A., Levit, L. A., Dale, W., Mohile, S. G., Muss, H. B., Fehrenbacher, L., ...Cohen, H. J. (2015). Improving the evidence base for treating older adults with cancer: American Society of Clinical Oncology Statement. *American Society of Clinical Oncology.* doi:10.1200/JCO.2015.63.0319

Ikeda, A. K. (2016). Tumor lysis syndrome [Abstract]. *Medscape*. Retrieved from http://emedicine.medscape.com/article/282171-overview

James, A. H. (2014). Sickle cell disease in pregnancy. *Contemporary OB/GYN*. Retrieved from: http://contemporaryobgyn.modernmedicine.com/contemporary-obgyn/news/sickle-cell-disease-pregnancy?page=full

Jha, P., Ramasundarahettige, C., Landsman, V., Rostron, B., Thun, M., Anderson, R. N., . . . Peto, R. (2013). 21st-century hazards of smoking and benefits of cessation in the United States. *New England Journal of Medicine, 368*(4), 341–350. doi:10.1056/NEJMsa1211128

Johnson, S. R., & Taylor, M. A. (2012). Identification and management of malignant skin lesions among older adults. *Journal for Nurse Practitioners, 8*(8), 610–616. Retrieved from http://www.medscape.com/viewarticle/770978

Kanter, J., & Kruse-Jarres, R. (2013). Management of sickle cell disease from childhood through adulthood. *Blood Reviews, 27*(2013), 279–287. http://dx.doi.org/10.1016/j.blre.2013.09.001

Karve, S. J., Price, G. L., Davis, K. L., Pohl, G. M., Nash Smyth, E., & Bowman, L. (2014). Comparison of demographics, treatment patterns, health care utilization, and costs among elderly. *BMC Health Services Research, 14*(555). Retrieved from http://search.proquest.com.proxy092.nclive.org/central/docview/1627796683/fulltextPDF/B33BE1C88C2A4C20PQ/1?accountid=14003

Khodaverdi, S., Valeshabad, A. K., & Khodaverdi, M. (2013). Case report: A case of colorectal cancer during pregnancy: A brief review of the literature. *Case Reports in Obstetrics and Gynecology, 2013*. http://dx.doi.org/10.1155/2013/626393

Kravits, K. G. (2013). An overview of non-pharmacological therapies for palliative cancer care. In W. C. Cho (Ed.), *Evidence-based non-pharmacological therapies for palliative cancer care*. London, United Kingdom: Springer: Retrieved from https://books.google.com/books?id=DPF7WcmWYqgC&pg=PA4-IA1&dq=Cho+2013+evidence+based+non+pharmacological+therapies+for+palliative+cancer+care&hl=en&sa=X&ved=0ahUKEwiGgrHDsqrNAhUFOSYKHZs7BKAQ6AEINDAA#v=onepage&q=Cho%202013%20evidence%20based%20non%20pharmacological%20therapies%20for%20palliative%20cancer%20care&f=false

Leukemia and Lymphoma Society (LLS). (2015a). *Types of CAM therapies*. Retrieved from http://www.lls.org/treatment/integrative-medicine-and-complementary-and-alternative-therapies/types-of-cam-therapies

Leukemia and Lymphoma Society (LLS). (2015b). *Integrative medicine and complementary and alternative therapies*. Retrieved from https://www.lls.org/treatment/integrative-medicine-and-complementary-and-alternative-therapies

Lichtin, A. (2013). Iron deficiency anemia. *Merck Manual Professional Version*. Retrieved from http://www.merckmanuals.com/professional/hematology-and-oncology/anemias-caused-by-deficient-erythropoiesis/iron-deficiency-anemia

Maakaron, J. (2015). Sickle cell anemia treatment and management. *Medscape*. Retrieved from http://emedicine.medscape.com/article/205926-treatment

Mayo Clinic. (2014a). *Sickle cell anemia—Symptoms and causes*. Retrieved from http://www.mayoclinic.org/diseases-conditions/sickle-cell-anemia/basics/symptoms/con-20019348

Mayo Clinic. (2014b). *Polycythemia vera—Complications*. Retrieved from http://www.mayoclinic.org/diseases-conditions/polycythemia-vera/basics/complications/con-20031013

Mayo Clinic. (2014c). *Polycythemia vera—Treatments and drugs*. Retrieved from http://www.mayoclinic.org/diseases-conditions/polycythemia-vera/basics/treatment/con-20031013

Mayo Clinic. (2014d). *Sickle cell anemia—Diagnosis*. Retrieved from http://www.mayoclinic.org/diseases-conditions/sickle-cell-anemia/basics/tests-diagnosis/con-20019348

Mayo Clinic. (2015a). *Cancer prevention: 7 tips to reduce your risk*. Retrieved from http://www.mayoclinic.org/healthy-lifestyle/adult-health/in-depth/cancer-prevention/art-20044816

Mayo Clinic. (2015b). *Breast cancer: Treatments*. Retrieved from http://www.mayoclinic.org/diseases-conditions/breast-cancer/basics/treatment/con-20029275

Mayo Clinic. (2016a). *Leukemia*. Retrieved from http://www.mayoclinic.org/diseases-conditions/leukemia/basics/treatment/con-20024914

Mayo Clinic. (2016b). *Breast cancer prevention: How to reduce your risk*. Retrieved from http://www.mayoclinic.org/healthy-lifestyle/womens-health/in-depth/breast-cancer-prevention/art-20044676

McNeil, C. (2013, May 1). Does every melanoma patient with a positive sentinel node need more lymph nodes removed? *The ASCO Post*. Retrieved from http://www.ascopost.com/issues/may-1-2013/does-every-melanoma-patient-with-a-positive-sentinel-node-need-more-lymph-nodes-removed

Medeiros, B. (2015). Ask the hematologist: Treatment of elderly patients with acute myeloid leukemia. *American Society of Hematology: The Hematologist ASH News and Reports, 12*(1). Retrieved from http://www.hematology.org/Thehematologist/Ask/3615.aspx

MedlinePlus. (2013). *Antioxidants*. Retrieved from http://www.nlm.nih.gov/medlineplus/antioxidants.html

Medline Plus. (2014a). *Lactate dehydrogenase test*. Retrieved from http://www.nlm.nih.gov/medlineplus/ency/article/003471.htm

MedlinePlus. (2014b). *Graft-versus-host disease*. Retrieved from http://www.nlm.nih.gov/medlineplus/ency/article/001309.htm

MedlinePlus. (2015). *Breast self-exam*. Retrieved from http://www.nlm.nih.gov/medlineplus/ency/article/001993.htm

Miller, A. B., Wall, C., Baines, C. J., Sun, P., To, T., & Narod, S. A. (2014, Feb 11). Twenty five year follow-up for breast cancer incidence and mortality of the Canadian National Breast Screening Study: Randomised screening trial. *BMJ, 348*, g366. doi:10.1136/bmj.g366

Mitou, S., Petrakis, D., Fotopoulos, G., Zarkavelis, G., & Pavlidis, N. (2016). Lung cancer during pregnancy: A narrative review. *Journal of Advanced Research, 7*(4), 571–574.

Molica, S., Brugiatelli, M., Morabito, F., Ferrara, F., Iannitto, E., Di Renzo, N., ...Di Raimondo, F. (2013). Treatment of elderly patients with chronic lymphocyte leukemia: An unmet clinical need. *Expert Review of Hematology, 6*(4), 441–449. Retrieved from https://www.ncbi.nlm.nih.gov/pubmed/23991930

Nadpara, P., Madhavan, S., & Tworek, C. (2015). Guideline-concordant timely lung cancer care and prognosis among elderly patients in the United States: A population-based study. *Cancer Epidemiology, 93*(6), 1136–1144. Retrieved from http://search.proquest.com.proxy092.nclive.org/central/docview/1746588972/fulltextPDF/D9A2282E72FC4D1DPQ/1?accountid=14003

National Cancer Institute (NCI). (2012a). *Psychological stress and cancer*. Retrieved from http://www.cancer.gov/about-cancer/coping/feelings/stress-fact-sheet

National Cancer Institute (NCI). (2012b). *Breast cancer risk in American women*. Retrieved from http://www.cancer.gov/cancertopics/factsheet/detection/probability-breast-cancer

National Cancer Institute (NCI). (2012c). *Prostate-specific antigen (PSA) test*. Retrieved from http://www.cancer.gov/types/prostate/psa-fact-sheet

National Cancer Institute (NCI). (2015a). *Cancer treatment: Types of treatment—Surgery*. Retrieved from http://www.cancer.gov/about-cancer/treatment/types/surgery

National Cancer Institute (NCI). (2015b). *Cancer treatment: Types of treatment—Radiation therapy*. Retrieved from http://www.cancer.gov/about-cancer/treatment/types/radiation-therapy

National Cancer Institute (NCI). (2015c). *Pediatric supportive care (PDQ)—Patient version*. Retrieved from http://www.cancer.gov/types/childhood-cancers/pediatric-care-pdq

National Cancer Institute (NCI). (2015d). *Children with cancer: A guide for parents*. Retrieved from http://www.cancer.gov/publications/patient-education/children-with-cancer.pdf

National Cancer Institute (NCI). (2015e). *BRCA1 and BRCA2: Cancer risk and genetic testing*. Retrieved from http://www.cancer.gov/about-cancer/causes-prevention/genetics/brca-fact-sheet

National Cancer Institute (NCI). (2015f). *Causes and prevention: Risk factors—Diet*. Retrieved from http://www.cdc.gov/cancer/prostate/statistics/race.htm

National Cancer Institute (NCI). (2015g). *Unusual cancers of childhood treatment (PDQ)—Patient version*. Retrieved from http://www.cancer.gov/types/childhood-cancers/patient/unusual-cancers-childhood-pdq#section/_58

National Cancer Institute (NCI). (2016a). *Cancer genetics overview (PDQ): Familial cancer susceptibility syndromes*. Retrieved from http://www.cancer.gov/cancertopics/pdq/genetics/overview/healthprofessional/page3

National Cancer Institute (NCI). (2016b). *Acupuncture—Health professional version (PDQ)*. Retrieved from http://www.cancer.gov/about-cancer/treatment/cam/patient/acupuncture-pdq

National Cancer Institute (NCI). (2016c). *Late effects of treatment for childhood cancer (PDQ)—Patient version*. Retrieved from http://www.cancer.gov/types/childhood-cancers/late-effects-pdq

National Cancer Institute (NCI). (2016d). *Topics in integrative, alternative and complementary therapies (PDQ)—Health professional version*. Retrieved from http://www.cancer.gov/about-cancer/treatment/cam/hp/cam-topics-pdq

National Cancer Institute (NCI). (2016e). *PDQ cancer information summaries: Screening/detection (testing for cancer)*. Retrieved from http://www.cancer.gov/publications/pdq/information-summaries/screening

National Cancer Institute (NCI). (2016f). *Male breast cancer treatment PDQ—Patient version*. Retrieved from http://www.cancer.gov/types/breast/patient/male-breast-treatment-pdq

National Center for Complementary and Integrative Health (NCCIH). (2014a). *Cancer in depth—What science says about the safety and side effects of complementary health approaches for cancer*. Retrieved from https://nccih.nih.gov/health/cancer/camcancer.htm?nav=gsa#science

National Center for Complementary and Integrative Health (NCCIH). (2014b). *Cancer in depth—Use of complimentary health approaches for cancer*. Retrieved from https://nccih.nih.gov/health/cancer/camcancer.htm#use

National Center for Complementary and Integrative Health (NCCIH). (2014c). *Cancer in depth—What the science says about the effectiveness of complimentary health approaches for cancer*. Retrieved from https://nccih.nih.gov/health/cancer/camcancer.htm?nav=gsa.#hed1

National Center for Complementary and Integrative Health (NCCIH). (2015). *Vitamin E supplements increase incidence of prostate cancer, according to SELECT study*. Retrieved from http://nccih.nih.gov/research/results/spotlight/101111.htm?nav=gsa

National Center for Complementary and Integrative Health (NCCIH). (2016). *Antioxidants: In depth*. Retrieved from https://nccih.nih.gov/health/antioxidants/introduction.htm

National Heart, Lung, and Blood Institute (NHLBI). (2012a). *Explore aplastic anemia*. Retrieved from http://www.nhlbi.nih.gov/health/health-topics/topics/aplastic/treatment

National Heart, Lung, and Blood Institute (NHLBI). (2012b). *What are thalassemias?* Retrieved from http://www.nhlbi.nih.gov/health/health-topics/topics/thalassemia

National Heart, Lung, and Blood Institute (NHLBI). (2012c). *What causes aplastic anemia?* Retrieved from http://www.nhlbi.nih.gov/health/health-topics/topics/aplastic/causes

National Heart, Lung, and Blood Institute (NHLBI). (2016). *What is sickle cell disease?* Retrieved from https://www.nhlbi.nih.gov/health/health-topics/topics/sca

NIH U.S. National Library of Medicine. (2017). *What is gene therapy? Genetics Home Reference*. Retrieved from https://ghr.nlm.nih.gov/primer/therapy/genetherapy.

Nelson, R. (2014). Unlikely to benefit, older adults still get cancer screening. *Medscape*. Retrieved from http://www.medscape.com/viewarticle/830092

Newman, T. (2016). Psychoneuroimmunology: Laugh and be well. *Medical News Today*. Retrieved from http://www.medicalnewstoday.com/articles/305921.php

News Medical. (2016). *Older adults experience greater survival rates after lung cancer surgery*. Retrieved from http://www.news-medical.net/

news/20160505/Older-adults-experience-greater-survival-rates-after-lung-cancer-surgery.aspx

Oancea, S. C., Brinkman, T. M., Ness, K. K., Krull, K. R., Smith, W. A., Srivastava, D. K., … Gurney, J. G. (2014). Emotional distress among adult survivors of childhood cancer. *Journal of Cancer Survivorship, 8*(2), 293–303. Retrieved from http://link.springer.com/article/10.1007/s11764-013-0336-0

Oncology Nursing Society (ONS). (2016a). *Ensuring healthcare workers safety when handling hazardous drugs.* Retrieved from https://www.ons.org/sites/default/files/Safe%20Handling.pdf

Oncology Nursing Society (ONS). (2016b). *Oncology Nursing Society position paper on access to quality cancer care.* Retrieved from http://www.ons.org/advocacy-policy/Positions/policy/access

Osborn, K. S., Wraa, C. E., Watson, A., & Holleran, R. S. (2013). *Medical-surgical nursing: Preparation for practice* (2nd ed.). Upper Saddle River, NJ: Pearson.

Papamichael, D., Audisio, R. A., Glimelius, B., de Gramont, A., Glynne-Jones, R., Haller, D., … Aapro, M. (2015). Treatment of colorectal cancer in older patients: International Society of Geriatric Oncology (SIOG) consensus recommendations 2013. *Annals of Oncology, 26*(3), 463–476. doi:10.1093/annonc/mdu253

Paul, D. A. (2013). Perinatal anemia. *Merck manual professional version.* Retrieved from http://www.merckmanuals.com/professional/pediatrics/perinatal-hematologic-disorders/perinatal-anemia#v1087415

Phillips, R. M. (2012). The mystery of leukemia in older adults. *Nursing Made Incredibly Easy, 10*(1), 39–45. Retrieved from http://www.nursingcenter.com/cearticle?tid=1284528

Porth, C., & Grossman, G. (2013). *Pathophysiology: Concepts of altered health states* (9th ed.). Philadelphia, PA: Lippincott Williams & Wilkins.

Powers, J. M., & Buchanan, G. R. (2014). Iron deficiency anemia in toddlers to teens: How to manage when prevention fails. *Contemporary Pediatrics.* Retrieved from http://contemporarypediatrics.modernmedicine.com/contemporary-pediatrics/content/tags/american-academy-pediatrics/iron-deficiency-anemia-toddlers-tee?page=full

Rampton, D., Folkerson, J., Fishbane, S., Hedenus, M., Howladt, S., Locatelli, F., … Weiss, G. (2014). Hypersensitivity reactions to intravenous iron: Guidance for risk minimization and management. *Haematologica, 99*(11), 1671–1676. doi:10.3324/haematol.2014.111492

Roberts, A. (2016). *The complete human body: The definitive visual guide* (2nd ed.). New York, NY: DK Publishing.

Rozzi, A., Lanzetta, G., & Salerno, M. (2014). Treatment of cancer pain: New drugs and same old questions? *Journal of Palliative Care Medicine, 4*(2). Retrieved from http://dx.doi.org/10.4172.2165-7386.1000e129

Salim, S. (2014). Oxidative stress and psychological disorders [Abstract]. *Current Neuropharmacology, 12*(2), 140–147. Retrieved from http://www.ncbi.nlm.nih.gov/pmc/articles/PMC3964745/pdf/CN-12-140.pdf

Shanafelt, T. (2013). Treatment of older patients with chronic lymphocytic leukemia: Key questions and current answers. *Hematology, 2013*(1), 158–167. Retrieved from http://asheducationbook.hematologylibrary.org/content/2013/1/158.full

Santacroce, L. (2015). Paraneoplastic syndromes. *Medscape.* Retrieved from http://emedicine.medscape.com/article/280744-overview#a3

Schapira, L., & Muss, H. (2013). Issues in treating older women with breast cancer. *Medscape.* Retrieved from http://www.medscape.com/viewarticle/781526_2

Selye, H. (1984). *The stress of life* (2nd ed. rev.). New York, NY: McGraw-Hill.

Shalkow, J. (2014). Pediatric colorectal tumors. *Medscape.* Retrieved from http://emedicine.medscape.com/article/993170-overview

Simon, S. (2012a). *Study links marijuana use to testicular cancer.* Retrieved from the American Cancer Society website: https://www.cancer.org/latest-news/study-links-marijuana-use-to-testicular-cancer.html

Simon, S. (2012b). *Can cancer be treated during pregnancy?* Retrieved from the American Cancer Society website: https://www.cancer.org/latest-news/cancer-can-be-treated-during-pregnancy.html

Simon, S. (2015c). *The ugly truth about indoor tanning.* Retrieved from the American Cancer Society website: http://www.cancer.org/cancer/news/features/the-ugly-truth-about-indoor-tanning

Skin Cancer Foundation. (n.d.a). *Sunburn.* Retrieved from http://www.skincancer.org/prevention/sunburn

Skin Cancer Foundation. (n.d.b). *Prevention guidelines.* Retrieved from http://www.skincancer.org/prevention

Smith, Y. (2015a). Thalassemia prevalence. *News Medical.* Retrieved from http://www.news-medical.net/health/Thalassemia-Prevalence.aspx

Smith, Y. (2015b). Thalassemia treatment. *News Medical.* Retrieved from http://www.news-medical.net/health/Thalassemia-Treatment.aspx

Stabler, S. P. (2013). Vitamin B_{12} deficiency. *New England Journal of Medicine, 368,* 149–160.

Steinberg, G. D. (2017). Overview of BCG immunotherapy. *Medscape.* Retrieved from http://emedicine.medscape.com/article/1950803-overview

Sung, L., Aplenc, R., Alonzo, T. A., Gerbing, R., & Gamis, A. S. (2012). Predictors and short-term outcomes of hyperleukocytosis in children with acute myeloid leukemia: A report from the Children's Oncology Group. *Haematologica, 97*(11), 1770–1773.

Surveillance, Epidemiology, and End Results Program (SEER). (2017). Cancer stat facts: Cancer of any site. *National Cancer Institute.* Retrieved from https://seer.cancer.gov/statfacts/html/all.html

University of Maryland Medical Center (UMMC). (2013a). *Anemia—Causes.* Retrieved from http://umm.edu/health/medical/reports/articles/anemia

University of Maryland Medical Center (UMMC). (2013b). *Sickle cell disease.* Retrieved from http://umm.edu/health/medical/reports/articles/sickle-cell-disease

University of Michigan Cancer Center. (2014). *Prostate cancer in younger men— More frequent and more aggressive?* Retrieved from http://www.mcancer.org/news/archive/prostate-cancer-young-men-more-frequent-and-more-aggressive

University of Texas MD Anderson Cancer Center. (2016a). *Cancer screening guidelines.* Retrieved from https://www.mdanderson.org/prevention-screening/get-screened.html

University of Texas MD Anderson Cancer Center. (2016b). *Childhood melanoma.* Retrieved from https://www.mdanderson.org/cancer-types/childhood-melanoma.html

U.S. Department of Health and Human Services. (2014). *Healthy people 2020: Cancer.* Retrieved from http://www.healthypeople.gov/2020/topics-objectives/topic/cancer

Vanneman, M., & Dranoff, G. (2012). Combining immunotherapy and targeted therapies in cancer treatment. *Nature Reviews: Cancer,* 12:232–251.

Volkow, N. D., Baler, R. D., Compton, W. M., & Weiss, S. R. (2014). Adverse effects of marijuana use. *New England Journal of Medicine, 370*(23), 2219–2227. doi:10.1056/NEJMra1402309

Welch, H. G., & Robertson, D. J. (2016). Colorectal cancer on the decline: Why screening can't explain it all. *New England Journal of Medicine, 374,* 1605–1607. doi:10.1056/NEJMp1600448

Wilson, B. A., Shannon, M. T., & Shields, K. M. (2016). *Pearson nurse's drug guide.* Upper Saddle River, NJ: Pearson.

Module 3
Comfort

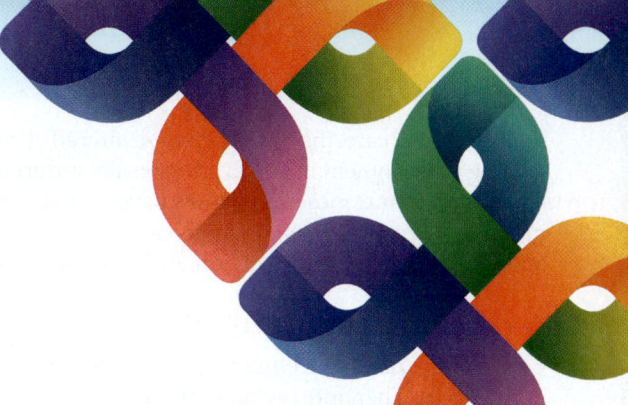

Module Outline and Learning Outcomes

The Concept of Comfort

Normal Presentation of Comfort
3.1 Analyze the physiology of comfort in the body.

Alterations to Comfort
3.2 Differentiate alterations in comfort.

Concepts Related to Comfort
3.3 Outline the relationship between comfort and other concepts.

Health Promotion
3.4 Explain the promotion of comfort.

Nursing Assessment
3.5 Differentiate common assessment procedures and tests used to examine comfort.

Independent Interventions
3.6 Analyze independent interventions nurses can implement for patients with alterations in comfort.

Collaborative Therapies
3.7 Summarize collaborative therapies used by interprofessional teams for patients with alterations in comfort.

Lifespan Considerations
3.8 Differentiate considerations related to the assessment and care of patients with alterations in comfort throughout the lifespan.

Comfort Exemplars

Exemplar 3.A Acute and Chronic Pain
3.A Analyze acute and chronic pain as they relate to comfort.

Exemplar 3.B End-of-Life Care
3.B Analyze end-of-life care as it relates to comfort.

Exemplar 3.C Fatigue
3.C Analyze fatigue as it relates to comfort.

Exemplar 3.D Fibromyalgia
3.D Analyze fibromyalgia as it relates to comfort.

Exemplar 3.E Sleep–Rest Disorders
3.E Analyze sleep–rest disorders as they relate to comfort.

» The Concept of Comfort

Concept Key Terms

Acute fatigue, **149**	Chronic pain, **149**	Imagery, **156**	Pain, **148**	Sleep apnea, **149**
Acute pain, **149**	Comfort, **147**	Insomnia, **149**	Parasomnia, **149**	Sleep hygiene, **154**
Breathing exercises, **156**	End-of-life care, **149**	Movement techniques, **156**	Polysomnography (PSG), **153**	Sleep loss, **149**
Chronic fatigue, **149**	Fatigue, **149**	Muscle relaxation, **156**	Restless legs syndrome (RLS), **149**	Tender points, **149**
Chronic fatigue syndrome, **149**	Fibromyalgia, **149**	Narcolepsy, **149**		

omfort in healthcare is defined by Katharine Kolcaba's Comfort Theory as "the immediate state of being strengthened by having the needs for relief, ease, and transcendence addressed in the four contexts of holistic human experience: physical, psychospiritual, sociocultural, and environmental." In this definition, patients achieve *relief* when their needs are met, *ease* from a state of contentment, and *transcendence*, which allows patients to rise above their problems. In addition, *physical* comfort is related to bodily sensations and homeostatic mechanisms, *psychospiritual* comfort is related to

the individual awareness of oneself and one's relationship to a higher being, *sociocultural* comfort is related to family and societal relationships, and *environmental* comfort is related to the external surroundings (Kolcaba, Tilton, & Drouin, 2006).

Emotional and physical comfort can relate to anxiety, fears, and relationships with hospital staff as well as overall comfort of the environment. Parlour and colleagues (2014) found that an environment that promoted person-centeredness increased patient satisfaction. According to Brownie and Nancarrow (2013), improvements in patient care were realized with care that was person-centered. Providing a healing environment in which stressors are reduced through adequate comfort measures allows patients to maintain normal vital signs, receive adequate sleep–rest and nutrition, and feel a sense of control over their healing process.

Normal Presentation

Comfort is a relative feeling based on expectations and past experiences. Therefore, a "normal" level of comfort may be different for every patient. However, there are some elements of comfort that are common to all individuals.

Physiology Review

An individual experiences comfort when each level of Maslow's hierarchy of needs is fulfilled (**Figure 3–1** ⟫). Once the most basic physiologic needs of oxygen, shelter, food, water, and sleep are met, the individual feels safe and free from anxiety, fear, and pain. The individual who experiences true comfort senses love and belonging from family and friends. For individuals seeking healthcare, comfort also includes participating in a healthy nurse–patient relationship. In addition, individuals experience comfort in the areas of self-esteem and self-actualization by giving and receiving respect, feeling confident, and accepting reality.

Because comfort is subjective, the nurse should aim to understand what is "comfortable" or "normal" for the patient. Some patients have difficulty articulating this or have such a high tolerance for discomfort that it is difficult to determine an appropriate baseline. For example, a woman who has worked for the Peace Corps in Africa for several years may be unperturbed by an extra day's stay in the hospital, but an Olympic athlete might find the extra day of confinement and rest intolerable.

Signs of comfort can sometimes be determined from patient assessment for sympathetic nervous system responses such as heart and respiratory rate, blood pressure, and body and skin temperature. However, "normal" vital signs are not always reliable indicators of comfort. A number of other criteria are also usually associated with a patient's comfort level, such as the presence or absence of pain; degree of sleep and rest; balance of nutrition and fluids; and sensory perceptions of heat, cold, odor, and noise. Body language, such as grimacing or guarding, is also an important indicator of comfort level. Age-related issues for assessing pain are covered in the Lifespan Considerations section.

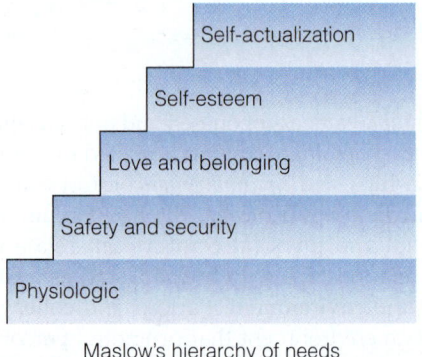

Maslow's hierarchy of needs

Figure 3–1 ⟫ Maslow's hierarchy of needs.

Focus on Diversity and Culture
Pain

Regardless of the degree of pain experienced, multiple studies have shown that Black and Hispanic populations are less likely to receive adequate treatment for pain and are more likely than white populations to receive nonopioid analgesics rather than opioid analgesics (Meghani, Byun, & Gallagher, 2012). This applies to children as well as adults (Goyal et al., 2015). All patients have the right to receive adequate comfort care using pharmacologic and nonpharmacologic methods. When caring for patients, nurses must be culturally competent in dealing with the patients' needs. Cultural competency begins with nurses identifying and acknowledging their own biases when conducting patient assessment. Assessment of the patients' use of traditional remedies, such as poultices or herbs, as well as pharmacologic treatments is essential (Spector, 2017). Factors that influence expression of pain, regardless of culture, include the patient's level of trust with the healthcare provider, the patient's ability to cope with pain, and the patient's skill at reporting pain and discomfort (Andrews & Boyle, 2016).

Sources: Data from Andrews, J. (2013). *Culture, ethnic, and religious reference manual for health care providers.* Kernersville, NC: Jamarda Resources; Carteret, M. (2011). *Cultural aspects of pain management. Dimensions of culture: Cross cultural communications for health care professionals.* Retrieved from: http://www.dimensionsofculture.com/2010/11/cultural-aspects-of-pain-management/; Giger, J. N. (2012). *Transcultural nursing: Assessment and intervention* (6th ed.). St. Louis, MO: Elsevier; Spector, R. E. (2017). Cultural Diversity in Health and Illness (9th ed.). New York, NY: Pearson Education.

Alterations to Comfort

Comfort is a desirable outcome from nursing care, yet very few people meet the criteria for comfort stated by Kolcaba (1995). What aspects of discomfort are most commonly encountered by nurses? This chapter focuses on five common sources of discomfort: pain, end-of-life care, fatigue, fibromyalgia, and sleep–rest disorders.

Alterations and Manifestations

Pain, fatigue, and sleep–rest disorders are basic alterations in comfort caused by disease, illness, or injury; fibromyalgia is a classic example of a disease characterized by these three types of discomfort. Discomfort is also a reality at the end of life, and nurses must provide comfort for patients and families during end-of-life care. These alterations in comfort will be summarized here and explored in depth in the exemplar sections (also see the Alterations and Therapies feature).

Pain

The International Association for the Study of Pain (2014) has defined **pain** as "an unpleasant sensory and emotional experience associated with actual or potential tissue damage, or described in terms of such damage." Because pain is a perceptual and emotional experience, patients can provide only a subjective description of their pain. Most individuals view pain as a negative, but pain can also be positive in that it provides a warning of injury, illness, and disease. Although it has sometimes been referred to as the fifth vital sign, pain assessment is indicated by patient history and clinical presentation and priorities for patient treatment are individualized to each patient's needs.

Pain may be described in terms of location, duration, intensity, quality, and etiology. *Duration* establishes the difference between acute and chronic pain. **Acute pain** is defined as pain that lasts only through the expected recovery period, which is usually 30 days to 6 months. Acute pain typically has a sudden onset related to injury, surgery, or illness. In contrast, **chronic pain** lasts longer than 6 months and persists beyond the expected period of healing.

According to The Joint Commission (2016), patients in pain have the right to receive adequate assessment and management of their pain. In conjunction with this patient right, The Joint Commission has provided pain management standards that require healthcare organizations to recognize the right to assessment and management of pain and educate both patients and providers about pain and pain management (2016).

End-of-Life Care

End-of-life care is nursing care given to a patient who is near death as well as care provided to the patient's family. Although frequently associated with older adults, end-of-life care may be needed by patients of all ages. The National Cancer Institute (2012) states that "end-of-life care provides physical, mental, and emotional comfort, as well as social support, to people who are living with and dying of advanced illness." Those who care for family members in the end stages of life have identified that pain management is one of the most common stressors (Syrjala et al., 2014). Nurses contribute to the quality of this care, particularly as it pertains to education, use of evidence-based practices, patient advocacy, and evaluation of care. Nursing interventions associated with end-of-life care include helping patients perform daily activities such as bathing and toileting; relieving pain and providing comfort; providing information and emotional and spiritual support to the patient and family; and helping the family make ethical decisions about life-sustaining interventions.

Fatigue

Fatigue is a lack of energy and motivation. Although drowsiness can be associated with fatigue, the two terms are not interchangeable. Fatigue is often accompanied by apathy. Like pain, fatigue can be characterized as acute or chronic. **Acute fatigue** manifests as normal tiredness associated with a single event, such as a poor night's sleep, a stressful experience, or an acute infection. Symptoms of acute fatigue usually begin quickly and are also resolved quickly by adequate sleep–rest and resolution of the underlying cause of fatigue.

In contrast, **chronic fatigue**, is more intense and lasts longer than acute fatigue, and may be exacerbated by physical and mental activity (Centers for Disease Control and Prevention [CDC], 2015a). Chronic fatigue is often caused by long-term illnesses or medications used to treat chronic disease. Chronic fatigue that lasts more than 6 months and is accompanied by muscle and joint pain, headaches, and sleep and memory problems may be **chronic fatigue syndrome** (CFS) (CDC, 2015a). Children may also have CFS. Chronic fatigue syndrome is usually diagnosed after all other causes of fatigue have been ruled out and if the fatigue does not diminish with adequate sleep–rest.

Fibromyalgia

Fibromyalgia is a disease that is often associated with other rheumatoid conditions and is characterized by widespread musculoskeletal pain, fatigue, sleep disturbances, and psychologic distress. Additional symptoms can include irritable bowel syndrome, numbness and tingling in extremities, headaches, and cognitive problems (CDC, 2015b). Its existence is often determined by a test of the tenderness at 18 **tender points** located throughout the neck, shoulder, chest, hip, knee, and elbow regions. Because no cure for fibromyalgia exists, treatment is symptomatic. According to the National Fibromyalgia Association (2016), an estimated 10 million Americans and a total of 3%–6% of the world's population have fibromyalgia.

Sleep and Rest Disorders

According to Maslow, sleep is one of the basic physiologic needs of life. Sleep is characterized by a state of unconsciousness and a decreased responsiveness to external stimuli. During sleep, the human body enters a phase of restoration, as manifested by enhanced wound healing, a boost in the immune system, anabolic metabolism, and energy conservation. In infants and children, sleep is also necessary for brain development.

Despite knowing the physiologic importance of sleep, approximately 40% of adults do not get enough sleep and unintentionally fall asleep during the day (National Heart, Lung and Blood Institute [NHLBI], 2015). Sleep deprivation hinders daily functioning and adversely affects health, contributing to diseases such as diabetes, cardiovascular disease, and depression. Sleep deprivation is also linked to an increased risk for motor vehicle crashes (NHLBI, 2015). The prevalence of sleep disorders and sleep deprivation caused the Institute of Medicine (IOM, 2006) to make several recommendations, including increasing the awareness of the general public about the problems caused by sleep loss and sleep disturbances and educating and training healthcare professionals about sleep medicine.

The Institute of Medicine's (IOM, 2006) report focused on the most common sleep disturbances, including sleep loss, sleep-disordered breathing, insomnia, narcolepsy, parasomnias, restless leg syndrome, and several others. **Sleep loss** refers to a duration of sleep shorter than the recommended 7–8 hours per night for adults. Sleep-disordered breathing, or **sleep apnea**, occurs when an individual experiences breathing pauses during sleep. **Insomnia** is characterized by difficulty falling asleep or maintaining sleep or by a short sleep duration even with adequate time spent attempting to sleep. **Narcolepsy** is a condition in which the individual experiences excessive daytime sleepiness even with adequate nighttime sleep, resulting in sleep attacks and cataplexy. **Parasomnias** are unpleasant or undesirable behaviors (e.g., sleepwalking, sleep terrors) that occur at any point during sleep. **Restless legs syndrome (RLS)** is a neurologic disorder that results in an irresistible urge to move the legs or other body parts, often resulting in impaired sleep habits.

Genetic Considerations and Nonmodifiable Risk Factors

Genetics plays a major role in an individual's susceptibility to a number of diseases associated with discomfort. For example, cancer, amyotrophic lateral sclerosis (ALS), Marfan syndrome, and sickle cell disease are related to genetic

Alterations and Therapies
Comfort

ALTERATION	DESCRIPTION/ DEFINITION	MANIFESTATIONS	INTERVENTIONS AND THERAPIES
Acute pain	Pain of varying severity, location, and etiology that lasts fewer than 6 months	▪ Elevated blood pressure ▪ Increased heart rate ▪ Nausea and vomiting ▪ Sweating ▪ Rapid/shallow respirations ▪ Anxiety ▪ Decreased function in activities of daily living	***Pharmacologic pain management:*** ▪ Opioid analgesics ▪ Nonsteroidal anti-inflammatory drugs (NSAIDs) ▪ Nonopioid analgesics ***Nonpharmacologic therapy:*** ▪ Massage ▪ Diversionary therapies (music, involvement in hobbies, aroma therapy) ▪ Application of heat and cold
Chronic pain	Pain of varying severity, location, and etiology that lasts 6 months or more (even if intermittent)	▪ Depression ▪ Irritability ▪ Impaired mobility and/or activity ▪ Sleep disturbance	***Pharmacologic pain management:*** ▪ Nonopioid analgesics ▪ Antidepressants ▪ NSAIDs ▪ Muscle relaxants ▪ Opioid analgesics ***Nonpharmacologic therapy:*** ▪ Guided imagery ▪ Massage ▪ Nerve stimulation units ▪ Chiropractic interventions ▪ Physical therapy ▪ Relaxation techniques ▪ Positioning
End-of-life care	Care that takes place when death is imminent	▪ Loss of muscle tone ▪ Slowing of circulation ▪ Change in respirations ▪ Sensory impairments ▪ Impaired metabolic processes	▪ Palliative or aggressive care as chosen by patient and family ▪ Maintenance of comfort ▪ Maintenance of hygiene ▪ Psychosocial support for patient and family
Fatigue	Lack of energy or motivation with or without drowsiness	▪ Tiredness ▪ Depression ▪ Anxiety ▪ Irritability ▪ Decreased cognition	***Pharmacologic therapy:*** ▪ Sleeping aids ▪ Stimulants ▪ Antidepressants ▪ Pain management ***Nonpharmacologic therapy:*** ▪ Improved sleep hygiene ▪ Nutritional supplements ▪ Relaxation techniques ▪ Complementary health approaches
Fibromyalgia	Widespread muscular and joint pain	▪ Tenderness in the neck, spine, shoulders, and hips ▪ Muscle spasm or stiffness ▪ Chronic fatigue ▪ Sleep disturbances	▪ Warm compresses or heat packs ▪ Massage ▪ Stretching exercises ▪ Fibromyalgia drugs ▪ Good sleep hygiene
Sleep–rest disorders	The inability to fall asleep or stay asleep, or a sleep disturbance that causes lack of adequate rest	▪ Sleep loss ▪ Insomnia ▪ Narcolepsy ▪ Sleep apnea ▪ Parasomnias	▪ Improved sleep hygiene ▪ Pharmacologic therapies ▪ Relaxation techniques ▪ Assistive breathing devices (e.g., continuous positive airway pressure [CPAP])

abnormalities. In addition, some genetic mutations directly affect an individual's ability to perceive pain. For example, certain mutations of the *SCN9A* gene are associated with an increased risk for chronic pain disorders such as paroxysmal extreme pain disorder, inherited erythromelalgia (a disease that causes intense burning sensations in the hands and/or feet), and fibromyalgia (Goldberg et al., 2012; Vargas-Alarcon et al., 2012). In contrast, other forms of *SCN9A* mutation cause congenital insensitivity to pain (National Institutes of Health, 2013). Genetic mutations can also cause sleep disturbances, depression, and anxiety. Genetic mutations are associated with both narcolepsy and fatal familial insomnia (National Center for Advancing Translational Sciences [NCATS], 2014). Multiple psychiatric disorders, including autism, anxiety, panic disorder, and other mood disorders, are believed to be genetic in origin (Cross-Disorder Group of the Psychiatric Genomics Consortium, 2013).

Case Study » Part 1

April Daves is a 34-year-old woman who was in a severe motor vehicle crash 6 months ago. All of her injuries have healed, but when she continues to have chronic pain in several of her joints and muscles, her primary care physician refers her to an orthopedic specialist. As the nurse at the orthopedic clinic, you are responsible for obtaining Ms. Daves's medical history and making the initial assessment. You learn that Ms. Daves broke her left fibula near the knee, dislocated her left shoulder, and sustained whiplash. She reports almost constant burning pain and stiffness in her left knee, shoulder, and neck, but sometimes she also feels pain in her right knee and in her hips. She figures it is just "sympathy pain," but the combined pain makes movement difficult. She rates her current pain at a 5 on a scale of 0–10, but if she has to move around a lot, it increases to a 7. Her vital signs are temperature 97.2°F oral; pulse 86 bpm; respirations 20/min; and BP 146/82 mmHg. Ms. Daves reports she has been trying to manage her pain with acetaminophen and ibuprofen. However, they aren't always effective, and she often has trouble sleeping at night because of the pain. Her boss is starting to notice a drop in productivity at work because she has trouble staying awake when sitting at her desk.

After the orthopedic specialist reviews Ms. Daves's health history and performs a physical assessment, he sends her for x-rays on her left knee and shoulder. Although the x-rays do not show any obvious abnormalities, he suspects Ms. Daves may have developed osteoarthritis. The orthopedic specialist asks you to schedule Ms. Daves for a CT scan of her left knee and left shoulder. He prescribes meloxicam (Mobic) as an analgesic and recommends that the patient return for a follow-up visit after her CT scans are completed.

Clinical Reasoning Questions Level I

1. During her patient history, what alterations in comfort does Ms. Daves reveal?
2. Based on Ms. Daves's vital signs, what assumptions can you make about her level of discomfort?
3. Why might Ms. Daves's other joints be feeling "sympathy pain," as she describes it?

Clinical Reasoning Questions Level II

4. What nonpharmacologic therapies could you suggest for pain management? Fatigue?
5. What possible conditions could Ms. Daves have other than osteoarthritis?
6. What additional assessments may be beneficial for Ms. Daves's care?

Concepts Related to Comfort

Promotion of comfort is an integral part of nursing care. The exemplars included in this module explore several common manifestations of discomfort, including pain, fatigue, and sleep–rest disorders. However, alterations in comfort are not limited to these specific manifestations. The concept of comfort is interrelated with numerous other physiologic and psychosocial concepts. For example, one of the classic symptoms of inflammation is pain. Therefore, nurses can offer comfort to patients with inflammation by administering pain medications as ordered and providing nonpharmacologic comfort measures such as cold therapy. Patients with pain, especially joint pain, lower back pain, or trauma pain, often experience decreased mobility. Nursing interventions for these patients may include ambulation assistance and hygiene care. Impaired tissue integrity is a common cause of discomfort and can also lead to more serious complications such as infection. Comfort measures may include assessing the patient for infection, providing hygiene care for the wound, and assisting with repositioning for immobile patients.

Promotion of comfort includes both physical and psychosocial wellness. Individuals experiencing grief over a lost loved one or lost personal health may need emotional comfort in the form of therapeutic communication or referrals to support groups. Comfort care is also closely tied to ethical issues for many patients, such as individuals with drug addiction who need opioid treatment for severe pain or the family deciding about withdrawing or withholding life-sustaining treatments for a patient at the end of life. The Concepts Related to Comfort feature links some, but not all, of the concepts related to comfort. They are presented in alphabetical order.

Health Promotion

Promotion of comfort includes teaching patients about lifestyle changes that can help decrease their symptoms of pain, depression, or fatigue. Three basic independent categories of teaching include sleep hygiene, psychosocial well-being, and relaxation therapy. These are discussed further in the Independent Interventions section.

Personal preferences, lifestyle habits, and culture are all factors in the development of chronic diseases and can contribute to alterations in comfort. Only the patient can change behaviors that increase the risk of discomfort related to these factors. However, nurses provide essential patient education that can encourage patients to change their behaviors to decrease the risk of developing a chronic disease or experiencing an acute illness or injury.

Lifestyle habits that predispose individuals to chronic health alterations, such as poor nutrition, smoking, excessive alcohol consumption, and poor sleep hygiene, all increase an individual's risk for experiencing illness and discomfort. Providing information to patients regarding healthy diets in combination with practices of good sleep hygiene can help prevent the development of many chronic diseases that lead to symptoms of discomfort.

Smoking, alcohol consumption, and illicit drug use can also lead to alterations in comfort. Because nicotine, alcohol, and illicit drugs are addictive, quitting drug use is associated with withdrawal symptoms. Emotional withdrawal symptoms

Concepts Related to
Comfort

CONCEPT	RELATIONSHIP TO COMFORT	NURSING IMPLICATIONS
Cognition	Altered cognition changes the patient's perception of comfort and the ability to notify the caregiver that the patient is in pain.	■ Utilize family members to assist with identification of behaviors that might indicate pain in their loved one. ■ Visual or numeric pain rating scales can be used.
Ethics	Physicians may be reluctant to prescribe opioids based on history of addiction or personal biases.	■ Advocate for the provision of adequate pain relief to all patients; provide culturally sensitive care; offer nonpharmacologic comfort measures to all patients.
Inflammation	Inflammation leads to pain.	■ Assess pain in patients with inflammation; provide pharmacologic treatments as ordered. ■ Offer comfort measures such as ice or heat; promote adequate sleep and rest.
Mobility	Decreased mobility is often caused by pain, injury, or disease.	■ Assist with ambulation and activities of daily living; encourage adequate sleep and rest. ■ Offer pharmacologic treatments as ordered.
Oxygenation	Pain increases respiratory rate.	■ Monitor respiratory status ■ Utilize pharmacologic and nonpharmacologic strategies to improve comfort level.
Safety	Having a safe environment can help provide comfort for patients and their families.	■ Ensure that safety measures are in place (e.g., call light, bed in low position) ■ Reassure patients that you will be making rounds on a routine basis to check on their status and their comfort level.
Tissue Integrity	Decreased tissue integrity means increased risk for pain, inflammation, and infection.	■ Assess for skin breakdown; promote mobility. ■ Assist with repositioning as needed; monitor for signs and symptoms of infection.

include anxiety, irritability, insomnia, and depression. Physical withdrawal symptoms include sweating, palpitations, nausea, and difficulty breathing. Nurses should assess patients for risk of substance abuse and provide education related to prevention, especially related to using healthy coping mechanisms and obtaining appropriate treatment for existing mental health disorders such as depression.

Occupations that require heavy lifting, long hours, or repetitive movement can result in an increased risk of injury and fatigue (**Figure 3–2 》**). Participation in physical activities such as team sports or extreme sports also increases susceptibility to injury and consequent comfort alterations. Nurses should teach proper body mechanics for lifting, urge use of good ergonomics for those who work at computers all day, and encourage athletes to use appropriate safety gear.

Nursing Assessment

The nursing assessment should explore not only the patient's level of discomfort but also the degree to which discomfort is affecting the patient's daily life. Some patients may not even realize the extent to which discomfort is affecting their lifestyle and overall well-being.

Observation and Patient Interview

Every assessment should begin with observing the patient at first encounter. Look for obvious signs of discomfort such as

altered mobility, grimacing, or guarding (Stites, 2013). The nurse should then proceed with reviewing the patient's health history, followed by interviewing the patient regarding any complaints related to discomfort, including pain, fatigue, anxiety, or depression. If the patient reports an alteration in comfort, the interview and physical examination should be further targeted to address the specific areas of

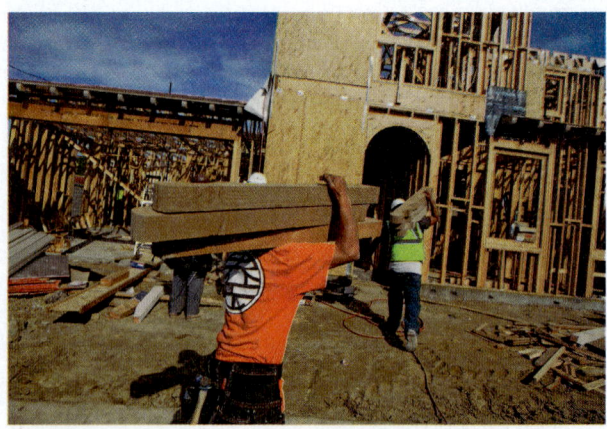

Source: Bloomberg/Getty Images.

Figure 3–2 》 Occupations that require heavy lifting, such as construction work, can result in an increased risk of injury and fatigue.

concern. Questions that can be asked during the patient interview include:

Current Problem

- When did your discomfort start?
- How would you describe your discomfort?
- On a scale of 0–10, with 0 meaning no pain and 10 meaning the worst pain you can imagine, how would you rate your current pain intensity?
- Which activities make the discomfort better or worse?
- How long have you had this discomfort?
- How does this discomfort affect your activities of daily living?
- What do you do to alleviate your discomfort?
- Are you currently taking any medications to alleviate your discomfort?
- Does your discomfort affect your sleep pattern or your mood?
- Does your discomfort affect your appetite?
- Does eating or drinking make your discomfort better or worse?
- Do you feel that your discomfort is related to another disease or condition?
- Do you feel sad frequently?
- Do you have trouble motivating yourself to participate in daily activities?
- Have you had thoughts of suicide?
- Have you had any changes in daily habits that increased your symptoms of discomfort?

Patient History

- Have you had this discomfort in the past?
- How often does this symptom of discomfort occur?
- Have you taken medications for this problem in the past?
- Have you had past experiences that affect the way you view this discomfort?

Lifestyle

- Do you drink alcohol? If so, how much? Do you feel this contributes to your symptoms?
- Do you smoke? If so, how much? Do you feel this contributes to your symptoms?
- Do you exercise? Is your condition related to your participation in physical activity?
- Describe your average daily food and drink intake. Do you feel that your diet contributes to your symptoms?
- What is your occupation? Do you feel this contributes to your symptoms of pain and discomfort?

Physical Examination

Physical examination of the patient who has discomfort is guided by the age, ethnicity, and severity of discomfort. Observations associated with discomfort include posturing, abnormal gait, facial grimaces, verbal complaints, and guarding. The interview should specifically focus on the onset, cause, length, relieving factors, and factors that create more discomfort for the

patient. Using the physical assessment, then, the nurse assesses the patient to validate the information the nurse has already obtained so that a plan of care can be developed.

Diagnostic Tests

Diagnostic tests may be ordered to determine if there is an underlying biological cause of the patient's discomfort, as well as to gain additional assessment data. X-rays may be useful for determining whether a physical injury is present. Blood tests may also be conducted. For example, a white blood cell (WBC) count may be useful in identifying infection, and hemoglobin and hematocrit measurements can be used to determine if fatigue is caused by iron-deficiency anemia. Abnormal urine analysis may indicate illness or malnutrition. A **polysomnography (PSG)**, or sleep study, is often used to diagnose sleep disorders.

Case Study >> Part 2

Two days before April Daves is scheduled to return to her orthopedic physician, she is awakened by severe pain. Because she is unable to get out of bed, Ms. Daves calls 911. She is transferred to the hospital by ambulance. As her emergency department (ED) nurse, you assess Ms. Daves. Her only complaint is pain, which she rates as a 9 on a scale of 1 to 10. Ms. Daves reports she has been taking her NSAIDs as prescribed. Her heart rate, respiratory rate, and blood pressure are all slightly elevated. Ms. Daves further reports that the pain has prevented her from sleeping more than 3–4 hours each night. Aside from her motor vehicle crash, Ms. Daves has no history of illness or trauma. You report your findings to the ED physician.

After reviewing Ms. Daves's medical history and performing a physical assessment, the ED physician orders a complete blood count (CBC) and a urinalysis, the results of which are normal. He also obtains the results of Ms. Daves's CT scans, which are normal. The ED physician suspects that Ms. Daves may have fibromyalgia. Using the 2010 fibromyalgia criteria, the ED physician determines that Ms. Daves's widespread pain index is 8, and her symptom severity scale score is 9. The ED physician diagnoses Ms. Daves with fibromyalgia and prescribes milnacipran (Savella). He instructs her to visit her primary care physician for follow up as soon as possible.

Clinical Reasoning Questions Level I
1. What causes fibromyalgia?
2. What nursing interventions can you implement immediately to help relieve Ms. Daves's pain?
3. For the patient with fibromyalgia, what findings would you expect to be revealed by the CBC and urinalysis?

Clinical Reasoning Questions Level II
4. Refer to Exemplar 3.D on Fibromyalgia. Based on your knowledge of Ms. Daves's clinical signs and symptoms, what somatic symptoms is she likely to be experiencing?
5. Why did the physician choose milnacipran instead of duloxetine or pregabalin for Ms. Daves's fibromyalgia?
6. What patient teaching topics should you review with Ms. Daves before her discharge?

Independent Interventions

For the patient experiencing alterations in comfort, initial interventions are directed at identifying the source of the discomfort. While pain relief for the patient with physical pain is a priority, masking the pain through analgesic administration can make identifying the underlying cause much

Comfort Assessment

ASSESSMENT/ METHOD	NORMAL FINDINGS	ABNORMAL FINDINGS	LIFESPAN OR DEVELOPMENTAL CONSIDERATIONS
Interview/Patient History			
Patient description of symptoms Pain scale Depression assessment	Patient should report no signs or symptoms of discomfort.	▪ Patient reports mild to severe pain. ▪ Patient reports disrupted sleep patterns. ▪ Patient reports or displays signs of nausea or vomiting. ▪ Patient reports lack of appetite or ravenous appetite. ▪ Patient reports lack of motivation, feelings of despair, or feelings of anxiety.	▪ Look for nonverbal signs of discomfort such as crying, shielding an injured area, lack of affect, or withdrawal in nonverbal children and patients with mental impairments. ▪ Signs of depression and anxiety in children may indicate abuse, and assessment of the child in the absence of the parent(s) may be warranted. ▪ Gastrointestinal (GI) discomfort can be a physiologic response to disease or it can be a side effect of medication. Check patient history for current medications and known drug allergies. ▪ Depression and anxiety can be primary or secondary conditions. Be sure to assess patients who have depression or anxiety for symptoms of chronic conditions.
Physical Assessment			
Vital signs Visual inspection	Patient should have normal vital signs and no obvious external injuries or infections.	▪ Severe pain may be accompanied by sympathetic nervous system findings such as increased heart rate, sweating, and nausea. ▪ Patient appears depressed, nervous, or confused.	▪ Children may be fearful of physical assessment. To promote comfort, allow the child to sit on the parent's or guardian's lap during the assessment. ▪ When conducting physical assessment, take into consideration biophysical changes that occur in older adults.

more difficult. For this reason, especially until the cause of the patient's discomfort is identified, interventions to promote comfort may focus on nonpharmacologic measures. These include simple interventions such as applying heat or cold as appropriate and providing distractions (e.g., reading material, music, crossword puzzles, humor); patient teaching related to sleep hygiene, repatterned thinking, and relaxation therapy; and collaborative interventions including complementary health approaches.

Sleep Hygiene

Discomfort associated with illness or injury often causes sleep disturbances. Therefore, education should include teaching about the importance of sleep hygiene. **Sleep hygiene** refers to a variety of sleep practices that help individuals attain good-quality sleep at night so they can be alert during the day. Good sleep hygiene includes maintaining a regular sleep and awake pattern, performing bedtime rituals, providing a restful environment, and promoting comfort and relaxation. If the patient takes medications to promote sleep, teaching should include the

appropriate use of pharmacologic agents and their side effects. More details on good sleep hygiene are provided in the Patient Teaching feature.

For patients in the hospital, sleep disturbances may be related to the hospital environment rather than physical or emotional discomfort. Whenever possible, schedule procedures, medications, meals, and other activities around patients' normal sleep schedules. Nurses should assess patients' individual circadian rhythm, because patients who normally go to sleep late may develop sleep disturbances if forced to attempt sleep before their normal bedtime. In contrast, patients who are early risers may prefer to have physical therapy first thing in the morning.

Once a sleep schedule is identified, bedtime rituals may include assisting the patient with hygiene activities such as toileting and a hand and face wash, offering a warm beverage or massage, and retrieving fresh pillows or extra blankets. Reduce environmental distractions such as noise and external light sources, as outlined in **Box 3–1 »**. If good sleep hygiene still does not produce a restful night of sleep, it may be appropriate to request an order for a sedative/hypnotic to help the patient sleep.

Patient Teaching

Sleep Hygiene

Fatigue is often the result of inadequate sleep. Nurses should promote and teach good sleep hygiene to all patients with fatigue, sleep–rest disorders, and acute and chronic illnesses that could cause fatigue. Good sleep hygiene includes:

- Establishing a regular bedtime and wake-up time to enhance biological rhythms
- Practicing bedtime rituals that are calming, such as reading, taking a bath, praying, and listening to music
- Maintaining a restful environment that is free of distractions (e.g., lights and noise), is a comfortable temperature, and has appropriate ventilation
- Avoiding dealing with office work or family problems before bedtime
- Wearing loose-fitting sleepwear
- Sleeping on a comfortable mattress and pillows, and using clean and dry linens

- Sleeping in a position that aids in muscle relaxation and supports injured areas
- Scheduling medications to promote sleep (i.e., taking medications that cause alertness in the morning and medications that cause drowsiness at night)
- Avoiding naps during the day
- Avoiding stimulants such as caffeine and alcohol, especially in the evening; also avoiding heavy meals late in the evening
- Using the bed for sleep and sexual activity, not other activities such as watching TV
- Exercising in the morning or afternoon rather than the evening
- Using sleeping medications only as a last resort
- Taking analgesics before bedtime to ease aches and pains.

Psychosocial Well-Being

Patients both in and out of a hospital environment who experience alterations in comfort will benefit from the promotion of optimal psychosocial well-being. Laughter helps relieve pain, reduces stress, boosts immunity, improves mood, and strengthens relationships. A positive attitude can also help ease distress (Wooten, 2013). It can decrease depression and stress, increase cardiovascular health, and help patients develop essential coping skills. Patients should be encouraged to participate in enjoyable activities such as gardening, crafting, reading, or playing games; interacting with a pet; listening to or performing music; spending time in nature; and volunteering to help others (Wooten, 2013). Patients who expend energy on enjoyable activities and on helping others tend to focus less on their own discomfort and instead develop a sense of self-worth and purpose in life.

The patient's psychosocial well-being may also be enhanced through interacting with family and friends. Family and friends can help lift the burden of an acute or chronic condition by assisting with activities of daily living and by helping patients feel they are not alone. They can encourage the patient to persist in following healthcare suggestions and pharmacologic therapies and to seek medical help when needed. A supportive group of family and friends is important not only for patients, but also for caregivers, especially when they are caring for someone with a debilitating disease or at the end of life.

Box 3–1

Minimizing Environmental Stimuli in the Hospital Setting

Noise

- Place patients in single-bed rooms when possible instead of multiple-bed rooms. If a patient must be in a semiprivate or larger room, close the curtains between patients.
- Keep the patient's door closed to reduce hallway noise.
- Reduce excess noise during specified quiet hours (e.g., turn off televisions, lower the ringtone of telephones, reduce the volume or discontinue use of the paging system).
- Minimize noise from staff interactions and minimize use of the public address system.
- Perform only essential activities in the patient's room during sleeping hours.

Light

- Adjust window coverings to block outside lights at night and to allow natural light during the day.
- At night, use a night-light or turn on bathroom lights instead of overhead lighting.
- When entering a patient's darkened room, use a flashlight instead of turning on the room lights.

Surroundings

- Pleasant surroundings and color schemes can produce a calming environment, producing comfort and improved outcomes.
- Decrease use of bold, abstract picture hangings, as this can enhance agitation and inability to sleep.

Sources: Based on Berman, A., Snyder, S. J., & Frandsen, G. (2016). Sleep. In *Kozier and Erb's fundamentals of nursing: Concepts, process, and practice* (10th ed., p. 1078, Box 45–5). New York, NY: Pearson Education; Thompson, D. R., Hamilton, D. K., Cadenhead, C. D., Swoboda, S. M., Schwindel, S. M., Anderson, D. C., . . . & Petersen, C. (2012). Guidelines for intensive care unit design. *Critical Care Medicine 40*(5). doi:10.1097/CCM.0b013e3182413bb2; Massachusetts General Hospital. (n.d.). *Addressing quietness on units: Best practice implementation guide.* Retrieved from http://www.mghpcs.org/eed_portal/Documents/PatExp/addressing-quietness.pdf

Focus on Integrative Health
Relaxation Therapies

Breathing exercises are used to slow the breathing rate by focusing on taking regular and deep breaths from the diaphragm. This process increases oxygen intake and therefore increases oxygen delivery throughout the body.

Muscle relaxation involves tightening and then relaxing each muscle group, usually spending between 5–15 seconds in the contraction phase and up to 30 seconds in the relaxation phase. It is most beneficial to relax muscles progressively either from head to toe or from toe to head. This technique helps patients recognize the difference between tension and relaxation so that they learn to consciously relax muscles that become tense due to stress or discomfort (NCCIH, 2013).

Imagery, or guided imagery, involves focusing on pleasant images, such as a beach or garden, to replace negative images, such as pain and darkness. Imagery can be directed by the individual or by a practitioner who uses storytelling or descriptions to guide the patient into a more relaxed state. Soothing music or nature sounds may be used to enhance the imagery. Imagery creates a connection between the mind and the body and enhances the patient's coping skills. In addition, guided imagery can counteract panic, anger, pain, depression, and insomnia and can decrease recovery time (Cleveland Clinic, 2016). Imagery can also be used as a nursing intervention to help alleviate pain and depression in patients with fibromyalgia (Onieva-Zafra, García, & del Valle, 2015).

Movement techniques include yoga and tai chi. Yoga postures stretch specific muscle groups, and tai chi is a series of slow movements that follow a set pattern. Tai chi has been shown to improve strength and balance, and reduce pain (Fransen et al., 2015) and may improve cognitive function (Zheng et al., 2015).

Relaxation Therapy

Relaxation techniques reduce stress by slowing the heart and respiratory rates, lowering blood pressure, and increasing blood flow to major muscles. Relaxation techniques can also be used to induce sleep, reduce pain, and calm emotions (NCCIH, 2013).

In addition, relaxation techniques are beneficial in the treatment of several symptoms of discomfort, including anxiety, depression, headache, and pain. Some of the major benefits of relaxation therapy are that the techniques can be learned with very little training, they are relatively inexpensive to practice, and they can be performed without the help of a healthcare provider (NCCIH, 2013).

The four major categories of relaxation techniques are breathing, muscle relaxation, imagery, and movement (see the Focus on Integrative Health feature). Other forms of relaxation include massage, acupuncture, meditation, and biofeedback. Relaxation techniques can be combined for maximum effectiveness. For example, imagery is often combined with deep breathing exercises. The choice of relaxation techniques depends on the patient's individual preferences.

Collaborative Therapies

Collaborative therapies for patients experiencing discomfort include both pharmacologic and nonpharmacologic interventions. Pharmacologic interventions involve the administration of medications, examples of which are listed in the Medications features. Nonpharmacologic therapies may be complementary health approaches, such as acupuncture, herbal supplements, or biofield therapy (see the Focus on Integrative Health feature). Other collaborative therapies may include use of exercise programs, physical therapy, and pain clinics (Wilsey et al., 2013). Use of aquatic therapy has more recently been found to aid recovery in patients with fibromyalgia, chronic low back pain, and osteoarthritis (Mooventhan & Nivethitha, 2014; Rewald et al., 2015). The use of eHealth and mHealth, electronic health and mobile health applications, such as texting, mobile apps, and social media for pain assessment and management offer promise to patients with chronic pain (Palermo & Jamison, 2015). Use of medical marijuana has become more popular in states where it has been legalized for helping patients with neuropathic pain.

Focus on Integrative Health
Use of Biofield Therapies for Patients with Cancer

Individuals with cancer have many symptoms as a result of their disease process and treatments. Traditional care is focused on symptom management and the acute needs of patients, often without taking a holistic approach to meet patients' needs. Some recent evidence supports the use of biofield therapies to help patients deal with the painful experiences. Biofield therapy is a complementary health approach used to balance the energy fields in the body that are disrupted by psychologic and physiologic imbalances. The three types of biofield therapy include Reiki, therapeutic touch, and healing touch. Gonella (2014) conducted a review of the literature related to biofield therapy and found that there is not enough rigorous evidence to have identifiable outcomes attributable to the use of biofield therapies. However, their use for patients has not shown side effects or interactions with medications or other treatments. Anderson and Taylor (2012) found similar results, identifying that though there is clinical efficacy in the use of these modalities, additional research needs to be done.

Medications
Pain

CLASSIFICATION AND DRUG EXAMPLES	MECHANISMS OF ACTION	NURSING CONSIDERATIONS
Nonopioids *Drug examples:* Acetaminophen	Act in the central nervous system (CNS) to increase the pain threshold. *May also be used as:* ■ Antipyretic	■ Acetaminophen causes hepatotoxicity; intake should be carefully monitored, especially in malnourished individuals or individuals who have consumed alcohol. ■ Acetaminophen is included in many drug mixtures, so be sure the patient is not accidentally overdosing. ■ Assess hepatic function for chronic acetaminophen users or in suspected overdose.
NSAIDs *Drug examples:* Aspirin Ibuprofen Naproxen Diclofenac Indomethacin Celecoxib	Block prostaglandin synthesis by inhibiting COX-1 and/or COX-2. *May also be used as:* ■ Antiplatelet ■ Anti-inflammatory ■ Antipyretic	■ Aspirin should be used cautiously in children and should never be given to children with chicken pox or flu-like symptoms. ■ NSAIDs may interfere with clinical tests such as pregnancy tests, urine tests, and liver function tests. ■ Patients should be monitored for GI distress and allergic reactions. ■ NSAIDs should be used cautiously in patients receiving anticoagulant therapy.
Opioids Full agonist Mixed agonist/antagonist Partial agonist *Drug examples:* Morphine Fentanyl Oxycodone Methadone	Activate opioid receptors to decrease the perception of pain. *May also be used for:* ■ Treatment of dyspnea related to acute left ventricular failure (morphine) ■ Treatment of pulmonary edema and pain of myocardial infarction (morphine) ■ Narcotics withdrawal symptoms (methadone)	■ Monitor patients for respiratory depression. ■ If opioid reversal is indicated, administer incremental doses of the reversal agent (naloxone) until symptoms of overdose are resolved. Opioid reversal may produce withdrawal symptoms. ■ Constipation is one of the most common side effects of opioid use; provide stool softeners or laxatives as needed.

Source: Data from Adams, M. P., Holland, L. N., & Urban, C. (2017). *Pharmacology for nurses: A pathophysiologic approach* (5th ed.). Hoboken, NJ: Pearson Education.

Medications
Sleep

CLASSIFICATION AND DRUG EXAMPLES	MECHANISMS OF ACTION	NURSING CONSIDERATIONS
Hypnotics/Sedatives Benzodiazepines Nonbenzodiazepines *Drug examples:* Temazepam Zolpidem Eszopiclone	Produces CNS depression by acting on the limbic, thalamic, and hypothalamic regions of the CNS (benzodiazepines). Interacts with GABA receptor (nonbenzodiazepines).	■ Monitor older adults for paradoxic reaction. ■ Do not use in patients who are depressed, suicidal, or pregnant. ■ Tolerance and addiction may result from benzodiazepine use; slowly taper dosage when discontinuing therapy; drugs should not be used for more than 4–6 months.

Source: Data from Adams, M. P., Holland, L. N., & Urban, C. (2017). *Pharmacology for nurses: A pathophysiologic approach* (5th ed.). Hoboken, NJ: Pearson Education.

Case Study » Part 3

Ms. Daves has been visiting her primary care provider as recommended for follow-up care. Six months after beginning treatment with milnacipran (Savella), Ms. Daves returns for a regular checkup. As you review her chart, you note that Ms. Daves's primary care physician confirmed the ED physician's diagnoses of fibromyalgia. Upon assessment, Ms. Daves's vital signs are normal, and her pain intensity is a 3 on a scale of 0–10. She also reports that she is sleeping better at night, although she occasionally has insomnia even though the pain is manageable. When you ask how Savella is working for her, she says that it has helped her pain and stiffness, but her mouth has been really dry since she started taking it, and she sometimes has slight nausea.

Clinical Reasoning Questions Level I

1. What suggestions can you give Ms. Daves to help decrease her dry mouth and nausea?
2. What further assessment should be included to help determine the cause of Ms. Daves's insomnia?
3. Can you suggest other therapies to help decrease Ms. Daves's pain even further?

Clinical Reasoning Questions Level II

4. What nursing interventions can you implement to help prevent future flare-ups of Ms. Daves's fibromyalgia?
5. What information should you give Ms. Daves about milnacipran (Savella) and drug–drug interactions?
6. What coping techniques would be useful for Ms. Daves as she deals with fibromyalgia?

Lifespan Considerations

Age and developmental stage affect the ability to accurately describe discomfort. Patients' culture also plays a major role in how they perceive discomfort, as some cultures expect flamboyant descriptions of discomfort while other cultures value stoicism. Cultural differences in expressions of pain are further discussed in the Focus on Diversity and Culture feature in the exemplar on Acute and Chronic Pain.

Discomfort in Infants and Toddlers

Infants verbalize discomfort by crying. Ask the parents for descriptions of the infant's manifestations of pain, including suspected location and how the pain influences eating, sleeping, and behavior. Discomfort in otherwise healthy infants may be related to milk components. Bottle-fed infants may need a specialized formula. For breastfed infants, the mother's diet may need to be modified.

Infants and toddlers should be comforted by being held or rocked, and murmuring soothing words, or rubbing/patting the torso or extremities. Many pain medications have no dosing instructions for children under 2 years old. Warn parents to follow physician's orders for all medications given to infants and toddlers.

Discomfort in Children

When caring for a child, involve the child in describing any discomfort, but also ask the parent(s) or guardian about the child's behaviors related to discomfort. Before performing any procedures or tests, explain the procedure to the child to help decrease anxiety. When possible, it may also help to demonstrate the procedure on the parent before performing the procedure on the child. If you must perform a painful procedure such as an injection, engage the parent in the child's care by asking the parent to offer comfort or distraction. For older school-age children, drawings of anatomic body parts and simple explanation may help decrease anxiety.

Depending on age and personality, children may be comforted by being held, hugging, holding hands, or receiving a treat like a sticker or small toy.

Discomfort in Adolescents

Adolescents may respond to treatment and comfort better if you interact with them as adults rather than as children. Some adolescents may reject any offer of comfort.

Discomfort in Adults

Comfort is a subjective experience, so listen carefully when patients describe any feelings of discomfort, and care for the patients accordingly. Adults diagnosed with a chronic or fatal disease may find comfort in knowledge. Take the time to describe the disease and what to expect for tests, medications, and other interventions, and to answer any questions they have.

Discomfort in Pregnant Women

Pregnant women, especially first-time mothers, may be very anxious about their health and the health of their baby. Take time to explain the expected growth and development of the fetus and expected maternal changes. Answer any questions.

Provide tips about self-care, physical activity, and sleeping positions that will help ease discomfort. Encourage adequate nutrition, hydration, and sleep–rest.

Discomfort in Older Adults

Older adults are more likely to have chronic conditions such as diabetes, chronic pain, heart disease, cancer, and arthritis. Provide a safe and comfortable environment for regular appointments, and foster a healthy nurse–patient relationship to promote comfort.

Explain procedures and medications at each visit; some older adult patients have memory deficits. Provide written instructions and explanations. Provide assistance with movement as needed, especially for patients with chronic pain or arthritis.

Discomfort at the End of Life

When caring for patients at the end of life, make sure to provide adequate pain relief with pharmacologic agents as ordered. Nurses can promote psychosocial comfort by offering to arrange a visit from a spiritual leader and/or loved ones. Facilitate referrals for grief counseling for the family and other loved ones, and make certain to honor the patient's and family's decisions about end-of-life care.

REVIEW The Concept of Comfort

RELATE Link the Concepts

Linking the concept of comfort with the concept of oxygenation:

1. What assessments would you make to help you differentiate increased respirations from pain versus increased respirations from a respiratory tract infection?

2. What comfort measures would you implement for a patient in labor who is breathing rapidly from the pain associated with childbirth?

Linking the concept of comfort with the concept of elimination:

3. How can you help patients with "embarrassing" symptoms such as bowel incontinence feel more comfortable talking about their condition?

4. Describe comfort measures for a patient who requires catheterization for treatment of urinary retention.

Linking the concept of comfort with the concept of trauma:

5. Explain the psychosocial considerations related to promoting comfort during the care and assessment of a rape victim.

6. When assessing a child who is believed to have been abused, what comfort measures can be used to reduce the child's anxiety and promote trust?

READY Go to Volume 3: Clinical Nursing Skills

- SKILL 3.1   Pain in Newborn, Infant, Child, or Adult: Assessing
- SKILL 3.2   Pain Relief: Back Massage
- SKILL 3.3   Pain Relief: Complementary Health Approaches
- SKILL 3.6   Sleep Promotion: Assisting

- SKILL 3.7   Cooling Blanket: Applying
- SKILL 3.8   Dry Cold: Applying
- SKILL 3.9   Dry Heat: Applying
- SKILL 3.10   Moist Pack and Tepid Sponge: Applying
- SKILL 3.12   Sitz Bath: Assisting
- SKILL 3.13   Physiologic Needs of the Dying Patient: Managing
- SKILL 3.14   Postmortem Care: Providing

REFER Go to Pearson MyLab Nursing and eText

- Additional review materials

REFLECT Apply Your Knowledge

You are caring for a 4-year-old boy who is 3 days post appendectomy via laparoscopy. He spiked a fever on day 2, so he remained hospitalized for longer than he and his family anticipated. The hand-off you receive from the nurse going off duty is that he has been resistant to move during the previous few days and wants to be in his mother's lap most of the time. Using a visual pain scale, he tells you that his pain level is at a 4. This is higher than was reported to you. You find that he has some guarding of his abdomen when you assess him. The mother tells you he does not like the oral pain medication, so he has not had anything for pain for a while. You check the physician's prescriptions and administer a safe dose of IV Tylenol.

1. What assessments, in addition to the assessment of pain, would be important to make in this child?

2. What additional information would you want to review in the child's chart as you begin to care for him?

» Exemplar 3.A
Acute and Chronic Pain

Exemplar Learning Outcomes

3.A Analyze acute and chronic pain as it relates to comfort.

- Describe the pathophysiology of acute and chronic pain.
- Describe the etiology of acute and chronic pain.
- Compare the risk factors and prevention of acute and chronic pain.
- Identify the clinical manifestations of acute and chronic pain.
- Summarize diagnostic tests and therapies used by interprofessional teams in the collaborative care of an individual with acute and chronic pain.
- Differentiate care of patients with acute and chronic pain across the lifespan.
- Apply the nursing process in providing culturally competent care to an individual with acute and chronic pain.

Exemplar Key Terms

Acute pain, *162*
Breakthrough pain, *164*
Central pain, *164*
Chronic pain, *162*
Co-analgesic, *167*
End-of-dose medication failure, *164*
Gate control theory, *162*
Idiopathic pain, *164*
Incident pain, *164*
Narcotics, *169*
Nerve block, *173*
Neuropathic pain, *162*
Nociceptive pain, *162*
Nociceptors, *161*
Opioids, *169*
Pain, *160*
Pain threshold, *175*
Pain tolerance, *175*
Phantom pain, *164*
Psychogenic pain, *164*
Referred pain, *162*
Sensitization, *175*
Somatic pain, *162*
Visceral pain, *162*

Overview

The International Association for the Study of Pain (2014) defines **pain** as "an unpleasant sensory and emotional experience associated with actual or potential tissue damage, or described in terms of such damage." This definition has several implications for nurses. First, pain is both a physical (sensory) experience and an emotional experience. As a physical experience, the degree of pain a patient feels depends both on the magnitude of stimuli and on the ability of the individual to transmit neuronal pain signals. As an emotional experience, the degree of pain a patient feels depends on the patient's mental state; for example, depression makes pain seem more severe, whereas laughter may appear to decrease pain. Second, pain is a result of actual or potential tissue damage. Therefore, pain can result from tissue damage that has already happened, such as a fractured bone, or as a warning that tissue damage may occur, such as when touching a hot surface. Third, pain can be described by the patient (Berman et al., 2016). This concept is consistent with McCaffery's (1968) classic definition of pain, which states that "pain is whatever the experiencing person says it is, existing whenever he says it does."

Each patient's description of pain depends on that individual's perception of that pain. However, some patients will not describe their pain unless asked, which is why a thorough pain assessment is vital to nursing care.

SAFETY ALERT The inability of a patient to verbalize pain does not necessarily reflect an absence of pain.

Describing Pain

Pain can be described in terms of location, intensity, quality, and duration. Duration was discussed previously, under "The Concept of Comfort," which detailed the difference between acute pain and chronic pain. The other three descriptors of pain are discussed in this section. Medically, pain can also be described based on its etiology, discussed later in the exemplar.

Location

A description of where the pain is located may give a primary indication of the patient's underlying problem. For example, lower back pain may indicate a bulging or herniated disc. Following surgery or traumatic injury, reports of pain in areas other than at the affected site should be thoroughly explored. For example, chest pain after a total joint replacement may indicate a blood clot and should be assessed and treated immediately. Pain may also radiate to other body regions, such as lower back pain that extends to the legs, or it may be referred based on nerve pathways. For example, jaw pain may actually be cardiac in origin.

Intensity

Pain intensity is often described as mild, moderate, or severe. Pain can also be rated on visual analog scales, such as the Wong-Baker FACES Pain Rating Scale, which is especially useful for young or illiterate patients (**Figure 3–3 »**). A numeric scale from 1 to 10, where 1 indicates no pain and 10 indicates the worst possible pain, can be useful in adults experiencing pain. According to the classic study by Serlin and colleagues (1995), mild pain correlates with a rating of 1–4, moderate pain correlates with a rating of 5–6, and severe pain correlates with a rating of 7–10. The intensity of the pain score is often consistent with the degree to which pain interferes with functioning.

Quality

The quality of pain can be expressed with common descriptors. A patient with sharp pain may say it feels like

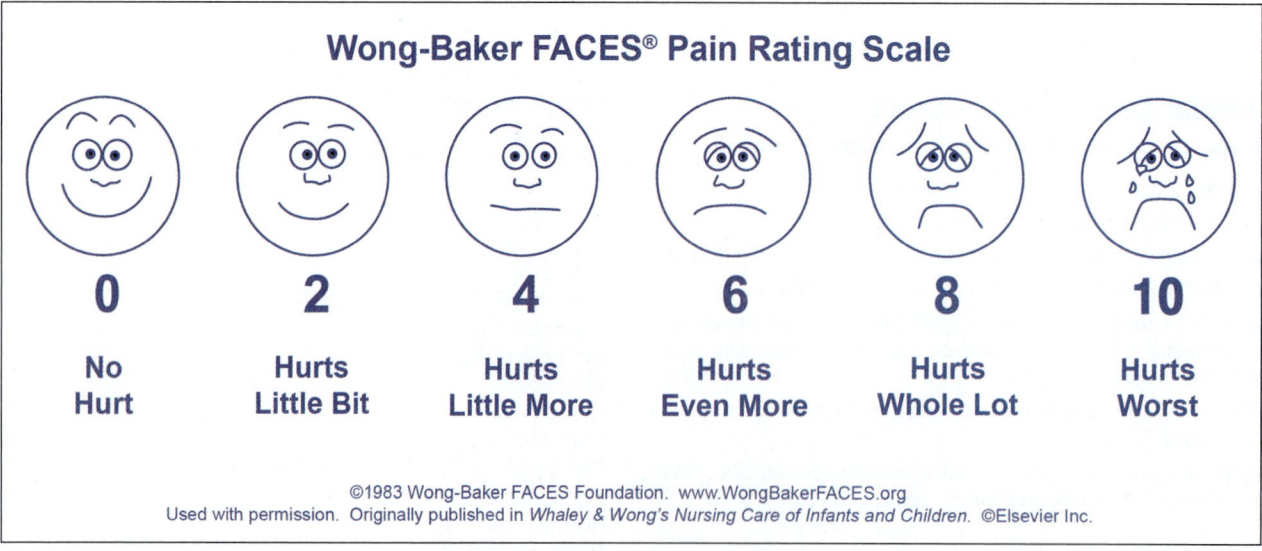

Wong-Baker FACES® Pain Rating Scale

0	2	4	6	8	10
No Hurt	Hurts Little Bit	Hurts Little More	Hurts Even More	Hurts Whole Lot	Hurts Worst

©1983 Wong-Baker FACES Foundation. www.WongBakerFACES.org
Used with permission. Originally published in *Whaley & Wong's Nursing Care of Infants and Children*. ©Elsevier Inc.

Source: © 1983 Wong-Baker FACES Foundation. www.WongBakerFACES.org. Used with permission. Originally published in *Whaley & Wong's Nursing Care of Infants and Children*. © Elsevier Inc.

Figure 3–3 » The Wong–Baker FACES Rating Scale.

being stabbed, and a patient with burning pain may say it feels like being on fire. Some descriptions of pain provide clues to whether the pain is superficial (e.g., itchy, tingling, cold) or deep (e.g., cramping, aching, dull). Other descriptors include *tender, sensitive, shooting, numb, radiating, throbbing,* and *heavy.* Descriptions of pain quality vary, depending on each patient's pain perception, vocabulary, personality, and culture.

Pathophysiology and Etiology

Pain is triggered by the peripheral nervous system, which lies outside the brain and spinal cord. There are two types of neurons in the peripheral nervous system: sensory and motor neurons. **Nociceptors**, or sensory receptors that respond to pain, send a signal along the sensory neurons to the spinal cord, where the signal is transmitted to the brain for interpretation. The brain then sends a signal back to the site of pain via motor neurons, causing the body to respond to the painful stimuli. This process happens so rapidly that the individual may reflexively withdraw from the painful stimuli even before becoming aware of the pain.

Nociceptors (**Figure 3–4** ≫) are specialized pain receptors that are present on all body tissues, with the exception of the brain. Skin and muscles contain many nociceptors, whereas internal organs have relatively few nociceptors.

TABLE 3–1 Types of Pain Stimuli

Category	Example
Biological	Bacteria Viruses
Mechanical	Shearing forces Fractures
Thermal	Extreme heat (burn) Extreme cold (frostbite)
Electrical	Electrical burn Electrical shock
Chemical	Cleaning solutions Tobacco smoke Acids/bases

Categories of pain stimuli include biological, mechanical, thermal, electrical, and chemical (**Table 3–1** ≫). The duration of exposure and magnitude of the stimuli determine the intensity of the pain response.

In addition to being stimulated by external factors, cellular injury can trigger the local release of biochemicals that stimulate nociceptors, including prostaglandins, serotonin, bradykinin, and hydrogen ions. These mediators act on ion channels and G protein–coupled receptors

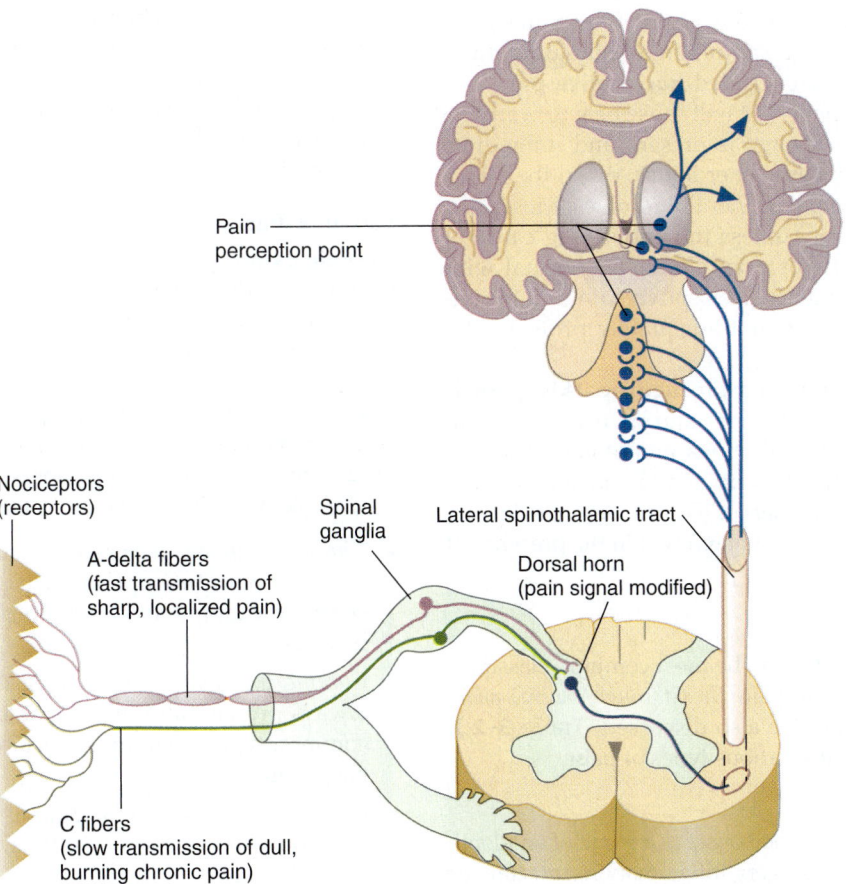

Pain perception point

Nociceptors (receptors)

A-delta fibers (fast transmission of sharp, localized pain)

Spinal ganglia

Lateral spinothalamic tract

Dorsal horn (pain signal modified)

C fibers (slow transmission of dull, burning chronic pain)

Figure 3–4 ≫ Physiology of pain perception.

to directly or indirectly initiate a pain impulse (Fein, 2012). These inflammatory mediators act to excite the pain neurons.

Pain Theories

Three theories about pain include the specificity theory, the peripheral pattern theory, and the gate control theory.

- The *specificity theory* states that pain is a specific sensation that uses sensory neurons separate from other sensations such as heat and touch.

- The *peripheral pattern theory* states that all sensory nerve fiber endings are the same, and pain is felt only when the fibers are intensely stimulated. It is the responsibility of the brain to decipher differences in signals coming from these nerve fibers.

- The **gate control theory** (Melzack & Wall, 1965) is the most widely accepted pain theory to date, although it still does not completely encompass all aspects of pain. The gate theory states that stimulation of small-diameter (pain) fibers causes gates to open, whereas stimulation of large-diameter (heat, cold, and mechanical) fibers causes gates to close. The amount of activity in the small fibers versus the large fibers controls the overall perception of pain. Factors that control the gates include physical factors, emotional factors, and behavioral factors.

Etiology

Pain can be classified based on the origin of the pain signal. Pain resulting from external stimuli on an uninjured, fully functional nervous system is called **nociceptive pain**. For example, a sunburn or paper cut will cause pain to warn the individual that tissue damage is present and immediate action is needed to prevent further injury. When the injury is treated or healed, the pain generally resolves. Most nociceptive pain is temporary unless the underlying cause of the pain is not treated. For example, an individual with osteoarthritis may experience nociceptive pain due to contact between bones that are not adequately protected by joint cartilage.

In contrast to nociceptive pain, **neuropathic pain** is caused by nerve malfunction or injuries resulting from trauma, disease, chemicals, infections, and tumors. The consequent spontaneous pain may be due to damage of either peripheral nerves or central nerves (Gilron, Baron, & Jensen, 2015). Nociceptive pain is often magnified in the presence of neuropathic pain.

Types of Pain

There are several types of pain, the most common classifications being *acute* and *chronic* pain. *Breakthrough, central, phantom,* and *psychogenic* pain are also discussed. **Table 3–2 ≫** provides a summary of the various types of pain.

Acute Pain

Acute pain usually has a sudden onset as a result of an identifiable tissue injury, such as surgery, inflammation, or traumatic injury. The duration of acute pain is short, lasting only until the injury has completely healed. Depending on the type of injury, acute pain could persist for a few minutes up to 6 months. Acute pain initiates the autonomic fight-or-flight response, causing physiologic responses such as increased breathing and heart rate, increased blood pressure, sweating, pallor, dilated pupils, and anxiety. The three primary categories of acute pain are somatic pain, visceral pain, and referred pain (International Association for the Study of Pain [IASP], 2014).

- **Somatic pain** originates from nociceptors located in the skin and musculoskeletal tissues. It is typically localized and described as being sharp. Somatic pain may be accompanied by swelling, cramping, or bleeding, and it usually responds well to mild analgesics. Examples of somatic pain are a cut finger or an overstretched muscle.

- **Visceral pain** originates from internal body organs and the linings of body cavities in the chest, abdomen, and pelvic areas. Because internal organs have relatively few nociceptors, visceral pain is usually described as dull, deep, or aching. In contrast to surface nociceptors, nociceptors on internal organs respond to inflammation, stretching, and ischemic changes rather than to lacerations or extreme temperatures. Visceral pain often manifests as radiating or referred pain, and it responds best to opioid treatment. Examples are myocardial ischemia and urinary colic resulting from renal stones.

- **Referred pain** is sensed in a region other than the site of origin. It occurs when nerve fibers that innervate the injured region and nerve fibers from other regions of the body converge at the same level in the spinal cord (**Figure 3–5 ≫**). Examples of referred pain are back pain from pancreatitis and shoulder pain from myocardial ischemia.

Chronic Pain

Chronic pain is pain that lasts beyond the expected time of healing, usually for at least 6 months; it does not always have a known cause. Pain can range from mild to severe, and autonomic responses decrease over time as the body adapts to the persistent pain impulses. However, autonomic responses may be present during severe flare-ups of pain. In addition, pain may evoke hormonal stress responses even in the absence of autonomic responses.

Chronic pain has three main categories.

- *Chronic recurrent pain* is characterized by intense episodes of pain interspersed with periods of no pain. A common example of chronic recurrent pain is migraine headaches.

- *Chronic intractable benign pain* is chronic pain that is always present, although the intensity varies. The most common type of chronic intractable benign pain is lower back pain.

- *Chronic progressive pain* is pain associated with a chronic condition that worsens over time, such as cancer or rheumatoid arthritis.

TABLE 3–2 Summary of Types of Pain

Type of Pain	Description	Examples
Acute Pain: Pain with Sudden Onset as a Result of an Identifiable Tissue Injury		
Somatic pain	▪ Originates from nociceptors in the skin and musculoskeletal tissues ▪ Typically localized and described as sharp	▪ Bursitis ▪ Muscle strain
Visceral pain	▪ Originates from internal organs and linings of body cavities ▪ Usually described as dull, deep, aching	▪ Appendicitis ▪ Gastroenteritis
Referred pain	▪ Pain that is sensed in a region other than the site of origin	▪ Sinusitis referred to upper jaw/teeth ▪ Cardiac pain referred to left arm
Chronic Pain: Pain that Lasts Beyond Expected Time of Healing, Usually for at Least 6 Months		
Chronic recurrent pain	▪ Characterized by intense episodes of pain interspersed with periods of no pain	▪ Migraines
Chronic intractable benign pain	▪ Pain that is always present ▪ Intensity varies	▪ Back injuries ▪ Fibromyalgia
Chronic progressive pain	▪ Pain associated with a chronic condition that worsens over time	▪ Osteoarthritis ▪ Fibromyalgia
Breakthrough Pain: Pain that Manifests Between Regularly Scheduled Doses of Pain Medication		
Incident pain	▪ Short-term, predictable pain associated with movement or activity	▪ Cancer pain
Idiopathic pain	▪ Pain with no known cause	▪ Typical in patients with back pain ▪ Often made worse by stress
End-of-dose pain	▪ Pain experienced at the end of one dose of medication and before the next dose	▪ Typically seen in patients who are on regular doses of pain medication, such as those with cancer
Central Pain: Pain from the CNS		
	▪ May occur shortly after injury or be delayed ▪ Described as pins and needles, aching, lacerating	▪ Spinal cord injury ▪ Multiple sclerosis
Phantom Pain: Pain Felt in an Amputated Body Part		
	▪ Described as shooting, stabbing, squeezing, throbbing, burning	▪ Amputation of limb ▪ Mastectomy
Psychogenic Pain: Pain Associated with Psychologic Factors		
	▪ Psychogenic pain is not an official medical diagnosis	▪ Headaches ▪ Stomach pain ▪ Back pain

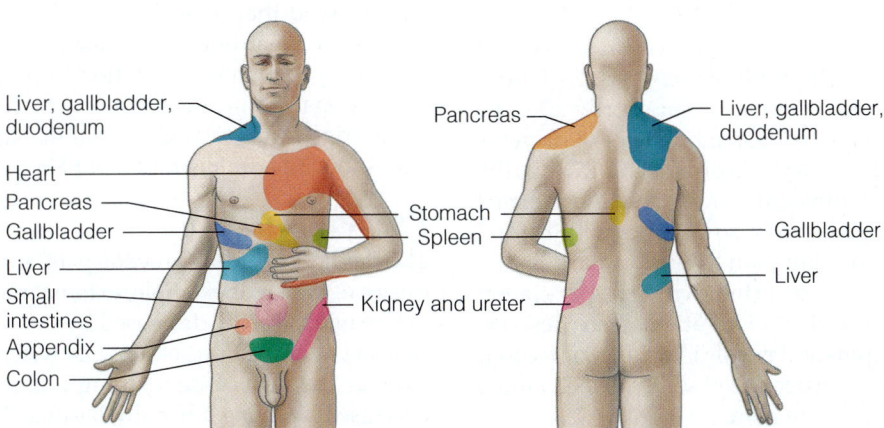

Figure 3–5 》 Referred pain is the result of the convergence of sensory nerves from certain areas of the body before they enter the brain for interpretation. For example, a toothache may be felt in the ear, pain from inflammation of the diaphragm may be felt in the shoulder, and pain from ischemia of the heart muscle (angina) may be felt in the left arm.

Many conditions cause chronic pain. For example, arthritis, which develops when cartilage in the joint disintegrates, allowing the bones to rub together, is characterized by inflammation in one or more joints. Cancer usually is associated with chronic pain as a result of the enlarging tumor, which causes nerve compression, visceral expansion, duct obstruction, or bone metastasis. The tumor may also produce biochemicals that stimulate pain, and pain often results from treatments such as chemotherapy and radiation. Neuralgia is a sharp pain that follows the path of a nerve. It is due to nerve damage and is often associated with a disease, trauma, or medication. Common examples of neuralgia include shingles and trigeminal neuralgia.

Breakthrough Pain

Breakthrough pain is defined as "a transient exacerbation of pain that occurs either spontaneously, or in relation to a specific predictable or unpredictable trigger, despite relatively stable and adequately controlled background pain" (Margarit et al., 2012). There are three main types of breakthrough pain: incident pain, idiopathic pain, and end-of-dose medication failure.

- **Incident pain** is short-term, predictable pain that accompanies a movement or activity. It can be caused by voluntary acts such as movement, involuntary acts such as coughing, or procedural events such as changing a wound dressing.

- **Idiopathic pain** is not associated with any known cause. It occurs unpredictably and is therefore harder to treat. Idiopathic pain usually lasts longer than incident pain.

- **End-of-dose medication failure** is pain experienced at the end of one dose of medication before the next dose is scheduled. Although end-of-dose medication failure has traditionally been considered breakthrough pain, some experts now believe that it is not breakthrough pain because it indicates that the background pain is not adequately controlled. End-of-dose medication failure can be prevented by shortening the time between doses or increasing the medication dose.

Central Pain

Central pain is caused by damage to nerves in the central nervous system due to stroke, multiple sclerosis, Parkinson disease, or trauma. Central pain may occur shortly after the causative injury, or it may be delayed for weeks or years (National Organization for Rare Disorders [NORD], 2015). Dysfunction of the spinothalamic tract causes abnormal temperature and pain perception, so patients with central pain often experience constant pain as well as pain paroxysms, evoked pain, or allodynia (International Association for the Study of Pain [ISAP], 2014.). Patients may describe their pain as burning, "pins and needles," aching, or lacerating. Patients may also have a decreased ability to feel normal touch as a result of the constant pain.

Phantom Pain

Phantom pain is pain felt in an amputated limb or body part. Phantom pain is usually recurring rather than constant, and patients often describe their pain sensations as shooting, stabbing, squeezing, throbbing, or burning. Some patients may feel that the amputated limb is being forced into an uncomfortable position. Phantom pain is associated with neurologic activity in portions of the brain that were once connected to the amputated body part.

Psychogenic Pain

Psychogenic pain is pain associated with psychologic factors, including mental or emotional problems, rather than physiologic factors, such as injury or disease. Although patients with psychogenic pain are often stigmatized as hypochondriacs, the pain they feel is no less real than pain caused by physical injury. Treatment for psychogenic pain should include interventions for both pain and emotional distress.

Risk Factors

Acute and chronic pain associated with a physiologic cause, such as illness or injury, are linked to a variety of internal and external factors and depend on the illness or injury that causes the pain. For example, adolescent boys who perform tricks on bicycles are at higher risk of pain associated with a fractured arm or leg than boys who ride a bicycle without performing tricks. Likewise, obese individuals are at higher risk of developing type 2 diabetes and associated complications such as diabetic neuropathy than individuals who are not obese.

Preoperative anxiety, younger age, and chronic pain are associated with severe postoperative pain. Patients who are vulnerable to stress and have an impaired cortisol response are more susceptible to persistent pain following a motor vehicle accident. Risk factors for lower back pain include a previous history of lower back pain, lifting weights, lack of exercise, emotional distress, obesity, nicotine dependence, alcohol abuse, and depressive disorders (American Academy of Orthopaedic Surgeons [AAOS], 2015). Age, gender, and genetic polymorphisms also contribute to a patient's risk of developing acute or chronic pain conditions.

In addition to risk factors that make patients more susceptible to pain, barriers exist that prevent patients from getting adequate pain relief, including barriers from the perspective of the patient, financial barriers, health infrastructure, and healthcare providers (see **Box 3–2** ⟫). Lewis and colleagues (2014) found that intensive care unit (ICU) nurses' lack of knowledge regarding pain management created a barrier to providing adequate medication to patients. Use of a small professional group discussion with ICU nurses increased knowledge levels related to pain management and reduced biases toward administration of pain medication.

Prevention

The methods used to prevent pain are as numerous as the causes of pain. For example, external risk factors, such as the risk of injury, can be decreased by safety precautions such as wearing a seatbelt or helmet. Likewise, internal risk factors, such as the risk of developing a chronic disease, can be decreased by living a healthy lifestyle. Many patients unfortunately live without considering how their lifestyle could contribute to the development of acute or chronic diseases or injuries. Therefore, nurses are responsible for providing pain relief for patients once they are already experiencing pain.

For patients with acute or chronic pain, the best way to prevent future pain is to provide adequate pain relief through

Box 3–2
Barriers that Prevent Patients from Getting Adequate Pain Relief

Barriers from the Perspective of the Patient Include:

- Reluctance to report pain to avoid taking the treatment focus off the primary disease
- Reluctance to discuss pain because the patient fears it indicates a progression of disease
- A belief that pain is inevitable, so there is nothing that can be done
- A belief that bearing pain is admirable or beneficial
- Cultural expectations that demand they not report pain
- A desire to be seen as a "good" patient
- A fear of becoming an addict or being perceived as an addict (especially in minority populations)
- Worries about side effects associated with pain medications
- A belief that minority populations do not get treated for pain adequately even when pain is reported
- Financial barriers.

Barriers from the Perspective of the Healthcare Provider Include:

- Regulatory issues related to controlled substances (opioids)

- A delay in giving pain medication to the patient until after the diagnosis
- Prescribing only small amounts of drugs upon discharge to prevent misuse
- Inadequate knowledge about pain management
- A poor assessment of pain
- A fear of adverse effects associated with analgesics
- A fear of tolerance and/or addiction.

Barriers from the Perspective of the Healthcare Infrastructure Include:

- A strict regulatory environment that discourages physicians from prescribing controlled substances in the appropriate dosage
- Lack of availability of controlled substances
- Low priority given to cancer pain management
- Inadequate reimbursement for pain treatment.

Sources: National Cancer Institute. (2013). *Pain (PDQ®).* Retrieved from http://www.cancer.gov/cancertopics/pdq/supportivecare/pain/HealthProfessional/page1; Lewis, C. P., Corley, D. J., Lake, N., Brockopp, D., & Moe, K. (2014). Overcoming barriers to effective pain management: The use of professionally directed small group discussion. *Pain Management Nursing, 16*(2), 121–127. doi:http://dx.doi.org/10.1016/j.pmn.2014.05.002; International Association for the Study of Pain (IASP). (2009). *Barriers to cancer pain treatment.* Retrieved from http://www.iasp-pain.org/files/Content/ContentFolders/GlobalYearAgainstPain2/CancerPainFactSheets/Barriers_Final.pdf

pharmacologic and nonpharmacologic therapies. Patients with acute pain should take their pain medications as prescribed until they are completely healed. In addition, patients with chronic pain should take their pain medications on schedule, even in the absence of severe pain. Pain medications are more effective at preventing pain when taken regularly than at reducing pain that has already become severe.

Clinical Manifestations

Often, the body responds to severe, acute pain by activating the sympathetic nervous system's fight-or-flight response. The sympathetic response causes an increase in blood pressure, pulse, and respiratory rate; diaphoresis; pallor; and dilated pupils. Nurses may also recognize visible symptoms of pain such as crying, grimacing, shielding the site of injury, compensatory posturing, and slow movements. In addition, the patient may express anxiety about the condition that is causing acute pain. Some patients may not manifest physiologic or behavioral signs of pain even while experiencing moderate to severe pain, and not all patients have the same physiologic response to the same intensity of pain.

As the body adapts to pain, visible and physiologic symptoms of pain may be harder to detect. The sympathetic response returns to baseline levels unless the patient experiences breakthrough pain and some visible signs of pain, such as crying, cease. Pain fibers may become sensitized so that the intensity and perception of pain increase over time. Therefore, clinical manifestations of chronic pain may include compensatory posturing, muscle spasms or tense muscles, limited mobility, groaning during movements, and clenched teeth. Chronic pain is also often accompanied by psychosocial manifestations, such as depression, withdrawal from previously enjoyable activities, fatigue, and resignation to dealing with constant pain.

Uncontrolled pain has multiple detrimental effects on the body. Compensatory posturing can lead to muscle atrophy, neuropathies, and contractures. To make up for this weakened area, the body overuses another area, occasionally causing pain in that area as well. In addition, lack of pain control in postsurgical patients can lead to pulmonary, digestive and mobility alterations (Stasiowska et al., 2015). Other effects of uncontrolled pain include changes in appetite, sleep disruption, decreased circulating oxygen levels, and increased risk of thrombosis. If allowed to continue, uncontrolled pain will decrease the quality of life for both the patient and the patient's family.

Developmental Considerations

Pain can be manifested differently according to age, developmental level, and degree of pain. Nurses must have a fundamental knowledge of growth and development to understand how individuals at various ages respond to pain and discomfort. Likewise, interventions must be based on the developmental level of the patients. Further information regarding clinical manifestations of pain can be found in the Lifespan Considerations section.

Cultural and Personal Considerations

Cultural and personal factors that influence an individual's pain experience include ethnic and cultural values, views about the meaning of pain, environment, availability of support, and past pain experiences.

Cultural and Ethnic Influences

Patients' ethnic and cultural values play an important role in their perception and description of pain (see the Focus on Diversity and Culture feature). Patients from stoic cultures rarely vocalize pain through groans or crying, and they may avoid showing a behavioral reaction to pain. They may tolerate a higher level of pain without requesting pain relief or even mentioning their pain. In contrast, individuals from expressive cultures routinely moan or scream when faced with pain, and they expect others to care for them to help relieve the pain (Carteret, 2011). Despite the variation in verbal and behavioral responses to pain, ethnic or cultural background does not affect the pain threshold so that people of different cultures experience similar pain sensations physiologically. It is simply their response to pain that differs (Carteret, 2011).

Patients' culture also affects how they describe pain. Words may have different connotations in different cultures. For example, individuals from certain cultures may use the words *ache*, *discomfort*, or *sore* rather than *pain*, and some words may not translate correctly into the English word *pain* despite the presence of a competent translator.

Culture may also affect the methods of treatment that a patient is willing to undergo. Individuals who believe that pain is punishment or that pain builds character may refuse pain treatment. Patients from stoic cultures are likely to refuse pharmacologic treatments to avoid admitting weakness. Some patients may prefer to treat pain with herbal medicines and complementary health approaches rather than pharmacologic agents (see the Focus on Integrative Health feature).

Because of the critical role culture plays in pain expression and management, nurses must approach each patient with cultural competence. Nurses must understand their own cultural beliefs about pain, and they must put aside those beliefs to provide culturally competent care. Nurses should discuss culturally acceptable ways of treating pain with the patient and the patient's family and suggest ways in which the patient can receive pain relief within those parameters.

Focus on Integrative Health
Comfort

Culture influences response to and beliefs about pain and comfort. The National Center for Complementary and Integrative Health (NCCIH, 2016a) estimates that 59 million Americans spend money on out-of-pocket integrative therapies each year. The National Center for Complementary and Alternative Medicine (NCCAM) published a special report in 2014 that estimates that approximately 36% of adults in the United States use integrative therapies for comfort, but the numbers vary among cultural groups at the following rates (NCCAM, 2014):

- American Indian/Native Alaskan: 50.3%
- Non-Hispanic White Americans: 43.1%
- Asian Americans: 39.9%
- Black Americans: 25.5%
- Hispanic Americans: 23.7%

The 10 most common integrative therapies used by adults and children are (NCCIH, 2016a, 2016b):

Integrative Therapy	Percentage of Adults Who Use Therapy	Percentage of Children Who Use Therapy
Natural products	17.7%	3.9%
Deep breathing	12.7%	2.2%
Meditation	9.4%	1%
Chiropractic and osteopathic therapies	8.6%	2.8%
Massage	8.3%	1%
Diet-based therapies	3.6%	0.8%
Progressive relaxation	2.9%	0.5%
Guided imagery	2.2%	—
Homeopathic treatment	1.8%	1.3%
Yoga	6.1%	2.1%
Traditional healers	—	1.1%

Other integrative therapies that patients may be using or that the healthcare team can discuss with the patient in pain include:

- **Acupuncture.** A procedure that uses thin, metallic needles that penetrate the skin to stimulate specific points on the body. It is a key component of traditional Chinese medicine, a holistic healthcare approach that was started in ancient China over 2500 years ago. Many other cultures and healthcare treatments have incorporated traditional Chinese medicine in their practices, including cupping, movement therapies, and herbal therapies.
- **Acupressure.** A component of traditional Chinese medicine that uses precise finger placement and pressure on specific parts of the body.
- **Ayurveda.** One of the world's oldest medical systems, it originated in India and includes varied approaches such as herbs, massage, and specialized diets.
- **Biofeedback.** A relaxation technique that measures body functions and gives patients feedback so they can learn to control the functions, such as muscle tension.
- **Cupping.** A traditional Chinese medicine practice that involves placing heated glass cups on the body to create suction, which increases blood flow and promotes healing.
- **Hypnosis.** A therapy that uses guided relaxation, intense concentration, and focused attention to achieve a heightened state of awareness, which is sometimes called a trance.
- **Movement therapy.** Practices such as the Feldenkrais method, the Alexander technique, and Pilates are psychophysical therapies.
- **Qi gong and tai chi.** These mind and body practices involve specific postures and gentle movements with mental focus, breathing, and relaxation.

Sources: National Center for Complementary and Integrative Health. (2016). *Americans spend $30 billion a year out-of-pocket on complementary health approaches.* Retrieved from https://nccih.nih.gov/research/results/spotlight/americans-spend-billions; National Center for Complementary and Integrative Health. (2016). *The use of complementary and alternative medicine in the United States.* Retrieved from https://nccih.nih.gov/research/statistics/2007/camsurvey_fs1.htm#children; National Center for Complementary and Alternative Medicine (NCCAM). (2014). *Special report.* Retrieved from http://nccam.nih.gov/sites/nccam

The Meaning of Pain

Depending on a patient's cultural beliefs, pain can take on many meanings. For patients who have undergone surgery, pain is a sign that treatment has occurred. Mothers in labor view pain as a temporary inconvenience compared to the precious gift of a new baby. Patients who see pain positively usually have a higher tolerance of pain and are less likely to develop depression and anxiety about their pain.

In contrast, many patients, especially patients with chronic pain, view pain negatively. Unrelenting pain must be endured, leaving feelings of hopelessness, depression, and anxiety. These patients tend to view pain as something that is preventing them from enjoying life. They are more likely to depend on others to care for them and may become angry at the pain for stealing their independence. Patients who give a negative meaning to pain tend to have a lower quality of life physically, emotionally, and socially.

Patients who have strong spiritual beliefs often give a spiritual meaning to pain; pain may be viewed as punishment, a test, or a gift from God. Nurses must respect these beliefs when providing care.

Environmental and Social Support

A patient's environment can influence the perceived intensity of pain. Patients in a hospital may perceive a greater pain stimulus because of the unfamiliar environment and the numerous sources of disruption. Children can be especially frightened their first time in the hospital, and the fright can intensify pain responses. Providing a more relaxed and welcoming environment will ease anxiety and decrease patients' perception of pain.

Patients who surround themselves with a support network often experience decreased pain sensations. Individuals who have no help in dealing with pain may perceive pain as more severe, whereas individuals who have ample family and friends to provide distractions, a positive environment, and a helping hand may tolerate pain better. Family members who are tasked with caregiving responsibilities should be included in patient education about pain management.

Previous Experience with Pain

Patients' previous experiences with pain play a major role in their perception of pain. Patients who have undergone a procedure without adequate pain management tend to experience more pain during future procedures even in the presence of adequate pain control. Patients who have seen a loved one experience severe pain associated with a disease will experience more anxiety and have an exaggerated perception of pain if diagnosed with the same disease compared to patients who have no previous experience with the disease.

Patients' past experience with a treatment plan also influences how they perceive the efficacy of future similar treatments. For example, an individual with severe pain who has tried several drugs or nonpharmacologic remedies unsuccessfully is less likely to believe that new treatments will be effective in managing the pain. When assessing a patient for pain, nurses need to ask about past pain experiences and how those experiences might influence the patient's current treatment plan.

Collaboration

In order to treat pain effectively, nurses collaborate with other healthcare providers. Pharmacologic therapies are nonopioids, NSAIDs, opioids, and co-analgesics. Nonpharmacologic therapies include nerve blocks, spinal cord stimulation, physical therapy, and nutritional supplements, among others. For patients with severe chronic pain, pain clinics offer the expertise needed to discover the right combination of treatments to provide consistent pain relief.

Diagnostic Tests

While laboratory and diagnostic tests may be performed to determine the cause of pain, no laboratory tests are available to directly measure a patient's pain level. Instead, pain scales such as a faces pain scale or a numeric pain scale are available to help gauge a patient's pain level. Changes in vital signs can also be an indication of pain, although these changes are also seen with other conditions. In addition, the body releases stress hormones in response to pain, which may be detected by blood tests. The most prevalent stress hormones are cortisol and catecholamines.

Surgery

Depending upon the pain's etiology, surgery may be a viable treatment option. For example, surgical repair of a bone fracture may be the first major step toward alleviating severe pain. Recovery from surgery often brings about its own pain, but that pain is usually short-lived compared to the pain that would result from not performing the surgery. In addition, patients may cope with pain better if they know the surgery was necessary to prevent more severe pain and health risks.

For chronic pain that cannot be managed by pharmacologic or nonpharmacologic therapies, surgery may be the last resort. Disrupting pain conduction pathways using surgical procedures is permanent, so it should be used only for intractable pain, such as pain related to cancer. Surgical procedures used to relieve pain vary depending on the source and location of the pain.

Pharmacologic Therapy

Pharmacologic therapies for pain include nonopioids/nonsteroidal anti-inflammatory drugs and opioids (see **Box 3–3 》**). **Co-analgesic** drugs, or drugs that are used primarily for another purpose but also have some analgesic properties, can also be used to treat pain alone or in combination with other analgesic drugs.

World Health Organization (WHO) Three-Step Approach

The three-step approach to treating pain developed by the World Health Organization in 1986 and updated in 1996 has been and continues to be invaluable in pain management for patients (**Figure 3–6 》**). The first step involves administering a nonopioid drug (e.g., aspirin, acetaminophen) with or without a co-analgesic drug and nonpharmacologic interventions. If pain is not adequately controlled with this mild intervention, patients should advance to step 2 and receive a mild opioid (e.g., codeine) in combination with the same or new nonopioid drugs, co-analgesics, and nonpharmacologic

Box 3–3
Categories and Examples of Analgesics

Nonopioid Analgesics/NSAIDs

- Acetaminophen/paracetamol (Tylenol, many others)
- Aspirin/acetylsalicylic acid (Bayer, many others)
- Celecoxib (Celebrex)
- Choline magnesium trisalicylate (Trilisate)
- Diclofenac sodium (PENNSAID, Voltaren), diclofenac potassium (Cataflam)
- Etodolac
- Ibuprofen (Advil, Motrin)
- Indomethacin (Indocin)
- Ketorolac (Toradol)
- Meloxicam (Mobic)
- Naproxen (Naprosyn), naproxen sodium (Aleve)

Weak or Partial Opioid Analgesics

- Buprenorphine hydrochloride (Buprenex)
- Butorphanol tartrate (generic)
- Codeine (Codeine)
- Hydrocodone bitartrate (Vicodin)
- Tramadol hydrochloride (Ultram)

Mixed Opioid Analgesics

- Codeine (Tylenol No. 3, Empirin No. 3)

- Nalbuphine hydrochloride (Nubain)
- Pentazocine hydrochloride (Talwin)

Strong Opioid Analgesics

- Fentanyl citrate (Actiq, Sublimaze)
- Hydromorphone hydrochloride (Dilaudid)
- Levorphanol tartrate (Levo-Dromoran)
- Meperidine hydrochloride (Demerol)
- Methadone hydrochloride (Dolophine, Methadose)
- Morphine sulfate (Avinza, Roxanol)
- Oxycodone hydrochloride (OxyContin)
- Remifentanil hydrochloride (Ultiva)

Co-analgesics

- Antidepressants (imipramine, milnacipran, nortriptyline)
- Anticonvulsants (gabapentin, pregabalin)
- Antihypertensives (clonidine)
- Antipruritics (hydroxyzine)
- Corticosteroids (prednisone, hydrocortisone)
- Topical local anesthetics (benzocaine, lidocaine)

Source: Data from Adams, M. P., Holland, L. N., & Urban, C. (2017). *Pharmacology for nurses: A pathophysiologic approach* (5th ed.). Hoboken, NJ: Pearson Education.

therapies. If the patient is still experiencing pain, the mild opioid should be replaced with a stronger opioid (e.g., morphine) in step 3. Pain-relieving drugs should be given "by the clock" (every 3–6 hours) rather than on demand to maintain freedom from pain. According to the WHO (2016), the three-step approach to administering pain relief is relatively inexpensive and 80%–90% effective.

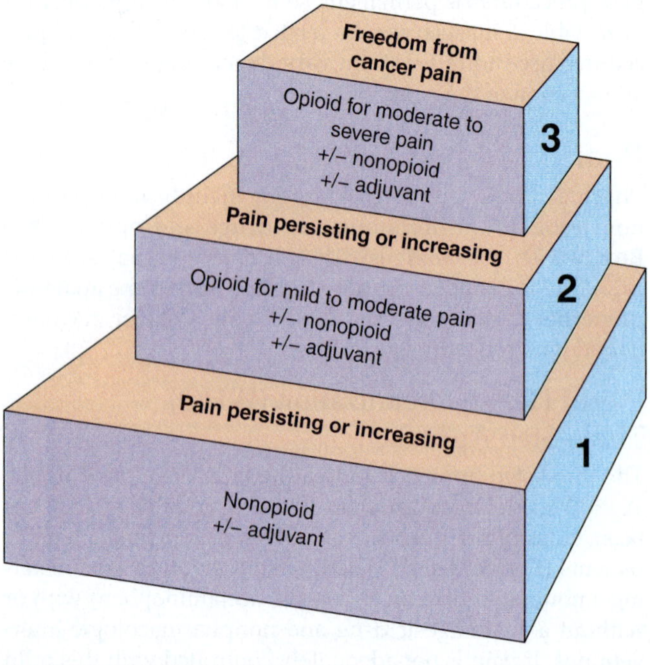

SAFETY ALERT If a patient is experiencing moderate to severe pain (pain rated 4–10 on a scale of 0–10), it may be appropriate to skip step 1 and proceed directly to step 2 or 3, depending on the condition of the patient. For example, a patient with severe burns over a large portion of the body will not receive adequate pain control with acetaminophen; in this case, treatment should start at step 3. Starting a patient's pain treatment at step 2 or 3 depends on the patient's pain report and the judgment of the healthcare provider.

This three-step approach allows the healthcare provider to give increasingly potent combinations of analgesic drugs until the patient's pain is managed effectively. For pain relief, a polypharmaceutical regimen combines multiple medications with different mechanisms of actions in order to obtain the best pain relief for the patient. This combination can allow the healthcare provider to use lower doses of opioids and other analgesics to minimize dependence and toxicity (WHO, 2016). The benefits of combining opioid and nonopioid analgesics are often overlooked. Because these drugs have different mechanisms of action and toxicity profiles, giving a nonopioid drug at the same time as or alternating with an opioid drug creates a synergistic effect with minimal side effects.

SAFETY ALERT When treating patients with multiple medications, healthcare providers must always be aware of potential drug–drug interactions that may cause additional, and sometimes life-threatening, side effects. In addition, when treating patients with combination drugs, healthcare providers must avoid giving duplicate drugs (e.g., acetaminophen in a combination analgesic plus acetaminophen for fever plus acetaminophen in a cold-and-flu preparation) to prevent an unintentional overdose.

Figure 3–6 »The World Health Organization (WHO) three-step analgesic ladder.

Nonopioids/NSAIDs

Nonopioids are analgesic and antipyretic drugs, including acetaminophen and NSAIDs, the most common of which are aspirin, ibuprofen, and naproxen. NSAIDs have anti-inflammatory properties, whereas acetaminophen does not. NSAIDs reduce pain and inflammation by inhibiting cyclooxygenase (COX) signaling pathways, which produce prostaglandins and thromboxane. These inflammatory mediators enhance both the transduction and the transmission of pain signals (Adams, Holland, & Urban, 2017). In 2005, the Food and Drug Administration (FDA) highlighted the risk of heart attacks and strokes from the use of NSAIDs. This warning label requirement was strengthened in 2015 to include the warning label on all prescription NSAIDs (FDA, 2005, 2015).

Nonopioid drugs have a *ceiling effect*; that is, once the patient consumes a specific dosage level, consuming more of the drug will not produce a greater analgesic effect but may increase toxic effects. Nonopioid drugs also have a narrow *therapeutic index*, meaning they have a very small efficacy range without being toxic. Given the increased risk for GI bleeding and prolonged bleeding times, repeatedly consuming NSAIDs at doses higher than are recommended could be life-threatening (see Patient Teaching feature). **Table 3–3** contains a list of common misconceptions related to nonopioid medications and their associated truths.

The mechanism of action and the side effects of acetaminophen differ from those of the NSAIDs. Large doses or long-term use can cause severe liver and kidney toxicity.

Acetaminophen is the most common drug associated with drug overdoses, and acetaminophen toxicity is the leading cause of acute liver failure in the Western world. Untreated, acetaminophen-induced acute liver failure can cause death within days. The maximum recommended dosage of acetaminophen for adults is 4 g per day. If a patient consistently takes slightly higher doses (5–6 g per day) or takes one large dose (10–12 g), liver toxicity is likely to occur. The risk for liver toxicity is heightened by alcohol consumption, so patients should be discouraged from drinking alcohol while taking acetaminophen. In addition, patients with liver or kidney disease should take lower doses of acetaminophen (2.5 g per day or less).

When taken in appropriate doses, acetaminophen is well tolerated. Healthcare professionals should not underestimate the effectiveness of acetaminophen and NSAIDs such as aspirin. For example, Craig and colleagues (2012) showed that morphine administration did not provide significantly more pain relief than acetaminophen, especially when both are administered via IV. In addition, acetaminophen is associated with fewer adverse events than morphine. Because of the safety profile of acetaminophen, it is included in many over-the-counter combination drugs, especially cold, cough, and allergy preparations, as well as in combination with narcotics for pain relief (**Table 3–4**). However, many patients do not realize that their combination medications contain acetaminophen; the result is inadvertent drug overdose when they take additional medications containing acetaminophen. Nurses and other healthcare professionals must be knowledgeable about the acetaminophen content in each drug and teach patients about acetaminophen content to prevent overdose.

Opioids

Opioids are drugs that act on one or more of three opioid receptors: mu, delta, and kappa. Opioids are also commonly referred to as **narcotics**, a term that means they are morphine-like drugs that have potential for abuse. Therefore, they are controlled substances. When activated, opioid receptors in the peripheral and central nervous systems produce an analgesic response (Adams et al., 2017). Opioid

TABLE 3–3 Misconceptions About Nonopioids

Misconception	Truth
Over-the-counter (OTC) nonopioids are safe for long-term use.	OTC nonopioids are associated with severe side effects, especially when taken long term. NSAIDs can produce GI toxicity and prolong bleeding times, and acetaminophen can produce liver and kidney toxicity.
OTC nonopioids do not have serious side effects; therefore, they can be taken at a higher dose than recommended.	The risk of internal GI bleeding and acute liver failure is significantly increased when nonopioids are taken at high doses. In addition, nonopioids have a ceiling effect, so taking a higher dose will not produce a greater analgesic effect.
A patient should not take both a nonopioid and an opioid.	For patients with moderate to severe pain, WHO recommends that both opioid and nonopioid medications be given.
Nonopioids should not be used for severe pain.	While nonopioids are rarely effective alone for severe pain, they may produce a synergistic effect to relieve pain when combined with an opioid.
Gastric distress from NSAIDs should be relieved by antacids.	Antacids may relieve gastric distress, but they also reduce the absorption of NSAIDs. Antacids can change the flora of the gut, increasing the risk of developing gastric ulcers from *Helicobacter pylori* infection.
An NSAID-induced gastric ulcer will always cause gastric distress.	Peptic ulcers caused by NSAIDs are less likely to produce gastric distress than other causes of peptic ulcers.

TABLE 3–4 Acetaminophen Content in Common Combination Narcotic Medications

Drug Name	Narcotic	Acetaminophen Content
Tylenol with Codeine (#1–4)	Codeine (7.5–60 mg/tablet)	300 mg
Capital with Codeine	Codeine (12 mg)	120 mg/5 mL
Anexsia	Hydrocodone (5–7.5 mg)	325–650 mg/tablet
Hydrocet	Hydrocodone (5 mg)	500 mg/capsule
Norco	Hydrocodone (7.5–10 mg)	325 mg/tablet
Vicodin	Hydrocodone (5–10 mg)	500–750 mg/tablet
Percocet	Oxycodone (2.5–10 mg)	325–650 mg/tablet
Roxicet	Oxycodone (5 mg)	325 mg/tablet or 5 mL syrup
Talacen	Pentazocine (25 mg)	625 mg/tablet

Source: Data from Adams, M. P., Holland, L. N., & Urban, C. (2017). *Pharmacology for nurses: A pathophysiologic approach* (5th ed.). Hoboken, NJ: Pearson Education.

drugs can be classified as weak or partial agonists, full agonists, or mixed agonists.

Weak or Partial Agonists

Weak opioid agonists, such as codeine and hydrocodone, have a low affinity for the opioid receptors (see Box 3–3). Partial agonists have high affinity for the opioid receptors but produce only a partial effect. Both weak and partial agonists have a ceiling effect. Prevention and management of common side effects is outlined in **Box 3–4 ≫**.

Full Agonists

Full agonists bind with high affinity to mu opioid receptors in the peripheral and central nervous systems and produce a strong analgesic effect. Examples are fentanyl, hydromorphone, methadone, morphine, and oxycodone (see Box 3–3).

As the most potent class of pain relievers, they should be used for patients in severe pain or when other medications have failed to control pain. Full opioid agonists do not have a ceiling effect. Therefore, full opioid agonists can be given in increasing doses until pain is relieved or side effects become intolerable. Full agonists are known to produce euphoria, respiratory depression, and tolerance. Euphoria may help the patient feel more comfortable even with uncontrolled pain, but respiratory depression may be a life-threatening side effect. Patients who develop tolerance to opioids are likely to experience withdrawal symptoms when the drug is discontinued, so they should be taken off opioids gradually.

Mixed Opioids

There are two types of mixed opioid agonists: mixed agonist–antagonist opioids (e.g., nalbuphine hydrochloride

Box 3–4
Prevention and Management of Common Opioid Side Effects

Constipation

- Increase fluid intake if patient is dehydrated.
- Dietary fiber intake should not increase unless the patient is fiber-deficient; opioids cause decreased peristalsis, which could result in bowel obstruction if fiber is increased.
- Daily stool softeners (e.g., docusate sodium [Colace]) and laxatives (e.g., bisacodyl USP [Dulcolax]) may be offered as a prophylactic or treatment for constipation.
- Severe constipation may be treated with suppositories, rectal irrigation, or manual evacuation.

Nausea and Vomiting

- Nausea can be treated with antiemetics such as antipsychotics (e.g., Haldol), prokinetic agents (e.g., metoclopramide [Reglan]), or serotonin antagonists (e.g., ondansetron [Zofran]).

Sedation

- Patients may be given psychostimulants (e.g., methylphenidate [Ritalin]) for persistent sedation.
- Sedation may be a sign of respiratory depression, so patients with sedation should be monitored for respiratory rate and pulse oximetry.

Pruritus

- Apply moisturizers or bathe in tepid water.
- Administer antihistamine medications (e.g., diphenhydramine).

Sexual Dysfunction

- Opioid-induced sexual dysfunction may be treated with androgen replacement therapies (i.e., testosterone for men and dehydroepiandrosterone, or DHEA, for women).

Sources: Based on Portenoy, R. K., Mehta, Z., & Ahmed, E. (2016). *Cancer pain management with opioids: Prevention and management of side effects*. Retrieved from http://www.uptodate.com/contents/cancer-pain-management-with-opioids-prevention-and-management-of-side-effects; Manchikanti, L., Abdi, S., Atluri, S., Balog, C. C., Benyamin, R. M., Boswell, M. V., . . . Wargo, B. W. (2012). American Society of Interventional Pain Physicians (ASIPP) guidelines for responsible opioid prescribing in chronic non-cancer pain: Part 2—Guidance. *Pain Physician*, *15*(Suppl. 3), S67–S116; Sloot, S., Boland, J., Snowden, J., Ezaydi, Y. L., Foster, A., Gethin, A. L., . . . Ahmedza, S. H. (2014). Side effects of analgesia may significantly reduce quality of life in symptomatic multiple myeloma: A cross-sectional prevalence study. *Supportive Care in Cancer*, *23*(3), 671–678.

Focus on Diversity and Culture
Codeine

Codeine and other opioids are converted to the active form morphine by the CYP2D6 enzyme. Approximately 7%–10% of Caucasians lack the CYP2D6 enzyme, so codeine is ineffective for them. In addition, although 99% of the Chinese population has a functional CYP2D6 enzyme, over 55% of the population contains a polymorphism (i.e., *CYP2D6*10*) that renders it less effective (< 30%). Almost 40% of the Japanese population carries the *CYP2D6*10* allele as well. Approximately 20% of African Americans carry the *CYP2D6*17* allele, which also has a decreased effect (80%) compared to the normal CYP2D6 enzyme (Haufroid & Hantson, 2015).

In contrast, 1%–7% of Caucasians and more than 25% of Ethiopians have three or more copies of CYP2D6, causing codeine to be more effective with greater side effects (Haufroid & Hantson, 2015). For these patients, alternative medications, such as morphine and hydromorphone, which do not rely on the activity of CYP2D6 may be prescribed (Haufroid & Hantson, 2015).

[Nubain]) and opioids mixed with nonopioids (e.g., opioid with acetaminophen, aspirin, ibuprofen). Mixed agonist–antagonist drugs act as an agonist at one opioid receptor (usually the kappa receptor) and as an antagonist at a different opioid receptor (usually the mu receptor). Because of the antagonist effect on the mu receptor, mixed agonist–antagonist opioids should be given only as the first opioid. If given after another opioid, the antagonist properties of the drug may cause withdrawal symptoms. Mixed agonist–antagonist drugs have a ceiling effect and should not be used for severe pain or in terminally ill patients.

Opioids can be mixed with nonopioid analgesic drugs or with a variety of other drugs, such as cough medicine, caffeine, and muscle relaxers. Codeine is the opioid available in the widest range of combination drugs (see Focus on Diversity and Culture feature). Pain medicines that contain both an opioid and a nonopioid are more efficacious than either drug alone. This greater efficacy allows the patient to take a lower dose of each medication, thus decreasing the risk of side effects. When using combination drugs, nurses and other healthcare providers must be aware of the daily dose limits of all ingredients in the combination.

Opioid Side Effects

Of all the side effects associated with opioids, the most life-threatening is severe respiratory depression. Respiratory depression is likely to occur when initial opioid doses are too high or are used in combination with other drugs that also cause respiratory depression (Manchikanti et al., 2012). Respiratory depression is also more common in patients with respiratory disorders such as chronic obstructive pulmonary disease (COPD), asthma, or obstructive sleep apnea (Manchikanti et al., 2012). Patients on opioids must be carefully monitored for respiratory depression. Sedation normally precedes respiratory depression; therefore, a sedation scale such as the Pasero Opioid-Induced Sedation Scale (POSS) (**Table 3–5 »**) can be used to monitor sedation and guide clinical responses to respiratory depression. Respiratory depression is also accompanied by increased $PaCO_2$, periods of apnea, and confusion.

SAFETY ALERT All patients on opioids should be monitored for sedation and respiratory depression during the first 24 hours (especially after surgery), during the peak effect, after increasing or decreasing a dose, before additional doses of opioids are given, or when changing opioids or routes of administration. If the respiratory rate falls below 8–10/min, the patient should be aroused and naloxone therapy should be considered (Kim & Nelson, 2015).

Common side effects of opioid use are outlined in Box 3–4. Many of these side effects, especially nausea and sedation, will decrease within 3–5 days as the patient develops tolerance for the drug. If sedation interferes with quality of life, stimulants can be taken in the morning to counteract daytime sedation. However, stimulants should be used with caution because of potential side effects and lack of usefulness in clinical trials. Tolerance to constipation usually does not develop. Therefore, medical interventions will be needed to prevent or treat constipation.

TABLE 3–5 Pasero Opioid-Induced Sedation Scale (POSS)

Scale	Description
S = Sleep, easy to arouse	Acceptable; no action necessary; may increase opioid dose if needed
1 = Awake and alert	Acceptable; no action necessary; may increase opioid dose if needed
2 = Slightly drowsy, easily aroused	Acceptable; no action necessary; may increase opioid dose if needed
3 = Frequently drowsy, arousable, drifts off to sleep during conversation	Unacceptable; monitor respiratory status and sedation level closely until sedation level is stable at less than 3 and respiratory status is satisfactory; decrease opioid dose 25%–50% (per opioid analgesic orders or hospital protocol) or notify prescriber (e.g., physician, nurse practitioner) or anesthesiologist for orders; consider administering a nonsedating, opioid-sparing nonopioid, such as acetaminophen or an NSAID, if not contraindicated.
4 = Somnolent, minimal or no response to verbal or physical stimulation	Unacceptable; stop opioid; consider administering naloxone (mix 0.4 mg of naloxone and 10 mL of normal saline in syringe and administer this dilute solution very slowly [0.5 mL over 2 minutes] while observing the patient's response; hospital protocols should include the expectation that a nurse will administer naloxone to any patient suspected of having life-threatening opioid-induced sedation and respiratory depression); notify prescriber or anesthesiologist; monitor respiratory status and sedation level closely until sedation level is stable at less than 3 and respiratory status is satisfactory.

Source: From Pasero, C. (2009). American Society of Perianesthesia Nurses: Assessment of sedation during opioid administration for pain management. *Journal of PeriAnesthesia Nursing 24*(3), 186–190.

Box 3–5
Pain Management for the Patient with a History of Drug Abuse

According to the National Institute on Drug Abuse (2012), 1.8 million Americans are addicted to prescription pain medications, and another 23 million are addicted to alcohol, marijuana, and other drugs. Therefore, healthcare providers will encounter patients with pain who are addicted to at least one drug. Healthcare providers unfortunately have a tendency to order nonopioids or lower doses of opioids for patients with a history of abuse; the result is undertreatment and increased drug-seeking behavior. For several reasons, it is critical to provide adequate pain relief in addicted patients, especially patients who are addicted to opioids.

1. Patients who are addicted to opioids have developed drug tolerance. Therefore, they require a *higher* dose to produce an analgesic effect, not a lower dose.
2. Opioid tolerance is often associated with *hyperalgesia*, or an increased physiologic response to pain. Therefore, patients

with a history of opioid abuse feel pain more extensively than non-abusers.
3. Abusers whose drug of choice is withheld during their hospital stay will go through withdrawal, which exacerbates pain symptoms, prohibits healing, and increases the length of the hospital stay.

Patients should be given adequate pain control during the acute phase of pain, regardless of their drug abuse history. This should be seen as a medical issue, not an ethical or moral issue. The patients can undergo detoxification after they are no longer in pain. Communication among healthcare providers is critical when treating patients with a history of drug abuse to ensure that increases in dosage are related to pain control and not addictive behavior. Pain levels and a need for prescription opioids should be reassessed frequently throughout treatment.

Source: Based on National Institute on Drug Abuse. (2012). *DrugFacts: Nationwide trends.* Retrieved from http://www.drugabuse.gov/publications/drugfacts/nationwide-trends

Most opioids are excreted via the kidneys, so a reduction in renal function may increase toxic effects. For this reason, morphine should be used with caution in older adults, and meperidine should not be used at all. Instead, hydromorphone, which has greater potency than morphine and is metabolized by the liver, can be used (Tracy & Morrison, 2013).

Opioid use is often associated with tolerance and addiction, and therefore many physicians are reluctant to prescribe opioids and patients are reluctant to take them even when in severe pain. Tolerance to opioids, in which a higher dose of medication is needed to produce the same analgesic effect, is expected with long-term use. Addiction is different from tolerance in that it can affect the individuals' behavior in addition to their physiologic response to the drug. Very few patients exhibit patterns of addiction when opioids are used as recommended. However, if physicians prescribe inadequate doses of opioids because they fear tolerance and addiction, patients may exhibit drug-seeking behaviors simply because their pain medication is ineffective. This situation strains the trust relationship between the patient and the healthcare provider. Nurses and other healthcare providers must become adept at recognizing behaviors of addiction compared to behaviors associated with inadequate pain control (see **Box 3–5 »**).

Clinical Manifestations and Therapies
Acute and Chronic Pain

ETIOLOGY	CLINICAL MANIFESTATIONS	CLINICAL THERAPIES
Acute pain	<ul><li>Patient report of acute pain</li><li>Elevated vital signs</li><li>Nausea and vomiting</li><li>Restlessness and anxiety</li><li>Behavioral indications (crying, grimacing, shielding)</li></ul>	<ul><li>Pharmacologic therapy</li><li>Heat/ice</li><li>Movement restriction</li><li>Distraction</li><li>Family support</li></ul>
Chronic pain	<ul><li>Patient report of chronic pain</li><li>Normal vital signs</li><li>Depression</li><li>Irritability</li><li>Impaired mobility and/or activity</li><li>Sleep disturbances</li></ul>	<ul><li>Pharmacologic therapy</li><li>Injections</li><li>Surgery</li><li>Massage</li><li>Chiropractic interventions</li><li>Cognitive–behavioral therapy</li><li>Positive attitude</li><li>Religious rituals</li><li>Support (family, friends, groups)</li></ul>

Focus on Integrative Health
Pain Control

Numerous types of complementary health approaches for pain control are available for use either alone or in conjunction with pharmacologic therapies. Many complementary therapies for pain are independent nursing interventions, such as repositioning a patient to relieve pain or providing patient education. Many patients ask about the use of acupuncture for pain. Acupuncture involves the stimulation of anatomic points on the body, often by using very thin, metallic needles. Although additional research is needed, the National Center for Complementary and Integrative Health reports some evidence that acupuncture can be helpful in treating chronic back pain and pain associated with osteoarthritis (NCCIH, 2016). Results from a retrospective study examining who uses integrative therapies found that the majority of those who do not use integrative therapies lack knowledge of the therapies. The alternative therapies included were acupuncture, chiropractic care, natural products, and yoga. The study participants either did not know about the integrative therapies or felt they did not need them (Burke, Nahin, & Stussman, 2015). A meta-analysis of 31 randomized controlled trials (RCT) showed that the use of acupuncture compared to sham-acupuncture (placebo) and no acupuncture (control) reduced pain outcomes for patients with chronic pain (Vickers, Phil, & Linde, 2014).

Some complementary methods are intended to provide physiologic pain relief, such as heat or ice, movement restriction, and chiropractic therapy. Some therapies are used to help the mind and spirit overcome the sensations of pain, such as guided imagery, cognitive–behavioral therapy, and religious rituals. Social methods include using support from family and friends, laughter, and a focus on others to help minimize pain. Dietary and herbal supplements can be used as an alternative therapy for pain, but current studies suggest that they may be no better than placebos at providing pain relief (Henrotin, Mobasheri, & Marty, 2012), and they may produce dangerous drug–herb interactions (NCCIH, 2016a).

Co-analgesics

Co-analgesics are drugs that have analgesic properties, potentiate the effects of pain medications, relieve other discomforts, or reduce the side effects of analgesic drugs. They are especially effective at reducing neuropathic pain. Examples of co-analgesic drugs are antidepressants, anticonvulsants, antihypertensives, antipruritics, corticosteroids, and local anesthetics (see Box 3–3).

- Antidepressants (e.g., imipramine) act to prevent the reuptake of serotonin and norepinephrine, slowing the transmission of pain signals.

- Anticonvulsants (e.g., gabapentin) may produce their analgesic effects through blocking sodium channels and enhancing gamma-aminobutyric acid (GABA) function.

- Antihypertensives (e.g., clonidine) are α_2-adrenergic receptor agonists that modulate ascending pain sensations.

- Antipruritics (e.g., hydroxyzine) are antihistamines that may relieve pruritus, nausea, and anxiety.

- Corticosteroids (e.g., prednisone) inhibit phospholipase A_2 and COX-2 as well as reduce pain associated with inflammation, and they are effective in treating nausea and vomiting.

- Local anesthetics (e.g., benzocaine, lidocaine) block the transmission of pain signals.

Nonpharmacologic Therapy

In addition to pharmacologic pain management, many nonpharmacologic therapies can be used to help control pain. These include both invasive and noninvasive therapies.

Invasive Therapies

Invasive therapies include injections, such as nerve blocks or radioablation, or surgeries, such as implantation of electrotherapy devices or interruption of pain conduction pathways. A **nerve block** is an injection of a local anesthetic around nerves to temporarily block nerve activity. Nerve blocks are often associated with dental procedures but may also be used to treat pain associated with musculoskeletal injuries, sciatica, shingles, or cancer. Nerve blocks can be administered through single injections, multiple injections over time, or continuous infusions. Permanent nerve blocks use alcohol or phenol, cryoanalgesia, or radioablation to destroy nerve tissue. Pain may return if nerve fibers regenerate over time.

Lifespan Considerations

In each patient, a unique set of factors influences how they perceive pain. In addition to physiologic factors such as transmission of pain signals, other factors may include the patient's developmental stage, ethnic and cultural values, environment, support from family and friends, past experiences with pain, and views on the meaning of pain. In 2001, The Joint Commission issued standards related to pain assessment and management for patients of all ages, which were updated in 2011 and clarified in 2016 (see **Box 3–6 》**).

Patients' age and developmental level influence how they express and respond to pain. The influence of age on pain perception and behavior, as well as some related nursing interventions, are described in **Table 3–6 》**. Additional information about nursing care for patients in pain is covered in the following sections.

Neonates and Pain

Neonates are routinely subjected to painful stimuli (**Figure 3–7 》**). The American Academy of Pediatrics (Fein, Zempsky, & Cravero, 2012) recommends the use of environmental, pharmacologic, and nonpharmacologic interventions

Box 3–6
The Joint Commission Pain Management Standards

In 1999, The Joint Commission approved pain assessment and management standards for accredited ambulatory care facilities, behavioral healthcare organizations, home care providers, hospitals, office-based surgery practices, and long-term care providers. These were updated in 2011 and advocate that patients have the right to appropriate assessment and management of pain. All patients should be screened for pain in the initial assessment and reassessed for pain as required. This assessment should include effectiveness and side effects of the patient's current treatment. In addition, the healthcare organization should provide adequate training in pain assessment and management to healthcare providers, and patients with pain and their families should be educated about effective and safe pain management. A new pediatric standard added in 2011 states that pediatric patients should receive both pharmacologic therapy and nonpharmacologic comfort measures before a procedure to reduce stress and pain related to the procedure. In addition, the family of the patient may be asked to assist in identifying pain in children.

Starting in 2015, The Joint Commission clarified their pain management standard to "affirm that organizations' treatment strategies may consider both pharmacologic and nonpharmacologic approaches, as well as the benefits and risks to patients, when determining the most appropriate interventions."

Sources: Based on The Joint Commission. (2011a). *Facts about pain management*. Retrieved from http://www.jointcommission.org/assets/1/18/pain_management.pdf; Joint Commission Resources. (2012). *Pain management: A systems approach to improving quality and safety*. Retrieved from http://www.jcrinc.com/pain-management-a-systems-approach-to-improving-quality-and-safety/; The Joint Commission. (2014). *Clarification of the pain management standard*. Retrieved from https://www.jointcommission.org/assets/1/18/Clarification_of_the_Pain_Management__Standard.pdf

TABLE 3–6 Influence of Age on Pain Perception and Behavior

Developmental Stage	Response to Pain	Sample Nonpharmacologic Interventions
Infant	Exhibits body rigidity or thrashing. Exhibits facial expression of pain. Cries inconsolably. Exhibits hypersensitivity or irritability. Has poor oral intake. Is unable to sleep.	Offer a pacifier. Swaddle infant. Rock infant. Allow the parent to hold the infant. Offer distractions such as music or a small toy. Breastfeed the infant.
Toddler and preschooler	May describe pain through basic words or gestures. May be verbally aggressive. May cry intensely. Exhibits physical resistance by pushing away painful stimulus. Guards painful area of body. May see pain as punishment. May request emotional support from parent.	Offer distractions such as toys, books, or treats. Allow the parent to hold the child. Teach the child what to expect when encountering a painful procedure. Play games (blow bubbles, pinwheel, peek-a-boo). Encourage the parent to be calm, as children can sense a parent's anxiety.
School-age child	Should be able to accurately describe their pain. Attempts to be brave in response to pain. May exhibit stalling behaviors. Exhibits muscle rigidity and other behaviors in anticipation of pain. May revert to earlier developmental stage with persistent or severe pain.	Simulate/act out the procedure beforehand. Encourage a parent to be present to provide support. Videos Guided imagery Give the child a book to read or an activity to do. Encourage cultural practices such as prayer.
Adolescent	May deny pain in the presence of peers. Exhibits changes in sleep patterns or appetite. Exhibits body control. May regress to earlier developmental stage in the presence of a trusted adult.	Discuss pain as with an adult patient. Maintain privacy. Encourage distractions such as music or TV to deal with pain. Allow parents to be present if so requested by adolescent.
Adult	May exhibit gender-specific behaviors learned as a child. May ignore pain in order to be a "good" patient. May ignore pain to prevent appearing weak. May deny pain based on fear that the condition has worsened.	Discuss the patient's misconceptions about pain. Address the patient's symptoms of fear and anxiety. Focus on providing adequate pain control based on the patient's description of pain intensity.
Older adult	Pain may result from multiple conditions. May view pain as being inherent in aging. May have increased pain threshold compared to younger adults. Manifestations of pain may include decreased energy level, loss of appetite, and general lethargy. May deny pain to prevent becoming dependent on others.	Spend time discussing the patient's health status, including pain, with the patient. This will give the patient a feeling of self-worth and credibility. Dispel myths related to age and pain. Promote the highest possible level of independence.

Sources: Based on Berman, A., Snyder, S. J., & Frandsen, G. (2016). Pain management. In *Kozier and Erb's fundamentals of nursing: Concepts, process, and practice* (10th ed., p. 1094, Table 46-3). Hoboken, NJ: Pearson Education; Wanless, S., Cohen, S. M., & Danford, C. A. (2015). The assessment and non-pharmacologic treatment of procedural pain from infancy to school age through a developmental lens: A synthesis of evidence with recommendations. *Journal of Pediatric Nursing*. doi:10.1016/j.pedn.2015.09.002; Kaheni, S., Reza, M.S., Bagheri, M., & Goudarzian, A.H. (2016). The effect of distraction technique on the pain of dressing change among 3–6 year old children. *International Journal of Pediatrics, 4*(4), 1603–1610.

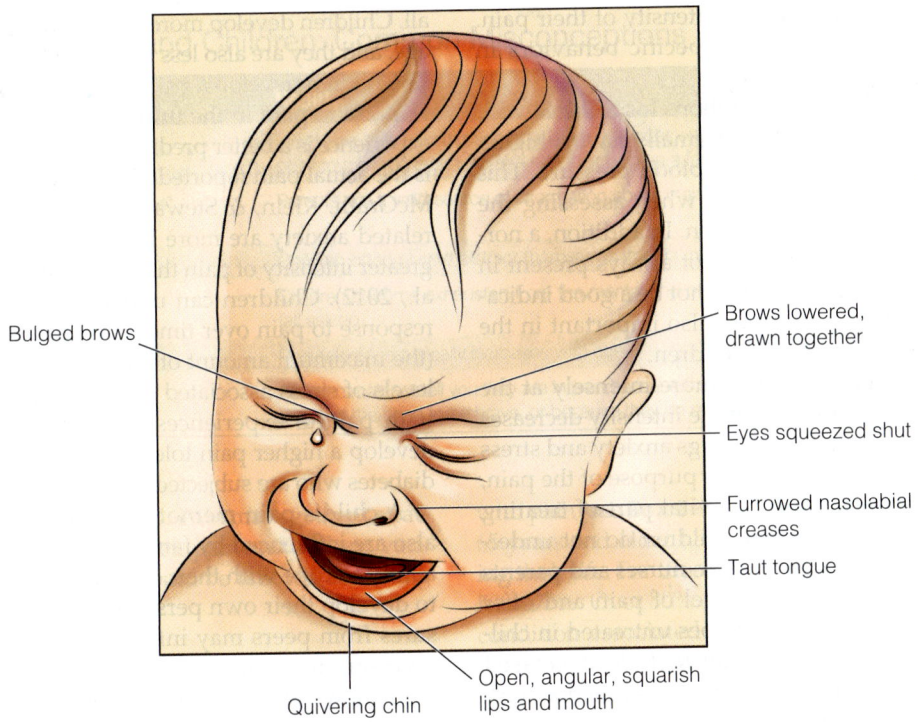

Bulged brows

Brows lowered, drawn together

Eyes squeezed shut

Furrowed nasolabial creases

Taut tongue

Open, angular, squarish lips and mouth

Quivering chin

Figure 3–7 ❯❯ Neonatal characteristic facial responses to pain include bulged brow, eyes squeezed shut, furrowed nasolabial creases, open lips, stretched mouth, taut tongue, and quivering chin.

to reduce pain in neonates. Environmental recommendations include the use of a dedicated pediatric area with a calming and child-friendly environment that includes colorful walls and ceilings and toys for distraction. Pharmacologic interventions for minor procedures include the use of topical anesthetics for venipuncture and circumcision and the use of a 12–25% sucrose solution to decrease the response to a noxious stimulus such as a heel stick. Nonpharmacologic interventions include the use of a pacifier, skin-to-skin contact (kangaroo care), and breastfeeding (American Academy of Pediatrics (AAP), 2016; IASP, 2011).

Swaddling is also an effective way to reduce the pain response in neonates. Reducing the number of painful procedures performed on each infant is a way to reduce pain (Fein et al., 2012; AAP, 2016).

Uncontrolled pain has many serious effects on newborns, including exhausting energy resources that should be used for growth and healing, decreasing oxygen saturation, changing the **pain threshold** (the point at which pain is initially felt), influencing the infant's future perception of pain, and decreasing the infant's **pain tolerance** (the maximum amount of pain a patient will tolerate). Unrelieved pain in neonates can also lead to **sensitization**, or an increased response to pain over time. Doesburg and colleagues (2013) found that neurocognitive alterations were present in school-age children who were born very prematurely (< 32 weeks, gestation) and who were exposed to procedural pain. These and other studies demonstrate that inadequate pain control in neonates can have long-term consequences, and they establish the importance of effective pain relief in this population.

Infants and Pain

Determining an infant's comfort level is complicated because infants are not yet able to verbalize specific complaints related to discomfort. Infants are likely to respond similarly to pain, fear, hunger, dirty diapers, and many other conditions, and deciphering the true cause of an infant's discomfort can be challenging. Previously held beliefs that children, particularly preverbal children, do not experience pain has been challenged by research that has shown that preverbal children have intact neural pathways of pain transmission, and older infants and toddlers have more of an ability to localize the pain (Manocha & Taneja, 2015). Assessing pain in newborns and infants can be challenging. Symptoms of pain in newborns and young infants include crying, lethargy, hypertension, hypotension, tachycardia, bradycardia, and apnea. Because of the wide array of symptoms that can indicate pain in the infant, any change in the child's condition should result in the nurse's consideration of a possible relationship to pain. Wanless, Cohen, and Danford (2015) identified that assessing the parent–infant bond in addition to using assessment tools to judge children's pain is also important. Infants who have a strong bond with their parents are likely to be more readily comforted by swaddling from the parents because of the flow of reciprocity between parents and their infant. Comforting from the parent may relieve some of the pain in the infant, thus altering how to proceed with nursing care related to pain management.

Children and Pain

Children are less able than adults to accurately describe their pain. However, children as young as 3 years old can give a

Nursing Care Plan (continued)

IMPLEMENTATION

The nurses caring for Mr. Crandall implement the following interventions:

- Administer medications, nutrition, and oxygen as ordered.
- Bathe patient and change linens as needed to maintain patient comfort.

- Provide oral care every 2 hours.
- Encourage family to express feelings about patient's terminal condition.
- Prepare family for signs and symptoms of impending death.

EVALUATION

Shortly after the family's arrival, Mr. Crandall died with family members surrounding him. Without regaining consciousness, he died peacefully with a gradual decrease in respirations and heart rate. His family members expressed appreciation that they had had the opportunity to tell him they loved him one last time.

CRITICAL THINKING

1. What recommendation or request would you make of the healthcare provider regarding Mr. Crandall's tube feedings? Explain your answer.
2. Mr. Crandall's daughter asks if he will be placed on a mechanical ventilator to support his breathing. How would you respond to this question?

3. Would you recommend that Mr. Crandall or his healthcare proxy agree to a DNR order? Why or why not?

REVIEW End-of-Life Care

RELATE Link the Concepts and Exemplars

Linking the exemplar of end-of-life care with the concept of family:

1. What is the priority nursing diagnosis for the family of the patient with a terminal illness requiring end-of-life care?
2. What teaching points would you provide the family of a terminal patient regarding end-of-life care?

Linking the exemplar of end-of-life care with the concept of grief and loss:

3. How can the nurse support the family's need to prepare for loss of a family member while meeting the patient's need for end-of-life care?
4. Describe your plan of care for helping the family of a school-age child with terminal illness provide end-of-life care for the child while meeting the family's need to grieve.

READY Go to Volume 3: Clinical Nursing Skills

REFER Go to Pearson MyLab Nursing and eText

- Additional review materials

REFLECT Apply Your Knowledge

Pam Allen is a middle-age woman who recently experienced a recurrence of colon cancer. She is dying. Mrs. Allen and her husband have elected for her to stay at home. Mrs. Allen's healthcare team includes a hospice nurse, a social worker, and her treating physician. Friends and church members have been bringing food for the Allen family. Mr. Allen has discussed his fears about Mrs. Allen's death with the social worker.

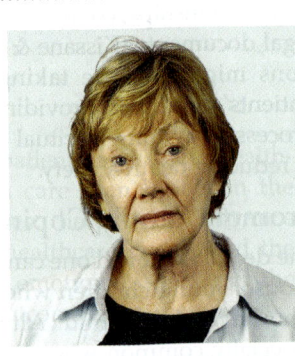

Mrs. Allen has had very little to eat or drink this week and is rarely urinating. The hospice nurse notices that she has abdominal fullness (ascites) due t the accumulation of fluid in the peritoneal cavity and appear more jaundiced. Her pain continues. She is agitated and has di ficulty speaking. At today's visit, the hospice nurse records th following vital signs: T_O 98°F; P 99 bpm; R 30/min (shallow); B 100/66 mmHg.

1. What is the priority of care for Mrs. Allen on this visit?
2. Based on the current assessment, what information would yo provide Mr. Allen?
3. Would you consider notifying the physician of your current fin ings? Why or why not?

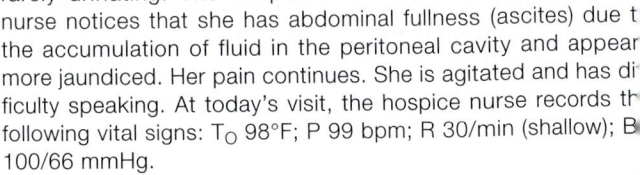

» Exemplar 3.C
Fatigue

Exemplar Learning Outcomes

3.C Analyze fatigue as it relates to comfort.

- Describe the pathophysiology, etiology, risk factors, and prevention of fatigue.
- Identify the clinical manifestations of fatigue.

- Summarize diagnostic tests and therapies used by interprofe sional teams in the collaborative care of an individual with fatigu
- Differentiate considerations for care of patients with fatigue acro the lifespan.
- Apply the nursing process in providing culturally competent care an individual with fatigue.

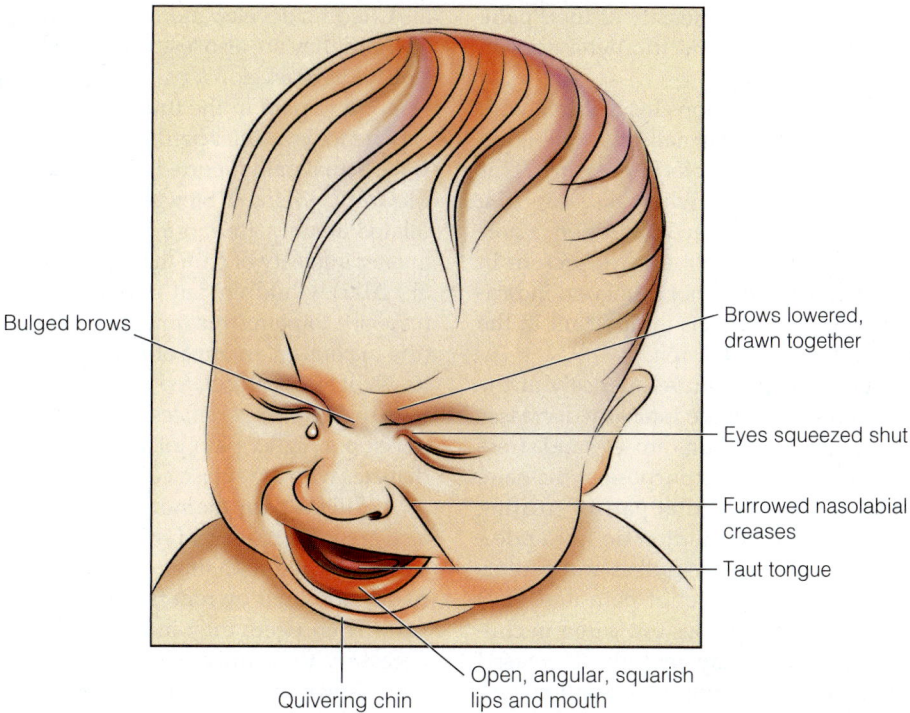

Bulged brows

Brows lowered, drawn together

Eyes squeezed shut

Furrowed nasolabial creases

Taut tongue

Quivering chin

Open, angular, squarish lips and mouth

Figure 3–7 ›› Neonatal characteristic facial responses to pain include bulged brow, eyes squeezed shut, furrowed nasolabial creases, open lips, stretched mouth, taut tongue, and quivering chin.

to reduce pain in neonates. Environmental recommendations include the use of a dedicated pediatric area with a calming and child-friendly environment that includes colorful walls and ceilings and toys for distraction. Pharmacologic interventions for minor procedures include the use of topical anesthetics for venipuncture and circumcision and the use of a 12–25% sucrose solution to decrease the response to a noxious stimulus such as a heel stick. Nonpharmacologic interventions include the use of a pacifier, skin-to-skin contact (kangaroo care), and breastfeeding (American Academy of Pediatrics (AAP), 2016; IASP, 2011).

Swaddling is also an effective way to reduce the pain response in neonates. Reducing the number of painful procedures performed on each infant is a way to reduce pain (Fein et al., 2012; AAP, 2016).

Uncontrolled pain has many serious effects on newborns, including exhausting energy resources that should be used for growth and healing, decreasing oxygen saturation, changing the **pain threshold** (the point at which pain is initially felt), influencing the infant's future perception of pain, and decreasing the infant's **pain tolerance** (the maximum amount of pain a patient will tolerate). Unrelieved pain in neonates can also lead to **sensitization**, or an increased response to pain over time. Doesburg and colleagues (2013) found that neurocognitive alterations were present in school-age children who were born very prematurely (< 32 weeks, gestation) and who were exposed to procedural pain. These and other studies demonstrate that inadequate pain control in neonates can have long-term consequences, and they establish the importance of effective pain relief in this population.

Infants and Pain

Determining an infant's comfort level is complicated because infants are not yet able to verbalize specific complaints related to discomfort. Infants are likely to respond similarly to pain, fear, hunger, dirty diapers, and many other conditions, and deciphering the true cause of an infant's discomfort can be challenging. Previously held beliefs that children, particularly preverbal children, do not experience pain has been challenged by research that has shown that preverbal children have intact neural pathways of pain transmission, and older infants and toddlers have more of an ability to localize the pain (Manocha & Taneja, 2015). Assessing pain in newborns and infants can be challenging. Symptoms of pain in newborns and young infants include crying, lethargy, hypertension, hypotension, tachycardia, bradycardia, and apnea. Because of the wide array of symptoms that can indicate pain in the infant, any change in the child's condition should result in the nurse's consideration of a possible relationship to pain. Wanless, Cohen, and Danford (2015) identified that assessing the parent–infant bond in addition to using assessment tools to judge children's pain is also important. Infants who have a strong bond with their parents are likely to be more readily comforted by swaddling from the parents because of the flow of reciprocity between parents and their infant. Comforting from the parent may relieve some of the pain in the infant, thus altering how to proceed with nursing care related to pain management.

Children and Pain

Children are less able than adults to accurately describe their pain. However, children as young as 3 years old can give a basic description of the location and intensity of their pain. In addition, most children exhibit specific behaviors in response to pain.

There are several special considerations for children with pain. Compared to adults, children normally have a higher pulse and respiratory rate and lower blood pressure. This needs to be taken into consideration when assessing the sympathetic response to pain in children. In addition, a normal sympathetic response to pain is not always present in children, so changes in vital signs may not be a good indicator of pain. Behavioral indicators are also important in the assessment of pain management in children.

Children tend to experience pain more intensely at the beginning of the painful episode, but the intensity decreases more rapidly than in an adult. Pain brings anxiety and stress to children, who do not understand the purpose of the pain, so providing emotional comfort is a vital part of treating pain in children. In addition, many children do not understand that they can ask for pain relief, so nurses and parents must attempt to gauge the child's level of pain and offer interventions as appropriate. If pain goes untreated in children, physiologic consequences may include decreased growth and development, decreased immune function, lack of appetite, hypertension, and increased sensitivity to future pain (Lundeberg, 2014; Simons, Sieberg, & Clarr, 2012).

Children display a variety of behaviors in response to pain. The most common behavioral responses to pain are crying and grimacing (**Figure 3–8**)). Other common pain behaviors related to age are detailed in Table 3–6. Changes in behavior are one of the best indicators of pain in nonverbal children, although verbal children also exhibit behavior changes in response to pain. For example, a child may sit quietly and play with a favorite toy for hours when in pain. Any behavior that is out of the ordinary may be an indicator of pain or discomfort, including both physical and emotional pain.

Children's behavioral responses to pain become more controlled as they age. For example, an infant cries inconsolably when experiencing pain, a school-age child may exhibit a restrained cry or whimper, and an adolescent may not cry at all. Children develop more advanced coping strategies as they age, and they are also less likely to admit needing comfort.

Children develop a pain memory that influences how they respond to pain in the future. A child's memory of a painful experience is a better predictor of future pain experiences than is the actual pain reported after a procedure (Noel, Chambers, McGrath, Klein, & Stewart, 2012), and children with pain-related anxiety are more likely to remember experiencing a greater intensity of pain than they initially reported (Simons et al., 2012). Children can undergo *sensitization* (an increased response to pain over time) that causes a lower *pain tolerance* (the maximum amount of pain a patient will tolerate), higher levels of stress associated with pain, and an inability to cope with painful experiences. In contrast, other children may develop a higher pain tolerance, such as children with type I diabetes who are subjected to repeated insulin injection.

A child's pain memory and reaction to painful stimuli also are influenced by family and peer experiences. Parents' ability to cope with their children's pain guides the children to develop their own personal response to pain. Social pressures from peers may influence a child to believe that it is necessary to be brave when facing pain and that admitting pain shows weakness. Past experiences may also lead children to believe that the nurse already knows they are in pain or that if they admit pain, they will be given an injection that will hurt more than the current pain.

Even with more advanced knowledge about how they respond to and perceive pain, children still receive less adequate treatment for pain than adults. Barriers to adequate pain relief in children are related to inadequate pain assessment and a lack of knowledge about how to treat a child's pain safely. Other barriers are related to misconceptions about pain in infants and children (**Table 3–7**)).

>> **Stay Current:** Visit http://www.who.int/medicines/areas/quality_safety/guide_perspainchild/en/ to retrieve the World Health Organization's brochures on guidelines for managing persistent pain in children.

Pain and Adolescents

How adolescents cope with pain can have effects on their physical and emotional functioning. Holm, Ljungman, Asenlof, and Soderland (2013) found that how children experience pain will influence their perception of pain-related disability and recommend that more biopsychosocial approaches be entertained in the care of children, rather than the biomedical care more commonly used. Results of a qualitative study (Lagerlov, Rosvoldl, Holager, & Helseth, 2016) classified adolescents according to their attitudes about pain and their pain management strategies. The four groups included those who found their "pain is manageable," "pain is communicable," "pain is inevitable," and "pain is all over." The adolescents' involvement with their parents seemed to have an impact on their perception of pain and ability to manage pain. For example, adolescents in the "pain is manageable" group typically were involved in school activities and sports and talked to their parents about their pain, but they had the ability to problem-solve ways to reduce their pain. In contrast the "pain is all over" group were typically girls who were involved in family issues and did not have a plan for reducing pain. They talked frequently with their parents about how to manage

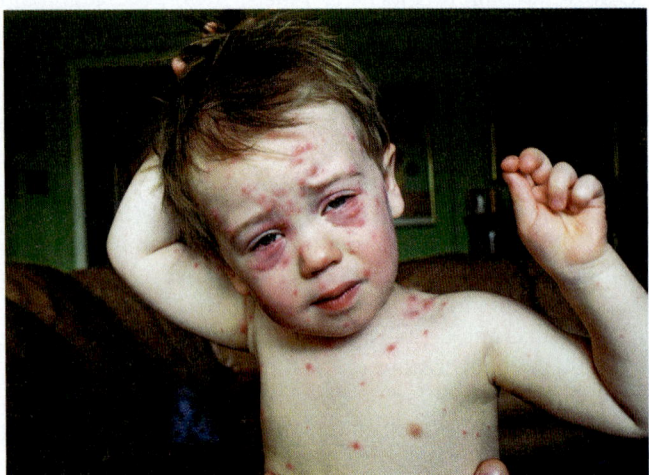

Source: Photofusion/Universal Images Group/Getty Images.

Figure 3–8)) The most common behavioral responses of children to pain are crying and grimacing.

TABLE 3–7 Pain in Infants and Children: Common Misconceptions

Myth	Reality
Infants and children cannot express pain.	Infants express pain through physiologic changes and behavioral responses. Children can accurately point to the area that hurts and rate their pain on a faces pain scale.
The patient's report is the only valid method of pain assessment.	Parents are a valid source of information about their child's pain, especially for nonverbal children.
Children in pain do not play.	Children often play to distract themselves from pain.
Children in pain do not sleep well.	Children become exhausted from the mental and physical stress of coping with pain and eventually fall asleep.
Children tolerate pain better than adults.	Pain tolerance typically increases with age.
Children will inform you of their pain.	Children may not tell you they are in pain because they are afraid of what will happen to them, because they feel the need to be brave, or because they do not understand why they have pain.

pain and were likely to be depressed. Pain management strategies to help adolescents manage their pain and address variables associated with their pain should be tailored according to the needs of each child.

Pain and Adults

Chronic pain is a widespread problem among adults, and conditions associated with chronic pain are more prevalent in women than in men. Approximately 80%–90% of fibromyalgia cases are women, and women are more likely to develop diseases that cause pain, such as osteoarthritis. This disparity may result from the fact that women have a lower *pain threshold* (the point at which pain is initially felt) and a lower pain tolerance than men (IASP, 2014).

Although women are at increased risk for chronic pain conditions, men are not exempt from chronic pain. Men are more likely to experience chronic pain from cluster headaches, coronary heart disease, gout, duodenal ulcer, and pancreatic disease (IASP, 2014).

Pain and Older Adults

Assessment of the older adult's comfort level may also be challenging. Some older adults believe chronic pain and sleep disorders are an inevitable part of the aging process and are therefore reluctant to report discomfort. The misconception that older adults feel less pain than younger adults may lead to undertreatment of pain and discomfort. Although older adults may have a higher pain threshold, their pain tolerance often is lower (Hallingbye, Martin, & Viscomi, 2011). Patients with cognitive impairment, such as Alzheimer disease, are unlikely to express even severe pain verbally, and the nurse must recognize behavioral cues as indicators of pain. Older adults are also more likely to have sleep disorders. A study by the American Academy of Sleep Medicine (2015) found that 34% of older adults had sleep-disordered breathing and 31% had short sleep duration. Treatment of sleep disorders and pain in older adults enhances their daytime functioning and quality of life.

≫ **Stay Current:** The Hartford Institute of Geriatric Nursing offers *Consult Geri*, a site with the most current information on assessment tools for use on older adults. https://consultgeri.org/

Estimates suggest that 72.1 million adults will be over age 65 by 2030 (American Nurses Association, 2012). As adults age, they develop chronic conditions that are associated

with pain (see **Box 3–7** ≫). In one estimate, 30%–50% of adults 65 years and older have two or more health problems affecting their life. For those 85 years and over, this statistic rises to 50%–75%. Over 80% of older adults have at least one chronic condition associated with pain, and approximately 20% of older adults have at least five coexisting chronic conditions. These statistics rise as the patient's age increases over 85 years (American Geriatrics Society, 2012; Rastogi & Meek, 2013). This increase in chronic conditions with pain, as well as sources of acute pain such as surgery, causes older adults to be the primary recipients of healthcare services.

Older adults undergo physiologic changes that affect how they perceive pain. They have decreased cerebral blood flow, neuronal loss, and a decreased synthesis of neurotransmitters and opioid receptors. These conditions may cause either an increased or a decreased pain response, depending on the patient's specific neuronal changes. A decrease in the descending inhibitory signal from the brain produces increased pain sensations, whereas a decrease in excitatory neurotransmitters, receptors, and neurons produces more mild pain sensations (Rastogi & Meek, 2013).

Changes in the GI and urinary systems cause decreased drug absorption, metabolism, and excretion. These changes alter the

Box 3–7
Disorders Linked to Pain in Older Adults

- Musculoskeletal pain
  - Back pain
  - Osteoarthritis
  - Rheumatoid arthritis
  - Joint pain (knees, hips, other)
  - Degenerative disc disease
  - Osteoporosis
- Neuropathic pain
  - Postherpetic neuralgia
  - Diabetic peripheral neuropathy
- Cancer-related pain (cancer and cancer treatments)
- Nighttime leg pain
- Secondary neuralgia
- Trauma
- Fibromyalgia
- Post stroke pain
- Cardiac disease/angina

pharmacokinetics of pain medications, producing either a reduced effect (inadequate pain control) or an amplified effect (increased side effects), depending on the unique changes within each patient. Drug interactions are also common in older adults who are taking multiple medications, leading to increased pain and discomfort and increased risk of life-threatening outcomes. Therefore, in order to prevent drug interactions, it is essential that nurses and pharmacists know and understand the complete list of drugs each patient is taking.

Older adults often face many barriers to effective pain management from both healthcare providers and personal preferences. Healthcare providers may lack the knowledge needed for appropriate assessment, diagnosis, and management of pain in the older population; they may fear that the patient will develop opioid dependence or that the provider will be scrutinized for regulatory reasons; or they may not have time to determine the best course of therapy for each patient. Personal barriers include misconceptions about aging, pain, and medication; fear of drug effects; noncompliance; religious beliefs; financial barriers; and comorbidities such as dementia.

Inadequate pain control can dramatically reduce patients' quality of life, decreasing their ability to perform activities of daily living and increasing their dependence on others. It can cause mood, sleep, and appetite disturbances; decreased mobility; falls; slow rehabilitation; and altered cognitive functioning (Rastogi & Meek, 2013). Decreased mobility can lead to deep vein thrombosis, pulmonary embolism, bone fractures, and reduced participation in social activities (Clarke et al., 2012). Altered cognitive functioning is a major contributor to poor pain management, as these patients are harder to assess for pain and are at increased risk for injury and therapeutic noncompliance. Older adults with chronic pain are also at greater risk for mood disorders (see **Box 3–8** 》). Therefore, adequate pain management, including patient teaching and the provision of effective and safe therapies, is essential in older adults.

》 **Stay Current:** Visit the American Society for Pain Management in Nursing at http://www.aspmn.org/ to learn more about optimal care for patients in pain.

Box 3–8
Chronic Pain in the Older Adult

As the population of older adults continues to grow, nurses will see more and more patients with chronic pain (Robeck, 2014). Older adults with chronic pain often endure their pain in silence because healthcare providers do not ask if they have pain. However, all individuals, including older adults, have the right to adequate pain assessment and effective pain management, including pharmacologic therapy.

Chronic pain conditions such as fibromyalgia, low back pain, and osteoarthritis are commonly comorbid with depression. These conditions inhibit the treatment of each other, causing faster progression of the disease and increased reliance on a caregiver. Depression is often accompanied by sleep disorders, anxiety, and cognitive impairment (National Institute of Mental Health, 2016). Therefore, older adults with chronic pain should be assessed for mood disorders in addition to the traditional pain assessment, and nursing care plans should integrate therapies to treat each condition and prevent development of additional comorbidities.

NURSING PROCESS

Pain causes physiologic, psychologic, social, and economic burdens for the patient as well as the family. In 2012, it was estimated that the cost of pain in America was more than $635 billion per year (Gaskin & Richard, 2012). Because of the overwhelming prevalence of pain, nurses are constantly caring for patients in pain.

Uncontrolled pain can lead to comorbidities such as depression, sleep disturbances, and obesity; changes in the nervous system's response to painful stimuli; accelerated disease progression; and increased length of hospital stay. Proper application of the nursing process provides information needed for appropriate care, attainable and measurable patient goals for pain management, effective nursing interventions for pain relief, and evaluation of the patient's pain level for potential revision of the nursing care plan.

Assessment

Unless a patient's physiologic needs require priority attention (e.g., severe burns, complex fracture, gunshot wound), all patients should be asked whether they are experiencing pain. Many patients do not voluntarily complain about pain even when pain is present, and persistent pain can contribute to a poor prognosis.

Observation

A visual assessment is the first component of a pain assessment. A visual assessment consists of observing a patient's behavior, such as facial expressions, body movement, and posture, to determine if the patient is in pain. Visual assessments are particularly important for neonates. Infants in pain have eyebrows that are lowered and drawn together, vertical furrows on the forehead with a bulge between the brows, tightly closed eyes, a deep nasolabial furrow, and an open mouth with a taut tongue (Arif-Rahu, Fisher, & Matsuda, 2012).

Patient Interview

The patient interview should begin with eliciting a description of the patient's pain. Asking the following questions will be helpful in identifying a plan for pain management for the patient.

- *Location.* "Where does it hurt?"
- *Intensity.* "On a scale of 1 to 10, with 1 representing no pain and 10 representing the worst possible pain, how would you rate the intensity of your pain now?"
- *Duration.* "How long have you had the pain, and how long does it usually last?"
- *Quality.* "Tell me what your pain feels like. Is it burning, throbbing, or stabbing?"

Find out when the pain started and what the patient believes caused the pain. Determine if any triggers make the pain worse and what methods help relieve the pain. Find out if the patient is taking any medications to relieve the pain. Ask if the patient experiences any other symptoms with the pain, such as nausea or dizziness, and if the pain is affecting activities of daily living. Inquire about use of herbal and dietary supplements.

When you have obtained a thorough description of the patient's current pain, continue the interview with questions about the patient's *pain history*. Have the patient describe previous diseases or injuries that caused pain, the methods used to control the pain (including the methods that have worked and those that have not), and how others' pain has influenced the patient's perception of pain. Find out if the patient places any significant meaning on the pain, such as whether it signifies disease progression, causes worry or fear, or affects the patient's relationships. Determine which methods the patient uses to cope with pain and if the pain is causing related discomforts such as depression or hopelessness.

As you perform a verbal pain assessment, keep in mind that pain is a subjective experience, and the patient is most qualified to describe the pain. Some patients, especially those with pain of an unknown etiology, may have been subjected to disdain and disbelief by others regarding their pain, so it is important to listen openly and nonjudgmentally.

Pain Rating Scales

Pain rating scales are reliable tools for helping patients report the intensity of their pain. There are multiple types of pain scales, including numeric pain scales, faces pain scales, verbal descriptor scales, and observational scales. The type of scale chosen will differ with the patient, but the same scale should be used for the same patient at each assessment to provide consistency throughout the treatment.

- **Numeric pain scales** use an 11-point rating scale (0–10) (**Figure 3–9** ≫). They are usually presented horizontally, with 0 on the left and 10 on the right. Numeric pain scales can be combined with other scales, such as the faces scale or the verbal descriptor scale; can be colored, which is helpful for children; or can be presented vertically, which may help patients from cultures who read vertically. To use a numeric pain scale, ask the patient to rate the pain on a scale of 0 to 10, with 0 representing no pain and 10 indicating the worst possible pain.

- **Verbal descriptor scales** include words to help describe the pain intensity, such as *mild*, *moderate*, or *severe*. They are helpful for patients who find it difficult to rate their pain numerically. Verbal descriptor scales may include a description of the extent to which pain interferes with activities of daily living. For example, is the patient aware of pain only when paying attention to it (mild pain), or is the patient constantly aware of pain that impairs the ability to function (severe pain)? The degree to which pain interferes with functioning is considered a good indication of pain intensity. To use a verbal descriptor scale, read each of the descriptions and ask the patient to choose the description that best fits the pain.

- The **faces pain scale** is most commonly used for children starting at age 3. It can also be helpful for patients who do not speak English or who have trouble relating to the numeric pain scales. The most common faces pain scales are the Wong–Baker FACES Rating Scale (see Figure 3–3) and the Faces Pain Scale–Revised by the International Association for the Study of Pain Faces; pain scales may include numeric values or verbal descriptions represented by each face. To use a faces pain scale, explain the pain scale using the verbal descriptions while pointing to each of the faces. Then ask the patient to point to the face that most represents the level of pain.

- An **observational or behavioral pain scale** is used to determine pain intensity for patients who are unable to provide a verbal report. Observational pain scales include the FLACC (Face, Legs, Activity, Cry, Consolability) scale, CHEOPS (Children's Hospital Eastern Ontario Pain Scale), and BOPS (Behavioral Observational Pain Scale). These pain scales use a numeric scale (usually 0–2 or 0–3) to rate patients for various behaviors, such as facial expression, leg movement, crying, and body position (see the Lifespan Considerations feature). An observational pain scale is also available that is specifically for patients with cognitive impairments. It contains areas of assessment similar to those in the pain scales designed for infants, such as facial expression, vocal complaints, and bracing behaviors. To use an observational or behavioral pain scale, the nurse observes the patient and rates the patient's behavior according to the descriptions provided. In addition, do not assume that patients with cognitive impairments are unable to provide a description of pain using numeric, descriptor, or faces pain scales.

Patients should understand the pain scale and the importance of accurately rating their pain. The pain intensity described by patients guides the healthcare team in choosing the appropriate interventions to help manage their pain. It also helps nurses track changes in pain even after shift changes, and it helps determine the effectiveness of the interventions. Nurses should remind patients that the goal of most therapeutic interventions is not to reduce pain to 1. Most patients find a reduction of 33%–50% meaningful, even if that reduction corresponds to a decrease of only 1 or 2 points on the numeric pain scale. This decrease in pain intensity usually corresponds to an increase in functioning and a higher quality of life.

In some cases, pain scales do not accurately represent patients' pain experience. Patients in pain may notice changes in pain depending on movement, the time of day, the weather, or the amount of their exertion throughout the day. Therefore, some patients prefer to describe their pain rather than choosing a number on a scale. These descriptions are an important component of the pain assessment because they help the nurse determine if there are any factors that may be affecting the pain, such as activity, state of consciousness, or distractions.

Management of pain is a continuous process that begins with assessment of pain, includes the administration of appropriate pharmacologic and nonpharmacologic therapies, and continues with reassessment of pain following the therapies. Assessment and documentation of pain severity have been shown to increase the adequacy of pain treatment (Zoega et al., 2015).

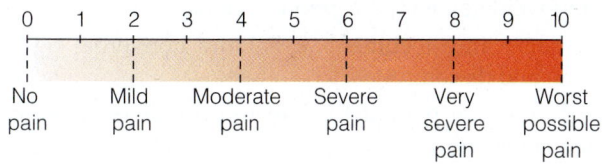

Figure 3–9 ≫ A universal pain assessment tool with an 11-point numerical pain scale with word modifiers.

Physical Examination

A physical examination includes taking vital signs. Acute pain and exacerbations in chronic pain can manifest in an increased sympathetic response, including increased blood pressure, pulse, and respiratory rate. A physical assessment also includes inspecting for any injuries that could be sources of pain, such as cuts, protruding bones, and ulcers. Any wound that impairs skin integrity is a potential source of pain and infection and should be treated immediately. If the patient has specified the location that is producing pain, superficial or deep palpation can pinpoint the exact location of the pain.

Diagnosis

NANDA-I has approved two nursing diagnoses directly related to pain: *Acute Pain* and *Chronic Pain*. The diagnosis should include a statement of the location of the pain (e.g., lower back, left knee, right occipital headache). Pain is often accompanied by physiologic and psychologic factors that may also be appropriate for nursing diagnoses (NANDA-I, 2014). Nursing diagnoses should include statements of related factors, which are specific for each patient.

General nursing diagnoses for patients in acute and chronic pain may include:

- *Mobility: Physical, Impaired*
- *Fatigue*
- *Activity Intolerance*
- *Knowledge, Deficient*
- *Anxiety.*

  (NANDA-I © 2014)

For acute pain, possible nursing diagnoses include:

- *Sleep Pattern, Disturbed*
- *Infection, Risk for*
- *Skin Integrity, Impaired.*

  (NANDA-I © 2014)

For chronic pain, possible nursing diagnoses include:

- *Insomnia*
- *Hopelessness*
- *Nutrition, Imbalanced: Less/More Than Body Requirements*
- *Social Isolation*
- *Self-Care Deficit.*

  (NANDA-I © 2014)

For patients who have been prescribed opioids, diagnoses may include:

- *Constipation, Risk for*
- *Breathing Pattern, Ineffective*
- *Fear*
- *Nausea.*

  (NANDA-I © 2014)

For parents who have children experiencing pain, diagnoses may include:

- *Family Processes, Interrupted*
- *Fear*
- *Caregiver Role Strain*
- *Stress Overload.*

  (NANDA-I © 2014)

Planning

During the planning phase, the nurse develops patient goals and nursing interventions for each nursing diagnosis. Nurses then prioritize the outcomes to determine the order in which to implement nursing interventions. For example, a patient with *Acute Pain* in the right ankle, *Impaired Physical Mobility* related to right ankle pain, and *Deficient Knowledge* about pain management may have the following expected outcomes:

- Patient will report a 50% reduction in pain.
- Patient will obtain adequate pain relief to allow for mobility.
- Patient will demonstrate skill at using crutches.
- Patient will repeat instructions for managing pain, including elevating ankle, applying ice, and taking pain medication as prescribed.

A patient-centered practice involves consulting with patients about their goals, cultural practices, and health beliefs. Patient input in the planning process increases patients' motivation to adhere to the care plan and assists in the development of the therapeutic nurse–patient relationship. (Also see the Evidence-Based Practice feature.)

Implementation

Many patients with pain are cared for in the community or in the home. Acute exacerbations may create a need for them to seek help from their healthcare provider or be admitted to the hospital.

Community-Based Care

Patients with chronic pain have to live at home and care for themselves in spite of their pain. Teaching patients and their families how to administer medications, watch for side effects, and perform nonpharmacologic interventions will help enhance both the patients' and the caregivers' lives. See **Table 3–8 》** for an overview of medications used for the management of chronic pain.

Hospital-Based Care

Nursing care of patients who have pain while hospitalized encompasses the interventions identified previously, as well as interventions aimed at reducing more acute pain, or an acute exacerbation of chronic pain. These interventions include:

- Listen carefully to the patients' description of their pain, and validate their perception of pain.
- Observe and document verbal and nonverbal signs of pain and discomfort.
- Advocate on patients' behalf to provide effective pain management.
- Monitor the patient's vital signs.
- Assess pain, the 5th vital sign, using an appropriate pain scale.

Evidence-Based Practice
Overcoming Barriers to Adequate Pain Management

Problem

Pain is a major reason that patients seek healthcare and take medications, and it accounts for a substantial portion of lost work productivity and disability. However, patients in pain are often underdiagnosed and undertreated, especially racial and ethnic minorities, people of lower socioeconomic status, women, children, older adults, military veterans, surgery and cancer patients, incarcerated men and women, and people at the end of life (IOM, 2011).

Evidence

Pain management remains ineffective because of attitudes and educational deficits of healthcare providers and patients and limitations of pharmacologic agents. Attitudes of healthcare providers can be influenced by both medical evidence and patients' psychosocial influences. In particular, providers are more likely to suggest that patients are feigning pain in the absence of medical evidence, and they are less likely to take patients' report of pain into account, if psychosocial influences are present (De Ruddere, Goubert, Stevens, Williams, & Crombez, 2013). Methods of pain management also need to be improved. Using multiple pain medications with different mechanisms of action and side effects will improve efficacy in relieving pain and decrease the incidence of adverse reactions compared to single drug therapies (Registered Nurses' Association of Ontario, 2013). In addition, compared to no intervention, physical and psychosocial nonpharmacologic interventions for pain can significantly improve patients' pain level (Park & Hughes, 2012).

Implications

Healthcare professionals need to have a better understanding of pain and pain management. The perception of pain involves both physiologic and psychosocial aspects, and pain management should include adequate pharmacologic interventions as well as complementary nonpharmacologic methods to reduce physiologic pain and increase psychosocial well-being. Education for healthcare providers should include training programs that offer standardized information about pain, guidelines related to caring for patients in pain, and experience in caring for patients in pain (IOM, 2011).

Critical Thinking Application

1. Do you have any biases that may hinder your ability to provide adequate pain management for patients? Think about a variety of situations that may present opportunities for bias, including caring for patients of different cultures, patients with drug addiction, young children and older adults, and patients at the end of life.

2. You are caring for a 72-year-old woman with osteoarthritis who is receiving inadequate pain control. How will you act as an advocate to provide better pain management for your patient?

3. You are caring for a 19-year-old man who is a known gang member. During a recent altercation, he sustained a stab wound. He is sleeping restlessly and moaning. It is time for his next dose of opioids, but your nurse manager tells you to give him only half the prescribed dose because he is probably a drug addict and giving him a full dose will feed his addiction. What should you do?

4. What are three ways in which you can stay up to date on current pain management nursing standards?

TABLE 3–8 Overview of Medications Used in the Management of Chronic Pain

Route	Drug	Nursing Implications
Oral	Hydromorphone (Exalgo)	To avoid medication errors, be aware that Exalgo is available in both immediate-release and extended-release tablets.
Oral	Methadone (Dolophine)	Evaluate patient for continued need for methadone for pain. Methadone has cumulative effects over time, so dosage may be reduced after long-term use.
Oral	Morphine (Kadian, Avinza)	Morphine is formulated as extended-release capsules. Do not chew or crush. If patient cannot swallow the capsule, pellets may be sprinkled over food and swallowed without chewing.
Oral	Oxycodone (OxyContin)	Oxycodone is available in a timed-release formulation for 12-hour dosing. Timed-release formulation must be swallowed whole. Fast-acting formulations (OxyFAST) can be used for breakthrough pain.
Transdermal	Fentanyl (Duragesic)	Patch should be placed on flat surface. Clip, do not shave, hair at site of application. Patch should be changed every 3 days. Transdermal fentanyl has slow onset effect (12–24 hours) and slow decay after discontinuation.
Transdermal	Lidocaine (Lidoderm)	Transdermal lidocaine is a patch used for postherpetic neuralgia. Apply one to three patches on most painful area for up to 12 hours per 24-hour period.
Transmucosal	Fentanyl (Actiq)	Transmucosal fentanyl is a lozenge formulation used for treatment of breakthrough pain. Patient should not suck or chew the lozenge. Lozenge should be consumed over 15 minutes.

Source: Data from Adams, M. P., Holland, L. N., & Urban, C. (2017). *Pharmacology for nurses: A pathophysiologic approach* (5th ed.). Hoboken, NJ: Pearson Education.

Patient Teaching
Managing Chronic Pain at Home

Many children and adults must learn to manage their pain while continuing their activities of daily living. Teaching patients aspects of pain management is an important part of nursing.

- Describe the drugs that are to be taken, including dose, frequency, route of administration, side effects, and potential drug, food, or herbal interactions.
- Discuss the importance of taking drugs around the clock rather than only when necessary.
- Dispel any myths or misconceptions about opioid analgesics, including teaching patients that the risk of addiction is very low when pain medications are taken as prescribed.
- Teach patients with pain and their families about proper medication administration, medication side effects, and nonpharmacologic methods of pain relief.

- Educate the patient about nonpharmacologic management of pain, such as sleep hygiene, progressive relaxation, repositioning, distraction, and integrative therapies. Combining pharmacologic and nonpharmacologic techniques provides enhanced pain control and increased quality of life. Involving family or friends increases patient support and well-being.
- Teach patients and their families the importance of adequate sleep and rest and not overusing the area in pain.
- Provide information about community resources, including support groups and pain clinics. If needed, supply resources for home care, financial assistance, support groups, and counseling.

- Administer analgesics as prescribed. (*Note:* Analgesics should be administered around the clock or by self-administration with a patient-controlled analgesic (PCA) pump to keep the pain from becoming severe.)
- Re-assess the patient's pain within 15–20 minutes of administering a pain medication. (*Note:* 15–20 minutes is

a general guideline. Intravenous narcotic analgesics act faster than oral pain medication).
- Regularly monitor patients to determine the effectiveness of analgesics and nonpharmacologic interventions.
- When administering opioids, monitor the patient for signs of respiratory depression. Slowly titrate opioid

Nursing Care Plan
A Patient with Chronic Pain

James Grier, age 28, visits the pain clinic with chronic low back pain. He states that he worked in a warehouse 3 years ago and injured his back while lifting heavy boxes. Although he was treated for the initial injury, he has had chronic back pain since then. During severe flare-ups, he can barely move, and he misses work approximately 5 days per month because of his back pain.

ASSESSMENT	DIAGNOSES	PLANNING
In an interview with Kenneth Hill, RN, regarding his pain, Mr. Grier rates his pain as a 7 on a scale of 0–10. Flare-ups usually last about a week before his pain is controlled to a 5. Mr. Grier describes his constant pain as a dull ache, but it throbs during flare-ups, with sharp piercing sensations during movement. Nothing seems to relieve the pain except lying completely still, although the pain keeps him from falling asleep. He is currently taking ibuprofen as needed, which is usually 400 mg every 4 hours. In the past, he has taken Vicodin, 5–10 mg every 4–6 hours, with moderate success, although it gives him slight nausea and drowsiness. Upon observation, Mr. Hill notes that Mr. Grier has no obvious external sources of pain, but he does have beads of sweat on his forehead. Mr. Hill also notices that Mr. Grier grimaces and holds his breath during movement, and his movements are very slow. A physical assessment indicates temperature 100.8°F oral; pulse 92 bpm; respirations 20/min with shallow breaths; and blood pressure 130/84 mmHg.	- *Chronic Pain* related to lower back pain as evidenced by behavioral and sympathetic reactions and the patient's report. - *Impaired Physical Mobility* related to severe lower back pain as evidenced by slow movements and grimacing during movement. - *Disturbed Sleep Pattern* related to lower back pain as evidenced by patient's report. - *Readiness for Enhanced Knowledge* about pain management. - *Fear* about potential job loss. (NANDA-I © 2014)	- After 3 days on the pain medication, the patient will report a decrease in pain intensity from a 7 to a 3 or 4 on the numeric scale. - The patient will report increased physical mobility with no increase in pain intensity over baseline during movement. - The patient will demonstrate an understanding of good sleep hygiene and will report receiving adequate sleep. - The patient will demonstrate knowledge about nonpharmacologic methods of pain relief. - The patient will choose three methods of nonpharmacologic pain relief to implement. - The patient will report decreased pain as a result of nonpharmacologic therapies. - The patient will report a decrease in lost workdays as a result of lower back pain.

Nursing Care Plan (continued)

IMPLEMENTATION

- Consult with a physician about opioid and nonopioid analgesic therapies for Mr. Grier.
- Teach Mr. Grier the importance of taking pain medications around the clock.
- Teach Mr. Grier about nonpharmacologic interventions, including heat, distractions, acupuncture, massage, and mild exercise.
- Encourage Mr. Grier to talk about his pain, and validate his pain experience. *Rationale: Through validation, the nurse is able to*

support and authenticate the patient's pain experience. Validation decreases the patient's anxiety, which will improve the patient's pain experience.

- Provide Mr. Grier with contact information for the pain clinic and encourage him to call the clinic if his prescribed therapies are ineffective.
- Encourage Mr. Grier to set regular follow-up appointments to help manage his pain effectively over time.

EVALUATION

Four days after Mr. Grier's appointment, Mr. Hill calls Mr. Grier to assess his pain. Mr. Grier reports that he has been taking his pain medications as prescribed. He is applying heat to his back for 30 minutes three times a day, and he is performing strengthening exercises for his back. When the pain is most severe, he listens to music to help distract him from the pain. Mr. Grier reports that with this new therapy, his pain is now a 4 on a scale of 0–10.

One month after his appointment, Mr. Grier returns to the pain clinic for a follow-up appointment. He reports that his pain

has been a 2 or 3 for the past week, and he has missed only one day of work in the past month. He continues to take the nonopioid analgesics as instructed and performs strengthening exercises three times a week. His boss has noticed an increase in his work productivity. To maintain pain control without opioids, Mr. Hill recommends alternating acetaminophen and ibuprofen and adding a monthly back massage to Mr. Grier's therapeutic regimen.

CRITICAL THINKING

1. Mr. Grier asks you why he needs to continue the strengthening exercises and include back massages in his therapy. What do you tell him?

2. If Mr. Grier reports excessive nausea in response to his opioid medication, what suggestions will you give him to decrease his nausea and provide comfort?

3. How would you adapt this care plan to a patient with knee pain instead of back pain?

---

antagonists (naloxone) to reduce the effects of the opioid agonist if prescribed.

- Help patients with self-care measures, such as bathing, toileting, and oral care.
- Provide comfort measures, such as offering snacks or drinks; changing bed linens; keeping noise, light, and room temperature at appropriate levels; and giving back massages.

Evaluation

Evaluation of the effectiveness of pain control measures begins with asking patients if they have experienced relief and, if so,

to what degree. A consistent pain rating scale should be used throughout the course of care. The nurse should also evaluate behavioral signs of continued pain. The time to onset for pain medication is highly dependent on the route of analgesic administration, the type of nonpharmacologic intervention, and the patient's pain level prior to initiation of therapy. Oral medications may take up to an hour to provide relief, while intravenous medications should begin working within minutes. If pain is still present, the nurse must evaluate the care plan, suggest changes to pharmacologic therapy, and implement changes to nonpharmacologic therapy.

REVIEW   Acute and Chronic Pain

RELATE Link the Concepts and Exemplars

Linking the exemplar of acute and chronic pain with the concept of culture and diversity:

1. How might understanding of the culture of a patient who appears to be in pain but denies it help you interpret the dichotomy between body language and reported pain?

2. How might interpretations and interventions for pain differ among cultures?

Linking the exemplar of acute and chronic pain with the concept of stress and coping:

3. What alterations in stress and coping would you anticipate when a patient experiences chronic pain?

4. A mother with acute pain over the past few weeks relates that she has not had the energy to deal with her children. How is pain affecting this patient's ability to cope with her children's needs?

READY Go to Volume 3: Clinical Nursing Skills

REFER Go to Pearson MyLab Nursing and eText

- Additional review material

REFLECT Apply Your Knowledge

Mr. Sharp is a 48-year-old Cherokee Indian. His history includes nicotine abuse, lung cancer, arthritis in both knees, and headaches.

Mr. Sharp has trouble breathing, especially after exertion. During a routine checkup, the nurse's assessment reveals that Mr. Sharp is experiencing severe pain in his right side when inhaling, and he has painful mouth sores as a result of his chemotherapy treatment. Between the chemotherapy and the mouth sores, Mr. Sharp is losing weight because of inadequate food intake.

1. What cultural influences do you need to consider when assessing Mr. Sharp's pain?

2. Should Mr. Sharp's history of nicotine abuse influence which pharmacologic agents are prescribed for his pain? Why or why not? How can you advocate for Mr. Sharp if inadequate pain medications are prescribed?

3. What cultural practices can you recommend as nonpharmacologic therapy for Mr. Sharp's pain?

≫ Exemplar 3.B
End-of-Life Care

Exemplar Learning Outcomes

3.B Analyze end-of-life care as it relates to comfort.

- Summarize the needs of patients at the end of life.
- Identify the clinical manifestations seen in patients at the end of life.
- Describe legal and ethical issues that inform care of patients at the end of life.
- Contrast palliative and hospice care.
- Differentiate considerations for the care of children and adolescents who are at the end of life.
- Differentiate therapies used by interprofessional teams in the collaborative care of an individual at the end of life.
- Apply the nursing process in providing culturally competent care to an individual at the end of life.

Exemplar Key Terms

Advance healthcare directive, *187*
Assisted suicide, *187*
Death anxiety, *193*
Do-not-intubate (DNI) order, *187*
Do-not-resuscitate (DNR) order, *187*
Durable power of attorney, *187*
End of life, *184*
Euthanasia, *187*
Healthcare proxy, *187*
Hospice care, *188*
Living will, *187*
Palliative care, *188*

Overview

The 2015 publication from the Institute of Medicine titled *Dying in America: Improving Quality and Honoring Individual Preferences Near the End of Life* provides a comprehensive report regarding the current care provisions for people who are nearing death and need comprehensive care surrounding their medical condition. This report outlines education, practice, and research pertinent to providing palliative and end-of-life care to patients as well as providing ways to integrate person- and family-centered care into a team-based approach. This report serves as a valuable reference for nurses who are caring for those who are approaching this period in their life.

Around the world, people are living longer, but there is a higher incidence of diseases, such as cancer, that bring about an early death. **End of life** refers to the final weeks of life just before death. Nurses who are educated about palliative and end-of-life care can make the end-of-life experience as comfortable as possible for the patient and family members. Through their compassion, skills in provision of care, and communication skills, nurses are able to provide a holistic, individualized approach to assist families through these difficult times (Hospice and Palliative Nurses Association, 2015; Sherman & Free, 2015).

As skilled clinicians, nurses must understand the technical aspects of managing the physiologic changes associated with end-of-life care. As advocates, nurses must ensure that the patient is receiving the best possible care by collaborating with other healthcare providers and adjusting the plan of care as needed. As guides, nurses must use communication and intuition to support patients and their families through the dying process (Sherman & Free, 2015).

Dying and Death

According to the Centers for Disease Control and Prevention (CDC, 2015d), the top 10 leading causes of death in 2013 included heart disease; malignant neoplasms; chronic lower respiratory disease; cerebrovascular diseases; accidents (unintentional injuries); Alzheimer disease; diabetes mellitus; influenza and pneumonia; nephritis, nephrotic syndrome, and nephrosis; and intentional self-harm (suicide). These 10 causes of death accounted for nearly 75% of all deaths in the United States in 2015. In addition, 23,000 infants died in 2015 (CDC, 2015d). The top five leading causes of infant death were congenital malformations, complications related to short gestation and low birth weight, sudden infant death syndrome, maternal complications of pregnancy, and accidents (CDC, 2015d).

A majority (70%–80%) of Americans claim that they would prefer to die at home. In 2013, according to the CDC, 27% of Americans died in their home, approximately 21% died in a long-term care facility, and 29% died in the hospital (Stanford School of Medicine, 2016). Americans age 65 and older have a 40% chance of entering a long-term care facility, and most of those individuals will die either at the long-term care facility or shortly after transfer to a hospital. However, studies indicate that families are less than satisfied with the care their dying loved ones receive, stating concerns about insufficient treatment of symptoms, lack of communication with physicians, inadequate emotional

Box 3–9
The Dying Person's Bill of Rights

- I have the right to be treated as a living human being until I die.
- I have the right to maintain a sense of hopefulness, however changing its focus may be.
- I have the right to express my feelings and emotions about my approaching death in my own way.
- I have the right to participate in decisions concerning my care.
- I have the right to expect continuing medical and nursing attention even though cure goals must be changed to comfort goals.
- I have the right not to die alone.
- I have the right to be free from pain.
- I have the right to have my questions answered honestly.
- I have the right not to be deceived.
- I have the right to have help from and for my family in accepting my death.
- I have the right to die in peace and with dignity.
- I have the right to retain my individuality and not be judged for my decisions that may be contrary to the beliefs of others.
- I have the right to be cared for by caring, sensitive, knowledgeable people who will attempt to understand my needs and will be able to gain some satisfaction in helping me face my death.

Source: From Barbus, A. J. (1975). The Dying Person's Bill of Rights, created at the workshop *The Terminally Ill Patient and the Helping Person*. Lansing: South Western Michigan Inservice Education Council.

support, and not being treated with respect. These concerns were more likely to occur in hospitals and other institutions than in home hospice care.

Regardless of setting, nurses are in a unique position to ensure that patients and their families receive appropriate care as the patient approaches death. The Dying Person's Bill of Rights (see **Box 3–9** ⟫) reflects the needs of individual patients during the dying process. Note that this document reflects the dying individual's need for a combination of physical comfort, emotional support, personal autonomy, and respect from those caring for the individual and his or her family.

Clinical Manifestations

Various signs and symptoms of death can present themselves up to 3 months before a patient's death. Some of these are changes in attitude, while others involve physiologic changes such as decreasing blood pressure and abnormal breathing. If patients have accepted their illness, they may be more willing to acknowledge the signs of death. Family members of patients are sometimes not as willing to accept these signs. The nurse is responsible for keeping patients informed about their condition and about any changes they can expect. Keeping the family informed (with patients' permission) about expected changes in patients can also be beneficial. For example, individuals who have accepted the terminal nature of their illness often become withdrawn for a time. If the nurse is able to alert the family to this potential common response or explain it when it occurs, it may make this period of withdrawal easier for both the patient and the family.

Physiologic Changes

A number of physiologic changes occur when an individual's body begins to stop functioning. Some of these changes can be of great concern to the patient and/or the patient's family, so the nurse should make them aware of such alterations. Nurses should inform the patient and the family about the normal progression of physiologic symptoms, depending on the patient's illness; this will help them prepare for what to expect in the coming days or weeks.

Dyspnea

Dyspnea occurs when the patient has trouble breathing normally. This can be caused by a number of factors, including chemotherapy, heart failure, abdominal ascites, and infection. The treatment will depend on the patient's desires for medical interventions during end-of-life care. Oxygen via nasal cannula can be used to lessen the symptoms of breathlessness. If the patient permits pharmacologic interventions, opioids can be administered, as well as benzodiazepines for any underlying anxiety. Of the opioids, morphine is the most commonly administered medication for patients receiving end-of-life care. Nonpharmacologic nursing interventions may include positioning the patient with the upper body elevated to a level of improved comfort, using an overhead or bedside fan to keep air moving over the patient, and teaching the patient relaxation techniques to reduce anxiety.

Hypotension

Low blood pressure, or hypotension, occurs as a patient's body begins to near death. This is often accompanied by cool skin and an irregular pulse rate. Hypotension can lead to blurry vision, as well as confusion and dizziness; however, etiologies other than low blood pressure may also be the source of these symptoms.

Anorexia, Nausea, and Dehydration

Anorexia involves a patient's loss of appetite and desire to eat. This may be a symptom of the patient's illness, but it is also a common occurrence in patients at the end of life. Loss of appetite often will be of less concern to patients than to their families. Nurses should explain that anorexia is normal at this stage in the individual's illness. Patients may consider trying to eat their favorite meals, which should be prepared with strong spices, as these will help the meal to be more appealing to the patient.

Nausea is also very common at the end of life. Nausea may result from a variety of causes, including medications, constipation, anxiety, or overwhelming odors. Nonpharmacologic interventions include sipping ginger ale, eating crackers, and practicing relaxation techniques. If the patient allows pharmacologic interventions, an antiemetic may be prescribed to reduce nausea.

Dehydration is rarely a cause for distress in patients at this stage. Often the patient will complain of a dry mouth, for which nurses should assess and provide care every 2 hours. Small sips of water should be offered. Intravenous fluids are not recommended, as they will generally make the patient more uncomfortable.

Most families are unfamiliar with the signs of dying and may take some of them as a sign that the patient is "giving up." Families should be reassured that symptoms such as loss of appetite and nausea are a normal part of the dying process.

Altered Levels of Consciousness

Patients at the end of life may experience confusion as the result of infection, electrolyte abnormalities, medications, illness progression, and pain, as well as from many other causes. During periods of altered consciousness, the patient may begin rambling or acting contrary to normal behaviors; concentration is also poor during these periods. If patients' actions become uncontrollable or put the patients at risk, sedation may be necessary. In cases such as this, haloperidol or chlorpromazine generally is used. Patients in their last hours who have altered levels of consciousness can also be treated with morphine. It is helpful for these patients to be surrounded with familiar family and staff, as changes will only cause more confusion.

Pain

Pain and pain management are primary concerns for the patient in need of end-of-life care. If a patient is dying from a terminal illness or an untreatable injury or condition, the patient will also likely have pain. At this stage in the patient's care, pain medication should be administered as needed, as there is no longer a concern about long-term effects or addiction. Nurses conduct a thorough pain assessment to ensure appropriate interventions. (See the exemplar on Acute and Chronic Pain). Morphine or other opioids are the most common pain medications used, but co-analgesic drugs and nerve blocks may also be considered. To be effective, pain management should be reassessed at least twice a day, with modifications in treatment and dosage being made as needed.

Psychosocial Needs

Each patient and family will exhibit different emotional responses and have different psychosocial needs. Nurses can provide essential support by promoting healthy coping, ensuring that patients have the opportunity to make final preparations whenever possible, and providing nursing presence during the time of death.

Anticipatory Grief

Anticipatory grief can affect both the patient who is dying and the patient's family. This type of grief is experienced in advance of an individual's death. When anticipatory grief is experienced by patients who are dying, this grief is not only directed at their own death, but also at the loss of everything they love that will soon be gone. Anticipatory grieving can be a catalyst for saying good-bye to loved ones and resolving any unfinished affairs. However, it can also result in the patients' distancing themselves from friends and family members in an effort to decrease the pain of loss (Walsh, 2012). Patients' family members may also experience anticipatory grieving, which in some cases could help to lessen the intensity of grief after the patients' death. Not all individuals who know of a loved one's death will experience anticipatory grieving, but it is common. If possible, nurses can try to encourage patients and family members to be honest with one another about how they are feeling.

Final Preparations

As patients approach death, nurses should encourage the patient and family to say good-bye and make any final arrangements in accordance with the patient's final wishes. This stage can be very difficult for the patient's family, so nurses should explain that it benefits the patient to have as much resolution as possible before dying. Any final cultural or religious practices should also be arranged in accordance with the patient's requests.

Emotional Support

When a patient dies, nurses may be present with both the patient and family members. In nursing homes and memory care centers, for example, it is not uncommon for nurses and other staff members who have cared for the patient to be in the room with the patient and family as the patient dies. This can provide great comfort to the family, especially when nurses have taken the time to build a therapeutic relationship with both the patient and the family.

Once the patient has died, family members may desire to spend time alone with the deceased. Allowing this time is important. In particular, nurses can encourage parents of a child or adolescent to hold their child and take as much time as they need to say good-bye. Families should also be allowed time and space to observe cultural and spiritual practices (see Focus on Diversity and Culture: Culture and the Dying Patient).

Focus on Diversity and Culture
Culture and the Dying Patient

- Cultural and religious beliefs and traditions are often of paramount importance for end-of-life patients and their families. Nurses should work to facilitate requests to every extent possible. For example, some cultures (such as those who practice the Islamic faith) observe a ritual of cleansing the body immediately after death. Others may call for a priest or spiritual leader to say prayers with the patient who is dying and family members.
- If a nurse is uncomfortable with the cultural practices and traditions of the patient, then another nurse who is of similar background or who is comfortable with the patient's traditions, should be asked to work with that patient.
- For patients who do not speak English, nurses should seek the assistance of a qualified interpreter to ensure that they understand the patient's and family's needs, and that the patient and family understand the care being provided.
- The parents' decision to tell a child who is terminally ill of impending death may also be based on cultural practices; some cultures consider it imperative that the dying, especially the very young and the very old, not be told of their illnesses (Walsh, 2012).
- Expressions of grief also may be culturally influenced. Some cultures see it as a sign of weakness to grieve or cry openly. Other cultures see loud wailing and/or crying to be a respectful expression of grief. Nurses must refrain from assuming that loved ones are not grieving simply because they do not show grief to others.

Legal and Ethical Considerations

When caring for patients at the end of life, nurses are faced with legal and ethical issues, including honoring patients' wishes, finding out who should make medical decisions for the patient if the patient is unable to make decisions, and deciding how to deal with families that disagree about the course of treatment. Patients who have legal documents specifying their wishes, such as advance directives and do-not-resuscitate (DNR) orders, have the right to expect care based on these documents. Other ethical issues, such as euthanasia, must follow state and federal laws.

Advance Directives

Advance healthcare directives, or advance directives, are legal documents that allow individuals to choose their preferred treatment plan while they are mentally able to ensure that their wishes will be carried out even when they are unable to make decisions themselves. These directives take the form of living wills and durable powers of attorney (see **Table 3–9 ≫**). All advance directives must be in writing, signed by the patient, witnessed, and notarized. Advance directives may be used in the event the patient becomes incapacitated and is unable to direct his or her own care. For detailed information, refer to the exemplar on Advance Directives in the module on Legal Issues.

The American Nurses Association (ANA, 2012) has issued a position statement about the impact of DNR and allow natural death (AND) decisions on nursing care. The ANA recommends that nurses play an active role in initiating discussions about DNR/AND with patients, families, and healthcare team members to prevent confusion about the patients' and family's wishes about end-of-life care. With this responsibility, nurses have the duty to educate patients and their families about procedures and treatments used at the end of life, to inform patients about advance directives and ensure the documentation and implementation of existing advance directives, to encourage patients to think about their preferences for end-of-life treatment, to communicate patients' end-of-life decisions to the healthcare team, and to advocate for patients' decisions about end-of-life care in spite of differing opinions by the healthcare proxy or physician. Regardless of patients' DNR/AND status, nurses have

the responsibility to provide palliative care and other medical treatments for all patients.

A variation of the DNR/AND order is the "comfort measures only" (CMO) order. A CMO order indicates that the patient prefers to receive maximum comfort while progressing through the natural dying process. A CMO order is *not* equivalent to a DNR/AND order, although they are often issued simultaneously. Patients with a CMO order should receive effective pain and symptom management, spiritual care, food and fluids as the patient is able, and hygiene care.

Euthanasia and Assisted Suicide

Euthanasia and assisted suicide are controversial legal and ethical issues that face nurses caring for patients at the end of life. Both **euthanasia** and **assisted suicide** refer to intentionally ending a life in order to relieve pain and suffering. The difference between the two is who performs the final act that causes death. In euthanasia, the physician or other healthcare provider performs the last act, usually in the form of an intentional drug overdose. In contrast, assisted suicide occurs when the physician or another healthcare team member provides the lethal dose of medication but the patient administers the medication to herself or himself. As of 2016, assisted suicide is legal (or in the process of being legalized) in Oregon, Washington, Montana, California, and Vermont.

There are various terms related to euthanasia, and the ethical and legal ramifications of different types of euthanasia are widely debated. Euthanasia can be voluntary, nonvoluntary, or involuntary, and it can be passive or active. *Voluntary* euthanasia occurs when the patient or the patient's family gives consent for the actions that will result in death for the patient. *Nonvoluntary* refers to euthanasia that occurs when the patient and the patient's family are unable or unavailable to give consent. *Involuntary* euthanasia is defined as euthanasia performed against the wishes of the patient or the patient's family. In addition, *passive* euthanasia is performed by the withdrawal or withholding of life-sustaining treatments, whereas *active* euthanasia is performed by the administration of drugs that will cause death.

In 1994, the ANA drafted its original position statement indicating that nurses should not participate in voluntary, nonvoluntary, or involuntary active euthanasia because it is

TABLE 3–9 Advance Healthcare Directives

Document	Function
Living will	Describes the patient's treatment preferences for life-prolonging procedures such as the use of feeding tubes, mechanical ventilation, and resuscitation.
Durable power of attorney	Designates an individual to make medical, legal, and financial decisions for the patient in the event the patient is unable to do so.
Healthcare proxy (healthcare power of attorney)	Designates an individual to make healthcare decisions for the patient in the event the patient is unable to do so.
Do-not-resuscitate (DNR) order (or "no code" order)	A medical order written by a physician that states the patient's wishes to withhold cardiopulmonary resuscitation (CPR) in the event of respiratory or cardiac arrest. It covers only CPR; it does not pertain to other treatments such as medications or nutrition.
Do-not-intubate (DNI) order	An order that prohibits endotracheal intubation in the event of severe respiratory failure or respiratory arrest. The DNI order is separate and distinct from the DNR order, in that the DNI order applies to situations in which the individual is not in cardiopulmonary arrest.

in direct violation of the *Code for Nurses with Interpretive Statements,* and in 2013, the ANA reaffirmed this position (ANA, 2013). In addition, active euthanasia is illegal in all 50 states. In contrast, passive voluntary euthanasia is considered an acceptable medical practice and occurs often for patients with DNR orders or living wills specifying that the patient does not want mechanical breathing, feeding tubes, and other life-prolonging procedures.

Palliative and Hospice Care

When death is inevitable, many patients and families choose palliative care rather than pursuing aggressive treatments aimed at regaining health. According to the WHO, **palliative care** is an approach to patient care "that improves the quality of life of patients and their families facing the problem associated with life-threatening illness, through the prevention and relief of suffering by means of early identification and impeccable assessment and treatment of pain and other problems, physical, psychosocial and spiritual" (WHO, 2015).

During palliative care, the nurse is responsible for caring for patients and their family in eight domains (see **Box 3–10** ») (National Consensus Project for Quality Palliative Care, 2013).

Palliative care should be provided to all patients, especially older adults with an acute life-threatening illness (e.g., stroke, myocardial infarction, trauma) or a chronic progressive illness (e.g., end-stage dementia, liver or kidney failure, terminal cancer). Palliative care for children with a chronic disorder (e.g., cystic fibrosis, hemophilia, muscular dystrophy) should begin at the time of diagnosis. It should provide total care of the child's body, mind, and spirit as well as support for the family (WHO, 2014).

Nursing approaches to providing palliative care include relieving pain and other distressing symptoms, affirming life, viewing death as a normal process, integrating psychologic and spiritual aspects of care, offering a support system for both patients and their family, and using a team to address the needs of patients and families. Palliative care providers may become more involved as patients near death and cannot perform basic comfort measures, such as hygiene care and nutrition intake, for themselves. This kind of care allows patients to die with dignity, and it assures the family that the patient was as comfortable as possible throughout the dying process.

Most Americans who have an illness that is no longer responding to treatment prefer to die at home, free from pain, surrounded by loved ones. Hospice care makes this preference a reality (Hospice Foundation of America, 2013). Hospice does not seek to lengthen life or hasten death. Instead, **hospice care** provides comfort and dignity for patients' last days by offering care provided by a team-oriented group of trained professionals with a specialized knowledge of pain management. Hospice also provides emotional, social, and spiritual support for patients and their family as well as bereavement and counseling services for the family for 1 year after the patients' death. In many cases, hospice is provided by the patients' health insurance or Medicare policy. In 2014, an estimated 1.6–1.7 million patients used hospice services, 84% of those patients being over the age of 65 (National Hospice and Palliative Care Organization, 2015). To be eligible for hospice care, patients need to be diagnosed by a physician as having 6 months or less to live. In addition, patients and their families must be comfortable with the patients' receiving only comfort care rather than curative care. Patients can receive hospice care for two 90-day periods and an unlimited number of 60-day periods with continued recertification by a physician or a hospice medical director. In most cases, hospice care is offered through routine visits to the patients' home, although continuous care is available for patients in crisis. Hospice care can also take place in hospice centers, hospitals, nursing homes, and other long-term care facilities. Hospice care also supports the involvement of family in patients' care and is available to help ease the burden of primary caregivers.

Box 3–10
Eight Domains of Palliative Care

1. **Structure and processes of care**
   - Identify patients' and their family's values and goals.
   - Provide an interprofessional team knowledgeable about palliative care.
2. **Physical aspects of care**
   - Administer pain medications as needed to provide comfort.
   - Provide hygiene care (e.g., oral care, skin care, change of bed linens).
3. **Psychologic and psychiatric aspects of care**
   - Promote psychologic services for patient.
   - Provide grief counseling for family.
4. **Social aspects of care**
   - Call family to be present at end of life.
   - Refer to social services (e.g., hospice care).
5. **Spiritual, religious, and existential aspects of care**
   - Facilitate visits with clergy.
   - Allow practice of religious rituals.
6. **Cultural aspects of care**
   - Hire culturally diverse staff that is representative of surrounding population.
   - Administer care that is culturally competent.
7. **Care of the imminently dying patients**
   - Communicate signs of impending death to family.
   - Provide comfort to patients and family during last minutes of life.
8. **Ethical and legal aspects of care**
   - Consider legal and ethical aspects of care, such as advance directives and DNR orders.
   - Respect patient and families wishes within the legal and ethical constraints of practice.

Lifespan Considerations
End-of-Life Care for Children

Having a child who is in need of palliative care or facing the death of a child can be a life-altering experience for families. It is estimated that each year, around the world, 7 million children could benefit from palliative care (WHO, 2014). The rate of deaths in children in 2010 was 45,000, and more than half of them were under the age of 1 year (CDC, 2015c). Too often, children who die fail to receive competent and compassionate care that meets their physical, emotional, and spiritual needs. Nurses play a vital role in improving care for children facing a life-threatening medical condition.

Clinical Manifestations and Therapies
End-of-Life Care

ETIOLOGY	CLINICAL MANIFESTATIONS	CLINICAL THERAPIES
Muscle control	<ul><li>Decreased food and fluid intake resulting from difficulty swallowing and decreased GI activity</li><li>Bladder and bowel incontinence</li><li>Increased periods of sleep</li></ul>	<ul><li>Provide nutrients and hydration artificially if requested by the healthcare team and/or patient and family.</li><li>Provide oral care regularly.</li><li>Provide hygiene care as needed.</li></ul>
Circulation	<ul><li>Cyanosis of extremities</li><li>Decreased body temperature</li><li>Slower and weaker pulse</li><li>Decreased blood pressure</li></ul>	<ul><li>Provide warm blankets.</li><li>Gently massage to stimulate circulation.</li></ul>
Respiration	<ul><li>Cheyne-Stokes breathing</li><li>Noisy breathing (the "death rattle")</li><li>Apnea</li></ul>	<ul><li>Administer oxygen through nasal cannula if needed.</li><li>Provide mechanical ventilation if needed and desired.</li></ul>
Sensation	<ul><li>Blurred vision</li><li>Impaired taste and smell</li><li>Increased confusion and disorientation</li></ul>	<ul><li>Provide palliative care.</li><li>Maintain patient safety.</li></ul>

Children with life-limiting conditions should receive palliative care in much the same way it is provided to adults. However, palliative care is often neglected for infants and very young children. Nursing care should be based on the best interests of the child, not on the best interests of the parents. However, parents must be involved in the decision making regarding their child's care and should receive complete, timely, understandable information about the diagnosis, prognosis, treatments, and palliative care options for their child. Parents should be allowed to spend as much time as possible with their child, and nursing staff should provide privacy for the family as needed.

The National Hospice and Palliative Care Organization (NHPCO) identified that palliative care and hospice care (PC/HC) for children should be instituted from the time a child is diagnosed with a life-limiting condition until the time of death. The PC/HC team must be able to care for children with a wide range of disease trajectories, diagnoses, and developmental levels (Friebert & Williams, 2015). Palliative care is especially important for children who have a disease for which no treatment has been shown to alter progression toward death and for which medical technology creates a larger burden than benefit for the patient. Many barriers exist to providing effective care for children with life-limiting conditions and their families, including:

1. Provider-related barriers, such as lack of formal pediatric palliative care (PPC) education, uncertainty about a prognosis, and concern regarding timing of palliative care
2. Patient- and family-related barriers such as misperceptions between the child's and parents' beliefs about palliative care and the providers' beliefs about palliative care, and concern over the ability of community PPC to be provided at the level of satisfaction of hospital care

3. Resource-related barriers such as lack of community palliative service for children, lack of referrals to a PPC team, financial barriers, and cultural barriers (Kaye et al., 2015).

Advance care planning for children is most appropriate early in the course of the child's disease, when the child is not in crisis, so rational decisions can be made based on all available options in collaboration with the child, parents, and healthcare team. This timing allows the care plan to be altered to meet the child's individual physical, psychologic, and spiritual needs, improving the quality of care and providing satisfaction and relief for the caregivers. If advance care planning begins early, then the care plan can be modified as the child's disease progresses to enhance the child's quality of life (Kaye et al., 2015).

The top three barriers to advance care planning for children are unrealistic parent expectations, differences in the understanding of the child's prognosis between clinicians and patient/parents, and lack of parent readiness to have the discussion. Other barriers included ethical considerations, a lack of importance of advance care planning to clinicians, and not knowing what to say. Addressing these barriers may help healthcare providers become more proficient in discussing advance care planning for pediatric patients (Durall, Zurakowski, & Wolfe, 2012).

End-of-Life Care for Adolescents

Adolescents with a serious medical condition are more capable of making treatment decisions than most teenagers. Although the Patient Self-Determination Act of 1990 limits the legal rights of individuals younger than 18 to make their own healthcare decisions, adolescents have the cognitive skills to participate in discussions regarding their own care. Most adolescents desire autonomy, so the healthcare team should discuss all choices for healthcare with them, including legal and ethical issues. If adolescents state a desire to withdraw from or refuse treatment, the parents and healthcare team should discuss the reasons for their decision and help them understand the implications of their decision and any treatment alternatives that may influence their choice. When adolescents have made this decision based on facts, it may be easier for the parents and the healthcare team to accept their decision.

Ethical Issues Surrounding a Child's Death

Making healthcare decisions for dying children can be an emotionally charged experience for both the parents and the healthcare providers. Misunderstandings and conflicts between the child, the parents, and the clinicians based on differences in clinical understanding, personal and religious preferences, and strong emotions are common. Sometimes these conflicts lead to ethical issues, including withdrawing or withholding treatments, parental refusal of treatment, and DNR orders (see the Evidence-Based Practice feature).

Nurses and other healthcare providers have the responsibility to accurately portray the child's health condition and the benefits versus the burden of treatment. Some parents may resist the recommendation to withdraw or withhold a treatment, while other parents may refuse a recommended treatment or test. This refusal may be based on religious beliefs or on the belief that children should not be subjected to the side effects of the treatment. Parental refusal of treatment may also be based on the parents' understanding that their child will die in the near future and they want to avoid

prolonging the child's suffering and to provide a peaceful death for the child (Diekema, 2014).

A physician who feels that withholding a medical treatment based on parental preferences is detrimental to the child's well-being can request legal intervention to remove decision-making rights from the parents on the grounds of child neglect. If the lifesaving treatment is urgent, the healthcare team will not be held liable for providing the treatment without a court order and over parental objections. Instead, withholding a clearly beneficial treatment could lead to prosecution as a criminal offense, even if the decision to withhold treatment was based on parental wishes. In cases such as these, the nurse should provide adequate care for the child while seeking to resolve the conflict with the family.

Collaboration

Spiritual and religious beliefs shape the context of death for many individuals. Patients may feel that death is a punishment, a release from an evil world, or God's will. Spiritual beliefs may cause individuals to feel regret or peace, and religious practices may bring comfort during their last days. Any requests for spiritual support should be quickly fulfilled and respected. If nurses have conflicting beliefs and feel they cannot assist patients in their spiritual needs, they should find another member of the healthcare team or religious staff to fulfill that role for the patient.

Collaboration between healthcare providers is essential to providing quality care at the end of life. Nurses interact with patients most frequently, so they are responsible for communicating any changes in the patient's condition that

Evidence-Based Practice

Improving the Quality of End-of-Life Care in the Pediatric Intensive Care Unit

Problem

Communication between care providers of children in pediatric intensive care units is essential so that the wishes of the dying child and parents can be met. Sanderson (2013) identified that over 60% of the physicians who work in intensive and cardiac care units felt that a DNR order should be executed only during a cardiac arrest. Clearly, decisions regarding care at end of life take a collaborative effort between healthcare providers and parents.

Evidence

Healthcare professionals need to play seven major roles when helping parents make end-of-life care decisions for their children: *family supporter* (addresses the emotional, spiritual, and informational needs of the family), *family advocate* (helps articulate the family's wishes to the healthcare team), *information giver* (provides parents with medical information and options), *general care coordinator* (facilitates interactions among professionals), *decision maker* (influences the plan of action), *end-of-life care coordinator* (organizes care directly before, during, and after death), and *point person* (develops a unique trusting relationship with parents) (Michelson et al., 2013). Having a team of healthcare professionals working together with the parents to provide end-of-life care and help with decision making serves five general functions: facilitating understanding of a complex situation, clarifying and organizing important information and values, serving as a decision-making compass, communicating with others about complex topics, and

justifying decisions (Renjilian et al., 2013). When parents have a supportive team around them and share the decision-making process with the healthcare team, they tend to have less grief over time than parents who either had no involvement or had the sole burden of making decisions about the care of their child (Caeymaex et al., 2013).

Implications

At a time when anxious and grieving parents feel that everything is uncertain, adequate communication and support from the healthcare team can help reduce their stress and bring them relief. Regular communication from a single familiar individual about the child's condition, options for treatment, and the benefits and burdens of treatment will reduce the risk of receiving conflicting information and help parents make informed decisions that they will not regret years later.

Critical Thinking Application

1. What is the most important role for a nurse to play when caring for a family in which a newborn has only a few hours to live?

2. Suggest two methods of communication other than a face-to-face discussion that may be advantageous to parents with a terminally ill child.

3. Of the seven necessary roles played by healthcare providers, which role would you be most comfortable playing? Which would be least comfortable for you?

would warrant a change in the care plan. This responsibility may involve communicating with physicians about the need for medication changes, religious staff about the need for spiritual support, social workers or psychologists for emotional and social support, and family to determine which care plan to implement based on the patients' condition.

As stated by the IOM (2015), an integrative, comprehensive approach to end-of-life care should be provided to all patients:

> This care should be provided by nurses, geriatricians, social workers, chaplains and other healthcare team members as deemed appropriate by the patients' needs. This care should be provided to the patient and family across a variety of settings, including the hospital, nursing care facility, and the home setting. This care should be family oriented, of high quality, and should incorporate the patient and families wishes, including declining medical care or social services.

Pharmacologic Therapy

The most common symptom at the end of life is pain, so end-of-life care must include pain management. Other symptoms common at the end of life include anxiety, constipation, delirium, dyspnea, nausea, sleep disturbances, and loss of skin integrity (Crozier & Hancock, 2012).

Pain

Pain medications are given at low doses initially to minimize discomfort, and then they are gradually increased to provide adequate pain relief 24 hours a day, 7 days a week. The dose of medication should allow patients to function as normally as possible and maintain the desired quality of life. Because the fear of addiction or tolerance is not an issue at the end of life, strong opioid agonists such as morphine should be given continuously for pain, as tolerated by the patients, and fast-acting pain medications such as OxyFAST and fentanyl lozenges can be given for breakthrough pain. For patients in a hospital or long-term care facility who are confined to a bed, patient-controlled analgesia through IV infusion is a typical method of controlling end-of-life pain.

Other Symptoms

Palliative care includes the relief of pain and other symptoms, including depression and anxiety, dyspnea, constipation, delirium, nausea, sleep disturbances, and loss of skin integrity. Each of these symptoms should be treated through classical methods as desired by the patient and the family. For example, dyspnea can be treated with oxygen, constipation can be relieved with stool softeners and laxatives, and nausea can be treated with antiemetics. Relief of symptoms may also include disease-specific medications, such as digoxin for congestive heart failure and dialysis for kidney failure. The goal of pharmacologic treatment is to give patients a high quality of life for the time they have left.

Nonpharmacologic Therapy

The use of nonpharmacologic therapies such as feeding tubes, mechanical respiration, and cardiopulmonary resuscitation are common at the end of life. Nurses must communicate clearly with patients and their families about the benefits and burdens of these therapies and discuss the desires of patients and their families to use these life-sustaining interventions.

Feeding Tubes

Patients at the end of life are often unable to take in food and fluids by mouth. Therefore, artificial nutrition and hydration (ANH) often is implemented via a feeding tube for nutrition and IV infusion of fluids for hydration. Withdrawing ANH for patients near death is an ethically controversial issue. Nutrition and hydration are essential to life, and patients, families, and clinicians are often reluctant to withdraw nutrition because they believe that starvation and dehydration are an agonizing way to die. However, clinical evidence suggests that patients who die after ANH withdrawal do not experience feelings of hunger and thirst, and they die peacefully (Arenella, 2015).

ANH does not improve the quality of life or the chance of recovery in terminally ill patients. In contrast, it may cause more discomfort for the patients, including increasing the patients' risk for esophageal perforation, infiltration of formula into the lung, infection, and edema (Alivizatos, Gavala, Alexopoulos, Apostolopoulos, & Bajrucevic 2012). In patients unable to take in food or drink by mouth, oral care in the form of applying moisture to the mouth and lips is adequate to relieve dry mouth, regardless of the hydration status of the patient.

Cardiopulmonary Resuscitation

Cardiopulmonary resuscitation (CPR) is the provision of artificial ventilation and external cardiac compressions to an individual who demonstrates cardiac and respiratory arrest. Current CPR training incorporates application of an automated external defibrillator (AED) for detection and treatment of certain cardiac dysrhythmias. AEDs are designed to deliver an electrical impulse (shock) to the heart based upon the AED's analysis of the cardiac rhythm. Advanced techniques of CPR include endotracheal intubation, which allows for both manual and mechanical ventilation. In patients with medical conditions such as metastatic cancer, dementia, or renal disease, CPR is often ineffective. In addition, patients age 65 or older have a continually decreasing chance of surviving CPR as they age (Hoyce & Reich, 2015).

SAFETY ALERT Patients with frail health are susceptible to damage during CPR, including rib fractures, heart contusions, airway and pulmonary complications, and liver and spleen lacerations.

For patients without a DNR order, CPR must be administered by default, even if it is not in the best interest of the patient. Therefore, the desire of the patient and family to have CPR performed should be an ongoing discussion as the patient's condition changes. The nurse should remind the patient and family that agreeing to a DNR order is not equivalent to condemning the individual to die, and DNR orders can be reversed at any time.

Complementary Health Approaches

There are many opportunities for nurses to use integrative therapies when caring for patients at the end of life. Selected examples include gentle touch therapy, music therapy, massage, and animal-assisted therapy (Dorfman, Denduluri, Walseman, & Bregman, 2012).

NURSING PROCESS

Nursing care for patients at the end of life must encompass all facets of the individual. Physical care includes pain and symptom management and hygiene care. Emotional care incorporates therapeutic communication. Spiritual care includes making provisions for a visit from clergy or religious rituals, and social care involves encouraging visits from family and friends.

Assessment

End-of-life nursing assessments include: assessing the patient's pain level; determining the patient's awareness of dying; assessing for signs of approaching death (see the Clinical Manifestations and Therapies feature); asking the patient and family about a living will, a healthcare proxy, and DNR status; and asking the patient and family about any physical, emotional, or spiritual needs.

It may be helpful to interview patients or their families to find out more about the patient in order to provide personalized means of comfort. Enabling personal preferences related to activities, daily routines, and spiritual practices can bring great comfort to patients and their family members. Encourage close family members and friends to call or visit as often as possible, and encourage placement of pictures and reminders in the room where the patients can see or hold them.

State of Awareness

Glaser and Strauss (1965) developed an awareness-of-dying model that describes four contexts of patients' awareness of their condition: closed awareness, suspected awareness, mutual pretense awareness, and open awareness.

- **Closed awareness.** The patients are unaware of their impending death, even though the healthcare team and family have the information. This may be the preference of the patients' family or culture, or the healthcare team may believe it will help the patients maintain hope. Closed awareness is difficult to maintain for an extended length of time.
- **Suspected awareness.** No one directly tells the patients about their condition, but they begin to suspect that they are near death. Suspected awareness may result in a lack of trust between the patients and their healthcare providers.
- **Mutual pretense awareness.** The patients, family, and healthcare team all know that the patients' condition is terminal, but no one discusses it, perhaps because of the discomfort discussing death or to protect the patients or family from emotional distress. Mutual pretense gives the patients privacy, but it also prevents the dying individuals from confiding in anyone.
- **Open awareness.** The patients, family, and healthcare team know about the patients' impending death and openly discuss it as needed. Open awareness provides the patients with the opportunity to participate in finalizing their affairs, and it gives nurses the opportunity to communicate freely with the patients and assist in the grieving process.

Diagnosis

Nursing diagnoses that may be appropriate for patients nearing death include:

- *Swallowing, Impaired*
- *Urinary Incontinence, Functional*
- *Bowel Incontinence*
- *Sleep Pattern, Disturbed*
- *Tissue Perfusion, Risk for Ineffective*
- *Confusion, Acute*
- *Anxiety, Death*
- *Skin Integrity, Risk for Impaired*
- *Pain, Acute.*

(NANDA-I © 2014)

Nursing diagnoses that may be appropriate for family members of patients near death include:

- *Hopelessness*
- *Caregiver Role Strain*
- *Coping: Family, Compromised*
- *Grieving*
- *Decisional Conflict.*

(NANDA-I © 2014)

Planning

The nurse collaborates with the patient, family, and healthcare team to develop a written care plan based on the patient's and family's preferences; the patient's advance directives; the decisions of the healthcare proxy; and the patient's physical, spiritual, and emotional needs. For the patient near death, appropriate outcomes may include:

- The patient will remain free of discomfort as much as possible.
- The family will verbalize feelings and understanding of events associated with the death process.
- The patient will remain free of complications (e.g., loss of skin integrity).
- The patient will demonstrate decreased anxiety.

Implementation

For patients who require end-of-life care, interventions incorporate both physiologic and psychosocial concerns. In addition to pain management, key interventions address death anxiety and compromised family coping.

Promote Physical Comfort

All terminally ill patients reach a point when they can no longer care for themselves. Nurses are responsible for implementing caring interventions to prevent impairments in skin integrity, prevent and alleviate pain, and maintain patient hygiene. Nursing care for patients who are comatose or have a very low level of consciousness or cognition includes:

- Using artificial tears if the patient does not blink
- Keeping lights at a low level

- Keeping the patient's skin clean and dry
- Covering the patient only with a light blanket
- Using adult incontinence pads or pants for incontinence
- Turning the patient every 2 hours and maintaining joint positions.

Promote Emotional Well-Being

Death anxiety, or anxiety associated with impending death, may stem from the patient's concerns for self or for others. Likewise, anxiety may be experienced by those close to the one who is dying and who fear that their loved one will suffer. It can also affect healthcare workers who care for dying patients. Interventions to reduce death anxiety include methods to reduce suffering and loneliness, as those are two factors that contribute to death anxiety (Sherman, Norman, & McSherry, 2010). Implementing pain and symptom management and basic palliative care can reduce suffering. Encouraging family and friends to visit the patient can reduce loneliness.

Patients may be encouraged to leave memories for the family. This activity is particularly important for parents who are leaving behind young children. Nurses may suggest leaving notes or videos for the child to open on special occasions such as birthdays and graduations. Nurses may also encourage patients to reminisce about their life, maintain relationships, continue spiritual practices, and complete legal documents (Kissane & Parnes, 2014). Simple interventions might include taking time to listen, holding the patients' hand, and providing information about the dying process. Providing spiritual support to patients is also vital in reducing death anxiety.

Promote Family Coping

The death of a loved one can be particularly difficult for the spouse, young children who have lost a parent, or parents who have lost a child. Alterations in family coping are especially common when the death is unexpected. Nurses can help families cope with impending or recent death by providing emotional support and information about the patient's condition. Interventions may include referring the family to hospice, funeral homes, grief counseling, and support groups. If the family is caring for the patient at home, hospice can assist the caregivers by providing respite services. Additional supportive interventions may include the following:

- Refer the patient and family to social services and other agencies that provide financial support.
- Provide bedside activities and distractions to decrease boredom and to limit obsessing about death. Schools, churches, and civic organizations are excellent sources of volunteers who read, play cards or board games, sit with and pray, or simply listen to music with the patient.
- Encourage the patient (if able) to form a support group to discuss fears and ways to alleviate them.

Perform Postmortem Care

Postmortem care centers around three major nursing functions: care of the body, care of valuables, and completion of paperwork. Care of the body should not take place until the patient is pronounced dead. Uncleanliness and discoloration of the body can be disconcerting to the family, so nurses should make sure the body is clean and discoloration is minimized. Valuables from the patient should be returned to the family or designated other soon after the death. Documentation should be thorough and timely. Above all, nurses should provide compassionate care to the family, ensuring that family members are comfortable and feel that their loved one has died with dignity.

Evaluation

Patient care is evaluated based on the following expected outcomes:

- Patient's comfort is maintained throughout the dying process.
- Patient is supported by nursing and/or family presence at time of death.
- Family members are informed and prepared for patient's dying process.

Nursing Care Plan
A Patient at the End of Life

Tom Crandall is a 75-year-old man with advanced Alzheimer disease. Three weeks ago, he became very agitated and began having difficulty swallowing. He was transferred from his assisted living facility to a hospital with a psychiatric gerontology unit.

ASSESSMENT	DIAGNOSES	PLANNING
Once transferred, Mr. Crandall experienced a steady decline in health, and he was transferred to the acute care area of the facility after experiencing a major stroke. He is arousable but seems unaware of his surroundings. He is currently receiving oxygen via a face mask and enteral nutrition. The treating physician has called his family and asked them to come to the hospital, advising them that Mr. Crandall is unlikely to live much longer.	■ Confusion, Chronic ■ Breathing Pattern, Ineffective ■ Swallowing, Impaired ■ Self-care Deficit: Bathing (NANDA-I © 2014)	■ The nursing plan of care includes the following goals: ■ Patient will remain safe and free from harm. ■ Patient will remain normoxemic. ■ Family will verbalize feelings and understanding of events associated with the death process. ■ Patient will remain free from aspiration. ■ Patient will remain comfortable.

(continued on next page)

Nursing Care Plan (continued)

IMPLEMENTATION

The nurses caring for Mr. Crandall implement the following interventions:

- Administer medications, nutrition, and oxygen as ordered.
- Bathe patient and change linens as needed to maintain patient comfort.
- Provide oral care every 2 hours.
- Encourage family to express feelings about patient's terminal condition.
- Prepare family for signs and symptoms of impending death.

EVALUATION

Shortly after the family's arrival, Mr. Crandall died with family members surrounding him. Without regaining consciousness, he died peacefully with a gradual decrease in respirations and heart rate. His family members expressed appreciation that they had had the opportunity to tell him they loved him one last time.

CRITICAL THINKING

1. What recommendation or request would you make of the healthcare provider regarding Mr. Crandall's tube feedings? Explain your answer.
2. Mr. Crandall's daughter asks if he will be placed on a mechanical ventilator to support his breathing. How would you respond to this question?
3. Would you recommend that Mr. Crandall or his healthcare proxy agree to a DNR order? Why or why not?

REVIEW End-of-Life Care

RELATE Link the Concepts and Exemplars

Linking the exemplar of end-of-life care with the concept of family:

1. What is the priority nursing diagnosis for the family of the patient with a terminal illness requiring end-of-life care?
2. What teaching points would you provide the family of a terminal patient regarding end-of-life care?

Linking the exemplar of end-of-life care with the concept of grief and loss:

3. How can the nurse support the family's need to prepare for loss of a family member while meeting the patient's need for end-of-life care?
4. Describe your plan of care for helping the family of a school-age child with terminal illness provide end-of-life care for the child while meeting the family's need to grieve.

READY Go to Volume 3: Clinical Nursing Skills

REFER Go to Pearson MyLab Nursing and eText

- Additional review materials

REFLECT Apply Your Knowledge

Pam Allen is a middle-age woman who recently experienced a recurrence of colon cancer. She is dying. Mrs. Allen and her husband have elected for her to stay at home. Mrs. Allen's healthcare team includes a hospice nurse, a social worker, and her treating physician. Friends and church members have been bringing food for the Allen family. Mr. Allen has discussed his fears about Mrs. Allen's death with the social worker.

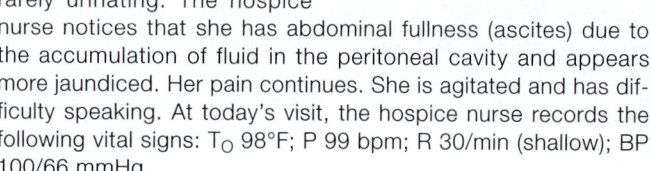

Mrs. Allen has had very little to eat or drink this week and is rarely urinating. The hospice nurse notices that she has abdominal fullness (ascites) due to the accumulation of fluid in the peritoneal cavity and appears more jaundiced. Her pain continues. She is agitated and has difficulty speaking. At today's visit, the hospice nurse records the following vital signs: T_O 98°F; P 99 bpm; R 30/min (shallow); BP 100/66 mmHg.

1. What is the priority of care for Mrs. Allen on this visit?
2. Based on the current assessment, what information would you provide Mr. Allen?
3. Would you consider notifying the physician of your current findings? Why or why not?

 # Exemplar 3.C
Fatigue

Exemplar Learning Outcomes

3.C Analyze fatigue as it relates to comfort.

- Describe the pathophysiology, etiology, risk factors, and prevention of fatigue.
- Identify the clinical manifestations of fatigue.
- Summarize diagnostic tests and therapies used by interprofessional teams in the collaborative care of an individual with fatigue.
- Differentiate considerations for care of patients with fatigue across the lifespan.
- Apply the nursing process in providing culturally competent care to an individual with fatigue.

Overview

Fatigue is characterized by tiredness, exhaustion, apathy, and lack of motivation. Fatigue is a subjective symptom that points to an underlying cause, such as illness, sleep deprivation, or intense physical or mental exertion. In addition, fatigue may occur because the individual feels the cultural pressure to perform a certain role, such as a mother who works outside the home and was up all night caring for a sick child or a husband who works three jobs to provide for his family. Fatigue usually is relieved by adequate sleep and rest and by treatment of the underlying condition causing the fatigue.

Pathophysiology and Etiology
Pathophysiology

Fatigue is associated with a decrease in the body's energy reserves that affects all basic body functions, including muscle contraction, neural transmission, and cellular regulation. Any physical condition that requires extracellular energy, such as illness, infection, sleep deprivation, malnutrition, and overexertion, can deplete energy and cause fatigue. Excessive cognitive demands, such as studying for an exam or working long hours, can also deplete energy reserves.

Fatigue associated with a chronic illness may result from a dysregulation of corticotropin-releasing hormone (CRH) and the hypothalamic–pituitary–adrenal (HPA) axis. The stress response, proinflammatory cytokines, and serotonin and norepinephrine neurotransmitter systems are all linked to CRH and HPA control, so any disruption in these systems can cause fatigue (CDC, 2015a). Fatigue is also associated with mood disorders such as depression and anxiety, which are also linked to changes in neurotransmitter regulation.

Etiology

According to the National Library of Medicine (2013), fatigue has many causes, including:

- Anemia (including iron deficiency anemia)
- Depression or grief
- Medications such as sedatives or antidepressants
- Persistent pain
- Sleep disorders such as insomnia, obstructive sleep apnea, and narcolepsy
- Hyper- or hypothyroidism
- Regular use of alcohol or illicit drugs
- Chronic diseases such as arthritis, cancer, diabetes, fibromyalgia, and liver or kidney disease.

Acute fatigue is mental or physical exhaustion associated with a temporary change in life circumstances, such as acute illness, planning a major event (e.g., a wedding), studying for an exam, starting a new job, or recovering from a natural disaster. Acute fatigue is normally resolved by the completion of the event and a good night of sleep. In contrast, **chronic fatigue** is mental or physical exhaustion associated with a chronic condition or situation that is not resolved quickly, such as a chronic illness or medications taken for a chronic illness, a single mother working to care for her family, or poor lifestyle habits. Caregivers for family members with a chronic or terminal illness are also susceptible to developing chronic fatigue.

Risk Factors

In addition to an acute or chronic illness or condition, other risk factors for fatigue include lifestyle factors (e.g., alcohol abuse, excessive physical activity, inactivity, lack of sleep), medications (e.g., antihistamines, pain medications, heart medications), medical procedures (e.g., surgery, chemotherapy), and mood disorders (e.g., depression, grief, stress) (CDC, 2015a).

Genetics also plays a role in fatigue. Individuals with alterations in the HPA axis and in neurotransmitter signaling are more susceptible to fatigue (CDC, 2015a). Women also tend to be highly susceptible to fatigue (see **Box 3–11** »).

Prevention

Fatigue resulting from lifestyle choices can be prevented by a balanced diet, daily exercise (see the Evidence-Based Practice feature), good sleep hygiene (see the Patient Teaching feature in The Concept of Comfort), and stress reduction. Eating several small meals each day instead of fewer large

---

Box 3–11
Fatigue and Women: Associated Conditions and Lifestyle Factors

- **Anemia.** Deficient iron intake can cause menstruating women to develop anemia and fatigue.
- **Poor nutrition.** Women who go on crash diets or consume high-fat, low-carbohydrate foods are subject to malnutrition, causing lethargy. When poor nutrition is coupled with water pills, hypokalemia can produce fatigue. Use of alcohol or drugs can also cause fatigue.
- **Endocrine gland function.** Hypothyroidism and loss of adrenal function can both lead to increased fatigue. Approximately 70% of the population with hypothyroidism are women.
- **Depression.** Clinical depression can cause fatigue, and more women than men are diagnosed with depression each year.
- **Heart failure.** Heart failure deprives tissues of oxygen and thus leads to fatigue.
- **Chronic fatigue syndrome.** Chronic fatigue syndrome is characterized by overwhelming fatigue that can last for months or years and does not get better with rest.
- **Liver disease.** Fatigue, along with nausea, vomiting, pain, and jaundice, is a symptom of liver disease.

Sources: Data from Mayo Clinic. (2016). *Symptoms of fatigue.* Retrieved from http://www.mayoclinic.org/symptoms/fatigue/basics/causes/sym-20050894; Wedro, B. (2013). *Fatigue related diseases and conditions.* Retrieved from http://www.medicinenet.com/fatigue/related-conditions/index.htm; CDC. (2015a). *Chronic fatigue syndrome.* Retrieved from: http://www.cdc.gov/cfs/causes/index.html

Evidence-Based Practice
Exercise and Fatigue

Problem

Americans often lead a sedentary lifestyle, spending much of their time at a desk or watching TV. This lifestyle can lead to fatigue and other health complications. In addition, many chronic health problems and the treatments they require cause fatigue.

Evidence

Fatigue has shown to be reduced with the use of mild to moderate exercise post-therapy in patients with multiple types of cancer, including prostate, breast cancer, and other solid tumors (Cramp & Byron-Daniel, 2012). Exercise also reduces fatigue in other chronic conditions, such as obstructive sleep apnea (Kline et al., 2012), multiple sclerosis (Kargarfard, Etemadifar, Baker, Mehrabi, & Hayatbakhsh, 2012), and depression (Cooney, Dwan, & Meak, 2015). Kiecolt-Glaser and colleagues (2014) showed that yoga can reduce fatigue associated with mood and inflammation in women. Those who have chronic fatigue syndrome and those who have been inactive from chronic health conditions should consider graded exercise therapy (GET). This type of exercise begins slowly and gradually increases over time as the patient gains strength and stamina (CDC, 2013; Kargarfard et al., 2012).

Implications

Patients who report persistent fatigue should be encouraged to begin a physician-approved mild to moderate exercise regimen. Higher-intensity exercise does not appear to produce a greater reduction in fatigue, so patients should be instructed to avoid intense workouts that may increase feelings of fatigue. In particular, conflicting results of exercise therapy are seen in patients with chronic fatigue syndrome (CDC, 2013), so these individuals should use exercise therapy with caution.

Critical Thinking Application

1. Why does a sedentary lifestyle contribute physiologically to fatigue? How does mild activity reverse these physiologic changes?
2. For what conditions (other than chronic fatigue syndrome) may an exercise program be contraindicated?
3. Develop a mild exercise program for a patient who has recently completed chemotherapy for breast cancer and is experiencing cancer-related fatigue.

meals helps prevent fatigue. Good hydration is also part of a balanced diet (six to eight 8-oz. glasses of water daily). Healthy diets limit refined sugar and fried and processed foods. In addition, avoiding caffeine, alcohol, and tobacco products can also help prevent fatigue.

Practicing good coping techniques is vital to preventing stress-related fatigue. Stressful situations that contribute to fatigue should be identified, and patients should determine ways to reduce or remove those situations. If the cause of stress cannot be removed, relaxation techniques such as deep breathing, meditation, or massage may help reduce feelings of stress. Counseling sessions may also help patients cope with stress.

Clinical Manifestations

The most common symptoms associated with fatigue are drowsiness, exhaustion, and lack of motivation. Fatigue is also associated with a variety of physical signs and symptoms, including lethargy, muscle weakness, palpitations, dizziness and dyspnea upon mild exertion, loss of appetite, slow movements, and blurry vision. Neurologic symptoms of fatigue include difficulty concentrating, impaired decision-making abilities, confusion, impaired coordination, and slowed reflexes. In addition, fatigue can be characterized by sleep disturbances, loss of interest in previously pleasurable activities, and a depressed mood.

SAFETY ALERT In 2011, The Joint Commission issued a *sentinel event alert* identifying nurses who work longer than 12.5 hours have a threefold increase of making mistakes in patient care (Joint Commission, 2011b). Taking short breaks can reduce fatigue and improve performance. Nurses should be vigilant about taking adequate breaks (i.e., 10 minutes every 2 hours, 30 minutes for meals, free of patient care responsibilities) to prevent fatigue and errors that may occur because of fatigue.

Chronic fatigue syndrome, also called *myalgic encephalomyelitis*, occurs when an individual experiences severe tiredness that lasts more than 6 months, is not caused by a primary condition (e.g., drug dependence, immune disorders, heart

Focus on Diversity and Culture
Culture Shock

Another common type of fatigue is culture fatigue or culture shock. Changing cultures demands an adjustment period that can cause fatigue regardless of whether the individual is moving from a foreign country, a different city within the United States, or back home after being away. Differences between cultures may include changes in population size, language, nonverbal communication, religions, transportation systems, food, presence of family and friends, and climate. Small changes build over time to cause physical and mental fatigue, which should decrease the longer the individual lives within the new culture. Nurses should encourage individuals with cultural fatigue to maintain a positive attitude, learn as much as possible about the new culture, and to share their experiences and struggles with family and friends.

Clinical Manifestations and Therapies
Fatigue

ETIOLOGY	CLINICAL MANIFESTATIONS	CLINICAL THERAPIES
Iron-deficiency anemia	▪ Mild anemia may be asymptomatic. ▪ Moderate anemia may cause fatigue, irritability, headaches, and difficulty concentrating. ▪ Severe anemia may cause pale skin, brittle nails, shortness of breath, and lightheadedness upon standing.	▪ Iron supplements ▪ Erythropoietin ▪ Monitoring hemoglobin and hematocrit ▪ Nutrition counseling
Hypothyroidism	▪ Increased sensitivity to cold ▪ Hoarseness ▪ Unexplained weight gain ▪ Muscle weakness/tenderness ▪ Joint stiffness ▪ Depression	▪ Thyroid hormone supplementation (e.g., levothyroxine)
Infection	▪ Loss of appetite ▪ Fever ▪ Coughing ▪ Body aches ▪ Nausea and vomiting ▪ Pain	▪ Antiviral agents ▪ Antibacterial drugs ▪ Antitubercular agents ▪ Antifungals

disease, depression, cancer, sleep disorders), and is not relieved by stress reduction. In addition to these conditions, chronic fatigue syndrome is diagnosed only if it is accompanied by at least four of the following symptoms: malaise lasting longer than 24 hours after exercise, feeling unrefreshed after adequate sleep, forgetfulness, confusion, inability to concentrate, joint pain with no swelling, headaches not previously experienced, irritability, mild fever, muscle aches, muscle weakness, sore throat, and sore lymph nodes.

Lifespan considerations of fatigue are covered in a later section. Cultural considerations have an effect as well (see the Focus on Diversity & Culture feature).

Collaboration

Acute fatigue is usually resolved with sufficient sleep and healing of the cause of fatigue. Fatigue associated with an illness is more complicated and requires the support of a healthcare team. For example, fatigue related to a mood disorder such as depression or anxiety may require both pharmacologic treatment and counseling. Some patients may need extensive testing to determine the underlying cause of the fatigue.

Diagnostic Tests

Diagnostic tests are often ordered to find the underlying cause of fatigue. Typical causes of fatigue include anemia; changes in endocrine, kidney, or liver function; and infection. Therefore, initial diagnostic tests may focus on these physiologic areas. A sleep study, or polysomnography, may also be ordered to determine if a sleep disorder is the cause of fatigue.

Surgery

If fatigue is related to a change in thyroid function, specifically hyperthyroidism or thyroid cancer, surgery may be scheduled to remove part or all of the thyroid. Fatigue as a sign of cancer may prompt a biopsy and subsequent surgical removal of a solid tumor.

Pharmacologic Therapy

Pharmacologic therapy depends on the cause of fatigue. For example, patients with fatigue related to iron-deficiency anemia should receive iron supplements and/or erythropoietin (e.g., epoetin alfa [Procrit, Epogen]) to stimulate the production of hemoglobin and red blood cells. To be effective, the pharmacologic therapy must be tailored to the patient's specific condition.

Nonpharmacologic Therapy

Nonpharmacologic therapies for fatigue include good sleep hygiene, mild to moderate exercise, and cognitive–behavioral therapy. Graded exercise programs may be especially beneficial by helping the patient gradually build stamina for exercise. Suggesting activities the patient enjoys promotes adherence to the exercise program. Cognitive–behavioral therapy focuses on the patient's thoughts and their relationship to the presenting problem. It helps patients identify stressors that contribute to symptoms and to take personal responsibility for change. Nurses can assist patients in minimizing fatigue by determining the patients' best time of day and scheduling more challenging activities during that time. Complementary health approaches for fatigue include acupuncture, massage, and relaxation techniques. Herbal and dietary supplements may include ginseng, NADH, and

L-carnitine. However, no complementary health approach is consistently supported by clinical studies.

Lifespan Considerations

Fatigue in Children

Fatigue in children is generally the result of stress, illness, insufficient sleep, or improper nutrition. Infections and allergies are two common illnesses in children that can cause fatigue, but fatigue can also be a sign of anemia, diabetes, thyroid disorders, depression, sleep apnea, or leukemia. If proper diet and adequate sleep do not correct fatigue in children, nurses should encourage parents to keep a journal of the child's sleep patterns, food intake, and activities that lead to fatigue. This journal may help a physician diagnose the underlying condition causing fatigue.

Fatigue During Pregnancy

Fatigue is also a common occurrence during pregnancy. The body uses large amounts of energy to build the placenta in the first trimester and to support rapid fetal growth in the third trimester. Hormonal changes can also contribute to pregnancy fatigue. In addition, as the baby grows, it increases the mother's physical stress and disrupts sleep, adding to the feelings of fatigue. Pregnant women should be encouraged to rest when they feel tired, allow others to help with everyday tasks, cut out unnecessary commitments, sleep more, consume a healthy diet, take in adequate water, and get regular exercise. If fatigue persists, it may be a sign of iron-deficiency anemia. Expectant mothers should be encouraged to eat more protein, including lean meats and beans, and to take an iron supplement. Vitamin C increases iron absorption, so pregnant women should be encouraged to eat fruits and vegetables that contain high amounts of vitamin C, including citrus fruits, melons, strawberries, tomatoes, broccoli, potatoes, and spinach.

Fatigue in Older Adults

Fatigue is extremely common in older adults; 43% of older adults report feeling tired most of the time. Fatigue tends to increase with age, especially in patients with a chronic illness. In addition, fatigue is associated with worse health, decreased physical activity, functional decline, and loss of independence. Increased fatigue at baseline is also associated with an increased mortality rate in older adults (National Institute of Aging, 2015). Therefore, assessment and treatment of fatigue are essential for older adults, especially those with one or more chronic condition.

NURSING PROCESS

An important component in treating a patient with fatigue is determining the underlying cause. Thorough assessment of the patient's symptoms, along with measures to promote rest, are priority areas of focus.

Assessment

A nursing assessment for patients with fatigue includes observation, a health history, and a physical examination.

- ***Observation and patient interview.*** Observe the patient and assess for symptoms of fatigue, including slumped posture, inability to focus on the current topic, poor skin turgor, and slow movements. Equally important to note are observations associated with other health conditions that may cause the patient to experience fatigue, such as those identified in the Clinical Manifestations and Therapies feature. The health history should include questions about the duration, timing, and quality of the fatigue; how the fatigue affects activities of daily living and relationships with family members; diet, sleep, and exercise habits; any medications or medical conditions that may contribute to fatigue; and cognitive effects associated with fatigue.

- ***Physical examination.*** Physical assessment includes assessment of the patient's vital signs, mobility, hydration, and muscle strength. Fever and changes in pulse rate may indicate infection or stress. Dyspnea upon exertion is often a sign of fatigue, and decreased muscle strength can be a sign of muscular or nervous system defects. In addition, poor hydration, as indicated by poor skin turgor, is a source of fatigue. Changes in skin tone, including jaundice and cyanosis, may indicate liver, cardiac, or pulmonary disease.

Diagnosis

Nursing diagnoses related to fatigue may include:

- *Insomnia*
- *Sleep Deprivation*
- *Fatigue*
- *Activity Intolerance*
- *Coping: Readiness for Enhanced*
- *Stress Overload.*

(NANDA-I © 2014)

Patients with chronic fatigue syndrome may have more severe symptoms that indicate other nursing diagnoses, such as:

- *Self-Neglect*
- *Coping, Ineffective.*

(NANDA-I © 2014)

Planning

A plan of care for patients with fatigue may include the following outcomes:

- The patient will verbalize an understanding and practice of good sleep hygiene.
- The patient will verbalize feelings of increased energy.
- The patient will indicate an increased ability to perform activities of daily living.
- The patient will participate in a mild exercise program.
- The patient will experience increased motivation.
- The patient will explain the relationship of fatigue to a disease process and activity level.

It is important to incorporate the patient's goals and preferences into the plan of care. Providing patient-centered care increases the likelihood that the patient will succeed in following the therapeutic regimen.

Implementation

When implementing care to reduce fatigue, it is important to consider the patient's cultural and developmental needs regarding sleep rituals. Fatigue is a subjective symptom, so careful attention must be given to the patient's assessment of how he or she feels. Interventions may include patient teaching related to the importance of adequate rest and sleep, structuring activities to coincide with the patient's peak energy level, and assisting the patient with self-care activities.

Promote Effective Coping

For patients with chronic conditions, inadequate coping mechanisms may contribute to prolonged feelings of fatigue. Several interventions may enhance patients' ability to cope:

- Assess patients' normal methods of coping and social support network to identify more effective methods of coping.

- Establish rapport with patients' families and significant others and encourage them to participate in establishing the plan of care.

- Encourage patients to be involved in the decision-making process to increase their feelings of self-worth.

- Facilitate the process of setting short-term and long-term goals. Short-term goals provide a sense of accomplishment, and long-term goals help patients adhere to the suggested therapy.

Evaluation

Evaluate patients with fatigue periodically to determine if the medical and nursing interventions are effective. Evaluations should include both subjective and objective data to reveal if the patient goals are being met. If the interventions are ineffective, modify the therapy by finding more effective therapies. Further diagnostic tests may also be needed to determine if additional physiologic factors are contributing to fatigue.

REVIEW Fatigue

RELATE Link the Concepts and Exemplars

Linking the exemplar of fatigue with the concept of infection:

1. How does infection and/or inflammation put an individual at risk for fatigue?
2. Is fatigue more likely to be acute or chronic as the result of infection?

Linking the exemplar of fatigue with the concept of oxygenation:

3. How does uncontrolled asthma put patients at risk for fatigue?
4. What strategies could patients with asthma use to decrease their risk for fatigue?

READY Go to Volume 3: Clinical Nursing Skills

REFER Go to Pearson MyLab Nursing and eText

- Additional review materials

REFLECT Apply Your Knowledge

Mr. Joe Harmon is an 87-year-old man. He is a World War II veteran who had a massive anteroseptal myocardial infarction (MI) at the age of 57. His MI was secondary to asbestosis. Since the age of 57, he has been hospitalized three times for COPD and congestive heart failure (CHF). His skin color is ruddy, his conjunctivas are pale pink, he walks with a stooped posture, and he experiences dyspnea after walking 100 feet. He states that he feels "OK, just tired most of the time."

1. When obtaining Mr. Harmon's vital signs, what readings would you anticipate?
2. What diagnostic tests do you anticipate might be useful to determine the cause of Mr. Harmon's fatigue?
3. What nursing diagnoses would be appropriate for Mr. Harmon's plan of care?
4. Develop a teaching plan to discuss with Mr. Harmon and his wife.

≫ Exemplar 3.D Fibromyalgia

Exemplar Learning Outcomes

3.D Analyze fibromyalgia as it relates to comfort.

- Describe the pathophysiology, etiology, risk factors, and prevention of fibromyalgia.
- Identify the clinical manifestations of fibromyalgia.
- Summarize diagnostic tests and therapies used by interprofessional teams in the collaborative care of an individual with fibromyalgia.

- Differentiate considerations for care of patients with fibromyalgia across the lifespan.
- Apply the nursing process in providing culturally competent care to an individual with fibromyalgia.

Exemplar Key Terms

Fibromyalgia, *199*
Tender points, *199*

Overview

Fibromyalgia is a chronic syndrome characterized by widespread musculoskeletal pain, stiffness, fatigue, sleep disturbances, and difficulty concentrating. Pain usually occurs in specific **tender points** that occur in the neck, spine, shoulders, hips, elbows, and knees. Fibromyalgia affects approximately 10 million Americans, about 75%–90% of whom are women, although men and children can also develop fibromyalgia. Diagnosis of fibromyalgia usually occurs between ages 20 and 50, and the incidence rises with age (National Fibromyalgia Association, 2016).

Pathophysiology and Etiology

Pathophysiology

Fibromyalgia is a disorder of pain processing. Pain associated with fibromyalgia results from central amplification of pain signals, including spontaneous nerve activity, enlarged receptive fields, and abnormal levels of neurotransmitters. Hyperalgesia, or an increased response to painful stimuli, is mediated by *N*-methyl-D-aspartate receptors in the dorsal horn. Patients with fibromyalgia also experience *allodynia*, or sensitivity to stimuli that are not normally painful. Descending inhibitory pain pathways are inhibited in fibromyalgia so that the central amplification is exacerbated (Bellato et al., 2012; Gracely & Ambrose, 2012). Sleep disturbances result from changes in the HPA axis, particularly elevated cortisol levels in the evening. The fourth stage of sleep is the most disrupted as a result of deficiencies in growth hormone and insulin-like growth factor-1 (Bellato et al., 2012).

Etiology

The exact cause of fibromyalgia is unknown; over 70% of patients with fibromyalgia have no precipitating factor for the disease. However, infections such as hepatitis C virus (HCV), HIV, Coxsackie B, and parvovirus may lead to fibromyalgia. Physical trauma (e.g., acute illness, surgery, motor vehicle crashes), psychosocial stressors (e.g., chronic stress, abuse), vaccinations, and chemical substances can all be causative factors (Bellato et al., 2012).

Risk Factors

The overwhelming majority of individuals with fibromyalgia are middle-aged women, so being a woman between the ages of 20 and 50 is considered a risk factor for fibromyalgia. Other risk factors include a family history of fibromyalgia, having a psychiatric disorder such as attention-deficit/hyperactivity disorder (ADHD) or depression, or having a medical disorder such as irritable bowel syndrome or rheumatoid arthritis. Genetic abnormalities may also predispose individuals to fibromyalgia, including polymorphisms in the *5-HTT* and *SCN9A* genes (Vargas-Alarcon et al., 2012).

Prevention

There is no known way to prevent fibromyalgia. However, in the absence of triggering factors and comorbid conditions, maintaining a healthy lifestyle is the best way to decrease the risk of developing fibromyalgia. In addition, prompt diagnosis and treatment of fibromyalgia symptoms can reduce flare-ups and help manage the widespread pain and fatigue characteristic of fibromyalgia.

Clinical Manifestations

The primary clinical symptoms associated with fibromyalgia are widespread pain and fatigue. Widespread pain is

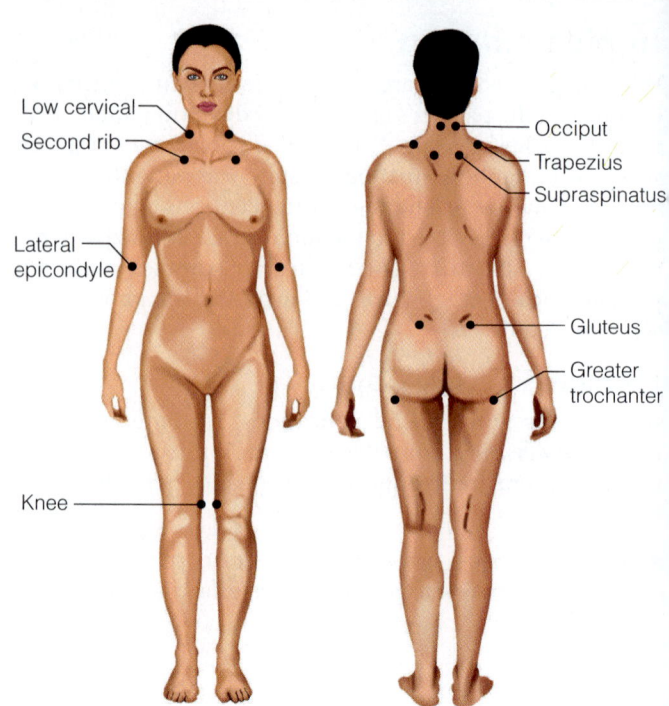

Figure 3–10 » Location of 18 paired "tender points" in fibromyalgia.

defined as pain above and below the waist and on the right and left sides of the body. Pain is often localized to 18 tender points located in the neck, spine, shoulders, hips, elbows, and knees (see **Figure 3–10 »**). Pain is typically described as deep, gnawing, stabbing, or burning, and it is not the result of inflammation or damage. Patients may also exhibit enhanced sensitivity to heat, cold, and pressure (Bradley, 2009). Pain and stiffness are often worse in the morning or after excessive physical activity.

Fatigue is likely the result of sleep disturbances, especially insomnia. Other sleep disturbances may include nonrestorative sleep, early morning awakening, and poor quality of sleep (Bradley, 2009). Systemic symptoms include mood disorders and cognitive dysfunction (often called *fibro fog*). Other symptoms associated with fibromyalgia include headaches, numbness in the hands and feet, irritable bowel syndrome, restless leg syndrome, and painful menstrual periods.

Collaboration

Fibromyalgia is difficult to treat. A combination of pharmacologic and nonpharmacologic therapies is needed to control pain and fatigue. Individuals with fibromyalgia are often referred to a rheumatologist for specialty care. In addition, treatment must address comorbidities such as depression, cognitive impairments, and irritable bowel syndrome.

The underlying cause of fibromyalgia is often unknown, so treatment directed at eliminating the source of pain is limited. A therapy or group of therapies that work for one patient may not be effective for another patient. Therefore, consistent evaluation of the patient's symptoms and the effectiveness of therapy and revision of the care plan are necessary to provide maximal relief from pain and fatigue associated with fibromyalgia. Patients who are having difficulty finding an effective treatment should be encouraged to keep trying new therapies until they find a treatment that allows them to cope with the disease and maintain an active lifestyle.

Diagnostic Tests

Diagnosis of fibromyalgia is based on criteria set by the American College of Rheumatology. The initial criteria, defined in 1990, stated that the patient must have widespread pain in all four quadrants of the body and a painful response to pressure on 11 of 18 tender points (Wolfe et al., 1990). The 2010 updated criteria (see **Box 3–12** ») define fibromyalgia as a widespread pain index of 7 or more, a symptom severity scale score of 5 or more, the presence of symptoms for at least 3 months, and the absence of a disorder that would otherwise explain the pain (Wolfe et al., 2010).

All laboratory and diagnostic tests are negative for individuals with fibromyalgia. Therefore, patients with positive blood tests, abnormal hormone levels, and abnormal imaging scans may have another underlying cause for their pain and fatigue. Symptoms associated with fibromyalgia are common to many diseases. So similar diseases, such as rheumatoid arthritis and hypothyroidism, should be ruled out before fibromyalgia is diagnosed.

Pharmacologic Therapy

Three drugs have been approved by the FDA for the treatment of fibromyalgia: duloxetine (Cymbalta), milnacipran (Savella), and pregabalin (Lyrica). Duloxetine and milnacipran are selective serotonin and norepinephrine reuptake inhibitors (SSNRIs). They are given orally at low doses initially. The drug dosage can then be increased to manage the patient's comfort. Common side effects of the drugs are nausea, dry mouth, constipation, dizziness, hot flashes, and insomnia. Both duloxetine and milnacipran interact with many drugs, so the healthcare team should carefully survey the patient's medications before initiating therapy (Wilson, Shannon, & Shields, 2016). Duloxetine is recommended for patients with significant depression, whereas milnacipran is recommended for patients with significant fatigue or cognitive dysfunction (Bellato et al., 2012).

Pregabalin is a GABA analog with anticonvulsant, analgesic, and anxiolytic properties. To begin therapy, it is given orally at a low dose; the dose can be titrated to a maximum dosage of 450 mg/day. Common side effects are ataxia, dizziness, somnolence, weight gain, and blurry vision (Adams et al., 2017).

Other pharmacologic therapies for fibromyalgia pain are acetaminophen and NSAIDs. Tricyclic antidepressants such as amitriptyline have also been used with some success, although SSNRIs are more commonly used. Tramadol may also be effective in providing pain and sleep relief (Bellato et al., 2012).

Box 3–12
2010 Fibromyalgia Diagnostic Criteria

A patient who exhibits the following three conditions satisfies the diagnostic criteria for fibromyalgia:

1. Widespread pain index (WPI) ≥ 7 and symptom severity (SS) scale score ≥ 5, or WPI 3–6 and SS scale score ≥ 9
2. Symptoms have been present at a similar level for at least 3 months
3. The absence of a disorder that would otherwise explain the pain.

Ascertainment

1. WPI: Note the number areas in which the patient has had pain over the last week. In how many areas has the patient had pain? Score will be between 0 and 19.

Shoulder girdle, left or right	Jaw, left or right
Upper arm, left or right	Chest
Lower arm, left or right	Abdomen
Hip (buttock, trochanter), left or right	Upper or lower back
Upper leg, left or right	Neck
Lower leg, left or right	

2. SS scale score:

   Fatigue

   Waking unrefreshed

   Cognitive symptoms

For each of the 3 symptoms above, indicate the level of severity over the past week using the following scale:

0 = no problem

1 = slight or mild problems, generally mild or intermittent

2 = moderate, considerable problems, often present and/or at a moderate level

3 = severe: pervasive, continuous, life-disturbing problems

Considering somatic symptoms in general, indicate whether the patient has*

0 = no symptoms

1 = few symptoms

2 = a moderate number of symptoms

3 = a great many symptoms

The SS scale score is the sum of severity of the three symptoms (fatigue, waking unrefreshed, and cognitive symptoms) plus the extent (severity) of somatic symptoms in general. The final score is between 0 and 12.

*Somatic symptoms that might be considered: muscle pain, irritable bowel syndrome, fatigue/tiredness, thinking or remembering problem, muscle weakness, headache, pain/cramps in the abdomen, numbness/tingling, dizziness, insomnia, depression, constipation, pain in the upper abdomen, nausea, nervousness, chest pain, blurred vision, fever, diarrhea, dry mouth, itching, wheezing, Raynaud phenomenon, hives/welts, ringing in the ears, vomiting, heartburn, oral ulcers, loss of/change in taste, seizures, dry eyes, shortness of breath, loss of appetite, rash, sun sensitivity, hearing difficulties, easy bruising, hair loss, frequent urination, and bladder spasms.

Source: From Wolfe, F., Clauw, D. J., Fitzcharles, M-A., Goldenberg, D. L., Katz, R. S., Mease, P., . . . Yunus, M. B. (2010). The American College of Rheumatology preliminary diagnostic criteria for fibromyalgia and measurement of symptom severity. *Arthritis Care and Research, 62*(5), 600–610. doi:10.1002/acr.20140

Evidence-Based Practice
Aerobic Exercise and Strength Training for Fibromyalgia

Problem

Patients with fibromyalgia experience a decrease in physical activity because of pain and fatigue. The combined effects of pain, fatigue, and activity intolerance dramatically reduce patients' quality of life.

Evidence

Aerobic training improves peak oxygen uptake and decreases pain intensity and fatigue (Hooten, Qu, Townsend, & Judd, 2012), and strength training increases muscle strength, health status, and current pain intensity in patients with fibromyalgia (Larsson et al., 2015). In addition, a more recent study conducted by Sevimli, Kozanoglu, Guzel, and Doganay (2015) found that aquatic therapy for fibromyalgia may be more effective than a gym-based aerobic exercise program or an isometric strength and stretching exercise program.

Implications

Patients with fibromyalgia should perform aerobic exercise of low to moderate intensity two or three times per week. Exercise should begin at a low level of intensity, and intensity and duration should increase as the patient builds physical fitness. To increase adherence, exercises should be a land- or water-based activity that the patient enjoys. Patients may see a short-term increase in pain and fatigue, but this increase should be manageable and will decrease over time. More research is needed to determine which type of exercise is most beneficial based on age, specific diagnoses, and health status (Sevimli et al., 2015).

Critical Thinking Application

1. Develop an exercise regimen for a 38-year-old female patient with fibromyalgia. How would it differ for a 15-year-old female patient? A patient with asthma?
2. Prepare a patient teaching brochure describing exercise suggestions for patients with fibromyalgia, including references for locations where the exercise can be performed.
3. What modifications in an exercise program would you recommend to a patient who complains of increased joint stiffness after exercise?

Nonpharmacologic Therapy

The two primary nonpharmacologic therapies linked to successful treatment of fibromyalgia are aerobic exercise and strength training (see the Evidence-Based Practice feature). Aquatic exercises may be helpful, and tai chi has been shown to improve symptoms (NCCIH, 2016b), physical function, quality of sleep, self-efficacy, and mobility.

Cognitive–behavioral therapy and relaxation therapy produce a moderate effect in short-term pain reduction and sleep problems compared to other psychologic treatments (Bellato et al., 2012). According to the National Center for Complementary and Integrative Health (NCCIH), there is insufficient research to support the use of "natural" products, including dietary supplements (NCCIH, 2016b).

Clinical Manifestations and Therapies
Fibromyalgia

ETIOLOGY	CLINICAL MANIFESTATIONS	CLINICAL THERAPIES
Pain	■ WPI ≥ 7 and SS scale score ≥ 5, or WPI 3–6 and SS scale score ≥ 9 ■ Pain lasting longer than 3 months ■ Pain not associated with any other condition	■ Duloxetine ■ Milnacipran ■ Pregabalin ■ NSAIDs ■ Aerobic exercise ■ Strength training ■ Massage
Fatigue	■ Chronic fatigue ■ Acute fatigue associated with increased activity	■ Milnacipran ■ Good sleep hygiene ■ Relaxation therapy ■ Tai chi
Sleep disruptions	■ Insomnia ■ Restless leg syndrome ■ Nonrestorative sleep ■ Early morning awakening ■ Poor quality of sleep	■ Duloxetine ■ Milnacipran ■ Pregabalin ■ Tramadol ■ Good sleep hygiene

Lifespan Considerations

Although fibromyalgia is most common in middle-age women, children and adolescents may develop a form of fibromyalgia called *juvenile primary fibromyalgia syndrome* (JPFS). JPFS is most commonly diagnosed in girls between the ages of 13 and 15. Triggers and symptoms of JPFS are similar to those of adult fibromyalgia. More than 80% of children who have JPFS will have fibromyalgia that persists into adulthood (Kashikar-Zuk et al., 2014).

NURSING PROCESS

The primary goals of fibromyalgia treatment are to reduce pain, increase restorative sleep, and improve physical function. Patients require a great deal of support as they seek a diagnosis because fibromyalgia is often diagnosed only after other diagnoses are ruled out.

Assessment

A nursing assessment for patients with symptoms of fibromyalgia includes a patient history and a physical assessment. Base the patient history on the 2010 criteria shown in Box 3–12 for the diagnosis of fibromyalgia. Also assess the family's history of fibromyalgia and other rheumatic disorders. A physical assessment should include testing the trigger points associated with the widespread pain index.

Diagnosis

Nursing diagnoses that may be appropriate for inclusion in the plan of care for the patient with fibromyalgia include:

- *Insomnia*
- *Sleep, Readiness for Enhanced*
- *Fatigue*
- *Activity Intolerance*
- *Knowledge, Readiness for Enhanced*
- *Hopelessness*
- *Anxiety*
- *Coping, Ineffective*
- *Pain, Chronic.*

(NANDA-I © 2014)

Planning

Possible goals of the nursing care plan are

- Patient will report decreased pain.
- Patient will report fewer sleep disturbances.
- Patient will improve activity tolerance.
- Patient's score on a symptom severity scale will be less than 5.

Implementation

Nursing interventions for fibromyalgia pertain to pain management, fatigue reduction, and increased activity tolerance. Interventions related to pain management include education about proper use of medications and nonpharmacologic methods to reduce pain, including massage, exercise, distractions, and family support. Interventions to reduce fatigue include encouraging enjoyable but quiet activities such as reading, listening to music, and participating in hobbies. Nurses should also teach patients good sleep hygiene to increase their restorative sleep and to reduce their fatigue. Interventions to increase activity tolerance include encouraging the patient to alternate periods of activity with periods of rest, delegating responsibilities to other members of the family, and encouraging a mild exercise program to build strength and physical fitness. Nursing interventions should also provide information on coping mechanisms for living with fibromyalgia (see Patient Teaching feature).

Evaluation

The evaluation of patient care is based on the following suggested expected outcomes:

- Patient is able to reduce pain sufficiently to allow periods of activity and sleep.
- Patient voices feelings related to chronic condition.
- Patient obtains adequate follow-up.
- Patient avoids use of narcotics or addictive substances to prevent substance addiction.

Patient Teaching
Coping with Fibromyalgia

Patients often have trouble coping with their diagnosis of fibromyalgia, possibly because they do not know what caused the fibromyalgia, because other people do not know what fibromyalgia is, or because other people do not believe the patients are sick since pain and fatigue have no outward signs. Nurses are instrumental in teaching patients with fibromyalgia how to cope with their syndrome. In teaching coping techniques:

- Validate patients' perception of their symptoms.
- Teach patients about the disease, and answer questions.
- Remind patients that the disease is nonprogressive and not life-threatening.
- Emphasize the importance of a positive attitude.
- Recommend a mild to moderate exercise program, or refer patients to a personal trainer.
- Teach patients basic sleep hygiene methods.
- Encourage patients to see a specialist in fibromyalgia.
- Explain the importance of self-efficacy, or the belief that patients can influence the course of the disease by specific behavior that meets health-related goals.
- Identify stressors that make pain and fatigue worse; then develop strategies to avoid those stressors or to minimize symptoms when those stressors occur. Such strategies include distractions, relaxation techniques, a warm bath, or writing in a journal.
- Encourage patients to develop a strong support network of family and friends and to ask for help when needed.
- Refer patients to community resources for more about fibromyalgia or encourage them to join a support group.

REVIEW Fibromyalgia

RELATE Link the Concepts and Exemplars

Linking the exemplar of fibromyalgia with the concept of development:

1. How might the pain of fibromyalgia affect the developmental tasks of the patient?

2. What would you expect your findings to be when you perform a developmental assessment of a 32-year-old with fibromyalgia?

Linking the exemplar of fibromyalgia with the concept of addiction:

3. What factors put the patient with fibromyalgia at risk for the development of addiction?

4. What would you plan for the patient with fibromyalgia to assist in the prevention of addiction?

READY Go to Volume 3: Clinical Nursing Skills

REFER Go to Pearson MyLab Nursing and eText

- Additional review materials

REFLECT Apply Your Knowledge

Nancy Franklin is a 49-year-old physical therapist with a history of alcoholism. She has not had a drink in 10 years. She was recently in a car accident and sustained whiplash of the shoulders and neck. After 3 months of treatment, Ms. Franklin's pain has not improved, so the physician refers her to a specialist who diagnoses her with fibromyalgia. Ms. Franklin now has trouble getting out of bed in the morning, sleeps most of the morning, and takes naps in the afternoon. The parents of several of the children that she treats have complained because she is chronically late or does not show up for appointments at all. Ms. Franklin is returning to the fibromyalgia clinic today for a follow-up visit; she is 30 minutes late.

1. What is your priority nursing diagnosis for Ms. Franklin?

2. What referral might you recommend for Ms. Franklin?

3. What is your plan of care to assist Ms. Franklin in coping with the diagnosis of fibromyalgia?

» Exemplar 3.E
Sleep–Rest Disorders

Exemplar Learning Outcomes

3.E Analyze sleep–rest disorders as they relate to comfort.

- Describe the pathophysiology, etiology, risk factors, and prevention of sleep–rest disorders.
- Identify the clinical manifestations of sleep–rest disorders.
- Summarize diagnostic tests and therapies used by interprofessional teams in the collaborative care of an individual with a sleep–rest disorder.
- Differentiate considerations for care of patients with sleep–rest disorders across the lifespan.
- Apply the nursing process in providing culturally competent care to an individual with a sleep–rest disorder.

Exemplar Key Terms

Bi-level positive air pressure (BiPAP), *208*
Continuous positive airway pressure (CPAP), *207*
Hypersomnia, *205*
Insomnia, *205*
Narcolepsy, *205*
Parasomnias, *204*
Polysomnography (PSG), *206*
Restless legs syndrome (RLS), *205*
Sleep apnea, *205*
Sleep loss, *209*

Overview

Sleep is essential to normal physiologic functioning. Adults need 7–9 hours of sleep each night. But many adults consistently sleep less than 7 hours, resulting in daytime drowsiness and fatigue. Sometimes the causes of this lack of sleep are busy schedules and poor planning. However, a sleep–rest disorder prevents some individuals from getting adequate sleep. Knowledge of common sleep disorders can help nurses to assess patients with drowsiness and fatigue and to develop nursing interventions that may increase sleep effectiveness.

Pathophysiology and Etiology

Sleep is divided into REM sleep and non-REM sleep. Non-REM sleep is divided into four stages, each stage representing a progressively deeper sleep. Each stage of sleep is associated with specific brain wave patterns and eye movements. The physiology of normal sleep is discussed further in the exemplar on Normal Sleep–Rest Patterns in the module on Health, Wellness, Illness, and Injury.

Pathophysiology

Sleep disorders can lead to disrupted activities of daily living, impair ability to complete tasks, affect the ability to drive safely, lead to other health-related problems, and alter physiologic functioning. Normal sleep patterns can be disrupted by several sleep–rest disorders, including, sleep-disordered breathing, insomnia, narcolepsy, and **parasomnias** (unpleasant or undesirable behaviors that occur at any point during sleep) such as restless legs syndrome.

- Sleep-disordered breathing, or **sleep apnea**, is characterized by repetitive periods of complete or partial airway obstruction that cause five or more apneic events (i.e., short pauses in breathing) per hour; more than 30 events per hour characterize severe apnea. Breathing pauses typically last between 10 and 20 seconds and are followed by a loud snore and/or awakening. Decreased oxygenation and repeated awakenings produce nonrestorative sleep and daytime drowsiness. The three types of sleep apnea are obstructive, central, and mixed. Obstructive sleep apnea occurs when the airway is blocked by the soft palate, tongue, and uvula. Snoring is one of the primary signs of obstructive sleep apnea, although it does not always indicate apnea. Central sleep apnea occurs when the muscles of the chest and diaphragm fail temporarily. Mixed sleep apnea has characteristics of both obstructive and central sleep apnea.

- **Insomnia**, the most common sleeping disorder, occurs when an individual has trouble falling asleep or staying asleep. Insomnia can be either a primary disorder or secondary to another condition or to a medication. In addition, insomnia can be acute, lasting a few days to a few weeks, or it can be chronic, lasting for a month or more. Insomnia causes daytime drowsiness, irritability, and fatigue. Severe insomnia may cause cognitive deficits and increase the risk of accidents.

- In **hypersomnia**, the individual obtains sufficient sleep but still has extreme daytime drowsiness. A severe form of hypersomnia is **narcolepsy**, which is characterized by daytime sleep attacks that last from a few seconds to several minutes. Other symptoms of narcolepsy are dreamlike hallucinations, sleep paralysis, and cataplexy. Narcolepsy is a nervous system disorder in which the brain is unable to regulate sleep–wake cycles; in some patients it is linked to a deficiency in hypocretin, a brain neurotransmitter. The onset of symptoms usually occurs between ages 15 and 30. However, narcolepsy has been reported in children (Baumann et al., 2014; Ratcliffe & Kallappa, 2015).

- Dyssomnias include restless leg syndrome and periodic limb movement disorder. They are a subset of parasomnias. **Restless legs syndrome (RLS)** is a neurologic sensorimotor disorder that is characterized by an overwhelming urge to move the legs when at rest. Periodic limb movements are repetitive movements that occur every 20–40 seconds and manifest as muscle twitches and jerking movements, usually of the legs. The International Restless Legs Syndrome Study Group (IRLSSG) updated the diagnostic criteria for this disorder to include five areas (IRLSSG, 2012). There is some suggestion that menopausal women are more prone to RLS. Researchers examined the relationship between RLS in postmenopausal women and onset of postmenopausal symptoms. Their findings indicate that the hypoestrogenemia associated with menopause may serve as a risk factor for RLS symptoms (Unaldi Karaer, Kaplan, Kurt, & Demirturk, 2014).

>> **Stay Current:** Visit the website of The International Restless Legs Syndrome Study Group at http://irlssg.org/diagnosticcriteria/ to find the full diagnostic criteria for restless leg syndrome.

Etiology

Many factors contribute to sleep disorders, including physical, medical, psychiatric, and environmental factors. Physical factors include injuries, ulcers, aging, and excessive weight; medical factors include conditions such as fibromyalgia, asthma, chronic pain, and genetic polymorphisms. Psychiatric factors include depression, anxiety, and life stresses. Environmental factors include alcohol, medications, and extreme temperatures.

Risk Factors

Risk factors for insomnia include being a woman, being over age 60, and having a mental health disorder. The primary risk factor for obstructive sleep apnea is obesity. Other risk factors are a large neck circumference, a narrow airway, and smoking. Among non-Hispanic Blacks and Hispanic Latinos, there is a twofold increase in obstructive sleep apnea (Ramos, Seixas, & Dib, 2015). Children are likely to have parasomnias such as sleepwalking. Drug or alcohol abuse contributes to night terrors in adults. Restless leg syndrome occurs more frequently with age and stress and in individuals with chronic conditions such as kidney disease, diabetes, and Parkinson disease.

Prevention

Good sleep hygiene is the main preventive measure for sleep–rest disorders. See the section on Sleep Hygiene and corresponding Patient Teaching feature in The Concept of Comfort.

Clinical Manifestations

Manifestations of sleep disorders vary from sleeplessness, to excessive sleepiness and fatigue, to irritability, distractibility, and morning headaches. Because lack of sleep is associated with the onset of a number of chronic conditions, the nurse should thoroughly assess any patient reporting frequent difficulty in sleeping or staying awake. A thorough assessment elicits information that may indicate the presence of either a sleep disorder or another developing medical condition. Cultural issues should be taken into consideration (see the Focus on Diversity and Culture feature).

Focus on Diversity and Culture
Ethnicity and Sleep

Studies related to the effects of ethnicity on sleep have determined that black populations are more likely to have shorter sleep duration, lower sleep efficiency, and higher sleep latency than white populations (Chen et al., 2015). A secondary analysis of the data from 542 midlife women in the United States (157 non-Hispanic Whites, 127 Hispanics, 135 African Americans, and 123 Asian Americans) using the Sleep Index for Midlife Women identified that there were more sleep-related symptoms for Hispanics compared to non-Hispanics. Sleep problems were also associated with depression, anxiety, restless legs syndrome, and musculoskeletal pain (Im et al., 2014).

Clinical Manifestations and Therapies
Sleep–Rest Disorders

ETIOLOGY	CLINICAL MANIFESTATIONS	CLINICAL THERAPIES
Insomnia	■ Inability to fall asleep or remain asleep ■ Drowsiness ■ Fatigue ■ Irritability ■ Cognitive deficits	■ Improved sleep hygiene ■ Stimulus control therapy ■ Sleep restriction therapy ■ Pharmacologic therapy ■ Cognitive–behavioral therapy ■ Exercise therapy ■ Relaxation techniques
Obstructive sleep apnea	■ Snoring ■ Five or more apneic episodes per hour that last 10–20 seconds each ■ Gasping during sleep ■ Frequent nighttime awakenings ■ Daytime drowsiness ■ Morning headache	■ Weight reduction ■ Avoiding alcohol ■ Nasal continuous positive airway pressure (CPAP) or bilevel positive airway pressure (BiPAP) ■ Surgery to remove obstruction ■ Modafinil
Narcolepsy	■ Daytime drowsiness ■ Sleep attacks ■ Cataplexy ■ Sleep paralysis ■ Hypocretin deficiency	■ Modafinil ■ Sodium oxybate ■ Antidepressants ■ Good sleep hygiene ■ Counseling and support groups
Restless legs syndrome	■ Overwhelming urge to move the legs ■ Unpleasant sensations in the legs ■ Nighttime leg twitching	■ Pharmacologic therapy ■ Massage ■ Gentle stretching ■ Exercise therapy ■ Good sleep hygiene

Collaboration

The treatment of sleep disorders is complicated by their complex and often unknown etiologies. Therefore, sleep disorders are best treated by a team of healthcare professionals, including the patient's primary care physician, nurses, sleep specialists, nutritionists, and others, depending on the patient's underlying medical conditions.

Diagnostic Tests

The primary diagnostic test for sleep disorders is a **polysomnography (PSG)**, or sleep study. A PSG records the patient's blood oxygen levels, heart rate, breathing, and eye and leg movements. An electroencephalogram (EEG) is also conducted to monitor brain waves associated with NREM and REM sleep patterns. The patient may also be monitored by video and audio equipment. An analysis of the sleep patterns identifies sleep disorders. Heart rate, breathing, and blood oxygen levels as well as audio monitoring can detect snoring and breathing changes that suggest sleep apnea. The monitoring of leg movements detects periodic limb movement disorder and restless leg syndrome (National Institute of Neurological Disorders and Stroke [NINDS], 2014). Audio and video equipment can also detect parasomnias such as sleepwalking, sleep talking, and night terrors.

Surgery

For patients with obstructive sleep apnea, surgery to remove the obstruction may be a treatment option, especially if the obstruction is caused by the tonsils (tonsillectomy) or adenoids (adenoidectomy). An adenotonsillectomy is commonly performed to treat obstructive sleep apnea in children. Partial removal of the soft palate, uvula, and posterior lateral pharyngeal wall (uvulopalatopharyngoplasty) may also be a treatment option. Surgery is usually considered only if CPAP therapy is not tolerated.

SAFETY ALERT Partners of patients with sleep apnea often become aware of apneic episodes because of a pause in snoring. Patients who undergo surgery, such as removing the tonsils, to prevent snoring are at an increased risk for adverse events associated with apnea because there is no warning that apnea is occurring.

Pharmacologic Therapy

The primary pharmacologic agents used to treat sleep–rest disorders are the sedative-hypnotics, including anxiolytics,

TABLE 3–10 Selected Medications Used for Sleep–Rest Disorders

Medication	Half-Life (Hours)	Sleep–Rest Disorder	Drug Class
Chloral hydrate (Noctec)	8–11	Short term for insomnia	Anxiolytic
Clonazepam (Klonopin)	18–40	Restless legs syndrome	Benzodiazepine, anticonvulsant
Diphenhydramine hydrochloride (Benadryl)	8–9	Intractable insomnia	Anti-Parkinson, antihistamine
Estazolam (Prosom)	10–24	Short term for insomnia	Anxiolytic, benzodiazepine
Eszopiclone (Lunesta)	5–6	Insomnia	Sedative-hypnotic
Flurazepam (Dalmane)	47–100	Insomnia	Anxiolytic, benzodiazepine
Gabapentin enacarbil (Horizant)	5–6	Restless legs syndrome	Anticonvulsant
Modafinil (Provigil)	15	Narcolepsy, obstructive sleep apnea	CNS stimulant
Pramipexole dihydrochloride (Mirapex)	8–12	Restless legs syndrome	Anti-Parkinson
Quazepam (Doral)	39	Insomnia	Sedative-hypnotic, anxiolytic, benzodiazepine
Ramelteon (Rozerem)	1–2.5	Insomnia	Melatonin receptor agonist
Ropinirole hydrochloride (Requip)	6	Restless legs syndrome	Anti-Parkinson
Sodium oxybate (Xyrem)	0.5–1	Cataplexy in patients with narcolepsy	CNS depressant
Temazepam (Restoril)	8–24	Insomnia	Anxiolytic, benzodiazepine
Zaleplon (Sonata)	1	Short term for insomnia	Sedative-hypnotic, anxiolytic
Zolpidem (Ambien)	1.7–2.5	Short term for insomnia	Anxiolytic

Source: Data from Adams, M. P., Holland, L. N., & Urban, C. (2017). *Pharmacology for nurses: A pathophysiologic approach* (5th ed.). Hoboken, NJ: Pearson Education.

barbiturates, and benzodiazepines. Anti-Parkinson drugs, opioids, and anticonvulsants also are occasionally prescribed for sleep–rest disorders. For insomnia drugs, the half-life of the drug is important for determining its effectiveness (see **Table 3–10** ⟩⟩). Drugs with short half-lives are helpful for patients who have trouble falling asleep but not for patients who have problems staying asleep. In contrast, drugs with longer half-lives are effective for patients who have periods of wakefulness during the night, but they may also produce daytime drowsiness. In addition, many sleep aids produce addiction/tolerance, so the risks of taking a sleep aid should be discussed with the patient prior to use.

Several side effects are shared by multiple sleep aids, including headache, dizziness, residual drowsiness, somnolence, and nausea. Other selected side effects include sleep attacks (ropinirole, pramipexole), dyspepsia (ropinirole), tachycardia (eszopiclone, diphenhydramine), and postural hypotension (pramipexole). Side effects are often amplified in older adults, especially dizziness, hallucinations, hypotension, impaired coordination, ataxia, and vertigo. These side effects put older adults at higher risk for injury during ambulation, so safety measures should be implemented, and older adults should be supervised if ambulating during the night. In addition, all patients should be warned to avoid driving, handling machinery, or participating in dangerous activities after taking sleep aids. Some sleep aids should not be used by patients with cardiac, respiratory, kidney, or liver disorders or by pregnant or breastfeeding women, so check patient history and contraindications before giving sleep aids to patients.

Drug, food, and herbal interactions with sleep aids are also common. The most common drug interactions are with alcohol and other CNS depressants, CYP3A4 inhibitors, and cimetidine. Cimetidine is known to increase plasma levels of multiple sleep aids. Many other drug interactions exist, so nurses and other healthcare team members should carefully review patients' current medications to avoid adverse drug reactions. Common food interactions are grapefruit juice (estazolam, ramelteon), high-fat meals (ramelteon, sodium oxybate), and food in general (zolpidem); all of these interactions decrease absorption of the medication. Common herbal interactions include kava and valerian (benzodiazepines), St. John's wort (eszopiclone), and melatonin (zaleplon), which increase drug levels or produce additional sedative effects.

Sleep aids can induce tolerance, so dosages may need to be increased over time. Some medications, such as chloral hydrate, estazolam, and zolpidem, should be used only for short-term management of insomnia because of tolerance issues. When treatment with sleep aids is stopped, dosages should be tapered down over a week or more to prevent withdrawal symptoms, including delirium, convulsions, dizziness, GI upset, and parasomnias. Patients should be warned that rebound insomnia may occur after they stop these medications.

Nonpharmacologic Therapy

Nonpharmacologic therapies that may be beneficial in the treatment of sleep–rest disorders include cognitive–behavioral therapy, good sleep hygiene, physical exercise, and relaxation techniques. Nasal strips can also be used to open the nasal passageways and prevent snoring that is not accompanied by airway obstruction.

For obstructive sleep apnea, the most common therapies are weight reduction, avoiding alcohol, avoiding the supine position for sleeping, and using a **continuous positive airway**

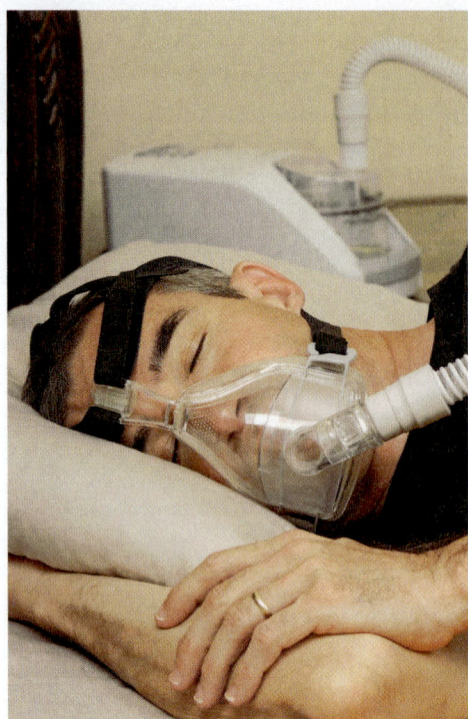

Source: Brian Chase/Shutterstock.

Figure 3–11 » A patient using a nasal mask and CPAP to treat sleep apnea.

pressure (CPAP) or a **bi-level positive air pressure (BiPAP)** machine to help the airway open (see **Figure 3–11** » and the Patient Teaching feature). A CPAP or BiPAP machine consists of a generator that produces positive air pressure administered by a close-fitting mask around the mouth and nose. The positive air pressure prevents collapse and obstruction of the airway to relieve apneic episodes. The BiPAP differs from the CPAP in that it produces less pressure during exhalation and more pressure during inhalation, thus causing less resistance to exhalation. The most common side effect of CPAP or BiPAP therapy is a dry mouth and airway, so an in-line or room humidifier is recommended. CPAP can be used for children with obstructive

Patient Teaching
CPAP and BiPAP Machines

Patient teaching for a CPAP or BiPAP machine should include:

- Proper fitting of the mask to the face, including wearing the right size mask and keeping the straps tight.
- The importance of getting used to wearing the mask. Step 1: Wear the mask *without* air pressure when awake. Step 2: Wear the mask *with* air pressure when awake. Step 3: Wear the mask *with* air pressure when asleep.
- The method of adjusting the air pressure of the machine to minimize difficulty exhaling.
- The importance of using a humidifier and nasal sprays to minimize dry mouth and nose.
- Relaxation exercises to reduce the claustrophobic feelings caused by wearing the mask.

Evidence-Based Practice
Sleep Restriction
Problem

Insomnia causes individuals to lie in bed for long periods without falling asleep or drifting between stage 1 NREM sleep and drowsy wakefulness. As a result, individuals believe they are getting less sleep than they actually are, and daytime drowsiness then decreases productivity and increases the risk of falling asleep during work or while driving.

Evidence

Research suggests that sleep restriction therapy (SRT) can help reduce primary chronic insomnia. Sleep restriction limits the amount of time in bed to maximize sleep efficiency, then gradually increases the time in bed until the individual is receiving adequate sleep. When sleep restriction therapy begins, time in bed should be close to the estimated time of actual sleep each night but no less than 4–5 hours. The morning wake time should remain constant throughout therapy. Each week, sleep efficiency is calculated from the total sleep time versus the time spent in bed. When sleep efficiency exceeds 90%, the patient should increase time in bed by 15–20 minutes (National Institutes of Health, 2015). Sleep restriction reduces the gap between the total sleep time and time in bed by decreasing sleep onset latency and improving total sleep time (Lande & Gragnani, 2010; Miller et al., 2014). Patients who utilized SRT were found to have reduced fatigue and higher sleep quality than those who were treated with sleep hygiene only (Falloon, Elley, Fernando, Lee, & Arrol, 2015). It is noteworthy that sleep restriction is comparable to stimulus control therapy as an effective treatment for primary chronic insomnia in older adults as measured by sleep onset latency, waking after sleep onset, and sleep efficiency (Epstein, Sidani, Bootzin, & Belyea, 2012).

Implications

For patients with chronic insomnia, sleep restriction helps increase sleep efficiency. It may be especially beneficial for older adults who have adverse side effects when using sedative-hypnotic drugs. Patients may be reluctant to try sleep restriction because of the misconception that time spent in bed is the same as receiving adequate sleep. However, time spent in bed not sleeping actually contributes to multiple sleep disturbances. Another barrier to sleep restriction therapy is the need to induce mild sleep deprivation, which may initially cause increased daytime drowsiness and decreased productivity. This therapy takes 4–8 weeks to achieve maximum effectiveness. Sleep education should also be included as an important part of sleep deprivation therapy.

Critical Thinking Application

1. You meet with a patient who wants to quit after 1 week on sleep restriction because of increased daytime drowsiness. What suggestions would encourage this patient to remain on the therapy?

2. How would you explain the importance of sleep efficiency to the patient who believes that time spent in bed is equivalent to receiving adequate sleep?

3. What recommendations would you make about timing sleep deprivation therapy for a working adult? A teenager in school? A retired older adult? A single parent?

Focus on Integrative Health

Herbal Supplements for Sleep Disorders

Herbal supplements may be an alternative for individuals who do not tolerate pharmacologic therapy because of side effects. Two herbs that are traditionally used to aid sleep are valerian (*Valeriana officinalis*) and chamomile (*Matricaria recutita*). Valerian usually has to be taken for 2 or 3 weeks before it produces an effect, and clinical trials have not proven its effectiveness. Possible side effects of valerian include indigestion, headache, palpitations, and dizziness. Chamomile, often taken as a tea, has a soothing effect that may induce sleep and decrease restlessness, although this effect has not been proven in clinical studies. It is safe for both adults and children except individuals who are allergic to ragweed or daisies.

Melatonin is a sleep hormone produced by the pineal gland. Synthetic melatonin is sold in many pharmacies and health food stores and may be taken to regulate sleep patterns. It is often helpful for sleep disturbances related to shift work or jet lag. It has been proven effective in treating sleep disorders in children with autism and children with ADHD. It may also be helpful for older adults with insomnia when combined with magnesium and zinc supplements (NCCIH, 2015).

sleep apnea and for patients with surgical contraindications or with persistent apnea after adenotonsillectomy, as often occurs in children with Down syndrome, craniofacial abnormalities, or neuromuscular disorders. Pressure levels may need to be adjusted as the child grows.

According to Schutte-Rodin and colleagues (2008), nonpharmacologic therapies for sleep–rest disorders include stimulus control, relaxation training, cognitive–behavioral therapy, and sleep restriction (see the Evidence-Based Practice feature).

Stimulus control therapy involves using the bed only for sleep and sex, not for other activities, such as watching TV, reading, or working. Cognitive–behavioral therapy in conjunction with room modification, temperature, and light and dark exposure has been helpful in chronic insomnia (Schutte-Rodin et al., 2008.)

Lifespan Considerations

The prevalence of specific sleep–rest disorders changes over the life course. For example, young children may have enuresis, adolescents may have delayed sleep phase syndrome, young parents may have **sleep loss** (duration of sleep shorter than the recommended 7–8 hours per night for adults) related to having a newborn, and older adults may have insomnia related to chronic health problems.

Children and Sleep

Sleep disturbances in children can be manifested in many ways, including bed wetting (nocturesis), teeth grinding (bruxism), nightmares, and sleepwalking. School-age children are more likely to have sleepwalking and sleep terrors, which can cause anxiety for the parents. In general, these disorders will decrease or be ameliorated as the child matures. However, if they persist, parents are encouraged to seek help from their healthcare provider (American Academy of Child

and Adolescent Psychiatry, 2013). Calhoun and colleagues (2013) conducted a study to identify the prevalence and risk factors for insomnia among young children and preadolescents. Parent questionnaires, body mass index (BMI), and a 9-hour sleep study was conducted on 700 children. The results of this study showed that approximately one-fifth of young and preadolescent children have insomnia. Insomnia was highest among girls age 11–12 years.

Adolescents and Sleep

Adolescents experience changes in the body's internal clock associated with puberty. In approximately 7%–16% of adolescents, these changes cause a delay in melatonin release each night; the result is delayed sleep phase syndrome. Signs of delayed sleep phase syndrome include an inability to fall asleep and wake up at the desired time; daytime sleepiness; difficulty learning, listening, and problem solving; behavioral problems; and unhealthy eating (National Sleep Foundation, 2016b). Much of the research done on sleep unfortunately is conducted on adults and extrapolated to adolescents. According to Vriend and Corkum (2011) the use of sleep hygiene, sleep restriction therapy, and relaxation techniques can be beneficial.

Pregnant Women and Sleep

Pregnant women often develop sleep disorders associated with physical discomfort and changing hormone levels. Insomnia in pregnant women may also be related to emotions and anxiety about labor and delivery, becoming a mother, and how the infant will change the mother's relationship with her spouse. Restless legs syndrome and gastroesophageal reflux disease are often worse during pregnancy, and the risk for developing sleep apnea is increased in pregnant women, especially if the woman is obese. Frequent urination can also disrupt sleep. Later in the pregnancy, it is more difficult to find a comfortable position in which to sleep, and decreased lung capacity may contribute to difficulties falling asleep. Because many medications can harm the developing fetus, the best treatment for pregnant women with sleep disorders is practicing good sleep hygiene. Continuous positive air pressure (CPAP) is also a safe and effective treatment for pregnant women with obstructive sleep apnea (National Sleep Foundation, 2016a).

Older Adults and Sleep

Sleep–rest disorders increase in prevalence with increasing age, especially as older adults develop chronic health problems such as hypertension, depression, and cardiovascular disease. In contrast, individuals with a sleep disorder are at higher risk of developing these chronic diseases (National Sleep Foundation, 2013). Other conditions linked to sleep disorders include menopause, pulmonary disease, arthritis, chronic pain, and Alzheimer disorder. Medications used for chronic medical conditions, such as beta-blockers, corticosteroids, diuretics, and selective serotonin reuptake inhibitors (SSRIs), also can contribute to sleep disturbances. Because sleep disorders are associated with chronic conditions and multiple medications, nurses must conduct a thorough patient history to determine if the sleep disorder is a primary condition or related to another medical condition.

Changes in sleep patterns in older adults include long periods of wakefulness, decreased total sleep time, reduced sleep efficiency, and decreased time spent in stages 3 and 4 NREM sleep and in REM sleep. These changes in nighttime sleep patterns are followed by increased daytime napping (National Sleep Foundation, 2013), which may in turn contribute to difficulty sleeping at night. When older adults do not get sufficient sleep, a sleep deficit occurs that results in loss of daytime functioning and decreased quality of life. When daytime activities are limited, older adults lose physical strength; strength loss further disrupts the sleep–wake cycle.

Other physiologic changes that may contribute to sleep disorders in older adults are changes in circulation, metabolism, and body tissue density. These changes limit the older adult's ability to generate heat and maintain a comfortable body temperature. Nursing interventions used to promote warmth and sleep for older adults include warming the bed with an electric or prewarmed blanket, using flannel sheets instead of cotton or polyester, encouraging the patient to wear warm clothing to bed, and providing extra blankets.

Older adults in long-term care facilities are at increased risk for developing sleep disorders. Similar to community-dwelling older adults, patients in long-term care facilities have precipitating factors such as pain, gastroesophageal reflux, nocturia, dyspnea, and dementia, and they are often taking multiple medications that interfere with sleep. In contrast to community-dwelling adults, individuals in long-term care facilities must also deal with environmental factors that interfere with sleep, such as limited interaction with the community, reduced bright light exposure, physical inactivity, and nighttime noise and sleep disruptions (National Sleep Foundation, 2013).

NURSING PROCESS

Patients experiencing sleep disorders often report a great deal of frustration and annoyance about their sleepless nights. However, sleep disorders are more than just an annoyance: Risks of injury increase dramatically in tired people. In addition to care of patients' sleeplessness, it is important for nurses to promote injury prevention by teaching strategies to reduce risk such as not driving when tired, using caution with potentially dangerous equipment, and preventing fires if patients smoke.

Assessment

- **Observation and patient interview.** A nursing assessment for sleep–rest disorders begins with observation and a patient interview, including a sleep history. Observation can indicate the presence of fatigue, decreased cognitive functioning and coordination, dark circles under the eyes, and irritability. If the patient is married, a spouse may provide additional helpful information about the patient's sleep habits. Parents may also provide information about a child's sleep habits. The interview and sleep history may include items such as:

  Do you have trouble falling asleep at night?

  How often do you wake up during the night? Do you have trouble falling asleep once you have woken up?

  How do you feel when you wake up in the morning?

  Describe your normal sleep schedule.

  Has anyone ever told you that you snore, walk, scream, stop breathing, or jerk in your sleep?

  Do you have daytime drowsiness? Does it interfere with your daily activities?

  Do you sleep in strange positions?

  Does your child wet the bed?

  Do you experience morning headaches?

  Does anything unusual happen when you laugh or get angry?

  Do you drink caffeinated beverages or alcohol or smoke? If so, how often and how much?

  Has anything happened lately to change your sleep patterns? Medical condition, medications, life stresses?

  What have you been doing to deal with your sleep problem? Does it help?

  How do your sleep habits affect your relationships, work, school, and activities?

  Assessment tools, such as the Epworth Sleepiness Scale, can help determine if an individual has a sleep–rest disorder (University of Maryland Medical Center, 2013). Scores between 0 and 10 are considered normal, and scores between 11 and 24 indicate a sleep disorder. Sleep scales are available that are specific for patients with Parkinson disease, pediatric patients, teachers, women, and others.

- **Physical examination.** The physical can indicate the presence of fatigue and a possible sleep–rest disorder. Indicators include abnormal vital signs, lack of muscle tone and reflexes, and decreased cognitive functioning and coordination. Polysomnography should be conducted for patients with a suspected sleep disorder.

Diagnosis

Nursing diagnoses related to sleep–rest disorders include:

- *Insomnia*
- *Sleep Deprivation*
- *Sleep, Readiness for Enhanced*
- *Sleep Pattern, Disturbed*
- *Fatigue*
- *Wandering* related to somnambulism
- *Ineffective Breathing Pattern* related to sleep apnea
- *Ineffective Coping*
- *Stress Overload*
- *Risk for Injury* related to sedative-hypnotic effects
- *Deficient Knowledge* related to sleep hygiene.

  (NANDA-I © 2014)

Planning

Appropriate goals for the patient with a sleep disturbance include:

- The patient will sleep through the night.
- The patient will use relaxation techniques 30–45 minutes prior to bedtime.

- The patient will maintain a consistent bedtime.
- The patient will use good sleep hygiene.
- The patient will reduce or remove environmental distractions from the bedroom.
- The patient will have sufficient energy for normal daily activities.
- The patient will report improved quality and quantity of sleep.
- The patient's spouse will report decreased snoring.
- The patient's spouse will report no apneic episodes.

Implementation

Nursing interventions for sleep–rest disorders should include the patient, the patient's spouse or parents, and the healthcare team. Possible interventions include:

- Educating the patient about the factors associated with impaired sleep–rest patterns.

- Instructing the patient in the proper use of assistive devices (e.g., BiPAP).
- If a pharmacologic treatment has been prescribed, teaching the patient about the proper use of the medication as well as its potential side effects and interactions.
- Teaching the patient about the principles of good sleep hygiene.

Evaluation

Evaluation should include collection of data about the quality and duration of the patient's sleep and how the patient feels upon awakening and throughout the day. If outcomes were not achieved, reassess the patient to determine if etiologic factors were correctly identified, if the patient has had any changes in medical conditions or medications, if the patient followed the instructions for good sleep hygiene, if the patient has avoided daytime napping, and if any pharmacologic or nonpharmacologic therapies have been implemented with success.

Nursing Care Plan

A Patient with Obstructive Sleep Apnea

Charles Huston visits his primary care physician because his wife, Amy, told him he stops breathing frequently during the night.

ASSESSMENT	DIAGNOSES	PLANNING
While speaking with the nurse, Mr. Huston says that he experiences mild drowsiness during the day, and if he sits for too long with no stimulation, he easily falls asleep. His wife reports that Mr. Huston snores heavily, but when he stops snoring he also stops breathing. The condition is worse when he is lying on his back, which Mr. Huston claims is his most comfortable sleeping position.	▪ *Breathing Pattern, Ineffective* ▪ *Gas Exchange, Impaired* ▪ *Sleep, Readiness for Enhanced* ▪ *Imbalanced Nutrition: More than Body Requirements* ▪ *Lifestyle, Sedentary* ▪ *Activity Intolerance.* (NANDA-I © 2014)	▪ Patient will breathe consistently through the night. ▪ Patient will feel refreshed upon awakening. ▪ Patient will demonstrate understanding of the use of a BiPAP machine. ▪ Patient will begin a mild exercise program of walking for 30 minutes three times a week, which will increase in intensity as the patient loses weight. ▪ Patient will meet with a nutritionist to develop a healthy eating plan. ▪ Patient will lose 10 pounds in the next 3 months and 70 pounds in the next year.
Physical Examination Height: 188 cm (74 in.) Weight: 130.2 kg (287 lb) Temperature: 38.2°C (100.8°F) Pulse: 88 bpm Respirations: 16/min Blood pressure: 149/89 mmHg **Diagnostic Data** A polysomnography reveals an apnea–hypoapnea index of 28.		

IMPLEMENTATION

- Teach Mr. Huston how to use the BiPAP machine (see Patient Teaching feature).
- Instruct Mr. Huston on good sleep hygiene techniques.
- Encourage his verbalization of his feelings, perceptions, and fears.
- Refer Mr. Huston to a nutritionist for a healthy eating plan.

- Refer Mr. Huston to a personal trainer or physical fitness facility for an exercise program.
- Refer Mr. and Ms. Huston to a support group for weight loss.
- Schedule regular follow-up appointments to evaluate Mr. Huston's weight loss, fitness, and control of his obstructive sleep apnea.

(continued on next page)

Nursing Care Plan *(continued)*

EVALUATION

Mr. Huston returns for a follow-up appointment 1 week after starting the BiPAP machine. He reports regular use of the BiPAP machine and feeling more refreshed during the day. Mr. and Ms. Huston have met with a nutritionist, and Ms. Huston has begun to prepare more healthy meals. Mr. Huston has joined the local YMCA and has met with a personal trainer once. He has lost 2 pounds in the first week. On subsequent follow-up appointments, Mr. Huston continues losing weight, but his progress stalls after 6 months at a 40-pound overall weight loss. The care plan is modified to include a more strenuous exercise program and a lower daily calorie intake.

CRITICAL THINKING

1. What suggestions would you make if Mr. Huston complained of a dry mouth, nose, and throat after using his BiPAP machine?

2. Outline two other methods of weight loss that Mr. Huston could incorporate to help him get past his stall in weight loss at 6 months.

3. What other conditions related to Mr. Huston's obesity could increase his daytime drowsiness?

REVIEW Sleep–Rest Disorders

RELATE Link the Concepts and Exemplars

Linking the exemplar of sleep–rest disorders with the concept of development:

1. How do requirements for sleep vary across the developmental stages?

2. What assessment differences might you expect in sleep deprivation across the lifespan?

Linking the exemplar of sleep–rest disorders with the concept of sexuality:

3. How might sleep–rest disorders affect the patient's sexual relationship with a significant other?

4. What interventions would you initiate for the couple when one of the partners has a sleep–rest disorder?

READY Go to Volume 3: Clinical Nursing Skills

REFER Go to Pearson MyLab Nursing and eText

- Additional review materials

REFLECT Apply Your Knowledge

Jennifer Leno is a 30-year-old nursing student who works 20 hours each week, carries a full-time academic load, and has an 8-year-old child. She begins to drink energy drinks at night to stay awake to study. However, after 2 months of 5 hours of sleep a night and three energy drinks each day, she begins to have problems going to sleep. Her friend Janie offers Ms. Leno zolpidem (Ambien) to help her relax.

1. What might be causing Ms. Leno's insomnia?

2. What is zolpidem, and is it likely to be effective in treating Ms. Leno's symptoms?

3. If you were a friend of Ms. Leno's as well, what advice would you give her?

References

Adams, M. P., Holland, L. N., & Urban, C. (2017). *Pharmacology for nurses: A pathophysiologic approach* (5th ed.). Hoboken, NJ: Pearson Education.

Alivizatos, V., Gavala, V., Alexopoulos, P., Apostolopoulos, A., & Bajrucevic, S. (2012). Feeding tube-related complications and problems in patients receiving long-term home enteral nutrition. *Indian Journal of Palliative Care, 18*(1), 31–33 doi:10.4103/0973-1075.97346

American Academy of Child and Adolescent Psychiatry. (2013). *Children's sleep problems.* Retrieved from https://www.aacap.org/AACAP/Families_and_Youth/Facts_for_Families/FFF-Guide/Childrens-Sleep-Problems-034.aspx

American Academy of Orthopaedic Surgeons (AAOS). (2015). *Low back pain risk factors identified.* Retrieved from https://www.sciencedaily.com/releases/2015/03/150325082726.htm

American Academy of Pediatrics. (2016). Prevention and management of procedural pain in the neonate: An update. *Pediatrics, 137*(2).

American Academy of Sleep Medicine. (2015). *Sleep disturbances are common, influenced by race and ethnicity.* Retrieved from https://www.sciencedaily.com/releases/2015/06/150619141605.htm

American Geriatrics Society. (2012). *Geriatrics health professionals leading change. Improving care of older adults.* Retrieved from http://www.americangeriatrics.org/files/documents/Adv_Resources/PP_Priorities.pdf

American Nurses Association. (2012). *Position statement: Nursing care and do not resuscitate (DNR) and allow natural death (AND) decisions.* Retrieved from http://nursingworld.org/dnrposition

American Nurses Association. (2013). *Position statement: Euthanasia, assisted suicide and aid in dying.* Retrieved from the American Nurses Association website: http://nursingworld.org/euthanasiaanddying

Anderson, J. G., & Taylor, A. G. (2012). Biotherapies and cancer pain. *Clinical Journal of Oncology Nursing, 16*(1). doi:10.1188/12.CJON.43-4

Andrews, M. M., & Boyle, J. S. (2016). *Transcultural concepts in nursing care.* (7th ed.). Philadelphia, PA: Wolters Kluwer.

Arenella, C. (2015). *Artificial nutrition and hydration at the end of life: Beneficial or harmful?* Retrieved from http://americanhospice.org/caregiving/artificial-nutrition-and-hydration-at-the-end-of-life-beneficial-or-harmful/

Arif-Rahu, M., Fisher, D., & Matsuda, Y. (2012). Biobehavioral measures for pain in the pediatric patient. *Pain Management Nursing, 13*(3), 157–168. doi:10.1016/j.pmn.2010.10.036

Barbus, A. J. (1975). The dying person's bill of rights, created at the workshop *The Terminally Ill Patient and the Helping Person.* Lansing: South Western Michigan Inservice Education Council.

Baumann, C. R., Mignot, E., Lammers, G. J., Overeem, S., Arnulf, I., Rye, D., . . .Scammell, T. E. (2014). Challenges in diagnosing narcolepsy without cataplexy: A consensus statement. *Sleep, 37*(6), 1035–1042. doi:10.5665/sleep.3756

Bellato, E., Marini, E., Castoldi, F., Barbasetti, N., Mattei, L., Bonasia, D. E., & Blonna, D. (2012). Fibromyalgia syndrome: Etiology, pathogenesis, diagnosis, and treatment. *Pain Research and Treatment*, Article 426130. doi:10.1155/2012/426130

Berman, A., Snyder, S. J., & Frandsen, G. (2016). Pain management. In *Kozier and Erb's fundamentals of nursing: Concepts, process, and practice* (10th ed.). Hoboken, NJ: Pearson Education.

Bradley, L. A. (2009). Pathophysiology of fibromyalgia. *American Journal of Medicine, 122*(12 Suppl.), S22. doi:10.1016/j.amjmed.2009.09.008

Brownie, S., & Nancarrow, S. (2013). Effects of person-centered care on residents and staff in aged-care facilities: A systematic review. *Clinical Interventions in Aging, 8*, 1–10. doi:10.2147/CIA.S38589

Burke, A., Nahin, R., & Stussman, B. (2015). Limited health knowledge as a reason for non-use of four common complementary health practices. *PLOS*. doi:10.1371/journal.pone.0129336

Caeymaex, L., Jousselme, C., Vasilescu, C., Danan, C., Falissard, B., Bourrat, M. M., . . . Speranza, M. (2013). Perceived role in end-of-life decision making in the NICU affects long-term parental grief response. *Archives of Disease in Childhood. Fetal and Neonatal Edition, 98*(1), F26–F31. doi:10.1136/archdischild-2011-301548

Calhoun, S. L., Fernandez-Mendoza, J., Vgontzas, A. N., Liao, D., & Bixler, E.O. (2013). Prevalence of insomnia symptoms in a general population sample of young children and preadolescents: Gender effects. *Sleep Medicine, 15*(1), 91–95. doi:10.1016/j.sleep.2013.08.787

Carteret, M. (2011). Cultural aspects of pain management. *Dimensions of Culture: Cross Cultural Communications for Health Care Professionals*. Retrieved from http://www.dimensionsofculture.com/2010/11/cultural-aspects-of-pain-management/

Centers for Disease Control and Prevention (CDC). (2015a). *Chronic fatigue syndrome*. Retrieved from http://www.cdc.gov/cfs/causes/index.html

Centers for Disease Control and Prevention (CDC). (2015b). *Fibromyalgia*. Retrieved from http://www.cdc.gov/arthritis/basics/fibromyalgia.htm

Centers for Disease Control and Prevention (CDC). (2015c). *Infant Mortality*. Retrieved from: http://www.cdc.gov/reproductivehealth/MaternalInfantHealth/InfantMortality.htm

Centers for Disease Control and Prevention (CDC). (2015d). *Leading causes of death*. Retrieved from http://www.cdc.gov/nchs/fastats/leading-causes-of-death.htm

Chen, X., Wang, R., Zee, P., Lutsey, P. S., Javaheri, S., Alcantara, C., . . . Redline, W. (2015) Racial/ethnic differences in sleep disturbances: The multi-ethnic study of atherosclerosis (MESA). *Sleep, 38*(6), 877–888. doi:10.5665/sleep.4732

Clarke, A., Anthony, G., Gray, D., Jones, D., McNamee, P., Schofield, P., . . . Martin, D. (2012). "I feel so stupid because I can't give a proper answer . . ." How older adults describe chronic pain: A qualitative study. *BMC Geriatrics, 12*, 78. doi:10.1186/1471-2318-12-78

Cleveland Clinic. (2016). *Guided imagery*. Retrieved from http://my.clevelandclinic.org/departments/integrativemedicine/guided_imagery_facts.aspx

Cooney, G., Dwan, K., & Meak, G. (2015). Exercise for depression. *Journal of American Medical Association, 311*(23), 2432–2433. doi:10.1001/jama.2014.4930

Craig, M., Jeavons, R., Probert, J., & Benger, J. (2012). Randomised comparison of intravenous paracetamol and intravenous morphine for acute traumatic limb pain in the emergency department. *Emergency Medicine Journal, 29*, 37–39. doi:10.1136/emf.2010.104687

Cramp, F., & Byron-Daniel, J. (2012). Exercise for the management of cancer-related fatigue in adults. *Cochrane Database of Systematic Reviews, 11*, CD006145. doi:10.1002/14651858.CD006145.pub3

Cross-Disorder Group of the Psychiatric Genomics Consortium. (2013). Genetic relationship between five psychiatric disorders estimated from genome-wide SNPs (single nucleotide polymorphisms). *Nature Genetics*. Retrieved from http://www.nature.com/ng/journal/v45/n9/full/ng.2711.html

Crozier, F., & Hancock, L. E. (2012). Pediatric palliative care. *Pediatric Nursing, 38*(4), 198–203.

De Ruddere, L., Goubert, L., Stevens, M., Williams, A. C., & Crombez, G. (2013). Discounting pain in the absence of medical evidence is explained by negative evaluation of the patient. *Pain*. doi:10.1016/j.pain.2012.12.018

Diekema, D. S. (2014). Ethics in medicine: Parental decision making. *University of Washington School of Medicine*. Retrieved from https://depts.washington.edu/bioethx/topics/parent.html

Doesburg, S. M., Chau, C. M., Cheung, T. P., Moiseev, A., Ribary, U., Herdman, A. T., . . . Grunau, R. E. (2013). Neonatal pain-related stress, functional cortical activity and visual-perceptual abilities in school-age children born at extremely low gestational age. *Pain, 154*(10), 1946–1952. doi:10.1016/j.pain.2013.04.009

Dorfman, J., Denduluri, S., Walseman, K., & Bregman, B. (2012). The role of complementary and alternative medicine in end-of-life care. *Psychiatry Annals, 4*, 150–155.

Durall, A., Zurakowski, D., & Wolfe, J. (2012). Barriers to conducting advance care discussions for children with life-threatening conditions. *Pediatrics, 129*(4), e975–982. doi:10.1542/peds.2011-2695

Epstein, D. R., Sidani, S., Bootzin, R. R., & Belvea, M. J. (2012). Dismantling multicomponent behavioral treatment for insomnia in older adults: A randomized controlled trial. *Sleep, 35*(6), 797–805. doi:10.5665/sleep.1878

Falloon, K., Elley, C.R., Fernando, A., Lee, A.C., & Arrol, B. (2015). Simplified sleep restriction for insomnia in general practice: a randomised controlled trial. *British Journal of General Practice*. doi:10.3399/bjgp15X686137

Fein, A. (2012) *Nociceptors and the perception of pain*. Retrieved from http://cell.uchc.edu/pdf/fein/nociceptors_fein_2012.pdf

Fein, J. A., Zempsky, W. T., & Cravero, J. P. (2012). Relief of pain and anxiety in pediatric patients in emergency medical systems. *Pediatrics, 130*(5), e1391–e1405. doi:10.1542/peds.2012-2536

Food and Drug Administration (FDA). (2005). *COX-2 selective (includes Bextra, Celebrex, and Vioxx) and non-selective non-steroidal anti-inflammatory drugs (NSAIDs)*. Retrieved from http://www.fda.gov/drugs/drugsafety/postmarketdrugsafetyinformationforpatientsandproviders/ucm103420.htm

Food and Drug Administration (FDA). (2015). *FDA drug safety communication: FDA strengthens warning that non-aspirin nonsteroidal anti-inflammatory drugs (NSAIDs) can cause heart attacks or strokes*. Retrieved from http://www.fda.gov/Drugs/DrugSafety/ucm451800.htm

Fransen, M., McConnell, S., Harmer, A. R., Van der Esch, M., Simic, M., & Bennell, K. L. (2015). Exercise for osteoarthritis of the knee. *Cochrane Database of Systematic Reviews, 2015*(1). doi:10.1002/14651858.CD004376

Friebert, S., & Williams, C. (2015). *National Hospice and Palliative Care Organization's (NPHCO) facts and figures: Pediatric palliative and hospice care in America*. Retrieved from http://www.nhpco.org/sites/default/files/public/quality/Pediatric_Facts-Figures.pdf

Gaskin, D. J., & Richard, P. (2012). The economic costs of pain in the United States. *The Journal of Pain, 13*(8), 715. doi:10.1016/j.jpain.2012.03.009

Gilron, I., Baron, R., & Jensen, T. (2015). Neuropathic pain: Principles of diagnosis and treatment. *Mayo Clinic Proceedings, 90*(4), 532–545. doi:10.1016/j.mayocp.2015.01.018

Glaser, B. G., & Strauss, A. L. (1965). *Awareness of dying*. Chicago, IL: Aldine.

Goldberg, Y. P., Pimstone, S. N., Namdari, R., Price, N., Cohen, C., Sherrington, R. P., & Hayden, M. R. (2012). Human Mendelian pain disorders: A key to discovery and validation of novel analgesics. *Clinical Genetics, 82*(4), 367–373. doi:10.1111/j.1399-0004.2012.01942.x

Gonella, S. S. (2014). Biofield therapies and cancer related symptoms: A review. *Clinical Journal of Oncology Nursing, 18* (5) 568–576. doi:10.1188/14.CJON.568-576

Goyal, M. K., Kuppermann, N., Cleary, S. D., Teach, S. J., & Chamberlain, J. M. (2015). Racial disparities in pain management of children with appendicitis in emergency departments. *JAMA Pediatrics, 169*(11), 996–1002. doi:10.1001/jamapediatrics.2015.1915

Gracely, R. H., & Ambrose, K. R. (2012). Exploring the pathophysiology of fibromyalgia. *Medscape education rheumatology*. Retrieved from http://www.medscape.org/viewarticle/763941

Hallingbye, T., Martin, J., & Viscomi, C. (2011). Acute postoperative pain management in the older patient. *Aging Health, 7*(6), 813–828.

Haufroid, V., & Hantson, P. (2015). CYP2D6 genetic polymorphisms and their relevance for poisoning due to amphetamines, opioid analgesics and antidepressants. *Clinical Toxicology, 53*(6). doi:10.3109/15563650.2015.1059025

Henrotin, Y., Mobasheri, A., & Marty, M. (2012). Is there any scientific evidence for the use of glucosamine in the management of human osteoarthritis? *Arthritis Research and Therapy, 14*(1), 201. doi:10.1186/ar3657

Herdman, T. H. & Kamitsuru, S. (Eds.). *Nursing Diagnoses—Definitions and Classification 2015–2017*. Copyright © 2014, 1994–2014 NANDA International. Used by arrangement with John Wiley & Sons, Inc. Companion website: www.wiley.com/go/nursingdiagnoses

Holm, S., Ljungman, G., Asenlof, P., & Soderland, A. (2013). How children and adolescents in primary care cope with pain and the biopsychosocial factors that correlate with pain related disability. *Acta Pediatrica, 102*, 1021–1026. doi:10.111/apa.12352

Hooten, W. M., Qu, W., Townsend, C. O., & Judd, J. W. (2012). Effects of strength vs. aerobic exercise on pain severity in adults with fibromyalgia: A randomized equivalence trial. *Pain, 153*(4), 915–923. doi:10.1016/j.pain.2012.01.020

Hospice and Palliative Nurses Association. (2015). *Position statement: Value of the nurse in and palliative care*. Retrieved from http://hpna.advancingexpertcare.org/wp-content/uploads/2015/08/Value-of-the-Professional-Nurse-in-Palliative-Care.pdf

Hospice Foundation of America. (2013). *What is hospice?* Retrieved from http://www.hospicefoundation.org/

Hoyce, M., & Reich, J. (2015). Critical care issues in the geriatric client. *Anesthesiology Clinics, 33*(3), 551–561.

Im, E. O., Teng, H., Lee, Y., Kang, Y., Ham, O. K., Chee, E., & Chee, W. (2014). Physical activities and sleep-related symptoms in four major racial/ethnic groups of midlife women. *Family and Community Health, 37*(4), 307–316. doi:10.1097/FCH.00000000000000

Institute of Medicine. (2006). *Sleep disorders and sleep deprivation: An unmet public health problem.* Washington, DC: National Academies Press.

Institute of Medicine. (2011). *Relieving pain in America.* Washington, DC: National Academies Press.

Institute of Medicine. (2015). *Dying in America: Improving quality and honoring individual preferences near the end of life.* Retrieved from http://www.nap.edu/catalog/18748/dying-in-america-improving-quality-and-honoring-individual-preferences-near. Published by National Academy of Sciences, © 2015.

International Association for the Study of Pain (IASP). (2009). *Barriers to cancer pain treatment.* Retrieved from http://www.iasp-pain.org/files/Content/ContentFolders/GlobalYearAgainstPain2/CancerPainFactSheets/Barriers_Final.pdf

International Association for the Study of Pain (IASP). (2011). *Acute pain management in newborn infants.* Retrieved from http://www.iasp-pain.org/PublicationsNews/NewsletterIssue.aspx?ItemNumber=2075

International Association for the Study of Pain (IASP). (2014). *IASP taxonomy.* Retrieved from http://www.iasp-pain.org/Taxonomy?navItemNumber=576#Pain

International Restless Legs Syndrome Study Group. (2012). *Diagnostic criteria.* Retrieved from http://irlssg.org/diagnostic-criteria/

Joint Commission. (2011a). *Facts about pain management.* Retrieved from http://www.jointcommission.org/pain_management

Joint Commission. (2011b). *Sentinel event ALERT: Health care worker fatigue and patient safety.* Retrieved from http://www.jointcommission.org/assets/1/18/SEA_48.pdf

Joint Commission. (2014). *Clarification of the pain management standard.* Retrieved from https://www.jointcommission.org/assets/1/18/Clarification_of_the_Pain_Management__Standard.pdf

Joint Commission. (2016). *Joint Commission statement on pain management.* Retrieved from https://www.jointcommission.org/topics/pain_management.aspx

Kaheni, S., Reza, M. S., Bagheri, M., & Goudarzian, A. H. (2016). The effect of distraction technique on the pain of dressing change among 3–6 year old children. *International Journal of Pediatrics, 4*(4), 1603–1610.

Kargarfard, M., Etemadifar, M., Baker, P., Mehrabi, M., & Hayatbakhsh, R. (2012). Effect of aquatic exercise training on fatigue and health-related quality of life in patients with multiple sclerosis. *Archives of Physical Medicine and Rehabilitation, 93*(10), 1701–1708. doi:10.1016/j.apmr.2012.05.006

Kashikar-Zuk, S., Cunningham, N., Sil, S., Bromberg, M. H., Lynch-Jordan, A. M., Strotman, D., . . . Arnold, L. M. (2014). Long-term outcomes for adolescents with juvenile-onset fibromyalgia in early adulthood. *Pediatrics, 133*(3). doi:10.1542/peds.2013-2220

Kaye, E. C., Rubenstein, J., Levine, D., Baker, J. N., Dabbs, D., & Friebert, S. E. (2015). Pediatric palliative care in the community. *Cancerjournal.com.* doi:10.3322/caac.21280

Kiecolt-Glaser, J. K., Bennett, J. M., Andridge, R., Peng, J., Shapiro, C. L., Malarkey, W. B., . . . Glaser, R. (2014). Yoga's impact on inflammation, mood, and fatigue in breast cancer survivors: A randomized controlled trial. *Journal of Clinical Oncology, 51*, 8860. Retrieved from http://jco.ascopubs.org/content/early/2014/01/21/JCO.2013.51.8860.abstract

Kim, H. K., & Nelson, L. S. (2015). Reducing the harm of opioid overdose with the safe use of naloxone: A pharmacologic review. *Drug Safety Evaluation, 14*(7), 1137–1146. doi:10.1517/14740338.2015.1037274

Kissane, D. W., & Parnes, F. (2014). *Bereavement care for families.* New York, NY: Routledge.

Kline, C. E., Ewing, G. B., Burch, J. B., Blair, S. N., Durstine, J. L., Davis, J. M., & Yongstedt, S. D. (2012). Exercise training improves selected aspects of daytime functioning in adults with obstructive sleep apnea. *Journal of Clinical Sleep Medicine, 8*(4), 357–365. doi:10.5664/jcsm.2022

Kolcaba, K. (1995). Comfort as process and product, merged in holistic nursing art. *Journal of Holistic Nursing, 13*(2), 117–131.

Kolcaba, K., Tilton, C., & Drouin, C. (2006). Comfort theory: A unifying framework to enhance the practice environment. *Journal of Nursing Administration, 36*(11), 538–544.

Lagerlov, P., Rosvoldl, E., Holager, T., & Helseth, S. (2016). How adolescents experience and cope with pain in daily life: A qualitative study on ways to cope and the use of over-the-counter analgesics. *British Medical Journal, 6*, e010184. doi:10.1136/bmjopen-2015-010184

Lande, R. G., & Gragnani, C. (2010). Nonpharmacologic approaches to the management of insomnia. *Journal of the American Osteopathic Association, 110*(12), 695–701.

Larsson, A., Palstam, A., Lofgren, M., Ernberg, M., Bjersing, J., Bileviciute-Ljungar, I, . . . Mannerkorpi, K (2015). Resistance exercise improves muscle strength, health status and pain intensity in fibromyalgia—a randomized controlled trial. *Arthritis Research and Therapy, 17*, 161. doi:10.1186/s13075-015-0679-1

Lewis, C. P., Corley, D. J., Lake, N., Brockopp, D., & Moe, K. (2014). Overcoming barriers to effective pain management: The use of professionally directed small group discussion. *Pain Management Nursing, 16*(2), 121–127. doi:10.1016/j.pmn.2014.05.002

Lundeberg, S. (2014). Pain in children: Are we accomplishing the optimum pain treatment? *Pediatric Anesthesia.* doi:10.1111/pan.12539

McCaffery, M. (1968). *Nursing practice theories related to cognition, bodily pain, and man-environment interactions.* Los Angeles, CA: University of California at Los Angeles Students' Store.

Manchikanti, L., Abdi, S., Atluri, S., Balog, C. C., Benyamin, R. M., Boswell, M. V., . . . Wargo, B. W. (2012). American Society of Interventional Pain Physicians (ASIPP) guidelines for responsible opioid prescribing in chronic non-cancer pain: Part 2—Guidance. *Pain Physician, 15*(Suppl. 3), S67–S116.

Manocha, S., & Taneja, N. (2015). Assessment of pediatric pain: A critical review. *Journal of Basic Physiology and Pharmacology.* doi:10.1515/jbcpp-2015-0041

Margarit, C., Julia, J., Lopez, R., Anton, A., Escobar, Y., Casas, A., . . . Zaragoza, F. (2012). Breakthrough cancer pain—still a challenge. *Journal of Pain Research, 5*, 559–566. doi:10.2147/JPR.S36428

Massachusetts General Hospital. (n.d.). *Addressing quietness on units: Best practice implementation guide.* Retrieved from http://www.mghpcs.org/eed_portal/Documents/PatExp/ADDRESSING-QUIETNESS.pdf

Mayo Clinic. (2016). *Symptoms of fatigue.* Retrieved from http://www.mayoclinic.com/symptoms/fatigue/basics/causes/sym-20050894

Meghani, S. H., Byun, E., & Gallagher, R. M. (2012). Time to take stock: A meta-analysis and systematic review of analgesic treatment disparities for pain in the United States. *Pain Medicine, 13*(2), 150–174. doi:10.1111/j.1526-4637.2011.01310.x

Melzack, R., & Wall, P. D. (1965). Pain mechanisms: A new theory. *Science, 150*(3699), 971–979.

Michelson, K. N., Patel, R., Haber-Barker, N., Emanuel, L., & Frader, J. (2013). End-of-life care decisions in the PICU: Roles professionals play. *Pediatric Critical Care Medicine, 14*(1), e34–e44. doi:10.1097/PCC.0b013e31826e7408

Miller, C. B., Espie, C. A., Epstein, D. R., Friedman, L., Morin, C. M., Pigeon, W. R., . . . Kyle, S. D. (2014). The evidence base of sleep restriction therapy for treating insomnia disorder. *Sleep Medicine Reviews, 18*(5), 415–424. doi:10.1016/j.smrv.2014.01.006

Mooventhan, A., & Nivethitha, L. (2014). Scientific evidence-based effects of hydrotherapy on various systems of the body. *North American Journal of Medical Science, 6*(5), 199–209. Retrieved from http://www.ncbi.nlm.nih.gov/pmc/articles/PMC4049052

National Cancer Institute. (2012). *End-of-life care for people who have cancer.* Retrieved from http://www.cancer.gov/cancertopics/factsheet/Support/end-of-life-care. Published by U.S. Department of Health and Human Services.

National Cancer Institute. (2013). *Pain (PDQ®).* Retrieved from http://www.cancer.gov/cancertopics/pdq/supportivecare/pain/Health-Professional/page1

National Center for Advancing Translational Sciences (NCATS). (2014). *Genetic and Rare Diseases Information Center.* Retrieved from: https://rarediseases.info.nih.gov/gard/6429/fatal-familial-insomnia/resources/1

National Center for Complementary and Alternative Medicine (NCCAM). (2014). *Special report.* Retrieved from http://nccam.nih.gov/sites/nccam

National Center for Complementary and Integrative Health (NCCIH). (2013). *Relaxation techniques for health: An introduction.* Retrieved from https://nccih.nih.gov/sites/nccam.nih.gov/files/relaxation_introduction.pdf

National Center for Complementary and Integrative Health (NCCIH). (2016). *Acupuncture for pain.* Retrieved from https://nccih.nih.gov/node/2422

National Center for Complementary and Integrative Health (NCCIH). (2016a). *Understanding drug-supplement interactions.* Retrieved from https://nccih.nih.gov/health/know-science/how-medications-supplements-interact

National Center for Complementary and Integrative Health (NCCIH). (2016b). *Fibromyalgia: In depth.* Retrieved from https://nccih.nih.gov/health/pain/fibromyalgia.htm

National Consensus Project for Quality Palliative Care. (2013). *Clinical practice guidelines for quality palliative care* (3rd ed.). Pittsburgh, PA: National Consensus Project for Quality Palliative Care.

National Fibromyalgia Association. (2016). *Prevalence*. Retrieved from http://www.fmaware.org/about-fibromyalgia/prevalence/

National Heart, Lung and Blood Institute (NHLBI). (2015). *Why is sleep important?* Retrieved from http://www.nhlbi.nih.gov/health/health-topics/topics/sdd/why

National Hospice and Palliative Care Organization. (2015). *NHPCO facts and figures: Hospice care in America*. Retrieved from http://www.nhpco.org/sites/default/files/public/Statistics_Research/2015_Facts_Figures.pdf

National Institute of Aging. (2015). *Fatigue: More than being tired*. Retrieved from https://www.nia.nih.gov/health/publication/fatigue

National Institute of Mental Health. (2016). *Depression*. Retrieved from https://www.nimh.nih.gov/health/topics/depression/index.shtml

National Institute of Neurological Disorders and Stroke. (2014). *Brain basics: Understanding sleep*. Retrieved from http://www.ninds.nih.gov/disorders/brain_basics/understanding_sleep.htm

National Institutes of Health. (2013). *Genetics home reference: SCN9A*. Retrieved from http://ghr.nlm.nih.gov/gene/SCN9A

National Institutes of Health. (2015). *What are sleep deprivation and deficiency?* Retrieved from http://www.nhlbi.nih.gov/health/health-topics/topics/sdd

National Library of Medicine. (2013). *Fatigue*. Retrieved from https://www.nlm.nih.gov/medlineplus/ency/article/003088.htm

National Organization for Rare Disorders. (2015). *Central pain syndrome*. Retrieved from https://rarediseases.org/rare-diseases/central-pain-syndrome/

National Sleep Foundation. (2013). *Does exercise help sleep in the elderly?* Retrieved from https://sleepfoundation.org/ask-the-expert/does-exercise-help-sleep-the-elderly

National Sleep Foundation. (2016a). *Pregnancy and sleep*. Retrieved from http://www.sleepfoundation.org/article/sleep-topics/pregnancy-and-sleep

National Sleep Foundation. (2016b). *Teens and sleep*. Retrieved from https://sleepfoundation.org/sleep-topics/teens-and-sleep

Noel, M., Chambers, C. T., McGrath, P. J., Klein, R. M., & Stewart, S. H. (2012). The influence of children's pain memories on subsequent pain experience. *Pain, 153*(8), 1563–1572. doi:10.1016/j.pain.2012.02.020

Onieva-Zafra, M. D., García, L. H., & del Valle, M. G. (2015). Effectiveness of guided imagery relaxation on levels of pain and depression in patients diagnosed with fibromyalgia. *Holistic Nursing Practice, 29* (1), 13–21. doi:10.1097/HNP.000000000000006

Palermo, T., & Jamison, R. N. (2015). Innovative delivery of pain management interventions. *Journal of Clinical Pain, 31*(6), 467–469.

Park, J., & Hughes, A. K. (2012). Nonpharmacological approaches to the management of chronic pain in community-dwelling older adults: A review of empirical evidence. *Journal of the American Geriatric Society, 60*(3), 555–568. doi:10.1111/j.1532-5415.2011.03846.x

Parlour, R., Slater, P., McCormack, B., Gallen, A., & Kavanagh, P. (2014). The relationship between positive patient experience in acute hospitals and patient-centered care. *International Journal of Research in Nursing, 5*(1), 24–36. doi:10.3844/ijrnsp.2014.27.36

Pasero, C. (2009). *American Society of Perianesthesia Nurses: Assessment of sedation during opioid administration for pain management*. Retrieved from http://www.mghpcs.org/eed_portal/Documents/Pain/Assessing_opioid-induced_sedation.pdf

Portenoy, R. K., Mehta, Z., & Ahmed, E. (2016). *Cancer pain management with opioids: Prevention and management of side effects*. Retrieved from http://www.uptodate.com/contents/cancer-pain-management-with-opioids-prevention-and-management-of-side-effects

Ramos, A. R., Seixas, A., & Dib, S. I. (2015). Obstructive sleep apnea and stroke: Links to health disparities. *Sleep Health, 1*(4), 244–248.

Rastogi, R., & Meek, B. D. (2013). Management of chronic pain in elderly, frail patients: Finding a suitable, personalized method of control. *Journal of Clinical Interventions in Aging, 8*, 37–46. doi:10.2147/cia.s30165

Ratcliffe, A., & Kallappa, C. (2015). G69(P) narcolepsy—an important but rare pediatric diagnosis. *Archives of Diseases in Children, 100*(A29). doi:10.1136/archdischild-2015-308599.68

Registered Nurses' Association of Ontario. (2013). *Assessment and management of pain* (3rd ed.). Toronto, Canada: Author.

Renjilian, C. B., Womer, J. W., Carroll, K. W., Kang, T. I., & Feudtner, C. (2013). Parental explicit heuristics in decision-making for children with life-threatening illnesses. *Pediatrics, 131*(2), e566–e572. doi:10.1542/peds.2012-1957

Rewald, S., Mesters, I., Emans, P., Arts, C., Lenssen, A. F., & Bie, R. A. (2015). Aquatic circuit training including aqua-cycling in patients with knee osteoarthritis: A feasibility study. *Journal of Rehabilitative Medicine, 47*(4), 376–381. doi:10.2340/16501977-1937

Robeck, I. (2014). *Chronic pain in the elderly: Special challenges*. Retrieved from http://www.practicalpainmanagement.com/pain/chronic-pain-elderly-special-challenges

Sanderson, A. (2013). *DNR orders and end-of-life decisions for children: The elephant in the room*. Retrieved from Boston Children's Hospital website: http://vector.childrenshospital.org/2013/09/dnr-orders-and-end-of-life-decisions-for-children-the-elephant-in-the-room/

Schutte-Rodin, S., Broch, L., Buysse, D., Dorsey, C., & Sateia, M. (2008). Clinical guideline for the evaluation and management of chronic insomnia in adults. *Journal of Clinical Sleep Medicine, 4*(5), 487–504.

Serlin, R. C., Mendoza, T. R., Nakamura, Y., Edwards, K. R., & Cleeland, C. S. (1995). When is cancer pain mild, moderate, or severe? Grading pain severity by its interference with function. *Pain, 61*(2), 277–284. doi:10.1016/0304-3959(94)00178-H

Sevimli, D., Kozanoglu, E., Guzel, R., & Doganay, A. (2015). The effects of aquatic, isometric strength-stretching and aerobic exercise on physical and psychological parameters of female patients with fibromyalgia syndrome. *Journal of Physical Therapy Science, 27*(6), 1781–1786. doi:10.1589/jpts.27.1781

Sherman, D. W., & Free, D. C. (2015). Nursing and palliative care. In N. Cherny, M. Fallon, S. Kaasa, R. Portenoy, & D. Currow (Eds.), *Oxford textbook of palliative medicine* (5th ed., 154–163). New York, NY: Oxford University Press.

Sherman, D. W., Norman, R., & McSherry, C. B. (2010). A comparison of death anxiety and quality of life of patients with advanced cancer or AIDS and their family caregivers. *Journal of the Association of Nurses in AIDS Care, 21*(2), 99–112. doi:10.1016/j.jana.2009.07.007

Simons, L. E., Sieberg, C. B., & Clarr, R. L. (2012). Anxiety and functional disability in a large sample of children and adolescents with chronic pain. *Pain Research and Management, 17*(2), 93–97.

Sloot, S., Boland, J., Snowden, J., Ezaydi, Y. L., Foster, A., Gethin, A. L., . . . Ahmedza, S. H. (2014). Side effects of analgesia may significantly reduce quality of life in symptomatic multiple myeloma: A cross-sectional prevalence study. *Supportive Care in Cancer, 23*(3), 671–678. doi:10.1007/s00520-014-2358-1

Spector, R. E. (2017). *Cultural diversity in health and illness* (9th ed.). Hoboken, NJ: Pearson Education.

Stanford School of Medicine. (2016). *Palliative care: Where do Americans die?* Retrieved from https://palliative.stanford.edu/home-hospice-home-care-of-the-dying-patient/where-do-americans-die

Stasiowska, M. K., Ng, S. C., Gubbay, A. N., & Cregg, R. (2015). Postoperative pain management. *British Journal of Hospital Medicine, 76*(10), 570–575. doi:10.12968/hmed.2015.76.10.570

Stites, M. (2013). Observational pain scales in critically ill adults. *Critical Care Nurse, 33*(3), 68–78. Retrieved from http://www.aacn.org/wd/cetests/media/c1333.pdf

Syrjala, K. L., Jensen, M. P., Mendoza, M. E., Hi, J. C., Fisher, H. M., & Keefe, F. J. (2014). Psychological and behavioral approaches to cancer pain management. *Journal of Clinical Oncology, 32*(16). doi:10.1200/JCO.2013.54.4825

Tracy, B., & Morrison, S. R. (2013). Pain management in older adults. *Clinical Therapy, 35*(11). doi:10.1016/j.clinthera.2013.09.026

Unaldi Karaer, H., Kaplan, Y., Kurt, S., & Demirturk, F. (2014). Prevalence and features associated with restless leg syndrome in postmenopausal females. *Journal of Neurologic Science, 31*(3), 578–585.

University of Maryland Medical Center. (2013). *Sleepiness scale*. Retrieved from http://umm.edu/programs/sleep/health/quizzes/sleepiness

Vargas-Alarcon, G., Alvarez-Leon, E., Fragoso, J. M., Vargas, A., Martinez, A., Vallejo, M., & Martinez-Lavin, M. (2012). A SCN9A gene-encoded dorsal root ganglia sodium channel polymorphism associated with severe fibromyalgia. *BMC Musculoskeletal Disorders, 13*, 23. doi:10.1186/1471-2474-13-23

Vickers, A. J., Phil, D., & Linde, K. (2014). Acupuncture for chronic pain. *Journal of the American Medical Association, 311*(9), 955–956. doi:10.1001/jama.2013.285478

Vriend, L., & Corkum, P. (2011). Clinical management of behavioral insomnia of childhood. *Psychological Research and Behavior Management, 4*, 69–70. Retrieved from http://www.ncbi.nlm.nih.gov/pmc/articles/PMC3218792/

Walsh, K. (2012). *Grief and loss: Theories and skills for the helping profession* (2nd ed.). New York, NY: Pearson.

Wanless, S., Cohen, S. M., & Danford, C. A. (2015). The assessment and non-pharmacologic treatment of procedural pain from infancy to school age through a developmental lens: A synthesis of evidence with recommendations. *Journal of Pediatric Nursing*. doi:10.1016/j.pedn.2015.09.002

Wilsey, B., Marcotte, T., Deutsch, R., Gouaux, B., Sakai, S., & Donaghe, H. (2013). Low-dose vaporized cannabis significantly improves neuropathic pain. *Journal of Pain, 14*(10), 136–148.

Wilson, B., Shannon, M., & Shields, K. (Eds.). (2016). *Pearson nurse's drug guide*. New York, NY: Pearson Education.

Wolfe, F., Clauw, D. J., Fitzcharles, M-A., Goldenberg, D. L., Katz, R. S., Mease, P., . . . Yunus, M. B. (2010). The American College of Rheumatology preliminary diagnostic criteria for fibromyalgia and measurement of symptom severity. *Arthritis Care and Research, 62*(5), 600–610. doi:10.1002/acr.20140

Wolfe, F., Smythe, H. A., Yunus, M. B., Bennett, R. M., Bombardier, C., Goldenberg, D. L., . . .

Sheon, R. P. (1990). The American College of Rheumatology 1990 criteria for the classification of fibromyalgia. *Arthritis and Rheumatism, 33*(2), 160–172. doi:10.1002/art.1780330203

Wong, D. L., Hockenberry-Eaton, M., Wilson, D., Winkelstein, M. L., & Schwartz, P. (2001). *Wong's essentials of pediatric nursing* (6th ed., p. 1301). St. Louis, MO: Mosby.

Wooten, P. (2013). Humor, laughter and play. In B. M. Doosey & L. Keegan (Eds.), *Holistic nursing: A handbook for practice*. Burlington, MA: Jones and Bartlett.

World Health Organization (WHO). (2014). *Global atlas of palliative care at the end of life*. Retrieved from http://www.thewhpca.org/resources/global-atlas-on-end-of-life-care

World Health Organization (WHO). (2015). *WHO definition of palliative care*. Retrieved from http://www.who.int/cancer/palliative/definition/en/

World Health Organization (WHO). (2016). *WHO's cancer pain ladder for adults*. Retrieved from http://www.who.int/cancer/palliative/painladder/en/

Zheng, G., Liu, F., Li, S., Huang, M., Tao, J., & Chen, L. (2015). Tai Chi and the protection of cognitive ability: A systematic review of prospective studies in healthy adults. *American Journal of Preventative Medicine, 49*(1), 89–97. doi:10.1016/j.amepre.2015.01.002

Zoega, S., Ward, S., Sigurdsson, G. H., Aspelund, T., Sveinsdottir, H., & Gunnarsdottir, S. (2015). Quality pain management practices in a university hospital. *Pain Management Nursing, 16*(3), 198–210.

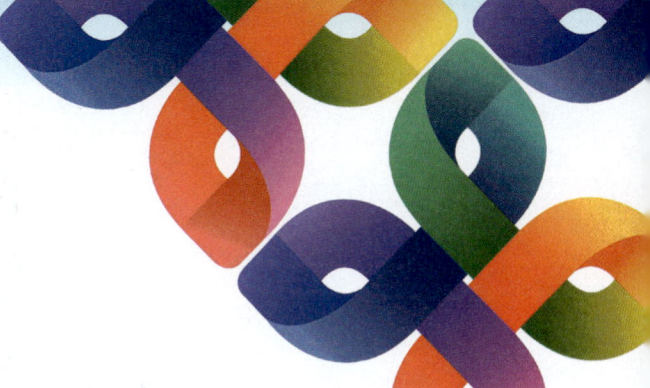

Module 4
Digestion

Module Outline and Learning Outcomes

The Concept of Digestion

Normal Digestion
4.1 Analyze the physiology of digestion in the body.

Alterations to Digestion
4.2 Differentiate alterations in digestion.

Concepts Related to Digestion
4.3 Outline the relationship between digestion and other concepts.

Health Promotion
4.4 Explain the promotion of healthy digestion.

Nursing Assessment
4.5 Differentiate common assessment procedures and tests used to examine digestion.

Independent Interventions
4.6 Analyze independent interventions nurses can implement for patients with alterations in digestion.

Collaborative Therapies
4.7 Summarize collaborative therapies used by interprofessional teams for patients with alterations in digestion.

Lifespan Considerations
4.8 Differentiate considerations related to the assessment and care of patients with alterations in digestion throughout the lifespan.

Digestion Exemplars

Exemplar 4.A Gastroesophageal Reflux Disease
4.A Analyze GERD as it relates to digestion.

Exemplar 4.B Hepatitis
4.B Analyze hepatitis as it relates to digestion.

Exemplar 4.C Malabsorption Disorders
4.C Analyze malabsorption disorders as they relate to digestion.

Exemplar 4.D Pancreatitis
4.D Analyze pancreatitis as it relates to digestion.

Exemplar 4.E Pyloric Stenosis
4.E Analyze pyloric stenosis as it relates to digestion.

❯❯ The Concept of Digestion

Concept Key Terms

Absorption, 218	Enteral nutrition, 230	Heartburn, 219	Nausea, 219	Total parenteral nutrition (TPN), 232
Acid indigestion, 219	Enzymes, 218	Hepatitis, 219	Nutrients, 218	Vomiting, 219
Anorexia, 219	Fluoroscope, 228	Malabsorption, 219	Pancreatitis, 219	
Digestion, 217	Gastroesophageal reflux	Maldigestion, 219	Probiotics, 234	
Emesis, 219	disease (GERD), 219	Motility, 218	Pyloric stenosis, 219	

Digestion is the conversion of food into absorbable substances in the gastrointestinal (GI) tract. It occurs through the mechanical and chemical breakdown of food into smaller molecules, with the help of glands located inside and outside the stomach. Digestion is an integrated process that affects the entire human body. Alterations in digestion occur when one or more of the processes that break down food and absorb nutrients are impaired. Impairments in digestion may be caused by changes in nutritional status, structural (anatomic) alterations, or the effects of one or more medications. Because of the widespread prevalence of alterations in digestion, nurses must be knowledgeable about

different alterations and their risk factors and be able to assess how alterations in digestion affect other physiologic processes. By utilizing the nursing process to care for patients who are experiencing alterations in digestion, nurses can engage with patients to optimize their health and well-being.

Normal Digestion
Physiology Review
The digestive system consists of the mouth, pharynx, esophagus, stomach, small intestine, and large intestine (see **Figure 4–1** ❯❯). Accessory organs such as the liver, gallbladder, and

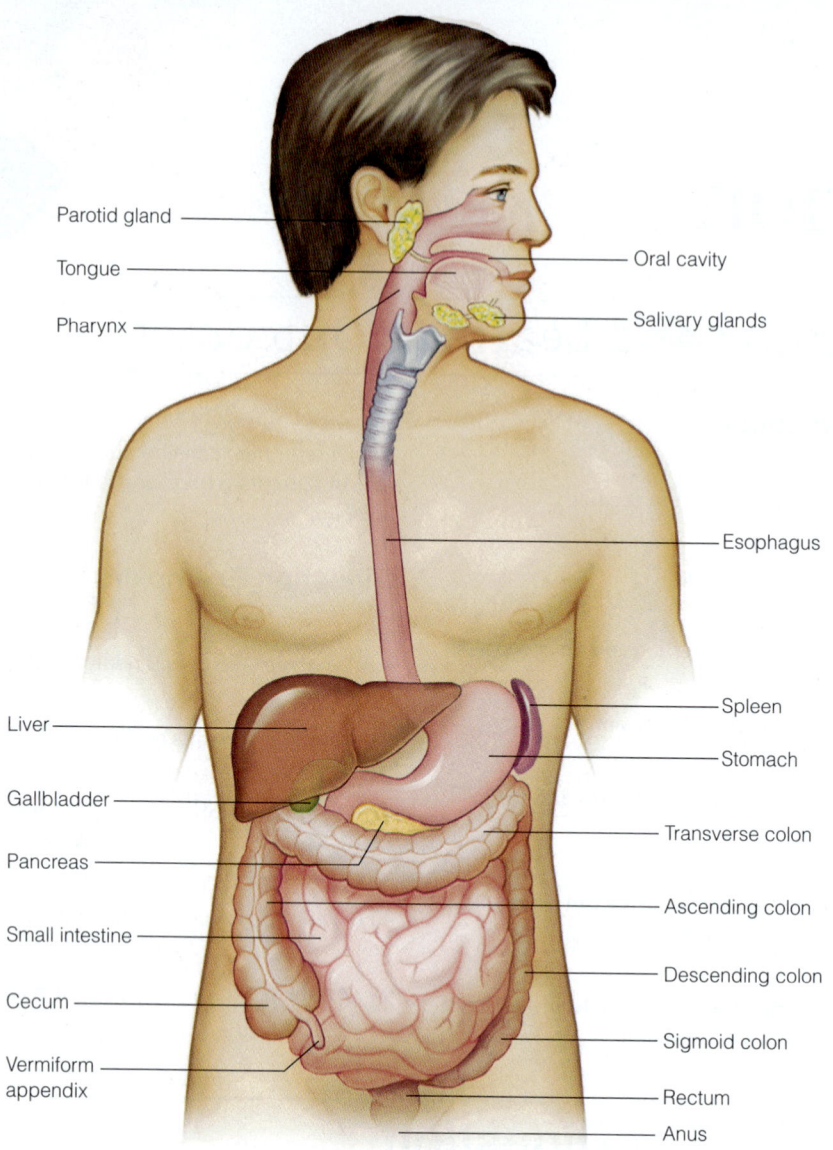

Parotid gland
Tongue
Pharynx
Oral cavity
Salivary glands
Esophagus
Liver
Gallbladder
Pancreas
Small intestine
Cecum
Vermiform appendix
Spleen
Stomach
Transverse colon
Ascending colon
Descending colon
Sigmoid colon
Rectum
Anus

Figure 4–1 ⟩⟩ Organs of the alimentary canal and related accessory organs.

pancreas assist in the normal digestive process. **Nutrients** are substances found in food that are used by the body to promote normal growth, maintenance, and repair. They include carbohydrates, proteins, fats, vitamins, minerals, and water. The digestive system provides the body with nutrition, balancing fluids and electrolytes, and eliminating waste products. It works congruently with the metabolic system for secretion of digestive **enzymes**, which assist in digestion of nutrients. Appropriate amounts and proper utilization of nutrients allow the body to function at optimal ability. For example, utilization of glucose allows the brain to function, whereas a deficiency in protein may delay wound healing. See the module on Nutrition for more information on nutrients.

⟩⟩ Go to **Pearson MyLab Nursing and eText** for a more detailed look at the physiology of digestion.

Alterations to Digestion

Disorders of motility and absorption can affect the functioning of the digestive system. **Motility** of the gastrointestinal

(GI) tract moves food and fluid from the mouth to the anus. The rate and strength of peristalsis are regulated by the autonomic nervous system. Disorders of gastric motility occur when coordination of the digestive muscles is interrupted in some way (International Foundation for Functional Gastrointestinal Disorders [IFFGD], 2015). Inflammation, infection, tumors, obstructions, or changes in structure can affect motility. Direct and indirect factors can influence motility. Food intake and bacteria can affect the number and consistency of stools. Stress and postponement of defecation can influence motility. Some disorders affecting motility include gastroesophageal reflux, impaired esophageal motility, pyloric stenosis, diarrhea, constipation, irritable bowel syndrome, and encopresis.

Absorption is the process by which nutrients from food move out of the intestine and into the bloodstream for distribution throughout the body (American College of Gastroenterology, n.d.). Absorption occurs through active transport and diffusion. Various medical or surgical conditions can affect absorption of nutrients, resulting in malabsorption.

Some disorders affecting absorption include pernicious anemia, lactose intolerance, celiac disease, Crohn disease, acute and chronic pancreatitis, and liver failure.

Alterations and Manifestations

Common symptoms that indicate a possible alteration of the digestive system are nausea and vomiting. **Nausea** is a vague but unpleasant subjective sensation of sickness or queasiness. It may or may not be accompanied by (and possibly relieved by) vomiting. **Vomiting** is the forceful expulsion of the contents of the upper GI tract resulting from contraction of muscles in the gut and abdominal wall. Nausea and vomiting are symptoms of underlying disorders. Food, stress, medications, smells, and tastes are common causes of nausea, vomiting, and diarrhea. Nausea and vomiting are commonly associated with food poisoning, drug and alcohol overuse, and infectious gastroenteritis. Individuals typically avoid foods, tastes, and smells and use stress reduction strategies to relieve these symptoms. Many times this is enough to resolve the underlying source of distress.

Nausea occurs when the vomiting center in the medulla of the brain is stimulated. Distention of the duodenum is a common stimulus for nausea. The vomiting center can be stimulated by input from several different sources:

- The GI tract produced by distention, irritation, or infection
- The vestibular system of the ear
- Higher central nervous system centers in response to certain sights, smells, or emotional experiences
- Chemoreceptors outside the blood–brain barrier that are stimulated by drugs, chemotherapeutic agents, toxins, systemic disorders, and pregnancy
- Disorders such as acute myocardial infarction and heart failure, which commonly produce nausea and vomiting, possibly due to direct stimulation of the vomiting center by hypoxia
- Increased intracranial pressure (e.g., due to intracranial bleeding or a tumor), which produces vomiting that may or may not be accompanied by nausea.

Anorexia (loss of appetite) commonly precedes nausea, just as nausea frequently precedes vomiting. Vomiting is coordinated by the brainstem. **Emesis** (or *vomitus*) is produced when inspiratory muscles of the thorax (including the diaphragm) and abdomen contract, increasing intrathoracic and intra-abdominal pressures. The gastroesophageal sphincter relaxes, and the larynx moves upward to facilitate oral expulsion of gastric contents.

In addition to the subjective sensation of queasiness, nausea frequently is accompanied by autonomic nervous system manifestations such as pallor, sweating, tachycardia, and increased salivation. Vomiting, which stimulates the vagus nerve and parasympathetic nervous system, may be accompanied by dizziness, light-headedness, hypotension, and bradycardia.

In **gastroesophageal reflux disease (GERD)**, stomach contents flow back up into the esophagus. This causes pyrosis or **heartburn**, a burning sensation in the chest or throat. It may also cause **acid indigestion**, which occurs when the individual can taste the stomach acid (National Institutes of Health [NIH], 2015c). Treatment ranges from symptom management through diet and lifestyle management to pharmacologic therapy and, for some patients, surgery.

Inflammation of the liver is termed **hepatitis**. In hepatitis, the inflammatory process may be triggered by a virus, alcohol, medications, toxins, autoimmune disorder, or other pathogens; the resulting inflammation affects the liver's ability to function normally. Hepatitis can be acute or chronic. Viral hepatitis is the most common type of hepatitis. Treatment of hepatitis is focused on finding the cause, treating the symptoms, and limiting liver damage.

Malabsorption is a condition in which the intestinal mucosa is unable to absorb nutrients, resulting in nutrients being excreted in the stool. Common systemic manifestations of malabsorption are weight loss, weakness, malaise, muscle cramps, bone pain, abnormal bleeding, and anemia. Selected causes of malabsorption include acute enteritis, AIDS-related opportunistic infections, celiac disease, Crohn disease, intestinal ischemia or infarction, scleroderma, and short bowel syndrome.

Maldigestion is a condition in which the preparation of chyme for absorption of nutrients is inadequate, resulting in malabsorption. Selected causes of maldigestion include biliary obstruction, chronic pancreatitis, cirrhosis, cystic fibrosis, gastrectomy, hepatitis, lactose intolerance, pancreatic cancer, and Zollinger-Ellison syndrome. See Exemplar 4.C on Malabsorption Disorders for a discussion of celiac disease, lactase deficiency, and short bowel syndrome.

Pancreatitis, or inflammation of the pancreas, is a condition in which pancreatic cells release pancreatic enzymes into the tissues of the pancreas. Clinical manifestations include abdominal pain, nausea, vomiting, fever, sweating, chills, and fatty stools. Pancreatitis can be acute or chronic. Acute pancreatitis usually presents with upper abdominal pain. Severe episodes can cause dehydration and low blood pressure. Untreated bleeding in the pancreas or organ failure may result. Patients with acute pancreatitis require immediate medical attention (NIH, 2015b). Repeat episodes of acute pancreatitis can lead to chronic pancreatitis (NIH, 2013b).

Chronic pancreatitis presents with upper abdominal pain and chronic weight loss. Common causes of chronic pancreatitis include chronic alcohol abuse, trauma, cystic fibrosis, hyperparathyroidism, and certain medications (e.g., corticosteroids, estrogens, thiazide diuretics). Other conditions can also result in chronic pancreatitis.

Pyloric stenosis is a thickening of the pyloric muscle resulting in a narrowing of the pyloric sphincter between the stomach and small intestine. The condition typically occurs before 6 months of age and is usually diagnosed by 12 weeks of age. Symptoms such as projectile vomiting usually begin around 3 weeks of age, although the onset may vary from 1 week to 5 months of age (Mayo Clinic, 2015b).

Prevalence

Nausea, vomiting, and diarrhea are common in all age groups. Twenty percent of the U.S. population exhibits weekly symptoms of GERD (NIH, 2014a). New cases of viral hepatitis vary by type: In 2013, there were 3500 new cases of hepatitis A, 19,800 new cases of hepatitis B, and 29,700 new cases of hepatitis C. Somewhere between 3 and 4 million individuals are living with chronic hepatitis (Centers for Disease Control and Prevention [CDC], 2015c).

Alterations and Therapies
Digestion

ALTERATION	DESCRIPTION	MANIFESTATIONS	INTERVENTIONS AND THERAPIES
Nausea	Uneasy feeling in the stomach, usually preceding vomiting	■ Distaste for food ■ May be accompanied by the urge to vomit ■ Abdominal discomfort	■ Monitor complaints of nausea, remembering that nausea is a subjective sensation best described by the patient. ■ Monitor vital signs, skin turgor and condition, and weight. ■ Maintain accurate intake and output records. ■ Monitor amount, color, and specific gravity of urine. ■ Be aware that nausea can result in dehydration even when not accompanied by vomiting. ■ Give antiemetics as ordered. ■ Teach deep breathing to suppress vomiting reflex. ■ Encourage intake of small quantities of clear fluids and dry foods at separate times to reduce nausea stimuli.

Vomiting	Emptying of stomach contents through the mouth	■ Expelling stomach contents through the mouth
		■ Diaphoresis
		■ Preceding nausea
			■ Withhold foods initially; give clear liquids in small quantities to prevent dehydration.
			■ For pediatric patients, administer fluid and electrolyte solution (e.g., Pedialyte). Milk-based infant formula may need to be withheld until symptoms subside.
			■ Once nausea and vomiting have stopped:
			  • Give clear liquids as tolerated; give dry foods (e.g., soda crackers) to reduce nausea and promote comfort.
			  • Introduce bland foods (e.g., rice, applesauce, toast) slowly. Avoid dairy products until symptoms disappear.
			  • Reassess need for antiemetic medications.

Gastroesophageal reflux disease (GERD)	Backward flow of stomach contents	■ Chest discomfort
		■ Heartburn
		■ Acid indigestion
			■ Treatment varies according to severity of the disorder but may include:
			  • Dietary and lifestyle management
			  • Medications
			  • Surgery.

Hepatitis	Inflammation of the liver	■ Abdominal pain ■ Dark urine ■ Nausea and vomiting ■ Jaundice ■ Fever	■ Underlying cause and type of hepatitis will dictate treatment. ■ Acute hepatitis is managed by supportive treatments; chronic hepatitis involves pharmacologic agents that eradicate the virus and prevent further liver damage (Medicine.Net, 2013).
Malabsorption disorders	Intestinal mucosa cannot absorb nutrients, which results in the nutrients being excreted in stool	■ Diarrhea ■ Weight loss	■ Underlying cause dictates treatment. In many cases, nutrition management plays an important role in treatment.

Alterations and Therapies (continued)

ALTERATION	DESCRIPTION	MANIFESTATIONS	INTERVENTIONS AND THERAPIES
Pancreatitis	Inflammation of the pancreas characterized by release of pancreatic enzymes into the pancreatic tissue; may be acute or chronic	■ Upper left or midabdominal pain worsening after eating or drinking, especially foods with high fat content ■ Fever ■ Nausea and vomiting ■ Diaphoresis ■ Clay-colored stools if bile duct obstruction occurs	■ Acute pancreatitis is often mild and self-limiting. ■ Treatment focuses on: • Reducing pancreatic secretions by having the patient NPO (nothing by mouth) • Providing supportive care • Eliminating causative factor after resolving inflammation. ■ Opioid analgesics, fluid replacement, and prophylactic antibiotics may be prescribed. ■ Chronic pancreatitis treatment focuses on managing pain and treating malabsorption and malnutrition: • Manage opioid analgesics carefully to avoid side effects. • Prescribe pancreatic enzyme supplements. • Prescribe H_2-blockers and proton pump inhibitors to neutralize and reduce gastric secretions.
Pyloric stenosis	Hypertrophic obstruction of the circular muscle of the pyloric canal	■ Projectile vomiting ■ Constant hunger ■ Weight loss or inability to gain weight ■ Notable peristaltic wave in abdomen immediately before vomiting occurs	■ Restore fluid and electrolyte balance. Follow with surgery to split the pyloric muscle to allow passage of food and fluid.

Genetic Considerations and Risk Factors

Genetics plays a role in diseases of the digestive system, affecting digestion and absorption of nutrients. Gene and chromosomal alterations in the digestive system can result in Crohn disease, which is discussed in detail in the exemplar on Inflammatory Bowel Disease in the module on Inflammation. The healthcare team should consider genetic and nonmodifiable risk factors when caring for individuals with digestive disorders. Early identification of risk factors leads to early intervention and disease prevention or lessens the severity of the disease processes. Genetics may play a role in GERD, pyloric stenosis, celiac disease, and pancreatitis. Approximately 10% of individuals with celiac disease have first-degree family members with the same condition. These family members may wish to be screened (National Digestive Diseases Information Clearinghouse, 2012). A genetic mutation on a gene associated with cystic fibrosis may play a role in pancreatitis. Those with a family history of pancreatitis, African Americans, and women who have gallstones are all at increased risk for pancreatitis (NIH, 2013a). The cause of pyloric stenosis is unknown, but genetics may play a role. It is more common in White, male, first-born infants with a family history of pyloric stenosis.

Case Study ›› Part 1

Jack Zambrano, a 9-year-old boy, came home from his afterschool program feeling sick. When his mother asked him what was wrong, he said, "I feel sick to my stomach, I'm tired, and my head hurts." Jack's mother helped him to bed and took his temperature, which was 102°F. Jack refused to eat his dinner after a couple of bites. His mother calls the health clinic where you work.

While conducting the assessment, you learn Jack's parents are Hispanic and came to live in the United States when Jack was 2 years old. Jack and his family travel annually to Mexico to visit his grandparents and extended family members. The family returned from Mexico 2 weeks ago. Jack's immunization record is incomplete.

Clinical Reasoning Questions Level I
1. What data point to a possible cause of Jack's illness?
2. What is the priority nursing diagnosis for Jack at this time?

Clinical Reasoning Questions Level II
3. How does Jack's immunization record relate to his signs and symptoms?
4. What independent nursing intervention can you discuss with Jack's mother to help Jack feel more comfortable?
5. What antipyretic medication should you tell Jack's mother to avoid giving to him?

Concepts Related to Digestion

Digestion plays an essential role in the body's well-being. Digestive processes provide energy and nutrients to the body, and they allow the body to access and absorb essential building blocks such as amino acids. Impairments in digestion may result in fluid and electrolyte imbalances and problems such as vomiting or diarrhea. Nutrition, metabolism, growth and development, elimination, and fluids and electrolytes are all directly related to digestion.

Proper nutrition—including lean meats, foods high in fiber, vitamins, minerals, and water—is essential for healthy digestion and normal growth and development. Malnutrition can impair digestion and increase the risk for impaired growth and development. Eating disorders may result in malnutrition. The altered eating behaviors associated with these disorders disrupt normal digestive patterns. Evidence suggests that these disruptions may be associated with alterations in production of digestive enzymes and changes in gut flora (Scarlata & Anderson, 2014). The following feature links some, but not all, of the concepts related to digestion. They are presented in alphabetical order.

Health Promotion

Digestive health involves three primary aspects: consumption, elimination, and prevention. As a result, digestive health promotion involves lifestyle choices and management. Foods that support good overall health are essential for healthy digestion. Fruits and vegetables, whole grains, and lean meats all support normal digestion, while highly processed foods and those with high fat content can have

Concepts Related to Digestion

CONCEPT	RELATIONSHIP TO DIGESTION	NURSING IMPLICATIONS
Development	Healthy nutrition and digestion → normal physical and mental function	■ Assess height, weight, and mental functioning in developing children. Be alert for children with low height/weight percentages and/or slow mental development. ■ Assess elimination, including diarrhea frequency and other signs indicating digestive abnormalities.
Elimination	Indigestible food products → out of the body through elimination	■ Assess recent changes to the typical elimination pattern. ■ Assess frequency, consistency, and urgency of stools. Be alert for diarrhea or constipation. ■ Assess pain or discomfort associated with bowel movements. Be alert for discomfort caused by hemorrhoids, which may be a result of straining during bowel movements. ■ Assess for fecal impaction, particularly in cases of chronic untreated constipation or frequent laxative use. Breathing problems, increased heart rate, and low blood pressure are all associated with impaction. ■ Assess for bowel obstruction, especially if the patient has a condition or history that may lead to formation of adhesions. Stomach cramping and pain, vomiting, and bloating are all indicative of obstruction.
Fluids and Electrolytes	↑ Frequency or amount of diarrhea → fluid and electrolyte imbalances	■ Assess pattern of bowel elimination. ■ Assess for signs of dehydration, including lethargy, poor skin turgor, and low urinary output. ■ Anticipate serum electrolyte tests and electrolyte and fluid supplements.
Metabolism	Food molecules broken down by digestive processes → bloodstream and are metabolized by cells	■ Assess sleep patterns and stress levels. Lack of sleep and high levels of stress slow metabolism. ■ Assess recent unexplained weight gain or loss. Gain can signal low metabolism, while loss can signal high metabolism. ■ In female patients, assess regularity of menses and the presence of reproductive issues. Both are associated with slow metabolism. ■ Anticipate blood tests to assess function of the thyroid gland and hormone levels in the bloodstream.
Nutrition	Nutrients → growth, development, and repair	■ Assess for unplanned weight loss, low body mass index (BMI), infection, and other signs and symptoms of malnutrition. ■ Assess bowel elimination for diarrhea and other malabsorption or digestive problems.
Self	Eating disorders → altered eating behaviors → digestive problems	■ Assess for eating disorder behaviors, such as patterns of food restriction, binge eating, and purging. Consider fiber and fluid intake. ■ Assess digestive patterns to determine whether they existed before an eating disorder or are a result of an eating disorder. ■ Assess laxative use. Frequent use alters digestion and can lead to fecal impaction.

detrimental effects. Some cooking techniques—such as frying—lessen the benefits of healthy foods. Beverages also affect digestion. Alcoholic and caffeinated beverages negatively affect digestive health, while adequate water consumption helps to maintain healthy digestive processes. Safe food and beverage storage and preparation practices are important for avoiding foodborne illnesses.

Fiber, water intake, and daily physical activity promote healthy elimination. In addition, responding to the urge to move the bowels is important for maintaining bowel health; postponing bathroom visits can lead to elimination issues. Some medications can alter elimination. Over-the-counter enemas and laxatives should be avoided, unless recommended by a medical professional. Prescription medication use should be monitored for side effects that can affect elimination.

Finally, avoiding or minimizing risk factors in daily life helps to promote healthy digestion. Identifying causes of a digestive disorder can help in determining plans of action to reduce risks. Because digestive disorders have varying etiologies, prevention methods vary. For example, taking steps to prevent conditions that may lead to pancreatitis, such as gallstones and alcoholism, will help to prevent the condition (NIH, 2013a). Immunizations (on schedule as recommended for children; before traveling to developing countries for adults) can help to prevent infections with the hepatitis A virus (HAV) and hepatitis B virus (HBV). Collaboration with healthcare providers and compliance with health plans to maintain healthy digestion will lessen or prevent complications that can occur with digestive disorders.

Modifiable Risk Factors

Individuals can reduce their risks of developing a digestive disorder through lifestyle choices. Modifiable risk factors can be controlled or altered to reduce the potential for digestive disorders. For example, GERD can be prevented by maintaining a healthy weight; eliminating smoking; limiting alcohol; and avoiding foods such as chocolate, caffeine, onions, citrus fruits, and spices. Modifiable risk factors for viral hepatitis include unsafe sex, improper hand hygiene, sharing personal items such as toothbrushes and razors, and traveling to developing countries without getting the proper vaccinations. There is a link between pyloric stenosis and early use of antibiotics (erythromycin) for whooping cough (Mayo Clinic, 2015b).

Screenings

A number of tests are available to screen for digestive disorders. The appropriate test for an individual depends upon symptoms, risk factors, and history. For example, individuals in whom celiac disease is suspected can be screened through blood tests. The primary healthcare provider may test blood for specific autoantibodies including anti-tissue transglutaminase antibodies (tTGA) or anti-endomysium antibodies (EMA). Other blood tests may be needed to confirm a celiac disease diagnosis.

One relatively common blood test is hepatitis screening. Screening in individuals with suspected hepatitis is important for early diagnosis and treatment, prevention of liver damage and other complications, and prevention of spread of the infection. Individuals who should be screened for hepatitis infection include all pregnant women, individuals

born outside the United States, individuals who use or have used illegal drugs via injection, individuals who received clotting factors before 1987, individuals who receive long-term hemodialysis, and healthcare workers after needlestick or mucosal exposure to hepatitis C positive blood (U.S. Preventive Services Task Force, 2013). Other types of digestive screening include colonoscopy and endoscopy.

Care in the Community

At the individual level, patients may rely on interventions in the home to treat digestive issues or disorders. The appropriateness of these interventions depends upon the type and severity of the problem. Bland foods are appropriate for individuals who are experiencing nausea; patients should avoid greasy or fried foods and sweets. Eating small, frequent meals may also help. For individuals with nausea, vomiting, and diarrhea, the **BRAT** diet is generally well tolerated.

Bananas
Rice
Applesauce
Toast

Other bland foods such as saltine crackers, boiled potatoes, and broths may also be appropriate. Individuals should drink water, sports drinks, and Nursery® water (distilled water with fluoride added) to avoid dehydration associated with vomiting or diarrhea. Juices and carbonated soft drinks increase the risk of dehydration. If the condition persists or becomes chronic, the patient should consult a healthcare professional.

Mild or moderate heartburn may be treated with over-the-counter antacids or acid reducers. Antacids are typically taken after heartburn has occurred; acid reducers are taken in advance of eating foods that may trigger heartburn. Decreasing pressure on the abdomen is also beneficial. Losing weight, wearing loose clothing, and maintaining proper posture all decrease abdominal pressure in patients with heartburn (Mayo Clinic, 2014a). Patients who experience nighttime heartburn should avoid eating within several hours of going to bed and should elevate the head of the bed. They should also avoid spicy foods and foods with high acidity, as well as cigarettes. Patients should see a healthcare professional if heartburn symptoms persist or occur regularly, if swallowing is difficult, or if appetite decreases or weight loss occurs as a result of heartburn symptoms.

Nursing Assessment

Thorough assessment is necessary to determine the underlying cause of a patient's presenting signs and symptoms. Patients who present with nausea and vomiting require assessment to rule out the possibility of an underlying systemic disease or acute illness that may require immediate care, such as a bowel obstruction. When the cause is known and if there are no other acute symptoms, nursing interventions focus on promoting comfort and preventing complications.

Observation and Patient Interview

The nurse begins the assessment by explaining the process to the patient, inquiring about family or patient history of GI disorders, and eliciting information about the patient's past and current health status and symptoms. Factors to assess include changes in appetite, weight, bowel habits, flatulence, and pain. The nurse listens for cues related to function of the GI system, taking into account age, gender, race, culture and cultural practices, environment, health practices, and any current therapies used, both pharmacologic and complementary health approaches. The nurse should tailor questions related to any changes identified by the patient. Suggested questions include the following:

Health History

- Describe your current problem.
- Do you currently have difficulty swallowing, nausea, vomiting, constipation, or diarrhea?
- Have you noticed any change in the frequency or the size of your stools? Bright red blood or black tarry stools?
- Do you drink alcohol?
- Have you ever been diagnosed with digestive problems? If so, when?
- What treatments were prescribed? Were they helpful?
- Has the disease or problem ever recurred? If so, how many times or how often?
- How are you managing this disease or problem now?

Appetite

- How would you describe your appetite?
- Have you experienced any changes in your appetite recently? In the past few months? The past year? What do you think is causing the changes?
- Have you experienced weight loss or gain in response to your appetite in the past 6 months?
- Has anything else occurred along with the changes in your appetite?

Symptoms of Abdominal Discomfort

- Are you or have you been experiencing feelings or symptoms of bloating or gas? What do you think may be causing these symptoms?
- What do you do to relieve the symptoms?
- Do you take any antacids or over-the-counter medications to relieve bloating or gas? Any prescription medications? If so, what do you take, and how often?
- How much water do you drink each day?
- How often do you exercise?

Family History

- Is there anyone in your family with a history of digestive problems? What disease or problem does he or she have?
- Do you know when it was diagnosed and what treatments were prescribed?

Physical Examination

Techniques required for physical assessment include inspection, auscultation, percussion, and palpation (see the Digestion Assessment feature). It is important to auscultate the

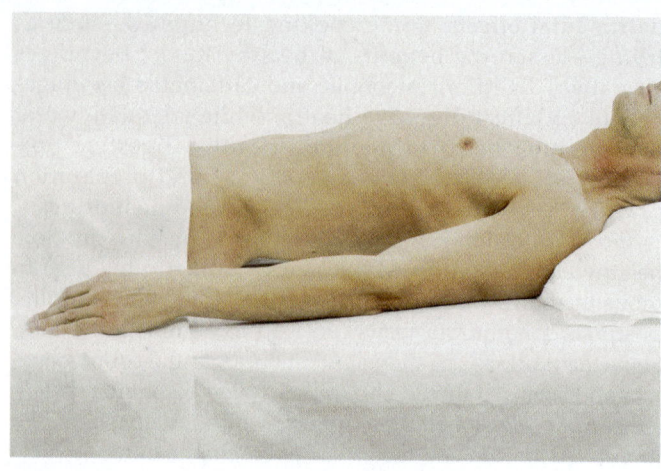

Figure 4–2 ❯❯ Patient positioned and draped.

digestive system prior to conducting any touch-based assessments, because percussion and palpation can disrupt bowel sounds. Palpation should be conducted last because it is the most invasive of the assessment techniques and can lead to abnormalities in other assessments.

The nurse should assess for findings of malnutrition throughout the assessment (see the Malnutrition Assessment feature). Position the patient supine with a small pillow beneath the head and knees and provide privacy, exposing the body as needed (see **Figure 4–2 ❯❯**). Begin with inspection by looking for abnormalities of the nails, hair, skin, eyes, nervous system, musculoskeletal system, cardiovascular system, and GI system.

Following inspection, the nurse auscultates the abdomen by listening with the diaphragm of the stethoscope to the bowel sounds in at least four quadrants (see **Figure 4–3 ❯❯**). Auscultation of bowel sounds should begin in the right lower quadrant and then proceed through the remaining quadrants (see **Figure 4–4 ❯❯**). The nurse should listen for a minimum of 60 seconds to bowel sounds. Hyperactive bowel sounds occur when a patient has an infection or diarrhea. Hypoactive bowel sounds are common after abdominal surgery or a bowel obstruction. Absent bowel sounds may be indicative of a paralytic ileus and should be confirmed by listening over each quadrant for a minimum of 3–5 minutes.

Next, the nurse uses percussion to assess the abdomen, liver, spleen, and gastric bubble. The nurse should tap the

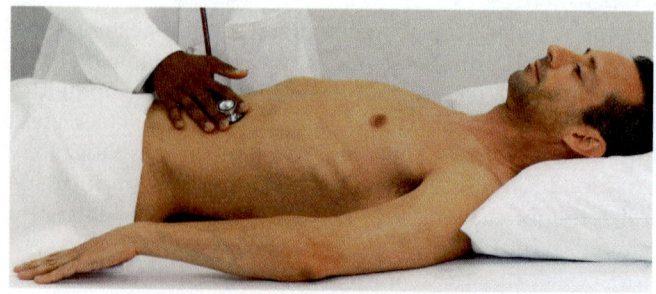

Figure 4–3 ❯❯ Auscultating the abdomen for bowel sounds.

Digestion Assessment

ASSESSMENT/ METHOD	NORMAL FINDINGS	ABNORMAL FINDINGS	LIFESPAN OR DEVELOPMENTAL CONSIDERATIONS
Inspection	The abdomen is symmetrical, and its contours are flat, rounded, or scaphoid. The abdomen is free of masses. The umbilicus is centered and may be protruding or inverted. A consistent skin color with macules and moles is considered to be normal (Barbarito & D'Amico, 2012).	■ Asymmetrical contours ■ Marked pulsations ■ Engorged veins ■ Marked distention ■ Bruising around the umbilicus (Cullen sign) or bruising of the flanks (Grey Turner sign) indicative of pancreatic necrosis with retroperitoneal or intra-abdominal bleeding	■ Inspection of a pediatric patient: a sunken abdomen is abnormal and may indicate dehydration. ■ Assess the midline of the abdomen for depression or bulging, which could indicate separation of the rectus abdominis muscle. As growth occurs, the separation usually becomes less prominent. ■ Infants and children up to age 6 breathe with the diaphragm, causing the abdomen to rise in inspiration and fall with expiration. ■ Abdominal movements such as peristaltic waves are considered abnormal and may indicate intestinal obstruction or pyloric stenosis (Ball, Bindler, Cowen, & Shaw, 2017).
Auscultation	Normal bowel sounds are irregular, high-pitched gurgling sounds that occur 5–30 times a minute.	■ Hyperactive bowel sounds (may be loud, higher pitched, and rushing) ■ Hypoactive bowel sounds (slow and sluggish) ■ Absent bowel sounds ■ Bruits and venous hums ■ Friction rubs over the liver and spleen	■ For infants, take advantage of opportunities presented when the infant is sleeping or quiet to listen to abdomen (Ball et al., 2017). ■ Toddlers and preschoolers should be allowed to touch and play with the stethoscope.
Percussion	Tympany is a loud hollow sound heard over the abdomen.	■ Dullness in the left lower quadrant (can indicate stool in the colon) ■ Dullness over the bladder (may indicate distention) ■ Dullness over the liver or spleen (may indicate hepatic or splenic enlargement)	■ Percussion of a pediatric patient: different tones, such as dullness, are expected over the liver, spleen, and full bladder. Dullness in the intestinal region could indicate obstruction (Ball et al., 2017).
Palpation	The abdomen is soft and nontender. It is pain-free on palpation.	■ Tightness, guarding, or discomfort with palpation ■ Crepitus ■ Irregularities of the abdominal wall such as hernias ■ Tenderness or pain	■ Palpation of a pediatric patient should be done last. Begin with light palpation to build the child's trust and check for tenseness of the abdomen. Use deep palpation to assess for masses and tenderness in the abdomen. Distractions such as toys may help gain the cooperation of younger children. Older children may want to "assist" by placing their hand on top of yours. Monitor the child's face and manner during palpation for indications of discomfort (James, Nelson, & Ashwill, 2014).

Malnutrition Assessment

ASSESSMENT/ METHOD	NORMAL FINDINGS	ABNORMAL FINDINGS	LIFESPAN OR DEVELOPMENTAL CONSIDERATIONS
Nails	The nails are strong and smooth with pink undertones and instant capillary refill.	■ Nails will be soft and spoon shaped when iron deficiency is present. ■ Splinter hemorrhages indicate vitamin C deficiency.	■ In older adults, nails may become thicker, yellow tinged, harder, opaque, and more brittle.
Hair	Hair is symmetrical in placement (even distribution) and color, with texture being fine to coarse. Hair may be thick, thin, straight, wavy, or curly.	■ Dull, dry, scarce hair is seen with deficiencies of protein, zinc, linoleic acid. ■ Gray patches or asymmetrical graying may indicate protein or copper deficiency.	■ In older adults, the hair grays and becomes thinner and coarser, especially on the face.
Skin	The skin is warm and moist, and the color is consistent. The skin is free from edema and lesions.	■ Flaky, dry skin may indicate deficiency of vitamin A, B, and/or linoleic acid. ■ Cracks and hyperpigmentation indicate niacin deficiency. ■ Bruising may indicate deficiency of vitamin C or K. ■ Abnormalities in abdominal skin color, contour, symmetry, pulsations, and movement should be noted.	■ Newborns have lanugo, which is replaced within months by vellus hair. ■ Adolescents have increased oil and sweat gland production and development of axillary and pubic hair. ■ In older adults, the skin becomes more thin and fragile (Barbarito & D'Amico, 2012).
Eyes	The eyeball is firm and moist with white sclera and pink conjunctivae. The cornea is clear and symmetrical.	■ Inadequate levels of vitamin A cause eyes to become dry and soft. ■ Pale conjunctivae indicate iron deficiency; red conjunctivae indicate insufficient levels of riboflavin.	■ In pregnant women, dry eyes are a common problem. ■ In older adults, a whitish-yellow color around the cornea indicates fat deposits.
Nervous system	Cranial nerves and reflexes are intact. The patient has congruent mood, language, mental status, and affect.	■ Patients deficient in thiamine will present with decreased reflexes and may experience peripheral neuropathies. ■ Irritability and/or disorientation also may be seen with thiamine deficiency.	■ Reflexes in infants include tonic neck reflex and Babinski reflex until age 2. ■ In older adults, reflexes, reflex reactions, and coordination are reduced.
Musculoskeletal system	The patient has smooth movement without pain, steady gait, and symmetrical posture. The patient is free from tremors, muscle spasms, and pain.	■ Muscle wasting is seen with deficits in protein, carbohydrate, and fat metabolism. ■ Calf pain occurs with thiamine deficiency; joint pain may occur with vitamin C deficiency. Low potassium levels can cause muscle cramping, especially in the legs.	■ In older adults, reduced bone mass results from low calcium and vitamin D intake.
Cardiovascular system	Blood pressure is within normal range (based on age) with 2+ peripheral pulses. Capillaries instantly refill. The patient has symmetrical color and is free from edema.	■ Heart size and rate may increase with thiamine deficiency. ■ Diastolic blood pressure may be increased with a high intake of fat. ■ Lowered cardiac output and decreased blood pressure may occur with caloric deficiencies over a long period.	■ In pregnant women, the heart may be displaced upward and to the left due to the enlarging fetus. Preexisting murmurs may become more prominent.
GI system	Tongue is smooth, moist, and pink. Membranes are moist and intact. Swallowing is intact.	■ Cheilosis (sores at corner of mouth) is seen in vitamin B–complex deficiencies, especially riboflavin. ■ Stomatitis and spongy, bleeding gums may also be seen in malnutrition. ■ Gingivitis can be caused by vitamin C deficiency.	■ In the older adult, the gums, buccal mucosa, and lips become more thin and pale.

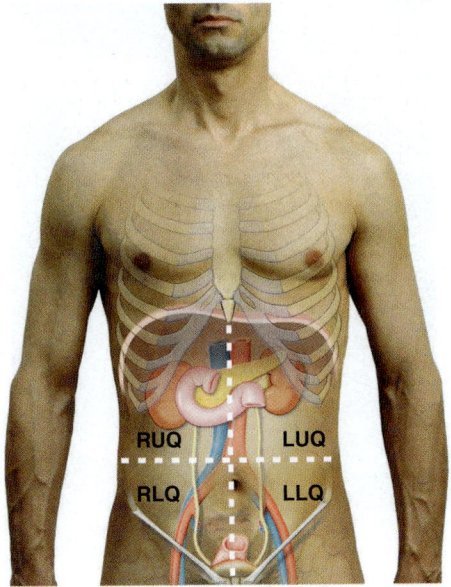

Right Upper Quadrant	Left Upper Quadrant
Liver and gallbladder	Left lobe of liver
Pylorus	Spleen
Duodenum	Stomach
Head of pancreas	Body of pancreas
Right adrenal gland	Left adrenal gland
Portion of right kidney	Portion of left kidney
Hepatic flexure of colon	Splenic flexure of colon
Portions of ascending and transverse colon	Portions of transverse and descending colon
Right Lower Quadrant	**Left Lower Quadrant**
Lower pole of right kidney	Lower pole of left kidney
Cecum and appendix	Sigmoid colon
Portion of ascending colon	Portion of descending colon
Bladder (if distended)	Bladder (if distended)
Right ovary and salpinx	Left ovary and salpinx
Right spermatic cord	Uterus (if enlarged)
Right ureter	Left spermatic cord
	Left ureter

Midline

Aorta

Bladder

Uterus

◯ = Umbilicus

Figure 4–4 》 The four quadrants of the abdomen.

patient's abdomen as shown in **Figure 4–5 》**. Tympany is a loud, hollow sound heard over the abdomen and is a normal finding. Dullness is often heard over organs such as the liver, spleen, or distended bladder. Dullness in the left lower quadrant can indicate stool in the colon (Barbarito & D'Amico, 2012).

Palpation of the abdomen is useful to determine organ size, muscle tone, masses, and presence of fluid. If patients have identified a painful area prior to the assessment, palpate this area last. Follow facility policy regarding whether deep palpation is allowed. If patients experience muscle tightness or guarding with palpation, this finding could indicate peritonitis. Advise patients to indicate if they experience any discomfort during the palpation, and watch patients for signs of pain, such as facial expressions or guarding. Palpation of the abdomen requires using both light and deep palpation (see **Figure 4–6 》**).

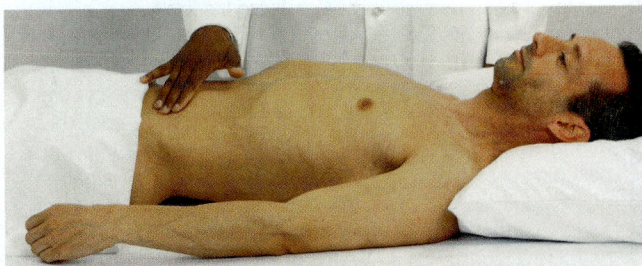

A

B

Figure 4–6 》 ***A,*** Light palpation of the abdomen. ***B,*** Deep palpation of the abdomen.

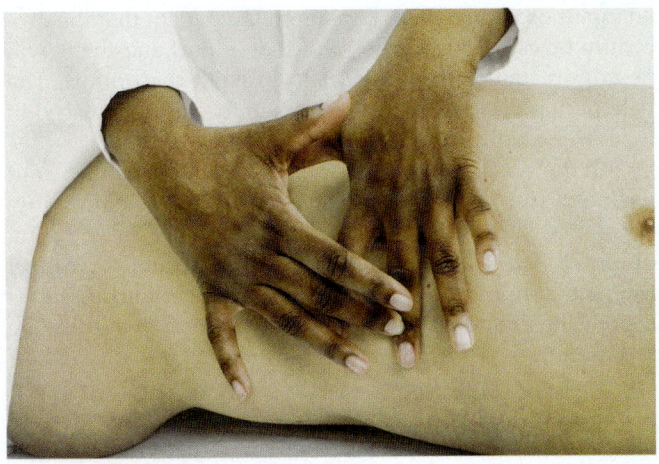

Figure 4–5 》 Percussing the spleen.

SAFETY ALERT Palpation is contraindicated in patients in whom appendicitis, dissecting aortic aneurysm, or polycystic kidneys is suspected. It is also contraindicated in patients who have had an organ transplant.

Diagnostic Tests

The results of diagnostic tests of nutritional status and GI function are used to support the diagnosis of a specific disease, to provide information to identify or modify the appropriate treatment, and to help the nurse monitor the patient's responses to treatment and nursing care interventions.

Upper GI Series (Barium Swallow)

An upper GI series is conducted to diagnose esophageal varices, inflammation, ulcerations, hiatal hernia, foreign bodies, polyps, diverticula, and tumors of the esophagus, stomach, and duodenal bulb. The patient should have nothing by mouth (NPO) before the test. The duration of NPO time will depend on the age of the patient, being less for infants and young children. The patient drinks 16–20 ounces of liquid barium sulfate or meglumine before the exam. These radiologic studies are done by observing movement of a contrast medium with a **fluoroscope**, an instrument with a screen that uses x-rays to show the internal structure of the body (see **Figure 4–7 》》**).

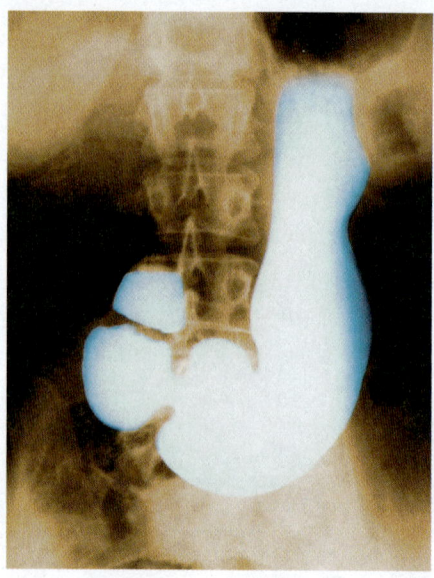

Source: Biophoto Associates/Science Source.

Figure 4–7 》》 A barium x-ray of a healthy stomach.

Nurses should instruct the patients who are to undergo an upper GI series not to smoke, eat, or drink fluids before the test for 8–12 hours for an adult and 4–6 hours for an infant or young child. Tell the patient not to take narcotics or anticholinergic medications for 24 hours pretest and not to take any medications for 8 hours pretest. Following the test, ensure that the patient eliminates the barium by taking laxatives and drinking fluids unless contraindicated.

Endoscopy

An upper GI endoscopy directly visualizes the mucous membrane lining of the esophagus, stomach, and duodenum. A flexible fiber optic endoscope is used to visualize inflammation, ulcerations, tumors, or varices, and video imaging may illustrate gastric mobility. The endoscopy may also be combined with an ultrasound examination by attaching an ultrasound transducer to the endoscope.

Schedule the endoscopy at least 2 days after an upper GI series or barium swallow. The patient should remove dentures and eyeglasses and not eat food or drink fluids before the procedure for 6–8 hours for an adult and 4–6 hours for an infant or young child. Explain to the patient that the procedure takes 20–30 minutes and that a local anesthetic will be administered to the throat to prevent discomfort. The patient may feel some pressure when the scope is placed in the lower esophagus and stomach.

Tell the patient to contact the physician after the examination if the patient experiences difficulty swallowing; epigastric, substernal, or shoulder pain; fever; or vomiting of blood. After the procedure, keep the patient NPO until the gag reflex returns; the patient may eat and drink as soon as he or she can swallow safely. Depending upon the sedation regimen used, the patient may experience different after effects of the procedure. If sedation is achieved using a combination of benzodiazepines and opioid agonists, such as midazolam (Versed) and fentanyl, the patient may experience mild bloating, belching, or flatulence. If sedation is achieved using propofol (Diprivan), aftereffects

---

Focus on Diversity and Culture
Patients with Digestive Disorders

Dietary practices linked to culture or religion are particularly important to consider in patients with digestive disorders. Some religions restrict or prohibit the consumption of certain foods or types of foods. For example, some followers of Judaism and Islam do not consume pork or shellfish, and many adherents of Buddhism and Hinduism follow a vegetarian diet. In addition, a number of religions observe fast or feast days during which the amount and types of food consumed are based on customary practices. For example, during Ramadan, many adult Muslims fast from sunrise to sunset. Research suggests that GERD symptoms like acid indigestion and heartburn tend to increase during this month-long period of daily fasting. In addition, complications with peptic ulcers may increase during Ramadan. These symptoms may be particularly pronounced in patients with diabetes who observe the fast (Abbas, 2015).

Patients with culturally based dietary practices may be less likely to adhere to dietary recommendations that do not take their cultural practices into account. When healthcare providers develop the care plan in partnership with the patient, rather than for the patient, the patient will be more likely to adhere to the care plan and avoid behaviors that increase symptoms or risks (Berman, Snyder, & Frandsen, 2016). Returning to the Ramadan example, working with patients to plan appropriate meals during nonfasting hours may reduce the occurrence of digestive issues. Patients should be encouraged to avoid overeating when breaking their fast and to avoid consuming fatty and spicy foods that may aggravate symptoms. Medications such as proton pump inhibitors may help with symptom management (Abbas, 2015).

are minimal and recovery time tends to be faster (Lera dos Santos et al., 2013).

Abdominal X-ray

An abdominal x-ray may be ordered for a patient to assist in diagnosing obstructions, perforations, and structural abnormalities. The x-ray is usually performed with two views with the patient supine and then standing.

CT Scan

A computed tomographic (CT) scan is a noninvasive tool that takes many views of the digestive tract from many different angles to produce cross-sectional images of the organs and soft tissues. CT scan images can provide much more information than x-rays.

SAFETY ALERT Assess patient for allergies to iodine or contrast medium before tests that use these chemicals.

Amylase

The serum blood test that measures the amount of amylase secreted from the pancreas is useful in diagnosing acute pancreatitis. Normal amylase levels for an adult are 60–160 Somogyi units/dL (Osborn et al., 2014). Amylase levels peak 24 hours after the start of the illness and usually drop to normal in 48–72 hours. No special preparation is needed for this test, though alcohol should be avoided prior to testing (NIH, 2013a).

Lipase

The serum blood test that measures the secretion of lipase by the pancreas is useful in diagnosing pancreatitis. The normal lipase level for all age groups is 20–180 international units/L (Osborn et al., 2014). Patients should fast for 8 hours before the test (NIH, 2013e).

Case Study » Part 2

The next day, you follow up with Jack Zambrano, the 9-year-old boy whose mother called the clinic yesterday. You call his parents and talk with Jack's father. You ask how Jack is doing. His father states, "His fever is about the same. He hasn't eaten much of anything, and he says his stomach hurts, although it isn't worse than yesterday. My wife said Jack's urine was really dark this morning, but Jack hasn't been drinking anything to speak of." You make an appointment for Jack to see the primary healthcare provider later this afternoon. Before the appointment, you talk with the primary healthcare provider and report Jack's condition, recent trip to Mexico, and incomplete immunization record. The primary healthcare provider sees Jack in the afternoon and suspects acute viral hepatitis. He orders a blood test to confirm the diagnosis.

Clinical Reasoning Questions Level I
1. Which assessment data concern you the most?
2. What other questions should you ask about Jack's condition?
3. What specific diagnostic tests would confirm the primary healthcare provider's diagnosis of viral hepatitis?

Clinical Reasoning Questions Level II
4. How does Jack's dark urine relate to a decrease in fluid intake?
5. Why is dark urine significant in the suspected diagnosis of viral hepatitis?

6. What risk factors do Jack and his parents have for viral hepatitis?
7. What measures should be taken at Jack's school or after-school program or with Jack's family to protect them against viral hepatitis A?

Independent Interventions

In individuals with digestive disorders, monitoring and early intervention and treatment help to prevent potential complications associated with fluid and electrolyte imbalances and nutritional imbalances. The assessment of pain assists in diagnosis of digestive disorders and provides data regarding the efficacy of interventions and treatments. Although interventions will vary based on the underlying cause of the patient's presenting symptoms, ensuring fluid and electrolyte balance, nutritional balance, and patient comfort are necessary to promote adherence to the treatment plan and prevent complications. In most cases, nausea and vomiting are self-limiting.

Nurses can be essential in identifying individuals who have digestive concerns and referring them for further evaluation and treatment. Severe vomiting or vomiting in the presence of other symptoms may require immediate attention to determine the underlying problem and prevent complications.

Promote Fluid and Electrolyte Balance

Encourage patients to restrict intake to small quantities of clear liquids (tea, apple juice, broth, Jell-O) and dry foods such as soda crackers to help reduce nausea and prevent vomiting. Teach patients to avoid food-preparation odors if they produce nausea. Instruct them to restrict fluid intake for 1 hour before and after meals; otherwise stress the need to maintain fluid intake to prevent dehydration. Also stress the importance of seeking additional medical help if unable to take in fluids or keep food down. Provide information about electrolyte replacement solutions such as sports drinks and commercially available electrolyte replacement solutions.

Provide Patient Education

Patient education should focus on promotion of healthy digestion and management of digestive disorder symptoms. For patients with general digestive issues not linked to a specific disorder, encourage healthy digestive habits such as sitting upright when eating, exercising regularly, and maintaining a healthy weight. Discuss foods to help avoid digestion problems and the importance of proper hydration. Discuss the effects of excessive alcohol on digestion, digestion-related organs, and nutritional status.

For patients with digestive disorders, education will be specific to the disorder; however, information about healthy digestive habits will be useful to most patients. In addition, patients will need to make lifestyle changes to reduce symptoms and prevent long-term effects of their particular disorder. Involving family and social support systems in the discussion can help the individual achieve health goals.

Collaborative Therapies

Collaborative care for digestive disorders may include pharmacologic therapies, nutrition and lifestyle management, and surgery. In addition to the primary care provider, other healthcare providers with whom the nurse may collaborate include nutritionists and dietitians, who assist in the nutritional assessment and plan of care for patients, and mental health providers. Mental health providers can provide support to patients with chronic conditions who need assistance with coping skills. They can also assist with alcohol assessment if indicated.

Pharmacologic Therapy

A variety of pharmacologic therapies are available to patients with digestive disorders. As with any medications, whether over-the-counter or prescribed, patient education focuses on proper administration, potential adverse effects, and when to contact the healthcare provider if symptoms do not resolve. Common pharmacologic therapies for digestion-associated disorders may include antacids, histamine$_2$-receptor (H$_2$-receptor) agonists, proton pump inhibitors, antiemetics, and dopamine receptor agonists.

Antacids

Antacids are alkaline substances that are commonly used to relieve simple acid indigestion (Mayo Clinic, 2014b). They are available over the counter in compound preparations that include aluminum, magnesium, sodium, or calcium (Wilson, Shannon, & Shields, 2013). Inexpensive and readily available, antacids are an appropriate treatment for infrequent symptoms of heartburn. Although the liquid forms work more quickly, many people prefer to take antacids in tablet or pill form. Patients with daily symptoms, or symptoms that do not resolve with use of antacids, should consult with their healthcare provider. Recurring symptoms, painful symptoms, or symptoms accompanied by fever may indicate a more serious condition (NIH, 2014c). Examples of antacids are calcium carbonate (TUMS), magnesium hydroxide (Milk of Magnesia), aluminum hydroxide (AlternaGEL), and sodium bicarbonate (Alka-Seltzer).

H$_2$-Receptor Antagonists

H$_2$-receptor antagonists are useful in the treatment of gastroesophageal reflux disease and peptic ulcer disease because they help to suppress volume and acidity of parietal cell secretions (Wilson et al., 2013). H$_2$-receptor agonists are usually administered twice daily or more often and can be used long term for recurring mild symptoms. Most H$_2$-receptor antagonists are available over the counter (Mayo Clinic, 2015a). Examples of H$_2$-receptor agonists are famotidine (Pepcid) and ranitidine hydrochloride (Zantac).

Proton Pump Inhibitors

Proton pump inhibitors bind the acid-secreting enzyme (H$^+$,K$^+$-ATPase) that functions as the proton pump, disabling it for up to 24 hours. Proton pump inhibitors are useful in short-term treatment of gastroesophageal reflux, gastric ulcers, and hypersecretory disorders (Wilson et al., 2013). Although it may take several days for patients to experience relief, side effects are rare; headache, diarrhea, abdominal pain, and nausea and vomiting are the most common adverse effects (Wilson et al., 2013). Commonly used proton pump inhibitors include omeprazole (Prilosec) and lansoprazole (Prevacid).

Antiemetics

Unless vomiting is associated with pregnancy, antiemetic medications may be prescribed to prevent or control nausea and vomiting. These drugs, which fall into a number of different classes, often are more effective when given in combination with other medications. See the Medications feature for more information.

Because of the sedating effect of many antiemetics, nursing considerations focus on patient safety. Sedated or drowsy patients may require interventions to prevent risk for falls, and patients who are heavily sedated and vomiting may need suction with a nasogastric tube. Antiemetics are contraindicated in patients who are comatose, have bone marrow depression, or have a history of hypersensitivity to these drugs (Wilson et al., 2013). Patient teaching should include cautioning patients against driving and explaining the importance of immediately reporting vomiting of blood or severe abdominal pain.

Metoclopramide Hydrochloride

Metoclopramide hydrochloride (Reglan) is a potent dopamine receptor agonist that promotes motility by enhancing esophageal clearance and gastric emptying. It is useful both as an antiemetic for chemotherapy patients and for treating GERD, but long-term use is not recommended because serious adverse effects can occur. Contraindications include sensitivity or intolerance to the drug, lactation, allergy to sulfites, ileus, and mechanical GI obstruction or perforation (Wilson et al., 2013).

Nutrition Therapy

Patients who are unable to achieve adequate nutrition through food consumption may require supplementary nutrition. The thought of using enteral or parenteral nutrition can be intimidating for both the patient and family. Nurses provide appropriate interventions related to providing enteral and parenteral nutrition and patient and family education and support.

Enteral Nutrition

Enteral nutrition, or tube feeding, may be used to meet calorie and protein requirements in patients who are unable to

Medications

Drugs Used as Antiemetics

CLASSIFICATION AND DRUG EXAMPLES	MECHANISMS OF ACTION	NURSING CONSIDERATIONS
Antihistamines *Drug examples:* Meclizine (Antivert) Hydroxyzine (Vistaril, Atarax) Dimenhydrinate (Dramamine)	Primarily used to treat nausea and vomiting due to motion sickness	▪ Advise patients to take 30–60 minutes prior to travel. ▪ Drowsiness can occur. ▪ Monitor for injury and falls. ▪ Use with caution for patients with narrow-angle glaucoma, urinary retention, and bowel obstruction.
Serotonin Receptor Agonists *Drug example:* Ondansetron (Zofran)	Very effective for patients experiencing nausea and vomiting due to chemotherapy; effective when given only once or twice a day	▪ Administer orally or intravenously. ▪ Headache is a common side effect. ▪ If giving frequently, monitor liver function and clotting abilities.
Dopamine Agonists *Drug examples:* Prochlorperazine (Compazine) Thiethylperazine (Torecan) Haloperidol (Haldol) Metoclopramide (Reglan)	Effective for patients experiencing nausea and vomiting, but can cause extrapyramidal symptoms, sedation, and hypotension	▪ These drugs can have sedative effects. ▪ Monitor older patients closely for adverse effects such as confusion.
Cannabinoids *Drug examples:* Dronabinol (Marinol) Nabilone (Cesamet)	Approved to treat the nausea and vomiting associated with chemotherapy, but may produce unpleasant psychiatric effects such as dissociation and dysphoria and are contraindicated in patients with psychiatric disorders	▪ Change positions slowly to prevent dizziness. ▪ These drugs are most effective when given 1–3 hours before nausea-inducing procedures. ▪ Tachycardia and hypotension are possible side effects.
Neurokinin Receptor Agonists *Drug example:* Aprepitant (Emend)	A new class of antiemetics primarily used to prevent nausea and vomiting associated with chemotherapy	▪ These drugs are not for long-term use. ▪ Monitor international normalized ratio (INR) levels for patients taking warfarin (Coumadin). ▪ Aprepitant can reduce the effectiveness of oral contraceptives. Women of childbearing age taking oral contraceptives should use a second form of birth control while taking this medication and for a month after the last dose. ▪ Monitor liver studies.

Source: Data from Adams, M. P., Holland, L. N., & Urban, C. (2017). *Pharmacology for nurses: A pathophysiologic approach* (5th ed.). Hoboken, NJ: Pearson Education.

consume enough food to meet the requirements. Tube feeding may be necessary for patients with impairment of the GI tract, difficulty swallowing, unresponsiveness, oral or neck surgery or trauma, anorexia, or serious illness. Enteral feedings provide nutrients directly to the stomach or small intestine. Tube feedings may provide all or part of patients' nutritional requirements.

Tube feedings usually are administered through a soft, small-caliber nasogastric or nasoduodenal tube that may have a weighted tip (see **Figure 4–8 ⟩⟩**). They also can be administered through a gastrostomy or jejunostomy tube. After insertion, proper position is verified through x-ray and by aspirating the tube and checking the pH of aspirated contents. A pH < 4 indicates placement in the stomach; pH > 6 indicates the tube is in the jejunum. Small-bore feeding tubes are easily displaced, so tube placement should be checked before each feeding (or every 4 hours if continuous feedings are being administered) and before administration of medications. Reassess tube placement if the patient vomits or retches, requires oropharyngeal suctioning, complains of discomfort or reflux into the mouth, or develops signs of respiratory distress.

Most tube feeding formulas provide 1 kcal/mL with approximately 14% of the calories from protein, 60% from carbohydrates, and 25%–30% from fat. Administering 1500 mL per day provides the recommended daily intake of all

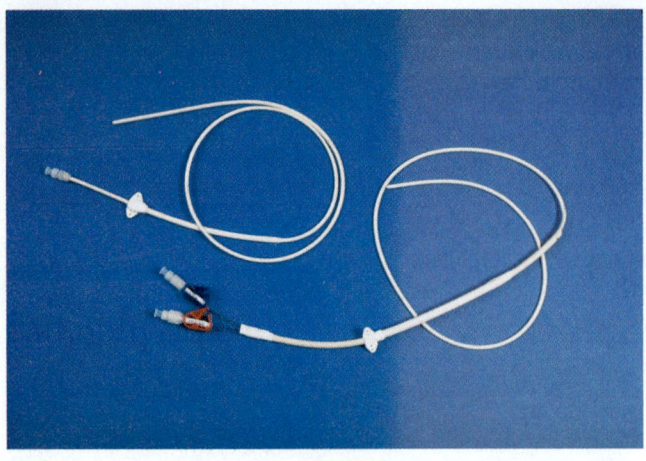

Figure 4–8 》 A nasoduodenal tube and a jejunostomy tube.

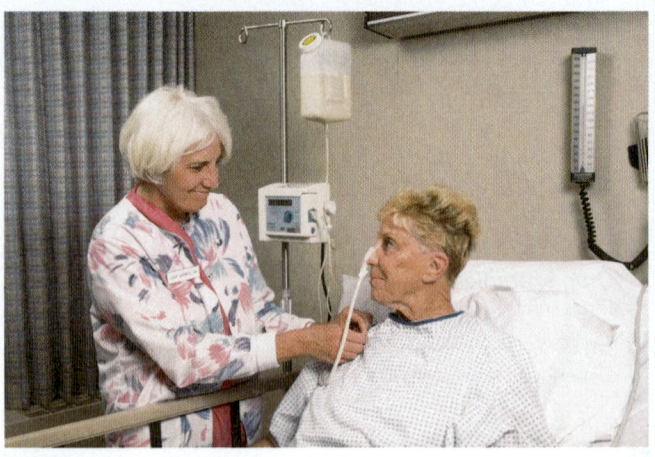

Figure 4–9 》 The nurse secures the feeding tube of a patient receiving continuous enteral feeding.

vitamins and minerals. Formulas that provide more calories per milliliter, more grams of protein, added fiber, or lower fat also are available (see **Table 4–1** 》). Commercial products provide instructions for initiating therapy. Enteral feedings may initially be started with smaller volumes or diluted per physician orders to prevent diarrhea, with the volume gradually increased to provide the required calories for maintenance and healing. Formulas may be administered as a bolus feeding or as a continuous-drip feeding regulated by a feeding pump (see **Figure 4–9** 》).

Aspiration and diarrhea are the most common complications of enteral feedings. Procedures and interventions that reduce the risk for aspiration include the following:

- Continuous infusion of the formula
- Placing the feeding tube in the jejunum rather than the stomach
- Elevating the head of the bed at least 30 degrees during feeding and for at least 1 hour after feeding
- Dual-lumen tubes that allow gastric suction with simultaneous instillation of an enteral feeding into the jejunum.

Formulas that contain fiber can reduce the incidence of diarrhea. Monitor fluid and electrolyte status carefully, and administer additional water as needed.

Total Parenteral Nutrition

Total parenteral nutrition (TPN) is the intravenous (IV) administration of amino acids, often with added carbohydrates, fats, electrolytes, vitamins, and minerals. These hypertonic solutions usually are administered through a central vein, such as the subclavian vein (see **Figure 4–10** 》), particularly when therapy may be prolonged. A peripherally inserted central catheter (PICC) line may be used for short-term TPN.

TPN is initiated when a patient's nutritional requirements cannot be met through diet or enteral feedings. It may be used concurrently with enteral nutrition. Patients who have undergone major surgery or trauma or who are seriously undernourished are often candidates for TPN. TPN is used for both short- and long-term management of nutritional deficiencies. Many patients are discharged to home with TPN and monitored by home health nurses.

TABLE 4–1 Selected Enteral Feeding Formulas

Formula Type	Contains	Examples
Complete—suitable for most patients requiring enteral feedings	1 kcal/mL Protein: ~14% total kcal Fat: ~30% total kcal Carbohydrate: ~60% total kcal Recommended daily intake of all minerals and vitamins is 1500 mL/day	Compleat, Ensure, Isocal, Nutren, Isolan, Sustacal, Resource
High-calorie complete—appropriate for patients on fluid restriction	As above; provides 1.5–2 kcal/mL	Ensure Plus, Sustacal HC, Comply, Nutren 1.5, Resource Plus, Isocal HCN, Magnacal, TwoCal HN
Complete lactose-free, high-residue—used to prevent/treat diarrhea, constipation	As above; provides fiber	Jevity, Profiber, Nutren 1.0 with fiber, Fiberlan, Sustacal with fiber, Ultracal, Ensure with fiber, Fibersource, Accupep HPF, Reabfin
Disease-Specific Formulas		
Renal failure	Essential amino acids	Amin-Aid, Travasorb Renal, Aminess
Respiratory failure	Fat: >50% total kcal	Pulmocare, NutriVent
Liver failure with hepatic encephalopathy	High amounts of branched-chain amino acids	Hepatic-Acid II, Travasorb Hepatic

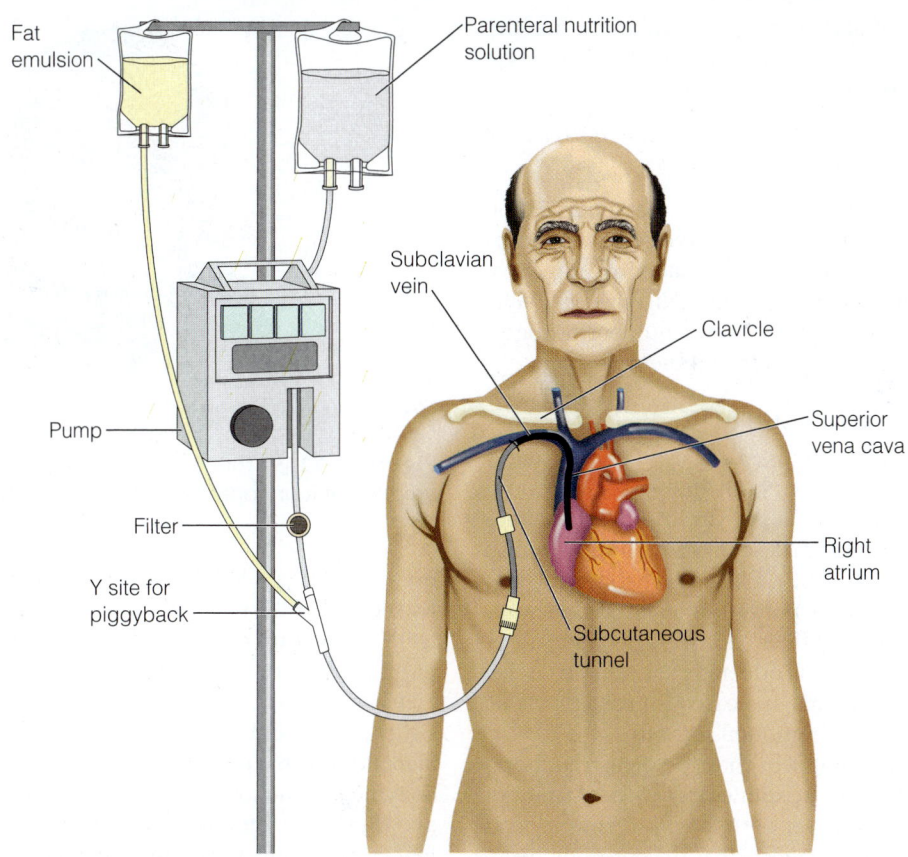

Fat emulsion

Parenteral nutrition solution

Subclavian vein

Clavicle

Superior vena cava

Pump

Right atrium

Filter

Y site for piggyback

Subcutaneous tunnel

Figure 4–10 》 Parenteral nutrition infused through a catheter in the right subclavian vein.

To begin TPN therapy, a peripheral or central venous catheter is inserted under aseptic conditions. The location of the catheter tip is confirmed by x-ray. Parenteral nutrition solutions are mixed in the pharmacy using sterile technique under a laminar-flow air hood. Solutions commonly contain 3–11.4% amino acids (a mixture of essential and nonessential amino acids); 10% or more dextrose; and added electrolytes, minerals, and vitamins. Fat emulsions (lipids) may be added to the solution, although often they are administered separately. The sterility of the solution is maintained, and no medication is added to the solution after it is mixed or to the lumen through which the TPN is being administered. When given separately, fat emulsions may be administered either through a peripheral vein or via the same IV catheter as TPN. TPN solutions are always administered with an infusion pump to ensure the correct rate of infusion.

The patient receiving TPN is at risk for infectious, metabolic, and mechanical complications. Disruption of the skin barrier and administration of a solution that is high in glucose present risks for infection, which may be local—limited to the insertion site or the catheter itself—or systemic. Meticulous sterile technique in inserting the catheter, preparing and administering TPN solutions, and caring for the site and catheter reduces the risk for infection. Using a catheter impregnated with antiseptics and an in-line filter also reduces the risk for infection. The nurse monitors the insertion site and the patient's temperature for evidence of infection. If infection is suspected, the nurse may obtain cultures of the solution, catheter, and blood.

Patients may develop glucose intolerance, particularly early in the course of TPN. The physician might increase the concentration of glucose in TPN solutions to reduce this risk. Laboratory personnel measure blood and urine glucose levels every 6 hours until insulin production adjusts to the increased glucose load. Patients with impaired kidney function or liver disease may develop excessively high blood urea nitrogen (BUN) levels or metabolic acidosis. Hyperlipidemia is a common complication of fat infusions; these solutions are given intermittently to allow fats to clear from the blood between infusions. Fluid overload or dehydration may develop, particularly in older adults; therefore, the nurse should assess lung sounds and check for edema frequently. In addition, TPN formulas can cause electrolyte shifts, with resulting imbalances.

Pneumothorax, brachial plexus injury, and improper positioning are possible mechanical complications of central venous catheter insertion. Once the catheter is in place, a thrombus (clot) or fibrin sheath may form within or around it. The catheter also can become mechanically occluded or may dislodge, leak, or break and become an embolus.

Diet

A healthy diet that is low in fat, cholesterol, and sugar and includes a variety of fruits, vegetables, grains, and protein sources is recommended for optimal digestive health. The U.S. Department of Agriculture and the U.S. Department of Health and Human Services issued new dietary guidelines for Americans in 2015. They include a healthy Mediterranean-style eating pattern and a healthy vegetarian eating pattern as well as the healthy U.S.-style eating pattern from the 2010 edition.

≫ **Stay Current:** Read the 2015–2020 USDA dietary guidelines at http://health.gov/dietaryguidelines/2015/guidelines.

When patients have a digestive disease, diet modification should be implemented on the basis of the patient's symptoms and treatment plan. Patients who have inflammatory diseases often benefit from a bland diet. Nicotine, caffeine, spicy foods, and alcohol can exacerbate a number of digestive disorders, and patients should avoid them.

Nonpharmacologic Therapy

Many patients with digestive disorders use nonpharmacologic therapies in conjunction with pharmacologic and nutritional therapies. Common nonpharmacologic therapies include lifestyle changes and complementary health approaches (Lahner et al., 2013). Lifestyle changes include alterations to diet and exercise patterns. Increased consumption of fruits, vegetables, and fiber and decreased consumption of fatty or processed foods may be effective for improving digestive symptoms. Increased exercise may also be effective (see the Health Promotion section).

Complementary health approaches for digestive disorders include hypnotherapy, acupuncture, and a variety of herbal remedies, including peppermint oil, turmeric, and ginger. Emerging evidence suggests that patients may benefit from these approaches, although there is not currently a strong body of research supporting their use (NCCIH, 2015). One increasingly popular complementary health approach for a number of different digestive symptoms is the use of probiotics. **Probiotics** are microorganisms that aid in digestion and help to protect the body from harmful bacteria. They may be taken along with prebiotics, which act as food for probiotics. Probiotics and prebiotics may be found in dietary supplements as well as a number of foods. Yogurt is a common source of probiotics; whole grains, bananas, and honey are good sources of prebiotics. Research suggests that probiotics and prebiotics can help with treatment of diarrhea and irritable bowel syndrome (IBS) and promote faster recovery from intestinal infections (Mayo Clinic, 2014c).

Lifespan Considerations

Normal digestion differs across the lifespan because growth and development of the individual affect digestive ability. In addition, variations in the digestive system tend to change with age. A number of acute and chronic illnesses of the digestive tract can affect children, adolescents, pregnant women, and older adults, causing difficulty with absorption of nutrients or motility, thereby affecting overall health.

Digestion in Infants and Children

The digestive system in a newborn is immature because, until birth, the placenta provides nutrients and removal of waste products. Voluntary control over swallowing does not occur until about 6 weeks of age. The infant's tongue is larger than that of a child or adult in comparison to the nasal and oral passages. The stomach capacity of a newborn is quite small, holding only 10–20 mL at a time, requiring fre-

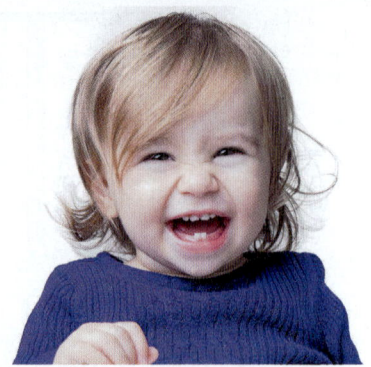

Source: Ozgur Coskun/Shutterstock.

Figure 4–11 ≫ This 1-year-old child shows a typical tooth eruption of four upper teeth and two lower teeth.

quent feedings. Teeth begin to erupt around 6 months of life. By the end of the first year, the infant usually has six to eight teeth (see **Figure 4–11 ≫**). Most children have a complete set of primary teeth by 3–6 years of age.

Infants have a deficiency of the amylase, lipase, and trypsin enzymes. Enzymes from the pancreas will not be sufficient to aid in digestion until 4–6 months in age. Lack of enzyme production results in frequent abdominal distention and flatulence. Infants have an immature liver. After the first few weeks of life, the infant's liver is able to conjugate bilirubin and excrete bile. Gluconeogenesis, ketone formation, vitamin storage, and myelination remain immature during the first year of life.

By the age of 2, a child's digestive processes generally are complete, and the infant can adapt to a typical schedule of three meals per day, with one or two snacks per day. Myelination of the spinal cord allows the child to begin to achieve control over elimination, typically resulting in complete voluntary control by the age of 3.

Gas, constipation, diarrhea, and vomiting commonly occur in children and may be the result of eating habits, diet, or infection. Smaller, more frequent meals may be helpful in alleviating symptoms. A food diary may also help identify certain foods that make symptoms worse. If the child is vomiting or has diarrhea, he or she should be monitored closely and be offered plenty of clear liquids.

Functional GI disorders may also develop during childhood. These conditions are the result of GI tract sensitivity coupled with changes in GI motility (American College of Gastroenterology, 2013). These common disorders sometimes run in families and are often found in healthy children who do not manifest typical symptoms such as bloody stool or weight loss. Common functional GI disorders in children include functional abdominal pain, which manifests as severe recurrent pain in the middle of the abdomen; functional dyspepsia, which is pain in the upper abdomen; and irritable bowel syndrome (IBS), which involves abdominal bloating and mucus in the stool (American College of Gastroenterology, 2013). Functional GI disorders are often treated with a combination of medication and dietary changes.

Digestive health promotion in infants and children relies on educating parents about healthy practices. Nurses should teach parents of newborns how to position the infant and use burping strategies to reduce acid reflux. They should also teach parents how to recognize hunger cues and signs of fullness in infants (American Academy of Pediatrics, 2015a). As children grow, parents should offer them a variety of foods that are high in fiber and protein and low in fat and added sugar (NIH, 2012a). Parents should offer foods repeatedly, even if children reject them, as tastes and preferences change with age. Regular exercise is also important to trigger normal intestinal peristalsis (NIH, 2012a).

Digestion in Adolescents

A period of growth—sometimes referred to as the adolescent growth spurt—begins in late childhood and continues into adolescence. This period of growth is accompanied by rapid gains in height and weight. Bodily demands for calories and nutrients increase dramatically during this time. Adolescent girls require about 2200 calories per day, and adolescent boys require about 2800 calories per day. Roughly 50% of calories should come from complex carbohydrates, 30% from fats, and 20% from proteins (American Academy of Pediatrics, 2015b). Many adolescents exceed fat intake recommendations and do not consume adequate amounts of other nutrients or vitamins, minerals, and fiber. Increased freedom in food choices along with taste preferences, lack of education about proper nutrition, and easy access to low-cost high-fat foods are the primary causes of these discrepancies. Dissatisfaction with personal appearance as a result of developmental changes may also increase incidence of disordered eating in some adolescents (California Department of Public Health, 2013). Improper nutrition in adolescence can negatively affect physical and cognitive development and give rise to digestive issues like acid reflux and constipation.

In children and teens, inability to absorb essential nutrients can result in slow growth and short stature, delayed puberty, and weak dental enamel (NIH, 2015a). One cause of this inability is celiac disease, which is believed to have a genetic component, and roughly 50% of people with celiac disease have a family member with the disease (NIH, 2015a).

Digestive health promotion focuses on teaching adolescents how to make healthy choices. Nurses should teach adolescents to differentiate between high-calorie, low-nutrient foods and those that contain nutrients essential for growth and development. Nurses should also discuss drink choices, encouraging water or low-fat milk in place of sugar-sweetened beverages. They should introduce portion control as well as methods for making healthier choices when eating away from home. Dieting and meal skipping for weight loss should be discouraged in favor of gradual changes to eating and exercise habits (NIH, 2012c).

Digestion in Pregnant Women

Nutritional requirements change during pregnancy, and gradual weight gain is expected. Pregnant women should gain between 2 and 4 pounds per month during the first trimester and 1 pound per week for the remainder of the pregnancy. Total weight gain should be between 11 and 40 pounds, based on the patient's prepregnancy weight category (Institute of Medicine, 2009).

Both hormonal changes and fetal growth affect digestion in pregnant women. Nausea and vomiting are one of the most common digestive issues of pregnancy and are believed to be the result of increases in human chorionic gonadotropin (HCG) and other hormones. Commonly referred to as morning sickness, nausea and vomiting can occur at any time of day and are typically experienced between the 6th and 12th weeks of pregnancy (NIH, 2012b).

Pregnancy hormones slow the movement of digestive muscles, slowing the movement of food through the digestive tract. Muscles in the bowels also relax as a result of high hormone levels. This combination of slowed digestion and muscle relaxation often results in constipation. Increasing fiber and water consumption may be useful for treating or preventing constipation.

Hormones also relax the valve that separates the esophagus from the stomach, allowing food and stomach acid to move back into the esophagus. This results in heartburn, which often becomes more frequent in late pregnancy as the uterus pushes on the stomach. Eating multiple small meals throughout the day and avoiding spicy, fatty, and greasy foods may alleviate mild heartburn symptoms. More severe symptoms may require medication (American Pregnancy Association, 2015).

For more information on factors affecting maternal nutrition and maternal weight gain in pregnancy, see the exemplar on Antepartum Care in the module on Reproduction.

Digestion in Older Adults

In older adults, decreases in lean body mass and metabolic rate result in lowered nutritional requirements. In addition, taste can become less acute as a result of the natural atrophy of the tongue. Tooth enamel can become more brittle, and loss of bone supporting teeth may result in loss of some or all permanent teeth. Saliva production can decrease by as much as one third, which may increase chewing and swallowing time. Esophageal motility may decrease, and a weaker gag reflex can cause discomfort in swallowing, increasing the risk of aspiration. Mucosa in the stomach atrophies, and a reduction in the production of hydrochloric acid and pepsin leads to a higher pH in the stomach, which can increase the incidence of gastric irritation and alteration in medication breakdown. All of these changes increase the risk for malnutrition in older adults.

A number of subtle changes also take place in the GI tract. For most people, a loss of nerve cells causes digested food to move more slowly along the intestinal pathway; this often leads to constipation. Surface area of the intestines decreases slightly, and the small intestine is less able to absorb some nutrients. Secretions from the small intestine decrease, as do secretions from the stomach, liver, and pancreas. The liver becomes smaller and less able to clear the body of waste, increasing the time required for the body to eliminate medications and other substances (Mayo Clinic, 2012).

People over age 50 are at increased risk of developing diverticular disease, in which small sacs called diverticula form and push outward through weak spots in the wall of the colon. The diverticula may become inflamed or infected, and bleeding may occur if blood vessels in the sac wall burst. The most common symptom of diverticular disease is sudden pain or cramping in the lower abdomen that worsens over the course of several days. Constipation, diarrhea, nausea, and vomiting may also occur. Blood tests, CT scans, x-rays of the lower GI tract, or colonoscopy may be used to diagnose diverticular disease. Treatment typically involves a high-fiber diet, medication, and probiotics (NIH, 2013c).

Gallstones also become more common between the ages of 50 and 60. Gallstones are small, hard deposits that form in the gallbladder when there is an excess of cholesterol or bilirubin in the bile (Mayo Clinic, 2016b). Gallbladder disorders are covered in detail in an exemplar in the module on Inflammation.

Digestive health promotion in older adults should focus on healthy diet and regular physical activity. The nurse should stress consumption of dietary fiber and fluids as a means of preventing constipation, which is a common complaint of older adults. The nurse should encourage older adults to eat moderate portions at regular intervals to promote regular function of the digestive system. In addition, the nurse should discuss the importance of eating slowly; rushing through meals can place undue stress on the digestive system. Older adults may also benefit from learning stress reduction strategies. Stress affects digestive nerves and can slow digestive processes, causing bloating and constipation. Smoking can also exacerbate digestive issues, and patients who smoke should be counseled about cessation (Gastroenterological Society of Australia [GESA], 2017).

Case Study >> Part 3

Jack Zambrano's diagnosis is confirmed as viral hepatitis type A (HAV). Two days after his appointment with the primary healthcare provider, you follow up with Jack and his parents. As you talk with Jack's mother, she begins to cry. She states, "I'm so worried about Jack. Will he have liver damage?" You reassure her that HAV does not typically cause chronic hepatitis or liver damage and that Jack will recover fully. His mother becomes calm and less tearful. You spend time talking with Jack, asking him how he feels and teaching him strategies to promote his health. Jack tells you he is eating only "a couple of bites," but he is drinking some fluids. Jack's mother confirms his intake. She states, "His urine is darker, and the whites of his eyes look yellowish."

Clinical Reasoning Questions Level I

1. What strategies should Jack and his parents use to prevent the spread of HAV?
2. What does "recover fully" mean in terms of the liver?
3. Why are Jack's sclera yellow? How does this phenomenon relate to HAV?

Clinical Reasoning Questions Level II

4. What independent nursing interventions should you teach Jack and his parents to provide comfort to Jack?
5. What education should you provide to Jack and his parents about following up with his primary healthcare provider about his condition?

REVIEW The Concept of Digestion

RELATE Link the Concepts

Linking the concept of digestion with the concept of acid–base balance:

1. What type of acid–base imbalance could occur in a patient experiencing nausea and vomiting?
2. What independent caring interventions might the nurse implement for a patient with nausea and vomiting to prevent an acid–base imbalance?

Linking the concept of digestion with the concept of fluids and electrolytes:

3. Healthy individuals are able to balance fluid intake with fluid loss. How do nausea and vomiting affect fluid balance?
4. How can the nurse promote normal fluid and electrolyte balance in the patient with digestive abnormalities?

Linking the concept of digestion with the concept of nutrition:

5. How do digestive disorders affect the nutritional status of an individual?
6. What collaborative care strategies could the nurse use to promote healthy digestion to aid in nutritional absorption?
7. Explain how collaborative care strategies, used long term, could have a negative impact on nutrition. (*Hint:* Consider the medications used for GERD.)

READY Go to Volume 3: Clinical Nursing Skills

- SKILL 1.10 Abdomen: Assessing
- SKILL 1.25 Skin: Assessing
- SKILL 3.1 Pain in Newborn, Infant, Child, or Adult: Assessing
- SKILL 5.1 Intake and Output: Measuring
- SKILL 10.2 Diet, Therapeutic: Managing
- SKILL 10.5 Nutrition: Assessing
- SKILL 10.9 Nasogastric Tube: Feeding
- SKILL 10.10 Nasogastric Tube: Flushing and Maintaining
- SKILL 10.12 Nasogastric Tube: Removing
- SKILL 13.1 Preoperative Patient Teaching
- SKILL 13.6 Surgical Patient: Preparing

REFER Go to Pearson MyLab Nursing and eText

- Additional review materials
- Minimodule: Physiology Review of Digestion

REFLECT Apply Your Knowledge

Greta Rasmussen is a 26-year-old woman who is 10 weeks pregnant with her first child. Ms. Rasmussen started experiencing nausea during the eighth week of pregnancy. At first, she would vomit once or twice each morning, but the nausea would subside over the course of the day. Her nausea gradually worsened, and for the past 3 days, she has been vomiting in excess of six times per day. Ms. Rasmussen states that she is constantly nauseous and that the smell of cooking food makes her nausea worse. She states that her urinary output has been minimal, and she describes the color of her urine as very dark. She also tells you that ginger ale is the only thing she has been able to keep down for the past 48 hours. She does not have a fever, but you observe that she is pallid and shaky.

1. What manifestations does Ms. Rasmussen exhibit to support a diagnosis of hyperemesis gravidarum?

2. How does hyperemesis gravidarum differ from normal nausea and vomiting during pregnancy?

3. What are the priority interventions for a patient presenting with hyperemesis gravidarum?

4. What priority nursing diagnoses would you choose for a patient who presents with hyperemesis gravidarum?

≫ Exemplar 4.A
Gastroesophageal Reflux Disease

Exemplar Learning Outcomes

4.A Analyze GERD as it relates to digestion.

- Describe the pathophysiology of GERD.
- Describe the etiology of GERD.
- Compare the risk factors and prevention of GERD.
- Identify the clinical manifestations of GERD.
- Summarize diagnostic tests and therapies used by interprofessional teams in the collaborative care of an individual with GERD.

- Differentiate care of patients with GERD across the lifespan.
- Apply the nursing process in providing culturally competent care to an individual with GERD.

Exemplar Key Term

Gastroesophageal reflux disease (GERD), *237*

Overview

In **gastroesophageal reflux disease (GERD)**, the gastric contents flow backward into the esophagus, causing the patient to experience heartburn. Many people with GERD have few symptoms; others develop inflammatory esophagitis as a result of exposure to gastric juices. GERD is a common GI disorder, affecting 15–20% of adults. Up to 7% of people experience daily symptoms such as heartburn, regurgitation, and indigestion. GERD is one of the most common digestive disorders affecting children. Until the age of 12, children with GERD may not experience heartburn; common manifestations may include dry cough, asthma, sore throat, recurrent pneumonia, or difficulty swallowing. Infants and young children may manifest with irritability and arching of the back associated with feedings. As a result of these varying signs and symptoms, GERD may be overlooked initially (Johns Hopkins Children's Center, n.d.). Factors that increase risk for GERD in the pediatric population include premature birth, being male, neurologic impairments, trisomy 21, bronchopulmonary dysplasia, and esophageal atresia (Lightdale & Gremse, 2013).

Pathophysiology and Etiology

Pathophysiology

The lower esophageal sphincter normally remains closed except during swallowing. Pressure differences between the stomach and the lower esophagus prevent reflux (backflow) of gastric contents into the esophagus. The diaphragm, the lower esophageal sphincter, and the location of the gastroesophageal junction below the diaphragm help maintain this pressure difference (see **Figure 4–12 ≫**).

Etiology and Risk Factors

Gastroesophageal reflux may result from transient relaxation of the lower esophageal sphincter, an incompetent lower esophageal sphincter, or increased pressure within the stomach. Factors contributing to gastroesophageal reflux include increased gastric volume (e.g., after meals), positioning that allows gastric contents to remain close to the gastroesophageal junction (e.g., bending over, lying down), and increased gastric pressure (e.g., obesity, wearing tight clothing).

Risk factors for GERD include obesity, excessive alcohol consumption, smoking, hiatal hernia, and pregnancy. Gastric juices contain acid, pepsin, and bile, which are corrosive substances. Esophageal peristalsis and bicarbonate in salivary secretions normally clear and neutralize gastric juices in the esophagus. During sleep, however, and in patients with impaired esophageal peristalsis or decreased salivation, the esophageal mucosa is damaged by gastric juices, causing an inflammatory response (see **Figure 4–13 ≫**). With prolonged exposure, reflux esophagitis develops. In nonerosive reflux disease, the mucosa remains normal or mildly inflamed. Erosive esophagitis, however, is characterized by red, friable (easily torn) mucosa and superficial ulcers. If it goes untreated, scarring occurs, and esophageal stricture may develop.

Prevention

The prevention of GERD entails behavioral and routine changes associated with eating and lifestyle. Individuals can prevent heartburn or symptoms of GERD by following these dietary and lifestyle guidelines:

1. Eat smaller and more frequent meals to prevent increasing pressure in the stomach and on the lower esophageal sphincter associated with larger meals.
2. Avoid or minimize eating foods that stimulate acid production in the stomach, such as orange juice, tomatoes, coffee, wine, and chocolate.
3. Avoid eating close to bedtime or naptime to prevent reflux into the esophagus.

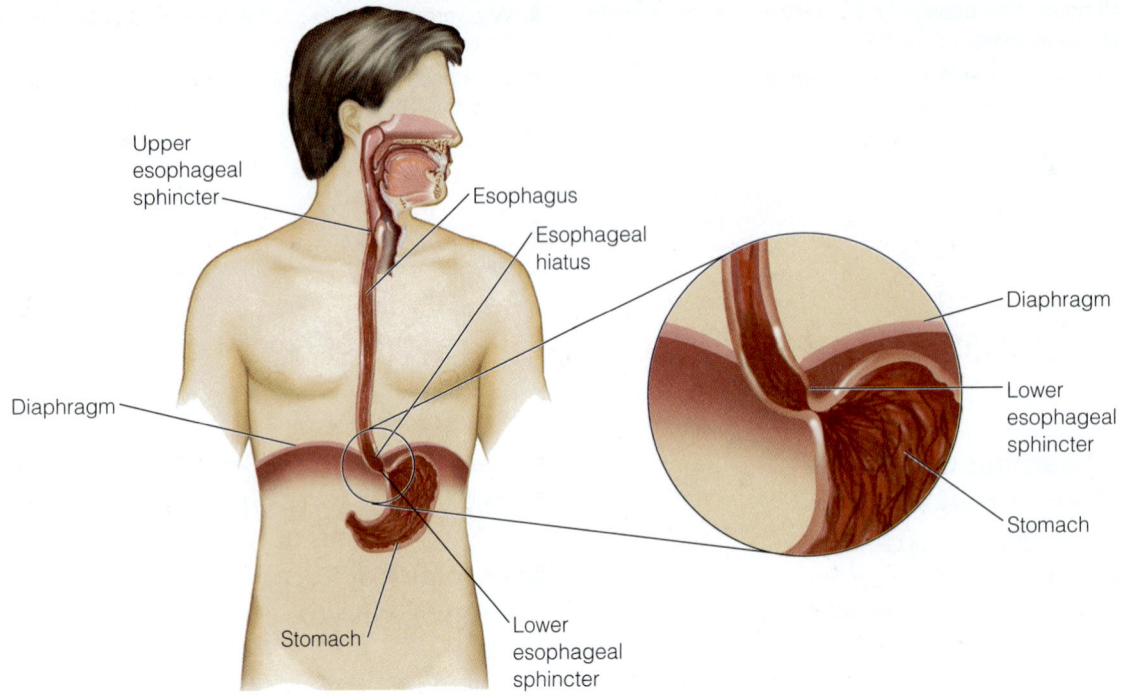

Figure 4–12 ⟩⟩ The esophagus. The inset shows a closer view of the lower esophageal sphincter.

4. Elevate the head of the bed to help prevent the stomach from pressing on the lower esophageal sphincter.
5. Avoid wearing tight-fitting clothing or accessories around the abdomen or any area that will squeeze on the stomach, pushing contents upward to the esophagus.

6. Avoid smoking and alcohol consumption because they increase stomach acid. In addition, smoking weakens the lower esophageal sphincter's ability to stay closed.
7. Maintain nearly ideal or ideal body weight. Obesity increases stomach pressure, causing the lower esophageal sphincter to open and allow stomach contents, including acid, to reflux into the esophagus (NIH, 2013d).

Clinical Manifestations

Adults with GERD complain primarily of heartburn, which usually occurs after meals, when bending over, or when reclining. Regurgitation of sour material into the mouth or difficulty and pain with swallowing may develop. Other manifestations may include atypical chest pain, sore throat, tooth enamel erosion, and hoarseness. Aspiration of gastric contents can also cause respiratory symptoms. GERD may manifest differently in infants and children (see the Lifespan Considerations section).

Complications include esophageal strictures and Barrett esophagus. Strictures, caused by scar tissue, edema, and spasm, can lead to dysphagia. Barrett esophagus is characterized by changes in the cells lining the esophagus and an increased risk of developing esophageal cancer (Cleveland Clinic, 2014a).

Collaboration

GERD often is diagnosed on the basis of the patient's symptom history and predisposing factors, such as smoking or caffeine use. Collaborative care focuses on diet and lifestyle changes. Pharmacologic therapy may be used for more severe cases. Patients who develop serious complications may require surgery.

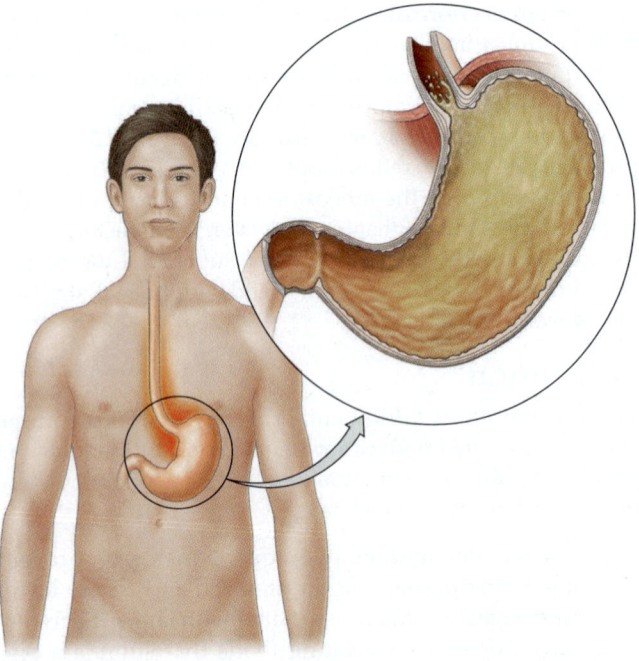

Figure 4–13 ⟩⟩ In gastroesophageal reflux disease, reflux of corrosive gastric secretions into the lower esophagus causes inflammation of esophageal mucosa.

Focus on Diversity and Culture
Patients with GERD

GERD occurs across all ethnic groups. In a population-based study by Yuen, Toner, Cobb, et al. (2010), they found that 50% of Hispanics, 37% of Caucasians, 31% of African Americans, and 20% of Asians experienced heartburn at least once a month. There are many home remedies for GERD such as eating mint, lying down after a meal, or taking bitter orange. None of these is effective. Eating mint and lying down after eating may exacerbate symptoms, and there are reports of individuals fainting and having heart attacks and strokes after ingesting bitter orange in conjunction with caffeine (NICCH, 2016).

Nurses should carefully interview all patients to determine whether they have GERD, and if so, how they are treating it at home. Community-based patient education directed at appropriate home and over-the-counter remedies is necessary to ensure that all patients are able to manage their symptoms. Using translators or providing documents in patients' native language is important for ensuring understanding and building trust (Juckett, 2013).

Diagnostic Tests

Diagnostic tests that may be ordered for patients with manifestations of GERD include the following:

- *Barium swallow* evaluates the esophagus, stomach, and upper small intestine.

- *Upper endoscopy* permits direct visualization of the esophagus. Tissue may be obtained for biopsy to establish the diagnosis and rule out malignancy.

- In the *Bernstein test*, saline and dilute acid solutions are instilled into the esophagus. In patients with GERD, the acid solution produces symptoms of heartburn, whereas the saline solution does not; neither solution produces symptoms in patients who do not have GERD.

- *24-hour ambulatory pH monitoring* may be performed to establish the diagnosis of GERD. For this test, a small tube with a pH electrode is inserted through the nose into the esophagus. The electrode is attached to a small box worn on the belt that records the data. The data are later analyzed by computer.

- *Esophageal manometry* measures pressures of the esophageal sphincters and esophageal peristalsis.

Pharmacologic Therapy

Antacids, such as calcium carbonate (TUMS) or commercial preparations of a combination of antacids (e.g., Mylanta), relieve mild or moderate symptoms by neutralizing stomach acid and are often tried first by the patient at home before the patient seeks healthcare.

Proton pump inhibitors (PPIs) such as omeprazole (Prilosec) and lansoprazole (Prevacid) reduce gastric secretions. PPIs promote healing of erosive esophagitis and also relieve symptoms. These are available over the counter. An 8-week course of treatment is typically recommended, although some patients may require 3–6 months

of therapy. Relapse is common after PPI therapy is discontinued; using a step-down approach to gradually discontinue therapy may reduce the likelihood of relapse in the immediate term, as may transitioning to treatment with H_2-receptor blockers or antacids (MedicineWise News, 2015). Although these drugs have minimal side effects, they may interfere with absorption of calcium and vitamin B_{12}. A study by Khalili and colleagues (2012) indicates that chronic use of PPI therapy is related to an increased risk of hip fractures. The risk was increased especially in women who had a history of smoking. Although there is a lack of causal evidence, emerging observational evidence suggests that overuse of PPIs may be related to increased risk of chronic kidney disease and dementia (Anderson, 2016; Kelly, 2016).

H_2-receptor blockers reduce gastric acid production and are effective in treating GERD symptoms. When treating GERD, H_2-receptor blockers are usually given twice a day or more frequently for a prolonged period of time. Several H_2-receptor blockers approved by the U.S. Food and Drug Administration (FDA) for the treatment of GERD are available over the counter. A study by Cea Soriano and colleagues (2014) showed that high doses of H_2-receptor blockers for GERD also increase the risk of hip fracture.

A promotility agent, such as metoclopramide (Reglan), may be ordered to enhance esophageal clearance and gastric emptying. Metoclopramide is used to treat patients with regurgitation, symptoms of indigestion, and nighttime symptoms. However, it is not recommended for long-term use. See the Medications feature for the nursing considerations to be aware of for drugs used to treat GERD.

SAFETY ALERT Long-term use of PPIs can affect the body's ability to absorb key vitamins and minerals and lead to anemia. Patients who have taken PPIs for an extended period of time should be assessed for fatigue, dizziness, abnormal heart rate, and other indicators of anemia.

Nutrition and Lifestyle Management

Although infants may outgrow GERD once the lower esophageal sphincter matures, in adults, GERD often is a chronic condition. Dietary and lifestyle changes help to reduce symptoms and long-term effects of the disorder. Topics for patient education and health promotion were discussed in the section on Prevention.

Surgery

Surgery may be necessary for patients who do not respond to pharmacologic and lifestyle interventions. Antireflux surgeries increase pressure in the lower esophagus, inhibiting gastric content reflux. Laparoscopic fundoplication, a procedure in which the gastric fundus is wrapped around the distal esophagus, narrowing the diameter of the lower esophageal sphincter, is the treatment of choice for GERD. As an alternative, an open surgical procedure known as Nissen fundoplication may be done (see **Figure 4–14** >>). Other laparoscopic procedures to tighten the lower esophageal sphincter may include use of an endoscopic suturing system or burning spots on the muscle surrounding the sphincter to

Medications
Gastroesophageal Reflux Disease

CLASSIFICATION AND DRUG EXAMPLES	MECHANISMS OF ACTION	NURSING CONSIDERATIONS
Antacids *Drug examples:* Aluminum hydroxide (Alu-Cap, AlternaGEL)	Neutralize stomach acid secretions Used for gastroesophageal reflux, peptic ulcers, gastritis	■ Monitor for metabolic alkalosis and electrolyte imbalances such as hypercalcemia and hypophosphatemia. ■ Antacids reduce the absorption abilities of other medications. Teach the patient to take the antacid 1–2 hours before or 1–2 hours after other medications (2 hours for quinolone antibiotics). ■ Avoid calcium- and magnesium-based antacids in patients with renal disease.
Proton Pump Inhibitors *Drug examples:* Esomeprazole (Nexium) Lansoprazole (Prevacid) Omeprazole (Prilosec) Pantoprazole (Protonix) Rabeprazole (AcipHex)	Block gastric acid secretion by inhibiting the hydrogen-potassium-ATPase pump in the stomach Are the drugs of choice for severe GERD	■ Administer 30 minutes before breakfast (and at bedtime if ordered twice a day). ■ Do not crush tablets. ■ Monitor liver function tests for possible abnormal values, including increased aspartate transaminase, alanine transaminase, alkaline phosphatase, and bilirubin levels. Health Education for the Patient and Family ■ Take as directed for full course of therapy, even if symptoms improve. ■ Do not crush, break, or chew tablets. ■ Increase calcium intake because PPIs can interfere with calcium absorption. ■ Avoid cigarette smoking, alcohol, aspirin, and nonsteroidal anti-inflammatory drugs (NSAIDs) because these substances may interfere with healing. ■ Report black, tarry stools; diarrhea; or abdominal pain to your primary care provider.
H$_2$-Receptor Blockers *Drug examples:* Cimetidine (Tagamet) Ranitidine (Zantac) Famotidine (Pepcid) Nizatidine (Axid)	Block histamine, thus reducing the release of hydrogen ion secretion from the parietal cells, causing the pH to increase in the stomach Used for acid-related disorders including gastroesophageal reflux and peptic ulcer disease	■ H$_2$-receptor blockers are given orally or intravenously. Both prescription and over-the-counter preparations are available. ■ To ensure absorption, do not give an antacid within 1 hour before or after giving an H$_2$-receptor blocker. ■ When administering intravenously, do not mix with other drugs. Administer in 20–100 mL of solution over 15–30 minutes. Rapid IV injection as a bolus may cause dysrhythmias and hypotension. ■ Monitor for interaction with such drugs as oral anticoagulants, beta-blockers, benzodiazepines, and tricyclic antidepressants. H$_2$-receptor blockers may inhibit the metabolism of other drugs, increasing the risk of toxicity. Health Education for the Patient and Family ■ Take the drug as directed, even if pain and gastric discomfort are relieved early in the course of therapy. ■ Take at bedtime if once-a-day dosing is ordered. If spaced through the day, take before meals. Avoid taking antacids for 1 hour before and 1 hour after taking this drug. ■ To promote healing, avoid cigarette smoking (which increases gastric acid secretion) and gastric mucosal irritants such as alcohol, aspirin, and NSAIDs. ■ Long-term use of these drugs can lead to gynecomastia (breast enlargement) and impotence in men and breast tenderness in women. Discontinuing the drug will reverse these effects. ■ Report possible adverse effects such as diarrhea, confusion, rash, fatigue, malaise, or bruising to your primary care provider.

Medications *(continued)*

CLASSIFICATION AND DRUG EXAMPLES	MECHANISMS OF ACTION	NURSING CONSIDERATIONS

Promotility Agents
 	
Drug examples:
GI stimulant or prokinetic agent
Metoclopramide (Reglan)
	Increase the tone of the lower esophageal sphincter and stomach contractions to move food through the stomach and small intestine
	   Used for gastroesophageal reflux and gastroparesis
	   Unlabeled use includes hiccups
		▪ Avoid using in patients who have intestinal obstruction or women who are lactating.
		 ▪ Teach patients to take 30 minutes before meals and 30 minutes before bedtime.
		 ▪ Should be stored in light-resistant bottles.
		 ▪ Monitor for common adverse effects including fatigue, extrapyramidal symptoms, diarrhea, and, in rare cases, hypertensive crisis.

Source: Data from Adams, M. P., Holland, L. N., & Urban, C. (2017). *Pharmacology for nurses: A pathophysiologic approach* (5th ed.). Hoboken, NJ: Pearson Education.

create scar tissue. Surgery or ablation therapy also is recommended to reduce the risk of esophageal cancer in patients with persistent cell changes in the distal esophagus.

》 Stay Current: It is essential that the nurse prepare the patient for what to expect from surgery for GERD and the recovery. One source of useful information is the website of the Society of Thoracic Surgeons at http://www.sts.org/patient-information/esophageal-surgery/gastroesophageal-reflux-disease.

Lifespan Considerations

GERD can occur in patients during all stages of life, though prevalence varies from age group to another. In some age groups, such as infants, GERD may resolve itself over the course of natural growth and development. In addition, different groups experience different severity of symptoms and likelihood of lasting effects on the esophagus.

GERD in Infants and Children

GERD affects a large percentage of children. Approximately 50% of infants exhibit symptoms of GERD at 4 months, though the number gradually declines to around 10% at 12 months.

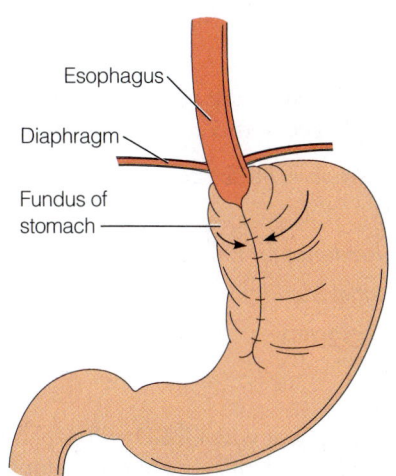

Figure 4–14 》 Nissen fundoplication. The fundus of the stomach is wrapped around the lower esophagus and the edges are sutured together.

An estimated 10–20% of children and adolescents also experience symptoms of GERD (Lightdale & Gremse, 2013).

Clinical manifestations of GERD in children younger than 1 year may include spitting up, vomiting, irritability, poor weight gain, and arching of the back during feedings. Respiratory symptoms such as choking, wheezing, and coughing may also occur. Children ages 1–5 may vomit, have abdominal pain, exhibit poor weight gain, and refuse to eat or have an aversion to food. Older children and adolescents may have symptoms similar to those of adults (Lightdale & Gremse, 2013).

History and physical examination are typically used to diagnose GERD in infants and children, particularly if there are no complications or potential for esophageal damage. In more complicated cases, diagnostic tests may be used. The most commonly used tests include upper GI imaging, esophageal pH monitoring, and endoscopy (Schwarz & Hebra, 2015).

In infants, GERD is treated primarily with feeding and position changes. An association between GERD and cow's milk allergy has been established, and restrictions on dairy consumption for nursing mothers and use of amino acid–based formulas for bottle-fed babies may ease symptoms (Lightdale & Gremse, 2013). Prethickened formulas may also ease symptoms. Infants with GERD should be burped after every 1–2 ounces consumed and should be held upright for a minimum of 30 minutes after feeding.

Children and adolescents with GERD may benefit from lifestyle modifications similar to those used in adults. Patients should avoid caffeine, chocolate, and spicy foods and should avoid eating close to bedtime. In addition, patients may benefit from weight loss and avoidance of tight-fitting clothes. Antacids, H_2-receptor blockers, and PPIs may also be prescribed. If GERD is chronic and persists in spite of lifestyle and pharmacologic treatment, surgery may be indicated.

GERD in Pregnant Women

GERD is very common during pregnancy; an estimated 30–50% of pregnant women experience symptoms (Gerson, 2012). Symptoms tend to worsen as weight gain and fetal size increase. Older maternal age and preexisting GERD also increase the likelihood of symptoms.

Symptoms of GERD in pregnancy are similar to those of the rest of the adult population; they include heartburn, acid taste in the mouth, and regurgitation. A burning sensation or pain behind the breastbone may also occur. Frequency and severity of symptoms tends to increase during the second and third trimesters of pregnancy (Malfertheiner et al., 2012).

For patients with mild-to-moderate GERD, lifestyle modifications may be enough to control symptoms. Eating small, frequent meals and avoiding foods that trigger symptoms may help. For patients who experience nighttime GERD, avoiding food within 3 hours of bed and elevating the head of the bed may be useful. Over-the-counter antacids and H_2-receptor blockers may be appropriate if lifestyle modifications are insufficient. For patients with severe or persistent GERD, PPIs may be prescribed. The majority of PPIs are considered safe for use by pregnant women; the exception is omeprazole. The FDA has concerns about fetal safety associated with maternal omeprazole use (Gerson, 2012). Pregnant patients should discuss these concerns with their physicians. Where indicated, laparoscopic surgery may be an option for treating severe GERD.

SAFETY ALERT Antacids that contain sodium bicarbonate can lead to fluid retention, and pregnant women should avoid using them. Antacids that contain calcium carbonate, which do not cause fluid retention, may be an appropriate alternative.

GERD in Older Adults

An estimated 6–17% of older adults experience symptoms of GERD. Physiologic changes of the esophagus that occur with aging can increase the likelihood of GERD in older adults. In addition, common age-related conditions and the medications prescribed for those conditions can predispose older adults to GERD (Achem & DeVault, 2014).

While some older adults have symptoms similar to other adult populations, others are asymptomatic. This is particularly true of individuals who have experienced GERD for a number of years. Other patients may develop atypical symptoms, including respiratory symptoms like wheezing and chronic cough, and GI symptoms like rapid weight loss and vomiting. Lack of typical GERD symptoms does not correlate with the severity of the condition in older adults; in fact, research suggests that while symptoms decrease with age, complications become more frequent and severe (Scholl, Dellon, & Shaheen, 2011). Visualization of the esophagus may be helpful for determining the extent of damage.

Some older adults produce little stomach acid or very weak stomach acid; as a result, antacids are not useful for alleviating GERD symptoms in these older adults. For these individuals, lifestyle and dietary changes may be useful, though these modifications may be difficult for some older adults to make because of habit, preference, and socioeconomic situation. PPIs and H_2-receptor blockers may be useful for addressing symptoms in some older adults, though the risk for hip fracture may be a concern in some patients. There are also concerns that use of PPIs increase the likelihood of community-acquired pneumonia in older adults (Scholl et al., 2011). Older adults should be monitored for medication side effects, such as diarrhea, abdominal pain, and constipation, as well as interactions with other medications.

NURSING PROCESS

Nursing care for patients with GERD focuses on alleviating symptoms and providing patient education regarding nutrition and lifestyle management. Appropriate interventions will, to some extent, depend upon the frequency with which symptoms are experienced. For example, a patient who experiences symptoms once per week may simply be able to avoid trigger foods, whereas a patient who experiences symptoms three or four times per week may require pharmacologic therapy.

Assessment

- ***Observation and patient interview.*** Assess health history and manifestations such as heartburn and atypical chest pain. Determine when pain occurs (night or day) and under what circumstances (before meals or after). Inquire about the patient's ability to tolerate acidic, spicy, or fatty foods. Record the patient's description of regurgitation of gastric acids, and note whether symptoms increase when the patient is bending, lying down, or wearing tight clothing. Inquire about difficulty swallowing. Inquire about soreness in the throat or mouth and any changes in appetite. Assess the use of antacids and other over-the-counter heartburn medicines.
- ***Physical examination.*** Assess vital signs, weight, and nutritional status. Inspect the abdomen, making note of distention and epigastric tenderness. Auscultate bowel sounds, making note of character and frequency. Assess the mouth and throat for sores and note the condition of teeth and gums. Note any unpleasant breath odor.

Diagnosis

Nursing diagnoses that may be appropriate for the patient with gastroesophageal reflux include the following:

- *Health Maintenance, Ineffective*
- *Pain, Acute*
- *Nutrition, Readiness for Enhanced*
- *Gastrointestinal Motility, Dysfunctional.*

(NANDA-I © 2014)

Planning

Planning for the patient with GERD will depend on the triggers of GERD, the patient's age and developmental level, and the severity and type of symptoms. Potential goals may include the following:

- The patient will exhibit decreased discomfort associated with GERD.
- The patient will work with the nurse to develop a plan for managing symptoms of GERD.
- The patient will modify lifestyle and eating habits to prevent symptoms and esophageal damage.
- The patient will verbalize understanding of the long-term consequences of GERD.
- The patient will achieve and maintain a healthy weight for age.

Implementation

The epigastric pain associated with GERD can be severe, interfering with rest and causing anxiety. Nurses can help patients reduce pain by providing the following education:

- Instruct patients to eat small, frequent meals to reduce pressure in the stomach, thereby reducing reflux symptoms.
- Refer patients who smoke to a smoking cessation program. Smoking interferes with healing and increases gastric acidity.
- Instruct patients on the proper use of H_2-receptor blockers, antacids, and PPIs. Remind patients to continue taking medications as prescribed even after symptoms improve.
- Coach patients on the importance of long-term changes in lifestyle, such as limiting intake of fat, acidic foods, alcohol, and coffee in order to promote continued health and manage symptoms over time.

See the Patient Teaching feature for additional information.

Patient Teaching
Gastroesophageal Reflux Disease

GERD can be a lifelong condition the patient does not outgrow with physical development. However, the patient and family can manage through a variety of strategies, including dietary changes, remaining upright after meals, and avoiding eating for at least 3 hours before bedtime. Additional strategies that patients may find helpful include the following:

- Elevating the head of the bed by 6 inches by placing wooden blocks under the legs
- Avoiding tight-fitting garments and belts
- Reducing stress
- Losing weight (if patient is overweight) (Mayo Clinic, 2014b).

Evaluation

The nurse evaluates the patient's adherence to the plan of care and the extent to which symptoms improve. Appropriate patient outcomes may include the following:

- The patient expresses freedom from heartburn.
- The patient is free from pain.
- The patient verbalizes knowledge of GERD and appropriate changes to diet and lifestyle.
- The patient demonstrates ability to manage symptoms.

If patient outcomes are not met, it may be necessary to change the patient's medication. If changing the patient's medication is not sufficient to reduce symptoms, surgery such as laparoscopic fundoplication may be indicated.

» Go to **Pearson MyLab Nursing and eText** to see Chart 1: Nursing Care Plan: A Patient with GERD.

REVIEW Gastroesophageal Reflux Disease

RELATE Link the Concepts and Exemplars

Linking the exemplar of GERD with the concept of inflammation:

1. How does the management of GERD affect inflammation?
2. What measures can the patient initiate to prevent or reduce inflammation from GERD?

Linking the exemplar of GERD with the concept of nutrition:

3. What role does patient nutrition play in the development of GERD symptoms?
4. What nutritional interventions can the nurse provide to the patient to improve the patient's symptoms of GERD?

READY Go to Volume 3: Clinical Nursing Skills

REFER Go to Pearson MyLab Nursing and eText

- Additional review materials
- Chart 1: Nursing Care Plan: A Patient with GERD

REFLECT Apply Your Knowledge

Waverly Shubert is a healthy but overweight 19-year-old woman who lives with her mother and younger brother and attends a local college. Ms. Shubert frequently goes out with her friends at night, eating popcorn and pizza and drinking soda. Sometimes they drink beer. She often eats before going to bed. Her mother comments frequently that she wears clothing that is too tight around the waist.

1. What risk factors for GERD does Ms. Shubert exhibit?
2. You are one of Waverly's friends. She asks you what she should do to be healthier. How would you respond?
3. What resources would you recommend Ms. Shubert use to assist her in achieving a healthier lifestyle?
4. Create a diet plan for Ms. Shubert.

» Exemplar 4.B
Hepatitis

Exemplar Learning Outcomes

4.B Analyze hepatitis as it relates to digestion.

- Describe the pathophysiology of hepatitis.
- Describe the etiology of hepatitis.
- Compare the risk factors and prevention of hepatitis.
- Identify the clinical manifestations of hepatitis.
- Summarize diagnostic tests and therapies used by interprofessional teams in the collaborative care of an individual with hepatitis.

- Differentiate care of patients with hepatitis across the lifespan.
- Apply the nursing process in providing culturally competent care to an individual with hepatitis.

Exemplar Key Term

Hepatitis, *244*

Overview

The liver produces bile, which helps the body break down and absorb fat. Bile is stored in the gallbladder and is released into the small intestine when needed. The liver also handles and processes nutrients that are carried from the small intestine via the blood. Inflammation of the liver, known as **hepatitis**, impedes the processes or functions of the liver. Hepatitis is a prevalent condition throughout the world that generally results from an underlying infectious agent or virus. It may also result from autoimmune disorders, alcohol or drug abuse or misuse, and exposure to industrial chemicals such as carbon tetrachloride (Mayo Clinic, 2016c). Hepatitis may be acute or chronic, mild or life threatening: the degree of inflammation and impairment depends on the underlying cause of the inflammation and how quickly it develops.

Pathophysiology and Etiology

Pathophysiology

The inflammatory process of hepatitis, whether caused by a virus, toxin, or other mechanism, damages hepatic cells and disrupts liver function. Cell-mediated immune responses damage hepatocytes and Kupffer cells, leading to hyperplasia, necrosis, and cellular regeneration. The flow of bile through bile canaliculi and into the biliary system can be impaired by the inflammatory process, leading to jaundice (see **Figure 4–15** »). When the inflammatory process is mild (e.g., hepatitis A), the liver parenchyma is not significantly damaged. However, the inflammatory processes associated with hepatitis B and hepatitis C can lead to severe liver damage (see **Figure 4–16** »). The metabolism of nutrients, drugs, alcohol, and toxins and the process of bile elimination are disrupted by the inflammation of hepatitis.

Etiology

Because of the diverse functions of the liver, the effects of hepatitis may occur locally throughout the liver, or they may occur as a systemic disease. See **Table 4–2** » for a comparison of the different types of viral hepatitis, modes of transmission, onset, carrier state, complications, and laboratory findings.

Nonviral forms of hepatitis may be associated with exposure to toxic substances or with disease states. Alcoholic hepatitis and drug-induced hepatitis are two examples of toxin-related hepatitis. Alcoholic hepatitis is the result of damage to the liver that occurs over many years of heavy drinking. It may lead to cirrhosis and other permanent liver damage. Drug-induced hepatitis may appear any time during drug treatment and in most cases can be reversed by discontinuing the drug (University of Maryland Medical Center, 2012).

Autoimmune hepatitis and metabolic-disorder hepatitis are associated with disease states. In autoimmune hepatitis, the body attacks the liver. The condition is often associated with other autoimmune disorders. In the case of metabolic-disorder hepatitis, hereditary metabolic disorders that lead to accumulation of certain substances in the liver result in liver damage and inflammation. Hemochromatosis and Wilson disease are two disorders that may lead to this condition. Nonalcoholic fatty liver disease (NAFLD) may occur in patients with diabetes or obesity. It is slow to progress and has other features similar to alcoholic hepatitis but occurs in patients who consume little or no alcohol (University of Maryland Medical Center, 2012).

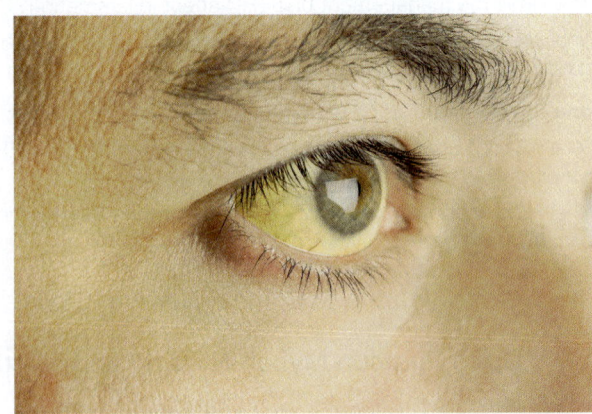

Source: Oktay Ortakcioglu/E+/Getty Images.

Figure 4–15 » A patient with jaundice.

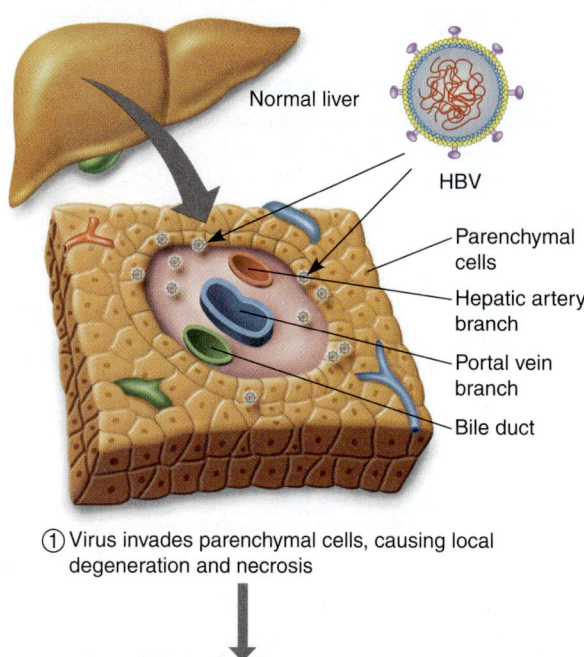

① Virus invades parenchymal cells, causing local degeneration and necrosis

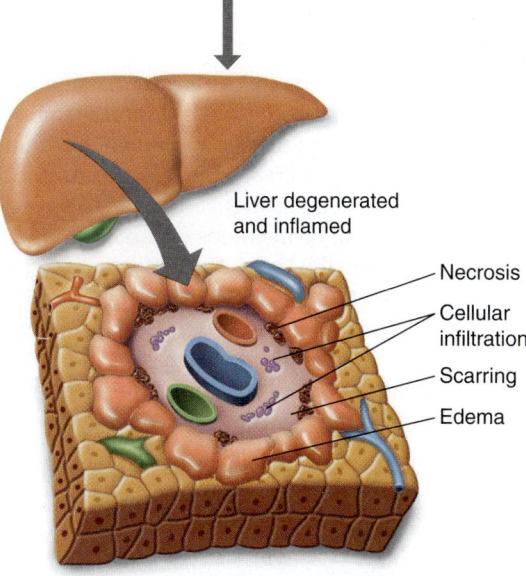

② Infiltration by lymphocytes, macrophages, and other white blood cells causes inflammation that blocks drainage

③ Structural changes occur in parenchymal cells, resulting in altered liver function:

| Impaired bile excretion | Elevated ALT and alkaline phosphatase levels | Decreased albumin synthesis |

Figure 4–16 ❯❯ The hepatitis virus causes degeneration and necrosis of the liver, which result in abnormal liver function and illness.

SAFETY ALERT If the causative agent is unknown or the individual has chronic hepatitis B or hepatitis C, healthcare providers should use standard precautions and personal protective equipment to prevent the spread of hepatitis.

Risk Factors and Prevention

Risk factors and preventive actions vary according to the type of hepatitis. Risk factors for nonviral hepatitis include having an autoimmune disorder, alcoholism, obesity, diabetes, high doses of acetaminophen, and toxins such as poisonous mushrooms. Risk factors for viral hepatitis include male-to-male sexual contact (A, B, D), illicit drug use and sharing of needles (A, C, D), drinking contaminated water or eating undercooked food (A, E), traveling in areas with high rates of infection (A, E), being HIV-positive (A, C), living with an infected individual (A, B), and assorted other factors such as being on hemodialysis, getting tattoos or body piercings, and being a healthcare worker.

Prevention primarily focuses on healthy lifestyle choices, such as practicing safe sex and avoiding drugs and alcohol. Safe food and water preparation practices are also important, particularly for individuals traveling in developing countries or visiting areas in which hepatitis infection is common. Other prevention strategies include practicing good personal hygiene and avoiding use of other people's personal care items. Finally, receiving vaccinations is important for preventing viral hepatitis; vaccines are currently available for hepatitis A and hepatitis B.

❯❯ Go to **Pearson MyLab Nursing and eText** for Chart 2: Risk Factors and Preventive Actions for Hepatitis

❯❯ **Stay Current:** Hepatitis A and B vaccines are important for decreasing morbidity and mortality in all age groups. Stay up to date on the latest recommendations by visiting http://www.vaccines.gov/diseases/hepatitis_a and http://www.cdc.gov/vaccines/vpd-vac/hepb

Focus on Diversity and Culture
Refugees with Hepatitis B

A large number of refugees entering the United States come from countries with high prevalence rates of hepatitis B (HBV) infection. Infection rates among refugees typically reflect the infection rates in their countries of origin. Individuals from Asia, Latin America, the South Pacific, and sub-Saharan Africa have the greatest risk for chronic infection. In those areas, new infections are most common in young children and are the result of perinatal or household transmission (CDC, 2014).

The nurse should review the vaccination records of patients who are refugees or whose parents are refugees and should offer HBV testing to individuals who have not been vaccinated, particularly if their countries of origin have high rates of infection. The nurse should make sure HBV vaccination is administered to individuals who are not infected and who are at an increased risk of infection (e.g., they live in a household with an infected individual). The number of refugees who have initiated the vaccine series before arriving in the United States is increasing, and the patient may have already received a dose of vaccine. If this is the case, the nurse should complete the series according to the Advisory Committee on Immunization Practices (ACIP) schedule (CDC, 2014).

TABLE 4–2 Comparison of Types of Viral Hepatitis

	Hepatitis A (HAV)	Hepatitis B (HBV)	Hepatitis C (HCV)	Hepatitis D (HDV)	Hepatitis E (HEV)
Mode of transmission	Fecal–oral	Blood and body fluids; perinatal	Blood and body fluids	Blood and body fluids; perinatal	Fecal–oral
Incubation (in weeks)	2–7	6–23	2–25	3–7	3–8
Onset	Abrupt	Slow	Slow	Abrupt	Abrupt
Carrier state	No	Yes	Yes	Yes	Yes
Possible complications	Rare	Chronic hepatitis; cirrhosis; liver cancer	Chronic hepatitis; cirrhosis; liver cancer	Chronic hepatitis; liver cancer; fulminant hepatitis	Chronic hepatitis; fulminant hepatitis; may be severe in pregnant women
Laboratory findings	Anti-HAV antibodies present	Positive HBsAg (HBV surface antigen); anti-HBV antibodies present	Anti-HCV antibodies present	Positive HDVAg (delta antigen) early; anti-HDV antibodies later	Anti-HEV antibodies present

Source: Centers for Disease Control and Prevention. (2015a). *The ABCs of hepatitis.* Retrieved from http://www.cdc.gov/hepatitis/Resources/Professionals/PDFs/ABCTable.pdf; Hepatitis B Foundation. (2014a). *ABC's of viral hepatitis.* Retrieved from http://www.hepb.org/hepb/abc.htm; World Health Organization. (2016a). *Hepatitis D.* Retrieved from http://www.who.int/mediacentre/factsheets/hepatitis-d/en; World Health Organization. (2016b). *Hepatitis E.* Retrieved from http://www.who.int/mediacentre/factsheets/fs280/en.

Clinical Manifestations

Clinical manifestations of acute and chronic hepatitis generally are similar regardless of the underlying etiology. Acute and chronic hepatitis can manifest with no symptoms or nonspecific symptoms to debilitating symptoms (see the Clinical Manifestations and Therapies feature). With acute viral hepatitis, patients usually are asymptomatic during the incubation period. HBeAg (hepatitis B e antigen) in the blood indicates a high degree of HBV infection. As the incubation period progresses, HBsAg (hepatitis B surface antigen) appears. Once the incubation period ends, the course of viral hepatitis involves three phases: the prodromal phase, the icteric phase, and the convalescent phase (recovery).

Prodromal Phase

The prodromal phase of acute hepatitis occurs between exposure to the virus and the appearance of clinical manifestations such as jaundice (yellowing of the skin, mucous membranes, and eyes) resulting from increased levels of bilirubin in the blood. The prodromal phase starts about 2 weeks after exposure to the virus and can be insidious or rapid in onset. Some of the symptoms mimic those of influenza: nausea, vomiting, malaise, and fatigue. Patients may experience frequent episodes of myalgia and arthralgia. Anorexia (loss of appetite) usually occurs early in the prodromal phase. Mild but chronic abdominal pain in the right upper quadrant or epigastrium and a low-grade fever may be present (Buggs, 2014).

Clinical Manifestations and Therapies
Hepatitis

ETIOLOGY	CLINICAL MANIFESTATIONS	CLINICAL THERAPIES
Acute hepatitis	■ No symptoms if mild ■ Fever ■ Malaise and fatigue ■ Jaundice ■ Pruritus ■ Abdominal pain in right upper quadrant or epigastrium area ■ Anorexia ■ Nausea/vomiting ■ Myalgia and arthralgia	■ Supportive therapy including rest, nutrition, vitamin supplements, and avoidance of alcohol
Chronic hepatitis	■ No symptoms if mild ■ Fatigue and malaise ■ Arthralgia ■ Right upper quadrant abdominal pain or pressure from the enlarged liver ■ Jaundice	■ Supportive therapy for lifelong management ■ Interferons and antiviral medications ■ Liver transplantation if liver failure occurs

Icteric Phase

The icteric phase begins with the onset of jaundice, approximately 5–10 days after initial symptoms manifest, although some patients will never develop jaundice. The urine may be dark during the icteric phase owing to increased levels of conjugated bilirubin, which results from the breakdown of hemoglobin conjugated by hepatocytes and excreted in the bile (Buggs, 2014).

Convalescent Phase

The convalescent, or recovery, phase brings an increased sense of well-being, usually following 2–3 weeks of acute illness. Signs of improvement include disappearance of abdominal pain and jaundice as well as increased levels of energy and improved appetite. Complete recovery times vary depending on the type of hepatitis. HAV typically resolves itself in less than 2 months but may last as long as 6 months (CDC, 2015b). Recovery from HBV may also take up to 6 months (Hepatitis B Foundation, 2014b).

Collaboration

Collaborative care by an interprofessional team that includes nurses, an infectious disease specialist, a gastroenterologist, a nutritionist, and the primary care provider ensures appropriate care for the various challenges faced by the patient with hepatitis. A social worker may also be helpful in accessing resources for the patient. Open communication between clinicians and the patient and family is essential in developing and evaluating the patient's plan of care. Treatment for hepatitis is primarily supportive, regardless of the cause. Supportive therapy includes rest, proper diet and nutrition, and avoiding alcohol. Increased protein may be necessary, depending on the level of functional impairment of the liver. A nutritionist or dietitian helps the patient develop a plan that includes low-fat proteins such as egg whites, beans, tofu, and fat-free dairy products.

Patient education includes discussions related to prevention and long-term management, including the need to avoid alcohol and substances that are toxic to the liver. Patients who acquire hepatitis as a result of IV drug use will need counseling and additional resources to overcome their addiction. Additional treatment and further assessment may be necessary for patients who acquire hepatitis through sexual activity. Social services may be helpful in identifying additional resources for patients with a history of drug abuse or sexually risky behaviors. Nurses facilitate patient education on these topics as well as education related to pharmacologic management and follow-up care.

Diagnostic Tests

The following diagnostic tests may be used to determine the extent of liver impairment: alanine aminotransferase (ALT), alkaline phosphatase (ALP), lactic dehydrogenase (LDH), aspartate aminotransferase (AST), gamma-glutamyltransferase (GGT), serum bilirubin, and liver biopsy.

For a list of specific tests for viral antigens, antibodies, or the virus itself, see **Table 4–3 »**.

Pharmacologic Therapy

Nearly all individuals with acute viral hepatitis recover fully without pharmacologic treatment. The Medications feature describes medications that may be used for preventing hepatitis A and hepatitis B, for providing prophylaxis for hepatitis A and hepatitis B (postexposure), and for treating chronic viral hepatitis. Also see the Evidence-Based Practice feature.

Lifespan Considerations

Although hepatitis can occur at any age, certain types of viral hepatitis are more prevalent in certain age groups. For example, in the United States, an estimated 50% of all hepatitis A cases are acquired by adults traveling to other

TABLE 4–3 Specific Tests for Viral Hepatitis

Hepatitis A	■ HAV-RNA is viral RNA that is found in stool; RNA is detected in feces up to 2 weeks before symptoms begin.
	■ Anti-HAV immunoglobulin M (IgM) is found in serum during acute illness, peaking about 1–3 months after exposure and slowly decreasing. It is usually gone by 1 year after exposure.
	■ Anti-HAV IgG is found in serum during recovery and indicates immunity to the virus. It remains elevated for years.
Hepatitis B	■ HBV-DNA is viral DNA that is found in serum just before the second month and disappears by the fifth month.
	■ HBeAg is a marker for viral replication and appears about 2 months after exposure.
	■ HBsAg is the surface antigen on the virus and is usually detected 2 weeks after exposure and 1 week before HBeAg; it usually disappears by the fifth month. Persistent levels indicate either a chronic or a carrier state.
	■ Anti-HBc IgM is antibody to HBcAg and is found during acute illness and convalescence but may persist for years.
	■ Anti-HBs IgM indicates acute illness and infectivity.
	■ Anti-HBs IgG and Anti-HBc IgG both indicate recovery from acute illness.
Hepatitis C	■ HCV-RNA is viral RNA and indicates a replicating virus.
	■ Anti-HCV is antibody to the virus but does not indicate immunity.
Hepatitis D	■ HDV-RNA is viral RNA and indicates acute infection.
	■ HDAg is hepatitis D antigen and indicates acute infection.
Hepatitis E	■ Anti-HEV is antibody and indicates infection.

Source: Osborn, K. S., Wraa, C. E., Watson, A. B., & Holleran, R. (2014). *Medical-surgical nursing: Preparation for practice* (2nd ed.). Upper Saddle River, NJ: Pearson Education.

Medications
Hepatitis

CLASSIFICATION AND DRUG EXAMPLES	MECHANISMS OF ACTION	NURSING CONSIDERATIONS
Immunizations *Drug examples:* Hepatitis A vaccine (Havrix)—two doses Recombinant Hepatitis B vaccine (Engerix-B)—three doses OR Combined hepatitis A and hepatitis B vaccine (Twinrix)—three doses	These immunizations promote active immunity to hepatitis A and hepatitis B infection (Lilley, Collins, & Snyder, 2014). They provide active immunity to HBV.	For Hepatitis A Vaccine ■ Given intramuscular (IM) in adults and children (1–18 years of age). ■ Avoid administration to individuals with hypersensitivity to vaccine components or sensitivity to neomycin. For Hepatitis B Vaccine ■ Given IM in adults and children (1–18 years of age). ■ Avoid administration to individuals with hypersensitivity to vaccine components or sensitivity to yeast.
Postexposure Prophylaxis *Drug examples:* Standard immune globulin Hepatitis B immune globulin (HBIG) (HepaGam B)	These drugs promote passive immunity to hepatitis A and hepatitis B infection (Lilley et al., 2014). They provide passive immunity to HBV.	■ *Hepatitis A postexposure:* Standard immune globulin. Must be given within 2 weeks of exposure. Given IM in large muscle mass. ■ *Hepatitis B postexposure:* Hepatitis B immune globulin (HBIG). Must be given within 24 hours of exposure. Given IM in large muscle mass. Begin concurrent hepatitis B vaccine series.
Interferon Alfa *Drug examples:* *Conventional interferons:* Interferon alfa-2a (Roferon-A) Interferon alfa-2b (Intron A) Interferon alfacon-1 (Infergen) *Long-lasting interferons:* Peginterferon alfa-2a (Pegasys) Peginterferon alfa-2b (PEG-Intron)	Human interferons have antiviral, immunosuppressive, and antineoplastic activity. Interferon alfa interferes with viral replication by blocking the virus from entering host cells, inhibiting syntheses of viral RNA and proteins, and viral release from host cells. Conventional interferons have a short half-life and must be administered several times weekly. Long-acting preparations, however, have a higher incidence of adverse effects.	■ Administer by subcutaneous injection. Monitor for manifestations of hypersensitivity (e.g., angioedema or bronchoconstriction); immediately notify physician and administer emergency treatment as needed to maintain cardiorespiratory status. ■ Monitor complete blood count (CBC), platelet count, and renal and liver function studies. Frequently assess mental status. Health Education for the Patient and Family: ■ This drug may cause flu-like symptoms with fever, fatigue, body aches, headaches, and chills. These symptoms tend to diminish over time with continued use of the drug. If approved by your physician, acetaminophen may be used to promote comfort. Notify your physician immediately if you become severely depressed or develop thoughts of suicide, have severe chest pain or difficulty breathing, notice unusual bleeding or bruising or have bloody diarrhea, notice a change in your vision, develop severe stomach or lower back pain, or notice a new or worsening skin condition. Keep all appointments for lab tests and follow-up visits to your physician. Women: Use a reliable means of birth control, and notify your physician immediately if you become pregnant.
Antiretroviral Drugs (Nucleoside/Nucleotide Analogs) *Drug examples:* Lamivudine (Epivir-HBV) Adefovir (Hepsera) Entecavir (Baraclude) Tenofovir (Viread) Telbivudine (Tyzeka)	These drugs inhibit synthesis of viral DNA. Therapy with antiretroviral drugs may be prolonged, as relapse is common when the drug is stopped. Viral resistance to the drug also is a concern. The nucleoside/nucleotide analog antiretroviral drugs were originally developed for treating HIV infection and now also are approved for HBV treatment, although the recommended doses differ for these two uses.	■ Administer by mouth as ordered. ■ Monitor baseline and periodic renal and liver function tests, CBC (complete blood count) with differential, blood chemistries, and serum electrolytes. Notify the physician of significant changes. ■ Lactic acidosis is a risk with these drugs; monitor for manifestations such as hyperventilation, lethargy, and arterial blood gas (ABG) values indicative of metabolic acidosis. Withhold the drug, and notify the physician if manifestations of lactic acidosis develop. Health Education for the Patient and Family: ■ Take the drug as prescribed. Notify your physician if you develop severe abdominal pain, nausea, vomiting, or anorexia or if you become jaundiced. Symptoms of recurrent hepatitis B may develop after you stop taking this drug; notify your physician if this occurs.

Source: Data from Adams, M. P., Holland, L. N., & Urban, C. (2017). *Pharmacology for nurses: A pathophysiologic approach* (5th ed.). Hoboken, NJ: Pearson Education.

Evidence-Based Practice

New Medications for Hepatitis C

Problem

For a number of years, standard treatment for hepatitis C virus (HCV) has involved a 24- to 48-week regimen of subcutaneous interferon and oral ribavirin. The success rate of this combination therapy is estimated to be between 10% and 50%. Recent advances in HCV therapy are promising, and a number of directly acting antiviral agents (DAAs) have entered the marketplace in the past 5 years. DAAs require an 8- to 12-week regimen of oral medication and have a success rate close to 90%, but they are not widely used at this time. How do these newer therapies compare to standard HCV therapy, and what factors limit their use?

Evidence

New oral therapies for HCV are faster acting, are simpler to use, and have higher success and patient adherence rates than interferon–ribavirin therapy. According to Mohamed and colleagues (2015), DAAs have fewer side effects and fewer contraindications than interferon–ribavirin therapy, making them a promising HCV treatment option for patients with comorbidities such as depression, epilepsy, and autoimmune thyroid disorders. Waheed (2015) highlights the potential of these new drugs to stem the global pandemic of HCV but cites their high price as a key limiting factor. In the United States, a cycle of standard HCV therapy costs about $4,000, whereas a cycle of DAA therapy costs between $85,000 and $110,000. This price tag—coupled with the fact that 80% of individuals with HCV live in low- and middle-income countries—puts the drug out of reach for most individuals. Enomoto and Nishiguchi (2015) further point out that in spite of its negative side effects, interferon offers protective benefits against hepatocellular carcinoma to older adults and those at risk of liver fibrosis. These benefits are lost when patients are treated with DAAs.

Implications

The evidence suggests that DAAs have the capability to drastically reduce 130–175 million estimated global cases of chronic HCV through their superior efficacy, shortened duration, and decreased side effects and contraindications as compared with standard HCV therapy. Their ability to be truly effective on a global scale depends upon a reduction in the cost of these therapies. Pharmaceutical companies and governments must search for ways to make DAAs more affordable to affected populations, in much the same way that they have sought to make HIV treatments more affordable and readily available in low-income countries. Furthermore, appropriate assessment of patient risk for hepatocellular carcinoma and fibrosis should be taken into consideration in prescribing DAAs and should be balanced against the risk for negative side effects associated with interferon use.

Critical Thinking Application

Consider patients with hepatitis C, insurance companies, and community leaders in your practice setting.

1. How would you assess the appropriateness and affordability of DAAs for individual patients?

2. How would you discuss issues of DAA affordability and necessity with a claims specialist for an insurance company?

3. Develop an education program for community leaders that explains the importance of improving affordability of and access to DAAs for community members with HCV.

---

countries, and roughly half of chronic hepatitis B infections occur in individuals born to mothers who are infected with the virus (CDC, 2013). Care is primarily supportive, regardless of age or type of infection.

Hepatitis in Infants and Children

All types of hepatitis can occur in children. Hepatitis A is the most common and is often spread at daycare centers where children are in diapers or are being potty trained. In the majority of cases, hepatitis A is mild, causes flulike symptoms, and rarely has long-term consequences. Hepatitis B may be spread to children by infected mothers; the likelihood of transmission depends upon the mother's viral load. Hepatitis B can also be spread through blood or bodily fluids or by sharing personal care items with individuals who are infected. Younger patients may be asymptomatic, whereas adolescents may experience more severe symptoms. Like hepatitis B, hepatitis C is most commonly spread to children via vertical transmission, though it can also be spread through blood and fluids. Infected individuals usually have mild symptoms. Hepatitis B and hepatitis C outcomes vary; some acute cases cause no long-term damage, while others lead to chronic infection.

Hepatitis D and hepatitis E are less common than other types. Hepatitis D can occur only in the presence of hepatitis B. It is rarely seen in children born in the United States because of widespread administration of the hepatitis B vaccine in infancy (University of Rochester Medical Center [URMC], 2015). Hepatitis E, which is similar to hepatitis A, is less common in the United States than in less-developed countries.

The onset of acute hepatitis in children is generally rapid. Symptoms include fever, nausea and vomiting, decreased appetite, and sore muscles. As the disease progresses, stool may become clay colored, and urine may become dark. Jaundice may occur at later stages of the disease. Treatments for hepatitis vary depending upon the underlying cause, the child's age and health history, and the extent of the disease. In addition to supportive care, antiviral or immune drugs may be given, as well as medications to relieve pain and any skin lesions that develop. Regardless of treatment method, the ultimate goal of care is to alleviate symptoms and prevent damage to the liver (Stanford Children's Health, 2015).

Hepatitis in Pregnant Women

The flulike symptoms of hepatitis, particularly the presence of jaundice, tend to be more severe during pregnancy. Because jaundice can be indicative of pregnancy complications such as preeclampsia, laboratory tests are essential to obtain a correct diagnosis. Once hepatitis infection has been confirmed, care is similar to that for other populations and focuses on comfort and nutritional balance (Contag & Arrabal, 2014).

Pregnant women with hepatitis B or C can pass it to their babies during birth, though administration of the hepatitis B vaccine after birth decreases the likelihood of hepatitis B infection. Children born to mothers with hepatitis B should receive the vaccine and a dose of hepatitis B immune globulin within 12 hours after birth; this is followed up with two or three additional vaccinations over the course of 15 months. A mother with hepatitis B can safely breastfeed an infant who has been vaccinated (Office on Women's Health, 2012). All pregnant women should be tested for hepatitis B to help prevent vertical transmission. There is currently no preventive treatment for vertical transmission of hepatitis C. Hepatitis A, D, and E can also be passed through vertical transmission, though this method of transmission is extremely rare (Contag & Arrabal, 2014).

Hepatitis in Older Adults

The likelihood of complications of hepatitis is higher in older adults than in other populations. Morbidity rates are also higher as a result of diminished immune response, nutritional deficiencies, and cumulative toxin exposure. Acute hepatitis A is more clinically severe in older adults than in other populations, and older adults are more likely to experience complications. Acute hepatitis B, by contrast, tends to be asymptomatic in older adults, though the rate of progression to chronic hepatitis B is higher than in other populations (Carrion & Martin, 2012).

Hepatitis C infections also occur in older adults, though to a lesser degree than in younger populations that may engage in more risk-taking behaviors. Older adults with hepatitis C typically experience more complications of cirrhosis than other groups, and scar tissue formation is more rapid in older adults (Carrion & Martin, 2012). Hepatitis D and E may also occur, though they are less prevalent than hepatitis A, B, and C.

Hepatitis care for older adults is similar to that for other populations and includes supportive interventions as well as immune and antiviral drugs. Antiviral therapy is contraindicated in many older adults with hepatitis C, however, because of age and other medical conditions. Older adults should also be encouraged to receive hepatitis A and B vaccinations, particularly those who live in nursing homes or other community settings where the disease can spread rapidly.

NURSING PROCESS

As was stated earlier, nursing care of patients with hepatitis focuses primarily on supportive measures and patient education. Many patients do not require medications and can manage their care at home; however, patients with chronic hepatitis that has progressed to cirrhosis, liver cancer, or liver failure and patients with fulminant hepatitis do require hospitalization.

Assessment

- ***Observation and patient interview.*** Assess for a history of chronic liver disease. Record the patient's description of nausea, vomiting, anorexia, joint pain, and malaise. Assess transmission risk and patient knowledge related to transmission of hepatitis to others. Discuss alcohol and drug use.
- ***Physical examination.*** Assess vital signs, weight, and nutritional status. Palpate the abdomen and assess epigastric pain. Examine skin for areas of redness or breakdown and note the presence of angioma or distended abdominal veins. Note the presence of jaundice. Examine nail beds and note the presence of silver-white discoloration (Terry's nails).

Diagnosis

Nursing diagnoses that may be appropriate for the individual with hepatitis include the following:

- *Imbalanced Nutrition: Less than Body Requirements*
- *Skin Integrity, Impaired*
- *Infection, Risk for*
- *Fatigue*
- *Knowledge, Deficient*
- *Nausea.*

(NANDA-I © 2014)

Planning

Planning for the patient with hepatitis will depend on the age of the patient, the type of hepatitis, and the symptoms the patient is experiencing. Expected outcomes may include the following:

- The patient will exhibit decreased discomfort associated with hepatitis.
- The patient will verbalize understanding of modes of transmission and infection.
- The patient will modify lifestyle to reduce the risk for transmission or infection.
- The patient will achieve and maintain a healthy weight for age.
- The patient will work with the nurse to develop a plan for management of chronic hepatitis.

Implementation

Nursing interventions to promote comfort, restore nutritional status, and promote skin integrity will help support patient health during acute episodes of hepatitis and will help manage chronic hepatitis. Preventing transmission of hepatitis is also important. Patient teaching is particularly important for proper implementation because many patients with hepatitis will receive care in the community. See the Patient Teaching feature for more information about appropriate interventions.

Promote Comfort

Pain associated with hepatitis can interfere with rest and cause anxiety. Educate patients who have abdominal or epigastric pain about over-the-counter medications they should avoid because some medications, such as acetaminophen (Tylenol), aspirin, and ibuprofen (Motrin), may be toxic to the liver. In addition, the nurse should do the following:

- Remind patients that fatigue and possible weakness are common in acute hepatitis.
- Explain that adequate periods of rest throughout the day and limitation of activities may be necessary, although bed rest is rarely indicated.
- Suggest using level of fatigue to determine activity level, with gradual resumption of activities as fatigue and sense of well-being improve.

Restore Nutritional Status

Encourage the individual with hepatitis to eat a healthy diet and follow recommendations from a nutritionist. Adequate nutrition is important for healthy immune function and healing in patients with acute or chronic hepatitis. To aid the patient in this process, the nurse should:

- Help to plan a diet of appealing foods that provides a high-kilocalorie intake of approximately 16 carbohydrate kilocalories per kilogram of ideal body weight per day
- Discuss eating smaller meals and using between-meal snacks to maintain nutrient and calorie intake
- Instruct patient to avoid alcohol and diet drinks
- Encourage use of nutritional supplements such as Ensure or instant breakfast drinks.

Prevent Transmission

An important goal in caring for patients with acute viral hepatitis is preventing spread of the infection. Effective means for doing so include:

- Encouraging prophylactic treatment of all members of the patient's household and intimate sexual contacts
- Using standard precautions with all patients, and for patients with HAV or HEV, using contact isolation if fecal incontinence is present
- Practicing meticulous hand hygiene.

SAFETY ALERT If the patient diagnosed with hepatitis A is employed as a food handler or child care worker, contact the local health department to report possible exposure of patrons. Maintain confidentiality. Prophylactic treatment of people who may have been exposed to the virus can prevent a local epidemic of the disease.

Patient Teaching

Hepatitis

When providing discharge teaching to patients with hepatitis and their families for home care, the nurse should include the following:

- Explain the recommended prophylactic treatment.
- Teach infection control measures such as frequent hygiene, not sharing eating utensils, avoiding food handling or preparation activities by the patient with hepatitis A, abstaining from sexual relations during acute infection, and using barrier protection if the patient or the patient's partner is a carrier or has a chronic infection.
- Promote management of fatigue and limited activity.
- Teach management of pruritus and maintenance of skin integrity. The patient should use warm, not hot, water when bathing; use mild or no soap; limit the duration of baths and showers; pat, do not rub, the skin dry; apply an alcohol-free lotion soon after bathing to retain skin moisture; wear loose cotton garments that allow moisture to evaporate from skin; reduce room temperature, especially at night, to prevent overheating; keep the fingernails short; and wear cotton mittens or gloves as needed to prevent scratching during sleep.
- Promote good nutrition, eating smaller meals, and avoiding hepatic toxins such as alcohol and acetaminophen.
- Recommend follow-up visits with the healthcare provider.

If chronic hepatitis B or C is being treated with medications, teach the patient how to administer the drug, its dosing schedule, precautions, and management of adverse effects. Stress the importance of keeping follow-up appointments, including recommended laboratory testing.

Evaluation

Outcomes and evaluation parameters include the following:

- The patient is free from abdominal or epigastric pain.
- The patient is free from anorexia, nausea, and vomiting.
- The patient is able to maintain weight.
- The patient's skin is intact and without pruritus.
- The patient verbalizes knowledge about hepatitis and prevention of spreading the infection.
- The patient is free from fatigue.

When patients start to feel less tired and weak, they may attempt to resume normal activities. If they do so too soon, they may prolong their recovery time. In addition, the high-kilocalorie demands of recovery can be difficult to meet. If patients struggle to recover from hepatitis or report prolonged feelings of fatigue and weakness, assess their activity levels and their nutritional status to ensure that their rest and nutrition needs are being met.

Nursing Care Plan
A Patient with Hepatitis

Abalonie Gertrush is a 45-year-old man. He presents to the emergency department with right upper quadrant abdominal pain and jaundice and is diagnosed with alcohol-induced hepatitis.

ASSESSMENT	DIAGNOSES	PLANNING
The nurse conducts a health history, health interview, and physical assessment. The nurse notes the following abnormal assessment data: Yellowish tinge to skin, mucous membranes, and sclera with pruritus Tender and enlarged liver on abdominal palpation Myalgia/arthralgia Temperature 38.3°C (101°F) oral; pulse 84 bpm; respirations 24/min; and blood pressure 142/86 mmHg Nausea and anorexia; no vomiting Fatigue Frequent social drinking; up to 6 beers/day	▪ *Acute Pain* related to inflammation of the liver ▪ *Risk for Impaired Skin Integrity* related to pruritus ▪ *Fatigue* related to disease state, nutritional status ▪ *Deficient Knowledge* related to new diagnosis of nonviral hepatitis and associated causes (NANDA-I © 2014)	Together, the nurse and Mr. Gertrush develop the following goals for his plan of care: ▪ The patient will express freedom from pain. ▪ The patient will remain free of skin breakdown. ▪ The patient will use strategies to decrease fatigue. ▪ The patient will understand the relationship between alcohol intake and liver disease.

IMPLEMENTATION

- Teach Mr. Gertrush about pain medication administration after alternative pain reduction measures are unsuccessful.
- Teach Mr. Gertrush strategies to prevent skin breakdown, including cool temperature in the environment, use of mild or no soap, wearing loose-fitting cotton clothing, and application of moisturizing lotions.

- Teach Mr. Gertrush to alternate activities with rest periods to decrease fatigue and increase tolerance.
- Discuss the effects of alcohol intake on liver functioning and its impact on daily life.

EVALUATION

In a follow-up visit to the primary healthcare provider after 3 days, Mr. Gertrush states that his pain is better and is being relieved with alternative strategies. He is wearing loose-fitting cotton clothing and has minimal red "scratch" marks on his arms and abdomen without skin breaks. Mr. Gertrush states that he is still working on not getting too tired. He is rearranging his schedule to include more rest periods during the day, especially in the late morning and early afternoon. He has begun contacting Alcoholics Anonymous because he wants "to be around for his kids."

CRITICAL THINKING

1. Is Mr. Gertrush's hepatitis contagious to others? Would his family members have to be given prophylactic medications or be taught transmission prevention strategies? Would healthcare providers have to take preventive measures to prevent transmission?
2. How would you handle protecting Mr. Gertrush through a plan to stop alcohol intake?
3. How has Mr. Gertrush's alcohol intake affected his nutritional status?
4. What complications could occur if Mr. Gertrush continues with his usual alcohol intake?

REVIEW Hepatitis

RELATE Link the Concepts and Exemplars

Linking the exemplar of hepatitis with the concept of digestion:

1. How does hepatitis affect digestion and absorption of nutrients?
2. What dietary changes, if any, should a patient with hepatitis make to ensure adequate nutritional balance?
3. What lifestyle changes should the patient with chronic hepatitis consider making to prevent liver damage?

Linking the exemplar of hepatitis with the concept of family:

4. What actions should the patient be taught to prevent the spread of hepatitis to family members and intimate partners?

5. How can the family members promote their health while caring for someone who has hepatitis A, hepatitis B, or hepatitis C?
6. Discuss strategies for teaching young children to prevent the spread of infection at day care facilities, schools, and home.

Linking the exemplar of hepatitis with the concept of safety:

7. What actions should healthcare providers implement to ensure workplace safety relating to caring for patients with hepatitis?
8. Discuss strategies for reviewing and updating policies and procedures for preventing the spread of infection within healthcare facilities.

READY Go to Volume 3: Clinical Nursing Skills

REFER Go to Pearson MyLab Nursing and eText

- Additional review materials
- Chart 2: Risk Factors and Preventive Actions for Hepatitis

REFLECT Apply Your Knowledge

Anna Majewski, a 28-year-old registered nurse, was caring for a patient who presented to the emergency department (ED) with a draining abdominal wound sustained from an auto accident 3 weeks ago. The patient stated, "I have been treating it like the doctor said, but it is getting worse every day." The ED physician ordered the wound to be irrigated. As Ms. Majewski irrigated the wound, the spray inadvertently squirted over Ms. Majewski's face shield and into her eyes. Ms. Majewski flushed her eyes according to agency protocol. The nurse taking the patient's medical history elicited that the patient has a positive recent history of hepatitis B.

1. What is the next step for Ms. Majewski?
2. How could this situation be prevented from occurring in the future?
3. What are the priority interventions for the patient and for Ms. Majewski?
4. Discuss the care needed for the patient and for Ms. Majewski in relation to preventing and treating hepatitis.

≫ Exemplar 4.C
Malabsorption Disorders

Exemplar Learning Outcomes

4.C Analyze malabsorption disorders as they relate to digestion.

- Describe the pathophysiology of malabsorption disorders.
- Describe the etiology of malabsorption disorders.
- Compare the risk factors and prevention of malabsorption disorders.
- Identify the clinical manifestations of malabsorption disorders.
- Summarize diagnostic tests and therapies used by interprofessional teams in the collaborative care of an individual with a malabsorption disorder.

- Differentiate care of patients with malabsorption disorders across the lifespan.
- Apply the nursing process in providing culturally competent care to an individual with a malabsorption disorder.

Exemplar Key Terms

Celiac disease, 254
Lactase deficiency, 257
Lactose intolerance, 257
Malabsorption, 253
Short bowel syndrome, 258

Overview

Malabsorption is a condition in which the intestinal mucosa ineffectively absorbs nutrients, resulting in their excretion in the stool. Many bowel disorders can lead to malabsorption. Among the most common are celiac disease, lactase deficiency, and short bowel syndrome.

Regardless of the cause, malabsorption causes common manifestations resulting from impaired absorption of chyme and the nutrients it contains (see **Table 4–4 ≫**). Predominant GI manifestations include anorexia; abdominal bloating; diarrhea with loose, bulky, foul-smelling stools; and steatorrhea (fatty stools). Weight loss, weakness, general malaise, muscle cramps, bone pain, abnormal bleeding, and anemia are common systemic manifestations of malabsorption. These manifestations result from malnutrition and fluid loss due to poor absorption.

TABLE 4–4 Local and Systemic Manifestations of Malabsorption

Category	Manifestation	Cause
Local (GI)	Diarrhea	Disruption of bowel mucosa, which impairs absorption of fluid and electrolytes, leading to excess water in the stool
	Abdominal distention	Gas formation from fermentation of undigested carbohydrates
	Steatorrhea	Impaired fat absorption leading to excess fat in feces
Systemic	Weight loss	Carbohydrate, protein, and fat deficit
	Weakness and malaise	Kilocalorie deficit; impaired absorption of micronutrients (vitamins and minerals) leading to nutrient deficiencies and anemia; fluid and electrolyte losses
	Anemia	Vitamin B_{12}, folic acid, and iron deficits leading to impaired erythropoiesis
	Bone pain	Calcium and vitamin D deficits leading to bone demineralization
	Muscle cramps, paresthesia (sensation of tingling or burning in the skin)	Protein wasting, and vitamin B_{12} and electrolyte deficits, which impair neuromuscular function
	Easy bruising and bleeding	Vitamin K deficit
	Glossitis (inflammation of the tongue), cheilosis (scaling and fissures of the lips)	Iron, folic acid, and vitamin B_{12} deficits

CELIAC DISEASE
Pathophysiology and Etiology

Celiac disease, also known as celiac sprue or nontropical sprue, is a chronic immune-mediated disorder of the small intestine in which the absorption of nutrients, particularly fats, is impaired. It is characterized by sensitivity to the gliadin fraction of gluten, a cereal protein. Gluten is found in wheat, rye, barley, and oats; it is also used as a filler in many prepared foods and in medications. Manifestations of celiac disease often develop in childhood but may develop at any age. The severity of the disease depends on the extent of mucosal involvement in the intestine and the duration of the disease.

Pathophysiology

Most absorption of nutrients occurs in the small intestine. The mucosa of the small intestine is arranged in microscopic folds, which in turn contain even smaller finger-like projections called villi. The cells of the villi are covered with microscopic hairs, microvilli, projecting from the cell membrane. The folds, villi, and microvilli of the intestinal mucosa provide a huge surface area for nutrient absorption. Cells of the intestines are specialized to absorb different nutrients. Readily digested nutrients are absorbed in the proximal intestine; others are absorbed more distally in the intestines. Nutrients are absorbed by the processes of simple diffusion (water and small lipids), facilitated diffusion (water-soluble vitamins), and active transport (glucose and amino acids). Once absorbed into the cells of the villi, nutrients enter the blood or lymph for systemic distribution.

Etiology

In celiac disease, the intestinal mucosa is damaged by an immunologic response. Gliadin acts as an antigen (a substance that induces the formation of antibodies that interact specifically with it), prompting an inappropriate T-cell–mediated immune response. People with celiac disease have increased antibodies to other antigens as well. The immune response prompts an inflammatory response in the small bowel, resulting in loss of villi and microvilli. The villi shorten and atrophy, resulting in loss of intestinal folds. With the loss of villi, intestinal absorptive surface is lost, and production of digestive enzymes, including disaccharidase and particularly lactase, is reduced. The proximal small bowel is affected to the greatest extent, likely because of its greater exposure to dietary gluten.

Risk Factors

The cause of celiac disease is unknown; however, genetic and immune factors are known to play a role in its development. In the past, people of European descent were believed to be most commonly affected, but research suggests that celiac disease has been underdiagnosed in other populations and in non-Western countries (Gujral, Freeman, & Thomson, 2012). Having a first-degree relative with celiac disease significantly increases risk. High-risk populations have been identified in familial forms of celiac disease, including individuals with iron-deficiency anemia, those with osteopenic bone disease,

children who have insulin-dependent diabetes, and individuals with genetic disorders, including Down syndrome and Turner syndrome (Gujral et al., 2012).

Clinical Manifestations

Local manifestations of celiac disease include abdominal bloating and cramps, diarrhea, and steatorrhea. Systemic manifestations result from the effects of malabsorption and resulting deficiencies. Anemia is common. Patients with celiac disease are often small in stature and may have delayed maturity. Other signs of nutrient deficiencies include tetany, vitamin deficiencies, muscle wasting, and rickets (impaired bone development). When gluten is removed from the diet, the manifestations typically resolve.

Gastrointestinal malignancies and intestinal lymphoma are potential complications of celiac disease. Other complications include intestinal ulceration and development of refractory disease, or disease that no longer responds to a gluten-free diet.

Collaboration

Once a diagnosis of celiac disease has been confirmed, the focus of patient care revolves around the patient's adoption of a gluten-free diet. Pharmacologic therapy may be necessary to treat specific deficiencies.

Diagnostic Tests

Laboratory and diagnostic tests are used to make the differential diagnosis for various causes of malabsorption syndromes and to determine the severity of nutrient deficiencies.

An enteroscopy permits direct examination of intestinal mucosa and collection of a tissue specimen for biopsy. Tissue biopsy is necessary to establish the diagnosis of celiac disease. An upper GI series with small-bowel follow-through may be done to evaluate the structures of the upper GI tract. With celiac disease, the typical "feathery" pattern of barium in the small bowel is lost, and the barium may precipitate and clump.

Evidence-Based Practice
Celiac Disease, Family Attitudes, and Dietary Adherence

Problem

A diagnosis of celiac disease affects both patients and their families. This is particularly true when young children are diagnosed with celiac disease, because responsibility for maintaining a therapeutic diet falls largely to the parents. Parental outlook on healthcare, nutrition, and dietary supplementation affect a child's attitude about and adherence to a gluten-free diet. In addition, a child's condition and care requirements affect parents' perception of quality of life. How do these factors have an impact on patient outcomes related to celiac disease?

Evidence

Consumption of a gluten-free diet is the primary treatment for celiac disease. Because celiac disease cannot be cured and cannot be outgrown, lifelong dietary abstinence from gluten is essential for maintaining health. According to Hoffman and colleagues (2016), parental attitudes toward dietary maintenance and micronutrient supplementation are important indicators of gluten-free diet adherence. Their research suggests that parents who adhered to a healthy lifestyle and who consumed vitamin supplements prior to a celiac diagnosis in their children were more likely to ensure that their children with celiac disease maintained a therapeutic diet that included vitamin supplements.

Dietary adherence itself is only one aspect of a celiac diagnosis, however. Khurana and colleagues (2015) explored the quality-of-life aspects associated with a celiac diagnosis. Their research revealed a positive correlation between children's physical health and gluten-free diet adherence but suggests a negative correlation between adherence and parents' quality of life. Bacigualupe and Plocha (2015) suggest that social isolation and misunderstanding of celiac disease contribute to quality-of-life issues and present barriers to dietary adherence. The presence of institutional and societal supports for families with children who have celiac disease as well as positive family processes for coping with dietary requirements are associated with both improved adherence to the dietary regimen and overall satisfaction with the lifestyle it requires.

Implications

Evidence suggests that knowledge of celiac disease and gluten-free diets is not the only contributor to positive outcomes for families with celiac children. Acceptance of a healthy lifestyle in general improves the likelihood of adherence to a gluten-free regimen. In addition, positive social experiences improve familial satisfaction with a gluten-free lifestyle. This suggests that health education at the family level and education about celiac disease at the school and community level will improve health and quality of life for children with celiac disease and their parents.

Critical Thinking Application

1. Why is it important to consider familial and parental quality of life when working with children with celiac disease and their families?

2. Develop a strategy for teaching families of children with celiac disease about gluten-free diets and a healthy lifestyle in general.

3. Develop a schoolwide education program for elementary students that explains what celiac disease is and why children with this condition should adhere to a gluten-free diet. Consider the developmental age of your audience and issues related to perceived differences in classmates with celiac disease.

Laboratory tests are used to identify pathophysiologic effects of the disease. Because the fat content of stool is increased in many malabsorptive disorders, including celiac disease, fecal fat is measured to document the presence of steatorrhea. Serologic testing for IgA endomysial antibodies, and IgG and IgA antigliadin antibodies are used to diagnose celiac disease and evaluate compliance with the prescribed gluten-free diet. Serum levels of protein, albumin, cholesterol, electrolytes, and iron may be ordered to evaluate for nutrient deficiencies. The hemoglobin, hematocrit, and RBC indices are used to evaluate anemia. Prothrombin time is increased in vitamin K deficiency.

Pharmacologic Therapy

Patients with severe nutritional deficits may require vitamin and mineral supplements, as well as iron and folic acid to correct anemia. Vitamin K may be administered parenterally if the prothrombin time is prolonged. In patients whose disease fails to respond to dietary management, corticosteroids may be ordered to suppress the inflammatory response.

Nutrition Management

The patient with celiac disease is placed on a gluten-free diet. This treatment generally is successful, as long as the patient avoids gluten completely. Consultation with a dietitian and detailed dietary instructions are necessary. Patients need to become aware of hidden sources of gluten and to analyze dietary labels. Gluten is so widely used in prepared foods that eliminating gluten from the patient's diet may be no easy task; however, many grocery stores are providing more gluten-free foods.

>> **Stay Current:** A list of common sources of gluten, including foods to avoid, can be found at http://www.mayoclinic.org/diseases-conditions/celiac-disease/basics/lifestyle-home-remedies/con-20030410.

The prescribed diet for a patient with celiac disease is high in calories and protein to correct nutrient deficits. To minimize steatorrhea, fat content is restricted. The diet usually is restricted in lactose as well to compensate for the loss of lactase-containing microvilli. Foods containing lactose may be reintroduced once remission has occurred. Patients with refractory disease may need IV nutrition (National Digestive Diseases Information Clearinghouse, 2012).

NURSING PROCESS

Nursing care for the patient with celiac disease focuses on the effects of the disorder on health and nutrition, as well as the patient's ability to manage the disease.

Assessment

- **Observation and patient interview.** Assess for the onset, duration, and severity of manifestations. Inquire about current treatment and diet. Determine the patient's level of understanding of the disease and whether there is a need for additional patient teaching.

- **Physical examination.** Assess vital signs, weight, and nutritional status. Assess skin and mucosa and note the presence of any lesions or bruises. Be alert for signs of severe vitamin and mineral deficiencies such as diminished reflexes, muscle spasm, bone tenderness, and bone pain. Note pallor, as this may indicate anemia.

Diagnosis

Nursing diagnoses that may be appropriate for patients with celiac disease include the following:

- *Fluid Volume, Risk for Imbalanced*
- *Diarrhea*
- *Pain, Chronic*
- *Imbalanced Nutrition: Less Than Body Requirements.*

(NANDA-I © 2014)

Planning

Expected outcomes for patients with celiac disease may include the following:

- The patient will provide input into the plan of care.
- The patient will verbalize management techniques for celiac disease.
- The patient will adhere to a gluten-free diet.
- The patient will report less diarrhea and steatorrhea.
- The patient will achieve and maintain a normal weight for age.

Implementation

Nursing interventions to improve bowel function, restore nutritional status, and maintain a therapeutic diet will help the patient with celiac disease to achieve and maintain a normal weight and to improve the quality of life. If corticosteroids have been prescribed, stress the importance of taking the medication as ordered. Emphasize the importance of not stopping the medication abruptly and the need to notify all caregivers that a corticosteroid is part of the patient's medication regimen. Instruct the patient or parent to frequently monitor weight. A weight gain of 5 lb (2.3 kg) or more in less than a week usually reflects fluid gain, a possible adverse effect of corticosteroids, and requires immediate clinical attention.

Restore Nutritional Status

Celiac disease is a chronic condition. With continuing malabsorption, multiple nutrient deficits may occur, increasing the likelihood of impaired growth and development, impaired healing, muscle wasting, bone disease, and electrolyte imbalances. Patients with these conditions may be hospitalized. When working with these patients, the nurse should do the following:

- Maintain accurate dietary records to document adherence to prescribed diet as well as the adequacy of nutrient intake.
- Monitor laboratory results to confirm nutritional status and guard against development of secondary conditions, such as anemia.

- Assess weight often, depending on the severity and control of the disease.
- Provide the prescribed high-kilocalorie, high-protein, low-fat, gluten-free diet.
- For the patient who is unable to absorb enteral nutrients, provide parenteral nutrition as ordered. This will help to reverse nutritional deficits and promote weight gain for patients with acute manifestations.

Improve Bowel Function

Steatorrhea and diarrhea typically occur with celiac disease because fat, water, and other nutrients are poorly absorbed, and some of them remain in the bowel to be eliminated in the stool. Diarrhea can interfere with lifestyle, activities of daily living, skin integrity, and fluid and electrolyte balance. The nurse should encourage the patient to do the following to help maintain proper bowel function:

- Assess for fluid balance by weighing daily, monitoring intake and output, and assessing skin and mucous membranes for signs of dehydration.
- Monitor perianal skin for breakdown due to frequent episodes of steatorrhea and diarrhea.

Maintain a Therapeutic Diet

Nursing care centers on teaching the importance of a gluten-free diet to the patient and family. To aid in this process, the nurse should do the following:

- Explain that lifelong dietary modifications are necessary and should not be discontinued when symptoms improve. Reinforce that discontinuing the diet in children increases the risk for growth retardation and for GI cancers in adulthood.
- Patient and family teaching includes explaining how to identify gluten-containing commercial products by reading labels and lists of ingredients and encouraging the purchase and use of a gluten-free cookbook.
- Encourage children and families to see a dietitian several times during the patient's childhood and to measure the patient's height and weight often. Advise patients and parents to get a dietary prescription, which will enable them to deduct the cost of special ingredients and commercially prepared products as a medical expense.

Evaluation

An outcome evaluation for an individual with celiac disease includes the following:

- The patient is free of abdominal discomfort including bloating, gas, indigestion, nausea, and vomiting.
- The patient is able to maintain normal or routine bowel habits.
- The patient is able to maintain adequate nutritional status.

Any residual signs of celiac disease should be reported for further treatment. If signs persist, assess the patient's understanding and adherence to dietary restrictions.

Nursing Care Plan

A Patient with Celiac Disease

Spencer Pacey is an 8-month-old boy. He has been eating solid foods for 2 weeks and has had diarrhea since the start of solid food intake. Spencer's parents called for an appointment at the pediatri-cian's office. Diagnosis of celiac disease has been confirmed through fecal fat content and through serum screening tests for transglutaminase and IgA antiendomysial antibodies.

ASSESSMENT	DIAGNOSES	PLANNING

At the time of the appointment, the nurse conducts a health history, health interview, and physical assessment and notes the following abnormal assessment data:
 	
    Diarrhea since solid food has been introduced
    Lack of appetite
    Lack of energy; one parent states, "He is taking two naps instead of his usual one afternoon nap."
    Abdominal distention
	■ *Imbalanced Nutrition: Less Than Body Requirements* related to malabsorption
	■ *Deficient Knowledge* related to new diagnosis of celiac disease
	
	(NANDA-I © 2014)
		Together the nurse and Spencer's parents develop the following goals for Spencer's plan of care:
		
		■ The patient's nutritional requirements will be met.
		■ The patient's parents will acknowledge understanding of celiac disease and nutritional strategies to prevent symptoms.

IMPLEMENTATION

■ Teach Spencer's parents about celiac disease: underlying causes, how it affects nutritional needs of the body and growth and development, and dietary treatment.

■ Explain to Spencer's parents about lifelong dietary modifications that are needed to prevent symptoms and complications of celiac disease.

■ Begin Spencer on a gluten-free diet as ordered.

■ Encourage follow-up visits with the pediatrician and dietitian.

■ Monitor Spencer's growth and development, naptimes, and energy levels.

EVALUATION

Spencer has been on the gluten-free diet for 2 weeks and has been without diarrhea for the past 7 days. His abdomen is no longer distended. His parents are feeding him gluten-free solid foods, as planned with the dietitian. Spencer's parents state that he is a "happier" baby and is more energetic. Spencer's weight and development are on target.

CRITICAL THINKING

1. Why might it be important to include family members in nutrition education for an adult patient with celiac disease?

2. What challenges would the patient with celiac disease face when attending school or leaving home to live in a college dorm? What would you include in health teaching for this type of patient?

3. If a patient with celiac disease requires corticosteroid therapy, why is it important for the patient to taper off corticosteroids rather than stopping abruptly?

Encourage the patient to meet with a dietitian to help with identification and preparation of gluten-free food options. If weight loss persists, nutritional supplementation may be necessary. In some circumstances, enteral or parenteral feedings may be indicated.

LACTOSE INTOLERANCE

Pathophysiology and Clinical Manifestations

Pathophysiology and Etiology

For carbohydrates to be absorbed from the small intestine, they must first be broken down into simple sugars, or mono-saccharides. Lactose is the primary carbohydrate in milk and milk products. It is a disaccharide, requiring the protein enzyme lactase for digestion and absorption. **Lactase deficiency** occurs when there is an insufficient amount of this enzyme in the body, which hinders the body's ability to chemically break down and metabolize lactose. Lactase deficiency is usually genetic in origin, but it also occurs secondarily to celiac disease, Crohn disease, and other disorders affecting the mucosa of the small intestine.

The malabsorption disorder lactase deficiency causes lactose intolerance. **Lactose intolerance** is the inability of adults and children to digest milk and dairy products. The condition causes uncomfortable side effects.

Risk Factors

Risk factors for lactose intolerance include previous radiation therapy for abdominal cancer, history of celiac disease or Crohn disease, premature birth, and increasing age. Lactose intolerance is not common in young children or in infants. Ethnicity also plays a role in lactose intolerance; it is more common in Native Americans, Asians, Hispanics, and African-Americans (Mayo Clinic, 2016b).

Clinical Manifestations

Many people with lactase deficiency are asymptomatic. They may be able to tolerate small to moderate amounts of milk (one to two 8-ounce glasses). Manifestations of lactose intolerance include lower abdominal cramping, pain, and diarrhea following milk ingestion. Undigested lactose ferments in the intestine, forming gases that contribute to bloating and flatus. Lactic and fatty acids produced by this fermentation irritate the bowel, leading to increased motility and abdominal cramping. The undigested lactose draws water into the intestine, which contributes to increased motility and diarrhea. The diarrhea associated with lactose intolerance can be explosive.

Collaboration and Nursing Care

The diagnosis of lactose intolerance usually is based on a history of negative reactions to milk and milk products and on a trial of a lactose-free diet. If manifestations resolve when lactose intake is eliminated, the diagnosis of lactose intolerance is confirmed. Diagnostic tests may also aid in the diagnosis of lactose intolerance.

Diagnostic Tests

The lactose breath test is a noninvasive test that may be used to diagnose lactose intolerance. Expired hydrogen gas (H_2) is measured following oral administration of 50 g of lactose. If lactose is digested and absorbed normally, then little change occurs in the amount of exhaled H_2 between fasting and post lactose administration. With lactose intolerance, exhaled H_2 increases following lactose administration as the sugar ferments in the bowel.

For the lactose tolerance test, 100 g of lactose solution is orally administered, followed by measurement of blood glucose levels at intervals of 30, 60, and 120 minutes. If lactose is digested and absorbed normally, the blood glucose rises more than 20 mg/dL. The expected blood glucose elevation does not occur in lactose intolerance.

Pharmacologic Therapy

Nonprescription lactase enzyme preparations are available to improve milk tolerance. Yogurt that contains bacterial lactases may be well tolerated. Calcium supplements are often recommended, particularly for women on a reduced-lactose or lactose-free diet. Supplements for vitamin D, riboflavin, and protein may need to be considered.

Nutrition Management

A lactose-free or reduced-lactose diet relieves the manifestations of the disorder. Some patients require total elimination of milk and milk products from the diet. Many can tolerate limited amounts of lactose. Milk pretreated with lactase is readily available.

SAFETY ALERT Some medications contain lactose and may cause symptoms in people with severe lactose intolerance. Review all prescription and over-the-counter medications with patients who are lactose-intolerant.

Nursing Care

Nursing care for the patient with lactose intolerance focuses on providing education and support. Discuss sources of lactose: Milk, ice cream, and cottage cheese are high in lactose; aged cheese and yogurt contain much smaller amounts. Potential hidden sources of lactose include sherbets, desserts made from milk and milk chocolate, sauces and gravies, baked goods, and cream soups. Suggest a trial of lactase-treated milk or lactase enzyme supplements. Emphasize the importance of obtaining nutrients contained in dairy products from other sources. Proteins may be obtained from meats, eggs, legumes, and grains. Other sources of calcium include sardines, oysters, and salmon, as well as plant sources such as beans, cauliflower, rhubarb, and green leafy vegetables.

SHORT BOWEL SYNDROME

Pathophysiology and Clinical Manifestations

Pathophysiology and Etiology

The small bowel may be resected because of tumors, infarction of bowel mucosa, incarcerated hernias, Crohn disease, trauma, and enteropathy resulting from radiation therapy. Resection of significant portions of the small intestine may result in a condition known as **short bowel syndrome**.

Resection of the small intestine affects the absorption of water, nutrients, vitamins, and minerals. Transit time of ingested foods and fluids is reduced, and digestive processes are impaired. The bowel undergoes an adaptive process in which the remaining villi enlarge and lengthen to increase absorptive surface following resection. For many patients, absorption and bowel function return to preoperative or near-normal levels. Others have continued significant impairment of digestion and absorption, leading to nutrient deficiencies, weight loss, and diarrhea. Short bowel syndrome also is associated with an increased risk for kidney stones and gallstones.

Clinical Manifestations

The severity of the disorder depends on the total amount of bowel resected, as well as the portions of bowel removed. Removal of the proximal portions, including the duodenum, jejunum, and proximal ileum, and the distal portion of the ileum is associated with more severe malabsorption and manifestations than is resection of midportions of the ileum.

Collaboration and Nursing Care

Management of short bowel syndrome focuses on alleviating manifestations. Patients often simply require frequent, small, high-kilocalorie, high-protein feedings.

Diagnostic Tests

Laboratory and diagnostic studies are used to evaluate nutrient deficiencies. Total serum proteins and albumin are reduced, as are serum levels of folate, iron, vitamins, minerals, and electrolytes. Anemia and a prolonged prothrombin time (indicative of vitamin K deficiency) may develop.

Pharmacologic Therapy

Multivitamin and mineral supplementation is frequently necessary for the patient with short bowel syndrome. Antidiarrheal medications can reduce bowel motility, allowing more time for nutrient absorption. Some patients are affected by gastric hypersecretion following bowel resection. For these patients, a proton pump inhibitor such as omeprazole (Prilosec) may be ordered.

Nutrition Management

Patients with severe manifestations of short bowel syndrome may require total parenteral nutrition (TPN). TPN can be very stressful for children. Children with short bowel syndrome often require insertion of multiple central lines over time, resulting from either infection or occlusion of the line.

SAFETY ALERT Central lines are used to deliver TPN to patients with short bowel syndrome. Recurrent infections of central lines can lead to life-threatening infections and necessitate their removal. It is essential to maintain sterile conditions in preparing TPN solution and in changing tubing or dressings.

Nursing Care

Nursing care for the patient with short bowel syndrome focuses on the problems of potential fluid volume deficit, malnutrition, and diarrhea. Fluid losses are generally greatest in the initial periods after surgery, so the closest attention is warranted at that time. Close monitoring of vital signs, intake and output, daily weights, skin turgor, and condition of mucous membranes is vital. The risk is also high when other abnormal fluid losses occur through, for example, fever, draining wounds, or excess perspiration.

Assessment includes documentation of nutritional status, including weight, anthropometric measurements, laboratory values, and kilocalorie intake. Nursing interventions include providing nutritional supplementation with enteral feedings as needed, maintaining central lines and TPN, and using aseptic technique.

For diarrhea, the nurse documents the number and character of stools and administers antidiarrheal medications as ordered. Interventions include limiting the intake of milk and milk products for patients who are lactose-intolerant and providing good skin care of the perianal region to prevent breakdown from frequent bowel movements. Refer to the discussion of nursing care for the patient with celiac disease for other measures for altered nutrition and diarrhea.

Patient and family education is critical. Because there is no way to cure or replace the lost bowel at this time, the patient must manage the disorder on a day-to-day basis. For the patient with short bowel syndrome, the nurse must provide education on the following topics:

- Educate patients on the recommended diet and medication regimen
- Stress the importance of maintaining an adequate fluid intake, particularly in hot weather or during strenuous exercise
- Describe the need for the patient to monitor weight frequently and report changes
- Refer the patient to a dietitian or counselor who can help the patient cope with what may be a lifelong problem.

Lifespan Considerations

Nutrition management is critical for patients with malabsorption disorders, regardless of the root cause or specific disorder. This can be particularly challenging in working with pediatric and older adult patients, who carry a number of risk factors for malnutrition and fluid imbalance. Close monitoring often is necessary until symptoms are controlled successfully and is particularly important for patients who are at increased risk of malnutrition due to malabsorption.

Malabsorption Disorders in Children and Adolescents

Children with malabsorption disorders may be at increased risk for vitamin D deficiency, so the nurse should closely monitor their serum concentration of vitamin D. Vitamin D deficiency in children is a risk factor for rickets and other bone-related conditions (NIH, 2014d).

Irritability and behavioral issues are common symptoms of celiac disease in children, as are bloating, gas, diarrhea, and vomiting. In some cases, rashes may also develop. Children with celiac disease tend to have decreased appetite and poor weight gain. In infants and small children, this can lead to failure to thrive; in older children, this can result in delayed growth or puberty. Nutritional deficiencies may also lead to weak bones that are prone to fractures (Celiac Disease Foundation, 2015).

Age-appropriate patient teaching is important for school-age children and adolescents with celiac disease. Nurses should teach them the importance of consuming gluten-free foods in the school cafeteria, during extracurricular activities, and at special events such as birthday parties as well as how to identify foods that may contain gluten and how to identify suitable gluten-free alternatives outside of the home. School-age patients may benefit from coping strategies (U.S. Department of Health and Human Services, 2014).

Lactose intolerance in children may be the result of either primary or secondary lactase deficiency. Primary lactase deficiency is a rare hereditary condition in which infants are born with deficient or absent lactase. Infants born with this condition require special formula that is lactose-free. Secondary lactase deficiency can be caused by celiac disease, Crohn disease, or infection of the GI tract that damages the lining of the small intestine. Lactose intolerance associated with secondary lactase deficiency typically resolves itself with proper treatment of the causative condition (American College of Gastroenterology, 2012).

Dietary changes and supplements that aid in digestion of lactose are common treatments for lactose intolerance associated with lactase deficiency. Patients and their parents need to understand sources of lactose, including nondairy products that contain milk or milk products. Nurses should closely monitor calcium intake in children with lactose intolerance, and patients may need calcium and vitamin D supplements to ensure adequate intake.

Short bowel syndrome in children can be the result of a congenital condition or of surgery to remove portions of the large intestine. One common cause of such surgery is necrotizing enterocolitis, an acute inflammatory disease that involves damage, necrosis, and perforation of the intestinal tract in premature infants (Cleveland Clinic, 2015). Diarrhea, bloating, poor appetite, and inability to gain weight are common in children with short bowel syndrome. Patients with the condition are also prone to dehydration and vitamin, mineral, and electrolyte imbalances.

Malabsorption Disorders in Pregnant Women

Malabsorption disorders can present special challenges for pregnant patients who face increased nutritional demands associated with fetal growth and development. Failure to meet these demands can have negative outcomes for both mother and child.

Research suggests that female infertility and amenorrhea are linked to celiac disease. In addition, poor pregnancy outcomes and intrauterine growth restrictions are associated with this condition (Wakim-Fleming, 2012). Women with celiac disease are at increased risk for miscarriage and stillbirth, and perinatal morbidity is more likely in children born to women with celiac disease. These outcomes are thought to be related to the malabsorption of iron and folate, which causes vitamin deficiency (Moleski et al., 2015). Preterm delivery and low infant birth weight are also more prevalent among mothers with celiac disease than among the general population.

Testing at-risk patients for celiac disease and teaching about celiac dietary restrictions are especially important for improving patient outcomes. Studies suggest that negative outcomes in mothers and their children are often the result of undiagnosed celiac disease. Adherence to a strict gluten-free diet after diagnosis may improve outcomes for patients with celiac-related infertility, miscarriage, and stillbirth. Birth weights of children born to mothers with celiac disease who follow a gluten-free diet may also be higher than those of mothers who do not (Moleski et al., 2015).

Calcium is critical for fetal bone development, and pregnant women should consume around 1000 mg of calcium per day. The body's ability to digest lactose often improves during pregnancy; as a result, lactose-intolerant patients may be better able to digest dairy products during pregnancy and may experience few digestive symptoms (Harms, 2015).

Patients whose symptoms persist during pregnancy should focus on consuming other sources of calcium. These include calcium-rich foods like sardines, salmon, broccoli, and spinach. Calcium supplements and lactose-free products are other viable options. In addition, yogurt and cheese are often well tolerated by patients who are lactose-intolerant (Harms, 2015). Pregnant or nursing patients should check with their physician before using commercially available lactase additives. These products come in tablet or liquid form and are typically taken before consuming dairy products (NIH, 2014b).

In general, women who have had bowel resection surgery prior to becoming pregnant do not experience specific pregnancy-related complications of short bowel syndrome (Crohn & Colitis Foundation of America, 2013). The primary concern for these patients is consumption of sufficient vitamins and nutrients to support maternal and fetal health. If maternal vitamin deficiencies are severe, birth defects can occur (Grabosh et al., 2013).

Nutritional status of pregnant patients with short bowel syndrome should be regularly evaluated and supplemented as necessary. Regular consultation between the patient's gastroenterologist and other members of the healthcare team can improve patient outcomes (Grabosh et al., 2013).

Malabsorption Disorders in Older Adults

A number of factors, including GI disease, dementia, side effects of medications, and financial considerations, may increase the older adult's risk for malnutrition. Nurses working with older adults should understand the additional risks these patients carry for malnutrition related to malabsorption. Nurses should intervene early by monitoring older adult patients carefully and working collaboratively with dietitians and healthcare providers to ensure that patients' nutritional needs are met (Ali, 2012).

An increasing number of older adults are being diagnosed with celiac disease, with an estimated 30% of new diagnoses occurring in people over age 60 (National Foundation for Celiac Awareness, 2017). Symptoms in older adults are less severe than those in other age groups. Furthermore, symptoms of celiac disease are similar to the results of other, normal age-related changes to the body. These factors lead to underdiagnosis of celiac disease in older adults (Lerner & Matthias, 2015).

Older adults with celiac disease are at increased risk of malnutrition and poor bone health; osteopenia is commonly diagnosed in older celiac patients. Iron deficiency anemia is also very prevalent. As with other age groups, a gluten-free diet is recommended. However, this may be especially problematic for older adults. They may be resistant to changing their dietary habits or may lack the financial or social resources to access gluten-free options (Lerner & Matthias, 2015). These patients need information about appropriate resources. In addition, many older adults take prescription medications, some of which may contain gluten. The nurse should teach patients with celiac disease to ask their doctor or pharmacist about gluten-free alternatives (National Foundation for Celiac Awareness, 2017).

As individuals age, they experience a normal decline in the amount of lactase found in the small intestine. For some older adults, this leads to acquired lactase deficiency, which manifests as an increasing intolerance to lactose over time (American College of Gastroenterology, 2012). In addition, illness or injury to the small intestine may result in decreased production of lactase.

Management for lactose intolerance is generally dietary. Depending upon the patient's level of lactose intolerance, he or she may be able to consume some lactose-containing products or small amounts of foods such as milk, yogurt, and cheese. In addition, lactose-free and lactose-reduced foods are readily available in stores, though the FDA does not regulate the use of these terms (FDA, 2015). Bone loss is a concern for older adults, particularly women; therefore, nurses must teach older patients who are lactose-intolerant the proper methods for dietary management and calcium supplementation.

Some medical conditions, such as cancer, that tend to occur with age may result in surgical resection of portions of the small intestine. The severity of short bowel syndrome depends upon the amount and portions of the small intestine that have been removed. It is also affected by how well the remaining portions of small intestine function and how well the other digestive organs function. Normal aging and other medical conditions may decrease GI function, increasing the severity of short bowel syndrome in older adults (NIH, 2015d).

A number of older patients take medication for other health conditions, some of which affect the body's ability to absorb nutrients. For patients with short bowel syndrome in particular, the nurse should review medications and side effects on absorption.

REVIEW Malabsorption Disorders

RELATE Link the Concepts and Exemplars

Linking the exemplar of malabsorption disorders with the concept of elimination:

1. How is bowel function affected by celiac disease? By lactose intolerance? By short bowel syndrome?

2. In caring for a patient with a malabsorption disorder, what precautions must the nurse implement related to bowel elimination?

Linking the exemplar of malabsorption disorders with the concept of development:

3. How does cognitive development affect the treatment of malabsorption disorders?

4. How do changes in growth and development affect the treatment plan of a malabsorption disorder across the lifespan?

READY Go to Volume 3: Clinical Nursing Skills

REFER Go to Pearson MyLab Nursing and eText

- Additional review materials

REFLECT Apply Your Knowledge

Chris Basham is a 16-month-old boy who is brought into the clinic by his mother. Chris was born healthy at 6 pounds 4 ounces. His weight currently is 15 pounds. During the past 3 months, his mother has noticed abdominal distention, irritability, and loose stools. Chris appears pale and slightly lethargic. His pediatrician confirms a diagnosis of celiac disease.

1. What assessment data would alert the nurse to a digestive problem?

2. What additional information would the nurse obtain from the mother?

3. Why is Chris pale?

4. What priority nursing diagnosis would you consider for Chris?

≫ Exemplar 4.D
Pancreatitis

Exemplar Learning Outcomes

4.D Analyze pancreatitis as it relates to digestion.

- Describe the pathophysiology of pancreatitis.
- Describe the etiology of pancreatitis.
- Compare the risk factors and prevention of pancreatitis.
- Identify the clinical manifestations of pancreatitis.
- Summarize diagnostic tests and therapies used by interprofessional teams in the collaborative care of an individual with pancreatitis.

- Differentiate care of patients with pancreatitis across the lifespan.
- Apply the nursing process in providing culturally competent care to an individual with pancreatitis.

Exemplar Key Terms

Acute pancreatitis, *262*
Chronic pancreatitis, *262*
Pancreatitis, *261*
Steatorrhea, *263*

Overview

The normal function of the pancreas involves the release of pancreatic enzymes in the duodenum to assist in the digestion of proteins, starches, and fatty acids. Food entering the small intestine stimulates release of the pancreatic enzymes; however, in **pancreatitis** (inflammation of the pancreas), the pancreatic enzymes are activated early and digest the pancreas and surrounding tissues, a process called autodigestion.

Pancreatitis can be acute or chronic. There are between 13 and 45 newly diagnosed cases of acute pancreatitis for every 100,000 individuals worldwide every year. Approximately 5–12 cases of chronic pancreatitis occur per 100,000 individuals worldwide per year. These numbers may not fully represent the population with chronic pancreatitis because many individuals affected by this disorder do not exhibit classic manifestations; furthermore, the majority of available data come from the United States, Europe, and Japan (Yadav & Lowenfels, 2013).

Pathophysiology and Etiology

Knowledge of the normal structure and functions of the exocrine pancreas is important for understanding how inflammation affects the pancreas and the patient. The exocrine pancreas consists of lobules of acinar cells. The acinar cells secrete digestive enzymes and fluids (pancreatic juices) into ducts that empty into the main pancreatic duct (the duct of Wirsung). The pancreatic duct joins the common bile duct and empties into the duodenum through the ampulla of Vater (in some people the main pancreatic duct empties directly into the duodenum). The epithelial lining of the pancreatic ducts secretes water and bicarbonate to modify the composition of the pancreatic secretions. Pancreatic enzymes are secreted primarily in an inactive form and are activated in the intestine, a modification that prevents digestion of pancreatic tissue by its own enzymes (American Pancreatic Association, 2014). The pancreatic enzymes, with related functions, are as follows:

- Proteolytic enzymes, including trypsin, chymotrypsin, carboxypolypeptidase, ribonuclease, and deoxyribonuclease, which break down dietary proteins
- Pancreatic amylase, which breaks down starch
- Lipase, which breaks down fats into glycerol and fatty acids.

Acute Pancreatitis

Acute pancreatitis is an inflammatory disorder that involves self-destruction of the pancreas by its own enzymes through autodigestion. The milder form of acute pancreatitis, *interstitial edematous pancreatitis*, leads to inflammation and edema of pancreatic tissue. It often is self-limiting. The more severe form, *necrotizing pancreatitis*, is characterized by inflammation, hemorrhage, and ultimately necrosis of pancreatic tissue.

Acute pancreatitis is most common in middle-age adults. Gallstones and alcoholism account for the majority of the cases of acute pancreatitis in the United States (Yadav & Lowenfels, 2013). Younger patients with cystic fibrosis may also develop acute pancreatitis. Some patients with acute pancreatitis recover completely, others experience recurring attacks, and still others develop chronic pancreatitis. The mortality and symptoms depend on the severity and type of pancreatitis, as well as the patient's age and general health.

Although the exact cause of acute pancreatitis is not known, the gallstones may activate pancreatic enzymes within the pancreas, leading to autodigestion, inflammation, edema, and/or necrosis. Alcohol causes duodenal edema and may increase pressure and spasm in the sphincter of Oddi, obstructing pancreatic outflow. It also stimulates pancreatic enzyme production, thus raising pressure within the pancreas.

Other factors associated with acute pancreatitis include tissue ischemia or anoxia, trauma or surgery, pancreatic tumors, third-trimester pregnancy, infectious agents (viral, bacterial, or parasitic), elevated calcium levels, and hyperlipidemia. Some medications have been linked with this disorder, including thiazide diuretics, estrogen, steroids, salicylates, and NSAIDs.

Regardless of the precipitating factor, the pathophysiologic process begins with the release of activated pancreatic enzymes into pancreatic tissue. Activated proteolytic enzymes, trypsin in particular, digest pancreatic tissue and activate other enzymes such as phospholipase A, which digests cell membrane phospholipids, and elastase, which digests the elastic tissue of blood vessel walls. This leads to protein breakdown, edema, vascular damage and hemorrhage, and necrosis of parenchymal cells. Cellular damage and necrosis release activated enzymes and vasoactive substances that produce vasodilation, increase vascular permeability, and cause edema. A large volume of fluid may shift from circulating blood into the retroperitoneal space, the peripancreatic spaces, and the abdominal cavity. In these cases, acute pancreatitis results in vascular changes, fat and coagulation necrosis, and swelling of the pancreas.

Chronic Pancreatitis

Chronic pancreatitis is characterized by chronic inflammation, fibrosis, and gradual destruction of functional pancreatic tissue. In contrast to acute pancreatitis, which is reversible, chronic pancreatitis is an irreversible process that eventually leads to pancreatic insufficiency. Alcoholism is the primary risk factor for chronic pancreatitis in the United States. Malnutrition is a major worldwide risk factor. About 10–20% of cases of chronic pancreatitis are idiopathic, with no identified cause. A genetic mutation on a gene associated with cystic fibrosis may play a role in these cases. Children or young adults with cystic fibrosis may develop chronic pancreatitis as well.

In chronic pancreatitis related to alcoholism, pancreatic secretions have an increased concentration of insoluble proteins. These proteins calcify, forming plugs that block pancreatic ducts and the flow of pancreatic juices. This blockage leads to inflammation and fibrosis of pancreatic tissue. In other cases, a stricture or stone may block pancreatic outflow, causing chronic obstructive pancreatitis. In chronic pancreatitis, recurrent episodes of inflammation eventually lead to fibrotic changes in the parenchyma of the pancreas, with loss of exocrine function. This leads to malabsorption from pancreatic insufficiency. If endocrine function is disrupted as well, clinical diabetes mellitus may develop.

Risk Factors and Prevention

Men are more likely to develop pancreatic cancer than women, and African Americans are slightly more likely to develop it than Caucasians (Yadav & Lowenfels, 2013; American Cancer Society, 2016). Alcoholism and gallstones are the primary known risk factors for acute pancreatitis; however, the etiology of about 30% of cases is unclear. Lifestyle choices aimed at managing modifiable risks can prevent acute pancreatitis.

Risk factors for chronic pancreatitis include alcohol abuse, autoimmune disorders, cystic fibrosis, hypertriglyceridemia, hyperparathyroidism, and medications such as estrogens, corticosteroids, and thiazide diuretics (Mount Sinai Hospital, 2015). Health promotion strategies in managing lifestyle choices can assist the individual in reducing risk factors for chronic pancreatitis.

Clinical Manifestations

Acute pancreatitis develops suddenly, typically with an abrupt onset of continuous severe epigastric and abdominal pain. This pain commonly radiates to the back and is relieved somewhat by sitting up and leaning forward. The pain often is initiated by a fatty meal or excessive alcohol intake.

Other manifestations of acute pancreatitis include nausea and vomiting; abdominal distention and rigidity; decreased bowel sounds; tachycardia; hypotension; elevated temperature; and cold, clammy skin. Within 24 hours, mild jaundice may appear. Retroperitoneal bleeding may occur 3–6 days after the onset of acute pancreatitis; signs of bleeding include bruising in the flanks (Turner sign) or around the umbilicus (Cullen sign). See the Clinical Manifestations and Therapies feature.

Systemic complications of acute pancreatitis include intravascular volume depletion with shock, acute tubular necrosis and renal failure, and acute respiratory distress syndrome (ARDS). Hypovolemic shock and acute renal failure usually develop within 24 hours after the onset of acute pancreatitis. Manifestations of ARDS may be seen 3–7 days after the onset of pancreatitis, particularly in patients who have experienced severe volume depletion.

Localized complications include pancreatic necrosis, abscess, pseudocysts, and pancreatic ascites. Pancreatic necrosis causes an inflammatory mass that may be infected. It may lead to shock and multiple organ failure. Pancreatic pseudocysts, encapsulated collections of fluid, may develop both within the pancreas itself and in the abdominal cavity (see **Figure 4–17**). They may impinge on other structures or may rupture, causing generalized peritonitis. Rupture of a pseudocyst or of the pancreatic duct can lead to pancreatic ascites. An infected pancreatic pseudocyst becomes a pancreatic abscess. A pancreatic abscess may also form as areas in damaged and infected pancreatic tissue become encapsulated (Cleveland Clinic, 2014b). Pancreatic ascites is signaled by gradually increasing abdominal girth and persistent elevation of the serum amylase level without abdominal pain.

Chronic pancreatitis typically causes recurrent episodes of epigastric and left upper abdominal pain that radiates to

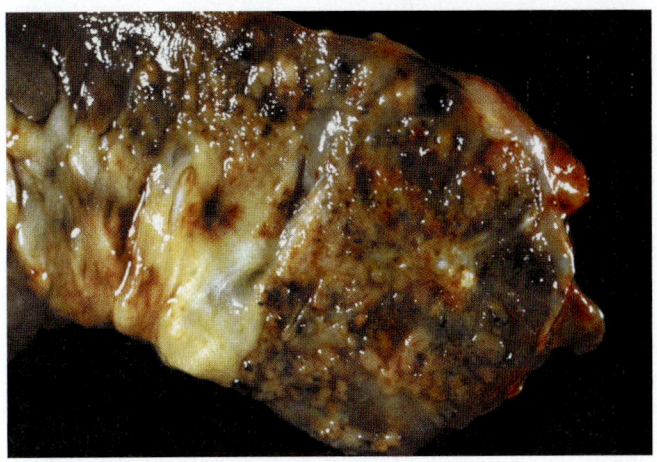

Source: CNRI/Science Source.

Figure 4–17 Acute pancreatitis. Gross clinical specimen of a pancreas affected by acute pancreatitis. A pseudocyst, a pus-filled bleb seen as the yellow area (lower left center), is a potential complication of acute pancreatitis.

the back. This pain may last for days to weeks. As the disease progresses, the interval between episodes of pain becomes shorter. Other manifestations include anorexia, nausea and vomiting, weight loss, flatulence, constipation, and **steatorrhea** (fatty, frothy, foul-smelling stools caused by a decrease in pancreatic enzyme secretion).

Complications of chronic pancreatitis include malabsorption, malnutrition, and possible peptic ulcer disease. A pancreatic pseudocyst or abscess may form, or stricture of the common bile duct may develop. Diabetes mellitus may develop, and there is an increased risk for pancreatic cancer. Opioid addiction related to frequent, severe pain episodes is common.

Clinical Manifestations and Therapies
Pancreatitis

ETIOLOGY	CLINICAL MANIFESTATIONS	CLINICAL THERAPIES
Acute pancreatitis	▪ Severe epigastric and abdominal pain ▪ Nausea and vomiting ▪ Abdominal distention and rigidity ▪ Decreased bowel sounds ▪ Tachycardia ▪ Hypotension ▪ Elevated temperature ▪ Cold and clammy skin	▪ NPO ▪ IV hydration ▪ Analgesics ▪ Antibiotics
Chronic pancreatitis	▪ Gastric and left upper abdominal pain radiating to the back ▪ Anorexia ▪ Weight loss ▪ Nausea and vomiting ▪ Constipation ▪ Steatorrhea	▪ Low-fat diet ▪ Abstaining from alcohol ▪ Surgery to relieve obstruction ▪ Pancreatectomy

Collaboration

Because acute pancreatitis often is a mild, self-limiting disease, treatment focuses on reducing pancreatic secretions and providing supportive care. Treatment to eliminate the causative factor begins after the acute inflammatory process resolves. Treatment for chronic pancreatitis often focuses on managing pain and treating malabsorption and malnutrition. Severe necrotizing pancreatitis puts patients at an increased risk of sepsis and may require intensive care management, including antibiotic therapy, nutritional support, and aggressive IV fluid replacement. In some cases, surgical drainage of the pancreas may be necessary.

Diagnostic Tests

The laboratory tests that may be ordered when pancreatitis is suspected are summarized in **Table 4–5 》**. Diagnostic studies include the following:

- **Ultrasonography** can identify gallstones, a pancreatic mass, or pseudocyst.
- **Endoscopic ultrasonography** can detect changes indicative of chronic pancreatitis in the pancreatic duct and parenchyma.
- **Contrast-enhanced CT scan** may be ordered to identify pancreatic enlargement, ductal calcifications, fluid collections in or around the pancreas, and perfusion deficits in areas of necrosis.
- **Magnetic resonance cholangiopancreatography (MRCP)** is a noninvasive test that allows visualization of the bile and pancreatic ducts.
- **Endoscopic retrograde cholangiopancreatography (ERCP)** may be performed to diagnose chronic pancreatitis and to differentiate inflammation and fibrosis from carcinoma.
- **Percutaneous fine-needle aspiration biopsy** may be performed to differentiate chronic pancreatitis from cancer of the pancreas; the cells that are aspirated are examined for malignancy.

》 Stay Current: For the latest information about acute and chronic pancreatitis and guidelines for the treatment of these conditions, visit the American Pancreatic Association website at http://www.american-pancreatic-association.org/.

Pharmacologic Therapy

The treatment of acute pancreatitis is largely supportive. Opioid analgesics such as morphine sulfate or hydromorphone (Dilaudid) may be used to control pain. Prophylactic antibiotics are prescribed for patients with severe or necrotizing pancreatitis to prevent infection.

Patients with chronic pancreatitis may also require analgesics but must be closely monitored to prevent drug dependence. Pancreatic enzyme supplements are given to manage abdominal pain and reduce steatorrhea (see the Medications feature). Patients with chronic pancreatitis may need to remain on pancreatic enzyme supplements for life. H_2-blockers such as cimetidine (Tagamet) and ranitidine (Zantac) and proton pump inhibitors such as omeprazole (Prilosec) may be given to neutralize or decrease gastric secretions.

Nutrition Management

Oral food and fluids generally are withheld during acute episodes of pancreatitis to reduce pancreatic secretions and allow the organ to rest. A nasogastric tube may be inserted and connected to suction. Administer IV fluids to maintain vascular volume, and initiate total parenteral nutrition (TPN). Begin oral food and fluids once the serum amylase levels have returned to normal, bowel sounds are present, and pain disappears. Order a low-fat diet, and strictly prohibit alcohol intake.

Surgery

If the pancreatitis is the result of a gallstone lodged in the sphincter of Oddi, an endoscopic transduodenal sphincterotomy may be performed to remove the stone. When cholelithiasis is identified as a causative factor, a cholecystectomy is performed once the acute pancreatitis has resolved. Surgical procedures to promote drainage of pancreatic enzymes into the duodenum or resection of all or part of the pancreas may be done to provide pain relief in patients with chronic pancreatitis. Large pancreatic pseudocysts may be drained endoscopically or surgically.

Lifespan Considerations

Pancreatitis occurs in patients of all ages, though it is less common in certain groups than in others. Mortality rates

TABLE 4–5 Laboratory Tests in Exocrine Pancreatic Disorders

Test	Normal Value	Significance
Serum amylase	60–160 Somogyi units/dL, 30–170 units/L (SI units)	Levels rise within 2–12 hours of onset of acute pancreatitis to two to three times normal. Levels return to normal in 3–4 days.
Serum lipase	20–180 international units/L	Levels rise in acute pancreatitis; they remain elevated for 7–14 days.
Urine amylase	6.5–48 units/hr (SI units); 4–37 units/L/2 hr	Urine amylase levels rise in acute pancreatitis.
Serum glucose (fasting)	70–110 mg/dL	Patient may have transient elevation of serum glucose in acute pancreatitis.
Serum bilirubin	0.1–1.2 mg/dL	Compression of the common duct may increase bilirubin levels in acute pancreatitis.
Serum alkaline phosphatase (ALP)	42–136 units/L	Compression of the common duct may increase levels in acute pancreatitis.
Serum calcium	9–11 mg/dL or 4.5–5.5 mEq/L	Hypocalcemia develops in up to 25% of patients with acute pancreatitis.
White blood cells	4500–10,000 μL (mm^3)	Leukocytosis indicates inflammation and is usually present in acute pancreatitis.

Medications

Chronic Pancreatitis

CLASSIFICATION AND DRUG EXAMPLES	MECHANISMS OF ACTION	NURSING CONSIDERATIONS
Pancreatic Enzyme Replacement *Drug example:* Pancrelipase (Lipancreatin)	Pancrelipase enhances the digestion of starches and fats in the GI tract by supplying an exogenous source of the enzymes protease, amylase, and lipase. The drug promotes nutrition and decreases the number of bowel movements.	▪ Assess for allergy to pork protein. ▪ Monitor frequency and consistency of stools. ▪ Weigh every other day. Record weights. ▪ Give with meals; if not enteric-coated, H_2-receptor antagonists or antacids may be given concurrently to prevent destruction of the enzymes by hydrochloric acid. ▪ Monitor for side effects: rash, hives, respiratory difficulty, hematuria, hyperuricemia, or joint pain. Health Education for the Patient and Family ▪ Take with meals or snacks. ▪ If medicine is enteric-coated, do not crush, chew, or mix with alkaline foods (e.g., milk, ice cream). ▪ Be sure to follow prescribed diet. ▪ Continue taking this drug until or unless advised by physician that it is no longer necessary.

Source: Data from Adams, M. P., Holland, L. N., & Urban, C. (2017). *Pharmacology for nurses: A pathophysiologic approach* (5th ed.). Hoboken, NJ: Pearson Education.

differ from age group to age group, and manifestations are somewhat variable among groups.

Pancreatitis in Children and Adolescents

Pancreatitis occurs in pediatric patients, though it is uncommon and the etiology is much more diverse than it is in adults. Nearly a quarter of cases of pancreatitis in children are the result of abdominal trauma; pancreatic anomalies, multisystem disease, medications, infections, and hereditary disorders are other potential causes of pancreatitis in children (Hebra, Adams, & Vargas, 2014). Children with pancreatitis typically present with abdominal pain, vomiting, and abdominal tenderness and distention. Fever, jaundice, and nausea may also be present. Treatment of pancreatitis in children is similar to that of adults with pancreatitis, though the differing etiology and differing clinical manifestations in children can make it difficult to determine the most appropriate course of treatment (Suzuki, Sai, & Shimizu, 2014).

Pancreatitis in Pregnant Women

Acute pancreatitis in pregnancy is relatively rare, occurring in roughly 3 of every 10,000 pregnancies (Juneja et al., 2013). The majority of cases are the result of gallstones that obstruct pancreatic outflow. Increased triglyceride levels can also lead to pancreatitis in pregnant patients. The hormonal changes of pregnancy are believed to impact gallstone formation and triglyceride levels (Gardner, 2014). Pregnant patients may present with epigastric pain, back pain, anorexia, and jaundice. Nausea and vomiting are also common. Sonography is the imaging method of choice in pregnant patients because it is safe for the fetus and has a high sensitivity to gallstones (Sahu et al., 2013). Maternal and fetal outcomes associated with pancreatitis have improved greatly in recent years; today, the mortality rate is below 5% for both mother and child (Štimac & Štimac, 2012).

Pancreatitis in Older Adults

The incidence of pancreatitis increases with age, with a 200-fold increase occurring after age 65 (Spangler et al., 2014). Gallstones are the most common cause of acute pancreatitis in older adults; alcoholism is the most common cause of chronic pancreatitis (Kim et al., 2012). Medications and hormone replacement therapy may also give rise to acute pancreatitis in this population.

Older adults may present with abdominal pain that varies in intensity from mild to severe. Low-grade fever and tachycardia are common. Confusion, shock, hypotension, and tachypnea may also occur (Spangler et al., 2014). Normal age-related changes to the pancreas such as dilation of pancreatic ducts can complicate diagnosis, as can formation of pancreatic cysts and calculi. Treatment for older adults is similar to that for other populations, though aggressive use of IV fluids is more likely to lead to edema in older adults and may not have the desired effect on renal function (Tenner et al., 2013). Mortality rates among older patients with pancreatitis are significantly higher than in younger patients, at 17.0% and 5.9%, respectively. This difference is thought to be associated with an increased likelihood of organ failure in older patients with pancreatitis (Machado, Pinheiro da Silva, & Coelho, 2015).

NURSING PROCESS

Nursing care for the patient with pancreatitis focuses on promoting comfort, controlling nausea and vomiting, and administering IV fluids to maintain proper hydration. Patients should also receive teaching about lifestyle changes for preventing pancreatitis in the future.

Assessment

- *Observation and patient interview.* Observe the patient's abdomen for distention and auscultate bowel sounds, which are usually hypoactive. Note the presence of jaundice. Record the patient's description of any nausea, vomiting, and flatus, as well as information about the patient's last bowel movement. For patients reporting pain, assess the location, nature, duration, and precipitating factors. Inquire about alcohol consumption, dietary intake, and family history of pancreatitis. Assess for previous illnesses, surgery, and current medications (including over-the-counter and complementary health approaches).

- *Physical examination.* Assess vital signs, weight, and nutritional status. Palpate the abdomen, making note of tenderness or guarding in the upper abdomen. Auscultate lung sounds for shallow, rapid respirations indicative of inflammation of the diaphragm, pleural effusions, or respiratory compromise. Assess the skin of the abdomen for the Grey Turner sign and the Cullen sign, which are indicative of bleeding. Be alert for signs of dehydration.

Diagnosis

The following nursing diagnoses may be appropriate for patients with pancreatitis:

- *Pain, Acute*
- *Fluid Volume, Deficient*
- *Nausea*
- *Imbalanced Nutrition: Less Than Body Requirements.*

(NANDA-I © 2014)

Planning

Planning for patients with pancreatitis will depend on whether the inflammation is chronic or acute and on the severity of symptoms. Potential nursing outcomes may include the following:

- The patient will exhibit decreased pain associated with pancreatitis.
- The patient will improve nutritional status.
- The patient will maintain adequate hydration.
- The patient will verbalize understanding of recommended dietary and lifestyle modifications.
- The patient will seek support for lifestyle modifications after discharge.

Implementation

For the patient with pancreatitis, nursing interventions to manage pain, restore nutritional status, and restore and maintain fluid and electrolyte balance will help reduce the patient's risk for a life-threatening event and increase the patient's chances for success in meeting and maintaining a healthy lifestyle and therapeutic regimen following discharge.

Promote Comfort

Managing pain will include obtaining pain levels using an appropriate pain scale and administering opioid analgesics as ordered. When administering medication, the nurse should do the following:

- Administer analgesics on schedule rather than waiting for pain to increase. This will result in better pain management for the patient.
- Offer frequent oral hygiene for patients who are NPO.
- Maintain nasogastric tube patency as ordered.

Restore Nutritional Status

The nurse administers antiemetics as ordered, weighs the patient daily, and monitors patient intake and output. In addition, the nurse should do the following:

- Provide ongoing assessment of bowel sounds.
- Note the frequency color, odor, and consistency of stools in a stool chart.
- Monitor lab values.
- Administer IV fluids or parenteral nutrition until oral intake resumes.
- Offer small, frequent meals once the patient can resume eating.

See the Patient Teaching feature for more information.

Meet Fluid and Electrolyte Needs

The patient with acute pancreatitis is at risk for a fluid shift from the intravascular space into the abdominal cavity (third spacing), which may cause hypovolemic shock, affecting cardiovascular function, respiratory function, renal function, and mental status.

- For these patients, the nurse assesses cardiovascular status every 4 hours or as indicated, including vital signs, cardiac rhythm, central venous and pulmonary artery

Patient Teaching

Pancreatitis

Before discharge, the nurse provides information about the disease and how to prevent further episodes of inflammation to the patient and family. The following topics should be covered:

- Alcohol can cause stones to form, blocking pancreatic ducts and the outflow of pancreatic juice. The patient should avoid alcohol entirely.
- Smoking and stress stimulate the pancreas, and the patient should avoid them.
- If pancreatic function has been severely impaired, the nurse should discuss appropriate use of pancreatic enzymes, including timing, dose, and potential side effects.
- A low-fat diet is recommended. The nurse should provide a list of high-fat foods to avoid. Crash dieting and binge eating also should be avoided. Spicy foods, coffee, tea, colas, and gas-forming foods stimulate gastric and pancreatic secretions and may precipitate pain.
- The patient should report symptoms of infection (fever of 38.8°C [102°F] or higher, pain, rapid pulse, malaise) because a pancreatic abscess can develop after initial recovery.
- Refer patients as needed to nutritionists, alcohol treatment programs, and home health agencies.

pressures, peripheral pulses and capillary refill, and temperature, color, moisture, and turgor of the skin.

- Patients who are at risk for fluid and electrolyte imbalance require ongoing monitoring of renal function. The nurse assesses urine output hourly, reporting if it is less than 30 mL/hr.

- In addition, the nurse should monitor neurologic function, mental state, level of consciousness, and behavior. This monitoring is essential because hypotension and hypoxia can decrease cerebral perfusion.

SAFETY ALERT Regularly assess respiratory status (at least every 4–8 hours), including respiratory rate, depth, and pattern; breath sounds; and oxygen saturation and arterial blood gas results. Report tachypnea, adventitious or absent breath sounds, oxygen saturation levels below 92%, PaO_2 less than 70 mmHg, or $PaCO_2$ greater than 45 mmHg. Severe abdominal pain causes shallow respirations and hypoventilation and suppresses cough effectiveness, which can lead to pooling of secretions, atelectasis, and pneumonia.

Evaluation

Outcome and evaluation parameters will include the following:

- The patient experiences reduction or elimination of pain.
- The patient is able to resume eating.
- The patient remains free from alterations in fluid and nutrition status.
- The patient is free from nausea.

If patient outcomes are not met with supportive care, the patient should be assessed for the presence of pseudocysts. If pseudocysts are present, surgery may be indicated. The type of surgery depends upon the location of the cyst. If cysts are not present, the patient should be assessed for pancreatic ascites and pancreatic necrosis.

≫ Go to **Pearson MyLab Nursing and eText** to see Chart 3: Nursing Care Plan: A Patient with Acute Pancreatitis.

REVIEW Pancreatitis

RELATE Link the Concepts and Exemplars

Linking the exemplar of pancreatitis with the concept of metabolism:

1. How does pancreatitis influence the normal process of metabolism?
2. What interventions by the patient can reduce the long-term effects of pancreatitis?

Linking the exemplar of pancreatitis with the concept of comfort:

3. How can the nurse utilize appropriate pain assessment instruments when caring for a patient with pancreatitis?
4. How can the nurse incorporate complementary health approaches in the care of a patient with pancreatitis?

READY Go to Volume 3: Clinical Nursing Skills

REFER Go to Pearson MyLab Nursing and eText

- Additional review materials
- Chart 3: Nursing Care Plan: A Patient with Acute Pancreatitis

REFLECT Apply Your Knowledge

Charles Johnson is a 28-year-old man. Mr. Johnson has been experiencing abdominal pain, but he has not seen his healthcare provider about it. On Saturday night, Mr. Johnson attended a party, staying until almost 2:00 a.m. As Mr. Johnson was driving home, he lost control of his car, and the vehicle rolled four times. Mr. Johnson, who was not wearing his seat belt, was ejected from the car. On arrival at the emergency department, Mr. Johnson was observed to be highly intoxicated. Mr. Johnson admitted to the physician that he has been drinking frequently and had acute pancreatitis in the past.

1. What additional assessment data would the nurse want to obtain from Mr. Johnson?
2. Mr. Johnson asks the nurse to explain the difference between acute and chronic pancreatitis. When and how would you provide education to Mr. Johnson about his diagnosis?
3. What priority interventions would you implement at this time?

≫ # Exemplar 4.E
Pyloric Stenosis

Exemplar Learning Outcomes

4.E Analyze pyloric stenosis as it relates to digestion.

- Describe the pathophysiology of pyloric stenosis.
- Describe the etiology of pyloric stenosis.
- Compare the risk factors and prevention of pyloric stenosis.
- Identify the clinical manifestations of pyloric stenosis.
- Summarize diagnostic tests and therapies used by interprofessional teams in the collaborative care of an individual with pyloric stenosis.

- Differentiate care of patients with pyloric stenosis across the lifespan.
- Apply the nursing process in providing culturally competent care to an individual with pyloric stenosis.

Exemplar Key Terms

Projectile vomiting, 268
Pyloric stenosis, 268

Overview

Pyloric stenosis, narrowing of the pyloric orifice, directly affects the structure and function of the digestive tract, preventing food within the stomach from passing through the pylorus into the duodenum. This impairs digestion and absorption of food, resulting in dehydration and malnutrition. Pyloric stenosis generally affects infants within the first month of life, causing regurgitation and poor feeding. Pyloric stenosis is rare in adults.

Pathophysiology and Etiology

Pathophysiology

The pylorus is the narrow, cone-shaped transition point from the stomach to the small intestine. Its primary functions are controlling the amount and size of food particles entering the intestine and preventing intestinal contents from reentering the stomach. The pylorus consists of circular muscle tissue with a mucous-membrane lining. In pyloric stenosis, the muscles of the pylorus become enlarged, narrowing the pyloric opening. Gastric contents of the stomach cannot empty into the small intestines through the narrowed pylorus and must exit the stomach as vomit.

Etiology and Risk Factors

For unknown reasons, the pyloric orifice may thicken from inflammation and edema, causing a partial or full obstruction between the stomach and duodenum (see **Figure 4–18 》**). As the pyloric orifice becomes narrower, vomiting becomes more forceful. As the obstruction progresses, the individual becomes dehydrated and electrolytes are depleted, resulting in metabolic imbalances.

Genetics may play a role in pyloric stenosis. Children with parents who had pyloric stenosis are more likely to have the condition. Pyloric stenosis is more common in male patients than in female patients. Antibiotics given in late pregnancy or in the first few weeks of life may be associated with an increased risk of pyloric stenosis (Mayo Clinic, 2015b).

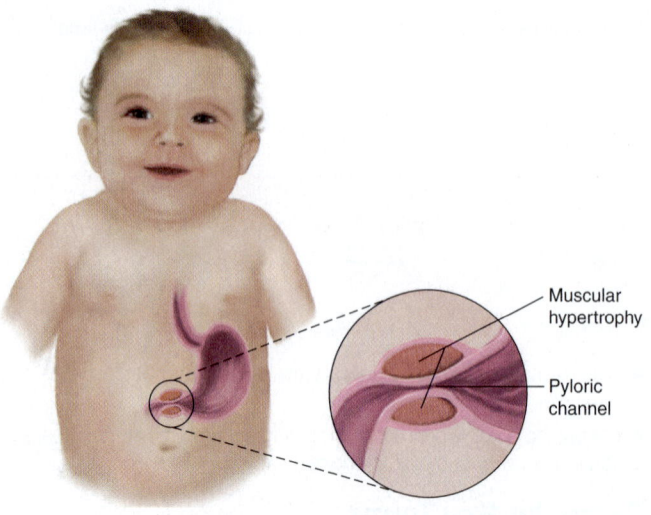

Muscular hypertrophy

Pyloric channel

Figure 4–18 》 In pyloric stenosis, the hypertrophied pyloric muscle causes symptoms of projectile vomiting and visible peristalsis.

Clinical Manifestations

Symptoms usually become evident 3–6 weeks after birth. Babies with pyloric stenosis feed normally and then vomit within 30 minutes. As the pyloric stenosis worsens, the vomiting becomes projectile. With **projectile vomiting**, the emesis may be spewed up to 2–3 feet out of the baby's mouth. At times the vomit may contain small amounts of blood. After vomiting, the baby is hungry and may want to feed again. Persistent hunger is a common symptom of pyloric stenosis. Parents may notice a wavelike ripple across the baby's abdomen after feeding and immediately before the child vomits. This peristaltic wave is the body's attempt to push the food through the pylorus. Frequent vomiting can easily lead to dehydration and malnutrition. Changes in the stool are common as the baby becomes constipated, and the baby is unable to gain weight or may even lose weight. Parents should contact the primary healthcare provider if the baby exhibits frequent vomiting, projectile vomiting, irritability due to dehydration, or failure to gain weight.

Collaboration

Diagnostic Tests

An abdominal ultrasound to determine the diameter and length of the pyloric muscle is usually performed to confirm the diagnosis. An upper gastrointestinal (UGI) study may also be performed. If the infant has pyloric stenosis, the UGI study will reveal a narrowing of the pyloric channel that prevents the passage of the contrast medium. Blood tests determine the degree of dehydration, electrolyte imbalance, and anemia. Early diagnosis decreases the severity of electrolyte alterations.

Surgery

Surgery is performed as soon as possible after the infant's fluid and electrolyte balance is restored. Open pyloromyotomy is performed though a periumbilical incision or through a small, transverse upper abdominal incision. Recovery time from a laparoscopic pyloromyotomy is faster than recovery from an open pyloromyotomy (Mayo Clinic, 2015c). With both procedures, the pyloric muscle is split to allow the passage of food and fluid.

The prognosis is good. The infant usually takes fluids within a few hours following surgery and is discharged on full-strength formula within 24 hours after surgery.

Lifespan Considerations

Pyloric stenosis is typically seen in infants and rarely occurs in adults. When it does occur in adults, pyloric stenosis may be classified as primary or secondary. The primary type can occur without an apparent cause. The secondary type is the result of other problems in the GI tract such as ulcer, hernia, a malignancy, or gastritis. There is typically little or no enlargement of the pyloric muscle in secondary pyloric stenosis. Adult pyloric stenosis occurs most commonly in middle-age men. Individuals who had pyloric stenosis as infants are believed to have an increased risk of developing it as adults (Lin, Lin, & Kuo, 2015).

Symptoms of adult pyloric stenosis include weight loss, easy satiety, loss of appetite, and gradual increase of upper abdominal pain. Nausea and vomiting are also common. Individuals with the secondary type often have a long history of peptic ulcers or other digestive disorders (Gurvits, Tan, & Volkov, 2013). Diagnosis of adult pyloric stenosis typically includes barium x-rays that reveal an elongated, thickened pylorus and increased gastric emptying time. Blood and urine analyses are also used to determine electrolyte balance and the extent of dehydration. Endoscopy may also be performed (Lin et al., 2015). As in infants, pyloric stenosis in adults is treated surgically.

NURSING PROCESS

Nursing care for the patient with pyloric stenosis focuses on correcting electrolyte and acid–base imbalances and replacing lost fluids, often in preparation for surgery. Care should also focus on minimizing parent anxiety related to the condition or the treatment. This is especially important if surgery is scheduled for the same day that the condition was diagnosed, which is common (Mayo Clinic, 2015c).

Assessment

- *Observation and patient interview.* Observe the infant's abdomen for the presence of peristaltic waves and auscultate bowel sounds, which are usually hyperactive on auscultation. Palpation reveals an olive-shaped mass in the right upper quadrant of the abdomen. Record the parents' description of the infant's history of vomiting. Assess the parents' level of anxiety related to the child's condition. The child is usually hungry and tries to feed. The parents frequently observe crying and general discomfort.

- *Physical examination.* Assess vital signs, weight, and nutritional status. Assess skin turgor, fontanel, mucous membranes, urinary output (weigh diapers), and urine specific gravity to determine whether hydration is adequate. Note vomiting episodes and estimated emesis amount. Be alert for signs of an electrolyte imbalance, particularly low levels of serum chloride, sodium, and potassium and an elevated pH. (See the module on Fluids and Electrolytes for a discussion of these electrolyte imbalances.)

Diagnosis

The following are some of the nursing diagnoses that might be appropriate for the child with pyloric stenosis:

- *Fluid Volume, Deficient*
- *Imbalanced Nutrition: Less Than Body Requirements*
- *Sleep Pattern, Disturbed*
- *Parental Anxiety.*

  (NANDA-I © 2014)

Planning

Planning for the infant patient with pyloric stenosis will focus on the parents. Outcomes may include the following:

- The patient's parents will receive sufficient explanation of treatment options.

- The patient's parents will provide input into the plan of care.
- The patient's parents will take part in pre- and postoperative infant care.

Implementation

Nursing care focuses on meeting the infant's fluid and electrolyte needs, minimizing weight loss, promoting rest and comfort, preventing infection, and providing supportive care for parents.

Meet Fluid and Electrolyte Needs

Because projectile vomiting will continue until the obstruction is relieved surgically, oral feedings should be withheld. In addition, the nurse should do the following:

- Emphasize to the infant's parents the importance of maintaining an NPO status preoperatively.
- Administer IV therapy to correct fluid and electrolyte imbalances and to maintain adequate hydration.
- Maintain patency of the nasogastric tube and measure aspirated contents.
- Inform the infant's parents that all diapers will be weighed to measure the infant's output of urine and stool.

Minimize Weight Loss

The infant loses weight because of frequent vomiting. When caring for the infant, the nurse should do the following:

- Monitor weight daily both preoperatively and postoperatively.
- Begin feedings postoperatively according to healthcare provider orders.

Some surgeons prefer an NPO period following pyloromyotomy, with slow, incremental increases in volume and strength of feedings once feeding has resumed. Others will implement an earlier postoperative feeding approach.

Promote Rest and Comfort

The infant will have discomfort before and after surgery.

- During the preoperative period the infant is hungry and cries often. To reduce discomfort, the nurse should swaddle the infant to maintain warmth and provide comfort, encourage the parents to hold and cuddle the infant, and provide a pacifier to meet the infant's need to suck.
- During the postoperative period, the nurse should administer analgesics as prescribed to relieve discomfort associated with the surgical incision; instruct the parents to avoid pressure on the incision; and when diapering the infant, slide the diaper gently under the buttocks rather than lifting the legs.

Prevent Infection

Postoperatively the incision is covered with collodion or Steri-Strips. These strips should be kept clean and dry. In addition, the nurse should do the following:

- Inspect the incision site for redness, swelling, or discharge
- Monitor the infant's temperature every 4 hours
- Auscultate the lungs to assess for any adventitious sounds.

Provide Supportive Care and Home Care Teaching

The need for hospitalization, surgery, and home care creates anxiety for parents. To ease parental anxiety, the nurse should do the following:

- Encourage the parents to participate in the infant's care and to discuss their fears and concerns.
- Provide simple and clear explanations about the infant's condition and care.
- Advise the parents that occasional vomiting may occur after surgery and that this is normal.
- Provide instructions about feeding to ensure the infant gets sufficient intake.

See the Patient Teaching feature for more information.

Evaluation

Expected outcomes of care include the following:

- The patient will exhibit adequate pain control
- The patient will be able to take in the recommended amount of fluid and food with absence of vomiting
- The patient will exhibit normal growth patterns.

If patient outcomes are not met, assess the infant for incomplete myotomy, as this is a common cause of persistent symptoms after surgery. In addition, assess the patient for GERD, as it can present with similar symptoms in infants. If normal growth patterns do not manifest after surgery and cessation of vomiting, assess the patient for malabsorption disorders.

>> **Stay Current:** Surgery on an infant is very upsetting to the parents. The nurse must provide reliable, easy-to-understand resources that the parents can review before their child's procedures. The American Pediatric Surgical Association's Parent and Family Resource Center offers information about pyloric stenosis and pylorotomy at http://www.pediatricsurgerymd.org/AM/Template.cfm?Section=Conditions&template=/CM/ContentDisplay.cfm&ContentID=4310.

Patient Teaching

Home Care Instructions Following Pyloromyotomy

After a pyloromyotomy, the infant is generally discharged home the day following surgery. The nurse should partner with the family to provide home feeding and care instructions:

- The infant may be bottle-fed or breastfed.
- The infant may vomit after some feedings following surgery. This does not mean that the surgical correction was unsuccessful.
- If the infant vomits, the parents should offer a bottle or breast as soon as the infant is interested in feeding again.
- The parents should burp the infant after every 1–2 ounces during feeding, or every 5–10 minutes if breastfeeding.
- After feeding, the parents should hold the infant in an upright position for 30 minutes.
- The infant should not play or be rocked for 30 minutes following feedings.
- The parents should administer analgesics as prescribed. They should inform the healthcare provider if they believe the infant is not obtaining adequate pain relief.
- The surgical wound area must be kept clean and dry. The bandage or strips may fall off; this is normal. If they do not fall off, they will be removed at the follow-up visit.
- The infant should be sponge bathed only. Tub baths are not allowed until the wound has healed or as instructed by the healthcare provider.
- The parents should notify the healthcare provider if the infant is inconsolable or demonstrates redness, drainage, bleeding, or swelling at the surgical site; has a fever of 38.1°C (100.6°F) or higher; or vomits the majority of two feedings in a row.

Nursing Care Plan

A Patient with Pyloric Stenosis

Adam Zorkowski is a 2-month-old boy. He presents to the primary healthcare provider with irritability, projectile vomiting, and constipation.

ASSESSMENT	DIAGNOSES	PLANNING
Adam has had recurrent episodes of projectile vomiting. His parents state, "He only vomits once in a while, it comes flying out, and then he wants to eat again." In reviewing the patient record, the nurse notes Adam weighs the same as he did at 6 weeks of age. The nurse asks his parents about elimination patterns. They both agree that Adam has required less frequent diaper changes and seems to be constipated. On abdominal auscultation, Adam has hyperactive bowel sounds, and on palpation, an olive-shaped mass in the right upper quadrant of the abdomen is noted. The diagnosis is pyloric stenosis. A laparoscopic pyloromyotomy is performed.	■ *Acute Pain* related to surgical procedure ■ *Imbalanced Nutrition: Less Than Body Requirements* related to recurrent episodes of vomiting ■ *Risk for Aspiration* due to vomiting. (NANDA-I © 2014)	Together the nurse and Adam's parents develop the following goals for Adam's plan of care: ■ The patient will have no outward symptoms of pain. ■ The patient will gain 2.2 lb (1 kg) per month. ■ The patient will not exhibit signs of aspiration.

Nursing Care Plan *(continued)*

IMPLEMENTATION

- Administer pain medications when Adam begins to demonstrate outward signs of pain.
- Following surgery, slowly increase the amount of feeding as Adam tolerates. Report any vomiting episodes.
- Encourage the parents to position Adam upright when feeding, keep Adam upright after feeding or lay him on his right side with the head of bed elevated, and avoid overfeeding.

EVALUATION

After recovery from the laparoscopic pyloromyotomy, Adam is discharged home. He had minimal signs of pain during hospitalization, and these were treated effectively with acetaminophen. Before discharge, Adam was able to tolerate full-strength breast milk without vomiting. His parents successfully demonstrated strategies to prevent aspiration when feeding Adam. The nurses taught the parents how to minimize pain when changing diapers and clothing Adam, as well as how to care for the laparoscopic insertion sites. The parents verbalized understanding and demonstrated a diaper change preventing pressure on the laparoscopic sites.

CRITICAL THINKING

1. What assessment data would you monitor to ensure Adam's nutritional status is adequate for his growth and development?
2. Besides weight gain, what concerns do you have in relation to episodes of vomiting and Adam's growth and development?
3. What strategies promote comfort and minimize acute pain for an infant?
4. What role does the nurse play in preoperative, perioperative, and postoperative care of an infant versus an adult?

REVIEW Pyloric Stenosis

RELATE Link the Concepts and Exemplars

Linking the exemplar of pyloric stenosis with the concept of acid–base balance:

1. What type of acid–base imbalance can occur with pyloric stenosis?
2. What caring interventions might be implemented in a patient with pyloric stenosis to prevent an acid–base imbalance?

Linking the exemplar of pyloric stenosis with the concept of development:

3. How would pyloric stenosis affect an infant's development?
4. How could pyloric stenosis affect the infant's cognitive growth?

READY Go to Volume 3: Clinical Nursing Skills

REFER Go to Pearson MyLab Nursing and eText

- Additional review materials

REFLECT Apply Your Knowledge

Kanye Long is a 3-week-old boy with a history of vomiting for 3 days. Kanye vomits only after being fed. The vomitus resembles partially digested formula without blood or bile. He feeds well but vomits 1–2 hours after the feeding. The emesis is forceful. His mother describes it as being able to project about 30 cm rather than just dribbling down his mouth. He has already vomited five times today. Kanye has also had two loose stools (no mucus, no blood, not foul). There is no history of irritability, fever, or ill contacts. His birth history is unremarkable.

1. What manifestations does Kanye exhibit to support a diagnosis of pyloric stenosis?
2. How do pyloric stenosis and GERD differ?
3. What are the priority interventions for a patient who has had surgery to correct the stenosis?
4. What priority nursing diagnoses would you choose for the preoperative and postoperative period?

References

Abbas, Z. (2015). Gastrointestinal health in Ramadan with special reference to diabetes. *Journal of the Pakistan Medical Association, 65*(5). Retrieved from http://jpma.org.pk/supplement_details.php?article_id=195

Achem, S., & DeVault, K. (2014). Gastroesophageal reflux disease and the elderly. *Gastroenterology Clinics, 43*(1), 147–160. doi:10.1016/j.gtc.2013.11.004

Adams, M. P., Holland, L. N., & Urban, C. (2017). *Pharmacology for nurses: A pathophysiologic approach* (5th ed.). Hoboken, NJ: Pearson Education.

Ali, N. (2012). *Failure to thrive in elderly adults.* Retrieved from http://emedicine.medscape.com/article/2096163-overview#a3

American Academy of Pediatrics. (2015a). *How often and how much should your baby eat?* Retrieved from https://www.healthychildren.org/English/ages-stages/baby/feeding-nutrition/Pages/How-Often-and-How-Much-Should-Your-Baby-Eat.aspx

American Academy of Pediatrics. (2015b). *Teenager's nutritional needs.* Retrieved from https://www.healthychildren.org/English/ages-stages/teen/nutrition/Pages/A-Teenagers-Nutritional-Needs.aspx

American Cancer Society. (2016). *Pancreatic cancer risk factors.* Retrieved from https://www.cancer.org/cancer/pancreatic-cancer/causes-risks-prevention/risk-factors.html

American College of Gastroenterology. (n.d.). *Understanding your GI tract.* Retrieved from http://patients.gi.org/topics/understanding-your-gi-tract/

American College of Gastroenterology. (2012). *Lactose intolerance in children.* Retrieved from http://patients.gi.org/topics/lactose-intolerance-in-children/

American College of Gastroenterology. (2013). *Functional gastrointestinal disorders in pediatric and* adolescent patients. Retrieved from http://patients.gi.org/topics/functional-gastrointestinal-disorders-in-pediatric-and-adolescent-patients/

American Pancreatic Association. (2014). *Pancreapedia: Anatomy and histology of the pancreas.* Retrieved from http://www.pancreapedia.org/reviews/anatomy-and-histology-of-pancreas

American Pregnancy Association. (2015). *Pregnancy and heartburn.* Retrieved from http://americanpregnancy.org/pregnancy-health/heartburn-during-pregnancy/

American Society of Clinical Oncologists. (2016). Nausea and vomiting. *Cancer.net.* Retrieved from http://www.cancer.net/navigating-cancer-care/side-effects/nausea-and-vomiting

Anderson, P. (2016). *Proton pump inhibitors linked to dementia.* Retrieved from http://www.medscape.com/viewarticle/858909

Bacigalupe, G., & Plocha, A. (2015). Celiac is a social disease: Family challenges and strategies. *Families, Systems & Health: The Journal of Collaborative Family Healthcare, 33*(1), 46–54. doi:10.1037/fsh0000099

Ball, J. W., Bindler, R. C., Cowen, K., & Shaw, M. (2017). *Principles of pediatric nursing: Caring for children* (7th ed.). Hoboken, NJ: Pearson Education.

Barbarito, C., & D'Amico, D. (2012). *Health and physical assessment in nursing* (2nd ed.). Upper Saddle River, NJ: Pearson Education.

Berman, A., Snyder, S. J., & Frandsen, G. (2016). *Kozier and Erb's fundamentals of nursing: Concepts, process, and practice* (10th ed.). Hoboken, NJ: Pearson Education.

Buggs, A. (2014). *Viral hepatitis clinical presentation.* Retrieved from http://emedicine.medscape.com/article/775507-clinical#b2

California Department of Public Health. (2013). *California nutrition and physical activity guidelines for adolescents.* Retrieved from http://www.cdph.ca.gov/programs/NutritionandPhysicalActivity/Documents/MO-NUPA-AdolescentNutrition-Handouts.pdf

Carrion, A., & Martin, P. (2012). Viral hepatitis in the elderly. *American Journal of Gastroenterology, 107,* 691–697. doi:10.1038/ajg.2012.7

Cea Soriano, L., Ruigómez, A., Johansson, S., & Garcia Rodríguez, L. (2014). Study of the association between hip fracture and acid-suppressive drug use in a UK primary care setting. *Pharmacotherapy, 34*(6), 570–581. doi:10.1002/phar.1410

Celiac Disease Foundation. (2015). *Celiac disease symptoms.* Retrieved from https://celiac.org/celiac-disease/symptomssigns/

Centers for Disease Control and Prevention (CDC). (2013). *Surveillance for viral hepatitis—United States, 2011.* Retrieved from http://www.cdc.gov/hepatitis/statistics/2011surveillance/commentary.htm

Centers for Disease Control and Prevention (CDC). (2014). *Screening for hepatitis during the domestic medical examination.* Retrieved from http://www.cdc.gov/immigrantrefugeehealth/guidelines/domestic/hepatitis-screening-guidelines.html

Centers for Disease Control and Prevention (CDC). (2015a). *The ABCs of hepatitis.* Retrieved from http://www.cdc.gov/hepatitis/Resources/Professionals/PDFs/ABCTable.pdf

Centers for Disease Control and Prevention (CDC). (2015b). *Hepatitis A questions and answers for the public.* Retrieved from http://www.cdc.gov/hepatitis/hav/afaq.htm

Centers for Disease Control and Prevention (CDC). (2015c). Action plan for the prevention, care and treatment of viral hepatitis. Retrieved from http://www.cdc.gov/hepatitis/hhs-actionplan.htm

Cleveland Clinic. (2014a). *Disease & conditions: Long-term complications of GERD.* Retrieved from https://my.clevelandclinic.org/health/diseases_conditions/hic_gastroesophageal_reflux_disease_GERD/hic_Long-Term_Complications_of_GERD

Cleveland Clinic. (2014b). *Disease & conditions: Pancreatic cysts and pseudocysts.* Retrieved from https://my.clevelandclinic.org/health/diseases_conditions/hic_Pancreatitis/hic-pancreatic-cysts-and-pseudocysts

Cleveland Clinic. (2015). *Short bowel syndrome in children.* Retrieved from https://my.clevelandclinic.org/childrens-hospital/health-info/diseases-conditions/hic-short-bowel-syndrome-in-children

Contag, S., & Arrabal, P. (2014). *Hepatitis in pregnancy.* Retrieved from http://emedicine.medscape.com/article/1562368-overview#a2

Crohn & Colitis Foundation of America. (2013). *Short bowel syndrome and Crohn disease.* Retrieved from http://www.ccfa.org/assets/short-bowel-syndrome-and.pdf

Enomoto, H., & Nishiguchi, S. (2015). Factors associated with the response to interferon-based antiviral therapies for chronic hepatitis C. *World Journal of Hepatology, 7*(26), 2681–2687. doi:10.4254/wjh.v7.i26.2681

Gardner, T. (2014). *Acute pancreatitis in pregnancy.* Retrieved from https://www.pancreasfoundation.org/patient-information/acute-pancreatitis/pancreatits-and-pregnancy/

Gastroenterological Society of Australia (GESA). (2017). *Maintaining a healthy digestive systems.* Retrieved from http://www.gesa.org.au/index.cfm/resources/patients/maintaining-a-healthy-digestive-system/

Gerson, L. (2012). Treatment of gastroesophageal reflux disease during pregnancy. *Gastroenterology & Hepatology, 8*(11), 763–764. Retrieved from http://www.ncbi.nlm.nih.gov/pmc/articles/PMC3966174/

Grabosh, S., Pennycook, J., Pakravan, A., & Mostello, D. (2013). Short bowel syndrome causing bleeding diathesis and profound vitamin deficiency in pregnancy. *Obstetrics & Gynecology, 121,* 434–436. doi:10.1097/ACOG.0b013e31827e5ab3

Gujral, N., Freeman, H., & Thomson, A. (2012). Celiac disease: Prevalence, diagnosis, pathogenesis, and treatment. *World Journal of Gastroenterology, 18*(42), 6036–6059. doi:10.3748/wjg.v18.i42.6036

Gurvits, G., Tan, A., & Volkov, D. (2013). Video capsule endoscopy and CT enterography in diagnosing adult hypertrophic pyloric stenosis. *World Journal of Gastroenterology, 19*(37), 6292–6295. doi:10.3748/wjg.v19.i37.6292

Harms, R.W. (2015). *Healthy lifestyle: Pregnancy week by week.* Retrieved from http://www.mayoclinic.org/healthy-lifestyle/pregnancy-week-by-week/expert-answers/pregnancy-and-lactose-intolerance/faq-20119824

Hebra, A., Adams, S., & Vargas, J. (2014). *Pediatric pancreatitis.* Retrieved from http://emedicine.medscape.com/article/2014039-overview#a7

Hepatitis B Foundation. (2014a). *ABC's of viral hepatitis.* Retrieved from http://www.hepb.org/hepb/abc.htm

Hepatitis B Foundation. (2014b). *Recovery.* Retrieved from http://www.hepb.org/patients/recovery.htm

Herdman, T. H. & Kamitsuru, S. (Eds.). *Nursing Diagnoses—Definitions and Classification 2015–2017.* Copyright © 2014, 1994–2014 NANDA International. Used by arrangement with John Wiley &

Sons, Inc. Companion website: www.wiley.com/go/nursingdiagnoses

Hoffman, M. R., Alzaben, A. S., Enns, S. E., Marcon, M. A., Turner, J., & Mager, D. R. (2016). Parental health beliefs, socio-demographics, and healthcare recommendations influence micronutrient supplementation in youth with celiac disease. *Canadian Journal of Dietetic Practice and Research, 77*(1), 47–23. doi:10.3148/cjdpr-2015-035

Institute of Medicine. (2009). *Weight gain during pregnancy: reexamining the guidelines.* Washington, DC: National Academies Press.

International Foundation for Functional Gastrointestinal Disorders (IFFGD). (2015). *GI disorders.* Retrieved from http://www.iffgd.org/site/gi-disorders/

James, S., Nelson, K., & Ashwill, J. (2014). *Nursing care of children: principles and practice* (4th ed.). St. Louis, MO: Elsevier Saunders.

Johns Hopkins Children's Center. (n.d.). *Gastroesophageal reflux disease.* Retrieved from http://www.hopkinschildrens.org/tpl_rlinks_nav1up.aspx?id=5066

Juckett, G. (2013). Caring for Latino patients. *American Family Physician, 87*(1):48–54. Retrieved from http://www.aafp.org/afp/2013/0101/p48.html

Juneja, S. K., Gupta, Sh. Virk, S. S., Tandon, P., & Bindal, V. (2013). Acute pancreatitis in pregnancy: A treatment paradigm based on our hospital experience. *International Journal of Applied Basic Medical Research, 3*(2), 122–125. doi:10.4103/2229-516X.117090

Kelly, J. C. (2016). *Proton pump inhibitors may increase risk for kidney disease.* Retrieved from http://www.medscape.com/viewarticle/857060#vp_1

Khalili, H., Huang, E. S., Jacobson, B. C., Camargo, C. A., Feskanich, D., & Chan, A. T. (2012). Use of proton pump inhibitors and risk of hip fracture in relation to dietary and lifestyle factors: A prospective cohort study. *BMJ.* doi:10.1136/bjm.e372

Khurana, B., Lomash, A., Khalil, S., Bhattacharya, M., Rajeshwar, K., & Kapoor, S. (2015). Evaluation of the impact of celiac disease and its dietary manipulation on children and their caregivers. *Indian Journal of Gastroenterology, 34*(2), 112–116. doi:10.007/s12664-015-0563-6

Kim, J. E., Hwang, J. H., Lee, S. H., Cha, B. H., Park, Y. S., Kim, J. W., . . . Lee, D. H. (2012). The clinical outcome of elderly patients with acute pancreatitis is not different in spite of the different etiologies and severity. *Archives of Gerontology and Geriatrics, 54*(1), 256–260. doi:10.1016/j.archger.2011.01.004

Lahner, E., Bellentani, S., De Bastiani, R., Tosetti, C., Cicala, M., Esposito, G., . . . Annibale, B. (2013). A survey of pharmacological and nonpharmacological treatment of functional gastrointestinal disorders. *United European Gastroenterology Journal, 1*(5), 385–393. doi:10.1177/2050640613499567

Lera dos Santos, M.E., Maluf-Filho, F., Chaves, D.M., Matuguma, S.E., Ide, E., de Oliveira Luz, G., . . . Sakai, P. (2013). Deep sedation during gastrointestinal endoscopy: Propofol-fentanyl and midazolam-fentanyl regimens. *World Journal of Gastroenterology, 19*(22), 3439–3446. doi:10.3748/wjg.v19.i22.3439

Lerner, A., & Matthias, T. (2015). Increased knowledge and awareness of celiac disease will benefit the elderly. *International Journal of Celiac Disease, 3*(3), 112–114. doi:10.12691/ijcd-3-3-6

Lightdale, J., & Gremse, D. (2013). Gastroesophageal reflux: Management guidance for the pediatrician. *Pediatrics, 131*(5). Retrieved from http://pediatrics.aappublications.org/content/131/5/e1684

Lilley, L. L., Collins, S. R., & Snyder, J. S. (2014). *Pharmacology and the nursing process* (7th ed.). St. Louis, MO: Elsevier.

Lin, H., Lin, Y., & Kuo, C. (2015). Adult idiopathic hypertrophic pyloric stenosis. *Journal of the Formosan Medical Association, 114*(7), 659–662. doi:http://dx.doi.org/10.1016/j.jfma.2012.07.001

Machado, M. C. C., Pinheiro da Silva, F., & Coelho, A. M. M. (2015). Do elderly patients with acute pancreatitis need a special treatment strategy? In L. Rodrigo (Ed.), *Acute and chronic pancreatitis.* doi:10.5772/58916. Retrieved from http://www.intechopen.com/books/howtoreference/acute-and-chronic-pancreatitis/do-elderly-patients-with-acute-pancreatitis-need-a-special-treatment-strategy-

Malfertheiner, S., Malfertheiner, M., Kropf, S., Costa, S. B., & Malfertheiner, P. (2012). A prospective longitudinal cohort study: Evolution of GERD symptoms during the course of pregnancy. *BMC Gastroenterology, 12*(131). doi:10.1186/1471-230X-12-131

Mayo Clinic. (2012). *Gut feelings: The effects of aging on your digestive system.* Minneapolis, MN: Author.

Mayo Clinic. (2014a). *Disease and conditions: Heartburn.* Retrieved from http://www.mayoclinic.org/diseases-conditions/heartburn/basics/definition/con-20019545

Mayo Clinic. (2014b). *Diseases and conditions: GERD.* Retrieved from http://www.mayoclinic.org/diseases-conditions/gerd/basics/lifestyle-home-remedies/con-20025201

Mayo Clinic. (2014c). *Do I need to include probiotics and prebiotics in my diet?* Retrieved from http://www.mayoclinic.org/healthy-lifestyle/consumer-health/expert-answers/probiotics/faq-20058065

Mayo Clinic. (2015a). *Histamine H2 antagonist (oral route, injection route, intravenous route).* Retrieved from http://www.mayoclinic.org/drugs-supplements/histamine-h2-antagonist-oral-route-injection-route-intravenous-route/description/drg-20068584

Mayo Clinic. (2015b). *Pyloric stenosis: Symptoms and causes.* Retrieved from http://www.mayoclinic.org/diseases-conditions/pyloric-stenosis/symptoms-causes/dxc-20163857

Mayo Clinic. (2015c). *Pyloric stenosis: Treatment.* http://www.mayoclinic.org/diseases-conditions/pyloric-stenosis/diagnosis-treatment/treatment/txc-20163881

Mayo Clinic. (2016a). *Gallstones.* Retrieved from http://www.mayoclinic.org/diseases-conditions/gallstones/home/ovc-20231394

Mayo Clinic. (2016b). *Lactose intolerance.* Retrieved from http://www.mayoclinic.org/diseases-conditions/lactose-intolerance/basics/definition/con-20027906

Mayo Clinic. (2016c). *Toxic hepatitis.* Retrieved from http://www.mayoclinic.org/diseases-conditions/toxic-hepatitis/home/ovc-20251578

Medicine.Net. (2013). *Viral hepatitis.* Retrieved from http://www.medicinenet.com/viral_hepatitis/page6.htm#what_is_the_treatment_for_viral_hepatitis

MedicineWise News. (2015). *Proton pump inhibitors—too much of a good thing?* Retrieved from http://www.nps.org.au/publications/health-professional/medicinewise-news/2015/proton-pump-inhibitors

Mohamed, A., Elbedwy, T., El-Serafy, M., El-Toukhy, N., Ahmed, W., & Ali El Din, Z. (2015). Hepatitis C virus: A global view. *World Journal of Hepatology, 7*(26), 2676–2680. doi:10.4254/wjh.v7.i26.2676

Moleski, S. M., Lindenmeyer, C. C., Veloski, J. J., Miller, R. S., Miller, C. L., Kastenberg, D., & DiMarino, A. (2012). Increased rates of pregnancy complications in women with celiac disease. *Annals of Gastroenterology, 28*(2), 236–240. Retrieved from http://www.ncbi.nlm.nih.gov/pmc/articles/PMC4367213/

Mount Sinai Hospital. (2015). *Chronic pancreatitis.* Retrieved from http://www.mountsinai.org/patient-care/health-library/diseases-and-conditions/chronic-pancreatitis

National Center for Complementary and Integrative Health (NCCIH). (2015). *6 tips: IBS and complementary health practices.* Retrieved from https://nccih.nih.gov/health/tips/IBS

National Center for Complementary and Integrative Health (NCCIH). (2016a). *Ginger.* Retrieved from https://nccih.nih.gov/health/ginger

National Center for Complementary and Integrative Health (NCCIH). (2016b). *Relaxation techniques for health.* Retrieved from https://nccih.nih.gov/health/stress/relaxation.htm#hed3

National Center for Complementary and Integrative Health. (2016c). *Bitter orange.* Retrieved from https://nccih.nih.gov/bitterorange

National Digestive Diseases Information Clearinghouse. (2012). *Celiac disease.* Retrieved from http://digestive.niddk.nih.gov/ddiseases/pubs/celiac

National Foundation for Celiac Awareness. (2017). *Celiac disease in the older adult.* Retrieved from http://www.celiaccentral.org/SiteData/docs/NFCACeliac/6f2ff901663872f1/NFCA_CeliacDiseaseintheOlderAdult.pdf

National Institutes of Health (NIH). (2012a). *Helping your child: Tips for parents.* Retrieved from http://www.niddk.nih.gov/health-information/health-topics/weight-control/helping-your-child-tips-parents/Pages/helping-your-child-tips-for-parents.aspx

National Institutes of Health (NIH). (2012b). *Morning sickness.* Retrieved from https://www.nlm.nih.gov/medlineplus/ency/article/003119.htm

National Institutes of Health (NIH). (2012c). *Take charge of your health: A guide for teenagers.* Retrieved from http://www.niddk.nih.gov/health-information/health-topics/weight-control/take-charge-your-health/Pages/take-charge-your-health.aspx

National Institutes of Health (NIH). (2013a). *Amylase—blood.* Retrieved from https://www.nlm.nih.gov/medlineplus/ency/article/003464.htm

National Institutes of Health (NIH). (2013b). *Chronic pancreatitis.* Retrieved from http://www.ncbi.nlm.nih.gov/pubmedhealth/PMH0001268

National Institutes of Health (NIH). (2013c). *Diverticular disease.* Retrieved from http://www.niddk.nih.gov/health-information/health-topics/digestive-diseases/diverticular-disease/Pages/facts.aspx

National Institutes of Health (NIH). (2013d). *GERD.* Retrieved from http://www.nlm.nih.gov/medlineplus/gerd.html

National Institutes of Health (NIH). (2013e). *Lipase test.* Retrieved from https://www.nlm.nih.gov/medlineplus/ency/article/003465.htm

National Institutes of Health (NIH). (2014a). *Digestive diseases statistics for the United States.* Retrieved from http://www.niddk.nih.gov/health-information/health-statistics/Pages/digestive-diseases-statistics-for-the-united-states.aspx

National Institutes of Health (NIH). (2014b). *Lactose intolerance.* Retrieved from http://www.niddk.nih.gov/health-information/health-topics/digestive-diseases/lactose-intolerance/Pages/facts.aspx

National Institutes of Health (NIH). (2014c). *Taking antacids.* Retrieved from https://www.nlm.nih.gov/medlineplus/ency/patientinstructions/000198.htm

National Institutes of Health (NIH). (2014d). *Vitamin D: Fact sheet for health professionals.* Retrieved from https://ods.od.nih.gov/factsheets/VitaminD-HealthProfessional/#h7

National Institutes of Health (NIH). (2015a). *Celiac disease.* Retrieved from http://www.niddk.nih.gov/health-information/health-topics/digestive-diseases/celiac-disease/Pages/facts.aspx

National Institutes of Health (NIH). (2015b). *Pancreatitis.* Retrieved from http://www.ncbi.nlm.nih.gov/pubmedhealth/PMH0078022/

National Institutes of Health (NIH). (2015c). *GERD.* Retrieved from http://www.nlm.nih.gov/medlineplus/gerd.html

National Institutes of Health (NIH). (2015d). *Short bowel syndrome.* Retrieved from http://www.niddk.nih.gov/health-information/health-topics/digestive-diseases/short-bowel-syndrome/Pages/facts.aspx

Office on Women's Health, U.S. Department of Health and Human Services. (2012). *Viral hepatitis fact sheet.* Retrieved http://www.womenshealth.gov/publications/our-publications/factsheet/viral-hepatitis.html#m

Osborn, K. S., Wraa, C. E., Watson, A. B., & Holleran, R. (2014). *Medical-surgical nursing: Preparation for practice* (2nd ed.). Upper Saddle River, NJ: Pearson Education. Reprinted and Electronically reproduced by permission of Pearson Education, Inc., New York, NY.

Oza, S., Akbari, M., Kelly, C., Hansen, J., Teethira, T., Tariq, S., . . . Leffler, D. (2015). Socioeconomic risk factors for celiac disease burden and symptoms. *Journal of Clinical Gastroenterology.* Retrieved from http://www.ncbi.nlm.nih.gov/pubmed/26084006

Sahu, S., Raghuvanshi, S., Bahl, D., & Sachan, P. (2013). Acute pancreatitis in pregnancy. *Internet Journal of Surgery, 11*(2). Retrieved from http://ispub.com/IJS/11/2/8706

Scarlata, K., & Anderson, M. (2014). Eating disorders and GI symptoms—Understand the link between them and how to treat patients. *Today's Dietician, 16*(10), 14. Retrieved from http://www.todays-dietitian.com/newarchives/100614p14.shtml

Scholl, S., Dellon, E., & Shaheen, N. (2011). Treatment of GERD and proton pump inhibitor use in the elderly: Practical approaches and frequently asked questions. *American Journal of Gastroenterology, 106*, 386–392. doi:10.1038/ajg.2010.409

Schwarz, S., & Hebra, A. (2015). *Pediatric gastroesophageal reflux treatment & management.* Retrieved from http://emedicine.medscape.com/article/930029-treatment

Spangler, R., Pham, T. V., Khouzah, D., & Martinez, J. P. (2014). Abdominal emergencies in the geriatric patient. *International Journal of Emergency Medicine, 7*(43). doi:10.1186/s12245-014-0043-2

Stanford Children's Health. (2015). *Hepatitis in children.* Retrieved from http://www.stanfordchildrens.org/en/topic/default?id=hepatitis-in-children-90-P02517

Štimac, T., & Štimac, D. (2012). Acute pancreatitis during pregnancy. In L. Rodrigo (Ed.), *Acute pancreatitis.* Retrieved from http://cdn.intechopen.com/pdfs-wm/26185.pdf

Suzuki, M., Sai, J. K., & Shimizu, T. (2014). Acute pancreatitis in children and adolescents. *World Journal of Gastroenterology, 5*(4): 416-426.

Tenner, S., Baillie, J., DeWitt, J., & Swaroop, S. (2013). *Management of acute pancreatitis.* Retrieved from http://gi.org/guideline/acute-pancreatitis/

University of Maryland Medical Center. (2012). *Hepatitis.* Retrieved from http://umm.edu/health/medical/reports/articles/hepatitis

University of Rochester Medical Center (URMC). (2015). *Hepatitis in children.* Retrieved from https://www.urmc.rochester.edu/encyclopedia/content.aspx?ContentTypeID=90&ContentID=P02517

U.S. Department of Health and Human Services. (2014). *Children and celiac disease: Going back to school*. Retrieved from http://www.celiac.nih.gov/BacktoSchool.aspx

U.S. Food and Drug Administration (FDA). (2015). *Problems digesting dairy products?* Retrieved from http://www.fda.gov/forconsumers/consumerupdates/ucm094550.htm

U.S. Preventive Services Task Force. (2013). Hepatitis C screening: Summary of recommendations. Retrieved from https://www.uspreventiveservicestaskforce.org/Page/Document/UpdateSummaryFinal/hepatitis-c-screening

Waheed, Y. (2015). Hepatitis C eradication: A long way to go. *World Journal of Gastroenterology, 21*(43), 12510–12512. doi:10.3748/wjg.v21.i43.12510

Wakim-Fleming, J. (2012). *Celiac disease and malabsorptive disorders*. Retrieved from http://www.clevelandclinicmeded.com/medicalpubs/diseasemanagement/gastroenterology/celiac-disease-malabsorptive-disorders/#top

Whyte, L., Kotecha, S., Watkins, W., & Jenkins, H. (2014). Coeliac disease is more common in children with high socio-economic status. *Acta Paediatrica, 103*(3), 289–294. doi:10.1111/apa.12494

Wilson, B. A., Shannon, M. T., & Shields, K. M. (2013). *Pearson nurse's drug guide 2013*. Upper Saddle River, NJ: Pearson/Prentice Hall.

World Health Organization. (2016a). *Hepatitis D*. Retrieved from http://www.who.int/mediacentre/factsheets/hepatitis-d/en

World Health Organization. (2016b). *Hepatitis E*. Retrieved from http://www.who.int/mediacentre/factsheets/fs280/en

Yadav, D., & Lowenfels, A. (2013). The epidemiology of pancreatitis and pancreatic cancer. *Gastroenterology, 144*(6), 1252–1261. doi:10.1053/j.gastro.2013.01.068

Yuen, E., Romney, M., Toner, R., Cobb, N., Katz, P., Spodic, M., & Goldfarb, N. (2010). Prevalence, knowledge and care patterns for gastro-oesophageal reflux disease in United States minority populations. *Alimentary Pharmacology and Therapeutics, 32*(5), 645–654. doi:10.1111/j.1365-2036.2010.04396.x

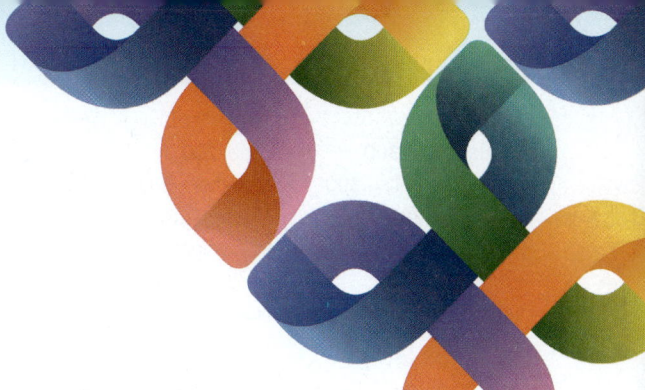

Module 5
Elimination

Module Outline and Learning Outcomes

The Concept of Elimination

Urinary Elimination

Normal Urinary Elimination
5.1 Analyze the physiology of urinary elimination in the body.

Alterations in Urination
5.2 Differentiate alterations in urinary elimination.

Nursing Assessment
5.3 Differentiate common assessment procedures and tests used to examine urinary elimination.

Independent Interventions
5.4 Analyze independent interventions nurses can implement for patients with alterations in urinary elimination.

Collaborative Therapies
5.5 Summarize collaborative therapies used by interprofessional teams for patients with alterations in urinary elimination.

Lifespan Considerations
5.6 Differentiate considerations related to the assessment and care of patients with alterations in urinary elimination throughout the lifespan.

Bowel Elimination

Normal Bowel Elimination
5.7 Analyze the physiology of bowel elimination in the body.

Alterations in Bowel Elimination
5.8 Differentiate alterations in bowel elimination.

Nursing Assessment
5.9 Differentiate common assessment procedures and tests used to examine bowel elimination.

Independent Interventions
5.10 Analyze independent interventions nurses can implement for patients with alterations in bowel elimination.

Collaborative Therapies
5.11 Summarize collaborative therapies used by interprofessional teams for patients with alterations in bowel elimination.

Lifespan Considerations
5.12 Differentiate considerations related to the assessment and care of patients with alterations in bowel elimination throughout the lifespan.

Concepts Related to Elimination
5.13 Outline the relationship between elimination and other concepts.

Health Promotion
5.14 Explain the promotion of healthy elimination.

Elimination Exemplars

Exemplar 5.A Benign Prostatic Hyperplasia
5.A Analyze benign prostatic hyperplasia (BPH) as it relates to elimination.

Exemplar 5.B Bladder Incontinence and Retention
5.B Analyze bladder incontinence and retention as they relate to elimination.

Exemplar 5.C Bowel Incontinence, Constipation, and Impaction
5.C Analyze bowel incontinence, constipation, and impaction as they relate to elimination.

Exemplar 5.D Urinary Calculi
5.D Analyze urinary calculi as they relate to elimination.

 ## The Concept of Elimination

Concept Key Terms

(continued on next page)

Elimination refers to the secretion and excretion of physiologic waste products by the kidneys and intestines. Nurses are frequently the first healthcare professionals to determine that a patient is experiencing problems with elimination, so they must be familiar with the different alterations in elimination, the contributing risk factors, and how these alterations affect other physiologic processes.

The concept of elimination can be divided into two distinct methods of elimination based on the path in which the waste travels and where it is expelled from the body. Urinary elimination requires structures of the urinary tract. The urinary tract performs processes that eliminate solute waste transported in the blood supply. Excess liquid not needed for homeostasis is also eliminated through the structures of the urinary tract. For bowel elimination to occur, solid ingested material travels through the alimentary canal as the process of digestion takes place until the unused portions are finally expelled through the anus.

URINARY ELIMINATION

Urinary elimination serves to control blood concentration and composition and to rid the body of excess fluid and electrolytes. Proper regulation of this system is essential to health. If the urinary system is working correctly, urination can be postponed for only so long before the urge becomes too great to control.

Normal Urinary Elimination

Through intricate processes, the urinary system filters the blood to remove fluid and electrolytes, reabsorb nutrients to maintain the optimal concentration of each, and eliminate the excess. This process helps maintain the concentration of ions needed for neuronal and muscle function, bone strength, and cellular regulation. It also helps maintain homeostatic regulation of blood pressure to ensure adequate circulation of oxygen and nutrients throughout the body.

Physiology Review

Urinary elimination depends on effective functioning of the upper urinary tract (kidneys and ureters) and the lower urinary tract (urinary bladder, urethra, and pelvic floor). **Figure 5–1** ⟫ shows the anatomical structures of the urinary tract.

⟫ *Go to* **Pearson MyLab Nursing and eText** *to see a review of the anatomy and physiology of urinary elimination.*

Urination

Micturition, **voiding**, and **urination** all refer to the process of emptying the urinary bladder. Urine collects in the bladder until pressure stimulates special sensory nerve endings, called *stretch receptors,* in the bladder wall. This stimulation occurs when the adult bladder contains between 250 and 450 mL of urine. In children, a considerably smaller volume (50–200 mL) stimulates these nerves.

The stretch receptors transmit impulses to the spinal cord—specifically to the voiding reflex center located at the level of the second to fourth sacral vertebrae—causing the internal sphincter to relax and stimulate the urge to void. If the time and place are appropriate for urination, the conscious portion of the brain relaxes the external urethral sphincter muscle, and urination occurs. If the time and place are inappropriate and the conscious portion of the brain chooses to delay urination, the micturition reflex usually subsides until the bladder becomes more filled and the reflex is stimulated again.

Voluntary control of urination is possible only if the nerves supplying the bladder and urethra, the neural tracts of the spinal cord and brain, and the motor area of the cerebrum are all intact. The individual must be able to sense that the bladder is full. Injury affecting these key areas of nerve conduction, such as a cerebral hemorrhage or a spinal cord injury above the level of the sacral region, results in intermittent involuntary emptying of the bladder. Older adults whose cognition is impaired may not be aware of the need to urinate or may not be able to respond to this urge appropriately.

Although patterns of urination are highly individual, most people void about five or six times a day. They usually void when they first awaken in the morning, before they go to bed, and around mealtimes. **Table 5–1** ⟫ lists the average urinary output per day at different ages.

Factors Affecting Urinary Elimination

Numerous factors affect the volume and characteristics of the urine produced and the manner in which it is excreted.

TABLE 5–1 Average Daily Urine Output by Age

Age	Amount (mL)
1–2 days	15–60
3–10 days	100–300
10 days to 2 months	250–450
2 months to 1 year	400–500
1–3 years	500–600
3–5 years	600–700
5–8 years	700–1000
8–14 years	800–1400
14 years through adulthood	1500
Older adulthood	1500 or less

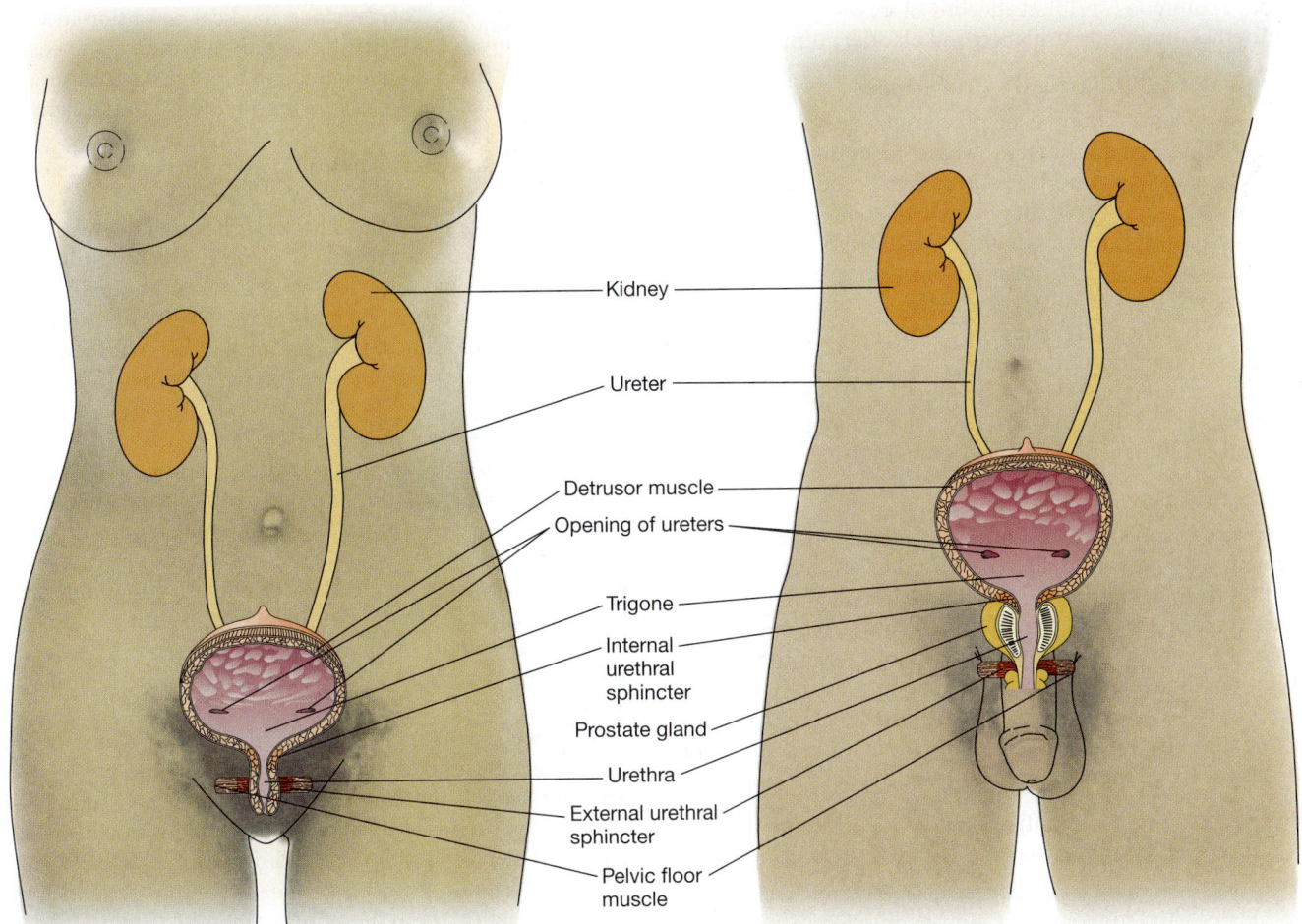

Source: Custom Medical Stock Photo, Inc.

Figure 5–1 >> Female and male urinary bladders and urethras, showing sphincter muscles.

These factors include fluid and food intake, muscle tone, psychosocial factors, pathologic conditions, surgical and diagnostic procedures, and medications.

Fluid and Food Intake

The healthy body maintains a balance between the amount of fluid ingested and the amount of fluid eliminated. When the amount of fluid intake increases, the fluid output normally increases accordingly. Certain fluids, such as alcohol, increase fluid output by inhibiting the production of antidiuretic hormone (ADH). By contrast, food and liquids high in sodium may cause fluid retention.

Muscle Tone

Good muscle tone maintains the elasticity and contractility of the **detrusor muscle**, allowing the bladder to fill adequately and empty completely. Patients who require long-term use of a retention (or Foley) catheter may develop poor bladder muscle tone because continuous drainage of urine prevents the bladder from filling and emptying normally. Pelvic muscle tone also contributes to the ability to store and empty urine.

Psychosocial Factors

Stimulation of the micturition reflex may be affected by a need for privacy, positioning, sufficient time, and the sound or feel of running water. Absence of the patient's familiar environmental conditions may produce anxiety and muscle tension that prevent the individual from relaxing the abdominal and perineal muscles, thereby interfering with relaxation of the external urethral sphincter. Individuals may also voluntarily suppress urination because of perceived time pressures; for example, nurses often ignore the urge to void until they are able to take a break. This behavior increases the risk of urinary tract infections (UTIs).

Pathologic Conditions

Some renal diseases and conditions affect the formation and excretion of urine. Glomerular dysfunction may lead to the presence of abnormal amounts of protein or blood cells in the urine. **Renal failure** is the term used when the kidneys cease to produce urine. Heart and circulatory disorders, such as heart failure, shock, or hypertension affect blood flow to the kidneys, interfering with urine production. When abnormal amounts of fluid are lost through another route (e.g., vomiting, high fever), the kidneys retain water, and urinary output decreases.

Processes that interfere with the flow of urine from the kidneys to the urethra also affect urinary excretion. A urinary stone (calculus) may obstruct a ureter, blocking urine flow from the kidney to the bladder. Hyperplasia of the prostate gland, a common condition affecting older men, may obstruct the urethra, impairing urination and bladder emptying.

Surgical and Diagnostic Procedures

Some surgical and diagnostic procedures can affect the passage of urine. The urethra may swell after cystoscopy (endoscopy of the urinary bladder), and surgical procedures on any part of the urinary tract may result in some postoperative bleeding (which can cause the urine to be pink or red) or the formation of blood clots during the recovery phase.

Anesthesia, especially when delivered through a spinal route, will affect the passage of urine because of the decreased sensation and awareness of the need to void. Swelling related to trauma sustained during surgery on structures of or adjacent to the urinary tract (e.g., the uterus) can cause complete or partial retention of urine.

Medications

Diuretics (e.g., chlorothiazide, furosemide) increase urine formation by preventing the reabsorption of water and electrolytes from the tubules of the kidney into the bloodstream. Some medications alter the color of the urine. If a medication alters the color of urine, the nurse should teach the patient about this side effect to reduce the patient's anxiety.

Many medications, particularly those affecting the autonomic nervous system, interfere with the normal urination process, leading to the retention of urine. These include:

- Anticholinergic and antispasmodic medications, such as atropine and papaverine
- Antidepressant and antipsychotic agents, such as phenothiazines and monoamine oxidase inhibitors
- Antihistamine preparations, especially those containing pseudoephedrine (e.g., Claritin-D, Sudafed)
- Antihypertensive agents, such as hydralazine (Apresoline) and methyldopa (Aldomet)
- Antiparkinsonism drugs, such as levodopa, trihexyphenidyl (Artane), and benztropine mesylate (Cogentin)
- Beta-adrenergic blockers, such as propranolol (Inderal)
- Opioids, such as hydrocodone (Vicodin)

Alterations in Urination

Alterations in urination are common throughout the lifespan due to age-related changes, as well as acute and chronic diseases and associated treatments. Understanding potential alterations in urinary elimination and responding with appropriate nursing interventions will assist the nurse in providing high-quality patient-centered care.

Alterations and Manifestations

Many diseases and processes of the body have the potential to interfere with blood flow to the kidneys, ultimately affecting urine production, storage, and elimination.

Altered Urine Production

Polyuria (or **diuresis**) is the production of abnormally large amounts of urine by the kidneys—often several liters more than the patient's usual daily output. Polyuria can occur after excessive fluid intake, or it may be associated with diseases such as diabetes mellitus, diabetes insipidus, and chronic nephritis. **Polydipsia**, a medical condition in which extreme thirst leads to compulsive intake of excessive amounts of fluid, is associated with polyuria. Polyuria can cause excessive fluid loss, leading to intense thirst, dehydration, and weight loss.

Anuria is an absence of urine production, whereas **oliguria** is scant urine output, usually less than 500 mL/day or 30 mL/hour for an adult. Although oliguria may result from abnormal fluid losses or a lack of fluid intake, it may indicate impaired blood flow to the kidneys or impending renal failure; oliguria should be reported promptly to the primary healthcare provider. Rapid restoration of renal blood flow and urinary output may prevent renal failure.

Altered Urinary Elimination

Despite normal production of urine, a number of factors or conditions can affect elimination. Urinary frequency, nocturia, urgency, and dysuria often are manifestations of underlying conditions such as a UTI. Enuresis, incontinence, retention, and neurogenic bladder may be either a manifestation of an underlying condition or the primary problem affecting elimination of urine. Selected factors associated with altered patterns of urinary elimination are identified in **Table 5–2** ≫.

Urinary frequency is voiding at frequent intervals. Frequency is determined when voiding occurs more often than an individual's typical pattern, or more than four to six times a day. Increased fluid intake causes some increase in the frequency of voiding. Total fluid volumes of intake and output (I&O) may be normal over a 24-hour period though voiding smaller amounts more frequently. Conditions such as UTI, stress, and pregnancy can cause frequent voiding of small quantities (50–100 mL) of urine. **Nocturia** is voiding at night or during usual sleep time. Nocturia can be expressed in terms of the number of times the individual gets out of bed to void, for example, "nocturia × 4." The exception is when accurate measurement of urinary output is required to monitor the patient's status.

Urgency is the sudden strong desire to void. Regardless of urine volume, the individual feels a need to void immediately. Urgency, which is an abnormal finding, can accompany psychologic stress and irritation of the trigone and urethra. Urgency is also common in individuals who have poor external sphincter control and unstable bladder contractions.

Dysuria refers to voiding that is either painful or difficult. It can be caused by a stricture, in which a portion of the urethra is decreased in diameter, a UTI, or an injury to the bladder and urethra. Patients may say that they have to "push" to void or burning accompanies or follows voiding. They may describe the burning sensation as severe, like a hot poker, or more subdued, like a sunburn. **Urinary hesitancy** is a delay and difficulty in initiating micturition and is often associated with dysuria.

Impaired neurologic function can interfere with the normal mechanisms of urinary elimination, resulting in a **neurogenic bladder**. The patient with a neurogenic bladder does not perceive a sensation indicating bladder fullness and is unable to control the urinary sphincters. The bladder may become flaccid and distended, or spastic, with frequent involuntary urination. For additional details, see the Alterations and Therapies feature.

TABLE 5–2 Selected Factors Associated with Altered Urinary Elimination

Pattern	Selected Associated Factors
Polyuria	Ingestion of fluids containing caffeine or alcohol
	Use of diuretics
	May lead to thirst, dehydration, and weight loss
	History of diabetes mellitus, diabetes insipidus, or kidney disease
Oliguria, anuria	Decrease in fluid intake
	Dehydration
	Presence of hypotension, shock, or heart failure
	History of kidney disease
	Presence of elevated BUN (blood urea nitrogen) and serum creatinine
	Edema, hypertension (retention of fluids)
Frequency or nocturia	Pregnancy
	Increase in fluid intake
	UTI
Urgency	Presence of psychologic stress
	UTI
Dysuria	Urinary tract inflammation, infection, or injury
	Hesitancy, hematuria, pyuria (pus in the urine), and frequency
Enuresis	Family history of enuresis
	Difficult access to toileting facilities
	Psychologic stress
Incontinence	Bladder inflammation or associated disease process
	Difficulties in independent toileting (mobility impairment)
	Leakage when coughing, laughing, or sneezing
	Cognitive impairment
Retention	Distended bladder on palpation and percussion
	Pain to suprapubic region, restlessness, frequent small volume voiding, or loss of consciousness
	Recent anesthesia
	Recent perineal surgery
	Presence of perineal swelling
	Medications
	Lack of privacy or other factors inhibiting micturition

Prevalence

According to Litwin and Saigal (2012), the economic impact of bladder, prostate, and other urinary tract diseases is estimated to be over $35 billion a year based on annual healthcare charges. In addition, a review of the literature revealed that up to 50% of all women and 5% of men under age 65 report symptoms of urinary incontinence each year (Campbell et al., 2012; Nambiar, Cody, & Jeffery, 2014). An estimated 60% of men over age 60 report urinary incontinence related to having had treatment for an enlarged prostate (Silva et al., 2014). Although urinary retention is less prevalent than urinary incontinence, it is experienced by more men than women and increases with age, related to enlargement of the prostate. Urinary retention is uncommon in women unless resulting from a neurogenic problem affecting the structures of the bladder (National Institute of Diabetes and Digestive and Kidney Diseases [NIDDK], 2012a).

In a study conducted by van Breda and colleagues (2015), data were collected from young (mean = 22 years), presumably healthy nulligravid female medical school students. The subjects were surveyed with a written scoring system about lower urinary tract symptoms (LUTS) and level of bother related to each symptom. The results were surprising in that 94.3% reported some type of LUTS or urinary incontinence symptoms. The incidence of nocturia at least 1–2 times each night was reported by 18.2%. Micturition frequency of 7–8 times/day was reported by 19.5%, 9–10 times/day was reported by 8.2%, and 11–12 times/day was reported by 1.3%. Involuntary loss of urine was reported by 20.1% from 0 to 2 times weekly. Of the respondents, only 5.7% indicated having no problems. In a similar study conducted on presumably healthy young men with no identifiable prostate enlargement, 7% reported moderate to severe LUTS.

Genetic Considerations and Risk Factors

The presence of physical, cognitive, or developmental disability and familial history of incontinence may increase an individual's risk of urinary incontinence. Genetic conditions such as myelomeningocele or spina bifida and conditions associated with aging, such as Parkinson disease, can also contribute to urinary problems. Conditions affecting cognitive function, such as Alzheimer disease, will increase the risk of developing elimination problems as functional ability declines with the progression of the disease process.

Aging is a risk factor for both urinary incontinence and retention. The excretory function of the kidneys diminishes with age, but function usually does not diminish significantly below normal levels unless caused by a contributing disease process. Arteriosclerosis can reduce blood flow and impair renal function. Conditions that alter normal fluid I&O, such as influenza or surgery can compromise the kidney's ability to filter, balance acid–base homeostasis, regulate blood pressures, and maintain optimal electrolyte levels in older adults. In addition, the recovery time for any acute process increases as an individual ages. Decreased kidney function and infrequent voiding intervals increase the risk of medication toxicity, especially in pediatric and geriatric populations.

Among age-related changes, those regarding urgency and frequency are most noticeable. In men, these changes are often caused by an enlarged prostate gland. For women, they may be caused by weakened muscles supporting the bladder or the urethral sphincter. The capacity of the bladder and its ability to empty both decrease with aging. In part, this decrease explains the need for older adults to awaken at night to void (nocturia) and the increase in residual urine retention. The increased risk of residual urine retention predisposes the older adult to potential bladder infections.

Nursing Assessment

Identification of signs and symptoms related to urinary incontinence or retention is vital to the proper treatment of the patient's condition. The nursing assessment includes conducting a patient interview and obtaining a health history as well as performing a physical assessment. Documentation of the information obtained during these assessments is a critical part of the nursing process.

Alterations and Therapies
Urinary Elimination Problems

ALTERATION	DESCRIPTION/ DEFINITION	MANIFESTATIONS	INTERVENTIONS AND THERAPIES
Urinary incontinence	Involuntary leakage of urine	■ Incontinence associated with stress (e.g., coughing, lifting, sneezing) ■ Incontinence related to urgency (i.e., inability to get to a toilet fast enough) ■ Incontinence related to neurologic deficits (e.g., after spinal cord injury)	■ Pelvic floor exercises ■ Surgery ■ Bladder training ■ Pharmacologic agents ■ Vaginal devices
Urinary retention	Inability to completely empty the bladder	■ Complete lack of voiding ■ Incomplete bladder emptying ■ Overflow incontinence ■ Pain ■ Constant urge to urinate ■ Weak urinary flow	■ Credé maneuver ■ Urinary catheter insertion ■ Discontinuing medications that cause retention ■ Surgery ■ Urethral dilation
Prostatic hyperplasia	Enlargement of the prostate—may be benign or malignant	■ Urinary retention ■ Dribbling at the end of urination ■ Incontinence ■ Nocturnal enuresis ■ Pain	■ Surgical removal ■ Medications ■ Pelvic floor exercises ■ Scheduled attempts to void ■ Extended time to empty bladder ■ Limits on alcohol and caffeine
Cancer of structures in urinary tract	Abnormal cellular growth within the organs of the urinary tract	■ Blood in urine ■ Frequent urination ■ Painful urination ■ Back or pelvic pain	■ Surgery ■ Chemotherapy ■ Radiation therapy
Kidney stones	Formation of calculi within the calyx of the kidney	■ Mild to severe pain in the side and back, in the abdomen, or during urination ■ Cloudy or foul-smelling urine ■ Frequent urination ■ Nausea and vomiting ■ Hematuria ■ UTI	■ Analgesics ■ Lithotripsy ■ Dietary alteration to reduce risk of recurrence ■ Increased fluid intake
Renal failure	Insufficient or absent kidney function	■ Decreased urine output ■ Fluid retention ■ Shortness of breath ■ Confusion ■ Chest pain or pressure	■ Administration of diuretics if some kidney function remains ■ Dialysis (hemodialysis or peritoneal dialysis) ■ Kidney transplantation
Urinary tract infection	Invasion of the bladder, ureter, or kidney by microorganisms	■ Persistent urge to urinate (frequency) ■ Burning sensation during urination ■ Cloudy, red, or strong-smelling urine ■ Pelvic or rectal pain	■ Administration of antibiotics if infection is caused by bacterium ■ Increased fluid intake

Observation and Patient Interview

The nurse will develop and use observation skills to anticipate potential problems with urination. It is common for individuals to become anxious or lose focus when experiencing the urge to void, especially when the bladder is full.

If the patient presents with the odor of urine, it can alert the nurse about potential problems with urinary incontinence. The nurse may observe incontinence products in use by the patient. Some older women may put other items, such as wash clothes or paper towels, in their undergarments to absorb urine because of the high cost of disposable products. These and any other nursing observations can create an opening for the nurse to discuss urinary problems during the assessment interview.

The nurse's assessment interview provides critical information about urinary function. The nurse should be direct and polite, recognizing that urinary function is not openly discussed in many cultures and can cause patients varying degrees of embarrassment. In many cases, the nurse will gain most of the assessment data about elimination from subjective information. The nurse can ask patients to describe their frequency of urination and any associated problems. The nurse should allow patients to describe in their own words their understanding of any potential problems. During the remainder of the interview, the nurse should use vocabulary that is understood by the patients. The nurse should assess the patients' use of prescription and over-the-counter medications that affect elimination. The nurse should inquire about all medication use, as patients may not be aware that some medications can alter elimination.

Voiding Pattern

- How many times do you urinate during a 24-hour period?
- Has this pattern changed recently?
- Do you need to get out of bed to void at night? How often?

Description of Urine and Any Changes

- How would you describe your urine in terms of color, clarity (clear, transparent, or cloudy), and odor (faint or strong)?

Urinary Elimination Problems

- What problems have you had or do you now have with passing your urine?
- Are you passing smaller amounts of urine than usual?
- Are you voiding at intervals that are more frequent?
- Do you have trouble getting to the bathroom in time or do you feel an urgent need to void?
- Do you have painful voiding?
- Do you have frequent dribbling of urine or a feeling of bladder fullness associated with voiding small amounts of urine?
- Do you have difficulty starting or reducing the force of your urine stream?
- Do you have accidental leakage of urine? If so, when does this occur (e.g., when coughing, laughing, or sneezing; at night; during the day)?
- Does the urge to void wake you up when sleeping?
- Have you experienced any past urinary tract illness, such as infection of the kidney, bladder, or urethra; urinary calculi; or surgery of kidney, ureters, or bladder?

Factors Influencing Urinary Elimination

- *Fluid intake.* What amount and kind of fluid do you take each day (e.g., six glasses of water, two cups of coffee, three cola drinks with or without caffeine)?
- *Environmental factors.* Do you have any problems with toileting (mobility, removing clothing, toilet seat too low, need for grab bars)?

- *Stress.* Are you experiencing any major stress? If so, what are the stressors? Do you think these affect your urinary pattern?
- *Disease.* Have you had or do you have any illnesses that may affect urinary function, such as hypertension, heart disease, neurologic disease, cancer, enlarged prostate, or diabetes?
- *Diagnostic procedures and surgery.* Have you recently had a cystoscopy or anesthesia?

Physical Examination

Although most of the assessment information about elimination will be subjective, assessment of the abdomen, genitalia, and perianal areas will provide meaningful information. Assessment of the abdomen includes inspection, auscultation, percussion, and palpation. Palpation of the abdomen is required, with careful observation in the lower midline suprapubic area, noting any pain, tenderness, or bladder distention. Palpation of the abdomen is always last as it can alter baseline peristalsis. The nurse uses percussion and palpation on the flank area of the lower back for assessment of the kidneys. The nurse should note any flank tenderness or pain, including any differences bilaterally. Inspection of soft tissues of, or tissues surrounding, the genitalia and perianal areas is necessary since this is a high-risk area for impairment related to exposure to excess moisture or fecal material. Inspection of the urethral meatus for swelling, discharge, and inflammation may also be indicated (Berman, Snyder, & Frandsen, 2016). Inspection of feces and urine is required by noting volume, color, consistency, odor, and presence of blood or mucus. The nurse should screen the patient's fluid volume status by assessing skin turgor, vital signs, and pertinent lab values.

Diagnostic Tests

Results of diagnostic tests for urinary elimination will lead to the diagnosis of specific diseases, provide information to identify or modify the appropriate medication or therapy for the disease, and help nurses monitor the patient's responses to treatment and nursing care interventions.

>> Go to **Pearson MyLab Nursing and eText** to see Appendix B for diagnostic tests to assess the structures and functions of the urinary system.

Diagnostic tests to assess the structures and functions of the urinary system are summarized below:

- Urine may be tested for characteristics and components through urinalysis, urine culture, and presence of post-void residual urine. Urine may be collected for 24 hours to test for total volume and other specific substances such as creatinine, potassium, urea, nitrogen, protein and sodium, that may be passed during a full day. Test results may serve as baseline data, support the diagnosis of various health problems, and allow for evaluation of bladder emptying and renal function (see **Table 5–3 >>**).
- Bladder emptying may be evaluated by an ultrasonic bladder scan to examine for residual urine; uroflowmetry to measure the volume of urine voided per second; and cystometrography to evaluate bladder capacity, neuromuscular functions of the bladder, urethral pressures, and causes of bladder dysfunction.

Urinary Assessment

ASSESSMENT/METHOD	NORMAL FINDINGS	ABNORMAL FINDINGS	LIFESPAN OR DEVELOPMENTAL CONSIDERATIONS
Skin Assessment			
Inspect the skin and mucous membranes, noting color, turgor, and excretions.	The color of skin and mucous membranes should be even and appropriate to the age and race of the patient; skin should be dry with no visible excretions.	▪ Pallor of the skin and mucous membranes may indicate anemia, which can be caused by kidney disease. ▪ Decreased skin turgor may indicate dehydration. Changes in skin turgor may indicate renal insufficiency with either excess fluid loss or retention. ▪ Edema (generalized or in the lower extremities) may indicate fluid volume excess. ▪ An accumulation of uric acid crystals, called *uremic frost*, may be seen on the skin of the patient with late-stage renal failure.	▪ Newborns often have lanugo and vernix present. The hands and feet may appear purple or bluish. ▪ Older adults have thinner, drier, more fragile skin with wrinkles; therefore, dehydration may be more difficult to detect in this population. An older individual's perineal skin is more susceptible to breakdown related to urinary incontinence. ▪ Turgor should be assessed on tissue that is centrally located.
Abdominal Assessment			
The patient should be in a supine position. Inspect the abdomen, noting size, symmetry, masses or lumps, swelling, distention, glistening, or skin tightness.	The abdomen should be slightly concave, symmetrical, without distention or masses.	▪ Enlargements or asymmetry may indicate a hernia or abnormal tissue mass. ▪ If the urinary bladder is distended, it rises above the symphysis pubis as a rounded mass. ▪ Distention, glistening, or skin tightness may be associated with fluid retention.	▪ It is normal for an infant's abdomen to appear distended and firm, especially if the infant has eaten recently. ▪ Young children may mistake an abdominal assessment as tickling; allow the child to "help" with the initial palpation to get used to the sensation. Parents can also help hold the child still and provide reassurance and emotional support. ▪ Limit the time older adults with arthritis or cardiovascular problems are in the supine position, which may cause back pain or shortness of breath. Use pillows to prop up the patient if needed; propping up may cause the abdomen to appear distended.
Urinary Meatus Assessment			
For the male patient: With the patient in a sitting or standing position, compress the tip of the glans penis with your gloved hand to open the urinary **meatus**.	The urinary meatus should be midline and free of redness, lesions, or discharge.	▪ Increased redness, swelling, or discharge from the urinary meatus may indicate infection or sexually transmitted infection. ▪ Hypospadias is displacement of the urinary meatus to the ventral surface of the penis. ▪ Epispadias is displacement of the urinary meatus to the dorsal surface of the penis.	▪ For pediatric patients, a parent should be present during assessment of the urinary meatus. ▪ Explain the procedure thoroughly to patients of all ages, but especially children and adolescents. ▪ The urinary meatus is usually partially or completely obscured in uncircumcised male patients and completely visible in circumcised male patients. Uncircumcised male patients may be at higher risk for UTI.

Urinary Assessment *(continued)*

ASSESSMENT/METHOD	NORMAL FINDINGS	ABNORMAL FINDINGS	LIFESPAN OR DEVELOPMENTAL CONSIDERATIONS
For the female patient: With the patient in the dorsal lithotomy position, spread the labia with your gloved hand to expose the urinary meatus.		■ Ulceration of the urinary meatus may indicate a sexually transmitted infection.	■ Adolescents and adults often prefer to have a nurse of the same gender perform this assessment. Be aware of and sensitive to privacy issues. ■ Newborn girls and postpartum women may have swollen labia. ■ Because of loss of skin elasticity, the urethral meatus may be difficult to distinguish from the clitoris in older women.

Kidney Assessment

Auscultate the renal arteries by placing the bell of the stethoscope lightly in the areas of the renal arteries, located in the left and right upper abdominal quadrants.
    Percuss the kidneys for tenderness or pain.
    Palpate the kidneys. The lower pole of the right kidney may be found on deep palpation; the remaining right kidney and the left kidney are normally not palpable.
	Bruits are not normally heard over the renal arteries.
	    No tenderness or pain should be elicited.
	    If palpable, they should be nontender, bilaterally of appropriate size and density, and without palpable masses.
		■ Systolic bruits ("whooshing" sounds) may indicate renal artery stenosis.
		■ Tenderness and pain on percussion of the costovertebral angle suggest glomerulonephritis or glomerulonephrosis.
		■ A mass or lump may indicate a tumor or cyst.
		■ Tenderness or pain on palpation may suggest an inflammatory process.
		■ A soft kidney that feels spongy may indicate chronic renal disease.
		■ Bilaterally enlarged kidneys may suggest polycystic kidney disease.
		■ Unequal kidney size may indicate hydronephrosis.
			■ Kidneys may be palpable in a normal newborn.
			■ Kidneys decrease in mass with older age.
			■ Do not palpate kidneys of individuals who have undergone renal transplantation or children with Wilms tumor.

Bladder Assessment

Percuss the bladder for tone and position.
    Palpate the bladder (over the symphysis pubis and abdomen) for distention.
	The bladder should be midline without dullness.
	    The bladder is normally not palpable.
		■ A dull percussion tone over the bladder of a patient who has just urinated may indicate urinary retention.
		■ A distended bladder may be palpated at any point from the symphysis pubis to the umbilicus and is felt as a firm, rounded organ. It indicates urinary retention.
			■ Palpation of a distended bladder may produce overflow incontinence in older adults.

- Radiologic examinations include intravenous pyelography (IVP), retrograde pyelography, and renal arteriography or angiography. These examinations are useful in visualizing (via radiographs) the urinary tract to identify abnormal size, shape, and function of the kidneys, kidney pelvis, and ureters, and to detect renal **calculi** (stones), tumors, or cysts.

- Cystoscopy allows direct visualization of the bladder wall and urethra. During this procedure, small stones can be removed, a sample of tissue may be taken for biopsy, and retrograde pyelography may be done. If a contrast dye is instilled in the bladder, then fistulas, tumors, or ruptures can be identified.

- Noninvasive tests include renal ultrasound, CT, MRI, and renal scan. These tests are used to identify and evaluate kidney size and structure as well as renal or perirenal masses and obstructions. In addition, a renal scan may be used to evaluate kidney blood flow, perfusion, and urine production.

TABLE 5–3 Normal and Abnormal Findings: Urinalysis

Characteristic	Normal	Abnormal	Nursing Considerations
Amount in 24 hours (adult)	1200–1500 mL	Less than 1200 mL A large amount over intake	Normal urinary output is approximately equal to fluid intake. Output of less than 30 mL/hr may indicate decreased blood flow to the kidneys and should be reported immediately.
Color	Light straw to amber yellow	Dark amber Dark orange Red or dark brown	Dark yellow to brownish urine is concentrated and may indicate dehydration, fever, or first urination in the morning.
			Dilute urine may appear almost clear or very pale yellow and may be caused by over-hydration, kidney disease, alcohol ingestion, or diabetes insipidus.
			Red or red brown urine may be caused by sulfisoxazole-phenazopyridine (Azo Gantri-sin), phenytoin (Dilantin), cascara, chlorpromazine (Thorazine), docusate calcium, and phenolphthalein (Doxidan), and by carrots, rhubarb, and food coloring.
			Orange urine is caused by fever, urobilin, phenazopyridine (Pyridium), amidopyrine, nitrofurantoin, sulfonamides, carrots, beets, and food coloring.
			Blue or green urine is caused by pseudomonas, amitriptyline (Elavil), methylene blue, methocarbamol (Robaxin), and yeast concentrate.
			Brown or black urine is caused by Lysol poisoning, melanin, bilirubin, methemoglobin, porphyrin, cascara, and injectable iron.
			Red blood cells (RBCs) in the urine (hematuria) may be evident as pink, bright red, or rusty brown urine.
			Menstrual bleeding also can color urine but should not be confused with hematuria.
Appearance/clarity	Transparent, clear	Cloudy Mucous plugs, viscous, thick	Hazy or cloudy urine indicates bacteria, pus, RBCs, white blood cells (WBCs), phosphates, prostatic fluid spermatozoa, or urates.
			Milky urine is the result of fats or pyuria.
			Yellow foam results from bilirubin, bile, or severe cirrhosis of the liver.
Odor	Faint, aromatic	Offensive	The odor of ammonia increases with the time the urine is outside the body.
			UTI causes a foul or unpleasant odor, depending on the causative organism.
			Mousy odors result from phenylketonuria.
			Sweet or fruity odors occur in starvation and diabetic ketoacidosis (high glucose).
Sterility	No microorganisms present	Microorganisms present	Urine in the bladder is sterile. Urine specimens, however, may be contaminated by bacteria from the perineum during collection.
pH	4.5–8	Greater than 8 or less than 4.5	Freshly voided urine is somewhat acidic.
			Alkaline urine may indicate a state of alkalosis, a UTI, bacteriuria, antibiotics, sulfonamides, sodium bicarbonate, acetazolamide, potassium citrate, or a diet high in fruits and vegetables.
			More acidic urine (low pH) is found in starvation, with diarrhea, with a diet high in protein foods or cranberries, in metabolic or respiratory acidosis, and with increased ammonium chloride and mandelic acid concentrations.
Specific gravity	1.005–1.030	Greater than 1.030 or less than 1.005	Concentrated urine has a higher specific gravity; diluted urine has a lower specific gravity. *Less than 1.005:* diabetes insipidus, overhydration, renal disease, severe potassium deficit *More than 1.030:* dehydration, fever, diabetes mellitus, vomiting, diarrhea, contrast media
Protein	2–8 mg/dL	More than 8 mg/dL	High protein indicates proteinuria, exercise, fever, stress, acute infection, kidney disease, lupus erythematosus, leukemia, multiple myeloma, cardiac disease, preeclampsia, septicemia, lead, mercury, neomycin, barbiturates, or sulfonamides.
Glucose	Not present	Present	Glucose in the urine (greater than 15 mg/dL or +4) indicates high blood glucose levels (greater than 180 mg/dL) and may indicate undiagnosed or uncontrolled diabetes mellitus. Glucose is also high in stroke, Cushing syndrome, anesthesia, glucose infusions, severe stress, infections, ascorbic acid, aspirin, cephalosporins, and epinephrine.
Ketone bodies (acetone)	Not present	Present	Ketones, the end product of the breakdown of fatty acids, are not normally present in the urine. They may be present (+1 to +3) in the urine of patients who have uncontrolled diabetes mellitus, those in a state of starvation, or who have ingested excessive amounts of aspirin.
RBCs	None	Greater than 2 per low-power field	Blood in urine indicates kidney trauma, kidney diseases, renal calculi, cystitis, excess aspirin, anticoagulants, sulfonamides, menstrual contamination, or bleeding from the urinary tract.
WBCs	3–4 per low-power field	Greater than 4 per low-power field	High WBCs in urine indicate UTI, fever, strenuous exercise, or kidney diseases.
Casts	Occasional hyaline	Fatty, granular, renal tubular epithelial, waxy casts	Casts may indicate fever, kidney diseases, or heart failure.

Note: Urine outputs below 30 mL/hr may indicate low blood volume or kidney malfunction. Nurses monitor urine output and should notify the primary provider if urine output averages less than 30 mL/hr over 4 hours.

- A kidney biopsy is done to obtain tissue for use in diagnosing or monitoring abnormal cells found in kidney disease such as cancer.

Regardless of the type of diagnostic test, the nurse is responsible for explaining the procedure and any special preparations needed as well as assessing for medication use that may affect the outcome of the tests. The nurse must ensure that the patient fully understands the conditions under which the test will be administered and which preparations the patient may need to make in advance (e.g., fasting) for tests to be accurate and successful. The nurse also supports the patient during the examination as necessary, documents the procedures as appropriate, and monitors the results of the tests.

Measurement of blood levels of urea and creatinine is useful for evaluation of renal function. Both substances are normally eliminated by the kidneys through filtration and tubular secretion. Urea, the end product of protein metabolism, is measured as BUN. Creatinine is produced in relatively constant quantities by the muscles. The **creatinine clearance** test uses 24-hour urine and serum creatinine levels to determine the glomerular filtration rate (GFR), a sensitive indicator of renal function.

Independent Interventions

Independent interventions are those that can be performed by the nurse without obtaining a medical order. Independent nursing interventions may include monitoring I&O, catheter care, managing dialysis, urine specimen collection, and patient teaching.

Independent nursing interventions to manage urinary problems should be patient-centered and require the nurse to understand the cause and severity of the primary problem. Patients with reduced urine output secondary to dehydration will require increased fluid intake. The nurse will encourage oral intake and monitor daily I&O in addition to any dependent interventions. Determining the cause of urinary incontinence by conducting a thorough assessment interview will lead to appropriate treatment and management. Patients requiring catheterization for treatment of urinary retention or wound management will require catheter care and extensive teaching if the patient will perform self-catheterization.

The tissues potentially affected by urinary problems will require protection to avoid breakdown. First and foremost, the skin must be kept clean and dry. This may also be referred to as *incontinence care* and also encompasses incontinence of fecal matter. Prompt cleansing of the skin after incontinence must be performed along with replacing soiled clothing and linens with clean ones. Barrier creams and skin treatments are a collaborative treatment but are often outlined in protocols adopted by the facility's medical staff for the nursing staff to use as needed. These protocols are often written by certified wound, ostomy, and continence nurses (CWOCN) and sent to the medical staff for review and approval. At the point of care, teaching patients and caregivers to provide prompt and appropriate skin care requires the nurse to be proficiently knowledgeable of basic principles for preventive skin care.

Aseptic technique is essential during any procedure that could introduce bacteria into the blood or urinary tract to decrease the incidence of ascending bladder contamination and subsequent UTI. It is the nurse's responsibility to implement best practice guidelines related to personal hand hygiene, patient perineal hygiene, catheter bag placement, use of sterile gloves, maintenance of a closed urinary system, and other aspects of catheter care. Education regarding these guidelines should be provided regularly to update nursing staff, and policies should be put in place to ensure that the guidelines are followed.

Collaborative Therapies

In the acute care setting, collaboration with other professionals is largely guided by the nature of the elimination problem. Collaborating with an expert nurse or one who has specialized in an area such as infection control may be of assistance for a patient who experiences chronic infections or is required to perform self-catheterizations to empty the bladder for relief of urinary retention. A radiologist is often included on the interprofessional team as a consultant to a primary care provider or urologist.

Referring the patient to professionals who can either prepare the patient for discharge or provide care after discharge will allow the patient optimal health maintenance or management. Examples include referral to a wound and ostomy nurse for patients with chronic wounds or a diversional ostomy and referrals to occupational therapists to help patients regain optimal functional status. For continuity of care, follow-up appointments should be made for patients to visit urologists and primary care providers. Patients with long-term teaching needs may qualify for home health nursing care. Referrals to medical supply companies for durable medical equipment required in the home may include safety devices such as grab bars, raised toilet seats, and bedside toileting chairs. Additional supplies required may be incontinence products such as adult briefs and bed pads, ostomy supplies, or catheters.

The importance of collaborating with the patient and family members or caregivers providing care in the home or at a facility is a responsibility that should not be overlooked. Collaboration of team members is equally necessary to provide needed equipment or supplies related to elimination for the patient who resides in a long-term care or assisted living facility.

Pharmacologic Therapy

Pharmacologic therapy for urinary elimination may include diuretics to increase urine production. Anticholinergic medications are used to reduce urinary frequency and treat urinary incontinence. Cholinergic medications are used to stimulate bladder contractions, promoting urination, especially in patients with difficulty voiding. See the Medications feature for additional information.

Diuretics are classified by their mechanism of action. Loop diuretics work in the loop of Henle by blocking reabsorption of sodium and chloride. Thiazide diuretics act on the distal tubule to block sodium reabsorption and

Evidence-Based Practice
Catheter Care and Infection Prevention

Problem

Urinary incontinence and urinary retention are often managed with the insertion of a catheter. The use of a catheter significantly increases the risk of developing a UTI, and that risk increases with every subsequent day of use. Each year in America, more than 560,000 individuals develop a UTI related to having an indwelling urinary catheter (ANA, 2017). Between 25 and 31% of hospitalized patients require catheterization, and at least 10% of those individuals will develop a catheter-associated urinary tract infection (CAUTI) (Centers for Disease Control and Prevention [CDC], 2015). Many of these patients do not require a catheter, but the catheter remains because of convenience, misunderstanding of its necessity, and lack of orders for removal (Greene et al., 2014; Oman et al., 2012). Between 5 and 10% of patients in long-term care facilities will require treatment with an indwelling catheter. Up to 30% of those patients requiring indwelling catheterization will develop a CAUTI each year (Nicolle, 2012).

Evidence

The CDC has issued guidelines for proper catheter use and care based on clinical evidence (National Healthcare Safety Network [NHSN], 2016). The consistent implementation of these guidelines have proven to reduce CAUTI. According to these guidelines, catheter use should be limited to appropriate situations and only for as long as needed. Duration of use should be minimal in patients with high risk of mortality from infection, including women, older adults, and patients with impaired immunity. In addition, catheters should not be used for nursing home residents simply to manage incontinence. Alternatives to indwelling catheters should be utilized when possible, including external catheters in male patients without urinary retention or bladder outlet obstruction and intermittent catheterization for patients with long-term catheterization needs (e.g., those with spinal cord injury or neurogenic bladder). In patients undergoing intermittent catheterization, the use of a portable ultrasound device to assess urine volume eliminates the need for catheter insertions to assess bladder volume. In addition, the CDC recommends that catheter care should be performed only by individuals with proper training. Catheters should be changed as clinically indicated (e.g., infection, obstruction, system compromise) and not at regular intervals. Bladder irrigation is not recommended unless obstruction is anticipated. Hand hygiene should always be performed immediately before and after catheter insertion.

Evidence indicates that facility-wide education can reduce the number of catheter-days and assist patients to achieve either continence or to use alternative strategies to manage incontinence (Felix et al., 2013). One hospital reported a reduction in the number of catheter-days after implementing facility-wide education, higher quality product usage, and newer equipment availability (Oman et al., 2012). A second hospital reported implementing education about appropriate device utilization and device removal, which decreased device utilization from 0.5 catheter-days/patient-days to 0.3 catheter-days/patient-days and subsequently reduced the CAUTI rate from 1.8/1000 catheter-days to 0.7/1000 catheter-days (Revello & Gallo, 2013).

Implications

Nurse education related to catheter use and care is essential to reduce the CAUTI rate. Based on education about indications for catheter use, nurses must learn to analyze each patient's situation for the necessity of catheter use and to recognize patients for whom catheter use is not indicated.

As the patient's advocate, it is the nurse's responsibility to approach the provider about removing the catheter when the risk of infection outweighs the benefit of having the catheter in place. It can be challenging to depend on the prevalence of routine face-to-face communication between the nurse and medical provider, especially on units that have higher nurse-to-patient ratios, such as general medical or postsurgical. Removal of a catheter that no longer meets medical necessity may be best accomplished with routine stop orders, medical protocols, or written reminders built into the patient's medical record (Fakih et al., 2013; Meddings et al., 2013).

Critical Thinking Application

Describe circumstances in which an older woman who has undergone hip replacement surgery would need a urinary catheter before or on day 1, 7, or 21 after surgery. Differentiate between conditions that require indwelling or intermittent catheterization and no catheterization. Visit http://nursingworld.org/ANA-CAUTI-Prevention-Tool and download a free copy of the American Nurses Association CAUTI Prevention Tool and the Companion Guide Document. Develop an educational session to provide nurses and other healthcare workers with an update on the latest guidelines for catheter use and care in an effort to reduce CAUTI (American Nurses Association, 2015).

---

increase potassium and water excretion. Potassium-sparing diuretics, which work in the distal tubule, allow sodium to be excreted while inhibiting potassium excretion, thereby preventing the large potassium loss caused by other types of diuretics. Finally, diuretics that cannot be otherwise classified make up a miscellaneous group; this group includes carbonic anhydrase inhibitors and osmotic diuretics.

Dialysis

For patients with severely reduced or absent renal function, some mechanism of filtering the blood is necessary to prevent illness and death. This filtering is done through renal **dialysis**, a technique by which fluids and molecules pass through a semipermeable membrane according to the rules of osmosis. The two types of dialysis are hemodialysis and peritoneal dialysis. In **hemodialysis**, the patient's blood flows through vascular catheters, passes by the dialysis solution in an external machine, and then returns to the patient. In **peritoneal dialysis**, the dialysis solution is instilled into the abdominal cavity through a catheter, allowed to rest there while the fluid and molecules exchange, and then removed from the abdomen through the catheter. Both hemodialysis and peritoneal dialysis must be performed at frequent intervals until the patient's kidneys can resume the filtering function. Depending upon the type of dialysis indicated, a specially trained nurse may administer or monitor the dialysis procedure.

Medications
Urinary Elimination

CLASSIFICATION AND DRUG EXAMPLES	MECHANISMS OF ACTION	NURSING CONSIDERATIONS
Anticholinergics *Drug examples:* Cxybutynin, tolterodine, darifenacin, solifenacin, trospium, fesoterodine	These drugs reduce urgency and frequency by blocking muscarinic receptors in the detrusor muscle of the bladder, thereby inhibiting contractions and increasing storage capacity. *May also be used for:* ■ Gastrointestinal disorders ■ Respiratory disorders	■ Anticholinergics are used to relieve symptoms associated with voiding in patients who have neurogenic bladder, reflex neurogenic bladder, or urge urinary incontinence. ■ Monitor for constipation, dry mouth, urinary retention, blurred vision, and (in older adults) mental confusion. Symptoms may be dose related. ■ Start with small doses for patients older than 75 years. ■ Anticholinergics are contraindicated in patients with urinary retention, gastrointestinal motility problems (partial or complete gastrointestinal obstruction, paralytic ileus), or uncontrolled narrow-angle glaucoma.
Cholinergic Agents or Parasympathomimetics *Drug examples:* Bethanechol chloride	These medications stimulate bladder contraction and facilitate voiding. *May also be used for:* ■ Gastroesophageal reflux disease ■ Ileus	■ Do not administer to patients with gastrointestinal or urinary tract obstructions, asthma, bradycardia, hypotension, or Parkinson disease. ■ These drugs may increase serum aspartate aminotransferase, amylase, and lipase levels. ■ Effect of medications is antagonized by angel's trumpet, jimson weed, or scopolia. ■ Overdose is treated with atropine sulfate.
Diuretics ■ Loop ■ Thiazide ■ Potassium-sparing ■ Miscellaneous *Drug examples:* Bumetanide, furosemide, chlorothiazide, metolazone, spironolactone	Each type of diuretic works in a specific place within the nephron to increase fluid excretion and prevent fluid reabsorption. *May also be used for:* ■ Heart failure ■ Edema ■ Polycystic ovary syndrome ■ Diabetes insipidus ■ Female hirsutism ■ Osteoporosis	■ Monitor hydration and electrolyte balance. ■ Monitor vital signs, and be alert for signs of hypotension secondary to fluid loss. ■ Monitor serum BUN, creatinine, electrolyte, and other pertinent laboratory values. ■ Patients taking potassium-sparing diuretics should avoid salt substitutes.

Source: Data from Adams, M. P., Holland, L. N., & Urban, C. (2017). *Pharmacology for nurses: A pathophysiologic approach* (5th ed.). Hoboken, NJ: Pearson Education.

Case Study » Part 1

Dennis Welborn is a 52-year-old man who visits his primary care physician with complaints of severe pain in his back and abdomen and painful urination with hematuria. As the nurse working at the clinic, you take Mr. Welborn's medical history and make a preliminary assessment. Mr. Welborn is 6'2" tall and weighs 265 pounds. His vital signs include temperature 100.8°F oral, pulse 95 bpm, respirations 22/min, and BP 140/92 mmHg. Mr. Welborn rates his back and abdominal pain as 9 on a scale of 0–10, and his midline abdominal pain level is a 7 when he is urinating. When asked about his diet, Mr. Welborn admits that as a widower, he often eats out with coworkers for lunch and picks up fast food on the way home for his evening meal. He usually drinks three cups of coffee in the morning and diet soda throughout the afternoon and evening. When he gets heartburn, he chews several antacid tablets for relief. An abdominal assessment reveals a distended bladder. Mr. Welborn states he delays urination as long as possible because of the pain. When he does urinate, he has noticed that he has a weak stream and continues to feel the urge to urinate when he has finished. The medical care provider orders lab tests, so a blood

and urine sample are obtained for analysis. Mr. Welborn is transferred to the radiology department to have an abdominal x-ray. The x-ray reveals a large stone (1.2 cm) in Mr. Welborn's proximal right ureter, and the urinalysis indicates the presence of small calcium crystals, RBCs, and bacteria. The blood test also detects high blood calcium levels.

Clinical Reasoning Questions Level I
1. What risk factors does Mr. Welborn have for developing urinary calculi?
2. Other than a distended bladder, what findings might you discover in your assessment of Mr. Welborn?
3. How would the stone in Mr. Welborn's ureter contribute to urinary retention?

Clinical Reasoning Questions Level II
4. What is the priority nursing diagnosis for Mr. Welborn?
5. What nursing interventions can you implement to help manage Mr. Welborn's pain?
6. *Refer to Exemplar 5.D on Urinary Calculi.* What is a likely treatment option to clear the stone from Mr. Welborn's ureter?

TABLE 5–4 Changes in Urinary Elimination Through the Lifespan

Stage	Variations
Fetal	The fetal kidney begins to excrete urine between the 11th and 12th weeks of development.
Infancy	The ability to concentrate urine is minimal; therefore, urine appears light yellow.
	Because of neuromuscular immaturity, voluntary urinary control is absent.
Childhood	Kidney function reaches maturity between the first and second year of life; urine is concentrated effectively and appears a normal yellow to amber color.
	Between 18 and 24 months of age, the child starts to recognize bladder fullness and is able to hold urine beyond the urge to void.
	At approximately 2.5–3 years of age, the child can perceive bladder fullness, hold urine after the urge to void, and communicate the need to urinate.
	Daytime urinary control is achieved by about 3 years of age.
	Full urinary control usually occurs at 4 or 5 years of age; daytime control is usually achieved by 3 years of age.
	The kidneys grow in proportion to overall body growth.
Adulthood	The kidneys reach maximum size between 35 and 40 years of age.
	After 50 years, the kidneys begin to diminish in size and function. Most shrinkage occurs in the cortex of the kidney as individual nephrons are lost.
Geriatric	An estimated 30% of nephrons are lost by 80 years of age.
	Renal blood flow decreases because of vascular changes and a decrease in cardiac output.
	The ability to concentrate urine declines.
	Bladder muscle tone diminishes, causing increased frequency of urination and nocturia (voiding two or more times at night).
	Diminished bladder muscle tone and contractility may lead to residual urine in the bladder after voiding, increasing the risk of bacterial growth and infection.
	Urinary incontinence may occur because of mobility problems or neurologic impairments.

Lifespan Considerations

Factors specific to infants, preschoolers, school-age children, pregnant women, and older adults can affect the elimination of urine (see **Table 5–4 》》**). Also see the Lifespan or Developmental Considerations column in the Urinary Assessment feature.

Urinary Elimination in Newborns

The GFR of the newborn's kidney is lower than the adult's. Because of immature function, the newborn's kidney is unable to rapidly excrete excess fluid; as a result, the newborn is at particular risk for fluid volume overload. Full-term newborns are less able to concentrate urine because the tubules are short and narrow. The limited tubular reabsorption of water and limited excretion of solutes (primarily sodium, potassium, chloride, bicarbonate, urea, and phosphate) in the growing newborn also reduce the ability to concentrate urine, making the effect of excessive insensible water loss or restricted fluid intake unpredictable. The newborn's kidneys are also limited in their ability to

dilute urinary output. These limitations regarding concentration and dilution are important considerations in monitoring fluid therapy to prevent dehydration or overhydration. The newborn attains the ability to efficiently concentrate urine by 3 months of age.

Healthy newborns usually void within the first 24 hours. The delivery room nurses must make a focused effort to witness and record the first void after birth; otherwise, it may go unnoticed because of other excess fluids from the birth process. The newborn who has not voided within 48 hours following delivery should be assessed for adequacy of fluid intake, bladder distention, restlessness, and symptoms of pain. The primary healthcare provider should be notified of any deviation from normal elimination.

The initial bladder volume ranges between 6 and 44 mL of urine. Unless edema is present, normal urinary output is limited and will remain low until fluid intake increases. For the first 2 days after birth, the newborn voids from 2 to 6 times daily, with a urine output of 15 mL/kg per day. The newborn subsequently voids from 5 to 25 times every 24 hours, with a volume of 25 mL/kg per day. Urine output varies according to fluid intake and gradually increases up to between 250 and 500 mL per day during the first year.

After emptying the bladder for the first time, the newborn's urine is frequently cloudy (because of mucus content) and has a high specific gravity, which decreases as fluid intake increases. Harmless pink stains ("brick dust spots"), which are caused by urates, occasionally appear on the diaper. During early infancy, urine is normally straw-colored and almost odorless. In these patients, odor can result from certain medications, metabolic disorders, or infection.

Urinary Elimination in Toddlers and Preschoolers

Most children develop urinary control between 2 and 5 years of age and are able to take responsibility for independent toileting shortly thereafter. Control during the daytime normally precedes nighttime control. Parents must realize that accidents occur and should never punish a child for a toileting accident. Because children at this age often forget to wash their hands or flush the toilet, they require reminders and appropriate adult modeling. Young children also require instruction in wiping themselves. Girls should be taught to wipe from front to back to prevent fecal contamination of the urinary tract.

Urinary Elimination in School-Age Children

A child's elimination system reaches maturity during early school age. The kidneys double in size between the ages of 5 and 10. During this period, the child urinates six to eight times a day.

Enuresis, the involuntary passing of urine when control should be established (approximately 5 years of age), is a problem for some school-age children. Although it is more prevalent in children, adults may also experience enuresis. Diurnal (daytime) enuresis may be persistent and pathologic in origin. It affects women and girls more frequently than it does men and boys. The occurrence of enuresis after achieving voluntary bladder control should be reported to the primary care provider.

Nocturnal enuresis (NE), or bedwetting, is the involuntary passing of urine during sleep. It is especially prevalent in children who are reported to be deep sleepers, although it can occur at any stage of sleep. The incidence of NE decreases as the child matures and should not be considered a problem until after 7 years of age. See the Exemplar 5.B on Bladder Incontinence and Retention for more information.

Urinary Elimination in Pregnant Women

During the first trimester of pregnancy, the enlarging uterus remains in the pelvis and presses against the bladder, increasing urinary frequency. This symptom decreases during the second trimester; when the uterus becomes larger and is contained in the abdominal cavity, pressure against the bladder decreases. Urinary frequency reappears during the third trimester, when the presenting part of the uterus descends into the pelvis and again presses on the bladder, thus reducing bladder capacity, contributing to hyperemia, and irritating the bladder. The ureters, especially the right ureter, elongate and dilate above the pelvic brim. The GFR rises by as much as 50% beginning in the second trimester, and it remains elevated until birth. To compensate for this increase, renal tubular reabsorption also increases. However, **glycosuria** (excretion of carbohydrates into the urine) is present during pregnancy because of the kidneys' inability to reabsorb all the glucose filtered by the glomeruli. Glycosuria may be normal or may indicate gestational diabetes and warrants further testing. The presence of protein, blood, or WBCs in the urine is always considered abnormal and should be evaluated.

The postpartum woman is at risk for overdistention, incomplete bladder emptying, and buildup of **residual urine** (urine that remains in the bladder after voiding) due to swelling and bruising of the tissue around the urethra, decreased sensitivity to fluid pressure, and decreased sensation of bladder filling. Women who have had an anesthetic block have inhibited neural functioning of the bladder and are more susceptible to bladder distention, difficulty with voiding, and bladder infections. In addition, immediate postpartum use of oxytocin (to facilitate uterine contractions following expulsion of the placenta) has an antidiuretic effect. After oxytocin is discontinued, women will experience rapid bladder filling.

Urinary output increases during the early postpartum period (first 12–24 hours) because of puerperal diuresis. The kidneys must eliminate an estimated 2000–3000 mL of extracellular fluid retained during a normal pregnancy, causing rapid filling of the bladder. As a result, adequate urinary elimination is an immediate concern. Women with preeclampsia, chronic hypertension, or diabetes experience greater fluid retention during pregnancy than other women, and postpartum diuresis increases accordingly. The risk of UTI increases with urinary retention because of bacteriuria and the presence of dilated ureters and renal pelvis. This risk will persist for approximately 6 weeks until the dilated ureters and renal pelvis return to pregravid functioning. A full bladder may also increase the tendency of the uterus to relax by displacing the uterus

and interfering with its contractility, resulting in an increased risk for hemorrhage.

Urinary Elimination in Older Adults

Renal function begins to decline around 40 years of age but usually does not create significant issues for an otherwise healthy individual until the ninth decade of life. By this time, GFR, renal blood flow, maximal urinary concentration, and response to sodium loss are significant. GFR declines at a rate of approximately 6.3 mL/min/1.73 m^2 per decade, and by age of 90 the individual's GFR is approximately half of what is expected for a 20-year-old (Denic, Glasscock, & Rule, 2016; Miller, 2016). The average weight of the kidney is about 400 g at age 40 and declines to 250 g at age 80. The change in size is a result of a decrease of functional nephrons related to a decline in blood supply.

Blood flow to the kidney decreases as a result of atrophy in the supplying blood vessels, particularly in the renal cortex. In addition, the proximal tubules decrease in number and length. Compared with a young adult, an older adult usually has a lower creatinine clearance, has urine that is more dilute (having a lower specific gravity), and typically excretes lower levels of glucose, acid, and potassium. As these changes progress, the BUN increases from 10–15 mg/dL at age 20 to 21 mg/dL by age 70 (Miller, 2016). In addition, the kidneys of older adults excrete more fluid and electrolytes during nighttime hours than during the day, resulting in increased urine formation during sleep, which often interrupts sleep patterns.

One important consequence of these changes is impaired excretion of drugs and their metabolites. Older adults become susceptible to drug overdose and other adverse effects of medication even when medications are prescribed and administered within the recommended dose range. This impairment is of particular concern when an individual has multiple health impairments that require several types of pharmacologic therapy. Another consequence of age-related changes is an increased probability of hyperkalemia, particularly when potassium-sparing diuretics, angiotensin-converting enzyme inhibitors, nonsteroidal anti-inflammatory drugs (NSAIDs), or beta-blockers are prescribed (Lederer et al., 2013).

The older adult's decreased ability to concentrate urine results in an increased susceptibility to dehydration, a problem that is further complicated by a decline in the thirst response; therefore, the older individual may not feel thirsty even if he or she is significantly dehydrated. In addition, an older adult who has concerns about incontinence may choose not to drink for fear of incontinence. These changes also produce a decline in the ability of older adults to increase urine production in response to fluid volume overload.

Changes in the bladder and urethra also occur with aging. The bladder becomes more fibrous, with a consequent decrease in storing capacity and increase in residual urine. The decrease in autonomic regulation of the bladder by the nervous system with aging affects contraction of both the detrusor muscle and the external sphincter. With age, the detrusor muscle becomes somewhat unstable and loses its ability to contract proficiently. As a result, the older adult is subject to an inability to completely empty the bladder. Age-related weakening also occurs in the voluntary muscles of the pelvic floor, which are important in controlling the release of urine from the urethra. These changes make older adults more likely to have difficulty delaying urination and predispose them to urinary incontinence and UTI. The nurse should understand that age-related anatomical and physiologic changes make incontinence more probable with aging, although urinary incontinence is not a normal condition of aging and may be treatable.

Older adults generally have normal to higher basal levels of ADH than younger adults. Although ADH is released as a response to hypotension and hypovolemia, its action is not as efficient in the aging kidney. More ADH is required to achieve an adequate antidiuretic effect; otherwise, the production of urine is poorly concentrated and high in sodium, predisposing the older adult to an increased risk of **hyponatremia**. Prescription diuretic use for treatment of hypertension and cardiac conditions is common in older adults and can further complicate inefficiencies in concentration of urine and regulation of electrolytes.

BOWEL ELIMINATION

Like urinary elimination, formation and expulsion of feces is a complex process that promotes the retention of nutrients and important compounds while removing waste products from the body. The digestive system is often taken for granted when functioning properly. However, alterations in bowel elimination can lead to conditions that range in severity from mild to fatal.

Normal Bowel Elimination

Ingested food that is not digestible moves through the gastrointestinal system and is eliminated from the bowel as **feces**. **Defecation** is the expulsion of feces from the anus and rectum. It is also referred to as a *bowel movement* or **stool**. The frequency of defecation is highly individual, varying from several times a day to bi-weekly. Fecal volume and consistency will vary based on dietary consumption and intestinal transit time.

Physiology Review

Peristalsis refers to the wavelike muscular contractions that propel food and digestive products through the digestive tract. Food travels from the mouth to the stomach, where is it broken down into a thick, semifluid mass called *chyme*. Peristalsis propels the mass of chyme through the small bowel and the colon. During transport through the bowels, nutrients and water are absorbed into the bloodstream and transported to the liver for processing via the hepatic portal vein. The portion of chyme that cannot be absorbed continues through the large intestine until it reaches the colon and rectum and is finally expelled through the anus (see **Figure 5–2** ≫).

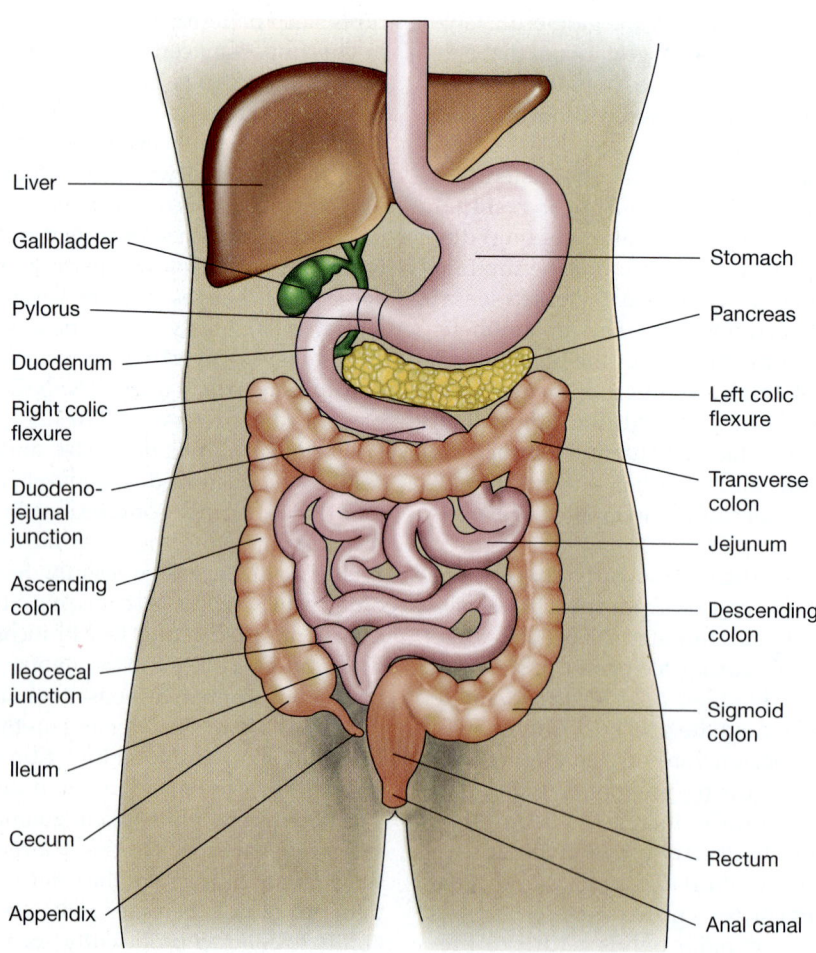

Figure 5–2 ≫ Digestive organs involved in the process of bowel elimination.

Normal feces are made up of approximately 75% water and 25% solid materials. They are soft but formed. Very quick propulsion of the feces along the large intestine allows inadequate time for most of the water in the chyme to be absorbed, and the feces are more fluid, containing perhaps 95% water. Normal feces require a normal fluid intake; feces that contain less water may be hard and difficult to expel. Feces normally are brown because of the presence of bile and bilirubin, which is a breakdown product of dead RBCs. The action of bacteria, such as *Escherichia coli* or *Staphylococcus* sp., which normally are present in the large intestine, also affects fecal color. The action of microorganisms on chyme is responsible for the odor of feces.

An adult usually forms 7–10 L of **flatus** (gas) in the large intestine every 24 hours. The gases include carbon dioxide, methane, hydrogen, oxygen, and nitrogen. Some are swallowed with food and fluids taken by mouth. Others are formed through the action of bacteria on the chyme in the large intestine. Still other gas diffuses from the blood into the gastrointestinal tract.

Factors Affecting Bowel Elimination

Many factors affect bowel elimination, including diet, fluid I&O, activity, defecation habits, medications, medical procedures, pathologic conditions, and psychologic factors.

Diet

Sufficient bulk (cellulose, fiber) in the diet is necessary to provide fecal volume. Bland diets and low-fiber diets lack bulk and therefore create insufficient residue of waste products to stimulate the reflex for defecation. Low-residue foods, such as rice, eggs, and lean meats, move more slowly through the intestinal tract. Increasing fluid intake with such foods increases their rate of movement.

Some foods are difficult, or even impossible, for people to digest. Foods that are difficult to digest can alter the usual transit time through the bowel, resulting in problems with elimination. Irregular eating schedules can affect regular defecation patterns. Individuals who eat at the same times every day usually have a regularly timed physiologic response to food intake and a regular pattern of peristaltic activity in the colon.

Spicy foods produce diarrhea and flatus in some individuals. Excessive sugar also can cause diarrhea. Other foods that may influence bowel elimination include the following:

- Gas-producing foods, such as cabbage, onions, cauliflower, bananas, and apples
- Laxative-producing foods, such as bran, prunes, figs, chocolate, and alcohol
- Constipation-producing foods, such as cheese, pasta, eggs, and lean meat.

Fluid

Healthy fecal elimination requires a daily fluid intake of 2000–3000 mL, but even when fluid intake is inadequate or output (e.g., urine, vomitus) is excessive, the body continues to reabsorb fluid from the chyme as it passes along the intestinal tract. The chyme becomes drier than normal, and the result is hard feces. In addition, reduced fluid intake slows the passage of chyme along the intestines, further increasing the absorption of fluid. If, on the other hand, chyme moves abnormally quickly through the large intestine, the decreased time available for fluid absorption results in softer, loose, or watery feces.

Activity

Activity stimulates peristalsis, facilitating the movement of chyme through the colon. Weak abdominal and pelvic muscles often are ineffective in increasing the intra-abdominal pressure during defecation or in controlling defecation. Weak muscles can result from lack of exercise, immobility, or impaired neurologic functioning. Patients confined to bed often experience constipation resulting from decreased peristalsis.

Defecation Habits

Early bowel training may establish the habit of defecating at a regular time. Many individuals defecate after breakfast, when the gastrocolic reflex causes mass peristaltic waves in the large intestine. If an individual ignores the urge to defecate, water continues to be absorbed, and the feces become hard and difficult to expel. When the normal defecation reflexes are inhibited or ignored, these conditioned reflexes tend to weaken progressively. When habitually ignored, the urge to defecate is ultimately lost. Adults may ignore these reflexes because of the pressures of time or obligations. Hospitalized patients may suppress the urge because of embarrassment about using a bedpan or lack of privacy or because defecation is too uncomfortable.

Medications

Some drugs have side effects that interfere with normal elimination. Large doses of tranquilizers and repeated administration of morphine or codeine decreases gastrointestinal activity, causing constipation. Iron tablets, which have an astringent effect, act more locally on the bowel mucosa to cause constipation. A variety of drugs can cause diarrhea.

Some medications directly affect elimination. **Laxatives** are medications that stimulate bowel activity and promote fecal elimination. Stool softeners facilitate defecation by drawing water into the feces. Antidiarrheal medications work by suppressing peristaltic activity.

Medications also affect the appearance of the feces. Any drug that causes gastrointestinal bleeding (e.g., aspirin products) can cause the stool to be red or black. Iron salts cause black stool because of the oxidation of the iron. Antibiotics may cause a gray-green discoloration. Antacids can cause a whitish discoloration or white specks in the stool. Bismuth subsalicylate, a common over-the-counter drug, causes stools to be black.

Diagnostic Procedures

Before certain diagnostic procedures, such as visualization of the colon (colonoscopy or sigmoidoscopy), the patient is restricted from ingesting food or fluid. Laxatives may be prescribed to be taken on the day prior to the procedure. The patient may also be given a cleansing enema before an examination. In these instances, normal defecation does not usually occur until eating resumes.

Anesthesia and Surgical Procedures

General anesthetics cause the normal colonic movements to cease or slow by blocking parasympathetic stimulation to the muscles of the colon. Patients who have regional or spinal anesthesia are less likely to experience this problem.

Surgery that involves direct handling of the intestines can cause temporary cessation of intestinal movement; this is referred to as an **ileus** or *paralytic ileus* and usually lasts from 24 to 48 hours postoperatively. Proper auscultation of bowel sounds that reflect intestinal motility is an important nursing assessment skill, especially following an abdominal surgery.

Pathologic Conditions

Spinal cord and head injuries can reduce the sensory stimulation for defecation. Impaired mobility may limit the patient's ability to respond to the urge to defecate, and the patient may experience constipation as a result. A patient may also experience fecal incontinence because of a poorly functioning anal sphincter.

Pain

Patients who experience discomfort when defecating (e.g., following hemorrhoid surgery or anal fissure repair) often suppress the urge to defecate to avoid increased pain. These patients can experience constipation as a result. Patients taking narcotic analgesics for pain also experience constipation as a side effect of the medication.

Psychologic Factors

Anxiety or anger may lead to increased peristaltic activity and consequent nausea or diarrhea. In contrast, depression may cause slowed intestinal motility, resulting in constipation. An individual's response to these emotional states is the result of variations in the response of the enteric nervous system to vagal stimulation from the brain.

Alterations in Bowel Elimination

Impaired peristalsis leads to alterations in bowel elimination. Manifestations may include anal leakage of loose, watery fecal material without stimulation or hardened fecal material that is difficult to expel.

Alterations and Manifestations

Four common problems are related to fecal elimination: diarrhea, flatulence, constipation, and bowel incontinence. Bowel incontinence and constipation are discussed in depth in Exemplar 5.C on Bowel Incontinence, Constipation, and Impaction. For more details, see the Alterations and Therapies feature.

Diarrhea

Diarrhea, the passage of liquid feces with increased frequency, results from rapid movement of fecal contents through the large intestine. Rapid passage of chyme reduces the time available for the large intestine to absorb water and electrolytes. The individual with diarrhea finds it difficult or impossible to maintain control of the urge to defecate. Often, spasmodic cramps are associated with diarrhea. Bowel sounds become more frequent because of increased transit

TABLE 5–5 Major Causes of Diarrhea

Cause	Physiologic Effect
Psychologic stress (e.g., anxiety)	Increased intestinal motility and secretion of mucus
Infection	Overgrowth or breakdown of pathogenic microorganisms in the intestines, causing inflammation of the mucosa
Medications	Irritation and inflammation of the mucosa
Antibiotics	Irritation of intestinal mucosa and imbalance of good and bad intestinal bacteria
Iron	Irritation of intestinal mucosa
Cathartics	Incomplete digestion of food or fluid
Allergy to food, fluid, or drugs	Increased intestinal motility and secretion of mucus
Intolerance of food or fluid	Reduced absorption of fluids
Diseases of the colon (e.g., malabsorption syndrome, Crohn disease)	Inflammation of the mucosa, often leading to ulcer formation

time. With persistent diarrhea, irritation of the anal region, which can extend to the perineum and buttocks, generally results. Fatigue, weakness, malaise, and emaciation are the results of prolonged diarrhea.

Diarrhea is thought to be a protective flushing mechanism caused by irritants in the intestinal tract. However, it can create serious fluid and electrolyte losses in the body, and these losses can develop quickly, particularly in infants, small children, and older adults. **Table 5–5** »» lists some of the major causes of diarrhea and the physiologic responses of the body.

The irritating effects of diarrheal stools increase the risk for skin breakdown. The area around the anal region should be kept clean and dry and protected with a skin barrier containing zinc oxide. In addition, a rectal tube with a collection bag can be inserted.

Flatulence

Most gases that are swallowed are expelled orally by eructation (belching). Large amounts of gases can accumulate in the stomach resulting in gastric distention. The gases that form in the large intestine are chiefly absorbed through the intestinal capillaries into the circulation. **Flatulence** is the presence of excessive flatus in the intestine that leads to inflation and stretching of the intestines (intestinal distention). Flatus has three primary sources: action of bacteria on the chyme in the large intestine, swallowed air, and gas that diffuses between the bloodstream and the intestine. In addition, flatulence can occur in the colon from a variety of causes, including foods (e.g., cabbage, onions), abdominal surgery, or narcotics. If the gas is propelled by increased colon activity before it can be absorbed, it may be expelled through the anus. If excessive gas cannot be expelled through the anus, it may be necessary to insert a rectal tube to relieve the pressure.

Constipation

Constipation is characterized by the passage of fewer than three bowel movements per week or by difficulty in passing stools. Manifestations of this condition may include the absence of stool passage or the passage of dry, hardened stool. In most cases, constipation is due to decreased motility and slow movement of feces through the large intestine. Constipation may reflect a primary problem, or it may indicate an underlying disorder.

Bowel Incontinence

Bowel incontinence or **fecal incontinence** is the inability to voluntarily control the passing of fecal contents and

intestinal gas through the anal sphincter. In most cases, fecal incontinence is a manifestation of another disorder. Numerous conditions may cause fecal incontinence, including neurologic disorders; depression; traumatic injuries; an inflammatory process affecting the bowel; and masses, hemorrhoids, or deformity in the anus. Episodes of incontinence may be unpredictable, or they may occur at specific intervals, such as following meals. For patients who experience fecal incontinence, embarrassment and shame may lead to social isolation.

Alterations and Therapies
Bowel Elimination

ALTERATION	DESCRIPTION/ DEFINITION	MANIFESTATIONS	INTERVENTIONS AND THERAPIES
Constipation	Infrequent passage of hard stool	Straining with defecation; Lumpy or hard stools; Sensation of incomplete emptying; Fewer than three bowel movements per week	Increase fluid and fiber intake. Increase activity level. Administer enema. Constipation may require medications (e.g., stool softeners, laxatives, cathartics). Evaluate medication profile for gastrointestinal side effects.
Diarrhea	Passage of liquid stools	Frequent, runny stools; Hyperactive bowel sounds; Bowel incontinence; Abdominal cramps; Fever; Dehydration	Increase fluid intake. Administer antidiarrheal medications. Assess for cause (medications, diet, infection).
Bowel incontinence	Inability to control release of feces	Leakage of feces from the anus; Loss of pelvic muscle control; Lack of ability to respond to urge to defecate	Administer bowel training. Treat with surgery (sphincter repair and fecal diversion or colostomy). Remove fecal impaction if present. Diet adjustment (e.g., avoid alcohol and caffeine; increase fiber). Administer medications (e.g., antidiarrheal drugs).
Impaction	Mass or collection of hardened feces in the folds of the rectum	Constipation; Fecal incontinence; Abdominal cramping; Straining during defecation; Small, liquid stools; Loss of bladder control	Manual removal may be necessary. Administer enema as necessary. Increase fluid and fiber intake, stool softeners, and increase activity to prevent recurrence. Evaluate medication profile for gastrointestinal side effects. Improve defecation habits, and reduce constipation.
Bowel cancer	Abnormal growth of cells in the bowel	Early cancer: possibly no symptoms; Blood in the stool; Change in the diameter of stools; Persistent change in bowel habits; Abdominal pain; Unexplained weight loss; Anemia; Bowel obstruction; Vomiting	Take preventive measures, and make an early diagnosis. Remove surgically. Administer chemotherapy or radiation therapy.
Obstruction	Blockage in the bowel preventing or reducing the passage of fecal material	Abdominal distention and cramping; Abdominal fullness; Constipation or diarrhea; Vomiting; Inability to pass gas	Remove blockage surgically. Use nasogastric tube to relieve abdominal pressure.

Prevalence

The prevalence of bowel problems varies based on etiology. Adults in the United States usually have one episode of acute diarrhea each year, on average, whereas children usually have two per year (NIDDK, 2012b). The prevalence of constipation in adult populations ranges from 2.6 to 26.9%, a median of 15.4% (Schmidt & Santos, 2014). Children have a prevalence of bowel problems between 0.1 and 30% worldwide (Nurko & Zimmerman, 2014). In addition, approximately 5.6–29% of patients admit to fecal incontinence when specifically questioned (Alsheik et al., 2012).

Genetic Considerations and Risk Factors

Age is a major risk factor for bowel problems. Both young children and older adults are at higher risk for diarrhea, constipation, and fecal incontinence than individuals in other age groups. Women are at higher risk than men for fecal incontinence, especially after pregnancy. Immobility or disability and chronic diseases such as multiple sclerosis and diabetes are major risk factors for constipation.

Nursing Assessment

Assessment of a patient with potential bowel elimination problems is vital to understanding the causative factor, its impact on health and wellness, and the treatment options. Nursing assessment includes collecting information about health history, physical assessment, and results from diagnostic tests. Assessment of fecal elimination includes obtaining subjective information; conducting an objective physical examination of the abdomen, rectum, and anus; and inspecting the feces.

SAFETY ALERT Never use deep palpation in a patient who has had a pulsatile abdominal mass, renal transplant, or polycystic kidneys or on a patient who is at risk for hemorrhage.

Observation and Patient History

During the assessment, the nurse will observe the patient's behavior for cues of abdominal discomfort such as grimacing, guarding, or frequent position changes. If in a home environment or the patient's room, the nurse can conduct a quick assessment of the environment to note any odor, soiling on clothing, or excess linens. The nurse can use these cues as an opener to discuss any issues with elimination.

Collecting data regarding fecal elimination helps the nurse to identify the patient's normal pattern. The nurse should obtain a description of usual defecation and any recent changes. The nurse should also collect information about any past or current problems with elimination, presence of an ostomy, and factors influencing the elimination pattern. Each person's defecation patterns are dependent on many variables that affect the time of day of defecation, the amount and consistency of feces expelled, and the frequency of defecation. The individual's usual bowel routines may develop primarily from early toilet training and out of convenience.

Examples of questions to elicit this information are listed below. The number of questions to ask is adapted to the individual patient, according to the patient's responses in the first three categories listed.

Defecation Pattern

- What time of the day do you usually have a bowel movement?
- Has this pattern changed recently?

Description of Feces and Any Changes

- Have you noticed any changes in the color, texture (hard, soft, watery), shape, or odor of your stool recently?

Fecal Elimination Problems

- What problems have you had or do you now have with your bowel movements (constipation, diarrhea, excessive flatulence, leaking of feces, or incontinence)?
- When and how often do they occur?
- What do you think causes these problems (food, fluids, exercise, emotions, medications, disease, surgery)?
- What have you tried to solve the problems, and how effective was it?

Factors Influencing Elimination

- ***Use of elimination aids.*** What routines do you follow to maintain your usual defecation pattern? Do you use natural aids such as specific foods or fluids (e.g., a glass of hot lemon juice before breakfast), laxatives, or enemas to maintain elimination?
- ***Diet.*** What foods do you believe affect defecation? What foods do you typically eat? What foods do you avoid? Do you take meals at regular times?
- ***Fluid.*** What amount and kind of fluid do you take each day (e.g., six glasses of water, two cups of coffee)?
- ***Exercise.*** What is your usual daily exercise pattern? (Obtain specifics about exercise rather than asking whether it is sufficient; ideas of what is sufficient will vary among individuals.)
- ***Medications.*** Have you taken any medications that could affect the intestinal tract (e.g., iron, antibiotics)? (Note the name and specific dosage of all medications because the patient may not be aware what medications may affect elimination.)
- ***Stress.*** Are you experiencing any stress? Do you think it affects your defecation pattern? If so, how?

Presence and Management of Ostomy

- What is your usual routine with your colostomy/ileostomy?
- What type of appliance do you wear, and did you bring a spare with you?
- What problems, if any, do you have with it?
- How can the nurses help you manage your colostomy/ileostomy?

Physical Examination

Physical examination of the abdomen in relation to fecal elimination problems includes inspection, auscultation, percussion, and palpation with specific reference to the intestinal tract (see the Bowel Assessment feature). Auscultation precedes palpation, because palpation can alter peristalsis. Examination of the rectum and anus includes inspection and palpation (see **Figure 5–3 »**). Observe the patient's stool for color, consistency, shape, amount, odor, and presence of abnormal constituents.

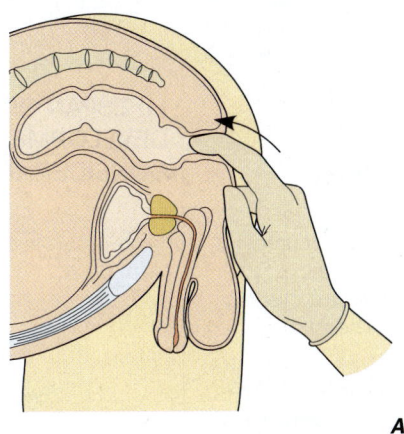 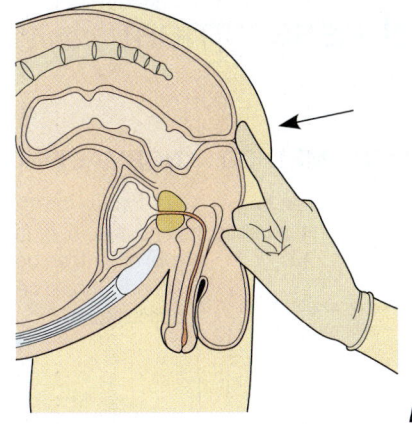

A   B

Figure 5–3 >> Digital examination of the **A**, rectum and **B**, anus.

Bowel Assessment

ASSESSMENT/METHOD	NORMAL FINDINGS	ABNORMAL FINDINGS	LIFESPAN OR DEVELOPMENTAL CONSIDERATIONS
Abdominal Assessment			
Inspect abdominal contour, skin integrity, and venous pattern and for aortic pulsation.	Abdomen should be slightly concave with intact skin. There should not be distended veins or obvious aortic pulsations.	■ Generalized abdominal distention may be seen in gas retention or obesity. ■ Lower midline abdominal distention is seen in bladder distention or ovarian mass. ■ General distention and an inverted umbilicus are seen with ascites and/or tumors. ■ A scaphoid (sunken) abdomen is seen in malnutrition or when fat is replaced with muscle. ■ **Striae** (white or silvery colored stretch marks) are seen in obesity. ■ Spider angiomas may be seen in liver disease. ■ Dilated veins are prominent in cirrhosis of the liver, ascites, portal hypertension, or obstructed vena cava. ■ Pulsation is visible with aortic aneurysm and may be significant.	■ Pregnant women have lower abdominal distention to accommodate the growing fetus and may have striae and linea nigra. ■ Infants and toddlers may have normal age-related abdominal distention, especially after feeding. ■ Allow young children to sit or lie on a parent's lap during the assessment if needed.
Auscultate all four quadrants of the abdomen with the diaphragm of the stethoscope. Begin in the lower right quadrant, where bowel sounds are almost always present.	Normal bowel sounds (gurgling or clicking) occur every 5–15 seconds. Listen for at least 5 minutes in each of the four quadrants to confirm the absence of bowel sounds.	■ **Borborygmus** (high-pitched, tinkling, rushing, or growling bowel sounds) will be hyperactive with diarrhea or at the onset of bowel obstruction. ■ Bowel sounds may be absent in late bowel obstruction, with an inflamed peritoneum, and/or following surgery of the abdomen.	■ Pregnant women may have decreased bowel sounds.

(continued on next page)

Bowel Assessment (continued)

ASSESSMENT/METHOD	NORMAL FINDINGS	ABNORMAL FINDINGS	LIFESPAN OR DEVELOPMENTAL CONSIDERATIONS
Auscultate the abdomen for vascular sounds with the bell of the stethoscope.	No sounds (bruits, venous hum, or friction rub) other than bowel sounds should be auscultated.	<ul><li>**Bruits** (blowing sound due to restriction of blood flow through vessels) may be heard over constricted arteries. A bruit over the liver may be heard in hepatic carcinoma.</li><li>A venous hum (continuous medium-pitched sound) may be heard over a cirrhotic liver.</li><li>Friction rubs (rough grating sounds) may be heard over an inflamed liver or spleen.</li></ul>	
Percuss the abdomen in all four quadrants.	Normally, is heard over the stomach and gas-filled bowels.	<ul><li>Dullness is heard when the bowel is displaced by fluid or tumors or filled with a fecal mass.</li></ul>	
Palpate the abdomen in all four quadrants. Use a circular motion to move the abdominal wall over underlying structures. Feel for masses, and note any tenderness or pain the patient may have during this part of the exam. Palpate lightly at first (0.5–0.75 inch), then more deeply (1.5–2 inch) with caution. If a mass is palpated, ask the patient to raise head and shoulders.	There should be no abdominal masses or pain on palpation.	<ul><li>A mass in the abdomen may become more prominent when the head and shoulders are raised, as will a ventral abdominal wall hernia. If it becomes nonpalpable the mass is deeper within the abdomen.</li><li>In cases of peritoneal inflammation, palpation causes abdominal pain and involuntary muscle spasms.</li><li>Abnormal masses include aortic aneurysms, neoplastic tumors of the colon or uterus, and a distended bladder or distended bowel due to obstruction.</li><li>A rigid, board-like abdomen is palpable when the patient has a perforated duodenal ulcer.</li></ul>	<ul><li>Children may complain of abdominal pain because of stressful events (e.g., tests) or emotional trauma (e.g., bullying, abuse).</li></ul>
Palpate for rebound tenderness. Press the fingers into the abdomen slowly and release the pressure quickly.	Releasing pressure should not cause or increase pain.	<ul><li>In peritoneal inflammation, pain occurs when the fingers are withdrawn.</li><li>Right upper quadrant pain occurs with acute cholecystitis.</li><li>Upper middle abdominal pain occurs with acute pancreatitis.</li><li>Right lower quadrant pain at McBurney's point occurs with acute appendicitis.</li><li>Left lower quadrant pain is seen in acute diverticulitis.</li></ul>	

Inguinal Area Assessment

ASSESSMENT/METHOD	NORMAL FINDINGS	ABNORMAL FINDINGS	LIFESPAN OR DEVELOPMENTAL CONSIDERATIONS
Inspect the inguinal area for bulges after asking the patient to bear down.	The inguinal area is normally free of bulges.	<ul><li>Bulges that appear in the inguinal area when the patient bears down may indicate a **hernia** (a defect in the abdominal wall that allows abdominal contents to protrude outward).</li></ul>	<ul><li>Inguinal hernias in infants are most obvious when the infant is crying, coughing, or straining during a bowel movement.</li><li>Male patients are more likely than female patients to develop inguinal hernias, regardless of age.</li></ul>

Bowel Assessment *(continued)*

ASSESSMENT/METHOD	NORMAL FINDINGS	ABNORMAL FINDINGS	LIFESPAN OR DEVELOPMENTAL CONSIDERATIONS
Palpate the inguinal area with a gloved hand. Ask the patient to shift weight to the left to palpate the right inguinal area and vice versa. Place your right index finger upward into the inguinal area and ask the patient to bear down or cough.	Bulging or masses are normally not palpable.	◾ A bulge or mass may indicate a hernia.	

Perianal Assessment

Inspect the perianal area. Wearing gloves, spread the patient's buttocks apart. Observe the area, and ask patient to bear down as if trying to have a bowel movement.	The perianal area should be intact, without obvious lesions.	◾ Swollen, painful, longitudinal breaks in the anal area may appear in patients with anal fissures. (These are caused by the passing of large, hard stools or by diarrhea.) ◾ Dilated anal veins appear with hemorrhoids. ◾ A red mass may appear with prolapsed internal hemorrhoids. ◾ Doughnut-shaped red tissue at the anal area may appear with a prolapsed rectum.	◾ A parent or guardian should be present during rectal examination of all minors. ◾ Some patients prefer to have the examination performed by a clinician of the same gender. ◾ Expect the possibility of fecal elimination when the patient bears down, especially in older adults with fecal incontinence.
Palpate the anus and rectum. Lubricate the gloved index finger, and ask the patient to bear down. Touch the tip of your finger to the patient's anal opening. Flex the index finger, and slowly insert it into the anus, pointing the finger toward the umbilicus (see Figure 5–3). Rotate the finger in both directions to palpate any lesions or masses.	There should be no masses in the anus or rectum.	◾ Movable, soft masses may be polyps. ◾ Hard, firm, irregular embedded masses may indicate carcinoma.	◾ Digital rectal examination (DRE) is often not tolerated well by children or their parents. It also has limited usefulness in assessing constipation in children. ◾ Be aware of skin fragility in older adults when performing a DRE.

Fecal Assessment

Inspect the patient's feces. After palpating the rectum, withdraw finger gently. Inspect any feces on the glove. Note color and/or presence of blood. Also use gloved fingers to determine consistency.	Stool should be soft with no blood present, either on the stool or as occult blood.		◾ Neonatal feces are referred to as meconium and are dark-green, almost black in color and sticky. Meconium can be difficult to clean from the neonatal skin. After 2–3 days the meconium will pass, and the feces will become yellow, tan, or light-green.
Test the feces for occult blood. Use an occult blood testing kit, and follow facility protocol for procedure.	There should be no blood in the feces.	◾ A positive occult blood test requires further testing for colon cancer or gastrointestinal bleeding due to peptic ulcers, ulcerative colitis, or diverticulosis.	
Note the odor of the feces.	No distinctly foul odors should be present.	◾ Distinctly foul odors may be noted with stools containing blood or extra fat or in cases of colon cancer.	

Diagnostic Tests

Diagnostic tests for bowel elimination problems include blood and fecal tests. Blood tests may be used to determine whether bowel problems have a systemic cause, and fecal tests can determine whether the problem is related to infection and detect the presence of blood or toxins. A DRE is performed to reveal abnormalities in the rectum and evaluate the strength of the sphincter muscles. A colonoscopy is often used to visualize the colon and rectum to screen for polyps, cysts, tumors, lesions, diverticula, inflammation, bleeding, and the general integrity of the mucosal lining. Tissue samples can be obtained for biopsy during a colonoscopy. X-ray imaging, including barium enema x-ray and defecography, can be performed to visualize the colon and part of the small intestine to determine how efficiently feces is evacuated. An anorectal manometry procedure is used to evaluate anal sphincter muscle function, and a colorectal transit study is used to determine how food moves through the colon.

Independent Interventions

Patients with bowel elimination problems require prompt and thorough nursing care. Both independent and collaborative interventions are beneficial for treating patients with diarrhea, constipation, bowel incontinence, and flatulence.

For patients with constipation, interventions include encouraging increased intake of fluid and fiber and teaching about the impact of dietary choices on bowel elimination. Bowel training using strategies such as digital stimulation can be implemented by the nurse or taught to the patient to help establish a regular schedule for bowel movements. (For discussion of digital stimulation, see Exemplar 5.C on Bowel Incontinence, Constipation, and Impaction.) Pelvic floor exercises and biofeedback can also be used to help the patient strengthen rectal muscles. Instruct the patient to use caution when straining the abdominal muscles during defecation, because it may close the anal sphincter rather than allowing feces to pass through. For patients with fecal incontinence, nursing care may include providing personal hygiene for the patient, especially if the patient is immobile. Regular assessment of the anal area is necessary to detect skin breakdown or other problems. If the patient has an ostomy, nursing care will require assisting the patient as needed to keep the pouch clean and the stoma free of infection or tissue excoriation.

Collaborative Therapies

Many bowel elimination problems are treated in collaboration with healthcare providers and surgeons. Healthcare providers may prescribe medications such as laxatives, antidiarrheal agents, or stool softeners. Medications may be given to promote bowel movement, to promote absorption of excess fluid in the intestine, or to coalesce gas or reduce the production of gas. For details regarding medications, see the Medications feature.

Patients with more acute problems, such as obstruction, ulceration, perforation, or cancer, may require surgical resection of the bowel with or without creation of an ostomy.

Medications
Bowel Elimination

CLASSIFICATION AND DRUG EXAMPLES	MECHANISMS OF ACTION	NURSING CONSIDERATIONS
Laxatives ■ Bulk-forming agents ■ Stool softeners ■ Stimulants ■ Saline or osmotic laxatives ■ Herbal agents ■ Miscellaneous agents *Drug examples:* Psyllium hydrophilic mucilloid, methylcellulose, docusate sodium, senna, mineral oil, Epsom salts	Promote bowel movement	■ Use is contraindicated in patients with nausea, cramps, colic, vomiting, or undiagnosed abdominal pain. Use is also contraindicated in patients after abdominal surgery. ■ Laxatives should not be used continuously, because they weaken the bowel's natural response to fecal distention, affecting peristalsis. ■ Before administration, assess abdomen for distention, bowel sounds, and bowel patterns. ■ Teach patients preventive measures for constipation to avoid overdependence on laxatives.
Antidiarrheal Agents *Drug examples:* Diphenoxylate with atropine, camphorated opium tincture, difenoxin with atropine, loperamide, bismuth salts, furazolidone	Slow motility of the intestines or promote absorption of excess fluid in the intestine	■ Monitor fluid and electrolyte status. ■ Use is contraindicated in patients with severe dehydration, electrolyte imbalance, liver and renal disorders, and glaucoma. ■ Teach patients to seek medical care if diarrhea does not subside in 2 days, fever develops, or dehydration occurs.
Antiflatulent Agents *Drug examples:* Simethicone	Coalesce gas bubbles and facilitate passage	■ Teach patients to seek medical care if symptoms persist or recur. ■ Side effects include bloating, constipation, diarrhea, and heartburn.

Source: Data from Adams, M. P., Holland, L. N., & Urban, C. (2017). *Pharmacology for nurses: A pathophysiologic approach* (5th ed.). Hoboken, NJ: Pearson Education.

Case Study » Part 2

Mr. Welborn's physician consults with a urologist, who suggests that Mr. Welborn be admitted to the hospital for a percutaneous nephrolithotomy. The urologist prescribes intravenous (IV) morphine for pain and schedules the surgery for 8:00 the next morning. The procedure is successful, without complications, and a urinary catheter and nephrostomy tube are put in place during surgery to drain urine. Postoperative pain is again managed with IV morphine, and Mr. Welborn states that his pain is manageable. He is confined to bed until 1 day postsurgery. The day after surgery, Mr. Welborn reports that he did not have his normal morning bowel movement. When he sat on the toilet, he was unable to defecate, and he was afraid to push too hard because of his surgery. He was also unable to have a bowel movement the previous morning because of anxiety about the surgery, and his abdomen is feeling full. Abdominal assessment reveals diminished bowel sounds and dullness to percussion.

Clinical Reasoning Questions Level I

1. What factors may have contributed to Mr. Welborn's constipation?
2. What independent nursing interventions can you implement to help Mr. Welborn eliminate feces?
3. What patient teaching can you provide to help Mr. Welborn prevent constipation in the future?

Clinical Reasoning Questions Level II

4. What effects might Mr. Welborn's constipation have on his urinary problems?
5. What complications may develop as a result of Mr. Welborn's constipation? What assessments should you perform to detect these complications?
6. What side effects of the percutaneous nephrolithotomy may Mr. Welborn experience related to his urinary system?

Lifespan Considerations

Defecation patterns vary at different stages of life. Altered elimination patterns may occur in newborns and infants, toddlers, school-age children, pregnant women, and older adults. Also see the Bowel Assessment Feature for additional lifespan and development considerations.

Bowel Elimination in Newborns and Infants

Term newborns usually pass meconium within 8–24 hours of life and almost always within 48 hours. **Meconium** is formed in utero from the amniotic fluid contents, intestinal secretions, and shed mucosal cells. It can be recognized by its thick, tarry black or dark green appearance (see **Figure 5–4A »**). Transitional (thin brown to green) stools consisting of part meconium and part fecal material are passed for the next day or two, and then the stools become entirely fecal.

Frequency of bowel movement in infants varies but ranges from one every 2 or 3 days to as many as 10 movements daily. Totally breastfed infants may have a bowel movement with every feeding for the first several weeks, then gradually progress to fewer bowel movements. Formula-fed infants also have frequent bowel movements, but not as frequently as breastfed infants, usually 4 or 5 movements per day. Between 1 and 2 months of age, the infant's bowel movement pattern changes. Infants may defecate from one or more times a day to once every 1–2 weeks. Mothers should be counseled that the newborn is not constipated as long as the bowel movement remains soft. Formula-fed infants are more likely to experience constipation than breastfed infants.

Because the intestine is immature, water is not well absorbed, and the stool is soft and liquid. Stools from breastfed infants are usually mustard yellow and may have a seedy appearance (see Figure 5–4B). Formula-fed infants have stools that range from tan to yellow to green (see Figure 5–4C). As long as blood is not present, any color is normal. The formula-fed infant has stool that is slightly firmer than that of a breastfed infant.

When the intestine matures, bacterial flora increase. After solid foods are introduced, the stool becomes firmer and less frequent. The odor that accompanies a bowel movement is more offensive once the infant starts to eat solid food.

Bowel Elimination in Toddlers

Some control of defecation starts between 1.5 and 2 years of age. By this time, children have learned to walk, and their

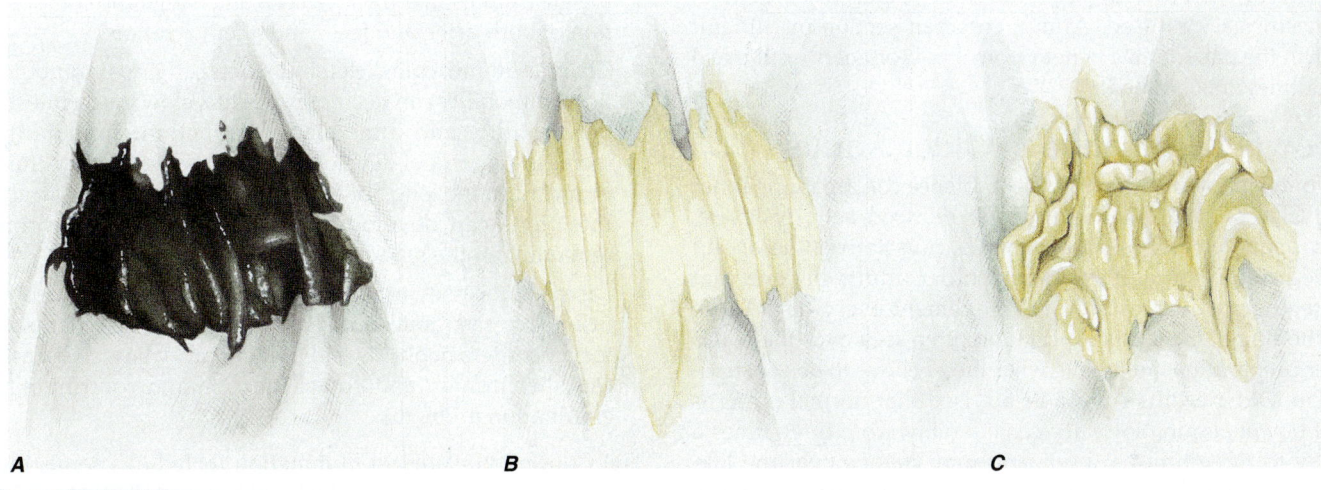

Source: Brigitte Hall.

Figure 5–4 » Newborn stool samples. ***A,*** Meconium, ***B,*** Breastfed newborn stool, ***C,*** Formula-fed newborn stool.

nervous and muscular systems are sufficiently well developed to permit bowel control. A desire to control daytime bowel movements and to use the toilet generally starts when the child becomes aware of the discomfort caused by a soiled diaper and the sensation that indicates the need for a bowel movement. Daytime control is typically attained by 2.5 years of age, after a process of toilet training.

Bowel Elimination in School-Age Children and Adolescents

School-age children and adolescents have bowel habits similar to those of adults. Patterns of defecation vary in frequency, quantity, and consistency. Some school-age children may delay defecation for play or another activity.

Bowel Elimination in Pregnant Women

During pregnancy, elevated progesterone levels cause smooth muscle relaxation, resulting in delayed gastric emptying and decreased peristalsis. As a result, the pregnant woman may complain of bloating and constipation. These symptoms are aggravated as the enlarging uterus displaces the stomach upward and the intestines are moved laterally and posteriorly. The cardiac sphincter also relaxes, and heartburn (pyrosis) may occur as a result of **gastric reflux**, a backward flow of acidic secretions into the lower esophagus. Hemorrhoids frequently develop in late pregnancy from constipation and from pressure on vessels below the level of the uterus.

The bowels tend to be sluggish following birth because of the lingering effects of progesterone, decreased abdominal muscle tone, and bowel evacuation associated with the labor and birth process. A woman who has had an episiotomy, lacerations, or hemorrhoids may delay elimination for fear of increasing her pain or because she believes her stitches will be torn if she bears down. In refusing or delaying the bowel movement, the woman may cause increased constipation and pain when bowel elimination finally occurs.

The woman who has had a cesarean birth may experience some initial discomfort from flatulence, which can be relieved by early ambulation and use of antiflatulent medications. Chamomile or peppermint tea may also be helpful in reducing discomfort from flatulence. It may take a few days for the bowel to regain its tone, especially if general anesthesia was used. After a cesarean section or difficult birth the patient may benefit from stool softeners until usual routines are obtained.

Bowel Elimination in Older Adults

Up to half of all older adults experience constipation (Toner & Claros, 2012). Causes include reduced activity levels, inadequate fluid and fiber intake, muscle weakness, and medication side effects. Many older adults believe that "regularity" means a bowel movement every day. Those who do not meet this expectation often seek over-the-counter preparations to relieve what they believe to be constipation. Older adults should be advised that normal patterns of bowel elimination vary considerably, from three times a day to three times a week, and may change over the lifespan. Adequate roughage in the diet, adequate exercise, and six to eight glasses of fluid daily are essential measures

to prevent constipation. A cup of hot water, coffee, or tea at a regular time in the morning is also helpful for some. Responding to the **gastrocolic reflex** (increased peristalsis of the colon after food has entered the stomach) is an important consideration as well. For example, toileting is recommended 5–15 minutes after meals—especially after breakfast, when the gastrocolic reflex is strongest (McKay, Fravel, & Scanlon, 2012).

The nurse should advise older adults that consistent use of laxatives inhibits natural defecation reflexes and will eventually cause chronic constipation. Habitual use of laxatives will eventually require stronger and increasing doses to obtain the intended effects. Laxatives may also interfere with the body's electrolyte balance and reduce the absorption of various vitamins. The nurse should carefully evaluate any complaints of constipation. A change in bowel habits over several weeks with or without weight loss, pain, or fever should be referred to a primary care provider for a complete medical evaluation.

Concepts Related to Elimination

Elimination processes are an indirect gauge of general health. Alterations in elimination may reflect impaired function of other body systems, side effects from medications, or improper levels of hydration or nutrition. Alterations that may affect elimination include:

- Changes in neurologic function, such as those associated with multiple sclerosis, Parkinson disease, or spinal cord injury, affect innervation of the urinary and gastrointestinal muscles and can lead to absent or inadequate control of the bladder and bowels.

- Increased or decreased food and fluid intake, as well as unhealthy food and drink choices, can alter urine and fecal volume and composition, ultimately contributing to elimination problems.

- Changes in respiratory and cardiovascular function can cause alterations in urinary pH, renal blood flow, and glomerular pressure in the kidney, all of which contribute to alterations in urine composition and volume.

- Changes in liver and gallbladder function alter the body's ability to digest fats and utilize nutrients absorbed from the gastrointestinal tract, which can change the composition of both urine and feces and alter excretion.

- Changes in musculoskeletal function can impair ambulation; immobility can decrease appetite, slow gastrointestinal motility, and alter bladder function. Immobility increases the risk of developing urinary calculi as calcium drains from the long bones and pools in the urinary tract. Infections can develop from postvoid residual urine remaining in the bladder.

- Disease processes, especially disorders directly related to urinary or gastrointestinal function such as the inflammatory disorders nephritis and inflammatory bowel disease, can alter urinary and bowel function and contribute to elimination problems.

The Concepts Related to Elimination table links some, but not all, of the concepts integral to elimination. They are presented in alphabetical order.

Concepts Related to
Elimination

CONCEPT	RELATIONSHIP TO ELIMINATION	NURSING IMPLICATIONS
Cognition	↓ Cognition = ↓ intake of H_2O and ↓ mobility ↓ Cognition = ↓ functional status ↓ Cognition = ↓ awareness of elimination patterns	■ Monitor I&O. ■ Encourage oral intake of fluids by providing beverages that are accessible and appealing to the patient. ■ Prompt the patient to drink fluids frequently. ■ Assist the patient to consume a healthy diet high in fiber. ■ Assist the patient in maintaining a healthy elimination pattern by prompting and providing assistive devices as needed to access the toilet.
Fluid and Electrolytes	↓ Renal function = ↑ medication toxicity ↓ Renal function = ↑ electrolytes ↓ Renal function = ↑ H_2O and ↑ BP ↑ Urination = ↓ electrolytes ↑ Urination (> intake) = ↓ BP ↑ Urination (> intake) = ↓ H_2O ↓ H_2O = constipation Diarrhea = ↓ H_2O and ↓ electrolytes Diarrhea = ↓ H_2O and ↓ BP Chronic diarrhea = ↓ H_2O and ↓ K^+ ↑ H_2O (> output) = edema, SOB ↑ Medications → impaired renal function	■ Monitor and record I&O, especially for patients with kidney disease, catheters, UTI, diarrhea, and chronic constipation. ■ Monitor and record vital signs, report unexpected or abnormal values. ■ Assess for dehydration: dry mouth and skin, fatigue, ↓ skin turgor, ↑ thirst, ↓ urine output, constipation, headache, dizziness, and tachycardia. ■ Assess for ↑ fluid volume: edema, weight gain, shortness of breath, fluid intake > output, ↑ BP. ■ Review medications and medical history. ■ *Anticipate:* Lab tests = CBC, electrolyte levels, and report abnormal values.
Infection	↑ IV antibiotic use = *Clostridium difficile* *C. diff* = diarrhea, strict isolation, ↑ hand washing, do not use hand sanitizers ↓ H_2O = ↑ UTI ↑ diarrhea = ↑ risk of UTI ↑ Urinary catheter = ↑ CAUTI	■ Assess for diarrhea in patients treated with long-term and multiple IV antibiotics (↑ risk of antibiotic-induced enterocolitis, e.g., *C. diff*). ■ If *C. diff*: follow isolation guidelines; wash hands with soap and water (no alcohol-based hand sanitizers). ■ ↑ Perineal care ■ See the Evidence-Based Practice box for CAUTI. ■ *Anticipate:* NOT administering antidiarrheal medications for infectious diarrheas until cause has been treated.
Inflammation	If: [↑ inflammation = ↑ elimination] then: [↑ elimination = ↓ H_2O, ↓ electrolytes, ↓ absorption of nutrients, ↓ comfort]	■ Monitor urine and feces for blood. ■ Monitor lab results for electrolyte levels, CBC, urinalysis, and report abnormal levels. ■ Assess for pain, diarrhea, frequent elimination. ■ Assess for imbalanced nutrition. ■ *Anticipate:* Total parenteral nutrition (TPN) when NPO.
Mobility	↓ Mobility = ↓ peristalsis ↓ Peristalsis = ↑ constipation ↑ Constipation = ↑ diverticular disease ↑ Constipation = ↑ impaction ↑ Constipation = ↑ bowel obstruction	■ Monitor urinary and fecal output for patients. ■ Administer prophylactic stool softeners or laxatives as prescribed. ■ Catheter care ■ *Anticipate:* Referrals to physical/occupational therapies & assistive devices.
Teaching and Learning	Elimination problems are often related to chronic conditions, so patients will need to learn self-care for discharge home. Elimination problems are common among older adults and hospitalized patients, so staff must be educated about nursing interventions appropriate for these patients.	■ Patient teaching; • Appropriate care for ostomy, catheter, or fecal pouch • Bladder and bowel training methods • Strategies to reduce psychosocial issues related to incontinence • Proper use & side effects of medications • Complications to report to healthcare provider • Proper handling of body waste, hand washing, skin care & perineal hygiene. ■ Teach staff members: • ↑ Privacy when providing bladder or bowel care • Communication techniques that will elicit pertinent information while decreasing shame and embarrassment for patient.

Health Promotion

Healthy lifestyle habits, such as maintaining a healthy weight, exercising regularly, and using good toileting habits can prevent or delay the onset of elimination problems. Good toileting habits include not delaying urination and defecation, not using pelvic floor muscles to force urine flow, and preventing constipation. Refraining from tobacco use, maintaining adequate fluid intake, and avoiding food and drinks that contain bladder irritants (e.g., alcohol, caffeine, high acidity) will help prevent many elimination problems. The patient should maintain pelvic floor muscle strength by performing pelvic floor exercises regularly, especially during pregnancy.

Regular exercise and consuming adequate amounts of fluid and fiber in the diet can prevent constipation and consequent fecal impaction. Patients who have an increased risk of developing constipation, such as those taking opioids, may prevent it by taking daily stool softeners. Fecal incontinence can also be prevented by treating constipation or diarrhea as it occurs.

Modifiable Risk Factors

Obesity is an independent risk factor for urinary incontinence, and evidence indicates that even moderate weight loss can reduce risk for urinary incontinence (Subak, Richter, & Hunskaar, 2009; Vissers et al., 2014). Pregnancy is a risk factor for elimination problems because of the weight of the expanding uterus on the elimination structures contained within the pelvic region. Other risk factors for loss of bladder control include UTIs, increased consumption of bladder irritants, and poor lifestyle habits. Individuals with bowel problems such as constipation are also at higher risk for developing urinary problems.

Medical conditions, procedures, and treatments can increase the risk of developing elimination problems. Medical procedures, especially surgical procedures that require anesthesia, can influence bowel and bladder control. Diarrhea and constipation are common possible side effects for many medications, including antibiotics, proton pump inhibitors, blood pressure medications, opioids, antihistamines, and iron supplements. Conditions such as diabetes, benign prostatic hyperplasia, arthritis, back problems, multiple sclerosis, Parkinson disease, Alzheimer disease, pain, stroke, and spinal cord injury increase the individual's risk of developing elimination problems. Lower socioeconomic status and lower educational levels are risk factors for constipation and diarrhea, most likely because of less access to a healthy diet and clean water, and a higher exposure to disease.

Poor hygiene, especially poor hand hygiene after coming into contact with fecal matter, is a risk factor for diarrhea. Individuals can prevent diarrhea from infection by cleansing hands thoroughly, especially after contacting fecal material (e.g., after defecating or changing an infant's diaper). Diarrhea from rotavirus can be prevented by administration of a rotavirus vaccine (RotaTeq, Rotarix).

Cooking all food completely and storing and handling food correctly can prevent diarrhea. Consuming a poor diet that is low in fiber and fluids is one of the greatest modifiable risk factors for bowel problems in general. Routinely practicing hand hygiene prior to handling food can decrease the spread of infectious elimination problems.

An additional modifiable risk factor for diarrhea is traveling, especially to developing countries that may have poor sanitation and contaminated food and water. When traveling to a foreign country, individuals should use commercially bottled water; should not use ice; and should avoid raw fruits, vegetables, and meat. It is not unusual for people to develop elimination problems simply by eating foods that contain new or unique ingredients, especially if eaten in excess. Local residents may have either built a tolerance to traditional foods or found routine ways of counteracting the distressing side effects.

Screenings

Other than written screening tools or verbal questioning during a nursing assessment or medical examination, there are not many standard screening procedures for elimination problems; therefore, many patients can be left untreated. Screening for elimination problems includes endoscopic procedures, mainly as a screening for colon cancer, though incidentally other conditions are routinely discovered during the process. A routine urinalysis can be performed to screen for infection or abnormal contents that indicate further investigation is warranted.

Basic verbal screening for abnormal symptoms should be included at each regular checkup, especially for older adults. Simple questions such as "Do you have difficulty holding your urine?" and "Do you have problems starting your urine stream?" could identify elimination problems that would otherwise be missed during the assessment. Many older adults believe that most elimination problems are simply the result of the aging process, but bowel and bladder incontinence and retention are never considered normal at any age once toilet training has been accomplished. Patients are more likely to report other medical problems, but elimination problems require a more direct manner of questioning.

Case Study » Part 3

After 3 days in the hospital, Mr. Welborn is discharged to home. His urinary catheter has been removed, and he states that he can urinate without pain. However, the nephrostomy tube remains in place. In addition, his IV morphine has been discontinued, and he now receives acetaminophen (1000 mg q6h). With consistent ambulation and discontinuation of morphine, Mr. Welborn had two bowel movements before discharge.

Clinical Reasoning Questions Level I

1. What methods can you teach Mr. Welborn to help prevent future renal calculi?
2. Describe the patient teaching you will provide Mr. Welborn about caring for his nephrostomy tube.
3. What assessment should be performed on Mr. Welborn before discharge?

Clinical Reasoning Questions Level II

4. What medications might the healthcare provider prescribe for Mr. Welborn upon discharge?
5. What follow-up appointments should you schedule for Mr. Welborn? Why?
6. How would a referral to a nutritionist benefit Mr. Welborn?

REVIEW   The Concept of Elimination

RELATE Link the Concepts

Linking the concept of elimination with the concept of infection:

1. What changes in urinary elimination indicate the presence of a UTI?

2. List the effects viral gastroenteritis has on bowel elimination.

Linking the concept of elimination with the concept of communication:

3. How can therapeutic communication be beneficial when assessing patients with urinary or bowel elimination problems?

4. Describe the importance of accurate documentation when caring for a hospitalized patient with urinary or bowel elimination problems.

READY Go to Volume 3: Clinical Nursing Skills

- SKILL 1.10   Abdomen: Assessing
- SKILL 2.25   Rectal Medication: Administering
- SKILLS 4.1–4.5   Elimination: Assessment—Collecting Specimens
- SKILLS 4.6–4.16   Elimination: Bladder Interventions
- SKILLS 4.17–4.23   Elimination: Bowel Interventions
- SKILLS 4.24–4.27   Elimination: Dialysis
- SKILL 6.1   Hand Hygiene: Performing

REFER Go to Pearson MyLab Nursing and eText

- Additional review materials
- MiniModule: Anatomy and Physiology of Urinary Elimination

REFLECT Apply Your Knowledge

Tony Norwinski is a 7-year-old boy in the second grade. He and his 4-year-old sister, Nyla, live at home with their mother, Diane Norwinski.

Ms. Norwinski is a single parent who works in the cafeteria at the high school. Tony has a problem with wetting the bed occasionally and is too embarrassed to discuss it with anyone. Ms. Norwinski thinks Tony wets the bed because of emotional problems caused by his father leaving them when he was so young. Ms. Norwinski does not want to try anything new to help with the bedwetting because she is afraid it will cause Tony more embarrassment and emotional upset. They try not to talk about the bedwetting because Ms. Norwinski thinks it will make matters worse for Tony and prolong the problem.

Today, both children have an appointment for an annual physical examination with the nurse practitioner prior to starting the new school year. Tony is soft spoken and reserved when questioned about his general heath. Ms. Norwinski is a good historian and offers complete answers about Tony's health history. The nurse notices the odor of urine on Tony's undergarments during the initial assessment. When questioned, Tony looks at his mother and does not answer. Ms. Norwinski looks away and does not answer right away. The nurse remains silent, waiting for a response to the questions.

After a period of silence, Ms. Norwinski reassures Tony and answers the nurse's questions about the odor. Though embarrassed, Tony appears to trust the nurse because he helps his mother explain about the bedwetting.

1. What therapeutic communication techniques could the nurse use to facilitate a full disclosure of the problem?

2. What are some questions the nurse could ask Tony and his mother to obtain the most pertinent information about Tony's situation? What nursing diagnosis would best describe the priority problem?

3. List four other possible nursing diagnoses the nurse may want to incorporate in the plan of care.

Exemplar 5.A
Benign Prostatic Hyperplasia

Exemplar Learning Outcomes

5.A Analyze benign prostatic hyperplasia (BPH) as it relates to elimination.

- Describe the pathophysiology of BPH.
- Describe the etiology of BPH.
- Compare the risk factors and prevention of BPH.
- Identify the clinical manifestations of BPH.
- Summarize diagnostic tests and therapies used by interprofessional teams in the collaborative care of an individual with BPH.
- Differentiate care of patients with BPH across the lifespan.
- Apply the nursing process in providing culturally competent care to an individual with BPH.

Exemplar Key Terms

Androgen, *304*
Benign prostatic hyperplasia (BPH), *304*
Continuous bladder irrigation (CBI), *309*
Detrusor muscles, *305*
Digital rectal examination (DRE), *305*
Dihydrotestosterone (DHT), *304*
Diverticula, *305*
Hydronephrosis, *305*
Hydroureter, *305*
Hyperplasia, *304*
Hypertrophy, *304*
Prostate-specific antigen (PSA), *305*
Prostatitis, *304*
Prostatodynia, *304*
Transurethral incision of the prostate (TUIP), *306*
Transurethral needle ablation (TUNA), *306*
Transurethral resection of the prostate (TURP), *306*
TURP syndrome, *309*
Uroflowmetry, *307*

Overview

Prostatitis refers to inflammatory disorders of the prostate gland. **Prostatodynia** is a condition in which the patient experiences the symptoms of prostatitis but shows no evidence of inflammation or infection. **Benign prostatic hyperplasia (BPH)** is a nonmalignant enlargement of the prostate gland commonly seen in the aging man.

BPH can be a cause of anxiety in the aging patient who fears loss of his virility and ability to maintain a satisfying sex life. Radical surgeries, which were once the only treatment choice, often left men impotent, and the stories from those days still circulate as current fact. Patient education and support play an important role in providing nursing care to patients diagnosed with BPH.

BPH is the most common benign neoplasm in men. It is characterized by a nonmalignant enlargement of the prostate gland that decreases the outflow of urine by obstructing the urethra, ultimately resulting in difficult urination. Although BPH typically begins in the fourth decade, the patient may not experience symptoms until much later, depending on how the individual's condition progresses. BPH is not considered a precursor to prostate cancer.

Pathophysiology and Etiology

Pathophysiology

The prostate gland borders the urethra near the lower part of the bladder. About the size of a chestnut (2 cm), it is partially palpable through the anterior wall of the rectum. The prostate is composed of glandular structures that continuously secrete a milky alkaline solution. During sexual intercourse, glandular activity increases and the alkaline secretions flow into the urethra. Because sperm motility is reduced in an acidic environment, these secretions aid sperm transport. In addition, the prostate gland produces about one third of all semen.

BPH begins as small nodules in the periurethral glands, which are the inner layers of the prostate. The nodules are formed from **hyperplasia** (increase in the number of cells) of the stromal and epithelial cells in the prostate gland rather than **hypertrophy** (increase in the size of individual cells). The terms *hyperplasia* and *hypertrophy* are used interchangeably because they both contribute to the problem. Hyperplasia of prostatic cells occurs over a long period of time, making BPH more common in older men. The pathophysiologic effects result from a combination of factors, including urethral resistance to the effects of BPH, intravesical pressure during voiding, detrusor muscle strength, neurologic functioning, and general physical health.

Etiology

An **androgen** is a type of hormone that stimulates the development and maintenance of male sex characteristics. The androgen testosterone signals the prostate to produce **dihydrotestosterone (DHT)**, which mediates prostatic growth. Although androgen levels decrease in aging men, the aging prostate appears to become more sensitive to available DHT. Estrogen, produced in small amounts in men, appears to sensitize the prostate gland to the effects of DHT. Increasing estrogen levels associated with aging or a relative increase in estrogen related to testosterone levels contributes to prostatic hyperplasia.

Risk Factors

The two main risk factors for developing BPH are age and the presence of testosterone. BPH rarely causes symptoms before age 40, greater than 50% of men have some symptoms of LUTS by their sixth decade. The NIDDK (2014), a division of the National Institutes of Health (NIH), predicts up to 90% of men over the age of 80 will experience symptoms of BPH and almost all men will develop BPH if they live long enough (NIDDK, 2012c). The prevalence of PBH is similar in African American and Caucasian men, but it tends to be more severe and progressive in African American men. (Deters, 2016).

SAFETY ALERT Urinary retention in men with BPH can be precipitated by several classes of medications, including those with anticholinergic properties and over-the-counter medications for the common cold, such as decongestants.

Prevention

Because the overgrowth of prostate cells leading to enlargement is indirectly caused by the presence of testosterone, other than castration at an early age, there is no known prevention for BPH. There is new evidence suggesting a connection between metabolic syndrome and BPH (Fleshner & Bhindi, 2014; Pashootan et al., 2015; Ryl et al., 2015). In light of this new evidence, the best advice for decreasing the risk of BPH is to maintain a healthy lifestyle, control body weight within the recommended ranges for stature, exercise daily, and maintain blood glucose levels with proper management of diet in combination with necessary treatment for hyperglycemia. Over the past 2 decades, multiple studies have attempted to prove the efficacy of using dietary supplements containing antioxidant and anti-inflammatory properties to treat BPH, producing no clearly meaningful or consistent results.

Clinical Manifestations

Although the symptoms of BPH are sometimes referred to as nuisances, they can have a profound effect on daily living. The expanding prostatic tissue compresses the urethra (see **Figure 5–5 》**) and causes partial or complete obstruction of

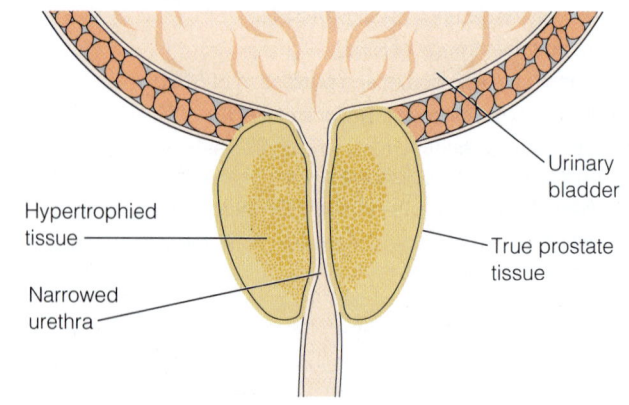

Figure 5–5 》 Benign prostatic hyperplasia.

Clinical Manifestations and Therapies
Benign Prostatic Hyperplasia

ETIOLOGY	CLINICAL MANIFESTATIONS	CLINICAL THERAPIES
Voiding BPH	Weak or intermittent urinary stream, hesitancy, incomplete emptying, dribbling at the end of urination, straining during urination	▪ Pharmacologic therapy ▪ Lifestyle changes
Storage BPH	Frequency, urgency, incontinence, nocturia, dysuria, bladder pain	▪ Pharmacologic therapy ▪ Lifestyle changes
Urinary retention	Bladder distention, diverticula, ureter obstruction, bladder or kidney infection, hydroureter, hydronephrosis, renal insufficiency	▪ Surgery

the outflow of urine from the urinary bladder. Even though the **detrusor muscle** (the muscle in the wall of the bladder that contracts during urination to release urine) becomes hypertrophic to compensate for increased resistance to urinary flow, decreased bladder capability and bladder instability will eventually result. LUTS will manifest as two main types: (1) voiding, such as weak urinary stream, increased time to void, hesitancy, incomplete bladder emptying, and postvoid dribbling; or (2) storage, such as frequency, urgency, incontinence, nocturia, dysuria, and bladder pain. These symptoms are often used to classify BPH. Urinary retention may become chronic, resulting in overflow incontinence with an increase in intra-abdominal pressure. Patients often report the sensation of incomplete bladder emptying. There is little correlation between the size of the prostate gland and the urinary manifestations.

Unless the enlarging mass is reduced, multiple complications may occur. As urine is retained, the bladder will become increasingly distended. **Diverticula** are saclike outward projections of mucosa protruding through the muscular layer of the bladder wall, developing from the pressure of urinary retention. The distention may also obstruct the ureters. Infection, which is more common in retained urine and in diverticula, may ascend from the bladder to the kidneys. Possible complications include **hydroureter** (distention of the ureter with urine), **hydronephrosis** (accumulation of urine in the renal pelvis as a result of obstructed outflow), and renal insufficiency.

Collaboration

Care of patients with BPH will focus on: (1) diagnosing the disorder, (2) correcting or minimizing the urinary obstruction, and (3) preventing or treating complications. Treatment is determined by the severity of the manifestations and the presence of complications. Mild cases are often monitored over time, and symptoms may remain stable, or with management, improvement may occur.

Diagnostic Tests

The most common diagnostic test for BPH is a **digital rectal examination (DRE)** (see **Figure 5–6 »**): The physician inserts a gloved and lubricated finger into the rectum to palpate the prostate gland and determine its size and condition. Several urine tests may be performed, including a urine flow rate test, a postvoid residual urine test, and a pressure flow

study. A urinalysis and urine culture may be done to check for blood or infection. A serum **prostate-specific antigen (PSA)** test may be performed to rule out prostate cancer. In addition, cystoscopy may be performed to visualize the bladder and urethra to rule out other causes of urinary symptoms and to visualize the degree of ureter obstruction (NIDDK, 2012c).

Surgery

Men who have urinary retention, recurrent UTI, hematuria, bladder stones, or renal insufficiency secondary to BPH are candidates for surgical intervention. Surgical treatment may be performed by minimally invasive surgery or through transurethral, open, or laser surgery.

Minimally Invasive Surgery

Not all cases of BPH respond to medications. Therefore, a number of procedures that are less invasive than traditional surgery have been developed to relieve the manifestations of BPH. *Transurethral microwave thermotherapy* uses microwaves to heat and destroy excess prostate tissue. During the

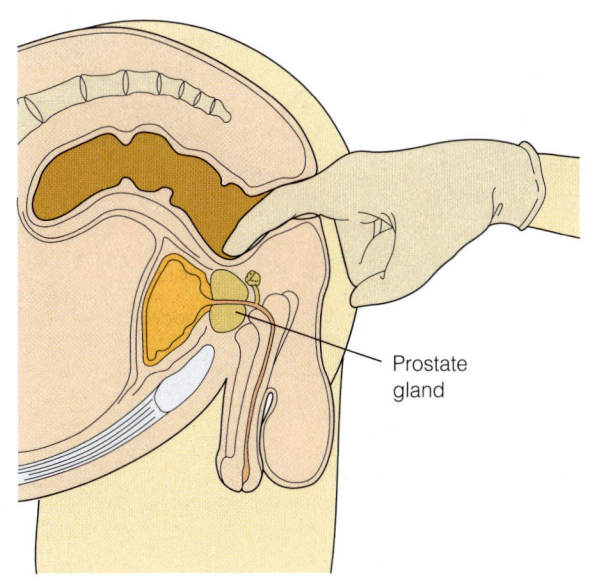

Prostate gland

Figure 5–6 » Digital rectal examination to palpate the prostate gland.

procedure, a cooling system protects the urinary tract. The procedure takes about an hour and can be performed on an outpatient basis. Although microwave procedures do not cure BPH, they do reduce urinary manifestations. These procedures do not cause impotence or incontinence.

The **transurethral needle ablation (TUNA)** uses low-level radio frequency through twin needles to burn away a region of the enlarged prostate. Shields protect the urethra during the procedure. TUNA improves the flow of urine through the urethra. TUNA does not cause impotence or incontinence.

Transurethral Surgery

Transurethral resection of the prostate (TURP) is the surgical procedure used most often. The resectoscope is inserted through the urethra, and the obstructing prostate tissue is excised with an electrocautery wire loop (see **Figure 5–7 》**). No external incision is necessary. During the procedure, the surgeon uses the resectoscope to remove obstructing tissue in several segments. The segments of tissue are then flushed into the bladder with irrigation solution, where they are stored until the end of the surgery and then flushed out of the body. This surgery has potential postoperative complications, including hemorrhage, clot retention, inability to void, and UTI. Possible long-term complications are incontinence, impotence, and retrograde ejaculation.

In the **transurethral incision of the prostate (TUIP)**, small incisions are made in the smooth muscle where the prostate is attached to the bladder neck. The gland is split to reduce pressure on the urethra. No tissue is removed, so this procedure is most appropriate for men with smaller prostate glands. TUIP can be done on an outpatient basis, and it has the additional advantage of lower risk of postoperative retrograde ejaculation than is associated with TURP and other prostatectomy procedures.

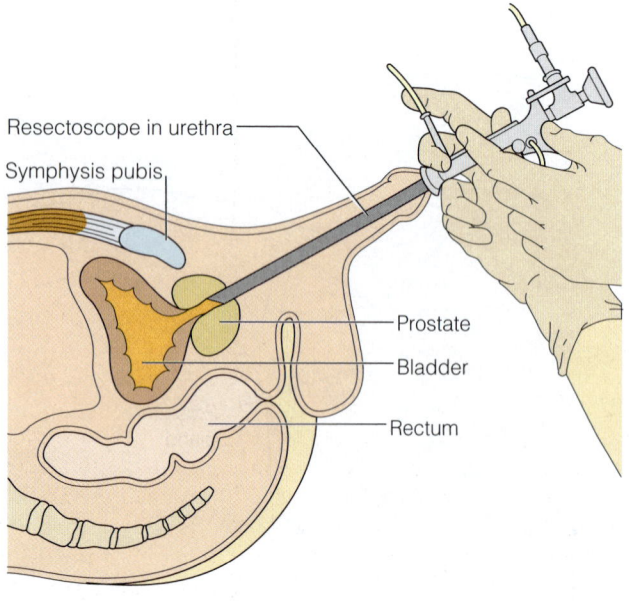

Figure 5–7 》 In a transurethral resection of the prostate, a resectoscope inserted through the urethra is used to remove excess prostate tissue.

Open Surgery

When the prostate gland is very large, an open prostatectomy may be required. This procedure is discussed in the exemplar on Prostate Cancer in the module on Cellular Regulation.

Laser Surgery

In laser surgery, the surgeon uses a cystoscope to pass the yttrium-aluminum-garnet (YAG) laser fiber through the urethra into the prostate and then vaporizes obstructing prostate tissue with several short bursts of energy. Advantages of laser surgery include decreased blood loss and a more rapid recovery time. However, this method may not be as effective for larger prostates.

New Treatments

Prostatic urethral lift (PUL) is a minimally invasive procedure for the treatment of LUTS caused by BPH. The PUL procedure involves placement of implants that retract the obstructing prostatic lobes. PUL offers rapid, though moderate, improvement in both voiding and storage LUTS. Improvements in quality of life, urinary flow rate, and preservation of sexual function continued to be reported 12 months after intervention (Bozkurt et al., 2016).

Pharmacologic Therapy

Medications such as alpha-blockers and 5-alpha reductase inhibitors have dramatically reduced the need for surgery to control the symptoms of BPH. Treatment with medications is based on two considerations: The hyperplastic tissue is androgen-dependent, and smooth muscle contraction within the prostate can exacerbate urinary obstruction (see **Table 5–6 》**). The first consideration is usually addressed by treatment for mild prostate enlargement with finasteride (Proscar) or dutasteride (Avodart), both of which are 5-alpha reductase inhibitors (antiandrogen agents) that inhibit the conversion of testosterone to DHT and cause the enlarged prostate to shrink in size. The use of 5-alpha reductase inhibitors decreases prostate size and decreases serum PSA levels by 50%, although it takes at least 3–6 months (Pearson & Williams, 2014). Potential side effects include impotence, decreased libido, and decreased volume of ejaculate.

Anticholinergic agents such as tolterodine (Detrol) block the effects of acetylcholine on muscarinic receptors in the bladder, resulting in decreased bladder contractions. A combination of anticholinergic and alpha-blocker therapy compared with alpha-blocker monotherapy demonstrated greater reduction in LUTS (Pearson & Williams, 2014).

SAFETY ALERT Pregnant women should not handle crushed tablets of 5-alpha reductase inhibitors because the drug may be absorbed through the skin and can harm a male fetus.

Excessive smooth muscle contraction in BPH is treated with alpha blockers alfuzosin (Uroxatral), doxazosin (Cardura), tamsulosin (Flomax), and terazosin, which are first-line treatments for men with bothersome, moderate to severe LUTS. These medications relax the smooth muscle of the prostate and bladder neck to relieve obstruction and increase the flow of urine. Because they may also cause

TABLE 5–6 Agents for Benign Prostatic Hyperplasia

Drug	Route and Adult Dose (Maximum Dose Where Indicated)	Adverse Effects
Alpha-Adrenergic Blockers		
Doxazosin (Cardura)	po; 1–8 mg/day	*Orthostatic hypotension, headache, dizziness*
Prazosin (Minipress)	1 mg qid or bid	<u>First-dose phenomenon</u> (severe hypotension and syncope), tachycardia
Tamsulosin (Flomax)	po; 0.4 mg 30 min after a meal (max: 0.8 mg/day)	
Terazosin (Hytrin)	po; start with 1 mg at bedtime, then 1–5 mg/day (max: 20 mg/day)	
5-Alpha Reductase Inhibitors		
Dutasteride (Avodart)	po; 0.5 mg/day	*Sexual dysfunction, decreased libido, decreased ejaculate volume*
Finasteride (Proscar)	po; 5 mg/day	No serious adverse effects

Note: Italics indicates common adverse effects; underlining indicates serious adverse effects.

orthostatic hypotension, patient/family teaching should include: (1) careful and slow position changes to prevent dizziness and accidental falls; (2) taking and recording blood pressures daily; and (3) checking with the healthcare provider before taking any medications for coughs, colds, or allergies (as these may contain an adrenergic agent).

Certain commonly used over-the-counter medications will worsen symptoms of BPH. Alpha-adrenergic agents, found in decongestants such as pseudoephedrine and phenylephrine, may activate alpha$_1$-adrenergic receptors in the bladder neck, causing restriction of urine flow. Drugs with anticholinergic side effects such as antihistamines, tricyclic antidepressants, and phenothiazines could also adversely affect BPH. Testosterone and other anabolic steroids may increase prostate enlargement, subsequently increasing the physical obstruction of the urethra. Older men who may have more bothersome LUTS should avoid drugs that are known to worsen these symptoms.

Nonpharmacologic Therapy

Patients with mild BPH are often treated with "watchful waiting" and lifestyle changes. A third of these individuals may experience relief of symptoms without treatment, but all patients with mild BPH should be regularly monitored. Lifestyle changes that are appropriate for men with mild BPH include (NIDDK, 2012c, 2014):

- Urinating at the first urge
- Avoiding alcohol and caffeine
- Drinking small amounts of fluids spread throughout the day
- Avoiding drinking fluids within 2 hours of bedtime
- Avoiding over-the-counter cold and sinus medications that contain decongestants or antihistamines
- Exercising regularly, including pelvic floor exercises
- Reducing stress.

NURSING PROCESS

The nurse who is caring for a patient with BPH must be sensitive to his concerns and fears while providing education and support. Therapeutic communication helps the nurse obtain a thorough history and assist the patient with discussing sensitive topics.

Assessment

Men over the age of 40 should be assessed for possible BPH and, depending on their health history, should be screened for prostate cancer. Assessment includes a health history, physical assessment, and diagnostic tests.

The health history includes risk factors, urinary elimination patterns and manifestations, hematuria, and pain. Symptoms of BPH can be assessed with the International Prostate Symptom Score (IPSS). The IPSS uses a scale of 0 (*not at all*) to 5 (*almost always*) to collect data about several subjective factors, including feeling as though the bladder did not empty with toileting; needing to urinate within 2 hours after urinating; starting and stopping the stream several times while urinating; and straining to urinate. This questionnaire also asks how many times during the night the patient needs to urinate and how he feels about having the disorder.

>> **Stay Current:** To view the IPSS online, visit http://www.usrf.org/questionnaires/AUA_SymptomScore.html

The physical examination usually includes a DRE of the external surface of the prostate for size, symmetry, firmness, and nodules. In BPH, the prostate is asymmetrical and enlarged. Note that a DRE is an advanced nursing assessment (see Figure 5–6). Abnormal findings include tenderness, masses, nodules, hardness, or overly soft. Nodules may be characteristic of prostate cancer, while tenderness usually indicates prostatitis.

Several diagnostic tests are used in the assessment of BPH. The patient's urine is examined for WBCs, RBCs, and bacteria. Urinary function is assessed by measuring residual urine (amount of urine remaining in the bladder after voiding) with ultrasonography or postvoid catheterization (more than 100 mL is considered high) and through **uroflowmetry**, which measures urine flow rate (normal is greater than 14 mL/sec). A finding of less than 10 mL/sec indicates obstruction. Creatinine levels of the blood are assessed for kidney damage. PSA levels are obtained to rule out prostate cancer. PSA is a glycoprotein produced only in the cytoplasm of benign and malignant prostate cells; the serum level corresponds with the volume of both benign and malignant prostate tissue.

Diagnosis

Examples of nursing diagnoses that may be considered for patients with BPH include the following:

- *Impaired Urinary Elimination* related to urinary retention
- *Ineffective Sexuality Pattern* related to urinary retention and overflow incontinence (discomfort or urine leaking during intimacy)
- *Risk for Infection* related to urinary retention
- *Overflow Urinary Incontinence* related to urinary retention secondary to enlarged prostate impinging flow of urine
- *Acute Pain* related to bladder distention
- *Deficient Knowledge* related to effects surgery or procedures may have on sexual function.

(NANDA-I © 2014)

Planning

The nursing plan of care should be individualized to meet the needs of each patient. Examples of potentially applicable goals are:

- The patient will regain urinary continence within 1 week after catheter removal (individualize time frame).
- The patient will verbalize the rationale for performing postoperative exercise at the close of the nurse-led teaching session.
- The patient will verbalize the need for continued follow-up care with a urologist (or other healthcare provider) prior to discharge.
- The patient will verbalize warning signs of UTI at the close of the nurse-led teaching session.
- The patient will report pain as less than or equal to 3/10 within 30 (45, 60) minutes after receiving prescribed IV (IM, PO) analgesics (individualize route and expected time frame).
- The patient describes signs and symptoms to report to the healthcare provider at the close of nurse-led teaching session.
- The patient lists over-the-counter medications to avoid at the close of the nurse-led teaching session.
- The patient will utilize prescribed medications as directed for pain to remain at or below a 3/10 until his postop follow-up appointment on (date).
- The patient will realize a decrease in LUTS as evidenced by an American Urological Association Symptom Index (AUASI) score less than or equal to (number) within 4 weeks of the procedure.
- The patient will be fully continent within 6 months after TURP (individualize time frame and procedure).

Implementation

Care of the patient with BPH differs based on treatment decisions and indications for surgical intervention. If the patient does not need surgical intervention, nursing care

includes primarily patient teaching about topics such as self-care, proper administration of medications, medication side effects, symptoms to report to the physician, and nutrition. Nursing care of all patients involves answering the patient's questions and providing emotional support. Patients who need surgical intervention will require more in-depth nursing care.

Preoperative Care

Sensitive and thorough preoperative care, education, and support are critical to the patient's subjective view of the surgery as well as to objective outcomes.

- Patients may be confused about the surgical approach because there are several different methods. Patient teaching will help reduce patient anxiety related to fear of the unknown and increase patient participation in postoperative care. Men may be anxious about the outcome of their surgery and its potential long-term effects on their sexuality. The nurse will communicate willingness to address any concerns or anxiety by maintaining a professional approach and creating a trusting relationship.
- The nurse should verify that the informed consent form has been signed. The nurse should explain to the patient that he will have a urinary catheter when he returns from surgery and that he may have a drain in his incision, depending on the type of surgery performed. The nurse should also explain that the patient will be treated prophylactically for venous thromboembolism, possibly by wearing sequential pneumatic compression stockings after the surgery. A bowel preparation such as an enema is ordered usually with a 2% neomycin solution to cleanse inside the intestinal lumen in the event of a perineal approach.

Postoperative Care

Nursing care of the patient after prostate surgery involves pain management, monitoring for complications, implementation of methods to prevent complications, and hygiene care. The nurse should do the following:

- Monitor vital signs closely for the first 24 hours and regularly thereafter to assess for early manifestations of hemorrhage or infection.
- Maintain accurate I&O records, including amounts of irrigating solution used. Frequently assess patency of any catheters and drains.
- Monitor color and character of urine. Catheters may become occluded by blood clots or when the catheter tubing becomes bent, interfering with urinary drainage and increasing the risk of hemorrhage.
- Assess and manage the patient's pain, which may include incisional pain, bladder spasms, or abdominal cramps due to intestinal gas. Analgesics are administered on a routine and as-needed basis to control incisional pain. Bladder spasms may be accompanied by strong urges to void and urine leakage around the catheter. Belladonna and opium (B&O) rectal suppositories may be used to relieve bladder spasms.
- Maintain venous thromboembolus prophylaxis with medications, thromboembolus disease/device stockings,

and sequential compression devices as ordered. Assist with leg exercises and ambulation as ordered. These are important preventive measures because the patient who has had prostate surgery is at risk for developing thromboembolism.

- Encourage the patient to maintain a liberal fluid intake of 2–3 L a day, and explain that increased fluids reduce burning upon urination after catheter removal, as well as decrease the risk of UTI.

- For the first 24–48 hours, a patient with a TURP should be monitored for hemorrhage, evidenced by bright red bloody urine, presence of large blood clots, decreased urinary output, increased bladder spasms, decreased hemoglobin and hematocrit, tachycardia, and hypotension. Notify the physician of any of these manifestations. Postoperative hemorrhage may be arterial or venous and may be precipitated by movement, bladder spasms, or obstructed urinary drainage.

- Instruct the patient with a three-way indwelling catheter with traction to keep his leg straight while the traction is in place. A No. 18–22 French three-way catheter with a 30–45 mL balloon usually is inserted following a TURP. The inflated balloon is pulled down into the prostatic fossa, and the catheter tubing is pulled down and taped to the patient's leg to apply pressure against the operative site, preventing bleeding.

- Pressure on the urethra by the large catheter and on the internal sphincter by the catheter's balloon stimulates the micturition reflex. Explain that although the presence of a urinary catheter will cause the sensation of needing to void, it is important not to strain, try to void around the catheter, or void when having a bowel movement. Straining to void or to have a bowel movement may stimulate bladder spasms and increase pain; it also may increase the risk for bleeding.

- Explain the possibility of bladder spasms, experienced as lower abdominal pressure or pain and a desire to urinate. Teach the patient to expect this sensation and what medications will help alleviate this discomfort.

- **Continuous bladder irrigation (CBI)** prevents the formation of blood clots, which can obstruct urinary output. If the patient has CBI, assess the catheter and the drainage tubing at regular intervals. Maintain the rate of flow of irrigating fluid to keep the output light pink or colorless. Assess the urinary output every 1–2 hours for color, consistency of amount, and presence of blood clots. Assess the patient for bladder spasms and pain.

- Bladder distention resulting from output obstruction increases the risk of bleeding because as the bladder stretches there will be pressure on the expanding tissue. Irrigating fluids are continuously infused and drained at a rate that keeps urine light pink or colorless. The flow rate of the irrigation solution is titrated, based on the volume, color, and consistency of the output in the tubing and collection bag. The fluid in the collection bag is an accumulation over time and may be deceptive about changes. The tubing will contain the most recent urine and should be considered to assess current color. A change in the flow rate is necessary for complaints of bladder spasms, bright

red hematuria, presence of multiple or large blood clots, or decrease in urinary output, as these conditions indicate possible urinary hemorrhage and obstruction.

- Assess for fluid volume excess and hyponatremia, called **TURP syndrome**, which is manifested by hyponatremia, decreased hematocrit, hypertension, bradycardia, nausea, and confusion. If these manifestations occur, notify the physician. TURP syndrome results from the absorption of irrigating fluids during and after surgery. Untreated, it may result in dysrhythmias and/or seizures.

- If the patient does not have CBI, follow agency procedure and physician orders for irrigating the indwelling catheter (for hematuria, presence of multiple large blood clots or increase in bladder spasms). In most instances, using sterile technique, gently irrigate the catheter with 50 mL of irrigating solution at a time until the obstruction is relieved or the urine is clear. Ensure equal input and output of irrigating fluid. Intermittent irrigation may be used to prevent obstruction of urinary drainage.

- Following catheter removal, assess the amount, color, and consistency of urine. Explain to the patient that he may experience burning upon urination, dribbling after urination is a common experience, and the urine may contain small blood clots after catheter removal. The CBI and catheter usually are removed in the 24–48 hours following surgery. To improve urinary control, teach the patient to start and stop the urine stream several times during each voiding, and have him practice pelvic floor exercises. Regaining full control may take up to 1 year.

- If the patient had a retropubic prostatectomy, assess the abdominal incision for the presence of urine or purulent drainage and if present, report to the surgeon. Because the bladder is not entered during a retropubic prostatectomy, no urine should be found on the dressing.

- If the patient had a suprapubic prostatectomy, assess urinary output from both the suprapubic and the urethral catheters. The patient with a suprapubic prostatectomy often has two separate closed drainage systems: one from a suprapubic incision and one in the urethra. Assess the abdominal dressing for urinary drainage, and change saturated dressings frequently. Consult with a skin care specialist if saturated dressings result in skin irritations. Following removal of the urethral catheter (usually 2–4 days after surgery) and based on the healthcare provider's orders, clamp the suprapubic catheter, and encourage the patient to void. Assess residual urine by unclamping the suprapubic catheter, and measure the remaining urine drained from the bladder. The order to remove the suprapubic catheter will depend on the volume of postvoid residual urine. Once the volume of postvoid residual urine is consistently 75 mL or less after voiding several times, the suprapubic catheter may be removed.

- The patient with a perineal prostatectomy should be assessed for perineal drainage and manifestations of infection. Rectal temperatures and enemas are contraindicated because they may precipitate bleeding. Use a T-binder or padded scrotal support to hold the dressing in place. (The location of the dressing makes application difficult.) Following removal of the dressing and perineal

Patient Teaching
Caring for Catheters and Drainage Bags

Teaching a patient or caregiver how to care for the catheter and drainage bag includes the following information:

- Change from the smaller leg drainage bag to a larger bedside drainage bag. A larger bag suspended from the bed frame at night permits gravity drainage of urine and prevents reflux of urine into the bladder.
- Avoid securing the leg bag too tightly, which can decrease venous return and increase risk for thrombophlebitis (swelling of the veins) and embolic complications such as pulmonary emboli.
- Place a soft cloth between the leg bag and thigh to decrease friction and to absorb perspiration under the bag, reducing the risk of skin irritation.
- Empty the leg bag every 3–4 hours during waking hours to prevent overfilling.
- Promptly report to the urologist any unexpected changes in urine color, urine consistency, urine odor, hematuria, evidence of frank bleeding, or large blood clots, as well as a lack of or significant decrease in urine output.

sutures, heat lamps or sitz baths may be used to provide heat and promote healing. Teach the patient to perform perineal irrigations with sterile normal saline as ordered and as instructed after each bowel movement. Because of the proximity of the incision to the anus, thorough wound care is necessary to prevent infection.

- Home care may involve care of an indwelling urinary catheter (see the Patient Teaching feature). Postoperative patients being discharged to home may or may not require temporary assistance from a home health nurse for additional teaching for postoperative care procedures. For patients who require a great deal of assistance and choose to recover at home, referral to an agency that provides caregiver respite or home health services may be helpful to assist if family members are providing care. Assessing the postoperative needs of the patient and the patient's ability to manage the recovery process successfully is essential. See **Box 5–1 >>** for discharge instructions to provide to the patient and family.

Evaluation

A patient's individualized plan of care is developed in collaboration with the patient and includes identifying outcomes based on the patient's participation. The patient's condition is regularly evaluated on the basis of the planned outcomes. If an outcome is not met, the nurse reviews the plan of care with the patient to determine necessary changes to either the plan or the chosen outcomes. Questions to consider to determine outcome include the following:

- Did the patient report the pain remained equal to or less than 3/10? Question the patient about adherence with prescribed pain medications. If needed, contact the healthcare provider for changes in prescribed medications.
- Is the patient continent? Is the incontinence expected within a range of time? If expected, further teaching and reassurance may be beneficial for the patient.
- Did the patient report a AUASI score at the desired level? What are the remaining symptoms? Are there nursing interventions that can assist in resolving them? Should the healthcare provider be notified? If not, is a referral applicable?

Box 5–1
Discharge Instructions After Prostate Surgery

Activity

The healing period lasts from 4 to 8 weeks. Avoid strenuous activity and heavy lifting. Except for short rides, do not drive for 2 weeks. Continue or begin nonstrenuous exercise such as walking, and remember to take stairs slowly and carefully. Continue exercises that you did in the hospital to prevent blood clots in the legs. You can take showers, but avoid tub baths while the catheter is in place.

Bleeding

Bleeding can occur any time after surgery. It is fairly common after a bowel movement, coughing, or increased exercise. If you notice blood in the urine, increase fluids and rest until the urine is clear. Report to your medical provider immediately if there is heavy bleeding or you are unable to empty the bladder. Avoid aspirin and NSAIDs for at least 2 weeks or as instructed by your medical provider.

Bowel Movements

Keep bowel movements regular and soft to prevent pressure on the prostate area. Drink fruit juices and take stool softeners as ordered.

Diet

Resume your normal diet. Increase fluids to 10 glasses (8 oz) daily. Avoid alcohol unless otherwise advised by your medical provider.

Sexual Intercourse

To prevent bleeding, do not have sex for 6 weeks after surgery. You may still have erections, even with the catheter in place. When you resume sexual activity, expect ejaculate to flow back into the bladder, so you will express little or no semen, and urine may appear cloudy after intercourse.

Urination

After your catheter is removed, you may experience some burning, stinging, or leakage for several weeks, and you may pass small blood clots occasionally. These symptoms will disappear as the area heals. It is best to use pads or adult briefs to control leakage.

Work

If work is not strenuous, you may return in 4 weeks; otherwise, wait 6–8 weeks or as directed by the healthcare provider.

Please Call Immediately If:

- You are unable to urinate or if you experience bladder pain and a substantial decrease in urine.
- Bleeding is not controlled by increasing your fluid intake and resting or if bleeding is excessive.
- You have chills and fever or severe abdominal pain.
- Your scrotum becomes swollen and tender.
- You have pain in one calf, chest pain, or difficulty breathing.

- Has the patient verbalized importance of follow-up with the surgeon (or urologist)? Further teaching and open discussion may be required. Is a referral required? If so, is follow-up attainable for the patient (directions, appointments, transportation, financial assistance, work release, baby sitter)?

- Has the patient followed the treatment regimen? Has the patient avoided over-the-counter medications as recommended? The patient may require further teaching and written instructions in the preferred or native language.

Nursing Care Plan

A Patient with Benign Prostatic Hyperplasia

William Turner is a 71-year-old man living with his wife in a small retirement community in Florida. His wife had a stroke 2 years ago, and Mr. Turner does all of the cooking and housework. He has been in good health for most of his life and reports some mild pain from osteoarthritis in his knees and hands. He has noticed a gradual onset of urinary urgency and frequency over the past 2 years and has found it increasingly difficult to initiate urination. During a routine checkup, the nurse practitioner at the local health clinic performs a DRE and finds Mr. Turner's prostate enlarged. Mr. Turner's PSA is within the normal range, so he is referred to a urologist, who diagnoses him with BPH. Mr. Turner chooses to have the recommended surgery, a TURP. Following surgery, his recovery is uncomplicated. However, the nurse caring for Mr. Turner is concerned about his ability to care for his indwelling catheter because of his arthritis and his wife's physical disabilities after having a stroke. The nurse makes a referral to a home health agency to ensure that Mr. Turner can manage his care at home. An initial home health assessment is scheduled for the day after Mr. Turner is discharged from the hospital.

ASSESSMENT

The home health nurse notes that the house is clean and neat. Mr. Turner is still wearing his bedside urinary drainage bag even though it is 1:00 p.m. Mr. Turner tells the nurse that his main problem is shopping for groceries because he is embarrassed to be seen with the drainage bag. He says that he has not been able to remove the drainage bag and attach the leg bag because of his arthritis. Physical assessment reveals no tenderness in his calves, chest pain, or shortness of breath. The urine is yellow, without odor or sedimentation. Mr. Turner states that he sees no need for the pelvic exercises, since he is no longer in the hospital.

DIAGNOSES

- *Stress Urinary Incontinence* related to surgical procedure
- *Ineffective Health Maintenance* related to inability to care for the urinary drainage system, lack of understanding about the need for postoperative exercises, and questions about follow-up care
- *Disturbed Body Image* related to urinary drainage bag in public view

(NANDA-I © 2014)

PLANNING

Planning care is done in collaboration with Mr. Turner to improve outcomes and includes the following goals:

- Mr. Turner will regain urinary continence within 90 days after having the TURP.
- Mr. Turner will change the urinary drainage bag with the appropriate assistance by the end of the nurse lead teaching session.
- Mr. Turner will verbalize the rationale for performing postoperative exercise at the close of the nurse-lead teaching session.
- Mr. Turner will verbalize the need for continued follow-up care with his urologist during each home health visit.
- Mr. Turner will verbalize relief of embarrassment when using the leg drainage bag in place of the larger bedside bag while out in public.

IMPLEMENTATION

- Discuss the possibility of stress incontinence after the catheter is removed.
- Reinforce the need for pelvic floor exercises while the catheter is still in place.
- Explore Mr. Turner's support system to identify individuals who can assist him with catheter care; arrange a teaching session with members of his support system.
- Teach Mr. Turner what follow-up care is recommended and how to obtain it.
- Refer Mr. Turner to a support group for individuals with BPH.

EVALUATION

The nurse evaluates Mr. Turner's care based on the goals of care established during the planning phase. Mr. Turner's friends from his church have assisted him with care of his drainage bag and reminded him to do his pelvic floor exercises several times a day while the catheter is in place. When the catheter is removed, Mr. Turner has a small amount of urine leaking out after voiding. He understands that it may take several weeks for the leaking to resolve. Efforts to help him understand the need for continued medical care are less successful. Mr. Turner continues to state that he is cured, his wife needs him, and he sees no reason to return to the doctor.

CRITICAL THINKING

1. Outline a teaching plan for Mr. Turner's risk of altered skin integrity related to urinary incontinence.
2. As a result of Mr. Turner refusing to have ongoing medical care, he might be labeled noncompliant. Would you make this nursing diagnosis? Why or why not?
3. If you were the home health nurse making a visit and found Mr. Turner had no urinary drainage for 16 hours, what assessments would you make? How would you handle this problem?

REVIEW Benign Prostatic Hyperplasia

RELATE Link the Concepts and Exemplars

Linking the exemplar of BPH with the concept of sexuality:

1. What communication strategies would the nurse use to discuss the impact BPH will have on sexuality without making an older man feel uncomfortable?

2. How can you assess his concerns, fears, and knowledge regarding the impact of BPH on his sexuality?

Linking the exemplar of BPH with the concept of infection:

3. What pathophysiology of BPH could increase the risk of UTIs?

4. What nursing interventions will reduce the risk of UTIs?

READY Go to Volume 3: Clinical Nursing Skills

REFER Go to Pearson MyLab Nursing and eText

- Additional review materials

REFLECT Apply Your Knowledge

Clifford Allen is a middle manager for a small manufacturing company where he has worked for the last 20 years. Overall, Mr. Allen is in good health, although he has been undergoing treatment recently for BPH. He has a history of depression, for which he does not seek treatment because he fears the social stigma connected to the diagnosis. Mr. Allen has been considering retiring within the next few years so he and his wife can travel, but mostly to escape his stressful work environment. He enjoys bowling and is involved in activities at church. He and his wife go for a walk each evening after supper.

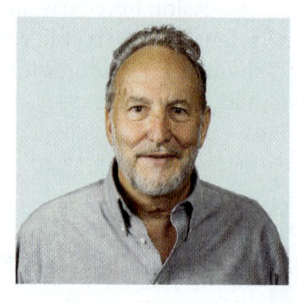

One evening while bowling, he notices that his bladder feels somewhat full. Mr. Allen calls to make an appointment to see his urologist for a follow-up examination. He has been taking finasteride (Proscar) for the last 6 months but does not believe it has been particularly effective. He still has trouble urinating and believes that his symptoms are worse than before he started taking the drug. When he sees the urologist 2 weeks later, he reports that he often feels his bladder is full after voiding, he has difficulty starting his stream of urine, and his stream is weak once started. He gets up frequently at night to void. His score on the AUASI is 28, which has increased from his score of 18 six months ago. The urologist confirms that the medication has not been effective and schedules further tests, including uroflowmetry, check postvoid residual, a PSA blood test, and a urinalysis. Results from the uroflowmetry and postvoid residual test show a significant obstruction of urinary flow. The serum PSA is negative, and the urinalysis is consistent with bladder inflammation. A TURP is recommended in the upcoming weeks.

1. To determine Mr. Allen's understanding of the procedure, what will the nurse want to ask him upon admission to the surgical center?

2. What teaching will the nurse prepare regarding postoperative self-care?

3. Design a nursing plan of care for this patient postoperatively.

≫ Exemplar 5.B
Bladder Incontinence and Retention

Exemplar Learning Outcomes

5.B Analyze bladder incontinence and retention as they relate to elimination.

- Describe the pathophysiology of bladder incontinence and retention.
- Describe the etiology of bladder incontinence and retention.
- Compare the risk factors and prevention of bladder incontinence and retention.
- Identify the clinical manifestations of bladder incontinence and retention.
- Summarize diagnostic tests and therapies used by interprofessional teams in the collaborative care of an individual with bladder incontinence or retention.

- Differentiate care of patients with bladder incontinence and retention across the lifespan.
- Apply the nursing process in providing culturally competent care to an individual with bladder incontinence or retention.

Exemplar Key Terms

Bladder training, *322*
Habit training, *322*
Scheduled toileting, *322*
Urinary incontinence, *312*
Urinary retention, *317*

Overview

When caring for patients with urinary tract disorders, it is important to consider the patient's modesty in voiding, embarrassment about discussing genitals or being exposed for examination and testing, and fear of changes in body image or function. These psychosocial issues may interfere with the patient's willingness to seek help, discuss treatment, and learn about preventive measures. Nursing interventions for patients with urinary tract disorders are directed toward

primary prevention, early detection, and management of the disorder through health teaching and nursing care.

URINARY INCONTINENCE

Urinary incontinence, or involuntary urination, is a symptom, not a disease. It is the most common manifestation of impaired bladder control. It can have a significant impact on the patient's life, creating physical problems, such as skin breakdown, and leading to psychosocial problems, including embarrassment, isolation, ineffective coping, and social withdrawal.

The incidence of urinary incontinence is estimated to be between 10 million and 13 million individuals in the United States and 200 million individuals worldwide. The estimated annual cost of managing urinary incontinence in the United States is $16.3 billion, 75% of which is spent on treating women (Vasavada, 2015). Although urinary incontinence is especially common among older patients, it is not a normal consequence of aging, and it can be treated. An estimated 30% or more of older women living in the community experience urinary incontinence. In long-term care, assisted living, and homebound populations, the incidence is between 50% and 80%. Despite these statistics, the actual prevalence of urinary incontinence is nearly impossible to determine. Embarrassment and the availability of products to protect clothing and prevent detection contribute to patients not seeking evaluation and treatment for incontinence.

Pathophysiology and Etiology

Pathophysiology

Urinary continence requires a bladder that is able to expand and contract and sphincters that can maintain a urethral pressure higher than that of the bladder. Incontinence results when the pressure within the urinary bladder exceeds urethral resistance, allowing urine to escape. Any condition causing higher-than-normal bladder pressures or reduced urethral resistance can result in incontinence. Three examples of conditions that can cause higher-than-normal bladder pressures are: (1) the increased volume of urine in the bladder from use of diuretics, (2) the growing size of the uterus during pregnancy that puts pressure on the bladder, and (3) a weakened urethral sphincter related to decreasing levels of estrogen during menopause. Relaxation of the pelvic musculature, disruption of control related to cerebral or neuronal dysfunction, and disturbances of the bladder and its musculature are also common contributing factors.

Etiology

Incontinence may be an acute, self-limited disorder, or it may be chronic. It may be congenital or acquired, reversible or irreversible. Urinary incontinence is acute and reversible if it is associated with partial or complete resolution. Reversible factors include polyuria, exposure to irritants, urinary retention, stool impaction or constipation, restricted mobility or dexterity, psychologic conditions, delirium, medications (e.g., diuretics, sedatives), and UTI. Some causes of urinary incontinence, such as acute confusion, may or may not be reversible, depending on the underlying cause of the confusion.

Chronic or irreversible causes of urinary incontinence are often associated with congenital or nervous system disorders. Congenital disorders associated with incontinence include epispadias (absence of the upper wall of the urethra) and meningomyelocele (a neural tube defect in which a portion of the spinal cord and its surrounding meninges protrude through the vertebral column). Central nervous system or spinal cord trauma, stroke, and chronic neurologic disorders, such as multiple sclerosis and Parkinson disease, are examples of acquired, irreversible causes of incontinence.

Risk Factors

Age is a primary risk factor for the development of urinary incontinence; older individuals experience more frequent incontinence than younger individuals. Incontinence can be experienced at any age. In all age groups, women are much more susceptible to urinary incontinence than men, especially women who are homebound or who live in a long-term care facility. Obesity, smoking, diabetes, inactivity, pregnancy, depression, and neurologic disorders (e.g., stroke) are all risk factors for urinary incontinence. Individuals who experience two or more UTIs per year or who take medications that affect the adrenergic system, diuretics, and calcium-channel blockers are at higher risk for urinary incontinence.

Prevention

Lifestyle modification is the best method of preventing urinary incontinence. Maintaining a healthy weight can help prevent urinary incontinence; this includes weight loss for individuals who are obese. Eating a diet that is high in fiber can help prevent constipation, which is a risk factor for urinary incontinence. Avoiding bladder irritants such as alcohol, caffeine, and acidic or spicy food can also help prevent urinary incontinence. Adequate fluid intake is necessary for normal bladder function; individuals should not drink less than six to eight 8-oz glasses of water daily. Likewise, drinking too much water can lead to rapid bladder filling and consequent urinary incontinence. Other prevention methods include regular exercise, refraining from tobacco use, reviewing medications for increased risk of urinary incontinence, and reducing physical barriers to toileting for patients with limited functional ability.

Clinical Manifestations

Symptoms of urinary incontinence include the inability to avoid urinating until a bathroom can be used, increased rate of urination, leakage, uncontrollable wetting, and frequent bladder infections. Incontinence is commonly categorized as stress incontinence, urge incontinence (i.e., overactive bladder), reflex urinary incontinence, overflow incontinence, and functional incontinence (see the Clinical Manifestations and Therapies feature). Mixed incontinence, when two or more types of incontinence are present, is common. Total incontinence, which may be due to a variety of etiologies, is loss of all voluntary control over urination: Urine loss occurs without stimulus and in all positions. The treatment of total urinary incontinence depends upon the medically diagnosed cause of the condition.

Collaboration

Diagnosis and treatments focus on identifying and treating the underlying cause of incontinence. Diagnosis and treatment are performed in collaboration with other healthcare professionals, including physicians, urologists, and surgeons.

Diagnostic Tests

Bladder diaries, urinalysis, and blood tests are commonly used for patients experiencing urinary incontinence. The bladder diary is used to record how much the patient drinks,

Clinical Manifestations and Therapies
Urinary Incontinence

ETIOLOGY	CLINICAL MANIFESTATIONS	CLINICAL THERAPIES
Stress incontinence. Relaxation of the pelvic musculature and weakness of the urethra and surrounding muscles and tissue lead to decreased urethral resistance.	Loss of a small amount of urine when sneezing, coughing, or lifting; uncontrollable wetting; weakness of urethra and pelvic muscles; increased pressure on the bladder from pregnancy, obesity, cystocele, or urethrocele	▪ Surgery ▪ Imipramine ▪ Pelvic floor exercises ▪ Behavioral modifications ▪ Absorbent pads or diapers ▪ Pessary device ▪ Urethral insert
Urge incontinence. This condition usually results from a hypertonic or overactive detrusor muscle, leading to increased pressure within the bladder and inability to inhibit voiding.	Involuntary loss of urine associated with a strong urge to void, increased rate of urination, inability to avoid urinating until a bathroom is available, overactive detrusor muscle, nocturia	▪ Oxybutynin ▪ Tolterodine ▪ Pelvic floor exercises ▪ Behavioral modifications ▪ Absorbent pads, adult briefs
Reflex incontinence. This condition results from disruption to neuronal control of the pontine and/or sacral micturition centers due to neurologic impairment or tissue damage.	Complete emptying of bladder at a predictable bladder volume, neurologic deficits, frequency, nocturia, inability to sense full bladder or initiate or inhibit voiding	▪ Medication ▪ Neuromodulation ▪ Surgery ▪ Catheterization ▪ Absorbent pads, adult briefs
Overflow incontinence. This condition results from outlet obstruction or lack of normal detrusor activity, leading to overfilling of the bladder and increased pressure.	Loss of urine associated with an overdistended bladder and urinary retention, urinary obstruction, BPH	▪ Surgery ▪ Catheterization ▪ 5-alpha reductase inhibitors ▪ Absorbent pads, adult briefs
Functional incontinence. This condition results when the ability to respond to the need to urinate is impaired, as is seen in dementia, some physical disabilities, and patients with impaired mobility.	Loss of urine associated with physical impairments that prevent the patient from reaching the toilet in time, mobility impairment, cognitive deficits	▪ Catheterization when the benefit outweighs the risk of infection ▪ Absorbent pads or diapers ▪ Home modifications for easy access for toileting ▪ Physical or occupational therapy ▪ Assistive devices ▪ Nonrestrictive clothing

when the patient urinates and how much urine is produced, if the patient felt the urge to urinate, how many incontinence episodes the patient experienced, and what the patient was doing at the time of incontinence. The bladder diary can help the healthcare provider to distinguish between stress, urge, reflex, overflow, and functional incontinence, and to understand the patient's bladder functioning. A urinalysis detects appearance, color, blood, infection, glucose, specific gravity, presence of stones, and other characteristics of urine to identify the underlying cause of incontinence, such as a UTI or calculi. Various blood tests likewise will identify potential hormonal or chemical causes of incontinence, such as diabetes mellitus.

Other urine tests that may be used for patients with urinary incontinence are a 24-hour urine sample, postvoid residual measurement, urodynamic testing, and a stress test. The 24-hour urine sample reveals the volume of urine a patient produces in 1 day, and various tests are performed to provide data about kidney and bladder function. The postvoid residual measurement shows the amount of residual urine left in the patient's bladder after voiding, and bladder volume. A large postvoid volume may indicate obstruction and nerve or muscle damage. Urodynamic testing measures the bladder pressure at rest and while filling. Filling is simulated by the insertion of a catheter and filling the bladder with water. This test measures bladder strength and urinary sphincter health. During a stress test, the patient is asked to bear down while the physician or nurse watches for urine loss.

Imaging tests may also be performed to reveal the cause of urinary incontinence. A pelvic ultrasound is used to visualize structures in the pelvic region and any structural abnormalities. Cystography uses a radioactive dye inserted into the bladder through a catheter to show bladder abnormalities and postvoid volume. In cystoscopy, the physician inserts a cystoscope to visualize the urinary tract, detect abnormalities, and obtain tissue samples to be sent for pathology tests.

Surgery

Surgery may be used to treat stress incontinence associated with cystocele (prolapsed bladder) or urethrocele (prolapsed urethra) and overflow incontinence associated with an enlarged prostate gland. Suspension of the bladder neck, a technique that brings the angle between the bladder and urethra closer to normal, is effective in treating stress incontinence associated with urethrocele in 80–95% of patients. A laparoscopic, vaginal, or abdominal approach may be used to perform this surgery.

>> Go to **Pearson MyLab Nursing and eText** to see Chart 1: Nursing Care of the Patient Undergoing Bladder Neck Suspension.

Prostatectomy, using either the transurethral or the suprapubic approach, is indicated for the male patient who is experiencing overflow incontinence as a result of an enlarged prostate gland and urethral obstruction.

Other surgical procedures of potential benefit in the treatment of incontinence are implantation of an artificial sphincter, formation of a urethral sling to elevate and compress the urethra, augmentation of the bladder with bowel segments to increase bladder capacity, implantation of nerve stimulators, and injection of collagen along the urethra to narrow the urinary passageway and support more normal urethral positioning.

Pharmacologic Therapy

Both stress and urge incontinence may improve with drug treatment. Some medications target the underlying cause of urinary incontinence, such as alpha-blockers and 5-alpha reductase inhibitors for men with BPH and antibiotics for individuals with a UTI. Drugs that contract the smooth muscles of the bladder neck may reduce episodes of mild stress incontinence. Imipramine (Tofranil), an antidepressant, is an effective therapy. It can make individuals drowsy, however, so it typically is taken at night. Adverse effects, such as dizziness and irregular heartbeat, and contraindications with a number of other medications may limit its use.

When incontinence is associated with postmenopausal atrophic vaginitis, estrogen therapy may be effective. Options include systemic estrogens and local creams. Patients with urge incontinence may be treated with preparations that increase bladder capacity. The primary drugs used to inhibit detrusor muscle contractions and increase bladder capacity include oxybutynin (Ditropan and the extended-release form, Ditropan XL), an anticholinergic drug, and tolterodine (Detrol and its longer-acting form, Detrol LA), a more specific antimuscarinic agent. These drugs can be taken once or twice a day and have fewer side effects than less-specific anticholinergic drugs. Drugs with anticholinergic effects are contraindicated for the patient with acute glaucoma. Urinary retention is a potential side effect that must be considered when these drugs are used.

Nonpharmacologic Therapy

To reduce the incidence of urinary incontinence, the nurse should teach all patients to perform pelvic floor muscle (Kegel) exercises (see the Patient Teaching feature) to improve perineal muscle tone. Kegel exercises are most often used for women with urinary incontinence, but they may also benefit men who experience urinary incontinence following prostatectomy for BPH or prostate cancer. Assistive devices, such as vaginal cones, and biofeedback may be useful for patients who have difficulty identifying appropriate muscle groups (Herbison & Dean, 2013).

Behavioral modification is a classic method for treating urinary incontinence. Behavioral techniques include scheduled toileting, habit training, and bladder training. *Scheduled toileting* is toileting at regular intervals (e.g., every 2–4 hours).

Patient Teaching
Pelvic Floor Muscle (Kegel) Exercises

Exercises for pelvic floor muscles, when performed correctly and regularly, will enable this muscle group to accomplish the task of supporting the structures in the pelvis. Everyone can benefit from exercising this muscle group. The nurse will include teaching interventions when planning care for women with urinary stress incontinence, men with urinary stress incontinence after prostate surgery, and anyone with bowel incontinence problems (Anderson et al., 2015; Lombrana et al., 2013).

- Identify the pelvic muscles with these techniques:
  1. Stop the flow of urine during voiding, and hold for a few seconds. Patients who have difficulty emptying the bladder completely should not stop urine flow while voiding in order to identify the pelvic floor muscles. Repeated interruption of micturition can interfere with complete bladder emptying and increase the risk for UTI.
  2. Women should tighten the muscles at the vaginal entrance around a gloved finger or tampon.
  3. Both women and men should tighten the muscles around the anus as though resisting defecation or passing flatulence.
  4. They will work to lift and contract as a group. You should be able to feel the lift when tightening these muscles.
- Always begin each exercise session with an empty bladder.
- Perform exercises by tightening pelvic muscles, holding for 3–10 seconds, and then relaxing for 10–15 seconds. Continue the sequence (tighten, hold, relax) for 10 repetitions.
- Keep abdominal muscles and breathing relaxed while performing exercises.
- Exercises initially should be performed twice a day, increasing frequency to four times a day.
- Exercise at a specific time each day or in conjunction with another daily activity (e.g., bathing, watching the news). Establish a routine, because these exercises should be continued for life.
- If the abdomen or buttocks becomes uncomfortable or sore, you have not been contracting the correct muscles. Try again to locate the correct muscles.

Habit training is toileting the patient on a schedule that corresponds with the normal pattern. *Bladder training* gradually increases the bladder capacity by increasing the time between voiding intervals and resisting the urge to void between scheduled times. Bladder training may also involve double voiding, or voiding once and then voiding a few minutes later to release residual urine; regulating fluid intake; avoiding dietary bladder stimulators; and performing relaxation and distraction techniques to overcome the urge to void (Vasavada, 2015).

Additional nonpharmacologic methods of treating urinary incontinence include using absorbent products such as pads or adult briefs; inserting a pessary, urethral insert, or a bladder support; or using a catheter. A pessary is a stiff ring that is inserted into the vagina to hold up the bladder and prevent urine leakage. Pessaries are generally used for patients with a prolapsed bladder. A urethral insert is a tampon-like device that is inserted into the urethra to act as a plug for leaks. A bladder support is made of flexible silicone and inserted into the vagina; it is shaped to support the bladder to decrease stress incontinence. Urethral inserts are usually used during specific activities that may cause incontinence. Catheters are used for patients with overflow incontinence due to bladder retention or for patients with neurologic damage that affects bladder muscle control. Intermittent self-catheterization is the preferred catheterization method because it significantly decreases the risk of developing a UTI. If the patient is unable to perform self-catheterization or has no control of bladder muscles (e.g., patient with paraplegia), an indwelling Foley catheter or suprapubic catheter may be necessary. Use of a catheter increases the risk for UTI.

SAFETY ALERT Limiting total fluid intake to less than 1.5–2.0 L per day is not recommended for patients with urinary incontinence. Inadequate fluid increases urine concentration, which leads to bladder wall irritation and possibly increases problems of urge incontinence.

Patient teaching is also an essential part of nursing care for patients with urinary incontinence. To learn more about teaching topics, see the Patient Teaching feature.

Lifespan Considerations

In addition to older adults, two population groups that are highly susceptible to urinary incontinence are children and pregnant women.

Urinary Incontinence in Children

The age at which a child attains urinary continence varies. Therefore, diurnal enuresis (daytime incontinence) is not diagnosed until age 5 or 6, and NE (nighttime incontinence) is not diagnosed until age 7. More than 90% of children are continent during the day by age 5, but nighttime continence takes longer to achieve. Most cases of urinary incontinence in children clear up spontaneously with no treatment. Potential causes of diurnal enuresis include bladder irritability, weak detrusor muscle, constipation, structural abnormalities, sexual abuse, UTI, and infrequent voiding (e.g., voluntarily holding urine to avoid using toilets at school or interrupting play) (Figueroa, 2012; NIDDK, 2012d).

Patient Teaching
Preventing UTIs and Urinary Incontinence

Patient teaching is essential for patients who experience problems with urinary incontinence and for their caregivers or family members. The nurse should discuss the following points with patients to help prevent UTI and urinary incontinence:

- Maintain a generous fluid intake. Reduce or eliminate fluid intake or using diuretics after the evening meal to reduce nocturia.
- Wear comfortable clothing that is easy to remove for toileting.
- Maintain good hygiene, but do not bathe more often than necessary. Frequent bathing and use of feminine hygiene sprays or douches may dry perineal tissues, increasing the risk of UTI or urinary incontinence.
- Perform pelvic floor muscle exercises several times a day to increase perineal muscle tone.
- Reduce consumption of caffeine-containing beverages (e.g., coffee, tea, colas), citrus juices, and beverages containing some artificial sweeteners.
- Use behavioral techniques to reduce the frequency of incontinence.
- See your primary care provider regularly for a pelvic or prostate examination.
- For women, discuss possible benefits and risks of hormone replacement therapy, physical therapy, or surgery to treat incontinence.
- Report any change in urine color, odor, or clarity or symptoms such as burning, frequency, or urgency to your primary care provider.

NE is more common than diurnal enuresis. Almost 30% of children at age 4 have NE, 10% at age 7, 3% at age 12, and 1% at age 18 (NIDDK, 2012d). NE is more common in boys than in girls. Although it is more prevalent in children, 0.5–1% of the adult population experience NE, and there is a lack of evidence exploring NE in geriatric populations (Howlett et al., 2016).

NE is referred to as primary NE when a person has never achieved nighttime urinary control. When NE appears after the child has achieved nighttime dryness for 6 consecutive months, it is considered secondary NE (Holloway, 2014; Prynn, 2012). Often, secondary NE is related to another problem, such as constipation, stress, illness (e.g., diabetes mellitus), or developmental delay, and may resolve when the cause is eliminated. A young child may temporarily regress in ability to use the toilet successfully during times of emotional trauma or stress. When NE is related to temporary toileting regression, treatment for secondary NE is not necessary as NE will usually resolve as emotional recovery occurs.

Etiology of NE is not fully understood; it appears to have multiple antecedents. Recent research indicates that NE is associated with daytime incontinence, encopresis (fecal incontinence), fecal impaction, bladder dysfunction, and male gender. Genetic studies have linked the decrease of ADH production to chromosome 22, along with tendencies for behavior disorders and ADHD (Fatouh et al., 2013; Friedman & Palmer, 2014).

NE can be a source of anxiety, stress, and decreased self-esteem, resulting in reduced quality of life. NE can also generate a financial burden from frequent laundering of bed linens, mattress replacement, and prolonged and multiple medical treatments.

Of the successful treatment options, biofeedback has an approximate success rate of 64% (Ebiloglu et al., 2016). Studies indicate that acupuncture may provide benefit, with better outcomes observed when the practitioner has a deep understanding of traditional Chinese medicine (TCM). Meta-analysis has brought to light that acupuncture is significantly more effective than placebo and monotherapy with both TCM and meclofenoxate (Lv et al., 2015).

Other interventions include bladder training, moisture alarms, and medication (e.g., desmopressin, imipramine, oxybutynin). Children can also benefit from behavioral modification techniques similar to those used for adults. A common modification technique for children with diurnal enuresis is urgency containment exercises. These exercises include having the child prepare to go to the bathroom when the urge occurs, and then sit on the toilet and hold the urine for as long as possible. When starting to urinate, the child is encouraged to start and stop the urine stream to gain control over the pelvic floor muscles and strengthen the sphincters. This process also gives the child confidence to hold the urine until reaching a bathroom, to avoid having an accident (Figueroa, 2012).

Urinary Incontinence in Pregnant Women

Pregnant women often experience stress incontinence because of hormonal changes and the excess weight of the growing uterus pressing on the bladder. After a vaginal delivery, postpartum women may have urinary incontinence, either temporary or long term, secondary to edema from local trauma, weakened bladder muscles, and damage to nerves and supporting structures. Prolapse of the pelvic floor may develop, pushing the pelvic organs toward the vagina. This abnormal pressure on the urethral sphincter will prohibit proper closure, and incontinence will occur. Pelvic floor exercises and bladder training throughout the pregnancy are not invasive and are effective for treatment and prevention of urinary incontinence during pregnancy and postpartum.

Urinary Incontinence in Older Adults

Functional incontinence may be the predominant problem in older adults living in institutions. Limited mobility, impaired vision, dementia, lack of access to toileting facilities, and privacy are considered contributory factors for functional incontinence. Tight staffing patterns increase the risk for incontinence in previously continent residents. The primary problem in functional incontinence is an outside factor that interferes with the ability to respond normally to the urge to void. An immobilized patient may wet the bed if a call light is not within reach; a patient with Alzheimer disease may perceive the urge to void but be unable to interpret its meaning or respond by seeking a bathroom. For these patients, self-care deficit in toileting is a primary problem.

Box 5–2
Strategies for Promoting Independence in Older Adults with Alterations in Elimination

- Provide assistive devices such as raised toilet seats, grab bars, a bedside commode, or nightlights as needed to facilitate independence. Fostering independence in toileting enhances self-concept and maintains a positive body image.
- Plan a toileting schedule based on the patient's normal elimination patterns to achieve a urine output of approximately 300 mL with each voiding. Allowing the bladder to fill to a point at which the urge to void is experienced and then emptying it completely helps to maintain normal bladder capacity and bacteriostatic functions.
- Position the patient for ease of voiding—sitting for women, standing for men—and provide privacy. Normal positioning, usual toileting facilities, and privacy all enhance the ability to void on a schedule and empty the bladder completely.
- Adjust fluid intake so that the majority of fluids are consumed during times of the day when the patient is capable of remaining continent. Unless fluids are restricted, maintain a fluid intake of at least 1.5–2.0 L per day. An adequate fluid intake is vital to promote hydration and urinary function. Overly concentrated urine can irritate the bladder, increasing incontinence.
- Promote use of clothing that is easily removed (e.g., elastic-waist pants, loose dresses). Hook and loop or zipper fasteners may be easier to use than snaps and buttons. Clothing that is difficult to remove can increase the risk of incontinence in patients with mobility problems or impaired dexterity. Provide assistance to patients when needed.

In addition to ensuring a thorough assessment, nurses can use the strategies outlined in **Box 5–2** ≫ to promote independence in elimination among older adults.

URINARY RETENTION

Urinary retention is the inability to empty the bladder. It is most common in men with BPH, but other factors also can contribute to urinary retention. Urinary retention can be acute, in which the patient is unable to urinate at all, or chronic, in which the bladder constantly contains a small residual volume of urine. Although urinary retention is less common than urinary incontinence, it can become a medical emergency if the patient is unable to void.

Pathophysiology and Etiology

Pathophysiology

When bladder emptying is impaired, urine accumulates and the bladder becomes overdistended. Overdistention causes poor contractility of the detrusor muscle, further impairing urination. If the problem persists, more serious problems, such as hydronephrosis (accumulation of urine in the renal pelvis as a result of obstructed outflow) or vesicoureteral reflux (backflow of urine from the bladder to the kidney) can result.

Etiology

Either mechanical obstruction of the bladder outlet or a functional problem can cause urinary retention. BPH is a common cause leading men to seek medical care with complaints of difficulty initiating and maintaining the flow of urine. Acute inflammation associated with infection or trauma to the bladder, urethra, or perineal tissues may also interfere with bladder elimination. Scarring caused by repeated UTIs subsequently leads to urethral stricture and produces mechanical obstruction. Although renal calculi at any location in the urinary tract can cause urinary retention from obstruction, calculus in the bladder may block the opening to the urethra. The unintended effects of anesthesia may cause individuals to experience urinary retention perioperatively. Side effects from various routine prescription and over-the-counter medications can also contribute to urinary retention.

Risk Factors

Individuals who have undergone surgery are also at higher risk for urinary retention as a result of anesthesia and limited mobility. Patients who have undergone abdominal or pelvic surgery are at especially high risk if the surgery disrupts the function of the detrusor muscle. Accidents to or infections of the brain or spinal cord can increase a patient's risk for urinary retention. According to Johansson and colleagues (2013) general risk factors for the development of urinary retention include advanced age, male gender, cognitive impairment or confusion, diabetes, constipation, immobility, and emotional distress. A history of UTI, urinary incontinence, prostatitis, or previous prostate, bladder, or voiding problems also increases risk for urinary retention.

Patients who take medications that interfere with detrusor muscle function are at increased risk of developing urinary retention. Anticholinergic medications, such as atropine, glycopyrrolate (Robinul), propantheline bromide (Pro-Banthine), and scopolamine hydrochloride (Transderm Scop), can lead to acute urinary retention and bladder distention. Many other drug groups have anticholinergic side effects and may cause urinary retention. Among these are antianxiety agents, such as diazepam (Valium); antidepressant and tricyclic drugs, such as imipramine (Tofranil); antiparkinsonism drugs (L-dopa); antipsychotic agents; and some sedative/hypnotic drugs. In addition, antihistamines, such as diphenhydramine (Benadryl), are a common ingredient in over-the-counter cough, cold, allergy, and sleep-promoting drugs; they have anticholinergic effects and may interfere with bladder emptying.

Voluntary urinary retention, which is particularly common among nurses, may lead to overfilling of the bladder and a loss of detrusor muscle tone. These individuals are also at increased risk of developing chronic urinary retention.

Prevention

The first step in preventing urinary retention is identifying patients who may be at risk for urinary retention (Johansson et al., 2013). Further diagnostic testing should be performed if risk factors are identified. Teaching and behavioral modifications should be implemented for all patients at risk for urinary retention. Timed voiding is especially helpful for patients with cognitive impairment. If needed, patients should be assisted to the toilet, provided a bedside commode, or taught intermittent self-catheterization to prevent urinary distention and the associated complications. For

men with BPH, urinary retention may be prevented by administering 5-alpha reductase inhibitors.

Clinical Manifestations

The patient with urinary retention is unable to empty the bladder completely and may continue to feel the urge to void after toileting. Urinary retention can be classified as either acute or chronic. Acute retention is the sudden and painful inability to void despite having a full bladder; this is a medical emergency. It may be accompanied by bloating. It is commonly caused by surgical procedures, medications, UTIs, excessive fluid or alcohol intake, or BPH (NIDDK, 2012a).

Chronic urinary retention is painless and is associated with an increase in the residual urine volume. Patients with chronic urinary retention may have difficulty starting and maintaining urination and may be able to produce a weak flow. The individual may feel the urge to void and toilet frequently but have little results with voiding, or continue to feel a need to void after toileting (NIDDK, 2012a). Overflow voiding or incontinence may occur, with 25–50 mL of urine eliminated at frequent intervals.

Assessment of patients with urinary retention reveals a firm, distended bladder that may be displaced to one side of midline. Percussion of the lower abdomen yields a dull tone, reflective of fluid in the bladder. Urinary retention is confirmed with a bladder scan or the insertion of a urinary catheter (if possible) and measurement of the urine output. The accuracy of using a bladder scan to predict the volume of urine in the bladder is comparable to draining the bladder with a urinary catheter (Nusee et al., 2014) and reduces the risk of UTI by avoiding catheterization.

Severe urinary retention with resulting bladder distention impairs the ability of the vesicoureteral junction to prevent backflow of urine into the ureters (see **Figure 5–8 »**). Reflux of urine from the distended bladder distends the ureters (hydroureter) and kidneys (hydronephrosis). Hydronephrosis impairs renal function, and acute renal failure can result.

Collaboration

The nurse can independently perform some treatments for urinary retention, such as catheter care. However, the nurse must collaborate with other healthcare team members for other aspects of care for patients with urinary retention, including diagnostic tests, surgery, and pharmacologic therapy.

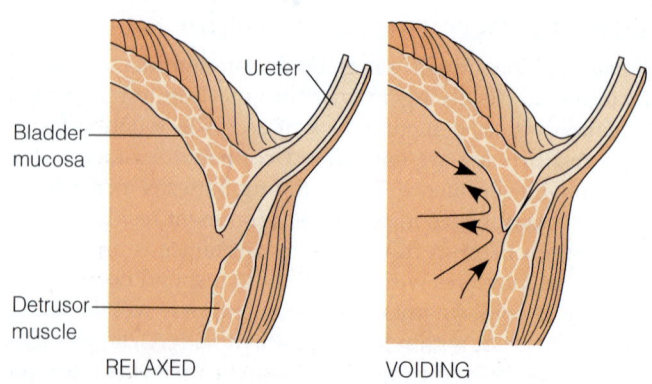

Figure 5–8 » A competent vesicoureteral junction.

Clinical Manifestations and Therapies
Urinary Retention

ETIOLOGY	CLINICAL MANIFESTATIONS	CLINICAL THERAPIES
Acute urinary retention	Inability to urinate, bladder distention, hydronephrosis, vesicoureteral reflux, pain, abdominal distention, dull sound upon abdominal percussion	■ Catheterization ■ Review and change medication (if indicated) ■ Antibiotics ■ Surgery
Chronic urinary retention	Large postvoid residual volume, bladder distention, urinary obstruction, poor detrusor muscle contractility, urinary inflammation, difficulty starting and maintaining stream, weak flow, frequent urination, little success at voiding, urge to urinate after voiding, overflow incontinence	■ Catheterization ■ Change in medication therapy ■ Surgery ■ Bethanechol chloride

Diagnostic Tests

Diagnostic tests for patients with urinary retention are similar to tests for urinary incontinence and include blood and urine tests. Imaging scans such as x-rays, CT scans, bladder scans, and cystoscopy are also used to detect urinary retention. Bladder scans use ultrasound images to detect the amount of residual urine in the bladder. Chronic urinary retention is diagnosed when the individual has more than 100 mL of residual urine left in the bladder after voiding.

Surgery

Mechanical obstructions are removed or repaired when possible. Resection of the prostate gland may be performed to detect urinary retention related to BPH. Bladder calculi are removed, and measures to prevent new formation are instituted. Surgery may also be performed to correct a cystocele or rectocele.

Pharmacologic Therapy

Cholinergic medications, such as bethanechol chloride (Urecholine), promote contraction of the detrusor muscle, and emptying of the bladder may be used. A medication with no anticholinergic side effects may be substituted when urinary retention is related to drug therapy.

Nonpharmacologic Therapy

Urinary retention should be immediately treated with complete emptying of the bladder by catheterization. An indwelling urinary catheter or intermittent straight catheterization may be necessary to prevent future urinary retention and overdistention of the bladder until the underlying problem is corrected.

Lifespan Considerations

Urinary Retention in Infants and Children

Common causes of urinary retention in infants are related to either physical deformity of structures of the urinary tract causing urine to be retained or a postsurgical complication. Congenital bladder or paraurethral diverticula are unusual but not uncommon in children. The diverticula can fill and retain urine, and based on location, can present the risk of completely blocking the opening of the urethra (Bhat et al., 2012; Hossain, Hasan, & Siddiqui, 2012; Singh et al., 2013). Postsurgical complications can be caused by anesthesia administered for an unrelated problem such as cleft palette (Alfheim et al., 2016) or after circumcision if inflammation impedes the opening of the urethra. Although not limited to infants and children, there is an increased risk of urinary retention related to genital infection and scarring in cultures that practice ceremonial circumcisions and genital mutilation of either gender (Rouzi et al., 2014).

Urinary Retention in Pregnant Women

Urinary retention for women during pregnancy may occur as a result of childbirth and other obstetrical procedures. In particular, vaginal delivery presents a lower risk of peripartum urinary retention through routine episiotomies (Mulder et al., 2016). Epidural analgesia and the birth weight of the child are independent risk factors contributing to urinary dysfunction. In addition, emergency cesarean delivery, prolonged operation time, and postoperative analgesia are the main causative risks related to cesarean delivery. If urinary retention can be detected early, it may not lead to permanent kidney damage and long-term voiding problems (Johansson et al., 2013; Stephansson et al., 2016). The duration of the second stage of labor, previous caesarean deliveries, and general maternal condition related to the pregnancy and delivery will potentially affect urinary elimination during the postpartum period. In addition to childbirth, urinary retention can be a significant postoperative problem for women undergoing any uro-gynecologic surgeries (Buchko, Robinson, & Bell, 2013; Geller, 2014).

Urinary Retention in Older Adults

As with incontinence, older adults are at a higher risk for urinary retention simply because they have the highest incidence of chronic disease and polypharmacy. Older adults are more likely to have a history of or require various surgical interventions. Postoperative urinary retention is a common perioperative issue (Buchko & Robinson, 2012; Buchko et al., 2013), not only in gynecologic procedures, but also in a wide range of abdominal, pelvic, and orthopedic procedures, largely related to the proximity to the urinary structures. Pelvic organ prolapse repairs and procedures to correct detrusor muscle function can result in detrusor underactivity (Geller, 2014; Juma, 2014). Detrusor underactivity can be difficult to identify if symptoms of other urinary problems exist. Detrusor underactivity is generally observed by the presence of a particularly weak stream of urine, straining to void, and a history of urinary retention. The underactive bladder may arise from a combination of faulty neuronal signaling to or from the bladder in combination with ischemia and weakened muscular functioning of the bladder (Cohn et al., 2016).

NURSING PROCESS

Understanding how to care for patients with urinary incontinence or retention is vital to nursing practice, because patients of any age may experience urinary problems related to physiologic changes and medical conditions or treatments. Nursing care of patients with bladder problems involves emptying the bladder, preventing complications, maintaining skin integrity, and providing emotional support.

Assessment

Because problems with urinary elimination can increase the patient's risk for other alterations—such as social isolation, disruption of sexually intimate relationships, impaired skin integrity, and disturbed body image—prompt assessment, diagnosis, and treatment are necessary to ensure that the patient returns to full health and functioning as soon as possible.

The preliminary assessment and identification of the symptoms of urinary incontinence and retention are within the scope of nursing practice. The nurse should ask all patients about their voiding patterns. Patients with mild symptoms may not even realize that they are experiencing a problem. Older adults who are incontinent while in their home or who manage to contain or conceal their incontinence from others do not consider themselves incontinent. Therefore, the nurse may need to ask about incontinence in several ways using different terminology to determine whether the individual is experiencing incontinence. The nurse may need to humanize the problem by asking questions such as, "Do you ever have trouble making it to the bathroom on time?" If incontinence is determined, a thorough history and an assessment are indicated to capture the extent and probable cause of incontinence.

A complete assessment of a patient's urinary function includes the following:

- **Observation and patient interview.** Observe for signs and symptoms of urinary incontinence, such as the odor of urine, soiled clothing, and the use of incontinence products. The patient may appear anxious in locating a toilet or may request frequent bathroom breaks in an attempt to avoid incontinence. A good tool to assist in the assessment process is a voiding diary that includes frequency of urination, volume of urine output, and activities associated with incontinence. Inquire about methods used to deal with incontinence, use of pelvic floor exercises or medications, any chronic diseases, medications, complementary health approaches, related surgeries, and effects of incontinence or retention on usual activities, including social activities.

- **Physical examination.** Assess the patient's physical and mental status, including any physical limitations or impaired cognition. Inspect, palpate, and percuss the abdomen for bladder distention. Inspect perineal tissues for redness, irritation, or tissue breakdown. Observe for bulging of the bladder into the vagina when bearing down. Perform DRE for prostate size. Assess pelvic muscle tone as indicated and hydration status. Examine the patient's urine.

Diagnosis

NANDA-I (2014) includes one general diagnostic label for urinary elimination problems: *Impaired Urinary Elimination.* More specific, NANDA-I nursing diagnoses related to urinary elimination include the following:

- *Urinary Incontinence, Functional*
- *Urinary Incontinence, Overflow*
- *Urinary Incontinence, Reflex*
- *Urinary Incontinence, Stress*
- *Urinary Incontinence, Urge*
- *Urinary Incontinence, Risk for Urge*
- *Urinary Elimination, Readiness for Enhanced*
- *Self-Care Deficit, Toileting*
- *Urinary Tract Injury, Risk for*

(NANDA-I © 2014)

Planning

Goals established for a patient depend on the diagnosis and defining characteristics. These goals of nursing care should be individualized, along with a realistic time frame to meet each goal. Examples of overall goals for patients with urinary elimination problems include the following:

- The patient will maintain or restore a normal voiding pattern (add a time frame, e.g., by discharge).
- The patient will regain normal urine output (time frame, e.g., on the first postoperative day).
- The patient will prevent associated risks, such as infection, skin breakdown, fluid and electrolyte imbalance, and lowered self-esteem (time frame, e.g., during the hospital stay).
- The patient will perform toileting activities independently, with or without assistive devices (time frame, e.g., upon discharge).
- The patient will contain urine with the appropriate device, catheter, ostomy appliance, or absorbent product (time frame, e.g., during social activity).

Implementation

Patients with urinary incontinence or retention may receive primary care in a hospital, in a long-term care facility, or at home. Nursing interventions for each of these patients' individual circumstances will depend on the patient's type of incontinence or retention, physical mobility status, cognitive status, and location.

Independent nursing interventions for patients with urinary problems may include (a) a behavior-oriented continence training program such as bladder training, habit training, prompted voiding, pelvic floor exercises, and positive reinforcement; (b) appropriate skin care; and (c) catheter care or patient teaching about intermittent self-catheterization. Other interventions include promoting adequate fluid intake, maintaining normal voiding habits, and assisting with toileting. For all patients, the nurse should assess and provide opportunities to promote independence to the greatest degree possible. Patients who are receiving home care must be alert and physically able or have caregivers who can assist with implementing the plan of care.

Some patients, including and especially some adults living in institutions, may require assistance with toileting. The nurse should assist these patients to the bathroom and remain with them if they are at risk for falling. The bathroom should contain an easily accessible call signal to summon help if needed. The nurse should encourage patients to use handrails placed near the toilet. For patients who are unable to use bathroom facilities, the nurse should provide urinary equipment close to the bedside (e.g., urinal, bedpan, bedside commode) and assist as necessary.

Maintain Normal Voiding Patterns

Many prescribed medical therapies interfere with a patient's normal voiding habits. When a patient's urinary elimination pattern is adequate, the nurse helps the patient adhere to normal voiding habits as much as possible (see **Box 5–3** »).

Promote Effective Urination

Nursing measures to promote urination include placing the patient in normal voiding position and providing privacy. Additional measures include running water, placing the patient's hands in warm water, pouring warm water over the perineum, and providing a warm sitz bath.

In acute urinary retention, catheterization may be necessary to relieve bladder distention and prevent hydronephrosis. The nurse should use a relatively small catheter (16 French for a man, 14 French for a woman). A coudé tip catheter is passed more easily in the older man with an enlarged prostate. The use of 2% lidocaine gel injected into the urethra will provide lubrication and topical analgesia. Providing adequate analgesia promotes pelvic muscle relaxation and decreases the risk of trauma to the lumen of the urethra, therefore possibly reducing catheter-associated infection. The nurse should carefully observe the patient as the distended bladder drains (Coffield & Willette, 2012).

SAFETY ALERT Some patients experience a vasovagal response, becoming pale, sweaty, and hypotensive if the bladder is rapidly drained. Draining urine in 500-mL increments and clamping the catheter for 5–10 minutes between increments may prevent this response. Hematuria, the presence of blood in the urine, also may occur with rapid bladder decompression. Promptly notify the physician if hematuria develops.

Maintain Skin Integrity

Skin that is continually moist becomes macerated (softened by liquid). Urine that accumulates on the skin is converted to ammonia, which is very irritating to the skin. Because both skin irritation and maceration predispose the patient to skin breakdown and ulceration, the individual who is incontinent requires appropriate skin care. To maintain skin integrity, the nurse cleanses or assists the patient to cleanse the perineal area with mild soap and water or a commercially prepared no-rinse cleanser after episodes of incontinence, rinses thoroughly if soap and water is used, dries gently and thoroughly, and provides clean, dry clothing or bed linen. The nurse applies or assists the patient to apply barrier ointments or creams to protect the skin from contact with urine. If incontinence products are necessary, the nurse should use or provide products that absorb wetness and leave a dry surface in contact with the skin. When skin care is complete, the nurse will provide clean, dry clothing and bed linens. Patients returning home or to another care facility should be instructed in techniques for maintaining skin integrity.

Box 5–3
Maintaining Normal Voiding Habits

Positioning

- If necessary, encourage the patient to push over the pubic area with the hands or to lean forward to increase intra-abdominal pressure and external pressure on the bladder.
- If the patient is unable to ambulate to the lavatory, use a bedside commode for women and a urinal for men at the bedside.
- Assist the patient to a normal position for voiding: standing for male patients; for female patients, squatting or leaning slightly forward when sitting. These positions enhance movement of urine through the tract by gravity.

Relaxation

- Suggest that the patient read or listen to music.
- Provide privacy for the patient. Many individuals cannot void in the presence of another individual.
- Allow the patient sufficient time to void.
- Provide sensory stimuli that may help the patient relax. Pour warm water over the perineum of a female patient or have the patient sit in a warm bath to promote muscle relaxation. Applying a hot water bottle to the lower abdomen of both men and women may also foster muscle relaxation.

- Turn on running water within hearing of the patient to stimulate the voiding reflex and to mask the sound of voiding for individuals who find it embarrassing.
- To decrease muscle tension, provide ordered analgesics and emotional support to relieve physical and emotional discomfort.

Timing

- Assist patients who have the urge to void immediately. Delays only increase the difficulty in starting to void, and the desire to void may pass.
- Offer toileting assistance to the patient at usual times of voiding, for example, on awakening, before or after meals, and at bedtime.

For Patients Who Are Confined to Bed

- Warm the bedpan. A cold bedpan may prompt contraction of the perineal muscles and inhibit voiding.
- Elevate the head of the patient's bed to Fowler position, place a small pillow or rolled towel at the lower back to increase physical support and comfort, and have the patient flex the hips and knees. This position simulates the normal voiding position for women.

Specially designed incontinence draw sheets, which provide significant advantages over standard draw sheets, may be used for patients who are incontinent and confined to bed. These sheets are like a standard draw sheet but are double layered, with a quilted upper nylon or polyester surface and an absorbent viscose rayon layer below. The rayon soaker layer generally has a waterproof backing on its underside. Fluid (i.e., urine) passes through the upper quilted layer and is absorbed and dispersed by the viscose rayon, leaving the quilted surface dry to the touch. This absorbent sheet helps maintain skin integrity; it does not stick to the skin when wet, decreases the risk of decubitus ulcers, and reduces odor.

Plan for Home Care

Successful home care for a patient with urinary incontinence involves a combination of the following strategies:

- Education involves the patient, family, and any nonfamily caregivers, including private nursing service personnel and respite caregivers. The Patient Teaching feature addresses the learning needs for patient care.

- **Bladder training** requires the patient to postpone voiding, resist or inhibit the sensation of urgency, and void according to a timetable rather than according to the urge to void. The goal is to gradually lengthen the interval between urination to correct the patient's frequent urination, to stabilize the bladder, and to diminish urgency. This form of training may be used for patients who have bladder instability and urge incontinence. Delayed voiding produces larger voided volumes and longer intervals between instances of voiding. Voiding may initially be encouraged every 1–2 hours except during sleep, and then every 3–4 hours. A vital component of bladder training is inhibiting the urge-to-void sensation: Every time the patient has a premature urge to void, repeat the instruction to practice deep, slow breathing until the urge diminishes or disappears.

- **Habit training** and **scheduled toileting** attempt to keep the patient dry by voiding on a schedule that corresponds to the patient's normal pattern or at regular intervals. With habit training and scheduled toileting, no attempt is made to motivate the patient to delay voiding if the urge occurs. Scheduled toileting can be effective for children who are experiencing urinary dysfunction. Biofeedback therapy can assist in pelvic floor muscle training (Barrie, 2015).

- Prompted voiding supplements habit training by prompting the patient to use the toilet (prompting) and reminding the patient when to void.

- Pelvic floor exercises are isometric exercises to strengthen the pelvic floor muscles for increased support of the neighboring organs (see Box 5–3 for a full explanation). Pelvic floor exercises can be performed any time, anywhere, sitting or standing and when voiding.

The nurse should instruct all patients who have experienced urinary retention to avoid over-the-counter drugs that affect micturition, especially those with an anticholinergic effect (allergy and cold medications, many nonprescription sleep aids). Home care measures include double-voiding (urinate, remain on the toilet for 2–5 minutes, and then urinate

again); scheduled voiding; or when other measures fail, an indwelling catheter. When an indwelling catheter is necessary, the nurse should teach the patient and family to use clean technique when changing from an overnight bag to a leg bag and to report any signs of UTI promptly to the primary care provider.

For hospitalized patients who are being discharged home, the nurse must consider the patient's needs for teaching and assistance with care in the home, including assessment of patient and family resources and abilities for self-care, available financial resources, and need for referrals and home health services.

Prevent Social Isolation

Urinary incontinence increases the risk for social isolation because of embarrassment, fear of not having ready access to a bathroom, body odor, or other factors. In turn, social isolation can increase problems of incontinence because normal cues and relationships are lost and the need to remain dry becomes less of a concern. To assist patients in the area of social isolation, the nurse should do the following:

- Assess for reasons and the extent of social isolation. Verify the degree of social isolation with the patient or significant other. Do not assume that social isolation is related to urinary incontinence without exploring other causes. Other problems associated with aging (e.g., a hearing deficit, decline in vision) may also be primary or contributing factors.

- Refer the patient for urologic examination and incontinence evaluation. Patients who assume that urinary incontinence is a normal part of the aging process may not be aware of treatment options.

- Explore alternative coping strategies with the patient, the significant other, staff, and other healthcare team members. Protective pads or adult briefs, good perineal hygiene, scheduled voiding, and clothing that does not interfere with toileting can enhance continence. Promote patient independence as much as possible (see Box 5–2).

Evaluation

Using the overall goals and desired outcomes identified in the planning stage, the nurse collects data to evaluate the effectiveness of nursing interventions. If the desired outcomes are not achieved, the nurse should explore the reasons before modifying the care plan or revising goals. The following are examples of questions that must be considered if the outcome "Remains dry between voiding and at night" is not met:

- What is the patient's perception of the problem? Is the patient's perception consistent with the actual problem? Is the patient following the healthcare instructions and treatment plan? Further patient teaching regarding the nature of the patient's problem or the treatment plan may be necessary.

- Is the patient experiencing any impediments to toileting or accessing the toilet? Assess and provide resources or modifications as necessary (e.g., make referrals for assistive devices or incontinence aids, relocate the patient to a room or bed closer to the toilet, make arrangements for alternative clothing).

Patient Teaching
Urinary Elimination in the Home Setting

Facilitating Urinary Elimination Self-Care

In addition to using the strategies outlined in Box 5–2, do the following:

- Suggest graduated lighting for nighttime voiding: a nightlight in the bedroom and adequate lighting in the pathways to the bathroom.
- Provide instruction for safe transfer techniques. Contact physical therapy or occupational therapy to provide assessment for training and strengthening exercises as needed.

Promoting Urinary Elimination

- Instruct the patient to respond to the urge to void as soon as possible; avoid voluntary urinary retention.
- Teach the patient to empty the bladder completely at each voiding.
- Emphasize the importance of drinking eight to ten 8-oz. glasses of water daily if not on a fluid restriction.
- Teach the patient about pelvic floor exercises to strengthen perineal muscles.
- Teach the patient to report any of the following to the primary care provider promptly: pain or burning on urination, changes in urine color or clarity, malodorous urine, or changes in voiding patterns (e.g., nocturia, frequency, dribbling).

Asepsis

- Teach the patient to maintain personal hygiene, cleansing with soap and water daily and cleansing the anal and perineal area after defecating.
- Instruct the female patient to wipe from front to back (from the urinary meatus toward the anus) after voiding and to discard toilet paper after each swipe.
- Teach the patient with an indwelling catheter and caregivers about care measures such as cleaning the urinary meatus, managing and emptying the collection device, and maintaining a closed system.
- For the patient with a urinary diversion, teach about care of the stoma, drainage devices, and surrounding skin. For continent diversions, teach the patient how to catheterize the stoma to drain urine.
- For the patient with an indwelling catheter or urinary diversion, emphasize the importance of maintaining a generous fluid intake (2.5–3 L daily) and of promptly reporting changes in urinary output; signs of urinary retention, such as abdominal pain or urine has stopped draining into the collection bag; and manifestations of UTI, such as malodorous urine, abdominal discomfort, fever, or confusion.

Medications

- Emphasize the importance of taking medications as prescribed. Instruct the patient to take the full course of antibiotics ordered to treat a UTI, even though symptoms have been relieved.
- Stress the importance of follow-up care to evaluate the effectiveness of medications.
- Inform the patient and family about any expected changes in urine color or odor associated with prescribed medications.
- For the patient with urinary retention, emphasize the need to contact the primary care provider before taking any medication (even over-the-counter medications such as antihistamines) that may exacerbate symptoms.
- For the patient taking medications that may damage the kidneys (e.g., aminoglycoside antibiotics), stress the importance of maintaining a generous fluid intake while taking the medication.
- Suggest measures to reduce anticipated side effects of prescribed medications, such as increasing intake of potassium-rich foods when taking a potassium-depleting diuretic such as furosemide.

Dietary Alterations

- Instruct the patient that calcium from food does not increase the risk of kidney stones. Calcium supplements may increase the risk of stones forming, especially if not taken with food. Foods rich in oxalate, such as spinach, rhubarb, nuts, and wheat bran, may need to be avoided to decrease oxalate in the urine (NIDDK, 2013a).
- Instruct the patient with stress or urge incontinence to limit the intake of caffeine, alcohol, citrus juices, and artificial sweeteners because these are bladder irritants that may increase incontinence. Also, teach the patient to limit fluid intake and not to take diuretics in the evening to reduce the risk of nighttime incontinence.

Measures Specific to Urinary Problems

- Provide instructions for patients with specific urinary problems or treatments such as timed urine specimens, urinary incontinence, urinary retention, and retention catheters.

Referrals

- Make appropriate referrals to home health agencies, community agencies, or social services for assistance with necessary equipment, such as grab bars and raised toilet seats; providing wheelchair access to bathrooms; obtaining toileting aids such as commodes, urinals, or bedpans; and securing services such as home health aides for assistance with activities of daily living (ADLs). Problems with elimination can affect sexual relationships and put a strain on the significant other; refer the patient and partner for counseling as needed.

- Is the patient performing pelvic floor muscle exercises appropriately as scheduled? If not, further teaching may be required. Assistance for reminders may need to be secured from friends or family members.
- Is the patient's fluid intake adequate? Does the timing of fluid intake require adjustment (e.g., should it be restricted after dinner)? Suggest easy ways for the patient to measure fluid intake throughout the day, such as by premeasuring a container and instructing the patient how many times to fill it each day to obtain the recommended volume.
- Is the nursing care goal realistic and attainable? If not, why? Collaborate with the patient and family and revise the goal as needed.

>> Go to **Pearson MyLab Nursing and eText** to see a nursing care plan for a patient with impaired urinary elimination.

REVIEW Bladder Incontinence and Retention

RELATE Link the Concepts and Exemplars

Linking the exemplar of bladder incontinence and retention with the concept of fluids and electrolytes:

The nurse admits an 83-year-old patient with a medical diagnosis of congestive heart failure, chronic renal failure, and diabetes mellitus. While the nursing history is being taken, the patient says she takes her diuretic in the morning and then spends the next few hours in the bathroom, because if she goes too far away, she ends up wetting her pants and then has to clean up the mess. She admits feeling so thirsty in the afternoon, and she drinks several glasses of water but stops drinking fluids after 6 p.m. to avoid "wetting the bed." The patient's skin turgor is poor, and assessment reveals possible dehydration.

1. What recommendations and patient teaching should the nurse provide this patient to prevent further dehydration?

2. What lab values should the nurse review to confirm potential dehydration?

Linking the exemplar of bladder incontinence and retention with the concept of self:

A busy 41-year-old executive of a thriving small business informs you that she has been experiencing bladder incontinence when she laughs, coughs, or sneezes and that it is causing her embarrassment at work. She blames it on having had five children.

3. What impact is bladder incontinence having on this patient's self-image?

4. What recommendations might you make for this patient to reduce her feelings of shame and self-consciousness?

READY Go to Volume 3: Clinical Nursing Skills

REFER Go to Pearson MyLab Nursing and eText

- Additional review materials
- Chart 1: Nursing Care of the Patient Undergoing Bladder Neck Suspension
- Nursing Care Plan for a Patient with Impaired Urinary Elimination

REFLECT Apply Your Knowledge

Justin Gardner is a 26-year-old man who fractured his third thoracic vertebra when he fell while rock climbing. In preparation for transfer to a rehabilitation center, the doctor orders discontinuation of the patient's indwelling urinary catheter and prn straight catheterization to reduce urinary retention.

1. What assessment data will the nurse collect to determine the presence of urinary retention?

2. What signs and symptoms would the nurse recognize as indicative of the need for straight catheterization?

3. What nursing diagnosis would be appropriate for this patient?

4. What patient teaching will this patient require, related to urinary retention, before discharge if he is to provide safe home care for himself?

» Exemplar 5.C
Bowel Incontinence, Constipation, and Impaction

Exemplar Learning Outcomes

5.C Analyze bowel incontinence, constipation, and impaction as they relate to elimination.

- Describe the pathophysiology of bowel incontinence, constipation, and impaction.
- Describe the etiology of bowel incontinence, constipation, and impaction.
- Compare the risk factors and prevention of bowel incontinence, constipation, and impaction.
- Identify the clinical manifestations of bowel incontinence, constipation, and impaction.
- Summarize diagnostic tests and therapies used by interprofessional teams in the collaborative care of an individual with bowel incontinence, constipation, or impaction.

- Differentiate care of patients with bowel incontinence, constipation, and impaction across the lifespan.
- Apply the nursing process in providing culturally competent care to an individual with bowel incontinence, constipation, or impaction.

Exemplar Key Terms

Constipation, *325*
Encopresis, *333*
Fecal impaction, *326*
Fecal incontinence, *330*

Overview

Disorders of intestinal absorption and bowel elimination can affect not only functional elimination status but also other functional health patterns. Bowel function can be affected by inflammation, infections, tumors, obstructions, or changes in structure.

Patients with intestinal disorders often face extensive diagnostic testing, surgery, and potential permanent changes in physical appearance and lifestyle. Nursing care is directed toward returning to or maintaining homeostasis, meeting the patient's physiologic needs, providing emotional support, and educating the patient to adapt to changes in lifestyle.

Few body functions respond as readily to internal and external influences as defecation. Factors affecting the gastrointestinal tract directly, such as food intake and bacterial population, affect the number and consistency of stools. Indirect factors, such as psychologic stress or voluntary postponement of defecation, also affect elimination. It is important to evaluate each patient's bowel elimination issues against that patient's usual patterns.

CONSTIPATION

Constipation may be defined as fewer than three bowel movements per week or difficult passage of stools. This term implies either the passage of dry, hard stool or no passage of stool at all. It occurs when the movement of feces through the large intestine is slow, allowing time for additional absorption of fluid from the large intestine. Difficult evacuation of stool and increased effort or straining of the voluntary muscles during defecation are associated with constipation. The individual may have a feeling of incomplete stool evacuation after defecation. Careful assessment of a patient's usual elimination pattern is necessary before a diagnosis of constipation is made.

Pathophysiology and Etiology
Pathophysiology

Constipation may be a primary problem or a manifestation of another disease or condition. Acute constipation, a definite change in the bowel elimination pattern, is often caused by an organic process (i.e., anatomical, neuromuscular, metabolic, or endocrine changes). A change in bowel patterns that persists or becomes more frequent or severe may be caused by a tumor or other partial bowel obstruction. With chronic constipation, functional causes that impair storage, transport, and evacuation mechanisms impede the normal passage of stools.

Constipation can cause other problems for some patients. Straining associated with constipation is often combined with taking in a deep breath and holding it. This combination can present problems for individuals with heart disease, brain injuries, or respiratory disease. When a deep breath is taken and held while straining to have a bowel movement, physiologic changes occur in the body. With normal respiratory effort there is moderate inflation of the lungs during inspiration, and the heart rate increases slightly due to a decrease in vagal nerve signaling. When the lungs expand to accommodate large volumes, reflex bradycardia occurs because of increased vagal nerve signaling. Vagal stimulation causes local release of acetylcholine, which acts at the sinus node in the heart, resulting in a slowed rate of impulse formation. Acetylcholine also acts at the atrioventricular node in the heart to slow conduction velocity and lengthen the refractory period (Wilcox, Kansagra, & Richards, 2013). Constipation should be carefully monitored and avoided when possible for patients with underlying conditions that affect profusion and gas exchange.

Constipation may also predispose children, older adults, and pregnant women to development of a UTI. Pressure placed on the bladder, ureters, or urethra by the colon when it contains a large amount of hard stool may cause structures of the urinary tract to develop a partial obstruction. When urine is allowed to pool in one area for an extended amount of time, bacteria can grow and cause infection (NIDDK, 2012e).

Etiology

Constipation can result from any condition that slows intestinal peristalsis. Psychologic problems that can influence

TABLE 5–7 Selected Causes of Constipation

Factor	Related Cause
Behavioral	
Activity	Inactivity, lack of exercise routines
Dietary	Highly processed food and ↓ fiber intake, ↓ fluid intake, alcohol abuse, mineral deficiencies, malnutrition, ↓ residue, ↓ intake of solids, eating disorders
Toileting	Voluntary stool retention, perceived need to defecate on a schedule, attempt to avoid discomfort related to defecation, time constraints, scheduling conflicts
Physiologic	
Structural	Partial obstruction, changes in colorectal or anal structure or function, tumors, advanced age, pregnancy, physical disabilities causing limited mobility or immobility
Neurogenic	Trauma affecting spinal cord, multiple sclerosis, cerebrovascular accident
Metabolic	Hypothyroidism, uremia, porphyria
Medication	Antacids containing aluminum or calcium salts; narcotic analgesics; anticholinergic agents; antidepressants, tranquilizers, and sedatives; antihypertensive agents; ganglionic blockers, calcium-channel blockers, beta-adrenergic blockers, and diuretics; iron salts; aftereffects of chronic laxative, cathartic, and enema use
Psychologic	
Somatic	Somatic pain or illnesses arising from physical, emotional, or sexual abuse or trauma (Elimination problems are common in sexual abuse survivors.)
Anxiety	Generalized or situational interference with regular elimination regimen
Depression	↓ Motivation, ↓ self-care, and ↓ desire for health or healthy lifestyle

intestinal motility usually stem from a somatic origin, anxiety, or depression. Behaviors found to be an underlying cause for constipation include unhealthy lifestyle choices, and voluntary stool retention related to: (1) prior uncomfortable defecation and (2) lack of opportunity, such as time and proper facilities. Physiologic conditions and abnormalities that restrict intestinal motility can be neurogenic, affecting sensory or motor function, or related to the structure of passageways. **Table 5–7 »** lists selected causes of constipation.

Risk Factors

Many factors increase a patient's risk for constipation, including insufficient activity, immobility, irregular defecation habits, changes in daily routines, lack of privacy, chronic use of laxatives or enemas, irritable bowel syndrome, pelvic floor dysfunction or muscle damage, and poor motility or slow transit. Older adults are at increased risk for constipation.

Constipation can also result from a neurologic condition, such as Parkinson disease, stroke, or paralysis; an emotional or cognitive disturbance, such as depression or mental confusion; or as a side effect of certain medications (e.g., opioids, iron supplements, antihistamines, antacids, antidepressants).

Prevention

Several strategies can help individuals prevent constipation. Dietary methods include eating foods high in fiber, limiting foods that are low in fiber, and drinking plenty of fluids. Fiber supplements may also be useful for preventing constipation, but they should be consumed with plenty of water. Behavioral methods include exercising regularly and not ignoring the urge to defecate. Stool hardens based on the length of time it remains in the intestinal tract because water is continuously absorbed; therefore, ignoring the urge to defecate can contribute to constipation. For patients with a risk of acute constipation, stool softeners and laxatives may be used to prevent constipation. However, stimulant laxatives should not be used for extended periods of time because they can lead to diarrhea with subsequent dehydration, possible fluid and electrolyte imbalances, and malnutrition. Overuse of stimulant laxatives can also cause the bowel to become dependent on medications to activate peristalsis.

Clinical Manifestations

Constipation

The manifestations of constipation include having bowel movements less often than the usual pattern, frequent flatus, abdominal discomfort, diminished appetite, straining to have a bowel movement, and the passage of hard, dry stools. Upon examination, the abdomen may appear somewhat distended, and the patient may have reduced bowel sounds.

To be diagnosed with chronic constipation, adults must experience two or more of the following symptoms for at least 12 weeks in the preceding 12 months (McKay et al., 2012):

- Straining with defecation more than 25% of the time
- Lumpy or hard stools more than 25% of the time
- Sensation of incomplete emptying more than 25% of the time
- Manual maneuvers used to facilitate emptying in more than 25% of defecations (e.g., digital evacuation, support of the pelvic floor)
- Fewer than three bowel movements per week.

Fecal Impaction

Fecal impaction is a mass or collection of hardened feces in the folds of the rectum or colon. Impaction results from prolonged retention and accumulation of fecal material. In severe impactions, the feces accumulate and extend well up into the sigmoid colon and beyond. Fecal impaction can be recognized by the passage of liquid, foul-smelling fecal (diarrhea) material in the absence of formed stool. This occurs as the liquid portion of the feces seeps out around the impacted mass. Impaction also can be assessed by digital examination of the rectum, during which the hardened mass can often be palpated.

Along with odorous liquid leaking and constipation of solid stool, rectal pain and a frequent nonproductive desire to defecate are usually present. Impaction will eventually cause a generalized feeling of illness. The patient will become anorexic, and the abdomen will become distended, increasing the probability of nausea and vomiting. The patient usually experiences abdominal cramping and a sensation of fullness in the rectal area.

Common causes of fecal impaction are poor defecation habits, including long-term dependence on laxatives or enemas, and constipation. Barium used in radiologic examinations of the upper and lower gastrointestinal tracts may also be a cause. After these examinations, laxatives or enemas can be used to ensure removal of the barium.

Digital examination of the impaction through the rectum should be performed gently and carefully. Although DRE is within the scope of nursing practice, some agency policies require a primary care provider's order for manual manipulation and removal of a fecal impaction.

Fecal impaction can be prevented, although there are occasions when treatment is necessary. When fecal impaction is suspected, healthcare providers may prescribe an oil retention enema; a cleansing enema 2–4 hours later; and then daily additional cleansing enemas, suppositories, or stool softeners until the impaction is cleared. If these measures fail, manual removal may be required to facilitate passage of the hard dry stool.

Collaboration

Simple or chronic constipation is treated with education (a daily bowel movement is not necessary for health), modification of diet, and exercise routines. More severe constipation may require diagnostic testing and pharmacologic treatment. Most patients with constipation do not require surgery. However, patients who do not respond to medication or who have rectal abnormalities that contribute to constipation (e.g., rectal prolapse, colonic inertia) may undergo surgery to correct the problem or remove the problematic portion of the colon.

Diagnostic Tests

The initial diagnostic exam for constipation is a DRE. If constipation is acute or does not resolve, a diagnostic examination may be ordered. This may include a barium enema examination to identify bowel structure, tumors, or diverticula. If the problem is acute, a sigmoidoscopy or colonoscopy may be used for evaluation and to obtain tissue samples for biopsy. Rectal muscle contractions and completeness of bowel eliminations can be tested by defecography and anorectal manometry. A colorectal transit study can determine how efficiently food moves through the patient's gastrointestinal tract.

Pharmacologic Therapy

Laxative and cathartic preparations are used to promote stool evacuation (see the Medications feature). Milder preparations generally are known as laxatives, whereas cathartics have a stronger effect. Most laxatives are appropriate only for short-term use; nurses should encourage patients to use over-the-counter constipation remedies no longer than 7 days before consulting with a healthcare provider. Cathartics and enemas interfere with normal bowel reflexes and should not be used for simple constipation. Laxatives should never be given to patients with appendicitis, enteritis, ulcerative colitis, diverticulitis, intestinal obstruction, fecal impaction, or undiagnosed abdominal pain (Spratto & Woods, 2012). When the bowel is obstructed, laxatives or cathartics may cause serious mechanical damage and may perforate the bowel.

Medications
Constipation

CLASSIFICATION AND DRUG EXAMPLES	MECHANISMS OF ACTION	NURSING CONSIDERATIONS
Bulk-forming Laxatives *Drug examples:* Calcium polycarbophil (FiberCon) Psyllium (Metamucil) methylcellulose (Citrucel)	These fiber supplements increase bulk and promote passage of stool. *May also be used for:* ▪ Treating diarrhea	▪ These drugs can interfere with the absorption of some medications; bulk-forming laxatives should be taken 2 hours before or after other medications. ▪ Always take these drugs with sufficient water; if not, they may cause gastrointestinal obstruction. ▪ The drugs may cause increased bloating and abdominal pain. ▪ Sugar-free options are available for patients with diabetes. ▪ These drugs should not be taken long term. ▪ Some preparations are made to be more appealing to children.
Stimulants (Cathartics) *Drug examples:* Bisacodyl (Dulcolax, Senokot)	Stimulants cause rhythmic muscle contractions in the intestines.	▪ An ingredient in some stimulants, phenolphthalein, may increase the risk of cancer. ▪ These drugs produce a bowel movement in 6–12 hours. ▪ Do not use within 1 hour of taking an antacid or milk. ▪ Stimulants may cause stomach discomfort, nausea, diarrhea, cramps, and fluid and electrolyte loss.
Osmotics and Saline Laxatives *Drug examples:* Lactulose (Chronulac) Polyethylene glycol (MiraLAX) Magnesium hydroxide (Milk of Magnesia) Sodium biphosphate (Fleet Phospho-Soda)	These drugs increase the amount of water in the intestines to soften stools.	▪ These drugs are often used for patients with idiopathic constipation. ▪ They may cause abdominal cramping and diarrhea. ▪ Patients with diabetes should be monitored for electrolyte imbalances. ▪ Expect bowel movement within 24–72 hours. ▪ These drugs may interfere with some antibiotics. ▪ Do not use if pregnant or breastfeeding. ▪ Magnesium hydroxide can increase risk of hypomagnesemia, resulting in cardiac dysthymias and respiratory failure.
Stool Softeners *Drug examples:* Docusate (Colace, Dulcolax)	Stool softeners moisten the stool and help prevent dehydration.	▪ These drugs are suggested for use in patients who should avoid straining. ▪ Prolonged use may cause an electrolyte imbalance. ▪ Stool softeners generally produce a bowel movement in 12–72 hours. ▪ Do not use in the presence of a bowel obstruction.
Lubricants *Drug examples:* Mineral oil (Fleet, Zymenol)	These drugs grease the stool, allowing it to move through the intestine more quickly.	▪ Lubricants typically stimulate a bowel movement within 8 hours. ▪ They are useful for constipation associated with dry, hard stools. ▪ They can be administered orally or rectally. ▪ They may increase the risk of aspiration and pneumonia in older patients who are frail.
Herbal Agent Castor oil (Emulsoil, Neoloid) Senna (Ex-lax, Senokot)	Castor oil lubricates the feces to facilitate bowel movement. Senna is an herb that irritates the lumen of the bowel, which stimulates peristalsis.	▪ These drugs may cause abdominal cramping and diarrhea.
Chloride Channel Activators *Drug examples:* Lubiprostone (Amitiza)	These drugs activate chloride channels to promote fluid release into the intestines.	▪ These drugs can be used safely for 6–12 months. ▪ They are used to treat chronic idiopathic constipation and irritable bowel disorder in women. ▪ Do not use if bowel obstruction is suspected. ▪ The drugs may cause fetal harm; do not take during pregnancy. ▪ Patients may experience nausea or diarrhea. ▪ These drugs cause bowel movement within 24 hours of the first dose.

(continued on next page)

Medications *(continued)*

CLASSIFICATION AND DRUG EXAMPLES	MECHANISMS OF ACTION	NURSING CONSIDERATIONS
Miscellaneous *Drug examples:* Naloxegol (Movantik) Methylnaltrexone (Relistor)	These drugs block the mu receptors in the gastrointestinal tract without affecting the opioid-induced analgesia.	■ These drugs may cause abdominal pain, nausea, vomiting, diarrhea, and flatulence. ■ They are used for patients who are in advanced stages of illness requiring opioid pain control. ■ There is a slight chance of opioid withdrawal symptoms or decreased pain control.
Enemas *Drug examples:* Fleet (saline) Fleet (mineral oil)	Liquid saline or medicine is inserted into the rectum to draw water into the colon and promote bowel movement.	■ Body positioning may be embarrassing for many patients; respect the patient's privacy at all times. ■ Self-administered enemas are available if desired. ■ Enemas can be used to clear the bowels before colonoscopy if the polyethylene glycol-electrolyte (PEG-ES) solution does not empty the bowels completely. ■ These drugs are used for significant constipation or fecal impaction on a short-term basis.
Suppositories *Drug examples:* Docusate, glycerin	Suppositories stimulate muscles in the bowel to promote defecation.	■ Suppositories produce a bowel movement in 15 minutes to 1 hour. ■ They are only for rectal use; they should not be given orally or vaginally.

Source: Data from Adams, M. P., Holland, L. N., & Urban, C. (2017). *Pharmacology for nurses: A pathophysiologic approach* (5th ed.). Hoboken, NJ: Pearson Education.

When choosing a medication, the healthcare team should consider which will be the most effective for evacuating the stool while causing the patient the least amount of discomfort and anxiety. Suppositories and enemas can cause fear in children. Polyethylene glycol-electrolyte solution can be administered orally or instilled via a nasogastric tube to promote stool evacuation. Electrolyte-free polyethylene glycol 3350 (MiraLAX) has been used effectively in children (Portalatin & Winstead, 2012). Once the stool has been evacuated, methods to prevent accumulation of stool in the bowel may be implemented, including eating foods or supplements high in fiber, introducing behavioral methods, and taking stool softeners.

Nonpharmacologic Therapy

Most patients can manage constipation with nonpharmacologic interventions, including education, nutrition, behavioral therapy, and biofeedback. In addition, impacted stool may be manually removed in severe cases.

Education

Education of the patient and family is the first step in treating constipation. A description of the pathophysiology of the condition and nonpharmacologic therapies to prevent constipation is essential. The nurse should provide education about any over-the-counter or prescription medications, including their use and therapeutic and side effects. If the patient needs treatment by manual removal of stool or surgical intervention, the nurse should provide education about what to expect before, during, and after the procedure.

Nutrition

Foods high in fiber are recommended for patients experiencing constipation. Vegetable fiber is largely indigestible and cannot be absorbed, so it increases stool bulk. Fiber also helps draw water into the fecal mass, softening the stool and making defecation easier. Bran and raw fruits and vegetables are good sources of dietary fiber, as is cereal bran. Patients can use 2–3 teaspoons of unprocessed bran with meals (sprinkled on fruit or cereal), or up to 1/4 cup daily, to supply adequate fiber. Removing constipating foods (e.g., bananas, rice, cheese) from the diet also reduces constipation.

Adequate fluid intake is important in maintaining bowel motility and soft stools. The patient should drink 6–8 glasses of fluid per day. The nurse should advise the patient to increase fluid intake when dietary fiber is initially increased to decrease flatus and help maintain softer stools. Constipation in young infants can usually be corrected by increasing the amount of fluids or adding 2 oz of pear or apple juice to daily intake.

Behavior Management and Bowel Training

Behavior modification may prove beneficial in managing constipation. Inactivity is a major contributor to constipation, so encouraging patients to exercise regularly can help decrease constipation and promote defecation.

According to Tabbers and colleagues (2014), evidence does not support the use of behavioral therapy in the treatment of childhood constipation. There may be a benefit to referring children with constipation and behavioral abnormalities to a mental health provider.

Biofeedback

Biofeedback uses visual or auditory feedback about a specific body function. In patients with bowel problems, biofeedback is used to strengthen the rectal sphincter and other rectal muscles. A rectal plug monitors the strength of the muscles, and an electrode is attached to the abdomen. The plug and electrode then record muscle contractions. The patient is taught how to squeeze the rectal muscles using the computer display to confirm correct technique, allowing the patient to control the muscles more effectively during bowel movements (Dugdale & Longstreth, 2012). Evidence does not support the use of biofeedback in the treatment of childhood constipation (Tabbers et al., 2014).

Manual Removal of Stool

Patients with fecal impaction may need to have the hard mass of stool broken up manually. This procedure involves a trained nurse or healthcare provider inserting one or two gloved fingers into the rectum to break up the mass into smaller pieces. Suppositories or enemas are then used to clear out the stool; several suppositories or enemas over a period of days may be necessary for the impaction to completely clear. This process is done in small increments to prevent injury to the mucosal lining of the bowel or the anus. See Volume 3 for Nursing Skill 4.21 Fecal Impaction: Removing.

Lifespan Considerations

Constipation is common throughout the lifespan. Specific developmental and aging changes contribute to constipation in children, pregnant women, and older adults.

Constipation in Children and Adolescents

Constipation is a common complaint in the pediatric population and accounts for up to 20–25% of gastrointestinal complaints. Because defecation patterns vary among children, identification of an abnormal pattern is sometimes difficult.

Pathophysiology and Etiology

Infants usually have several bowel movements a day. Breastfed infants may have bowel movements as frequently as every feeding or just one bowel movement in several days. Firm or hard stools are often seen when the breastfed infant is changed to infant formula or after the introduction of solid foods. Constipation is reported in 9.4% of infants that are exclusively given standard baby formula with no prebiotic or probiotic supplementation. Hard stools are reported more frequently in infants fed with formulas containing palm olein oil or palm oil as the main source of fat (Vandenplas et al., 2015).

One bowel movement each day may be normal for one child, and another child may normally have three to four bowel movements per day. As the child grows, three to four bowel movements a week may become a normal pattern. According to Rome III criteria, children must have two or more of the following symptoms to be diagnosed with functional constipation (Osatakul & Puetpaiboon, 2014).

- Two or fewer defecations in the toilet per week
- At least one episode of fecal incontinence per week
- History of retentive posturing or excessive volitional stool retention

- History of painful or hard bowel movements
- Presence of a large fecal mass in the rectum
- History of large diameter stools that may obstruct the toilet.

Constipation in children is influenced by a variety of factors, including but not limited to the following:

- **Physical factors:** Anal and rectal disorders or malformations, fecalith, poor rectal sensation, diseases that influence gastrointestinal or neurologic systems (e.g., celiac disease, cerebral palsy), obesity, stool withholding, some medications, decreased activity or mobility
- **Psychologic factors:** Embarrassment or shame related to soiling or lack of privacy, reluctance to sit on the toilet, premature toilet training, fear of pain from a hard stool, being too busy to use the bathroom, being restricted from using the bathroom by adults or circumstance, parental anger or shaming related to soiling or toileting refusal.

Inactivity is a risk factor for constipation to occur at any age. Infants and children with severe mental or physical disabilities such as multiple sclerosis are at a high risk for chronic constipation. Constipation may temporarily follow surgery or may last longer when the patient is immobilized during the healing phase, such as when non–weight-bearing, requiring traction, or wearing a body cast.

Constipation during infancy is uncommon, and is usually attributed to mismanagement of the diet. The transition from formula to cow's milk and solid foods may cause a transient constipation, because the bowel must adjust to the increased protein content of cow's milk.

Constipation occurs most frequently in toddlers and preschoolers and is often associated with learning to control body functions. Many toddlers do not like the sensations of a bowel movement and may begin withholding stool or hiding from parents until the urge to defecate has passed. The stool accumulates in and dilates the rectum until the next urge to defecate, often after the next meal. Stool withholding can lead to hard stools and painful defecation, causing the child to avoid the experience. Passing the hard stool could be traumatic, causing a tear in the mucosal tissue of the rectum or anus.

Constipation may occur as a result of limited time for toileting. Busy school-age children may delay toileting to participate in other activities, and adolescents participating in sports or other extracurricular activities may have limited time for toileting. Children may also be hesitant to use an unfamiliar bathroom.

Constipation in toddlers, school-age children, and adolescents may result in overflow fecal incontinence. The parents may think the overflow fecal incontinence is diarrhea and seek medical care to find out the incontinence is liquid stool leaking around the fecal impaction (Xinias & Mavroudi, 2015) or as the fecal matter moves toward the anus.

Interventions and Therapies

Encouragement from parents and relaxation of bathroom privileges at school promote regularity and healthy bowel patterns. Behavior modification is a helpful strategy for younger children to recover from functional constipation. The reflex for defecation usually happens in the morning about 1 hour after eating. It is helpful to schedule routine toilet sitting time for 3–10 minutes after breakfast and possibly a second time after the evening meal. To encourage good positioning, parents can use a footstool to support the child's legs effectively to increase intra-abdominal pressure (Valsalva maneuver). Parents should give positive feedback and reward for defecation and offer no negative or punitive response if there are no results during the scheduled sitting time (Xinias & Mavroudi, 2015).

A balanced diet that includes grains, fruits, and vegetables is recommended as part of the treatment of constipation in children. Fruit juice does not take the place of fruit, although prune, pear, and apple juices can cause increased motility and water content in stools. Cow's milk in excess may cause constipation; children without lactose intolerance usually tolerate milk without issue. A limited temporary trial removing cow's milk may be tried if other measures to correct constipation fail (Xinias & Mavroudi, 2015).

Laxatives containing polyethylene glycol (PEG) are currently the treatment of choice for children with constipation. PEG can be administered with or without additional electrolytes, depending on the child's risk for electrolyte imbalance. Other laxatives can also be used, depending on the child's condition, the effectiveness of PEG for that child, and any adverse experience in the child. Mineral oil may be an equally effective choice for children who do not tolerate PEG.

Constipation in Pregnant Women

Constipation is a common complaint of pregnant women. In pregnancy, mechanical pressure from the growing uterus contributes to displacement of the small intestine and reduces motility. The increased secretion of progesterone further reduces motility because of decreased gastric tone and increased smooth muscle relaxation; thus, the emptying time of the stomach and bowel is prolonged. Constipation is a side effect of iron supplementation found in prenatal vitamins. Hemorrhoids (swollen and inflamed veins in the anus and rectum) frequently develop in late pregnancy from constipation and from pressure on structures below the level of the uterus, causing the pregnant woman further discomfort.

The initial treatment for constipation during pregnancy is the same as for any other adult; increase activity, fluid, and dietary fiber intake. If the initial measures do not relieve constipation, adding a laxative may produce results. Infrequent and short-term use of laxatives does not absorb readily from the bowel lining and should not cause any risk to a developing fetus. Bulk-forming, osmotic, stimulant, and lubricant laxatives along with stool softeners are safe to use sparingly during pregnancy (Trottier, Erebara, & Bozzo, 2012).

Constipation in Older Adults

Constipation affects older adults more frequently than younger adults. Constipation affects between 24 and 50% of older adults. In this population, 10–18% of individuals in the community setting use laxatives daily. In the extended care setting, as many as 74% receive daily laxatives (Rao, 2013). Although fecal transit in the large intestine slows with aging, the increased incidence of constipation in older adults is thought to relate more to impaired general health status, increased medication use, and decreased physical activity. Factors contributing to increased risk for constipation include lack of teeth or ill-fitting, broken, or lost dentures; periodontal disease; and lack of fresh produce or other sources of bulk or fiber. The older adult may self-limit daily fluid intake, especially water, to decrease frequency of urination, or episodes of incontinence, unintentionally increasing the potential for constipation.

Cultural influences and advertising lead many older adults to believe that a daily bowel movement is important for health. This belief contributes to an increased incidence of perceived constipation in older adults. Because of this perception, the older adult may come to rely on laxatives, suppositories, or enemas to facilitate regular bowel movements. These external aids to defecation can further impair the ability to maintain a bowel movement of soft-formed stool every 2–3 days.

FECAL INCONTINENCE

Fecal incontinence, or bowel incontinence, is the loss of the voluntary control of fecal and gaseous discharges through the anal sphincter. It occurs less frequently than urinary incontinence but is no less distressing to the patient. The incontinence may occur at specific times, such as after meals, or it may occur irregularly. Patients often do not reveal fecal incontinence in discussing health concerns, so treatment of this condition is often overlooked, though the personal impact is devastating on the quality of life. Studies indicate that patient reporting of fecal incontinence increases fivefold when the patient is asked directly about the issue by the healthcare worker rather than being expected to report incontinence voluntarily (Alsheik et al., 2012; Bharucha et al., 2015). Therefore, nurses should be diligent in asking the patient about fecal incontinence during the health history interview, especially for older adults and other individuals at high risk for incontinence.

Pathophysiology and Etiology
Pathophysiology

Fecal incontinence is generally associated with impaired functioning of the anal sphincter or its nerve supply, such as in some neuromuscular diseases, spinal cord trauma, and

---

Focus on Integrative Health
Herbal Laxative Use in Children

In many cultures, herbal laxatives are used as therapies for a variety of health problems. Safety and effectiveness of herbal laxatives are not well documented for use in children. One study reviewed found that psyllium, an ingredient in bulk-forming laxatives, is effective for treatment of constipation in children in combination with acacia fiber and fructose. No clinically significant side effects were observed during the 8-week study. Compliance was found to be better for PEG + electrolytes than for psyllium (Quitadamo et al., 2012). Cascara sagrada and senna are stimulant laxatives that have been approved by the U.S. Food and Drug Administration for use to treat constipation in children older than 2 years. Stimulant laxatives should be used rarely and with caution in children because they can lead to dependency and cause abdominal pain.

tumors of the external anal sphincter muscle. Bowel incontinence is usually considered a manifestation of a disorder rather than being a disorder itself. The two types of bowel incontinence are partial and major. Partial incontinence is the inability to control flatus or to prevent minor soiling. Major incontinence is the inability to control feces of normal consistency.

The rate of fecal incontinence among older adults living in the community has been reported to be 7–17%, compared with 2.6% in the young adult population and 33–65% in older nursing home residents (Bharucha et al., 2015; Shah, Chokhavatia, & Rose, 2012; Townsend et al., 2012). Fecal incontinence is an emotionally distressing problem that ultimately can lead to social isolation. To minimize the embarrassment associated with soiling, individuals with fecal incontinence withdraw to their home or, if in the hospital or nursing home, the confines of their room.

Etiology

Multiple factors, both physiologic and psychologic, contribute to fecal incontinence. The most common causes of fecal incontinence are those that interfere with either sensory or motor control of the rectum and anal sphincters. If the external sphincter is paralyzed as a result of spinal cord injury or disease, defecation occurs automatically when the internal sphincter relaxes with the defecation reflex. If sphincter muscles have been damaged or excessive pelvic floor relaxation has occurred, it may not be possible to override the defecation reflex with voluntary control.

Diarrhea, stool impaction, tumors, pelvic floor relaxation, or loss of sphincter tone can all cause fecal incontinence. Other causes of fecal incontinence include the following:

- *Neurologic.* Spinal cord injury or disease; head injury, stroke, or brain tumor; degenerative neurologic diseases such as multiple sclerosis, amyotrophic lateral sclerosis, or dementia; diabetic neuropathy
- *Local trauma.* Obstetrical tears, anorectal injury, anorectal surgery with sphincter damage
- *Inflammatory processes.* Infection, radiation
- *Psychologic.* Depression, confusion, delirium.

Risk Factors

Individuals with nerve damage, including multiple sclerosis, spinal cord injury, or long-term diabetes, are at greatest risk of developing fecal incontinence because they are unable to control the muscles in the bowel and anus. Older age and female gender are also risk factors for fecal incontinence. Age-related changes in anal sphincter tone and response to rectal distention increase the risk for fecal incontinence in older adults. Resting and maximal anal sphincter pressures are decreased, particularly in older women. In addition, less rectal distension is needed to produce sustained relaxation of the anal sphincter in older women.

Dementia and physical disability are also associated with increased fecal incontinence, either because the individual does not comprehend the urge to defecate or because the individual is unable to reach the bathroom before defecation occurs.

Prevention

Methods to prevent fecal incontinence involve controlling the cause of incontinence, including constipation and diarrhea. Methods to prevent constipation include increasing physical activity, fiber consumption, and fluid intake. Treating or eliminating the cause of diarrhea, such as an intestinal infection, can help prevent fecal incontinence. In addition, patients should be taught to avoid straining during bowel movements, which can eventually weaken the anal sphincter muscles and cause nerve damage. Pelvic floor exercises can also help strengthen the sphincter muscles to prevent fecal incontinence.

Clinical Manifestations

Fecal incontinence is characterized by the loss of voluntary bowel control, causing stool or mucus to leak out of the anus at unwanted times. This effect can be minor, in which case the patient passes gas or a small amount of liquid fecal material soils the undergarments; or it can be major, when the patient loses the entire contents of the bowel. It often occurs as a result of nerve or muscle damage that affects control of the rectal muscles. Fecal incontinence may be accompanied by constipation, diarrhea, gas, bloating, abdominal cramping, and urinary incontinence. Emotional distress, including shame and embarrassment, is also common in patients with fecal incontinence.

Collaboration

Treatment of fecal incontinence and encopresis depends on the underlying cause of the incontinence. Many therapies are similar to the treatment of constipation, if constipation is the primary cause of incontinence. In addition, a need for psychologic treatment may be based on the patient's emotional response to the problem. The nurse plays a key role in treatment and management of patients with fecal incontinence through education, implementation of nonpharmacologic therapies, emotional support, and referral to other healthcare workers.

For the patient with bowel elimination issues, collaboration frequently involves a nutritionist, who can help support the patient in making any needed changes in diet or dietary patterns. Nurses may consult with the patient's pharmacist, who can provide additional information regarding medications and supplements in use and any related side effects. Physical therapists may offer important points on exercise within the patient's range of motion that can promote bowel health and management. Nurses working with children who have problems with bowel elimination should encourage parents to work with teachers and dietitians to assist the child with forming dietary habits that support healthy bowel elimination.

Diagnostic Tests

The diagnosis of fecal incontinence includes patient history and physical examination of the pelvic floor and anus to evaluate muscle tone and rule out a fecal impaction. Impaired sphincter muscles may be palpable on digital examination. Anorectal manometry or a rectal motility test may be used to evaluate the functional ability of the sphincter

Clinical Manifestations and Therapies
Bowel Elimination

ETIOLOGY	CLINICAL MANIFESTATIONS	CLINICAL THERAPIES
Acute constipation	Fewer than three bowel movements per week; difficult passage of stools; dry, hard stools; straining; feelings of incomplete evacuation; an abrupt change in bowel elimination patterns; bowel obstruction; UTI; diminished appetite; reduced bowel sounds	■ High-fiber diet or fiber supplements ■ Adequate fluid intake ■ Behavioral modification ■ Pharmacologic therapy ■ Digital stimulation
Chronic constipation	Storage, transport, or evacuation impairment; abdominal discomfort; frequent flatus; straining more than 25% of the time; passage of hard, dry stools more than 25% of the time; abdominal distention; ↓ bowel sounds; manual maneuvers needed to facilitate emptying; fewer than three bowel movements per week; symptoms of constipation for at least 12 weeks in the preceding 12 months	■ High-fiber diet or fiber supplements ■ Adequate fluid intake ■ Behavioral modification ■ Pharmacologic therapy ■ Surgery ■ Education ■ Biofeedback ■ Digital stimulation
Fecal impaction	Similar to symptoms of constipation, plus a mass of hardened feces in the rectum and leakage of liquid fecal material around the fecal mass; rectal pain; a frequent nonproductive desire to defecate; distended abdomen; nausea and vomiting; abdominal cramping	■ Manual evacuation of stool ■ Oil retention enema ■ Cleansing enema ■ Suppositories ■ Prevention methods after successful evacuation
Stool withholding	Most common in children; manifestations include tightening of the external sphincter and gluteal muscles, squatting, rocking, stiff walking on tiptoes, crossing legs, sitting with heels against the perineum, stretching of the rectum and lower colon, stool retention, soiling by involuntary overflow	■ Polyethylene glycol 3350 with or without electrolytes ■ High-fiber diet or fiber supplements ■ Adequate fluid intake ■ Behavioral modification ■ Education ■ Rewards for defecation ■ Child and family psychotherapy
Partial fecal incontinence	Inability to control flatus; minor soiling; constipation; social isolation; bloating; abdominal cramping; urinary incontinence	■ Treatment of constipation ■ Pelvic floor exercises ■ Education ■ Surgery to correct bowel defect ■ Behavioral modification ■ Instructions for self-care techniques
Major fecal incontinence	Evacuation of the entire bowel contents at an inappropriate time and place; impaired functioning of the anal sphincter or nerve supply; inability to control feces of normal consistency; diarrhea; gastrointestinal infection; social isolation; urinary incontinence	■ Pelvic floor exercises ■ Colostomy ■ Antidiarrheal drugs ■ Antimicrobial agents ■ Teaching self-care techniques
Encopresis	Recurrent soiling at inappropriate times by a child who should have achieved bowel continence; constipation; withholding behavior; small, hard, and painful bowel movements; emotional withdrawal	■ Psychologic treatment ■ Collaboration with school nurses and teachers ■ Pharmacologic treatment of constipation ■ High-fiber diet ■ Behavioral modification

muscles. In this test, a small, flexible balloon catheter is introduced into the rectum, and pressures are measured in the rectum and internal and external sphincters. Rectal dilatation normally causes the internal sphincter to relax and the external sphincter to contract. Sigmoidoscopy is used to examine the rectum and anal canal if visualization of the bowel lumen is required.

A thorough history; physical examination; and possibly a barium enema, CT scan, or other diagnostic radiographic studies are necessary to rule out organic causes and anatomical abnormalities related to encopresis. Examination of mental health and cognitive functioning may be indicated. Information about the child's toilet training habits and the parents' attitudes concerning toilet training should be evaluated. A dietary history, including eating habits and types of foods eaten, often is helpful as well. One purpose of palpating the lower abdomen during a nursing assessment or the healthcare provider's physical examination is to reveal any nontender mass or structural abnormality in the patient's anatomy.

Surgery

When damage to the sphincter or a rectal prolapse (protrusion of rectal mucous membrane through the anus) is the cause of fecal incontinence, surgical repair is the treatment of choice. Surgery also may be indicated when conservative measures have not been effective. Permanent colostomy (the creation of an opening from the large bowel on the abdominal wall) is a last-choice option for some patients, but it can control fecal output when other measures fail.

Pharmacologic Therapy

Management of fecal incontinence is directed toward the identified cause. Medications to relieve diarrhea or constipation may be prescribed (see the Medications feature on constipation). Drugs to control diarrhea include loperamide (Imodium) and bismuth subsalicylate (Kaopectate, Pepto-Bismol). Diarrhea from an infection may also be treated with an appropriate antimicrobial agent. Treatment of encopresis may include the temporary use of lubricants, bulk-forming laxatives, or stool softeners to clear the bowel of impacted stool and encourage normal defecation.

Nonpharmacologic Therapy

Several nonpharmacologic therapies can be used to treat fecal incontinence. A high-fiber diet, ample fluids, and regular exercise are helpful for many patients. Exercises to improve sphincter and pelvic floor muscle tone (pelvic floor exercises) may be of long-term benefit. Biofeedback therapy may be used for mentally alert patients with intact sphincter muscles but low muscle tone. The nurse may also teach the patient self-care techniques that should be used to keep the anal area clean after fecal incontinence.

Lifespan Considerations

Fecal Incontinence in Children and Adolescents

Children with bowel incontinence require special care based on their developmental level. Nurses should partner with parents to teach toilet training techniques, emphasizing the child's developmental readiness. The nurse should encourage parents to praise the child for successes and to avoid punishment and power struggles. The nurse should encourage high-fiber diets and regular times for elimination.

Encopresis

Encopresis is an abnormal elimination pattern characterized by recurrent soiling or passage of stool at inappropriate times by a child who should have achieved bowel continence. An estimated 1–2% of children younger than 10 years have encopresis, approximately 80% of those children being boys. In addition, 80–95% of children with encopresis have a history of constipation (Borowitz, 2013). Children with primary

encopresis have never achieved bowel control. Children with secondary encopresis have had bowel continence for several months.

Encopresis usually is associated with voluntary or involuntary retention of stool in the lower bowel and rectum. This leads to constipation, dilation of the lower bowel, and incompetence of the inner sphincter. The retention of stool usually is a result of being "too busy": The child puts off going to the bathroom because leaving the current activities would be an inconvenience. The retention of stool leads to constipation that is untreated and chronic. Loose stool leaks around the hard feces, and the child becomes unaware of a need to eliminate. Soiling may occur during the day or night. Bowel movements are irregular, painful, small, and hard. The child may be ridiculed by peers because of offensive odor. This rejection leads to withdrawal and behavioral problems, often resulting in altered school performance and attendance. The child continues to hold stool because the passage has become painful. Parents commonly seek healthcare, believing that the child has diarrhea or constipation.

The underlying constipation that leads to encopresis may be caused by the stress of environmental changes (e.g., birth of a sibling, moving to a new house, attending a new school), issues of anger and control related to bowel training, diet, a full schedule of activities, or a genetic predisposition.

Interventions and Therapies

The focus of nursing care centers on educating the child and parents about the disorder, treatment, and on providing emotional support. The nurse should explain the treatment plan, including dietary changes and use of laxatives or stool softeners. The nurse should reassure the child that he or she has a healthy body and, with treatment, will achieve normal functioning. The nurse should also monitor the child for at least 6 months to be certain new patterns become established.

Treatment of encopresis may include behavior modification techniques, dietary changes, and psychotherapy. Behavior modification programs that reward and reinforce appropriate toileting habits can be successful for some children. Dietary changes include incorporating high-fiber foods, such as fruits, vegetables, and whole-grain cereal, into the diet. Limiting intake of refined and highly processed foods and hard cheeses may be helpful. The child should sit on the toilet for several minutes after the morning and evening meals. It takes several months for the bowel to be retrained to respond to sphincter stimulation. Psychotherapy involving the child and family may be indicated in instances of dysfunctional parent–child relationships or in cases of suspected sexual abuse.

Fecal Incontinence in Pregnant women

The prevalence of fecal incontinence in pregnancy varies from 3 to 29%. Determining the true incidence is often difficult because many women consider it a personal matter and are too embarrassed to discuss incontinence with anyone. Women were more incontinent late in pregnancy than 6 months after delivery; therefore, these findings suggest that pregnancy itself may be a risk factor. It is possible the hormonal changes in pregnancy and the weight of the uterus, alterations in the pelvic floor, and changes in anal and perineal anatomy play a role in the pathophysiology of fecal incontinence in pregnancy. Pregnancy after 20 weeks, regardless of mode of delivery, greatly increases the prevalence of major pelvic floor dysfunction, including all types of incontinence (Naidoo, 2014). Anal canal volume (ACV) increases by 20% between 18 and 28 weeks of pregnancy, and there is significant association between ACV and incontinence scores (Olsen, Wilsgaard, & Kierud, 2012).

If there is stool present in the sigmoid colon or rectum during labor and delivery, fecal incontinence is probable. During peripartum, the perineum swells, subsequently increasing pressure on the rectum and anus. Incontinence during labor and birth is due to the close proximity of the birth canal to the rectum and anus, coupled with the pressure of the fetus in the lower pelvis during the labor and birth process.

Many of the problems associated with postpartum changes in the pelvic floor may be attributed to biomechanical changes occurring in pregnancy (Olsen et al., 2012). Many of the problems specific to postpartum fecal incontinence may be attributed to changes in function of the rectum and anus during pregnancy. Sphincter disruption and nerve damage are complications of childbirth and possibly the primary contributory factors in development of postpartum fecal incontinence, though there is no correlation between symptoms of fecal incontinence and anal sphincter injury. Symptoms of flatus and fecal incontinence are commonly present in early pregnancy and consistently predictive for the same women reporting similar symptoms after delivery (Naidoo, 2014).

Fecal Incontinence in Older Adults

The etiology of fecal incontinence is multifactorial, involving a delicate balance between stool consistency and physical integrity of the anatomical structures involved in bowel elimination (Alavi et al., 2015). Fecal incontinence is abnormal and should not be considered a normal change of aging. Attributes related to structural integrity of the intestinal tract can include: decreasing muscle tone and rectal sensation from cumulative local trauma resulting from childbirth, constipation, rectal impaction, or other conditions that can affect the structures of the intestinal tract. Older adults are at increased risk for fecal incontinence due to chronic disease, polypharmacy, and fecal impaction from inactivity or immobility and reduced fluid intake.

Fecal incontinence presents a significant direct and indirect burden on patients, their caregivers, and the healthcare system. Older adults who are cognitively intact and physically able should be considered for treatment to alleviate the psychosocial effects associated with fecal incontinence and the undue burden to care providers and healthcare systems (Razjouyan, Prasad, & Chokhavatia, 2015).

NURSING PROCESS

The nurse plays a fundamental role in the care of patients with bowel problems. Assessment, education, administration of medications, hygiene care, monitoring of food and fluid intake, and emotional support are all interventions the nurse can implement to provide care to patients with constipation, fecal impaction, and fecal incontinence.

Assessment

- **Observation and patient interview.** During the patient interview the nurse should observe for signs and symptoms of bowel elimination problems. Frequent, urgent, or untimely requests to use the bathroom would be a reason to question the patient further about elimination problems. The presence of fecal odor or soiled clothing may be a sign of bowel elimination problems. Many patients become distracted, anxious, and possibly appear agitated when withholding stool, especially if discomfort, odorous flatulence, or the fear of incontinence is present.

  The nurse should discuss the extent, onset, and duration of constipation, impaction, or incontinence; contributing factors; history of spinal cord or anorectal injury or surgery; pregnancy; chronic diseases, such as diabetes, multiple sclerosis, or other neurologic disorders; medications and use of alternative therapies; nutrition; and hydration patterns.

- **Physical examination.** The nurse palpates the abdomen for firmness or tenderness as well as for the presence of any mass (retained stool). Bowel sounds should also be assessed. If a DRE is performed, the nurse assesses for the presence of stool in the rectum. The nurse also assesses for hemorrhoids, anal fissures, or other abnormalities of the abdomen or perineum.

Diagnosis

Nursing diagnoses that may be appropriate for inclusion in the plan of care for the patient with impaired fecal elimination include the following:

- *Bowel Incontinence*
- *Constipation*
- *Functional Constipation, Chronic*
- *Constipation, Perceived*
- *Constipation, Risk for*
- *Gastrointestinal Motility, Dysfunctional*
- *Gastrointestinal Motility, Risk for Dysfunctional*
- *Diarrhea*
- *Self-care deficit, Toileting.*

  (NANDA-I © 2014)

Fecal elimination problems may affect many other areas of human functioning and, as a consequence, may be the etiology of other NANDA-I nursing diagnoses. Examples are the following:

- *Anxiety*
- *Skin Integrity, Risk for Impaired*
- *Fluid Volume Deficient (or Risk for)*
- *Pain, Acute*
- *Sleep Pattern, Disturbed*
- *Self-Esteem, Chronic Low*
- *Knowledge, Deficient.*

  (NANDA-I © 2014)

Planning

Goal planning for patients with fecal elimination problems requires a patient-centered approach. Goals will be dependent on each patient's unique set of circumstances. The primary areas to consider are included in the following examples:

- The patient will have a brown soft-formed stool within 4 hours of receiving the prescribed laxative.

- The patient will have a brown soft-formed stool at least two times a week while receiving prescribed (medication).

- The patient will maintain or restore normal bowel elimination patterns prior to discharge (or other patient-centered time frame).

- The patient will maintain or regain normal stool consistency prior to discharge (or other patient-centered time frame).

- The patient will prevent associated risks: (fluid and electrolyte imbalance, skin breakdown, falls, or other patient-centered risk factors).

- The patient will list at least four foods high in dietary fiber by the end of a nurse-led teaching session.

Implementation

Nursing interventions will be directed toward achieving each of the goals of care. These interventions can include: promoting regular defecation, perineal skin care, bowel training programs, digital removal of fecal impaction, and use of a fecal incontinence pouch. The Patient Teaching feature also addresses aspects of fecal elimination.

Promote Regular Defecation

The nurse can assist the patient to achieve regular defecation by providing for and encouraging:

- *Privacy.* During defecation it is extremely important to most individuals to have privacy. The nurse should provide as much privacy as possible for such patients but may need to stay with those who are too weak to be left alone. Some patients also prefer to wipe, wash, and dry themselves independently after defecating. The nurse may need to provide water, a washcloth, and a towel for this purpose.

- *Timing.* The patient should be encouraged to defecate when the urge is recognized. To establish regular bowel elimination, the patient and nurse can discuss when peristalsis normally occurs and provide time for defecation. Many individuals have well-established routines. Other activities, such as bathing and ambulating, should not interfere with the defecation time.

- *Nutrition and fluids.* The diet required for regular, normal elimination varies depending on the kind of feces the patient currently has, the frequency of defecation, and the types of foods that the patient finds assist with normal defecation.

For constipation, the patient should increase daily fluid intake and drink hot liquids and fruit juices, especially prune juice. The patient can increase dietary fiber by adding foods such as raw fruit, bran products, and whole-grain cereals and bread. The nurse should caution the patient to increase fluid intake when dietary fiber is initially increased to decrease flatus and help maintain softer stools.

To decrease flatulence, the patient should limit carbonated beverages, the use of drinking straws, and chewing gum, all of which increase the ingestion of air. Gas-forming foods, such as cabbage, beans, onions, and cauliflower, should be avoided as well.

- *Regular exercise.* Exercise assists in developing a regular defecation pattern. Weak abdominal and pelvic muscles contribute to irregular defecation patterns. The patient may be able to strengthen these muscles with the following isometric exercises:
  - In a supine position, the patient tightens the abdominal muscles as though pulling them inward, holding them for about 10 seconds and then relaxing them. This exercise should be repeated 5–10 times each session and four times a day, depending on the patient's health.
  - Again in a supine position, the patient can contract the thigh muscles and hold them contracted for about 10 seconds, repeating the exercise 5–10 times each session four times a day. This exercise helps the patient confined to bed gain strength in the thigh muscles that makes it easier to use a bedpan.

- *Positioning.* Although the squatting position best facilitates defecation, some patients have good results by leaning forward while sitting on the toilet seat.

For patients who have difficulty sitting down on and getting up from the toilet, an elevated toilet seat can be used to raise a regular toilet. A higher toilet seat decreases the distance patients will need to lower onto and lift themselves up from the seat. Elevated toilet seats can be purchased for use in the home. In addition, manufacturers offer a "comfort" height, which is higher than a standard toilet.

Maintain Skin Integrity

Good skin care is vital for the patient with fecal incontinence. Stool contains enzymes and other irritating substances that promote skin breakdown when they are not promptly removed. Skin breakdown can lead to decubitus ulcer, particularly when a neurologic disorder (e.g., spinal cord injury, dementia, stroke) impairs mobility.

Skin care should include the following:

- Cleanse the skin thoroughly with mild soap and water after each bowel movement. Toilet tissue may be more irritating to the skin and less effective in removing fecal material.

- Apply a skin barrier cream or ointment after each bowel movement. These help protect the skin from irritating substances in the feces.

- If incontinence pads or briefs are used, check frequently for soiling, and change the pad or brief when feces are noted. Although these help to protect bedding and clothing from soiling, they can contribute to skin breakdown if they are not checked and changed frequently.

For further information, see Volume 3, Chapter 2, Caring Interventions and Skill 2.8 Perineal-Genital Area: Caring for.

Facilitate Bowel Training Programs

For patients who have chronic constipation, frequent impactions, or fecal incontinence, bowel training programs may be helpful. The program is based on factors within the patient's control and is designed to help the patient establish normal defecation. Matters such as food and fluid intake, exercise, and defecation habits are all considered. Before beginning a bowel training program, patients must understand it and want to be involved. The major phases of the program are as follows:

■ Determine the patient's usual bowel habits and factors that help and hinder normal defecation.

■ Design a plan with the patient that includes fluid intake of approximately 2500 mL per day; increase fiber in the diet; intake of warm beverages, especially just before the usual defecation time; and an increase in exercise.

■ Maintain the following daily routine for 2–3 weeks:
  a. To stimulate peristalsis, administer a suppository (e.g., Dulcolax) 30 minutes before the patient's defecation time.
  b. When the patient experiences the urge to defecate, assist the patient to the toilet or commode or onto a bedpan. Note the length of time between the insertion of the suppository and the urge to defecate.
  c. Provide the patient with privacy for defecation and a time limit (30–40 minutes is usually sufficient).
  d. Teach the patient to lean forward at the hips, to apply pressure on the abdomen with the hands, and to gently bear down for defecation. These measures increase pressure on the colon. Straining should be avoided because it can cause hemorrhoids.

■ Offer support and encouragement, and convey that patience often is required. Many patients require weeks or months of training to achieve success.

■ Provide room odor control with deodorizer tablets, sprays, or other devices. Controlling odor is important to preserve the patient's self-esteem.

Provide Manual Removal of Fecal Impaction as Ordered

Manual removal of a fecal impaction is described in Volume 3. This procedure can be painful. The nurse should plan for adequate pain control prior to beginning.

Maintain a Fecal Incontinence Pouch

To collect and contain large volumes of liquid feces, the nurse may place a rectal tube and fecal incontinence collector pouch around the anal area. The purpose of the pouch is to prevent progressive perianal skin irritation and breakdown as well as the frequent linen changes necessary from incontinence. In many agencies, the pouch is replacing the more traditional approach of inserting a large Foley catheter into the patient's rectum and inflating the balloon to keep it in place, a practice that may damage the rectal sphincter and rectal mucosa. A rectal catheter also increases peristalsis and incontinence by stimulating sensory nerve fibers in the rectum.

A fecal collector is secured around the anal opening and may or may not be attached to drainage. Pouches are best applied before the perianal skin becomes excoriated. If perianal skin excoriation is present, the nurse either (a) applies a dimethicone-based moisture-barrier cream or an alcohol-free barrier film to the skin to protect it from feces until it heals and then applies the pouch or (b) applies a skin barrier or hydrocolloid barrier underneath the pouch to achieve the best possible seal.

Nursing responsibilities for patients with a rectal tube and fecal pouch include (a) regularly assessing and documenting the perianal skin status, (b) changing the bag every 72 hours, or less if leakage occurs, (c) maintaining the drainage system, and (d) providing explanations and support to the patient and support people.

Some patients (e.g., those with quadriplegia or paraplegia, those who have experienced trauma or stroke) may be treated for fecal incontinence by surgical repair of a damaged sphincter or an artificial bowel sphincter. The artificial sphincter consists of three parts: a cuff around the anal canal, a pressure-regulating balloon, and a pump that inflates the cuff. The cuff is inflated to close the sphincter, maintaining continence. To have a bowel movement, the patient deflates the cuff. The cuff automatically inflates again in 10 minutes. Management of this device is specific to the model being used. The nurse should follow manufacturer instructions for details. Administering enemas and rectal medications may be harmful with this device in place.

Provide Patient Education for Home Care

Managing fecal incontinence is a challenging problem for the patient, family, and caregivers. For the patient with adequate cognition, it can be psychologically devastating. The patient may become socially isolated for fear of odor or soiled clothing. The patient may experience a decrease in self-esteem if control over body functions is lost, especially if there is an inability to provide self-care. The nurse should stress that incontinence is not a normal age-related problem and is often treatable. The nurse can encourage the patient to seek medical evaluation of the problem.

See the Patient Teaching feature for topics to include in patient and family education:

Evaluation

The goals established during the planning phase are evaluated according to the specific desired outcomes. If the desired outcomes are not achieved, the nurse should explore the reasons. The nurse might consider some or all of the following questions:

■ Were the patient's fluid intake and diet appropriate? If not, additional teaching is required. Also consider a referral to a dietitian.

■ Was the patient's activity level appropriate? Assess the patient's level of activity and make further recommendations accordingly. What are the obstacles: inclement weather, need for assistive devices, safety, or lack of transportation? Many people walk in a local mall or large grocery store to avoid exercising in extreme weather and to feel safer than in some neighborhoods. Referrals may be needed for transportation or assistive devices such as a walker with wheels.

■ Are prescribed medications or other factors affecting gastrointestinal function? A full review of medications in use should be discussed with the patient and caregiver with each assessment and evaluation of outcomes.

Patient Teaching
Fecal Elimination

Nurses should do the following for the patient to facilitate successful fecal elimination.

Facilitating Toileting

- Ensure safe and easy access to the toilet. Make sure lighting is appropriate, scatter rugs are removed or securely fastened, and so forth.
- Facilitate instruction as needed about transfer techniques.
- Suggest ways that garments can be adjusted to make disrobing easier for toileting (e.g., Velcro closing on clothing).

Monitoring Bowel Elimination Pattern

- Instruct the patient, if appropriate, to keep a record of time and frequency of stool passage, any associated pain, and color and consistency of the stool.
- Discuss the recommended bowel training program, including techniques for digital anal stimulation, inserting suppositories, or administering enemas as recommended.

Dietary Alterations

- Provide information about required food and fluid alterations to promote defecation or manage diarrhea.

Medications

- Discuss medications with the patient at each healthcare interaction. Discussions should address problems associated with overuse of laxatives, if appropriate, and the use of alternatives to laxatives, suppositories, and enemas.
- Discuss the addition of a fiber supplement if the patient is taking a constipating medication.

Exercise and Self-Care

- Discuss the need for regular exercise to stimulate bowel peristalsis and regular evacuation.
- Emphasize the importance of appropriate skin care, particularly if neurologic impairment is present.

Community Agencies and Other Sources of Help

- Provide appropriate referrals to home care or community care for assistance with resources such as installation of grab bars and raised toilet seats, structural alterations for wheelchair access, homemaker or home health aide services to assist with ADLs, and an enterostomal therapy nurse for assistance with stoma care and selection of ostomy appliances.
- Provide information about companies from which durable medical equipment (e.g., raised toilet seats, commodes, bedpans, urinals) can be purchased, rented, or obtained free of charge and supplies (e.g., incontinence pads, ostomy irrigating supplies and appliances) can be obtained.
- Discuss additional sources of information and help, such as ostomy self-help and support groups or clubs.

- Do the patient and family understand instructions well enough to comply with the required therapy? If not, further teaching may be necessary. If the caregiver is older, such as a spouse, consider teaching a younger family member such as an adult child. Translation to the patient or caregiver's native language may be required to clear up misunderstandings.
- Was sufficient physical and emotional support provided? If not, consider additional referrals for home health or programs providing in-home caregivers for ADLs. If there is not adequate physical and emotional support in the home setting, then the nurse or case manager should explore options for admission to a rehabilitation facility, an assisted living facility, or long-term care.

≫ Go to **Pearson MyLab Nursing and eText** to see a nursing care plan for a patient with altered bowel elimination.

REVIEW Bowel Incontinence, Constipation, and Impaction

RELATE Link the Concepts and Exemplars

Linking the exemplar of bowel incontinence, constipation, and impaction with the concept of mobility:

1. What impact does the concept of mobility have on elimination?
2. How can the nurse promote normal bowel elimination in the patient with altered mobility?

Linking the exemplar of bowel incontinence, constipation, and impaction with the concept of metabolism:

3. When caring for a patient with liver disease, what special precautions must the nurse implement related to bowel elimination?
4. When caring for a patient diagnosed with hypothyroidism, what nursing implementations can be initiated to reduce the impact of this disorder on bowel elimination?

READY Go to Volume 3: Clinical Nursing Skills

REFER Go to Pearson MyLab Nursing and eText

- Additional review materials
- Nursing Care Plan: A Patient with Altered Bowel Elimination

REFLECT Apply Your Knowledge

Justin Gardner is a 26-year-old man who fractured his third thoracic vertebra when he fell while rock climbing. He is incontinent of feces secondary to sensory loss and the inability to feel the need to defecate.

1. What nursing interventions can be implemented to promote adequate bowel elimination for this patient? Explain your answer.
2. What skin care precautions will the nurse implement to maintain skin integrity?
3. What nursing diagnosis would be appropriate for this patient?
4. What patient teaching will this patient require, related to bowel continence, before discharge if he is to provide effective home care for himself?

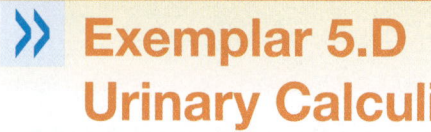

Exemplar 5.D
Urinary Calculi

Exemplar Learning Outcomes

5.D Analyze urinary calculi as they relate to elimination.

- Describe the pathophysiology of urinary calculi.
- Describe the etiology of urinary calculi.
- Compare the risk factors and prevention of urinary calculi.
- Identify the clinical manifestations of urinary calculi.
- Summarize diagnostic tests and therapies used by interprofessional teams in the collaborative care of an individual with urinary calculi.
- Differentiate care of patients with bowel incontinence, constipation, and impaction across the lifespan.
- Apply the nursing process in providing culturally competent care to an individual with urinary calculi.

Exemplar Key Terms

Calcium oxalate, *339*
Calcium phosphate, *339*
Extracorporeal shock wave lithotripsy (ESWL), *341*
Hydronephrosis, *340*
Lithiasis, *338*
Lithotripsy, *341*
Nephrolithiasis, *338*
Nephrolithotomy, *341*
Nucleation, *338*
Pyelolithotomy, *341*
Renal colic, *339*
Staghorn calculi, *339*
Struvite calculi, *339*
Ureterolithotomy, *341*
Uric acid stones, *339*
Urinary calculi, *338*
Urolithiasis, *338*

Overview

Urinary calculi, often referred to as kidney stones, are caused by the development of one or more crystals ranging in size from very small to large enough to fill the renal calyces. These calculi can lodge anywhere in the urinary tract and may cause obstruction and kidney damage. The excruciating pain associated with renal calculi occurs when the multifaceted crystal scrapes against the lining of the ureter, causing extreme irritation. As a result, pain management is an important consideration in caring for patients with this disorder.

Urinary calculi are the most common cause of upper urinary tract obstruction (Kim, 2016). The term **lithiasis** means "stone formation." When the stones form in the kidney, the condition is known as **nephrolithiasis**; when they form elsewhere in the urinary tract (e.g., the bladder), the condition is called **urolithiasis**. Stones may form and obstruct the urinary tract at any point (see **Figure 5–9** »). In the United States and other industrialized countries, formation of renal (or kidney) calculi is common.

Pathophysiology and Etiology

Pathophysiology

A balance normally exists in the kidneys between the need to conserve water and the need to eliminate poorly soluble materials such as calcium salts. This balance is affected by factors such as diet, environmental temperature, and activity. Protective inorganic and organic substances in the urine, such as pyrophosphate, citrate, and glycoproteins, normally inhibit stone (calculi) formation.

Three factors contribute to urolithiasis: supersaturation, **nucleation** (formation of a crystal from a liquid), and lack of inhibitory substances in the urine. When the concentration of an insoluble salt in the urine is very high (i.e., when the urine is supersaturated), crystals may form. These crystals usually disperse and are eliminated because the bonds holding them

together are weak. However, a nucleus of crystals may develop stable bonds to form a stone. More often, crystals form around an organic matrix, or mucoprotein nucleus, to become a stone. The stimulus required to initiate crystallization in supersaturated urine may be minimal. Things as simple as ingesting a meal high in insoluble salt or decreased fluid intake, as occurs during sleep, allow the concentration to increase to the point where precipitation occurs and stones form and grow. When fluid intake is adequate, no stone growth occurs. The acidity or

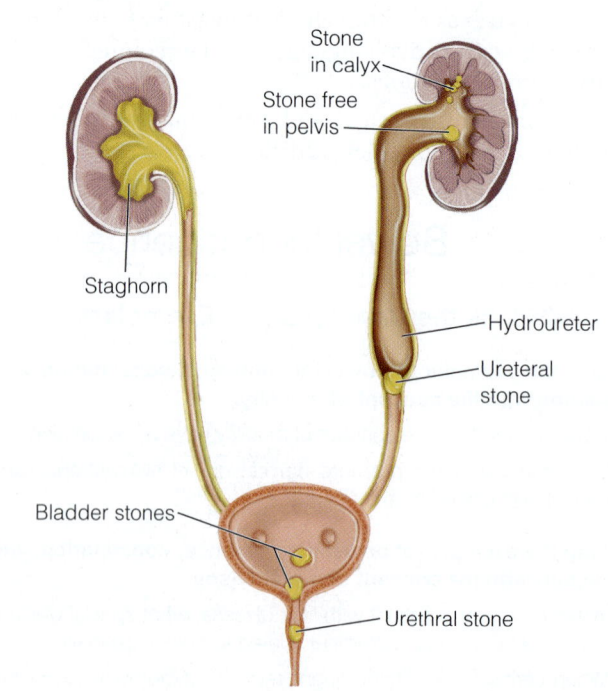

Figure 5–9 » Development and location of calculi in the urinary tract.

alkalinity of the urine and the presence or absence of calculus-inhibiting compounds also affect lithiasis.

Most kidney calculi (75–80%) are composed of **calcium oxalate** and/or **calcium phosphate**. These calculi are generally associated with high concentrations of calcium in the blood or urine. **Uric acid stones** develop when the urine concentration of uric acid is high. They are more common in men and may be associated with gout. Genetic factors contribute to the development of calculi comprised of uric acid and calcium. **Struvite calculi** are associated with UTI caused by urease-producing bacteria such as *Proteus.* These stones can become very large, filling the renal pelvis and calyces. They are often called **staghorn calculi** because of their shape. Cystine stones, which are rare, are associated with a genetic defect. The types of renal calculi, contributing factors, and recommended dietary modifications and other treatments are listed in **Table 5–8 ≫**.

Etiology

Most urinary calculi form in the renal pelvis and are composed primarily of calcium salts. Urolithiasis affects up to 720,000 individuals annually in the United States (Papadakis & McPhee, 2013). In the United States, the incidence varies by region, with the highest frequency in Southern and Midwestern states. Male patients in general are affected 1 or 2 times more often than female patients. Calculi are more common among Caucasians than African-Americans. Most individuals affected are in young or middle adulthood (Roudakova & Monga, 2014).

Risk Factors

Although the majority of urinary stones are idiopathic (having no demonstrable cause), a number of risk factors have been identified. The greatest risk factor for stone formation is a prior personal or family history of urinary calculi. A genetic predisposition to the accumulation of certain mineral substances in the urine or a congenital lack of protective factors may explain the familial link. Other identified risk factors include dehydration with resultant increased urine concentration; immobility; and excess dietary intake of calcium, oxalate, or proteins. Gout, hyperparathyroidism, and urinary stasis or repeated infections also contribute to calculus formation. Loss of calcium from the bones (e.g., due to immobility) and dehydration are major risk factors for urinary stones.

Prevention

Adequate fluid intake is the most important intervention for preventing all types of kidney stones. In addition, specific measures can be taken to prevent each type of kidney stone. Calcium stones can be prevented by reducing sodium and animal protein intake, getting enough calcium from food, and avoiding foods high in oxalate (e.g., spinach, nuts, wheat bran). Uric acid stones can be prevented by limiting animal protein intake (NIDDK, 2013a). For individuals with a history of kidney stones, medications may help prevent future stone formation. For example, thiazide diuretics are used to prevent calcium stones, allopurinol is used to prevent uric acid stones, and antibiotics may help prevent struvite stones (Mayo Clinic, 2012).

Clinical Manifestations

The symptoms caused by urinary calculi vary with their size and location. (See the Clinical Manifestations and Therapies feature.) Manifestations develop from obstructed urine flow resulting in distention and from tissue trauma caused by passage of the rough-edged crystalline stone.

Calculi affecting the kidney calyces and pelvis may cause few symptoms. If the stone has gradually or partially obstructed urinary flow, dull, aching flank pain may be present, but renal calculi are often without symptoms. Bladder calculi may cause few symptoms other than dull suprapubic pain with exercise or after voiding.

Renal colic (acute, severe flank pain on the affected side) develops when a stone obstructs the ureter, causing ureteral spasm. The pain of renal colic may radiate to the suprapubic region, groin, and external genitals (the scrotum or labia). The severity of the pain often causes a sympathetic response with associated nausea; vomiting; pallor; and cool, clammy skin.

Manifestations of UTI, including chills and fever, frequency, urgency, and dysuria, may accompany urinary calculi at any level. Calculi may cause trauma to the urinary tract, resulting in gross or microscopic hematuria. Gross hematuria is often the only sign of bladder stones.

TABLE 5–8 Risk Factors and Interventions for Renal Calculi

Stone Type and Incidence	Risk Factors	Management
Calcium phosphate and/or oxalate 75–80%	Hypercalciuria and hypercalcemia: hyperparathyroidism, immobility, bone disease, vitamin D intoxication, multiple myeloma, renal tubular acidosis, prolonged steroid intake, alkaline urine, dehydration, inflammatory bowel disease	*Pharmacology:* Thiazide, diuretics, phosphates, calcium-binding agents *Dietary:* Limited foods high in calcium and oxalate, increased foods that acidify urine *Other:* Increased hydration, exercise
Struvite 15–20%	UTIs, especially *Proteus* infections	*Pharmacology:* Antibiotic therapy for UTI *Other:* Surgical intervention or lithotripsy to remove stone
Uric acid 5–10%	Gout, increased purine intake, acid urine	*Pharmacology:* Potassium citrate, allopurinol *Dietary:* Low purine diet *Other:* Increased hydration
Cystine (uncommon)	Genetic defect, acid urine	*Pharmacology:* Penicillamine, sodium bicarbonate *Dietary:* Sodium restriction *Other:* Increase hydration

Complications

Urinary stones may obstruct urine flow at any point in the urinary tract, causing complications such as hydronephrosis and urinary stasis with subsequent infection.

Obstruction

Stones can obstruct the urinary tract from the calyces of the kidney to the distal urethra, impeding the outflow of urine. If the obstruction develops slowly, there may be few or no symptoms, whereas sudden obstruction (e.g., blockage of a ureter by a passing stone) may cause severe manifestations. Urinary tract obstruction can ultimately lead to renal failure. The degree of obstruction, its location, and the duration of impaired urine flow determine the effect on renal function.

Hydronephrosis

The kidneys continue to produce urine, causing increased pressure and distention of the urinary tract behind the obstruction. **Hydronephrosis** (accumulation of urine in the renal pelvis as a result of obstructed outflow) and hydroureter (distention of the ureter with urine) are possible results. If the pressure is not relieved, damage to the collecting tubules, proximal tubules, and glomeruli of the kidney causes a gradual loss of renal function.

Acute hydronephrosis typically causes colicky pain on the affected side. The pain may radiate into the groin. Chronic hydronephrosis develops slowly and may have few manifestations other than dull, aching back or flank pain. When hydronephrosis is significant, a palpable mass may be felt in the flank region. Hematuria and signs of UTI such as pyuria, fever, and discomfort may occur. Gastrointestinal symptoms such as nausea, vomiting, and abdominal pain may accompany hydronephrosis.

Infection

The urinary stasis associated with partial or complete obstruction increases the risk of UTI. Upper or lower UTIs may develop. See the exemplar on UTIs in the module on Infection.

Clinical Manifestations and Therapies
Urinary Calculi

ETIOLOGY	CLINICAL MANIFESTATIONS	CLINICAL THERAPIES
Acute hydronephrosis caused by the development of a sudden obstruction of urine flow	■ Acute, colicky pain; may radiate into groin ■ Hematuria, pyuria ■ Fever ■ Nausea, vomiting, abdominal pain	■ Lithotripsy or surgical removal of the stone ■ IV therapy ■ Thiazide diuretics if stone is caused by excess calcium ■ Dietary modification ■ Monitoring of BUN and creatinine to determine extent of kidney damage ■ Patient teaching to reduce risk factors and prevent recurrence
Chronic hydronephrosis caused by gradual development of obstruction of urine flow	■ Possibly asymptomatic until complete obstruction develops ■ Dull, aching flank pain ■ Hematuria, pyuria ■ Fever ■ Palpable flank mass	■ Lithotripsy or surgical removal of the stone ■ Evaluation of kidney function ■ Dietary modification ■ IV therapy ■ Patient teaching to reduce risk of recurrence
Kidney stones	■ Often asymptomatic ■ Dull, aching flank pain ■ Microscopic hematuria ■ Manifestations of UTI	■ Hydration ■ Thiazide diuretics ■ Monitoring of hemoglobin and hematocrit ■ Limits on foods high in calcium ■ Calcium-binding agents
Ureteral stones	■ Renal colic ■ Acute, severe flank pain on affected side ■ Likelihood of pain radiating to suprapubic region, groin, and external genitals ■ Nausea; vomiting; pallor; cool, clammy skin	■ Hydration ■ Monitoring of hemoglobin and hematocrit ■ Limits on foods high in calcium ■ Calcium-binding agents ■ Analgesics for pain (morphine sulfate); NSAIDs (indomethacin) ■ Thiazide diuretics ■ IV fluids
Bladder stones	■ Possibly asymptomatic ■ Dull suprapubic pain, possibly associated with exercise or voiding ■ Gross or microscopic hematuria ■ Manifestations of UTI	If asymptomatic, often no treatment other than increasing hydration and monitoring for hematuria

Collaboration

Collaborative care for patients diagnosed with urinary calculi focuses on relieving acute symptoms, destroying or removing stones, and preventing further stone formation. Asymptomatic stones (those not causing pain, infection, or obstruction) are treated conservatively.

Diagnostic Tests

The following laboratory and diagnostic tests may be ordered when urinary calculi are suspected:

- Urinalysis assesses for hematuria and the possible presence of WBCs and crystal fragments. Urine pH is helpful in identifying the type of stone.

- Chemical analysis of any stones passed in the urine determines the type of stone and suggests measures to prevent further stone formation. Retrieving stones or teaching the patient to do so is a nursing responsibility. All urine is strained and may be saved. Any visible stones or sediment is sent for analysis.

- Urine calcium, uric acid, and oxalate levels measure the amount of these substances excreted over a 24-hour period and may be assessed to help identify possible causes of lithiasis. Elevated calcium levels occur in hyperparathyroidism, Cushing syndrome, and osteoporosis, all of which may contribute to lithiasis. Uric acid levels may be elevated in patients with gout and those at risk for forming uric acid calculi. Urine oxalate excretion may help to differentiate calcium oxalate from calcium phosphate stones.

- Serum calcium, phosphorus, and uric acid levels may be obtained to help identify factors contributing to calculus formation.

- A KUB (kidneys, ureters, and bladder x-ray) may be used to identify calculi as opacities in the kidneys, ureters, and bladder.

- Renal ultrasonography may be used to detect stones and evaluate the kidneys for possible hydronephrosis.

- CT scan of the kidney, with or without contrast medium, may be used to provide a computer-generated photograph that shows calculi, ureteral obstruction, and other renal disorders.

- IVP may be done to visualize the kidneys, ureters, and bladder after injection of a contrast medium. This procedure is of particular importance when KUB, renal ultrasonography, and CT scan fail to demonstrate clear evidence of urinary calculi.

- Cystoscopy is used to visualize and possibly remove calculi from the urinary bladder and distal ureters.

Surgery

Surgical intervention for removal of calculi is usually indicated if there is severe obstruction, recurring infection, intractable pain, or heavy bleeding. The decision to perform surgery also depends on the location and accessibility of the stone, and the patient's general state of health.

Lithotripsy, using sound or shock waves to crush a stone, is the preferred treatment for urinary calculi. There are several lithotripsy techniques available. **Extracorporeal shock**

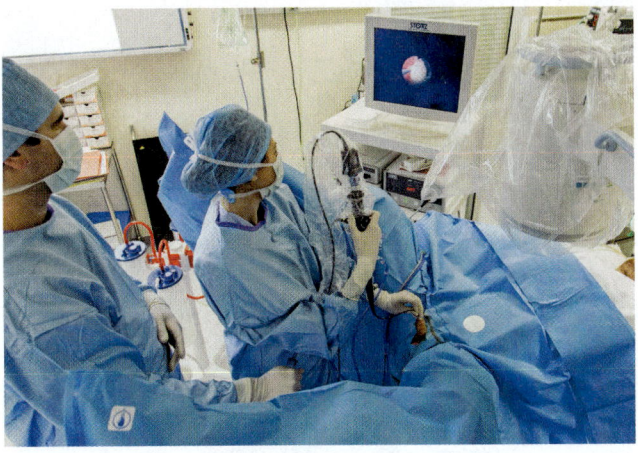

Source: GARO/Phanie/Alamy Stock Photo

Figure 5–10 》》 Extracorporeal shock wave lithotripsy. Acoustic shock waves generated by the shock wave generator travel through soft tissue to shatter the urinary stone into fragments, which are then eliminated in the urine.

wave lithotripsy (ESWL) is a noninvasive technique for fragmenting kidney stones by using shock waves generated outside the body. Acoustic shock waves are aimed at the stone under fluoroscopic guidance (see **Figure 5–10 》》**). These shock waves travel through soft tissue without causing damage and shatter the stone, as its greater density stops their progress. Repeated shock waves pulverize the stone into fragments that are small enough to pass through the urinary tract in the flow of urine. Lithotripsy can be performed during an office visit or as an outpatient procedure (NIDDK, 2013b).

》》 Go to **Pearson MyLab Nursing and eText** for Chart 4: Nursing Care of the Patient Having Lithotripsy.

Lithotripsy may also be performed with a percutaneous ultrasonic or laser technique. Percutaneous ultrasonic lithotripsy uses a nephroscope inserted into the kidney pelvis through a small flank incision (see **Figure 5–11 》》**). A small ultrasonic transducer fragments the stone, and the fragments are removed through the nephroscope. Laser lithotripsy is an alternative to ultrasonic lithotripsy. Laser beams are used to disintegrate the stone without damaging soft tissue. A nephroscope or a ureteroscope passed up the ureter from the bladder during cystoscopy is used to guide the laser probe into direct contact with the stone. A double J stent may be inserted into the affected ureter to maintain its patency following ESWL or other lithotripsy procedures.

On rare occasions, surgical intervention is necessary to remove a calculus in the renal pelvis or ureter. **Ureterolithotomy** is an incision made in the affected ureter to remove a calculus. **Pyelolithotomy** is an incision into the kidney pelvis and removal of a stone. A staghorn calculus that invades the calyces and renal parenchyma may require a **nephrolithotomy** for removal. Bladder stones may be removed by an instrument passed through a cystoscope to crush the stones. The remaining stone fragments are then irrigated out of the bladder with an acid solution that counteracts the alkalinity that precipitated stone formation.

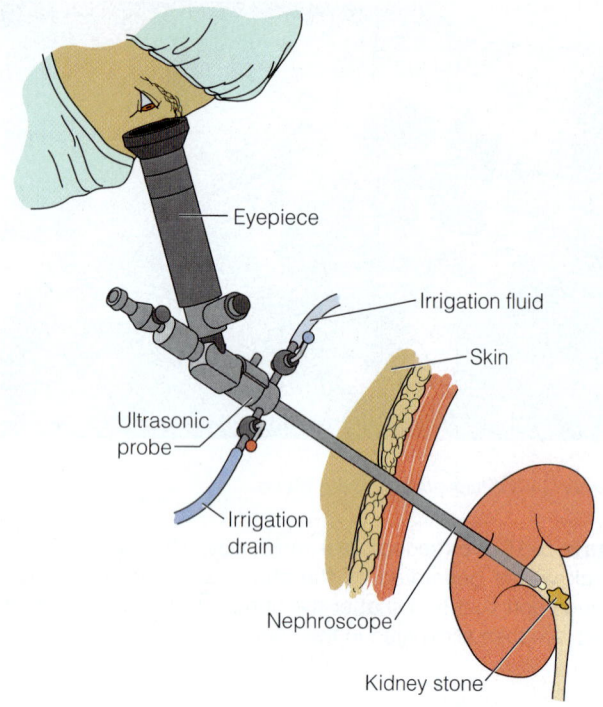

Figure 5–11 ❯❯ Percutaneous ultrasonic lithotripsy. A nephroscope is inserted into the renal pelvis, and ultrasonic waves are used to fragment the stone. Then, the fragments are removed through the nephroscope.

Pharmacologic Therapy

An acute episode of renal colic is treated with analgesia and hydration. A narcotic analgesic such as morphine sulfate is given, often intravenously, to relieve pain and reduce ureteral spasm. Indomethacin, a NSAID, given as a suppository, may reduce the amount of narcotic analgesia required for acute renal colic. Increased fluid intake reduces the risk of further stone formation and promotes urine output.

After analysis of the calculus, various medications may be ordered to inhibit or prevent further lithiasis. A thiazide diuretic, frequently prescribed for calcium calculi, acts to reduce urinary calcium excretion and is very effective in preventing further stones. Potassium citrate alkalinizes urine (raises the pH) and is often prescribed to prevent stones that tend to form in acidic urine (uric acid, cystine, and some forms of calcium stones). See Table 5–8 for other preparations related to types of stones. Nursing responsibilities focus on teaching the patient about the importance in preventing further stone formation by taking prescribed medications and potential adverse effects.

Nonpharmacologic Therapy

Small kidney stones are treated conservatively with increased water intake. The nurse should encourage the patient to drink at least 2 L of water per day. This increases urine production and helps flush out the urinary system. Activity, such as walking, is encouraged because it plays a therapeutic role by increasing metabolism enough to assist by increasing thirst and urination. After the stone has passed, dietary changes to prevent recurrence of kidney

Focus on Integrative Health
Urinary Calculi

A number of complementary health approaches are popular in the prevention of urinary calculi, including cranberry supplements, oral probiotics, and herbal preparations such as teas and tinctures. Four traditional herbal remedies and their regions of origin are summarized here.

Two areas in India have been identified as a "stone belt" a geographical region with a higher concentration of patients per capita treated for urolithiasis. An ethnobotanical study conducted in and around the Bhopal district of Madhya Pradesh revealed a total 67 plant species belonging to 40 families being used in the treatment of urolithiasis. The highest therapeutic value was found to be from the species *Boerhavia diffusa L.* (Agarwal & Varma, 2015).

In Taiwan, the Chinese medicine formulas Jia-Wei-Xiao-Yao-San and Ji-Sheng-Shen-Qi-Wan extracts in powder form have been reported to slow down the progression of renal failure and alleviate flank pain and tenderness for patients with urolithiasis (Lin et al., 2016). Zhou (2013) presented a compelling scientific abstract in support of using Chinese herbs to treat urolithiasis. Zhou's conclusion was reported as: "This Chinese herb tea formula dissolved the kidney stone and prevented a new stone from recurring."

A flower found in Turkey, Helichrysum (Asteraceae), is widely used to dissolve renal calculi and as a diuretic. Extracts from the Helichrysum flower are considered an alternative therapy in place of potassium citrate in treating urolithiasis consisting of calcium oxalate (Onaran et al., 2016).

The spice plant Nigella sativa is widely used to treat and prevent many illnesses in Muslim countries and worldwide. According to a recent study, Nigella sativa and its components are considered useful for prevention and curing of nephrolithiasis and reversing subsequent renal damage (Hayatdavoudi et al., 2016).

stones include reduced intake of oxalate-rich foods, salt, and animal protein.

Lifespan Considerations

Urolithiasis in Newborns and Infants

Although urolithiasis in newborns and infants is considered rare in the United States (Saitz et al., 2016), other countries by comparison have recently reported a relatively large number of infants requiring treatment for urolithiasis. An 11-year longitudinal study in Iran included 1172 infants diagnosed with urolithiasis. All subjects were under 12 months old, and 77 were under 60 days old. Hypercalciuria was the most common metabolic renal issue among the subjects. Of the 1172 infants, 49.4% had a familial history of urolithiasis (Naseri, 2015). In Turkey, urolithiasis diagnosed in infants is not considered rare. The clinical manifestations for infants are nonspecific, but most commonly vomiting and restlessness are reported (Baştuğ et al., 2013).

Urolithiasis in Children and Adolescents

The incidence of kidney stones in children is increasing, although it is difficult to know if it is worldwide because there is a lack of a centralized database and consistent reporting. In children and adolescents, clinical manifestations of urolithiasis include dysuria, hematuria, and pain in the back or lower abdomen. Pain may be short or long in duration and may be accompanied by nausea and vomiting. Some children with small stones may pass the stones with no symptoms. Kidney stones are more likely to develop in children with defects in the urinary tract or with metabolic disorders such as hypercalciuria (NIDDK, 2012f). Research in Korea suggests a difference in metabolic conditions present in the urine of children who have been treated for urolithiasis. The recommended follow-up care for the children previously treated for urolithiasis is diligent screening for risk factors by collection of a 24-hour urine sample to evaluate the presence of hypercalciuria, hyperuricosuria, hypomagnesuria, hyperoxaluria, and hypocitraturia, to prevent renal insufficiency.

Urolithiasis in Pregnant Women

Pregnant women also require special consideration in assessing and treating urinary calculi. Symptoms of urolithiasis are common during pregnancy, and the symptoms are often misdiagnosed as appendicitis, diverticulitis, or placental abruption. If kidney stones do not pass spontaneously, numerous complications can occur, including premature labor, intractable pain, urosepsis, and interruption of normal progression of labor. Treatment of pregnant women is also complicated by the inability to use radiation, anesthesia, and surgery. Renal ultrasonography is the imaging modality of choice for pregnant women, and conservative management, ureteroscopy, or nephrostomy can be used for invasive treatment of larger stones (Wayment & Schwartz, 2015).

Urolithiasis in Older Adults

Older adults usually present with atypical or no pain, fever, diarrhea, pyuria, UTIs, and bacteremia. Determining a diagnosis of urolithiasis in older adults is often delayed because of differences in presentation and increased incidence of other conditions such as UTIs and diarrhea. A higher suspicion for urolithiasis in the older adult population may be required for earlier diagnosis and intervention that consequently improves treatment outcomes and prognosis. Uric acid stone and atypical stone composition is associated with older age. Older individuals are not as likely to pass a stone spontaneously and are more likely to require surgical intervention (Krambeck et al., 2013).

NURSING PROCESS

Nursing care for the patient with urolithiasis is directed at providing comfort during acute renal colic, assisting with diagnostic procedures, ensuring adequate urinary output, and teaching the patient information necessary to prevent future stone formation.

Assessment

The nurse should obtain the following subjective and objective assessment data specific to urolithiasis:

- **Observation and patient interview.** The nurse may observe the patient grimacing, moaning, or guarding the

flank area on either side of the lower back. The patient may bend over at the waist to guard the pain. The patient may pace the floor or request to sit or lay down, occasionally in unusual positions. Some patients will become pale and stoic, whereas others may cry or cry out as the pain becomes intense.

- **Pain assessment.** During the assessment interview, questions should be directed toward obtaining information about flank, back, or abdominal pain and a description of radiation, characteristics, timing, and aggravating or relieving factors. Further questioning should elicit additional symptoms such as nausea and vomiting, possible contributing factors such as dehydration, previous or family history of kidney stones, and current or previous treatment measures.

Note that pain caused by calculi (stones) in the kidney or upper ureter is unique and different in character, severity, and duration from that caused by kidney enlargement. This pain occurs as calculi travel from the kidney to the ureters and the urinary bladder. Some patients experience no pain, and others feel excruciating pain. A stationary stone causes a dull, aching pain. As stones travel down the urinary tract, spasms occur. These spasms produce sharp, intermittent, colicky pain (often accompanied by chills, fever, nausea, and vomiting) that radiates from the flanks to the lower quadrants of the abdomen and, in some cases, the upper thigh and scrotum or labium.

- **Physical examination.** The nurse should note general appearance, including position, vital signs, skin color, temperature, moisture, and turgor; abdominal, flank, or costovertebral tenderness; and amount, color, and characteristics of urine (pH and presence of hematuria, bacteria, and pyuria).

Assessment guidelines for percussion and palpation of the kidneys are demonstrated in the Assessment feature. Note that the kidneys of an older patient are more difficult to palpate abdominally because the mass of the adrenal cortex decreases with age. The nurse should omit blunt percussion in a frail older individual. Instead, palpation of the costovertebral angles and flanks can be used to reveal any pain or tenderness. In some clinical settings, the primary care provider will perform the kidney assessment.

When conducting the assessment, note that flank color and symmetry must be carefully correlated to other diagnostic cues as the assessment proceeds. If ecchymosis is present (Grey Turner sign), there may be other signs of trauma, such as blunt, penetrating wounds or lacerations.

Diagnosis

Possible nursing diagnoses for the patient with urolithiasis include the following:

- *Acute Pain* related to inflammation from renal calculi in the urinary tract (state location)
- *Impaired Urinary Elimination* related to partial (or full) obstruction of urine flow from inflammation (or calculi lodged in ureter or urethra)
- *Deficient Knowledge* related to process of passing calculi (e.g., procedures, lithotripsy, surgery, pain control, diet)

Kidney Assessment

ASSESSMENT/METHOD	NORMAL FINDINGS	ABNORMAL FINDINGS	LIFESPAN OR DEVELOPMENTAL CONSIDERATIONS
General Survey			

Abbreviations: RUQ = right upper quadrant, LUQ = left upper quadrant, RLQ = right lower quadrant, LLQ = left lower quadrant

A quick survey of the patient enables the nurse to identify any immediate problem as well as the patient's ability to participate in the assessment.
 	
1. *Instruct the patient.*
2. *Position the patient.*
   ■ Begin the examination with the patient in a supine position with the abdomen exposed from the nipple line to the pubis (see **Figure 5–12 》**).
3. *Assess the general appearance.*
   ■ Assess general appearance, and inspect the patient's skin for color, hydration status, scales, masses, indentations, or scars.
4. *Inspect the abdomen for color, contour, symmetry, and distention.*
   ■ It may be helpful to stand at the foot of the exam table and inspect the abdomen from there (see **Figure 5–13 》**).
	The patient should not show signs of acute distress and should be mentally alert and oriented.
	
	The patient's abdomen normally is not distended; is relatively symmetrical; and is free of bruises, masses, and swellings.
	
	In most cases, no sounds are heard upon auscultation of the renal arteries.
		■ Patients with kidney disorders frequently look tired and complain of fatigue. If a kidney disorder is suspected, it is important to look for signs of circulatory overload (pulmonary edema) or peripheral edema (puffy face or fingers), or indications of pruritus (scratch marks on the skin).
		■ Elevated nitrogenous wastes (azotemia) in the blood contribute to mental confusion.
		■ A distended bladder may be visible in the suprapubic area, indicating that it is full.
			■ Explain that you will be looking, listening, touching, and tapping on parts of the abdomen. Tell the patient you will explain each procedure as it occurs. Tell the patient to report any discomfort and that you will stop the examination if the procedure is uncomfortable.
			■ Children may benefit from a demonstration on a doll.
			■ An upper abdominal bruit is occasionally heard in young adults and is considered normal.
			■ On a thin adult, renal artery pulsation may be auscultated.

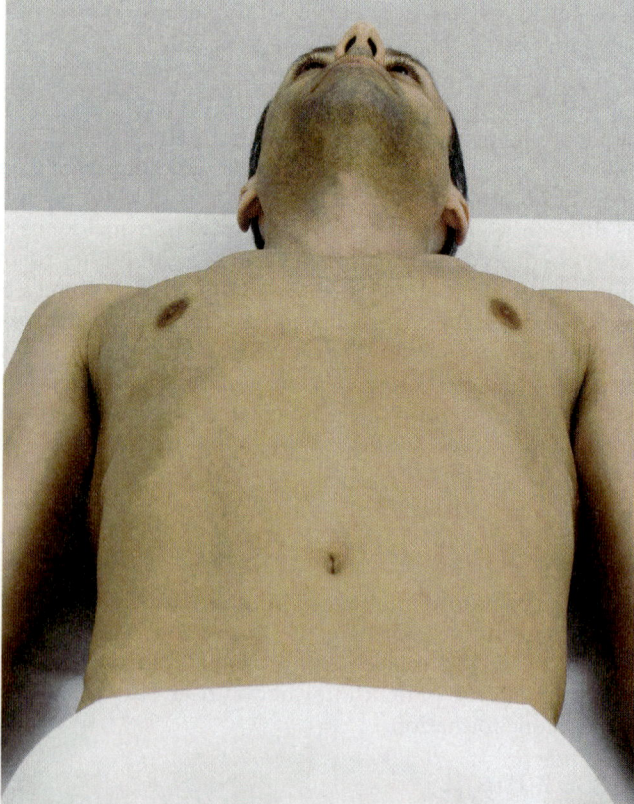

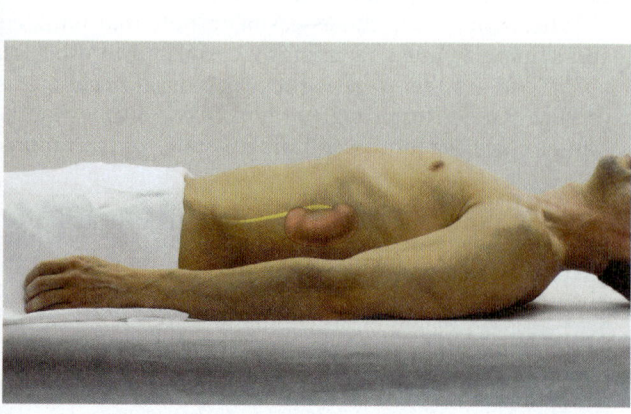

Figure 5–12 》 Position the patient.

Figure 5–13 》 Inspecting the abdomen from the foot of the bed.

Kidney Assessment *(continued)*

ASSESSMENT/METHOD	NORMAL FINDINGS	ABNORMAL FINDINGS	LIFESPAN OR DEVELOPMENTAL CONSIDERATIONS
5. *Auscultate the right and left renal arteries to assess circulatory sounds.* 　■ Gently place the bell of the stethoscope over the extended midclavicular line (MCL) on either side of the abdominal aorta, which is located above the level of the umbilicus (see **Figure 5–14 》**). 　■ Be sure to auscultate both the right and left sides, and over the epigastric and umbilical areas.		■ Many diseases contribute to abdominal distention. These include renal conditions such as polycystic kidney disease and enlarged kidneys, as seen in acute pyelonephritis.	

The Kidneys and Flanks

1. *Position the patient.* 　■ Place the patient in a sitting position, facing away from you with the back exposed. 2. *Inspect the left and right costovertebral angles for color and symmetry.* 3. *Inspect the flanks (the side areas between the hips and the ribs) for color and symmetry.* 4. *Gently palpate the area over the left costovertebral angle (see* **Figure 5–15 》**).	The costovertebral angles and flanks should be symmetrical and even in color; the color should be consistent with the rest of the back. The patient should not experience discomfort upon palpation of the costovertebral angles.	■ A protrusion or elevation over a costovertebral angle occurs when the kidney is grossly enlarged or when a mass is present.	■ Palpation in children can be done over the child's hand if the child resists the assessment.

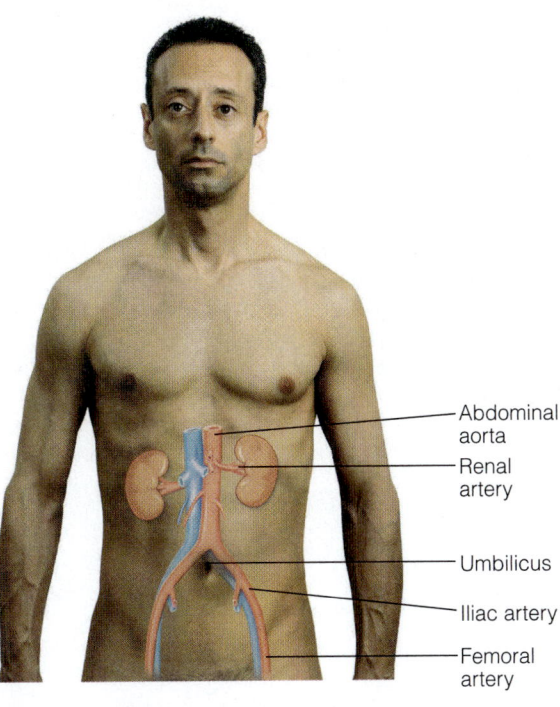

Abdominal aorta
Renal artery
Umbilicus
Iliac artery
Femoral artery

Figure 5–14 》 Auscultating the renal arteries.

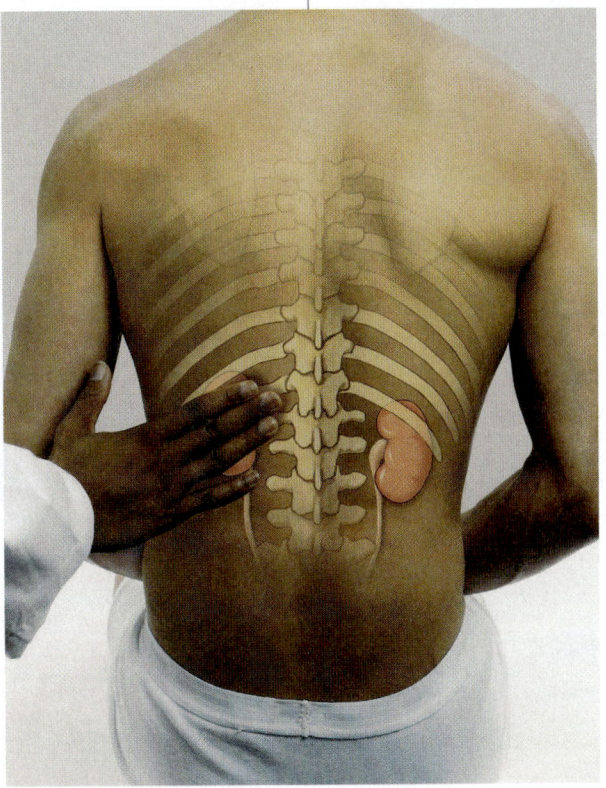

Figure 5–15 》 Palpating the costovertebral angle.

(continued on next page)

Kidney Assessment *(continued)*

ASSESSMENT/METHOD	NORMAL FINDINGS	ABNORMAL FINDINGS	LIFESPAN OR DEVELOPMENTAL CONSIDERATIONS
■ Watch the reaction, and ask the patient to describe any sensation the palpation causes. 5. *Use blunt or indirect percussion to further assess the kidneys.* ■ Place your left palm flat over the left costovertebral angle. ■ Thump the back of your left hand with the ulnar surface of your right fist, causing a gentle thud over the costovertebral angle (see **Figure 5–16 »**). ■ Repeat the procedure on the right side. Ask the patient to describe the sensation as you examine each side.	The patient should feel no pain or tenderness with pressure or percussion.	■ Pain, discomfort, or tenderness from an enlarged or diseased kidney may occur over the costovertebral angle, flank, and abdomen. When questioned, the patient complains of a dull, steady ache. This type of pain is associated with polycystic formation, pyelonephritis, and other disorders that cause kidney enlargement. In the patient with polycystic kidney disease, a sharp, sudden, intermittent pain may mean that a cyst in the kidney has ruptured. If the costovertebral angle is tender, red, and warm, and the patient is experiencing chills, fever, nausea, and vomiting, the underlying kidney could be inflamed or infected. ■ If the patient reports severe pain, hematuria (blood in the urine) or oliguria (diminished volume of urine), and nausea and vomiting, it is important to be alert for hydroureter, which can lead to shock, infection, and impaired renal function. If the nurse suspects hydroureter or obstruction at any point in the urinary tract, medical collaboration must be sought immediately. ■ Pain or discomfort during and after blunt percussion suggests kidney disease. This finding is correlated with other assessment findings.	■ Do not percuss or palpate the patient who reports pain or discomfort in the pelvic region. Do not percuss or palpate the kidney if a tumor of the kidney is suspected, such as a neuroblastoma or Wilms tumor. Palpation increases intra-abdominal pressure, which may contribute to intraperitoneal spreading of the neuroblastoma. Deep palpation should be performed only by experienced practitioners.

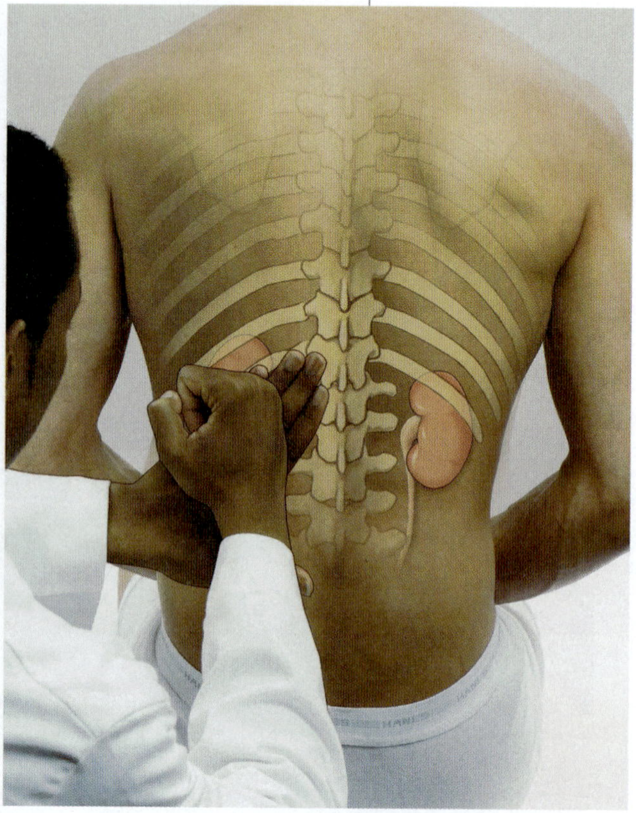

Figure 5–16 » Blunt percussion over the left costovertebral angle.

Kidney Assessment *(continued)*

ASSESSMENT/METHOD	NORMAL FINDINGS	ABNORMAL FINDINGS	LIFESPAN OR DEVELOPMENTAL CONSIDERATIONS
The Left Kidney 1. *Attempt to palpate the lower pole of the left kidney.* ▪ Although it is not usually palpable, attempt to palpate the lower pole of the kidney for size, contour, consistency, and sensation. Note that the rib cage obscures the upper poles. ▪ Place the patient in a supine position. All palpation should be performed from the patient's right side. ▪ While standing on the patient's right side, reach over the patient and place your left hand between the posterior rib cage and the iliac crest (the left flank). ▪ Place your right hand on the LUQ of the abdomen lateral and parallel to the left rectus muscle just below the costal margin. ▪ Instruct the patient to take a deep breath. As the patient inhales, lift the patient's left flank with your left hand and press deeply with your right hand (approximately 4 cm) to attempt to palpate the lower pole of the kidney (see **Figure 5–17 »**). 2. *Attempt to capture the left kidney.* ▪ Because of its position deep in the retroperitoneal space, the left kidney is not normally palpable. The capture maneuver may enable you to palpate it. This maneuver is possible because the kidneys descend during inspiration and slide back into their normal position during exhalation. ▪ Standing on the patient's right side, place your left hand under the patient's back to elevate the flank as before. Place your right hand on the LUQ of the abdomen lateral and parallel to the left rectus muscle with the fingertips just below the left costal margin. Instruct the patient to take a deep breath and hold it. As the patient inhales, attempt to capture the kidney between your two hands.	Left kidneys are rarely palpable in healthy individuals. If palpable upon capture, the kidney surface should be rounded, smooth, firm, and nontender.	▪ When enlargement occurs in the presence of conditions such as neoplasms and polycystic disease, the kidneys may be palpable. ▪ An enlarged, palpable kidney could be painful for the patient. This suggests tumor, cyst, or hydronephrosis.	▪ Because deep kidney palpation can cause tissue trauma, novice nurses should not attempt either deep palpation or capture of the kidney unless supervised by an experienced nurse or nurse practitioner. Deep kidney palpation should not be done in patients who have undergone recent kidney transplantation or have an abdominal aortic aneurysm. ▪ Care must be taken not to mistake an enlarged spleen for an enlarged left kidney. An enlarged kidney feels smooth and rounded, whereas an enlarged spleen feels sharper, with a more delineated edge.

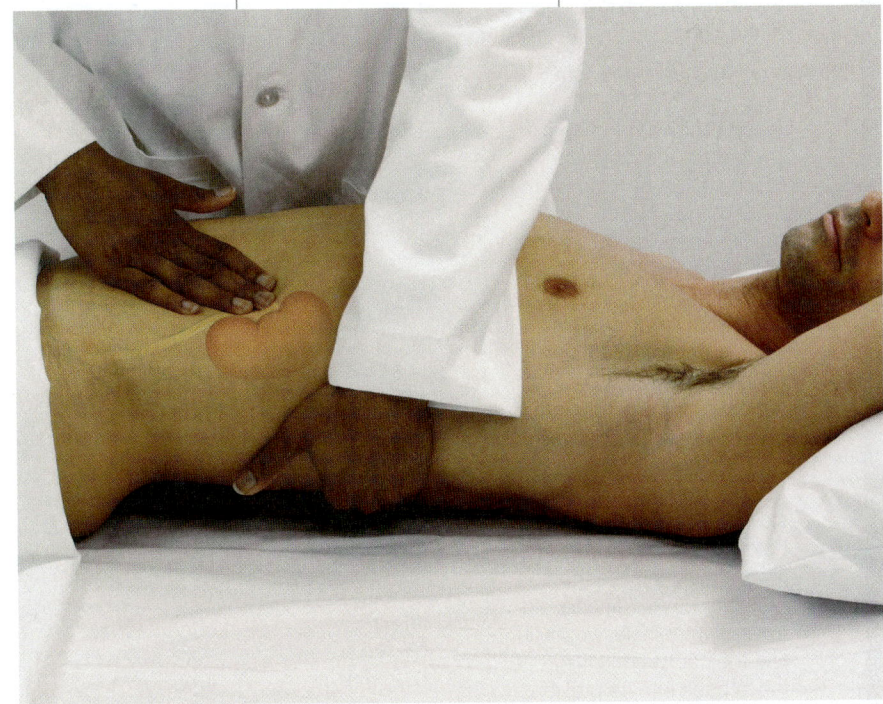

Figure 5–17 » Palpating the left kidney.

(continued on next page)

Kidney Assessment *(continued)*

ASSESSMENT/METHOD	NORMAL FINDINGS	ABNORMAL FINDINGS	LIFESPAN OR DEVELOPMENTAL CONSIDERATIONS
▪ Ask the patient to exhale slowly and then to briefly hold the breath. At the same time, slowly release the pressure of your fingers. As the patient exhales, you will feel the captured kidney move back into its previous position.			

The Right Kidney

ASSESSMENT/METHOD	NORMAL FINDINGS	ABNORMAL FINDINGS	LIFESPAN OR DEVELOPMENTAL CONSIDERATIONS
1. *Attempt to palpate the lower pole of the right kidney.* ▪ Standing on the patient's right side, place your left hand under the back parallel to the right 12th rib (about halfway between the costal margin and iliac crest) with your fingertips reaching for the costovertebral angle. Place your right hand on the RUQ of the abdomen lateral to the right rectus muscle and just below the right costal margin. ▪ Instruct the patient to take a deep breath. As the patient inhales, lift the flank with your left hand and use deep palpation to feel for the lower pole of the kidney. 2. *Attempt to capture the right kidney.* ▪ Place your left hand under the patient's right flank. Place your right hand on the RUQ of the abdomen with the fingertips lateral and parallel to the right rectus muscle just below the right costal margin. ▪ Instruct the patient to take a deep breath and hold it. As the patient inhales, attempt to capture the kidney between your two hands. ▪ Ask the patient to exhale slowly and then to briefly hold the breath. At the same time, slowly release the pressure of your fingers. As the patient exhales you will feel the captured kidney move back into its previous position.	The kidney surface should be rounded, smooth, firm, and nontender. If palpable, the lower pole of the kidney has a smooth, firm, uninterrupted surface.	▪ It is important not to mistake an enlarged liver for an enlarged right kidney. An enlarged kidney feels smooth and rounded, whereas an enlarged liver is closer to the midline and has a more distinct border. Polycystic kidney disease or carcinoma should be suspected when there is gross enlargement of the kidney. The kidneys may be 2 or 3 times their normal size in patients with polycystic disease.	▪ The lower pole of the right kidney is palpable in some individuals, especially in thin, relaxed women. ▪ During the capture maneuver, some patients describe a nonpainful sensation as the kidney slides between the nurse's fingers back into its normal position.

- *Anxiety* related to fear of urolithiasis reoccurring (procedures, surgery, passing the stone)
- *Readiness for Enhanced Nutrition* related to dietary modifications to control urolithiasis reoccurrences
- *Risk for Infection* related to trauma to the urinary tract from renal calculi moving through the urinary tract.

(NANDA-I © 2014)

Planning

Goals appropriate for the patient with urolithiasis must be individualized to meet each patient's specific needs and may include:

- The patient will request analgesics as needed at onset of pain and report effective pain relief within 30 minutes of parenteral analgesic administration.
- The patient will maintain urine output of 2500 mL in each 24-hour period while hospitalized.
- The patient will remain without signs of infection during the hospital stay.
- The patient will remain without signs of urinary obstruction during the hospital stay.
- The patient will verbalize understanding of disease process by the end of a nurse-lead teaching session.
- The patient will verbalize understanding of dietary changes that may reduce the risk of recurrence of calculi formation by the end of a nurse-lead teaching session.
- The patient will demonstrate reduced anxiety as evidenced by nonverbal gestures and return of vital signs to baseline after preprocedure teaching.

Implementation

In collaboration with the healthcare team, the nurse will provide culturally competent interventions to ensure the comfort of the patient and promote continuing health following discharge. While treating the patient's pain may be the most immediate intervention, patient teaching and health promotion help the patient maintain urinary health beyond the current need for healthcare intervention.

Manage Pain

Pain is the primary outward manifestation of urolithiasis, particularly when a calculus becomes immovable in a ureter, causing acute obstruction and distention. Invasive and noninvasive procedures to remove or crush stones also may be painful. Patients undergoing surgery also experience incisional pain. The intensity of renal colic pain can cause a vasovagal response with resulting hypotension and syncope. Patient safety is the first priority. The nurse should do the following:

- Unless contraindicated, encourage fluid intake and ambulation in the patient with renal colic. Increased fluids and ambulation will increase urinary output, facilitating movement of the calculus through the ureter and subsequently decreases the pain. Encourage and assist with ambulation as needed, and closely monitor the patient for dizziness or other complications that may increase the risk for impaired mobility.

- Use nonpharmacologic measures such as positioning, moist heat, relaxation techniques, guided imagery, and diversion as adjunctive therapy for pain relief. Adjunctive pain relief measures can enhance the effectiveness of analgesics and other prescribed treatment.

- Assess pain using a standard pain scale, and include characteristics of the pain. Administer analgesia as ordered, and monitor its effectiveness. Administering an ordered NSAID to reduce inflammation on a routine schedule may significantly decrease the need for narcotic analgesia in patients with renal colic.

- If surgery has been performed, monitor urinary output, catheters, incision, and wound drainage. Pain may be a symptom of proximal distention due to a blocked catheter. Infection or hematoma at the surgical site can increase pain significantly.

Monitor Urinary Output

Obstruction of the urinary tract is the primary problem associated with urolithiasis. A stone that completely obstructs the ureter can lead to hydronephrosis and kidney damage on the affected side. The nurse should report symptoms of hydronephrosis, such as dull flank pain or aching and changes in renal function studies (BUN and serum creatinine level). Because the other kidney continues to function, urine output may not fall significantly with obstruction of one ureter. A rising BUN and serum creatinine may be early signs of renal failure. Obstruction can ultimately lead to stasis, infection, or irreversible renal damage. The nurse should do the following:

- Monitor amount and character of urine output. If the patient is catheterized, measure output hourly. Urine volume reflects possible urinary tract obstruction and adequacy of hydration. Strain all urine for stones, saving any recovered stones for laboratory analysis. Analysis of calculi recovered from the urine can direct measures used to prevent further lithiasis. Document hematuria, dysuria, frequency, urgency, and pyuria. Hematuria, gross or microscopic, is often associated with calculi and with procedures used to remove stones, such as cystoscopy or lithotripsy. A change in the amount of hematuria may indicate stone passage or a complication. Dysuria, frequency, urgency, and cloudy urine are symptoms of UTI, often associated with urolithiasis. Antibiotic therapy may be required.

- Maintain patency and integrity of any catheter systems. Secure catheters well, label if there are more than one, and use sterile technique for all ordered irrigations or other invasive procedures. A kinked or plugged catheter, particularly a ureteral catheter or nephrostomy tube, may damage the urinary system. Labeling catheters can prevent mistakes such as inappropriate irrigation and clamping. Any catheter increases the risk of infection; aseptic technique in all procedures reduces this risk.

Provide Patient Teaching

The patient with urolithiasis has multiple learning needs. These include information about the disease and its possible consequences, understanding of any diagnostic or therapeutic procedures performed, and strategies to prevent future lithiasis. The nurse working with a patient with urolithiasis should do the following:

- Assess the patient's understanding and previous learning. Relating information to previously learned material enhances retention and understanding.

- Present all material in a manner appropriate to the patient's knowledge base, developmental and educational levels, and current needs. Tailor teaching to the individual's learning style and needs. Knowledge and understanding will encourage the patient's involvement and compliance with the care plan.

- Provide teaching in regard to all diagnostic and treatment procedures. Knowing what to expect reduces anxiety, enhances compliance, and hastens recovery.

- If the patient will be managed at home or in the community, teach the patient to:
  a. Collect and strain all urine, saving any stones.
  b. Report stone passage to the physician, and bring in the stone for analysis.
  c. Report to the physician any changes in the amount or character of urine output.
  When pain can be managed with oral analgesics, urolithiasis is managed at home or in the community. The patient needs to know how and why to collect the calculus as well as what the indicators of complications are, such as reduced urine output and cloudy or bloody urine.

- Teach measures to prevent further urolithiasis, including the need to increase fluid intake to 2500–3500 mL per day, follow recommended dietary guidelines, take medications as prescribed, and maintain activity level to prevent urinary stasis and bone resorption (loss).
  The risk of recurrent urolithiasis is approximately 50%; however, this risk can be reduced through measures used to prevent conditions favoring stone formation.

- Teach about the relationship between renal calculi and UTI, emphasizing preventive measures and the importance of prompt treatment. UTI promotes urolithiasis and thus requires prompt treatment to reduce this risk.

Promote Health and Wellness

The nurse should discuss with all patients the importance of maintaining an adequate fluid intake. The nurse should also stress the need to increase fluid intake during warm weather and strenuous exercise or physical labor. The nurse should discuss the relationship between weight-bearing activity and retention of calcium in the bones. The nurse should encourage all patients to remain as physically active as possible to prevent bone resorption and possible hypercalciuria.

The nurse should instruct patients with known gout to maintain a generous fluid intake to produce at least 2 L of urine every day. The nurse should also discuss the risk of lithiasis with patients who have frequent UTIs and teach measures to reduce the incidence of UTI and the risk for lithiasis.

Prepare the Patient for Discharge

The patient with urinary calculi needs to know how to manage existing stones and what will reduce the risk of future lithiasis. The nurse should discuss the following topics to prepare the patient and family for home care:

- Importance of maintaining a fluid intake adequate to produce 2.0–2.5 L of urine per day
- Prescribed medication management, and potential adverse effects
- Dietary recommendations
- Prevention, recognition, and management of UTI
- Management of treatment measures.

When the patient is to be discharged with dressings, a nephrostomy tube, or a catheter, the nurse should teach the patient and family about the following:

- How to change dressings, maintaining aseptic technique
- How to assess the wound and skin for healing and possible complications such as infection or skin breakdown
- How to manage drainage systems and maintain their patency
- How to empty drainage bags and assess urine output
- When to contact the physician and what the recommendations are for follow-up care.

Evaluation

The patient is evaluated on the basis of the selected outcomes and nursing diagnoses, and the plan of care is amended depending on the patient's response to interventions. While straining of the patient's urine may indicate that the stone has passed, the nurse should assess the patient for possible complications such as infection or kidney damage. Expected outcomes include the following:

- The patient rates pain at 3 (or a level acceptable to the patient) or less on a 0–10 scale and is comfortable enough to perform ADLs. If pain is not 3 or below, the nurse should assess patient adherence to the treatment plan and the effectiveness of pain medication. Further teaching may be required for additional nonpharmacologic comfort measures.

- The patient remains free from signs and symptoms of infection. If signs and symptoms of infection are present, the healthcare provider should be notified, and the nurse should expect an order for a urinalysis.

- The patient chooses an appropriate diet to prevent the recurrence of renal calculi. If the patient is not able to choose the appropriate diet: (1) further teaching should be provided, (2) teaching should include a family member if one is responsible for meal planning at home, and (3) a referral to a dietitian may be required.

- The patient demonstrates adequate fluid intake. If the patient's intake is not adequate, the nurse should ascertain the reason for the deficit. Once the reason has been determined, the nurse should stress the importance of adequate hydration, and further teaching may be required. The patient may need assistance in making a strategy for meeting this goal such as planning ahead for the day with an adequate supply of water, or measuring out the required amount in the morning and continuing to drink until the goal is reached.

Nursing Care Plan
A Patient with Urinary Calculi

Richard Leton, age 44, owns a small business. He is admitted to the medical unit from the emergency department after awakening at 4 a.m. with severe right-sided pain. His CBC is normal, and urinalysis reveals microscopic hematuria but no protein or bacteria. A renal ultrasound shows a 4–5 mm stone partially obstructing the right ureter.

Stephen Phillips, Mr. Leton's admitting nurse, notes that Mr. Leton is pale, diaphoretic, and very anxious. Mr. Leton complains of nausea and asks for an emesis basin. Mr. Leton received 4 mg of IV morphine sulfate shortly after admission to the emergency department, approximately 2.5 hours ago. He denies pain at this time but says, "I'm scared to death that it'll come back—I couldn't even move, it hurt so bad."

ASSESSMENT

Mr. Leton's history reveals no previous episodes of renal calculi. He felt well until the pain awakened him during the night. He reports that he has been working under a deadline to complete a construction project and that he probably has not been drinking enough fluids "considering how hot it's been." Physical assessment findings include temperature 38.0°C (100.4°F), pulse 98 bpm, respirations 24/min, and BP 160/86 mmHg. Color is pale to ashen; skin is cool and moist. Abdomen is firm, with moderate tenderness in the right upper outer quadrant. The emergency department physician orders an IV of 5% dextrose in 1/2 normal saline at 200 mL/h until nausea is relieved, then PO fluids of at least 3000 mL/24 h; morphine sulfate (MS) 2–10 mg IV prn severe pain; indomethacin (Indocin) 50 mg per rectal suppository q8h; promethazine (Phenergan) 25 mg PO or per suppository q6h prn nausea; activity to tolerance; and strain all urine, sending recovered stones for analysis.

DIAGNOSES

- *Anxiety* related to anticipation of recurrent severe pain
- *Risk for Imbalanced Nutrition: Less Than Body Requirements* related to nausea.
- *Acute Pain* related to partial obstruction of right ureter by calculus.
- *Impaired Urinary Elimination* related to partial obstruction of ureter by calculus
- *Deficient Knowledge* related to lack of information about disease process, contributing factors, and management

(NANDA-I © 2014)

PLANNING

To return to health and achieve expected outcomes, Mr. Leton's goals for care include the following:

- He will demonstrate reduced anxiety while hospitalized as evidenced by relaxed facial expression, vital signs within his normal range, and the ability to rest when not disturbed.
- He will consume at least 50% of his prescribed diet while hospitalized.
- He will receive 100% of ordered fluids while hospitalized.
- He will remain free of nausea and vomiting within 30 minutes of receiving prescribed antiemetics.
- He will request analgesia as needed at onset of pain.
- His pain will be less than 3/10 in 20 minutes after receiving IV morphine.
- He will maintain urine output of 2500 mL/24 h while hospitalized.
- He will be free of complications such as increased pain, dysuria, pyuria, or hematuria.
- He will relate an understanding of the process of urolithiasis and contributing factors by the end of a nurse-lead teaching session.
- He will verbalize dietary and fluid intake and other measures to reduce risk of future stone formation by the end of a nurse-lead teaching session.

IMPLEMENTATION

The nurse caring for Mr. Leton should do the following:

- Reassure Mr. Leton that measures to prevent further episodes of renal colic are being implemented and that medication is available to relieve pain promptly.
- Administer all medications as prescribed.
- Assess the effectiveness of analgesia and its adverse effects, especially nausea. Collaborate with healthcare provider for unrelieved nausea, vomiting, or if pain is not controlled at or below a level acceptable for Mr. Leton.
- Maintain IV as prescribed until oral fluid intake exceeds 200 mL of fluid per hour while awake.

- Measure and strain all urine. Assess urine for color, clarity, and odor. Collaborate with the healthcare provider for any abnormal findings.
- Teach about urolithiasis and its risk factors, especially as they relate to Mr. Leton.
- Teach Mr. Leton the importance of maintaining a high fluid intake, especially when working outdoors in hot weather; recommended dietary modifications and their rationale; ordered medications and their effects; ways to identify and prevent UTI; and symptoms that should be reported to his healthcare provider.

EVALUATION

Mr. Leton's care is evaluated based on the planned goals of nursing care. Mr. Leton passes the obstructing stone the evening after admission and is discharged the following day. On discharge, he denies pain or nausea, his urine is clear and pale yellow, and urinalysis is normal. Laboratory analysis shows that the calculus was calcium. Mr. Leton is able to state the importance of continuing a high fluid intake. He verbalizes that he will reduce his intake of calcium-rich foods such

as milk and milk products and that he will increase his intake of foods to acidify his urine. He is able to list foods to include in his diet. He states, "You'd better believe I'll follow my diet, drink my water, so the stones don't come back and I don't get an infection. I hope to never feel pain like that again!" Based on Mr. Leton's response to the nursing care implemented, the planned goals were met, indicating the nurse developed a successful care plan.

(continued on next page)

Nursing Care Plan (continued)

CRITICAL THINKING

1. What factors contributed to the onset and timing of Mr. Leton's ureteral colic?

2. What is the rationale for administering indomethacin, an NSAID, to a patient with ureteral colic?

3. Why did Mr. Phillips include a nursing intervention to assess for a relationship between Mr. Leton's nausea, his pain, and the ordered analgesic agent?

REVIEW Urinary Calculi

RELATE Link the Concepts and Exemplars

Linking the exemplar of urinary calculi with the concept of comfort:
You are caring for a patient with urinary calculi who is experiencing severe pain that he rates as an 11 on the 0–10 scale, with 10 being the worst pain he has ever felt.

1. Describe both pharmacologic and nonpharmacologic strategies you would use to relieve the patient's pain.

2. What expected outcomes would you assess as indicating that pain management techniques were successful?

Linking the exemplar of urinary calculi with the concept of culture and diversity:

3. How would you respond if a patient with urinary calculi informed you of a website he looked at last night that recommended increasing magnesium intake to cure kidney stones instead of following the therapy recommended by his provider?

4. A patient with urinary calculi has already been seen several times for the same diagnosis. What cultural assessment would you perform to determine whether there is a cultural link to the recurrent diagnosis?

READY Go to Volume 3: Clinical Nursing Skills

REFER Go to Pearson MyLab Nursing and eText

- Additional review material
- Chart 4: Nursing Care of the Patient Having Lithotripsy

REFLECT Apply Your Knowledge

Guy Markson, age 28, is a business executive with a sedentary lifestyle. His wife says that he is always telling her that he needs to exercise more, but business meetings and job responsibilities seem to get in the way of his plans to work out. As of late, he has been even busier than usual and sometimes forgets to eat lunch or dinner unless he has a business lunch, which is usually red meat and wine.

Mr. Markson called his healthcare provider today, reporting excruciating pain under his rib cage on the left side of his back, saying that when his urine looked bloody, he knew he had to do something. The physician ordered a renal ultrasound, serum laboratory testing (calcium, uric acid, BUN, creatinine, phosphorus), and urinalysis to include urine calcium and instructed Mr. Markson to go to the emergency department, which would coordinate the ordered tests and inform him of the results.

When Mr. Markson arrives at the hospital, the nurse administers morphine sulfate for pain and indomethacin by suppository and initiates IV normal saline at 150 mL/hour. A renal ultrasound is performed, and Mr. Markson receives a diagnosis of a 6-mm stone completely obstructing the left ureter, with resulting acute hydronephrosis. Diagnostic tests lead to the suspicion that the stone is a uric acid stone, although further testing will be performed on it when removed. The doctor recommends ESWL as the initial treatment and admits Mr. Markson to the acute care facility.

1. As the nurse admitting this patient to the unit, what preparations will you make for the patient while awaiting his arrival from the emergency department?

2. What nursing diagnosis would be appropriate for this patient?

3. Following successful lithotripsy and confirmation that the stone was composed of uric acid, what discharge teaching will you provide the patient and his wife?

References

Adams, M. P., Holland, L. N., & Urban, C. (2017). *Pharmacology for nurses: A pathophysiologic approach* (5th ed.). Hoboken, NJ: Pearson Education.

Agarwal, K., & Varma, R. (2015). Ethnobotanical study of antilithic plants of Bhopal district. *Journal of Ethnopharmacology, 174*, 17–24. doi:10.1016/j.jep.2015.08.003

Alavi, K., Chan, S., Wise, P., Kaiser, A. M., Sudan, R., & Bordeianou, L. (2015). Fecal incontinence: Etiology, diagnosis, and management. *Journal of Gastrointestinal Surgery, 19*(10), 1910–1921. doi:10.1007/s11605-015-2905-1

Alfheim, H. B., Steenfeldt-Foss, A., Hanem, S., & Rosseland, L. A. (2016). High risk of postoperative urinary retention in 1-year-old cleft palate patients: An observational study. *Journal of PeriAnesthesia Nursing, 31*(1), 41–48. doi:10.1016/j.jopan.2014.05.016

Alsheik, E. H., Coyne, T., Hawes, S. K., Merikhi, L., Naples, S. P., Kanagarajan, N., . . . Ahmad, A. S. (2012). Fecal incontinence: Prevalence, severity, and quality of life data from an outpatient gastroenterology practice (Article ID 947694). *Gastroenterology Research and Practice*. Retrieved from http://www.hindawi.com/journals/grp/2012/947694/

American Nurses Association. (2015). *Streamlined evidence-based RN tool: Catheter associated urinary tract infection (CAUTI) prevention* [Decision-making instrument]. Retrieved from http://nursingworld.org/ANA-CAUTI-Prevention-Tool

American Nurses Association. (2017). *ANA CAUTI prevention tool*. Retrieved from http://nursingworld.org/ANA-CAUTI-Prevention-Tool.

Anderson, C. A., Omar, M. I., Campbell, S. E., Hunter, K. F., Cody, J. D., & Glazener, C. M. (2015). *Conservative management for postprostatectomy urinary incontinence* (Art. No. CD001843). Retrieved from Cochrane Database of Systematic Reviews website: http://onlinelibrary.wiley.com/doi/10.1002/14651858.CD001843.pub5/full

Barrie, M. (2015). Identifying urinary incontinence in community patients. *Journal of Continence Nursing, (29)6,* 45–52.

Baştuğ, F., Gündüz, Z., Tülpar, S., Poyrazoğlu, H., & Düşünsel, R. (2013). Urolithiasis in infants: Evaluation of risk factors. *World Journal of Urology, 31*(5), 1117–1122. doi:10.1007/s00345-012-0828-y

Berman, A., Snyder, S., & Frandsen, G. (2016). Pain Management. In *Kozier & Erb's fundamentals of nursing: Concepts, processes, and practice* (10th ed.). Hoboken, NJ: Pearson Education.

Bharucha, A. E., Dunivan, G., Goode, P. S., Lukacz, E. S., Markland, A. D., Matthews, C. A., . . . Hamilton, F. A. (2015). Epidemiology, pathophysiology, and classification of fecal incontinence: State of the science summary for the National Institute of Diabetes and Digestive and Kidney Diseases (NIDDK) workshop. *American Journal of Gastroenterology, 110*(1), 127–136. doi:10.1038/ajg.2014.396

Bhat, A., Bothra, R., Bhat, M. P., Chaudhary, G. R., Saran, R. K., & Saxena, G. (2012). Congenital bladder diverticulum presenting as bladder outlet obstruction in infants and children. *Journal of Pediatric Urology, 8*(4), 348–353. doi:10.1016/j.jpurol.2011.07.001

Borowitz, S. (2013). Encopresis. *Medscape Reference.* Retrieved from http://emedicine.medscape.com/article/928795

Bozkurt, A., Karabakan, M., Keskin, E., Hirik, E., Balci, M., & Nuhoglu, B. (2016). Prostatic urethral lift: A new minimally invasive treatment for lower urinary tract symptoms secondary to benign prostatic hyperplasia. *Urologia Internationalis, 96*(2), 202–206. doi:10.1159/000441850

Buchko, B. L., & Robinson, L. E. (2012). An evidence-based approach to decrease early post-operative urinary retention following urogynecologic surgery. *Urologic Nursing, 32*(5), 260–264, 273.

Buchko, B. L., Robinson, L. E., & Bell, T. D. (2013). Translating an evidence-based algorithm to decrease early post-operative urinary retention after urogynecologic surgery. *Urologic Nursing, 33*(1), 24–28.

Campbell, S. E., Glazener, C. M. A., Hunter, K. F., Cody, J. D., & Moore, K. N. (2012). *Conservative management for postprostatectomy urinary incontinence* (Art. No. CD001843). Retrieved from Cochrane Database of Systematic Reviews website: http://onlinelibrary.wiley.com/doi/10.1002/14651858.CD001843.pub5/full

Centers for Disease Control and Prevention (CDC). (2015). *Catheter-associated urinary tract infections (CAUTI).* Retrieved from https://www.cdc.gov/hai/ca_uti/uti.html

Coffield, S., & Willette, P. (2012). Current trends in the management of difficult urinary catheterizations. *Western Journal of Emergency Medicine, 13*(6), 472–478. doi:10.5811/westjem.2011.11.6810

Cohn, J. A., Brown, E. T., Kaufman, M. R., Dmochowski, R. R., & Reynolds, W. S. (2016). Underactive bladder in women: Is there any evidence? *Current Opinion in Urology, 26*(4), 309–314. doi:10.1097/MOU.0000000000000280

Denic, A., Glasscock, R., & Rule, A. (2016). Structural and functional changes with the aging kidney. *Advances in Chronic Kidney Disease, 23*(1), 19–28. doi:10.1053/j.ackd.2015.08.004

Deters, L. A. (2016). *Benign prostatic hypertrophy.* Retrieved from http://emedicine.medscape.com/article/437359-overview

Dugdale, D. C., III, & Longstreth, G. F. (2012). Bowel retraining. *MedlinePlus.* Retrieved from http://www.nlm.nih.gov/medlineplus/ency/article/003971.htm

Ebiloglu, T., Ergin, G., Irkilata, H. C., & Kibar, Y. (2016). The biofeedback treatment for non-monosymptomatic enuresis nocturna. *Neurourology and Urodynamics, 25*(1), 58–61.

Fakih, M., Rey, J., Pena, M., Szpunar, S., & Saravolatz, L. (2013). Sustained reductions in urinary catheter use over 5 years: Bedside nurses view themselves responsible for evaluation of catheter necessity. *American Journal of Infection Control, 41*(3), 236–239. doi:10.1016/j.ajic.2012.04.328

Fatouh, A. A., Motawie, A. A., Abd Al-Aziz, A. M., Hamed, H. M., Awad, M. A., El-Ghany, A. A., . . . Eid, M. M. (2013). Anti-diuretic hormone and genetic study in primary nocturnal enuresis. *Journal of Pediatric Urology, 9*(6, Pt. A), 831–837. doi:10.1016/j.jpurol.2012.11.009

Felix, H., Thostenson, J., Bursac, Z., & Bradway, C. (2013). Effect of weight on indwelling catheter use among long-term care facility residents. *Urologic Nursing, 33*(4), 194–200.

Figueroa, T. E. (2012). *Urinary incontinence in children.* Retrieved from the Merck Manual for Health Care Professionals website: http://www.merckmanuals.com/professional/pediatrics/incontinence_in_children/urinary_incontinence_in_children.html

Fleshner, N., & Bhindi, B. (2014). Metabolic syndrome and diabetes for the urologist. *Canadian Urological Association Journal, 8*(7–8), 159–161. Retrieved from http://dx.doi.org/10.5489/cuaj.2314

Friedman, A. A., & Palmer, L. S. (2014). Enuresis in children: Have we made therapeutic progress? *AUANews, 19*(11), 17–18.

Geller, E. J. (2014). Prevention and management of postoperative urinary retention after urogynecologic surgery. *International Journal of Women's Health, 2014*(6), 829–838. doi:https://dx.doi.org/10.2147/IJWH.S55383

Greene, M. T., Kiyoshi-Teo, H., Reichert, H., Krein, S., & Saint, S. (2014). Urinary catheter indications in the United States: Results from a national survey of acute care hospitals. *Infection Control and Hospital Epidemiology, 35*(S3).

Hayatdavoudi, P., Khajavi Rad, A., Rajaei, Z., & Hadjzadeh, M. A. (2016). Renal injury, nephrolithiasis and Nigella sativa: A mini review. *Avicenna Journal of Phytomedicine, 6*(1), 1–8. Retrieved from http://www.ncbi.nlm.nih.gov/pmc/articles/PMC4884213/

Herbison, G. P., & Dean, N. (2013). *Weighted vaginal cones for urinary incontinence* (Art. No. CD002114). Retrieved from https://www.ncbi.nlm.nih.gov/pubmed/23836411

Herdman, T. H. & Kamitsuru, S. (Eds.). *Nursing Diagnoses—Definitions and Classification 2015–2017.* Copyright © 2014, 1994–2014 NANDA International. Used by arrangement with John Wiley & Sons, Inc. Companion website: www.wiley.com/go/nursingdiagnoses

Holloway, C. A. (2014). Bedwetting. In B. C. Auday, M. A. Buratovich, G. F. Marrocco, & P. Moglia (Eds.), *Magill's medical guide* (7th ed.). New York, NY: Greyhouse Publishing.

Hossain, M. Z., Hasan, G. Z., & Siddiqui, T. H. (2012). Congenital bladder diverticulum causing acute urinary retention in an infant. *Mymensingh Medical Journal, 21*(2), 360–362.

Howlett, M., Gibson, W., Hunter, K., Chambers, T., & Wagg, A. (2016). Nocturnal enuresis in older people: Where is the evidence and what are the gaps? *Journal of Wound, Ostomy and Continence Nursing, 43*(4), 401–406. doi:10.1097/WON.0000000000000234

Johansson, R. M., Malmvall, B. E., Andersson-Gare, B., Larsson, B., Erlandsson, I., Sund-Levander, . . . Christensson, L. (2013). Guidelines for preventing urinary retention and bladder damage during hospital care. *Journal of Clinical Nursing, 22*(3–4), 347–355. doi:10.1111/j.1365-2702.2012.04229.x

Juma S. (2014). Urinary retention in women. *Current Opinion in Urology, 24*(4), 375–379. doi:10.1097/MOU.0000000000000071

Kim, E. D. (2016). Urinary tract obstruction. *Medscape.* Retrieved from http://emedicine.medscape.com/article/438890-overview#a8

Krambeck, A. E., Lieske, J. C., Li, X., Bergstralh, E. J., Melton, L. J., Andrew, D., & Rule, A. D. (2013). Effect of age on the clinical presentation of incident symptomatic urolithiasis in the general population. *Journal of Urology, 189*(1), 158–164. doi:http://dx.doi.org/10.1016/j.juro.2012.02.2420

Lederer, E., Nayak, V., Alassauskas, Z. C., & Mackelaite, L. (2013). Hyperkalemia. *Medscape Reference.* Retrieved from http://emedicine.medscape.com/article/240903-overview

Lin, P. H., Lin, S. K., Hsu, R. J., Cheng, K. C., & Liu, J. M. (2016). The use and the prescription pattern of traditional Chinese medicine among urolithiasis patients in Taiwan: A population-based study. *Journal of Alternative and Complementary Medicine, 22*(1), 88–95. doi:10.1089/acm.2015.0116

Litwin, M. S., & Saigal, C. S. (Eds.). (2012). *Urologic diseases in America. U.S. Department of Health and Human Services, Public Health Service, National Institutes of Health, National Institute of Diabetes and Digestive and Kidney Diseases* (NIH Publication No. 12-7865, pp. 464–496). Washington, DC: U.S. Government Printing Office.

Lombrana, M., Izquierdo, L., Gomez, A., & Alcaraz, A. (2013). Impact of a nurse-run clinic on prevalence of urinary incontinence and everyday life in men undergoing radical prostatectomy. *Journal Wound Ostomy Continence Nursing, 40*(3), 309–312. doi:10.1097/WON.0b013e31828f5e22

Lv, Z-T., Song, W., Wu, J., Yang, J., Wang, T., Wu, C-H., . . . Li, M. (2015). Efficacy of acupuncture in children with nocturnal enuresis: A systematic review and meta-analysis of randomized controlled trials. *Evidence-Based Complementary and Alternative Medicine.* Retrieved from https://www.hindawi.com/journals/ecam/2015/320701/

Mayo Clinic. (2012). *Kidney stones.* Retrieved from http://www.mayoclinic.com/health/kidney-stones/DS00282

McKay, S. L., Fravel, M., & Scanlon, C. (2012). Management of constipation. *Journal of Gerontological Nursing, 38*(7), 9–15. doi:10.3928/00989134-20120608-01

Meddings, J., Rogers, M. A., Krein, S. L., Fakih, M. G., Olmsted, R. N., & Saint, S. (2013). Reducing unnecessary urinary catheter use and other strategies to prevent catheter-associated urinary tract infection: An integrative review. *BMJ Quality & Safety, 23*(4), 277–289. Retrieved from http://qualitysafety.bmj.com/content/23/4/277.long

Miller, P. (2016). *Basic geriatric nursing* (6th ed., p. 54). St. Louis, MO: Elsevier.

Mulder, F. E., Rengerink, K. O., Van der Post, J. A., Hakvoort, R. A., & Roovers, J. W. (2016). Delivery-related risk factors for covert postpartum urinary retention after vaginal delivery. *International Urogynecology Journal, 27,* 55–60. doi:10.1007/s00192-015-2768-8

Naidoo, T. D. (2014). Post-partum anal incontinence in SA: A myth or reality? *Obstetrics & Gynaecology Forum, 24*(3), 24–28.

Nambiar, A., Cody, J. D., & Jeffery, S. T. (2014). *Single-incision sling operations for urinary incontinence in women* (Art. No. CD008709). Retrieved from Cochrane Database of Systematic Reviews website: http://onlinelibrary.wiley.com/doi/10.1002/14651858.CD008709.pub2/abstract;jsessionid=26D E2053E50AD809F22D31CB696C8C4B.f02t01

Naseri, M. (2015). Urolithiasis in the first 2 months of life. *Iran Journal of Kidney Diseases, 9*(5), 379–385.

National Healthcare Safety Network (NHSN). (2016). *Surveillance definitions: Central line associated bloodstream infection (CLABSI) & related sites.* Retrieved from http://www.msic-online.org/pdf/NHSN_Definitions_CLABSI.pdf

National Institute of Diabetes and Digestive and Kidney Diseases (NIDDK). (2012a). *Urinary retention.* Retrieved from http://kidney.niddk.nih.gov/kudiseases/pubs/UrinaryRetention/

National Institute of Diabetes and Digestive and Kidney Diseases (NIDDK). (2012b). *Diarrhea.* Retrieved from http://digestive.niddk.nih.gov/ddiseases/pubs/diarrhea/

National Institute of Diabetes and Digestive and Kidney Diseases (NIDDK). (2012c). *Prostate enlargement: Benign prostatic hyperplasia.* Retrieved from http://kidney.niddk.nih.gov/kudiseases/pubs/prostateenlargement/

National Institute of Diabetes and Digestive and Kidney Diseases (NIDDK). (2012d). *Urinary incontinence in children.* Retrieved from http://kidney.niddk.nih.gov/kudiseases/pubs/uichildren/

National Institute of Diabetes and Digestive and Kidney Diseases (NIDDK). (2012e). *What I need to know about my child's urinary tract infection.* Retrieved from https://www.niddk.nih.gov/health-information/health-topics/urologic-disease/urinary-tract-infection-in-children/Pages/ez.aspx

National Institute of Diabetes and Digestive and Kidney Diseases (NIDDK). (2012f). *Kidney stones in children.* Retrieved from http://kidney.niddk.nih.gov/kudiseases/pubs/stoneschildren/

National Institute of Diabetes and Digestive and Kidney Diseases (NIDDK). (2013a). *Eating, diet, & nutrition for kidney stones.* Retrieved from http://kidney.niddk.nih.gov/kudiseases/pubs/kidneystonediet/

National Institute of Diabetes and Digestive and Kidney Diseases (NIDDK). (2013b). *Kidney stones in adults* (NIH Publication No. 13-2495). Retrieved from http://www.niddk.nih.gov/health-information/health-topics/urologic-disease/kidney-stones-in-adults/Pages/facts.aspx

National Institute of Diabetes and Digestive and Kidney Diseases (NIDDK). (2014). *Prostate enlargement: Benign prostatic hyperplasia* (NIH Publication No. 14-3012). Retrieved from http://www.niddk.nih.gov/health-information/health-topics/urologic-disease/benign-prostatic-hyperplasia-bph

Nicolle, L. E. (2012). Urinary catheter infections. *Infectious Disease Clinics in North America, 26*(1), 13–28. doi:10.1016/j.idc.2011.09.009

Nurko, S., & Zimmerman, L. (2014). Evaluation and treatment of constipation in children and adolescents. *American Family Physician, 90*(2),

82–90. Retrieved from http://www.aafp.org/afp/2014/0715/p82.html

Nusee, Z., Ibrahim, N., Mohd Rus, R., & Ismail, H. (2014). Is portable three-dimensional ultrasound a valid technique for measurement of postpartum urinary bladder volume? *Taiwanese Journal of Obstetrics and Gynecology, 53*(1), 12–16. Retrieved from http://dx.doi.org/10.1016/j.tjog.2013.01.028

Olsen, I. P., Wilsgaard, T., & Kierud, T. (2012). Development of the maternal anal canal during pregnancy and the postpartum period: A longitudinal and functional ultrasound study. *Obstetrics & Gynecology, 39,* 690–697. doi:10.1002/uog.11104

Oman, K. S., Makic, M. B. F., Fink, R., Schraeder, N., Hulett, T., Keech, T., & Wald, H. (2012). Nurse-directed interventions to reduce catheter-associated urinary tract infections. *American Journal of Infection Control, 40*(6), 548–553. doi:10.1016/j.ajic.2011.07.018

Onaran, M., Orhan, N., Farahvash, A., Ekin, H. N., Kocabıyık, M., Gönül, İ. I., . . . Aslan, M. (2016). Successful treatment of sodium oxalate induced urolithiasis with Helichrysum flowers. *Journal of Ethnopharmacology, 186,* 322–328. doi:10.1016/j.jep.2016.04.003

Osatakul, S., & Puetpaiboon, A. (2014). Use of Rome II versus Rome III criteria for diagnosis of functional constipation in young children. *Pediatrics International, 56,* 83–88. doi:10.1111/ped.12194. Published by Japan Pediatric Society, © 2015.

Papadakis, M. A., & McPhee, S. J. (Eds.). (2013). *Current medical diagnosis and treatment* (52nd ed.). New York, NY: McGraw-Hill.

Pashootan, P., Ploussard, G., Cocaul, A., De Gouvello, A., & Desgrandchamps, F. (2015). Association between metabolic syndrome and severity of lower urinary tract symptoms: Observational study in a 4666 European men cohort. *BJU International, 116*(1), 124–130. doi:10.1111/bju.12931

Pearson, R., & Williams, P. (2014). Common questions about the diagnosis and management of benign prostatic hyperplasia. *American Family Physician, 90*(11), 769–774. Retrieved from http://www.aafp.org/afp/2014/1201/p769.html

Portalatin, M., & Winstead, N. (2012). Medical management of constipation. *Clinics in Colon and Rectal Surgery, 25*(1), 12–19. doi:10.1055/s-0032-1301754

Prynn, P. (2012). Nocturnal enuresis in children and adolescents. *Practice Nurse, 42*(6), 20–24.

Quitadamo, P., Coccorulio, P., Guannetti, E., Romano, C., Chiaro, A., Campanozzi, A., . . . Staiano, A. (2012). A randomized, prospective, comparison study of a mixture of acacia fiber, psyllium fiber, and fructose vs polyethylene glycol 3350 with electrolytes for the treatment of chronic functional constipation in childhood. *Journal of Pediatrics, 161*(4), 710–715. doi:10.1016/j.peds.2012.04.043

Rao, S. S. (2013). Constipation in the older adult. In T. W. Post (Ed.), *UpToDate.* Retrieved from http://www.uptodate.com/contents/constipation-in-the-older-adult?source=search_result&search=constipation&selectedTitle=4~150

Razjouyan, H., Prasad, S., & Chokhavatia, S. (2015). Clinical challenges of fecal incontinence in the elderly. *Current Treatment Options in Gastroenterology, 13*(3), 287–300. doi:10.1007/s11938-015-0060-0

Revello, K., & Gallo, A. M. (2013). Implementing an evidence-based practice protocol for prevention of catheterized associated urinary tract infections in a progressive care unit. *Journal of Nursing Education and Practice, 3*(1), 99–107. doi:10.5430/jnep.v3n1p99

Roudakova, K., & Monga, M. (2014). The evolving epidemiology of stone disease. *Indian Journal of Urology, 30*(1), 44–48. doi:10.4103/0970-1591.124206

Rouzi, A. A., Sahly, N., Alhachim, E., & Abduljabbar, H. (2014). Type I female genital mutilation: A cause of completely closed vagina. *Journal of Sexual Medicine, 11*(9), 2351–2353. doi:10.1111/jsm.12605

Ryl, A., Rotter, I., Miazgowski, T., Słojewski, M., Dołęgowska, B., Lubkowska, A., & Laszczyńska, M. (2015). Metabolic syndrome and benign prostatic hyperplasia: Association or coincidence? *Diabetolgy Metablolic Syndrome, 7*(94). doi:10.1186/s13098-015-0089-1

Saitz, T., Mongoue-Tchokote, M., Sharadin, C., Giel, D., Corbett, S., & Bayne, A. (2016). MP43-07 factors associated with recurrent pediatric urolithiasis: A multi-institutional analysis (Suppl.). *Journal of Urology, 195*(4), e580–e581. Retrieved from http://dx.doi.org/10.1016/j.juro.2016.02.216

Schmidt, F. M., & Santos, V. L. (2014). Prevalence of constipation in the general adult population: An integrative review. *Journal of Wound, Ostomy & Continence Nursing, 41*(1), 70–76. doi:10.1097/01.WON.0000438019.21229.b7

Shah, B. J., Chokhavatia, S., & Rose, S. (2012). Fecal incontinence in the elderly: FAQ. *American Journal of Gastroenterology, 107,* 1635–1646. doi:10.1038/ajg.2012.284

Silva, L. A., Andriolo, R. B., Atallah, Á. N., & da Silva, E. M. (2014). *Surgery for stress urinary incontinence due to presumed sphincter deficiency after prostate surgery* (Art. No. CD008306). Retrieved from Cochrane Database of Systematic Reviews website: http://onlinelibrary.wiley.com/doi/10.1002/14651858.CD008306.pub3/full

Singh, B. P., Nagathan, D. S., Sankhwar, S., & Yadav, R. (2013). Hutch diverticulum presenting as acute urinary retention in early life (bcr2013200528). *BMJ Case Reports.* doi:10.1136/bcr-2013-200528. Retrieved from http://www.ncbi.nlm.nih.gov/pmc/articles/PMC3794219/

Spratto, G. R., & Woods, A. L. (2012). *Delmar nurse's drug handbook.* Clifton Park, NY: Delmar Cengage Learning.

Stephansson, O., Sandström, A., Petersson, G., Wikström, A. K., & Cnattingius, S. (2016). Prolonged second stage of labour, maternal infectious disease, urinary retention and other complications in the early postpartum period. *BJOG, 123*(4), 608–616. doi:10.1111/1471-0528.13287

Subak, L. L., Richter, H. E., & Hunskaar, S. (2009). Obesity and urinary incontinence: Epidemiology and clinical research update. *Journal of Urology, 182*(6 Suppl.) S2–S7.

Tabbers, M. M., DiLorenzo, C., Berger, M. Y., Faure, C., Langendam, M. W., Nurko, S., . . . Benning, M. A. (2014). Evaluation and treatment of functional constipation in infants and children: Evidence-based recommendations from ESPGHAN and NASPGHAN. *JPGN, 58*(2), 258–274. doi:10.1097/MPG.0000000000000266

Toner, F., & Claros, E. (2012). Preventing, assessing, and managing constipation in older adults. *Nursing, 42*(12), 32–39. doi:10.1097/01.NURSE.0000422642.83383.17

Townsend, M. K., Matthews, C. A., Whitehead, W. E., & Grodstein, F. (2012). Risk factors for fecal incontinence in older women. *American Journal of Gastroenterology, 108,* 113–119. doi:10.1038/ajg.2012.364

Trottier, M., Erebara, A., & Bozzo, P. (2012). Treating constipation during pregnancy. *Canadian Family Physician, 58*(8), 836–838. Retrieved from http://www.ncbi.nlm.nih.gov/pmc/articles/PMC3418980/?report=reader

van Breda, H. M., Laetitia, R. B., & de Kort, M. O. (2015). Hidden prevalence of lower urinary tract symptoms in healthy nulligravid young women. *International Urogynecology Journal, 26,* 1637–1643. doi:10.1007/s00192-015-2754-1

Vandenplas, Y., Alarcon, P., Alliet, P., De Greef, E., De Ronne, N., Hoffman, I., . . . Hauser, B. (2015). Algorithms for managing infant constipation, colic, regurgitation and cow's milk allergy in formula-fed infants. *Foundation Acta Pædiatrica, 104,* 449–457. doi:10.1111/apa.12962

Vasavada, S. P. (2015). Urinary incontinence. *Medscape Reference.* Retrieved from http://emedicine.medscape.com/article/452289

Vissers, D., Neels, H., Vermandel, A., De Wachter, S., Tjalma, W. A. A., Wyndaele, J. J., & Taeymans, J. (2014). The effect of non-surgical weight loss interventions on urinary incontinence in overweight women: A systematic review and meta-analysis. *Obesity Reviews, 15*(7), 541–617.

Wayment, R. O., & Schwartz, B. F., (2015). Pregnancy and urolithiasis. *Medscape Reference.* Retrieved from http://emedicine.medscape.com/article/455830-overview

Wilcox, S., Kansagra, K., & Richards, J. (2013). Profound bradycardia with decreased PEEP.

Respiratory Care, 58(11), e138–e143. doi:10.4187/respcare.02437

Xinias, I., & Mavroudi, A. (2015). Constipation in childhood: An update on evaluation and management. *Hippokratia, 19*(1), 11–19.

Zhou, X. (2013). Chinese herbs cured a kidney calculus: A retrospective case report [Scientific abstracts presented at the International Congress for Clinicians in Complementary & Integrative Medicine 2013. *Global Advances in Health and Medicine, 2*(Suppl.), 18C. doi:10.7453/gahmj.2013.097CP.S18C. Published by Global Advances in Health and Medicine, © 2013.

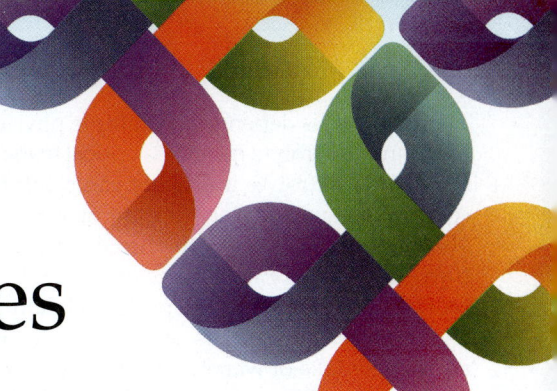

Module 6
Fluids and Electrolytes

Module Outline and Learning Outcomes

The Concept of Fluids and Electrolytes

Normal Fluids and Electrolytes

6.1 Analyze the physiology of fluids and electrolytes in the body.

Alterations to Fluids and Electrolytes

6.2 Differentiate alterations in fluids and electrolytes.

Concepts Related to Fluid and Electrolyte Balance

6.3 Outline the relationship between fluids and electrolytes and other concepts.

Health Promotion

6.4 Explain the promotion of maintaining fluid and electrolyte balance.

Nursing Assessment

6.5 Differentiate among common assessment procedures and tests used to examine fluid and electrolyte balance.

Independent Interventions

6.6 Analyze independent interventions nurses can implement for patients with alterations in fluid and electrolyte balance.

Collaborative Therapies

6.7 Summarize collaborative therapies used by interprofessional teams for patients with alterations in fluid and electrolyte balance.

Lifespan Considerations

6.8 Differentiate considerations related to the care of patients with alterations in fluid and electrolyte balance throughout the lifespan.

Fluids and Electrolytes Exemplars

Exemplar 6.A Fluid and Electrolyte Imbalance

6.A Analyze fluid and electrolyte imbalance and its effect on the body.

Exemplar 6.B Acute Kidney Injury

6.B Analyze acute kidney injury (AKI) as it relates to fluids and electrolytes.

Exemplar 6.C Chronic Kidney Disease

6.C Analyze chronic kidney disease (CKD) as it relates to fluids and electrolytes.

» The Concept of Fluids and Electrolytes

Concept Key Terms

Active transport, 360	Diffusion, 360	Hematocrit, 372	Insensible fluid loss, 362	Oncotic pressure, 360
Anions, 358	Edema, 360	Hydrostatic pressure, 360	Interstitial fluid, 359	Osmolality, 359
Body surface area (BSA), 374	Electrolytes, 357	Hyperkalemia, 373	Intracellular fluid (ICF), 358	Osmosis, 359
Cations, 358	Extracellular fluid (ECF), 359	Hypernatremia, 373	Intravascular fluid, 359	Osmotic pressure, 360
Colloid osmotic pressure, 360	Filtration, 360	Hypertonic, 360	Ions, 358	Saline, 360
Colloids, 359	Fluid volume deficit (FVD), 372	Hypodermoclysis, 373	Isotonic, 360	Solutes, 358
Crystalloids, 359	Fluid volume excess (FVE), 372	Hypokalemia, 373	Milliequivalent, 358	Solvent, 359
Dehydration, 361		Hyponatremia, 373	Obligatory losses, 362	Tonicity, 360
		Hypotonic, 360		Transcellular fluid, 359

he body is composed largely of fluid in many forms: blood, serum, albumin, urine, bile, hormones, and cerebrospinal fluid—these are just a few of the fluids required for homeostasis, a part of the delicate balance of fluids and electrolytes that promotes the body's functions.

Within each of these fluids are **electrolytes**, charged ions capable of conducting electricity, in various concentrations and combinations. Learning what fluids contain specific electrolytes can help nurses identify causes of electrolyte imbalances in patients and specifically design care to restore homeostasis.

Homeostasis depends on multiple physiologic processes. Fluid and electrolyte balance is critical to maintaining health. Fluid and electrolyte imbalance can result from a variety of conditions, such as dehydration or renal failure, and can also negatively affect both chronic and acute illnesses. In turn, almost every illness has the potential to threaten this crucial balance. Even in the process of daily living, excessive temperatures or vigorous activity can disturb the balance if adequate intake of water and electrolytes is not maintained. Therapeutic measures can also disturb the body's homeostasis unless water and electrolytes are replaced.

Normal Fluids and Electrolytes

The proportion of the human body composed of fluid is surprisingly large. Approximately 60% of the average healthy adult's weight is water, the primary body fluid. When an individual is healthy, this volume, reflected in body weight, remains relatively constant, and the individual's weight varies by less than 0.2 kg (0.5 lb) in 24 hours, regardless of the amount of fluid ingested.

Total body water is affected by gender and body size. Because fat cells contain little or no water and lean tissue has a high water content, individuals with a higher percentage of body fat have less body fluid. Women have proportionately more body fat and less body water than men. Water accounts for approximately 60% of an adult man's weight but only 52% for an adult woman. In an individual with obesity, this percentage may be even less, water being responsible for only 30–40% of the individual's weight.

Water is vital to health and normal cellular functioning, serving as a medium for metabolic reactions within cells; a transporter for nutrients, waste products, and other substances; a lubricant; an insulator and shock absorber; and one means of regulating and maintaining body temperature.

Distribution and Composition of Body Fluids

The body's fluid is divided into two major compartments: intracellular and extracellular (see **Figure 6–1** »). Both of these contain oxygen from the lungs, dissolved nutrients from the gastrointestinal (GI) tract, excretory products of metabolism such as carbon dioxide, and charged particles called **ions**. The composition of fluids varies from one body compartment to another.

Many salts dissociate in water; that is, they break up into electrically charged ions. The salt sodium chloride breaks up into one ion of sodium (Na^+) and one ion of chloride (Cl^-). These charged particles are called electrolytes because they are capable of conducting electricity. The number of ions that carry a positive charge, called **cations**, and the number of ions that carry a negative charge, called **anions**, should be equal. Examples of cations are sodium (Na^+), potassium (K^+), calcium (Ca^{2+}), and magnesium (Mg^{2+}). Examples of anions are chloride (Cl^-), bicarbonate (HCO_3^-), phosphate (HPO_4^{2-}), and sulfate (SO_4^{2-}).

Electrolytes generally are measured in milliequivalents per liter of water (mEq/L) or milligrams per 100 mL (mg/100 mL). The term **milliequivalent** refers to the chemical combining power of the ion, or the capacity of cations to combine with anions to form molecules. This combining activity is measured in relation to the combining activity of the hydrogen ion (H^+). Thus, 1 mEq of any anion equals 1 mEq of any cation. The milliequivalent system is most often used clinically. However, nurses need to be aware that different systems of measurement may be found in interpretations of laboratory results. For example, calcium levels frequently are reported in milligrams per deciliter (1 dL = 100 mL) instead of milliequivalents per liter. It also is important to remember that laboratory tests are usually performed using blood plasma, an extracellular fluid (ECF). Although these results may reflect what is happening in the intracellular fluid (ICF), it generally is not possible to directly measure electrolyte concentrations within the cell.

Intracellular Fluid

Intracellular fluid (ICF) is found within the cells of the body. It constitutes approximately two thirds of the total body fluid in adults. ICF is vital to normal cell functioning. It contains **solutes** (substances that dissolve in liquid) such as oxygen, electrolytes, and glucose, and it provides a medium in which metabolic processes of the cell take place.

The composition of ICF differs significantly from that of ECF. Potassium and magnesium are the primary cations

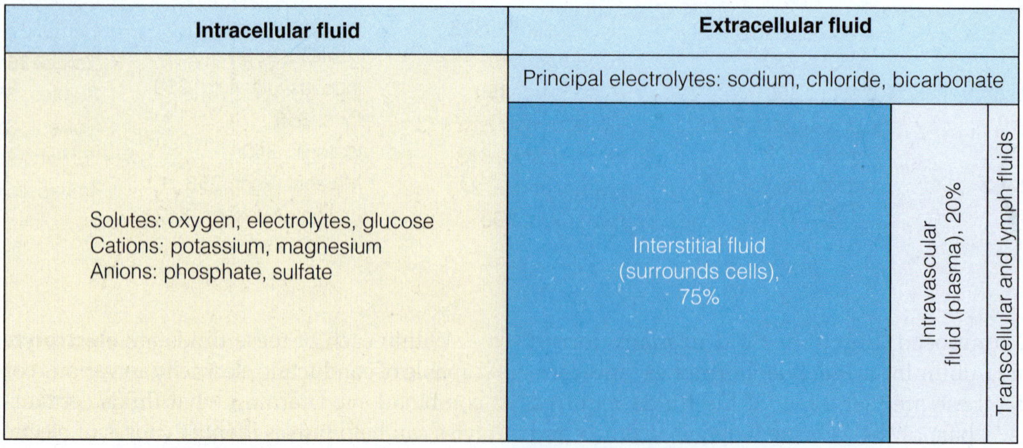

Figure 6–1 » Electrolyte composition (cations and anions) of body fluid compartments.

present in ICF, and phosphate and sulfate are the major anions. As in ECF, other electrolytes are present within the cell, but in much smaller concentrations.

Extracellular Fluid

Extracellular fluid (ECF) is found outside the cells and accounts for about one third of total body fluid. It is subdivided into compartments. The two main compartments of ECF are intravascular and interstitial. **Intravascular fluid**, or plasma, accounts for approximately 20% of the ECF and is found within the vascular system. **Interstitial fluid**, accounting for approximately 75% of the ECF, surrounds the cells. The other compartments of ECF are the lymph and transcellular fluids. Examples of **transcellular fluid** are cerebrospinal, pericardial, pancreatic, pleural, intraocular, biliary, peritoneal, and synovial fluids.

In ECF, the principal electrolytes are sodium, chloride, and bicarbonate. Other electrolytes (e.g., potassium, calcium, magnesium) are also present, but in much smaller quantities. Plasma and interstitial fluid, the two primary components of ECF, contain essentially the same electrolytes and solutes, with the exception of protein. Plasma is a protein-rich fluid, containing large amounts of albumin; interstitial fluid contains little or no protein. Although ECF is in the smaller of the two compartments, it is the transport system that carries nutrients to and waste products from the cells. Interstitial fluid transports wastes from the cells by way of the lymph system as well as directly into the blood plasma through capillaries.

Maintaining a balance of fluid volumes and electrolyte compositions in the fluid compartments of the body is essential to health. Normal and unusual fluid and electrolyte losses must be replaced if homeostasis is to be maintained.

Other body fluids, such as gastric and intestinal secretions, also contain electrolytes. Excessive loss of these fluids from the body (e.g., with severe vomiting or diarrhea, when gastric suction removes the gastric secretions) is of particular concern, as fluid and electrolyte imbalances can result. **Table 6–1** ≫ shows electrolyte concentrations in body fluid compartments.

Movement of Body Fluids

The body fluid compartments are separated from one another by cell membranes and the surrounding capillary membrane. Whereas these membranes are completely per-

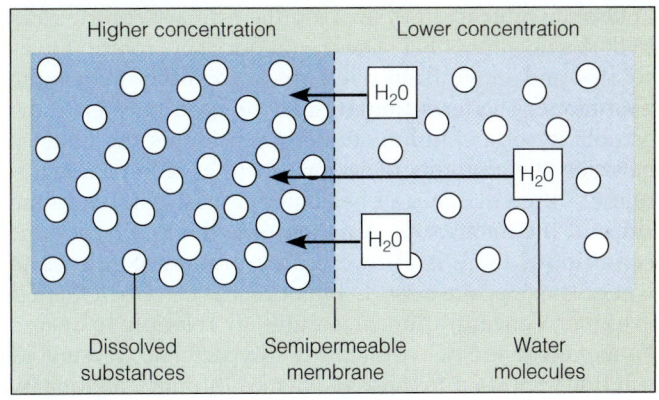

Figure 6–2 ≫ Osmosis: Water molecules move from the less concentrated area to the more concentrated area in an attempt to equalize the concentration of solutions on two sides of a membrane.

meable to water, they are considered to be selectively permeable to solutes, as substances move across them with varying degrees of ease. Small particles (e.g., ions, oxygen, carbon dioxide) move easily across these membranes; larger molecules, such as glucose and proteins, have more difficulty moving among fluid compartments. The methods by which electrolytes and other solutes move are osmosis, diffusion, filtration, and active transport.

Osmosis

Osmosis is the movement of water across cell membranes, from the less concentrated solution to the more concentrated solution (see **Figure 6–2** ≫). In other words, water moves toward the higher concentration of solute to equalize the concentrations on either side of the membrane.

Solutes may be **crystalloids** (salts that dissolve readily into true solutions) or **colloids** (substances such as large protein molecules that do not readily dissolve into true solutions). A **solvent** is the component of a solution that can dissolve a solute. An example of the solute–solvent relationship is sugar added to coffee: Sugar is the solute, and coffee is the solvent.

In the body, water is the solvent; the solutes include electrolytes, oxygen and carbon dioxide, glucose, urea, amino acids, and proteins. Osmosis occurs when the concentration of solutes is higher on one side of a selectively permeable membrane, such as the capillary membrane, than on the other side. For example, a marathon runner loses a significant amount of water through perspiration, increasing the concentration of solutes in the plasma because of water loss. This higher solute concentration draws water from the interstitial space and cells into the vascular compartment to equalize the concentration of solutes in all fluid compartments. Osmosis is an important mechanism for maintaining homeostasis and fluid balance.

The concentration of solutes in body fluids is usually expressed as the **osmolality**. Osmolality is determined by the total solute concentration within a fluid compartment and is measured as parts of solute per kilogram of water.

Osmolality is reported as milliosmoles per kilogram (mOsm/kg). Sodium is by far the greatest determinant of osmolality of ECF, with glucose and urea also contributing.

TABLE 6–1 Electrolyte Concentrations in Body Fluid Compartments

Components	Extracellular Fluid (ECF) Vascular	Extracellular Fluid (ECF) Interstitial	Intracellular Fluid (ICF)
Na^+	High	High	Low
K^+	Low	Low	High
Ca^{2+}	Low	Low	Low (higher than ECF)
Mg^{2+}	Low	Low	High
PO_4^-	Low	Low	High
Cl^-	High	High	Low
Proteins	High	Low	High

Potassium, glucose, and urea are the primary contributors to the osmolality of ICF. These substances are referred to as solutes and move from one side to the other across the membrane. The term **tonicity** may be used to refer to the osmolality of a solution. Tonicity represents the balance between the amounts of water on either side of a membrane. Different states of balance can exist relative to the sides of the membrane. A patient may be in a hypotonic condition if there is a lower concentration of solutes to water. The opposite exists in hypertonic states when there is a higher concentration of solutes in relation to water. Patients who are dehydrated have hypertonia. Crystalloid solutions are used to manage balance through the tonicity of the solution. An **isotonic** solution has the same osmolality as body fluids. Isotonic solutions do not result in any movement across the membrane through osmosis or diffusion. Normal **saline**, 0.9% sodium chloride, and lactated Ringer's solution are isotonic solutions. They are indicated in patients with hypotensive and hypovolemic states, since these patients require volume expansion. **Hypertonic** solutions have a higher level of solutes and include fluids such as 3% sodium chloride, D_5NS (5% dextrose in normal saline), and D_5LRS (5% dextrose in lactated Ringer's solution). Hypertonic fluids pull fluid from the cells into the vascular space; these solutions are used in patients with elevated intracranial pressure. **Hypotonic** solutions have less solutes than isotonic fluids. Examples of hypotonic fluids include 0.45% normal saline, referred to as one half normal saline (0.45% sodium chloride) or D_5 0.45% NS. Hypotonic solutions cause fluid to move into the cells and are indicated in patients with dehydration or hypernatremia (McClelland, 2014; McLafferty et al., 2014).

Osmotic pressure is the power of a solution to draw water across a semipermeable membrane. When two solutions of different solute concentrations are separated by a semipermeable membrane, the solution of higher solute concentration exerts a higher osmotic pressure, drawing water across the membrane to equalize the concentrations of the solutions. For example, infusing a hypertonic intravenous (IV) solution such as 3% sodium chloride will draw fluid out of red blood cells (RBCs), causing them to shrink. On the other hand, a hypotonic solution administered intravenously will cause the RBCs to swell as water is drawn into the cells by their higher osmotic pressure. In the body, plasma proteins exert an osmotic draw called **colloid osmotic pressure** or **oncotic pressure**, pulling water from the interstitial space into the vascular compartment. This is an important mechanism in maintaining vascular volume.

Diffusion

Diffusion is the continual intermingling of molecules in liquids, gases, or solids brought about by the random movement of the molecules. For example, two gases become mixed by the constant motion of their molecules. The process of diffusion occurs even when two substances are separated by a thin membrane. In the body, diffusion of water, electrolytes, and other substances occurs through the "split pores" of capillary membranes.

The rate of diffusion of substances varies according to (a) the size of the molecules, (b) the concentration of the solution, and (c) the temperature of the solution. Larger mole-

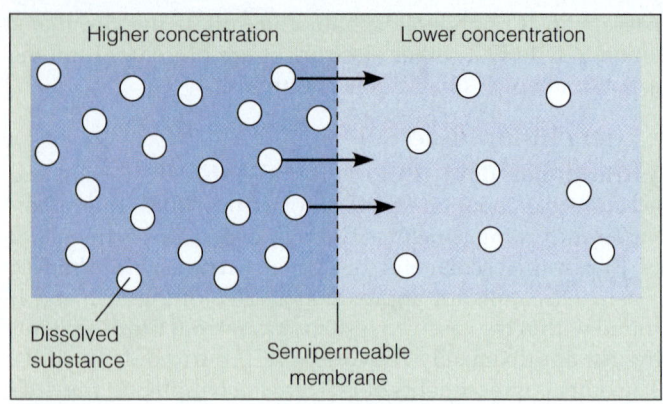

Figure 6–3 ›› Diffusion: Molecules move through a semipermeable membrane from an area of higher concentration to an area of lower concentration.

cules move less quickly than smaller ones because they require more energy to move about. With diffusion, the molecules move from a solution of higher concentration to a solution of lower concentration (see **Figure 6–3** ››). Increases in temperature increase the rate of motion of molecules and therefore the rate of diffusion.

Filtration

Filtration is a process whereby fluid and solutes move together across a membrane from one compartment to another. The movement is from an area of higher pressure to one of lower pressure. An example of filtration is the movement of fluid and nutrients from the capillaries of the arterioles to the interstitial fluid around the cells. The pressure in the compartment that results in the movement of the fluid and substances dissolved in fluid out of the compartment is called filtration pressure. **Hydrostatic pressure** is the pressure a fluid exerts within a closed system on the walls of its container. The hydrostatic pressure of blood is the force blood exerts against the vascular walls (e.g., the artery walls). The principle involved in hydrostatic pressure is that fluids move from the area of greater pressure to the area of lesser pressure. Using the example of the blood vessels, the plasma proteins in the blood exert a colloid osmotic or oncotic pressure (see the earlier section on Osmosis) that opposes the hydrostatic pressure and holds the fluid in the vascular compartment to maintain the vascular volume. When the hydrostatic pressure is greater than the osmotic pressure, the fluid filters out of the blood vessels, which can lead to the development of **edema**, swelling caused by excess fluid trapped in body tissues. The filtration pressure in this example is the difference between the hydrostatic pressure and the osmotic pressure (see **Figure 6–4** ››).

Active Transport

Substances can move across cell membranes from a less concentrated solution to a more concentrated one by **active transport** (see **Figure 6–5** ››). This process differs from diffusion and osmosis in that metabolic energy is expended. In active transport, a substance combines with a carrier on the outside surface of the cell membrane, and together they move to the inside surface of the cell membrane. Once inside, they separate, and the substance is released to the

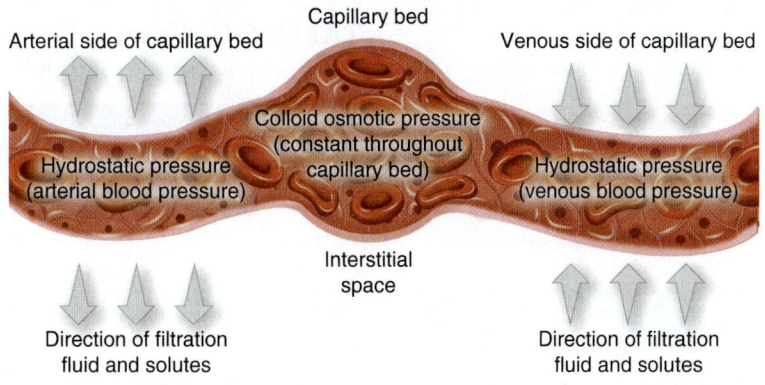

Figure 6–4 >> Schematic of filtration pressure changes within a capillary bed. On the arterial side, arterial blood pressure exceeds colloid osmotic pressure so that water and dissolved substances move out of the capillary into the interstitial space. On the venous side, venous blood pressure is less than colloid osmotic pressure so that water and dissolved substances move into the capillary.

inside of the cell. Each substance requires a specific carrier, active transport requires enzymes, and energy is expended.

Active transport is particularly important in maintaining the differences in sodium and potassium ion concentrations of ECF and ICF. Under normal conditions, sodium concentrations are higher in the ECF, and potassium concentrations are higher inside the cells. To maintain these proportions, the active transport mechanism (the sodium-potassium pump) is activated, moving sodium out of the cells and potassium into the cells.

Regulating Body Fluids

In a healthy individual, the volumes and chemical composition of the fluid compartments stay within narrow, safe limits. Fluid intake and fluid loss are normally balanced. Illness can upset this balance so that the body has too little or too much fluid. Fluid imbalance can result in a number of illnesses and conditions. The most common example is

dehydration, a condition that occurs when a body does not take in as much water as it loses or lacks sufficient reserves to maintain proper function. Edema and hypervolemia occur when the body has excess fluid.

Fluid Intake

During periods of moderate activity at moderate temperature, the average adult drinks about 1500 mL per day but needs 2500 mL per day, an additional 1000 mL. This added volume is acquired from foods and the oxidation of these foods during metabolic processes. The water content of food is relatively large, contributing about 750 mL per day. The water content of fresh vegetables is approximately 90%, that of fresh fruits about 85%, and that of lean meats around 60% (prior to cooking).

Water as a by-product of food metabolism accounts for most of the remaining fluid volume required. This quantity is approximately 200 mL per day for the average adult (see **Table 6–2** >>).

The thirst mechanism is the primary regulator of fluid intake. The thirst center is located in the hypothalamus of the brain. A number of stimuli trigger this center, including the osmotic pressure of body fluids, vascular volume, and angiotensin (a hormone released in response to decreased blood flow to the kidneys). For example, a long-distance runner loses significant amounts of water through perspiration and rapid breathing during a race, increasing the concentration of solutes and the osmotic pressure of body fluids. This increased osmotic pressure stimulates the thirst center, causing the runner to experience the sensation of thirst and the desire to drink to replace lost fluids.

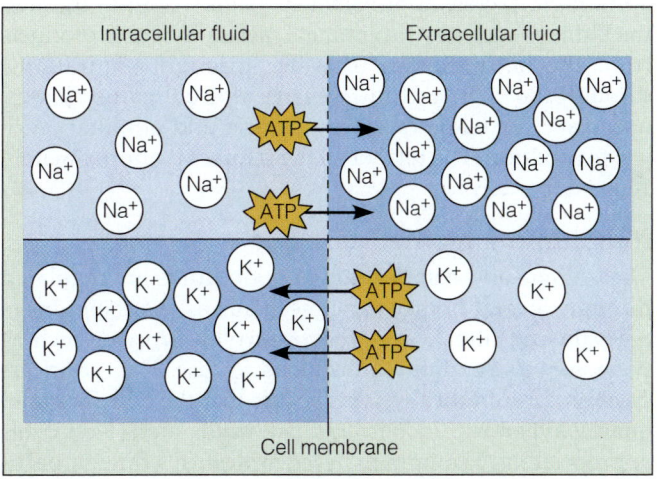

Figure 6–5 >> Active transport: Energy (ATP) is used to move sodium molecules and potassium molecules across a semipermeable membrane against sodium's and potassium's concentration gradients (i.e., from areas of lesser concentration to areas of greater concentration).

TABLE 6–2 Average Daily Fluid Intake for an Adult

Source	Amount (mL)
Oral fluids	1200–1500
Water in foods	750
Water as by-product of food metabolism	200
Total	2150–2450

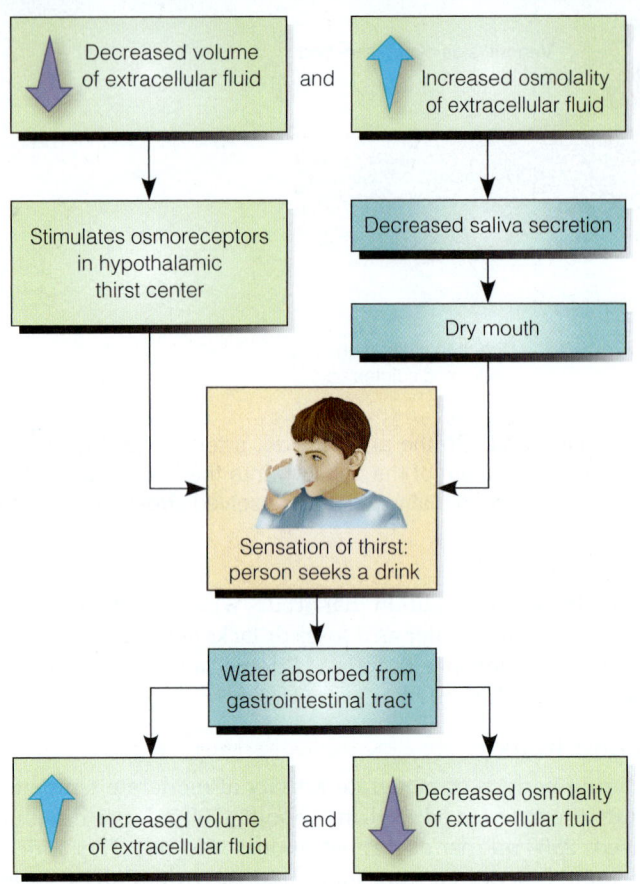

Figure 6–6 ❱❱ Factors stimulating water intake through the thirst mechanism.

Thirst is normally relieved immediately after drinking a small amount of fluid, even before the fluid is absorbed in the GI tract. However, this relief is only temporary, and thirst returns in about 15 minutes. Thirst is again temporarily relieved after the ingested fluid distends the upper GI tract. These mechanisms protect the individual from drinking too much, because it takes from 30 minutes to 1 hour for the fluid to be absorbed and distributed throughout the body (see **Figure 6–6** ❱❱).

Fluid Output

Fluid losses from the body counterbalance the adult's 2500-mL average daily intake of fluid, as shown in **Table 6–3** ❱❱. The four routes of fluid output are:

1. Urine
2. Insensible loss through the skin as perspiration and through the lungs as water vapor in the expired air
3. Noticeable loss through the skin
4. Loss through the intestines in feces.

Urine formed by the kidneys and excreted from the urinary bladder is the major avenue of fluid output. Normal urine output for an adult is 1400–1500 mL per 24 hours, or at least 0.5 mL/kg per hour. In healthy people, urine output may vary noticeably from day to day. Urine volume automatically increases as fluid intake increases. If fluid loss through perspiration is large, however, urine volume decreases to maintain fluid balance in the body.

TABLE 6–3 Average Daily Fluid Output for an Adult

Route	Amount (mL)
Urine	1400–1500
Insensible losses	
Lungs	300–400
Skin	300–400
Sweat	100
Feces	100–200
Total	2200–2600

Insensible fluid loss occurs through the skin and lungs. It is called insensible because it usually is not noticeable and cannot be measured. Insensible fluid loss through the skin occurs in two ways: through diffusion and perspiration. Water loss through diffusion is not noticeable but normally accounts for 300–400 mL per day. This loss can significantly increase if the protective layer of the skin is lost due to burns or large abrasions. Water loss through perspiration is noticeable, but not measurable. It varies depending on factors such as environmental temperature and metabolic activity. Fever and exercise increase metabolic activity and heat production, thereby increasing fluid losses through the skin.

Another type of insensible loss is the water in exhaled air. In an adult, this is normally 300–400 mL per day. When the respiratory rate accelerates owing to changes such as exercise or an elevated body temperature, this loss can increase.

The chyme that passes from the small intestine into the large intestine contains water and electrolytes. The volume of chyme entering the large intestine in an adult is normally about 1500 mL per day. Of this amount, all but about 100 mL is reabsorbed in the proximal half of the large intestine. The rest is excreted as feces.

Certain fluid losses are required to maintain normal body function. These are known as **obligatory losses**. An adult must excrete approximately 500 mL of fluid through the kidneys each day to eliminate metabolic waste products from the body. Losses of water through respirations, through the skin, and in feces are also obligatory losses, necessary for temperature regulation and elimination of waste products. The total of all these losses is approximately 1400 mL per day.

Maintaining Homeostasis

The volume and composition of body fluids are regulated through several homeostatic mechanisms. As the kidneys regulate and filter waste, they return electrolytes such as potassium and sodium to the blood for use. The cardiovascular and respiratory systems ensure that the body has adequate oxygen to function and use fluids and electrolytes appropriately. The immune system destroys foreign particles and pathogens that can undermine homeostasis. Hormones such as antidiuretic hormone (ADH; also known as arginine vasopressin, or AVP), the renin-angiotensin-aldosterone system, and atrial natriuretic factor (ANF) are involved, as are mechanisms to monitor and maintain vascular volume.

Illness or injury to any one system can negatively affect homeostasis. Some illnesses and diseases, such as cancer, affect fluid and electrolyte balance directly by their destructive presence in the body. They also have an indirect impact by the nature of the treatments required to rid the body of the illness. Chemotherapy, which can wreak havoc on fluid and electrolyte balance, is a prime example of such a treatment.

The kidneys are the primary regulator of body fluids and electrolyte balance. They regulate the volume and osmolality of ECF by regulating water and electrolyte excretion. The kidneys adjust the reabsorption of water from plasma filtrate and ultimately the amount excreted as urine. Although 135–180 L of plasma per day is normally filtered in an adult, only about 1.5 L of urine is excreted. Electrolyte balance is maintained by selective retention and excretion by the kidneys. The kidneys also play a significant role in acid–base regulation, excreting hydrogen ions (H^+) and retaining bicarbonate.

ADH, which regulates water excretion from the kidney, is synthesized in the anterior portion of the hypothalamus and acts on the collecting ducts of the nephrons. When serum osmolality rises, ADH is produced, causing the collecting ducts to become more permeable to water. This increased permeability allows more water to be reabsorbed into the blood. As more water is reabsorbed, urine output falls and serum osmolality decreases because the water dilutes body fluids. If serum osmolality decreases, ADH is suppressed, the collecting ducts become less permeable to water, and urine output increases. Excess water is excreted, and serum osmolality returns to normal. Other factors also affect the production and release of ADH, including blood volume, temperature, pain, stress, and some drugs such as opiates, barbiturates, and nicotine (see **Figure 6–7 》**).

Specialized receptors in the juxtaglomerular cells of the kidney nephrons respond to changes in renal perfusion. This initiates the renin-angiotensin-aldosterone system. If blood flow or pressure to the kidney decreases, renin is released. Renin causes the conversion of angiotensinogen to angiotensin I, which is then converted to angiotensin II by angiotensin-converting enzyme (ACE) released from the lungs. Angiotensin II acts directly on the vasculature and promotes vasoconstriction; it also acts on the nephrons to promote sodium and water retention. In addition, it stimulates the release of aldosterone from the adrenal cortex. Aldosterone also promotes sodium retention in the distal nephron. The net effect of the renin-angiotensin-aldosterone system is to restore blood volume (and renal perfusion) through sodium and water retention.

ANF is a peptide hormone released from cells in the atrium of the heart in response to excess blood volume and stretching of the atrial walls. Acting on the nephrons, ANF promotes sodium wasting and acts as a potent diuretic, thus reducing vascular volume. ANF also inhibits thirst, reducing fluid intake.

Regulating Electrolytes

Electrolytes are present in all body fluids and fluid compartments. Just as maintaining the fluid balance is vital to normal body function, so is maintaining electrolyte balance. Although the concentration of specific electrolytes differs

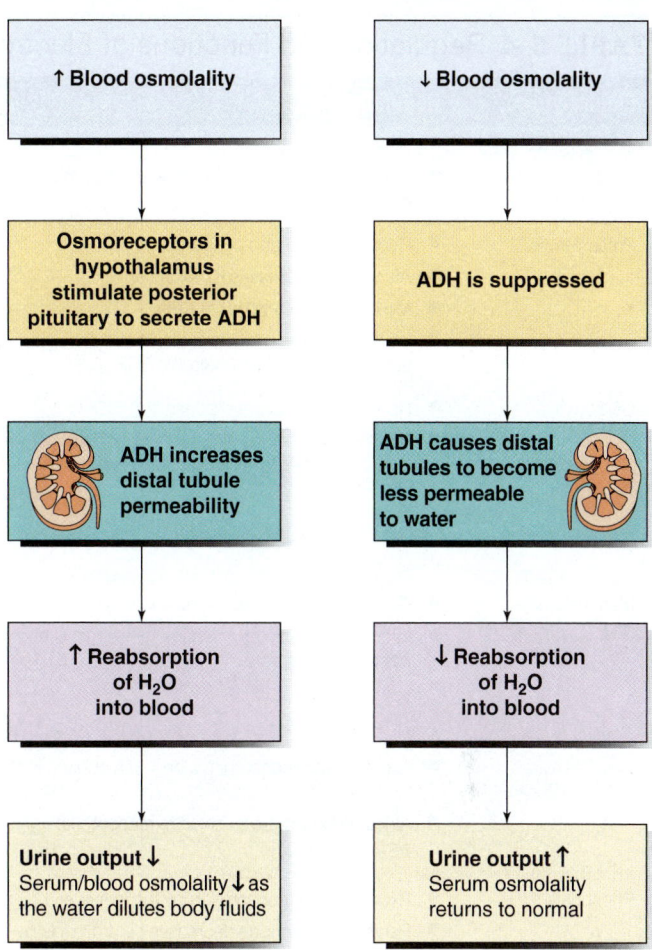

Figure 6–7 》 Antidiuretic hormone (ADH) regulates water excretion from the kidneys.

between fluid compartments, a balance of cations (positively charged ions) and anions (negatively charged ions) always exists. Electrolytes are important for the following:

- Maintaining fluid balance
- Contributing to acid–base regulation
- Facilitating enzyme reactions
- Transmitting neuromuscular reactions.

Most electrolytes enter the body through dietary intake and are excreted in the urine. The body does not store some electrolytes, such as sodium and chloride, which must be consumed daily to maintain normal levels. Potassium and calcium, on the other hand, are stored in the cells and bone, respectively. When serum levels drop, ions can shift out of the storage "pool" and into the blood to maintain adequate serum levels for normal functioning. The regulatory mechanisms and functions of the major electrolytes are summarized in **Table 6–4 》**.

Sodium (Na^+)

Sodium is the most abundant cation in ECF and a major contributor to serum osmolality. Normal serum sodium levels are 135–145 mEq/L. Sodium functions largely in controlling and regulating water balance. When sodium is reabsorbed from the kidney tubules, chloride and water are reabsorbed

TABLE 6–4 Regulation and Functions of Electrolytes

Electrolyte	Regulation	Function
Sodium (Na^+)	■ Renal reabsorption or excretion ■ Aldosterone increases Na^+ reabsorption in collecting duct of nephrons	■ Regulating ECF volume and distribution ■ Maintaining blood volume ■ Transmitting nerve impulses and contracting muscles
Potassium (K^+)	■ Renal excretion and conservation ■ Aldosterone increases K^+ excretion ■ Movement into and out of cells ■ Insulin helps move K^+ into cells; tissue damage and acidosis shift K^+ out of cells into ECF	■ Maintaining ICF osmolality ■ Transmitting nerve and other electrical impulses ■ Regulating cardiac impulse transmission and muscle contraction ■ Skeletal and smooth muscle function ■ Regulating acid–base balance
Calcium (Ca^{2+})	■ Redistribution between bones and ECF ■ Parathyroid hormone and calcitriol increase serum Ca^{2+} levels; calcitonin decreases serum levels	■ Forming bones and teeth ■ Transmitting nerve impulses ■ Regulating muscle contractions ■ Maintaining cardiac pacemaker (automaticity) ■ Blood clotting ■ Activating enzymes such as pancreatic lipase and phospholipase
Magnesium (Mg^{2+})	■ Conservation and excretion by kidneys ■ Intestinal absorption increased by vitamin D and parathyroid hormone	■ Intracellular metabolism ■ Operating sodium-potassium pump ■ Relaxing muscle contractions ■ Transmitting nerve impulses ■ Regulating cardiac function
Chloride (Cl^-)	■ Excreted and reabsorbed along with sodium in the kidneys ■ Aldosterone increases chloride reabsorption with sodium	■ HCl production ■ Regulating ECF balance and vascular volume ■ Regulating acid–base balance ■ Buffering oxygen–carbon dioxide exchange in RBCs
Phosphate (PO_4^-)	■ Excretion and reabsorption by the kidneys ■ Parathyroid hormone decreases serum levels by increasing renal excretion ■ Reciprocal relationship with calcium: increasing serum calcium levels decrease phosphate levels; decreasing serum calcium increases phosphate	■ Forming bones and teeth ■ Metabolizing carbohydrate, protein, and fat ■ Cellular metabolism; producing adenosine triphosphate (ATP) and DNA ■ Muscle, nerve, and RBC function ■ Regulating acid–base balance ■ Regulating calcium levels
Bicarbonate (HCO_3^-)	■ Excretion and reabsorption by the kidneys ■ Regeneration by the kidneys	■ Major body buffer involved in acid–base regulation

with it, thus maintaining ECF volume. Sodium is found in many foods, including bacon, ham, processed and canned foods, processed cheeses, and table salt.

Suggested sodium intake is 1500–2300 mg per day or less. According to the Centers for Disease Control and Prevention (CDC; 2013), average sodium intake in the United States is more than 3400 mg per day. Studies have indicated that certain ethnic groups, such as African Americans, have greater sensitivity to sodium compared to other populations. This salt sensitivity is primarily manifested by significant elevations in hypertension and by continued elevations of blood pressure throughout the night. In addition, salt sensitivity has been linked to the need for higher dosages of antihypertensive medications in this population.

Potassium (K^+)

Potassium is the major cation in ICFs, with only a small amount found in plasma and interstitial fluid. ICF levels of potassium are usually 125–140 mEq/L, whereas normal

Focus on Diversity and Culture
Sodium Use

To adapt teaching about low-sodium diets to the cultural practices of a family, ask the family members what types of food they usually eat. Help them to choose low-sodium foods from their diets and to avoid high-sodium foods. This approach is more effective than giving the same list of restricted foods to each family.

For example, some families use monosodium glutamate to flavor foods. They should be encouraged to add this at the table for family members who can have extra sodium rather than to use it during cooking. Many Americans consume too much sodium. Encourage patients to look for low-sodium foods. Low-sodium milk is available and is a good option for young children. Canned foods tend to be high in sodium, so teach all families to use fresh or frozen produce rather than canned when possible. Be mindful of the fact that some families live in areas where there are fewer food options, so shopping for low-sodium products may be difficult.

serum potassium levels are 3.5–5.3 mEq/L. The ratio of intracellular to extracellular potassium must be maintained for neuromuscular response to stimuli. Potassium is a vital electrolyte for skeletal, cardiac, and smooth muscle activity. It is involved in maintaining acid–base balance as well, and it contributes to intracellular enzyme reactions. Potassium must be ingested daily because the body does not conserve it. Many fruits and vegetables, meat, fish, and other foods contain potassium.

Calcium (Ca^{2+})

The vast majority (99%) of calcium in the body is in the skeletal system, with a relatively small amount in ECF. Although the calcium found outside the bones and teeth amounts to only about 1% of the total calcium in the body, it is vital in regulating muscle contraction and relaxation, neuromuscular function, and cardiac function. ECF calcium is regulated by a complex interaction of parathyroid hormone, calcitonin, and calcitriol, a metabolite of vitamin D. When calcium levels in the ECF fall, parathyroid hormone and calcitriol cause calcium to be released from bones into ECF and increase the absorption of calcium in the intestines, thus raising serum calcium levels. Calcitonin conversely stimulates the deposition of calcium in bone, reducing the concentration of calcium ions in the blood.

With aging, the intestines absorb calcium less effectively, and more calcium is excreted via the kidneys. Calcium shifts out of the bone to replace these ECF losses, increasing the risk of osteoporosis and fractures of the wrists, vertebrae, and hips. Lack of weight-bearing exercise (which helps to keep calcium in the bones) and vitamin D deficiency (usually due to inadequate exposure to sunlight) contribute to this risk.

Milk and milk products are the richest sources of calcium; other foods such as dark green leafy vegetables and canned salmon contain smaller amounts. Many patients benefit from calcium supplements.

Calcium levels are often reported in two ways, based on how the calcium circulates in the blood. Approximately 50% of blood calcium circulates in a free, ionized, or unbound form. The other 50% circulates in the blood bound to either plasma proteins or other nonprotein ions. Blood calcium is typically measured from the serum rather than total blood. The normal total serum calcium levels, which range from 9 to 11 mg/dL, represent both bound and unbound calcium. The normal ionized serum calcium, which ranges from 4.25 to 5.25 mg/dL, represents calcium circulating in the free, or unbound, form.

Magnesium (Mg^{2+})

Magnesium is found primarily in the skeleton and ICF. It is the second most abundant intracellular cation, with normal serum levels of 1.5–2.5 mEq/L. It is important for intracellular metabolism, particularly in the production and use of adenosine triphosphate (ATP). Magnesium also is necessary for protein and DNA synthesis within the cells. Only about 1% of the body's magnesium is in ECF, where it is involved in regulating neuromuscular and cardiac function. Maintaining and ensuring adequate magnesium levels is an important part of care of patients with cardiac disorders. Cereal grains, nuts, dried fruit, legumes, and green leafy vegetables are good sources of magnesium in the diet, as are dairy products, meat, and fish.

Chloride (Cl^-)

Chloride is the major anion of ECF, and normal serum levels are 95–105 mEq/L. Chloride functions with sodium to regulate serum osmolality and blood volume. The concentration of chloride in ECF is regulated secondarily to sodium; when sodium is reabsorbed in the kidney, chloride usually follows. Chloride is a major component of gastric juice, as hydrochloric acid (HCl), and is involved in regulating acid–base balance. It also acts as a buffer in the exchange of oxygen and carbon dioxide in RBCs. Chloride is found in the same foods as sodium.

Phosphate (PO_4^-)

Phosphate is the major anion of ICF. It also is found in ECF, bone, skeletal muscle, and nerve tissue. Normal adult serum levels of phosphate range from 2.5 to 4.5 mg/dL. Children have much higher phosphate levels than adults, that of a newborn being nearly twice that of an adult. Higher levels of growth hormone and a faster rate of skeletal growth probably account for this difference. Phosphate is involved in many chemical actions of the cell; it is essential for functioning of muscles, nerves, and RBCs. It is also involved in the metabolism of protein, fat, and carbohydrate. Phosphate is absorbed from the intestine and is found in many foods such as meat, fish, poultry, milk products, and legumes.

Bicarbonate (HCO_3^-)

Bicarbonate is present in both ICFs and ECFs. Its primary function is regulating acid–base balance as an essential component of the carbonic acid–bicarbonate buffering system. Extracellular bicarbonate levels are regulated by the kidneys: Bicarbonate is excreted when too much is present, but if more is needed, the kidneys both regenerate and reabsorb bicarbonate ions. Unlike other electrolytes that must be consumed in the diet, bicarbonate is produced through metabolic processes in amounts that are adequate to meet the body's needs.

Alterations to Fluids and Electrolytes

Many health conditions cause changes in body fluids that must be regulated and managed. Sometimes management of fluid status in the home or in a short-term ambulatory facility can prevent more serious illness or hospitalization.

Alterations and Manifestations

Examples of conditions that commonly require fluid, electrolyte, or acid–base balance interventions include gastroenteritis, burns, kidney disorders, oral fluid restriction for surgery, anorexia or bulimia, and dehydration and electrolyte imbalances that can result from athletics in hot weather. Common alterations to fluid and electrolyte balance, their manifestations, and interventions and therapies for them are outlined in the Alterations and Therapies feature.

Compensation

The body continuously attempts to compensate for a fluid and electrolyte imbalance by shifting fluid and electrolytes from one component to another. Therefore, it is rare for only one type of imbalance to occur; the fluid and electrolyte status

Alterations and Therapies
Fluids and Electrolytes

ALTERATION	DESCRIPTION	MANIFESTATIONS	INTERVENTIONS AND THERAPIES
Fluid volume deficit (dehydration)	Fluids are lost secondary to diarrhea, vomiting, inability to take in fluids, excessive perspiration, or increased basal metabolic rate due to fever, hyperthyroidism, or medications.	■ Dry to tenting skin ■ Dry mucous membranes ■ Increased hemoglobin and hematocrit ■ Thirst ■ Decreased urine output ■ Weight loss	■ Administer fluids via either the oral or IV route, and treat the underlying cause.
Fluid volume excess	Too much fluid in the body may be caused by excessive fluid intake (IV fluid administration, water intoxication), or inadequate fluid excretion (e.g., kidney failure, poor perfusion to the kidneys secondary to congestive heart failure, low cardiac output, hypertension).	■ Edema ■ Pitting edema ■ Weight gain ■ Ascites ■ Adventitious lung sounds ■ Increased central venous pressure	■ Administer diuretics to increase fluid excretion, reduce fluid intake, and elevate the head of the bed if dyspnea results from pulmonary edema.
Elevated electrolyte level	Any electrolyte level may be elevated. Hypernatremia and hyperkalemia are the most common and significant extracellular findings.	■ Hyperkalemia: fatigue, nausea, muscle weakness, cardiac irregularities ■ Hypernatremia: swelling, irritability, muscle spasms, thirst, confusion, coma ■ Hypercalcemia: nausea and vomiting, excessive thirst, frequent urination, constipation, muscle pain	■ Limit intake of the elevated electrolyte. ■ Administer glucose and insulin to lower serum potassium levels by driving potassium from the extracellular space into the intracellular space. ■ Diuretics will increase potassium and sodium loss but will also remove fluid.
Low electrolyte level	Any electrolyte level can decrease, but hypokalemia (low potassium) is the most common result of diuretics unless a potassium-sparing diuretic is administered.	■ Cardiac arrhythmias ■ Weakness ■ Muscle twitching ■ Blood pressure changes ■ Confusion ■ Seizures ■ Numbness ■ Sleep disturbances ■ Constipation	■ Administer an electrolyte supplement, monitor serum electrolyte levels, and monitor for symptoms associated with electrolyte imbalance. For example, low potassium levels can cause cardiac arrhythmias, and the patient should be placed on a cardiorespiratory monitor.
Chronic kidney disease (CKD)	Damage to the kidney over time causes progressive decline in kidney function; CKD may be caused by diabetes mellitus, hypertension, or cardiac disease.	■ Confusion ■ Fluid retention	■ CKD initially may be treated with diuretics. It progresses to the need for dialysis or kidney transplantation.
Acute kidney injury (AKI)	Rapidly progressive loss of kidney function is characterized by oliguria, (voiding less than 500 mL per day) and fluid and electrolyte imbalances. AKI can be the result of disturbed blood supply to the kidneys, toxins, or kidney trauma; it may be reversible or permanent.	■ Oliguria ■ Fluid and electrolyte imbalances ■ Fluid retention ■ Drowsiness ■ Dyspnea ■ Fatigue ■ Confusion ■ Nausea	■ Administer dialysis, monitor fluid and electrolyte balance, and treat the underlying cause. Kidney transplantation may be necessary.

and symptoms are constantly changing, requiring ongoing assessment and management by the nurse.

Prevalence

Electrolyte disorders are found on a consistent basis among certain populations. Results of a study by Liamis and colleagues (2013) suggest that 15% of those surveyed had at least one electrolyte disorder, with hyponatremia (7.7%) and hypernatremia (3.4%) being most common. The disorders of diabetes mellitus and hypertension were associated with hyponatremia, hypomagnesemia, and hypokalemia. The use of diuretics was independently associated with electrolyte imbalances, as were medications such as benzodiazepines. Because even mild electrolyte disorders are associated with significant illness and mortality, the nurse must monitor electrolyte balance on an ongoing basis and discuss with the patient and physician the need for discontinuation of problematic drugs.

Case Study » Part 1

Hope Balan, a 22-year-old woman, presents at the university clinic where you work with complaints of fever, chills, and a sore throat for more than 48 hours. She has been nauseated and, because of the severity of her sore throat, has been limiting her fluid intake. Data collected during assessment identifies dry mucous membranes with cracked lips, a very red throat with patches of white, temperature 102.8°F, pulse 120 bpm, and blood pressure 120/72 mmHg. Her skin is warm and very dry. She is tired and has not been sleeping well.

Clinical Reasoning Questions Level I

1. Why is Ms. Balan's pulse rate high?
2. At this time, what are the priorities for care?
3. What additional assessment or diagnostic information would be helpful in planning care for Ms. Balan?

Clinical Reasoning Questions Level II

4. Would you expect to see an elevation in Ms. Balan's hemoglobin and hematocrit? Why or why not?
5. What would you expect her urine specific gravity to be?
6. What risk factors do college students have for fluid or electrolyte imbalance?

Concepts Related to Fluid and Electrolyte Balance

Because fluid and electrolyte balance is critical to maintaining homeostasis, it both affects and is affected by other body systems. Throughout the day, the body makes adjustment to changes in temperature through fluid retention or excretion. To illustrate this adjustment, think about an athlete during a basketball game. As the game progresses, more and more sweating occurs. The body is getting rid of excess heat built up by acceleration in metabolism. As more and more heat is lost and the external temperature rises, the body could respond with hyperthermia, which can be a life-threatening occurrence. (For further discussion, see the module on Thermoregulation.)

Imbalance of fluids and electrolytes can severely affect cognition. Moderate to severe dehydration can result in confusion in the healthiest adult. Fluid and electrolyte imbalance can also be a factor in delirium, and best practice dictates that fluid and electrolyte levels be assessed through diagnostic testing when a patient presents with symptoms of delirium. (For further discussion, see the module on Cognition with a focus on confusion.) Cognitive factors may also affect fluid status. Individuals with impaired function due to dementia, other brain disease, or certain drugs that depress the central nervous system may experience impairment of the thirst mechanism, increasing their risk for fluid imbalance.

Patients with an imbalance in fluid and electrolytes, particularly increases in fluid and sodium, can experience overload in the extravascular space, resulting in stress on the cardiovascular system. This is especially important for the patient with congestive heart failure. Patients in overload and with resulting perfusion disorders are frequently placed on medications that can cause a fluid or electrolyte imbalance through gains or losses. For information on heart failure, see the module on Perfusion.

Because of the critical relationship between fluid and electrolyte balance and homeostasis, thorough assessment is necessary to determine the underlying cause of any imbalance and prevent or address potential complications. The Concepts Related to Fluid and Electrolyte Balance feature lists some, but not all, of the concepts integral to maintaining balance of fluids and electrolytes. They are presented in alphabetical order.

Health Promotion

Lifestyle factors such as fluid intake, diet, exercise, and stress affect fluid and electrolyte balance. Appropriate replacement of fluids throughout the day to maintain hydration benefits the heart, lungs, and kidneys. The delicate balance of fluids and electrolytes is also affected by foods consumed. Regular weight-bearing exercise and other physical exercise such as walking, running, or bicycling has a helpful effect on calcium and phosphorus balance. Individuals who maintain a healthy lifestyle are less likely to experience fluid and electrolyte imbalance.

Modifiable Risk Factors

Stress can increase cellular metabolism, blood glucose concentration, and catecholamine levels. In addition, stress can increase production of ADH, which in turn promotes retention of fluid and decreased urine output. Intake should be adjusted accordingly.

SAFETY ALERT Medications may contribute to fluid and electrolyte imbalance. Diuretics are most often implicated, but patients taking antipsychotic agents are often at risk for alterations in fluid intake because of the effect on thirst mechanisms. Even drugs for conditions such as overactive bladder alter balances. Patients taking vasoconstrictors, beta-blockers, and certain stimulants are at increased risk of fluid imbalance resulting from heat stroke, as these medications can impair the body's thermoregulation processes. Patient education regarding specific side effects and appropriate intervention can foster health promotion regarding fluid and electrolyte balance.

Heat-Related Illness

In the United States, approximately 7000 people annually are treated in emergency departments for heat-related illness

Concepts Related to
Fluid and Electrolyte Balance

CONCEPT	RELATIONSHIP TO FLUID AND ELECTROLYTE BALANCE	NURSING IMPLICATIONS
Assessment	Assists in identifying the underlying source of the imbalance and addressing potential complications.	■ Assess vital signs, intake and output (I&O), daily weights, skin turgor (except in older adults), and mentation. ■ See the Fluid and Electrolyte Assessment feature for more information.
Cellular Regulation	Acute hemorrhage → fluid imbalance manifested by hypovolemia.	■ Be alert to signs and symptoms of blood loss, fatigue, tachycardia, low hemoglobin, and hematocrit. ■ Anticipate the need for fluid replacement, administration of whole blood, packed cells, or colloids.
Cognition	Electrolyte loss or excess can lead to changes in cognition. Confusion and coma may result if loss is severe.	■ Assess mentation. ■ Rule out acute brain trauma before considering other causes.
Communication	Some patients may be unable to communicate thirst needs. Effective nurse–patient communication is an essential aspect of healthcare.	■ Offer fluids to patients frequently throughout the day, even if not requested. ■ Place fluids within reach and easy access.
Elimination	Certain alterations (e.g., diarrhea) → fluid and electrolyte loss.	■ Be alert for symptoms of sodium and chloride loss. Evaluate the patient for the degree of dehydration. ■ Children become dehydrated more quickly than adults, so patient education and quick response time are essential.
Perfusion	Fluid loss leads to decreased perfusion.	■ Assess perfusion, including pulses, nail beds, color, body position for comfort, and orientation. ■ Administer oxygen as ordered. ■ Anticipate the need for pharmacotherapy to improve cardiac output.
Thermoregulation	Fluid loss can lead to alterations in thermoregulation as the body loses its ability to regulate its heat loss because of hypovolemia.	■ Replace fluids. Move the patient to air conditioning or shade. Consider electrolyte replacement fluid.

(CDC, 2013). Individuals with an illness and those participating in strenuous activity are at risk for fluid and electrolyte imbalances when the environmental temperature is high. Fluid losses through sweating increase in hot environments as the body attempts to dissipate heat.

Both salt and water are lost through sweating. When only water is replaced, the individual is at risk for salt depletion. Symptoms include fatigue, weakness, headache, and GI symptoms such as loss of appetite and nausea. The risk of adverse effects increases if lost water is not replaced; the individual becomes at risk for heat exhaustion or stroke. Older adults, small children, athletes, laborers, and those who are ill are at greater risk.

Health promotion begins with education. As warmer temperatures approach, nurses can advise patients to (CDC, 2017):

■ Limit outdoor activity during the hottest part of the day.

■ Take frequent breaks for rest and water.

■ Drink water before they begin to feel thirsty.

■ Wear lightweight clothes.

■ Work or exercise with others when engaging in activity outside.

See the module on Thermoregulation for more information.

Nursing Assessment

Evaluating patients for fluid and electrolyte status is an important nursing care function. Components of the assessment include the nursing history and physical assessment of the patient, clinical measurements, and review of laboratory test results.

Observation and Patient Interview

Before seeking information from the patient's history and performing a more invasive exam, the nurse can use skills of observation to identify alterations in fluid and electrolyte balance. Patients may demonstrate edema of the lower extremities or the hands and face. The patient may look flushed with redness to the face, neck, and arms. Dehydration may be observable with dry, cracked lips; dry mucous membranes; dry skin; and a sunken look to the eyes. Infants may demonstrate depressed fontanels and dry mucous membranes.

The nursing history follows and is important for identifying patients who are at risk for fluid and electrolyte imbalances. The current and past medical history reveals conditions such as chronic cardiac disease or diabetes mellitus that can disrupt normal balances. Medications prescribed to treat acute or chronic conditions (e.g., diuretic therapy for hypertension) also may put the patient at risk for altered homeostasis. Functional, developmental, and socioeconomic factors must also be considered when assessing the patient's risk. Older adults and very young children, patients who must depend on others to meet their needs for food and fluid intake, and people who cannot afford or do not have the means to cook food for a balanced diet (e.g., people who are homeless) are at greater risk for fluid and electrolyte imbalances.

When obtaining the nursing history, the nurse needs not only to recognize risk factors but also to obtain data about the patient's food and fluid intake and fluid output and the presence of signs or symptoms that suggest altered fluid and electrolyte balance. The following are examples of questions designed to elicit information regarding fluid and electrolyte balance.

Current and Past Medical History

- Are you currently seeing a healthcare provider for treatment of any chronic diseases such as kidney disease, heart disease, high blood pressure, diabetes insipidus, or thyroid or parathyroid disorders?
- Have you recently experienced any acute conditions such as gastroenteritis, severe trauma, head injury, or surgery? If so, describe the condition(s).

Medications and Treatments

- Are you currently taking any medications on a regular basis such as diuretics, steroids, potassium supplements, calcium supplements, hormones, salt substitutes, or antacids?
- Have you recently undergone any treatments such as dialysis, parenteral nutrition, or tube feedings or been on a ventilator? If so, when and why?

Food and Fluid Intake

- How much and what type of fluids do you drink each day?
- Describe your diet for a typical day. (Pay particular attention to the patient's intake of foods that are high in sodium as well as intake of protein, whole grains, fruits, and vegetables.)
- Have you made any recent changes in your food or fluid intake, for example, as a result of following a weight-loss program?
- Are you on any type of restricted diet?
- Has your food or fluid intake recently been affected by changes in appetite, nausea, or other factors such as pain or difficulty breathing?

Fluid Output

- Have you noticed any recent changes in the frequency or amount of urine output?
- Have you recently experienced any problems with vomiting, diarrhea, or constipation? If so, when and for how long?
- Have you noticed any other unusual fluid losses, such as excessive sweating?

Fluid and Electrolyte Imbalances

- Have you gained or lost weight in recent weeks?
- Have you recently experienced any symptoms such as excessive thirst, dry skin or mucous membranes, dark or concentrated urine, or low urine output?
- Do you have problems with swelling of your hands, feet, or ankles? Do you ever have difficulty breathing, especially when lying down or at night? How many pillows do you use to sleep?
- Have you recently experienced any of the following symptoms: difficulty concentrating or confusion; dizziness or feeling faint; muscle weakness, twitching, cramping, or spasm; excessive fatigue; abnormal sensations such as numbness, tingling, burning, or prickling; abdominal cramping or distention; or heart palpitations?

Physical Examination

Physical assessment to evaluate a patient's fluid and electrolyte status focuses on the skin, the oral cavity and mucous membranes, the eyes, the cardiovascular and respiratory systems, and neurologic and muscular status. Often, the agency will use a standardized form or computer software to help the nurse make sure that certain elements of physical assessment are conducted consistently between visits and from one patient to the next. In addition to these important tools, the nurse should also make note of anything unusual in the patient's physical appearance. For example, edema may be readily observed in a patient's extremities and recorded during the physical assessment. Data from the physical assessment are used to expand and verify information obtained in the nursing history.

Three simple clinical measurements that the nurse can initiate without a primary care provider's order are daily weights, vital signs, and fluid intake and output (I&O). See the Fluid and Electrolyte Assessment feature for guidelines for completing a focused assessment.

Daily Weights

Daily weight measurements provide a relatively accurate assessment of a patient's fluid status. Significant changes in weight over a short time (e.g., more than 5 lb in a week or less) indicate acute fluid changes. Each kilogram (2.2 lb) of weight gained or lost is equivalent to 1 L of fluid gained or lost. Such fluid gains or losses indicate changes in total body fluid volume rather than in any specific compartment. Rapid losses or gains of 5–8% of total body weight indicate moderate to severe fluid volume deficits (FVDs) or excesses (FVEs). Regular assessment of weight is particularly important for patients in the community and in extended care facilities who are at risk for fluid imbalance. For these patients, measuring I&O may be impractical because of lifestyle or problems with incontinence. Regular weight measurement, taken daily, every other day, or weekly, provides valuable information about the patient's fluid volume status.

Vital Signs

Changes in the vital signs may indicate, or in some cases precede, fluid, electrolyte, and acid–base imbalances. For example, elevated body temperature may be a result of dehydration or a cause of increased body fluid losses.

Tachycardia is an early sign of hypovolemia. Pulse volume will decrease if an FVD is present and increase in the case of an FVE. Irregular pulse rates may occur with electrolyte imbalances.

Blood pressure, a sensitive measure to detect blood volume changes, may fall significantly with FVD and hypovolemia or increase with FVE. Postural, or orthostatic, hypotension may also occur with FVD and hypovolemia.

Fluid Intake and Output

The measurement and recording of all fluid I&O during a 24-hour period provides important data about the patient's fluid and electrolyte balance.

Most agencies have a form for recording I&O, usually a bedside record on which the nurse lists all items measured and the quantities per shift. Some agencies have another form for recording the specifics of IV fluids, such as the type of solution, additives, time started, amounts absorbed, and amounts remaining per shift.

The nurse should inform patients, family members, and all caregivers that accurate measurements of the patient's fluid I&O is essential, especially in infants, children, and older adults, who are particularly vulnerable to slight changes in fluid balance. The nurse should explain and emphasize the need to use a bedpan, urinal, commode, or in-toilet collection device (unless a urinary drainage system is in place). The patient should not put toilet tissue into the container with urine. Patients who wish to be involved in recording fluid intake measurements need to be taught how to compute the values and which foods are considered fluids.

To measure fluid intake, the patient or nurse must record each volume of fluid consumed or provided on the I&O form, specifying the time and type of fluid. All of the following fluids need to be recorded:

- Oral fluids
- Ice chips
- Foods that are or tend to become liquid at room temperature
- Tube feedings
- Parenteral fluids
- IV medications
- Catheter or tube irrigants.

Fluid and Electrolyte Balance Assessment

The following table summarizes normal and abnormal findings relative to the assessment of fluid and electrolyte balance. Developmental considerations are also included; additional information can be found in the Lifespan Considerations section.

ASSESSMENT/ METHOD	NORMAL FINDINGS	ABNORMAL FINDINGS	LIFESPAN OR DEVELOPMENTAL CONSIDERATIONS
Inspection			
View general appearance of skin.	Skin is appropriate color for ethnicity. Skin is firm, warm, and moist.	▪ Skin is flushed, warm, or very dry. ▪ Skin is very moist or diaphoretic or cool and pale.	Skin of older adults is thinner and less elastic.
Turgor: Gently pinch up a fold of skin over the sternum or inner aspect of thigh for adults.	Pinched tissue immediately returns to normal.	▪ Skin remains tented for several seconds instead of immediately returning to normal position.	▪ Gently pinch up a fold of skin on the abdomen or medial thigh for children. ▪ Turgor is difficult to assess in very old individuals because of loss of skin elasticity. Use other methods to assess turgor.
Mucous membranes: Assess for dryness and cracking.	Membranes are moist in appearance.	▪ Membranes are dry or cracking.	Infants may have a decrease in the number of diapers, and the urine may appear dark with crystals forming in the diaper. Tenting is not an accurate sign in the older adult.
Edema: Assess for pitting by depressing skin over tibia or on top of foot.	No swelling is noted. Depressed skin rebounds immediately.	▪ Depression remains when tissue is depressed ("pitting").	Edema in older adults may be indicative of heart failure. Rule out lymphedema characterized by nonpitting (Trayes et al., 2013).
Eyes: Gently palpate eyeball with lid closed.	Eyeball is soft.	▪ Eyeball is firm to touch.	Eyes may appear sunken in infants and children with dehydration.
Fontanels: Inspect and gently palpate anterior fontanel.	Fontanel is soft, flush with scalp.	▪ Fontanel is bulging. ▪ Fontanel is sunken.	Infection can lead to bulging fontanels in infants.

Fluid and Electrolyte Balance Assessment (continued)

ASSESSMENT/ METHOD	NORMAL FINDINGS	ABNORMAL FINDINGS	LIFESPAN OR DEVELOPMENTAL CONSIDERATIONS
Cardiovascular Assessment			
Heart rate and peripheral pulses	Rate and rhythm are regular. Pulses are equal.	▪ Tachycardia or bradycardia is present. ▪ Dysrhythmias are present. ▪ Pulse is weak or thready.	▪ Remember to evaluate vital signs in the normal range for children based on age.
Blood pressure	Blood pressure is normal for age.	▪ Hypotension or postural hypotension is present. ▪ Hypertension is present.	▪ Remember to evaluate vital signs in the normal range for children based on age.
Capillary refill: Assess for venous filling.	Refill is quick, less than 2–3 seconds.	▪ Refill is prolonged, sluggish.	A refill time of 3 seconds or more is considered abnormal in children (Fleming et al., 2015).
Respiratory Assessment			
Assess rate and rhythm and lung sounds.	Rate is normal for age. Lungs are clear to auscultation.	▪ Tachypnea, rales, wheezing, and frothy sputum are present. ▪ Cyanosis is a late sign.	▪ Remember to evaluate vital signs in the normal range for children based on age.
Neurologic Assessment			
Assess level of consciousness (LOC), orientation, cognition.	The patient is awake and arousable. The patient is alert and oriented to person, place, and time.	▪ The patient has decreased LOC, lethargy, stupor, or coma. ▪ The patient is disoriented or confused; the patient has difficulty concentrating.	Infants may demonstrate irritability or sleepiness.
Motor Function Assessment			
Strength and movement	The patient is able to move all extremities as directed, has a firm grip, and has 2+ deep tendon reflexes.	▪ Weakness and decreased motor strength are present. ▪ Hyperactive or depressed deep tendon reflexes are present.	Infants may demonstrate irritability and be difficult to console.
Chvostek sign: Tap over facial nerve about 2 cm anterior to tragus of ear.	No response	▪ The patient experiences facial muscle twitching, including eyelids and lips on the side of stimulus.	Chvostek sign could indicate hypomagnesemia in the very young.
Trousseau sign: Inflate a blood pressure cuff on the upper arm to 20 mmHg greater than the systolic pressure; leave in place for 2–5 minutes.	No response	▪ The patient experiences carpal spasm: contraction of hand and fingers on affected side.	Trousseau sign may demonstrate hypomagnesemia in children.

To measure fluid output, the patient or nurse measures the following fluids (remembering to observe appropriate infection control precautions):

- Urinary output
- Vomitus and liquid feces (The amount and type of fluid and the time of output need to be specified.)
- Tube drainage, such as gastric or intestinal drainage
- Wound drainage and draining fistulas.

Fluid I&O measurements are totaled at intervals according to agency protocol or physician instruction, and the totals are recorded in the patient's permanent record. To determine whether the fluid output is proportional to fluid intake or whether there are any changes in the patient's fluid status, the nurse (a) compares the total 24-hour fluid output measurement with the total fluid intake measurement and (b) compares both to previous measurements. Urinary output is normally equivalent to the amount of fluids ingested; the usual range is 1500–2000 mL in 24 hours, or 40–80 mL in 1 hour (0.5 mL/kg per hour). Patients whose output substantially exceeds intake are at risk for **fluid volume deficit (FVD)**. By contrast, patients whose intake substantially exceeds output are at risk for **fluid volume excess (FVE)**. In assessing the patient's fluid balance, the nurse should consider additional factors that may affect I&O. The patient who is extremely diaphoretic or who has rapid, deep respirations has fluid losses that cannot be measured but must be considered in evaluating fluid status.

When a significant discrepancy is noticed between intake and output or when fluid intake or output is inadequate (e.g., a urine output of less than 500 mL in 24 hours or less than 0.5 mL/kg per hour in an adult), this information should be reported to the charge nurse or primary care provider.

Diagnostic Tests

Many laboratory studies may be conducted to determine the patient's fluid and electrolyte status. Some of the more common tests are discussed here.

Serum Electrolytes

Serum electrolyte levels are often routinely ordered for any patient admitted to the hospital as a screening test for electrolyte imbalances. The most commonly ordered serum tests are for sodium, potassium, chloride, magnesium, and bicarbonate ions. Normal values of commonly measured electrolytes are shown in **Box 6–1 》**. Some primary care providers use a diagram format (see **Figure 6–8 》**) for keeping track of the patient's electrolytes when documenting in their progress notes.

Complete Blood Count

The complete blood count (CBC), another basic screening test, includes information about the hematocrit (Hct). The **hematocrit** measures the volume (percentage) of whole blood that is composed of RBCs. Because the hematocrit is a measure of the volume of cells in relation to plasma, it is affected by changes in plasma volume. Thus, the hematocrit

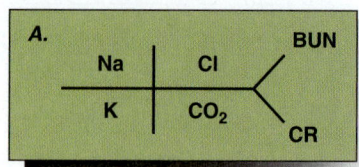

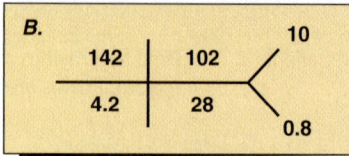

Figure 6–8 》 A, Format for a diagram of serum electrolyte results. **B,** Example that may be seen in a primary care provider's documentation notes.

increases with severe dehydration and decreases with severe overhydration. Normal hematocrit values are 40–54% (men) and 36–46% (women).

Osmolality

Serum osmolality is a measure of the solute concentration of the blood. The particles included are sodium ions, glucose, and urea (blood urea nitrogen, or BUN). Serum osmolality can be estimated by doubling the serum sodium, because sodium and its associated chloride ions are the major determinants of serum osmolality. Serum osmolality values are used primarily to evaluate fluid balance. Normal values are 280–300 mOsm/kg. An increase in serum osmolality indicates an FVD; a decrease reflects an FVE.

Urine osmolality is a measure of the solute concentration of urine. The particles included are nitrogenous wastes, such as creatinine, urea, and uric acid. Normal values average 200–800 mOsm/kg H_2O in children and adults. An increased urine osmolality indicates an FVD; a decreased urine osmolality reflects an FVE.

Urine Specific Gravity

Specific gravity is an indicator of urine concentration that can be performed quickly and easily by nursing personnel. Normal specific gravity ranges from 1.005 to 1.030 (usually 1.015–1.024). When the concentration of solutes in the urine is high, the specific gravity rises; in very dilute urine with few solutes, it is abnormally low.

Case Study 》 Part 2

It has been 2 weeks since Hope Balan was seen at the university clinic. She now presents to the emergency department, where you are the admitting nurse. Ms. Balan states that she awoke this morning with severe pain in her back, fever, and chills. You note that her face, hands, and feet are swollen. When you ask about prior medical history, she tells you she was well until 2 weeks ago when she had to visit the university clinic because she had a very sore throat and nausea. She tells you that she was diagnosed with strep throat and given amoxicillin clavulanate (Augmentin) to take for 10 days. She says that she completed half of her prescription, began to feel better, and did not finish the antibiotics. You take her

---

Box 6–1
Normal Electrolyte Values for Adults*

Venous Blood

Sodium	135–145 mEq/L
Potassium	3.5–5.3 mEq/L
Chloride	95–105 mEq/L
Calcium (total)	4.5–5.5 mEq/L or 9–11 mg/dL
Calcium (ionized)	50% of the total calcium (2.2–2.5 mEq/L or 4.25–5.25 mg/dL)
Magnesium	1.5–2.5 mEq/L or 1.8–3.0 mg/dL
Phosphate (phosphorus)	1.7–2.6 mEq/L or 2.5–4.5 mg/dL
Serum osmolality	280–300 mOsm/kg

Note: Normal laboratory values vary from agency to agency.

blood pressure, which is 140/100 mmHg, and her pulse rate is 92 bpm. Her temperature is 101.2°F. You ask her to provide a urine sample and note that her urine is dark in color. Ms. Balan's lab work reveals blood in her urine. The primary care provider makes a diagnosis of glomerulonephritis.

Clinical Reasoning Questions Level I

1. What would you expect to be the etiology of Ms. Balan's edema?
2. What is the etiology of hematuria?

Clinical Reasoning Questions Level II

3. What patient teaching is essential for Ms. Balan at this time?
4. What will the treatment plan include to reduce the edema and help Ms. Balan's kidneys heal?

Independent Interventions

Alterations in fluid and electrolytes may occur as a primary event or as a secondary response to a preexisting disease state or a sudden traumatic event. When alterations of fluid and electrolytes exceed the narrow limits consistent with good health, the body needs to adjust quickly. Independent nursing interventions for patients experiencing fluid and electrolyte balance include the following:

- Compare intake with output on a frequent basis.
- Assess the choice and types of fluid consumed, especially those that contain caffeine and may exert a diuretic effect.
- Weigh the patient daily.
- Engage the patient in the plan of care, particularly with regard to meal planning if the patient requires dietary modifications, such as sodium restriction.
- Provide patient education as indicated, especially with regard to medication regimens and side effects and prevention measures.

SAFETY ALERT Consider the outcomes that could occur with inaccurate documentation and recording of I&O. First, underestimates could lead to increased fluids being administered, which could result in fluid overload. Overestimates could lead to fluid restriction, which could result in additional adverse effects. For example, given the cellular intensity of chemotherapeutic agents, fluid restriction could lead to toxicity due to dehydration of the patient's extravascular space.

Collaborative Therapies

Many patients are avid exercisers, and the use of electrolyte replacement fluid is common in exercise arenas and sports complexes. In most instances, these fluids are used appropriately to replace lost water and electrolytes. It is important that patients understand that these fluids contain electrolytes that could alter the dynamic balance of individual electrolytes. Some runners and high-intensity athletes may also add additional sodium through the use of salt tablets to maintain sodium levels. One study found that some adolescents and young adults take salt tablets to maintain cognitive focus (Ross et al., 2013). Nurses must provide ongoing education regarding appropriate fluid and electrolyte replacement in all populations.

In cases of significant loss, the severity of fluid and electrolyte imbalance determines whether treatment will consist of oral replacements or the initiation of IV therapy. IV fluids may be ordered for the patient with an FVD if oral fluids cannot be taken in sufficient quantity. In some patients, when IV access proves problematic and management of dehydration becomes a concern, **hypodermoclysis** (fluid administered subcutaneously) may be used as a fluid delivery method, especially among older adults. Electrolyte supplements may be used to replace electrolyte deficits. Diuretics may be ordered to reduce FVE.

Pharmacologic Therapy

Pharmacologic therapies are aimed at replacing what has been lost or depleting what may be excessive in order to restore a normal balance to the body's fluid and electrolytes. Fluids are replaced in an attempt to put back what is lost, so blood loss is replaced with blood transfusions, albumins, or other large-molecule protein solutions (colloids). Fluids lost secondary to excessive diuresis, perspiration, inadequate intake, or insensible water losses are replaced by using crystalloids.

Electrolyte correction is highly dependent on the specific electrolyte and whether the body is in deficit or in excess. For example, elevated potassium levels (sometimes referred to as **hyperkalemia**) are ultimately corrected by dialysis, but treatments such as administration of glucose and insulin can help to drive potassium back into the cell, where elevated levels will create less risk. A deficit in potassium is known as **hypokalemia** and is frequently a side effect of diuretics.

Sodium excess, known as **hypernatremia**, is often seen in patients with reduced production of ADH; it may be corrected by administration of ADH. Sodium deficiency, known as **hyponatremia**, may be treated with oral supplementation, or if the deficiency is severe or life-threatening, IV supplementation may be administered. See the Medications feature for more information.

Case Study » Part 3

Hope Balan is admitted to the hospital because her condition has not improved. Her urinary output has continued to decrease to oliguria, and her edema continues. The nurse also notes the presence of ascites. Ms. Balan's blood pressure is now 148/104 mmHg. Her respiratory rate has increased, and she complains of being short of breath. She also complains of a metallic taste in her mouth. The results of urinalysis demonstrate proteinuria. A diagnosis of AKI is made.

Clinical Reasoning Questions Level I

1. What type of kidney injury does Ms. Balan have: prerenal, intrinsic, or postrenal? Why?
2. What is the etiology of the metallic taste Ms. Balan is experiencing?
3. What additional signs of AKI would the nurse expect to find upon assessment?

Clinical Reasoning Questions Level II

4. What is the reason for ascites?
5. What medications would you expect the provider to order?

Medications

Fluids and Electrolytes

CLASSIFICATIONS AND DRUG EXAMPLES	MECHANISMS OF ACTION	NURSING CONSIDERATIONS
Electrolyte Supplements *Drug examples:* Sodium chloride (sodium supplement) Potassium chloride (potassium supplement)	Electrolyte supplements replace lost electrolytes and return to homeostasis. Oral or IV routes may be used.	▪ Monitor serum electrolyte levels, I&O, and vital signs.
Colloids *Drug examples:* Serum albumin Dextran 40	Colloids expand the ECF volume through replacement of proteins, starches, or other large molecules. IV routes are used.	▪ Carefully monitor patient's condition, laboratory values, and renal function. Fluid overload can occur.
Crystalloids *Drug examples:* 5% dextrose and water Normal saline solution Lactated Ringer's solution 5% dextrose and 1/2 normal saline solution	IV solutions that contain electrolytes and other agents that mimic the body's ECF are used to replace depleted fluid and promote urine output. They represent different tonicities.	▪ Monitor patient's fluid and electrolyte status.
Diuretics *Drug examples:* Furosemide Hydrochlorothiazide Spironolactone (Aldactone)	Some diuretics block sodium and water reabsorption and thus promote urine output. Some inhibit aldosterone and inhibit fluid reabsorption. Some deplete potassium; some spare it.	▪ Monitor I&O, daily weight, serum electrolytes, and hydration status. ▪ Assess for changes in hearing. ▪ Thiazides are ineffective if the glomerular filtration rate is low.

Source: Data from Adams, M. P., Holland, L. N., & Urban, C. (2017). *Pharmacology for nurses: A pathophysiologic approach* (5th ed.). Hoboken, NJ: Pearson Education.

Lifespan Considerations

Age, sex, and body fat affect total body water. Infants have the highest proportion of water, accounting for 70–80% of their body weight. The proportion of body water decreases with aging. In individuals older than 60 years of age, water represents only about 50% of the total body weight. Women have a lower percentage of body water than men. Women and older adults have less body water because they have a lower muscle mass and a greater percentage of fat tissue. Fat tissue is essentially free of water, whereas lean tissue contains a significant amount of water.

The ability of the body to adjust fluid and electrolyte balance is influenced by age, gender and body size, and ethnicity.

Fluid and Electrolyte Balance in Infants and Young Children

Infants and young children differ physiologically from adults in ways that make them more vulnerable to fluid and electrolyte imbalances. Infants lose more fluid through the kidneys because immature kidneys are less able to conserve water than are adult kidneys. The **body surface area (BSA)** of infants (the relationship between height and weight measured in square meters) is proportionally greater than that of adults, increasing insensible fluid losses. This greater percentage of

BSA also puts infants and young children at greater risk when they sustain burns. In addition, infants' respirations are more rapid, which also increases insensible fluid losses.

The percentage of body weight that is composed of water also varies with age (see **Figure 6–9** »). The percentage is highest at birth (and higher in premature than in full-term infants) and decreases with age (see **Figure 6–10** »). Neonates and young infants have a proportionately larger ECF volume than older children and adults because their brain and skin (both rich in interstitial fluid) constitute a greater proportion of their body weight. Because much of the body's ECF is exchanged each day, infants have a high daily fluid requirement with little fluid volume reserve, making them vulnerable to dehydration. As an infant grows, the proportion of water inside the cells increases, the extracellular amount decreases in comparison, and the risk of fluid imbalance begins to decrease.

Infants and children under 2 years of age lose a greater proportion of fluid each day than do older children and adults and are thus more dependent on adequate intake. Respiratory illnesses, stomach viruses resulting in vomiting or diarrhea, and burns can all result in fluid or electrolyte imbalance in an infant or young child, increasing the risk for serious complications (Milanovic & Groselj-Grenc, 2014). A nurse working with parents of a young child presenting with these conditions

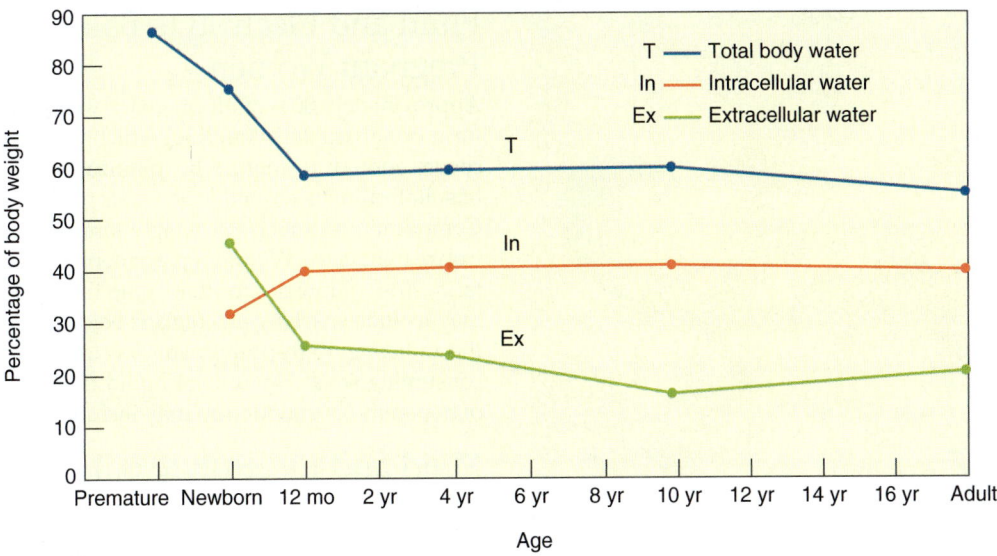

Figure 6–9 ›› The major body fluid compartments at various ages. *Extracellular fluid* (ECF) is composed mainly of vascular fluid (fluid in blood vessels) and interstitial fluid (fluid between the cells and outside the blood and lymphatic vessels). *Intracellular fluid* (ICF) is found within cells.

should take time to explain the importance of monitoring the child's hydration until the child returns to health.

In addition, respiratory and metabolic rates are high during early childhood. These factors lead to greater water loss from the lungs and greater water demand to fuel the body's metabolic processes (see **Figure 6–11** ››). Because of these factors, the exercising child dehydrates easily and must consume more fluid during physical activity, particularly during hot weather.

When fluid status is compromised, a number of body mechanisms activate to help restore balance. Several of these mechanisms occur in the kidneys. The kidneys conserve water and needed electrolytes while excreting waste products and drug metabolites. In children under 2 years of age, however, the glomeruli, tubules, and nephrons of the kidneys are immature. They are therefore unable to conserve or excrete water and solutes effectively. Because more water is generally excreted, the infant and young child can become

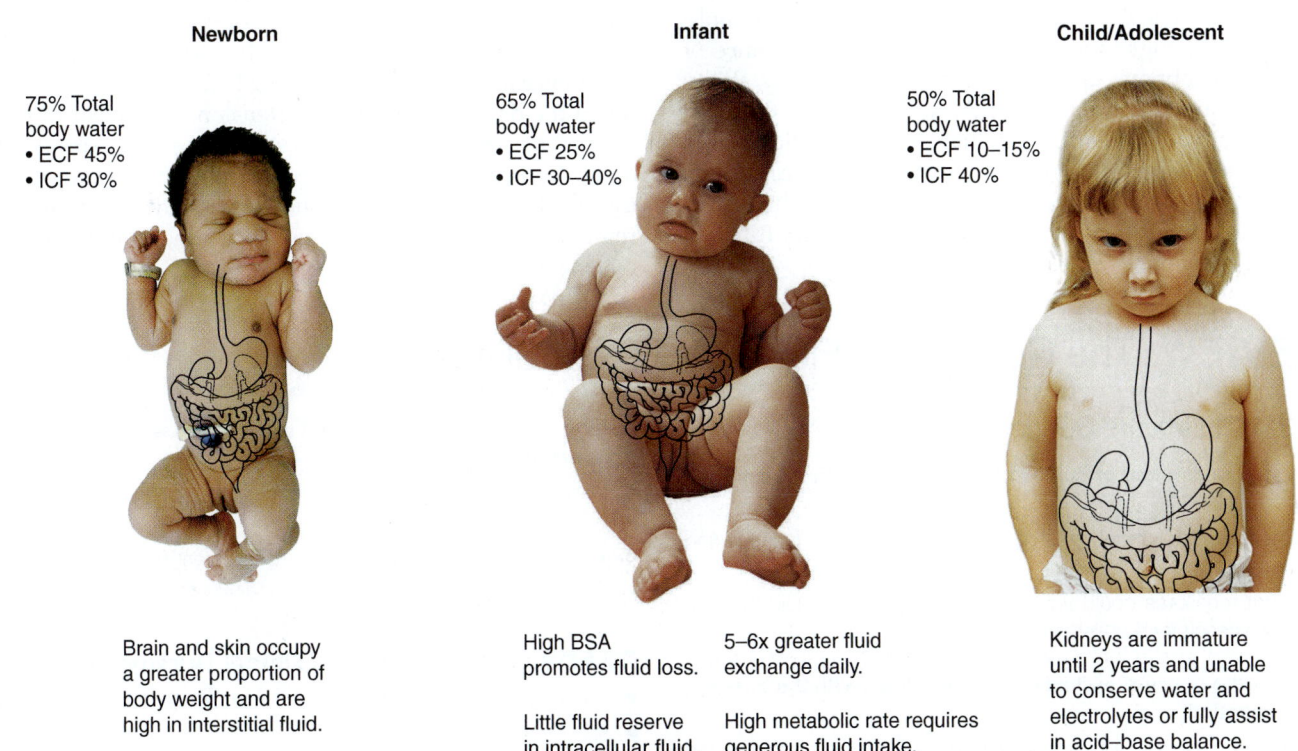

Newborn

75% Total body water
• ECF 45%
• ICF 30%

Infant

65% Total body water
• ECF 25%
• ICF 30–40%

Child/Adolescent

50% Total body water
• ECF 10–15%
• ICF 40%

Brain and skin occupy a greater proportion of body weight and are high in interstitial fluid.

High BSA promotes fluid loss.

Little fluid reserve in intracellular fluid.

5–6x greater fluid exchange daily.

High metabolic rate requires generous fluid intake.

Kidneys are immature until 2 years and unable to conserve water and electrolytes or fully assist in acid–base balance.

Figure 6–10 ›› The newborn and infant have a high percentage of body weight composed of water, especially extracellular fluid, which is lost from the body easily. Note the small stomach size, which limits ability to rehydrate quickly.

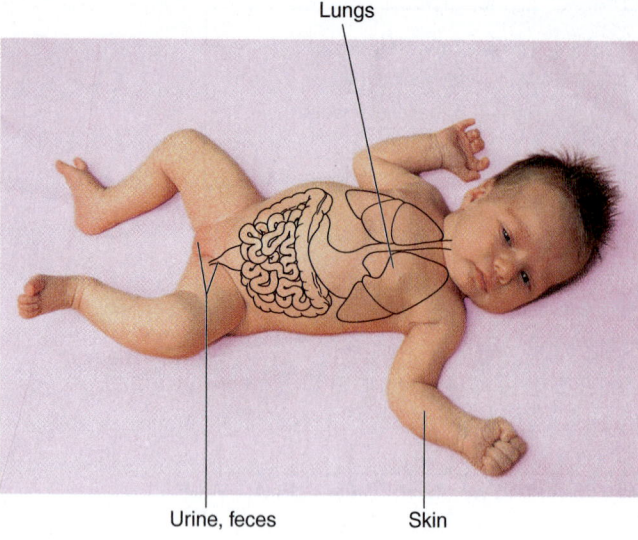

Figure 6–11 》 Normal routes of fluid excretion from infants and children.

dehydrated or develop electrolyte imbalances quickly. Children under 2 years of age also have difficulty regulating electrolytes such as sodium and calcium. Renal response to high solute loads is slower and less developed, with function improving gradually during the first year of life.

Fluid and Electrolyte Balance in School-Age Children and Adolescents

Gastroenteritis and diarrhea are the most common causes of fluid imbalance in children (Al Sabbagh, 2013). Although weight change is the most accurate of the assessment tools, other clinical signs include capillary refill, appearance of mucous membranes, quality of pulses, skin elasticity, ability to make tears, and urine output (Al Sabbagh, 2013). Children with chronic diseases such as diabetes and cystic fibrosis may normally present with some alterations in electrolytes; additional assessments may be required in these children to diagnose dehydration, such as evaluation of kidney function (Scurati-Manzoni et al., 2014).

Fluid and Electrolyte Balance in Pregnant Women

Approximately 80% of all pregnant women experience some form of nausea and vomiting, which can range from mild to severe enough to require hospitalization. Nausea requiring hospitalization is termed *hyperemesis gravidarum* (Dean, 2014). Complications can include weight loss, dehydration, and electrolyte imbalance. IV fluid replacement is often indicated (Fantasia, 2014). Strategies for managing the mild forms of nausea may include snacking on crackers before getting out of bed in the morning, high-protein snacks throughout the day, and consuming small amounts of liquid frequently. Management of hyperemesis gravidarum may include antiemetics.

Fluid and Electrolyte Balance in Older Adults

In older adults, the normal aging process may affect fluid balance. Age-related factors include diminished thirst, a decline in kidney function, and reduced fluid reserve. For community-dwelling older adults, isolation may reduce social interaction normally associated with drinking, and reduced availability or access to preferred fluids may also be factors (Uribe & Schub, 2015). At particular risk are older adults either living at home or in long-term care centers and are dependent on others for fluid replacement (Goldberg et al., 2014).

ADH levels remain normal in older adults or may even be elevated, but the nephrons become less able to conserve water in response to ADH. Increased levels of ANF seen in older adults may also contribute to this impaired ability to conserve water. These normal changes of aging increase the risk of dehydration. When combined with the increased likelihood of heart diseases, impaired renal function, and multiple drug regimens, the older adult's risk for fluid and electrolyte imbalance is significant. In addition, older adults experience increased sensitivity to salt, and this can be a factor in the development of hypertension. Salt sensitivity is defined as a rise in blood pressure when salt is consumed and a drop when salt is restricted. At each interaction within the healthcare system, nurses should take the opportunity to remind older adults and caregivers of the importance of adequate hydration.

REVIEW The Concept of Fluids and Electrolytes

RELATE Link the Concepts

Linking the concept of fluids and electrolytes with the concept of perfusion:

1. Describe the pathophysiology of fluid and electrolyte balance and how it affects perfusion.

2. What measures could you implement to promote fluid balance when caring for a patient with heart failure?

Linking the concept of fluids and electrolytes with the concept of elimination:

3. Describe the pathophysiology of fluid and electrolyte balance and how it affects elimination.

4. What assessment findings would you expect to see when a patient with benign prostatic hypertrophy experiences an alteration in fluid balance?

Linking the concept of fluids and electrolytes with the concept of tissue integrity:

5. Describe the pathophysiology of fluid and electrolyte balance and how it affects tissue integrity.

6. What fluid and electrolyte balance assessment findings would you expect to see in a patient who has experienced burns over 40% of his body?

READY Go to Volume 3: Clinical Nursing Skills

- SKILL 1.4   Weight: Newborn, Infant, Child, Adult, Measuring
- SKILLS 1.5–1.9   Vital Signs
- SKILL 5.1   Intake and Output: Measuring
- SKILL 5.6   Infusion Device: Discontinuing
- SKILL 5.7   Infusion Flow Rate Using Controller or IV Pump: Regulating

SKILL 5.8   Infusion Intermittent Device: Maintaining

- SKILL 5.9   Infusion: Initiating
- SKILL 5.10   Infusion: Maintaining
- SKILL 5.11   Infusion Pump and "Smart" Pump: Using
- SKILL 5.12   Infusion Syringe Pump: Using
- SKILL 6.1   Hand Hygiene: Performing
- SKILL 10.5   Nutrition: Assessing

REFER Go to Pearson MyLab Nursing and eText

- Additional review materials

REFLECT Apply Your Knowledge

Five-year-old Emma Ozaki is brought to the walk-in clinic with a 2-day history of profuse diarrhea. Her parents have administered over-the-counter antidiarrheal agents with little result. Emma is listless, lying in her mother's lap. The child answers questions by nodding or shaking her head yes or no. Her skin turgor is poor, and her eyes are soft and sunken with dark circles present below her eyes. Her parents report decreasing urination and that the urine has been dark in color. Ms. Ozaki says that the child was not producing tears when crying. Emma's pulse is 114 bpm apically; respirations are 22/min; and BP is 98/66 mmHg. A fingerstick identifies a hematocrit of 58%. Lungs are clear upon auscultation, and the abdomen is soft and nontender in all quadrants. Bowel sounds are significantly hyperactive. No new foods were included in the diet over the past few days, and Emma has been drinking only electrolyte solutions and water for the past 48 hours. The healthcare provider orders stat electrolytes, urinalysis, and a stool culture.

1. Identify the assessment findings indicative of FVD.
2. What is the pathophysiology underlying the elevation in hematocrit?
3. What electrolyte findings would the nurse expect to find in this child?
4. What is the rationale for the healthcare provider's order of a stool culture?

» Exemplar 6.A
Fluid and Electrolyte Imbalance

Exemplar Learning Outcomes

6.A Analyze fluid and electrolyte imbalance and its effect on the body.

- Describe the pathophysiology of fluid volume deficit (FVD) and dehydration.
- Describe the etiology of FVD and dehydration.
- Compare the risk factors for and prevention of FVD and dehydration.
- Identify the clinical manifestations of FVD and dehydration.
- Summarize diagnostic tests and therapies used by interprofessional teams in the collaborative care of an individual with FVD and dehydration.
- Differentiate considerations for care of patients with FVD and dehydration across the lifespan.
- Apply the nursing process in providing culturally competent care to an individual with FVD or dehydration.
- Describe the pathophysiology of fluid volume excess (FVE).
- Describe the etiology of FVE.
- Compare the risk factors for and prevention of FVE.
- Identify the clinical manifestations of FVE.
- Summarize diagnostic tests and therapies used by interprofessional teams in the collaborative care of an individual with FVE.
- Differentiate considerations for care of patients with FVE across the lifespan.
- Apply the nursing process in providing culturally competent care to an individual with FVE.

Exemplar Key Terms

Anasarca, *387*
Anorexia, *384*
Ascites, *387*
Dehydration, *378*
Dyspnea, *387*
Fluid volume deficit (FVD), *378*
Fluid volume excess (FVE), *385*
Hypercalcemia, *394*
Hyperchloremia, *394*
Hypermagnesemia, *394*
Hypertonic dehydration, *378*
Hypervolemia, *385*
Hypocalcemia, *394*
Hypochloremia, *394*
Hypomagnesemia, *394*
Hypotonic dehydration, *378*
Iatrogenic, *387*
Isotonic dehydration, *378*
Isotonic fluid volume deficit, *378*
Isotonic imbalances, *378*
Oncotic pressure, *386*
Orthopnea, *387*
Osmolar imbalances, *378*
Polyuria, *387*
Third spacing, *378*

Exemplar Overview

The balance of fluids and electrolytes is delicate and easily disrupted by illness, injury, stress, or strenuous activity. Mild imbalances are resolved quickly by the body, often without any outside intervention. If intervention is required for a mild fluid or electrolyte imbalance, there is seldom any residual effect. However, more severe imbalances that are complicated by disease processes or that last a significant time can result in short-term and long-term effects. The body needs and expects a balance, and its chemistry leaves little room for error.

Factors such as illness, trauma, surgery, and medications can affect the body's ability to maintain fluid and electrolytes. Patients who are confused, experiencing dementia, or unable to communicate their needs are at greater risk for inadequate fluid intake. Vomiting, diarrhea, or nasogastric suction can also lead to fluid and electrolyte imbalance. The kidneys play a major role in maintaining fluid and electrolyte balance, and renal disease is a significant cause of imbalance.

Tissue trauma, such as burns or crush injury, causes fluid and electrolytes to be lost from damaged cells. Decreased blood flow to the kidneys as a result of impaired cardiac function stimulates the renin-angiotensin-aldosterone system, causing sodium and water retention. Medications such as diuretics or corticosteroids can result in abnormal losses of electrolytes and in fluid loss or retention. Complications from diabetes, cancer, and head injury may also lead to electrolyte imbalances. Fluid and electrolyte imbalances can be classified in terms of FVD, FVE, and electrolyte imbalance.

Fluid imbalances are of two basic types: isotonic and osmolar. **Isotonic imbalances** occur when water and electrolytes are lost or gained in equal proportions, so the osmolality of body fluids remains constant. **Osmolar imbalances** involve the loss or gain of only water, so the osmolality of the serum is altered. Thus, four categories of fluid imbalances may occur:

1. Fluid volume deficit
2. Fluid volume excess
3. Dehydration or hyperosmolar imbalance
4. Overhydration or hypo-osmolar imbalance.

FLUID VOLUME DEFICIT AND DEHYDRATION

Overview

Fluid volume deficit (FVD) is a decrease in intravascular, interstitial, and/or intracellular fluid in the body. FVD is a relatively common problem that may exist alone or in combination with other electrolyte or acid–base imbalances. **Dehydration** refers to loss of fluid alone, even though the term often is used interchangeably with FVD.

Pathophysiology and Etiology

Pathophysiology

FVD can develop slowly or rapidly, depending on the type of fluid loss. Loss of ECF volume can lead to hypovolemia (decreased circulating blood volume). Often, electrolytes are lost along with fluid, resulting in an **isotonic fluid volume deficit**. When both water and electrolytes are lost, the serum sodium level remains normal, although levels of other electrolytes, such as potassium, may fall. Fluid is drawn into the vascular compartment from the interstitial spaces as the body attempts to maintain tissue perfusion. This eventually depletes fluid in the intracellular compartment as well.

Hypovolemia stimulates regulatory mechanisms to maintain circulation. The sympathetic nervous system is stimulated, as is the thirst mechanism. ADH and aldosterone are released, prompting sodium and water retention by the kidneys. Severe fluid loss can lead to cardiovascular collapse.

Another classification of FVD is by location of the deficiency, whether extracellular or intracellular. Extracellular

FVD occurs when there is not enough fluid in the extracellular compartment (vascular and interstitial). Depending on the cause of the deficit, sodium may be at a normal, low, or elevated level. Each level is described as a specific type of dehydration:

- **Isotonic dehydration** or *isonatremic dehydration:* This type of dehydration is the most common and occurs when fluid loss is not balanced by intake and the losses of water and sodium are in proportion. The serum sodium is therefore within normal limits even though the circulating blood volume is lowered. Most of the fluid lost is from the extracellular component. This type of dehydration is commonly manifested through such symptoms as vomiting and diarrhea or hemorrhage.

- **Hypotonic dehydration** or *hyponatremic dehydration:* This occurs when fluid loss is characterized by a proportionately greater loss of sodium than of water. Serum sodium is below normal levels. Compensatory fluid shifts occur from the extracellular to intracellular components in an attempt to establish normal proportions, thus leading to even greater extracellular dehydration. Hypotonic dehydration may result from severe and prolonged vomiting and diarrhea, burns, and renal disease. Administering IV fluid without electrolytes as treatment for dehydration increases patient risk for hypotonic dehydration.

- **Hypertonic dehydration** or *hypernatremic dehydration:* This occurs when sodium loss is proportionately less than water loss. Serum sodium is above normal levels. Compensatory fluid shifts from the intracellular to extracellular components occur as the body attempts to establish normal proportions. The extracellular component therefore remains fairly normal, delaying the onset of signs and symptoms of dehydration until the condition is quite serious. Neurologic symptoms reflecting intracellular imbalance may occur simultaneously with more common symptoms of dehydration. The condition may result from health problems, such as end-stage renal disease (ESRD), diabetes insipidus, or administration of IV fluid or tube feedings with high electrolyte levels.

Fluid and electrolyte balance is essential to supporting vascular function. A shift of fluid from the vascular space into an area where it is not available to support normal physiologic processes is known as **third spacing**. The trapped fluid represents a volume loss and is unavailable for normal physiologic processes. Fluid may be sequestered in the abdomen or bowel or in other actual or potential body spaces, such as the pleural or peritoneal space. Fluid may also become trapped within soft tissues following trauma or burns.

In many cases, fluid is sequestered in interstitial tissues and unavailable to support cardiovascular function. For example, surgery triggers adaptive stress responses and the release of stress hormones (adrenocorticotropic hormone, cortisol, and catecholamines). These hormones increase blood glucose levels to provide increased fuel for metabolic processes and lead to vasoconstriction that redistributes blood to vital organs (the heart and brain). Renal blood flow falls, stimulating the renin-angiotensin-aldosterone system. This promotes sodium and water retention to maintain intravascular volume. The blood vessel and tissue damage caused by surgery stimulate the release of inflammatory mediators, such as histamine and prostaglandins. These substances lead to local vasodilation and increased capillary permeability, allowing fluid to accumulate in interstitial tissues. Third spacing is difficult to assess because it may not be reflected in measurable data.

Etiology

FVDs may be the result of excessive fluid losses, insufficient fluid intake, or failure of regulatory mechanisms and fluid shifts within the body. The most common cause of FVD is excessive loss of GI fluids, which can result from vomiting, diarrhea, GI suctioning, intestinal fistulas, or intestinal drainage. Other causes of fluid losses include the following:

- Excessive renal losses of water and sodium from diuretic therapy, renal disorders, or endocrine disorders
- Water and sodium losses during sweating from excessive exercise or increased environmental temperature
- Hemorrhage
- Chronic abuse of laxatives and/or enemas.

Inadequate fluid intake may result from lack of access to fluids, inability to request or to swallow fluids, oral trauma, or altered thirst mechanisms. Excessive exercise during very hot weather without sufficient fluid replacement can lead to fluid and electrolyte imbalance. Athletes and those whose jobs require them to expend enormous amounts of energy in hot climates, such as military personnel and ROTC candidates, are frequently at risk for fluid imbalance.

Burns of the skin usually involve a huge loss of body fluids, including water and electrolytes, particularly sodium. Hypotonic dehydration is the type most commonly seen in the initial period after a burn. Because serum proteins are also lost, body fluid is more likely to leak into interstitial spaces, causing edema and further contributing to the fluid deficit. The kidneys decrease urine production because of their decreased blood flow, which leads to lowered urinary output. While the fluid imbalance of burns is therefore very complicated, the first imbalance encountered often is that of dehydration with accompanying hyponatremia.

For burns, gastroenteritis, and other illnesses, initial dehydration in the first 3 days reflects a high loss of ECF. Approximately 80% of the fluid loss is extracellular, and only approximately 20% is intracellular. Over time the relationship begins to change so that in illnesses lasting longer than 3 days, approximately 60% of fluid loss is extracellular while 40% is intracellular. Because the electrolyte composition of ECFs and ICFs differs, electrolyte management needs to be adapted in long-term conditions.

Risk Factors

Risk factors for FVD include any factors that prevent normal intake or lead to increase loss. Factors that prevent normal intake include NPO status; dysphagia; lack of potable water; inaccurate fluid replacement compared to loss; and fluid shifts due to burns, albuminuria, or diabetes insipidus. Factors that lead to increased fluid loss include diarrhea (especially in infants and children), burns, nausea and vomiting, acute and chronic renal failure, hemorrhage, and diabetic ketoacidosis.

Prevention

FVD may occur in normal daily life, not only in cases of illness, burns, and other circumstances discussed previously. Some important factors to keep in mind are the following:

- A significant amount of fluid is lost to the body through sweating and perspiration, especially in hot or humid weather, or in cold weather when sweating occurs under heavy clothing.
- Some artificially heated indoor air can cause skin to lose moisture, requiring replacement.
- Altitudes greater than 8200 feet increase the need for water because the air becomes drier, and the increased breathing rate stimulated by high altitudes increases water loss through respiration.
- Fluid loss through respiration may also become significant if the individual is exposed to a very cold, dry environment for an extended period of time.

Prevention of fluid loss in such situations involves drinking enough water and other fluids to replace fluid lost to environmental factors. Electrolyte fluids should be drunk in moderation, rather than just water. Individuals working with younger children need to encourage water breaks and water consumption. Older adults and those who work with them must pay special attention to drinking enough fluids, since older adults may lose the internal cues for thirst.

Clinical Manifestations

Symptoms of dehydration relate to the severity or degree of the body water deficit. They result from both the decreased fluid (e.g., diminished turgor and mucous membrane moisture) and the body's response to the fluid deficit (e.g., pulse and blood pressure changes). A water loss of as little as 1–2% impairs cognition and physical performance. Loss of 7% of body water can lead to circulatory collapse. With a rapid fluid loss (e.g., hemorrhage, uncontrolled vomiting), manifestations of hypovolemia develop rapidly. When the loss of fluid occurs more gradually, the patient's fluid volume may become very low before symptoms develop.

Initial symptoms may be as simple as thirst. As fluid loss increases, however, lethargy, dry mucous membranes, reduced urine output, and weakness develop. Manifestations of acute fluid loss are similar to those associated with hypovolemic shock and include hypotension, tachycardia, tachypnea, decreased or absent urine output, and decreased cardiac output (see the Clinical Manifestations and Therapies feature). Coma and death may result if treatment is not initiated. See the Multisystem Effects of Fluid Volume Deficit feature.

SAFETY ALERT Because rapid weight loss is a good indicator of FVD, it is critical to weigh patients who are at risk for FVD daily. Each liter of body fluid weighs approximately 1 kg (2.2 lb). The severity of the FVD can be estimated by the percentage of rapid weight loss:

- A loss of 2–5% of total body weight represents mild FVD.
- A loss of 6–9% represents moderate FVD.
- A loss of 10% or greater represents severe FVD.

Multisystem Effects of
Fluid Volume Deficit

Mucous Membranes

- Dry; may be sticky
- ↓ tongue size, longitudinal furrows ↑

Neurologic

- Altered mental status
- Anxiety, restlessness
- Diminished alertness/cognition
- Possible coma (severe FVD)

Integumentary

- Diminished skin turgor
- Dry skin
- Pale, cool extremities

Cardiovascular

- Tachycardia
- Orthostatic hypotension (moderate FVD)
- Falling systolic/diastolic pressure (severe FVD)
- Flat neck veins
- ↓ venous filling
- ↓ pulse volume
- ↓ capillary refill
- ↑ hematocrit

Potential complication

- Hypovolemic shock

Urinary

- ↓ urine output
- Oliguria (severe FVD)
- ↑ urine specific gravity

Musculoskeletal

- Fatigue

Metabolic processes

- ↓ body temperature (isotonic FVD)
- ↑ body temperature (dehydration)
- Thirst
- Weight loss
  2–5% mild FVD
  6–9% moderate FVD
  >10% severe FVD

Clinical Manifestations and Therapies
Fluid Volume Deficit and Dehydration

ETIOLOGY	CLINICAL MANIFESTATIONS	CLINICAL THERAPIES
Decreased cardiac output	■ Hypotension (may be orthostatic or postural initially) ■ Tachycardia ■ Weak pulse ■ Tachypnea ■ Reduced urine output or very concentrated urine with high specific gravity	■ Administer fluid replacement. ■ Administer isotonic IV solutions. ■ Monitor vital signs frequently. ■ Monitor I&O. ■ Assess serum electrolytes and hematocrit. ■ Conduct urine specific gravity and osmolality. ■ Monitor CVP.
Inadequate fluid supply to the tissues	■ Dry, cracked skin ■ Dry mucous membranes ■ Increased hematocrit ■ Poor skin turgor ■ Weight loss	■ Administer isotonic or mildly hypotonic solutions. ■ Measure weight daily. ■ Monitor serum electrolytes and serum osmolality. ■ Monitor hemoglobin and hematocrit.
Third spacing	■ Edema ■ Symptoms of FVD ■ No weight loss	■ Administer hypertonic IV fluid.

Loss of interstitial fluid causes skin turgor (the skin's ability to return to normal shape after being pinched) to diminish. When pinched, the skin of a patient with FVD remains elevated. Loss of skin elasticity with aging makes this assessment finding less accurate in older adults. Tongue turgor is not generally affected by age; therefore, assessing the size, dryness, and longitudinal furrows of the tongue may be a more accurate indicator of FVD.

Postural or orthostatic hypotension is a sign of hypovolemia. A drop of more than 15 mmHg in systolic blood pressure when changing from a lying to standing position often indicates loss of intravascular volume. Venous pressure falls as well, causing flat neck veins, even when the patient is recumbent. Loss of intravascular fluid causes the hematocrit to increase.

Compensatory mechanisms to conserve water and sodium and maintain circulation account for many of the manifestations of FVD, such as tachycardia; pale, cool skin (vasoconstriction); and decreased urine output. The specific gravity of urine increases as water is reabsorbed in the tubules.

Collaboration

The diagnosis of dehydration is best accomplished by clinical observations. The major observation that provides clues to the degree of dehydration is the percentage of weight loss. In cases of mild impairment, interprofessional care typically is not required. For patients with moderate to severe fluid loss, collaborative care will depend on the underlying cause of the imbalance, presenting symptoms, and assessment of the patient's care needs.

Diagnostic Tests

The serum electrolyte panel may be helpful in severe and continuing dehydration that is complicated by electrolyte imbalance or acidosis. The panel includes serum electrolytes, creatinine, and glucose tests. Elevated BUN (5–25 mg/dL) and low serum bicarbonate (less than 16 mmol/L) are also useful in identifying moderate and severe dehydration (Mayo Clinic, 2014). The results can be used to target the fluid type and amount to best meet the imbalances identified. Urine specific gravity may provide useful information in adults and older children who are dehydrated. However, because of the inability of the child under 2 years of age to concentrate urine effectively, a rising specific gravity may not be seen as definitively in the younger child who is dehydrated.

Clinical Therapies

Medical management depends on accurate identification of the degree of dehydration. The treatment for extracellular FVD is administration of fluid containing sodium. This may be accomplished by oral rehydration therapy or by IV fluids.

Oral Rehydration

Oral rehydration is the safest and most effective treatment for FVD in alert patients who are able to take oral fluids. Adults require a minimum of 1500 mL of fluid per day for maintenance, or approximately 30 mL/kg body weight. (Ideal body weight is used to calculate fluid requirements for patients who are obese.) Fluids are replaced gradually, particularly in older adults, to prevent too rapid rehydration of the cells. In general, fluid deficits are replaced at a rate of approximately 30–50% of the deficit per 24 hours.

With mild fluid deficits, in which the loss of electrolytes has been minimal (e.g., moderate exercise in warm weather), fluid replacement may be accomplished with water alone. When the fluid deficit is more severe and when electrolytes have also been lost (e.g., FVD caused by vomiting or diarrhea, strenuous exercise for longer than an hour or two), a carbohydrate/electrolyte solution, such as a sports drink, ginger ale, or a rehydrating solution (e.g., Pedialyte, Rehydralyte), is more appropriate. These solutions provide sodium, potassium, chloride, and calories to help meet metabolic needs.

Intravenous Fluids

When the fluid deficit is severe or the patient is unable to ingest fluids, the IV route is used to administer replacement fluids. Isotonic electrolyte solutions (0.9% NaCl or Ringer's solution) are used to expand plasma volume in patients who are hypotensive or to replace abnormal losses, which are usually isotonic in nature. Normal saline (0.9% NaCl) tends to remain in the vascular compartment, increasing blood volume. When administered rapidly, however, this solution can precipitate acid–base imbalances, so balanced electrolyte solutions, such as lactated Ringer's solution, are preferred to expand plasma volume. Often, lactated Ringer's solution is administered intravenously, followed or accompanied by dilute saline, such as one half or one quarter normal saline. This fluid combination replenishes the ECF volume and adds solutes to return the body fluid to normal.

A mixture of 5% dextrose in water or 0.45% NaCl (one half normal saline) is given to treat total body water deficits. The D_5W mixture is isotonic (similar in tonicity to the plasma) when administered and thus does not provoke hemolysis of RBCs. The dextrose is metabolized to carbon dioxide and water, leaving free water available for tissue needs. Hypotonic saline solution (0.45% NaCl with or without added electrolytes) or 5% dextrose in 0.45% sodium chloride may be used as a maintenance solution. These solutions provide additional electrolytes (e.g., potassium), a buffer (lactate or acetate) as needed, and water. When dextrose is added, they also provide a minimal number of calories.

A fluid challenge (the rapid administration of a designated amount of IV fluid) may be performed to evaluate fluid volume when urine output is low and cardiac or renal function is questionable. A fluid challenge helps to prevent fluid volume overload resulting from IV fluid therapy when cardiac or renal function is compromised.

Lifespan Considerations

FVD in Children and Adolescents

Sources of Fluid Loss in Children

A number of conditions may contribute to fluid imbalance in pediatric patients. Low-birth-weight infants who are kept under radiant warmers to maintain heat may experience FVD through increased water loss (see **Figure 6–12**). Their high BSA puts them at risk of dehydration as a result of insensible fluid loss through the skin. Radiant heat (phototherapy) used to treat hyperbilirubinemia increases insensible water loss through the skin. The increased respiratory rate of pediatric patients increases insensible water loss from the lungs.

Children are at increased risk for fever, which increases the metabolic rate and, therefore, the water demands of metabolism (for each degree Celsius increase above 37°C,

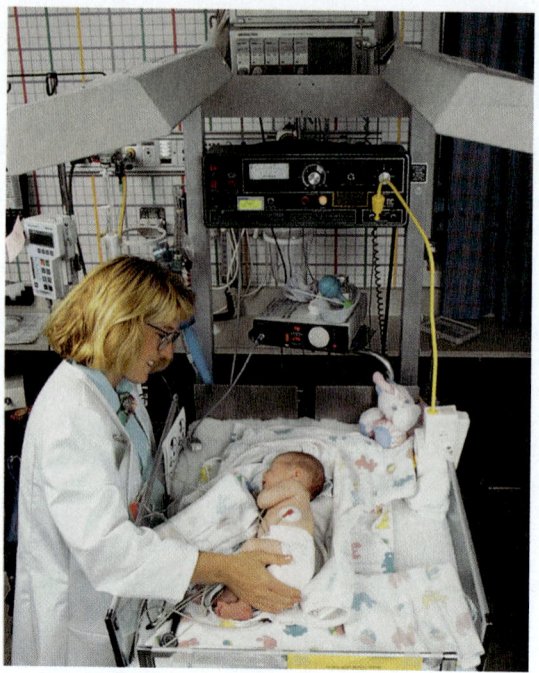

Figure 6–12 Use of an overhead warmer or phototherapy with an infant increases insensible fluid excretion through the skin, thus increasing the infant's required fluid intake.

0.42 mL/kg/hr of additional fluid is needed). Vomiting and diarrhea are other common causes of fluid imbalance in children. One of the primary causes of gastroenteritis in children is rotavirus. In the United States, it is a major source of morbidity and hospitalization in children younger than 5 years of age. It accounts for approximately 300 deaths, more than 1.5 million outpatient visits, and 200,000 hospitalizations annually (Payne et al., 2013; Tam et al., 2014). The annual hospital admission rate for children experiencing fluid and electrolyte imbalance is 400 for 100,000 in the United States (Waddell, McGrath, & Maude, 2014).

Children are more likely than adults to experience imbalance from exercise. Because of their larger BSA, children can gain more heat from the environment when it is hot and lose more heat when it is cold (Waddell et al., 2014). In addition, the high metabolic rate of children is further increased during exercise so that fluid lost in metabolism is significant. Children may not feel thirsty and so may fail to drink, even when dehydrated (Wong & Sun, 2014).

Adrenal insufficiency, accumulation of ECF in a third space (e.g., the peritoneal cavity), and overuse of diuretics may also result in FVD in children. Overuse of diuretics is most often seen in adolescents with bulimia.

Assessment and Treatment Considerations

Symptoms of dehydration relate to the severity or degree of the body water deficit (see **Table 6–5**). Mild dehydration is hard to detect in pediatric patients, because children with mild dehydration appear alert and have moist mucous membranes. Infants may become irritable, and older children may become thirsty. In moderate dehydration, the child is often lethargic and sleepy. Children, especially infants, may experience periods of restlessness and irritability. Skin

TABLE 6–5 Severity of Clinical Dehydration in Pediatric Patients

Clinical Assessment	Mild	Moderate	Severe
Percent of body weight lost	Less than 5% (40–50 mL/kg)	6–9% (60–90 mL/kg)	10% or greater (100 mL/kg or greater)
Level of consciousness	Alert, restless, thirsty	Infants and very young children: irritable or lethargic Older children and adolescents: alert, thirsty, restless	Infants and very young children: lethargic to comatose Older children and adolescents: often conscious, apprehensive
Blood pressure	Normal	Normal or low Older children and adolescents: postural hypotension	Low to undetectable
Pulse	Normal	Normal or rapid	Tachycardia or bradycardia
Skin turgor	Normal	Poor	Very poor
Mucous membranes	Moist	Dry	Parched
Urine	May appear normal	Decreased output (less than 1 mL/kg/hr), dark color; increased specific gravity	Very decreased or absent output
Thirst	Slightly increased	Moderately increased	Greatly increased unless lethargic
Fontanel (in infants)	Normal	Sunken	Sunken
Extremities	Warm; normal capillary refill	Delayed capillary refill (more than 2 sec)	Cool, discolored, delayed capillary refill (more than 3–4 sec)
Respirations	Normal	Normal or rapid	Changing rate and pattern
Eyes	Normal	Slightly sunken, decreased tears	Deeply sunken, absent tears

turgor is diminished, mucous membranes appear dry, and urine is dark in color and diminished in amount. Pulse rate is usually increased, and blood pressure can be normal or low. Severe dehydration is manifested by increasing lethargy or nonresponsiveness, markedly decreased blood pressure, rapid pulse, poor skin turgor, dry mucous membranes, seizure activity, and markedly decreased or absent urinary output.

For children with mild to moderate dehydration, oral rehydration therapy is the first intervention, given in frequent, small amounts. A useful guideline for starting oral rehydration is 1–3 tsp of fluid every 5–15 minutes. For the first 2–4 hours of treatment, 50 mL of fluid for each kilogram of weight should be the target intake. Hospitalized children and those with severe hydration usually require IV fluids following careful assessment of the type of imbalance.

In children under 2 years of age, the glomeruli, tubules, and nephrons of the kidneys are immature. They are thus unable to conserve or excrete water and solutes effectively. Because more water is generally excreted, infants and young children can become dehydrated or develop electrolyte imbalances quickly. In addition, infants have a weaker transport system for ions and bicarbonate, placing them at greater risk for acidosis and acid–base imbalances. Children under 2 years of age also have difficulty regulating electrolytes, such as sodium and calcium. Renal response to high solute loads is slower and less developed, with function improving gradually during the first year of life. As a result, fluid challenge must be administered with caution in young children.

Children and adolescents may experience fluid loss with exercise, especially if exercising or playing outdoors for long periods of time or in warm or hot weather. See the Evidence-Based Practice feature for information on fluid replacement following exercise.

FVD in Pregnant Women

Pregnancy carries risk for FVD, especially during the first trimester, when vomiting from morning sickness and blood loss during a spontaneous abortion (miscarriage) are most likely to occur. During the first prenatal visit, the nurse should provide patient teaching on how to avoid dehydration, the proper fluids to consume, and the importance of avoiding caffeine, alcohol, and diet drinks.

FVD in Older Adults

Because older adults have fewer intracellular reserves, they are at increased risk for rapidly becoming dehydrated. A blunted thirst perception and altered hormone response also contribute to the development of dehydration in the older adult. Changes in mentation or cognition resulting from altered health status or adverse effects of medications can increase the risk for an imbalance. It is important to teach older adult patients to drink fluids even though they may not be thirsty.

Older adults who live in extended care homes and those who live at home but require assistance with activities of daily living are particularly vulnerable. Older adults who have limited mobility may voluntarily restrict their fluids for fear of incontinence or if they do not want to burden others with helping them with toileting or are embarrassed to have help. These factors increase their risk for inadequate fluid consumption and chronic dehydration. See **Box 6–2 »** for dehydration risk factors and symptoms common in older adults.

Manifestations of FVD may be more difficult to recognize in the older adult. A change in mental status, memory, or attention may be an early sign. Skin turgor is less reliable as an indicator of dehydration, although assessing turgor over the sternum or on the inner aspect of the thigh may be more

Box 6–2

Dehydration Risk Factors and Symptoms in the Older Adult

Dehydration Risk Factors

Physical changes of aging:

- ↓ Total body water
- ↓ Lean body mass
- ↓ Thirst from aging, medication, or disease
- Impaired angiotensin production

Lack of free access to fluids:

- Dependency on others
- Cognitive impairment
- Physical impairment

Voluntary fluid restriction to manage:

- Incontinence
- Nocturia
- Diuretic side effect
- Limited physical movement due to mobility or pain issues

Increased insensitive fluid losses:

- Sweating from fever or climate
- ↑ Respiratory rate
- Vomiting
- Diarrhea
- Polyuria
- Exudative wound or fistula

Symptoms of Dehydration

Darkened urine
↓ Urine output
Confusion
Lethargy
Headache
Lightheadedness
Sunken eyes
Dry mucous membranes
Dry axillae
Long tongue furrows
Postural changes in pulse and blood pressure

effective. Dry oral mucous membranes and tongue furrows also are indicative of dehydration. Chronic dehydration may result in dry, itchy skin; dull-appearing, brittle hair; and loss of thirst reflex.

SAFETY ALERT Orthostatic, or postural, hypotension may be unrelated to hydration status, and vital signs may not demonstrate typical changes in the older adult who is dehydrated. Other common signs of dehydration, such as dry oral membranes and upper body weakness, may be better indicators of dehydration in the older adult.

Many medications lead to dehydration in the older adult. Complicating this fact are the age-related changes in decreased kidney function, decreased sense of thirst, self-limiting intake on the part of older adults to decrease instances of incontinence, and changes in taste. Dehydration can develop more quickly in frail older adults as well as older adults with cognitive impairment (McCrow et al., 2016).

NURSING PROCESS

Nurses are responsible for identifying patients at risk for FVD, initiating and carrying out measures to prevent and treat FVD and reduce the risk of complications, and monitoring the effects of therapy. Health promotion activities focus on teaching patients to prevent FVD, including instructing patients who are ill regarding the importance of maintaining fluid intake, particularly during periods of fever.

Assessment

The nurse should carefully monitor patients at risk for abnormal fluid losses through routes such as vomiting, diarrhea, nasogastric suction, increased urine output, fever, or wounds. The nurse should monitor fluid intake in patients with decreased LOC, disorientation, nausea, **anorexia** (loss of appetite), and physical limitations. The nurse should also assess hydration by looking at skin for dryness, flakiness, or scaling as well as tenting when skin is pinched (skin turgor). The nurse should check oral mucous membranes for dryness.

The nurse should collect the following assessment data through the health history interview and physical examination:

- ***Observation and patient interview.*** Risk factors, such as medications and acute or chronic renal or endocrine disease; precipitating factors, such as hot weather, extensive exercise, lack of access to fluids, and recent illness (especially if accompanied by fever, vomiting, and/or diarrhea); and onset and duration of symptoms

- ***Physical examination.*** Weight; vital signs, including orthostatic blood pressure and pulse; peripheral pulses and capillary refill; jugular neck vein distention; skin color, temperature, and turgor; LOC and mentation; urine output. (See the Lifespan Considerations feature for physical assessment of the older adult.)

Diagnosis

Appropriate nursing diagnoses may include the following:

- *Fluid Volume, Deficient*
- *Ineffective Peripheral Tissue Perfusion* related to hypovolemia
- *Risk for Injury* related to postural hypotension
- *Confusion*
- *Activity Intolerance.*

(NANDA-I © 2014)

Planning

Appropriate outcomes, planned together with patients and caregivers, may include the following:

- The patient will achieve electrolyte and fluid balance.
- The patient will drink 1500 mL of fluid per day.
- The patient will relate the need to replace fluids lost during exercise with sports drinks.
- The patient will return to normal hydration status and not develop hypovolemic shock.

For pediatric patients:

- The parents will relate strategies for preventing the child from becoming dehydrated.
- The parents will describe appropriate home management of fluid replacement for diarrhea and vomiting.
- The parents will describe when to seek healthcare if a child's condition worsens.

Implementation

The focus of care for the patient with FVD is on managing the effects of the deficit and preventing complications. The nurse should do the following:

- Record I&O accurately; on occasion, hourly I&O may be indicated.
- Weigh the patient daily at the same time with the same scale and in the same or similar clothing. (Young children should be weighed without clothing.) Compare to past weights, and calculate weight loss or gain.
- Take vital signs, CVP, and peripheral pulse volume at least every 4 hours.
- Administer and monitor intake of fluids as prescribed.
- Administer IV fluid using an electronic infusion pump.
- Monitor laboratory values (electrolytes, BUN, creatinine, osmolality, and urine specific gravity).
- Monitor for changes in LOC and mental status.
- Reposition the patient every 2 hours if the patient is unable to move independently.
- Initiate safety precautions to avoid falls secondary to dizziness or loss of balance.
- Teach the patient and family how to reduce orthostatic hypotension:
  a. Move from one position to another in stages; for example, raise the head of the bed before sitting up, and sit for a few minutes before standing.
  b. Avoid prolonged standing.
  c. Rest in a recliner rather than in bed during the day.
  d. Use assistive devices to pick up objects from the floor rather than stooping.
- Teach the importance of maintaining adequate fluid intake (at least 1500 mL/day).
- Teach how to prevent fluid deficit:
  a. Avoid exercising during extreme heat.
  b. Increase fluid intake during hot weather.
  c. If vomiting, take frequent small amounts of ice chips or clear liquids, such as flat cola or ginger ale.
  d. Reduce intake of coffee, tea, and alcohol, all of which increase urine output and can cause fluid loss.

Sugar facilitates the absorption of sodium in oral rehydration fluids. The nurse should teach parents not to give diet beverages for oral rehydration, because they contain no sugar and will not be effectively absorbed. However, if an oral rehydration solution is too concentrated, it can worsen the diarrhea. Juice and cola are highly concentrated and should be diluted to half strength when given to a child who has diarrhea. The nurse should encourage parents to keep an oral rehydration solution in liquid or powder form on hand at all times and to use this solution rather than juice or soda when the child first develops diarrhea.

Evaluation

The nurse should evaluate the patient's progress toward meeting the outcomes created in collaboration with the patient and adjust the nursing plan of care as indicated. The condition of a patient with severe FVD should be evaluated every few minutes to hourly until progress is made.

Expected outcomes of nursing care for the patient with dehydration include the following:

- The patient has water and electrolytes that are balanced in intracellular and extracellular compartments as measured by serum electrolytes, hematocrit, and assessment findings.
- The patient's urinary output is within normal limits.
- The patient's fluid intake is adequate to meet maintenance needs.
- The patient's vital signs are within normal limits.

If patient outcomes are not met, more aggressive intervention is indicated. If factors such as nausea and vomiting prohibit oral intake, IV fluids with electrolyte replacement will be considered. If oliguria is present, the healthcare provider may initiate a fluid challenge with 250–500 mL of lactated Ringer's or normal saline.

FLUID VOLUME EXCESS

Overview

Fluid volume excess (FVE) results when both water and sodium are retained in the body. FVE may be caused by fluid overload (excess water and sodium intake) or by impairment of the mechanisms that maintain homeostasis, leading to excess intravascular fluid (**hypervolemia**) and excess interstitial fluid (edema).

Pathophysiology and Etiology

Pathophysiology

ECF volume excess occurs when there is too much fluid in the extracellular compartment (vascular and interstitial). This imbalance may also be called saline excess or extracellular volume overload. An increase in total body sodium content causes an increase in total body water. Because the increase in sodium and water is isotonic, the serum sodium and osmolality remain normal, and the excess fluid remains in the extracellular space.

Stress responses activated before, during, and immediately after surgery commonly lead to increased ADH and aldosterone levels, leading to sodium and water retention. In the immediate postoperative period, however, this additional fluid tends to be sequestered in interstitial tissues and is thus unavailable to support cardiovascular and renal function (see the earlier discussion of third spacing in this module). This sequestered fluid is reabsorbed into the circulation within approximately 48–72 hours after surgery. Although it is then normally eliminated through a process of diuresis, patients with heart or kidney failure are at risk for developing fluid overload.

Interstitial FVE, or edema, is an abnormal increase in the volume of the interstitial fluid. It may be caused by an extracellular FVE, or it may result from other causes.

The causes of edema are best understood in the context of normal capillary dynamics. Fluid moves between the vascular and interstitial compartments by the process of filtration. Filtration is the net result of forces that tend to move fluid in opposing directions. The strongest forces will determine the direction of fluid movement.

At the capillary level, two forces (blood hydrostatic pressure and interstitial osmotic pressure) tend to move fluid from the capillaries into the interstitial fluid, while two other forces (blood colloid osmotic pressure and interstitial fluid hydrostatic pressure) tend to move fluid in the opposite direction (from the interstitial fluid into the capillaries). The net result of these forces usually moves fluid from the capillaries into the interstitial compartment at the arterial end of the capillaries and fluid from the interstitial compartment back into the capillaries at the venous end of the capillaries. This process brings oxygen and nutrients to the cells and removes carbon dioxide and other waste products.

Edema occurs if the balance of these four forces is altered so that excess fluid either enters or leaves the interstitial compartment. This may occur through increased blood hydrostatic pressure, decreased blood colloid osmotic pressure, increased interstitial fluid osmotic pressure, or blocked lymphatic drainage. Various clinical conditions are associated with these altered forces (see **Box 6–3** ≫):

1. ***Increased blood hydrostatic pressure.*** When extracellular FVE occurs, the increased fluid volume in the vascular compartment congests the veins. The pressure against the sides of the capillary is increased, and more fluid then enters the interstitial compartment.
2. ***Decreased blood colloid osmotic pressure.*** Much of the osmotic pressure that pulls fluid into the capillaries results from the presence of albumin and other plasma proteins made by the liver. The part of the blood osmotic pressure that is caused by plasma proteins is often called **oncotic pressure**, or blood colloid osmotic pressure. Any condition that decreases plasma proteins will decrease blood colloid osmotic pressure and cause edema. For example, if a clinical condition causes large amounts of albumin to leak into the urine, the liver will not be able to make albumin fast enough to replace it. As a result, the plasma protein level will fall, decreasing the blood osmotic pressure. Without this pulling force to return fluid to the capillaries, edema will occur. This is the cause of the edema that occurs in patients who have nephrotic syndrome. Another cause is prolonged surgical procedures with significant blood loss. IV fluids and blood may be infused during surgery to replace these losses, but plasma proteins are lost and not fully restored by infusion, causing edema in the postoperative period.
3. ***Increased interstitial fluid osmotic pressure.*** Only a few small proteins ordinarily enter the interstitial fluid, and the interstitial fluid osmotic pressure is small. If the capillary becomes abnormally permeable to proteins, however, the influx of large amounts of proteins into the interstitial fluid causes a dramatic increase in interstitial fluid osmotic pressure. This increased pulling force keeps an abnormal amount of fluid in the interstitial compartment. This mechanism plays an important part in edema caused by a bee sting or a sprained ankle. It occurs to a greater extent in burns, leading to swelling at the same time that there is a great loss of fluid volume through the burned skin.
4. ***Blocked lymphatic drainage.*** The lymph vessels normally drain small proteins and excess fluid from the interstitial compartment and return them to the blood vessels. If this process is blocked, fluid accumulates in the interstitial compartment. This may occur when a tumor blocks lymphatic drainage.

Edema causes swelling, which may be localized or generalized. The swelling of tissue may cause pain and restrict motion. Edema that results from ECF volume excess or right-sided heart failure usually occurs in the dependent portion of the body, often observed in the ankles. In a patient who is supine in bed, it is seen in the sacral area or in the scrotal area in men. The skin over an edematous area often appears thin and shiny.

Box 6–3
Clinical Conditions that Cause Edema

Edema Caused by Increased Blood Hydrostatic Pressure
Increased Capillary Blood Flow
- Inflammation
- Local infection

Venous Congestion
- ECF volume excess
- Right heart failure
- Venous thrombosis
- External pressure on vein
- Muscle paralysis

Edema Caused by Decreased Blood Osmotic Pressure
Increased Albumin Excretion
- Nephrotic syndrome (albumin leaks into urine)
- Protein-losing enteropathies (excess albumin in feces)

Decreased Albumin Synthesis
- Kwashiorkor (low-protein, high-carbohydrate starvation diet provides too few amino acids for liver to make albumin)
- Liver cirrhosis (diseased liver unable to make enough albumin)

Edema Caused by Increased Interstitial Fluid Osmotic Pressure
Increased Capillary Permeability
- Inflammation
- Toxins
- Hypersensitivity reactions
- Burns

Edema Caused by Blocked Lymphatic Drainage
- Tumors
- Goiter
- Parasites that obstruct lymph nodes
- Surgery that removes lymph nodes

Etiology

FVE usually results from conditions that cause retention of both sodium and water. These conditions include heart failure, cirrhosis of the liver, renal failure, adrenal gland disorders, corticosteroid administration, and stress conditions causing the release of ADH and aldosterone. Other causes include an excessive intake of sodium-containing foods, drugs that cause sodium retention, and the administration of excess amounts of sodium-containing IV fluids (e.g., 0.9% NaCl, Ringer's solution). This **iatrogenic** (induced by the effects of treatment) cause of FVE primarily affects patients with impaired regulatory mechanisms.

Risk Factors

An increase in fluid volume is anticipated with normal pregnancy, but conditions such as preeclampsia may cause abnormal retention of fluid, resulting in increased stress on the body. Pregnant women with preeclampsia are taught that mild to moderate edema of the lower extremities (dependent edema) is to be anticipated, but edema of the face or hands or severe edema of the lower extremities must be reported to the provider immediately.

Patients with heart disease, kidney dysfunctions, or diabetes with peripheral vascular disease are at increased risk. Any disease that impairs blood flow to the kidney, such as hypertension, can potentially cause FVE. Any patient receiving IV therapy is at risk if the infusion rate and type of solution are not carefully monitored.

Prevention

Prevention of FVE focuses on those disease states that lead to overload. Taking medications such as diuretics and antihypertensives keeps fluids in balance between the intra- and extracellular spaces. Weighing daily helps with early identification of fluid retention. Careful intake of sodium and avoidance of any added salt to foods helps prevent edema. When sitting, the patient should elevate the lower extremities as this promotes venous return and lowers venous hydrostatic pressure facilitating fluid remaining in or returning to the vascular space.

Clinical Manifestations

The following manifestations of FVE relate to both the excess fluid and its effects on circulation:

- The increase in total body water causes weight gain (greater than 5% of body weight) over a short time.
- Circulatory overload causes manifestations such as:
  a. A full, bounding pulse
  b. Distended neck and peripheral veins (distended neck veins are difficult to assess in infants)
  c. Increased CVP (more than 11–12 cm of water)
  d. Cough, **dyspnea** (labored or difficult breathing), and **orthopnea** (difficulty breathing when supine)
  e. Moist crackles (rales) in the lungs or, if severe, pulmonary edema (excess fluid in pulmonary interstitial spaces and alveoli)
  f. **Polyuria** (greatly increased urine output)
  g. **Ascites** (excess fluid in the peritoneal cavity)
  h. Peripheral edema or, if severe, **anasarca** (severe, generalized edema).

- Dilution of plasma by excess fluid causes a decreased hematocrit and BUN.
- Possible cerebral edema (excess water in brain tissues) can lead to altered mental status and anxiety.

Heart failure is not only a potential cause of FVE, but it is also a potential complication of the condition if the heart is unable to increase its workload to handle the excess blood volume. Severe fluid overload and heart failure can lead to pulmonary edema, a medical emergency.

Collaboration

Managing FVE focuses on prevention in patients at risk, treating the manifestations of FVE, and correcting the underlying cause. Management includes limiting sodium and water intake and administering diuretics. A consultation with a dietitian or nutritionist may help the patient to make appropriate food choices and provide the staff with a better understanding of patient food preferences.

Diagnostic Tests

The following laboratory tests may be ordered:

- *Serum electrolytes* and *serum osmolality* are measured. Serum sodium and osmolality usually remain within normal limits.
- *Serum hematocrit* and *hemoglobin* often are decreased because of plasma dilution from excess ECF.

Additional tests of renal and liver function (e.g., serum creatinine, BUN, liver enzymes) may be ordered to help determine the cause of FVE if it is unclear.

Pharmacologic Therapy

Diuretics are commonly used to treat FVE. They inhibit sodium and water reabsorption, increasing urine output. The three major classes of diuretics, each of which acts on a different part of the kidney tubule, are as follows:

1. *Loop diuretics*, which act in the ascending loop of Henle
2. *Thiazide-type diuretics*, which act on the distal convoluted tubule
3. *Potassium-sparing diuretics*, which affect the distal nephron.

Fluid Management

Fluid intake may be restricted in patients who have FVE. The amount of fluid allowed per day is prescribed by the primary care provider. All fluid intake must be calculated, including fluid consumed at meals and that used to administer medications orally or intravenously. Some foods may be higher in fluid content (e.g., watermelon, oranges, soups) and must be considered as well. **Box 6–4 ⟫** provides guidelines for patients with a fluid restriction.

Dietary Management

Because sodium retention is one of the dietary-related causes of FVE, a sodium-restricted diet often is prescribed. Americans typically consume more than 4–5 g of sodium every day, though the recommended sodium intake is 500–2400 mg/day.

Clinical Manifestations and Therapies
Fluid Volume Excess

ETIOLOGY	CLINICAL MANIFESTATIONS	CLINICAL THERAPIES
Congestive heart failure	<ul><li>Dependent edema</li><li>Distended neck veins</li><li>Pulmonary edema</li><li>Tachycardia</li><li>Dyspnea</li><li>Hypoxia</li><li>Respiratory crackles</li><li>White or pink foamy sputum</li><li>Liver enlargement</li><li>Loss of appetite</li><li>Nausea</li><li>Weakness</li><li>Fatigue</li><li>Decreased activity tolerance</li><li>Nocturia</li><li>Paroxysmal nocturnal dyspnea</li><li>Ascites</li><li>Cardiogenic shock</li></ul>	<ul><li>Diuretics</li><li>Fluid restrictions</li><li>Fowler or high Fowler position</li><li>Oxygen</li><li>Medications, including cardiac glycosides, ACE inhibitors, phosphodiesterase inhibitors, and β-adrenergic agonists (particularly dobutamine)</li><li>Monitoring of lab values: serum electrolytes, brain natriuretic peptide, BUN, creatinine, urinalysis, alanine aminotransferase, aspartate aminotransferase, lactate dehydrogenase, bilirubin, total protein, albumin levels, thyroid function tests, and arterial blood gas</li><li>Chest x-ray</li><li>Electrocardiography</li><li>Hemodynamic monitoring</li><li>Intra-arterial pressure monitoring</li><li>CVP monitoring</li></ul>
Liver cirrhosis	<ul><li>Weight loss</li><li>Weakness</li><li>Anorexia</li><li>Disrupted bowel function</li><li>Portal hypertension</li><li>Bleeding</li><li>Ascites</li><li>Jaundice</li><li>Neurologic changes</li><li>Peripheral edema</li><li>Anemia</li><li>Esophageal varices</li></ul>	<ul><li>Avoidance of hepatotoxic drugs</li><li>Diuretics</li><li>Lactulose and neomycin</li><li>Beta-blocker</li><li>Ferrous sulfate and folic acid</li><li>Antacid</li><li>Antianxiety drugs</li><li>Low-sodium, low-ammonia diet with vitamin and mineral supplements</li><li>Paracentesis</li><li>Hemodynamic monitoring</li></ul>
Adrenal tumor	<ul><li>Increased aldosterone production</li><li>Water and sodium retention</li><li>Edema</li><li>FVE</li></ul>	<ul><li>Removal of the tumor</li><li>Diuretics</li><li>Monitoring of serum electrolytes, hemoglobin, and hematocrit</li><li>Cardiorespiratory monitoring</li><li>Oxygen</li></ul>
Overadministration of IV fluids	<ul><li>Edema</li><li>Pulmonary edema</li><li>Shortness of breath</li><li>Orthopnea</li><li>Hypertension</li><li>Reduced peripheral perfusion</li></ul>	<ul><li>Administration of diuretics</li><li>Elevating head of bed</li><li>Cardiorespiratory and oxygen saturation monitoring</li><li>Administration of oxygen</li><li>Daily weights</li><li>Accurate measurement of I&O</li><li>Fluid restriction</li></ul>

Lifespan Considerations

FVE in Infants and Children

In children who are healthy, FVE is due to overhydration, with newborns being at greatest risk because the kidneys' filtering mechanism is too immature to maintain fluid balance as older infants do. Breast milk or formula provides all the fluids a healthy baby needs. Water should be given slowly, sparingly, and only during extremely hot weather. Symptoms of FVE include a change in behavior and drowsiness. Treatment includes limiting intake and use of diuretics if the FVE is severe. FVE can also be associated with serious injury or illness. Ingelse and colleagues (2016) suggest that FVE occurs in the pediatric intensive care unit because intervention includes the use of fluids, and that balancing intake is difficult. These researchers also identified that excess fluid is associated with increased risk for AKI and mortality.

FVE in Pregnant Women

FVE in pregnancy is associated with pregnancy-induced hypertension, preeclampsia, or eclampsia. The disorders are manifested by an increase in peripheral edema with pitting present, an increase in proteinuria, and hypertension. These disorders are addressed in the exemplar on Hypertensive Disorders in Pregnancy in the module on Perfusion. In addition, a disorder known as polyhydramnios, in which an excess of amniotic fluid exists, can be noted in pregnancy. This disorder can indicate fetal abnormalities and is addressed in the module on Reproduction.

FVE in Older Adults

FVE in older adults is most frequently manifested as a result of heart failure or kidney disease. Age-related changes in the heart itself lead to a decrease in output. The stretch of fibers decreases, and "snap back" is less; thus, the heart does not empty as well as it did previously, and the heart may enlarge in size. This leads to backup of blood in the venous system with resultant edema in the lower extremities as well as the spleen and liver. Age-related changes in the kidneys can affect the concentration of urine and may lead to fluid

excess. This is less common than dehydration. Additional factors include the use of antacids such as sodium bicarbonate for gastric distress, as the sodium is systemically absorbed and can lead to further movement of water into the vascular space, further adding to volume excess.

NURSING PROCESS

Nursing care focuses on preventing FVE in patients at risk and on managing problems resulting from its effects. Health promotion related to FVE focuses on teaching preventive measures to patients who are at risk (e.g., patients who have heart or kidney failure). The nurse should discuss the relationship between sodium intake and water retention. The nurse should also provide guidelines for a low-sodium diet and teach patients to carefully read food labels to identify "hidden" sodium, particularly in processed foods. The nurse should instruct patients who are at risk to weigh themselves on a regular basis, using the same scale, and to notify their primary care provider if they gain more than 5 lb in a week or less.

The nurse should carefully monitor patients receiving IV fluids for signs of hypervolemia. If hypervolemia develops, the nurse should reduce the flow rate and promptly report manifestations of fluid overload to the physician.

Assessment

The nurse should collect assessment data through the health history interview and physical examination:

- ***Observation and patient interview.*** Risk factors, such as medications, heart failure, and acute or chronic renal or endocrine disease; precipitating factors, such as a recent illness, change in diet, or change in medications; recent weight gain; complaints of persistent cough, shortness of breath, swelling of feet and ankles, or difficulty sleeping when lying down.

- ***Physical examination.*** Daily weight, preferably using the same scale and wearing the same or similar clothing; vital signs; peripheral pulses and capillary refill; jugular neck vein distention; edema; lung sounds (crackles or wheezes), dyspnea, cough, and sputum; urine output; and mental status.

A focused assessment includes checking for edema of the legs by pressing the skin for at least 5 seconds over the tibia, behind the medial malleolus, and over the dorsum of each foot (see **Figure 6–13** ≫). If edema is present, it may be graded

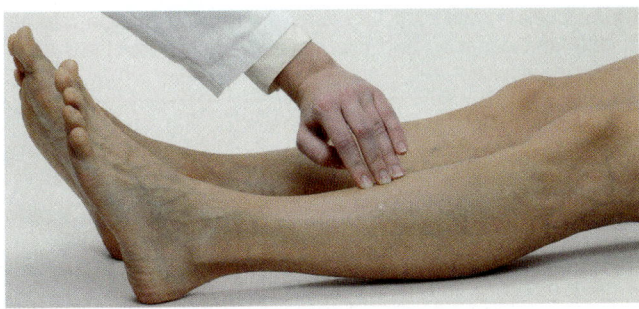

Figure 6–13 ≫ Palpating for edema over the tibia.

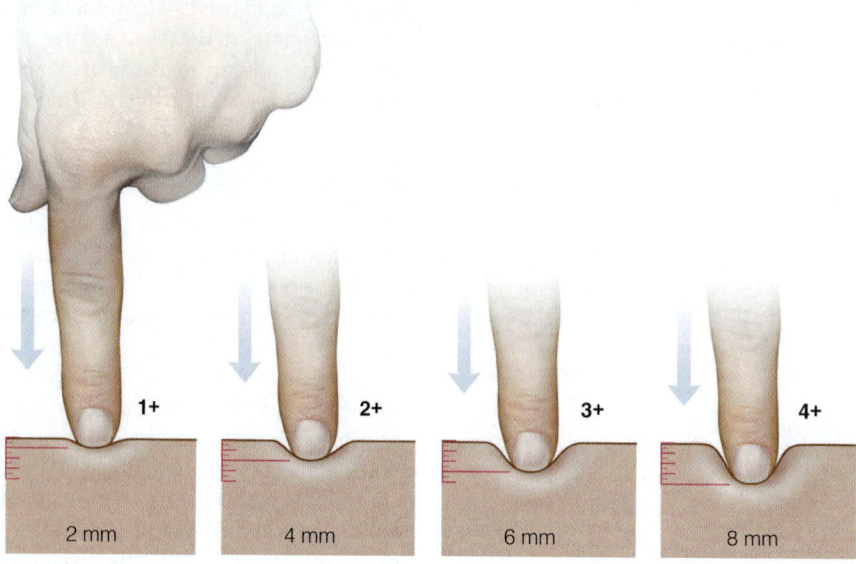

Figure 6–14 >> Grading pitting edema.

on a scale of 1+ (mild) to 4+ (severe) (see **Figure 6–14** >>). The nurse should assess for periorbital edema, swollen puffy eyelids that may result from crying or FVE. Men may experience scrotal edema, because the scrotum is in the dependent position when sitting.

The nurse should measure the patient's I&O. Output of infants is measured by weighing the diapers. Sudden weight gain (e.g., 0.5 kg [1 lb] in 1 day) is caused by the accumulation of fluid. A gain of 0.5 kg overnight is caused by retention of approximately 500 mL of fluid.

The nurse should assess the character of the pulse and observe for neck vein distention when the patient is sitting (usually visible only in adults and older children). The nurse should also monitor for signs of pulmonary edema (an indication of severe imbalance) by listening to lung sounds in the dependent lung fields (crackles) and assessing for respiratory distress (rapid respiratory rate, use of accessory muscles of respiration). Finally, the nurse should observe for edema.

SAFETY ALERT The potential for a patient (especially a small child) to develop a fluid overload is present whenever an isotonic IV solution containing sodium is being administered. Careful assessment of infusion rates is essential to all patient care but especially when caring for pediatric patients. Therefore, monitor the infusion rate frequently and carefully, and use a pump when possible to aid in accurate administration.

Diagnosis

Appropriate nursing diagnoses may include the following:

- *Fluid Volume, Excess*
- *Skin Integrity, Impaired*
- *Gas Exchange, Impaired*
- *Intolerance, Activity*
- *Health Maintenance, Ineffective.*

  (NANDA-I © 2014)

Planning

Outcomes are designed in collaboration with the patient and may include the following:

- The patient will regain fluid balance.
- The patient will have clear lung fields with eupneic (normal) breathing patterns.
- The patient will maintain skin integrity.
- The patient will tolerate increased levels of activity.
- The patient will make appropriate food choices to limit sodium.

Implementation

Nursing interventions for the patient with FVE vary depending on the patient's specific needs and treatment. However, interventions generally include the following:

- Weigh the patient daily.
- Maintain I&O records.
- Administer oral fluids carefully.
- Perform oral hygiene at least every 2 hours.
- Teach the patient and significant others about a sodium-restricted diet (see the Patient Teaching feature on low-sodium diets).
- Administer prescribed diuretics, and monitor the patient's response to therapy.
- Report significant changes in serum electrolytes or osmolality.

Patient Teaching
Low-Sodium Diet

- Reducing sodium intake helps the body excrete excess sodium and water.
- The body needs less than one tenth of a teaspoon of salt per day.
- Approximately one third of sodium intake comes from salt added to foods during cooking and at the table, one fourth to one third comes from processed foods, and the rest comes from food and water naturally high in sodium.
- Sodium compounds are used in foods as preservatives, leavening agents, and flavor enhancers.
- Many nonprescription drugs (e.g., analgesics, cough medicine, laxatives, antacids), toothpastes, and mouthwashes contain high amounts of sodium.
- Low-sodium salt substitutes are not sodium free; they may contain half as much sodium as regular salt.
- Use salt substitutes sparingly; larger amounts often taste bitter instead of salty.
- The preference for salt will eventually diminish.
- Salt, monosodium glutamate, baking soda, and baking powder contain substantial amounts of sodium.
- Read labels.
- In place of salt or salt substitutes, use herbs, spices, lemon juice, vinegar, and wine as flavoring when cooking.

Focus on Diversity and Culture
Dehydration in Infants

Early in their education, nursing students learn that a sunken fontanel is a sign of dehydration. Water balance is more fragile in infants than adults, so a sunken fontanel indicates the need for intervention. In Latin American countries, however, such a finding is called *caida de la mollera* (fallen fontanel) (Pachter et al., 2015). One traditional belief is that the fontanel is pulled down by suction caused when the infant is pulled too suddenly off the nipple (the mother's or a bottle). Another belief is that it is caused by a sudden bump or fall.

Traditional "cures" for *caida de la mollera* include pressing upward on the soft palate in an attempt to reshape the affected area, sucking on the outside of the fontanel, and holding the baby upside down, sometimes gently shaking and tapping the feet. Other treatments include the application of various poultices and ointments. Treatment of dehydration is not considered.

The National Library of Medicine, however, indicates that *caida de la mollera* is a medical emergency and is usually a sign the infant is severely dehydrated or malnourished (Gillette, 2013). Understanding the cultural impact of beliefs and etiologies of disease is an essential piece of assessment and intervention as nurses interact with patients from cultures different from their own.

- Teach the patient how to safely self-administer diuretics after discharge.
- Reposition the patient every 2 hours.
- Reduce shearing or friction to the skin.
- Provide a low-pressure alternative mattress, foot cradle, heel protectors, and other devices to reduce pressure on tissues.
- Place the patient in Fowler position if dyspnea or orthopnea is present.
- Monitor oxygen saturation and arterial blood gas results.
- Elevate area of edema (if possible) to encourage fluid reabsorption into ECF compartment.
- Assess for cultural practices that may affect the patient's dietary practices (see the Focus on Diversity and Culture feature).

Evaluation

The nurse should evaluate changes in weight, respirations, edema, and activity tolerance to determine the patient's response to treatment. To evaluate patient understanding of dietary teaching, the nurse should encourage the patient to participate in making appropriate diet choices from the menu. The nurse should revise the nursing plan of care as indicated on the basis of the patient's progress toward meeting outcomes. Expected outcomes may include the following:

- The patient maintains fluid balance, as evidenced by lack of edema and laboratory diagnostic results.
- The patient is able to participate in desired activities.
- The patient maintains skin integrity.

If the expected outcomes are unmet, the patient may need referral to other specialties, such as physical therapy to assist with activity and gaining strength. If alterations in skin integrity occur, the patient should be referred to the healthcare provider for follow-up with skin care treatment. Continued presence of edema should also be reported to the healthcare provider for possible additional medication intervention.

Nursing Care Plan
A Patient with FVE

Dorothy Radliffe is a 45-year-old Native American woman hospitalized with AKI that developed as a result of acute glomerulonephritis. She is expected to recover, but she has very little urine output.

Ms. Radliffe is a single mother of two teenage sons. Until her illness, she was active in caring for her family, her career as a high school principal, and community activities.

(continued on next page)

Nursing Care Plan (continued)

ASSESSMENT

Ms. Radliffe's nurse notes that she is in the oliguric phase of AKI and that her urine output for the previous 24 hours was 250 mL; this low output has been constant for the past 8 days. Ms. Radliffe gained 1 lb (0.45 kg) in the past 24 hours. Laboratory test results from that morning are as follows: sodium, 155 mEq/L (normal, 135–145 mEq/L); potassium, 5.6 mEq/L (normal, 3.5–5.3 mEq/L); calcium, 7.6 mg/dL (normal, 9–11 mg/dL); and urine specific gravity, 1.008 (normal, 1.010–1.030). Ms. Radliffe's serum creatinine and BUN are high; however, her arterial blood gases are within normal limits.

The nurse's assessment of Ms. Radliffe yields the following:

- T_O 37°C (98.6°F); P 102 bpm, with obvious neck vein distention; R 28/min, with crackles and wheezes; BP 160/92 mmHg. Head of bed elevated 30°.
- Periorbital and sacral edema present; 3+ pitting bilateral pedal edema; and skin cool, pale, and shiny.
- Alert, oriented, and responds appropriately to questions.
- Patient states she is thirsty, slightly nauseated, and extremely tired.

Ms. Radliffe is receiving IV furosemide and is on a 24 hr fluid restriction of 500 mL plus the previous day's urine output to manage her FVE.

DIAGNOSES

- *Excess Fluid Volume* related to AKI
- *Risk for Impaired Skin Integrity* related to fluid retention and edema
- *Risk for Impaired Gas Exchange* related to pulmonary congestion
- *Activity Intolerance* related to FVE, fatigue, and weakness

(NANDA-I © 2014)

PLANNING

- The patient will regain fluid balance, as evidenced by weight loss, decreasing edema, and normal vital signs.
- The patient will experience decreased dyspnea.
- The patient will maintain intact skin and mucous membranes.
- The patient will increase activity levels as prescribed.

IMPLEMENTATION

- Weigh at 6:00 a.m. and 6:00 p.m. daily.
- Assess vital signs and breath sounds every 4 hours.
- Measure I&O every 4 hours.
- Obtain urine specific gravity every 8 hours.
- Restrict fluids as follows: 375 mL from 7:00 a.m. to 3:00 p.m.; 250 mL from 3:00 p.m. to 11:00 p.m.; and 125 mL from 11:00 p.m. to 7:00 a.m. Patient prefers water or apple juice.
- Turn every 2 hours, following schedule posted at head of bed. Inspect and provide skin care as needed; avoid vigorous massage of pressure areas.

- Provide oral care every 2–4 hours (patient can brush her own teeth; caution patient not to swallow water); use moistened applicators as desired.
- Elevate head of bed to 30–40°; patient prefers to use own pillows.
- Assist to recliner chair at bedside for 20 minutes two or three times a day. Monitor ability to tolerate activity without increasing dyspnea or fatigue.

EVALUATION

At the end of the shift, the nurse evaluates the effectiveness of the plan of care and continues all diagnoses and interventions. Ms. Radliffe gained no weight, and her urinary output during this shift is 170 mL. Her urine specific gravity remains at 1.008. Her vital signs are unchanged, but her crackles and wheezes have decreased slightly. Her skin and mucous membranes are intact. Ms. Radliffe tolerated sitting in the bedside chair without dyspnea or fatigue.

CRITICAL THINKING

1. What is the pathophysiologic basis for Ms. Radliffe's increased respiratory rate, blood pressure, and pulse?
2. Explain how elevating the head of the bed 30° facilitates respirations.
3. Suppose Ms. Radliffe says, "I would really like to have all my fluids at once instead of spreading them out." How would you reply, and why?
4. Outline a plan for teaching Ms. Radliffe about diuretics.

ELECTROLYTE IMBALANCE

Overview

All body fluids contain electrolytes in varying concentrations, depending on whether the electrolyte is prominent in the ICF or ECF environment. Measurements of serum electrolyte values provide information about the concentration of that electrolyte in the blood. Such measurements reflect the concentration of the electrolyte in other body compartments.

Electrolytes are normally gained and lost in relatively equal amounts, so the body remains in balance. However, when a patient has an abnormal route of loss, such as vomiting, wound drainage, diuretic administration, or nasogastric suction, electrolyte balance can be uneven. Monitoring for signs of imbalance is an important part of nursing care for all patients, but especially for those at risk.

Signs and symptoms of electrolyte imbalance can be very subtle if the imbalance is minimal. Moderate to severe electrolyte imbalance often produces multisystem effects and can lead to death if not reversed. In caring for patients, the nurse must consider the role of electrolytes in maintaining homeostasis and assess for signs of imbalance. It is often important to assess a patient's new symptoms in light of a possible electrolyte imbalance.

Electrolytes and Imbalances

Nurses must understand the interactions among electrolytes and that an imbalance rarely occurs with only one electrolyte. For example, if sodium is lost, chloride is often lost with it; FVE often dilutes other electrolytes, resulting in lower serum levels; and gastric suctioning causing hypokalemia also causes loss of magnesium, sodium, and chloride as well as acid–base imbalance. In this section, we outline the etiology, manifestation, and indicated interventions for each of the electrolytes and provide information relative to excesses and deficits.

Sodium

Sodium is the most abundant electrolyte in ECF. Normal serum values for sodium are 135–145 mEq/L. The role of sodium in the body is to assist with maintenance of osmotic pressure and acid–base balance and with the conduction of nerve impulses. Aldosterone is the principal mineralocorticoid that assists in regulating serum sodium balance. It does this by stimulating the kidneys to conserve sodium and to excrete potassium when serum sodium levels fall below normal. Water follows the sodium, and blood volume rises. When ECF osmolality increases, ADH is secreted, leading to additional water reabsorption. The atria detect this rise in ECF volume and secrete atrial natriuretic peptide (ANP) to reverse the aldosterone process and promote sodium and water excretion to return the ECF to balance.

Sodium balance is also affected by food intake. Most Americans consume far more sodium than is necessary for maintaining sodium balance. This can lead to sodium excess and contribute to health concerns. The primary dietary sources of sodium are foods that are naturally high in sodium and processed foods and condiments.

>> **Stay Current:** Guidelines for patient teaching list of low- and high-sodium foods can be found at https://www.ucsfhealth.org/education/guidelines_for_a_low_sodium_diet.

Education to assist patients and their families with maintaining appropriate sodium intake includes reducing the amount of salt in recipes, avoiding adding salt during meals, and limiting intake of foods that contain high levels of sodium (either naturally or because of processing). In moderately and severely sodium-restricted diets, salt is avoided altogether, as are all foods containing significant amounts of sodium.

Hypernatremia

Hypernatremia occurs when serum sodium levels are greater than 145 mEq/L. Critical values occur at levels greater than 160 mEq/L. Etiologies include impaired thirst mechanism, profuse sweating, diarrhea, diabetes insipidus, Cushing syndrome, and inappropriate use of oral electrolyte solutions. Hypernatremia is manifested by hyperosmolality of the ECF; cellular dehydration; excessive thirst; elevated temperature; dry, sticky membranes; and restlessness. Management is aimed toward fluid replacement at a rate not to exceed 0.5–1 mEq/hr to prevent intracranial fluid shifts and cerebral edema. Nurses must observe for headache, nausea, and vomiting; increasing blood pressure; and confusion.

Hyponatremia

Hyponatremia occurs when serum sodium levels fall below 135 mEq/L. Critical values occur at levels below 115 mEq/L, although some studies suggest that 120 mEq/L should be the lowest point (Geoghegan et al., 2015). Etiology includes diuretic use, renal disease, adrenal insufficiency, vomiting, diarrhea, excessive GI suctioning, irrigation of nasogastric tubes with water rather than saline, repeated tap-water enemas, burns, heart failure, and administration of hypotonic IV fluid replacement. Hyponatremia is manifested by edema, muscle cramps, weakness, fatigue, anorexia, nausea and vomiting, and abdominal cramps. At very low levels, symptoms include headache, depression, personality changes, lethargy, hyperreflexia, muscle twitching, and tremors. If levels drop below 120 mEq/L, convulsions, coma, and death can occur. These symptoms may also be present at higher sodium levels if the serum level reduction is rapid. Management consists of administration of sodium-containing fluids, increased intake of sodium-rich fluids, and promotion of safety.

Potassium

Potassium is primarily an intracellular cation, with 98% of all potassium found within the cell. Potassium plays a role in cellular depolarization and repolarization. As a component of the potassium pump, it assists in the movement of potassium into the cell while sodium moves out of the cell. Both hyperkalemia and hypokalemia can lead to deadly cardiac dysrhythmias.

Hyperkalemia

Hyperkalemia is a serum potassium level of greater than 5.3 mEq/L. Critical values occur at levels greater than 7.0 mEq/L. Etiologies include renal failure, potassium-sparing diuretic use, excessive potassium intake, adrenal insufficiency, acidosis, severe tissue trauma (including burns), starvation, and medications such as trimethoprim. Hyperkalemia is manifested by tall, peaked T waves and widened QRS, dysrhythmias, cardiac arrest, nausea and vomiting, abdominal cramping, diarrhea, and paresthesias. Management consists of administration of calcium gluconate, administration of insulin and glucose, and sodium polystyrene sulfonate (Kayexalate) orally or by enema. Diuretics may be indicated if renal excretion is normal.

Hypokalemia

Hypokalemia is a serum potassium level of less than 3.5 mEq/L. Critical values occur at levels below 2.5 mEq/L. Etiologies include potassium-depleting diuretic use, corticosteroid use, antibiotics such as amphotericin B, severe vomiting, gastric suctioning, alkalosis, and long-term IV fluid replacement without the addition of potassium. Hypokalemia is manifested by dysrhythmias, flat or inverted T waves, anorexia, decreased bowel sounds, ileus, muscle cramps, increased risk for digoxin toxicity, and suppressed insulin secretion. Management consists of potassium salts replacement.

Chloride

Chloride is most prevalent in the ECF. It is found with sodium, and together they maintain the electricity of the body in a neutral state. Chloride is also found in combination with hydrogen to form the hydrochloric acid found in the stomach as an aid to digestion. It also plays a role in the maintenance of acid–base balance, especially in the measurement of the anion gap.

Hyperchloremia

Hyperchloremia is a serum chloride level greater than 105 mEq/L. Etiologies include diarrhea, renal failure, overactive parathyroid glands, use of carbonic anhydrase inhibitors, metabolic acidosis, and respiratory alkalosis. Manifestations include the presence of Kussmaul respirations, weakness, and increased thirst. Management consists of diuretics, increased IV fluids, treatment of the underlying cause, and dialysis.

Hypochloremia

Hypochloremia is a serum chloride level of less than 95 mEq/L. Although it is not a common disorder, when it does occur, its etiologies include loss of body fluid, vomiting, and diarrhea. Manifestations include paresthesias of the face and extremities, muscle spasm, and tetany. The abdomen may be distended. Management consists of increasing salt in the diet, adding chloride to IV fluids, and treating underlying causes.

Calcium

Calcium has several major functions in the body, including neuromuscular transmission and control of muscle contraction, blood clotting, bone and tooth formation, and cellular membrane functioning. Only 2% of calcium is found in the blood serum. Calcium levels are controlled by vitamin D, calcitonin, and parathyroid hormone.

Hypercalcemia

Hypercalcemia is a serum calcium of greater than 11 mg/dL. Etiologies include hyperparathyroidism, bone malignancy, and drug toxicity (e.g., from thiazide diuretics, lithium carbonate, vitamins A and D). Manifestations include fatigue, weakness, decreased deep tendon reflexes, headache, impaired cognition, anorexia, nausea and vomiting, lethargy, polyuria, renal calculi, anorexia, constipation, cardiac dysrhythmias, muscle weakness, and conjunctival calcifications. Management includes partial parathyroidectomy, discontinuation of thiazide diuretics and vitamin and mineral supplements, and a low-calcium diet.

Hypocalcemia

Hypocalcemia is a serum calcium level below 9 mg/dL. Etiologies include transfusion of a large volume of citrated blood, decreased parathyroid hormone, elevated serum phosphorus, decreased magnesium levels, hypoalbuminemia, and alkalosis. Hypocalcemia often results from accidental removal of the parathyroid glands during thyroidectomy. Manifestations are based on the speed at which the calcium level drops. Bradycardia and hypotension can occur. Patients experience numbness and tingling of the fingers, hyperactive reflexes, muscle cramps, laryngeal spasms, tetany, confusion, and possible seizures. Pathologic fractures can occur. Patients may also exhibit Trousseau sign and Chvostek sign, in which case IV replacement of calcium is indicated. Rates should not exceed 60 mg of elemental calcium per minute.

Magnesium

As the fourth most abundant cation and located in the cell similar to potassium, magnesium is an essential element in all living cells. The bones contain 60% of the body's magnesium, and the muscles contain 40%. Magnesium plays a role in energy production, protein synthesis, and neuromuscular function. Serum levels range from 1.8 to 3.0 mg/dL for adults. A balanced diet provides the necessary intake of magnesium needed for bodily functioning.

Hypermagnesemia

Hypermagnesemia, a serum magnesium level above 3.0 mg/dL, occurs rarely. When manifested, it generally occurs in patients with bowel disorders, from overconsumption of magnesium-containing antacids, and renal insufficiency. Older adults are also at risk because of poor kidney function. Patients with hypermagnesemia display flaccid muscle tone and decreased response in deep tendon reflexes. In addition to discontinuing any intervention containing magnesium, the treatment involves calcium gluconate, and at very high magnesium levels, hemodialysis may be indicated (Karahan et al., 2015).

Hypomagnesemia

Hypomagnesemia is defined as a magnesium level of less than 1.8 mg/dL. Malabsorption and renal wasting are the two most common causes. Poor dietary intake and side effects of medication are other causes. Hypomagnesemia is often misdiagnosed and can lead to neurologic and cardiac complications (Lewis, 2016). Symptoms include muscle cramps and tremors. They become evident when the level drops to less than 1.24 mg/dL. A positive Chvostek sign may be evident. When magnesium deficiency is symptomatic or persistently less than 1.25 mg/dL, treatment with magnesium salts is indicated (Lewis, 2016).

Phosphorus

Next to calcium, phosphorus is the most abundant mineral in the body. It works closely with calcium to maintain bone and tooth integrity. Approximately 85% of the body's phosphorus is in bones and teeth. Hypophosphatemia can be caused by alcoholism; excessive antacid intake; low vitamin D intake; and certain medications such as acetazolamide, foscarnet, imatinib, and pentamidine. It can also be caused by hyperparathyroidism. Hyperphosphatemia is rare, is considered asymptomatic, and is related to excessive intake.

Evidence-Based Practice
Sodium Intake: A Focus on Children

Problem

Is there a relationship between sodium intake and hypertension in children and adolescents?

Evidence

In a study of 6235 U.S. children and adolescents ages 8–18 years, daily sodium intake was measured by using dietary recall. Although reporting in dietary recall is acknowledged not to be 100% accurate, these findings suggested that these children consumed, on average, 3387 mg/day of sodium (Yang et al., 2012). In addition, the study outcome suggested that sodium intake increased with age. The presence of overweight or obesity was 39%, and pre–high blood pressure and existing high blood pressure were 14.9%, much of which was attributed to sodium intake. Children with hypertension are predisposed to hypertension in adulthood. The researchers in this study concluded that increased sodium intake was directly related to a rise in systolic blood pressure.

Implications

According to many sources (CDC, 2012), Americans eat too much salt. In addition, there is a direct correlation between sodium intake and increasing blood pressure numbers throughout the United States (Moshfegh et al., 2012). Education of parents and children regarding appropriate salt intake and avoidance of added salt and foods high in sodium may help to prevent significant hypertension as children mature into adults.

Critical Thinking Application

1. What foods that children and adolescents typically like are lower in sodium?

2. Design a health promotion activity for adolescents related to sodium intake. Include strategies for ways that adolescents can eat healthier foods.

Lifespan Considerations

Electrolyte Imbalance in Children and Adolescents

Most electrolyte imbalances that occur in children and adolescents are due to illnesses such as diarrhea or gastroenteritis that lead to FVD and dehydration. The Evidence-Based Practice feature suggests that significant sodium intake is connected with obesity and high blood pressure in children and adolescents and with hypertension later in life.

Electrolyte Imbalance in Pregnant Women

During pregnancy, the increased blood volume in pregnant women makes it particularly important to get the necessary additional electrolytes. Leg cramps can be a symptom of electrolyte deficit. A common cause of electrolyte imbalance during pregnancy is vomiting due to morning sickness, which is particularly common during the first 3 months of pregnancy. Hyperemesis gravidarum is the most severe form of nausea and vomiting in pregnant women and requires hospitalization in 0.3–2% of pregnancies (Ogunyemi, 2015). Clinical manifestations of hyperemesis gravidarum include persistent nausea and vomiting, excessive salivation, fatigue, weakness, dizziness, and weight loss greater than 5% of prepregnancy weight.

Treatment of nausea and vomiting in pregnant women ranges from dietary changes to nonpharmacologic interventions such as avoiding triggers to pharmacologic intervention, which is done in a stepwise progression using drugs that have the best maternal–fetal safety profile (Smith, Refuerzo, & Ramin, 2016). Pregnant women who have been unable to keep down food or fluids for 12 hours, and who have lightheadedness, dizziness, faintness, or tachycardia, should be evaluated in the emergency department. Treatment may include rehydration and antiemetic therapy on an outpatient basis, or hospital admission for longer treatment and even enteral and parental nutrition for those with severe hyperemesis gravidarum (Smith et al., 2016).

Electrolyte Imbalance in Older Adults

Changes in renal function and filtration can affect electrolyte balance in older adults. There is a reduction in glomerular filtration and a concurrent decrease in the ability to concentrate urine. In addition, total body water is reduced by 10–15%. Older adults also experience a decrease in thirst sensation and can experience a greater insensible loss in warm weather. Age-related changes also include reduction of renin secretion and aldosterone and an increase in ANP, making sodium imbalance (hyponatremia or hypernatremia) a possibility. The changes in renal tubular functioning result in hyperkalemia (El-Sharkawy et al., 2014). Medication intervention such as diuretics can also affect electrolytes.

NURSING PROCESS

Almost all body systems are sensitive to changes in fluid and electrolyte balance. Care of the patient experiencing an electrolyte imbalance requires the nurse to have a thorough understanding of the etiology, signs and symptoms, and suggested treatment of both excesses and deficiencies in specific electrolytes. Deficiencies can develop quickly and may require immediate intervention. These interventions may include simple replacement of water losses or intricate minute-by-minute monitoring of complex signs and symptoms, including laryngeal edema, Chvostek sign, cardiac rhythm, or urine output.

Assessment

Although each electrolyte imbalance has specific assessment components, general assessment of the patient with suspected electrolyte imbalance includes a review of the lab data for specific electrolyte excess or deficit, ECG, urinalysis, hemoglobin and hematocrit, and arterial blood gases. These findings should be followed by assessment of subjective data such as abnormal thirst, frequent urination, presence of anorexia or nausea, pain, problems with muscle cramping, and diarrhea. Objective data include vital signs, a mental status exam, deep tendon reflexes, presence of diarrhea or vomiting, heart and lung sounds, and presence of edema. A dietary review should also be performed, with emphasis on foods high in sodium or potassium and frequent intake of fluids with added electrolytes.

Diagnosis

Nursing diagnoses applicable to fluid and electrolyte imbalance include:

- *Fluid Volume: Deficit*
- *Electrolyte Imbalance, Risk for*
- *Cardiac Output, Decreased.*

(NANDA-I © 2014)

Planning

Outcomes are designed in collaboration with the patient and may include the following:

- The patient will maintain electrolyte levels within normal limits as determined by serum electrolyte findings and results of other laboratory diagnostics.
- The patient will be free of symptoms of electrolyte or acid–base imbalance.
- The patient will maintain regular heart rhythm.
- The patient will maintain electrolyte balance; for instance, the patient will have normal potassium levels in the presence of medication therapy such as diuretics.
- The patient will relate indications of imbalance that need to be reported to the healthcare provider.

Implementation

Nursing interventions to address specific electrolyte imbalances are identified in the discussions of specific electrolyte deficit or excess. General interventions include the following:

- Monitor sodium, potassium, chloride, and magnesium levels daily; monitor more frequently if levels are significantly elevated or decreased.
- Monitor I&O as indicated by agency policy.
- Observe for signs and symptoms of dehydration.
- Observe for signs and symptoms of fluid and electrolyte excess or deficiency.

Promote Adequate Nutrition and Hydration

- Provide nutritional teaching to maintain balance despite the side effects of medication therapy (e.g., foods high in potassium in patients receiving furosemide or thiazide diuretics).

- Provide teaching for parents, teachers, coaches, and caregivers regarding early recognition of symptoms of dehydration and the need for ongoing fluid replacement. Include the need for water as well as electrolyte solutions.
- Incorporate cultural or ethnic principles into the nutritional teaching for patients who are at risk for fluid and electrolyte imbalance.

Evaluation

Achievement of expected outcomes for patients with electrolyte imbalance may include the following:

- The patient's electrolyte status returns to appropriate levels as evidenced by normal serum electrolytes, normal urinalysis, and the absence of edema and other symptoms associated with excess or deficit.
- The patient maintains appropriate weight for age and height.
- The patient maintains equality of I&O as evidenced by direct measurement (hospital setting) or measurement of intake and documentation of food intake via journals (home setting).
- The patient consumes food and/or fluids to maintain fluid and electrolyte balance during times of exercise or to replenish fluids and electrolytes lost during drug therapy.

On the basis of these findings, the nurse may revise the nursing care plan as needed to facilitate the patient's progress toward meeting outcomes.

Patient Teaching
The Patient Taking Diuretics

Diuretics are often the first-line therapy for hypertension, and these medications can lead to significant electrolyte imbalances. Information given to patients should include:

- Diuretics can increase serum glucose and cholesterol levels.
- Thiazide or loop diuretics can result in hypokalemia, and patients should report muscle weakness, irritability, and confusion. Foods that are high in potassium include beans, baked potato with the skin on, apricots, and fish.
- Patients taking potassium-sparing diuretics should report muscle twitching or changes in pulse rate.
- Patients should take diuretics in the morning to avoid waking at night to void.
- Patients should stand up slowly to minimize the risk of dizziness from orthostatic hypotension.
- Patients should weigh themselves daily at the same time using the same scale and wearing similar clothing. They should report an unusual weight gain, such as 3 lb in 3 days.
- Diuretics should never be stopped abruptly (Qavi, Kamal, & Schrier, 2015).

REVIEW   Fluid and Electrolyte Imbalance

RELATE Link the Concepts and Exemplars

Linking the exemplar of fluid and electrolyte imbalance with the concept of cognition:

1. What impact might the nurse anticipate a fluid and electrolyte imbalance to have on an older patient's cognition?

2. What expected outcomes are appropriate for the patient with confusion and hyperkalemia?

Linking the exemplar of fluid and electrolyte imbalance with the concept of elimination:

3. You are caring for a patient with acute nausea, vomiting, and diarrhea. What impact do you anticipate these symptoms will have on the patient's fluid and electrolyte balance? How can you minimize this impact?

4. What focused assessment is a priority for the patient with CKD who has a potassium level of 5.7?

READY Go to Volume 3: Clinical Nursing Skills

REFER Go to Pearson MyLab Nursing and eText

- Additional review materials

REFLECT Apply Your Knowledge

Pamela Allen is a 65-year-old woman who has been married to Clifford for 40 years. Their only child, Gary, has Down syndrome

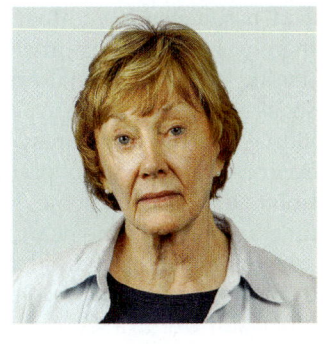

and lives with them. Mrs. Allen stopped working outside the home after Gary was born to care for him. She has recently been diagnosed with advanced colorectal cancer and had surgery last month (colectomy and colostomy). Because the tumor extended into the perineum and lymph nodes, she has been advised to start radiation and chemotherapy. She underwent treatment for endometrial cancer at age 50 but did not receive chemotherapy or radiation at that time.

1. When caring for Mrs. Allen during administration of chemotherapy, what issues might you anticipate could result in fluid and electrolyte imbalance?

2. If Mrs. Allen experiences dehydration after chemotherapy administration, what suggestions could you make to improve her fluid status?

3. As a result of chemotherapy and radiation causing bowel irritation, Mrs. Allen develops severe acute diarrhea. What changes would you recommend regarding Mrs. Allen's fluid intake to maintain adequate fluid balance and normal electrolyte levels?

≫ Exemplar 6.B Acute Kidney Injury

Exemplar Learning Outcomes

6.B Analyze acute kidney injury (AKI) as it relates to fluids and electrolytes.

- Describe the pathophysiology of AKI.
- Describe the etiology of AKI.
- Compare the risk factors for and prevention of AKI.
- Identify the clinical manifestations of AKI.
- Summarize diagnostic tests and therapies used by interprofessional teams in the collaborative care of an individual with AKI.
- Differentiate considerations for care of patients with AKI across the lifespan.
- Apply the nursing process in providing culturally competent care to an individual with AKI.

Exemplar Key Terms

Overview

The kidneys control fluid and electrolyte balance as well as acid–base balance, and they help to control blood pressure, thereby helping to maintain homeostasis. Only one functioning kidney is normally necessary to maintain homeostasis, as is frequently seen in patients with a single transplanted kidney. When both kidneys fail to function properly, fluids accumulate in atypical locations within the body, and electrolyte levels, hemoglobin, hematocrit, and BUN and creatinine are altered. The heart rate increases in an attempt to accommodate excess fluid, and muscle function is affected by electrolyte imbalance. Cerebral edema may occur. Death will result within a few days without appropriate treatment.

Renal failure is a condition in which the kidneys are unable to remove accumulated metabolites from the blood, resulting in altered fluid, electrolyte, and acid–base balance. The cause may be a primary kidney disorder, or renal failure may be secondary to a systemic disease or other urologic defects (Connell & Laing, 2015; Schetz, Gunst, & Van den Berghe, 2014). Renal failure may be either acute or chronic. When acute, renal failure has an abrupt onset and may be reversed with prompt intervention.

CKD is a silent disease, progressing slowly with few symptoms until the kidneys are severely damaged and unable to meet the excretory needs of the body. Both AKI and CKD are characterized by **azotemia** (increased levels of nitrogenous wastes in the blood). This exemplar discusses the acute form of renal failure.

Acute kidney injury (AKI), previously referred to as **acute renal failure (ARF)**, is a rapid decline in renal function, particularly the glomerular filtration rate (GFR), due to a decrease in the excretion function of the kidneys with concurrent increases in creatinine and urea levels (Ellis & Jenkins, 2014). The disorder affects 13–18% of patients admitted to the hospital. The most common causes of AKI are **ischemia** (insufficient blood supply) and exposure to **nephrotoxins** (substances that damage nerves or nerve tissue). Because of the amount of blood that passes through them, the kidneys are particularly vulnerable to these factors. A fall in blood pressure or volume can cause ischemia of kidney tissues. Nephrotoxins in the blood damage renal tissue directly. Other causes of AKI include major surgery, sepsis, and severe pneumonia (Mizokamia & Mizuno, 2015; Uettwiller-Geiger & McPherson, 2015).

Pathophysiology and Etiology
Pathophysiology

The causes and pathophysiology of AKI are commonly categorized as prerenal, intrinsic, or postrenal. Prerenal AKI is the most common, accounting for approximately 55% of cases. In prerenal AKI, **hypoperfusion** (decreased blood flow) leads to AKI without directly affecting the integrity of kidney tissues. Intrinsic (or intrarenal) AKI, caused by direct damage to functional kidney tissue, is responsible for another 40%. Urinary tract obstruction with resulting kidney damage is the precipitating factor for postrenal AKI, the least common form (approximately 5%). **Table 6–6 》** summarizes the causes of AKI, and **Figure 6–15 》** outlines the pathophysiology of AKI.

Prerenal AKI

Prerenal AKI results from conditions that affect renal blood flow and perfusion. Any disorder that significantly decreases vascular volume, cardiac output, or systemic vascular resistance can affect renal blood flow. Prerenal AKI is common, particularly in patients who experience trauma or surgery or are critically ill. The kidneys normally receive 20–25% of the cardiac output to maintain the **glomerular filtration rate (GFR)**, the rate at which fluid is filtered through the kidneys. A drop in renal blood flow to less than 20% of normal causes the GFR to fall. As the filtration of substances by the glomeruli is reduced, less reabsorption of substances in the tubule is required. As a result, kidney cells require less energy and oxygen, and their metabolism slows. Prerenal AKI is rapidly reversed when blood flow is restored and the renal parenchyma remains undamaged. Unresolved ischemia can lead to tubular cell necrosis and significant nephron damage. Intrinsic AKI caused by ischemic injury may result.

Intrarenal (Intrinsic) AKI

Intrinsic or intrarenal failure is characterized by acute damage to the renal parenchyma and nephrons. Causes include diseases of the kidney itself and acute tubular necrosis (ATN), the most common intrarenal cause of AKI.

In acute glomerulonephritis, glomerular inflammation can reduce renal blood flow and cause AKI. Vascular disorders affecting the kidney, such as vasculitis (inflammation of the blood vessels), malignant hypertension, and arterial or venous occlusion, can damage nephrons sufficiently to result in AKI.

TABLE 6–6 Causes of Acute Kidney Injury

	Cause	Examples
Prerenal	Hypovolemia	Hemorrhage, dehydration, excess fluid loss from GI tract, burns, wounds
	Low cardiac output	Heart failure, cardiogenic shock
	Altered vascular resistance	Sepsis, anaphylaxis, vasoactive drugs
Intrarenal	Glomerular/microvascular injury	Glomerulonephritis, disseminated intravascular coagulation, vasculitis, hypertension, toxemia of pregnancy, hemolytic uremic syndrome
	Acute tubular necrosis	Ischemia resulting from conditions associated with prerenal failure; toxins, such as drugs and heavy metals; **hemolysis** (destruction of RBCs); rhabdomyolysis (muscle cell breakdown)
	Interstitial nephritis	Acute pyelonephritis, toxins, metabolic imbalances, idiopathic
Postrenal	Ureteral obstruction	Calculi, cancer, external compression
	Urethral obstruction	Prostatic enlargement, calculi, cancer, stricture, blood clot

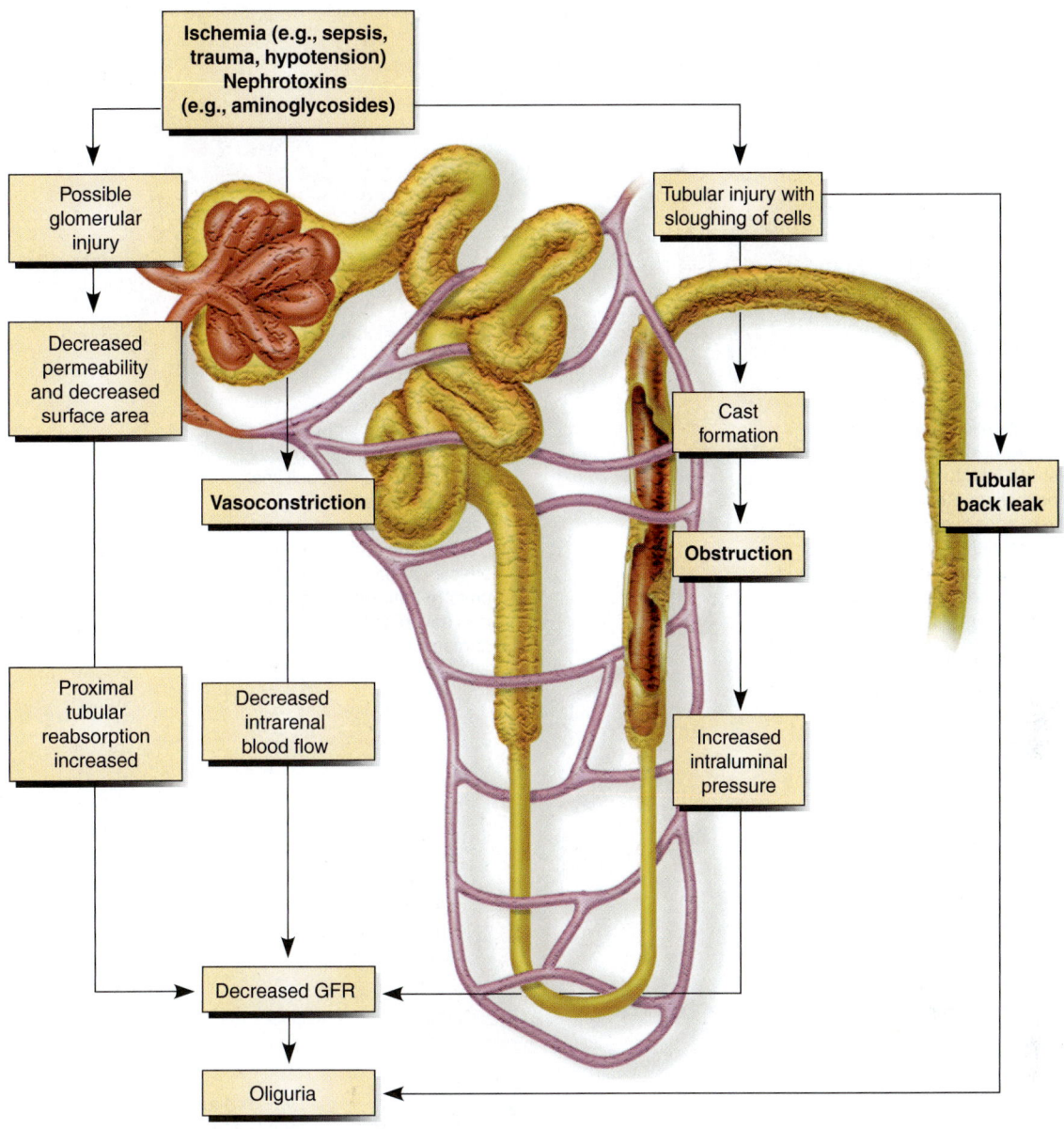

Figure 6–15 》 The pathophysiology of acute kidney injury.

Postrenal AKI

Obstructive causes of AKI are classified as postrenal. Any condition that prevents urine excretion can lead to postrenal AKI. Benign prostatic hypertrophy is the most common precipitating factor. Others include renal or urinary tract calculi and tumors. Children with AKI may experience **oliguria** (decreased urine output) or normal or increased urine output. Renal failure without oliguria usually indicates a less severe renal injury.

Acute Tubular Necrosis

Nephrons are especially susceptible to injury from ischemia or exposure to nephrotoxins. **Acute tubular necrosis (ATN)** (the destruction of tubular epithelial cells) causes an abrupt and progressive decline of renal function. Prolonged ischemia is the primary cause of ATN. When ischemia and nephrotoxin exposure occur concurrently, the risk for ATN and tubular dysfunction is especially high. See **Figure 6–16 》** for the pathogenesis of AKI caused by ATN. Risk factors for ischemic ATN include major surgery, severe **hypovolemia** (decreased circulating blood volume), sepsis, trauma, and burns. The impact of ischemia resulting from vasodilation and fluid loss in sepsis, trauma, and burns often is compounded by toxins released by bacteria or from damaged tissue. Injury to the tubule resulting in ATN is the most frequent cause of intrinsic renal failure in children.

Ischemia lasting more than 2 hours causes severe and irreversible damage to kidney tubules, with patchy cellular necrosis and sloughing. The GFR is significantly reduced as a result of ischemia, activation of the renin-angiotensin system, and tubular obstruction by cellular debris, which raises the pressure in the glomerular capsule.

Common nephrotoxins associated with ATN include the aminoglycoside antibiotics and radiologic contrast media.

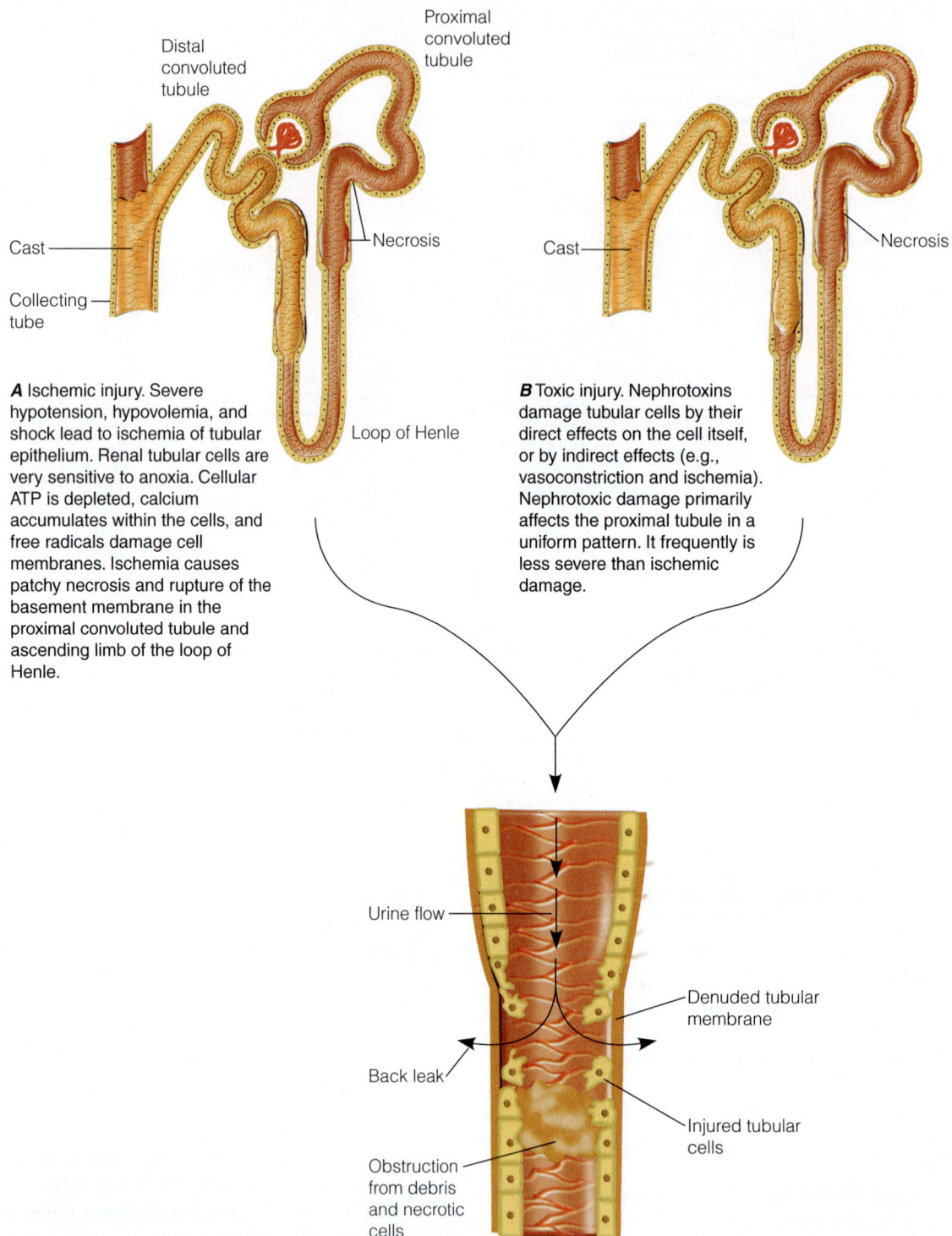

A Ischemic injury. Severe hypotension, hypovolemia, and shock lead to ischemia of tubular epithelium. Renal tubular cells are very sensitive to anoxia. Cellular ATP is depleted, calcium accumulates within the cells, and free radicals damage cell membranes. Ischemia causes patchy necrosis and rupture of the basement membrane in the proximal convoluted tubule and ascending limb of the loop of Henle.

B Toxic injury. Nephrotoxins damage tubular cells by their direct effects on the cell itself, or by indirect effects (e.g., vasoconstriction and ischemia). Nephrotoxic damage primarily affects the proximal tubule in a uniform pattern. It frequently is less severe than ischemic damage.

C Injured tubular cells release intracellular debris, which combines with proteins within the tubules to form casts. These casts, together with sloughed necrotic cells, occlude the tubular lumen, increasing tubular pressure and disrupting the flow of glomerular filtrate. The increased pressure pushes filtrate out of the damaged tubule into interstitial tissues (back leak). Renal blood flow and glomerular filtration may be further reduced by intrarenal angiotension II release and vasoconstriction.

Figure 6–16 》 Acute tubular necrosis (ATN). In ATN, tubular epithelial cells are destroyed by either ischemic or toxic injury.

Many other drugs (e.g., nonsteroidal anti-inflammatory drugs [NSAIDs], some chemotherapeutic drugs), heavy metals (e.g., mercury, gold), and some common chemicals (e.g., ethylene glycol [antifreeze]) also are potentially toxic to the renal tubule. Ibuprofen and acetaminophen are particularly problematic in children. The risk for ATN is higher when nephrotoxic drugs are given to older patients or to patients with preexisting renal insufficiency and when used in combination with other nephrotoxins (Mizokami & Mizuno, 2015). Dehydration increases the risk by increasing the toxin concentration in nephrons.

Nephrotoxins destroy tubular cells by both direct and indirect effects. As tubular cells are damaged and lost through necrosis and sloughing, the tubule becomes more permeable. This increased permeability results in filtrate reabsorption, further reducing the ability of the nephron to eliminate wastes.

Etiology

Approximately 5% of all hospitalized patients develop AKI, including 4.5% of children cared for in pediatric intensive care units and up to 8% of infants cared for in neonatal intensive care units (Stojanović et al., 2014). The incidence increases proportionally with the severity of the patient's illness. The mortality rate for AKI in seriously ill patients may reach 75%. This high death rate is probably more related to the populations affected by AKI—older patients and the critically ill—than to the disorder itself (Joslin et al., 2015).

AKI can occur at any point throughout an individual's life. Etiologies that can lead to AKI are outlined in **Table 6–7 »** by their occurrence in relation to the kidney and prerenal, intrarenal, and postrenal causes.

Risk Factors

Risk factors for AKI include major trauma or surgery, infection, hemorrhage, severe heart failure, severe liver disease, and lower urinary tract obstruction. Drugs and radiologic contrast media that are toxic to the kidney also increase the risk for AKI.

Older adults develop AKI more frequently because of their higher incidence of serious illness, hypotension, major surgeries, diagnostic procedures, and treatment with nephrotoxic drugs (Mizokami & Mizuno, 2015). Decrease in kidney function associated with aging also puts older adults at greater risk for kidney failure.

Children with **renal insufficiency** (decrease in the kidneys' ability to conserve sodium and concentrate the urine) are at greater risk for fluid loss with illness. In cases of acute GI illness, these children are at greater risk for dehydration and AKI.

Prevention

Contrast-induced nephropathy is the third most common cause of hospital-acquired AKI, after decreased renal perfusion and administration of nephrotoxic medications. Identification of patients at risk and implementation of preventive strategies can decrease the incidence of this nephropathy. Prevention strategies focus on counteracting vasoconstriction, enhancing blood flow through the nephron, and providing protection against injury by oxygen free radicals. Knowledge of the adverse effects associated with infusion of contrast media, identification of patients at risk for contrast-induced nephropathy, and application of evidence-based prevention strategies allow nurses to assist in the prevention of contrast-induced nephropathy (Jorgenson, 2013).

Clinical Manifestations

The course of AKI typically includes three phases: initiation, maintenance, and recovery.

Initiation Phase

The initiation phase may last hours to days. It begins with the initiating event (e.g., hemorrhage) and ends when tubular injury occurs. If AKI is recognized and the initiating event is treated effectively during this phase, the prognosis is good. The initiation phase of AKI is often asymptomatic, however, making it difficult to identify AKI before the appearance of the manifestations of the maintenance phase.

Maintenance Phase

The maintenance phase of AKI is characterized by a significant fall in GFR and tubular necrosis. Oliguria may develop, although many patients continue to produce normal or near-normal amounts of urine (nonoliguric AKI). Even though urine may be produced, the kidney cannot efficiently eliminate metabolic wastes, water, electrolytes, and acids from the body during the maintenance phase of AKI. Azotemia, fluid retention, electrolyte imbalances, and metabolic acidosis develop. These abnormalities are more severe in the patient

TABLE 6–7 Etiologies of Acute Kidney Injury

Prerenal Causes	Intrarenal Causes	Postrenal Causes
Dehydration	Acute glomerulonephritis	Benign prostatic hyperplasia
Shock	Aminoglycoside antibiotics	Prostate cancer
Vomiting and diarrhea	Sepsis	Bladder cancer
Surgery	Acute pyelonephritis	Calculi
Cardiac failure	Aneurysm	Fecal impaction
Diuretics	Cholesterol embolus	Bladder outlet obstruction
Nonsteroidal anti-inflammatory drugs (NSAIDs)	Allergic response to radio contrast media	Gynecologic cancers
Angiotensin-converting enzyme (ACE) inhibitors	Intratubular obstruction	
Liver failure	Exposure to nephrotoxic drugs	
Hypovolemia	Diabetic nephropathy	

Sources: Based on Elliott, R. W. (2012). Demographics of the older adult and chronic kidney disease. *Nephrology Nursing Journal, 39*(6), 491–496; Mayo Clinic. (2016). *Acute kidney failure.* Retrieved from http://www.mayoclinic.com/health/kidney-failure/DS00280/DSECTION=causes; Yue, Z., Jiang, P., Sun, H., & Wu, J. (2014). Association between excess risk of AKI and a concomitant use of ibuprofen and acetaminophen in children: Retrospective analysis of a spontaneous reporting system. *European Journal of Clinical Pharmacology, 70,* 479–482.

with oliguria than in the patient without oliguria, leading to a poorer prognosis with oliguria.

During the maintenance phase, salt retention and water retention cause edema, increasing the risk for heart failure and pulmonary edema. Impaired potassium excretion leads to hyperkalemia (increased levels of potassium in the blood). When the serum potassium level is greater than 6.0–6.5 mEq/L, manifestations of its effect on neuromuscular function develop, including muscle weakness, nausea and diarrhea, electrocardiographic changes, and possible cardiac arrest. Other electrolyte imbalances include **hyperphosphatemia** (increased blood levels of phosphate) and **hypocalcemia** (decreased blood levels of calcium). Metabolic acidosis results from impaired hydrogen ion elimination by the kidneys.

Anemia develops after several days of AKI because of suppressed erythropoietin secretion by the kidneys. Immune function may be impaired, increasing the risk for infection. Other manifestations of the maintenance phase include the following:

- Confusion, disorientation, agitation, or lethargy; hyperreflexia; and possible seizures or coma because of azotemia and electrolyte and acid–base imbalances
- Anorexia (loss of appetite), nausea, vomiting, and decreased or absent bowel sounds
- Uremic syndrome (if AKI is prolonged; see Exemplar 6.C on Chronic Kidney Disease).

Recovery Phase

The recovery phase of AKI is characterized by a process of tubule cell repair and regeneration and gradual return of the GFR to normal or pre-AKI levels. **Diuresis** (excretion of abnormally large quantities of urine) may occur as the nephrons and GFR recover, promoting the excretion of retained salt, water, and solutes. Serum creatinine, BUN, potassium, and phosphate levels remain high and may continue to rise in spite of increasing urine output. Renal function improves rapidly during the first 5–25 days of the recovery phase and continues to improve for up to 1 year.

Collaboration

Preventing AKI is a goal in caring for all patients, especially those in high-risk groups. Maintaining adequate vascular volume, cardiac output, and blood pressure is vital to preserving kidney perfusion, as is avoiding nephrotoxic drugs whenever possible. When a nephrotoxic drug or substance must be used, the risk of AKI can be reduced by using the minimum effective dose, maintaining hydration, and eliminating other known nephrotoxins from the medication regimen.

SAFETY ALERT When discharging a patient with instructions to avoid nephrotoxic drugs, the nurse should encourage the patient to contact his or her pharmacist. Adding that information to the patient's pharmacy history will help the patient to avoid nephrotoxic drugs that may be prescribed in the future.

Clinical Manifestations and Therapies
Acute Kidney Injury

ETIOLOGY	CLINICAL MANIFESTATIONS	CLINICAL THERAPIES
Anemia	- Fatigue - Pallor - Dizziness, confusion, lethargy - Tachycardia, tachypnea, hypotension	- Iron supplementation - Administration of epoetin - Blood transfusion - Therapies aimed at treating the underlying cause of AKI
Fluid volume excess	- Dependent **pitting edema** (edema that retains indentation caused by pressure) - Respiratory crackles - Dyspnea, pulmonary edema, hypoxemia - Weight gain - Tachycardia - Jugular vein distention	- Fluid restriction - Sodium-restricted diet - Diuretics - Dialysis
Hyperkalemia	- Ventricular arrhythmias - Tall, peaked T waves; widened QRS - Cardiac arrest - Smooth muscle hyperactivity - Nausea and vomiting - Abdominal cramping - Diarrhea - Muscle weakness - Paresthesias - Flaccid paralysis	- Removal of all potassium from IV solutions - Low-potassium diet - Administration of glucose and insulin to drive potassium into the cell - Potassium-absorbing enema solutions - Dialysis

If a patient develops AKI, maintaining the fluid and electrolyte balance is a key goal in managing the condition. Other goals in the treatment of AKI include the following:

1. Identifying and correcting the underlying cause
2. Preventing additional kidney damage
3. Restoring the urine output and kidney function
4. Compensating for renal impairment until kidney function is restored.

Diagnostic Tests

Diagnostic tests are used to identify the cause of AKI and monitor its effects on homeostasis. These tests include the following:

- *Urinalysis* often shows the following abnormal findings in AKI:
  a. A fixed specific gravity of 1.010 (equal to the specific gravity of plasma), because the tubules are unable to concentrate the filtrate
  b. *Proteinuria* (excess protein in urine) if glomerular damage is the cause of AKI
  c. The presence of RBCs (caused by glomerular dysfunction), WBCs (related to inflammation), and renal tubular epithelial cells (indicating ATN)
  d. Cell casts, which are protein and cellular debris molded in the shape of the tubular lumen (In AKI, RBCs, WBCs, and renal tubular epithelial casts may be present; brownish-pigmented casts and positive tests for occult blood indicate hemoglobinuria or myoglobinuria.)

- *Serum creatinine* and *BUN* are used to evaluate renal function. In AKI, serum creatinine levels increase rapidly, within 24–48 hours of onset. Creatinine levels generally peak within 5–10 days. Creatinine and BUN levels tend to increase more slowly when urine output is maintained. The onset of recovery is marked by a halt in the rise of the serum creatinine and BUN.

- *Serum electrolytes* are monitored to evaluate the fluid and electrolyte status. The serum potassium rises at a moderate rate and is often used to indicate the need for dialysis. Hyponatremia is common because of the water excess associated with AKI.

- *Arterial blood gas* studies often show a metabolic acidosis caused by the kidneys' inability to adequately eliminate metabolic wastes and hydrogen ions.

- *Complete blood count (CBC)* shows reduced RBCs, moderate anemia, and a low hematocrit. AKI affects erythropoietin secretion and RBC production. Iron and folate absorption may also be impaired, further contributing to anemia.

- *Renal ultrasonography* is used to identify obstructive causes of renal failure and to differentiate AKI from ESRD. In AKI, the kidneys may be enlarged, whereas in CKD, they typically appear small and shrunken.

- *Computed tomographic scan (CT)* may be done to evaluate kidney size and identify possible obstructions.

- *IV pyelography, retrograde pyelography, or antegrade pyelography* may be used to evaluate kidney structure and function. Radiologic contrast media are used with extreme caution because of their potential nephrotoxicity.

Retrograde pyelography, in which contrast dye is injected into the ureters, and antegrade pyelography, in which the contrast medium is injected percutaneously into the renal pelvis, are preferred, because they have fewer nephrotoxic effects than IV pyelography.

- *Renal biopsy* may be necessary to differentiate between acute and chronic kidney disease.

- *Radiographic studies* may be helpful in determining AKI in pediatric patients, because these studies will indicate the size of the kidney. A common cause of AKI in children is **osteodystrophy** (a complex bone disease process of CKD in which increased resorption of bone is caused by chronic hyperparathyroidism).

Pharmacologic Therapy

The primary focus in drug management for AKI is to restore and maintain renal perfusion and to eliminate from the treatment regimen any drugs that are nephrotoxic. IV fluids and blood volume expanders are given as needed to restore renal perfusion. Dopamine (Intropin), administered in low doses by IV infusion, increases renal blood flow. Dopamine is a sympathetic neurotransmitter that improves cardiac output and dilates blood vessels of the mesentery and kidneys when given in low therapeutic doses.

If restoration of renal blood flow does not improve urinary output, a potent loop diuretic, such as furosemide (Lasix), or an osmotic diuretic, such as mannitol, may be given with IV fluids. The purpose for giving a potent diuretic is twofold. First, if nephrotoxins are present, the combination of fluids and potent diuretics may, in effect, "wash out" the nephrons, reducing the toxin concentration. Second, establishing urine output may prevent oliguria and reduce the degree of azotemia and fluid and electrolyte imbalances. Furosemide also may be used to manage the salt and water retention that is associated with AKI.

Aggressive management of hypertension limits renal injury when AKI is associated with disorders such as toxemia and pregnancy-induced hypertension. ACE inhibitors or other antihypertensive medications are used to control arterial pressures.

All drugs that either are directly nephrotoxic or may interfere with renal perfusion (e.g., potent vasoconstrictors) are discontinued. NSAIDs, nephrotoxic antibiotics, and other potentially harmful drugs are avoided throughout the course of AKI.

The patient with AKI has an increased risk of GI bleeding, probably related to the stress response and impaired platelet function. Regular doses of antacids (although not ones that are magnesium based), histamine H_2-receptor antagonists (e.g., famotidine, ranitidine), or a proton pump inhibitor (e.g., omeprazole [Prilosec]) are often ordered to prevent GI hemorrhage.

Hyperkalemia may require active intervention as well as restricted potassium intake. Serum levels greater than 6.5 mEq/L are treated to prevent the adverse cardiovascular effects of hyperkalemia. With significant hyperkalemia, calcium chloride, bicarbonate, and insulin and glucose may be given intravenously to reduce serum potassium levels by moving potassium into the cells. A potassium-binding exchange resin, such as sodium polystyrene sulfonate (Kayexalate, SPS Suspension), may be given orally or by enema. This agent removes potassium from the body by exchanging sodium for potassium, primarily in the large intestine. When given orally, it is often combined with sorbitol to prevent constipation. Rectally, it is instilled as a retention enema, allowed to remain in the bowel for approximately 30–60 minutes, and then irrigated out using a tap-water enema.

Aluminum hydroxide (ALternaGEL, Amphojel, Nephrox), an antacid, is used to control hyperphosphatemia in renal failure. It binds with phosphates in the GI tract, which are then excreted in the feces.

Because many drugs are eliminated from the body by the kidney, drug dosages may need to be adjusted for the patient with AKI. Doses within the usual range can lead to potentially toxic blood levels, because their elimination is slowed and their half-life is prolonged. Nursing implications for medications commonly prescribed for the patient with AKI are summarized in the Medications feature.

Fluid Management

Once vascular volume and renal perfusion have been restored, fluid intake usually is restricted. The restricted daily fluid intake is calculated by allowing 500 mL for insensible losses (respiration, perspiration, and bowel losses) and adding the amount excreted as urine (or lost in vomitus) during the previous 24 hours. For example, if a patient with AKI excretes 325 mL of urine in 24 hours, the nurse should allow the patient a fluid intake (including oral and IV fluids) of 825 mL for the next 24 hours. The nurse should carefully monitor fluid balance by using accurate weight measurements and the serum sodium as the primary indicators.

Nutrition Management

Renal insufficiency and the underlying disease process increase the rate of catabolism and decrease the rate of anabolism (body tissue repair). The patient with AKI needs adequate nutrients and calories to prevent catabolism. Proteins

Medications
Acute Kidney Injury

CLASSIFICATION AND DRUG EXAMPLES	MECHANISMS OF ACTION	NURSING CONSIDERATIONS

Loop Diuretics
 	
Drug examples:
 	
Bumetanide (Bumex)
 	
Ethacrynic acid (Edecrin)
 	
Furosemide (Lasix)
 	
Torsemide (Demadex)
	The loop diuretics, named for their primary site of action in the loop of Henle, are high-ceiling diuretics (the response increases with increasing doses). These are highly effective diuretics used in early AKI to reestablish urine flow and convert oliguric renal failure to nonoliguric renal failure. Loop diuretics may be given with IV dopamine to promote renal blood flow. In ATN caused by a nephrotoxin, loop diuretics are used to clear the toxin from the nephrons more rapidly. Loop diuretics cause potassium wasting, which is generally not a concern in AKI because renal failure impairs normal potassium elimination.	■ Assess weight and vital signs for baseline data.
		■ Monitor I&O, daily weight (or more frequently as ordered), vital signs, skin turgor, and other indicators of fluid volume status frequently.
		■ Assess for orthostatic hypotension; these potent diuretics can lead to hypovolemia.
		■ Monitor laboratory results, especially serum electrolyte, glucose, BUN, and creatinine levels.
		■ Administer as ordered:
		  a. Furosemide, undiluted at a rate of no more than 20 mg/min
		  b. Ethacrynic acid, 50 mg diluted with 50 mL of normal saline, at a rate of no more than 10 mg/min
		  c. Bumetanide, undiluted over at least 1 min or diluted in lactated Ringer's solution, normal saline, or 5% dextrose in water for infusion
		  d. Torsemide, undiluted over at least 2 min.
		■ Assess response. Urine output typically increases within 10 min after IV administration.
		■ Monitor hearing and for complaints such as tinnitus. High doses of loop diuretics, especially ethnacrynic acid, increase the risk of ototoxicity in particular. These effects may be reversible if they are detected early and the drug is discontinued.
		■ Avoid administering concurrently with other ototoxic agents, such as aminoglycoside antibiotics and cisplatin.
		■ Patient teaching for the patient and family:
		  a. Unless contraindicated, maintain a fluid intake of 2–3 L per day.
		  b. Rise slowly from lying or sitting positions, because a fall in blood pressure may cause lightheadedness.
		  c. Take in the morning and, if ordered twice a day, in the late afternoon to avoid sleep disturbance.
		  d. Take with food or milk to prevent gastric distress.
		  e. NSAIDs interfere with the effectiveness of loop diuretics and should be avoided.

Medications *(continued)*

CLASSIFICATION AND DRUG EXAMPLES	MECHANISMS OF ACTION	NURSING CONSIDERATIONS
Osmotic Diuretics *Drug examples:* Mannitol (Osmitrol, Isotel) Urea (Ureaphil)	The osmotic diuretics act by increasing the osmotic draw in the blood and urine. In the blood, the effect is to pull extracellular water into the vascular system, increasing the GFR. These substances are then freely filtered in the glomerulus and increase the osmotic draw of the urine, inhibiting water reabsorption. The effect is to increase urine volume and flow. In addition, osmotic diuretics dilute waste products in the urine, decreasing the risk of renal damage because of excess concentrations.	■ Assess urine output. Osmotic diuretics are used in early renal failure to maintain urine output but are contraindicated in **anuria** (inability of kidneys to produce urine). A test dose may be administered; urine output of 30 mL/hr following the test dose shows an adequate response. ■ Do not give these diuretics to patients who have heart failure or are severely dehydrated. These drugs increase vascular volume and may worsen heart failure. They are not effective unless extracellular volume is adequate. ■ Administer mannitol intravenously, diluting before use if indicated. Check solution for crystallization. Dissolve crystals by warming the solution slightly. Infuse 15–25% mannitol solutions through a filter over 30–90 min. ■ Administer urea intravenously, diluting in 100 mL of 5 or 10% dextrose in water for every 30 g of urea. Administer no faster than 4 mL/min through a filter. ■ Monitor vital signs, breath sounds, and urinary output. ■ Discontinue the drug if signs of heart failure or pulmonary edema develop or if renal function continues to decline. ■ Patient teaching for the patient and family: Report shortness of breath, headache, chest pain, or dizziness immediately.

Electrolytes and Electrolyte Modifiers
 	
Drug examples:
Calcium chloride
Calcium gluconate
Sodium bicarbonate
Sodium polystyrene sulfonate (Kayexalate)
	Calcium chloride or gluconate and sodium bicarbonate are administered intravenously in the initial management of hyperkalemia. Calcium is also administered to correct hypocalcemia and reduce hyperphosphatemia. (Calcium and phosphate have a reciprocal relationship in the body; as the level of one rises, the level of the other falls.) Sodium bicarbonate helps to correct acidosis and move potassium back into the intracellular space. Sodium polystyrene sulfonate is not used to replace an electrolyte but to remove excess potassium from the body by exchanging sodium for potassium in the large intestine.	■ Assess serum electrolyte levels before and during therapy. Report rapid shifts or adverse responses to the physician.
		■ Administer as appropriate:
		  a. IV calcium chloride at less than 1 mL/min; IV calcium gluconate at 0.5 mL/min. Inject into a large vein through a small-bore needle; avoid infiltration, because extravasation of IV solution will cause tissue necrosis.
		  b. IV sodium bicarbonate infusion over 4–8 hr; oral tablets as prescribed.
		  c. Sodium polystyrene sulfonate as an oral solution mixed with sorbitol to prevent constipation, or as a retention enema mixed with warm water. Leave in the bowel for 30–60 min, irrigate using a small tap-water enema.
		■ Monitor for adverse reactions, such as dysrhythmias, electrolyte imbalances, and metabolic alkalosis.
		■ Patient teaching for the patient and family:
		  a. IV calcium may make you light-headed; remain in bed for at least 30 min after administration.
		  b. Chew sodium bicarbonate tablets and follow with 8 oz of water. Do not take with milk.
		  c. Retain the sodium polystyrene sulfonate enema as long as possible.

Source: Based on Adams, M. P., Holland, L. N., & Urban, C. (2017). *Pharmacology for nurses: A pathophysiologic approach* (5th ed.). Hoboken, NJ: Pearson Education.

are limited to 0.6 g/kg of body weight per day to minimize the degree of azotemia. Dietary proteins should be of high biological value (rich in essential amino acids). Carbohydrates are increased to maintain adequate calorie intake and provide a protein-sparing effect. For additional information, refer to the module on Nutrition.

Parenteral nutrition providing amino acids, concentrated carbohydrates, and fats may be instituted when the patient cannot consume an adequate diet (e.g., because of nausea, vomiting, or underlying critical illness). The disadvantages of parenteral nutrition in the patient with AKI are the high volume of fluid required and the risk for infection through the venous line.

Renal Replacement Therapy

Manifestations of uremia (urea in the blood), organ dysfunction caused by accumulated metabolic wastes, severe fluid overload, hyperkalemia, or metabolic acidosis in a patient

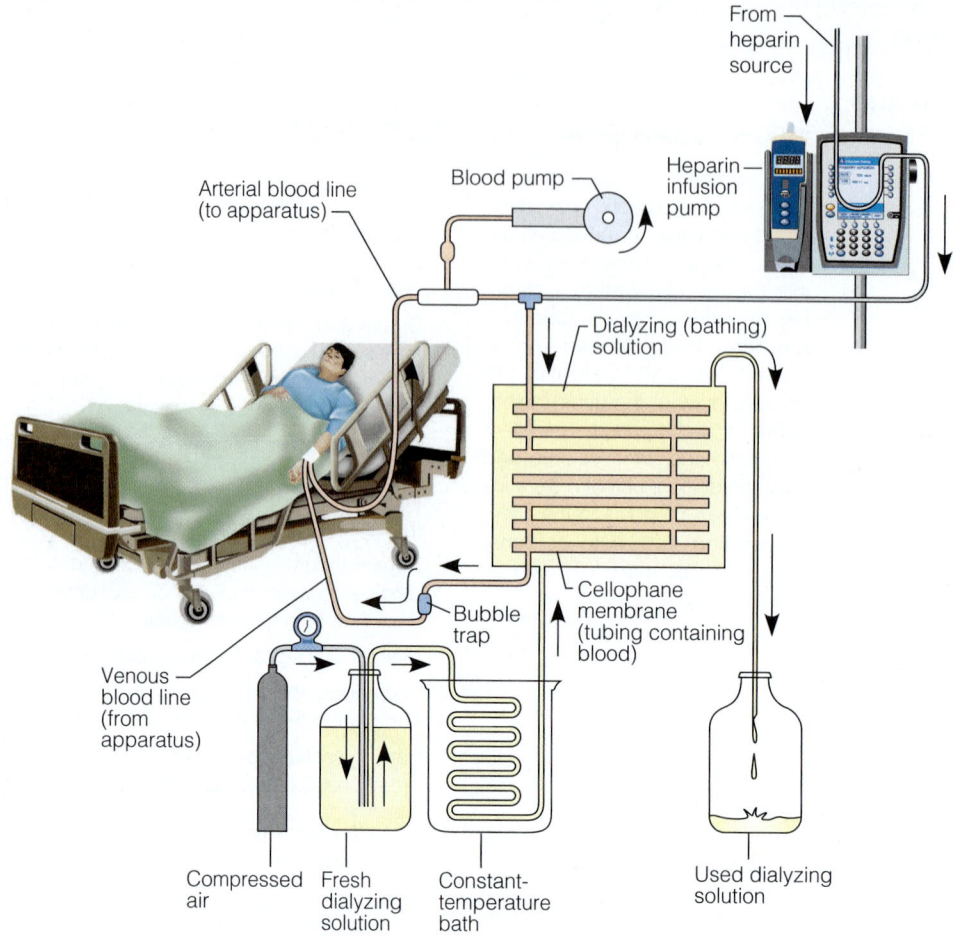

Arterial blood line
(to apparatus)

Blood pump

From heparin source

Heparin infusion pump

Dialyzing (bathing) solution

Cellophane membrane (tubing containing blood)

Venous blood line (from apparatus)

Bubble trap

Compressed air

Fresh dialyzing solution

Constant-temperature bath

Used dialyzing solution

Figure 6–17 ›› The components of a hemodialysis system.

with renal failure indicate a need to replace renal function. **Dialysis** is the diffusion of solute molecules across a semipermeable membrane from an area of higher solute concentration to one of lower concentration according to the rules of osmosis. It is used to remove excess fluid and metabolic waste products in renal failure. Dialysis may also be used to rapidly remove nephrotoxins in ATN. Although dialysis compensates for lost renal elimination functions, it does not replace lost erythropoietin production. Anemia is a continuing problem for the patient receiving dialysis.

In dialysis, blood is separated from a dialysis solution (**dialysate**) by a semipermeable membrane. The two most common forms of dialysis used to treat AKI are **hemodialysis**, a procedure in which the patient's blood flows through vascular catheters, is pumped through the dialyzer unit, and then is returned to the patient, and **peritoneal dialysis**, which uses the peritoneum surrounding the abdominal cavity as the dialyzing membrane. **Continuous renal replacement therapy (CRRT)**, in which blood is continuously circulated through a highly porous hemofilter from artery to vein or from vein to vein, is a newer form of dialysis that may be used to treat AKI.

Hemodialysis

Hemodialysis uses the principles of diffusion and ultrafiltration to remove electrolytes, waste products, and excess water from the body. Blood is taken from the patient via a vascular

access and is pumped to the dialyzer (see **Figure 6–17** ››). The porous membranes of the dialyzer unit allow small molecules (e.g., water, glucose, electrolytes) to pass through but block larger molecules (e.g., serum proteins, blood cells). The dialysate, a solution of approximately the same composition and temperature as normal ECF, passes along the other side of the membrane. Small solute molecules move freely across the membrane by diffusion. The direction of movement for any substance is determined by the concentrations of that substance in the blood and the dialysate. Electrolytes and waste products (e.g., urea, creatinine) diffuse from the blood into the dialysate. If it is necessary to add something to the blood, such as calcium to replace depleted stores, it can be added to the dialysate to diffuse into the blood. Excess water is removed by creating a hydrostatic pressure of the blood moving through the dialyzer that is higher than that of the dialysate, which flows in the opposite direction. This process is known as **ultrafiltration**.

Patients with AKI typically undergo daily hemodialysis initially. As their condition improves, they may change to three to four sessions per week as indicated. Hemodialysis is not used if the patient is hemodynamically unstable (e.g., with hypotension or low cardiac output). The following complications are associated with hemodialysis:

- Hypotension, the most frequent complication during hemodialysis, may result from changes in serum osmolality, rapid removal of fluid from the vascular compartment, vasodilation, and other factors.

- Bleeding may result from altered platelet function associated with uremia and the use of heparin during dialysis.

- Infection (local or systemic) may result from WBC damage and immune system suppression. *Staphylococcus aureus* septicemia is commonly associated with contamination of the vascular access site. Patients on chronic hemodialysis have higher rates of hepatitis B, hepatitis C, cytomegalovirus, and HIV infection than the general population.

》》 *Go to* **Pearson MyLab Nursing and eText** *to see Chart 1: Nursing Care for the Patient Undergoing Hemodialysis.*

Continuous Renal Replacement Therapy

Patients with AKI may be unable to tolerate hemodialysis and rapid fluid removal if their cardiovascular status is unstable (e.g., because of trauma, major surgery, or heart failure). Continuous renal replacement therapy (CRRT), which allows more gradual fluid and solute removal, often is used for these patients. In CRRT, blood is continuously circulated from an artery to a vein or from a vein to a vein through a highly porous hemofilter for a period of 12 hours or more. Excess water and solutes, such as electrolytes, urea, creatinine, uric acid, and glucose, drain into a collection device. Fluid may be replaced with normal saline or a balanced electrolyte solution as needed during CRRT. This slower process helps to maintain hemodynamic stability and avoid complications associated with rapid changes in composition of the ECF. The most common CRRT techniques are outlined in **Table 6–8** 》》.

CRRT is typically performed in an intensive care unit (ICU) or specialized nephrology unit. Both arterial and venous lines are required for some types of CRRT (see **Figure 6–18** 》》); for others, a double-lumen venous catheter is used. Strict aseptic technique is vital in caring for vascular access sites to reduce the risk of infection.

Vascular Access for Hemodialysis and Continuous Renal Replacement Therapy

Acute or temporary vascular access for hemodialysis or CRRT usually is gained by inserting a double-lumen catheter into the subclavian, jugular, or femoral vein. The double-lumen catheter has a central partition separating the blood-withdrawal side of the catheter from the return side. Blood is drawn into the catheter through small openings in the proximal

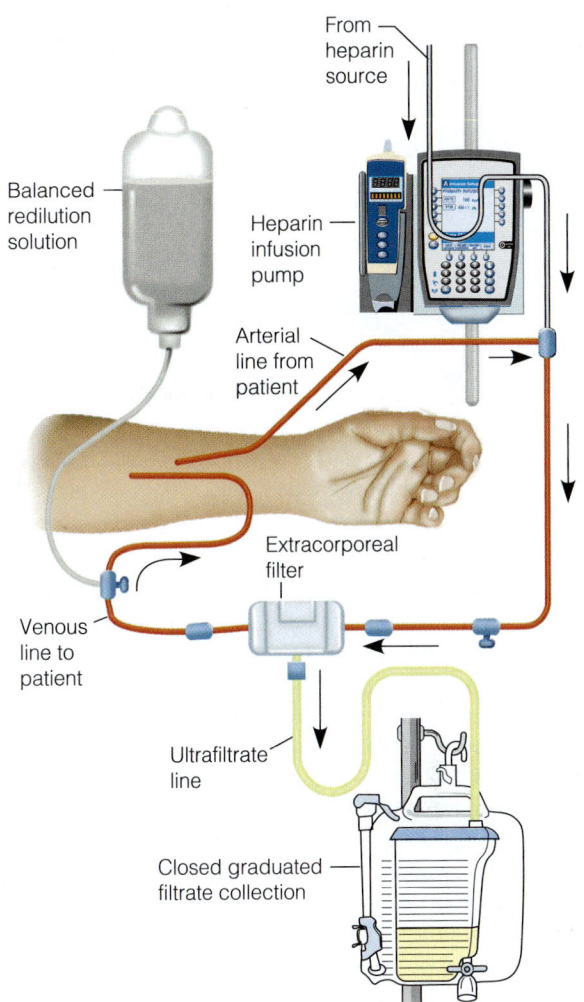

Figure 6–18 》》 Continuous arteriovenous hemofiltration.

portion of the catheter, and it is returned to the circulation through an opening in the distal end of the catheter to avoid withdrawing the blood that has just been dialyzed.

For longer-term vascular access, an **arteriovenous (AV) fistula** (an artificial connection between a vein and an artery) is created (see **Figure 6–19** 》》). In preparation for fistula formation, the nondominant arm is not used for venipuncture or blood pressure measurement during renal failure. The fistula is created by surgical anastomosis of an artery and vein, usually the radial artery and cephalic vein. It takes about a month for the fistula to mature so that it can be used

TABLE 6–8 Continuous Renal Replacement Therapies

Type	Indications	Description
Continuous arteriovenous hemofiltration (CAVH)	Removes fluid and some solutes	Arterial blood circulates through a hemofilter, then returns to the patient through a venous line; ultrafiltrate collects in a drainage bag.
Continuous arteriovenous hemodialysis (CAVHD)	Removes fluid and waste products	Arterial blood circulates through a hemofilter surrounded by dialysate, then returns to the patient through a venous line; ultrafiltrate collects in a drainage bag.
Continuous venovenous hemodialysis (CVVHD)	Removes fluid and waste products	Venous blood circulates through a hemofilter surrounded by dialysate, then returns to the patient through a double-lumen venous catheter; ultrafiltrate collects in a drainage bag.

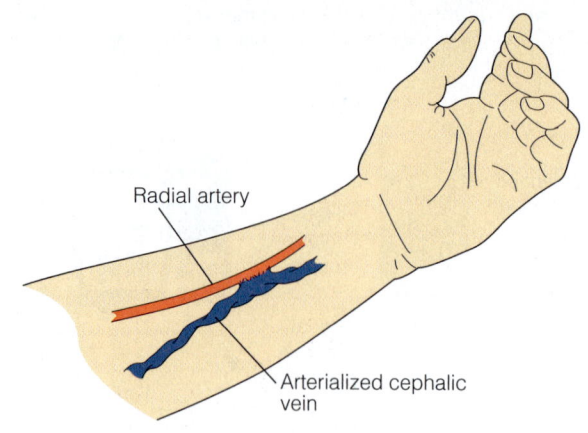

Figure 6–19 》 An arteriovenous fistula.

for taking and replacing blood during dialysis. A functional AV fistula has a palpable pulsation and a bruit on auscultation. The nurse should avoid venipunctures and blood pressures on the arm with the fistula.

In CKD, an AV graft is most often used for vascular access. The graft, a tube made of Gore-Tex, is surgically implanted and connects the artery and the vein. Blood flows through the graft from the artery to the vein. On occasion, an external AV shunt connecting a peripheral artery with a peripheral vein is used for vascular access. An AV fistula or graft ideally is created as soon as the potential need for long-term renal replacement therapies is identified (Al-Jaishi et al., 2016).

The rate of complications and mortality associated with catheter access is higher than with AV fistulas or grafts; however, localized AV fistula, graft, or shunt problems can occur. Infection and clotting or thrombosis are the most common shunt problems. Aneurysms may also develop. Both infection and thrombosis can lead to systemic manifestations, such as septicemia and embolization. These local complications may cause the fistula or graft to fail, necessitating development of a new site. The psychologic impact of AV fistula or graft failure is significant, often causing depression and low self-esteem.

Peritoneal Dialysis

In peritoneal dialysis, the highly vascular peritoneal membrane serves as the dialyzing surface (see **Figure 6–20** 》). Warmed, sterile dialysate is instilled through a catheter inserted into the peritoneal cavity. Metabolic waste products and excess electrolytes diffuse into the dialysate while it remains in the abdomen. The used fluid is then drained by gravity out of the peritoneal cavity into a sterile bag and disposed of. This process of dialysate infusion, dwell time of the solution in the abdomen, and drainage is repeated at prescribed intervals.

Because excess fluid and solutes are removed more gradually in peritoneal dialysis, this type of renal replacement therapy poses less risk than other methods for patients who are unstable; however, this slower rate of metabolite removal can be a disadvantage in patients with AKI, as it reduces waste removal. Peritoneal dialysis increases the risk for developing peritonitis, and it is contraindicated for patients

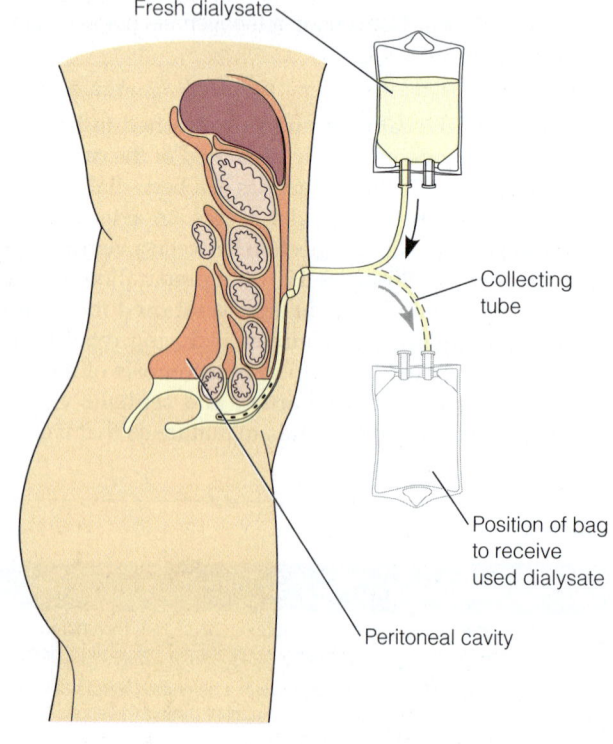

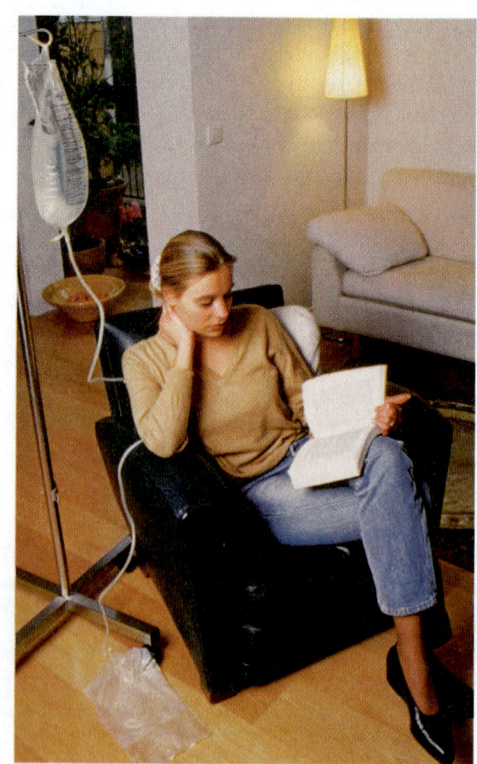

Source: Philippe Garo/Science Source.

Figure 6–20 》 **A,** Peritoneal dialysis. **B,** Woman receiving peritoneal dialysis.

who have had recent abdominal surgery, significant lung disease, or peritonitis.

>> Go to **Pearson MyLab Nursing and eText** to see Chart 2: Nursing Care for the Patient Undergoing Peritoneal Dialysis.

Lifespan Considerations

AKI in Infants

AKI in infants most commonly occurs in preterm infants. In fact, AKI can occur in up to 56% of infants in the neonatal intensive care unit. Potential causes include hemolytic uremic syndrome, acute glomerulonephritis, sepsis, poisoning, hypovolemia, obstructive uropathy, and complication of cardiac surgery. Predisposing factors include a low Apgar score, hypothermia, nephrotoxic drugs, dehydration, and congenital anomalies of the heart, especially a patent ductus arteriosus (PDA). Low birth weight is also a predisposing factor (Carmody et al., 2014). Asphyxia before and during delivery is also a causative factor (Saboute et al., 2016). Hematologic-oncologic complications, bone marrow transplantation, and respiratory failure have recently become more common causes of AKI in children. In some cases, a combination of factors leads to the development of AKI. AKI is associated with high mortality in preterm newborns. Children who recover from AKI may have residual kidney damage and compromised renal function (Stojanović et al., 2014).

AKI in Children and Adolescents

Pediatric manifestations of AKI characteristically begin with a healthy child who suddenly becomes ill with nonspecific symptoms that indicate a significant illness or injury. These symptoms may include any combination of the following: nausea, vomiting, lethargy, edema, gross **hematuria** (blood in the urine), oliguria, and hypertension. These manifestations result from electrolyte imbalances (see **Table 6–9 >>**), uremia (excessive amounts of urea in the blood), and fluid overload. The child appears pale and lethargic.

Initial emergency treatment of children with fluid depletion associated with AKI focuses on rapid fluid replacement with 20 mL/kg of saline or lactated Ringer's solution given over 5–10 minutes and repeated as needed. This ensures that renal perfusion and stabilizes blood pressure. Albumin may also be administered when blood loss is the cause of the patient's circulatory depletion. If oliguria persists after restoration of adequate fluid volume, intrinsic renal damage is suspected.

SAFETY ALERT The unexpected and acute nature of a child's hospitalization creates anxiety for both parents and the child. Assess for feelings of anger, guilt, or fear associated with the hospitalization. Such feelings are likely if AKI developed as a result of dehydration, a preventable injury, or poisoning. Assess coping mechanisms, family support systems, and level of stress.

AKI in Pregnant Women

During pregnancy, glomerular filtration rate increases significantly, perhaps by as much as 50%. This leads to a decrease in baseline serum creatinine and other changes associated with the increased blood volume that pregnancy brings. AKI in pregnant woman is often related to the same etiologies as are identified in the general population. However, there are unique etiologies that manifest themselves throughout the pregnancy cycle. Over 90% of women develop a physiologic hydronephrosis of pregnancy, and this can promote urinary stasis, lead to urinary tract infection, and ultimately lead to AKI (Machado et al., 2012). In addition, in the first trimester, hyperemesis gravidarum and placenta previa may lead to AKI, and as pregnancy progresses, pregnancy-induced hypertension, preeclampsia, and eclampsia stress the kidneys, leading to proteinuria, hydronephrosis, and AKI (Bajwa et al., 2013). It should be noted that the incidence of AKI and mortality worldwide is associated with sepsis that can follow illegal

---

TABLE 6–9 Electrolyte Imbalances in Acute and Chronic Kidney Disease in Children

Electrolyte Imbalance	Cause	Clinical Manifestations
Hyperkalemia (excess potassium in the blood)	Hyperkalemia results from the inability to adequately excrete potassium derived from diet and catabolized cells. In metabolic acidosis, potassium also moves from ICF to ECF.	■ Peaked T waves, widening of QRS waves on electrocardiogram ■ Dysrhythmias: ventricular dysrhythmias, heart block, ventricular fibrillation, cardiac arrest ■ Diarrhea ■ Muscle weakness
Hyponatremia (decreased sodium in the blood)	In the acute oliguric phase, hyponatremia is dilutional, related to the accumulation of fluid in excess of solute.	■ Change in LOC ■ Muscle cramps ■ Anorexia ■ Abdominal reflexes, depressed deep tendon reflexes ■ Cheyne-Stokes respirations ■ Seizures
Hypocalcemia (decreased calcium in the blood)	Phosphate retention (hyperphosphatemia) caused by impaired renal function depresses the serum calcium concentration. Calcium is deposited in injured cells. Hyperkalemia and metabolic acidosis may mask the common clinical manifestations of severe hypocalcemia.	■ Muscle tingling ■ Changes in muscle tone ■ Seizures ■ Muscle cramps and twitching ■ Positive Chvostek sign (contraction of the facial muscles after tapping the facial nerve just anterior to the parotid gland)

abortion. Puerperal sepsis and postpartum hemorrhage are the leading causes of AKI in the postpartum period (Krishna et al., 2015).

AKI in Older Adults

Advancing age is a risk factor for AKI. Decreased renal reserve and declining function interfere with the kidney's ability to recover from AKI (Kane-Gill et al., 2015). Structural changes, including reduction in cortical mass, hyperfiltration of the glomerulus associated with hypertrophy, and thickening of the renal artery lead to decreased blood flow and further risk of AKI in older adults (Hain & Paixao, 2015). In the critical care setting, there is a 20% greater rate of AKI among older adults than younger adults. Etiology of AKI in older adults includes sepsis and the presence of polypharmacy, especially nephrotoxic drugs such as NSAIDs. Older adults who have undergone lifesaving cardiac care, such as heart valve or bypass surgery, are also at high risk for AKI (Cho et al., 2015).

NURSING PROCESS

AKI often can be prevented by measures that maintain fluid volume and cardiac output and reduce the risk of exposure to nephrotoxins. The nurse should carefully monitor critically ill, postoperative, and other at-risk patients for early signs of hypovolemia (low urine output; altered mental status; and changes in vital signs, skin color, or temperature). The nurse should promptly report a fall in urine output to less than 30 mL/hr in adult patients and other evidence of decreased cardiac output. In addition, the nurse should maintain IV fluids as ordered. The nurse should also alert the healthcare provider if the patient is receiving more than one nephrotoxic drug or if a nephrotoxic drug is ordered for a patient who is dehydrated. The nurse should closely observe patients receiving blood or blood components for early signs of transfusion reaction and intervene appropriately as needed.

Assessment

Both subjective and objective data are useful in assessing the patient with AKI. The patient's history and physical assessment can provide clues about the initiating event for AKI. Impaired perfusion for as few as 30 minutes may cause significant renal ischemia, so obtaining a thorough history is essential. For pediatric and older patients, assessments should include input from immediate family members or caregivers.

- **Observation and patient interview.** Ask patients about complaints of anorexia, nausea, weight gain, or edema; recent exposure to a nephrotoxin, such as an aminoglycoside antibiotic or radiologic procedure using an injected contrast medium; previous transfusion reaction; and chronic diseases, such as diabetes, heart failure, or kidney disease.
- **Physical examination.** Assess vital signs, including temperature; urine output (amount, color, clarity, specific gravity, presence of blood cells or protein); weight; skin color; peripheral pulses; presence of edema (periorbital or dependent); and lung, heart, and bowel sounds.

Diagnosis

The patient with AKI has numerous nursing care needs related both to the renal failure and to the underlying condition that precipitated it. Priority nursing care needs relate to fluid volume alterations, appetite and nutrition, and teaching/learning. Appropriate nursing diagnoses may include any of the following:

- *Fluid Volume: Excess*
- *Imbalanced Nutrition: Less than Body Requirements*
- *Perfusion: Renal, Risk for Ineffective*
- *Skin Integrity, Risk for Impaired*
- *Tissue Perfusion: Cardiac, Risk for Decreased*
- *Infection, Risk for*
- *Family Coping, Compromised.*

(NANDA-I © 2014)

Planning

Nursing care focuses on preventing complications, maintaining fluid balance, administering medications, meeting nutritional needs, preventing infection, and providing emotional support to the patient and family. Possible outcomes, created in collaboration with the patient and family, include the following:

- The patient's weight will return to baseline measurement.
- The patient's urine output will be greater than 30 mL/hr.
- The patient's hemoglobin and hematocrit values will be within normal limits.
- The patient's serum electrolytes will be within normal limits.
- The patient's pulse rate, volume, and rhythm will return to baseline.

Implementation

The care of each patient will vary on the basis of the cause of AKI and the specific needs of the individual patient. Ensuring compliance with the treatment plan is the best way to prevent complications. Careful monitoring of vital signs, I&O, serum electrolytes, and LOC can alert the nurse to changes that indicate potential complications. The nurse should be sensitive to any cultural or religious practices, even if it means scheduling appointments or nursing activities around scheduled prayer times. The nurse should do the following:

- Maintain hourly I&O records. Accurate I&O records help to guide therapy, especially fluid restrictions.
- Weigh the patient daily or more frequently as ordered. Use standard technique (same scale, clothing, or coverings) to ensure accuracy. Rapid weight changes are an accurate indicator of fluid volume status, particularly in the patient with oliguria.
- Assess vital signs at least every 4 hours. Hypertension, tachycardia, and tachypnea may indicate excess fluid volume.
- Assess breath and heart sounds, neck veins for distention, and back and extremities for edema; report abnormal findings.

- If not contraindicated, place patient in semi-Fowler position to enhance cardiac and respiratory function.
- Report abnormal serum electrolyte values and manifestations of electrolyte imbalance. The patient with AKI is at particular risk for the following electrolyte imbalances:
  a. **Hyperkalemia** caused by impaired potassium excretion. Manifestations include irritability, nausea, diarrhea, abdominal cramping, cardiac dysrhythmias, and electrocardiographic changes.
  b. **Hyponatremia** caused by water retention. Manifestations include nausea, vomiting, and headache, with possible central nervous system manifestations of lethargy, confusion, seizures, and coma. If the serum sodium concentration rises and the patient's weight falls, insufficient fluids are being administered. If the serum sodium level falls and the patient's weight increases, excessive fluids are being administered.
  c. **Hyperphosphatemia** caused by decreased phosphate excretion. Manifestations include hyperreflexia, paresthesias, and possible **tetany** (tonic muscle spasms). AKI impairs electrolyte and water excretion, causing multiple electrolyte imbalances.
- Turn the patient frequently, and provide good skin care. Edema decreases tissue perfusion and increases the risk of skin breakdown, especially in patients who are older or debilitated.
- Restrict fluids as ordered. Provide frequent mouth care, and encourage use of hard candies to decrease thirst. If ice chips are allowed, include the water content (approximately half the total volume) as intake. Fluids are restricted to minimize fluid retention and complications of FVE.
- Administer medications with meals. Giving oral medications with meals minimizes ingestion of excess fluids.

Address Nutrition Imbalances

Anorexia and nausea associated with renal failure often interfere with food intake and good nutrition. In addition, the disease process leading to AKI may contribute to increased nutritional needs for healing concurrently with decreased food intake. Interventions for patients experiencing inadequate nutrition include the following:

- Monitor and record food intake, including the amount and type of food consumed. A detailed intake record helps to guide decisions about nutritional status and necessary supplements.
- Weigh the patient daily. Weight changes over time (days to weeks) reflect nutritional status, whereas rapid weight changes are more reflective of fluid volume status. In AKI, weight may remain stable or increase because of fluid retention even though tissue mass is being lost.
- Arrange for consultation with a dietitian. A registered dietitian can assist in planning meals within prescribed limitations that consider the patient's food preferences, especially if the patient follows cultural or religious mandates regarding foods. Diets restricted in protein, salt, and potassium can be unpalatable; intake and

appetite improve when preferred foods are included as allowed.
- Engage the patient in planning daily menus. Participation in meal planning increases the patient's sense of control and autonomy.
- Allow family members to prepare meals within dietary restrictions. Encourage family members to eat with the patient. Familiar foods and social interaction encourage eating and increase enjoyment of meals.

SAFETY ALERT Remember that AKI requires nutritional intervention. In children and adolescents with AKI, these interventions must take into consideration the particular nutritional needs brought about by growth and development, which may include additional calorie intake as well as consideration of increasing protein foods of high biologic value such as eggs, poultry, or fish.

- Provide frequent, small meals or between-meal snacks. These measures promote food intake in the patient who is fatigued or anorectic.
- Administer antiemetics as ordered, and provide mouth care before meals. Nausea and a metallic taste in the mouth, common manifestations of uremia, can decrease food intake.
- Administer parenteral nutrition as ordered if the patient is unable to eat or tolerate enteral nutrition. Preventing or slowing tissue **catabolism** (the breakdown of body proteins) is important for the patient with AKI.

Provide Patient Teaching

Patient teaching is essential to resolving AKI and preventing any further complications. Before providing any information, the nurse should assess the patient's anxiety level and ability to comprehend instructions; the patient with AKI may be critically ill or be experiencing uremic effects that hinder learning. During the initial stages of AKI, it may be necessary to limit information to immediate concerns, such as treatment of the underlying cause of kidney failure. The nurse should tailor the information and presentation to the patient's developmental level as well as physical, mental, and emotional status. The nurse should do the following:

- Assess knowledge and understanding. To enhance understanding and retention, relate the information presented to previous learning.
- Teach the patient and immediate family about diagnostic tests and therapeutic procedures. Teaching reduces anxiety and improves understanding and cooperation.
- Discuss dietary and fluid restrictions. These measures may be continued after discharge.
- If the patient is discharged before the recovery phase of AKI, teach the signs and symptoms of complications, including FVE or FVD, heart failure, and electrolyte imbalances. Explain to the patient that urine output increases as kidney function returns, but that the concentrating ability of the nephrons and electrolyte excretion remain impaired. This impaired function increases the

risk of excess fluid loss, possible dehydration, orthostatic hypotension, and electrolyte imbalance.

- Teach the patient how to monitor weight, blood pressure, and pulse. These are important means of assessing fluid status.

- Instruct the patient to avoid nephrotoxic drugs and chemicals for up to 1 year following an episode of AKI. During recovery, nephrons are vulnerable to damage by nephrotoxins, such as NSAIDs, some antibiotics, radiologic contrast media, and heavy metals. Because alcohol can increase the nephrotoxicity of some materials, discourage alcohol ingestion.

Evaluation

Evaluation of the patient with AKI is based on resolution of symptoms and prevention of complications. Data to be evaluated include weight, cardiac rhythm, vital signs, breath sounds, oxygen saturation, serum electrolyte levels, I&O, and hemoglobin and hematocrit. The patient should be evaluated for response to treatment as well as for under-

standing of the disease process and self-care requirements. Expected outcomes of nursing care include the following:

- The patient maintains fluid, electrolyte, and acid–base balance, as evidenced by absence of signs and symptoms of imbalance.

- The patient's nutritional needs are met, as evidenced by dietary recall, return to appropriate weight, and absence of signs and symptoms of nutrition imbalance.

- The patient acquires no secondary infections.

If the expected outcomes are unmet, the patient may need referral to other specialists, such as a dietitian. Should symptoms of infection arise (e.g., elevated body temperature, rise in WBC counts, general complaints of increasing malaise), the patient should be referred to the healthcare provider. Psychologic support may also be necessary, and the nurse can refer the patient to a social worker or perhaps a chaplain or clergy. It will be important to include family members in these discussions as well.

Nursing Care Plan

A Patient with AKI

Judy Devak was driving home late one evening when she lost control of her car while trying to avoid a deer in the road. Her car struck a tree and rolled into a deep ditch beside the road, out of sight of passing cars. The wreck was not discovered until 2 hours later. On arrival at the accident scene, the paramedics found Ms. Devak

hypotensive: pulse 120 bpm, respirations 24/min, BP 90/60 mmHg. She was alert and in severe pain, with a fractured right femur. After immobilizing Ms. Devak's neck and back and extricating her from the car, the paramedics applied a traction splint to her leg and transported her to the local hospital.

ASSESSMENT	DIAGNOSES	PLANNING
On Ms. Devak's admission to the ICU, Katie Leaper, RN, obtains a nursing history. Ms. Devak indicates that she has been healthy, having experienced only minor illnesses and chickenpox as a child. She has never been hospitalized and has no known allergies to medications. She is not currently taking prescription or nonprescription drugs. Physical assessment findings include temperature 36.3°C (97.4°F) oral, pulse 100 bpm, respirations 18/min, and BP 124/68 mmHg. Ms. Devak's skin is pale, cool, and dry, with multiple scrapes, minor abrasions, and bruises on her face and extremities. Nurse Leaper notes a linear bruise on Ms. Devak's chest and abdomen from the seat belt. Ms. Devak's lung sounds are clear, heart tones normal, and abdomen tender but soft to palpation. Right leg alignment is maintained with skeletal traction. One unit of whole blood was infused before ICU admission; a second unit is currently infusing. An indwelling urinary catheter and a nasogastric tube are in place. During the first few hours after admission, Nurse Leaper notes that Ms. Devak's hourly output has dropped from 55 to 45 to 28 mL of clear yellow urine. The physician orders a 500 mL IV fluid challenge, STAT urinalysis, BUN, and serum creatinine. The fluid challenge elicits only a slight increase in urine output. Urinalysis results show a specific gravity of 1.010 and the presence of WBCs, red and white cell casts, and tubular epithelial cells in the sediment. Ms. Devak's BUN is 28 mg/dL; her serum creatinine is 1.5 mg/dL. The physician diagnoses probable AKI and orders a nephrology consultation. In addition, the physician orders aluminum hydroxide, 10 mL every 2 hours via nasogastric tube, and ranitidine, 50 mg intravenously every 8 hours.	▪ *Acute Pain* related to injuries sustained in the accident ▪ *Anxiety* related to being in the ICU ▪ *Risk for Excess Fluid Volume* related to impaired renal function ▪ *Impaired Physical Mobility* related to skeletal traction ▪ *Ineffective Protection* related to injuries and invasive procedures (NANDA-I © 2014)	▪ The patient will report adequate pain control. ▪ The patient will verbalize reduced anxiety. ▪ The patient will maintain stable weight and vital signs within normal range. ▪ The patient will maintain skin integrity. ▪ The patient will use the trapeze appropriately to adjust her position in bed while maintaining body alignment. ▪ The patient will remain free of infection, bleeding, or respiratory distress.

Nursing Care Plan *(continued)*

IMPLEMENTATION

- Maintain patient-controlled anesthesia.
- Assess frequently for pain control and response to analgesia.
- Encourage expression of thoughts, feelings, and fears about the patient's condition and placement in the ICU.
- Document vital signs and heart and lung sounds at least every 4 hours.
- Weigh every 12 hours.
- Document hourly I&O.

- Restrict fluids as ordered, including diluent for all IV medications as intake.
- Assist with mouth care every 3–4 hours; allow frequent rinsing of mouth and ice chips as allowed.
- Assist with position changes at least every 2 hours; teach use of the overhead trapeze.
- Monitor frequently for signs of infection, bleeding, or respiratory distress.

EVALUATION

After just over 3 days of oliguria, Ms. Devak's urine output increases. By the end of the fourth day, she is excreting 60–80 mL/hr of urine. Although her BUN, serum creatinine, and potassium levels remain high, they never reach a critical point, and dialysis is not required. She is transferred from the ICU on the fifth day after admission. When Ms. Devak is able to begin eating, she is placed on a low-potassium diet and restricted to 50 g of protein. Her renal function gradually improves. By discharge, results of her renal function studies, including BUN and serum creatinine, are nearly normal. Ms. Devak verbalizes an understanding of the need to avoid nephrotoxins, such as NSAIDs, until allowed by her physician.

CRITICAL THINKING

1. What was the most likely specific precipitating factor for Ms. Devak's AKI? Did anything else contribute to her risk?
2. Why did the physician prescribe aluminum hydroxide and ranitidine? Consider both the AKI and Ms. Devak's placement in the ICU.
3. Ms. Devak is at risk for respiratory distress related to potential FVE. How does her fractured femur further contribute to her risk for respiratory distress?
4. Develop a care plan for Ms. Devak for the nursing diagnosis of *Deficient Diversional Activity*.

REVIEW Acute Kidney Injury

RELATE Link the Concepts and Exemplars

Linking the exemplar of AKI with the concept of elimination:

1. Nurses often are so busy that they do not take time to use the restroom until they can no longer postpone urination. Explain how this behavior increases the risk of AKI.
2. How would you teach a patient who reported this behavior to reduce the patient's risk of AKI?

Linking the exemplar of AKI with the concept of acid–base balance:

3. What laboratory results would you review to determine the acid–base balance of the patient with AKI?
4. What acid–base finding would you anticipate when caring for a patient with AKI?

READY Go to Volume 3: Clinical Nursing Skills

REFER Go to Pearson MyLab Nursing and eText

- Additional review materials
- Chart 1: Nursing Care for the Patient Undergoing Hemodialysis
- Chart 2: Nursing Care for the Patient Undergoing Peritoneal Dialysis

REFLECT Apply Your Knowledge

Missy Sengstadt is a healthy 4-year-old who seems to be in perpetual motion. She came home from preschool yesterday and told her mother she was tired and wanted to take a nap. Ms. Sengstadt immediately sensed that there was something wrong, because Missy never volunteers to take a nap. Missy's appetite was diminished at dinner, and although she appeared pale, she went to bed that night without complaint.

This morning, Missy looked very ill, refused to get out of bed, and had not urinated since 8 p.m. the evening before. Ms. Sengstadt brought Missy to the pediatrician's office, where Missy was diagnosed with ATN. Her pediatrician admitted Missy to the local acute care facility. You are the nurse admitting Missy to the pediatric unit.

1. What questions would you ask Ms. Sengstadt to determine contributory factors to the development of ATN in Missy?
2. What orders would you anticipate from the healthcare provider to prevent the development of AKI?
3. What independent nursing orders would you develop to provide holistic, family-centered care for Missy?
4. What nursing diagnosis would be appropriate for Missy's plan of care?

» Exemplar 6.C
Chronic Kidney Disease

Exemplar Learning Outcomes

6.C Analyze chronic kidney disease (CKD) as it relates to fluids and electrolytes.

- Describe the pathophysiology of CKD.
- Describe the etiology of CKD.
- Compare the risk factors for and prevention of CKD.
- Identify the clinical manifestations of CKD.
- Summarize diagnostic tests and therapies used by interprofessional teams in the collaborative care of an individual with CKD.
- Differentiate considerations for care of patients with CKD across the lifespan.

- Apply the nursing process in providing culturally competent care to an individual with CKD.

Exemplar Key Terms

Chronic kidney disease (CKD), *414*
End-stage renal disease (ESRD), *414*
Nephrectomy, *422*
Paresthesias, *418*
Uremia, *416*
Uremic fetor, *418*
Uremic frost, *419*

Overview

The internal environment of the body normally remains in a relatively constant or homeostatic state. The kidneys help maintain homeostasis by regulating the composition and volume of ECF. They excrete excess water and solutes and, when deficits occur, can conserve water and solutes. In addition, the kidneys help to regulate acid–base balance, and they excrete metabolic wastes. Regulation of blood pressure is also a key function of the kidneys.

Both primary kidney disorders (e.g., glomerulonephritis) and systemic diseases (e.g., diabetes mellitus) can affect renal function. In North America, more than 26 million individuals have CKD, and 73 million (1 in 3 individuals) are at increased risk for some type of kidney disease (National Kidney Foundation, 2013). Every year, approximately 3.6 of every 1000 individuals in the United States develop **end-stage renal disease (ESRD)**, the final phase of **chronic kidney disease (CKD)**, in which little or no kidney function remains. CKD is a major cause of lost work time and wages (U.S. Renal Data System, 2016). Ironically, the increased prevalence of CKD in recent years is partially related to the success of dialysis and transplantation.

Renal function is dependent on an adequate supply of blood. Blood supports renal cell metabolism and is vital to kidney function, the nephron in particular. Only with sufficient blood supply can the kidney regulate fluid, electrolyte, and acid–base balance and serve as a major organ of excretion. Vascular disorders, therefore, can have a significant impact on renal function. Hypertension causes arteriosclerotic lesions in the afferent (leading into) and efferent (going out of) arterioles and the glomerular capillaries. The GFR declines, and tubular function is affected, resulting in proteinuria and microscopic hematuria. Approximately 10% of deaths attributed to hypertension result from renal failure (Yang et al., 2014).

Although the kidneys usually recover from acute injury, many chronic conditions can lead to progressive renal tissue destruction and loss of function. Nephron units are lost, and renal mass decreases, with progressive deterioration of glomerular filtration, tubular secretion, and reabsorption. CKD may progress slowly for many years without being recognized. The kidneys eventually are unable to excrete metabolic wastes and to regulate fluid and electrolyte balance adequately—the condition known as ESRD. Because of the increasing prevalence of CKD and ESRD, *Healthy People 2020* selected CKD as one of its focus areas (see **Box 6–5** »).

Box 6–5
Healthy People 2020: **Chronic and End-Stage Renal Disease**

Prevalence	Objectives	Actions
<ul><li>In 1999–2004, 15.1% of the U.S. population had CKD. The 2020 target is to reduce that rate to 13.6% (Office of Disease Prevention and Health Promotion, 2017).</li><li>ESRD results from chronic damage to the kidneys over a decade or more.</li><li>Diabetes and hypertension increase the risk for ESRD.</li><li>The number of new cases of ESRD is increasing and correlates to an increase in cases of type 2 diabetes mellitus.</li><li>African Americans are at the highest risk for renal disease.</li><li>American Indians, Native Alaskans, Asians, and Pacific Islanders also have increased risk.</li><li>Mexicans have a high risk for renal disease related to a higher incidence of type 2 diabetes mellitus.</li></ul>	<ul><li>Reduce the proportion of U.S. citizens with CKD.</li><li>Improve the cardiovascular care of people with CKD.</li><li>Reduce the number of deaths among people with CKD.</li><li>Reduce the number of new cases of ESRD.</li><li>Reduce kidney failure related to diabetes.</li><li>Increase the proportion of patients with a chronic disease receiving care from a nephrologist at least 12 months before the start of renal replacement therapy.</li></ul>	<ul><li>Early identification of people at risk</li><li>Control of diabetes and hypertension</li><li>Education related to diet and exercise</li></ul>

TABLE 6–10 Pathophysiology of Chronic Kidney Disease

Cause	Examples
Diabetic nephropathy	Initial increases in glomerular flow rate lead to hyperfiltration with eventual glomerular damage and thickening and sclerosis of the glomerular basement membrane and the glomerulus; gradual destruction of nephrons leads to a fall in GFR.
Hypertensive nephrosclerosis	Long-standing hypertension leads to sclerosis and narrowing of renal arterioles and small arteries with subsequent reduction of blood flow. This leads to ischemia, glomerular destruction, and tubular atrophy.
Chronic glomerulonephritis	Chronic interstitial inflammation of renal parenchyma leads to obstruction and damage to the tubules and capillaries that surround them, affecting glomerular filtration and tubular secretion and reabsorption, with gradual loss of entire nephrons.
Chronic pyelonephritis	Chronic infection commonly associated with an obstructive or neurologic process and vesicoureteral reflux leads to scarring and deformity of renal calyces and pelvis, resulting in intrarenal reflux and nephropathy.
Polycystic kidney disease	Multiple bilateral cysts gradually compress renal tissue, impairing renal perfusion and leading to ischemia, renal vascular remodeling, and release of inflammatory mediators, which damage and destroy normal kidney tissue.
Systemic lupus erythematosus	Immune complexes form in capillary basement membrane leading to inflammation and sclerosis, with focal, local, or diffuse glomerulonephritis.

Pathophysiology and Etiology

Pathophysiology

The pathophysiology of CKD varies depending on the underlying disease process and involves gradual destruction of entire nephron units. In the early stages, as nephrons are lost, remaining functional nephrons hypertrophy (enlarge as a result of an increase in size of the constituent cells). Glomerular capillary flow and pressure increase in these nephrons, and more solute particles are filtered to compensate for lost renal mass. This increased demand predisposes the remaining nephrons to glomerular sclerosis (scarring), resulting in their eventual destruction. Proteinuria resulting from glomerular damage is thought to contribute to tubular injury. This process of continued loss of nephron function may persist even after the initial disease process has resolved (Noone & Licht, 2014). **Table 6–10** ⟫ outlines common pathologic processes leading to nephron destruction and ESRD.

The course of CKD is variable, progressing over a period of months to many years. In the early stage, known as decreased renal reserve, unaffected nephrons compensate for the lost nephrons. The GFR is approximately 50% of normal, and the patient is asymptomatic, with normal BUN and serum creatinine levels. As the disease progresses and the GFR falls further, hypertension and some manifestations of renal insufficiency may be seen. Any further insult to the kidneys (e.g., infection, dehydration, exposure to nephrotoxins, urinary tract obstruction) at this stage can further reduce function and precipitate the onset of renal failure or overt uremia. The serum creatinine and BUN levels rise sharply (see **Figure 6–21** ⟫), the patient becomes oliguric, and manifestations of uremia are seen. Finally, in ESRD, the GFR is less than 10–15% of normal, and renal replacement therapy is necessary to sustain life. **Table 6–11** ⟫ summarizes the stages of CKD.

Etiology

Twenty-six million American adults have CKD, the precursor to ESRD, and millions more are at increased risk. Kidney disease is the ninth leading cause of death in the United States. An estimated 31 million people have CKD (American Kidney Fund, 2015). ESRD rates are more than 3 times

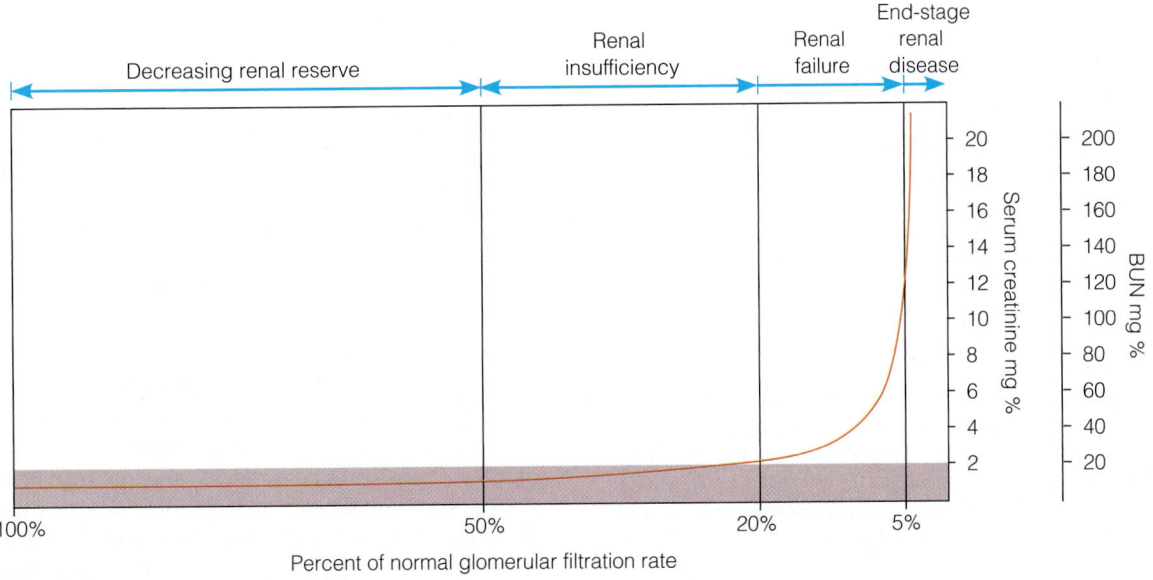

Figure 6–21 ⟫ The relationship of renal function to BUN and serum creatinine values through the course of chronic renal disease.

TABLE 6–11 Stages of Chronic Kidney Disease

Stage	Glomerular Filtration Rate	Description and Manifestations
Stage 1	>90 mL/min/1.73 m^2	Kidney damage with normal or increased GFR
		Asymptomatic; normal BUN and creatinine
Stage 2	60–89 mL/min/1.73 m^2	Mildly decreased GFR
		Asymptomatic, possible hypertension; blood work generally within normal limits
Stage 3	30–59 mL/min/1.73 m^2	Moderate GFR decrease
		Hypertension; possible anemia and fatigue, anorexia, possible malnutrition, bone pain; slight elevation of BUN and serum creatinine
Stage 4	15–29 mL/min/1.73 m^2	Severely decreased GFR
		Hypertension, anemia, malnutrition, altered bone metabolism; edema, metabolic acidosis, hypercalcemia; possible uremia; azotemia with increasing BUN and serum creatinine levels
Stage 5	<15 mL/min/1.73 m^2	ESRD
		Kidney failure with azotemia and overt uremia

Based on Renal Association. (2013). *The stages of kidney disease.* Retrieved from http://www.renal.org/information-resources/the-uk-eckd-guide/ckd-stages#sthash.epEDkCW7.dpbs

higher for African Americans than for Caucasians (Kazley et al., 2014), especially patients with hypertension (National Kidney Foundation, 2016a; Tanner et al., 2015). (See the Focus on Diversity and Culture feature.) The incidence of ESRD is increasing most rapidly in older adults. Although many patients report satisfaction with their quality of life, patients on dialysis are often unable to work, treatment regimens are time consuming and costly, and family structures may disintegrate under the strain (National Kidney and Urologic Diseases Information Clearinghouse [NKUDIC], 2012).

Risk Factors

Conditions that cause CKD typically involve diffuse, bilateral disease of the kidneys with progressive destruction and scarring of the entire nephron. Diabetes is the leading cause of ESRD in all population groups in the United States. Hypertension closely follows diabetes as a major cause of ESRD; in many patients, these disorders coexist (U.S. Renal Data System, 2016).

Focus on Diversity and Culture
African Americans and Kidney Disease

African Americans are nearly three times as likely to develop kidney disease as white populations. Among new patients with kidney disease resulting from high blood pressure, more than half are African American. Among new patients with kidney disease resulting from diabetes, more than one third are African American. Considering that African Americans make up approximately 12% of the population of the United States, these figures are significant. Because kidney disease resulting from diabetes or high blood pressure accounts for 70% of new cases, nurses working with African American patients who have high blood pressure or diabetes should take the opportunity for patient teaching at every healthcare visit. It is critical for African American patients with high blood pressure or diabetes to understand the risk for kidney disease and the importance of following their treatment regimens (Kazley et al., 2014; Tanner et al., 2015).

Prevention

According to the National Kidney Foundation, prevention of both ESRD and CKD should focus on aggressive management of chronic disease states, especially diabetes and hypertension. In addition, patients should consume diets low in sodium, exercise regularly, keep healthcare provider appointments, avoid smoking, and limit alcohol intake (American Kidney Fund, 2013; Mayo Clinic, 2016).

Clinical Manifestations

CKD often is not identified until its final, uremic stage is reached. **Uremia**, which literally means "urea in the blood," refers to the syndrome or group of symptoms associated with ESRD. In uremia, fluid and electrolyte balance is altered, the regulatory and endocrine functions of the kidney are impaired, and accumulated metabolic waste products affect essentially every other organ system (Connell & Laing, 2015). Early manifestations of uremia include nausea, apathy, weakness, and fatigue—symptoms that typically are dismissed as a viral infection or influenza. As the condition progresses, frequent vomiting, increasing weakness, lethargy, and confusion develop (Connell & Laing, 2015). See the Multisystem Effects of Uremia feature.

Fluid and Electrolyte Effects

Loss of functional kidney tissue impairs the kidneys' ability to regulate fluid, electrolyte, and acid–base balance. In the early stages of CKD, impaired filtration and reabsorption lead to proteinuria, hematuria, and decreased urine-concentrating ability. Salt and water are poorly conserved, and risk for dehydration increases. Polyuria, nocturia, and a fixed specific gravity of 1.008–1.012 are common. As the GFR decreases and renal function deteriorates further, sodium and water retention may occur, necessitating salt and water restrictions.

Hyperkalemia develops as renal failure progresses. Manifestations of hyperkalemia, such as muscle weakness, paresthesias, and electrocardiographic changes, are not usually seen until the GFR is less than 5 mL/min. Phosphate excretion is also impaired, leading to hyperphosphatemia and hypocalcemia. Reduced calcium absorption caused by

Multisystem Effects of
Uremia

Endocrine
- Hyperparathyroidism
- Glucose intolerance

Respiratory
- Pulmonary edema
- Pleuritis
- Kussmaul respirations

Urinary
- Proteinuria
- Hematuria
- Fixed specific gravity
- Nocturia
- Oliguria, anuria

Gastrointestinal
- Anorexia
- Nausea and vomiting
- Gastroenteritis
- Hiccups
- Abdominal pain
- Uremic fetor

Potential complications
- Peptic ulcer
- GI bleeding

Musculoskeletal
- Osteodystrophy
- Bone pain
- Spontaneous fractures

Immune System
- Diminished leukocyte count
- ↑ susceptibility to infection

Metabolic Processes
- Azotemia (↑BUN and serum creatinine)
- Hyperkalemia
- Hyperphosphatemia
- Hypocalcemia
- Hypermagnesemia
- Acidosis
- Hyperlipidemia
- Hyperuricemia
- Malnutrition

Neurologic
- Apathy
- Lethargy
- Headache
- Impaired cognition
- Insomnia
- Restless leg syndrome
- Gait disturbances
- Paresthesias

Potential complications
- Seizures
- Decreased LOC
- Coma

Cardiovascular
- Hypertension
- Edema
- Coronary heart disease
- Dysrhythmias

Potential complications
- Pericarditis
- Pericardial effusion
- Cerebrovascular disease
- Heart failure

Hematologic
- Anemias
- Impaired clotting

Reproductive
- Amenorrhea (female)
- Impotence (male)

Potential complication
- Spontaneous abortion

Integumentary
- Pallor
- Uremic skin color (yellow-green)
- Dry skin, poor turgor
- Pruritus
- Ecchymoses
- Uremic "frost"

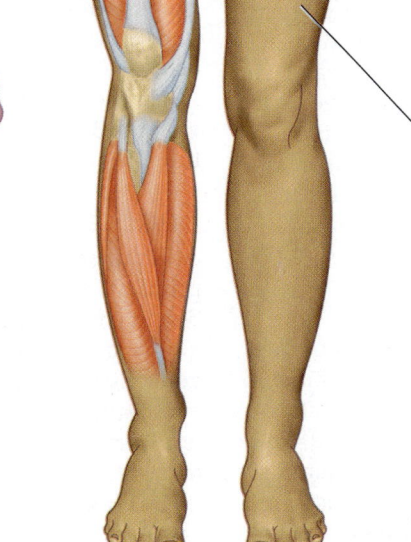

impaired vitamin D activation also contributes to hypocalcemia. Because hypermagnesemia develops with advancing renal failure, patients with renal failure should avoid magnesium-containing antacids.

As renal failure advances, hydrogen ion excretion and buffer production become impaired, leading to metabolic acidosis. Respiratory rate and depth (Kussmaul respirations) increase to compensate for metabolic acidosis. Although metabolic acidosis is often asymptomatic, possible manifestations include general malaise, weakness, headache, nausea and vomiting, and abdominal pain.

Cardiovascular Effects

Cardiovascular disease resulting from accelerated atherosclerosis is a common cause of death in ESRD. Hypertension, hyperlipidemia, and glucose intolerance all contribute to the process. Cerebral and peripheral vascular manifestations of atherosclerosis are also seen.

Systemic hypertension is a common complication of ESRD. Hypertension results from excess fluid volume, increased renin-angiotensin activity, increased peripheral vascular resistance, and decreased prostaglandins. Increased ECF volume also can lead to edema and heart failure. Pulmonary edema may result from heart failure and increased permeability of the alveolar capillary membrane.

Retained metabolic toxins can irritate the pericardial sac, causing an inflammatory response and signs of pericarditis. Cardiac tamponade, a potential complication of pericarditis, occurs when inflammatory fluid in the pericardial sac interferes with ventricular filling and cardiac output. Once a common complication of uremia, pericarditis is less common when dialysis is initiated early.

Hematologic Effects

Anemia, which is common in patients with uremia, is caused by multiple factors. The kidneys produce erythropoietin, a hormone that controls RBC production. In renal failure, erythropoietin production declines. Retained metabolic toxins further suppress RBC production and contribute to a shortened RBC lifespan. Nutritional deficiencies (iron and folate) and increased risk for blood loss from the GI tract also contribute to anemia. Anemia contributes to manifestations such as fatigue, weakness, depression, and impaired cognition. It also affects cardiovascular function, and it may be a major contributing factor in heart failure associated with ESRD (Zadrazil & Horak, 2015). Renal failure also impairs platelet function, increasing the risk of bleeding disorders, such as epistaxis and GI bleeding. The mechanism of impaired platelet function associated with renal failure is poorly understood but is thought to be due, in part, to uremia.

Immune System Effects

Uremia increases the risk for infection. High levels of urea and retained metabolic wastes impair all aspects of inflammation and immune function. The WBC count declines, humoral and cell-mediated immunity are impaired, and phagocyte function is defective. Both the acute inflammatory response and delayed hypersensitivity responses are affected (Imig & Ryan, 2013). Fever is suppressed, often delaying the diagnosis of infection. This increased risk for infection is a growing concern.

Gastrointestinal Effects

Anorexia, nausea, and vomiting are the most common early symptoms of uremia. Hiccups also are common, as is gastroenteritis. Ulcerations may affect any level of the GI tract and contribute to an increased risk of GI bleeding. Peptic ulcer disease is particularly common in patients with uremia. **Uremic fetor** (a urine-like breath odor often associated with a metallic taste in the mouth) may develop. Uremic fetor can further contribute to anorexia.

Neurologic Effects

Uremia alters both central and peripheral nervous system function. Central nervous system manifestations occur early and include changes in cognitive processing, such as difficulty concentrating, fatigue, and insomnia. Psychotic symptoms, seizures, and coma are associated with advanced uremic encephalopathy.

Peripheral neuropathy is also common in advanced uremia. Both the sensory and motor tracts are involved. The lower limbs are initially affected. Restless leg syndrome, which involves sensations of crawling, prickling, or itching of the lower legs with frequent leg movement, increases during rest. **Paresthesias** (skin sensations such as prickling or numbing) and sensory loss typically occur in a "stocking and glove" pattern (i.e., as if one were wearing long stockings and long gloves; American Academy of Neurology, 2016). As uremia progresses, motor function is also impaired, causing muscle weakness, decreased deep tendon reflexes, and gait disturbances.

Musculoskeletal Effects

Hyperphosphatemia and hypocalcemia associated with uremia stimulate parathyroid hormone secretion. Parathyroid hormone causes increased calcium resorption from bone. In addition, osteoblast (bone-forming) and osteoclast (bone-destroying) cell activity are affected. Combined with decreased vitamin D synthesis and decreased calcium absorption from the GI tract, the resulting bone resorption and remodeling lead to renal osteodystrophy, also known as renal rickets. Osteodystrophy is characterized by osteomalacia (softening of the bones) and osteoporosis (decreased bone mass). Bone cysts may develop. Manifestations of osteodystrophy include bone tenderness, pain, and muscle weakness. Patient with osteodystrophy (including children with the disorder) are at increased risk for spontaneous fractures (Wesseling-Perry & Salusky, 2013).

Endocrine and Metabolic Effects

Accumulated waste products of protein metabolism are a primary factor in the effects and manifestations of uremia. Serum creatinine and BUN levels are significantly elevated. Uric acid levels increase, contributing to an increased risk of gout. Tissues become resistant to the effects of insulin in uremia, leading to glucose intolerance. High blood triglyceride levels and lower-than-normal levels of high-density lipoprotein contribute to the accelerated atherosclerotic process.

CKD affects reproductive function. Pregnancies are rarely carried to term, and menstrual irregularities are common. Reduced testosterone levels, low sperm counts, and impotence affect male patients with ESRD.

Clinical Manifestations and Therapies
Chronic Kidney Disease

ETIOLOGY	CLINICAL MANIFESTATIONS	CLINICAL THERAPIES
Uremia	■ Hyperparathyroidism ■ Glucose intolerance ■ Pulmonary edema ■ Pleuritis ■ Kussmaul inspirations ■ Proteinuria ■ Hematuria ■ Fixed specific gravity ■ Nocturia ■ Oliguria ■ Anorexia, nausea, vomiting, gastroenteritis ■ Hiccups ■ Abdominal pain, peptic ulcer, GI bleeding ■ Uremic fetor ■ Osteodystrophy, bone pain, spontaneous fractures ■ Apathy, lethargy, headache, impaired cognition, insomnia, restless leg syndrome, gait disturbances ■ Hypertension, edema, coronary heart disease or failure ■ Anemias, impaired clotting ■ Pallor, uremic skin color, dry skin, poor skin turgor, pruritus	■ Serum electrolytes, BUN, creatinine, arterial blood gas (pH), lipid level monitoring ■ Cardiorespiratory monitoring ■ Accurate I&O ■ Diuretic administration ■ Fluid restriction ■ Dietary consult if needed to improve nutrition status ■ Dialysis (often the only option)
Anemia	■ Fatigue ■ Pallor ■ Dizziness, confusion, lethargy ■ Tachycardia, tachypnea, hypotension	■ Iron supplementation ■ Administration of epoetin ■ Blood transfusion ■ Therapies aimed at treating the underlying cause of renal failure
Fluid volume excess	■ Dependent pitting edema ■ Respiratory crackles ■ Dyspnea, pulmonary edema, hypoxemia ■ Weight gain ■ Tachycardia ■ Jugular vein distention	■ Fluid restriction ■ Sodium-restricted diet ■ Diuretics ■ Dialysis
Hyperkalemia	■ Ventricular arrhythmias ■ Tall, peaked T waves; widened QRS ■ Cardiac arrest ■ Smooth muscle hyperactivity ■ Nausea and vomiting ■ Abdominal cramping ■ Diarrhea ■ Muscle weakness ■ Paresthesias ■ Flaccid paralysis	■ Removal of all potassium from IV solutions ■ Low-potassium diet ■ Administration of glucose and insulin to drive potassium into the cell ■ Potassium-absorbing enema solutions ■ Dialysis

Dermatologic Effects

Anemia and retained pigmented metabolites cause pallor and a yellowish hue to the skin in patients with uremia. Dry skin with poor turgor, a result of dehydration and sweat gland atrophy, is common. Bruising and excoriations are common as well. Metabolic wastes not eliminated by the kidneys may be deposited in the skin, contributing to itching or pruritus. In advanced uremia, high levels of urea in the sweat may result in crystallized deposits of urea on the skin, known as **uremic frost** (Saardi & Schwartz, 2016).

Collaboration

Early management of CKD focuses on eliminating factors that may further decrease renal function and on measures to slow the progression of the disease to ESRD. Treatment goals for patients in all stages of development include the following:

- Maintain nutritional status while minimizing the accumulation of toxic waste products and manifestations of uremia.
- Identify and treat complications of CKD.
- Prepare for renal replacement therapies such as dialysis or renal transplantation.

Treatment of CKD should be modified for the older adult. The restrictions on fluid intake and dietary protein should be less stringent, because most older adults have already decreased their protein and sodium intakes as well as their fluid intake. Constipation, a concern for many older adults, especially those who curb their own fluid intake, may exacerbate the hyperkalemia that accompanies CKD. Nursing and medical management for regularity are important contributions to the treatment plan. Thinning and dry skin is a common concern for all older adults, and the pruritus of CKD can present a real challenge. The older patient will very much appreciate careful skin care by the nurse.

Diagnostic Tests

Diagnostic tests are used both to identify CKD and to monitor kidney function. A number of tests may be performed to determine the underlying renal disorder. Once the diagnosis has been established, renal function is monitored primarily through blood levels of metabolic wastes and electrolytes.

- *Urinalysis* is done to measure urine specific gravity and detect abnormal urine components. In CKD, the specific gravity may be fixed at approximately 1.010, equivalent to that of plasma. This fixed specific gravity is the result of impaired tubular secretion, reabsorption, and urine-concentrating ability. Abnormal proteins, blood cells, and cellular casts may also be noted in the urine.
- *Urine culture* is ordered to identify any urinary tract infection that may hasten the progress of CKD.
- *BUN* and *serum creatinine* values are obtained to evaluate kidney function in eliminating nitrogenous waste products. Levels of both are monitored to assess the progress of renal failure. A BUN of 25–50 mg/dL signals mild azotemia; levels greater than 100 mg/dL indicate severe renal impairment. Uremic symptoms are seen when the BUN is around 200 mg/dL or higher. Serum creatinine levels of greater than 4 mg/dL indicate serious renal impairment.
- *Creatinine clearance* evaluates the GFR and renal function. In early CKD (renal insufficiency), the GFR is more than 20% of normal, and the creatinine clearance is 30 mL/min or greater. As the disease progresses and the stage of renal failure is reached, the GFR is reduced to less than 20% of normal and the creatinine clearance to 15–29 mL/min. In ESRD, the GFR is less than 10–15% of normal, and the creatinine clearance is less than 15 mL/min.

- *Serum electrolytes* are monitored throughout the course of CKD. The serum sodium may be within normal limits or low because of water retention. Potassium levels are elevated but usually remain below 6.5 mEq/L. Serum phosphate is elevated, and the calcium level is decreased. Metabolic acidosis is identified by a low pH, low CO_2, and low bicarbonate levels.
- *Complete blood count (CBC)* reveals moderately severe anemia with a hematocrit of 20–30% and a low hemoglobin. The numbers of RBCs and platelets are reduced.
- *Renal ultrasonography* is done to evaluate kidney size. In CKD, kidney size decreases as nephrons are destroyed and kidney mass is reduced.
- *Kidney biopsy* may be done to identify the underlying disease process if this is unclear. It is also used to differentiate acute from CKD. Kidney biopsy may be performed in surgery or done percutaneously using needle biopsy.

Pharmacologic Therapy

CKD affects both the pharmacokinetics and pharmacodynamics of drug therapy. Most medications are excreted primarily by the kidney. The half-life and plasma levels of many drugs increase in CKD. Drug absorption may decrease when phosphate-binding agents are administered concurrently. Proteinuria can significantly reduce plasma protein levels, leading to manifestations of toxicity when highly protein-bound drugs are given. In addition, any potentially nephrotoxic agent should be used with extreme caution. Avoid drugs eliminated by the kidney, such as meperidine, metformin (Glucophage), and other oral hypoglycemic agents.

Furosemide or other loop diuretics may be prescribed to reduce ECF volume and edema. Diuretic therapy also can reduce hypertension and cause potassium wasting, lowering serum potassium levels (see **Figure 6–22** »).

Other antihypertensive agents are used to maintain the blood pressure within normal levels, slow the progress of renal failure, and prevent complications of coronary heart disease and cerebral vascular disease. ACE inhibitors are preferred, although any class of antihypertensive agent may be prescribed.

Other drugs may be used to manage electrolyte imbalances and acidosis. Sodium bicarbonate or calcium carbonate may be used to correct mild acidosis. Oral phosphorus-binding agents, such as calcium carbonate or calcium acetate, are given to lower serum phosphate levels and normalize serum calcium levels. Aluminum hydroxide may be used in acute treatment of hyperphosphatemia. It is limited to short-term use, however, because of complications such as encephalopathy and osteodystrophy associated with long-term administration of aluminum-containing preparations. Vitamin D supplements may be given to improve calcium absorption.

If the patient's serum potassium rises to dangerously high levels, a combination of bicarbonate, insulin, and glucose may be given intravenously to promote potassium movement into the cells. Sodium polystyrene sulfonate (Kayexalate), a potassium-ion exchange resin, can be given either orally or rectally (as an enema).

Folic acid and iron supplements are given to combat anemia associated with CKD. A multiple vitamin preparation is

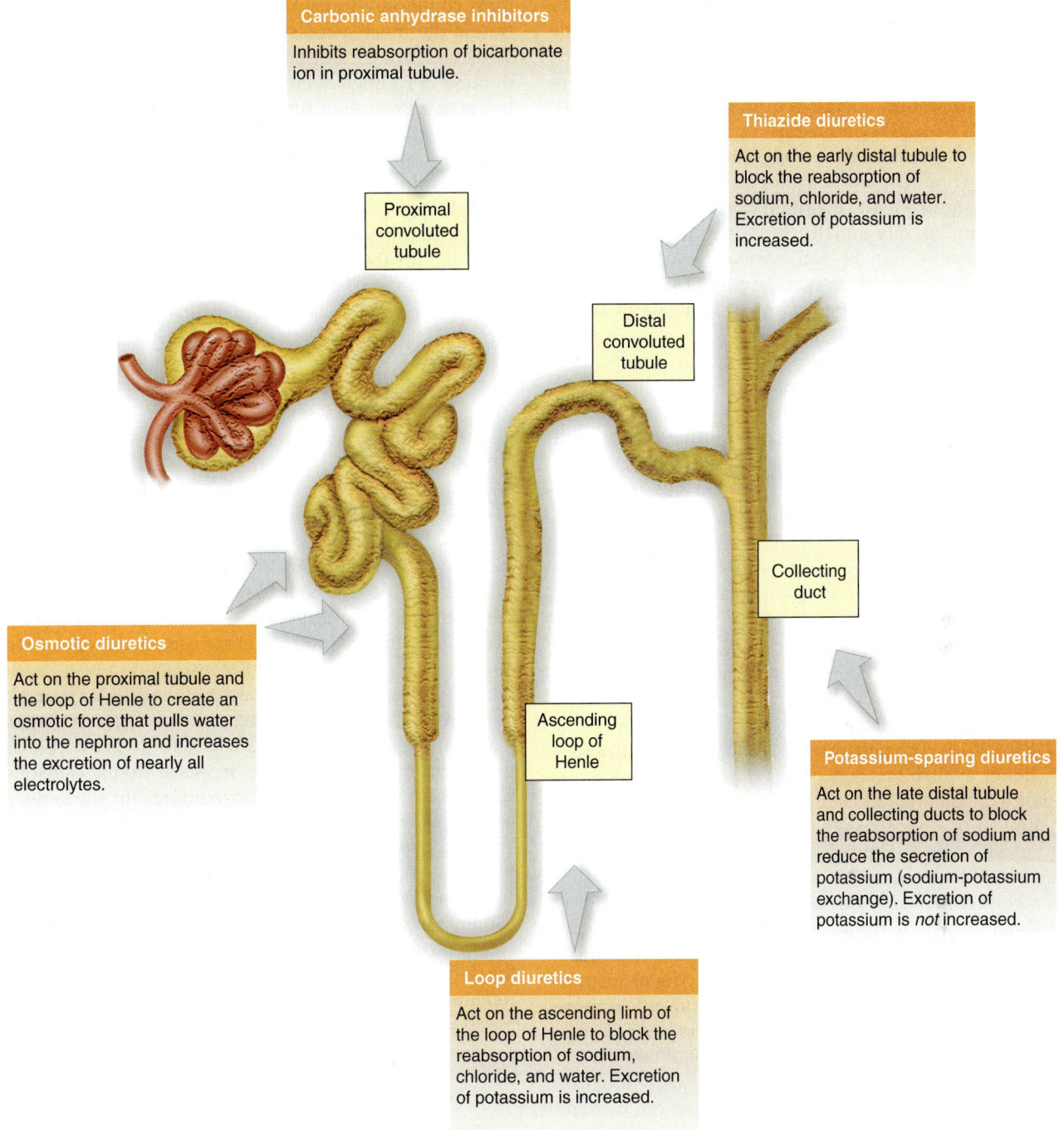

Carbonic anhydrase inhibitors
Inhibits reabsorption of bicarbonate ion in proximal tubule.

Proximal convoluted tubule

Thiazide diuretics
Act on the early distal tubule to block the reabsorption of sodium, chloride, and water. Excretion of potassium is increased.

Distal convoluted tubule

Collecting duct

Osmotic diuretics
Act on the proximal tubule and the loop of Henle to create an osmotic force that pulls water into the nephron and increases the excretion of nearly all electrolytes.

Ascending loop of Henle

Potassium-sparing diuretics
Act on the late distal tubule and collecting ducts to block the reabsorption of sodium and reduce the secretion of potassium (sodium-potassium exchange). Excretion of potassium is *not* increased.

Loop diuretics
Act on the ascending limb of the loop of Henle to block the reabsorption of sodium, chloride, and water. Excretion of potassium is increased.

Source: From Adams, M. P., & Urban, C. (2016). *Pharmacology: Connections to Nursing Practice* (3ed.). Pearson Education, Inc.

Figure 6–22 ❱❱ Sites of action of diuretics.

also often prescribed, because anorexia, nausea, and dietary restrictions may limit nutrient intake.

Nutrition and Fluid Management

As renal function declines, the elimination of water, solutes, and metabolic wastes is impaired. Accumulation of these wastes in the body leads to uremic symptoms. Instituted early in the course of CKD, dietary modifications can slow the progress of nephron destruction, reduce uremic symptoms, and help prevent complications.

Although it can store carbohydrates and fats, the body cannot store excess proteins. Unused dietary proteins are degraded into urea and other nitrogenous wastes, which are then eliminated by the kidneys. Protein-rich foods also contain inorganic ions, such as hydrogen ion, phosphate, and sulfites, that are eliminated by the kidneys. Research has shown that restricting dietary protein intake slows the progression of CKD and reduces uremic symptoms. A daily protein intake of 0.6 g/kg of body weight, or approximately 40 g/day for all patients, provides the amino acids necessary for tissue repair. Proteins should be of high biological value, rich in the essential amino acids. Examples of proteins with high biological value include eggs, poultry, and fish (Nephron Information Center, 2012). Carbohydrate intake is increased to maintain energy requirements and provide approximately 35 kcal/kg each day.

Water and sodium intake are regulated to maintain the ECF volume at normal levels. Water intake of 1–2 L/day is generally recommended to maintain water balance. Sodium is restricted to 2 g/day initially. More stringent water and sodium restrictions may be necessary as renal failure progresses. The nurse should instruct the patient to monitor his or her weight daily and to report any weight gain in excess of 5 lb over a 2-day period.

In later stages of CKD, potassium and phosphorus intake are also restricted. Potassium intake is limited to less than 60–70 mEq/day (normal intake is approximately 100 mEq/day). The nurse should caution the patient and caregivers to avoid using salt substitutes, which typically contain high levels of potassium chloride. Foods high in phosphorus include eggs, dairy products, and meat.

Renal Replacement Therapies

When pharmacologic and dietary management strategies are no longer effective to maintain fluid and electrolyte balance and prevent uremia, dialysis or kidney transplantation is considered. The most common therapies for ESRD in the United States are hemodialysis performed in a dialysis center, followed by peritoneal dialysis and kidney transplant (NKUDIC, 2012). The patient's age, concurrent health problems, donor availability, and personal preference influence the choice of renal replacement therapy.

A number of other considerations also affect the choice of long-term treatment. Hemodialysis and peritoneal dialysis each have advantages and disadvantages. Establishing vascular access for hemodialysis may take several months. Planning ahead to develop the access before dialysis is necessary can ease the transition to dialysis. Also, when dialysis treatments will be performed at home, starting patient instruction before the treatments are required can result in more effective learning. If a family member will serve as a dialysis helper, training should begin before the onset of uremia.

If transplantation is being considered, tissue typing and identification of potential living related donors can be done before the onset of ESRD. To make an informed decision, both the patient and the potential donor need to understand the risks, benefits, and options available. If the decision for transplantation is made early, dialysis can potentially be avoided.

Dialysis

Both hemodialysis and peritoneal dialysis can be done in the home, but few patients use home hemodialysis. An important factor is that hemodialysis for ESRD is done three times a week for a total of 9–12 hours.

>>*See Renal Replacement Therapy in the Collaboration section of Exemplar 6.B on AKI for more information about dialysis.*

Kidney Transplantation

Kidney transplantation has become the treatment of choice for many patients with ESRD. Kidneys are the solid organ most commonly transplanted; to date, kidney transplantation is the most successful of transplantation procedures. The first kidney transplantation was performed in 1954; the donor and recipient were identical twins. Kidney transplantation as a treatment for ESRD is limited primarily by the availability of organs. In 2014, 17,197 kidney transplantations took place. According to the National Kidney Foundation there are currently over 121,678 people awaiting kidney transplantations (National Kidney Foundation, 2016b).

Kidney transplantation improves both survival and quality of life for the patient with ESRD. Today, the patient on dialysis has a great probability of surviving after 3–5 years of dialysis; the transplant recipient has a greater than 90% probability of survival after 2 years. At 5 years, the difference is even greater: 33% for dialysis compared with almost 90% for those who receive a transplant. Organs come from both living and deceased sources. In 2014, 5537 kidneys came from live donors; over 11,570 came from a deceased donor, with deceased donors donating two kidneys (National Kidney Foundation, 2016c). Quality of life improves dramatically once the patient is no longer tethered to a dialysis catheter, machine, or center. Dietary and fluid restrictions are reduced, and the body image is more "whole."

With both deceased and living donor transplants, a close match between blood and tissue type is desired. Human leukocyte antigens are compared between the donor and recipient; six antigens in common is considered to be a "perfect" match. The success of well-matched living donor transplants is better than that for deceased donor organ transplants, with a 1-year graft survival of 95.1% for living donor transplants compared to 89% for deceased donor transplants. Close tissue matching probably accounts for the better outcome with living donors. People with normal kidneys who are in good physical health may donate a kidney. Figures from the National Kidney Foundation in 2014 outlined that the majority of donors are siblings or spouses (National Kidney Foundation, 2016b). Predonation counseling is vital. **Nephrectomy** (removal of a kidney) is major surgery, and the donor faces the risk that trauma or disease may affect the remaining kidney in the future. If the transplant fails, the psychologic impact on the donor can be significant.

>>*Go to Pearson MyLab Nursing and eText to see Chart 3: Nursing Care of the Patient Having a Nephrectomy.*

Deceased donor kidneys are obtained from people who meet the criteria for brain death, are younger than 65 years, and are free of systemic disease, malignancy, or infection, including HIV and hepatitis B or C. Kidneys are removed after brain death has been determined and are preserved by hypothermia or a technique called continuous hypothermic pulsatile perfusion. A kidney preserved by hypothermia must be transplanted within 24–48 hours. Continuous hypothermic pulsatile perfusion, however, allows up to 3 days before transplantation.

>>**Stay Current:** For more information on how deceased donor kidneys are allocated for transplant, visit the website of the United Network for Organ Sharing (UNOS) at http://www.unos.org/transplantation/matching-organs.

The donor kidney is placed in the lower abdominal cavity of the recipient, and the renal artery, vein, and ureter are

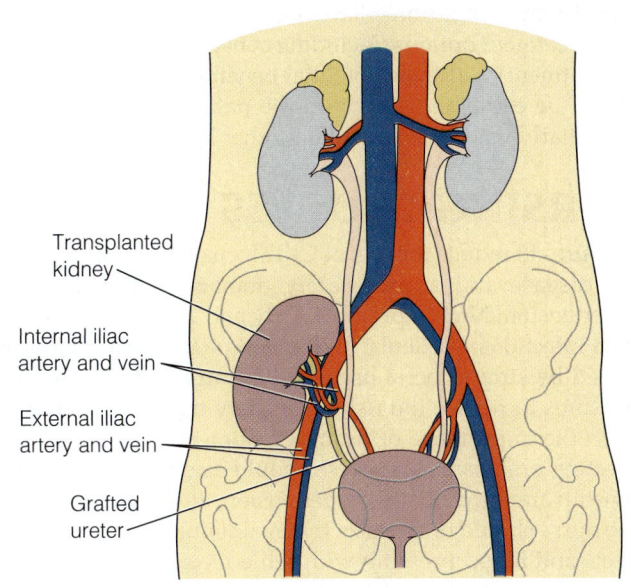

Figure 6–23 ❯❯ Placement of a transplanted kidney in the iliac fossa with anastomosis to the hypogastric artery, iliac vein, and bladder.

anastomosed (see **Figure 6–23 ❯❯**). The renal artery of the donor kidney is connected to the hypogastric artery, and the renal vein is connected to the iliac vein. The ureter is connected to one of the recipient's ureters or directly to the bladder, using a tunnel technique to prevent reflux.

❯❯ *Go to* **Pearson MyLab Nursing and eText** *to see Chart 4: Nursing Care of the Patient Undergoing Kidney Transplantation.*

Unless the donor and recipient are identical twins, the grafted organ stimulates an immune response to reject the transplanted organ. Immunosuppressive drugs minimize this response. Azathioprine or mycophenolate mofetil are commonly used, often in combination with prednisone, a corticosteroid. Cyclosporine, a potent immunosuppressive, also may be used. These drugs suppress a portion of the immune system and the inflammatory response, increasing the risk for infections and cancers with long-term therapy.

Glucocorticoids such as prednisone and methylprednisolone are used for maintenance immunosuppression and to treat acute rejection episodes. Side effects of long-term corticosteroid use include impaired wound healing, emotional disturbances, osteoporosis, and Cushingoid effects on glucose, protein, and fat metabolism.

Cyclosporine primarily affects cellular immunity, the helper T cells in particular. Among its many adverse effects, which include hepatotoxicity and hirsutism, nephrotoxicity is a primary concern for the patient undergoing kidney transplantation.

Even with immunosuppressive therapy, however, the transplanted kidney can be rejected at any time. Either acute or chronic rejection may develop. Acute rejection develops within months of the transplantation. It is caused by a cellular immune response with T-lymphocyte proliferation. Few manifestations may be apparent other than a rise in serum creatinine and possible oliguria. Methylprednisolone, a glucocorticoid, and OKT3 monoclonal antibody are used to

manage acute rejection episodes. OKT3 can cause severe systemic reactions, including chills, fever, hypotension, headache, and possible pulmonary edema. Chronic rejection, which may develop months to years following the transplantation, is a major cause of graft loss. Both humoral and cellular immune responses are involved in chronic rejection. Chronic rejection does not respond to increased immunosuppression. The presenting manifestations of chronic rejection—progressive azotemia, proteinuria, and hypertension—are those of progressive renal failure.

Hypertension is a possible complication of kidney transplantation, resulting from graft rejection, renal artery stenosis, or renal vasoconstriction. Patients may develop glomerular lesions and manifestations of nephrosis. Hypertension and altered blood lipids (increased low-density lipoprotein and decreased high-density lipoprotein levels) increase the risk of death from myocardial infarction and stroke following transplantation (Cross & Webster, 2016).

Long-term immunosuppression has adverse effects as well. Infection is a continuing threat. Bacterial and viral infections may develop, as well as fungal infections of the blood, lungs, and central nervous system. Tumors are also common, with carcinoma in situ of the cervix, lymphomas, and skin cancers most prevalent. The risk of congenital anomalies is increased in infants whose mothers have undergone immunosuppressive therapy. Corticosteroid use may lead to bone problems, GI disorders (e.g., peptic ulcer disease), and cataract formation.

Complementary Health Approaches

Patients with CKD should avoid herbal supplements, which can contain minerals that may be harmful to the kidneys or contraindicated with one or more medications the patient might be taking (Crow, 2016). Nurses should encourage patients and their caregivers to discuss the use of any over-the-counter or complementary health approaches with the physician. Making small changes in the diet can help kidney performance. Foods that may help increase kidney function are sprouts, garlic, legumes, beans, potato, banana, papaya, watermelon, yogurt, green vegetables, and whole grains. Drinking unsweetened cranberry juice maintains urine acidity. Palliative care can provide emotional support for both patients and their families, and can provide additional therapies such as massages and relaxation techniques stress. Spiritual support can also be advantageous (National Kidney Foundation, 2016d).

Lifespan Considerations

CKD in Children and Adolescents

Physical activity is important to help children maintain optimal health and self-esteem. Nurses should encourage children with CKD to participate in developmentally appropriate activities as tolerated. Nurses may partner with children to establish routine plans for physical activity as tolerated that will help to promote strong bones. Nurses should encourage parents to promote children's participation in age-appropriate activities to minimize the psychologic consequences of coping with a chronic disease.

CKD in Pregnant Women

The rate of preterm delivery, which is 1.2% in the general population, increases to 16.3% in women with CKD. Similar increases are seen in the occurrence of preeclampsia: from 2.9% in the general population to 40.1% in women with CKD. The rate of neonatal death when the mother has CKD is 2.1%, whereas that in newborns of women with normal renal function is 0.2%. The rate of small for gestational age neonates is 9.3% in women without CKD and 33.9% in women with CKD (Merrill et al., 2016).

Care of the pregnant patient with CKD is multifaceted. First, serum albumin levels must be maintained at normal levels throughout the pregnancy to promote normal growth of the fetus, and blood pressure must be well controlled to prevent ongoing kidney damage. The maintenance of blood pressure at a normal level helps to maintain fetal and placental circulation. Most individuals with CKD, pregnant or not, have chronic hypertension and may require multiple medications. However, it is advantageous for the pregnant patient to maintain pressure with a single agent. For women who are undergoing dialysis, the dialysis may need to occur at least five times per week during pregnancy. All patients with CKD have problems with anemia, and this is an area of particular concern in pregnant women. The use of higher doses of iron and erythropoietin replacement may help in preventing preterm birth. It should be noted that despite rigorous intervention, preeclampsia is a frequent occurrence (Chang et al., 2016).

Some authors suggest that rather than CKD leading to preeclampsia, preeclampsia leads to CKD (Topf, Sparks, & August, 2015). These researchers suggest that preeclampsia can have effects that last far longer than originally thought. Hypertension, ischemic heart disease, and cardiovascular death were much higher in women with preeclampsia than in women with normal pregnancies. Having a low-birth-weight infant or an early delivery was also associated with CKD. Findings from the research outlined that a clear relationship of increased risk for CKD exists with additional occurrences of preeclampsia in future pregnancies. In addition, having preeclampsia later in the pregnancy was associated with greater risk than if it occurred earlier in pregnancy.

CKD in Older Adults

Structural and functional changes occur in the aging kidney. Structurally, the number of nephrons decreases. Functionally, the GFR decreases, resulting in decreased renal clearance of drugs. Urine-concentrating ability decreases, and the kidney is less able to conserve sodium. Renal compensation for acid–base imbalances takes longer. Despite these changes, the kidney retains its ability to regulate fluid and electrolyte homeostasis remarkably well unless additional stresses are added. Any additional stressors, such as hypotension, exposure to nephrotoxic drugs, or an inflammatory process such as glomerulonephritis, may precipitate renal failure in the older adult.

The manifestations of renal failure often are missed in older adults (e.g., edema may be attributed to heart failure or high blood pressure to preexisting hypertension). Serum creatinine levels may rise slowly. Because older adults have less muscle mass, they produce less creatinine, a by-product of muscle cell metabolism. Likewise, the BUN may remain within normal limits.

The same measures used to treat renal failure in younger people are used for older adults. Hemodialysis, peritoneal dialysis, and renal transplantation are appropriate if necessary. Treatment options (including conservative treatment or no treatment) and their potential benefits and ramifications should be explained clearly to the patient and caregivers, particularly when the patient has other health challenges.

NURSING PROCESS

Measures to reduce the risk of CKD focus on preventing kidney disease and appropriately managing diabetes and hypertension. Nurses promote early and effective treatment of all infections, particularly skin and pharyngeal infections caused by streptococcal bacteria. The nurse should discuss measures to reduce the risk for urinary tract infections and stress the importance of prompt treatment to eradicate the infecting organism. The nurse should also discuss the relationship among diabetes, hypertension, and kidney disease. The nurse should emphasize that maintaining blood glucose levels and blood pressure within the recommended ranges reduces the risk of adverse effects on the kidneys. The nurse should ensure that all patients with less-than-optimal renal function are well hydrated, particularly when a nephrotoxic drug is prescribed or anticipated. Finally, the nurse should encourage the patient with ESRD to investigate options for early transplantation to avoid long-term dialysis.

Assessment

Both subjective and objective data are used to assess the patient with CKD:

- ***Observation and patient interview.*** Complaints of anorexia, nausea, weight gain, or edema; current treatment (if any), including type and frequency of dialysis or previous kidney transplantation; chronic diseases, such as diabetes, heart failure, or kidney disease
- ***Physical examination.*** Mental status; vital signs, including temperature, heart and lung sounds, and peripheral pulses; urine output (if any); weight; skin color, moisture, and condition; presence of edema (periorbital or dependent); bowel tones; and presence and location of an AV fistula, shunt, or graft, or peritoneal catheter.

Diagnosis

Nursing diagnoses for patients with CKD may include the following:

- *Perfusion: Renal, Risk for Ineffective*
- *Nutrition, Imbalanced: Less than Body Requirements*
- *Fluid Volume: Excess*
- *Skin Integrity, Impaired*
- *Infection, Risk for*
- *Body Image, Disturbed.*

(NANDA-I © 2014)

Planning

The plan of care, made in collaboration with the patient, may include the following goals:

- The patient will verbalize fluid allotment allowed throughout the day.

- The patient's weight will decrease and approach baseline level.
- The patient will breathe comfortably, with clear breath sounds.
- The patient will remain free of infection.
- The patient will share feelings regarding change in body image.

Implementation

Whether the patient with ESRD is facing long-term dialysis or renal transplantation, a number of nursing care needs can be identified. This section focuses on nursing care related to impaired renal function, nutritional deficits caused by dietary restrictions and nausea, increased risk for infection, and changes in body image. See the Nursing Care Plan feature that follows for additional potential nursing diagnoses and interventions for the patient with CKD.

Promote Effective Tissue Perfusion

Capillaries are an integral part of the nephron. As nephrons are destroyed, kidney perfusion progressively declines. As renal perfusion and nephron function fall, the kidney is less able to maintain fluid and electrolyte balance and to eliminate waste products from the body. The nurse should do the following:

- Monitor I&O; vital signs, including orthostatic blood pressures; and weight. Weight changes are a more accurate indicator of fluid volume status in the patient with oliguria or anuria than I&O measurements. These provide important data to identify changes in fluid volume.
- Restrict fluids as ordered. As renal function declines, the ability to eliminate excess fluid is impaired.
- Monitor respiratory status, including lung sounds, every 4–8 hours. Fluid volume overload may lead to heart failure and possible pulmonary edema.
- Monitor BUN, serum creatinine, pH, electrolytes, and CBC. Report significant changes. As renal function declines, progressive azotemia with increasing BUN and serum creatinine appears. Metabolic acidosis develops because the kidney is unable to eliminate hydrogen ions and conserve bicarbonate. Hyponatremia, hyperkalemia, hyperphosphatemia, and hypocalcemia are associated with renal failure. The RBC count, hemoglobin, and hematocrit decline because of deficient erythropoietin to stimulate cell production in the bone marrow. An acute fall in hemoglobin and hematocrit may indicate GI bleeding, a risk in patients with ESRD.
- Report manifestations of electrolyte imbalances, such as cardiac dysrhythmias and other electrocardiographic changes.
- Administer antihypertensive medications as ordered. Hypertension management is an important factor in slowing the progression of CKD.

SAFETY ALERT Time activities and procedures to allow rest periods for the patient. The anemia associated with CKD may cause significant fatigue and activity intolerance.

Promote Balanced Nutrition

Anorexia, nausea, and vomiting are common manifestations of ESRD and uremia. The metallic taste associated with uremia combined with a diet restricted in protein and sodium will compound loss of appetite. This increases the risk that food intake will be insufficient to meet metabolic needs. Catabolism exacerbates azotemia and uremia, resulting in muscle tremors and possible tetany, and Kussmaul respirations. Manifestations of electrolyte imbalance may indicate the need for intervention. The nurse should do the following:

- Administer medications to treat electrolyte imbalances as ordered. Carefully monitor for desired and adverse effects. Impaired renal function affects drug elimination and increases the risk for toxic effects. Medications may be prescribed to help maintain electrolyte and acid–base balance and prevent adverse effects of imbalances.
- Monitor food and nutrient intake as well as episodes of vomiting. Careful monitoring helps to determine the adequacy of intake.
- Weigh the patient daily before breakfast. This provides the most accurate measurement. Remember that a gain of 2 lb or more over a 24-hour period is more likely to reflect fluid retention than a gain in body mass.
- Administer antiemetic agents 30–60 minutes before eating. Antiemetics reduce nausea and the risk of vomiting with food intake.
- Assist with mouth care before meals and at bedtime. Mouth care improves taste, stimulates the appetite, and maintains the integrity of oral mucous membranes.
- Serve small meals, and provide between-meal snacks. Small meals are less likely to prompt nausea and will help to improve food intake.
- Arrange for a dietary consultation. Provide preferred foods to the extent possible, and involve the patient in planning daily menus. Encourage family members to bring food as dietary restrictions allow. Providing preferred foods within restrictions promotes intake.
- Monitor nutritional status by tracking weight; laboratory values, such as serum albumin and BUN; and anthropometric measurements. Indicators of impaired nutrition develop gradually and may be subtle. Careful assessment is important.
- Administer parenteral nutrition as prescribed. Routinely monitor blood glucose levels, and use strict aseptic technique when handling the solution and venous access site. Parenteral nutrition may be necessary to prevent catabolism and increasing azotemia. Hyperglycemia and infection are risks associated with parenteral nutrition. Immune system suppression associated with renal failure further increases the risk for infection.

Reduce Risk for Infection

CKD affects the immune system and leukocyte function, increasing susceptibility to infection. Invasive devices required for hemodialysis or peritoneal dialysis add to this risk. The patient who has undergone kidney transplantation remains on immunosuppressive therapy for life, further depressing the immune system and increasing the risk for infection. The nurse should do the following:

- Use standard precautions and good hand cleansing technique at all times. Hand hygiene is a primary means of preventing the transfer of organisms. Patients who are on hemodialysis or who have had multiple blood transfusions to treat anemia have an increased risk for hepatitis B, hepatitis C, and HIV infection.

- Monitor temperature and vital signs at least every 4 hours. A low-grade fever or increased pulse rate may indicate an infection in the patient who is immunosuppressed.

- Monitor WBC count and differential. Increased WBCs may indicate a bacterial infection; decreased WBCs may indicate viral infection. A shift in the differential showing more immature WBCs (bands) in circulation is another indicator of infection.

- Culture urine, peritoneal dialysis fluid, and other drainage as indicated. Culture is performed to verify the presence of pathogens.

- Monitor clarity of dialysate return. Dialysate should return clear in the patient undergoing peritoneal dialysis. Cloudy dialysate may indicate peritonitis, the most common complication of peritoneal dialysis, and should be reported and cultured.

- Provide good respiratory hygiene, including position changes, coughing, and deep breathing. These measures improve clearance of respiratory secretions, reducing the risk for infection.

- Restrict visits from people who are obviously ill. Teach the patient and family about the risk for infection and measures to reduce the spread of infection.

SAFETY ALERT Because the patient's resistance to infection is impaired, extra caution is required to prevent unnecessary exposures.

Promote Healthy Body Image

Chronic disease and impaired kidney function can affect the patient's body image. Hemodialysis requires an AV fistula or shunt, and peritoneal dialysis requires a permanent peritoneal catheter. Although kidney transplantation can restore an image of wholeness, a visible scar remains, and the patient may perceive the organ as "foreign." The nurse should do the following:

- Involve the patient in care, including meal planning; dialysis; and catheter, port, or incision care to the extent possible. Involvement improves acceptance and stimulates discussion about the effect of the disease and treatment measures on the patient's life.

- Encourage expression of feelings and concerns, accepting perceptions and feelings without criticism. Self-expression enhances the patient's sense of self-worth and acceptance.

- Include the patient in decision making, and encourage self-care. Increased autonomy enhances the patient's sense of control, independence, and self-worth.

- Support positive gains, but do not support denial. The patient may have difficulty accepting the renal failure, but adaptation to the loss is important.

- Help the patient develop and achieve realistic goals. Realistic goals allow the patient to see progress.

- Provide positive reinforcement and feedback. These measures support growth and adaptation.

- Reinforce effective coping strategies. Reinforcement helps the patient develop positive versus negative strategies for coping.

- Facilitate contact with a support group or other community members affected by renal failure. The patient benefits by providing and receiving support in a group of people going through similar circumstances.

- Refer the patient for mental health counseling as indicated or desired. Counseling can help the patient develop effective coping and adaptation strategies.

The nurse should refer the patient to a dietitian for diet planning and counseling. If home hemodialysis is planned, the nurse should refer the designated dialysis helper for formal training. Both the National Kidney Foundation and the American Association of Kidney Patients may be able to provide support and educational materials for the patient with ESRD. Local and state chapters of these organizations can provide additional support.

Nurses should assess both fluid and nutritional intake in the older adult. Older patients may consciously or unconsciously decrease fluid intake because of a blunted thirst mechanism, fear of incontinence or nocturia, or lack of access to beverages due to lack of mobility or other factors. Embarrassment also may be a factor for the older patient who needs assistance with toileting. Dehydration may lead to confusion, digestion problems, constipation, and bladder infections. The nurse should encourage older adults to drink fluids even when they do not feel thirsty. In addition, the nurse should educate caregivers to make fluids available throughout the day, and to take into account the older adult's preferences in providing fluids.

Patient Teaching
Home Care for the Patient with CKD

Teaching for home care includes the following topics:

- Nature of the kidney disease and renal failure, including expected progression and effects
- Monitoring weight, vital signs, and temperature
- Prescribed dietary and fluid restrictions (Involve the patient, a dietitian, and the family member who is usually responsible for cooking. Include strategies to manage nausea and relieve thirst within allowed fluid limits.)
- How to assess and protect a fistula or shunt for hemodialysis (or the extremity to be used if one is anticipated)
- Peritoneal catheter care and the procedure for peritoneal dialysis as indicated (Include a family member or significant other, in case the patient is unable to perform the procedure independently at some time.)

Evaluation

CKD and ESRD are long-term processes that require management by the patient. No matter what treatment option the patient chooses (hemodialysis, peritoneal dialysis, or renal transplantation), day-to-day management falls to the patient and family. When evaluating the patient, an important aspect to consider is the patient and family's readiness to assume self-care and management (see **Box 6–6** ≫). Expected outcomes may include the following:

- The patient remains free from infection.
- The patient maintains an appropriate weight.
- The patient demonstrates the ability to participate in self-care, either independently or with assistance.
- The patient is able to participate in desired activities.

If the expected outcomes are unmet, the patient may need referral to other specialists, such as a dietitian or physical therapist. Psychologic support may also be necessary, and the nurse can suggest referrals to the social worker or perhaps a chaplain or clergy. It will be important to include family members in these discussions as well.

Box 6–6
Assessing for Home Care for Patients with Kidney Disease

A number of factors should be considered in assessing the patient's ability to manage treatment such as dialysis at home:

- Does the patient have reasonable access to a dialysis center or outpatient unit? Is transportation available?
- Would home hemodialysis be appropriate? Is a caregiver available who can be trained to manage dialysis? Does the patient's home have appropriate electrical and plumbing fixtures?
- Would continuous ambulatory peritoneal dialysis (CAPD) be appropriate? Does the patient have the manual dexterity, will, and cognitive ability to manage dialysis infusions? If not, would intermittent peritoneal dialysis using a dialyzing machine be more appropriate?
- Are family members or other support people available to assist the patient as needed?

Nursing Care Plan
A Patient with ESRD

Walter Cohen, 45 years old, is the print shop manager at a local community college. He has had type 1 diabetes mellitus since the age of 20 and was diagnosed with diabetic nephropathy 10 years ago. Despite blood pressure control with antihypertensive medications and frequent blood glucose monitoring with insulin coverage, he developed overt proteinuria 5 years ago and has now progressed to ESRD. He enters the nephrology unit for temporary hemodialysis to relieve uremic symptoms. While there, a CAPD catheter will be inserted. Mr. Cohen's desire to continue working is the primary factor in his choice of CAPD over hemodialysis.

ASSESSMENT	DIAGNOSES	PLANNING
Richard Gonzalez, Mr. Cohen's care manager, obtains a nursing assessment. Mr. Cohen states that his diabetes has always been difficult to control. He has had numerous hypoglycemic episodes and has been hospitalized "four or five times" for ketoacidosis. Recently, he has developed symptoms of peripheral neuropathy and increasing retinopathy. He attributed his lack of appetite and his nausea, vomiting, and fatigue over the past month to "a touch of the flu." His weight remained stable, so he did not worry about not eating much. Physical assessment findings include temperature 36.5°C (97.8°F) oral, pulse 96 bpm, respirations 20/min, and BP 178/100 mmHg. His skin is cool and dry, with minor excoriations on forearms and lower legs. His breath odor is fetid. Scattered fine rales are noted in bilateral lung bases, and a soft S_3 gallop is noted at cardiac apex. Bilateral pitting edema of lower extremities to just below the knees is observed; fingers and hands are also edematous. Abdominal assessment is essentially normal, with hypoactive bowel sounds. Urinalysis shows a specific gravity of 1.011, gross proteinuria, and multiple cell casts. CBC results are as follows: RBCs, 2.9 million/mm^3; hemoglobin, 9.4 g/dL; hematocrit, 28%. Blood chemistry abnormalities include the following: BUN, 198 mg/dL; creatinine, 18.5 mg/dL; sodium, 125 mEq/L; potassium, 5.7 mEq/L; calcium, 7.1 mg/dL; and phosphate, 6.8 mg/dL. A temporary jugular venous catheter will be placed for hemodialysis the next day, followed by peritoneal catheter insertion later in the week.	- *Excess Fluid Volume* related to failure of kidneys to eliminate excess body fluid - *Imbalanced Nutrition: Less than Body Requirements* related to effects of uremia - *Impaired Skin Integrity* of lower extremities related to dry skin and itching - *Risk for Infection* related to invasive catheters and impaired immune function (NANDA-I © 2014)	- The patient will adhere to the prescribed fluid restriction of 750 mL/day. - The patient will demonstrate reduced ECF volume by weight loss, decreased peripheral edema, clear lung sounds, and normal heart sounds. - The patient will consume and retain 100% of prescribed diet, including snacks. - The patient will have healing of lower extremity skin lesions. - The patient will remain free of infection. - The patient will demonstrate appropriate peritoneal catheter care and CAPD.

(continued on next page)

Nursing Care Plan *(continued)*

IMPLEMENTATION

- Space fluid administration, allowing 350 mL from 7 a.m. to 3 p.m., 250 mL from 3 p.m. to 11 p.m., and 100 mL from 11 p.m. to 7 a.m.
- Provide mouth care at least every 4 hours and before every meal.
- Keep sugarless hard candy and ice chips at the bedside; include ice consumed as fluid intake.
- Weigh daily before breakfast; monitor vital signs and heart and lung sounds every 4 hours.
- Document I&O every 4 hours.

- Arrange dietary consultation for menu planning.
- Administer prescribed antiemetic 1 hour before meals.
- Monitor food intake, noting percentage and types of food consumed.
- Clean lesions on lower extremities every 8 hours, and assess healing.
- Teach CAPD procedure and peritoneal catheter care.

EVALUATION

Mr. Cohen was hospitalized for 2 weeks, undergoing four hemodialysis sessions to reduce uremic symptoms. An AV fistula was created in his left arm in case he should need hemodialysis in the future. He began peritoneal dialysis the second week, and by discharge, he has been able to manage the catheter care and dialysis runs with the help of his wife. His heart and lung sounds are normal, and he has minimal peripheral edema on discharge. The excoriations on his legs have healed. His temperature is normal, and no evidence of infection is noted. Mr. Cohen remains anorectic and slightly nauseated but is eating most of his prescribed diet and snacks. He has lost 10 lb with excess fluid removal by dialysis, but his weight remains stable during the second week. Mr. Cohen and his wife have been introduced to another patient who has been on CAPD for several years and promises to help them with problem solving.

CRITICAL THINKING

1. How does diabetes mellitus damage the kidneys and lead to ESRD? Why is this more significant for a patient with type 1 diabetes mellitus than for someone with type 2 diabetes mellitus?

2. Why do high levels of urea in the blood often cause changes in cognition and mental status? What manifestations of encephalopathy would you expect to see?

3. How might Mr. Cohen's insulin dosage and diet need to be changed with the institution of peritoneal dialysis? Why?

4. Develop a care plan for Mr. Cohen for the nursing diagnosis *Disturbed Body Image*.

REVIEW Chronic Kidney Disease

RELATE Link the Concepts and Exemplars

Linking the exemplar of CKD with the concept of perfusion:

1. When providing health promotion education to the community, what information would you provide to improve overall perfusion and, as a result, reduce the risk of kidney damage resulting in CKD?

2. What impact would CKD have on the cardiovascular system of the patient? What assessments would indicate that the patient is experiencing cardiovascular complications?

Linking the exemplar of CKD with the concept of development:

3. How does CKD impact a pediatric patient's development?

4. What nursing interventions may be helpful in promoting normal development in the pediatric patient with CKD?

READY Go to Volume 3: Clinical Nursing Skills

REFER Go to Pearson MyLab Nursing and eText

- Additional review materials
- Chart 3: Nursing Care of the Patient Having a Nephrectomy
- Chart 4: Nursing Care of the Patient Undergoing Kidney Transplantation

REFLECT Apply Your Knowledge

Joe Jenkins is a 45-year-old man who has been a long-distance truck driver for the past 20 years. He is admitted to the hospital with complaints of nausea for several weeks, weakness, fatigue, and loss of appetite. He has been feeling very depressed. He has a past medical history of type 1 diabetes mellitus, hypertension, and diabetic nephropathy. On admission, his vital signs are T_O 37.1°C (98.7°F); P 96 bpm; R 20/min; BP 170/110 mmHg. He has bilateral pitting edema of the lower extremities. His fingers and hands are also edematous. He complains of dry and itching skin. His urine is dark, frothy, and scant. A specimen is collected for a urinalysis, and blood is drawn and sent to the laboratory. Urinalysis results show a specific gravity of 1.011, gross hematuria, and 3+ protein. His blood work reveals a BUN of 198 mg/dL and creatinine of 12.5 mg/dL. Based on his past medical history of diabetes, hypertension, and diabetic nephropathy and on the current findings, a medical diagnosis of CKD is established. Based on Mr. Jenkins's assessment and past medical history, the nursing diagnosis of *Impaired Urinary Elimination* is identified as the highest priority for planning nursing care.

1. What would be the priority nursing interventions when admitting Mr. Jenkins to the acute care facility?

2. What teaching will this patient need considering his prediagnosis lifestyle?

3. What alterations will Mr. Jenkins need to make in his life if daily dialysis is required?

References

Adams, M. P., Holland, L. N., & Urban, C. (2017). *Pharmacology for nurses: A pathophysiologic approach* (5th ed.). Hoboken, NJ: Pearson Education.

Al Sabbagh, M. (2013). The accuracy of clinical signs in detecting dehydration in children. *Middle East Journal of Family Medicine, 11*(8), 28–40.

Al-Jaishi, A. A., Jain, A. K., Garg, A. X., Zhang, A. C., & Moist, L. M. (2016). Hemodialysis vascular access creation in patients switching from peritoneal dialysis to hemodialysis: A population-based retrospective cohort. *American Journal of Kidney Disease, 67*(5), 813–816.

American Academy of Neurology. (2016). *Peripheral neuropathy.* Retrieved from http://patients.aan.com/disorders/?event=view&disorder_id=1034

American Kidney Fund. (2013). *Kidney failure/ESRD.* Retrieved from http://www.kidneyfund.org/kidney-health/kidney-failure/end-stage-renal-disease.html#.Uh9RGxuTgoo

American Kidney Fund. (2015). *2015 kidney disease statistics.* Retrieved from http://www.kidneyfund.org/assets/pdf/kidney-disease-statistics.pdf

Bajwa, S. J., Kwatra, I. S., Bajwa, S. K., & Kaur, M. (2013). Renal diseases during pregnancy: Critical and current perspectives. *Journal of Obstetrics Anesthesia Critical Care, 3*(1), 7–15.

Carmody, J. B., Swanson, J. R., Rhone, E. T., & Charlton, J. R. (2014). Recognition and reporting of AKI in very low birth weight infants. *Clinical Journal the American Society of Nephrology, 9*(12), 2036–2043.

Centers for Disease Control and Prevention (CDC). (2012). *Where's the sodium: There's too much in many common foods.* Retrieved from http://www.cdc.gov/vitalsigns/Sodium/index.html

Centers for Disease Control and Prevention (CDC). (2013). *Sodium: The facts.* Retrieved from http://www.cdc.gov/salt/pdfs/sodium_fact_sheet.pdf

Centers for Disease Control and Prevention (CDC). (2017). *Keep your cool in hot weather.* Retrieved from http://www.cdc.gov/features/extremeheat

Chang, J. Y., Jang, H., Chung, B. H., Youn, A. Y., Sung, I. K., Kim, Y. S., & Yang, C. W. (2016). The successful clinical outcomes of pregnant women with advanced chronic kidney disease. *Kidney Research and Clinical Practice, 35*(2), 84–89.

Cho, C., Perez, R., Shearer, R., Kate, R., Mazumdar, D., & Nilakartan, V. (2015). Predictors of acute kidney injury for elderly patients who undergo cardiac procedure. *Journal of the American Journal of Cardiology, 65*(10–S).

Connell, A., & Laing, C. (2015). Acute kidney injury. *Clinical Medicine, 15*(6), 581–584.

Cross, N. B., & Webster, A. C. (2016). Angiotensin-converting enzyme inhibitors: Beneficial effects seen in many patient groups may not extend to kidney transplant recipients. *Transplantation, 100*(3), 472–473.

Crow, S. (2016). *What you need to know post-transplant: Common nutrient and herbal interactions.* Retrieved from https://www.kidney.org/transplantation/transaction/TC/winter14/What_You_Need_to_Know_PostTx

Dean, C. (2014). Helping women prepare for hyperemesis gravidarum. *British Journal of Midwifery, 22*(12), 847–852.

Ellis, P., & Jenkins, K. (2014). An overview of NICE guidance: Acute kidney injury. *British Journal of Nursing, 23*(16), 904–909.

El-Sharkawy, A. M., Sahota, O., Maughan, R. J., & Lobo, D. N. (2014). The pathophysiology of fluid and electrolyte balance in the folder adult surgical patient. *Clinical Nutrition, 13*(2014), 6–13.

Fantasia, H. C. (2014). A new pharmacologic treatment for nausea and vomiting. *Nursing for Women's Health, 18*(1), 73–77.

Fleming, S., Gill, P., Jones, C., Taylor, J. A., Van den Bruel, A., Heneghan, C., . . . Thompson, M. (2015). Validity and reliability of measurement of capillary refill time in children: A systematic review. *Archives of Disease in Childhood, 100*, 239–249.

Geoghegan, P., Harrison, A. M., Thongprayoon, C., Kashyap, R., Ahmed, A., & Dong, Y. (2015). Sodium correction practice and clinical outcomes in profound hyponatremia. *Mayo Clinic Proceedings, 90*(1), 1348–1355.

Gillette, H. (2013, Aug. 21). Latino folk illnesses: Exploring "caida de la mollera." *Saluidiy.* Retrieved from http://newstaco.com/2013/08/21/latino-folk-illnesses-exploring-caida-de-la-mollera/

Goldberg, L. R., Heiss, C. J., Parsons, S. D., Foley, A. S., Mefferd, A. S., Hollinger, D., . . . Patterson, J. (2014). Hydration in older adults: The contribution of bioelectric impedance analysis. *International Journal of Speech-Language Pathology, 16*(3), 273–281.

Hain, D., & Paixao, R. (2015). The perfect storm: Older adults and acute kidney injury. *Critical Nursing Quarterly, 38*(3), 271–279.

Herdman, T. H. & Kamitsuru, S. (Eds.). *Nursing Diagnoses—Definitions and Classification 2015–2017.* Copyright © 2014, 1994–2014 NANDA International. Used by arrangement with John Wiley & Sons, Inc. Companion website: www.wiley.com/go/nursingdiagnoses

Imig, J. D., & Ryan, M. J. (2013). Immune and inflammatory role in renal disease. *Comprehensive Physiology, 3*(2), 957–976.

Ingelse, S. A., Wösten-van Asperen, R. M., Lemson, J., Daams, J. G., Bem, R. A., & van Woensel, J. B. (2016). Pediatric acute respiratory distress syndrome: Fluid management in the PICU. *Frontiers in Pediatrics, 4*, 21. http://doi.org/10.3389/fped.2016.00021

Jorgenson, A. L. (2013). Contrast induced nephropathy: Pathophysiology and preventive strategies. *Critical Care Nurse, 33*(1), 37–47.

Joslin, J., Wilson, H., Zubli, D., Gauge, N., Kinirons, M., Hopper, A., . . . Ostermann, M. (2015). Recognition and management of acute kidney injury in hospitalized patients can be partially improved with the use of a care bundle. *Clinical Medicine, 15*(5), 431–436.

Kane-Gill, S. L., Sileanu, F. E., Murugan, R., Trietley, G. S., Handler, S. M., & Kellum, J. A. (2015). Risk factors for acute kidney injury in older adults with critical illness: A retrospective cohort study. *American Journal of Kidney Diseases, 65*(6), 860–869.

Karahan, M. A., Kucuk, A., Buyukfirat, E., & Yalcin, F. (2015). Acute respiratory and renal failure due to hypermagnesemia, induced by counter laxatives in an elderly man. *Journal of Clinical and Diagnostic Research, 90*(2), 1.

Kazley, A. S., Johnson, E. E., Simpson, K. N., Chavin, K. D., & Baliga, P. (2014). Health care provider perception of chronic kidney disease: Knowledge and behavior among African American patients. *BMC Nephrology, 15*, 112. doi:10.1186/1471-2369-15-112

Krishna, A., Singh, R., Prasad, N., Gupta, A., Bhadauria, D., Kaul, A., . . . Kapoor, D. (2015). Maternal, fetal and renal outcomes of pregnancy-associated acute kidney injury requiring dialysis. *Indian Journal of Nephrology, 25*(2), 77–81. http://doi.org/10.4103/0971-4065.136890

Lewis, J. L. (2016). Hypomagnesemia. *Merck Manual.* Retrieved from https://www.merckmanuals.com/professional/endocrine-and-metabolic-disorders/electrolyte-disorders/hypomagnesemia

Liamis, G., Rodenberg, E. M., Hoffman, A., Zietse, R., Stricker, B. H., & Hoorn, E. J. (2013). Electrolyte disorders in community subjects: Prevalence and risk factors. *American Journal of Medicine, 126*(3), 256–263.

Machado, S., Figueiredo, N., Borges, A., São José Pais, M., Freitas, L., Moura, P., . . . Campos, M. (2012). Acute kidney injury in pregnancy: A clinical challenge. *Journal of Nephrology, 25*(1), 19–30.

Mayo Clinic. (2014). *Dehydration.* Retrieved from http://www.mayoclinic.org/diseases-conditions/dehydration/basics/definition/con-20030056

Mayo Clinic. (2016). *Chronic kidney disease.* Retrieved from http://www.mayoclinic.org/diseases-conditions/kidney-disease/basics/definition/con-20026778

McClelland, M. (2014). IV therapies for patients with fluid and electrolyte imbalances. *MEDSURG Nursing, 23*(5), S4–S8. Retrieved from Academic OneFile: http://go.galegroup.com/ps/anonymous?id=GALE%7CA389798024&sid=googleScholar&v=2.1&it=r&linkaccess=fulltext&issn=10920811&p=AONE&sw=w&authCount=1&isAnonymousEntry=true

McCrow, J., Morton, M., Travers, C., Harvey, K., & Eeles, E. (2016). Associations between dehydration, cognitive impairment, and frailty in older hospitalized patients: An exploratory study. *Journal of Gerontological Nursing, 42*(5), 19–27.

McLafferty, E., Johnstone, C., Hendry, C., & Farley, A. (2014). Fluid and electrolyte balance. *Nursing Standard, 28*(29), 42–49.

Merrill, M., Aviram, A., Niu, B., Ameel, B., & Caughey, A. (2016). Outcomes of pregnancies complicated by maternal chronic renal disease. *American Journal of Obstetrics and Gynecology, 214*(1), S328.

Milanovic, D., & Groselj-Grenc, M. (2014). Fluid balance in critically ill neonates—ways to improve it. *Signa Vitae, 9*(1), 33–36. doi:10.22514/sv91.042014.5

Mizokami, F., & Mizuno, T. (2015). Acute kidney injury induced by antimicrobial agents in the elderly: Awareness and mitigation strategies. *Drugs and Aging, 32*, 1–12.

Moshfegh, A. J., Holden, J. M., Cogswell, M. E., Kuklina, E. V., Patel, S. M., Gunn, J. P., . . . Galuska, D. A. (2012). Vital signs: Food categories contributing the most to sodium consumption. *Morbidity & Mortality Weekly Report, 61*(5), 92–98.

National Kidney and Urologic Diseases Information Clearinghouse (NKUDIC). (2012, June). *Kidney disease statistics for the United States* (NIH Publication No. 12-3895). Retrieved from http://kidney.niddk.nih.gov/KUDiseases/pubs/kustats/KU_Diseases_Stats_508.pdf

National Kidney Foundation. (2013). *About chronic kidney disease.* Retrieved from http://www.kidney.org/kidneydisease/aboutckd.cfm#facts

National Kidney Foundation. (2016a). *African Americans and kidney disease.* Retrieved from https://www.kidney.org/news/newsroom/factsheets/African-Americans-and-CKD

National Kidney Foundation. (2016b). *Organ donation and transplant statistics.* Retrieved from https://www.kidney.org/news/newsroom/factsheets/Organ-Donation-and-Transplantation-Stats

National Kidney Foundation. (2016c). *Organ donation and transplantation statistics.* Retrieved from https://www.kidney.org/news/newsroom/factsheets/Organ-Donation-and-Transplantation-Stats

National Kidney Foundation. (2016d). *Palliative care helps patients with kidney disease.* Retrieved from https://www.kidney.org/atoz/content/palliative-care-helps-patients-kidney-disease

Nephron Information Center. (2012). *Dietary protein for the person with chronic kidney disease.* Retrieved from http://nephron.com/nephsites/adp/index.htm/protein_ckd.htm

Noone, D., & Licht, C. (2014). Chronic kidney disease: A new look at pathogenetic mechanisms and treatment options. *Pediatric Nephrology, 29,* 771–784.

Office of Disease Prevention and Health Promotion. (2017). Chronic kidney disease. *Healthy People 2020.* Retrieved from https://www.healthypeople.gov/2020/topics-objectives/topic/chronic-kidney-disease

Ogunyemi, D. A. (2015). Hyperemesis gravidarum. *Medscape.* Retrieved from http://emedicine.medscape.com/article/254751-overview

Pachter, L. M., Weller, S. C., Baer, R. D., Garcia, J. E. G., Glazer, M., Trotter, R., . . . Gonzalez, E. (2015, Aug.). Culture and dehydration: A comparative study of caida de la mollera (fallen fontanel) in three Latino populations. *Journal of Immigrant Minority Health, 2015,* 1–39.

Payne, D. C., Vinje, J., Szilagv, P. G., Edwards, K. M., Staat, M. A., Weinberg, G. A., . . . Parashar, U. D. (2013). Norovirus and medically attended gastroenteritis in U.S. children. *New England Journal of Medicine, 366*(12), 1121–1130.

Qavi, A. H., Kamal, R., & Schrier, R. W. (2015). Clinical use of diuretics in heart failure, cirrhosis, and nephrotic syndrome. *International Journal of Nephrology* (Article ID 975934). doi:10.1155/2015/975934

Renal Association. (2013). *The stages of kidney disease.* Retrieved from http://www.renal.org/information-resources/the-uk-eckd-guide/ckd-stages#sthash.epEDkCW7.dpbs

Ross, A. J., Medow, M. S., Rowe, P. C., & Stewart, J. M. (2013). What is brain fog? An evaluation of the symptom in postural tachycardia syndrome. *Clinical Autonomic Research, 23*(6), 305–311.

Saardi, K. M., & Schwartz, R. A. (2016). Uremic frost: A harbinger of impending renal failure. *International Journal of Dermatology, 55*(1), 17–20. doi:10.1111/ijd.12963

Saboute, B., Parvini, N., Khalessi, N., Kalbassi, Z., Kalani, M., & Khosravi, N. (2016). The prevalence of acute kidney injury in neonates with asphyxia. *Journal of Pediatric Nephrology, 4*(1), 30–32.

Schetz, M., Gunst, J., & Van den Berghe, G. (2014). The impact of using estimated GFR versus creatinine clearance on the evaluation of recovery from acute kidney injury in the ICU. *Intensive Care Medicine, 40*(11), 1709–1717.

Scurati-Manzoni, E., Fossali, E. F., Agostoni, C., Riva, E., Simonetti, G. D., Zanolari-Calderari, M., . . . Lava, S. A. G. (2014). Electrolyte abnormalities in cystic fibrosis: Systematic review of the literature. *Pediatric Nephrology, 29*(6), 1015–1023.

Smith, J. A., Refuerzo, J. S., & Ramin, S. M. (2016). Treatment and outcome of nausea and vomiting of pregnancy. *UpToDate.* Retrieved from http://www.uptodate.com/contents/treatment-and-outcome-of-nausea-and-vomiting-of-pregnancy

Stojanović, V., Barišić, N., Milanović, B., & Doronjski, A. (2014). Acute kidney injury in preterm infants admitted to a neonatal intensive care unit. *Pediatric Nephrology, 29*(11), 2213–2220.

Tam, R. K., Wong, H., Plint, A., Lepage, N., & Filler, G. (2014). Comparison of clinical and biochemical markers of dehydration with the clinical dehydration scale in children: A case comparison trial. *BMC Pediatrics, 14,* 149.

Tanner, R. M., Shimbo, D., Dreisbach, A. W., Carson, A. P., Fox, E. R., & Muntner, P. (2015). Association between 24-hour blood pressure variability and chronic kidney disease: A cross-sectional analysis of African Americans participating in the Jackson heart study. *BMC Nephrology, 16.* doi.org/10.7916/D8CV4HQ6

Topf, J., Sparks, M., & August, P. (2015, March 2). Preeclampsia due to CKD vs CKD due to preeclampsia. *NephMadness 2015: Obstetric Nephrology Region.* Retrieved from http://www.medscape.com/viewarticle/840394_3

Trayes, K. P., Studdiford, J. S., Pickle, S., & Tully, A. S. (2013). Edema: Diagnosis and management. *American Family Physician, 88*(2), 102–110.

Uettwiller-Geiger, D., & McPherson, P. (2015). Acute kidney injury: New biomarkers detect risk for this silent killer. *Medical Laboratory Observer.* Retrieved from https://www.mlo-online.com/acute-kidney-injury-new-biomarkers-detect-risk-for-this-silent-killer.php

Uribe, L. M., & Schub, M. M. (2015). *Hydration: Maintaining oral hydration in older adults. Evidence-based care sheet.* Glendale, CA: Cinahl Information Systems.

U.S. Renal Data System. (2016). *USRDS: Annual data report, 2016.* Retrieved from https://www.usrds.org/adr.aspx

Waddell, D., McGrath, I., & Maude, P. (2014). The effect of a rapid rehydration guideline in emergency department management of gastroenteritis in children. *International Emergency Nursing, 22*(3), 159–164.

Wesseling-Perry, K., & Salusky, I. B. (2013). Chronic kidney disease: Mineral and bone disorder in children. *Seminars in Nephrology, 33*(2), 169–179. Retrieved from https://www.ncbi.nlm.nih.gov/pubmed/23465503

Wong, S. H. S., & Sun, F. H. (2014). Effect of beverage flavor on body hydration in Hong Kong Chinese children exercising in a hot environment. *Pediatric Exercise Science, 26*(2), 177–186.

Yang, F., Zhang, L., Wu, H., Zou, H., & Du, Y. (2014). Clinical analysis of cause, treatment and prognosis in acute kidney injury patients. *PLoS ONE, 9*(2), e85214. https://doi.org/10.1371/journal.pone.0085214

Yang, Q., Zhang, A., Kuklina, E. V., Fang, J., Ayala, C., Hong, Y., . . . Merrit, R. (2012). Sodium intake and blood pressure among U.S. children and adolescents. *Pediatrics, 120*(4), 611–619.

Yue, Z., Jiang, P., Sun, H., & Wu, J. (2014). Association between excess risk of acute kidney injury and a concomitant use of ibuprofen and acetaminophen in children: Retrospective analysis of a spontaneous reporting system. *European Journal of Clinical Pharmacology, 70,* 479–482.

Zadrazil, J., & Horak, P. (2015). Pathophysiology of anemia in chronic kidney diseases: A review. *Biomedical Papers, 159*(2), 197–202.

Module 7
Health, Wellness, Illness, and Injury

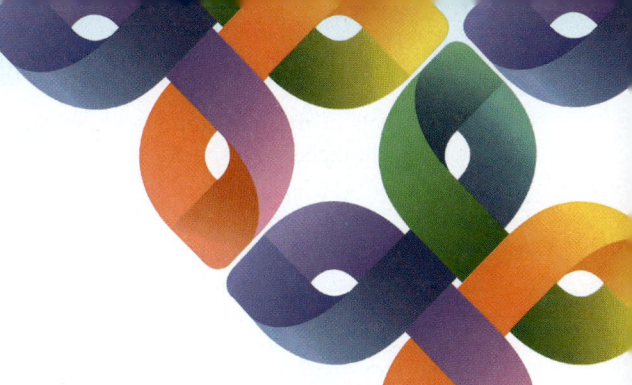

Module Outline and Learning Outcomes

» The Concept of Health, Wellness, Illness, and Injury

Concept Key Terms

Acute illness, **434**	Disease, **434**	Illness, **434**	Positive reinforcement, **445**	Self-concept, **441**
Alternative medicine, **443**	Exacerbation, **434**	Illness behavior, **434**	Primary prevention, **438**	Sick-role behavior, **434**
Autonomy, **435**	External locus of control, **442**	Injury, **434**	Remission, **434**	Tertiary prevention, **438**
Chronic illness, **434**	Health, **432**	Integrative health, **442**	Risk factors, **441**	Well-being, **433**
Complementary health approaches, **442**	Health beliefs, **442**	Internal locus of control, **442**	Secondary prevention, **438**	Wellness, **432**
	Health promotion, **435**	Lifestyle choices, **441**		

Nurses' understanding of health and wellness largely determines the scope and nature of nursing practice. Patients' health beliefs also influence health practices. Some individuals think of health and wellness as the same thing or, at the very least, as accompanying one another. However, health may not always accompany well-being. An individual who has a terminal illness may have a sense of well-being; another person conversely may lack a sense of well-being, yet be in a state of good health.

For many years, the concept of disease was the yardstick by which health was measured. In the late 19th century, the "how" of disease (pathogenesis) was the major concern of health professionals. The 20th century focused on finding cures for diseases. Healthcare providers today are increasing their emphasis on promoting health and wellness in individuals, families, and communities.

Health, Wellness, and the Health Continuum

Health, wellness, and well-being have many definitions and interpretations. Nurses should be familiar with the most common aspects of these concepts and consider how they may be individualized with specific patients.

Health

Health has traditionally been defined as the presence or absence of disease. Nightingale (1859/1969) defined *health* as a state of being well and using every power the individual possesses to the fullest extent. The World Health Organization (WHO, 1948) takes a more holistic view of health. Its constitution defines *health* as "a state of complete physical, mental, and social well-being, and not merely the absence of disease or infirmity." This definition serves the following purposes:

- It reflects concern for the individual as a total person, functioning physically, psychologically, and socially. Mental processes determine individuals' relationships with their physical and social surroundings, their attitudes about life, and their interaction with others.

- It places health in the context of the environment. Individuals' lives, and therefore their health, are affected by everything they interact with—not only environmental influences, such as climate and the availability of food, shelter, clean air, and water to drink, but also other individuals, including family members, lovers, employers, coworkers, friends, and associates. See the exemplar on Environmental Quality in the module on Advocacy for more details.

In 1980, the American Nurses Association (ANA) defined *health* in its social policy statement as "a dynamic state of being in which the developmental and behavioral potential of an individual is realized to the fullest extent possible" (1980, p. 5). In this definition, health is more than a state or the absence of disease; it includes striving toward optimal functioning. In 2004, the ANA also stated that health was "an experience that is often expressed in terms of wellness and illness, and may occur in the presence or absence of disease or injury" (2004, p. 48).

Personal Definitions of Health

Health is a highly individual perception. Consider the following examples of individuals who would probably say they are healthy, even though they have physical impairments that some people would consider illnesses or injuries:

- A 15-year-old boy with diabetes takes injectable insulin each morning. He plays on the school soccer team and is editor of the high school newspaper.

- A 32-year-old man is paralyzed from the waist down after a car accident and needs a wheelchair for mobility. He is taking an accounting class at a nearby college and uses a specially designed automobile for transportation.

- A 72-year-old woman takes antihypertensive medications to treat high blood pressure. She bowls once a week, is a member of the neighborhood golf club, makes handicrafts for a local charity, and travels 2 months each year.

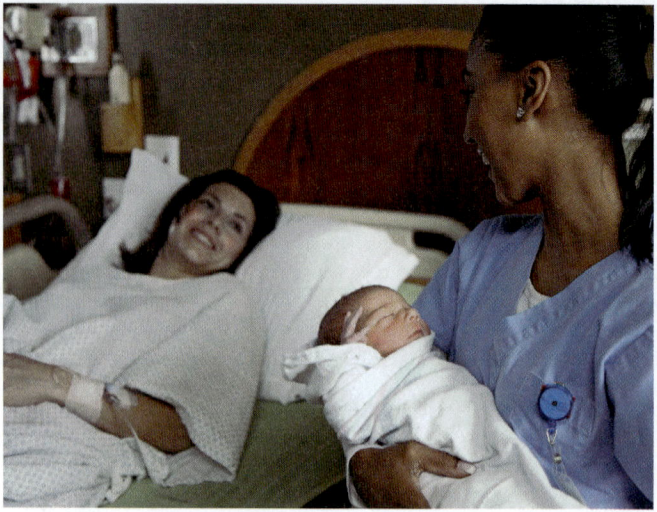

Source: RubberBall Productions/Brand X Pictures/Getty Images.

Figure 7–1 》 Satisfaction with work enhances a sense of well-being and contributes to wellness.

Many individuals describe health as being free as possible from symptoms of disease and pain, being able to be active, and being in good spirits most of the time. These characteristics indicate that health is not a state that an individual achieves suddenly at a specific time. It is an ongoing process, a way of life through which an individual develops. Every aspect of the body, mind, and emotions strives to interrelate as harmoniously as possible.

Many factors affect individual definitions of health: the individual's previous experiences, expectations of self, age, and sociocultural influences. Nurses should be aware of their personal definitions of health and appreciate that other individuals also have their own definitions. Individuals' definitions of health influence their behavior related to health and illness. By understanding patients' perceptions of health and illness, nurses can better help them to attain or regain a state of health.

Wellness and Well-Being

Wellness is a state of well-being. Basic aspects of wellness include self-responsibility; an ultimate goal; a dynamic, growing process; and daily decision making in the areas of nutrition, stress management, physical fitness, preventive healthcare, and emotional health. Most important, wellness focuses attention on the whole being of the individual (see **Figure 7–1 》**).

Anspaugh, Hamrick, and Rosato (2010) propose seven components of wellness (see **Figure 7–2 》**). To realize optimal health and wellness, individuals must deal with the factors within each component:

1. **The environmental component** involves the ability to promote health measures that improve the standard of living and quality of life in the community and includes influences such as food, water, and air.

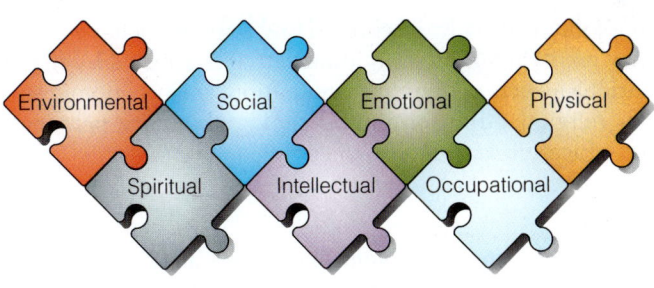

Figure 7–2)) The seven components of wellness.

2. **The occupational component** is the ability to achieve a balance between work and leisure time. Individuals' beliefs about education, employment, and home influence their personal satisfaction and relationships with others.

3. **The intellectual component** includes the ability to learn and use information effectively for personal, family, and career development. Intellectual wellness involves striving for continued growth and learning to deal effectively with new challenges.

4. **The spiritual component** is the belief in some force (nature, science, religion, or a higher power) that serves to unite human beings and provide meaning and purpose to life. It includes individuals' own morals, values, and ethics.

5. **The physical component** is the ability to carry out daily tasks, achieve fitness (e.g., pulmonary, cardiovascular, gastrointestinal), maintain adequate nutrition and proper body fat levels, avoid abusing drugs and alcohol or using tobacco products, and generally practice positive lifestyle habits.

6. **The emotional component** is the ability to manage stress and to express emotions appropriately. Emotional wellness involves individuals' ability to recognize, accept, and express their feelings and to accept their limitations.

7. **The social component** is the ability of individuals to interact successfully with other people and within their environment, to develop and maintain intimacy with significant others, and to develop respect and tolerance for those with different opinions and beliefs.

The seven components overlap to some extent, and factors in one component often directly affect factors in another. For example, an individual who learns to control daily stress levels from a physiologic perspective is also helping to maintain the emotional stamina needed to cope with a crisis. Wellness involves working on all aspects of the model.

Well-being is a component of health. The Centers for Disease Control and Prevention (CDC, 2013b) defines *well-being* as "the presence of positive emotions and moods (e.g., contentment, happiness), the absence of negative emotions (e.g., depression, anxiety), satisfaction with life, fulfillment and positive functioning, judging life positively and feeling good."

The Health Continuum

Health can be conceptualized as a continuum (see **Figure 7–3**)). Wellness is located at the opposite end of the health continuum from the disabling effects of illness or injury. Beginning at a high level of wellness, an individual can move through good health, normal health, poor health, extremely poor health, and eventually to death. Individuals move back and forth within this continuum day by day. There is no distinct boundary across which individuals move from wellness to illness or injury, or a threshold that moves them back to wellness. How individuals perceive themselves and how others see them in terms of wellness and illness or injury also affect their placement on the continuum.

Illness and Injury

The terminology of illness and injury is important for nurses to make part of their everyday vocabulary. Nurses use these terms in talking with patients, their families and significant others, and the entire range of healthcare professionals. These definitions apply regardless of the specialty of the clinical professional.

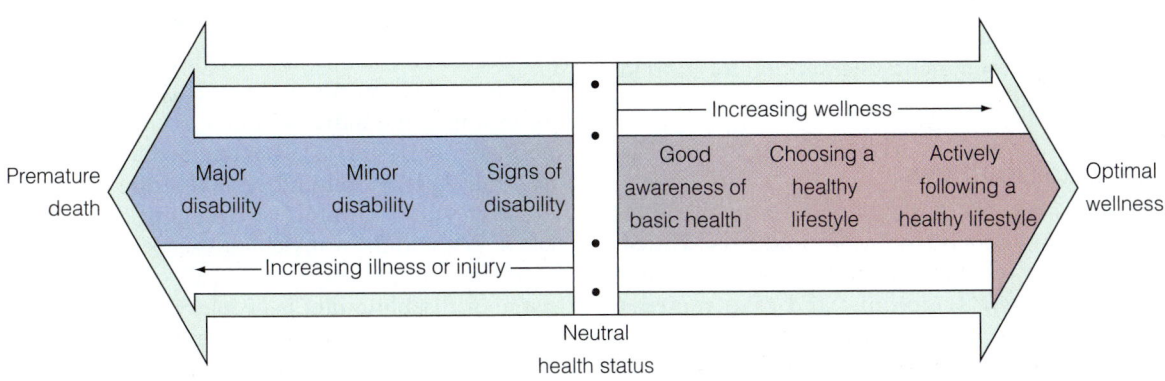

Figure 7–3)) The health continuum.

Illness and Disease

Illness is a highly personal state in which the individual's physical, emotional, intellectual, social, developmental, or spiritual functioning is diminished. It is not synonymous with disease, and it may or may not be related to disease. One individual can have a disease, such as a growth in the stomach, and not feel ill. Another individual can feel ill—that is, feel uncomfortable—and yet have no discernible disease.

Disease can be described as an alteration in body functions that reduces the capacities or shortens the normal lifespan. Some diseases mainly affect the individual's physical condition; others affect the individual's mental status. Disease results from many causes, such as infection, inflammation, biochemical imbalances, stress, environmental factors, or genetic factors. Its presence is usually signaled by identifiable signs and symptoms. Some diseases can be contracted by other people; some are noncommunicable.

Illness and disease can be classified in many ways. The terms *acute* and *chronic* are commonly used. **Acute illness** is typically characterized by severe symptoms of relatively short duration. The symptoms often appear abruptly and subside quickly and, depending upon the cause, may or may not require intervention by healthcare professionals. Some acute illnesses are serious (e.g., appendicitis may require surgery). But many acute illnesses, such as colds, subside without medical intervention or with only over-the-counter medications. Following an acute illness, most individuals return to their normal level of wellness.

A **chronic illness** is one that lasts for an extended period, usually 6 months or longer, and often for the duration of the individual's life. Chronic illnesses usually have a slow onset and often have periods of **remission**, when the symptoms disappear, and **exacerbation**, when the symptoms reappear.

Examples of chronic illnesses include arthritis, heart and lung diseases, and diabetes mellitus. Nurses care for individuals of all ages with chronic illness in many settings—patients' homes, nursing homes, hospitals, clinics, and other institutions. Care focuses on promoting the highest possible level of independence, sense of control, and wellness. Patients with chronic illness often need to modify their activities of daily living, social relationships, and perception of self and body image. In addition, many patients must learn how to live with increasing physical limitations and discomfort. Teaching compliance with medications and treatment plans, even when the patient feels well, is an essential nursing intervention for individuals with chronic illnesses.

Health Behavior in Illness

When individuals become ill, they often use two kinds of coping mechanisms described by sociologists. **Illness behavior** involves ways that individuals describe, monitor, and interpret their symptoms, and take remedial actions (Kasl & Cobb, 1966a). An example would be a patient eating a family recipe for chicken soup when flu symptoms start. **Sick-role behavior** often includes using the healthcare system for help and may involve dependent behaviors, such as avoiding usual responsibilities (Kasl & Cobb, 1966b). An example would be a patient staying in bed for an extended rest and not doing housework, going to a job, or attending school. How patients behave when they are ill is highly individualized. It is affected by many variables such as age, sex, occupation, socioeconomic status, religion, ethnic origin, psychologic stability, personality, education, and modes of coping.

Injury

An **injury** is an act or event that causes damage, harm, or loss to a body's functioning. No matter how healthy individuals are, regardless of their optimum lifestyle habits and genetic background, they can experience unexpected accidents that cause injury. They can also be involved in intentionally violent activities that result in physical or mental trauma. Either way, the outcomes can range from minor, self-healing wounds to life-threatening and life-altering catastrophes. See the module on Trauma for more details, including independent and collaborative interventions for patients with injuries.

Effects of Illness and Injury on the Patient and Family

When individuals become ill or are injured, the full effect of the alteration to their wellness is experienced by the whole family. The impact of the changes depends on the nature, severity, and duration of the events; attitudes toward the precipitating factor by the patient and others; the associated financial costs; the required lifestyle changes; and the significant adjustments in usual roles.

Four types of situations have a universally significant-enough effect on the family system to characterize them as crises:

1. Chronic illness
2. Major injuries
3. Mental illness
4. Pediatric illness.

These events often greatly disrupt normal family functioning. Dealing with these challenges is an integral part of designing an individualized plan of care. See the exemplar on Family Response to Health Alterations in the module on Family for more information about how to include the family in treatment.

Patients who are ill or injured may experience behavioral and emotional changes, changes in self-concept and body image, and lifestyle changes (see **Figure 7–4 》》**). Behavioral and emotional changes associated with short-term illness or quickly healed injuries are generally mild and short-lived. For example, the individual may become irritable and lack the energy or desire for usual interactions with family members or friends. More acute responses are likely with severe, life-threatening, chronic, or disabling diagnoses. Anxiety, fear, anger, withdrawal, denial, a sense of hopelessness, and feelings of powerlessness are all common responses to severe or disabling illness or injury. For example, a patient experiencing a heart attack or a car accident fears for her life and the financial burden it may place on the family. Another patient diagnosed with cancer or told about a need for limb amputation may, over time, experience episodes of denial, anger, fear, and hopelessness. For a patient with a lifelong chronic illness or permanent disabilities, these feelings can recur with acute attacks or new life challenges. Additional

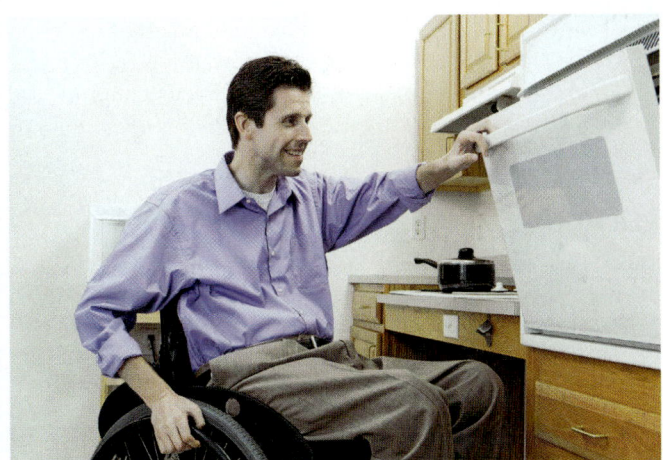

Source: Huntstock/Brand X Pictures/Getty Images.

Figure 7–4 》 Customized home environments, illustrated by the lowered countertops and pull-out cabinet shelves of this kitchen, allow people with major injuries to function independently.

financial expenses and the resulting emotional strain can greatly stress both the patient and the family.

Certain illnesses or injuries can also change the patient's body image or physical appearance, especially those that involve severe scarring or loss of a limb or a sense organ. The patient's self-esteem and self-concept may also be affected. Many factors play a part in low self-esteem and a disturbance in self-concept, including loss of body parts and function, pain, disfigurement, dependence on others, unemployment, financial problems, inability to participate in social functions, strained relationships with others, and spiritual distress. Nurses must help patients express their thoughts and feelings, as well as provide care that helps patients cope effectively with changes.

Individuals who are ill or injured are vulnerable to loss of **autonomy**, the state of being independent and self-directed without outside control. Family interactions may change so that patients are no longer involved in making family decisions or even in making decisions about their own healthcare. Nurses must support patients' right to self-determination and autonomy. Patients need sufficient information to participate in decision-making processes and to maintain a feeling of being in control.

Illness and injury often necessitate radical changes in both an individual's and a family's lifestyle. In addition to participating in treatments and taking medications, the patient may need to change diet, activity and exercise, and rest and sleep patterns. Nurses can help patients and families in the following ways:

- Providing explanations about necessary lifestyle adjustments and accommodations to all involved individuals, including their role in helping the patient recover

- Making arrangements whenever possible to balance negative effects on the patient's and the family's lifestyles

- Encouraging other health professionals to become aware of the patient's lifestyle and to support healthy aspects of that lifestyle

- Reinforcing desirable changes with a goal of making them a permanent part of the patient's and family's lifestyles.

Case Study 》 Part 1

Bette Smithers is a 30-year-old woman who visits her primary care physician with complaints of double vision, leg muscle cramps, lumbar back pain, and increasing fatigue. As the nurse working at the clinic, you are tasked with taking Ms. Smithers' medical history and preliminary assessment. She is 5'4" tall and weighs 180 pounds. Her vital signs include temperature 98.2°F oral; pulse 60 bpm; respirations 16/min; and BP 130/98 mmHg. Ms. Smithers rates her back pain as 3 on a scale of 0–10, but adds that it was an 8 when she got out of bed this morning. Per the physician's orders, a blood sample and urine sample are obtained for analysis. When asked about her diet, Ms. Smithers admits that she visits a coffee shop every day on her way to work for a latte and a roll. She skips lunch "to save money and calories" and has a salad, soup, and sandwich for dinner. She explains her muscle cramps, back pain, and fatigue as starting around the time she moved from the Midwest to the West Coast. "I have lifted a lot of heavy boxes," she explained. "And I don't get a lot of sleep in my new apartment."

Clinical Reasoning Questions Level I

1. What risk factors does Ms. Smithers have for developing the symptoms that brought her to the clinic?
2. Other than tenderness in her lumbar region of her spine, what findings might you discover in your assessment of Ms. Smithers?
3. What is your professional opinion of Ms. Smithers' explanation of the cause of her symptoms? How would you respond to her speculation?

Clinical Reasoning Questions Level II

4. What is the priority nursing diagnosis for Ms. Smithers?
5. What nursing interventions can you implement to help manage Ms. Smithers' pain and her lack of sleep?
6. How would you explain to Ms. Smithers your calculation of her body mass index (BMI) and its contribution to her position on the health continuum?

Concepts Related to Health, Wellness, Illness, and Injury

All nursing concepts relate to health, wellness, illness, and injury. Thus, nurses should think about how each concept affects the patient's and the family's overall well-being. A disturbance in one part of the body has an impact on the entire person.

For example, a patient with chronic obstructive pulmonary disease (COPD) may have altered cognition because his brain is not getting enough oxygen. He may have issues with safety because he is using supplemental oxygen (which is flammable) at home, and he still wants to smoke. He may have altered fluid and electrolyte levels because he is not drinking enough liquids. He does not respond to his wife's and his nurse's encouragement to increase his fluid intake because his mobility is limited. He has trouble getting to the kitchen and to the bathroom. His wife may have alterations in stress and coping due to the physical, emotional, and financial stresses of caring for her husband. The nurse may have difficulty with communication because the patient's cognition is altered. The Concepts Related to Health, Wellness, Illness, and Injury feature links some, but not all, of the concepts related to health, wellness, illness, and injury. They are presented in alphabetical order.

Health Promotion

The national vision of **health promotion** was initially expressed in 1979 with the U.S. Surgeon General's report *Healthy People,*

Concepts Related to
Health, Wellness, Illness, and Injury

CONCEPT	RELATIONSHIP TO HEALTH, WELLNESS, ILLNESS, AND INJURY	NURSING IMPLICATIONS
Advocacy	Nurses advocate for healthy individuals, populations, nations, and the planet.	■ Assess all patients' health literacy abilities to encourage full participation in their healthcare. ■ Educate vulnerable populations about their legal rights and ways to give input to their healthcare providers. ■ Be informed about the current national and global health and wellness issues.
Assessment	A nursing assessment identifies habits of health and wellness and effects of illness and injury.	■ Become adept in the four primary techniques used in physical examinations: inspection, palpation, percussion, and auscultation. ■ Review documentation of patient interviews to produce a complete nursing health history. ■ Keep updated with the current literature about evidence-based assessments.
Family	Illness and injury affect the well-being of the whole family, not just the individual patient.	■ Include family members in the patient education process, especially when making discharge plans. ■ Be aware of the impact that recent family crises, such as divorce or death, can have on the recovery of patients. ■ Include a family health history in the assessment of patients, using a genogram if indicated.
Infection	Infections cause illnesses and can be dangerous complications of injuries.	■ Use good infection prevention measures to reduce the risk of spread of infection, especially healthcare-associated infections. ■ Promptly recognize the early signs of an infected wound and immediately respond. ■ Teach patients and caregivers good hygiene habits and compliance with taking antimicrobial medications.
Mobility	Treatment for illnesses and injuries, such as prolonged bedrest, can cause mobility problems.	■ Teach patients the proper way to use crutches, canes, and walkers to avoid the complication of falling. ■ Perform range-of-motion exercises on patients who are immobile. ■ Adapt physical fitness exercises to the limitations posed by musculoskeletal disorders, such as doing stretches while sitting in a chair.
Reproduction	Hormones in pregnant women maintain the health and wellness of their fetuses.	■ Prepare the patient and significant others for the profound physical and psychologic changes of pregnancy. ■ Emphasize the value of keeping routine visits for prenatal care for the health of the mother and the baby. ■ Individualize care for the pregnant adolescent and the pregnant woman over 35 years old.
Trauma	Trauma can cause both physical and emotional injuries. Recovery can produce a sense of well-being.	■ When caring for a trauma victim, prioritize assessment of health by using the ABCDEs. (A = airway, B = breathing, C = circulation, D = disability and neurologic assessment, E = exposure and environmental control) ■ To help prevent the trauma of abuse, identify patients' high-risk situations and review their strengths and coping skills.

which emphasized health promotion and disease prevention. Every decade since then, the Surgeon General has updated the report, establishing benchmarks and monitoring progress.

Healthy People 2020

Healthy People 2020: Improving the Health of Americans (U.S. Department of Health and Human Services, 2015) presents a comprehensive 10-year agenda with four goals:

1. Attain high-quality, longer lives free of preventable disease, disability, injury, and premature death
2. Achieve health equity, eliminate disparities, and improve the health of all groups

3. Create social and physical environments that promote good health for all
4. Promote quality of life, healthy development, and healthy behaviors across all life stages.

To support these goals, *Healthy People 2020* is organized into 42 topic areas, 13 of which are newly added targets for this decade (see **Box 7–1** »). *Healthy People 2020* also established a set of 12 types of health indicators, which reflect the current major public health concerns in the United States. Healthcare professionals are expected to develop matching action plans for these health indicators to improve the health of both individuals and communities. *Nursing: A Concept-Based Approach to Learning, Third Edition,* covers all 12 types (see **Table 7–1** »).

TABLE 7–1 The 12 Types of Health Indicators in *Healthy People 2020*

Health Indicators	Description	Covered in This Program
1: Access to health services	Strong predictors of access to quality healthcare services include having health insurance (1 in 5 Americans under age 65 do not have that) and a regular primary care provider or other source of ongoing healthcare (almost 1 in 4 Americans do not have that).	Exemplar on Access to Healthcare in the module on Healthcare Systems
2: Clinical preventive services	Clinical preventive services, such as early prenatal care, and routine disease screening are key to reducing death and disability. Vaccines are among the greatest public health achievements of the 20th century. Immunizations can prevent disability and death from infectious diseases and can help control the spread of infections within communities.	Health Promotion is a main heading with an accompanying learning outcome in every Concept.
3: Environmental quality	An estimated 25% of all deaths and the total disease burden world-wide can be attributed to environmental factors. Nearly 1 in 10 children and 1 in 12 adults in the United States have asthma. That condition is caused, triggered, and exacerbated by air pollution and secondhand smoke.	Exemplar on Environmental Quality in the module on Advocacy
4: Injury and violence	For Americans age 1–44, injuries are the leading cause of death. Annually, more than 29 million individuals seek emergency department treatment for injuries. More than 180,000 individuals die from injuries each year, and about 51,000 deaths result from violence.	Module on Trauma
5: Maternal, infant, and child health	The rate of preterm births has risen by more than 20% from 1990 to 2006. That rate is one factor in the high American infant death rate; in 2011, the rate was higher than in 46 other countries.	Every Concept and most Exemplars have a Lifespan Considerations section and accompanying learning outcomes.
6: Mental health	Approximately 25% of the adult U.S. population is affected by mental illness during a given year; no one is immune. One in seventeen has been diagnosed with a serious mental illness. Of all mental illnesses, depression and anxiety are the most common. Major depression is the leading cause of disability and is the cause of more than two thirds of suicides each year. Suicide is the 11th leading cause of death in the United States for all age groups. For individuals age 25–34, it is the second leading cause of death. *Note:* Serious mental illnesses (SMIs) are those that cause persistent or recurrent impairments in functioning or significant disability. SMIs include major depressive disorder, schizophrenia, bipolar disorder, posttraumatic stress disorder (PTSD), obsessive–compulsive disorder, panic disorder, and borderline personality disorder.	Module on Addiction Module on Cognition Module on Grief and Loss Module on Mood and Affect Module on Self Module on Stress and Coping Module on Trauma
7: Nutrition, physical activity, and obesity	Regular physical activity throughout life is important for maintaining a healthy body, enhancing psychologic well-being, and preventing premature death. A majority of adults (81.6%) and adolescents (81.8%) do not get the recommended amount of physical activity. Being overweight or obese is a major contributor to many preventable causes of death. On average, higher body weights are associated with higher death rates. The number of overweight children, adolescents, and adults has risen since the 1970s. About 1 in 3 adults (34.0%) and 1 in 6 children and adolescents (16.2%) are obese. Obesity-related conditions include heart disease, stroke, and type 2 diabetes.	Module on Nutrition Exemplar on Obesity Exemplar on Physical Fitness and Exercise
8: Oral health	Poor oral health, especially gum disease, is linked to chronic diseases such as diabetes, heart disease, and stroke. In pregnant women, poor oral health is associated with preterm births and low birth weight. In 2007, only about half of individuals age 2 and older had seen a dentist in the past year.	Exemplar on Oral Health
9: Reproductive and sexual health	Unintended pregnancies and sexually transmitted diseases (STDs), including infection with HIV, which causes AIDS, can result from unprotected sexual behaviors. About 19 million new cases of STDs are diagnosed in the United States each year, almost half among young adults age 15–24. Out of every 5 individuals with HIV, 1 is unaware of having it.	Module on Sexuality Module on Reproduction
10: Social determinants	This new leading indicator recognizes the critical role of the environment in improving health. It focuses attention on home, school, workplace, neighborhood, and community.	Module on Culture and Diversity Focus on Culture and Diversity features in every module
11: Substance abuse	Alcohol and illicit drug use are associated with many serious problems, including family disruptions, financial debt, school failure, domestic violence, child abuse, and crime.	Module on Addiction Exemplar on Substance Abuse
12: Tobacco use	Cigarette smoking is the single most preventable cause of disease, disability, and death in the United States. More deaths result from tobacco use than all deaths from HIV, illegal drugs, alcohol, car accidents, suicides, and murders combined.	Module on Addiction Exemplar on Nicotine Use

Source: Data from U.S. Department of Health and Human Services, Office of Disease Prevention. (2015). *Healthy People 2020: Improving the health of Americans.* Retrieved from http://www.healthypeople.gov/2020/

Box 7–1
The 13 New Topic Areas in *Healthy People 2020*

These 13 topic areas were not evaluated in *Healthy People 2010* but were added for measurement in the next decade:

1. Adolescent Health
2. Blood Disorders and Blood Safety
3. Dementias, Including Alzheimer's Disease
4. Early and Middle Childhood
5. Genomics
6. Global Health
7. Healthcare-Associated Infections
8. Health-Related Quality of Life and Well-Being
9. Lesbian, Gay, Bisexual, and Transgender Health
10. Older Adults
11. Preparedness
12. Sleep Health
13. Social Determinants of Health

Critical Thinking Questions

1. Which topics most interest you?
2. Why do you think national health promotion experts added these specific topic areas?
3. Which topics are priorities for your community? For your family? For you?

Source: From *2020 Topics and Objectives – Objectives A–Z.* Published by U.S. Department of Health & Human Services.

>> **Stay Current:** Visit http://www.healthypeople.gov to learn more about the *Healthy People 2020* goals.

The foundation for *Healthy People 2020* is the belief that individual health is closely linked to community health, and vice versa. For example, community health is affected by the beliefs, attitudes, and behaviors of the individuals who live in the community. As a result, partnerships and collaborations are important to improving individual and community health. Businesses; local government; and civic, professional, and religious organizations can all participate. Examples include sponsoring health fairs, establishing fitness programs, beginning community recycling, and printing immunization schedules.

Types of Preventive Services

The original *Healthy People* report from 1979 laid the foundation for a national prevention agenda. Today's healthcare system tries to avoid hospital stays, moving from a focus on curing activity to one of promoting wellness and preventing illness and injury. **Primary prevention** services focus on health promotion and illness prevention. **Secondary prevention** services include the diagnosis and treatment of disease. **Tertiary prevention** services seek to restore health following

an illness or accident and include rehabilitation and palliative services. See **Table 7–2** >> and the module on Healthcare Systems for more information on preventive healthcare.

Health Promotion Across the Lifespan

In either independent or collaborative health promotion approaches, the nurse may work with individuals of all age groups and diverse family units. The nurse may also concentrate on a specific population, such as pregnant women, elementary school-age children, or older adults. When focusing on a particular audience, the nurse needs to take condition-relevant or age-appropriate factors into consideration.

Factors that might affect a choice of health promotion approaches during pregnancy could include:

- Age of the mother
- Commitment to and availability of prenatal care
- Presence of a supportive significant other, spouse, friend, or family member
- Events surrounding the fertilization process (pregnancy by choice, rape, incest)
- Presence of other physical impairments (e.g., gestational diabetes) or mental conditions (e.g., schizophrenia)
- Previous pregnancy experiences and outcomes
- Mother's choice of childbirth setting (hospital, home delivery)
- Cultural or ethnic factors; for example, attitudes toward and access to flu shots during pregnancy (Ahluwalia et al., 2014).

Childhood obesity is a serious health problem. Data collected from 2011 to 2012 by the CDC show that 17% of American children ages 2–19 years are obese. On a positive note, the prevalence of obesity among children age 2–5 years decreased significantly, from 13.9% in 2003–2004 to 8.4% in 2011–2012 (CDC, 2015c, 2015e). Children who are obese or overweight can develop long-term health problems such as high blood pressure, high cholesterol, sleep apnea, asthma, and psychologic stress.

Specific causes of obesity and strategies to reduce weight vary from child to child, but healthy eating habits and exercise patterns form the overall basis for normal growth and prevention of obesity in children. School administrators, teachers (especially those instructing physical education classes), parents, and caregivers share responsibility for providing children with healthy food choices and environments that make eating a pleasure. All stakeholders can work together to make use of recent research findings. For example, a research study increased the portion sizes of fruits and vegetables in an elementary school cafeteria

TABLE 7–2 Levels of Prevention Activities

Level	Description	Example
Primary prevention	Activity to block disease or injury before it ever occurs	■ Campaign to encourage children to wear seat belts and not smoke ■ Promoting use of sunscreen
Secondary prevention	Activity to reduce the impact of existing disease or injury	■ Screening tests to detect early-stage diseases ■ Modified physical requirements for return-to-work after back injuries
Tertiary prevention	Activity to lessen the impact of ongoing illness or injury	■ Chronic disease management programs ■ Retraining in another career for injured workers

lunch program. That change in turn significantly increased the consumption of those healthy foods by children who chose them (Miller et al., 2015).

Older adults need to learn to adapt to and live with increasing changes and limitations. Maximizing strengths continues to be of prime importance in maintaining optimal function and quality of life. Several factors indicate a need for additional information or resources, including:

- Increase in physical limitations
- Presence of one or more chronic illnesses
- Change in cognitive status
- Difficulty gaining access to healthcare services due to transportation problems

- Inadequacy of support systems
- Need for environmental modifications for safety and maintaining independence
- Attitude of hopelessness and depression, which decreases the motivation to use resources or learn new information.

The optimum focus of health promotion activities varies widely across the lifespan of individuals. Each age group needs specific examinations and screenings, vaccinations, and health and wellness education. Because the activities are so important to maximize well-being across the lifespan, it is risky to skip over activities recommended for each age group. See **Table 7–3 ≫** and **Table 7–4 ≫** for recommended health promotion activities across the lifespan.

TABLE 7–3 Recommended Health Promotion Activities from Birth to Adolescence

Age Group	Recommended Health Promotion Activities by Age Group
Newborn and infant	<ul><li>Screening of newborns for congenital heart disease and for hearing loss (American Academy of Pediatrics [AAP], 2015b)</li><li>Health examinations at 2 weeks and at 2, 4, 6, 9, and 12 months</li><li>Immunizations: diphtheria, tetanus, acellular pertussis (DTaP), inactivated poliovirus vaccine (IPV), pneumococcal (PVC), *Haemophilus influenzae* type b (HIB), hepatitis B (HepB), hepatitis A (HepA), rotavirus, and influenza vaccines (over 6 months of age) as recommended. Varicella and measles–mumps–rubella (MMR) are not given before 12 months of age.</li><li>Fluoride supplements for infants over 6 months of age if there is inadequate water fluoridation (less than 0.3 parts per million)</li><li>Screening for metabolic conditions including phenylketonuria (PKU)</li><li>Denver Developmental Screening Test (DDST-II) or other developmental screening</li><li>Education about infant–parent attachment and bonding, playful activities to stimulate development, safety promotion, and injury control</li></ul>
Toddler	<ul><li>Health examinations at 15 and 18 months and then as recommended by the pediatrician</li><li>Dental visits starting at tooth formation, with fluoride varnish application from age 6 months through 5 years</li><li>Immunizations: continuing DTaP, IPV, pneumococcal, MMR, varicella, HIB, HepA, HepB, annual influenza vaccines (CDC, 2015g), and meningococcal vaccines as recommended</li><li>Risk assessment at age 15 months and 30 months to detect iron deficiency</li><li>Fluoride supplements if there is inadequate water fluoridation (less than 0.6 parts per million)</li><li>Education about nutrition, rest and exercise, safety promotion, and injury control</li></ul>
Preschool	<ul><li>Health examinations every 1–2 years</li><li>Immunizations: continuing DTaP, IPV, MMR, HepA and HepB, pneumococcal, varicella, annual influenza vaccines (CDC, 2015g), and other immunizations as recommended</li><li>Vision and hearing screening</li><li>Dental visits regularly with fluoride varnish application through age 5 years</li><li>Education about nutrition, rest and exercise, safety promotion, and injury control</li></ul>
School-age	<ul><li>Annual physical examination or as recommended</li><li>Immunizations as recommended, e.g., human papilloma virus [HPV] can be given as early as 9 years old (CDC, 2015b), MMR, meningococcal, tetanus–diphtheria [Tdap], and annual influenza vaccines (CDC, 2015g)</li><li>Screening for blood cholesterol level between 9 and 11 years to reduce risks of obesity (AAP, 2015a)</li><li>Periodic vision, speech, and hearing screenings</li><li>Education about nutrition and obesity prevention, rest and exercise, safety promotion, and injury control</li><li>Prediabetes screening, if in high-risk group (American Diabetes Association, 2015)</li><li>Regular dental screenings and fluoride treatments</li></ul>
Adolescent	<ul><li>Health examination as recommended by the primary care provider</li><li>Immunizations as recommended, such as adult Tdap vaccine, MMR, pneumococcal, HPV (recommended for 11- and 12-year-olds; CDC, 2015b), annual influenza vaccines (CDC, 2015g), and HepB vaccine</li><li>HIV screening between ages 16 and 18 years old (AAP, 2015a)</li><li>Periodic vision and hearing screenings</li><li>Regular dental assessments</li><li>Assessing for depression annually for ages 11–21 (AAP, 2015a)</li><li>Use of CRAFFT (Car, Relax, Forget, Friends, Trouble) screening questionnaire for drug and alcohol use (AAP, 2015a)</li><li>Education about hormonal changes, peer group influences, self-concept and body image, sexuality, safety promotion, and accident prevention</li><li>Prediabetes screening, if in high-risk group (American Diabetes Association, 2015)</li></ul>

TABLE 7–4 Recommended Health Promotion Activities for Adults

Age Group	Recommended Health Promotion Activities for Adults
Young adults	■ Routine physical examination (every 1–3 years for women; every 5 years for men) ■ Immunizations as recommended, such as tetanus–diphtheria boosters every 10 years, meningococcal vaccine if not given in early adolescence, annual influenza vaccines (CDC, 2015g), and hepatitis B vaccine ■ HPV vaccine for women up to 26 years old who have not yet received or completed the vaccine series (CDC, 2015b) ■ Regular dental assessments (every 6 months) ■ Risk-based assessment of vision at age 18 (AAP, 2015a) ■ Professional breast examination every 1–3 years for women ■ Screening for cervical dysplasia for women starting at 21 years old (AAP, 2015a) Pap test pattern: every 3 years for women age 21–29; every 3 years or Pap and HPV test every 5 years for women age 30–65 (American Cancer Society, 2015) ■ Testicular examination every year for men ■ Screening for cardiovascular disease (e.g., cholesterol test every 5 years if results are normal; blood pressure to detect hypertension; baseline electrocardiogram at age 35) ■ Diabetes mellitus screen every 3 years, if in high-risk group (American Diabetes Association, 2015) ■ Smoking: history and counseling, if needed ■ Education about career efforts and personal balance, stress management, sexuality, safety promotion, and accident prevention
Middle-aged adults	■ Physical examination (every 3–5 years until age 40, then annually) ■ Immunizations as recommended, such as a tetanus booster every 10 years and annual influenza vaccines (CDC, 2015g). ■ Regular dental assessments (e.g., every 6 months) ■ Tonometry for signs of glaucoma and other eye diseases every 2–3 years or annually if indicated ■ Breast examination for women annually by primary care provider. For ages 40–44, choice of getting mammogram; for ages 45–54, annual mammogram; age 55 and older, choice of mammogram annually or every 2 years (American Cancer Society, 2015). ■ Screen women for cervical dysplasia with a Pap test until age 65 every 3 years or Pap and HPV test every 5 years (American Cancer Society, 2015) ■ Testicular examination for men annually by primary care provider. Prostate-specific antigen (PSA) testing starting at age 50, or age 45 for African Americans with positive history (American Cancer Society, 2015) ■ Screenings for cardiovascular disease (e.g., blood pressure measurement, electrocardiogram and cholesterol test as directed by primary care provider) ■ Diabetes mellitus screen every 3 years, if in high-risk group (American Diabetes Association, 2015) ■ Starting at age 50, screenings for colorectal cancer: choice of flexible sigmoidoscopy every 5 years, colonoscopy every 10 years, double-contrast barium enema every 5 years, or CT colonography (virtual colonoscopy) every 5 years (American Cancer Society, 2015) ■ Smoking: history and counseling, if needed. Starting at age 55, low-dose CT chest scan with contrast annually if 30 pack-year smoking history, current smoker, or quit smoking within the last 15 years (American Cancer Society, 2015) ■ Education about adequate sleep, weight control, medication compliance, and accident prevention
Older adults	■ Regular dental assessments (e.g., every 6 months) ■ Tonometry for signs of glaucoma and other eye diseases every 2–3 years or annually if indicated ■ Total cholesterol and high-density lipoprotein measurement every 3–5 years until age 75 ■ Aspirin, 81 mg, daily, if in high-risk group ■ Diabetes mellitus screen every 3 years, if in high-risk group (American Diabetes Association, 2015) ■ Smoking: history and counseling, if needed. Until age 74, low-dose CT chest scan with contrast annually if 30 pack-year smoking history, current smoker, or quit smoking within the past 15 years (American Cancer Society, 2015) ■ Breast examination for women annually by primary care provider. Mammogram annually or every 2 years (American Cancer Society, 2015) ■ Pap smear for women, only if previous abnormal smears, serious cervical precancer, or hysterectomy for malignancy (American Cancer Society, 2015) ■ Annual digital rectal exam ■ Testicular examination for men annually by primary care provider. PSA testing by choice, with repeat frequency depending on PSA level (American Cancer Society, 2015) ■ Annual guaiac-based fecal occult blood test (gFOBT), fecal immunochemcial test (FIT), or stool DNA test (sDNA) every 3 years (American Cancer Society, 2015) ■ Screenings for colorectal cancer: choice of flexible sigmoidoscopy every 5 years, colonoscopy every 10 years, double-contrast barium enema every 5 years, or CT colonography (virtual colonoscopy) every 5 years (American Cancer Society, 2015) ■ Visual acuity and hearing screen annually ■ Depression screen and family violence screen periodically ■ Height and weight measurements annually ■ Sexually transmitted disease testing, if in high-risk group ■ Annual flu vaccine if over 65 or in high-risk group (CDC, 2015g). ■ Two pneumococcal vaccines, PCV13 and PPSV23, at age 65 (CDC, 2015a) ■ Single dose of shingles vaccine starting at 60 years ■ Tetanus booster every 10 years ■ Education about restful sleep, adequate nutrition, maximization of strengths, medication compliance, and accident prevention

Variables Influencing Health Choices

Patients' decisions about health choices are influenced by their individual health status, beliefs, and behaviors or practices. These factors may or may not be under conscious control. Individuals can usually control their health behaviors and can choose healthy or unhealthy activities (external variables), but they have little or no choice about their genetic makeup, age, sex, or culture and sometimes their geographic environment (internal variables).

Internal variables are often described as nonmodifiable variables because, for the most part, they cannot be changed. Examples include genetic factors, such as race or history of heart disease; mental illness; and disorders of cognition such as autism spectrum disorder. However, when internal variables link to health problems, the nurse and patient must work together even more diligently to influence external variables (e.g., exercise, diet). Social support systems to encourage health choices can vary by culture (see the Focus on Diversity and Culture feature).

There are several factors influencing health choices. Psychologic (emotional) factors include awareness of mind–body interactions and self-concept. Cognitive (intellectual) factors include lifestyle choices, health beliefs, and spiritual and religious beliefs. One choice that combines both types of factors is the use of nontraditional health providers.

Awareness of Mind–Body Interactions

Mind–body interactions can affect health status either positively or negatively. Increasing attention is being given to the mind's ability to direct the body's functioning because emotional responses to stress affect body function. For example, a student who is extremely anxious before a test may experience urinary frequency or diarrhea. An individual who is worried about the outcome of surgery or about the behavior of a teenager may chain-smoke. Prolonged emotional distress may increase susceptibility to organic disease or precipitate it. Emotional distress may influence the immune system through central nervous system and endocrine alterations. Alterations in the immune system are related to the incidence of infections, cancer, and autoimmune diseases. Emotional reactions also occur in response to body conditions. For example, an individual diagnosed with a terminal illness may experience fear and depression.

Self-Concept

Self-concept is how an individual feels about the self (self-esteem) and perceives the physical self (body image) and his needs, roles, and abilities. Self-concept affects how individuals view and handle situations. Such attitudes can affect health practices, responses to stress and illness, and treatment seeking. An example is the anorexic woman who deprives herself of needed nutrients because she believes she is too fat, even though she is well below an acceptable weight level. Self-perceptions are also associated with an individual's definition of health. For example, a 75-year-old man who can no longer move large objects may need to redefine his concept of health in view of his current abilities.

Lifestyle Choices

Lifestyle choices refer to an individual's general way of life, including living conditions and individual patterns of behavior, which are influenced by sociocultural factors and personal characteristics. In brief, lifestyle is often considered the behavior and activities over which individuals have control.

Lifestyle assessment focuses on the personal lifestyle and habits as they affect the patient's health. Categories of lifestyle generally assessed include physical activity; nutritional practices; stress management; and habits such as smoking, alcohol consumption, and drug use. The goals of lifestyle assessment are to provide an opportunity for patients to evaluate their present lifestyle and to have a basis for decisions about desired behavior and lifestyle changes.

Lifestyle choices may have positive or negative effects on health. Practices with potentially negative effects on health are often referred to as **risk factors**. For example, overeating, getting insufficient exercise, and being overweight are closely related to the incidence of heart disease, arteriosclerosis, diabetes, and hypertension. Excessive use of tobacco is implicated in lung cancer, emphysema, and cardiovascular diseases. See **Box 7–2** ›› for examples of healthy lifestyle choices.

Many interrelated factors affect whether individuals will make and maintain changes in their lifestyle choices to improve health or prevent disease. To help patients succeed in implementing behavior changes, nurses need to understand the stages of change. Then, they can choose effective interventions that focus on helping patients progress through the stages of change (Prochaska, Norcross, & DiClemente, 2007). **Figure 7–5** ›› shows ways to identify patients' stage of change and suggested strategies relevant to that stage.

Focus on Diversity and Culture
Cultural Aspects of Social Support

Individuals from many cultures participate in extended family networks in which related individuals outside the immediate family provide some aspect of social, emotional, or spiritual support. In many cases, these extended family members can be helpful in responding to a patient's illness or injury, assisting in providing care during the immediate recovery period, bringing food, and running errands. All patient situations, however, are not the same. Some families may insist that a patient use traditional healing methods that the family has followed for generations, and one or more of these methods may conflict with the patient's prescribed treatment regimens. Some families may have had negative experiences with the modern healthcare system and may be reluctant to encourage a loved one to continue with treatment or return for a follow-up appointment (Spector, 2017).

Nurses should assess each patient's social support network and the extent to which the network will assist the patient in following the treatment regimen and returning to maximum health. Nurses working with patients who wish to integrate traditional remedies (e.g., acupuncture, poultices, herbs) should assess the congruence or contraindications of these remedies with the proposed or current treatment plan (Spector, 2017).

Box 7–2

Examples of Healthy Lifestyle Choices

- Exercising regularly
- Controlling weight
- Avoiding saturated fats
- Avoiding alcohol and tobacco
- Using seat belts
- Using bike helmets
- Updating immunizations
- Having regular dental checkups
- Having regular health maintenance visits for screening examinations or tests

Health Beliefs

Health beliefs are concepts about health that individuals believe are true. They may or may not be founded in fact. Some beliefs are influenced by culture, such as the belief that health and wellness are closely associated with the amount and quality of blood in the body. For example, in the American South, some individuals use the phrase "high blood" to mean they have too much blood in the body, causing headaches and dizziness. Another example is the racial/ethnic disparity in flu vaccination rates for older adults. Groom, Zhang, Fisher, and Wortley (2014) found that the percentage of adults receiving such vaccinations mirrored their differing beliefs in its effectiveness (66% for white populations, 50% for black populations).

Health beliefs can affect whether patients are likely to engage in health promotion or to follow a treatment plan. Social learning theory makes an effort to capture this likelihood through its explanation of locus of control. Individuals who believe that they can affect their own health and well-being are said to have an **internal locus of control**. These individuals are more likely to take control over their own health, follow therapeutic regimens, and engage in health promotion and prevention activities, including exercise and dietary modifications. Individuals who believe their health is controlled by forces outside their control (e.g., chance, fate, others) are said to have an **external locus of control**. For example, a research study of adults over age 80 examined individuals who attributed their current health status to uncontrollable "old age." Stewart, Chipperfield, Perry, and Weiner (2012) found that, compared to the control subjects, those individuals reported more perceived health symptoms, poorer health maintenance behaviors, and a greater likelihood of mortality at 2-year follow-up.

Spiritual and Religious Beliefs

Spiritual and religious beliefs can significantly affect health behavior. For example, Jehovah's Witnesses oppose blood transfusions; some fundamentalists believe that a serious illness is a punishment from God; some religious groups are strict vegetarians; and religious Jews perform circumcision on the eighth day of a male baby's life. The influence of spirituality and religion is discussed further in the module on Spirituality.

Use of Complementary Health Approaches

Complementary health approaches include practices and products of nonmainstream origin. Some of the more common ones are listed in **Table 7–5 ≫**. **Integrative health** describes the process of incorporating complementary health approaches into mainstream Western healthcare.

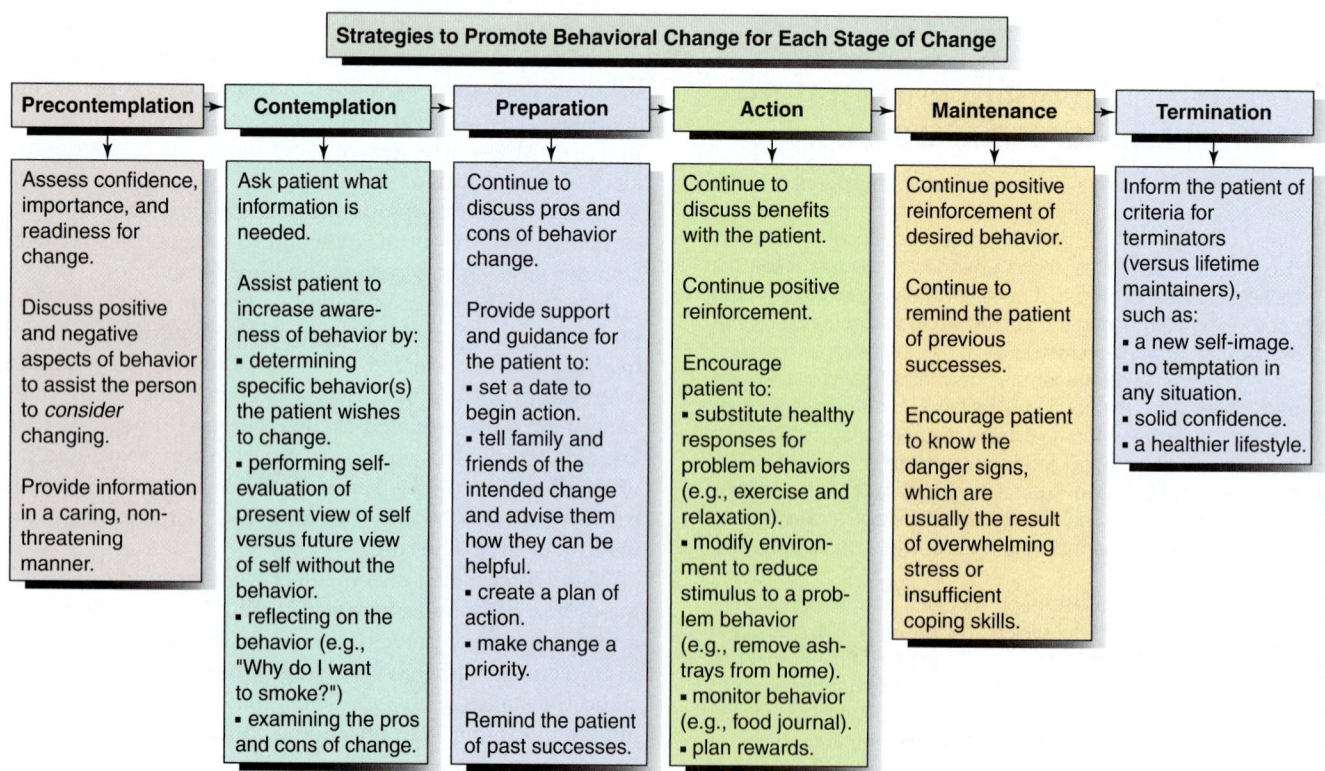

Figure 7–5 ≫ Strategies for behavioral change.

TABLE 7–5 Complementary Health Treatments

Term	Definition	Example
Acupuncture	Stimulation of points on the body by penetrating the skin with thin, solid, metallic needles	Acupuncture needles manipulated by hands or electrical stimulation
Ayurvedic medicine	Traditional Hindu medicine that uses foods, herbs, and breathing exercises	Osteoarthritis treated with a compound derived from *B. serrata* gum resin
Biofeedback	Use of electronic devices to measure body functions, giving information to encourage changes	Equipment measures muscle tension to increase awareness of need for, and sense of, relaxation
Chiropractic medicine	Practitioners perform adjustments (manipulations) to the spine or other parts of the body to support the body's natural ability to heal itself	Use of hands to apply a controlled, sudden force to a joint, pushing it beyond its usual range of motion
Deep breathing	Taking slow, deep, and even inhalations and exhalations	Listening to music with a slow beat and breathing in and out to the rhythm
Dietary and herbal supplements	Substances taken by mouth to add to the nutrition of food products	Oral intake of vitamins, minerals, herbs, or amino acids
Homeopathy	Treatments designed in the late 1700s in Germany, based on principles such as "like cures like"	Use of minute doses of a substance that cause symptoms to stimulate the body's self-healing response
Massage therapy	Therapists press, rub, and manipulate muscles and soft body tissues	Swedish massage uses a light touch; deep massage is more vigorous
Meditation	Becoming mindful of thoughts, feelings, and sensations, and observing them in a nonjudgmental way	Mindfulness meditation
Naturopathy	Noninvasive treatments to help the body do its own healing	Use of massage, acupuncture, herbal remedies, exercise, and lifestyle counseling
Osteopathic medicine	Belief that the musculoskeletal system influences the condition of all other body systems	Treating individuals as a whole instead of specific symptoms
Traditional Chinese medicine (TCM)	Methods used in China for over 5000 years	Treatment for asthma using acupuncture, herbal formulas, or both
Yoga	Practice of physical postures, breathing techniques, and meditation or relaxation	Hatha yoga's emphasis on postures (*asanas*) and breathing exercises (*pranayama*)

Sources: Data from American Osteopathic Association. (2015). *About osteopathic medicine.* Retrieved from http://www.osteopathic.org/osteopathic-health/about-dos/about-osteopathic-medicine/Pages/default.aspx; Mayo Clinic. (2014). *Consumer health: Complementary and alternative medicine.* Retrieved from http://www.mayoclinic.org/healthy-lifestyle/consumer-health/in-depth/alternative-medicine/art-20045267; Mayo Clinic. (2015a). *Chiropractic adjustment.* Retrieved from http://www.mayoclinic.org/tests-procedures/chiropractic-adjustment/basics/what-you-can-expect/prc-20013239; National Center for Complementary and Integrative Health (NCCIH). (2012). *Chiropractic: An introduction.* Retrieved from https://nccih.nih.gov/health/chiropractic/introduction.htm; National Center for Complementary and Integrative Health (NCCIH). (2015a). *Ayurvedic medicine: An introduction.* Retrieved from https://nccih.nih.gov/health/ayurveda/introduction.htm; National Center for Complementary and Integrative Health (NCCIH). (2015b). *Complementary, alternative, or integrative health: What's in a name?* Retrieved from https://nccih.nih.gov/health/integrative-health

Alternative medicine, which substitutes nonmainstream approaches in place of conventional medicine, is uncommon. An example of alternative medicine is treating cancer with a special diet rather than with chemotherapy, radiation, or surgery.

≫ Stay Current: Visit https://nccih.nih.gov for up-to-date information about nontraditional health provision.

Nontraditional treatment methods are undergoing intensive research efforts to support their use, with leadership at the federal government level. An organization set up for that purpose, the National Center for Complementary and Alternative Medicine (NCCAM) recently changed its name to the National Center for Complementary and Integrative Health (NCCIH).

Meanwhile, relaxation, meditation, and biofeedback techniques are gaining wider recognition among patients and healthcare professionals. For example, women often use relaxation techniques to decrease pain during childbirth. A highly stressed executive can meditate during office hours to better respond to work-life challenges. Acupuncture or hypnosis can provide pain relief when other routes have failed (see **Figure 7–6 ≫**). Other individuals may learn biofeedback skills to reduce hypertension.

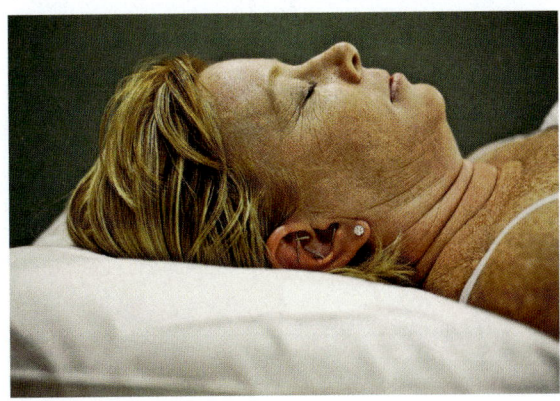

Source: Jacob Langston/Orlando Sentinel/MCT/Tribune News Service/Getty Images.

Figure 7–6 ≫ In traditional Chinese medicine, acupuncture is used to balance the flow of energy in the body (chi). Western healthcare providers often view acupuncture as a means of stimulating nerves, muscles, and connective tissue. Acupuncture can also be used to treat pain. This patient is being treated for breast cancer, and her oncologist recommended acupuncture to help control the associated discomforts.

SAFETY ALERT Individuals with generalized anxiety disorder have increasingly turned to herbal remedies for a variety of reasons: ease of access, labels of "natural products," individual treatment choices. However, the benefits have not been proven by research findings while the risks are evident. Some examples are:

- Chamomile can set off allergic responses in people who are allergic to ragweed, marigolds, daisies, and chrysanthemums.
- Kava can seriously damage liver cells, even with short-term use.
- Lavender can have side effects of constipation and headache.
- Lemon balm can result in nausea and abdominal pain.
- Passionflower can cause drowsiness, dizziness, and confusion.
- Valerian can trigger headaches and drowsiness.

In addition to being aware of these shortcomings, patients should make sure to inform their healthcare provider of their use of herbal products (Hall-Flavin, 2015).

Case Study » Part 2

Ms. Smithers's blood and laboratory tests come back with normal values. When contacted to share the results, Ms. Smithers says that she has developed a tingling sensation in her face and arms, down to her fingers. Her double vision continues. Her physician refers her to a neurologist, who suggests a series of tests: a neurologic exam, an eye exam, and a spinal tap. The spinal tap fluid test results come back with a note that protein was found consistent with a diagnosis of multiple sclerosis. The neurologist orders an MRI study of Ms. Smithers's brain. When she returns to her primary care physician, Ms. Smithers shares with you her frustration of the long time it is taking to get closer to a final diagnosis. "The stress of waiting is making it harder than ever to get a good night's sleep," she admits. "My leg cramps and back pain are making me stumble when I walk."

Clinical Reasoning Questions Level I

1. What factors may have contributed to Ms. Smithers's insomnia?
2. What independent nursing interventions can you implement to help Ms. Smithers sleep better?
3. What effects might Ms. Smithers's insomnia have on her other symptoms?

Clinical Reasoning Questions Level II

4. What patient teaching can you provide to help Ms. Smithers feel prepared for undergoing an MRI of her brain?
5. What complications may develop as a result of Ms. Smithers's insomnia and mobility issues? What assessments should you perform to detect these complications?
6. What therapeutic communication approaches can you take to help Ms. Smithers?

NURSING PROCESS

The nursing process provides a framework for nurses to organize their efforts, either independent or collaborative, in providing promotion activities and programs.

Assessment

A thorough assessment of the individual's health status is basic to health promotion. As nurses move toward greater autonomy in patient care, expanded assessment skills will provide more meaningful data.

Observation and Patient Interview

The nursing assessment begins with careful observation of the patient. Some characteristics to note: the patient's posture, facial expression, and nonverbal response to the beginning of the interview. Document vital signs, and include a thorough health history during the patient interview to detect existing problems. Review previous methods used to address those problems to identify the most effective ways to proceed in the future.

Lifestyle Assessment

Health risk appraisal and wellness assessment approaches are used to teach individuals about the risk factors inherent in their lifestyles. This education is meant to motivate them to reduce specific risks and develop positive health habits. Wellness assessment activities are focused on more positive methods of enhancement, in contrast to the risk factor approach used in the health appraisal. A variety of tools are available to facilitate these assessments; some are computer-based and can therefore be offered to educational institutions and workplaces at a reasonable cost.

Physical Fitness Assessment

During an evaluation of physical fitness, the nurse assesses several components of the body's physical functioning: muscle endurance, flexibility, body composition, and cardiorespiratory endurance. See Exemplar 7.A on Physical Fitness and Exercise.

Spiritual Health Assessment

Spiritual health is individuals' ability to develop their inner being to its fullest potential, including the ability to discover and articulate their basic purpose in life; to learn how to experience love, joy, peace, and fulfillment; and to help themselves and others achieve their fullest potential (Pender, Murdaugh, & Parsons, 2015). Spiritual beliefs can affect individuals' interpretation of life events. Therefore, an assessment of spiritual well-being is a part of evaluating patients' overall health. (See the module on Spirituality for more information.)

Social Support Systems Review

Understanding the social context in which a patient lives and works is important in health promotion. Individuals and groups, through interpersonal relationships, can provide comfort, assistance, encouragement, and information. Social support fosters successful coping and promotes satisfying and effective living.

Social support systems contribute to health by creating an environment that encourages healthy behaviors, promotes self-esteem and wellness, and provides feedback for actions leading to desirable outcomes. Examples of social support systems are family, peer support groups (including Internet-based support groups), community-organized religious support systems (e.g., churches), and self-help groups (e.g., Mended Hearts, Weight Watchers). The Focus on Diversity and Culture feature addresses aspects of social support within the context of culture.

Life Stress Review

There is abundant research about the impact of stress on mental and physical well-being. A variety of stress-related assessment instruments can be found in the clinical literature.

>> **Stay Current:** Visit the following websites to see current information about the impact of stress on mental health and physical well-being:

National Institute of Mental Health (NIMH) home page, to search for specific topics, at http://www.nimh.nih.gov/index.shtml

NIMH Fact Sheet on Stress, at http://www.nimh.nih.gov/health/publications/stress/fact-sheet-on-stress.shtml

U.S. National Library of Medicine Medline Plus home page, to search for specific topics, at http://www.nlm.nih.gov/medlineplus/

Diagnosis

Nurses can choose from 26 nursing diagnoses accepted by NANDA-I as the basis for health promotion interventions. Selection of an appropriate diagnosis depends upon nurses making clinical judgments, having heard or read clearly expressed motivation to increase health and well-being. Nurses cannot impose their opinion of what would be good for patients and their family, group, or community. Patients must actually express "a readiness to enhance specific health behaviors." For this reason, a health promotion nursing diagnosis begins with the phrase, "Expresses desire to enhance…" (NANDA-I © 2014).

Planning

Health promotion plans are developed according to the needs, desires, and priorities of the patient. The patient decides on health promotion goals, activities or interventions to achieve those goals, frequency and duration of the activities, and method of evaluation of outcomes. During the planning process, the nurse acts as a resource person, rather than as an adviser or counselor. The nurse provides information when asked, emphasizes the importance of small steps to behavioral change, and reviews the patient's goals and plans to make sure they are realistic, measurable, and acceptable to the patient.

Steps in Planning

Pender and colleagues (2015, pp. 105–118) outlined nine steps to develop a joint health promotion–illness prevention plan. These steps actively involve both the nurse and the patient from the start:

1. *Review and summarize data from assessment.* The nurse summarizes the data collected from the various assessments (e.g., physical health and fitness status, nutrition, sources of stress, spirituality, health practices).
2. *Emphasize strengths and competencies of the patient.* The nurse and the patient come to consensus about areas in which the patient is doing well and areas that need further development.
3. *Identify health goals and related behavioral-change options.* The patient selects the top-priority personal health goals and selects behavior-change options.
4. *Identify behavioral or health outcomes that indicate success from the patient's perspective.* The focus is on how to achieve the desired outcome. For example, to reduce the risk of cardiovascular disease, the patient may need to stop smoking, lose weight, and increase activity level.
5. *Develop a behavior change plan based on patient preferences and current knowledge about effective interventions.* A constructive program of change is based on patient ownership of those behavior changes selected for implementation within everyday life. The nurse may need to assist the patient in examining value–behavior inconsistencies and in selecting the most appealing behavioral change. The patient's priorities will reflect personal values, activity preferences, and expectations for success.
6. *Reiterate benefits of change, concentrating on patient-approved incentives.* The positive benefits are more likely to be achieved if the patient is routinely reminded of them, even if the patient is totally motivated to change. The nurse should encourage the patient to keep reminders of the health-related and non–health-related benefits visible to provide motivation.
7. *Address environmental and interpersonal facilitators and barriers to change.* Use environmental and interpersonal factors that support positive change to reinforce the patient's efforts to change lifestyle. All individuals experience barriers, some of which can be anticipated and planned for, thereby making change more likely to occur.
8. *Determine a time frame for implementation.* A time frame allows the patient to develop appropriate knowledge and skills before a new behavior is implemented. The time frame may be several weeks or months. Scheduling short-term goals and rewards can encourage the patient to achieve long-term objectives.
9. *Formalize commitment to behavior change plan goals, and provide needed support.* In the past, commitments to changing behaviors were usually informal and verbal. Now, formal and written behavior contracts are being used to motivate patients to follow through with selected actions. Motivation to follow through is provided by a **positive reinforcement** or reward stated in the contract. Contracting is based on the belief that all individuals have the potential for growth and the right of self-determination.

Implementation

While patient teaching efforts often occur independently, on a one-to-one basis, health promotion efforts generally involve collaborative relationships with patients, primary care providers, multidisciplinary specialists, and other support personnel, often in groups. The role of the nurse is to work *with* these individuals, not *for* them—that is, to act as a facilitator of the process of assessing, evaluating, and understanding health. The nurse may act as an advocate, a consultant, a teacher, or a coordinator of services using a variety of approaches described next.

Information Dissemination

Information dissemination is the most basic type of health promotion approach. It uses a variety of media to offer information to the public about the risk of particular lifestyle choices and personal behavior. It also spells out the specific benefits of changing that behavior and improving the quality of life. Billboards, posters, brochures, newspaper features, books, and health fairs all offer opportunities for disseminating health promotion information. Information dissemination is a useful strategy for raising individuals' and groups' level of knowledge and awareness about health habits.

When planning information dissemination, it is important to consider factors such as culture, age group, and literacy level. Knowing the best place and method for distributing information increases its effectiveness. For example, churches often provide older adults with social support while serving as a spiritual home, especially in African American communities. The church is often the appropriate place to hold health fairs or even small group discussions on various health topics. It offers a stepping-stone to providing information and suggesting resources for sensitive individual needs—all done in a comfortable, nonthreatening environment.

It is just as critical to know where individuals get misinformation. Sending multiple mailings has become a marketing ploy for advertising "miracle" vitamins, herbs, and food supplements. These are heavily directed toward older adults, who are often not informed about current evidence-based therapies and may choose this route to purchase items if they have transportation problems.

Lifestyle and Behavior Change Plans

Lifestyle- and behavior-change plans require the participation of the individual. They are geared toward enhancing the quality of life and extending the lifespan. Individuals generally consider lifestyle changes after they have been informed of the need to change their health behavior and have become aware of the potential benefits of the process. Many formal programs are available to the public, on both a group and an individual basis. Topics may include stress management, nutrition awareness, weight control, smoking cessation, and exercise.

Environmental Control Programs

Environmental control programs have been developed in response to the continuing increase of contaminants of human origin in the environment. The amount of contaminants already present in the air, food, and water will affect the health of future generations. The most common concerns of community groups are toxic and nuclear wastes, nuclear power plants, air and water pollution, and herbicide and pesticide use.

Facilitation of Social Support

Social networks, such as family and friends, can facilitate or impede efforts directed toward health promotion and illness prevention. The nurse's role is to assist the patient to assess, modify, and develop the social support necessary to achieve the desired change. To provide the necessary support, families must communicate effectively, be aware of and support each other's needs and goals, and provide help to achieve those goals. The patient may wish the nurse to meet with the family or significant others to enlist their understanding and support.

Evaluation

Evaluation is ongoing, monitoring both short- and long-term goals. The healthcare team and patient write goals during the planning phase, along with target dates for attaining the specific desired results or behaviors. During evaluation, the healthcare team should examine both positive and negative outcomes. Even if the final results are not completely satisfying to the patient, the nurse can discuss the patient's movement along the continuum of stages of change. Knowing the current stage, the nurse can work together with the patient to find ways to advance to the next stage of change (see Figure 7–5). The patient may decide to continue with the plan, reorder priorities, change strategies, or revise the health promotion contract. Evaluation of the plan is a collaborative effort between the nurse and the patient.

Case Study >> Part 3

The neurologist ordered a mild sedative before Ms. Smithers entered the MRI machine. "Not only did it help me feel less anxious," she reports to you on her next visit to her primary care physician, "but it also relieved much of my back pain. Good thing! That was a cold, hard table to lie on." She holds in her hands the results from the MRI scan. Her hand is shaky, so the paper rattles. "They only found a couple of lesions," she explains, "so they think the MS is in the early stages. Thank God they found it as soon as they did. I have started on medication to prevent further damage to my nerves."

Clinical Reasoning Questions Level I

1. What patient teaching can you provide to help Ms. Smithers understand the concepts of "relapsing" and "remission"?
2. What factors might contribute to Ms. Smithers's acceptance of her diagnosis?
3. Where would you place Ms. Smithers on the health continuum? Where do you expect she would place herself?

Clinical Reasoning Questions Level II

4. What is your current primary nursing diagnosis for Ms. Smithers? Did it change from your original diagnosis? Why or why not?
5. What nursing interventions can you implement to help Ms. Smithers deal with a chronic disease? For which future situations would you prepare her? Who else should be involved in designing her care plan?
6. In light of her diagnosis, would you make any changes in your original suggestions to help Ms. Smithers sleep better? Eat more healthy foods?

REVIEW The Concept of Health, Wellness, Illness, and Injury

RELATE Link the Concepts

Linking the concept of health, wellness, illness, and injury with the concept of comfort:

1. Your patient has a diagnosis of rheumatoid arthritis. What kinds of exercise would you suggest for the days the patient experiences severe joint pain?

2. Your patient started a yoga class and states that some poses cause her intermittent backache to increase in intensity. The patient's attitude is "No pain, no gain." Do you agree? What will you discuss with the patient?

3. Your patient fractured his wrist when he broke his fall, tripping over a discarded toy. "It's nothing," he claims. Do you agree? What will you discuss with the patient?

Linking the concept of health, wellness, illness, and injury with the concept of stress and coping:

4. Your patient with PTSD has difficulty sleeping and complains that he is too tired to exercise. How could you apply your knowledge of the stages of change to help him?

5. After her child's epileptic seizure has ended, your patient (the mother) states that she feels "all beat up." What suggestions do you have for her, after she deals with the immediate crisis?

6. Your patient with a whiplash injury due to a car accident complains that the cervical collar is uncomfortable to wear. It reminds him of his helplessness in not being able to avoid being hit. What suggestions do you have for him?

Linking the concept of health, wellness, illness, and injury with the concept of teaching and learning:

7. You supervise a team of nurses, who share ongoing stresses. You find that they are not taking full advantage of the recreation benefits provided by the organization. How can you educate or mentor them to change?

8. Your nursing colleague injured his back while lifting by himself a patient who was obese. Your clinical team has access to lifting equipment and attends instructional sessions on how to use it. What is a workable approach to help your colleague prevent further injury?

READY Go to Volume 3: Clinical Nursing Skills

- SKILL 1.1 — Appearance and Mental Status: Assessing
- SKILLS 1.5–1.9 — Vital Signs
- SKILLS 1.10–1.27 — Physical Assessment
- SKILL 2.7 — Mouth: Regular and for the Unconscious or Debilitated Patient, Caring for
- SKILL 3.3 — Pain Relief: Complementary Health Approaches
- SKILL 3.6 — Sleep Promotion: Assisting

REFER Go to Pearson MyLab Nursing and eText

- Additional review materials

REFLECT Apply Your Knowledge

Susanna Randolph is a 40-year-old single mother, living in a suburban townhouse with her 10-year-old son, Jeff, who has autism. She keeps in regular contact with Jeff's father, who runs a high-tech start-up company. Ms. Randolph pursued a successful career as a medical technologist until her son's diagnosis. After she resigned her post as a laboratory supervisor, she was able to get a position working at home as an instructional designer for a nearby laboratory.

When Ms. Randolph gets stressed, she finds that she tends to decrease her physical activity rather than increase her exercise time or intensity. Her sleep pattern mirrors that of her son; when he sleeps well, she sleeps well. When he has insomnia, she stays up with him. Ms. Randolph and Jeff enjoy brushing their teeth together in their small bathroom, looking in the mirror at their images.

You are the public health nurse who has Ms. Randolph and her son on your home visit schedule.

1. What questions would you ask Ms. Randolph about her wellness routine that might lead to positive changes?

2. How does her concern for her son affect her plans for her own health? What factors can you use to motivate her?

3. What priorities would you assign to your work with this family?

≫ Exemplar 7.A
Physical Fitness and Exercise

Exemplar Learning Outcomes

7.A Analyze physical fitness and exercise as they relate to health, wellness, illness, and injury.

- Describe the benefits of physical fitness.
- Contrast the types of exercise.
- Outline the effects of exercise on body systems.
- Summarize the recommendations for physical activity across the lifespan.

Exemplar Key Terms

Activity–exercise pattern, *448*
Activity tolerance, *448*
Aerobic exercise, *449*
Anaerobic exercise, *449*
Exercise, *448*
Functional strength, *448*
Hypertrophy, *449*
Isokinetic exercise, *449*
Isometric exercise, *448*
Isotonic exercise, *448*
Physical activity, *448*
Physical fitness, *448*

Overview

The role of physical fitness in health promotion and wellness is gaining both attention and credibility. For example, exercise, in particular walking, is increasingly "prescribed" to patients with Parkinson disease. There is evidence that it combats progression of the condition and that it assist patients to build strength, stability, and endurance (Harvard University, 2012). The CDC defines **physical fitness** as:

> the ability to carry out daily tasks with vigor and alertness, without undue fatigue, and with ample energy to enjoy leisure-time pursuits and respond to emergencies. Physical fitness includes a number of components consisting of cardiorespiratory endurance (aerobic power), skeletal muscle endurance, skeletal muscle strength, skeletal muscle power, flexibility, balance, speed of movement, reaction time, and body composition (CDC, 2015f).

Benefits of Physical Fitness

There are many benefits of physical fitness, including (CDC, 2015f):

- Improving mood and overall mental health
- Reducing the risk for cardiovascular disease
- Strengthening bone and muscle
- Reducing the risk of some illnesses, such as type 2 diabetes, and some cancers
- Improving stability and reducing risk of falling in older adults.

Many *Healthy People 2020* objectives pertain to exercise and activity. Following are some of these objectives:

- Retained from *Healthy People 2010:* Reduce the proportion of adults who engage in no leisure-time physical activity. Increase the proportion of schools that require daily physical education.
- Modified from *Healthy People 2010:* Increase the proportion of adults and adolescents who engage in aerobic physical activity. Increase the proportion of children and adolescents who do not exceed recommended limits for screen time.
- New for *Healthy People 2020:* Increase regularly scheduled elementary school recess.

A strong, well-developed body of research evidence supports the role of exercise in improving the health status of individuals with cardiovascular disease, pulmonary dysfunction, disabilities of aging, and depression. Integrating well-researched exercise protocols with conventional nursing and medical approaches results in optimal treatment of these common disorders. Evidence shows that exercise can prevent and even reverse many of the chronic diseases experienced by aging adults. As stated earlier, a growing body of research supports the preventive and therapeutic effects of exercise on a number of conditions, including diabetes, cancer, arthritis, chronic fatigue syndrome, cystic fibrosis, fibromyalgia, menopause, urinary incontinence, Parkinson disease, Alzheimer disease, and HIV/AIDS

(Micozzi, 2015; van de Weert-van Leeuwen, Arets, van der Ent, & Beekman, 2013).

An **activity–exercise pattern** refers to an individual's routine of exercise, activity, leisure, and recreation. It includes: (a) activities of daily living (ADLs) that require energy expenditure, such as hygiene, dressing, cooking, shopping, eating, working, and home maintenance, and (b) the type, quality, and quantity of exercise, including sports.

Individuals often define their health and physical fitness by their activity. Mental well-being and the effectiveness of body functioning depend largely on mobility status. For example, when an individual is upright, the lungs expand more easily, intestinal activity (peristalsis) is more effective, and the kidneys are able to empty completely. In addition, motion is essential for proper functioning of bones and muscles.

Physical Activity and Exercise

The CDC (2015e) defines physical activity and exercise as follows:

- **Physical activity** is any bodily movement produced by skeletal muscle contraction that increases energy expenditure above a basal level.
- **Exercise** is a type of physical activity that is planned, structured, repetitive, and purposive. It refers to bodily movement performed to improve or maintain one or more components of physical fitness.

Individuals participate in exercise programs to decrease risk factors for cardiovascular disease and to increase their health and well-being. **Activity tolerance** is the type and amount of exercise or daily living activities an individual is able to perform without experiencing adverse effects. **Functional strength** is another goal of exercise, and it is defined as the body's ability to perform work.

Exercise involves the active contraction and relaxation of muscles. Exercises can be classified according to the type of muscle contraction (isotonic, isometric, or isokinetic) and the source of energy (aerobic or anaerobic).

In **isotonic exercises**, which are dynamic exercises, the muscle shortens to produce muscle contraction and active movement (see **Figure 7–7** »). Most physical conditioning exercises—running, walking, swimming, cycling, and other such activities—are isotonic, as are ADLs and active range-of-motion (ROM) exercises (those initiated by the patient). Examples of isotonic bed exercises are pushing or pulling against a stationary object, using a trapeze to lift the body off the bed, lifting the buttocks off the bed by pushing with the hands against the mattress, and pushing the body to a sitting position.

Isotonic exercises increase muscle tone, mass, and strength and maintain joint flexibility and circulation. During isotonic exercise, both heart rate and cardiac output quicken to increase blood flow to all parts of the body.

In **isometric exercises**, which are static or setting exercises, muscles contract without moving the joint (muscle length does not change). These exercises involve exerting pressure against a solid object and are useful for strengthening abdominal, gluteal, and quadriceps muscles used in ambulation; for maintaining strength in immobilized

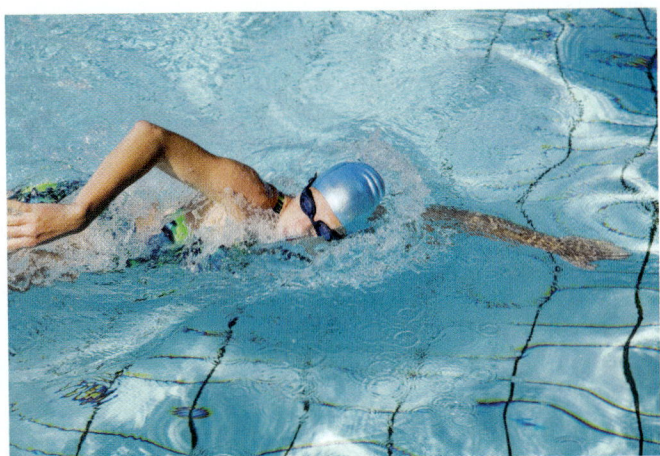

Source: Westend61/Getty Images.

Figure 7–7 》 Isotonic exercise involves moving the joints and muscles through their ranges of motion using low resistance, such as water.

muscles in casts or traction; and for endurance training. These are often called "quad sets." Isometric exercises produce a mild increase in heart rate and cardiac output but no appreciable increase in blood flow to other parts of the body.

Isokinetic exercises, which are resistive exercises, involve muscle contraction or tension against resistance; thus they can be either isotonic or isometric. During isokinetic exercises, the individual moves (isotonic) or tenses (isometric) against resistance. Special machines or devices provide the resistance to the movement. These exercises are used in physical conditioning and are often done to build up certain muscle groups. For example, the pectorals (chest muscles) may be increased in size and strength by weight lifting (see **Figure 7–8 》**).

During **aerobic exercise**, the amount of oxygen taken into the body is greater than that used to perform the activity. Aerobic exercises use large muscle groups that move repetitively. Aerobic exercises improve cardiovascular con-

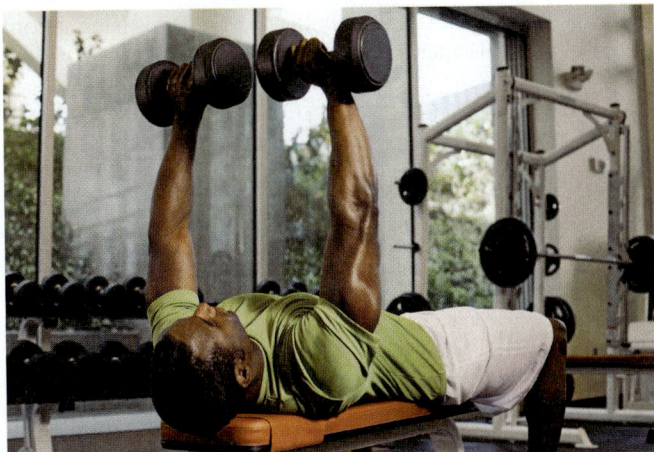

Source: Fuse/Corbis/Getty Images.

Figure 7–8 》 Isokinetic exercise is performed using specialized apparatus that allows the individual to control resistance. Most isokinetic exercises use only body weight or very light weights.

ditioning and physical fitness and bring more oxygen into the body than is used to perform the activity.

1. ***Target heart rate.*** The goal is to work up to and sustain a target heart rate during exercise; the target rate is based on the individual's age. To determine target heart rate, first calculate the individual's maximum heart rate by subtracting her current age in years from 220. Then, obtain the target heart rate by taking 60%–85% of the maximum. Because heart rates vary among individuals, the talk test is one of several tests being used to replace this measure.

2. ***Talk test.*** This test is easier to implement and keeps most individuals at 60% of maximum heart rate or higher. The test is simple: When exercising, an individual should experience labored breathing, yet still be able to carry on a conversation.

During **anaerobic exercise**, the muscles cannot draw out enough oxygen from the bloodstream, and anaerobic pathways are used to provide additional energy for a short time. This type of exercise, such as weight lifting and sprinting, is used in endurance training for athletes.

Effects of Exercise on the Mind and Body

In general, regular exercise is essential for maintaining optimum mental and physical health. It can have effects on cognitive function and on the musculoskeletal, cardiovascular, respiratory, gastrointestinal, metabolic/endocrine, elimination, immune, and psychoneurologic systems. In short, everything!

Cognitive Function

Some recent research supports the positive effects of physical exercise on cognitive functioning, in particular decision making and problem solving, planning, and paying attention. Physical exertion is theorized to induce cells in the brain to strengthen and build neuronal connections. Other research indicates that physical exercise is associated with positive effects in individuals with Parkinson and Alzheimer diseases (Brown, Peiffer, & Martins, 2012; Grazina & Massano, 2013).

Other research is questioning those findings, however. For example, Barnes and colleagues (2013) looked at inactive older adults with cognitive complaints participating in 12 weeks of physical or mental activities. They found no difference between intervention and active control groups. A Cochrane Database System Review by Young, Angevaran, Rusted, and Tabet (2015) looked at adults over 55 without cognitive impairment. They analyzed 12 randomized controlled trials of over 700 people and found that physical exercise did improve cardiorespiratory fitness but not cognition functioning.

Musculoskeletal System

The size, shape, tone, and strength of muscles (including the heart muscle) are maintained with mild exercise and increased with strenuous exercise. With strenuous exercise, muscles **hypertrophy** (enlarge), and the efficiency of muscular contraction increases. Hypertrophy is commonly seen in the arm muscles of a tennis player, the leg muscles of a skater, and the arm and hand muscles of a carpenter.

Joints lack a discrete blood supply and receive nourishment through activity. Exercise increases joint flexibility, stability, and range of motion.

Bone density and strength are maintained through weight bearing. The stress of weight-bearing and high-impact movement maintains a balance between osteoblasts (bone-building cells) and osteoclasts (bone-resorption and breakdown cells). Weight-bearing activity is particularly important for individuals at risk for osteoporosis. Examples of weight-bearing activity are walking, dancing, and weight lifting. Non–weight-bearing exercises offer great benefit for individuals with a variety of health considerations. Examples of non–weight-bearing exercise are swimming and bicycling.

The CDC (2015f) believes that exercise improves stability and decreases the risk of falls in older adults. One Cochrane Database System Review supports this viewpoint; it showed positive results in fall risk and fall incidence reduction for older adults living in the community (Gillespie et al., 2012). Another more recent Cochrane Database System Review did not confirm evidence-based results of reducing fear of falling, its risk, or its frequency after exercise interventions with the same population (Kendrick et al., 2014). Alvarez and colleagues (2015) found that strength training did reduce the frequency of falls in assisted-living residents; however, Barker and colleagues (2016) found that exercise did not reduce the risk of falls or lessen injuries sustained in a fall in individuals staying in hospitals.

Cardiovascular System

The American Heart Association's collaboration with the American Stroke Association describes the most recent guidelines for primary prevention of stroke and cardiovascular disease, placing great emphasis on physical activity (American Heart Association & American Stroke Association, 2014). Adequate moderate-intensity exercise (40%–60% of maximum capacity such as walking a mile in 15–20 minutes) increases the heart rate, the strength of heart muscle contraction, and the blood supply to the heart and muscles through increased cardiac output. In two studies with male participants, levels of "good" (high-density lipoprotein [HDL]) cholesterol were increased through regular endurance (walking/jogging) exercise. Exercise also promotes heart health by mediating the harmful effects of stress. The types of exercise that provide cardiac benefit vary. They include aerobic exercise such as walking and cycling. Recent research supports the benefits of yoga practice in cardiovascular health. Statistically significant effects include lowered systolic and diastolic blood pressure, improved oxygen uptake, improved heart rate variability, improved circulation, and self-reported stress reduction (Fontaine, 2014).

Respiratory System

Ventilation (air circulating into and out of the lungs) and oxygen intake increase during exercise, thereby improving gas exchange. More toxins are eliminated with deeper breathing, and problem solving and emotional stability are enhanced by increased oxygen to the brain. Adequate exercise also prevents pooling of secretions in the bronchi and bronchioles, decreasing breathing effort and risk of infection. Attention to exercising muscles of respiration (by deep breathing) throughout activity as well as during rest enhances oxygenation (improving stamina) and circulation of lymph (improving immune function). A strong body of evidence supports the use of lower-extremity exercise forms (e.g., walking, treadmill, stationary bike, stair climbing) for treating individuals with COPD. Increasing research reports cite the benefits of yogic breathing and postures for individuals with asthma (Fontaine, 2014; Micozzi, 2015).

Gastrointestinal System

Exercise improves the appetite and increases gastrointestinal tract tone, facilitating peristalsis. Activities such as rowing, swimming, walking, and sit-ups work the abdominal muscles and can help relieve constipation (Fontaine, 2014). Abdominal compressive exercise, such as with twisting and forward bending yoga postures, has been shown to improve symptoms of irritable bowel syndrome (Fontaine, 2014; Micozzi, 2015).

Metabolic/Endocrine System

Exercise elevates the metabolic rate, thus increasing the production of body heat, waste products, and calorie use. During strenuous exercise, the metabolic rate can increase to as much as 20 times the normal rate. This elevation lasts after exercise is completed. Exercise increases the use of triglycerides and fatty acids, resulting in a reduced level of serum triglycerides and cholesterol. Weight loss and exercise stabilize blood sugar and make cells more responsive to insulin. The Diabetes Prevention Program, a large 3-year study, showed that even a modest 5% decrease in body weight (about 10 pounds in most participants) achieved through exercise and dietary modification reduced the risk of diabetes by a striking 58%. In those over 60 years of age, the reduction was 71% (National Institutes of Health (NIH), National Institute of Diabetes and Digestive Health and Kidney Diseases, 2013).

Elimination System

As adequate exercise promotes efficient blood flow and increases peristalsis, the body excretes wastes more effectively. In that way, adequate exercise helps prevent stasis (stagnation) of urine in the bladder and constipation in the colon.

Focus on Diversity and Culture
Children's Physical Fitness and Socioeconomic Status

Researchers looked at data from over 1.6 million fifth-, seventh-, and ninth graders who took a physical fitness test in California. Fitness was measured on a scale from 0 (least healthy) to 6 (most healthy). The average fitness score was 4.45. The purpose of the study was to assess the association between family income and the children's fitness test results. About half (56%) of the children were eligible for the National School Lunch Program, a marker of lower family income. Regardless of belonging to a specific racial/ethnic group (American Indian, Asian, Pacific Islander, Filipino, Hispanic/Latino, African American, and White), lower family income was associated with a lower fitness score (Jin & Jones-Smith, 2015).

Immune System

As respiratory and musculoskeletal effort increase with exercise and as gravity is enlisted with postural changes, lymph fluid is more efficiently pumped from tissues into lymph capillaries and vessels throughout the body. Circulation through lymph nodes, where destruction of pathogens and removal of foreign antigens can occur, also improves.

While moderate exercise seems to enhance immunity, strenuous exercise may reduce immune function, leaving a window of opportunity for infection during the recovery phase. Adequate rest is important after vigorous training to allow the body to recover (Edelman, Kudzma, & Mandle, 2013).

Psychoneurologic System

Mental disorders such as depression or chronic stress may affect an individual's desire to move. A patient with depression, for example, may lack enthusiasm for taking part in any activity and may even lack energy for usual hygiene practices. Chronic stress can deplete the body's energy reserves to the point that the resulting fatigue discourages the desire to exercise, even though muscular exertion (especially with movement modalities such as yoga and t'ai chi) could help release stored stress (see **Figure 7–9 》**).

Researchers have studied the effect of exercise on clinical depression. They found that exercise produced a more positive effect than relaxation, meditation, or placebo (Cooney et al., 2013). However, exercise was not more effective than medication or psychologic therapy (Cooney, Dwan, & Mead, 2014).

Regular exercise improves the quality of sleep for most individuals. Previous research verified the positive effect that high levels of physical exercise can have on older adults with chronic insomnia. Recent research has established a minimum level of physical activity required for good results. Gathering data on over 900 adults older than age 65, researchers found that participants walking at least 150 minutes per week reported fewer problems with onset of sleep and better sleep maintenance. Follow-up contact 4 years later showed that the benefits were maintained over time (Hartescu, Morgan, & Stevinson, 2015).

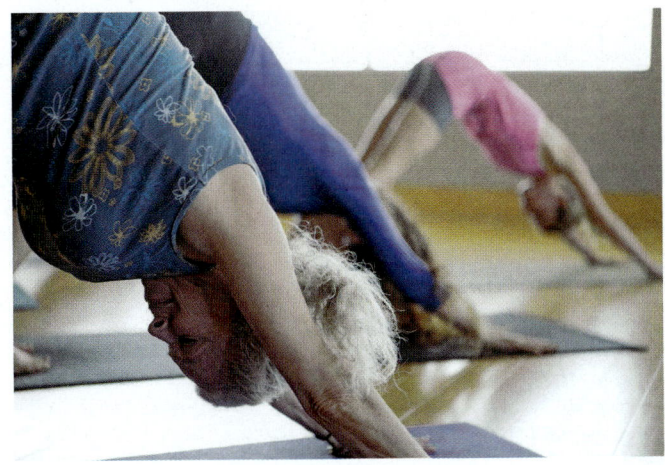

Figure 7–9 》 Yoga helps individuals relax, manage stress, and improve fitness. Yoga can be performed solo or in a group, and anywhere—at home, on the beach, or in a studio.

TABLE 7–6 Ideal Duration of Exercise by Age Group

Age Group	Ideal Duration of Exercise
Infants (birth to 1 year)	■ Outside two to three times a day, as tolerated
Toddlers (1–3 years)	■ 60–90 minutes of outdoor play daily
Preschoolers (3–6 years)	■ 60–90 minutes of outdoor play daily
Children (6–17 years)	■ 60 minutes of physical activity daily, most of it aerobic activity ■ Some vigorous intensity, some muscle and bone strengthening 3 days a week
Adults (18–64 years)	■ 150 minutes of moderate-intensity aerobic activity each week ■ OR 75 minutes of vigorous-intensity activities ■ OR a mix of equivalent intensities ■ 2 days a week, muscle-strengthening
Older adults (65 years and older)	■ 150 minutes of moderate-intensity aerobic activity each week ■ OR 75 minutes of vigorous-intensity activities ■ OR a mix of equivalent intensities ■ 2 days a week, muscle-strengthening
Pregnant or postpartum women	■ 150 minutes of moderate-intensity aerobic activity each week ■ Vigorous activity if already engaged ■ Discuss with healthcare provider

Sources: Information from National Resource Center for Health and Safety in Child Care and Early Education. (2015). *Caring for our children.* Retrieved from http://www.cfoc.nrckids.org/StandardView/3.1.3.1; Information from Centers for Disease Control and Prevention (CDC). (2015d). *Physical activity basics.* Retrieved from http://www.cdc.gov/physicalactivity/basics/index.htm and http://www.cdc.gov/physicalactivity/everyone/guidelines

Lifespan Considerations

During the course of an individual's lifetime, the recommendations for physical activity change by age group, and they take into account weather conditions. **Table 7–6 》** shows the ideal amounts of time for exercise by age group.

SAFETY ALERT   While walking is good exercise, talking on a cell phone at the same time increases the risk of injuries. Researchers identified over 300 visits to an emergency department (ED) for "cell-phone-induced distraction" between 2000 and 2011. Most were female (68%) and under the age of 40 (54%). The primary reason for medical attention was a fall (74%), and most people (85%) were discharged straight from the ED. The researchers found that each year the numbers increased significantly more than the previous year ($p < 0.001$ for trend). They predicted that smartphones, with their engaging features, would trigger even more injuries in the future (Smith, Schreiber, Saltos, Lichenstein, & Lichenstein, 2013).

Nursing Management

Nurses can initiate many interventions to help patients improve and maintain their optimum physical activity levels:

1. Model healthy exercise attitudes and behaviors. Nurses should know how their physical activity patterns measure up against the recommendations for movement and strength training. Even if they are not

tracking their own data, nurses should be familiar with ways that patients can record their efforts, such as exercise diaries and step pedometers.

2. Facilitate patient involvement in setting specific, reasonable physical activity goals. Set target deadlines for evaluation of efforts, such as "by the next check-up visit."

3. Teach patients self-care strategies to enhance fitness and to be ready to deal with the possible aches and pains of increasing exercise. Have visual aids handy to show how to perform stretching exercises before more rigorous activities.

4. Assist individuals, families, and communities to increase their physical activities. This might mean advocating places to do indoor exercises, such as a gym, or outside exercises, such as hiking trails.

5. Educate patients to be effective consumers of products to assist with exercise, such as yoga mats, dumbbells, and exercise machines.

6. Reinforce patients' personal and family health-promoting exercises.

7. Advocate in the community for changes that promote physical fitness in a healthy environment.

REVIEW Physical Fitness and Exercise

RELATE Link the Concepts and Exemplars

Linking the exemplar physical fitness and exercise with the concept of metabolism:

1. Identify the benefits of physical activity for a patient with type 2 diabetes and osteoporosis.

2. What teaching plan will you implement for the obese patient regarding exercise and nutrition?

Linking the exemplar physical fitness and exercise with the concept of mobility:

3. A patient with rheumatoid arthritis is interested in beginning a weight-lifting program. What are your teaching priorities for this patient?

4. You are caring for a patient who normally exercised daily before fracturing his leg. How can you help to meet the patient's exercise needs when he is placed in traction for 6 weeks?

Linking the exemplar of physical fitness and exercise with the concept of cognition:

5. How does the presence of a chronic illness or a negative change in cognitive status affect the ability of older adults to engage in exercise? What modifications could the nurse suggest?

6. You are working with the parent of a teenager with schizophrenia who has recently gained significant weight. What suggestions could you make to the parent? How could you involve the teenager in the formulation of a care plan?

READY Go to Volume 3: Clinical Nursing Skills

REFER Go to Pearson MyLab Nursing and eText

- Additional review materials

REFLECT Apply Your Knowledge

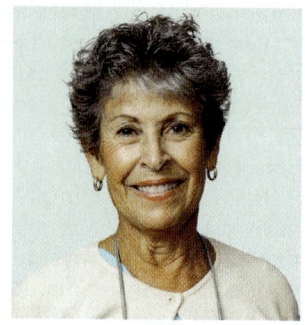

Mary Martin is a 75-year-old woman who was recently widowed. She has limited income because her husband's pension terminated when he died, so she has moved in with her son, his wife, and their three teenage children. Mary has cataracts and glaucoma, for which she regularly sees an ophthalmologist, but otherwise she is in good health. Mary recently learned she has low bone density.

1. What kind of physical activity and exercise is appropriate for Mary?

2. What are the benefits of these activities on body systems?

3. What are your expected outcomes for Mary?

4. What safety teaching will you provide Mary and her family?

›› Exemplar 7.B
Oral Health

Exemplar Learning Outcomes

7.B Analyze oral health as it relates to health, wellness, illness, and injury.

- Describe the functions of the oral cavity and normal oral health.
- Identify commonly occurring alterations in oral health.
- Describe the significance of oral hygiene across the lifespan.
- Outline nursing management of oral health including identifying patients at risk and promoting oral hygiene.

Exemplar Key Terms

Dental caries, *453*
Dentifrice, *454*
Enamel, *453*
Gingiva, *453*
Gingivitis, *454*
Halitosis, *455*
Periodontal disease, *453*
Plaque, *453*
Pyorrhea, *454*
Tartar, *453*
Xerostomia, *455*

Overview

The year 2014 marked the issuance of the first Surgeon General's Report on Oral Health. The report emphasized the importance of oral health with four themes:

1. *Oral health means much more than healthy teeth.* It means that the oral cavity is free of pain, cancers, lesions, and birth defects.
2. *Oral health is integral to general health.* Research has identified associations of chronic oral infections with health and lung diseases, strokes, diabetes, and low-birth-weight, premature births.
3. *Interventions can improve oral health and prevent disease.* These include daily oral hygiene, community water fluoridation, tobacco cessation programs, application of dental sealants, and examinations for cancers.
4. *Other factors, such as tobacco use and poor diets, negatively affect oral health.* The cost to the nation is a dental bill exceeding $60 billion (National Institute of Dental and Craniofacial Research, 2014).

Normal Oral Health

Figure 7–10 ❯❯ shows the parts of the oral cavity, more often called the mouth. From the top right of the image, the *hard palate* covers the bone in the roof of the mouth. It serves to give a hard surface for the tongue to bring food further into the mouth. The *soft palate* extends backward from the hard palate and is primarily muscle. The soft palate ends in a fold at the back of the mouth called the *uvula*, a small, finger-shaped piece of tissue. The *tonsils*, made of lymphatic tissue, are located on either side of the uvula. Coming forward to the front of the mouth, the *dorsum of the tongue* is its upper surface; the lower surface is very vascular and covered with a thin membrane. The *teeth*, which are set in the **gingiva** (gum), have three parts:

- Crown, uppermost exposed part of the tooth, outside the gum, covered with a hard substance called **enamel**
- Pulp cavity, center of tooth containing the blood vessels and nerves
- Root, lowest part of the tooth embedded in the jaw and covered by bony tissue.

The lips and cheeks keep food in the mouth during chewing. The tongue mixes food with saliva during chewing. Saliva moistens food and provides enzymes such as amylase that begin to digest starches. The teeth break down food into smaller parts. When the food is swallowed, the soft palate rises to direct food into the esophagus.

Teeth usually appear 5–8 months after birth. By the time children are 2 years old, they usually have all 20 of their deciduous (temporary) teeth. At about age 6 or 7, children start losing their deciduous teeth, which are gradually replaced by 33 permanent teeth. By age 25, most individuals have the rest of their permanent teeth, including wisdom teeth. As individuals age, their teeth enamel wears away, making the teeth susceptible to damage and decay. That results in 30% of people losing their natural teeth between the ages of 65 and 74.

Alterations of Oral Health

The mouth and teeth can have a wide variety of problems that could cause discomfort and eventually a loss of teeth, as well as serious medical conditions elsewhere in the body. The most commonly encountered problems in community settings are described in the following text. Ten problems more often seen in institutional environments are listed in the Clinical Manifestations and Therapies feature.

The most common problems are **dental caries** (cavities) and **periodontal disease** (gum disease). Dental cavities develop when teeth are exposed to bacteria that use the sugars and starches in foods or drinks to produce acids. Over time these acids weaken the tooth enamel and destroy its smooth surface. This results in the permanent damage of tooth decay. Two materials can reverse the process: Minerals, such as calcium and potassium in a person's saliva, and fluoride from toothpaste or other sources can restore the enamel (American Dental Association, 2014b).

Both dental caries and periodontal disease are commonly associated with plaque and tartar deposits. **Plaque** is in invisible soft film that adheres to the enamel surface of teeth; it consists of bacteria, molecules of saliva, and remnants of epithelial cells and leucocytes. When plaque is unchecked, **tartar** (dental calculus) is formed. Tartar is a

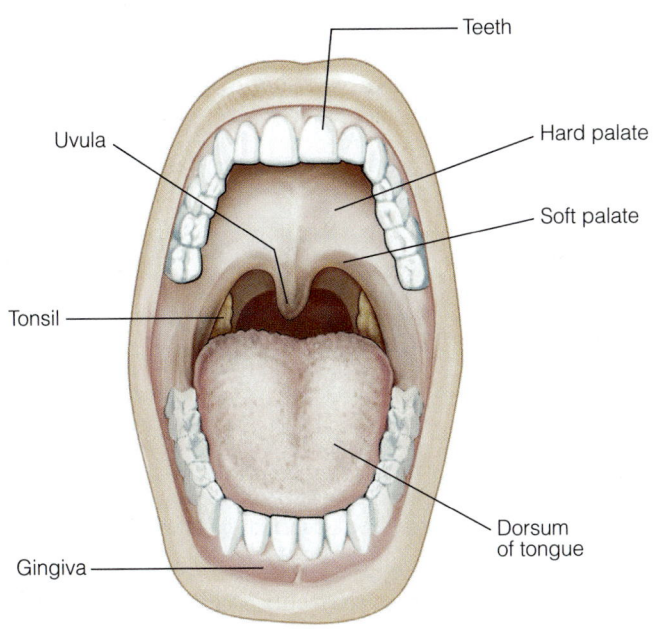

Teeth

Uvula

Hard palate

Soft palate

Tonsil

Dorsum of tongue

Gingiva

Figure 7–10 ❯❯ Oral cavity.

visible, hard deposit of plaque and dead bacteria that forms at the gum lines. Tartar buildup can alter the fibers that attach the teeth to the gums, and eventually disrupt bone tissue. Periodontal disease is characterized by **gingivitis** (red, swollen gingiva), bleeding, receding gum lines, and the formation of pockets between the teeth and gums. In **pyorrhea** (advanced periodontal disease), the teeth are loose and pus is evident when the gums are pressed.

SAFETY ALERT Thirty thousand telephone calls to poison control centers in the United States concern ingested fluoride, as reported in a classic oral science monograph. The usual source is **dentifrice** (a paste or powder for cleaning the teeth). Children are attracted by ease of access and the pleasant flavors of children's toothpaste, but a 10-year-old child swallowing under 2 ounces of dentifrice (5 mg/kg body weight) could suffer a toxic dose (Whitford, 2011).

Lifespan Considerations

A major role of the nurse in promoting oral health is teaching patients about specific oral hygiene measures across the lifespan.

Oral Health for Infants and Toddlers

Most dentists recommend that dental hygiene begin when the first tooth erupts and be practiced after each feeding. Cleaning can be accomplished by using a wet washcloth or small gauze moistened with water.

Dental caries occur frequently during the toddler period, often as a result of the excessive intake of sweets or a prolonged use of bottle feeding during naps and at bedtime. The nurse should give parents the following instructions to promote and maintain dental health:

- Beginning at about 18 months of age, brush the child's teeth with a soft toothbrush. Use only a toothbrush moistened with water at first and introduce toothpaste later. Use toothpaste that contains fluoride.

- Give a fluoride supplement daily or as recommended by the primary care provider or dentist, unless the drinking water is fluoridated.

- Schedule an initial dental visit for the child at age 6 months, to discuss fluoride varnish applications through age 5 years. This is to prevent the most common chronic disease affecting young children, dental cavities (AAP, 2015a).

Clinical Manifestations and Therapies
Problems of the Mouth

CLINICAL TERM AND ETIOLOGY	CLINICAL MANIFESTATIONS	CLINICAL THERAPIES
Baby-bottle syndrome: Carbohydrates in solutions demineralize tooth enamel, causing tooth decay	Decay of all of the upper teeth and the lower posterior teeth (AAP, 2016)	Educate parents about the risks. Suggest substitutes to soothe the child, such as pacifiers.
Burning mouth syndrome: Estrogen deficiency due to menopause and other conditions	Unpleasant tingling sensation in the mouth; sometimes changes in taste perception	Use over-the-counter medicated creams or lozenges or prescribed oral medications.
Cheilosis: Bacteria, fungus infections, nutritional deficiencies	Cracking of lips	Address the cause of the condition; lubricate lips; use antimicrobial ointment.
Glossitis: Allergic response	Inflammation of the tongue; tongue can change color or look smooth	Encourage regular oral hygiene, recognizing the difficulty of cleaning the tongue.
Granulomas: Hormones of pregnancy	Benign tumor-like growths on gums	Refer to a dentist for ruling out other causes.
Hairy leukoplakia: Early sign of HIV infection	Fuzzy white patch on the tongue	Refer for clinical testing to confirm diagnosis.
Parotitis: Mumps causing inflammation	Swelling of one or both of the parotid glands or other salivary glands	Encourage regular oral hygiene, even though brushing and flossing can be difficult.
Reddened or excoriated mucosa: Friction against soft tissue	Mouth mucous membranes irritated with some bleeding	Check for ill-fitting dentures, dental bridges, or other irritants.
Sordes: Debilitating diseases with protracted low fever	Crusts on teeth and lips	Remove crusts, and apply ointments to keep lips lubricated; keep teeth clean.
Stomatitis: Trauma, allergy, vitamin deficiency, infection	Inflammation of the oral mucous membranes	Respond to the cause of inflammation; encourage regular effective oral hygiene.

- Seek professional dental attention for any problems like discoloring of the teeth, chipping, or signs of infection such as redness and swelling.

Oral Health for Preschoolers and School-Age Children

Because deciduous teeth guide the entrance of permanent teeth, dental care is essential to keep these deciduous teeth in good repair and to establish good dental habits early. Abnormally placed or lost deciduous teeth can cause misalignment of permanent teeth. Fluoride remains important at this stage to prevent dental caries. Preschoolers need to be taught to brush their teeth after eating and to limit their intake of refined sugars. Parental supervision may be needed to ensure the completion of these self-care activities. Regular dental checkups are required during these years when permanent teeth appear.

Oral Health for Adolescents and Adults

Proper diet and tooth and mouth care should be evaluated and reinforced for adolescents and adults. Specific measures to prevent tooth decay and periodontal disease are listed in the Patient Teaching feature. Smokers should be made aware of the latest research on their smoking habit and the risk of losing teeth. Researchers looking at data from over 20,000 study participants found that those who smoked at least 15 cigarettes per day were much more likely to lose their teeth. Male smokers were more than 3 times as likely, and female smokers more than 2 times as likely to lose their teeth as nonsmokers. After 10–20 years of smoking cessation, the risk decreased to the level of nonsmokers (Dietrich et al., 2015).

Oral Health for Pregnant Women

A pregnant woman's progesterone level rises, and other hormones change after conception. The effect in the woman's mouth can be gingivitis, increased or decreased saliva, or granulomas on the gums. The stomach contents, coming through the mouth with morning sickness, also bring up gastric acids. This can hasten tooth decay (Healthline, 2014).

The incidence of periodontal disease (gum disease) increases during pregnancy because the rise in female hormones affects gingival tissue and increases its reaction to bacterial plaque. Many pregnant women experience more bleeding from the gingival sulcus during brushing and increased redness and swelling of the gingiva (gum).

Oral Health for Older Adults

Nurses have an important role in promoting optimal geriatric oral healthcare. Good oral health can have a positive effect on the older adults' ability to eat nutritious meals and other good health habits. They are often at risk for dental cavities and periodontal disease because they cannot maintain their oral hygiene practices and/or may not be able to visit the dentist routinely.

Lack of fluoridated water and preventive dentistry during their developmental years can contribute to tooth and gum problems in older adults (Edelman et al., 2013). As a result, about 25% of adults 60 years old and older no longer have any natural teeth. About 23% of 65- to 74-year-olds have severe gum disease (CDC, 2013c). Loss of teeth occurs mainly because of periodontal disease rather than dental caries.

Oral care may be difficult for certain older adults to perform due to problems with dexterity or dementia. Nurses can help by problem-solving with caregivers ways to remove residual food debris, including rinsing the mouth after meals. Even using plain water can reduce bacteria by 30%. Use of an electric toothbrush might be useful (Periodontitis, 2013).

Xerostomia (severe dryness of the mouth) is common in older adults. Drinking at least 7 glasses of water per day can trigger the production of more saliva (Periodontitis, 2013). See the Patient Teaching feature for other suggestions.

Nursing Management

Assessment of the patient's mouth and hygiene practices includes: (a) observation and patient interview, (b) physical examination of the mouth, and (c) identification of patients at risk for developing oral problems.

Observation and Patient Interview

Observation may show a coated tongue, missing teeth, or a dry mucous membrane. The color of the teeth and of the gums and the number of cavities filled will be evident. Lack of tooth flossing and brushing might be discovered by seeing food trapped between teeth. The patient's breath might smell like the most recent meal or be unpleasant from **halitosis** (bad breath). The patient might be dealing with the need to thoroughly clean teeth while using appliances such as braces, dental bridges, or dentures (American Dental Association, 2014a).

Interview questions for an adult may include:

- What are your usual mouth care and/or denture care practices?
- What oral hygiene products do you routinely use (e.g., mouthwash, type of toothpaste, dental floss, denture cleaner)?
- When was your last dental examination, and how often do you see your dentist?

Patient Teaching
Measures to Prevent Tooth Decay

- Brush teeth thoroughly after meals and at bedtime. Fluoride toothpaste is often recommended because of its antibacterial protection. If the teeth cannot be brushed after meals, vigorously rinse the mouth with water.
- Floss teeth daily.
- Ensure an adequate intake of nutrients, particularly calcium, phosphorus, fluoride, and vitamins A, C, and D.
- Avoid sweet foods and drinks between meals. Take them in moderation at meals.
- Eat coarse, fibrous foods (cleansing foods), such as fresh fruits and raw vegetables.
- Have topical fluoride applications as prescribed by a dentist. This treatment is useful for adults and teens in cases of dry mouth, gum disease, frequent cavities, braces, crowns, and bridges (WebMD, 2016).
- Have a checkup by a dentist every 6 months.

Patient Teaching
Suggestions for Relieving Dry Mouth

Offer the following suggestions to patients to help relieve xerostomia:

- Drink water frequently.
- Avoid mouthwash rinses that contains alcohol.
- Limit fluids with caffeine and alcohol.
- Sip water or sugar-free fluids, or let ice chips melt in your mouth for moisture.
- Drink water during meals to help with chewing and swallowing.
- Eat soft, moist, room-temperature food.
- Avoid salty or dry foods.
- Enjoy sugar-free hard candies or chew sugar-free gum. Be aware that they might contain xylitol, which can cause diarrhea or abdominal cramps.
- Try over-the-counter saliva substitutes.
- Consciously breathe through your nose, not your mouth.
- Sleep next to a room humidifier.
- Moisturize lips with an ointment.

Sources: Data *from* Cleveland Clinic. (2016). *Diseases and conditions: Dry mouth treatments.* Retrieved from https://my.clevelandclinic.org/health/diseases_conditions/hic_Dry_Mouth_Treatments; Mayo Clinic. (2015b). *Dry mouth.* Retrieved from http://www.mayoclinic.org/diseases-conditions/dry-mouth/basics/definition/con-20035499; Periodontitis. (2013). *The New York Times.* Retrieved from http://www.nytimes.com/health/guides/disease/periodontitis/prevention.html#

- Do you have any problems managing your mouth care?
- Have you had or do you have any problems such as bleeding, swollen or reddened gums, ulcerations, lumps, or tooth pain?

Interview questions of parents of young children may include:

- Do you share spoons, forks and other utensils with your baby?
- Do you put your young child to bed with a bottle of milk, formula, juice, or other product that contains sugar?
- Does your local water supply contain fluoride? Do you use bottled water for cooking or drinking?
- Is your child exposed to cigarette smoke?
- Do you know whom to contact in case your child knocks out or breaks a tooth?
- Does your child suck her fingers or thumb?

Physical Examination

A lot of useful information about patients' health can be obtained by examining their mouths. The following checklist is efficient and effective and prevents nurses from missing important areas. In general, the assessment should move from the front to the back:

- *Lips:* Are they a normal color and without breaks in the surface?
- *Tongue:* Is it pink, smooth, and muscular?
- *Mucosa (the lining of the mouth):* Is it moist, without surface breaks, and of appropriate color?

- *Teeth:* Do they show evidence of food collecting on them? Are particles caught between them?
- *Gums:* Are they of even color without being swollen?
- *Throat:* Is it a healthy color, similar to the tongue? Does it have a coating over it? Is the surface smooth or bumpy and swollen?
- *Tonsils (if present):* Are they a similar color and not swollen? Do they have an exudate?
- *Patient's breath:* Does the patient's breath have any unusual or foul odor?

SAFETY ALERT When examining the mouth, wash your hands before donning and after doffing gloves. Be aware that gloves can have small, unseen defects, or become compromised during the oral health examination (CDC, 2013a).

Identifying Patients at Risk

Certain patients are prone to oral problems because of lack of knowledge or the inability to maintain oral hygiene. Among these are patients who are seriously ill, confused, comatose, depressed, illiterate, or dehydrated. In addition, patients with nasogastric tubes and patients receiving oxygen are likely to develop dry oral mucous membranes, especially if they breathe through their mouths. Patients who have had oral or jaw surgery must maintain meticulous oral hygiene to prevent the development of infections.

Healthy-appearing individuals, too, may be at risk. High-risk variables such as inadequate nutrition, lack of money and/or insurance for dental care, excessive intake of refined sugars, and family history of periodontal disease also need to be identified. Some older individuals may also be at risk, for example, those who choose salty and enamel-eroding sugary foods because of a decline in their number of taste buds. Decreased saliva production in older adults, which produces a dry mouth and thinning of the oral mucosa, is another factor.

A dry mouth can be aggravated by poor fluid intake, heavy smoking, alcohol use, high salt intake, anxiety, and many medications. Medications that can cause dryness of the mouth include diuretics; laxatives, if used excessively; and tranquilizers, such as diazepam (Valium). Some chemotherapeutic agents used to treat cancer also cause oral dryness and lesions. A common side effect of the anticonvulsant drug phenytoin (Dilantin) is gingival hyperplasia. Optimal oral hygiene (e.g., brushing with a soft toothbrush, flossing) is necessary for patients taking these medications.

Patients who are receiving or have received radiation treatments to the head and neck may have permanent damage to salivary glands. Their very dry mouth can be treated with a thick liquid called *artificial saliva.* Some patients prefer to sip liquids to moisten their mouth. Radiation can also damage teeth and jaw structure.

Patients in long-term care are at high risk for oral health problems. The nurse must assess patients' oral health and teach the importance of and methods to promote oral hygiene.

Promoting Oral Hygiene

Good oral hygiene includes daily stimulation of the gums, mechanical brushing and flossing of the teeth, and flushing of the mouth. The nurse frequently is in a position to help individuals maintain oral hygiene by helping or teaching them to clean the teeth and oral cavity, by inspecting whether patients (especially children) have done so, or by actually providing mouth care to patients who are ill or incapacitated. The nurse can also identify problems that require the intervention of a dentist or oral surgeon and can arrange a referral.

Individuals with artificial dentures need to clean them regularly, at least once a day. They can be removed from the mouth, scrubbed with a toothbrush, rinsed, and reinserted. A dentifrice or a commercial cleaning compound can be used. Most individuals prefer privacy when they remove their artificial teeth to clean them. Many do not like to be seen without their teeth; often the first request of many postoperative patients is "May I have my teeth in, please?"

For the patient who is debilitated or unconscious or who has excessive dryness, sores, or irritations of the mouth, it may be necessary to clean the oral mucosa and tongue in addition to the teeth. If the patient cannot tolerate the use of a soft-bristled toothbrush, the nurse can use an oral swab or gauze soaked with saline to clean the teeth and tongue. Saliva substitutes can also help moisturize the oral cavity. Agency practices differ in regard to special mouth care and its frequency. Depending on the health of the patient's mouth, special care may be needed every 2–8 hours.

REVIEW Oral Health

RELATE Link the Concepts and Exemplars

Linking the exemplar of oral health with the concept of development:

1. What are the different dental concerns of each developmental stage across the lifespan?
2. Design a teaching plan for a group of young mothers regarding oral health and nutrition for their toddlers.
3. If a patient fears visiting a dentist, what possible motivational factors could the nurse point out?

Linking the exemplar of oral health with the concept of oxygenation:

4. You are caring for a 6-year-old child diagnosed with cystic fibrosis. How would you adapt your teaching about oral health to meet this child's needs?

Linking the exemplar of oral health with the concept of comfort:

5. While working as a hospice nurse you are caring for a patient requiring end-of-life care. What oral care will be of particular importance to provide this patient?
6. What will you teach the patient with chronic mouth pain about oral care?

READY Go to Volume 3: Clinical Nursing Skills

REFER Go to Pearson MyLab Nursing and eText

- Additional review materials

REFLECT Apply Your Knowledge

Tyler Martin is a 2-year-old boy. Since he was 4 weeks old, Tyler has been going to various babysitters while his parents work. He and his father have recently moved in with Tyler's grandparents. Tyler loves living at his grandfather's home because of all the attention he gets. Tyler also no longer has to go to day care.

Tyler has generally been in good health; he is of normal weight and has a good appetite. Tyler still loves his bottle, and each night he is given a bottle of milk or juice to help him go to sleep. If he does not receive a bottle to sleep with, he screams until someone gives in and brings him one.

1. Are there any concerns in this scenario that require intervention and teaching?
2. What dental visits and tooth care does Tyler require?
3. How would you teach Tyler to brush his teeth? Can he be taught how to floss at this stage? Explain your answer.

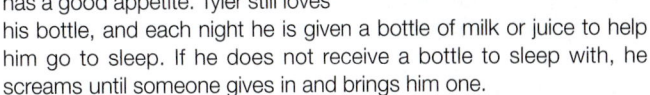

>> **Exemplar 7.C**
Normal Sleep–Rest Patterns

Exemplar Learning Outcomes

7.C Analyze sleep and rest as they relate to health, wellness, illness, and injury.

- Describe the physiology and functions of sleep.
- Describe variations in sleep patterns across the lifespan.
- Outline factors affecting sleep.
- Plan interventions that promote normal sleep.

Exemplar Key Terms

Biological rhythms, *458*
Circadian rhythm, *458*
Nocturnal emissions, *461*
NREM (non–REM) sleep, *459*
REM sleep, *459*
Sleep, *458*

Overview

Sleep is a basic human need; it is a universal biological process common to all individuals. Humans spend about one third of their lives asleep. We require sleep for many reasons: to cope with daily stresses, to prevent fatigue, to conserve energy, to restore the mind and body, and to enjoy life more fully. Sleep enhances daytime functioning. It is vital not only for optimal psychologic functioning but also for physiologic functioning.

Sleep is an important factor in quality of life, yet sleep disorders and sleep deprivation are an unmet public health problem. Clinical studies have found a clear minimum requirement of sleep continuity to ensure optimal sleep-dependent memory processes (Djonlagic, Saboiskyh, Carusona, Stickgold, & Malhotra, 2012). Numerous *Sleep in America* polls by the National Sleep Foundation show that Americans, from infants to older adults, need more sleep. Over 40 million Americans are undiagnosed, misdiagnosed, or untreated for sleep disorders (Salas et al., 2013). An additional 20 million people have occasional sleeping difficulties. Added together, their direct cost is an estimated $16 billion in medical costs annually. Indirect costs of lost productivity are thought to be even more expensive (American Sleep Association, 2015).

Furthermore, many members of the general public and health professionals are unaware that sleep disorders are commonly associated with other major medical problems, such as cardiovascular disease, depression, obesity, and Type 2 diabetes (CDC, 2013d).

See the exemplar on Sleep Disorders in the module on Comfort for more information.

>> **Stay Current:** To see the latest information on sleep, visit the National Sleep Foundation at http://www.sleepfoundation.org.

Physiology of Sleep

Sleep historically was considered a state of unconsciousness. In recent years, sleep has come to be considered an altered state of consciousness in which the individual's perception of and reaction to the immediate environment are decreased. Sleep is characterized by minimal physical activity, variable levels of consciousness, changes in the body's physiologic processes, and decreased responsiveness to external stimuli. Some environmental stimuli, such as a smoke detector alarm, will usually awaken a sleeper, whereas many other noises will not. It appears that individuals respond to meaningful stimuli while sleeping and selectively disregard nonmeaningful stimuli. For example, a mother may respond to her own baby's crying but not to the crying of another baby.

The cyclical nature of sleep is controlled by centers located in the lower part of the brain. Neurons within the reticular formation, located in the brainstem, integrate sensory information from the peripheral nervous system and relay the information to the cerebral cortex. The upper part of the reticular formation consists of a network of ascending nerve fibers called the *reticular activating system (RAS)*, which is involved in the sleep–wake cycle. An intact cerebral cortex and reticular formation are necessary for the regulation of sleep and waking states.

Neurotransmitters, located within neurons in the brain, affect the sleep–wake cycle. For example, serotonin is thought to lessen the response to sensory stimulation, and gamma-aminobutyric acid (GABA) is believed to shut off the activity in the neurons of the RAS. Another key factor in sleep is exposure to darkness. Darkness and preparing for sleep cause a decrease in RAS stimulation. During this time, the pineal gland in the brain begins actively to secrete the natural hormone melatonin, and the individual feels less alert. During sleep, the growth hormone is secreted, and cortisol is inhibited.

With the beginning of daylight, melatonin is at its lowest level in the body and the stimulating hormone cortisol is at its highest. Wakefulness is also associated with high levels of acetylcholine, dopamine, and noradrenaline. Acetylcholine is released in the reticular formation, dopamine in the midbrain, and noradrenaline in the pons. These neurotransmitters are localized within the reticular formation and influence cerebral cortical arousal.

Circadian Rhythms

Biological rhythms are daily cycles in many of our physiologic functions and activities: sleep, body temperature, alertness, neurotransmitter levels, and so on. They are controlled within the body and are synchronized with environmental factors such as light and darkness. The most familiar biological rhythm is the **circadian rhythm** (**Figure 7–11** >>). The term *circadian* is from the Latin *circa dies,* meaning "about a day." Although sleep and waking cycles are the best known of the circadian rhythms, body temperature, heart activity, blood pressure, oxygen consumption, metabolism, and many other physiologic functions also follow a circadian pattern (University of Utah, 2015).

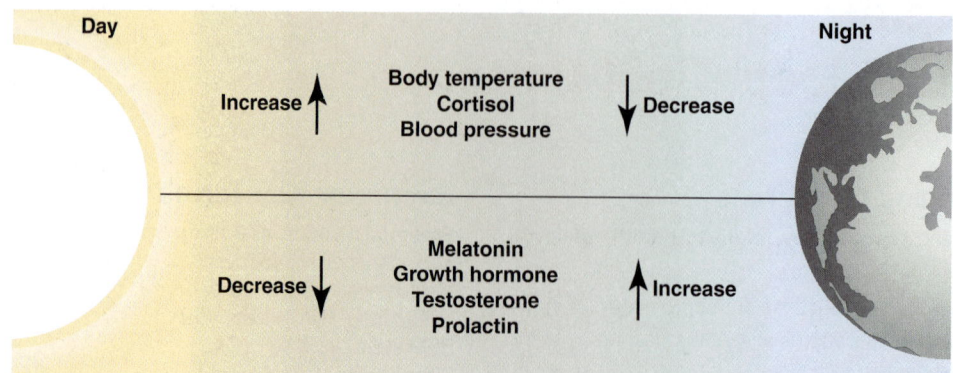

Figure 7–11 >> Many physiologic functions follow a circadian pattern through the course of day and night.

Sleep is a complex biological rhythm. An individual whose biological clock coincides with the sleep–wake cycle is said to be in circadian synchronization, that is, awake when the body temperature is highest and asleep when the body temperature is lowest. Circadian regularity begins to develop by the sixth week of life, and by 3–6 months most infants have a regular sleep–wake cycle.

The Sleep Cycle

There are two types of sleep: **NREM (non-REM) sleep** and **REM sleep**. During a healthy adult's sleep, NREM and REM sleep alternate every 90–110 minutes for complete sleep cycle. The healthy adult sleeper usually experiences four to six cycles of sleep during 7–8 hours (National Institute of Neurological Disorders and Stroke [NINDS], 2014).

NREM Sleep

About 80% of sleep during a night is NREM sleep. NREM sleep is divided into four stages, each associated with distinct brain and body activity. Stage N1 is the stage of light sleep and lasts only a few minutes. During this stage, the eyes move very slowly, and the muscle activity slows. The sleeper can be easily awakened, and if roused, often remembers fragmented visual images.

Stage N2 is the stage of light sleep during which body processes continue to slow down. Eye movements stop, and brain waves become slower. Bursts of rapid brain waves sometimes occur. Stage N2 constitutes 50% of total sleep,

Stages N3 and N4 are together called deep sleep. In stage N3, extremely slow brain waves appear, punctuated with smaller, faster waves. In stage N4, delta waves predominate. In either stage of deep sleep, the sleeper is difficult to arouse. The eyes do not move, and muscle activity ceases. People awakened during deep sleep often feel disoriented. Some children wet their beds, have night terrors, or sleepwalk during deep sleep (NINDS, 2014).

REM Sleep

The first REM sleep usually occurs about 70–90 minutes after sleep begins. Most dreams take place during REM sleep. A healthy adult sleeper typically spends more than 2 hours each night dreaming.

During REM sleep, the body and brain are highly active. Distinctive eye movements occur; breathing becomes more rapid, irregular, and shallow; and voluntary muscle tone is dramatically decreased. The heart rate increases, blood pressure rises, and men develop penile erections. Researchers think that the regions of the brain used in learning, thinking, and organizing information are stimulated during REM sleep (NINDS, 2014).

Functions of Sleep

The effects of sleep on the body are not completely understood. Sleep exerts physiologic effects on both the nervous system and other body structures. Sleep in some way restores normal levels of activity and normal balance among parts of the nervous system. Sleep is also necessary for protein synthesis, which allows repair processes to occur.

The role of sleep in psychologic well-being is best noticed by the deterioration in mental functioning related to sleep loss. Individuals with inadequate amounts of sleep tend to become emotionally irritable, have poor concentration, and experience difficulty making decisions.

SAFETY ALERT In a recent study, after 24 hours of sleep deprivation, healthy individuals showed symptoms of psychosis. The effects were similar to those of people with schizophrenia. The study confirmed the severe effect of insomnia on cognitive functioning (Melville, 2014).

Lifespan Considerations

Although researchers used to believe that maintaining a regular sleep–wake rhythm was more important than the number of hours actually slept, recent research has shown that sleep deprivation is associated with significant cognitive and health problems. Early impairment in cognitive function usually manifests as difficulty with concentration and memory. More significant impairment may manifest in a decreasing ability to perform tasks requiring speed and accuracy (e.g., driving) and in an increasing engagement in risk-taking behaviors. Sleep deprivation has also been found to play a role in obesity, type 2 diabetes, depression, and cardiovascular health (CDC, 2013d).

To prevent sleep deprivation, nurses should compare the patient's reported sleep time with the data in **Figure 7–12 》**.

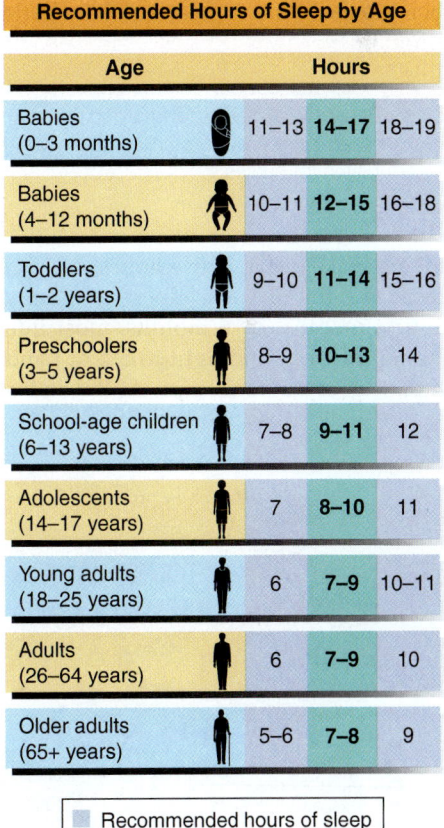

Recommended Hours of Sleep by Age			
Age	**Hours**		
Babies (0–3 months)	11–13	**14–17**	18–19
Babies (4–12 months)	10–11	**12–15**	16–18
Toddlers (1–2 years)	9–10	**11–14**	15–16
Preschoolers (3–5 years)	8–9	**10–13**	14
School-age children (6–13 years)	7–8	**9–11**	12
Adolescents (14–17 years)	7	**8–10**	11
Young adults (18–25 years)	6	**7–9**	10–11
Adults (26–64 years)	6	**7–9**	10
Older adults (65+ years)	5–6	**7–8**	9

☐ Recommended hours of sleep
■ May be appropriate

Source: Data from "The National Sleep Foundation's Sleep Time Duration Recommendations: Methodology and Results Summary" by Max Hirshkowitz, Steven M. Albert, Kaitlyn Whiton and Cathy Alessi et al. in Sleep Health, Volume 1, Issue 1, pp. 40–43. Copyright © 2015 by National Sleep Foundation.

Figure 7–12 》 The National Sleep Foundation recommends optimum sleep duration throughout the lifespan as illustrated here.

That chart shows the recommended duration of sleep for individuals across the lifespan (Hirshkowitz et al., 2015).

Sleep and Newborns

Newborns sleep on an irregular schedule with periods of 1–3 hours spent awake. Unlike older children and adults, newborns enter REM sleep (called *active sleep* during the newborn period) immediately. Rapid eye movements are observable through closed lids, and body movements and irregular respirations may be observed. NREM sleep (also called *quiet sleep* during the newborn period) is characterized by regular respirations, closed eyes, and the absence of body and eye movements. Newborns spend nearly 50% of their time in each of these states, and the sleep cycle is about 50 minutes (**Figure 7–13 >>**).

It is best to put newborns to bed when they are sleepy but not asleep. Newborns can be encouraged to sleep less during the day by exposure to light and by being played with more during the daytime hours. As evening approaches, the environment can be made less bright and quieter, with less activity (National Sleep Foundation, 2015b).

Nurses should teach new parents and caregivers of newborns to put their babies "back to sleep," which is to make sure newborns sleep on their backs, because babies who sleep on their stomachs are at greater risk for sudden infant death syndrome.

>> Stay Current: Visit the Safe to Sleep website at https://www.nichd.nih.gov/sts/Pages/default.aspx for more information, including free brochures for healthcare providers and patients and information on continuing education for nurses.

Sleep and Infants

At first, infants wake every 3 or 4 hours, eat, and then go back to sleep. Periods of wakefulness gradually increase during the first months. By 6 months, most infants sleep through the night (from midnight to 5 a.m.) and begin to establish a pattern of daytime naps. At the end of the first year, an infant usually takes two naps per day.

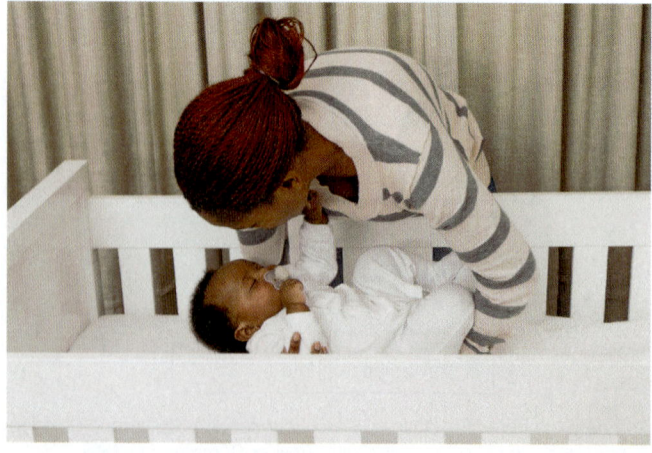

Source: BFG Images/Getty Images.

Figure 7–13 >> This newborn's mother is following the Safe to Sleep recommendations: The baby is being put in his crib on his back, wearing warm clothes, sleeping on a firm mattress, and with no blankets, bumpers, toys, or other objects in the crib.

About half of the infant's sleep time is spent in light sleep. During light sleep, the infant exhibits a great deal of activity, such as movement, gurgles, and coughing. Parents need to make sure that infants are truly awake before picking them up for feeding and changing. Putting infants to bed when they are drowsy but not asleep helps them to become "self-soothers"; that is, they fall asleep independently, and if they do awake at night, they can put themselves back to sleep. Infants who become used to parental assistance at bedtime may become "signalers" and cry for their parents to help them return to sleep at night (National Sleep Foundation, 2015b).

Sleep and Toddlers

Most children 1–3 years of age still need an afternoon nap, but the need for midmorning naps gradually decreases. The toddler may exhibit a great deal of resistance to going to bed and may awaken during the night. Nighttime fears and nightmares are also common. A security object such as a blanket or stuffed animal may help. Parents need assurance that if the child has had adequate attention from them during the day, maintaining a daily sleep schedule and consistent bedtime routine will promote good sleep habits for the entire family (National Sleep Foundation, 2015b).

Sleep and Preschoolers

The sleep needs of the preschool child (3–5 years of age) fluctuate in relation to activity and growth spurts. Many children this age dislike bedtime and resist by requesting another story, game, or television program. However, the 4- to 5-year-old may become restless and irritable if sleep requirements are not met (National Sleep Foundation, 2015b).

Parents can help children who resist bedtime by maintaining a regular and consistent sleep schedule. It also helps to have a relaxing bedtime routine that ends in the child's room. Preschool children wake up frequently at night, and they may be afraid of the dark or experience night terrors or nightmares. Often, limiting or eliminating TV reduces the number of nightmares (National Sleep Foundation, 2015b).

Sleep and School-Age Children

Most school-age children (6–13 years of age) receive less-than-optimal sleep because of increasing demands (e.g., homework, sports, social activities). They may also be spending more time at the computer and watching TV. Some may be drinking caffeinated beverages. All of these activities can lead to difficulty falling asleep and fewer hours of sleep. Nurses can teach parents and school-age children about healthy sleep habits, such as a regular and consistent sleep schedule and bedtime routine.

Sleep and Adolescents

Few teens (14–18 years of age) get adequate sleep. One research study reported that only 15% of teens slept 8½ hours on school nights. In adolescence, normal biological sleep patterns shift to both sleeping later and waking up later. It is natural not to be able to fall asleep before 11 p.m. (National Sleep Foundation, 2015d). Many schools, however, start at 7 a.m., a time that is in conflict with the adolescent's sleep patterns and

Box 7–3
Sleep Deprivation and Sleep Problems in Teens

A sleep-deprived teen may:

- Have difficulty waking in the morning for school
- Fall asleep in class or during quiet times of the day
- Increase the use of caffeinated beverages such as cola, coffee, and energy drinks
- Feel tired enough to have trouble initiating or persisting in projects, such as school assignments
- Be irritable and anxious and anger easily on days after less sleep
- Sleep extra-long periods of time on the weekend.

Focus on Diversity and Culture
Population Sleep Differences

Researchers have examined data about sleep differences in minority populations, such as African Americans and Hispanics, and individuals of lower socioeconomic status to check for a possible correlation with increased risk of cardiometabolic diseases. These conditions include obesity, diabetes, hypertension, and cardiovascular disease. Several studies found a correlation between people's ethnicity and socioeconomic status and their decreased sleep duration and lower quality of sleep. Researchers theorize that these factors combine to produce suboptimal sleep and are associated with increased risk of cardiometabolic diseases (Rangaraj & Knutson, 2015).

needs and contributes to their sleep deprivation (National Sleep Foundation, 2015c).

Nurses can teach parents to recognize signs and symptoms that their teen is not getting enough sleep (see **Box 7–3** »).

During adolescence, boys begin to experience **nocturnal emissions** (orgasm and emission of semen during sleep), known as *wet dreams*, several times each month. Boys need to be informed about this normal development to prevent embarrassment and fear.

Sleep and Pregnant Women

A pregnant woman will usually find that she needs more sleep during the first trimester of her pregnancy. Her progesterone level and her metabolism rate are rising. Her blood pressure becomes lower, and her blood production is increasing. After the first trimester, her body becomes used to her new condition. Then, at the end of the pregnancy, the size of the baby can interfere with finding a comfortable resting position. Recommendations about getting better sleep include sleeping on the left side, using pillows between the knees and under the abdomen, and elevating the head of the bed (Mayo Clinic, 2013).

Sleep and Adults

Healthy adults ages 18–64 years old vary in sleep needs. Some adults may be able to function well (e.g., without sleepiness or drowsiness) with 6 hours of sleep, and others may need 10 hours to function optimally. Signs that indicate an individual may not be getting enough sleep include falling asleep or becoming drowsy during a task that is not fatiguing (e.g., listening to a boring or monotonous presentation), not being able to concentrate or remember information, and being unreasonably irritable.

SAFETY ALERT Drowsy driving caused 72,000 crashes in 2013, resulting in 44,000 injuries and 800 deaths (National Highway Traffic Safety Administration, 2016).

The National Sleep Foundation (2014) reports that certain adults are particularly vulnerable to getting insufficient sleep: shift workers, travelers, and individuals suffering from other clinical disorders, such as acute stress, depression, or chronic pain. Unhealthy sleep habits and certain medications can interfere with sleep. Adults working long hours or multiple jobs may find their sleep less refreshing. Sleep specialist Dr. William C. Dement estimates that

parents of newborns lose about 2 hours of sleep each night until their baby is 5 months old. Then, for the next year and a half, parents continue to lose an hour of sleep each night (Ding, 2016). Also, the sleep habits of children have an impact on the adults caring for them. Parents and caregivers whose children get the least amount of sleep are twice as likely to say they sleep less than 6 hours a night (National Sleep Foundation, n.d.). Parents of infants lose the most sleep—nearly an hour on a typical night. A National Sleep Foundation poll (2009) revealed that women have more difficulty than men falling and staying asleep. Thus, women experience more daytime sleepiness. In addition, women may experience more disrupted sleep during pregnancy, menses, and the perimenopausal period (National Sleep Foundation, 2015e).

Sleep and Older Adults

A hallmark change with age is a tendency toward earlier bedtime and wake times. Older adults (65–75 years) usually awaken 1.3 hours earlier and go to bed approximately 1 hour earlier than younger adults (ages 20–30). Older adults may show an increase in disturbed sleep that can create a negative impact on their quality of life, mood, and alertness. Although sleeping becomes more difficult, the need to sleep does not decrease with age (National Sleep Foundation, 2015a).

The National Sleep Foundation's ongoing research polls looked at the sleep habits of Americans between the ages of 55 and 84. It found that older adults are sleeping 7–9 hours on both weeknights and weekends. Of interest, however, was the striking relationship between the older adult's health and quality of life and the individual's sleep quantity and quality. The poll found that the better the health of older adults, the more likely they are to sleep well, and, conversely, the more diagnosed medical conditions they have, the more likely they are to report sleep problems (National Sleep Foundation, 2015a). Older adults who have several medical conditions and complain of having sleeping problems should consult with their primary care provider: They may have a major sleep disorder that is complicating treatment of the other conditions. Nurses should teach about the connection between sleep, health, and aging.

Some older adult patients with dementia may experience *sundown syndrome*. Although not a sleep disorder directly, it

TABLE 7–7 Factors Affecting Sleep

Factor	Explanation of Reason for Effect
Emotional stress	Individual is preoccupied with personal problems (e.g., school- or job-related pressures, financial difficulties, family or marriage problems). Anxiety increases norepinephrine blood levels, resulting in less deep sleep and REM sleep and more stage changes and awakenings.
Stimulants and alcohol	Caffeine-containing beverages stimulate central nervous system. Alcohol may hasten onset of sleep, but it disrupts REM sleep.
Diet	Weight gain is associated with reduced total sleep time, interrupted sleep, and earlier awakening. Weight loss is associated with increase in total sleep time and fewer interruptions of sleep. Dietary L-tryptophan found in cheese and milk may induce sleep.
Smoking	Nicotine is a stimulant. Smokers often have more difficulty falling asleep than nonsmokers. They are usually easily aroused and often describe themselves as light sleepers. Smokers can try not smoking after the evening meal.
Motivation for alertness and boredom	Motivation can increase alertness when a tired individual wants to stay awake. Motivation alone is insufficient to overcome normal circadian rhythm or sleepiness due to insufficient sleep. When insufficient sleep combines with boredom, sleep is likely to occur.
Medications	Hypnotics can interfere with deep sleep and suppress REM sleep. Beta-blockers can cause insomnia and nightmares. Narcotics such as meperidine hydrochloride (Demerol) and morphine suppress REM sleep and cause frequent awakenings and drowsiness. Tranquilizers interfere with REM sleep. Although antidepressants suppress REM sleep, this effect is therapeutic, resulting in immediate but transient improvement in mood. Patients taking hypnotic medications and antidepressants may experience REM rebound (increased REM sleep) when medications are discontinued.
Environment	Sounds, lighting, and comfort of bedding can contribute to or hinder onset and maintenance of sleep.
Pain, illness, and injury	Medical conditions can disturb regular sleep.

refers to a pattern of symptoms (e.g., agitation, anxiety, aggression, sometimes delusions) that occur in the late afternoon (thus the name). These symptoms can last throughout the night, further disrupting sleep (National Sleep Foundation, 2015a).

Factors Affecting Sleep

Both the quality and the quantity of sleep are affected by a number of factors. *Sleep quality* is a subjective characteristic and is often determined by whether or not an individual wakes up feeling energetic. *Quantity of sleep* is the total time the individual sleeps.

Following an irregular morning and nighttime schedule can affect sleep. Moderate exercise in the morning or early afternoon usually is conducive to sleep, but exercise late in the day can delay sleep. The individual's ability to relax before retiring is an important factor affecting the ability to fall asleep. Patients should, therefore, avoid doing homework or office work before or after getting into bed.

Night shift workers frequently obtain less sleep than other workers and have difficulty falling asleep after getting off work. Wearing dark wraparound sunglasses during the drive home and using light-blocking shades can minimize the alerting effects of exposure to daylight, thus making it easier to fall asleep when body temperature is rising.

Common factors affecting sleep are outlined in **Table 7–7** ».

Nursing Management

Nurses need to teach adults the importance of obtaining sufficient sleep. They can do the following to promote sleep and help the patient wake up feeling restored or refreshed:

■ Make evidence-based suggestions to help the patient get more hours of restful sleep.

■ Ask the patient: Is your difficulty falling asleep, or maintaining sleep during the night? Or both problems?

■ Suggest that the patient keep a sleep diary to see the patterns of her sleep habits.

■ Emphasize that the most important change to make in a bedtime routine is to set a routine mandatory time to go to bed and set a routine mandatory time to get out of bed. The patient needs to train his mind and body to expect to sleep on this schedule.

■ Assure the patient that the rigidity of the new schedule and food intake changes will become more comfortable over time and will give the best opportunity for restful sleep.

For more suggestions, see the Sleep Hygiene feature in the module on Comfort.

REVIEW Normal Sleep–Rest Patterns

RELATE Link the Concepts and Exemplars

Linking the exemplar of normal sleep–rest patterns with the concept of cognition:

1. How would you expect a postpartum patient's cognition to be affected if the patient is being woken up every 2–4 hours by the newborn's cry and need to eat?

2. The daughter of an 80-year-old patient who has early dementia complains to the nurse that the patient is up and ready to go at 4:30 in the morning. She is concerned that lack of sleep will eventually affect her mother's dementia. What teaching would you provide this patient's daughter?

Linking the exemplar of normal sleep–rest patterns with the concept of infection:

3. What is your priority of care for the patient with pneumonia who sleeps 4 hours a night?

4. What interventions would you initiate to promote normal sleep patterns for a patient with septicemia who is in the intensive care unit?

5. What measures could you suggest to parents of a toddler with an ear infection to promote restful sleep for all of them?

READY Go to Volume 3: Clinical Nursing Skills

REFER Go to Pearson MyLab Nursing and eText

- Additional review materials

REFLECT Apply Your Knowledge

Ms. Iliana Smith, a 70-year-old woman, reports that she is having difficulty falling asleep at night. She enjoys a hearty bedtime snack of chocolate sweets. Her grandson recently gave her a large-screen TV. Sometimes she falls asleep in her recliner, missing the end of the TV show or movie. She says, "I am so tired in the mornings, I can hardly get out of bed."

1. Which assessment tools might be used to determine her problem?

2. Identify lifespan and environmental issues that might be influencing her condition.

3. What will Ms. Smith report if your interventions are successful?

References

Ahluwalia, I. B., Ding, H., Harrison, L., D'Angelo, D., Singleton, J. A., Bridges, C., & PRAMS Influenza Working Group. (2014). Disparities in influenza vaccination coverage among women with live born infants: PRAMS surveillance during the 2009–2010 influenza season. *Public Health Reports, 129*(5), 408–416.

Alvarez, K. J., Kirchner, S., Chu, S., Smith, S., Winnick-Baskin, W., & Mielenz, T. J. (2015). Falls reduction and exercise training in an assisted living population. *Journal of Aging Research, 957598.* doi:10.1155/2015/957598.

American Academy of Pediatrics (AAP). (2015a). *AAP releases summary of updated preventive healthcare screening and assessment schedule for children's checkups.* Retrieved from https://www.aap.org/en-us/about-the-aap/aap-press-room/pages/AAP-Releases-Summary-of-Updated-Preventive-Health-Care-Screening-and-Assessment-Schedule-for-Children's-Checkups.aspx

American Academy of Pediatrics (AAP). (2015b). *Early hearing detection and intervention (EHDI).* Retrieved from https://www.aap.org/en-us/advocacy-and-policy/aap-health-initiatives/PEHDIC/pages/early-hearing-detection-and-intervention.aspx#sthash.WX52dlT1.dpuf

American Academy of Pediatrics (AAP). (2016). *How to prevent tooth decay in your baby.* Retrieved from https://www.healthychildren.org/English/ages-stages/baby/teething-tooth-care/Pages/How-to-Prevent-Tooth-Decay-in-Your-Baby.aspx

American Cancer Society. (2015). *American Cancer Society guidelines for the early detection of cancer.* Retrieved from http://www.cancer.org/healthy/findcancerearly/cancerscreeningguidelines/american-cancer-society-guidelines-for-the-early-detection-of-cancer

American Dental Association. (2014a). *Brushing your teeth.* Retrieved from http://www.mouthhealthy.org/en/az-topics/b/brushing-your-teeth

American Dental Association. (2014b). *Toothpaste.* Retrieved from http://www.mouthhealthy.org/en/az-topics/t/toothpaste

American Diabetes Association (2015). Standards of medical care in diabetes—2015. *Diabetes Care, 38*(Suppl. 1), S1–S93.

American Heart Association & American Stroke Association. (2014). *Guidelines for the prevention of stroke in patients with stroke or transient ischemic attack.* Retrieved from http://stroke.ahajournals.org/content/early/2014/04/30/STR.0000000000000024

American Nurses Association. (1980). *Nursing: A social policy statement.* Kansas City, MO: Author.

American Nurses Association. (2004). *Nursing: Scope and standards of practice.* Washington, DC: Author.

American Osteopathic Association. (2015). *About osteopathic medicine.* Retrieved from http://www.osteopathic.org/osteopathic-health/about-dos/about-osteopathic-medicine/Pages/default.aspx

American Sleep Association. (2015). *What is sleep?* Retrieved from https://www.sleepassociation.org/patients-general-public/what-is-sleep/

Anspaugh, D. J., Hamrick, M. H., & Rosato, F. D. (2010). *Wellness: Concepts and applications* (8th ed.). New York, NY: McGraw-Hill.

Barker, A. L., Morello, R. T., Wolfe, R., Brand, C. A., Haines, T. P., Hill, K. D., … Kamar, J. (2016). 6-PACK programme to decrease fall injuries in acute hospitals: Cluster randomised controlled trial. *British Medical Journal (BMJ), 352*, h6781. doi:10.1136/bmj.h6781

Barnes, D. E., Santos-Modesitt, W., Poelke, G., Kramer, A. F., Castro, C., Middleton, L. E., & Yaffe, K. (2013). The mental activity and exercise (MAX) trial: A randomized controlled trial to enhance cognitive function in older adults. *JAMA Internal Medicine, 173*(9), 797–804. doi:10.1001/jamainternmed.2013.189

Brown, B. M., Peiffer, J. J., & Martins, R. N. (2012). Multiple effects of physical activity on molecular and cognitive signs of brain aging: Can exercise slow neurodegeneration and delay Alzheimer's disease? *Molecular Psychiatry.* doi:10.1038/mp.2012.162

Centers for Disease Control and Prevention. (2013a). *Division of oral health: Infection control.* Retrieved from http://www.cdc.gov/oralhealth/infection-control/faq/protective_equipment.htm

Centers for Disease Control and Prevention. (2013b). *Health-related quality of related (HRQOL): Well-being concepts.* Retrieved from http://www.cdc.gov/hrqol/wellbeing.htm

Centers for Disease Control and Prevention. (2013c). *Oral health for older Americans.* Retrieved from http://www.cdc.gov/oralhealth/publications/factsheets/adult_oral_health/adult_older.htm

Centers for Disease Control and Prevention. (2013d). *Sleep and chronic disease.* Retrieved from http://www.cdc.gov/sleep/about_sleep/chronic_disease.html

Centers for Disease Control and Prevention. (2015a). *Adults: Protect yourself with pneumococcal vaccines.* Retrieved from http://www.cdc.gov/features/adult-pneumococcal/

Centers for Disease Control and Prevention. (2015b). *HPV vaccination information for young women.* Retrieved from http://www.cdc.gov/std/hpv/stdfact-hpv-vaccine-young-women.htm

Centers for Disease Control and Prevention. (2015c). *Obesity and overweight.* Retrieved from http://www.cdc.gov/nchs/fastats/obesity-overweight.htm

Centers for Disease Control and Prevention (CDC). (2015d). *Physical activity basics.* Retrieved from http://www.cdc.gov/physicalactivity/basics/index.htm and http://www.cdc.gov/physicalactivity/everyone/guidelines

Centers for Disease Control and Prevention. (2015e). *Prevalence of childhood obesity in the Unites States, 2011–2012.* Retrieved from http://www.cdc.gov/obesity/data/childhood.html

Centers for Disease Control and Prevention. (2015f). *Physical activity.* Retrieved from http://www.cdc.gov/physicalactivity/

Centers for Disease Control and Prevention. (2015g). *Key facts about seasonal flu vaccine.* Retrieved from http://www.cdc.gov/flu/protect/keyfacts.htm

Centers for Disease Control and Prevention. (2017). *Disparities in oral health.* Retrieved from https://www.cdc.gov/oralhealth/oral_health_disparities/index.htm

Cleveland Clinic. (2016). *Diseases & conditions: Dry mouth treatments.* Retrieved from https://my.clevelandclinic.org/health/diseases_conditions/hic_Dry_Mouth_Treatments

Cooney, G., Dwan, K., & Mead, G. (2014). Exercise for depression. *Journal of the American Medical Association, 311*(23), 2432–2433. doi:10.1001/jama.2014.4930

Cooney, G. M., Dwan, K., Greig, C. A., Lawlor, D. A., Rimer, J., Waugh, F. R., … Mead, G. E. (2013). Exercise for depression. *Cochrane Database for Systematic Reviews, 9*, CD004366. doi:10.1002/14651858.CD004366.pub6

Dietrich, T., Walter, C., Oluwagbemigun, K., Bergmann, M., Pischon, T., … Boeing, H. (2015). Smoking, smoking cessation, and risk of tooth loss. *Journal of Dental Research, 94*(10), 1369–1375. doi:10.1177/0022034515598961

Ding, K. (January 2016). *Sleep deprivation and new parents.* Retrieved from http://consumer.healthday.com/encyclopedia/parenting-31/parenting-health-news-525/sleep-deprivation-and-new-parents-643886.html

Djonlagic, I., Saboisky, J., Carusona, A., Stickgold, R., & Malhotra, A. (2012). Increased sleep fragmentation leads to impaired off-line consolidation of motor memories in humans. *PLoS One, 7*(3). doi:10.1371/journal.pone.0034106

Edelman, C. L., Kudzma, E. C., & Mandle, C. L. (2013). *Health promotion throughout the lifespan* (8th ed.). St. Louis, MO: Mosby.

Fontaine, K. L. (2014). *Complementary and alternative therapies for nursing practice* (4th ed.). Upper Saddle River, NJ: Prentice Hall.

Gillespie, L. D., Robertson, M. C., Gillespie, W. J., Sherrington, C., Gates, S., Clemson, L. M., & Lamb, S. E. (2012). Interventions for preventing falls in older people living in the community. *Cochrane Database Systematic Reviews*, 9. CD007146. doi:10.1002/14651858.CD007146.pub3

Grazina, R., & Massano, J. (2013). Physical exercise and Parkinson's disease: Influence on symptoms, disease course and prevention. *Reviews in the Neurosciences*, 1–14. doi:10.1515/revneuro-2012-0087

Groom, H. C., Zhang, F., Fisher, A. K., & Wortley, P. M. (2014). Differences in adult influenza vaccine-seeking behavior: the roles of race and attitudes. *Journal of Public Health Management and Practice*, 20(2), 246–250. doi:10.1097/PHH.0b013e318298bd88

Hall-Flavin, D. K. (2015). *Generalized anxiety disorder: Is there an effective herbal treatment for anxiety?* Retrieved from http://www.mayoclinic.com/diseases-conditions/generalized-anxiety-disorder/expert-answers/herbal-treatment-for-anxiety/faq-20057945

Hartescu, I., Morgan, K., & Stevinson, C. D. (2015). Increased physical activity improves sleep and mood outcomes in inactive people with insomnia: a randomized controlled trial. *Journal of Sleep Research*, 24(5), 526–534. doi:10.1111/jsr.12297

Harvard University. (2012). *Another reason to get out there and get moving!* Retrieved from http://www.health.harvard.edu/newsletters/Harvard_Health_Letter/2012/March/another-reason-to-get-out-there-and-get-moving

Healthline. (2014). *Preventing oral health problems.* Retrieved from http://www.healthline.com/health/dental-oral-health-prevention#Overview1

Herdman, T. H. & Kamitsuru, S. (Eds.). *Nursing Diagnoses—Definitions and Classification 2015–2017.* Copyright © 2014, 1994–2014 NANDA International. Used by arrangement with John Wiley & Sons, Inc. Companion website: www.wiley.com/go/nursingdiagnoses

Hirshkowitz, M., Whiton, K., Albert, S. M., Alessi, C., Bruni, O., DonCarlos, L., ... Adams Hillard, P. J. (2015). National Sleep Foundation's sleep time duration recommendations: Methodology and results summary. *Sleep Health*, 1(1), 40–43. doi:10.1016/j.sleh.2014.12.010

Jin, Y., & Jones-Smith, J. C. (2015). Associations between family income and children's fitness and obesity in California, 2010-2-12. *Preventing Chronic Disease*, 12(E17). doi:10.5888/pcd12.140392

Kasl, S. V., & Cobb, S. (1966a). Health behavior, illness behavior, and sick-role behavior: I. Health and illness behavior. *Archives of Environmental Health*, 12(2), 246–266.

Kasl, S. V., & Cobb, S. (1966b). Health behavior, illness behavior, and sick-role behavior: I. Sick-role behavior. *Archives of Environmental Health*, 12(4), 531–541.

Kendrick, D., Kumar, A., Carpenter, H., Zijlstra, G. A., Skelton, D. A., Cook, J. R., ... Delbaere, K. (2014). Exercise for reducing fear of falling in older people living in the community. *Cochrane Database of Systematic Reviews*, 11, CD009848. doi:10.1002/14651858.CD009848.pub2

Mayo Clinic. (2013). *Sleep during pregnancy: Follow these tips.* Retrieved from http://www.mayoclinic.org/healthy-lifestyle/pregnancy-week-by-week/in-depth/sleep-during-pregnancy/art-20043827

Mayo Clinic. (2014). *Consumer health: Complementary and alternative medicine.* Retrieved from http://www. mayoclinic.org/healthy-lifestyle/consumer-health/in-depth/alternative-medicine/art-20045267

Mayo Clinic. (2015a). *Chiropractic adjustment.* Retrieved from http://www.mayoclinic.org/tests-procedures/chiropractic-adjustment/basics/what-you-can-expect/prc-20013239

Mayo Clinic. (2015b). *Dry mouth.* Retrieved from http://www.mayoclinic.org/diseases-conditions/dry-mouth/basics/definition/con-20035499

Melville, N. A. (2014). Sleep deprivation mimics psychosis. *Medscape.* Retrieved from http://www.medscape.com/viewarticle/828576

Micozzi, M. S. (2015). *Fundamentals of complementary and alternative medicine* (5th ed.). St. Louis, MO: Saunders.

Miller, N., Reicks, M., Redden, J. P., Mann, T., Mykerezi, E., & Vickers, Z. (2015). *Appetite, 91,* 426–430. doi:10.1016/j.appet.2015.04.081

NANDA-I. (2016). Glossary of terms. Retrieved from http://www.nanda.org/nanda-international-glossary-of-terms.html

National Center for Complementary and Integrative Health (NCCIH). (2012). *Chiropractic: An introduction.* Retrieved from https://nccih.nih.gov/health/chiropractic/introduction.htm

National Center for Complementary and Integrative Health (NCCIH). (2015a). *Ayurvedic medicine: An introduction.* Retrieved from https://nccih.nih.gov/health/ayurveda/introduction.htm

National Center for Complementary and Integrative Health (NCCIH). (2015b). *Complementary, alternative, or integrative health: What's in a name?* Retrieved from https://nccih.nih.gov/health/integrative-health

National Highway Traffic Safety Administration. (2016). *Research on drowsy driving.* Retrieved from http://www.nhtsa.gov/Driving+Safety/Drowsy+Driving

National Institute of Dental and Craniofacial Research. (2014). *Executive summary.* Retrieved from http://www.nidcr.nih.gov/DataStatistics/SurgeonGeneral/sgr/execsum.htm

National Institutes of Health (NIH), National Institute of Diabetes and Digestive Health and Kidney Diseases. (2013). *Diabetes Prevention Program (DPP).* Retrieved from http://www.niddk.nih.gov/about-niddk/research-areas/diabetes/diabetes-prevention-program-dpp/Pages/default.aspx

National Institute of Neurological Disorders and Stroke (NINDS). (2014). *Brain basics: Understanding sleep.* Retrieved from http://www.ninds.nih.gov/disorders/brain_basics/understanding_sleep.htm

National Resource Center for Health and Safety in Child Care and Early Education. (2015). *Caring for our children.* Retrieved from http://www.cfoc.nrckids.org/StandardView/3.1.3.1

National Sleep Foundation. (2014). *What is insomnia?* Retrieved from https://sleepfoundation.org/insomnia/content/what-is-insomnia

National Sleep Foundation. (2015a). *Aging and sleep.* Retrieved from http://www.sleepfoundation.org/sleep-topics/aging-and-sleep

National Sleep Foundation. (2015b). *Children and sleep.* Retrieved from http://www.sleepfoundation.org/article/sleep-topics/children-and-sleep

National Sleep Foundation. (2015c). *School start time and sleep.* Retrieved from http://www.sleepfoundation.org/sleep-news/school-start-time-and-sleep

National Sleep Foundation. (2015d). *Teens and sleep.* Retrieved from http://www.sleepfoundation.org/sleep-topics/teens-and-sleep

National Sleep Foundation. (2015e). *Women and sleep.* Retrieved from http://www.sleepfoundation.org/sleep-topics/women-and-sleep

Nightingale, F. (1969). *Notes on nursing: What it is, and what it is not.* New York, NY: Dover Books. (Originally published in 1859.)

Pender, N. J., Murdaugh, C. L., & Parsons, M. A. (2015). *Health promotion in nursing practice* (7th ed.). Upper Saddle River, NJ: Prentice Hall.

Periodontitis. (2013). *The New York Times.* Retrieved from http://www.nytimes.com/health/guides/disease/periodontitis/prevention.html#

Prochaska, J. O., Norcross, J., & DiClemente, C. (2007). *Changing for good: A revolutionary six-stage program for overcoming bad habits and moving your life positively forward.* New York, NY: William Morrow.

Rangaraj, V. R., & Knutson, K. L. (2015). Association between sleep deficiency and cardiometabolic disease: implications for health disparities. *Sleep Medicine*, ii, S1389-9457(15)00648-6. doi:10.1016/j.sleep.2015.02.535

Salas, R. E., Gamaldo, A., Collop, N. A., Gulyani, S., Hsu, M., David, P. M., ... Gamaldo, C. E. (2013). A step out of the dark: Improving the sleep medicine knowledge of trainees. *Sleep Medicine*, 14(1), 105–108. doi:10.1016/j.sleep.2012.09.013

Smith, D. C., Schreiber, K. M., Saltos, A., Lichenstein, S. B. & Lichenstein, R. (2013). Ambulatory cell phone injuries in the United States: An emerging national concern. *Journal of Safety Research*, 47, 19–23. doi:10.1016/j.jsr.2013.08.003

Spector, R. E. (2017). *Cultural diversity in health and illness* (9th ed.). Hoboken, NJ: Pearson Education.

Stewart, T. L., Chipperfield, J. G., Perry, R. P., & Weiner, B. (2012). Attributing illness to "old age": Consequences of a self-directed stereotype for health and mortality. *Psychology and Health*, 27(8), 881–897.

University of Utah. (2015). *Time of our lives.* Retrieved from http://learn.genetics.utah.edu/content/inheritance/clockgenes/

U.S. Department of Health and Human Services (DHHS), Office of Disease Prevention and Health Promotion. (2015). *Healthy people 2020: Improving the health of Americans.* Washington, DC: U.S. Government Printing Office. Retrieved from http://www.healthypeople.gov

U.S. Department of Health & Human Services. 2020 Topics and Objectives—Objectives A–Z. van de Weert-van Leeuwen, P. B., Arets, H. G., van der Ent, C. K., & Beekman, J. M. (2013). Infection, inflammation and exercise in cystic fibrosis. *Respiratory Research*, 14, 32. doi:10.1186/1465-9921-14-32

WebMD. (2016). *Dental health and fluoride treatment.* Retrieved from http://www.webmd.com/oral-health/guide/fluoride-treatment

Whitford, G. M. (2011). Acute toxicity of ingested fluoride. *Monographs of Oral Science*, 22, 22–66. doi:10.1159/000325146

World Health Organization. (1948, June 19–22). *Preamble to the constitution of the World Health Organization as adopted by the International Health Conference.* New York, NY.

Young, J., Angevaren, M., Rusted, J., & Tabet, N. (2015). Aerobic exercise to improve cognitive function in older people without known cognitive impairment. *Cochrane Database of Systematic Reviews*, 4, CD005381. doi:10.1002/14651858.CD005381.pub4

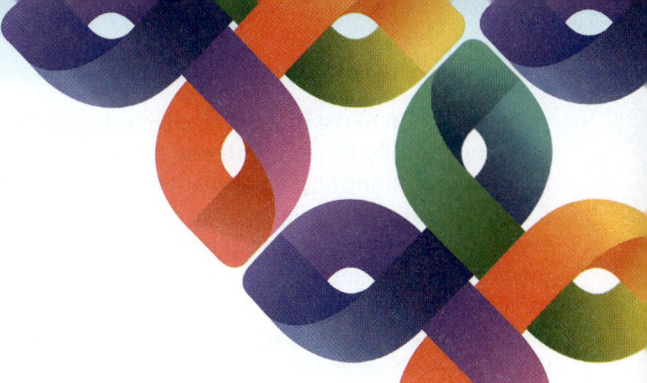

Module 8
Immunity

Module Outline and Learning Outcomes

The Concept of Immunity

Normal Presentation
8.1 Analyze the physiology of immunity in the body.

Alterations to Immunity
8.2 Differentiate alterations in immunity.

Concepts Related to Immunity
8.3 Outline the relationship between immunity and other concepts.

Health Promotion
8.4 Explain the promotion of healthy immune function.

Nursing Assessment
8.5 Differentiate common assessment procedures and tests used to examine immune function.

Independent Interventions
8.6 Analyze independent interventions nurses can implement for patients with alterations in immunity.

Collaborative Therapies
8.7 Summarize collaborative therapies used by interprofessional teams for patients with alterations in immunity.

Lifespan Considerations
8.8 Differentiate considerations related to the assessment and care of patients with alterations in immunity throughout the lifespan.

Immunity Exemplars

Exemplar 8.A HIV/AIDS
8.A Analyze HIV/AIDS as they relate to immunity.

Exemplar 8.B Hypersensitivity
8.B Analyze hypersensitivity as it relates to immunity.

Exemplar 8.C Rheumatoid Arthritis
8.C Analyze rheumatoid arthritis (RA) as it relates to immunity.

Exemplar 8.D Systemic Lupus Erythematosus
8.D Analyze systemic lupus erythematosus (SLE) as it relates to immunity.

>> The Concept of Immunity

Concept Key Terms

The human body is continually threatened by foreign substances, infectious agents, and abnormal cells. Recent years have seen the emergence of resistant microorganisms, such as methicillin-resistant *Staphylococcus aureus* (MRSA), and altered strains of familiar diseases, such as multidrug-resistant tuberculosis. Chronic diseases such as Lyme disease and human immunodeficiency virus (HIV) result in extensive human and financial costs. The body's major weapon against these threats is the immune system.

The function of the immune system is to protect the body from invasion by foreign **antigens** (foreign substances that trigger the immune response), to identify and destroy potentially harmful cells, and to remove cellular debris. Lymphoid organs and specifically designed lymphocytes accomplish these actions through the processes of antibody-mediated immune response and cell-mediated immune response. The immune system recognizes any foreign substances within the body—in simple terms, it distinguishes "nonself" from "self"—and attempts to eliminate foreign substances as efficiently as possible.

Immunity is the body's natural or induced response to infection and its associated conditions. Patients who are **immunocompetent** have immune systems that identify antigens and effectively destroy or remove them. When the immune system functions ineffectively, the result may be an overreaction or an immunodeficiency. Overreaction of the immune system to an antigen or antigens is termed **hypersensitivity**. In **autoimmune disorders**, for example, the immune system loses the ability to recognize its own tissues and begins to attack them. An **immunodeficiency** can develop when the immune system is incompetent or unable to respond effectively. **Acquired immunodeficiency syndrome (AIDS)** is an immune system deficit that is induced by infection with HIV and is characterized by **opportunistic infections** (infections that would normally not affect people with intact immune systems).

Scientific understanding of the components of the immune system and specific immune responses is growing. Having a thorough knowledge of the immune system increases understanding of the local and systemic inflammatory response, resistance to infectious disease, and the importance of immunization. This foundation helps nurses teach patients and families to follow recommended treatment regimens, to promote and maintain health, and to prevent disease. In addition, nurses can prescribe appropriate rehabilitative measures, such as increased rest and attention to optimal nutrition. Therefore, nurses must understand the foundations of the immune system and the immune response.

Normal Presentation

The immune system is a complex and intricate network of specialized cells, tissues, and organs. Cells of the immune system seek out and destroy damaged cells and foreign tissue, yet recognize and preserve host cells (Porth & Grossman, 2013). The immune system performs the following functions:

- Defends and protects the body from **infection** (an invasion of the body tissue by microorganisms)
- Removes and destroys damaged or dead cells
- Identifies and destroys malignant cells, thereby preventing their further development into tumors.

The immune system is activated by external agents. External agents include microorganisms; minor injuries, such as small lacerations or bruises; and major injuries, such as burns, surgeries, and systemic diseases (e.g., pneumonia). The response of the immune system may be nonspecific or specific. Nonspecific responses prevent or limit the entry of invaders into the body, thereby limiting the extent of tissue damage and reducing the workload of the immune system. Inflammation is a nonspecific response.

When the inflammatory process is unable to destroy invading organisms or toxins, the body's more specific *immune response* is activated.

There are two types of immunity: active and passive. **Active immunity** can occur through exposure to disease or through vaccination. In the case of exposure to a disease (e.g., varicella), the causative organism triggers the production of antibodies by the immune system to that disease (natural immunity). Vaccination (e.g., the measles-mumps-rubella [MMR] vaccine) involves introducing a weakened or killed form of the disease into the body (vaccine-induced immunity). Despite the way active immunity is acquired, the results are long lasting and often lifelong but usually take several weeks to develop.

Passive immunity occurs when individuals receive antibodies from another person rather than by producing them through their own immune system. This type of immunity can be acquired through the passing of antibodies between mother and newborn via the placenta and/or breast milk (the only physiologic example) or through the administration of blood products that contain an antibody such as immune globulin to protect against a specific disease. Passive immunity has a major advantage over active immunity in that protection is immediate; however, it only lasts for a few weeks or months (Abbas, Lichtman, & Pillai, 2014; Centers for Disease Control and Prevention [CDC], 2014).

Physiology Review

The immune system consists of molecules, cells, and organs that produce the immune response (see **Table 8–1 »**). These components may be involved in the nonspecific inflammatory response, the specific immunologic response, or both.

Leukocytes

Leukocytes, or white blood cells (WBCs), are the primary cells involved in both nonspecific and specific immune system responses. Like all blood cells, leukocytes derive from stem cells (hemocytoblasts) in the bone marrow (see **Figure 8–1 »**). Unlike red blood cells (RBCs), which are confined to the circulatory system, leukocytes can transport themselves to the site of an inflammatory or immune response. As the mobile units of the immune system, leukocytes detect, attack, and destroy anything that is recognized as "foreign." They are able to move through tissue spaces, where they locate damaged tissue and infection by responding to chemicals released by other leukocytes and damaged tissue.

The normal number of circulating leukocytes is 4500–10,000 cells per cubic millimeter (mm^3) of blood. Many more leukocytes are marginated; that is, they adhere to vascular epithelial cells along the vessel walls, in other tissue spaces, or in the lymph system. In the presence of an attack such as an infection, the bone marrow releases additional WBCs. As these WBCs move out of the bone marrow into the blood, the bone marrow increases its production of additional leukocytes. This process leads to a WBC count of greater than $10,000/mm^3$, a condition known as **leukocytosis**. A decrease in the number of circulating leukocytes, known as **leukopenia**, occurs when bone marrow activity is suppressed or when leukocyte destruction increases.

Leukocytes are divided into three major groups: granulocytes, monocytes, and lymphocytes. The granulocytes and monocytes derive from the myeloid stem cells of the bone

TABLE 8–1 Cells and Tissues of the Immune System

Component	Location	Function
Leukocytes		
Granulocytes		
Neutrophils	Circulatory system	Phagocytosis and chemotaxis
Eosinophils	Circulatory system, respiratory tract, and gastrointestinal (GI) tract	Phagocytosis Protection against parasites Involvement in allergic response
Basophils	Circulatory system	Release of chemotactic substances
Monocytes and Macrophages	Circulatory system (monocytes) and body tissue, such as skin (histiocytes), liver (Kupffer cells), alveoli, spleen, tonsils, lymph nodes, bone marrow, and brain	Trapping and phagocytosis of foreign substances and cellular debris Secretion of interleukin-1 to stimulate lymphocyte growth
Lymphocytes		
T cells (mature in thymus gland)	Circulatory system, lymph system, and tissues	Activation of T and B cells Control of viral infections and destruction of cancer cells Involvement in hypersensitivity reactions and graft tissue rejection
B cells (mature in bone marrow)	Circulatory system and spleen	Production of antibodies (immunoglobulins) to specific antigens
Natural Killer (NK) Cells	Circulatory system	Cytotoxicity (killing of tumor cells, fungi, viral-infected cells, and foreign tissue)
Lymphoid Tissues		
Primary or central lymphoid structures	Bone marrow and thymus gland	Production of immune cells; sites for cell maturation
Secondary or peripheral lymphoid structures	Lymph nodes, spleen, tonsils, intestinal lymphoid tissue, and lymphoid tissue in other organs	Sites for activation of immune cells by antigens

marrow and are instrumental in the inflammatory response. Lymphocytes derive from the lymphoid stem cells of the bone marrow and are the primary cells involved in the specific immune response. In laboratory tests, the WBC count indicates the total number of circulating leukocytes. The WBC differential identifies the portion of the total represented by each type of leukocyte.

Granulocytes

Granulocytes constitute 60–80% of the total number of normal blood leukocytes. Their cytoplasm has a granular appearance, and their nuclei are distinctively multilobular (see Figure 8–1). Granulocytes have a short lifespan, measured in hours to days, compared with the lifespan of monocytes, which is measured in months to years. Granulocytes play a key role in protecting the body from harmful microorganisms during acute inflammation and infection. There are three types of granulocytes: neutrophils, eosinophils, and basophils.

- **Neutrophils,** also called *polymorphonuclear leukocytes* (or *polys*), are the most plentiful of the granulocytes, constituting 55–70% of the total number of circulating leukocytes. Neutrophils are phagocytic cells, responsible for engulfing and destroying foreign agents, particularly bacteria and small particles. Drawn by chemicals released by damaged tissue and invading organisms, neutrophils are the first phagocytic cells to arrive at the site of invasion. Neutrophils are produced in the bone marrow and released into the circulation when they mature. Segmented neutrophils (or segs) are mature forms and usually account for approximately 55% of total leukocytes. Bands are immature neutrophils and usually comprise 5% of leukocytes. As neutrophils mature, their nucleus

changes from round to kidney-bean–shaped (banded), and then the nucleus separates into small, attached segments—thus the designations *banded* versus *segmented* neutrophils. A neutrophil takes approximately 10 days to mature and be released into the circulation. Once released, neutrophils have a circulating half-life of 6–10 hours. They cannot replicate and must be replaced constantly to maintain adequate numbers in the circulation. They do not return to the bone marrow.

- **Eosinophils** account for 1–4% of the total number of circulating leukocytes. They mature within the bone marrow in 3–6 days before being released into the circulation. Eosinophils have a circulating half-life of 30 minutes and a tissue half-life of 12 days. They, too, are phagocytic cells, but they are less efficient at this process than neutrophils. Eosinophils are found in large numbers in the respiratory and GI tracts, where they are thought to be responsible for protecting the body from parasitic worms, including tapeworms, flukes, pinworms, and hookworms. Eosinophils surround the parasite and release toxic enzymes from their cytoplasmic granules. The parasite, although too large to be phagocytized, is destroyed. Eosinophils also are involved in a hypersensitivity response, inactivating some of the inflammatory chemicals released during the inflammatory response.

- **Basophils** constitute approximately 0.5–1% of the circulating leukocytes. These cells are not phagocytic. Granules within basophils contain proteins and chemicals, such as heparin, histamine, bradykinin, serotonin, and a slow-reacting substance of anaphylaxis (leukotrienes). These substances are released into the bloodstream during an acute hypersensitivity reaction or stress response.

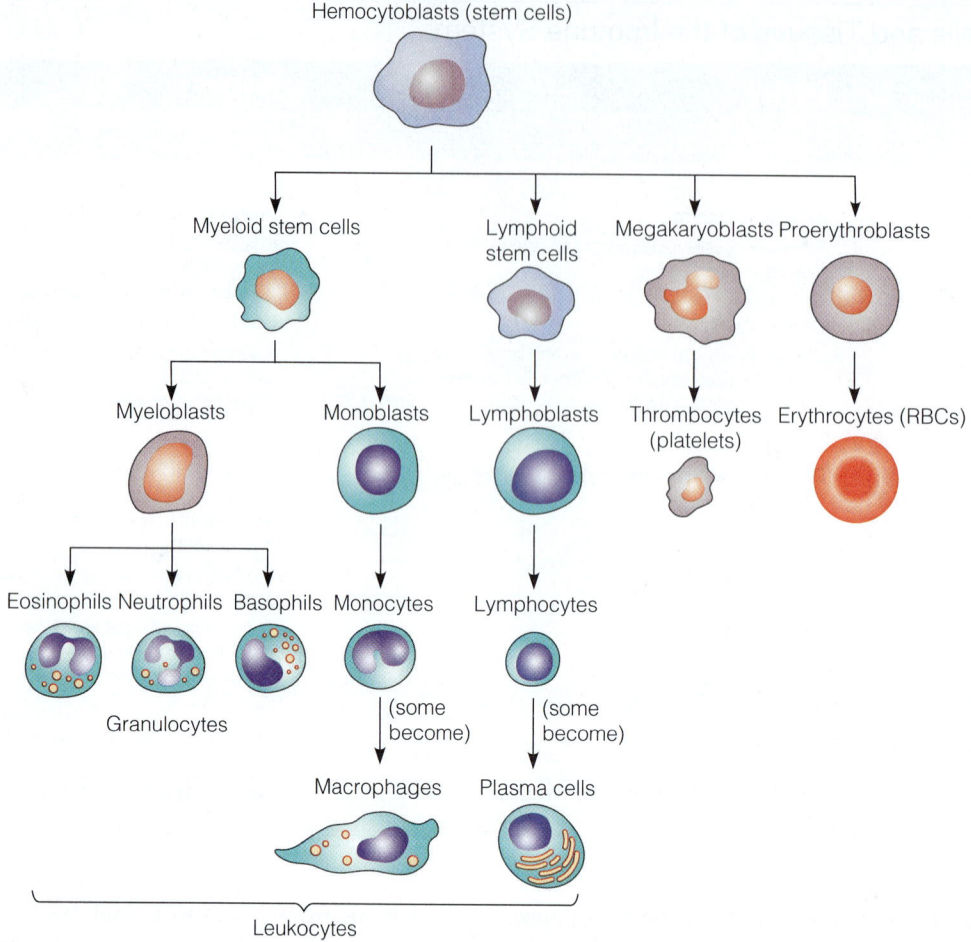

Figure 8–1 ❯❯ The development and differentiation of leukocytes from hemocytoblasts.

Monocytes, macrophages, and dendritic cells are the mediators of immunity. They recognize foreign matter (from molecules to cells), initiate immune responses, and are actively phagocytic, with the capacity to phagocytize large foreign particles and cellular debris.

Monocytes

Monocytes are the largest of the leukocytes and constitute 2–3% of circulating leukocytes. After their release from the bone marrow, monocytes are in circulation for 1–2 days. They then migrate to various tissues throughout the body, attach themselves to the tissues, and remain for months or even years until they are activated. Monocytes activate the immune response against chronic infections such as tuberculosis, viral infections, and certain intracellular parasitic infections.

■ After settling into the tissues, monocytes mature into **macrophages**, which are differentiated by the tissues in which they reside. Histiocytes are tissue macrophages in loose connective tissue, Kupffer cells are found in the liver, alveolar macrophages are found in the lungs, and microglia are found in the brain. Tissue macrophages also can be found in the spleen, tonsils, lymph nodes, and bone marrow. Once they are in the tissue, macrophages can multiply to encapsulate and trap foreign matter that cannot be phagocytized. Like neutrophils, macrophages

are drawn to an inflamed area by chemicals released from damaged tissue, a process known as *chemotaxis*. Like monocytes, macrophages activate the immune response against chronic infections, such as tuberculosis, viral infections, and certain intracellular parasitic infections.

■ ***Dendritic cells*** are star-shaped cells that originate in both the myeloid and the lymphoid cell lines. These antigen-presenting cells (APCs) have long processes that can capture antigens and migrate to lymphoid tissue. They serve as sentinels for antigens in most organs, including the heart, lungs, liver, kidney, and GI tract (Rockefeller University, 2013). Langerhans cells are specialized dendritic cells (DCs) in the skin. These cells originate from stem cells in the bone marrow and migrate into the epithelium, where they perform the function of antigen recognition. Studies have shown that these dendritic cells, though similar in origin, will differentiate in response to their environmental stimuli to perform even more distinct functions (Jaitley & Saraswathi, 2012). Additional research has provided insight into the relationship between dendritic cells and autoimmune diseases such as systemic lupus erythematosus (SLE), rheumatoid arthritis (RA), and multiple sclerosis. These diseases can develop when the normal function of the DCs is suppressed and they become too tolerant. This tolerance can also create an environment for chronic infections such as HIV to develop (Rockefeller University, 2016).

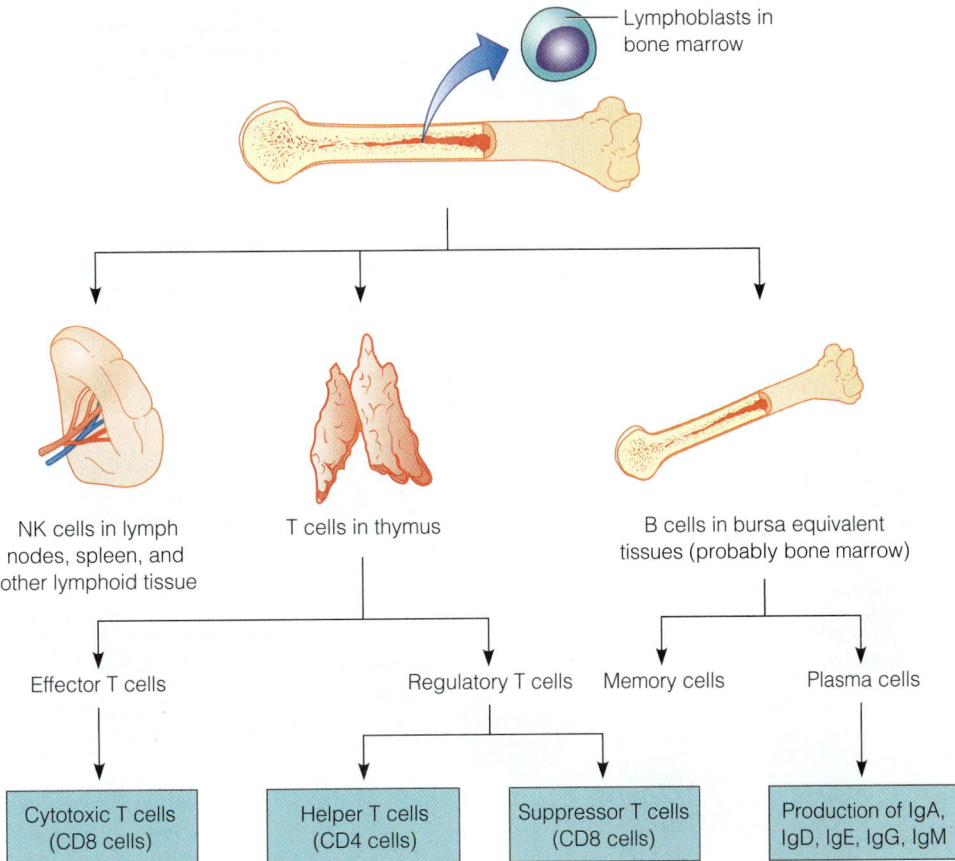

Lymphoblasts in bone marrow

NK cells in lymph nodes, spleen, and other lymphoid tissue

T cells in thymus

B cells in bursa equivalent tissues (probably bone marrow)

Effector T cells

Regulatory T cells

Memory cells

Plasma cells

| Cytotoxic T cells (CD8 cells) | Helper T cells (CD4 cells) | Suppressor T cells (CD8 cells) | Production of IgA, IgD, IgE, IgG, IgM |

Figure 8–2 ›› The development and differentiation of lymphocytes from lymphoid stem cells (lymphoblasts).

Lymphocytes

Like other leukocytes, **lymphocytes** derive from the stem cells in the bone marrow (see **Figure 8–2** ››). Small and nondescript, these cells account for 20–40% of circulating leukocytes and are the principal effector and regulator cells of specific immune responses to protect the body from microorganisms, foreign tissue, and cell mutations or alterations. Through a process known as *immune surveillance,* lymphocytes monitor the body for cancerous cells and attempt to destroy them.

Lymphocytes constantly circulate, then return in a "homing" pattern to concentrate in lymphoid tissues, where they often mature into memory cells. Memory cells stay inactive, sometimes for years, but activate immediately with subsequent exposure to the same antigen. They then proliferate rapidly, producing an intense immune response. Memory cells are responsible for providing **acquired immunity** (resistance to an antigen resulting from previous exposure to that antigen).

Although difficult to distinguish by appearance, lymphocyte types have distinct differences in how and where they mature as well as in life cycle, surface characteristics, and function. The three types of lymphocytes are **T lymphocytes (T cells)**, **B lymphocytes (B cells)**, and **natural killer cells (NK cells** or **null cells)**. None of these cells act independently; their functions are closely interrelated.

- **T cells** mature in the thymus gland and are integral to the specific immune response. On contact with APCs,

T lymphocytes mature into active helper T cells, cytotoxic T cells, or memory T cells.

- **B cells** complete their maturation in the bone marrow and, like T cells, are integral to the specific immune response. On contact with an antigen, B lymphocytes are activated and mature into either plasma cells, which secrete antibodies, or memory cells.

- **Natural killer (NK) cells** are large, granular cells found in the spleen, lymph nodes, bone marrow, and blood. They constitute 15% of circulating lymphocytes. NK cells provide immune surveillance and resistance to infection, and they play an important role in the destruction of early malignant cells. Like B cells and T cells, NK cells are cytotoxic, but unlike T cells, they do not require connection with an APC to become activated and kill cancer cells, virus-infected cells, or cells infected with microbes (Porth & Grossman, 2013). Fortunately, NK cells are inhibited when contact is made with normal host cells.

Antigens

Antigens provoke a specific immune response when introduced into the body. They are typically large protein molecules, although polysaccharides, polypeptides, and nucleic acids also may be antigenic. Many antigens are proteins found on the cell membrane or cell wall of microorganisms or tissues (e.g., transplanted tissue or organs), incompatible blood cells, vaccines, pollen, egg white, animal dander, and insect or snake venom.

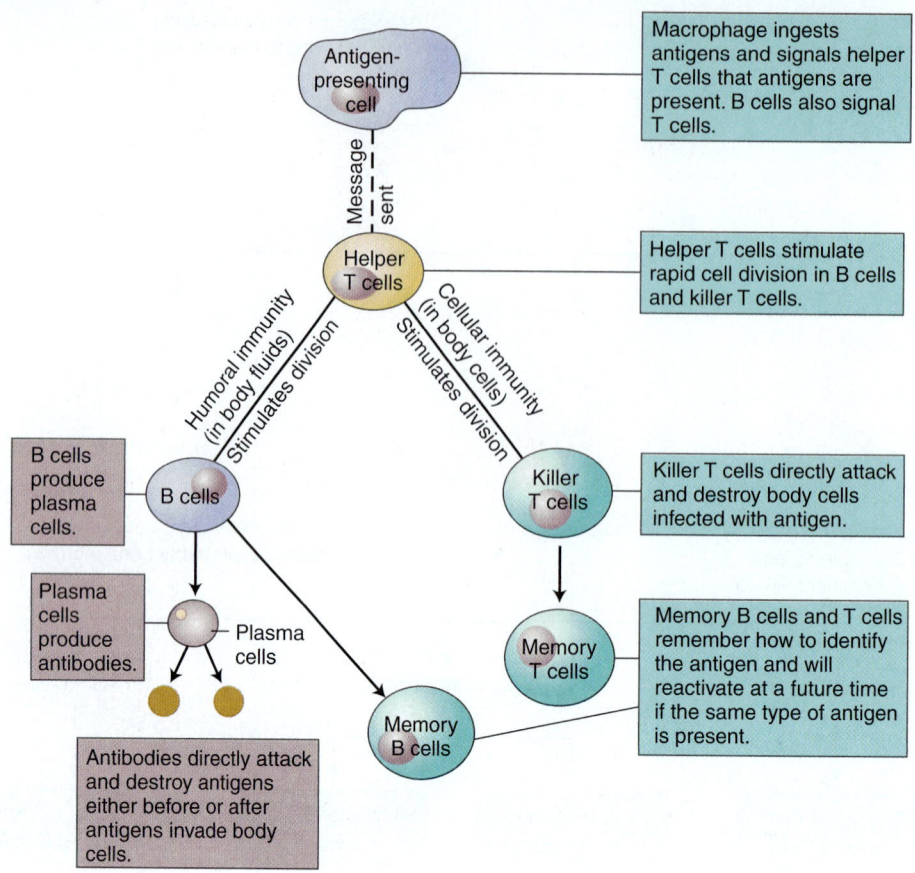

Macrophage ingests antigens and signals helper T cells that antigens are present. B cells also signal T cells.

Antigen-presenting cell

Message sent

Helper T cells

Helper T cells stimulate rapid cell division in B cells and killer T cells.

Humoral immunity (in body fluids)
Stimulates division

Cellular immunity (in body cells)
Stimulates division

B cells produce plasma cells.

B cells

Killer T cells

Killer T cells directly attack and destroy body cells infected with antigen.

Plasma cells produce antibodies.

Plasma cells

Memory T cells

Memory B cells and T cells remember how to identify the antigen and will reactivate at a future time if the same type of antigen is present.

Memory B cells

Antibodies directly attack and destroy antigens either before or after antigens invade body cells.

Figure 8–3 ❯❯ The primary immune response encompasses a cascade of events that involve humoral immunity and cellular immunity.

The portion of an antigen that incites a specific immune response is called its *antigenic determinant site* (or *epitope*). Complete antigens (also known as *immunogens*) typically are large molecules with multiple antigenic determinant sites; examples are proteins and certain polysaccharides. Complete antigens have two characteristics:

1. *Immunogenicity,* or the ability to stimulate a specific immune response
2. *Specific reactivity,* or the ability to stimulate specific immune system components.

Small molecules that cannot evoke an antigenic response alone (e.g., chemical toxins, drugs, dust) may link to proteins to function as complete antigens. The proteins to which they link are known as haptens.

When they encounter an antigen in the body, two major groups of cells—lymphocytes and APCs—generate an effective immune response. A specific receptor on the lymphocytes recognizes the APCs, and those lymphocytes generate an immune response. Depending on the antigen itself and the type of immune cell activated by contact with the antigen, two separate but overlapping immune responses may occur. The B cell, or humoral branch of the immune system, mainly eliminates extracellular antigens, such as bacteria, bacterial toxins, and free viruses, through the production of **antibodies** (molecules that bind with the antigen and inactivate it). Antibodies are found in serum, body fluids, and certain tissues. When an individual is first

exposed to an antigen, the B lymphocyte system begins to produce antibodies that react specifically to that antigen (see **Figure 8–3 ❯❯**). It takes approximately 3 days for this process, known as the **primary immune response**, to occur. Subsequent encounters with the antigen trigger memory cells, and the result is a **secondary immune response** within 24 hours.

There are five classes of antibodies, called **immunoglobulins**: IgM, IgG, IgA, IgD, and IgE. Together, these proteins make up the **antibody-mediated (humoral) immune response**. The functions of the five major types of immunoglobulins are as follows:

- *IgM* antibodies are produced 48–72 hours after an antigen enters the body and are responsible for primary immunity. IgM produces antibody activity against rheumatoid factors, gram-negative organisms, and the ABO blood group. IgM activates the complement system by destroying antigenic substances. Because it does not pass the placental barrier, the serum value of IgM is low in newborns; however, it is produced early in life and the level increases after 9 months of age.
- *IgG* is the major immunoglobulin. IgG results from secondary exposure to the foreign antigen and is responsible for antiviral and antibacterial activity. This antibody passes through the placental barrier and provides early immunity for the newborn. The IgG response is longer and stronger than that of the other immunoglobulins.

- *IgA* is found in the secretions of the respiratory, GI, and genitourinary tracts; tears; and saliva. Its purpose is to protect mucous membranes from invading organisms (viruses, certain bacteria—*Escherichia coli* and *Clostridium tetani*). IgA does not pass the placental barrier. Those having congenital IgA deficiency are prone to autoimmune disease.

- The role of *IgD* is unknown.

- *IgE* increases during allergic reactions and anaphylaxis. It is important in defense against parasitic disease (Stokes & Casale, 2016).

Intracellular pathogens, such as virus-infected cells, cancer cells, and foreign tissue, activate T lymphocytes, which are the primary agents of the **cell-mediated (cellular) immune response**. In this immune response, the lymphocytes themselves, in the form of helper T cells, cytotoxic T cells, and NK cells, inactivate the antigen, either directly or indirectly.

Cell-mediated immunity acts at the cellular level by attacking antigens directly and by activating B cells. T lymphocytes comprise the cell-mediated immune response and are subdivided into effector cells and regulatory cells. The cytotoxic cell or killer T cell is the primary effector cell. Regulatory T cells are divided into two subsets, known as *helper T cells* and *suppressor T cells*.

Helper T cells initiate the immune response, whereas suppressor T cells limit it. Helper T cells accomplish their role by promoting growth of additional T cells, by stimulating proliferation of B cells, and by activating killer T cells. Suppressor T cells are believed to be important in preventing autoimmune disorders. Proper immune system function depends on the correct balance between helper and suppressor T cells.

Complement is a component of blood serum consisting of 11 protein compounds. It is an inactive enzyme that activates in response to antigen–antibody functions, causing a generalized inflammatory reaction that kills foreign cells. It also plays a role in causing some autoimmune disorders.

Immune cells also secrete proteins, called **cytokines**, that carry messages for immune system function. Lymphocytes, monocytes, and macrophages all secrete cytokines that have a variety of effects on the target cells. These effects may include stimulation of growth through cell proliferation, differentiation of cellular actions, production of inflammation, sensitization to pain, and other actions. Interleukins, a type of cytokine, were identified first in WBCs but are present in many cells. Many types of interleukins have been identified, and some are known to influence the function of the immune system.

In addition to destroying viruses and bacteria, cytotoxic T lymphocytes also attack malignant cells and are responsible for the rejection of transplanted organs and grafted tissues.

Lymphoid System

The lymphoid system consists of the lymph nodes, spleen, thymus, tonsils, lymphoid tissue scattered in connective tissues and mucosa, and bone marrow. The thymus and bone marrow, in which T cells and B cells mature, are considered central lymphoid organs. The spleen, lymph nodes, tonsils, and other peripheral lymphoid tissue are considered peripheral lymphoid organs (see **Figure 8–4** »).

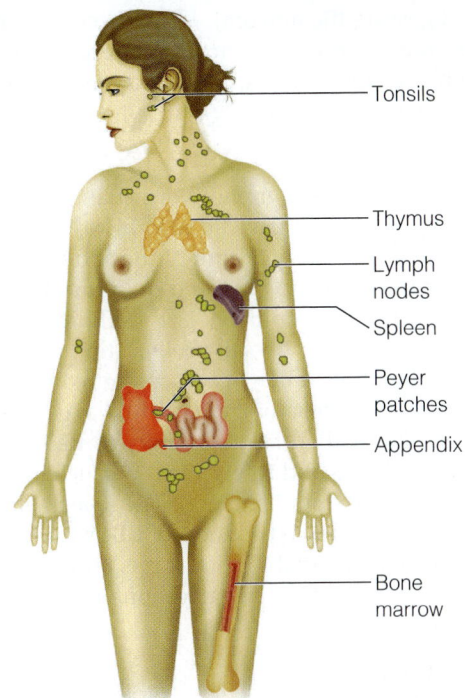

Figure 8–4 » The lymphoid system, showing the central organs of the thymus and bone marrow and the peripheral organs, including the spleen, tonsils, lymph nodes, and Peyer patches.

Tonsils

Thymus

Lymph nodes

Spleen

Peyer patches

Appendix

Bone marrow

This system exists to recover proteins for the vascular system and to protect the bloodstream from invading organisms. Cells of the immune system, such as neutrophils, macrophages, and dendritic cells, carry antigens from the interstitial space to the lymph nodes for immune surveillance in the lymphatic circulation. Unlike the vascular tree, which has tight epithelial junctions, lymphatic epithelium is replete with open junctions that promote lymphocyte access and effectively protect the bloodstream from antigen entry.

Lymph Nodes

The most numerous elements of the lymphoid system, lymph nodes are small, round, or bean-shaped bodies that are encapsulated and vary in size from 1 mm to 2 cm. Distributed throughout the body, lymph nodes generally occur in groups at the junction of the lymphatic vessels. They can be found in the neck, axillae, abdomen, and groin and have two specific functions:

1. To filter foreign products or antigens from the lymph
2. To house and support proliferation of lymphocytes and macrophages.

Lymph, a clear, protein-containing fluid transported within lymph vessels, enters the node through afferent lymphatic vessels. Inside the node, the lymph flows through sinuses in the cortex of the lymph node (where T lymphocytes, B lymphocytes, and macrophages are abundant) and then through sinuses of the medulla of the lymph node, which contains macrophages and plasma cells. The presence of a foreign antigen stimulates lymphocytes and macrophages to proliferate in the lymph nodes. Macrophages destroy the antigen by **phagocytosis** (engulfing and then digesting the antigen). Immune cells and lymph then leave the lymph node through efferent vessels. An abundant blood supply to the node also facilitates lymphocyte movement.

Spleen

The spleen is the largest lymphoid organ in the body—and the only lymphoid organ that can filter blood. The spleen is located in the upper left quadrant of the abdomen and has two kinds of tissue: white pulp and red pulp. White pulp, in which B cells predominate, is lymphoid tissue that serves as a site for lymphocyte proliferation and immune surveillance. Blood filtration occurs in the red pulp, where phagocytic cells dispose of damaged or aged RBCs and platelets in blood-filled venous sinuses. Red pulp also removes other debris and foreign matter, such as bacteria, viruses, and toxins, from the blood. The spleen also stores blood and the breakdown products of RBCs for future use. The spleen is not essential for life; if it is removed because of disease or trauma, the liver and bone marrow assume its functions.

Thymus Gland

The thymus gland is located in the superior anterior mediastinal cavity beneath the sternum. During fetal life and childhood, the thymus serves as a site for the maturation and differentiation of thymic lymphoid cells, the T cells. After puberty, the thymus gland begins to atrophy slowly. Thymosin, an immunoregulatory hormone of the thymus, stimulates lymphopoiesis, the formation of lymphocytes or lymphoid tissue.

Bone Marrow

Bone marrow is soft organic tissue found in the hollow cavity of the long bones, particularly the femur and humerus, as well as in the flat bones of the pelvis, ribs, and sternum. Bone marrow produces and stores hematopoietic stem cells, from which all cellular components of the blood are derived (see Figure 8–2).

Lymphoid Tissues

Lymphoid tissues are located at key sites of potential invasion by microorganisms: the submucosa of the genitourinary, respiratory, and GI tracts and the skin. Plasma cells in these lymphoid tissues defend the body against bacterial invasion at areas exposed to the external environment. In general, these tissues are known as mucosa-associated lymphoid tissue (MALT) and include bronchial/tracheal-associated lymphoid tissue (BALT), nose-associated lymphoid tissue (NALT), vulvovaginal-associated lymphoid tissue (VALT) and gut-associated lymphoid tissue (GALT) (Grethlein, 2014).

Ingestion and absorption of solid foodstuffs and liquids continually expose the lining of the gut to resident microflora and infectious pathogens. Unlike peripheral lymph nodes, which respond to pathogens with acute inflammatory responses, GALT processes common intestinal antigens without producing acute inflammation. GALT is comprised of collections of immune cells known as Peyer patches, making it the largest accumulation of immune cells in the body. Beneath the basement membrane of gut epithelium lie an abundance of T cells and mature plasma cells, which are sources of IgA. As naive B cells and T cells migrate through Peyer patches, which hold dense collections of lymphocytes, the cells are sensitized to specific antigens. In mesenteric lymph nodes, these sensitized cells multiply and circulate throughout the vascular tree, where they produce secretory IgA. Secretory IgA coats mucosal cells and prevents attachment of intraluminal bacteria in the intestine, upper respiratory tract, bronchi, mammary ducts, and salivary glands. Thus, the collection of immune cells in GALT effectively protects mucosa throughout the body as the mucosa are exposed to resident and foreign pathogens.

Tonsils and Adenoids

Tonsils and adenoids protect the body from inhaled or ingested foreign agents. These skin-associated lymphoid tissues contain lymphocytes and dendritic cells, such as Langerhans cells, in the epidermis, which transport antigens to regional lymph nodes for destruction and development of specific immunity to the antigen.

Nonspecific Inflammatory Response

Barrier protection is the body's first line of defense against infection. The skin is the primary barrier; when intact, it prevents invasion by external organisms. The membranes lining the inner surfaces of the body are protected by a barrier of mucus, which traps microorganisms and other foreign substances. These can then be removed by other protective mechanisms, such as ciliary movement or the washing action of tears or urine. In addition, many body fluids contain bactericidal substances that provide barrier protection. These include acid in gastric fluid; zinc in prostatic fluid; and lysozyme in tears, nasal secretions, saliva, and sweat (Haase & Rink, 2013; Porth & Grossman, 2013).

When these first-line defenses are breached, the resulting tissue damage or foreign material entering the body induces a nonspecific immune response known as **inflammation**, an adaptive response to what the body sees as harmful. Inflammation brings fluid, dissolved substances, and blood cells into the interstitial tissues where the invasion or damage has occurred. (The inflammatory response is described in more detail in the module on Inflammation.) The inflammatory response is called a nonspecific response because the same events occur regardless of what causes the inflammatory process. The inflammatory reaction neutralizes and eliminates the invader, removes destroyed tissue, and initiates the process of healing and repair.

Genetic and Lifespan Considerations

Immune function changes across the lifespan. The developing immune function of infants and children makes them susceptible to infection until their systems reach maturity in late childhood. On the contrary, the declining immune function of older adults makes them more prone to infection as well. These developmental processes occur naturally but may be helped or hindered by a number of influencing factors. Genetics ranks among these factors, though its role is difficult to pinpoint outside of infancy. The role of the immune system across the lifespan is covered in the Lifespan Considerations sections.

TABLE 8–2 Selected Autoimmune Disorders

Organ Specificity	Disorder	Description
More organ-specific	Hashimoto thyroiditis	A chronic, progressive inflammatory disease of the thyroid, with lymphocyte infiltration and gradual destruction of the gland
	Addison disease	Atrophy and hypofunction of the adrenal cortex, probably autoimmune in origin
	Goodpasture syndrome	A type II hypersensitivity disorder, with pulmonary hemorrhage and progressive glomerulonephritis characterized by circulating antiglomerular basement membrane antibodies
	Active chronic hepatitis	A serious liver disease often resulting in hepatic failure and/or cirrhosis; may be autoimmune, with infiltration by T cells and plasma cells
Less organ-specific	Ulcerative colitis	A chronic inflammatory disease of the colon mucosa, possibly of autoimmune origin
	Sjögren syndrome	A systemic inflammatory disorder characterized by dryness of the mouth, eye, and other mucous membranes, with lymphocyte infiltration of affected tissues
	Scleroderma	Diffuse fibrosis, degenerative changes, and vascular abnormalities of the skin, joint structures, and internal organs; probably of autoimmune origin

Alterations to Immunity

Considering the complexity of the immune system, it is not surprising that abnormal or harmful responses occur. Altered immune system responses include those characterized by hyperresponsiveness of the immune system and those characterized by an impaired immune response. Allergies, autoimmune disorders, and reactions to organ or tissue transplants are all examples of hyperresponsive immune function. AIDS and other immunodeficiency disorders result from impairment of the immune system. **Table 8–2 »** outlines selected autoimmune disorders; other alterations related to the endocrine system but not discussed here are Graves disease, Hashimoto disease, myasthenia gravis, and urticaria.

Alterations and Manifestations

Allergic reactions, also called *hypersensitivity reactions*, are immune responses that lead to tissue damage. There are four types of allergic reactions:

- **Type I, or immediate hypersensitivity.** This response is characterized by rapid development of symptoms after exposure to an antigen. These symptoms can range from minor (e.g., sneezing, runny nose, itchy eyes) to causing death. Reactions usually occur within 15–30 minutes after antigen exposure and may involve the skin, eyes, nasopharynx, bronchopulmonary tissues, and GI tract. There can sometimes be a delayed onset of symptoms ranging from 10–12 hours. Anaphylaxis is the most severe form of an immediate hypersensitivity reaction.

- **Type II, or cytotoxic hypersensitivity.** This response includes the rupture of cells targeted by the immune response that may affect a variety of organs and tissues. Reaction time can be from minutes to hours and is primarily mediated by IgM or IgG antibodies. Examples include transfusion reaction, Rh incompatibility, Hashimoto thyroiditis, and Goodpasture syndrome.

- **Type III, or immune complex reaction.** This reaction includes inflammatory response in the targeted tissues that leads to tissue damage. The reaction may occur 3–10 hours after antigen exposure and be general or involve individual organs. Autoimmune disorders such as SLE and RA are included in this type of reaction.

- **Type IV, or delayed-type hypersensitivity.** This response involves a major histocompatibility complex and is characterized by tissue damage at the site of antigen contact within 24–48 hours after exposure. The classic example is the tuberculin (Mantoux test) reaction; allergic contact dermatitis is another example (Family Practice Notebook, 2015; Ghaffar, 2014).

Autoimmune diseases occur when the immune system attacks components of its own body because the immune system loses its ability to distinguish self from other. These disorders have no definitive cause, although bacteria, genetics, viruses, and environmental factors may play a role (American Autoimmune Related Diseases Association [AARDA], 2015b). Diseases may be localized or generalized, tend to occur more often in women, and often run in families.

Transplant reactions occur when a recipient's body has an immune reaction to newly transplanted organs or tissues. Antigens on the organs or tissues—including the major histocompatibility complex (MHC)—activate the recipient's T cells and stimulate an inflammatory reaction. This reaction can lead to transplant rejection. There are three types of transplant rejection:

- **Hyperacute rejection.** This type occurs minutes or hours after transplantation. It is characterized by organ swelling, clot formation, and hemorrhage.

- **Acute rejection.** This reaction occurs in the weeks following transplantation. In the case of kidney transplant, a decrease in urine output, swelling, pain, and blood and protein in the urine are common.

- **Chronic rejection.** This type occurs months after transplantation. Slow, insidious organ failure occurs as a result of immune-mediated damage.

Finally, immune deficiencies lead to dysfunction in either the primary or the secondary immune response. Primary immune deficiencies are congenital and may affect T cells, B cells, or both. Defects in WBCs may also lead to primary immune deficiencies. Acquired later in life, secondary immune deficiencies lead to decreased immune function and increased susceptibility to infection and malignancies. Many types of trauma or stress—including some cancer

Alterations and Therapies
Immunity

ALTERATION	DESCRIPTION	INTERVENTIONS AND THERAPIES
Hypersensitivity reaction	Hypersensitivity reaction is an altered immune response to an antigen, resulting in harm to the patient ranging from simple allergic rhinitis (e.g., watery eyes, runny nose) to anaphylactic shock.	■ Antihistamines for mild reactions ■ Epinephrine and corticosteroids in life-threatening reactions ■ Maintain airway
Rheumatoid arthritis (RA)	RA is a chronic, systemic autoimmune disorder that causes inflammation of connective tissue.	■ Nonsteroidal anti-inflammatory drugs (NSAIDs) ■ Low-dose corticosteroids ■ Antirheumatic drugs, including immunosuppressive and cytotoxic drugs
HIV/AIDS	AIDS results from a retrovirus (HIV) that is transmitted by direct contact with infected blood and body fluids. HIV infection weakens the immune system, leaving patients vulnerable to opportunistic infections.	■ Prevention of opportunistic infections ■ Ensuring adequate respiratory function and perfusion ■ Stimulating hematopoietic response ■ Antiviral treatment if CD antigen count falls below 200/mm^3 or patient exhibits severe disease symptoms
Systemic lupus erythematosus (SLE)	SLE is a chronic inflammatory disease that involves many organ systems.	■ Dependent on severity of the disease ■ Aspirin or NSAIDs for arthralgias, arthritis, fever, or fatigue ■ Antimalarial drugs ■ High-dose corticosteroids ■ Immunosuppressive agents

therapies—can lead to secondary deficiencies, though the best-known example, AIDS, comes from HIV. HIV attacks and depletes helper T cells, causing immune dysfunction. When lymphocyte levels fall below 200, opportunistic infections develop; when this occurs, the patient has progressed from HIV to AIDS (Mayo Clinic, 2015).

Prevalence

In the United States, an estimated 8% of children have food allergies (American Academy of Allergy Asthma and Immunology [AAAI], 2016b). Current data have shown that of these children, non-Hispanic Blacks were more likely to report having a food allergy. However, it was also suggested that Black and Asian children were less likely to report having received a formal diagnosis of food allergy (Dyer & Gupta, 2013).

Approximately 14.7 to 23.5 million Americans are affected by autoimmune disease, and nearly 80% of affected individuals are female (National Institutes of Health [NIH], 2012). In fact, autoimmune diseases are one of the leading causes of death in young and middle-age women. Lupus is one of the most common autoimmune diseases, affecting 1.5 million Americans; 90% of these individuals are women. Prevalence rates for lupus vary from 164 Caucasian women to 406 African American women per 100,000 in the U.S. (Schur & Hahn, 2017). RA, multiple sclerosis, and scleroderma are also common and tend to affect more women than men (NIH, 2012; U.S. Department of Health and Human Services, Office on Women's Health, 2012).

Over 29,000 organ and tissue transplantations were performed in the United States in 2014; the prevalence of transplant rejection is difficult to determine, however, because

rejection can occur long after transplantation (U.S. Department of Health and Human Services [USDHHS], 2017). Finding a perfect tissue match is difficult because the odds of two individuals having identical antigens are roughly 1 in 100,000 (National Institute of Allergy and Infectious Diseases [NIAID], 2012; USDHHS, 2017). As a result, all transplant recipients receive lifelong antirejection therapies in the form of immunosuppressive medications.

Primary immune deficiencies affect about 500,000 people in the United States (Kobrynski, Powell, & Bowen, 2014; NIAID, 2012). Secondary immune deficiencies are much more common than primary deficiencies (Fernandez, 2013). This category includes the 1.2 million people in the United States with HIV or AIDS; globally this number exceeds 37 million (NIAID, 2017). Regardless of type, immune deficiencies are debilitating, and morbidity and mortality rates for affected individuals are high.

Genetic Considerations and Risk Factors

Genetics is a key component in a number of immune disorders and deficiencies. Evidence suggests that children are at increased likelihood of developing sensitivities to certain allergens if their parents or older siblings are allergic. Children are also more prone to developing allergies in general if one or both of their parents have allergies (Healthychildren.org, 2016). Autoimmune diseases are also due—in part—to a genetic predisposition in conjunction with the presence of an environmental trigger (American Autoimmune Related Diseases Association [AARDA], 2015b). Inherited genetic mutations are the cause of primary immune deficiencies, though secondary immune deficiencies do not have a genetic component. Genetic

Focus on Diversity and Culture
Autoimmune Diseases

Many cultures demonstrate increased prevalence for autoimmune diseases. African American, Native American, and Hispanic women have been identified as being more susceptible to specific autoimmune diseases than women of other ethnicities. African Americans and Native Americans exhibit an increased prevalence for more severe scleroderma compared to people of other cultures (Johns Hopkins Scleroderma Center, 2016). African American, Hispanic, Asian, and Native American women tend to have a higher prevalence of SLE than white women. Multiple factors such as genetics, environmental risk, and metabolism may contribute to the differences in disease prevalence between these groups (AARDA, 2015a).

which you administer. Within 30 minutes after administration of the medications, Marisol's breathing is improving and her hives appear to be slightly diminished. The pediatrician instructs Ms. Jimenez to follow up with an allergist for further evaluation of Marisol's allergies.

Clinical Reasoning Questions Level I
1. What symptoms of hypersensitivity does Marisol have?
2. Why might Marisol's blood pressure be low and her heart rate rapid?
3. What age-appropriate education about peanut allergies can you provide Marisol?

Clinical Reasoning Questions Level II
4. What is the priority nursing diagnosis for Marisol at this time?
5. What independent nursing interventions can you perform to help make Marisol more comfortable while she waits for the corticosteroid injection to provide some relief of her discomfort?
6. Given Marisol's history, what is the significance of her respiratory symptoms?

counseling is recommended for patients with primary immune deficiencies who are considering becoming pregnant.

Gender is also an important factor in immune disease, and a number of conditions are more prevalent in women than in men; this is particularly evident in autoimmune disease. The explanation for this prevalence is unclear, though evidence suggests that estrogen can increase the immune response. Some autoimmune diseases may be triggered by pregnancy; however, pregnancy can cause some autoimmune diseases to go into remission (AARDA, 2015a).

As individuals age, they are more likely to be exposed to the stress, environmental factors, and bodily insults that lead to secondary immune conditions. Studies have shown that people over age 55 are also more prone to transplantation problems (Hricik et al., 2016). Race may also play a role in transplantation rejection in that African American patients tend to experience higher rejection rates than Caucasian patients (Suryanarayana et al., 2014; Taber et al., 2014).

Case Study » Part 1

Marisol Jimenez is a 7-year-old girl who was diagnosed with a peanut sensitivity as a toddler. She presents at her pediatrician's office at 8:30 Monday morning after her mother, Luisa, called to report that Marisol had developed urticaria and tightness in her throat Sunday night. As the nurse working with Marisol's pediatrician, you conduct an initial assessment and patient interview with Marisol and Ms. Jimenez. Ms. Jimenez reports that Marisol developed a similar rash last year after eating peanut butter cookies at a friend's birthday party; the throat tightness is a new symptom, however. Ms. Jimenez limits Marisol's exposure to peanuts, but Marisol's grandmother recently emigrated from Mexico and speaks little English. Ms. Jimenez is having difficulty getting her to understand Marisol's "peanut problems." As a result, the grandmother served Marisol sopapillas fried in peanut oil at dinner last night. Ms. Jimenez has given Marisol two 12.5-mg doses of diphenhydramine (Benadryl) 6 hours apart, one at 2100 hours last night and the other at 0300 this morning, per the doctor's previous instructions for treating Marisol's sensitivity. In the past, her symptoms cleared up after the second dose, but Marisol tells you that the itchiness "just won't stop" and that her throat "feels like something is squeezing it."

You observe patchy red welts on Marisol's face, some of which are irritated and open due to Marisol's scratching. Her lips appear slightly swollen. On assessment of Marisol's vitals, you note that her blood pressure is slightly decreased and her heart rate is rapid. When you auscultate her lungs, you hear faint stridor. The pediatrician orders a corticosteroid injection and albuterol (4 puffs) via inhaler to Marisol,

Concepts Related to Immunity

Due to its role in protecting the body, the immune system affects and is affected by a number of other conceptual areas. The rapid, dramatic nature of immune response can lead to a variety of localized and systemic discomforts. Given the skin's role as the body's primary barrier to foreign bodies and antigens, discomforts of the skin are very common and stem from a variety of sources, including allergic reaction, inflammation, and wound healing.

Individuals are continuously in contact with microorganisms in the environment, and decreased immunity can increase their risk for developing infection. Proper nutrition and fluid intake, good personal hygiene, adequate sleep, vaccines, and reduction of stress are ways to reduce risk of infection. Nurses should carefully assess for signs and symptoms of infection and use good hand hygiene and proper aseptic/sterile technique for all procedures.

Inflammation is a reaction of the local circulatory system to an insult, injury, or antigen. It involves movement of fluid and cells out of the bloodstream to the affected tissue in an effort to eliminate infectious agents. Inflammation often resolves itself once the threat is eliminated; it may, however, lead to abscess, scar formation, and persistent inflammation that leads to chronic inflammation.

Tissue integrity has a two-way relationship with immunity: Impaired skin integrity can trigger an immune response, and certain immune responses can lead to impaired skin integrity. Burns, traumatic injuries, and some cancer therapies can impair skin integrity, allowing infectious agents to enter the body. On the contrary, allergic reactions can result in manifestations such as contact dermatitis. The Concepts Related to Immunity feature links some, but not all, of the concepts integral to immunity. They are presented in alphabetical order.

Health Promotion

Two types of prevention promote healthy immune systems: the prevention of immune disorders themselves and the use of vaccines to prevent infectious diseases. Educating patients about modifiable risk factors and encouraging routine vaccination are important prevention initiatives aimed at improving the health of the U.S. population.

Concepts Related to
Immunity

CONCEPT	RELATIONSHIP TO IMMUNITY	NURSING IMPLICATIONS
Comfort	Painful conditions, such as swelling and skin reactions, often occur during immune response.	▪ Assess related symptoms, such as edema, rash, malaise, loss of appetite, and trouble sleeping. ▪ Be alert to topical and latex allergies that could worsen symptoms. ▪ *Anticipate:* Additional assessments, comfort measures
Infection	Patients with alterations in immunity can experience acute or chronic infections.	▪ Assess area of suspected infection (see Infection Assessment section in the module on Infection). ▪ Educate patients regarding the importance of immunizations and encourage their use. ▪ Educate patients regarding the importance of avoiding situations that could increase exposure to infection. ▪ Practice standard precautions, proper hand hygiene, and aseptic/sterile technique with all procedures. ▪ Assess complete blood count (CBC) results; be alert for elevated WBC count.
Inflammation	Movement of fluid and cells to the site of injury or infection causes inflammation during an immune response.	▪ Assess for fever, skin warmth and redness, edema, and generalized pain. ▪ Be alert for abscess formation, purulent exudate, and increased WBC count. ▪ *Anticipate:* Aspirin, antipyretics, cold packs
Managing Care	Patients with alterations in their immune system can greatly benefit from participating in managed care and have more positive health outcomes.	▪ Assess the needs of patients to identify actual or potential problems related to care. ▪ Advocate for patients in relation to their care needs.
Spirituality	Patients experiencing an alteration in their immune system can have their spirituality challenged or can question their beliefs.	▪ Be sensitive to the spiritual needs of patients. ▪ Observe for cues related to patients' religion or spiritual preference (e.g., Bible, rosary, Koran). ▪ Avoid imposing personal spiritual beliefs on patients. ▪ Refer for spiritual guidance as appropriate.
Tissue Integrity	Impaired skin integrity triggers immune response; some immune responses lead to impaired skin integrity.	▪ Tissue integrity is important in burns, traumatic injury, cancer therapies, and skin and allergic disorders. ▪ Educate patients about care measures for impaired skin. ▪ *Anticipate:* Antibiotics, medications for pain relief, altered sensation or pain

Reducing the number of preventable childhood illnesses is one of the major goals of *Healthy People 2020,* and nurses are important partners in this effort. The incidences of the following infectious diseases are targeted for elimination or reduction (U.S. Department of Health and Human Services, Office of Disease Prevention and Promotion, 2014):

▪ **Elimination.** Rubella, congenital rubella syndrome, and polio

▪ **Reduction.** Pertussis, hepatitis A, hepatitis B, hepatitis C, tuberculosis, varicella, *Haemophilus influenzae* type b (Hib), measles, mumps, meningococcal diseases, and pneumococcal infections.

To accomplish this goal, a national public health initiative aims to increase the numbers of children protected against vaccine-preventable diseases and to monitor immunization status.

>> **Stay Current:** Visit the *Healthy People 2020* website at https://www.healthypeople.gov/2020/topics-objectives/topic/immunization-and-infectious-diseases to see the specific goals for immunizations.

Modifiable Risk Factors

A number of modifiable factors put people at risk for immune disorders across the lifespan. Nutrition is of particular interest, especially as it relates to the development of food allergies in children. Unlike food intolerance, which is associated with conditions such as celiac disease and lactose intolerance, food allergies are immune-mediated allergic responses. For the individual with a food allergy, sensitization to proteins in certain foods, such as peanuts, triggers the production of IgE antibodies and may progress to anaphylaxis. Research suggests that early introduction of solid foods decreases the likelihood of food sensitization during early childhood (Abrams & Becker, 2013). There is, however, some debate about the right age at which to introduce certain foods, such as peanuts, eggs, and cow's milk. This debate centers on the question of whether early exposure increases or decreases the likelihood of sensitivity to these common allergens. It has been recommended by the American Academy of Pediatrics (AAP) not to introduce solid foods to infants younger than 4–6 months of age and to breastfeed for as long as possible. The timing of introducing certain foods is also being investigated as a means of preventing food allergies (AAP, 2015a). In the United States and other Western countries, the general practice of delaying the introduction of certain foods in the first year may not help the child tolerate the food (American College of Allergy, Asthma and Immunology [ACAAI], 2016). Protein-energy malnutrition and lipid, vitamin, and mineral deficiencies are all believed to impair the immune response (Calder, 2013).

Weight is a factor closely related to nutrition, and research suggests that being either underweight or overweight can have an impact on the immune system, causing alterations in leukocyte counts and the cell-mediated immune responses (de Heredia, Gomez-Martinez, & Marcos, 2012). Malnutrition, either deficiency or excess, has been identified as the most common cause of immunodeficiency in the world. Individuals who are undernourished may have inadequate intake of certain micronutrients needed for adequate immune function. The immunocompetence of an individual can also be altered by overnutrition, another form of malnutrition, and obesity. Studies have indicated a link between obesity and an inflammatory response (Linus Pauling Institute Micronutrient Information Center, 2016). Following a healthy diet, maintaining a healthy weight, avoiding the use of tobacco products, controlling blood pressure, consuming alcohol in moderation, and getting adequate sleep are ways to positively improve immune function (Harvard Medical School, 2016).

Stress is another modifiable risk factor. Chronic stress leads to heightened endocrine response; this response simultaneously suppresses the immune response, which decreases the immune system's ability to respond to threats (Sizemore, 2012). Stress management strategies to aid in reduction may prove beneficial to the immune system of individuals exposed to prolonged stress (Mayo Clinic, 2014b).

Alcohol, drug, and cigarette use can also increase susceptibility to immune diseases. These substances act as toxins in the body; these toxins can, in turn, act as environmental triggers for individuals with genetic predisposition to autoimmune disorders.

Unprotected vaginal and anal sex with multiple partners is also a key risk factor for HIV. Intravenous (IV) drug use and risky sexual behaviors as modifiable risk factors are explored more thoroughly in Exemplar 8.A on HIV/AIDS.

Immunizations

One of the great breakthroughs of modern medicine was the development and widespread availability of vaccines. The average infant born today receives immunizations for 16 diseases during childhood. Diseases for which vaccines are routinely recommended include measles, mumps, rubella, polio, pertussis (whooping cough), diphtheria, tetanus, *Haemophilus influenzae* type b, hepatitis A and B, pneumococcus, varicella (chickenpox), and influenza (CDC, 2016d). In 2006 and 2008, new rotavirus vaccines were approved for administration to infants. In addition, vaccines have been developed recently for older children, adolescents, and adults to protect against pertussis, meningococcus, human papillomavirus, and shingles. Administering these vaccines greatly improves health and reduces the familial burden of caring for ill children and older relatives.

Immunization introduces an antigen into the body, allowing immunity against a disease to develop naturally. The immunized individual then produces antibodies in

response to the antigens. In *active immunity* (which stimulates antibody production without causing clinical disease), an antigen is given in the form of a **vaccine**.

When an individual requires antibodies faster than the body can develop them, *passive immunity* may be induced. In this approach, antibodies are produced in another human or animal host and then given to the child. This approach also is used with at-risk individuals after a single exposure to a disease in an attempt to prevent the disease from occurring or to reduce its severity. For example, if a child who has never had a tetanus immunization steps on a rusty nail, the child needs immediate protection (passive immunity) from tetanus. Tetanus immunoglobulin is given by injection to combat the tetanus toxin produced when bacterial spores are introduced by the nail. Passive immunity does not confer lasting immunity. So, the tetanus toxoid vaccine also is administered to start the process of antibody development (active immunity).

Types of Vaccines

Types of vaccines used in the United States include the following:

- *Killed virus vaccine.* A vaccine that contains a microorganism that has been killed but is still capable of inducing the human body to produce antibodies (e.g., inactivated poliovirus vaccine)
- *Toxoid.* A toxin that has been treated (by heat or chemical) to weaken its toxic effects but retain its antigenicity (e.g., tetanus toxoid)
- *Live virus vaccine.* A vaccine that contains a microorganism in live but attenuated (weakened) form (e.g., measles and varicella vaccines)
- *Recombinant forms.* An organism that has been genetically altered for use in vaccines (e.g., hepatitis B and acellular pertussis vaccine, which uses proteins from pertussis rather than the whole cell to stimulate the process of active immunity)
- *Conjugated forms.* An altered organism joined with another substance to increase the immune response (e.g., *Haemophilus influenzae* type b vaccine is conjugated with a protein carrier like tetanus toxoid; however, this specific vaccine brand confers no immunity to tetanus).

Improvements in vaccine technology continue to increase the safety and efficacy of immunization against an increasing number of diseases. Today's vaccines often are produced synthetically by means of recombinant DNA technology or genetic engineering.

SAFETY ALERT Thimerosal, a bacteriostatic agent that contains ethyl mercury, was previously used to prevent contamination of vaccines in multidose vials. Vaccine manufacturers worked to remove thimerosal from vaccines. Most vaccines now have either no thimerosal or only trace amounts (Food and Drug Administration [FDA], 2015c).

Responses to Vaccines

Individuals who have received vaccines may have a variety of responses as the body responds to the injected antigen stimulating the immune system. Depending on the specific immunization, up to 50% of vaccine recipients have a local reaction that includes erythema, swelling, pain, and induration at the site of the injection. Systemic reactions that often occur include fever, fussiness or irritability, malaise, and loss of appetite. With some vaccines, other systemic reactions include a rash or arthralgia. The nurse provides guidelines for managing expected mild reactions at home and makes sure patients or their parents have the correct dosage information for the acetaminophen or ibuprofen formulation that is in the home.

Other serious reactions to vaccines occur in rare instances. The range of illnesses and disabilities that may occur include anaphylaxis, encephalopathy, bacterial neuritis, chronic arthritis, thrombocytopenia purpura, and death. Each of these reactions must be reported to the local health authority as well as the National Vaccine Injury Compensation Program.

Local allergic reactions, such as a wheal and urticaria, can occur in minutes to hours after the injection. A severe local allergic reaction is manifested by warmth, erythema, edema, petechiae, or ulceration occurring 2–8 hours after vaccination. A non–life-threatening systemic allergic reaction, such as generalized urticaria or transient petechiae, may occur within minutes. Anaphylaxis is a life-threatening allergic reaction that may result in shock and death. Its manifestations include hypotension, generalized urticaria, and angioedema. Laryngeal edema has occurred in rare cases with nearly every vaccine.

SAFETY ALERT   Be prepared for potential vaccine anaphylaxis and keep epinephrine (1:1000) and resuscitation equipment immediately available. The standard dose for epinephrine (aqueous 1:1000) is 0.01 mg/kg body weight, up to 0.5 mg maximum single dose in children and 0.5 mg maximum single dose in adolescents intramuscularly. The dose can be repeated every 5–15 minutes, up to a total of three doses, until symptoms subside or other emergency care interventions are initiated (Immunization Action Coalition, 2015).

Immunization Schedule

The recommended schedule for immunization is updated at least annually to reflect new vaccines and the need for repeat immunization. The Advisory Committee on Immunization Practices (ACIP) of the Centers for Disease Control and Prevention (CDC), the AAP, and the American Academy of Family Practitioners (AAFP) collaborate to provide a uniform vaccination schedule. The ACIP publishes vaccination schedules for children, adolescents, and adults in both a technical edition for healthcare professionals and an easy-to-read edition for laypeople. Immunization schedules take the form of charts that show the ages at which common vaccines are recommended.

》 Stay Current: To view the most current technical and lay immunization schedules for children and adults, visit the CDC's website at http://www.cdc.gov/vaccines/schedules/downloads/child/0-18yrs-child-combined-schedule.pdf; http://www.cdc.gov/vaccines/parents/downloads/parent-ver-sch-0-6yrs.pdf; http://www.cdc.gov/vaccines/schedules/downloads/adult/adult-schedule.pdf; http://www.cdc.gov/vaccines/schedules/downloads/adult/adult-schedule-easy-read.pdf and the ACIP website at http://www.cdc.gov/vaccines/hcp/acip-recs/index.html

Children (Birth to 18 Years)

Vaccines should be administered to children at specific ages and intervals. The timing for first immunizations is determined by the age at which **transplacental immunity** (passive immunity transferred from mother to infant) decreases or

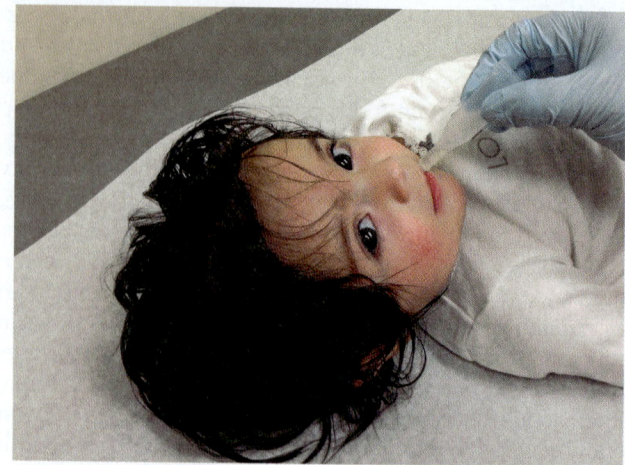

Source: Centers for Disease Control and Prevention (CDC).

Figure 8–5 》 Six-month-old girl receiving her oral rotavirus vaccine.

disappears and the age at which the infant or child develops the ability to make antibodies in response to the vaccine. Most vaccines for infants and children are started between the age of 2 and 18 months, depending on the vaccine (see **Figure 8–5 》》**). If vaccines are not given at the recommended age, catch-up immunizations can be given throughout childhood and into adolescence as needed. Current vaccines specifically recommended to begin in adolescence include papillomavirus vaccine (for both boys and girls) and meningococcal vaccine (CDC, 2013a).

Scientists also continue to study the duration of protection from vaccines. Some do not confer lifelong immunity. For example, it was determined recently that a second dose of varicella vaccine is necessary for immunity (CDC, 2016c). Many other childhood vaccines also require multiple doses, including DTaP (diphtheria, tetanus, pertussis), pneumococcal vaccine, MMR (measles, mumps, rubella), and hepatitis A and B vaccines.

Adults

Immunization recommendations for adults include boosters of childhood vaccines (e.g., MMR, TDaP), annual vaccines (e.g., influenza), vaccines for older adults (e.g., herpes zoster), and immunizations for individuals at high risk of infection. The CDC recommends that many adult vaccinations, such as HPV and hepatitis A and C, be administered via a multiple-dose series, like in childhood vaccinations. In addition, some immunizations are contraindicated in specific populations, especially during pregnancy or in individuals who are immunocompromised (CDC, 2013b, 2016e).

The risk of developing herpes zoster (shingles) increases as a person ages with a major increase after age 50. The herpes zoster vaccine was licensed by the ACIP in 2006 and recommended in 2008 for the prevention of herpes zoster and its complications in adults ages 60 and older. The FDA approved vaccine use in 2011 for adults ages 50–59 but did not recommend it. Protection offered by the vaccine has been shown to diminish within 5 years after receiving it, and to date, no long-term studies related to effectiveness have been performed (CDC, 2014).

Contraindications

Contraindications for immunizations may include an acute illness with high fever, a hypersensitivity reaction to specific vaccine components, immunoglobulin therapy in the past 3–6 months, cancer treatment, and pregnancy (AAP, 2015a).

Parent Education and Informed Consent

An increasing number of parents are choosing not to immunize their children for a number of reasons, some of which are related to religious beliefs or lack of access to healthcare. Other reasons articulated by parents include (Brunson, 2013; Immunization Action Coalition, 2016; Luthy et al., 2012):

- Concerns related to the danger of overwhelming the child's developing immune system with multiple antigens at a young age
- Doubts about the efficacy of vaccines
- Belief that "herd immunity" of vaccinated children will protect their child
- Belief that natural healing methods are superior to vaccines
- Previous negative vaccine reactions in family members or friends
- Concerns about perceived associations between vaccinations and development of chronic disease.

The healthcare provider is often the most trusted source of health information for parents and the manner in which the provider initiates conversation about recommended vaccines is important (Immunization Action Coalition, 2016; Opel et al., 2013). This conversation should contain "balanced" information related to the risks and benefits about immunizations and provide parents with an opportunity to have their questions answered before giving consent for immunization (Glanz, Kraus, & Daley, 2015). Legislation requiring parental consent for vaccine administration is controlled at the state level and varies from state to state. Conversation with the provider that better relates to informed consent, rather than implied or simple consent, is more appropriate (Opel et al., 2013). The federal government, however, requires that Vaccine Information Statements (VISs) be given to parents or guardians prior to the vaccination of a minor. These statements explain the benefits and risks of a vaccine.

In most healthcare settings, the nurse is responsible for informing the parents or the child's legal guardian, supplying literature, and obtaining written consent before the vaccine is administered. The nurse has a legal obligation to ensure that consent is obtained from an individual who has the legal authority to give consent (see the Patient Teaching feature).

Nursing Assessment

Unlike body systems that are composed of a few closely related organs, the immune system is diverse and scattered. Optimal immune function depends on intact skin and mucous membrane barriers, adequate blood cell production and differentiation, a functional system of lymphatics and the spleen, and the ability to differentiate foreign tissue and pathogens from normal body tissue and flora. Because of this diversity of organs and functions, assessment of the

Patient Teaching
Immunizations

Parental education should include discussion of the vaccine risks and benefits. Many times parents hear dramatic stories about the consequences of vaccines; therefore, correct information is required in order to help them make informed decisions. The nurse has the responsibility to provide the most current VIS to the parents related to the vaccines to be administered, assess for understanding of the information provided, and answer any questions from the parents or caregiver.

Multiple studies have failed to find a relationship between the measles, mumps, and rubella vaccine and the development of autism (AAP, 2013; Maglione et al., 2014). In addition, other studies have not revealed a relationship between vaccines and disorders such as leukemia (Maglione et al., 2014), seizure disorder, attention-deficit/hyperactivity disorder (Luthy et al., 2012), sudden infant death syndrome (Neeman, 2013), and type 1 diabetes mellitus (CDC, 2015w). The nurse should identify the vaccines to be given at each visit so that the parents know their child's immunization status. It may save time to give parents the VIS about the next vaccines to take home and review before the next visit.

Parents have the right to refuse immunizations, but if a disease outbreak occurs, the child who is not immunized must be kept out of child care or school. If the parent chooses not to have the child receive a particular vaccine, the nurse should document an informed refusal.

» Stay Current: Visit the CDC at http://www.cdc.gov/vaccines/hcp/conversations/downloads/talk-infants-bw-office.pdf and Every Child by Two at http://vaccinateyourfamily.org/files/resources/Interactive_Vaccine_Preventable_Disease_eBook_ECBT.pdf for topics to cover with parents.

immune system often is integrated throughout the health history and physical examination.

Observation and Patient Interview

Before conducting the interview, review the patient's biographical data, including age, sex, race, and ethnic background. Observe the general appearance of the patient, and note whether the patient's stated and apparent age coincide. Family history also is important because the etiology of many disorders affecting the immune system includes a genetic component. Many interview questions related to the immune system and the disorders that affect it are of a sensitive nature. Be sure to provide privacy for the interview. If family members are present, request that they leave as well. Establish a trusting relationship with the patient before asking the most sensitive questions (e.g., those related to the use of illicit drugs or sexual activity). Interview questions may include:

- When were you last immunized for diphtheria, tetanus, poliomyelitis, rubella, measles, influenza, hepatitis, and pneumococcal pneumonia? Do you have a record of your immunizations?
- When did you last have a tuberculin skin test?
- What infections have you had in the past, how were these treated, and have they recurred?

- Does anyone in your family have an immune disorder?
- Are you taking any antibiotics, anti-inflammatory medications, or medications for cancer?
- Have you had any recent invasive procedures or radiologic examinations?
- Do you have any allergies to food, medications, or any other substance, such as latex, bees, or pollen? If so, what happens when you come in contact with this substance?
- On a scale of 1–10, how would you rate the stress you have experienced during the past 6 months?
- Do you have any chronic conditions?

As with all patient interviews, individualize the specific terms used and the examples given to the patient.

Patients who are immunocompromised are at greater risk for infection and other disease conditions; the severity of risk depends on the degree of immunosuppression. Healthcare providers need to maintain a high alert with these patients in monitoring for infection and disease. In addition to manifestations of infection, patients may present with various noninfectious manifestations (i.e., impaired kidney function; liver disease; cardiopulmonary dysfunction; psychosocial, dermatologic, and neurologic disorders). These noninfectious manifestations may be directly related or unrelated to the degree of immunosuppression.

The GI tract in patients who are immunocompromised is particularly at risk for infectious and noninfectious injuries because of the disruption of the normal defenses. This can lead to various conditions, including mucosal injury and ulceration, biliary tract diseases, diverticular disease, pancreatitis, and malignancy. The infections in the GI tract may be viral, bacterial, fungal, or parasitic. Patients experiencing any of these disorders may present with oral lesions, oral or esophageal candidiasis, diarrhea, and/or abdominal pain (Okafor, 2012).

Physical Examination

Begin the physical examination by assessing height, weight, and body type for apparent weight loss or wasting. Check vital signs. An elevated temperature may indicate an infection or inflammatory response.

Diagnostic Tests

Diagnostic and laboratory tests are ordered according to the type of immune disorder that is suspected. Possible tests include:

- Enzyme immunoassay (EIA)
- Enzyme-linked immunosorbent assay (ELISA)
- Immunoglobulins
- Polymerase chain reaction
- Rapid HIV tests
- Radioallergosorbent test
- Skin reactions
- Western blot test
- CBC
- Complement.

>> *Go to* **Pearson MyLab Nursing and eText** *to see Appendix B for information on diagnostic values and laboratory tests.*

Case Study >> Part 2

Marisol Jimenez recovered from her hypersensitivity reaction quickly. After discharge, several months passed during which she was not exposed to peanuts or peanut products. Then, late in the school year, Marisol's class went on a field trip and the children brought picnic lunches. Marisol was not happy about the turkey sandwich in her lunch, so she traded it with a friend for what she thought was a jelly sandwich. However, the sandwich had both peanut butter and jelly in it. After a couple of bites, Marisol started gasping for air and clutching her throat. Her friend alerted the teacher, who called 911.

Marisol was transported to the emergency department (ED), where you are the admitting nurse. The paramedics give you their field report: 7-year-old girl with an anaphylactic reaction to peanut butter. Vital signs include temperature within normal limits; pulse 115 bpm; respirations 29/min; and blood pressure 85/50 mmHg. Paramedics administered 0.2 mL (1:1000) IM epinephrine and 10 L oxygen by face mask en route to the hospital. Initial pulse oximeter readings were 91% but improved to 95% with oxygen. Marisol is continued on 10 L oxygen by face mask in the ED and placed on a cardiac monitor. IV access is established, and she is given 115 mg of IV hydrocortisone. She is aware of her surroundings and resting comfortably, but she is very scared and asking for her mother. You are called away to another patient, so you ask a hospital volunteer to sit with Marisol and keep her calm until Ms. Jimenez arrives.

Thirty minutes later, the volunteer calls you back to Marisol's room. Marisol is suddenly having difficulty breathing, her skin has become very pale, and she is confused. You perform a respiratory assessment and note significant stridor. Pulse oximeter readings have fallen to 90%. You notify the physician of the change in Marisol's condition. Because of Marisol's respiratory distress and declining level of consciousness, the physician orders another dose of epinephrine 1:1000 0.2 mL IM STAT, then epinephrine 1:1000 0.2 mL IM every 5–15 minutes as needed. The physician also orders a one-time administration of racemic epinephrine via nebulizer to reduce laryngeal edema.

Ms. Jimenez arrives, and the physician discusses Marisol's condition with her. Because there is no significant improvement in Marisol's condition, the use of continuous positive airway pressure (CPAP) has become necessary. Marisol will be admitted to the pediatric unit for observation.

Clinical Reasoning Questions Level I

1. What might be the reason behind the sudden deterioration of Marisol's condition?
2. What independent interventions can you perform to help ease Marisol's fears?
3. Why did the paramedics administer epinephrine to Marisol?

Clinical Reasoning Questions Level II

4. Why is Marisol given hydrocortisone after her arrival at the hospital?
5. *Referring to the concept of acid–base balance:* Would a blood gas analysis be useful in Marisol's case? Why or why not?
6. *Referring to the concept of oxygenation:* What does Marisol's 91% pulse oximeter rating reflect? What is the relationship between Marisol's breath sounds and her pulse oximetry measurements?

Immune System Assessment

ASSESSMENT/METHOD	NORMAL FINDINGS	ABNORMAL FINDINGS	LIFESPAN OR DEVELOPMENTAL CONSIDERATIONS
Family History			
Review history of allergy in family members. Review history of HIV or immune disorder in mother and other family members.	Lack of history eliminates primary immune deficiencies and may also eliminate other disorders that run in families or have a congenital component.	▪ Increased likelihood of allergies if parents have allergies ▪ Maternal HIV (give prophylactic treatment to the child)	▪ Parents or guardians may provide history for children and adolescents.
Growth and Development (Children)			
Plot height and weight during each visit. Assess appetite and eating habits. Assess achievement of developmental milestones.	Growth and weight gain are steady. Appetite is healthy, and normal amounts of food are consumed for age. Development is appropriate for age.	▪ Delayed growth ▪ Failure to thrive ▪ Lack of appetite ▪ Lethargy ▪ Lack of energy ▪ Delayed development	▪ Developmental delays in toddlers may be secondary to serious illness.
Skin and Mucous Membranes			
Examine skin and mucous membranes for lesions and other injuries.	Skin and mucous membranes are intact. When lesions and injury occur, they heal quickly without additional infection.	▪ Frequent and easy bruising ▪ Slow healing ▪ Frequent infection ▪ Frequent allergic response ▪ Pale, boggy (edematous) nasal mucosa (often associated with chronic allergies) ▪ Petechiae, white patches, or lacy white plaques in the oral mucosa (may indicate hemolysis or immunodeficiency)	▪ The skin of older adults is more fragile than that of younger adults and children. ▪ Physiologic changes of age increase older adults' susceptibility to skin disorders.
Assess skin color, temperature, and moisture.	Skin color is even and appropriate to the age and race of the patient. Skin is warm and dry.	▪ Pale or jaundiced skin (may indicate a hemolytic reaction) ▪ Pallor (may indicate bone marrow suppression with accompanying immunodeficiency)	▪ In darker skin tones, an ashy appearance indicates dryness. ▪ Temperature regulation in infants is inefficient; skin may feel warm or cool in the absence of inflammation or decreased blood flow.
Evidence of Disease			
Assess for frequency and type of infections. Assess respiratory function.	Infection occurs infrequently. When infection does occur, causes are common and easily treatable.	▪ Frequent infection ▪ Infection caused by unusual or uncommon infectious agents ▪ Respiratory infection ▪ Untreatable ear infection	▪ Ear infections are common among preschool-age children.
Cervical Lymph Nodes			
Inspect and palpate the cervical lymph nodes (see **Figure 8–6** ⟫); palpate the nodes of the axillae and groin as well.	Normal cervical lymph nodes are <2 cm and soft. Normal axilla and inguinal lymph nodes are <3 cm and soft.	▪ Lymphadenopathy (swelling) or tenderness (indicates presence of infection)	▪ Because children may have frequent viral infections, their cervical lymph nodes may be enlarged.

(continued on next page)

Immune System Assessments (continued)

ASSESSMENT/METHOD	NORMAL FINDINGS	ABNORMAL FINDINGS	LIFESPAN OR DEVELOPMENTAL CONSIDERATIONS

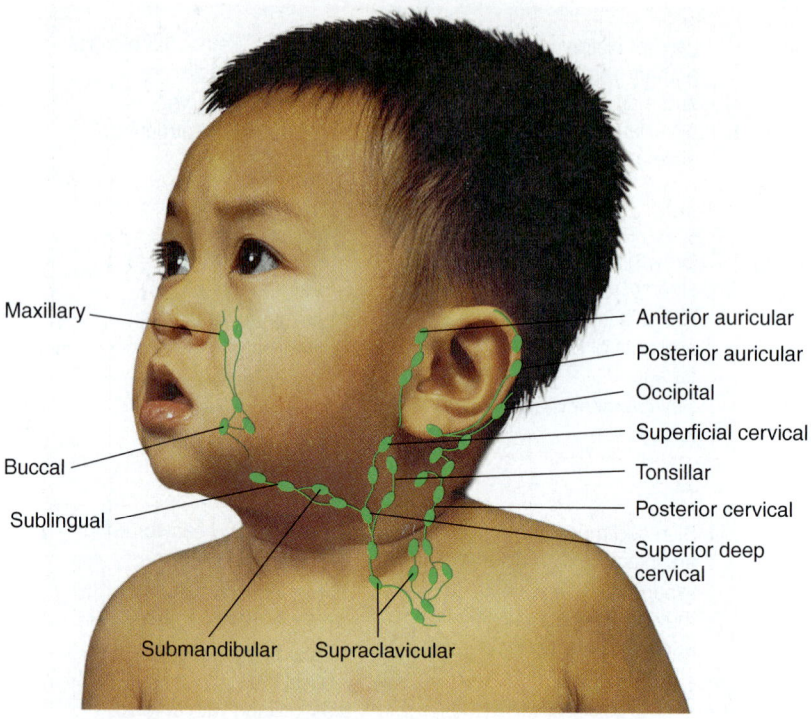

Maxillary
Buccal
Sublingual
Submandibular   Supraclavicular

Anterior auricular
Posterior auricular
Occipital
Superficial cervical
Tonsillar
Posterior cervical
Superior deep cervical

Figure 8–6 》 Lymph nodes that can be assessed by palpation.

Musculoskeletal System

Inspect and palpate the joints.	There is no visible inflammation or deformity. Joints have no tenderness, pain, warmth, or crepitation.	■ Redness, swelling, tenderness, or deformity (may indicate an autoimmune disorder such as RA or SLE)	■ Palpate swollen joints gently; they can be quite painful. ■ Older adults will often have some degree of cartilage loss (osteoarthritis).
Check joint range of motion (ROM), including that of the spine.	Patient has ease of movement and shows no evidence of stiffness or difficulty moving.	■ Evident fatigue or weakness (may indicate acute or chronic illness or immunodeficiency)	■ Older adults may naturally have less flexibility of joints compared to children and young adults.

Independent Interventions

The immune system is affected by both physical and psychologic factors. These factors affect both independent nursing care and the collaborative efforts of the interprofessional healthcare team. While vaccinations and other pharmacologic agents can be crucial to promoting a healthy immune system, lifestyle factors also have a significant impact on immune function.

Proper nutrition, adequate exercise, and a good night's sleep are profoundly important in maintaining an effective immune system. Nurses can assist with proper nutrition by assessing patient nutritional intake and providing nutrition counseling for under- or overweight individuals. They can also provide patients with valuable resources such as online and community programs that assist with healthy eating

behaviors and weight management (see the Independent Interventions section in the module on Nutrition). Moderate exercise has been shown to prevent and even reverse many chronic disease processes. It also has a positive effect on the immune system by causing lymph fluid to be pumped more efficiently throughout the body. While moderate exercise seems to enhance immunity, strenuous exercise may reduce immune function, leaving a window of opportunity for infection during the recovery phase. Adequate rest is important after vigorous training to allow the body to recover (Gleeson & Walsh, 2012). Nurses should educate patients regarding the positive benefits of exercise on the immune system.

Sleep is a basic human need. Inadequate amounts of sleep can have an impact on the immune system. Individuals who are deprived of non–rapid eye movement (NREM) sleep can experience immunosuppression and have increased susceptibility to infection. Nurses need to assess patients' sleep patterns and habits and educate them about the importance of good sleep hygiene. More details on sleep hygiene are provided in a section on the topic and a Patient Teaching feature in the module on Comfort.

Stress reduction and stress management also play a role. The normal stress response allows the body to compensate for the impact of stressors and either maintain or regain homeostasis. If there is prolonged overexposure to stressors, the immune system can be compromised, and illness can result. Nurses can assist patients in managing stress by first assessing the stressors that are present and then identifying strategies and coping mechanisms to manage these stressors (see the module on Stress and Coping).

Collaborative Therapies

The goals of medical management are to restore immune function and to prevent further stress on the immune system. Treatment may be supportive for those with only mild manifestations.

Pharmacologic Therapy

Anti-inflammatories, such as NSAIDs and corticosteroids, are a staple in the management of alterations in immune function, because pain and swelling are frequent manifestations.

Prevention and prompt treatment of infection are essential. Antibiotic therapy targets infectious agents. Patients also need antibiotic prophylaxis and specific immunization recommendations for immunodeficiency. Patients with T-cell deficiencies should receive cytomegalovirus-negative, irradiated blood products because of the risk of infection and graft-versus-host disease posed by lymphocytes in donor blood (Gaspar et al., 2013). IV immunoglobulin may be administered to provide protection until humoral immunity can be established. Consider hematopoietic stem cell transplantation if T-cell function cannot be restored by other methods. Biologic therapies also show promise (see **Box 8–1 ▶▶**).

Nonpharmacologic Therapy

Gene transfer appears promising, and long-term observation of patients suggests that this therapy is safe and effective.

Medications
Immunity

CLASSIFICATION AND DRUG EXAMPLES	MECHANISMS OF ACTION	NURSING CONSIDERATIONS
Antibiotics Aminoglycosides Macrolides Tetracyclines Cephalosporins Penicillins Sulfonamides **Drug examples:** Cefaclor, erythromycin, penicillin, tobramycin	Antibiotics may be used prophylactically to prevent infection or to treat existing bacterial infection in patients who are immunodeficient. Specific antibiotics are chosen based on the infection-causing pathogen. **May also be used for:** ■ Treatment of *Staphylococcus* infections ■ Prophylaxis for ophthalmia neonatorum	■ Teach patients the importance of taking the entire prescribed amount. ■ Encourage adequate fluid intake. ■ Monitor for signs of allergic reaction. ■ Assess renal and hepatic function and vital signs. ■ Advise against chewing or crushing tablets.
Anti-inflammatories NSAIDs Corticosteroids **Drug examples:** Aspirin, ibuprofen, naproxen, oxaprozin, prednisone, hydrocortisone, methylprednisolone	Anti-inflammatories may be used to manage pain and swelling common with immune function alterations. NSAIDs block prostaglandin synthesis that leads to inflammation; corticosteroids modify immune response to various stimuli. **May also be used for:** ■ Treatment of fever ■ Prophylaxis for stroke and heart attack	■ Monitor for signs of allergic reaction and renal problems. ■ Encourage patients to take with a full glass of water, milk, or small snack to avoid GI distress. ■ Assess for blood-clotting problems. ■ Advise against abrupt discontinuation of drugs.
Immunizations **Drug examples:** Haemophilus b conjugate vaccine, hepatitis A vaccine, meningococcal diphtheria toxoid conjugate, bacillus Calmette-Guérin vaccine, herpes zoster vaccine live	Immunizations may be used to provide active or passive immunity to patients with a likelihood of contracting certain illnesses due to immunodeficiency. **May also be used for:** ■ Prophylaxis against infectious disease in the general population	Review specific immunization recommendations for immunodeficiency. ■ Assess for hypersensitivity to the vaccine and its components. ■ Evaluate for advanced immunodeficiency. ■ Monitor for vaccine reaction.

Source: Data from Adams, M. P., Holland, L. N., & Urban, C. (2017). *Pharmacology for nurses: A pathophysiologic approach* (5th ed.). Hoboken, NJ: Pearson Education.

Box 8–1
Targeted Biologic Therapies

The use of biologic therapies as adjunct to disease-modifying antirheumatic drugs (DMARDs) is rapidly expanding because of their efficacy and safety (Ding & Gordon, 2013; Rosman, Shoenfeld, & Zandman-Goddard, 2013). Targeted therapy use with autoimmune diseases is also growing because these therapies are generally well tolerated. The major targets of most biologic therapies are cytokines, B cells, and co-stimulation molecules: some are useful in treatment of more than one disease, whereas others are disease-specific. The availability of various biological therapies allows their use to be tailored to the needs of the individual patient. Biological and targeted therapies have not been widely used as first-line treatment because of the increased cost, inconvenience of IV administration, and adverse events. However, recent phase III clinical trials have given way to new advances in biological therapy, enabling self-administration, which substantially decreases delivery costs, and promoting the extension of this therapy to additional conditions (Ward & Bodmer, 2014). Examples of biological agents approved for use in autoimmune disease in the United States include infliximab (Remicade), etanercept (Enbrel), adalimumab (Humira), and abatacept (Orencia).

The majority of patients experience improved immune function and quality of life (Bersenev & Levine, 2012).

Complementary Health Approaches

Many patients with immune disorders have begun trying complementary health approaches to relieve symptoms. Individuals with HIV may use acupuncture to alleviate symptoms such as fatigue, insomnia, and night sweats, and to minimize side effects of antiretroviral mediations. Some have also found it beneficial in relieving peripheral neuropathy (University of Maryland Medical Center, 2016). Research related to the benefits of complementary health approaches such as dietary supplements, mind and body practices, and acupuncture for treating conditions like RA is limited. These may be more beneficial as integrative health therapies, used as part of the overall treatment plan along with pharmacologic and other therapies (National Center for Complementary and Integrative Health, 2016b).

Integrative health therapies designed to bolster the immune system are of particular interest. These therapies seek to increase antibody production or improve other areas of the immune response; this kind of therapy is sometimes referred to as *immune stimulation*. For example, vitamin A, C, D, and E regimens and plant-based therapies have all been studied for their efficacy as immune stimulants and have shown varying degrees of effectiveness in the treatment of asthma and inflammatory diseases (National Center for Complementary and Integrative Health, 2016a).

Some of the available complementary health approaches have undergone careful evaluation and have been found to be safe and effective while others have been found to be ineffective or potentially harmful. Not as much information is known about many of the complementary health approaches, and research in these areas is slower because of regulatory issues; timing; funding; and difficulties finding institutions, unbiased subjects, and researchers to participate in the studies (National Institutes of Health, National Institute on Aging, 2015).

Lifespan Considerations

The immune system changes with age. At birth, the immune system of newborns is not fully developed; however, some antibodies are present because they crossed the placenta from the mother during pregnancy. They protect newborns against infections until their own immune system becomes fully developed. Breast milk also contains antibodies from the mother, and newborns who are breastfed can receive antibodies in this manner. The immune system becomes less effective with age. The ability to distinguish self from non-self decreases, and autoimmune disorders become more common. The ability of macrophages, T cells, and leukocytes to respond quickly to and defend against antigens decreases, contributing to the greater susceptibility of older adults to certain infections and cancers (Delves, 2014).

Considerations for Infants and Children

Immune system development is a complex and multifactorial process. Early in utero experiences, environmental exposures after birth, and other factors influence this important feedback system. While the immune system protects children from harmful diseases, it also can lead to conditions such as asthma, food allergies, or skin atopy.

Infants and children have differing amounts of some immunoglobulins. IgG is the only immunoglobulin that crosses the placenta; as a result, a newborn's levels are similar to those of the mother. This maternal IgG disappears by 6–8 months of age. The infant's IgG level then increases gradually, until mature levels are reached at 7–8 years. IgM levels are low at birth, rise markedly at 1 week of age, and then continue to increase until adult levels are reached at about 1 year. IgA and IgE are not present at birth. Manufacture of these immunoglobulins begins by 2 weeks of age; however, normal values are not achieved until 6–7 years. Thus, it is easy to see why children under 6 years of age become ill so often: They do not have a full complement of immunoglobulins.

In contrast, cell-mediated immunity achieves full function early in life. Early in fetal life, the thymus begins producing T cells, and by birth many of these cells are present. After puberty is reached, the thymus begins to slowly shrink and becomes replaced by fat. By puberty, all the T cells an individual will need have been produced (Sargis, 2014). Other lymphoid tissues, such as the spleen and tonsils, also are comparatively large in young children. Because of well-developed cellular immunity, any blood infused into newborns generally is irradiated to prevent **graft-versus-host disease** (a series of immunologic reactions in response to transplanted cells) as a result of transfused lymphocytes (see **Figure 8–7 »**).

Newborns are the most prone to development of infection, particularly when they are born prematurely, because they have lower levels of their own immune protections as well as fewer antibodies (IgG) obtained from the mother because these antibodies do not cross the placenta until late in pregnancy (Delves, 2015). Newborns have been found to have comparable to higher percentages of NK cells in their peripheral blood than older adults; however, evidence has suggested that there is an impaired ability of these NK cells to adhere to

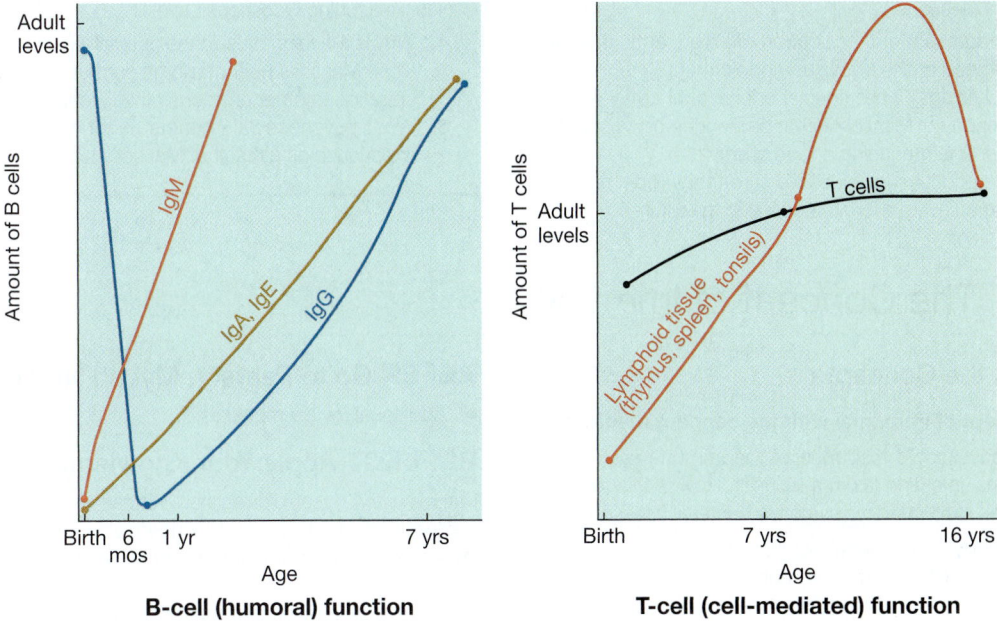

Figure 8–7 ›› Different types of immunoglobulins mature at different times throughout childhood. Children have high levels of some types of immunoglobulins, whereas the levels of other types may be low at certain periods during development.

their target cells (Lee & Lin, 2013). Nurses play an important role by following infection-control practices with newborns and promptly identifying infections in children of all ages.

Considerations for Adolescents

The immune system is constantly maturing during the adolescent period. Studies have found that adolescents who use marijuana may cause serious long-term damage to their immune systems. This damage may result in the development of chronic inflammatory and autoimmune diseases such as inflammatory bowel disease, multiple sclerosis, and RA during adulthood (Federation of American Societies for Experimental Biology, 2014).

Considerations for Pregnant Women

During pregnancy, the immune system experiences a brief decline in maternal cell-mediated immunity in order to prevent rejection of the fetus while also maintaining sufficient maternal host defense mechanisms to fight infection (Brazão et al., 2015). A study by the Cincinnati Children's Hospital Medical Center (2015) further supports this by suggesting that pregnant women are especially susceptible to infection because their immune system is performing a delicate balancing act of sustaining protection against infection while trying not to harm the fetus from overreactive immune responses.

This immune system "balancing act" is what places pregnant women at greater risk for developing viral and bacterial infections. For this reason, women who are considering becoming pregnant and those who are pregnant must be up to date on their immunizations. Some immunizations, such as influenza, pertussis, and hepatitis B, can and should be given during pregnancy if necessary. The influenza virus is especially dangerous to pregnant women because of the changes in their immune system. A study by Stanford University offers persuasive data that this is not due to immune suppression, but to a strong immune reaction. These results strengthen the argument for pregnant women receiving the influenza vaccine (Sanders, 2014).

Considerations for Older Adults

Although in some older adults the immune system is as effective as in younger individuals, normal changes associated with aging demonstrate a decrease in immune response and lowered resistance to infection, with poor response to immunizations. T cells are less responsive to antigens, while B cells produce fewer antibodies. Immune system changes may precipitate insulin resistance, and the hypersensitivity response is reduced or delayed.

Because the antibody response to foreign antigens is diminished in older adults, autoantibodies (antibodies that react to the patient's own tissues) are more common. Immunologic theories of aging propose that a decrease in immune function may result in an increase in autoimmune responses, causing the body to produce antibodies that attack the body itself.

Case Study ›› Part 3

Marisol Jimenez has been hospitalized for 2 days. Within 2 hours of receiving IM and aerosolized epinephrine, aerosolized albuterol, and corticosteroids, she was removed from the CPAP. She has experienced no further reactions to her exposure, her airways are no longer swollen, and she is maintaining oxygen saturation of 95% without supplemental oxygenation.

You are preparing Marisol and her mother for discharge. Discharge instructions include a self-injectable form of epinephrine, or EpiPen. You explain that the pen should be used immediately to inject epinephrine into Marisol's thigh muscle if she experiences an anaphylactic episode. Marisol should keep the pen with her at all times and should understand how and when to use it. Ms. Jimenez should inform school officials, including Marisol's teachers and the school nurse, about Marisol's allergy and the fact that she has the EpiPen. Marisol will be followed at home by her allergist. She has a follow-up appointment scheduled in 1 week.

Clinical Reasoning Questions Level I

1. What additional patient education do you anticipate Ms. Jimenez will need at the follow-up appointment?
2. Because of her age, what special educational considerations should be made for Marisol? What challenges do you foresee for a child her age managing a food allergy?
3. What are the priorities for Marisol's care that will decrease her risk of having a severe allergic reaction in the future?

Clinical Reasoning Questions Level II

4. Why is the thigh muscle the optimal injection site for the EpiPen?
5. Does Marisol's peanut allergy put her at increased risk for sensitization to other allergens? If so, which ones?
6. What psychosocial impacts might Marisol and Ms. Jimenez experience as a result of Marisol's allergy?

REVIEW The Concept of Immunity

RELATE Link the Concepts

Linking the concept of immunity with the concept of infection:

1. Describe the physiologic response of the immune system to a localized bacterial infection (as in a wound). How is this response different from the response to a systemic bacterial infection?
2. How does the body's immune response to the first exposure to an infectious disease differ from its immune response to a second exposure to that disease? What is the reason for this difference?

Linking the concept of immunity with the concept of development:

3. You are caring for a 4-year-old who was just diagnosed with a type I hypersensitivity to shellfish after experiencing an anaphylactic reaction. How can you explain her condition to her in a developmentally appropriate way? How would your explanation be different if she was 8 years old? If she was 12 years old?
4. What aspects of psychologic and psychosocial development should you consider when explaining age-related changes in the immune system to a patient in his 60s?

READY Go to Volume 3: Clinical Nursing Skills

- SKILL 1.8   Respirations: Newborn, Infant, Child, Adult, Obtaining
- SKILL 1.23   Nose and Sinuses: Assessing
- SKILL 1.25   Skin: Assessing
- SKILL 1.27   Thorax and Lungs: Assessing
- SKILL 2.31   Injection, Intramuscular: Administering
- SKILL 2.32   Injection, Subcutaneous: Administering
- SKILL 3.1   Pain in Newborn, Infant, Child, or Adult: Assessing
- SKILL 3.3   Pain Relief: Complementary Health Approaches
- SKILL 3.8   Dry Cold: Applying
- SKILL 3.9   Dry Heat: Applying
- SKILL 9.2   Range-of-Motion Exercises: Assisting
- SKILL 10.5   Nutrition: Assessing

REFER Go to Pearson MyLab Nursing and eText

- Additional review materials

REFLECT Apply Your Knowledge

Patricia is a 42-year-old registered nurse working in a large, southern California medical center. The hospital is located in an area with a large population of immigrants from Southeast Asia, and she has cared for many of these patients on the medical unit during her 12 years of employment at the facility.

Patricia recently transferred from the medical unit to the facility's home health agency to work with patients in hospice. Patricia lost her mother to breast cancer approximately 6 months earlier. She has been hoping to have a more regular schedule that will allow her to spend more time with her teenage son. During the same time as her mother's death, her husband was "downsized" from his position as an aerospace engineer. It was a difficult time for the entire family. Patricia tried to compensate for all that was occurring in their lives. Not only was she trying to deal with the loss of her mother and give attention to her father, husband, and son, but she was also trying to perform well in her new job and work extra hours to help with their financial shortcomings.

In late November, Patricia developed a cold that progressed to bronchitis and seemed to hang on forever. She was often awake at night either coughing or having drenching night sweats. In March, she finally went to her primary care provider to have her condition assessed.

Tests confirmed that Patricia had developed tuberculosis (TB), and she was started on the appropriate medication. She was shocked by this diagnosis and embarrassed to tell anyone because, how could she, a nurse who should know universal precautions technique, develop a contagious disease?

1. What modifiable risk factor in Patricia's recent history could have contributed to her development of tuberculosis? Explain.
2. Why did Patricia not develop tuberculosis after her initial exposure? Explain.
3. What independent nursing interventions would be appropriate for you to initiate?

≫ Exemplar 8.A
HIV/AIDS

Exemplar Learning Outcomes

8.A Analyze HIV/AIDS as they relate to Immunity.

- Describe the pathophysiology of HIV/AIDS.
- Describe the etiology of HIV/AIDS.
- Compare the risk factors and prevention of HIV/AIDS.

- Identify the clinical manifestations of HIV/AIDS.
- Summarize diagnostic tests and therapies used by interprofessional teams in the collaborative care of an individual with HIV/AIDS.
- Differentiate care of patients with HIV/AIDS across the lifespan.
- Apply the nursing process in providing culturally competent care to an individual with HIV/AIDS.

Overview

In 1981, five cases of *Pneumocystis carinii* pneumonia (PCP) and 26 cases of a rare cancer, Kaposi sarcoma, were diagnosed in young, previously healthy gay men in Los Angeles and New York City. The term **acquired immunodeficiency syndrome (AIDS)** was given to this new phenomenon to describe the immune system deficits associated with these opportunistic disorders. Before this time, both PCP and Kaposi sarcoma had been seen only in older adults, patients who were debilitated, or those with severe immunodeficiency.

Research to identify the cause of this apparently new disease progressed feverishly, and in 1983 a common antibody was identified in patients with AIDS. In 1984, the **human immunodeficiency virus (HIV)**, a retrovirus (meaning that it carries its genetic information in RNA) that is transmitted by direct contact with infected blood and body fluids, was isolated. It then became apparent that the chronic disease known as AIDS was the final, fatal stage of infection with HIV, transmitted via sexual contact with carriers of the infection (CDC, 2015s).

HIV is an example of an emerging infectious agent that jumped from animal to human, probably in the 1950s. The widespread organ involvement associated with the infection has caused much human suffering and death. Like so many previous **epidemics** (widespread outbreaks of infectious disease with many infected people), the HIV/AIDS epidemic began with a few isolated cases and has now become a worldwide concern. See the accompanying Focus on Diversity and Culture feature. The virus invaded modern life in ways not previously imagined—testing scientific knowledge, probing private values, and eluding a vaccine or a cure.

Focus on Diversity and Culture
HIV/AIDS

An estimated 36.9 million people are infected with HIV/AIDS worldwide, with virtually every country in the world reporting cases of HIV/AIDS (CDC, 2015h; WHO, 2015). The highest incidence is found in the regions of Africa, Southeast and Central Asia, the Americas, and Eastern Europe. Other regions significantly affected by HIV/AIDS include the Pacific, Latin America, and the Caribbean. Approximately 70% of all people who are infected with HIV or who have AIDS live in the African region. The most common mode of transmission globally is heterosexual intercourse. The co-occurring factors of general health status, presence of other sexually transmitted diseases, and number of sexual partners correlate with incidence (CDC, 2015t; WHO, 2016).

Since its first appearance, progression of HIV-positive status to AIDS has slowed, because of the effectiveness of **antiretroviral therapy (ART)**, which combines the administration of at least three medications that inhibit HIV replication (CDC, 2016c; World Health Organization [WHO], 2013a). The change these medications have caused in HIV's progression to AIDS makes monitoring of AIDS less useful as an indicator of infected cases. For this reason, the CDC has developed new surveillance methods based on infection rates in high-risk populations.

Pathophysiology and Etiology
Pathophysiology

AIDS is caused by HIV (specifically, HIV-1), which destroys the body's ability to fight infection. Significant concentrations of the virus are present in blood, semen, preseminal fluid, rectal fluid, vaginal and cervical secretions, and cerebrospinal fluid of infected individuals. The virus is also found in breast milk and saliva. Sexual contact is the primary mode of transmission. However, HIV also can be transmitted through contact with infected blood via needle sharing during drug injection. Before mandatory screening of blood and blood products was instituted in 1985, some individuals received HIV through transfusions of infected blood. Today, rigorous testing of the U.S. blood supply has made transmission via transfusion extremely rare (CDC, 2015r).

On entry into the body, the HIV virus infects cells that have the CD4 antigen. Once inside the cell, the virus sheds its protein coat and uses an enzyme called *reverse transcriptase* to convert the viral RNA to DNA. This viral DNA is then integrated into host cell DNA and duplicated during normal processes of cell division. Within the cell, the virus may remain latent or become activated to produce new RNA and to form **virions** (virus particles that are unable to grow and reproduce outside a host cell). The virus then buds from the cell surface, disrupting its cell membrane and leading to destruction of the host cell.

Although the virus may remain inactive in infected cells for years, antibodies are produced to its proteins, a process known as **seroconversion**. The antibodies usually are detectable 6 weeks to 6 months after the initial infection. Although helper T or CD4 cells are the primary cells infected by HIV, the virus also infects macrophages and certain cells of the central nervous system (CNS). **Helper T cells** play a vital role in normal function of the immune system, recognizing foreign antigens and infected cells and activating antibody-producing B cells. They also direct cell-mediated immune activity and influence the phagocytic activity of monocytes and macrophages. The loss of these helper T cells leads to

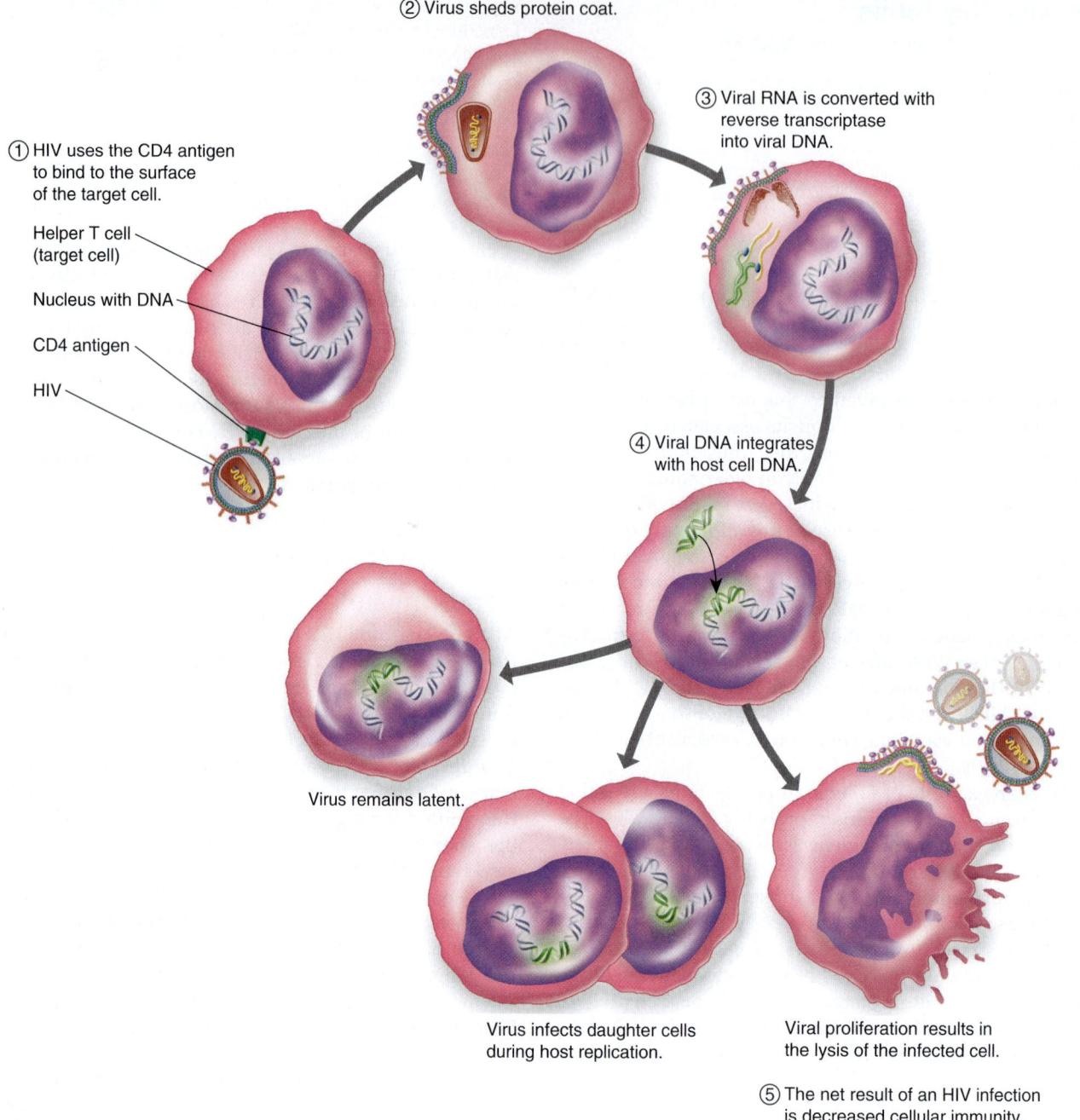

② Virus sheds protein coat.

③ Viral RNA is converted with reverse transcriptase into viral DNA.

① HIV uses the CD4 antigen to bind to the surface of the target cell.

Helper T cell (target cell)

Nucleus with DNA

CD4 antigen

HIV

④ Viral DNA integrates with host cell DNA.

Virus remains latent.

Virus infects daughter cells during host replication.

Viral proliferation results in the lysis of the infected cell.

⑤ The net result of an HIV infection is decreased cellular immunity.

Figure 8–8 》 The HIV virus gains entry into helper T cells, uses the cell DNA to replicate, interferes with normal function of the T cells, and destroys the normal cells.

the immunodeficiencies seen with HIV infection (Porth & Grossman, 2013). **Figure 8–8 》** illustrates the typical course of HIV infection.

Etiology

HIV carries a significant impact in the United States. According to the CDC, 1.2 million people in the United States age 13 years and older were living with HIV at the end of 2016, and 1 in 8 patients did not know their HIV-positive status yet (AIDS.gov, 2016a). In 2014, an estimated 44,073 new cases of HIV/AIDS were diagnosed in the United States with confidential name-based reporting (CDC, 2015n). Men still make

up the majority of infected individuals; women account for approximately 23% (CDC, 2015h). The major transmission categories are identified in **Figure 8–9 》**. Among women, the majority of HIV infections result from heterosexual contact. African American and Hispanic women accounted for 79% of all new female HIV cases in 2010 (CDC, 2015q; 2015v). Transgender individuals are among those at highest risk for acquiring HIV infection (CDC, 2015u).

Current trends of which nurses should be aware include the following:

- Among risk groups, the most rapid increases in recent years have been noted in young gay and bisexual men,

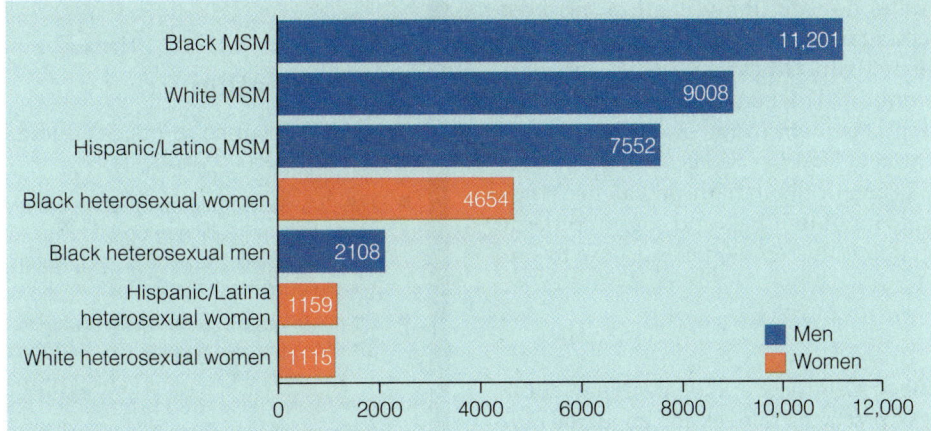

Source: Data from Centers for Disease Control and Prevention. (2015). *HIV in the United States: At a glance.* Retrieved from http://www.cdc.gov/hiv/statistics/overview/ataglance.html

Figure 8–9 》 Estimated new HIV diagnoses in the United States for the most-affected populations, 2014.
MSM = men who have sex with men.

followed by women and inner-city injection drug users, especially African Americans and Hispanics (AIDS.gov, 2016a).

- The rapid increase of AIDS cases among women is of special concern; those numbers increased from 7% of cases in 1985 to 20% of newly reported cases in 2013; a decrease of 3% since 2009 (CDC, 2015q).

- The rates of infection have decreased by 90% for children under 13 years, thanks to improved interventions during the perinatal period (CDC, 2015f). However, the number of cases in children older than 13 remains a concern because of the increasingly early age of sexual initiation, the prevalence of substance abuse, and that age group's general lack of awareness of the risks associated with HIV/AIDS.

- The number of patients age 50 and older with HIV/AIDS has been increasing in recent years. In 2013, the most recent year for which the CDC has statistics, 21% of new HIV/AIDS diagnoses occurred in this age group. In addition, 44% of people living with AIDS were 50–54 years old, a significant increase from 2001, when only 17% of affected individuals were in this group. One major reason for this increase is the effectiveness of ART (antiretroviral therapy), which has increased the life expectancy of patients with HIV (CDC, 2015i).

- Current research suggests the possibility of developing a "functional cure" for patients with HIV. A functional cure theoretically would suppress viral replication to the point where the symptoms go into remission, even without complete eradication of the virus. Additional research is needed to establish the viability of this emerging treatment approach (Vanham & Van Gulck, 2012).

Risk Factors

The risk factors for HIV infection are primarily behavioral, such as having sex without a condom or sharing needles or injection drug use equipment with others. Other risk factors involve hemophilia and blood transfusions, healthcare

as an occupation, poverty, pregnancy and breastfeeding, and older age.

Among adults in the United States, 83% of reported cases are in men who have sex with other men (AIDS.gov, 2016a). Unprotected anal intercourse is the major route of transmission in these cases (CDC, 2015l). Illegal drug use is another risk factor, due to sharing of needles and drug paraphernalia and to the increased likelihood of impaired judgment and risky sexual behaviors while under the influence of drugs (CDC, 2015k). Heterosexual intercourse with an infected partner and injection drug use are major risk factors for women (CDC, 2015t).

Current blood-screening methods use antibody testing, and the small risk of HIV transmission through blood supplies arises from donors in the so-called window period between contracting the virus and the development of detectable antibodies (CDC, 2015t). This window period usually lasts from 6 weeks to 6 months; in rare cases, it lasts up to 1 year. Those in the window period are able to transmit HIV to others even though they do not yet test positive for HIV.

A small but real occupational risk exists for healthcare workers. Percutaneous exposure to infected blood or body fluids through a needlestick injury or nonintact skin is the primary route of transmission. Documented evidence indicates that parenteral exposure poses less than a 1% risk of becoming HIV-positive (CDC, 2015a). Mucosal exposures, such as splashing in the eyes or mouth, pose a much smaller risk.

Findings show no significant differences in HIV prevalence by race or ethnicity among low-income urban populations. This finding is surprising considering the racial and ethnic disparities that characterize the U.S. HIV/AIDS epidemic in general (CDC, 2015h).

Prevention

Preventing AIDS involves preventing new cases of HIV infection, as well as treating opportunistic infections in patients diagnosed with HIV to stop conversion of the virus to AIDS. To date, no safe immunization has been developed to protect against HIV infection. Education, counseling, and behavior modification are the primary tools for AIDS prevention. The benefit of education and behavior modification is evident in the gay male population. The incidence of new HIV infections within this population has declined dramatically in high-prevalence cities. Nurses play a vital role for individuals and communities in providing education about this epidemic and how to prevent infection.

Education

Nurses should educate sexually active adolescents and adults about the importance of practicing safe sex and about the ramifications of high-risk sexual behaviors and injecting drugs. In fact, all sexually active individuals need to know how HIV is spread and how to practice safer sex (see the Patient Teaching feature). For guidelines on safer sex, see the section on Responsible Sexual Behaviors in the module on Sexuality.

When possible, nurses provide education regarding the use of autologous transfusion (using the blood patients themselves donate before an anticipated surgery). Seeking donations from family members is not encouraged for several reasons. Family members may have engaged in high-risk behaviors but lie about their risk because of embarrassment or fear of discovery. Furthermore, the family member may have a different blood type or other contraindications to transfusion.

Patients who are HIV-positive should refrain from donating blood, organs, or sperm. They should understand the tactics used to avoid exchange of body fluids: not sharing needles or other drug paraphernalia, not sharing razors, and not getting a tattoo. Stress the importance of informing all medical personnel providing direct care (especially anyone performing a dental, surgical, or obstetric procedure) about the diagnosis.

Patient Teaching
HIV Prevention

Patient education should include the following to help patients reduce their risk of contracting HIV:

- The only *totally* safe sex practices are no sex (abstinence); long-term, mutually monogamous sexual relations between two uninfected individuals; and mutual masturbation without direct contact.

- Do not engage in unprotected sex, especially if the HIV status of the partner is unknown. Condoms must be used with every sexual encounter involving vaginal, oral, or anal intercourse; they also need to be applied and removed properly. A female condom also is available for use.

- Injection drug users should never share needles, syringes, or other drug paraphernalia. Use sterile supplies from needle-exchange programs. A fresh solution of household bleach and water in a 1:10 ratio is effective to clean paraphernalia when sterile supplies are not available.

Standard Precautions

Healthcare workers can prevent most exposures to HIV by using standard precautions. With standard precautions, healthcare professionals treat all patients alike, eliminating the need to know patients' HIV status. Treat all high-risk body fluids as if they are infectious, and use barrier precautions to prevent skin, mucous membrane, or percutaneous exposure to these fluids. Also follow standard precautions when caring for newborns of mothers who are HIV-positive, as the status of the infant's blood is not known until after discharge. **Table 8–3 »** outlines issues for caregivers of infants who are at risk for HIV/AIDS. More information about standard precautions can be found in the module on Infection.

TABLE 8–3 Issues for Caregivers of Infants at Risk for HIV/AIDS

Resuscitation	For suctioning use a bulb syringe, mucus extractor, or meconium aspirator with wall suction on low setting. Use masks, goggles, and gloves.
Admission care	Remove blood from baby's skin as soon as possible after admission; give a warm water–mild soap bath using gloves.
Hand washing	Wash hands thoroughly before and after caring for the infant. Wash hands immediately if they come in contact with blood or body fluids. Wash hands after removal of gloves.
Gloves	Wear gloves during all diaper changes and examinations of the baby, especially when it is necessary to touch blood or other high-risk fluids. Also wear gloves when handling newborns before and during their initial baths, cord care, eye prophylactics, and vitamin K administration.
Mask, goggle, and gown	These are not routinely needed unless it is necessary to come into contact with placenta or the blood and amniotic fluid on the skin of the newborn.
Needles and syringes	Do not recap or bend used needles; dispose of them in a puncture-resistant plastic container belonging specifically to that baby. After the newborn is discharged discard the container.
Specimens	Double-bag blood and other specimens and/or seal them in an impervious container and label them according to agency protocol.
Equipment and linen	Discard articles contaminated with blood or body fluids or bag them according to isolation or facility protocol.
Body fluid spills	Clean blood and body fluid spills promptly with a solution of 5.25% sodium hypochlorite (household bleach) diluted 1:10 with water. Apply for at least 30 seconds, then wipe after the minimum contact time.
Exempted personnel	Staff who are immunologically compromised (pregnant women may be included in this group) and who are possibly infectious should not care for these infants.

Sources: Based on American Academy of Pediatrics, Committee on Pediatric AIDS and Committee on Infectious Diseases. (1999). Issues related to human immuno-deficiency transmission in schools, child care, medical settings, the home, and community. *Pediatrics, 104*(2), 318–324; Calles, N. R., & Cazacu, A. C. (2010). *Standard precautions and HIV post exposure prophylaxis in the healthcare setting in HIV curriculum for the healthcare professional* (pp. 128–137). Retrieved from http://www.bipai.org/HIV-curriculum/; Centers for Disease Control and Prevention (2011). *Human immunodeficiency virus in healthcare settings.* Retrieved from http://www.cdc.gov/HAI/organisms/hiv/hiv.html

Pre-exposure Prophylaxis (PrEP)

Pre-exposure prophylaxis is a treatment approach that allows individuals who are currently HIV negative but at high risk for becoming infected with HIV, to reduce their risk of HIV infection by taking one pill every day. Truvada (a combination of tenofovir and emtricitabine) is the current drug of choice for PrEP therapy, having greater than 90% efficacy when taken daily, and is an even more powerful prevention tool when combined with the use of condoms and other prevention methods. Truvada works by blocking important pathways that HIV uses to set up an infection. Everyone does not qualify for the use of PrEP. Federal guidelines recommend that PrEP be considered for individuals who are HIV-negative and at very high risk for becoming infected with HIV, including men who have sex with both men and women, a heterosexual man or woman who does not regularly use condoms during sex with high-risk partners of unknown HIV status, or individuals not in mutually monogamous relationships with partners who recently tested HIV-negative. This medication can be prescribed only by a healthcare provider, and patients need to be instructed that they must take it as directed for it to be effective (HIV/AIDS Basics, 2016).

Postexposure Prophylaxis

Healthcare workers exposed to HIV infection or adults who experience a high-risk exposure to HIV may choose postexposure prophylaxis (PEP). Risk of exposure for healthcare workers may be through needlesticks or cuts with a sharp object or contact with mucous membranes or nonintact skin; semen; vaginal secretions; fluids contaminated with visible blood; cerebrospinal fluid; synovial fluid; and pleural, peritoneal, pericardial, or amniotic fluids.

PEP needs to begin within 72 hours of an exposure and consists of two to three antiretroviral medications that must be taken for 28 days. The healthcare provider will determine the medications to be used for treatment based on how the individual was exposed to HIV. Follow-up appointments and additional HIV testing are required (AIDS.gov, 2015; CDC, 2016a).

>> **Stay Current:** For up-to-date information on HIV/AIDS prevention, go to the Centers for Disease Control and Prevention at http://www.cdc.gov/hiv/guidelines and Aids.gov at https://www.aids.gov/hiv-aids-basics/index.html

Clinical Manifestations

The clinical manifestations of HIV infection range from no symptoms at all to severe immunodeficiency with multiple opportunistic infections and cancers. The majority of patients develop an acute, mononucleosis-type illness within days to weeks after contracting the virus. Typical manifestations include fever, sore throat, arthralgias and myalgias, headache, rash, and lymphadenopathy. The patient also may experience nausea, vomiting, and abdominal cramping. Patients often attribute this initial manifestation of HIV infection to a common viral illness, such as influenza, upper respiratory infection, or stomach virus. Pathologic changes also are noted in the CNS of many individuals who are infected, although the mechanism of neurologic dysfunction is unclear.

Following this acute illness, patients enter a long-lasting, asymptomatic period. Although the virus is present and can be transmitted to others, the individual who is infected has few or no symptoms. The majority of individuals who are infected with HIV are in this stage of the disease. The length of the asymptomatic period varies widely, but its mean duration is estimated to be 8–10 years.

Some patients with few other symptoms following HIV infection develop persistent generalized lymphadenopathy, defined as enlargement of two or more lymph nodes outside the inguinal chain, with no other illness or condition to account for the lymphadenopathy.

The move from asymptomatic disease or persistent lymphadenopathy to AIDS often is not clearly defined. The patient may complain of general malaise, fever, fatigue, night sweats, and involuntary weight loss. Persistent skin dryness and rash may be a problem. Diarrhea is common, as are oral lesions, such as hairy leukoplakia, candidiasis, and gingival inflammation and ulceration. The development of advanced HIV occurs between 10 and 15 years after initial infection; the length of time varies according to the viral load, rate of disease progression, and development of resistance to antiretroviral therapy (WHO, 2013a).

Characteristic manifestations of AIDS are the development of significant constitutional disease, neurologic manifestations, or opportunistic infections or cancers. At this stage, the patient has a very poor prognosis. HIV/AIDS may be classified using either the CDC's disease staging system or the WHO's Clinical Staging and Disease Classification System (see **Box 8–2** >>). The CDC's staging system assesses the severity of HIV disease by CD4 cell counts and the presence of specific HIV-related conditions. In contrast, the WHO's Classification System can be used in situations with limited resources when access to CD4 cell count measurements or other diagnostic testing methods may not be available. HIV infection may be classified in one of four infection stages (stage 1, stage 2, stage 3, and stage 4). Stages are defined by the severity of infection as determined by T-lymphocyte count, percentage of total lymphocytes, or the presence of an AIDS-defining condition. When T-lymphocyte counts fall below $200/mm^3$, T-lymphocyte percentage falls below 14%, or an AIDS-defining condition is documented, the patient has stage 3 HIV, or AIDS (Guide for HIV/AIDS Clinical Care, 2014a).

AIDS dementia complex is the most common cause of changes in mental status for patients with HIV infection. This dementia results from a direct effect of the virus on the brain and affects cognitive, motor, and behavioral functioning. Fluctuating memory loss, confusion, difficulty concentrating, lethargy, and diminished motor speed are typical manifestations of AIDS dementia complex. Patients become apathetic, losing interest in work as well as social and recreational activities. As the complex progresses, the patient develops severe dementia with motor disturbances such as ataxia, tremor, spasticity, incontinence, and paraplegia (Porth & Grossman, 2013; University of California, 2016).

Infections and lesions that are common in patients with AIDS also may affect the CNS. **Toxoplasmosis** and non-Hodgkin lymphoma are space-occupying lesions that may cause headache, altered mental status, and neurologic deficits. Cryptococcal meningitis and cytomegalovirus infection

Box 8–2
Clinical Staging of Adult HIV Infection

HIV Infection, Clinical Stage 1 (Acute)

- Asymptomatic or persistent generalized lymphadenopathy
- Lack of an AIDS-defining condition and either a CD4+ T-lymphocyte count higher than 500/mm^3 or a percentage of total lymphocytes of more than 29%
- Greatest risk of transmission

HIV Infection, Clinical Stage 2 (Chronic/Latency)

- Virus present but may not be producing symptoms
- Lack of an AIDS-defining condition and either CD4+ T-lymphocyte count between 200 and 499/mm^3 or a percentage of total lymphocytes between 14% and 28%
- Moderate unexplained weight loss (less than 10% of presumed or measured body weight)
- Recurrent respiratory infections (sinusitis, tonsillitis, otitis media, and pharyngitis)
- Herpes zoster
- Recurrent oral ulceration
- Papular pruritic eruptions
- Seborrheic dermatitis
- Fungal nail infections

HIV Infection, Clinical Stage 3 (AIDS)

- Presence of an AIDS-defining condition (e.g., Kaposi sarcoma, PCP, tuberculosis) or a CD4+ T-lymphocyte count lower than 200/mm^3 or a percentage of total lymphocytes less than 14%
- Unexplained severe weight loss (greater than 10% of presumed or measured body weight)
- Unexplained chronic diarrhea for more than 1 month
- Unexplained persistent fever for more than 1 month (greater than 37.6°C, intermittent or constant)
- Persistent oral candidiasis (thrush)

- Oral hairy leukoplakia
- Pulmonary tuberculosis (current)
- Severe presumed bacterial infections (e.g., pneumonia, bone or joint infection, meningitis)
- Acute necrotizing ulcerative stomatitis, gingivitis, or periodontitis
- Unexplained anemia (hemoglobin less than 8 g/dL)
- Neutropenia (neutrophils less than 500 cells/μL)
- Chronic thrombocytopenia (platelets less than 50,000 cells/μL)

HIV Infection, Clinical Stage 4

- HIV wasting syndrome, as defined by the CDC (involuntary weight loss greater than 10% of baseline body weight associated with either chronic diarrhea for 1 month or more or chronic weakness and documented fever for 1 month or more)
- *Pneumocystis jiroveci* pneumonia
- Recurrent severe bacterial pneumonia
- Chronic herpes simplex infection (orolabial, genital, or anorectal site for more than 1 month or visceral herpes at any site)
- Esophageal candidiasis (or candidiasis of trachea, bronchi, or lungs)
- Extrapulmonary tuberculosis
- Kaposi sarcoma
- Cytomegalovirus infection (retinitis or infection of other organs)
- CNS toxoplasmosis
- HIV encephalopathy
- Progressive multifocal leukoencephalopathy
- Chronic cryptosporidiosis (with diarrhea)
- Lymphoma (cerebral or B-cell non-Hodgkin)
- Invasive cervical carcinoma
- Symptomatic HIV-associated nephropathy
- Symptomatic HIV-associated cardiomyopathy

Source: Based on Guide for HIV/AIDS Clinical Care. (2014a). *HIV classification: CDC and WHO staging systems.* Retrieved from http://aidsetc.org/guide/hiv-classification

also are common in patients with AIDS. CNS complications have declined with the use of ART (AIDS.gov, 2016a).

Peripheral nervous system manifestations also are common in patients infected with HIV. Sensory neuropathies manifesting in numbness, tingling, and pain in the lower extremities affect approximately 30% of patients with AIDS. A Guillain-Barré type of inflammatory demyelinating polyneuropathy can occur as well, resulting in progressive weakness and paralysis.

Opportunistic Infections

Opportunistic infections are the most common manifestations of AIDS and often occur simultaneously. The risk of opportunistic infections can be predicted by the patient's T4 or CD4 cell count. The normal CD4 cell count is higher than 1000/mm^3. When the CD4 count falls below 500/mm^3, manifestations of immunodeficiency develop. With a CD4 count of lower than 200/mm^3, opportunistic infections and cancers are likely.

Pneumocystis jiroveci Pneumonia

***Pneumocystis jiroveci* pneumonia (PCP)** (previously called *Pneumocystis carinii* pneumonia) is the most common

opportunistic infection affecting patients with AIDS and is a common cause of death in patients with AIDS. PCP is caused by a common environmental fungus that is not pathogenic in patients with intact immune systems.

The manifestations of PCP are nonspecific and may progress insidiously. Patients often present with fever, cough, dyspnea, tachypnea, and tachycardia. Complaints of mild chest pain also may be present. Breath sounds initially may be normal. With severe disease, the patient may present with cyanosis and significant respiratory distress.

Tuberculosis

Patients with AIDS also may develop tuberculosis. In some patients, active tuberculosis results from reactivation of a previous infection; in others, it is a new, primary disease facilitated by impaired immune function. Rapid progression, diffuse pulmonary infiltrates, and disseminated disease occur more commonly in patients with AIDS. For more information on tuberculosis, see the exemplar in the module on Infection.

Candidiasis

Candida albicans infection, or **candidiasis**, is a common, opportunistic fungal infection in patients with AIDS. It

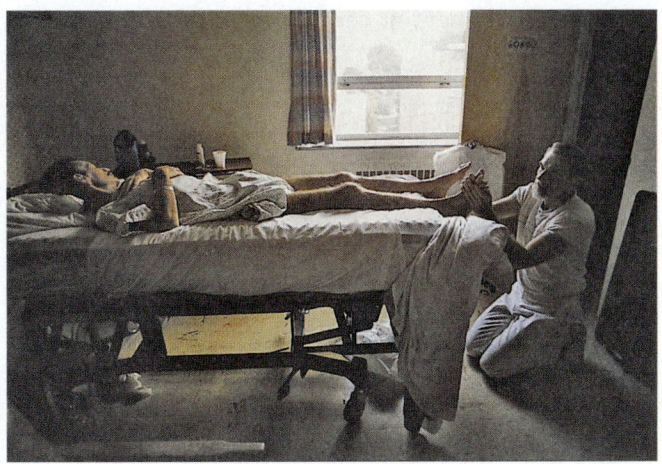

Figure 8–10 ❯❯ Wasting syndrome in a patient with AIDS.

usually manifests as oral thrush or esophagitis. Oral thrush presents as white, friable plaques on the buccal mucosa or tongue and, in the patient with HIV infection, often is the first indication of progression to AIDS. Patients with esophagitis have difficulty swallowing as well as substernal pain or burning that increases with swallowing. In women with AIDS, vaginal candidiasis is frequent and often recurrent.

Mycobacterium avium Complex

Mycobacterium avium complex (MAC) affects many patients with AIDS and typically occurs late in the course of the disease, when CD4 cell counts are less than $50/\text{mm}^3$. MAC is more common in women than in men. It is caused by organisms commonly found in food, water, and soil and is a major cause of "wasting syndrome" in individuals with AIDS (see **Figure 8–10** ❯❯). Manifestations of MAC include chills and fever, weakness, night sweats, abdominal pain and diarrhea, and weight loss. Nearly every organ can be infected, and most people with MAC develop disseminated disease.

Other Infections

Herpesvirus infections are common in patients with AIDS and may be severe. Cytomegalovirus can affect the retina, GI tract, or lungs. Disseminated herpes simplex or herpes zoster infection may occur, although severe mucocutaneous manifestations are more common.

Parasitic infections with *Toxoplasma gondii* and *Cryptococcus neoformans* commonly affect the CNS. Toxoplasmosis occurs as encephalitis or an intracerebral mass lesion. Changes in mental status, focal neurologic signs, and seizures may result. *Cryptococcus* infection may present as either meningitis or disseminated disease, primarily affecting the lungs. *Cryptosporidium*, a protozoan affecting the GI tract, is an important cause of prolonged diarrhea in patients with AIDS. Bacterial salmonella infections also are a relatively common cause of diarrhea.

Women with AIDS have a high incidence of pelvic inflammatory disease (PID). Although the pathogens appear to be the same as those in PID affecting women who are not

infected with HIV, the disease is more severe. Inpatient treatment with IV antibiotics often is necessary.

Secondary Cancers

As cell-mediated immune function declines, the risk of malignancy increases. The CDC classification of AIDS currently includes four cancers: Kaposi sarcoma, two lymphomas (non-Hodgkin lymphoma and primary lymphoma of the brain), and invasive cervical carcinoma.

Kaposi Sarcoma

Often the presenting symptom of AIDS, **Kaposi sarcoma (KS)** remains the most common cancer associated with the disease. KS may progress slowly or rapidly, and it is an indicator of late-stage HIV disease. The average survival time after diagnosis of KS is 18 months.

Kaposi sarcoma is related to a secondary viral infection with the *KS-associated herpesvirus*, also known as *human herpesvirus 8* (HHV-8). This virus appears to be transmitted mainly through sexual contact, although cases have been reported in injection drug users. Men who have sex with men not only have a risk for HIV infection but also have a higher risk for infection with the virus responsible for KS. Women who have sex with these men have a risk for HIV infection and KS as well. Individuals whose immune system is suppressed because they have received an organ transplant also have an increased risk of developing KS (American Cancer Society, 2014).

Arising from the cells that line the lymph or small blood vessels, KS presents as vascular macules, papules, or violet lesions affecting the skin and viscera (see **Figure 8–11** ❯❯). A common site for skin lesions is the face, especially the tip of the nose and pinnae of the ears. Common sites for visceral disease include the GI tract, lungs, and lymphatic system.

The lesions of KS usually are painless initially, but they may become painful as the disease progresses. The tumors may obstruct organ function or cause bleeding. When the lungs are involved, gas exchange may be severely impaired, and the result is pulmonary hemorrhage.

Lymphomas

Lymphomas are malignancies of the lymphoid tissue, including lymphocytes, lymph nodes, and the lymphoid organs such as the spleen and bone marrow. In patients with

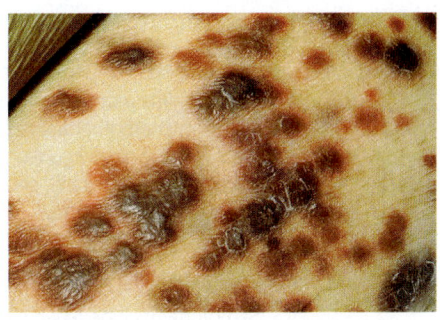

Source: Mediscan/Alamy Stock Photo.

Figure 8–11 ❯❯ Kaposi sarcoma lesions.

AIDS, two lymphomas are common: non-Hodgkin lymphoma (including Burkitt lymphoma) and primary lymphoma of the CNS, which starts in the brain or spinal cord. Hodgkin disease also occurs five times more frequently in patients with HIV infection than in those without it. The CNS is the usual site for these lymphomas, but they also may be found in the bone marrow, GI tract, liver, skin, and mucous membranes. These malignancies are aggressive tumors that grow and spread rapidly. Headache and changes in mental status are common early symptoms of lymphomas affecting the CNS.

Cervical Cancer

Cervical dysplasia is common in women infected with HIV. Cervical cancer develops frequently and tends to be aggressive. Women with concurrent HIV infection and cervical cancer usually die of the cervical cancer, not AIDS. Therefore, it is recommended that women with HIV infection have a Papanicolaou (Pap) smear every 6 months and

aggressive treatment of cervical dysplasia with colposcopy and conization.

Collaboration

Although multiple research studies are under way to identify a cure for HIV/AIDS, no cure is currently available. This fact and the apparent universally fatal nature of the disease make prevention a vital strategy in HIV care.

The goals of care for the patient with HIV infection are early identification of the infection, promotion of health maintenance activities to prolong the asymptomatic period for as long as possible, prevention of opportunistic infections, treatment of disease complications such as cancer, and provision of emotional and psychosocial support.

Diagnostic Tests

Diagnostic testing is used to screen and identify HIV infection as well as to monitor the patient's disease and immune

Clinical Manifestations and Therapies
HIV/AIDS

ETIOLOGY	CLINICAL MANIFESTATIONS	CLINICAL THERAPIES
Opportunistic infections		
Kaposi sarcoma (KS)	KS is the most common AIDS-related cancer and is frequently seen in gay and bisexual men. It usually manifests as red to purple lesions on the skin but also can be found on internal organs, including the lymph nodes, mouth, GI tract, and lungs. The CDC considers this an AIDS-defining condition.	■ Treatment may include liposomal daunorubicin or liposomal doxorubicin. ■ Recombinant human interferon alfa may be used if the patient's CD4 count is less than 200/mm^3. ■ Radiation therapy may also be used.
Cytomegalovirus (CMV)	While 50% of adults are infected with CMV, the normal immune system usually can keep it under control. In patients with AIDS and with ineffective immune systems, CMV can infect the eyes, brain, throat, large intestines, stomach, or spinal cord.	■ Preventive therapy or treatment may include administration of cidofovir, ganciclovir, foscarnet, or fomivirsen. ■ Approximately 10% of patients with CMV have a strain resistant to ganciclovir.
Candidiasis	Candidiasis is the most common HIV-related fungal infection, involving the mucous membranes around the mouth, vagina, esophagus, and skin. It manifests as white bumps, dry mouth, difficulty swallowing, and altered sense of taste. The CDC considers this an AIDS-related complex (ARC) disease.	■ Oral thrush is treated with fluconazole, clotrimazole, ketoconazole, or nystatin. ■ Esophageal candidiasis is treated with fluconazole, ketoconazole, or itraconazole. ■ Vaginal candidiasis is treated with over-the-counter antifungal remedies, clotrimazole, or miconazole.
Aspergillosis	Aspergillosis is a fungal pathogen found in soil and decaying plant life. It is more commonly seen in patients with cancer receiving chemotherapy and patients receiving a transplant but it may be seen in patients with HIV infection. It manifests with cough, chest pain, shortness of breath, facial pain, fever, and night sweats.	■ Treatment may include amphotericin B or itraconazole.
Histoplasmosis	This infection occurs from inhaling the fungus, which infects the lungs, but it can also affect other internal organs. Symptoms include fever, skin lesions, breathing problems, weight loss, and liver enlargement. The CDC considers this an AIDS-defining condition.	■ Clinical trials are under way to study the effect of itraconazole as prophylaxis therapy. ■ Treatment may include amphotericin B or itraconazole and requires long-term maintenance therapy.

Clinical Manifestations and Therapies (continued)

ETIOLOGY	CLINICAL MANIFESTATIONS	CLINICAL THERAPIES
Mycobacterium avium complex	In patients who are not HIV-positive, this infection normally involves only the lungs, but in patients with HIV infection, the disease usually disseminates. It is often seen in patients with late-stage AIDS involving the liver, spleen, and bone marrow. Resulting symptoms include night sweats, fevers, unintentional weight loss, diarrhea, low RBCs and WBCs, elevated alkaline phosphate, and painful intestines.	■ Treatment may include clarithromycin, azithromycin, ethambutol, rifampin, rifabutin, ciprofloxacin, or amikacin.
Tuberculosis (TB)	This infection occurs from contact with patients who are TB-positive and often occurs early in the course of HIV infection, months or years before other opportunistic infections occur. In later stages of HIV infection, TB often infects other organs outside the lungs. Multidrug-resistant TB is of particular concern.	■ Prophylaxis usually is isoniazid. ■ Treatment may include multiple drugs, including some combination of isoniazid, rifampin, pyrazinamide, and ethambutol.
Oral hairy leukoplakia	Oral hairy leukoplakia is often the first opportunistic infection to appear. Symptoms include white lesions on the edges of the tongue caused by Epstein-Barr virus. The infection occurs almost exclusively in men and indicates serious damage to the immune system.	■ Treatment may include acyclovir or topical podophyllin resin.

Neurologic Disorders

ETIOLOGY	CLINICAL MANIFESTATIONS	CLINICAL THERAPIES
AIDS dementia complex	This disorder is caused directly by the HIV infection, but the patient's CNS also can be damaged by opportunistic infections or the toxic effects of drug treatments. Early symptoms include dementia, apathy, and loss of interest in surroundings. Later symptoms involve cognitive and motor problems, resulting in memory loss and mobility issues.	■ Treatment includes zidovudine.
Peripheral neuropathy	This disorder is characterized by severe burning and aching pain in the feet and legs that may prevent walking. It is most commonly seen as sensory neuropathy (distal symmetric polyneuropathy). A less frequent but more severe type is acute or chronic inflammatory demyelinating polyneuropathy. Drug-induced or toxic neuropathies can be very painful.	■ Acetylcarnitine from vitamin stores may reduce symptoms.

Gastroesophageal Disorders

ETIOLOGY	CLINICAL MANIFESTATIONS	CLINICAL THERAPIES
Diarrhea	Diarrhea may be caused by infection, lactose intolerance, pancreatic issues, medications, or emotional stress.	■ The patient should avoid diarrhea-causing foods, such as dairy, fatty or spicy foods, and foods high in insoluble fiber. ■ The patient should eat bananas, plain white rice, applesauce, cream of wheat, toasted white bread, crackers, plain pasta, boiled eggs, oatmeal, mashed potatoes, or yogurt. Soluble fiber reduces therapy-related diarrhea. ■ Over-the-counter products may help treat the symptoms; calcium supplements also are helpful.
Malabsorption	Malabsorption is fairly common with advanced AIDS and reduces absorption of nutrients and medications taken orally. It is caused by GI infections and other health problems and leads to weight loss, fatigue, anemia, and malnutrition.	■ Careful monitoring of nutritional status, administration of vitamin supplements, increased intake of calories, and administration of IV total parenteral nutrition may help to improve nutritional status.

Sources: Adapted from Centers for Disease Control and Prevention. (2016b). *Opportunistic infections.* Retrieved from http://www.cdc.gov/hiv/basics/livingwithhiv/opportunisticinfections.html; Guide for HIV/AIDS Clinical Care. (2014a). *HIV classification: CDC and WHO staging systems.* Retrieved from http://aidsetc.org/guide/hiv-classification; Shah, I. (2012). *HIV in children: HIV and clinical manifestations.* Retrieved from http://www.hivinchildren.org/Diagnosis/hiv_clinicalmanisfest.aspx

status (CDC, 2015p). Screening tests should also be administered to women in labor who do not know their HIV status and who received little or no prenatal care. The likelihood that a positive screening test will truly indicate the presence of HIV infection decreases as HIV prevalence in the tested population becomes lower. Therefore, false-positive HIV test results are more likely in settings where the tested population prevalence is lower than in settings where the tested population prevalence is higher. When explaining to patients a positive result from a preliminary rapid diagnostic test, use phrases like "a good chance of being infected" or "very likely infected" to indicate the likelihood of HIV infection, qualified by the HIV prevalence in that particular setting and the patient's individual risk.

Rapid Diagnostic Tests

Rapid diagnostic tests are widely used because the results can be given immediately (see **Box 8–3** »). Immediate notification of results is critical because many patients who are tested for HIV do not return to learn the results and then cannot be located to be given the test results and educated about safe behaviors regardless of their HIV status. Although confirmation of results requires testing with a second source, such as an enzyme-linked immunosorbent assay or a Western blot test, learning the results immediately gives patients more information to make wise choices about their behaviors and self-care.

Further testing is always required to confirm a reactive or rapid screening test result. The following diagnostic tests may be ordered:

- *Enzyme-linked immunosorbent assay (ELISA).* This test is the most widely used screening test for HIV infection. ELISA tests for HIV antibodies; it does not detect the virus itself. Therefore, a patient may have a negative ELISA test early in the course of infection, before detectable antibodies have developed. The test has a sensitivity of 99.5% or higher when performed at least 13 weeks after infection. This means that more than 99.5% of tests performed on blood containing HIV antibodies show a positive result. False-positive results can occur, however, so

an individual who has an initial positive result is always tested repeatedly, and the results are confirmed by use of a different method of antibody detection, usually the Western blot. The enzyme immunoassay (EIA) was developed after the ELISA and works in much the same way as the ELISA. EIA tests that are positive are repeated, and following a second positive test, a Western blot test is performed (Osborn et al., 2013).

- *Western blot antibody testing.* This test is more reliable than ELISA but is more time consuming and more expensive. When it is combined with ELISA, however, a specificity of greater than 99.9% is achieved. Specificity is a measure of the probability that a negative test result indicates no antibodies are present. In this test, the patient's serum is mixed with HIV proteins to reveal a reaction. If antibodies to HIV are present, a detectable antigen–antibody response will occur.

- *HIV viral load tests.* These tests measure the amount of actively replicating HIV. Levels correlate with disease progression and with response to antiretroviral medications. Levels higher than 5000–10,000 copies/mL indicate the need for treatment.

- *CBC.* This test is performed to detect anemia, leukopenia, and thrombocytopenia, which often are present in patients with HIV infection. Lymphopenia (low levels of lymphocytes) is especially common in patients with this disease.

- *CD4 cell count.* This test is the most widely used one to monitor progress of the disease and to guide therapy. The CD4 cell count correlates very closely with the immunodeficiency disorders seen in patients with AIDS. Today, AIDS is defined not only by the presence of opportunistic infections and other diseases indicative of immunodeficiency but also by a CD4 count of less than $200/mm^3$ or a percentage of CD4 lymphocytes of less than 14%. CD4 counts are recommended every 3–6 months for all individuals with HIV disease.

Other Diagnostic Tests

In addition to these widely used tests, other tests may be ordered that are both general and specific to the patient's manifestations:

- *Tuberculin skin testing* to detect possible tuberculosis infection
- *MRI* of the brain to identify lymphomas
- *Specific cultures and serologic examinations for opportunistic infections* such as PCP and toxoplasmosis
- *Pap smears* for early detection of cervical cancer in women. For women younger than 30 years old, screening is recommended within the first year after onset of sexual activity but no later than age 21; women ages 21–29 years should be screened at the time of initial diagnosis and, if the results are normal, then again in 12 months. (Some experts recommend every 6 months). After three consecutive normal screenings, follow-up testing can be done every 3 years. Guidelines for women age 30 or older are similar, and screenings should continue throughout their lifetime (Panel on Opportunistic Infections in HIV-Infected Adults and Adolescents, 2016).

Box 8–3
HIV Testing

Many individuals who are at risk of HIV infection do not have access to regular healthcare. To reduce barriers to early detection of the virus, rapid HIV tests can be purchased without a prescription over the internet or through local pharmacies (CDC, 2015c). Specimens are obtained from saliva or fingerstick for a blood sample. Oral fluids are obtained by gently swabbing both the upper and lower outer gum of the mouth. Some options include OraQuick Rapid HIV-1/2 Antibody Test, Reveal Rapid HIV-1 Antibody Test, Uni-Gold Recombigen HIV Test, and Multispot HIV-1/HIV-2 Rapid Test (CDC, 2015j). When rapid HIV tests are administered as part of a healthcare interaction, counseling is provided in the same session. Positive results require confirmation through traditional methods. Individuals choosing to test themselves at home are encouraged to follow up with a healthcare provider (AIDS.gov, 2016a).

Pharmacologic Therapy

Pharmacologic treatment of HIV disease has four primary foci: (1) to suppress the infection itself, decreasing symptoms and prolonging life; (2) to provide prophylaxis of opportunistic infections; (3) to stimulate hematopoietic response; and (4) to treat opportunistic infections and malignancies. Treatment approaches that are likely to be successful use a minimum of three antiretroviral agents.

SAFETY ALERT Patients undergoing retroviral therapy are still infectious. Patient teaching should include measures to prevent transmission.

Effectiveness of treatment is monitored by viral load and CD4 cell counts; positive results are indicated by a reduction in viral load along with preserving the CD4 count above $350/mm^3$. Treatment is recommended when the CD4 count falls below $200/mm^3$. Patients with symptoms of severe disease are treated regardless of their CD4 level or viral load, so monitoring these individuals may reveal higher levels of CD4 or lower viral load. Initiating therapy in asymptomatic individuals with higher CD4 levels did not show a protective effect and was thought to perhaps increase viral resistance. Today, in order to help patients adhere to medication administration schedules, the drugs have been combined and the dosing schedules simplified.

Four classes of drugs used in antiretroviral treatment include nucleoside analog reverse-transcriptase inhibitors (NRTIs or NARTIs), nonnucleoside reverse-transcriptase inhibitors (NNRTIs), protease inhibitors (PIs), and entry inhibitors (EIs); as more antiretroviral medications have been developed, a wide array of options have emerged. ART combines three or four antiretroviral drugs to reduce the incidence of drug resistance. It generally includes zidovudine (Retrovir, AZT); one or two NRTIs, such as didanosine or lamivudine; and an NNRTI, such as nevirapine, or a PI, such as indinavir, ritonavir, or saquinavir. Combination therapies increase the likelihood of decreasing viral load and symptoms but also burden patients with complicated and expensive medication schedules. Patients beginning the ART protocol must understand the benefits, risks, costs, and effects on daily life. ART does not eradicate HIV infection, and the medications are expensive. Newer combinations, such as Triumeq or Stribild, cost upwards of $2550–$2950 for a 30-day supply of 30 doses, or over $30,600–$35,400 per year, and this sum does not cover medications to prevent or treat opportunistic infections or cancer (Panel on Opportunistic Infections in HIV-Infected Adults and Adolescents, 2016). If a combination product is not used, these medications can be scheduled for specific times throughout the day, so leading a normal life becomes a challenge. In addition, all ART medications cause major adverse reactions, leading to less-than-perfect adherence, as with most chronic diseases. In this case, however, the outcome can be fatal.

Each patient must be able to adhere to the treatment regimen. It may be preferable to delay therapy until the patient can agree to adhere to it, to prevent viral resistance caused by irregular dosing. Some providers gauge patient ability to follow the ART regimen by the patient's success with prophylaxis for an opportunistic infection.

Several methods to promote and ensure adherence are being used and studied. One approach uses electronic monitoring devices. Electronic monitoring provides real-time data about the time, date, and frequency of medication dosing. The concept is not new, and there is no guarantee that the medication is taken every time the pill container is opened; however, newer generations of the technology have improved the accuracy and usefulness of this kind of tracking. These improved devices include pill box organizers; alarms that alert patients when it is time to take medications; and programmable journals that allow patients to chart medication ingestion, side effects, and symptoms. The transmission of these data to providers via a phone connection makes it easier to detect missed doses and to improve adherence (Haberer et al., 2012). Smartphone apps have been developed to remind patients when it is time to take medication (Healthline, 2016).

Some patients undergoing ART develop body composition changes and metabolic abnormalities associated with the therapy, especially therapy involving PIs. The body composition changes include increased fat deposition in the midsection, breasts, and neck; atrophy in the face, buttocks, and extremities; and metabolic abnormalities including increased low-density lipoprotein cholesterol and triglycerides as well as insulin resistance. The combination of changes is consistent with metabolic syndrome, which increases the risk of cardiovascular disease and diabetes. These conditions commonly are treated with medications.

Nucleoside Reverse-Transcriptase Inhibitors

The NRTIs (also called *nucleoside analogues*) inhibit the action of viral reverse transcriptase, a retroviral enzyme that catalyzes the substrates for converting and copying viral RNA to DNA sequences. This enzyme is necessary for viral integration into cellular DNA and replication. The nucleoside analogues act as a chemical decoy for building blocks in the formation of the DNA copy, preventing the RNA from being copied into DNA. Each drug substitutes for a particular nucleoside base at different points on the chain. See the Medications feature for an overview of this group of drugs.

Zidovudine was the first antiretroviral agent approved for use with HIV infection. It remains in widespread use and has been shown to decrease symptoms and prolong the lives of patients with AIDS. Zidovudine often is given to patients with a CD4 cell count of less than $500/mm^3$ because of evidence that it slows the progression to severe disease. Zidovudine also may be used prophylactically following a documented parenteral exposure to HIV. It is used in combination with didanosine, ddC, or 3TC (see the Medications feature).

Protease Inhibitors

Protease is a viral enzyme used in the formation of specific viral protein for viral assembly and maturation. PIs bond chemically with protease to block the function of the enzyme and result in the production of immature, noninfectious viral particles. When combined with other antiviral drugs, these chemicals increase the chance of eliminating the virus by interfering with different stages of its life cycle. Viral resistance occurs rather quickly, however. PIs inhibit and induce metabolism of other drugs, so their use with other

Medications
Antiretroviral Nucleoside Analogues

CLASSIFICATION AND DRUG EXAMPLES	MECHANISMS OF ACTION	NURSING CONSIDERATIONS
Nucleoside and Nucleotide Reverse-Transcriptase Inhibitors Zidovudine *Drug examples:* AZT Azidothymidine	Zidovudine was the first antiretroviral agent developed to treat HIV infection. It interferes with reverse transcriptase, thus inhibiting replication of the virus. The usual dose is 300 mg twice daily. It is administered orally. Dose-limiting side effects are anemia and neutropenia.	■ Assess for possible contraindications to therapy, including allergic response or a CD4 count of greater than 350/mm^3. ■ Administer by mouth, instructing the patient to swallow capsules whole. ■ Assess for adverse effects. Nausea and headache are common. ■ Assess CBC with differential and creatine phosphokinase. Notify the physician of significant changes. Health Education for the Patient and Family ■ Zidovudine will not cure HIV infection, but it will slow its progress and reduce significant symptoms. ■ Take the drug at least a half hour before or 1 hour after meals if tolerated. ■ Notify the physician if signs of an infection or adverse response to zidovudine develop: sore throat, swollen lymph glands, and fever; unusual fatigue or weakness; easy bruising, bleeding gums, or an injury that will not heal; persistent or intractable nausea; and muscle pain or wasting. ■ Continue all scheduled follow-up visits and laboratory studies to monitor for drug toxicity. ■ Check with the physician before taking any other prescription or over-the-counter drug.
Didanosine *Drug examples:* Ddl Videx EC	Like zidovudine, didanosine does not kill HIV; rather, the drug inhibits its replication within the cells. Its activity is similar to that of zidovudine. Didanosine is used alone for patients who are intolerant or resistant to zidovudine. It also is used with zidovudine in combination therapy regimens. Didanosine does not cause the anemia associated with zidovudine, but it may cause neutropenia. Didanosine also is associated with an increased risk of pancreatitis, peripheral neuropathy, and dry mouth.	■ Assess for possible contraindications, including previous episodes of pancreatitis and impaired renal or liver function. ■ Administer as directed. ■ Administer with caution to patients taking vincristine, rifampin, pentamidine, ethambutol, or metronidazole; the action of both drugs may be affected by concurrent administration. IV pentamidine and trimethoprim-sulfamethoxazole taken concurrently may increase the risk of acute and fatal pancreatitis. ■ Didanosine interferes with the absorption of ketoconazole and dapsone. Doses of these drugs should be scheduled at least 2 hours before or after doses of didanosine. ■ Evaluate for therapeutic response and possible adverse effects. Notify the physician if manifestations of peripheral neuropathy, diarrhea, depression, or other adverse effects develop. ■ Stop the drug and notify the physician immediately if the patient develops manifestations of pancreatitis or hepatic failure, including nausea and vomiting, severe abdominal pain, elevated bilirubin, or elevated serum enzymes (e.g., amylase, aspartate aminotransferase, alanine aminotransferase). Health Education for the Patient and Family ■ Take the drug as directed. The prescribed two-tablet dose always must be taken with the amount of antacid required to prevent destruction of the drug by stomach acid. ■ Take on an empty stomach, at least 1 hour before or 2 hours after meals. ■ Do not use alcohol while taking didanosine; alcohol may increase the risk of pancreatitis. ■ Stop the drug and call the doctor immediately if nausea, vomiting, abdominal pain, or diarrhea develops. Any of these may indicate pancreatitis. ■ Call the doctor if extremity pain, weakness, numbness, or tingling occurs. These side effects usually disappear when didanosine is discontinued. ■ Other side effects to report to the physician are unusual bleeding or bruising, fatigue, weakness, fever, or persistent sore throat.

Medications *(continued)*

CLASSIFICATION AND DRUG EXAMPLES	MECHANISMS OF ACTION	NURSING CONSIDERATIONS
Abacavir	Abacavir is a nucleoside analogue that acts against some HIV strains that are resistant to other nucleoside drugs. It is prepared in combination with dolutegravir and lamivudine (Triumeq), and one tablet is taken daily. This combination drug is composed of two nucleoside analogues and an integrase strand transfer inhibitor; it lacks NNRTIs or PIs. Therefore, it is less effective at decreasing viral load and allowing immune system enhancement, but the ease of administration makes it a useful drug for patients who cannot adhere to more complex regimens. The main toxicity is a hypersensitivity response in approximately 5% of patients, which manifests with flulike symptoms; avoid repeated use in those individuals.	■ Assess for possible hypersensitivity reactions, anemia, and neutropenia. ■ Evaluate for the desired effect of increased CD4 counts and lower blood levels of p24 antigen. ■ Notify the physician if the patient develops evidence of pancreatitis, impaired hepatic function, or painful peripheral neuropathy. Health Education for the Patient and Family ■ Take without regard to food or water. ■ Check with the physician before taking any other prescription or over-the-counter medication. ■ Report all signs and symptoms of hypersensitivity to this drug. ■ Report any signs of infection or changes in condition.

Source: Data from Adams, M. P., Holland, L. N., & Urban, C. (2017). *Pharmacology for nurses: A pathophysiologic approach* (5th ed.). Hoboken, NJ: Pearson Education.

medications as well as the dosage of those medications must be carefully planned. Some drugs will circulate longer because their metabolism is inhibited; others will be rapidly metabolized and eliminated.

PIs and nucleoside analogues are associated with serious metabolic derangements. These include elevated cholesterol and triglycerides, insulin resistance and diabetes mellitus, and changes in body fat composition, which are particularly distressing to patients. These body fat changes are primarily abdominal obesity and skeletal wasting; this set of symptoms is referred to as *lipodystrophy* (Robles, 2013). Elevated cholesterol should be treated with pravastatin or atorvastatin. Lovastatin and simvastatin react to PIs, so they should be avoided. Dietary sources of cholesterol should be reduced.

■ Saquinavir (Invirase), Ritonavir (Norvir), and Indinavir (Crixivan) are used in combination with nucleoside analogues to treat progression of the disease.

■ Nelfinavir (Viracept) is used in patients with failure of or intolerance to other PIs.

■ Amprenavir (Agenerase) is the newest PI.

■ Lopinavir/ritonavir (Kaletra) is the first combination of PIs active against some HIV strains resistant to other PIs.

Nonnucleoside Reverse-Transcriptase Inhibitors

Nevirapine (Viramune), delavirdine (Rescriptor), and efavirenz (Sustiva) are NNRTIs that may be used in combination with nucleoside analogues and PIs. However, one limitation to NNRTIs is the high incidence of cross-resistance to NRTIs. Some studies have shown that nevirapine and efavirenz may significantly reduce serum levels of the PIs. Only one NNRTI should be used at a time. Nevirapine has a reported risk for liver toxicity and Stevens-Johnson syndrome (Wilson, Shannon, & Shields, 2013).

Entry Inhibitors

Entry or fusion inhibitors, such as enfuvirtide (Fuzeon), prevent HIV from entering target cells by binding to the protein envelope that surrounds the virus. When bound to the drug, the virus cannot transform to fit and adhere to cell membranes. The effectiveness of an entry or fusion inhibitor is measured by improved CD4 counts and reduced viral loads (Wilson et al., 2013).

Agents Used in Combination with Antiretroviral Therapy

Other agents may be administered in combination with antiretroviral therapy. Interferons, which are naturally occurring lymphokines, have been used alone and in combination. Interferon alfa may be used to treat KS and, in combination with zidovudine, to slow disease progression. Gamma-interferon also is used. As more drugs become available, the burden of choosing the best regimen increases for the healthcare provider. As mentioned, the most important limiting factor in the choice of a regimen is patient adherence. Second to that is selecting an effective combination of drugs without

TABLE 8–4 Pharmacologic Treatment of Common Opportunistic Infections and Malignancies in HIV Disease

Condition	Treatment	Potential Adverse Effects
Infections		
Pneumocystis jiroveci pneumonia	Trimethoprim-sulfamethoxazole pentamidine	Rash, neutropenia, anemia, thrombocytopenia, Stevens-Johnson syndrome, hypotension, altered blood glucose levels, hypocalcemia, anemia and leukopenia, liver and renal toxicity, pancreatitis
Tuberculosis	Combination drug therapy using isoniazid, rifampin, ethambutol, pyrazinamide, or streptomycin	Multiple (see the module on Infection for an exemplar on this diagnosis)
Candidiasis (oral thrush)	Clotrimazole troches nystatin suspension	Few toxic responses noted
Esophagitis or recurrent vaginitis	Ketoconazole fluconazole amphotericin b	Hepatitis, adrenal insufficiency, bone marrow toxicity, acute renal or hepatic failure, nausea and vomiting, chills, fever, headache
Mycobacterium avium complex	Combination therapy using: clarithromycin, plus clofazimine, ethambutol, rifampin, ciprofloxacin, amikacin	Hepatitis, nausea and vomiting, diarrhea, skin discoloration, pruritus, thrombocytopenia, hepatitis, optic neuritis, bone marrow depression, renal failure, ototoxicity
Cytomegalovirus	Ganciclovir and foscarnet in combination	Bone marrow depression, fever, renal failure, electrolyte imbalances, seizures
Herpes simplex or herpes zoster	Acyclovir	Nausea and vomiting, diarrhea, CNS effects, renal failure
Toxoplasmosis	Pyrimethamine, plus sulfadiazine or clindamycin and folinic acid (leucovorin)	Bone marrow depression, rash, respiratory failure, nausea and vomiting, abdominal pain, hematuria
Malignancies		
Kaposi sarcoma	Intralesional vinblastine	Inflammation and pain at injection site
Lymphoma	Combination chemotherapy	Nausea and vomiting, bone marrow toxicity, alopecia

overlapping toxicities and without toxicities so debilitating that adherence will be further impaired.

A number of pharmacologic agents are used to prevent and treat opportunistic infections and malignancies in patients with HIV. These agents are outlined in **Table 8–4 »**.

All patients infected with HIV receive pneumococcal, influenza, hepatitis B, and *Haemophilus influenzae* type B vaccines. Individuals with a positive PPD and negative chest x-ray are given prophylactic isoniazid. When the patient's CD4 cell count falls to less than 200/mm^3, prophylactic treatment for PCP is begun, usually with trimethoprim-sulfamethoxazole. Patients with a CD4 count of less than 100/mm^3 are started on prophylactic treatment for MAC.

SAFETY ALERT Patients may require an implanted venous access device to facilitate blood sampling, IV medication administration, transfusions, and parenteral nutrition when frequent IV access is needed. However, because of the patient's altered immune response, strict infection control principles should be followed to prevent the introduction of pathogens into the bloodstream.

SAFETY ALERT Patients with HIV/AIDS may need to take a number of medications on a routine basis, and regular consultation with a pharmacist will help to ensure a patient is not taking any medications that are contraindicated. Nurses should encourage patients with HIV/AIDS to use a single pharmacy to fill prescriptions to decrease the possibility of taking contraindicated medications.

Nonpharmacologic Therapy

Collaboration among physicians, nurses, and other health-care team members treating patients with HIV/AIDS is essential in care management. Nurses may find themselves collaborating with homeless shelter directors and other non-profit managers to provide preventive education to communities whose members have an unusually high risk for contracting HIV/AIDS. Counselors and religious leaders can provide support and leadership to patients with HIV infection and their families.

Nurses also may collaborate with child care directors and teachers, school staff, and even camp personnel to ensure the health and safety not only of a child with HIV/AIDS but also of the center's personnel. Nurses should instruct staff in these centers about the use of standard precautions in handling blood and body fluids. Nurses also should assist child care centers in establishing procedures to notify all parents when a child with an infectious disease has been at the center. Parents of children who are immunocompromised can then take any necessary precautions to minimize the chances of their children becoming ill. Parents of children with HIV infection must be very careful to limit the exposure of their children to infectious diseases.

Complementary Health Approaches

Complementary health approaches have been shown to help decrease side effects of certain medical treatments and to increase patient comfort related to acute exacerbations. However, the National Institutes of Health (NIH) has issued warnings against the use of garlic supplements with HIV medications (NIH, 2016). The use of St. John's wort also is contraindicated for patients receiving antiretroviral therapy (National Center for Complementary and Integrative Health, 2015, 2016b). Any patient with HIV/AIDS should be encouraged to consult his or her treating physician before beginning any therapy involving integrative therapy.

Lifespan Considerations

HIV/AIDS can affect individuals ranging in age from the very young to older adults. The approach to care should include prevention and lifecycle changes as they relate to each age group for individuals who are uninfected or at risk for infection. Healthcare providers also need to be aware of how the needs and priorities of those living with HIV/AIDS change as they mature or grow older. Overall, increased attention needs to be placed on the changing care needs and priorities associated with HIV/AIDS occurring during each stage of life.

HIV/AIDS in Pregnant Women and Newborns

Infants can acquire HIV by **vertical transmission** from their mothers, either transplacentally or during delivery. Risk factors for perinatal transmission include cigarette smoking, illicit drug use, sexually transmitted infections, and unprotected sexual intercourse with multiple partners (AIDS.gov, 2016a). Transmission can also occur during birth from blood, amniotic fluid, and exposure to genital tract secretions.

Asymptomatic pregnant women should be advised that pregnancy is not believed to accelerate the progression of HIV/AIDS. In addition, taking most HIV medications (Retrovir, AZT) during pregnancy is safe and significantly reduces the risk of transmitting HIV-1 to the fetus. Delivery by cesarean section also decreases the risk of transmission. Following birth, infants often have a positive antibody titer, which reflects the passive transfer of maternal antibodies and does not indicate HIV infection. However, prophylactic treatment with antiretroviral therapy can decrease the risk of active infection for all newborns of mothers who are HIV-positive. Transmission can also occur through breastfeeding (WHO, 2013b). The CDC recommends that women infected with HIV living in developed countries not breastfeed because of this risk. Therefore, if a viable alternative method of feeding is available, it should be used (AIDS.gov, 2016a).

Without these interventions, between 15% and 45% of infants born to mothers with HIV are infected perinatally; the rate drops below 2% when mothers receive appropriate care (CDC, 2016e). Because of the high rate of transmission from mother to infant, HIV counseling and voluntary testing are encouraged for all pregnant women. In 2001, the CDC recommended including HIV screening as a routine part of prenatal care. In 2006, the CDC recommended HIV screening for patients in all healthcare settings unless the patient declines such testing. In areas with elevated HIV rates, pregnant women should be offered repeat HIV screening during the third trimester (CDC, 2015f).

Caring for the Pregnant Woman with HIV

Assessment of the pregnant woman with HIV should include assessment for sexually transmitted infections and secondary infections commonly seen in women with HIV such as tuberculosis and cervical dysplasia. When assessment results for an infection are positive, treatment should be initiated in consultation with both the woman's obstetrician and infectious disease specialist. Vaccinations for pneumonia and influenza are also recommended, as is the hepatitis B vaccine, provided the woman has no history of hepatitis B. In addition to routine laboratory tests, baseline platelet count and CBC with differential are essential at the first healthcare interaction. These tests should be repeated each trimester to identify secondary conditions associated with HIV and HIV treatment, such as anemia, leukopenia, and thrombocytopenia.

When a woman with HIV who is under treatment becomes pregnant, she should continue her existing HIV treatment regimen if it is effective but should not receive any medications that are teratogenic, such as efavirenz (EFV) (Panel on Antiretroviral Therapy and Medical Management of HIV-Infected Children, 2013). If a pregnant woman with HIV is not already in treatment, or does not yet need treatment because of her health status, she should be tested for antiviral drug resistance before beginning treatment. Note that the treatment regimen will be based on recommended protocols and on an individual risk-versus-benefit analysis made in consultation with the patient.

At each prenatal visit, women with HIV who are asymptomatic are monitored for early signs of complications, such as fever or weight loss during the second or third trimester. Assessment should include inquiring about signs of vaginal infection (i.e., itching, irritation, unusual discharge or odor); inspecting the patient's mouth for signs of infections, such as thrush (candidiasis) or hairy leukoplakia; auscultating the patient's lungs for signs of pneumonia; and palpating the patient's lymph nodes, liver, and spleen for signs of enlargement. In addition, during each trimester, the woman should have a visual examination and a funduscopic examination to detect complications, such as toxoplasmosis retinitis.

The woman with HIV also should be assessed regularly for serologic changes that indicate progression of the disease. Progression is determined by the absolute CD4 T-lymphocyte count, which provides the number of helper T4 cells. When the CD4 counts fall to $200/mm^3$ or lower, opportunistic infections (e.g., PCP) are more likely to develop. Recommendations for treatment may change based on either the progression of the pregnancy or the progression of the disease state.

A pregnancy complicated by HIV infection, even if asymptomatic, is considered high risk, and the fetus is monitored closely. These women may have increased rates of pregnancy loss and neonatal mortality than women without HIV (Kim et al., 2012). Weekly nonstress testing is begun at 32 weeks' gestation, and serial ultrasounds are performed to detect intrauterine growth restriction. Biophysical profiles also are indicated. Invasive procedures such as amniocentesis are avoided when possible to prevent contamination of a noninfected fetus. To reduce the risk of perinatal transmission, intrapartum IV zidovudine is indicated for all pregnant women regardless of their prenatal therapy regimen.

Intrapartum and Postpartum Care

Scheduled cesarean birth at 38 weeks' gestation and before rupture of the membranes is recommended for women with elevated viral loads (CDC, 2016e). Women who are HIV-positive have an increased risk for complications such as intrapartum or postpartum hemorrhage, postpartum infection, poor wound healing, and infections of the genitourinary tract. Thus, they need careful monitoring and appropriate therapy as indicated. Following childbirth, women who are HIV-positive should be referred to a physician knowledgeable in the treatment of individuals with HIV infection. Clinics located in areas with a large HIV-positive population may require routine HIV screening of all prenatal patients (CDC, 2015b).

Caring for Newborns of Women with HIV

Medical management of the infant begins with prevention of the spread of HIV from mother to newborn. Because of the rapidity of disease progression in perinatally transmitted HIV infection, early identification of infected infants is important to ensure the most effective treatment. Like their HIV-positive mothers, these infants should undergo periodic laboratory testing as described previously. All infected mothers should receive oral zidovudine (AZT) after the first trimester of pregnancy and IV AZT during labor, preferably 6–12 hours prior to delivery. In addition, for term infants of infected mothers, AZT is started prophylactically 4 mg/kg PO twice daily, beginning as soon after birth as possible (Panel on Treatment of HIV-Infected Pregnant Women and Prevention of Perinatal Transmission, 2016). If the infant is confirmed to be HIV-positive, AZT is changed to a multidrug antiretroviral regimen.

All infants of infected mothers should start prophylaxis against PCP (a commonly serious or fatal outcome in infants) by 4–6 weeks of age. Prophylaxis should continue to 12 months unless two of the three HIV PCR tests (at 48 hours, 1–2 months, and 2–4 months) are documented as negative.

HIV/AIDS in Infants and Children

The neonate with HIV infection is asymptomatic at birth. The time period for development of opportunistic infections varies; however, the interval is shorter for children infected during the prenatal period compared to children infected through blood product transfusion.

Opportunistic diseases such as gram-negative sepsis and problems associated with prematurity are the primary causes of mortality in babies infected with HIV. Some infants infected by maternal–fetal transmission experience severe immunodeficiency, and HIV disease progresses more rapidly during the first year of life. Many newborns exposed to HIV/AIDS in utero can experience prematurity, low birth weight, or both and show evidence of failure to thrive during the neonatal and infant periods (Kourtis et al., 2013). These infants can show signs and symptoms of disease within 2–3 months after birth. Signs that may be seen during early infancy include enlarged spleen and liver, swollen glands, recurrent respiratory infections, rhinorrhea, interstitial pneumonia (rarely seen in adults), recurrent GI manifestations (diarrhea and weight loss) and urinary system infections, persistent or recurrent oral candidiasis infections, and loss of achieved developmental milestones (Ball, Bindler, Cowen, & Shaw, 2017). They also have a high risk of acquiring *Pneumocystis jiroveci* pneumonia.

Most children with AIDS have nonspecific findings, including lymphadenopathy, hepatosplenomegaly, nephropathy, oral candidiasis, failure to thrive and weight loss, diarrhea, chronic eczema and dermatitis, and fever. Specific symptoms often appear within approximately 2 years of infection and include conjunctivitis, ear infections, and tonsillitis.

Bacterial and opportunistic infections, such as *Streptococcus*, *Haemophilus influenzae*, *Salmonella*, and PCP, as well as malignancies, such as lymphoma, frequently occur in children as the disease progresses. Lymphocytic interstitial pneumonitis is a common manifestation of pediatric AIDS, and children often develop encephalopathy, resulting in developmental delay or a deterioration of motor skills and intellectual functioning. Approximately 26% of all new cases of HIV occurred in adolescents in 2010, with African Americans accounting for 57% of this group (CDC, 2015g).

Children with HIV should be immunized as soon as they reach the age recommended for diphtheria, tetanus, and acellular pertussis; inactivated poliovirus; *Haemophilus influenzae* type b; hepatitis B; pneumococcal vaccine; and annual influenza vaccine. Vaccines with inactivated viruses can be used in children with weakened immune systems with no increased risk, but the effectiveness may be reduced in some cases (AAP, 2015a). Live measles-mumps-rubella vaccine is administered at 12 months of age unless the child is severely immunocompromised, because measles raises the risk of serious outcomes. Live varicella vaccine should be administered if the child has no or mild symptoms of HIV. If the child is exposed to varicella, the parents should notify their healthcare professional, because the child may need varicella zoster immunoglobulin (VZIG) within 96 hours of exposure. If exposed to measles, the child may need vaccination within 72 hours of exposure. Tuberculosis is more common in children with AIDS, so they should have annual skin tests (AAP, 2015b).

Prior to the development of ART, the prognosis for children born with HIV infection was poor. Today, the majority of children born with HIV infection can live well beyond the age of 5 years (Weinberg, 2015). Younger children are more likely to die of pulmonary diseases or infection, while children who survive past 10 years of age are more likely to die of cardiac disease, wasting syndrome, encephalopathy, and infection with *Mycobacterium avium* complex. However, as treatment improves, more children are living longer with the disease. Many adolescent and adult women infected perinatally intend to become pregnant in spite of the risk of transmission to offspring. These women are at higher risk for preterm birth, so the risk of complications in the newborn is increased (Badell & Lindsay, 2012).

Early identification of infants who have HIV infection or are at risk for HIV/AIDS is essential during the newborn period. However, the ELISA and Western blot tests cannot distinguish between infant and maternal antibodies; therefore, these tests are inappropriate for infants before 18 months of age (Ball et al., 2017). HIV DNA polymerase chain reaction (PCR) and HIV RNA assays are the preferred method of testing. The first DNA PCR test should be performed on the newborn of a mother with HIV infection during the first 48 hours after birth. Note that use of umbilical cord blood for tests can be misleading because HIV-positive umbilical cord blood represents maternal infection (Rivera &

Clinical Manifestations and Therapies
Pediatric HIV

ETIOLOGY	CLINICAL MANIFESTATIONS	CLINICAL THERAPIES
Frequent, chronic, or unusual infections because of poor immune response	▪ Chronic bilateral otitis media ▪ Oral candidiasis ▪ *Pneumocystis jiroveci* pneumonia ▪ Skin disorders ▪ Fever	▪ Use vigorous antimicrobial therapy for treatment of infections. ▪ Limit exposure to groups of people. ▪ Obtain recommended immunizations.
Poor nutritional intake because of lack of appetite resulting from disease and medications	▪ Failure to thrive (eating disorder of childhood) ▪ Weight and body mass index below 10th percentile ▪ Chronic diarrhea ▪ Skin irritation	▪ Monitor growth. ▪ Use supplemental intake such as enteral feedings at night, and total parenteral nutrition (TPN) if needed. ▪ Practice meticulous skin care to prevent breakdown.
Immune system overgrowth to compensate for lack of proper immune response	▪ Hepatosplenomegaly ▪ Lymphadenopathy	▪ Assess abdomen frequently. ▪ Teach about safe transport to avoid injury to liver and spleen.

Frye, 2015). Infants with known perinatal HIV exposure should receive virologic diagnostic testing at ages 14–21 days, 1–2 months, and 4–6 months. Absolute exclusion of HIV infection in infants who are non-breastfed is based on two or more negative virologic tests, with one obtained at age 1 month or older and one at age 4 months or older, or two negative HIV antibody tests from separate specimens obtained at age 6 months or older (NIH, 2015; Panel on Treatment of HIV-Infected Pregnant Women and Prevention of Perinatal Transmission, 2016).

When the infant has had two negative tests, testing with ELISA (for HIV antibody) should be done at 12, 15, and 18 months. Most clinicians confirm the absence of HIV infection with a negative HIV antibody assay result at 12–18 months of age (Ball et al., 2017). In addition, a CBC and a CD4 T-cell subset count are performed at 3–6 months of age. A quick-response HIV test using saliva is available for use in certain circumstances as well; positive results are checked with blood studies. The CDC considers children under 13 years of age to be infected if their symptoms meet the CDC criteria for AIDS, if they have HIV in their blood or tissues, or if they have antibodies to HIV. The CDC criteria address two issues: the diagnosis of HIV and the clinical classification of children infected with HIV (see **Box 8–4** »).

Nurses should encourage parents and family members to bond with the baby. They may need to be reassured that there are no documented cases of individuals contracting HIV/AIDS from routine care of infected babies. The nurse should remind family members to hold the baby during feedings, because the infant benefits from frequent gentle touch, and to speak to the infant to provide auditory stimulation.

HIV/AIDS in Adolescents

Older children and adolescents currently make up the largest percentage of the HIV-infected pediatric group being cared for in pediatric HIV clinics in the United States. It has been estimated by the CDC that approximately 60% of this group have undiagnosed infections and are unaware that they are infected with HIV. The majority of adolescents who acquire HIV are infected through risky sexual behavior and have been infected recently. There are, however, a number of adolescents infected with HIV who are long-term survivors

Box 8–4
Clinical Staging of Pediatric HIV Infection

The 1994 Revised HIV Pediatric Classification System remains the standard for determining clinical staging and related treatment for children with HIV. Classifications of children, when infected, are as follows:

▪ *Category N*—not symptomatic
▪ *Category A*—mildly symptomatic with two or more of the following:
  – lymphadenopathy/hepatomegaly/splenomegaly/dermatitis/parotitis/recurrent or persistent upper respiratory infection, sinusitis, or otitis media
▪ *Category B*—moderately symptomatic with symptoms additional to those previously listed, such as:
  – anemia/bacterial meningitis, pneumonia, sepsis/candidiasis/cardiomyopathy/cytomegalovirus/diarrhea/hepatitis/herpes simplex virus, herpes zoster/leiomyosarcoma/nephropathy/persistent fever/toxoplasmosis
▪ *Category C*—severely symptomatic, manifested by:
  – Multiple, recurrent infections/encephalopathy/kaposisarcoma/lymphoma/wasting syndrome

Source: Adapted from Panel on Antiretroviral Therapy and Medical Management of HIV-Infected Children. (2013). *Guidelines for the use of antiretroviral Agents in pediatric HIV infection* (pp. E3–E4). Retrieved from http://aidsinfo.nih.gov/contentfiles/lvguidelines/pediatricguidelines.pdf.

of HIV infection that was acquired perinatally or in infancy via blood products. These adolescents have usually been exposed to ART, and their clinical course may significantly differ from that of adolescents infected later in life.

Adolescents are at a point in their lives when their needs for autonomy and independence are competing with their concrete thinking processes, risk-taking behaviors, and need to fit in with peers. These struggles make it challenging for them to sustain focus on maintaining their health, especially when dealing with chronic illness. Other potential challenges encountered with adolescents include denial and fear of their HIV infection, adherence to their medical regimen, low self-esteem, misinformation, unstructured and chaotic lifestyles, and lack of familial and social support.

HIV/AIDS in Older Adults

Adults older than age 55 account for approximately 26% of cases of HIV/AIDS in the United States, a number that is increasing every year (AIDS.gov, 2016b). Older patients who have been in monogamous relationships earlier in their lives often find themselves newly single as a result of divorce or death of a partner; when these patients resume sexual relations, they may not understand the risks for HIV because of lack of knowledge about its transmission. They may not take preventive measures, such as using condoms, or may not feel comfortable discussing HIV/AIDS risk or condom use with their new partners. Individuals in this age group may also not be aware of the importance of getting tested for HIV or discussing it with their healthcare provider. Educators and healthcare workers frequently do not discuss HIV/AIDS prevention with the older population; conversations related to their sex lives or other risk-taking behaviors are also not initiated by healthcare providers. In addition, manifestations of HIV may be overlooked by healthcare professionals, being attributed to normal age-related physiologic changes or being masked by other chronic diseases common to aging, errors that can lead to a delayed diagnosis and increased severity of the disease.

As a result of these combined factors, patients in the age group of 50 and over have been called the "invisible population" in terms of HIV prevention (CDC, 2015i; NIH National Institute on Aging, 2015). Polypharmacy is common in the older adult population, and those with HIV are at greater risk for drug-to-drug interactions when starting antiretroviral medications. The potential for drug-to-drug interactions must be regularly assessed and is especially important when beginning or changing antiretroviral and related medications (Panel on Opportunistic Infections in HIV-Infected Adults and Adolescents, 2016).

NURSING PROCESS

The patient with HIV/AIDS has many care needs and requires both physical and psychosocial support. Because no cure or effective treatment currently exists for HIV disease, many of these needs fall within the realm of nursing to promote knowledge and understanding, self-care, comfort, and quality of life. Like the course of many diseases with an ultimately fatal outcome, the course of HIV infection may well be affected by the patient's social support systems, perceived self-efficacy in management, and coping mechanisms.

As the epidemic continues, nurses are providing care for increasing numbers of patients with HIV infection at various stages of disease. These patients are not only in special care settings but also in general units, maternal–child units, hospices, long-term care facilities, and home settings. As patients with HIV disease live longer, nurses will increasingly encounter those in whom HIV disease is a secondary diagnosis, with another primary diagnosis such as seizures, heart disease, diabetes mellitus, or an operative procedure.

Assessment

Collect the following data through the health history and physical examination. Further focused assessments are described in the Implementation section that follows.

- **Observation and patient interview.** Observe the patient carefully and collect a thorough initial history because this provides the best opportunity to obtain a complete overview of the patient's current disease status, comorbid conditions, and physical and emotional state. This is also the opportunity for the nurse to establish an ongoing, therapeutic relationship with the patient. The nurse should observe the patient's general appearance, affect, demeanor, and body language throughout the interview process. The nurse should determine current HIV status; risk factors (transfusion, unprotected sex, and needle exposure); treatment status; presence of any HIV-related illnesses or infections (sexually transmitted infections, hepatitis, and tuberculosis); current medications (including antiretroviral therapy); recreational drug use; and history of foreign travel (Guide for HIV/AIDS Clinical Care, 2014b).

- **Psychosocial assessment.** The nurse should determine the patient's developmental age and ability to understand the diagnosis, coping mechanisms, and support systems, as well as access to and availability of resources in order to provide competent care.

- **Physical examination.** The initial physical examination will provide baseline information against which future data can be compared. The physical assessment should include vital signs; height, weight, and body mass index; nutrition status; vision; oral cavity and mucous membranes; skin; lymph nodes; heart and lung sounds; abdomen for tenderness; extremities and musculoskeletal system; cranial nerves; deep tendon reflexes; genitourinary examination; and mental status (Guide for HIV/AIDS Clinical Care, 2014c).

Assessment centers on observation and evaluation of potential sites of infection. Assess breath sounds, respiratory status, arterial blood gases, level of consciousness, and mental status. Report any evidence of lymphocytic interstitial pneumonitis or neurologic abnormalities. Assess the patient's height and weight frequently, assess for anemia, and look for *Candida* infections in the mouth or, in young children, the diaper area. Note any developmental delays in motor skills or intellectual functioning, which could result from encephalopathy and poor nutrition and can signal an increasing severity in symptom level. Older adults can develop certain observable properties such as decreases in muscle mass, weight, physical strength, energy, and activity level (Panel on Opportunistic Infections in HIV-Infected Adults and Adolescents, 2016). Assess infants and young children, as well as older adults, for failure to thrive. These observations and any indicators of failure to thrive (in both young children and older adults) should be reported so that further medical evaluation can be carried out.

Diagnosis

Patient needs change throughout the course of the disease, so nurses amend plans of care and diagnoses frequently, sometimes with every visit. Possible appropriate nursing diagnoses include the following:

- *Coping, Ineffective*
- *Skin Integrity, Impaired*
- *Nutrition, Imbalanced: Less than Body Requirements*
- *Fluid Volume: Deficient, Risk for*
- *Infection, Risk for*
- *Anxiety*
- *Fear*
- *Knowledge, Deficient.*

(NANDA-I © 2014)

Specific disease-related diagnoses may include the following:

- *Diarrhea* related to GI infection, malignancy, or drug reactions
- *Gas Exchange, Impaired,* related to pulmonary disease
- *Coping: Family, Compromised, Risk for,* related to life-threatening illness.

(NANDA-I © 2014)

Planning

The first step in dealing with HIV infection is prevention. Nurses must be active in evaluating test results and in teaching measures to prevent transmission of HIV to others. Adequate testing, prophylaxis for HIV and PCP, and follow-up visits to evaluate the general health of those at risk for the disease are advised. Guidelines from the AAP recommend that pediatricians offer HIV testing and counseling to adolescents who are sexually active or involved in substance abuse (CDC, 2015g). The United Nations Educational, Scientific, and Cultural Organization (2013) recommends inclusion of HIV/AIDS education in comprehensive health education for children ages 5 and up (see the Patient Teaching feature). Nurses can implement these policies and counsel teens about the dangers of and prevention measures for HIV.

The needs of patients with HIV infection change over the course of the disease, and therefore care priorities change as well. Preventive healthcare measures, health maintenance activities, education, counseling, and support of coping mechanisms are important during the early stages of the disease. As the disease progresses and the patient experiences more physical symptoms, the need for psychosocial support continues, but direct care needs become more important.

Patient Teaching
HIV/AIDS Education for Children

The United Nations Educational, Scientific, and Cultural Organization recommends that HIV and AIDS education be part of health education for children ages 5 and above. School nurses should be educated about HIV/AIDS, ethics, testing, and counseling. Nurses can enhance these efforts by doing the following:

- Promote an understanding of the need for HIV/AIDS education and raise awareness of the sexual health issues affecting children and adolescents.
- Protect the rights of students or staff with HIV infection or AIDS.
- Define what HIV/AIDS education is and what it is intended to do; prepare teachers to cover sensitive issues of sexuality and infection in class; and offer guidance about age-appropriate, socially relevant HIV/AIDS education at all levels.
- Provide guidance to administrators about building support for HIV/AIDS education in the community; answer questions about transmission of HIV, symptoms of HIV, and testing for HIV.

Source: Data from United Nations Educational, Scientific, and Cultural Organization. (2013). *International technical guidance on sexuality education.* Retrieved from http://unesdoc.unesco.org/images/0018/001832/183281e.pdf

---

Acute exacerbation of opportunistic infections may necessitate hospitalization, but typically the patient's care is managed at home.

Implementation

Nursing interventions are directed toward specific nursing diagnoses selected on the basis of patient needs. Nurses will find that many patients require interventions to prevent secondary infection, promote adherence to the treatment plan, and promote successful coping.

Prevent Secondary Infections in Those with HIV/AIDS

Bacteria as well as other organisms that are common in the environment can infect patients who are immunosuppressed.

- Children with HIV should be immunized as soon as they reach the age recommended for diphtheria, tetanus, and acellular pertussis; inactivated poliovirus; *Haemophilus influenzae* type b; hepatitis B; pneumococcal vaccine; and annual influenza vaccine. Annual tuberculosis testing is also recommended (see Lifespan Considerations for Infants and Children).
- Nurses should educate patients about how to prevent opportunistic, sexually transmitted, and other infections. They should recommend frequent hand hygiene and limiting exposure to individuals with upper respiratory or other infections to protect the patient with HIV from acquiring other infections.
- Nurses should avoid invasive procedures in the newborn and encourage the mother to formula-feed the baby rather than breastfeed (CDC, 2016e).

Promote Adherence to Medication Regimen

The treatment regimen of antiretroviral therapies for the patient with HIV/AIDS may be complex and time consuming, presenting an overwhelming challenge to patients and their families. Nonadherence to the prescribed antiretroviral treatment regimen is likely to result in increased morbidity and mortality. Some common reasons for nonadherence are frequent dosing, patients' lack of confidence in the efficacy of the treatment, and the side effects of the treatment, such as nausea and rashes. Other influences include patients' social situation and relationship with the healthcare provider (Panel on Opportunistic Infections in HIV-Infected Adults and Adolescents, 2016).

- Nonadherence to treatment regimens may be intentional or unintentional. Patients' attitude toward therapy—particularly their belief, or lack of belief, in its effectiveness—has a big impact on adherence. Assessing the patients' readiness for and attitudes toward therapy and preparing them for the effects of ART may reduce intentional nonadherence. Nurses should also address unintentional nonadherence as best they can.
- Nursing strategies for achieving optimal management of the treatment regimen include educating patients regarding the purpose of the medication, tailoring the medication regimen to patients' routines, and explaining the potential consequences of failing to adhere to the regimen. Using technology such as smartphone apps may be especially useful for adolescents and young adults.
- The type of clinical setting has been found to influence the success or failure with adherence to therapy. Healthcare facilities that deliver comprehensive interprofessional or integrated care have had greater success because of the support provided. A patient–provider relationship that is nonjudgmental and uses motivational strategies and supportive care appears to have the most influence on adherence (Panel on Opportunistic Infections in HIV-Infected Adults and Adolescents, 2016).
- If problems exist in the management of the treatment regimen, nurses should carefully listen to patients to help determine the cause. They should collaborate with patients to establish goals to help meet the prescribed treatment regimen, and they should consider the effect of cultural beliefs on medication adherence. If further intervention is required, options include direct observational therapy, home visits, and use of electronic monitoring devices.

Promote Effective Coping

Once they receive the test results indicating seropositive status, individuals with HIV infection face multiple issues that only rarely affect other patients. First and foremost, HIV is a disease with no known cure, one that is almost universally thought to be fatal. Social support systems, family relationships, and the ability to obtain and retain useful work and health insurance may be disrupted by the disease. In addition, patients may feel guilty about their lifestyle and how they contracted the disease. As the disease progresses, social isolation, fatigue, changes in body image, medication side effects, and many other issues affect patients' abilities to cope.

If possible, a primary nurse should be assigned, whether the setting is home healthcare, hospice, or acute care. Assigning a nurse helps to promote a therapeutic and trusting relationship and provides for continuity of care. Appropriate interventions include the following:

- Determine patient perception of the current situation. This can help the nurse to identify cultural beliefs and previous experiences that may affect responses to the present situation and provides a foundation for planning care and appropriate interventions.
- Assess the patient's social support network and usual methods of coping. This assessment will help both the nurse and the patient identify individuals and mechanisms that can help the patient cope more effectively with the disease.
- Plan for consistent, uninterrupted time with the patient. Time and a consistent presence encourage the patient to express feelings and work through issues related to HIV infection.
- Support the patient's social network. Nontraditional families may offer more support than the traditional family, necessitating a liberal interpretation of the term *family* if unit policy is immediate family only.
- Promote interaction between the patient, significant others, and family. The result of hospitalization and manifestations of HIV disease may be isolation from others and a decrease in the patient's ability to cope.
- Encourage the patient's involvement in making care decisions. This participation in planning gives the patient a greater sense of self-worth and more control over the situation and thus increases the patient's coping abilities.
- Support positive coping behaviors, decisions, actions, and achievements. As self-esteem is enhanced, coping improves (Gulanick & Myers, 2014).

Caring for a loved one with HIV/AIDS can cause a family to experience increased stress and social isolation. It is essential that nurses offer families information about support groups, available counseling, and information resources.

>> **Stay Current:** Healthcare providers and families can access current therapeutic information about HIV through the AIDS Clinical Trials Information Service (1-800-448-0440) or by visiting the U.S. Department of Health and Human Services AIDSinfo website (https://aidsinfo.nih.gov).

Maintain Skin Integrity

Dryness, malnutrition, immobility from fatigue, and skin lesions on pressure sites contribute to impaired integrity of the skin of the patient with HIV disease. Maintaining skin integrity is important because of HIV's progressive and debilitating nature. Also, the skin is both the first line of defense against infection in a patient with immunosuppression and a site for secondary manifestations (e.g., KS, herpes).

- Monitor the skin frequently for lesions and areas of breakdown. Early identification of impaired skin integrity allows prompt intervention.

- Monitor lesions for signs of infection or impaired healing. Infection or poor tissue perfusion not only impairs healing but also may lead to further skin breakdown.

- Use strategies to relieve pressure on bony prominences and improve circulation. Turn the hospitalized patient at least every 2 hours, and more frequently if necessary. Prevent skin shearing by using a turnsheet and adequate personnel when repositioning. Use pressure-relieving devices, such as pressure and egg-crate mattresses, or sheepskin pads for elbows and heels. Massage around, but not over, affected pressure sites to increase circulation to surrounding tissue. Massaging over affected sites can cause skin breakdown.

- Keep skin clean and dry by using mild, nondrying soaps or oils for cleansing. Frequent cleansing with nondrying products discourages bacterial growth, reducing the risk of infection. Night sweats and diarrhea, if present, can cause breakdown and damage to the skin. Applying protective creams to reddened areas in the rectal area protects skin from the caustic effects of diarrhea.

- If you see blisters, leave them intact, and dress them with a hydrocolloid (DuoDERM) dressing. Blisters provide natural sterile coverings for damaged tissue, improving healing and preventing bacterial invasion.

- Caution the patient against scratching. Scratching and skin damage allow bacteria to be introduced into lesions, increasing the risk of infection. Mitts or restraints may be used with a patient who is confused, but check the circulation of the patient's hands and fingers frequently. Tight or restrictive restraints or mitts may compromise circulation.

- Avoid the use of heat or occlusive dressings. Heat can further dry and damage the skin; occlusive dressings may impair circulation and lead to ulceration.

- Encourage ambulation if possible; if the patient is confined to bed, encourage active or passive ROM exercises. Activity increases circulation, decreases pressure and skin breakdown, and helps to maintain muscle tone.

Promote Adequate Nutrition

Many factors associated with HIV disease, including manifestations of the disease itself, put the patient at risk for altered nutrition and weight loss. Nausea and anorexia may be manifestations of the disease or the result of antiretroviral therapy. Chronic diarrhea is a common manifestation of constitutional HIV disease. Wasting syndrome also is common. The exact cause of wasting syndrome is unclear, but the diarrhea and fatigue contribute, as does the increased metabolic rate associated with fever. Oral and esophageal candidiasis and KS of the GI tract may cause painful swallowing, making eating difficult and thereby contributing to anorexia. Poor nutritional status in the patient with HIV ultimately can result in altered comfort, change in body image, muscle wasting, increased risk for infection, and higher mortality and morbidity.

- Assess nutritional status, including weight, body mass, caloric intake, and laboratory studies, such as total protein and albumin levels, hemoglobin, and hematocrit.

The baseline provided by these factors allows a determination of the effectiveness of interventions.

- Identify possible causes of altered nutrition to provide direction for planned interventions.

- Administer prescribed medications for candidiasis and other manifestations as ordered. Eliminating this opportunistic infection improves comfort and facilitates food intake. Topical viscous anesthetic can help to reduce pain and improve oral intake.

- Administer antidiarrheal medications after stools, and administer antiemetics before meals. Provide antipyretics as needed to control fever. Reducing diarrhea improves nutrient absorption; preprandial medication with an antiemetic reduces nausea and improves food intake. Reduction of fever lowers the body's metabolic demands.

- Involve the patient in meal planning, and encourage significant others to bring favorite foods from home.

- Provide a diet high in protein and kilocalories. A high-protein, high-kilocalorie diet provides the necessary nutrients to meet metabolic needs as well as requirements for tissue healing. Offer soft foods (which are easy to digest) and serve small portions (which may be more appealing). Provide supplementary vitamins and enteral feedings, such as Ensure. These improve nutritional status and caloric intake.

- Administer appetite stimulants, such as megestrol (Megace) and dronabinol (Marinol), as ordered. Both drugs may increase appetite and promote weight gain.

Address Ineffective Sexuality Patterns

The diagnosis of HIV infection can significantly alter the patient's expressions of sexuality. Guilt over the diagnosis may interfere with libido, and the patient may fear spreading the disease to others via sexual relations. The patient also may be angry with a significant other or partner who was the probable source of infection. As the disease progresses, its manifestations can affect body image and self-esteem, and other symptoms, such as nausea, fatigue, and weakness, may interfere with libido and sexual satisfaction as well.

- Examine your own feelings about sexuality, your role in dealing with a patient's sexuality, and the patient's lifestyle and sexual preferences. To deal effectively with the patient's concerns, you must be comfortable with your own feelings and be able to accept the patient's lifestyle and sexual expression.

- Establish a trusting, therapeutic relationship through the use of time, active listening, and caring. Maintain a nonthreatening, nonjudgmental attitude toward the patient. Sexuality is a private issue that will be uncomfortable or impossible for the nurse and patient to discuss without a mutually trusting relationship.

- Provide factual information about HIV infection and its effects. Facts help the patient to separate fears and myths from reality.

- Discuss safer sex practices, including hugging, cuddling, nonsexual contact, use of latex condoms and spermicidal

Nursing Care Plan
A Patient with HIV Infection

Sara Lu is a 26-year-old elementary school teacher who lives with her parents and two younger sisters. Ms. Lu is very close to her parents and sisters; they share everything with each other.

During the required physical for admission to graduate school, Ms. Lu tells her physician that lately she has felt fatigued. She also states that she has had a persistent sore throat, intermittent bouts of diarrhea, and mild shortness of breath for about a month. She takes no routine medications other than a daily multivitamin and an occasional acetaminophen tablet for a headache. She is active in a drama club in her community, and she jogs 3 miles three to four times a week. She is engaged to be married in 6 months, and her fiancé is the only individual with whom she has had sexual relations. Her sexual activity has been unprotected. Ms. Lu also has a history of open heart surgery 7 years ago to correct a congenital valve defect. She has been physically healthy since that time until about a month or two ago.

The physician orders a mononucleosis test, enzyme-linked immunosorbent assay (ELISA), Western blot analysis, CD4 cell count, a p24 antigen test, and an erythrocyte sedimentation rate (ESR). Ms. Lu is asked to return in 1 week for follow-up.

ASSESSMENT

On Ms. Lu's follow-up visit, Carole Kee, RN, obtains her health history. Ms. Lu continues to have flulike symptoms but has improved somewhat. She states that she has not been as active as usual and is worried about her health. Her appetite has decreased because of soreness in her mouth, and she has noted some whitish patches on her tongue and cheeks.

A chest film reveals no abnormality. The results of her laboratory tests are as follows:

- *ELISA:* positive for antibodies against HIV
- *Western blot analysis:* positive for antibodies against HIV
- *p24 antigen test:* positive for circulating HIV antigens
- *Erythrocyte sedimentation rate (ESR):* increased to 25 mm/hr (normal range: women, 15–20 mm/hr; men, 10–15 mm/hr)
- *CD4 cell count:* 599/mm^3 (normal range, 600–1200 mm^3)

Ms. Lu's physical examination reveals that she has enlarged lymph nodes in her neck and white patches on her oral mucosa. Her skin is warm to the touch. Her vital signs are as follows: T$_O$ 99.9°F (37.7°C); P 84 bpm; R 20 16/min; BP 120/78 mmHg.

Ms. Lu is told of the results of her laboratory tests and the medical diagnosis of HIV infection. Ms. Lu is obviously distressed and wants to know how this happened, what it means, whether she has infected her loved ones, and whether she will get better.

DIAGNOSES

Nursing diagnoses that may be appropriate for Ms. Lu are the following:

- *Imbalanced Nutrition: Less Than Body Requirements* related to soreness in mouth
- *Deficient Fluid Volume, Risk for,* related to decreased fluid intake and diarrhea
- *Infection, Risk for,* related to altered immune protection
- *Anxiety* related to diagnosis and fear
- *Deficient Knowledge* about the HIV disease

(NANDA-I © 2014)

PLANNING

The goals for care specify that Ms. Lu will:

- Maintain adequate nutrition for optimal body and cellular function.
- Consume at least 2500 mL of fluid per day.
- Remain free of infections and their complications.
- Verbalize anxiety and use appropriate coping mechanisms.
- Verbalize and demonstrate knowledge of HIV disease.
- Verbalize measures, including safer sex practices, to prevent transmission of HIV to others.

IMPLEMENTATION

The following nursing interventions may be appropriate for Ms. Lu:

- Monitor daily weight as well as intake and output.
- Monitor dietary habits, anthropometric measurements, and serum albumin levels.
- Teach Ms. Lu the importance of consuming a nutritionally balanced diet and of maintaining adequate fluid intake. Include Ms. Lu and her family in meal planning; suggest small, frequent meals and snacks of nutritionally dense, nonacidic foods.
- Suggest strategies for coping with anorexia and nausea, such as limiting foods that induce nausea and/or vomiting, scheduling medications between meals, removing noxious environmental stimuli, and using antiemetics and appetite stimulants as prescribed.
- Provide referral for dietary consultation.
- Encourage oral care before and after meals.
- Assess bowel sounds, and monitor elimination pattern.
- Administer antiemetic and antimotility medications as ordered.
- Monitor for signs of dehydration, such as poor skin turgor, oliguria, and orthostatic hypotension.

Nursing Care Plan *(continued)*

- Increase fluid intake to 2500 mL daily.
- Use strict aseptic technique for all invasive procedures.
- Teach Ms. Lu to avoid exposure to infection and people with known illnesses.
- Administer antiretroviral medications and antibiotics as prescribed, and monitor response.
- Encourage maintenance of regular physical exercise.

- Provide opportunities for Ms. Lu to verbalize her feelings; avoid false reassurances.
- Provide appropriate and adequate information about HIV/AIDS.
- Teach patient and family measures to prevent transmission of HIV such as use of proper hand hygiene, use of personal protective equipment, washing of laundry, and safer sex practices.
- Teach anxiety-controlling techniques, such as deep breathing and meditation.

EVALUATION

Ms. Lu is eager to learn about her illness and wants her family to come with her for further explanation. She states that she is sure her fiancé will be available as well. Ms. Lu is taking home antifungal medication, diet plans, and a schedule for increased exercise. She will return in 1 week for counseling and in 1 month for a follow-up physical.

CRITICAL THINKING

1. How does age affect the body's response to fighting HIV? What other factors affect the risk for HIV infection and its progression?
2. Are the laboratory results for Ms. Lu a true indication that she is HIV-positive? What additional tests might be ordered?
3. What is the most likely source of Ms. Lu's infection? What measures could have been used to reduce this risk, and how did she contract HIV? What is another possible source of Ms. Lu's HIV infection?
4. Ms. Lu says that her fiancé would like to have a child. How will you counsel her regarding pregnancy and childbearing?

---

lubricant, and mutual masturbation. Alternative forms of sexual activity and expressing affection can allow the patient and significant other to remain close.

- Encourage discussion of fears and concerns with the significant other, if any. Open communication helps a couple to deal with issues related to sexuality.
- For the patient without a significant other, stress the need to continue meeting people and developing social relationships while practicing safer sex. The patient with HIV infection has a high risk of isolation, and relationships with others help the patient to cope with the disease.

Address Knowledge Deficits

Both the patient and the significant other/family have extensive teaching needs. The primary need is current, factual information about the disease, its spread, and its expected course. This information will help them to plan realistically and to combat myths, misperceptions, and prejudices. At the same time, it is important to include information about current research and progress in treating the disease to maintain a sense of hope.

Discuss the following topics with the patient and family to prepare for home care:

- Guidelines for safer sex practices
- Nutrition, rest and exercise, stress reduction, lifestyle changes, and maintaining a positive outlook
- Infection prevention and transmission, including hand hygiene and wearing gloves when handling patient's secretions or excretions
- Importance of regular medical follow-up and monitoring of immune status

- Signs and symptoms of opportunistic infections and malignancies, as well as other symptoms that should be reported
- Medications and adverse effects
- Use and care of implanted venous access devices, total parenteral nutrition, IV pumps and continuous medication delivery systems, and IV or aerosolized medications
- Cessation of smoking, alcohol, and recreational or illicit drug use
- Community resources, such as support groups, social agencies, and counselors.

Evaluation

There are many desired outcomes of care for the patient with HIV/AIDS. Expected outcomes of nursing care include the following:

- The patient remains free from secondary infection.
- The patient has adequate respiratory function and perfusion.
- The patient has adequate nutritional intake.
- The patient demonstrates adequate coping with the stress of chronic disease.
- The child or adolescent with HIV is able to attend school and receive other supports in the educational process.

Secondary interventions are aimed at preventing the spread of disease, controlling disease progression and preventing the development of opportunistic infections (OI). Chemoprophylaxis therapy can be initiated along with ART to prevent OI development in susceptible patients. All patients with HIV need to be screened for hepatitis A, B, and C; follow-up is related to the test results. Screening for sexually transmitted infection is also recommended (Kloser & Nakata, 2016).

REVIEW HIV/AIDS

RELATE Link the Concepts and Exemplars

Linking the exemplar of HIV/AIDS with the concept of stress and coping:

1. How might excessive stress affect the patient with HIV and/or AIDS?

2. What nursing interventions could you implement to improve a patient's coping methods in order to reduce complications related to HIV infection?

Linking the exemplar of HIV/AIDS with the concept of grief and loss:

3. You are caring for a patient who is newly diagnosed as being HIV-positive with no symptoms of AIDS. Why might this patient experience grief and loss?

4. What nursing interventions might you initiate to help the patient through the grieving process?

Linking the exemplar of HIV/AIDS with the concept of collaboration:

5. What actions can you take when developing a plan of care for a patient with stage 3 HIV to promote her involvement in her own care and encourage a sense of autonomy and equality with others on her care team?

6. You have been asked to work with the health education teacher at a local high school to create an HIV/AIDS education program suitable for 10th-grade students. What kinds of information and guidance would you need from the teacher? What kinds of information and guidance should you provide to the teacher?

READY Go to Volume 3: Clinical Nursing Skills

REFER Go to Pearson MyLab Nursing and eText

- Additional review materials

REFLECT Apply Your Knowledge

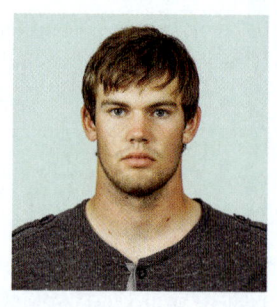

Casey Holmes is a physically fit 23-year-old man who had a troubled youth. His parents divorced when he was very young, and he bounced back and forth between them. Both parents remarried. Growing up, he often saw his father hit his stepmother when she made him angry. As an adolescent, Casey was involved with a gang and arrested on a couple of occasions for petty crimes, such as shoplifting and vandalism. He never finished high school and moved out on his own at the age of 18. Since that time, he has held a number of odd jobs and has made an effort to stay out of trouble. He currently works for a landscape contractor. He hates his job because he has to work too hard and is underpaid, but he has not attempted to look for other jobs.

Casey lives with his pregnant girlfriend, Jessica Riley, and her 10-month-old son, Ryan. Casey does not particularly like Ryan and thinks that Jessica spoils him. However, he is very proud of the fact that Jessica is pregnant with his baby. He is controlling of Jessica and does not want anybody else looking at her.

On most days after work and into the evening, Casey drinks beer and smokes marijuana with his buddies. He is irritated that Jessica does not party with him as much as she did when they first met. Casey also uses other drugs when he can afford to buy them. He sometimes worries about the possibility of getting caught in a random drug screen but figures he can always get another job.

1. What factors in Casey's lifestyle place him at risk for HIV infection?

2. What teaching might you provide Casey to help him reduce his risk of HIV infection?

3. What teaching might be indicated for Jessica to reduce her risk of HIV infection related to her relationship with Casey?

≫ Exemplar 8.B
Hypersensitivity

Exemplar Learning Outcomes

8.B Analyze hypersensitivity as it relates to immunity.

- Describe the pathophysiology of hypersensitivity.
- Describe the etiology of hypersensitivity.
- Compare the risk factors and prevention of hypersensitivity.
- Identify the clinical manifestations of hypersensitivity.
- Summarize diagnostic tests and therapies used by interprofessional teams in the collaborative care of an individual with hypersensitivity.
- Differentiate care of patients with hypersensitivity across the lifespan.
- Apply the nursing process in providing culturally competent care to an individual with hypersensitivity.

Exemplar Key Terms

Allergen, *511*
Allergy, *511*
Anaphylaxis, *511*
Antigen, *511*
Cell-mediated immune responses, *515*
Hypersensitivity, *511*
Localized response, *512*
Serum sickness, *514*
Systemic response, *511*
Transfusion reaction, *513*

Overview

Hypersensitivity is an altered immune response to an **antigen** (a foreign substance triggering the immune response) that results in harm to the patient. When the antigen is environmental, or exogenous, the response is called an **allergy**, and the antigen is referred to as an **allergen**. The tissue response to a hypersensitivity reaction may be simply irritating or bothersome, such as a runny nose or itchy eyes, or it may be life-threatening, leading to blood cell hemolysis or laryngospasm.

Hypersensitivity reactions are classified primarily by the type of immune response to contact with the allergen. Reactions are also classified as immediate or delayed hypersensitivity responses. Anaphylaxis and transfusion reactions are examples of immediate hypersensitivity reactions; contact dermatitis is a typical delayed response. The names of allergies sometimes refer to the organ system affected (e.g., allergic rhinitis) or the allergen involved (e.g., hay fever). However, classification by immunologic response is the preferred means of categorizing allergies. Although more than one type of reaction may occur simultaneously, it is practical and insightful to study and treat allergy by classified types.

An estimated 50 million people in the United States (or 1 in every 5) are diagnosed with some form of hypersensitivity. The incidence of hypersensitivity has been on the increase since the early 1980s. Hypersensitivity is the fifth leading chronic disease in the United States among all age groups and the third most common in children under 18 years of age. Hypersensitivity reactions account for more than 17 million outpatient office visits a year. Each year, nearly 400 people die from penicillin reactions; 200 from food allergies; and 100 from allergies to insects. In 2008, 10 deaths were attributed to latex reactions (Asthma and Allergy Foundation of America, 2016).

Pathophysiology and Etiology

In a hypersensitivity reaction, an antigen–antibody or antigen–lymphocyte interaction causes a response that is damaging to body tissues. Antigen–antibody responses characterize types I, II, and III hypersensitivity, which are also known as *immediate hypersensitivity responses* (see **Table 8–5** ≫). Type IV hypersensitivity is an antigen–lymphocyte reaction resulting in a delayed hypersensitivity response.

Type I (IgE-Mediated) Hypersensitivity

Common hypersensitivity reactions, such as allergic asthma, allergic rhinitis (hay fever), allergic conjunctivitis, hives, and anaphylactic shock, are typical of type I, or IgE-mediated, hypersensitivity. This type of hypersensitivity response is triggered when an allergen interacts with free IgE, causing IgE to bind to mast cells and basophils. This antigen–antibody complex prompts release of histamine and other chemical mediators, complement, acetylcholine, kinins, and chemotactic factors (see **Figure 8–12** ≫). Exposure to an allergen that initiates a type I hypersensitivity reaction can occur through ingestion of a food or medication, injection of a medication, inhalation of a triggering substance, or absorption via skin contact.

When a potent allergen enters the bloodstream and triggers a widespread antibody–antigen reaction and response to these chemical mediators, a **systemic response**, such as anaphylaxis, urticaria, or angioedema, results.

Anaphylaxis is an acute systemic type I response that may result in shock and death. It occurs in highly sensitive individuals following exposure to a specific antigen, usually through injection or ingestion. The reaction begins within minutes of exposure to the allergen and may be almost instantaneous. The release of histamine and other mediators causes vasodilation and increased capillary permeability, smooth muscle contraction, and bronchial constriction. These chemical mediators cause the patient to experience the typical manifestations of anaphylaxis. At first, the patient notes a sense of foreboding or uneasiness, light-headedness, and itching palms and scalp. Hives may develop, along with angioedema (localized tissue swelling) of the eyelids, lips, tongue, hands, feet, and genitals. Swelling also can affect the uvula and larynx, impairing breathing; this response is further complicated by bronchial constriction. The patient exhibits air hunger, stridor and wheezing, and a barking

TABLE 8–5 Types of Hypersensitivity Reactions

Type	Etiology	Clinical Manifestations	Examples
Type I: Localized or systemic reactions	Antibodies bind to certain cells, causing release of chemical substances that produce inflammation.	Hypotension, wheezing, GI or uterine spasm, stridor, and urticaria	Extrinsic asthma, allergic rhinitis (hay fever), and food allergies
Type II: Tissue-specific reactions	Antibodies cause activation of a complement system that leads to tissue damage.	Variable; may include dyspnea or fever	Transfusion reaction, ABO incompatibility, and hemolytic disease of the newborn
Type III: Immune-complex–mediated reactions	Immune complexes are deposited in tissues, where they activate complement; the result is a generalized inflammatory reaction.	Urticaria, fever, and joint pain	Acute glomerulonephritis and serum sickness
Type IV: Delayed reactions	Antigens stimulate T cells, which release lymphokines that cause inflammation and tissue damage.	Variable; may include fever, erythema, and itching	Contact dermatitis, tuberculin skin test, and graft-versus-host disease

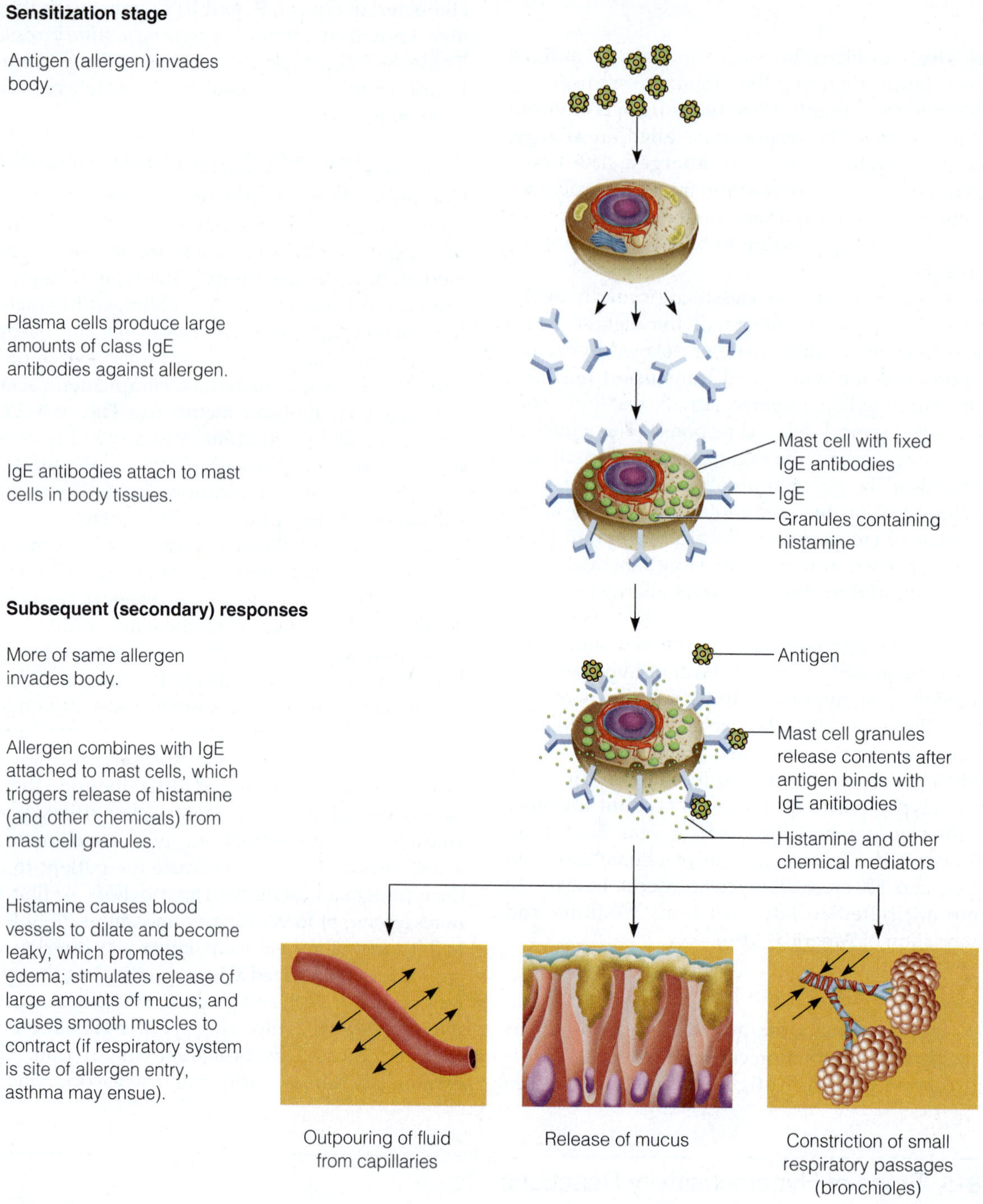

Sensitization stage

Antigen (allergen) invades
body.

Plasma cells produce large
amounts of class IgE
antibodies against allergen.

IgE antibodies attach to mast
cells in body tissues.

Subsequent (secondary) responses

More of same allergen
invades body.

Allergen combines with IgE
attached to mast cells, which
triggers release of histamine
(and other chemicals) from
mast cell granules.

Histamine causes blood
vessels to dilate and become
leaky, which promotes
edema; stimulates release of
large amounts of mucus; and
causes smooth muscles to
contract (if respiratory system
is site of allergen entry,
asthma may ensue).

- Mast cell with fixed
  IgE antibodies
- IgE
- Granules containing
  histamine

- Antigen

- Mast cell granules
  release contents after
  antigen binds with
  IgE anitbodies
- Histamine and other
  chemical mediators

Outpouring of fluid
from capillaries

Release of mucus

Constriction of small
respiratory passages
(bronchioles)

Figure 8–12 ›› Type I (IgE-mediated) hypersensitivity response.

cough. These respiratory effects can be lethal if the reaction is severe and intervention is not immediately available. Vasodilation and fluid loss from the vascular system can lead to impaired tissue perfusion and hypotension, a condition known as *anaphylactic shock*. Substances known to trigger anaphylaxis are summarized in **Box 8–5** ››.

A **localized response** is a more common manifestation of type I hypersensitivity. Localized responses typically are atopic; that is, they have a strong genetic predisposition. Atopic reactions are the result of localized, rather than systemic, IgE-mediated responses to an allergen.

They are prompted by contact of the allergen with IgE in the bronchial tree, the nasal mucosa, and the conjunctival tissues. Chemical mediators are released locally, producing symptoms such as asthma, allergic rhinitis (hay fever), conjunctivitis, or atopic dermatitis. Allergens commonly associated with atopic reactions of this type include pollens, fungal spores, house dust mites, animal dander, and feathers (Porth & Grossman, 2013). Food allergens also may cause localized responses, such as diarrhea or vomiting. If the GI mucosa is altered by a local allergic response, then the allergen may be absorbed, and the resulting reaction

Box 8–5

Substances Known to Trigger Anaphylaxis in Sensitized Individuals

Hormones
- Insulin
- Vasopressin
- Parathormone

Enzymes
- Trypsin
- Chymotrypsin
- Penicillinase

Pollens
- Ragweed
- Grass
- Trees

Foods
- Eggs
- Seafood
- Nuts and nut by-products
- Grains
- Beans
- Cottonseed oil
- Chocolate

Vitamins
- Thiamine
- Folic acid

Insect Venom
- Yellow jacket
- Hornet
- Paper wasp
- Honey bee

Occupational Agents
- Rubber products
- Industrial chemicals (ethylenes)

Antibiotics
- Penicillins
- Cephalosporins
- Amphotericin b
- Nitrofurantoin

Local Anesthetics
- Procaine
- Lidocaine

Medical Diagnostic Agents
- Sodium dehydrocholate
- Sulfobromophthalein

Antiserum
- Antilymphocyte gamma globulin

maybe systemic. Urticaria (hives) is the most common systemic response to food allergies.

Type II (Cytotoxic) Hypersensitivity

A hemolytic **transfusion reaction** to blood of an incompatible type is characteristic of a type II, or cytotoxic hypersensitivity, reaction. IgG- or IgM-type antibodies are formed to a cell-bound antigen, such as the ABO or Rh antigen. The binding of these antibodies with the antigen activates the complement cascade, resulting in destruction of the target cell (see **Figure 8–13** ≫). This type of reaction causes hemolytic disease of the newborn.

Type II reactions may be stimulated by an exogenous antigen, such as foreign tissue or cells, or by a drug reaction, in which the drug forms an antigenic complex on the surface of a blood cell, stimulating the production of antibodies. The resulting antigen–antibody reaction destroys the affected cell; for example, the administration of certain drugs, such as penicillins, may cause a condition known as drug-induced hemolytic anemia. Withdrawal of the drug stops the reaction and cell destruction.

Endogenous antigens (which are produced by the body) also can stimulate a type II reaction, resulting in an autoimmune disorder such as Goodpasture syndrome, in which antigens form to specific tissues in the lungs and kidneys. Hashimoto thyroiditis and autoimmune hemolytic anemia are additional examples of autoimmune type II reactions.

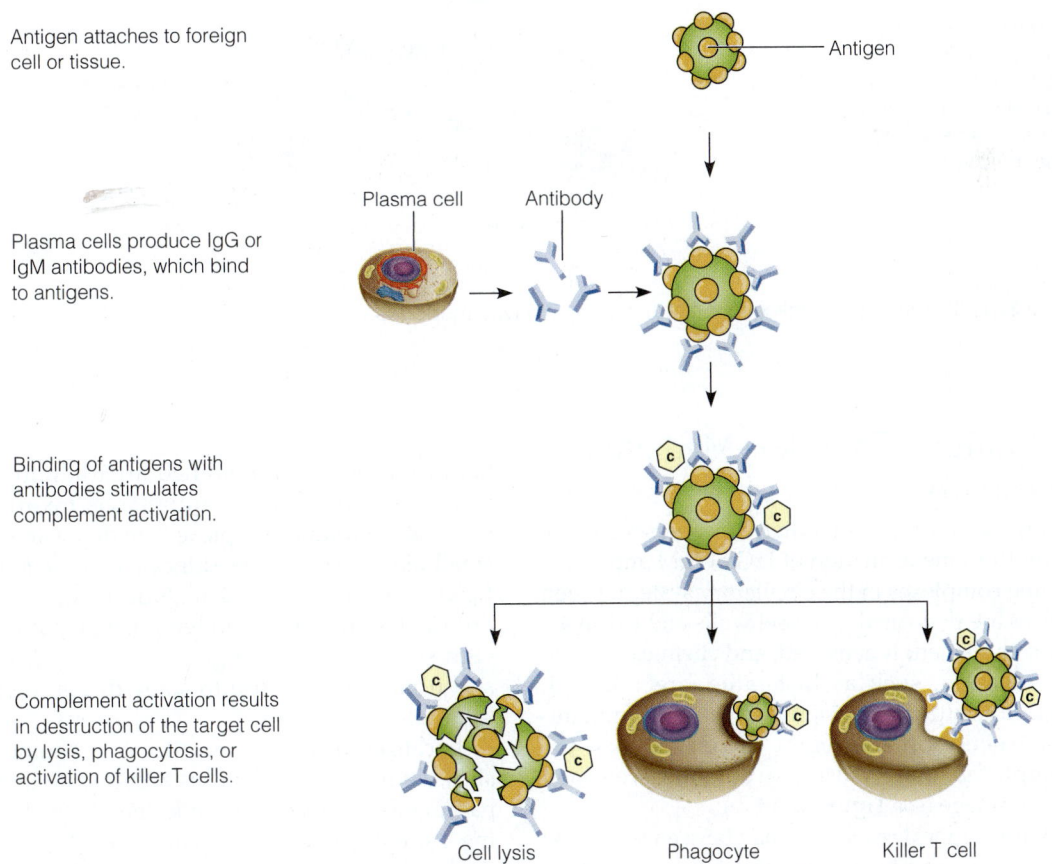

Antigen attaches to foreign cell or tissue.

Plasma cells produce IgG or IgM antibodies, which bind to antigens.

Binding of antigens with antibodies stimulates complement activation.

Complement activation results in destruction of the target cell by lysis, phagocytosis, or activation of killer T cells.

Antigen

Plasma cell   Antibody

Cell lysis   Phagocyte   Killer T cell

Figure 8–13 ≫ Type II (cytotoxic) hypersensitivity response.

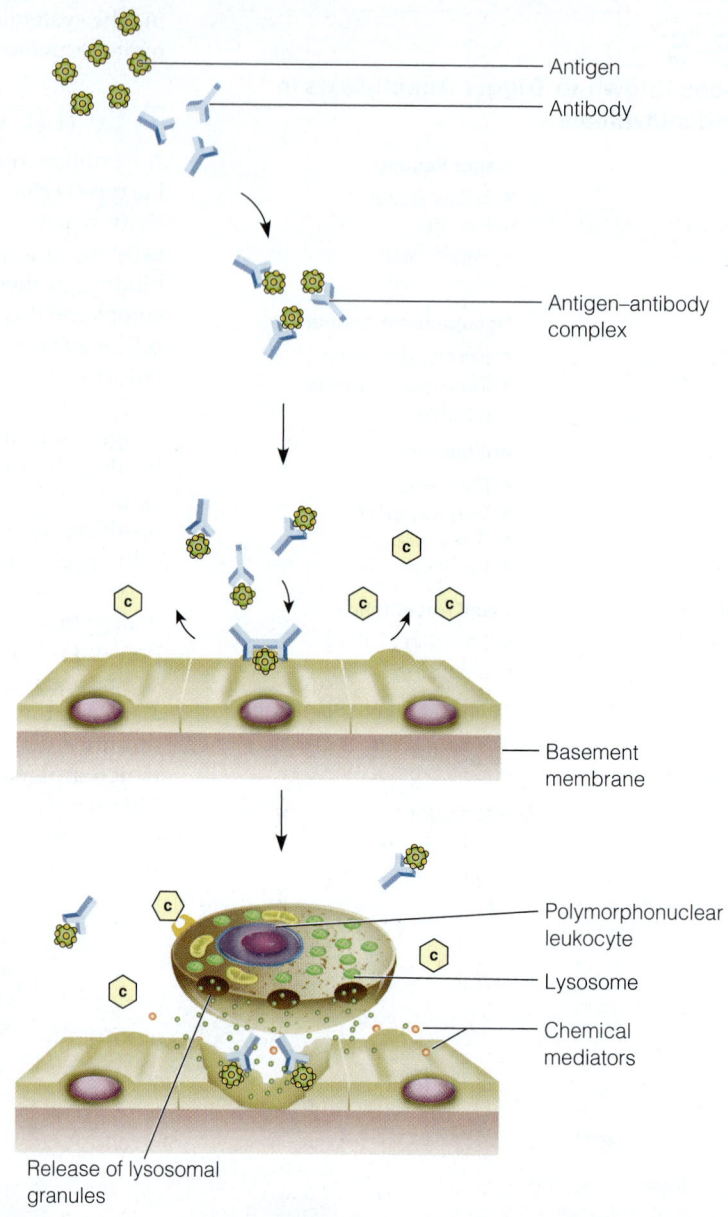

Antigens invade body and bind to antibodies in circulation. Antigen–antibody complexes are formed.

Antigen

Antibody

Antigen–antibody complex

Antigen–antibody complexes are deposited in the basement membrane of vessel walls and other body tissues, activating complement.

Basement membrane

Complement activation leads to release of inflammatory chemical mediators. Infiltration of polymorphonuclear leukocytes (PMNs) is followed by release of lysozymes. Tissue damage may be extensive.

Polymorphonuclear leukocyte

Lysosome

Chemical mediators

Release of lysosomal granules

Figure 8–14 » Type III (immune complex–mediated) hypersensitivity response.

Type III (Immune Complex–Mediated) Hypersensitivity

Type III, or immune complex–mediated, hypersensitivity reactions result from the formation of IgG or IgM antibody–antigen immune complexes in the circulatory system. When these complexes are deposited in vessel walls and extravascular tissues, complement is activated, and chemical mediators of inflammation, such as histamine, are released. Chemotactic factors attract neutrophils to the site of inflammation. When neutrophils attempt to phagocytize the immune complexes, the lysosomal enzymes released increase tissue damage (see **Figure 8–14** »).

Either systemic or local responses may be seen with type III reactions. For example, **serum sickness**, so named because it was first identified after administration of foreign serum (e.g., horse antitetanus toxin), is a systemic response. Immune complexes are deposited in the walls of small blood vessels, the kidneys, and the joints. Manifestations of serum sickness include fever, urticaria or rash, arthralgias, myalgias, and lymphadenopathy. Although foreign serums are no longer administered, serum sickness still occurs in response to some drugs, such as penicillin and sulfonamides.

Localized responses may occur at a number of different sites. As immune complexes accumulate in the glomerular basement membrane of the kidneys—for example, following a streptococcal infection or with SLE—glomerulonephritis develops. When an antigen such as dust from moldy hay

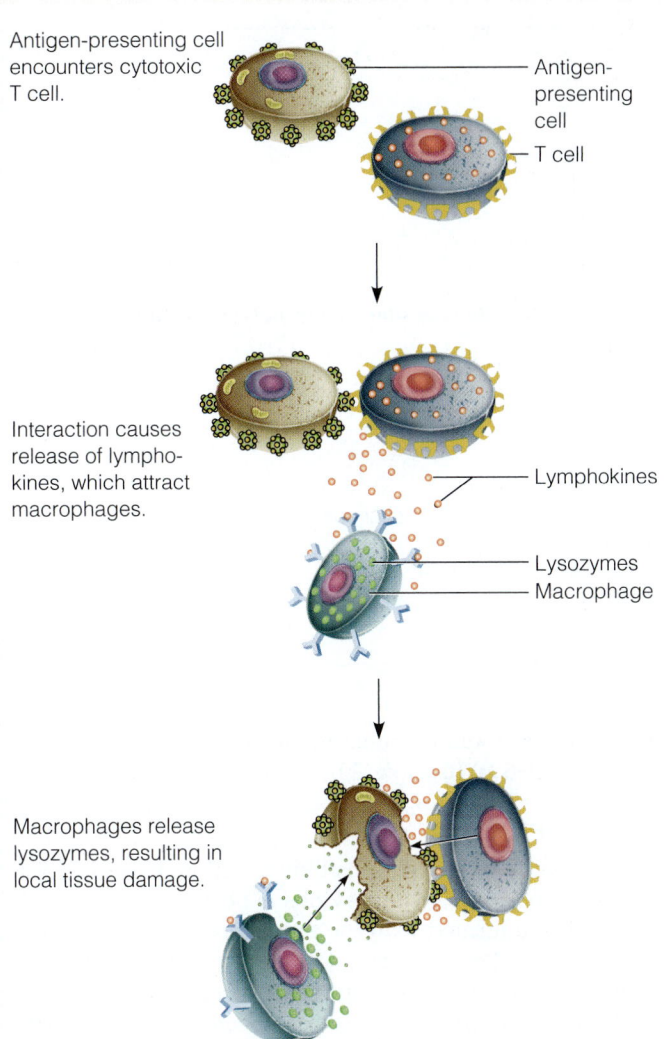

Antigen-presenting cell encounters cytotoxic T cell.

Antigen-presenting cell

T cell

Interaction causes release of lympho-kines, which attract macrophages.

Lymphokines

Lysozymes

Macrophage

Macrophages release lysozymes, resulting in local tissue damage.

Figure 8–15 》 Type IV (delayed) hypersensitivity response.

is inhaled, an acute alveolar inflammatory response can occur. This condition can develop in agricultural workers.

Type IV (Delayed) Hypersensitivity

Type IV reactions differ from other hypersensitivity responses in two ways. First, they are **cell-mediated immune responses**, not antibody-mediated responses, and involve T cells of the immune system. Second, type IV reactions are delayed rather than immediate, developing 24–48 hours after exposure to the antigen.

Type IV hypersensitivity responses result from an exaggerated interaction between an antigen and normal cell-mediated mechanisms. This exaggerated interaction results in the release of soluble inflammatory and immune mediators (from the lysozymes within the macrophages) and recruitment of killer T cells, causing local tissue destruction (see **Figure 8–15 》**).

Contact Dermatitis

Contact dermatitis is a classic example of a type IV reaction. Intense redness, itching, edema, and thickening affect the skin in the area exposed to the antigen. Fragile vesicles often

are present as well. Many antigens can provoke this response; poison ivy is a prime perpetrator. In the healthcare setting, an allergic response to latex also can produce contact dermatitis (see the Latex Allergy section). Other examples of cell-mediated responses are a positive tuberculin test and episodes of graft rejection.

Latex Allergy

Within the hospital environment, healthcare workers and patients can be exposed to a variety of items that frequently contain natural rubber latex (NRL). These items may include, but are not limited to, Band-Aids™, blood pressure cuffs, bulb syringes, Fleet enemas, sterile gloves, IV bags, personal protective equipment (PPE), reflex hammers, and tourniquets (Spina Bifida Association, 2015). In addition, chemicals used in the manufacture of latex products may be irritating. Products such as balloons, condoms, and rubber bands commonly are made of latex. **Box 8–6 》** addresses latex use in the hospital and the home.

Sensitivity to NRL develops without the user's awareness until a rash appears. Type IV hypersensitivity (contact dermatitis) can progress to type I systemic allergic reactions without previous symptoms signaling an escalation. It is important to protect both patients and healthcare workers who are allergic to NRL. Prevention of allergic reactions is aided by employers' selection of products that are not made with NRL. Workers should be screened periodically for symptoms of allergy and should be educated about latex sources. Hand hygiene after using latex products limits exposure (National Institute for Occupational Safety and Health, 2012).

An estimated 8–12% of healthcare workers are latex-sensitive (FDA, 2015a). Among these individuals the symptoms can range from mild (sneezing and runny nose) to severe (chest tightness, wheezing or shortness of breath). These symptoms may progress to life threatening (anaphylaxis) if the exposure to latex continues.

Latex allergy also is common among patients with certain health conditions. Children and adults most at risk for latex allergy include those with spina bifida; congenital urologic, GI, and tracheoesophageal defects; multiple surgeries; diabetes requiring insulin; and a history of atopy. Individuals who are allergic to latex also have a high incidence of allergy to certain foods, including kiwi fruit, bananas, tomatoes, bell peppers, stone fruits, and avocados (American Latex Allergy Association, 2016).

Box 8–7 》 describes measures to protect against latex allergy.

》 Stay Current: For a list of medical products that are not made with NRL, visit the American Latex Allergy Association at http://latexallergyresources.org/medical-products

Etiology

Hypersensitivity classifications have different causational factors. Immediate or type I hypersensitivity is facilitated by IgE with the primary cellular component being the mast cell or basophil. The reaction initially involves the production of IgE in response to certain antigens and is intensified by the release of histamine and other mediators from the mast cells.

Box 8-6
Latex in the Hospital and Home Environment

Any number of products used in both hospital and home environments may contain NRL. Nurses must be aware of these products and be knowledgeable about the alternatives offered in the settings in which they work. Nurses must also be able to provide appropriate education to patients with latex allergy.

Products in the Hospital that Frequently Contain Latex:

- Band-Aids
- Anesthesia circuits, bags, and oxygen masks
- Blood pressure cuffs and tubing
- Various types of catheters
- Cardiopulmonary resuscitation (CPR) mannequins and training aids
- Some types of dressings
- Earplugs
- Elastic wrap
- Endotracheal tubes, airways
- Gloves

- IV access materials
- Pulse oximeters
- Thermometer probes
- Suction tubing
- Vascular stockings

Products in the Home or Community that May Contain Latex:

- Art supplies
- Balloons
- Balls and toys
- Carpet backing, floor sealant
- Chewing gum
- Elastic in clothing
- Condoms, diaphragms, sponges
- Diapers, rubber pants
- Pacifiers, feeding nipples
- Beach toys and equipment, including sandals
- Gloves used for cleaning or hair coloring

Type II reactions are primarily mediated by IgM or IgG antibodies that are bound to cell surface antigens. Immune complex, or type III, hypersensitivity reactions are mediated by soluble immune complexes and mostly involve IgG. Antigens causing a type III reaction may be exogenous (bacterial, viral or parasitic) or endogenous (autoimmune disease, e.g., SLE). Type IV hypersensitivity reactions are mediated by T cells rather than antibodies and are involved in the development of many autoimmune and infectious diseases (see **Table 8-6** ❯❯) (Buelow, 2015; Ghaffar, 2014).

Risk Factors

Anyone can have a hypersensitivity reaction. However, risk generally increases with previous exposure, because antigens must be formed with the first exposure before hypersensitivity is likely to occur. Age, sex, concurrent illnesses such as asthma or other respiratory disease, and previous reactions to related substances have been identified as having a role in the risk for hypersensitivity (Mirone et al., 2015). According to the American Academy of Allergy, Asthma and Immunology (2013) and Mustafa (2015), factors associated with the development and severity of anaphylaxis

Box 8-7
Measures to Protect Against Latex Allergy

Healthcare personnel are at high risk of developing latex allergy because of intense exposure to products containing NRL. For protection from allergic reactions:

- Check products in your healthcare facility for this FDA label—"Caution: This product contains natural rubber latex, which may cause allergic reactions"—and avoid those products.
- Use nonlatex gloves whenever possible (especially for tasks involving blood and body fluids).
- If using latex gloves, use ones that are powder-free (the powder is a carrier of the latex allergen, which can be inhaled).
- When wearing latex gloves, do not use oil-based lotions on the hands because these preparations break down the latex.
- When symptoms of sensitivity to latex occur on exposure (e.g., rash, hives, nasal congestion, conjunctivitis, cough, wheezing), contact the employee health department of your facility.
- If you are diagnosed with an NRL allergy, avoid contact with NRL; alert your physician, dentist, and employer; and wear a medical identification bracelet.

❯❯ **Stay Current:** Visit the FDA's website for the most current information on latex allergy: http://www.fda.gov/ForConsumers/ConsumerUpdates/ucm342641.htm

TABLE 8-6 Characteristic Findings in Patients with Allergies

System	Characteristic Findings
Respiratory	Asthma, rhinitis (seasonal and perennial), serous otitis media, cough, pneumonia, croup, and edema of glottis
Gastrointestinal	Abdominal pain and colic, stomatitis, constipation, diarrhea, bloody stools, geographic tongue, and vomiting
Skin	Angioedema, urticaria, eczema, atopic dermatitis, erythema multiforme, purpura, drug and food rashes, and contact dermatitis
Nervous	Headache, tension, fatigue, convulsions, Ménière disease, and tremor
Eye	Conjunctivitis, cataract, ciliary spasm, and iritis
Blood	Thrombocytopenic purpura, hemolytic anemia, leukopenia, and agranulocytosis
Musculoskeletal	Arthralgia, myalgia, RA, and torticollis
Genitourinary	Dysuria, vulvovaginitis, and enuresis
Miscellaneous	Anaphylactic shock, serum sickness, and autoimmune disorders

include older age, lung disease, antigen's route of entry, amount of antigen introduced, rate of absorption for the antigen, and degree of individual hypersensitivity.

Having a family member with an allergy increases the chance that an individual will have an allergy, even to different allergens or by showing different bodily manifestations. If one parent has an allergy of any type, chances are one in three that each child will have an allergy (Asthma and Allergy Foundation of America, 2016).

Clinical Manifestations

Hypersensitivity can manifest in a number of ways, and symptoms can range from mild to severe or life-threatening. They can be either localized or systemic. Hypersensitivity reactions require a presensitization to the antigen and are classified into four types:

- **Type I:** Type I reactions are localized. Typical manifestations occur as hypotension, wheezing, GI or uterine spasm, stridor, or urticaria.
- **Type II:** Type II reactions are tissue-specific and the manifestations vary. They usually include dyspnea or fever.
- **Type III:** Type III reactions are immune-mediated and manifest with urticaria, fever, and joint pain.
- **Type IV:** Type IV reactions are delayed and are variable. They may include fever, erythema, and itching.

Characteristic findings in patients with hypersensitivity are summarized in Table 8–6.

Mild hypersensitivity responses can cause discomfort, fatigue, and even embarrassment to the patient. These may last for a few hours to a day or two and normally resolve either by themselves or with over-the-counter treatments. Acute exacerbations of allergic rhinitis or asthma lasting beyond a day or two may result in a localized infection. Localized pain and inflammation; difficulty breathing; and loss of smell, taste, and appetite are associated with moderate to severe respiratory hypersensitivity responses. Moderate hypersensitive responses of the skin include urticaria and atopic and contact dermatitis. Moderate reactions from food allergies include urticaria and GI symptoms. Severe reactions, regardless of the antigen's means of entry or the location of the initial reaction, may lead to respiratory distress or death.

Care for patients with allergic responses focuses on minimizing exposure to the allergen; preventing a hypersensitivity response; and providing prompt, effective interventions for allergic responses when they occur. Identifying allergens for the individual to reduce the likelihood of exposure is a key aspect of management. Obtain a complete history of the patient's allergies, including medications, foods, animals, plants, and other materials, and document the type of hypersensitivity response, its onset, its manifestations, and the usual treatment.

When a documented or suspected hypersensitivity reaction occurs, the allergen (e.g., an IV medication or a transfusion) is withdrawn immediately. With a type I hypersensitivity response, managing the patient's airway takes highest priority, followed by maintaining cardiac output. Type II hypersensitivity responses may necessitate aggressive management of bleeding or renal failure. A type III

(immune complex–mediated) reaction is treated by removing the offending antigen and interrupting the inflammatory response.

With a hypersensitivity response, supportive care is important to relieve discomfort. It often involves the administration of selected antihistamine or anti-inflammatory medications. Other therapies, such as plasmapheresis, may be prescribed in selected instances.

Collaboration

Due to technological advances and continued research, a variety of diagnostic tests and treatment protocols are available to patients with suspected or known hypersensitivity. Treatment protocols generally include pharmacotherapy. Individuals with hypersensitivity may need to avoid certain herbal supplements and should be counseled regarding the need to adhere to the care plan in order to decrease the risk for severe reactions.

Diagnostic Tests

The healthcare team may order laboratory tests to identify possible allergens and hypersensitivity reactions. The team may order skin tests to determine causes of hypersensitivity reactions.

Laboratory Testing

The following laboratory tests may be ordered to identify possible allergens or hypersensitivity reactions:

- **WBC count with differential.** This test can detect high levels of circulating eosinophils. Eosinophils normally constitute a very small percentage (1–4%) of the total of WBCs. Eosinophilia, however, often is present in patients with type I hypersensitivities.
- **Radioallergosorbent test (RAST).** This test measures the amount of IgE directed toward specific allergens. Test results are compared with control values and used to identify hypersensitivities. RAST poses no risk for an anaphylactic reaction. It is particularly useful in detecting allergies to some occupational chemicals and toxic allergens (Mayo Clinic, 2014c).
- **Blood type and crossmatch.** These tests are ordered before any anticipated transfusions. They determine the patient's ABO blood group and Rh status. Two major antigens, designated A and B, may be present on RBCs. Patients with the A antigen are designated as blood type A; those with the B antigen are designated as blood type B. When neither antigen is found on the RBCs, the individual is identified as type O. A third major RBC antigen is the Rh antigen. Individuals with this antigen are called Rh-positive; those without are called Rh-negative. Because a blood transfusion is actually a transplantation of living tissue, antigen matching is vital to prevent significant hypersensitivity reactions. Once blood type is determined, a sample of the patient's blood is mixed with a sample of matching donor blood and observed for antigen–antibody reactions in the crossmatch portion of this test. Although this procedure greatly reduces the risk of a

Clinical Manifestations and Therapies
Hypersensitivity

ETIOLOGY	CLINICAL MANIFESTATIONS	CLINICAL THERAPIES
Serum sickness is a reaction to proteins in antiserum derived from animals.	◾ Manifestations develop up to 2 weeks after exposure and may include rash, pruritus, arthralgia, fever, lymphadenopathy, hypotension, splenomegaly, glomerulonephritis, or proteinuria.	◾ Serum sickness often does not require medical intervention. Severe reactions may be treated with corticosteroids, antihistamines, and/or plasmapheresis.
Allergic rhinitis is a seasonal response to pollens of specific plants but also may result from exposure to dust mites, danders, or molds at any time of year.	◾ Rhinorrhea, watery eyes, itchy throat, hives, sore throat, nasal congestion, and headache are common manifestations. Facial edema is also possible; if the patient does not respond to initial treatment, a severe reaction may occur.	◾ The most effective treatment is reducing exposure to the allergen by remaining indoors, showering on entering the house to remove pollen, keeping doors and windows closed, using special filters on air conditioners, and maintaining a clean, dust-free environment. ◾ Pharmacologic therapies include decongestants, antihistamines, antileukotrienes, and immunotherapy. A tapered dose of oral steroids may be necessary to resolve an acute exacerbation.
Graft-versus-host disease results as an immune response to organ, bone marrow, or stem cell transplants.	◾ This disease is acute if it occurs within the first 3 months after transplantation. Manifestations include a skin rash, nausea, vomiting, diarrhea, cramping, abdominal pain, and jaundice. ◾ It is chronic if it occurs after the first 3 months. Manifestations include dry eyes and dry mouth, difficulty swallowing, fatigue and muscle weakness, skin reactions, liver disease, shortness of breath, and genitourinary symptoms (Cleveland Clinic, 2014).	◾ Immunosuppressant drugs are the standard therapy. ◾ Carefully assess patients who have received a transplant. ◾ Educate the patient regarding symptoms to report immediately.
Allergic asthma is the most common type of asthma and is caused by the same allergens that cause allergies in some people.	◾ Allergic asthma is characterized by bronchoconstriction and airway inflammation. Patients may report having shortness of breath, chest pain, or a feeling like "an elephant is sitting on my chest."	◾ Prevention and treatment are similar to those for allergic rhinitis, with inhaled medications such as albuterol and inhaled corticosteroids being among the most effective treatments. Patients with severe allergic asthma may require antibiotics and oral steroids if an exacerbation continues beyond 2–3 days, trapping mucus and resulting in an infection.

hemolytic transfusion reaction (type II hypersensitivity), it does not totally eliminate it.

- **Indirect Coombs test.** This test detects the presence of circulating antibodies (other than ABO antibodies) against RBCs. The patient's serum is mixed with the donor's RBCs. If the patient's serum contains antibodies to an RBC antigen, agglutination (clumping together) will occur. This is called a positive response. The normal value is negative (no agglutination). This test is also part of the crossmatch of a blood "type and crossmatch."

- **Direct Coombs test.** This test detects antibodies on the patient's RBCs that damage and destroy the cells. This test is used following a suspected transfusion reaction, to detect antibodies coating the transfused RBCs. It also can identify hemolytic anemia when the cause is unknown. In the direct Coombs test, the patient's RBCs are mixed with Coombs serum, which contains antibodies to IgG and several complement components. Agglutination occurs if the patient's RBCs are coated with antibodies; it means the test is positive. As with the indirect Coombs test, the normal test result is negative (no agglutination).

- **Immune complex assays.** These tests may be performed to detect the presence of circulating immune complexes in suspected type III hypersensitivity responses. These

Assessment

The nurse should collect the following data:

- *Observation and patient interview.* Observe the patient for the presence of rhinorrhea, sneezing, pruritus, urticaria, or atopic eczema. Inquire as to the frequency, onset, and duration of the symptoms. Ask the patient about known risk factors for hypersensitivities (e.g., medications, household dust, bee stings); reaction signs and symptoms (rash, hives, difficulty breathing); type of treatment for hypersensitivity reactions; allergy skin testing; history of asthma, hay fever, or dermatitis; and use of herbal supplements and over-the-counter and prescription medications.

- *Physical examination.* Assess the mucous membranes of the nose and mouth; assess the skin for lesions or rashes; and assess eyes (tearing and redness), respiratory rate, and breath sounds.

Further focused assessments are described in the Implementation section that follows.

Diagnosis

Priority nursing diagnoses vary according to the type of hypersensitivity reaction. Because nurses are most likely to see a patient experiencing a type I or type II response, this section focuses on diagnoses for these patients.

Airway, breathing, and circulation (the ABCs) are of greatest importance for the patient with an anaphylactic reaction. When a hemolytic reaction to an incompatible blood transfusion occurs, the patient is at risk for injury. Possible high-priority nursing diagnoses are the following:

- *Airway Clearance, Ineffective*
- *Cardiac Output, Decreased*
- *Injury, Risk for*
- *Ventilation: Spontaneous, Impaired*
- *Shock, Risk for.*

(NANDA-I © 2014)

Planning

Of key importance in planning nursing care is prevention of hypersensitivity reaction through thorough data collection to help the patient avoid exposure to known allergens. Priority goals for the patient with hypersensitivity may include the following:

- Patient will avoid known substances that provoke hypersensitivity response.

- Patient will describe self-care to reduce symptoms of seasonal allergies.

- Patient will describe proper self-administration of medications prescribed by the primary care provider or specialist.

- Patient will help determine substances that cause hypersensitivity by keeping an accurate food journal.

Implementation

Nursing implementations depend on the patient's individual needs and the nursing diagnoses selected.

Patient Teaching
Patient and Family Care for Hypersensitivity

Educate patients and family members about:

- When and how to use an anaphylaxis kit containing epinephrine and antihistamines in injectable, inhaled, and oral forms
- When to seek medical attention
- How to use and look for adverse reactions to prescription and nonprescription antihistamines and decongestants
- How to prevent an immune complex reaction, such as glomerulonephritis
- What skin care can prevent contact dermatitis, including exposing affected areas to air and sun as much as possible; avoiding direct contact with people who have an infection; wearing cool, light, nonrestrictive clothing of natural fibers to avoid irritating affected areas; avoiding exposure to extremes of heat or cold; using bath oils or plain water instead of soaps and detergents; taking tub baths in cool to lukewarm water rather than showers; decreasing pruritus by maintaining a cool environment and avoiding exercising; and trimming fingernails to reduce the risk of skin damage.

Provide Patient and Family Education

The vast majority of hypersensitivity responses are appropriately treated by the patient or family members, with little or no medical intervention. Therefore, teaching is a vital component of care. If the patient is at risk for anaphylaxis, involving the family in teaching is essential because the rapidity of the response may keep the patient from providing self-care. When teaching the patient and family about managing hypersensitivities, include the points outlined in the Patient Teaching features.

Patients with type I hypersensitivities often are misunderstood and even mistreated by their families and community. "Are you really sick, or is it just your allergies?" is not an uncommon response to children returning to school or adults returning to work after being out sick because of an allergic reaction. Sometimes even family members express these negative attitudes. Nurses can help patients who are getting the "it's all in your head" treatment by giving them language, print media, and other resources to help them teach family members, fellow students, and coworkers about this sometimes life-threatening condition.

Maintain a Patent Airway

Maintaining a patent airway (or establishing airway clearance in the event of anaphylactic shock) is the highest priority in caring for the patient experiencing a hypersensitivity response. Placing the patient in Fowler or high Fowler position allows optimal lung expansion and ease of breathing (see Figure 15–11 in the module on Oxygenation).

For mild to moderate reactions, the nurse will do the following:

- Assess respiratory rate and pattern, level of consciousness and anxiety, nasal flaring, use of accessory muscles of res-

Patient Teaching

Using an Epinephrine Autoinjector

If the patient has had a severe or systemic reaction in the past, the nurse ensures that the patient and family or caregivers know how to handle an anaphylactic reaction if another one occurs:

- Inform the patient that kits with syringes of premeasured epinephrine are available by prescription. It is recommended by the NIAID that two epinephrine autoinjectors (i.e., two doses of epinephrine) be prescribed. Two different types of epinephrine autoinjectors are the EpiPen and Adrenaclick. Because each type uses a slightly different mechanism of injection, the FDA has ruled that they are not therapeutically equivalent, so a prescription for one cannot be substituted for the other. Depending on insurance coverage, Adrenaclick may cost up to 80% less than the EpiPen (Miller, 2017; FDA, 2016). Nurses should work with patients, families, and insurance providers to help determine affordability and accessibility and ensure that patients who need to carry epinephrine autoinjectors do not go without them due to financial considerations.

- Ensure that the patient, family members, and caregivers understand how to use the kit.

- Encourage the patient to wear a medical alert bracelet or tag.

- Instruct the patient and family on proper storage of the kit, avoiding exposure to sun or high temperature.

- Instruct the patient and family to frequently check the expiration date of the EpiPen.

- Emphasize to the patient and family that a kit should be readily available in all settings where the patient studies, works, or plays, including school, camp, work, and child care. In addition to the patient, someone else should always know how to use the kit as well.

- Emphasize to the patient and family that if an anaphylactic reaction occurs, the patient should seek emergency medical attention even if symptoms resolve after use of the epinephrine auto-injector; secondary reactions may occur (biphasic reaction) within 8 and 72 hours after the initial reaction. The healthcare professional can give the patient additional medications such as corticosteroids to prevent a biphasic reaction.

Sources: Data from Miller, M. (2017). *The cheaper, generic "EpiPen" is great. Slate.* Available from: http://www.slate.com/articles/health_and_science/medical_examiner/2017/01/cvs_announces_plans_to_stock_an_alternative_to_the_notoriously_expensive.html; U.S. Food and Drug Administration. (2016). *Prescribing information for Adrenaclick.* Available from: http://www.accessdata.fda.gov/drugsatfda_docs/label/2016/020800s034lbl.pdf

piration, chest wall movement, and audible stridor; palpate for respiratory excursion; and auscultate lung sounds and any adventitious sounds, such as wheezes. Extreme anxiety or agitation, nasal flaring, stridor, and diminished lung sounds indicate air hunger and possible airway obstruction, necessitating immediate intervention.

In anaphylactic reactions, the airway obstruction may be a result of facial angioedema, bronchospasm, or laryngeal edema. In these cases, the nurse will:

- Administer oxygen per nasal cannula at a rate of 2–4 L/min. Apply oxygen emergently, and obtain a physician order for oxygen administration to increase the alveolar oxygen and its availability to cells of the body.

- Insert a nasopharyngeal or oropharyngeal airway, and arrange for immediate intubation as indicated. Ensuring an adequate airway is vital to preserve life.

- Administer subcutaneous epinephrine 1:1000, 0.3–0.5 mL, as prescribed. This may be repeated in 5–15 minutes if necessary. Also, administer parenteral diphenhydramine (deep intramuscular or IV) as prescribed. Epinephrine is a potent vasoconstrictor and bronchodilator, counteracting the effects of histamine. Diphenhydramine is an antihistamine that blocks histamine receptors and their effect. These medications can rapidly reverse manifestations of anaphylaxis.

- Provide calm reassurance. Hypoxemia and air hunger terrify the patient. Anxiety can impair the patient's ability to cooperate with treatment and can increase the respiratory rate, making breathing less effective. Comfort measures may be helpful when attempting to calm small children and may include distraction (e.g., reading a story, singing to the child), letting the child hold a soft or beloved object, and allowing the child to sit on the parent's lap when possible.

Monitor Cardiac Status

Peripheral vasodilation and increased capillary permeability resulting from the release of histamine can significantly impair cardiac output. In all cases in which a patient is exhibiting a hypersensitivity reaction, the nurse should:

- Monitor vital signs frequently, noting fall in blood pressure, decreasing pulse pressure, tachycardia, and tachypnea. These changes in vital signs may indicate shock.

- Assess skin color, temperature, capillary refill, edema, and other indicators of peripheral perfusion. As cardiac output falls, peripheral vessels constrict, and tissue perfusion is impaired.

- Monitor level of consciousness. A change in level of consciousness (lethargy, apprehension, or agitation) often is the first indicator of decreased cardiac output.

When cardiac output falls to where tissue perfusion is impaired and hypoxia results, a state of anaphylactic shock exists. In this event, the nurse should:

- Insert one or more large-bore (18 gauge or larger) IV catheters. It is important to insert IV catheters as soon as possible to provide sites for rapid fluid replacement.

- Administer warmed IV solutions of lactated Ringer or normal saline as prescribed. These isotonic solutions help to maintain intravascular volume. Solutions are warmed to prevent hypothermia from the rapid administration of large amounts of fluid at room temperature (~70°F [21.1°C]).

- Insert an indwelling catheter, and monitor urinary output frequently. As the cardiac output drops, the glomerular filtration rate falls. With an output of less than 0.5 mL/kg/hr in less than 6 hr, the patient is at risk for acute renal failure from ischemia (Hughes, 2014).

- Place a tourniquet above the site of an injected venom (e.g., a bee sting), and infiltrate the site with epinephrine as prescribed. Use of a tourniquet and the vasoconstriction resulting from epinephrine infiltration reduce further absorption of the allergen.

- Once normal breathing is established, place the patient flat with the legs elevated. This position enhances perfusion of the central organs, such as the brain, heart, and kidneys.

SAFETY ALERT Aggressive infusion of IV fluids may lead to hypervolemia and pulmonary edema. Assess for shortness of breath and crackles in the lungs.

Reduce Risk for Injury

As noted, the potential for hypersensitivity responses is high in patients subjected to medical treatments. Because a blood transfusion is a transplantation of living tissue, the risk for adverse immunologic response and injury is particularly significant.

- Obtain and record a thorough history of previous blood transfusions and any reactions experienced, *no matter how mild.* Alert the physician if previous transfusion reactions have occurred. The patient who has received prior blood transfusions is at increased risk for a hypersensitivity reaction, because antibody production may have been stimulated by previous exposure to antigens.

- Check for signed informed consent to administer blood or blood products. It is important to obtain informed consent for such invasive and risky procedures.

- Using two licensed healthcare professionals, double-check patient identity, blood type, Rh factor, crossmatch, and expiration date for all blood and blood components received from the blood bank with the patient's data. This is an important safety measure to reduce the risk of a hemolytic transfusion reaction as a result of incompatible blood types.

- Take and record vital signs within 15 minutes before initiating the blood infusion. This information provides a baseline for evaluating any changes related to the blood transfusion.

- Administer the prescribed acetaminophen and diphenhydramine prior to beginning a blood transfusion to decrease inflammation and increase patient comfort. These medications will not mask serious reactions.

- Infuse blood into a site separate from that of any other IV infusion, using a catheter of at least 20 gauge to promote flow. This procedure reduces the risk of damage to the blood cells because of incompatibility with other IV solutions or physical trauma.

- Administer blood with normal saline to prime IV tubing. When blood is administered with dextrose solutions (e.g., D_5W, D_5NS), blood cell hemolysis and aggregation occur; administration with lactated Ringer can cause agglutination of cells.

- Administer 50 mL of blood during the first 15 minutes of the transfusion. Reactions generally occur within the first 15 minutes.

- During transfusion, monitor for reports of back or chest pain, increase in temperature of more than 1.8°F, chills, tachycardia, tachypnea, wheezing, hypotension, hives, rashes, or cyanosis. These signs may indicate an adverse reaction to the blood transfusion.

- Stop the blood transfusion immediately if a reaction occurs, no matter how mild. Remove the blood bag and the tubing with blood in it. Flush new IV tubing with normal saline, keeping the IV line open. Notify the physician and the blood bank.

- If a reaction is suspected, send the blood and administration set to the laboratory with a freshly drawn blood sample and urine specimen from the patient. These will be used to identify the cause of the reaction as well as its effect on the patient.

- If no adverse reaction occurs, administer the transfusion over 2–4 hours. This time frame is important to limit the risk of bacterial growth.

Evaluation

Patients are evaluated based on their progress in meeting goals set during the planning stage. Potential outcomes may include the following:

- Patient exhibits decreased symptoms and decreased frequency of hypersensitivity responses.

- Patient demonstrates proper technique when using an epinephrine autoinjector.

- Patient provides accurate and thorough information in food or activity and symptom journal.

Secondary interventions should also be evaluated to determine if progression has been made toward meeting these potential outcomes. These outcomes may include:

- Patient/family will develop an action plan and share with appropriate contacts if there is potential for severe allergic reaction or life-threatening episode.

- Patient will wear medical alert identification.

- Patient will avoid intentional exposure to known allergens.

REVIEW Hypersensitivity

RELATE Link the Concepts and Exemplars

Linking the exemplar of hypersensitivity with the concept of oxygenation:

1. You are caring for a patient who is having a severe hypersensitivity response. How do you assess the patient's oxygenation status?

2. What nursing care can you provide to improve the patient's oxygenation status?

Linking the exemplar of hypersensitivity with the concept of comfort:

3. You are caring for a patient with seasonal hypersensitivity resulting in rhinorrhea, sore throat, and sinus congestion. What actions will improve the patient's comfort?

4. What patient teaching would you provide to improve this patient's comfort?

Linking the exemplar of hypersensitivity with the concept of teaching and learning:

5. You are working with an adult patient who has developed a type I hypersensitivity to insect venom and who has limited English proficiency. What teaching techniques would be most appropriate for addressing his learning needs? What other resources could you call upon for assistance?

6. What learner characteristics and learning factors would you need to address in order to improve compliance in a 15-year-old woman who experiences contact dermatitis when exposed to sodium lauryl sulfate in cosmetics?

READY Go to Volume 3: Clinical Nursing Skills

REFER Go to Pearson MyLab Nursing and eText

■ Additional review materials

REFLECT Apply Your Knowledge

Ron Jackson is a 12-month-old child born to Martha Jackson. Ms. Jackson has a history of multiple allergies, including drugs, food, pine pollen, and environmental hypersensitivities. She has brought Ron to the clinic today for a well-baby checkup and to receive his 1-year immunizations. His vital signs are within normal limits, he is meeting developmental milestones, and his growth charts are within the 50th percentile. Ms. Jackson reports that Ron has had several upper respiratory tract infections this spring and that she has been treating them with over-the-counter medications, such as acetaminophen (Tylenol) for fever and discomfort and saline nasal spray to reduce nasal congestion. Ron is currently asymptomatic, bright, and alert.

1. When administering immunizations, what special precautions would you take based on Ron's history?

2. What teaching would you provide to Ms. Jackson regarding his risk for hypersensitivity?

3. What symptoms related to potential hypersensitivity would you teach Ms. Jackson to report?

›› Exemplar 8.C
Rheumatoid Arthritis

Exemplar Learning Outcomes

8.C Analyze rheumatoid arthritis (RA) as it relates to immunity.

■ Describe the pathophysiology of RA.
■ Describe the etiology of RA.
■ Compare the risk factors and prevention of RA.
■ Identify the clinical manifestations of RA.
■ Summarize diagnostic tests and therapies used by interprofessional teams in the collaborative care of an individual with RA.
■ Differentiate care of patients with RA across the lifespan.
■ Apply the nursing process in providing culturally competent care to an individual with RA.

Exemplar Key Terms

Arthrodesis, *531*
Arthroplasty, *531*

Autoimmune disorder, *526*
Boutonnière deformities, *537*
Immunosuppression, *532*
Juvenile idiopathic arthritis (JIA), *535*
Orthotic devices, *533*
Osteoarthritis, *527*
Pannus, *527*
Pauciarticular arthritis, *535*
Plasmapheresis, *535*
Polyarticular arthritis, *536*
Range of motion (ROM) exercises, *538*
Rheumatoid arthritis (RA), *526*
Swan-neck deformity, *528*
Synovectomy, *531*
Systemic arthritis, *535*
Total lymphoid irradiation, *535*

Overview

Rheumatoid arthritis (RA) is a chronic systemic **autoimmune disorder** (a disease caused by abnormal, overactive functioning of the immune system that produces a response against the body's own cells and tissues, normally resulting in damage to the tissues). RA causes inflammation of connective tissue, primarily in the joints (CDC, 2015m). The course and severity of the disease are variable. Manifestations of RA may be minimal, with mild inflammation of only a few joints and little structural damage, or relentlessly progressive, with multiple inflamed joints and marked deformity. RA contributes to disability and tends to shorten life expectancy. Most patients exhibit a pattern of symmetric involvement of multiple peripheral joints and periods of remission and exacerbation.

Patients diagnosed with RA must cope with chronic pain, experience alterations in body image, and often

require specially modified tools to allow them to perform activities of daily living (ADLs). Holistic care is of particular importance in helping these patients meet physical, psychosocial, and safety needs.

Pathophysiology and Etiology
Pathophysiology

Long-term exposure to an unidentified antigen is believed to cause an aberrant immune response in a patient who is genetically susceptible. As a result, normal antibodies (immunoglobulins) become autoantibodies and attack host tissues. The transformed antibodies usually present in individuals with RA are called *rheumatoid factors*. The self-produced antibodies bind with their target antigens in blood and synovial membranes, forming immune complexes.

Leukocytes are attracted to the synovial membrane from the circulation, where neutrophils and macrophages ingest the immune complexes and release enzymes that degrade synovial tissue and articular cartilage. Activation of B lymphocytes and T lymphocytes results in increased production of rheumatoid factors and enzymes that, in turn, increase and continue the inflammatory process.

The synovial membrane is damaged by the inflammatory and immune processes. It swells from infiltration of the leukocytes, and it thickens as cells proliferate and enlarge abnormally. The inflammation then spreads and involves synovial blood vessels. Small venules are occluded, and vascular flow to the synovial tissue decreases. As blood flow decreases and metabolic needs increase (because of the increased number and size of cells), hypoxia and metabolic acidosis occur. Acidosis stimulates synovial cells to release hydrolytic enzymes into surrounding tissues, starting erosion of the articular cartilage and inflammation of the supporting ligaments and tendons. The damage to cartilage that occurs in RA results from at least three processes:

1. Neutrophils, T cells, and other synovial fluid cells are activated and degrade the surface layer of the articular cartilage.
2. Cytokines, especially interleukin-1 (IL-1) and tumor necrosis factor alpha (TNF-α), cause the chondrocytes to attack the cartilage.
3. The synovium digests nearby cartilage, releasing inflammatory molecules containing IL-1 and TNF-α.

The inflammation also causes hemorrhage, coagulation, and deposits of fibrin on the synovial membrane, in the intracellular matrix, and in the synovial fluid. **Pannus** tissue, which is an abnormal tissue layer that includes newly formed blood vessels, may develop within the synovial membrane, leading to greater loss of bone and cartilage (Osborn et al., 2013). The formation of pannus leads to scar tissue formation that immobilizes the joint (**Figure 8–17 》**).

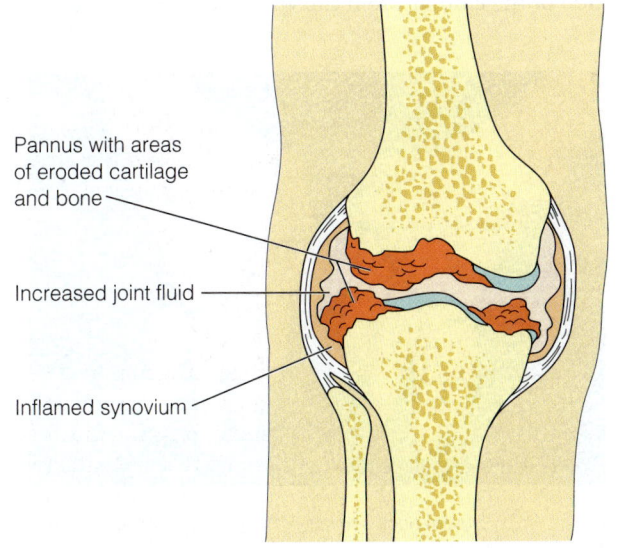

Pannus with areas of eroded cartilage and bone

Increased joint fluid

Inflamed synovium

Figure 8–17 》 Joint inflammation and destruction in rheumatoid arthritis. Note the synovial inflammation with pannus formation and the erosion of cartilage and underlying bone.

Etiology

Osteoarthritis is the most common form of arthritis in older adults. It is caused by chronic degenerative changes in the cartilage and synovial membranes of the joints. However, RA is the most common form of autoimmune arthritis, affecting from 1% to 2% of the worldwide population and all races of people. RA affects three times as many women as men, and while the typical age of onset is between 40 and 60 years, this disease strikes people of all ages (American College of Rheumatology, 2016a; Mayo Clinic, 2016). In children under 16 years of age, juvenile idiopathic arthritis (JIA; formerly called *juvenile rheumatoid arthritis*) is the most common form of arthritis (Mayo Clinic, 2014a). Remissions are most likely to occur in the first year of the disease: Approximately 10% of patients diagnosed with RA experience long-term remission within 1 year. Following the onset of RA, an estimated 60% of individuals whose disease does not enter remission within approximately 10 years will be disabled to the extent of being unable to maintain employment (Ruffing & Bingham, 2012).

The cause of RA is unknown. Genetic, environmental, hormonal, and immunologic factors are thought to be involved. Infectious agents, such as bacteria, mycoplasmas, and viruses (especially Epstein-Barr virus), may play a role in initiating the autoimmune processes in RA. Genetic factors are believed to account for 50% of the risk of developing RA, and approximately 60% of patients in the United States with the disease have been found to carry a specific genetic marker of the human leukocyte antigen (HLA)-DR4 cluster (Temprano, 2015a).

Risk Factors and Prevention

Individuals with a family history of RA may be at increased risk. Researchers have discovered that individuals with the specific HLA-DR4 genetic marker are five times more likely to develop RA than those who do not. Several studies have also found that heavy smokers are at increased risk for developing RA, but that the risk can be reduced if the individual stops smoking. Obesity; physical or emotional trauma; or exposure to air pollution, insecticides, and occupational exposures (i.e., mineral oil and silica) may also play a role in the development of RA (Arthritis Foundation, 2017). It is important to note that absence of risk factors does not preclude diagnosis of the disease.

Clinical Manifestations

Although the onset and manifestations of RA are much the same in older and younger patients, differentiating between RA and osteoarthritis in the older adult may be difficult. Establishing an accurate diagnosis is important, however, because the management of these disorders differs significantly. Clinical features distinguishing RA from osteoarthritis are listed in **Table 8–7 》**.

In addition to the characteristic joint deformity commonly seen in RA, signs and symptoms usually include redness, warmth, pain, and swelling at the affected sites. During exacerbations, when the disease is more active, patients may also experience fever, loss of appetite (anorexia), fatigue, and symmetrical joint deformity. RA may be polyarticular (affecting more than one joint), and in most cases, the hands

TABLE 8–7 Comparison of the Manifestations of Rheumatoid Arthritis and Osteoarthritis

Feature	Rheumatoid Arthritis	Osteoarthritis
Onset	Usually insidious, may be abrupt	Insidious
Course	Generally progressive, characterized by remissions and exacerbations	Slowly progressive
Pain and stiffness	Predominant on arising, lasting less than 1 hour; also occurs after prolonged inactivity	Pain with activity; stiffness following periods of immobility, generally relieved within minutes
Affected joints	Appear red, hot, and swollen; "boggy" and tender to palpation; decreased ROM; weakness	Affected joints may appear swollen; cool and bony hard on palpation; decreased ROM
	Multiple joints affected in symmetrical pattern; proximal interphalangeal, metacarpophalangeal, wrists, knees, ankles, and toes often involved	One or several joints affected, including hips, knees, lumbar and cervical spine, proximal interphalangeal and distal interphalangeal, wrist, and first metatarsophalangeal joint
Systemic manifestations	Fatigue, weakness, anorexia, weight loss, fever; rheumatoid nodules; anemia	Fatigue

and feet are affected. However, note that the destruction associated with this disease is not limited to the joints; RA can affect the blood, leading to anemia, as well as potentially damaging all organs of the body (Osborn et al., 2013). See the Multisystemic Effects of Rheumatoid Arthritis feature.

Over time, the inflammatory process associated with RA produces characteristic joint deformities. Sleep patterns, psychosocial well-being, and overall quality of life are negatively affected as well. In the most severe cases, the progressive, severe effects of RA lead to complete disability and even death.

Joint Manifestations

The pattern of joint involvement typically is polyarticular (involving multiple joints) and symmetrical, but the rate at which joint deformities develop can fluctuate. The proximal interphalangeal (PIP) and metacarpophalangeal (MCP) joints of the fingers, the wrists, the knees, the ankles, and the toes are most frequently involved, although RA can affect any joint. Stiffness is most pronounced in the morning and typically lasts more than 1 hour. It may also occur with prolonged rest during the day and may be more severe following strenuous activity. Swollen, inflamed joints feel "boggy" or spongelike on palpation because of synovial edema. ROM is limited in affected joints, and weakness may be evident (see **Figure 8–18 》**).

The persistent inflammation of RA causes deformities of the joint itself and of the supporting structures, such as ligaments, tendons, and muscles. As the joint is destroyed, ligaments, tendons, and the joint capsule are weakened or destroyed. Joint cartilage and bone also are destroyed. Weakening or destruction of these supporting structures results in lack of opposition to muscle pull, causing deformity.

Hands and Fingers

Characteristic changes in the hands and fingers are ulnar deviation of the fingers and subluxation at the MCP joints. **Swan-neck deformity** is characterized by hyperextension of the PIP joints with compensatory flexion of the distal interphalangeal (DIP) joints. A flexion deformity of the PIP joints with extension of the DIP joints is called a *boutonnière deformity* (see **Figure 8–19 》**). The ability to pinch is limited by hyperextension of the interphalangeal joint and flexion of the metacarpophalangeal joint of the thumb.

Wrists and Elbows

Wrist involvement is nearly universal, leading to limited movement, deformity, and carpal tunnel syndrome. Inflammation of the elbows often causes flexion contracture.

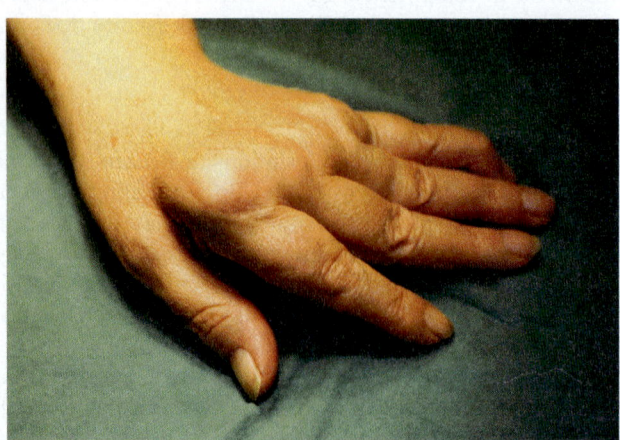

Source: Mediscan/Alamy Stock Photo.

Figure 8–18 》 Swelling and inflammation of the second and third PIP joints of the hand in a patient with rheumatoid arthritis.

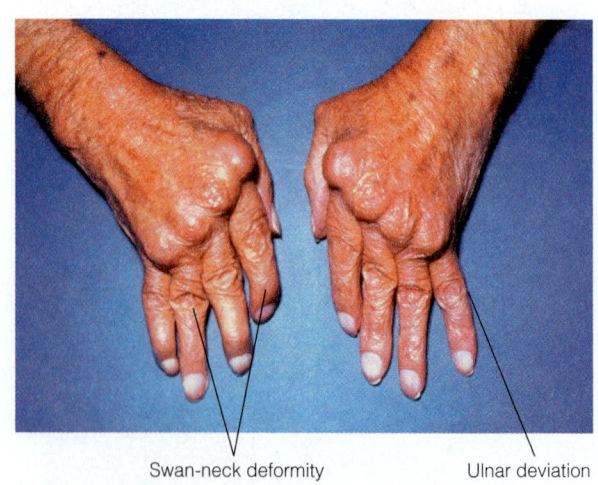

Swan-neck deformity   Ulnar deviation

Source: James Stevenson/Science Source.

Figure 8–19 》 Typical hand deformities associated with rheumatoid arthritis.

Multisystem Effects of
Rheumatoid Arthritis

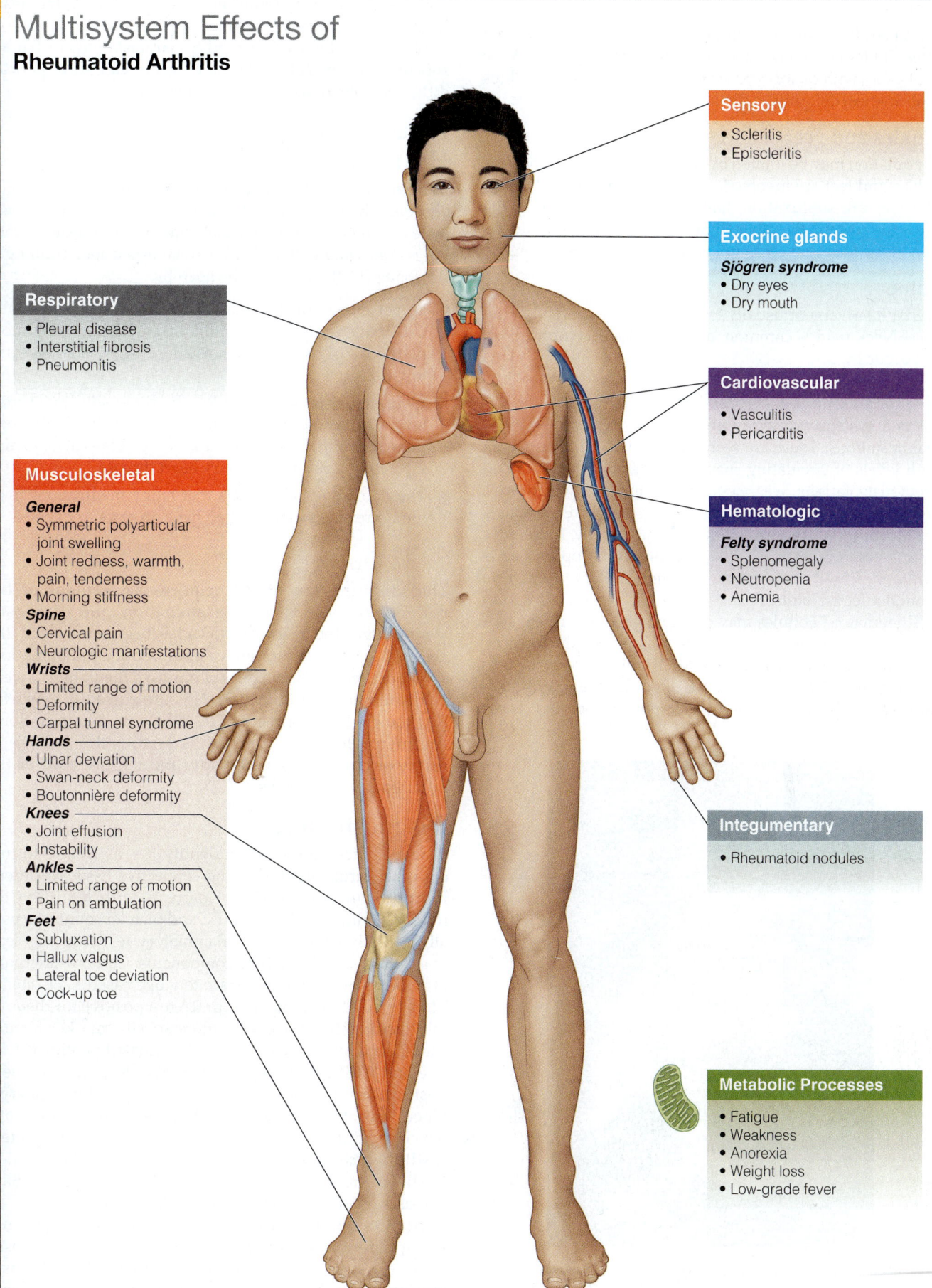

Sensory
- Scleritis
- Episcleritis

Exocrine glands

Sjögren syndrome
- Dry eyes
- Dry mouth

Cardiovascular
- Vasculitis
- Pericarditis

Hematologic

Felty syndrome
- Splenomegaly
- Neutropenia
- Anemia

Integumentary
- Rheumatoid nodules

Metabolic Processes
- Fatigue
- Weakness
- Anorexia
- Weight loss
- Low-grade fever

Respiratory
- Pleural disease
- Interstitial fibrosis
- Pneumonitis

Musculoskeletal

General
- Symmetric polyarticular joint swelling
- Joint redness, warmth, pain, tenderness
- Morning stiffness

Spine
- Cervical pain
- Neurologic manifestations

Wrists
- Limited range of motion
- Deformity
- Carpal tunnel syndrome

Hands
- Ulnar deviation
- Swan-neck deformity
- Boutonnière deformity

Knees
- Joint effusion
- Instability

Ankles
- Limited range of motion
- Pain on ambulation

Feet
- Subluxation
- Hallux valgus
- Lateral toe deviation
- Cock-up toe

Knees

The knees frequently are affected in RA, and visible swelling often obliterates the normal contours. Instability of the knee joint along with quadriceps atrophy, contractures, and valgus (knock-knee) deformities can lead to significant disability.

Ankles and Feet

Ambulation may be limited by pain and deformity when the ankles and feet are involved. Typical deformities of the feet and toes are subluxation, hallux valgus (deviation of the great toe toward the other digits of the foot), lateral deviation of the toes, and cock-up toes (turned-up toes).

Spine

Spinal involvement usually is limited to the cervical vertebrae. Neck pain is common, and neurologic complications can occur.

Extra-articular Manifestations

RA is a systemic disease with a variety of extra-articular manifestations. These are seen particularly in patients with high levels of circulating rheumatoid factor. As mentioned previously, fatigue, weakness, loss of appetite, weight loss, and low-grade fever are common when the disease is active. In addition, anemia resistant to iron therapy frequently affects patients with RA. Skeletal muscle atrophy also is common, usually being most apparent in the musculature around affected joints.

Rheumatoid nodules may develop, generally in the subcutaneous tissue of areas subject to pressure: on the forearm, in the olecranon bursa, over the MCP joints, and on the toes (see **Figure 8–20 》**). Rheumatoid nodules are granulomatous lesions that are firm and either movable or fixed. These

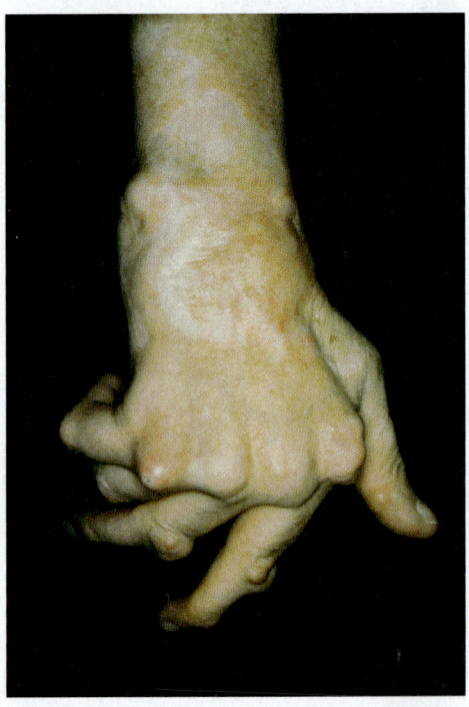

Figure 8–20 》 Rheumatoid nodules.

nodules also may be found in viscera, including the heart, lungs, intestinal tract, and dura.

Other possible extra-articular manifestations of RA are subcutaneous nodules, pleural effusion, vasculitis, pericarditis, and splenomegaly (enlargement of the spleen).

Increased Risk of Coronary Heart Disease

Individuals with RA have an increased risk of developing coronary heart disease. In turn, coronary heart disease increases the risk for myocardial infarction and death; in fact, RA is associated with a shortened life expectancy (Ruffing & Bingham, 2012). RA affects the heart by:

- Direct effects on the blood vessels, with measures of C-reactive proteins (inflammatory markers) being more predictive of future cardiovascular disease than levels of low-density lipoprotein
- Increased risk for having low high-density lipoprotein level, high cholesterol and triglyceride levels, high blood pressure, and high homocysteine levels—all of which increase the risk for coronary heart disease
- The damaging side effects that many medications (e.g., methotrexate, steroids) often have on coronary vessels.

Collaboration

The identification of RA requires assessment of the patient's history, physical examination, and diagnostic testing. Once the diagnosis of RA has been established, the goals of therapy are to relieve pain, reduce inflammation, slow or stop joint damage, and improve the patient's well-being and ability to function. No cure currently exists for RA; the goal of treatment is to relieve its manifestations. An interprofessional approach is used, with a balance of rest, exercise, physical therapy, and suppression of the inflammatory processes.

Diagnostic Tests

Diagnostic tests are used to identify RA, as well as to rule out other forms of arthritis and connective tissue disorders. In approximately 25–35% of patients with RA, the CBC reveals a mild anemia. The WBC and platelet counts are usually normal; however, the inflammatory response may lead to an increase in both these components. Certain subgroups of patients may also demonstrate a decreased WBC count. More than 70% of patients with RA test positive for rheumatoid factor (RF). However, a more specific marker for this condition is antibodies to cyclic citrullinated peptide (CCP). The anti-CCP test detects these antibodies and may yield positive results even years before RA symptoms emerge. Blood tests also include the erythrocyte sedimentation rate, which typically is elevated with RA, and C-reactive protein (CRP), which is a nonspecific indicator of inflammation (National Institute of Arthritis and Musculoskeletal Skin Diseases [NIAMS], 2014; Ruffing & Bingham, 2012).

In the earliest stages of RA, when bone damage is not yet apparent, x-rays are not of great use for diagnosis. Even so, x-rays may help to rule out other potential causes of joint pain and may be useful for monitoring the disease's progression (Ruffing & Bingham, 2012). Examination of

Clinical Manifestations and Therapies
Rheumatoid Arthritis

ETIOLOGY	CLINICAL MANIFESTATIONS	CLINICAL THERAPIES
Coronary heart disease (CHD)	■ Elevated C-reactive protein, low high-density lipoprotein, elevated cholesterol and triglycerides, and high homocysteine ■ Hypertension	■ Treatment is similar to that of any patient with CHD but must include management of RA, with additional goal of reducing inflammation that exacerbates risk for worsening CHD.
Pleural effusion (collection of fluid in the pleural space)	■ Shortness of breath and hypoxia ■ Pain, fever, and heat at the site if fluid becomes infected	■ Therapeutic aspiration may be sufficient; the patient may require chest tube insertion for continuous drainage. ■ Perform chemical or surgical pleurodesis, in which two pleural surfaces are adhered to each other to prevent recurrence of fluid accumulation. ■ Place a PleurX catheter with one-way valve for daily drainage of fluid. ■ Management of the inflammatory process resulting from RA can reduce the risk of development or reduce reaccumulation of fluid.
Vasculitis (inflammation of veins and/or arteries)	■ Fever, weight loss, palpable purpura, livedo reticularis, myalgia or myositis, mononeuritis multiplex, stroke, myocardial infarction, hypertension, gangrene, nosebleeds, bloody cough, pulmonary infiltrates, abdominal pain, bloody stools, perforations, and glomerulonephritis	■ Reduce the inflammatory process. ■ Use immune suppression. ■ Administer cortisone. ■ Use specific treatments aimed at the organ system involved.
Pericarditis (inflammation of the pericardium)	■ Chest pain radiating to the back that is relieved by sitting up and leaning forward and worsened by lying down ■ Dry cough, fever, and anxiety ■ Auscultated friction rub, ST-segment elevation, PR-interval depression in all leads, cardiac tamponade, congestive heart failure, jugular vein distention, and peripheral edema	■ Perform pericardiocentesis. ■ Prescribe antibiotics if the cause is believed to be infectious (unlikely when associated with RA). ■ Prescribe steroids to reduce inflammation. ■ Prescribe colchicine. ■ Emergency surgery may be required to restore normal heart function if other treatments fail.
Uveitis (inflammation of the middle layer of the eye; most commonly a complication of juvenile RA)	■ Redness of the eye, blurred vision, sensitivity to light, dark floating spots along the visual field, and eye pain	■ The condition has a good prognosis if treated promptly. ■ Prescribe glucocorticoid steroids (oral or topical eye drops) after ruling out any corneal ulcers. ■ Prescribe topical cycloplegics to reduce eye swelling. ■ Antimetabolite medications are used for harder-to-treat or more aggressive cases.

the synovial fluid will demonstrate changes associated with inflammation, including increased turbidity (cloudiness), decreased viscosity, and increased protein and WBC levels.

Surgery

Patients with RA may receive surgical intervention at a variety of disease stages. Early in the course of the disease, **synovectomy** (excision of synovial membrane) provides temporary relief of inflammation, relieves pain, and slows the destructive process, thus helping to preserve joint function. **Arthrodesis** (joint fusion) may be used to stabilize joints such as cervical vertebrae, wrists, and ankles. **Arthroplasty** (total joint replacement) may be necessary in cases of gross deformity and joint destruction.

Pharmacologic Therapy

The four general approaches used in the pharmacologic management of RA are (1) nonsteroidal anti-inflammatory drugs (NSAIDs) for reduction of inflammation and pain; (2) low-dose oral corticosteroids for reduction of inflammation and pain, as well as for slowing disease progression; (3) disease-modifying antirheumatic drugs (DMARDs) to relieve disease-related symptoms and to slow disease progression; and (4) intra-articular steroid injection for localized relief of pain and inflammation.

Nonsteroidal Anti-inflammatory Drugs

The NSAIDs include aspirin and numerous other drugs (see the Medications feature). While a risk for GI toxicity is associated with all NSAIDs, aspirin's incidence of GI toxicity is particularly high. In the treatment of RA, aspirin is also linked to other undesirable characteristics, including the need for multiple doses per day and a narrow therapeutic window, which means that even minor dosage increases can be toxic. For these reasons, other NSAIDs and/or a combination of medications may be preferable to aspirin in the treatment of RA (Ruffing & Bingham, 2012).

Included within the NSAIDs is a special group of drugs called cyclooxygenase 2 (COX-2) inhibitors. These NSAIDs work by selectively blocking the synthesis of prostaglandins generated by way of COX-2 enzymes (Ruffing & Bingham, 2012). In the United States, celecoxib (Celebrex) is the only available medication in this class. Although the COX-2 inhibitors carry fewer GI-related risks than do traditional NSAIDs, the potential increased risk for stroke and heart attack associated with these drugs has prompted removal of two of them—rofecoxib (Vio8) and valdecoxib (Bextra)—from the U.S. market.

The most common side effects of NSAIDs involve the GI system and may include stomach lining irritation, erosions, and bleeding ulcers. Taking these medications with food may reduce the symptoms; however, the risk for GI bleeding is not decreased. Concurrent administration of medications known as proton pump inhibitors (e.g., esomeprazole [Nexium], lansoprazol [Prevacid], pantoprazole [Protonix], and rabeprazole [Aciphex]), along with misoprostol (Cytotec), which is believed to have protective effects on the stomach mucosa, may reduce the risk for GI bleeding due to NSAIDs. Arthrotec combines both diclofenac (an NSAID) and misoprostol (Ruffing & Bingham, 2012). All NSAIDs are potentially nephrotoxic, meaning that they can cause kidney damage. In addition, they can cause blood pressure alterations that may be particularly dangerous for patients with cardiovascular disorders. NSAIDs may be contraindicated for patients with renal impairment and/or cardiac disease, depending upon the severity of the alteration. The drugs are extensively metabolized in the liver and are contraindicated in patients with liver disease.

In past years, aspirin or other analgesic drugs were the initial treatment of choice for RA, with more powerful medications added to the regimen only when the disease progressed. However, studies have shown that early treatment with more powerful medications (as well as medication combinations) may be more effective in decreasing or preventing the extensive damage associated with RA (NIAMS, 2014).

Corticosteroids

Systemic corticosteroids can dramatically decrease both inflammation and immune reactions and appear to slow the progression of joint destruction in RA. However, long-term use of corticosteroids is associated with multiple side effects (see Box 10–2 in the module on Inflammation). Ingestion of exogenous steroids can cause a decrease in the body's production of endogenous steroids. Abrupt discontinuation of exogenous steroids may have disastrous consequences and may even be fatal. Patients who discontinue systemic corticosteroids should do so under the direct supervision of a healthcare professional, as tapering (weaning) is required for prevention of the severe physiologic effects associated with sudden cessation of exogenous steroid administration.

Examples of corticosteroids used in the treatment of RA are prednisone and cortisone. Certain steroids (e.g., methylprednisolone, triamcinolone) may be injected directly into the affected joint.

Disease-modifying Antirheumatic Drugs

DMARDs are a diverse group of medications that modify immune and inflammatory responses, such as gold salts, antimalarial agents, and sulfasalazine (see the Medications feature). However, they share characteristics that make them useful in the treatment of RA. Beneficial effects are not apparent for several weeks or months following the initiation of therapy, but these drugs can produce both clinical improvement and evidence of decreased disease activity. Because their anti-inflammatory effect is minimal, NSAIDs are continued during therapy with DMARDS. As many as two thirds of patients taking these drugs show improvement, although such therapy has not been shown to slow bone erosion or facilitate healing. All of these drugs are fairly toxic, and close monitoring is necessary during the course of therapy.

Immune and Inflammatory Agents

Immunosuppression (suppression of the immune response) helps to reduce the body's autoimmune response, thereby limiting the effects of the autoimmune disease process. Immunosuppressive or cytotoxic drugs are increasingly employed in the management of RA. Indeed, many healthcare providers now consider methotrexate the treatment of choice for patients with aggressive RA. Methotrexate may be used along with NSAIDs in the initial treatment plan. A weekly dose can produce a beneficial effect in as few as 2–4 weeks. Gastric irritation and stomatitis are the most frequent side effects associated with methotrexate, but side effects may be better controlled if folic acid is taken at the same time. Alcoholism, diabetes, obesity, advanced age, and renal disease increase the risk of toxic effects (e.g., hepatotoxicity, bone marrow suppression, interstitial pneumonitis). Other immunosuppressive agents, such as cyclosporine, azathioprine, and monoclonal antibodies, also have been employed in the treatment of patients with severe, progressive, and crippling disease who have failed to respond to other measures.

Tumor necrosis factor (TNF) inhibitors used to treat patients with RA include etanercept (Enbrel), which inhibits the binding of TNF to receptor sites. Infliximab (Remicade) is a biological response modifier and a TNF-α receptor antagonist. Given by IV infusion, this drug is administered to reduce infiltration of inflammatory cells and production of TNF-α. Adalimumab (Humira) is a biological response modifier that is given to individuals with RA to reduce the inflammatory events of polyarthritis and to slow the progression of joint damage. Given by subcutaneous injection, the drug cannot be administered if the individual has an acute or chronic infection in any part of the body. Before the drug is initiated, the patient should be tested for tuberculosis.

Gold Salts

Gold salts may be administered by mouth, but the intramuscular route is more effective. The mode of action of gold is unknown, but it may produce clinical remission in some patients and decrease new bony erosions. Unless toxic reactions occur, weekly therapy is continued until significant improvement is noted. Patients experiencing benefit from gold therapy may be continued on monthly injections for several years. About one third of patients on gold therapy experience toxic reactions, including dermatitis, stomatitis, bone marrow depression, and proteinuria. Mild skin reactions do not always necessitate discontinuation of therapy.

Antimalarial Agents

Hydroxychloroquine (Plaquenil) is an antimalarial agent sometimes employed in the treatment of RA. The desired response requires 3–6 months of therapy, and many patients do not experience significant benefit. Although hydroxychloroquine has a relatively low toxicity, it can cause pigmentary retinitis and vision loss. Because chloroquine is associated with high risk for eye toxicity, this drug is not commonly prescribed (Ruffing & Bingham, 2012). Patients receiving this drug require a thorough vision examination every 6 months.

Sulfasalazine

Sulfasalazine, a drug regularly prescribed for chronic inflammatory bowel disease, also may be prescribed for RA. It is used with other drugs, rest, and physical therapy in patients who have not responded to other medications (salicylates and NSAIDs).

For patients not responding to the previously mentioned preparations, penicillamine may be prescribed. Although this agent may be effective in the management of RA, toxic reactions, including bone marrow suppression, proteinuria, and nephrosis, are common and can be severe.

Including the patient's pharmacist as a member of the healthcare team helps to ensure that contraindicated medications are not being prescribed and minimizes any potential side effects. Patients with RA should be encouraged to get all their prescriptions filled at a single pharmacy to reduce the chance of contraindicated medications being prescribed by multiple physicians.

Steroid Injections

Corticosteroids can be injected directly into joints to provide relief. Injections work faster than systemic corticosteroids to decrease inflammatory cells and swelling in the joint, which reduces pain. Intra-articular corticosteroids are effective for controlling local flare-ups without changing a patient's overall drug regimen (Johns Hopkins Arthritis Center, 2016).

Nonpharmacologic Therapy

The primary objectives in treating the patient with RA are to reduce pain and inflammation, preserve function, and prevent deformity. Therapies in this area include rest and exercise, physical and occupational therapy, heat and cold, assistive devices and splints, and nutrition, as well as complementary health approaches.

Patients benefit from collaboration among many healthcare providers, including physicians, nurses and nurse practitioners, physical and occupational therapists, and nutritionists or dietitians. Working together, the healthcare team and the patient can find a more effective combination of treatments that will result in minimum discomfort and maximum function for the patient.

Rest and Exercise

A balanced program of rest and exercise is an important component in the management of RA. During an acute exacerbation of the disease, the patient may be hospitalized or prescribed a short period of complete bedrest. For most patients, regular rest periods during the day are beneficial to reduce manifestations of the disease. In addition, splinting of inflamed joints reduces unwanted motion and provides local joint rest (see the Orthotic and Assistive Devices section).

Patients must balance rest with a program of physical therapy and exercise to maintain muscle strength and joint mobility. ROM exercises are prescribed to maintain joint function and prevent contractures. Isometric exercises help preserve muscle strength without increasing joint stress. Isotonic exercises help to improve muscle strength and preserve function. Low-impact aerobic exercises, such as swimming and walking, have been shown to benefit patients with RA without adversely affecting joint inflammation or prompting acute episodes.

Physical and Occupational Therapy

Physical and occupational therapists can design and monitor individualized programs of activity and rest. Physical therapy is aimed at improving mobility and preventing the complications of inactivity. Occupational therapy works to create modifications in practices and tools needed to perform ADLs and promote as normal a lifestyle as possible.

Heat and Cold

Heat and cold are used for their analgesic and muscle-relaxing effects. Moist heat generally is most effective and can be provided by a tub bath. Some patients relieve joint pain through the application of cold.

Orthotic and Assistive Devices

A variety of **orthotic devices** (orthopedic devices that may include splints or braces applied to reduce strain on a joint) are available to help maintain function. Splints provide joint rest and prevent contractures. Night splints for the hands and/or wrists should maintain the extremity in a position of maximum function. The best "splint" for the hip is lying prone for several hours a day on a firm bed. In general, splints should be applied for the shortest period needed, made of lightweight materials, and easily removed to perform ROM exercises once or twice a day. Assistive devices, such as canes, walkers, and raised toilet seats, are most useful for patients with significant hip or knee arthritis.

Nutrition

For most patients with RA, an ordinary, well-balanced diet is recommended. Some patients may benefit from substitution of usual dietary fat with omega-3 fatty acids found in certain fish oils. Inactivity can lead to obesity, which places excess strain on the joints and can exacerbate pain. Patients should receive adequate calories and nutrients while adapting calorie intake to meet activity levels.

Medications
Rheumatoid Arthritis

CLASSIFICATION AND DRUG EXAMPLES	MECHANISMS OF ACTION	NURSING CONSIDERATIONS
Nonprescription NSAIDs Aspirin Ibuprofen (Motrin, Advil, Nuprin) Naproxen (Aleve) **Prescription NSAIDs** Diclofenac (Arthrotec, Cataflam, Voltaren) Diflunisal (Dolobid) Etodolac (Lodine) Indomethicin (Indocin) Ketoprofen (Orudis, Oruvail) Meloxicam (Mobic) Nabumetone (Relafen) Oxaprozin (Daypro) Piroxicam (Feldene) Sulindac (Clinoril) Tolmetin (Tolectin)	NSAIDs reduce inflammation and pain by blocking the synthesis of prostaglandins through inhibition of cyclooxygenase enzymes; specifically, COX-1 and COX-2 enzymes.	■ Monitor for signs and symptoms of GI toxicity, including GI bleeding (e.g., bloody/tarry stools) and gastric distress. ■ Aspirin increases bleeding time and should not be given to patients receiving anticoagulant therapy (i.e., warfarin, heparin). ■ Monitor for impaired kidney function, including decreased urine output, unexplained weight gain, and swelling due to fluid retention. ■ If long-term use is indicated, monitor CBC, electrolytes, and kidney and liver function studies. ■ Inquire about the use of herbal supplements such as feverfew, garlic, ginger, or ginkgo, which may increase bleeding.
COX-2 Inhibitors Celecoxib (Celebrex)	COX-2 inhibitors selectively block prostaglandin synthesis by inhibiting COX-2 enzymes.	■ Use caution with celecoxib due to FDA review.
Immunosuppressant/ Cytotoxic DMARDs *Drug examples:* Methotrexate Azathioprine Cyclosporine Monoclonal antibodies	These drugs have various mechanisms of action; for methotrexate, the mechanism appears to involve interruption of adenosine and possibly interference with other pathways of inflammation and immunoregulation, as well. Methotrexate inhibits an enzyme (dihydrofolate reductase) needed for metabolism of folic acid.	■ Monitor CBC with differential, platelets, kidney, and liver function studies, and chest x-rays. ■ Be alert for indicators of thrombocytopenia, such as unusual bleeding, bruising, and petechiae. ■ Teach patients taking methotrexate to avoid supplements that contain folate or its derivatives, as this alters the medication's effects. ■ Patients taking methotrexate should use contraception during and for a minimum of 3 months following therapy. ■ Grapefruit juice can increase cyclosporine levels by 50–200%. ■ Herbal supplements astragalus and echinacea may interfere with immunosuppression. ■ DMARDs should be administered only by healthcare providers experienced in immunosuppressive therapy.
Sulfasalazine *Drug example:* Azulfidine	Sulfasalazine is believed to produce anti-inflammatory effects through conversion of intestinal flora. In the GI tract, it affects prostaglandins and fluid and electrolyte absorption.	■ Prior to use, patients must be screened for glucose-6-phosphate dehydrogenase (G6PD) deficiency, which may increase risk for RBC destruction, hemolysis, and anemia. ■ Monitor CBC and liver function studies.
Antimalarials *Drug examples:* Chloroquine Hydroxychloroquine (Plaquenil)	Unknown	■ Monitor patients for visual changes and weakness. ■ Monitor CBC. ■ Administer medication with food or milk to reduce GI distress.

Medications *(continued)*

CLASSIFICATION AND DRUG EXAMPLES	MECHANISMS OF ACTION	NURSING CONSIDERATIONS
TNF Inhibitors *Drug examples:* Etanercept (Enbrel) Infliximab (Remicade) Adalimumab (Humira)	These drugs inhibit tumor necrosis factor (TNF), which is a cytokine that mediates joint damage and destruction.	■ TNF inhibitors increase susceptibility to routine and opportunistic infection; monitor for indicators of infection.
Gold Salts *Drug examples:* Gold sodium Auranofin (Ridaura) Thiomalate (Myochrysine)	Unknown	■ Monitor for indicators of hypersensitivity, ranging from rash and itching to anaphylaxis. ■ Monitor CBC and urinalysis for indicators of toxicity. ■ Gold salts are contraindicated in patients with renal disease, hepatic dysfunction, congestive heart failure, and diabetes mellitus.

Source: Data from Adams, M. P., Holland, L. N., & Urban, C. (2017). *Pharmacology for nurses: A pathophysiologic approach* (5th ed.). Hoboken, NJ: Pearson Education.

Plasmapheresis and Irradiation

Several newer treatments not yet in widespread use may be employed for patients with progressive RA. **Plasmapheresis** has been used to remove circulating antibodies and thereby moderate the autoimmune response. **Total lymphoid irradiation** decreases total lymphocyte levels, although serious adverse effects are associated with this treatment and its continued efficacy has not been established.

Complementary Health Approaches

The patient and healthcare team may consider complementary health approaches if the patient continues to experience discomfort from RA despite adherence to more traditional therapies. While many patients have reported improvement of pain and swelling with acupuncture or hydrotherapy, these therapies have yet to be proven clinically beneficial. Nutritional supplements such as fish oils may be used if they are not contraindicated. Because a cure is not available and traditional therapies are not always fully effective, the patient with RA is vulnerable to quackery. Many nontraditional treatments, including diets, topical preparations, vaccines, hormones, plant extracts, and copper bracelets, have been put forth. These treatments often are costly, and none has been shown to be effective. The nurse should ask the patient at each healthcare interaction about any nontraditional therapies being used.

Lifespan Considerations

RA affects approximately 40 per 100,000 individuals, women more frequently than men, and can occur in all races and ethnic groups (Gabriel & Crowson, 2016). Even though the disease is often diagnosed in middle age and frequently occurs in older individuals, older teenagers and young adults may also be diagnosed with RA. Children and younger teenagers are not exempt from this disease process and may be diagnosed with a similar condition known as juvenile idiopathic arthritis.

Juvenile Idiopathic Arthritis

Juvenile idiopathic arthritis (JIA) is a chronic inflammatory autoimmune juvenile disorder characterized by joint inflammation resulting in decreased mobility, swelling, and pain. It is similar to RA diagnosed in adults. JIA occurs slightly more often in girls than in boys and typically occurs between ages 3 and 6 and at or around puberty. Although no national studies have been conducted to determine the incidence of JIA in the United States, an estimated 1 in 1000 children in this country develop some form of juvenile arthritis. Many children do not complain of pain when symptoms first develop; observable symptoms such as joint swelling and unusual patterns of walking are early key indicators. Treatment is similar to that provided for adults with RA. Aspirin is often used to treat JIA because it is fast acting and inexpensive, but, because of the risk of Reye syndrome, it should be discontinued if the child develops chickenpox or flulike symptoms. Exercise is important for slowing the progression of JIA; however, joint soreness and discomfort may limit the intensity of exercise. JIA may enter remission; occasionally it continues as a chronic disease (CDC, 2015o; Sherry, 2016).

Remission may last for months, years, or a lifetime. JIA affects joints and surrounding tissues and has the potential to affect other organs, such as the heart, lungs, liver, and eyes. During the course of JIA, the child may experience pain, impaired mobility, and interference with normal growth and development. However, 70% of children with JIA experience permanent remission by adulthood. In rare cases, the disease is unresponsive to treatment, or the child may have lasting impairment, such as bone and joint changes. Children with an early onset of JIA have a better prognosis for complete recovery.

The three types of JIA are pauciarticular, systemic, and polyarticular. **Pauciarticular arthritis** primarily affects the knees, ankles, and elbows. It occurs more frequently in female patients. **Systemic arthritis** affects male and female patients equally, with characteristic manifestations of high fever, polyarthritis, and rheumatoid rash. Systemic arthritis also affects internal organs and joints. **Polyarticular arthritis** involves many joints (five or more), particularly the small joints of the hands and fingers. It also may affect the hips, knees, feet, ankles, and neck.

Like RA, the cause of JIA is unknown, but it is thought to have an autoimmune basis. Inflammation begins in the joint and leads to pain and swelling. Scar tissue eventually develops, resulting in limited ROM. This may be restricted to a few joints, or it may be systemic, involving multiple joints. Symptoms can include fever, rash, lymphadenopathy, splenomegaly, and hepatomegaly. The child may develop a limp or may obviously favor one extremity over the other. A slow rate of growth or uneven growth of extremities also may be noted. Pain, stiffness, loss of motion, and swelling occur in the large joints, such as the knees. Older children may develop symmetrical involvement of the small joints of the hand. The disease frequently is chronic, extending over several years after an initial manifestation with pain and other symptoms. However, remissions and exacerbations are characteristic.

Complications such as eye chronic uveitis, which results from chronic inflammation, may occur in children with JIA, especially those with pauciarticular arthritis. Children with polyarticular and systemic JIA should be examined by an ophthalmologist for uveitis every 6 months, and children with pauciarticular arthritis should be examined every 3 months.

As mentioned, interference with normal growth is another potential complication. JIA may result in bone growth disturbance, such as contractures or effusions. Treatment with corticosteroids also can inhibit growth.

Pregnant Women with RA

Many women diagnosed with RA experience a remission during pregnancy, often followed by a relapse after delivery. Reasons for the improvement of RA during pregnancy remain unknown. Multiple changes that occur during pregnancy, including hormonal changes, the effect on cell-mediated immunity, elevated levels of anti-inflammatory cytokines, and altered neutrophil function may play a role in the decreased disease severity. After delivery, during the postpartum period, elevated levels of prolactin and a decrease in the anti-inflammatory steroid levels are believed to be responsible for relapse.

During pregnancy, a diet low in fat and high in fiber and carbohydrates is recommended. Extra rest is encouraged, particularly to relieve weight-bearing joints, and continuation of ROM exercises is important as well. Routine consumption of oral calcium and vitamin D supplementation is also recommended. Medications used for the treatment of RA carry safety risks when used during pregnancy, and careful assessment of the risks and benefits should be considered. During remission, medication may be stopped because salicylates may prolong labor and may induce teratogenic effects. If salicylate therapy is continued, anemia may be present during the postpartum period as a result of blood loss. Corticosteroids, in

low doses, are designated as pregnancy category B. However, they may increase maternal risk for the development of hypertension, edema, gestational diabetes, osteoporosis, premature rupture of membranes, and delivery of a small-for-gestational-age baby. It is not uncommon for women diagnosed with RA to have prolonged gestations; however, cesarean delivery does not appear to be performed more commonly in these women (Temprano, 2015b).

Older Adults with RA

For older adults, RA is managed much as it is for younger individuals. Prolonged bedrest or inactivity is not prescribed for acute episodes, however, because it may result in irreversible immobility in the older adult. Medications are used with greater caution with this population because of the increased risk of toxicity. In many cases, less emphasis is placed on preventing joint deformity in older adults and more emphasis is placed on maintaining functional status, which benefits from an interprofessional team approach.

NURSING PROCESS

Patients with chronic, progressive, systemic disorders such as RA have multiple needs involving many functional health patterns. Physical manifestations of the disease often result in acute and chronic pain, fatigue, impaired mobility, and difficulty performing routine tasks. The disease also has many psychosocial effects. The patient has an incurable, chronic disease that may lead to severe crippling. Pain and fatigue can interfere with the patient's ability to perform expected roles, such as home maintenance or job responsibilities. Even though the patient's hands may appear swollen or deformed, other people may not understand the systemic nature of the disease or realize the difference between RA and osteoarthritis. Information about arthritis self-management is found in the Patient Teaching feature, and a Nursing Care Plan for a patient with RA is found later in this section.

Assessment

A careful history is important, because the history sometimes is the primary mode of diagnosis. Collect the following data:

- **Observation and patient interview.** Observe the patient's gait and posture. Look for any noticeable redness, swelling, deformities, or contractures of the joints. Inquire about the presence of pain; stiffness; fatigue; joint problems, including location, duration, onset, and effect on function; fever; sleep patterns; past illnesses or surgery; and ability to carry out ADLs and self-care activities.

- **Physical examination.** Assessment should begin with obtaining height and weight. Assess all joints for symmetry, size, shape, color, appearance, temperature, ROM, and pain. The skin assessment should include inspection and palpation for nodules and purpura. Respiratory system assessment should note the presence of cough and/or crackles. The cardiovascular assessment should also be completed, noting presence of pericardial friction rub, apical bradycardia, and/or S_3 (third heart sound).

Patient Teaching
Arthritis Self-Management

Nurses can help individuals with RA to become arthritis self-managers. Patients can help to prevent deformities and the effects of arthritis by following prescriptions for exercise, rest, weight management, posture, and positioning. The following are suggestions for patients with RA (Gecht-Silver & Duncombe, 2015):

- Do not attempt any activity you cannot stop immediately if you find you cannot complete it without pain or injury.
- Pain is a sign that you should change your action or way of doing things. Use tools or equipment (e.g., handles, jar openers) as necessary, and alternate periods of activity with rest.
- Use the strongest joints possible to complete tasks. For example, use your palm or the crook of your elbow, not your fingers, to grasp and carry items.
- Avoid activities requiring a tight grip, such as writing with a pen or pencil or screwing/unscrewing objects.

General examination includes assessing for joint swelling and deformities, fever, nodules under the skin, growth delays in children, and enlarged lymph nodes. During the physical examination, examine the hands for swan-neck contractures, which present as hyperextension of the PIP joints with the distal joint in a state of fixed flexion. **Boutonnière deformities**, which present as extreme flexion of the PIP, may also be observed (see Figure 8–19). Painless, hard nodules along the proximal and distal IP joints may be noted as well. Assessment of the lower extremities and feet may reveal nodules or tenderness around the Achilles tendon (Osborn et al., 2013).

Diagnosis

Many nursing diagnoses may be appropriate for the patient with RA. Those focusing on predominant manifestations and their effect on the patient's life are the following:

- *Pain, Chronic*
- *Fatigue*
- *Role Performance, Ineffective*
- *Body Image, Disturbed*
- *Mobility: Physical, Impaired*
- *Anxiety*
- *Activity Intolerance*
- *Self-Care Deficit.*

(NANDA-I © 2014)

The diagnosis of RA is based on the patient's history, physical assessment, and diagnostic tests. Diagnostic criteria developed by the American College of Rheumatology and the European League against Rheumatism may be used (Aletaha et al., 2010). This system classifies "definite" arthritis if there is the confirmed presence of synovitis in at least one joint, there is no alternative diagnosis for the observed arthritis, and there is a score of at least 6 from the following ranges:

- Number and site of involved joints (0–5)
- Serologic abnormalities (0–3)
- Elevated acute phase response (0–1)
- Two levels of symptom duration (0–1).

Planning

Outcomes are individualized to each patient's needs. These outcomes may include the following:

- Patient will report effectiveness of pain management techniques, maintaining pain at tolerable levels by (*specific date*).
- Patient will perform ADLs independently (or with minimal assistance, depending on degree of impairment) using tools modified by occupational therapy.
- Patient will express feelings about diagnosis of chronic disease and display progression through the grieving process.

Implementation

Nursing care focuses on promoting mobility, encouraging adequate nutrition, and teaching the patient and family about the disease and its management (see the Evidence-Based Practice feature). Most care will occur in the community, including physical therapy, with only occasional hospitalizations at the time of an exacerbation of the disease.

Monitor and Treat Chronic Pain

Pain is a constant feature of RA when the disease is active. It accompanies both acute inflammation and lower levels of chronic inflammation. Some patients say the pain in joints and surrounding tissue is like a deep, constant toothache. Pain can significantly affect the patient's ability to provide self-care and maintain daily activities. It also contributes to the patient's fatigue.

- Monitor the pain level and duration of morning stiffness. Pain and morning stiffness are indicators of disease activity. Increased pain may necessitate changes in the therapeutic treatment plan.
- Encourage the patient to relate pain to activity level and adjust his or her activities accordingly. Teach the importance of joint and whole-body rest in relieving pain. Pain is an indicator of excess stress on inflamed joints. Increasing pain indicates a need to decrease activity levels.
- Teach the use of heat and cold applications to provide pain relief. The patient may apply heat by showering

Evidence-Based Practice

Patient-Centered Care for Patients with Rheumatoid Arthritis

Problem

RA is a disease that can occur at any age, but it is seen most often in older adults. RA causes physical, emotional, and economic difficulties, but appropriate management can do much to reduce pain and disability, increase a sense of control, and improve quality of life. In the past, physicians were at the center of care and patients were expected to be compliant with instructions given by healthcare providers. With the current shift toward patient-centered care, there is greater desire for patients to have more involvement in planning their care and to participate in making important medical decisions.

Evidence

Recent examination of patient-centered care in RA has indicated that involving the patient has a relevant impact on the safety, effectiveness, and cost of treatment. The patient-centered approach also empowers patients to take more personal responsibility for their treatment. This new patient role in their treatment involves patient education, shared decision making, self-management, and involvement of family and friends who provide physical and emotional support. Patient-centered care is viewed as higher quality care because of the collaboration of healthcare professionals and patients jointly working to restore or maintain patient health status.

Participation in treatment planning gives patients ownership of their illness (National Council on Aging, 2016). As a consequence, they require knowledge of the disease, symptoms, treatment options, and possible outcomes. These patients also require the necessary skills to allow them to self-manage their disease and participate in decision making. Last, they require the

power to believe in their ability to self-manage their disease and be able to influence treatment decisions. Evidence has shown that the amount of participation by patients in their care has a significant impact on the treatment quality in regard to safety and effectiveness. The healthcare system may also benefit from this participation in the financial aspect. Studies have indicated that patients participating in patient-centered care show improved experience with healthcare, lower dependence on healthcare services, better adherence to treatment, and occasionally measurable improvements in health outcomes. This approach to care is agreed upon and supported by the WHO (Voshaar et al., 2015).

Implications

Patients who experience patient-centered care exhibit a decreased dependence on healthcare services and greater safety and efficacy of treatment. Patients who are empowered to make informed decisions about their care, manage their disease properly at home, and learn as much as they can about their illness and its treatment are likely to achieve greater adherence to their treatment regimens and better health outcomes overall.

Critical Thinking Application

1. What strategies would you consider in providing patient teaching to older adults with RA? What information would you need to have before implementing a patient teaching session for one or more older adults?

2. In providing information to older adults about RA, what internet sites would you recommend and why?

---

or taking tub baths or by using warm compresses or other local applications, such as paraffin dips. For patients who find that heat increases pain and swelling during periods of acute inflammation, cold packs may be more effective.

- Teach about the use of prescribed anti-inflammatory medications and the relationship of pain and inflammation. Anti-inflammatory agents reduce chemical mediators of inflammation and swelling, relieving pain.

- Encourage the use of nonpharmacologic pain relief measures, such as visualization, distraction, meditation, and progressive relaxation techniques. These techniques can reduce muscle tension and help the patient focus away from the pain, decreasing the intensity of the pain experience.

Prevent Fatigue

The pain and chronic inflammatory processes associated with RA lead to fatigue, but other factors contribute as well. Discomfort often disrupts the patient's sleep patterns. Anemia, muscle atrophy, oxygenation, and poor nutrition play a role in the development of fatigue. The patient with RA also may experience depression or hopelessness, with associated

manifestations of fatigue. Interventions to help patients prevent fatigue include:

- Encourage a balance of periods of activity with periods of rest. Both joint rest and whole-body rest are important in reducing the inflammatory response. Stress the importance of planned rest periods during the day. Rest is vital during acute exacerbations of the disease and is also important for the patient in remission.

- Help the patient to prioritize activities, encouraging the performance of the most important ones early in the day. Assigning priorities helps the patient to avoid performing relatively unimportant activities at the expense of more meaningful and important ones.

- Encourage regular physical activity in addition to prescribed **range of motion (ROM) exercises** (exercises designed to take each joint through all possible movements to maintain flexibility and movement in the joint). Aerobic exercise promotes a sense of well-being and restful sleep patterns.

Address Ineffective Role Performance

Fatigue, pain, and the crippling effects of RA can interfere with the patient's ability to pursue an education or career and to fill other life roles, such as parent, spouse, or homemaker. As the patient's roles change, so must the roles of other family members. These role changes contribute to changes in family processes, increased stress in the family, and further difficulty in coping with the effects of the disease. Nursing interventions to promote effective role performance include:

- Discuss the effects of the disease on the patient's career and other life roles. Encourage the patient to identify changes brought on by the disease. Discussion helps the patient to accept the changes and begin to identify strategies for coping with them.

- Encourage the patient and family to discuss their feelings about role changes and to grieve over lost roles or abilities. Verbalization allows family members to validate and accept feelings about losses and changes, helping them to move into new roles.

- Help the patient and family to identify strengths they can use to cope with role changes. Identifying strengths helps the patient and family to consider role changes that maintain self-esteem and dignity.

- Encourage the patient to make decisions and assume personal responsibility for management of the disease. Patients who assume a personal and active role in managing their disease maintain a greater sense of self-control and self-esteem.

Promote a Healthy Body Image

The acute and long-term effects of RA can affect the patient's body image and thus lead to feelings of hopelessness and powerlessness, social withdrawal, and difficulty adapting to changes. When inflammation and joint deformity occur despite compliance, the patient may have difficulty accepting the need to continue therapeutic measures, particularly those that have side effects or are costly or time consuming. In addition, unproven alternative treatment strategies and quackery may become increasingly attractive. Nursing interventions to promote a healthy body image include:

- Encourage the patient to talk about the effects of the disease, both the physical effects and the effects on life roles. Verbalization helps the patient to identify feelings and gives the nurse an opportunity to validate these feelings.

- Encourage the patient to maintain self-care and usual roles to the extent possible. Discuss the use of clothing and adaptive devices that promote independence. Independence enhances the patient's self-esteem.

- Refer the patient to self-help groups, support groups, and other agencies that provide assistive devices and literature. These groups and agencies can help the patient develop adaptive strategies to cope with the effects of RA, enhancing the patient's self-concept, body image, and independence.

- Encourage children with RA to maintain contact with peers and to attend school when possible. Children require social interaction and education to meet developmental milestones, and changes in body image can make them feel self-conscious or awkward and thus lead to isolation.

- For children with JIA, plot growth carefully, and watch for changes in growth percentiles. Growth must be carefully monitored for early detection of problems and prevention of long-term complications.

Provide Support Related to Impaired Mobility

Nurses can help patients with impaired mobility by encouraging them to perform ADLs. Medications may be given to reduce joint swelling and inflammation. In addition, warm or cold compresses applied to involved joints may provide pain relief.

- Physical therapists play an essential role in the patient's treatment. The goals of physical therapy are to maintain joint function, strengthen muscles, increase tone, maintain body alignment, and prevent permanent deformities, such as contractures. ROM exercises, stretching, hydrotherapy, and swimming all help to prevent deformities.

- Occupational therapists can help the patient to continue performing ADLs. Tools with larger handles can reduce the pain of gripping, and longer handles on implements reduce reaching. The goal is for the patient to maintain independence in performing daily activities.

- Teach the patient and family about the condition, prognosis, and importance of optimizing activity levels. The patient needs to understand that overexertion may lead to exacerbation of the disease and that activities should be within tolerable limits.

Evaluation

RA typically is a chronic, progressive disease. As with most diseases of this nature, involvement of the patient and family in its management is vital. Evaluation of nursing care is a continuous and ongoing part of meeting the patient's needs to determine if the current plan of care is effective. Expected outcomes of nursing care for the patient include the following:

- The patient maintains joint mobility.
- The patient expresses comfort and freedom from pain.
- The patient develops or maintains a positive body image.
- The patient is free from infection.
- The patient and family display adequate understanding, support, and management of the therapeutic regimen.

Secondary intervention evaluation may include:

- The patient will use medication for pain prior to planned activities or exercise as appropriate.
- The patient will use stress management techniques such as progressive relaxation or guided imagery to enhance coping abilities.
- The patient will have an active role in planning care and managing the disease.

Nursing Care Plan

A Patient with Rheumatoid Arthritis

Janice James is a 42-year-old high school science teacher who began noticing vague joint pain, fatigue, poor appetite, and general malaise, which she initially attributed to a case of the flu. However, her symptoms continued, and she began to notice aching in her hands and wrists, which she attributed to the quilting she loves to do in the evenings. She made an appointment with her family physician when she noticed that her knuckles and finger joints were not just achy but also swollen and hot. She reports feeling very stiff in the mornings, often taking until 10:00 or 11:00 a.m. to begin to feel "normal."

Noting that Ms. James has lost 10 pounds since her last visit and has mild anemia and a significantly elevated erythrocyte sedimentation rate, the physician refers her to the rheumatology clinic for further evaluation. Following examination and laboratory and radiologic testing, the rheumatologist establishes a diagnosis of RA and initiates a multidisciplinary team conference to plan the management of Ms. James's condition.

ASSESSMENT

Cathy Greenstein, RN, completes an assessment of Ms. James. She notes that Ms. James is well groomed and answers questions readily. However, she appears fatigued and ill. Ms. James relates that her job has been extremely stressful, because teacher layoffs have resulted in larger class sizes and fewer teaching assistants. Despite symptoms, she continues to teach full time but says she feels unable to keep up with all her responsibilities because of her fatigue.

Ms. James states that she is allergic to penicillin. Her medical history reveals only the usual childhood diseases and three uncomplicated pregnancies, resulting in the births of her children, ages 14, 11, and 9. Physical assessment findings include: T_O 37.8°C (100.2°F); P 82 bpm regular; R 18/min; BP 124/78 mmHg. There is swelling of the PIP and MCP joints of both hands; second and third PIP and second MCP joints on right hand are red, shiny, hot, spongy, and tender to palpation. Ms. James is able to extend her fingers to 180° but cannot make a complete fist with either hand, with flexion limited to less than 90°. Her grip strength is weak bilaterally; her wrist ROM is limited in all directions. Her knees are swollen, and flexion is slightly limited. There is a positive bulge sign in the right knee. Diagnostic findings are an erythrocyte sedimentation rate of 52 mm/hr, a hematocrit of 30%, and positive for rheumatoid factor. Few changes other than soft-tissue swelling are evident on hand and wrist x-rays.

DIAGNOSES

Nursing diagnoses that may be appropriate for Ms. James include the following:

- *Pain, Chronic,* related to joint inflammation
- *Home Maintenance, Impaired,* related to fatigue
- *Activity Intolerance* related to the effects of inflammation
- *Knowledge, Deficient,* regarding her therapeutic regimen

(NANDA-I © 2014)

PLANNING

The expected outcomes for the plan of care specify that Ms. James will:

- Verbalize effective pain management strategies.
- Use assistive devices to minimize joint stress with ADLs.
- Verbalize a plan to reduce responsibilities for home maintenance.
- Express willingness to plan rest breaks during the day.
- Demonstrate understanding of the prescribed therapeutic regimen and its importance for both short- and long-term benefit.

IMPLEMENTATION

The following nursing interventions may be appropriate for Ms. James:

- Teach techniques for relieving pain and morning stiffness, including: scheduling NSAIDs at equal intervals throughout the day; taking morning NSAID dose with milk and crackers approximately 30 minutes before rising; performing ROM exercises while seated in the shower or tub; applying local heat with paraffin dip or compress; using cold packs as needed; and learning techniques to minimize joint stress while performing ADLs.

- Provide Arthritis Foundation literature and information.
- Discuss ways to delegate household tasks to other family members.
- Explore ways to incorporate 30-minute rest breaks into work schedule.
- Provide information about the disease process and its manifestations, prescribed medications and their desired and adverse effects, and the importance of balancing rest and activity.

Nursing Care Plan (continued)

EVALUATION

The initial treatment regimen of aspirin, rest, exercise, and physical therapy succeeded in partially relieving the acute manifestations of RA in Ms. James. However, complete remission has not been achieved. She has had difficulty scheduling rest periods at work and has had to struggle to delegate household tasks. "I don't look sick to the kids, and they seem to think housecleaning is a terrible imposition on their time. It's often easier to just do it myself than to fight about it. Besides, that way it gets done right." Ms. James has faithfully followed the prescribed medication regimen and exercise routines, and she has kept her scheduled appointments and maintained contact with the treatment team.

CRITICAL THINKING

1. Ms. James is 42 years old. Would your nursing interventions differ if she were 72 years old? If so, how?
2. RA is a chronic illness. What are the physical, emotional, and economic implications of an illness that results in chronic pain and deformity?
3. Develop a nursing care plan for Ms. James using the nursing diagnosis *Ineffective Role Performance*.

REVIEW Rheumatoid Arthritis

RELATE Link the Concepts and Exemplars

Linking the exemplar of rheumatoid arthritis with the concept of inflammation:

1. What role does inflammation play in the disease process of RA?
2. What nursing care (independent or collaborative) can you provide that will slow the inflammatory process?
3. What signs and symptoms of RA indicate the inflammatory process?

Linking the exemplar of rheumatoid arthritis with the concept of safety:

4. When caring for a patient with RA affecting both knees, what nursing care can you provide to improve the patient's safety?
5. What risks for injury would RA in both knees create?

Linking the exemplar of rheumatoid arthritis with the concept of mobility:

6. What are the foreseeable impacts of RA on ADLs at different stages in the lifespan? Why could these be particularly problematic for individuals with JIA?
7. You are caring for a 63-year-old patient with RA who recently sustained a broken leg during a car accident. What special considerations should you give to selecting an assistive device to allow her to ambulate while her leg heals?

READY Go to Volume 3: Clinical Nursing Skills

REFER Go to Pearson MyLab Nursing and eText

- Additional review materials

REFLECT Apply Your Knowledge

Justine Belamo is a 48-year-old woman who has been married to Gil Belamo for 18 years. Ms. Belamo has a daughter, Majel, from a previous marriage, and she has two teenage children, Mark and Maria, with Gil. Ms. Belamo works as a grocery store clerk. Although she finds her job monotonous, she appreciates the steady income and family health insurance.

Ms. Belamo is overweight and has tried to lose weight most of her adult life. She frequently diets and, in the past, has lost a great deal of weight, but she just cannot seem to keep the weight off. She blames menopause for her most recent weight gain.

1. What factors place Ms. Belamo at risk for development of RA?
2. When talking with Ms. Belamo, what interview questions might you ask to determine whether she has any early signs of RA?
3. If Ms. Belamo were to be diagnosed with RA, what teaching might you provide to reduce joint damage?

›› Exemplar 8.D
Systemic Lupus Erythematosus

Exemplar Learning Outcomes

8.D Analyze systemic lupus erythematosus (SLE) as it relates to immunity.

- Describe the pathophysiology of SLE.
- Describe the etiology of SLE.
- Compare the risk factors and prevention of SLE.
- Identify the clinical manifestations of SLE.
- Summarize diagnostic tests and therapies used by interprofessional teams in the collaborative care of an individual with SLE.
- Differentiate care of patients with SLE across the lifespan.
- Apply the nursing process in providing culturally competent care to an individual with SLE.

Overview

The generalized disorder known as **systemic lupus erythematosus (SLE)** is a chronic, inflammatory, **connective tissue** disease of unknown origin that affects almost all body systems, including the musculoskeletal system. SLE is characterized by remissions and exacerbations. It can range from a mild, episodic disorder to a rapidly fatal disease process. Manifestations are widely variable; can affect the joints, skin, brain, lungs, kidneys, and blood vessels; and are thought to result from cell and tissue damage caused by deposition of antigen–antibody complexes in connective tissues. The majority of cases are diagnosed during the teenage and early adult years.

Pathophysiology and Etiology

Pathophysiology

The pathophysiology of SLE involves production of a large variety of **autoantibodies** (antibodies that react to the patient's own tissues) against normal body components, such as nucleic acids, erythrocytes, coagulation proteins, lymphocytes, and platelets. Autoantibody production results from hyperreactivity of B cells (**humoral immune response**) because of disordered T-cell function (**cellular immune response**). These autoantibodies may be present in an individual for many years prior to the first onset of symptoms. One long-standing theory related to the development of autoantibodies involves a defect in apoptosis that causes increased cell death and a disturbance in immune tolerance. T cells in individuals with this disease have been found to show defects in both signaling and effector functioning; they also secrete less interleukin-2 (Bartels, 2015).

The SLE autoantibodies react with their corresponding antigen to form immune complexes, which are then deposited in the connective tissue of blood vessels, lymphatic vessels, and other tissues. These deposits trigger an **inflammatory response** (a chain reaction leading to inflammation described in detail in the module on Inflammation), which leads to local tissue damage. The kidneys are a frequent site of complex deposition and damage; other affected tissues include the musculoskeletal system, brain, heart, spleen, lung, GI tract, skin, and peritoneum. The autoantibodies produced and their target tissues determine the manifestations of SLE.

Etiology

Although the exact etiology of SLE is unknown, genetic, ethnic, environmental, and hormonal factors play a role in its development. Twin studies and a familial pattern of the disease point to a genetic component, as does an increased incidence of other connective tissue diseases in relatives of individuals with SLE. In addition, certain **human leukocyte antigen (HLA)** genes (a major histocompatibility complex) are seen more frequently in individuals with SLE.

Researchers believe that individuals are born with a genetic predisposition for developing lupus. Exposure to environmental factors then triggers manifestation of the disease (Lupus Foundation of America [LFA], 2016a). Environmental factors believed to play a role in activating the pathologic mechanisms of SLE include viruses, bacterial antigens, chemicals, drugs, and ultraviolet light.

Sex hormones also are thought to influence the development of SLE. Women with SLE have reduced levels of several active androgens that are known to inhibit antibody responses. In addition, estrogens have been shown to enhance antibody responses and to have an adverse effect in patients with SLE.

Risk Factors and Prevention

In 2014, the CDC estimated the annual incidence of SLE to range from 1.8 to 7.6 per 100,000 individuals in the United States, with women comprising 90% of the affected population (Bartels, 2015). While SLE can develop at any point in life, it is most common among women of childbearing age. SLE is more common in African Americans, Hispanics, Native Americans, Native Hawaiians, and Asians than it is in Caucasians (LFA, 2016b).

A clear genetic component has been established with SLE, and the risk for sibling development of the disease ranges from 8 to 29 times higher than for the general population (Bartels, 2015). Patients who have other autoimmune conditions have a risk for developing SLE. In patients with no other risk factors for the disease, a number of drugs can cause a syndrome that mimics lupus (drug-induced lupus). These symptoms usually occur 3–6 months after starting a medication and disappear when the medication is discontinued (CDC, 2015d). Procainamide (Procan-SR, Pronestyl) and hydralazine (Apresoline, Hydralyn) are the most commonly implicated drugs, along with isoniazid (INH). Renal and CNS manifestations of SLE rarely occur with drug-induced lupus, but arthritic and other systemic symptoms are common. The development of this disease cannot be prevented, and there is no known cure. However, patients can prevent disease flare-ups by avoiding excessive sun exposure, reducing stress, exercising regularly, receiving influenza and pneumococcal vaccines, and avoiding the use of high-dose birth control pills, penicillin, and sulfonamides (University of Maryland Medical Center, 2015).

Clinical Manifestations

There are three major classifications of SLE. In addition to *drug-induced lupus,* there are two major classifications of SLE. *Systemic lupus* involves one or more of the following systems: cardiovascular, central nervous, hematologic, kidneys, lungs, and musculoskeletal. *Cutaneous* or *discoid lupus* is limited to the skin.

The course of SLE is mild in most patients, with periods of remission and exacerbation. The number and severity of exacerbations tend to decrease with time. In some patients, however, SLE is a virulent disease, with significant organ system involvement.

Patients with active disease have an increased risk for infections, which often are opportunistic and severe. Infections such as pneumonia and septicemia are the leading cause of death in patients with SLE, followed by the effects of renal or CNS involvement (see the Multisystem Effects feature).

Multisystem Effects of
Systemic Lupus Erythematosus

Integumentary

- Butterfly rash on face
- Photosensitivity
- Maculopapular rash on exposed body surfaces
- Discoid lesions
- Erythematous fingertip lesions
- Splinter hemorrhages
- Alopecia
- Ulcers (lip, mouth, nose)

Endocrine

- Thyroid abnormalities
- Hyperparathyroidism
- Glucose intolerance

Respiratory

- Pleurisy
- Pleural effusion
- Pneumonitis
- Interstitial fibrosis

Urinary

- Proteinuria
- Cellular casts
Potential complications
- Nephrotic syndrome
- Renal failure

Gastrointestinal

- Anorexia
- Nausea
- Abdominal pain
- Diarrhea
- Hepatomegaly

Musculoskeletal

- Arthralgias
- Symmetric polyarthritis
- Joint swelling and effusion
- Morning stiffness

Neurologic

- Neuropathies (peripheral and central)
- Seizures
- Depression
- Psychosis
Potential complications
- Stroke
- Organic brain syndrome
  - Intellectual impairment
  - Memory loss
  - Personality changes
  - Disorientation

Sensory

- Conjunctivitis
- Photophobia
- Retinal vasculitis with transient blindness
- Cotton-wool spots on retina

Cardiovascular

- Pericarditis
- Myocarditis
- Endocarditis
- Vasculitis
- Venous or arterial thrombosis

Hematologic

- Anemia
- Leukopenia
- Thrombocytopenia
- Splenomegaly

Reproductive

- Pregnancy-induced hypertension, edema, and proteinuria
- Fetal loss

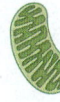

Metabolic Processes

- Low-grade fever
- Malaise
- Weight loss

Typical early manifestations of SLE mimic those of RA, including systemic manifestations of fever, loss of appetite, malaise, and weight loss, and musculoskeletal manifestations of multiple arthralgias and symmetric polyarthritis. Joint symptoms affect more than 90% of patients with SLE. Although synovitis may be present, the arthritis associated with SLE is rarely deforming.

Most individuals affected by SLE have skin manifestations at some point during their disease. In fact, SLE originally was described as a skin disorder and was named for the characteristic red butterfly rash across the cheeks and bridge of the nose (see **Figure 8–21 »**). Many patients with SLE are photosensitive; a diffuse, maculopapular rash on skin exposed to the sun is common. Other cutaneous manifestations include **discoid lesions** (raised, scaly, circular lesions with an erythematous rim), hives, erythematous fingertip lesions, and splinter hemorrhages. Alopecia is common in patients with SLE, although the hair usually grows back. Painless mucous membrane ulcerations may occur on the lips or in the mouth or nose. Common manifestations of SLE include painful or swollen joints, muscle pain, unexplained fever, red rash (especially on the face), unusual loss of hair, pale or cyanotic fingers or toes, sensitivity to the sun, edema in legs and around the eyes, ulcers in the mouth, enlarged glands, and extreme fatigue.

Approximately 50% of individuals with SLE experience renal manifestations of the disease, including proteinuria, cellular casts, and nephrotic syndrome. Up to 10% develop renal failure as a result of the disease.

Hematologic abnormalities, such as anemia, leukopenia, and thrombocytopenia, are common with SLE. Cardiovascular disorders, such as pericarditis, vasculitis, and Raynaud phenomenon, often occur. Less frequently, myocarditis, endocarditis, and venous or arterial thrombosis may develop. Pleurisy, pleural effusions, and lupus pneumonitis are common pulmonary manifestations of SLE.

Many patients with SLE develop transient nervous system involvement, often within the first year of the disease. Manifestations of organic brain syndrome include decline in intellect, memory loss, and disorientation. Other possible neurologic manifestations include psychosis, seizures, depression, and stroke. Ocular manifestations of SLE include conjunctivitis, photophobia, and transient blindness due to retinal vasculitis.

GI manifestations of SLE, such as anorexia, nausea, abdominal pain, and diarrhea, may affect up to 45% of patients with the disease. The liver may be enlarged, and liver function tests may yield abnormal results.

Although SLE was once considered a fatal disease, the survival rate has improved through earlier diagnosis and better treatment options. In the 1950s, the 5-year survival rate associated with SLE was approximately 50%. Because of more effective and aggressive treatment, the survival rate for individuals at the 10-year mark has increased to 90% (Wallace, 2015).

Prognosis depends on the severity of the internal organ involvement. Kidney failure is managed by hemodialysis or peritoneal dialysis. Renal transplantation has been very successful for treatment of renal failure secondary to lupus nephritis, a common complication of SLE. See the Lifespan Considerations section for a discussion about SLE and pregnancy.

Collaboration

As with RA, effective management of SLE requires teamwork, with active participation by both the patient and members of the healthcare team. Depending on the severity of a patient's manifestations, nurses may want to collaborate with dietitians and physical therapists to help the patient develop a nutrition and exercise plan. Referrals to counselors can help the patient and caregivers learn to manage stress.

Diagnostic Tests

Because of the diversity of both organ system involvement and manifestations of SLE, diagnosis can be difficult. No one specific test is available to confirm the presence of this disease in all individuals who are suspected of having it. Instead, the diagnosis is based on the patient's history and physical assessment, as well as laboratory studies.

The multiple autoantibodies produced in SLE cause a number of abnormalities in laboratory studies. The following tests may be helpful in confirming the presence of SLE:

- **Anti-DNA antibody testing.** This test is a more specific indicator of SLE, because these antibodies are rarely found in any other disorder.

- **Erythrocyte sedimentation rate.** This value typically is elevated, occasionally to 100 mm/hr or greater.

- **Serum complement levels.** These values usually are decreased as complement is consumed or "used up" by the development of **antigen–antibody complexes**.

- **CBC.** Abnormalities in the CBC include moderate to severe anemia, leukopenia, lymphocytopenia, and possible thrombocytopenia.

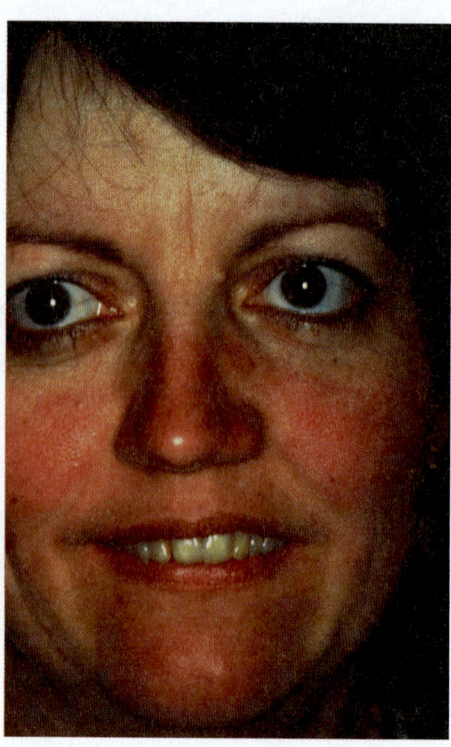

Figure 8–21 » The butterfly rash of systemic lupus erythematosus.

Clinical Manifestations and Therapies
Systemic Lupus Erythematosus

ETIOLOGY	CLINICAL MANIFESTATIONS	CLINICAL THERAPIES
Organic brain syndrome, resulting from neurologic involvement	This general term refers to many disorders causing impaired mental function. Manifestations include confusion with impaired memory, judgment, and cognition. Symptoms may include agitation, withdrawal, or depression.	Treatment varies and is aimed at treating the underlying cause of the condition, in this case SLE.
Anemia	Manifestations range from absence of clinical signs and symptoms to more life-threatening, depending on the severity of the condition. Common manifestations include: ■ Weakness ■ Fatigue ■ Poor concentration ■ Shortness of breath ■ Dyspnea ■ Palpitations ■ Intermittent claudication ■ Symptoms of heart failure.	Initial treatment is aimed at restoring normal RBC counts as well as treating the underlying cause. Treatment to increase RBC counts includes: ■ Increased iron intake in diet ■ Iron supplementation ■ Medications to stimulate red cell production, such as erythropoietin. In severe cases, blood transfusions may be administered.
Leukopenia	The most common manifestation is frequent infections resulting from inadequate immune response caused by low WBC count.	Treatment to increase WBC counts is predominantly aimed at treating the underlying cause of leukopenia. Supportive treatment to resolve infections and prevent further infection may include antibiotics, protective isolation, and strict aseptic technique.
Thrombocytopenia (may occur spontaneously but is more commonly associated with medications used to treat SLE)	Manifestations generally do not arise until the platelet count falls to significant levels of less than 50,000 per mL. Common manifestations include: ■ Bruising ■ Petechiae ■ Purpura ■ Nosebleeds ■ Bleeding gums.	Treatment is guided by the etiology and severity and may include: ■ Corticosteroids ■ IV IgG ■ Splenectomy ■ Administration of IV platelet transfusion.
Pericarditis	Common manifestations include: ■ Chest pain radiating to the back relieved by sitting forward and worsening when lying down ■ Dry cough ■ Fever ■ Fatigue ■ Anxiety ■ Friction rub ■ ST elevation and PR depression.	Treatment may include: ■ Pericardiocentesis to remove fluid produced by the inflammatory process, especially if it is restricting function ■ Antibiotics if pericarditis is infectious ■ Corticosteroids to reduce inflammation ■ Colchicine.
Renal involvement	Common manifestations include: ■ Proteinuria ■ Cellular casts ■ Nephrotic syndrome ■ Renal failure.	Treatment is aimed at correcting the underlying cause and relieving stress on the kidney. Dialysis may be indicated if renal failure results.
Skin involvement (most common result of SLE)	Common manifestations include photosensitivity with a diffuse maculopapular rash on skin exposed to the sun, discoid lesions, hives, erythematous fingertip lesions, alopecia, and splinter hemorrhages.	Treatment may include: ■ Corticosteroids ■ Immunosuppressants ■ Disease-modifying antirheumatic drugs ■ Low-fat, mostly vegetarian, wholesome diet (may lessen symptoms).

- **Urinalysis.** This test shows mild proteinuria, hematuria, and blood cell casts during exacerbations of the disease when the kidneys are involved. Renal function tests including *serum creatinine* and *blood urea nitrogen (BUN)* may also be ordered to evaluate the extent of renal disease.
- **Kidney biopsy.** This test may be performed to assess the severity of renal lesions and to guide therapy.

Surgery

Although there is no surgical treatment for SLE, damage caused by SLE can lead to other conditions that require surgery. The kidneys are particularly vulnerable to injury. Patients with lupus nephritis who progress to develop end-stage renal disease are treated with hemodialysis or peritoneal dialysis and kidney transplantation.

Pharmacologic Therapy

The patient with mild or remittent SLE may need little or no therapy other than supportive care. Arthralgias, arthritis, fever, and fatigue often can be managed with aspirin or other NSAIDs. Aspirin is particularly beneficial for patients with SLE, because its antiplatelet effects help to prevent thrombosis. However, it may cause liver toxicity and hepatitis.

Skin and arthritic manifestations of SLE may be treated with antimalarial drugs, such as hydroxychloroquine (Plaquenil). Hydroxychloroquine also has been shown to be effective in reducing the frequency of acute episodes of SLE in individuals with mild or inactive disease. Retinal toxicity and possibly irreversible blindness are the primary concerns with this drug. For this reason, patients taking hydroxychloroquine should undergo an ophthalmologic examination every 6 months.

Topical corticosteroids may be used to treat skin lesions. Some physicians recommend avoiding the use of oral contraceptives, because estrogen can trigger an acute episode.

Patients with severe and life-threatening manifestations of SLE (e.g., nephritis, hemolytic anemia, myocarditis, pericarditis, CNS manifestations) require corticosteroid therapy in high doses. At first, such patients may need 40–60 mg of prednisone per day. The dosage is then tapered as rapidly as the patient's disease allows, although lowering the dosage may precipitate an acute episode. Some patients with SLE require long-term corticosteroid therapy to manage symptoms and prevent major organ damage. These patients are at increased risk for corticosteroid side effects, such as cushingoid effects, weight gain, hypertension, infection, accelerated osteoporosis, and hypokalemia.

Certain cytotoxic or antineoplastic drugs are as effective as immunosuppressive agents and may be used either alone or in combination with corticosteroids to treat patients with active SLE or lupus nephritis. These agents act by decreasing the proliferation of cells within the immune system and are widely used to prevent rejection following a tissue or organ transplant. They are usually administered concurrently with corticosteroid therapy, allowing lower doses of both preparations and resulting in fewer side effects. Examples include azathioprine (Imuran), cyclophosphamide (Cytoxan), and cyclosporine (Sandimmune).

The patient receiving immunosuppressive agents is at increased risk for infection, malignancy, bone marrow depression, and toxic effects specific to the drug prescribed. Nursing responsibilities for patients on immunosuppressants include:

- Monitor blood count, with particular attention to the WBC and platelet counts. Notify the physician if WBCs fall below 4000 or platelets below 75,000.
- Monitor renal and liver function studies, including creatinine, blood urea nitrogen, creatinine clearance, and liver enzyme levels. Report abnormal levels to the physician.
- Administer oral preparations with food to minimize GI effects.
- Increase fluids to maintain good hydration and urinary output; monitor intake and output.
- Monitor for signs of abnormal bleeding (e.g., bleeding gums, petechiae, joint pain, hematuria, and black or tarry stools).
- Use meticulous hand hygiene and other appropriate measures to prevent infection; assess for signs of infection.
- Pulmonary fibrosis is a potential adverse effect of cyclophosphamide. Monitor the results of pulmonary function studies and be alert for dyspnea or cough.

For patients receiving immunosuppressive agents, careful teaching is required to make sure both patients and family members understand appropriate precautions to take while on these medications as well as ways to protect themselves against the threat of infection (see the Patient Teaching feature). Note that women may not experience menstruation while taking cyclophosphamide; menses will resume once the drug is discontinued.

Patient Teaching
Precautions to Reduce Infection Risk

Teach patients to:

- Avoid large crowds and situations that increase exposure to infection.
- Report signs of infection, such as chills, fever, sore throat, fatigue, or malaise to the healthcare provider.
- Refrain from taking aspirin or ibuprofen, which may increase the risk of bleeding. Report any signs of bleeding to the physician.
- Do not use oral contraception to prevent pregnancy, as these drugs may increase the risk of birth defects.
- Report difficulty breathing or cough to the physician if taking cyclophosphamide.
- Use sunscreen with an SPF rating of 15 or higher when outdoors.

Nonpharmacologic Therapy

Patients with SLE should be counseled to avoid smoking. Among numerous other negative effects, smoking can exacerbate the risks of cardiovascular damage linked to SLE, as well as increasing susceptibility to infection, especially in the lungs. During periods of known or suspected infection, these patients should be advised to consult with their healthcare provider prior to receiving any immunizations. While there is no standard recommended diet for patients with SLE, they should be encouraged to consume a healthy diet that includes oily fish, as omega-3 fatty acids appear to offer protection against cardiovascular disease. Before adding any herb, vitamin, or supplement to the diet, these patients should consult their healthcare provider. Some dietary supplements are associated with known undesirable effects; for example, alfalfa tablets are linked to lupus flares (acute episodes) (LFA, 2016e).

Exacerbations of SLE have been linked to stress (LFA, 2016f). Counseling that emphasizes stress reduction and enhanced coping strategies has been linked to fewer pain-related complaints, while also improving social and physical function in individuals with SLE (Williams et al., 2014).

Lifespan Considerations

Roughly 20% of patients with SLE develop the disease before the age of 20, though it is rare in children younger than 5 years (American College of Rheumatology, 2016b; Tucker & Watcher, 2013). The number of childhood cases is roughly equal across genders; after puberty, however, significantly more adolescent girls are affected than adolescent boys (Arthritis Foundation, 2013).

Pregnant Women and Newborns with SLE

For women with SLE, all pregnancies are considered high risk. The majority of these pregnancies are not associated with any complications; however, the risk for complications is higher for pregnant women with active SLE than for those whose SLE is in remission. Pregnancy-related complications associated with this disease include preeclampsia, the syndrome known as HELLP (hemolysis, elevated liver function, and low platelets), and a higher rate of spontaneous abortion (LFA, 2016c). During pregnancy, if anti-SSA/Ro antibodies are transferred from mother to fetus through the placenta, neonatal lupus may develop. Neonatal lupus is rare, occurring in only 2% of first-time mothers who test positive for anti-SSA/Ro antibodies. While symptoms seen in infants born with neonatal lupus may be minimal and resolve spontaneously, such as rashes or mild liver involvement, the potentially fatal condition of congenital heart block (CHB) may also occur. If indicated, fetal echocardiography may be used to assess for CHB. This test usually is performed during the second trimester. The prognosis for CHB varies, depending upon when CHB is detected. With treatment, early CHB may be reversible. However, late CHB may require insertion of a pacemaker at the time of delivery (LFA, 2016d).

Children and Adolescents with SLE

Studies have found lupus nephritis to be more prevalent in patients who have an earlier onset of the disease, which would be the adolescent population. This group is more likely to have higher incidence of active disease and receive more intensive drug therapy, which can result in greater risk for renal damage. Among those who respond to treatment, prognosis is better for younger patients despite the risk for renal damage (Sato et al., 2012).

Children and teens with SLE need to be encouraged to live as normal a life as possible by continuing to go to school, playing with friends, eating healthily, exercising and continuing family activities (Tucker & Watcher, 2013). The side effects of the corticosteroids, immunosuppressants, and antimalarial drugs used in the treatment of SLE are significant and include hair loss, susceptibility to infection, "moon face," retinal damage, and bone loss. These are significant side effects for adolescent patients, who commonly are concerned about appearance. Special teaching, guidance, and support may be needed for teens with SLE. The nurse should encourage teens to find methods to explain the side effects and appearance. For example, a science or health teacher may allow the adolescent the opportunity to present information about the disease and treatment. The adolescent also may benefit from peer interaction with others who have similar experiences. Support groups or internet chat rooms may be helpful.

Older Adults with SLE

There is little known about the older adult and SLE, but it is becoming more common to encounter an older individual with this disease as the population ages. Late-onset SLE clearly differs from early-onset in its clinical, epidemiologic, and serologic features. It is also frequently misdiagnosed as other forms of rheumatic disease or drug-induced SLE. With misdiagnosis comes a delay in proper identification and treatment. The prevalence of female-to-male ratio declines significantly to 4:1 in the older adult population and has been attributed to the decrease in sex hormones. Another significant difference between late and early onset SLE is Caucasian predominance. Older adults present with nonspecific symptoms such as weight loss, arthralgias, weakness, fatigue, fever, and cognitive or affective changes; the more specific clinical manifestations tend to occur later. Although individuals with late-onset SLE also tend to have less major organ involvement and lower disease activity, their outcomes tend to be poor because more damage generally occurs. This has been attributed to the negative impact of age and associated comorbidities. Higher mortality rates have been observed in this age group than in those with early-onset SLE.

The therapeutic approach appears to be the same regardless of age at onset of disease. However, it is important to remember that older adults may be taking multiple medications. Pharmacokinetics and drug-to-drug interactions need to be considered prior to initiation of medications commonly used to treat SLE. These individuals may also have decreased renal function; this should also be taken into account prior to initiation of medication therapy.

NURSING PROCESS

Nursing management focuses on thorough assessments (because of the multitude of systems that can be affected by SLE) and on teaching patients to enhance general health practices. Patients with severe disease, however, have diverse nursing needs that vary according to the organ systems involved. Because of the close link between RA and

SLE, many of the nursing diagnoses and interventions identified for patients with arthritis may be appropriate for patients with SLE. Patients with lupus nephritis or end-stage renal disease have the nursing care needs outlined in the exemplar on Chronic Renal Failure in the module on Fluids and Electrolytes, and in the exemplar on Nephritis in the module on Inflammation.

Assessment

Active SLE may involve any organ system. Thorough assessment is essential based on the variety of patient presentations that may be encountered. The nurse should collect the following data:

- *Observation and patient interview.* Assess the patient's nutritional status, including baseline weight and history of recent weight loss or weight gain. Observe for the presence of any dermatologic manifestations, visible musculoskeletal deformities, or cognitive dysfunction during the interview process. Ask if the patient has experienced fatigue, nausea, anorexia, generalized pain, or photosensitivity.
- *Physical examination.* Assess the skin for rashes, ulcers, photosensitivity, ecchymosis, petechiae, cyanosis, and hair loss. Respiratory assessment includes breath sounds and respiratory rate as well as assessment for pleural effusion or pleuritis. Cardiovascular assessment includes vital signs, heart tones, and symptoms of pericarditis or friction rub. Musculoskeletal assessment includes joint pain, joint deformity, pain, weakness, and ability to perform ADLs. Neurologic assessment includes changes in affect or cognitive abilities and seizure activity. GI assessment includes splenomegaly.
- *Psychosocial assessment.* Because SLE is a chronic disease that can affect quality of life, psychosocial assessment is indicated. Assess family interactions, and explore stressful situations, such as divorce or trauma. Treatment-related restrictions and changes in appearance can lead to withdrawal, depression, and suicidal tendencies. Perform psychologic assessments periodically as the patient adapts to the disorder or faces new challenges with a chronic disease.

Diagnosis

Nursing diagnoses will depend on the severity of the disease process and organ involvement but are likely to include the following:

- *Infection, Risk for*
- *Fluid Volume: Deficient, Risk for*
- *Nutrition, Imbalanced: Less than Body Requirements, Risk for*
- *Tissue Perfusion, Peripheral, Ineffective, Risk for*
- *Skin Integrity, Risk for Impaired*
- *Activity Intolerance, Risk for*
- *Body Image, Disturbed, Risk for*
- *Coping: Family, Compromised.*

(NANDA-I © 2014)

Planning

The goals of nursing care are to assist patients (especially children) to manage and cope with a chronic disease, prevent infection, promote nutrition, facilitate a remission, and recognize and avoid triggers for flares. Goals are created with input from the patient based on needs, current status, and severity of disease, including organ involvement. Goals should be specific and contain a time frame for attainment. Goals may include the following:

- Patient will be able to verbalize skin care needs to reduce the risk of altered skin integrity at the end of the teaching session.
- Patient will demonstrate proper hand hygiene techniques before discharge.
- Patient will verbalize the impact of the diagnosis to the healthcare provider.
- Patient will verbalize methods for preventing infection, including use of prophylactic antibiotics and home infection-control measures.

Implementation

The priority nursing interventions for the patient with SLE are focused on problems with impaired skin integrity, ineffective protection, and impaired health maintenance. The Lifespan Considerations section provides information regarding treatment of children and adolescents with SLE.

Prevent Infection

Infections are a leading cause of death for patients with SLE. Prophylactic antibiotics may be required for dental work and surgical procedures. Instruct the patient and family to inform all healthcare providers of the disease in order to plan for prophylactic measures. Educate the patient and family on the importance of adhering to the immunization schedule and obtaining a yearly influenza vaccine to prevent infection. Instruct the patient on hand hygiene and infection-control measures in the home, and warn patients about the dangers of tattooing and body piercing because of the risk of infection.

SLE puts the patient at increased risk for infection and multiple organ system problems. In addition, treatment with corticosteroids or immunosuppressive agents further impairs immune responses and the ability to fight infection. The following interventions are appropriate for inclusion in the care of the hospitalized patient:

- Teach the patient the importance of good hand hygiene after using the bathroom and before eating. Hand hygiene reduces the risk of infection by endogenous organisms.
- Monitor for potential adverse effects of medications, including thrombocytopenia and possible bleeding, fluid retention with edema and possible hypertension, loss of bone density, osteoporosis, and possible pathologic fractures, renal or hepatic toxicity, and cardiac effects, particularly in the patient with fluid retention and hypervolemia. Medications used to treat SLE have many potential adverse effects that can impair normal protective and homeostatic mechanisms.

- Use strict aseptic technique in caring for IV lines and indwelling urinary catheters or in performing any wound care. Aseptic technique offers protection against external and resident host microorganisms.

- Assess the patient frequently for infection. Monitor temperature and vital signs every 4 hours. Assess for signs of cellulitis, including tenderness, redness, swelling, and warmth. Report signs of infection to the physician promptly. Therapy can suppress usual responses, such as elevated temperature and inflammation. The fever of infection may be mistaken for the fever commonly associated with SLE. The patient receiving immunosuppressive therapy for the disease has an even higher risk for infection.

- Monitor laboratory values, including CBC and tests of organ function; report changes to the physician. An elevation in the WBC count with a shift to the left (increased numbers of immature leukocytes in the blood) may be an early indication of infection. Changes in liver function studies, renal function studies, myocardial enzymes, or other laboratory values may indicate organ system involvement.

- Initiate reverse or protective isolation procedures as indicated by the patient's immune status. These procedures provide further protection from infection for patients who are severely immunocompromised.

Promote Fluid Balance and Adequate Nutrition

Because many patients with SLE have renal involvement, it is important for the nurse to monitor intake and output and frequently evaluate fluid and electrolyte status. Renal dysfunction can manifest itself by edema, muscle cramps, diarrhea, tetany, and convulsions.

There are currently no specific dietary plans for the patient with SLE; however, the diet may be altered according to renal involvement, weight gain, weight loss, or other complications. The patient is at risk for weight gain associated with treatment involving steroids and a decreased activity level during exacerbations of this disease. Encourage a well-balanced, nutritious diet as well as appropriate fluid intake.

Promote Skin Integrity

Skin lesions are a common manifestation of SLE. A rash or discoid lesion interrupts the integrity of the skin, which is the first line of protection against infection, so the patient's already high risk for infection is increased. These lesions, which usually appear on exposed parts of the skin, also can be disfiguring and cause the patient emotional distress. The nurse can promote skin integrity through the following interventions:

- Recommend limited use of cosmetics. Cosmetics can irritate the skin and increase the risk of integumentary symptoms.

- Recommend the patient avoid fluorescent lighting. Exacerbations of SLE have been reported following such exposure (LFA, 2016e).

- Assess the patient's knowledge of SLE and its possible effects on the skin. Assessment allows the nurse to base teaching and information on the patient's existing knowledge, thereby improving learning and retention.

- Discuss the relationship between sun exposure and disease activity. Teach appropriate strategies for limiting sun exposure, such as avoiding outdoor activity between 10:00 a.m. and 3:00 p.m. and applying sunscreen 30 minutes prior to going out in the sun.

- Encourage the patient to keep skin clean and dry and to apply therapeutic creams or ointments to lesions as prescribed. These measures promote healing and reduce the risk of infection.

- Provide instructions on oral care to maintain intact oral mucosa. Alterations in skin integrity, including those in the oral cavity, can increase the risk of acute exacerbations of SLE.

- Provide instructions on the care of the head if alopecia occurs. Alopecia, especially in women, can be very traumatic, so care of the skin on the head is important because the patient cannot wear a wig when skin integrity is affected.

Manage Medication Side Effects

Observe the patient for any side effects of medications used for treatment, and teach the patient and family about these effects. For example, immunosuppressant drugs can promote infection anywhere in the body, and NSAIDs commonly cause gastric distress and bleeding of the GI tract. The antimalarial drug hydroxychloroquine can cause serious vision changes; thus, frequent eye examinations are needed.

Provide Emotional Support

Patients may have an altered body image as a result of rash, alopecia, arthritic changes in the joints, and chronic disease. Referral to a lupus support group, the local Department of Social Services, or counseling may be helpful. The patient needs ongoing support and information to deal with the complexity of the disease.

>> **Stay Current:** The American Lupus Society and the Lupus Foundation of America (http://www.lupus.org) can provide information to help patients and family members adjust to the disease. The Arthritis Foundation (http://www.arthritis.org) also publishes a useful pamphlet: Meeting the Challenge: A Young Person's Guide to Living with Lupus.

Promote Health Maintenance

- Educate the patient on self-care (see the Patient Teaching feature).

- Assess the patient's ability to maintain optimal health, identifying physical and psychosocial factors that may affect health maintenance. Before intervening to improve the patient's health maintenance, the nurse must identify and understand the factors affecting it.

- Initiate an interprofessional care conference with the patient and family. In this care conference, the expression of a number of perspectives will improve the planning of strategies for health maintenance activities.

Patient Teaching
Self-Care for Patients with Systemic Lupus Erythematosus

Teaching is a critical factor in preparing patients with SLE for self-care at home. Address the following topics:

- The disease and its potential effects. Promote an optimistic outlook, stressing that the majority of patients do not require long-term corticosteroid therapy and that the disease may improve over time.
- The triggers of flares, warning signs of flares (which include increased fatigue, pain or abdominal discomfort, rash, headache, fever, and dizziness), and preventative measures (e.g., avoiding stress, alcohol, smoking, and drugs)
- The importance of skin care
- The importance of avoiding exposure to infection
- The need to follow the prescribed treatment plan, including rest and exercise, medications, and follow-up appointments. Discuss manifestations of an acute episode, and stress the importance of contacting the healthcare provider promptly if any of these manifestations occur.

- The significance of wearing a medical alert bracelet or tag that identifies their condition and therapy (e.g., corticosteroids, immunosuppressives)
- Family planning with the patient and spouse. The use of oral contraceptives may be contraindicated for the patient; if appropriate, provide information about alternative means of birth control. Pregnancy is not contraindicated for most women with SLE. However, the pregnant patient requires close monitoring, because acute episodes sometimes accompany pregnancy.
- The need for preventive healthcare for both men and women with SLE. Women should have gynecologic and breast examinations and men should have prostate examinations each year. Both men and women should have regular screenings for cholesterol and blood pressure. Annual influenza vaccinations are important, as are pneumococcal vaccinations for older patients. If patients are taking corticosteroids or antimalarial medications, annual eye examinations should be conducted to screen for and treat any ocular problems.

Evaluation

Successful outcomes of nursing care involve management of this chronic disease. Expected outcomes include the following:

- Patient maintains normal intake and output levels, with demonstrated fluid and electrolyte balance.
- Patient maintains healthy, intact skin.
- Patient maintains a balance of rest and activity to promote health.

- Patient maintains medication regimen to promote health and prevent side effects.
- Patient develops or maintains a positive body image.

Secondary outcomes also require evaluation and may include:

- Patient identifies methods to reduce stress.
- Patient elicits assistance from family members to reduce levels of stress.
- Patient keeps a log of situations that precipitate disease exacerbations.

REVIEW Systemic Lupus Erythematosus

RELATE Link the Concepts and Exemplars

Link the exemplar of systemic lupus erythematosus with the concept of inflammation:

1. Describe the inflammatory reaction and explain the role this process plays in SLE.
2. What types of treatment for inflammation would also be useful in treating SLE?

Link the exemplar of systemic lupus erythematosus with the concept of health, wellness, and illness:

3. Why would the patient with SLE be less likely to have acute exacerbations if he or she made healthy lifestyle choices?
4. Create a teaching plan explaining healthy behaviors that promote fewer acute exacerbations of SLE.

Link the exemplar of systemic lupus erythematosus with the concept of self:

5. How would a diagnosis of SLE affect a patient's self-concept? Why might these effects be especially pronounced in male patients with SLE?
6. What interventions would be appropriate for enhancing the self-esteem of an adolescent SLE patient?

READY Go to Volume 3: Clinical Nursing Skills

REFER Go to Pearson MyLab Nursing and eText

- Additional review materials

REFLECT Apply Your Knowledge

Yvonne Johnson is 35 years old, and she is a single parent to her 15-year-old son, Randall. Ms. Johnson has had relationships with men off and on, but she is not currently involved with anybody. Ms. Johnson completed a bachelor's degree in marketing 5 years ago but has been unable to break into the marketing field locally. Instead, she has been working full time as an administrative assistant for a large company. Her parents and siblings live nearby, and she maintains a close relationship with them.

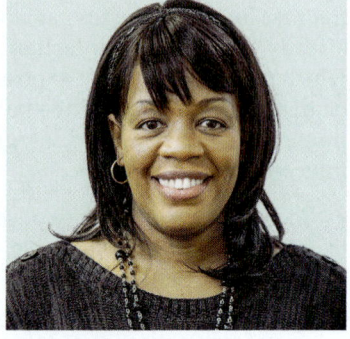

Over the past 4 years, Ms. Johnson has noticed mild swelling in her hands and feet every morning. The symptoms began subtly not long after she graduated from college. She has always attributed the symptom to her sedentary lifestyle and being somewhat overweight. More recently, she has been experiencing pain along with the swelling in her hands and feet.

Ms. Johnson saw her healthcare provider, Dr. Rowe, and told her that she had had pain in her hands for the past several months. When asked about other symptoms, she mentioned the swelling in her hands and feet for the past 4 years. Dr. Rowe thought that the pain was likely occupational (from typing) and suggested that Ms. Johnson take over-the-counter pain relievers, such as ibuprofen. Dr. Rowe noticed that Ms. Johnson's blood pressure was slightly elevated (134/92 mmHg) but attributed this to her race and diet. She suggested that Ms. Johnson lose a little weight and reduce her salt intake.

Ms. Johnson has been trying to follow Dr. Rowe's advice for the past 3 months. Although she has lost approximately 5 pounds, has avoided salty foods, and has been taking ibuprofen three times a day, she continues to have pain in her hands and swelling in her hands and feet. She also wonders whether the symptoms are really associated with her work.

1. What diagnosis do you suspect for Ms. Johnson? Explain the basis of your answer.

2. What diagnostic testing would you anticipate to confirm this diagnosis? Explain your answers.

3. If you are the nurse admitting Ms. Johnson to her provider's office, what specific assessments would you perform to help you confirm the suspected diagnosis?

References

Abbas, A. K., Lichtman, A. H., & Pillai, S. (2014). *Basic immunology: Functions and disorders of the immune system* (Chapters 1 & 2). Retrieved from https://books.google.com/books?hl=en&lr=&id=jOwdl_MEr7sC&oi=fnd&pg=PP1&dq=active+vs+passive+immunity+in+humans&ots=U6RMmMALR9&sig=rcE84bwe_J6B5oU-8_44PHR7AbM#v=onepage&q=active%20vs%20passive%20immunity%20in%20humans&f=false

Abrams, E. M, & Becker, A. B. (2013). Introducing solid food: Age of introduction and its effect on risk of food allergy and other atopic diseases. *Canadian Family Physician, 59*(7). Retrieved from http://www.ncbi.nlm.nih.gov/pmc/articles/PMC3710027

Adams, M. P., Holland, L. N., & Urban, C. (2017). *Pharmacology for nurses: A pathophysiologic approach* (5th ed.). Hoboken, NJ: Pearson Education.

AIDS.gov. (2015). *Post exposure prophylaxis.* Retrieved from https://www.aids.gov/hiv-aids-basics/prevention/reduce-your-risk/post-exposure-prophylaxis/

AIDS.gov. (2016a). *HIV/AIDs basics.* Retrieved from https://www.aids.gov/hiv-aids-basics

AIDS.gov. (2016b). *Newly diagnosed: Older adults.* Retrieved from https://www.aids.gov/hiv-aids-basics/just-diagnosed-with-hiv-aids/overview/aging-population

Aimmune Therapeutics. (2016). *Working toward an FDA approved treatment for food allergies.* Retrieved from http://www.aimmune.com/clinical-trials

Aletaha, D., Neogi, T., Silman, A. J., Funovits, J., Felson, D. T., Bingham, C. O., . . . Hawker, G. (2010). 2010 rheumatoid arthritis classification criteria. *Arthritis & Rheumatism, 62*(9), 2569–2581. Retrieved from http://www.rheumatology.org/Portals/0/Files/2010_revised_criteria_classification_ra.pdf

American Academy of Allergy Asthma and Immunology. (2013). *Swish or swallow? Comparing oral and sublingual immunotherapy for peanut allergy.* Retrieved from http://www.aaaai.org/global/latest-research-summaries/Current-JACI-Research/oral-sublingual-immunotherapy-peanut-allergy.aspx

American Academy of Allergy Asthma and Immunology. (2015). *Peanut patch to treat allergy in the works.* Retrieved from http://www.medscape.com/viewarticle/840734

American Academy of Allergy Asthma and Immunology. (2016a). *Food allergy overview.* Retrieved from http://www.aaaai.org/conditions-and-treatments/allergies/food-allergies

American Academy of Allergy Asthma and Immunology. (2016b). *Allergy statistics.* Retrieved from http://www.aaaai.org/about-the-aaaai/newsroom/allergy-statistics.aspx

American Academy of Allergy Asthma and Immunology. (2016c). *SLIT treatment (allergy tablets) for allergic rhinitis nothing to sneeze about.* Retrieved from http://www.aaaai.org/conditions-and-treatments/library/allergy-library/sublingual-immunotherapy-for-allergic-rhinitis.aspx

American Academy of Pediatrics. (2013). Vaccine safety: Examine the evidence. Retrieved from https://www.aap.org/en-us/documents/immunization_vaccine_studies.pdf

American Academy of Pediatrics. (2015a). *Red book: 2015 Report of the committee on infectious disease* (30th ed.). Elk Grove Village, IL: Author.

American Academy of Pediatrics. (2015b). *Tuberculosis.* Retrieved from https://www.healthychildren.org/English/health-issues/conditions/chest-lungs/Pages/Tuberculosis.aspx?nfstatus=401&nftoken=00000000-0000-0000-0000-000000000000&nfstatusdescription=ERROR%3a+No+local+token

American Autoimmune Related Diseases Association. (2015a.). *Autoimmunity: A major women's health issue.* Retrieved from http://www.aarda.org/autoimmune-information/autoimmune-disease-in-women/

American Autoimmune Related Diseases Association. (2015b). *Patient education courses: Basic autoimmunity module.* Retrieved from http://www.aarda.org/autoimmune-information/educational-modules

American Cancer Society. (2014). *How are HIV and AIDS related to cancer?* Retrieved from http://www.cancer.org/cancer/cancercauses/othercarcinogens/infectiousagents/hivinfectionandaids/hiv-infection-and-aids-hiv-aids-and-cancer

American College of Allergy, Asthma and Immunology (ACAAI). 2016. *Prevention of allergies and asthma in children.* Retrieved from https://www.aaaai.org/conditions-and-treatments/library/at-a-glance/prevention-of-allergies-and-asthma-in-children

American College of Rheumatology. (2016a). *Rheumatoid arthritis.* Retrieved from http://www.rheumatology.org/practice/clinical/patients/diseases_and_conditions/ra.asp

American College of Rheumatology. (2016b). *Systemic lupus erythematosus (juvenile).* Retrieved from http://www.rheumatology.org/I-Am-A/Patient-Caregiver/Diseases-Conditions/Systemic-Lupus-Erythematosus-Juvenile

American Latex Allergy Association. (2016). About latex allergy. Retrieved from http://latexallergyresources.org/about-latex-allergy

Arthritis Foundation. (2013). *Disease center: Systemic lupus erythematosus (lupus) in children and adolescents.* Retrieved from http://www.arthritis.org/conditions-treatments/disease-center/systemic-lupus-erythematosus-lupus-in-children-and-adolescents/

Arthritis Foundation. (2017). *How to prevent arthritis.* Retrieved from http://www.arthritis.org/about-arthritis/understanding-arthritis/arthritis-prevention.php

Asthma and Allergy Foundation of America. (2016). *Allergy facts and figures.* Retrieved from http://www.aafa.org/display.cfm?id=9&sub=30

Badell, M. L., & Lindsay, M. (2012). Thirty years later: Pregnancies in females perinatally infected with human immunodeficiency virus-1. *AIDS Research and Treatment, 2012,* 418630. doi:10.1155/2012/418630

Ball, J. W., Bindler, R. C., Cowen, K., & Shaw, M. (2017). *Principles of pediatric nursing: Caring for children* (7th ed.). Hoboken, NJ: Pearson Education.

Bartels, C. M. (2015). Systemic lupus erythematous. *Medscape.* Retrieved from http://emedicine.medscape.com/article/332244-overview

Berin, C. M., & Sampson, H. A. (2013). Food allergy: An enigmatic epidemic. *Trends in Immunology, 34*(8), 390–397. Retrieved from http://dx.doi.org/10.1016/j.it.2013.04.003

Bersenev, A., & Levine, B. L. (2012). Convergence of gene and cell therapy. *Regenerative Medicine, 7*(6s), 50–56.

Brazão, V., Kuehn, C., Domingues dos Santos, C., Bronzon da Costa, C., Clóvis do Prado Júnior, J., & Carraro-Abrahão, A. (2015). Endocrine and immune system interactions during pregnancy. *Immunobiology, 220*(1), 42–47. doi:10.1016/j.imbio.2014.09.005

Brunson, E. K. (2013). How parents make decisions about their children's vaccinations. *Vaccine, 31*(46), 5466–5470. Retrieved from http://dx.doi.org/10.1016/j.vaccine.2013.08.104

Buelow, B. (2015). Immediate hypersensitivity reactions: Background. *Medscape.* Retrieved from http://emedicine.medscape.com/article/136217-overview

Business Wire. (2016). *Aimmune enrolls first patient in phase III PALISADE trial of AR101 for the treatment of peanut allergy.* Retrieved from http://www.businesswire.com/news/home/20160111005391/en/Aimmune-Therapeutics-Enrolls-Patient-Phase-3-PALISADE

Calder, P. C. (2013). Feeding the immune system. *Proceedings of the Nutrition Society, 72*(3), 299–309. Retrieved from http://dx.doi.org/10.1017/S0029665113001286

Centers for Disease Control and Prevention. (2013a). Advisory Committee on Immunization Practices recommended immunization schedule for persons aged 0 through 18 years—United States, 2013. *Morbidity and Mortality Weekly Report, 62*(1), 2–8.

Centers for Disease Control and Prevention. (2013b). Advisory Committee on Immunization Practices recommended immunization schedule for adults aged 19 years and older—United States, 2013. *Morbidity and Mortality Weekly Report, 62*(1), 9–19.

Centers for Disease Control and Prevention. (2014). *Vaccines and immunizations.* Retrieved from http://www.cdc.gov/vaccines/vac-gen/immunity-types.htm

Centers for Disease Control and Prevention. (2015a). *Occupational HIV transmission and prevention among healthcare workers.* Retrieved from http://cdc.gov/hiv/workplace/occupational.html

Centers for Disease Control and Prevention. (2015b). *Rapid HIV testing of women in labor and delivery.* Retrieved from http://www.cdc.gov/hiv/testing/clinical/women.html

Centers for Disease Control and Prevention. (2015c). *HIV testing in nonclinical settings.* Retrieved from http://www.cdc.gov/hiv/testing/nonclinical/

Centers for Disease Control and Prevention. (2015d). *Systemic lupus erythematosus (SLE).* Retrieved from http://www.cdc.gov/arthritis/basics/lupus.htm

Centers for Disease Control and Prevention. (2015e). *Healthy schools: Food allergies in schools.* Retrieved from: http://www.cdc.gov/healthyschools/foodallergies/index.htm

Centers for Disease Control and Prevention. (2015f). *HIV among pregnant women, infants and children.* Retrieved from http://www.cdc.gov/hiv/group/gender/pregnantwomen/index.html

Centers for Disease Control and Prevention. (2015g). *HIV among youth.* Retrieved from http://www.cdc.gov/hiv/group/age/youth/index.html

Centers for Disease Control and Prevention. (2015h). *Statistics overview.* Retrieved from http://www.cdc.gov/hiv/statistics/overview/index.html

Centers for Disease Control and Prevention. (2015i). *HIV among people age 50 and older.* Retrieved from http://www.cdc.gov/hiv/group/age/olderamericans/index.html

Centers for Disease Control and Prevention. (2015j). *Home tests.* Retrieved from http://www.cdc.gov/hiv/testing/hometests.html

Centers for Disease Control and Prevention. (2015k). *HIV and injection drug use in the United States.* Retrieved from http://www.cdc.gov/hiv/group/gender/transgender/index.html

Centers for Disease Control and Prevention. (2015l). *Condom fact sheet in brief.* Retrieved from http://www.cdc.gov/condomeffectiveness/brief.html

Centers for Disease Control and Prevention. (2015m). *Rheumatoid arthritis.* Retrieved from http://www.cdc.gov/arthritis/basics/rheumatoid.htm

Centers for Disease Control and Prevention. (2015n). *About HIV/AIDS: Statistics.* Retrieved from http://www.cdc.gov/hiv/basics/statistics.html

Centers for Disease Control and Prevention. (2015o). *Childhood arthritis.* Retrieved from http://www.cdc.gov/arthritis/basics/childhood.htm

Centers for Disease Control and Prevention. (2015p). *HIV testing.* Retrieved from http://www.cdc.gov/hiv/testing/

Centers for Disease Control and Prevention. (2015q). *HIV among women.* Retrieved from http://www.cdc.gov/hiv/group/gender/women/index.html

Centers for Disease Control and Prevention. (2015r). *HIV and the law.* Retrieved from http://www.cdc.gov/hiv/policies/law/risk.html

Centers for Disease Control and Prevention. (2015s). *About HIV/AIDS.* Retrieved from http://www.cdc.gov/hiv/basics/whatishiv.html

Centers for Disease Control and Prevention. (2015t). *About HIV/AIDS: Transmission.* Retrieved from http://www.cdc.gov/hiv/basics/transmission.html

Centers for Disease Control and Prevention. (2015u). *HIV among transgendered people.* Retrieved from http://www.cdc.gov/hiv/group/gender/transgender/index.html

Centers for Disease Control and Prevention. (2015v). *HIV in the United States: At a glance.* Retrieved from http://www.cdc.gov/hiv/statistics/overview/ataglance.html

Centers for Disease Control and Prevention. (2015w). *Preventing diabetes.* Retrieved from http://www.cdc.gov/diabetes/consumer/prevent.htm

Centers for Disease Control and Prevention. (2016a). *PEP.* Retrieved from http://www.cdc.gov/hiv/basics/pep.html

Centers for Disease Control and Prevention. (2016b). *Opportunistic infections.* Retrieved from http://www.cdc.gov/hiv/basics/livingwithhiv/opportunisticinfections.html

Centers for Disease Control and Prevention. (2016c). *HIV treatment.* Retrieved from http://www.cdc.gov/actagainstaids/campaigns/hivtreatmentworks/stayincare/treatment.html

Centers for Disease Control and Prevention. (2016d). *Chickenpox (varicella): Vaccination.* Retrieved from http://www.cdc.gov/chickenpox/vaccination.html

Centers for Disease Control and Prevention. (2016e). *HIV among pregnant women, infants, and children in the United States.* Retrieved from http://www.cdc.gov/hiv/group/gender/pregnantwomen/

Cincinnati Children's Hospital Medical Center. (2015). *Mother's own immune system may cause pregnancy complications.* Retrieved from http://www.cincinnatichildrens.org/news/release/2015/prematurity-pregnancy-complications-03-09-2015/

Cleveland Clinic. (2014). *Graft vs host disease: An overview in bone marrow transplant.* Retrieved from http://my.clevelandclinic.org/health/treatments_and_procedures/hic_bone_marrow_and_transplantation/hic-graft-vs-host-disease-an-overview-in-bone-marrow-transplant

Daniels, R. (2015). Allergen skin testing. In *Delmar's guide to laboratory and diagnostic tests* (3rd ed.). Boston, MA: Cengage Learning.

de Heredia, F. P., Gomez-Martinez, S., & Marcos, A. (2012). Obesity, inflammation and the immune system. *The Proceedings of the Nutrition Society, 71*(2): 332-338.

Delves, P. J. (2014). Geriatric essentials. *Merck Manual.* Retrieved from http://www.merckmanuals.com/professional/immunology;-allergic-disorders/biology-of-the-immune-system/overview-of-the-immune-system

Delves, P. J. (2015). Effects of aging on the immune system. *Merck Manual.* Retrieved from http://www.merckmanuals.com/home/immune-disorders/biology-of-the-immune-system/effects-of-aging-on-the-immune-system

Ding, H. J., & Gordon, C. (2013). New biologic therapy for systemic lupus erythematosus. *Current Options in Pharmacology.* Available from http://dx.doi.org/10.1016/j.coph.2013.04.005

Dyer, A. A., & Gupta, R. (2013). Epidemiology of childhood food allergy. *Pediatric Annals, 42*(6), 91–95. Retrieved from http://search.proquest.com.proxy092.nclive.org/pqcentral/docview/1355950539/FD0AF21923B4763PQ/1?accountid=14003

Family Practice Notebook. (2015). *Hypersensitivity reaction.* Retrieved from http://www.fpnotebook.com/ent/exam/HyprsnstvtyRctn.htm

Federation of American Societies for Experimental Biology. (2014). Adolescent exposure to THC may cause immune systems to go up in smoke. *Science Daily.* Retrieved from http://www.sciencedaily.com/releases/2014/09/140930113117.htm

Fernandez, J. (2013). Overview of immunodeficiency disorders. *Merck Manual.* Retrieved from http://www.merckmanuals.com/professional/immunology;-allergic-disorders/immunodeficiency-disorders/overview-of-immunodeficiency-disorders

Food Allergy Research and Education. (2015a). *Results of new peanut allergy trials presented at EAACI meeting.* Retrieved from http://blog.foodallergy.org/2015/06/15/results-of-new-peanut-allergy-trials-presented-at-eaaci-meeting/

Food Allergy Research and Education. (2015b). *Where we stand today.* Retrieved from https://www.foodallergy.org/research/overview

Food and Drug Administration. (2015a). *Don't be misled by "latex free" claims.* Retrieved from http://www.fda.gov/ForConsumers/ConsumerUpdates/ucm342641.htm

Food and Drug Administration. (2015b). *FDA approves Nucala to treat severe asthma.* Retrieved from http://www.fda.gov/NewsEvents/Newsroom/PressAnnouncements/ucm471031.htm

Food and Drug Administration. (2015c). *Thimerosal in vaccines.* Retrieved from http://www.fda.gov/BiologicsBloodVaccines/SafetyAvailability/VaccineSafety/ucm096228.htm

Gabriel, S. E., & Crowson, C. S. (2016). *Epidemiology of, risk factors for, and possible causes of rheumatoid arthritis. Up to Date.* Retrieved from http://www.uptodate.com/contents/epidemiology-of-risk-factors-for-and-possible-causes-of-rheumatoid-arthritis

Gaspar, H. B., Qasim, W., Davies, E. G., Rao, K., Amrolia, P. J., & Veys. (2013). How I treat severe combined immunodeficiency. *Blood Journal, 122*(23), 3749–3758. Retrieved from http://www.bloodjournal.org/content/122/23/3749?rss=1&variant=short&sso-checked=true

Gecht-Silver, M. R., & Duncombe, A. M. (2015). Patient information: Arthritis and exercise beyond the basics. *UpToDate.* Retrieved from http://www.uptodate.com/contents/arthritis-and-exercise-beyond-the-basics

Ghaffar, A. (2014). Hypersensitivity reactions. In *Immunology* (Chapter 17). Retrieved from http://www.microbiologybook.org/ghaffar/hyper00.htm

Glanz, J. M., Kraus, C. R., & Daley, M. F. (2015). Addressing parental vaccine concerns: Engagement, balance and timing. *Academic Pediatrics, 13*(8), 481–488. http://dx.doi.org/10.1016/j.acap.2013.05.030

Gleeson, M., & Walsh, N. P. (2012). The BASES expert statement on exercise, immunity, and infection. *Journal of Sports Sciences, 30*(3), 321–324.

Grethlein, S. (2014). Mucosa-associated lymphoid tissue. *Medscape.* Retrieved from http://emedicine.medscape.com/article/207891-overview

Guide for HIV/AIDS Clinical Care. (2014a). *HIV classification: CDC and WHO staging systems.* Retrieved from http://aidsetc.org/guide/hiv-classification

Guide for HIV/AIDS Clinical Care. (2014b). *Initial history.* Retrieved from http://aidsetc.org/guide/initial-history

Guide for HIV/AIDS Clinical Care. (2014c). *Initial physical examination.* Retrieved from http://aidsetc.org/guide/initial-physical-examination

Gulanick, M., & Myers, J. L. (2014). *Nursing care plans: Diagnoses, interventions and outcomes* (8th ed.). Philadelphia, PA: Elsevier. Available from https://www.scribd.com/doc/287304249/Nursing-Care-Plans-Nursing-Diagnosis-and-Intervention-8E-Gulanick-Meg-Myers-Judith-L#

Haase, H., & Rink, L. (2013). Zinc signals and immune function. *BioFactors, 40*(1), 27–40. doi:10.1002/biof.1114

Harvard Medical School. (2016). *Staying healthy: How to boost your immune system.* Retrieved from Harvard Health Publications website: http://www.health.harvard.edu/staying-healthy/how-to-boost-your-immune-system

Healthline. (2016). The best HIV/AIDS apps of 2016. Retrieved from http://www.healthline.com/health/hiv-aids/top-iphone-android-apps#1

Healthychildren.org. (2016). *Allergy causes in children: What parents can do.* Retrieved from https://www.healthychildren.org/English/health-issues/conditions/allergies-asthma/Pages/Allergy-Causes.aspx

Herdman, T. H. & Kamitsuru, S. (Eds.). *Nursing Diagnoses—Definitions and Classification 2015–2017.* Copyright © 2014, 1994–2014 NANDA International. Used by arrangement with John Wiley & Sons, Inc. Companion website: www.wiley.com/go/nursingdiagnoses

HIV/AIDS Basics. (2016). *Pre-exposure prophylaxis (PrEP).* Retrieved from http://www.aids.gov/hiv-aids-basics/prevention/reduce-your-risk/pre-exposure-prophylaxis

Hricik, D. E., Ojo, A. D., Solez, K., Kasiske, B. L., Lober, M. I., Flechner, S. M., & Kaplan, B. (2016). Modifiable and nonmodifiable donor and recipient factors as targets for preservation of renal function. *Medscape.* Retrieved from http://www.medscape.org/viewarticle/494040

Hughes, P. J. (2014). Classification systems for acute kidney injury. *Medscape.* Retrieved from http://emedicine.medscape.com/article/1925597-overview#a2

Immunization Action Coalition. (2015). *Medical management of vaccine reactions in children and teens.* Retrieved from http://www.immunize.org/catg.d/p3082a.pdf

Immunization Action Coalition. (2016). *Talking about vaccines.* Retrieved from http://www.immunize.org/talking-about-vaccines

Jaitley, S., & Saraswathi, T. R. (2012). Pathophysiology of Langerhans cells. *Journal of Oral and Maxillofacial Pathology, 16*(2), 239–244. Retrieved from http://www.ncbi.nlm.nih.gov/pmc/articles/PMC3424941

Johns Hopkins Arthritis Center. (2016). *Rheumatoid arthritis treatment.* Retrieved from https://www.hopkinsarthritis.org/arthritis-info/rheumatoid-arthritis/ra-treatment/#cor

Johns Hopkins Scleroderma Center. (2016). *Understanding scleroderma: Who gets scleroderma.* Retrieved from http://www.hopkinsscleroderma.org/scleroderma

Kasper, D. L., Fauci, A., Hauser, S., Longo, D., Loscaizo, J., & Jamison, J. L. (2015). *Harrison's principles of internal medicine* (19th ed.). New York, NY: McGraw-Hill.

Kim, H. Y., Kasonde, P., Myiya, M., Thea, D. M., Kankasa, C., Kinkala, M., . . . Kuhn, L. (2012). Pregnancy loss and role of infant HIV status on perinatal mortality among HIV infected women. *BMC Pediatrics.* doi:10.1186/1471-2431_12-138

Kloser, P., & Nakata, K. (2016). What is good practice? HIV care beyond art. *Center for Continuing & Outreach Education.* Retrieved from http://ccoe.rbhs.rutgers.edu/online/ARCHIVE/11HC07/article3.htm

Kobrynski, L., Powell, R. W., & Bowen, S. (2014). Prevalence and morbidity of primary immunodeficiency diseases, United States 2001-2007. *Journal of Clinical Immunology, 34*(8): 954-961.

Kourtis, A. P., Wiener, J., Kayira, D., Chasela, C., Ellington, S. R., Hyde, L., . . . Jamieson, D. J. (2013). Health outcomes of HIV-exposed uninfected African infants. *AIDS, 13;* 27(5), 749–759. doi:10.1097/QAD.0b013e32835ca29f

Lee, Y-C., & Lin, S-J., (2013). Neonatal natural killer cell function: Relevance to antiviral immune defense. *Journal of Immunological Research.* Retrieved from https://www.hindawi.com/journals/jir/2013/427696

Linus Pauling Institute Micronutrient Information Center. (2016). *Overnutrition and obesity.* Retrieved from Oregon State University website: http://lpi.oregonstate.edu/mic/micron3utrients-health/immunity

Lupus Foundation of America. (2016a). *What is lupus?* Retrieved from http://www.lupus.org/answers/entry/what-is-lupus

Lupus Foundation of America. (2016b). *What are the risks for developing lupus?* Retrieved from http://www.lupus.org/answers/entry/risks-for-developing-lupus

Lupus Foundation of America. (2016c). *Pregnancy and lupus.* Retrieved from http://www.lupus.org/podcasts/entry/pregnancy-and-lupus

Lupus Foundation of America. (2016d). *A clue to congenital heart block.* Retrieved from http://www.lupus.org/webmodules/webarticlesnet/templates/new_researchupdates.aspx?articleid=1688&zoneid=33

Lupus Foundation of America. (2016e). *Should I be following a specific diet or nutrition plan for my lupus?* Retrieved from http://www.lupus.org/answers/entry/lupus-diet-and-nutrition

Lupus Foundation of America. (2016f). *What are common triggers for a lupus flare?* Retrieved from http://www.lupus.org/answers/entry/what-are-common-triggers-for-a-lupus-flare

Luthy, K. E., Beckstrand, R. L., Callister, L. C., & Cahoon, S. (2012). Reasons parents exempt children from receiving immunizations. *Journal of School Nursing, 28*(2), 153–60. doi:10.1177/1059840511426578

Maglione, M. A., Das, L., Raaen, L., Smith, A., Chari, R., Newberry, S., . . . Gidengil, C. (2014). Safety of vaccines used for routine immunization of U.S. children: A systematic review. *Pediatriacs, 134*(2), 325–37. doi:10.1542/peds.2014-1079

Mayo Clinic. (2014a). *Juvenile rheumatoid arthritis.* Retrieved from http://www.mayoclinic.org/diseases-conditions/juvenile-rheumatoid-arthritis/basics/definition/con-20014378

Mayo Clinic. (2014b). *Healthy lifestyle: Stress management.* Retrieved from http://www.mayoclinic.org/healthy-lifestyle/stress-management/basics/stress-basics/hlv-20049495

Mayo Clinic. (2014c). *Diseases and conditions: Allergies.* Retrieved from http://www.mayoclinic.org/diseases-conditions/allergies/basics/definition/con-20034030

Mayo Clinic. (2015). *Diseases and conditions: HIV/AIDS.* Retrieved from http://www.mayoclinic.org/diseases-conditions/hiv-aids/basics/definition/con-20013732

Mayo Clinic. (2016). *Diseases and conditions: Rheumatoid arthritis.* Retrieved from http://www.mayoclinic.org/diseases-conditions/rheumatoid-arthritis/home/ovc-20197388

Miller, M. (2017). *The cheaper, generic "EpiPen" is great. Slate.* Available from: http://www.slate.com/articles/health_and_science/medical_examiner/2017/01/cvs_announces_plans_to_stock_an_alternative_to_the_notoriously_expensive.html

Mirone, C., Preziosi, D., Mascheri, A., Micarelli, G., Farioli, l., Balossi, L. G., . . . Pastorello, E. A. (2015). Identification of risk factors of severe hypersensitivity reactions in general anesthesia. *Clinical and Molecular Allergy, 13*(1). doi:10.1186/s12948-015-0017-9

Mustafa, S. S. (2015). Anaphylaxis. *Medscape.* Retrieved from http://emedicine.medscape.com/article/135065-overview

Nath, I. (2015a). Peanut patch shows promise for treatment of allergy. *Allergic Living.* Retrieved from http://allergicliving.com/2015/03/19/peanut-patch-shows-promise-for-treatment-of-allergy/

Nath, I. (2015b). FDA labels peanut OIT treatment "breakthrough therapy." *Allergic Living.* Retrieved from http://allergicliving.com/2015/07/08/fda-designates-peanut-treatment-breakthrough-therapy

National Center for Complementary and Integrative Health. (2015). *Herb-drug interactions.* Retrieved from https://nccih.nih.gov/health/providers/digest/herb-drug

National Center for Complementary and Integrative Health. (2016a). *Herbs at a glance: Chamomile.* Retrieved from https://nccih.nih.gov/health/chamomile/ataglance.htm

National Center for Complementary and Integrative Health. (2016b). *Safe use of complementary health products and practices.* Retrieved from https://nccih.nih.gov/health/safety

National Council on Aging. (2016). *Chronic disease self-management: Facts.* Retrieved from https://www.ncoa.org/news/resources-for-reporters/get-the-facts/chronic-disease-facts/

National Institute of Allergy and Infectious Diseases. (2016). *Health and research topics A to Z: Allergic diseases.* Retrieved from https://www.niaid.nih.gov/diseases-conditions/allergic-diseases

National Institute of Allergy and Infectious Diseases. (2017). HIV/AIDS. Retrieved from https://www.niaid.nih.gov/diseases-conditions/hivaids

National Institute of Arthritis and Musculoskeletal Skin Diseases. (2014). *Handout in health: Rheumatoid arthritis.* Retrieved from http://www.niams.nih.gov/Health_Info/Rheumatic_Disease/default.asp

National Institute of Occupational Safety and Health. (2012). *Home healthcare workers: How to prevent latex allergies.* Publication no. 2012-119. Retrieved from http://www.cdc.gov/niosh/docs/2012-119/pdfs/2012-119.pdf

National Institutes of Health. (2012). *Report of the director of the National Institutes of Health, Chapter 3.* Retrieved from https://report.nih.gov/pdf/NIH_Biennial_Report_2012.pdf

National Institutes of Health. (2015). *HIV and women: Preventing mother-to-child transmission of HIV after birth.* Retrieved from https://aidsinfo.nih.gov/education-materials/fact-sheets/24/71/preventing-mother-to-child-transmission-of-hiv-after-birth

National Institutes of Health. (2016). *Dailymed: Invirase.* Retrieved from https://dailymed.nlm.nih.gov/dailymed/drugInfo.cfm?setid=c00d1607-ac36-457b-a34b-75ad74f9cf0a

National Institutes of Health, National Institute on Aging. (2015). *HIV, AIDS, and older people.* Retrieved from http://www.nia.nih.gov/health/publication/hiv-aids-and-older-people

Neeman, K. (2013). Kawasaki disease and sudden infant death syndrome: Any connection to vaccination? In Chatterjee, A. (Ed.), *Vaccinophobia and vaccine controversies of the 21st century* (Chapter 19). Retrieved from http://link.springer.com/chapter/10.1007/978-1-4614-7438-8_19#

Okafor, U. H. (2012). Pattern of clinical presentations in immunocompromised patient. In Metodiev, K. (Ed.), *Immunology and microbiology* (Chapter 7). Retrieved from http://www.intechopen.com/books/immunodeficiency/pattern-of-clinical-presentations-in-immunocompromised-patient

Opel, D. J., Heritage, J., Taylor, J. A., Mangione-Smith, R., Salas, H. S., DeVere, V., . . . Robinson, J. D. (2013). The architecture of provider-parent vaccine discussion at health supervision visits. *Pediatrics, 132*(6), 1–10. doi:10.1542/peds.2013-2037

Osborn, K. S., Wraa, C. E., Watson, A., & Holleran, R. S. (2013). *Medical-surgical nursing: Preparation for practice* (2nd ed.). Upper Saddle River, NJ: Pearson.

Panel on Antiretroviral Therapy and Medical Management of HIV-Infected Children. (2013). *Guidelines for the use of antiretroviral agents in pediatric HIV infection.* Retrieved from http://aidsinfo.nih.gov/contentfiles/lvguidelines/pediatricguidelines.pdf

Panel on Opportunistic Infections in HIV-Infected Adults and Adolescents. (2016). *Guidelines for the prevention and treatment of opportunistic infections in HIV-infected adults and adolescents: Recommendations from the Centers for Disease Control and Prevention, the National Institutes of Health, and the HIV Medicine Association of the Infectious Diseases Society of America.* Retrieved from http://aidsinfo.nih.gov/contentfiles/lvguidelines/adult_oi.pdf

Panel on Treatment of HIV-Infected Pregnant Women and Prevention of Perinatal Transmission. (2016). *Recommendations for use of antiretroviral drugs in pregnant HIV-1-infected women for maternal health and interventions to reduce perinatal HIV transmission in the United States.* Retrieved from http://aidsinfo.nih.gov/contentfiles/lvguidelines/PerinatalGL.pdf

Porth, C., & Grossman, S. (2013). *Pathophysiology: Concepts of altered health states* (9th ed.). Philadelphia, PA: Lippincott Williams & Wilkins.

Rivera, D. M., & Frye, R. E. (2015). Pediatric HIV infection. *Medscape.* Retrieved from http://emedicine.medscape.com/article/965086-overview#a6

Robles, D. T. (2013). Lipodystrophy in HIV. *Medscape.* Retrieved from http://emedicine.medscape.com/article/1082199-overview

Rockefeller University. (2013). *Ralph Steinman: Introduction to dendritic cells.* Retrieved from http://lab.rockefeller.edu/steinman/dendritic_intro

Rockefeller University. (2016). *Ralph Steinman: Dendritic cells initiate the immune response.* Retrieved from http://lab.rockefeller.edu/steinman/

Rosman, Z., Shoenfeld, Y., & Zandman-Goddard, G. (2013). Biologic therapy for autoimmune diseases: An update. *BMC Medicine, 11*(88), 1–12. doi:10.1186/1741-7015-11-88

Ruffing, V., & Bingham, C. O. (2012). *Rheumatoid arthritis signs and symptoms.* Retrieved from http://www.hopkinsarthritis.org/arthritis-info/rheumatoid-arthritis/ra-symptoms

Sanders, L. (2014). Pregnant women's immune systems overreact to the flu. *Science Direct.* Retrieved from https://www.sciencenews.org/blog/growth-curve/pregnant-women%E2%80%99s-immune-systems-overreact-flu

Sargis, R. M. (2014). *An overview of the thymus gland: The gland that protects you long after its gone.* Retrieved from http://www.endocrineweb.com/endocrinology/overview-thymus

Sato, V. A. H., Marques, I. D. B., Goldenstein, P. T., Carmo, L. P. F., Jorge, L. B., Titan, S. M. O., . . . Woronik, V. (2012). Lupus nephritis is more severe in children and adolescents than in older adults. *Lupus, 21*(9), 978–983. doi:10.1177/0961203312443421

Schur, P.H., & Hahn, B.H. (2017). Epidemiology and pathogenesis of systemic lupus erythematosus. *UpToDate.* Retrieved from https://www.uptodate.com/contents/epidemiology-and-pathogenesis-of-systemic-lupus-erythematosus

Sherry, D. D. (2016). Juvenile idiopathic arthritis. *Medscape.* Retrieved from http://emedicine.medscape.com/article/1007276-overview#a5

Sizemore, R. C. (2012). How does stress affect the immune response? *Cell Developmental Biology, 1*(e101).

Spina Bifida Association. (2015). *Latex in the hospital environment.* Retrieved from http://spinabifidaassociation.org/wp-content/uploads/2015/07/latex-in-the-hospital-environment-eng.pdf

Stokes, J., & Casale, T. B. (2016). *The biology of IgE.* Retrieved from http://www.uptodate.com/contents/the-biology-of-ige

Suryanarayana, P. G., Copeland, H., Friedman, M., & Copeland, J. G. (2014). Cardiac transplantation in African Americans: A single-center experience. *Clinical Cardiology, 37*(6), 331–336. doi:10.1002/clc.22275

Taber, D. J., Douglas, K., Srinivas, T., McGillicuddy, J. W., Bratton, C. F., Chavin, K. D., . . . Egede, L. E. (2014). Significant racial difference in the key factors associated with early graft loss in kidney transplant recipients. *American Journal of Nephrology, 40,* 19–28. doi:10.1159/000363393

Temprano, K. (2015a). Rheumatoid arthritis. *Medscape.* Retrieved from http://emedicine.medscape.com/article/331715-overview#a4

Temprano, K. (2015b). Rheumatoid arthritis and pregnancy. *Medscape.* Retrieved from http://emedicine.medscape.com/article/335186-overview

Tucker, L., & Watcher, S. (2013). Systemic lupus erythematosus. *American College of Rheumatology.* Retrieved from http://www.rheumatology.org/I-Am-A/Patient-Caregiver/Diseases-Conditions/Systemic-Lupus-Erythematosus-Juvenile

United Nations Educational, Scientific, and Cultural Organization. (2013). *International technical guidance on sexuality education.* Retrieved from http://unesdoc.unesco.org/images/0018/001832/183281e.pdf

University of California. (2016). Symptom management guidelines: Delirium/dementia. *HIV InSite.* Retrieved from http://hivinsite.ucsf.edu/InSite?page=kb-03-01-06#S8X

University of Maryland Medical Center. (2015). *Systemic lupus erythematosus.* Retrieved from http://umm.edu/health/medical/altmed/condition/systemic-lupus-erythematosus

University of Maryland Medical Center. (2016). *Complementary and alternative medicine guide: HIV/AIDS complementary and alternative therapies: Acupuncture.* Retrieved from https://umm.edu/health/medical/altmed/condition/hiv-and-aids

U.S. Department of Health and Human Services. (2016). The need is real: Data. *Organdonor.gov.* Retrieved from http://www.organdonor.gov/about/data.html

U.S. Department of Health and Human Services, Office of Disease Prevention and Promotion. (2014). Immunization and infectious disease. *Healthy People 2020.* Retrieved from http://www.healthypeople.gov/2020/topics-objectives/topic/immunization-and-infectious-diseases

U.S. Department of Health and Human Services, Office on Women's Health. (2012). *Who gets autoimmune diseases?* Retrieved from http://womenshealth.gov/publications/our-publications/fact-sheet/autoimmune-diseases.html#c

U. S. Food and Drug Administration. (2016). *Prescribing information for Adrenaclick.* Available from: http://www.accessdata.fda.gov/drugsatfda_docs/label/2016/020800s034lbl.pdf

Vanham, G., & Van Gulck, E. (2012). Can immunotherapy be useful as a "functional cure" for infection with human immunodeficiency virus-1? *Retrovirology, 9*(1).

Voshaar, M. J. H., Nota, I., van de Laar, M. A. F. J., & van den Bemt, B. J. F. (2015). Patient-centered care in established rheumatoid arthritis. *Best Practice & Research Clinical Rheumatology, 29,* 643–663. Retrieved from http://dx.doi.org/10.1016/j.berh.2015.09.007

Wallace, D. (2015). Patient education: Systemic lupus erythematosus (SLE). *UpToDate.* Retrieved from http://www.uptodate.com/contents/systemic-lupus-erythematosus-sle-beyond-the-basics

Ward, P., & Bodmer, M. (2014). Antibodies in phase III studies for immunological disorders. In *Handbook of therapeutic antibodies* (Ch. 29). Retrieved from https://www.researchgate.net/publication/278313174_Antibodies_in_Phase_III_Studies_for_Immunological_Disorders

Weinberg, G. A. (2015). Human immunodeficiency virus (HIV) infection in children. *Merck Manual.* Retrieved from https://www.merckmanuals.com/home/children's-health-issues/human-immunodeficiency-virus-(hiv)-infection-in-children/human-immunodeficiency-virus-(hiv)-infection-in-children

Williams, E. W., Kamen, D., Penfield, M., & Oates, M. (2014). Stress intervention and disease in African American lupus patients: The balancing lupus experiences with stress strategies (BLESS) study. *Health, 6*(1), 7–79. doi:10.4236/health.2014.61011

Wilson, B. A., Shannon, M. T., & Shields, K. M. (2013). *Nurse's drug guide, 2013.* Upper Saddle River, NJ: Prentice Hall.

World Health Organization. (2013a). *Antiretroviral therapy.* Retrieved from http://www.who.int/topics/antiretroviral_therapy/en/

World Health Organization. (2013b). *HIV/AIDS: Mother-to-child transmission of HIV.* Retrieved from http://www.who.int/hiv/topics/mtct/en/index.html

World Health Organization. (2015). *HIV/AIDS fact sheet.* Retrieved from http://www.who.int/mediacentre/factsheets/fs360/en/

World Health Organization. (2016). *Global health observatory: HIV/AIDS.* Retrieved from http://www.who.int/gho/hiv/en/

Module 9
Infection

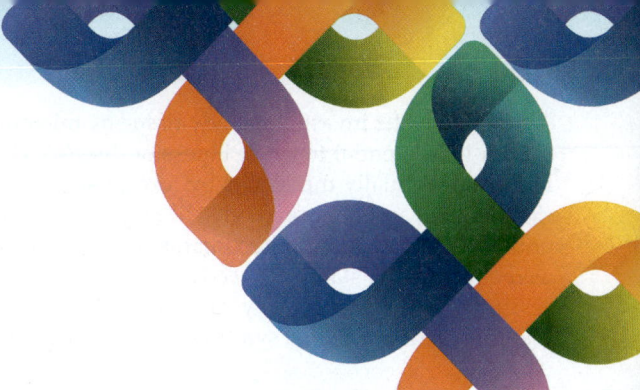

Module Outline and Learning Outcomes

The Concept of Infection

Normal Presentation
9.1 Analyze the process of infection in the body.

Alterations
9.2 Differentiate alterations that occur as a result of the infectious process.

Concepts Related to Infection
9.3 Outline the relationship between infection and other concepts.

Health Promotion
9.4 Explain health promotion and infection prevention.

Nursing Assessment
9.5 Differentiate common assessment procedures and tests used to examine the individual's infection status.

Independent Interventions
9.6 Analyze independent interventions nurses can implement for patients with infection.

Collaborative Therapies
9.7 Summarize collaborative therapies used by interprofessional teams for patients with infections.

Lifespan Considerations
9.8 Differentiate considerations related to the assessment and care of patients with infections throughout the lifespan.

Infection Exemplars

Exemplar 9.A Cellulitis
9.A Analyze cellulitis as it relates to infection.

Exemplar 9.B Conjunctivitis
9.B Analyze conjunctivitis as it relates to infection.

Exemplar 9.C Influenza
9.C Analyze influenza as it relates to infection.

Exemplar 9.D Otitis Media
9.D Analyze otitis media as it relates to infection.

Exemplar 9.E Pneumonia
9.E Analyze pneumonia as it relates to infection.

Exemplar 9.F Sepsis
9.F Analyze sepsis as it relates to infection.

Exemplar 9.G Tuberculosis
9.G Analyze tuberculosis as it relates to infection.

Exemplar 9.H Urinary Tract Infection
9.H Analyze urinary tract infection as it relates to infection.

 # The Concept of Infection

Concept Key Terms

Acute infections, **557**
Airborne precautions, **570**
Antibody, **593**
Antiseptics, **569**
Asepsis, **556**
Bacteremia, **557**
Bacteria, **557**
Bactericidal agent, **569**
Bacteriostatic agent, **569**
Bloodborne pathogens, **570**

Body substance isolation (BSI), **570**
Carrier, **557**
Chronic infection, **557**
Clean, **557**
Colonization, **557**
Communicable disease, **556**
Compromised host, **559**
Contact precautions, **571**
Dirty, **557**
Disease, **556**
Disease surveillance, **566**

Disinfectants, **569**
Droplet nuclei, **559**
Droplet precautions, **571**
Endogenous, **564**
Endotoxins, **562**
Exogenous, **564**
Exotoxins, **562**
Fungi, **557**
Healthcare-associated infection (HAI), **563**
Iatrogenic infections, **564**
Infection, **556**

Infectious disease, **556**
Isolation, **570**
Local infection, **557**
Medical asepsis, **557**
Occupational exposure, **576**
Opportunistic pathogen, **556**
Parasites, **557**
Pathogen, **556**
Pathogenicity, **556**
Reservoirs, **557**

Sepsis, **557**
Septicemia, **557**
Specific defenses, **559**
Sterile field, **574**
Sterile technique, **557**
Sterilization, **570**
Surgical asepsis, **557**
Systemic infection, **557**
Universal precautions (UP), **570**
Virulence, **556**
Viruses, **557**

555

Infection is the invasion of body tissue by microorganisms with the potential to cause illness or disease. The human body is continually threatened by foreign substances, infectious agents, and abnormal cells. In response to widespread antibiotic use, resistant microorganisms have emerged, such as methicillin-resistant *Staphylococcus aureus* and multidrug-resistant tuberculosis. New diseases have also emerged, including irritable bowel syndrome and Heartland virus.

Normal Presentation

The immune system is the body's major defense mechanism against infectious organisms and abnormal or damaged cells. Any illness or injury can result in an infection if it is left untreated or if the body's immune system is compromised in some way. Nurses must think about infection prevention all the time. They know that if they move from patient room to patient room with contaminated hands or equipment, they risk infecting everyone they touch. The effectiveness of other care provided does not matter if nurses are not protecting patients against infection. Therefore, nurses are always directly involved in providing a biologically safe environment. Infection-control is central to delivering high-quality nursing care. This concept explains what steps to take to prevent the spread of infection, how infection is shared, and what impact an infection can have on the human body.

Microorganisms exist everywhere: in water, in soil, and on body surfaces such as the skin, intestinal tract, and other areas open to the environment (e.g., mouth, upper respiratory tract, vagina, lower urinary tract). Most microorganisms are harmless, and some are even beneficial, performing essential functions in the body. Some microorganisms found in the intestines (e.g., enterobacteria) produce substances called *bacteriocins*, which are lethal to related strains of bacteria. Others produce substances that repress the growth of other microorganisms. Some microorganisms are normal resident flora (the collective vegetation in a given area) in one part of the body, yet produce infection in another. For example, *Escherichia coli* is a normal inhabitant of the large intestine but a common cause of infection of the urinary tract. **Table 9–1 》** provides a list of common resident microorganisms by body area.

Recall that an infection is an invasion of body tissue by microorganisms. If the microorganisms produce no clinical evidence of disease, the infection is *asymptomatic* or *subclinical*. **Disease** occurs when the microorganisms produce a detectable alteration in normal tissue function. A **communicable disease** is an illness that is directly transmitted from one individual or animal to another by contact with body fluids or indirectly transmitted by contact with contaminated objects, airborne particles, or vectors (e.g., ticks, mosquitoes, other insects). An **infectious disease** is any communicable disease that is caused by microorganisms that are commonly transmitted from one individual or animal to another or from an animal to an individual. Infectious and communicable diseases are a major cause of disease and death in infants and children in the United States. Some subclinical infections can cause considerable damage. For example, cytomegalovirus (CMV) infection in a pregnant woman can lead to significant disease in the unborn child.

TABLE 9–1 Examples of Common Resident Microorganisms

Body Area	Resident Microorganisms
Skin	*Staphylococcus epidermidis*
	Staphylococcus aureus
	Corynebacterium xerosis
	Micrococcus luteus
Nasal passages	*Staphylococcus aureus*
	Staphylococcus epidermidis
Oropharynx	*Streptococcus pneumoniae*
	Streptococcus salivarius
	Neisseria meningitidis
Mouth	*Streptococcus mutans*
	Streptococcus mitis
	Lactobacillus
	Actinomyces
	Spirochetes
Intestine	*Staphylococcus aureus*
	Bacteroides
	Bifidobacterium bifidum
	Eubacterium
	Clostridium
	Lactobacillus
	Escherichia coli
Anterior urethra	*Staphylococcus epidermidis*
	Streptococcus viridians
	Corynebacterium
Vagina	*Lactobacillus*
	Candida albicans

Infectious diseases are a major cause of death worldwide. Efforts are made on the international, national, state, community, and individual levels to control the spread of microorganisms and to protect people from communicable diseases and infections. The World Health Organization (WHO) is the major regulatory agency at the international level. In the United States, the Centers for Disease Control and Prevention (CDC) is the principal public health agency concerned with disease prevention and control at the national level. State and county or city health departments track epidemics and illnesses as reports are made throughout those areas.

Microorganisms vary in **pathogenicity** (ability to produce disease); thus, a **pathogen** is a microorganism that causes disease. Many microorganisms that are normally harmless can cause disease under certain circumstances. A "true" pathogen causes disease or infection in a healthy individual, whereas an **opportunistic pathogen** causes disease only in susceptible individuals. Microorganisms also vary in their **virulence**, or severity of the diseases they produce, and in their degree of communicability. For example, the common cold virus is more readily transmitted than the bacillus that causes leprosy (*Mycobacterium leprae*).

Asepsis is the absence of disease-causing microorganisms. Aseptic technique decreases the possibility of transferring microorganisms from one place to another. There are two basic types of asepsis: medical and surgical. **Medical asepsis** includes all practices intended to confine a specific microorganism to a specific area, thus limiting the number, growth, and transmission of microorganisms. In medical asepsis, objects are referred to as **clean**, which means that almost all microorganisms are absent, or **dirty** (soiled, contaminated), which means that microorganisms are likely to be present, some of which may be capable of causing infection.

Surgical asepsis, or **sterile technique**, refers to practices that keep an area or object free of all microorganisms; it includes practices that destroy all microorganisms and spores (microscopic dormant structures formed by some pathogens that are very hardy and often survive common cleaning techniques). Surgical asepsis is used for all procedures involving sterile areas of the body. **Sepsis** is a whole body inflammatory process resulting in acute illness; however, the term is often used generally to refer to the state of infection.

Types of Microorganisms that Cause Infections

Four major categories of microorganisms cause infection in humans: bacteria, viruses, fungi, and parasites. **Bacteria** are by far the most common infection-causing microorganisms. Several hundred species of bacteria can cause disease in humans and can live and be transported through air, water, food, soil, body tissues and fluids, and inanimate objects. Most of the microorganisms listed in Table 9–1 are bacteria. **Viruses** consist primarily of nucleic acid and therefore must enter living cells to reproduce. Common virus families include the rhinovirus (causes the common cold), hepatitis, herpes, and HIV. **Fungi** include yeasts and molds. *Candida albicans* is a yeast considered normal flora in the human vagina. **Parasites** live on other organisms. They include protozoa, such as the one that causes malaria, helminths (worms), and arthropods (mites, fleas, ticks).

Types of Infections

Colonization is the process by which strains of microorganisms become resident flora. In this state, the microorganisms may grow and multiply, but they do not cause disease. Infection occurs when newly introduced or resident microorganisms succeed in invading a part of the body where the host's defense mechanisms are ineffective, and the pathogen causes tissue damage. The infection becomes a disease when the signs and symptoms of the infection are unique, can be differentiated from other conditions, and alter bodily function or processes.

Infections can be local or systemic. A **local infection** is limited to the specific part of the body where the microorganisms remain. Examples of local infections include otitis media and urinary tract infection (UTI). If the microorganisms spread and damage different parts of the body, the result is a **systemic infection**. Examples of systemic infections include cellulitis and sepsis. When a culture of the individual's blood reveals bacteria, the condition is called **bacteremia**. When bacteremia results in systemic infection,

it is referred to as **septicemia**. These infections have unfortunately become more common recently.

Infections are also classified as acute or chronic. **Acute infections**, such as influenza or pneumonia, generally appear suddenly and last a short time. A **chronic infection**, such as tuberculosis, may develop slowly, over a very long period, and often persists for months and sometimes years.

An individual does not need to have an identified infection to transmit potentially infective microorganisms to another individual. Even microorganisms that are normal for one individual can infect another individual.

Chain of Infection

The chain of infection consists of six links (see **Figure 9–1** »): the etiologic agent, or microorganism; the place where the organism naturally resides (reservoir); a portal of exit from the reservoir; a method (mode) of transmission; a portal of entry into a susceptible host; and a susceptible host.

Etiologic Agent

The extent to which any microorganism is capable of producing an infectious process depends on the number of microorganisms present, the virulence (potential for causing harm) and pathogenicity of the microorganisms, the ability of the microorganisms to enter the body, the susceptibility of the host, and the ability of the microorganisms to live in the host's body.

Some microorganisms, such as the smallpox virus, can infect almost all susceptible people after exposure. By contrast, microorganisms such as *Mycobacterium tuberculosis* infect a relatively small number of the population who are susceptible and exposed. Those at risk are usually people who are poorly nourished or living in crowded conditions, or those whose immune systems are less competent (e.g., older adults, individuals with HIV or cancer).

Reservoir

There are many **reservoirs**, or sources of microorganisms. Common sources are other humans, the patient's own microorganisms, plants, animals, and the general environment. People are the most common source of infection for others and for themselves. For example, an individual with an influenza virus frequently spreads it to others. A **carrier** is a human or animal reservoir of a specific infectious agent that usually does not manifest any clinical signs of disease. For example, the *Anopheles* mosquito reservoir carries the malaria parasite (*Plasmodium* spp.) but is unaffected by it. The carrier state may also exist in individuals with a clinically recognizable disease, such as a dog with rabies. Under either circumstance, the carrier state may be of short duration (temporary or transient carrier) or long duration (chronic carrier). Food, water, and feces can also be reservoirs.

Portal of Exit from Reservoir

Before an infection can establish itself in a host, the microorganisms must leave the reservoir. Common human reservoirs and their associated portals of exit are summarized in **Table 9–2** ».

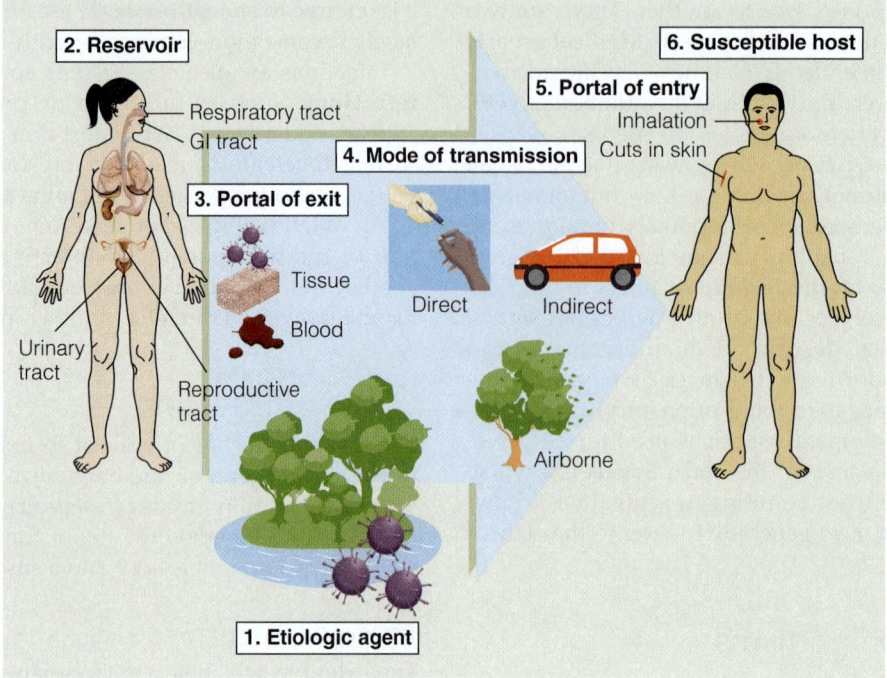

Figure 9–1 ›› The chain of infection.

Method of Transmission

After a microorganism leaves its source or reservoir, it requires a means of transmission to reach another host through a receptive portal of entry. There are three modes of transmission:

1. **Direct transmission.** Direct transmission involves the immediate and direct transfer of microorganisms from one individual to another through touching, biting, kissing, or sexual intercourse. Droplet spread is also a form of direct transmission, but it occurs only if the source and the host are within 3 ft of each other. Sneezing, coughing, spitting, singing, or talking can project droplet spray into the conjunctiva or onto the mucous membranes of the eye, nose, or mouth of another individual.

TABLE 9–2 Human Body Area Reservoirs, Common Infectious Microorganisms, and Portals of Exit

Body Area Reservoir	Common Infectious Microorganisms	Portals of Exit
Respiratory tract	Parainfluenza virus *Mycobacterium tuberculosis* *Staphylococcus aureus*	▪ Nose or mouth through sneezing, coughing, breathing, or talking
Gastrointestinal tract	Hepatitis A virus *Salmonella* species *Clostridium difficile*	▪ Mouth: saliva, vomitus ▪ Anus: feces, ostomies
Urinary tract	*Escherichia coli,* enterococci *Pseudomonas aeruginosa*	▪ Urethral meatus and urinary diversion
Reproductive tract	*Neisseria gonorrhoeae* *Treponema pallidum* Herpes simplex virus type 2 Hepatitis B virus	▪ Vagina: vaginal discharge ▪ Urinary meatus: semen, urine
Blood	Hepatitis B virus HIV *Staphylococcus aureus* *Staphylococcus epidermidis*	▪ Open wound, needle puncture site, any disruption of intact skin or mucous membrane surfaces
Tissue	*Staphylococcus aureus* *Escherichia coli* *Proteus* species *Streptococcus,* beta-hemolytic A or B	▪ Drainage from cut or wound

2. ***Indirect transmission.*** Indirect transmission can be either vehicle-borne or vector-borne.

   a. ***Vehicle-borne transmission.*** A *vehicle* is any substance that serves as an intermediate means to transport and introduce an infectious agent into a susceptible host through a suitable portal of entry. Fomites (inanimate materials or objects), such as handkerchiefs, toys, soiled clothes, cooking or eating utensils, and surgical instruments or dressings, can act as vehicles. Water, food, blood, serum, and plasma are also vehicles. For example, food can become contaminated by a food handler who carries the hepatitis A virus, and the food may then be ingested by a susceptible host.

   b. ***Vector-borne transmission.*** A *vector* is an animal or flying or crawling insect that serves as an intermediate means of transporting the infectious agent. Transmission can occur by injection of salivary fluid during biting or by the deposit of feces or other materials on the skin through the bite wound or a traumatized skin area.

3. ***Airborne transmission.*** Airborne transmission involves droplets or dust. **Droplet nuclei**, the residue of evaporated droplets emitted by an infected host, such as an individual with tuberculosis, can remain in the air for long periods of time. Dust particles containing the infectious agent (e.g., *Clostridium difficile* spores from the soil) can also become airborne. The material is transmitted by air currents to a suitable portal of entry on another individual, usually the respiratory tract.

Portal of Entry to the Susceptible Host

Before an individual can become infected, microorganisms must enter the body. The skin is a barrier to infectious agents; however, any break in the skin can readily serve as a portal of entry. Often, microorganisms enter the body of a host by the same route they used to leave the source. For example, an airborne infection escapes its host or carrier via sneezing or coughing and is transmitted to a new host who inhales the microorganism through the nose or mouth. The mouth, throat, nose, ears, eyes, and genitalia are open to outside exposure and thus are the most frequent portals of entry for microorganisms. Cuts and tears in the skin also provide portals through which microorganisms enter and cause disease.

Susceptible Host

A susceptible host is any individual who is at risk for infection. Infants and young children are often susceptible hosts. Their immune systems have not fully matured, and they have not yet developed antibodies to many agents. Therefore, their bodies cannot defend against infectious and communicable diseases as well as those of older children and adults. A **compromised host** is an individual at increased risk, that is, one who, for one or more reasons, is more likely than others to acquire an infection. Impairment of the body's natural defenses and a number of other factors affect susceptibility to infection. Examples are age (the very young or the very old), receiving immune suppression treatment for cancer or chronic illness or following a successful organ transplantation, and immune deficiency conditions.

Table 9–3 ❯❯ outlines nursing interventions that break the chain of infection, including their rationales.

Physiology Review

Individuals normally have defenses that protect the body from infection. Nonspecific defenses include anatomical and physiologic barriers and the inflammatory response. **Specific defenses** involve the immune system when an antigen induces a state of sensitivity and antibodies respond to contain or destroy the antigen.

Intact skin and mucous membranes are the body's first line of defense against invading microorganisms. Unless the skin and mucosa become cracked and broken, they act as an effective barrier against bacteria. Fungi can live on the skin, but they cannot penetrate it. The dryness of the skin also is a deterrent to bacteria. Bacteria are most plentiful in moist areas of the body, such as the perineum and axillae. Resident bacteria of the skin also prevent other bacteria from multiplying. The resident bacteria use up the available nutrients, and the end products of their metabolism inhibit other bacterial growth. Normal secretions make the skin slightly acidic and thus also inhibit bacterial growth.

The nasal passages have a defensive function. As entering air follows the tortuous route of the nasal passages, it comes in contact with moist mucous membranes and cilia. These structures trap microorganisms, dust, and foreign materials. The lungs have alveolar macrophages (large phagocytes) that ingest microorganisms, other cells, and foreign particles.

Each body orifice also has protective mechanisms. The oral cavity regularly sheds mucosal epithelium to rid the mouth of colonizers. The flow of saliva and its partially buffering action help prevent infections. Saliva contains microbial inhibitors, such as lactoferrin, lysozyme, and secretory immunoglobulin A (IgA). The eye is protected from infection by tears, which continually wash microorganisms away and contain inhibiting lysozyme. The vagina also has natural defenses against infection. When a girl reaches puberty, lactobacilli ferment sugars in the vaginal secretions, creating a vaginal pH of 3.5–4.5. This low pH inhibits the growth of many disease-producing microorganisms. The entrance to the urethra normally harbors many microorganisms, including *Staphylococcus epidermidis* coagulase (from the skin) and *Escherichia coli* (from feces). The urine flow is believed to have a flushing and bacteriostatic action that keeps the bacteria from ascending the urethra. An intact mucosal surface also acts as a barrier.

The gastrointestinal tract also has defenses against infection. The high acidity of the stomach normally prevents microbial growth. The resident flora of the large intestine help prevent the establishment of disease-producing microorganisms. Peristalsis also tends to move microbes out of the body.

Genetic Considerations

A patient's susceptibility to infection is affected by age and heredity. Heredity also influences the development of infection in that some people have a genetic susceptibility to certain infections. For example, some individuals are deficient in serum immunoglobulins, which play a significant role in

TABLE 9–3 Nursing Interventions that Break the Chain of Infection

Link in Chain of Infection	Interventions	Rationales
Etiologic agent (microorganism)	▪ Educate patients and support them and their families in using appropriate methods to clean, disinfect, and sterilize articles.	▪ Knowledge of ways to reduce or eliminate microorganisms reduces the number of microorganisms present and the likelihood of transmission.
	▪ Ensure that articles are correctly cleaned and disinfected or sterilized before use.	▪ Correct cleaning, disinfecting, and sterilizing reduce or eliminate microorganisms.
Reservoir (source)	▪ Change dressings and bandages when they are soiled or wet.	▪ Moist dressings are ideal environments for microorganisms to grow and multiply.
	▪ Assist patients to carry out appropriate skin and oral hygiene.	▪ Hygienic measures reduce the number of resident and transient microorganisms and the likelihood of infection.
	▪ Dispose of damp, soiled linens appropriately.	▪ Damp, soiled linens harbor more microorganisms than dry linens.
	▪ Dispose of feces and urine in appropriate receptacles.	▪ Urine and feces in particular contain many microorganisms.
	▪ Ensure that all fluid containers, such as bedside water jugs and suction and drainage bottles, are covered or capped.	▪ Prolonged exposure increases the risk of contamination and promotes microbial growth.
	▪ Empty suction and drainage bottles at the end of each shift, before they become full, or according to agency policy.	▪ Drainage harbors microorganisms that, if left for long periods, proliferate and can be transmitted to others.
Portal of exit from the reservoir	▪ Avoid talking, coughing, or sneezing over open wounds and sterile fields, and cover the mouth and nose when coughing and sneezing.	▪ These measures limit the number of microorganisms that escape from the respiratory tract.
Method of transmission	▪ Cleanse hands between patient contacts, after touching body substances, and before performing invasive procedures or touching open wounds.	▪ Hand cleansing is an important means of controlling and preventing the transmission of microorganisms.
	▪ Instruct patients and support them and their families in hand hygiene before handling food or eating, after eliminating, and after touching infectious material.	▪ Hand hygiene helps prevent the transfer of microorganisms from one individual to another.
	▪ Wear gloves when handling secretions and excretions.	▪ Gloves prevent soiling of the hands and clothing.
	▪ Wear gowns if there is danger of soiling clothing with body substances.	▪ Gowns prevent soiling of clothing.
	▪ Place discarded soiled materials in moisture-proof refuse bags.	▪ Moisture-proof bags prevent the spread of microorganisms to others.
	▪ Hold used bedpans steadily to prevent spillage, and dispose of urine and feces in appropriate receptacles.	▪ Urine and feces in particular contain many microorganisms.
	▪ Initiate and implement aseptic precautions for all patients.	▪ All patients harbor potentially infectious microorganisms that can be transmitted to others.
	▪ Wear masks or respirators, and use eye protection when in close contact with patients who have infections transmitted by droplets from the respiratory tract or when sprays of body fluid are possible (e.g., during irrigation procedures).	▪ Masks, respirators, and eyewear provide protection from airborne droplets and microorganisms in patients' body substances.
Portal of entry to the susceptible host	▪ Use sterile technique for invasive procedures (e.g., injections, catheterizations).	▪ Invasive procedures penetrate the body's natural protective barriers to microorganisms.
	▪ Use sterile technique when exposing open wounds and handling dressings.	▪ Open wounds are vulnerable to microbial infection.
	▪ Place used disposable needles and syringes in puncture-resistant containers for disposal.	▪ Injuries from needles contaminated by blood or body fluids from an infected patient or carrier are a primary cause of hepatitis B virus and HIV transmission to healthcare workers.
	▪ Provide all patients with their own personal care items.	▪ People have less resistance to another individual's microorganisms than to their own.
Susceptible host	▪ Maintain the integrity of patients' skin and mucous membranes.	▪ Intact skin and mucous membranes protect against invasion by microorganisms.
	▪ Ensure that patients receive a balanced diet.	▪ A balanced diet supplies proteins and vitamins necessary to build and maintain body tissues.
	▪ Educate the public about the importance of immunizations.	▪ Immunizations protect people against virulent infectious diseases.

the internal defense mechanism of the body. Mutations in inflammatory proteins, such as proteins in the interleukin-12, interleukin-23, and interferon-gamma signaling pathways, can also increase an individual's susceptibility to mycobacterial infection (Chapman & Hill, 2012). See the Lifespan Considerations section for more information.

Itan and colleagues (2014) described the human gene connectome server (HGCS), which is an online format that enables researchers to explore and prioritize genes according to the phenotype of interest. Researchers must identify the genotypes underlying human disease phenotypes as this is an essential step in human genetics and medicine. For example, platelet activation and aggregation play important roles in ischemic event occurrences in individuals with coronary artery disease. Identifying patients with the phenotype for this platelet activation may reduce the risk of a future cardiac crisis (Tantry et al., 2013). Further research on these types of medical concerns will influence the methods for managing patients' prevention of illness and well as post-acute care.

Alterations

Microorganisms often invade the human body and proliferate when they are undetected, uncontrolled, or not eliminated by the inflammatory and immune responses. In most cases, contact between humans and microorganisms is incidental and may even be beneficial to both organisms. However, many microorganisms are pathogens.

Modern medicine, antibiotic therapy, immunizations, and other public health measures to protect food and water supplies have significantly reduced the prevalence of infectious diseases in many parts of the world. In spite of these advances, many infections, including malaria, typhoid, and tuberculosis, remain prevalent in developing nations. Sexually transmitted infections rage through modern cities and industrialized populations. New varieties and strains of pathogens, called emerging infectious pathogens, evolve to cause disease. Two examples are Ebola and the Zika virus.

To a certain extent, modern medicine has contributed to the development of infectious diseases caused by antibiotic-resistant strains of microorganisms. For example, tuberculosis is on the rise in the United States, partially because organisms have become resistant to standard therapies. Following organ or tissue transplantation and in the treatment of neoplasms, patients receive immunosuppressive therapy, which makes them more susceptible to infection. The implantation of metal and plastic prosthetic devices provides potential sites for colonization of disease-producing organisms (Osmon et al., 2013). Many diseases that were long considered unrelated to microorganisms may also actually be infectious; for example, colonization of the gastric mucosa with *Helicobacter pylori* is the predominant cause of peptic ulcer disease, and oncogenic viruses can transform normal cells into malignant cells.

Poor hygiene behaviors of young children and their caregivers facilitate transmission of infectious diseases in child care settings and other environments, including hospitals, clinics, and healthcare providers' offices. The fecal-oral and respiratory routes are the most common modes of transmission in children. Children often do not wash their hands after toileting unless they are closely supervised. They put toys and their hands in their mouths and then rub their noses and eyes. They often need help in caring for a runny nose. Diapers may leak stool and provide exposure to fecal organisms. In addition, caregivers in child care centers, other people caring for children, and healthcare professionals may not use proper hand hygiene. All of these behaviors promote the transmission of infection.

Pathogens

Pathogens capable of infecting and causing disease in susceptible hosts include bacteria, viruses, fungi, and parasites, such as protozoa, helminths (worms), and arthropods (see **Figure 9–2 »** and **Box 9–1 »**). Each organism causes a different specific reaction in the host.

Box 9–1
Pathogenic Organisms

Bacteria
Bacteria are single-celled organisms capable of autonomous reproduction. Bacteria have different characteristics and growth requirements: *Aerobes* require oxygen for survival, whereas *anaerobes* cannot survive in the presence of oxygen; *gram-positive* bacteria stain purple when subjected to crystal violet stain, whereas *gram-negative* bacteria do not stain with crystal violet stain but turn red when subjected to safranin stain, and the colonies formed by replicating bacteria differ from one another.

Mycoplasma
Mycoplasma are very small bacteria that have no cell wall, making them resistant to antibiotics that inhibit cell wall synthesis, such as the penicillins.

Rickettsia and Chlamydia
Rickettsia and *Chlamydia* are obligate intracellular parasites with a rigid cell wall; they use vitamins, nutrients, and products of metabolism (e.g., ATP) from the host. *Chlamydia* are transmitted by direct contact, whereas *Rickettsia* infect the cells of arthropods (e.g., fleas, ticks, lice) and are transmitted from these vectors to humans.

Viruses
Viruses are obligate intracellular parasites that are incapable of reproducing outside a living cell. Some viruses are shed continuously from infected cell surfaces; others, after inserting their genetic material into that of the infected cell, remain latent until they are stimulated to replicate. Viruses may or may not cause lysis and death of the host cell during replication. Oncogenic viruses are able to transform normal cells into malignant cells.

Fungi
Fungi are prevalent throughout the world, but few are capable of causing disease in humans. Most fungal infections are self-limited, affecting the skin and subcutaneous tissue. Some fungi, such as *Pneumocystis jiroveci*, can cause life-threatening opportunistic infections in hosts who are immunocompromised.

Parasites
The term *parasite* is typically applied to members of the animal kingdom that infect and cause disease in other animals. Protozoa, helminths, and arthropods are considered parasites. Protozoa are single-celled organisms transmitted via direct or indirect contact or by an arthropod vector. Helminths are wormlike parasites. Roundworms, tapeworms, and flukes are examples. They gain entry into humans primarily through ingestion of fertilized eggs or penetration of larvae through the skin or mucous membranes. Arthropod parasites, such as scabies (mites), lice, and fleas, typically infest external body surfaces, causing localized tissue damage and inflammation. Transmission is by direct contact with the arthropod or its eggs.

Sources: Data from Adams, M. P., Holland, L. N., & Urban, C. (2017). *Pharmacology for nurses: A pathophysiologic approach* (5th ed.). Hoboken, NJ: Pearson Education; Centers for Disease Control and Prevention. (2015m). *CDC's Infection Disease National Centers.* Retrieved from http://www.cdc.gov/oid/centers.html; Porth, C., & Grossman, S. (2014). *Pathophysiology: Concepts of altered health states* (9th ed.). Philadelphia, PA: Lippincott Williams & Wilkins.

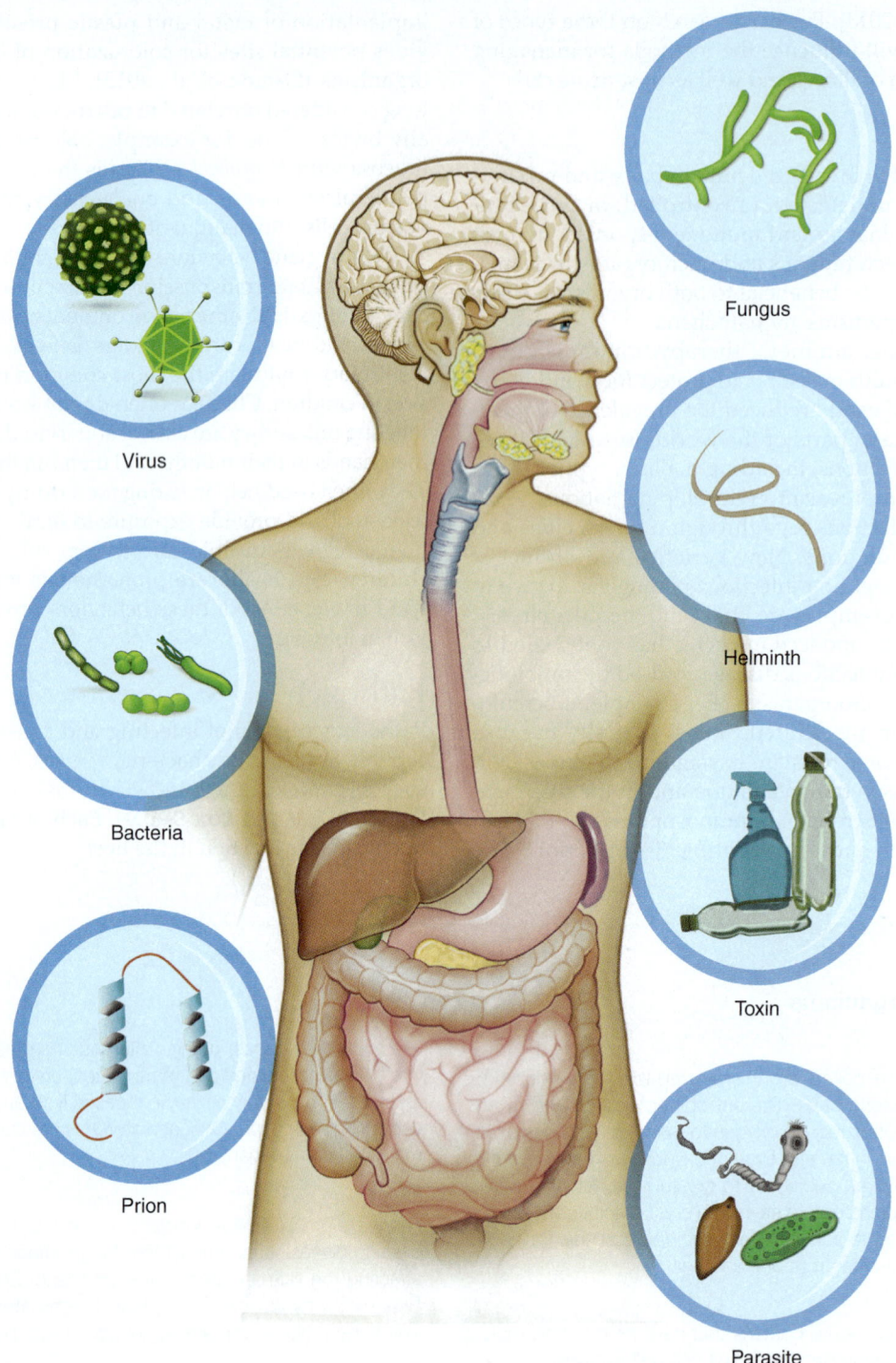

Virus

Fungus

Bacteria

Helminth

Prion

Toxin

Parasite

Figure 9–2 》 Pathogens.

A number of mechanisms have evolved in pathogens to facilitate their transmission and increase their ability to invade the host and cause disease. Factors influencing the transmission of an organism include its resistance to drying and to variations in environmental temperature. For example, spore-forming organisms are extremely resistant to drying.

Pathogens are often capable of producing toxins or enzymes that alter or destroy the normal function of host cells and promote colonization, proliferation, and invasion by the pathogen. Adhesion factors produced by or incorporated into the cell wall or membrane of the pathogen improve its ability to attach to and colonize the host. Toxins often increase the disease-producing capability of the pathogen and, in some cases, are totally responsible for it. For example, cholera, tetanus, and botulism result from bacterial toxins, not from the direct effects of the infection. **Exotoxins** are soluble proteins that the microorganisms secrete into surrounding tissue. Exotoxins are highly poisonous, causing cell death or dysfunction. **Endotoxins** are found in the cell wall of gram-negative bacteria and are released only when the cell is disrupted. They have less specific effects than exotoxins but can activate many human regulatory systems, producing fever, inflammation, and potentially clotting, bleeding, or hypotension when released in large quantities. Pathogens may also produce enzymes to enhance their spread to local tissues, chemicals to block specific immune processes or deplete neutrophils and macrophages, or extracellular capsules to discourage phagocytosis.

Stages of the Infectious Process

When infectious disease develops in a host, it typically follows a predictable course, with stages based on the progression and intensity of manifestations. Stages include:

1. Incubation period
2. Prodromal stage
3. Illness stage
4. Convalescent stage

The initial stage is the *incubation period*, during which the pathogen begins active replication but does not yet cause symptoms. Depending on the organism and host factors, the incubation period may last from hours, as with *Salmonella*, to years, as with HIV infection.

In the *prodromal stage*, symptoms begin to appear. At this stage, symptoms are often nonspecific and include general malaise, fever, myalgias, headache, and fatigue.

Maximal impact of the infectious process occurs during the *illness stage* as the pathogen proliferates and disseminates rapidly. Toxic by-products of microorganism metabolism and cell lysis, along with the immune response, produce tissue damage and inflammation during this stage (Porth & Grossman, 2014). Manifestations are more pronounced and specific to the infecting organism and site. Fever and chills may be significant during this phase. However, patients who are alcoholics and older adults may respond to severe infection by becoming hypothermic. Patients in the illness stage of infection are often tachycardic and tachypneic because of increased metabolic demands. Localized manifestations include redness, heat, swelling, pain, and impaired function. When the infectious disease affects an internal organ, manifestations are related to inflammatory changes in that organ and surrounding tissue. Patients may experience tenderness to palpation over the site or show signs of impaired function, such as the hematuria and proteinuria that are characteristic of renal infections.

If the infectious process is prolonged, manifestations of the continuing immune response may become apparent. Catabolic and anorexic effects of the infection can lead to muscle wasting and loss of body fat. Immune complexes may be deposited at sites other than that of the primary infection, the result being an inflammatory process. Glomerulonephritis (e.g., following strep throat) and vasculitis are possible results. Another possible consequence of prolonged infection and immune response is the triggering of an autoimmune disease process, such as rheumatic cardiomyopathy or celiac disease. Type 1 diabetes mellitus is thought to be the result of such a response (Porth & Grossman, 2014).

As the infection is contained and the pathogen eliminated, the *convalescent stage* of the disease occurs. During this stage, affected tissues are repaired and manifestations resolve. Resolution of the infection is total elimination of the pathogen from the body without residual manifestations.

If a balance between organism and host factors occurs, with neither predominating, chronic disease may develop, or the organism may be driven into a protected site, such as an abscess. A *carrier state* develops when host defenses eliminate the infectious disease, but the organism continues to multiply on mucosal sites (Longo et al., 2012).

Alterations and Manifestations

Infections cause predictable diseases depending on the infecting microorganism, and they often respond predictably to the right treatment. However, complications can occur if the infection spreads to other parts of the body, if the infecting organism develops resistance to treatment, or if the host's immune system is unable to fight off the infection. In addition, infectious agents can be used as biological threats to communities, causing widespread panic and a demand on resources that may prevent adequate treatment.

Complications of Infectious Diseases

Multiple and varied complications are associated with infectious diseases. They are typically specific to the infecting organism and the body system affected.

One life-threatening complication is sepsis, which is a severe reaction to infection. Bacteremia, or the presence of bacteria in the blood, may not have serious effects; however, if the infection becomes severe or if the microorganisms produce toxins, they can cause septicemia. Septicemia may lead to septic shock, a state of life-threateningly low blood pressure caused by overwhelming infection. Unless treated aggressively, septic shock leads to diffuse cell and tissue injury and potentially to organ failure. Older adults are at a higher risk of developing sepsis than younger individuals. Approximately two thirds of the individuals hospitalized for sepsis are over the age of 65, and the rate of septicemia hospitalization is four times higher for patients over the age of 85 than for patients between the ages of 65 and 74 (Rhee, Gohil, & Klompas, 2014).

Healthcare-Associated Infections

Healthcare-associated infections (abbreviated as HAIs or HCAIs) are classified as infections that are associated with the delivery of healthcare services in a facility such as a hospital or nursing home. HAIs add hospital days, reduce admissions by occupying available beds, and increase the cost of healthcare (Goodman, 2013). HAIs can either develop during a patient's stay in a facility or manifest after discharge. They typically manifest after 48 hours of hospitalization. Infections that manifest during the first 48 hours of hospitalization are attributed to community sources.

Respiratory complications have become a common type of HAI. Healthcare-associated pneumonia has a mortality rate of 38–70% (Rhee et al., 2014) and is most often associated with mechanical ventilators, tracheostomies, and endotracheal intubation (Porth & Grossman, 2014). Ventilator-associated pneumonia (VAP) is defined as pneumonia that occurs in patients who are intubated and ventilated at the time of, or within 48 hours before, the onset of the pneumonia. VAP accounts for more than 80% of healthcare-associated pneumonias. VAP is associated with increased mortality rates, longer hospital stays, increased hospitalization costs, and increased morbidity (deJuilio, Rivera, & Huml, 2012). In addition to

VAP, adult respiratory distress syndrome (ARDS) is a critical concern in acute care and intensive care areas. This illness is further discussed in the exemplar on ARDS in the module on Oxygenation.

UTI is the most common type of HAI and the most frequent cause of gram-negative septicemia in hospitalized patients. Surgical site infections and pneumonia are the other two of the top three HAIs. Bacteremia is associated with intravascular and urinary catheters. Because of the risk of infection, insertion of central lines and urinary catheters is conducted as a sterile procedure with careful attention to preventing contamination. *Clostridium difficile*–associated diarrhea is a frequently acquired HAI. Associated with antibiotic use, this infection's risk increases with length of hospital stay, especially in an intensive care unit (ICU). Healthcare personnel working in the facility can also acquire HAIs, which can cause significant illness and time lost from work.

HAIs have received increasing attention in recent years. They are believed to involve approximately 1.7 million patients per year, cause 90,000 deaths, and add $28–$33 billion in excess healthcare costs annually (Close Up Media, 2013). The Joint Commission (2012), an independent, not-for-profit organization that accredits and certifies healthcare organizations and programs in the United States, included reducing the risk of HAIs as one of the 2013 National Patient Safety Goals. The most common settings where HAIs develop are hospital surgical units and medical ICUs. The microorganisms that cause HAIs can originate from the patients themselves (an **endogenous** source) or from the hospital environment and hospital personnel (**exogenous** sources). Most HAIs appear to have endogenous sources. *Escherichia coli, Staphylococcus aureus,* and *Enterococci* are the most common infecting microorganisms.

>> **Stay Current:** Visit The Joint Commission website every year to see the latest National Patient Safety Goals: http://www.jointcommission.org/standards_information/npsgs.aspx

A number of factors contribute to HAIs. **Iatrogenic infections** are the direct result of diagnostic or therapeutic procedures. One example of an iatrogenic infection is the bacteremia that results from insertion of an intravascular line. Not all HAIs are iatrogenic, nor are they all preventable.

Another factor that contributes to the development of HAIs is the compromised host, that is, a patient whose normal defenses have been lowered by surgery or illness. Patients entering hospitals are often the least able to mount immune defenses to infection. Immunologic responses may be compromised and normal defenses impaired in patients with, for example, cancer or chronic diseases, pressure ulcers, or organ transplants (Papadakis & McPhee, 2013). HAIs also occur when antibiotic therapy has altered the body's natural defenses and impaired resistance to harmful microorganisms. Endogenous organisms outside their normal habitats (e.g., *E. coli* in the urinary tract) become a threat to the patient. Other pharmacologic and therapeutic procedures, such as chemotherapy, the use of corticosteroids, and radiation therapy, also contribute to HAIs. Gram-negative enteric bacteria and gram-positive *S. aureus* are the most common bacteria responsible.

Invasive procedures and altered immune defenses are the main contributors to infection. Urinary catheterization is the number one cause; cardiac catheterization, insertion of peripheral and central intravenous (IV) lines, respiratory care procedures such as mechanical ventilation, and surgical procedures are also closely linked to HAIs. As a consequence, the urinary tract, surgical wounds, the respiratory tract, and invasive catheter sites on the skin are most often affected by HAIs. Organisms causing the infection are often resistant to many drugs and may not respond to antibiotics that are usually effective in treating infections acquired outside the hospital. **Table 9–4 >>** outlines the most common microorganisms responsible for HAIs and their causes.

Hands are a common vehicle for the spread of microorganisms, and insufficient hand hygiene is an important factor contributing to the spread of HAIs. For routine patient care, the CDC (2015b) recommends scrubbing and rinsing for 40–60 seconds using plain granule soap, soap-filled sheets, or liquid soap when hands are visibly soiled, after using the restroom, after removing gloves, before handling invasive devices (e.g., IV tubing), and after contact with medical equipment or furniture. Antimicrobial

TABLE 9–4 Causes of Healthcare-Associated Infections

Site of Infection	Most Common Microorganisms	Causes
Urinary tract	*Escherichia coli*	Improper catheterization technique
	Enterococcus species	Contamination of closed drainage system
	Pseudomonas aeruginosa	Inadequate hand hygiene
Surgical sites	*Staphylococcus aureus* (including methicillin-resistant strains—MRSA)	Inadequate hand hygiene
	Enterococcus species (including vancomycin-resistant strains—VRE)	Improper dressing change technique
	Pseudomonas aeruginosa	
Bloodstream	Coagulase-negative staphylococci	Inadequate hand hygiene
	Staphylococcus aureus	Improper IV fluid, tubing, and site care technique
	Enterococcus species	
Pneumonia	*Staphylococcus aureus*	Inadequate hand hygiene
	Pseudomonas aeruginosa	Improper suctioning technique
	Enterobacter species	

soaps are usually provided in high-risk areas, such as the newborn nursery, and are frequently supplied in dispensers at the sink. Wearing gloves does not eliminate the need for hand hygiene.

Soap and water are often inadequate to sufficiently remove pathogens. The CDC (2015b) recommends use of alcohol-based antiseptic hand rubs (rinses, gels, or foams) before and after direct patient contact. Studies have shown that the convenience of antimicrobial foams and gels, which do not require soap and water, may increase healthcare workers' adherence to hand hygiene (Ji & Jeong, 2013). Previous concerns that ready access to antimicrobial foams and gels represented a fire hazard have been addressed in the regulations.

Performing hand hygiene with either soap or alcohol-based cleansers can damage the skin through the drying effect of the detergents or chemicals. If the nurse develops dermatitis, the patient may be at higher risk for infection, because hand hygiene does not decrease bacterial counts on skin with dermatitis. The nurse is also at higher risk because the normal skin barrier has been broken. The use of hand lotions and creams to replace skin lipids can help prevent and treat dermatitis caused by hand hygiene products (CDC, 2015b).

Antibiotic-Resistant Bacteria

Antibiotic-resistant microorganisms are increasing at an alarming rate, primarily because of the prolonged and inappropriate use of antibiotic therapy. Bacteria with genetic mutations or genes that confer resistance survive antibiotic therapy, and the resulting reproduction of a colony of resistant bacteria can be spread to other organisms. Horizontal gene transfer can also produce resistance in previously susceptible bacteria (AHRQ, 2015). Other bacteria produce enzymes that inactivate drugs, change drug-binding sites, or alter their cell membrane to prevent drug absorption.

Some of the current resistant strains include: methicillin-resistant *S. aureus* (MRSA), multidrug-resistant tuberculosis (MDR-TB), penicillin-resistant *Streptococcus pneumoniae* (PRSP), fluoroquinolone-resistant *Neisseria meningitides*, vancomycin-resistant *Enterococcus* (VRE), and vancomycin-intermediate or resistant *S. aureus* (VISA or VRSA) (CDC, 2013a), extended-spectrum beta-lactamase (ESBL)–producing *Enterobacteriaceae*, carbapenem-resistant *Enterobacteriaceae* (e.g., *Klebsiella*), and multidrug-resistant *Pseudomonas aeruginosa* (Shime, Kosaka, & Fujita, 2013).

MRSA is becoming more prevalent in community settings in which young people, such as children in day care and amateur and professional athletes, share equipment. MRSA colonizes in the nares and skin. It is transmitted primarily by direct physical contact, not through respiratory droplets (Perovic et al., 2015). Healthcare personnel often unknowingly transmit *S. aureus* on their hands. Most *S. aureus* strains resist treatment by methicillin and similar drugs, which are the treatment of choice for *S. aureus* infections. Vancomycin and a semisynthetic derivative, telavancin, are the most uniformly effective drugs for both hospital-acquired and community-acquired MRSA (Morgan, 2015), although community-acquired MRSA may also be successfully treated by other antibiotics, such as rifampin

and clindamycin (Morgan, 2015). Soft-tissue infections with MRSA may manifest as abscesses, furuncles, or cellulites and may be mistaken for spider bites.

In 1997, a new form of *S. aureus* emerged with resistance to vancomycin, known as vancomycin-intermediate *S. aureus* (VISA) or vancomycin-resistant *S. aureus* (VRSA). Both VISA and VRSA are resistant to methicillin. Patients with MRSA, VISA, or VRSA are isolated in a private room, and caregivers use contact precautions (which are covered in Box 9–2).

Enterococci are part of the normal flora of the gastrointestinal and female genital tracts. Frequent use of vancomycin causes *Enterococci* to develop resistance, leading to VRE. Direct transmission occurs on the hands of healthcare personnel and from contact with contaminated equipment. In cases of infection, stringent infection-control measures are instituted, care is provided with contact precautions, and patients are placed either alone or with other patients with VRE infection.

Streptococcus pneumoniae, the most common cause of community-acquired pneumonia, has developed into its resistant form, penicillin-resistant *S. pneumoniae* (PRSP). Unlike MRSA and VRE, PRSP is transmitted by droplets from the respiratory tract and requires transmission-based droplet precautions (which are covered in Box 9–2).

C. difficile is an organism that has developed very resistant and highly morbid strains associated with frequent use of broad-spectrum antibiotics in hospitals. A common cause of healthcare-associated diarrhea, it is usually treated with metronidazole for mild to moderate cases or vancomycin for severe cases (Barclay, 2013). An even more virulent strain has been identified that is resistant to both metronidazole and vancomycin (Perovic et al., 2015).

Extended-spectrum beta-lactamase–producing microorganisms are resistant to third-generation cephalosporins and include gram-negative *Klebsiella* and *E. coli*. These organisms colonize indwelling urinary catheters and gastrostomies, as well as mechanical ventilators. They spread by direct and indirect contact.

SAFETY ALERT Universal precautions, the most important being hand hygiene, and modest use of antibiotics are critical in stopping the spread of antibiotic-resistant bacteria. The nurse should restrict equipment such as stethoscopes, blood pressure cuffs, and thermometers to use with the particular patient identified with one of these diseases. Disposing appropriately of used personal protective gear is another important safeguard. Universal precautions are discussed in the Prevention section.

Certain antibiotics can also induce resistance in some strains of organisms. This resistance has become so widespread that the CDC (2016a) has created a 12-step Campaign to Prevent Antimicrobial Resistance in Healthcare Settings, which consists of four strategies: preventing infection, diagnosing and treating infection effectively, using antimicrobials wisely, and preventing transmission.

Biological Threat Infections

Since the terrorist attacks on September 11, 2001, and the anthrax attacks by mail later that year, concern about the possible use of biological weapons has increased in the United

States. The most likely pathogens to be used for this purpose are anthrax, smallpox, botulism, pneumonic plague, and viral hemorrhagic fevers.

>> **Stay Current:** For more information about the numerous bioterrorism agents and their associated effects, view the CDC resource available at http://emergency.cdc.gov/agent/agentlist.asp

As with any potential large-scale infectious disease, state public health systems are charged with the responsibility of identifying cases, controlling the spread of infection, and preparing local and state responses for caring for the potentially large numbers of ill adults and children. As a part of this responsibility, public health authorities conduct **disease surveillance**, monitoring patterns of disease occurrence from the cases of infectious and communicable diseases reported by healthcare workers to state health officials. Disease surveillance procedures may be followed for any type of communicable and infectious disease, from *Shigella* to H1N1 influenza to a biological threat infection.

The Alterations and Therapies feature covers the infectious illnesses or diseases that a nurse encounters most frequently. Others are, but are not limited to, bacterial meningitis, bacterial endocarditis, giardiasis, chlamydia, tetanus, streptococcus A, *Shigella*, hepatitis, and HIV.

Prevalence

Using proper precautions with general medical asepsis, appropriately using personal protective equipment (PPE) (e.g., gloves, masks, respirators, gowns, goggles, special resuscitative equipment), and vigilance in the clinical area will place the nurse at significantly less risk for infection. The chance of a healthcare worker becoming infected from exposure to pathogens varies widely; estimates range from 30% for hepatitis B (nonimmune workers), to 1.8% for hepatitis C, to 0.3% for HIV (CDC, 2012c). The CDC has delineated measures to be taken in cases of possible exposure to these viruses. Hepatitis C, a worldwide epidemic with a higher prevalence than HIV (CDC, 2012c), has become a significant concern to all healthcare workers because there is currently no vaccine against the virus and there is no postexposure prophylaxis. Prevention remains the primary goal.

The Occupational Safety and Health Administration (OSHA) requires that healthcare employers make the hepatitis B vaccine and vaccination series available to all employees. Other vaccinations may also be made available (e.g., nurses working in an obstetric area should be vaccinated against rubella to protect pregnant patients and their fetuses).

Genetic Considerations and Risk Factors

Some medical therapies may predispose an individual to infection. For example, radiation treatments for cancer destroy not only cancerous cells but also some normal cells, thereby rendering the patient more vulnerable to infection. Some diagnostic procedures may also predispose the patient to infection, especially when the skin is broken or sterile body cavities are penetrated during the procedure.

Certain medications also increase susceptibility to infection. Antineoplastic (anticancer) medications can depress bone marrow function, the result being production of white blood cells (WBCs) that is inadequate to combat infections. Anti-inflammatory medications such as adrenal corticosteroids inhibit the inflammatory response, which is an essential defense against infection. Even some antibiotics used to treat infections can have adverse effects. Antibiotics can kill resident flora, allowing for the proliferation of strains that would not normally grow and multiply in the body. An important example is *C. difficile*–associated disease, an infection of the colon that is almost always caused initially by treatment with an antibiotic for another infection (Barclay, 2013).

Any disease that lowers the body's defenses against infection places the patient at risk. Examples are chronic pulmonary disease, which impairs ciliary action and weakens the mucous barrier; peripheral vascular disease, which restricts blood flow; burns, which impair skin integrity; chronic or debilitating diseases, which deplete protein reserves; and immune system diseases such as leukemia and aplastic anemia, which alter the production of WBCs. Diabetes mellitus is a major underlying disease that predisposes patients to infection because compromised peripheral vascular status and increased serum glucose levels increase susceptibility. Older adults who have multiple chronic diseases, particularly individuals over the age of 75 years, are also at greater risk of acquiring an infection than younger people.

Case Study >> Part 1

Sam Werner is a 58-year-old man who comes to the emergency department because he is coughing up blood. As the nurse assigned to care for him, you conduct a patient history and preliminary physical assessment. You find that Mr. Werner is undergoing chemotherapy for colorectal cancer, having been diagnosed 4 months ago. He has been having fatigue and sweats, but he attributes these symptoms to side effects of the chemotherapy. However, the fatigue has been worse the past couple days, and he has started coughing as well. His cough has got progressively worse, and today he has started coughing up blood and having chest pains. He also thinks he has a fever, because he is alternately chilled and sweating. Your physical assessment indicates T 104.3°F; P 92 bpm; R 20/min; BP 122/74 mmHg. You can hear that his breathing is labored. During your assessment, Mr. Werner has another coughing spell and coughs up more bloody sputum. After conducting his exam, the healthcare provider orders a complete blood cell count (CBC) and chest x-ray, which indicate that Mr. Werner has bacterial pneumonia. Because he is immunocompromised from his chemotherapy treatment, Mr. Werner is admitted to the hospital.

Clinical Reasoning Questions Level I

1. What physical symptoms indicate that Mr. Werner has an infection?
2. What nursing interventions can you implement to lessen the effects of the chills and sweating?
3. What safety precautions should you take to clean up the bloody sputum?

Clinical Reasoning Questions Level II

4. What results would you expect from the CBC?
5. What other diagnostic tests could be performed to help diagnose Mr. Werner?
6. *Refer to Exemplar 9.E on Pneumonia:* What medication is the healthcare provider likely to prescribe?

Alterations and Therapies
Infections

ALTERATION	DESCRIPTION/ DEFINITION	MANIFESTATIONS	INTERVENTIONS AND THERAPIES
Cellulitis	Acute bacterial infection of the dermis and underlying connective tissue	■ Fever ■ Inflammation in area of infection ■ Skin sore or rash	■ Antibiotics ■ Antipyretics ■ Palliative care ■ Fluid administration
Urinary tract infection	Infection of any part of the urinary tract: kidneys, ureters, urinary bladder, or urethra	■ Pain or burning when urinating ■ Fever ■ Urge to urinate often ■ Cloudy or malodorous urine	■ Antibiotics per culture results ■ Antipyretics ■ Fluid management
Viral pneumonia	Infection of the lung, often causing fluid accumulation in one or more lobes	■ Cough with mucus (may be bloody) ■ Fever ■ Chills ■ Chest pain when breathing deeply or coughing ■ Loss of appetite ■ Fatigue	■ Treatment based on symptoms ■ Cough suppressant, expectorant ■ Rest ■ Encouraging breathing ■ Support for respiratory effort, which may include oxygen, Fowler position, respiratory hygiene
Otitis media	Inflammation of the middle ear	■ Ear pain ■ Redness of the eardrum ■ Pus or fluid in the ear ■ Fever ■ Difficulty hearing	■ Palliative care ■ Antibiotics only if symptoms do not resolve after 48–72 hours
Influenza	Highly contagious viral respiratory disease	■ Fever over 100°F ■ Aching muscles ■ Chills and sweats ■ Dry cough ■ Fatigue and weakness ■ Nasal congestion	■ Antipyretics ■ Rest ■ Fluid management ■ Monitoring for respiratory rate and pattern, and for effective airway clearance ■ Antiviral medications to reduce duration and severity of symptoms ■ Prevention through vaccination of at-risk individuals
Conjunctivitis	Highly contagious inflammation of the conjunctiva	■ Blurred vision ■ Crusts that form on eyelids ■ Eye pain ■ Redness of the eyes ■ Sensitivity to light ■ Increased tears	■ Antibiotics ■ Palliative care
Tuberculosis	Chronic, recurrent infectious disease caused by *Mycobacterium tuberculosis*	■ Cough with mucus (may be bloody) ■ Fever ■ Excessive sweating ■ Fatigue ■ Breathing difficulty ■ Fluid around the lungs	■ Fluid management ■ Monitoring of vital signs, especially temperature ■ Antipyretics and analgesics ■ Antitubercular medications ■ Respiratory support as dictated by symptoms ■ Isolation
Sepsis	Whole-body inflammatory process resulting in acute critical illness	■ Change in mental status ■ Fast breathing ■ Fever or hypothermia ■ Lightheadedness ■ Tachycardia ■ Skin rash	■ Reversal of underlying cause ■ Protection of respiratory and cardiovascular systems ■ Fluid management ■ Monitoring of neurologic status and vital signs

Concepts Related to Infection

All individuals develop infections throughout their lifetime; the type of infection determines its clinical manifestations. For example, an infection in the gastrointestinal tract may produce diarrhea, whereas an eye infection is likely to produce purulent drainage. Once an individual becomes infected, the infection may cause an inflammatory response, leading to redness, swelling, and pain. Because of the prevalence of infections in the clinic, hospital, and other healthcare facilities, nursing education is essential to the prevention of infection.

Oxygenation problems are a concern in respiratory infections. Congestion can lead to inefficient airway clearance and may result in difficulty protecting their airway. Patients facing an infectious process may experience an alteration in self-concept. They may experience shame or embarrassment with their illness and the resulting restrictions on their social activities. Such patients would benefit from thorough nursing assessment, as well as referral to psychosocial resources such as a social worker or a chaplain in the acute care setting. The Concepts Related to Infection feature links some, but not all, of the concepts integral to infection. They are presented in alphabetical order.

Health Promotion

Individuals are constantly in contact with microorganisms in the environment. The body's natural defenses normally ward off the development of an infection. Some individuals are more susceptible to infections than others. Susceptibility is the likelihood of an organism's causing an infection in that individual. The following measures can reduce an individual's susceptibility to infection:

- *Hygiene.* Intact skin and mucous membranes are one barrier against microorganisms entering the body. In addition, good oral care, including flossing the teeth, reduces the likelihood of an oral infection. Regular and thorough bathing and shampooing remove microorganisms and dirt that can result in an infection.

- *Nutrition.* A balanced diet enhances the health of all body tissues, helps keep the skin intact, and promotes the skin's ability to repel microorganisms. Adequate nutrition enables tissues to maintain and rebuild themselves and helps keep the immune system functioning well. In addition, because antibodies are proteins, inadequate nutrition can impair the body's ability to synthesize them, especially when protein reserves are depleted (e.g., as a result of injury, surgery, or debilitating diseases such as cancer). Nurses can teach patients and their families ways to improve patients' nutritional status to help prevent infection.

- *Fluid.* Fluid intake permits fluid output, which flushes out the bladder and urethra, removing microorganisms that could cause an infection.

Concepts Related to
Infection

CONCEPT	RELATIONSHIP TO INFECTION	NURSING IMPLICATIONS
Elimination	GI infection ↑ damage to intestines and a ↓ in absorption, leading to diarrhea. ↑ Abnormal gut flora may lead to constipation. UTIs and yeast infections can cause painful and/or frequent urination.	▪ Be aware of the risk for dehydration and inadequate nutrition especially in children and older adults. ▪ Watch for signs of kidney infection in patients with UTIs. ▪ Provide comfort measures related to elimination problems (e.g., hygiene care, pharmacologic interventions, safety interventions). ▪ Use proper biohazard precautions when handling urine and feces.
Inflammation	↑ Infection leads to ↑ inflammation, including pain, swelling, and redness.	▪ Provide hygiene care for wounds to prevent infection and inflammation. ▪ Provide comfort care (e.g., pain medication, cool compress/ice).
Oxygenation	Congestion from increased secretions → ineffective airway clearance.	▪ Assess temperature. ▪ Assess respiratory rate. ▪ Assess lung sounds. ▪ Assess pulse oximetry. ▪ Teach self-airway protection.
Sexuality	↑ Sexual partners = ↑ increased risk of STI.	▪ Provide patient education about STIs, especially for adolescents.
Teaching and learning	↑ Education = ↑ prevention habits = ↓ risk of infection.	▪ Attend classes to learn about infection prevention. ▪ Teach patients about good hygiene to prevent infection. ▪ Teach staff members proper protocols for handling potentially infectious materials.
Tissue integrity	↓ Tissue integrity = ↑ risk of infection.	▪ Provide wound care to prevent infection. ▪ Turn patients who are bedridden to prevent pressure ulcers. ▪ Cover wounds with antibiotic ointment and sterile gauze.

- *Sleep.* Adequate sleep is essential to maintaining health and renewing energy.
- *Stress.* Excessive stress predisposes people to infections. Nurses can help patients to learn stress-reducing techniques. The nature, number, and duration of physical and emotional stressors can influence susceptibility to infection. Stressors elevate blood cortisone, and the prolonged elevation of blood cortisone decreases anti-inflammatory responses, depletes energy stores, leads to a state of exhaustion, and decreases resistance to infection. For example, an individual recovering from a major operation or injury is more likely to develop an infection than a healthy individual.

The use of immunizations has dramatically decreased the incidence of infectious diseases. Pediatric immunizations should begin shortly after birth and be completed throughout childhood (except for boosters). Pediatric immunizations against diphtheria, tetanus, and pertussis are usually started at 2 months, when the infant's immune system can respond. Immunizations may be given by injection, inhalation, oral solutions, or nasal sprays. They are frequently given in combination to minimize multiple injections. Because of the prevalence of influenza and its potential for causing death, the CDC recommends annual immunization against influenza for all individuals but highly recommends immunization for older adults and individuals with chronic cardiac, respiratory, metabolic, and renal disease. Pneumococcal vaccine is recommended for older adults who were last vaccinated more than 5 years previously and for individuals who are immunocompromised or have risk factors such as chronic pulmonary, liver, or cardiac disease.

>> **Stay Current:** CDC recommendations for immunizations change frequently. Updated immunization schedules for all age groups can be found on the CDC website at http://www.cdc.gov/vaccines/schedules/

Prevention

Everyone, including healthcare workers and patients, can play a role in preventing infections. Among the many techniques available to help prevent infection are good hand hygiene, getting immunizations, preventing airborne droplets from spreading, and taking precautions when handling potentially contaminated materials.

Prevention of infection is a vital nursing role. Nurses and other healthcare workers can take multiple precautions to prevent infection, both for patients and for themselves.

Disinfecting and Sterilizing

The first two links in the chain of infection, the etiologic agent and the reservoir, are interrupted by the use of **antiseptics** (agents that inhibit the growth of some microorganisms) and **disinfectants** (agents that destroy pathogens other than spores), and by sterilization.

Disinfecting

A disinfectant is a chemical preparation, such as phenol or iodine compounds, used on inanimate objects. Disinfectants are frequently caustic and toxic to tissues. An antiseptic is a chemical preparation used on skin or tissue. Disinfectants and antiseptics often have similar chemical components, but disinfectants are more concentrated.

Both antiseptics and disinfectants have bactericidal or bacteriostatic properties. A **bactericidal agent** destroys bacteria, whereas a **bacteriostatic agent** prevents the growth and reproduction of some bacteria. Select an agent that is known to be effective against the specific bacteria. For example, spore-forming bacteria such as *C. difficile,* which is a frequent cause of healthcare-associated diarrhea, and *Bacillus anthracis* (anthrax) may be inhibited by only a few of the agents normally effective against other forms of bacteria. **Table 9–5 >>** lists commonly used antiseptics and disinfectants.

When disinfecting articles, nurses need to follow agency protocol and consider the following factors:

1. *The type and number of infectious organisms.* Some microorganisms are readily destroyed; others require longer contact with the disinfectant.
2. *The recommended concentration of the disinfectant and duration of contact.*
3. *The presence of soap.* Some disinfectants are ineffective in the presence of soap or detergents.
4. *The presence of organic materials.* The presence of saliva, blood, pus, or excretions can readily inactivate many disinfectants.
5. *The surface areas to be treated.* The disinfecting agent must come into contact with all surfaces and areas.

TABLE 9–5 Commonly Used Antiseptics and Disinfectants: Their Effectiveness and Use

Agent	Effective Against					Use On
	Bacteria	**Tuberculosis**	**Spores**	**Fungi**	**Viruses**	
Isopropyl and ethyl alcohol	X	X		X	X	Hands, vial stoppers
Chlorine (bleach)	X	X	X	X	X	Blood spills
Hydrogen peroxide	X	X	X	X	X	Surfaces
Iodophors	X	X	X	X	X	Equipment, intact skin, and tissues if diluted
Phenol	X	X		X	X	Surfaces
Chlorhexidine gluconate (Hibiclens)	X				X	Hands
Triclosan (Bacti-Stat)	X					Hands, intact skin

Sterilizing

Sterilization is a process that destroys all microorganisms, including spores and viruses. Four commonly used methods of sterilization are moist heat, gas, boiling water, and radiation.

- *Moist heat.* To sterilize with moist heat (e.g., in an autoclave), steam under pressure is used to attain temperatures higher than the boiling point. It cannot be used for items that can be damaged by heat, moisture, or high pressure, a major disadvantage.
- *Gas.* Ethylene oxide gas destroys microorganisms by interfering with their metabolic processes. It is also effective against spores. Its advantages are good penetration and effectiveness for heat-sensitive items. Its major disadvantage is its toxicity to humans.
- *Boiling water.* This is the most practical and inexpensive method for sterilizing in the home. The main disadvantage is that this method does not kill spores and some viruses. Boiling for a minimum of 15 minutes is advised to disinfect articles in the home.
- *Radiation.* Both ionizing (e.g., alpha, beta, x-rays) and nonionizing (ultraviolet light) radiation are used for disinfection and sterilization. The main drawback to ultraviolet light is that the rays do not penetrate deeply. Ionizing radiation is used effectively in industry to sterilize foods, drugs, and other items that are sensitive to heat. Its main advantage is that it is effective for items difficult to sterilize, and its chief disadvantage is that the equipment is very expensive.

Isolation Precautions

Isolation refers to measures designed to prevent the spread of infection or potentially infectious microorganisms to health personnel, patients, and visitors. Several sets of guidelines have been used in hospitals and other healthcare settings.

Category-specific isolation precautions use seven categories: strict isolation, contact isolation, respiratory isolation, tuberculosis isolation, enteric precautions, drainage/secretions precautions, and blood/body fluid precautions.

Disease-specific isolation precautions do exactly that: provide precautions to protect against a specific disease. These precautions call for use of private rooms with special ventilation, sharing of rooms only with other patients infected with the same organism, and gowning to prevent gross soilage of clothes for specific infectious diseases (CDC, 2015c).

Universal precautions (UP) are techniques to be used with all patients to decrease the risk of transmitting unidentified pathogens (CDC, 2015c). Universal precautions obstruct the spread of **bloodborne pathogens**, microorganisms carried in blood and body fluids that are capable of infecting other individuals with serious and difficult-to-treat viral infections, namely, hepatitis B virus, hepatitis C virus, and HIV. The CDC recommends not that universal precautions replace disease-specific or category-specific precautions, but that they be used in conjunction with them.

The **body substance isolation (BSI)** system employs generic infection-control precautions for all patients, except those with the few diseases transmitted through the air. The BSI system (Vayas, 2014) is based on three premises:

1. All people have an increased risk for infection from microorganisms entering through mucous membranes and nonintact skin.
2. All people are likely to have potentially infectious microorganisms in all of their moist body sites and substances.
3. An unknown portion of patients and healthcare workers will always be colonized or infected with potentially infectious microorganisms in their blood and other moist body sites and substances.

The term *body substance* refers to blood, some body fluids, urine, feces, wound drainage, oral secretions, and any other body product or tissue.

In addition to other actions and precautions discussed in this concept, significant emphasis is placed on avoiding injury from sharp instruments, taking measures in cases of exposure to bloodborne pathogens, and communicating information about biohazards to employees. In most cases, federal regulations require that warning labels be affixed to containers of regulated waste and to refrigerators and freezers containing blood or other potentially infectious materials. The labels required are fluorescent orange or orange-red and feature the biohazard legend shown in **Figure 9–3 ❱❱**.

CDC (HICPAC) Isolation Precautions (2015)

The Hospital Infection-Control Practices Advisory Committee (HICPAC) of the CDC presented updated guidelines for isolation precautions in 2015 (CDC, 2015c). These guidelines designate two tiers of precautions: (1) standard precautions, and (2) transmission-based precautions.

Standard precautions are used in the care of all hospitalized individuals regardless of their diagnosis or possible infection status. *Transmission-based precautions* are used in addition to standard precautions for patients with known or suspected infections that are spread by contact or by airborne or droplet transmission. The three types of transmission-based precautions may be used alone or in combination but always *in addition to* standard precautions. They encompass all of the conditions or diseases previously listed in the category-specific or disease-specific classifications developed by the CDC in 1983.

Airborne precautions are used for patients who are known to have or suspected of having serious illnesses transmitted by airborne droplet nuclei smaller than 5 microns. Examples of such illnesses are measles (rubeola),

Figure 9–3 ❱❱ Biohazard alert.

varicella (including disseminated zoster), and tuberculosis. The CDC has prepared special guidelines for preventing the transmission of tuberculosis.

>> **Stay Current:** The most current information can be found on the CDC Division of Tuberculosis Elimination website: http://www.cdc.gov/tb/

Droplet precautions are used for patients who are known to have or suspected of having serious illnesses transmitted by particle droplets larger than 5 microns. Examples of such illnesses are diphtheria (pharyngeal); *Mycoplasma pneumoniae*; pertussis; mumps; rubella; influenza virus; streptococcal pharyngitis, pneumonia, and scarlet fever in infants and young children; and pneumonic plague.

Contact precautions are used for patients who are known to have or suspected of having serious illnesses that are easily transmitted by direct patient contact or by contact with items in the patient's environment. According to the CDC (CDC, 2015c), such illnesses include gastrointestinal, respiratory, skin, or wound infections or colonization with multidrug-resistant bacteria; specific enteric infections, such as *C. difficile*, enterohemorrhagic *Escherichia coli* O157:H7, *Shigella*, and hepatitis A, in patients who wear diapers or are incontinent; respiratory syncytial virus, parainfluenza virus, and enteroviral infections in infants and young children; and highly contagious skin infections, such as herpes simplex virus, impetigo, pediculosis, and scabies.

Box 9–2 >> lists recommended isolation precautions for use in hospitals.

Isolation Practices

The initiation of practices to prevent the transmission of microorganisms is generally a nursing responsibility that is based on a comprehensive assessment of the patient. This assessment takes into account the status of the patient's normal defense mechanisms, the patient's ability to implement necessary precautions, and the source and mode of transmission of the infectious agent. Nurses decide whether to wear gloves, gowns, masks, and protective eyewear. *In all patient situations, nurses must cleanse their hands before and after providing care.*

In addition to the precautions cited in this concept, nurses implement aseptic precautions when performing many specific therapies that are described in other modules. The following are examples of aseptic precautions:

- Use strict aseptic technique when performing any invasive procedure (e.g., inserting an IV needle or catheter) and when changing surgical dressings.
- Change IV tubing and solution containers according to hospital policy (e.g., every 48–72 hours).
- Check all sterile supplies for expiration date and intact packaging.
- Prevent urinary infections by maintaining a closed urinary drainage system with a downhill flow of urine. Keep the drainage bag and spout off the floor.
- Implement measures to prevent impaired skin integrity and accumulation of secretions in the lungs (e.g., encourage the patient to move, cough, and breathe deeply at least every 2 hours).

Personal Protective Equipment

All healthcare providers must apply clean or sterile gloves, gowns, masks, respirators, and protective eyewear according to the risk of exposure to potentially infective materials.

Gloves

Gloves are worn for three reasons:

1. Gloves protect the hands when nurses are likely to handle any body substances.
2. Gloves reduce the likelihood of nurses transmitting their own endogenous microorganisms to individuals receiving care. Nurses who have open sores or cuts on the hands must wear gloves for protection.
3. Gloves reduce the chance that nurses' hands will transmit microorganisms or a fomite from one patient to another patient.

In all situations, nurses must change gloves between patient contacts. Nurses should clean their hands each time they remove gloves for two primary reasons: The gloves may have imperfections or may have been damaged during wearing, allowing microorganism entry, and the hands may become contaminated during glove removal.

Some of the gloves used in infection-control are made of latex, as are various other items used in healthcare (e.g., catheters, blood pressure cuffs, rubber sheets, IV tubing, stockings and binders, adhesive bandages, dental dams). Because of the frequent use of gloves, healthcare workers and some patients with chronic illnesses have increasingly reported allergic reactions to latex. Latex gloves that are lubricated by powder or cornstarch are particularly allergenic because the latex allergen adheres to the powder, which is aerosolized during glove use or removal of gloves and is then inhaled by the user. Latex gloves that are labeled "hypoallergenic" still contain measurable latex and should not be used by or on individuals with known latex sensitivity. OSHA estimates that 8–12% of healthcare personnel have some level of latex allergy (OSHA, 2016). The individuals at greatest risk for developing latex allergies are those with other allergic conditions and those who have had frequent or long-term exposure to latex. Even though most hospitals have eliminated latex products wherever possible and established a "latex-free environment" goal, patients and healthcare workers should be assessed for possible allergies to latex.

Gowns

Nurses wear clean or disposable impervious (water-resistant) gowns or plastic aprons during procedures when their uniforms are likely to become soiled. Sterile gowns may be indicated when nurses change the dressings of a patient with extensive wounds (e.g., burns). *Single-use gown technique* (using a gown only once before it is discarded or laundered) is the usual practice in hospitals. After gowns have been worn, nurses discard them (if they are paper) or place them in a laundry hamper. Before leaving the patient's room, nurses cleanse their hands. An *isolation gown* is meant to be worn only one time. It is donned prior to entering the patient's room to provide bedside care and removed at the conclusion of care. The gown prevents contamination of the care provider's uniform by a patient's infection. It is important to review

Box 9–2
Recommended Isolation Precautions in Hospitals

Standard Precautions

- These precautions are designed for all patients in the hospital.
- They apply to (a) blood; (b) all body fluids, excretions, and secretions except sweat; (c) nonintact (broken) skin; and (d) mucous membranes.
- They are designed to reduce the risk of transmission of microorganisms from recognized and unrecognized sources.

1. Perform proper hand hygiene after contact with blood, body fluids, secretions, excretions, and contaminated objects, whether or not gloves are worn.
   a. Perform proper hand hygiene immediately after removing gloves.
   b. Use a nonantimicrobial product for routine hand cleansing.
   c. Use an antimicrobial agent or an antiseptic agent for the control of specific outbreaks of infection.
2. Wear clean gloves when touching blood, body fluids, secretions, excretions, and contaminated items (e.g., soiled gowns).
   a. Clean gloves can be unsterile unless their use is intended to prevent the entrance of microorganisms into the body. (See point b, on sterile gloves.)
   b. Remove gloves before touching noncontaminated items and surfaces.
   c. Perform proper hand hygiene immediately after removing gloves.
3. Wear a mask, eye protection, or a face shield if splashes or sprays of blood, body fluids, secretions, or excretions can be expected.
4. Wear a clean, nonsterile gown if patient care is likely to result in splashes or sprays of blood, body fluids, secretions, or excretions. The gown is intended to protect clothing.
   a. Remove a soiled gown carefully to avoid the transfer of microorganisms to other individuals (e.g., patients, other healthcare workers).
   b. Cleanse hands after removing gown.
5. Carefully handle patient care equipment that is soiled with blood, body fluids, secretions, or excretions to prevent the transfer of microorganisms to other individuals and the environment.
   a. Ensure reusable equipment is cleaned and reprocessed correctly.
   b. Dispose of single-use equipment correctly.
6. Handle, transport, and process linen that is soiled with blood, body fluids, secretions, or excretions so as to prevent contamination of clothing and the transfer of microorganisms to other individuals and to the environment.
7. Prevent injuries from used scalpels, needles, and other equipment, and place in puncture-resistant containers.
8. Use respiratory hygiene/cough etiquette.
   a. Educate healthcare facility staff, patients, and visitors.
   b. Post signs in languages appropriate to the population served, with instructions to patients and accompanying family members or friends.
   c. Use source-control measures (e.g., covering the mouth/nose with a tissue when coughing, disposing of used tissues promptly, using surgical masks on the coughing individual when tolerated and appropriate).
   d. Use good hand hygiene after contact with respiratory secretions.
   e. Individuals with respiratory infections should be separated from others by at least 3 ft in common waiting areas.

9. Use safe injection practices by using needles only once, especially when obtaining medication from a multiple-dose vial or solution container or when injecting multiple patients.
10. Wear a face mask during catheter placements or when injecting material into the spinal or epidural space.

Transmission-Based Precautions
Airborne Precautions
Use standard precautions, as well as the following:

1. Place the patient in a private room that has negative air pressure, 6–12 air changes per hour, and either discharge of air to the outside or a filtration system for the room air.
2. If a private room is not available, place the patient with another patient who is infected with the same microorganism.
3. Wear a respiratory device (N95 respirator) when entering the room of a patient who is known to have or suspected of having primary tuberculosis.
4. A respiratory protection program should be in place that provides education about the use of respirators, fit-testing, and user seal checks.
5. Susceptible people should not enter the room of a patient who has rubeola (measles) or varicella (chickenpox). If they must enter, they should wear a respirator.
6. Limit movement of the patient outside the room to essential purposes. Place a surgical mask on the patient during transport.

Droplet Precautions
Use standard precautions, as well as the following:

1. Place the patient in a private room.
2. If a private room is not available, place the patient with another patient who is infected with the same microorganism. The curtain should be drawn between patient beds.
3. Wear a mask if working within 3 ft of the patient.
4. Limit movement of the patient outside the room to essential purposes. Place a surgical mask on the patient during transport.

Contact Precautions
Use standard precautions, as well as the following:

1. Place the patient in a private room.
2. If a private room is not available, consult with infection-control personnel to assess the risks associated with other placement options. Beds should be separated by more than 3 ft.
3. Wear gloves as described in standard precautions.
   a. Change gloves after contact with infectious material.
   b. Remove gloves before leaving the patient's room.
   c. Cleanse hands immediately after removing gloves, using an antimicrobial agent. *Note:* If the patient is infected with *C. difficile*, do *not* use an alcohol-based hand rub, as it may not be effective on these spores. Use soap and water.
   d. After hand cleansing, do not touch possibly contaminated surfaces or items in the room.
4. Wear a gown (see Standard Precautions) when entering a room if there is a possibility of contact with infected surfaces or items or if the patient is incontinent or has diarrhea, a colostomy, or wound drainage that is not contained by a dressing.
   a. Remove the gown in the patient's room.
   b. Make sure the uniform does not contact possible contaminated surfaces.
5. Limit movement of the patient outside the room.
6. Dedicate the use of noncritical patient care equipment to a single patient or to patients with the same infecting microorganisms.

Source: Based on Siegel, J. D., Rhinehart, E., Jackson, M., Chiarello, L., & the Healthcare Infection-Control Practices Advisory Committee. (2007). *Guideline for Isolation Precautions: Preventing Transmission of Infectious Agents in Healthcare Settings.* Retrieved from http://www.cdc.gov/hicpac/pdf/isolation/isolation2007.pdf

the agency's protocol for correct use of the type of isolation gown provided by the agency.

SAFETY ALERT Providers should not wear a patient hospital gown over their uniform because it does not serve any infection-control purpose. They should wear isolation gowns to prevent contamination of their uniform or clothes, and remove the gowns at the end of the healthcare interaction.

Face Masks

Masks are worn to reduce the risk of transmitting organisms by the droplet contact and airborne routes, and by splatters of body substances. The CDC (2015c) recommends that masks be worn by the following individuals:

1. Individuals close to the patient if the infection (e.g., measles, mumps, or acute respiratory diseases in children) is transmitted by large-particle aerosols (droplets). Large-particle aerosols are transmitted by close contact and generally travel short distances (about 1 m, or 3 ft).
2. All individuals entering the room if the infection (e.g., pulmonary tuberculosis, SARS-CoV) is transmitted by small-particle aerosols (droplet nuclei). Small-particle aerosols remain suspended in the air and thus travel greater distances by air. Special masks that provide a tighter face seal and better filtration may be used for these infections.

Various types of masks differ in their filtration effectiveness and fit. Single-use disposable surgical masks are effective for use while the nurse provides care to most patients, but they should be changed if they become wet or soiled. These masks are discarded in the waste container after use. Disposable particulate respirators of different types may be effective for droplet transmission, splatters, and airborne microorganisms.

During performance of certain techniques requiring surgical asepsis (sterile technique), masks are worn (a) to prevent droplet contact transmission of exhaled microorganisms to the sterile field or to a patient's open wound and (b) to protect the nurse from splashes of body substances from the patient.

Respirators

Some respirators now available are effective in preventing inhalation of tuberculin organisms. The National Institute for Occupational Safety and Health (NIOSH) tests and certifies such respirators. The category N respirator at 95% efficiency (referred to as an *N95 respirator*) meets tuberculosis and SARS control criteria (CDC, 2012g).

Eyewear

Protective eyewear (goggles, glasses, or face shields) and masks are indicated in situations in which body substances may splatter the face. If the nurse wears prescription eyeglasses, goggles must be worn over the glasses to extend around the sides of the glasses.

Disposal of Soiled Equipment and Supplies

Many pieces of equipment are supplied for single use only and disposed of afterward. Some items, however, are reusable.

Agencies have specific policies and procedures for handling soiled equipment (e.g., disposal, cleaning, disinfecting, sterilizing), and nurses need to become familiar with the practices of the employing agency. Appropriate handling of soiled equipment and supplies is essential to prevent inadvertent exposure of healthcare workers and patients to articles contaminated with body substances and to contamination of the environment.

Bagging

Articles that are contaminated or likely to have been contaminated with infective material such as pus, blood, body fluids, feces, or respiratory secretions need to be enclosed in a sturdy bag impervious to microorganisms before they are removed from the room of any patient. Some agencies use labels or bags of a particular color that designates them as infective waste.

Linens

Soiled linens should be handled as little as possible and with the least agitation possible before being placed in a laundry hamper. This minimal handling prevents gross microbial contamination of the air and of the individuals dealing with the linen. The bag is closed before being sent to the laundry in accordance with agency practice.

Laboratory Specimens

Laboratory specimens, if placed in a leakproof container with a secure lid and labeled as a biohazard, need no special precautions. Use care when collecting specimens to avoid contaminating the outside of the container. To prevent personnel from having hand contact with potentially infective material, place containers that are visibly contaminated on the outside in a sealable plastic bag before sending them to the laboratory.

Dishes

Dishes require no special precautions. Prevent soiling of dishes by encouraging patients to cleanse their hands before eating. Some agencies use paper dishes for convenience; these are disposed of in the refuse container.

Blood Pressure Equipment

Blood pressure equipment needs no special precautions unless it becomes contaminated with infective material. If it does become contaminated, the agency policy should be followed to decontaminate it. Cleaning procedures vary according to whether the equipment is a wall or portable unit. A disposable cuff should be used for patients placed on contact precautions.

Disposable Needles, Syringes, and Sharps

Place needles, syringes, and sharps (e.g., lancets, scalpels, broken glass) in a puncture-resistant container. To avoid puncture wounds, use approved safety or needleless systems, and do not detach needles from the syringe or recap them before disposal.

Disposable Equipment and Supplies

Place garbage and soiled *disposable* equipment, including dressings and tissues, in the plastic bag that lines the waste container. Some agencies separate dry and wet waste material and incinerate dry items, such as paper towels and disposable items. No special precautions are required for disposable equipment that is not contaminated. Federal rules protecting the privacy of personal health information may extend to the patient labels placed on disposable supplies such as IV fluid containers. Agencies may require that these be returned to the pharmacy so that personal information can be removed before disposal. Check agency policy.

Nondisposable Equipment and Supplies

Place *nondisposable* or *reusable* equipment that is visibly soiled in a labeled bag before removing it from the patient's room or cubicle, and then send it to a central processing area for decontamination. Some agencies may require that glass bottles or jars and metal items be placed in separate bags from rubber and plastic items. Glass and metal can be sterilized in an autoclave, but rubber and plastic are damaged by this process and must be cleaned by other methods, such as gas sterilization.

Transporting Patients with Infection

Avoid transporting patients with infections outside their own rooms unless it is absolutely necessary. If patients must be moved, the nurse follows agency protocol to implement appropriate precautions and measures to prevent soilage of the environment. For example, the nurse ensures that any draining wound is securely covered or that patients who have an airborne infection wear a surgical mask during transport. In addition, the nurse notifies personnel at the receiving area of any infection risk so that they can maintain necessary precautions.

Sterile Technique

An object is sterile only when it is free of all microorganisms. Sterile technique is practiced in operating rooms and special diagnostic areas. It is also employed for many procedures in general care areas, such as administering injections, changing wound dressings, performing urinary catheterizations, and administering IV therapy. In these situations, all of the principles of surgical asepsis are applied, as in the operating and delivery rooms; however, not all of the sterile techniques that follow are always required. For example, before an operating room procedure, the scrub nurse generally puts on a mask and cap, performs a surgical hand scrub, and then dons a sterile gown and gloves. In a general care area, the nurse may only perform hand cleansing and don sterile gloves. The basic principles of surgical asepsis and practices that relate to each principle are outlined in **Table 9–6 》**.

Sterile Field

A **sterile field** is a microorganism-free area. Nurses often establish a sterile field by using the innermost side of a sterile wrapper or by using a sterile drape. When the field is established, sterile supplies and sterile solutions can be placed on it. Sterile forceps are often used to handle and transfer sterile supplies.

So that sterility can be maintained, supplies may be wrapped in a variety of materials. Commercially prepared items are frequently wrapped in plastic, paper, or glass.

Liquids are preferably packaged in amounts adequate for one use only. Any leftover liquid is discarded.

Sterile Gloves

Latex and latex-free (e.g., nitrile and vinyl) sterile gloves are available to protect nurses from contact with blood and body fluids. Latex and nitrile are more flexible than vinyl, mold to the wearer's hands, allow freedom of movement, and have the added feature of resealing tiny punctures automatically. Therefore, the nurse should wear latex or nitrile gloves when performing tasks that (a) demand flexibility, (b) place stress on the material (e.g., turning stopcocks, handling sharp instruments or tape), and (c) involve a high risk of exposure to pathogens. Vinyl gloves are best for tasks that are unlikely to stress the glove material, require minimal precision, and carry a minimal risk of exposure to pathogens.

Sterile gloves may be donned by the open method or the closed method. The open method is most frequently used outside the operating room because the closed method requires that the nurse wear a sterile gown. Gloves are worn during many procedures to maintain the sterility of equipment and protect a patient's wound. Sterile gloves are packaged with a cuff of approximately 5 cm (2 in.) and with the palms facing upward when the package is opened. The package usually indicates the size of the glove (e.g., size 6 or $7\frac{1}{2}$).

Sterile Gowns

Sterile gowning and closed gloving are carried out chiefly in operating and delivery rooms, where surgical asepsis is necessary. The closed method of gloving can be used only when a sterile gown is worn because the gloves are handled through the sleeves of the gown. Before these procedures, the nurse dons a hair cover and a mask and performs a surgical hand cleanse.

Preventing Healthcare-Associated Infections

Prevention is the most important control measure for HAIs. The pathogens causing these infections are transmitted primarily by contact with hospital personnel and contaminated inanimate objects (CDC, 2015c). *Effective hand hygiene is the single most important measure in infection-control.* Although infections can also be transmitted by the airborne route, via contaminated equipment, and from the environment, these are less significant routes. Invasive procedures and equipment should be used only when absolutely necessary; for example, it is not appropriate to insert an indwelling catheter when the only indication is incontinence. The use of antimicrobial dressings and antimicrobial venous catheters is central to CDC guidelines for the prevention of HAIs. In addition, a daily audit should be performed to determine whether a central line is necessary or can be removed.

Meticulous use of medical and surgical asepsis is necessary to prevent transport of potentially infectious microorganisms. Many HAIs can be prevented by proper hand hygiene techniques, environmental controls, sterile technique when warranted, and identification and treatment

TABLE 9–6 Principles and Practices of Surgical Asepsis

Principles	Practices
All objects used in a sterile field must be sterile.	■ Before use, all articles are sterilized appropriately by dry or moist heat, chemicals, or radiation. ■ Always check a package containing a sterile object for intactness, dryness, and expiration date. Sterile articles can be stored for only a prescribed time; after that, they are considered unsterile. Any package that appears already open, torn, punctured, or wet is considered unsterile. ■ Storage areas should be clean, dry, off the floor, and away from sinks. ■ Always check chemical indicators of sterilization before using a package. The indicator is often a tape used to fasten the package or contained inside the package. The indicator changes color during sterilization, indicating that the contents have undergone a sterilization procedure. If the color change is not evident, the package is considered unsterile. Commercially prepared sterile packages may not have indicators but may be marked with the word *sterile*.
Sterile objects become unsterile when touched by unsterile objects.	■ Handle sterile objects that will touch open wounds or enter body cavities only with sterile forceps or sterile gloved hands. ■ Discard or resterilize objects that come into contact with unsterile objects. ■ Whenever the sterility of an object is questionable, assume the article is unsterile.
Sterile items that are out of vision or below the waist or table level are considered unsterile.	■ Once left unattended, a sterile field is considered unsterile. ■ Sterile objects are always kept in view. Nurses do not turn their backs on a sterile field. ■ Only the front part of a sterile gown, from shoulder to waist (or table height, whichever is higher), and the cuff of the sleeves to 2 in. above the elbows are considered sterile. ■ Always keep sterile gloved hands in sight and above waist/table level; touch only objects that are sterile. ■ Sterile draped tables in the operating room or elsewhere are considered sterile only at surface level.
Sterile objects can become unsterile by prolonged exposure to airborne microorganisms.	■ Keep doors closed and traffic to a minimum in areas where a sterile procedure is being performed, because moving air can carry dust and microorganisms. ■ Keep areas in which sterile procedures are carried out as clean as possible by frequent damp cleaning with detergent germicides to minimize contaminants in the area. ■ Keep hair clean, and keep it short or enclose it in a net to prevent hair from falling on sterile objects. Microorganisms on the hair can make a sterile field unsterile. ■ Wear surgical caps in operating rooms, delivery rooms, and burn units. ■ Refrain from sneezing or coughing over a sterile field. Droplets containing microorganisms from the respiratory tract can travel 1 m (3 ft), making a sterile field unsterile. Some agencies recommend that masks covering the mouth and the nose should be worn by anyone working over a sterile field or an open wound. ■ Nurses with mild upper respiratory tract infections should refrain from carrying out sterile procedures or should wear masks. ■ When working over a sterile field, keep talking to a minimum. Avert the head from the field if talking is necessary. ■ To prevent microorganisms from falling into a sterile field, refrain from reaching over a sterile field unless sterile gloves are worn. Refrain from moving unsterile objects over a sterile field.
Fluids flow in the direction of gravity.	■ Unless gloves are worn, always hold wet forceps with the tips below the handles. When the tips are held higher than the handles, fluid can flow onto the handle and become contaminated by the hands. When the forceps are again pointed downward, the contaminated fluid can flow back down and contaminate the tips. ■ During a surgical hand cleanse, hold the hands higher than the elbows to prevent contaminants from the forearms from reaching the hands.
Moisture that passes through a sterile object draws microorganisms from unsterile surfaces above or below the sterile surface by capillary action.	■ Sterile, moisture-proof barriers are used beneath sterile objects. Liquids (sterile saline or antiseptics) are frequently poured into containers on a sterile field. If they are spilled onto the sterile field, the barrier keeps the liquid from seeping beneath it. ■ Keep the sterile covers on sterile equipment dry. Damp surfaces can attract microorganisms in the air. ■ Replace sterile drapes that do not have a sterile barrier underneath when they become moist.
The edges of a sterile field are considered unsterile.	■ A 2.5-cm (1-in.) margin at each edge of an opened drape is considered unsterile because the edges are in contact with unsterile surfaces. ■ Place all sterile objects more than 2.5 cm (1 in.) inside the edges of a sterile field. ■ Any article that falls outside the edges of a sterile field is considered unsterile.
The skin cannot be sterilized and is unsterile.	■ Use sterile gloves or sterile forceps to handle sterile items. ■ Prior to a surgical aseptic procedure, cleanse the hands to reduce the number of microorganisms on them.
Conscientiousness, alertness, and honesty are essential qualities in maintaining surgical asepsis.	■ When a sterile object becomes unsterile, it does not necessarily change in appearance. ■ The individual who sees a sterile object become contaminated must correct or report the situation. ■ Do not set up a sterile field ahead of time for future use.

of patients at risk for infection. Many research studies have investigated the effectiveness of aseptic technique. A number of studies have shown a link between artificial fingernails and infection transmission, especially fungal infections. In addition, skin underneath rings is more highly colonized than other skin, and organisms can remain under the ring for months without proper hand hygiene (CDC, 2015b). In any case, nurses use critical thinking and agency policy in implementing infection-control procedures.

Infection-Control Oversight

The National Institute for Occupational Safety and Health (NIOSH) is part of the CDC and is a research agency of the U.S. Department of Health and Human Services. It investigates potentially hazardous working conditions and publishes recommendations for preventing workplace illnesses and injuries. For example, in 1999, NIOSH published a study that found that the majority of needlestick injuries in healthcare settings were preventable. This finding, in part, led to the Needlestick Safety and Prevention Act, which went into effect in April 2001.

OSHA, an agency of the U.S. Department of Labor, publishes and enforces regulations to protect healthcare workers from occupational injuries, including exposure to bloodborne pathogens in the workplace. **Occupational exposure** is defined as skin, eye, mucous membrane, or parenteral contact with blood or other potentially infectious materials that may result from the performance of an employee's duties.

There are three major modes of transmission of infectious materials in the clinical setting:

1. Puncture wounds from contaminated needles or other sharps
2. Skin contact, which allows infectious fluids to enter through wounds and broken or damaged skin
3. Mucous membrane contact, which allows infectious fluids to enter through mucous membranes of the eyes, mouth, or nose.

All healthcare organizations are required to have interprofessional infection-control committees that may include representatives from the clinical laboratory, housekeeping, maintenance, dietary, and patient care areas. One important member of this committee is the infection-control nurse. This nurse is specially trained in the latest research and practices in preventing, detecting, and treating infections. All infections are reported to the infection-control nurse in a manner that permits recording and analyzing statistics that can assist in improving infection-control practices. In addition, the infection-control nurse may be involved in employee education and implementation of the control plan for bloodborne pathogen exposure mandated by OSHA.

Nursing Assessment

Assessment of patients for infection is vital to treating the patients as well as preventing the spread of infection. Assessment for infection is also important for patients at risk of infection, such as patients with IV lines, indwelling catheters, and surgical wounds.

Observation and Patient Interview

During the nursing history, the nurse assesses the degree to which a patient is at risk for developing an infection and any patient complaints suggesting the presence of an infection. To identify patients at risk, the nurse reviews the patient's chart and structures the patient interview to collect data regarding the factors that influence the development of infection, especially existing disease process, history of recurrent infections, current medications and therapeutic measures, current emotional stressors, nutritional status, and history of immunizations. Prior to the interview, the nurse must make observations of the patient's current condition. This observation should

include: visually assessing the skin, the scalp, the eyes, and the presence or absence of a foul odor; assessing for signs and symptoms of an elevated temperature, including but not limited to shivering, sweating, or complaints of feeling too warm; observing for signs or symptoms of respiratory difficulty, such as elevated respiratory rate, coughing, wheezing, or shortness of breath. In addition, the nurse should observe the patient for signs or symptoms of pain, such as facial expressions or guarding, or indications that the patient is unable to remain comfortable in the chair or bed. These observations provide data with which to then conduct the patient interview. As with all history taking, the nurse must individualize the specific terms used, examples given to the patient, and teaching techniques used to validate agreement on the meaning of words according to the patient's culture, language spoken, and education or intellectual abilities. Interview questions may include:

- Have you recently traveled to a foreign country? If so, please explain.
- When were you last immunized for diphtheria, tetanus, poliomyelitis, rubella, measles, influenza, hepatitis, and pneumococcal pneumonia?
- When did you last have a tuberculin skin test?
- What infections have you had in the past, and how were these treated? Have any of these infections recurred?
- Are you taking any antibiotics, anti-inflammatory medications such as aspirin or ibuprofen, or medications for cancer?
- Have you had any recent diagnostic procedure or therapy that penetrated your skin or a body cavity?
- What past surgeries have you had?
- Do you take vitamins? Do you take any nonprescription supplements, such as herbal remedies?
- On a scale of 0–10, how would you rate the stress you have experienced in the past 6 months?
- On a scale of 0–10, how would you rate the pain you have today?
- Have you experienced any loss of energy, loss of appetite, nausea, headache, or other signs associated with specific body systems (e.g., difficulty urinating, urinary frequency, sore throat)?

Physical Examination

Signs and symptoms of an infection vary according to the body area involved (see the Infection Assessment feature). For example, sneezing, watery or mucoid discharge from the nose, and nasal stuffiness commonly occur with an infection of the nose and sinuses, and urinary frequency and cloudy or discolored urine often occur with a urinary infection. The skin and mucous membranes are commonly involved in a local infectious process, resulting in localized swelling and redness, pain or tenderness with palpation or movement, palpable heat in the infected area, and loss of function of the body part affected, depending on the site and extent of involvement.

In addition, open wounds may exude drainage of various colors. Signs of systemic infection include fever, increased pulse and respiratory rate if the fever is high, malaise and loss of energy, loss of appetite, nausea and vomiting, and enlargement and tenderness of lymph nodes that drain the area of infection.

Infection Assessment

ASSESSMENT/ METHOD	NORMAL FINDINGS	ABNORMAL FINDINGS	LIFESPAN OR DEVELOPMENTAL CONSIDERATIONS
Vital Signs			
	Normal pulse, respiratory rate, temperature, and blood pressure	■ Rapid pulse ■ Rapid respiratory rate ■ Fever or hypothermia	■ Infants or toddlers who are sick or in pain may be easier to assess when comforted or held by a parent. ■ Vital signs in children are different than in adults; vital signs should be compared to normal for the patient's specific age group.
Ear Assessment			
	Intact ear canal and tympanic membrane, ear canal the same color as complexion, pearly gray tympanic membrane, no fluid or pus, possibly earwax, responsiveness to sound	■ Ruptured tympanic membrane ■ Pus or fluid in ear ■ Ear pain ■ Not responsive to sound, or report that sound is muffled ■ Redness or bulging of the eardrum	■ Infants and children with cleft lip/palate are at an increased risk of developing ear infections. ■ Infants or toddlers with ear pain may resist an ear assessment; distraction with toys or other objects may be helpful. ■ Children's tugging or rubbing the ear(s) may be a sign of otitis media.
Oral Cavity Assessment			
	Mucous membranes pink, smooth, moist, and intact	■ Bleeding or discolored gums ■ Cherry red or dry lips ■ Bright red or enlarged tonsils, white or yellow exudates on the tonsils ■ Bright red throat	■ Tonsils may be removed in some individuals. ■ Demonstrate for children how to open their mouth, stick out their tongue, and say "ah" for the assessment.
Eye Assessment			
	White sclera, normal amount of tears, clear of crusts	■ Red sclera ■ Crusts on eyelids ■ Excessive tears ■ Eye pain or itching	■ Abnormal findings in older adults may be related to glaucoma or other eye disorders rather than infection.
Lymph Node Assessment			
	Cervical nodes less than 1 cm, movable, soft, and nontender; often nonpalpable	■ Enlarged nodes ■ Asymmetrical nodes ■ Tender nodes	■ Cervical nodes may not be palpable in healthy infants and adolescents; they are often small but palpable in children between the ages of 1 and 11. ■ The frequency of palpable cervical nodes decreases with age.
Respiratory Assessment			
	Normal respiratory rate and breath sounds	■ Rapid breathing ■ Abnormal respiratory sounds (e.g., wheezing, crackles, stridor)	■ Warm your hands and stethoscope before auscultating infants to help prevent resistance to the procedure; a pacifier may also be used. ■ Use a stethoscope with an appropriately sized diaphragm for infants. ■ Patients with lung diseases such as chronic obstructive pulmonary disease (COPD) or asthma may have abnormal breath sounds and respiratory rate in the absence of infection.

(continued on next page)

Infection Assessment *(continued)*

ASSESSMENT/ METHOD	NORMAL FINDINGS	ABNORMAL FINDINGS	LIFESPAN OR DEVELOPMENTAL CONSIDERATIONS
Skin Assessment			
	Normal complexion depending on race, skin intact, dry, and warm	▪ Rash ▪ Open wounds with inflammation and/or pus ▪ Pallor ▪ Redness ▪ Increased warmth ▪ Sweating ▪ Itching or burning	▪ Warm your hands before touching bare skin, especially when assessing infants. ▪ Individuals with skin conditions such as psoriasis may have abnormal skin findings in the absence of infection. ▪ Older adults may have fragile skin that is highly susceptible to infection. ▪ Patients with diabetes mellitus may develop neuropathy that decreases sensation and increases the risk of infection; poor circulation may increase the time of healing for skin wounds.
Urinary Assessment			
	Clear or yellow urine with normal smell, no pain or itching	▪ Frequent urination ▪ Pain or burning during urination ▪ Cloudy, bloody, or foul-smelling urine	▪ If a urinary sample is needed from infants, a catheter may be used. ▪ Children may need help obtaining a clean-catch urine sample. ▪ UTIs are rare in men, so all cases require further investigation. ▪ Be aware of privacy issues, especially for adolescents.

Diagnostic Tests

To assess the patient's response to infection, identify the infecting organism, and monitor the progress of therapy, the following diagnostic tests may be ordered:

▪ *WBC count* provides clues about the infecting organism and the body's immune response to it (see **Table 9–7 》**).

▪ *WBC differential* is also ordered (see Table 9–7). Neutrophilia, or increased numbers of circulating neutrophils (or PMNs), is a common response to infection, as the bone marrow responds to an increased need for phagocytes. Along with neutrophilia, a shift to the left is common in acute infection. This means that there are more immature neutrophils in circulation than normal (see **Figure 9–4 》**), indicating an appropriate bone marrow response.

▪ *Procalcitonin (CTpr)* is a precursor of the hormone calcitonin. Procalcitonin increases dramatically during infection and sepsis and is accepted as both a marker of sepsis

Focus on Diversity and Culture
Infection

Culture can play a role in the exposure of individuals to specific infections as well as their beliefs about the cause of disease. In some cultures, infectious diseases are seen as punishment for sin or the result of curses or evil spirits. For example, many Native Americans traditionally view illnesses as the result of disharmony with nature (Spector, 2017). They may or may not believe in the germ theory of disease causation. In another example, one study found that perceptions of the risk of contracting HIV infection varied among Spanish and Mexican men and women (Giménez-García et al., 2013).

The culture of the healthcare agency caring for the patient is critically important. Healthcare agencies can provide culturally competent care to their staff and their patients by having a code of ethics and values that meet the community's needs (Anonymous, 2012). However, some healthcare entities have moved toward retail rather than open agency operations. Donovan (2015) described the change of hospitals looking similar to retail agencies. A corporate culture that fails to recognize and respect the cultural health traditions of its community may fail to meet the health needs of those living in the community. Regardless of an organization's corporate culture, nurses ask patients how their illness affects them and their family, what cultural practices are part of their daily lives, and how the staff can best support their health and cultural needs.

TABLE 9–7 White Blood Cell Count and Differential for Adults

Cell Type and Normal Value	Increased	Decreased
Total WBCs: 4500–10,000 per mm³	*Leukocytosis:* Infection or inflammation, leukemia, trauma or stress, tissue necrosis	*Leukopenia:* Bone marrow depression, overwhelming infection, viral infections, immunosuppression, autoimmune disease, dietary deficiency
Neutrophils (segs, PMNs, or polys): 50–70%	*Neutrophilia:* Acute infection or stress response, myelocytic leukemia, inflammatory or metabolic disorders	*Neutropenia:* Bone marrow depression, overwhelming bacterial infection, viral infection, Addison disease
Eosinophils (eos): 1–3%	*Eosinophilia:* Parasitic infections, hypersensitivity reactions, autoimmune disorders	*Eosinopenia:* Cushing syndrome, autoimmune disorders, stress, certain drugs
Basophils (basos): 0.4–1%	*Basophilia:* Hypersensitivity responses, chronic myelogenous leukemia, chickenpox or smallpox, splenectomy, hypothyroidism	*Basopenia:* Acute stress or hypersensitivity reactions, hyperthyroidism
Monocytes (monos): 4–6%	*Monocytosis:* Chronic inflammatory disorders, tuberculosis, viral infections, leukemia, Hodgkin disease, multiple myeloma	*Monocytopenia:* Bone marrow depression, corticosteroid therapy
Lymphocytes (lymphs): 25–35%	*Lymphocytosis:* Chronic bacterial infection, viral infections, lymphocytic leukemia, pertussis, mononucleosis, tuberculosis	*Lymphopenia:* Bone marrow depression, immunodeficiency, leukemia, Cushing syndrome, Hodgkin disease, renal failure

Source: Based on Corbett, J. V., & Banks, A. D. (2013). *Laboratory tests and diagnostic procedures with nursing diagnoses* (8th ed.). Upper Saddle River, NJ: Pearson Education; Dugdale, D. C., III. (2011). Blood differential. *MedlinePlus.* Retrieved from http://www.nlm.nih.gov/medlineplus/ency/article/003657.htm; Pagana, K. D., & Pagana, T. J. (2013). *Diagnostic and laboratory test reference* (11th ed.). St. Louis, MO: Elsevier-Mosby.

and a harmful mediator in lower respiratory tract and systemic infections (Mortazavi & Ghojazadeh, 2014).

- *Cultures of the wound, blood, or other infected body fluids* are used to identify probable microorganisms by their characteristics, such as shape, growth patterns, and Gram-staining qualities. After the organism is cultured, it is subjected to various antibiotics known to be effective against its particular strain to determine which antibiotic is likely to be most effective. This process is known as sensitivity testing. In general, 24–48 hours are required to grow the organism, potentially delaying initiation of therapy. Because antibiotics (and possibly oxygen therapy) can alter the ability to culture an organism, obtain specimens before instituting therapy.

- *Serologic testing* provides an indirect means of identifying infecting agents by detecting antibodies to the suspected organism. When the antibody titer against a specific organism rises during the acute phase of an infectious disease and begins to fall during convalescence, the diagnosis is supported. Although it is not as accurate as culture, serology is particularly useful for organisms that cannot easily be cultured, such as hepatitis B and HIV (Porth & Grossman, 2014).

- *Direct antigen detection methods* are in the process of being developed. These tests use monoclonal antibodies (see **Box 9–3 》**), which are purified antibody forms, to detect antigens in specimens from a diseased host (Porth & Grossman, 2014). These tests offer rapid and accurate identification of the offending microorganism.

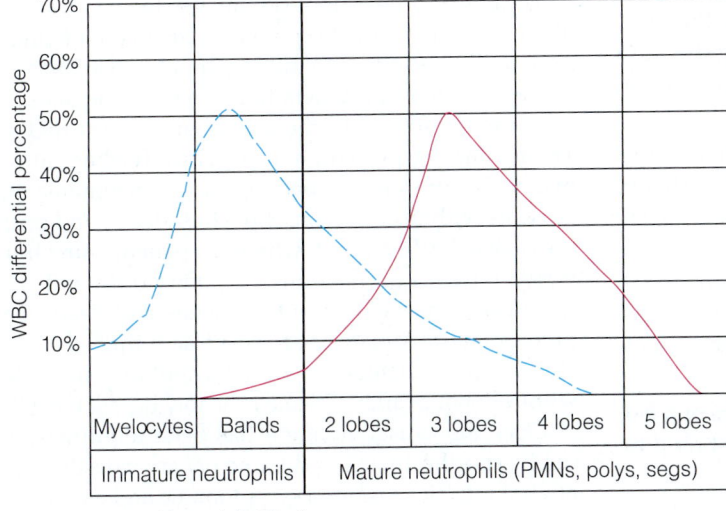

Type of WBC	Normal differential	Shift to left
Myelocytes	0%	Present
Band neutrophils (bands)	3–5%	Increased
Segmented neutrophils (segs, polys, PMNs)	50–65%	May be stable, increased, or decreased

Figure 9–4 》 Neutrophils by stage of maturity and normal distribution in the blood.

Box 9–3
Monoclonal Antibodies

Antigens typically have numerous antigenic determinant sites, each capable of stimulating a different subset of B cells. Each clone secretes a slightly different antibody from the others. The immunoglobulin produced is therefore *polyclonal*, with multiple different antibodies. In 1975, researchers devised a technique for making a single clone of "immortal" B cells that could be maintained indefinitely in a laboratory and would produce a single antibody to a specific antigen. This pure antibody, known as a *monoclonal* antibody, offers the following advantages:

- It can target specific antigens.
- It has a single, constant binding affinity for the antigen.
- It can be diluted to a specific titer or concentration, because it is not mixed with other antibodies.
- It can be purified to avoid adverse responses (Arvanitis et al., 2014).

In addition to providing passive protection from disease, monoclonal antibodies are being used in a variety of other ways, including the diagnosis and treatment of cancer, immunosuppression to prevent rejection of transplanted tissue or organs, immune response analysis, imaging techniques for diagnostic uses, and the early detection of viral infections (Arvanitis et al., 2014; Itan et al., 2014).

- *Antibiotic peak and trough levels* monitor therapeutic blood levels of the prescribed medication(s). The therapeutic range—that is, the minimum and maximum blood levels at which the drug is effective—is known for a given drug. By measuring blood levels at the predicted peak (1–2 hours after oral administration, 1 hour after intramuscular administration, and 30 minutes after IV administration) and trough (lowest level, usually a few minutes before the next scheduled dose), healthcare personnel can determine whether the patient is maintaining a level within the therapeutic range at all times, ensuring maximal effect from the drug. Measuring blood levels of a prescribed medication also helps determine whether the drug is reaching a toxic or harmful level during therapy, an unintended result that can increase the likelihood of adverse effects.

- *Radiologic examination of the chest, abdomen, or urinary system* may be ordered to detect organ abnormalities that indicate an inflammatory response or tissue damage.

- *Lumbar puncture* is performed to obtain cerebrospinal fluid (CSF) for examination and culture if a central nervous system (CNS) infection, such as meningitis or encephalitis, is suspected.

- *Ultrasonic examination, such as echocardiography or renal ultrasonography,* is a noninvasive diagnostic test used to evaluate organ function.

- *Urinalysis* is a noninvasive test used to assess for the presence of bacteria or blood in the urine.

- *Stool culture* is a noninvasive test used to assess for the presence of bacteria or parasites in the stool.

Case Study » Part 2

Mr. Werner is prescribed acetaminophen for his fever and IV fluids to prevent dehydration. His cultures indicated a *Streptococcus pneumoniae* infection, so he is placed on high-dose amoxicillin and levofloxacin. He is also placed in a room with humidified air. You begin caring for Mr. Werner on his third day in the hospital. You have been assigned to perform a vital signs and respiratory assessment every 4 hours. Your first assessment indicates that Mr. Werner's pulse and blood pressure are normal, but his breathing rate and temperature are still slightly elevated at 18/min and 101.8°F. Auscultation of his lungs indicates rales in the lower right lobe, and the lower right lobe is dull to percussion. Mr. Werner reports that he still coughs up sputum regularly, but he is no longer coughing up blood.

Clinical Reasoning Questions Level I

1. What is the purpose of the humidified air in Mr. Werner's treatment?
2. What other assessments are important to conduct regularly for someone in Mr. Werner's condition?
3. Mr. Werner will be in the hospital for several more days. What can you do to prevent feelings of isolation and boredom?

Clinical Reasoning Questions Level II

4. Why did the healthcare provider not prescribe a cough suppressant?
5. What effect does Mr. Werner's immunocompromised state have on his level of care?
6. What nursing interventions can reduce the risk of the infection spreading to the blood?

Independent Interventions

The goals of care for the patient with an infection are to identify the organ system affected by the infection, identify the causative agent, and achieve a cure by the least toxic, least expensive, and most effective means. Most infectious diseases are fortunately self-limiting and will resolve with little or no medical care. However, medical treatment may be required for an overwhelming infection or immunocompromised host.

The body part or organ system affected by the infection is often obvious from the patient's history and presenting signs and symptoms. Identifying the system involved allows nurses and other providers to narrow the range of possible infecting organisms to those known to affect that system. The manner of presentation provides further clues to the diagnosis. For example, pneumococcal pneumonia typically presents with the acute onset of chills, fever, and cough in a previously healthy adult, whereas a patient with viral pneumonia relates a gradual onset of symptoms, with systemic manifestations such as muscle aches and headache often predominant. A history of recent activities also provides clues. Family members who all vomit and have diarrhea within 12 hours after a picnic probably do not have the flu.

Once the causative agent has been identified, therapy can be specifically tailored to the patient's needs. Treatment of viral infections is often symptomatic and entails supportive care, such as promoting rest and encouraging oral intake of fluids. Skin infections may respond to treatment with a topical agent, which prevents potential adverse effects from one administered systemically.

Prevent Transmission of Infection

All skills and treatments, whether administering medications or preparing patients for discharge, are performed in a manner that prevents possible infection of patients. Some nursing skills are specific to preventing infection, recognizing signs and symptoms of infection, and treating patients who are diagnosed with an infection. Nursing skills used in preventing infection and caring for patients diagnosed with infection include hand hygiene, basic medical asepsis, use of standard precautions, isolation techniques, sterile field, and use of PPE and decontamination.

Promote Psychosocial Needs of Patients in Isolation

Patients requiring isolation precautions can develop several problems as a result of the special precautions taken in their care and their separation from other people. Two of the most common are sensory deprivation and decreased self-esteem related to feelings of inferiority. Sensory deprivation occurs when the environment lacks normal stimuli for the patient, such as communication with others. Nurses should be alert to common clinical signs of sensory deprivation, such as boredom, inactivity, slowness of thought, daydreaming, increased sleeping, thought disorganization, anxiety, hallucinations, and panic.

A patient's feeling of inferiority can stem from perception of the infection itself or from the required precautions and related isolation. In North America, many people place a high value on cleanliness, and the idea of being "soiled," "contaminated," or "dirty" can make patients feel as if they are at fault and substandard. Although this is obviously not true, infected individuals may feel "not as good" as others and blame themselves. An appropriate nursing diagnosis may be risk for situational low self-esteem.

Nurses need to provide care that prevents or addresses sensory deprivation and feelings of inferiority. Related nursing interventions include:

1. Assess the individual's need for stimulation.
2. Initiate measures to help meet the need for stimulation, including regular communication with the patient and diversionary activities, such as toys for a child and books, television, or radio for an adult. Provide a variety of foods to stimulate the patient's sense of taste, and stimulate the patient's visual sense by providing a view or an activity to watch.
3. Explain the infection and the associated procedures to help patients, their families, and caregivers understand and accept the situation.
4. Demonstrate warm, accepting behavior. Avoid conveying to the patient any sense of annoyance about the precautions or any feelings of revulsion about the infection.
5. Do not use stricter precautions than are indicated by the diagnosis or the patient's condition.

Collaborative Therapies

Many interventions for infection must be performed in collaboration with the healthcare provider or other healthcare professionals. For example, a healthcare provider may order a specimen collection of blood or urine for diagnostic testing. The nurse may be responsible for collecting these specimens from the patient and delivering them to the laboratory for testing. The nurse may also be asked to retrieve the laboratory results and inform the healthcare provider of them. Once a diagnosis has been made, the nurse may be involved in administering medications ordered by the healthcare provider, especially in a hospital setting.

Pharmacologic Therapy

Once the causative agent and affected body system have been identified, specific therapy to cure the infectious disease can begin. The perfect anti-infective agent destroys pathogens while preserving host cells, is effective against many organisms while not promoting the development of resistance, distributes to necessary tissues, and remains in the body for relatively long periods.

Because no available antimicrobial meets all these criteria, healthcare providers look for an agent that is effective, has little toxicity, can be administered with relative convenience, and is cost effective. In the process of selection, characteristics of both the patient and the infecting organism are considered. See the Medications feature.

SAFETY ALERT Nurses should encourage patients to take the full regimen of antibiotics as prescribed. Bacterial resistance often results from incomplete antibiotic therapy, which can lead to more serious and resistant infections in the future. Lack of adherence to the antibiotic regimen may also increase the risk of recurrent infections, producing further complications. In addition, patients who have leftover antibiotics from one infection may tend to self-medicate using those antibiotics for another infection even if the infection is caused by a different organism. Using antibiotics for nonsusceptible organisms is another major cause of bacterial resistance.

Nonpharmacologic Therapy

In addition to the medical regimen commonly associated with treating infections, there are common nonpharmacologic therapies important to patient care. Some of these include elevating the affected area, rest, hydration to ensure adequate fluid intake, sterile saline dressings on a wound, and the use of cold or warm compresses on an affected site.

Surgery

Surgical interventions are used when an infectious process must be eradicated in order to ensure other therapies will prevent further infection. For example, a myringotomy is conducted to remove infected inner ear drainage and to prevent further recurrence of infection. Wound irrigation and debridement are done to remove dead tissue, slough, and debris from the wound bed. Wound debridement is an important factor in the healing process, and after debridement a special dressing is applied to keep the site moist and ensure appropriate healing (Brown, 2013). Other surgical interventions, such as amputation of a toe or foot with gangrene, may be used, depending on the site of the infection.

Complementary Health Approaches

Various nontraditional methods may be used by individuals in the management of an infectious process. For example,

Medications
Antimicrobial Agents

CLASSIFICATION AND DRUG EXAMPLES	MECHANISMS OF ACTION	NURSING CONSIDERATIONS
Antibiotics - Amino-glycosides - Macrolides - Tetracyclines - Cephalosporins - Penicillins - Sulfonamides - Fluoroquinolones *Drug examples:* Cefaclor, erythromycin, penicillin, tobramycin, trimethoprim-sulfamethoxazole	Antibiotics may be used prophylactically to prevent infection or used to treat existing bacterial infection. A specific antibiotic is chosen on the basis of the pathogen causing the infection.	- Teach patients the importance of taking the entire prescribed amount. - Encourage adequate fluid intake. - Monitor for signs of allergic reaction. - Assess renal and hepatic function and vital signs.
Antifungal *Drug examples:* Amphotericin B, anidulafungin, caspofungin acetate, flucytosine, micafungin, fluconazole, nystatin	These drugs are selective for fungal plasma membranes. They inhibit ergosterol synthesis.	- Carefully monitor the patient's condition. - Use cautiously in patients with renal impairment and severe bone marrow suppression as well as patients who are pregnant. - Closely monitor kidney function (intake and output, BUN, creatinine, daily weights). - Monitor serum electrolytes.
Antipyretic, Analgesic *Drug example:* Acetaminophen	These drugs relieve pain and reduce fever.	- Monitor temperature. - Assess pain level. - Teach proper administration.
Antipyretic, Analgesic, Anti-inflammatory *Drug examples:* Aspirin, ibuprofen	These drugs reduce fever and inflammation, in addition to relieving pain.	- Monitor temperature. - Assess pain level. - Teach proper administration.
Antimalaria *Drug examples:* Atovaquone, proguanil, chloroquine, hydroxychloroquine sulfate, mefloquine, primaquine phosphate, pyrimethamine, quinine	Antimalaria drugs interrupt the complex life cycle of plasmodium, with greater success early in the course of the disease.	- Carefully monitor the patient's condition. - Provide education about the prescribed drug treatment. - Do not use in patients with hematologic disorders or severe skin disorders such as psoriasis or in patients who are pregnant. - Assess lab results (CBC, liver and renal function tests, G5PD deficiency). - Obtain a baseline electrocardiogram. - Monitor for gastrointestinal side effects and changes in cardiac rhythm.
Antihelminthic *Drug examples:* Albendazole, diethyl-carbamazine, ivermectin, mebendazole, praziquantel, pyrantel	These drugs target killing the parasites locally in the intestine and systemically in the tissues and organs the parasites have invaded.	- Monitor vital signs, CBC, and liver function studies after obtaining a baseline. - Identify specific worm or parasite before initiating therapy. - Educate on nature of parasite infestation to prevent future reinfestation. - Warn patients if bowel elimination of the worm is anticipated. - Assess for gastrointestinal symptoms. - Monitor for CNS side effects.

Medications *(continued)*

CLASSIFICATION AND DRUG EXAMPLES	MECHANISMS OF ACTION	NURSING CONSIDERATIONS
Antiretroviral ■ Nonnucleoside reverse transcriptase inhibitors ■ Nucleoside and nucleotide reverse transcriptase inhibitors ■ Protease inhibitors ■ Fusion and integrase inhibitors *Drug examples:* Delavirdine, efavirenz, abacavir, didanosine, amprenavir, atazanavir, darunavir, enfuvirtide, raltegravir, acyclovir, cidofovir, docosanol, idoxuridine, penciclovir	These drugs target specific phases of the HIV replication cycle, requiring multiple drugs taken concurrently.	■ Patients require extensive teaching regarding pharmacotherapy, disease process, and prevention of contaminating others. ■ Psychosocial issues must be addressed to improve compliance with treatment regimen. ■ Use a nonjudgmental approach. ■ Assess for side effects that can dramatically affect the patient's life. ■ Assess T-cell count and patient response to pharmacotherapy.

Source: Data from Adams, M. P., Holland, L. N., & Urban, C. (2017). *Pharmacology for nurses: A pathophysiologic approach* (5th ed.). Hoboken, NJ: Pearson Education.

over-the-counter (OTC) echinacea and goldenseal, herbal supplements purported to eliminate upper respiratory infections, have been used for many years by the general public (Weiss, Tessema, & Brown, 2013). These are only two simple supplements commonly in use. There are multiple other supplements and therapies in the nontraditional domain that a patient may be using, and their use often depends on the traditions and beliefs of the patient's particular cultural group (Magge & Wolf, 2013).

SAFETY ALERT Many patients do not mention use of these supplements during a medical appointment or nursing assessment. The nurse must ask in a nonjudgmental tone what other therapies a patient may be using and document this information in the patient's record.

Lifespan Considerations

A patient's susceptibility to infection is affected by age and heredity. Newborns and older adults have reduced defenses against infection. Infections are a major cause of death in newborns, who have immature immune systems and are protected only for the first 2 or 3 months by immunoglobulins passively received from the mother. Infants begin to synthesize their own immunoglobulins between 1 and 3 months of age.

Infections in Infants, Children, and Adolescents

Infections are a normal part of childhood, and most children experience some kind of infection from time to time. The majority of these infections are caused by viruses, and for the most part they are transient and relatively benign and can be overcome by the body's natural defenses and supportive care. One example is otitis media, or an ear infection, which is one of the most frequent reasons parents take children to the doctor. In some cases, however, severe and even life-threatening infections

occur. Considerations related to infants, children, and adolescents include the following:

■ Newborns may not be able to respond to infections because of an underdeveloped immune system. As a result, in the first few months of life, infections may not be associated with typical signs and symptoms (e.g., an infant with an infection may not have a fever).

■ Newborns have some naturally acquired immunity that is transferred from the mother across the placenta at birth.

■ Breastfed infants enjoy higher levels of immunity against infections than infants fed with formula.

■ Fevers of less than 39°C (102.2°F) in children should not be treated, except for comfort of the child (Mayo Clinic, 2014).

■ Children between 6 months and 5 years of age are at higher risk for fever-induced (febrile) seizures. Febrile seizures are not associated with neurologic seizure disorders (e.g., epilepsy).

■ Children who are immune compromised (e.g., by leukemia or HIV) or have a chronic health condition (e.g., cystic fibrosis, sickle cell disease, congenital heart disease) need additional precautions to prevent exposure to infectious agents.

■ Hand hygiene, comprehensive immunizations, proper nutrition, adequate hydration, and appropriate rest are essential to preventing and/or treating infections in children.

■ Hand cleansing and good hygiene in child care centers and schools are important to prevent the spread of infections.

■ Adolescents are at high risk for sexually transmitted diseases and should be well educated about how to prevent infections.

Infections manifest in a variety of ways in newborns, infants, and children. See **Table 9–8 ⟩⟩** for a list of the clinical manifestations of infection in infants and children by body system. Infants and children also need special considerations during the assessment. Nurses should make sure that their hands and other instruments are warm before touching children's bare skin. In addition, nurses should explain procedures before the

TABLE 9–8 Clinical Manifestation of Infection in Infants and Children

Body System	Infants	Children
Central nervous system	Irritability Decreased responsiveness Lethargy Bulging anterior fontanel High-pitched cry Muscle weakness *Additional signs in newborns:* Seizures Subtle changes in muscle tone, or hypotonia	Irritability or combativeness Stiff neck Back pain Decreased responsiveness Photophobia Brudzinski sign Kernig sign Malaise
Cardiovascular system	Tachycardia Decreased perfusion Weak peripheral pulses Pallor or mottled skin Flushed, dry skin Delayed capillary refill time *Additional signs in newborns:* Cyanosis Hypotension Bradycardia	Tachycardia Decreased perfusion Weak peripheral pulses Pallor or flushed, dry skin Delayed capillary refill time
Respiratory system	Tachypnea Increased work of breathing with retractions, nasal flaring Crackles Cough Stridor Decreased oxygen saturation Irregular breathing *Additional signs in newborns:* Apnea (new onset or increased episodes) Increased or new-onset oxygen requirement Grunting	Tachypnea Dyspnea Retractions Nasal flaring Crackles Cough Stridor Decreased oxygen saturation
Gastrointestinal system	Vomiting Diarrhea Abdominal distention Poor feeding *Additional signs in newborns:* Abdominal wall discoloration Paralytic ileus Bloody stool Jaundice or hepatosplenomegaly	Nausea and vomiting Diarrhea Abdominal discomfort Abdominal distention Poor appetite
Renal system	WBCs and bacteria in urine *Additional signs in newborns:* Decreased urine output Hematuria, proteinuria	WBCs and bacteria in urine
Hematopoietic system	Neutropenia Increased immature WBCs (bands) in bacterial infections Lymphocytosis in viral infections *Additional signs in newborns:* Fraction of band cells greater than 0.2 Thrombocytopenia	Leukocytosis Increased immature WBCs (bands) in bacterial infections Lymphocytosis in viral infections
Metabolic system	Hyperthermia or hypothermia Hypoglycemia or hyperglycemia	Hyperthermia Chills Hypothermia in septic shock
Other systems	Rash Dry mucous membranes Poor skin turgor Sunken anterior fontanel Petechiae and/or purpura	Rash Petechiae and/or purpura Dry mucous membranes Poor skin turgor

assessment to children who are old enough to understand. Infants and toddlers may feel more secure if they are held by a parent during the assessment. Distractions such as a pacifier or toy for infants and toys, books, or treats for toddlers and children may calm the children and aid in the assessment process. Nurses may also talk with verbal children about non-assessment–related topics to provide distraction. Other special considerations for specific assessments are provided in the Infection Assessment feature earlier in this module.

Pediatric Infectious and Communicable Diseases

Reducing the number of vaccine-preventable diseases is a major national goal in *Healthy People 2020*, and nurses are important partners in this effort. Specific objectives targeted at reducing or eliminating specific infectious diseases (U.S. Department of Health and Human Services, 2013) include:

- *Elimination.* Rubella and congenital rubella syndrome, serogroup A meningitis, and neonatal tetanus.
- *Reduction.* Pertussis, hepatitis B, varicella, measles, and other vaccine-preventable diseases, as well as other illnesses, such as foodborne pathogens and HIV infection.

Common preventable infectious diseases are a significant public health problem. The national health objectives reflect the significance of these preventable diseases as a public health problem. **Table 9–9 》** lists selected infectious and communicable diseases in children.

Infections in Pregnant Women

Pregnant women need special considerations if they contract an infection that may cause birth defects, such as rubella, cytomegalovirus (CMV), parvovirus, and chicken pox. CMV is the most common infection that causes birth defects. Pregnant women should be educated about the risks of infection and ways to prevent infection during pregnancy. If a pregnant woman has an infection, it can be transmitted to the newborn. Infections that can be transmitted from the mother to the newborn include HIV, group B *Streptococcus*, cytomegalovirus, and listeriosis. Precautions such as antiviral treatment for HIV infections, antibiotics during labor for group B *Streptococcus*, good hygiene techniques, and not eating potentially contaminated foods are all ways to prevent the transmission of the infection to the fetus or newborn.

Infection in Older Adults

Normal aging may predispose older adults to increased risk of infection and delayed healing. As the body ages, changes take place in the skin, respiratory tract, gastrointestinal system, kidneys, and immune system. If unchallenged, these systems work well to maintain the individual's homeostasis, but if compromised by stress, illness, infections, treatments, or surgeries, these defense systems cannot provide adequate protection. Recognizing these changes in older adults is important for the early detection and treatment of infections and delayed healing. Special considerations for older adults include the following:

- Nutrition is often poor in older adults. Certain nutritional components, especially adequate protein, are necessary to build up and maintain the immune system. In addition, lack of proper intake of necessary vitamins and minerals challenges the older adult immune system.

- Diabetes mellitus, which occurs frequently in older adults, increases the risk of infection and delayed healing by causing an alteration in nutrition and impaired peripheral circulation, which in turn decrease oxygen transport to the tissues.
- The immune system reacts slowly to the introduction of an antigen, allowing the antigen to reproduce itself several times before the immune system recognizes it.
- The normal inflammatory response is delayed, and this delay often causes atypical responses to infection, with unusual presentations. Instead of the redness, swelling, and fever that are usually associated with infections, atypical symptoms, such as confusion and disorientation, agitation, incontinence, falls, lethargy, and general fatigue, are often seen first in the older adult.

With advancing age, multiple physiologic changes cause increased susceptibility to infection. Physiologic changes of aging that put older adults at increased risk for infection include the following:

- *Cardiovascular changes.* Decreased cardiac output, loss of capillaries, and decreased tissue perfusion delay inflammatory response and healing.
- *Respiratory system changes.* Decreased mucociliary escalator, decreased elastic recoil, and a diminished cough reflex lead to decreased clearance of respiratory secretions.
- *Genitourinary changes.* Loss of muscle tone, reduced bladder contractility, altered bladder reflexes, and prostatic hypertrophy in men lead to reduced bladder capacity and incomplete emptying.
- *Gastrointestinal system changes.* Impaired swallow reflex, decreased gastric acidity, and delayed gastric emptying increase the risk of aspiration.
- *Skin and subcutaneous tissue changes.* Thinning of skin, decreased cushioning, and decreased sensation lead to increased risk of injury and ulceration.
- *Immune changes.* Decreased phagocytosis, reduced inflammatory response, and slowed or impaired healing processes lead to reduced immunity.

In addition to these physiologic changes, the following factors contribute to an older adult's increased risk for infectious disease:

- Decreased activity level related to musculoskeletal, neurologic, or balance problems
- Poor nutrition and an increased risk of dehydration
- Chronic diseases, such as diabetes mellitus, cardiac disease, and renal disease
- Long-term medication use
- Lack of recent immunizations against preventable infectious diseases
- Altered mental status and dementias
- Hospitalization or residence in a long-term care facility
- Presence of invasive devices, such as indwelling urinary catheters and gastric tubes.

The thymus gland also atrophies, and by age 50–60 years, thymic hormone levels are undetectable. Although the exact

TABLE 9–9 Selected Infectious and Communicable Diseases in Infants, Children, and Adolescents

Disease	Clinical Manifestations	Clinical Therapy	Nursing Management
Diphtheria*⁺			
Causal agent: Corynebacterium diphtheriae *Epidemiology:* Occurs mostly in the colder months in unimmunized or partially immunized children and immunized children with waning immunity. Cases of cutaneous and wound diphtheria occur sporadically in the tropics. Maternal immunity lasts up to 6 months after birth. The disease is endemic in areas where immunization is no longer routine, such as Russia. *Transmission:* Contact with nasal or eye discharge or skin lesions, or, less commonly, by indirect contact with contaminated items. Unpasteurized milk has served as a vehicle. *Incubation period:* 2–7 days or longer *Period of communicability:* Usually 2–4 weeks or until 4 days after antibiotics are started	Symptoms can be mild or severe with a gradual onset over 1–2 days. Low-grade fever, anorexia, malaise, rhinorrhea (runny nose) with a foul odor, cough, sore throat, hoarseness, stridor or noisy breathing, cervical lymphadenitis, and pharyngitis may be present. In more severe cases, the membranes of the tonsils, pharynx, and larynx are affected. The characteristic membranous lesion is a thick, bluish white to grayish black patch that covers the tonsils. It can spread to cover the soft and hard palates and the posterior portion of the pharynx. Attempts to remove the membrane result in bleeding. *Complications:* Diphtheria produces an endotoxin that causes myocarditis and peripheral neuropathy (diplopia, slurred speech, difficulty swallowing, or paralysis of the palate) or ascending paralysis similar to Guillain-Barré syndrome.	Diagnostic tests include a culture from any mucosal or cutaneous lesion. Administer IV antitoxin and antibiotics within 3 days of onset of symptoms. The child must be tested for sensitivity to horse serum before being given the antitoxin. When diphtheria is suspected, antibiotic therapy (penicillin G or erythromycin) should be initiated without waiting for laboratory results. Removal of the membrane may be needed to treat airway obstruction. *Prognosis:* With treatment, prognosis is good. If untreated, death can occur due to airway obstruction. *Prevention:* Diphtheria is a vaccine-preventable disease. Booster doses are needed every 10 years after the primary series. This is a reportable disease.	■ Use droplet precautions for pharyngeal disease and contact precautions for cutaneous disease. ■ Monitor closely for signs of increasing respiratory distress, as well as cardiac and neurologic complications. Provide humidified oxygen as necessary. ■ Have emergency airway equipment available. ■ Administer antibiotics. Give no medications containing caffeine or other stimulants. ■ Use oral suction gently as necessary. ■ Allow children to use mouthwash if desired. Gargling is not permitted because it can irritate the pharyngeal surfaces. ■ Encourage liquids as tolerated. IV fluids may be necessary. ■ Provide emotional support to the family. ■ Initiate the search for patient contacts to give antibiotics and immunization boosters.
Erythema Infectiosum (Fifth Disease)			
Causal agent: Human parvovirus B-19 *Epidemiology:* Occurs worldwide, most often in winter and spring. The disease also occurs in epidemics, with peak activity every 6 years. The incidence is highest in children between the ages of 5 and 14 years. *Transmission:* Respiratory secretions and blood *Incubation period:* 6–21 days *Period of communicability:* Believed to be highest the week before symptom onset 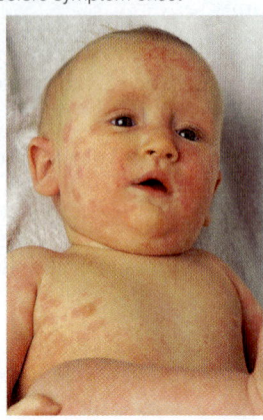	Stage 1 begins as a flulike illness (headache, chills, malaise, nausea, body ache) lasting 2–3 days. A symptom-free period of 1–7 days follows. Stage 2 occurs 1 week later with a fiery-red rash on the cheeks, giving a "slapped face" appearance. Circumoral pallor is seen. In 1–4 days a lacelike, symmetric, erythematous, maculopapular rash appears on the trunk and limbs, spreading proximal to distal but sparing the palms and soles (see **Figure 9–5 ≫**). Stage 3 lasts 1–3 weeks as the rash fades but can reappear if the skin is irritated or exposed to sunlight. The rash can be mildly pruritic. *Complications:* Children with hemolytic conditions can have transient aplastic crisis. Arthritis and arthralgia can occur.	Diagnosis is made by physical signs or a serologic test for immunoglobulin M (IgM) parvovirus B-19–specific antibody. Medical treatment is supportive, and recovery is usually spontaneous. Children with hemolytic conditions may need blood transfusions if an aplastic crisis occurs. Patients who are immunodeficient may develop a chronic infection for which IV immune globulin therapy is often effective (Pickering et al., 2012). *Prognosis:* Fetal infection can occur, resulting in fetal hydrops or spontaneous abortion. *Prevention:* Avoid contact with infected individuals.	■ Children with aplastic crisis are often hospitalized. ■ Use standard and droplet precautions. Isolation is needed only for children with aplastic crisis or who are immunosuppressed. ■ Nonaspirin antipyretics may be given to control fever. ■ Use soothing oatmeal or Aveeno baths if the rash is pruritic. Antipruritics may also help to relieve itching. ■ Encourage rest and offer frequent fluids. ■ Keep children out of direct sunlight if possible. Provide protective, light, loose clothing if exposure to sunlight cannot be avoided. ■ Provide quiet diversionary activity. There is no reason to keep the immune-competent child out of school or child care once he or she is no longer infectious. ■ Explain the three stages of rash development to parents.

Note: *Indicates that a vaccine or antitoxin is available for use in high-risk or as-needed situations. ⁺Indicates that the disease has a safe and effective vaccine.

Source: Loisjoy Thurstun/Alamy Stock Photo.

Figure 9–5 ≫ Lace-like, erythematous, maculopapular rash with erythema infectiosum.

TABLE 9–9 Selected Infectious and Communicable Diseases in Infants, Children, and Adolescents *(continued)*

Disease	Clinical Manifestations	Clinical Therapy	Nursing Management
Haemophilus influenzae, Type b+			
Causal agent: Coccobacilli *H. influenzae* bacteria, which have several serotypes and may or may not be encapsulated (surrounded by a protective outer covering) *Epidemiology:* Occurs most often in the spring and summer. Infants and young children in child care centers are most commonly affected. Low-birth-weight children and children with chronic illnesses have an increased susceptibility. *Transmission:* Direct contact or droplet inhalation. The organism is frequently asymptomatically colonized in the respiratory tract. *Incubation period:* Unknown *Period of communicability:* 3 days from onset of symptoms	The disease begins with a viral upper respiratory infection. The organism passes through the mucosal barrier to directly invade the bloodstream. It can cause several severe invasive illnesses, including meningitis, epiglottitis, pneumonia, septic arthritis, and cellulitis. It is also a cause of sepsis in infants. Other illnesses include sinusitis, otitis media, bronchitis, and pericarditis. Each disease has very specific clinical manifestations. Invasive disease has decreased 99% since the introduction of the vaccine (Pickering et al., 2012). *Complications:* Illness caused by *H. influenzae* type b responds to antibiotic therapy. If it is left untreated, severe sequelae and death, especially in young infants, can occur from conditions such as meningitis, epiglottitis, sinusitis, pneumonitis, and cellulitis.	Diagnosis is made by culture of blood, CSF, or middle ear aspirate. Treatment consists of antibiotic therapy. Rifampin may be given to unprotected household contacts (not pregnant women), if another child has not completed immunizations, within 1 week after diagnosis. *Prognosis:* With rapid diagnosis and treatment, recovery is good, but highly dependent on the disease the organism has caused. When treatment is delayed, the prognosis for full recovery becomes much more guarded. *Prevention:* H. influenzae type b vaccine is available.	■ Use droplet precautions until 24 hours after the initiation of antibiotics. ■ Antibiotic therapy is administered intravenously for severe infections. Infections such as otitis media can be managed with oral antibiotics. ■ Unimmunized children under the age of 4 years are at increased risk for developing disease from *H. influenzae*. Specific prophylactic measures for susceptible children may be ordered by the healthcare provider. ■ Administer antipyretics to help the child feel more comfortable. ■ Closely monitor IV sites for patency and infiltration. ■ Perform nursing care measures specific to the illness. ■ Inform family members that rifampin turns urine and other body fluids orange, and it will cause stains.
Influenza			
Causal agent: Orthomyxoviridae, types A and B *Epidemiology:* Prevalent in the United States from October to March, but the virus is active in other parts of the world year-round. During annual epidemics, 10–40% of healthy children are infected, and 1% are hospitalized (Pickering et al., 2012). *Transmission:* Spreads by aerosolized particles and direct contact with respiratory secretions *Incubation period:* 1–4 days *Period of communicability:* 1 day before symptoms until 5 days after onset of illness	Influenza has abrupt onset of fever (38–40°C), chills, cough, runny nose, sore throat, malaise, aches, headache, and anorexia. Children can have nausea and vomiting, diarrhea, and abdominal pain. Children may also present with croup, bronchiolitis, conjunctivitis, or other nonspecific febrile illness. *Complications:* Otitis media and exacerbations of chronic lung conditions such as asthma and cystic fibrosis can occur. Pneumonia, croup, bronchiolitis, and wheezing can occur in up to 25% of children. Myositis, myocarditis, encephalitis, transverse myelitis, Reye syndrome, and Guillain-Barré syndrome are all potential complications.	Diagnostic tests may include viral culture, rapid antigen testing from throat or nasopharynx, polymerase chain reaction, and immunofluorescence. Treatment is supportive. Antiviral therapy (oseltamivir and zanamivir) may be given to children 1 year of age or older who are at high risk of complications. Zanamivir is approved for children 5 years and older (Food and Drug Administration, 2013). Amantadine and rimantadine should not be used because of viral resistance (Food and Drug Administration, 2013). Follow updated antiviral therapy guidelines on http://www.cdc.gov/flu. When antiviral medication is initiated within 2 days of symptoms, the duration of symptoms may be reduced by 1–1.5 days. *Prevention:* Influenza vaccine is now recommended for infants and children over 6 months of age.	■ Use droplet and contact precautions for hospitalized infants and children. ■ The child is usually cared for at home. Encourage parents to use proper hand hygiene and to reduce exposure of other family members to the infected child. ■ Provide fluids to keep nasal secretions moist and prevent dehydration. ■ Provide acetaminophen or ibuprofen for fever management and mild pain. ■ If antiviral medications are given, be alert for nausea and vomiting. Zanamivir can exacerbate asthma. ■ Provide rest and quiet diversionary activities. ■ Teach parents to be alert to signs of complications from the viral infection. ■ Nurses should be familiar with pandemic influenza plans for the local area and state (http://www.pandemicflu.gov).
Measles (Rubeola) ++			
Causal agent: Morbillivirus, a member of the *Paramyxovirus* group *Epidemiology:* Occurrence peaks in the late winter and early spring. In developed countries, measles occurs mostly in outbreaks among unimmunized children, or possibly those with declining immunity. It spreads by direct contact with droplets or by the airborne route. Passive maternal immunity lasts until the infant is age 12–15 months. In developing countries, measles remains an endemic disease and is a significant cause of infant and child morbidity and mortality.	Children are quite ill in the prodromal phase of 3–5 days, with symptoms including high fever, conjunctivitis, coryza, cough, anorexia, and malaise. Koplik spots (small, irregular, bluish white spots on a red background) appear on the buccal mucosa about 2 days before and after the rash appears. The characteristic red, blotchy maculopapular rash that becomes confluent usually appears 2–4 days after onset of prodromal phase. The rash begins on the face and spreads to the trunk and extremities (see **Figure 9–6 »**). Symptoms gradually subside in 4–7 days.	Diagnosis can be made by a serologic test for IgM measles antibody. Treatment is supportive. No antiviral therapy is available. Antibiotics are used for secondary bacterial infections. *Prognosis:* Recovery is generally good with supportive care. *Prevention:* Measles is a vaccine-preventable disease. Immune globulin, administered up to 6 days after exposure, can be helpful in preventing the disease in susceptible individuals (immunocompromised children, infants less than 1 year of age, pregnant women). All healthcare workers should have documented immunity.	■ If the child is hospitalized, maintain airborne precautions during the contagious period. ■ Use a cool-mist vaporizer to help clear respiratory passages. ■ Suction nose and oral cavity very gently as necessary. ■ Give nonaspirin antipyretics for fever and antipruritics for itching. ■ Assess lungs carefully, especially in young children in whom pneumonias are a common complication. ■ Antitussives may be ordered to control coughing. ■ Keep lights dim and cover windows if the child has photophobia.

(continued on next page)

TABLE 9–9 Selected Infectious and Communicable Diseases in Infants, Children, and Adolescents *(continued)*

Disease	Clinical Manifestations	Clinical Therapy	Nursing Management
**Measles (Rubeola) ** *(continued)*			

Transmission: Airborne, respiratory droplets and contact with infected individuals

Incubation period: Approximately 8–12 days

Period of communicability: Begins 3–5 days before the rash until 4 days after the rash appears

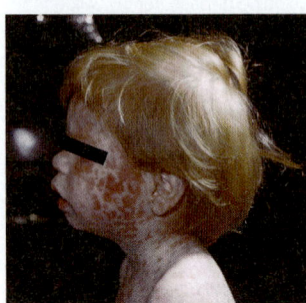

Source: Centers for Disease Control and Prevention.

Figure 9–6 ›› Confluent maculopapular rash with measles.

Other symptoms include anorexia, malaise, fatigue, and generalized lymphadenopathy.

Complications: Diarrhea, otitis media, pneumonia, bronchitis, laryngotracheobronchitis, encephalitis, and death may occur. Complications and sequelae occur most often in children who are malnourished, medically fragile, and immunosuppressed. The younger the child, the greater the risk for complications.

This is a reportable disease. A total of 222 cases and 17 outbreaks (defined as an incidence of 3 or more linked cases) were reported in the United States in 2011. Of these cases, 200 were importations from another country (CDC, 2012b).

- Elevate the head of the bed. Keep the room cool with good air circulation. Provide light and nonirritating blankets.
- Keep skin clean and dry. No soaps should be used.
- Maintain fluid intake. Offer cool liquids frequently in small amounts. Blended, pureed, and mashed foods are most easily tolerated.
- Maintain bedrest. Visitors should be immune to measles.
- Provide diversions such as music, stories, and favorite toys.

| **Meningococcus** | | | |

Causal agent: Neisseria meningitides, a gram-negative diplococcus

Epidemiology: Most often in winter or early spring. It is spread by respiratory droplets from human carriers. The majority of infections in the United States are caused by serogroups B, C, and Y. Serogroup B infections are most common in infants younger than 1, while children over 11 and adults are more likely to be infected by C, Y, or W serogroups (CDC, 2015a). The highest rates are in children under 2 years, with incidence of infection dropping drastically after age 2 (CDC, 2015a). African Americans and individuals of low socioeconomic status are at higher risk. Outbreaks have occurred in child care centers, college dormitories, and military recruit camps.

Transmission: Direct contact with droplet respiratory secretions

Incubation period: 1–10 days

Period of communicability: Until 24 hours after antibiotic is started

Meningococcus causes abrupt onset of flulike symptoms of fever, chills, malaise, muscle aches, vomiting, and prostration (extreme exhaustion).

Neurologic meningitis signs include drowsiness, disorientation, hallucinations, and convulsions.

Meningococcemia: An urticarial, maculopapular, or petechial rash also appears that may progress to purpura (see **Figure 9–7** ››). The condition may further deteriorate to shock, hypotension, disseminated intravascular coagulation, and coma.

Complications: Loss of digits or limbs due to necrosis, hearing loss, arthritis, myocarditis, pericarditis, ataxia, seizures, hemiparesis, cranial nerve palsies, and obstructive hydrocephalus may occur. Up to 10% of children and 25% of adolescents with invasive meningococcal disease die (Pickering et al., 2012).

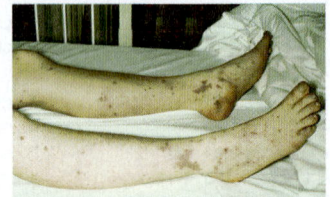

Source: John Radcliffe Hospital/Science Source.

Figure 9–7 ›› Purpura with meningococcemia.

Diagnostic tests include cultures of the blood and CSF. Gram stain of petechial skin scrapings may also be done.

Treatment: IV penicillin G is given. (cefotaxime, ceftriaxone, and ampicillin are alternative antibiotics.)

Chloramphenicol is used for children allergic to penicillin. The child is treated aggressively in the ICU to maintain the airway, assist ventilation, and manage shock with IV fluids and vasopressors. Plasma, blood, or platelets are used to treat the disseminated intravascular coagulation.

Prevention: A vaccine has been approved for adolescents 11 years and older. A vaccine is available for children over 2 years old with asplenia and other high-risk conditions. Close contacts are given medication (rifampin, ceftriaxone, or ciprofloxacin) for prophylaxis. Health professionals exposed to oral secretions need prophylaxis (Pickering et al., 2012).

This is a reportable disease.

- The child will be hospitalized. Use standard precautions and droplet precautions until the antibiotic has been administered for 24 hours.
- Disease onset is abrupt and rapidly progresses to life-threatening. Be alert for development of shock and respiratory compromise. Have emergency equipment available, and be prepared to perform resuscitation.
- When giving IV fluids and blood products, make sure the child does not get overloaded with fluids, and monitor for evidence of increased intracranial pressure.
- Keep the family informed of the child's status and treatment as the disease progresses. Help the family to mobilize its support system.
- The child who survives will likely need rehabilitation. Work with the social worker or case manager to transition the child to long-term care.
- Help identify close contacts who should receive prophylactic antibiotics and educate them about the expected side effects (e.g., orange urine with rifampin).
- Teach close contacts to be observant for signs of illness and to seek healthcare promptly if they occur.

Note: *Indicates that a vaccine or antitoxin is available for use in high-risk or as-needed situations. ⁺Indicates that the disease has a safe and effective vaccine.

TABLE 9–9 Selected Infectious and Communicable Diseases in Infants, Children, and Adolescents *(continued)*

Disease	Clinical Manifestations	Clinical Therapy	Nursing Management
Mononucleosis			
Causal agent: Epstein-Barr virus (EBV), a member of the herpesvirus group *Epidemiology:* Occurs worldwide in no seasonal pattern. Infection commonly occurs early in life, and it often spreads among family members. *Transmission:* Direct contact with infected oropharyngeal and genital tract secretions. EBV can survive in saliva for several hours outside the body. EBV can also be transmitted by blood transfusion. *Incubation period:* Estimated to be 30–50 days *Period of communicability:* Indeterminate, asymptomatic carriage is common (Pickering et al., 2012)	In very young children, mononucleosis can cause irritability but be otherwise asymptomatic. A maculopapular rash may be seen in a few cases. In other children, the disease is characterized by malaise, headache, anorexia, abdominal pain, fatigue, and fever for 2–3 days, followed by lymphadenopathy and a sore throat. Hepatosplenomegaly can occur. Pain from swelling of the tonsils and lymph nodes may be significant. The syndrome typically lasts 2–3 weeks and is self-limited. Weakness and lethargy may continue for several months. *Complications:* Rare side effects include CNS symptoms, such as encephalitis, aseptic meningitis, and Guillain-Barré syndrome. Splenic rupture, respiratory failure, and hematologic complications such as thrombocytopenia can also occur. In children who are immunodeficient, fatal infections or lymphomas can develop.	Diagnostic tests include the serologic monospot test or a heterophil antibody response test. Greater than 10% atypical lymphocytes and a positive heterophil antibody response test are diagnostic (Pickering et al., 2012). Treatment is supportive. Corticosteroids may be used to control tonsillar swelling and pain when there is impending airway obstruction, massive splenomegaly, myocarditis, or hemolytic anemia. Ampicillin and amoxicillin should be avoided, as a nonallergic rash often develops (Pickering et al., 2012). *Prognosis:* After recovery, the virus remains latent in the lymphoid system. It can be reactivated during periods of immunosuppression. *Prevention:* There is no known prevention.	▪ Children are usually treated at home. Standard precautions should be used. ▪ Give antipyretics and analgesics for fever and sore throat. Offer warm saltwater for gargling. Offer soft foods and encourage fluids. ▪ Maintain bedrest during acute phase. ▪ Give adolescents a sense of responsibility by involving them in decisions about care whenever possible. Be sure to include parents and adolescents in discussions. ▪ Reassure adolescents who may be worried about keeping up with schoolwork that they can return to school when the fever is gone and swallowing is normal. ▪ Teens should avoid kissing until the fever has been gone for several days. ▪ Contact sports should be avoided until the liver and spleen are normal, usually in about 4 weeks. ▪ If splenomegaly is present, alcohol should be avoided for 3 months after liver function test results return to normal.
Mumps (Parotitis)⁺			
Causal agent: Rubulavirus in the Paramyxoviridae family *Epidemiology:* Occurs worldwide in unvaccinated children, most often in winter and spring. Infection and vaccination induce lifelong immunity. Maternal antibodies begin to disappear in infants at the age of 12–15 months. *Transmission:* Contact with respiratory tract secretions *Incubation period:* 12–25 days *Period of communicability:* 1–2 days before parotid swelling until 9 days after swelling occurs 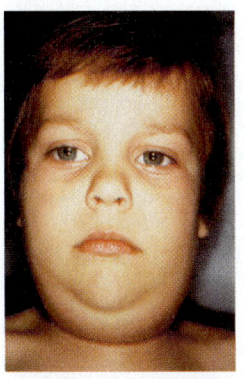 *Source:* Centers for Disease Control and Prevention. **Figure 9–8 ≫** Parotid gland swelling with mumps.	Malaise, low-grade fever, earache, headache, pain with chewing, and decreased appetite and activity; followed by bilateral or unilateral parotid gland swelling (see **Figure 9–8 ≫**). Swelling peaks around the third day. Meningeal signs (stiff neck, headache, and photophobia) occur in about 15% of patients. *Complications:* Orchitis (inflammation of the epididymis, pain on testicular palpation, and scrotal swelling—most often unilateral) may occur in postpubertal men; sterility is relatively rare (Pickering et al., 2012). Oophoritis, pancreatitis, glomerulonephritis, myocarditis, thrombocytopenia, cerebellar ataxia, and hearing impairment are sometimes seen.	Diagnostic tests include a viral culture from a throat washing, urine, or CSF. Serum mumps IgM antibody titer may also be performed. Therapy is supportive, focused on symptom relief. *Prognosis:* Mumps is usually self-limiting. *Prevention:* Mumps is a vaccine-preventable disease. This is a reportable disease. In 2009–2010 an outbreak of more than 3500 cases of mumps occurred in the upper Northeast United States. The infection was originally imported from the United Kingdom (Barskey et al., 2012).	▪ Use standard and droplet precautions for hospitalized children while contagious. ▪ Children are usually cared for at home. They are generally uncomfortable but are rarely very ill. ▪ Avoid exposure to immunocompromised or susceptible individuals. ▪ Give nonaspirin analgesics and antipyretics to control fever and pain. ▪ Encourage fluid intake. Swallowing and chewing may be painful. Offer soft and blended foods. Avoid foods and beverages that increase salivary flow (citrus, spices, and candies), because they cause pain. ▪ Talking may be painful. Provide a bell or other attention-getting device. ▪ Apply warm or cool compresses, whichever is preferred, to the parotid area. ▪ Be alert for signs of complications. Headache, stiff neck, vomiting, and photophobia may indicate meningeal irritation. ▪ Provide scrotal supports if testicular swelling occurs. ▪ Reassure children that the facial swelling will go away. ▪ Keep children out of school or child care until 9 days after parotid swelling occurs. Encourage diversionary activities.

(continued on next page)

TABLE 9–9 Selected Infectious and Communicable Diseases in Infants, Children, and Adolescents *(continued)*

Disease	Clinical Manifestations	Clinical Therapy	Nursing Management
Pertussis (Whooping Cough)⁺			

Causal agent: Bordetella pertussis

Epidemiology: Occurs worldwide. It is most common in children under 6 months of age. Epidemic cycles occur every 3–4 years. Pertussis can occur in healthcare workers, adolescents, and adults who have waning immunity, and these individuals can spread the disease to unimmunized children. Pertussis immunity may last 10 years following immunization, but there is concern about diminishing efficacy of the vaccine following the last childhood booster (Klein et al., 2012).

Transmission: Respiratory droplets and direct contact with discharge from the respiratory membranes

Incubation period: 7–10 days

Period of communicability: Begins about 1 week after exposure. It is communicable for 5–7 days after antibiotic therapy is initiated. The disease is most contagious before the paroxysmal cough stage.

The onset is insidious.

Catarrhal stage: The disease begins with nasal congestion, a runny nose, low-grade fever, and a mild nonproductive cough, lasting about 2 weeks.

Paroxysmal stage: The cough is more severe at night, with coughing spasms when the child attempts to expel a thick mucoid plug. A forceful inspiration through a narrowed glottis and stridor, or "whooping," follows. Young infants may have apnea rather than the "whooping." Sucking on a bottle may trigger the coughing spell. Coughing may be accompanied by flushing; cyanosis; vomiting; and profuse drainage from the nose, eyes, and mouth. Paroxysmal coughing can last 1–6 weeks or more. Dehydration may result from decreased oral intake.

Convalescent stage: This stage lasts up to 6 weeks, when paroxysms gradually subside.

Adolescents and adults often have symptoms of an upper respiratory infection with persistent coughing spasms lasting longer than 7 days.

Complications: Pneumonia, atelectasis, otitis media, encephalopathy, seizures, and death may occur. The highest mortality rate and complication rate is in infants under 1 year.

Diagnostic tests include culture and polymerase chain reaction (PCR) testing.

Treatment includes macrolide antibiotics (erythromycin, azithromycin, and clarithromycin); corticosteroids, if ordered; and supportive care.

Prognosis: The disease is most severe in infants under 1 year of age, and most deaths occur in this age group.

Prevention: Pertussis is a vaccine-preventable disease. Close contacts should be treated with macrolide antibiotics for prophylaxis. Vaccine protection wanes after 5–10 years.

This is a reportable disease. In 2012, more than 41,000 cases of pertussis were reported in the United States (CDC, 2013c).

- Use droplet precautions until 5–7 days after antibiotics are initiated. Most hospitalized cases occur in children under the age of 5 years.
- Use a cardiac monitor and pulse oximeter to continuously assess respirations and oxygen saturation. The smaller the child, the greater the risk for respiratory distress and apnea.
- Remain with the child during coughing spells, when hypoxic and apneic episodes are most likely. Give oxygen if ordered. Have emergency equipment available.
- Provide humidification. Gentle suctioning may be necessary.
- Give nonaspirin antipyretics as needed for fever.
- Encourage frequent rest periods.
- Allow the child to eat desired foods in small, frequent feedings.
- Encourage the child to take fluids. The child may need IV hydration if oral intake is not tolerated.
- Provide emotional support to parents.
- Teach parents to watch for signs of respiratory failure and dehydration if the child is treated at home.

Disease	Clinical Manifestations	Clinical Therapy	Nursing Management
Pneumococcal Infection⁺			

Causative agent: Streptococcus pneumoniae, a gram-positive diplococcus

Epidemiology: The organism is found in the nasopharynx of healthy people. Outbreaks occur in the winter and spring among people in crowded settings. In temperate climates, 8 of 90 serotypes account for most of the invasive pediatric infections. The disease is more common in infants, young children, African Americans, Native Americans, and Alaskan Natives. Of particular concern is the development of penicillin- and multidrug-resistant strains.

Transmission: Respiratory secretions and droplets

Period of communicability: Unknown; probably less than 24 hours after beginning effective antibiotic therapy

The signs and symptoms are related to the focal area of infection. The organism causes otitis media, sinusitis, pharyngitis, laryngotracheobronchitis, pneumonia, meningitis, and bacteremia.

In otitis media, upper respiratory infection, fever, ear pain, and decreased appetite are seen.

In bacteremia, there is unexplained fever and no localized infection site.

In pneumonia, fever, chills, chest pain, dyspnea, malaise, and a productive cough are seen.

In meningitis, inconsolable crying, increased irritability, lethargy, refusal to eat, nausea, vomiting, diarrhea, myalgia, photophobia, and seizures are seen.

Complications: Prior to the introduction of a vaccine, it caused 30–50% of acute otitis media and was a major cause of sinusitis, meningitis, bacteremia, and pneumonia. Other complications include septic arthritis, osteomyelitis, endocarditis, and brain abscess.

Diagnostic tests include bacterial culture from the site of infection.

Symptomatic care is provided. Antibiotic selection is based on susceptibility of the organism to penicillin, macrolides, and other agents. Up to 50% of pneumococcal strains are penicillin resistant. Third-generation cephalosporins (cefotaxime or ceftriaxone) may be used. Vancomycin and rifampin are used in combination when strains are resistant to the antibiotics listed above (Pickering et al., 2012).

Prevention: Many serotypes are preventable with immunization. A significant reduction in invasive disease and antibiotic-resistant strains caused by serotypes in the vaccine has occurred since vaccination of infants was initiated (CDC, 2015e).

- If the child is hospitalized, maintain standard precautions.
- Provide nonaspirin antipyretics for control of fever and comfort.
- Encourage fluids, and monitor intake and output.
- Monitor vital signs and level of consciousness to identify signs of worsening condition.
- Educate parents about the need for the vaccine, as the unimmunized child could become infected repeatedly with different serotypes.
- Many children with mild disease are treated at home. Educate parents about the need for proper medication administration and comfort measures for the child and about signs indicating a need to seek additional medical care.
- Individuals with congenital asplenia or traumatic splenectomy, malignancy, sickle cell disease, and nephrotic syndrome are at higher risk for invasive disease with this organism.
- Additional factors that increase risk of pneumococcal disease include poverty, crowded housing, homelessness, and exposure to tobacco smoke.

Note: *Indicates that a vaccine or antitoxin is available for use in high-risk or as-needed situations. ⁺Indicates that the disease has a safe and effective vaccine.

TABLE 9–9 Selected Infectious and Communicable Diseases in Infants, Children, and Adolescents *(continued)*

Disease	Clinical Manifestations	Clinical Therapy	Nursing Management
Poliomyelitis[+]			
Causal agent: Poliovirus is an enterovirus with three serotypes. *Epidemiology:* Occurs worldwide. Polio primarily affects children and immunocompromised or unimmunized adults caring for infants who received live poliovirus vaccine. The vaccine induces lifelong immunity. Most cases of polio in the United States are contracted from individuals who were given the oral vaccine in another country. The oral poliovirus vaccine may induce vaccine-associated paralytic polio, but cases are very rare in the United States because the oral vaccine is no longer used. The most recent case of vaccine-associated paralytic polio in the United States occurred in 2009 (CDC, 2015g). *Transmission:* Primarily by the fecal-oral route, but also the respiratory route *Incubation period:* Usually 7–10 days (range, 3–21) *Period of communicability:* Greatest shortly before and right after clinical symptoms develop when the virus is in the throat; excreted in the feces for several weeks.	The disease affects the CNS. Less severe infections may be limited to fever and stiffness in the neck and back, headache, vomiting, and sore throat. In other cases, fever, headache, stiff neck, Kernig or Brudzinski sign, decreased deep tendon reflexes, and progressive weakness occur. With cranial nerve involvement, there may be respiratory tract muscle paralysis. An increased respiratory rate may interfere with the ability to talk, because frequent pauses are needed. Onset of paralysis may be sudden, over hours, or gradual over 3–5 days. Paralysis results from damage to motor neurons. *Complications:* Permanent motor paralysis, respiratory arrest, myocardial failure, aseptic meningitis, and postpolio syndrome may occur.	Diagnosis is made by cell culture from stool or throat swabs. Treatment is supportive. No chemotherapeutic agents that directly kill the poliovirus are available. *Prognosis:* Respiratory complication is life-threatening and involves 5–10% of all cases. Respiratory paralysis can lead to death, and motor paralysis can result in long-term disability. *Prevention:* Poliomyelitis is a vaccine-preventable disease. This is a reportable disease.	▪ Use standard and contact precautions in the hospital, and keep the child on strict bedrest. ▪ Observe closely for respiratory paralysis (ineffective cough, talking with frequent pauses, shallow and rapid respiratory rate). Have emergency equipment at bedside. Assist ventilations as needed until mechanical ventilation is set up. ▪ Administer sedatives and nonaspirin analgesics as ordered to allow for rest and comfort. Moist hot packs may relieve discomfort. ▪ Encourage fluids. ▪ Position the child to promote body alignment. ▪ Perform range-of-motion exercises to prevent contractures after the acute phase. ▪ Provide emotional support. ▪ Patients are alert and aware. Tell them what is happening to them. ▪ Some children may need long-term orthopedic (physical therapy) support.
Roseola (Exanthem Subitum, Sixth Disease)			
Causal agent: Human herpesvirus type 6 (HHV-6) *Epidemiology:* Occurs worldwide, primarily in children 6–24 months of age (after maternal antibodies decline); no seasonal pattern *Transmission:* Likely to be from respiratory secretions of healthy individuals *Incubation period:* Appears to be 9–10 days *Period of communicability:* Lifelong persistent viral shedding in healthy individuals (Pickering et al., 2012).	The disease causes sudden high fever up to 40.5°C (105°F) for 3–8 days, during which the child does not appear toxic (normal appetite and behavior). The fever phase is followed by a characteristic pale pink, discrete, maculopapular rash that starts on the trunk and spreads to the face, neck, and extremities. The rash can last for 1–2 days. The child's appetite is normal. *Complications:* Children may have febrile seizures during the high fever stage. Encephalopathy can develop in rare cases.	Roseola is self-limiting, and treatment is supportive. *Prognosis:* Roseola is benign in most cases. Nearly all children over 2 years of age have an antibody titer to HHV-6 (Pickering et al., 2012).	▪ Children are rarely hospitalized, but if they are, use standard precautions. ▪ Give nonaspirin antipyretics to control fever. ▪ Observe closely for any seizure activity, especially during the acute febrile periods. ▪ Encourage fluids. ▪ Reassure parents that the rash will disappear in a few days.
Rotavirus			
Causal agent: Group A, B, and C rotaviruses *Epidemiology:* Occurs during late fall to early spring in yearly diarrhea epidemics in the United States. It is the most common cause of severe diarrhea in children under 5 years. *Transmission:* Fecal-oral route *Incubation period:* 2–4 days *Period of communicability:* Virus is present in stool before onset and may persist up to 21 days after onset of symptoms.	The disease manifests with acute onset of low-grade fever and vomiting followed by watery diarrhea 1–2 days later. Up to 10–20 diarrheal stools occur a day. Symptoms last 3–8 days. *Complications:* Dehydration and electrolyte disturbances may occur. Death occurs in rare circumstances.	Diagnosis is by enzyme immunoassay or latex agglutination assay to detect (group A rotavirus antigen). Treatment involves adequate fluid and electrolyte replacement with oral rehydration solution. Introducing a regular diet within a few hours of rehydration shortens the duration of the disease (Parez et al., 2014). In severe dehydration, IV fluid resuscitation is performed. No antiviral therapy is available. *Prevention:* Naturally acquired infection protects against reinfection that causes severe diseases. A new vaccine has been approved for infants.	▪ Use standard and contact precautions. ▪ Hand hygiene with soap and water removes 75% of virus from contaminated hands. Use of alcohol-based hand sanitizers after washing with soap and water increases effectiveness (Parez et al., 2014). ▪ Clean contaminated surfaces followed by disinfection with an alcohol-containing disinfectant (Parez et al., 2014). ▪ Assess hydration status frequently. ▪ Breastfeeding is continued during oral rehydration therapy. Formula feeding can begin 12–24 hours after oral rehydration therapy is started. ▪ Older children can be fed complex carbohydrates and lean meats, yogurt, fruits, and vegetables 12–24 hours after oral rehydration therapy is started.

(continued on next page)

TABLE 9–9 Selected Infectious and Communicable Diseases in Infants, Children, and Adolescents *(continued)*

Disease	Clinical Manifestations	Clinical Therapy	Nursing Management
Rubella (German Measles)+			

Causal agent: An RNA virus, member of the family Togaviridae, genus *Rubivirus*

Epidemiology: Occurs worldwide and is most prevalent in the winter and spring. Maternal antibodies disappear about 6–9 months after birth. Most U.S. cases occur among foreign-born children and adults from countries that do not have rubella vaccination programs. Congenital rubella syndrome is thought to occur because of lack of immunization. Three cases were reported in 2009 in the United States (National Center for Health Statistics, 2012).

Transmission: Droplet spread, direct contact with infected individuals, or contact with articles soiled by nasal secretions

Incubation period: 14–21 days (most commonly 16–18)

Period of communicability: 7 days before until 7 days after the onset of rash. Infants with congenital rubella may shed the virus for months after birth.

Rubella is generally a mild disease with a characteristic pink, nonconfluent, maculopapular rash. The rash appears on the face; progresses to the neck, trunk, and legs; and disappears in the same order. Prodromal symptoms occur 1–5 days before the rash and include low-grade fever, headache, malaise, coryza, sore throat, and anorexia. Forchheimer spots (discrete, erythematous pinpoint or larger lesions on the soft palate) are seen during the prodromal phase. Generalized lymphadenopathy involving the postauricular, suboccipital, and posterior cervical areas is common up to 7 days before the rash. Many cases are asymptomatic.

Neonatal signs of congenital rubella syndrome include growth retardation, radiolucent bone disease, hepatosplenomegaly, thrombocytopenia, and purpuric skin lesions (giving a "blueberry muffin" appearance) (see **Figure 9–9** ≫≫).

Complications: Complications are rare but include arthritis in adolescents and encephalitis.

Diagnostic tests include cell culture from a nasal swab and detection of IgM or IgG antibodies.

Treatment is supportive. Rubella is generally self-limiting in children.

Prognosis: The disease is usually mild and benign. The major risk is for the fetus if the mother is infected in the first trimester. Congenital rubella syndrome is associated with ophthalmologic, cardiac, auditory, and neurologic anomalies.

Prevention: Rubella is a vaccine-preventable disease. Women of child-bearing age need to be immunized to reduce the risk for congenital rubella syndrome. All healthcare workers should have documented immunity.

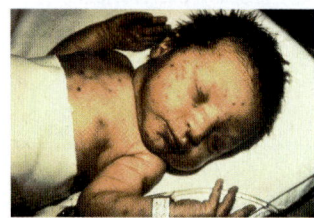

Source: Centers for Disease Control and Prevention.

Figure 9–9 ≫ "Blueberry muffin" appearance in infant with congenital rubella syndrome.

- Maintain standard and droplet precautions for contagious children.
- Maintain contact precautions for infants with congenital rubella syndrome until 1 year of age unless nasopharyngeal and urine cultures are repeatedly negative after 3 months of age (Pickering et al., 2012).
- Children are usually treated at home. They should be isolated from pregnant women.
- Give nonaspirin analgesics and antipyretics for any pain and fever.
- Allow children to choose what they would like to eat and drink. Encourage fluids.
- Provide quiet activities.
- Keep children out of child care or school for 7 days after onset of rash. School and child care facilities should be notified of the child's illness.

Streptococcus A			

Causal agent: Group A streptococci (GAS)

Epidemiology: The illness is caused by various M-protein groups of group A beta-hemolytic streptococci. Different strains are associated with pharyngeal and pyodermal infections, and also rheumatic fever and acute glomerulonephritis (Pickering et al., 2012). Pharyngeal infections tend to occur more in late fall, winter, and spring. Pyodermal infections tend to occur in warmer seasons because of the association with minor skin trauma and insect bites.

Transmission: Contact with respiratory secretions for pharyngitis or skin lesions for pyoderma

Incubation period: Pharyngeal: usually 2–5 days; Pyodermal: usually 7–10 days

Period of communicability: 4 weeks in untreated pharyngeal infections; noncontagious within 24 hours of starting antibiotics.

Pharyngeal: Abrupt onset with a sore throat, dysphagia, malaise, high fever, chills, headache, abdominal pain, anorexia, and vomiting. A beefy red pharynx with exudate (strep throat) and tender cervical nodes are seen. Palatal petechiae may be seen. Cough and rhinitis are absent in most cases.

GAS respiratory tract infection: Children under 3 years may develop serous rhinitis and a respiratory illness with moderate fever, irritability, and anorexia rather than pharyngitis.

Scarlet fever: A characteristic erythematous, "sandpaper" rash that blanches with pressure appears in some cases 12–48 hours after onset of symptoms, concentrates in flexor skin creases, and spares the circumoral area. In 3–4 days, the rash begins to fade, and the tips of the toes and fingers begin to peel. The classic strawberry tongue is seen on days 4–5.

Diagnosis can be made by a rapid strep antigen test or culture of secretions from the pharynx and tonsils. Cultures of skin lesions are not indicated (Pickering et al., 2012).

Prompt antibiotic treatment is effective. Penicillin V is the drug of choice. Erythromycin is used if the child is allergic to penicillin. Uncomplicated impetigo is treated with mupirocin ointment. Invasive strains causing necrotizing fasciitis or myositis need IV antibiotics and surgical intervention (exploration and debridement of dead tissue).

Prognosis: Recovery is usually good with antibiotic therapy. It is possible for healthy children to become chronic carriers.

Prevention: None

- Children with uncomplicated infections are usually cared for at home.
- Promote bedrest during the febrile stage.
- Give nonaspirin antipyretics to control fever. Teach parents important signs of a worsening condition.
- For pharyngeal infections, offer warm saltwater for gargling, a soft diet, and nonacidic beverages. Encourage fluids. Provide cool, clear liquids. Swallowing may be difficult.
- Explain to parents the importance of giving the child the full course of antibiotics.
- Encourage family members with sore throats to have throat cultures taken.
- For impetigo, teach the parents to wash the skin, remove crusts, and apply antibiotic ointment.
- If the child is hospitalized, maintain droplet precautions for pharyngeal infections and contact precautions for skin lesions for 24 hours after beginning antibiotics. Monitor vital signs, especially temperature. Administer antibiotics as ordered.

TABLE 9–9 Selected Infectious and Communicable Diseases in Infants, Children, and Adolescents *(continued)*

Disease	Clinical Manifestations	Clinical Therapy	Nursing Management
Streptococcus A (continued)			

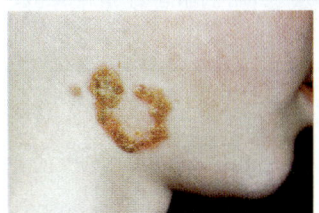

Source: Mediscan/Alamy Stock Photo

Figure 9–10 ≫ Impetigo.

| | *Pyodermal:* Lesions (impetigo) are honey-colored crusts at the site of open lesions (see **Figure 9–10** ≫).

Complications: If untreated, acute otitis media, sinusitis, peritonsillar or retropharyngeal abscess, cervical lymphadenitis, acute rheumatic fever, or acute glomerulonephritis may occur. Invasive disease with toxic shock syndrome, bacteremia, and necrotizing fasciitis or myositis can be fatal. | | ▪ If the child develops invasive streptococcal infection, use standard precautions. The child with toxic shock syndrome will need intensive care to manage shock and fluid and electrolyte imbalances. |

Tetanus			
Causal agent: Clostridium tetani or tetanus bacillus *Epidemiology:* The bacillus is common and exists as a spore in soil, dust, and animal excretions. The organism produces an endotoxin that affects the CNS. *Transmission:* The organism is transmitted to humans through puncture wounds or broken skin. Newborns can acquire tetanus via the umbilical cord if they are born in an unclean area, a contaminated implement is used to cut the cord, or clay is applied to the umbilical cord as a ritual in some Middle Eastern cultures. *Incubation period:* 3 days to 3 weeks (average, 8 days) *Period of communicability:* Not communicable to other individuals except through skin wounds	Stiffness of the neck and jaw, with painful facial spasms and difficulty chewing and swallowing over a few days, and headache. Noise and sudden movements can stimulate spasms. Spasms of facial muscles may produce a grinning expression (risus sardonicus). Localized prolonged and painful muscle contraction may occur at the site of the wound. Eventually rigidity of the abdomen and trunk produce *opisthotonos* (rigid hyperextension of the entire body). Spasms and fever occur, along with difficulty swallowing the increased oral secretions. Respiratory muscles can be affected and cause airway obstruction and suffocation. Newborns have difficulty with sucking, progressing to an inability to suck, irritability, and nuchal rigidity. *Complications:* Laryngospasm, respiratory distress, or death may occur.	Tetanus immune globulin is given to unimmunized individuals as soon as possible. Tetanus toxoid is given at the same time at a separate site. Medications are provided to treat muscle spasms. Intensive care is provided, with cardiorespiratory monitoring, assisted ventilation, IV metronidazole or penicillin G, nutrition, and supportive care. Wound cleansing and debriding are performed. Survival beyond 4 days indicates an increased chance of recovery. Paroxysms become less frequent, and complete recovery may take weeks. *Prognosis:* The disease has 30% mortality; mortality is much higher in newborns. Intensive care has improved mortality. *Prevention:* Tetanus is a vaccine-preventable disease. Tetanus boosters are updated every 10 years, or, if a potentially contaminated wound occurs, in 5 years. Proper surgical debridement of wounds decreases the chance of infection.	▪ Prevent the disease by checking immunization records and administering immunizations as necessary. ▪ Give immune globulin to unimmunized individuals. ▪ Assist with wound debridement. ▪ Use standard precautions, as the child with tetanus is hospitalized. ▪ Monitor the child's condition. Handle the child as little as possible. Reduce stimulation by placing the child in a quiet, darkened room. ▪ Offer skin and respiratory care. The child may need an endotracheal tube, suctioning, and supplemental oxygen for airway support. ▪ Provide feedings via total parenteral nutrition or feeding tube. ▪ Maintain hydration with IV fluids and electrolytes. ▪ Try to reduce the child's anxiety, as mental status may be unaffected. ▪ Prepare the family for a possible poor prognosis.

Note: *Indicates that a vaccine or antitoxin is available for use in high-risk or as-needed situations. †Indicates that the disease has a safe and effective vaccine.

relationship of these events to T-cell function is unclear, some T-cell populations decrease or decline in function as the individual ages. The ability of T cells to proliferate following activation also declines with advancing age, and a portion of T cells cannot be activated in older adults (Porth & Grossman, 2014). With these changes, cell-mediated immune function declines, and the patient has reduced resistance to antigens, such as *Mycobacterium tuberculosis*, influenza and varicella-zoster viruses, malignant cells, and tissue grafts.

Although immunoglobulin levels remain relatively stable, primary and secondary **antibody** responses decline with aging. This diminished antibody production has clinical implications in that immunizations (single-dose and booster) may not produce the expected protective immune response.

Older adults are not only at increased risk for infection but also may not exhibit the classic manifestations of inflammation and infection. They are likely to take nonsteroidal anti-

inflammatory drugs (NSAIDs) and corticosteroids, which interfere with inflammation and healing. The cardinal signs of inflammation—redness, heat, and swelling—tend to be diminished or absent in older adults. The classic signs of infection—fever and chills—may be absent altogether because of age-related changes in the immune system, loss of central temperature control mechanisms, decreased muscle mass, and loss of shivering ability. The older adult may have only subtle signs of sepsis, such as changes in mental status, disorientation, and tachypnea (Porth & Grossman, 2014).

Case Study ≫ Part 3

After 1 week in the hospital, Mr. Werner is finally going home. His vital signs have stabilized, he is no longer coughing up sputum, and his rales are barely audible. He was able to continue his chemotherapy treatments in the hospital, and he now has only one treatment left. He still feels fatigued from the chemotherapy, but the fatigue is not as severe as during the acute infection. You are providing discharge teaching for Mr. Werner.

Clinical Reasoning Questions Level I

1. What patient teaching can you perform to help decrease Mr. Werner's risk of infection while he is still immunocompromised?
2. The healthcare provider has prescribed an additional regimen of oral antibiotics. What should you emphasize about the importance of completing the therapeutic regimen?

3. What warning signs should Mr. Werner watch for that may indicate another infection?

Clinical Reasoning Questions Level II

4. To what other opportunistic infections may Mr. Werner be susceptible?
5. What nursing diagnoses apply to Mr. Werner upon his discharge?
6. What nutritional requirements does Mr. Werner have now that he is going home?

REVIEW The Concept of Infection

RELATE Link the Concepts

Linking the concept of infection with the concept of metabolism:

1. How does an infection such as hepatitis affect metabolism in the liver?
2. What physiologic changes related to obesity increase an individual's risk for infection?

Linking the concept of infection with the concept of reproduction:

3. Describe the links between infection during pregnancy and congenital disorders.
4. Which infections are most likely to occur in neonates in the first few days of life?

READY Go to Volume 3: Clinical Nursing Skills

- SKILLS 1.5–1.9   Vital Signs
- SKILL 1.13   Ears: Hearing Acuity, Assessing
- SKILL 1.14   Eyes: Visual Acuity, Assessing
- SKILL 1.23   Nose and Sinuses: Assessing
- SKILL 1.27   Thorax and Lungs: Assessing
- SKILL 2.3   Eyes and Contact Lenses: Caring for
- SKILL 2.17   Ear Medication: Administering
- SKILL 2.19   Eye Medication: Administering
- SKILL 2.24   Oral Medication: Administering
- SKILL 3.1   Pain in Newborn, Infant, Child, or Adult: Assessing
- SKILL 4.3   Urine Specimen, Clean-Catch, Closed Drainage System for Culture and Sensitivity: Obtaining
- SKILL 4.11   Urinary Catheter: Caring for and Removing
- SKILL 5.1   Intake and Output: Measuring
- SKILLS 6.1–6.9   Medical Asepsis and PPE and Isolation Precautions
- SKILL 11.8   Oxygen Delivery Systems: Using

- SKILL 11.14   Suctioning, Oropharyngeal and Nasopharyngeal: Newborn, Infant, Child, or Adult
- SKILL 11.17   Tracheostomy: Caring for
- SKILL 16.4   Dressing, Dry: Changing
- SKILL 16.9   Surgical Wound: Caring for

REFER Go to Pearson MyLab Nursing and eText

- Additional review materials

REFLECT Apply Your Knowledge

Randy Sonderburgh, a 5-year-old boy, woke up during the night crying, coughing, and complaining of feeling hot. His mother, Sharon, observed that he had watery eyes and a runny nose. Ms. Sonderburgh checked his temperature and noted it was near 101.3°F at 4:00 a.m. She told her son not to touch his eyes or face with his hands, and she gave him liquid acetaminophen for his fever.

Within 2 hours, Randy complained of a worsening sore throat and his temperature climbed to 102.2°F at 6:00 a.m. He was unable to drink more than a few sips of water before he began to cry. Ms. Sonderburgh was concerned and called the clinic's on-call advice nurse. The nurse asked multiple questions, including any travel or flights taken in the last week or two. Ms. Sonderburgh mentioned that they had been at Disneyland 10 days earlier, visiting her sister and other family members who live in Southern California. The nurse alerted Ms. Sonderburgh to the possible contact to someone with rubeola. Ms. Sonderburgh asked what that meant, and the nurse told her that measles were very contagious and it would be best if Randy was seen by medical staff as soon as the clinic opened.

1. How many days after a person is infected are you likely to see symptoms of measles?
2. Why is it important that Randy see someone at the clinic the next day?
3. What patient teaching needs to be done with Sharon, Randy's mother?

» Exemplar 9.A Cellulitis

Exemplar Learning Outcomes

9.A Analyze cellulitis as it relates to infection.

- Describe the pathophysiology of cellulitis.
- Describe the etiology of cellulitis.
- Compare the risk factors and prevention of cellulitis.

- Identify the clinical manifestations of cellulitis.
- Summarize diagnostic tests and therapies used by interprofessional teams in the collaborative care of an individual with cellulitis.
- Differentiate care of patients with cellulitis across the lifespan.
- Apply the nursing process in providing culturally competent care to an individual with cellulitis.

Overview

Infection can occur in a small localized area, affect an entire organ system, or attack the entire body, as in the case of septicemia. Cellulitis is an example of an infection that can be small and well contained, but if not treated promptly, it can develop into a life-threatening septicemia.

Cellulitis is an acute bacterial infection of the dermis and underlying connective tissue. It is characterized by red or lilac, tender, warm, edematous skin with a well-defined, non-elevated border. Cellulitis usually occurs on the face and lower extremities as a result of trauma or a compromised skin barrier. Its chief symptom is **inflammation**, which includes intense pain, heat, redness, and swelling. It may appear in a localized area as a complication of a wound infection, or it may involve an entire limb. In severe infections, fever may be present, as well as an increase in **white blood cells (WBCs)** and tender lymph nodes (**lymphadenopathy**). Elevated WBCs and fever, though common signs of infection, may not be present in frail, older adults.

Pathophysiology and Etiology

Pathophysiology

Normal flora gain entry into the dermis through a break in the skin. There, they multiply, causing an inflammatory response with classic signs of inflammation, including **erythema** (redness), pain, warmth at the site, and edema. The wound is generally irregular in shape with well-defined borders. As the organisms grow in number, they can overwhelm the immune response that normally contains and localizes inflammation. This condition allows cellular debris to accumulate, the result being enlarged areas of involvement.

Erysipelas, a superficial cellulitis of the skin caused by group A Streptococcus, usually affects the lower extremities or the face (see **Figure 9–11 》**). The involved area is bright red

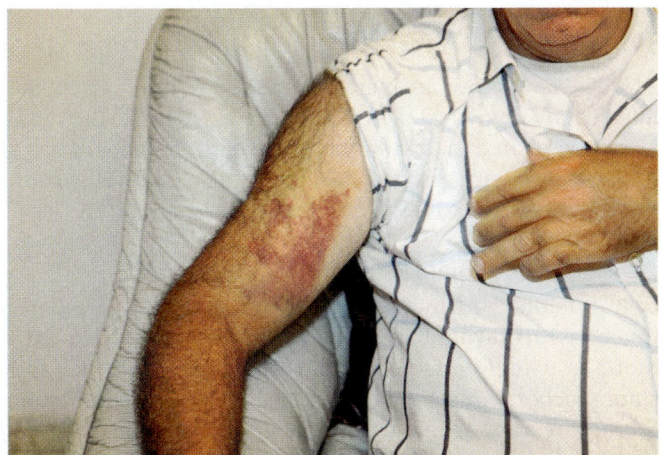

Source: Oren Shalev/PhotoStock-Israel/Alamy Stock Photo

Figure 9–11 》 Erysipelas, a superficial cellulitis of the skin caused by group A streptococcus.

and raised with well-defined borders. If treated promptly, the prognosis is generally very good. Skin infections such as this can predispose the individual to septicemia and septic shock if treatment is delayed. Although antibiotic therapy is effective, the most important method of therapy is prevention.

Etiology

The most common causative organism is *Staphylococcus aureus*, followed by group A *Streptococcus* (Herchline, 2016). Cellulitis can also result from a nearby abscess or sinusitis. Onset is usually rapid.

Risk Factors

Children with cellulitis often have a history of trauma, impetigo, folliculitis, untreated tooth decay, or recent otitis media. As the skin becomes thinner and less elastic with age, older adults become more susceptible to injury and breakdown of tissue, which can result in cellulitis. Peripheral neuropathy with decreased sensation and circulation can lead to abrasions, burns, and stasis ulcers that can become infected. Reduced physical activity, malnutrition, dehydration, and other systemic illnesses are also predisposing factors. Any interruption of skin integrity can lead to infection, especially with organisms that are part of the normal skin flora.

Other factors that increase the risk for cellulitis include any illness that compromises skin integrity such as diabetes mellitus, obesity, a previous history of cellulitis, peripheral vascular disease, tinea pedis, and a weakened immune system (Mayo Clinic, 2015). Patients with **tinea pedis** (fungal infection of the feet) or lymphatic obstruction are most vulnerable to cellulitis and may experience recurrent infections over time.

Prevention

Any individual with a skin wound is at a high risk of developing cellulitis. Good wound care is a vital part of cellulitis prevention. This care includes washing the wound carefully with soap and water and applying an antibiotic cream or ointment daily, covering the wound with a bandage to maintain adequate moisture (see the Evidence-Based Practice feature), and monitoring the wound for signs of infection. Skin protection is also an important part of cellulitis prevention. It is particularly important for individuals at risk for loss of skin integrity or infection, such as individuals with diabetes, HIV, or cancer. Methods of skin protection include keeping the skin moist with lotion, wearing shoes that fit properly, having good nail hygiene, and wearing protective equipment when participating in work or sports (Mayo Clinic, 2015).

SAFETY ALERT Individuals with diabetes may develop peripheral neuropathy, which decreases sensations in the feet. Therefore, individuals with diabetes are at higher risk for developing skin infections because they do not realize they have been injured. Individuals with diabetes should be taught to check their skin regularly for signs of injury and infection, and superficial skin infections should be treated immediately to prevent complications (Mayo Clinic, 2015).

Evidence-Based Practice
Moist Wound Management

Problem

Individuals with open wounds are more susceptible to contracting a skin infection such as cellulitis. Many individuals believe that wounds should be kept dry and should not be covered until a scab forms. However, this slows wound healing and leaves the wound exposed to potential pathogens if the scab comes off.

Evidence

Many studies indicate that keeping a wound moist can promote healing by preventing cell death, improving the rate of re-epithelialization, and protecting the wound from infection. Proper wound moisture management can also reduce pain and improve the cosmetic outcome. In particular, three cleansing techniques can be used individually or in combination to keep the wound moist and help remove any pathogens and debris: compression, pressure irrigation, and soaking. Compression involves pressing excess moisture from a gauze or cloth on the wound and removing the cloth after wound contact, irrigation involves running a steady flow of clean water or saline solution across the wound surface, and soaking involves immersing the wound in clean solution or applying an overhydrated cloth to the wound (Niederauer, Michalek, & Armstrong, 2015). Proper use of a wound covering is also vital to moist wound management. Many modern wound dressings help maintain a moist environment for nondraining wounds and help remove excess fluid through absorption or evaporation for wounds draining fluid or pus. Wound covering helps maintain a moist healing environment while avoiding maceration and breakdown of adjacent skin, which could lead to infection (Lachenbruch & VanGilder, 2012). Using an ointment is also an important part of moist wound care. Antibiotic ointments and white petrolatum are equally effective at maintaining wound moisture, promoting healing, and preventing infection. For uncomplicated wounds, white petrolatum is recommended to prevent the development of resistant organisms (Morton & Phillips, 2012).

Implications

Nurses caring for patients with wounds should implement three methods for keeping a wound moist: cleansing techniques, proper wound covering, and ointment application. These methods of moist wound management promote a healing environment and prevent infections such as cellulitis. Allowing a wound to remain dry or applying a dry wound covering may slow the healing process and increase the risk of infection.

Critical Thinking Application

1. What are the physiologic principles that support the need for a moist environment for effective wound healing?
2. How does wound care differ for patients with small acute wounds versus wounds that cover a significant portion of the body, such as a burn?
3. What nursing interventions can you implement when changing a wound dressing and performing irrigation for a toddler who was bitten by a dog?

Clinical Manifestations

Cellulitis may occur quickly in patients, with symptoms suddenly changing. Emergency department observation beds are often utilized to rapidly identify and treat patients with cellulitis. Because most emergency departments do not currently allow longer than a 24-hour stay, these patients are usually admitted to the acute care area for continued care (Volz et al., 2013). The presence of an elevated blood lactate level and fever also limit outpatient or observation level of care (Herchline, 2016) and indicate admission to the acute care level of care. Patients with cellulitis experience a rapid onset and appear ill. Classic signs and symptoms include erythema, edema of the face or infected limb, and warmth and tenderness around the infected site.

Other symptoms include fever, chills, malaise, and enlargement and tenderness of regional lymph nodes (also see the Clinical Manifestations and Therapies feature). **Lymphangitis** (inflammation of a lymph vessel) may be present. In some cases, a rapidly progressive lesion can lead to septicemia.

Individuals with darker skin tones may have more difficulty identifying the characteristic redness associated with cellulitis. Therefore, presenting symptoms may be focused on fever, pain, and edema of the affected area. Carefully inspect the area to determine the spread of infection.

Collaboration

Treatment of cellulitis is aimed at reducing the infection, promoting comfort, and preventing complications such as septicemia. Care is provided in collaboration with family members and other members of the healthcare team. The wound care nurse plays a central role in the promotion of a positive wound care plan (Varga & Holloway, 2016). This specialist collaborates with the patient and the care team to create recommendations for wound care in an acute care agency as well as for home care. Recovery from an extensive wound that impairs use of an extremity or limb for an extended period of time may require consultation with an occupational or physical therapist. If the face is involved, referral to a dentist may be necessary.

Diagnostic Tests

A CBC may show an increase in WBCs. Fluid from the affected area may be taken for cultures to identify the causative organism. Blood cultures are taken if the patient has a toxic (very ill) appearance. A blood lactic acid level is commonly measured to identify possible sepsis.

Pharmacologic Therapy

Cellulitis on the trunk, limbs, or perianal area is usually treated with oral antibiotics on an outpatient basis. The antibiotic is usually effective against both streptococcal and staphylococcal infections. If the face is involved, antibiotic therapy is administered to prevent serious complications such as periorbital cellulitis. Patients with severe cases or a large affected surface area may be treated with systemic antibiotics and analgesics in the hospital to prevent sepsis. Recovery begins within 48 hours, but therapy should continue for at least 10 days. Untreated cellulitis or cellulitis that

Clinical Manifestations and Therapies
Cellulitis

ETIOLOGY	CLINICAL MANIFESTATIONS	CLINICAL THERAPIES
Fever	Tachycardia, tachypnea, elevated temperature, lethargy, chills	■ Maintain adequate hydration. ■ Administer antipyretics. ■ Treat underlying cause.
Skin inflammation	Redness, pain, warmth, edema	■ Administer antibiotics. ■ Maintain bedrest. ■ Provide adequate nutrition to promote healing. ■ Manage pain using both pharmacologic and nonpharmacologic therapies.
Septicemia	Whole-body inflammation manifested by fever, altered WBC count (may be high or low), and hemodynamic alterations (tachycardia, tachypnea, decreased cardiac output); elevated lactic acid level.	■ Monitor hemodynamic status. ■ Administer antibiotic therapy. ■ Provide fluid management. ■ Provide supportive care based on symptoms. ■ Measure vital signs frequently.

does not respond to treatment can lead to osteomyelitis, arthritis, or serious systemic infection.

Nonpharmacologic Therapy

Common nonpharmacologic therapies associated with cellulitis are adequate rest, elevation of the affected area above the heart to reduce swelling, and infection-control measures. Sterile saline dressings can also be applied to reduce edema and promote drainage. Complementary health approaches should not be used in lieu of pharmacologic therapy, and nurses should assess for use of complementary health practices to prevent patients from inadvertently engaging in a practice or use a substance that may increase the risk for an adverse outcome.

Lifespan Considerations

Children with wounds or insect or animal bites often have difficulty not picking at the wounds or scratching bites that itch. Picking and scratching can increase the risk of developing cellulitis, which is frequently caused by bacteria already present on the skin. Children with wounds or insect bites should be monitored carefully for rapidly progressing inflammation and growing sites of infection, and they should be educated about the risks associated with touching sores. Infants with cellulitis may be more susceptible to sepsis because their immune systems cannot protect them from infection. Facial cellulitis is most common in children under 3 years of age and in adults over age 50. Facial cellulitis may lead to the development of meningitis, so patients with facial cellulitis should be closely monitored.

One study reviewed the incidence of fetal demise in pregnant women with submandibular cellulitis (Mukherjee, Sharma, & Maru, 2013). Poor hygiene that results in cellulitis in a pregnant woman presents a challenge to safe care, and untreated infection can potentially result in fetal septicemia. Cellulitis in a pregnant woman requires an interprofessional team for management and treatment.

Older adults and adults with poor circulation, diabetes, or a weakened immune system may develop cellulitis without loss of skin integrity. These individuals are more likely to develop severe cellulitis with complications than are younger adults with no medical conditions. Older adults and those with poor circulation are also more likely to get recurrent cellulitis. Complications from sinus infections can lead to orbital and periorbital cellulitis, which can lead to loss of vision if not treated aggressively.

NURSING PROCESS

The nurse plays an important role in assessing the status of the patient and teaching self-care to prevent complications.

Assessment

Assessment centers on recognizing infection, documenting location and related symptoms, and monitoring vital signs. The nurse should assess the patient's health history to determine whether the patient has any underlying conditions that may increase susceptibility to cellulitis.

■ **Observation and patient interview.** The health history should include a patient interview to determine the cause of any skin wound, such as a cut, bite, or other injury. It is also important to determine whether the wound has been exposed to contaminated water, such as a wound that occurred while swimming in a lake. This may help to determine the causative organism and affect the choice of antibiotic. The nurse should conduct an overall observation of the patient's current status, such as skin color, malaise, fatigue, ability to fully answer questions, and the patient's understanding of the reason for the visit to the clinic or hospital setting. Other observations are included in the physical examination below. Inquire when the patient noticed the infection and how rapidly the affected area has spread. During the health history, also assess additional symptoms such as pain, muscle aches, stiffness, and nausea. Note any history of other conditions that may increase susceptibility to infection, such as diabetes, poor circulation, HIV, cancer treatments, and immunosuppression.

- **Physical examination.** A physical examination should include assessment of vital signs, especially fever, and a thorough assessment of the affected area. The assessment should include observation of redness, swelling, warmth, and size of the affected area. For patients in the hospital, the nurse should assess the affected site frequently (at least every 2 hours), including tracing along the border with a marker so that any change in size can be clearly recognized. In the event of change, the nurse places a new mark so that future care providers can clearly see if the wound enlarges. Physical assessment may also include observation of lines radiating from the site, indicating involvement of the lymphatic system, and obtaining blood and wound drainage specimens for diagnostic testing.

Diagnosis

Nursing diagnoses that may be appropriate for a patient with cellulitis:

- *Skin Integrity, Impaired*
- *Pain, Acute*
- *Family Processes, Interrupted*

  (NANDA-I © 2014)

Planning

Planning care for the patient with cellulitis is directed at pain management, patient teaching related to self-care, and infection resolution without progression to systemic infection. Potential outcomes may include the following:

- The patient will report pain of 3 or lower, on a scale of 0–10.
- The patient will describe situations requiring contact with the provider.
- The patient will explain how to take antibiotics and analgesics properly.

- The patient will demonstrate understanding of proper wound care and infection-control processes.

Implementation

Because of the risk of sepsis, cellulitis is managed carefully. The nurse should administer prescribed oral or IV antibiotics as scheduled. Supportive care includes warm compresses to the affected area four times daily, elevation of the affected limb, and bedrest. Outpatient follow-up is crucial to ensure positive response to therapy.

Advise the patient about possible complications, such as abscess formation, and to contact the healthcare provider if any of the following signs develop:

- Spread of the infected area in the 24- to 48-hour period after the start of treatment
- Temperature over 38.3°C (101°F)
- Increased lethargy.

Reinforce with the patient and caregivers the importance of compliance with the treatment regimen and the seriousness of the possible complications.

Because it is anticipated that the patient will need to take part in self-care of the cellulitis, patient teaching is particularly important. Patient teaching begins early in the acute care stay, as soon as the appropriate treatment plan has been identified and discharge plans are in place (Herchline, 2016). Patients being transferred to a skilled facility will rely upon agency staff for much of their wound care, but they will still need to maintain infection-control practices on their own. Patients who are going home need to fully understand safe practices concerning infection-control and self-care. See the Patient Teaching feature for more information.

Evaluation

Outcomes developed in collaboration with the patient are evaluated to determine the patient's progress. The provider should be notified if the cellulitis enlarges or spreads.

Patient Teaching

Infection-Control in Patients with Cellulitis

Infection-control in patients with cellulitis includes hand hygiene and wound care.

Hand Hygiene

- Scrub hands with soap and water for 20 seconds before and after touching the infected area; wash under rings, around cuticles, between fingers, and under fingernails. Dry hands thoroughly after washing.
- Do not touch the affected area and then touch another susceptible area such as an uninfected wound or mucous membranes such as the eyes, mouth, or anus.
- Wash hands before, during, and after handling food, including eating.
- Wash hands after toileting or changing a child's diaper.
- Wash hands after touching the eyes, nose, or mouth.
- Wash hands after touching waste products, including household garbage, animal waste, and contaminated materials.

Wound Care

- Wash the wound with soap and water at least once daily.
- Using cleansing techniques, clear away any dead skin or purulent drainage.
- Apply an antibiotic ointment and sterile bandage to the wound after washing.
- Do not touch the wound unless medically necessary, such as when washing or assessing the wound.
- Dispose of all contaminated materials properly.
- Monitor the size of the affected area to assess treatment effectiveness.
- Keep the wound at a proper moisture as instructed; wet or moist wounds heal faster than dry wounds.

Possible expected outcomes include

- The patient reports pain of 3 or lower, on a scale of 0–10.
- The patient describes situations that require alerting the healthcare provider.
- The patient adheres to the medication schedule.
- The patient demonstrates understanding of proper wound care and infection-control processes.

If the infection continues to spread and current wound care practices are not demonstrating improvement in the wound site, the patient may need to be hospitalized. This is a concern in the modern healthcare environment, as a patient readmission within 30 days for the same diagnostic issue may result in hospital financial risk, particularly if the patient is a Medicare recipient (Bushnell, 2014). Older adults are at increased risk of readmission, which makes concise discharge instruction and timely follow-up important to reduce readmission. In the case of cellulitis, a patient would be evaluated upon admission for further diagnostic workup and possible change to the antibiotic therapies (Herchline, 2016). In addition, medical evaluation may include possible surgical intervention for loss of limb integrity or gangrene in the wound site.

Nursing Care Plan
A Patient with Cellulitis

Maria Gonzalez is a 74-year-old widow who lives in an assisted living facility in a small town in central Pennsylvania. Her family includes three daughters and two sons who live out of state and a son who lives within 5 miles of Ms. Gonzalez's home. While visiting his mother, the son who lives locally notices a red area on her lower leg and asks her about it. She says it developed earlier today and is very painful. She's been treating it with wet compresses, but that does not seem to be helping much. Her son takes her to the local emergency department, where the nurse admits her to one of the examination rooms.

ASSESSMENT

Ms. Gonzalez speaks Spanish and is able to communicate only minimally in English. Although this arrangement is not ideal, her son acts as an interpreter when necessary. Ms. Gonzalez's history reveals diabetes mellitus with complications of peripheral vascular disease and neuropathy in the right leg, hypertension, coronary artery disease with angina, and cataracts in both eyes. She says she is allergic to penicillin and sulfa drugs. She denies ever having had a similar wound and describes the pain as a 7 on a scale of 0–10.

Physical examination of the painful right leg reveals an irregularly shaped, flat area that is red, warm, and painful, extending from just below the knee to mid-shin, and wrapping medially from midline to the back of the leg. The wound measures 6 in. by 5 in. at its widest point. Her vital signs are T 100.8°F oral, P 88 bpm, R 16/min, and BP 122/74 mmHg.

The healthcare provider orders laboratory studies that reveal an elevated WBC count. Because of Ms. Gonzalez's age and medical history, the healthcare provider orders blood cultures and admits her to the facility for IV antibiotics and monitoring.

DIAGNOSES

- *Impaired Skin Integrity* related to the infectious process
- *Acute Pain* related to the inflammatory process secondary to cellulitis
- *Deficient Knowledge* of the cause of the skin disorder and recommended treatment
- *Anxiety* related to the need to be admitted to the hospital and inability to communicate with staff
- *Impaired Verbal Communication* related to the inability to speak English

(NANDA-I © 2014)

PLANNING

- Skin will heal without evidence of a secondary infection or complication of sepsis.
- The patient will obtain relief of pain with the proper use of medications.
- The patient will verbalize an understanding of the disease process and participate in the treatment plan.
- The patient will describe proper home care, including self-administration of medication after discharge.
- The patient's anxiety will be reduced after orientation to the hospital environment and speaking with staff members who also speak Spanish.
- Communication will be improved when a Spanish-speaking nurse is assigned and the hospital's translation services are used.

IMPLEMENTATION

- Provide orientation to facility and treatment plan (IV therapy, warm soaks) in Spanish.
- Keep the right leg elevated, and explain the need to stay in bed.
- Trace the outer border of the wound with black marker, and avoid washing off marks to allow for assessment every 2 hours. Report any increase in size to the provider.
- Provide verbal and written instructions (in Spanish) for self-care after discharge, including the following:
  a. Take all antibiotics prescribed until they are gone.
  b. Take medications as prescribed for pain.
  c. Take the antibiotic every 6 hours, even during nighttime hours, for 10 days.
  d. Monitor the size of the wound and notify the healthcare provider if there is any increase or if fever returns.
  e. Apply warm, moist heat to the wound four times a day.
  f. Wash hands carefully before applying warm, moist compresses.
  g. Reduce activity to bathroom privileges only and keep the right leg elevated.
  h. Monitor oral temperature and take two acetaminophen (Tylenol) for a temperature higher than 100°F orally.

(continued on next page)

Nursing Care Plan *(continued)*

EVALUATION

Ms. Gonzalez's wound decreased in size over the next 48 hours. She was discharged with a prescription for antibiotics to be taken orally for 10 days and pain medication, although she reported that the pain was almost gone by the time she went home. Her fever subsided within 36 hours of beginning treatment. Ms. Gonzalez will see her healthcare provider at the completion of oral antibiotics and says she will call the office sooner if the wound increases in size or her fever returns.

CRITICAL THINKING

1. Identify barriers to care in this case, including those related to communication. What nursing interventions can be initiated to overcome these barriers?

2. What further assessments and interventions might have been indicated if the wound had shown little improvement or the pain had remained severe?

3. If Ms. Gonzalez were unable to provide self-care after discharge, what options might the nurse have recommended for her?

REVIEW Cellulitis

RELATE Link the Concepts and Exemplars

Linking the exemplar of cellulitis with the concept of comfort:

1. What teaching interventions will you provide the patient with cellulitis of the leg who is taking a narcotic for pain?

2. What nonpharmacologic interventions will you implement for the patient experiencing pain from cellulitis?

Linking the exemplar of cellulitis with the concept of perfusion:

3. How will you assess perfusion in the patient with cellulitis of the thigh?

4. What symptoms of perfusion will you teach the patient with cellulitis to report to the healthcare provider immediately?

READY Go to Volume 3: Clinical Nursing Skills

REFER Go to Pearson MyLab Nursing and eText

- Additional review materials

REFLECT Apply Your Knowledge

Norma James is a 65-year-old widow who lives alone. Although she has lived in the neighborhood for years, she is somewhat socially isolated. She has two adult sons with whom she has limited contact because they live out of state and rarely call. She has only a few individuals she considers friends; she does not particularly like many people and prefers the company of her six cats.

Ms. James has a long history of type 2 diabetes mellitus and hypertension. In more recent years, she has been diagnosed with atrial fibrillation. She has multiple healthcare providers and takes multiple medications, including glipizide, 10 mg, twice a day; captopril, 50 mg, twice a day; digoxin, 125 mcg, once a day; and coumadin, 5 mg, once a day. Ms. James has a known drug allergy to penicillin.

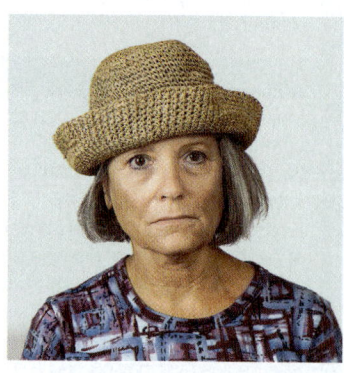

Ms. James does not work; she has very limited savings and relies on Social Security benefits for income. She smokes about half a pack of cigarettes a day and has been a smoker since she was in her 20s. She drinks alcohol "a couple times a year, usually a glass of wine at a special dinner."

She does not drive and relies on her friends, neighbors, or the city bus for transportation. She lives near a grocery store and prides herself on being able to get most things she needs without assistance. She spends most of her time alone at home and occupies herself by watching television, reading, and doing crossword and jigsaw puzzles.

Ms. James noticed a small, tender area on her ankle yesterday and, remembering what the cashier at the convenience store told her, decided to apply butter to the wound.

1. What factors in Ms. James's history put her at risk for cellulitis?

2. What do you suspect may be the outcome of applying butter to this wound?

3. What patient teaching would you provide Ms. James?

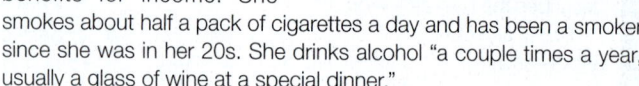

≫ Exemplar 9.B
Conjunctivitis

Exemplar Learning Outcomes

9.B Analyze conjunctivitis as it relates to infection.

- Describe the pathophysiology of conjunctivitis.
- Describe the etiology of conjunctivitis.
- Compare the risk factors and prevention of conjunctivitis.
- Identify the clinical manifestations of conjunctivitis.
- Summarize diagnostic tests and therapies used by interprofessional teams in the collaborative care of an individual with conjunctivitis.

- Differentiate care of patients with conjunctivitis across the lifespan.
- Apply the nursing process in providing culturally competent care to an individual with conjunctivitis.

Overview

The conjunctiva—the thin, transparent membrane that covers the anterior surface of the eye and lines the inner surfaces of the eyelids—is vulnerable to inflammation and infection because of its constant exposure to the environment. **Conjunctivitis** (inflammation of the conjunctiva) is the most common eye disease. It can be caused by bacteria and viruses that are transmitted to the eye by direct contact (e.g., hands, tissues, towels). Allergens, chemical irritants, and exposure to radiant energy, such as ultraviolet light from the sun or tanning devices, can also lead to this common condition. Conjunctivitis caused by allergens, irritants, or radiant energy exposure is not contagious; however, viral and bacterial conjunctivitis can be easily spread from person to person and can cause epidemics (CDC, 2014). The severity of conjunctivitis can range from mild irritation with redness and tearing to conjunctival edema, hemorrhage, or a severe necrotizing process with tissue destruction. While viral and bacterial conjunctivitis appear more frequently among neonates and children, this infection can occur at any age, and parents of children with conjunctivitis are at risk for exposure (Shultz & Adam, 2015). See the Lifespan Considerations section for more information.

Pathophysiology and Etiology

Pathophysiology

There are several types of conjunctivitis, depending on the cause of inflammation. Bacteria, viruses, allergies, trauma, or irritants cause the conjunctiva to become edematous, inflamed, and reddened, with a yellow or white discharge (see **Figure 9–12** »). Patients commonly

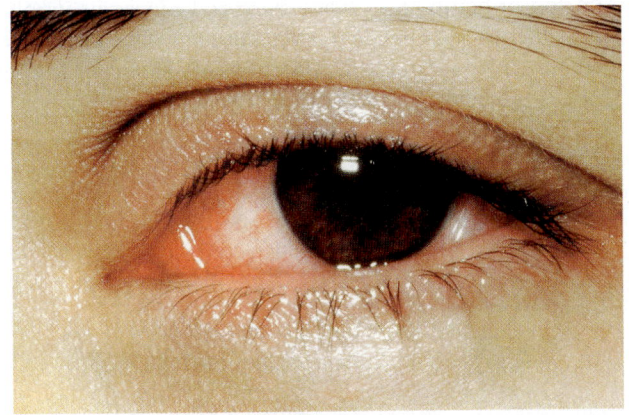

Source: Mediscan/Alamy Stock Photo.

Figure 9–12 » Acute conjunctivitis. The major difference between bacterial and viral conjunctivitis is that bacterial conjunctivitis has a purulent discharge that may result in crusting, whereas the discharge from viral conjunctivitis is serous (watery). Allergic conjunctivitis produces watery to thick drainage and is characterized by itching.

refer to conjunctivitis as "pink eye." The cause of the redness, swelling, itching, and discomfort is inflammation or injury of the conjunctiva (CDC, 2014).

Etiology

Redness of the eye may result from various conditions (see **Table 9–10** »), so do not assume that redness always signals conjunctivitis. Common bacteria that cause conjunctivitis include *Staphylococcus aureus*, *Haemophilus* species, *Streptococcus pneumoniae*, and *Pseudomonas aeruginosa* (CDC, 2012a). Hand-to-eye contact causes most cases. The disease can spread rapidly when groups of youth spend time together, such as young children and adolescents in schools and child care centers and college students in dormitories or on sports teams. The infection can be bilateral but is more commonly unilateral.

Viruses can cause other infections in newborns and children. Viral conjunctivitis is commonly bilateral. Adenovirus is a common cause and spreads hand-to-eye from respiratory adenovirus infection.

Herpes simplex virus (HSV) can also cause infections, either by transfer to a neonate during birth from a mother with herpes infection, or by contact of infants or children of any age with an infected individual. Any age group can contract an HSV infection in the eye, with some reports noting it is more common in adults in their 30s–40s (American Association for Pediatric Ophthalmology and Strabismus, 2014). Ophthalmic herpes infection is often accompanied by characteristic vesicular lesions on the skin of the face. A culture of the lesion is performed for diagnosis, and any accompanying conjunctivitis is assumed to be caused by herpes virus. The infection caused by HSV needs prompt and vigorous treatment to prevent eye injury or blindness, which can occur in children with recurrent herpes virus infections as a result of antibody reaction to the viral antigen. Older adults who contract HSV infection will have a prior history of herpes virus (American Association for Pediatric Ophthalmology and Strabismus, 2014). Herpes virus infections commonly recur, so periodic treatment and sometimes prophylaxis may be needed.

Allergic conjunctivitis is a common cause of eye discomfort. When conjunctivitis is caused by an allergy, the patient complains of intense itching. Examination reveals reddened eyes with watery discharge and conjunctivae with a "cobblestone" appearance. The eyes may also appear edematous.

Risk Factors

Patients who wear contact lenses, especially extended-wear lenses, are at higher risk for conjunctivitis. Others at risk include young children in school and child care settings and patients with compromised immune response. The most common occurrence of viral conjunctivitis is seen in children with viral upper respiratory infections.

TABLE 9–10 Possible Causes of Acute Red Eye

	Acute Conjunctivitis	Corneal Trauma or Infection	Acute Uveitis	Acute Angle-Closure Glaucoma
Incidence	Very common	Common	Common	Rare
Pain	Mild	Moderate to severe	Moderate	Severe
Vision	Normal	Blurred	Blurred	Markedly blurred
Discharge	May be copious	Watery, may be purulent	None	None
Conjunctival Erythema	Diffuse	Primarily around cornea	Primarily around cornea	Primarily around cornea
Cornea	Clear	Depends on cause	Usually clear	Cloudy
Pupils	Normal size, response to light	Normal size, response to light	Small, minimal response to light	Moderately dilated, fixed

Prevention

Bacterial and viral conjunctivitis is highly contagious; therefore, infection-control strategies are vital to the prevention of conjunctivitis. For individuals who are infected, transmission to others can be decreased by good hand hygiene techniques, avoiding touching the eyes, washing discharge from the eyes several times daily, washing linens frequently, not sharing towels or other objects that have touched the eyes, and not sharing eyedrop dispensers between infected and uninfected eyes. For an individual who is around someone with conjunctivitis, prevention techniques include thorough hand hygiene, especially after contact with an infected individual, and avoiding sharing with the infected individual any items that touch the face, such as towels, makeup, or pillows (CDC, 2014).

Although no vaccine is available that protects against all types of conjunctivitis, vaccines are available for conjunctivitis related to rubella, measles, chickenpox, shingles, *Streptococcus pneumoniae,* and *Haemophilus influenzae* type b (CDC, 2014).

Clinical Manifestations

Redness and itching of the affected eye are common manifestations of acute conjunctivitis. The patient may also complain of a scratchy, burning, or gritty sensation. Although pain is not common, **photophobia** (sensitivity to light) may occur. Tearing and discharge accompany the inflammatory process. The discharge may be watery, purulent, or mucoid, depending on the cause of the conjunctivitis. The patient may have associated manifestations, such as pharyngitis, fever, malaise, and swollen preauricular lymph nodes.

Early manifestations of **trachoma**, which is a chronic conjunctivitis caused by *Chlamydia trachomatis,* include redness, eyelid edema, tearing, and photophobia. Small conjunctival follicles develop on the upper lids. The inflammation also causes superficial corneal vascularization and infiltration with granulation tissue. The sclera will have a cobblestone appearance due to inflammation (Shultz & Adam, 2015). Scarring of the conjunctival lining of the lid causes **entropion** (inversion of the eyelid) (see **Figure 9–13 »**). The lashes then abrade the cornea, eventually causing ulceration and scarring. The opacity of the scarred cornea results in loss of vision (see the Focus on Diversity and Culture feature).

Collaboration

Collaboration with an ophthalmologist may be indicated if involvement of the cornea is suspected. A nurse in a pediatric practice who observes a number of children from a single school or child care setting presenting with conjunctivitis may want to contact the school or child care nurse or health coordinator to discuss increased prevention and student education.

Diagnostic Tests

Accurate diagnosis of conjunctivitis is especially important, because other potentially vision-threatening conditions, such as acute **uveitis** (inflammation of the middle layer of the eye, called the *uvea*) or acute angle-closure glaucoma, can also cause a red eye (see Table 9–10). In most cases, a diagnosis of the cause of conjunctivitis is based on the patient's history and presenting symptoms.

In severe cases, diagnostic procedures may include the following:

- *Culture and sensitivity* of exudates to determine presence of an infection and identify the infecting organism. Cultures are taken especially in infants or in cases suspected of being an unusual bacterial illness or involving herpes viruses. A Gram stain of discharge and conjunctival scraping for potential *Chlamydia* or herpes

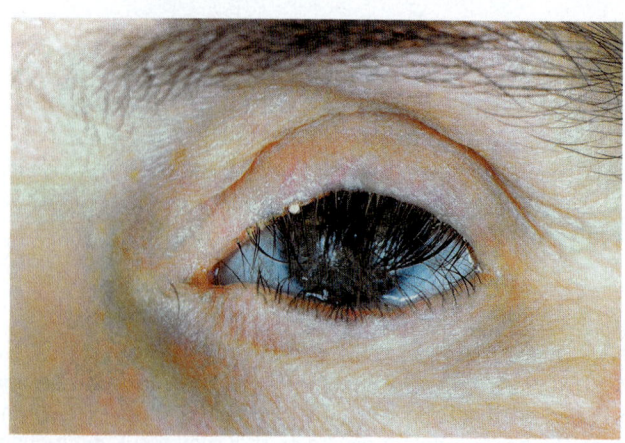

Source: Mediscan/Alamy Stock Photo.

Figure 9–13 » Entropion.

Focus on Diversity and Culture
Trachoma

Trachoma is a chronic conjunctivitis caused by *Chlamydia trachomatis* that is endemic in 41 countries and has caused the blinding or visual impairment of 1.9 million people worldwide. The World Health Organization (n.d.) launched the WHO Alliance for the Global Elimination of Trachoma by the year 2020 (GET2020) in 1997 to eliminate this public health problem. The methods used are improving access to water and sanitation, encouraging facial cleanliness, treating infected individuals with antibiotics, and providing surgery for those who have reached the blinding stage of the disease.

virus is performed. Cultures, if ordered, should be obtained before the start of treatment.

- *Fluorescein stain* with slit-lamp examination to identify possible corneal ulcerations or abrasions, which appear green with staining.
- *Conjunctival scrapings*, which are examined microscopically or cultured to identify the organisms.

Additional laboratory testing, such as blood counts or antibody titers, may be used to identify underlying infectious or autoimmune processes.

Pharmacologic Therapy

Conjunctivitis is treated with antibiotic, antiviral, or anti-inflammatory drugs as appropriate. Topical anti-infectives, applied as either eyedrops or ointment, may include erythromycin, azithromycin, gentamicin, tobramycin, neomycin, ciprofloxacin, ofloxacin, bacitracin, sulfacetamide sodium, amphotericin B, or trifluridine. The fluoroquinolones (e.g., ciprofloxacin, ofloxacin) are broad-spectrum antibiotics that are effective against both gram-positive and gram-negative organisms. For severe infections or cellulitis, anti-infectives may be administered orally, by

subconjunctival injection, or by systemic IV infusion (see the Medications feature).

SAFETY ALERT In July 2016, the Food and Drug Administration issued a safety warning regarding the fluoroquinolones and their association with disabling and potentially permanent side effects and to limit their use in patients with less serious bacterial infections. A safety review by the Food and Drug Administration found that both oral and injectable fluoroquinolones are associated with disabling side effects involving tendons, muscles, joints, nerves, and the CNS (Food and Drug Administration, 2016). Retrieved from: http://www.fda.gov/NewsEvents/Newsroom/PressAnnouncements/ucm513183.htm

Viral infections are usually not treated with pharmacologic therapy, except for herpes simplex infections. Individuals with herpes simplex conjunctivitis should be taught how to look for characteristic herpes simplex lesions and to report all lesions immediately.

SAFETY ALERT Conjunctivitis due to herpes simplex virus infection can cause scarring of the cornea that leads to a permanent loss of vision. Therefore, all HSV eye infections should be treated with antiviral medications (e.g., acyclovir) and infection-control techniques to prevent the spread of HSV to others.

Nonpharmacologic Therapies

Frequent eye irrigations may be ordered to remove the copious purulent discharge associated with bacterial conjunctivitis. Soaking the lids with warm saline compresses before cleansing promotes comfort and facilitates the removal of crusts and exudate in conjunctivitis. Viral conjunctivitis may be treated by use of a warm clean cloth to clean drainage away and by avoiding bright lights and reading. Cool compresses applied to the eyes help to relieve the feeling of eye irritation.

Clinical Manifestations and Therapies
Conjunctivitis

ETIOLOGY	CLINICAL MANIFESTATIONS	CLINICAL THERAPIES
Allergic conjunctivitis	Redness, itching	Topical antihistamines; topical NSAIDs
Bacterial conjunctivitis	Redness, purulent drainage, burning/irritation, sore throat, photophobia	▪ Antibiotic eyedrops or ointment ▪ Soaking eyelids with warm cloth ▪ Eye irrigation to remove discharge ▪ Avoiding bright lights ▪ Infection-control techniques ▪ Cool compresses
Viral conjunctivitis	Redness, serous drainage, burning/irritation, sore throat, photophobia	▪ Antiviral drugs (HSV only) ▪ Cool compresses ▪ Avoiding bright lights ▪ Infection-control techniques ▪ Removing discharge with wet cloth

Lifespan Considerations

As mentioned previously, conjunctivitis occurs in all age groups, from neonates to older adults (CDC, 2014). Treatment and management of this infection depends, in part, on the age of the patient.

Conjunctivitis in Neonates and Infants

All neonates born in the United States receive prophylactic treatment to prevent conjunctivitis. By federal law, all infants are given prophylactic eye treatment soon after delivery. The nurse is responsible for administering this eye ointment. Erythromycin is the most common ointment used, but penicillin, tetracycline, or povidone-iodine ointments may also be used. Sometimes an infant develops chemical conjunctivitis due to the prophylactic eye ointment. A chemical reaction should be considered as a possible cause when conjunctivitis develops within 24–48 hours after instillation of this medication.

Conjunctivitis in an infant under 30 days of age is called *ophthalmia neonatorum*. These infections are usually acquired from the mother during vaginal delivery as a result of contact with vaginal discharge containing bacterial organisms such as *Chlamydia trachomatis* and *Neisseria gonorrhoeae*. Contact with genital secretions infected with *Gonococcus* species can cause gonococcal conjunctivitis, a medical emergency that can lead to corneal perforation. Ceftriaxone is recommended for gonococcal conjunctivitis in newborns because that particular disease is resistant to penicillin. Chlamydial infections are treated with oral erythromycin or tetracycline. Herpes simplex virus infections of the eye are treated promptly by an ophthalmologist, neonatologist, or others who are trained in this serious disease. Neonatal HSV is treated vigorously with parenteral acyclovir for 14 days (or longer if lumbar puncture reveals CNS involvement) and with topical ophthalmic medication (trifluridine, iododeoxyuridine, or vidarabine). Careful total evaluation of the newborn with any type of conjunctivitis is important to show any other signs of infection.

In infants who have frequent tearing and mattering (eyelid discharge that has formed a crust) on awakening, a plugged lacrimal duct may be mimicking conjunctivitis.

Conjunctivitis in Children

Bacterial conjunctivitis is common in older children. It is characterized by edema of the eyelid, reddened conjunctiva, and enlarged preauricular lymph glands. Mucopurulent discharge causes matting and makes the eyes difficult to open upon awakening. Older children with conjunctivitis complain of itching or burning, mild photophobia, and a feeling of scratching under the lids. The close contact children commonly have in child care and school settings allows easy infection with conjunctivitis. Children are also less likely to cleanse their hands after touching objects or other people prior to putting their fingers in their eyes or mouth (CDC, 2014).

Conjunctivitis in Older Adults

Older adults may experience conjunctivitis secondary to problems with their immune system or other chronic illnesses influencing their immunity. Close contact with young family members at home or visitors in a long-term care facility may result in viral or bacterial conjunctivitis. Exposure to irritants and strong odors, such as cleaning products or chemical solutions, can cause allergic conjunctivitis (Shultz & Adam, 2015).

NURSING PROCESS

The nursing role in treating conjunctivitis is primarily one of education to prevent both the disorder itself and its spread when it does occur. Education is a vital strategy for preventing conjunctivitis. Teach all patients about proper eye care, including the importance of not sharing towels, makeup, or contact lenses, as well as avoiding rubbing or scratching the eyes. Instruct patients to avoid using old eye makeup, which can cause eye infections.

Assessment

Collect the following data through the health history and physical examination of patients with conjunctivitis:

- **Observation and patient interview.** To assess for the presence of conjunctivitis, check for the presence of redness, discomfort, tearing, photophobia, and drainage. Also, ask patients to describe in their own terms how the symptoms feel to them. Interview the patients to ascertain the symptoms and possible contact that could have caused the infection. Ask the patients to describe the symptom onset and how long between each symptom was noticed, such as redness, itching, pain, and so forth. Then ask the patients to describe current care measures in use at home. Nurses need to know if patients report routine use of contact lenses, and plan accordingly for patient education. To ascertain exposure to "pink eye," ask about recent contacts with others who may have had symptoms and also any recent travel. Ask patients to list all known allergies, as well as previous history of conjunctivitis. Ask patients about the presence of any chronic diseases, and identify what those diseases are and medications taken to manage those diseases.

- **Physical examination.** To complete the physical examination, determine visual acuity, which can be done by having patients read from a paper and/or follow a pen in your hand as you move it up and down. Be sure to don gloves prior to each assessment. Inspect the eyelids, the conjunctiva, the sclera, and the cornea. This assessment concerns the color and the texture of the various parts of the eye as well as the presence and type of discharge (i.e., serous versus purulent). In addition, collect vital signs, including temperature, pulse, and blood pressure.

Diagnosis

Nursing diagnoses relevant to the plan of care for patients with conjunctivitis may include the following:

- *Infection, Risk for*
- *Comfort, Impaired*
- *Knowledge, Readiness for Enhanced.*

(NANDA-I © 2014)

Planning

Goals are created on the basis of each patient's needs and may include the following:

- The patient will demonstrate proper hand hygiene.
- The patient will avoid contaminating unaffected eye and other family members.
- The patient will experience no visual complications following recovery.

Implementation

Nursing care of the patient with conjunctivitis focuses primarily on preventing complications and on preventing the spread of infection to the other eye or to other individuals in close contact with the patient. Individualize care on the basis of specific needs of the patient.

Prevent Infection

Acute conjunctivitis is highly contagious. While most patients experience no more than discomfort from the disease, the infection carries a risk for scarring and damage to the delicate cornea of the eye. Preventing the spread of this infection is a vital nursing role.

When conjunctivitis is diagnosed in an infant in the neonatal ICU, the infant is isolated to prevent the spread of the disease to other infants. However, patients with conjunctivitis are typically treated in the community, where effective teaching for home care is required to prevent transmission of infection. Bacterial infectious conjunctivitis is extremely contagious.

The nurse can take the following steps to help prevent infection:

- Teach the patients to cleanse hands thoroughly before and after instilling eye medications. Hand hygiene is the single most important means of preventing transmission of infection.
- Instruct the patient to avoid touching or rubbing the eyes to reduce the risk of corneal trauma and spreading the infection. Mittens can be put on a young child to prevent spreading the infection.
- Advise the patient to use a new, clean, cotton-tipped swab or cotton ball for cleaning each eye, to prevent cross-contamination.
- Tell parents that the child should not return to child care or school until antibiotics have been taken for 24 hours.
- Advise the patient to avoid sharing towels.
- Teach the patient how to administer eye ointments and eyedrops as ordered (see the Patient Teaching box in the exemplar on Eye Injuries in the module on Sensory Perception). Prescribed medications reduce inflammation and eliminate infection.
- Discuss the importance of avoiding contact lens use until the infection has cleared.
- Teach contact lens users appropriate care of the lenses and lens case (see the Patient Teaching feature).

Promote Comfort

Nursing interventions to promote comfort in patients with conjunctivitis include gently washing drainage from the eyes

---

Patient Teaching
Contact Lens Care

- Cleanse hands thoroughly before handling contact lenses.
- Keep the storage case clean and replace it every 3 months.
- Remove lenses every night before sleep.
- Clean and store the lenses as recommended by the manufacturer.
- Use cleaning and wetting solutions recommended by an eye care professional or the lens manufacturer. Do not use water, saliva, or homemade solutions for wetting or cleaning lenses.
- If eye redness, tearing, vision loss, discharge, or pain occurs, remove lenses and contact an eye care professional as soon as possible. Using contact lenses during an eye infection can lead to further damage and interfere with healing.
- Do not share contact lenses or allow another individual to "try on" your lenses.

Source: Food and Drug Administration, 2015.

---

with a warm cloth; applying a cool compress to reduce itching, burning, or other discomforts; and administering pain medications and anti-infective agents as prescribed. If photophobia accompanies conjunctivitis, the nurse can recommend that the patient avoid high-acuity activities and use dark sunglasses with ultraviolet protection when outdoors or in bright light.

Community-Based Care

The patient with conjunctivitis typically is treated in the community, so the patient needs effective teaching for home care. The nurse should emphasize to the family ways to prevent transmission of infection. If the patient is unable to administer eye medications, the nurse should involve the family in teaching, including the following topics:

- Safety and medical asepsis when cleansing the eye
- Instillation of prescribed eyedrops and ointments
- Comfort measures such as reducing lighting intensity and wearing sunglasses
- Avoidance of activities such as excessive reading while the eye is inflamed.

Evaluation

Patients are evaluated on the basis of the outcomes created during the planning process. Resolution of the infection is indicated by return of conjunctiva to a normal white color, absence of drainage, and elimination of symptoms. Expected outcomes may include that

- The patient demonstrates proper hand hygiene.
- The patient avoids contaminating the unaffected eye and other family members.
- The patient experiences no visual complications following recovery.

REVIEW Conjunctivitis

RELATE Link the Concepts and Exemplars

Linking the exemplar of conjunctivitis with the concept of development:

1. What strategies can you use to stop eye rubbing in children with conjunctivitis who are in different developmental stages?

2. What cognitive developmental issues will the nurse anticipate for a child with recurrent conjunctivitis?

Linking the exemplar of conjunctivitis with the concept of health, wellness, and illness:

3. What strategies could the school nurse teach students to prevent conjunctivitis?

4. When teaching infant care to a group of new parents, what important strategy will you demonstrate to reduce the risk of conjunctivitis?

READY Go to Volume 3: Clinical Nursing Skills

REFER Go to Pearson MyLab Nursing and eText

- Additional review materials

REFLECT Apply Your Knowledge

Marcus Young is a typical 6-year-old boy who is enrolled in first grade. He likes his teacher at school and has many friends. He has a stable home life and is close to his parents, Angie and Steve, and his sister, Kelsey. He loves to read and to go to the park and play on the playground equipment. He is very interested in sports and wants to play football and baseball someday. He takes piano lessons but is not interested in this activity at all.

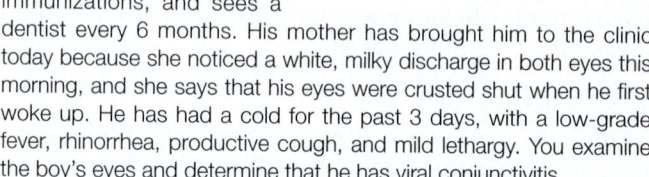

Marcus is normally healthy, is up to date on his immunizations, and sees a dentist every 6 months. His mother has brought him to the clinic today because she noticed a white, milky discharge in both eyes this morning, and she says that his eyes were crusted shut when he first woke up. He has had a cold for the past 3 days, with a low-grade fever, rhinorrhea, productive cough, and mild lethargy. You examine the boy's eyes and determine that he has viral conjunctivitis.

1. What patient teaching will you provide this family to prevent others from contracting this infection?

2. What teaching will you provide to Mrs. Young regarding how to care for Marcus's conjunctivitis?

3. Develop a nursing plan of care for Marcus.

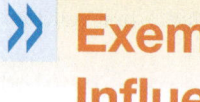

Exemplar 9.C
Influenza

Exemplar Learning Outcomes

9.C Analyze influenza as it relates to infection.

- Describe the pathophysiology of influenza.
- Describe the etiology of influenza.
- Compare the risk factors and prevention of influenza.
- Identify the clinical manifestations of influenza.
- Summarize diagnostic tests and therapies used by interprofessional teams in the collaborative care of an individual with influenza.
- Differentiate care of patients with influenza across the lifespan.
- Apply the nursing process in providing culturally competent care to an individual with influenza.

Exemplar Key Terms

Antigenic drift, *607*
Antigenic shift, *607*
Atelectasis, *611*
Avian influenza, *606*
Coryza, *606*
Epidemic, *606*
H1N1 influenza, *606*
Influenza, *606*
Malaise, *606*
Pandemic, *606*
Rhinorrhea, *607*

Overview

Influenza, or "the flu," is a highly contagious, viral respiratory disease characterized by **coryza** (inflammation of the mucous membranes lining the nose, usually associated with nasal discharge), fever, cough, and systemic symptoms, such as headache and **malaise** (a vague feeling of physical discomfort). Influenza tends to be mild and self-limited in healthy adults. Children under the age of 5, older adults, those with compromised immune systems, pregnant women, and people with chronic heart or pulmonary disease, however, have a high incidence of complications (e.g., pneumonia) and a higher risk for mortality related to the disease and its complications (CDC, 2017a).

Influenza usually occurs as an **epidemic** (widespread outbreak of an infectious disease) or a **pandemic** (global epidemic), although sporadic cases do occur. Localized outbreaks of influenza usually occur approximately every 1–3 years. The most recent pandemic incidence of influenza occurred in 2009 with the outbreak of H1N1. **H1N1 influenza** (popularly but incorrectly known as "swine flu") is a form of the virus that consists of avian genes, human genes, and genes from flu viruses typically found in pigs from Asia and Europe. H1N1, like all flu viruses, spreads from human to human via airborne droplets (Townsend, 2014).

Avian influenza (bird influenza) has also raised concerns about a potential future pandemic. The avian flu virus has demonstrated limited ability to spread between humans; however, the possibility that it will mutate to allow wider individual-to-individual spread is a concern. This viral strain has a mortality rate of greater than 50% in people who have been infected as a result of close association with infected birds. (See **Box 9–4** >> for more information about avian influenza.)

Pathophysiology and Etiology

Pathophysiology

The incubation period for influenza is short, only 18–72 hours. The virus infects the respiratory epithelium. It rapidly replicates in infected cells and is released to infect neighboring cells. The resulting inflammation leads to necrosis and shedding of serous and ciliated cells of the respiratory tract, a process that allows extracellular fluid to escape, producing **rhinorrhea** (runny nose). With recovery, serous cells are replaced more rapidly than ciliated cells, and the result is continued cough and coryza. Systemic symptoms of influenza are likely caused by release of inflammatory mediators (Longo et al., 2012) as the influenza infection activates humoral and cell-mediated immune responses.

The respiratory epithelial necrosis caused by influenza increases the risk for secondary bacterial infections. Sinusitis and otitis media are frequent complications of influenza. Tracheobronchitis (inflammation of the trachea and bronchi) may develop. Although tracheobronchitis is not a serious health risk, its manifestations may persist for up to 3 weeks.

Influenza is clearly linked to an increased risk for pneumonia, particularly in young children and older adults. Narrower airways and underdeveloped alveoli increase the risk for pneumonia in young children. Changes in respiratory function associated with aging, including decreased effectiveness of cough and increased residual lung volume (the volume of air remaining in the lung after exhalation), pose little risk in the healthy older adult but greatly increase the risk for pneumonia when associated with influenza. Primary influenza viral pneumonia, while uncommon, is a serious complication that may be fatal. It typically develops within 48 hours after the onset of influenza, often in patients with preexisting heart valve or pulmonary disease. Influenza pneumonia progresses rapidly and can cause hypoxemia and death within a few days. Bacterial pneumonia is more likely to occur in older at-risk adults but also may affect otherwise healthy adults. It usually presents as a relapse of influenza, with a productive cough and evidence of pneumonia on the chest x-ray. (See Exemplar 9.E on Pneumonia for more information.) Other respiratory complications of influenza include exacerbation of COPD, chronic bronchitis, or asthma.

Reye syndrome is a rare but potentially fatal complication of influenza. A neurologic disease that typically occurs following a viral infection, it is more likely to affect children but also has been identified in older adults. It is associated with administration of aspirin products to children with any viral infection, including influenza. Most often associated with influenza B virus, Reye syndrome develops within 2–3 weeks after the onset of influenza. It has a 30% mortality

Box 9–4
Focus on Influenza and its Potential for Pandemic

Influenza viruses are common in nature and found in wild birds, such as ducks and shore birds, and in some animals, such as pigs. Although wild birds and animals carry the virus, they usually are not harmed by it. Movement of the virus into domesticated animals, however, can be devastating to that animal population.

Three major strains of the virus have been identified as influenza A virus, influenza B virus, and influenza C virus. Type A influenza viruses are subclassified by two proteins found on the surface of the virus: hemagglutinin (HA) and neuraminidase (NA). HA allows the virus to attach to a cell and initiate an infection, whereas NA allows the virus to exit the host cell after replicating. Only three known subtypes of influenza A (H1N1, H1N2, and H3N2) are circulating currently among humans. The H5N1 virus, commonly called avian influenza, is particularly virulent and is spread by migratory birds. Almost all cases of H5N1 infection in people have been associated with close contact with infected live or dead birds, or H5N1-contaminated environments. The virus does not infect humans easily, and spread of the virus from person to person appears to be unusual (WHO, 2015). Influenza viruses are prone to undergoing small, continuous changes as well as occasional large and abrupt changes.

Antigenic drift is the term for small changes that occur continuously as a virus makes copies of itself. These changes help a virus elude the immune system and necessitate the production of new vaccines every year. Sudden, dramatic changes occur when two different strains of influenza virus (e.g., avian influenza and human influenza) infect the same cell and exchange genetic material. These changes, called **antigenic shift**, create a new subtype of a virus to which people have little or no immunity.

On April 29, 2009, the WHO raised its Influenza Pandemic Alert from Phase 4 to Phase 5 (indicating individual-to-individual contact of the virus in at least two countries of the same region) based on reported instances of H1N1 flu from around the world. By the next week, 23 countries had reported 1490 cases of H1N1 flu. It is important to note that the cases reported probably represent the most seriously ill people; milder infections may not be reflected in reported numbers. Early symptoms of H1N1 flu include runny nose, fever, cough, headache, muscle and joint pain, and, in some cases, gastrointestinal symptoms, such as diarrhea (MedicineNet. com, 2015). The vaccine for H1N1 is now included in the seasonal flu vaccine. An H5N1 vaccine is also available for high-risk patients, but it is not yet available in sufficient quantities should a pandemic occur. While the H1N1 flu is not considered a pandemic as of this writing, the CDC continues to monitor reports of this virus (Townsend, 2014).

A severe pandemic of any type of influenza could disrupt all aspects of life, causing not only severe illness and death but also overwhelming the healthcare system, affecting social services, and causing significant economic loss. Advance preparations such as those currently being undertaken by the WHO and the United States and other countries can reduce the impact of a pandemic.

>> **Stay Current:** Visit the CDC's website for updates on flu epidemics at http://www.cdc.gov/flu/

rate. Hepatic failure and encephalopathy develop rapidly in patients with Reye syndrome.

Other potential complications of influenza, while uncommon, include myositis (inflammation of skeletal muscles), myocarditis (inflammation of the heart muscle), and CNS disorders, such as encephalitis and Guillain-Barré syndrome.

Etiology

Influenza virus is transmitted by airborne droplet and direct contact. Influenza A is responsible for most infections and for the most severe outbreaks of influenza. This is primarily a result of its ability to alter its surface antigens, bypassing previously developed immune defenses to the virus. New strains of influenza virus are named according to the strain, geographic origin, and year the strain was identified (e.g., A/Taiwan/89). Surface antigens of the specific virus may be used to further differentiate influenza A viruses. Outbreaks of influenza B virus are generally less extensive and less severe than those caused by influenza A virus. Illness associated with influenza C virus is mild and often goes unrecognized.

Type A influenza viruses are found in birds, pigs, whales, and humans and are believed to have caused four pandemics (in 1918, 1957, 1968, and 2009). Type B influenza viruses are commonly found among humans and often are responsible for influenza outbreaks, but not pandemics. Type C influenza viruses, found in humans, pigs, and dogs, typically cause mild respiratory infections (Townsend, 2014).

Risk Factors

Individuals at increased risk for influenza or its complications include infants, young children, and anyone age 50 or older. Residents of nursing homes or other long-term care facilities are at increased risk because of their age as well as the increased risk of exposure from others (residents, visitors, and healthcare providers). Patients with chronic disorders, especially diabetes and cardiac, renal, or pulmonary diseases, are more susceptible as well. Pregnant women, particularly during the second and third trimesters, are also at increased risk of complications. As with any infection, patients with weakened or compromised immune systems, such as those diagnosed with AIDS, receiving treatment for cancer, or taking immunosuppressive medications, are at greatest risk. Healthcare providers who work in a facility where they are likely to be exposed to the influenza virus and child care providers or others who have close contact with infants and young children also face greater risk.

Prevention

Preventing community outbreaks and protecting vulnerable populations (e.g., older adults, individuals with chronic diseases) are the primary focus for interprofessional care related to influenza. Influenza vaccine is recommended for all individuals. The predominant strain of influenza virus varies from year to year. Therefore, a new vaccine formulation is prepared yearly, which incorporates antigens of the influenza strains predicted to be the most prevalent for the upcoming flu season (typically the winter months). The vaccine contains egg protein and is not recommended for

people who have a severe allergy to eggs or have previously experienced a severe hypersensitivity response to the vaccine. The vaccine is given in the fall, before the annual winter outbreak. Live attenuated vaccine, administered by intranasal spray, is available for healthy people under age 50. The effectiveness of the vaccine varies from year to year. The 2012–2013 seasonal flu vaccine, which contained vaccines against two influenza A viruses and one influenza B virus, was estimated to have a vaccine effectiveness rate of 56%, with effectiveness in the older population (age 65 and older) of only 9% (CDC, 2013b).

Although the CDC has recently changed its recommendations to include all individuals for annual influenza immunization, annual immunization is especially recommended for at-risk patients, including people older than the age of 65, residents of nursing homes, adults and children with chronic cardiopulmonary disorders (e.g., asthma) or chronic metabolic diseases (e.g., diabetes), and healthcare workers who have frequent contact with high-risk patients. In addition, family members of an at-risk patient should be vaccinated to reduce the patient's risk of exposure.

Although the vaccine is readily available and inexpensive, not everyone who is at risk will get the vaccine. Many may fear a reaction from the vaccine, even though these vaccines are highly purified and reactions are rare. Approximately 5% of individuals who are vaccinated experience mild symptoms of low-grade fever, malaise, or myalgia for up to 24 hours after vaccination. Serious adverse reactions to influenza vaccine are rare. *Guillain-Barré syndrome*, an acute neurologic disorder characterized by muscle weakness and distal sensory loss, has been associated with certain batches of vaccine.

Clinical Manifestations

Infection with influenza virus produces one of three syndromes: (1) uncomplicated nasopharyngeal inflammation, (2) viral upper respiratory infection followed by bacterial infection, or (3) viral pneumonia. The onset is rapid; profound malaise may develop in a matter of minutes.

Manifestations of influenza include abrupt onset of chills and fever, malaise, muscle aches, and headache. Respiratory manifestations include cough, sore throat, substernal burning, and coryza. The cough may be severe and either dry and nonproductive or productive. Acute symptoms subside within 2–3 days, although fever may last as long as a week. Along with fatigue and weakness, the cough can persist for days or several weeks.

Collaboration

Medical treatment of influenza focuses on establishing the diagnosis, providing symptomatic relief, and preventing complications. Collaborative partners include local health departments, hospitals and urgent care centers, primary care and infectious disease clinics, school nurses, and other medical providers.

Diagnostic Tests

The diagnosis of influenza is based on history, clinical findings, and knowledge of an influenza outbreak in the community. A chest x-ray and WBC count may be done to rule

Clinical Manifestations and Therapies
Influenza

ETIOLOGY	CLINICAL MANIFESTATIONS	CLINICAL THERAPIES
Uncomplicated nasopharyngeal inflammation	Dry cough, sore throat, coryza, fever, chills, myalgia, headache, malaise, rhinitis	■ Rest ■ Antipyretics ■ Antivirals ■ Decongestants ■ Antitussives at night ■ Increased fluid intake
Viral upper respiratory infection followed by bacterial infection	Dry cough, fever, myalgia, coryza, sore throat, wheezing, shortness of breath	■ Rest and fluids ■ Antivirals ■ Antibiotics ■ Antipyretics ■ Analgesics ■ Cough expectorant
Viral pneumonia	Fever, productive cough, coryza, myalgia, headache, chest pain, loss of appetite, fatigue, shortness of breath	■ Rest and fluids ■ Antivirals ■ Humidified air ■ Oxygen
Reye syndrome (linked to children with a virus who are receiving aspirin)	Acute noninflammatory encephalopathy with an altered level of consciousness, hepatic failure with liver biopsy showing fatty metamorphosis, increase in alanine aminotransferase and aspartate aminotransferase, CSF with WBCs, cerebral edema with or without inflammation Initial symptoms include the following: ■ Persistent or recurrent vomiting ■ Listlessness ■ Personality changes and alteration in level of consciousness ■ Seizures	■ IV therapy with D10/NS ■ Maintenance of patent airway and brain oxygenation ■ Monitoring of cardiorespiratory function (be prepared for potential cardiac arrest) ■ Assessment for hyperventilation to reduce cerebral edema ■ Osmotic diuretics to reduce intracranial pressure ■ Possible liver transplantation if extensive liver damage results
Guillain-Barré syndrome (possible complication of influenza)	Progressive paralysis of the muscles that may include muscles of respiration	■ Supportive care to prevent complications such as assistance with activities of daily living, frequent repositioning, and artificial airway with mechanical ventilation to support oxygenation ■ IV therapy as ordered ■ Nasogastric tube to meet nutritional needs if swallowing is impaired ■ Rehabilitation after disease recovery to restore baseline functioning

out complications, such as pneumonia. The WBC count is commonly decreased in patients with influenza; bacterial infections usually cause an increased WBC count. If there is a local outbreak of respiratory infections, an influenza rapid diagnostic test can be used to determine whether influenza is the cause of the outbreak or whether influenza is prevalent in a specific patient population. Nasal, throat, or nasopharyngeal swabs or washes can be used to obtain specimens for diagnostic testing. Specimens should be obtained as early in the course of disease as possible. Rapid diagnostic tests can produce results in 10–15 minutes (CDC, 2012e).

Pharmacologic Therapy

The CDC (2012b) is currently recommending the use of two antiviral drugs, zanamivir (Relenza) and oseltamivir (Tamiflu), for the treatment and prophylaxis of influenza. These drugs prevent the release of newly formed virus from the surface of infected cells and inhibit the replication of influenza A and B viruses (Wilson, Shannon, & Shields, 2013). Zanamivir is given by inhalation, whereas oseltamivir is given orally. Other antiviral drugs that are available include amantadine (Symmetrel), rimantadine (Flumadine), and ribavirin (Virazole).

Antiviral treatment should continue for 5 days; patients with severe illness may be treated longer. For prophylaxis, those who have been exposed to influenza but not vaccinated should receive the vaccine along with the antiviral drug. Antivirals should be administered for 7 days after exposure; in long-term care facilities, treatment should continue for at least 2 weeks or until 1 week after the last case has been identified.

Over-the-counter analgesics, such as aspirin, acetaminophen, and NSAIDs, provide symptomatic relief of fever and muscle ache. As mentioned earlier, aspirin should never be given to children because of the risk of Reye syndrome. Antitussives may decrease cough, promoting rest. Antibiotics are not indicated unless secondary bacterial infection occurs.

Nonpharmacologic Therapy

In most patients, influenza is a self-limiting infection. Therefore, nonpharmacologic therapy should include bedrest to alleviate fatigue and malaise, boost the immune system, and prevent the spread of infection. Adequate fluid intake in the form of water, juice, warm tea, and soup is essential to prevent dehydration and reduce cough. Hygiene interventions to prevent the spread of infection include adequate hand hygiene, proper disposal of infected waste materials such as tissues, and covering the nose and mouth when coughing or sneezing. Complementary health approaches that ease symptoms may be used as long as they are not contraindicated against any over-the-counter or pharmacologic therapy that the patient is already using.

Lifespan Considerations

Individuals who are very young (i.e., less than 5 years old), or older (i.e., older than 65) are at higher risk for developing complications related to influenza infection, including viral and bacterial pneumonia, myositis, Reye syndrome, and exacerbation of chronic respiratory diseases. These complications increase the risk of mortality in these age groups, and mortality increases with age in the older population.

Influenza in Pregnant Women

Flu is more likely to cause severe illness in pregnant women than in women who are not pregnant. Changes in the immune system, heart, and lungs during pregnancy make pregnant women (and women up to 2 weeks postpartum) more prone to severe illness from flu, as well as to hospitalizations and even death (CDC, 2015j). Pregnant women with flu also have a greater chance for serious problems for their unborn baby, including premature labor and delivery. The CDC recommends that the best prevention is a flu shot, with no indication of harm to the unborn child.

Influenza in Children

According to the CDC (2015i), flu is more dangerous than the common cold for children, and flu places a large burden on the health and well-being of children and their families.

Annual influenza vaccination is the best method for preventing flu and its potentially severe complications in children.

Influenza in Older Adults

According to the CDC (2015l), individuals 65 years and older are at greater risk of serious complications from the flu compared with young, healthy adults because human immune defenses become weaker with age. While flu seasons can vary in severity, during most seasons adults 65 years and older bear the greatest burden of severe flu disease. In recent years, for example, it is estimated that between 80% and 90% of seasonal flu-related deaths have occurred in people 65 years and older, and between 50% and 70% of seasonal flu-related hospitalizations occurred among people in that age group (CDC, 2015l; Townsend, 2014). Therefore, influenza is often quite serious for adults 65 and older.

NURSING PROCESS

Stress the importance of yearly influenza vaccination for all patients. Teach about the spread of the disease, including measures to reduce the risk for contracting influenza, such as thorough and timely hand hygiene and avoiding crowds and people who are ill.

Assessment

Unless there is a known outbreak of influenza in the community, it can be difficult to differentiate the manifestations of influenza from those of other upper respiratory infections. A thorough nursing assessment should provide clues to help determine whether a patient's symptoms can be attributed to influenza. The assessment should include the following:

- ***Observation and patient interview.*** Observe the patient for respiratory or cardiac symptoms to include the presence of dyspnea, the presence or absence of chest pain, and the nature of any productive cough. Assess and observe for facial pain or pressure in the patient's sinus areas. Ask the patient about known exposure to influenza. Ask the patient to describe current symptoms, onset, and duration. Also ask about all current medications and known medication allergies, the patient's history of influenza vaccine, and the presence of chronic diseases, such as heart disease, COPD, or diabetes.

- ***Physical examination.*** Much information can be obtained through the physical examination. Observe the patient's general appearance, including skin color, skin temperature, and any presence of fatigue or malaise. Obtain vital signs, including temperature, respiratory and heart rate. Assess thorough lung sounds and perform an abdominal exam.

Influenza pandemics within the past century have originated in the United States, Asia, and Mexico. Infections that started outside the United States were transported here by infected immigrants and visitors or by U.S. residents who were traveling in infected areas and then returned home. Therefore, one aspect of a patient history should be a history of recent travel and interaction with potentially infected animals. Testing and documentation of the type of influenza may be necessary to detect emerging strains of influenza virus.

Diagnosis

Nursing diagnoses may differ based on the patient's comorbid conditions and any complications that may develop. Suggested nursing diagnoses for patients with influenza include the following:

- *Airway Clearance, Ineffective*
- *Breathing Pattern, Ineffective*
- *Infection, Risk for*
- *Thermoregulation, Ineffective*
- *Sleep Patterns, Disturbed*
- *Fatigue*
- *Coping: Community, Ineffective.*

(NANDA-I © 2014)

Planning

Outcomes are individualized on the basis of each patient's condition and baseline health patterns. Suggested outcomes include the following:

- The patient's temperature will remain within normal limits.
- The patient will maintain normal fluid balance by increasing fluid intake.
- The patient's oxygen saturation will remain within acceptable limits.
- The patient will maintain a patent airway.

Implementation

Severe disease or complications of influenza may necessitate hospitalization for respiratory support and management. For these patients, nursing care focuses on maintaining a clear airway, ensuring adequate ventilatory patterns, reducing the risk for infection, and promoting adequate rest.

Maintain Airway Patency

Swelling and congestion of mucous membranes, extracellular fluid exudate, and impaired ciliary action as a result of cell damage increase the risk of impaired airway clearance during influenza. Older adults are at particular risk because of normally reduced ciliary activity and increased lung compliance. The nurse's role in maintaining a patent airway may include the following:

- Assist the patient to maintain adequate hydration. Assess mucous membranes and skin turgor for evidence of dehydration. Fever and decreased oral fluid intake may lead to dehydration and increased viscosity of secretions. Thick, viscous secretions are more difficult to expectorate.
- Increase the humidity of inspired air with a bedside humidifier. Increasing the water content of inhaled air helps to loosen thick secretions and soothe mucous membranes.
- Teach effective cough techniques. Administer analgesics as ordered. The huff cough (a series of small, low-pressure coughs) is effective to maintain open airways, and it spares energy. Relieving muscle ache increases the ability to cough effectively.

SAFETY ALERT Monitor the effectiveness of the cough and the ability to remove airway secretions. Fatigue and general malaise may impair the ability to cough effectively and mobilize secretions.

Ensure Effective Ventilation

Muscle aches, malaise, and elevated temperature may increase the respiratory rate and alter the depth of respirations, decreasing effective alveolar ventilation. Shallow respirations also increase the risk of **atelectasis** (the collapse of lung tissue affecting all or part of the lung, affecting the exchange of oxygen and carbon dioxide). Interventions that promote respiration and ventilation include:

- Planning activities to provide for periods of rest. Tachypnea increases the work of breathing, causing fatigue; fatigue, in turn, can further impair ventilation and reduce the effectiveness of coughing.
- Elevating the head of the bed. The upright position improves lung excursion (movement from the resting position) and reduces the work of breathing by lowering the diaphragm, moving abdominal contents downward, creating less resistance to diaphragmatic excursion, and slightly decreasing venous return.

Promote Sleep Hygiene

Airway congestion, malaise, muscle aches, and persistent cough may interfere with rest, increasing fatigue and prolonging recovery. To assist the patient in getting enough sleep, the nurse may do the following:

- Assess sleep patterns using subjective and objective information. The patient who appears to be sleeping may not be achieving normal sleep patterns because of influenza symptoms. Both subjective and objective data are important to accurately assess sleep.
- Provide antipyretic and analgesic medications to be taken at or shortly before bedtime. These drugs promote comfort by reducing fever and relieving muscle aches.
- If necessary, request a cough suppressant for nighttime use. Cough suppressants are not recommended during the day, because coughing promotes airway clearance. They may, however, be helpful at night to allow rest.

Prevent Infection

Infection-control measures are recommended to prevent individual-to-individual transmission of influenza and to control influenza outbreaks in healthcare facilities.

- Use standard precautions, and droplet precautions for patients with suspected or confirmed influenza, and encourage all staff and visitors to cleanse their hands frequently. Hand hygiene is a primary control measure for infections transmitted via respiratory secretions.
- Instruct patients and visitors to control respiratory secretions by using tissues and to maintain a distance of at least 3 ft from others when coughing or sneezing. Provide masks for patients and visitors who are unable to control secretions. Limiting the spread of aerosolized secretions by covering the nose and mouth and maintaining distance from other people can reduce the spread of the disease to vulnerable populations.

Community-Based Care

Although the symptoms of influenza are distressing, most people with the illness provide self-care and do not contact a healthcare provider. The nurse should encourage appropriate self-care for patients with influenza and discuss the following actions that patients should take related to home care:

- Increase rest during the acute, febrile phase of the illness.
- Maintain a liberal fluid intake, even if anorexic.
- Appropriate use over-the-counter medications can be helpful for symptom relief.
- Employ hygiene measures, such as using disposable tissues and frequent cleansing of hands, to reduce spread of the disease.
- Know the manifestations of potential complications of influenza that should be reported to the primary care provider.

Evaluation

Evaluate the patient for airway patency, breathing pattern, oxygenation, and thermoregulation. Expected potential outcomes may include:

- The patient's temperature remains within normal limits.
- The patient maintains normal fluid balance by increasing fluid intake.
- The patient's oxygen saturation remains within acceptable limits.
- The patient maintains a patent airway.

Consider appropriate alterations to the plan of care if the patient is not responding to therapy or develops complications.

REVIEW Influenza

RELATE Link the Concepts and Exemplars

Linking the exemplar of influenza with the concept of oxygenation:

1. Describe the pathophysiology that would cause influenza to diminish the body's ability to meet oxygen demands.

2. Would an older adult with COPD be at any greater risk for complications from influenza? Why or why not?

Linking the exemplar of influenza with the concept of cognition:

3. Why might the older adult who develops influenza display alterations in cognition?

4. What caring interventions can the nurse implement to reduce this impact on cognition when working in a long-term care facility with older adults?

READY Go to Volume 3: Clinical Nursing Skills

REFER Go to Pearson MyLab Nursing and eText

- Additional review materials

REFLECT Apply Your Knowledge

Courtney Hollis is a 34-year-old woman who is married and has three young children ages 6, 3, and 1. She was diagnosed with asthma when she was a child. Ms. Hollis sees her primary care healthcare provider with symptoms of a sore throat; fever; malaise; and severe, productive cough. She has been having trouble breathing because of the secretions in her lungs. Her vital signs are temperature 102.1°F oral; pulse 96 bpm; respirations 20/min; and blood pressure 112/78 mmHg. She reports that the flu has been going around her child's school, and her 6-year-old had mild flu symptoms last week. After a patient history and physical examination, Ms. Hollis is diagnosed with influenza A and prescribed oseltamivir (Tamiflu).

1. With the task of caring for three young children, Ms. Hollis admits that she will not be able to get bedrest during the day. What patient teaching can you provide to help Ms. Hollis rest during the day?

2. On the basis of Ms. Hollis's patient and family history, would you recommend that her three children receive the influenza vaccine? Why or why not?

3. What increased risks does Ms. Hollis face because of her history of asthma?

≫ Exemplar 9.D
Otitis Media

Exemplar Learning Outcomes

9.D Analyze otitis media as it relates to infection.

- Describe the pathophysiology of otitis media.
- Describe the etiology of otitis media.
- Compare the risk factors and prevention of otitis media.
- Identify the clinical manifestations of otitis media.
- Summarize diagnostic tests and therapies used by interprofessional teams in the collaborative care of an individual with otitis media.

- Differentiate care of patients with otitis media across the lifespan.
- Apply the nursing process in providing culturally competent care to an individual with otitis media.

Exemplar Key Terms

Audiologist, *615*
Eustachian tube, *613*
Hemotympanum, *614*

Overview

The ear can become infected in any of the three chambers. **Otitis externa** is inflammation of the ear canal (often called *swimmer's ear,* because it is most frequently found in people who spend significant time in the water). **Otitis interna**, also called **labyrinthitis**, is inflammation of the inner ear. **Otitis media**, the topic of this exemplar, is inflammation of the middle ear.

Usually referred to as an "ear infection," otitis media is one of the most common childhood illnesses and a common reason for office visits, but it is not always accompanied by an actual infection. Although otitis media is very common in children under the age of 5 years, it can occur at any age. Since 2003, an increased number of cases has been observed, and recent changes have been made in recommendations for treatment (Friedel et al., 2014; Lieberthal et al., 2013).

Pathophysiology and Etiology

Pathophysiology

The **tympanic membrane** (a thin, tense membrane that separates the middle ear from the external auditory canal) protects the middle ear from the external environment. However, the **eustachian tube** connects the middle ear with the nasopharynx to help equalize the pressure in the middle ear with the atmospheric pressure, and this connecting tube provides a route by which infectious organisms can enter the middle ear from the nose and throat, causing otitis media.

An upper respiratory infection often precedes the development of otitis media. An estimated 29–50% of all upper respiratory infections lead to acute otitis media (Friedel et al., 2014). This infection causes the mucous membranes of the eustachian tube to become edematous. As a result, air that normally flows to the middle ear is blocked, and the air in the middle ear is reabsorbed into the bloodstream. Fluid is pulled from the mucosal lining into the former air space, providing a medium for the rapid growth of pathogens. The tympanic membrane and the fluid behind it become infected.

Types of Otitis Media

The two primary forms of otitis media are serous and acute or suppurative; a chronic form can also develop. Both forms are associated with upper respiratory infection and eustachian tube dysfunction. The eustachian tube is narrow and flat, normally opening only during yawning and swallowing. Allergies or upper respiratory tract infections can cause edema of the tube lining, impairing its function.

Serous Otitis Media

Serous otitis media (also called *otitis media with effusion*) occurs when obstruction of the eustachian tube is prolonged, impairing equalization of air pressure in the middle ear. As the air within the middle ear space is gradually absorbed, the tube obstruction prevents more air from entering the middle ear. The resulting negative pressure in the middle ear causes sterile serous fluid to move from the capillaries into the space, a process that is known as **middle ear effusion**.

Acute Otitis Media

The eustachian tube also provides a route for the entry of pathogens into the normally sterile middle ear, resulting in acute, or suppurative, otitis media. Acute otitis media typically follows an upper respiratory infection. Edema of the eustachian tube impairs drainage of the middle ear, causing mucus and serous fluid to accumulate. This fluid is an excellent environment for the growth of bacteria, which may enter from the oronasopharynx via the eustachian tube.

Chronic Otitis Media

Chronic otitis media involves permanent perforation of the tympanic membrane, with or without recurrent pus formation. It usually is the result of recurrent acute otitis media and eustachian tube dysfunction, but it may also result from trauma or other diseases. Changes in the mucosa and bony structures (ossicles) of the middle ear often accompany chronic otitis media.

Marginal perforations, which usually occur in the posterosuperior portion of the tympanic membrane, are associated with more complications than central perforations. With marginal perforations, squamous epithelium may migrate from the ear canal into the middle ear, where it begins to desquamate and accumulate, forming a *cholesteatoma* (a benign and slow-growing cyst or mass filled with epithelial cell debris). The desquamating epithelium continues to accumulate until it fills the entire middle ear. It often remains infected, producing collagenases (enzymes) that progressively destroy the ossicles and erode into the inner ear. The inflammatory process impairs the blood supply to the stapes, causing its destruction, which results in conductive hearing loss. Its incidence is highest in children and young adults.

Tympanic membrane perforation can be repaired with a tympanoplasty to restore sound conduction and the integrity of the middle ear. Delicate surgery may be required to remove a cholesteatoma. If possible, radical mastoidectomy with removal of the tympanic membrane, ossicles, and tumor should be avoided.

Etiology

The most common causative organisms of acute otitis media are *Streptococcus pneumoniae, Haemophilus influenzae,* and *Moraxella catarrhalis* (Friedel et al., 2014). Invasion and colonization of the middle ear by bacteria and the resultant migration of WBCs cause pus formation. Accumulated pus can increase middle ear pressure sufficiently to rupture the tympanic membrane. The bacterial infection may also migrate internally, causing mastoiditis, brain abscess, or bacterial meningitis. A more common complication of otitis media is a persistent conductive hearing loss, which typically resolves when the middle ear effusion clears. Viral upper respiratory infection may also predispose the patient to acute otitis media, and an upper respiratory infection or allergies (e.g., hay fever) can lead to serous otitis media.

Eustachian tube dysfunction plays a major role in the development of otitis media because fluid cannot drain properly, so infection is allowed to develop. Patients with narrowed or edematous eustachian tubes may also be subject to barotrauma or barotitis media. In these patients, the middle ear cannot adapt to rapid changes in barometric pressure, such as those that occur during air travel or underwater diving.

Risk Factors

Risk factors for developing otitis media include being younger than age 2, participating in group care settings (e.g., child care, school), having seasonal allergies, or being exposed to poor air quality (Mayo Clinic, 2017).

Prevention

For infants and children, several practices help reduce the risk of otitis media: breastfeeding for 12 months or more if possible, bottle feeding in the upright position, keeping up to date with immunizations, and avoiding air pollution, especially secondhand smoke. Using a small child care or private child care rather than a large child care facility can also decrease the risk of otitis media in children.

Clinical Manifestations

Typical manifestations of serous otitis media in adults include decreased hearing in the affected ear and complaints of "snapping" or "popping" in the ear. On examination, the tympanic membrane demonstrates decreased mobility and may appear retracted or bulging. Fluid or air bubbles are often visible behind the drum. Severe pressure differences, such as those occurring with barotrauma, may cause acute pain, hemorrhage into the middle ear, rupture of the tympanic membrane, or even rupture of the round window, with sensory hearing loss and severe **vertigo** (a sensation of whirling or rotation). **Hemotympanum** (bleeding into or behind the tympanic membrane, see **Figure 9–14** ❯❯) may be observed when examining the ear with an **otoscope** (a handheld instrument with a light and a cone-shaped attachment known as the *ear speculum*).

The patient with acute otitis media typically experiences mild to severe pain in the affected ear. The patient's temperature is often elevated. Diminished hearing, dizziness, vertigo, and tinnitus are common associated complaints. Pus within the mastoid air cells often causes mastoid tenderness in acute otitis media. On otoscopic examination, the tympanic membrane appears red and inflamed or dull and bulging (see **Figure 9–15** ❯❯). Decreased movement of the membrane is demonstrated by tympanometry or air insufflation (blowing air into the ear). Spontaneous rupture of the tympanic membrane (see **Figure 9–16** ❯❯) releases a purulent

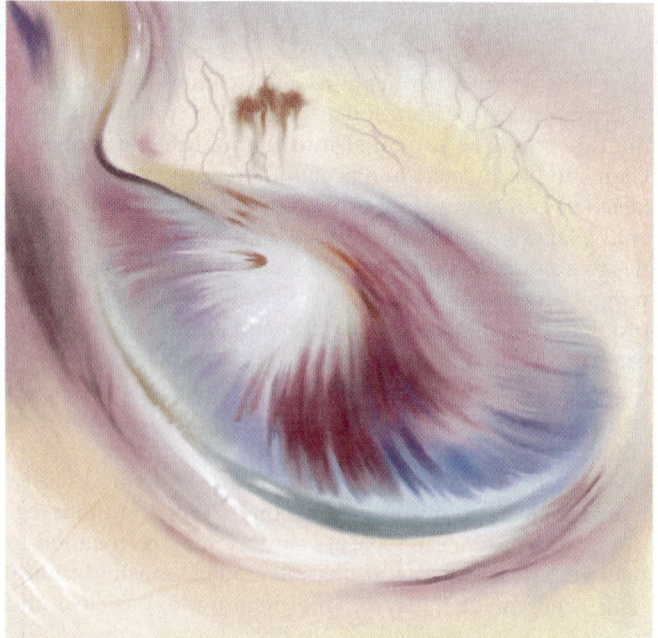
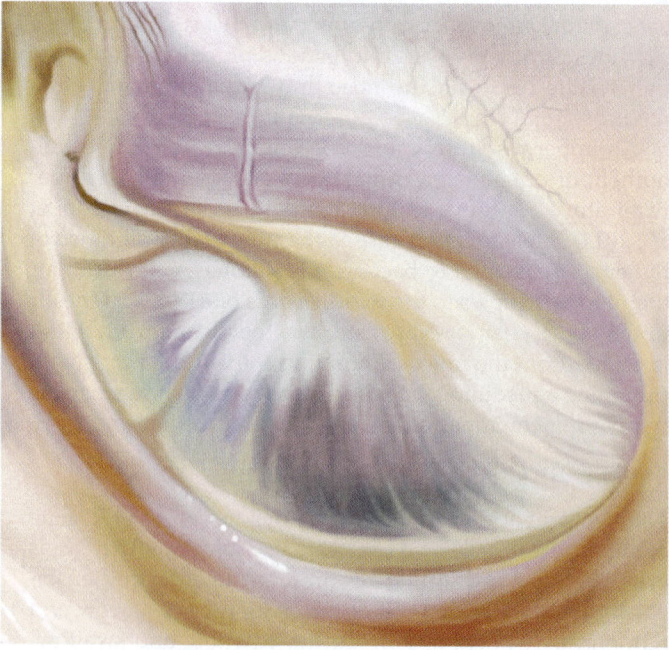

A   B

Source: Mediscan/Alamy Stock Photo.

Figure 9–14 ❯❯ *Hemotympanum* refers to the presence of blood in the tympanic cavity of the middle ear. This rare condition is characterized by discoloration of the tympanic membrane. ***A,*** Fresh blood often causes red coloration of the tympanic membrane. ***B,*** Old blood may produce a black-blue coloration of the tympanic membrane.

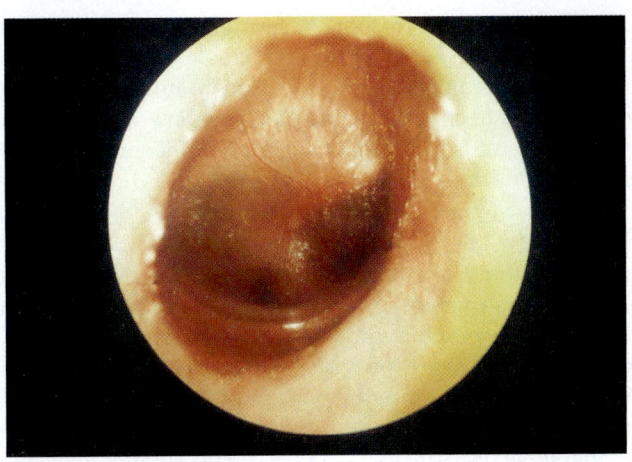

Source: © Mediscan/Alamy Stock Photo.

Figure 9–15 ❯❯ A red, bulging tympanic membrane of otitis media.

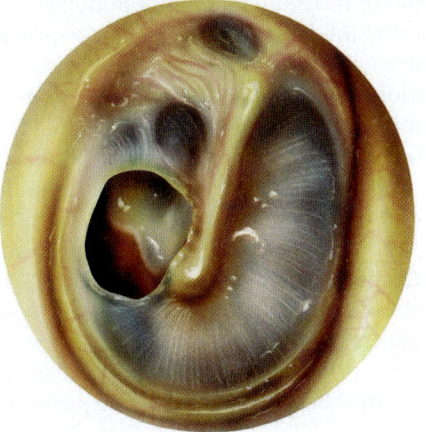

Source: Bo Veisland/Science Source.

Figure 9–16 ❯❯ Perforation of tympanic membrane.

discharge. A **myringotomy** (a surgical incision of the tympanic membrane) may be performed to relieve the pressure.

Collaboration

A number of professionals may provide support to a patient with recurrent otitis media. Both adults and children may meet with an audiologist. Either the nurse or an **audiologist**

(a healthcare professional specializing in identifying, diagnosing, treating, and monitoring disorders of the auditory and vestibular portions of the ear) can conduct a hearing screening. With a child, a speech-language pathologist may perform a screening to ensure the child's speech development is age-appropriate. If a child fails a hearing screening, the professional conducting the screening should refer the patient to an audiologist for further testing. For children

Clinical Manifestations and Therapies
Otitis Media

ETIOLOGY	CLINICAL MANIFESTATION	CLINICAL THERAPIES
Acute otitis media: Bacterial infection in the middle ear from pathogens transferred from the nasopharynx; most common infectious agents are *Streptococcus pneumoniae, Haemophilus influenzae,* and *Moraxella catarrhalis.*	*Behavioral:* Ear pain, rapid onset. Among children you may also see: pulling at ear, irritability, malaise, and poor feeding	■ Treatment of ear pain with local anesthetic, local herbal pain products, or systemic acetaminophen or ibuprofen
	Examination: Bulging tympanic membrane; air or fluid bubbles present behind tympanic membrane; immobile or poorly mobile tympanic membrane; red tympanic membrane, or other color change (e.g., white, gray, or yellow) as long as bulging is present; and reduced visibility of tympanic membrane landmarks with displaced light reflex	■ Observation of the patient's condition for 48–72 hours; if not improved, treatment with course of antibiotics
Otitis media with effusion: Collection of fluid in the middle ear behind the tympanic membrane, which is not infected with bacteria	*Behavioral:* Difficulty hearing or responding as expected to sounds. An adult may complain of not hearing the phone, the TV, or other people speaking to them.	■ Symptomatic treatment for pain
	Examination: Signs of acute inflammation NOT present; tympanic membrane retracted or neutral; immobile or partly mobile tympanic membrane; yellow or gray tympanic membrane; opaque or thickened tympanic membrane with visibility of landmarks reduced	■ Careful observation of hearing acuity over several months ■ In children: Speech assessment if loss of hearing acuity occurs Developmental assessment

who experience hearing loss or speech delays as a result of recurrent otitis media, the audiologist or speech language pathologist may collaborate with both the parents and the child's school or child care to strengthen strategies to promote communication at home and at school. This includes the importance of maintaining verbal communication, reading to the child regularly, input on individual education plans or accommodations (e.g., sitting at the front of the classroom) and facilitating access to assistive technology.

With both adults and children, the nurse and healthcare provider will assist the patient or caregivers with the appropriate treatment plan, clinical follow-up, and education concerning further hearing or infection concerns to be alert for. In some cases, surgery may be required to alleviate pressure in the ear.

Diagnostic Tests

Diagnostic tests that may be conducted in addition to physical examination include the following:

- *Impedance audiometry*, also known as tympanometry, is an accurate diagnostic test for serous otitis media. An audiometer with a sealed probe tip delivers a continuous tone to the tympanic membrane. Compliance of the tympanic membrane and middle ear is measured by a recording of the energy reflected from the membrane surface. With middle ear effusion, compliance is reduced.

- A *complete blood count (CBC)* may be done to assess for an elevated WBC count and increased numbers of immature cells indicative of acute bacterial infection.

- *Tympanocentesis* or *myringotomy* is performed if the tympanic membrane has ruptured. Drainage is cultured to determine the infecting organism.

- *Spectral gradient acoustic reflectometry* measures the condition of the middle ear by introducing a sound and then measuring the response of the tympanic membrane. A flat **tympanogram** (a test that provides a graph of the middle ear's ability to transmit sound), indicating absence of normal movement of the tympanic membrane, also suggests otitis media.

- *Culture and sensitivity tests* may be performed on fluid from the middle ear to determine causative organisms if drainage is noted secondary to rupture of the tympanic membrane. If the tympanic membrane is intact, a tympanocentesis may be done to aspirate some fluid from the middle ear through the tympanic membrane.

- *Audiologic testing* may be performed to determine hearing loss if serous otitis media persists for more than 3 months. Audiologic testing is conducted on both children and adults as part of a diagnostic workup. Children who fail the hearing test should be referred to an audiologist.

Pharmacologic Therapy

Acute otitis media in adults is usually treated with antibiotic therapy, especially amoxicillin, trimethoprim-sulfamethoxazole, cefaclor, or azithromycin, for 5–10 days. This course of treatment is long enough to ensure eradication of the infective organism yet short enough to reduce the incidence of bacterial resistance. Analgesics, antipyretics, antihistamines, and local application of heat may provide symptomatic relief. Referral to an audiologist may be neces-

sary if the adult reports loss of hearing following successful healing of infection.

Neither decongestants nor antihistamines have been shown to be effective in treating otitis media with or without effusion. Steroids also do not appear to have any long-term beneficial effect.

Surgery

A myringotomy or tympanocentesis may be performed to relieve excess pressure in the middle ear and prevent spontaneous rupture of the eardrum. To perform a **tympanocentesis**, the healthcare provider inserts a 20-gauge spinal needle through the inferior portion of the tympanic membrane, allowing aspiration of fluid and pus from the middle ear to relieve pressure and, if necessary, to obtain a specimen for culture. Myringotomy may be performed to relieve severe pain or when complications of acute otitis media, such as mastoiditis, are present. As soon as the pressure is released, pain subsides and hearing improves.

Myringotomy in adults is a less common procedure than in children, primarily because adults benefit from certain changes in the anatomy of the middle ear that occur after childhood. In particular, the adult ear is less likely to accumulate fluid because the eustachian tube, which connects the middle ear to the throat area, lies at about a 45-degree angle from the horizontal (Friedel et al., 2014). This relatively steep angle means that the force of gravity helps to keep disease-containing fluids from the throat out of the middle ear.

Lifespan Considerations

Older adults and pregnant women typically do not have any more serious risk for or complications from otitis media than the general adult population. Treatment for pregnant women should focus on nonpharmacologic and complementary health approaches, but if discomfort or symptoms worsen, the pregnant woman should consult with her obstetrician.

Young children are at greater risk for otitis media and for possible complications, and considerations for working with this population are outlined in the next section.

Otitis Media in Children

Approximately 17–20% of children develop acute otitis media within the first 2 years of life, and one third of children experience six or more episodes before age 7. Peak prevalence of otitis media is between the ages of 6 and 18 months, with a smaller peak at ages 4–5 when entering school. Over 80% of all cases of otitis media occur in children under the age of 6 (Friedel et al., 2014). Many young children are susceptible to recurrent acute otitis media, which is defined as three or more distinct episodes of acute otitis media within 6 months or four or more episodes within 12 months.

Otitis media occurs more frequently in children who attend child care centers, those with allergies, those exposed to tobacco smoke, and those who use pacifiers several hours daily. It is most common during the winter months. Children with conditions such as Down syndrome or cleft lip and palate experience otitis media more often because of eustachian tube dysfunction. To reduce the risk for otitis media, nurses should teach parents to feed infants in an upright position and not to put children to bed with a bottle. Breastfeeding appears to be protective against otitis media. Conditions such as enlarged adenoids or edema from allergic rhinitis can also obstruct the eustachian tube and lead to otitis media. Pacifier use can alter dental structure and promote eustachian tube dysfunction, and it also allows reflux of nasopharyngeal secretions into the middle ear from sucking (Seckman, 2013). Recurrent otitis media has an increased frequency in children of parents who smoke and in children who attend child care centers (Csakanyi et al., 2012).

Serous otitis media is not treated with antibiotics; instead it is evaluated periodically for the presence of an additional acute otitis media that needs treatment. Children with serous otitis media generally improve within 3 months. Since this type of otitis is more commonly associated with hearing loss and cochlear damage, follow-up with an audiologist is essential. When eustachian tube dysfunction and serous otitis media do not spontaneously resolve, or when they lead to hearing loss, a short course of an anti-inflammatory drug (e.g., oral prednisone for 7 days) may be prescribed to reduce mucosal edema of the tube and improve its patency.

If infection recurs despite antibiotic treatment for acute otitis media or if serous otitis media continues 4 months or more with persistent hearing loss, a myringotomy may be performed, and **tympanostomy tubes** (pressure-equalizing tubes) may be inserted to provide ventilation and drainage of the middle ear during healing. The tube is eventually extruded from the ear, and the tympanic membrane heals. While the tube is in place, research has shown that usual patient behavior (e.g., showering, swimming) is unlikely to affect treatment outcome (Conrad et al., 2014).

The *Haemophilus influenzae* type B (Hib) vaccine, which is routinely given to children beginning at 2 months of age, has been influential in reducing the incidence of diseases, such as otitis media, that are caused by *H. influenzae* type B. Another, more recently recommended immunization for pneumococcal disease has also decreased cases of otitis media from that pathogen.

Acute otitis media is diagnosed in pediatric patients when the child has acute onset of ear pain, marked redness of the tympanic membrane on otoscopy, and middle ear effusion. *Recurrent acute otitis media* refers to repeated bouts of acute otitis media, such as three in 6 months or four in 12 months. *Serous otitis media* is evidenced by fluid in the middle ear without inflammation, as demonstrated

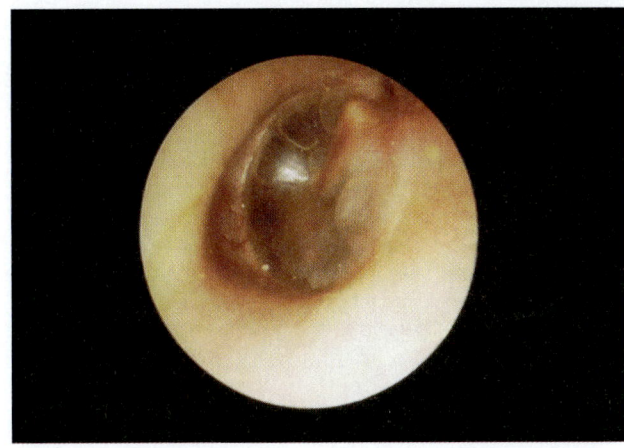

Source: Southern Illinois University/Getty Images.

Figure 9–17 ≫ Otitis media with effusion is noted on otoscopy by line of fluid or air bubbles. Pneumatic otoscopy or tympanometry shows a nonmobile tympanic membrane. Note that the light reflex is not in the expected position because of a change in tympanic membrane shape from air bubbles. Where would you expect to see the cone of light?

in **Figure 9–17** ≫. Serous otitis media sometimes becomes chronic (continuing for more than 3 months) and is more commonly associated with hearing loss.

Diarrhea, vomiting, and fever are typical of otitis media. In infants and young children, characteristic behaviors may indicate the presence of otitis media. Pulling at the ear is a sign of ear pain (see **Figure 9–18** ≫). Irritability and acting out may signal a related hearing impairment. The child with otitis media often awakens crying at night because ear pressure increases when the child is prone or supine.

Concern in the medical community has grown over the increasing appearance of drug-resistant bacteria as causative agents in otitis media. The American Academy of Pediatrics in 2009 updated their 2004 recommendations (Lieberthal et al., 2013). The updated recommendations suggest that the clinician should prescribe antibiotic therapy for acute otitis media (bilateral or unilateral) in children 6 months and older

Focus on Diversity and Culture
Otitis Media

Native American and Native Alaskan children have a very high rate of otitis media, perhaps related to differences in eustachian tube structure in these individuals (Lieberthal et al., 2013). These children are seen about three times more frequently in outpatient clinics for otitis media than are other U.S. children. Nurses should be alert for the common incidence in these population groups, plan prevention programs, and ensure prompt care and teaching about treatments for families of children affected.

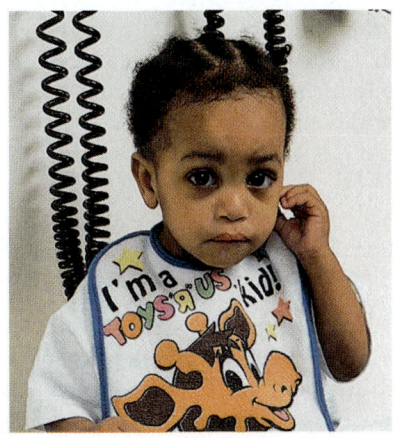

Figure 9–18 ≫ This young child is pulling at the ear and acting fussy, two important signs of otitis media. Ask the parents about the presence of fever and night awakenings, additional signs that are often observed in children with this condition.

Focus on Integrative Health
Otitis Media

Because many children with otitis media experience ear pain that can disrupt their sleep as well as that of family members, anesthetic eardrops have been used for their analgesic effect on the tympanic membrane. Because some families prefer to use natural remedies for ear pain, it is important to discuss such options with their healthcare provider. Naturopathic treatment protocols have included a botanical formula, nutritional supplementation, low-antigenic diet, and hydrotherapy (Barrett, 2012).

with severe signs or symptoms (i.e., moderate or severe otalgia or otalgia for at least 48 hours or temperature 39°C [102.2°F] or higher) (Lieberthal et al., 2013). Further delineation of therapy and watching and waiting is discussed in the updated recommendations at several levels and is too extensive and detailed to discuss here. Of note is that amoxicillin remains the drug of choice, with recommendations not to prescribe if the child has had this drug within the past 30 days.

When an antibiotic is prescribed, the choice of drug depends on the probable organism, ease of administration, cost, previous effectiveness, and any history of allergies. First-line therapy for children is amoxicillin at a dose of 80–90 mg/kg/day. Amoxicillin with clavulanate is a second-line drug. Other available antibiotics include azithromycin, cefdinir, cefpodoxime, ceftriaxone, cefuroximine, clarithromycin, clindamycin, and levofloxacin (Lieberthal et al., 2013). Patients who are allergic to penicillin should receive a cephalosporin, trimethoprim-sulfamethoxazole, or macrolides (Friedel et al., 2014). When the tympanic membrane is intact, topical anesthetic eardrops are sometimes prescribed for several days to provide pain relief.

NURSING PROCESS

Patients with otitis media are commonly treated in outpatient and community settings. The nursing role is primarily one of support and education. Health promotion for otitis media focuses on educating patients about the importance of seeking medical care for prolonged, severe ear pain, with or without drainage, combined with an upper respiratory tract infection. Untreated or repeated attacks of otitis media can progress to a chronic form, to acute mastoiditis, or to eardrum perforation.

Assessment

Collect assessment data through a health history and physical examination. The data collected should include observation, patient interview, and physical examination.

- *Observation and patient interview.* Observe the patient for indications of pain, and signs and symptoms of elevated temperature. Observe for signs of impaired hearing, such as difficulty hearing a whisper or soft sounds. The patient interview should include history of recent upper respiratory infection. Ask the patient to describe the presence, intensity, and nature of pain in the affected ear and any sense of fullness or pressure in the ear. Ask the patient to explain any change in hearing, or

any snapping or popping sensation in the affected ear, and ask if the patient has had any episodes of vertigo.

- *Physical examination.* Physical examination includes obtaining and assessing vital signs, such as temperature, pulse, and respiratory rate. A hearing test should be conducted as well as inspection of the tympanic membrane at each health promotion visit and during examinations for illness. The nurse or healthcare provider will examine the color, transparency, mobility, presence of landmarks, and light reflex. With children, ask the parents if the child has had a fever, been fussy, or pulled at the ears.

Physical examination of a young child may be complicated by the child's excessive movement. Parents or other healthcare workers should be enlisted to help hold the child's head steady (see **Figure 9–19 》**). The nurse should hold the pinna down and back to inspect the auditory canal and tympanic membrane of a child younger than 3 years old. To prevent injury, insert the speculum of the otoscope only 0.25–0.5 in. To examine adults, pull the pinna up and back to straighten the ear canal. To maximize vision of the ear canal choose the largest diameter speculum that will fit comfortably in the patient's ear (Berman, Snyder, & Frandsen, 2016). Inspect the tympanic membrane for color, gloss, transparency, mobility, bulging, presence of fluid or blood, perforation, and other abnormalities. A pneumatoscope (an otoscope with a bulb attachment that introduces air into the ear canal) can be used to test mobility of the eardrum. Normal tympanic membranes are pearly gray, semitransparent, shiny, and mobile and have a neutral position. Abnormal findings that may indicate otitis media include redness, reduced mobility, presence of fluid or blood, and bulging or retraction of the tympanic membrane. The tympanic membrane is white or yellow in the presence of acute otitis media and otitis media with effusion, whereas an amber-colored tympanic membrane indicates otitis media with effusion (Lieberthal et al., 2013).

SAFETY ALERT When assessing a patient's ears with an otoscope, hold the otoscope with your hand between the otoscope and the patient's head, using the patient's head to stabilize your hand. This position protects the eardrum and canal from injury if the patient moves the head.

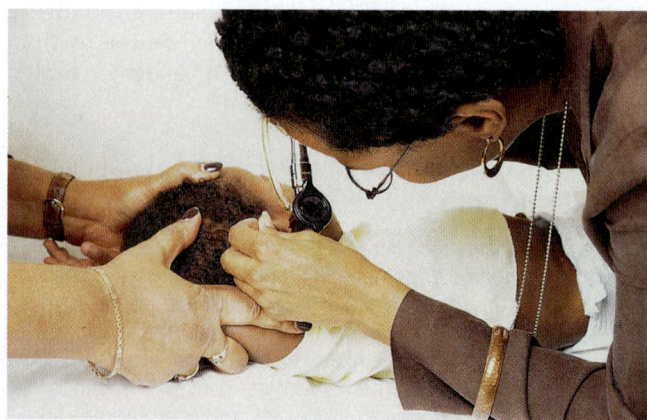

Figure 9–19 》 Parent restraint of a young child during examination of the ear.

Diagnosis

Nursing diagnoses that may apply to the patient with otitis media are the following:

- *Pain, Acute*
- *Infection*
- *Caregiver Role Strain, Risk for*
- *Knowledge, Deficient*
- *Growth: Disproportionate, Risk for*
- *Body Temperature: Imbalanced, Risk for*
- *Fatigue*
- *Verbal Communication, Impaired.*

(NANDA-I © 2014)

Planning

Most patients with otitis media do not require hospitalization; therefore, nursing management centers on planning care in the home. Potential outcomes include the following:

- The patient or parent will indicate absence of pain.
- The patient will be infection-free after finishing the course of treatment.
- Caregivers will manage the child's condition with minimal stress.
- The patient or parents will state their understanding of preventive measures.
- The patient will have normal hearing.
- The pediatric patient will have normal motor and language development.

Implementation

Nursing care is individualized based on the diverse needs presented by patients. It focuses on pain management, patient and family teaching, and preventing recurrence of infection. Screening for potential hearing loss is of particular importance in patients who contract otitis media repeatedly.

Manage and Control Pain

Tissue edema, effusion of the middle ear, and the resulting inflammatory response can affect the pain-sensitive tissues of the middle ear in otitis media, causing acute discomfort. This discomfort is increased by pressure changes, such as those that occur during air travel or underwater diving. A nurse working with a patient who reports pain associated with otitis media should:

- Assess the patient's pain for severity, quality, and location. A thorough assessment is important to determine the source of the pain. The pain of otitis media, unlike that of external otitis, is not aggravated by movement of the external ear.
- Encourage the patient to use mild analgesics, such as ibuprofen or acetaminophen, as needed to relieve pain and fever. Ibuprofen also has anti-inflammatory properties that may help to relieve inflammation of the ear.

- Advise the patient to apply heat to the affected side unless contraindicated. Heat dilates blood vessels, promoting the reabsorption of fluid and reducing swelling.
- Instruct the patient to avoid air travel, rapid changes in elevation, or diving. A rapid change in barometric pressure can increase the patient's pain significantly.
- Instruct the patient to promptly report to the primary care provider. Pain that subsides abruptly may indicate spontaneous perforation of the tympanic membrane, which relieves the pressure within the middle ear.
- Elevate the head of the bed to decrease pressure on the middle ear when the patient is in bed.

Support Caregivers

The chronic nature of otitis media in some children can create many problems for the family. Parents often become frustrated and disillusioned because the healthcare system is unable to cure the child, and they may fear a permanent hearing impairment. Nursing interventions include the following:

- Reassure parents that as the child grows older, the recurrent infections will eventually cease.
- Teach pain relief techniques, such as correct administration of eardrops, oral administration of acetaminophen, and positioning the baby or child with the head slightly elevated, a position that often decreases pressure and pain.

Provide Age-Appropriate Education to Patients and Family Members

Both the patient who has otitis media and the family benefit from learning about the disorder, its causes and prevention, and any specific treatment that is recommended or prescribed. Patient teaching typically includes the following:

- Discuss with the patient and family the antibiotic therapy (if prescribed) and potential side effects, and the importance of completing all ordered doses. Discuss the follow-up examinations in 2–4 weeks, and, if ventilation tubes are in place, the importance of avoiding diving, or submerging the head while bathing.
- Emphasize preventive measures. Exposure to secondhand smoke in the home increases the incidence of otitis media in children; therefore, parents who smoke should be encouraged to avoid smoking near the child or in the home. Use of wood burning stoves should also be avoided when possible. Breastfeeding provides some protection from the disease. Pacifier use may increase the incidence of otitis media and should be avoided in the infant with prior infections (Seckman, 2013).
- If surgical intervention is necessary, teach the patient and family members about the surgery and postoperative care. Provide instruction about any special postoperative precautions, such as avoidance of water in the ear canals and of sudden changes in air pressure.
- Inform parents that the child who is having tympanostomy tubes inserted is generally treated in a day surgery setting. Teach the child and parents about what to expect, and provide instructions for safe care upon discharge.

- Explain to parents and patients the problem of developing resistant strains of bacteria. Parents may not understand why the child with a possible infection is not given antibiotics. Explain that most children improve after 48–72 hours even without antibiotics, and that overuse of antibiotics contributes to drug resistance.

- Explain to parents of children with serous otitis media that antibiotics, steroids, and antihistamines/decongestants have not been effective and that most children improve in 3 months without medication. Assure parents that if the effusion continues beyond that time, the child will be tested for hearing acuity and, if indicated, for speech development.

Facilitate Communication

Nursing interventions for children with decreased hearing or hearing loss related to otitis media include encouraging parents to read and talk frequently with children with decreased hearing to prevent delayed development. Perform hearing and language assessments at regular intervals, and recommend an auditory specialist if hearing loss persists. For patients with permanent hearing loss, alternative methods of communication should be pursued, such as American Sign Language.

Evaluation

Expected outcomes of nursing care for the child with otitis media include the following:

- The patient or parent indicates absence of pain.
- The patient is infection-free after finishing the course of treatment.
- Caregivers manage the child's condition with minimal stress.
- The patient or parents are able to state their understanding of preventive measures.
- The patient has normal hearing.
- The pediatric patient has normal motor and language development.

If indicated, a child may require a tympanoplasty with tube placement to prevent further infection in the middle ear (Lieberthal, 2013). The child with tubes will be evaluated on a routine basis over the next year, and the implanted tubes usually fall out on their own or may be removed by a healthcare provider. The child's caregivers must understand the rationale for this intervention as well as the necessary medical visits following the surgery.

Nursing Care Plan
A Patient with Otitis Media

Melinda Jeffries is a 2-year-old toddler who lives with her mother, father, and 6-year-old sister. Melinda attends child care every day, because both parents work outside the home. The child care center is a large building with multiple classrooms for different age groups. There are approximately 15–20 students in her class on any given day. Melinda's recurrent diagnoses of otitis media include four infections over the course of the winter thus far.

Ms. Jeffries has brought Melinda to the pediatric nurse practitioner's office today because she has an axillary temperature of 102.6°F, has been pulling at her ear, and was awake most of last night crying in pain. The nurse practitioner diagnoses a left acute otitis media, prescribes amoxicillin and corticosteroid eardrops, and instructs the mother to administer ibuprofen every 6 hours for pain and fever control. Ms. Jeffries is concerned that these recurrent ear infections will result in hearing loss and asks about insertion of tubes to prevent further infections. The nurse practitioner explains that the occurrence of ear infections tends to be highest during the winter months; she recommends waiting to see if Melinda improves when the weather gets warmer. Ms. Jeffries agrees, saying that she noticed that pattern with her older child when she was this age.

ASSESSMENT	DIAGNOSES	PLANNING
Melinda is admitted to the provider's office by Sarah McKinney, RN. In her assessment, she finds Melinda irritable and less tolerant of separation from her mother than usual. Examination finds an orange-yellow tympanic membrane with decreased motility, warm dry skin, and vital signs including a temperature 99.8°F axillary, pulse 128 bpm, and respirations 26/min; blood pressure is deferred at this time because of Melinda's age and general good health. Neurologic, respiratory, cardiovascular, and abdominal assessments are essentially normal. Auditory examination reveals a slight decrease in hearing, most likely caused by the collection of fluid in the middle ear. Further testing will need to be done when Melinda is asymptomatic.	■ *Acute Pain* related to tympanic pressure secondary to fluid accumulation in the middle ear ■ *Deficient Knowledge* related to lack of information regarding indications for myringotomy and administration of eardrops ■ *Risk for Deficient Fluid Volume* related to hyperthermia ■ *Impaired Verbal Communication* related to decreased hearing (NANDA-I © 2014)	Goals for Melinda's care include: ■ Melinda will demonstrate improved hearing with resolution of otitis media. ■ Melinda will demonstrate reduced level of pain and increased ability to sleep at night. ■ Melinda's mother will be able to describe indications for performing myringotomy and to demonstrate administration of eardrops. ■ Melinda will take in fluid adequate to maintain hydration.

Nursing Care Plan *(continued)*

IMPLEMENTATION

- Schedule a return visit to retest hearing in 2–3 weeks.
- Encourage Ms. Jeffries to call the office if Melinda shows signs of discomfort uncontrolled by ibuprofen.
- Teach Ms. Jeffries nonpharmacologic pain relief measures, such as application of heat and elevation of the head of the bed at night to promote drainage from the middle ear via the eustachian tube.
- Teach the patient and Ms. Jeffries to keep the head elevated when she is resting in bed to reduce pressure on the middle ear.

- Instruct Ms. Jeffries on the importance of administering the entire dispensed quantity of antibiotics, calling the office if a rash or other sign of allergic reaction occurs, and encouraging fluid intake.
- Demonstrate the technique for administering eardrops, and then have Ms. Jeffries provide a return demonstration.
- Provide verbal and written instructions about ear care, including scheduled follow-up examinations.
- Teach Ms. Jeffries about potential complications, actions to take in response, and when to call the care provider.

EVALUATION

Melinda returns in 2 weeks and is found to be infection free. Her tympanic membrane is normal in appearance, and she is her usual happy self. Hearing tests reveal that her hearing is within the normal range, and consultation with an audiologist is not indicated.

CRITICAL THINKING

1. What are the indications for performance of a myringotomy? Why was this patient not a candidate?
2. What other medications might have been prescribed to treat Melinda's ear infection?
3. Had Melinda's hearing not improved after resolution of the infection, what actions could the audiologist have recommended to improve her hearing?
4. Develop a plan of care related to caregiver role strain secondary to Melinda's inability to sleep because of pain.

REVIEW Otitis Media

RELATE Link the Concepts and Exemplars

Linking the exemplar of otitis media with the concept of evidence-based practice:

1. What peer-reviewed research can you find supporting the evidence-based practice of not prescribing antibiotics routinely for all diagnosed otitis media?
2. On the basis of your findings, how would knowledge of this research affect your practice when caring for patients with otitis media?

Linking the exemplar of otitis media with the concept of health policy:

3. How has health policy changed in the treatment of otitis media?
4. Does this change in policy seem reasonable? Why or why not?

READY Go to Volume 3: Clinical Nursing Skills

REFER Go to Pearson MyLab Nursing and eText

- Additional review materials

REFLECT Apply Your Knowledge

Ryan Riley is the 1-year-old son of Jessica Riley. They live in a one-bedroom apartment with Ms. Riley's boyfriend, Casey Miller. Ryan has a history of hospital admission for dehydration, respiratory syncytial 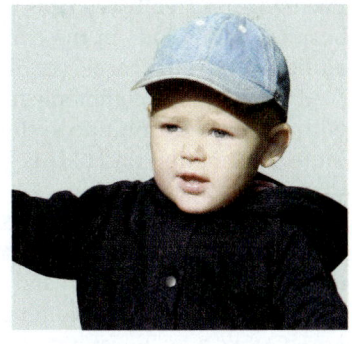 virus, and failure to thrive. Because he was found to be underweight and undernourished, social services made arrangements for him to attend Peanut Butter and Jelly Child Care during the day and to stay with his grandmother, Evelyn Sykes, in the evenings when his mother is working. He is seen for his 12-month immunizations and well-child exam, and his weight is 20 pounds, demonstrating good progress.

Fifteen-month-old Ryan has been running a fever and has a great deal of nasal drainage and congestion. He does not feel well at all. Worried about how ill he was last time he was sick, Ms. Sykes takes him to Neighborhood Pediatrics to be examined. Ryan is diagnosed with an upper respiratory infection. Mrs. Sykes is instructed to give Ryan plenty of fluids and children's Tylenol for the fever.

1. What factors place Ryan at risk for developing otitis media?
2. What teaching would you provide Ryan's grandmother to reduce the risk of otitis media?
3. While teaching Ms. Sykes about Ryan's care, what symptoms would you tell her need to be reported to the care provider, should they occur?

›› Exemplar 9.E Pneumonia

Exemplar Learning Outcomes

9.E Analyze pneumonia as it relates to infection.

- Describe the pathophysiology of pneumonia.
- Describe the etiology of pneumonia.
- Compare the risk factors and prevention of pneumonia.
- Identify the clinical manifestations of pneumonia.
- Summarize diagnostic tests and therapies used by interprofessional teams in the collaborative care of an individual with pneumonia.
- Differentiate care of patients with pneumonia across the lifespan.
- Apply the nursing process in providing culturally competent care to an individual with pneumonia.

Exemplar Key Terms

Overview

Inflammation of the lung parenchyma (the respiratory bronchioles and alveoli) as a result of infection is known as **pneumonia**. Despite significant advances in antibiotic therapy, pneumonia and influenza together are the eighth leading cause of death in the United States overall and the leading cause of death from infectious disease. In 2014, more than 50,000 deaths in the United States were attributed to pneumonia (CDC, 2016e). Its incidence and mortality rates are highest in older adults and people with debilitating diseases. Pneumonia currently accounts for approximately 3% of adult hospital admissions in the United States (CDC, 2015e). In addition, HAIs such as ventilator-associated pneumonia (VAP), occur more commonly in older adults and in patients with weakened immune systems (Arvanitis et al., 2014). More information on HAIs is provided in The Concept of Infection section.

The respiratory system is constantly open to the possibility of infection. The respiratory tree is exposed to the environment as air moves into and out of the lower respiratory tract. In addition, huge numbers of microorganisms in the oropharynx may be aspirated into the bronchial tree. Both anatomical and physiologic defenses help to maintain the sterility of the lower respiratory tract. When these defenses are impaired, the risk for infection increases. For example, drugs, alcohol, or neuromuscular disease may suppress the cough reflex; asthma can both narrow and inflame airways, trapping mucus and impairing oxygenation; and the influenza virus can leave the respiratory epithelium vulnerable to bacterial infection. Even in healthy people, microorganisms and other foreign material occasionally enter the bronchial tree and lung parenchyma.

Disorders affecting the lower respiratory system (below the larynx) can affect the ability to effectively move air into and out of the lungs (ventilation), exchange oxygen and carbon dioxide across the alveolar-capillary membrane (respiration), and maintain clear and patent airways and ventilate the lungs.

Organisms causing such disorders can enter the lung in several ways. The most common means of entry is aspiration of microbe-containing secretions from the oropharynx. Microorganisms may be inhaled following release when an infected individual coughs, sneezes, or talks. Inhalation of contaminated aerosolized water can result in viral and some other types of pneumonia. Bacteria also may spread to the lungs through the bloodstream from infection elsewhere in the body. Regardless of the means of entry, host defenses must be overwhelmed either by the number of organisms or by their **virulence** (disease-causing ability) for an infection to develop.

Pathophysiology and Etiology

Pathophysiology

When invading microorganisms colonize the alveoli, they initiate an inflammatory and immune response. The antigen–antibody response and endotoxins released by some organisms damage bronchial and alveolar mucous membranes, causing inflammation with vascular congestion and edema. Infectious debris and exudate can fill alveoli, interfering with ventilation and gas exchange (see **Figure 9–20** ››). Pneumonia may develop in any one of four distinct patterns (see **Table 9–11** ››): (1) lobar pneumonia, (2) bronchopneumonia, (3) interstitial pneumonia, and (4) miliary pneumonia.

The pathologic process, anatomical location, and manifestations of pneumonia vary according to the infective organism. Bacterial and viral pathogens act differently within the lungs:

- Bacterial pathogens circulate through the bloodstream to the lungs, where they damage cells. Cellular debris and mucus cause airway obstruction. Bacteria tend to be distributed evenly throughout one or more lobes of a single lung, a pattern termed **unilateral lobar pneumonia**.
- Viruses frequently enter from the upper respiratory tract, infiltrating the alveoli nearest the bronchi of one or both

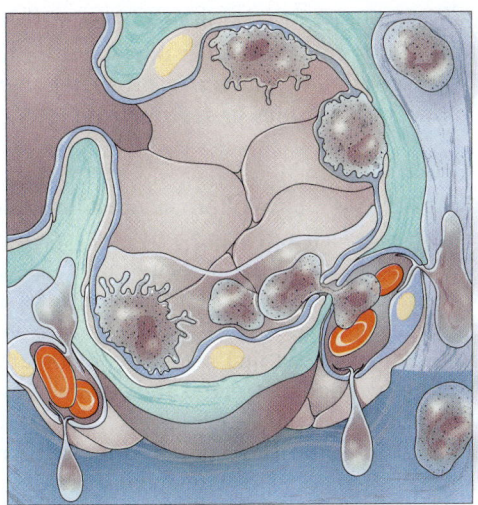

Figure 9–20 In pneumonia, the inflammatory response causes fluid to accumulate in the alveoli and edema to form as alveolar capillaries dilate and allow fluid to leak into interstitial tissues.

lungs. There, they invade the cells, replicate, and burst out forcefully, killing the cells and sending out cell debris. They rapidly invade adjacent areas, distributing themselves in the scattered, patchy pattern referred to as *bronchopneumonia*.

TABLE 9–11 Patterns of Lung Involvement in Pneumonia

Pattern of Involvement	Description
Lobar pneumonia	Lobar pneumonia typically involves an entire lobe of a lung. Early in the process, when the immune response is minimal, bacteria spread throughout the affected lobe by rapid accumulation of fluid exudate. As the immune and inflammatory responses develop, red blood cells and neutrophils, damaged epithelial cells, and fibrin accumulate in the alveoli and bronchioles, causing **consolidation** (solidification) of lung tissue. Purulent exudate containing neutrophils and macrophages also forms. The process finally resolves as enzymes destroy the exudate and residual debris is reabsorbed, phagocytized, or coughed out.
Bronchopneumonia	Bronchopneumonia usually involves dependent portions of lung tissue; characterized by patchy consolidation. Exudate tends to remain primarily in the bronchi and bronchioles, with less edema and congestion of the alveoli than with lobar pneumonia.
Interstitial pneumonia	The inflammatory process primarily involves the interstitium (the alveolar walls and connective tissue supporting the bronchial tree). Involvement may be patchy or diffuse as lymphocytes, macrophages, and plasma cells infiltrate the alveolar septa. While alveoli typically do not contain significant exudates, protein-rich hyaline membranes may line the alveoli, interfering with gas exchange.
Miliary pneumonia	In miliary pneumonia, the spread of the pathogen to the lungs via the bloodstream causes the development of numerous discrete inflammatory lesions. Miliary pneumonia is seen primarily in individuals who are severely immunocompromised. Because the immune response is poor, damage to pleural tissue may be significant.

- Aspiration of food, emesis, gastric reflux, or hydrocarbons causes a chemical injury and an inflammatory response. Materials with a lower pH cause more inflammation, which sets the stage for bacterial invasion.

Pneumonia may be either infectious or noninfectious. Bacteria, viruses, fungi, protozoa, and other microbes can lead to infectious pneumonia. Noninfectious causes include aspiration of gastric contents and inhalation of toxic or irritating gases. Pneumonias often are classified as community acquired, healthcare associated, or opportunistic. Different organisms are implicated in each of these classifications (see **Table 9–12**). The most common causative organism for community-acquired pneumonia is *Streptococcus pneumoniae* (also called *pneumococcus*), a gram-positive bacterium. This organism causes approximately 50% of the cases of community-acquired pneumonia leading to hospital admission. *Staphylococcus aureus* and gram-negative bacteria are often implicated as healthcare-associated causes of pneumonia. Organisms such as *Pneumocystis jiroveci* generally cause infections only in individuals who are immunocompromised (opportunistic infections).

Etiology

The several different classifications of pneumonia are based on the infecting organism, including acute bacterial pneumonia, Legionnaires disease, primary atypical pneumonia, viral pneumonia, *Pneumocystis jiroveci* pneumonia, and aspiration pneumonia.

Acute Bacterial Pneumonia

Of the bacterial pneumonias, the pathogenesis of pneumococcal (*Streptococcus pneumoniae*) pneumonia is best understood (see **Figure 9–21**). These bacteria reside in the upper respiratory tract of up to 70% of adults. They may be spread by direct individual-to-individual contact via droplets. In many cases, infection results from aspiration of resident bacteria. The typical pattern for pneumococcal pneumonia is lobar pneumonia (see Table 9–11), although it may present

TABLE 9–12 Common Organisms Causing Pneumonia in Adults

Community-Acquired	Healthcare-Associated	Opportunistic
Streptococcus pneumoniae	*Streptococcus pneumoniae*	*Pneumocystis jiroveci*
Staphylococcus aureus	*Staphylococcus aureus*	*Mycobacterium tuberculosis*
Mycoplasma pneumoniae	*Pseudomonas aeruginosa*	Cytomegalovirus
Haemophilus influenzae	*Haemophilus influenzae*	Atypical mycobacteria
Klebsiella pneumoniae	*Klebsiella pneumoniae*	Fungi
Influenza virus	*Escherichia coli*	
Chlamydia pneumoniae		
Legionella pneumophila		

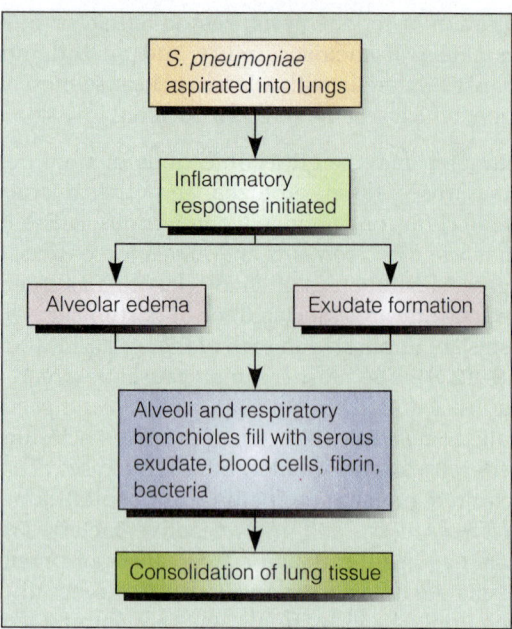

S. pneumoniae
aspired into lungs

↓

Inflammatory
response initiated

↓

Alveolar edema   Exudate formation

↓

Alveoli and respiratory
bronchioles fill with serous
exudate, blood cells, fibrin,
bacteria

↓

Consolidation of lung tissue

Figure 9–21 ❯❯ The pathogenesis of pneumococcal pneumonia.

in a pattern more typical of bronchopneumonia. The lower lobes of the lungs are usually affected because of gravity.

Pneumococcal pneumonia typically resolves uneventfully; normal lung structure is restored on completion of the process. Local extension of the infection to involve the pleura (**pleuritis**) is the most common complication. Pneumonias caused by *Staphylococcus aureus* and gram-negative bacteria often cause extensive parenchymal damage, with necrosis, lung abscess, and empyema, or **pleural effusion** (accumulation of excess fluid in the pleural cavity). Progressive destruction of lung tissue and functional impairment are possible consequences of *Klebsiella* pneumonia.

A **lung abscess** is a local area of necrosis and pus formation within the lung itself and is relatively uncommon. The manifestations of lung abscess develop slowly and include weight loss, malaise, night sweats, fever, and a productive cough. Sputum is foul smelling and tasting. Rupture of the abscess into a larger airway is heralded by production of copious amounts of purulent sputum.

Empyema is accumulation of purulent exudate in the pleural cavity. It is identified by chest x-ray or CT. **Thoracentesis** (insertion of a needle into the pleural space to remove fluid accumulation) may be done, or a chest tube may be inserted to allow continuous drainage of purulent exudates.

The presentation of bacterial pneumonia is usually acute, with rapid onset of shaking chills, fever, and cough that produces rust-colored or purulent sputum. Chest aching or **pleuritic pain** (sharp, localized chest pain that increases with breathing and coughing) is common. Limited breath sounds and fine crackles or rales are heard over the affected area of lung. A pleural friction rub may be audible. If the involved area is large and gas exchange is impaired, dyspnea and cyanosis may be noted.

A more insidious onset with low-grade fever, cough, and scattered crackles is more typical of bronchopneumonia. However, dyspnea is less common with bronchopneumonia. The older adult or patient who is debilitated may have atypical manifestations of pneumonia, with little cough, scant sputum, and minimal evidence of respiratory distress. Fever, tachypnea (rapid respirations), and altered mentation or agitation may be the primary presenting symptoms.

Legionnaires Disease

Legionnaires disease is a form of bronchopneumonia caused by *Legionella pneumophila*, a gram-negative bacterium widely found in water, particularly warm, standing water. Legionnaires disease occurs sporadically and in outbreaks, such as the one that occurred at an American Legion convention in 1976, when the disease was first recognized. Contaminated water-cooled air-conditioning systems and other water sources have been implicated in its spread. Smokers, older adults, and individuals with chronic diseases or impaired immune defenses are most susceptible to Legionnaires disease.

Symptoms of Legionnaires disease develop gradually, beginning 2–10 days after exposure. Dry cough, dyspnea, general malaise, chills and fever, headache, confusion, diminished appetite and diarrhea, myalgias, and arthralgias are common manifestations. Consolidation of lung tissue is patchy or lobar. Patients who develop Legionnaires disease while in the hospital have a mortality rate close to 50%. Patients who have additional diseases and who are immunocompromised are at higher risk for mortality from Legionnaires disease (Sakamoto, 2015).

Primary Atypical Pneumonia

Pneumonia caused by *Mycoplasma pneumoniae* is generally classified as *primary atypical pneumonia*, because its presentation and course differ significantly from those of other bacterial pneumonias. Mycoplasma infection often causes pharyngitis or bronchitis. When this type of pneumonia develops, patchy inflammatory changes occur in the alveolar septum and interstitial tissue of the lung. Alveolar exudate and consolidation of lung tissue are not features of atypical pneumonia. Young adults—college students and military recruits in particular—are the populations primarily affected.

Primary atypical pneumonia is highly contagious. Its manifestations resemble those of viral pneumonia; systemic manifestations of fever, headache, myalgias, and arthralgias often predominate. The cough associated with atypical pneumonia is dry, hacking, and nonproductive. Because of the typically mild nature and predominant systemic manifestations, mycoplasmal and viral pneumonia are often referred to as *walking pneumonias*.

Viral Pneumonia

Approximately 10% of pneumonias in adults are viral. Influenza virus and adenovirus are the most common organisms; however, the incidence of cytomegalovirus (CMV) pneumonia in those who are immunocompromised is on the rise. Other viruses, such as herpes viruses and measles virus, may also cause viral pneumonia. As in primary atypical pneumonia, lung involvement in viral pneumonia is limited to the alveolar septum and interstitial spaces.

Viral pneumonia is typically a mild disease that often affects older adults and people with chronic conditions. It usually occurs in community epidemics. Flulike symptoms of headache, fever, fatigue, malaise, and muscle aching are common, along with a dry cough.

Pneumocystis jiroveci Pneumonia

Individuals with AIDS and others who are significantly immunocompromised are at significant risk for developing an opportunistic pneumonia caused by *Pneumocystis jiroveci* (previously known as *P. carinii*), a common parasite found worldwide. Immunity to *P. jiroveci* is nearly universal, except in those who are immunocompromised. Opportunistic infection may develop in patients treated with immunosuppressive or cytotoxic drugs for cancer or who have undergone organ transplantation and in patients with genetic or acquired immunodeficiency.

Infection with *P. jiroveci* produces patchy involvement throughout the lungs, causing affected alveoli to thicken, become edematous, and fill with foamy, protein-rich fluid. Gas exchange is severely impaired as the disease progresses. *P. jiroveci* pneumonia has an abrupt onset, with fever, tachypnea, shortness of breath, and a dry, nonproductive cough. Respiratory distress can be significant, with intercostal retractions and cyanosis.

Aspiration Pneumonia

Aspiration of gastric contents into the lungs results in a chemical and bacterial pneumonia known as *aspiration pneumonia*. Major risk factors for aspiration pneumonia include emergency surgery in which the patient was not NPO 8 hours prior (e.g., emergency cesarean birth); depressed cough and gag reflexes; and impaired swallowing.

Older surgical patients and those with advanced dementia are at significant risk. Enteral nutrition by either nasogastric or gastric tube also increases the risk for aspiration pneumonia. Vomiting is not always apparent; silent regurgitation of gastric contents may occur when the level of consciousness is decreased. Measures to reduce the risk for aspiration pneumonia include elevating the head of the bed, minimizing the use of preoperative medications, promoting anesthetic elimination from the body, preventing nausea and gastric distention, serving thickened liquids, and performing swallowing tests, especially for patients who have had strokes.

The low pH of gastric contents causes a severe inflammatory response when aspirated into the respiratory tract. Pulmonary edema and respiratory failure may result. Common complications of aspiration pneumonia are abscesses, **bronchiectasis** (chronic dilation of the bronchi and bronchioles), and gangrene of pulmonary tissue.

Risk Factors

The immature immune systems of infants and young children increase their risk for pneumonia. Older adults are at increased risk because of diminished cough and gag reflexes as well as diminishing immune response. Anyone with a compromised immune system, such as those diagnosed with HIV/AIDS, individuals on medication to prevent rejection of a transplanted organ, and those receiving treatment for cancer such as chemotherapy or radiation therapy, is at increased risk for infection—and for pneumonia in particular. Patients in a debilitated or weakened condition from any cause, including chronic cardiac or respiratory conditions, diabetes mellitus, or alcoholism, also face increased risk. Patients at high risk for pneumonia also face a higher risk for adverse outcomes and complications.

Research indicates a high rate of pneumonia in patients with frequent exposure to cigarette smoke and alcohol or drug abuse. Smoking injures tissues in the airways and decreases the action of cilia. Chemicals in cigarettes have a numbing effect on the cough reflex. All of these actions diminish the lung's natural protective mechanisms. Alcohol interferes with the actions of macrophages, while injection drug users are at risk from infections that originate at the injection site and then spread through the bloodstream to the lungs.

Prevention

Prevention is a key component in managing pneumonia. Identifying vulnerable populations and instituting preventive strategies are measures to reduce the mortality and morbidity associated with the condition. With early identification of the infecting organism, appropriate treatment, and support of respiratory function, most patients recover uneventfully. However, pneumonia remains a serious disease with significant mortality, especially in older adults and individuals who are frail or have chronic diseases.

Vaccines offer some degree of protection against the most common bacterial and viral pneumonias. Pneumococcal vaccine, made of antigens from 23 types of pneumococcus, usually imparts lifetime immunity with a single dose. The vaccine is recommended for patients who have a high risk of adverse outcome from bacterial pneumonias, including all adults over the age of 65; individuals with chronic diseases such as heart conditions, lung disease, alcoholism, diabetes, and cirrhosis; individuals with chronic renal failure; individuals who are immunocompromised (e.g., those with malignancy, HIV/AIDS, organ transplant); individuals who smoke or have asthma; and individuals receiving chemotherapy with selected agents, radiation therapy, or long-term steroids. A one-time revaccination is recommended for selected populations, including individuals with immunosuppressive conditions and adults over age 65 who were immunized more than 5 years previously and before age 65 (CDC, 2015f).

SAFETY ALERT Annual influenza vaccination helps prevent pneumonia. Inquire about allergic responses to eggs or previous influenza vaccinations before administering influenza vaccine. A significant hypersensitivity response may occur in patients who are allergic to egg protein.

Clinical Manifestations

Infection of the lower respiratory tract has both local and systemic effects. Local effects include cough, excess mucus production, shortness of breath or **dyspnea** (difficult or labored breathing) and hypoxia that may proceed to apnea due to respiratory collapse, **hemoptysis** (bloody sputum), and chest pain. Systemic effects may include fever, diminished appetite and malaise, **cyanosis** (gray to blue or purple skin color caused by deoxygenated hemoglobin, secondary to hypoxia), and other manifestations of impaired gas exchange. **Table 9–13 》** compares the manifestations of infectious pneumonias.

Bacteremia can spread the infection to other tissues, leading to meningitis, endocarditis, or peritonitis and increasing the risk of mortality. Entry of the pathogens into the bloodstream can result in septicemia, leading to septic shock.

TABLE 9–13 Manifestations of Infectious Pneumonias

Type	Onset	Respiratory Manifestations	Systemic Manifestations
Pneumococcal or lobar pneumonia	Abrupt	Cough productive of purulent or rust-colored sputum; pleuritic or aching chest pain; decreased breath sounds and crackles over affected area; possible dyspnea and cyanosis	Chills and fever
Bronchopneumonia	Gradual	Cough, scattered crackles; minimal dyspnea and respiratory distress	Low-grade fever
Legionnaires disease	Gradual	Dry cough; dyspnea	Chills and fever; general malaise; headache; confusion; diminished appetite and diarrhea; myalgias and arthralgias
Primary atypical pneumonia	Gradual	Dry, hacking, nonproductive cough	Fever, headache, myalgias, and arthralgias predominate
Viral pneumonia	Sudden or gradual	Dry cough	Flulike symptoms
Pneumocystis jiroveci pneumonia	Abrupt	Dry cough; tachypnea and shortness of breath; significant respiratory distress	Fever

Collaboration

Collaboration in caring for an individual with pneumonia may include nurses, doctors, phlebotomists, respiratory therapists, radiologists, and speech-language pathologists to perform swallow tests. In some cases, consultation with an infectious disease specialist or a pulmonologist may be necessary. Patients who are gravely ill and their families may want the opportunity to talk with the hospital chaplain or their own minister, rabbi, or other spiritual leader.

Diagnostic Tests

The history and physical examination, along with diagnostic testing, are used to establish the diagnosis, determine the

Clinical Manifestations and Therapies
Pneumonia

ETIOLOGY	CLINICAL MANIFESTATIONS	CLINICAL THERAPIES
Presence of pathogens causes the hypothalamus to increase the set point of body temperature in an attempt to kill the invader	Fever	■ Increase fluid intake. ■ Administer antipyretics, such as ibuprofen or acetaminophen. Aspirin may be used in adults but is contraindicated in children because of the risk for Reye syndrome. ■ Minimize clothing and coverings. ■ Monitor temperature frequently. ■ Give a tepid bath if fever does not respond to other therapies or becomes too high.
Respiratory muscle fatigue	Apnea	■ Use a cardiorespiratory monitor. ■ Use measures to reduce the work of breathing, including assistance with airway clearance, positioning, and oxygen administration. ■ Recurrent or severe episodes of apnea indicate the need for intubation and mechanical ventilation.
Accumulation of fluid and debris in the airways	Cough	■ Increase fluid intake to liquefy secretions. ■ Frequently change position to prevent atelectasis and help drain different airways. ■ Use chest physiotherapy to promote airway clearance. ■ Use airway suctioning to promote airway clearance if the cough is weak or ineffective. ■ Administer mucolytics to promote sputum expectoration and bronchodilators to open airways, allowing movement of sputum.
Fluid accumulation in the airways impairing gas exchange	Hypoxia	■ Administer oxygen. ■ Encourage coughing and deep breathing to clear airways and promote gas exchange. ■ Monitor vital signs and oxygen saturation. ■ Position to promote airway clearance.

extent of lung involvement, and identify the causative organism. Diagnostic tests include the following:

- *Chest x-ray* is obtained to determine the extent and pattern of lung involvement. Fluid, infiltrates, consolidated lung tissue, and **atelectasis** (areas of alveolar collapse) appear as densities on the film.

- *CT* provides a more detailed image of pulmonary tissue and may be used when the chest x-ray is not diagnostic.

- *Sputum Gram stain* rapidly identifies the infecting organisms as gram-positive or gram-negative bacteria. Antibiotic therapy can then be directed at the predominant type of organism until culture and sensitivity results are obtained.

- *Sputum culture and sensitivity* are ordered to identify the infecting organism and determine the most effective antibiotic therapy. When obtaining sputum for culture, it is important to obtain secretions from the lower respiratory tract, not from the mouth and nasal passages.

- *Complete blood count (CBC) with WBC differential* shows an elevated WBC (greater than or equal to $10,000/\text{mm}^3$) with increased circulating immature leukocytes (a left shift) in response to the infectious process. WBC changes are minimal in viral and other pneumonias.

- *Serology testing* (blood tests to detect antibodies to respiratory pathogens) may be used to identify the infecting organism when blood and sputum cultures are negative.

- *Pulse oximetry,* a noninvasive method of measuring arterial oxygen saturation (SaO_2), is ordered to continuously monitor gas exchange. The SaO_2 normally is 95% or higher. An SaO_2 of less than 95% may indicate impaired alveolar gas exchange.

- *Arterial blood gas* may be ordered to evaluate gas exchange. Respiratory secretions or pleuritic pain can interfere with alveolar ventilation. Alveolar inflammation can interfere with gas exchange across the alveolar-capillary membrane, especially if exudate or consolidation is present. An arterial partial pressure of oxygen (PaO_2) of less than 75–80 mmHg indicates impaired gas exchange or alveolar ventilation.

- *Fiberoptic bronchoscopy* may be done to obtain a sputum specimen or remove secretions from the bronchial tree.

Pharmacologic Therapy

Medications used to treat pneumonia include antibiotics to eradicate the infection and bronchodilators to reduce bronchospasm and improve ventilation. Initial antibiotic therapy is based on the results of sputum Gram stain and the pattern of lung involvement shown on a chest x-ray. The presence of cardiovascular disease or residence in a long-term care facility is also considered in the initial antibiotic choice. A broad-spectrum antibiotic, such as a macrolide (e.g., clarithromycin, azithromycin, erythromycin), a penicillin or a second- or third-generation cephalosporin, or a fluoroquinolone (e.g., ciprofloxacin), is typically ordered until the results of sputum culture and sensitivity tests are available. **Table 9–14** ⟫ lists commonly prescribed antibiotics for selected pneumonias.

When an inflammatory response to the infection causes bronchospasm and constriction, bronchodilators may be ordered to improve ventilation and reduce hypoxia. Bronchodilators generally belong to one of two major groups: the sympathomimetic drugs, such as albuterol sulfate (Proventil) and the methylxanthines, such as theophylline and aminophylline.

A medication may be prescribed to "break up" mucus or reduce its viscosity. Acetylcysteine (Mucomyst), potassium iodide, and guaifenesin (a common ingredient in expectorant cough syrups) help to liquefy mucus, making it easier to expectorate. For many patients, however, increasing fluid intake is an effective means of liquefying mucus.

Oxygen therapy may be indicated for the patient who is tachypneic or hypoxemic. Inflammation of the alveolar–capillary membrane interferes with diffusion of gases across the membrane. Diffusion is affected by several other factors, including the partial pressure of gases on each side of the membrane. Increasing the percentage of inspired oxygen above that of room air (21%) increases the partial pressure of oxygen in the alveoli and enhances its diffusion into the capillaries. Supplemental oxygen therefore improves oxygenation of the blood and tissues in patients with pneumonia.

Depending on the degree of hypoxia, oxygen may be administered by either a low-flow or a high-flow system. Low-flow systems include the nasal cannula, simple face

TABLE 9–14 Antibiotic Therapy for Selected Pneumonias

Causative Organism	Antibiotic of Choice	Alternative Antibiotics
Streptococcus pneumoniae	Penicillin G, amoxicillin	Erythromycin, cephalosporins, doxycycline, fluoroquinolone, clindamycin, vancomycin, trimethoprim-sulfamethoxazole (TMP-SMZ), linezolid
Haemophilus influenzae	Second- or third-generation cephalosporins, doxycycline, azithromycin, TMP-SMZ	Fluoroquinolones, clarithromycin
Staphylococcus aureus	Penicillinase-resistant penicillin (e.g., nafcillin), vancomycin for methicillin-resistant organisms	Cephalosporins, vancomycin, clindamycin; ciprofloxacin, fluoroquinolones, TMP-SMZ
Mycoplasma pneumoniae	Erythromycin, doxycycline	Clarithromycin, azithromycin, fluoroquinolone
Klebsiella pneumoniae	Third-generation cephalosporin (with aminoglycoside if severe), metronidazole	Aztreonam, imipenem-cilastatin, fluoroquinolone
Legionella pneumophila	Macrolide + rifampin, fluoroquinolone	TMP-SMZ, doxycycline + rifampin
Pneumocystis jiroveci	TMP-SMZ, pentamidine + prednisone	Dapsone + trimethoprim, clindamycin + primaquine, trimetrexate + folinic acid
Chlamydia pneumoniae	Doxycycline	Macrolide, fluoroquinolone

mask, partial rebreathing mask, and nonrebreather mask (see **Figure 9–22** 》). A nasal cannula can deliver 24–45% oxygen concentrations with flow rates of 2–6 L/minute. The nasal cannula is comfortable and does not interfere with eating or talking. A simple face mask delivers 40–60% oxygen concentrations with flow rates of 5–8 L/minute. Up to 100% oxygen can be delivered by the nonrebreather mask, the

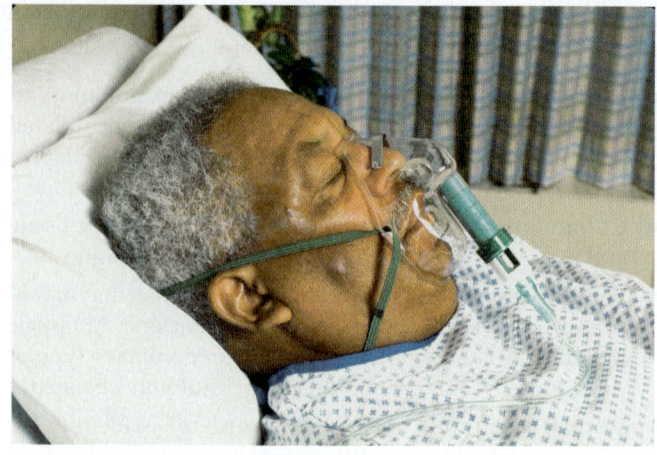

Figure 9–23 》 Venturi mask, a high-flow oxygen delivery system.

highest concentration possible without mechanical ventilation. When the amount of oxygen delivered must be precisely regulated, a high-flow system, such as a Venturi mask, is used (see **Figure 9–23** 》). The Venturi mask regulates the ratio of oxygen to room air, allowing precise regulation of the oxygen percentage delivered, from 24% to 50%. Severe hypoxia may necessitate intubation and mechanical ventilation.

Nonpharmacologic Therapy

Supportive care for all types of pneumonia includes airway management, fluids, and rest. When mucus secretions are thick and viscous, increasing fluid intake to between 2500 and 3000 mL/day helps to liquefy secretions, making them easier to cough up and expectorate. If the patient is unable to maintain an adequate oral intake, IV fluids and nutrition may be required.

Incentive spirometry may be used to promote deep breathing, coughing, and clearance of respiratory secretions. Endotracheal suctioning may be required if the cough is ineffective. On occasion, bronchoscopy is used to perform pulmonary hygiene and remove secretions.

Chest Physiotherapy

Chest physiotherapy, including percussion, vibration, and postural drainage, may be performed by a nurse, physiotherapist, respiratory therapist, or trained family member to reduce lung consolidation and prevent atelectasis. Perform *percussion* by rhythmically striking or clapping the chest wall with cupped hands (see **Figure 9–24A** 》), using rapid wrist flexion and extension. Cupping traps air between the palm and the patient's skin, setting up vibrations through the chest wall that loosen respiratory secretions. The trapped air also provides a cushion, preventing injury. When performed correctly, percussion produces a hollow, popping sound. Percussion may also be done using a mechanical percussion cup. The breasts, sternum, spinal column, and kidney regions are avoided during percussion.

Vibration facilitates the movement of secretions into larger airways. It usually is combined with percussion, although it may be used when percussion is contraindicated or poorly tolerated. Perform vibration by repeatedly

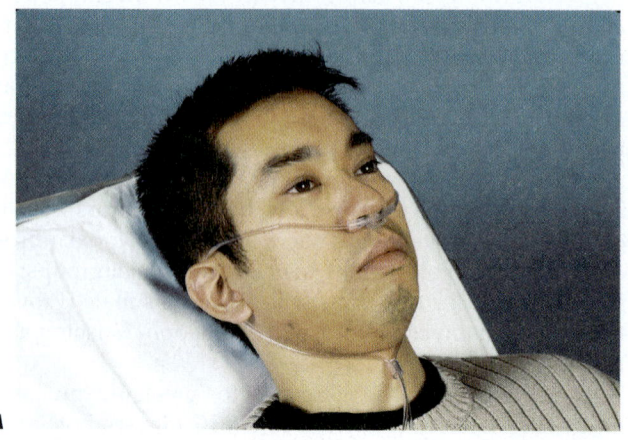

A

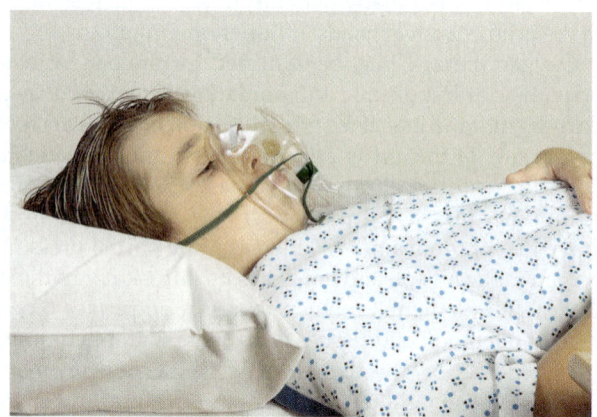

B

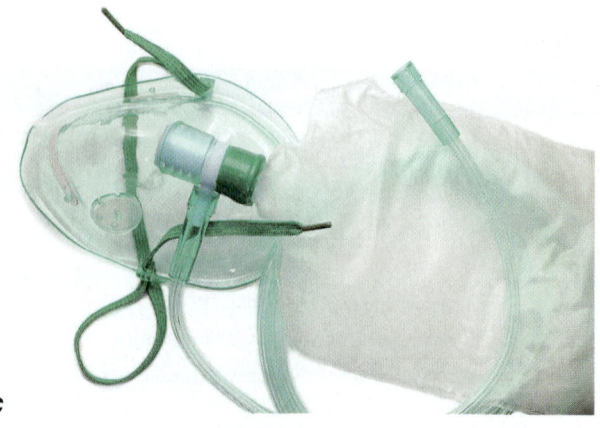

C

Source: **B**, Tony McConnell/Science Source.

Figure 9–22 》 Low-flow oxygen delivery devices: **A,** nasal cannula; **B,** simple face mask; **C,** nonrebreather mask.

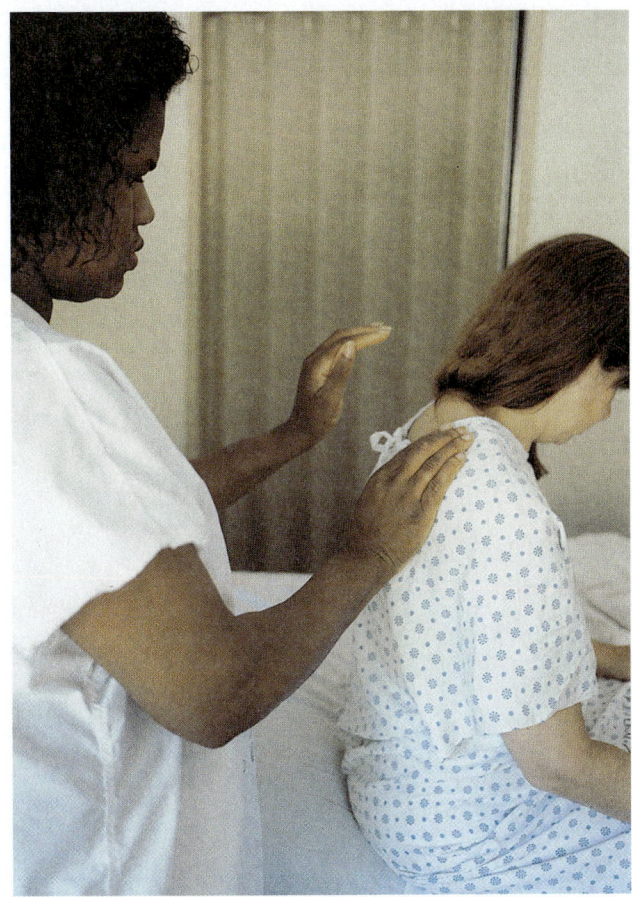 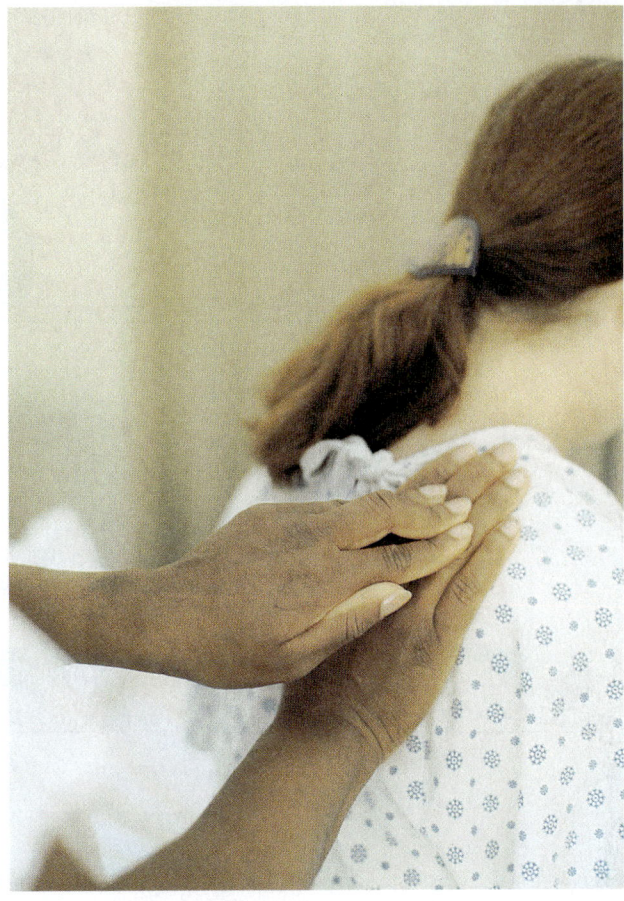

Figure 9–24 》 A, Percussing (clapping) the upper posterior chest. Notice the cupped position of the nurse's hands. **B,** Vibrating the upper posterior chest.

tensing the arm and hand muscles while maintaining firm but gentle pressure over the affected area with the flat of the hand (see Figure 9–24*B*).

Percussion and vibration are combined with *postural drainage*, which uses gravity to facilitate removal of secretions from a particular lung segment. The patient is positioned with the segment to be drained superior to or above the trachea or mainstem bronchus. Drainage of all lung segments requires a variety of positions (see **Figure 9–25 》**); rarely do all segments require drainage. Administer bronchodilators or nebulizer treatments as ordered before postural drainage. Perform postural drainage before meals to avoid nausea and vomiting.

Lifespan Considerations

The populations that are most susceptible to pneumonia include young children and older adults based on increased risk of airway obstruction and on physiologic changes in the airway that decrease airway clearance of infecting organisms. Pregnant women are at increased risk for pneumonia particularly if they have a history of smoking or recent or recurrent respiratory illnesses (Benoit et al., 2013).

Pneumonia in Children

The immature airway of the child makes children more susceptible to the development of pneumonia. The primary physiologic aspects of the immature lung that contribute to pneumonia severity are the size of the airways, number of alveoli, differential use of muscles for breathing, and higher oxygen consumption. For more information on the pediatric airway, see Figures 15–7 through 15–20 in the Lifespan Considerations section in the module on Oxygenation.

Oxygen consumption is higher in children than in adults because of children's greater metabolic rate. This rate of oxygen consumption increases further when the child is in respiratory distress. The child also has fewer muscle glycogen reserves, leading to more rapid muscle fatigue when accessory muscles must be used for breathing (Varman, 2015). As a result, children become hypoxic more quickly than adults. Tachypnea, retractions, nasal flaring (opening of the nares on inspiration in an attempt to draw in more air), and increased effort of breathing may tire the infant or young child and result in periods of **apnea** (absence of breathing).

Physiologic differences in children affect the clinical manifestations of pneumonia. Symptoms include fever, tachypnea, rhonchi, crackles, wheezes, cough, dyspnea, nasal flaring, restlessness, chest pain, and malaise. Decreased breath sounds may be present if consolidation exists. The child also may have poor oral intake, nausea, vomiting, and abdominal pain. In children over 12 months of age who have clinical manifestations associated with pneumonia, a respiratory rate greater than 50/min and an oxygen saturation of

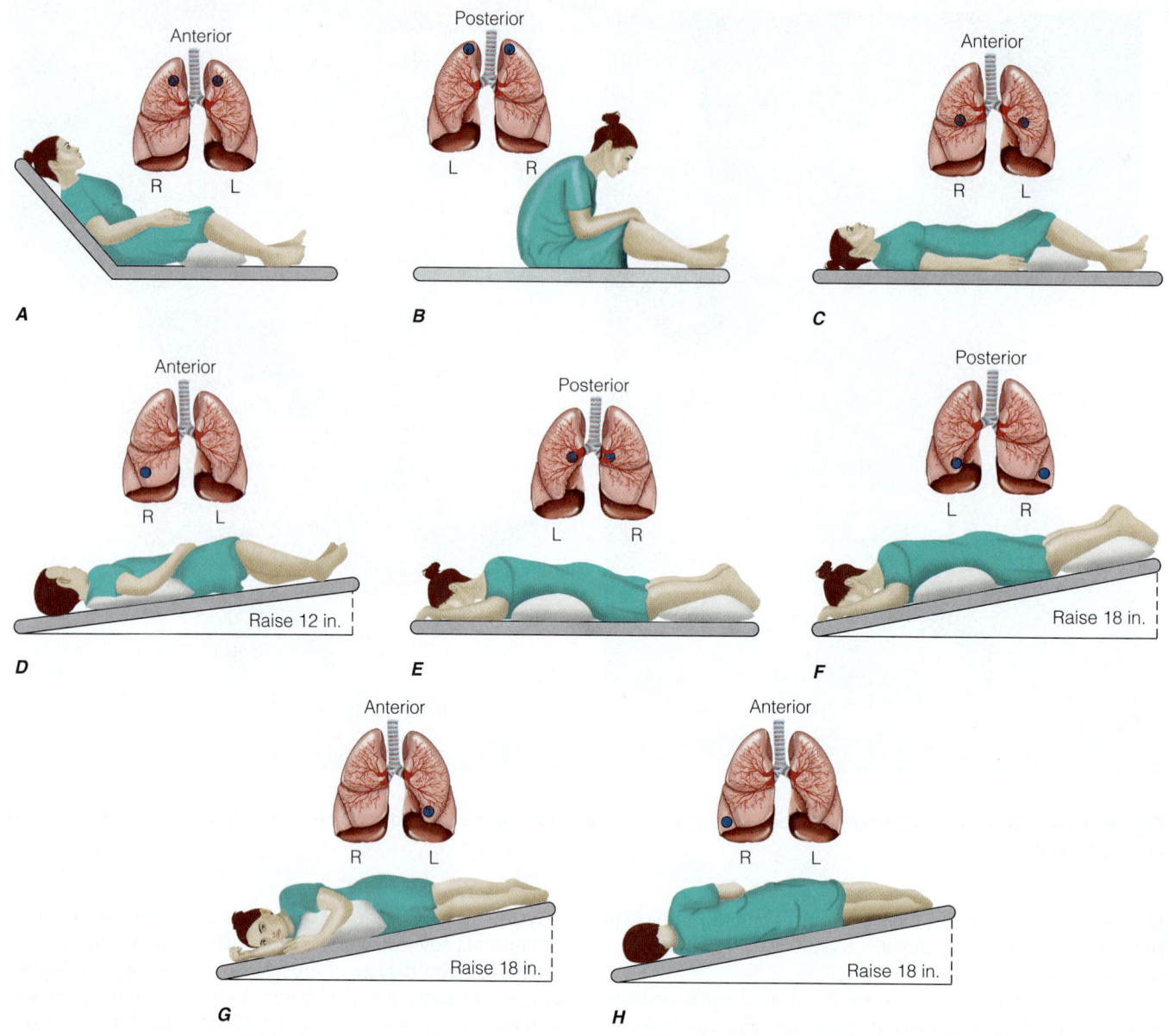

Figure 9–25 》 Positions for postural drainage. **A,** Left and right anterior apical. **B,** Left and right posterior apical. **C,** Left and right anterior upper. **D,** Right middle lobe. **E,** Superior lower lobes. **F,** Left and right lower posterior. **G,** Left lower lateral. **H,** Right lower lateral.

96% or less are more likely to be associated with a positive chest x-ray. In children under 12 months of age, nasal flaring is an important finding that is more likely to be associated with a positive chest x-ray (Varman, 2015). The older child may have dullness to chest percussion, increased fremitus (vibration felt on palpation), and egophony (increased resonance of voice sounds).

There is no clinical way to differentiate the bacterial from the viral cause of pneumonia, because it is difficult to get a sputum culture from a child. Blood cultures may be taken instead. In children older than 5 years, pneumonia is caused primarily by bacteria, such as *Streptococcus pneumoniae*. The child's age, severity of symptoms, and the presence of an underlying lung, cardiac, or immunodeficiency disease create varying responses. Children with a condition such as cystic fibrosis or immunosuppression are susceptible to many other bacterial, parasitic, or fungal infections. Pneumonia in children often resolves much sooner than in adults. The key is early recognition, enabling the child to be treated at home rather than in the hospital.

Because of the aforementioned differences in the child's anatomy and physiology and related manifestations of pneumonia, assessment of pediatric patients is different than that of adults. Assessment guidelines for pediatric patients are given in **Table 9–15 》**. See **Table 9–16 》** for fluid requirements of the pediatric patient. A liberal fluid intake helps to liquefy secretions and facilitate their clearance. In pediatric patients, rapid fluid replacement is indicated in sepsis conditions, as well as appropriate pharmacologic interventions (Normandin, 2015). Also, while aspirin may be used with adults, aspirin is never prescribed for the pediatric patient because of the risk of Reye syndrome.

TABLE 9–15 Assessment Guidelines for the Child with a Respiratory Condition

Assessment Focus	Assessment Guidelines
Position of comfort	■ Is the child comfortable lying down? ■ Does the child prefer to sit up or be in the tripod position (sitting forward with arms on knees for support and extending the neck)?
Vital signs	■ Assess the rate, depth, and ease of respirations. See Table 34–3 in the module on Assessment for expected respiratory rate ranges by age. ■ Assess the pulse for rate and strength. See Table 34–3 in the module on Assessment for expected heart rate ranges by age.
Lung auscultation	■ Are breath sounds bilateral, diminished, or absent? ■ Are adventitious sounds (wheezes, crackles, or rhonchi) present?
Respiratory effort (work of breathing)	■ Are there audible inspiratory and expiratory breath sounds or stridor? Is there grunting with expiration? ■ Is breathing labored? ■ Are **retractions** (visible appearance of the chest being drawn in on inspiration) present, or are accessory muscles used to breathe? ■ Is nasal flaring present? ■ Is **tachypnea** (abnormally rapid rate of respirations) present? ■ Can the child say a full sentence or is a breath needed every few words? Is the cry strong or weak? ■ Do the chest and abdomen rise simultaneously with inspiration, or is paradoxical breathing present in which the chest and abdomen do not rise simultaneously?
Color	■ What is the color of the mucous membranes (pink, pale, mottled, cyanotic)? ■ Does crying improve or worsen the color?
Cough	■ Is the cough dry (nonproductive), wet (productive, mucousy), brassy (noisy, musical), or croupy (barking, seal-like)? ■ Is the coughing effort forceful or weak?
Behavior change	■ Note any sudden behavior changes such as irritability, restlessness, or change in level of responsiveness.
Family history	■ Is there a family history of asthma or cystic fibrosis?

Pneumonia in Older Adults

Several changes associated with aging and disease affect respiratory function and airway clearance. As an individual ages, the number of cilia decreases, and the gag and cough reflexes diminish. The older adult is at greater risk for dehydration, leading to thick, viscous mucus that is difficult to expectorate. Immune function declines with aging as well. These factors increase the risk of pulmonary infection and reduce the older adult's ability to respond effectively to infectious processes.

Other factors also may increase the risk for and severity of lower respiratory infections in the older adult. These factors include immobility, smoking history, surgical procedures, use of multiple medications, malnutrition, and diseases such as COPD and heart disease. Pneumonia in the older adult can result in continued respiratory failure, organ failure, complications throughout the body such as sepsis, or even death (Benoit et al., 2013). There is an increased risk for hospitalization for community-acquired pneumonia in older adults with a chronic cardiac disease history (Shah et al., 2014). Pneumonia and the related complications in the older adult are one of the common reasons for an ICU admission and remain a concern in today's healthcare settings.

NURSING PROCESS

Pneumonia can quickly escalate from minor to severe disease if not treated properly. Adequate assessment and implementation of medical and nursing interventions are vital to the healing process. Frequent pulmonary assessment and aggressive interventions help to prevent problems. Restoring and maintaining mobility improve ventilation and help to mobilize secretions. Promoting adequate fluid intake is necessary, because fluid helps to liquefy secretions, making them easier to expectorate.

TABLE 9–16 Daily Maintenance Fluid Requirements for the Pediatric Patient

Standard formula	For the first 10 kg of body weight, administer 100 mL/kg/day.	For the second 10 kg of body weight, administer 50 mL/kg/day.	For all additional body weight over 20 kg, administer 20 mL/kg/day.
Example: For a child weighing 53 lb, which is equal to 24 kg	100 mL/kg/day = 100 mL × 10 kg = 1000 mL/day	50 mL/kg/day = 50 mL × 10 kg = 500 mL/day	24 kg − 20 kg = 4 kg over 20 kg 4 kg × 20 mL = 80 mL/day
Example total			This 53-lb child requires a total 1580 mL of fluid to be administered during a 24-hour period.

Assessment

Focused assessment of the patient with pneumonia includes the following:

- **Observation and patient interview.** Observe the patient for the presence of shortness of breath and/or difficulty breathing, as well as the presence and nature of cough, and the color and consistency of sputum. Also observe the patient's skin color and use of accessory muscles while breathing. Ask the patient to describe the current symptoms and their duration and assess for the presence of chest pain. Ask the patient about recent upper respiratory or other acute illness, as well as chronic diseases such as diabetes, chronic lung disease, or heart disease. Ask for a list of all current medications, the patient's medication allergies, and immunization status.

- **Physical examination.** Examine the patient's current presentation and any apparent distress. Assess the patient's level of consciousness, and collect and evaluate vital signs, including temperature. Examine skin color and temperature. Respiratory examination focuses on any respiratory excursion, use of accessory muscles of respiration, and thorough assessment of the patient's lung sounds. Examine the patient's current oxygen saturation reading as well, being alert to levels indicating hypoxia.

Ongoing respiratory assessments are important in the care of all patients with pneumonia. Frequency of assessment is determined by the clinical acuity of the patient and the severity of the symptoms displayed. Auscultation of breath sounds, measurement of vital signs and oxygen saturation, and general assessment should be performed at a minimum of every 4 hours for patients who are clinically stable.

Diagnosis

Patients with lower respiratory disorders such as pneumonia may have multiple nursing care needs, depending on the severity of the illness. Possible nursing diagnoses related to pneumonia include the following:

- *Airway Clearance, Ineffective*
- *Breathing Pattern, Ineffective*
- *Hyperthermia*
- *Activity Intolerance*
- *Anxiety* related to hypoxia
- *Imbalanced Nutrition: Less Than Body Requirements* related to altered breathing pattern
- *Disturbed Sleep Pattern* related to orthopnea.

(NANDA-I © 2014)

Planning

The goal of nursing care is to restore optimal respiratory function. Outcomes are determined in conjunction with patient and family and may include the following:

- The patient will maintain normal temperature for 24 hours.
- The patient will obtain adequate sleep and rest without interruption from coughing or orthopnea.
- The patient will maintain adequate fluid and caloric intake.
- The patient will demonstrate a strong cough sufficient to clear airway.
- The patient will maintain an oxygen saturation greater than 90%.
- The patient will not require supplemental oxygen to maintain oxygen saturations of greater than 90%.

Implementation

In addition to teaching the patient to take all antibiotics and other medications exactly as ordered, nursing care focuses on supporting optimal respiratory function, such as maintaining airway patency and an effective breathing pattern and promoting rest to reduce metabolic and oxygen needs. Nursing interventions are prioritized on the basis of the most important nursing diagnoses of *Ineffective Airway Clearance, Ineffective Breathing Pattern*, and *Activity Intolerance*.

Community-Based Care

If the patients are stable enough and managing their respiratory needs as expected for their age and health condition, they may go home after an acute care stay or following evaluation by the primary provider or specialist. Therefore, many patients with pneumonia will recover at home. Patient teaching is an important nursing intervention. Discuss the following topics when preparing patients and family for home care:

- The importance of completing the prescribed medication regimen as ordered; potential drug side effects and their management, including manifestations that necessitate stopping the drug and notifying the healthcare provider

---

Focus on Integrative Health
Herbal Supplements for Treating Pneumonia

The herb echinacea is widely used to stimulate immune function and treat upper respiratory infections. Because viral upper respiratory infections often precede pneumonia, echinacea may be helpful in preventing pneumonia. Recent research, however, shows mixed results for the effectiveness of echinacea in reducing the duration and severity of an upper respiratory infection (National Center for Complementary and Integrative Health [NCCIH], 2016). Goldenseal, which often is sold in combination with echinacea, is used to treat bacterial, fungal, and protozoal infections of the mucous membranes of the respiratory tract.

Ma huang contains the active ingredient ephedra, which has been used to relieve bronchospasm and ease breathing. The primary active ingredient in ephedra is epinephrine, a cardiac and CNS stimulant. Because of the dangers associated with its use, sale of dietary supplements containing ephedra has been banned. However, this ban does not apply to Chinese herbal remedies or herbal teas (NCCIH, 2016). If patients ask about the use of Chinese herbal remedies to reduce pneumonia symptoms, the nurse should inquire whether any of the products contain ma huang or ephedra and advise the patient to avoid such products. The nurse should also advise patients who have plant allergies to check with their allergist before taking any kind of herbal supplement.

- Recommendations for limiting activities and increasing rest
- The importance of maintaining adequate fluid intake to keep mucus thin for easier expectoration
- Ways to maintain adequate nutritional intake, such as small, frequent, well-balanced meals
- The importance of avoiding smoking or exposure to secondhand smoke to prevent further irritation of the lungs
- Manifestations to report to the healthcare provider, such as increasing shortness of breath; difficulty breathing; and increased fever, fatigue, headache, sleepiness, or confusion
- The importance of keeping all follow-up appointments to ensure disease cure.

Maintain Airway Patency

For the patient treated in the hospital, the focus will be on airway and infection management. Infections of the lower lungs can generate sputum that hinders respiration, decreasing SaO_2 and making it difficult for the patient to breathe. There are several nursing assessments that must be done for patients in the hospital with a respiratory illness. Nursing interventions to help maintain airway patency include the following:

- Assess the patient's respiratory status, including vital signs, breath sounds, SaO_2, and skin color at least every 4 hours. Early identification of respiratory compromise allows intervention before tissue hypoxia is significant.
- Assess the patient's cough and sputum (amount, color, consistency, and possible odor). Assessment of the cough and nature of sputum produced allows evaluation of the effectiveness of respiratory clearance and the response to therapy.
- Monitor the patient's arterial blood gas results; report increasing **hypoxemia** (deficient blood oxygenation) and other abnormal results to the healthcare provider. Blood gas changes may be an early indicator of impaired gas exchange caused by airway narrowing or obstruction.
- Place the patient in high-Fowler position. Encourage frequent position changes and ambulation as allowed. The upright position promotes lung expansion; position changes and ambulation facilitate the movement of secretions.
- Assist the patient to cough, deep-breathe, and use assistive devices. Provide endotracheal suctioning using aseptic technique as ordered. Coughing, deep breathing, and suctioning help to clear airways.
- Provide a fluid intake of at least 2500–3000 mL/day for adults.
- Work with the healthcare provider and respiratory therapist to provide pulmonary hygiene measures, such as postural drainage, percussion, and vibration. These techniques help to mobilize and clear secretions.
- Administer prescribed medications as ordered and monitor their effects. If the infecting organism is resistant to the prescribed antibiotic, little improvement may be seen with treatment. Bronchodilators help to maintain open airways but may have adverse effects such as anxiety and restlessness.

Ensure Effective Ventilation

Chest pain and fatigue associated with a lung infection may cause patients to take shallow breaths, which prevents adequate exhalation of carbon dioxide and inhalation of oxygen. Nursing interventions that promote effective ventilation include:

- Provide for rest periods. Rest reduces metabolic demands, fatigue, and the work of breathing, promoting a more effective breathing pattern.
- Assess the patient for pleuritic discomfort. Provide analgesics as ordered. Adequate pain relief minimizes splinting and promotes adequate ventilation. Analgesics, such as ibuprofen or acetaminophen, can have the added benefit of fever control and may aid in sleep.
- Teach the patient how to splint the chest by hugging a small pillow, or a teddy bear for the pediatric patient, to make coughing less painful. Pain may result from coughing and deep breathing as well as from accessory muscle fatigue.
- Provide reassurance during periods of respiratory distress. Hypoxia and respiratory distress produce high levels of anxiety, which tend to further increase tachypnea and fatigue and decrease ventilation.
- Administer oxygen as ordered. Oxygen therapy increases the alveolar oxygen concentration and facilitates its diffusion across the alveolar–capillary membrane, reducing hypoxia and anxiety.
- Teach the patient slow abdominal breathing. This breathing pattern promotes lung expansion.
- Teach the patient use of relaxation techniques, such as visualization and meditation. These techniques help to reduce anxiety and slow the breathing pattern.

SAFETY ALERT Assess respiratory rate, depth, and lung sounds at least every 4 hours for adults, and at least every 1–2 hours for children. Tachypnea and diminished or adventitious breath sounds may be early indicators of respiratory compromise.

Promote Balance Between Activity and Rest

Patients with pneumonia tire easily because breathing requires increased effort. Activity heightens this fatigue. Therefore, periods of activity should be alternated with periods of rest for patients with pneumonia. In the hospital, nurses should:

- Assess the patient's activity tolerance, noting any increase in pulse, respirations, dyspnea, diaphoresis, or cyanosis. These assessment findings may indicate limited or impaired activity tolerance.
- Assist the patient with self-care activities, such as bathing. Assistance with activities of daily living reduces energy demands.
- Schedule activities, planning for rest periods. Rest periods minimize fatigue and improve activity tolerance. Minor activities, such as taking vital signs and using the bathroom, may be grouped together. However, major activities, such as chest physiotherapy or showering, should be immediately followed by a period of rest.
- Provide assistive devices, such as an overhead trapeze. These assistive devices facilitate movement and reduce energy demands.

- Enlist the family's help to minimize stress and anxiety levels. Stress and anxiety increase metabolic demands and can decrease activity tolerance.

- Perform active or passive range-of-motion exercises. Exercises help to maintain muscle tone and joint mobility and to prevent contractures if bedrest is prolonged.

- Provide emotional support and reassurance that strength and energy will return to normal when the infectious process has resolved and the balance of oxygen supply and demand is restored. The patient may be concerned that activity intolerance will continue to be a problem after the acute infection is resolved.

SAFETY ALERT Activity intolerance may be an early sign of cardiorespiratory compromise, particularly in the older adult or patient with preexisting heart disease. New or worsening manifestations of activity intolerance should be reported to the healthcare provider.

Evaluation

Patients with pneumonia are usually treated in the community unless their respiratory status is significantly compromised (e.g., altered mental status, tachypnea, tachycardia, hypotension, hypo- or hyperthermia, altered blood gases) or if risk factors (e.g., advanced age and/or coexisting heart, kidney, or liver disease) are present. As a result, caregivers must be taught to evaluate the outcome of care and the signs and symptoms requiring immediate consultation with the primary care provider. Potential expected outcomes may include:

- The patient maintains normal temperature for 24 hours.

- The patient obtains adequate sleep and rest without interruption from coughing or orthopnea.

- The patient maintains adequate fluid and caloric intake.

- The patient demonstrates strong cough sufficient to clear airway.

- The patient maintains oxygen saturation greater than 90%.

Patients who are unable to demonstrate appropriate airway management will likely be admitted to the hospital for further treatments, including possible airway suctioning and further interventions. One of the causes of further issues is aspiration pneumonia, which occurs frequently with adults who are unable to manage their swallowing and protect their airway (Dibardino & Wonderlink, 2015). The goal of these interventions is to bring the patient back to the appropriate oxygen saturation level and to prevent further infections.

Nursing Care Plan
A Patient with Pneumonia

Mary O'Neal is a 35-year-old executive assistant and part-time college student. On returning home from class one evening, she began to feel chills. She alternated between chills and sweats all night. She stayed home from work the next day and remained in bed most of the day. Her fever continued, and she developed a cough and dull, aching chest pain. When the cough became productive of rust-colored sputum the following day, she decided to seek medical treatment from her family doctor.

ASSESSMENT	DIAGNOSES	PLANNING
Debby Kowalski, RN, the family practice clinic nurse, admits Ms. O'Neal to the clinic and obtains the nursing assessment. Ms. O'Neal denies any previous history of respiratory diseases "other than the usual colds, flu, and such." She also denies any history of smoking or medication allergies. She says her symptoms began abruptly, with an onset of the chills. She describes her chest pain as a dull ache that was initially substernal but now is localized in her lower lateral right chest. The pain increases with deep breathing, coughing, and moving. Her cough is increasing in frequency and severity, and her sputum appears rusty brown. Her vital signs include temperature 101.8°F oral; pulse 104 bpm; respirations 22/min; and blood pressure 116/74 mmHg. Her skin is warm and flushed, with no evidence of cyanosis. Her respirations are shallow and unlabored; respiratory excursion is equal. Breath sounds are diminished in the bases bilaterally, with crackles noted in the right posterior and lateral base. A Stat CBC shows a WBC of 18,900/mm^3; differential shows increased numbers of neutrophils and immature WBCs (bands). Ms. Kowalski has Ms. O'Neal rinse with an antiseptic mouthwash and then collects a sputum specimen for culture and Gram stain before Ms. O'Neal sees the healthcare provider. The healthcare provider orders a chest x-ray after examining Ms. O'Neal. Based on her history, examination, and chest x-ray, he makes the diagnosis of acute bacterial pneumonia, probably pneumococcal. He prescribes oral penicillin V, 500 mg every 6 hours for 10 days. He asks Ms. O'Neal to return for a follow-up appointment in 10 days and refers her back to Ms. Kowalski for appropriate teaching.	▪ *Ineffective Breathing Pattern* related to pleuritic chest pain ▪ *Hyperthermia* related to inflammatory process ▪ *Deficient Knowledge* about pneumonia and its treatment (NANDA-I © 2014)	Goals for Ms. O'Neal's care include: ▪ The patient will maintain normal pulmonary function. ▪ The patient will describe measures to minimize elevations in body temperature. ▪ The patient will identify a schedule for taking her medication that will facilitate compliance with the regimen. ▪ The patient will describe manifestations that should be reported to the healthcare provider.

Nursing Care Plan (continued)

IMPLEMENTATION

- Assess knowledge and understanding of pneumonia and its effects.
- Assist to develop a medication schedule that coordinates with normal daily routine.
- Teach the patient and family about the following:
  a. Importance of avoiding use of a cough suppressant except at night to facilitate rest
  b. Ways to increase fluid intake to reduce fever and maintain thin mucus for easy expectoration

  c. Beneficial effects of rest, especially during the acute phase of her illness
  d. Safe use of aspirin and acetaminophen to reduce fever
  e. Importance of taking all prescribed medication doses as scheduled
  f. Common side effects of penicillin V and their management
  g. Early manifestations of penicillin allergy that necessitate stopping the medication and notifying the healthcare provider
  h. Signs of complications or worsening pneumonia to report.

EVALUATION

The sputum culture confirms *Streptococcus pneumoniae* as the cause of Ms. O'Neal's pneumonia. When she returns for her follow-up appointment, she reports that she began to feel better after 2 days on the penicillin and returned to work the following Monday. Her examination reveals good breath sounds throughout, with no adventitious sounds. The follow-up sputum culture is free of pathogens.

CRITICAL THINKING

1. Do any of the factors identified in the case study increase Ms. O'Neal's risk for acute bacterial pneumonia? If so, which factors?
2. Ms. O'Neal's WBC differential showed increased neutrophil and band counts. Describe the reason for and effect of this change.
3. Even though Ms. O'Neal has no history of medication allergies, anaphylactic shock remains a potential risk. Describe the sequence of events leading to anaphylactic shock, its initial symptoms, and immediate nursing interventions.
4. If Ms. O'Neal had required hospitalization to treat her acute pneumonia, interruption of her usual activities and responsibilities could lead to anxiety. Develop a care plan for this situation, using the nursing diagnosis *Ineffective Role Performance* related to hospitalization.

REVIEW Pneumonia

RELATE Link the Concepts and Exemplars

Linking the exemplar of pneumonia with the concept of oxygenation:

1. Describe the pathophysiology of pneumonia related to how it affects oxygenation.
2. What measures could you implement when caring for a patient with pneumonia to improve oxygenation?

Linking the exemplar of pneumonia with the concept of development:

3. You are caring for a 6-year-old child diagnosed with cystic fibrosis who is hospitalized for recurrent pneumonia. How can you promote this child's normal development during hospitalization?

READY Go to Volume 3: Clinical Nursing Skills

REFER Go to Pearson MyLab Nursing and eText

- Additional review materials

REFLECT Apply Your Knowledge

Jimmy Bley is a 78-year-old man with moderate emphysema and hearing loss. He is a retired veteran who served as an electronics technician in the army for his entire career. In his retirement, Mr. Bley has taken an interest in computers. He spends most of his time surfing the internet or playing games on the computer; he also likes to build computers. Mr. Bley has been married for 56 years to his wife, Cecelia. They argue a lot, but they would not know what to do without one another. They have several grown children, grandchildren, and great-grandchildren who live in the same community. Mr. Bley often goes with his wife to the neighborhood senior center for bingo night.

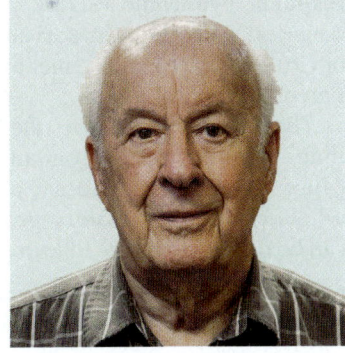

Mr. Bley considers himself healthy. He describes his hearing loss as mild. He has a hearing aid, but he does not like to wear it and therefore does not make changing the batteries a priority. He does not perceive his hearing loss to be much of a problem. Likewise, Mr. Bley describes his emphysema as "not that bad." However, he becomes short of breath with most activities; thus, it takes time for him to complete tasks. He compensates by taking his time to do most things. He has learned that he must pace himself; if he does not, he becomes exhausted and needs several days to recover. He continues to smoke and knows he should quit, but he enjoys it.

One night, Jimmy is awakened from sleep feeling as though he cannot catch his breath. He sits up, and his breathing becomes a little easier and he feels slightly less anxious. However, he also notices that he is hot. When he takes his temperature, he gets a reading of 101.2°F orally. He still feels a little bit short of breath and decides that he will call the clinic in the morning. In the meantime, he goes downstairs, sits in the recliner, and naps fitfully. When Mr. Bley gets to the clinic, the doctor performs a chest x-ray (patchy infiltrates in left lower lobe), CBC with differential (elevated WBC count, with differential showing a shift to the left, indicating a bacterial infection), and arterial blood gas (pH 7.32, PaO_2 52, $PaCO_2$ 48, HCO_3 30) and diagnoses Mr. Bley with pneumonia. Mr. Bley is taken to the local hospital and admitted with orders for IV fluids; a high-calorie, low-salt, low-fat diet; oxygen via nasal cannula at 2 L/min; cefaclor (Keflex, Ceclor), 500 mg IV q8h; aminophylline, 100 mg PO q8h; and Atrovent HFA 2 puffs qid.

1. What factors contributed to the decision to hospitalize Mr. Bley instead of treating him at home?

2. Why would the healthcare provider order oxygen at only 2 L/min instead of a 100% mask at 6 L/min? Provide a physiologic explanation for this order.

3. Develop a nursing plan of care for this patient.

›› Exemplar 9.F
Sepsis

Exemplar Learning Outcomes

9.F Analyze sepsis as it relates to infection.

- Describe the pathophysiology of sepsis.
- Describe the etiology of sepsis.
- Compare the risk factors and prevention of sepsis.
- Identify the clinical manifestations of sepsis.
- Summarize diagnostic tests and therapies used by interprofessional teams in the collaborative care of an individual with sepsis.
- Differentiate care of patients with sepsis across the lifespan.
- Apply the nursing process in providing culturally competent care to an individual with sepsis.

Exemplar Key Terms

Bacteremia, *637*
Ischemia, *640*
Refractory septic shock, *636*
Sepsis, *636*
Septic shock, *636*
Septicemia, *637*
Severe sepsis, *636*
Systemic inflammatory response syndrome (SIRS), *636*

Overview

Sepsis, septicemia, bacteremia, septic shock, blood poisoning—these are all terms that have been used at one time or another to describe the whole-body inflammatory process resulting in acute critical illness. The term **systemic inflammatory response syndrome (SIRS)** was coined in 1992 when the American College of Chest Healthcare providers and Society of Critical Care Medicine met to develop a consensus definition of this critical illness.

The term *SIRS* describes the body's response to a critical illness that can result from an infectious or noninfectious cause (e.g., burns, trauma, pancreatitis) precipitating a whole-body inflammatory process. Other common terms can be differentiated as follows:

- **Sepsis** is defined as SIRS resulting from an infection.
- **Severe sepsis** is defined as sepsis with acute associated organ failure.
- **Septic shock** is defined as a persistently low mean arterial blood pressure as a result of overwhelming infection despite adequate fluid resuscitation.
- **Refractory septic shock** is a persistently low mean arterial blood pressure despite vasopressor therapy and adequate fluid resuscitation.

This exemplar explores sepsis that occurs in response to infection-related SIRS.

Pathophysiology and Etiology
Pathophysiology

Sepsis is the leading cause of death in noncoronary ICUs and the 11th leading cause of death in the United States overall (CDC, 2016e). More than 70% of patients with sepsis have comorbidities, and more than 60% of cases occur in individuals over the age of 65 (Rhee et al., 2014). SIRS, which is a precursor to sepsis, can occur as a complication of virtually any infection of any body tissue. In infection-related SIRS, the infection triggers a systemic inflammatory response that leads to a series of adverse events, including vasodilation, increased capillary permeability, and hypercoagulability. SIRS also triggers the activation of certain types of cells that typically help the body during an immune or inflammatory reaction: platelets, neutrophils, macrophages, and endothelial cells. However, during SIRS, the function of these cells is exaggerated, and the uncontrolled cellular release of chemical mediators sparks a systemwide immune and inflammatory response (see the module on Immunity and the module on Inflammation).

When the SIRS response is severe, sepsis can develop. Disseminated intravascular coagulation (DIC) is a potential risk associated with sepsis. DIC is characterized by simultaneous bleeding and clotting throughout the vasculature. Sepsis injures blood cells, causing platelet aggregation and decreased blood flow. As a result, blood clots form throughout the microcirculation. The clotting slows circulation further while stimulating excess fibrinolysis. As the body's stores of clotting factors are depleted, generalized bleeding begins. For an illustration of the pathophysiology of sepsis that develops into septic shock, see **Figure 9–26** ››. The progression of sepsis may lead to severe sepsis, during which reduced organ perfusion can cause multiple-organ dysfunction syndrome (MODS) and ultimately death.

Patients with sepsis are very ill and require attentive monitoring and rapid intervention in response to even subtle changes in condition. Nurses play a pivotal role in caring for these patients, because they are with the patients constantly and are most competent to monitor their condition.

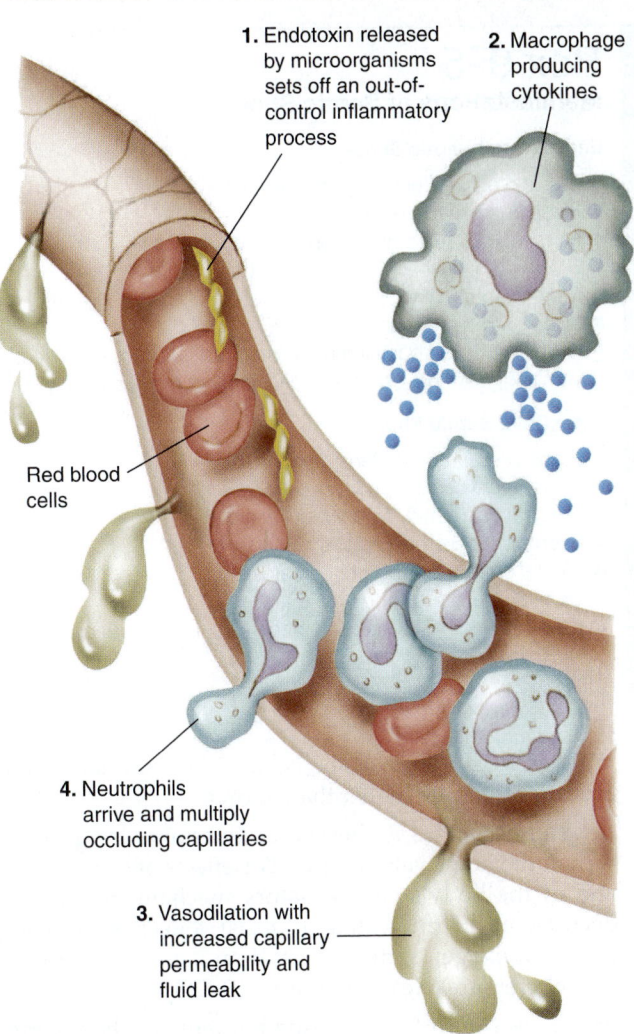

1. Endotoxin released by microorganisms sets off an out-of-control inflammatory process

2. Macrophage producing cytokines

Red blood cells

4. Neutrophils arrive and multiply occluding capillaries

3. Vasodilation with increased capillary permeability and fluid leak

Figure 9–26 » In septic shock, blood pools in the extremities. Blood flow is sluggish and amounts of oxygen received by the tissues are inadequate for cell metabolism.

Etiology

Sepsis due to infection begins with **septicemia** (the presence of pathogens and their toxins in the blood). Sources of infection include bacteria, viruses, and fungi. Rickets and certain types of protozoa may also lead to septic shock (Close Up Media, 2013). The presence of bacteria and their toxins in the bloodstream, which is a common cause of sepsis, is called **bacteremia**.

Sepsis is most often the result of gram-positive infections from *Staphylococcus* and *Streptococcus* bacteria but may also follow gram-negative bacterial infections (i.e., *Pseudomonas* spp., *Escherichia coli*, and *Klebsiella* spp.); 6% of cases are related to fungal infections (Rhee et al., 2014).

The incidence of gram-negative sepsis has greatly increased since 2003, with a 60% mortality rate despite treatment. The incidence of sepsis is increasing the most in older adults and non-White populations. The reason is believed to be an increase in invasive procedures, immunosuppressive therapy, and antimicrobial resistance (Rhee et al., 2014).

Portals of entry for infection that may lead to septic shock are:

- *Urinary system.* Catheterizations, suprapubic tubes, and cystoscopy

- *Respiratory system.* Suctioning, aspiration, tracheostomy, endotracheal tubes, respiratory therapy, and mechanical ventilators

- *Gastrointestinal system.* Peptic ulcers, ruptured appendix, and peritonitis

- *Integumentary system.* Surgical wounds, IV catheters, intra-arterial catheters, invasive monitoring, decubitus ulcers, burns, and trauma

- *Female reproductive system.* Elective surgical abortion, ascending infections from transmission of bacteria during the intrapartal and postpartal periods, tampon use, and sexually transmitted infections.

Risk Factors

Patients at risk for developing infections leading to septic shock include those who are hospitalized, have debilitating chronic illnesses, or have poor nutritional status. The risk is heightened after invasive procedures or surgery. Other patients at risk of septic shock include older adults and those who are immunocompromised.

During periods of immune suppression, the patient is vulnerable to overwhelming infection, which results in circulatory failure, hypothermia or hyperthermia, tachypnea, mental changes, inadequate tissue perfusion, and hypotension. Factors contributing to massive infection include inadequate neutrophil production, abnormal granulocytes (that are not able to be actively phagocytic), erosions through normal barriers (e.g., blood vessels, mucous membranes), and altered bone marrow production caused by chemotherapy and some forms of radiation. Such infections must be vigorously treated with antimicrobial therapy and hydration management.

Toxic shock syndrome is an especially virulent form of septic shock and occurs most frequently in menstruating women who use tampons improperly. Sliding a tampon into place in the vagina may make microscopic tears in the walls of the vagina, rupturing tiny blood vessels. A super-absorbent tampon—especially if it is left in place too long, or if it is used when the menstrual flow is light—can dry out the vagina, making such tearing even more likely. It is thought that bacterial toxins diffuse from the site of infection in the vagina into the circulation. The toxins then trigger a widespread inflammatory response and septic shock. The manifestations of toxic shock syndrome include extreme hypotension, hyperpyrexia, headache, myalgia, confusion, skin rash, vomiting, and diarrhea (Porth & Grossman, 2014).

Prevention

Any infant with an infectious process must be watched carefully for early signs of sepsis; thorough teaching of parents and regular caregivers is indicated. Individuals with cancer, especially those undergoing treatment with chemotherapy or radiation therapy, must be carefully monitored for symptoms of sepsis and may be placed on prophylactic antibiotics because their risk is so great.

Because complications from pneumonia are a major cause of sepsis, immunization against organisms that cause pneumonia, such as *H. influenzae* and *S. pneumoniae*, is a primary method of sepsis prevention. Infections from catheter and IV use are also a major cause of sepsis, so aseptic techniques and good hand hygiene techniques when inserting, removing, or caring for catheters and IV lines are vital to preventing sepsis.

Clinical Manifestations

Manifestations of sepsis include fever or hypothermia, tachycardia, tachypnea, peripheral vasodilation, septic shock, and mental status changes. Hemodynamic monitoring shows an increase in cardiac output. Lab results show an abnormal CBC (leukocytosis or leukopenia) and alteration in clotting factors (thrombocytosis or thrombopenia), which results in DIC, a critical illness that must be managed quickly. Elevated liver enzyme, C-reactive protein, and creatinine levels are likely. Hypophosphatemia and positive blood culture are anticipated.

Septic shock has an early phase and a late phase. In early septic shock (sometimes called the *warm phase*), vasodilation results in hypotension due to intense vasodilation and fluid shifts due to increased capillary permeability, weakness, and warm, flushed skin. Septicemia often causes high fever and chills. In late septic shock (sometimes called the *cold phase*), hypovolemia and activity of the compensatory mechanisms result in typical shock manifestations, including cold, moist skin; oliguria; and changes in mental status. Death may result from respiratory failure, cardiac failure, and/or renal failure. Manifestations of septic shock are listed in **Box 9–5 »**.

Collaboration

Septic shock can be fatal, but early and aggressive therapy improves outcomes (Mayo Clinic, 2016a). Collaborative care of the patient with sepsis includes active participation by a number of specialists, such as infectious disease specialists, phlebotomists, and respiratory therapists. Gerontologists and pediatricians may be required for patients in those respective age groups, especially in determining safety and side effects when multiple medications are recommended.

Diagnostic Tests

The following diagnostic tests can help to identify the cause of sepsis and assess the patient's physical status:

- *Hemoglobin and hematocrit* are tested, because changes in hematocrit concentrations usually occur in patients with septic shock as fluid leaks from the intravascular to the extravascular spaces. These changes reflect the body's response to endotoxins. In septic shock resulting from

intravascular fluid loss, the hemoglobin and hematocrit concentrations are higher than normal.

- *Arterial blood gas* is checked to determine oxygen and carbon dioxide levels and pH. The effects of septic shock and of the body's compensatory mechanisms cause a decrease in pH (indicating acidosis), a decrease in PaO_2 and total oxygen saturation, and an increase in arterial partial pressure of carbon dioxide ($PaCO_2$).

- *Serum electrolytes* are measured to monitor the severity and progression of septic shock. As septic shock progresses, glucose levels decrease, sodium levels decrease, and potassium levels increase.

- *Blood urea nitrogen, serum creatinine levels, urine specific gravity, and osmolality* are obtained to check renal function, which declines as reduced perfusion and microclotting damage the small renal arterioles. As perfusion of the kidneys is decreased and renal function is reduced, the blood urea nitrogen and creatinine levels increase, as does urine specific gravity and osmolality.

Box 9–5
Manifestations of Septic Shock

Early (Warm) Septic Shock
- *Blood pressure:* normal to hypotension
- *Pulse:* increased, thready
- *Respirations:* rapid and deep
- *Skin:* warm, flushed
- *Mental status:* alert, oriented, anxious
- *Urine output:* normal
- *Other:* increased body temperature; chills; weakness; nausea, vomiting, diarrhea; decreased central venous pressure (CVP)

Late (Cold) Septic Shock
- *Blood pressure:* hypotension
- *Pulse:* tachycardia, arrhythmias
- *Respirations:* rapid, shallow, dyspneic
- *Skin:* cool, pale, edematous
- *Mental status:* lethargic to comatose
- *Urine output:* oliguria to anuria
- *Other:* normal to decreased body temperature, decreased CVP.

Clinical Manifestations and Therapies
Sepsis

ETIOLOGY	CLINICAL MANIFESTATIONS	CLINICAL THERAPIES
Disseminated intravascular coagulation may develop as a result of altered coagulation.	Clinical manifestation varies from increased tendency to bleed to hemorrhage. Small clots may reduce blood flow to major organs; manifestations will be determined by organs affected. Prolonged clotting times, and reduced fibrinogen and platelet levels are possible. Spider angiomas or purpura are often seen on the patient's skin if the affected individual is acutely ill.	▪ Reverse the underlying cause (i.e., sepsis)—only effective treatment ▪ Platelet transfusions ▪ Fresh-frozen plasma administration ▪ Possible administration of antithrombin ▪ Activated protein—given only in the ICU to patients with severe sepsis

- *Blood cultures* are done to identify the causative organism in septic shock and to direct treatment toward destruction of the pathogen.
- *WBC count and differential* may initially show an increase or decrease in WBCs. As the body attempts to fight the infection, the WBC count may decrease as an increasing number of WBCs are destroyed. Elevated neutrophils indicate acute infection, increased monocytes indicate a bacterial infection, and increased eosinophils indicate an allergic response.
- *Serum enzymes*, such as lactate dehydrogenase, creatine kinase, and serum glutamic-oxaloacetic transaminase, are often elevated in later stages of septic shock as capillaries in the liver are damaged.
- *Hemodynamic monitoring* provides information about preload and cardiac output to direct fluid resuscitation needs. A pulmonary artery catheter may be inserted to monitor cardiac dynamics, fluid balance, and the effects of vasoactive medications.

Other diagnostic tests may be ordered to determine the extent of injury or damage. These tests might include x-ray studies, CT, MRI, endoscopic examinations, and echocardiograms. Newer diagnostic methods for hypoperfusion include gastric tonometry and sublingual $PaCO_2$. Gastric tonometry measures the $PaCO_2$ in the gastric lumen. The measurement of sublingual carbon dioxide correlates well with decreased mean arterial pressure (MAP) (Sole, Klein, & Moseley, 2013).

Pharmacologic Therapy

Antimicrobials are a primary pharmacologic treatment if the infection is caused by bacteria or fungi. Broad-spectrum antibiotics are generally used. The patient may be placed on several antibiotics to ensure adequate coverage of the pathogen until culture and sensitivity results return in 72 hours to indicate the best antibiotic. As antibiotics begin to take effect, the patient's condition may worsen initially as increasing numbers of toxins are released into the circulating bloodstream because of pathogen destruction, further activating the immune response.

When fluid replacement alone is not sufficient to reverse shock, vasoactive drugs (drugs causing vasoconstriction or vasodilation) and inotropic drugs (drugs improving cardiac contractility) may be administered. When used to treat shock, these drugs increase venous return through vasoconstriction of peripheral vessels; they also improve the pumping ability of the heart by facilitating myocardial contractility and dilating coronary arteries to increase perfusion of the myocardium. More information on pharmacologic treatment for shock can be found in the exemplar on Shock in the module on Perfusion.

Oxygen Therapy

Establishing and maintaining a patent airway and ensuring adequate oxygenation are critical interventions in reversing septic shock. All patients in septic shock (even those with adequate respirations) should receive oxygen therapy (usually by mask or nasal cannula) to maintain the PaO_2 at greater than 80 mmHg during the first 4–6 hours of care. If the patient's unassisted respiration cannot maintain PaO_2 at

this level, endotracheal intubation may be necessary. Care of the patient requiring ventilatory assistance is discussed in the module on Oxygenation.

Fluid Replacement

The most effective treatment for the patient in septic shock is the administration of IV fluids or blood. Various fluids may be administered alone or in combination as part of fluid replacement therapy. Whole blood or blood products increase the oxygen-carrying capacity of the blood and thus increase the oxygenation of cells. Fluid replacements, such as crystalloid and colloid solutions, increase circulating blood volume and tissue perfusion. Fluid replacements are administered in massive amounts through two large-bore peripheral lines or, most often, through a central line. More information about types of fluids can be found in the module on Fluid and Electrolytes.

SAFETY ALERT Optimal fluid balance is +3 L at 12 hours after presentation, with a CVP of less than 8 mmHg. A higher positive fluid balance and CVP correlates to a greater mortality rate in patients with sepsis.

Lifespan Considerations

Sepsis in Infants and Children

Manifestations of sepsis in infants include temperature instability, abdominal distention, poor feeding, lethargy, respiratory distress, hepatomegaly, vomiting, and/or jaundice. Children under 3 months of age with a temperature higher than 38°C (100.4°F) require diagnostic testing to rule out sepsis, because they are at increased risk due to immature immune systems and inadequate immune response to infection.

Septic shock may initially present with tachycardia, tachypnea, fever, warm extremities, bounding pulses, and rapid capillary refill. Urine output may be normal, but responsiveness may be altered. As shock progresses, capillary refill time becomes prolonged, pulses become weak, mental status changes, and urine output decreases. Hypotension and temperature instability presents (Ball et al., 2017).

Sepsis in Pregnant Women

A recent study in the United Kingdom suggests that pregnant women experience sepsis on an increasing basis worldwide regardless of the level of the available healthcare system (Acosta et al., 2014). This study reviewed more than 350 cases of sepsis and noted that a small percentage of the cases resulted in death of the mother and fetus. The study team recommends fast action to prevent further complications when any of the symptoms of SIRS begin to appear in a pregnant woman. Routine prenatal care is part of the prevention of sepsis for many women.

Sepsis in Older Adults

Cardiac changes associated with aging in adults may include a thickened left ventricular wall, decreased elasticity of the myocardium, and more rigid valves. These changes result in a decreased stroke volume and cardiac output, thus decreasing compensatory responses to septic shock. Decreased arterial wall elasticity and vasomotor tone reduce the older adult's ability to respond to a decrease in oxygenation. Decreased elasticity of the skin makes assessment of skin turgor, and thus dehydration status, more difficult. Decreased immune system response increases the risk of septic shock. Sepsis is a critical concern in adults who cannot respond appropriately to infections before SIRS begins (Rhee et al., 2014).

NURSING PROCESS

Nursing assessment is critical in reducing the complications associated with sepsis. Identifying patients at risk and performing focused assessments are essential.

Assessment

Sepsis affects the entire body. Patient assessment often includes continuous monitoring of vital signs, as well as monitoring of hemodynamic status, if a CVP monitoring device (or central line) or pulmonary artery catheter (PA catheter or Swan-Ganz catheter) is in place. Focused assessments are performed to monitor adequacy of ventilation, perfusion, and renal function.

As septic shock progresses, blood pressure decreases and the pulse becomes rapid, weak, and thready. As perfusion of the lungs decreases, crackles, wheezes, and dyspnea are commonly present. Capillary refill is prolonged, and peripheral pulses are weak or nonpalpable. Flattened neck veins that cannot be seen when the patient is in the supine position indicate decreased intravascular volume. CVP is very useful in evaluating the fluid balance status of the patient with sepsis. While normal CVP typically ranges from 2 to 8 mmHg, CVP will be decreased in patients experiencing septic shock.

Diagnosis

Priority nursing diagnoses for the patient with sepsis include the following:

- *Shock, Risk for*
- *Gas Exchange, Impaired*
- *Perfusion: Renal, Risk for Ineffective*
- *Tissue Perfusion: Peripheral, Ineffective*
- *Fluid Volume: Imbalanced, Risk for*

(NANDA-I © 2014)

Planning

Planning care for the patient with sepsis is very fluid, because the patient's condition and needs can change very quickly. Because the patient is critically ill, reassessment findings will often redirect the plan of care. Potential outcomes that may be appropriate for the patient with sepsis include the following:

- The patient will maintain oxygen saturation greater than 90% and PaO₂ within normal limits.
- The patient will maintain adequate renal perfusion to produce a minimum of 30 mL of urine per hour.

- The patient will respond to fluid resuscitation with mean arterial blood pressure that returns to normal range.

Implementation

Diminished tissue perfusion causes **ischemia** (inadequate blood supply) and hypoxia (insufficient oxygen) of major organ systems, with the potential for significant impact on the kidneys, brain, heart, lungs, and gastrointestinal tract. Nurses working with patients who have sepsis should do the following:

- Monitor the patient's skin color, temperature, turgor, and moisture. Decreased tissue perfusion is evidenced by the skin becoming pale, cool, and moist; as hemoglobin concentrations decrease, cyanosis occurs.
- Monitor the patient's cardiopulmonary function by assessing blood pressure (by auscultation or hemodynamic monitoring), rate and depth of respirations, lung sounds, pulse oximetry, and peripheral pulses (including presence, equality, rate, rhythm, and quality).
- Monitor the patient's jugular vein distention.
- Take the patient's CVP measurements.
- Monitor the patient's body temperature. An elevated body temperature increases metabolic demands, depleting reserves of bodily energy. It also increases myocardial oxygen demand and may place the patient with previous cardiac problems at even greater risk for hypoperfusion.
- Monitor the patient's urinary output per Foley catheter hourly, using a urometer. Urine output of 30 mL of urine per hour is a reliable indicator of renal perfusion.
- Assess the patient's mental status and level of consciousness. The appropriateness of the patient's behavior and responses reflect the adequacy of cerebral circulation. Restlessness and anxiety are common early in septic shock; in later stages, the patient may become lethargic and progress to a comatose state. Altered levels of consciousness are the result of both cerebral hypoxia and the effects of acidosis on brain cells.

Other nursing interventions appropriate for the patient with sepsis can be found in the exemplar on Shock in the module on Perfusion.

Evaluation

Potential expected outcomes may include:

- The patient maintains oxygen saturation greater than 90% and PaO₂ within normal limits.
- The patient maintains adequate renal perfusion to produce a minimum of 30 mL of urine per hour.
- The patient responds to fluid resuscitation with mean arterial blood pressure that returns to the normal range.

Patients with sepsis must be continuously and frequently reevaluated, sometimes as often as every few minutes, because their condition can change quickly. Following fluid administration, the patient's blood pressure and perfusion may improve. As fluid leaves the intravascular space, however, the patient's condition may decline again. As perfusion declines, renal, cardiac, pulmonary, and neurovascular status may change quickly.

Nursing Care Plan

A Patient with Septic Shock

Huang Mei Lan is a 43-year-old unmarried woman who lives alone in a major West Coast city. Ms. Huang came to the United States 15 years ago from China and now speaks English well. Her family still lives in China. She worked in a neighborhood sewing shop until 3 years ago, when she was diagnosed with breast cancer. Her treatment included mastectomy of the affected breast and follow-up chemotherapy.

Last month, Ms. Huang experienced a recurrence of cancer in the lymph glands of the affected side. Surgery to remove the glands was performed, and chemotherapy was started. Ms. Huang has a central line, a urinary catheter, and a surgical incision. She is underweight, weak, and depressed. Although she has multiple physical problems, she never complains or asks for any kind of medication.

ASSESSMENT

Ms. Huang's primary nurse, Robert O'Brien, enters her room early in the morning to make an initial assessment. He finds Ms. Huang huddled in the middle of the bed, shivering violently. Her vital signs are temperature 104°F oral; pulse 130 bpm; respirations 30/min; and blood pressure 88/42 mmHg. Her skin is hot, dry, and flushed with poor turgor. She is alert and oriented but is restless and appears anxious. Ms. Huang states she is nauseated and suddenly begins vomiting and is incontinent of liquid stool. Laboratory data indicate leukocytosis, respiratory alkalosis, and reduced platelet count. Blood cultures, as well as cultures of Ms. Huang's sputum, urine, and wound drainage, are conducted. She is diagnosed as having septic shock.

Hetastarch is ordered per IV line, and IV broad-spectrum antibiotics are begun until the organism and its portal of entry can be determined. Despite treatment, Ms. Huang's condition worsens. Her blood pressure continues to drop, her skin becomes cool and cyanotic, and she begins to have periods of disorientation. She is transferred to the critical care unit. As she is being prepared for the transfer, she begins to cry and asks, "Am I going to die?"

DIAGNOSES

- *Ineffective Breathing Pattern* related to rapid respirations and progression of septic shock
- *Ineffective Tissue Perfusion* related to progression of septic shock with decreased cardiac output, hypotension, and massive vasodilatation
- *Deficient Fluid Volume* related to vomiting, diarrhea, high fever, and shift of intravascular volume to interstitial spaces
- *Anxiety* related to feelings that illness is worsening and is potentially life-threatening and the transfer to the critical care unit

(NANDA-I © 2014)

PLANNING

Goals for Ms. Huang's care include:

- The patient will maintain adequate circulating blood volume.
- The patient will regain and maintain blood gas parameters within normal limits.
- The patient will regain and maintain stable hemodynamic levels.
- The patient will verbalize increased ability to cope with stressors.

IMPLEMENTATION

- Monitor respiratory status, including respiratory rate, rhythm, breath sounds, and oxygen saturation.
- Monitor cardiovascular status, including arterial blood pressure; rate, rhythm, and quality of pulses; CVP; pulmonary artery pressure; and cardiac output.
- Monitor urinary output hourly, reporting output of less than 0.5 mg/kg/hr or any sustained decrease in urine production.
- Monitor neurologic status, including mental status and level of consciousness.
- Monitor color and character of skin.
- Monitor results of arterial blood gas, blood counts, clotting times, and platelet counts.
- Monitor body temperature every 2 hours.
- Explain procedures and provide comfort measures (e.g., oral care, skin care, turning, positioning).

EVALUATION

Despite intensive nursing and medical care, Ms. Huang's condition remains critical. The interventions are continued.

CRITICAL THINKING

1. Vasopressors may be used in the treatment of septic shock. Explain the rationale for their use.
2. While monitoring Ms. Huang's arterial blood gas, the nurse notes that her PaO_2 is less than 60 mmHg and her $PaCO_2$ is greater than 50 mmHg. What do these findings indicate, and why have they occurred?
3. Ms. Huang has been given large amounts of colloids intravenously. Hemodynamic monitoring indicates a higher-than-normal CVP and pulmonary artery pressure. What do these findings indicate? What physical assessments would you make to confirm the changes?

REVIEW Sepsis

RELATE Link the Concepts and Exemplars

Linking the exemplar of sepsis with the concept of perfusion:

1. How is perfusion affected by sepsis?

2. What nursing interventions could you initiate to promote perfusion in the patient diagnosed with sepsis?

Linking the exemplar of sepsis with the concept of acid–base balance:

3. When analyzing the arterial blood gas of a patient in septic shock, what changes would you anticipate?

4. What interventions (both nursing and collaborative) could you implement to promote acid–base balance in the patient diagnosed with sepsis?

READY Go to Volume 3: Clinical Nursing Skills

REFER Go to Pearson MyLab Nursing and eText

■ Additional review materials

REFLECT Apply Your Knowledge

Frank Lauer is a 72-year-old man with moderate emphysema and hearing loss. He is a retired veteran who served as a medic in the army for his entire career. In his retirement, Mr. Lauer has taken an interest in electronics. Mr. Lauer has been married for 49 years to his wife, Marie. They have several grown children, grandchildren, and great-grandchildren who live within a few miles. Mr. Lauer occasionally goes with his wife to the senior center for Bingo night or to the local movies.

Mr. Lauer's daughter tells him about free flu shots being provided at the local clinic, but he is afraid a flu shot will make him sick, so he declines. A few weeks later, he feels tired and develops a nagging cough. He gets short of breath very easily. His children want him to see the healthcare provider immediately, but Mr. Lauer says it is just a cold and he will feel better in a few days without seeing the doctor. His cough becomes more severe at night, and he begins having trouble breathing but finds that sleeping in the recliner makes him feel better.

A few nights later, Mr. Lauer's cough is so severe that he feels as though he cannot catch his breath between coughing episodes. Mrs. Lauer sets up a humidifier next to his chair and encourages him to drink more fluids and see the doctor in the morning. He just laughs and tells her she is a worrier. His breathing improves, and he falls asleep in the chair. In the morning, he feels so weak that he has trouble walking to the bathroom. His temperature is elevated again, his breathing is rapid, and he feels awful. He consents to visiting the doctor, who diagnoses bacterial pneumonia. Blood cultures are drawn and the results indicate septicemia.

1. What factors increased Mr. Lauer's likelihood of being diagnosed with sepsis?

2. How would you explain his condition to Mr. and Mrs. Lauer?

3. Develop a nursing plan of care listing all potential nursing diagnoses and developing two of them to include goals, interventions, and expected outcomes.

≫ Exemplar 9.G Tuberculosis

Exemplar Learning Outcomes

9.G Analyze tuberculosis as it relates to infection.

■ Describe the pathophysiology of tuberculosis.

■ Describe the etiology of tuberculosis.

■ Compare the risk factors and prevention of tuberculosis.

■ Identify the clinical manifestations of tuberculosis.

■ Summarize diagnostic tests and therapies used by interprofessional teams in the collaborative care of an individual with tuberculosis.

■ Differentiate care of patients with tuberculosis across the lifespan.

■ Apply the nursing process in providing culturally competent care to an individual with tuberculosis.

Exemplar Key Terms

Anergic, *646*
Bacilli, *643*
Caseation necrosis, *643*
Cavitation, *643*
Dormant, *643*
Encapsulated, *643*
Extrapulmonary tuberculosis, *643*
Hematogenous spread, *643*
Hemoptysis, *646*
Miliary tuberculosis, *643*
Mycobacterium tuberculosis, *642*
Negative airflow room, *653*
Pneumothorax, *646*
Purified protein derivative (PPD), *644*
Tubercle, *643*
Tuberculosis, *642*

Overview

Tuberculosis is a chronic, recurrent, infectious disease caused by *Mycobacterium tuberculosis*, a relatively slow-growing, slender, rod-shaped, acid-fast organism with a waxy outer capsule that increases its resistance to destruction. Because tuberculosis most often affects the lungs, many people think of it as a pulmonary disease, but primary or secondary tuberculosis lesions may affect other body systems, such as the kidneys, genitalia, bone, and brain.

Tuberculosis was a major public health concern early in the 20th century before the development of effective sanitation measures and drug treatments. Although it remains prevalent worldwide, tuberculosis is currently uncommon in the United States, especially among young adults of European descent.

However, tuberculosis remains a significant public health threat because of the development of drug-resistant strains, susceptibility of individuals with HIV/AIDS, recent influxes of refugee populations, and inadequate access to healthcare for high-risk populations.

Pathophysiology and Etiology

Pathophysiology

Minute droplet nuclei containing one to three *M. tuberculosis* **bacilli** (rod-shaped bacteria) may elude upper airway defense systems, enter the lungs, and implant in an alveolus or respiratory bronchiole, usually in an upper lobe. As these bacteria multiply, they cause a local inflammatory response. The inflammatory response brings neutrophils and macrophages to the site. These phagocytic cells then surround and engulf the bacilli, isolating them and preventing their spread. The *M. tuberculosis* organisms continue to multiply slowly within the macrophage, however, and some of these bacilli enter the lymphatic system to stimulate a cell-mediated immune response. Neutrophils and macrophages isolate the bacteria but, again, cannot destroy them. A granulomatous lesion called a **tubercle** (a sealed-off colony of bacilli) is formed. Within the tubercle, infected tissue dies, forming a cheeselike center, a process called **caseation necrosis**.

After 2–12 weeks, once the organisms number from 1000 to 10,000, a cellular immune response can be elicited with the tuberculosis skin test. In infants younger than 6 months, because of their immature immune system, infection may progress to active tuberculosis even before the skin test becomes reactive (CDC, 2015h). If the immune response is adequate, scar tissue develops around the tubercle, and the bacilli remain **encapsulated** (enclosed). Although these lesions eventually calcify and become visible on x-ray, the patient will not develop tuberculosis disease. If the immune response is inadequate to contain the bacilli, the tubercle may rupture, allowing the bacilli to spread; the result is tuberculosis pneumonia. The infection occasionally progresses, causing extensive destruction of lung tissue. In *primary tuberculosis,* granulomatous tissue may erode into a bronchus or a blood vessel, allowing the disease to spread throughout the lung or other organs. This severe form of tuberculosis is uncommon in healthy adults (Longo et al., 2012).

A previously healed tuberculosis lesion may be reactivated. *Reactivation tuberculosis* occurs when the immune system is suppressed because of age, disease, or use of immunosuppressive drugs. The extent of lung disease can vary from small lesions to extensive cavitation of lung tissue. Tubercles rupture, spreading bacilli into the airways to form satellite lesions and produce tuberculosis pneumonia. Without treatment, massive lung involvement can lead to death, or a more chronic process of tubercle formation and **cavitation** (formation of a cavity or bubble) may result. Individuals with chronic disease continue to spread *M. tuberculosis* into the environment, potentially infecting others.

When primary disease or reactivation allows live bacilli to enter the bronchi, the disease may spread through the blood and lymph system to other organs and become **extrapulmonary tuberculosis**. These distant disease metastases may produce an active lesion, or they may become **dormant** (temporarily inactive but not dead) and reactivate at a later time. Extrapulmonary tuberculosis is especially prevalent in people with HIV/AIDS.

Miliary tuberculosis results from **hematogenous spread** (through the blood) of the bacilli throughout the body. Miliary tuberculosis causes chills and fever, weakness, malaise, and progressive dyspnea. Multiple lesions evenly distributed throughout the lungs are noted on x-ray, but the sputum rarely contains organisms. The bone marrow is usually involved, and the result is anemia, thrombocytopenia, and leukocytosis. Without appropriate treatment, the prognosis is poor.

The kidney and genitourinary tract are common extrapulmonary sites for tuberculosis. The organism spreads to the kidney through the blood, initiating an inflammatory process similar to the one in the lungs. Reactivation can occur years after the original infection. As the lesion then enlarges and caseates, a large portion of the renal parenchyma is destroyed. The infection then can spread to the rest of the urinary tract, including the ureters and bladder. Scarring and strictures commonly result. In men, the prostate, seminal vesicles, and epididymis may be involved. In women, tuberculosis may affect the fallopian tubes and ovaries. Manifestations of genitourinary tuberculosis develop insidiously. Symptoms of a UTI, including malaise, dysuria, hematuria, and pyuria, develop. Flank pain may be present. Men may develop manifestations of epididymitis or prostatitis: perineal, sacral, or scrotal pain and tenderness; difficulty voiding; and fever. Women may have manifestations of pelvic inflammatory disease, impaired fertility, or ectopic pregnancy.

Tuberculosis meningitis results when tuberculosis spreads to the subarachnoid space. In the United States, this complication most often affects older adults, usually from reactivation of latent disease. Manifestations develop gradually and include listlessness, irritability, diminished appetite, and fever. Headache and behavioral changes are common early symptoms in the older adult. As the disease progresses, the headaches increase in intensity, vomiting develops, and the level of consciousness decreases. Convulsions and coma may follow. Without appropriate treatment, neurologic effects may become permanent.

Tuberculosis of the bones and joints is most likely to occur during childhood, when bone epiphyses are open and their blood supply is rich. The organisms spread via the blood to vertebrae, the ends of long bones, and joints. Immune and inflammatory processes isolate the bacilli, and the disease often becomes evident years or even decades later. Tuberculous spondylitis usually involves the thoracic vertebrae, eroding vertebral bodies and causing them to collapse. Significant kyphosis (concave curvature of the spinal column) develops, and the spinal cord may be compressed. The large, weight-bearing joints (hips and knees) are most often affected by tuberculous arthritis, although other joints can also be affected, particularly if they have been previously damaged. The involved joint is painful, warm, and tender.

Epidemiology

Thanks to improved sanitation, surveillance, and treatment of people with active disease, the incidence of tuberculosis in the United States fell steadily until the mid-1980s. The late

1980s and early 1990s, however, saw a resurgence of the disease, attributed primarily to the HIV/AIDS epidemic; the emergence of multidrug-resistant (MDR) strains of tuberculosis; and social factors, such as immigration, poverty, homelessness, and drug abuse. Today, the number of people affected in the United States continues to decline, with a total of 9287 cases reported in 2016, the lowest number recorded since national reporting began in 1953 (CDC, 2017b); 89 of the cases were classified as multidrug resistant. (CDC, 2017c). The decline in new cases can be attributed to tuberculosis control programs that emphasize promptly identifying new cases and initiating and completing appropriate therapy.

Worldwide, tuberculosis continues to be a significant health problem, with an estimated 2 billion people (one third of the world's population) infected by *M. tuberculosis*. An estimated 10 million cases of tuberculosis develop annually, and approximately 80% of the reported cases occur in 22 countries, most of which are in Asia and sub-Saharan Africa. In the United States, more than 66% of new cases occur in individuals who are foreign born (CDC, 2017c). Tuberculosis accounted for 1.8 million deaths worldwide in 2015 (CDC, 2017c).

Some strains of *M. tuberculosis* have become resistant to the primary drugs used to treat the disease (isoniazid and rifampin). The number of MDR cases decreased slightly by from 2014 to 2015 (CDC, 2017c). Worldwide, approximately 3.7% of new tuberculosis cases and 20% of recurrent cases are MDR, demonstrating resistance to at least isoniazid and rifampin. Of MDR tuberculosis cases identified worldwide, 9% are extensively drug resistant (XDR) (WHO, 2012). XDR tuberculosis is resistant to isoniazid and rifampin, as well as all fluoroquinones and at least one of three second-line drugs (i.e., amikacin, kanamycin, and capreomycin). The prevalence of XDR tuberculosis in the United States is lower. Only 1 case of XDR was reported in the United States in 2015 (CDC, 2017c).

Risk Factors

Today in the United States, tuberculosis affects primarily immigrants, individuals with HIV/AIDS, and disadvantaged populations. Racial and ethnic minorities, foreign-born individuals, and those with altered immune function are more likely to develop tuberculosis than U.S.-born white populations (CDC, 2017c; see the Focus on Diversity and Culture feature).

Poor urban areas are hit the hardest with tuberculosis, as are areas that are also affected by the epidemics of injection drug use, homelessness (see the Evidence-Based Practice

feature), malnutrition, and poor living conditions. Overcrowded institutions also contribute to spread of the disease. Transmission has been documented in hospitals, homeless shelters, drug treatment centers, prisons, and residential facilities.

The risk for a new infection by *M. tuberculosis* is affected by characteristics of the infectious individual, extent of air contamination, duration of exposure, and susceptibility of the host. The number of microbes in the sputum, frequency and force of coughing, and behaviors such as covering the mouth when coughing affect the production of droplet nuclei. In a small, closed, or poorly ventilated space, droplet nuclei become more concentrated, increasing the risk of exposure. Prolonged contact, such as living in the same household, increases the risk. Less-than-optimal immune function, a problem for people in lower socioeconomic groups, injection drug users, the homeless, and individuals with alcoholism or HIV infection, increases the susceptibility of the host.

Once infection with *M. tuberculosis* has occurred, patients with HIV/AIDS are at high risk for developing active tuberculosis. HIV infection suppresses cellular immunity, which is vital to limiting the replication and spread of the bacilli.

Prevention

The tuberculin test is used to screen for tuberculosis infection. A cellular, or delayed hypersensitivity, response to *M. tuberculosis* develops within 3–10 weeks after the infection. Injecting a small amount of **purified protein derivative (PPD)** of tuberculin any time thereafter activates this response, attracting macrophages to the area and causing a pronounced local inflammatory response. The amount of induration surrounding the injection site, not the extended area of redness, is used to determine infection (see **Table 9–17** >> and **Figure 9–27** >>) (CDC, 2017b). It is important to remember that a positive response indicates that infection and a cellular (T-cell) response have developed; however, it does not mean that active disease is present or that the patient is infectious to others.

(see **Table 9–17** >> and **Figure 9–27** >>)

Focus on Diversity and Culture
Incidence of Tuberculosis

Rates of TB differ among racial and ethnic groups as follows (CDC, 2016c):

- Asians: 18.2 TB cases per 100,000 persons
- Blacks or African Americans: 5.0 TB cases per 100,000 persons
- Hispanics or Latinos: 4.8 TB cases per 100,000 persons
- Whites: 0.6 TB cases per 100,000 persons

TABLE 9–17 Interpreting Tuberculin Test Results

Area of Induration	Significance
Less than 5 mm	Negative response; does not rule out infection
5–9 mm	Positive for people who: ■ Are in close contact with a patient who has infectious tuberculosis ■ Have an abnormal chest x-ray ■ Have HIV infection or are immunocompromised ■ Have an organ transplant Negative for all others
10–15 mm	Positive for people who have other risk factors: ■ Birth in a high-prevalence country ■ Residents of high-risk congregate settings ■ Injection drug use ■ Infants, children, and adolescents exposed to adults in high-risk categories ■ Medical risk factors (e.g., malnutrition, diabetes)
More than 15 mm	Positive for all people

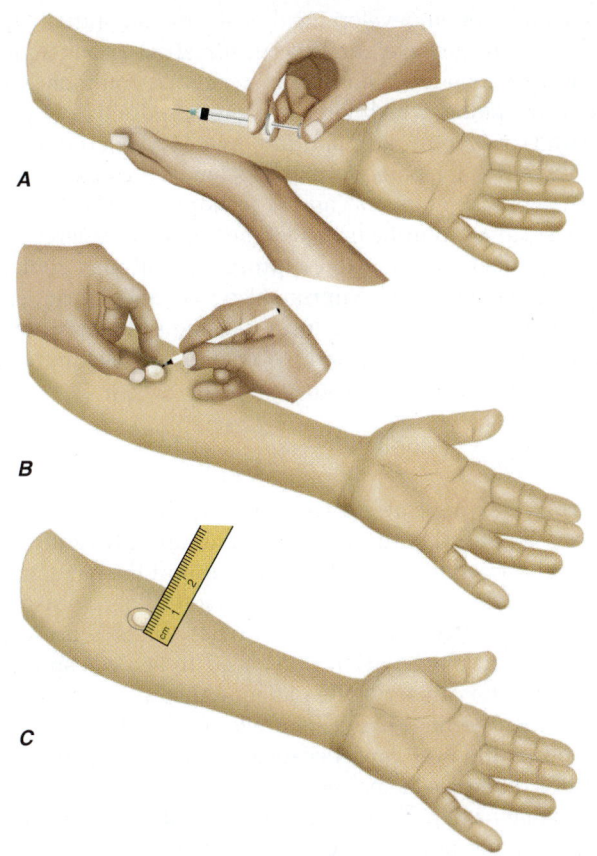

Figure 9–27 ›› **A,** Intradermal injection for tuberculin testing. **B,** The injection causes a local inflammatory response (wheal). **C,** Measurement of induration following tuberculin testing.

Skin tests and blood tests are available for tuberculin testing:

- **TB skin test (TST), also called a Mantoux test.** Injection of 0.1 mL of dPPD (5 tuberculin units) intradermally into the dorsal aspect of the forearm. The patient must return within 48–72 hours (the peak reaction period) for the TST to be read and recorded as the diameter of induration (raised area, not erythema) in millimeters.

- **Interferon-gamma release assays.** Two blood tests to screen for TB have been approved by the Food and Drug Administration: the QuantiFERON-TB test and the T-Spot test. Either can be used on patients who have received the tuberculosis vaccine, and they are useful for patients who may be unable to return to have a TST read (CDC, 2016b).

Although it is impractical and unnecessary to screen the entire population, the CDC recommends screening people in the following risk groups:

- People with or at high risk for HIV infection
- Close contacts of people who have or are suspected of having infectious tuberculosis
- People with medical risk factors, such as silicosis, chronic malabsorption, end-stage renal failure, diabetes mellitus, immunosuppression, and hematologic and other malignancies
- People born in countries with a high prevalence of tuberculosis

Evidence-Based Practice

Patients with Risk for Tuberculosis Problems

Problem

Homeless people and those living in homeless shelters have several identified risk factors for tuberculosis: a high incidence of drug and alcohol abuse, a high incidence of HIV infection, and crowded living conditions. Access to and participation in tuberculosis screening and completion of pharmacologic therapy, however, are often problematic.

Evidence

In the United States, only 1% of the population experiences homelessness in a given year, but more than 5% of individuals with tuberculosis reported being homeless within the year prior to diagnosis (CDC, 2013d). Studies in specific U.S. populations have indicated that as many as 43% of individuals with tuberculosis had a history of homelessness (Duval County, Florida; CDC, 2012d), and homeless and low-income populations were three times more likely than the general population to be infected with tuberculosis (Fitzpatrick, 2012). Major outbreaks also tend to cluster in homeless populations, such as an outbreak of 28 cases in Kane County, Illinois, in 2010–2011, all being associated with a specific homeless shelter (CDC, 2012f). Many of these individuals lack access to healthcare, including both screening and treatment. Of the two major screening tests for tuberculosis, the tuberculin skin test (TST) and the interferon-gamma release assay (IGRA), the TST was more cost effective in the homeless population (Fitzpatrick, 2012). Several states now have recommendations in place to offer free tuberculosis screening for individuals living and working at homeless shelters. Many homeless individuals choose to participate in the screening out of a desire to maintain good health and a recognition that homelessness and shelter life increase their risk of developing tuberculosis. Fear of the results and a desire "not to be bothered" had negative effects on participation. Women with children were least likely to participate in screening, citing fear of a diagnosis resulting in a loss of child custody (Fitzpatrick, 2012). Once an individual has been diagnosed with tuberculosis, homelessness is also associated with a risk of not completing the required pharmacologic therapy (Mitruka, Winston, & Navin, 2012), which can lead to recurrent infection and antibiotic resistance.

Implications

Outreach to homeless populations for health services, while difficult, has personal and public health benefits. The homeless often lack access to preventive and health promotion services, instead interacting with healthcare providers only when urgent care is needed. Shelter personnel are instrumental in getting individuals to participate in screening. Recruiting the support of these workers can improve resident participation. Regularly scheduling a nurse in a shelter can also improve participation in health promotion activities by allowing trust to develop.

Critical Thinking Application

1. Provide a rationale for the importance of tuberculosis screening and effective treatment for homeless individuals in light of the national goal to eliminate tuberculosis.

2. Develop a patient teaching strategy to increase the participation in free tuberculosis screening programs by homeless individuals and to increase medication adherence in those infected with tuberculosis.

3. What can you do personally to help provide tuberculosis screening, treatment, and follow-up for the local homeless population?

- Medically underserved, low-income populations, including racial and ethnic minorities and the homeless
- Individuals with alcoholism and injection drug users
- Residents and staff of long-term residential facilities, such as long-term care facilities, correctional institutions, and mental health facilities

False-negative responses are common in people who are immunosuppressed. A two-step procedure may be necessary to elicit a positive response. If the first test elicits a negative response, a second PPD test is given 1 week later. If the second test also is negative, the patient either is free of infection or is **anergic** (unable to react to common antigens). This two-step procedure is recommended for long-term care residents and employees.

If tuberculosis screening tests indicate the presence of tuberculosis infection, patients with latent infection should take precautions to prevent the development of active disease, and patients with active disease should take precautions to prevent the transmission of disease to others. Prophylactic pharmacologic therapy is indicated for treatment of latent disease, and pharmacologic therapy in addition to infection prevention techniques such as staying home during the first several weeks of therapy, covering the mouth and nose when coughing, wearing a mask in public places, and providing adequate room ventilation should be implemented for patients with active disease (Mayo Clinic, 2016b). For clinicians, infection-control methods include promptly identifying patients with active disease, using airborne precautions, and effectively treating individuals with suspected or confirmed disease (CDC, 2016d).

Clinical Manifestations

Initial infection with *M. tuberculosis* causes few symptoms and typically goes unnoticed until the tuberculin test becomes positive or calcified lesions are seen on a chest x-ray. Manifestations of primary progressive or reactivation

tuberculosis often develop insidiously and are initially nonspecific. Fatigue, weight loss, diminished appetite, low-grade afternoon fever, and night sweats are common. A dry cough develops, which later becomes productive of purulent and/or blood-tinged sputum (**hemoptysis**). It is often at this stage that the patient first seeks medical attention.

Tuberculosis empyema and bronchopleural fistula are the most serious complications of pulmonary tuberculosis. When a tuberculosis lesion ruptures, bacilli may contaminate the pleural space. Rupture also may allow air to enter the pleural space from the lung, causing **pneumothorax** (a partial lung collapse caused by air or gas collecting in the lung or pleural space that surrounds the lungs).

Collaboration

Interprofessional care focuses on early detection, accurate diagnosis, effective disease treatment, and preventing the spread of tuberculosis to others. To support the patient with active infection, collaboration with an infectious disease specialist may be necessary. A patient whose tuberculosis negatively affects oxygenation may need to see a respiratory therapist who can serve the patient either at home or in an institutional setting. The patient who is homeless may need additional medical care, because the diagnosis and treatment of tuberculosis may lead to the diagnosis of other illnesses that have not been previously identified or for which the patient has not been receiving treatment.

Diagnostic Tests

A positive tuberculin test alone does not indicate active disease. Sputum tests for the bacillus and chest x-rays are routinely used to diagnose and evaluate active disease. A series of three consecutive early-morning sputum specimens are typically examined for bacilli. The nurse should use special procedures or personal protective devices when obtaining

Clinical Manifestations and Therapies
Tuberculosis

ETIOLOGY	CLINICAL MANIFESTATIONS	CLINICAL THERAPIES
Rupture of tuberculosis lesion with contamination of the pleural space results in pneumothorax.	Shortness of breath, hypoxia, dry cough, cyanosis, chest pain, and subcutaneous emphysema	- Place a chest tube to water-seal. - Provide analgesics. - Provide continuous cardiorespiratory monitoring. - Monitor drainage from the chest tube. - Isolate the patient in a room with negative airflow.
Empyema and bronchopleural fistula are the most serious complications of tuberculosis. Empyema is a collection of pus within the pleural space that initiates an inflammatory response, leading to fibrous peel and trapped lung parenchyma. After resection of lung tissue, bronchopleural fistulas may develop because of inadequate healing of the stump, allowing bacteria to move into the pleural space and risking infection of the other lung.	Dyspnea with little exertion, low-grade fever, pleuritic chest pain, chest heaviness on affected side, purulent sputum, decreased breath sounds on involved side of chest, hemithorax, and opacification of the affected side on chest x-ray	- CT may be used to locate and direct drainage of the area. - The priority is to protect the healthy lung. - The patient may require intubation. - Antibiotics may be given both intravenously and directly into the infected cavity. - Analgesics for pain related to the condition and treatment may be required.

sputum specimens, including a mask capable of filtering droplet nuclei. If possible, collect specimens in a room equipped with airflow control devices, ultraviolet light, or both. As an alternative, the patient should step outside for collection of the specimen. Aerosol therapy, percussion, and postural drainage may help the patient to produce sputum. On occasion, endotracheal suctioning, bronchoscopy, or gastric lavage is necessary to obtain a specimen.

Diagnostic testing often proceeds as follows:

- A *sputum smear* is microscopically examined for acid-fast bacilli. *M. tuberculosis* resists decolorizing chemicals after staining. Therefore, *M. tuberculosis* is called *acid fast*. The acid-fast smear provides a rapid indicator of the tubercle bacillus.

- *Sputum culture* that is positive for *M. tuberculosis* provides the definitive diagnosis. However, *M. tuberculosis* is slow growing, requiring 4–8 weeks before it can be detected with traditional culture techniques. Automated radiometric culture systems (e.g., Bactec) allow detection of *M. tuberculosis* in several days.

- *Sensitivity testing* is performed to identify the appropriate drug therapy once the organism is detected.

- A *polymerase chain reaction* assay permits rapid detection of DNA from *M. tuberculosis*.

- A *chest x-ray* is ordered to diagnose and evaluate tuberculosis. Typical findings in pulmonary tuberculosis include dense lesions in the apical and posterior segments of the upper lobe and possible cavity formation.

Before initiating antituberculosis drug therapy, several additional diagnostic tests may be done to establish baseline data for monitoring potential adverse effects of the drugs:

- *Liver function tests* are obtained before treatment with isoniazid, because this drug is hepatotoxic.

- *A thorough vision examination* is done before treatment with ethambutol, a commonly used antituberculosis medication. Optic neuritis is a potential adverse effect of this drug. Periodic eye examinations are scheduled during the course of therapy.

- *Audiometric testing* is performed before streptomycin therapy is initiated. Ototoxicity is a significant adverse effect of streptomycin and other aminoglycoside antibiotics. Hearing also is evaluated periodically during the course of therapy to detect any hearing loss.

Pharmacologic Therapy

Antibiotics are used both to prevent and to treat tuberculosis infection. Goals of the pharmacologic treatment of tuberculosis are to make the disease noncommunicable to others, to reduce symptoms of the disease, and to effect a cure in the shortest possible time.

Prophylaxis

Prophylactic treatment is used to prevent active tuberculosis. Patients with a recent skin test conversion from negative to positive are often started on prophylactic therapy, especially when other risk factors are present. Prophylactic therapy also is used for people in close household contact with an individual whose sputum is positive for bacilli. Single-drug therapy is effective for prophylactic treatment, whereas treatment of active disease always involves two or more chemotherapeutic medications. For adults, isoniazid, 300 mg per day for a period of 6–12 months, is commonly used to prevent active tuberculosis. This therapy may also be used for individuals who are susceptible to tuberculosis infection, such as individuals with HIV.

When isoniazid prophylaxis is contraindicated, bacille Calmette-Guérin (BCG) vaccine may be prescribed. This vaccine is widely used in developing countries. BCG is made from an attenuated strain of *Mycobacterium bovis*, a closely related bacillus that causes tuberculosis in cattle. In the United States, BCG vaccine is recommended only for foreign-born infants and children as well as infants, children, and healthcare workers with a negative tuberculin test who are repeatedly exposed to untreated or ineffectively treated individuals who have active disease. After vaccination with BCG, a positive reaction to tuberculin testing is common. Periodic chest x-rays may be required for screening purposes.

Treatment of Active Disease

The tuberculosis bacillus mutates readily to drug-resistant forms when only one anti-infective agent is used. Active disease is always treated with concurrent use of at least two antibacterial medications to which the organism is sensitive. The primary antituberculosis drugs can prevent development of resistance, because all act by different mechanisms. However, the organism is protected within the tubercle, and 6 or more months of treatment are necessary to eradicate it.

Newly diagnosed tuberculosis is typically treated with an initial regimen of four oral antituberculosis drugs—isoniazid, rifampin, pyrazinamide, and ethambutol daily (or several times per week on a decreasing schedule of frequency)—for the first 2 months of treatment. This initial regimen is followed by at least 4 additional months of therapy with isoniazid and rifampin, given daily, twice per week, or weekly. In the presence of HIV infection, treatment is continued for at least 9 months. The most common antituberculosis drugs and their nursing implications are outlined in the Medications feature. If a drug-resistant strain is suspected, therapy is tailored to the resistance.

Adherence

Adherence to the prescribed regimen is evaluated during follow-up visits. The patient's urine can be examined for color changes characteristic of rifampin and tested for metabolites of isoniazid. When adherence is a problem, medications are administered under direct supervision. Twice-weekly therapy is more cost effective in this instance, with a public health nurse watching the patient take and swallow the prescribed medication.

Follow-up

Repeat sputum specimens and chest x-rays are used to evaluate the effectiveness of therapy. In most cases, sputum cultures for *M. tuberculosis* are negative within 2 months after the end of therapy; virtually all patients have negative sputum cultures within 3 months. If cultures remain positive at 3 months and beyond, treatment failure and drug resistance are suspected. In this case, cultures of the organism are tested for susceptibility to antituberculosis agents, and two or three previously unused drugs are added to the treatment regimen (Longo et al., 2012). Given adequate treatment, almost all patients are cured of tuberculosis. Nonadherence to the treatment regimen is the greatest barrier to the control of tuberculosis (CDC, 2015h).

Medications
Antituberculosis Drugs

CLASSIFICATION AND DRUG EXAMPLES	MECHANISMS OF ACTION	NURSING CONSIDERATIONS
First-Line Agents		
Ethambutol *Drug example:* Myambutol	Ethambutol (oral, 15–25 mg/kg/day) (max: 1600 mg per day) is added to the initial treatment regimen or substituted for isoniazid when an isoniazid-resistant strain of tuberculosis is suspected. Ethambutol is a bacteriostatic drug that reduces the development of resistance to the bactericidal first-line agents. Its principal toxic effect is optic neuritis, but this effect is reversible. Early signs of optic neuritis include decreased visual acuity and loss of red–green discrimination. This drug may be safe for use in pregnancy.	■ Record a baseline visual examination before therapy. Schedule periodic eye exams during the course of treatment. ■ Administer with meals to reduce gastrointestinal side effects. ■ Monitor liver and renal function studies and neurologic status while taking this drug. Notify the healthcare provider of abnormal findings or significant changes. Health Education for the Patient and Family ■ Monitor vision daily by reading newspapers and looking at the same blue object (using usual corrective lenses, if appropriate). Notify the healthcare provider of changes in vision or color perception.

Isoniazid
 	
Drug examples:
 	
Isoniazid
Laniazid
Nydrazid
	Isoniazid (oral, 5 mg/kd/day [max: 300 mg/day], or 900 mg twice weekly) is the drug of choice for tuberculosis prophylaxis and a first-line drug for treating active disease. It is effective against both intracellular and extracellular organisms. Isoniazid is used alone as a prophylactic medication and in combination with rifampin, ethambutol, or both. A fixed-dose combination form with 150 mg of isoniazid and 300 mg of rifampin (Rifamate) is available as well.	■ Administer on an empty stomach 1 hour before or 2 hours after meals for maximal effect if tolerated; it may be given with meals to reduce gastrointestinal effects.
		■ Administer pyridoxine (vitamin B_6) concurrently.
		■ Monitor for adverse effects:
		  a. Peripheral neuropathy
		  b. Hypersensitivity reactions
		  c. Evidence of anemia, bruising, bleeding, or infection related to agranulocytosis
		■ Isoniazid interferes with the metabolism of diazepam, phenytoin, and carbamazepine. Doses of these drugs may need to be reduced to prevent toxicity.
		Health Education for the Patient and Family
		■ Take the medication as prescribed for the entire treatment period to prevent incomplete eradication of the bacteria and development of resistant strains.
		■ Report adverse effects (diminished appetite, nausea, jaundice, allergic reaction) to the healthcare provider immediately.
		■ Take pyridoxine as prescribed to prevent peripheral neuropathy.
		■ Avoid alcohol and other agents that may be harmful to the liver.
		■ Use measures to prevent pregnancy while taking isoniazid; this drug may be harmful to the developing fetus.

Pyrazinamide *Drug example:* Tebrazid	Pyrazinamide (oral, 5–15 mg/kg/tid to qid [max: 2 g/day]) typically is given with isoniazid and rifampin for the first 2 months of tuberculosis treatment. Concurrent use of pyrazinamide allows a shorter course of therapy. Like many of the antituberculosis agents, pyrazinamide is toxic to the liver. Its other principal adverse effect is hyperuricemia. Gout, however, rarely develops.	■ Administer with meals to reduce gastrointestinal side effects. ■ Monitor liver function studies and serum uric acid levels. Notify the healthcare provider of any changes. Health Education for the Patient and Family ■ Notify the healthcare provider of loss of appetite, nausea, vomiting, jaundice, or symptoms of gout (a painful, red, hot, swollen joint, often the great toe or elbow). ■ While taking this drug, avoid using alcohol or other substances that may be harmful to the liver.

Medications *(continued)*

CLASSIFICATION AND DRUG EXAMPLES	MECHANISMS OF ACTION	NURSING CONSIDERATIONS
Rifabutin *Drug example:* Mycobutin	Rifabutin (oral 300 mg daily) is used for prophylaxis, or 5 mg/kg/day is used for active tuberculosis (max: 300 mg/day).	▪ Monitor CBC, liver function, and bleeding times for evidence of toxicity. ▪ While taking this drug, avoid using alcohol or other substances that may be harmful to the liver.
Rifampin *Drug examples:* Rifadin Rimactane	Rifampin (oral or IV, 600 mg daily; or 900 mg twice weekly for 4 months) is commonly used in combination with isoniazid and other antituberculosis drugs. Rifampin stimulates the microsomal enzymes of the liver, increasing the rate of metabolism of many drugs and decreasing their effectiveness.	▪ Administer on an empty stomach. ▪ Monitor CBC, liver function, and renal function for evidence of toxicity. ▪ Rifampin reduces the effect of oral contraceptives, quinidine, corticosteroids, warfarin, methadone, digoxin, and hypoglycemics. Monitor for the effectiveness of these drugs. Health Education for the Patient and Family ▪ Rifampin causes body fluids, including sweat, urine, saliva, and tears, to turn red-orange. This effect is not harmful. Avoid wearing soft contact lenses, because they may be permanently stained. ▪ Do not miss or skip doses; flulike syndrome and fever occur when the drug is resumed. ▪ Aspirin may interfere with rifampin absorption and should not be taken concurrently. ▪ Fever, flulike symptoms, excessive fatigue, sore throat, or unusual bleeding may indicate an adverse reaction to the drug and should be reported to the healthcare provider.
Rifapentine *Drug example:* Priftin	Rifapentine (oral, 600 mg) is used twice per week for 2 months then once a week for 4 months.	▪ Monitor CBC, liver function, and renal function for evidence of toxicity.
Second-Line Agents		
Amikacin *Drug example:* Amikin	Amikacin (IV/IM 5–7.5 mg/kg) is given as a loading dose; then 7.5 mg bid.	▪ Monitor for rash, fever, pain at injection site, nausea, diarrhea, tinnitus, and dizziness. ▪ Monitor urine output, weight, and renal function (including blood urea nitrogen and serum creatinine) to detect early signs of nephrotoxicity. Report significant changes to the healthcare provider. ▪ Monitor for tinnitus, hearing loss, or changes in hearing as irreversible damage may occur.
Streptomycin	An aminoglycoside antibiotic, streptomycin (intramuscular, 15 mg/kg/day [max: 1 g/day]) is highly effective in treating most mycobacterial infections. Resistance may develop if it is used alone. There are two primary drawbacks to streptomycin: First, it must be administered parenterally, because it is not absorbed in the gastrointestinal tract. Second, it has toxic effects on the kidneys and ears.	▪ Administer by deep intramuscular injection into a large muscle mass, rotating sites to minimize tissue trauma. ▪ Monitor urine output, weight, and renal function (including blood urea nitrogen and serum creatinine) to detect early signs of nephrotoxicity. Report significant changes to the healthcare provider. ▪ Maintain fluid intake at 2000–3000 mL per day to minimize the concentration of drug in the kidney tubules. ▪ Assess hearing and balance frequently. Have audiometric testing performed as indicated. Health Education for the Patient and Family ▪ Maintain a daily fluid intake of at least 2–3 liters. ▪ Weigh yourself on the same scale at least twice a week. Report any significant weight gain to the healthcare provider. ▪ Notify the healthcare provider of decreased hearing acuity, ringing or buzzing sensations in the ear, or vertigo.

Source: Based on Adams, M. P., Holland, L. N., & Urban, C. (2017). *Pharmacology for nurses: A pathophysiologic approach* (5th ed.). Hoboken, NJ: Pearson Education.

Lifespan Considerations

Tuberculosis in Pregnant Women and Newborns

When caring for a woman who is pregnant or who has recently delivered, the nurse must consider both the woman and the baby. If the new mother is found to have tuberculosis, prevent direct contact with the newborn until the mother is noninfectious. If maternal tuberculosis is inactive or the mother has been on therapy long enough to prevent infection of the newborn, the mother may breastfeed and care for her baby. Because the newborn has an immature immune response, the nurse must teach the mother how to reduce the infant's risk of infection.

None of the tuberculosis drugs has been proven to be teratogenic. While isoniazid crosses the placenta, most studies show no teratogenic effects. Rifampin crosses the placenta, and the possibility of teratogenic effects is still being studied. However, potential adverse effects on the fetus are weighed against the benefit to the mother before they are prescribed during pregnancy.

Tuberculosis in Children

Only children who have one or more risk factors, such as close contact with an individual diagnosed with tuberculosis, a compromised immune system, or recent immigration, should have an intradermal tuberculin skin test with PPD. Children with a positive PPD should then undergo further diagnostic testing to determine whether active disease is present. Children are more likely than adults to progress rapidly from infection to disease; progression to disease is influenced by age, nutritional and immune status, genetic factors, virulence of the organism, and magnitude of infection. Young age (less than 2 years) and HIV infection are the two greatest risk factors in children for progression to disease (Gao et al., 2015).

Infants, children, and adolescents with latent tuberculosis have no symptoms. Clinical manifestations of active tuberculosis in infants include a persistent cough, weight loss or failure to gain weight, and low-grade fever. Wheezing and decreased breath sounds may be present. Children with active disease may have fatigue, cough, diminished appetite, weight loss or growth delay, night sweats, chills, a low-grade fever, and enlarged lymph nodes.

According to the CDC (2015k), tuberculosis is a serious illness as infants and young children are more likely than older children and adults to develop life-threatening forms of the disease (e.g., disseminated tuberculosis, tuberculosis meningitis). Tuberculosis disease is treated by taking several antituberculosis medicines for 6–9 months. If a child stops taking the drugs before completion, the child can become sick again. In addition, if drugs are not taken correctly, the bacteria that are still alive may become resistant to those drugs. Tuberculosis that is resistant to drugs is harder and more expensive to treat, and treatment lasts much longer (up to 18–24 months) (CDC, 2015k).

Tuberculosis in Older Adults

Community-dwelling older adults as well as those in care facilities are susceptible to tuberculosis. The older adult with respiratory symptoms often is treated presumptively for pneumonia, without a sputum smear and Gram stain. Older adults living in the community may not have had a tuberculin test or chest x-ray for many years.

Nurses working with these patients typically assess risk factors for tuberculosis, such as the following:

- General health and nutritional status, including intake of specific nutrients, such as vitamin D (lack of vitamin D is associated with a higher risk of developing active tuberculosis)
- Presence of a chronic disease (e.g., silicosis, diabetes, alcoholism, HIV infection) or past history of a gastrectomy
- Past history of a positive tuberculin test that now has converted to negative
- Medications, such as corticosteroids or other immunosuppressive drugs.

Nurses may also assess living and social situations, such as the following:

- Natural light and ventilation in the home
- Access to clean water, cooking facilities, grocery stores, and other services
- Possible exposure to infected people, such as sharing a household with someone who has active tuberculosis, crowded living facilities, homelessness, frequent participation in activities for older adults, and volunteer work in residential care facilities or other institutional settings
- Access to healthcare.

Tuberculosis is typically treated in the community; hospitalization or institutionalization is rarely necessary or desirable. For the older adult being treated for active tuberculosis in the community, the nurse should assess the following:

- Knowledge and understanding of the disease and the prescribed treatment regimen
- Mental status and ability to follow both the prescribed regimen and precautions to avoid exposing others to the disease
- Transportation and regular access to healthcare services
- Financial resources to complete treatment and follow-up care
- Need for home health or social services to ensure adequate treatment.

Presenting symptoms of tuberculosis in the older adult are often vague, including coughing, weight loss, diminished appetite, and periodic fevers. These signs and symptoms should not be dismissed as a normal part of aging. The prevalence of active tuberculosis is significantly higher among older adults in the United States than among young adults (CDC, 2015h). Among older adults, approximately 90% of cases occur because of reactivation of a dormant bacterium. Older adults are at increased risk for reactivation tuberculosis as a result of age-related decreases in cell-mediated immunity. Chronic illnesses, poor nutrition, gastrectomy, alcoholism, or the long-term use of steroids and immunosuppressive agents may also reactivate dormant tuberculosis lesions.

Residents of nursing homes are at increased risk for acquiring tuberculosis because of their close proximity to each other. Yearly tuberculin skin testing with PPD is often required by state health departments for nursing home residents. If the initial test is negative, a repeat PPD in 1–2 weeks is recommended. This repetition improves sensitivity to the test so that silent cases of tuberculosis are not missed. A chest x-ray and sputum culture for acid-fast bacilli are obtained if the PPD is positive.

NURSING PROCESS

Nurses play a key role in maintaining public health. Education and tuberculosis screening are major nursing strategies to prevent tuberculosis. Nurses have an important role in identifying individuals with one or more risk factors for infection, such as foreign-born individuals, individuals with HIV, and individuals residing in states with a higher incidence of tuberculosis (California, Texas, New York, and Florida) (CDC, 2012i).

Public health teaching includes increasing awareness of tuberculosis as a reemerging threat. Teach patients in all settings how to reduce the spread of tuberculosis by covering their mouths when coughing or sneezing and disposing of sputum appropriately. Also include in public health education the benefit of screening programs to identify infected (though not necessarily infective) individuals.

Assessment

Focused assessment for the patient with suspected tuberculosis includes the following:

- **Observation and patient interview.** Observe the patient's general appearance and assess the patient for difficulty breathing, presence of cough and nature of the cough (productive or nonproductive), as well as general condition and skin color. Ask patients about complaints of fatigue, weight loss, night sweats, perceived difficulty breathing, and presence of a cough. In addition, inquire about any blood in the sputum (hemoptysis) and any symptoms of chest pain. Ask patients about any known exposure to tuberculosis and when they had their most recent tuberculin test and results. Last, ask patients to describe their living circumstances, as well as use of alcohol and recreational drugs.
- **Physical examination.** Obtain a full set of vital signs, including temperature. Assess the respiratory rate and lung sounds. Assess the patient's weight and observe for signs of malnutrition.

Use screening questions (**Box 9–6** ⟩⟩) to identify individuals at risk for latent infection. Screen infants and children at 1 month, 6 months, and 12 months and then annually (American Academy of Pediatrics, 2016).

Diagnosis

Nursing diagnoses for the patient with the medical diagnosis of tuberculosis may include the following:

- *Fatigue*
- *Imbalanced Nutrition: Less Than Body Requirements*

Box 9–6
Screening Questions to Identify Risk for Latent Tuberculosis Infection

- Determine the patient's understanding of tuberculosis.
- Collect demographic information so follow-up can be provided if needed.
- Review the patient's medical record, including laboratory and radiology findings.
- Question the patient's past tuberculosis history and exposure to others diagnosed with tuberculosis.
- Does the patient have any symptoms of tuberculosis?
- Determine the history of present illness and social history.
- If the patient was previously treated for tuberculosis, was the patient compliant with the treatment regimen?
- Was the patient born outside the country or has the patient traveled outside the country? Have immediate family members recently traveled outside the country?

Source: Based on Centers for Disease Control and Prevention. (2010). *Self-study modules on tuberculosis.* Retrieved from http://www.cdc.gov/tb/education/ssmodules/module8/ss8reading4.htm

- *Knowledge, Deficient*
- *Health Management, Ineffective*
- *Infection, Risk for*
- *Health: Community, Deficient*
- *Social Isolation.*

(NANDA-I © 2014)

Planning

Care planning is based on the needs of the patient, the resources and support available, the patient's general health status, and the patient's environment. Suggested outcomes include the following:

- The patient will demonstrate behaviors that reduce the risk of contamination of others.
- The patient will describe the required treatment and follow-up care required.
- The patient will have adequate resources available to obtain necessary medications and supplies.

Implementation

Nursing care related to tuberculosis focuses primarily on infection-control and compliance with prescribed treatment. See the Nursing Care Plan feature.

Provide Patient Education

Adequate knowledge and information are necessary to manage the disease and prevent its transmission to others. The patient needs to understand the reasons for prolonged drug therapy and the importance of complying with treatment and follow-up. Antituberculosis drugs are relatively toxic. The patient needs to know how to minimize toxicity. Interventions to promote the patient's understanding of disease transmission and management include the following:

- Assess the patient's knowledge about the disease process, and identify misperceptions and emotional reactions.

Teaching based on previous learning enhances understanding and retention of information.

- Assess the patient's ability and interest in learning, developmental level, and obstacles to learning. Assessment allows tailoring the presentation of information to the learning needs and style of the patient, promoting learning.

- Identify the patient's support systems, and include significant others in teaching. A knowledgeable significant other provides reinforcement of learning, confirmation of understanding, and encouragement for the patient. Including significant others also reduces the risk of inadvertent sabotage of the treatment plan.

- Establish a relationship of mutual trust with the patient and significant others. An atmosphere of trust increases receptiveness to teaching and learning.

- Develop mutually acceptable learning goals with the patient and significant other. Working together to identify learning needs and establish goals increases the patient's ownership of and interest in the process.

- Select appropriate teaching strategies, using learning aids such as literature and visual materials that are appropriate for age, level of education, and intellect. Teaching tailored to the patient is more effective and results in better learning.

- Document your teaching and the level of the patient's understanding. Reinforce teaching and learning as needed. Teaching is not complete until the patient can demonstrate learning of the information.

Specific topics to cover during the teaching session are outlined in the Patient Teaching feature.

Promote Effective Therapeutic Regimen Management

The populations at highest risk for developing active tuberculosis—the homeless and members of lower socioeconomic groups—are also at high risk for being unable to manage its complex treatment regimen. Three or more costly medications are prescribed that may have unpleasant or even dangerous side effects. Frequent medical follow-up is required. Infectious diseases such as tuberculosis also carry a stigma that may lead to denial of the disease or its seriousness. Individuals with alcoholism and those who use injection drugs need to withdraw from their addiction to be successful in treating the disease, and individuals with HIV infection face a potentially fatal disease and costly treatment that may well override their concerns about tuberculosis management. Nursing interventions may include the following:

- Assess the patient's self-care abilities and support systems. Assessment is used to help determine the patient's ability to follow the prescribed regimen.

- Assess the patient's knowledge and understanding of the disease, its complications, treatment, and risks to others. Provide additional teaching and reinforcement as indicated. Lack of understanding is a barrier to compliance with and management of the treatment regimen.

- Work collaboratively to identify barriers or obstacles to managing the prescribed treatment. Working collaboratively with the patient and other members of the healthcare team provides insight for overcoming identified barriers to effective treatment.

Patient Teaching
Managing Tuberculosis

Tuberculosis is a chronic disease requiring lengthy treatment with antituberculosis medications. Teaching focuses on treatment and on improving the patient's ability to self-manage the disease. A good understanding of the disease, its treatment, and the potential adverse effects of therapy prepares the patient to manage care. Teach the patient and family about tuberculosis and the prescribed treatment, including:

- Nature of the disease and its spread to others
- Purpose of treatment and follow-up procedures
- Measures to prevent spreading the disease to others
  a. Using disposable tissues to contain respiratory secretions, especially during the first 2 weeks of treatment, when the disease may be transmitted to others
  b. Avoiding exposure to crowds or individuals with infectious diseases
  c. Ensuring that housemates or others having frequent contact with the patient are tested and receive prophylactic treatment if indicated
- Importance of maintaining good general health by eating a well-balanced, high-protein, high-carbohydrate diet and balancing exercise with rest.
- Names, doses, purposes, and adverse effects of prescribed medications, with emphasis on the importance of taking all medications as prescribed

- The possible side effects of the prescribed medications and the importance of reporting them to healthcare providers. Possible side effects:
  a. Peripheral neuropathy (numbness, tingling, or a burning sensation of the extremities) may occur with isoniazid. Pyridoxine (vitamin B_6) often is prescribed to prevent this adverse effect.
  b. Both isoniazid and rifampin may cause hepatitis. Avoid alcohol while taking these drugs and report any manifestations, such as nausea and diminished appetite, jaundice, a change in urine or stool color, or pain in the upper right quadrant.
  c. Rifampin may cause an orange-red coloration of saliva and urine.
  d. Streptomycin can affect hearing and balance. Promptly report any changes, because they may be irreversible.
  e. Ethambutol may affect red–green color discrimination and visual acuity. Use caution when driving or walking in unfamiliar areas, and promptly report any vision changes.
- Importance of avoiding alcohol and other substances that may damage the liver while taking chemotherapeutic drugs
- Fluid intake needs of 2–3 L of fluid per day
- Manifestations to report to the healthcare provider: chest pain, hemoptysis, or difficulty breathing; diminished appetite, nausea, or vomiting; yellow tint to skin or sclera; sudden weight gain; swollen feet, ankles, legs, or hands; hearing loss, tinnitus, or vertigo; and change in vision or difficulty discriminating colors.

- Assist the patient, significant others (if available), and healthcare team members to develop a plan for managing the prescribed regimen. Including the patient in developing a plan to manage care increases the patient's sense of control and ownership and helps to ensure that personal, cultural, and lifestyle factors are considered. All of this increases the likelihood of compliance.

- Provide verbal and written instructions that are clear and appropriate for the patient's level of literacy, knowledge, and understanding. Clearly written directions provide support and reinforcement.

- Provide active intervention for homeless people, including shelter placement or other housing and ongoing follow-up by easily accessed healthcare providers (clinics and public health workers in the neighborhood that do not present transportation or access problems, either real or perceived). Simple referral does not ensure compliance, especially among disenfranchised populations. Active intervention is needed to help ensure treatment compliance.

- Refer patients who are unlikely to comply with the treatment regimen to the public health department for management and follow-up. Because tuberculosis presents a significant public health risk, public health follow-up is essential. In some cases, nurses must administer medications, observing the patient swallow all pills. Direct observation therapy may be needed for children as well as adults.

Reduce Risk for Infection

The spread of tuberculosis is a risk in any facility that houses many people. The risk is especially high in residential care facilities for older adults and for people with AIDS. The increasing incidence of tuberculosis among homeless people and members of lower socioeconomic groups increases the risk in hospitals, emergency departments, and public and urgent care clinics. Respiratory precautions are necessary to prevent the spread of the disease to other patients and to healthcare workers via microscopic airborne droplets. The following steps can help to lower the risk of spreading the infection:

- Place the patient in a private room with airflow control that prevents air within the room from circulating into the hallway or other rooms. A **negative airflow room** (a room where air flows out of the room) in which air is diluted by at least six fresh-air exchanges per hour is recommended. A negative flow room and multiple fresh-air exchanges dilute the concentration of droplet nuclei within the room and prevent their spread to adjacent areas.

- Use standard precautions and tuberculosis isolation techniques as recommended by the CDC, including wearing a respirator and gown when caring for patients with tuberculosis. These measures are important to prevent the spread of tuberculosis to others.

SAFETY ALERT Use personal protective devices to reduce the risk of transmission during patient care. OSHA requires use of a HEPA-filtered respirator for protection against occupational exposure to tuberculosis. Surgical masks are ineffective in filtering droplet nuclei, so the use of protective devices capable of filtering bacteria and particles smaller than 1 micron is necessary.

- Discuss with the patient the reasons for and importance of respiratory isolation procedures during initial hospitalization. When outpatient treatment is provided, instruct the patient to avoid crowds and close physical contact and to maintain ventilation in living facilities, particularly during the first 3 weeks of treatment. These measures help to protect others during initial treatment, when sputum is still likely to contain significant numbers of bacilli.

- Place a mask on the patient during transport to other parts of the facility for diagnostic or treatment procedures. Covering the patient's nose and mouth minimizes air contamination and the risk to visitors and personnel.

- Inform all personnel having contact with the patient of the diagnosis. This information allows personnel to take appropriate precautions.

- Assist visitors to mask before entering the room. Providing visitors with appropriate masks or respirators reduces their risk of infection.

- Teach the patient how to limit transmitting the disease to others:
  a. Always cough and expectorate into tissues.
  b. Dispose of tissues properly, placing them in a closed bag.
  c. Wear a mask if sneezing or unable to control respiratory secretions.
  d. The disease is not spread by touching inanimate objects, so no special precautions are required for eating utensils, clothing, books, or other objects used.
  e. How to collect sputum specimens to minimize healthcare personnel's risk of exposure.
  f. The importance of complying with the prescribed treatment for the entire course of therapy.

The nurse should provide referrals as appropriate:

- Smoking cessation clinics or support groups

- Alcohol treatment facilities, Alcoholics Anonymous, and other treatment programs or support groups

- Drug treatment facilities, Narcotics Anonymous, and other outpatient or inpatient treatment programs or support groups

- Low-cost community clinics and incentive programs for people with tuberculosis

- Counseling, support groups, and other community resources that provide additional assistance and support.

Evaluation

Compliance with prescribed therapies, resolution of symptoms, and improvement on chest x-ray are all positive evaluation findings. Patients are evaluated on progress toward outcomes, and the plan of care is amended as indicated. Expected outcomes of nursing care include the following:

- The patient with latent infection completes therapy and does not develop active tuberculosis.

- The patient's contacts are evaluated for tuberculosis and those infected are treated.

Nursing Care Plan
A Patient with Tuberculosis

Harry Facée, age 53, arrives at a metropolitan public health clinic complaining of aching chest pain that has lasted for the past few days. He says that his sputum also is bloody. He is afraid he might have lung cancer, so he came in to see a healthcare provider.

ASSESSMENT

Raj Kamil, RN, the public health nurse at the clinic, obtains an admission history and physical examination of Mr. Facée. Mr. Kamil notes that Mr. Facée is a homeless individual who has lived on the streets and in various shelters for the past "10 years or so." He usually prefers to sleep outdoors, taking refuge in shelters only during very cold or very wet weather. He has a small disability income but usually scrounges for food or eats with other homeless people at soup kitchens. Mr. Facée states that he has had a cough for a long time, which has become worse recently. It is now productive, especially in the mornings. He also admits that he has recently been waking up drenched with sweat in the middle of the night and is more tired than usual.

Although Mr. Facée's clothes are tattered, he is fairly clean. He answers questions appropriately and intelligently. Mr. Kamil does not detect any odor of alcohol on his breath. Mr. Facée is very thin, almost emaciated. His vital signs are temperature 37.8°C (100.2°F); pulse 92 bpm; respirations 20/min; and blood pressure 152/86 mmHg

Suspecting tuberculosis, Mr. Kamil obtains a sputum specimen for Gram stain and culture, administers a tuberculin test, and sends Mr. Facée for a chest x-ray before he sees the clinic healthcare provider. Although the chest x-ray is inconclusive, the Gram stain is positive for acid-fast bacilli. The diagnosis is probable active pulmonary tuberculosis. The healthcare provider prescribes daily isoniazid, 300 mg orally; rifampin, 600 mg orally; and pyrazinamide, 1500 mg orally for 2 months, to be followed by twice-weekly isoniazid, 900 mg orally, and rifampin, 600 mg orally. The healthcare provider also orders weekly sputum cultures for the first month.

DIAGNOSES

- *Ineffective Health Maintenance* related to homelessness
- *Risk for Noncompliance* with prescribed treatment related to lack of understanding and resources
- *Imbalanced Nutrition: Less Than Body Requirements* related to increased metabolic needs associated with infection

(NANDA-I © 2014)

PLANNING

Goals for Mr. Facée's care include:

- The patient will keep all follow-up appointments as scheduled.
- The patient will verbalize an understanding of the disease and its treatment.
- The patient will follow the prescribed plan of care.
- The patient will demonstrate measures to prevent the spread of the organism to others.
- The patient will gain 1–2 lb of weight per week.
- The patient will promptly report symptoms of peripheral neuropathy, including numbness, tingling, or burning sensations.

IMPLEMENTATION

- Teach the patient about tuberculosis, and provide a patient education pamphlet about the disease.
- Instruct the patient about the prescribed medications, potential adverse effects, and importance of completing the entire prescribed regimen.
- Emphasize the importance of continued follow-up.
- Teach and demonstrate sputum and droplet control measures.
- Escort the patient to the local incentive shelter program for directly observed medical therapy and meals.
- Identify verbally and in writing manifestations to report to the healthcare provider.

EVALUATION

Mr. Kamil successfully enrolls Mr. Facée in the local incentive shelter program. In this program, a healthcare worker administers Mr. Facée's medications daily, watching him swallow them. Mr. Facée is assigned a small individual room and can eat three daily meals at the shelter. He still prefers to sleep outside when the weather permits, but he complies with the requirement for supervised medication administration because he "likes the food there." Always a clean individual, Mr. Facée is able to demonstrate appropriate sputum-control measures and practices them faithfully. The sputum culture done after 2 months of treatment is negative for tubercle bacilli, and Mr. Facée's chest x-ray indicates no disease progression.

CRITICAL THINKING

1. Many homeless people have schizophrenia or other mental illnesses. How would you adapt the care plan for a homeless patient with schizophrenia and active tuberculosis?
2. Mr. Kamil was fortunate in having access to an incentive shelter with healthcare workers to supervise medication compliance. Identify available resources in your area for homeless patients infected with tuberculosis.
3. Develop a care plan for the nursing diagnosis *Ineffective Airway Clearance* related to mucopurulent sputum and weak cough.

REVIEW Tuberculosis

RELATE Link the Concepts and Exemplars

Linking the exemplar of tuberculosis with the concept of health policy:

1. What role does the government play in determining policies to mandate tuberculosis testing of those traveling to the United States from other countries, especially those countries with the highest number of cases?

2. What government reporting requirements must be followed when a patient is diagnosed with tuberculosis?

Linking the exemplar of tuberculosis with the concept of ethics:

3. You are working in a clinic and read as positive a PPD skin test done 2 days ago. While providing routine teaching, you inform the patient of the need to test those who have been in contact with the patient, and the patient says, "No, I will not tell you who I've been in contact with, and you have no right to share my personal medical information with others, especially the government." What legal rights does this patient have regarding privacy of information, and how would you handle this situation?

4. What information can you provide about the necessity for testing and treatment for a mother who is afraid of losing custody of her children if diagnosed with tuberculosis?

READY Go to Volume 3: Clinical Nursing Skills

REFER Go to Pearson MyLab Nursing and eText

- Additional review materials
- Pathogenesis of Tuberculosis

REFLECT Apply Your Knowledge

Ngong Lee is a 62-year-old woman who has been married to Daniel Lee for 42 years. Born and raised in Vietnam, Ms. Lee came to the United States after marrying her husband when she was 20. Their only child, John, died at age 22 in an automobile accident. His death devastated Ms. Lee, but over time, she adequately adjusted and coped with the loss. All of her brothers and sisters have passed away, but she has a few nieces and nephews who still live in Vietnam. She and Mr. Lee have no relatives nearby.

Ms. Lee has noticed a steady weight loss and lack of appetite over the past few weeks, ever since they returned from visiting relatives in Vietnam. At first, she was delighted with her new, slender figure, but as she continued to lose weight, she started to wonder whether she had cancer. This week she has been waking at night wet with perspiration, and this afternoon she took her temperature and has a slight fever. As she thinks about it, she realizes she has been tired lately and decides that it is time to see a healthcare provider. She makes an appointment at the local clinic and tells the nurse that she has lost 12 pounds in the past 3 weeks and describes her other symptoms. The nurse notices Ms. Lee coughing and asks when the cough started. Ms. Lee looks surprised and says that she had not noticed that she had been coughing. The healthcare provider orders a chest x-ray, CBC with differential, PPD, and sputum specimen for culture. The healthcare provider advises the nurse to take appropriate precautions, because tuberculosis is the suspected diagnosis.

1. How will the nurse collect the sputum specimen to reduce the spread of infection?

2. When Ms. Lee comes back in 48 hours, her PPD is negative. The chest x-ray ordered by the healthcare provider shows dense lesions in the apical and posterior segments of the lung consistent with a diagnosis of tuberculosis. Sputum culture results have not returned yet. What does the nurse anticipate will be ordered for this patient?

3. If Ms. Lee is confirmed to have tuberculosis, what teaching will the nurse provide?

4. Ms. Lee's sputum culture returns positive for the presence of bacilli. Why did her PPD come back negative? Will her family in Vietnam need to be tested? How will that testing be arranged? Who else will need to be tested secondary to exposure to Ms. Lee?

›› Exemplar 9.H
Urinary Tract Infection

Exemplar Learning Outcomes

9.H Analyze urinary tract infection as it relates to infection.

- Describe the pathophysiology of urinary tract infections.
- Describe the etiology of urinary tract infections.
- Compare the risk factors and prevention of urinary tract infections.
- Identify the clinical manifestations of urinary tract infections.
- Summarize diagnostic tests and therapies used by interprofessional teams in the collaborative care of an individual with a urinary tract infection.
- Differentiate care of patients with urinary tract infection across the lifespan.
- Apply the nursing process in providing culturally competent care to an individual with a urinary tract infection.

Exemplar Key Terms

Catheter-associated urinary tract infection (CAUTI), *657*
Cystitis, *656*
Cystoscopy, *659*

Dysuria, *659*
Enuresis, *661*
Gram stain, *659*
Hematuria, *659*
Hydronephrosis, *657*
Intravenous pyelography (IVP), *659*
Neurogenic bladder, *657*
Nocturia, *659*
Persistent bacteriuria, *664*
Pyelonephritis, *656*
Pyuria, *659*
Reflux, *656*
Reinfection, *664*
Unresolved bacteriuria, *664*
Ureteral stent, *660*
Ureteroplasty, *660*
Urgency, *659*
Urinary drainage system, *656*
Urinary tract infection (UTI), *656*
Vesicoureteral reflux, *656*
Voiding cystourethrography, *659*

Overview

The urinary tract includes the kidneys, ureters, urinary bladder, and urethra. Any part of this system can be affected by pathogens. A severe **urinary tract infection (UTI)** may involve multiple components of the urinary tract. Kidney infections can affect urine production and waste elimination and result in renal failure (explained in the module on Fluids and Electrolytes). Infection can interrupt the **urinary drainage system** (the organs required to drain urine from the kidneys, including the ureters, urinary bladder, and urethra), obstructing urine flow and affecting elimination.

- When caring for patients with UTIs, the nurse must consider the patient's modesty in voiding, possible difficulty in discussing the genitals, potential embarrassment about being exposed for examination and testing, and fear of changes in body function. These psychosocial issues can interfere with the patient's willingness to seek help, discuss treatment, and learn about preventive measures.

- Nursing interventions for patients with UTIs are directed toward primary prevention, early detection, and management of the disorder through health teaching and nursing care.

- Bacterial infections of the urinary tract are a common reason for seeking health services, second only to upper respiratory infections. More than 8 million people are treated annually for UTI (Porth & Grossman, 2014). Community-associated UTIs are common in young women but unusual in men under the age of 50.

- Most community-acquired UTIs are caused by *Escherichia coli*, a common gram-negative enteral bacterium. Approximately 5–15% of symptomatic UTIs are caused by *Staphylococcus saprophyticus*, a gram-positive organism. Catheter-associated UTIs often involve other gram-negative bacteria, such as *Proteus*, *Klebsiella*, *Serratia*, and *Pseudomonas*.

Pathophysiology and Etiology

Pathophysiology

The urinary tract is normally sterile above the urethra. Adequate urine volume, a free flow from the kidneys through the urinary meatus, and complete bladder emptying are the most important mechanisms of maintaining sterility. Pathogens that enter and contaminate the distal urethra are washed out during voiding. Other defenses for maintaining sterile urine include the normal acidity of urine itself and the bacteriostatic properties of the bladder and urethral cells.

The peristaltic activity of the ureters and a competent vesicoureteral junction help to maintain sterility of the upper urinary tract. As the ureter enters the bladder, the distal portion tunnels between the mucosa and muscle layers of the bladder wall (**Figure 9–28 》**). During voiding, increased intravesicular (within the bladder) pressure compresses the ureter, preventing **reflux**, the backflow of urine toward the kidneys. In men, a long urethra and the antibacterial effect of zinc in prostatic fluid also help prevent contamination of this normally sterile environment.

UTIs can be bacterial, viral, or fungal and may be categorized in several ways. Anatomically, UTIs may affect the lower or the upper urinary tract. Infections of the lower

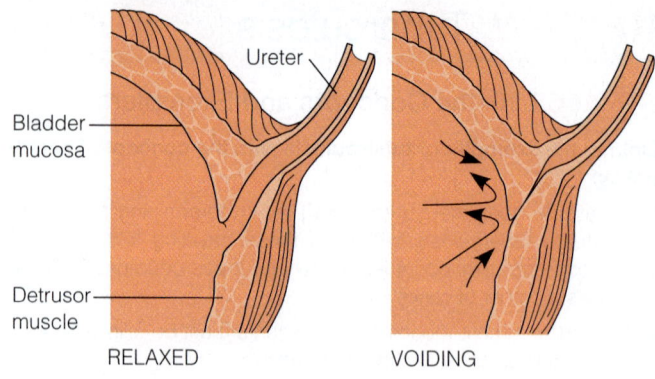

Figure 9–28 》 A competent vesicoureteral junction. Note how increased intravesicular pressure during voiding occludes the distal portion of the ureter, preventing reflux.

urinary tract include *urethritis*, inflammation of the urethra; *prostatitis*, inflammation of the prostate gland; and **cystitis**, inflammation of the urinary bladder. The most common upper UTI is pyelonephritis, inflammation of the kidney and renal pelvis. The infection can involve superficial tissues, such as the bladder mucosa, or invade other tissues, such as prostate or renal tissues.

Epidemiologically, UTIs are identified as community acquired or healthcare associated (often related to catheterization). UTIs can be further categorized as acute or chronic, the latter being either recurrent or persistent.

Cystitis is the most common UTI. This infection tends to remain superficial, involving the bladder mucosa. The mucosa becomes hyperemic (red) and may hemorrhage. The inflammatory response causes pus to form, a process that causes the classic manifestations associated with cystitis.

Pyelonephritis is inflammation of the renal pelvis and parenchyma, the functional kidney tissue. *Acute pyelonephritis* is a bacterial infection of the kidney, and *chronic pyelonephritis* is associated with nonbacterial infections and inflammatory processes that can be metabolic, chemical, or immunologic in origin (see the module on Inflammation).

Acute pyelonephritis usually results from an infection that ascends to the kidney from the lower urinary tract. Asymptomatic bacteriuria or cystitis can lead to acute pyelonephritis. Risk factors include pregnancy (due to slowed ureteral peristalsis), urinary tract obstruction, and congenital malformation. Urinary tract trauma, scarring, calculi (stones), kidney disorders such as polycystic or hypertensive kidney disease, and chronic diseases such as diabetes can also contribute to pyelonephritis. **Vesicoureteral reflux**, a condition in which urine moves from the bladder back toward the kidney, is a common risk factor in children who develop pyelonephritis and is also seen in adults when bladder outflow is obstructed.

The infection spreads from the renal pelvis to the renal cortex. The pelvis, calyces, and medulla of the kidney are primarily affected, with WBC infiltration and inflammation. The kidney becomes grossly edematous. Localized abscesses may develop on the cortical surface of the kidney. As with cystitis, *E. coli* is the organism responsible for 85% of the cases of acute pyelonephritis. Other organisms commonly found include *Proteus* and *Klebsiella*, bacteria that normally inhabit the intestinal tract.

The onset of acute pyelonephritis is typically rapid, with chills and fever, malaise, vomiting, flank pain, costovertebral tenderness, and urinary frequency. Symptoms of cystitis also may be present. The older adult may present with a change in behavior, acute confusion, incontinence, or a general deterioration in condition.

Etiology

UTIs are the second most common infections in children, after otitis media. An estimated 8% of girls and 2% of boys have a UTI by age 7 (Fisher & Steele, 2015). Most UTIs among newborns and young infants occur in boys, as obstructive structural defects that predispose infants to infection have a higher incidence in boys. The incidence of UTIs in older infants and children is higher in girls because the shorter female urethra (2 cm [1 in.] in young girls) has closer proximity to the anus and vagina, increasing the risk of contamination by fecal bacteria.

Pathogens usually enter the urinary tract by ascending from the mucous membranes of the perineal area into the lower urinary tract. Bacteria that have colonized the urethra, vagina, or perineal tissues are the usual source of infection (Porth & Grossman, 2014). From the bladder, bacteria can continue to ascend the urinary tract, eventually infecting the *parenchyma* (functional tissue) of the kidneys (Longo et al., 2012). Hematogenous spread of infection to the urinary tract is rare; infections introduced in this manner are usually associated with previous damage or scarring of the urinary tract. Bacteria introduced into the urinary tract can cause asymptomatic bacteriuria or an inflammatory response with manifestations of UTI.

At least 10–15% of hospitalized patients with indwelling urinary catheters develop bacteriuria. The longer the catheter remains in place, the greater the risk for infection. Bacteria, including *E. coli*, *Proteus*, *Pseudomonas*, and *Klebsiella*, reach the bladder either by migrating through the column of urine within the catheter or by moving up the mucous sheath of the urethra outside the catheter (Longo et al., 2012). **Catheter-associated urinary tract infection (CAUTI)** has become a major healthcare concern and is one of the major HAIs (Panchisin, 2016). Bacteria enter the catheter system at the connection between the catheter and the drainage system or through the emptying tube of the drainage bag. Colonization of perineal skin by bowel flora is a common source of infection in catheterized women. Because the Centers for Medicare and Medicaid Services is no longer reimbursing for CAUTIs, healthcare institutions are highly motivated to decrease CAUTI rates nationally.

Prevention of CAUTIs includes several decision-making and care guidelines criteria (Panchisin, 2016):

- Criteria for insertion
- Urinary retention and bladder emptying
- Consideration of alternatives to a urinary catheter
- Patient preparation and following CDC hygiene guidelines
- Best practice for maintenance, including timely removal, care and maintenance, and hygiene.

Another cause of UTI is vesicoureteral reflux (VUR), the backflow of urine from the bladder into the ureters during voiding. Bacteria in the urine swept up to the kidneys cause pyelonephritis. Vesicoureteral reflux also prevents complete emptying of the bladder, and because urine returns to the bladder, it creates a reservoir for bacterial growth (Mortazavi & Ghojazadeh, 2014). Vesicoureteral reflux can also result from a structural anomaly in which the ureters insert into the bladder in an abnormal position.

Renal scarring can result from **hydronephrosis** (accumulation of urine in the renal pelvis as a result of obstructed outflow) or pyelonephritis, due to the inflammatory and ischemic effects of the infection. Scars have been associated with hypertension, proteinuria, and kidney failure. The risk of kidney damage increases in the following cases:

- UTI in an infant less than 1 year of age
- Delay in diagnosis and effective antibacterial treatment for an upper UTI
- Anatomical obstruction or nerve supply interruption
- Recurrent episodes of upper UTIs.

Risk Factors

A variety of factors can predispose patients to UTI. Some risk factors cannot be changed (e.g., aging and a woman's short urethra). Cystitis occurs most frequently in adult women, usually because of colonization of the bladder by bacteria that are normally found in the lower gastrointestinal tract. These bacteria gain entry by ascending the short, straight female urethra. Wiping from back to front after urination can transfer bacteria from the anorectal area to the urethra.

Urinary stasis increases the risk of UTI. Stasis may be caused by abnormal anatomical structures or abnormal function (e.g., a **neurogenic bladder**, in which an interrupted nerve supply from meningomyelocele or a spinal cord trauma impairs the bladder voiding function and leads to incomplete bladder emptying). Children typically void five to six times a day. Infrequent voiding, which is common in school-age children, results in incomplete emptying of the bladder and urinary stasis. Voluntarily suppressing the desire to urinate is a predisposing factor, as retention overdistends the bladder and can lead to an infection.

Congenital and acquired factors that contribute to the risk of infection include urinary tract obstruction by tumors or calculi; benign prostatic hyperplasia, structural abnormalities such as strictures, impaired bladder innervation, bowel incontinence, or constipation; and chronic diseases such as diabetes mellitus. Instrumentation of the urinary tract (e.g., catheterization, cystoscopy) is a major risk factor for UTI. Even when performed under strict aseptic conditions, catheterization can result in bladder infection. Research indicates that the risk for CAUTI is reduced when anesthetic lubricating gels are inserted into the urethra prior to catheter insertion (Fisher & Steele, 2015). The placement of the catheter prevents the flushing action of voiding, and bacteria can ascend to the bladder through the catheter lumen or via exudate between the urethral mucosa and the catheter.

In women, including adolescents, sexual activity (e.g., intercourse, abuse, masturbation) increases the risk for UTI, because bacteria can be introduced into the bladder via the urethra during sexual intercourse. Use of spermicidal compounds with a diaphragm, cervical cap, or condom alters the normal bacterial flora of the vagina and perineal tissues, further increasing the risk for UTI. Diaphragms are not recommended for women with a history of UTIs because pressure from the diaphragm on the urethra can interfere with complete bladder emptying and lead to recurrent UTIs.

Some women lack a normally protective mucosal enzyme, and the resulting decreased levels of cervicovaginal antibodies to enterobacteria further increase their risk. Personal hygiene practices and voluntary urinary retention can contribute to the risk for UTI in women. Up to three UTIs annually are considered within normal limits for sexually active women and do not usually warrant additional diagnostic tests beyond urine culture. A woman who has had a UTI is susceptible to recurrent infection. If a pregnant woman develops an acute UTI, especially with a high temperature, amniotic fluid infection can develop and retard the growth of the placenta.

Asymptomatic bacteriuria (ASB; bacteria in the urine that actively multiply without accompanying clinical symptoms) is a condition that becomes significant if a woman is pregnant, because up to 40% of pregnant women with untreated ASB develop a kidney infection (MedlinePlus, 2012). ASB is almost always caused by a single organism, typically *E. coli.* If more than one type of bacteria is cultured, the possibility of urine-culture contamination must be considered.

Prostatic hypertrophy and bacterial prostatitis are risk factors among men. Circumcision appears to have a protective effect. Anal intercourse is also a risk factor for men. In healthy adult men, UTIs are unusual and may prompt additional diagnostic testing.

Prevention

The primary prevention of UTI is practice of good personal hygiene. See the Patient Teaching feature to learn important ways in which nurses can teach patients to prevent UTIs. Some healthcare providers may recommend prophylactic antibiotic treatment for patients with recurrent UTIs or with asymptomatic bacteriuria (see the Evidence-Based Practice feature).

Clinical Manifestations

The symptoms of UTI depend on the infection's location as well as the patient's age. Symptoms in a newborn tend to be nonspecific: unexplained fever, failure to thrive, poor feeding,

Patient Teaching
Prevention of Urinary Tract Infection

Patient teaching is a vital aspect of preventing primary and recurrent UTIs. Nurses should do the following:

- Encourage patients to maintain a generous fluid intake of 2.0–2.5 liters per day, increasing intake during hot weather and strenuous activity, as this helps clear bacteria from the urinary system.
- Discuss the need to avoid voluntary urinary retention by emptying the bladder every 3–4 hours.
- Instruct women to cleanse the perineal area from front to back after voiding and defecating, to prevent the transfer of gastrointestinal bacteria to the urethra.
- Teach patients to void and wash the perineal area before and after sexual intercourse to flush out bacteria introduced into the urethra and bladder.
- Teach measures to maintain the integrity of perineal tissues, such as avoiding bubble baths, feminine hygiene sprays, and vaginal douches, and wearing cotton briefs rather than underwear made from synthetic materials.
- Unless contraindicated, suggest the following measures to maintain acid urine: Drink two glasses of low-sugar cranberry juice daily; take ascorbic acid (vitamin C); and avoid excess intake of milk and milk products, other fruit juices, and sodium bicarbonate (baking soda).

vomiting and diarrhea, strong-smelling urine, and irritability. Any child younger than age 2 years with a fever of unknown origin should be tested for a UTI. The more "classic" symptoms of lower UTI, as shown in the following Clinical Manifestations and Therapies feature, are not seen until the toddler years. Approximately 40% of UTIs are asymptomatic.

Evidence-Based Practice
Vesicoureteral Reflux and Prophylactic Antibiotics

Problem

The presence of VUR, the backflow of urine from the bladder to the upper urinary tract, is a risk factor for the development of UTIs. Multiple studies indicate that 18–35% of children with a UTI also have VUR (Fisher & Steele, 2015).

Evidence

The standard of practice for many years has been to treat children with VUR with prophylactic antibiotics to prevent development of a UTI. Some studies support this practice, antibiotic prophylaxis being associated with lower UTI occurrence in girls with dilating VUR (Mortazavi & Ghojazadeh, 2014). However, other studies indicate that the risk of developing recurrent UTI is not significantly different between children with VUR who received prophylactic antimicrobial therapy and those who did not. In addition, children who received antimicrobial prophylaxis were more likely to develop antimicrobial-resistant UTIs (Fisher & Steele, 2015). Children with VUR on observation therapy were more likely to develop a UTI if they presented with more than one febrile UTI or were older at VUR diagnosis or prophylactic withdrawal (Drzewiecki et al., 2012).

Implications

Children with VUR are at increased risk for developing UTIs; however, prophylactic antibiotic treatment may cause more burden than benefit in some children. Prophylaxis is not consistently associated with a decreased risk of recurrent infection, but it increases the risk of developing resistant infections. Nurses need to conduct a thorough patient history of previous UTIs, age of VUR diagnosis, bowel and bladder dysfunction, and bowel and bladder control (i.e., toilet training). Some patients, such as patients with multiple previous UTIs or older age when VUR was diagnosed, may benefit from prophylactic therapy more than will younger patients with no history of recurrent UTI.

Critical Thinking Application

1. What symptoms would you teach parents to watch for and report if their child with VUR is on observation therapy?

2. On the basis of evidence presented here and in additional studies, what characteristics of a child with VUR would prompt you to recommend that that child be placed on prophylactic antibiotics?

3. Develop a nursing care plan for a 15-month-old child with VUR and one previous UTI.

Clinical Manifestations and Therapies
Urinary Tract Infection

ETIOLOGY	CLINICAL MANIFESTATIONS	CLINICAL THERAPIES
Lower UTI: cystitis	■ Frequency, dysuria, urgency, enuresis, strong-smelling urine, cloudy urine, hematuria, abdominal or suprapubic pain	■ Administer a 5- to 7-day course of trimethoprim or sulfamethoxazole or antibiotic matching the organism sensitivity; encourage oral fluids; administer analgesic such as acetaminophen or phenazopyridine.
Upper UTI: pyelonephritis	■ High fever, chills, abdominal pain, flank pain, costovertebral angle tenderness, persistent vomiting, moderate to severe dehydration ■ Infants may have nonspecific signs such as poor appetite, failure to thrive, lethargy, and irritability. ■ Older children may have signs of cystitis.	■ Administer antipyretics and IV antibiotics initially; then, transition to oral antibiotics matching the organism sensitivity for a total of 7–10 days. ■ Rehydration is essential.

Typical presenting symptoms of cystitis include **dysuria** (painful or difficult urination), urinary frequency and **urgency** (a sudden, compelling need to urinate), and **nocturia** (voiding two or more times at night). In addition, the urine may have a foul odor and appear cloudy (**pyuria**) or bloody (**hematuria**) because of mucus, excess white cells in the urine, and bleeding of the inflamed bladder wall. Suprapubic pain and tenderness also may be present. Cystitis is usually uncomplicated and readily responds to treatment. When left untreated, the infection can ascend to involve the kidneys. Severe or prolonged infection can lead to sloughing of bladder mucosa and ulcer formation. Chronic cystitis can lead to bladder stones.

Collaboration

Collaborative treatment of UTI focuses on eliminating the causative organism, preventing relapse or reinfection, and identifying and correcting any contributing factors. Drug treatment with antibiotics and urinary anti-infectives is common. In some cases, surgery may be indicated to correct contributing factors.

Diagnostic Tests

- Urinalysis assesses for pyuria, bacteria, and blood cells in the urine. A bacteria count greater than 100,000 (1.0×10^5) per milliliter indicates infection. Rapid tests for bacteria in the urine include using a *nitrite dipstick* (which turns pink in the presence of bacteria) and the *leukocyte esterase test*, an indirect method of detecting bacteria by identifying lysed or intact WBCs in the urine.

- Urine should be obtained as a midstream clean-catch specimen; if necessary, use straight catheterization or "mini-cath," with strict aseptic technique. Avoid catheterization if possible to reduce the risk of further infection. Urine from urine collection bags may be used to screen for UTIs in infants, but it cannot be used to confirm a UTI and should not be used for most patients because the specimen collection procedure is not sterile.

SAFETY ALERT Cleansing with nonsterile gauze moistened with tap water and mild soap is as effective as using a prepackaged sterile towelette and is gentler on the mucous membranes.

- **Gram stain** of the urine may be done to identify the infecting organism by shape and characteristic (gram-positive or gram-negative).

- Urine culture and sensitivity tests may be ordered to identify the infecting organism and the most effective antibiotic. Urine specimens collected for culture must be delivered to the laboratory within 1 hour, or the specimen must be refrigerated to prevent the growth of organisms that occur with prolonged room temperature exposure. Culture requires 24–72 hours, so treatment to eliminate the most common organisms often is initiated without culture. Urine cultures do not distinguish between upper and lower UTIs.

- WBC count with differential may be done to detect the typical changes associated with infection, such as leukocytosis (elevated WBC) and increased numbers of neutrophils.

In patients with recurrent infections or persistent bacteriuria, additional diagnostic testing may be ordered to evaluate for structural abnormalities, renal scarring, and other contributing factors. These tests include the following:

- **Intravenous pyelography (IVP)**, also known as *excretory urography*, is used to evaluate the structure and excretory function of the kidneys, ureters, and bladder. As the kidneys clear an intravenously injected contrast medium from the blood, the size and shape of the kidneys, their calyces and pelves, the ureters, and the bladder can be evaluated, and structural or functional abnormalities, such as vesicoureteral reflux, can be detected.

- **Voiding cystourethrography** involves instilling contrast medium into the bladder and then using x-rays to assess the bladder and urethra when filled and during voiding. This study can detect structural and functional abnormalities of the bladder and urethral strictures. This test has a lower risk of allergic response to the contrast dye than IVP.

- **Cystoscopy** (direct visualization of the urethra and a bladder through a cystoscope) can be used to diagnose conditions such as prostatic hypertrophy, urethral strictures, bladder calculi, tumors, polyps, diverticula, and congenital abnormalities. A tissue biopsy may be obtained during the procedure, and other interventions may be performed (e.g., stone removal or stricture dilation).

■ *Manual pelvic or prostate examinations* assess for structural changes of the genitourinary tract, such as prostatic enlargement, cystocele, or rectocele.

■ *Renal and bladder ultrasound and DMSA scintigraphy* are used to detect pyelonephritis and renal scarring (National Kidney and Urological Diseases Information Clearinghouse, 2012).

Surgery

Surgery may be indicated for recurrent UTI if diagnostic testing indicates calculi, structural anomalies, or strictures that contribute to the risk of infection. Stones, or *calculi*, in the renal pelvis or bladder are an irritant and provide a matrix for bacterial colonization. Treatment may include surgical removal of a large calculus from the renal pelvis or cystoscopic removal of bladder calculi. *Percutaneous ultrasonic pyelolithotomy* or *extracorporeal shock wave lithotripsy* (see the exemplar on Urinary Calculi in the module on Elimination) may be used instead of surgery to crush and remove stones.

Ureteroplasty, the surgical repair of a ureter, may be indicated for structural abnormality or stricture of a ureter. This may be combined with a ureteral reimplantation if vesicoureteral reflux is present. The patient returns from these surgeries with an indwelling urinary catheter (Foley or suprapubic) and a **ureteral stent** (a thin catheter inserted into the ureter to provide for urine flow and ureteral support), which remain in place for 3–5 days. **Box 9–7** >> describes nursing care of the patient with a ureteral stent in place.

Follow-up urine cultures should be obtained according to the frequency specified by agency guidelines. Patients with pyelonephritis may have to repeat urine cultures monthly for 3 months, every 3 months for 6 months, and then annually. Most reinfections occur within 1 year, and subsequent infections may be asymptomatic. Children with renal scarring should have their blood pressure monitored.

Pharmacologic Therapy

Most uncomplicated infections of the lower urinary tract can be treated with a short course of antibiotic therapy. Upper UTIs, in contrast, usually require longer treatment (2 or more weeks) to eradicate the infecting organism. Treatment should be initiated as soon as the UTI is diagnosed.

Antibiotics are selected based on the age of the patient, the sensitivity of the cultured organism, renal function, and the patient's signs and symptoms. Gender is a consideration in treatment choices, because men require longer periods of treatment than women. The longer urethra in men makes it

Box 9–7
Ureteral Stent

Ureteral stents are used to maintain patency and promote healing of the ureters (see **Figure 9–29** >>). A stent may be temporary, used during and after a surgical procedure, or it may be used for longer periods in patients with ureteral obstruction due to tumors, strictures, or other causes.

Stents may be positioned during surgery or cystoscopy. They are made of a nontoxic material such as silicone or polyurethane, with side drainage holes placed along the length of the stent. Stents are radiopaque for easy radiographic identification. One or both ends of the stent may be pigtail or J shaped to prevent migration.

In caring for a patient with a ureteral stent, the nurse should do the following:

■ Label all drainage tubes, including stents, for easy identification. Attach each catheter and stent to a separate closed drainage system. Careful labeling allows close monitoring of output from all sources and reservoirs. Separate drainage systems minimize the risk of infection.

■ If the stent has been brought to the surface, secure it and maintain its position. The stent is usually placed in the renal pelvis. Secure it well to prevent trauma to the kidney, inadvertent removal of the stent, and ureter obstruction.

■ Monitor urine output, including color, consistency, and odor. Monitor for signs of infection or bleeding, including fever, tachycardia, pain, hematuria, and cloudy or malodorous urine. The stent facilitates urine flow but can become obstructed by bleeding, calculi, or sediment. Obstruction can result in hydronephrosis and kidney damage. The stent itself is a foreign body in the urinary tract and can increase the risk of UTI.

■ Maintain fluid intake, encouraging fluids that acidify urine, such as low-sugar apple, cranberry, and blueberry juice. The stent can precipitate calculus formation as well as UTI.

Increasing fluid intake and acidifying the urine help prevent these complications.

■ For an indwelling stent, stress the need for regular follow-up to monitor for and prevent complications such as UTI and calculi. The patient with an indwelling stent may tend to forget that the stent is in place and become noncompliant with follow-up and preventive measures.

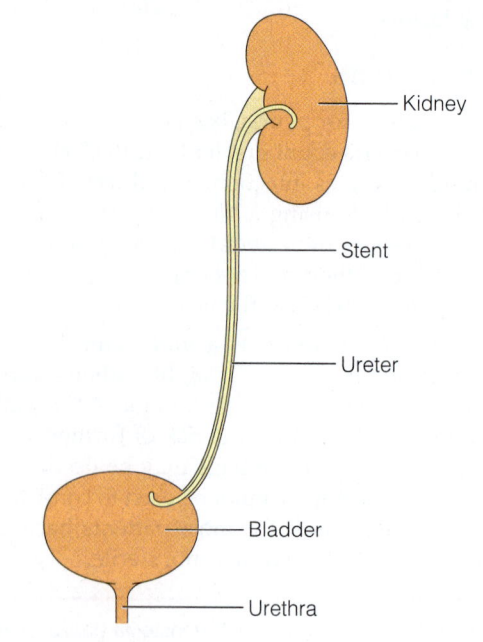

Figure 9–29 >> A ureteral stent.

less likely that bacteria can ascend into the bladder. However, when bacteria do reach the older man's bladder, the infection is considered complicated and requires a longer course of treatment. The antibiotic is changed if necessary after culture sensitivity is determined.

Follow-up cultures may be obtained 48–72 hours after drug therapy is started in the pediatric patient who is still febrile (Fisher & Steele, 2015). Children with pyelonephritis should be maintained on antibiotic prophylaxis until radiologic tests are performed to detect any structural defects.

Short-course therapy (either a single antibiotic dose or a 3-day course of treatment) reduces treatment cost, increases compliance, and has a lower rate of side effects. Single-dose therapy is associated with a higher rate of recurrent infection and continued vaginal colonization with *E. coli*, making a 3-day course of treatment the preferred option for uncomplicated cystitis. Oral trimethoprim-sulfamethoxazole (TMP-SMZ), TMP, or a quinolone antibiotic such as ciprofloxacin (Cipro) or enoxacin (Penetrex) may be ordered.

Men and women with pyelonephritis, urinary tract abnormalities or stones, or a history of previous infections with antibiotic-resistant infections require a 7- to 10-day course of TMP-SMZ, ciprofloxacin, ofloxacin (Floxin), or an alternative antibiotic. Patients with severe illness may need hospitalization. IV ciprofloxacin, gentamicin, ceftriaxone (Rocephin), or ampicillin may be prescribed for severe illness or sepsis associated with UTI.

Patients who experience frequent symptomatic UTIs may be treated with prophylactic antibiotic therapy. Drugs such as TMP-SMZ, TMP, and nitrofurantoin (Furadantin, Macrodantin, Macrobid) do not achieve effective plasma concentrations at recommended doses but do reach effective concentrations in the urine. Nitrofurantoin also may be used to treat UTI in pregnant women.

Antibiotics and urinary anti-infectives generally are not recommended to treat asymptomatic bacteriuria in patients who are catheterized. The preferred treatment for catheter-associated UTI is removal of the indwelling catheter, followed by a 10- to 14-day course of antibiotic therapy to eliminate the infection.

Nonpharmacologic Therapy

Nonpharmacologic therapies can be helpful in treating and preventing UTI. Drinking adequate fluids will increase urination and flush bacteria out of the urinary system. Drinking low-sugar cranberry juice in particular is recommended to help fight UTIs. However, fluids that may irritate the bladder, including caffeinated beverages, alcohol, and soft drinks with citrus juices, should be avoided.

Complementary Health Approaches

Complementary health approaches, such as aromatherapy or herbal preparations, may be used in conjunction with antibiotics to treat UTIs. Adding bergamot, sandalwood, lavender, or juniper oil to bath water may help relieve the discomfort of a UTI. Herbal supplements such as saw palmetto have a urinary antiseptic effect and may be beneficial in treating or preventing UTIs. The nurse should advise the patient to consult a qualified herbologist for recommended doses and appropriate use. Some aromatherapy and herbal preparations are contraindicated in patients with allergies; those patients should check with their allergist before participating in these types of therapies.

Lifespan Considerations

UTIs in Infants and Children

UTI in the newborn, which may occur as a result of exposure of the urethra to bacteria in the feces in the diaper, predisposes the neonate to hyperbilirubinemia (elevated serum bilirubin) and bacteremia.

Nursing assessment for a child with a suspected UTI involves assessing the infant or child for signs of acute or chronic illness, examining the genitourinary system, and collecting a urine specimen for culture. Assess the infant for toxic (very ill) appearance, fever, and oral fluid intake. Evaluate the child's oral fluid intake. Assess for quality, quantity, and frequency of voiding. Measure the child's height and weight, and plot the data on a growth curve to identify any change in growth pattern associated with a chronic illness. Take the infant's or child's blood pressure. Palpate the abdomen and suprapubic and costovertebral areas for masses, tenderness, and distention.

Children who appear ill and cannot tolerate oral antibiotics are often hospitalized because they need rehydration and parenteral antibiotic treatment until they have been afebrile for 24 hours (CDC, 2015d). Infants can develop permanent kidney damage or generalized sepsis if the UTI is not treated aggressively. If a structural defect is identified, surgical correction may be necessary to prevent recurrent infections that could lead to renal damage.

Because bladder training is such an important milestone for young children, any disorder that affects voiding can have developmental implications. A toddler who has been toilet trained may regress and require diapers temporarily because of incontinence related to the UTI. An older child may develop **enuresis** (the involuntary passage of urine after control has been established) after a prolonged period of being dry at night. A preschooler may perceive the infection as punishment for an imagined wrong, such as masturbation. Reassure parents that this temporary period of urinary incontinence is normal when associated with UTI, and emphasize that they should offer the child support rather than disapproval.

UTIs in Adolescents

Sexually active adolescents may deny having symptoms for fear of disclosing their sexual activity to their parents. Careful questioning may be necessary to elicit a response despite these concerns. The nurse should be open and approachable and give the patient and the family the chance to address their concerns.

UTIs in Pregnant Women

The risk for UTI increases during pregnancy, particularly during the second trimester, secondary to the pressure of the fetus, which causes urinary stasis and incomplete bladder emptying. The diagnosis of UTI in the pregnant woman carries significant risks for the mother and fetus. UTIs are associated with an increased risk of preeclampsia (Shoff, 2014). An increased risk of premature birth and intrauterine growth restriction is associated with acute pyelonephritis, which is often caused by ASB. Although the exact cause is unknown, an increased risk of premature rupture of membranes is associated with UTI. If urine stasis exists, the risk of UTI increases because of bacteriuria and the presence of dilated ureters and renal pelves, which persist for about 6 weeks after delivery.

The postpartal woman is at increased risk of developing urinary tract problems caused by the normal postpartal diuresis, increased bladder capacity, and decreased bladder sensitivity from stretching or trauma. Possible inhibited neural control of the bladder following the use of general or regional anesthesia and contamination from catheterization also puts the postpartal woman at risk for UTIs. These factors make it essential that the mother empty her bladder completely with each voiding.

UTIs in Older Adults

Older adults have an increased incidence of UTI. The greatest increase is seen in men, as the ratio of female-to-male UTI in older adults changes from 50:1 to less than 5:1. Although the bacteriostatic effect of prostatic fluid and a longer urethra provide an effective barrier to bladder infection for adult men, the hypertrophy of the prostate that is commonly associated with aging increases the risk of cystitis in older men. An enlarged prostate can impede urine flow and lead to incomplete bladder emptying and urinary stasis. Because bacteria are not completely flushed with voiding, colonization of the bladder may occur. An increased risk of urinary stasis, chronic disease states (e.g., diabetes mellitus), and an impaired immune response also contribute to the higher incidence of UTI in older adults. In older women, loss of tissue elasticity and weakening of perineal muscles often contribute to the development of a cystocele or rectocele. Resulting changes in bladder and urethral position increase the risk of incomplete bladder emptying.

UTI is one of the top two infections in patients in long-term care facilities and is common in both community-dwelling and facility-dwelling older adults. Older adults may not experience the classic symptoms of cystitis. Instead, they often present with nonspecific manifestations, such as nocturia, incontinence, confusion, behavior change, lethargy, loss of appetite, or "just not feeling right." Fever may be present; however, hypothermia also may develop in an older adult. Particularly in a long-term care setting, a change in behavior may be the only indicator of a UTI (Shlamovitz & Kim, 2013). The frustrated family members and healthcare team may easily suspect any number of other possible causes when an older adult presents with these symptoms.

The symptoms usually seen in younger adults with UTIs—urgency and frequency—are common age-related changes in the older adult and therefore lack diagnostic usefulness. However, if an older adult has not previously experienced urinary urgency and presents with a shortened period of time between the urge to void and actual urination or urinary frequency of more than seven voids per 24-hour period, these symptoms should be thoroughly investigated.

Studies have suggested that adults without catheters in long-term care facilities have a prevalence of 25–50% for asymptomatic bacteriuria (Toward Optimized Practice, 2015), which may also be called *asymptomatic UTI* by some clinicians and researchers. Asymptomatic UTI does not require treatment. In fact, treatment does not improve the morbidity or mortality in affected older adults (Toward Optimized Practice, 2015; Shlamovitz & Kim, 2013). Routine urinalysis for older adults without symptoms is neither appropriate nor cost effective.

Catheter-associated UTIs often are asymptomatic. Gram-negative bacteremia is the most significant complication associated with these UTIs. Most catheter-associated UTIs resolve quickly when the catheter is removed and a short course of antibiotic is administered. Intermittent catheterization carries a lower risk of infection than does an indwelling catheter and is preferred for patients who are unable to empty their bladder by voiding. UTIs in catheterized older adults tend to be polymicrobial and difficult to eradicate. Before an indwelling catheter is used, the potential benefits to the older adult must be carefully weighed against the serious risks posed.

NURSING PROCESS

The nursing process for UTI generally focuses on returning the patient to maximum health. To maintain optimum urinary health, nurses should be alert for opportunities to provide health promotion, teaching measures to prevent UTI to all patients, particularly to young, sexually active women (see the Patient Teaching feature in the Prevention section).

Assessment

Focused assessment data for the patient with a suspected UTI includes the following:

- ***Observation and patient interview.*** Observe the skin color of the patient, and observe for any indication of discomfort. Note the color, clarity, and odor of urine. Interview the patient about current symptoms, including urination frequency and urgency, burning on urination, and the number of voidings per night. Ask the patient about other manifestations, such as lower abdominal, back, or flank pain, nausea or vomiting, or fever. Have the patient describe the duration of symptoms and any treatment attempted, as well as a history of previous UTIs and their frequency. With women of childbearing age (including adolescents), ask about the possibility of pregnancy and type of birth control used. Last, ask the patient about chronic diseases such as diabetes, current medications, and any known allergies.

- ***Physical examination.*** Examine the patient's general health and collect vital signs, including temperature. Examine the patient's abdominal shape, contour, and tenderness to palpation (especially suprapubic), and percuss for costovertebral tenderness.

Diagnosis

Nursing diagnoses for patients with UTIs focus on comfort, urinary elimination, and teaching/learning needs and may include the following:

- *Pain, Acute*
- *Urinary Elimination, Impaired*
- *Knowledge, Deficient*
- *Growth: Disproportionate, Risk for* (pediatric patients)
- *Urinary Retention*
- *Fluid Volume, Deficient, Risk for*
- *Fear.*

(NANDA-I © 2014)

Planning

In planning and implementing nursing care for the patient with a UTI, the patient's general health, abilities for self-care, and risk factors that may contribute to UTI are considered. Outcomes, developed in collaboration with the patient, may include the following:

- The patient will describe pain as a 3 or lower on a 0–10 scale.
- The patient will regain normal voiding pattern and will produce normal urine without blood, bacteria, or protein.
- The patient will verbalize understanding of the disease process, proper method of taking medications, and required follow-up care.
- The patient will describe strategies for reducing the risk of another UTI.
- The patient will increase fluid intake and number of voidings each day.
- The patient will complete the prescribed course of antibiotic therapy.
- The patient will experience no recurrent UTIs for 1 year.
- The patient will incorporate preventive self-care measures into the daily regimen.

Implementation

Nursing care for the hospitalized patient with a complicated UTI focuses on administering prescribed medications, promoting rehydration, assessing renal function, and teaching the patient and family how to minimize the risk of future infection.

Manage Pain

Pain is a common manifestation of both lower and upper UTIs. Urinary tract pain is caused primarily by distention and increased pressure within the urinary tract. The severity of the pain is related to the rate at which inflammation and distention develop, not their degree.

SAFETY ALERT The older adult with a UTI may not complain of dysuria. Be alert for other manifestations of UTI, such as incontinence or cloudy or malodorous urine. Inflammatory and immune responses tend to diminish with aging, so the irritative symptoms of UTI are reduced.

In cystitis, inflammation causes a sensation of fullness; dull, constant suprapubic pain; and possibly low back pain. The inflamed bladder wall and urethra cause dysuria, pain, and burning on urination. Bladder spasms may develop, causing periodic severe, stabbing discomfort. Pain associated with pyelonephritis is often steady and dull, localized to the outer abdomen or flank region. Urologic disorders rarely cause central abdominal pain.

Nursing interventions for the patient experiencing pain include the following:

- Assess pain: timing, quality, intensity, location, duration, and aggravating and alleviating factors. A change in the nature, location, or intensity of the pain may indicate an extension of the infection or a related but separate problem.
- Teach or provide comfort measures, such as warm sitz baths, warm packs or heating pads, and balanced rest and activity. Use systemic analgesics, urinary analgesics, or antispasmodic medication as ordered. Warmth relaxes muscles, relieves spasms, and increases local blood supply. Because pain can stimulate a stress response and delay healing, it should be relieved when possible.
- Increase fluid intake unless contraindicated. Increased fluid dilutes urine, reducing irritation of the inflamed bladder and urethral mucosa.
- Instruct the patient to notify the primary care provider if pain and discomfort continue or intensify after therapy is initiated. Pain and discomfort in voiding typically are relieved within 24 hours of initiating antibiotic therapy. Continued discomfort may indicate a complicated UTI or other urinary tract disorder.

Provide Patient Education

Because both upper and lower UTIs are usually managed in the community, teaching is the most important nursing intervention. Provide instruction on the following topics:

- Risk factors for UTI and how to minimize or eliminate these factors through increased fluid intake, regular elimination, and personal hygiene measures
- Early manifestations of UTI and the importance of seeking medical intervention promptly
- Maintaining optimal immune system function by attending to physical and psychosocial stressors, such as lack of adequate rest, poor nutrition, and high levels of emotional stress
- The importance of completing the prescribed treatment and keeping follow-up appointments
- Minimizing the risk of UTI when an indwelling urinary catheter is necessary:
  a. Use alternatives to an indwelling catheter when possible. For urinary incontinence, try scheduled toileting, incontinence pads or diapers, and external catheters if possible. For urinary retention, teach the patient or a family member to perform straight catheterization every 3–4 hours using clean technique.
  b. When an indwelling catheter is necessary, teach care measures such as perineal care, managing and emptying the collection chamber, maintaining a closed system, and bladder irrigation or flushing if ordered.

Facilitate Effective Urinary Elimination

Inflammation of the bladder and urethral mucosa affects the normal process and patterns of voiding, causing frequency, urgency, and burning on urination, as well as nocturia. Urine may be blood tinged, cloudy, and malodorous. The patient with short- or long-term urinary retention requires additional measures to assess for and prevent UTI.

SAFETY ALERT Nurses who work with patients in hospitals and other institutional settings should provide easy access to a bedpan, urinal, commode, or bathroom. Make sure that lighting is adequate and that pathways are free from obstacles for patients getting up to use the bathroom. Frequency, urgency, and nocturia increase the risk of urinary incontinence and injury due to falls, particularly in patients who are older or debilitated.

Nursing interventions for patients with impaired urinary elimination include the following:

- Monitor (or instruct the patient to monitor) color, clarity, and odor of urine. Urine should return to clear yellow within 48 hours, unless drug therapy causes a change in the color of urine. If clarity does not return, further investigation may be necessary.

- Instruct patients with impaired urinary elimination to avoid caffeinated drinks, including coffee, tea, and cola; citrus juices; drinks containing artificial sweeteners; and alcoholic beverages. Caffeine, citrus juices, and artificial sweeteners irritate bladder mucosa and the detrusor muscle and can increase urgency and bladder spasms.

- Use strict aseptic technique and a closed urinary drainage system when inserting a straight or indwelling urinary catheter. Insert indwelling catheters to the full recommended length (4 in. or more in women and to the bifurcation in men) before inflating the balloon. Bacteria colonizing the perineal tissues or on the nurse's hands can be introduced into the bladder during catheterization. Aseptic technique reduces this risk. Inflating the balloon while it is in the urethra damages urethral tissues and can cause the patient significant discomfort.

- When possible, use intermittent straight catheterization to relieve urinary retention. Using intermittent straight catheterization allows the bladder to fill and completely empty more normally, maintaining physiologic function. Remove indwelling urinary catheters as soon as possible. The risk of infection associated with an indwelling catheter is about 3–6% and increases cumulatively with each day (Shlamovitz & Kim, 2013).

- Maintain the closed urinary drainage system, and use aseptic technique when emptying the catheter drainage bag. Maintain gravity flow to prevent reflux of urine into the bladder from the drainage system. Bacteria can enter the drainage system when its integrity is interrupted (e.g., when the catheter is disconnected from the drainage system) or during emptying of the drainage bag. These bacteria can ascend the column of urine to the bladder, causing UTI.

- Provide perineal care regularly and following defecation. Use antiseptic preparations only as ordered. Regular cleansing of perineal tissues reduces the risk of colonization by bowel or other bacteria. Although antiseptic solutions may be ordered for catheter care, they can dry perineal tissues and reduce normal flora, increasing the risk of colonization by pathogens, and they should not be used routinely.

Promote Effective Health Maintenance

Because patients with UTIs are at increased risk for future UTIs, they need to understand the disease process, risk factors, measures to prevent recurrent infection, diagnostic procedures, and best practices for home care. In addition, patients need to understand that, even when the manifestations of UTI are relieved, the treatment plan needs to continue. Failure to complete the full course of therapy and recommended follow-up can lead to continued bacteriuria and recurrent infections. In addition to interventions already mentioned, nursing interventions to promote effective health maintenance include the following:

- Teach patients how to obtain a midstream clean-catch urine specimen. Cleansing of the urinary meatus and perineal area reduces contamination of the specimen by external cells and bacteria; 90% of urethral bacteria are cleared in the first 10 mL of voided urine, so a midstream specimen is representative of urine in the bladder.

- Help the patient develop a plan for taking medications, such as taking them with meals (unless contraindicated) or setting out all doses for the day in the morning. Missed doses of antibiotic can result in subtherapeutic blood levels and reduced effectiveness. Taking medication in association with a regular daily activity such as meals helps patients remember doses.

- Instruct patients to keep appointments for follow-up and urine culture. Follow-up urine culture, often scheduled 7–14 days after completion of antibiotic therapy, is vital to ensure complete eradication of bacteria and prevent relapse or recurrence.

- Teach measures to prevent future UTI, as discussed at the beginning of this exemplar. Keeping urine dilute and acidic and voiding regularly help to flush bacteria out of the bladder and urethra. The proximity of the female urethral meatus to the vagina and anus increases the risk of bacterial contamination, especially during intercourse. Bubble baths, feminine hygiene sprays, synthetic fibers, and douches can dry and irritate perineal tissues, promoting bacterial growth.

Evaluation

The outcome of treatment for UTI may be determined by follow-up urinalysis and culture. Cure, as evidenced by the absence of pathogens in the urine, is the desired outcome. When therapy fails to eradicate bacteria in the urine, the condition is known as **unresolved bacteriuria**. **Persistent bacteriuria**, or *relapse,* occurs when a persistent source of infection causes repeated infection after the initial cure. **Reinfection** is the development of a new infection with a different pathogen following successful UTI treatment (Papadakis & McPhee, 2013). Patients are generally required to submit a urinalysis for culture 7–10 days after completing a course of antibiotics to ensure that bacteria have been eliminated.

Nursing Care Plan

A Patient with Cystitis

Miija Waisanen is a 25-year-old second-year nursing student. She was recently married, and she and her husband live in an apartment near the college she attends. Ms. Waisanen has never been pregnant, and she is using a diaphragm for birth control. She presents at the local urgent care clinic complaining of low back pain, frequency and urgency of urination, and burning on urination, which began yesterday.

ASSESSMENT

Patrice Ramiros, a nurse practitioner, admits Ms. Waisanen to the clinic. Ms. Waisanen denies having had similar symptoms in the past or ever having been diagnosed with a UTI. She describes her pain as a constant, dull ache that does not change with movement. She feels the need to urinate almost constantly but experiences difficulty in starting her stream and feels burning pain and cramping when voiding. She reports getting up four times last night to urinate. She denies painful intercourse and states that her last menstrual period began only 2 weeks ago. Physical examination reveals pulse 90 beats/minute and regular and blood pressure 112/68 mmHg. She is afebrile. Suprapubic tenderness is noted, but there is no flank or costovertebral angle tenderness. Clean-catch urine specimen shows hematuria, multiple WBCs, and a bacteria count greater than 105 /mL.

Ms. Ramiros prescribes trimethoprim-sulfamethoxazole (TMP-SMZ) 160 mg/800 mg PO two times a day for 3 days, and acetaminophen two pills every 4 hours as needed for pain. Ms. Waisanen is instructed to return to the clinic in 7 days for a follow-up urine culture, or sooner if her symptoms do not improve.

DIAGNOSES

- *Pain* related to infection and inflammatory process in the urinary tract
- *Impaired Urinary Elimination* related to inflammation, as evidenced by frequency, urgency, nocturia, and dysuria
- *Deficient Knowledge* related to lack of information about risk factors for UTI

(NANDA-I © 2014)

PLANNING

- The patient will report relief of low back pain and burning on urination.
- The patient will report a normal voiding pattern without frequency, urgency, nocturia, and abnormal urine characteristics.
- The patient will verbalize understanding of the disease process, related risk factors, follow-up instructions, and symptoms of recurrence that indicate the need for medical attention.

IMPLEMENTATION

- Teach comfort measures: warm sitz baths, a heating pad on low heat applied to the lower back or abdomen, rest, increased fluid intake, avoiding caffeinated beverages, and taking aspirin or acetaminophen as ordered.
- Advise the patient to refrain from sexual intercourse until the infection and inflammation have cleared to avoid further irritation of inflamed tissues.
- Discuss the possible relationship between using a diaphragm for birth control and UTIs in women.
- Discuss dietary and hygiene practices to prevent UTI symptoms.
- Discuss symptoms indicating the need for further intervention and the risks of undertreatment.

EVALUATION

Six months later, Ms. Waisanen rotates through the urgent care clinic for her community-based nursing experience. When Ms. Ramiros asks how she is doing, Ms. Waisanen reports that her symptoms and urine cleared within about a day after she started the antibiotic, and she has had no further problems. She has seen her women's healthcare nurse practitioner to change her birth control to oral contraceptives, increased her intake of fluid and vitamin C, and no longer puts off urinating until she "has time to go."

CRITICAL THINKING

1. What physiologic and psychosocial factors put Ms. Waisanen at risk for UTI?
2. Compare the benefits and drawbacks to short-course therapy versus conventional therapy for UTI.
3. Why was it appropriate for the nurse practitioner to use short-course therapy with the advice to return if symptoms did not clear?
4. Develop a care plan for Ms. Waisanen for the nursing diagnosis *Ineffective Health Maintenance*.

REVIEW Urinary Tract Infection

RELATE Link the Concepts and Exemplars

Linking the exemplar of urinary tract infection with the concept of evidence-based practice:

1. If you were caring for a patient with bacteria in the urine who denied any symptoms or problems, how would you explain the decision not to treat this patient?

2. What would you tell the patient who adamantly demands a prescription for an antibiotic after being informed that taking an antibiotic is not in her best interest?

Linking the exemplar of urinary tract infection with the concept of mobility:

3. What factors put the 90-year-old patient in a wheelchair at risk for a UTI?

4. To reduce the risk of UTIs, what preventive measures will you implement for the older adult who is confined to bed?

READY Go to Volume 3: Clinical Nursing Skills

REFER Go to Pearson MyLab Nursing and eText

- Additional review materials

REFLECT Apply Your Knowledge

Ms. James, who was introduced in Exemplar 9.A on Cellulitis, wakes up one day and does not feel well. She is taken by ambulance to the neighborhood hospital, where a diagnosis of stroke is made. She has a feeding tube and indwelling catheter placed. She later develops a fever and confusion. The urine in the drainage bag is cloudy. A urine specimen is collected and sent to the laboratory for urinalysis and culture and sensitivity. Results confirm the diagnosis of UTI.

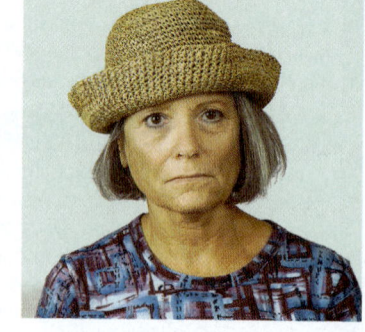

1. How will Ms. James's history of diabetes mellitus affect her risk for UTI and her response to treatment?

2. What risk factors does Ms. James have that place her at increased risk for UTI?

3. After Ms. James's indwelling catheter is removed and the UTI is treated with antibiotics for 7 days, urine culture reveals that bacteria remain in the urine. What does the nurse anticipate will be done next if the patient still experiences symptoms? How would the treatment differ if the patient did not have symptoms?

References

Acosta, C. D., Kurinczuk, J. J., Lucas, D. N., Tuffnell, D. J., Sellers, S., & Knight, M. (2014). *Severe maternal sepsis in the UK, 2011–2012: A national case-control study*. Retrieved from http://journals.plos.org/plosmedicine/article?id=10.1371%2Fjournal.pmed.1001672

Adams, M. P., Holland, L. N., & Urban, C. (2017). *Pharmacology for nurses: A pathophysiologic approach* (5th ed.). Hoboken, NJ: Pearson Education.

AHRQ. (2015). *AHRQ's healthcare-associated infections program*. Retrieved from http://www.ahrq.gov/professionals/quality-patient-safety/hais/index.html

American Academy of Pediatrics. (2016). *Recommendations for preventive pediatric health care*. Retrieved from https://www.aap.org/en-us/Documents/periodicity_schedule.pdf

American Association for Pediatric Ophthalmology and Strabismus. (2014). *Herpes eye disease*. Retrieved from http://www.aapos.org/terms/conditions/57

Anonymous. (2012). Heterogeneity exists in infectious disease prevalence rates in homeless people. *Infectious Disease News, 25*(9), 6. Retrieved from http://search.proquest.com.ezproxy.nu.edu/pqcentral/docview/1285165441/fulltextPDF/11081135AE74792PQ/5?accountid=25320

Arvanitis, M., Anagnostou, T., Kourkoumpetis, T. K., Ziakas, P. D., Desalermos, A., & Mylonakis, E. (2014). The impact of antimicrobial resistance and aging in VAP outcomes: Experience from a large tertiary care center. *PLoS One, 9*(2), e89984. doi:10.1371/journal.pone.008998

Ball, J. W., Bindler, R. C., Cowen, K., & Shaw, M. (2017). *Principles of pediatric nursing: Caring for children* (7th ed.). Hoboken, NJ: Pearson Education.

Barclay, L. (2013). Updated treatment guidelines for C difficile infection. *Medscape Drugs and Diseases*. Retrieved from http://www.medscape.org/viewarticle/813654

Barrett, R. (2012). A naturopathic treatment protocol for acute otitis media: A report of twenty-four cases. *BMC Complementary and Alternative Medicine, 12*(Suppl. 1), 12.

Barskey, A. E., Schulte, C., Rosen, J. B., Handschur, E. F., Rausch-Phung, E., Doll, M. K., … Gallagher, K. M. (2012). Mumps outbreak in Orthodox Jewish communities in the United States. *New England Journal of Medicine, 367*, 1704–1713. doi:10.1056/NEJMoa1202865

Benoit, S. R., Burkom, H., McIntyre, A. F., Kniss, K., Brammer, L., Finelli, L., & Jain, S. (2013). Pneumonia in US hospitalized patients with influenza-like illness: BioSense, 2007–2010. *Epidemiology of Infections, 141*, 805–815. doi:10.1017/S0950268812001549

Berman, A., Snyder, S. J., & Frandsen, G. (2016). Pain management. In *Kozier and Erb's fundamentals of nursing: Concepts, process, and practice* (10th ed.). Hoboken, NJ: Pearson Education.

Brown, A. (2013). The role of debridement in the healing process. *Nursing Times, 109*(40), 16–19. Retrieved from http://search.proquest.com.ezproxy.nu.edu/health/docview/1443920271/fulltextPDF/91AB0E006936432FPQ/5?accountid=25320

Bushnell, C. (2014). Study identifies risk factors for hospital readmissions. *American Journal of Medical Quality*. Retrieved from http://medicalxpress.com/news/2014-06-factors-hospital-readmissions.html

Centers for Disease Control and Prevention. (2012a). *Conjunctivitis (pink eye)*. Retrieved from http://www.cdc.gov/conjunctivitis/clinical.html

Centers for Disease Control and Prevention. (2012b). *Influenza antiviral medications: Summary for clinicians*. Retrieved from http://www.cdc.gov/flu/professionals/antivirals/summary-clinicians.htm

Centers for Disease Control and Prevention. (2012c). *Bloodborne infectious diseases: HIV/AIDS, hepatitis B, hepatitis C*. Retrieved from http://www.cdc.gov/niosh/topics/bbp/default.html

Centers for Disease Control and Prevention. (2012d). Notes from the field: Tuberculosis cluster associated with homelessness—Duval County, Florida, 2004–2012. *Morbidity and Mortality Weekly Report, 61*(28), 537–540.

Centers for Disease Control and Prevention. (2012e). *Rapid diagnostic testing for influenza*. Retrieved from http://www.cdc.gov/flu/professionals/diagnosis/rapidlab.htm

Centers for Disease Control and Prevention. (2012f). Tuberculosis outbreak associated with a homeless shelter—Kane County, IL, 2007–2011. *Morbidity and Mortality Weekly Report, 61*(11), 186–189.

Centers for Disease Control and Prevention. (2012g). *Interim domestic guidance on the use of respirators to prevent transmission of SARS*. Retrieved from http://www.cdc.gov/sars/clinical/respirators.html

Centers for Disease Control and Prevention. (2013a). *Diseases/pathogens associated with antimicrobial resistance: Outbreaks*. Retrieved from http://www.cdc.gov/drugresistance/DiseasesConnectedAR.html

Centers for Disease Control and Prevention. (2013b). Interim adjusted estimates of seasonal influenza vaccine effectiveness—United States, February 2013. *Morbidity and Mortality Weekly Report, 62*(07), 119–123.

Centers for Disease Control and Prevention. (2013c). *Pertussis (whooping cough): Outbreaks.* Retrieved from http://www.cdc.gov/pertussis/outbreaks/about.html

Centers for Disease Control and Prevention. (2013d). *TB in the homeless population.* Retrieved from http://www.cdc.gov/tb/topic/populations/Homelessness/default.htm

Centers for Disease Control and Prevention. (2014). *Preventing the spread of conjunctivitis.* Retrieved from http://www.cdc.gov/conjunctivitis/about/prevention.html

Centers for Disease Control and Prevention. (2015a). *2012 epidemiology and prevention of vaccine-preventable diseases.* Retrieved from http://www.cdc.gov/vaccines/ed/webinar-epv/index.html

Centers for Disease Control and Prevention. (2015b). *Hand hygiene in healthcare settings.* Retrieved from http://www.cdc.gov/handhygiene/

Centers for Disease Control and Prevention. (2015c). *Healthcare infection practices advisory committee (HICPAC).* Retrieved from http://www.cdc.gov/hicpac/index.html

Centers for Disease Control and Prevention. (2015d). *National Hospital Discharge Survey.* Retrieved from http://www.cdc.gov/nchs/nhds.htm

Centers for Disease Control and Prevention. (2015e). *Pneumococcal disease.* Retrieved from http://www.cdc.gov/pneumococcal/index.html

Centers for Disease Control and Prevention. (2015f). *Pneumococcal polysaccharide vaccine.* Retrieved from http://www.cdc.gov/vaccines/hcp/vis/vis-statements/ppv.html

Centers for Disease Control and Prevention. (2015g). *Polio eradication.* Retrieved from http://www.cdc.gov/polio/

Centers for Disease Control and Prevention. (2015h). *Tuberculosis.* Retrieved from http://www.cdc.gov/tb/default.htm

Centers for Disease Control and Prevention. (2015i). *Flu information for parents with young children.* Retrieved from http://www.cdc.gov/flu/parents/index.htm

Centers for Disease Control and Prevention. (2015j). *Pregnant women and influenza.* Retrieved from http://www.cdc.gov/flu/protect/vaccine/pregnant.htm

Centers for Disease Control and Prevention. (2015k). *TB in children in the United States.* Retrieved from http://www.cdc.gov/tb/topic/populations/TBinChildren/default.htm

Centers for Disease Control and Prevention. (2015l). *What you should know and do this flu season if you are 65 years and older.* Retrieved from http://www.cdc.gov/flu/about/disease/65over.htm

Centers for Disease Control and Prevention. (2015m). *CDC's Infection Disease National Centers.* Retrieved from http://www.cdc.gov/oid/centers.html

Centers for Disease Control and Prevention. (2016a). *Get smart for healthcare.* Retrieved from http://www.cdc.gov/getsmart/healthcare/

Centers for Disease Control and Prevention. (2016b). *Testing for TB infection.* Retrieved from http://www.cdc.gov/tb/topic/testing/tbtesttypes.htm

Centers for Disease Control and Prevention. (2016c). *Trends in tuberculosis.* Retrieved from https://www.cdc.gov/tb/publications/factsheets/statistics/tbtrends.htm

Centers for Disease Control and Prevention. (2016d). *Infection control in health care settings.* Retrieved from https://www.cdc.gov/tb/topic/infectioncontrol/default.htm

Centers for Disease Control and Prevention. (2016e). *Pneumonia.* Retrieved from https://www.cdc.gov/nchs/fastats/pneumonia.htm

Centers for Disease Control and Prevention. (2017a). *Influenza (flu).* Retrieved from https://www.cdc.gov/flu/about/disease/2015-16.htm

Centers for Disease Control and Prevention. (2017b). *Tuberculosis – United States, 2016. Morbidity and Mortality Weekly Report.* Retrieved from https://www.cdc.gov/mmwr/volumes/66/wr/mm6611a2.htm?s_cid=mm6611a2_w

Centers for Disease Control and Prevention. (2017c). *Tuberculosis (TB).* Retrieved from https://www.cdc.gov/tb/publications/factsheets/testing/skintesting.htm

Chapman, S. J., & Hill, A. V. S. (2012). Human genetic susceptibility to infectious disease. *Nature Reviews Genetics, 13*, 175–188. doi:10.1038/nrg3114

Close Up Media. (2013). *Sepsis Alliance rolls out response to U.S. government findings that most expensive condition to treat in hospitals is sepsis.* Retrieved from http://search.proquest.com.ezproxy.nu.edu/pqcentral/docview/1458634978/abstract/E1A6DB39F49749DFPQ/6?accountid=25320

Conrad, D. E., Levi, J. R., Theroux, Z. A., Inverso, Y., & Shah, U. K. (2014). Risk factors associated with postoperative tympanostomy tube obstruction. *JAMA Otolaryngology—Head & Neck Surgery, 140*(8), 727–730.

Corbett, J. V., & Banks, A. D. (2013). *Laboratory tests and diagnostic procedures with nursing diagnoses* (8th ed.). Upper Saddle River, NJ: Pearson Education.

Csakanyi, Z., Czinner, A., Spangler, J., Rogers, T., & Katona, G. (2012). Relationship of environmental tobacco smoke to otitis media (OM) in children. *International Journal of Pediatric Otorhinolaryngology, 76*(7), 989–993. doi:10.1016/j.ijporl.2012.03.017

deJuilio, P. A., Rivera, S. J., & Huml, J. P. (2012). A successful VAP prevention program. *RT: The Journal for Respiratory Care Practitioners, 25*(6), 26.

Dibardino, D. M., & Wonderlink, R. G. (2015). Aspiration pneumonia: A review of modern trends. *Journal of Critical Care, 30*(1), 40–48.

Donovan, S. (2015). The retailing of healthcare. *Healthcare Design 15*(9), 30. Retrieved from http://search.proquest.com.ezproxy.nu.edu/health/docview/1737443033/fulltextPDF/2F6DC03762924907PQ/41?accountid=25320

Drzewiecki, B. A., Thomas, J. C., Pope, J. C., IV, Adams, M. C., Brock, J. W., III, & Tanaka, S. T. (2012). Observation of patients with vesicoureteral reflux off antibiotic prophylaxis: Healthcare provider bias on patient selection and risk factors for recurrent febrile urinary tract infection. *Journal of Urology, 188*(Suppl. 4), 1480–1484. doi:10.1016/j.juro.2012.02.033

Dugdale, D. C., III. (2011). Blood differential. *MedlinePlus.* Retrieved from http://www.nlm.nih.gov/medlineplus/ency/article/003657.htm

Fisher, D. J., & Steele, R. W. (2015). Pediatric urinary tract infection. *Medscape Drugs and Diseases.* Retrieved from http://emedicine.medscape.com/article/969643-overview

Fitzpatrick, J. (2012). QNI Opening Doors Project—Improving health for homeless people and families. *Community Practitioner, 85*(2), 19–22.

Food and Drug Administration. (2013). *Influenza (flu) antiviral drugs and related information.* Retrieved from http://www.fda.gov/Drugs/DrugSafety/InformationbyDrugClass/ucm100228.htm

Food and Drug Administration. (2015). *Contact lens care.* Retrieved from http://www.fda.gov/ForConsumers/ByAudience/ForWomen/ucm118511.htm

Food and Drug Administration. (2016). *FDA updates warnings for fluoroquinolone antibiotics.* Retrieved from http://www.fda.gov/NewsEvents/Newsroom/PressAnnouncements/ucm513183.htm

Friedel, V., Zilora, S., Bogaard, D., Casey, J. R., & Pichichero, M. E. (2014). Five-year prospective study of paediatric acute otitis media in Rochester, NY: Modelling analysis of the risk of pneumococcal colonization in the nasopharynx and infection. *Epidemiology of Infection, 142*, 2186–2194. doi:10.1017/S0950268813003178

Gao, L., Lu, W., Bai, L., Wang, X., Xu, J., Catanzaro, A., … LATENTTB-NSTM Study Team. (2015). Latent tuberculosis in rural China: Baseline results of a population-based, multicenter, prospective cohort study. *Lancet Infectious Diseases.* doi:http://dx.doi.org.ezproxy.nu.edu/10.1016/S1473-3099(14)71085-0

Giménez-García, C., Ballester-Arnal, R., Gil-Llario, M. D., Cárdenas-López, G., & Duran-Baca, X. (2013). Culture as an influence on the perceived risk of HIV infection: A differential analysis comparing young people from Mexico and Spain. *Journal of Community Health, 38*(3), 434–442.

Goodman, B. (2013). Hospital-acquired infections cost $10 billion a year. *U.S. News & World Report, Health.* Retrieved from http://health.usnews.com/health-news/news/articles/2013/09/03/hospital-acquired-infections-cost-10-billion-a-year-study

Herchline, T. E. (2016). Cellulitis. *Medscape Drugs and Diseases.* Retrieved from http://emedicine.medscape.com/article/214222-overview

Herdman, T. H. & Kamitsuru, S. (Eds.). *Nursing Diagnoses—Definitions and Classification 2015–2017.* Copyright © 2014, 1994 -2014 NANDA International. Used by arrangement with John Wiley & Sons, Inc. Companion website: www.wiley.com/go/nursingdiagnoses

Itan, Y., Mazel, M., Mazel, B., Abhyankar, A., Nitschke, P., Quintana-Murci, L., … Casanova, J-L. (2014). HGCS: An online tool for prioritizing disease-causing gene variants by biological distance. *BMC Genomics, 15*(256), 2–7. Retrieved from http://www.biomedcentral.com/1471-2164/15/256

Ji, Y. J., & Jeong, J. S. (2013). Comparison of antimicrobial effect of alcohol gel according to the amount and drying time in health personnel hand hygiene. *Journal of Korean Academy of Nursing, 43*(3), 305–311. http://dx.doi.org/10.4040/jkan.2013.43.3.305

Joint Commission, The. (2012). *National patient safety goals effective January 1, 2013.* Retrieved from http://www.jointcommission.org/assets/1/18/NPSG_Chapter_Jan2013_HAP.pdf

Klein, N. P., Bartlett, J., Rowhani-Rahbar, A., Fireman, B., & Baxter, R. (2012). Waning protection after fifth dose of acellular pertussis vaccine in children. *New England Journal of Medicine, 367*(11), 1012–1019.

Lachenbruch, C., & VanGilder, C. (2012). Estimates of evaporation rates from wounds for various dressing/support surface combinations. *Advances in Skin and Wound Care, 25*(1), 29–36. doi:10.1097/01.ASW.0000410688.21987.1d

Lieberthal, A. S., Carroll, A. E., Chonmaitree, T., Ganiats, T. G., Hoberman, A., Jackson, M. A., … Tunkel, D. E. (2013). The diagnosis and management of acute otitis media. *Pediatrics, 131*(3), e965–e989. doi:10.1542/peds.2012-3488

Longo, D. L., Fauci, A. S., Kasper, D. L., Hauser, S. L., Jameson, J. L., & Loscalzo, J. (Eds.). (2012). *Harrison's principles of internal medicine* (18th ed.). New York, NY: McGraw-Hill.

Magge, S. S., & Wolf, J. L. (2013). Complementary and alternative medicine and mind-body therapies for treatment of irritable bowel syndrome in women. *Women's Health, 9*(6), 557–667. Retrieved from http://search.proquest.com.ezproxy.nu.edu/ health/docview/1446321636/fulltextPDF/4785D6 404D42444CPQ/1?accountid=25320

Mayo Clinic. (2014). *Fever*. Retrieved from http://www.mayoclinic.org/diseases-conditions/fever/basics/definition/con-20019229

Mayo Clinic. (2015). *Cellulitis*. Retrieved from http://www.mayoclinic.org/diseases-conditions/cellulitis/basics/definition/con-20023471

Mayo Clinic. (2016a). *Sepsis*. Retrieved from http://www.mayoclinic.org/diseases-conditions/sepsis/home/ovc-20169784

Mayo Clinic. (2016b). *Tuberculosis*. Retrieved from http://www.mayoclinic.org/diseases-conditions/tuberculosis/home/ovc-20188556

Mayo Clinic. (2017). *Ear infection (middle ear)*. Retrieved from http://www.mayoclinic.org/diseases-conditions/ear-infections/home/ovc-20199482

MedicineNet.com. (2015). *Swine flu: (Swine influenza A [H1N1 and H3N2v] virus)*. Retrieved from http://www.medicinenet.com/swine_flu/article.htm

MedlinePlus. (2012). *Asymptomatic bacteriuria*. Retrieved from http://www.nlm.nih.gov/medlineplus/ency/article/000520.htm

Mitruka, K., Winston, C. A., & Navin, T. R. (2012). Predictors of failure in timely tuberculosis treatment completion, United States. *International Journal of Tuberculosis and Lung Disease, 16*(8), 1075–1082. doi:10.5588/ijtld.11.0814

Morgan, D. J. (2015). *MRSA: New methicillin-resistant Staphylococcus aureus data have been reported by investigators at Virginia Commonwealth University: Reconsidering contact Precautions for endemic methicillin-resistant staphylococcus aureus and VRE*. Retrieved from http://search.proquest.com.ezproxy.nu.edu/pqcentral/docview/1725085635/fulltext/501C1F9C848B4F46PQ/18?accountid=25320

Mortazavi, F., & Ghojazadeh, M. (2014). Usefulness of serum procalcitonin level for prediction of vesicoureteral reflux in pediatric urinary tract infection. *Iranian Journal of Kidney Diseases, 8*(1), 37–41. Retrieved from http://search.proquest.com.ezproxy.nu.edu/pqcentral/docview/1503674506/fulltextPDF/7543C09F45 CA4837PQ/1?accountid=25320

Morton, L. M., & Phillips, T. J. (2012). Wound healing update. *Seminars in Cutaneous Medicine and Surgery, 31*, 33–37. doi:10.1016.j.sder.2011.11.007

Mukherjee, S., Sharma, S., & Maru, L. (2013). Poor dental hygiene in pregnancy leading to submandibular cellulitis leading to intrauterine fetal demise. *International Journal of Preventive Medicine, 4*(5), 603–606. Retrieved from http://search.proquest.com.ezproxy.nu.edu/health/docview/1368605259/fulltextPDF/BD8CB5E3A56 441B8PQ/1?accountid=25320

National Center for Complementary and Integrative Health. (2016). *Echinacea*. Retrieved from https://nccih.nih.gov/health/echinacea/ataglance.htm

National Center for Health Statistics. (2012). *Health, United States, 2011: With special features on socioeconomic status and health*. Hyattsville, MD: U.S. Department of Health and Human Services.

National Kidney and Urological Diseases Information Clearinghouse. (2012). *Pyelonephritis: Kidney infection*. Retrieved from http://kidney.niddk.nih.gov/kudiseases/pubs/pyelonephritis/#7

Niederauer, M. Q., Michalek, J. E., & Armstrong, D. G. (2015). Interim results for a prospective, randomized, double-blind multicenter study comparing continuous diffusion of oxygen

therapy to standard moist wound therapy in the treatment of diabetic foot ulcers. *Wound Medicine, 8*(1), 19–23.

Normandin, P. A. (2015). Pediatric infectious diseases. *Journal of Emergency Nursing, 41*(2), 160–161.

Occupational Safety and Health Administration. (2016). Latex allergy. *Safety and health topics*. Retrieved from https://www.osha.gov/SLTC/latexallergy/

Osmon, D. R., Berbari, E. F., Berendt, A. R., Lew, D., Zimmerli, W., Steckelberg, J. M., … Wilson, W. R. (2013). Diagnosis and management of prosthetic joint infection: Clinical practice guidelines by the Infectious Diseases Society of America. *Clinical Infectious Diseases, 56*(1), e1–e25.

Pagana, K. D., & Pagana, T. J. (2013). *Diagnostic and laboratory test reference* (11th ed.). St. Louis, MO: Elsevier-Mosby.

Panchisin, T. L. (2016). Improving outcomes with the ANA CAUTI Prevention Tool. *Nursing, 46*(3), 55–59.

Papadakis, M. A., & McPhee, S. J. (Eds.). (2013). *Current medical diagnosis and treatment 2013* (52nd ed.). New York, NY: McGraw-Hill.

Parez, N., Giaquinto, C., Du Roure, C., Martinon-Torres, F., Spoulou, V., Van Damme, P., & Vesikari, T. (2014). Rotavirus vaccination in Europe: Drivers and barriers. *Lancet Infectious Diseases, 14*(5), 416–425. Retrieved from http://search.proquest.com.ezproxy.nu.edu/health/docview/1518120988/full textPDF/49C9E586B7F4413DPQ/4?accoun tid=25320

Perovic, O., Iyaloo, S., Kularatne, R., Lowman, W., Bosman, N., Wadula, J., … Singh-Moodley, A. (2015). Prevalence and trends of *Staphylococcus aureus bacteraemia* in hospitalized patients in South Africa, 2010 to 2012: Laboratory-based surveillance mapping of antimicrobial resistance and molecular epidemiology. *PLoS One, 10*(12), e0145429. doi:10.1371/journal.pone.014542

Pickering, L. K., Baker, C. J., Kimberlin, D. W., & Long, S. S. (Eds.). (2012). *Red Book: 2012 Report of the Committee on Infectious Diseases*. Media, PA: American Academy of Pediatrics.

Porth, C., & Grossman, S. (2014). *Pathophysiology: Concepts of altered health states* (9th ed.). Philadelphia, PA: Lippincott Williams & Wilkins.

Rhee, C., Gohil, S., & Klompas, M. (2014). Regulatory mandates for sepsis care—reasons for caution. *New England Journal of Medicine, 370*(18), 1673–1676.

Sakamoto, R. (2015). Legionnaire's disease, weather and climate. *Bulletin of the World Health Organization, 93*(6), 435–436.

Seckman, C. H. (2013). Pacifiers and thumb sucking. *ProQuest Central, 46*, 76–78.

Shah, S., McArthur, E., Farag, A., Nartey, M., Fleet, J. L., Knoll, G. A., … Jain, A. K. (2014). Risk of hospitalization for community acquired pneumonia with renin-angiotensin blockade in elderly patients: A population-based study. *PLoS One, 9*(10), e110165. doi:10.1371/journal.pone.0110165

Shime, N., Kosaka, T., & Fujita, N. (2013). De-escalation of antimicrobial therapy for bacteremia due to difficult-to-treat Gram-negative bacilli. *Infection, 41*(1), 203–210.

Shlamovitz, G. Z., & Kim, E. D. (2013). Urethral catheterization in men. *Medscape Drugs and Diseases*. Retrieved from http://emedicine.medscape.com/article/80716-overview

Shoff, W. F. (2014). Asymptomatic bacteriuria. *Medscape Drugs and Diseases*. Retrieved from

http://emedicine.medscape.com/article/2059290-overview

Shultz, S., & Adam, P. (2015). What is the most effective topical treatment for allergic conjunctivitis? *Journal of Family Practice, 64*(5), 315–321.

Sole, M. L., Klein, D. G., & Moseley, M. J. (Eds.). (2013). *Introduction to critical care nursing* (6th ed.). St. Louis, MO: Elsevier.

Spector, R. E. (2017). *Cultural Diversity in Health and Illness* (9th ed.). Hoboken, NJ: Pearson Education.

Tantry, U. S., Jeong, Y., Navarese, E. P., Kubica, J., & Gurbel, P. A. (2013). Influence of genetic polymorphisms on platelet function, response to antiplatelet drugs and clinical outcomes in patients with coronary artery disease. *Expert Reviews in Cardiovascular Therapy, 11*(4), 447–462.

Toward Optimized Practice. (2015). *Diagnosis and management of urinary tract infection in long term care facilities. Clinical practice guideline*. Retrieved from http://www.topalbertadoctors.org/download/401/urinary_tract_infection_guideline.pdf

Townsend, A. (2014). *Focus on flu campaign*. Retrieved from http://www.cleveland.com/healthfit/index.ssf/2014/10/focus_on_flu_campaign_hospitals_city_and_county_health_officials_urging_residents_to_get_their_shots.html

U.S. Department of Health and Human Services, Office of Disease Prevention and Promotion. (2013). *Healthy People 2020*. Washington, DC. Retrieved from http://www.healthypeople.gov/2020/default.aspx

Varga, M., & Holloway, S. (2016). The lived experience of the wound care nurse in caring for patients with pressure ulcers. *International Wound Journal, 13*(2), 243–251.

Varman, M. (2015). Pediatric pneumococcal infections. *Medscape Drugs and Diseases*. Retrieved from http://emedicine.medscape.com/article/967694-overview

Vayas, J. M. (2014). Isolation precautions. *U.S. National Library of Medicine*. Retrieved from https://www.nlm.nih.gov/medlineplus/ency/patientinstructions/000446.htm

Volz, K. A., Canham, L., Kaplan, E., Sanchez, L. D., Shapiro, N. I., & Grossman, S. A. (2013). Identifying patients with cellulitis who are likely to require inpatient admission after a stay in an ED observation unit. *American Journal of Emergency Medicine, 31*(2), 360–364.

Weiss, J. R., Tessema, B., & Brown, S. M. (2013). Complementary and integrative treatments: Upper respiratory infection. *Otolaryngologic Clinics of North America, 46*(3), 335–344. doi:10.1016/j.otc.2012.12.007

Wilson, B. A., Shannon, M. T., & Shields, K. M. (2013). *Nurse's drug guide*. Upper Saddle River, NJ: Pearson Education.

World Health Organization. (n.d.). *Trachoma*. Retrieved from http://www.who.int/topics/trachoma/en/

World Health Organization. (2012). *Global tuberculosis report 2012*. Geneva, Switzerland: WHO Press.

World Health Organization. (2013). *Tuberculosis*. Retrieved from http://www.who.int/mediacentre/factsheets/fs104/en/

World Health Organization. (2015). *H5N1 influenza FAQs*. Retrieved from http://www.who.int/influenza/human_animal_interface/avian_influenza/h5n1_research/faqs/en/

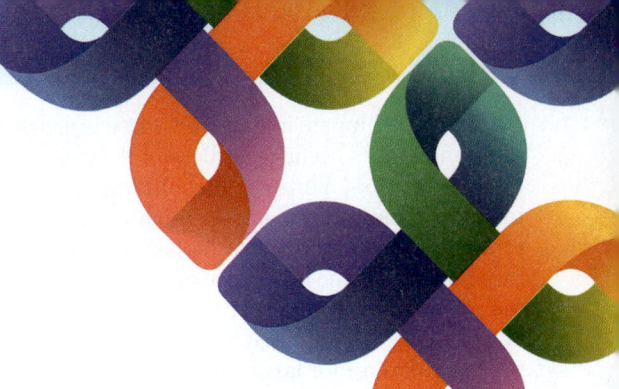

Module 10
Inflammation

Module Outline and Learning Outcomes

The Concept of Inflammation

Normal Presentation

10.1 Analyze the physiology of inflammation in the body.

Alterations Involving Inflammation

10.2 Differentiate alterations in inflammation.

Concepts Related to Inflammation

10.3 Outline the relationship between inflammation and other concepts.

Health Promotion

10.4 Explain the promotion of a healthy inflammatory response.

Nursing Assessment

10.5 Differentiate common assessment procedures and tests used to examine inflammation.

Independent Interventions

10.6 Analyze independent interventions nurses can implement for patients with inflammation.

Collaborative Therapies

10.7 Summarize collaborative therapies used by interprofessional teams for patients with inflammation.

Lifespan Considerations

10.8 Differentiate considerations related to the assessment and care of patients with inflammation throughout the lifespan.

Inflammation Exemplars

Exemplar 10.A Appendicitis

10.A Analyze appendicitis as it relates to inflammation.

Exemplar 10.B Gallbladder Disease

10.B Analyze gallbladder disease as it relates to inflammation.

Exemplar 10.C Inflammatory Bowel Disease

10.C Analyze inflammatory bowel disease as it relates to inflammation.

Exemplar 10.D Nephritis

10.D Analyze nephritis as it relates to inflammation.

Exemplar 10.E Peptic Ulcer Disease

10.E Analyze peptic ulcer disease as it relates to inflammation.

›› The Concept of Inflammation

Concept Key Terms

Anaphylaxis, 672	Exudate, 670	H_4 receptor, 672	Inflammation, 669	Margination, 670
Debridement, 670	Granulation tissue, 671	Histamine, 670	Leukocyte, 670	Mast cells, 671
Emigration, 670	H_1 receptor, 672	Hyperemia, 670	Leukocytosis, 670	Regeneration, 671

Inflammation is a nonspecific but complex response to reduce the effects of what the body sees as harmful. Inflammation may result from an injury such as an ankle sprain or from an underlying infection. Autoimmune diseases frequently cause inflammation sufficient to result in tissue damage. Other harmful agents include pathogens, damaged cells, and irritants such as cigarette smoke.

Under normal circumstances, inflammation acts as a protective process that stimulates healing and prevents further damage or progressive deterioration. The occasional uncomfortable symptoms of normal inflammation usually resolve successfully with palliative care. However, the inflammatory process can escalate and lead to complications such as autoimmune disorders (e.g., rheumatoid arthritis, psoriasis, asthma, and allergies). These conditions may require more aggressive care that includes pharmacotherapy.

Normal Presentation

Inflammation is an adaptive response to injury or illness that brings fluid (plasma), dissolved substances, and blood cells into the interstitial tissues where the invasion or damage has occurred. This innate immune response is *nonspecific* because the same events occur regardless of the cause of the inflammatory process. Through the inflammatory reaction, the invader is neutralized and eliminated, destroyed tissue is removed, and the process of healing and repair begins. Inflammation is the first phase of the healing process. During the inflammatory process, particulate matter, bacteria, damaged cells, and inflammatory exudate are removed through phagocytosis and a large number of potentially damaging chemicals and microorganisms may be neutralized. This process, called **debridement**, prepares the wound for healing. Adequate nutrition is essential for inflammation and healing to proceed.

Inflammation is characterized by five signs: (a) pain, (b) swelling, (c) redness, (d) heat, and (e) impaired function of the body part (if the injury is severe). Words with the suffix *-itis* typically describe an inflammatory process. For example, *appendicitis* means inflammation of the appendix; *gastritis* means inflammation of the stomach.

Injurious agents can be categorized as physical agents, chemical agents, and microorganisms. *Physical agents* include mechanical objects causing trauma to tissues, excessive heat or cold, and radiation. *Chemical agents* include external irritants (e.g., strong acids, alkalis, poisons, irritating gases) and internal irritants (substances manufactured within the body, such as excessive hydrochloric acid in the stomach). Microorganisms that can cause inflammation are bacteria and viruses.

The Inflammatory Process

Inflammation is a complex response of vascular tissues that is triggered by harmful stimuli. By isolating the damaged area and promoting repair of the surrounding tissue, the inflammatory response protects the body. Without this necessary and beneficial process, wounds and infections would never heal. Inflammation may be classified as either acute or chronic. During acute inflammation, the inflammatory response may occur within minutes of an injury such as a splinter or insect bite. On the other hand, a response to a bacterial infection may take a few hours. During the acute inflammatory response, the typical signs of inflammation (redness, swelling, pain, heat, and impaired function) occur. The acute process continues until the trauma or infection is neutralized. When the acute inflammatory response is unable to neutralize the harmful stimuli, the response may become chronic, continuing for months or years. Chronic inflammation ranges from seasonal allergic reactions to pollen to responses that damage healthy tissues in autoimmune diseases.

Stages of Inflammation

In simplest terms, the complex inflammatory process can be categorized into three stages: vascular and cellular responses, exudate production, and repair.

Vascular and Cellular Responses

Immediately after injury or infection, blood vessels temporarily constrict in the surrounding area. The injured tissues release **histamines**, kinins, and prostaglandins in response to the injury or infection. These substances serve as chemical mediators to dilate blood vessels, causing more blood

to flow to the injured area. This marked increase in blood supply is referred to as **hyperemia** and is responsible for the characteristic signs of redness and heat that accompany inflammation.

Vascular permeability increases at the site with dilation of the vessels. Fluid, proteins, and **leukocytes** (white blood cells [WBCs]) leak into the interstitial spaces, causing inflammatory swelling (edema) and pain. Pain is caused by the pressure of accumulating fluid on nerve endings and the irritating chemical mediators. Fluid pouring into areas such as the pleural or pericardial cavity can seriously affect organ function. In other areas, such as joints, accumulating fluid impairs mobility.

Slowed blood flow in the dilated vessels allows more leukocytes to arrive at the injured tissues. The leukocytes aggregate, or line up, along the inner surface of the blood vessels. This process is known as **margination**. Leukocytes then move through the blood vessel wall into the affected tissue spaces, a process called **emigration**.

In response to the exit of leukocytes from the blood, the bone marrow produces more leukocytes in even larger numbers and releases them into the bloodstream. This process is called **leukocytosis**. A normal leukocyte count of 4500–10,000 per cubic millimeter of blood can increase to 20,000 or more when inflammation occurs.

All these conditions result in the first stage of inflammation. Often individuals do not seek medical treatment for an acute inflammatory response unless it progresses to the second stage. Typical injuries for which an individual seeks treatment for stage 1 inflammation are sprained ankles and wrists, broken bones, and minor blunt force injuries (e.g., two children running into each other on a playground).

Exudate Production

In the second stage of inflammation, inflammatory **exudate** is produced. The term *exudate* comes from the Latin word meaning "to exude" or "to ooze." Exudate consists of fluid that escaped from the blood vessels, dead phagocytic and tissue cells, and the products they release.

The nature and amount of exudate vary according to the tissue involved and the intensity and duration of the inflammation. The major types of exudate are serous, purulent, and hemorrhagic (sanguineous). Serous exudate typically accompanies mild inflammation and presents as clear- or straw-colored with a thin, watery consistency. Purulent exudate is usually opaque, or milky. Commonly referred to as "pus," purulent exudate normally indicates the presence of infection and contains a large quantity of cells and necrotic debris. Because hemorrhagic exudate contains blood from ruptured blood vessels, it is red and thick. This type of exudate leaks from tissue or its capillaries as a result of infection or injury.

Whether the presence of exudate should be reported depends primarily on the underlying cause and the amount and degree of the exudate. A minor cut that exhibits either serous or hemorrhagic exudate may resolve with simple first aid. Exudate that appears over a larger surface or in conjunction with other symptoms, such as fever, warrants a greater degree of medical care.

Reparative Phase

The third stage of the inflammatory response involves the repair of injured tissues by regeneration or replacement with fibrous tissue (scar formation). **Regeneration** is the replacement of destroyed tissue cells by cells that are identical or similar in structure and function. Damaged cells are replaced one by one, and new cells are organized so that the architectural pattern and function of the tissue are restored. The ability to regenerate cells varies considerably from one type of tissue to another. For example, epithelial tissues of the skin and the digestive and respiratory tracts have a good regenerative capacity, as long as their underlying support structures are intact. The same is true of osseous, lymphoid, and bone marrow tissues. Tissues that have little regenerative capacity include nervous, muscular, and elastic tissues.

When regeneration is not possible, repair occurs by fibrous (scar) tissue formation. The inflammatory exudate with its interlacing network of fibrin provides the framework for this tissue to develop. Damaged tissues are replaced with the connective tissue elements of collagen, blood capillaries, lymphatics, and other tissue-bound substances. In the early stages of this process, the tissue is called **granulation tissue**. It is a fragile, gelatinous tissue that appears pink or red because of the many newly formed capillaries. Later in the process, the tissue shrinks (the capillaries are constricted, even obliterated), and the collagen fibers contract, leaving a firmer fibrous tissue. This is called a *cicatrix*, or scar tissue.

Mediators of Inflammation

The process of inflammation is initiated by the release of mediators from inflammatory cells such as macrophages and mast cells. **Mast cells** are leukocytes found in most tissues of the body, including the skin, respiratory system, and intestines. They are one of the principal sources of cell-derived

TABLE 10–1 Chemical Mediators of Inflammation

Mediator	Description
Bradykinin	Causes dilation of vessels, acts with prostaglandins to cause pain, increases vascular permeability, and stimulates histamine release
Complement	Comprises over 20 proteins, activated sequentially, and is responsible for dilation, permeability, chemotaxis, phagocytosis, and histamine release
Histamine	Stored and released by mast cells, contributes to early vasodilation and increased permeability, and chemically attracts eosinophils
Leukotrienes	Stored and released by mast cells and chemically attracts neutrophils and macrophages
Prostaglandins	Present in most tissues, stored and released by mast cells, and causes vasodilation

Source: Data from Delves, P. J. (2014). Overview of the immune system. *Merck manual: Health care professionals.* Retrieved from http://www.merckmanuals.com/professional/immunology_allergic_disorders/biology_of_the_immune_system/overview_of_the_immune_system.html

mediators of inflammation, including histamine and heparin (see **Table 10–1 》**).

In response to injury or contact with an antigen, histamine and heparin work together to increase blood flow to the injured site. Histamine causes the dilation of nearby blood vessels and increases their permeability, while heparin prevents blood clotting. This combined action allows blood to easily enter the affected tissue, resulting in the redness and swelling associated with inflammation. **Figure 10–1 》** illustrates the fundamental steps in acute inflammation.

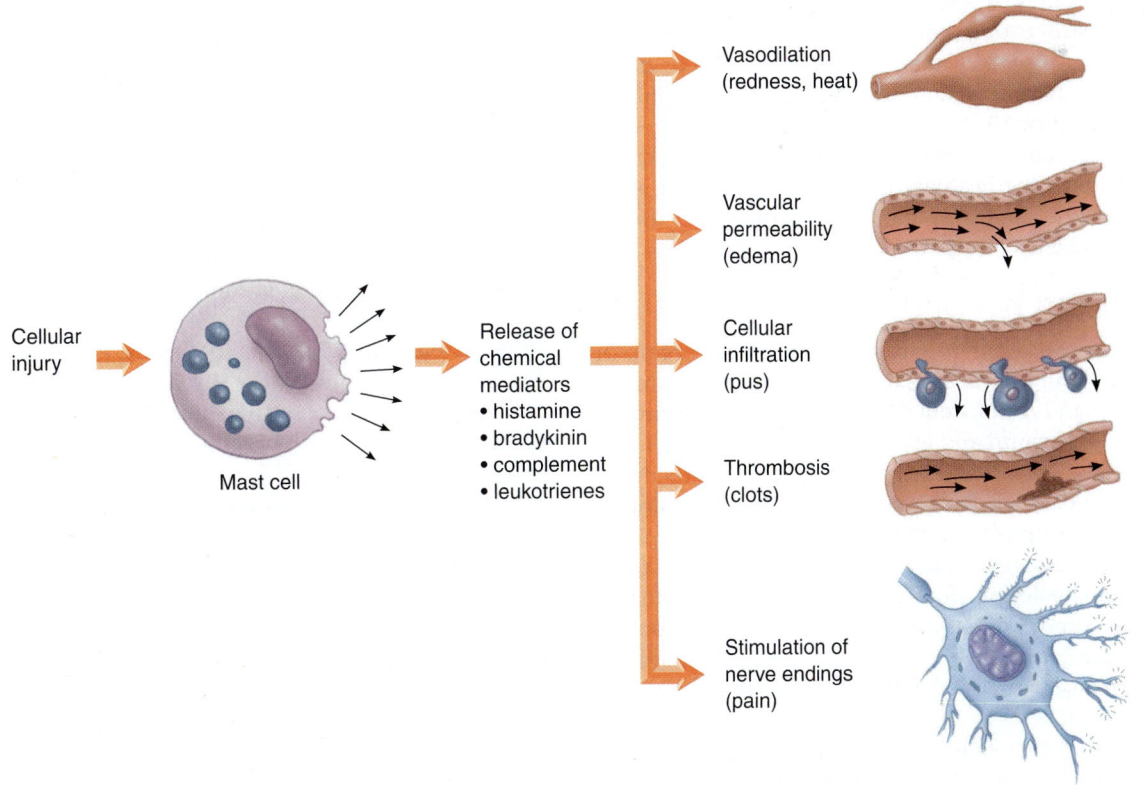

Figure 10–1 》 Steps in acute inflammation.

Box 10–1
Symptoms and Treatment of Anaphylaxis

Anaphylaxis is a life-threatening allergic reaction that develops extremely rapidly—in seconds to minutes—and requires immediate initiation of the emergency medical system (EMS) in out-of-hospital settings. In healthcare facilities, the nurse will initiate treatment immediately and call for the rapid response team. Signs and symptoms of anaphylaxis include the following:

- Inflammation of the airways, swelling of the throat (which can become severe enough to block the airway)
- Wheezing, labored breathing
- Abnormal heart rhythm
- Low blood pressure
- Weakness, light-headedness, dizziness
- Nausea, vomiting, or diarrhea
- Cyanosis due to decreased tissue oxygenation or pallor secondary to shock (advanced manifestations)
- Hives, itching.

Epinephrine is the first line of treatment for an anaphylactic reaction. Epinephrine dilates the airways and narrows the blood vessels, essentially counteracting the allergic response. While the intramuscular route is preferred, epinephrine may also be administered subcutaneously or intravenously. For intubated patients in whom no other option is available, epinephrine may be administered via an endotracheal tube (Vincent, 2014). Some individuals with allergies carry self-injectors with epinephrine (e.g., EpiPens) to use in the case of an anaphylactic response. In the event of an anaphylactic reaction, EMS should be called even for patients who carry and use an EpiPen. During and immediately following an anaphylactic response, airway protection is critical, so adjunctive medications may include beta-agonists, antihistamines, and corticosteroids. A severe reaction resulting in laryngeal swelling sufficient to close the airway may require a tracheotomy.

The four types of histamine receptors are H_1, H_2, H_3, and H_4. Of these, the H_1 and H_4 receptors are involved in the inflammatory response. **H_1 receptors** are primarily found on smooth muscle cells, on the endothelium, and in the central nervous system (CNS). Stimulation of these receptors results in vasodilation, bronchoconstriction, pain, itching, and hives. **H_4 receptors**, located in peripheral WBCs and mast cells, are also involved in immune responses (Ayuso et al., 2013). Antihistamines block histamine receptors on tissues, thus reducing the effect of histamine and the resultant allergic symptoms.

When a patient is exposed to an allergen that results in a rapid release of inflammatory mediators, anaphylaxis occurs. If left untreated, anaphylaxis may lead to death caused by airway obstruction or vascular collapse (Simons et al., 2013; see **Box 10–1** »). The most common triggers of anaphylaxis are food (including peanuts, shellfish, milk, and egg), insect stings, medications (particularly penicillin, anesthetic agents, and nonsteroidal anti-inflammatory drugs [NSAIDs]), and latex (Singla et al., 2013).

Alterations Involving Inflammation
Inflammation can occur in virtually any tissue, organ, or system. Many autoimmune disorders involve the inflammatory response and result from the body's misinterpreting its own tissues as harmful and needing to be destroyed or limited. Rheumatoid arthritis (RA), systemic lupus erythematosus (SLE), and Guillain-Barré syndrome are a few examples of autoimmune responses involving inflammation.

Additional disorders that involve an inflammatory component are allergic rhinitis, anaphylaxis, ankylosing spondylitis, appendicitis, asthma, osteoarthritis, contact dermatitis, Crohn disease, gallbladder disease, inflammatory bowel disease (IBD), nephritis, peptic ulcers, and ulcerative colitis.

Inflammation carries implications for nursing care in a number of areas. Patients with mild alterations (e.g., a sprain) may need simple palliative care, rest, and reminders related to safety and injury prevention. Infection, however, requires treatment, and the resulting acute inflammatory response may cause additional complications for patients.

Alterations and Manifestations
Classic signs of inflammation include redness and swelling. A healthy inflammatory response includes activation and recruitment of WBCs to the affected site. Localized responses are limited in terms of which sites are affected, while generalized responses can affect the entire body. Chronic inflammation of the intestines associated with inflammatory bowel disorders may result in structural changes. For example, Crohn disease results in fibrotic changes to the bowel wall; local obstruction, abscesses, and fistulas may develop. Malabsorption or malnutrition may result. In RA, discussed in the module on Immunity, the chronic inflammatory response affects the lining of the joints and can lead to joint deformity. RA is characterized by pain, swelling, and redness of the joint.

Ankylosing spondylitis is a form of arthritis that primarily involves the spine. With this condition, vertebral inflammation leads to severe, chronic pain and discomfort. The sacroiliac (SI) joints, which are located at the base of the spine where the spine joins the pelvis, are affected by disease progression. In severe disease, new bone formation occurs on the spine, causing spinal processes to fuse into a fixed, immobile position, sometimes creating a forward-stooped posture.

For an overview of additional disorders that incorporate an inflammatory component, see the Alterations and Therapies feature.

Prevalence
Millions of adults and children in the United States have inflammatory disorders. The typical onset of RA occurs in middle age with an increased incidence among older adults. However, RA also occurs in children and young adults. An estimated 1.3 million U.S. adults, or 0.6% of the population, have RA (National Institute of Arthritis and Musculoskeletal and Skin Diseases [NIAMS], 2014). (For further discussion of

this condition, refer to the exemplar on RA in the module on Immunity.)

Ankylosing spondylitis, which primarily affects the spine and SI joints, is another debilitating inflammatory disorder. The Centers for Disease Control and Prevention (CDC)'s National Health and Nutrition Examination Study (NHANES) estimates that at least 2.7 million adults in the United States have this form of inflammatory arthritis (Spondylitis Association of America, 2012).

Each year in the United States, 80,000 children develop appendicitis. In 50% of pediatric cases, the patient has a positive family history of appendicitis. The incidence of ruptured appendix is 30% in children, with a higher incidence in children under 5 years of age (Cleveland Clinic, 2013).

Alterations and Therapies
Inflammation

ALTERATION	DESCRIPTION/ DEFINITION	MANIFESTATIONS	INTERVENTIONS/TREATMENTS
Pain	An unpleasant feeling caused by damaging stimuli; subjective experience described by the patient	■ Acute or chronic pain; onset, location, intensity, etiology, aggravating, or alleviating factors described by patient or caregiver	■ Analgesics (acetaminophen, NSAIDs, opioids) ■ Treatment of underlying cause of pain ■ Heat/ice, distraction, massage, and relaxation techniques

Edema	Swelling caused by fluid in the body's tissues
	    Peripheral edema: swelling of the limbs
	    Ascites: edema of the abdomen
	    Pulmonary edema: fluid accumulation in the lungs
	    Pleural effusion: edema in the space around the lungs
		■ Swelling or puffiness of skin, stretched skin, shortness of breath (pulmonary edema), decreased mobility, dimple in skin after pressure	■ Diuretics
			■ Reduced salt intake
			■ Treatment of underlying cause of edema
			■ Assessment of medications for potential adverse effects
			■ Movement
			■ Elevation
			■ Compression

Heat	Increased local or systemic temperature	■ Elevated body temperature, localized skin warmth and redness	■ Antipyretics ■ Application of ice or cool packs
Impaired function	Inability to use the tissue or organ efficiently	■ Decreased mobility of joint, difficulty breathing, pain during use, altered mental status, decreased peripheral oxygenation, impaired sensory function, impaired nutrition, altered urination, fatigue	■ Treatment of underlying condition ■ Physical therapy ■ Analgesics ■ Adequate sleep/rest ■ Administration of oxygen ■ Administration of parenteral nutrition ■ Dialysis
Altered oxygenation	Inadequate oxygen intake, decreased ability to expel carbon dioxide, inadequate delivery of oxygen to tissues	■ Cyanosis, labored breathing, dyspnea, changes in arterial blood gas (ABG), abnormal lung sounds, chest tightness, inability to clear sputum from lungs, hypotension, heart arrhythmia, fatigue	■ Treatment of underlying condition (e.g., infection, heart condition, chronic lung disease) ■ Administration of oxygen, bronchodilators, and other medications as prescribed ■ Encouragement of expectoration ■ Adequate sleep/rest ■ Monitoring of ABG and vitals
Infection	Invasion of the body by microorganisms such as bacteria and viruses	■ Inflammation, pain, mucus production, purulent drainage, hyperthermia, malaise, nausea, vomiting, diarrhea, headache	■ Antibiotics or antivirals ■ Antipyretics ■ Analgesics ■ Adequate sleep/rest ■ Adequate fluids/nutrition ■ Good wound hygiene ■ Surgical removal of infected part (e.g., appendectomy, tonsillectomy, amputation)

Genetic Considerations and Nonmodifiable Risk Factors

Genetic considerations and risk factors vary depending on the nature of the inflammatory disorder. Native and Mexican Americans are at increased risk for gallstones. Family history and female gender are also associated with increased risk. African Americans are more likely than Caucasians to develop nephritis as a complication of SLE and tend to develop nephritis earlier in the course of disease (Brent, 2015). Family history is also associated with peptic ulcer disease (PUD), although diet and other modifiable risk factors typically are involved.

RA occurs among individuals of all races and ethnic groups. Recent research has identified a number of genes that may promote the development of RA in some individuals. Women are 2–3 times more likely than men to develop RA (NIAMS, 2014).

Concepts Related to Inflammation

When bacteria or a virus enters the body and causes an infection, it triggers the inflammatory response. The normal process of inflammation neutralizes the antigen and initiates healing. Widespread infection prompts a widespread inflammatory response, the manifestations of which include generalized pain and fever. A localized infection results in a limited inflammatory response that causes redness and tenderness at the affected site. An acute inflammatory response usually resolves when the invading pathogen is eradicated. When acute inflammation persists, chronic inflammation may develop. With chronic inflammation, the inflammatory response may be disproportionate to the initial insult and can lead to greater damage than would be expected from the initial cause. Examples of chronic inflammatory disorders include Crohn disease and ulcerative colitis.

Many of the blood cells and components of the inflammatory response are mediated by the immune system, which also protects the body from harm. In autoimmune diseases, inflammation and immune responses are mistakenly initiated against normal healthy tissue. The symptoms of an autoimmune disease depend on the tissue affected. In asthma, the inflammatory response causes constriction of smooth muscle in the airways and increased mucus production, resulting in decreased oxygenation (see the exemplar on Asthma in the module on Oxygenation). The narrowed airway requires the patient to exert more effort to move air in and out of the lungs. In gastrointestinal (GI) disorders such as IBD, ulcerative colitis, appendicitis, and cholecystitis patients may experience various symptoms related to inflammation. For example, the inflammation characteristic of appendicitis causes profuse lower abdominal pain and tenderness. Nausea and vomiting (often with sudden onset) are common (Kumamoto et al., 2015; National Library of Medicine, 2015; Samulkorpi, Mentula, & Leppaniemi, 2014). The renal system inflammatory diseases include nephritis, lupus nephritis, and glomerulonephritis, which may affect patients of all ages (Brent, 2015; Parmar, 2015).

The Concepts Related to Inflammation feature links some, but not all, of the concepts integral to inflammation. They are presented in alphabetical order.

Case Study » Part 1

Ryan Blake is a 29-year-old man. He is married with two children under the age of 5. Seven years ago, Mr. Blake was diagnosed with distal colitis characterized by inflammation below the descending colon. Mr. Blake has maintained remission of symptoms with the use of a mesalamine suppository nightly. As the nurse conducting the initial interview and assessment at his gastroenterologist's office, you ascertain that Mr. Blake is experiencing an acute onset of bloody diarrhea and for the past 7 days has experienced an average of five bowel movements per day. In addition, he has rectal urgency, tenesmus (chronic sense of needing to have a bowel movement), and abdominal pain. A complete blood count (CBC) revealed a hematocrit (HCT) of 39%. Vital signs are temperature 99.8°F oral; pulse 92 bpm; respirations 18/min; and BP 130/78 mmHg. Mr. Blake currently weighs 180 pounds, a loss of 6 pounds in the past 2 weeks.

Mr. Blake is prescribed mesalamine oral tablets in addition to continued use of the mesalamine suppository. Remission is not achieved, so prednisone (60 mg per day) is added until symptoms are controlled; then the dose is tapered to discontinuation. After remission, Mr. Blake will be started on maintenance mesalamine rectally and orally.

Clinical Reasoning Questions Level I

1. Why is a mesalamine suppository used daily instead of an oral preparation?
2. Why has Mr. Blake lost weight?
3. Why is prednisone prescribed for Mr. Blake?

Clinical Reasoning Questions Level II

4. Identify two nursing diagnoses that are appropriate for inclusion in the nursing plan of care for Mr. Blake.
5. Why has oral mesalamine been added to Mr. Blake's regimen?
6. What adverse effects associated with oral mesalamine should Mr. Blake understand?

Health Promotion

Preventing excessive inflammatory response generally involves avoidance. Individuals with hypersensitivity should avoid known triggers (e.g., dust, pollen, animal dander). Individuals with IBD or PUD should avoid foods or beverages that trigger inflammation. Hand hygiene is a primary method of preventing infection that can result in inflammation.

Modifiable Risk Factors

For Crohn disease, ways to lower the risk of triggering a flare-up include a diet low in refined sugars, increased fiber intake, and smoking cessation (National Institute of Diabetes and Digestive and Kidney Diseases [NIDDK], 2014). Gallstone formation risk can be lowered by maintaining an appropriate weight, consuming a diet high in fiber and low in fat, and avoiding rapid weight loss (NIDDK, 2012a). There are several risk factors for nephritis, including diabetes mellitus, hypertension, overuse of NSAIDs, and drug abuse. Patients with diabetes or hypertension can reduce their risk by following their treatment protocols, including maintaining a healthy diet.

Dietary Factors

While consumers have been told that a low-fat diet is a healthy diet, experts suggest that healthy fats are a necessary part of a healthy diet (McCulloch, 2014; Tweed, 2013) and that replacing the fats in low-fat foods with carbohydrates

Concepts Related to
Inflammation

CONCEPT	RELATIONSHIP TO INFLAMMATION	NURSING IMPLICATIONS
Immunity	Foreign substance activates an immune response; in abnormal response, body perceives normal tissue as a foreign object and initiates an attack against that tissue; inflammation is uncontrollable.	■ Be alert for signs and symptoms (S/Sx) of anaphylaxis: hives, itching, alterations in skin color, airway constriction, weak and rapid pulse, nausea, and dizziness. ■ Patient complains of (c/o) joint pain and stiffness, fatigue, and shortness of breath. ■ Assess for mentation, patent airway, and known allergies. ■ *Anticipate:* administration of epinephrine, oxygen, antihistamines, cortisone, beta-agonists, and analgesics; blood tests; x-ray to determine causative factor.
Infection	Pathogen triggers activation of inflammatory and immune responses; WBCs are attracted to pathogen with increased WBC production; goal is to destroy invading pathogen.	■ Be alert to S/Sx of hyperthermia, malaise, pain and discomfort, purulent drainage, and excess sputum production. ■ Of particular concern in patients with altered skin or tissue integrity are chronic respiratory disorders and neuropathy. ■ *Anticipate:* blood test for WBC and differential, culture, and serum albumin; treatment includes possible antipyretics and anti-infectives.
Mood and Affect	Corticosteroids, which many patients with inflammation may be prescribed, may cause mood changes, euphoria, depression, or severe mental instability (Adams, Holland, & Urban, 2017).	■ Be alert to signs of mood swings or unusual changes in mood. ■ Teach the family to be alert to and to promptly report the signs of excessive mood swings or unusual changes in mood.
Oxygenation	Exposure to allergen or infection (bronchitis, pneumonia) results in abnormal inflammatory response resulting in airway edema, bronchoconstriction, and increased mucus production.	■ Patient c/o coughing, wheezing, dyspnea, and chest tightness. ■ Be alert for S/Sx of inadequate oxygenation: cyanosis, changes in ABG, labored breathing, abnormal lung sounds, and inability to clear sputum. ■ *Anticipate:* administration of epinephrine, bronchodilators, antihistamines, and anti-inflammatory medications. ■ Continuously monitor oxygen saturation using pulse oximetry; administer oxygen as needed. ■ May assess airflow through use of pulmonary function testing.
Safety	If corticosteroids are abruptly stopped, adrenal insufficiency and crisis may occur with profound hypotension, tachycardia, and other adverse effects.	■ Teach the patient corticosteroid treatment protocol. ■ Teach the importance of gradual tapering of corticosteroids, as prescribed by the healthcare provider. ■ Teach the patient to contact the healthcare provider if unable to take medication for 1 day or longer due to an illness. ■ Be alert to signs of adverse effects in the event the medication has been abruptly stopped.

can result in blood glucose elevation. Food intolerances, which are different than food allergies, can result in inflammation appearing in various bodily systems, such as skin problems, headaches, joint pain, weight gain, and so forth (Yates, 2012). To identify what foods are causing inflammatory responses, a patient may try to keep track of foods in a daily diary, and may need to have bloodwork completed to identify the source of food intolerance (Yates, 2012).

"Whole food" categories such as omega-3 fats, slow-digested carbs, antioxidant-rich foods, probiotic foods and supplements, and spices and herbs are highly recommended to prevent inflammation (Harvard Women's Health Watch, 2015; McCulloch, 2014; Tweed, 2013). Some of the specific foods that are recommended for preventing inflammation include nuts, soy, dark green leafy vegetables, tomatoes, garlic, onion, tart cherries, berries, ginger, turmeric, healthy fats, beets, olive oil, and whole grains.

Screening

The goals of early identification and treatment of inflammatory diseases include reduced mortality and effective management of the disorder. For many acute disorders that have an inflammatory component, such as appendicitis, screening is not possible. However, for some conditions, such as allergic rhinitis, skin testing identifies the allergens that trigger an inflammatory response. Likewise, a thyroid stimulating hormone (TSH) test determines if an asymptomatic patient has Hashimoto thyroiditis.

Nursing Assessment

During assessment, the nurse obtains the patient's history, conducts the physical assessment, and gathers laboratory data. Assessment for inflammation, which can affect any of the body's tissues, is guided by the area of the body involved.

Observation and Patient Interview

Prior to conducting the patient interview, the nurse must make observations of the patient's current condition. This observation should include assessment of the skin; the scalp; the eyes; the presence or absence of discharge or inflammation; the signs and symptoms of an elevated temperature, including but not limited to shivering, sweating, or complaints of feeling too warm; and signs or symptoms of respiratory difficulty, such as elevated respiratory rate, a cough or wheezing, or shortness of breath. In addition, the nurse should observe the patient for signs or symptoms of pain, such as the patient's facial expression, or indications that the patient is unable to remain comfortable in the chair or bed. These observations provide data with which to then conduct the patient interview.

When taking the patient's medical history, the nurse assesses (a) the degree to which the patient is at risk of developing inflammation and (b) any patient reports that suggest the presence of inflammation. Because inflammation can involve any organ or organ system, a thorough history is required. To identify whether the patient is at risk, the nurse reviews the patient's medical record or electronic medical record (EMR) and structures the nursing interview to collect data regarding the factors influencing the development of inflammation, especially existing conditions.

Questions to ask as part of the assessment interview may include the following:

- Do you have any pain? (If yes, assess the pain for location, intensity, type, severity, current treatments, and effectiveness of treatment.)
- Are you taking any anti-inflammatory medications such as aspirin or ibuprofen, or medications for chronic conditions?
- Have you had any recent diagnostic procedure or therapy that penetrated your skin or a body cavity?
- What past surgeries have you had?
- How would you describe your eating habits? Do you eat a variety of types of foods?
- Do you take vitamins or dietary supplements?
- On a scale of 1 to 10, how would you rate the stress you have experienced in the past 6 months?
- Have you experienced any loss of energy, loss of appetite, nausea, headache, or other signs associated with specific body systems (e.g., difficulty urinating, urinary frequency, sore throat)?

As with all history taking, the nurse must individualize the specific terms used; give examples to the patient; and use teaching techniques to validate agreement on the meaning of words according to the patient's culture, language spoken, and education or intellectual abilities.

Physical Examination

Physical assessment of the patient involves a focus on either localized inflammation or more diverse symptoms. Localized inflammation requires assessment for localized edema, pain or tenderness with palpation or movement, redness or palpable heat at the inflamed area, and reduced or absent function in the body part involved. Conditions causing more widespread inflammation, such as nephritis or allergies, may cause more diverse symptoms. Systemic manifestations of inflammation include an oral temperature greater than 38°C (100.4°F) or less than 36°C (96.8°F), pulse greater than 90 bpm, respiratory rate greater than 20 per minute (tachypnea), and WBC greater than 12,000 or greater than 10% bands.

Diagnostic Tests

A primary laboratory test ordered to detect the presence of inflammation is the erythrocyte sedimentation rate (ESR), which measures how far the erythrocyte settles in a tube over a given period of time, usually 1 hour. Normal sedimentation rate is 0–15 mm/hr for men and 0–20 mm/hr for women. The sedimentation rate may be slightly elevated in older adults. When an inflammatory process is active, the increased proportion of fibrinogen causes red blood cells to stick to one another and settle faster, causing a higher reading.

Another important diagnostic laboratory test is C-reactive protein (CRP). CRP is a protein found in the blood that is produced by the liver and fat cells in response to the inflammatory process. In the absence of liver failure, a rise in CRP levels indicates an inflammatory process somewhere in the body. CRP can also be used to evaluate the effectiveness of treatment for inflammation. Research also indicates that the CRP level can be used to assess risk for cardiac disease, as it elevates in response to arterial damage.

Other laboratory tests for inflammation are ordered based on the cause, location, and type of inflammation suspected. A WBC count with differential may be ordered to determine the presence of an infection (see **Table 10–2 》**); serum protein electrophoresis may reveal increased gamma globulin and decreased albumin, indicating SLE; and routine chemistry panels may reveal kidney involvement, abnormal liver function, or increased muscle enzymes if the muscle is involved.

Case Study 》 Part 2

After experiencing a flare-up of his symptoms, Mr. Blake returns to see his gastroenterologist. Mr. Blake informs you he is averaging several bloody bowel movements daily and complains of abdominal pain. His complaints include severe fatigue and weight loss of 8 pounds. Mr. Blake shows you the large oozing lesions on his lower legs, which were preceded by bruising. He is frustrated by his disease and the negative impact it is having on his quality of life at home and at work. Mr. Blake is fearful his uncontrolled symptoms will interfere with his receiving a promotion at work. Laboratory diagnostic test results include HCT = 29%; K+ = 3.2 mEq/L (normal range = 3.5–5.3 mEq/L); and albumin 2.8 g/dL (normal range = 3.5–5.0 dg/L). Vital signs: temperature 100.1°F oral; pulse 95 bpm; respirations 18/min; and BP 132/82 mmHg. Mr. Blake has tried prednisone at home to try to regain remission, but the use of the oral corticosteroid has not helped. The gastroenterologist orders cephalexin for 2 months for the erythema nodosum. Mr. Blake is admitted to the hospital to receive IV methylprednisolone therapy. After 7 days only partial remission is achieved. Azathioprine is ordered, and remission of symptoms is achieved. Mr. Blake's drug regimen is now mesalamine rectally and oral with azathioprine.

Clinical Reasoning Questions Level I

1. What is the most likely cause of Mr. Blake's low potassium level?
2. What is the goal of adding azathioprine to Mr. Blake's drug regimen?
3. What are other potential sites of extraintestinal manifestations of ulcerative colitis?

Clinical Reasoning Questions Level II

4. What adverse effects associated with azathioprine should you discuss with Mr. Blake?
5. Describe three nursing interventions to address Mr. Blake's psychosocial considerations.

Independent Interventions

Management of inflammation due to injury generally aims to reduce movement of the involved area and elevate to reduce edema. Antipyretics may be used if fever is involved, and anti-inflammatory medications are used as appropriate. Other causes of inflammation necessitate other, more specific treatments. For example, antibiotics may be required to treat inflammation caused by infection, and steroids may be indicated for severe systemic inflammation. Patients who are prescribed antibiotics and/or oral steroids will require medication teaching to ensure appropriate management of the treatment. Nurses working with patients facing surgical interventions need to emphasize the preparations before surgery and what to expect postoperatively (perioperative care is covered in detail in the module on Perioperative Care). Nurses also need to review dietary intake with patients to be sure they are receiving adequate nutrients to support healing, including adequate protein, carbohydrates, and vitamins. Vitamin C in particular is important in cellular repair.

Nurses working with patients experiencing inflammation should emphasize the importance of preventing further injury, taking medications as prescribed to treat or prevent illness, and maintaining adequate intake of liquids and nutrients. Family teaching may be necessary if patients need assistance with changing dressings, preventing exposure of the inflamed area to water while bathing, or any other aspects of daily living until healing occurs. Additional patient teaching during the reparative phase may be necessary to ensure that the patient does not resume activity too quickly and continues treatment until healing is complete and the patient is released by the physician. Other independent interventions include those related to alleviating discomfort and reducing inflammation (e.g., positioning, application of heat or ice) and promoting coping during healing and recovery (acute) or exacerbations (for those with chronic inflammatory conditions).

Collaborative Therapies

A chronic inflammatory state is often associated with aging and obesity. These patients may benefit from a balanced diet and exercise, which may require collaboration with a nutritionist and physical therapist. A nutritionist can advise the patient on consuming an anti-inflammatory diet that contains omega-3 fatty acids, antioxidant vitamins, and probiotics (Calder et al., 2009), while decreasing consumption of pro-inflammatory foods that contain saturated fats, cholesterol, and a high glycemic index. A physical therapist can help patients build muscle strength and increase overall physical health by encouraging exercise and physical activity

---

TABLE 10–2 The White Blood Cell and Differential Counts

Children Younger than 11 Years
Normal ranges vary depending on the age of the child. Nurses should consult the diagnostic values provided by their agency or a current, reliable reference such as the Mayo Medical Laboratory's guide, available at http://a1.mayomedicallaboratories.com/webjc/attachments/110/30a2131-complete-blood-count-normal-pediatric-values.pdf.

Adult and Child Older than 11 Years

Cell Type and Normal Value	Cause of Increased Value	Cause of Decreased Value
Total WBCs: 4500–10,000/μL (mm³)	*Leukocytosis:* infection or inflammation, leukemia, trauma or stress	*Leukopenia:* bone marrow depression, viral infections, immunosuppression, autoimmune disease, dietary deficiency
Neutrophils (segs, PMNs, or polys): *Adults:* 50–70%	*Neutrophilia:* acute infection or stress response, myelocytic leukemia, inflammatory or metabolic disorders, tissue necrosis	*Neutropenia:* bone marrow depression, viral infection, Addison disease
Eosinophils (eos): 1–3%	*Eosinophilia:* parasitic infections, allergic reactions, autoimmune disorders	*Eosinopenia:* stress, certain drugs
Basophils (basos): 0.4–1%	*Basophilia:* hypersensitivity responses, leukemia, splenectomy, hypothyroidism	*Basopenia:* allergic reaction or acute infection (indicated by decreased basophils) *Note:* Because normal levels are low, decreased counts can only be detected by absolute counts.
Monocytes (monos): 4–6%	*Monocytosis:* chronic inflammatory disorders, infections, leukemia, Hodgkin disease	*Monocytopenia:* corticosteroid therapy
Lymphocytes (lymphs): 25–35%	*Lymphocytosis:* infections, viral infections, lymphocytic leukemia	*Lymphocytopenia:* bone marrow depression, immunodeficiency, Hodgkin disease

Source: Data from Kee, J. L. (2014). *Laboratory and diagnostic tests with nursing implications* (9th ed.). Upper Saddle River, NJ: Prentice Hall; Van Leeuwen, A. M., Poelhuis-Leth, D. J., & Bladh, M. L. (2013). *Laboratory diagnostic tests with nursing implications* (5th ed.). Philadelphia, PA: F. A. Davis.

Box 10–2
Management of Corticosteroids

Corticosteroids are powerful medications that need careful management. Patients must understand the need to take the medication as ordered, and to not miss any dosages, to prevent physical safety issues. Corticosteroids carry a risk of side effects that can be severe and even life threatening. The side effects vary depending on whether the corticosteroid is administered orally or by inhalation. Duration of therapy also is a factor.

Side effects of corticosteroids given orally as short-term therapy (and which typically resolve once therapy concludes) include glaucoma (elevated pressure in the eyes); fluid retention, which causes swelling in the lower legs; hypertension; mood swings; and weight gain (fat deposits in the abdomen, face, and the back of the neck).

Side effects of corticosteroids given by mouth for long-term treatment include cataracts (clouding of the lens in one or both eyes), hyperglycemia, increased risk of infections, osteoporosis, increased risk of fractures, suppression of adrenal gland hormone production, bruising, thin skin, delayed wound healing, and growth suppression in children.

Side effects of long-term steroid use may take additional time and adjunctive therapies to resolve. Some adverse effects, such as growth suppression and osteoporosis, may not resolve. Oral thrush and hoarseness may result from use of inhaled and nebulized corticosteroids. These can be avoided easily by rinsing and gargling with water following medication administration.

Patient teaching related to use of corticosteroids includes the following:

- Take medication as directed, and do not discontinue without consulting the provider.
- Notify the provider if adverse or Cushingoid effects occur.
- Take with food or milk to decrease GI effects.
- Monitor weight. Notify the provider of a gain of more than 5 pounds.
- Moderate salt intake, and avoid foods and snacks high in sodium. Increase intake of foods high in potassium, such as fruits and vegetables and lean meats.

Sources: Based on Adams, M. P., Holland, L. N., & Urban, C. (2017). *Pharmacology for nurses: A pathophysiologic approach* (5th ed.). Hoboken, NJ: Pearson Education; Cleveland Clinic. (2015). *Corticosteroids*. Retrieved from http://my.clevelandclinic.org/health/drugs_devices_supplements/hic_Corticosteroids; Mayo Clinic. (2016). *Corticosteroids*. http://www.mayoclinic.org/drugs-supplements/corticosteroid-oral-route-parenteral-route/description/drg-20070491

(Addison et al., 2012). Physical therapy can also help patients regain the use of limbs that have been underused because of loss of function related to inflammation.

Complementary Health Approaches

Management of nutrition is a vital part of managing GI inflammation as well as other similar illnesses that affect patients' ability to meet their appropriate nutritional needs. Along with dietary changes, some patients are helped with homeopathy that is effective in lowering inflammation, such as *Arnica montana* (Iannitti et al., 2016). Supplements that can help reduce inflammation include omega-3 fish oils; flaxseed oil; vitamins C, E, and D; and an anti-inflammatory plant oil called gamma-linolenic acid (GLA) (University of Maryland Medical Center, 2015). Mind–body medicine has been suggested for management of respiratory illnesses with children and adults (McClaffery, 2014). Patients who plan to add integrative therapy to their treatment management should discuss their plans with their primary healthcare provider.

Surgery

Treatment for many inflammatory conditions involves collaboration with surgeons. For example, patients with ulcerative colitis may require surgery to remove the colon and rectum. Patients with gallbladder inflammation caused by recurrent gallstones or other conditions may undergo a cholecystectomy. Patients with severe infection and inflammation of extremities may require amputation of the damaged part to avoid life-threatening sepsis. When a patient's condition is treated with surgery, the nurse is responsible for pre- and postoperative care and patient teaching.

Pharmacologic Therapy

Pharmacologic therapies are aimed at reducing the inflammatory response and reducing pain associated with the symptoms of inflammation. Common medications include NSAIDs, which have fewer adverse effects than the more powerful anti-inflammatory corticosteroids. NSAIDs, in addition to their anti-inflammatory actions, are also analgesics and antipyretics that help not only to reduce inflammation but also to minimize its effects. Corticosteroids are normally administered when inflammation is more severe or is life threatening, and their use must be managed carefully (see **Box 10–2 »**). See the Medications feature for a list of medications used to treat inflammation.

Case Study » Part 3

Mr. Blake's condition worsens, and he goes to the emergency department. As the triage nurse, you are admitting Mr. Blake. He reports that he is experiencing more than 10 bowel movements daily with continuous bleeding. His abdomen is distended, painful, and tender. Vital signs are temperature 101.1°F oral; pulse 110 bpm; respirations 22/min; and BP 120/60 mmHg. Lab results include HCT 28% and albumin 2.6 g/dL. You note that Mr. Blake is experiencing shortness of breath, and his extremities are cool to the touch. Results of an abdominal x-ray indicate 7 cm dilation of his transverse colon. Mr. Blake is admitted with the diagnosis of fulminant ulcerative colitis with toxic megacolon and is scheduled for emergency surgery. Prior to surgery Mr. Blake receives a blood transfusion and IV fluids to replenish electrolytes. Mr. Blake undergoes an ileal pouch–anal anastomosis (IPAA) procedure and recovers without complications.

Clinical Reasoning Questions Level I

1. Which of Mr. Blake's signs and symptoms indicate he will most likely be hospitalized?
2. Why does Mr. Blake have low HCT and albumin levels?

Clinical Reasoning Questions Level II

3. Explain why surgery can potentially cure ulcerative colitis but can offer only symptomatic relief in Crohn disease.
4. What are potential complications from the IPAA surgical procedure?
5. What type and frequency of cancer screening are recommended for patients with ulcerative colitis?

Medications
Inflammatory Diseases

CLASSIFICATION AND DRUG EXAMPLES	MECHANISMS OF ACTION/ DOSAGE	NURSING CONSIDERATIONS
NSAIDs *Drug examples:* Aspirin (ASA) Celecoxib (Celebrex) Ibuprofen Naproxen	Analgesic, antipyretic, and anti-inflammatory properties act by inhibiting the synthesis of prostaglandin precursors. NSAIDs block inflammation by reversibly inhibiting cyclooxygenase (COX-1 and COX-2), the key enzyme in the biosynthesis of prostaglandins. They are also used for colorectal polyps, ankylosing spondylitis, vascular headache, and Paget disease. *Dosages:* ASA: 350–650 mg Q4h orally (max: 4g/day) for pain or fever. 3.6–5.4 g/day in 4–6 divided doses for arthritis conditions Celecoxib (Celebrex): 100–400 mg bid oral (max: 800 mg/day) Ibuprofen: 400–800 mg tid–qid orally (max: 3200 mg/day) Naproxen: 200–500 mg bid orally (max: 1000 mg/day)	• Administer with food or milk. • These drugs are pregnancy category C. • They are contraindicated in patients with peptic ulcer disease or who are taking anticoagulants. • They may interact with certain diuretics, causing decreased effectiveness of NSAIDs. • They may increase clotting time. • Use cautiously in older adults because of their reduced kidney and liver function.

Corticosteroids (glucocorticosteroids)
 	
Drug examples:
Betamethasone
Dexamethasone
Hydrocortisone
Methylprednisolone
Prednisone
	These drugs have potent anti-inflammatory and immunosuppressant properties for severe inflammation.
	
	They mimic natural hormones secreted by the adrenal cortex and affect almost all body systems.
	
	They have short- and long-term use indications.
	
	They are also used as an antiemetic in chemotherapy regimens, lupus nephritis, and multiple sclerosis.
	
	Dosages:
	Betamethasone: 0.6–7.2 mg/day orally
	Cortisone: 20–300 mg/day orally or intramuscular (IM) in divided doses
	Dexamethasone: 0.25–4 mg/bid–qid orally
	Hydrocortisone: 10–320 mg/day orally, in 3–4 divided doses
	Methylprednisolone: 15–800 mg/day intravenous (IV) or IM, in 3–4 divided doses (max: 2g/day)
	Prednisone: 5–60 mg 1–4 times per day orally
		• These drugs are contraindicated in patients:
		  a. With a systemic infection (will reduce immune response)
		  b. With systemic fungal infections
		  c. When administered with live virus vaccines
		  d. With PUD, glaucoma or cataracts, diabetes, or psychiatric disorders.
		• Obtain baseline vital signs and weight; monitor both routinely during therapy. Do not discontinue abruptly.
		• Administer as ordered. For daily or alternate-day dosing, administer in the morning to reduce adrenal cortisone suppression.
		• These drugs are pregnancy category C.
		• If administered IM, give deep IM to avoid possible atrophy or abscess. Avoid deltoid muscle.
		• Monitor blood glucose levels, changes in mood, and signs of edema or Cushing syndrome if used long term.
		• Monitor for adverse effects:
		  a. Increased susceptibility to infection and masking of early signs of infection
		  b. Hyperglycemia, hypokalemia, hypertension, signs of heart failure
		  c. Peptic ulcer formation and possible GI hemorrhage.

Opioid Analgesics *Drug examples:* Hydromorphone Fentanyl Morphine Oxycodone	These drugs are potent analgesics. They block receptors in the brain to achieve analgesia.	• Take with food if GI upset occurs. • These drugs are pregnancy category C. • Reduce dose for renal impairment. • Monitor respiratory rate. See the module on Pain for further information about analgesics.
Natural Therapies *Drug examples:* Fish oil Omega-3	Natural therapies have anti-inflammatory activity. They are also used for elevated triglyceride levels.	• These drugs are pregnancy category C. • They interact with anticoagulants, aspirin, and other NSAIDs. • Adverse side effects include the potential for bruising and nosebleeds.

Source: Data from Adams, M. P., Holland, L. N., & Urban, C. (2017). *Pharmacology for nurses: A pathophysiologic approach* (5th ed.). Hoboken, NJ: Pearson Education.

Lifespan Considerations

Inflammation in Children and Adolescents

Several differences in anatomy and physiology influence the effects of inflammation on children compared to adults (Bagus, Kahar, & Wardhani, 2014; Murer et al., 2014; Nachalon et al., 2014):

- In pediatric patients, structural differences in the airway increase the risk for obstruction, especially in the event of airway inflammation. In comparison to adults, children have a larger tongue relative to the oral cavity, decreased airway muscle tone, a shorter epiglottis, a more anteriorly positioned larynx, a shorter and narrower trachea, and prominent adenoid and lymphoid tissue. These differences are especially evident when the child is supine; because of the child's proportionately larger head and occiput compared to those of adults, hyperflexion of the neck further narrows the airway.

- Fewer and smaller lung alveoli equate to a reduction in the surface area available for gas exchange in children. In addition, the decreased elastic recoil pressure of the alveoli increases the risk of alveolar collapse during respiratory distress. The increased energy needed to achieve adequate oxygenation during acute airway inflammation or anaphylaxis may lead to fatigue and respiratory failure in infants.

- Glomerular filtration, as well as the kidneys' ability to dilute and concentrate urine, is not fully developed in infants. As a result, the infant's renal system is less capable of compensating for fluctuations in fluid volume than is the adult's.

- Because of the small size of the child, absolute volumes of fluid loss represent a larger proportion of total body fluid. For example, a 1 L fluid loss in a 30 lb child represents 7.3% dehydration, whereas the same fluid loss in a 180 lb man represents only 1.2% dehydration.

- Changes in excitation–contraction coupling, left ventricular mass, and the high contractile state of the heart reduce the pediatric patient's sympathetic nervous system response to changes in blood volume and stress. While adults typically respond to hypovolemia with a compensatory increase in heart rate, tachycardia often is a late symptom of hypovolemia in children.

- GI inflammation that reduces nutrient absorption affects children more than adults. Children have higher metabolic rates and generally have less stored fat, so decreased absorption of nutrients has more immediate detrimental effects on growth, body weight, energy levels, bone and muscle strength, and overall health.

- The child's immune system response to insult differs significantly from that of the adult. In pediatric patients, macrophages are more responsive to pro-inflammatory molecules, increasing the production of additional inflammatory mediators. In addition, infants are less able than adults to produce anti-inflammatory mediators.

Inflammatory disorders are often related to internal organs, including the GI tract, kidneys, lungs, and gallbladder.

Children are often too young to understand the implications of assessment of internal organs, especially as it relates to the discomfort of invasive procedures. For example, assessment of adults with respiratory inflammation often involves bronchoscopy or bronchoalveolar lavage. These procedures are far too invasive and uncomfortable for regular use in children, so less invasive techniques, such as analysis of exhaled breath condensates, should be used if available and appropriate (Durani, 2014; van de Kant et al., 2012).

Negative blood tests should be interpreted with caution in children with potential inflammatory disorders. Normal blood test results are common for children with inflammatory disorders such as IBD (Kopylov et al., 2015) and acute glomerulonephritis (Welch, 2012). False positives may also occur for some laboratory tests, such as an increase in alkaline phosphatase in healthy children and adolescents who are still growing (Shaffer, 2012).

Likewise, IBD can be detected in children through sequencing of fecal microbiota rather than the more invasive colonoscopy, which many physicians are reluctant to perform on children (Papa et al., 2012). Fecal calprotectin is also a noninvasive diagnostic test for IBD in children (Wattanabe et al., 2014). Noninvasive techniques for analyzing kidney function include monitoring voiding for volume and frequency as well as analyzing urine for electrolytes, protein, and blood.

If visualization of the inflamed organ is necessary, ultrasound may be a viable option for many disorders rather than endoscopy, especially when used in conjunction with a contrast agent specific for inflammation such as microbubbles (Alzaraa et al., 2012). Other noninvasive imaging tools include x-ray, CT scan, and MRI. Visual examination via inspection is an appropriate option for inflammation of the skin, upper airway, ears, and eyes. Internal inflammation may also be evident upon external inspection based on the presence of edema, swelling, or jaundice.

Recent studies have explored the association between inflammation and children's illnesses. One study found that the surgical intervention of adenotonsillectomy results in enhanced somatic growth in young children that correlates with a decrease in systemic inflammation (Nachalon et al., 2014). The relationship between inflammation of adipose tissue in children who are obese and future insulin resistance was noted by Landgraf and colleagues (2015).

Inflammation in Pregnant Women

Recent research has focused on the influence of inflammation on pregnancy outcomes. One study found that maternal physical activity may reduce inflammation during pregnancy in women who are obese and that maternal lipid metabolism is related to systemic inflammation (Tinius et al., 2016). Preeclampsia is an inflammatory-mediated hypertensive disorder of pregnancy, and a recent study found that preeclampsia is associated with alterations in the inflammatory response postpartum, mostly independent of other cardiac risk markers (van Rijn et al., 2016). A relationship between an impaired inflammatory response due to chronic anxiety among African American women may contribute to race disparities in pregnancy outcomes (Catov et al., 2015). Wu, Chen, and Jiang (2015) found a relationship between pregnancy and the occurrence of gingival inflammation.

Inflammation in Older Adults

Inflammatory markers (e.g., C-reactive protein, IL-6, TNFα) may be increased in older adults and individuals who are obese; both of these states are associated with a low-grade pro-inflammatory condition. This increase in inflammation may not be linked to a specific disease (e.g., gallbladder disease, asthma, IBD) but instead is an indicator of poor overall health that makes these individuals more susceptible to chronic illnesses and cognitive decline (Akbaraly et al., 2013). A recent study found a significant association between frailty and a gene responsible for the inflammatory response (Ghezzi & Rajkumar, 2015). Another study found that coexisting depressive syndrome in patients with mild cognitive impairment through common inflammatory pathways may result in intensification of psychiatric disorders (Gorska-Ciebiada et al., 2015). Chronic inflammation has been associated with a range of unhealthy aging phenomenon and a decreased likelihood of successful aging (Akbaraly et al., 2013). Cognitive decline in older adults is associated with the presence of inflammation (Ghosh, Biswas, & Banerjee, 2015).

REVIEW The Concept of Inflammation

RELATE Link the Concepts

Linking the concept of inflammation with the concept of immunity:

1. Describe how inflammation affects the immune system.
2. What preventive measures would you recommend to reduce the risk of chronic inflammation?

Linking the concept of inflammation with the concept of oxygenation:

3. How does the inflammatory response adversely affect a patient's airway?
4. What type of medications would you anticipate administering to reduce inflammation and improve respiratory function?

READY Go to Volume 3 Clinical Nursing Skills

- SKILL 1.1 — Appearance and Mental Status: Assessing
- SKILLS 1.5–1.9 — Vital Signs
- SKILL 1.10 — Abdomen: Assessing
- SKILL 1.27 — Thorax and Lungs: Assessing
- SKILL 2.11 — Medications: Preparing and Administering
- SKILLS 2.36–2.38 — Intravenous Medications
- SKILL 3.1 — Pain in Newborn, Infant, Child, or Adult: Assessing
- SKILL 4.5 — Urine Specimen, Routine, 24-Hour: Obtaining
- SKILL 5.1 — Intake and Output: Measuring
- SKILL 10.2 — Diet, Therapeutic: Managing
- SKILL 10.5 — Nutrition: Assessing
- SKILLS 10.9–10.12 — Nasogastric Tube
- SKILL 11.8 — Oxygen Delivery Systems: Using

REFER Go to Pearson MyLab Nursing and eText

- Additional review materials

REFLECT Apply Your Knowledge

Mr. Alan Thomas, age 68, was admitted to the surgical unit following an open appendectomy. He had a urinary catheter placed while in the operating room. He is awake, alert, and oriented. Mr. Thomas has orders to get out of bed and ambulate, but he complains of severe pain in his lower abdomen, and his temperature is 100.5°F according to the last vital signs taken. The nurse checks Mr. Thomas's morning labwork and notes his WBC is elevated at 14.3. The nurse calls the surgeon, who orders an IV antibiotic to begin immediately and plans to assess the patient after her current surgery is completed.

1. Why would Mr. Thomas's WBC be elevated?
2. Why did the nurse call the surgeon after she assessed the patient?
3. During bedside shift report, what will the nurse recommend to the oncoming nurse if the patient continues to have pain and an elevated temperature?
4. If the fever continues in the next 24 hours, what will the nurse need to do next?

≫ Exemplar 10.A Appendicitis

Exemplar Learning Outcomes

10.A Analyze appendicitis as it relates to inflammation.

- Describe the pathophysiology of appendicitis.
- Describe the etiology of appendicitis.
- Compare the risk factors for and prevention of appendicitis.
- Identify the clinical manifestations of appendicitis.
- Summarize diagnostic tests and therapies used by interprofessional teams in the collaborative care of an individual with appendicitis.
- Differentiate care of patients with appendicitis across the lifespan.
- Apply the nursing process in providing culturally competent care to an individual with appendicitis.

Exemplar Key Terms

Appendectomy, *683*
Appendicitis, *682*
Fecalith, *682*
Perforation, *682*
Peritonitis, *682*

Overview

Appendicitis, inflammation of the vermiform appendix, is a common cause of acute abdominal pain. In many cases, appendicitis treatment involves emergency abdominal surgery. Appendicitis affects over 7% of the population; it can occur at any age, but it is more common in adolescents and young adults (Craig, 2015).

Pathophysiology and Etiology

Pathophysiology

The appendix is a tubelike pouch attached to the cecum just below the ileocecal valve. It is usually located in the right iliac region, in an area designated as McBurney point (see **Figure 10–2A ▶▶**). The function of the appendix is not fully understood, although it is regularly filled with and emptied of digested food.

Obstruction of the proximal lumen of the appendix is apparent in most acutely inflamed appendices. Following obstruction, the appendix becomes distended with fluid secreted by its mucosa. Pressure within the lumen of the appendix increases, impairs its blood supply, and leads to inflammation, edema, ulceration, and infection. The purulent exudate formed causes further distention of the appendix. If treatment is not initiated, tissue necrosis and gangrene result within 24–36 hours, leading to **perforation** (rupture). Perforation allows the contents of the GI tract to

flow into the peritoneal space of the abdomen, resulting in **peritonitis**, inflammation and bacterial infection of the entire abdominal area. Appendicitis is classified as simple, gangrenous, or perforated, depending on the stage in the process. In simple appendicitis, the appendix is inflamed but intact. In gangrenous appendicitis, areas of tissue necrosis and microscopic perforations are present in the appendix. A perforated appendix shows evidence of gross perforation and contamination of the peritoneal cavity.

Etiology

Appendicitis almost always results from an obstruction in the appendiceal lumen. The obstruction is often caused by a hard mass of feces (**fecalith**). Other obstructive causes include a calculus or stone, parasites (e.g., pinworms), edema of lymphoid tissue, a tumor, or a foreign body. Continued secretion of mucus following acute obstruction of the lumen increases pressure, causing ischemia, inflammation, cellular death, and ulceration.

Risk Factors and Prevention

Adolescent boys are at greatest risk, although fecaliths can occur in both genders at any age. Individuals whose diet is low in fiber or high in carbohydrates are at greater risk for developing fecaliths. GI infections also promote appendicitis.

Appendicitis cannot be prevented; however, certain dietary habits may reduce the risk of developing this condition. Eating foods that contain high fiber content, such as fresh fruits and vegetables, decreases the incidence of appendicitis (National Library of Medicine, 2015).

Clinical Manifestations

The initial characteristic manifestation of acute appendicitis is continuous, mild, generalized or upper abdominal pain. Over the next 4 hours, the pain intensifies and localizes in the right lower quadrant of the abdomen. Pain associated with appendicitis is aggravated by moving, walking, or coughing. On palpation, localized and rebound tenderness are noted at McBurney point. Rebound tenderness is demonstrated by relief of pain with direct palpation of McBurney point, followed by pain on release of pressure. Extension or internal rotation of the right hip increases the pain. In addition to pain, a low-grade fever, anorexia, nausea, and vomiting are often present.

Because of less acute pain and local tenderness in older adults, the diagnosis is delayed. The course of acute appendicitis is more virulent in older adults, so complications can develop sooner and result in increased mortality (Omari, et al., 2014). Pregnant women may develop right lower quadrant, periumbilical, or right subcostal (under the rib cage) pain due to possible displacement of the appendix by the distended uterus. In adolescent and young adult women, symptoms must be differentiated from those associated with ovulation (mittelschmerz), ruptured ectopic pregnancy, and pelvic inflammatory disease.

Possible complications related to acute appendicitis include perforation, peritonitis, and abscess (accumulation of pus). Perforation is manifested by increased pain and a high fever. It can lead to a small, localized abscess; local peritonitis; or significant generalized peritonitis.

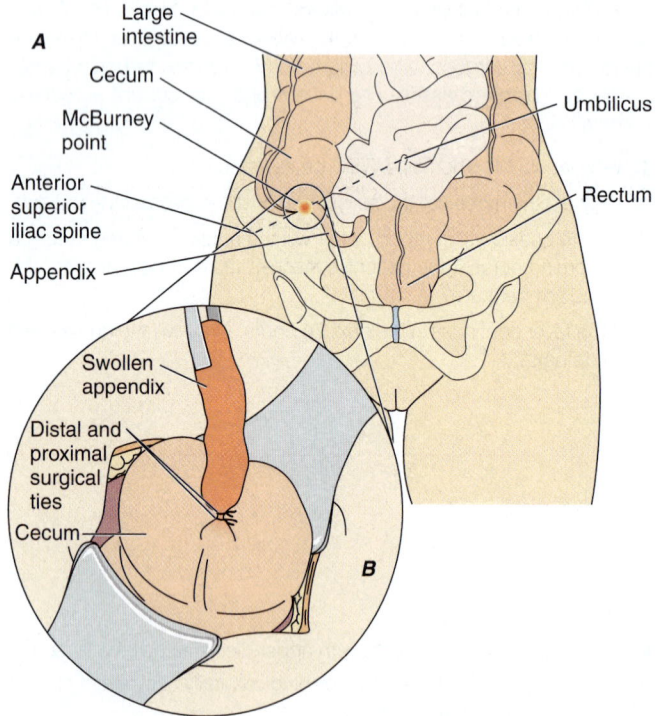

Figure 10–2 ▶▶ **A.** McBurney point, located midway between the umbilicus and the anterior iliac crest in the right lower quadrant. It is the usual side for localized pain and rebound tenderness due to appendicitis. **B.** In an appendectomy, the appendix and cecum are brought through the incision to the surface of the abdomen. The base of the appendix is clamped and ligated; the appendix is then removed.

Clinical Manifestations and Therapies
Appendicitis

ETIOLOGY	CLINICAL MANIFESTATIONS	CLINICAL THERAPIES
Peritonitis resulting from appendix rupture with bowel contents leaking into the abdominal cavity	■ High fever, acute severe abdominal pain, abdominal distention, resultant death if not treated aggressively and rapidly	■ Removal of the ruptured appendix ■ Antibiotics ■ Fluid resuscitation ■ Supportive treatment to maintain vital signs
Chronic appendicitis	■ Chronic recurrent abdominal pain over several months	■ Appendectomy ■ Pain management

A less common disorder is chronic appendicitis, characterized by chronic abdominal pain and recurrent acute attacks at intervals of several months or more. Other conditions, such as IBD and renal disorders, often cause manifestations attributed to chronic appendicitis.

Collaboration

The acutely inflamed appendix can perforate within 24 hours, so rapid diagnosis and treatment are important. Because of this urgency and the low incidence of surgical complications, diagnostic testing and preoperative treatment are limited. The patient is admitted to the hospital, and IV fluids are initiated. Oral food and fluids are withheld until a diagnosis is confirmed.

Diagnostic Tests

Diagnostic and laboratory tests help confirm the diagnosis and rule out other possible causes for the manifestations. Abdominal ultrasound is the most effective test for diagnosing acute appendicitis (Fallon et al., 2015). Ultrasound examination has reduced the incidence of exploratory surgery. It is particularly useful with patients who have atypical symptoms (e.g., older adults). Other diagnostic tests used to diagnose appendicitis and rule out other possible conditions include abdominal x-rays, IV pyelogram, urinalysis, and pelvic examination. In addition, a WBC count with differential is obtained. With appendicitis, the total WBC count is elevated, with an increased number of immature WBCs (bands).

Surgery

The treatment of choice for acute appendicitis is an **appendectomy**, surgical removal of the appendix. Either a laparoscopic approach (insertion of an endoscope to view abdominal contents) or laparotomy (surgical opening of the abdomen) is used for appendectomy. Laparoscopic appendectomy requires a very small incision, through which the laparoscope is inserted. This procedure has several advantages: (1) Direct visualization of the appendix allows definitive diagnosis without laparotomy, (2) postoperative hospitalization is short, (3) postoperative complications are infrequent, and (4) recovery and resumption of normal activities are rapid.

An open appendectomy is performed by laparotomy. A small transverse incision is made at McBurney point (see Figure 10–2A); the appendix is isolated and ligated (tied off) to prevent contamination of the site with bowel contents, and it is then removed (see Figure 10–2B). Laparotomy generally is used when the appendix has ruptured. It allows removal of contaminants from the peritoneal cavity by irrigation with sterile normal saline. The wound may occasionally be left unsutured for periodic irrigation. Recovery is generally uneventful.

Pharmacologic Therapy

Prior to surgery, IV fluids are given to restore or maintain vascular volume and prevent electrolyte imbalance. Antibiotic therapy with a third-generation cephalosporin, such as cefoperazone (Cefobid), cefotaxime (Claforan), ceftazidime (Fortaz), or ceftriaxone (Rocephin), is initiated prior to surgery. Third-generation cephalosporins are effective against many gram-negative bacteria. Antibiotic administration is repeated during surgery and continued for at least 48 hours postoperatively. The sudden disappearance of pain is an indication that the appendix has ruptured, so administration of strong analgesics is withheld preoperatively during assessment for this indicator. Once the diagnosis is established, an appendectomy is performed and analgesics are administered as ordered to maintain comfort.

Lifespan Considerations
Appendicitis in Children and Adolescents

Children under the age of 4 typically do not develop appendicitis. However, appendicitis in young children often progresses to rupture because they cannot accurately tell their parents how they feel and where it hurts (Boston Children's Hospital, n.d.). Common manifestations in infants include listlessness, inconsolability, vomiting, and a distended abdomen. Because appendicitis is rare in infants, its low diagnostic priority is linked to delay in diagnosis and an increase in rupture, complications, and death in the infant population (Minkes, 2013).

Cultural factors play a role in the progression of appendicitis in children. A recent study found that the perforation rate for White children was 26.7%; Black children, 35.5%; and Latino children, 36.5%. Only a small percentage of this difference was related to insurance status, income level, and age. The differences between appendicitis perforation rates that was not explained by measurable factors was two thirds for Black children and one third for Latino children compared to White children (Livingston & Fairlie, 2012).

Black children are less likely to receive adequate medication in emergency departments for pain during episodes of appendicitis (Goyal et al., 2015). Nurses should advocate for appropriate management of pain for all patients.

Appendicitis in Pregnant Women

Acute appendicitis is one of the most common surgical presentations in pregnant women, yet its management is not always clear. Appendicitis in pregnancy may be managed jointly by both the surgical and obstetric teams, which can lead to discrepant pathways that may be detrimental to the patient (Flexer, Tabib, & Peter, 2014). Therefore, appendicitis in the pregnant woman is seen as a complex problem that needs careful consideration (Kensuke et al., 2015).

One study found that MRI is useful in the diagnosis of suspected acute appendicitis during pregnancy (Burke et al., 2015). A recent study found that acute appendicitis during pregnancy can be managed successfully without any dangerous fetal outcomes (Kumamoto et al., 2015).

Appendicitis in Older Adults

Less than 30% of older adults who have appendicitis present with classic symptoms. Almost half of older patients are afebrile, half demonstrate no rebound or involuntary guarding, and one fourth have no lower right quadrant tenderness or pain (Tracy & Morrison, 2013). Instead, older adults are likely to present with confusion (Samulkorpi et al., 2014). Approximately 25–30% of older adults with appendicitis do not seek medical care until 3 or more days after the onset of symptoms. A new diagnostic scoring tool was found to prove fast and accurate in categorizing adults with suspected appendicitis and to roughly halve the need of diagnostic imaging (Samulkorpi et al., 2014).

NURSING PROCESS

Nursing management of the patient with appendicitis includes collaborative assessment, preoperative and postoperative care, and prevention of complications. Refer to the module on Perioperative Care for more information on taking care of patients who have undergone surgery for appendicitis.

Assessment

Because appendicitis can rapidly progress from inflammation to perforation, prompt assessment is vital. Obtain the following assessment data:

- *Observation and patient interview.* Current manifestations, including onset, duration, progression, and aggravating or relieving factors; most recent food or fluid intake; known medication or other allergies; current medications; and history of chronic diseases
- *Physical examination.* Vital signs, including temperature; apparent general health; abdominal shape and contour; bowel sounds; tenderness to light palpation.

SAFETY ALERT Keep the patient with suspected appendicitis NPO (nothing by mouth). Do not administer laxatives or enemas, which may cause perforation of the appendix. Do not apply heat to the abdomen, as this may increase circulation to the appendix and also cause perforation.

Diagnosis

The following nursing diagnoses may apply to the patient with appendicitis:

- *Gas Exchange, Impaired*
- *Fluid Volume, Risk for Deficient*
- *Infection, Risk for*
- *Pain, Acute*
- *Anxiety*
- *Fear.*

(NANDA-I © 2014)

Planning

The plan of care developed in collaboration with the patient and family may include the following:

- The patient will articulate any concerns about surgery prior to the event.
- The patient will articulate an understanding of the procedure, the reasons for it, and any preoperative instructions prior to arrival for surgery.
- The patient will verbalize relief from pain following administration of pain management.
- The patient will receive appropriate postoperative wound care.
- The patient will verbalize instructions for self-care prior to being discharged.

Implementation

Nursing management focuses on promoting comfort, maintaining hydration, providing emotional support, supporting respiratory function, providing care of the surgical site, and monitoring for symptoms of infection. For many patients, hospitalization for appendicitis may be their first experience with healthcare personnel beyond their usual provider. Anxiety may be heightened by the necessarily rapid-pace physical examination, diagnostic testing, and preoperative preparation. Preoperative education helps reduce anxiety. Encourage and answer any questions the patient or family may have, and provide emotional support as necessary.

Promote Effective Respiratory Gas Exchange

General anesthesia during surgery compromises respiratory function.

- The patient needs to turn, cough, and breathe deeply to prevent atelectasis.
- While the patient with uncomplicated appendicitis is usually willing to get out of bed and walk soon after

surgery, the patient with a ruptured appendix is generally hesitant to move and may need to be repositioned by family or staff. The patient must get out of bed as soon as his or her condition allows and walk two or three times a day to decrease recovery time and the risk of pulmonary complications.

- The nurse should encourage the patient to splint the incision area with a pillow during coughing to decrease pain.

- Incentive spirometry is frequently ordered for the patient. Young children may be resistant to (or too young to understand) this procedure. An effective alternative approach is to give the child bubbles to blow. Giving praise and rewards such as stickers each time the child completes the task is likely to increase compliance with the procedure and decrease the likelihood of complications.

Promote Fluid Volume Balance

- Monitor and continue the IV infusion that was initiated preoperatively until bowel function returns after surgery.

- Once bowel sounds return and after the nasogastric tube has been removed (if needed), offer water in small amounts, then other clear fluids.

- After introducing oral fluids, closely monitor the patient for nausea.

- Monitor intake and output. If the patient had a ruptured appendix and has a nasogastric tube after surgery, accurate assessment of the amount of output from the nasogastric tube is essential. The patient may have orders for the amount of fluid lost from the nasogastric tube to be replaced with additional IV fluids. The nurse should be alert to an increase in nasogastric drainage postoperatively, as this drainage should decrease over time. Promptly report any concerns to the physician.

Prevent Infection

Preventing complications during the preoperative and postoperative periods is a primary nursing care goal. Perforation and peritonitis are the most likely preoperative complications; postoperative complications include wound infection, abscess, and possible peritonitis.

- Monitor vital signs, including temperature. Tachycardia and rapid, shallow respirations may indicate perforation of the appendix with resulting peritonitis. Fever may develop as well; a decrease in blood pressure may indicate the presence of sepsis.

- Maintain IV infusion until oral intake is adequate. IV fluids are given to maintain vascular volume and to provide a route for antibiotic administration.

- Assess wound, abdominal girth, and postoperative pain. Swelling of the wound, increased abdominal girth, or an increase in pain may indicate infection or peritonitis.

Provide Effective Pain Management

The patient with appendicitis experiences pain before and after surgery. Analgesia is limited until the diagnosis is established. Postoperative pain is controlled by opioid or nonopioid analgesics.

- Assess pain, including its etiology, location, severity, and duration. Report any unexpected changes in the nature of pain. Both preoperatively and postoperatively, the patient's pain provides important clues about the diagnosis and possible complications, such as rupture of the appendix or peritonitis.

- Administer analgesics as ordered. Pain medication can be given preoperatively after a diagnosis is established. Provide analgesics postoperatively to maintain comfort and enhance mobility.

- Assess effectiveness of medication 30 minutes after administration. Report unrelieved pain. Pain unrelieved by the prescribed analgesic may indicate a complication or the need for further assessment. Abdominal distention may be monitored by measuring the abdominal girth every 4 hours or as indicated for the patient. In addition, continued abdominal discomfort and distention may indicate excess intestinal gas that may be better relieved by ambulation.

SAFETY ALERT Be alert to the child who does not complain of postoperative pain following surgery for a ruptured appendix. The child who does not verbally complain of pain may cry when approached and resist being moved or refuse to move in the bed. Proper pain management will facilitate the child's recovery and help prevent respiratory complications related to immobilization.

Provide Effective Patient Teaching

The patient whose appendix did not rupture is discharged once bowel function returns and the patient has a bowel movement. If the appendix was ruptured, the patient will be hospitalized for several days in order to administer IV antibiotics. Prior to discharge, the nurse should provide patient teaching (or parent education if the patient is a child; see the Patient Teaching feature).

Patient Teaching
The Patient with Appendicitis

Preoperative teaching may be limited by pain and the emergent nature of surgery. Explain why food and fluids are not permitted during this time. If time allows, teach postoperative turning, coughing, deep breathing, and pain management.

The patient with uncomplicated appendectomy often is discharged the day of surgery or the day following surgery. Postoperative teaching includes the following:

- Wound or incision care, including hand hygiene and dressing change procedures as indicated

- Instructions to report to the physician fever, increased abdominal pain, swelling, redness, drainage, bleeding, or warmth of the operative site

- Activity limitations (e.g., lifting, driving), if any

- Return to work if appropriate.

Evaluation

Expected outcomes of nursing care include the following:

- The patient demonstrates effective respiratory gas exchange, as evidenced by normal breath sounds, oxygen saturation of greater than or equal to 95%, and no indications of atelectasis.

- The patient demonstrates no signs or symptoms of secondary infection.

- Adequate hydration is achieved and maintained, as evidenced by balanced oral intake and output and by no signs or symptoms of fluid overload or dehydration.

- Using a predetermined pain rating scale, the patient rates pain at a level that is tolerable.

- The patient verbalizes decreased fear and anxiety associated with the hospitalization and procedures.

If the patient is unable to meet the expected outcomes, complete a thorough nursing assessment to determine whether the patient is having complications related to hydration, gas exchange, or pain management or is having psychosocial concerns. A patient who develops a secondary infection, for example, will demonstrate an elevated temperature and WBC count, as well as possible atelectasis or wound inflammation and redness. Notify the physician of such changes and related signs and symptoms, with further treatment plans likely involving IV antibiotics, IV fluids for hydration, wound care, and blood tests. If atelectasis is involved, supplemental oxygen and respiratory treatments would be added to the treatment protocol.

Nursing Care Plan

A Patient with Acute Appendicitis

Jamie Lynn is a 19-year-old college student majoring in physical therapy. Ms. Lynn arrives at the emergency department at 1 a.m. complaining of general lower abdominal pain that started the previous evening. By midnight, the pain was localized over the right lower quadrant. She also reports nausea and vomiting.

ASSESSMENT

Sue Grady, RN, completes the admission assessment in the emergency department. Ms. Lynn is complaining of nausea and severe abdominal pain, stating, "Walking makes my stomach hurt worse." Physical assessment findings include temperature 37.8°C (100.2°F) oral; pulse 84 bpm; respirations 16/min; and BP 110/70 mmHg. Skin is warm to the touch, and the abdomen is flat and guarded, with marked tenderness in the right lower quadrant. Ms. Lynn's CBC shows WBCs 14,000/mm^3, neutrophils 81.1%, and lymphocytes 12.5%. The diagnosis is acute appendicitis, and Ms. Lynn is transferred to surgery for a laparoscopic appendectomy.

DIAGNOSES

- *Infection, Risk for*
- *Skin Integrity, Impaired,* related to surgical incision
- *Pain, Acute,* related to surgical intervention
- *Anxiety* related to situational crisis

(NANDA-I © 2014)

PLANNING

- The incision will heal without infection or complications.
- The patient will verbalize adequate pain relief.
- The patient will verbalize decreased anxiety.
- The patient will return to preoperative activities.

IMPLEMENTATION

- Provide analgesics as needed.
- Teach pain management.
- Teach abdominal splinting as needed during coughing, turning, or ambulating.
- Teach home care of incision.
- Discuss activity limitations as ordered.
- Instruct patient to report fever or warmth, redness, or drainage from the incision.

EVALUATION

On discharge the following evening, Ms. Lynn is fully ambulatory. Her appetite has returned, and she is tolerating food and fluids well. Her temperature is normal. The nurse provides Ms. Lynn with written and verbal information on postoperative care following an appendectomy.

CRITICAL THINKING

1. What is the pathophysiologic basis for Ms. Lynn's elevated WBCs?

2. How would Ms. Lynn's postoperative care and teaching differ if she had undergone a laparotomy instead of a laparoscopic appendectomy?

3. Outline a teaching plan to give to patients for home care following an appendectomy.

4. Develop a care plan for Ms. Lynn for the nursing diagnosis *Anxiety* related to a situational crisis.

REVIEW Appendicitis

RELATE Link the Concepts and Exemplars

Linking the exemplar of appendicitis with the concept of infection:

1. How would you change or anticipate changing your nursing care for a patient whose appendix is believed to have ruptured preoperatively?

2. How would the pathophysiology of a patient with a ruptured appendix differ from a patient whose appendix is removed without rupturing?

Linking the exemplar of appendicitis with the concept of mobility:

3. When caring for a patient who required a laparoscopic appendectomy yesterday, what teaching would you provide to stress the importance of mobility?

4. The 14-year-old patient who is 1 day postoperative following an appendectomy is reluctant to ambulate for fear of pain. What strategies would you use to encourage ambulation?

READY Go to Volume 3: Clinical Nursing Skills

REFER Go to Pearson MyLab Nursing and eText

- Additional review material

REFLECT Apply Your Knowledge

Mike Mortimer is a healthy, active 9-year-old boy who lives with his father. His mother died 6 months ago from metastatic breast cancer. At first, everyone at school was really nice to him, but lately they have been teasing him about being a motherless orphan. He has started to wish he did not have to go to school. This morning he told his dad that he had a stomachache and asked to stay home, but his dad said he did not have a fever so he needed to get dressed and get going. The school nurse called his father at 11:30 to report that Mike had a fever and was feeling sick to his stomach. The nurse encouraged his dad to take him to the doctor.

When Mike arrives at the doctor's office, he reports severe pain in his lower right quadrant, nausea, and one emesis at school. Vital signs include the following: temperature 100.2°F oral; pulse 96 bpm; respirations 12/min; and BP 110/74 mmHg. Rebound tenderness is noted in McBurney point. CBC reveals a WBC count of 11,000/mm^3, and an ultrasound reveals an inflamed appendix. Mike is scheduled for surgery and admitted to the local acute care facility.

1. As you admit Mike to the pediatric unit, his father asks you to please give him something for pain. How do you respond?

2. Mike is scheduled to leave the unit for the operating room in 1 hour. What information will you gather to prepare him for surgery?

3. When Mike returns from the operating room, what priority assessments will you perform?

4. What teaching will you provide Mike and his dad prior to discharge?

» Exemplar 10.B
Gallbladder Disease

Exemplar Learning Outcomes

10.B Analyze gallbladder disease as it relates to inflammation.

- Describe the pathophysiology of gallbladder disease.
- Describe the etiology of gallbladder disease.
- Compare the risk factors and prevention of gallbladder disease.
- Identify the clinical manifestations of gallbladder disease.
- Summarize diagnostic tests and therapies used by interprofessional teams in the collaborative care of an individual with a gallbladder disease.
- Differentiate care of patients with gallbladder disease across the lifespan.
- Apply the nursing process in providing culturally competent care to an individual with gallbladder disease.

Exemplar Key Terms

Biliary colic, *688*
Cholangitis, *687*
Cholecystitis, *688*
Cholelithiasis, *687*
Empyema, *688*
Gallstone ileus, *688*
Laparoscopic cholecystectomy, *690*

Overview

Altered or obstructed bile flow through the hepatic, cystic, or common bile duct is a common problem. It often leads to inflammation and other complications. Gallstones are the most common cause of obstructed flow. Tumors and abscesses may also obstruct bile flow.

Cholelithiasis is the formation of stones (*calculi* or *gallstones*) in the gallbladder or biliary duct system. Cholelithiasis is a common problem in the United States, affecting 10–20% of the U.S. population; approximately 500,000 individuals require cholecystectomy each year (Heuman, 2016).

Pathophysiology and Etiology

Pathophysiology

Most gallstones are formed in the gallbladder. Their migration into the ducts (see **Figure 10–3** ») leads to **cholangitis** (duct inflammation). Although some individuals with cholelithiasis

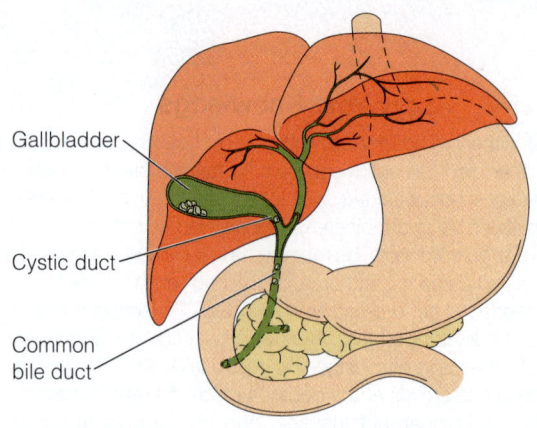

Gallbladder

Cystic duct

Common
bile duct

Figure 10–3 ›› Common locations of gallstones.

are asymptomatic, many develop manifestations. Early manifestations of gallstones may be vague: epigastric fullness or mild gastric distress after eating a large or fatty meal. Stones that obstruct the cystic duct or common bile duct lead to distention and increased pressure behind the stone, causing **biliary colic**, a severe, steady pain in the epigastric region or right upper quadrant (RUQ) of the abdomen. The pain may radiate to the back, right scapula, or shoulder. The pain often begins suddenly following a meal and may last as long as 5 hours. It is often accompanied by nausea and vomiting.

Obstruction of the common bile duct may cause bile reflux into the liver, leading to jaundice, pain, and possible liver damage. If the common duct is obstructed, pancreatic enzymes are unable to enter the small intestine, and pancreatitis becomes a potential complication.

Cholecystitis is inflammation of the gallbladder. *Acute cholecystitis* usually follows obstruction of the cystic duct by a stone. The resulting increased pressure in the gallbladder leads to ischemia of the gallbladder wall and mucosa. Chemical and bacterial inflammation often follows. The ischemia can lead to necrosis and perforation of the gallbladder wall.

Acute cholecystitis usually begins with an attack of biliary colic. The pain involves the entire RUQ and may radiate to the back, right scapula, or shoulder. Movement or deep breathing may aggravate the pain. The pain usually lasts longer than biliary colic, continuing for 12–18 hours. Anorexia, nausea, and vomiting are common. Fever is often present and may be accompanied by chills. The RUQ is tender to palpation.

Chronic cholecystitis may result from repeated bouts of acute cholecystitis or from persistent irritation of the gallbladder wall by stones. Bacteria may be present in the bile as well. Chronic cholecystitis often is asymptomatic.

Complications of cholecystitis include **empyema**, a collection of infected fluid in the gallbladder; gangrene and perforation with resulting peritonitis or abscess formation; formation of a fistula into an adjacent organ (e.g., duodenum, colon, stomach); and obstruction of the small intestine by a large gallstone (**gallstone ileus**).

Etiology

Gallstones form when several factors interact: abnormal bile composition, biliary stasis, and inflammation of the gallbladder. Most gallstones (80%) consist primarily of cholesterol; the rest contain a mixture of bile components. Excess cholesterol in bile is associated with obesity, a high-calorie and high-cholesterol diet, and drugs that lower serum cholesterol levels. Bile that is supersaturated with cholesterol can precipitate out to form stones. Biliary stasis, or slowed emptying of the gallbladder, contributes to cholelithiasis. Stones do not form when the gallbladder empties completely in response to hormonal stimulation. Slowed or incomplete emptying allows cholesterol to concentrate and increases the risk of stone formation. Finally, inflammation of the gallbladder allows excess water and bile salt reabsorption, increasing the risk for lithiasis.

Risk Factors

The incidence of gallstones varies among individuals of different ethnic backgrounds and other characteristics: Native Americans and Hispanics of Mexican origin are at greater risk for gallstones than other populations. Age, family history of gallstones, obesity, rapid weight loss, and being female are all risk factors. Other risk factors include biliary stasis (e.g., pregnancy, fasting, prolonged total parenteral nutrition) and certain diseases or conditions, such as cirrhosis, sickle cell disease, leukemia, hyperlipidemia, ileal disease or resection, and glucose intolerance.

Prevention

The modifiable risk factors that can be controlled or treated to reduce the occurrence of cholelithiasis include obesity, certain medications (estrogen and clofibrate), a high-fat diet, rapid weight loss, and dyslipidemia. Dyslipidemia is identified by a blood test that screens for increased total cholesterol, low-density lipids and triglycerides, or decreased high-density lipids. Risk factors that are nonmodifiable are age, gender, and ethnicity (Weerakoon et al., 2014).

Clinical Manifestations

Table 10–3 ›› compares the manifestations and complications of acute cholelithiasis with those of cholecystitis. The Clinical Manifestations and Therapies feature outlines signs, symptoms, and treatment of biliary colic, cholecystitis, choledocholithiasis, and cholangitis.

Focus on Diversity and Culture
Gallstones

Individuals of Northern European descent, those of Hispanic descent, and Native Americans have higher rates of gallstones than do individuals of Asian or African descent. Native Americans in both the Northern and Southern Hemispheres—and those of the Pima tribe of Arizona in particular—have a higher incidence of gallstones. This higher incidence is thought to result from a genetic predisposition to secrete high levels of cholesterol in the bile. Mexican American men and women of all ages also have elevated rates of gallstones (Heuman, 2016; NIDDK, 2012a).

TABLE 10–3 Manifestations and Complications of Cholelithiasis and Cholecystitis

Manifestations	Cholelithiasis	Cholecystitis
Pain	■ Abrupt onset ■ Severe, steady ■ Localized to epigastrium and RUQ of abdomen ■ May radiate to back, right scapula, and shoulder ■ Lasts 30 minutes to 5 hours	■ Abrupt onset ■ Severe, steady ■ Generalized in RUQ of abdomen ■ May radiate to back, right scapula, and shoulder ■ Lasts 12–18 hours ■ Aggravated by movement, breathing
Associated symptoms	■ Nausea, vomiting	■ Anorexia, nausea, vomiting ■ RUQ tenderness and guarding ■ Chills and fever
Complications	■ Cholecystitis ■ Common bile duct obstruction with possible jaundice and liver damage ■ Common duct obstruction with pancreatitis	■ Gangrene and perforation with peritonitis ■ Chronic cholecystitis ■ Empyema ■ Fistula formation ■ Gallstone ileus

Collaboration

Treatment of the patient with cholelithiasis or cholecystitis depends on the acuity of the condition and the patient's overall health status. When gallstones are present but asymptomatic and the patient has a low risk for complications, conservative treatment is indicated. However, when the patient experiences frequent symptoms, has acute cholecystitis, or has very large stones, the gallbladder and stones are usually surgically removed.

Diagnostic Tests

Diagnostic tests are ordered to identify the presence and location of stones, identify possible complications, and help differentiate gallbladder disease from other disorders.

■ *Serum bilirubin* is measured. Elevated direct (conjugated) bilirubin may indicate obstructed bile flow in the biliary duct system (see **Box 10–3**).

■ *CBC* may indicate infection and inflammation if the WBC count is elevated.

■ *Serum amylase and lipase* are measured to identify possible pancreatitis related to common duct obstruction.

■ *Abdominal x-ray* (flat plate of the abdomen) may show gallstones that have a high calcium content.

■ *Ultrasonography of the gallbladder* is a noninvasive exam that can accurately diagnose cholelithiasis. More accurate than a CT scan, it also can be used to assess emptying of the gallbladder.

■ *Oral cholecystogram* is performed with a dye administered orally to assess the gallbladder's ability to concentrate and excrete bile.

■ *Gallbladder scan,* such as cholescintigraphy, also known as a *hepatobiliary iminodiacetic acid (HIDA) scan*, uses an IV radioactive solution that is rapidly extracted from the blood and excreted into the biliary tree to allow diagnosis of cystic duct obstruction and acute or chronic cholecystitis.

Clinical Manifestations and Therapies
Gallbladder Disease

ETIOLOGY	CLINICAL MANIFESTATIONS	CLINICAL THERAPIES
Biliary colic	■ Severe steady ache in RUQ that begins suddenly and lasts for several hours; may radiate to right scapula or back; nausea/vomiting; fat intolerance	■ Analgesics; adequate rest; adequate nutrition; correction of electrolyte imbalances; antiemetics
Cholecystitis	■ RUQ or epigastric pain that progressively worsens; anorexia; nausea/vomiting; fever/chills; fat intolerance	■ Analgesics; adequate rest; adequate nutrition; IV antibiotic therapy; antiemetics; laparoscopic surgery, which may convert to open surgery with possible T-tube placement; if surgery is contraindicated or chronic, oral dissolution therapy or lithotripsy
Choledocholithiasis	■ RUQ pain; fever; jaundice; pruritus; abdominal tenderness	■ Analgesics; antihistamines; adequate nutrition; IV antibiotic therapy; antiemetics; surgery
Cholangitis	■ RUQ pain; fever; jaundice; pruritus; abdominal tenderness; clay-colored stools; dark urine; low blood pressure; lethargy	■ Analgesics; antihistamines; adequate nutrition; IV antibiotic therapy; antiemetics; surgery

Box 10–3
Sorting Out Total, Direct, and Indirect Bilirubin Levels

When serum bilirubin levels are drawn, the results usually are reported as total bilirubin, direct bilirubin, and indirect bilirubin levels. Most bilirubin is formed from hemoglobin as aging or abnormal red blood cells (RBCs) are removed from circulation and destroyed. Bilirubin is not water-soluble, so it must be bound to albumin before being transported to the liver. This albumin-bound bilirubin is called *indirect* or *unconjugated bilirubin*. Once in the liver, bilirubin is separated from albumin and conjugated to glucuronic acid. This water-soluble form of bilirubin is called *direct* or *conjugated bilirubin*. Conjugated bilirubin is then excreted in the bile.

- Total (serum) bilirubin, the total bilirubin in the blood, includes both indirect and direct forms. In adults, the normal total bilirubin is 0.1–1.2 mg/dL. Total bilirubin levels increase when more is being produced (e.g., by RBC hemolysis) or when its metabolism or excretion are impaired (e.g., by liver disease or biliary obstruction).
- The levels of direct (conjugated) bilirubin, normally 0.1–0.3 mg/dL in adults, rise when its excretion is impaired by obstruction in the liver (e.g., in cirrhosis, hepatitis, exposure to hepatotoxins) or in the biliary system.
- Indirect (unconjugated) bilirubin levels, normally less than 1.1 mg/dL in adults, rise in RBC hemolysis (e.g., sickle cell disease, transfusion reaction).

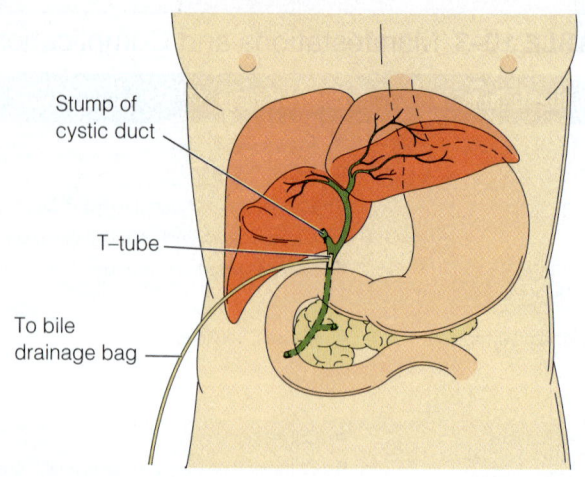

Figure 10–4 》》 T-tube placement in the common bile duct. Bile fluid flows with gravity into a drainage collection device below the level of the common bile duct.

Surgery

Laparoscopic cholecystectomy (removal of the gallbladder) is the treatment of choice for symptomatic cholelithiasis or cholecystitis (see the Evidence-Based Practice feature). This minimally invasive procedure has a low risk of complications and generally requires a hospital stay of less than 24 hours. Not all patients are candidates for laparoscopic cholecystectomy, however, and there is a risk that a laparoscopic cholecystectomy may need to be converted to a *laparotomy* (surgical opening into the abdomen) during the procedure.

When stones are lodged in the ducts, a cholecystectomy with common bile duct exploration may be done. A T-tube (see **Figure 10–4 》》**) is inserted to maintain patency of the duct and to promote bile passage while the edema decreases. Excess bile is collected in a drainage bag secured below the surgical site. If it is suspected that a stone has been retained following surgery, a postoperative cholangiogram via the T-tube or a direct visualization of the duct with an endoscope may be performed.

Some patients who are poor surgical risks and for whom laparoscopic cholecystectomy is inappropriate may have a *cholecystostomy* to drain the gallbladder or a *choledochostomy* to remove stones and position a T-tube in the common bile duct.

In some cases, shock wave lithotripsy may be used with drug therapy to dissolve large gallstones. In *extracorporeal shock wave lithotripsy*, ultrasound is used to align the stones with the source of shock waves and the computerized lithotripter. Positioning is of prime importance throughout the procedure, which usually takes an hour. Mild sedation may be given during the procedure. Nursing care after the proce-

dure includes monitoring for biliary colic, which can result when the gallbladder contracts to remove stone fragments; nausea; and transient hematuria. *Percutaneous cholecystostomy*, ultrasound-guided drainage of the gallbladder, may be done in high-risk patients to postpone or even eliminate the need for surgery.

Pharmacologic Therapy

Patients who refuse surgery or for whom surgery is inappropriate may be treated with a drug to dissolve the gallstones. Ursodiol (Actigall) and chenodiol (Chenix) reduce the cholesterol content of gallstones and lead to their gradual dissolution. These drugs act by reducing cholesterol production in the liver, thus reducing the cholesterol content of bile. As a consequence, these drugs are most effective in treating stones with high cholesterol content. They are less effective in treating radiopaque stones with high calcium salt content. Ursodiol is generally well tolerated but can cause diarrhea or constipation, whereas chenodiol has a high incidence of diarrhea at therapeutic doses and may require dose reduction. Chenodiol is also hepatotoxic, so periodic liver function studies are required during therapy. The primary disadvantages of pharmacologic treatment for gallstones are its cost, its long duration (up to 2 years), and the high incidence of recurrent stone formation when treatment is discontinued.

If infection is suspected, antibiotics may be ordered to cure the infection and reduce associated inflammation and edema. Patients with pruritus (itching) due to severe obstructive jaundice and an accumulation of bile salts on the skin may be given cholestyramine (Questran). This drug binds with bile salts to promote their excretion in the feces. A narcotic analgesic such as morphine may be required for pain relief during an acute attack of cholecystitis.

Nonpharmacologic Therapy

When food intake is eliminated during an acute attack of cholecystitis, a nasogastric tube is inserted to relieve nausea and vomiting. Dietary fat intake may be limited, especially if the patient is obese. If bile flow is obstructed, fat-soluble vitamins (A, D, E, and K) and bile salts may need to be administered.

Evidence-Based Practice
Pain Management Following Laparoscopic Cholecystectomy

Problem
Following ambulatory surgical procedures such as laparoscopic cholecystectomy, patients must manage their pain after discharge. In a study of analgesic use by ambulatory surgery patients, Han and colleagues (2014) found that patients did not always adhere to their analgesic regimens.

Evidence
Patients' intentional decision to endure moderate to severe pain by not taking the analgesics was influenced by patients' beliefs concerning pain, their analgesic use, and their previous pain experience. Patients feared the potential unknown side effects of the analgesics and did not believe taking multiple analgesics as part of a multimodal analgesic regimen was safe. The negative perception regarding morphine use was the fear of addiction. A factor that resulted in the patients' ultimately using their analgesic was reaching their pain threshold and no longer tolerating the pain. When the healthcare provider encouraged patients to take the analgesic regularly, patients were more likely to follow the prescribed analgesic regimen. Patient education regarding postoperative pain management and the effective use of analgesics underestimates the role of the patients' decision regarding analgesic use (Han et al., 2014).

Implications
Effective pain relief is known to promote healing and immune function following surgery (Stein & Kuchler, 2012). Research reveals a need to carefully prepare patients undergoing ambulatory surgery, including laparoscopic cholecystectomy, for pain management strategies. For example, in combination with additional analgesics, injection of local anesthetics at the surgical site significantly reduces pain following ambulatory surgery (Das et al., 2016). Effective postoperative pain management requires a combination of good preoperative education, discharge planning related to the patient's expectations of pain, and compliance of the patient with the physician's prescribed analgesic regimen.

Critical Thinking Application
1. Some patients in this study reported purposely not taking their analgesic prescription because of anticipated adverse effects of the drug. How can the nurse intervene to prevent this and to promote effective postoperative pain management?
2. Adjunctive pain relief measures (e.g., NSAIDs, application of heat or cold) may be recommended to supplement analgesic use. What adjunctive pain relief measures would be appropriate for the nurse to teach patients undergoing laparoscopic cholecystectomy?
3. Some patients in this study did not take the prescribed opioid analgesics because of concern about addiction. How should the nurse respond to a patient who expresses this concern?

SAFETY ALERT The herb goldenseal has been used in treating cholecystitis. However, the evidence is not sufficient to support the safe use of goldenseal, according to the National Center for Complementary and Integrative Medicine (2015). Berberine, one of the active ingredients in goldenseal, stimulates secretion of bile and bilirubin. It also inhibits the growth of many common pathogens, including those known to infect the gallbladder. Goldenseal can stimulate the uterus, so it is contraindicated for use during pregnancy. It also should not be used by nursing mothers.

Lifespan Considerations

Gallbladder Disease in Children and Adolescents

Biliary dyskinesia accounts for 81% of patients admitted with a gallbladder diagnosis. These admissions continue to increase, with a pronounced increase in the pediatric population (700% increase from 1997 to 2010) (Bielefeldt, 2013). Pediatric patients with sickle cell disease and any biliary abnormality often require cholecystectomy and may experience complications (Gale et al., 2015).

Gallbladder Disease in Pregnant Women

Diseases of the gallbladder have been reported as the most common cause for a hospitalization during the first year postpartum. According to Moghaddam and colleagues (2013), the incidence of biliary sludge and gallstones is significantly correlated with the number of pregnancies and higher age at pregnancy.

Gallbladder Disease in Older Adults

Variant ABCG8-D19H is the most widely recognized genetic risk factor for gallstone disease, and adults with this variant are more likely to have gallstone recurrence, a major long-term postoperative biliary complication (von Schonfels et al., 2013). Studies have considered whether abnormal lipid profiles are related to cholesterol in gallbladder disease, but no relationship was noted in a recent study (Weerakoon et al., 2014). In addition, research has shown that biliary dyskinesia is now a common cause of surgical intervention (cholecystectomy) for gallbladder disease (Bielefeldt, 2013).

NURSING PROCESS

Nursing care of the patient with gallbladder disease is focused on patient teaching, pain management, and instruction on healthy nutrition.

Assessment

Assessment data related to cholelithiasis and cholecystitis include the following:

- ***Observation and patient interview.*** The nurse should note current manifestations, including RUQ pain, its character and relationship to meals, duration, and radiation; nausea and vomiting; other symptoms; duration of symptoms; risk factors or previous history of symptoms; chronic diseases such as diabetes, cirrhosis, or IBD; current diet; and use of oral contraceptives or possibility of pregnancy

■ *Physical examination.* The nurse will assess current weight, color of skin and sclera, abdominal tenderness, and color of urine and stool.

Diagnosis

Priority nursing diagnoses for the patient with cholelithiasis or cholecystitis often include the following:

■ *Infection, Risk for*

■ *Pain, Acute*

■ *Imbalanced Nutrition: Less Than Body Requirements.*

(NANDA-I © 2014)

Planning

Goals of nursing care, developed in collaboration with the patient, may include the following:

■ The patient will demonstrate no signs or symptoms of infection.

■ The patient will report adequate pain control.

■ The patient will demonstrate understanding of low-fat diet with adequate intake of fat-soluble vitamins.

■ The patient will verbalize awareness of symptoms that require immediate notification of the healthcare provider.

Implementation

Prior to surgery, the nurse should assess the abdomen every 4 hours and as indicated (e.g., when pain level changes abruptly). Increasing abdominal tenderness or a rigid, boardlike abdomen may indicate rupture of the gallbladder, with peritonitis. Nursing interventions for the patient who has undergone a laparoscopic or open cholecystectomy are similar to those for other patients who have had abdominal surgery. The first interventions will therefore occur in the acute care environment, before the patient can be discharged to home.

Care for the Postoperative Patient

An acutely inflamed gallbladder may become necrotic and rupture, releasing its contents into the abdominal cavity. While the resulting infection often remains localized, peritonitis can result from chemical irritation and bacterial contamination of the peritoneal cavity. Following open cholecystectomy (laparotomy), the risk for pulmonary infection is significant because of the high abdominal incision.

■ Monitor vital signs, including temperature, every 4 hours. Promptly report vital sign changes or temperature elevation. Tachycardia, increased respiratory rate, or an elevated temperature may indicate an infectious process.

■ Assist with coughing and deep breathing or use incentive spirometer every 1–2 hours while the patient is awake. Splint the abdominal incision with a blanket or pillow during coughing. The high abdominal incision of an open cholecystectomy interferes with effective coughing and deep breathing, increasing the risk of atelectasis and respiratory infections such as pneumonia.

■ Place the patient in Fowler position, and encourage ambulation as allowed. Fowler position and ambulation promote lung expansion and airway clearance, reducing the risk of respiratory infections.

■ Administer antibiotics as ordered. Antibiotics may be given preoperatively to reduce the risk of infection from infected gallbladder contents; they may be continued postoperatively to prevent infection.

Care of the T-tube

■ Ensure that the T-tube is properly connected to a sterile container; keep the tube below the level of the surgical wound. This position promotes the flow of bile and prevents backflow or seepage of caustic bile onto the skin. The tube itself decreases biliary tree pressure.

■ Monitor drainage from the T-tube for color and consistency; record as output. The tube normally drains up to 500 mL in the first 24 hours after surgery; drainage decreases to less than 200 mL in 2–3 days and is minimal thereafter. Drainage may be blood-tinged initially, changing to green-brown. Report excessive drainage immediately. (After 48 hours, drainage greater than 500 mL is considered excessive.) Stones or edema and inflammation can obstruct ducts below the tube, requiring treatment.

■ Place the patient in Fowler position, which promotes gravity drainage of bile.

■ Assess skin for bile leakage during dressing changes. Bile irritates the skin; it may be necessary to apply barrier product for skin protection.

■ Teach the patient how to manage the tube when turning, ambulating, and performing activities of daily living (ADLs). Direct pulling or traction on the tube must be avoided.

■ If indicated, teach the patient how to take care of the T-tube, clamp it, and recognize signs of infection. The patient may be discharged home with the tube in place. Reporting early signs of infection facilitates prompt treatment.

Provide Effective Pain Management

The pain associated with cholelithiasis can be severe. Sometimes a combination of interventions is indicated:

■ Discuss the relationship between fat intake and pain. Teach ways to reduce fat intake. Fat entering the duodenum initiates gallbladder contractions, causing pain when gallstones are in the ducts.

■ Withhold oral food and fluids during episodes of acute pain. Insert a nasogastric tube, and connect it to low suction if ordered. Emptying the stomach reduces the amount of chyme entering the duodenum and the stimulus for gallbladder contractions, thus reducing pain.

■ For severe pain, administer morphine, meperidine, or another opioid analgesic as ordered. Recent research indicates that morphine is no more likely to cause spasms of the sphincter of Oddi than meperidine.

- Place the patient in Fowler position. Fowler position decreases pressure on the inflamed gallbladder.

Promote Balanced Nutrition

The patient with severe gallbladder disease may develop nutritional imbalances related to anorexia, pain, nausea following meals, and impaired bile flow that alters absorption of fat and fat-soluble vitamins (A, D, E, and K) from the gut.

- Assess nutritional status, including diet history, height and weight, and skinfold measurements. The patient with gallbladder disease may have an imbalanced diet or may have specific vitamin deficiencies, particularly of the fat-soluble vitamins.

- Evaluate laboratory results, including serum bilirubin, albumin, glucose, and cholesterol levels. Report abnormal results to the primary care provider. Elevated serum bilirubin may indicate impaired bilirubin excretion due to obstructed bile flow. A low serum albumin may indicate poor nutritional status. Glucose intolerance and hypercholesterolemia are risk factors for cholelithiasis.

- Refer the patient to a dietitian or nutritionist for diet counseling to promote healthy weight loss and to reduce pain episodes. A low-carbohydrate, low-fat, higher-protein diet reduces symptoms of cholecystitis. While fasting and very low-calorie diets are contraindicated, a moderate reduction in calorie intake and increased activity levels promote weight loss.

- Assist the patient in learning how to manage dietary restrictions related to gallbladder diagnosis.

- Administer vitamin supplements as ordered. The patient who does not absorb fat well because of obstructed bile flow may require supplements of the fat-soluble vitamins.

Evaluation

Patient progress toward goals may be evaluated based on the following expected outcomes:

- The patient reports adequate pain control to maintain comfort.

- The patient demonstrates food choices reflecting a diet low in fat and high in fat-soluble vitamins.

- The patient's temperature remains within normal limits, and patient displays no symptoms of infection.

If the patient does not progress satisfactorily to the expected outcomes, the nurse must complete a thorough assessment; particularly the patient's reported pain level, diet tolerance, and vital signs. Signs and symptoms of infection such as elevated temperature and increased pain will require notifying the patient's primary provider. Further diagnostic workup may include a CBC and blood cultures to rule out sepsis. IV fluids may be reinstated as well as IV pain medication, an NPO status and IV antibiotics. Surgical consult may be conducted.

Nursing Care Plan
A Patient with Cholelithiasis

Joyce Colbert is a 44-year-old married mother of three children. A member of the Chickasaw tribe, she is active in tribal activities and works part time as a cook at a community kitchen. Ms. Colbert has recently noticed a dull pain in her upper abdomen that gets worse after she eats fatty foods; nausea and sometimes vomiting accompany the pain. She had a similar pain after the birth of her last child. She is diagnosed with cholelithiasis and is admitted for a laparoscopic cholecystectomy, with an anticipated short length of stay.

ASSESSMENT	DIAGNOSES	PLANNING
David Corbin, RN, takes Ms. Colbert's admission history. It includes intolerance of fatty foods and intermittent "stabbing" abdominal pain that radiates to her back. Her usual diet includes tacos or fried bread and biscuits with gravy for breakfast. She reports "not wanting to eat much of anything lately." She states that she has never had surgery before and hopes "everything goes well." Physical assessment includes temperature 37.7°C (100°F) oral; pulse 88 bpm; respirations 20/min; and BP 130/84 mmHg. She has had a recent 5-lb weight loss and currently weighs 59 kg (130 lb). She is 160 cm (63 in.) tall. Abdominal examination elicits tenderness in the RUQ of the abdomen. She has no jaundice, chills, or evidence of complications.	■ *Infection, Risk for,* related to potential bacterial contamination of abdominal cavity ■ *Imbalanced Nutrition: Less Than Body Requirements* related to anorexia and recent weight loss ■ *Pain, Acute,* related to inflamed gallbladder and surgical incisions ■ *Anxiety* related to lack of information about perioperative experience (NANDA-I © 2014)	■ The patient will maintain present weight within 2.3 kg (5 lb) over the next 3 weeks. ■ The patient will resume regular diet, decreasing intake of foods high in fat. ■ The patient will verbalize adequate pain control after surgery and with activity resumption. ■ The patient will remain free of infection. ■ The patient will verbalize a decrease in anxiety before surgery.

(continued on next page)

Nursing Care Plan (continued)

IMPLEMENTATION

- Teach about the gallbladder and the function of bile.
- Discuss pre- and postoperative care, including self-care following discharge.
- Promote mobility as soon as allowed after surgery.
- Teach home care of incisions and recognition of signs of infection.
- Review specific high-fat foods to avoid and ways to maintain her weight.
- Provide analgesia as needed postoperatively. Teach appropriate analgesic use after discharge.

EVALUATION

Ms. Colbert is discharged the morning after her surgery. She is afebrile, has no signs of infection, and is able to appropriately care for her incisions. She identifies signs of infection and talks about ways to reduce her fat intake while keeping her weight stable. She verbalizes understanding of initial activity restrictions and resumption of normal activities. Ms. Colbert states, "It wasn't as bad as I thought it would be at first." She has an appointment to see her surgeon in 1 week.

CRITICAL THINKING

1. What is the rationale for a low-fat diet with cholelithiasis? Discuss nutritional practices as they relate to the medical problem and Ms. Colbert's culture.
2. How would your discharge teaching for Ms. Colbert differ if she had had an open cholecystectomy instead of a laparoscopic cholecystectomy?
3. Design a nursing care plan for Ms. Colbert for the nursing diagnosis *Fatigue*.

REVIEW Gallbladder Disease

RELATE Link the Concepts and Exemplars

Linking the exemplar of gallbladder disease with the concept of fluids and electrolytes:

1. How might gallbladder disease affect fluid homeostasis?
2. To prevent fluid and electrolyte imbalance, what nursing care might you initiate for the patient who reports severe, acute abdominal pain secondary to cholelithiasis?

Linking the exemplar of gallbladder disease with the concept of health, wellness, and illness:

3. What health promotion topics might you teach adults to prevent the development of cholelithiasis?
4. What group would you consider most at risk for development of gallbladder disease?

READY Go to Volume 3: Clinical Nursing Skills

REFER Go to Pearson MyLab Nursing and eText

- Additional review material

REFLECT Apply Your Knowledge

Helen Martin is a 48-year-old woman who has been married to Gil Martin for 18 years. Ms. Martin has a daughter (Tracie) from a previous marriage, and she has two teenage children with Gil (Anthony and Kristina). Ms. Martin works as a teller at a bank. Although she finds her job monotonous, she appreciates the steady income and family health insurance.

Ms. Martin is overweight and has tried to lose weight most of her adult life. She frequently diets and, in fact, has lost a great deal of weight in the past but has been unable to keep the weight off. She blames menopause for her most recent weight gain.

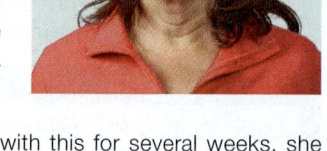

Ms. Martin experiences indigestion following a few meals. Over several weeks, the severity and frequency have increased. She takes an antacid, believing the problem is just heartburn. The discomfort is usually located in the upper right side of her abdomen, and sometimes it is quite painful. The pain may last up to a couple of hours and then subsides. She occasionally feels nauseated as well. After putting up with this for several weeks, she makes an appointment with her physician.

Based on Ms. Martin's symptoms, her physician suspects that she has cholelithiasis and orders an ultrasound scan of her abdomen. The ultrasound confirms the presence of gallstones. The physician tells Ms. Martin that she has two options: (1) conservative therapy that would involve a low-fat, reduced-calorie diet or (2) surgery to remove her gallbladder. Helen decides to try dietary modification.

1. What information would you include in your teaching plan for Ms. Martin about low-fat, low-calorie diets?
2. Based on your own likes and dislikes, design a 1-week diet plan, including all meals and snacks that would meet the low-fat, low-calorie requirements for Ms. Martin.
3. What is the rationale for beginning with conservative treatment rather than immediately initiating surgical intervention?
4. How will you evaluate the effectiveness of conservative treatment for Ms. Martin?

Exemplar 10.C
Inflammatory Bowel Disease

Exemplar Learning Outcomes

10.C Analyze inflammatory bowel disease as it relates to inflammation.

- Describe the pathophysiology of inflammatory bowel disease.
- Describe the etiology of inflammatory bowel disease.
- Compare the risk factors and prevention of inflammatory bowel disease.
- Identify the clinical manifestations of inflammatory bowel disease.
- Summarize diagnostic tests and therapies used by interprofessional teams in the collaborative care of an individual with inflammatory bowel disease.
- Differentiate care of patients with inflammatory bowel disease across the lifespan.

- Apply the nursing process in providing culturally competent care to an individual with inflammatory bowel disease.

Exemplar Key Terms

Colectomy, *700*
Crohn disease, *695*
Fulminant colitis, *699*
Ileostomy, *700*
Inflammatory bowel disease (IBD), *695*
Stoma, *700*
Ulcerative colitis, *695*

Overview

Approximately 1.4 million Americans have **inflammatory bowel disease (IBD)**, a collection of chronic inflammatory conditions of the intestines. With both ulcerative colitis and Crohn disease, the patient experiences periods of symptom-free remissions with sporadic periods of active disease (flares). Twice as many individuals develop ulcerative colitis as develop Crohn disease (CDC, 2014). **Ulcerative colitis** affects the mucosa and submucosa of the colon and rectum.

Classification of IBD is based on the severity of symptoms, primarily the number of bowel movements per day. Patients with mild disease (30% of cases) have fewer than four stools per day, and patients with moderate disease

(20%) experience four to six stools per day. Patients with ulcerative colitis who have more than six stools per day (2%) have severe disease. The remaining patients (48%) are in remission (CDC, 2014).

Crohn disease can affect any portion of the GI tract from the mouth to the anus, but it usually affects the terminal ileum and ascending colon. Areas of disease involvement appear as patches, leaving adjacent areas unaffected. Because any portion of the GI tract can be affected, disease activity and severity can fluctuate considerably over time. The extent of the inflammation in Crohn disease is deep and can extend through the entire bowel wall (CDC, 2014). A comparison of ulcerative colitis and Crohn disease is found in **Table 10–4 »**.

TABLE 10–4 Characteristics of Ulcerative Colitis and Crohn Disease

	Characteristic	Ulcerative Colitis	Crohn Disease
Clinical	Gender	Equal	Equal
	Age at onset	Any age, peaks in 15- to 30-year-olds	Any age, peaks in 15- to 30-year-olds
	Course of disease	Chronic disease with periods of remission of symptoms and active disease	Chronic disease with periods of remission of symptoms and active disease
	Diarrhea	5–30 stools per day with blood and mucus	Common, usually less severe than in colitis, with no obvious blood or mucus in stool
	Abdominal pain	Cramping in left lower quadrant; relieved by defecation	Cramping, or steady right lower quadrant or periumbilical pain; tenderness and mass noted in right lower quadrant
	Nutritional deficit	Common, involving anemia, hypoalbuminemia, and weight loss	Common and significant, involving anemia, weight loss, and multiple vitamin and mineral deficits
	Constitutional manifestations	Fever rare; possible associated arthritic, skin, or other organ involvement, such as erythema nodosum or uveitis	Fever, malaise, fatigue; possibly some associated conditions and urinary complications
Pathologic	Depth of involvement	Mucosa and submucosa	Transmural (entire bowel wall)
	Portion of bowel involved	Typically rectum and sigmoid colon, possibly extending to entire large bowel	Any portion of GI tract, terminal ileum and ascending colon involvement predominating
	Distribution	Continuous from rectum	Patchy; skip lesions
	Appearance of mucosa	Granular, dull, hyperemic, and friable; disease uniform in affected bowel; possibly pseudopolyps	Cobblestone appearance, with areas of normal tissue surrounded by ulceration and fissures
Complications	Acute	Toxic megacolon, perforation, massive hemorrhage	Obstruction, fistulization, abscess formation, malabsorption
	Long term	Colorectal cancer	Colon cancer

Sources: Data from Centers for Disease Control and Prevention. (2014). *Inflammatory bowel disease.* Retrieved from http://www.cdc.gov/ibd; Crohn and Colitis Foundation of America. (2014). *The facts about inflammatory bowel diseases.* Retrieved from http://www.ccfa.org/assets/pdfs/ibdfactbook.pdf

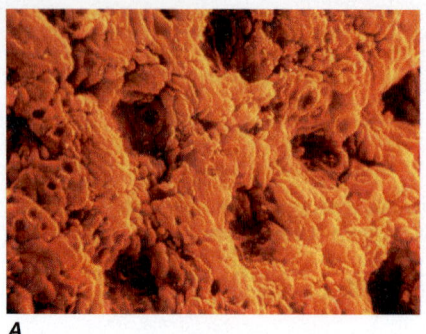
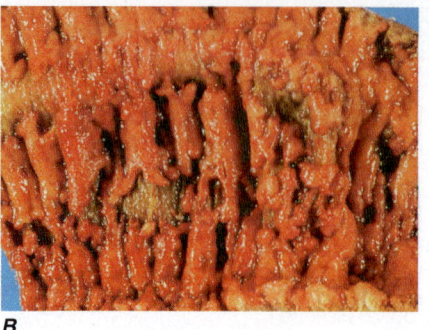
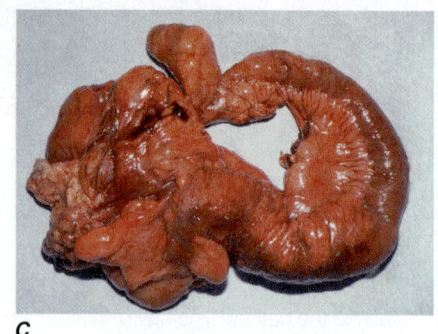

A

B

C

Source: A, CNRI/Science Source. *B,* Dr. E. Walker/Science Source, *C,* Biophoto Associates/Science Source.

Figure 10–5 》 A, Photomicrograph of the mucosa of the large intestine showing the entrances to the crypts of Lieberkühn. The crypts are the focal points for **B,** ulcerative colitis and **C,** Crohn disease.

Pathophysiology and Etiology

Pathophysiology

The inflammatory process of ulcerative colitis usually begins at the rectosigmoid area of the anal canal and progresses proximally. In most patients, the disease is confined to the rectum and sigmoid colon. It may progress to involve the entire colon, stopping at the ileocecal junction.

Ulcerative colitis begins with inflammation at the base of the crypts of Lieberkühn in the distal large intestine and rectal mucosa. Microscopic, pinpoint mucosal hemorrhages occur, and crypt abscesses develop (see **Figure 10–5 》**). These abscesses penetrate the superficial submucosa and spread laterally, leading to necrosis and sloughing of bowel mucosa. Further tissue damage is caused by inflammatory exudates and the release of inflammatory mediators such as prostaglandins and other cytokines. The mucosa becomes red and edematous because of vascular congestion, friable (easily broken), and ulcerated. It bleeds easily, and hemorrhage is common. Edema creates a granular appearance. Pseudopolyps, tonguelike projections of bowel mucosa into the lumen, may develop as the epithelial lining of the bowel regenerates. Chronic inflammation leads to atrophy, narrowing, and shortening of the colon, with loss of its normal haustra (small pouches or recesses into which the large intestine is divided).

Crohn disease typically begins as a small inflammatory *aphthoid lesion* (a shallow ulcer with a white base and an elevated margin, similar to a canker sore) of the mucosa and submucosa of the bowel. The initial lesions may regress, or the inflammatory process may progress to involve all layers of the intestinal wall. Deeper ulcerations, granulomatous lesions, and fissures (knifelike clefts that extend deeply into the bowel wall) develop. The inflammatory process involves the entire bowel wall (transmural).

The lumen of the affected bowel assumes a cobblestone appearance as fissures and ulcers surround islands of intact mucosa over edematous submucosa. The inflammatory lesions of Crohn disease are not continuous; rather, they often occur as "skip" lesions, with intervening areas of normal-appearing bowel. Some evidence suggests that despite its normal appearance, the entire bowel is affected by this disorder.

As the disease progresses, fibrotic changes in the bowel wall cause it to thicken and lose flexibility, taking on a rubber-hose-like appearance. The inflammation, edema, and fibrosis can lead to local obstruction, the development of abscesses, and the formation of fistulas between loops of bowel or between the bowel and other organs (see **Figure 10–6 》**). Fistulas between loops of bowel are known as *enteroenteric fistulas*; fistulas that occur between bowel and bladder are known as *enterovesical fistulas*; and fistulas that occur between bowel and skin are known as *enterocutaneous fistulas*. Perineal fistulas are relatively common, originating in the ileum.

Depending on the severity and extent of the disease, malabsorption and malnutrition may develop as the ulcers prevent absorption of nutrients. When the jejunum and ileum are affected, the absorption of multiple nutrients (including carbohydrates, proteins, fats, vitamins, and folate) may be impaired. Disease in the terminal ileum can lead to vitamin B_{12} malabsorption and bile salt reabsorption. The ulcerations also can lead to protein loss and chronic, slow blood loss with consequent anemia. See the Multisystem Effects of Inflammatory Bowel Disease feature.

Etiology

The etiology of both ulcerative colitis and Crohn disease is unknown. Genetic and environmental factors have been implicated in the development of IBD (see the Focus on Diversity and Culture feature). As of 2015, studies still indicate that the environment and biopsychosocial factors and neuropeptides influence the occurrence and progression of Crohn disease (El-Salhy & Hausken, 2016; Moum, Hovde, Høivik, 2014). Factors such as an infectious agent and altered immune responses are also thought to play a role in the development of IBD. Autoimmunity is thought to play a role, and lifestyle factors (e.g., smoking) also may affect its development.

Risk Factors

IBD occurs more frequently in the United States and in Northern European nations than it does in Southern Europe and countries in the Southern Hemisphere. American Jews of European descent are 4–5 times more likely to develop IBD, while African Americans and Whites are more likely to develop the disease than Hispanics or Asians (CDC, 2014).

Multisystem Effects of
Inflammatory Bowel Disease

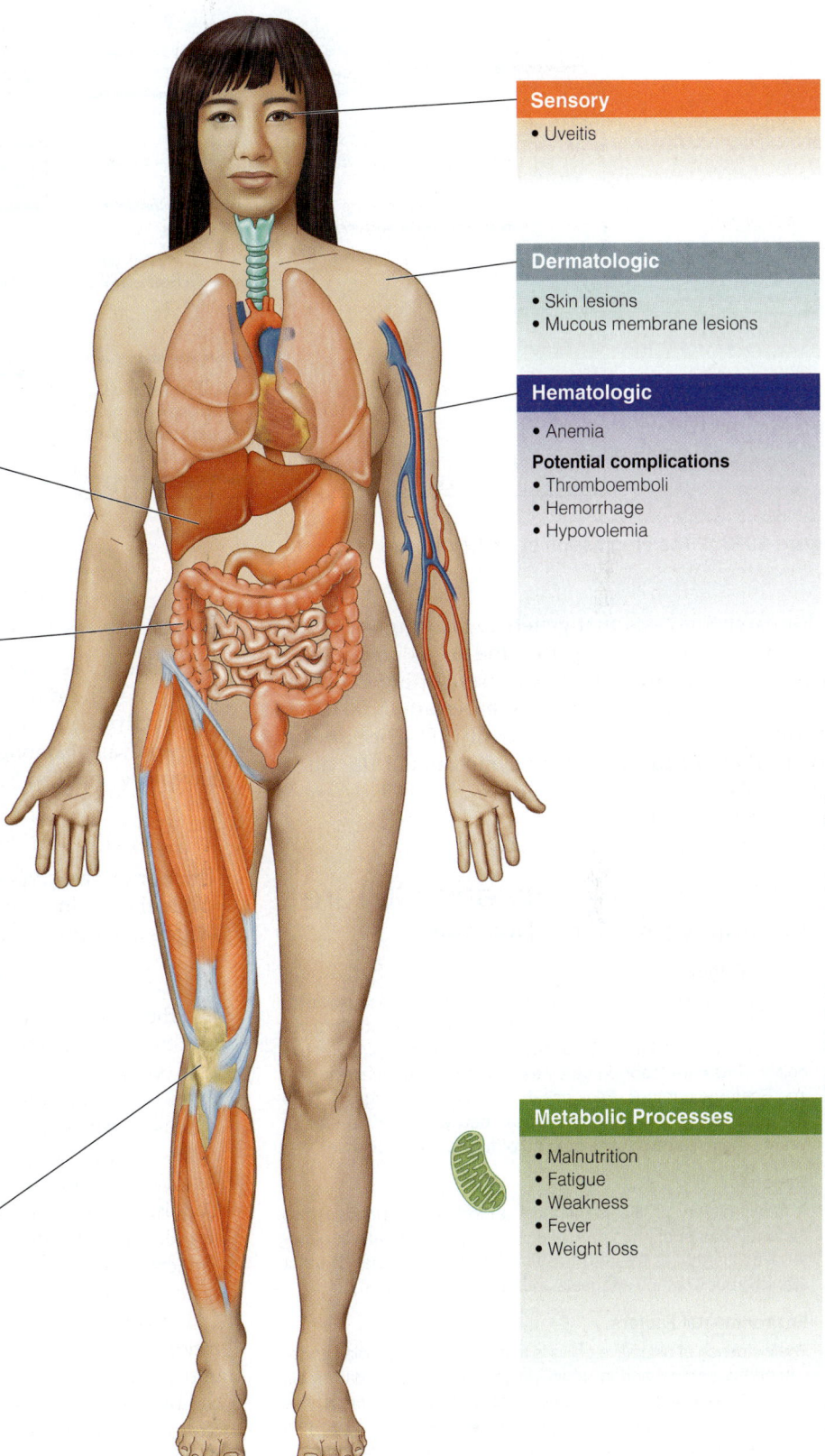

Sensory
- Uveitis

Dermatologic
- Skin lesions
- Mucous membrane lesions

Hematologic
- Anemia

Potential complications
- Thromboemboli
- Hemorrhage
- Hypovolemia

Hepatic
- Risk for sclerosing cholangitis

Gastrointestinal
- Diarrhea
- Blood and mucous in stool
- Intermittent rectal bleeding and mucous
- Fecal urgency
- Tenesmus
- Abdominal pain, tenderness, cramping, often relieved by defecation
- Anorexia
- Nausea, vomiting, epigastric pain
- Palpable right lower quadrant mass
- Anorectal lesions

Potential complications
- Toxic megacolon
- Perforation with peritonitis
- Obstruction
- Abscess
- Fistula formation

Musculoskeletal
- Arthritis of one or more joints
- Ankylosing spondylitis

Metabolic Processes
- Malnutrition
- Fatigue
- Weakness
- Fever
- Weight loss

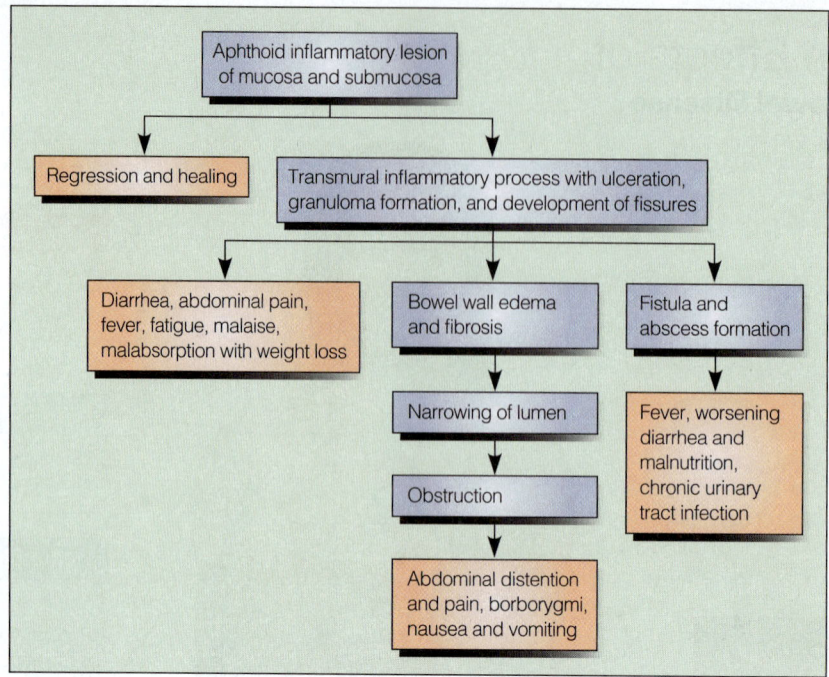

Figure 10–6 » The progression of Crohn disease.

Research suggests that genetics, the immune system, and environmental factors affect the development of IBD. Smoking can increase the risk of developing Crohn disease, and the use of medications, especially NSAIDs and antibiotics, can increase the risk of IBD. Diet does not trigger IBD but can aggravate symptoms of the disease (CDC, 2014).

Focus on Diversity and Culture
Inflammatory Bowel Disease

Epidemiology

Ulcerative colitis is more prevalent than Crohn disease. According to Ordas and colleagues (2012), North America and Northern Europe have the highest incidence and prevalence of ulcerative colitis. Rates are reported as lowest in the Southern Hemisphere and Eastern countries. Peak onset occurs between ages 15 and 30 years, with a second smaller peak between ages 50 and 70 years. These same studies note no difference regarding sex.

Genetics

A family history of IBD is the most important independent risk factor (Ordas et al., 2012). Ashkenazi Jews have a rate of ulcerative colitis that is three to five times higher than that of other ethnic groups, which suggests another genetic link.

Environmental Factors

The incidence of ulcerative colitis is higher in developed than undeveloped countries, and in urban versus rural areas (Ordas et al., 2012). Several environmental factors act as triggers or preventive factors, such as cigarette smoking, which is reported to protect against ulcerative colitis, with the disease becoming worse if patients stop smoking. Infection with a GI illness such as *Salmonella* or *Shigella* can trigger an ulcerative colitis development in patients with genetic possibility in their history. Some work has shown that breastfeeding prevents development of ulcerative colitis, as does an appendectomy in the early adult years (Ordas et al., 2012).

Prevention

Avoidance or cessation of smoking is a major factor in prevention of the development of IBD. Crohn disease more commonly occurs among smokers, while ulcerative colitis is more prevalent among former smokers and individuals who have never smoked (CDC, 2014).

Clinical Manifestations

There are several types of inflammatory intestinal disorders. While they share some of the same characteristics, their etiologies and clinical manifestations may vary.

Ulcerative Colitis

Diarrhea is the predominant manifestation of ulcerative colitis. Stools contain both blood and mucus. Nocturnal diarrhea may occur. Mild to moderate ulcerative colitis is characterized by six or fewer stools per day, intermittent rectal bleeding and mucus, and few systemic manifestations. Severe ulcerative colitis can lead to more than 6–10 bloody stools per day, extensive colon involvement, anemia, hypovolemia, and malnutrition. Rectal inflammation causes fecal urgency and tenesmus (a painful but ineffective urge to defecate). Left lower quadrant cramping relieved by defecation is common. Other manifestations include fatigue, anorexia, and weakness.

Patients with severe disease may have systemic manifestations such as arthritis involving one or several joints, skin and mucous membrane lesions, or *uveitis* (inflammation of the uvea, the vascular layer of the eye, which may involve the sclera and cornea as well). Some patients develop thromboemboli, with blood vessel obstruction due to clots carried from the site of their formation. Sclerosing cholangitis (inflammation leading to scarring and narrowing of the bile ducts) may occur; it is more common in men than in women, with an average age at diagnosis of 40 years (NIDDK, 2012b).

Intestinal complications of ulcerative colitis include hemorrhage, perforation, and rupture of the bowel, and **fulminant colitis**, which may advance to toxic megacolon. Hemorrhage, which is the most common complication, often results in anemia. Perforation occurs when the intestinal wall is weakened because of chronic inflammation and ulceration, resulting in the formation of an opening. This opening allows the intestinal contents to leak into the abdomen and cause peritonitis. Less than 10% of patients with ulcerative colitis develop fulminant colitis (Crohn and Colitis Foundation of America, 2012a). It occurs when damage to the entire thickness of the intestinal wall results in intestinal dilation with paralysis and abdominal distention. Toxic megacolon, a rare form of fulminant colitis, is the most severe complication of ulcerative colitis. In addition to the transverse colon dilating more than 6 cm, the resulting paralysis allows excessive amounts of intestinal gas to collect and causes severe abdominal distention. It may result in perforation of the bowel if left untreated. Causes of toxic megacolon include hypokalemia and the use of antidiarrheals, opiates, antispasmodics, and certain antidepressants (Sheth & LaMont, 2012).

According to American College of Gastroenterology (ACG) Practice Guidelines, patients with ulcerative colitis are at increased risk for colorectal cancer proportional to disease duration, extent of inflammation, and amount of colon involvement. After 8–10 years of disease, colonoscopies with multiple biopsies are recommended every 6–12 months (Kornbluth, Sachar, & the Practice Parameters Committee of the American College of Gastroenterology, 2010).

Crohn Disease

Because involvement of the GI system in Crohn disease can be so diverse, manifestations vary among patients. The majority of individuals with Crohn disease experience persistent diarrhea. Stools are liquid or semiformed and typically do not contain blood, although blood may be passed if the colon is involved. Abdominal pain and tenderness are common. The pain may be located in the right lower quadrant and relieved by defecation. A palpable right lower quadrant mass is often present. Systemic manifestations such as fever, fatigue, malaise, weight loss, and anemia are common. Anorectal lesions such as fissures, ulcers, fistulas, and abscesses are also common and may occur years before intestinal disease is apparent. If the stomach and duodenum are involved, nausea, vomiting, and epigastric pain may occur.

Certain complications of Crohn disease (e.g., intestinal obstruction, abscess, fistula) are so common that they are considered part of the disease process. For many patients, the disease initially presents with one of these complications. Intestinal obstruction is a common complication caused by repeated inflammation and scarring of the bowel that leads to fibrosis and stricture. Obstruction of the bowel lumen causes abdominal distention, cramping pain, and borborygmi (excessive loud and hyperactive bowel sounds). Nausea and vomiting may occur.

Fistulas may be asymptomatic, particularly if they occur between loops of small bowel. An abscess caused by fistulization produces chills and fever, a tender abdominal mass, and leukocytosis. A fistula between the small bowel and the colon may exacerbate diarrhea, weight loss, and malnutrition. When the bladder is involved, recurrent urinary tract infections (UTIs) occur.

Perforation of the bowel is uncommon but can lead to generalized peritonitis. Massive hemorrhage is also an uncommon complication of Crohn disease. Long-standing Crohn disease increases the risk of colorectal cancer.

Collaboration

Interprofessional care for IBD begins by establishing the diagnosis and the extent and severity of the disease. Treatment is supportive, including medications and dietary measures to decrease inflammation, promote intestinal rest and healing, and reduce intestinal motility. Many patients with IBD require surgery at some point to manage the disease or its complications. As a member of the healthcare team, the nurse plays an essential role by providing patient teaching about disease management, diagnostic tests, and surgical or other treatments.

Diagnostic Tests

Diagnostic testing establishes the diagnosis of IBD, assesses the extent of the disease, and evaluates the effects of the disorder. A sigmoidoscopy, colonoscopy, or barium upper and lower x-ray series inspect the bowel mucosa for characteristic changes of IBD.

Laboratory tests used to differentiate IBD and to identify effects and complications of the disease include a stool examination for blood and mucus and stool cultures to rule out infectious causes of bowel inflammation and diarrhea. CBC with hemoglobin and hematocrit shows anemia from chronic inflammation, blood loss, and malnutrition, as well as leukocytosis due to inflammation and possible abscess formation. The sedimentation rate is typically elevated during periods of acute inflammation. Serum albumin may decrease because of malabsorption, malnutrition, protein loss through intestinal lesions, and chronic inflammation. Folic acid and serum levels of most vitamins, including A, B complex, C, and the fat-soluble vitamins, often decrease because of malabsorption. Liver function tests may show elevated liver enzymes (e.g., ALT, alkaline phosphatase, AST, GGTP, LDH) and bilirubin levels if sclerosing cholangitis is present.

Surgery

Surgical interventions for IBD differ depending on the primary disease process and the portion of the bowel affected. Surgery is generally performed only when necessitated by complications of the disease or failure of conservative treatment measures.

Bowel obstruction is the leading indication for surgery in Crohn disease. Other complications that may require surgical intervention are perforation, internal or external fistula, abscess, and perianal complications. The usual treatment is resection of the affected portion of bowel with an end-to-end anastomosis to preserve as much bowel as possible. The disease process tends to recur in other areas following removal of affected bowel segments. The risk of fistula formation increases following surgery. Bowel strictures may be treated with a *strictureplasty*, in which longitudinal incisions are made in the narrowed segment to relieve the stricture while preserving bowel.

Clinical Manifestations and Therapies
Inflammatory Bowel Disease

ETIOLOGY	CLINICAL MANIFESTATIONS	CLINICAL THERAPIES
Hemorrhage	■ Pale mucous membranes, thirst, light-headedness, hypotension, reduced urine output	■ Blood transfusions ■ Iron supplements ■ IV fluid ■ Possibly surgery to remove damaged bowel ■ Possibly vasoconstrictive medications
Megacolon	■ Fever, tachycardia, hypotension, dehydration, abdominal tenderness and cramping, change in the number of stools per day	■ Fecal disimpaction ■ Enemas ■ Suppositories ■ Bowel decompression ■ Colonoscopic decompression ■ Bowel habit retraining ■ Total abdominal colectomy
Diarrhea	■ Frequent loose stools, abdominal cramping, abdominal tenderness, stool that may or may not contain blood, thirst, dehydration, hypovolemia, malnutrition	■ Monitoring of intake and output ■ IV fluid ■ Antidiarrheal medications (should be avoided in severe ulcerative colitis) ■ Possible guaiac testing
Fistulas	■ Possibly asymptomatic between bowel loops; between bowel and bladder—frequent UTIs; between bowel and abdominal cavity—abscess, chills and fever, a tender abdominal mass, leukocytosis; between small bowel and colon—weight loss, malnutrition, possible exacerbation of diarrhea	■ Symptomatic treatment: antibiotics, antidiarrheal medication, IV fluid support ■ Possible dissection of section of bowel with fistula if tissue cannot be repaired

Colectomy

Patients with extensive chronic ulcerative colitis may require a total **colectomy** (surgical resection and removal of the colon) to treat the disease itself; to eliminate complications such as toxic megacolon, perforation, or hemorrhage; or to serve as a prophylactic measure against the high colon cancer risk associated with extensive ulcerative colitis.

The surgical procedure of choice for extensive ulcerative colitis is a *total colectomy with an ileal pouch–anal anastomosis (IPAA)*. In this procedure, the entire colon and rectum are removed, a pouch is formed from the terminal ileum, and the pouch is brought into the pelvis and anastomosed (connected) to the anal canal (see **Figure 10–7 》**). A temporary or loop ileostomy (described under the heading Ostomy) is generally performed at the same time and is maintained for 2–3 months to allow the anal anastomosis to heal. When the healing is complete, the ileostomy is closed, and the patient has six to eight daily bowel movements through the anus. Advanced age, obesity, and other factors may preclude an IPAA. For these patients, a permanent ileostomy or continent ileostomy may be created.

Ostomy

An intestinal ostomy is a surgically created opening between the intestine and the abdominal wall that allows the passage of fecal material. The surface opening is called a **stoma** (see **Figure 10–8 》**). The precise name of the ostomy depends on

the location of the stoma. An **ileostomy** is an ostomy made in the ileum of the small intestine. In an ileostomy, the colon, rectum, and anus are usually completely removed (*total proctocolectomy with permanent ileostomy*). The anal canal is closed, and the end of the terminal ileum is brought to the

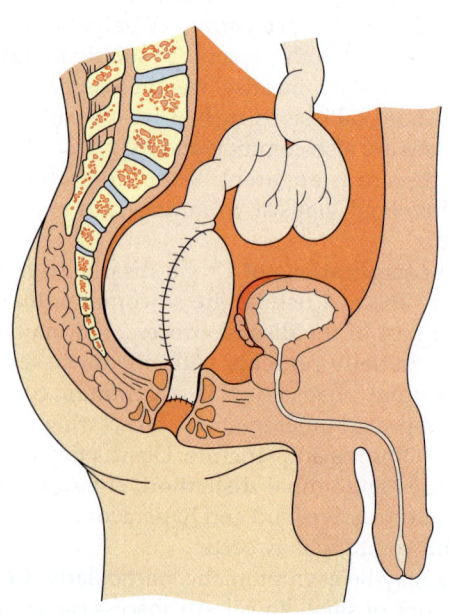

Figure 10–7 》 Ileal pouch–anal anastomosis (IPAA).

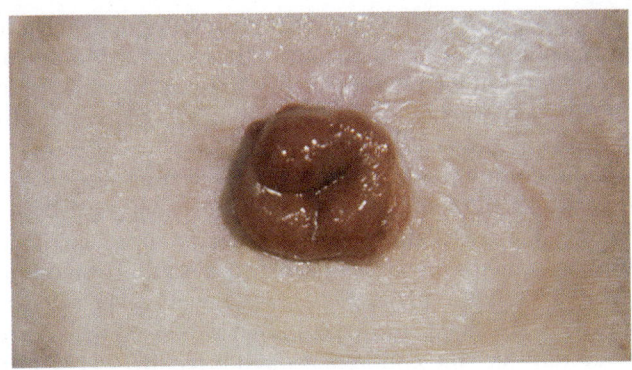

Figure 10–8 》 A healthy-appearing stoma.

body surface through the right abdominal wall to form the stoma. A temporary or *loop ileostomy* may be formed to eliminate feces and allow tissue healing for 2–3 months following an IPAA. A loop of ileum is brought to the body surface to form a stoma and allow stool drainage into an external pouch. When the ileostomy is no longer necessary, a second surgery is performed to close the stoma and repair the bowel, restoring fecal elimination through the anus.

In a *continent ileostomy* (see **Figure 10–9** 》), an intra-abdominal reservoir is constructed and a nipple valve is formed (the ileum is folded back on itself) from the terminal ileum before it is brought to the surface of the abdominal wall. Stool collects in the internal pouch; the nipple valve prevents it from leaking through the stoma. A catheter is inserted into the pouch to drain the stool.

》 *Go to **Pearson MyLab Nursing and eText** to see a chart outlining nursing care of the patient having an ileostomy.*

Pharmacologic Therapy

The ultimate goal of care is to terminate acute attacks as quickly as possible and to reduce the incidence of relapse. Drug therapy plays a key role in achieving this goal (see the Medications feature). Locally acting and systemic anti-inflammatory drugs are the primary medications used to manage mild to moderate IBD. Drugs to suppress the immune response may be used to treat patients with severe disease.

Sulfasalazine (Azulfidine) combines a sulfonamide antibiotic that is poorly absorbed from the GI tract with

mesalamine, which acts topically on the colonic mucosa to inhibit the inflammatory process. Mesalamine (5-amino-salicylic acid) is also available in preparations that do not contain sulfa but instead use other vehicles, such as olsalazine and balsalazide. They have the advantage of causing fewer adverse effects than sulfasalazine.

For acute exacerbations of IBD, corticosteroids are given to reduce inflammation and induce remission (see the Medications feature in The Concept of Inflammation for an overview of corticosteroids). For ulcerative colitis, the drug may be administered rectally as an enema, a suppository, or foam for its local effect and to minimize systemic effects. IV corticosteroids may be required to treat severe disease; oral preparations are used for less severe manifestations and long-term therapy. Many patients are unable to withdraw from steroid therapy without experiencing relapse and may need long-term low-dose therapy.

Mercaptopurine (6-MP, Purinethol) and other immunosuppressive agents such as azathioprine (Imuran) and cyclosporine (Sandimmune) can be used to treat patients who have not responded to other treatments or who require long-term steroid therapy. These drugs may allow withdrawal from corticosteroids, maintain remission, and facilitate healing. Long-term therapy may be required to produce a beneficial effect.

Newer treatments for IBD employ other immune response modifiers, such as the monoclonal antibodies infliximab (Remicade) and adalimumab (Humira), to suppress tumor necrosis factor (TNF, an inflammatory mediator substance) in patients with moderate to severe active Crohn disease who have not responded to standard therapies. Only infliximab is approved for use in ulcerative colitis (Ordas et al., 2012).

Although antibiotic therapy generally is not indicated in IBD, metronidazole (Flagyl) and ciprofloxacin (Cipro) are used when abscesses occur.

Antidiarrheal agents, such as loperamide and diphenoxylate, may be given to slow GI motility and reduce diarrhea. These drugs are safe for patients with mild, chronic manifestations, but they are not given during acute attacks because they may precipitate toxic dilation of the colon.

When working with patients who are prescribed pharmacologic therapy for IBD, reinforce the importance of adhering to a strict medication regimen. Emphasize that medications should be continued even when the patient is asymptomatic. Discuss the side effects of the drugs and what to do if any of the side effects occur. Teach the patient and family members how to recognize and respond to side effects of medications. Because immune status may be altered by steroid use, have the family of a patient taking steroids avoid risk of exposure to infectious diseases. Instruct them to report any diseases and fevers the patient experiences and to report the use of steroids to all healthcare providers. Immunization schedules for pediatric patients may need to be altered.

Nonpharmacologic Therapy

Antigens in the diet may stimulate the immune response in the bowel, exacerbating IBD. As a result, dietary management for IBD should be individualized. Some patients benefit from eliminating all milk and milk products from the diet. Increased dietary fiber may help reduce diarrhea and relieve rectal manifestations, but it is contraindicated for patients

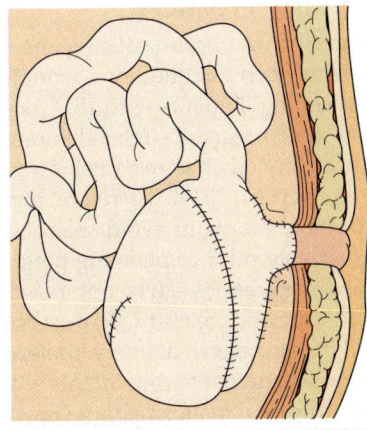

Figure 10–9 》 Continent (Kock) ileostomy.

with intestinal strictures caused by repeated inflammation and scarring. Current literature supports the need for a nutritionist to collaborate with the patient's medical provider to ensure that micronutrients needs are being met, as well as enough calories and protein to prevent undernourishment (Halmos & Gibson, 2015).

All food may be withheld to promote bowel rest during an acute exacerbation of Crohn disease. Nutritional status during this time is maintained by enteral or total parenteral nutrition (TPN). TPN carries a higher risk of complications than does enteral nutrition. An elemental diet such as Ensure, which contains all essential nutrients in a residue-free formula, may be prescribed. Elemental diets provide essential nutrients to the small intestine to support cell growth, but they are not always palatable.

Complementary Health Approaches

The chronic nature of IBD and the adverse effects of many prescribed treatments lead many patients with IBD to seek or use integrative therapies. There is some preliminary evidence that suggests some probiotics may improve symptoms of IBS; however, benefits have not been conclusively demonstrated, and not all probiotics have the same effects (National Center for Complementary and Integrative Health, 2015).

The lack of research to determine the effectiveness and safety of most alternative therapies in the treatment of IBD, especially herbal supplements, limits the use of these therapies by conventional practitioners (Crohn and Colitis Foundation of America, 2012b). In addition, many integrative therapies used by patients with IBD may interact with prescribed medications. Nurses should instruct the patient to discuss all potential therapies with the primary care provider.

Lifespan Considerations
IBD in Children and Adolescents

Although the occurrence of IBD peaks at 15–30 years of age, it also occurs in the pediatric population. The pediatric etiology differs from that of adult-onset IBD. For example, IBD is more common in boys than girls in the pediatric population, whereas equal numbers of adult men and women have IBD. In addition, children have Crohn disease more frequently than ulcerative colitis (2.8:1); the opposite is true of adults (0.85:1).

The location of disease is also different in children and adults. Whereas adults with Crohn disease usually present with terminal ileal disease without colonic involvement, the majority of pediatric patients have ileocolonic or colonic disease, increasing the incidence of hematochezia (blood in stool). In addition, children with Crohn disease usually present with inflammatory or nonstricturing, nonpenetrating disease, whereas adults often present with fistulizing or stricturing disease. Children with ulcerative colitis usually present with pancolitis, whereas adults more often present with left-sided colitis. Pediatric pancolitis is usually more aggressive, and first surgery often comes earlier for children than for adults (Buderus, Boone, & Lentz, 2015).

The primary objective in the management of pediatric ulcerative colitis is the induction and maintenance of disease remission. Experts note that induction is achieved primarily with aminosalicylates in patients with mild disease and with corticosteroids in those with moderate or severe disease

(Adis Medical Writers, 2014). Maintenance options include aminosalicylates, immunomodulators, and biological agents. Surgical interventions today focus on minimal laparoscopic approaches for children with ulcerative colitis (Perger et al., 2014).

An important pediatric consequence of malabsorption of adequate nutrition in this disease is failure to grow. It is not uncommon for children to receive dietary supplements in addition to medications to control their disease. The medications used to treat IBD in pediatric patients are the same as those used in adults; however, dosage is reduced when they are administered to children. As in adults, IBD in children may progress to the point of requiring surgery to remove a portion of the bowel. Children with IBD can also have lower bone density than children without the disease. Other manifestations of the disease are very similar to those experienced by an adult (Gaspareto & Guariso, 2013).

Provide emotional support and counseling to help the pediatric patient adjust to feeling "different" from peers. Inability to compete with peers and frequent absences from school can affect the patient's self-esteem. Collaborate with parents in the patient's care, and assist them in contacting their child's school to arrange for tutoring or home schooling in the case of extended absences from school. Patient teaching is a critical aspect of preparation for the young patient, as well as adult family members, to care for the disease appropriately. Patient teaching related to dietary instructions for a child with IBD includes providing the following information:

- Provide several small feedings each day, which may be better tolerated than three larger meals.
- Limit fiber intake to decrease intestine motility and inflammation. Peel fruits, and avoid large quantities of whole grains and nuts.
- Offer high-calorie meals if the child is not eating well. If lactose intolerance is not a problem, offer cream soups, milkshakes, puddings, and custards.
- Provide liquid dietary supplements to ensure that protein and caloric requirements are met.
- Watch for foods that cause intestinal problems for the individual child and avoid them.
- Prevent mealtimes from becoming a reason for family strife. Seek help of nurses and dietitians if needed.

IBD in Pregnant Women

The peak incidence of IBD occurs during the childbearing years, and so patients often ask questions about fertility, pregnancy, and breastfeeding. Patients with IBD receive twice as much information about pregnancy-related issues from gastroenterologists than from any other source (including the internet) (Hendy, Chadwick, & Hart, 2015). Therefore, the gastroenterologist must educate patients to avoid misconceptions and should do so proactively prior to planning pregnancy so that patients' health and medications can be optimized.

Women with IBD are at increased risk of severe preeclampsia, medically indicated preterm delivery, preterm premature rupture of membranes, and delivering infants with low Apgar scores and major congenital malformations (Boyd et al., 2015). These associations are only partly explained by severe disease as reflected by systemic corticosteroid use.

Medications
Inflammatory Bowel Disease

CLASSIFICATION AND DRUG EXAMPLES	MECHANISMS OF ACTION/DOSAGES	NURSING CONSIDERATIONS
5-Aminosalycylic Acid Medications (5-ASA) **Drug examples:** Sulfasalazine (Azulfidine) Olsalazine (Dipentum) Balsalazide (Colazal) Mesalamine (Asacol, Canasa, Lialda)	5-ASA medications are metabolized by colonic bacteria into active metabolites such as mesalamine. These medications are believed to act topically on the diseased portion of the gastrointestinal tract by inhibiting mediators of inflammation (prostaglandins, leukotrienes and others) and tumor necrosis factor. **Adult dosages:** Sulfasalazine: 3–4 g/day orally divided tid (ulcerative colitis; 3–6 g/day orally divided tid (Crohn disease) Olsalazine: 500 mg bid orally Balsalazide (Colazal): 2250 mg (capsule) PO tid for 8–12 weeks Mesalamine (Pentasa): 1 gm orally qid × 8 weeks	▪ Assess for contraindications to sulfasalazine including a history of hypersensitivity to sulfonamides or salicylates and intestinal or urinary tract obstruction. ▪ Assess baseline values for renal function tests, liver function tests, and CBC. ▪ Administer as ordered. Suppositories or retention enemas should be administered at bedtime. Administer oral forms with 8 ounces of water. ▪ Have resuscitation equipment available in the event of anaphylactic response. ▪ Evaluate for therapeutic response, including reduced number of stools, reduced mucus and blood, and improved stool consistency. ▪ Monitor for possible adverse effects including anorexia, headache, gastric distress, skin reactions, fatigue, oligospermia, urticaria, pruritus, hepatitis, myocarditis, blood dyscrasias.
Immunosuppressant Drugs **Drug examples:** Mercaptopurine (6-MP, Purinethol) Azathioprine (Imuran) Cyclosporine (Sandimmune) Methotrexate (MTX, Rheumatrex, Trexall)	Suppresses the action of the immune system linked to inflammation by impairing DNA and/or RNA biosynthesis and inhibiting cell proliferation or causing death **Adult dosages:** Mercaptopurine: 1-1.5 mg/kg PO Azathioprine: 2-3 mg/kg PO once daily (Chron); 1.5-2.5 mg/kg PO once daily (ulcerative colitis) Cyclosporine: individualized Methotrexate: 25 mg weekly SC or PO	▪ Advise patients to split azathioprine dose and take twice a day after eating. ▪ Methotrexate should not be used by women who may become pregnant. ▪ Monitor for side effects: infections, dry cough or shortness of breath; diarrhea, vomiting, white patches or sores in the mouth, blood in urine or stools, infrequent urination, fever, sore throat, headache.
Biologic Therapies Tumor necrosis factor inhibitors **Drug examples:** Infliximab (Remicade) Adalimumab (Humira) Certolizumab pegol (Cimzia) Golimumab (Simponi)	Monoclonal antibodies interrupt endogenous tumor necrosis factor alpha (TNFα) to suppress inflammation in the intestine. **Adult dosages:** Infliximab: 5 mg/kg IV at 0, 2, and 6 weeks, then every 8 weeks; may be increased to 10 mg/kg Adalimumab: Induction: 160 mg SC either as 4 injections of 40 mg on day 1 or as 2 injections of 40 mg daily on 2 consecutive days, then 80 mg SC 2 weeks later (day 15). Maintenance (beginning Week 4) 40 mg SC every 2 weeks. Certolizumab pegol: Initial: 200 mg SC BID; repeat at 2 and 4 weeks. Maintenance: 400 mg SC every 4 weeks Golimumab (Simponi): 200 mg SC at week 0 followed by 100 mg SC at week 2, then 100 mg SC every 4 weeks	▪ Not used for initial therapy. ▪ Infliximab is approved for Crohn disease and ulcerative colitis. ▪ Adalimumab and certolizumab pegol are approved for Crohn disease. ▪ Assess for redness, itching, bruising, pain, or swelling at the injection site; headache, fever, chills, hives and other rashes. ▪ For older adults, monitor for serious infections including TB and histoplasmosis. ▪ In pediatric patients, monitor for unusual cancers.
Alpha-4 Integrin Inhibitors **Drug examples:** Natalizumab (Tysabri) Vedolizumab (Entyvio)	Humanized monoclonal antibody target the adhesion molecule alpha-4 integrin **Adult dosages:** Natalizumab: 300 mg IV every 28 days Vedolizumab: 300 mg IV at weeks 0, 2 and 6 and then every 8 weeks	▪ Natalizumab is approved for Crohn disease and affects the entire body. ▪ Vedolizumab is specific to the GI tract and is approved for Crohn disease and ulcerative colitis. ▪ Natalizumab has a black box warning for progressive multifocal leukoencephalopathy. ▪ Monitor for side effects including infections, headache, bronchitis, rash, pain in extremities, arthralgia, diarrhea, nausea.

Source: Data from Adams, M. P., Holland, L. N., & Urban, C. (2017). *Pharmacology for nurses: A pathophysiologic approach* (5th ed.). Hoboken, NJ: Pearson Education.

IBD in Older Adults

Ulcerative colitis is becoming a disease of older adults, and approximately 10–30% of patients with ulcerative colitis are over the age of 60 (Baggenstos, Hanson, & Shaukat, 2013). In addition, while ulcerative colitis is often treated with immunosuppressive agents in older adults, insufficient evidence exists regarding the appropriate management of this illness (Baggenstos et al., 2013).

NURSING PROCESS

Although at this time IBD cannot be predicted or prevented, effective management may help the patient avoid complications of the disease. Stress the importance of complying with the prescribed treatment regimen and promptly reporting manifestations of exacerbations to the physician.

Assessment

A thorough assessment of the patient with IBD should include the following:

- **Observation and patient interview.** Current manifestations, including onset, duration, and severity (number of stools per day, presence of blood or mucus in stool, abdominal pain or cramping, tenesmus); usual diet, ability to maintain weight and nutrition, and food intolerances; associated manifestations such as arthralgias, fatigue, and malaise; current medications; and previous treatment and diagnostic tests
- **Physical examination.** General appearance; weight; vital signs, including orthostatic vitals and temperature; abdominal assessment, including shape, contour, bowel sounds, palpation for tenderness and masses, and presence of stoma or scars.

Diagnosis

When planning nursing care for the patient with IBD, it is vital to consider the chronic, recurrent nature of the disorder. Potential nursing diagnoses include the following:

- *Fluid Volume, Risk for Deficient*
- *Imbalanced Nutrition: Less Than Body Requirements*
- *Constipation*
- *Diarrhea*
- *Pain, Acute*
- *Pain, Chronic*
- *Body Image, Disturbed.*

(NANDA-I © 2014)

Planning

In planning care for the patient with IBD, review the patient's needs, including severity of disease process, age, frequency of exacerbations, and physical condition. Potential goals of care include the following:

- The patient will achieve resolution of discomfort from symptoms such as diarrhea.
- The patient will maintain adequate hydration.
- The patient will maintain optimal nutritional status.
- The patient will demonstrate positive, healthy coping skills.

- The patient will describe appropriate home self-care, including administering medication, making dietary choices, and preventing exacerbations.

Implementation

Teaching is a major aspect of care. Diarrhea and disturbed body image are significant problems for the patient with IBD. Children and adolescents often have specific needs, especially related to body image and the desire to fit in with peers. With severe disease, impaired nutrition must be considered a priority problem as well. As with other related GI disorders, the first interventions may occur within the acute care environment during an acute exacerbation of the disease, as the following discussion demonstrates.

Monitor Fluid Volume

During an acute exacerbation of IBD, diarrhea can be frequent and painful. The frequency of defecation and associated abdominal pain and cramping may interfere with ADLs and increase the risk for fluid volume deficit and impaired skin integrity. If a patient is hospitalized with IBD:

- Use a stool chart to record the frequency, amount, and color of stools. Measure and record liquid stool as output. The severity of diarrhea is an indicator of the severity of the disease and helps determine the need for fluid replacement.
- Monitor vital signs every 4 hours. Tachycardia, tachypnea, and fever may be indicators of fluid volume deficit.
- Weigh daily and record. Rapid weight loss (over days to a week) usually indicates fluid loss, whereas weight loss over weeks to months may indicate malnutrition.
- Assess for other indications of fluid deficit: warm, dry skin; poor skin turgor; dry, shiny mucous membranes; weakness; lethargy; complaints of thirst. The extent of fluid loss may not be readily evident with diarrhea, particularly if the patient uses the bathroom without assistance. Systemic manifestations of fluid volume deficit may be the first indicators of the problem.
- Maintain bowel rest by keeping NPO or limiting oral intake to elemental feedings as indicated. Bowel rest during an acute exacerbation of IBD promotes healing and reduces diarrhea and other manifestations.
- Administer prescribed anti-inflammatory and antidiarrheal medications as indicated. Anti-inflammatory medications reduce the extent of bowel inflammation and diarrhea. Unless contraindicated, antidiarrheal medications help reduce fluid loss and increase comfort.
- Maintain fluid intake by mouth or intravenously as indicated. The patient with IBD requires fluid to replace ongoing losses, as well as fluid to meet the usual daily needs of the body. If an elemental diet or total parenteral nutrition is prescribed, additional fluids may be required to meet fluid intake needs.
- Provide good skin care. Fluid deficit and tissue dehydration increase the risk for skin excoriations or breakdown.
- Assess perianal area for irritation or denuded skin from the diarrhea. Use gentle cleansing agents such as Peri-Wash or Tucks, diaper wipes, or cotton balls saturated with witch hazel. Apply a protective cream, such as a zinc

oxide–based preparation, to protect skin from the irritating effects of diarrheal stool. Digestive enzymes in the stool are very corrosive, increasing the risk of breakdown of the skin when it is exposed to diarrheal stool.

When patients are being discharged, remind them that the intestinal swelling associated with IBD may cause constipation.

- In addition to promoting adequate fluid intake, instruct the patient to take only laxatives recommended by the primary care provider. All laxatives should be avoided during a flare of the disease.

- Also explain nonpharmacologic interventions to help relieve constipation: These include mild exercise (30-minute walk), abdominal massage, and a warm bath (relaxes the rectal muscles).

- If these treatments are ineffective and the constipation continues for an extended time, contact the primary care provider. Inform the patient to take constipation seriously. In addition to the abdominal discomfort it causes, it may be a symptom of impaction or bowel obstruction.

SAFETY ALERT The patient should be taught to observe stools for obvious blood and test for occult blood as indicated. Report grossly bloody stools, which may indicate hemorrhage and necessitate emergency surgery.

Promote Healthy Body Image

The patient with IBD may experience frustration at not being able to control, or even predict, fecal elimination, particularly when the disease is severe. Diarrhea can interfere with the ability to complete tasks; maintain employment or engage in social activities; and even meet basic needs such as eating, sleeping, and having sex. Body image can suffer as a result. Treatment of IBD, be it total colectomy with IPAA, ileostomy, or chronic corticosteroid therapy, also can affect the patient's self-image.

Body image is a major concern for a child or adolescent with IBD. Corticosteroid therapy causes growth retardation and delayed sexual maturation. Encourage the patient to discuss feelings about these side effects. If a permanent colostomy or ileostomy is required, the nurse can assist the patient and family in understanding the need for surgical treatment.

- Accept the patient's feelings and self-perception. Negating or denying the reality of the patient's perception impairs trust.

- Encourage discussion of physical changes and their consequences as they relate to self-concept and close personal relationships. This encouragement demonstrates acceptance and provides an opportunity for the patient to describe the personal impact of the disease and its treatment.

- To increase the patient's sense of control over the disease and his or her future, encourage the patient to make choices and decisions regarding care.

- Discuss possible treatment options and their effects openly and honestly. Open discussion allows for more informed decisions.

- Teach coping strategies (e.g., odor control, dietary modifications) and support their use. These strategies facilitate healthy adaptation to the disease.

Promote Adequate Nutritional Intake

Ensuring adequate intake is part of acute care interventions, but is especially important while the patient is independent in his or her own home or any other care area outside of the hospital. Crohn disease can significantly alter the bowel's ability to absorb nutrients. In both forms of IBD, blood and protein-rich fluid may be lost in diarrheal stools. Malabsorption and continuing nutrient losses may cause multiple nutrient deficits that affect growth and development, healing, muscle mass, bone density, and electrolyte balances. Monitoring laboratory results assists in accurate assessment of nutritional status.

- Provide the prescribed diet: high-kilocalorie, high-protein, low-fat diet with restricted milk and milk products if lactose intolerance is present. Calories and protein are important to replace lost nutrients. Fat restriction helps reduce diarrhea and nutrient loss, particularly when significant portions of the terminal ileum have been resected.

- Provide parenteral nutrition as necessary if the patient is unable to absorb enteral nutrients. Parenteral nutrition can help reverse nutritional deficits and promote weight gain and healing in the patient with acute manifestations.

- Arrange for dietary consultation. Consider food preferences as allowed. Providing preferred foods in the prescribed diet increases intake and supports nutritional status.

- Provide or administer elemental enteral nutrition and supplements as ordered. Elemental enteral nutritional supplements support healing while providing for bowel rest. They can replace losses and improve nutritional status more rapidly than diet alone.

- Include family members, the primary food preparer in particular, in teaching and dietary discussions. Families can reinforce teaching and help the patient maintain the required restrictions or kilocalorie intake.

Evaluation

Expected outcomes of nursing care for the patient with IBD include the following:

- The patient demonstrates absence of GI distress.

- The patient and family demonstrate successful management of medications without side effects.

- The patient demonstrates no signs or symptoms of infection.

- The patient verbalizes attainment of a positive body image.

- The patient demonstrates integration of relaxation techniques into daily life.

If the patient does not progress satisfactorily to the expected outcomes, the nurse must complete a thorough assessment; particularly the patient's reported pain level, diet tolerance, and vital signs. Signs and symptoms of infection such as elevated temperature and increased pain will require notifying the patient's primary provider. Further diagnostic workup may include a CBC and blood cultures to rule out sepsis. IV fluids may be reinstated as well as IV pain medication, an NPO status and IV antibiotics. Surgical consult may be conducted.

Patient Teaching
Home Care for the Patient with IBD

Patient teaching may occur at all levels of care, within the acute care area, by a home health nurse, or in the patient's primary care practitioner office. IBD is a chronic condition for which the patient provides daily self-management. For this reason, teaching is a vital component of care. The patient and family members require instruction for total parenteral nutrition if it is used, as well as information about care of a central venous catheter, including dressing changes and sterile and nonsterile techniques. Instructions should also include how to recognize signs of infection, how to handle infusion pumps and tubing, and how to measure the patient's intake and output. Assist the patient in obtaining the equipment and supplies necessary for care. During home visits and appointments for healthcare, have the patient or parents demonstrate their mastery of care for the central venous catheter and their understanding of TPN techniques. Teach the patient and family about the following topics:

- The type of IBD affecting the patient, including the disease process, short- and long-term effects, the relationship of stress to disease exacerbations, and manifestations of complications
- Prescribed medications, including drug names, desired effects, schedules for tapering the doses if ordered (as with

corticosteroids), and possible side effects or adverse reactions and their management

- Recommended diet and the rationale for any specific restrictions
- Indicators of malabsorption and impaired nutrition; recommendations for self-care and when to seek medical intervention
- If discharged with a central catheter and home parenteral nutrition, written and verbal instructions on catheter care, troubleshooting, and TPN administration (have the patient and a family member demonstrate catheter care and TPN maintenance).
- Importance of maintaining a fluid intake of at least 2–3 quarts per day and increasing fluid intake during warm weather, exercise, or strenuous work and when fever is present
- Increased risk for colorectal cancer and the importance of regular bowel exams
- Risks and benefits of various treatment options.

Provide referrals to a dietary consultant or nutritionist, a community healthcare agency, home care services, and home IV care services as indicated. In addition, suggest resources such as the Crohn and Colitis Foundation of America and the United Ostomy Associations of America, Inc.

Nursing Care Plan
A Patient with Ulcerative Colitis

Cortez Lewis is a 42-year-old real estate agent and mother of three school-age children. She has had ulcerative colitis for 18 years and has been treated with prednisone and sulfasalazine. Over the past 4 months, she has been having abdominal pain and cramping and frequent bloody diarrhea stools. During the same period, she has lost 9 kg (20 lb), and she has had difficulty maintaining her career.

She recently developed several lesions of the lower leg, identified as erythema nodosum. A recent colonoscopy revealed extensive involvement of the entire colon. On admission, Ms. Lewis states, "I'm tired of fighting this disease. I'm a prisoner in my home because of the diarrhea." She is admitted for a total proctocolectomy and IPAA.

ASSESSMENT	DIAGNOSES	PLANNING
Janet Wheeler, RN, completes the admission assessment. Ms. Lewis now weighs 52.2 kg (115 lb). She complains of abdominal cramping, pain, and frequent bloody diarrhea stools. Several reddened lesions are noted on her lower legs. Physical assessment findings include temperature 36.6°C (98°F) oral; pulse 72 bpm; respirations 20/min; and BP 104/72 mmHg. Skin is cool and pale. Abnormal laboratory findings include hemoglobin 7.3 g/dL (normal 12–15), hematocrit 23.3% (normal 36–46), WBCs 15,580/mm^3 (normal 4500–10,000), platelet count 995,000/mm^3 (normal 150,000–400,000), serum protein 4.6 g/dL (normal 6–8), and serum albumin 2.4 g/dL (normal 3.5–5.0). Preparation for surgery is begun.	- *Imbalanced Nutrition: Less Than Body Requirements* related to impaired absorption - *Diarrhea* related to inflammation of bowel - *Fluid Volume, Risk for Deficient,* related to abnormal fluid loss - *Tissue Integrity, Impaired,* related to drainage from temporary ileostomy - *Pain, Acute,* related to surgical intervention - *Sexual Dysfunction* related to temporary ileostomy (NANDA-I © 2014)	- The patient will resume prescribed diet within 5 days after surgery. - The patient will demonstrate normal fecal elimination through the temporary ileostomy. - The patient will maintain adequate fluid balance. - The patient will demonstrate appropriate ostomy care prior to discharge. - The patient will report a tolerable level of discomfort. - The patient will verbalize feelings about sexuality and acknowledge the importance of discussing sexual issues with her husband.

IMPLEMENTATION

- Discuss dietary modifications related to nutritional status and the presence of ileostomy. Provide referral to a dietitian for diet planning and teaching.
- Teach manifestations of dehydration and the importance of maintaining a high fluid intake.
- Teach how to empty and change the ostomy pouch of choice.

- Teach stoma and peristomal skin assessment with each pouch change.
- Teach food blockage management.
- Refer to the local chapter of the United Ostomy Association.
- Provide a list of local medical suppliers for ostomy appliances.

Nursing Care Plan (continued)

EVALUATION

On discharge, Ms. Lewis is caring for her ileostomy by demonstrating her ability to empty, rinse, and change the pouch. The enterostomal therapy (ET) nurse has provided written and verbal instructions on ileostomy care. Ms. Lewis verbalizes her understanding of the recommended diet and the need to limit high-fiber food intake and avoid enteric-coated and timed-release medications. The ET nurse has discussed sexual aspects of having an ileostomy and has given Ms. Lewis a booklet, "Sex and the Female Ostomate," available through the United Ostomy Association. Ms. Lewis is looking forward to the planned surgery to close the temporary ileostomy.

CRITICAL THINKING

1. Why is the patient with an ileostomy at risk for dehydration? How can Ms. Lewis monitor her fluid status at home?

2. Why were Ms. Lewis's hemoglobin and hematocrit low on admission? If her hemoglobin had been low but her hematocrit normal on admission, what might be the explanation?

3. Outline a teaching plan that could be given to patients for home care of an ileostomy.

4. Develop a care plan for Ms. Lewis for the nursing diagnosis *Risk for Impaired Skin Integrity*.

REVIEW Inflammatory Bowel Disease

RELATE Link the Concepts and Exemplars

Linking the exemplar of irritable bowel disease with the concept of stress and coping:

1. What stress management techniques might you teach an adolescent diagnosed with IBD?

2. You are caring for a patient diagnosed with IBD who was just informed of the need for a colectomy with creation of an ileostomy. The patient is very upset and tells the doctor that death is preferable to walking around with "poop coming out of my stomach." What can you do to help this patient cope with the idea of an ileostomy?

Linking the exemplar of irritable bowel disease with the concept of elimination:

3. The patient with IBD is about to have surgery to create an ileostomy. The patient asks, "Will I need to wear a bag all of the time?" How do you respond? Explain your answer.

4. If the patient with IBD is to have a colostomy instead of an ileostomy, how do you respond to the same question: "Will I need to wear a bag all of the time?" Explain your answer.

READY Go to Volume 3: Clinical Nursing Skills

REFER Go to Pearson MyLab Nursing and eText

- Additional review material
- Chart: Nursing Care of the Patient Having an Ileostomy

REFLECT Apply Your Knowledge

Jodi Thompson is a 17-year-old who is a junior in high school. She is a cheerleader for the school, a member of the debate team, and an honor student. Jodi lives with her mother, Marie, and her two brothers, George (age 10) and Joe (age 8). Jodi's mom works full time, so Jodi is responsible for her brothers' care after school or for arranging care. Jodi's dad died of cirrhosis of the liver when Jodi was 10. Jodi is also responsible for caring for her brothers when her mom works weekends, and she is responsible for getting them off to school in the morning. Jodi is planning to take the SAT exam in a few weeks because she is interested in becoming a dentist. Jodi has come to the clinic today because she has been having abdominal pain and frequent loose stools.

1. What risk factors for IBD are apparent in Jodi's history?

2. What nutritional teaching will you plan for Jodi?

3. Create a plan of care for Jodi.

» Exemplar 10.D
Nephritis

Exemplar Learning Outcomes

10.D Analyze nephritis as it relates to inflammation.

- Describe the pathophysiology of nephritis.
- Describe the etiology of nephritis.
- Compare the risk factors and prevention of nephritis.
- Identify the clinical manifestations of nephritis.
- Summarize diagnostic tests and therapies used by interprofessional teams in the collaborative care of an individual with nephritis.
- Differentiate care of patients with nephritis across the lifespan.

- Apply the nursing process in providing culturally competent care to an individual with nephritis.

Exemplar Key Terms

Acute postinfectious glomerulonephritis (APIGN), *708*
Glomerulonephritis, *708*
Goodpasture syndrome, *709*
Lupus nephritis, *709*
Nephritis, *708*
Plasmapheresis, *711*

Overview

Nephritis is an inflammation of the kidneys. The different classifications of nephritis are based on the area of involvement or etiology. One example is **glomerulonephritis**, which is an inflammation of the glomerular capillary membrane. Another is **acute postinfectious glomerulonephritis (APIGN)**, which may develop as a response to a group A beta-hemolytic streptococcal infection of the skin (impetigo) or pharynx (strep throat). Other infecting organisms that cause APIGN are *Staphylococcus*, *Pneumococcus*, and *Coxsackie* virus. Patients with SLE are also at high risk for developing nephritis (called *lupus nephritis*) as a result of autoimmune attacks on the kidney.

Pathophysiology and Etiology

Pathophysiology

In *acute proliferative glomerulonephritis*, glomerular damage occurs as a result of an immune complex reaction that localizes on the glomerular capillary wall. The lodging of antibody–antigen complexes in the glomeruli leads to inflammation and obstruction. The glomerular membranes are thickened, and the obstruction of capillaries in the glomeruli by damaged tissue cells leads to a decreased glomerular filtration rate (GFR). Vascular permeability increases allow protein, red blood cells, and red cell casts to be excreted. The retention of sodium and water expands the intravascular and interstitial compartments, resulting in the characteristic finding of edema (see **Figure 10–10 »**).

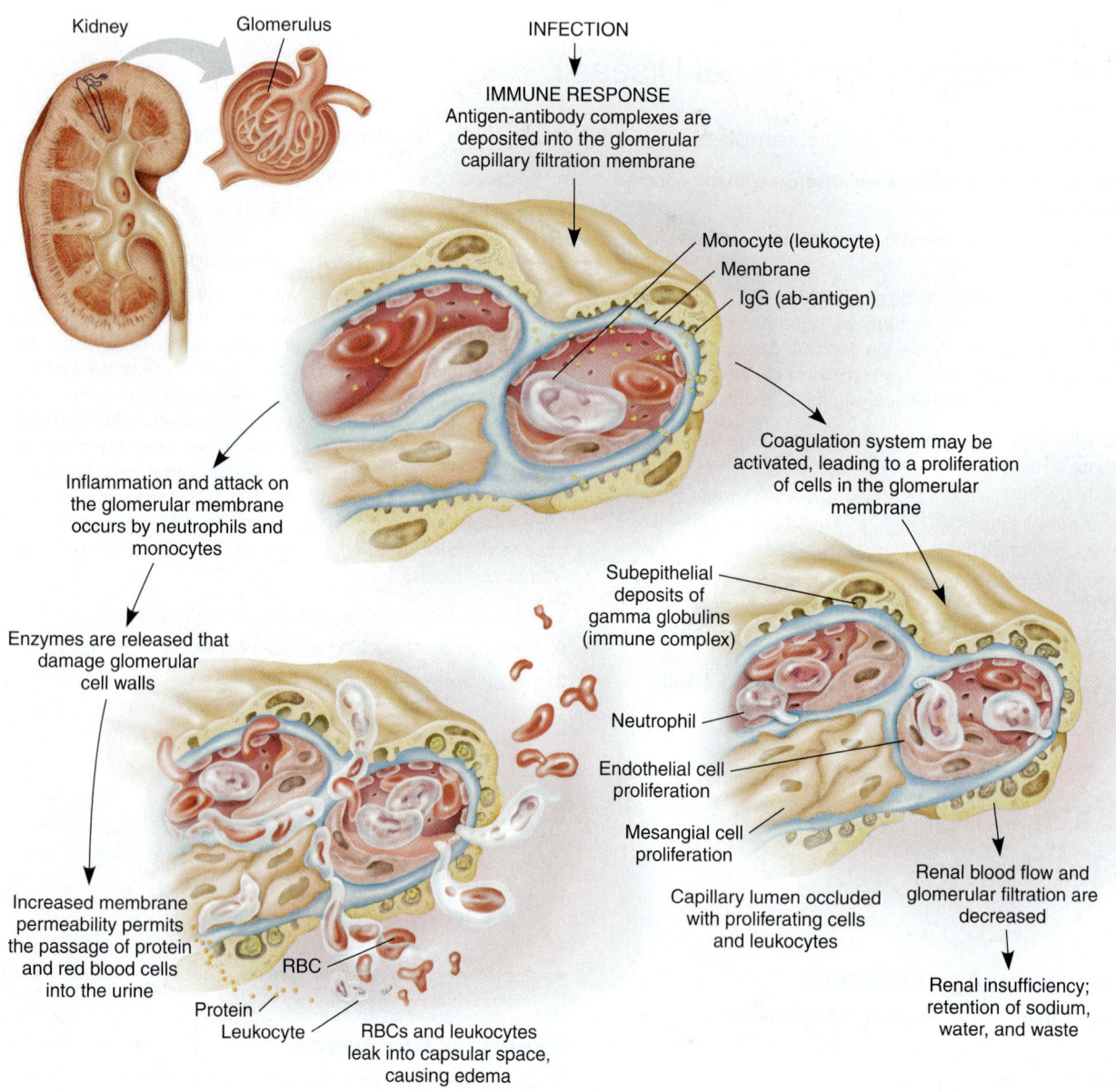

Figure 10–10 » Infection from group A beta-hemolytic *Streptococcus* leads to an immune response that causes inflammation and damage to glomeruli. Protein and red blood cells are allowed to pass through the glomeruli. Obstruction reduces blood flow to the glomeruli, and damaged cells and renal insufficiency lead to retention of sodium, water, and waste.

Chronic glomerulonephritis is typically the end stage of other glomerular disorders, such as rapidly progressive glomerulonephritis (RPGN), lupus nephritis, and diabetic nephropathy. In many cases, however, no previous glomerular disease has been identified. Slow, progressive destruction of the glomeruli and a gradual decline in renal function are characteristic of chronic glomerulonephritis. The kidneys decrease in size symmetrically, and their surfaces become granular or roughened. Entire nephrons are eventually lost. Symptoms develop insidiously, and the disease often is not recognized until signs of renal failure develop.

Lupus nephritis is one of the most severe consequences of SLE, an inflammatory autoimmune disorder affecting the connective tissue of the body (see the Focus on Diversity and Culture feature). Approximately 60% of patients with SLE develop nephritis, and as many as 22% advance to end-stage renal disease. Therefore, nephritis is a major cause of morbidity and mortality associated with SLE (Schwartzman-Morris & Putterman, 2012). Immune complexes that form in the glomerular capillary wall are the usual trigger for glomerular injury in SLE. Manifestations of lupus nephritis range from microscopic hematuria to massive proteinuria. Its progression may be slow and chronic or fulminant, with a sudden onset and the rapid development of renal failure.

Goodpasture syndrome is a rare autoimmune disorder of unknown etiology. It is characterized by formation of antibodies to the glomerular basement membrane. These antibodies may also bind to alveolar basement membranes, damaging alveoli and causing pulmonary hemorrhage. Goodpasture syndrome occurs most commonly in patients between the ages of 20 and 30 and again after the age of 60. It affects men more than women and is most prevalent in White populations (National Kidney Foundation, 2015).

Although the glomeruli may be nearly normal in appearance and function in Goodpasture syndrome, extensive cell proliferation and crescent formation characteristic of RPGN are common. Renal manifestations include hematuria, proteinuria, and edema. Progression to acute renal failure is frequently rapid. Alveolar membrane damage can lead to mild or life-threatening pulmonary hemorrhage. Cough, shortness of breath, and hemoptysis (bloody sputum) are early respiratory manifestations.

Etiology

Each form of nephritis has a distinct etiology. Lupus nephritis is the result of the inflammatory process caused by SLE and is an autoimmune disorder. Glomerulonephritis can result from infection, diabetes mellitus, or SLE. Tubulointerstitial nephritis results from injury to the renal tubules and interstitium, often secondary to glomerular damage (due to drugs, toxins, or radiation) and renovascular disease.

Risk Factors

Patients with diabetes mellitus and/or hypertension are at much higher risk for nephritis secondary to vascular damage to the fragile vessels in the nephron. Infections can travel from the bladder to the kidney or cause scarring that results in urine retention that can damage the nephron. Drug abuse and chronic overuse of over-the-counter painkillers increase risk of nephritis as well.

Focus on Diversity and Culture
Lupus Nephritis

Although the CDC has funded several smaller studies to capture incidence and prevalence of SLE and lupus nephritis, national data are lacking due to the expense involved in gathering and tracking this information and the difficulties determining year of onset (CDC, 2017). Over time, research has confirmed that SLE and the resulting complication of lupus nephritis differentially affect individuals of diverse racial and ethnic backgrounds (Brent, 2015):

- African Americans develop lupus more frequently than Caucasians, have a younger age at onset, and develop nephritis more frequently and at an earlier stage of the disease than Caucasians.
- Hispanic and Asian Americans have greater frequency and severity of nephritis than Caucasians.
- African Americans and Hispanics are more likely than Caucasians to progress to end-stage renal disease after nephritis.
- Mortality related to SLE and lupus nephritis is higher in African Americans and occurs at a younger age than in Caucasians.

Nephritis can also result from prematurity, trauma, or family history of kidney disease. Diseases such as SLE, sickle cell anemia, AIDS, and congestive heart failure can damage the kidney, causing nephritis.

Prevention

The exact cause of nephritis is unknown. Preventing viral infections through practicing good hygiene habits, maintaining adequate diabetes and blood pressure control, quitting smoking, and maintaining a healthy body weight reduce the risk of developing this disease (Parmar, 2015).

Clinical Manifestations

Many patients with acute glomerulonephritis are asymptomatic. The onset is abrupt in other patients, with flank or midabdominal pain, irritability, malaise, and fever. Microscopic hematuria is present in nearly all cases, and gross hematuria, resulting in tea-colored urine, is found in up to 50% of cases and may last for 1–2 weeks. Mild periorbital edema occurs early, along with dependent edema of the feet and ankles. Edema may progress in severity to cause pleural effusion manifested as dyspnea, cough, and crackles (Osborn et al., 2013). Acute hypertension may cause an encephalopathy that includes headache, nausea, vomiting, irritability, lethargy, and seizures. Oliguria may or may not be present.

Acute postinfectious glomerulonephritis is characterized by an abrupt onset of hematuria, proteinuria, salt and water retention, and evidence of azotemia (abnormally high levels of nitrogen waste products in the blood) occurring 10–14 days after the initial infection. The urine often appears brown or cola colored. Salt and water retention increases extracellular fluid volume, leading to hypertension and edema. The edema is noted primarily in the face, particularly around the eyes. Dependent edema, affecting the hands

Clinical Manifestations and Therapies
Nephritis

ETIOLOGY	CLINICAL MANIFESTATIONS	CLINICAL THERAPIES
Salt and water retention	<ul><li>Hypertension</li><li>Hematuria</li><li>Mild to moderate edema</li></ul>	<ul><li>Diuretics</li><li>Antihypertensives</li><li>Sodium restriction</li><li>Low-protein diet</li></ul>
Severe hypertension	<ul><li>Extremely high blood pressure with cerebral dysfunction</li></ul>	<ul><li>Emergency care that includes IV diazoxide, hydralazine, or labetalol</li></ul>
Progressive edema, acute inflammatory processes	<ul><li>Ascites</li><li>Pulmonary effusion</li></ul>	<ul><li>Immunosuppressive therapy (cyclophosphamide, azathioprine)</li><li>Corticosteroids</li><li>Sodium restriction</li></ul>
Encephalopathy resulting from acute hypertension	<ul><li>Headache</li><li>Nausea and vomiting</li><li>Irritability</li></ul>	<ul><li>Antihypertensives</li><li>Analgesics</li><li>Additional therapies as warranted</li></ul>
Presence of infection	<ul><li>Salt and water retention</li><li>Fever</li><li>Malaise</li><li>Edema</li></ul>	<ul><li>Antibiotics</li><li>Bedrest</li><li>Sodium restriction</li><li>Antipyretics</li></ul>

and upper extremities in particular, may also be noted. Other manifestations are fatigue, anorexia, nausea and vomiting, and headache.

Collaboration

Collaborative care of the patient with nephritis may include a nephrologist, primary care provider, nurses, pharmacists, dieticians or nutritionists, and (in the case of school-age children) parents, teachers, and the school nurse. The nurse's role includes patient teaching, follow-up, and coordination of referral services and communication between members of the healthcare team. Treatment focuses on relief of symptoms and supportive therapy.

Diagnostic Tests

Laboratory and diagnostic testing is valuable for identifying the cause of nephritis and to evaluate kidney function.

The following studies may be ordered to help identify the etiology:

- *Throat or skin cultures* detect infection by group A beta-hemolytic streptococci. Although poststreptococcal glomerulonephritis typically follows the acute infection by 1–2 weeks, treatment to eradicate any remaining organisms is initiated to minimize antibody production.
- *Antistreptolysin O (ASO) titer* and other blood tests detect streptococcal *exoenzymes* (bacterial enzymes that stimulate the immune response in acute postinfection glomerulonephritis). Other titers such as antistreptokinase (ASK) and antideoxyribonuclease B (ADNAase B) may be obtained as well.

- *Erythrocyte sedimentation rate (ESR)* is a general indicator of inflammatory response. It may be elevated in acute postinfection glomerulonephritis and in lupus nephritis.
- *KUB* (kidney, ureter, bladder) *abdominal x-ray* may be done to evaluate kidney size and to rule out other causes of the patient's manifestations. The kidneys may be enlarged in acute nephritis, whereas bilateral small kidneys are typical of late chronic glomerulonephritis.
- *Kidney scan,* a nuclear medicine procedure, allows visualization of the kidney after IV administration of a radioisotope. In glomerular diseases, the uptake and excretion of the radioactive material are delayed.
- *Biopsy,* a microscopic examination of kidney tissue, is essential and the most reliable diagnostic procedure for glomerular disorders. Biopsy helps determine the type of nephritis, the prognosis, and the appropriate treatment. Renal biopsy is usually done percutaneously, by inserting a biopsy needle through the skin into the kidney to obtain a tissue sample. Open biopsy, which requires surgery, may also be done.

The following studies are used to evaluate kidney function:

- *BUN* measures urea nitrogen, the end product of protein metabolism, which is created by the breakdown and metabolism of both dietary and body proteins. Urea is eliminated from the body by filtration in the glomerulus; minimal amounts are reabsorbed in the renal tubules. Glomerular diseases interfere with filtration and elimination of urea nitrogen, causing blood levels to rise. Increased protein catabolism (destruction), which may occur with GI bleeding or tissue breakdown, can also raise BUN. Levels up to 50 mg/dL or 17.7 mmol/L indicate mild azotemia, and levels higher than 100 mg/dL or 35.7 mmol/L indicate severe renal impairment.

- *Serum creatinine* measures the amount of creatinine in the blood. Creatinine also is a metabolic by-product, produced in relatively constant amounts by skeletal muscles. It is excreted entirely by the kidneys, making serum creatinine a good indicator of kidney function. Normal values are lower in the older adult because of decreased muscle mass. Levels greater than 4 mg/dL indicate serious impairment of renal function.

- *Urine creatinine* is also an indicator of renal function and the GFR. Urine creatinine levels decrease when renal function is impaired because creatinine is not effectively eliminated from the body.

- *Creatinine clearance* is a specific indicator of renal function used to evaluate the GFR. The *clearance,* or amount of blood cleared of creatinine in 1 minute, depends on the amount and pressure of blood being filtered and the filtering ability of the glomeruli. Levels normally decline with age as the GFR decreases in the older adult. Disorders such as nephritis affect glomerular filtration, decreasing the creatinine clearance.

- *Serum electrolytes* are evaluated because impaired kidney function alters their excretion. Monitoring serum electrolytes is particularly important to prevent complications associated with imbalances.

- *Urinalysis* often shows RBCs and proteins in the urine of patients with a glomerular disorder. These substances, normally too large to enter glomerular filtrate, escape because of increased porosity of glomerular capillaries in glomerular disorders. A 24-hour urine specimen is used to determine the amount of protein in the urine.

Pharmacologic Therapy

Although no drugs are available to cure glomerular disorders, medications are used to treat underlying disorders, reduce inflammation, and manage the symptoms.

Edema and mild to moderate hypertension should be treated with sodium restriction and a diuretic such as furosemide (Huang et al., 2013). Immediate emergency care is needed for severe hypertension with cerebral dysfunction; medication such as diazoxide or hydralazine is administered intravenously. Antibiotics are prescribed for the patient with acute postinfection glomerulonephritis to eradicate any remaining bacteria, removing the stimulus for antibody production. Nephrotoxic antibiotics, such as the aminoglycoside antibiotics and some cephalosporins, are avoided.

Aggressive immunosuppressive therapy is used to treat acute inflammatory processes such as RPGN, Goodpasture syndrome, and exacerbations of SLE. When begun early, immunosuppressive therapy significantly reduces the risk of end-stage renal disease and renal failure. Prednisone, a glucocorticoid, is prescribed in relatively large doses of 1 mg per kilogram of body weight per day (e.g., a 160-lb man would receive 70–75 mg per day) and tapered according to response. Other immunosuppressive agents such as cyclophosphamide (Cytoxan), azathioprine (Imuran), or mycophenolate (Cellcept) are prescribed in conjunction with corticosteroids (Vincent, 2014). Corticosteroid use in acute postinfectious glomerulonephritis may actually worsen the condition, so it is avoided.

Angiotensin-converting–enzyme (ACE) inhibitors or angiotensin receptor blockers (ARBs) may be ordered to reduce protein loss associated with nephrotic syndrome. These drugs reduce proteinuria and slow the progression of renal failure. They have a protective effect on the kidney in patients with diabetic nephropathy.

Antihypertensives may be prescribed to maintain blood pressure within normal levels. Blood pressure management is important because systemic and renal hypertension is associated with a poorer prognosis in patients with glomerular disorders.

Nonpharmacologic Therapy

Bedrest may be ordered during acute postinfectious glomerulonephritis. Fluid requirements are determined by careful monitoring of urinary output, weight, blood pressure, and serum electrolytes. At first, only insensible fluid losses are replaced until the status of renal function is known. Dietary restriction of sodium and potassium intake may be necessary; with severe azotemia, protein intake may have to be limited.

When the edema of nephrotic syndrome is significant or the patient is hypertensive, sodium intake may be restricted to 1–2 g per day. Dietary protein may be restricted if azotemia is present. When proteins are restricted, those included in the diet should be complete or high-value proteins. Complete proteins supply the essential amino acids required for growth and tissue maintenance; they include milk, eggs, cheese, meats, poultry, fish, and soy. Incomplete proteins either lack one or more essential amino acids or lack adequate proportions. They include breads, cereals and grains, legumes, seeds, and nuts.

Plasma exchange therapy (**plasmapheresis**), a procedure to remove damaging antibodies from the plasma, is used in conjunction with immunosuppressive therapy to treat RPGN and Goodpasture syndrome. Plasma and glomerular-damaging antibodies are removed with a blood cell separator. The RBCs are then returned to the patient along with albumin or human plasma to replace the plasma removed. This procedure is usually done in a series of treatments. It does have risks, and informed consent is required. Potential complications of plasma exchange therapy include those associated with IV catheters, fluid volume shifts, and altered coagulation.

Lifespan Considerations

Nephritis in Children

Acute focal bacterial nephritis, renal abscess, and pyonephrosis should be suspected in children with severe presentation and urologic history (Bitsori et al., 2015). In addition, appropriate imaging is critical for management planning with close follow-up regarding the prognosis.

Nephritis in Pregnant Women

A recent study explored the management of lupus nephritis in pregnancy; it showed that pregnancy may result in an increased risk of disease flare and adverse maternal and fetal outcomes, such as preeclampsia, fetal loss, and preterm delivery (Kattah & Garovic, 2015). Experts also ascertain that maternal disease activity and fetal well-being should be monitored closely by an interprofessional team throughout the patient's pregnancy (Brent, 2015).

Nephritis in Older Adults

Acute interstitial nephritis is seen as an important cause of acute kidney injury, and its prevalence in older adults may be increasing. In addition, the vast majority of acute interstitial nephritis cases in older adults are due to drugs (proton pump inhibitors [PPIs] and antibiotics), and older adults appear to have an increased risk of developing chronic kidney disease or end-stage renal disease as compared with younger patients, with the highest mortality risk if the condition develops during hospitalization (Murithi et al., 2014).

At the outset the older adult may have fewer apparent symptoms. Nausea, malaise, arthralgias, and proteinuria are common manifestations; hypertension and edema are seen less often. Pulmonary infiltrates may occur early in the disorder, often due to worsening of a preexisting condition such as heart failure.

NURSING PROCESS

Nursing care is supportive and educational. Monitoring renal function and fluid volume status are key components of care, as is protecting the patient from infection. Both manifestations of glomerular disorders and their treatment can interfere with a patient's ability to maintain usual roles and responsibilities.

Assessment

Focused assessment data related to glomerular disorders include the following:

- **Observation and patient interview.** Complaints of facial or peripheral edema or weight gain, fatigue, nausea and vomiting, headache, general malaise, and abdominal or flank pain; cough or shortness of breath; changes in amount, color, or character of urine (e.g., frothy urine); history of skin or pharyngeal streptococcal infection, diabetes, SLE, or kidney disease; and current medications
- **Physical examination.** General appearance; vital signs; weight; presence of periorbital, facial, or peripheral edema; skin for lesions or infection; throat to obtain culture as indicated; and urine specimen for color, character, and odor.

Diagnosis

Nursing diagnoses that may apply to the patient with nephritis include the following:

- *Infection, Risk for*
- *Fluid Volume, Excess*
- *Skin Integrity, Risk for Impaired*
- *Imbalanced Nutrition: Less Than Body Requirements*

- *Fatigue*
- *Role Performance, Ineffective.*

(NANDA-I © 2014)

Planning

Goals of nursing care should be developmentally appropriate and may include the following:

- The patient will demonstrate urinary output of at least 0.5 mL/kg/hr.
- The patient will demonstrate dietary intake that adequately meets nutritional and caloric needs.
- The patient will demonstrate no signs or symptoms of infection.
- The patient will demonstrate no alterations in skin integrity.

For pediatric patients, the following additional goals may be appropriate:

- The patient will remain on track to complete educational requirements.
- The patient will engage in diversional activities during periods of bedrest and activity restriction.

Implementation

Bedrest is required during the acute phase. Nursing care focuses on monitoring fluid status, preventing infection, preventing skin breakdown, meeting nutritional needs, and providing emotional support to the patient and family.

Prevent Infection

Impaired renal function puts the patient at risk for infection. Immunosuppressive drugs may mask the presence of infection. Monitor for signs of infection, including fever, increased malaise, and an elevated WBC count, which may be an early indicator of infection.

Avoid or minimize invasive procedures. If catheterization is required, use sterile intermittent straight catheterization or maintain a closed drainage system for an indwelling catheter. Prevent urine reflux from the drainage system to the bladder or the bladder to the kidneys by ensuring a patent gravity flow system.

Instruct the family in good hand hygiene. Limit visitors, and screen for upper respiratory infections. Screen family members for the presence of streptococcal infection and, if necessary, refer for treatment.

SAFETY ALERT Monitor vital signs, temperature, and mental status every 4 hours. Fever and elevated WBCs are common indicators of infection; anti-inflammatory drugs, however, may moderate this response. Patients taking anti-inflammatory drugs may exhibit tachycardia, increasing lethargy, or confusion as the initial signs of infection.

Protect Skin Integrity

Dependent areas or areas prone to pressure are vulnerable to skin breakdown. Turn the hospitalized patient frequently.

Pad bony prominences or susceptible areas with sheepskin, or protect skin with a transparent dressing. Make sure the patient's bed is free of crumbs. Keep sheets tight and free of wrinkles.

Promote Nutritional Balance

A team approach is often needed to meet the patient's nutritional needs. In most cases, the patient follows a no-added-salt and low-protein diet. Anorexia presents the greatest challenge to meeting daily nutritional requirements during the acute phase of the disease. To increase the patient's appetite, encourage family members to bring the patient's favorite foods from home, serve age-appropriate quantities to children, and allow the patient to eat with other patients or with family members.

Monitor and Maintain Fluid Volume Balance

Monitor vital signs, fluid and electrolyte status, and intake and output. Hypovolemia can occur as a result of fluid shifting from vascular to interstitial spaces despite the outward clinical signs of excess fluid retention. Monitor the degree of ascites by measuring abdominal girth. Document urine specific gravity.

Maintain fluid restriction as ordered. Offer ice chips (in limited and measured amounts) and frequent mouth care to relieve thirst. Make sure family members and visitors understand the need to limit fluids to prevent excessive intake. Arrange dietary consultation regarding sodium- or protein-restricted diets.

SAFETY ALERT Carefully monitor and regulate IV infusions; include fluid used to dilute IV medications as intake. Significant "hidden" fluid intake can occur with IV medication administration.

Prevent Unnecessary Fatigue

Fatigue is a common manifestation of nephritis. Anemia, loss of plasma proteins, headache, anorexia, and nausea compound this fatigue. The maintenance of usual physical and mental activities may be impaired.

Schedule activities and procedures to provide adequate rest and energy conservation. Assist with ADLs as needed. Reduce energy demands with frequent small meals and short periods of activity. Limit the number of visitors and visit length. Discuss with the patient and family the relationship between fatigue and the disease process.

Promote Healthy Self-Esteem

The manifestations and treatment of nephritis can affect the maintenance of usual roles and activities. Fatigue and muscle weakness may limit physical and social activities. Bedrest or activity limitations may be ordered to minimize the degree of proteinuria. If azotemia is present, malaise, nausea, and mental status changes can interfere with role function. Facial and periorbital edema affects the patient's self-esteem and may lead to isolation.

Encourage patient self-care and participation in decision making. Support coping skills, helping the patient identify personal strengths. Discuss the effect of the disease and treatments on roles and relationships, helping the patient identify potential changes in roles, relationships, and lifestyle. Help the patient and family develop a plan for alternative behaviors and relationships, encouraging the patient to maintain usual roles to the extent possible.

Provide accurate and optimistic information about the disorder and its short- and long-term effects. Evaluate the need for additional support and social services for the patient and family. Provide referrals as indicated.

Evaluation

Expected outcomes of nursing care include the following:

- The patient maintains or regains normal urine output.
- The patient develops no areas of redness, abrasions, or skin breakdown over pressure points.
- The patient's temperature remains within normal limits, and the patient is free of secondary infection.
- The patient maintains pre-illness weight and tolerates daily intake that meets nutritional requirements.
- The patient takes medications as prescribed.
- The patient's sodium and potassium levels reflect adherence to dietary restrictions.

If the patient does not progress satisfactorily to the expected outcomes, the nurse must complete a thorough assessment; particularly the patient's reported pain level, diet tolerance, and vital signs. Signs and symptoms of infection such as elevated temperature and increased pain will require notifying the patient's primary provider. Further diagnostic workup may include a CBC and blood cultures to rule out sepsis development secondary to the disease. IV fluids may be reinstated as well as IV pain medication, an NPO status and IV antibiotics. Surgical consult may be conducted.

Patient Teaching
Acute Nephritis

Acute postinfectious glomerulonephritis typically resolves following appropriate treatment. Other types of nephritis, however, may be progressive. In either case, the course of the disorder is difficult and may be lengthy, sometimes ranging from months to years. Self-management is essential. Provide instructions for the patient and family, including the following topics:

- Information about the disease and the prognosis
- Prescribed treatment, including activity and diet restrictions; the use and potential effects, both beneficial and adverse, of all medications
- Risks, manifestations, prevention, and management of complications such as edema and infection
- Signs, symptoms, and implications of improving or declining renal function
- Measures to prevent further kidney damage, such as avoiding nephrotoxic drugs
- Community resources such as home care providers, support groups, and (for children) home school teachers or tutoring programs.

Nursing Care Plan
A Patient with Acute Nephritis

Jung-Lin Chang is a 23-year-old graduate student in biology. He presents at the university health center with brown and foamy urine. The physician admits him to the infirmary and orders a throat culture, ASO titer, CBC, BUN, serum creatinine, and urinalysis.

ASSESSMENT

Connie King, the nurse admitting Mr. Chang, notes that his history is essentially negative for past kidney or urinary problems. He relates having had a "pretty bad" sore throat a couple of weeks before admission. However, it was during midterms, so he took a few antibiotics he had from a previous bout of strep throat, increased his fluids, and did not see a doctor. The sore throat resolved, and he felt well until noticing the change in his urine. He admits that his eyes seemed a little puffy, but he thought this was due to lack of sleep and fatigue. He has eaten little the past 2 days but was not alarmed because his food intake is irregular most of the time.

Physical assessment findings include temperature 37.1°C (98.8°F) oral; pulse 98 bpm; respirations 18/min; and BP 136/90 mmHg. His weight is 75 kg (165 lb), up from his normal of 72.5 kg (160 lb). BUN is 42 mg/dL, and serum creatinine is 2.1 mg/dL. Urinalysis reveals the presence of protein, RBCs, and RBC casts. A subsequent 24-hour urine protein analysis shows 1025 mg of protein (normal 25–150 mg/24 hours).

The physician diagnoses acute postinfectious glomerulonephritis and places Mr. Chang on bedrest with bathroom privileges. The physician orders fluid restriction (1200 mL/day) and a restricted sodium and protein diet.

DIAGNOSES

- *Fluid Volume, Excess,* related to plasma protein deficit and sodium and water retention
- *Imbalanced Nutrition: Less Than Body Requirements* related to anorexia
- *Anxiety* related to prescribed activity restriction
- *Self-Care, Readiness for Enhanced,* related to lack of information about nephritis and treatment

(NANDA-I © 2014)

PLANNING

- The patient will maintain blood pressure within normal limits.
- The patient will return to usual weight with no evidence of edema.
- The patient will consume adequate calories following prescribed dietary limitations.
- The patient will verbalize reduced anxiety regarding ability to continue studies.
- The patient will demonstrate an understanding of acute nephritis and the prescribed treatment regimen.

IMPLEMENTATION

- Take vital signs every 4 hours; notify the physician of significant changes.
- Weigh daily; monitor and record intake and output.
- Schedule fluids, allowing 650 mL on day shift, 450 mL on evening shift, and 100 mL on night shift.
- Arrange dietary consultation to plan a diet that includes preferred foods as allowed.
- Provide small meals with high-carbohydrate between-meal snacks.
- Encourage Mr. Chang to talk about his condition and its potential effects.
- Assist with problem solving and exploring options for maintaining studies.
- Enlist friends and family to listen and provide support.
- Teach Mr. Chang and his family about acute nephritis and the prescribed treatment.
- Instruct in appropriate antibiotic use.

EVALUATION

Mr. Chang is released from the infirmary after 4 days. He decides to return to his parents' home for the 6–12 weeks of convalescence prescribed by his doctor. Mr. Chang's renal function gradually returns to normal with no further azotemia and minimal proteinuria after 4 months. He verbalizes understanding the relationship between the strep throat, his inappropriate use of antibiotics, and the nephritis. He says, "I may not always remember to take every pill on time in the future, but I sure won't save them for the next time again!"

CRITICAL THINKING

1. How did Mr. Chang's use of "a few" previously prescribed antibiotics to treat his sore throat affect his risk for developing acute postinfectious glomerulonephritis?

2. What additional risk factors did Mr. Chang have for developing nephritis?

3. The initial manifestations of acute postinfectious glomerulonephritis and RPGN are very similar. What diagnostic test would the physician use to make the differential diagnosis? Develop a plan of care for a patient undergoing this examination.

REVIEW Nephritis

RELATE Link the Concepts and Exemplars

Linking the exemplar of nephritis with the concept of fluids and electrolytes:

1. If you are caring for a patient with nephritis whose kidney function is insufficient to eliminate adequate fluid and waste products from the body, what nursing care might you provide to maintain fluid and electrolyte homeostasis?

2. While caring for a patient with acute nephritis and reduced urine output, you review the laboratory studies and find that the patient's serum potassium is greater than 6 mg/dL. What are your priorities for care? What orders would you anticipate receiving when you notify the primary provider?

Linking the exemplar of nephritis with the concept of mobility:

3. If the patient with nephritis is required to maintain bedrest, how will you promote a return to ambulation when the time comes?

4. To promote future mobility, what nursing care can you provide the patient who requires bedrest?

READY Go to Volume 3: Clinical Nursing Skills

REFER Go to Pearson MyLab Nursing and eText

- Additional review material

REFLECT Apply Your Knowledge

Marina McCullough, 13 years old, comes home from school and tells her mother that she does not feel well. She complains of feeling tired, having pain in her left flank, and feeling warm. Her mother goes into the bathroom to get the electronic thermometer to check Marina's temperature and notices that Marina forgot to flush the toilet. When she reaches over to flush the toilet, she notices that the water looks like iced tea. She checks Marina's oral temperature and gets a reading of 100.8°F. She suspects a possible UTI and wonders if Marina is sexually active, but she decides not to approach the subject when Marina is not feeling well.

Ms. McCullough, Marina's mother, makes an appointment with Marina's pediatrician and takes her in later that afternoon. The nurse admits her, notes mild periorbital edema and +2 pitting edema in both feet, and collects a urine specimen that tests positive for blood and protein. Ms. McCullough administered acetaminophen earlier in the afternoon to treat both the fever and the pain. Marina's vital signs upon arrival at the pediatrician's office are temperature 99.4°F tympanic; pulse 92 bpm; respirations 18/min; and BP 138/86 mmHg. Her weight is 132 lb, which Marina reports is an 8-lb weight gain since she last checked it 3 days ago. Breath sounds reveal mild crackles in bases bilaterally, and the nurse notes a rattling productive cough. Marina reports pain rated 7 in the right flank area, persistent headache, and nausea and feeling tired.

Marina is diagnosed with nephritis and is admitted to the acute care facility on the adolescent unit. The doctor orders serum electrolytes, CBC with differential, BUN, serum creatinine, creatinine clearance, KUB, urine culture, and kidney scan. He also orders fluid restriction to 750 mL per day.

1. How will you ration Marina's fluids throughout a 24-hour day?

2. You are starting a 24-hour urine collection for creatinine. How will you instruct the patient to begin? What actions will you take to improve accuracy of the 24-hour collection?

3. What priority assessments will you perform when admitting Marina?

≫ Exemplar 10.E
Peptic Ulcer Disease

Exemplar Learning Outcomes

10.E Analyze peptic ulcer disease as it relates to inflammation.

- Describe the pathophysiology of peptic ulcer disease.
- Describe the etiology of peptic ulcer disease.
- Compare the risk factors and prevention of peptic ulcer disease.
- Identify the clinical manifestations of peptic ulcer disease.
- Summarize diagnostic tests and therapies used by interprofessional teams in the collaborative care of an individual with peptic ulcer disease.
- Differentiate care of patients with peptic ulcer disease across the lifespan.
- Apply the nursing process in providing culturally competent care to an individual with peptic ulcer disease.

Exemplar Key Terms

Duodenal ulcers, *715*
Gastric outlet obstruction, *717*
Gastric ulcers, *716*
Hemorrhage, *717*
Peptic ulcer disease (PUD), *715*
Peptic ulcers, *715*
Perforation, *717*
Steatorrhea, *717*
Ulcer, *716*
Zollinger-Ellison syndrome, *717*

Overview

Peptic ulcer disease (PUD) is a chronic health problem caused by a break in the mucous lining of the GI tract where it comes in contact with gastric juice. PUD affects over 14.5 million individuals in the United States yearly, resulting in 1.4 million ambulatory care visits and approximately 500,000 hospitalizations every year (NIDDK, 2014).

Peptic ulcers may occur in any area of the GI tract exposed to acid-pepsin secretions, including the esophagus, stomach, and duodenum. The most common are **duodenal ulcers**, which occur in the duodenum. They usually develop between the ages of 30 and 55 and are more common in men than in women. **Gastric ulcers**, which occur in the stomach, more often affect older patients between the ages of 55 and 70. Ulcers are more common in individuals who smoke and who are long-term users of NSAIDs. Alcohol and dietary intake do not seem to cause PUD, and the role of stress is uncertain.

Pathophysiology and Etiology

Pathophysiology

The innermost layer of the stomach wall, the gastric mucosa, consists of columnar epithelial cells supported by a middle layer of blood vessels and glands and a thin outer layer of smooth muscle. The mucosal barrier of the stomach, a thin coating of mucous gel and bicarbonate, protects the gastric mucosa. The mucosal barrier is maintained by bicarbonate secreted by the epithelial cells, by mucous gel production stimulated by prostaglandins, and by an adequate blood supply to the mucosa. An **ulcer** develops when the mucosal barrier is unable to protect the mucosa from damage by hydrochloric acid and pepsin, the gastric digestive juices.

Helicobacter pylori infection, found in about 70% of individuals who have PUD, is unique in colonizing the stomach. It is spread individual to individual (oral–oral or fecal–oral) and contributes to ulcer formation in several ways. The bacteria produce enzymes that reduce the efficacy of mucous gel in protecting the gastric mucosa. In addition, the host's inflammatory response to *H. pylori* contributes to gastric epithelial cell damage without producing immunity to the infection. Although the gastric mucosa is the usual site for *H. pylori* infection, this infection also contributes to duodenal ulcers. The reason may be increased production of gastric acid associated with *H. pylori* infection.

NSAIDs contribute to PUD through both systemic and topical mechanisms of injury. Prostaglandins are necessary for maintaining the gastric mucosal barrier. NSAIDs interrupt prostaglandin synthesis by disrupting the action of the two cyclooxygenase (COX) enzymes. COX-1 is necessary to maintain the integrity of the gastric mucosa, and COX-2 responds to inflammatory stimulation. The COX-2–selective NSAIDs may be less damaging to the gastric mucosa because they have less effect on the COX-1 enzyme. In addition to their systemic effect, aspirin and many other NSAIDs exert topical injury by crossing the lipid membranes of gastric epithelial cells, damaging the cells themselves.

The ulcers of PUD may affect the esophagus, stomach, or duodenum. They may be superficial or deep, affecting all layers of the mucosa. Duodenal ulcers, the most common, usually develop in the proximal portion of the duodenum, close to the pylorus (see **Figure 10–11** 》). They are sharply demarcated and usually less than 1 cm in diameter (see **Figure 10–12** 》). Gastric ulcers often are found on the lesser curvature and the area immediately proximal to the pylorus. Gastric ulcers are associated with an increased incidence of gastric cancer.

PUD may be chronic, with spontaneous remissions and exacerbations. Exacerbations of the disease may be associated with trauma, infection, or other physical or psychologic stressors.

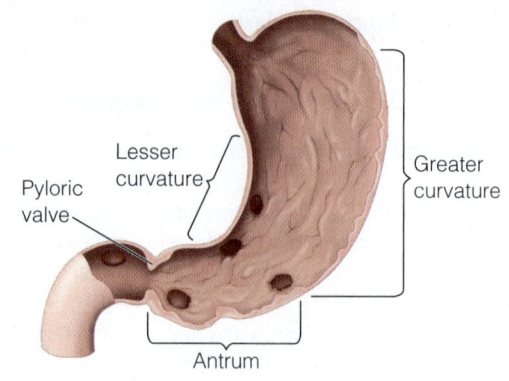

Figure 10–11 》 Common sites affected by peptic ulcer disease.

Etiology

H. pylori infections often occur in several members of a family, especially when the family's water supply is contaminated. Diet is usually not a major factor in the development of peptic ulcers, although caffeine and alcohol consumption may exacerbate the disease.

Risk Factors

Chronic *H. pylori* infection and chronic use of NSAIDs, including aspirin, are the major risk factors for PUD (NIDDK, 2015). Overall, an estimated 1 in 6 patients infected with *H. pylori* develops PUD. Of the NSAIDs, aspirin is the most ulcerogenic. Cigarette smoking is a significant risk factor, doubling the risk of PUD. Cigarette smoking inhibits the secretion of bicarbonate by the pancreas and may cause more rapid transit of gastric acid into the duodenum. Other risk factors include low socioeconomic status; crowded, unsanitary living conditions; unclean food or water; advanced age; history of ulcer or family history of PUD; and concurrent use of other drugs (e.g., glucocorticoids, bisphosphonates).

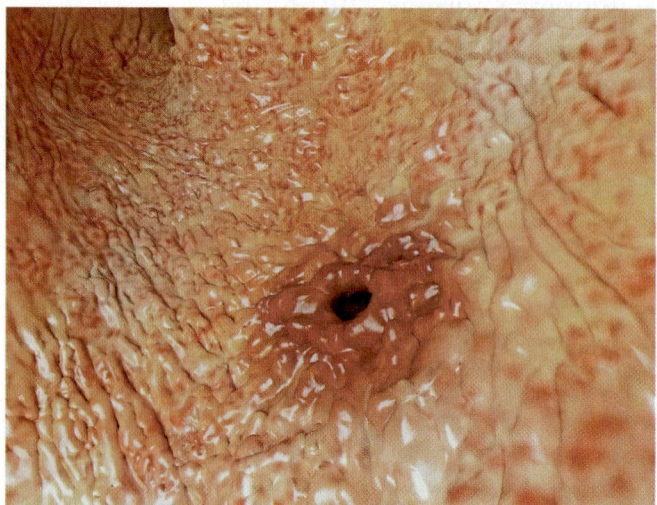

Source: Juan Gaertner/Shutterstock.

Figure 10–12 》 A superficial peptic ulcer.

Prevention

The etiology of the peptic ulcer determines what actions are possible to minimize the risk of developing the disease. Recommendations for prevention of *H. pylori* infection include meticulous hand hygiene and implementing all recommendations related to food preparation, including ensuring thorough cooking of meat. For patients whose history includes long-term NSAID use, recommendations include adding either a histamine receptor antagonist, PPI, or misoprostol (Cytotec) with the NSAID or changing treatment to a COX-2–selective NSAID to reduce the occurrence of peptic ulcers. All patients started on long-term therapy with nonselective NSAIDs should be tested for *H. pylori* regardless of their level of risk (He et al., 2014).

Clinical Manifestations

Abdominal pain is the classic symptom of PUD. The pain is typically described as gnawing, burning, aching, or hunger-like, and it is experienced in the epigastric region, sometimes radiating to the back. The pain occurs when the stomach is empty (2–3 hours after meals and in the middle of the night) and is relieved by eating, with a classic pain–food–relief pattern. The patient may complain of heartburn or regurgitation and may vomit.

The presentation of PUD in the older adult is often less clear, with vague and poorly localized discomfort, perhaps chest pain or dysphagia, weight loss, or anemia. In the older adult, a complication of PUD, such as upper GI hemorrhage or perforation of the stomach or duodenum, may be the presenting symptom.

The complications associated with peptic ulcers include hemorrhage, obstruction, and perforation. See **Box 10–4 »** for the manifestations of these complications.

Among individuals with PUD, 10–20% experience **hemorrhage** (rapid or excessive bleeding) as a result of ulceration

---

Box 10–4
Manifestations of Peptic Ulcer Disease Complications

Hemorrhage
- Occult or obvious blood in the stool
- Hematemesis
- Fatigue
- Weakness, dizziness
- Orthostatic hypotension
- Hypovolemic shock

Obstruction
- Sensations of epigastric fullness
- Nausea and vomiting
- Electrolyte imbalances
- Metabolic alkalosis

Perforation
- Severe upper abdominal pain radiating to the shoulder
- Rigid, boardlike abdomen
- Absence of bowel sounds
- Diaphoresis
- Tachycardia
- Rapid, shallow respirations
- Fever

---

and erosion into the blood vessels of the gastric mucosa. In the older adult, bleeding is the most frequent complication. When small blood vessels erode, blood loss may be slow and insidious, with occult blood in the stool the only initial sign. If bleeding continues, the patient becomes anemic and experiences symptoms of weakness, fatigue, dizziness, and orthostatic hypotension. Erosion into a larger vessel can lead to sudden and severe bleeding with hematemesis, melena, or hematochezia and signs of hypovolemic shock.

Gastric outlet obstruction (obstruction of the pyloric region of the stomach and duodenum that impairs gastric outflow) may result from edema surrounding the ulcer, smooth muscle spasm, or scar tissue. In general, obstruction is a gradual rather than an acute process. Symptoms include a feeling of epigastric fullness, accentuated ulcer symptoms, and nausea. If the obstruction becomes complete, vomiting occurs. Hydrochloric acid, sodium, and potassium are lost in vomitus, the potential result being fluid and electrolyte imbalance and metabolic alkalosis.

The most lethal complication of PUD is **perforation**, penetration of the ulcer through the mucosal wall. When perforation occurs, gastric or duodenal contents enter the peritoneum, causing an inflammatory process and peritonitis. Chemical peritonitis from the hydrochloric acid, pepsin, bile, and pancreatic fluid is immediate; within 6–12 hours bacterial peritonitis follows from gastric contaminants entering the normally sterile peritoneal cavity. When an ulcer perforates, the patient has immediate, severe upper abdominal pain radiating throughout the abdomen and possibly to the shoulder. The abdomen becomes rigid and boardlike, and bowel sounds are absent. Signs of shock may be present and include diaphoresis; tachycardia; and rapid, shallow respirations. Classic symptoms of perforation may not be present in an older adult. Instead, the older adult may present with mental confusion and other nonspecific symptoms. This atypical presentation can lead to delays in diagnosis and treatment, increasing the associated mortality rate.

Zollinger-Ellison syndrome is a form of PUD caused by a gastrinoma, or gastrin-secreting tumor. Gastrinomas may be benign, although they are usually malignant. Gastrin is a hormone that stimulates the secretion of pepsin and hydrochloric acid. The increased gastrin levels associated with these tumors result in hypersecretion of gastric acid, which in turn causes mucosal ulceration.

The peptic ulcers of Zollinger-Ellison syndrome most often affect the duodenum but may involve the stomach or jejunum. Characteristic ulcerlike pain is common. The high levels of hydrochloric acid entering the duodenum overwhelm the protective buffering mechanism; the result is diarrhea and **steatorrhea** (excess fat in the feces) from impaired fat digestion and absorption. Complications of bleeding and perforation are often seen with Zollinger-Ellison syndrome. Fluid and electrolyte imbalances also may result from persistent diarrhea, with resultant losses of potassium and sodium in particular.

Collaboration

Treatment for PUD focuses on treating its cause. Primary treatments include eradicating *H. pylori* infection and treating or preventing ulcers related to use of NSAIDs. The nurse

Clinical Manifestations and Therapies
Peptic Ulcer Disease

ETIOLOGY	CLINICAL MANIFESTATIONS	CLINICAL THERAPIES
H. pylori infection	■ Gnawing or burning pain in the epigastric region when stomach is empty ■ Possible heartburn or regurgitation ■ Manifestations in older adults possibly unapparent until complications arise	■ PPI in combination with two antibiotics to eliminate infection OR ■ Bismuth-containing product with two antibiotics and a PPI ■ If retreatment is required, use of different antibiotics (Lv et al., 2015)
NSAIDs	■ Pain in the epigastric region when stomach is empty ■ Possible heartburn or regurgitation ■ Manifestations in older adults possibly unapparent until complications arise	■ Discontinuation or reduction of dose of NSAIDs if possible or change to less ulcerogenic NSAID ■ PPIs, possibly twice-daily doses (He et al., 2014) ■ H_2-receptor agonists ■ Mucosa-protecting agents

plays an essential role on the healthcare team by providing ongoing assessment and patient teaching.

Diagnostic Tests

■ *Upper GI series* using barium as a contrast medium can detect 80–90% of peptic ulcers via x-ray. It commonly is the diagnostic procedure chosen first because it does not require sedation and is less costly and less invasive than gastroscopy. Small or very superficial ulcers may be missed, however.

■ *Gastroscopy* allows visualization of the esophageal, gastric, and duodenal mucosa and direct inspection of ulcers. Tissue also can be obtained for biopsy.

■ *Biopsy specimens* obtained during a gastroscopy can be tested for the presence of *H. pylori* by several different methods. In the *rapid urease test,* the specimen is placed on a gel containing urea. If urease from *H. pylori* is present, it will convert the urea to ammonia and carbon dioxide, increasing the pH of the gel. This action leads to a color change of the pH indicator in the gel to produce a positive result. Results are obtained within 1–24 hours. Biopsy specimen cells also can be microscopically examined or cultured for evidence of *H. pylori*. Although these tests are highly specific for *H. pylori* infection, their invasiveness, cost, and lack of availability in some areas limit their usefulness.

■ *Noninvasive methods* of detecting *H. pylori* infection include *serologic testing* (to detect *H. pylori*–specific IgG antibodies through ELISA), fecal antigen immunoassays (to detect antigens to *H. pylori* in the feces), and the *urea breath test.* In this test, radiolabeled urea is given orally. The urease produced by *H. pylori* bacteria converts the urea to ammonia and radiolabeled carbon dioxide, which can then be measured as the patient exhales. This test, as well as fecal antigen testing, can also be used to evaluate the effectiveness of treatment to eradicate *H. pylori*. Treatment with PPIs interferes with the urea breath test results, so these drugs should be discontinued for 14 days prior to testing (Van Leeuwen et al., 2013).

■ If Zollinger-Ellison syndrome is suspected, *gastric analysis* may be performed to evaluate gastric acid secretion. Stomach contents are aspirated through a nasogastric tube and analyzed. In Zollinger-Ellison syndrome, gastric acid levels are very high.

Surgery

The identification of *H. pylori* infection as the primary cause of PUD and the availability of drugs to effectively treat and heal peptic ulcers have dramatically decreased surgery as a treatment option for PUD. Older patients, however, may have undergone gastric resection surgery for PUD and may have long-term complications related to the surgery.

Pharmacologic Therapy

The medications used to treat PUD include agents to eradicate *H. pylori,* drugs to decrease gastric acid content, and agents that protect the mucosa.

Eradication of *H. pylori* depends on using drug regimens with proven effectiveness. Combination therapies that use two antibiotics with a PPI (known as triple therapy), or a PPI (or histamine receptor antagonist) with bismuth and two antibiotics (quadruple therapy) for 10–14 days are necessary. Antibiotics used in triple therapy are clarithromycin, amoxicillin, and metronidazole. The quadruple therapy usually utilizes metronidazole and tetracycline. Eradication rates vary by regimen used, duration of therapy (7 versus 10 versus 14 days), patient compliance, and antibiotic resistance (Yang & Huang, 2014).

In patients who have NSAID-induced ulcers, the NSAID in use should be discontinued if at all possible. If that is not possible, twice-daily PPIs, histamine receptor antagonists, or sucralfate should be used to promote ulcer healing (Lanza et al., 2009).

Medications that decrease gastric acid content include PPIs and the H_2-receptor antagonists.

■ PPIs inhibit the acid-secreting enzyme (H^+/K^+ ATPase) that functions as the proton pump of the parietal cells, disabling it for up to 24 hours. These drugs are very effective, resulting in more than 90% ulcer healing after 4 weeks.

Compared to the H₂-receptor blockers, the PPIs provide faster pain relief and more rapid ulcer healing.

■ Histamine₂-receptor blockers inhibit histamine binding to the receptors on the gastric parietal cells to reduce acid secretion. These drugs are well tolerated and have few serious side effects; however, drug interactions can occur. These drugs must be continued for 8 weeks or longer for ulcer healing.

Agents that protect the mucosa include sucralfate, bismuth, antacids, and prostaglandin analogs.

■ Sucralfate binds to proteins in the ulcer base, forming a protective barrier against acid, bile, and pepsin. Sucralfate also stimulates the secretion of mucus, bicarbonate, and prostaglandin.

■ Bismuth compounds (Pepto-Bismol) stimulate mucosal bicarbonate and prostaglandin production to promote ulcer healing. In addition, bismuth suppresses *H. pylori*. There are very few side effects, other than a harmless darkening of stools.

■ Antacids stimulate gastric mucosal defenses, thereby aiding in ulcer healing. They provide rapid relief of ulcer symptoms and are often used as needed to supplement other antiulcer medications. Antacids are inexpensive, but patients often have difficulty complying with a long-term regimen because the drugs must be taken frequently and may cause constipation (the aluminum-type antacids) or diarrhea (the magnesium-based antacids). Antacids also interfere with the absorption of iron, digoxin, some antibiotics, and other drugs.

■ Prostaglandin analogs (misoprostol) promote ulcer healing by stimulating mucus and bicarbonate secretions and by inhibiting acid secretion. Although not as effective as the other drugs discussed, misoprostol is used to prevent NSAID-induced ulcers. Diarrhea is a common side effect. Because of its uterotropic effect, misoprostol is contraindicated in pregnant women.

Nonpharmacologic Therapy

In addition to pharmacologic treatment, patients are encouraged to maintain good nutrition, consuming balanced meals at regular intervals. It is important to teach patients that bland or restrictive diets are no longer necessary. Mild alcohol intake is not harmful. Smoking is discouraged because it slows the rate of healing and increases the frequency of relapses.

Complementary Health Approaches

The main integrative health options include lowering the patient's stress by any healthy option they enjoy, such as yoga, walking, listening to music, and so forth. Also, increasing fiber in their diet to prevent further ulcers, and taking 25–50 mg of zinc each day to assist healing of ulcers.

Lifespan Considerations

PUD in Children and Adolescents

The incidence of peptic ulcer bleeding in the pediatric population in the United States is reported to range from 378 to 3250 cases per year (Park, 2012). Acutely ill children should be assessed for health disparities. For example, life-threatening GI bleeding in patients in the pediatric intensive care unit with complex chronic disease should be reviewed because the pediatric patient may be at risk for PUD.

PUD in Pregnant Women

While nausea and vomiting are common in pregnancy, the occurrence of atypical features such as epigastric discomfort and hematemesis or weight loss prompts further assessment (Frise & Nelson-Piercy, 2012). While historically PUD was rare during pregnancy, today's routine endoscopy provides further data. Treatment of PUD during pregnancy may include PPIs, which Frise and Nelson-Piercy suggest are safe and appropriate during pregnancy.

PUD in Older Adults

Among patients older than 65 years of age, PUD has been associated with NSAID use (He et al., 2014). The common co-therapy with NSAIDs to lower the risk of PUD is H₂-receptor antagonist (H2RA). In research, the high-dose H2RA showed greater effectiveness than its low-dose form in the prophylaxis of PUD in NSAID use in adults (He et al., 2014). The nurse working with such patients must remind them to discuss the co-therapy with their primary medical professional.

NURSING PROCESS

Nurses may identify patients with PUD by looking for the symptoms and noting family history of *H. pylori* infection. Nursing care centers on interventions to promote adequate nutritional intake, promote healing, and prevent recurrences.

Although it is difficult to predict which patients will develop PUD, nurses can promote health by advising patients to avoid risk factors such as excessive aspirin or NSAID use and cigarette smoking. In addition, nurses should encourage patients to seek treatment for manifestations of gastroesophageal reflux disease (GERD) or chronic gastritis, both of which also are associated with *H. pylori* infection.

Assessment

Collect the following subjective and objective data when assessing the patient with PUD:

■ *Observation and patient interview.* Complaints of epigastric or left upper quadrant pain, heartburn, or discomfort; its character, severity, timing, and relationship to eating; measures used for relief; nausea or vomiting; presence of bright blood or "coffee-grounds" appearing in vomitus; current medications, including use of aspirin or other NSAIDs; and cigarette smoking and use of alcohol or other drugs

■ *Physical examination.* General appearance, including height and weight relationship; vital signs, including orthostatic measurements; abdominal examination, including shape and contour, bowel sounds, and tenderness to palpation; and presence of obvious or occult blood in vomitus and stool.

Patient Teaching
Home Care for Patients with PUD

Provide information on the following topics when preparing the patient for home care:

- Prescribed medication regimen, including desired effects and potential adverse effects
- Importance of continuing therapy even when symptoms are relieved
- Relationship between peptic ulcers and factors such as NSAID use and smoking; if indicated, referral to a smoking cessation clinic or program
- Importance of avoiding aspirin and other NSAIDs and the necessity of reading the labels of over-the-counter medications for possible aspirin content
- Manifestations of complications that should be reported to the care provider, including increased abdominal pain or distention, vomiting, black or tarry stools, light-headedness, or fainting
- Stress and lifestyle management techniques that may help prevent exacerbation; referral to resources for stress management, such as classes, counseling, and formal or informal groups.

Diagnosis

Nursing diagnoses that are frequently appropriate for patients with PUD include the following:

- *Bleeding, Risk for*
- *Fluid Volume, Risk for Deficient*
- *Imbalanced Nutrition: Less Than Body Requirements*
- *Pain, Chronic*
- *Sleep Pattern, Disturbed.*

(NANDA-I © 2014)

Planning

Goals of treatment are developed in collaboration with the patient and may include the following:

- The patient will demonstrate no complications related to bleeding.
- The patient will demonstrate no signs or symptoms of infection.
- The patient will demonstrate fluid volume balance, including maintenance of urine output of at least 0.5 mL/kg/hr.
- The patient will demonstrate dietary intake that adequately meets nutritional and caloric needs.
- The patient will verbalize risk factors related to PUD exacerbation and recurrence.
- The patient will verbalize maintaining pain at a tolerable level.

Implementation

PUD is managed in home and community-based settings; only its complications typically require treatment in an acute care setting. The Patient Teaching feature outlines home care guidelines for patients with PUD.

The priorities of nursing care for the hospitalized patient with PUD include restoring and maintaining fluid volume balance, reducing discomfort, maintaining nutritional status, and preventing or rapidly identifying and intervening for potential complications. Priorities for patients with complications of PUD are described in **Box 10–5 »**.

Restore and Maintain Fluid Volume Balance

Erosion of a blood vessel with resultant hemorrhage is a significant risk for the patient with PUD. Acute bleeding can lead to hypovolemia and fluid volume deficit, which can lead

Box 10–5
Treatment for Complications of Peptic Ulcer Disease

The patient hospitalized with a complication of PUD (e.g., bleeding, GI obstruction, perforation and peritonitis) requires additional interventions to restore homeostasis.

In hemorrhage associated with PUD, initial interventions focus on restoring and maintaining circulation. Normal saline, lactated Ringer's, or other balanced electrolyte solutions are administered intravenously to restore intravascular volume if signs of shock (tachycardia, hypotension, pallor, low urine output, and anxiety) are present. Whole blood or packed RBCs may be administered to restore hemoglobin and hematocrit levels. A nasogastric tube is inserted to prevent aspiration of vomited gastric contents.

Gastroscopy with direct injection of a clotting or sclerosing agent into the bleeding vessel may be performed. Laser photocoagulation, which uses light energy, or electrocoagulation, which uses electric current to generate heat, can also be performed via gastroscopy to seal bleeding vessels.

The patient is kept NPO until bleeding is controlled. PPIs are administered intravenously [e.g., 40 mg of pantoprazole (Protonix) per IV push or admixture daily] to reduce the risk of rebleeding. Surgery may be necessary if medical measures are ineffective in controlling bleeding. Older adults who experience bleeding as a complication of PUD are more likely to rebleed or require surgery to control the hemorrhage.

Repeated inflammation, healing, scarring, edema, and muscle spasm can lead to gastric outlet (pyloric) obstruction. Initial treatment includes gastric decompression with nasogastric suction and administration of IV normal saline and potassium chloride to correct fluid and electrolyte imbalance. H_2-receptor blockers are given intravenously as well. Balloon dilation of the gastric outlet may be done via upper endoscopy. If these measures are unsuccessful in relieving obstruction, surgery may be required.

Gastric or duodenal perforation resulting in contamination of the peritoneum with GI contents often requires immediate intervention to restore homeostasis and minimize peritonitis. IV fluids maintain fluid and electrolyte balance. Nasogastric suction removes gastric contents and minimizes peritoneal contamination. Placing the patient in Fowler or semi-Fowler position allows peritoneal contaminants to pool in the pelvis. IV antibiotics aggressively treat bacterial infection from intestinal flora. Laparoscopic surgery or an open laparotomy may close the perforation.

to a decrease in cardiac output and impaired tissue perfusion. The care of a patient with PUD who is at risk of PUD bleeding starts in the acute area and then moves to outpatient, with the care in clinics and at home.

- Monitor stools and gastric drainage for overt and occult blood. Assess gastric drainage (vomitus or drainage from a nasogastric tube) to estimate the amount and rapidity of hemorrhage. Drainage is bright red with possible clots in acute hemorrhage and is dark red or the color of coffee grounds when blood has been in the stomach for a time. Hematochezia is present in acute hemorrhage; melena (black, tarry stool) is an indicator of less acute bleeding. When small vessels are disrupted, bleeding may be slow and not overtly evident. With chronic or slow GI bleeding, the risk of a fluid volume deficit is minimal; anemia and activity intolerance are more likely.

- Maintain IV therapy with fluid volume and electrolyte replacement solutions; administer whole blood or packed cells as ordered. Both fluids and electrolytes are lost through vomiting, nasogastric drainage, and diarrhea in an episode of acute bleeding. To prevent shock, it is essential to maintain a blood volume and cardiac output sufficient to perfuse body tissues. Whole blood and packed cells replace both blood volume and RBCs, providing additional oxygen-carrying capacity to meet cell needs.

- Insert a nasogastric tube and maintain its position and patency. At first, measure and record gastric output every hour, then every 4–8 hours. Nasogastric suction removes blood from the GI tract, preventing vomiting and possible aspiration. Gastric output is replaced milliliter for milliliter with a balanced electrolyte solution to maintain homeostasis.

- Monitor hemoglobin and hematocrit, serum electrolytes, BUN, and creatinine values. Report abnormal findings. Hemoglobin and hematocrit are lower than normal with acute or chronic GI bleeding. In acute hemorrhage, initial results may be within the normal range because both cells and plasma are lost. Loss of fluids and electrolytes with gastric drainage and diarrhea alters normal levels. Digestion and absorption of blood in the GI tract may result in elevated BUN and creatinine levels.

- Assess the abdomen, including bowel sounds, distention, girth, and tenderness, every 4 hours, and record findings. Borborygmi or hyperactive bowel sounds with abdominal tenderness are common with acute GI bleeding. Increased distention; increasing abdominal girth; absent bowel sounds; or extreme tenderness with a rigid, boardlike abdomen may indicate perforation.

- Maintain bedrest with the head of the bed elevated. Ensure safety. Loss of blood volume may cause orthostatic hypotension with resultant syncope or dizziness upon standing.

Manage Pain

The pain of PUD is often predictable and preventable. Pain is typically experienced 2–4 hours after eating, as high levels of gastric acid and pepsin irritate the exposed mucosa. Measures to neutralize the acid, minimize its production, or protect the mucosa often relieve this pain, minimizing the need for analgesics.

- Assess pain, including location, type, severity, frequency, and duration. Assess the relationship of pain to food intake or other contributing factors.

- Administer PPIs, H_2-receptor antagonists, antacids, or mucosal protective agents as ordered. Monitor for effectiveness and side effects or adverse reactions. The pain associated with PUD is generally caused by the effect of gastric juices on exposed mucosal tissue. These medications reduce pain and promote healing by reducing acid production, neutralizing acid, or providing a barrier for the damaged mucosa.

- Teach relaxation, stress reduction, and lifestyle management techniques. Refer for stress management counseling or classes as indicated. Although there is no clear relationship between stress and PUD, measures to relieve stress and promote physical and emotional rest help reduce the perception of pain and may reduce ulcer genesis.

SAFETY ALERT Avoid making assumptions about pain. Acute pain may indicate a complication, such as perforation (often manifesting as sudden, severe epigastric pain and a rigid, boardlike abdomen), or it may be totally unrelated to PUD (e.g., angina, gallbladder disease, pancreatitis).

Facilitate Adequate Rest

Prior to the patient being discharged to home, it is important to teach the patient about planning for appropriate rest. Nighttime ulcer pain, which typically occurs between 1 and 3 a.m., may disrupt the sleep cycle and result in inadequate rest. Anticipation of pain may lead to insomnia or other sleep disruptions. The following care will be mostly the patient's self-care at home, in the community.

- Emphasize the importance of taking medications as prescribed. The bedtime dose of PPI or H_2-receptor blocker minimizes hydrochloric acid production during the night, reducing nighttime pain.

- Instruct the patient to limit food intake after the evening meal, eliminating any bedtime snack. Eating before bedtime can stimulate the production of gastric acid and pepsin, increasing the likelihood of nighttime pain.

- Encourage the use of relaxation techniques and comfort measures such as soft music as needed to promote sleep. Once the pain associated with PUD has been controlled, these measures help reduce anxiety and reestablish a normal sleep pattern.

Promote Balanced Nutrition

In an attempt to avoid discomfort, the patient with PUD may gradually reduce food intake, sometimes jeopardizing nutritional status. Anorexia and early satiety are additional problems associated with PUD.

- Assess the patient's current diet, including pattern of food intake, eating schedule, and foods that precipitate pain or are being avoided in anticipation of pain.
- Refer the patient to a dietitian for meal planning to minimize PUD symptoms and meet nutritional needs.
- Monitor for complaints of anorexia, fullness, nausea, and vomiting. Adjust dietary intake or medication schedule as indicated. PUD and resultant scarring can lead to impaired gastric emptying, necessitating a treatment change.
- Monitor laboratory values for indications of anemia or other nutritional deficits. Monitor for therapeutic effects and side effects of treatment measures such as oral iron replacement. Instruct the patient taking oral iron replacement to avoid using an antacid within 1–2 hours of taking the iron preparation. Antacids bind with oral iron preparations, blocking absorption. Anemia can result from poor nutrient absorption or chronic blood loss in patients with PUD. Oral iron supplements may cause GI distress, nausea, and vomiting. If these side effects are intolerable, notify the physician for a possible change of therapy.

SAFETY ALERT Advise the patient to report increasing or persistent symptoms of anorexia, nausea and vomiting, or fullness to the healthcare provider.

Evaluation

Patient care may be evaluated for the following expected outcomes:

- The patient experiences no complications related to PUD, including uncontrolled or excessive bleeding.
- The patient demonstrates balanced oral intake and output and no signs or symptoms of fluid overload or dehydration.
- Using a predetermined pain rating scale, the patient rates pain at a tolerable level (as defined by the patient).
- The patient verbalizes attainment of adequate rest and sleep.
- The patient describes actions that will reduce the risk of recurrence of PUD.

If the patient does not progress satisfactorily to the expected outcomes, the nurse must complete a thorough assessment; particularly the patient's reported pain level, diet tolerance, and vital signs. Signs and symptoms of further bleeding such as abdominal pain and increased pain will require notifying the patient's primary care provider. Further diagnostic workup may include a CBC to review for a possible lowering of the patient's hemoglobin and hematocrit. IV fluids may be reinstated as well as IV pain medication, an NPO status, a nasogastric tube, and IV PPIs. Surgical or endoscopic consult may be conducted.

Nursing Care Plan
A Patient with Peptic Ulcer Disease

Sean O'Donnell is a 47-year-old stock broker who lives and works in a metropolitan area. Mr. O'Donnell has had heartburn and abdominal discomfort for years but thought they went along with his job. Last year, after becoming weak, light-headed, and short of breath, he was found to be anemic and was diagnosed as having a duodenal ulcer. He took omeprazole (Prilosec) and ferrous sulfate for 3 months before stopping both, saying he had "never felt better in his life." Mr. O'Donnell has now been admitted to the hospital with active upper GI bleeding.

ASSESSMENT	DIAGNOSES	PLANNING
Rachel Clark is Mr. O'Donnell's admitting nurse and case manager. On initial assessment, Mr. O'Donnell is alert and oriented, although very apprehensive about his condition. His skin is pale and cool. Vital signs include temperature 99.1°F oral; pulse 98 bpm; respirations 20/min; and BP 136/88 mmHg. Mr. O'Donnell's abdomen is distended and tender, with hyperactive bowel sounds; 200 mL of bright red blood is obtained on nasogastric tube insertion. Hemoglobin is 8.2 g/dL and hematocrit is 23% on admission. Mr. O'Donnell is taken to the endoscopy lab, where his bleeding will be controlled by capsule endoscopy and possible embolization, if indicated. On his return to the nursing unit, he receives 2 units of packed RBCs and IV fluids to restore blood volume. A 5-day course of high-dose IV omeprazole, most often as a bolus of 80 mg with a continuous dosage afterward, is ordered to prevent rebleeding, and Mr. O'Donnell is allowed to begin a clear liquid diet 24 hours after his endoscopy. Tissue biopsy obtained during endoscopy confirms the presence of *H. pylori* infection. Many gastroenterologists assert that IV PPI therapy maintains hemostasis more effectively than IV H2RA.	■ *Fluid Volume, Deficient,* related to acutely bleeding duodenal ulcer ■ *Injury, Risk for,* related to acute blood loss ■ *Fear* related to threat to well-being ■ *Health Management, Readiness for Enhanced,* related to lack of knowledge regarding PUD and its treatment (NANDA-I © 2014)	■ The patient will maintain normal blood pressure, pulse, and urine output (greater than 30 mL/hr). ■ The patient will remain free of injury. ■ The patient will seek information to reduce fear. ■ The patient will identify and use coping strategies to manage fear. ■ The patient will describe prescribed therapeutic regimen. ■ The patient will verbalize ability to manage prescribed regimen.

Nursing Care Plan *(continued)*

IMPLEMENTATION

- Place the call light within reach, and encourage the patient to ask for help when getting up or ambulating. Remind the patient to rise slowly from lying to sitting and from sitting to standing.

- Discuss the situation, and provide information about all procedures and treatments.

- Reassure the patient about the effectiveness of treatment in reducing the risk for further bleeding.

- Discuss current and planned treatment measures; stress the importance of completing the prescribed treatment to reduce the risk of further ulcer development.

- Encourage the patient to avoid using aspirin or NSAIDs in the future; suggest alternative medications such as acetaminophen.

- Discuss stress reduction techniques, and refer for stress reduction counseling or workshops as indicated.

EVALUATION

Mr. O'Donnell is discharged 48 hours after admission. He has had no further evidence of bleeding and has resumed a regular diet. His hemoglobin and hematocrit remain low, and he has a prescription for ferrous sulfate. He will complete the prescribed high-dose omeprazole regimen at home, then begin treatment with omeprazole, amoxicillin, and clarithromycin (Biaxin) to eradicate the *H. pylori* infection detected during endoscopy. After 2 weeks of this regimen, he will continue taking omeprazole at bedtime for 4–8 weeks. He verbalizes a good understanding of his treatment and the importance of completing the entire regimen. Mr. O'Donnell expresses concern about his ability to "keep his cool on the inside" when under stress. Ms. Clark, his case manager, gives him the names of several resources to help with stress management in case he wants help.

CRITICAL THINKING

1. How does *H. pylori* infection contribute to the development of peptic ulcers?
2. Describe the physiologic responses to fear and anxiety. Why is it important to alleviate fear and its physical consequences in patients with PUD?
3. What suggestions can you make to help Mr. O'Donnell manage his complex treatment regimen during the next 3 months?
4. Develop a teaching plan that includes stress reduction techniques that Mr. O'Donnell can use while performing his job as a stock broker.

REVIEW Peptic Ulcer Disease

RELATE Link the Concepts and Exemplars

Linking the exemplar of peptic ulcer disease with the concept of addiction:

1. When admitting a patient with acute PUD, you learn that the patient has a 20+ year history of smoking. How might this behavior contribute to PUD?

2. What teaching would you provide to motivate and support the patient to quit smoking?

Linking the exemplar of peptic ulcer disease with the concept of perfusion:

You are caring for a patient with acute PUD who has had profuse hemoptysis secondary to ulceration of the stomach lining. The patient has had significant blood loss, with approximately 3 L of bloody emesis measured over the past 24 hours. The provider orders iced lavages, which seem to have stopped the bleeding for now.

3. How will you assess this patient with regard to shock?

4. What actions, independent or collaborative, can you take to promote the patient's hemovascular stability?

READY Go to Volume 3: Clinical Nursing

REFER Go to Pearson MyLab Nursing and eText

- Additional review material

REFLECT Apply Your Knowledge

Raymond Combs, 38 years old, owns a chain of neighborhood convenience stores. He is married to his third wife, and they have two children by this marriage and are raising three children from former relationships. Mr. Combs often jokes that he prefers to stay at work because it is less stressful than being at home with the children and his wife.

For the past month, Mr. Combs has been noticing pain in his left upper abdomen approximately 2–3 hours after meals. He describes the pain as a burning, gnawing pain that goes away when he eats. He and his wife make plans to go out for dinner with their next door neighbors. Mr. Combs's wife suggests that he talk to the neighbor, who is a nurse, about the discomfort he's been feeling.

1. You are Mr. Combs's neighbor. When you go out for dinner with Mr. Combs and his wife, he describes the pain and asks what you think is happening. How do you respond?

2. Mr. Combs asks you what he can do to make his problem go away if it is, in fact, an ulcer. How do you respond?

3. Mr. Combs's wife says that she heard that a milk and dairy diet is good for ulcers. How do you respond?

References

Adams, M. P., Holland, L. N., & Urban, C. (2017). *Pharmacology for nurses: A pathophysiologic approach* (5th ed.). Hoboken, NJ: Pearson Education.

Addison, O., LaStayo, P. C., Dibble, L. E., & Marcus, R. L. (2012). Inflammation, aging, and adiposity: Implications for physical therapists. *Journal of Geriatric Physical Therapy, 35*(2), 86–94. doi:10.1519/JPT.0b013e3182312b14

Adis Medical Writers. (2014). Consider disease severity and response to corticosteroids when selecting agents to manage ulcerative colitis in children. *Drugs & Therapy Perspectives, 30*(11), 390–394. Retrieved from http://link.springer.com/article/10.1007%2Fs40267-014-0150-4

Akbaraly, T. N., Hamer, M., Ferrie, J. E., Lowe, G., Batty, G. D., Hagger-Johnson, G., … Kävimäki, M. (2103). Chronic inflammation as a determinant of future aging phenotypes. *CMAJ, 185*(16), E763–E770. Retrieved from http://search.proquest.com.ezproxy.nu.edu/health/docview/1476500581/fulltextPDF/AA95FEFC19444267PQ/1?accountid=25320

Alzaraa, A., Gravante, G., Chung, W. Y., Al-Leswas, D., Bruno, M., Dennison, A. R., & Lloyd, D. M. (2012). Targeted microbubbles in the experimental and clinical setting. *American Journal of Surgery, i*(3), 355–366. doi:10.1016/j.amjsurg.2011.10.024

Ayuso, P., Blanca, M., Cornejo-García, J. A., Torres, M. J., Doña, I., Salas, M., … García-Martín, E. (2013). Variability in histamine receptor genes HRH1, HRH2 and HRH4 in patients with hypersensitivity to NSAIDs. *Pharmacogenomics, 14*(15), 1871–1878. Retrieved from http://search.proquest.com.ezproxy.nu.edu/health/docview/1477548215/fulltextPDF/AF8C41B66E874F00PQ/13?accountid=25320

Baggenstos, B. R., Hanson, B. J., & Shaukat, A. (2013). Treatment of ulcerative colitis in the elderly: A systematic review. *Clinical Medicine Insights: Geriatrics, 6*, 1–26.

Bagus, E., Kahar, H., & Wardhani, P. (2014). Diagnostic values of immature granulocytes, eosinopenia and I/T ratio. *Folia Medica Indonesia, 50*(1), 43–47. Retrieved from http://search.proquest.com.ezproxy.nu.edu/health/docview/1652620628/fulltextPDF/A5772A5B671D4973PQ/14?accountid=25320

Bielefeldt, K. (2013). The rising tide of cholecystectomy for biliary dyskinesia. *Alimentary Pharmacology & Therapeutics, 37*, 98–106.

Bitsori, M., Raissaki, M., Maraki, S., & Galanakis, E. (2015). Acute focal bacterial nephritis, pyonephrosis and renal abscess in children. *Pediatric Nephrology, 30*, 1987–1993.

Boston Children's Hospital. (n.d.). *Appendicitis.* Retrieved from http://www.childrenshospital.org/az/Site2178/mainpageS2178P1.html

Boyd, H.A., Basit, S., Harpsøe, M. C., Wohlfahrt, J., & Jess, T. (2015). Inflammatory bowel disease and risk of adverse pregnancy outcomes. *PLoS One*. Retrieved from http://journals.plos.org/plosone/article?id=10.1371/journal.pone.0129567

Brent, L. H. (2015). Lupus nephritis. *Medscape Drugs & Diseases.* Retrieved from http://emedicine.medscape.com/article/330369-overview

Buderus, S., Boone, J. H., & Lentz, M. J. (2015). Fecal lactoferrin: Reliable biomarker for intestinal inflammation in pediatric IBD. *Gastroenterology Research and Practice.* Retrieved from http://search.proquest.com.ezproxy.nu.edu/health/docview/1709301436/fulltextPDF/E7246904785042CFPQ/2?accountid=25320

Burke, L. M., Bashir, M. R., Miller, F. H., Siegelman, E. S., Brown, M., Alobaidy, M., Jaffe, T. A., … Semelka, R. C. (2015). Magnetic resonance imaging of acute appendicitis in pregnancy: A 5-year multiinstitutional study. *American Journal of Obstetrics & Gynecology, 213*(5), 693.e1–693.e6. doi:10.1016/j.ajog.2015.07.026

Calder, P. C., Albers, R., Antione, J. M., Blum, S., Bourdet-Sicard, R., Ferns, G. A., … Zhao, J. (2009). Inflammatory disease processes and interactions with nutrition. *British Journal of Nutrition, 101*(Suppl. 1), S1–45. doi:10.1017/S0007114509377867

Catov, J. M., Flint, M., Lee, M., Roberts, J. M., & Abatemarco, D. J. (2015). The relationship between race, inflammation and psychosocial factors among pregnant women. *Maternal Child Health Journal, 19*, 401–409.

Centers for Disease Control and Prevention. (2014). *Inflammatory bowel disease (IBD).* Retrieved from http://www.cdc.gov/ibd/index.htm

Centers for Disease Control. (2017). *Lupus detailed fact sheet.* Retrieved from https://www.cdc.gov/lupus/facts/detailed.html

Cleveland Clinic. (2013). *Appendicitis in children.* Retrieved from http://my.clevelandclinic.org/childrens-hospital/health-info/diseases-conditions/hic-appendicitis-in-children

Cleveland Clinic. (2015). *Corticosteroids.* Retrieved from http://my.clevelandclinic.org/health/drugs_devices_supplements/hic_Corticosteroids

Craig, S. (2015). Appendicitis. *Medscape.* Retrieved from http://emedicine.medscape.com/article/773895-overview#a1

Crohn and Colitis Foundation of America. (2012a). *Intestinal complications.* Retrieved from http://www.ccfa.org/resources/intestinal-complications.html

Crohn and Colitis Foundation of America. (2012b). *Complementary and alternative medicine.* Retrieved from http://www.ccfa.org/resources/complementary-alternative.html

Crohn and Colitis Foundation of America. (2014). *The facts about inflammatory bowel diseases.* Retrieved from http://www.ccfa.org/assets/pdfs/ibdfactbook.pdf

Das, A., Dutta, S., Chattopadhyay, S., Chhaule, S., Mitra, T., Banu, R., … Chandra, M. (2016). Pain relief after ambulatory hand surgery: A comparison between dexmedetomidine and clonidine as adjuvant in axillary brachial plexus block: A prospective, double-blinded, randomized controlled study. *Saudi Journal of Anesthesia, 10*(1), 6–12. Retrieved from http://search.proquest.com.ezproxy.nu.edu/health/docview/1759999188/fulltextPDF/814ABA72FDCD4E9CPQ/8?accountid=25320

Delves, P. J. (2014). Overview of the immune system. *Merck manual: Health care professionals.* Retrieved from http://www.merckmanuals.com/professional/immunology_allergic_disorders/biology_of_the_immune_system/overview_of_the_immune_system.html

Durani, S. (2014). Management of asthma in school-aged children and adolescents. *Pediatric Annals, 43*(8), e184–e191. Retrieved from http://search.proquest.com.ezproxy.nu.edu/health/docview/1551986463/fulltextPDF/6145B5CBAEC3421CPQ/9?accountid=25320

El-Salhy, M., & Hausken, T. (2016). The role of the neuropeptide Y (NPY) family in the pathophysiology of inflammatory bowel disease (IBD). *Neuropeptides, 55*:137-144. doi:10.1016/j.npep.2015.09.005

Fallon, S. C., Orth, R. C., Guillerman, R. P., Munden, M. M., Zhang, W., Elder, S. C., … Bisset, G. S. (2015). Development and validation of an ultrasound scoring system for children with suspected acute appendicitis. *Pediatric Radiology, 45*(13), 1945–1952.

Flexer, S. M., Tabib, N., & Peter, M. B. (2014). Suspected appendicitis in pregnancy. *Surgeon 12*(3), 82–86.

Frise, C. J., & Nelson-Piercy, C. (2012). Peptic ulcer disease in pregnancy. *Journal of Obstetrics and Gynecology, 32*, 804–811.

Gale, H., Setty, B., Sprinz, P., & Doros, G. (2015). Implications of radiologic-pathologic correlation for gallbladder disease in children and young adults with sickle cell disease. *Emergency Radiology, 22*(5), 543–551.

Gasparetto, M., & Guariso, G. (2013). Highlights in IBD epidemiology and its natural history in the paediatric age. *Gastroenterology Research and Practice.* Retrieved from http://search.proquest.com.ezproxy.nu.edu/health/docview/1710265180/fulltextPDF/35A1147CF8BD4F0EPQ/9?accountid=25320

Ghezzi, P., & Rajkumar, C. (2015). Is frailty in the elderly linked to inflammation? *Age and Ageing, 44*(6), 913–914.

Ghosh, A., Biswas, A. K., & Banerjee, A. (2015). *Neurology India, 63*(4), 537–541.

Gorska-Ciebiada, M., Saryusz-Wolska, M., Borkowska, A., Ciebiada, M., & Loba, J. (2015). Serum soluble adhesion molecules and markers of systemic inflammation in elderly diabetic patients with mild cognitive impairment and depressive symptoms. *BioMed Research International, 15*, 1–8.

Goyal, M. K., Kuppermann, N., Clearly, S. D., Teach, S. J., & Chamberlain, J. M. (2015). Racial disparities in pain management of children with appendicitis in emergency departments. *JAMA Pediatrics, 169*(11), 996–1002. Retrieved from http://archpedi.jamanetwork.com/article.aspx?articleid=2441797

Halmos, E. P., & Gibson, P. R. (2015). Dietary management of IBD—insights and advice. *Nature Reviews Gastroenterology & Hepatology, 12*(3), 133–146.

Han, H., Lee, K. H., Lee, K. H., Ryu, J. S., Kim, Y. C., Park, S. W., … Ahn, J. S. (2014). A prospective, open-label, multicenter study of the clinical efficacy of extended-release hydromorphone in treating cancer pain inadequately controlled by other analgesics. *Support Care Cancer, 22*(3), 741–750.

Harvard Women's Health Watch. (2015). *Foods that fight inflammation.* Retrieved from http://www.health.harvard.edu/staying-healthy/foods-that-fight-inflammation

He, Y., Chan, E. W., Man, K. K., Lau, W. C., Leung, W. K., Ho, L. M., & Wong, I. C. (2014). Dosage effects of histamine-2 receptor antagonist on the primary prophylaxis of non-steroidal anti-inflammatory drug (NSAID)-associated peptic ulcers: A retrospective cohort study. *Drug Safety, 37*(9), 711–721. Retrieved from http://search.proquest.com.ezproxy.nu.edu/health/docview/1566321963/fulltextPDF/BEA204777BB14797PQ/3?accountid=25320

Hendy, P., Chadwick, G., & Hart, A. (2015). Republished curriculum based clinical review: IBD: Reproductive health, pregnancy and lactation. *Postgraduate Medical Journal, 91*(1074), 230–235.

Herdman, T. H. & Kamitsuru, S. (Eds.). *Nursing Diagnoses—Definitions and Classification 2015–2017.* Copyright © 2014, 1994–2014 NANDA International. Used by arrangement with John Wiley & Sons, Inc. Companion website: www.wiley.com/go/nursingdiagnoses.

Heuman, D. M. (2016). Gallstones (cholelithiasis). *Medscape.* Retrieved from http://emedicine.medscape.com/article/175667-overview#a1

Huang, C. C., Lehman, A., Albawardi, A., Satoskar, A., Brodsky, S., Nadasdy, G., … Nadasdy, T. (2013). IgG subclass staining in renal biopsies with membranous glomerulonephritis indicates subclass switch during disease progression. *Modern Pathology, 26*(6), 799–805. Retrieved from http://search.proquest.com.ezproxy.nu.edu/health/docview/1357565316/fulltextPDF/FFA9437C529B4EC9PQ/3?accountid=25320

Iannitti, T., Morales-Medina, J. C., Bellavite, P., Rottigni, V., & Palmieri, B. (2016). Effectiveness and safety of Arnica montana in post-surgical setting, pain and inflammation. *American Journal of Therapeutics, 23*(1):e184–e197. doi:10.1097/MJT.0000000000000036

Kattah, K. G., & Garovic, V. D. (2015). Pregnancy and lupus nephritis. *Seminars in Nephrology, 35*(5), 487–499.

Kee, J. L. (2014). *Laboratory and diagnostic tests with nursing implications* (9th ed.). Upper Saddle River, NJ: Prentice Hall.

Kensuke, K., Imaizumi, H., Hokama, N., Ishiguro, T., Ishibashi, K., Baba, K., … Ishida, H. (2015). Recent trend of acute appendicitis during pregnancy. *Surgery Today, 45*(12), 1521–1526.

Kopylov, U., Battat, R., Benmassaoud, A., Paradis-Surprenant, L., & Seidman, E. G. (2015). Hematologic indices as surrogate markers for monitoring thiopurine therapy in IBD. *Digestive Diseases & Sciences, 60*(2), 478–484. doi:10.1007/s10620-014-3362-5

Kornbluth, A., Sachar, D. B., & the Practice Parameters Committee of the American College of Gastroenterology. (2010). Ulcerative colitis practice guidelines in adults: American College of Gastroenterology, Practice Parameters Committee. *American Journal of Gastroenterology, 105*, 501–523.

Kumamoto, K., Imaizumi, H., Hokama, N., Ishiguro, T., Ishibashi, K., Baba, K., … Ishida, H. (2015). Recent trend of acute appendicitis during pregnancy. *Surgery Today, 45*(12), 1521–1528.

Landgraf, K., Rockstroh, D., Wagner, I. V., Weise, S., Tauscher, R., Schwartze, J. T., … Körner, A. (2015). Evidence of early alterations in adipose tissue biology and function and its association with obesity-related inflammation and insulin resistance in children. *Diabetes, 64*(4), 1249–1261.

Lanza, F. L., Chan, F. K. L., Quigley, M. M., & the Practice Parameters Committee of the American College of Gastroenterology. (2009). Guidelines for prevention of NSAID-related ulcer complications. *American Journal of Gastroenterology, 104*, 728–738.

Livingston, E. H., & Fairlie, R. W. (2012). Little effect of insurance status or socioeconomic condition on disparities in minority appendicitis perforation rates. *Archives of Surgery, 147*(1), 11–17. doi:10.1001/archsurg.2011.746

Lv, Z-F., Wang, F-C., Zheng, H-L., Wang, B., Xie, Y., Zhou, X-J., & Lv, N-H. (2015). Meta-analysis: Is combination of tetracycline and amoxicillin suitable for *Helicobacter pylori* infection? *World Journal of Gastroenterology, 21*(8), 2522–2533. Retrieved from https://www.ncbi.nlm.nih.gov/pmc/articles/PMC4342932/

Mayo Clinic. (2016). *Corticosteroids.* http://www.mayoclinic.org/drugs-supplements/corticosteroid-oral-route-parenteral-route/description/drg-20070491

McClaffery, H. (2014). An overview of integrative therapies in asthma treatment. *Current Allergy and Asthma Reports, 14*(10), 1–8.

McCulloch, M. (2014). 5 foods to help fight inflammation. *Environmental Nutrition, 37*(3), 4.

Minkes, R. K. (2013). Pediatric appendicitis. *Medscape Reference.* Retrieved from http://emedicine.medscape.com/article/926795-overview

Moghaddam, T. G., Fakheri, H., Abdi, R., Rostami, F. K., & Bari, Z. (2013). The incidence and outcome of pregnancy-related biliary sludge/stones and potential risk factors. *Archives of Iranian Medicine (AIM), 16*(1), 12–16.

Moum, B., Hovde, O., & Høivik, M. L. (2014). What have we learnt about the role of the environment and natural course of IBD in the new millennium? 20-year follow-up of the IBSEN cohort. *Digestive Diseases, 32*(Suppl. 1), 2–9. doi:10.1159/000367818

Murer, S. B., Aeberli, I., Braegger, C. P., Gittermann, M., Hersberger, M., Leonard, S. W., … Zimmermann, M. B. (2014). Antioxidant supplements reduced oxidative stress and stabilized liver function tests but did not reduce inflammation in a randomized controlled trial in obese children and adolescents. *Journal of Nutrition, 144*(2), 193–201. Retrieved from http://search.proquest.com.ezproxy.nu.edu/health/docview/1500943149/fulltextPDF/F9DDB02C84474591PQ/9?accountid=25320

Murithi, A. K., Leung, N., Valeri, A. M., Cornell, L. D., Sethi, S., Fidler, M. E., & Nasr, S. H. (2014). Clinical characteristics, causes and outcomes of acute interstitial nephritis in the elderly. *Kidney International, 87*, 458–464.

Nachalon, Y., Lowenthal, N., Greenberg-Dotan, S., & Goldbart, A. D. (2014). Inflammation and growth in young children with obstructive sleep apnea syndrome before and after adenotonsillectomy. *Mediators of Inflammation.* Retrieved from http://search.proquest.com.ezproxy.nu.edu/health/docview/1709454526/fulltextPDF/E9D0F140BED8440BPQ/17?accountid=25320

National Center for Complementary and Integrative Health. (2015). *Goldenseal.* Retrieved from https://nccih.nih.gov/health/goldenseal

National Institute of Arthritis and Musculoskeletal and Skin Diseases. (2014). *Handout on health: Rheumatoid arthritis.* Retrieved from http://niams.nih.gov/Health_Info/Rheumatic_Disease/rheumatoid_arthritis_ff.asp

National Institute of Diabetes and Digestive and Kidney Diseases. (2012a). *Gallstones.* Retrieved from http://digestive.niddk.nih.gov/ddiseases/pubs/gallstones/Gallstones_508.pdf

National Institute of Diabetes and Digestive and Kidney Diseases. (2012b). *Primary sclerosing cholangitis.* Retrieved from http://digestive.niddk.nih.gov/ddiseases/pubs/primarysclerosingcholangitis/Primary_Sclerosing_Cholangitis_508.pdf

National Institute of Diabetes and Digestive and Kidney Diseases. (2014). *Digestive diseases statistics for the United States.* Retrieved from http://www.niddk.nih.gov/health-information/health-statistics/Pages/digestive-diseases-statistics-for-the-united-states.aspx

National Institute of Diabetes and Digestive and Kidney Diseases. (2015). *H. pylori and peptic ulcers.* Retrieved from http://www.niddk.nih.gov/health-information/health-topics/digestive-diseases/peptic-ulcer/Pages/overview.aspx

National Kidney Foundation. (2015). *Goodpasture's syndrome.* Retrieved from https://www.kidney.org/atoz/content/goodpasture

National Library of Medicine. (2015). *Appendicitis.* Retrieved from http://www.ncbi.nlm.nih.gov/pubmedhealth/PMHT0022755/

Omari, A. H., Khammash, M. R., Qasaimeh, G. R., Shammari, A. K., Bani Yassen, M. K., & Hammori, S. K. (2014). Acute appendicitis in the elderly: Risk factors for perforation. *World Journal of Emergency Surgery.* 9:6. doi: 10.1186/1749-7922-9-6

Ordas, I., Eckmann, L., Talamini, M., Baumgart, D. C., & Sandborn, W. J. (2012). Ulcerative colitis. *Lancet, 380*, 1606–1619. Retrieved from http://search.proquest.com.ezproxy.nu.edu/health/docview/1139242474/fulltextPDF/E87EDDF4AE374A00PQ/12?accountid=25320

Osborn, K. S., Wraa, C. E., Watson, A. B., & Holleran, R. (2013). *Medical-surgical nursing* (2nd ed.). Upper Saddle River, NJ: Pearson.

Papa, E., Docktor, M., Smillie, C., Weber, S., Preheim, S. P., Gevers, D., … Alm, E. J. (2012). Non-invasive mapping of the gastrointestinal microbiota identifies children with inflammatory bowel disease. *PLoS One, 7*(6), e39242. doi:10.1371/journal.pone.0039242

Park, K. T. (2012). Clinical applicability of the incidence of pediatric peptic ulcer bleeding in the United States. *JPGN, 54*(6), 718.

Parmar, M. S. (2015). Acute glomerulonephritis. *Medscape Drugs & Diseases.* Retrieved from http://emedicine.medscape.com/article/239278-overview

Perger, L., Little, D. C., Muensterer, O. J., Chong, A. J., Mortellaro, V. E., & Harmon, C. M. (2014). Minimal access laparoscopic surgery for treatment of ulcerative colitis and familial adenomatous polyposis coli in children and adolescents. *Journal of Laparoendoscopic & Advanced Surgical Techniques, 24*(10), 731–734.

Samulkorpi, H. E., Mentula, P., & Leppaniemi, A. (2014). A new adult appendicitis score improves diagnostic accuracy of acute appendicitis—a prospective study. *BMC Gastroenterology, 14*, 114–121. Retrieved from http://search.proquest.com.ezproxy.nu.edu/health/docview/1543816152/fulltextPDF/97ADA53F65C848A9PQ/4?accountid=25320

Schwartzman-Morris, J., & Putterman, C. (2012). Gender differences in the pathogenesis and outcome of lupus and of lupus nephritis. *Clinical and Developmental Immunology.* doi:10.1155/2012/604892

Shaffer, E. A. (2012). Laboratory tests of the liver and gallbladder. *Merck manual: Health care professionals.* Retrieved from http://www.merckmanuals.com/professional/hepatic_and_biliary_disorders/testing_for_hepatic_and_biliary_disorders/laboratory_tests_of_the_liver_and_gallbladder.html

Sheth, S. G., & LaMont, J. T. (2012). Toxic megacolon. *Up to Date.* Retrieved from http://www.uptodate.com/contents/toxic-megacolon?source=search_result&search=megacolon&selectedTitle=1%7E66#H4

Simons, F. E., Ardusso, L. R. F., Dimov, V., Ebisawa, M., El-Gamal, Y. M., Lockey, R. F., …Worm, M. (2013). World Allergy Organization anaphylaxis guidelines: 2013 update of the evidence base. *International Archives of Allergy and Immunology, 162*, 193–204. doi:10.1159/000354543

Singla, A., Amini, M. R., Alpert, M. A., & Gornik, H. L. (2013). Fatal anaphylactoid reaction associated with heparin-induced thrombocytopenia. *Vascular Medicine, 18*(3), 136–138. Retrieved from http://search.proquest.com.ezproxy.nu.edu/health/docview/1356445510/fulltextPDF/53DB8A0B3F9D421BPQ/7?accountid=25320

Spondylitis Association of America. (2012). *Breaking news: New rate of prevalence of spondyloarthritis.* Retrieved from http://www.spondylitis.org/press/news/542.aspx

Stein, C., & Kuchler, S. (2012). Non-analgesic effects of opioids: Peripheral opioid effects on inflammation and wound healing. *Current Pharmaceutical Design, 18*(37), 6053–6069.

Tinius, R. A., Cahill, A. G., Strand, E. A., & Cade, W. T. (2016). Maternal inflammation during late pregnancy is lower in physically active compared with inactive obese women. *Applied Physiology, Nutrition & Metabolism, 41*(2), 191–199.

Tracy, B., & Morrison, S. (2013). Pain management in older adults. *Clinical Therapeutics, 35*(11), 1659–1668. Retrieved from http://search.proquest.com.ezproxy.nu.edu/health/docview/1473647895/fulltextPDF/D1A1067B45A047DFPQ/3?accountid=25320

Tweed, V. (2013). The secrets of health fats. *Health Source, 75*(7), 3–5.

University of Maryland Medical Center. (2015). *Gamma-linolenic acid.* Retrieved from http://umm.edu/health/medical/altmed/supplement/gammalinolenic-acid

van de Kant, K. D. G., Klaassen, E. M. M., van Aerde, K. J., Damoiseaux, J., Bruggeman, C. A., Stelma, F. F., … Dompeling, E. (2012). Impact of bacterial colonization on exhaled inflammatory markers in wheezing preschool children. *Journal of Breath Research, 6*(4), 046001. doi:10.1088/1752-7155/6/4/046001

Van Leeuwen, A. M., Poelhuis-Leth, D. J., & Bladh, M. L. (2013). *Laboratory diagnostic tests with nursing implications* (5th ed.). Philadelphia, PA: F. A. Davis.

van Rijn, B. B., Bruinse, H. W., Veerbeek, J. H., Post Uiterweer, E. D., Koenen, S. V., van der Bom, J. G., … Franx, A. (2016). Postpartum circulating markers of inflammation and the systemic acute-phase response after early-onset preeclampsia. *Hypertension, 67*(2), 404–415.

Vincent, J. L. (2014). *Annual update in intensive care and emergency medicine.* New York, NY: Springer.

von Shonfels, W., Buch, S., Wolk, M., Aselmann, H., & Egberts, J. H. (2013). Recurrence of gallstones after cholecystectomy is associated with ABCG5/8 genotype. *Journal of Gastroenterology, 48*(3), 391–396. Retrieved from http://search.proquest.com.ezproxy.nu.edu/health/docview/1324277858/8E56D0EE0D9D4252PQ/6?accountid=25320

Wattanabe, C., Komoto, S., Hokari, R., Kurihara, C., Okada, Y., Hozumi, H., … Miura, S. (2014). Prevalence of serum celiac antibody in patients with IBD in Japan. *Journal of Gastroenterology, 49,* 825–834. doi:10.1007/s00535-013-0838-6

Weerakoon, H. T., Ranasinghe, S., Navaratne, A., Sivakanesan, R., Galketiya, K. B., & Rosairo, S. (2014). Serum lipid concentrations in patients with cholesterol and pigment gallstones. *BMC Research Notes, 7,* 548. Retrieved from http://search.proquest.com.ezproxy.nu.edu/health/docview/1555419040/fulltextPDF/6BA939D98F924293PQ/16?accountid=25320

Welch, T. R. (2012). An approach to the child with acute glomerulonephritis. *International Journal of Pediatrics, 2012,* 426192. doi:10.1155/2012/426192

Wu, M., Chen, S., & Jiang, S. (2015). Relationship between gingival inflammation and pregnancy. *Mediators of Inflammation, 15,* 1–11. http://dx.doi.org/10.1155/2015/623427

Yang, Y., & Huang, Y. (2014). Effect of *Lactobacillus acidophilus* and *Bifidobacterium bifidum* supplementation to standard triple therapy on *Helicobacter pylori* eradication and dynamic changes in intestinal flora. *World Journal of Microbiology and Biotechnology, 30,* 847–853. doi:10.1007/s11274-013-1490-2

Yates, B. (2012). Food intolerances, inflammation, and weight gain. *Townsend Letter, 347,* 62–63.

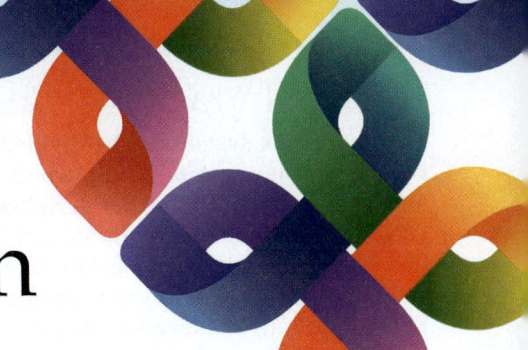

Module 11
Intracranial Regulation

Module Outline and Learning Outcomes

The Concept of Intracranial Regulation

Normal Intracranial Regulation

11.1 Analyze the physiology of intracranial regulation.

Alterations to Intracranial Regulation

11.2 Differentiate alterations to intracranial regulation.

Concepts Related to Intracranial Regulation

11.3 Outline the relationship between intracranial regulation and other concepts.

Health Promotion

11.4 Explain the promotion of healthy intracranial regulation.

Nursing Assessment

11.5 Differentiate common assessment procedures and tests used to examine intracranial regulation.

Independent Interventions

11.6 Analyze independent interventions nurses can implement for patients with alterations in intracranial regulation.

Collaborative Therapies

11.7 Summarize collaborative therapies used by interprofessional teams for patients with alterations in intracranial regulation.

Lifespan Considerations

11.8 Differentiate considerations related to the assessment and care of patients with alterations in intracranial regulation throughout the lifespan.

Intracranial Regulation Exemplars

Exemplar 11.A Increased Intracranial Pressure

11.A Analyze increased intracranial pressure (IICP) as it relates to intracranial regulation.

Exemplar 11.B Seizure Disorders

11.B Analyze seizure disorders as they relate to intracranial regulation.

Exemplar 11.C Traumatic Brain Injury

11.C Analyze traumatic brain injury as it relates to intracranial regulation.

» The Concept of Intracranial Regulation

Concept Key Terms

Aphasia, **740**
Arousal, **731**
Brain death, **734**
Brainstem, **729**
Central nervous system (CNS), **728**
Cerebellum, **729**
Cerebrospinal fluid (CSF), **728**

Cerebrum, **729**
Cognition, **731**
Consciousness, **731**
Decerebrate posturing, **732**
Decorticate posturing, **732**
Diencephalon, **729**
Doll's eye reflex, **732**

Fasciculations, **743**
Increased intracranial pressure (IICP), **734**
Intracranial regulation, **727**
Kinesthesia, **743**
Locked-in syndrome, **734**
Meninges, **728**

Monro-Kellie hypothesis, **734**
Neuron, **728**
Nystagmus, **732**
Oculocephalic reflex, **732**
Peripheral nervous system (PNS), **728**
Persistent vegetative state, **734**

Reflexes, **729**
Reticular activating system (RAS), **729**
Seizures, **734**
Spinal cord, **729**
Tremors, **744**
Vestibule-ocular reflex, **732**

Intracranial regulation refers to the processes that affect intracranial compensation and adaptive neurologic function. The neurologic system regulates and integrates all body functions, muscle movements, senses, mental abilities, and emotions. It collects, as sensory input, information from the internal and external environments, processes and interprets the input, and causes responses that manifest as motor or sensory output.

Normal Intracranial Regulation

The neurologic system can be divided into two parts: the **central nervous system (CNS)**, which consists of the brain and the spinal cord, and the **peripheral nervous system (PNS)**, which is made up of the cranial nerves and the spinal nerves. The somatic component of the PNS allows voluntary activities to occur, whereas the autonomic component of the PNS controls involuntary activities that are usually required to maintain life (e.g., breathing, heart rate).

The basic cell of the nervous system is the **neuron**. Neurons are highly specialized cells that send electrical impulses throughout the body. The information relayed by these impulses can travel in only one direction. If the transmission is to the brain, the information is transmitted via sensory neurons. In contrast, when the brain transmits information, it does so via motor neurons.

Myelin sheaths that cover many of the larger diameter and long nerves help speed the rate of conduction of nerve impulses. Although myelin is present in both the CNS and PNS, it is more commonly associated with the PNS. The myelin sheath that surrounds the larger diameter and longer nerve fibers throughout the PNS is discontinuous. The gaps in this sheath are referred to as nodes of Ranvier. As electrical signals travel from the brain via the neurons to specific points in the body, the impulses "jump" from one node of Ranvier to the next, thus speeding signal transmission.

Central Nervous System

The CNS consists of the brain and the spinal cord. The brain is the control center of the nervous system. It regulates homeostasis within the body, controls basic functions such as breathing, allows problem solving and judgment, forms memories and emotions, and regulates many more functions that allow life to continue and define who each individual is as a person. The brain is a sensitive organ covered by a protective coating of three connective tissue membranes, known as the **meninges**, that protect and nourish the CNS. The meninges from the outermost layer inward are the dura mater, the arachnoid mater, and the pia mater. In addition to being covered by the meninges, the brain is protected by the bony structure of the skull and cushioned by cerebrospinal fluid that lies in the subarachnoid space, between the arachnoid mater and the pia mater. **Cerebrospinal fluid (CSF)** cushions the brain and spinal cord and helps prevent injury to these tissues. (See **Box 11–1** ⟫ for more information). The CNS also contains myelin-producing cells called oligodendrocytes that allow for efficient transfer of electrical impulses between the neurons of the brain and spinal cord.

A specialized group of endothelial cells that are connected by tight junctions line the capillary beds of the brain. These endothelial cells form the blood-brain barrier. This barrier helps protect the CNS by preventing potential neurotoxins from passing out of the blood stream into the brain. However, important nutrients that the brain needs to function, such as glucose and amino acids, are able to cross the blood-brain barrier via active transport. In a similar fashion, water and oxygen can cross via passive diffusion. The blood-brain barrier becomes more permeable during times of inflammation, sometimes permitting viruses and bacteria to pass through. When infections of the CNS do occur, the

Box 11–1
Cerebrospinal Fluid

Most CSF is produced from arterial blood by a process of diffusion, active transport, and pinocytosis by the choroid plexuses within the ventricles of the brain; a small percentage is produced by the surfaces of the ventricles themselves. CSF is reabsorbed via the arachnoid villi into venous circulation, and in neonates (who have sparse distribution of arachnoid granulation), into lymphatic vessels that are near the spinal column and cranial vault. The CSF flushes out toxins and metabolic waste from around the brain and spinal cord as it is reabsorbed back into the body's circulatory system.

The brain closely regulates the amount of CSF that is produced and reabsorbed. In adults, there is typically 100–150 mL of CSF within the CNS at any given time. In infants, there is on average 50 mL of CSF at any given time. Between 500 and 600 mL of CSF is produced each day, so it is replaced multiple times throughout the day.

The composition of healthy CSF closely resembles that of the blood plasma from which it is derived. CSF has less protein, potassium, calcium, and magnesium than plasma, but it contains slightly more chloride. Whereas normal blood pH is around 7.4, normal CSF pH is slightly more acidic at around 7.3. CSF pressure can be measured by performing a lumbar puncture procedure with the patient lying on his or her side. Normal pressures are 8–10 cm H_2O (4.4–7.3 mmHg) in newborns and 10–18 cm H_2O (8–15 mmHg) in adults. In this side-lying position, CSF pressures closely correlate to intracranial pressures.

barrier also makes them more difficult to treat, because it prevents most antibiotics from permeating. In some cases, the only way to deliver antibiotics to the CNS may be by directly injecting them into the CSF.

The brain consists of four parts: the cerebrum, cerebellum, diencephalon, and brainstem (see **Figure 11–1** ⟫). The

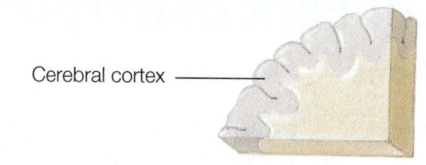

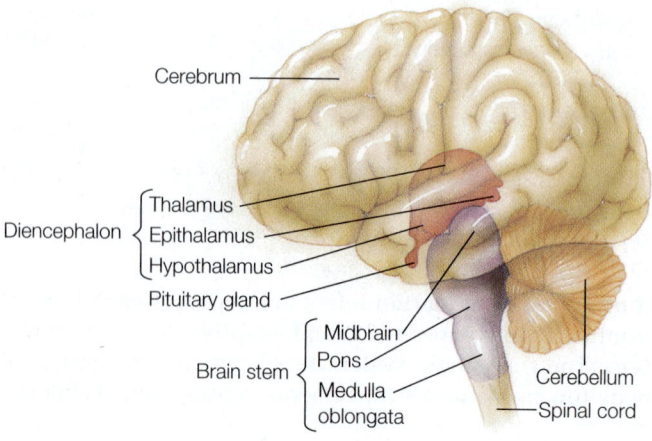

Figure 11–1 ⟫ Regions of the brain.

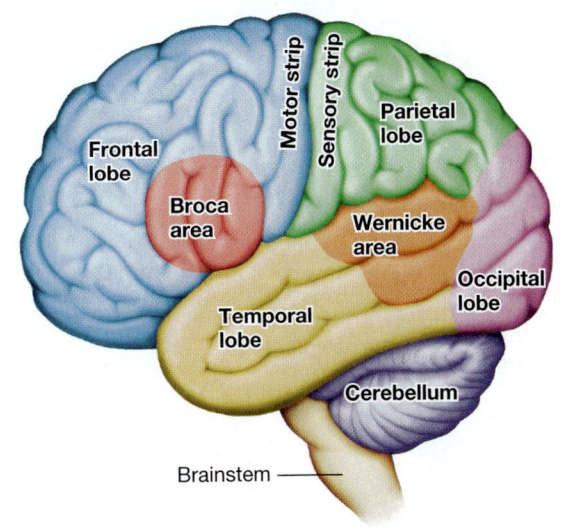

Figure 11–2 ⟩⟩ Lobes of the cerebrum.

cerebrum is the largest part of the brain; its two hemispheres account for most of the brain's mass. It is composed of an outer cortex of gray matter, an inner core of myelinated nerve fibers (white matter), and two hemispheres that are divided into four regions known as lobes (see **Figure 11–2** ⟩⟩). The frontal lobe is involved with speech, thought, learning, emotion, and voluntary movement. The prefrontal cortex of the frontal lobe controls more complicated cognitive processes, such as judgment, reasoning, and concern for others. The parietal lobe processes sensory information, including shapes, temperature, pain, and two-point discrimination. The occipital lobe, where the visual cortex is located, processes vision. Finally, the temporal lobe stores memory and interprets auditory stimuli. The cerebrum does not have a flat surface, but rather a highly convoluted surface composed of sulci (grooves) and gyri (ridges). This "folding" of the brain increases the amount of cerebral material that can fit into the skull.

The next largest part of the brain is the **cerebellum**. The cerebellum is made of gray and white matter and is responsible for controlling muscle movement and balance. The cerebellum coordinates stimuli from the cerebral cortex and the spinal cord, transmitting information required for skeletal muscle coordination and smooth movements. The surface of the cerebellum is covered with thin parallel grooves folded similar to an accordion. The extra surface area gained through this folding allows more neurons to increase signal-processing capabilities.

The **diencephalon** consists of the thalamus (sometimes called the dorsal thalamus), hypothalamus, epithalamus, and subthalamus. The thalamus is the brain's relay center; it takes all incoming nerve impulses and sends those signals to the correct region of the brain. The most important role of the hypothalamus is to link the endocrine system to the nervous system via the pituitary gland. The hypothalamus is the autonomic control center, and it is involved in regulating activities such as heart rate, blood pressure, respiratory rate and depth, pain, pleasure, and fear. The hypothalamus also controls body temperature, food and water intake and balance, sleep cycles, and digestive motility. The epithalamus

connects the limbic system (which controls emotions and forms memories) to other parts of the brain. It contains the pineal gland, which secretes melatonin, a hormone that controls circadian rhythms. The subthalamus is the part of the diencephalon that integrates the basal ganglia, which are responsible for motor movement.

The **brainstem** is made up of the midbrain, pons, and medulla oblongata. The brainstem controls reflexes and influences all basic life functions, including breathing, blood pressure, and heart rate. The brainstem also regulates activities such as vomiting, hiccupping, coughing, and sneezing. Ten of the twelve pairs of cranial nerves originate in the brainstem. The brainstem is where many connections between sensory and motor pathways that link the brain and the rest of the body reside. Some important pathways include the spinothalamic tract (crude touch, temperature, pain, and itch), the corticospinal tract (motor functions), and the posterior column–medial lemniscus pathway (proprioception, fine touch, and the sensation of vibration). The brainstem also contains the reticular formation. This network of ascending nerves relays information to the cerebral cortex about alertness and arousal mechanisms and directs the brain's attention to sensory events. This modulation of sleep–wake transitions is known as the **reticular activating system (RAS)**.

The **spinal cord** is an extension of the brainstem, specifically the medulla oblongata, through the foramen magnum at the base of the skull. In adults, the spinal cord is 40–50 cm long and 1.0–1.5 cm in diameter. It contains both gray and white matter. Like the brain, the spinal cord is protected by the meninges and CSF. The bony structure of the vertebrae also provides protection for the spinal cord, which ends at approximately L3 in infants and L1–L2 in adults. The spinal cord transmits impulses to and from the brain. The ventral roots of the spinal cord carry motor (efferent) nerve fibers, whereas the dorsal roots carry sensory (afferent) nerve fibers.

Peripheral Nervous System

The PNS contains 12 pairs of cranial nerves (see **Figure 11–3** ⟩⟩) and 31 pairs of spinal nerves (see **Figure 11–4** ⟩⟩). The cranial nerves all originate in the brain, with 10 pairs originating in the brainstem and 2 pairs originating in the anterior part of the brain. When assessing and documenting activity related to the cranial nerves, be sure to use the number rather than the name to avoid confusion. See **Table 11–1** ⟩⟩ for a summary of the cranial nerves.

The 31 pairs of spinal nerves are named by their location: 8 cervical pairs, 12 thoracic pairs, 5 lumbar pairs, 5 sacral pairs, and 1 pair of coccygeal nerves. All spinal nerves produce both motor and sensory activities. Each nerve is responsible for a different segment of the body, called a dermatome. Although each spinal nerve root has a specific dermatome distribution, overlap often exists between adjacent nerve roots.

Reflexes are involuntary, almost instantaneous motor responses to a stimulus. Reflex arcs are neural pathways that allow the sensory neuron to synapse in the spinal cord, which allows the lightning-fast result. The sensory input does reach the brain, but it does not require the brain to

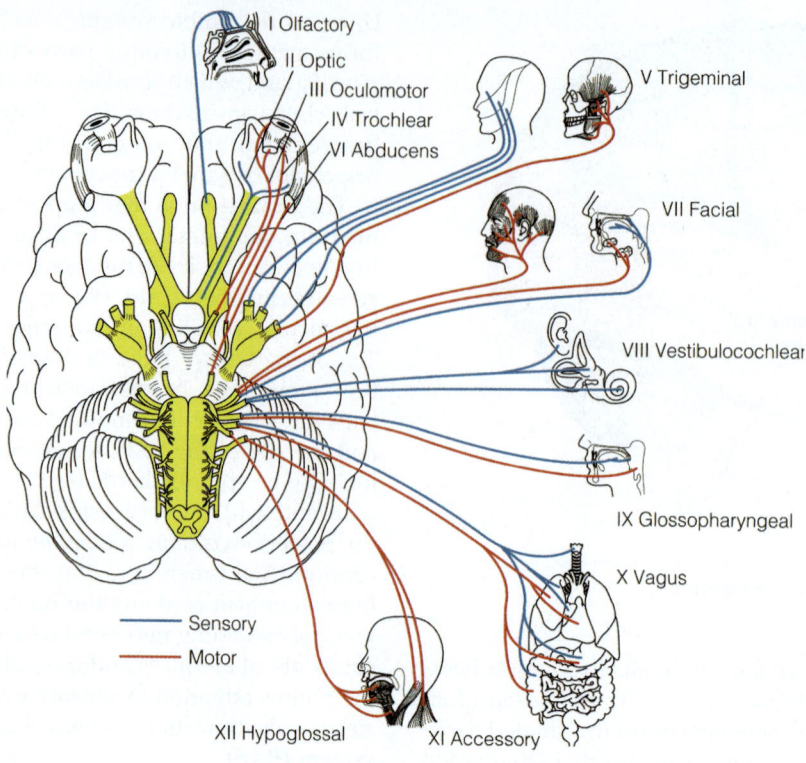

Figure 11–3 ≫ Cranial nerves.

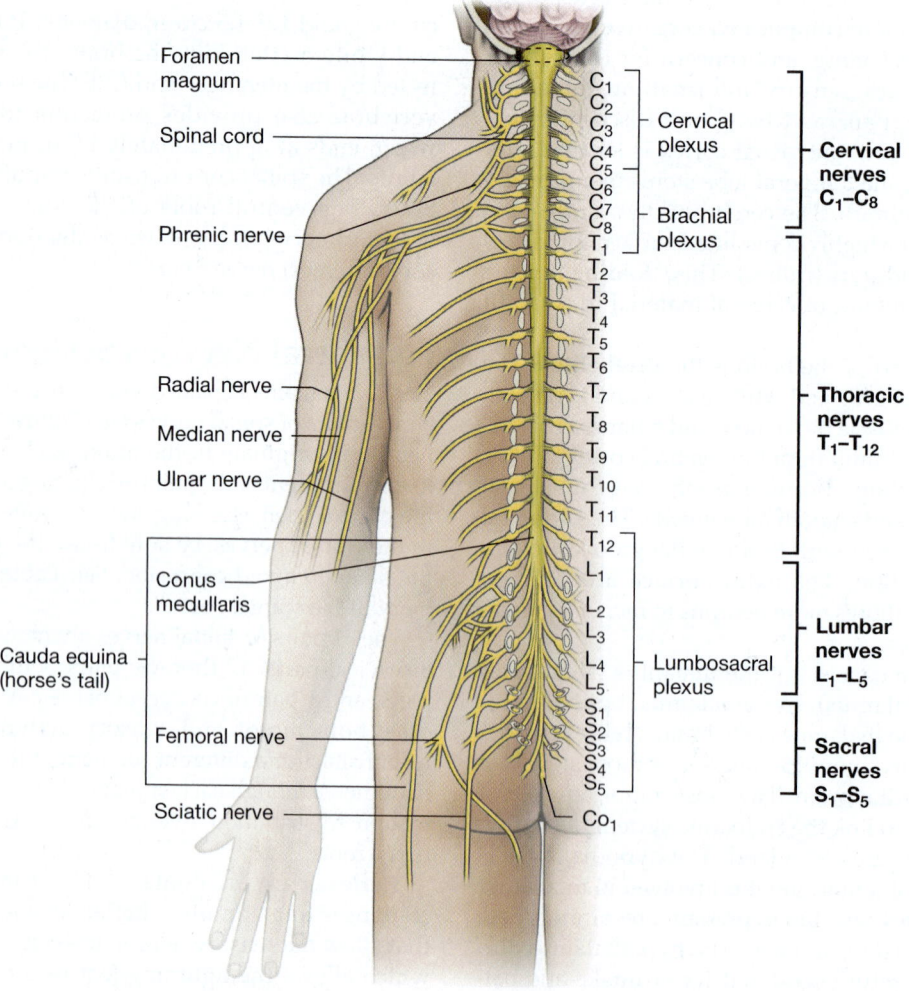

Figure 11–4 ≫ Spinal nerves.

TABLE 11–1 Cranial Nerves

Nerve Number and Name		Modality	Activity Function
I	Olfactory	Sensory	Smell
II	Optic	Sensory	Vision
III	Oculomotor	Motor	Pupillary reflex, eyelid movement, allows eye movement in every direction not controlled by cranial nerves IV and VI
IV	Trochlear	Motor	Turns eye downward and laterally
V	Trigeminal	Mixed	*Ophthalmic branch:* Sensory impulses from scalp, forehead, upper eyelid, nose, cornea, and lacrimal gland
			Maxillary branch: Sensory impulses from lower eyelid, cheek, nasal cavity, upper teeth, upper lip, and palate
			Mandibular branch: Sensory impulses from tongue, lower teeth, skin of chin, and lower lip; motor action includes teeth clenching, movement of mandible
VI	Abducens	Mixed	Controls outward lateral eye movement
VII	Facial	Mixed	Taste (anterior two-thirds of tongue); facial movements such as smiling, closing of eyes, and frowning; production of tears and saliva
VIII	Vestibulocochlear (acoustic)	Sensory	*Vestibular branch:* Aids equilibrium and provides information about balance, posture, and movement
			Cochlear branch: Hearing
IX	Glossopharyngeal	Mixed	Produces the gag and swallowing reflexes; taste (posterior third of the tongue); senses carotid blood pressure
X	Vagus	Mixed	Innervates voluntary muscles that allow coughing, swallowing, and speech; involuntarily senses aortic blood pressure, slows heart rate, and stimulates digestive organs
XI	Spinal accessory	Motor	Movement of the trapezius and sternocleidomastoid muscles; helps control swallowing
XII	Hypoglossal	Motor	Controls tongue movement involved in speech and swallowing

process the signal in order to elicit a motor response. A common example is the patellar (knee-jerk) reflex. This is a *somatic reflex* because it causes skeletal muscle contractions. There are also *autonomic reflexes*, which cause reactions from smooth muscles, cardiac muscles, or glands. A classic example of an autonomic reflex is the mammalian diving reflex: When cold water contacts the face, it causes bradycardia, peripheral vasoconstriction, and a shift in blood flow to more central organs. This reflex exists to help humans survive drowning.

Note that some reflexes are normal in newborns and infants but can be a sign of PNS or CNS damage if they exist in older children or adults. Examples include the sucking reflex (in which infants suck when the area around their mouth is touched); the grasp reflex (in which infants close their hand around a finger placed in their open palm, then grip the finger tighter when the individual attempts to remove it); and the Babinski reflex (in which stroking the outside of the sole of an infant's foot, starting at the heel and going towards the toes, causes the infant's big toe to extend and other toes to fan out).

Alterations to Intracranial Regulation

Alterations to intracranial regulation may occur because of illness or injury. Assessment of the patterns of an individual's signs and symptoms will help determine the extent of improvement or deterioration of intracranial regulation. A local brain injury or illness (in which only one area is affected) will cause a focal neurologic deficit but should not disrupt a patient's level of consciousness (LOC). For example, a brain tumor that is located near the vision center may cause a disruption in sight, but the patient should be fully conscious with no other noted neurologic deficits.

Consciousness requires both cerebral hemispheres and the RAS to be intact. The cerebral hemispheres are more susceptible to damage, and changes in behavior and alterations in levels of consciousness may be early signs of brain dysfunction. If damage to the brain continues, the patient will usually exhibit signs of that damage in a fairly predictable stepwise fashion, with higher brain functions failing first. Decreased consciousness, neurologic dysfunctions, and hemodynamic instabilities become apparent as damage progresses within the more primitive parts of the brain (midbrain and brainstem). Without successful intervention to stop this progression, death will occur. Manifestations of progressive deterioration of cerebral function are outlined in **Table 11–2 》**.

Intracranial regulation has important implications across all body systems and in a variety of areas. The Concepts Related to Intracranial Regulation section describes some of these relationships.

Alterations in Level of Consciousness

Consciousness is a condition in which the individual is aware of self and environment and is able to respond appropriately to stimuli. Full consciousness requires both normal arousal and full cognition.

- **Arousal**, or alertness, depends on the RAS, a diffuse system of neurons in the thalamus and upper brainstem.

- **Cognition** is a complex process by which an individual learns, stores, retrieves, and uses information. Cognitive processing involves all mental activities controlled by the cerebral hemispheres, including thought processes, memory, perception, communication, problem solving, and emotion.

These two components of consciousness depend on the normal physiologic functions of and connections between the

TABLE 11–2 Progression of Deteriorating Brain Function

Level of Consciousness	Clinical Signs Indicating Level of Consciousness
Full consciousness: The patient is alert and oriented to time, place, and person. ■ Intact brain function	■ **Pupillary responses.** The patient has brisk and equal reaction to light; the pupils are regular. ■ **Oculomotor responses.** The eyes move in the opposite direction as the head turns to the side. **Doll's eye reflex** (also called the **oculocephalic reflex**) is present (see **Figure 11–5 »**). Caloric testing (ear irrigation with air or water) produces **nystagmus**, rapid side-to-side movements of the eyes. With cold water, the eyes turn away from the ear being tested and back again. With warm water, the eyes turn toward the ear being tested and back again. This is also called the **vestibule-ocular reflex**. ■ **Motor responses.** The patient has purposeful movement and responds appropriately to commands. ■ **Breathing.** The patient has a regular breathing pattern with normal rate and depth.
The patient responds to verbal stimuli; shows decreased concentration and increased agitation, confusion, and/or lethargy; and is disoriented. ■ May reflect some damage to the cerebral cortex	■ **Pupillary responses.** The patient has brisk and equal reaction to light; the pupils are equal. ■ **Oculomotor responses.** The vestibulo-ocular reflex and oculocephalic reflex are intact. ■ **Motor responses.** The patient has purposeful movement in response to pain stimulus and may follow simple commands. ■ **Breathing.** The patient experiences yawning and sighing respirations.
The patient requires continuous stimulation to rouse. ■ Probable damage to diencephalon	■ **Pupillary responses.** The patient has small, reactive pupils. ■ **Oculomotor responses.** The oculocephalic reflex is intact. The patient probably has impaired vestibulo-ocular reflex with loss of nystagmus. ■ **Motor responses.** The patient has **decorticate posturing** (abnormal posture with the upper arms close to the sides and the elbows, wrists and fingers flexed; the legs extended and internally rotated; and the feet plantar flexed) with upper extremity flexion (see **Figure 11–6A »**). ■ **Breathing.** The patient has Cheyne-Stokes respirations with a crescendo–decrescendo pattern in rate and depth, followed by a period of apnea.
The patient displays reflexive positioning to pain stimulus. ■ Probable damage to midbrain	■ **Pupillary responses.** The pupils are fixed (nonreactive) in midposition. ■ **Oculomotor responses.** The patient has impaired oculocephalic reflex (doll's eye reflex absent). The patient probably has impaired vestibule-ocular reflex with loss of nystagmus. ■ **Motor responses.** The patient has **decerebrate posturing** (abnormal posture with the neck extended; the jaw clenched; arms pronated, extended, and close to the sides; legs extended; and feet plantar flexed) with adduction and rigid extension of upper and lower extremities (see Figure 11–6B). ■ **Breathing.** The patient may have central neurogenic hyperventilation with rapid, regular, and deep respirations or apneustic breathing (slow, deep breathing, holding the breath for 30–90 seconds before rapid exhalation) with prolonged inspiration and pauses at full inspiration and following expiration.
The patient shows no response to stimuli. ■ Probable damage to pons	■ **Pupillary responses.** The pupils are fixed in midposition and may be irregular. ■ **Oculomotor responses.** The oculocephalic reflex is absent. The vestibulo-ocular reflex is absent with loss of nystagmus. The corneal reflex (spontaneous closure of the eyelids when the eye is touched) is absent. ■ **Motor responses.** The patient has decerebrate posturing and hemiparesis/quadraparesis. ■ **Breathing.** The patient has apneustic breathing.
Coma: The patient has no response to stimulus. ■ Probable damage to medulla	■ **Pupillary responses.** The pupils are fixed and nonreactive. ■ **Oculomotor responses.** The oculocephalic reflex is absent. If the coma is due to diffuse damage to the cerebral cortex but the RAS is intact, cold caloric stimulation will produce eye movement toward the source of stimulus without nystagmus. If the coma is due to brainstem damage, there will be no response to caloric test. The corneal reflex is absent. ■ **Motor responses.** The body is flaccid with loss of protective cough and gag reflexes. The patient may have pathologic Babinski reflex. ■ **Breathing.** The patient has ataxic/apneic respirations (irregular breathing with long periods of no breath).

arousal mechanisms of the reticular formation and the cognitive functions of the cerebral hemispheres. Because arousal and cognition are independent components of consciousness, each can act separately on stimuli. For example, the RAS reacts to the discomfort of a full bladder by waking the individual in the middle of the night. Once the individual is awake, however, the frontal cortex alerts the individual that the bladder is full and prompts the individual to go to the bathroom and empty it.

An individual's LOC may be altered by processes that affect the arousal functions of the brainstem, the cognitive functions of the cerebral hemispheres, or both. The major causes of altered LOC are (1) lesions, infections, or injuries that affect the cerebral hemispheres directly and widely or that compress or destroy the neurons of the RAS; (2) metabolic disorders or diseases (these may occur outside the nervous system, such as severe heart failure); and (3) medications (e.g., psychoactive drugs), toxins, or alcohol consumption. Note that many of these causes involve disruption or alteration of blood flow to the brain. Normal brain function, especially in the cerebral hemispheres, depends on continuous blood flow with unimpeded supplies of oxygen and glucose. Processes that disrupt the flow of blood and nutrients may cause widespread damage, impairing arousal and cognition. Localized masses that displace normal structures and cause direct or indirect pressure on the same or opposite hemisphere or the brainstem also can affect LOC.

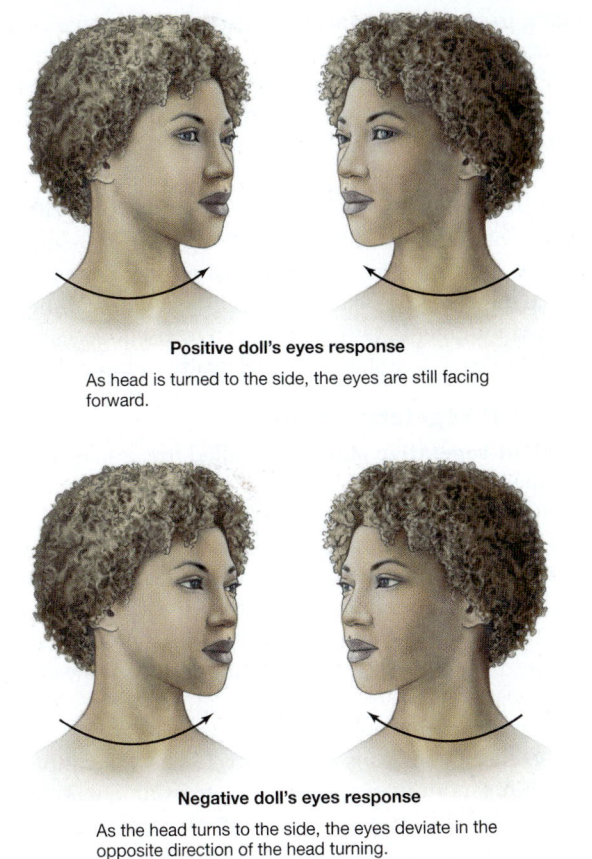

Positive doll's eyes response

As head is turned to the side, the eyes are still facing forward.

Negative doll's eyes response

As the head turns to the side, the eyes deviate in the opposite direction of the head turning.

Figure 11–5 » Doll's eye movements characteristic of altered LOC.

Consciousness is a dynamic state: A patient may pass from full consciousness to coma within hours or experience a slow diminishment of consciousness that does not become evident for weeks or months. Family members may notice this slow decline outside of a clinical setting and seek evaluation of the patient. The nurse can help provide effective care for a patient with an altered LOC by looking beyond the

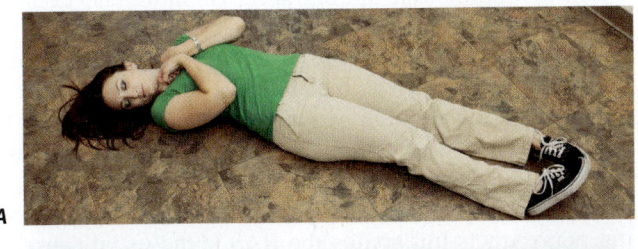

A

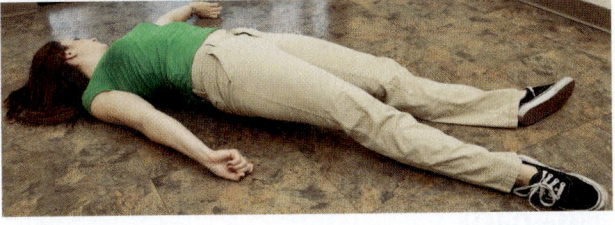

B

Figure 11–6 » **A,** Decorticate posturing, characterized by rigid flexion, is associated with lesions above the brainstem in the corticospinal tracts. **B,** Decerebrate posturing, distinguished by rigid extension, is associated with lesions of the brainstem.

diagnostic labels of consciousness and accurately assessing the patient's behavior and response to stimuli. The nurse should document assessment findings (e.g., "patient is not oriented to place or time") rather than a descriptive label (e.g., "patient is disoriented").

Disorders Affecting Level of Consciousness

As previously mentioned, both localized neurologic processes and systemic disorders can alter LOC. Processes occurring in the brain that may directly destroy or compress neurologic structures are numerous but include increased intracranial pressure (IICP), cerebral infarction, hematoma, hydrocephalus, intracranial hemorrhage, tumors, infections, traumatic brain injury (TBI)/concussion, seizure activity and recovery, and demyelinating disorders.

Any systemic condition that affects the delivery of blood, oxygen, and glucose to the brain or that alters cell membranes also may alter LOC. If cerebral blood flow is impaired or the patient becomes hypoxic or hypoglycemic, cerebral metabolism is impaired and LOC often declines rapidly. Severe hypoxia quickly leads to ischemia. Ischemia may be focal (e.g., following a stroke) or global (e.g., from cardiac arrest or hypovolemic shock). Patients at particular risk include those with poorly controlled diabetes and those with cardiac or respiratory failure.

Other metabolic alterations that can affect LOC include fluid and electrolyte imbalances and acid–base imbalances. Accumulated waste products and toxins from liver or renal failure can affect neuronal and neurotransmitter function, altering LOC. Exposure to hydrocarbons, toxic gases, or heavy metals (e.g., lead) may cause either an immediate decrease or slow decline in LOC or other evidence of neurologic or cognitive impairment. Drugs that depress the CNS (e.g., alcohol, analgesics, anesthetics) suppress metabolic and membrane activities in the RAS and cerebral hemispheres, thereby affecting LOC. Glutamate, the main excitatory neurotransmitter in the brain, may accumulate during prolonged ischemia, resulting in acute glutamate toxicity and cell death.

As the impairment of brain function progresses, more stimuli are required to elicit a response from the patient. The patient may initially rouse to verbal stimuli and respond appropriately to questions, remaining oriented to time, place, and person. With deterioration of neurologic function, the patient becomes more difficult to rouse and may become agitated and confused when awakened. Orientation to time is lost initially, followed by orientation to place and then to person. Continuous stimulation or vigorous shaking is required to maintain wakefulness as LOC further decreases. The individual eventually does not respond, even to deep, painful stimuli.

Increased Intracranial Pressure

The normal range for intracranial pressure (ICP) is typically 1.5–15 mmHg, but it can vary based on measurement techniques and age. Normal ranges across the lifespan are as follows:

- Infants: 1.5–6 mmHg
- Children: 3–7 mmHg
- Adults: 5–15 mmHg

Increased intracranial pressure (IICP) is defined as sustained elevated pressure (15 mmHg or higher in adults) in the cranial cavity (Gupta & Nosko, 2015). In adults, IICP greater than 20 mmHg warrants immediate treatment interventions.

Like blood pressure, ICP can be affected by routine activities such as sneezing, coughing, or even something as simple as sitting up. The body's compensatory mechanisms control for these minor alterations. However, when ICP rises dramatically or for a sustained period, significant tissue ischemia and damage to delicate neural tissue may result. The cranial vault has a fixed size (except in infants whose suture lines remain open, allowing for expansion) and only has room for a prescribed amount of blood (10%), CSF (5%), and brain matter (85%). The relationship among the three components is known as the **Monro-Kellie hypothesis** (Gupta & Nosko, 2015). As pressure within the cranial vault increases, CSF is reduced to make room, followed by decreasing blood perfusion, resulting in diminished oxygenation of neurons. Because the neurons in the cerebral cortex are most sensitive to oxygen deficits, changes in cortical function are the earliest manifestations of IICP, demonstrated by personality changes as well as impaired memory and judgment.

Another set of unique vital signs that nurses should know and understand related to ICP involves cerebral perfusion pressure (CPP). CPP depends on the patient's ICP and mean systemic arterial pressure (MAP). This relationship can be expressed as:

$$CPP = MAP - ICP,$$

where MAP = (1/3 systolic BP) + (2/3 diastolic BP).

The normal range for CPP is 50–100 mmHg. CPP can be reduced by decreasing blood pressure, increasing ICP, or both. If the patient's CPP is too low, it can be raised by increasing the blood pressure, decreasing the ICP, or both.

Seizures

Seizure activity commonly affects LOC. **Seizures** are periods of abnormal electrical discharges in the brain that may cause involuntary movement and/or behavior and sensory alterations. The spontaneous, disordered discharge of activity that occurs during a seizure exhausts energy metabolites or produces locally toxic molecules, altering LOC for a time after the seizure. Consciousness returns when the metabolic balance of the neurons is restored.

Concussion

A concussion is a minor loss of normal brain function caused by a head injury. It is a common result of sports injuries and falls. Concussions can be difficult to diagnose, as their symptoms may be minor or may not appear for days or even weeks after the occurrence. Some symptoms may include confusion, headache, or nausea. Concussion may be accompanied by a loss of consciousness, but this is not required for a concussion to occur.

Traumatic Brain Injury

TBI is a result of a violent blow to the head or an object penetrating the skull (e.g., a bullet) that causes brain dysfunction. Symptoms vary according to the severity of the injury, ranging from mild headache to death. Loss of consciousness may occur in mild, moderate, or severe traumatic injuries. The ability to recover consciousness varies widely based on the severity and location within the brain that the injury occurred (Mayo Clinic, 2014a).

Outcomes of Altered Level of Consciousness

Possible outcomes of altered LOC and coma include full recovery with no long-term residual effects; recovery with residual damage (e.g., learning deficits, emotional difficulties, impaired judgment); and more severe consequences such as persistent vegetative state (cerebral death) or brain death.

Persistent Vegetative State

Persistent vegetative state (also called *irreversible coma*) is a permanent condition of complete unawareness of self and the environment and loss of all cognitive functions. Usually the result of severe brain trauma or global ischemia, this condition results from death of the cerebral hemispheres with continued function of the brainstem and cerebellum. Although the homeostatic regulatory functions of the brain continue, the ability to respond meaningfully to the environment is lost.

The patient in a persistent vegetative state has sleep–wake cycles and retains the ability to chew, swallow, and cough but cannot interact with the environment. When the person is awake, the eyes may wander back and forth across the room, but they cannot track objects or individuals. In a minimally conscious state, the patient is aware of the environment and can follow simple commands, manipulate objects, gesture or verbalize to indicate yes/no responses, and make meaningful movements (e.g., blinking, smiling) in response to a stimulus. With appropriate supportive care, the patient may remain in this state for years (see the Focus on Diversity and Culture feature).

Locked-In Syndrome

Locked-in syndrome is distinctly different from a persistent vegetative state in that the patient is alert and fully aware of the environment and has intact cognitive abilities but is unable to communicate through speech or movement because of blocked efferent pathways from the brain. Motor paralysis affects all voluntary muscles, although the upper cranial nerves (I through IV) may remain intact, allowing the patient to communicate through eye movements and blinking. In essence, the patient is "locked" inside a paralyzed body while remaining fully conscious of self and environment.

Infarction or hemorrhage of the pons that disrupts outgoing nerve tracts but spares the RAS is the usual cause of locked-in syndrome. This condition also may result when the corticospinal tracts between the midbrain and pons are interrupted. Disorders of the lower motor neurons or muscles (e.g., acute polyneuritis, myasthenia gravis, amyotrophic lateral sclerosis) also may paralyze motor responses, leading to locked-in syndrome.

Brain Death

Brain death is the cessation and irreversibility of all brain functions, including those associated with the brainstem. Although the exact legal criteria for establishing brain death vary somewhat from state to state, brain death is generally

Focus on Diversity and Culture
Religion and Life Support

After a year of being in a persistent vegetative state, patients are classified as being in a "permanent vegetative state." In some states, life may be terminated at this time, although this is a highly controversial issue that is often left up to the patient's family. Families' different points of view on whether to keep someone in a permanent vegetative state are often informed by their religious principles. Religious leaders from every major faith have stated that doctors should not provide life support treatment if it will cause harm or will not be helpful to the patient. Catholicism, Pentecostalism, Mormonism, Hinduism, Islam, Buddhism, Judaism, and other faiths and religions all prohibit euthanasia while supporting the cessation of life support in specific cases where the prolongation of life may cause more harm than good. However, points of view within these religions vary considerably, and an individual family's desires for the continuation or suspension of life support may differ significantly from their religion's stated policy. Decisions about permanent vegetative states are made, ultimately, based on consideration of the patient's expressed wishes, the family's wishes, and applicable laws. The nurse and healthcare team should consult the family of the patient in a vegetative state many times over the course of the patient's treatment to understand and carry out the family's wishes.

Sources: Based on Pew Research Center. (2013). *Religious groups' views on end-of-life issues.* Retrieved from http://www.pewforum.org/2013/11/21/religious-groups-views-on-end-of-life-issues/; Royal Children's Hospital Melbourne. (n.d.). *Religion, culture, and life support.* Retrieved from http://www.rch.org.au/caringdecisions/Chapters/Religion,_culture_and_life_support/; Wickman, G. (2016). *The levels of coma.* Retrieved from http://www.healthguidance.org/entry/14188/1/The-Levels-of-Coma.html

considered to have occurred when there is no evidence of cerebral or brainstem function for an extended period (usually 6–24 hours) in a patient who has a normal body temperature and is not affected by a depressant drug or alcohol poisoning. Generally recognized criteria for brain death are as follows:

- Unresponsive coma with absent motor and reflex movements
- No spontaneous respiration (apnea)
- Pupils fixed (unresponsive to light) and dilated
- Absent ocular responses to head turning and caloric stimulation
- Flat electroencephalogram (EEG) and no cerebral blood circulation present on angiography (if performed)
- Persistence of these manifestations for 30 minutes to 1 hour and for 6 hours after onset of coma and apnea.

Apnea in the patient who is comatose is determined by the apnea test. There are no standardized protocols, and the procedure varies among agencies; however, it is imperative that the patient is monitored closely and continuously for hemodynamic deterioration throughout the procedure. During the apnea test, the ventilator is removed for approximately 8–10 minutes while oxygenation is maintained by endotracheal or tracheal cannula, allowing the $PaCO_2$ to increase to 60 mmHg or higher. This level of carbon dioxide is high enough to stimulate respiration if the brainstem is functional.

EEG may be used to establish the absence of brain activity when brain death is suspected. A flat (isoelectric) EEG over a period of 6–12 hours in a patient who is not hypothermic or under the influence of drugs that depress the CNS is generally accepted as an indicator of brain death.

Prognosis

The prognosis for patients with altered LOC and coma varies according to the underlying cause and pathologic process. Age and general medical condition also play a role in determining outcome. Young adults may fully recover following deep coma from head injury, drug overdose, or other causes. Recovery of consciousness within 2 weeks is associated with a favorable outcome. In general, the prognosis is poor for patients who lack pupillary reaction or reflex eye movements 6 hours after the onset of coma.

Prevalence

Alterations in intracranial regulation may result from disease processes or from trauma. In particular, TBIs are becoming more prevalent. According to the Centers for Disease Control and Prevention (CDC), TBIs account for 2.2 million emergency department visits each year. TBIs predominantly affect very young individuals (0–4 years old), older adults (age 65 and above), and men or boys (CDC, 2016a). Newborns and infants are especially vulnerable to TBI from "shaken baby syndrome" or other forms of child abuse (Mayo Clinic, 2014a). Interpersonal violence also contributes to brain trauma injuries.

Falls continue to be the leading cause of TBI (40%) in the United States, causing 55% of TBIs among children ages 0–14 and 81% of TBIs among adults ages 65 years or older (CDC, 2016a). In addition, concussion, often seen in athletes, occurs between 1.6 million and 3 million times per year (American College of Sports Medicine, 2012). Collisions involving motor vehicles, bicycles, and pedestrians are also a common cause of injury to the brain. Combat injuries and explosive blasts are common sources of brain injuries among military personnel. Beyond the obvious wounds from debris or shrapnel, pressure waves from the blast passing through brain tissue can significantly disrupt brain function (Mayo Clinic, 2014a).

Genetic Considerations and Risk Factors

IICP can be caused by some genetic mutations. Hydrocephalus can result from a blockage in the normal flow of CSF, which leads to increased CSF within the ventricular system. The ventricles can dilate somewhat to accommodate the extra fluid, but at a certain point they can no longer compensate, and brain damage can occur. Hydrocephalus is a common nervous system congenital anomaly, occurring in 0.3–2.5 per 1000 live births. Some conditions in which hydrocephalus occur include Chiari II malformations (most common cause), aqueductal stenosis, and Dandy-Walker malformation. To avoid further damage related to IICP, most neonates will undergo a shunting procedure shortly after delivery (Nelson, 2016).

Seizure disorders affect more than 2 million people in the United States. Although seizures have been identified

Alterations and Therapies
Intracranial Regulation

ALTERATION	DESCRIPTION	MANIFESTATIONS	INTERVENTIONS AND THERAPIES
Increased intracranial pressure (IICP)	Sustained elevated pressure (15 mmHg or higher) in the cranial cavity	▪ Oxygen deficit causes personality changes as well as impaired memory and judgment. ▪ IICP is a medical emergency.	▪ Maintain airway patency. ▪ Monitor neurologic status; assessment areas include LOC, behavior, motor/sensory function, pupillary size and reaction to light, and vital signs. ▪ Monitor IICP monitoring device or ventilator. ▪ Raise pads and bedrails, as seizures may occur. ▪ Elevate the head of the bed 30 degrees unless otherwise indicated. ▪ Monitor arterial blood gases, fluids and electrolytes, bladder distention, and bowel constipation. ▪ Provide emotional support as needed. ▪ Reduce stimuli, coughing, sneezing, and vagal maneuvers that increase ICP. ▪ Identify and treat the underlying cause of the disorder.
Seizure disorder	Periods of abnormal electrical discharges in the brain	▪ Seizure disorder involves involuntary movement as well as behavioral and sensory alterations. ▪ Seizures can be focal or generalized.	▪ Maintain airway patency. ▪ Ensure safety. ▪ Administer medications as ordered. ▪ Provide emotional support. ▪ Identify and treat the underlying cause of the disorder.
Status epilepticus	A continuous seizure that lasts for more than 30 minutes or a series of seizures during which time consciousness is not regained	▪ Status epilepticus involves involuntary movement as well as behavioral and sensory alterations. ▪ It may cause alterations in breathing, injury, or pain perception. ▪ Status epilepticus is a medical emergency.	▪ Maintain airway patency. ▪ Keep suction equipment at the bedside for excessive secretions. ▪ Give oxygen by mask. ▪ Monitor vital signs and circulation. ▪ Perform neurologic assessments frequently. ▪ Establish an intravenous (IV) line. ▪ Insert a nasogastric tube. ▪ Ensure safety. ▪ Manage thermoregulation. ▪ Administer medications as ordered; cumulative doses of drugs may produce apnea, so be prepared to assist with ventilations.
Concussion	Most common and least serious type of TBI	▪ Concussion can be difficult to diagnose, as symptoms vary widely and may not appear for weeks after injury. ▪ It may or may not involve a loss of consciousness. ▪ Symptoms may include confusion, nausea, headache, light or noise sensitivity, or memory loss.	▪ Encourage seeking medical evaluation, even if no symptoms are present. ▪ Consider the possibility of concurrent spinal cord injury. ▪ Perform neurologic assessment. ▪ Ensure safety. ▪ Monitor vital signs. ▪ Provide emotional support. ▪ Teach the need to be vigilant in noticing changes in neurologic status, as they may not occur until weeks afterward. ▪ Emphasize the need to seek medical help immediately for neurologic changes.
Traumatic brain injury (TBI)	Usually due to a violent blow to the head or an object (e.g., bullet) penetrating the skull	▪ Symptoms vary widely based on the amount and location of brain dysfunction. ▪ Even mild injury may cause loss of consciousness. ▪ Manifestations include confusion, slurred speech, headache, nausea, mood swings, loss of balance, decreased LOC, weakness, and death.	▪ Maintain airway patency. ▪ Keep suction equipment at the bedside for excessive secretions. ▪ Administer oxygen if needed. ▪ Perform frequent neurologic assessments, especially for signs of increasing ICP and decreasing LOC. ▪ Monitor vital signs. ▪ Consider the high probability of concurrent spinal cord injury. ▪ Ensure safety. ▪ Establish IV access. ▪ Administer medications as ordered. ▪ Provide emotional support.

as causing decreased LOC and many forms of seizures have been identified, etiologies of seizure disorders have been difficult to pinpoint. Approximately 70–80% of individuals with epilepsy have a genetic component to the disorder, but no single mutation has been found that explains a majority of cases. Instead, research has found multiple different genetic mutations, each of which contributes to epilepsy in a small number of individuals (Myers & Mefford, 2015). Still, the incidence of epilepsy within first-degree family members is reported to be two to four times higher than in the general population (International League Against Epilepsy, 2013).

Case Study » Part 1

Joshua Thomson is an active 13-year-old who was riding his bicycle with friends when he fell while attempting to jump over a ditch. His friends helped him home, and his mother has brought him to the urgent care center with complaints of a slight headache and a painful left wrist. As the triage nurse at the clinic, you interview Joshua and his mother. According to Joshua, he was attempting to jump the ditch when his bike tire caught on the curb. He flipped forward over the handlebars of his bike and landed on his back. He does not remember hitting his head on the ground but does remember putting his hands down to brace his fall. His biggest complaint at this moment is the pain he experiences when he moves his left wrist, but he is also nauseous and has a "small headache." Joshua's mother thinks that the headache and nausea may be due to the fact that Joshua has not eaten anything since 7:00 a.m. and it is now 4:00 p.m.

The attending physician orders an x-ray of Joshua's wrist and acetaminophen (Tylenol) 650 mg for pain. The x-ray shows that Joshua's left wrist is fractured. He is placed in a cast, given prescriptions for acetaminophen for the pain and ondansetron for the nausea, and sent home. As the nurse, you give Joshua's mother some discharge instructions for caring for the cast, using both the acetaminophen and ondansetron, and watching Joshua for any sign of neurologic damage.

Clinical Reasoning Questions Level I

1. What neurologic alterations would you educate Joshua's mother to watch for?
2. What should Joshua's mother do if she makes any of these observations?

Clinical Reasoning Questions Level II

3. What prevention education should be given to Joshua and his mother?
4. What focused assessment should you perform?
5. Why would the physician prescribe ondansetron (Zofran) for nausea instead of promethazine (Phenergan)?

Concepts Related to Intracranial Regulation

Alterations in intracranial regulation are often the result of trauma, but they may also be related to changes in acid–base balance, infection, inflammation and edema, and other causes. Often the earliest warning signs of alterations to intracranial regulation are changes in LOC and respirations. The increased CO_2 level associated with respiratory acidosis can result in vasodilation (lowering the blood pressure), leading to an increase in ICP. Patients with impaired intracranial regulation frequently experience changes in cognition. This may range from the mild, temporary confusion often associated with a minor fall to the complete unconsciousness associated with TBI.

IICP and damage to the brain can cause a decrease in LOC and in the brain's ability to perform vital functions. This may result in decreased mobility due to unconsciousness, coma, or paralysis; decreased respirations (apnea), leading to reduced oxygenation and perfusion; and decreased sensory perception. Decreased mobility can lead to reduced tissue integrity with the formation of pressure ulcers or wounds, and tissue integrity may also be compromised because of the traumatic injury that caused the change in ICP. If changes in intracranial regulation are the result of trauma, the awake patient may experience acute pain, requiring the nurse to understand interventions related to comfort for treating pain. Depending on the cause of the alteration to intracranial regulation, surgery may be required for treatment, requiring the nurse to be proficient in perioperative care. When caring for patients with alterations in intracranial regulation and their families, the nurse will need to be conscious of the patient's developmental level, the family's dynamics and cultural beliefs, and the ethics and legal issues that may apply to the patient's case. The nurse will likely need to provide patient teaching related to stress and coping, as changes in intracranial regulation are often sudden and life threatening, and they may produce physical changes (e.g., paralysis) that will require a change in lifestyle. The nurse will also need to provide for the safety of the patient, especially if the patient is experiencing a seizure.

The Concepts Related to Intracranial Regulation feature links some, but not all, of the concepts integral to intracranial regulation. They are presented in alphabetical order.

Health Promotion

Health promotion related to intracranial regulation generally involves anticipatory guidance related to the individual's age, development, and activities. For example, nurses provide information about protective equipment for outdoor activities and vehicle restraint systems.

Health promotion education for older adults includes fall prevention and adhering to cautions that accompany prescription medications. Older adults who are at risk for falls may benefit from a home safety assessment. Patients who have a disorder that affects their balance or mobility should also receive information about fall prevention.

Nurses can teach patients at risk for impaired intracranial regulation the importance of wearing a medical alert bracelet, discussing care plans at school or the workplace, and taking all medications as prescribed. For young children, health promotion may involve wearing a helmet to prevent head injury during a seizure.

Health promotion for patients with a history of stroke, seizure disorder, or brain injury also includes patient teaching related to following the treatment regimen. Nurses should review prescription and over-the-counter medications with all patients, making sure to discuss side effects that may affect intracranial regulation. For example, blood thinners may increase the risk of a hemorrhagic stroke, and

Concepts Related to
Intracranial Regulation

CONCEPT	RELATIONSHIP TO INTRACRANIAL REGULATION	NURSING IMPLICATIONS
Acid–Base Balance	$\uparrow CO_2 \rightarrow$ vasodilation $\rightarrow$ IICP	■ Assess LOC; act immediately to decrease ICP. ■ Underlying cause determines treatment.
Cognition	Alterations in intracranial regulation can lead to impaired cognitive function, ranging from mild confusion to lack of consciousness.	■ Assess LOC. ■ Assess vital signs. ■ Underlying cause (e.g., fall, seizure, disease) determines treatment.
Mobility	Patients will have different needs based on the underlying pathology. A patient who is comatose will need passive range-of-motion (ROM) exercises, whereas one with IICP should have stimulation kept at a minimum to avoid further increases in ICP.	■ Assess LOC. ■ Assess vital signs in response to interventions. ■ Consider involving physical or occupational therapy to minimize any deficits, if appropriate.
Oxygenation	$\downarrow$ LOC may result in $\downarrow$ respirations	■ Assess airway and respirations. ■ *Anticipate:* airway support. A nasopharyngeal airway may be sufficient for patients who are drowsy but arousable. Patients with more serious alterations in consciousness may require an oropharyngeal airway or endotracheal intubation and mechanical ventilation.
Safety	Patients may be awake and cooperative or confused and combative. Patients with seizures may unintentionally put themselves at risk of injury.	■ Assess LOC. ■ Identify etiology of any decrease in LOC. If SpO₂ is low, O₂ may help with confusion. ■ Reorient often as appropriate. ■ Be aware of potential drug side effects or drug–drug interactions that could harm the patient. ■ Educate the patient and/or family about care and prevention of future episodes as appropriate (e.g., teach patient with sports-related concussion about helmet use).
Stress and Coping	Neurologic disorders are often sudden, sometimes life threatening, and always life altering.	■ Allow the patient and family time to process situation. ■ Answer questions and assess reaction to situation. ■ Consider referral to a psychologist, support group, or clergy as appropriate.

many medications cause drowsiness or require changes in activity level. Nurses should also instruct patients to avoid alcohol, which can increase the risk for injury, and products that contain nicotine, which increase heart rate and blood pressure and cause vasoconstriction that can increase the patient's risk of stroke.

Nursing Assessment

A nursing assessment to determine problems with neurologic structure and/or function may be conducted during a health screening, may focus on a chief complaint (e.g., headaches), or may be part of a total health assessment. Nurses should complete neurologic assessments as early as possible in the assessment process.

If the patient has a problem with neurologic structure or function, the nurse should analyze the problem's onset,

characteristics, course, severity, precipitating and relieving factors, and any associated symptoms, noting the time and circumstances.

If the patient's LOC is altered, the nurse may need to rely on family members for information. The patient's LOC can be assessed using the Glasgow Coma Scale, as described in **Table 11–3 >>**.

Observation and Patient Interview

Some information about the patient's neurologic status can be gleaned just by careful observation on the part of the nurse. In out-of-hospital settings, notice the patient's appearance and dress. Does the patient look well groomed or disheveled? Some patients who have had a stroke may neglect the side of the body that was affected. Observe how the patient walks and whether the patient requires an assistive device or the help of a caregiver to walk. Does the

TABLE 11–3 Glasgow Coma Scale for Assessment of Coma in Infants, Children, and Adults

Category	Score	Infant and Young Child Criteria	Older Child and Adult Criteria
Eye opening	4	Spontaneous opening	Spontaneous
	3	To loud noise	To verbal stimuli
	2	To pain	To pain
	1	No response	No response
Verbal response	5	Smiles, coos, cries to appropriate stimuli	Oriented to time, place, and person; uses appropriate words and phrases
	4	Irritable; cries	Confused
	3	Inappropriate crying	Inappropriate words or verbal response
	2	Grunts, moans	Incomprehensible words
	1	No response	No response
Motor response	6	Spontaneous movement	Obeys commands
	5	Withdraws to touch	Localizes pain
	4	Withdraws to pain	Withdraws to pain
	3	Abnormal flexion (decorticate)	Flexion to pain (decorticate)
	2	Abnormal extension (decerebrate)	Extension to pain (decerebrate)
	1	No response	No response

Add the score from each category to calculate the total score. The maximum score is 15, indicating the best possible level of neurologic functioning. The minimum score is 3, indicating total neurologic unresponsiveness.

Sources: Data from Christensen, B. (2014). *Pediatric Glasgow Coma Scale.* Retrieved from http://emedicine.medscape.com/article/2058902-overview; Glasgow Coma Scale. (2014). *What is the Glasgow Coma Scale?* Retrieved from http://glasgowcomascale.org/what-is-gcs/; Jevon, P. (n.d.). *Annex 3.* Retrieved from http://www.sign.ac.uk/pdf/sign110_annex3.pdf

patient make any other movements that seem different from normal?

During the patient interview, observe facial movements and speech patterns as well as alertness or general comprehension of simple instructions such as where to sit or which forms to fill out. Do not draw any conclusions from these observations, but make sure to address any observed deviations from normal in the patient interview.

A thorough and accurate neurologic assessment requires the nurse to be attentive. Assessment is a skill that is developed through practice with much repetition. Nurses should develop a systematic approach to neurologic assessment to make sure no essential elements are left out. The following general interview questions may be employed as part of this approach:

1. Have you ever been diagnosed with a neurologic illness?
   - If so, when were you diagnosed?
   - What was the treatment plan?
   - What helped the problem? What made it worse?
   - What medications were you prescribed?

2. Do you have a history of fainting or seizures?
   - If so, when was your first episode? When was your last episode?
   - How long does it take you to recover from a seizure?
   - Describe your seizures.
   - What medication do you take to control your seizures?
   - When was your last blood work done?

3. Have you noticed any changes in your vision, hearing, or smelling? (See the module on Sensory Perception for specific questions.)

4. Have you noticed a change in your balance and coordination?
   - If so, can you describe these changes?
   - Do you notice tremors?
   - Do you feel that you are "clumsy"?
   - Are you able to bend over without falling over or getting dizzy?

5. Are you having pain? (If the patient reports pain, conduct a pain assessment following the guidelines recommended in the module on Comfort.)

6. Have you noticed any changes in your memory?
   - If yes, can you describe the changes?
   - Do you need to make lists to help you remember things?

Physical Examination

As discussed earlier, some parts of the physical examination portion of a neurologic assessment can be done by general observation rather than a formal process. The nurse should document all findings in a clear, concise manner to help other nurses and clinicians quickly note any change in neurologic status. For example, the nurse should document "The patient is alert and oriented to person and place but not time" rather than "The patient is alert and oriented × 2."

A thorough neurologic examination should ideally include assessment of the patient's cranial nerves, mental status, reflexes, muscle strength and coordination, and gait. The nurse should note lack of symmetry between sides of the body. A complete neurologic examination is usually not performed in otherwise healthy patients.

The physical examination with a neurologic focus is often one of the hardest assessment skills for new nurses to conduct proficiently. Strategies student nurses and new nurses can use to improve their skills in this area include practicing on fellow students and family members and carefully observing focused neurologic assessments conducted by more experienced clinicians. The neurologic examination only becomes efficient and accurate with practice and repetition.

Diagnostic Tests

Although a patient's history and physical examination often indicate the cause of alterations in LOC, several diagnostic tests may be useful in establishing the diagnosis. The results of diagnostic tests of neurologic structure and function are

Neurologic Assessment

ASSESSMENT/ METHOD	NORMAL FINDINGS	ABNORMAL FINDINGS	LIFESPAN OR DEVELOPMENT CONSIDERATIONS
Mental Status			
Assess appearance, including dress, hygiene, grooming, gait, and posture.	The patient should be appropriately dressed and clean, with normal gait and posture.	■ Unilateral neglect (inattention to one side of body) may occur in some patients who have had a stroke. ■ Poor hygiene and grooming may be seen in patients with dementia. ■ Abnormal gait and posture may be seen in transient ischemic attacks (TIAs), strokes, and Parkinson disease.	■ In older adults, poor hygiene or grooming may be a result of financial constraints or limited mobility, so always investigate unexpected findings.
Assess behavior, including actions and affect, content and quality of speech, and LOC. Use the Glasgow Coma Scale (see Table 11–3) to document findings.	A score of 15 on the Glasgow Coma Scale indicates that the patient is alert and oriented.	■ Emotional swings or changes in personality may be observed in patients who have had a stroke. ■ Apathy is often seen in patients with dementing disorders. ■ **Aphasia** (defective or absent language function) may occur in patients who experience TIAs and strokes. Aphasias are associated with damage to the left cerebral cortex, so they are more often observed in patients with strokes of the left hemisphere. ■ *Dysphonia* (change in the tone of the voice) is common in patients who have had strokes. Dysphonia is seen in patients with paralysis of the vocal cords (cranial nerve X). ■ *Dysarthria* (difficulty speaking) may be observed in patients with lesions of the upper and lower motor neurons, cerebellum, and extrapyramidal tract. ■ Drowsiness and decreased LOC may be associated with brain trauma, infections, TIAs, stroke, and brain tumors. ■ LOC is usually altered in patients who have had a stroke, and can range from confusion to coma.	■ Infants and children may be lethargic, irritable, and difficult to console. ■ Children may become scared and uncooperative in unknown settings or around strangers. ■ Older adults may also become easily overwhelmed in certain settings and have difficulty following simple directions even if they do not have an underlying disorder. Input from family members or friends may be especially helpful in clarifying a patient's baseline.

Assess cognitive function.
   Note orientation to time, place, and person.
   Note attention span and recent and remote memory.
Ask the patient to:
1. Repeat five to seven numbers.
2. Recall three items after 5 minutes.
3. Recall his or her address, breakfast, or birthday.
   Note ability to understand what is said and to express thoughts.
   Note ability to make logical and safe judgments.
	The patient should be oriented to time, place, and person; demonstrate attention and the ability to remember recent and past events; respond appropriately to questions; and be able to make judgments.	■ Disorientation to time and place may occur in patients with a stroke of the right cerebral hemisphere and in patients with dementia.
		■ Memory deficits are often seen in patients who have had a stroke.
		■ Perceptual deficits may be seen in patients with a history of stroke, brain injury, or dementia.
			■ Children's verbal skills and ability to follow directions should be appropriate for their age. (Refer to the module on Development for a review of age-appropriate behavior.)
			■ In older adults, assess the patient's ability to hear before making any assessment judgments regarding cognition.

Neurologic Assessment *(continued)*

ASSESSMENT/ METHOD	NORMAL FINDINGS	ABNORMAL FINDINGS	LIFESPAN OR DEVELOPMENT CONSIDERATIONS
Cranial Nerves (CNs) in the Conscious Patient (Note that CN 1 is not routinely tested) See **Table 11–4 »** for assessment of cranial nerves in the unconscious patient.			
Test CN II (optic). Assess vision in each eye with a Snellen chart.	Based on previous ability to see and use of visual aids, the patient should be able to see with both eyes.	▪ Blindness in one eye may be observed in patients with strokes or TIAs. Impaired vision or blindness in one side of both eyes (homonymous hemianopia) is associated with stroke. ▪ Impaired vision may occur in patients with strokes and brain tumors. Double vision may be noted in patients with strokes and TIAs.	▪ *Infants:* Shine a bright light in the eyes; a quick blink reflex and dorsal head flexion indicate light perception. ▪ *Children:* Test vision and visual fields; visual acuity should be appropriate for age. ▪ *Adults and older adults:* Test vision and visual fields; visual acuity should be appropriate for age.
Test CNs III, IV, and VI (oculomotor, trochlear, and abducens, respectively). Assess extraocular movements by asking the patient to follow your finger as you write an *H* in the air. Assess PERRL (pupils equal, round, and reactive to light) by covering one eye at a time and shining a bright light directly into the uncovered eye using a penlight or the ophthalmoscope. Assess for *ptosis* (drooping eyelids).	Extraocular movements should be present bilaterally, and pupils should be equal, round, and reactive to light. Eyelids should not droop.	▪ *Nystagmus* may be observed in patients who have experienced stroke. ▪ Constricted pupils are associated with impaired blood flow from a stroke. ▪ Ptosis occurs in patients with strokes, myasthenia gravis, and palsy of CN III.	▪ *Infants:* Shine a penlight in the eyes and move it side to side; infants should be able to focus and track the light. ▪ *Children and adults:* Move an object through the six cardinal points of gaze; patients should be able to track the object through all fields. ▪ *Older adults:* Bilateral ptosis may occur as part of the normal aging process.
Test CN V (trigeminal). Assess the ability to feel light, dull, and sharp sensations on the face. With the patient's eyes closed, check whether sensation is the same on both sides of the face. Stroke the cheek with a wisp of cotton for light touch, with a closed safety pin for dull touch, and with a tongue depressor for sharp touch. If the sharp point of a safety pin is used to assess sharp touch, avoid scratching the surface of the skin and discard the pin after use. Assess the corneal reflex by touching the corneal surface with a wisp of sterile cotton. The reflex may be absent or decreased in patients who wear contact lenses.	The ability to feel light, dull, and sharp sensations should be intact. The patient should blink when the corneal surface is touched.	▪ Changes in facial sensation are noted with impaired blood flow to the carotid artery. ▪ Decreased sensation in the face and cornea on the same side of the body, as well as numbness of the lip and mouth, occur in patients with strokes. ▪ Loss of facial sensation or contraction of the masseter and temporal muscles is seen in patients with lesions of CN V. ▪ The corneal reflex may be impaired in patients with lesions of CN V or VII.	▪ *Infants:* Stimulate the rooting and sucking reflexes to assess strength and pattern. ▪ *Children:* Observe the child chewing a cracker to assess bilateral jaw strength. Touch the forehead and cheeks with a cotton ball with the child's eyes closed; the child should push the cotton ball away. ▪ *Adults and older adults:* Test for light touch with a cotton ball, dull touch with a closed safety pin or tongue depressor, and sharp touch with an open safety pin or broken tongue depressor. Test all distribution areas of the nerve (forehead, cheek, and chin). Be careful not to scratch the patient, especially older adults with frail skin. Test the corneal reflex with a wisp of sterile cotton.

(continued on next page)

Neurologic Assessment *(continued)*

ASSESSMENT/ METHOD	NORMAL FINDINGS	ABNORMAL FINDINGS	LIFESPAN OR DEVELOPMENT CONSIDERATIONS
Test CN VII (facial). Assess the ability to taste sweet, sour, and salt on the anterior two thirds of the tongue by asking the patient to stick out the tongue and applying a salty, sweet, or sour substance. Assess the ability to frown, show teeth, blow out cheeks, raise eyebrows, smile, and close eyes tightly.	The ability to taste sweet, sour, and salt should be intact. The patient should be able to frown, show teeth, blow out cheeks, raise eyebrows, smile, and close eyes tightly. Muscle movement should be equal bilaterally.	▪ Loss of the ability to taste may occur in patients with brain tumors or nerve impairment. ▪ Asymmetry or decreased movement of facial muscles is noted in patients with lesions of the upper and lower motor neurons. ▪ Paralysis of the lower motor neurons from injury to CN VII results in an inability to close the eyes, a flat nasolabial fold, paralysis of the lower face, and the inability to wrinkle the forehead. ▪ Paralysis of the upper motor neurons due to stroke results in weakness of the eyelids and paralysis of the lower face. ▪ Pain, paralysis, and sagging of facial muscles is seen on the affected side in Bell palsy.	▪ *Older adults:* Taste diminishes as part of the normal aging process. Ask the patient about dietary habits to ensure nutritional needs are being met.
Test CN VIII (acoustic). Assess the ability to hear the ticking of a watch and whispered and spoken words.	The patient should be able to hear with both ears.	▪ Decreased hearing or deafness may occur in patients with strokes and/or tumors of CN VIII.	▪ *Infants:* The patient should blink, move the head toward the sound, or freeze position on hearing a loud sound. ▪ *Children, adults, and older adults:* Whisper in each ear; the patient should turn the head toward the sound and repeat words correctly. Allow patients with hearing aids to wear them.
Test CNs IX and X (glossopharyngeal and vagus, respectively). If the gag reflex is intact, observe the patient swallowing a small drink of water. Observe for a symmetric rise of the soft palate and uvula as the patient says "ah." Assess the gag reflex by touching the back of patient's throat with a tongue depressor. Assess the ability to taste salty, sweet, and sour substances on the posterior third of the tongue. (See previous description.)	The patient should be able to swallow without difficulty, have symmetrical rise of the soft palate, have intact gag reflex, and taste appropriately.	▪ *Dysphagia* (difficulty swallowing) is common in patients with impaired blood flow to the brain. ▪ Unilateral loss of the gag reflex occurs in patients with lesions of CNs IX and X.	▪ *Infants:* Observe swallowing during feeding.

Neurologic Assessment *(continued)*

ASSESSMENT/ METHOD	NORMAL FINDINGS	ABNORMAL FINDINGS	LIFESPAN OR DEVELOPMENT CONSIDERATIONS
Test CN XI (spinal accessory). Assess the patient's ability to shrug the shoulders while you exert downward pressure. Assess the patient's ability to turn the head to each side against the resistance of your hand. In both cases, observe for symmetry, strength, and size of muscles.	The patient should be able to shrug the shoulders and turn the head against resistance.	■ Muscle weakness is noted in patients with lower motor neuron disease. ■ *Contralateral hemiparesis* (muscle weakness on the side opposite the lesion or trauma) is seen with strokes.	■ *Infants:* Not tested. ■ *Children, adults, and older adults:* Ask the patient to raise the shoulders and turn the head side to side against resistance. Observe for good strength in the neck and shoulders.
Test CN XII (hypoglossal). Assess the patient's ability to stick out the tongue and move it from side to side against the resistance of a tongue depressor.	The patient should be able to stick out the tongue and move it from side to side against resistance.	■ Atrophy and **fasciculations** (twitches) of the tongue are seen in patients with lower motor neuron disease. ■ The tongue may deviate toward the involved side of the body.	■ *Infants:* Sucking and swallowing should be coordinated during feeding. ■ *Children, adults, and older adults:* Use a tongue depressor.

Body Systems

Assess the ability to perceive various sensations. Touch both sides of various parts of the body (chest, abdomen, arms, and legs) with one or more of the following: ■ Cotton wisp ■ Sharp object ■ Dull object Place a vibrating tuning fork on bony prominences.	The patient should be able to differentiate between soft and sharp and feel vibrations appropriately.	■ Decreased sensation of pain occurs in patients with injury to the spinothalamic tract. ■ Decreased vibratory sensation is seen in patients with injuries to the posterior column tract. ■ Transient numbness of the face, arm, or hand is seen in patients with TIAs. ■ Sensation may be impaired in patients with strokes, brain tumors, and spinal cord trauma or compression.	■ Infants and younger children will not be able to verbalize the sensations that they feel, but they should have a reaction to the sensations (e.g., withdrawal from noxious stimuli).
Assess sense of position (**kinesthesia**). Move the patient's finger or big toe up or down. Ask the patient to describe the movement.	The patient should be able to accurately describe the position of a finger or toe when it is moved up or down.	■ Lesions of the posterior column of the spinal cord may affect sense of position.	■ The test cannot be performed with infants and younger children because they cannot verbalize the position of a finger or toe.
Assess the ability to discriminate fine touch. Ask the patient to identify: 1. Object in hand, such as a coin or key (tests stereognosis) 2. Number written on hand (tests graphesthesia) (see **Figure 11–7 ≫**) 3. Two points of simultaneous pinpricks on the hand (tests two-point discrimination) (see **Figure 11–8 ≫**) 4. Where he or she is being touched (tests localization) 5. How many sensations are felt when the patient is touched simultaneously on both sides of the body (tests extinction).	The patient should be able to identify and discriminate fine touch.	■ Inability to discriminate fine touch (stereognosis, graphesthesia, two-point discrimination, point localization, and extinction) may occur in patients with injury to the posterior columns or sensory cortex.	■ The test cannot be performed with infants and younger children because the exam involves cooperation, the ability to understand and follow directions, and verbalization of results to the examiner.

(continued on next page)

Neurologic Assessment *(continued)*

ASSESSMENT/ METHOD	NORMAL FINDINGS	ABNORMAL FINDINGS	LIFESPAN OR DEVELOPMENT CONSIDERATIONS
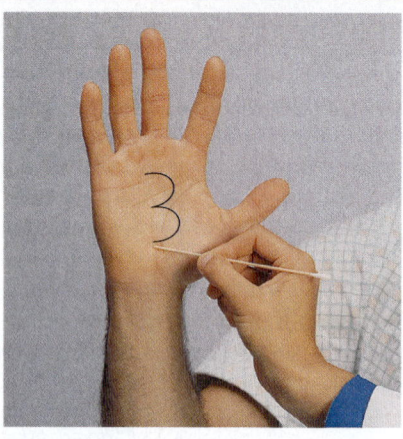 **Figure 11–7** ❯❯ Testing graphesthesia.		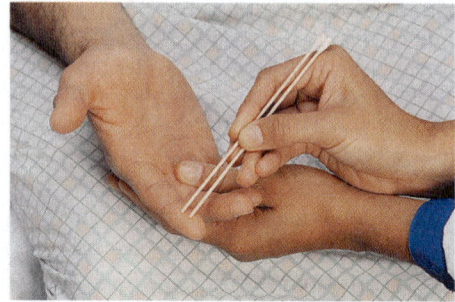 **Figure 11–8** ❯❯ Testing two-point discrimination.	
Assess bilateral symmetry and size of muscles. 　　Assess for **tremors** (rhythmic movements) and fasciculations (irregular movements). Observe movements as the patient is at rest (not making a purposeful movement) and with activity (making a purposeful movement, such as reaching for a glass of water).	Muscles should be bilaterally symmetrical and of equal size. Tremors or fasciculations should not be present.	▪ Atrophy of muscles is seen in patients with diseases of the lower motor neurons. ▪ Tremors that occur with activity are seen in patients with multiple sclerosis and diseases of the cerebellar system. ▪ Tremors that occur at rest and disappear with movement are common in patients with Parkinson disease.	▪ All age groups should have symmetry in muscles and lack tremors. ▪ Be aware that infants may have jerky, nonsmooth movements; these should not be confused with tremors.
Assess muscle tone.	Muscle tone should be appropriate.	▪ Muscle tone is decreased (*flaccidity*) in patients with diseases of or trauma to the lower motor neurons and early stroke. ▪ Muscle tone is increased (*spasticity*) in patients with diseases of the corticospinal motor tract. ▪ Muscles are rigid in patients with diseases of the extrapyramidal motor tract.	▪ Children with autism often have low muscle tone. ▪ Muscle tone should be symmetrical within all age groups.
Assess bilateral muscle strength and movement. 　　Ask the patient to: 1. Squeeze your hands 2. Push the feet against the resistance of your hands 3. Raise both legs off the bed	Muscle strength and movement should be bilaterally equal and strong.	▪ Weakness of the arms, legs, or hands is often seen in patients with TIAs. ▪ Hemiplegia (paralysis of one-half of the body vertically) is noted in patients with strokes. ▪ Flaccid paralysis is noted in patients with strokes. ▪ Paralysis or decreased movement is seen in patients with multiple sclerosis and myasthenia gravis. ▪ There is total loss of motor function below the level of injury in complete spinal cord transection and in injuries to the anterior portion of the spinal cord. ▪ Spasticity of muscles may occur as a result of incomplete spinal cord injuries.	▪ In newborns, bilateral upper extremity strength may be tested by utilizing the grasp reflex. ▪ Infants and young children may not be able to be assessed because of age-related difficulty in following instructions. ▪ In older children, teens, and all adults, movement and strength should be equal bilaterally. The hand-dominant side of the body may have slightly stronger findings.

Neurologic Assessment *(continued)*

ASSESSMENT/ METHOD	NORMAL FINDINGS	ABNORMAL FINDINGS	LIFESPAN OR DEVELOPMENT CONSIDERATIONS
Cerebellar Function			
Assess gait: Ask the patient to walk normally, then in a heel-to-toe fashion, then on toes, and finally on heels. Perform the Romberg test: Ask the patient to stand with feet together and eyes closed. (Stand close to the patient to prevent falling.)	The patient should have appropriate gait and be able to walk heel to toe, on toes, and on heels. The patient should exhibit minimal swaying for up to 20 seconds.	■ *Ataxia* is a lack of coordination and a clumsiness of movements, with staggering, wide-based, and unbalanced gait. Ataxia is often seen in patients with strokes and cerebellar tumors. ■ Swaying and falling (positive Romberg test) are seen in patients with cerebellar ataxia. ■ Inability to walk on toes, then heels, may indicate diseases of the upper motor neurons. ■ Spastic hemiparesis is often associated with strokes or upper motor neuron disease. Here, the patient walks with one leg stiffly dragging while the other leg circles out and forward. One arm is held flexed and close to the side. ■ Steppage gait is noted with diseases of the lower motor neurons. Here, the patient drags or lifts the foot high, then slaps the foot onto the floor. The patient cannot walk on the heels. ■ Sensory ataxia may be associated with polyneuropathy or damage to the posterior column. Here, the patient walks on the heels before bringing down the toes, and the feet are held wide apart. Gait worsens when the eyes are closed.	■ Assessment can be performed only if the patient can walk, cooperate, and understand and follow directions. ■ Ensure safety by standing close enough to catch the patient if he or she loses balance.
Assess coordination. Observe the ability to pat the knees, alternating front and back of hands and gradually increasing speed. Observe the ability to touch each finger of one hand to the thumb. Observe the ability to touch the nose, then one of your fingers, then the nose again. Observe the ability to run each heel down each shin while in a supine position (see **Figure 11–9 》**).	The patient should demonstrate coordinated movements. 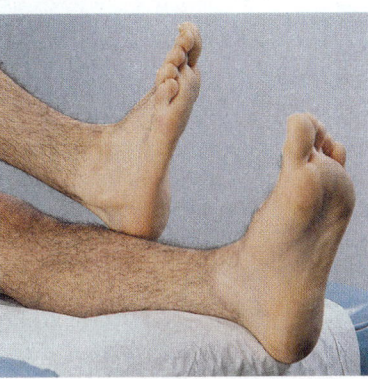 **Figure 11–9 》** Heel-to-shin test.	■ Ataxic movements are apparent in patients with cerebellar disease.	■ Assessment can be performed only if the patient can cooperate and understand and follow directions.

(continued on next page)

Neurologic Assessment *(continued)*

ASSESSMENT/ METHOD	NORMAL FINDINGS	ABNORMAL FINDINGS	LIFESPAN OR DEVELOPMENT CONSIDERATIONS
Assess for the Brudzinski sign: With the patient supine, flex the patient's head to the chest (see **Figure 11–10 »**).	There should be no flexion of the hips or knees.	■ Flexion of the hips and knees occurs in patients with meningeal irritation.	■ All age groups should exhibit the same response.
Assess for the Kernig sign: With the patient supine, flex the knees and hips, then straighten the knee (see **Figure 11–11 »**).	There should be no pain or resistance.	■ Excessive pain and/or resistance occurs in patients with meningeal irritation.	■ All age groups should exhibit the same response.
Assess for abnormal postures in patients who are unconscious.	There should be no abnormal posturing.	■ Observe for decorticate posturing, in which the upper arms are close to the sides; the elbows, wrists, and fingers are flexed; the legs are extended with internal rotation; and the feet are plantar (see Figure 11–6A). Decorticate posturing occurs with lesions of the corticospinal tracts. ■ Observe for decerebrate posturing, in which the neck is extended, with the jaw clenched; the arms are pronated, extended, and close to the sides; the legs are extended straight out; and the feet are plantar (see Figure 11–6B). Decerebrate posturing occurs with lesions of the midbrain, pons, or diencephalon.	■ All age groups should exhibit the same response.

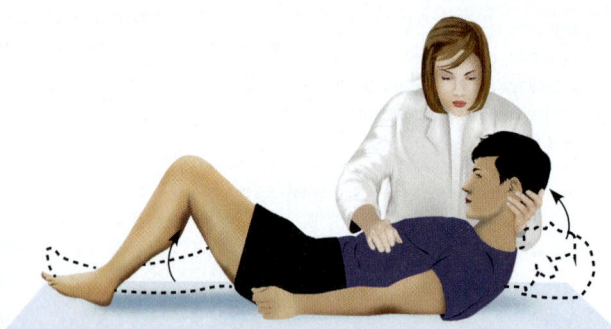

Figure 11–10 » Assessing the Brudzinski sign.

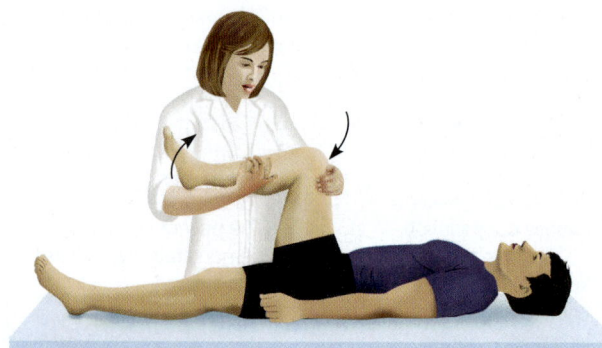

Figure 11–11 » Assessing the Kernig sign.

used to support the diagnosis of a specific injury or disease, to provide information to identify or modify the appropriate medications or therapy used to treat the problem, and to help nurses monitor the patient's responses to treatment and nursing care interventions.

Diagnostic tests used to assess the structure and function of the neurologic system include CT scan, MRI, x-ray, EEG, ultrasonography of the brain, brain echography, echoencephalography, cerebral angiography, positron emission tomography (PET) scan, nerve conduction studies, myelography, thermography, serum electrolytes, ICP monitoring,

CSF assessment, therapeutic drug level monitoring, antidiuretic hormone level monitoring, and serum glucose testing.

» *For more details about these diagnostic tests, go to **Pearson MyLab Nursing and eText** to access Appendix B.*

Case Study **»** Part 2

Joshua and his mother stop by the pharmacy to pick up Joshua's prescriptions. When they arrive home, Joshua's mother makes dinner and then helps her son get ready for bed. Joshua asks to watch

TABLE 11–4 Assessment of Cranial Nerves in the Unconscious Patient

Cranial Nerves	Reflex	Assessment Procedure	Normal Findings
II, III	Pupillary	Shine a light source in the eye.	Rapid, concentrically constricting pupils indicate intact CNs II and III.
II, IV, VI	Oculocephalic	Hold the eyes open and turn the head from side to side. _Precaution:_ Cervical spine injury must be ruled out before this assessment is performed.	Eyes gazing straight up or lagging slightly behind head motion indicates intact cranial nerves.
III, VIII	Oculovestibular	Place the head in a midline and slightly elevated position. Inject ice water into the ear canal. _Precautions:_ Cervical spine injury must be ruled out before this assessment is performed. The tympanic membrane must be intact; otherwise, the brain may be filled with bacteria-laden fluid. _Note:_ This assessment is usually performed by a physician.	Eyes deviating toward the irrigated ear indicate intact CNs III and VIII. (Note that this is opposite of the result in conscious patients.)
V, VII	Corneal	Gently touch the cornea with a sterile cotton swab.	A blink indicates intact CNs V and VII.
IX, X	Gag	Irritate the pharynx with a tongue depressor or cotton swab.	Gagging response indicates intact CNs IX and X.

some TV before bed, but he complains that the sound is too loud and he cannot see the picture clearly. His mother tells him that he has had a rough day, so he should get some sleep. As she tucks him into bed and kisses him, Joshua asks what day tomorrow is. His mother tells him that tomorrow is Sunday, and he can sleep in if he wishes.

The next morning, Joshua's mother goes in to check on him and he is sleeping peacefully. She goes about her business. At 10:00 a.m., she checks on him again and finds him still asleep. This time, she tries to wake him and has difficulty. After his mother shakes him for a minute, Joshua finally opens his eyes. He slurs his speech and has difficulty keeping his eyes open. Joshua's mother calls 9-1-1, and the paramedics take Joshua to the emergency department.

As the nurse on duty, you assess the Glasgow Coma Scale. In doing so, you find that Joshua arouses to painful stimuli; localizes pain and is confused; has slurred speech; and does not recognize his mother. He can follow simple commands. You give Joshua a score of 11 out of a possible 15. The emergency department physician calls for a neurologic surgery consult.

Clinical Reasoning Questions Level I

1. Why might Joshua be having difficulty arousing?
2. What signs or symptoms would indicate that Joshua's condition is deteriorating?
3. What does a Glasgow Coma Scale score of 11 mean for Joshua?

Clinical Reasoning Questions Level II

4. What medications would you anticipate having to administer to Joshua to prevent further increased pressure?
5. What education would you provide to Joshua's mother?
6. Who would you contact about the possibility of death in this patient?

Independent Interventions

The nurse must be able to recognize a change in the LOC of a patient and provide care immediately. The first step in care is to treat the underlying cause and prevent further deterioration. Primary interventions include maintaining a patent airway and initiating protocols to treat neurologic issues. The nurse may also need to prepare the patient for surgical interventions.

In addition to measuring vital signs, specific interventions initiated and performed by the nurse may include the following:

- Assessing LOC, pupil response, neurologic status
- Monitoring fluid intake and output
- Reducing environmental stimuli
- Raising the head of the bed 30 degrees to decrease ICP (if appropriate and there are no contraindications)
- Taking precautions for seizures, including padding side rails
- Monitoring CCP/ICP as indicated
- Deep vein thrombosis prophylaxis, such as graduated compression stockings or sequential compression devices
- Administering IV fluids as ordered.

Two additional interventions the nurse may perform are assessing for signs of Cushing triad and using hyperventilation to reduce ICP. Cushing triad is a set of clinical signs that indicate increasing ICP: bradycardia, irregular respirations, and a widening pulse pressure (i.e., increasing systolic blood pressure and decreasing diastolic blood pressure) (Gupta & Nosko, 2015). Hyperventilation to decrease ICP requires an intubated patient. The practice was quite common but has recently been called into question, as it can exacerbate cerebral ischemia. It is now only advocated as a short term (less than 16 hours) intervention while waiting until other methods of controlling IICP can be utilized (Rangel-Castilla et al., 2016).

Collaborative Therapies

Patients with altered LOC require support of their airways and assistance with respiration. For patients who are drowsy but capable of being aroused, a nasopharyngeal airway may be sufficient. Patients who are not easily aroused may tolerate an oropharyngeal airway. More severe alterations in LOC, however, may require endotracheal intubation to maintain a patent airway, particularly if the patient's cough and gag reflexes are absent. If the decrease in LOC is due to a concussion or TBI, be sure that the cervical spine is maintained in a neutral position during laryngoscopy unless a spinal cord injury has already been ruled out. Hypoventilation or apnea indicates the need for mechanical ventilation. Unless the patient has a do-not-resuscitate (DNR) order, the healthcare team should initiate mechanical ventilation even if it is not yet known if the disorder is reversible. Without sufficient support of ventilation, cerebral anoxia develops quickly and may result in brain death. Monitor arterial blood gases of patients on ventilation frequently to determine the adequacy of ventilation. Cautious hyperventilation ($PaCO_2$ of 30–35 mmHg) may be used to reduce $PaCO_2$ and promote cerebral vasoconstriction to reduce cerebral edema.

SAFETY ALERT Recent research has discouraged routine use of long-term hyperventilation. If done too aggressively, it can cause cerebral ischemia and produce a poor patient outcome. If hyperventilation is used, it should be only a temporary measure until another intervention to reduce IICP can be initiated. Note that hyperventilation has also been shown to lose its effectiveness after about 16 hours of continuous use (Rangel-Castilla et al., 2016).

Fluid Management

The nurse inserts an IV catheter and maintains a fluid balance using isotonic or slightly hypertonic solutions such as normal saline solution. The nurse should avoid hypotonic fluids, as they may cause an increase in cerebral edema and decrease serum osmolarity. The nurse should closely monitor the patient's response to fluid administration for evidence of increased cerebral edema.

Any underlying fluid and electrolyte imbalance is corrected by administering IV fluid containing appropriate electrolytes. For the patient who is hyponatremic and has a low serum osmolality, furosemide (Lasix) or an osmotic diuretic such as mannitol may be administered to promote water excretion, and fluid infusion may be minimized. In certain circumstances, a bolus of 3% NaCl (hypertonic saline) may be used. This strategy requires close monitoring of serum sodium and serum osmolarity (Ropper, 2012).

Surgery

There are a multitude of surgical procedures that may be appropriate for the patient experiencing alterations in intracranial regulation. These procedures are specific to the underlying cause of the alteration and are covered at length in the exemplars. The nurse should be aware that because intracranial regulation is such a dynamic system, the patient may deteriorate to the point that surgery is required at any time.

Pharmacologic Therapy

Pharmacologic therapy may be necessary to reduce or control seizures. Medications also play a role in the treatment of IICP and TBI/concussions.

Seizures

Medications are available to reduce/manage seizure activity by raising the seizure threshold or limiting the spread of abnormal activity in the brain. See the Medications feature in the Seizure exemplar.

The goals of medications for seizure disorders are to protect the patient from harm and to reduce or prevent seizure activity without impairing cognitive function or producing undesirable side effects. The lowest possible dose of a single medication that will control the patient's seizures should be prescribed. Often, however, several medications must be tried before the most effective one is identified, and a combination of drugs may be needed to manage the patient's seizures. Some medications have been found to be more effective in treating certain types of seizures than others.

Status epilepticus requires immediate intervention to preserve life. Establishing and maintaining the airway are priorities. A solution of 50% dextrose is administered intravenously to prevent hypoglycemia. Diazepam or lorazepam is given intravenously as a first-line agent. Phenytoin or fosphenytoin may be administered intravenously to control seizures for a longer period. Phenobarbital or pentobarbital also may be administered to patients in status epilepticus. On rare occasions in which none of these drugs stop the seizure activity, general anesthesia using IV propofol may be used.

Increased Intracranial Pressure

Medications play an important role in the management of IICP. Diuretics, particularly osmotic diuretics, are commonly used to reduce ICP and are the mainstays of pharmacologic treatment. Loop diuretics such as furosemide may be prescribed for some patients with IICP. Sedation and paralysis are used as chemical restraints to control restlessness and agitation because these movements increase blood pressure, ICP, and cerebral metabolism (NSGMED, 2014). Antipyretics such as acetaminophen are used alone or in combination with a hypothermia blanket to treat hyperthermia. (Hyperthermia increases the cerebral metabolic rate and exacerbates an existing increase in ICP.) Antiseizure drugs are often required to manage seizure activity associated with brain injury and IICP. Gastrointestinal prophylaxis with IV histamine H_2 antagonists or proton pump inhibitors is often used because patients with IICP are at increased risk for developing stress gastritis and ulcers (Liu et al., 2015). Corticosteroids are no longer recommended for routine use in decreasing ICP and have been shown to increase mortality (Spiegel, 2014).

IV fluids are usually necessary to maintain the patient's fluid and electrolyte balance as well as vascular volume. If the patient's blood pressure is unstable, vasoactive medications may be administered to maintain the mean arterial pressure (MAP) in a range that supports cerebral perfusion while minimizing increases in ICP.

TBI/Concussion

The presentation of TBI ranges widely, from very mild (e.g., mild concussion) to severe (e.g., gunshot wound with severe cerebral swelling, loss of brain tissue, loss of blood volume, and decreased LOC). Because there is such a dramatic range of injuries, there is also a dramatic range of pharmacologic treatments. Mild concussions may be treated with acetaminophen for pain control, whereas a gunshot wound to the head may require a drug-induced coma, vasoactive medications to support blood pressure and CPP, antibiotics to prevent infection, plasma expanders or blood products to replace lost blood volume, electrolytes to maintain homeostasis, and antiarrhythmics to prevent cardiac instability from the massive insult the body has just sustained.

Nonpharmacologic Therapy

The patient with alterations in intracranial regulation may have many needs based on the severity of the insult. Respiratory therapy will probably be required. If a patient is on a ventilator, the respiratory therapist will assist with ventilator weaning, ensure adequate oxygenation and ventilation, and maintain a patent airway with endotracheal tube or tracheostomy tube care and suctioning. Pulmonary hygiene is important, but it requires a delicate balance between activities that may cause IICP (coughing) and prevention of atelectasis and pneumonia (incentive spirometry).

Most patients will need the assistance of a physical therapist. The unconscious patient will require passive ROM exercises. Patients who have sustained paralysis due to intracranial processes will need physical therapy beginning early in their hospital admission and continuing after discharge. Specialized physical therapy such as vestibular rehabilitation may be required based on the site and extent of neurologic disruption the patient has experienced.

Occupational therapists may be helpful for patients who require assistance with more fine motor skills. Speech therapy may be required to teach the patient how to talk again or assist with feeding or swallowing. Of all of the systems in the body, an insult to the neurologic system can cause the most damage and require the most support of the patient and family during and after the event. Many patients will experience permanent alterations in their lifestyle after an illness or injury that affects intracranial regulation. They may require or benefit from the support of clergy members, social workers, mental health specialists, and support groups.

Nutrition Management

In patients with long-term alterations in consciousness (e.g., persistent vegetative state, locked-in syndrome), the healthcare team initiates measures to maintain nutritional status. Enteral feedings with a gastrostomy tube are preferred if the patient is unable to take enough food by mouth without aspirating. In some cases, total parenteral nutrition may be required.

Case Study >> Part 3

The neurosurgeon has placed a drain, and Joshua now has a Glasgow Coma Scale rating of 15 out of 15. Your orders for the day are to clamp the drain and to watch Joshua for signs of deterioration. You performed a focused assessment before clamping the drain. Joshua was oriented to time, place, and person, and he was watching TV. Four hours after the drain was clamped, you notice that Joshua is very sleepy and cannot tell you where he is. You unclamp the drain and inform the neurosurgeon that Joshua has failed the trial.

Clinical Reasoning Questions Level I
1. What other signs and symptoms would show that Joshua was failing the trial?
2. Are there other reasons that Joshua may be tired?

Clinical Reasoning Questions Level II
3. What are the priority nursing diagnoses for Joshua?
4. What nursing interventions are required when caring for a drain?
5. What other disciplines may need to be involved in providing care to Joshua?

Lifespan Considerations

Individuals are susceptible to alterations in intracranial regulation throughout their lifespan. Assessments may differ slightly and teaching modalities may need to be altered based on a patient's age and ability to understand the situation. (See the Lifespan Considerations column in the Neurologic Assessment feature for more information.) In addition, some interventions and therapies related to intracranial regulation are appropriate for specific patients across the lifespan.

Intracranial Regulation in Infants

At birth, babies have what are known as primitive reflexes. These are reflexes that arise in the spinal cord and do not require interpretation by the brain. Several of the common primitive reflexes present at birth are the stepping reflex, the startle reflex, the sucking reflex, and the Babinski reflex. (See Table 33–16 in the exemplar on Newborns in the module on Reproduction for further explanation.) Throughout the first 6 months of life, many of the primitive reflexes disappear, although the Babinski reflex is normal in children through the age of 2.

When assessing a newborn, the nurse should measure the head circumference and assess the anterior and posterior fontanels. Both fontanels are open at birth to accommodate the infant's head passing through the birth canal and then to accommodate ongoing brain growth and development. If intracranial edema or bleeding occur, the open fontanels also help accommodate expansion in the cranium. The anterior fontanel remains open for a year; the posterior closes at about 2 months. An abnormally large head circumference with fontanels that are spread apart is an indicator of IICP, which warrants immediate intervention. Other signs of IICP in infants are bulging fontanels; a shrill, "catlike" cry or a weak or absent cry; irritability and lethargy; and loss of previously acquired motor skills.

In otherwise healthy infants, IICP often results from child abuse, especially shaken baby syndrome. Another common cause of IICP in infants is congenital hydrocephalus, in which CSF builds up in the brain. Hydrocephalus can be caused by genetic abnormalities or developmental disorders, among other causes. For conditions such as hydrocephalus in which fluid accumulates in the brain, the most common treatment is insertion of a shunt to drain the fluid (National Institute of Neurological Disorders and Stroke [NINDS], 2016).

Intracranial Regulation in Children

Causes of IICP are similar in children as in other age groups, including trauma, infection, tumors, certain medications, or endocrine disorders; the condition may also be idiopathic. Signs of IICP in children include changes in behavior, difficulty waking, nausea, vomiting, stiff neck, uncoordinated movements, and changes in the eyes (e.g., droopy eyelids, crossed eyes, vision changes) (Nationwide Children's Hospital, 2015).

When beginning a neurologic assessment on a child, the nurse should consider the child's developmental age. Simpler interview questions and a shorter assessment may be necessary. When assessing children for neurologic deficits, the nurse should keep the following points in mind:

- Present the procedures as games whenever possible.
- A positive Babinski reflex is abnormal after the child ambulates or at 2 years of age.
- For children under 5 years of age, instruments are available to screen for developmental delays in cognition, communication, adaptive behavior, and fine and gross motor skills (see the module on Development).
- Note the child's ability to understand and follow directions.
- Assess immediate recall or recent memory by using names of cartoon characters. Normal recall in children is the ability to recall a number that is one less than the child's age in years; that is, a 5-year-old child should be able to recall four characters.
- Children should be able to walk backward by 2 years of age, balance on one foot for 5 seconds by 4 years of age, heel–toe walk by 5 years of age, and heel–toe walk backward by 6 years of age.
- The Romberg test is appropriate for use in children over 3 years of age.

Management of IICP is similar in children as in adults, with precautions taken for the child's age and developmental level. For example, if the child must be intubated, use an endotracheal tube size that is appropriate for the child. The nurse should also be familiar with normal levels of ICP for children when monitoring ICP, because pediatric ICP levels are lower than those for adults.

Intracranial Regulation in Pregnant Women

Pregnant women who experience alterations in intracranial regulation require close monitoring by their obstetrician and, in many cases, a neonatologist. With careful management, pregnant women who experience seizures, IICP, and other alterations can have safe and healthy pregnancies. However, severe trauma to the intracranial regulation in a pregnant patient may pose serious ethical dilemmas and may require the assistance of a multispecialty ethics committee to help resolve them. See the Lifespan Considerations sections of the exemplars for more information about caring for pregnant women with alterations in intracranial regulation.

Intracranial Regulation in Older Adults

Normal neurologic changes associated with aging often go unnoticed in the older adult. These include memory loss, subtle loss of coordination, and slower or diminished reflexes. Sensory changes may occur as well. Careful assessment of the older adult is recommended, because neurologic changes may result from a variety of factors, including medications, acute illness (e.g., infection), and progressive illness (e.g., Parkinson or Alzheimer disease). For older adults, an illness or injury that affects the neurologic system sometimes marks the end of their independence and is a source of depression for the patients and a great burden on the family.

When interviewing older adults, the nurse should allow time for them to think of a reply and to answer the question; the nurse should not assume that they do not know the answer. The nurse should also keep the following points in mind:

- A full neurologic assessment can be lengthy. Conduct the assessment in several sessions if indicated, and cease the tests if the patient is noticeably fatigued.
- Declines in mental status are not a normal result of aging. Changes are most often the result of an underlying disorder (e.g., fever, fluid and electrolyte imbalances, medications, progressive neurocognitive disorders). Acute, abrupt-onset mental status changes are usually caused by delirium, which is often reversible with treatment.
- Intelligence and learning ability are unaltered with age. Many factors, however, may inhibit learning (e.g., anxiety, illness, pain, cultural barriers).
- Short-term memory is often less efficient in older adults, but long-term memory is usually unaltered.
- Mood changes, weight loss, anorexia, constipation, and early morning awakening may all be manifestations of depression.
- The stress of being in unfamiliar situations can cause confusion in older adults.
- Although there is a progressive decrease in the number of functioning neurons in the CNS and in the sense organs, older adults usually function well because of abundant reserves in the number of brain cells.
- Impulse transmission and reaction to stimuli are slower in older adults.
- Many older adults have some impairment of hearing, vision, smell, temperature and pain sensation, memory, and/or mental endurance.
- Age-associated coordination changes include slower fine finger movements. Standing balance remains intact, and the Romberg test remains negative.
- When testing sensory function, the nurse needs to give older adults time to respond. Older adults have unaltered perception of light touch and superficial pain, decreased perception of deep pain, and decreased perception of temperature stimuli. Many also reveal a decrease or absence of position sense in the large toes.

The most common cause of IICP in older adults is falls, but these patients also experience alterations in ICP due to motor vehicle accidents, infections, and other illnesses, similar to other age groups. Treatment for the older adult with an alteration in intracranial regulation is similar to that for younger adults. However, with more serious alterations resulting from injuries and illnesses, the nurse should check to see whether the patient has a durable power of attorney for healthcare or a living will. Many older adults wish to have every medical and surgical intervention, whereas others prefer no heroic efforts to prolong their life. Check with the patient and family and have an honest, open dialogue about resuscitation status and efforts and reasonable expectations.

REVIEW The Concept of Intracranial Regulation

RELATE Link the Concepts

Linking the concept of intracranial regulation with the concept of perfusion:

1. What can the nurse do to provide adequate oxygenation to the patient with alteration in intracranial regulation?

2. Why should the nurse be concerned about the patient's MAP?

Linking the concept of intracranial regulation with the concept of safety:

3. What teaching should the nurse perform when talking with parents and children about sports injuries?

4. Does the teaching change when working with adults only?

Linking the concept of intracranial regulation with the concept of nutrition:

5. Why is it important to keep the patient's nutritional status up while the patient has IICP?

6. If the patient is unconscious, how would the nurse anticipate the patient will receive nutrition?

READY Go to Volume 3: Clinical Nursing Skills

- SKILL 1.1   Appearance and Mental Status: Assessing
- SKILL 1.3   Newborn's and Infant's Head, Chest, and Abdomen: Measuring
- SKILL 1.8   Respirations: Newborn, Infant, Child, Adult, Obtaining
- SKILL 4.11   Urinary Catheter: Caring for and Removing
- SKILL 5.1   Intake and Output: Measuring
- SKILL 7.1   Glasgow Coma Scale: Using

REFER Go to Pearson MyLab Nursing and eText

- Additional review materials

REFLECT Apply Your Knowledge

Lamont Jones is a 48-year-old man with a history of obesity and uncontrolled type II diabetes mellitus. Last week, Mr. Jones was hit by a falling beam at work, which fractured his skull. He was released from the hospital 3 days ago and has been healing well. Mr. Jones's wife, Deanna, brought him in to the emergency department this morning, reporting that she had a hard time waking him up earlier today. Once he was awake, he was confused and complained of a stiff neck and severe headache. The initial assessment indicated that Mr. Jones's vital signs are temperature 103.8°F, pulse 107 bpm, respirations 22/min, and blood pressure 153/87 mmHg. Based on these findings and Mrs. Jones's description of Mr. Jones's symptoms, the nurse suspects that Mr. Jones has developed bacterial meningitis.

1. What clinical tests might the nurse expect the physician to order based on her assessment?

2. How do uncontrolled diabetes and hypertension place Mr. Jones at risk for meningitis and IICP?

3. What immediate interventions should the nurse implement for Mr. Jones?

4. What neurologic assessments need to be performed for Mr. Jones?

5. What comfort interventions should be provided for Mr. Jones and his wife?

 # Exemplar 11.A
Increased Intracranial Pressure

Exemplar Learning Outcomes

11.A Analyze increased intracranial pressure (IICP) as it relates to intracranial regulation.

- Describe the pathophysiology of IICP.
- Describe the etiology of IICP.
- Compare the risk factors and prevention of IICP.
- Identify the clinical manifestations of IICP.
- Summarize diagnostic tests and therapies used by interprofessional teams in the collaborative care of an individual with IICP.

- Differentiate care of patients with IICP across the lifespan.
- Apply the nursing process in providing culturally competent care to an individual with IICP.

Exemplar Key Terms

Cerebral perfusion pressure (CPP), *754*
Compliance, *752*
Increased intracranial pressure (IICP), *751*
Intracranial hypertension, *751*
Monro-Kellie hypothesis, *752*

Overview

Increased intracranial pressure (IICP), also called **intracranial hypertension**, is sustained elevated pressure (15 mmHg or higher in adults) in the cranial cavity (Gupta & Nosko, 2015). An individual's ICP increases and decreases throughout the day depending on the type of activities in which the individual is engaged. Coughing, bending, sneezing, and straining are examples of activities that increase ICP. These typical, brief activities are not harmful; only sustained increased pressure will result in damage to tissue. Cerebral edema is the most frequent cause of sustained increases in ICP. Other common causes of IICP include hydrocephalus, brain tumors, CNS infections, hemorrhage, TBI, metabolic encephalopathy, cysts, and status epilepticus (Roytowski & Figaji, 2013).

Pathophysiology and Etiology

Pathophysiology

In adults, the rigid cranial cavity created by the skull is normally filled to capacity with three essentially noncompressible elements: the brain (85%), CSF (5%), and blood (10%). A state of dynamic equilibrium exists: If the volume of any of the three components increases, the volume of the others must decrease to maintain normal pressures in the cranial cavity. This relationship is known as the **Monro-Kellie hypothesis**. Venous blood or CSF will normally shift out of the cranium and into the spinal column in an effort to maintain a near constant ICP. The normal ICP is 5–15 mmHg in adults, 3–7 mmHg in children, and 1.5–6 mmHg in infants (measured intracranially with a pressure transducer while the patient is lying with the head elevated 30 degrees) (Gupta & Nosko, 2015).

Blood and CSF both contribute small percentages to normal intracranial volume, but vascular factors account for twice the amount of increase in ICP that CSF does. The brain requires a constant supply of oxygen and glucose to meet its metabolic demands; 15–20% of the resting cardiac output goes to the brain to meet its metabolic needs. Interruption of cerebral blood flow leads to ischemia and disruption of the cerebral metabolism.

Pressure and chemical autoregulation are compensatory mechanisms in which cerebral arterioles change diameter to maintain cerebral blood flow when ICP increases. In pressure autoregulation, stretch receptors in the small blood vessels of the brain cause the smooth muscle of the arterioles to contract. Increased arterial pressure stimulates these receptors, leading to vasoconstriction. When arterial pressure is low, stimulation of these receptors decreases, causing relaxation and vasodilation. Chemical, or metabolic, autoregulation works in much the same way as pressure autoregulation. In this case, however, the stimulus is a buildup of by-products of cell metabolism, including lactic acid, pyruvic acid, carbonic acid, and carbon dioxide. Carbon dioxide and increased hydrogen ion concentration are potent cerebral vasodilators that may act locally or systemically to increase cerebral blood flow. On the contrary, a fall in $PaCO_2$ causes cerebral vasoconstriction. Arterial oxygen tension (PaO_2) also affects cerebral blood flow, although it is a less powerful mechanism than that exerted by carbon dioxide and hydrogen ions.

Displacement of some CSF to the spinal subarachnoid space and increased CSF absorption are early compensatory mechanisms for IICP. The low-pressure venous system is also compressed, and cerebral arteries constrict to reduce blood flow. Brain tissue's ability to accommodate change is relatively restricted. The relationship between the volume of the intracranial components and ICP is known as **compliance**. When the capacity to compensate for IICP is exceeded, intracranial hypertension develops.

Autoregulatory mechanisms have a limited ability to maintain cerebral blood flow. When autoregulation fails, cerebrovascular tone is reduced and cerebral blood flow becomes dependent on changes in blood pressure. Autoregulation may be lost either locally or globally because of several factors, including increasing ICP, local or diffuse cerebral tissue ischemia or inflammation, prolonged hypotension, and hypercapnia or hypoxia.

Etiology

IICP may result from head injury, hydrocephalus, cerebral edema, excess CSF, brain tumors or abscesses, or intracranial hemorrhage. Hydrocephalus results from an imbalance between production and absorption of CSF, which causes too much CSF to accumulate in the brain and the ventricles to widen. Hydrocephalus may be congenital or acquired as a result of head trauma, infection, tumor, or other pathogenic processes. Head trauma results from different causes throughout the lifespan, which will be discussed in the section on Lifespan Considerations.

Abnormal cellular growth such as intracranial tumors, either benign or malignant, may compete for space in the cranial vault, resulting in IICP. Increases in CSF production as seen in hydrocephalus or tissue necrosis as the result of cerebrovascular accidents or aneurysms also may lead to IICP.

Risk Factors

Any factor that increases the patient's risk of trauma increases the risk of cerebral trauma resulting in IICP. Risk factors for cerebral trauma are plentiful but increase when normal safety considerations, such as wearing protective equipment, are ignored. Any trauma to the brain will also change the equilibrium of the Monro-Kellie hypothesis. Other factors that may influence this equilibrium include medications, poor nutrition, illnesses such as meningitis, and drug and alcohol abuse.

Prevention

The nurse can help prevent IICP by teaching the patient ways to prevent trauma. This includes providing guidance related to the use of personal protective equipment and other safety measures, including wearing seat belts and avoiding phone use while driving or in motion, to reduce risk for injury. Nurses who work with adolescents and young adults should emphasize avoidance of recreational drug and alcohol use. For all patients, but especially for older adults, patient teaching related to standard fall precautions is recommended. (See the Fall Prevention in Older Adults section in the exemplar on Fractures in the module on Mobility.) Other than trying to prevent cerebral trauma, there is really no means to prevent IICP.

Clinical Manifestations

With loss of autoregulation, ICP continues to rise and cerebral perfusion falls. Cerebral tissue becomes ischemic, and manifestations of cellular hypoxia appear. Because the neurons of the cerebral cortex are most sensitive to oxygen deficit, changes in cortical function are the earliest manifestations of increasing ICP. In some cases, however, the onset of symptoms may be delayed if the ICP rises steadily because of compensatory measures (i.e., displacement of blood and CSF). If there has been a slow onset of IICP, a decrease in LOC may not be the presenting symptom; instead, the patient may complain of visual disturbances (double vision), vomiting, or headache. A patient who presents with these symptoms requires a careful workup. If a lumbar puncture is performed in a patient who has had a slow onset of IICP, it could cause fatal brain herniation because the only thing left to displace out of the cranial vault is brain tissue. If a downward displacement of brain tissue into the spinal column occurs, the patient may exhibit signs of

Clinical Manifestations and Therapies
Increased Intracranial Pressure

ETIOLOGY	CLINICAL MANIFESTATIONS	CLINICAL THERAPIES

Cerebral edema, head trauma, tumors, abscesses, stroke, inflammation, and hemorrhage	■ Decreased LOC:
	  – *Early:* Confusion; restlessness and lethargy; disorientation, first to time, then to place and person
	  – *Late:* Comatose with no response to painful stimuli
	■ Pupillary dysfunction: Sluggish response to light, progressing to fixed pupils; with a localized process, pupillary dysfunction first noted on the ipsilateral side
	■ Oculomotor dysfunction: Inability to move eye(s) upward; ptosis (drooping) of the eyelid
	■ Visual abnormalities: Decreased visual acuity, blurred vision, diplopia
	■ Papilledema (may be late sign)
	■ Motor impairment:
	  – *Early:* Hemiparesis or hemiplegia of the contralateral side
	  – *Late:* Abnormal responses such as decorticate or decerebrate positioning; flaccidity
	■ Headache: Uncommon but may occur with processes that slowly increase ICP; worse upon rising in the morning and with position changes
	■ Projectile vomiting without nausea
	■ Cushing triad/response: Irregular respirations, widening pulse pressure, bradycardia
	■ Respirations: Altered respiratory pattern related to level of brain dysfunction
	■ Temperature (may be significantly elevated as compensatory mechanisms fail)
		■ Maintain airway patency.
		■ Monitor neurologic status; assessment areas include LOC, behavior, motor/sensory functions, pupillary size and reaction to light, and vital signs.
		■ Monitor IICP monitoring device or ventilator.
		■ Decrease stimuli.
		■ Raise pads and bedrails, as seizures may occur.
		■ Elevate the head of the bed 30 degrees unless otherwise indicated.
		■ Monitor arterial blood gases.
		■ Position the patient as prescribed.
		■ Prevent complications associated with immobility.
		■ Monitor fluid and electrolytes.
		■ Monitor bladder distention and bowel constipation.
		■ Provide emotional support as needed.
		■ Administer medications as ordered.

Cushing triad (irregular breathing, bradycardia, and widening pulse pressure) (Roytowski & Figaji, 2013). Behavior and personality changes occur; the patient may become irritable and agitated. Memory and judgment are impaired, and changes in speech pattern may be noted. Changes in gait may also occur. The patient's LOC eventually decreases. As cerebral hypertension and hypoxia progress, LOC continues to decrease in a predictable pattern to coma and unresponsiveness.

Collaboration

Treatment of the patient with IICP is directed toward identifying and treating the underlying cause of the disorder and controlling ICP to prevent herniation syndrome. Sustained ICP greater than 40 mmHg is a life-threatening emergency, and there is little time to complete lengthy diagnostic tests. The diagnosis must be made based on observation and neurologic assessment; even subtle changes may be clinically significant. The nurse, who often spends the most time caring for the patient, is most likely to assess any subtle changes in condition and must advocate for the patient's needs.

Diagnostic Tests

Diagnostic tests are used mainly to determine what might be the cause of IICP. A CT scan or MRI is generally the initial

test used to identify the possible causes of IICP (e.g., space-occupying lesions, hydrocephalus) and to evaluate therapeutic options. In general, a lumbar puncture is not performed when IICP is suspected because the sudden release of the pressure in the skull may cause cerebral herniation. Serum osmolality and arterial blood gases are also ordered and monitored. Electroencephalography (EEG), although more commonly used in diagnosing and treating seizures, may be used to monitor the depth of a coma or to diagnose brain death. Transcranial Doppler (TCD) is used to measure cerebral blood flow velocity. It is especially helpful in diagnosing and following patients who have vasospasms related to cerebral hemorrhage (Haddad & Arabi, 2012).

Surgery

Patients with IICP may undergo various intracranial surgical techniques to treat the underlying cause of their condition. In addition, infarcted or necrotic tissue may be resected to reduce brain mass. A drainage catheter or shunt may be inserted laterally via a burr hole into a ventricle to drain excess CSF and reduce hydrocephalus. The removal of even a small amount of CSF may dramatically reduce IICP and restore cerebral perfusion pressure.

Patients with chronic IICP caused by hydrocephalus may receive a permanent shunt. The shunt system contains a valve that allows for one-way flow and for CSF to be diverted only if the ICP rises past a certain level. The shunt is placed in a ventricle of the brain and empties the excess CSF into the peritoneal cavity (most common), atria of the heart, or pleural cavity. In rare circumstances, the shunt may empty into the gallbladder or urinary bladder. Shunts may be either programmable or fixed with how much CSF is allowed to drain (National Hydrocephalus Foundation, 2014).

Pharmacologic Therapy

Medications play an important role in the management of IICP. Diuretics, particularly osmotic diuretics such as mannitol, are commonly used to reduce ICP and are the mainstays of pharmacologic treatment. Osmotic diuretics work by increasing the osmolarity of the blood, thereby drawing water out of edematous brain tissue and into the vascular system for elimination via the kidneys. Loop diuretics such as furosemide (Lasix), the drug of choice, and ethacrynic acid (Edecrin) may be prescribed for some patients with IICP. Loop diuretics inhibit sodium and chloride reabsorption at the ascending loop of Henle. They cause a reduction in the rate of CSF production, thus reducing the ICP. Patients with ICP who are prescribed diuretics require close monitoring of electrolyte values, fluid status, and renal function.

Antipyretics, such as acetaminophen, are used alone or in combination with a hypothermia blanket to treat hyperthermia. (Hyperthermia increases the cerebral metabolic rate and exacerbates an existing increase in ICP.) Antiseizure drugs are often required to manage seizure activity associated with brain injury and IICP, especially if there has been damage to the temporal lobe. Antihypertensives, in particular beta blockers, may be used if the patient's MAP is high, whereas vasopressors may be used if the MAP is low. Gastrointestinal prophylaxis with IV H_2-receptor antagonists or proton pump inhibitors is often used because patients with IICP are at increased risk for developing stress gastritis and ulcers.

IV fluids are usually necessary to maintain the patient's fluid and electrolyte balance and vascular volume. Hypotonic IV fluids should be avoided because they can lead to cerebral swelling. If the patient's blood pressure is unstable, vasoactive medications may be administered to maintain the MAP in a range that supports cerebral perfusion while minimizing increases in ICP. When enteral feeding is not possible, total parenteral nutrition may be administered.

Nonpharmacologic Therapy

Nonpharmacologic therapies for patients with IICP may include ICP monitoring and mechanical ventilation. Continuous assessment is necessary to determine and respond to changes in the patient's condition. Maintaining a quiet environment with limited stimulation will help keep the patient's ICP lower. One of the simplest ways to decrease ICP is by raising the head of the bed to a 30-degree angle.

ICP Monitoring

Careful assessment is critical to preserving brain function and preventing secondary brain damage from IICP. Monitoring pressure with ICP monitors, measuring cerebral perfusion pressure, and measuring the oxygen levels of brain

tissue can provide useful information in guiding the care of patients with IICP. **Cerebral perfusion pressure (CPP)**, or the difference between MAP and ICP, can be readily calculated, allowing more precise manipulation of therapeutic measures to maintain cerebral perfusion and thereby prevent ischemia. The CPP should ideally be maintained between 50 and 100 mmHg in adults. When a patient's CPP falls below 50 mmHg, compensatory measures within the brain might not occur, and cerebral blood flow will decrease as CPP continues to decrease (Rangel-Castilla et al., 2016). The criteria for ICP monitoring depends on the patient's condition, but in general, patients whose condition is salvageable, who present with an abnormal CT scan, and have a Glasgow Coma Scale score of 8 or lower should be monitored. ICP monitoring is also recommended for patients with a normal CT scan if two or more of the following factors are present (Kirkman & Smith, 2014):

- Unilateral or bilateral motor posturing
- Systolic blood pressure less than 90 mmHg
- Age greater than 40.

Basic monitoring systems include an epidural probe, a subarachnoid bolt or screw, and an intraventricular catheter (see **Figure 11–12** 》). The intraventricular ICP catheter is the preferred technique whenever possible. It is inexpensive

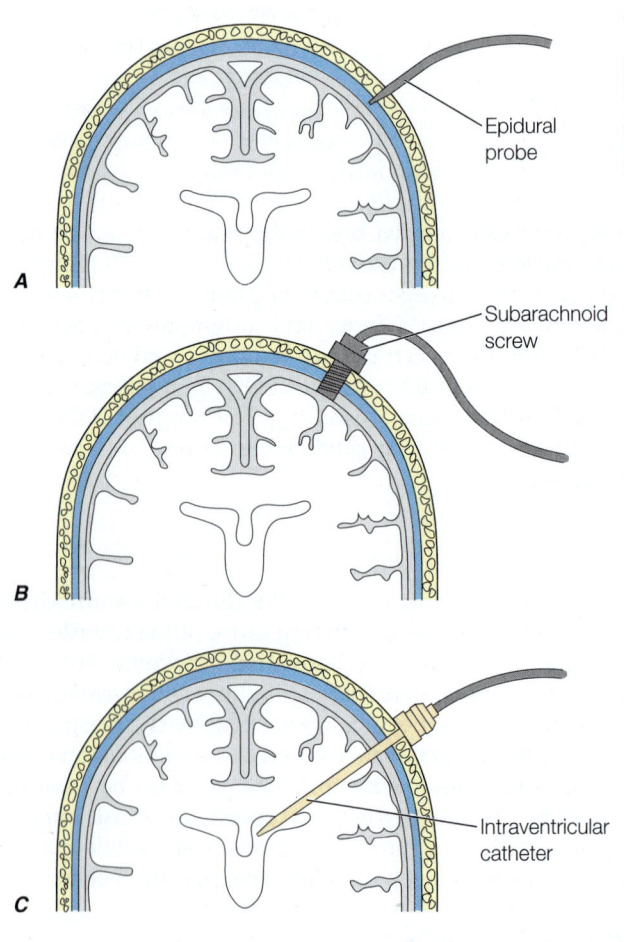

Figure 11–12 》 Types of ICP monitoring. **A,** Epidural probe. **B,** Subarachnoid screw. **C,** Intraventricular catheter.

and the most reliable and accurate way to measure ICP. In addition to measuring ICP, the intraventricular ICP catheter also allows drainage of CSF when ICP becomes elevated. The catheter is usually placed in the ventricle on the right side, because the right hemisphere is nondominant in the majority of the population. It is calibrated at the level of the tragus. The intraventricular ICP catheter allows for trials of "clamping" the drainage of CSF to evaluate what happens to the patient, in terms of both clinical symptoms and ICP values. Subarachnoid, epidural, and subdural monitors are less accurate and do not allow for CSF drainage (Haddad & Arabi, 2012). Microtransducer-tipped and fiber optic ICP monitoring devices may be placed into the subdural space or brain parenchyma (tissue). Neither of these devices allow for CSF drainage. Pressures can be very accurate, providing the catheter does not drift, is inserted into the correct area of the brain, and is calibrated properly prior to placement. There is no way to recalibrate these devices once they have been placed into the patient's cranial cavity (Kirkman & Smith, 2014). Factors that increase the risk for infection during ICP monitoring include open head trauma or neurosurgery; intracranial hemorrhage; use of an intraventricular catheter; and IP monitoring for more than 3–5 days or using an open system or frequent irrigation. Older adults are also at increased risk because of impaired immune defenses.

Transcranial blood flow is monitored with transcranial Doppler studies to measure the velocity of blood flow in the cerebral vessels. CPP is the pressure required for the heart to provide the brain with blood; it is calculated by subtracting the ICP from the MAP. Normal CPP is 50–100 mmHg. Monitoring of brain oxygenation may be conducted using a jugular bulb oxygen saturation ($SjvO_2$) monitor connected to a small fiber optic catheter inserted into the jugular vein. Normal $SjvO_2$ is 55–69% (Dhawan & DeGeorgia, 2012). Because $SjvO_2$ can provide information about cerebral metabolism and oxygenation, a reading below 50% can be an early indicator of ischemia long before clinical symptoms appear (Haddad & Arabi, 2012). Another device used to monitor brain tissue oxygenation is the Licox system, which includes information about oxygen status and temperature status in the brain tissue itself (McCarthy, 2013). In addition, cerebral microdialysis catheters can provide information about the nature of the cerebral interstitial fluid, although they are not frequently used.

Mechanical Ventilation

Patients with IICP often require intubation and are placed on a ventilator for airway protection and respiratory management. Mechanical ventilation may be used to maintain partial pressure of oxygen and carbon dioxide, thus preventing hypoxemia and hypercapnia, both of which can increase ICP. Maintaining adequate oxygenation with a partial pressure of arterial oxygen of about 100 mmHg and a partial pressure of arterial carbon dioxide of about 35 mmHg is important. The patient with IICP and signs of impending herniation may be judiciously hyperventilated to cause cerebral vasoconstriction; however, this option also increases cerebral ischemia, so it should only be used until another means to decrease IICP can be instituted (e.g., surgical intervention, medication). Mechanical ventilation is discussed in

greater detail in the exemplar on Acute Respiratory Distress Syndrome in the module on Oxygenation.

Other Therapies

Physical therapy to prevent muscle atrophy may be necessary for a patient who is unconscious or bedridden for more than a few days. Nurses must be diligent to prevent the formation of decubitus ulcers but cautious with their movement and stimulation of the patient so as not to further increase ICP. Occupational therapy can help the patient regain any motor skills needed to perform activities of daily living that may have been compromised. Respiratory therapy is necessary if a patient requires mechanical ventilation and during and after the ventilator weaning process. Speech therapy may be needed if the patient needs to learn how to eat or talk following damage to associated areas of the brain. Patients who have IICP and their families may also benefit from spiritual or psychologic counseling.

Lifespan Considerations

Increased Intracranial Pressure in Children

Infants born more than 10 weeks prematurely can sustain intraventricular hemorrhage (IVH). The earlier the delivery and the smaller the newborn, the higher the risk of IVH. All infants born at a gestational age earlier than 30 weeks should have a cranial ultrasound to assess for the presence of IVH. The blood vessels in the brains of premature infants are not yet fully developed, and this may be a factor in the development of IVH. If an infant experiences only minimal bleeding, there may be no permanent damage. Greater amounts of bleeding may put direct pressure on the brain and cause permanent damage. Manifestations of IVH in the newborn range from no visible signs or symptoms to decreased muscle tone; labile vital signs; and periods of apnea, lethargy, or seizure activity. Newborns with IVH may develop IICP, which may be relieved by performing a lumbar puncture or inserting a shunt system (see **Figure 11–13** »). Newborns with IICP require special handling to reduce further damage and should be cared for in the NICU (Lee, 2015). Refer to the exemplar on Prematurity in the module on Reproduction for more information.

The unique anatomy of the skull in infants allows the symptoms of IICP to present differently than in children or adults. Because the bones in the skull have not yet fused, an infant with IICP may have bulging fontanelles, separated sutures on the skull, drowsiness, or vomiting. In children, and as ICP increases in infants, the signs and symptoms of IICP present similarly to adults. Examination may reveal headaches, weakness, eye movement disturbances, behavioral changes, decreased LOC, or seizures (Kantor, 2015).

Infants and young children may experience IICP as the result of falling, abuse, or bumping their heads because of poor head control or depth perception. Preschool and school-age children are at risk for bicycle, swimming, or activity-related accidents that cause head trauma. Adolescents are at risk for motor vehicle–related crashes, addiction behavior, and trauma resulting from violence.

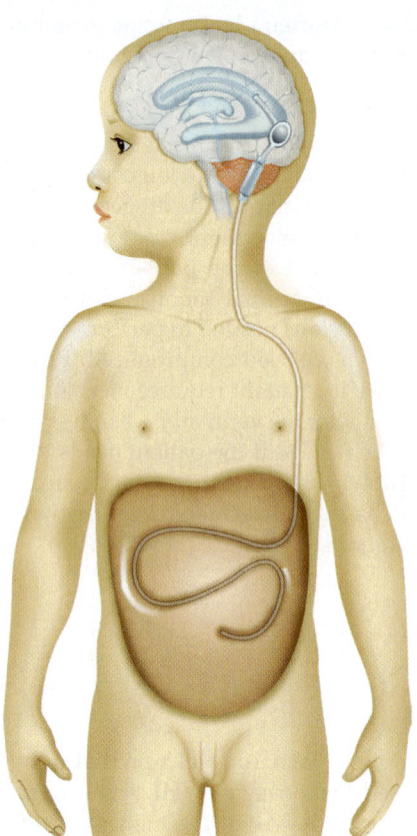

Source: Dorling Kindersley/Getty Images.

....

Figure 11–13 》 Cerebral shunt with valve inserted in brain to remove excess CSF with tube to carry it to the stomach.

Increased Intracranial Pressure in Pregnant Women

The physiologic status of pregnancy does not directly affect ICP. However, a condition called idiopathic intracranial hypertension (IIH) exists and is common in obese women of childbearing age. If the patient with IIH becomes pregnant, neurology and obstetrics should work together closely to ensure safety for both the mother and fetus. Medications to treat IIH can usually be taken throughout pregnancy, and patients can usually have a normal vaginal delivery. However, the safety profiles for some medications used to treat IIH are not known for all gestational ages, so medications should be taken only after discussing risks and benefits with the physician. For these women, pregnancy-related weight gain should be on the lower end (5–9 kg). If there are optic nerve dysfunctions, the second stage of labor should not be prolonged, but otherwise no special care must be provided to the pregnant woman with IIH (Mollan et al., 2014).

Increased Intracranial Pressure in Older Adults

Older adults are prone to falls that can result in IICP. As stated earlier, older adults may take medications that increase their risk for falls and trauma. Sensory losses and

instabilities can increase the risk for accidents. Increased blood pressure associated with hypertension may damage blood vessels, especially ones in the brain, and cause them to be more fragile, increasing the risk for hemorrhagic stroke and related IICP. Undiagnosed or poorly controlled cardiac arrhythmias may cause a decrease in cerebral blood flow, which can lead to vertigo and falls. Often arrhythmias originating in the atria are treated with medications that interfere with the clotting process, which can turn an otherwise simple fall into a catastrophic hemorrhage with IICP. In addition, brain tissue volume decreases with age (Society for Neuroscience, n.d.). As a result, there is more room in the cranial vault. A hemorrhage may have room to expand over a longer period before symptoms are noticed, and these symptoms may be more subtle than those from a hemorrhage that causes an abrupt increase in ICP.

In older adults, the empty space in the cranial vault may also become passively filled with CSF. Normal pressure hydrocephalus (NPH) causes enlarged ventricles without a dramatic increase in ICP because the patient has had time to adjust to the increase in CSF. The Hakim triad of dementia, gait apraxia, and incontinence are classic signs of NHP, which rarely occurs in patients under 60 years old. NPH is often treated with medications that decrease CSF secretion, but it may ultimately require a shunting procedure, as only 25% of patients can be treated with medications (Nelson, 2016).

NURSING PROCESS

The nursing care of patients with IICP involves identifying those at risk and managing factors known to increase ICP. A major focus is protecting the patient from sudden increases in ICP or decreases in cerebral blood flow.

Assessment

Proper assessment of the patient with IICP is vital. Not only should assessment involve neurologic tests, but it should also help identify the underlying cause of IICP to provide insights into the best treatment strategy. Observation, patient interview, and physical assessment are all key components of the nursing assessment. However, keep in mind that some patients, especially those with decreased LOC, will be unable to complete a patient interview, so the nurse will need to rely on just observation and physical assessment for these individuals.

■ ***Observation and patient interview.*** Observation of the patient with IICP begins by noting the patient's LOC using the Glasgow Coma Scale. Observation also includes noting any loss of motor control. During the patient interview, ask the patient (or a caregiver or friend if the patient is unable to respond) about the patient's primary complaints, including vision changes, presence of nausea or vomiting, headache, breathing problems, behavior changes, and any events leading up to the patient's current condition. Obtain the patient's basic medical history, including any comorbid conditions.

- *Physical examination.* For an alert patient presenting at the clinic, urgent care center, or emergency department after a fall or trauma, follow the assessment guidelines outlined in the Concept of Intracranial Regulation section. Assessment of neurologic status establishes the patient's clinical condition and provides a baseline for measuring changes. Assessment areas include LOC; behavior; motor/sensory functions; pupillary size and reaction to light; and vital signs, including temperature. An elevated temperature with increased oxygen consumption further increases ICP. Pupillary responses mirror the status of the midbrain and pons. Pressure on the brainstem may compromise the function of cranial nerves IX and X and protective mechanisms such as the gag and cough reflexes.

- *Ongoing monitoring.* Once IICP has been identified, assess for and report manifestations of IICP every 15 minutes to 1 hour and as necessary. Patients with unstable ICP may require continuous or more frequent monitoring. Look for trends, because vital signs alone do not correlate well with early deterioration. Sudden changes in neurologic signs often indicate deterioration. Any subtle change may indicate early signs of a declining neurologic condition.

- *Monitor pulse oximetry and arterial blood gas measurements.* Adequate air exchange to keep oxygen and carbon dioxide levels within normal ranges and maintenance of acid–base balance are critical to reduce the risk of hypoxemia and IICP. If adequate respiratory effort cannot be maintained, or if the patient cannot protect his or her own airway, mechanical ventilation will be necessary. If a device to measure IICP is in place, record the readings, assess the patency of the catheter, and monitor the insertion site for signs of infection.

SAFETY ALERT Often the earliest manifestations of a change in ICP are alterations in LOC and respirations. Therefore, the importance of assessing a patient's neurologic status cannot be overemphasized. Reduce environmental stimuli (including the number of visitors) and follow all safety protocols (e.g., keeping bedrails up, placing call lights within reach).

Diagnosis

Appropriate nursing diagnoses for the patient with IICP may include the following:

- *Airway Clearance, Ineffective*
- *Tissue Perfusion: Cerebral, Risk for Ineffective*
- *Breathing Pattern, Ineffective*
- *Infection, Risk for*
- *Body Temperature, Risk for Imbalanced.*

(NANDA-I © 2014)

Planning

Nursing care plans for the patient with IICP are highly individualized and depend on cause, treatment, and prognosis. Common goals include the following:

- The patient will maintain ICP less than 20 mmHg.

- The patient will experience no further complications as a result of IICP.

- The patient will not experience infection as the result of ICP monitoring.

- The patient will maintain adequate cerebral perfusion to prevent further cellular damage.

- Family members will demonstrate the ability to maintain a low-stimulus environment.

Implementation

Nursing interventions include maintaining airway patency, ensuring adequate oxygenation and ventilation, positioning and moving, preventing infection, and monitoring fluids and electrolytes. In addition, both patient and family need emotional support during this period.

Because occurrences of IICP are unplanned and usually happen suddenly, there is little opportunity for the patient or family to gain knowledge about the condition, treatment, or outcomes. Patient and family teaching prior to discharge is therefore important to help patients improve outcomes and/or prepare for life-altering changes. Teaching needs to be directed at both inpatient and outpatient care. Because of the stressful nature of this diagnosis, patient and their families may have difficulty comprehending and maintaining the information provided. Therefore, the nurse should assess their understanding; ask questions to validate their knowledge base; identify gaps; and allow the patient and family opportunities for repeated teaching regarding risks, prevention, and the treatment plan.

Ensure Adequate Oxygenation

Ensuring airway patency and adequate oxygenation is essential to maintaining the health of the patient with IICP. If the patient cannot breathe independently, a ventilator may be necessary to assist the patient's breathing. Patients may also need suctioning to remove secretions and maintain airway patency. For the patient who needs ventilation and suctioning, preoxygenate with 100% oxygen before suctioning to help maintain O_2 levels during suctioning. Limit suctioning to 10 seconds, because suctioning itself increases ICP. Suction gently and monitor arterial blood gases. If oxygen concentration is low, oxygen may be given or increased.

Reduce Intracranial Pressure

One simple way to reduce ICP is to elevate the head of the bed to 30 degrees, unless this is contraindicated. Some nursing interventions related to positioning the patient correctly to reduce ICP include:

- Maintain alignment of the head and neck to avoid hyperextension or exaggerated neck flexion.

- Avoid the prone position. Keeping the head of the bed elevated facilitates venous drainage from the cerebrum. Obstruction of jugular veins can impede venous drainage from the brain.

SAFETY ALERT If neck trauma is involved, the bed may need to be kept flat until x-rays of the cervical spine show no fractures and MRI confirms no soft tissue damage.

- If the patient is alert, assist in moving up in bed. Do not ask the patient to push with heels or arms or push against a footboard. Avoid a footboard and restraints. Moving up in bed requires pushing. Helping the patient move prevents initiation of the Valsalva maneuver, which increases ICP.

ICP can also be reduced by helping the patient maintain regular bowel movements and regularly empty the bladder, because constipation and bladder distention increase intrathoracic or intra-abdominal pressure and place the patient at risk for impaired venous drainage from the brain. In addition to monitoring bladder distention and bowel constipation:

- Administer stool softeners as needed.
- Use the Credé method (the method of applying pressure to the suprapubic region with the fingers of one or both hands) to empty the bladder. If the Credé method is not effective, evaluate the pros and cons of urinary catheterization if the bladder remains distended.
- Maintain fluid limitations if prescribed. Restricting fluids helps decrease cerebral edema by reducing total body water.

Reduce Environmental Stimulation

Patients who are overstimulated are at risk of increasing their ICP even further. Therefore, the nurse should strive to reduce environmental stimulation as much as possible to help reduce ICP. Steps for doing this include the following:

- Plan nursing care so that activities are not clustered together. Multiple procedures, including certain nursing care activities, can increase ICP. Individualized nursing care ensures optimal spacing of activities and rest.
- Provide a quiet environment and avoid activities or tasks that jar the patient or the bed.
- Maintain a calm, reassuring manner. Noxious stimuli and emotional upsets cause elevation of ICP.
- Educate family members to avoid exciting or unpleasant conversation around the patient.

Reduce Risk of Infection

Patients with an intracranial monitoring device will need specific nursing interventions to help reduce the risk of infection and maintain the patency of the monitoring system. Most clinical units have written protocols for managing these systems. The following nursing actions serve only as a general guide.

- Keep dressings over the catheter dry, and change dressings on a prescribed basis (usually every 24–48 hours). Wet dressings promote bacterial growth.
- Monitor the insertion site for leaking CSF, drainage, or infection. Manifestations of infection include changes in vital signs, chills, increased white blood counts (WBCs), lack of clarity in CSF, and positive cultures of drainage.

Close monitoring helps detect the earliest signs of infection and prevent major complications. Fever usually is considered the key assessment criterion. However, fever in a patient with a neurologic disorder may be due to damage to the hypothalamus. Headache, generalized muscle aches, shivering, and chills may also be seen in the patient with infection.

- Use strict aseptic technique when in contact with the drainage device, and check the system for loose connections. Using aseptic technique and monitoring drainage systems for loose connections help prevent nosocomial infections.
- Ensure that the device is properly functioning. Look for kinks along the lines. Calibrate according to which device is being used. Maintain transducers at proper anatomical locations (usually the tragus of the ear) depending on orders and the device being used. Remember to reposition the transducer if the patient's position has changed (change in head of bed elevation, elevating or dropping the height of the bed, or moving the patient from the bed to a chair).

Prepare the Patient and Family for Discharge

Although patients with IICP will usually be monitored in the hospital, many of them will eventually be discharged home. The nurse is responsible for providing teaching to the patient and family related to both detecting increases in ICP (see the Patient Teaching feature) and reducing the risk of injury for the patient at home. The nurse will facilitate scheduling a home safety assessment and discuss injury prevention through use of motor vehicle restraints and protective gear when participating in sports.

Patient Teaching
Patients Who Have or Are at Risk for IICP

Patients who are being discharged home after being in the hospital with IICP should be monitored carefully for any signs that their ICP has increased again. Because IICP can cause changes in LOC, the following measures should be taught to both the patient and a family member or friend who lives with the patient:

- Monitor the patient for decreased LOC. Even slight changes in neurologic status, such as increased confusion, can indicate that ICP is increasing.
- If the patient is difficult to awaken, call 9-1-1.
- If the patient complains of a stiff neck, severe headache, or nausea and vomiting, take the patient to the emergency department immediately.
- Monitor the patient for seizures, which are an indication of IICP. Also teach the patient's friend or family member how to help the patient during and after a seizure.
- Ask the patient to immediately report any changes in vision or motor control.
- Teach the patient to follow instructions to avoid coughing; blowing the nose (or to blow gently through one nostril at a time); straining to have a bowel movement; or performing isometric (muscle contracting exercises).
- Advise the patient to maintain head and neck alignment when turning in bed.
- Encourage the patient and family members to reduce environmental stimuli.

Evaluation

The patient with IICP should be evaluated based on the plan of care developed. Expected outcomes vary but often include the following:

- The patient's ICP returns to acceptable limits following treatment.
- The patient's LOC improves with reduction of ICP.
- The patient experiences no infection as the result of ICP monitoring.
- The patient's family describes appropriate outcome expectations related to the amount of cellular damage resulting from IICP.
- The patient and family institute and maintain adequate safety measures after discharge.

Some patients require days, weeks, or months of monitoring for ICP changes. In such cases, the nurse will continually need to reassess the plan of care to provide care that is relevant for the patient's current condition. This may include reporting oxygenation changes that indicate the patient either needs a ventilator or no longer needs a ventilator; reporting signs of infection; reporting changes in the patient's LOC; and discussing with the provider major changes such as the need for different medications, insertion of a shunt, or emergency surgery to reduce ICP. Because the nurse interacts with the patient more closely than any other healthcare professional, the nurse must be responsible for monitoring and reporting significant changes in the patient's condition.

REVIEW   Increased Intracranial Pressure

RELATE Link the Concepts and Exemplars

The nurse is caring for a patient who experienced severe head trauma in a motor vehicle crash. The patient is placed on a mechanical ventilator set to 28 breaths per minute and is completely nonresponsive to deep, painful stimuli. The patient's vital signs are T 101.2°F; P 112 bpm; R 28/min; and BP 100/88 mmHg. ICP readings are currently 16 mmHg but increase to 34–38 mmHg when touched and 52 mmHg when the endotracheal tube is suctioned.

Linking the exemplar of IICP with the concept of perfusion:

1. What nursing interventions can the nurse perform to optimize brain perfusion?
2. How would you interpret the patient's blood pressure and ICP readings to determine brain perfusion?

The family of the patient in the preceding scenario is told that if the patient survives, he is likely to experience significant neurologic losses and may remain in a chronic vegetative state. The patient's wife says, "I know him. He's a fighter, and he won't settle for anything less than full recovery." She then relates the story of a television show she saw the other day. The character on the show received this same prognosis and was back to normal within a few weeks.

Linking the exemplar of IICP with the concept of grief and loss:

3. In what stage of the grieving process is this family member?
4. What nursing care can you provide to support this woman's grieving process and to help her accept the likelihood of a less than complete recovery?

READY Go to Volume 3: Clinical Nursing Skills

REFER Go to Pearson MyLab Nursing and eText

- Additional review materials

REFLECT Apply Your Knowledge

Antwan, 7 years old, was injured when he was struck by a car and thrown several feet into the air. He was unconscious on admission to the emergency department and showed some signs of IICP (dilated and fixed pupils, lack of response to painful stimuli, irregular breathing pattern). Antwan was treated for shock, and his neurologic status and vital signs were assessed frequently. The initial evaluation revealed that Antwan had sustained several contusions of the brain but no skull fracture. He was intubated and medicated to manage the airway and IICP. After 7 days in the intensive care unit, Antwan was moved to a general care floor. He is still not fully conscious but quiets when his parents speak to him. He is moving all of his extremities, but he does not yet follow commands.

1. Describe the neurologic nursing assessment that should be performed on Antwan at regular intervals in the general care unit.
2. Identify age-appropriate sensory stimulation strategies that may help promote Antwan's awareness and improvement in LOC.
3. What would you teach Antwan's family to help promote neurologic improvement?
4. What changes in Antwan's condition would require immediate notification of the primary provider?

» Exemplar 11.B Seizure Disorders

Exemplar Learning Outcomes

11.B Analyze seizure disorders as they relate to intracranial regulation.

- Describe the pathophysiology of seizure disorders.
- Describe the etiology of seizure disorders.

- Compare the risk factors and prevention of seizure disorders.
- Identify the clinical manifestations of seizure disorders.
- Summarize diagnostic tests and therapies used by interprofessional teams in the collaborative care of an individual with a seizure disorder.

- Differentiate care of patients with seizure disorders across the lifespan.
- Apply the nursing process in providing culturally competent care to an individual with seizure disorders.

Exemplar Key Terms

Overview

Seizures are periods of abnormal electrical discharges in the brain that may cause involuntary movement and/or behavior and sensory alterations. The involuntary movements may encompass the whole body or just certain areas, such as the right arm. These involuntary movements are what most people think of when they think about seizures. However, seizure activity can manifest as altered level of consciousness (LOC), changes in behavior, or sensory alterations that only the patient can notice. An estimated 2.2 million people in the United States are affected with seizure disorders. Seizures can happen to anyone at any age, but they seem to occur more frequently in older adults and younger children. When seizure activity becomes chronic with recurrent episodes secondary to a CNS disorder, the affected individual is said to have **epilepsy** (Epilepsy Foundation, 2014a; National Institutes of Health, 2016).

Pathophysiology and Etiology

Pathophysiology

Seizures are believed to be the result of abnormal excessive concurrent electrical discharges from the cortical neuronal network of cells on the surface of the brain. Chemical changes in the neurons create an electrical negativity that enables the transfer of information between neurons. When an excessive number of these cells become excited, they discharge abnormally. These cells may be triggered by environmental or physiologic stimuli (e.g., emotional stress, anxiety, fatigue, infection, metabolic disturbances). Acute insults such as CNS infection, hypoxia, and brain trauma are the most common causes of seizures in children. Most seizures last between 30 seconds and 2 minutes.

Focal seizures (previously known as *partial seizures*) occur when abnormal electrical activity is contained to a limited area of the brain. They can be classified as focal aware or focal impaired. Focal aware seizures do not affect memory or awareness. In contrast, focal impaired seizures can affect behavior, awareness, or memory before, during, or after the seizure episode (International League Against Epilepsy [ILAE], 2017). Focal seizures can sometimes turn into generalized seizures, which affect the whole brain. This process is called secondary generalization (Shelat, 2015).

In contrast, **generalized seizures** are caused by abnormal electrical discharges that originate from both hemispheres of the brain (ILAE, 2017). When people think of seizure activity, most think of the dramatic tonic–clonic (grand mal) seizure. Although this is an example of a generalized seizure, it is not the only presentation of generalized seizures. Generalized seizures may also manifest as a blank stare, brief muscle twitches, or muscle stiffening (Mayo Clinic, 2015a).

Etiology

Some seizures are idiopathic; that is, they are not provoked by known stimuli. Genetic factors may lower the seizure threshold by making brain cells more vulnerable to abnormal electrical discharges. Acquired seizures may be caused by underlying pathologic conditions such as trauma, infection, hypoglycemia, hypotonic dehydration, electrolyte imbalance, endocrine dysfunction, toxins, tumors, or lesions that may be manifested at any time.

Febrile seizures usually occur in children as the result of a rapid temperature rise above 39°C (102.2°F, rectal), often in association with an acute illness. Most febrile seizures present as generalized seizures and last only a few minutes. Sometimes the fever can occur a few hours after the seizure. No evidence of intracranial infection or other definitive cause is found. Febrile seizures usually occur in children between the ages of 6 months and 5 years old, peaking in incidence during the second year of life. Infants and toddlers have a lower seizure threshold than adults, so they are more susceptible to seizures from minor stimuli such as fevers. There is often a family history of febrile seizures. In addition, children who have one febrile seizure have a 40% chance of experiencing more febrile seizures, especially if a relatively low temperature accompanied the seizure, the first febrile seizure occurred before the age of 18 months, or the seizure was the first sign of an illness (NINDS, 2015).

Risk Factors

The lifetime prevalence of epilepsy in children is 10 per 1000 (1%), with 6 per 1000 (0.6%) reporting a currently active seizure disorder. Prevalence is higher in low income families and in older, male children (Russ, Larson, & Halfon, 2012). In addition, about 1.8% of adults age 18 and older have had a seizure disorder, with 1% reporting a currently active seizure disorder (CDC, 2016b).

Other risk factors include being an infant who is small for gestational age, the presence of underlying neurologic conditions, brain tumors or infections of the brain, stroke, cerebral palsy, autism spectrum disorder, family history, or abuse of drugs (Epilepsy Foundation, 2014b). Risk factors and other considerations for older adults are described in the Lifespan Considerations section.

Children who have a seizure disorder are at higher risk for comorbid conditions, including depression, anxiety, attention-deficit/hyperactivity disorder (ADHD), developmental delay, autism spectrum disorder, and headaches. They are also more likely to have to repeat a school grade, have social difficulties, and have unmet medical needs (Russ et al., 2012).

Prevention

Everyone has a seizure threshold. When this threshold is exceeded, a seizure may occur. Some individuals have abnormally low seizure thresholds, increasing their risk for seizure activity. Others may experience seizures as the result of a pathologic process such as epilepsy. Prevention of seizures is difficult, but there are some steps individuals can take to reduce their risk for seizures or reduce the frequency of seizure activity.

Individuals with epilepsy often experience seizure activity upon exposure to a trigger. Triggers may be individualized (e.g., odors, flashing lights). General triggers include fatigue, hypoglycemia, fever, alcohol, hyperventilation, and menstruation. Individuals who are able to identify triggers may succeed in reducing their frequency. Maintaining good self-care (e.g., maintaining the therapeutic regimen, avoiding alcohol, eating properly, balancing rest and activity) is important for individuals with known seizure disorders. Certain drugs may predispose people to seizures. Alcoholics who attempt sudden withdrawal or engage in heavy binge drinking may experience seizures. Other drugs, such as cocaine or ecstasy, can cause a seizure episode in patients who do not have a seizure disorder (Epilepsy Foundation, 2014b).

Clinical Manifestations

The symptoms that occur with a seizure episode are important to note, because they play a critical role in helping define the type of seizure and guide treatment options. The initial manifestations of the **tonic phase** of a generalized seizure are unconsciousness and continuous muscular contraction. The basal metabolic rate rises during the peak of seizure activity, increasing the body's demand for oxygen and glucose. The patient may become pale or cyanotic as a result of hypoxia. The patient also may become hypoglycemic if glucose demand is excessive. The tonic phase is followed by the **clonic phase**, which is characterized by alternating muscular contraction and relaxation. During the **postictal period** following seizure activity, LOC is decreased and the patient is often sleepy but arousable. The length of the postictal period varies.

SAFETY ALERT   The belief that an individual can "swallow" his or her tongue during a tonic–clonic seizure is inaccurate. Many people have attempted to wedge apart the jaws of an individual experiencing a tonic–clonic seizure, but doing so can cause harm to the patient or actually cause airway obstruction.

The exact symptoms of a seizure depend on its type and the area of the brain from which the abnormal electrical discharges originated. Tonic–clonic seizures are the most common seizure type in children, characterized by alternating repetitive tonic–clonic activity. An **aura** may provide an early warning sign, especially for focal seizures, and may manifest as any type of sensory disturbance, such as auditory, visual, or abdominal. When patients recognize the pattern of an aura, they may have time to avoid injury by getting to the floor. **Automatisms** occur most commonly with focal seizures. They are unconscious movements such as lip smacking, picking at clothing, or other repetitive motions that may resemble tics. Patients experiencing automatisms are usually unaware of them after the seizure activity ends.

Collaboration

The healthcare team, composed of the nurse, physician or advanced practice nurse or nurse practitioner, family, and patient, works together to understand seizure care and prevention requirements. In the case of children, the teacher, school nurse, and other adults who work with the child are included as extensions of the child's healthcare team to ensure that care and prevention requirements are maintained during school and extracurricular activities. Referral to social workers and/or psychologic services may be appropriate for patients or families who are having difficulty coping. Occupational counseling may be needed for patients whose seizures cannot be well controlled to help find employment pathways that ensure safety and support. Many seizures are self-limiting and require no emergency intervention.

Diagnostic Tests

Laboratory tests that may be ordered for patients who are experiencing seizures include a complete blood cell count, blood chemistry, urine culture, and lumbar puncture. If the patient is taking any anticonvulsants, the serum drug level is monitored regularly. An EEG is usually ordered with the first occurrence of seizure activity, and it may be performed under conditions that lower the seizure threshold, such as sleep deprivation, hyperventilation, or exposure to flashing lights. EEG testing may be done either one time or over several days using a portable monitor. (See **Figure 11–14 ≫**.) An EEG is often performed at a follow-up visit between seizures. An example of what an EEG reading looks like can be found in **Figure 11–15 ≫**. A lead level, toxicology screening, and radiologic tests such as a CT scan or MRI and angiography may be performed to identify cerebral lesions or metabolic disorders in the brain.

Surgery

If a patient fails drug therapy and continues to have seizure activity that interferes with daily life, surgical intervention may be considered. Seizures that cannot be controlled are

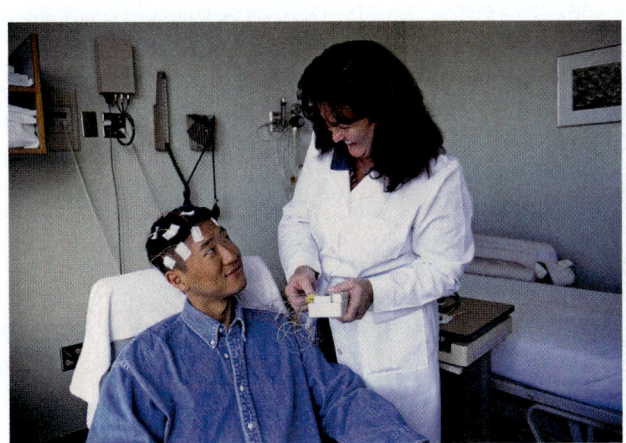

Source: Keith Brofsky/Photodisc/Getty Images.

Figure 11–14 ≫ EEG testing.

Clinical Manifestations and Therapies
Seizure Disorders

ETIOLOGY	CLINICAL MANIFESTATIONS	CLINICAL THERAPIES
Focal aware seizures Previously called *simple partial seizures*. Involve activation of only a restricted part of one cerebral hemisphere.	■ No alteration in consciousness occurs. ■ Typically only the motor portion of the cortex is affected, causing recurrent muscle contractions of the face or contralateral part of the body. Motor movement may be confined to one area. If it spreads sequentially to adjacent parts, it is called a Jacksonian march or Jacksonian seizure. ■ If the sensory portion of the cortex is involved, manifestations may include abnormal sensations such as tingling, numbness, or hallucinations. ■ Disruption in the autonomic nervous system may result in tachycardia, flushing, hypotension, or hypertension. ■ Psychic symptoms such as a sense of déjà vu or inappropriate fear or anger may be experienced. ■ Often, patients with focal aware seizures experience a remission of the disease around age 16.	■ Antiseizure medications may be prescribed. There is not one drug of choice for treating focal aware seizures. ■ Maintain patient safety during the seizure. ■ Assess the exact manifestations experienced by the patient and document them fully. ■ Gamma knife procedure, focal cortical resection, or thermal laser ablation may be tried if epilepsy is refractory to medications. ■ Vagal nerve stimulation therapy may be appropriate for patients who do not respond to medications and are poor surgical candidates.
Focal impaired seizures Previously called *complex partial seizures*. Involve activation of only a restricted part of one cerebral hemisphere, usually originating in the temporal lobe.	■ Focal impaired seizures are often proceeded by an aura, which can be psychic, somatosensory, auditory, visual, autonomic, abdominal, olfactory, or gustatory in nature. ■ Seizures typically last 30 seconds to 2 minutes. ■ Impaired consciousness continues for several hours before full consciousness is regained. ■ During a focal impaired seizure, the patient exhibits automatisms, such as lip smacking, aimless walking, or picking at clothing. ■ Amnesia is common after a focal impaired seizure.	■ Antiseizure medications (except ethosuximide [Zarontin]) may be prescribed. There is not one drug of choice for treating focal impaired seizures. ■ Maintain patient safety during and after the seizure. ■ Vagal nerve stimulation may be considered. ■ Resection of epileptogenic focus, such as the temporal lobe, may be considered.
Generalized seizures Involve both hemispheres of the brain as well as deeper structures such as thalamus, basal ganglia, and upper brainstem. Types: tonic-clonic, clonic, tonic, myoclonic, atonic, myoclonic-tonic-clonic, myoclonic-atonic, epileptic spasms, typical absence, atypical absence, myoclonic absence, eyelid myoclonia	■ The patient's LOC is impaired. ■ Sudden brief cessation of all motor activity is accompanied by blank stare and unresponsiveness. ■ This seizure type is more common in children. ■ Generalized seizures usually last 5–10 seconds, but can be as long as 30 seconds. ■ Frequency of generalized seizures varies from occasional to several hundred per day. ■ Warning aura does NOT proceed seizure activity. ■ Seizure involves sudden loss of consciousness and consists of tonic and clonic phases. *Tonic phase:* ■ Sharp tonic muscle contraction forces air out of the lungs, which may cause the patient to cry out. ■ Loss of postural control causes the patient to fall in opisthotonic posture (the head and feet are bent backward and the body is arched forward). ■ Muscles are rigid, with arms and legs extended and jaw clenched. ■ Urinary incontinence is common and may be accompanied by bowel incontinence. ■ Breathing ceases, and cyanosis develops. ■ Pupils are fixed and dilated.	■ Antiseizure medications may be prescribed. First-line medications to control absence seizures are ethosuximide (Zarontin) and valproic acid (Depakene, Depacon). ■ Maintain patient safety. ■ The ability to drive may not be granted. Prescribers must be aware of state laws. ■ Helmets may be recommended to prevent head injury until seizure activity is controlled. ■ Do not restrain the patient. ■ Pad bedrails.

Clinical Manifestations and Therapies (continued)

ETIOLOGY	CLINICAL MANIFESTATIONS	CLINICAL THERAPIES
	Clonic phase: ■ Alternating contraction and relaxation occur in muscles of all extremities. ■ Hyperventilation occurs. ■ The eyes roll back. ■ The patient froths at the mouth. ■ This phase varies in duration and subsides gradually, generally over 60–90 seconds. **Postictal phase:** ■ The patient remains unconscious and unresponsive to stimuli. ■ Breathing is relaxed and quiet. ■ The patient regains consciousness gradually and may be confused and disoriented on waking. ■ Headache, muscle ache, and fatigue are often reported. ■ The patient may sleep for several hours. ■ Amnesia is usual both for the seizure and for several minutes before seizure activity.	■ Diazepam, lorazepam, or phenobarbital may be administered during the seizure to limit the length of the seizure. ■ Vagal nerve stimulators are not approved by the Food and Drug Administration for treatment of tonic–clonic seizures, but some patients have experienced a reduction in tonic–clonic seizure activity after implantation of these devices.
Status epilepticus	■ This condition involves continuous seizure activity, with only short periods of calm between intense and persistent seizures. ■ Seizures may be any type but most often are generalized tonic–clonic. ■ The patient is in great danger of hypoxia, acidosis, hypoglycemia, hyperthermia, and exhaustion if seizure activity is not halted.	■ Provide immediate interventions to preserve life. ■ Establish and maintain an airway. ■ Administer 50% glucose to prevent hypoglycemia. ■ Administer diazepam or lorazepam IV; repeat every 10 minutes until seizure activity stops. ■ Administer antiseizure medications such as phenytoin or fosphenytoin. Phenobarbital may also be administered. ■ IV general anesthesia with propofol may be used as a last resort if seizure activity does not cease.

Sources: Data from Boggs, J. G. (2016). *Simple partial seizures.* Retrieved from http://emedicine.medscape.com/article/1184384-overview; Carroll, E., & Benbadis, S. R. (2016). *Complex partial seizures.* Retrieved from http://emedicine.medscape.com/article/1183962-overview; Ko, D. Y., & Sahai-Srivastava, S. (2015). *Generalized tonic-clonic seizures.* Retrieved from http://emedicine.medscape.com/article/1184608-overview; Roth, J. L., & Blum, A. S. (2016). *Status epilepticus.* Retrieved from http://emedicine.medscape.com/article/1164462-overview; International League Against Epilepsy (ILAE). (2017). New ILAE seizure classification. Retrieved from https://www.ilae.org/news-and-media/news-about-ilae/new-ilae-seizure-classification

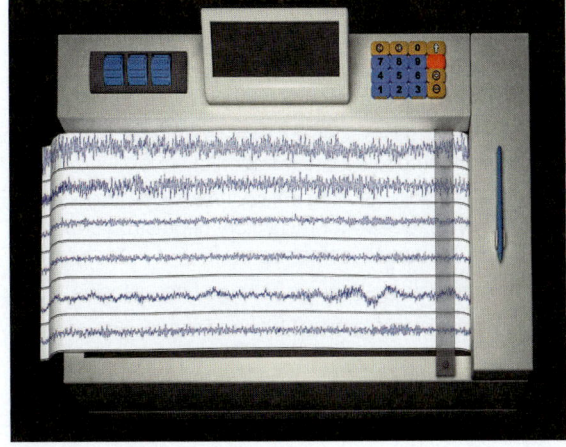

Source: Satori13/iStock/Getty Images.

Figure 11–15 ❯❯ An EEG reading.

called **intractable seizures**. These seizures occur in approximately 30% of patients with a seizure disorder. Surgery will be considered only if the area of seizure focus (where the seizure activity starts) can be identified and is not responsible for any critical functions such as movement, sensation, or speech. The evaluation and diagnostic testing involved in determining whether a patient is a candidate for surgery is quite extensive.

There are three main types of surgeries used in the treatment of seizure disorders. The most common type of surgery is a *resection*, in which the section of brain tissue that has been found to be the source of seizure initiation is removed (Epilepsy Foundation, 2013a). This can include a lobe, a portion of a lobe, or even an entire hemisphere of the brain (Mayo Clinic, 2015b). A *transection* interrupts the nerve pathways by which the seizure impulses are transmitted through the brain (Epilepsy Foundation, 2013a). One common type of transection is a corpus callosotomy, in which the neural connections between the right and left hemispheres of the brain are severed (Mayo Clinic, 2015b). The third type of surgery involves placing a vagus nerve stimulator in the chest. This procedure has been approved for patients who are age 12 and older and have focal seizure disorders (Mayo Clinic, 2015c).

Pharmacologic Therapy

Antiseizure drugs can reduce or control most seizure activity. (See the Medications feature for more information).

The goals of medications are to protect the patient from harm and to reduce or prevent seizure activity without impairing cognitive function or producing undesirable side effects. The lowest possible dose of a single medication that will control the patient's seizures should be prescribed; often, however, several medications must be tried before the most effective one is identified. In some cases, a combination of drugs may be needed to manage the patient's seizures.

Status epilepticus is a continuous seizure that lasts for more than 30 minutes or a series of seizures during which time consciousness is not regained. Status epilepticus requires immediate intervention to preserve life. Establishing and maintaining the airway is a priority. A solution of 50% dextrose is administered intravenously to prevent hypoglycemia. Diazepam (Valium) or lorazepam (Ativan) is given intravenously, and if necessary, the dose is repeated in 10 minutes to stop seizure activity. Phenytoin (Dilantin) is administered intravenously for longer-term control of seizures. Phenobarbital also may be administered to patients in status epilepticus. If seizures continue, IV general anesthesia using propofol (Diprivan) should be considered.

Complementary Health Approaches

Many conventional medical practitioners employ integrative health for patients with epilepsy. Complementary health approaches may confer tangible benefits via "indirect effects on anxiety, depression and other aspects of psychological wellbeing" (Baxendale, 2015). These complementary health approaches may work through the placebo effect, but as Baxendale relates, "the placebo effect is a real phenomenon that produces tangible, replicable results in a wide variety of patients, including those with epilepsy. The literature is clear: patients receiving placebos do better than those who receive no treatment at all." As with all treatment strategies, complementary health approaches, such as the mind and body practices listed below, should be used in consultation with the treating provider.

Patients who regularly use essential oils, whether massaged into the skin or inhaled for aromatherapy, should be cautioned that many essential oils can trigger seizures. Herbal preparations can also be problematic: ginkgo and St. John's wort have been found to decrease the effectiveness of antiseizure medications such as valproic acid and carbamazepine. Kava, passionflower, and valerian may increase the sedative effects of primidone and phenobarbital. Garlic can possibly increase antiseizure medication levels, whereas chamomile may prolong the effects of these medications (Krucik, 2014). At each healthcare interaction nurses should ask patients about all herbal preparations used.

Relaxation techniques, such a meditation and deep breathing, can help reduce stress and may help reduce seizures, but not for those patients whose seizures begin when they are deeply relaxed (Epilepsy Foundation, 2013b; Epilepsy Society, 2015).

Medications
Seizure Disorders

CLASSIFICATION AND DRUG EXAMPLES	MECHANISMS OF ACTION	NURSING CONSIDERATIONS
Antiseizure drugs *Drug examples:* Phenytoin (Dilantin) Phenobarbital Primidone (Mysoline) Carbamazepine (Tegretol) Valproic acid (Depakene) Ethosuximide (Zarontin) Clonazepam (Klonopin) Gabapentin (Neurontin) Lamotrigine (Lamictal) Tiagabine HCl (Gabitril) Eslicarbazepine (Aptiom) Lacosamide (Vimpat) Levetiracetam (Keppra) Pregabalin (Lyrica) Topiramate (Topamax)	These drugs act in the motor cortex of the brain to reduce the spread of electrical discharges from the rapidly firing epileptic foci in this area. These agents control seizures without impairing the normal functions of the CNS.	■ Monitor blood pressure, pulse, and respirations. ■ Note evidence of CNS side effects such as blurred vision, dimmed vision, slurred speech, nystagmus, or confusion. Gingival hyperplasia may be noted in patients taking phenytoin. ■ Recognize that patients on prolonged therapy may need a diet rich in vitamin D. ■ Monitor serum calcium level as ordered; phenytoin can contribute to demineralization of bone. ■ When administering antiseizure drugs intravenously, monitor closely for respiratory depression and cardiovascular collapse. ■ Administer gabapentin 2 hours after antacids. ■ Administer tiagabine HCl with food.

Neurofeedback (biofeedback) techniques may be specifically tailored to help individuals with epilepsy identify the warning signs of seizures to prevent a seizure from developing. Relaxation and behavior modification therapy are psychologic therapies that may help certain patients feel less anxious and better adjust to having epilepsy (Epilepsy Foundation, 2013b; Epilepsy Society, 2015).

Lifespan Considerations

Seizure disorders can strike any individual during the course of the lifespan. Epilepsy can be present from birth or develop at any point during an individual's life, or it may develop because of a secondary intracranial process such as brain tumors, injury, or IICP. Every year, more than 1 in 1000 individuals with epilepsy experience sudden, unexpected death. Individuals who are at greatest risk for **sudden unexpected death in epilepsy (SUDEP)** include those with poorly controlled seizures, frequent seizures, and generalized tonic–clonic seizures.

>> *Go to* **Pearson MyLab Nursing and eText** *to see Chart 1, and the Evidence-Based Practice feature about Sudden Unexpected Death in Epilepsy (SUDEP).*

Seizure Disorders in Children

Children with febrile seizures are usually not treated with antiseizure medications at the time of the seizure because febrile seizures typically abate before arrival at the emergency department or clinic. Acetaminophen is given to lower the child's temperature. Long-term antiseizure medication use is not recommended for simple febrile seizures. Following medical evaluation, the provider may suggest administration of antipyretics at home when fever appears, because children with a history of febrile seizure are at increased risk for having another episode. A head CT and EEG (usually with sleep deprivation and flashing lights) is typically done to rule out a pathologic origin of a seizure that occurs in a child with a fever.

Any child with a generalized seizure lasting longer than 10 minutes needs to be monitored for electrolytes, glucose, blood gases, increasing fever, and abnormal blood pressure. Most seizure disorders are managed with antiseizure drugs, which may be given intravenously or rectally. For children, a single medication (monotherapy) is preferred for seizure

Focus on Diversity and Culture
Seizures

Illness is not always experienced the same way in different cultures. For example, epilepsy has been misunderstood and stigmatized among people who have it and their families. This stigmatization has occurred over many centuries and across many cultures. The suddenness of the convulsions and their violent nature has caused many people to fear epilepsy or attribute it to supernatural causes, even during this modern era. In some Asian and Oceanic regions, many people regard epilepsy as a psychiatric disorder.

Nurses must assess whether there are any cultural barriers that may affect the care of a patient with any illness, not just epilepsy. They should approach the subject with respect and sensitivity to cultural differences, otherwise the conversation may end abruptly and the patient might not receive the correct medical care. Questions to ask to help elicit cultural practices related to the patient's health and perspectives and beliefs about health and healing address the patient's perceptions of the cause of the problem, anything the patient has done to try to ameliorate the problem, and how the problem is affecting the patient and family. For more information on culturally competent assessment, see the module on Culture and Diversity.

Sources: Based on Giger, J. N. (2013). *Transcultural nursing: Assessment and intervention* (6th ed.). St. Louis, MO: Elsevier/Mosby; Goh, S., & Ng, B. (2013). Epilepsy—A cross-cultural perspective. *ASEAN Journal of Psychiatry, 14*(2), 187–189; Spector, R. E. (2017). *Cultural diversity in health and illness* (9th ed.). Hoboken, NJ: Pearson Education.

control to minimize the potential for adverse effects such as sleepiness and difficulty with speech. An additional antiseizure drug may be used only if seizure control is not achieved with the first medication (Ko & Sahai-Srivastava, 2015). The child should be monitored for continued motor activity and the potential for status epilepticus. The postictal period ranges from 30 minutes to 2 hours. Management of status epilepticus is described in **Table 11–5** >>. Serum drug levels should be monitored to achieve therapeutic levels or to identify whether toxicity is possible. When tolerated, therapeutic ranges of medications may be exceeded to control seizures. Medication dosage adjustments are often needed in the pediatric patient as the child grows.

TABLE 11–5 Management of Status Epilepticus

Type of Care	Clinical Therapy
Emergency assessment and management	■ Maintain a patent airway. Muscle rigidity may compromise the airway. ■ Perform a jaw-thrust maneuver if the airway is obstructed. ■ Keep suction equipment at the bedside in case secretions are excessive. ■ Give oxygen by mask, because increased metabolic demands deplete oxygen stores. ■ Monitor vital signs and circulation with pulse oximeter, electrocardiogram, and blood pressure device. ■ Perform neurologic assessment as often as needed, especially when any changes in vital signs or LOC are noted.
Ongoing urgent interventions	■ Establish an IV line to administer any necessary fluids or medications. ■ Administer glucose if the child is hypoglycemic. (The physical stress of the seizure may result in declining glucose levels.) ■ Insert a nasogastric tube. This should be done only if head injury has been ruled out as a cause of the seizure. ■ Protect the child from injury. ■ Manage thermoregulation.
Medications	■ Administer benzodiazepines such as diazepam, lorazepam, or midazolam. If there is no response, the dose may be repeated. ■ Phenytoin or phenobarbital may be necessary if seizure activity continues. ■ Cumulative doses of drugs may produce apnea, so be prepared to assist with ventilations.

The primary healthcare provider should provide a seizure action plan for any child with a history of seizure activity who attends school or child care or who is cared for outside the home while the parents work. Nurses can assist parents in making sure that teachers and caregivers understand the action plan and know when and how to use it.

Children who experience refractory or intractable seizures (those that continue to occur despite medical management) should be referred to an epilepsy center for other potential treatments, such as a ketogenic diet, vagal nerve stimulation, or evaluation for surgical treatment.

A ketogenic diet is occasionally used for children under age 8 who experience myoclonic and absence seizures. This diet involves high intake of fat (up to 80% of calories), adequate intake of protein (1 g/kg), and low intake of carbohydrates. The medium-chain triglyceride (MCT) ketogenic diet is used extensively for treating refractory childhood epilepsy. This diet increases the plasma levels of medium straight-chain fatty acids (Chang et al., 2013). The child usually begins the diet in the hospital with a fast for 24 hours. The ketosis caused by the diet is believed to produce anticonvulsant effects. The diet is customized to the child to maintain ideal body weight, maximize ketosis, and achieve optimal seizure control. Motivation must be high for the family to prepare the food and maintain the child on the diet for several years; improved seizure control is directly related to compliance with the diet. The child's urine ketone values are monitored weekly or more frequently. The most common complications are constipation, hyperlipidemia, and kidney stones. Constipation can be treated with MCT oil and increased fluids. Kidney stones are treated by increasing fluid intake and alkalinizing the urine.

SAFETY ALERT When the child on a ketogenic diet is hospitalized, it is important to limit glucose and dextrose from all sources. Normal saline IV fluid should be used. Medications in elixirs or syrups cannot be used because of the sugar content. As an alternative, medications can be obtained in pill form, crushed, and mixed with an allowable food that has been approved by the pharmacy.

A trial of antiseizure medication withdrawal is often attempted for children who have been seizure free for 1–2 years, with medications tapered slowly over a period of months. Approximately 65% of children remain seizure free if they have not had a seizure within 2 years of stopping medication. Criteria that boost a child's chances of remaining seizure free after discontinuation of medication include easily controlled seizures, normal neurologic and developmental function, epilepsy with no identifiable cause, and no changes on EEG that are characteristic of epilepsy (Epilepsy Foundation, 2013c). Information on teaching for children and parents is included in the Patient Teaching feature.

Seizure Disorders in Pregnant Women

Every year, approximately 20,000 women with a seizure disorder give birth. With proper care, these women can have healthy pregnancies and healthy babies. However, several special considerations must be given to women with seizure disorders when they are planning to get pregnant.

One important consideration is the need for women with seizure disorders to discuss with their providers the risks

Patient Teaching
Seizures in School-Age Children and Adolescents

- Inform parents that their child's medications will need to be adjusted as the child ages and that their child's plasma levels will need to be monitored carefully in order to maintain the medication level within the therapeutic range.
- Provide both patients and parents with education about medication regimens (see Box 51–2 in the module on Safety). This includes safe administration of antipyretics. Teaching the older child to take medications without parental intervention gives the child a feeling of control.
- Discuss the importance of regular dental care because of phenytoin's effects on the gingiva.
- Encourage the family to work with school administrators to develop an individualized healthcare plan so the child can receive needed medications and care during school hours.
- Physical activity and exercise are important for all children and adolescents. Encourage participation in sports when adequate supervision is provided. Patients who are prone to seizures require one-to-one supervision during swimming and water activities.
- The child or adolescent may be afraid of having a seizure in front of friends. Reassure the child and family that taking medications regularly should control seizures.
- Summer camps for children with seizures can be a safe and comfortable place for the child to enjoy outdoor activities. Talk with parents about communicating with camp administrators and sharing health and action plans like they do with school administrators.
- Educate adolescent women about the potential teratogenicity of some antiseizure medications, such as valproic acid and carbamazepine, which are associated with neural tube defects and heart defects. Until pregnancy is desired, contraception should be used when the adolescent is sexually active.
- Discuss the complexity of contraception with adolescents. Some antiseizure medications cause a drug interaction with oral contraceptive pills that can lead to contraceptive failure.
- Provide teaching to patients and families about safety guidelines. Families of patients with severe seizure disorders need to develop an emergency care plan so that emergency personnel know about the need for care in advance.

versus benefits of taking certain antiseizure drugs during pregnancy. Most providers believe that the risk associated with fetal birth defects is minor compared to the potential complications associated with a tonic–clonic seizure during pregnancy. If the pregnant woman has a seizure during pregnancy, it could result in injury to the woman and fetus because of a fall, or it could result in decreased oxygen to the fetus, preterm labor, or preterm birth (American College of Obstetricians and Gynecologists [ACOG], 2013). In addition, many of these defects can be prevented by increasing the woman's dosage of folic acid to 4 mg/day before and during pregnancy (ACOG, 2013; Friel, 2014). In addition, risk of hemorrhagic disease in the newborn due to exposure to antiseizure medications can be reduced by increasing the pregnant woman's intake of vitamin D during pregnancy and administering vitamin K to the neonate (Friel, 2014).

Women with epilepsy who are contemplating pregnancy should be advised to coordinate their care with their neurologist and obstetrician; preferably, these providers will already have experience treating pregnant patients who have epilepsy. Both the pregnant patient and the fetus will need to be monitored closely throughout the pregnancy (Mayo Clinic, 2014b). Any medication changes should be made prior to conception to allow the woman and her provider to determine how effective the new medication regimen will be at controlling seizures without putting the fetus at risk (ACOG, 2013). Once the woman is pregnant, dosages may need to be further adjusted to maintain appropriate drug levels in the blood, because blood volume changes drastically during pregnancy (Friel, 2014).

Eclampsia is a seizure disorder associated with pregnancy. Pregnant women with extremely high blood pressure and rapid weight gain have preeclampsia, and eclampsia is simply preeclampsia plus seizures. The seizures associated with eclampsia are not related to a pre-existing brain condition. For more information on preeclampsia and eclampsia, see the exemplar on Hypertensive Disorders of Pregnancy in the module on Perfusion.

Seizure Disorders in Older Adults

Approximately 1.1% of older adults on Medicare have epilepsy, with the highest rate occurring in African Americans (Faught et al., 2012). Epilepsy in older adults is often caused by stroke, Alzheimer disease, heart disease, tumors, and injuries from falls. However, approximately half of the seizures seen in older adults are cryptogenic, meaning their cause cannot be identified (Epilepsy Foundation, 2014c). Epilepsy in older adults can threaten their independence and quality of life by increasing their risk for falls and fractures, forcing driving restrictions, increasing social isolation and depression, and causing low self-esteem and loss of employment (Austin & Abdulla, 2013).

The manifestations of seizures in older adults are often different from those in children and younger adults. Older adults more frequently have focal seizures rather than the classic tonic–clonic seizures. Older adults often present with a blank stare, brief unresponsiveness, language difficulties, confusion, and automatisms such as lip smacking. The postictal phase is also longer in older adults, sometimes lasting up to 2 weeks, with symptoms such as sleepiness and confusion. Older adults with epilepsy have a higher mortality rate than older adults without epilepsy (Austin & Abdulla, 2013).

Because of the symptoms associated with seizures in older adults, seizures are often misdiagnosed as stroke, dementia, or heart disease in this population. Diagnosis is complicated by both comorbid conditions and the fact that the standard diagnostic tool, the EEG, is often unreliable in older adults, because many healthy older adults have EEG changes. Epilepsy in older adults is usually controlled by antiseizure medication. However, care must be taken when choosing the right antiseizure medication for each older adult. First-generation antiseizure drugs such as phenytoin, carbamazepine, valproic acid, and phenobarbital have a greater incidence of drug interactions and adverse effects such as imbalance issues and confusion compared to the newer, second-generation antiseizure drugs such as lamotrigine, levetiracetam, and gabapentin (Austin & Abdulla, 2013).

NURSING PROCESS

Assessment

Nurses play an important role in the care of patients who have seizure disorders. The first priority is to ensure patient safety during a seizure. Accurate assessment and documentation of the seizure length, symptoms, and spread can help determine which type of seizure the patient is having (if not already known). It also provides ample opportunity for the nurse to teach patients and their support network about seizures, safety precautions, and medications.

- *Observation and patient interview.* After the patient's first seizure, obtain a thorough history from the parent, primary caretaker, or witnesses to the event. Take a description of the seizure and its length, in addition to whether an aura was present and whether the patient lost consciousness. If the nurse observes seizure activity, document the time the seizure started and finished, the symptoms involved, whether it was localized or spread or was generalized, whether the patient lost consciousness and for how long, and the duration of the postictal phase. If the patient loses consciousness, after the seizure the nurse can ask whether there was an aura and what the patient remembers about the event (**Table 11–6 》》**).

- *Physical examination.* Perform a complete physical and neurologic examination. Assess and monitor the patient's physiologic status. Observe the specific seizure activity, LOC, vital signs, and signs of hypoxia. During the postictal period, monitor vital signs, perform neurologic checks, and ensure safety. Once the patient is stable, a more definitive assessment can be made. LOC is one of the most important indicators of neurologic function. Remember that a lack of response may be the result of the postictal state.

To help determine the type of seizure, collect and analyze historical information about the seizure activity, clustering, auras, motor activity or changes in muscle tone, automatisms, and any changes in developmental performance. Assess the family's adaptation to the seizure disorder, including how well the family is coping with the uncertainty of when the next seizure will occur.

Diagnosis

Common nursing diagnoses for an individual with a seizure disorder include the following:

- *Breathing Pattern, Ineffective*
- *Trauma, Risk for*
- *Self-Esteem, Chronic Low*
- *Verbal Communication, Impaired*
- *Confusion, Acute.*

(NANDA-I © 2014)

Planning

Nursing care for the patient with a seizure disorder focuses on maintaining safety, ensuring a patent airway, preventing or controlling seizure activity, providing emotional support to the patient and family, and administering medications as ordered. Planning must include care of the patient in both

TABLE 11–6 Nursing Assessments Before, During, and After a Seizure

Assessment	Rationale
What was the patient's LOC? If consciousness was lost, at what point?	This indicates the area of the brain involved and the type of seizure.
What was the patient doing just before the attack?	This may suggest precipitating factors.
In what part of the body did the seizure start?	This may indicate the site of seizure activity in the brain tissue; for example, if jerking movements were first observed in the right hand, the seizure focus may be in the left motor cortex.
Was there an epileptic cry?	This cry usually indicates the tonic stage of a generalized tonic–clonic seizure.
Were any automatisms observed, such as eyelid fluttering, chewing, lip smacking, or swallowing?	Automatisms are often seen in focal and absence seizures.
How long did movements last? Did the location or character change (e.g., tonic to clonic)? Did movements involve both sides of the body or just one side?	This indicates areas in which the focal activity originated.
Did the head and/or eyes turn to one side? If so, which side?	This helps localize the focus of the seizure; during the seizure, the head and eyes typically turn away from the side of the epileptogenic focus.
Were there changes in pupillary reactions?	This indicates involvement of the autonomic nervous system.
If the patient fell, was the head hit?	Skull x-ray studies may be needed to rule out subdural hematoma or fracture.
Was there foaming or frothing from the mouth?	This usually indicates a tonic–clonic seizure.

the inpatient and outpatient setting. Nurses should help patients and their families find support groups or other available resources. Goals may include the following:

- The patient will not experience trauma or injury related to a seizure episode.
- The patient will maintain a patent airway and effective respiratory function during a seizure episode.
- The patient will experience no or a limited number of seizures through adequate administration of prescribed medications.
- The patient and family will have an adequate support system in place so that the patient can maintain a positive self-image.
- The patient and family will be aware of signs and symptoms that are specific to the patient and occur with seizure activity. Any precursors to seizure activity will be noted, and a seizure diary may be utilized.
- The patient and family will not experience a disruption of educational, social, or workplace opportunities due to the seizure disorder.

>> **Stay Current:** Sample seizure action plans and other resources are available on the Epilepsy Foundation's website: http://www. epilepsy.com/.

Implementation

Nursing interventions for patients with seizures include ensuring the patient's safety during and after the seizure, maintaining the patient's airway during the seizure, and providing information to the patient and family related to home management of seizures.

Provide for Patient Safety

Ensuring safety for the patient during a seizure is vital to reducing complications associated with the seizure. Nurses can help provide for patient safety by keeping the following points in mind:

- Place nothing in the patient's mouth during a seizure; loose teeth may be knocked out and aspirated.

- Do not restrain the patient during a seizure. This can result in injury or asphyxiation.
- Protect the patient from self-harm during violent seizures (see **Figure 11–16** >>). If the patient is in bed, the side rails should be padded to prevent injury.
- Children who have frequent, recurrent seizures should wear helmets to protect their heads during falls.
- All patients with seizure disorders should wear some form of medical alert identification.
- Discuss information regarding triggers and auras with the patient to help identify causes of seizures and when a seizure might occur. This allows the patient to avoid potential triggers and get in a safe place before a seizure begins.

Maintain the Airway

If a patient is having trouble breathing during or after a seizure, the nurse should perform actions to help maintain an adequate airway. Such actions may include the following:

- Position the patient on his or her side so secretions can drain.
- Maintain functioning suction at the bedside to clear the airway as necessary.

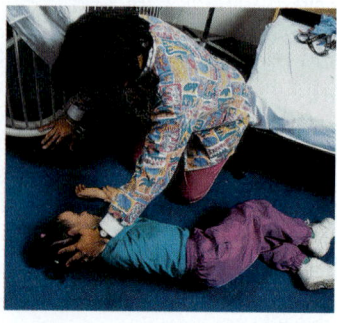

Figure 11–16 >> A patient who has a seizure when standing should be gently assisted to the floor and placed in a side-lying position. Clear the area of any objects that might cause harm.

- Monitor to ensure adequate oxygenation. Mucous membranes should be pink, heart rate should be at a normal or slightly elevated rate for age, and the pulse oximetry reading (SpO_2) should be greater than 95%. Oxygen is usually administered when the SpO_2 falls below 95%.

- Take special precautions when administering IV medications (diazepam, lorazepam, or phenytoin) for the emergency management of status epilepticus. Give these medications very slowly over several minutes to minimize the risk of respiratory or circulatory collapse.

Support Home Management

Individuals with epilepsy must learn how to manage their condition in the community. The nurse needs to perform patient teaching to support home management, which may include the following:

- Give medications orally for the ongoing management of seizures. Crushing pills and mixing them in a teaspoonful of applesauce, pudding, or other soft food may make them more palatable and easier for a child or older adult to swallow, but only if the pill is one that may be crushed.

- Make sure parents know how to administer medications and keep their child safe.

- Encourage patients and their families to express their fears and anxieties.

- Patients with seizures should have a seizure action plan to implement at school, work, or on trips in the community. Work with the patient or the patient's parents to create a successful seizure action plan, and ensure that the action plan is given to the appropriate individuals at the patient's school or work.

- Provide information related to seizure assistance dogs. These dogs can help alert the patient of an upcoming seizure, alert family members that a seizure is occurring, or help the patient to safety during a seizure.

- Answer questions honestly and refer patients and their families to organizations such as the Epilepsy Foundation, where they can get more information about the disorder.

- Refer the patient and family to support groups and counseling services if indicated.

Evaluation

Expected outcomes of nursing management include the following:

- The patient achieves good seizure control with medication, ketogenic diet, or surgical intervention.

- The patient's self-esteem is enhanced through participation in well-supervised sports and activities.

- The patient maintains a patent airway during seizure activity.

- The patient's safety is maintained during seizure activity.

- Medication administration reduces the frequency of seizure recurrence.

- The patient, family, and healthcare team create an appropriate seizure management plan.

For patients with recurrent seizures that are not controlled by the initial medication choice, discuss the possibility of replacing the medication with another antiseizure medication or adding a secondary antiseizure drug to the regimen. Most patients can control their seizures with antiseizure medication once the right medications and dosages are prescribed. If medication does not control the seizures, discuss with the provider the advantages and disadvantages of surgery. Continue to provide patient teaching for the patient and the patient's family to help identify triggers and recognize auras (if present) to reduce the risk of injury. Also provide patient teaching to as many family, friends, coworkers, teachers, and others as needed to help ensure proper care of the patient with a seizure disorder.

Nursing Care Plan
A Patient with a Seizure Disorder

Janet Carlson is a 19-year-old college student who lives with her parents and one younger sister. Although Ms. Carlson had seizures while she was in grade school, they have been controlled with medication. Yesterday, however, she had a tonic–clonic seizure and immediately made an appointment with her family physician. She is currently taking phenytoin (Dilantin) 300 mg/day as a maintenance medication to prevent seizures.

ASSESSMENT	DIAGNOSES	PLANNING
Evita Farias, RN, completes a health history for Ms. Carlson. During the history, Ms. Carlson says that she has been under stress because of difficulties in completing her course requirements this semester. She has not been sleeping as many hours at night, and sometimes she forgets to take her medication. Her serum phenytoin level is only 8 mcg/mL, even though her therapeutic level is 10–20 mcg/mL.	■ *Risk for Trauma* related to recurrence of generalized tonic–clonic seizure activity and low serum phenytoin levels ■ *Deficient Knowledge* of activities that may trigger seizure occurrence, the effect of stress on seizures, and medication information (NANDA-I © 2014)	■ Verbalize precipitating and triggering factors related to the onset of seizures. ■ Verbalize the relationship between emotional and physical stress and seizures. ■ Verbalize the importance of taking antiseizure drugs.

(continued on next page)

Nursing Care Plan (continued)

IMPLEMENTATION

Teach the patient and her family about the following subjects: Current information about seizures care during and after a seizure, medication protocols, factors and activities that can trigger seizures, and the importance of follow-up care.

The nurse should also:

- Refer the patient and her family to a local epilepsy support group.
- Recommend that the patient purchase and wear a medical ID bracelet.

EVALUATION

Ms. Carlson is instructed to continue taking Dilantin 300 mg/day. Ms. Farias teaches Ms. Carlson regarding the importance of nutrition, rest, and measures to reduce stress. She also discusses with Ms. Carlson the importance of maintaining proper blood levels of her medication, stating that too little or too much of the medication could cause problems. Ms. Carlson understands that the seizures recurred during a busy time in school when she had forgotten to take her medication. She is now wearing a medical ID bracelet. Ms. Farias provides the Carlsons with the telephone number of the Epilepsy Foundation.

CRITICAL THINKING

1. If you were the nurse, would your teaching differ if Ms. Carlson were living alone? If so, how? If not, why not?
2. Ms. Carlson tells you that although she knows she should not drive a car, she often drives herself to and from school. What would you say to Ms. Carlson about driving?
3. Ms. Carlson states, "It's embarrassing to wear a medical ID bracelet." How would you respond? What recommendation(s) would you make?

REVIEW Seizure Disorders

RELATE Link the Concepts and Exemplars

Linking the exemplar of seizures with the concept of legal issues:

1. When caring for an adult patient newly diagnosed with recurrent seizures, what legal obligation does the nurse have regarding the patient's driving privileges versus the obligation to maintain patient privacy?
2. If the patient says, "You don't have to report this to the DMV— I promise not to drive until I get medical clearance," is it permissible for the nurse to take the patient's word for it?

Linking the exemplar of seizures with the concept of thermoregulation:

3. The nurse is caring for a 14-month-old infant with a fever whose mother reports that the infant's two older siblings both experienced febrile seizures. What nursing interventions would you initiate with this child?
4. What would differ in your plan of care for a child with a fever if the child had a history of febrile seizures?

READY Go to Volume 3: Clinical Nursing Skills

REFER Go to Pearson MyLab Nursing and eText

- Additional review materials
- Chart 1: Evidence-Based Practice: Sudden Unexpected Death in Epilepsy (SUDEP) Problem

REFLECT Apply Your Knowledge

Joe Hill is a 77-year-old man admitted to the hospital with a diagnosis of new-onset seizure. His temperature is 97°F oral, pulse is 78 bpm, blood pressure is 154/90 mmHg, and O_2 sat is 99%. He appears confused and is unable to respond to questions. Mr. Hill's wife reports that her husband has a history of hypertension, but he is otherwise healthy. Mr. Hill is placed on seizure precautions, and his vital signs are monitored.

1. On the basis of this description, what kind of seizure might Mr. Hill have experienced?
2. What factors may have contributed to Mr. Hill's seizure?
3. What will the nurse include in the assessment of this patient?
4. What are the priority nursing interventions?

≫ Exemplar 11.C
Traumatic Brain Injury

Exemplar Learning Outcomes

11.C Analyze traumatic brain injury as it relates to intracranial regulation.

- Describe the pathophysiology of traumatic brain injury.
- Describe the etiology of traumatic brain injury.
- Compare the risk factors and prevention of traumatic brain injury.
- Identify the clinical manifestations of traumatic brain injury.

- Summarize diagnostic tests and therapies used by interprofessional teams in the collaborative care of an individual traumatic brain injury.
- Differentiate care of patients with traumatic brain injury across the lifespan.
- Apply the nursing process in providing culturally competent care to an individual with traumatic brain injury.

Exemplar Key Terms

Chronic traumatic encephalopathy (CTE), 773
Concussion, 771
Contusion, 771

Overview

Traumatic brain injury (TBI) results from an external physical force, such as a blow or jolt to the head, causing displacement of the brain within the skull and disruption of normal brain function. TBI can also be caused by a penetrating injury, such as a bullet through the brain. TBI can range from mild to severe; mild TBI is called a **concussion**. TBI accounts for approximately 2.2 million emergency department visits and 50,000 deaths every year in the United States (CDC, 2016a). The effects of TBI can last from a few minutes or hours to the rest of the patient's life, depending on severity and the areas of the brain that are damaged.

Pathophysiology and Etiology

Depending on the cause and severity of the trauma, the pathophysiology of TBI can vary greatly. The following sections take a closer look at the pathophysiology and etiology of various types of TBI.

Pathophysiology

TBI occurs when an external force causes some degree of impairment to brain structure or function. The damage caused by this external force is referred to as the *primary injury*. The energy associated with the external force then causes shearing of the tissues, which ruptures neurons, astrocytes, oligodendrocytes, and blood vessels. As a result, blood and cellular contents leak into the extracellular space and cause further damage to surrounding tissues. This damage is called the *secondary injury* (Kurland et al., 2012).

Primary Injuries

Primary injuries can be the result of either penetrating or nonpenetrating injuries. **Penetrating injuries** (also called *open injuries*) cause an open head wound with focal damage around the site of the injury. Such injuries are commonly caused by gunshots and sharp objects, including skull fragments. In contrast, **nonpenetrating injuries** (also called *closed injuries*) are associated with blunt-force injuries that do not result in the entrance of a foreign object into the brain.

The main types of primary injury include skull fracture, concussion (a mild form of TBI), contusion, hematoma and hemorrhage, laceration, and diffuse axonal injury (see **Table 11–7** ≫) (American Speech-Language-Hearing Association [ASHA], n.d.a). Penetrating injuries are more likely to cause skull fractures and lacerations in the brain tissue and meninges than nonpenetrating injuries. Nonpenetrating injuries are often associated with contusions and concussions. Patients can have more than one type of primary injury and should receive interventions related to each type of injury they experience.

TABLE 11–7 Selected Types of Primary Injury

Type of Injury	Description	Variables
Skull fracture	Occurs when an object hits the head with sufficient force to crack open the skull	The classification depends on the degree of skin damage, depression of the brain matter, and location of the fracture.
Contusion	Bruise on the brain	The severity of brain injury depends on the size and location. See **Box 11–2** ≫.
Hematoma	Collection of blood outside the blood vessel (e.g., blood clot)	Hematomas may be subdural, epidural, or intraparenchymal (located within the brain tissue). They are associated with IICP and increase the risk for death.
Hemorrhage	Bleeding from a blood vessel	Hemorrhaging can lead to IICP, deteriorating brain function, and hydrocephalus.
Laceration	Disruption of the brain tissue caused by the entrance of a foreign object such as a bullet, knife, or skull fragment	Entrance of a foreign object increases the patient's susceptibility to complications such as infection, IICP, hemorrhage, and herniation. Depending on its location, laceration may cause brain injury that affects other body functions.
Diffuse axonal injury	Occurs due to a rotational deceleration that is dramatic enough to cause damage to the brain's white matter in the form of widespread disruption of axon fibers and myelin sheaths	Diffuse axonal injury is often seen in shaken baby syndrome. It often results in long-term disability or persistent vegetative state.

Box 11–2
Classifications of Brain Contusions

Brain contusions are classified as coup or contrecoup (see **Figure 11–17** »). A **coup injury** occurs when the brain strikes the same side of the skull as the side of impact. A **contrecoup injury** occurs when the brain strikes the opposite side of the skull as the side of impact. A contusion then forms at the site where the brain struck the skull. In addition, individuals can have a **coup–contrecoup injury**, in which the brain strikes the coup side then bounces back and strikes the contrecoup side, resulting in contusions on both sides of the brain. It can take hours to days for contusions formed during coup–contrecoup injuries to enlarge. This expansion can cause neurologic deterioration and even death. Patients with brain contusions should be monitored closely for the first several days after injury.

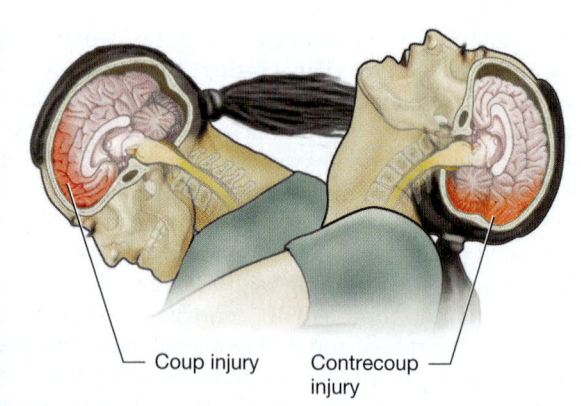

Coup injury   Contrecoup injury

Figure 11–17 » Coup and contrecoup injuries.

Secondary Injury

Secondary injuries can be caused by intracranial damage or systemic insults to the brain. Some examples of secondary injuries include cerebral ischemia, cerebral edema, IICP, infection, hypoxia, hypotension, fever, and hyponatremia (Rangel-Castilla et al., 2016). One of the most severe secondary injuries is hemorrhagic progression of a contusion, a process through which new, noncontiguous contusions appear in addition to the original contusion within several hours of the initial injury (Kurland et al., 2012). If damage from primary and secondary injuries causes an increase in ICP so that it equals the MAP, then the CPP becomes zero, resulting in complete ischemia and brain death (Wilberger & Dupre, 2013a).

Concussion

Concussion is a form of mild TBI caused by shaking of the brain. Concussion usually leads to rapid-onset but transient neurologic impairment, which may include confusion, unconsciousness, headache, loss of memory, impaired balance, and visual disturbances (Wilberger & Dupre, 2013b). An alteration in mental status may last from a few seconds to a few minutes, but usually lasts less than 6 hours

(Wilberger & Dupre, 2013a). Brain dysfunction related to concussion is thought to be due to excitotoxicity, or excessive release of the excitatory neurotransmitter glutamate (Wilberger & Dupre, 2013b).

SAFETY ALERT Despite common belief, individuals do not need to lose consciousness to sustain a concussion. Thus, any individual who experiences a jarring blow to the head followed by one or more common signs of concussion should be given a neurologic assessment.

The impact that causes a concussion does not result in pathologic changes to the brain; therefore, no changes will be seen upon neuroimaging studies (American Association of Neurological Surgeons [AANS], 2014). However, microscopic changes that are not visible in imaging studies may occur, including breakage of small blood vessels and nerve connections. Although concussions used to be graded as mild (grade 1), moderate (grade 2), or severe (grade 3), the American Academy of Neurology (AAN; 2013) has moved away from this grading system in its most recent guidelines. Instead, the AAN now recommends that decisions regarding a patient's return to normal activities should be made on an individual basis.

Concussion usually resolves spontaneously with no treatment. However, some individuals will experience postconcussion syndrome. **Postconcussion syndrome** is a series of concussion-like symptoms that occur 7–10 days after a concussion (Mayo Clinic, 2014c). It is evidenced by the presence of nausea, headache, dizziness, fatigue, memory problems, difficulty concentrating, insomnia, light and noise sensitivity, and/or personality changes. Postconcussion syndrome may be caused by either physiologic damage to the brain due to the primary insult or secondary emotional trauma related to the event (Mayo Clinic, 2014c). Postconcussion syndrome typically resolves spontaneously within a few weeks, but it can take a year or more for some patients to recover. Patients who have postconcussion syndrome are at risk for complications such as depression or migraines (Leddy et al., 2012).

Additional concerns for patients with concussion include second impact syndrome and cumulative concussions. **Second impact syndrome (SIS)** can occur when an individual receives a second concussion before the initial concussion is completely healed. Athletes who return to play too quickly after a head injury (particularly athletes who have postconcussion syndrome) and athletes who have undiagnosed concussions are at higher risk for SIS. SIS is accompanied by rapid swelling of the brain, which causes vascular congestion and IICP (AANS, n.d.). Because these symptoms appear suddenly and occur rapidly, the risk for sudden death is high (Mayo Clinic, 2014d). Although multiple concussions in a single individual are common, the severe symptoms associated with SIS are relatively rare.

A patient who has sustained one concussion is at higher risk of a second concussion even with less severe impact (Wilberger & Dupre, 2013b). For individuals who expose themselves to multiple concussions, especially boxers, football players, and members of the armed forces, these cumulative concussions can cause permanent brain damage. In particular, multiple concussions are associated with development of

chronic traumatic encephalopathy (CTE), which is a form of dementia. CTE results in a progressive decline of memory and cognition. Individuals with CTE may also experience depression, aggression, poor decision making and impulse control, personality change, parkinsonism, and suicidal behavior (Defense and Veterans Brain Injury Center, 2016; Wilberger & Dupre, 2013b). CTE triggers the buildup of an abnormal protein called tau in the brain, which can cause "memory loss, confusion, impaired judgment, impulse control problems, aggression, depression, and, eventually, progressive dementia" (BU CTE Center, n.d.).

Classification of TBI

The severity of TBI is measured using the Glasgow Coma Scale (see Table 11–3). Mild TBI is associated with a Glasgow Coma Scale score of 13–15, moderate TBI is associated with a score of 9–12, and severe TBI is associated with a score of 3–8 (American Psychiatric Association, 2013). A score of 3 indicates likely fatal damage. Higher scores predict a better recovery. Depending on the types of primary and secondary injuries the patient encounters, the patient's score may improve or decline over time. Therefore, the nurse should frequently assess the patient's Glasgow Coma Scale score.

TBI severity can also be measured by the length of time the patient was unconscious and the length of time amnesia is present. Loss of consciousness for less than 30 minutes or amnesia for less than 24 hours is associated with mild TBI; loss of consciousness for more than 30 minutes but less than 24 hours or amnesia for more than 24 hours but less than 7 days is associated with moderate TBI; and loss of consciousness for 24 or more hours or amnesia for more than 7 days is associated with severe TBI (American Psychiatric Association, 2013).

Etiology

Concussions and TBI share many causative factors. Falls, violence (interpersonal violence or child abuse), vehicle-related collisions (occurring as a driver, passenger, or pedestrian), explosive blasts and other combat injuries (penetrating wounds, blast pressure waves, direct blows to the head), and sports injuries are common causes of concussions and TBI. High-impact and extreme sports such as boxing, football, hockey, and skateboarding also carry a higher risk of concussion and TBI (Mayo Clinic, 2014a, 2014d).

Risk Factors

Because TBI is often the result of an accident, every individual is at risk for TBI. However, some individuals have a higher risk than others. Children, especially children under the age of 4, are at increased risk for TBI due to falls or abuse. Adolescents and young adults are at increased risk for TBI due to interpersonal violence and sports. Older adults are at increased risk for TBI due to falls, which are usually related to sensory perception changes or medication side effects (Mayo Clinic, 2014a). Other individuals who are at increased risk for TBI include individuals who do not use proper safety precautions in vehicles (e.g., safety belts, child safety seats), individuals who participate in high-impact or extreme sports (e.g., boxing, football, skateboarding), individuals who are frequently exposed to violence (e.g., victims

of abuse, individuals in gangs), and individuals who serve in the armed forces.

Prevention

Prevention of concussion and TBI revolves around safety measures already discussed, such as using vehicle restraint systems and wearing protective gear for sports activities. Provide patient teaching related to fall prevention (see the exemplar on Fractures in the module on Mobility). Institute safety precautions in hospital settings, including the following:

- Place call lights within reach.
- Follow medication administration protocols to prevent accidentally administering the wrong medication, the wrong dosage, or medications that are contraindicated with one another.
- Follow assessment protocols for patients taking medications that can cause confusion or altered mental status.

Refer to the exemplar on IICP to review ways of preventing secondary causes of TBI.

Clinical Manifestations

The clinical presentation of concussion and TBI will vary widely based on the cause and degree of damage to the brain. In general, the signs and symptoms associated with mild TBI or concussion are also associated with moderate to severe TBI, but they often manifest more severely in patients with a greater degree of brain injury. In addition, individuals with moderate to severe TBI will have symptoms reflective of greater impact, including skull fracture, bleeding in the brain, IICP, and lacerations. Depending on the cause of the injury, foreign objects may be embedded in the brain. These injuries produce not only physical changes to the brain and body, but also visual changes, auditory and vestibular changes, behavioral and cognitive changes, and language changes. For more information, see the Clinical Manifestations and Therapies feature and the Focus on Diversity and Culture feature.

As previously described, individuals with concussion are at risk for development of postconcussion syndrome. Based on the World Health Organization's ICD-10 criteria, manifestations of postconcussion syndrome include three or more of the following symptoms: headache, dizziness, fatigue, irritability, insomnia, difficulty concentrating, and memory difficulty (Leddy et al., 2012). Postconcussion syndrome may also include depression, apathy, anxiety, poor judgment, and personality changes (U.S. Department of Veterans Affairs [USDVA], 2015; Wilberger & Dupre, 2013a). Postconcussion syndrome is usually diagnosed if the signs and symptoms of concussion last longer than 2 weeks. SIS is an additional risk for individuals who participate in full-contact sports or military combat. SIS can be identified by a rapid increase in ICP and sudden loss of consciousness, which can potentially lead to death.

Individuals who are in the military are at increased risk for TBI related to gunshot wounds, blast injuries, falls, and motor vehicle collisions. Symptoms of TBI tend to last longer for members of the military than for most individuals, often persisting up to 18–24 months (USDVA,

Clinical Manifestations and Therapies
Concussion and TBI

ETIOLOGY	CLINICAL MANIFESTATIONS	CLINICAL THERAPIES
Physical changes	*Mild TBI/concussion:* ■ Possible loss of consciousness for 30 minutes or less ■ Nausea or vomiting ■ Headache, fatigue *Moderate/severe TBI:* ■ Loss of consciousness for a period of 30 minutes to several days or weeks ■ Skull fracture (may be evidenced by bleeding from facial orifices, Battle sign, raccoon eyes, drainage of CSF from ears or nose, and/or stiff neck; see **Figures 11–18 》** and **11–19 》**) ■ Bleeding in the brain ■ Increased ICP ■ Lacerations ■ Seizures ■ Loss of coordination, muscle weakness ■ Paralysis ■ Loss of bladder and bowel control ■ Difficulty breathing ■ Dysphagia	■ Administer acetaminophen. ■ Provide comfort measures to reduce environmental stimuli. ■ Surgery may be needed to repair skull fractures or remove hematomas. ■ Perform trauma responses: ensure airway, breathing, and circulation; stop bleeding of wounds; clean and bandage wounds; set fractured bones. ■ Monitor ICP. ■ Ensure the patient's safety during seizures. ■ Administer antiseizure medications. ■ Insert a urinary catheter as needed.

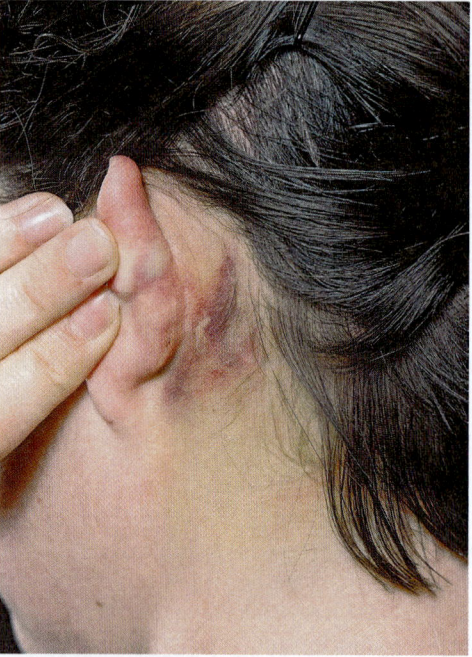

A

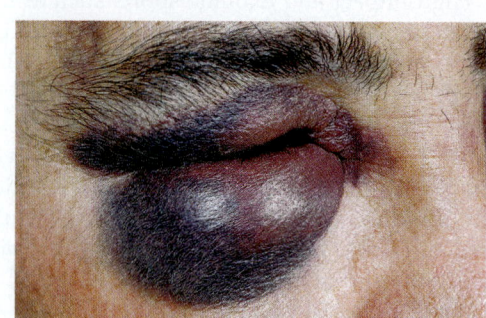

B

Source: Mediscan/Alamy Stock Photo.

Figure 11–19 》 *A,* Battle sign, and *B,* raccoon eyes.

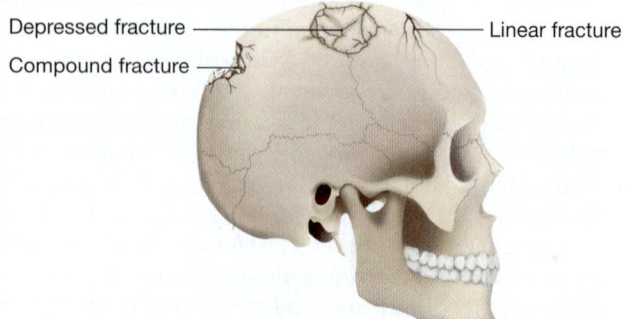

Depressed fracture

Compound fracture

Linear fracture

Figure 11–18 》 Types of temporal bone fractures.

Clinical Manifestations and Therapies *(continued)*

ETIOLOGY	CLINICAL MANIFESTATIONS	CLINICAL THERAPIES
Visual changes	*Mild TBI/concussion:* ▪ Double or blurred vision ▪ Sensitivity to light *Moderate/severe TBI:* ▪ Unequal pupils ▪ Pupils that are not reactive to light ▪ Loss of eye movement ▪ Problems with convergence and accommodation ▪ Blindness	▪ Monitor neurologic status frequently. ▪ Provide comfort measures. ▪ Clean wounds and place an eye patch over injured eyes. ▪ Prepare the patient for surgery if needed to repair eye damage.
Auditory and vestibular changes	*Mild TBI/concussion:* ▪ Sensitivity to sound ▪ Dizziness, impaired balance ▪ Tinnitus *Moderate/severe TBI:* ▪ Transient or permanent hearing loss ▪ Difficulty distinguishing words from background noise ▪ Mechanical injuries to ear structure	▪ Monitor neurologic status frequently. ▪ Provide comfort measures to reduce environmental noise. ▪ Use safety measures when the patient needs to stand or walk. ▪ Provide information about hearing aids, American Sign Language, and other aids as needed.
Behavioral changes	*Mild TBI/concussion:* ▪ Irritability *Moderate/severe TBI:* ▪ Depression ▪ Apathy ▪ Anxiety ▪ Personality changes ▪ Agitation ▪ Flat affect ▪ Aggression ▪ Problems with impulse control	▪ Monitor neurologic status frequently. ▪ Provide referrals to counselors as needed. ▪ Administer medications related to behavioral and emotional changes as prescribed.
Cognitive changes	*Mild TBI/concussion:* ▪ Confusion ▪ Trouble with memory or concentration ▪ Retrograde or anterograde amnesia ▪ Difficulty waking up *Moderate/severe TBI:* ▪ Poor judgment ▪ Reduced attention span ▪ Problems processing information ▪ Problems with short-term memory ▪ Deficits in orientation to person, place, and time ▪ Problems with self-care	▪ Monitor neurologic status frequently. ▪ Provide referrals to therapists who can help the patient regain cognitive skills. ▪ Provide orientation to person, place, and time as needed. ▪ Give the patient time to think through information and respond; it may take more time than usual to form a response. ▪ Provide teaching to the patient and/or family regarding how to perform hygiene care.
Verbal and language changes	*Mild TBI/concussion:* ▪ Slurred speech *Moderate/severe TBI:* ▪ Deficits in verbal and reading comprehension ▪ Decreased ability to articulate words ▪ Decreased knowledge about appropriate tone of voice ▪ Writing difficulty	▪ Provide referrals to speech therapists as needed. ▪ Be patient with the individual when communicating; allow the individual time to form thoughts and ideas and to verbalize or write them. ▪ Provide writing instruments and paper if the patient finds it easier to write than speak to communicate.

2015). Military personnel who experience a blast injury without other physical injury will often have TBI with auditory changes. The severity of these changes depends on the size of the blast, the distance from the blast, and the environment (ASHA, n.d.b). Approximately 7% of all military veterans have had a TBI, and of those, approximately 75% also have PTSD (Congressional Budget Office, 2012). Diagnosis is complicated by the fact that TBI and PTSD can have similar symptoms.

Collaboration

Care of the patient with concussion or TBI is likely to require collaboration among multiple healthcare providers. As with IICP, the nurse must be diligent and conduct careful and continuous neurologic assessments to help prevent further deterioration and/or loss of brain function. Depending on the cause and severity of the injury, the nurse may need to implement primary CAB protocols within the Basic Life Support guidelines and the ABC protocols within the Advanced Cardiac Life Support guidelines (these are protocols developed and taught by the American Red Cross and the American Heart Association that are required courses in emergency departments). Many times, TBI does not occur by itself, so the patient may have other injuries that take higher priority if neurologic presentation and evaluation indicate neurologic stability. (For discussion about diagnosis and treatment of injuries related to trauma to other body systems, see the module on Trauma.) Neurosurgeons, neurologists, general surgeons, orthopedic surgeons, craniofacial or maxillary surgeons, vascular surgeons, and/or hematologists may need to be consulted. As nurses assess the patient's and family's psychosocial and spiritual needs, they may need to offer assistance in calling a chaplain or spiritual advisor or make referrals to support groups and professional therapists.

Diagnostic Tests

Diagnostic tests depend heavily on the patient's presentation and the etiology of the injury.

Following the initial nursing and neurologic assessments, a CT scan or MRI scan (with proper cervical spine protection until cleared) of the head or other area of obvious injury may be ordered. A CT scan is vital to the diagnosis of TBI because it can detect the presence and location of skull fractures, contusions, hematomas, hemorrhage, and other brain damage. MRI scans are beneficial for providing more detailed brain images, including axonal injury, once the patient is stabilized (National Institute of Child Health and Human Development [NICHD], 2013). Any clear fluid that leaks from the patient's nose or ears should be assessed for CSF (glucose will be present), as this may be indicative of a basilar skull fracture. (Often Battle sign or raccoon eyes are also present.) Transcranial Doppler may be indicated for intracerebral hemorrhage and is especially useful with grading cerebral vasospasms that may accompany a subarachnoid hemorrhage. Any device that may be used to measure ICP may be utilized as needed. (For more information on measuring ICP, see the exemplar on IICP.)

In addition to diagnostic tests to assess the extent of the physical injury, the healthcare team should also perform cognition, neuropsychologic, and speech assessments. These tests should include patient or family interviews to determine the patient's cognitive and neurologic status before the injury as a baseline. Other tests may be needed to test the cranial nerves, depending on the location of the injury and the patient's presenting symptoms (see Table 11–1). These tests can help determine the extent of the patient's injury and the potential need for rehabilitation once the patient is stabilized.

Surgery

The patient's condition and the severity and type of injuries present will dictate what type of surgery may be required. Evacuation of a cerebral hematoma (especially an epidural hematoma) or contusion may be indicated. Skull, facial, or mandibular fractures may need surgical repair. Placement of a device to monitor ICP may be performed at the bedside or in the operating room if required. Removal of foreign bodies from the cranial vault may be necessary. Non-neurosurgical operations may also need to be performed and may be of higher priority than the insult sustained by the TBI.

Pharmacologic Therapy

Vasoactive medications may be required to keep the patient hemodynamically stable. Anesthesia may be necessary if the patient requires advanced airway management or surgery. Pain medications may be administered (see the module on Comfort), but doing so requires careful monitoring of neurologic, cardiovascular, and respiratory responses to prevent any deterioration of the patient. Medications to reduce IICP may be indicated (refer to Exemplar 11.A on IICP). Antiseizure medications may be used, especially if the patient is actively seizing or has an injury to the temporal lobe region, which carries a higher risk for seizure activity (refer to Exemplar 11.B on Seizure Disorders). Gastrointestinal prophylaxis should be initiated using H_2-receptor antagonists or proton pump inhibiting agents. Stool softeners and/or laxatives may be prescribed to prevent extension of cerebral injury if there is straining with bowel movements.

Nonpharmacologic Therapy

Individuals who have a TBI, especially a moderate or severe TBI, will likely need one or more types of rehabilitation or therapy depending on the extent of the patient's injury and alterations in functioning. Psychologists, social workers, and career counselors may be called in based on the extent of the TBI and the patient's ability to cope. In severe TBI, the family may need the help of clergy, grief counselors, or psychologists if the injury is severe enough to pose an immediate threat to life or has a bad prognosis. Rehabilitative facilities may be needed for short-term recovery after the acute phase of TBI, or assisted living or skilled nursing homes might be required for long-term or permanent residence based on the severity and outcome of the injury. Note that complementary health approaches are not recommended until the patient has had a medical evaluation and is cleared for discharge. Prior to discharge, the nurse should assess the patient to determine which complementary health approaches may be contraindicated based on the patient's current condition or medications.

Lifespan Considerations

Concussions and TBI can happen to any individual at any point in the lifespan. As outlined in the sections that follow, prevalence and risk factors vary. Note that falls and accidents (motor vehicle and otherwise) can affect all age groups, ethnic groups, races, and genders.

TBI in Infants and Toddlers

The primary cause of TBI in infants and toddlers is falls. Other causes include motor vehicle collisions (both passenger and pedestrian), accidental strikes to the head, and assault or child abuse. Assaults or child abuse is the leading cause of death for infants and children with TBI (CDC, 2016a). Injury patterns will depend on the cause of injury. For example, an infant who sustains a TBI from shaken baby syndrome will exhibit diffuse axonal injury, whereas a toddler who experiences a fall may have a local contusion with edema from a coup–contrecoup injury.

The types of injuries, treatment, and monitoring of ICP are similar for infants and toddlers as they are for adults. However, the Glasgow Coma Scale has been modified for infants who cannot respond verbally (see Table 11–3). In addition, the nurse should remember that infants and toddlers tend to express their discomfort in different ways than older children and adults. For example, an older child may be able to explain symptoms of nausea or pain, whereas a younger child may cry inconsolably, vomit, or be restless (Brain Injury Association of America [BIAA], n.d.). Therefore, the nurses should communicate with the child's parents to understand the child's normal activities and how those activities have changed since the brain injury. Infants and toddlers with TBI may experience a change in eating patterns or sleep habits, have seizures, become easily upset, be lethargic, or be uninterested in favorite toys (Mayo Clinic, 2014a). Of these changes, the appearance of seizures should be seen as a sign of severe injury and treated aggressively. In addition, retinal hemorrhage is often a sign of shaken baby syndrome and frequently associated with a subdural hematoma. Papilledema (optic disc swelling) is also a sign of IICP in young children and should be treated accordingly (Su, Huh, & Raghupathi, 2015).

TBI in Children and Adolescents

For school-age children and adolescents, common causes of TBI include falls, motor vehicle crashes, unintentional blunt trauma, sports-related injuries, and assaults. For children ages 5–14, falls are the leading cause of emergency department visits and hospitalization due to TBI. For adolescents ages 15–19, assaults are the leading cause of emergency department visits due to TBI, and motor vehicle collisions are the leading cause of hospitalization. Motor vehicle collisions are the leading cause of death due to TBI in both age groups. In addition, emergency department visits related to sports injuries continue to rise dramatically in this age group (CDC, 2016a).

Following TBI, the type of primary and secondary injuries sustained are similar in children and adults. However, children are more likely to have subdural hematomas and diffuse axonal injury than local contusions (Su et al., 2015). These injuries have similar symptoms and are diagnosed and treated similarly in all age groups. For younger children who are not able to describe their injuries, signs of TBI may be similar to those in infants and toddlers, including changes in eating or sleeping habits, irritability, depression, and lack of interest in favorite activities.

Adolescents present their own unique challenges when it comes to preventing TBI. Many adolescents, especially boys, are excited by dangerous and risky activities, including performing tricks on bicycles or skateboards, participating in full-contact sports, and driving too fast. All of these activities increase the risk for TBI, as do experimentation with drugs and alcohol. Adolescents often downplay their injuries or do not report them for fear of looking weak or being unable to participate in sports and other activities. This greatly increases their risk of being injured again and developing SIS, which can be fatal. Nurses play a vital role in helping prevent both first-time and repeated TBIs by providing appropriate patient teaching (see Patient Teaching feature).

Patient Teaching
Preventing TBI in Adolescents

Sports safety and community safety are vital to ensuring brain health for children, adolescents, and young adults. Some ways the nurse can help prevent TBI in adolescents include (American Academy of Pediatrics, 2016; American College of Sports Medicine, 2012; Children's Safety Network, 2013a; National Athletic Trainers' Association, 2013):

- Encourage the adolescent to have a full physical each year before participating in sports.
- Encourage the adolescent to always wear appropriate safety equipment when participating in sports or recreation, especially helmets. Helmets should be fitted properly based on the size of the adolescent's head.
- Teach adolescents the importance of avoiding plays that could cause TBI, including sliding headfirst (baseball/softball), tackling headfirst (football), and checking (hockey/lacrosse). This also includes performing dangerous tricks on bicycles, skateboards, and other recreational equipment.
- Teach adolescents the importance of learning proper techniques to use when playing sports in order to avoid head injuries; also teach them to follow the rules of the sport.
- Teach adolescents the importance of reporting all head injuries to a coach, physical trainer, parent, or other authority figure.
- Encourage adolescents to make sure a trusted adult with emergency training is present during activities, games, and practices to monitor for rough play and to respond to emergencies.
- Inform parents and adolescents about the risk of SIS if the adolescent returns to sports before the initial injury is healed.
- Teach parents and adolescents the signs and symptoms of TBI, concussion, and postconcussion syndrome, and their short- and long-term effects.
- Teach adolescents the importance of gradual return to full activity after a concussion: step 1: complete rest; step 2: light aerobic activity, no resistance training; step 3: sport-specific exercise and light resistance training; step 4: non-contact sports practice; step 5: full-contact sports practice; step 6: game play. If any symptoms return, revert to the previous step and progress again until no symptoms appear.

To help children and adolescents maintain safety before, during, and after a concussion, all 50 states and the District of Columbia have passed legislation regarding how to handle athletes with concussion. This legislation primarily states that athletes who sustain a concussion should be removed from play and not allowed to return until cleared by a physician. Some states also require coaches to complete a concussion management training program and recognize when a concussion has occurred. Most states also require schools to provide information to students and parents regarding concussion and to have students and parents sign that they have received this information. In a few states, these requirements are also applicable to private sports teams and public recreation facilities in addition to schools (Children's Safety Network, 2013b).

>> **Stay Current:** For more information about current legislation in each state regarding concussion and TBI, see http://www.ncsl.org/research/health/traumatic-brain-injury-legislation.aspx.

TBI in Pregnant Women

Women who experience TBI during pregnancy present both physical and ethical issues that must be considered during care. Because the medical personnel may not always know that the woman with TBI is pregnant, they should assume that all women of childbearing age are pregnant until this possibility has been ruled out. If a woman is known to be pregnant, fetal monitoring should begin immediately, because there is an increased risk to the fetus if the mother's TBI requires surgical intervention or compromises hemodynamics or oxygenation status (Schwaitzberg, Newton, & Mahoney, 2015). Refer to the module on Reproduction for more information on fetal monitoring.

In cases of severe TBI, the health and well-being of the mother and the fetus must be weighed against each other. If the fetus is not yet viable and the mother has the potential for being saved, the trauma team must focus solely on the health of the mother, because maternal death will lead to fetal death. If maternal death is imminent and the fetus is not yet viable, both may die as a result of the trauma. In this case, the family should be consulted about whether to maintain the mother on life support until the fetus is viable. For late-term pregnancy, delivery of the neonate by cesarean section may take priority over the health of the mother, especially if the mother has a poor expected outcome.

If both the mother and neonate survive the TBI, the mother will need additional support to care for her infant when she is discharged home, especially if she sustained a moderate to severe TBI with complications related to cognitive functioning, speech, or mobility. The nurse needs to assess the mother's injuries, long-term expected outcome, and support systems and help the mother make arrangements for additional help if needed.

TBI in Older Adults

Adults age 65 and older have the highest rates of hospitalizations and deaths due to TBI, with more than 80% of all TBIs in this age group being the result of falls (CDC, 2016a). The normal aging process causes comorbidities that increase fall risk, such as postural hypotension, poor eyesight, and impaired balance (Stippler, Holguin, & Nemoto, 2012). Older adults often have a worse outcome than younger individuals because of pre-existing complex conditions, polypharmacy, and susceptibility to complications. Falls that cause TBI also increase the incidence of hip fracture, which decreases the patient's independence and has a high rate of poor outcomes. In addition, some medications commonly used in older adults increase the risk of complications during TBI, in particular anticoagulant and antiplatelet drugs such as aspirin, warfarin, and clopidogrel. These drugs inhibit blood clotting, thus increasing the patient's risk for intracranial hemorrhage and death (Mak et al., 2012).

Mild TBI presents a challenging case in the older population. For individuals with mild dementia, signs of mild TBI are similar to signs of dementia and thus may go unnoticed. Mild TBI with a subdural hematoma may not cause noticeable symptoms for days or weeks in this population. Therefore, older adults with mild signs of TBI, especially those who are on anticoagulants, should be monitored for intracranial hemorrhage. Not surprising, individuals who experienced one or more TBIs at a younger age have an increased risk of developing dementia at an earlier age (Filer & Harris, 2015), putting these same individuals at higher risk for TBI later in life.

Older adults with moderate to severe TBI present both physical and ethical challenges. For many older adults with severe TBI, initial interventions may help save the life of the patient only to leave them in a persistent vegetative state, which may not be desired by the patient. Often the decision regarding whether to treat the patient aggressively is left up to the family. Prognostic outcomes based on the injury are often not good, and quality of life must be weighed against quantity of life (Stippler et al., 2012).

If older adults with TBI survive the initial injury, rehabilitation should begin immediately, even while they are still in the intensive care unit. Rehabilitation can help prevent complications such as skin breakdown, joint contractures, and pulmonary infections. Nurses should also be aware that manifestations of cognitive deficits in older adults may be due to either TBI or depression. Treatment of depression in older adults after TBI may improve cognitive outcomes (Stippler et al., 2012). Many older adults who survive to discharge will be placed in an inpatient rehabilitation center or long-term nursing care facility rather than released home.

NURSING PROCESS

Once patients with TBI and concussion are stabilized after the traumatic event, the major focus of care is preserving neurologic function that was not destroyed by the initial injury and preventing further brain damage from secondary injuries. The nurse must perform a complete and thorough neurologic examination that includes use of the Glasgow Coma Scale. Any change in or deterioration of the patient's neurologic status should be immediately conveyed to the physician.

Assessment

Thorough and rapid assessment of the patient with a TBI is necessary to determine the severity of the injury and to identify any comorbid complications or conditions. The assessment also helps identify potential complications that the nurse needs to monitor.

- **Observation and patient interview.** Patients with a mild TBI/concussion often show few visible signs of injury, although vomiting, confusion, impaired balance, and sensitivity to light may be observed by the nurse. Patients with moderate to severe TBI may have more noticeable symptoms, including unconsciousness, bleeding or drainage of CSF from facial orifices, Battle sign or raccoon eyes, protrusion of a foreign object, flat affect, reduced attention span, and decreased ability to articulate words. Some signs of a concussion or TBI may be known only after the patient interview, which may involve interviewing either the patient or the patient's family and friends, depending on the severity of the injury and the patient's LOC. Ask about the precipitating event, length of time the patient was unconscious, whether the patient has amnesia, and whether the patient has symptoms such as headache or vision or hearing problems.

- **Physical examination.** Once the patient is stabilized, the first priority for physical examination related to TBI or concussion is the Glasgow Coma Scale. Use of the scale provides a baseline for comparison to determine whether the patient is improving or deteriorating. The nurse may also need to prepare the patient for a CT scan shortly after entry to the emergency department. The nurse will eventually need to perform an accurate and complete neurologic examination, with assessment of cranial nerves, spinal nerves, and reflexes, especially focusing on vision and hearing difficulties. Depending on the injury, not all pieces of the examination may be able to be performed. Once a baseline is established, assessment and physical examination must be ongoing, ranging from every 15 minutes, to every hour, to every 2–4 hours depending on the patient's condition. This is a dynamic process, and the frequency of examination may change at any time based on the patient's status. Any changes in the patient's Glasgow Coma Scale score that indicate deterioration should be relayed to the physician accurately and immediately.

Diagnosis

Common nursing diagnoses for the patient with concussion (mild TBI) include:

- *Pain, Acute*
- *Confusion, Acute*
- *Memory, Impaired*
- *Nausea.*

(NANDA-I © 2014)

In addition to diagnoses appropriate for mild TBI, common nursing diagnoses for the patient with moderate to severe TBI include:

- *Bleeding, Risk for*
- *Tissue Perfusion: Cerebral, Ineffective*
- *Verbal Communication, Impaired*

- *Development, Risk for Delayed*
- *Post-Trauma Syndrome, Risk for.*

(NANDA-I © 2014)

Planning

Nursing care for the patient with a concussion or TBI focuses on maintaining homeostasis and stable vital signs, ensuring a patent airway, preventing or controlling further brain injury, providing emotional support to the patient and family, and administering medications as ordered. Planning should include care of the patient in the inpatient setting, a transitional setting, and the outpatient setting. Many patients may require extensive rehabilitative services to ensure they attain their best possible outcome. Nurses should help patients and their families find support groups or other available resources. Goals may include:

- The patient will not experience further brain injury related to hemodynamic instability.
- The patient will maintain a patent airway and effective respiratory function.
- The patient and their family will have adequate support to manage self-image, self-care, and role performance.
- The patient and family will be aware of realistic outcomes based on the severity of the brain injury.
- The patient and family will experience minimal disruption of educational, social, and workplace activities due to TBI to the greatest extent possible.
- The patient will articulate steps to reduce risk for injury after discharge.
- The patient will articulate signs and symptoms indicating the need to return for immediate assessment by the healthcare provider.

Implementation

Nursing interventions will vary widely depending on the severity and type of injury. In addition, because TBI is often accompanied by trauma to other body systems, nursing interventions may require the nurse to prioritize other interventions unrelated to the head injury.

Patients with moderate to severe TBI will require more extensive care than patients with mild TBI. Many of these interventions are similar to those needed for patients who have experienced trauma (see the module on Trauma) or who have IICP (Exemplar 11.A), including maintaining adequate oxygenation, monitoring and reducing ICP, and treating wounds. Similar to these patients, individuals with moderate to severe TBI will likely require diagnostic testing, particularly a CT scan, and they may need emergency surgery to remove a hematoma or repair a skull fracture.

The nursing interventions outlined below focus on caring for patients with a brain injury following stabilization.

Provide Patient Teaching Related to Concussion

Concussion often resolves itself with little to no intervention. Therefore, nurses are responsible for providing comfort measures for patients, such as administering acetaminophen and reducing environmental stimulation. In addition, nurses should provide patient teaching related to monitoring the patient at home and restricting activities. Appropriate actions may include the following:

- Provide patient teaching related to the signs of postconcussion syndrome, including headache, dizziness, irritability, and memory difficulty, among others. Inform the patient and patient's family or friends that they should seek medical care for the patient if these symptoms appear.

- Provide patient teaching related to appropriate activity levels. If no symptoms are present, the patient can return to work or school but should refrain from sports for at least 7–10 days for complete healing and to ensure that no postconcussion symptoms appear. Return to any physical activity that may increase ICP should be gradual, and the patient should be consistently monitored for returning symptoms throughout this process.

- Provide patient teaching related to SIS and the hazards of participating in sports and other activities that could cause a second concussion before the original concussion is healed.

Provide Emotional Support

Many patients who sustain moderate to severe TBI will either be permanently disabled or will die. The nurse should be available to provide emotional support to the patient and family in these circumstances.

Strategies for providing emotional support include discussing the patient's condition, prognosis, and limitations openly and honestly; listening to patient and family fears and concerns; providing an atmosphere that encourages patients and family members to discuss their feelings honestly in appropriate ways; and acknowledging feelings of patients and family members in a nonjudgmental manner. In addition, nurses can provide encouragement to the patient and family to promote the hard work of rehabilitation. Patients who are motivated to achieve will make more progress during rehabilitation than those who have an attitude of defeat and hopelessness. As always, provide referrals to a counselor or clergy member as appropriate.

Prepare the Patient and Family for Discharge

Patients with moderate to severe TBI who survive the initial injury and recover sufficiently to be discharged from the hospital will likely require months of rehabilitation. The nurse is responsible for discussing with the patient what to expect in the weeks and months to come.

- Provide information about what to expect from different types of therapy, including but not limited to physical therapy, occupational therapy, and speech therapy. Provide referrals or facilitate initial appointments as appropriate.

- Discuss potential needs for home care and provide patient teaching for the family related to these needs. For example, the nurse may provide patient teaching related to feeding the patient, bathing the patient, dressing the patient, and other daily activities.

- Educate patients to engage in light activity around the home, to keep their diet light if they experience nausea or vomiting, and to have an adult stay with them for 12–24 hours after leaving the emergency department.

- Teach patients that after discharge, sleep is okay, but for the first 12 hours after discharge, someone should wake them every 2–3 hours to ask simple questions and look for changes in the way they act.

- Inform patients that acetaminophen (Tylenol) is acceptable but that aspirin and nonsteroidal anti-inflammatories should be avoided.

- Educate patients to contact the health provider if any of the following signs or symptoms occur: stiff neck, fluid leaking from nose or ears, chronic sleepiness, worsening headache, fever, vomiting, problems walking or talking, problems thinking, seizures, or changes in vision.

Evaluation

The patient with a concussion or mild TBI should be evaluated based on the following expected outcomes:

- The patient verbalizes an understanding of activity limitations, including when to return to sports.

- The patient or the patient's caregiver verbalize understanding related to signs of postconcussion syndrome and worsening neurologic status.

- The patient shows no further signs of deterioration on the Glasgow Coma Scale.

The patient with moderate to severe TBI should also be evaluated on the following expected outcomes:

- The patient maintains a patent airway and does not sustain secondary brain injury due to hypoxia or lung injury due to aspiration.

- The patient and patient's family maintain a positive attitude about the patient's recovery while still feeling free to express feelings of grief and loss.

- The patient and patient's family have realistic goals for outcomes after brain injury.

- The patient and patient's family verbalize an understanding of available community resources.

- The patient attends all therapy sessions and makes progress toward recovery with each session.

- The patient's family demonstrate the ability to provide daily care for the patient, including bathing, dressing, and feeding.

Recovery from TBI is a lengthy process, and the patient's condition is likely to deteriorate at times, especially in the hours after the injury. The nurse's most important responsibility during this time is to maintain the patient's airway, breathing, and circulation. This may require adding mechanical ventilation, performing CPR, or defibrillating the patient's heart. The nurse should also prioritize efforts to stop any bleeding, to administer medications or blood products as ordered, and to provide emotional support to the patient's family. After the initial emergency is over, the nurse will be responsible for preventing complications, including but not limited to encouraging the use of antiembolism stockings, administering laxatives if needed for constipation, inserting a urinary catheter to prevent bladder distention, checking wounds and incisions for infection and drainage, and monitoring ICP.

Nursing Care Plan
A Patient with a Concussion

Tyler Galecko is a 14-year-old boy with no comorbidities. He has been skateboarding for 4 years and enjoys trying new tricks with his friends. He usually does not wear a helmet because none of his friends do. Tyler was trying a new jump and fell and hit his head on the concrete. His friends rushed over to him and found that he was complaining of nausea and a bad headache. After a few minutes, he said he wanted to go home because the hot sun was making his head hurt worse.

ASSESSMENT	DIAGNOSIS	PLANNING
When Tyler's friends brought him home, his mother was sufficiently concerned to bring him to the emergency department. On arrival at the emergency department, Tyler was awake and oriented to person, place, and time, although he kept his eyes closed because he said the light hurt them. He said he did not lose consciousness and that he remembered the events leading up to the accident. Tyler still complained of nausea, a headache, and sensitivity to light. He had a small bump on his head from where he hit the ground. His vital signs were HR 88 bpm, R 16/min, BP 112/72 mmHg, and SpO$_2$ 98% on room air. He had a Glasgow Coma Scale score of 14.	*Acute Pain* related to patient report of headache *Nausea* related to head injury *Risk for bleeding* related to unintentional blow to the head (NANDA-I © 2014)	■ The patient will reveal no bleeding on the CT scan. ■ The patient will report reduced pain and sensitivity to light. ■ The patient will report reduced nausea. ■ The patient will have a Glasgow Coma Scale score of 15 before discharge. ■ The patient and parent will report understanding related to the use of personal protective equipment while skateboarding.

IMPLEMENTATION

The nurse's primary role in this case is providing comfort measures and patient teaching related to skateboarding safety. Implementation includes:

■ Prepare the patient for a CT scan.

■ If no bleeding is present, administer acetaminophen as prescribed for acute pain.

■ Dim the lights as needed to reduce discomfort.

■ Provide an emesis basin for the patient.

■ Provide patient teaching related to the use of helmets and safety pads when skateboarding.

■ Provide patient teaching related to signs and symptoms of worsening brain injury and when to seek further medical attention.

■ Provide patient teaching related to when the patient can return to skateboarding.

EVALUATION

Tyler's CT scan revealed no bleeding. One hour after administration of acetaminophen and sitting in a dark room, Tyler states that his headache is less and he no longer feels nauseated. After turning on the room lights, Tyler states that the light does not hurt his eyes. His new Glasgow Coma Scale score is 15. After receiving patient teaching, Tyler and his mother state their understanding of the importance of wearing a properly fitting helmet and safety pads while skateboarding. Tyler also states that he will refrain from skateboarding for at least 1 week to allow his head to heal. Tyler's mother states her understanding of the signs and symptoms of postconcussion syndrome and when to seek medical care if Tyler's condition deteriorates.

CRITICAL THINKING

1. What interview questions should the nurse ask to help determine the extent of Tyler's injury?

2. What tests might have been ordered if Tyler was unresponsive, had HR 132 bpm, R 28/min, BP 134/88 mmHg, and SpO$_2$ 86% on room air?

3. What interventions could the nurse perform if Tyler presented with the symptoms in question 2?

REVIEW Traumatic Brain Injury

RELATE Link the Concepts and Exemplars

Linking the exemplar of traumatic brain injury with the concept of comfort:

1. What nursing interventions can be performed for the patient with TBI who is complaining of headache and photophobia?

2. If pain medication is ordered for this patient, what should the nurse assess for following medication administration?

Linking the exemplar of traumatic brain injury with the concept of mood and affect:

3. You are caring for a patient who has lost vision in one eye due to TBI. What questions could you ask to see how she is feeling about the loss?

4. What would be some signs, symptoms, or statements by the patient that would prompt you to seek additional support for this patient? What services would you seek?

Linking the exemplar of traumatic brain injury with the concept of ethics:

5. You are caring for an 87-year-old patient with multiple comorbidities and a rapidly decreasing LOC after a fall in her home. What questions should you ask the patient's family?

6. The family wants treatment that goes against the patient's wishes. What can you do?

READY Go to Volume 3: Clinical Nursing Skills

REFER Go to Pearson MyLab Nursing and eText

REFLECT Apply Your Knowledge

Cheryl Struthers is a married 23-year-old technical writer who just had her first child 2 months ago. The baby has been very fussy, and Cheryl has not been getting a lot of sleep. One night when she wakes up to feed the baby, Cheryl stumbles down eight steps and lands at the bottom. She loses consciousness. Cheryl's husband Mike hears the baby crying and gets up to see what is wrong. He sees Cheryl at the bottom of the steps. She opens her eyes only when Mike talks to her and seems able to follow commands. She does not remember having a baby or what she was doing before she fell.

1. Assign Cheryl a Glasgow Coma Scale score and explain how you came to your conclusion.

2. Name three priority nursing interventions for Cheryl.

3. Given this information, what tests would you anticipate being ordered for Cheryl?

References

American Academy of Neurology (AAN). (2013). *AAN issues updated sports concussion guideline: Athletes with suspected concussion should be removed from play.* Retrieved from https://www.aan.com/pressroom/home/pressrelease/1164

American Academy of Pediatrics. (2016). *2016 sports injury prevention tip sheet.* Retrieved from https://www.aap.org/en-us/about-the-aap/aap-pressroom/news-features-and-safety-tips/pages/sports-injury-prevention-tip-sheet.aspx

American Association of Neurological Surgeons (AANS). (n.d.). *Concussion.* Retrieved from http://www.aans.org/patient%20information/conditions%20and%20treatments/concussion.aspx

American Association of Neurological Surgeons (AANS). (2014). *Sports-related head injury.* Retrieved from http://www.aans.org/patient%20information/conditions%20and%20treatments/sports-related%20head%20injury.aspx

American College of Obstetricians and Gynecologists (ACOG). (2013). *Seizure disorders in pregnancy.* Retrieved from http://www.acog.org/~/media/For%20Patients/faq129.pdf

American College of Sports Medicine. (2012). *Sport-related concussions.* Retrieved from http://www.acsm.org/public-information/articles/2012/01/13/sport-related-concussions

American Psychiatric Association. (2013). *Diagnostic and statistical manual of mental disorders (DSM-5)* (5th ed.). Arlington, VA: Author.

American Speech-Language-Hearing Association (ASHA). (n.d.a). *Common classifications of TBI.* Retrieved from http://www.asha.org/Practice-Portal/Clinical-Topics/Traumatic-Brain-Injury-in-Adults/Common-Classifications-of-TBI/

American Speech-Language-Hearing Association (ASHA). (n.d.b). *Traumatic brain injury in adults.* Retrieved from http://www.asha.org/PRP-SpecificTopic.aspx?folderid=8589935337&section=Signs_and_Symptoms

Austin, J., & Abdulla, A. (2013). Identifying and managing epilepsy in older adults. *Nursing Times.* Retrieved from http://www.nursingtimes.net/clinical-archive/neurology/identifying-and-managing-epilepsy-in-older-adults/5053730.fullarticle

Baxendale, S. (2015). *Non-pharmacological treatments for epilepsy: The case for and against complementary and alternative medicines.* Retrieved from https://www.epilepsysociety.org.uk/sites/default/files/attachments/Chapter35Baxendale2015.pdf

Boggs, J. G. (2016). *Simple partial seizures.* Retrieved from http://emedicine.medscape.com/article/1184384-overview

Brain Injury Association of America (BIAA). (n.d.). *Brain injury in children.* Retrieved from http://www.biausa.org/brain-injury-children.htm

BU CTE Center. (n.d.). *What is CTE?* Retrieved from http://www.bu.edu/cte/about/what-is-cte/

Carroll, E., & Benbadis, S. R., (2016). *Complex partial seizures.* Retrieved from http://emedicine.medscape.com/article/1183962-overview

Centers for Disease Control and Prevention (CDC). (2016a). *TBI: Get the facts.* Retrieved from http://www.cdc.gov/traumaticbraininjury/get_the_facts.html

Centers for Disease Control and Prevention (CDC). (2016b). *Epilepsy fast facts.* Retrieved from http://www.cdc.gov/epilepsy/basics/fast-facts.htm

Chang, P., Terbach, N., Plant, N., Chen, P. E., Walker, M. C., & Williams, R. S. B. (2013). Seizure control by ketogenic diet-associated medium chain fatty acids. *Neuropharmacology, 69*(100), 105–114.

Children's Safety Network. (2013a). *Strategies for preventing sport-related concussions and subsequent injury.* Waltham, MA: Author.

Children's Safety Network. (2013b). *Legislation on sport-related concussions.* Waltham, MA: Author.

Christensen, B. (2014). *Pediatric Glasgow Coma Scale.* Retrieved from http://emedicine.medscape.com/article/2058902-overview

Congressional Budget Office. (2012). *The Veteran's Health Administration's treatment of PTSD and traumatic brain injury among recent combat veterans.* Retrieved from https://www.cbo.gov/sites/default/files/cbofiles/attachments/02-09-PTSD.pdf

Defense and Veterans Brain Injury Center. (2016). *Cumulative concussions.* Retrieved from http://dvbic.dcoe.mil/about-traumatic-brain-injury/article/cumulative-concussions

Dhawan, V., & DeGeorgia, M. (2012). Neurointensive care biophysiological monitoring. *Journal of Neurointerventional Surgery, 4*(6), 407–413.

Epilepsy Foundation. (2013a). *Types of surgeries.* Retrieved from http://www.epilepsy.com/learn/treating-seizures-and-epilepsy/surgery/types-surgeries

Epilepsy Foundation. (2013b). *Complementary health approaches.* Retrieved from http://www.epilepsy.com/learn/treating-seizures-and-epilepsy/complementary-health-approaches

Epilepsy Foundation. (2013c). *How long do children need seizure medicine?* Retrieved from http://www.epilepsy.com/learn/seizures-youth/about-kids/how-long-do=children-need-seizure-medicine

Epilepsy Foundation. (2014a). *Epilepsy statistics.* Retrieved from http://www.epilepsy.com/learn/epilepsy-statistics

Epilepsy Foundation. (2014b). *What are the risk factors?* Retrieved from http://www.epilepsy.com/learn/epilepsy-101/what-are-risk-factors

Epilepsy Foundation. (2014c). *Epilepsy and the senior community.* Retrieved from http://www.epilepsy.com/learn/age-groups/epilepsy-and-senior-community

Epilepsy Society. (2015). *Complementary therapies.* Retrieved from https://www.epilepsysociety.org.uk/complementary-therapies#.VyJABSMrIy4

Faught, E., Richman, J., Martin, R., Funkhouser, E., Foushee, R., Kratt, P., … Pisu, M. (2012). Incidence and prevalence of epilepsy among older US Medicare beneficiaries. *Neurology, 78*(7), 448–453.

Filer, W., & Harris, M. (2015). Falls and traumatic brain injury among older adults. *North Carolina Medical Journal, 76*(2), 111–114.

Friel, L. A. (2014). *Seizure disorders in pregnancy.* Retrieved from http://www.merckmanuals.com/professional/gynecology-and-obstetrics/pregnancy-complicated-by-disease/seizure-disorders-in-pregnancy

Giger, J. N. (2013). *Transcultural nursing: Assessment and intervention* (6th ed.). St. Louis, MO: Elsevier/Mosby.

Glasgow Coma Scale. (2014). *What is the Glasgow Coma Scale?* Retrieved from http://glasgowcomascale.org/what-is-gcs/

Goh, S., & Ng, B. (2013). Epilepsy—A cross-cultural perspective. *ASEAN Journal of Psychiatry, 14*(2), 187–189.

Gupta, G., & Nosko, M. G. (2015). *Intracranial pressure monitoring.* Retrieved from http://www.emedicine.medscape.com/article1829950-overview

Haddad, S. H., & Arabi, Y. M. (2012). Critical care management of severe traumatic brain injury in adults. *Scandinavian Journal of Trauma, Resuscitation and Emergency Medicine, 20*, 12.

Herdman, T. H. & Kamitsuru, S. (Eds.). Nursing *Diagnoses—Definitions and Classification 2015–2017.*

Copyright © 2014, 1994–2014 NANDA International. Used by arrangement with John Wiley & Sons, Inc. Companion website: www.wiley.com/go/nursingdiagnoses

International League Against Epilepsy. (2013). *Epilepsy and genetics: Things you want to know.* Retrieved from http://www.ilae.org/Commission/genetics/documents/Genetics-Pamphlet-2013.pdf

International League Against Epilepsy (ILAE). (2017). New ILAE seizure classification. Retrieved from https://www.ilae.org/news-and-media/news-about-ilae/new-ilae-seizure-classification

Jevon, P. (n.d.). *Annex 3.* Retrieved from http://www.sign.ac.uk/pdf/sign110_annex3.pdf

Kantor, D. (2015). *Increased intracranial pressure.* Retrieved from https://www.nlm.nih.gov/medlineplus/ency/article/000793.htm

Kirkman, M. A., & Smith, M. (2014). Intracranial pressure monitoring, cerebral perfusion pressure estimation, and ICP/CPP-guided therapy: A standard of care or optional extra after brain injury? *British Journal of Anaesthesia, 112*(1), 35–46.

Ko, D. Y., & Sahai-Srivastava, S. (2015). *Generalized tonic-clonic seizures.* Retrieved from http://emedicine.medscape.com/article/1184608-overview

Krucik, G. (2014). *Natural treatments for epilepsy.* Retrieved from http://www.healthline.com/health/natural-treatments-epilepsy

Kurland, D., Hong, C., Aarabi, B., Gerzanich, V., & Simard, J. M. (2012). Hemorrhagic progression of a concussion after traumatic brain injury. *Journal of Neurotrauma, 29*(1), 19–31.

Leddy, J. J., Sandhu, H., Sodhi, V., Baker, J. G., & Willer, B. (2012). Rehabilitation of concussion and post-concussion syndrome. *Sports Health, 4*(2), 147–154.

Lee, K. G. (2015). *Intraventricular hemorrhage of the newborn.* Retrieved from http://www.nlm.nih.gov/medlineplus/ency/article/007301.htm

Liu, B., Liu, S., Yin, A., & Siddiqi, J. (2015). Risks and benefits of stress ulcer prophylaxis in adult neo-critical care patients: A systematic review and meta-analysis of randomized controlled trials. *Critical Care, 19*, 409.

Mak, C. H. K., Wong, S. K. H., Wong, G. K., Ng, S., Wang, K. K. W., Lam, P. K., & Poon, W. S. (2012). Traumatic brain injury in the elderly: Is it as bad as we think? *Current Translational Geriatrics and Experimental Gerontology Reports, 1*(3), 171–178.

Mayo Clinic. (2014a). *Traumatic brain injury.* Retrieved from http://www.mayoclinic.org/diseases-conditions/traumatic-brain-injury/basics/definition/con-20029302

Mayo Clinic. (2014b). *Epilepsy and pregnancy: What you need to know.* Retrieved from http://www.mayoclinic.org/healthy-lifestyle/pregnancy-week-by-week/in-depth/pregnancy/art-20048417

Mayo Clinic. (2014c). *Post-concussion syndrome.* Retrieved from http://www.mayoclinic.org/diseases-conditions/post-concussion-syndrome/basics/definition/con-20032705

Mayo Clinic. (2014d). *Concussion.* Retrieved from http://www.mayoclinic.org/diseases-conditions/concussion/basics/definition/con-20019272

Mayo Clinic. (2015a). *Epilepsy.* Retrieved from http://www.mayoclinic.org/diseases-conditions/epilepsy/home/ovc-20117206

Mayo Clinic. (2015b). *Epilepsy surgery.* Retrieved from http://www.mayoclinic.org/tests-procedures/epilepsy-surgery/basics/definition/prc-20014204

Mayo Clinic. (2015c). *Vagus nerve stimulation.* Retrieved from http://www.mayoclinic.org/tests-procedures/vagus-nerve-stimulation/home/ovc-20167755

McCarthy, J. (2013). *Licox brain tissue oxygen monitoring system.* Retrieved from http://www.ele.uri.edu/Courses/bme181/S13/2_JeffreyM_2.pdf

Mollan, S. P., Markey, K. A., Benzimra, J. D., Jacks, A., Matthews, T. D., Burdon, M. A., & Sinclair, A. J. (2014). A practical approach to diagnosis, assessment and management of idiopathic intracranial hypertension. *Practical Neurology, 14*(6), 380–390.

Myers, C. T., & Mefford, H. C. (2015). Advancing epilepsy genetics in the genomic era. *Genome Medicine, 7*(1), 91.

National Athletic Trainers' Association. (2013). *National action plan for sports safety.* Retrieved from http://www.youthsportssafetyalliance.org/sites/default/files/docs/National-Action-Plan.pdf

National Hydrocephalus Foundation. (2014). *Treatment of hydrocephalus.* Retrieved from http://www.nhfonline.org/treatment-of-hydrocephalus.htm

National Institute of Child Health and Human Development (NICHD). (2013). *How do health care providers diagnose traumatic brain injury (TBI)?* Retrieved from https://www.nichd.nih.gov/health/topics/tbi/conditioninfo/Pages/diagnose.aspx

National Institute of Neurological Disorders and Stroke (NINDS). (2015). *Febrile seizures fact sheet.* Retrieved from http://www.ninds.nih.gov/disorders/febrile_seizures/detail_febrile_seizures.htm

National Institute of Neurological Disorders and Stroke (NINDS). (2016). *Hydrocephalus fact sheet.* Retrieved from http://www.ninds.nih.gov/disorders/hydrocephalus/detail_hydrocephalus.htm

National Institutes of Health. (2016). *Seizures.* Retrieved from http://www.nlm.nih.gov/medlineplus/seizures.html

Nationwide Children's Hospital. (2015). *Increased intracranial pressure.* Retrieved from http://www.nationwidechildrens.org/increased-intracranial-pressure-1

Nelson, S. (2016). *Hydrocephalus.* Retrieved from http://www.emedicine.medscape.com/article/1135286-overview

NSGMED. (2014). *Increased intracranial pressure, management.* Retrieved from http://www.nsgmed.com/neuro/increased-intracranial-pressure-part-4/

Pew Research Center. (2013). *Religious groups' views on end-of-life issues.* Retrieved from http://www.pewforum.org/2013/11/21/religious-groups-views-on-end-of-life-issues/

Rangel-Castilla, L., Salinas, P., Hanbali, F., & Gasco, J. (2016). *Closed head injury.* Retrieved from http://emedicine.medscape.com/article/251834-overview

Ropper, A. (2012). Hyperosmolar therapy for raised intracranial pressure. *New England Journal of Medicine, 367*, 746–752.

Roth, J. L., & Blum, A. S. (2016). *Status epilepticus.* Retrieved from http://emedicine.medscape.com/article/1164462-overview

Royal Children's Hospital Melbourne. (n.d.). *Religion, culture, and life support.* Retrieved from http://www.rch.org.au/caringdecisions/Chapters/Religion,_culture_and_life_support/

Roytowski, D., & Figaji, A. (2013). Raised intracranial pressure: What it is and how to recognize it. *Continuing Medical Education, 31*(3), 85–90.

Russ, S. A., Larson, K., & Halfon, N. (2012). A national profile of childhood epilepsy and seizure disorder. *Pediatrics, 129*(2), 256–264.

Schwaitzberg, S. D., Newton, E. R., & Mahoney, B. (2015). *Trauma and pregnancy.* Retrieved from http://emedicine.medscape.com/article/435224-overview

Segan, S. (2015). *Absence seizures.* Retrieved from http://reference.medscape.com/article/1183858-overview

Shelat, A. M. (2015). *Partial (focal) seizure.* Retrieved from http://www.nlm.nih.gov/medlineplus/ency/article/000697.htm

Society for Neuroscience. (n.d.). *Cerebral atrophy.* Retrieved from http://www.brainfacts.org/diseases-disorders/diseases-a-to-z-from-ninds/cerebral-atrophy/

Spector, R. E. (2017). *Cultural diversity in health and illness* (9th ed.). Hoboken, NJ: Pearson Education.

Spiegel, R. (2014). *A moratorium on steroids for TBI.* Retrieved from http://www.emlitofnote.com/2014/08/a-moratorium-on-steroids-for-tbi.html?m=1

Stippler, M., Holguin, E., & Nemoto, E. (2012). Traumatic brain injury in elders. *Annals of Long-Term Care, 20*(5).

Su, F., Huh, J. W., & Raghupathi, R. (2015). *Traumatic brain injury in children.* Retrieved from http://emedicine.medscape.com/article/909105-overview#a1

U.S. Department of Veterans Affairs (USDVA). (2015). *Traumatic brain injury and PTSD.* Retrieved from http://www.ptsd.va.gov/public/problems/traumatic_brain_injury_and_ptsd.asp

Wickman, G. (2016). *The levels of coma.* Retrieved from http://www.healthguidance.org/entry/14188/1/The-Levels-of-Coma.html

Wilberger, J. E., & Dupre, D. A. (2013a). *Traumatic brain injury.* Retrieved from http://www.merckmanuals.com/professional/injuries-poisoning/traumatic-brain-injury-tbi/traumatic-brain-injury

Wilberger, J. E., & Dupre, D. A. (2013b). *Sports-related concussion.* Retrieved from http://www.merckmanuals.com/professional/injuries-poisoning/traumatic-brain-injury-tbi/sports-related-concussion

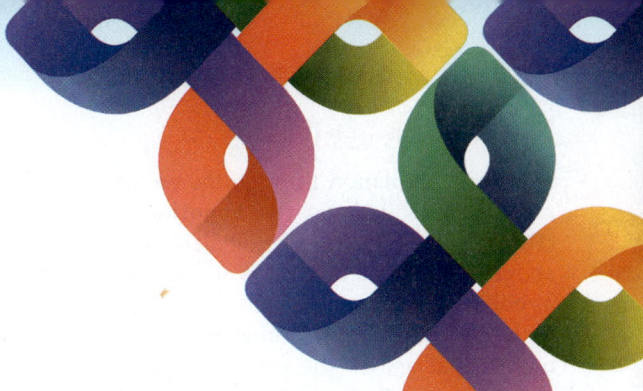

Module 12
Metabolism

Module Outline and Learning Outcomes

The Concept of Metabolism

Normal Metabolism
12.1 Analyze the physiology of metabolism in the body.

Alterations to Metabolism
12.2 Differentiate alterations in metabolism.

Concepts Related to Metabolism
12.3 Outline the relationship between metabolism and other concepts.

Health Promotion
12.4 Explain the promotion of healthy metabolism.

Nursing Assessment
12.5 Differentiate common assessment procedures and tests used to examine metabolism.

Independent Interventions
12.6 Analyze independent interventions nurses can implement for patients with alterations in metabolism.

Collaborative Therapies
12.7 Summarize collaborative therapies used by interprofessional teams for patients with alterations in metabolism.

Lifespan Considerations
12.8 Differentiate considerations related to the assessment and care of patients with alterations in metabolism throughout the lifespan.

Metabolism Exemplars

Exemplar 12.A Type 1 Diabetes Mellitus
12.A Analyze type 1 diabetes mellitus as it relates to metabolism.

Exemplar 12.B Type 2 Diabetes Mellitus
12.B Analyze type 2 diabetes mellitus as it relates to metabolism.

Exemplar 12.C Liver Disease
12.C Analyze liver disease as it relates to metabolism.

Exemplar 12.D Osteoporosis
12.D Analyze osteoporosis as it relates to metabolism.

Exemplar 12.E Thyroid Disease
12.E Analyze thyroid disease as it relates to metabolism.

» The Concept of Metabolism

Concept Key Terms

Acromegaly, **790**	Dwarfism, **801**	Hormones, **785**	Insulin, **789**	Type 1 diabetes (T1D), **791**
Addison disease, **791**	Exophthalmos, **799**	Hyperthyroidism, **790**	Metabolism, **785**	
Carpal spasm, **801**	Glucagon, **789**	Hypothalamic-pituitary axis (HPA), **786**	Tetany, **791**	Type 2 diabetes (T2D), **791**
Chvostek sign, **801**	Goiter, **790**		Trousseau sign, **801**	
Cushing syndrome, **791**	Gonadotropins, **789**	Hypothyroidism, **790**		

etabolism is a collection of biochemical reactions that occur in the body's cells to produce energy, repair cells, and maintain life. Much of the metabolic process takes place in the digestive system, as the body processes nutrients from food and drink and transports the nutrients across cell membranes for use throughout the body (see the module on Digestion and module on Nutrition for more information). Equally as important, the endocrine system controls the process of metabolism through the release of hormones. **Hormones** are chemical messengers that are secreted by endocrine glands. Their purpose is to regulate metabolism, growth, reproduction, fluid and electrolyte balance, gender differentiation, and other functions within the cells of the body.

Normal Metabolism

Hormone regulation through the endocrine system is primarily controlled via the **hypothalamic-pituitary axis (HPA)**. In the HPA, the hypothalamus, which is located just above the brain stem, detects signals from the brain as well as circulating hormone levels. If the hormone levels are too high or too low, the hypothalamus secretes regulatory hormones that act on the pituitary gland, which is located directly beneath the hypothalamus. When the pituitary gland detects hormones from the hypothalamus, it increases or decreases the secretion of additional hormones. Whereas the hormones secreted by the hypothalamus work primarily on the pituitary gland, the hormones secreted by the pituitary gland travel through the bloodstream to regulate multiple major endocrine glands (see **Figure 12–1 »**). The regulation of these endocrine glands by the HPA helps maintain homeostasis throughout the body.

Physiology Review

The human body contains nine endocrine glands: hypothalamus, pituitary gland, thyroid gland, parathyroid gland, adrenal glands, pancreas (specifically the islets of Langerhans), thymus, pineal gland, and gonads (ovaries in women and testes in men). The locations of these glands are illustrated in **Figure 12–2 »**. In addition to endocrine glands, other organs also secrete hormones. For example, the liver, kidneys, heart, and stomach all secrete hormones. The following sections will describe the function of each of these endocrine glands and organs.

Hypothalamus

The hypothalamus is often called the "master switchboard" of the endocrine system, because its function is to integrate signals from the endocrine and nervous systems to help control hormone production and secretion by the pituitary gland. This feedback system allows the body to maintain homeostasis, regulating heart rate, blood pressure, body temperature, fluid and electrolyte balance, sleep patterns, appetite, and other body functions. The hypothalamus produces 10 different hormones, most of which regulate production and secretion of hormones by the anterior pituitary (see **Table 12–1 »**). However, some of the hormones produced by the hypothalamus are stored in and released from the posterior pituitary.

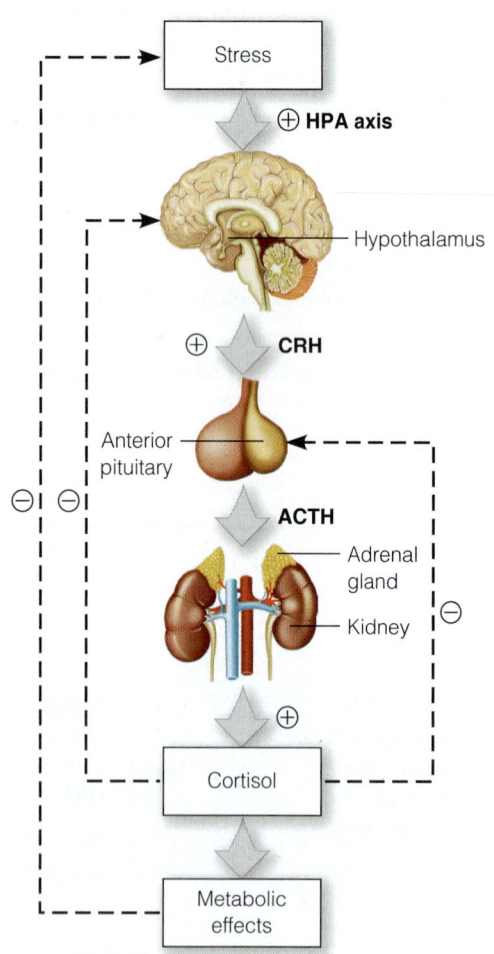

Figure 12–1 » Hypothalamic-pituitary axis (HPA). When the pituitary gland detects hormones from the hypothalamus, it increases or decreases the secretion of additional hormones. Whereas the hormones secreted by the hypothalamus work primarily on the pituitary gland, the hormones secreted by the pituitary gland travel through the bloodstream to regulate multiple major endocrine glands.

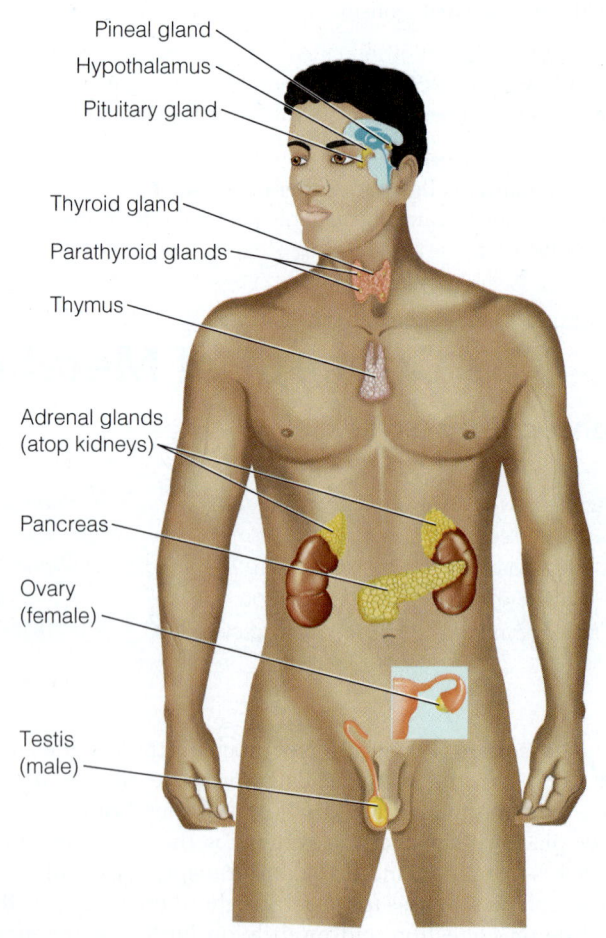

Figure 12–2 » Location of the major endocrine glands.

TABLE 12–1 Glands, Hormones, and Their Functions

Gland	Hormone	Function
Adrenal cortex	Cortisol (hydrocortisone)	Glucocorticoid; regulates metabolism of carbohydrates, fats, and proteins; activates anti-inflammatory responses to stressors; low levels stimulate secretion of corticotropin-releasing hormone from the hypothalamus, which prompts the pituitary to release ACTH, which then prompts the adrenal cortex to release cortisol
	Cortisone (corticosterone)	Glucocorticoid; suppresses the immune response to decrease inflammatory reactions, including pain and swelling
	Aldosterone	Mineralocorticoid; promotes reabsorption of sodium and water in the kidneys; promotes potassium excretion in the kidneys; increases blood pressure and blood volume
	Progesterone	Gonadocorticoid; development of reproductive organs
	Estrogen	Gonadocorticoid; development of reproductive organs
	Testosterone (and other androgens)	Gonadocorticoid; development of reproductive organs
	Dehydroepiandrosterone (DHEA)	Intermediate in the production of androgens and estrogens; stimulates adrenarche (development of secondary sexual characteristics)
Adrenal medulla	Adrenaline	Stimulates the heart; constricts blood vessels; inhibits visceral muscles; dilates bronchioles; increases respiration and metabolism; promotes hyperglycemia; secreted in response to stress
	Norepinephrine	Increases heart rate; induces release of glucose from energy stores; increases blood flow to muscles
Hypothalamus	Antidiuretic hormone	Produced in hypothalamus and stored in posterior pituitary
	Corticotropin-releasing hormone	Stimulates release of ACTH from the anterior pituitary; released in response to low cortisol levels
	Gonadotropin-releasing hormone	Stimulates release of gonadotropins from the pituitary gland
	Growth hormone–releasing hormone	Stimulates release of growth hormone from the pituitary gland; released in response to low growth hormone levels, hypoglycemia, increased amino acids, low fatty acids, and stress
	Growth hormone–inhibiting hormone (somatostatin)	Inhibits secretion of growth hormone and thyroid-stimulating hormone (TSH) from the pituitary gland
	Oxytocin	Produced in hypothalamus and stored in posterior pituitary; stimulates uterine contractions to prepare for labor
	Prolactin-releasing hormone	Stimulates release of prolactin from the pituitary gland
	Prolactin-inhibiting hormone (dopamine)	Inhibits prolactin production in the pituitary gland
	Thyrotropin-releasing hormone	Regulates synthesis and secretion of TSH in the pituitary gland; stimulates the release of prolactin from the pituitary gland
Ovaries	Estrogen (estradiol, estrone, estriol)	Development and maintenance of female reproductive system; prepares the uterus for menstruation; stimulates the pituitary gland to release oxytocin
	Progesterone	Development and maintenance of female reproductive system; prepares the uterus for menstruation; prepares the body for pregnancy; prevents uterine contractions; prepares breasts for lactation
	Relaxin	Released prior to giving birth; relaxes the pelvic ligaments in preparation for labor and delivery
	Inhibin	Signals the pituitary to inhibit the release of follicle-stimulating hormone
Pancreas	Insulin	Decreases blood glucose levels by increasing glucose uptake into cells and preventing glycogen breakdown; increases lipid formation and inhibits the breakdown of stored fat; promotes uptake of amino acids into cells
	Glucagon	Increases blood glucose levels by stimulating the release of glucose from glycogen stores in the liver
	Gastrin	Stimulates gastric acid secretion in the stomach; stimulates gastric motility; stimulates mucosal growth in the stomach
	Somatostatin	Inhibits secretion of glucagon and insulin
	Vasoactive intestinal peptide (pancreatic polypeptide)	Inhibits exocrine activity of the pancreas
Parathyroid	Parathyroid hormone	Increases blood calcium by stimulating bone resorption and increasing calcium reabsorption in the kidneys; increases phosphate secretion; activates vitamin D
Pineal gland	Melatonin	Maintains circadian rhythm and regulates reproductive hormones
Anterior pituitary	Growth hormone	Stimulates growth by signaling cells to increase protein production and by stimulating the epiphyseal plates of the long bones
	Prolactin	Stimulates the production of breast milk
	Adrenocorticotropic hormone (ACTH; corticotropin)	Stimulates the release of glucocorticoids (cortisol) from the adrenal cortex
	Melanocyte-stimulating hormone	Stimulates the production of melanin to increase skin pigmentation
	Thyroid-stimulating hormone (TSH)	Stimulates the synthesis and release of thyroid hormone (TH) from the thyroid gland
	Luteinizing hormone	Stimulates the ovaries and testes
	Follicle-stimulating hormone	Stimulates the ovaries and testes

(continued on next page)

TABLE 12-1 Glands, Hormones, and Their Functions *(continued)*

Gland	Hormone	Function
Posterior pituitary	Oxytocin	Plays a role in social recognition and bonding; active during labor, birth, maternal bonding, and lactation
	Antidiuretic hormone (vasopressin)	Retains water in the body (increases water absorption in kidney); constricts blood vessels
Testes	Testosterone	Development and maintenance of male reproductive system; stimulates development of secondary male characteristics; maintains libido, muscle strength, and bone density; stimulates sperm production
	Inhibin	Signals the pituitary to inhibit the release of follicle-stimulating hormone
Thymus	Thymosin	Stimulates development and maturation of T cells
	Thymopoietin	Stimulates the differentiation of lymphocytes to thymocytes
Thyroid	T_3 (triiodothyronine)	Very active form of TH
	T_4 (thyroxine)	Less active form of TH, but it has a longer half-life; converted to T_3 in target tissues
	Calcitonin	Decreases blood calcium by decreasing bone resorption and calcium reabsorption by the kidneys

Pituitary Gland

The pituitary gland, also called the hypophysis or "master gland," has two parts: the anterior pituitary and the posterior pituitary. The anterior pituitary is connected to the hypothalamus by a capillary network that transports regulatory hormones from the hypothalamus directly to the anterior pituitary without entering the larger circulatory system. Through this capillary network, the hypothalamus controls the production and secretion of seven different hormones from the anterior pituitary (see Table 12–1). When they are released, hormones from the anterior pituitary enter the circulatory system and regulate other endocrine glands.

In contrast, the posterior pituitary does not produce its own hormones. Instead, neurons in the hypothalamus produce antidiuretic hormone (ADH) and oxytocin (see Table 12–1) and transport the hormones along the neuronal axons into the posterior pituitary, where they are stored. When the hypothalamus detects that more ADH or oxytocin are needed, it sends a neuronal signal to the posterior pituitary to stimulate the release of hormones into the circulatory system.

Thyroid Gland

The thyroid gland is a butterfly-shaped gland with two lobes that is located anterior to the upper part of the trachea and inferior to the larynx. Cells within the follicles of the thyroid produce and secrete TH, a general name for two similar hormones: thyroxine (T_4) and triiodothyronine (T_3). The thyroid produces 20% T_3 and 80% T_4, but T_3 is approximately four times more active than T_4. In addition, T_4 is converted to T_3 in target tissues. The primary role of TH in adults is to increase metabolism. Secretion of TH is initiated by the release of TSH from the pituitary gland and is dependent on an adequate supply of iodine. The thyroid also secretes calcitonin, a hormone that decreases excessive levels of calcium in the blood by decreasing the bone resorption activity of osteoclasts and decreasing reabsorption of calcium in the kidneys.

Parathyroid Gland

The parathyroid glands (usually four in number) are embedded on the posterior surface of the lobes of the thyroid gland. They secrete parathyroid hormone (PTH), or parathormone.

When calcium levels in the blood fall, secretion of PTH increases. This increased secretion acts to maintain calcium levels by stimulating bone resorption and reabsorption of calcium in the kidney. In addition, PTH increases the activation of vitamin D, which is responsible for increasing the absorption of calcium from the gut. In this way, PTH works together with calcitonin to maintain blood calcium levels within an ideal range; PTH is more active when calcium levels are too low, and calcitonin is more active when calcium levels are too high. PTH also controls phosphate metabolism by increasing renal excretion of phosphate.

Adrenal Glands

The two adrenal glands are pyramid-shaped organs that sit on top of the kidneys (see Figure 12–2). Each gland consists of two distinct parts: the outer cortex and the inner medulla. The adrenal cortex secretes several hormones, all corticosteroids. These hormones are classified into three groups: mineralocorticoids, glucocorticoids, and gonadocorticoids.

Aldosterone is the primary mineralocorticoid released by the adrenal cortex. The release of aldosterone is controlled by the renin-angiotensin system. In this system, renin is released by kidney cells in response to hypotension or hyponatremia. Renin then activates angiotensinogen to angiotensin, which stimulates the release of aldosterone from the adrenal cortex. Aldosterone prompts the distal tubules of the kidneys to reabsorb water and sodium, thus increasing blood volume and pressure.

The glucocorticoids include cortisol and cortisone. Cortisol is the primary glucocorticoid, and it is regulated by the HPA; because of this relationship, the HPA is also sometimes called the hypothalamic-pituitary-adrenal axis. When cortisol levels are low, the hypothalamus releases corticotropin-releasing hormone, which travels to the anterior pituitary and stimulates the secretion of adrenocorticotropic hormone (ACTH). ACTH then stimulates the release of cortisol from the adrenal cortex. Cortisol affects carbohydrate metabolism by regulating glucose use in body tissues, mobilizing fatty acids from fatty tissue, and shifting the source of energy for muscle cells from glucose to fatty acids. Cortisol is also released during times of stress. Both cortisol and cortisone suppress the inflammatory response and inhibit the effectiveness of the immune system.

The primary gonadocorticoid released from the adrenal cortex is dehydroepiandrosterone (DHEA). DHEA is a precursor molecule to both testosterone and estrogen, which are more active than DHEA. However, DHEA is still active during adrenarche, which is an early sexual maturation stage that occurs in middle childhood as a precursor to puberty. In addition to DHEA, the adrenal cortex also releases small amounts of progesterone, estrogen, testosterone, and other androgens.

The adrenal medulla produces two hormones (also called catecholamines): epinephrine (adrenaline) and norepinephrine (noradrenaline). Epinephrine increases blood glucose levels and stimulates the release of ACTH from the pituitary; in turn, ACTH stimulates the adrenal cortex to release glucocorticoids. Epinephrine also increases the rate and force of cardiac contractions; constricts blood vessels in the skin, mucous membranes, and kidneys; and dilates blood vessels in the skeletal muscles, coronary arteries, and pulmonary arteries. Norepinephrine increases both heart rate and the force of cardiac contractions. It also constricts blood vessels throughout the body.

Pancreas

The pancreas, located behind the stomach between the spleen and the duodenum, is both an endocrine gland (producing hormones) and an exocrine gland (producing digestive enzymes). The endocrine cells of the pancreas are clustered in bodies called pancreatic islets (or islets of Langerhans) scattered throughout the gland, and they function primarily to produce hormones that control carbohydrate metabolism, including blood glucose levels. Pancreatic islets have at least four different cell types, three of which are the most common:

1. Alpha cells produce **glucagon**, which decreases glucose oxidation and promotes an increase in the blood glucose level by signaling the liver to release glucose from glycogen stores.
2. Beta cells produce **insulin**, which facilitates the uptake and use of glucose by cells and prevents excessive breakdown of glycogen in the liver and muscle.
3. Delta cells secrete somatostatin, which inhibits the secretion of glucagon and insulin by the alpha and beta cells.

Pineal Gland

The pineal gland is located deep in the center of the brain. The primary hormone produced and released by the pineal gland is melatonin, not to be confused with the skin pigment melanin. The secretion of melatonin is regulated by light; light decreases the secretion of melatonin, and darkness increases its secretion. Therefore, melatonin functions to maintain the circadian rhythm, which is responsible for regulating sleep/wake cycles. The pineal gland also regulates reproductive hormones. Melatonin specifically regulates the secretion of **gonadotropins** (luteinizing hormone and follicle-stimulating hormone) from the anterior pituitary.

Thymus

The thymus is located just in front of and above the heart and beneath the breastbone in the mediastinum. The thymus has two lobes and weighs a maximum of 1 ounce during puberty. However, the thymus gradually decreases in size as the individual ages into adulthood, and the gland is eventually replaced by fat. The primary purpose of the thymus during development is to stimulate the production and maturation of T lymphocytes (T cells). Two hormones produced by the thymus contribute to this process. Thymopoietin stimulates the differentiation of lymphocytes into thymocytes, and thymosin stimulates the development of thymocytes into T lymphocytes. T cells are active in preventing autoimmune reactions in the body and are involved in the long-term health of the individual.

Ovaries

The two ovaries are the major female reproductive glands. The ovaries are located in the pelvic area, one on each side of the uterus. The ovaries produce and secrete the female reproductive hormones, including estrogen and progesterone. In addition, the ovaries respond to the pituitary hormones follicle-stimulating hormone and luteinizing hormone to stimulate maturation and release of an ova during the menstrual cycle. The reproductive hormones and gonadotropins together regulate the menstrual cycle. The reproductive hormones are also involved in stimulating the development of secondary female sex characteristics and supporting reproduction. For more information, see the module on Sexuality and the module on Reproduction.

Testes

The two testes are the major male reproductive glands; they are housed in the scrotum, which lies just outside the main body cavity behind the penis. The testes produce and secrete the male reproductive hormone, testosterone. Testosterone is regulated by the HPA; the hypothalamus secretes gonadotropin-releasing hormone, which signals the pituitary gland to release gonadotropins, specifically luteinizing hormone. Luteinizing hormone then travels to the testes to stimulate testosterone production. As a feedback mechanism, testosterone inhibits the secretion of gonadotropin-releasing hormone and luteinizing hormone. Testosterone is responsible for maintaining the male reproductive system and stimulating the development of secondary male characteristics, among other roles (see Table 12–1). In addition, testosterone and follicle-stimulating hormone together regulate spermatogenesis, or the development and maturation of sperm.

Organs with Secondary Endocrine Functions

Several organs and tissues have secondary endocrine functions, including bones, kidneys, stomach, small intestine, liver, skin, heart, and adipose tissue. For example, leptin is a hormone secreted by adipose tissue that is involved in suppressing food intake and regulating body weight and energy homeostasis, among other roles. In contrast, ghrelin is a hormone secreted by the stomach that stimulates the appetite. Both ghrelin and leptin are regulated by the hypothalamus.

The liver secretes three hormones: angiotensinogen, insulin-like growth factor-1, and thrombopoietin. Angiotensinogen is involved in the renin-angiotensin pathway that regulates blood pressure. Insulin-like growth factor-1 has actions similar to insulin and regulates cell growth and development.

Thrombopoietin is involved in the development of platelets from the bone marrow. In addition, several hormones have an effect on the liver, including TH, growth hormone, adrenal hormones, and sex hormones.

Other hormones include erythropoietin and renin from the kidneys, secretin and cholecystokinin from the small intestine, atrial natriuretic peptide and brain natriuretic peptide from the heart, and osteocalcin from the bones, among many others.

Alterations to Metabolism

When the body secretes too much or too little hormone, the individual may develop an endocrine disorder that disrupts homeostasis and leads to complications. Alterations to hormone levels affect not only the organs or glands that the hormones act on, but they may also have more global effects on the body. Altered secretion of hormones from endocrine glands results in multiple disorders, depending on the gland and hormone affected. Some of the major endocrine disorders are reviewed in this section.

Disorders of the Hypothalamus

The primary disorder of the hypothalamus is called hypothalamic disease, which may result from surgery, trauma, tumors, or radiation. Symptoms can be varied and widespread depending on the hormones affected. For example, individuals may have growth problems, hypothyroidism, dizziness or weakness, loss of vision, or sleep or appetite disturbances.

Disorders of the Pituitary Gland

Manifestations of pituitary disorders depend on the hormone(s) affected. Disorders related to growth hormone include growth hormone deficiency, acromegaly, and gigantism. Growth hormone deficiency and gigantism are both found in children. Growth hormone deficiency results in slow growth, causing the child to be shorter than other children of a similar age and gender. Gigantism causes an increase in growth of the bones, organs, and muscles, resulting in a child who is much larger than other children of a similar age and gender. **Acromegaly** (continued growth of bone from growth hormone hypersecretion) is similar to gigantism, except it occurs in adults rather than children. Because it occurs after epiphyseal plates have closed, acromegaly may not be detected for many years.

Acromegaly is often the result of a pituitary adenoma that causes excess secretion of growth hormone. In general, secretory pituitary adenomas often result in hyperpituitarism, the excess secretion of one or more hormones from the pituitary gland. In addition to acromegaly, other complications that may result from pituitary adenomas include hyperprolactinemia (excess secretion of prolactin), hyperthyroidism (excess secretion of TSH), and Cushing disease (excess secretion of ACTH).

Some disorders of the pituitary gland result from too little secretion of one or more hormones (hypopituitarism). For example, diabetes insipidus results when the posterior pituitary does not release ADH. This causes excessive thirst (polydipsia) and excretion of large amounts of dilute urine (polyuria). Hormonal dysfunction of the pituitary gland may result from pituitary apoplexy, which is caused by acute hemorrhage or infarct of the pituitary gland, or nonsecretory pituitary adenomas that destroy glandular tissue.

Disorders of the Thyroid Gland

Disorders of the thyroid gland often result in either **hyperthyroidism** (too much TH) or **hypothyroidism** (too little TH). Hyperthyroidism is often referred to as thyrotoxicosis, although hyperthyroidism usually refers to physiologic increases in TH whereas thyrotoxicosis also includes too much supplemental TH. One of the most common causes of hyperthyroidism is Graves disease, which is an autoimmune disorder. The symptoms of Graves disease are representative of increased metabolism. If hyperthyroidism is complicated by infection or other stressors, the individual is susceptible to thyroid storm, which can be fatal.

Hypothyroidism has numerous causes. In countries other than the United States, iodine deficiency is the leading cause of hypothyroidism. In the United States and Europe, this deficiency is rare and the leading cause of hypothyroidism is autoimmune disease. Hypothyroidism occurs most frequently in middle-age and older women. The presenting symptoms are manifested as a slowing of the body's functions. If hypothyroidism is accompanied by an increase in TSH, thyroid tissue enlarges, forming a **goiter** (enlarged thyroid gland). Long-term, severe hypothyroidism can result in myxedema, a condition in which mucopolysaccharides are deposited in the dermis. Severe hypothyroidism with other insults (e.g., infection) can lead to myxedema coma, in which the individual experiences an altered mental state leading to coma. Infants born with a dysfunctional thyroid gland have congenital hypothyroidism, which can lead to cretinism if left untreated. Cretinism manifests as severe physical and mental retardation.

Some thyroid conditions can result in either hypothyroidism or hyperthyroidism, depending on the individual and the pathophysiology of their exact condition. These conditions include thyroid cancer, solitary thyroid nodules, and thyroiditis. The most common type of thyroid cancer is papillary carcinoma; these tumors tend to grow slowly and have a high treatment success rate. However, more rare types of thyroid cancer also exist, and some of them are much harder to treat. Solitary thyroid nodules can be either benign or malignant. Benign nodules are usually soft and nontender, whereas malignant tumors are usually hard. Thyroiditis results from inflammation of the thyroid, which can be caused by infection, trauma, or an autoimmune disorder. Hashimoto thyroiditis is the most common form, and it typically results in hypothyroidism. A less common form called De Quervain thyroiditis usually results in hyperthyroidism, and it generally resolves over several weeks.

Thyroid disease is covered in more detail in Exemplar 12.E.

Disorders of the Parathyroid Gland

Similar to the thyroid gland, disorders of the parathyroid gland are due to hyperparathyroidism (too much PTH) or hypoparathyroidism (too little PTH). Hyperparathyroidism can be either primary or secondary. Primary hyperparathyroidism results from overproduction of PTH by the parathyroid glands. Secondary hyperparathyroidism results from low levels of blood calcium that stimulate the parathyroid glands to release increased amounts of PTH. Because PTH stimulates bone resorption, it can lead to osteoporosis due to inadequate levels of calcium stored in the bones. In addition, it can cause hypercalcemia, increasing the risk for the formation of calcium-based renal calculi. Osteoporosis is covered in more detail in Exemplar 12.D. Renal calculi are covered in more detail in the exemplar on Urinary Calculi in the module on Elimination.

Hypoparathyroidism is rare and is often caused by trauma or removal during thyroid- or parathyroid-related surgeries. It can also be congenital, although this is rare. Symptoms of hypoparathyroidism can range from mild tingling of the upper extremities to limited muscle cramping to **tetany** (tonic muscle spasms), or whole body muscle cramping. These symptoms are directly related to low calcium levels in the blood due to inadequate PTH.

Disorders of the Adrenal Glands

Two disorders related to the adrenal glands are Addison disease and Cushing syndrome. **Addison disease** results from adrenal insufficiency, particularly a cortisol deficiency. Aldosterone may also be decreased. Symptoms associated with Addison disease include muscle weakness and joint pain, fatigue, weight loss, loss of appetite, hyperpigmentation, low blood pressure, hypoglycemia, depression, and sexual dysfunction. These symptoms often develop slowly over several months. If adrenal failure is acute, it may result in addisonian crisis, which causes pain in the lower back, abdomen, or legs; vomiting; diarrhea; dehydration; hyperkalemia; and loss of consciousness. Addison disease is often treated with oral or injected corticosteroids. Individuals with Addison disease should be instructed to wear a medical ID bracelet or other form of medical identification.

Cushing syndrome is the opposite of Addison disease in that it results from too much cortisol. It can develop in individuals who take too much exogenous glucocorticosteroid for asthma or other disorders, or it can develop as a result of the overproduction of endogenous cortisol due to a pituitary or adrenal tumor. Individuals with Cushing syndrome usually have moon face and central obesity. They may also develop striae on their abdomen, thin skin, bone pain, weak muscles, fatigue, a buffalo hump, and other symptoms. Treatment of Cushing syndrome due to glucocorticosteroid medications will include gradually decreasing the medication dosage. Treatment due to a tumor often requires surgery to remove the tumor and potential cortisol replacement therapy depending on the source of the tumor.

Other disorders related to the adrenal glands include congenital adrenal hyperplasia, adrenal tumors, and pheochromocytoma. In congenital adrenal hyperplasia, the adrenal glands cannot produce adequate levels of cortisol and aldosterone. In girls, this results in abnormal genitals at birth, abnormal menstrual periods, and excessive hair growth. In boys, this results in early puberty. Both boys and girls will be taller as children but shorter as adults compared to their peers. Severe forms can cause adrenal crisis, including dehydration, shock, or death.

Adrenal tumors can be either benign or malignant, and they almost always appear in the adrenal cortex. Benign tumors are more likely to result in high levels of aldosterone and thus increase blood pressure. However, most benign tumors have no symptoms. Most malignant tumors in the adrenal gland are the result of metastasis from other tumors. They may cause hormonal changes such as weight gain, fluid retention, and excess hair growth. Some tumors lead to a Cushing-like syndrome. Pheochromocytoma is a rare type of tumor that develops in the adrenal medulla. Due to the increased release of epinephrine and norepinephrine, pheochromocytoma often causes high blood pressure and headache. Pheochromocytomas are usually benign.

Disorders of the Pancreas

The most common disorder of the pancreas is diabetes mellitus (DM). Diabetes is a disorder of metabolism related to the body's production and use of the hormone insulin. In **type 1 diabetes (T1D)**, there is an absolute deficiency of insulin related to pancreatic beta cell destruction. This results in severe hyperglycemia and diabetic ketoacidosis (DKA), among other symptoms. **Type 2 diabetes (T2D)** has a more insidious onset and may develop over several years. There is relative deficiency of insulin, which may be related to insulin resistance and inadequate secretion of insulin to meet body needs. Both of these components are usually present at the time of diagnosis. The onset may be acute, with markedly elevated glucose levels resulting in nonketotic hyperglycemia that requires hospitalization for treatment. However, the more common presentation is mildly elevated glucose levels with weight gain and symptoms of hyperglycemia, such as thirst, frequent urination, and increased susceptibility to infections, blurred vision, and fatigue. Diabetes will be covered more thoroughly in Exemplars 12.A and 12.B.

Disorders of the Pineal Gland

Pineal gland disorders result in a disruption of melatonin homeostasis, interfering with normal circadian rhythms. This is often seen in individuals with jet lag, seasonal affective disorder, insomnia, and other similar disorders. The pineal gland can also develop life-threatening tumors that cause increased pressure in the brain and disrupt endocrine signaling through the hypothalamus and pituitary gland.

Disorders of the Thymus

Hodgkin lymphoma and non-Hodgkin lymphoma are two cancers that involve the lymphocytes and the lymphatic system, of which the thymus is a part. Although these cancers can start in the thymus, they more commonly start in the lymph nodes or spleen. However, one type of non-Hodgkin lymphoma that often starts in the thymus is precursor T-lymphoblastic lymphoma/leukemia. If a tumor develops in the thymus, it can press on the trachea and make breathing difficult. It can also block the superior vena cava, causing swelling of the arms and face. The other types of tumors that arise from the thymus are thymoma and thymic carcinoma. Thymoma is often linked to myasthenia gravis and other autoimmune diseases. They are usually benign and result in cough, chest pain, and difficulty breathing. Thymic carcinoma is malignant, and it is usually faster growing than thymoma. Symptoms of thymic carcinoma are similar to thymoma.

Other Endocrine Disorders

Obesity occurs when individuals consume more calories than they expend each day, and these excess calories are stored as adipose tissue. Although obesity in itself has few symptoms other than increased BMI (body mass index), adipose tissue secretes cytokines and hormones that increase the risk of hypertension, dyslipidemia, type 2 diabetes, coronary artery disease, stroke, fatty liver and gallbladder disease, sleep disorders, cancers, and dementia. Obesity is discussed further in the exemplar on Obesity in the module on Nutrition.

Osteoporosis is a metabolic bone disorder in which the rate of bone resorption increases and the rate of bone formation decreases. The result is decreased bone mass. It may be a primary disorder or secondary to another disease or medications. The presentation is loss of height with possible increased vertebral curvature, decreased exercise tolerance, and decreased spinal movement. The symptoms may occur over time and not be readily recognized as osteoporosis. Individuals with osteoporosis are at high risk for bone fracture and related complications. Osteoporosis will be discussed further in Exemplar 12.D.

Cirrhosis is characterized by widespread destruction of liver cells, which are replaced by less efficient fibrous cells. Cirrhosis has many causes, but all the manifestations are those of a dying liver. Early signs may be vague, such as loss of appetite, indigestion, nausea, vomiting, constipation, diarrhea, and jaundice. The patient may report bruising easily. Later symptoms are related to progression of cell damage and may include respiratory problems, central nervous effects, hematologic effects, skin effects, renal effects, and hepatic effects. Liver disease is discussed further in Exemplar 12.C.

Alterations and therapies for selected endocrine and metabolic disorders are shown in the Alterations and Therapies feature.

Prevalence

Although some metabolic disorders such as diabetes and obesity are fairly common, most metabolic disorders and disorders related to the endocrine system are rare. The following are prevalence rates for selected metabolic disorders:

- **Diabetes.** As of 2014, 21 million individuals in the United States have been diagnosed with diabetes, and an estimated 8.1 million have the disease but have not been diagnosed. Of individuals younger than 20 years of age, 208,000 (0.25% of this age group) have diabetes. Of all individuals age 20 or older, 28.9 million (12.3%) have diabetes; 15.5 million (13.6%) of men and 13.4 million (11.2%) of women in this age group have diabetes (Centers for Disease Control and Prevention [CDC], 2014a).

- **Obesity.** National data on obesity prevalence among U.S. adults, adolescents, and children show that almost 35% of adults and almost 17% of youth were obese in 2011–2012. Over 6% of adults were considered extremely obese (BMI greater than or equal to 40). In addition, 8.1% of children under the age of 2 had high weight (95th percentile) (Ogden et al., 2014).

- **Osteoporosis.** An estimated 10.2 million adults age 50 and over in the United States have osteoporosis (10.3%), and 43.4 million (43.9%) have low bone mass. Women are approximately four times more likely to develop osteoporosis than men, and the prevalence of osteoporosis increases with age (Wright et al., 2014). Approximately 50% of women and 20% of men age 50 or older will have an osteoporosis-related fracture in their lifetime. Approximately 2 million bone fractures each year are attributed to osteoporosis (National Osteoporosis Foundation, 2014).

- **Thyroid disorders.** Hyperthyroidism occurs in approximately 1% of the U.S. population. The most common causes of hyperthyroidism are Graves disease, thyroid nodules, and thyroiditis (National Institute of Diabetes and Digestive and Kidney Disease [NIDDK], 2012a). Graves disease, the most common form of hyperthyroidism, is more common in women and in individuals under the age of 40. The overall prevalence of hypothyroidism in the United States is 4.6% for individuals age 12 and over. The most common causes of hypothyroidism are Hashimoto disease, thyroiditis, congenital hypothyroidism, and surgical removal of all or part of the thyroid (NIDDK, 2013).

- **Addison disease.** Because of its low prevalence rate (1 in 20,000 individuals), healthcare providers must be aware of the signs of adrenal crisis, including fatigue, anorexia, nausea, joint pain, and salt craving (Michels & Michels, 2014).

- **Cushing syndrome.** Affecting only 10–15 people out of every 1 million (Guaraldi & Salvatori, 2012), Cushing syndrome is most common in individuals ages 20–50 years old.

- **Cirrhosis.** Liver cirrhosis is a major cause of death in the United Sates, and its prevalence is related to the cause of the liver disease. The overall prevalence of cirrhosis is 0.27%, affecting a total of over 630,000 individuals. Common causes of cirrhosis are alcohol abuse, hepatitis B or C, diabetes, and older age. Men are also more likely to develop cirrhosis than women (Scaglione et al., 2015).

Genetic Considerations and Risk Factors

Evidence can be found for the genetic nature of almost any disorder related to endocrine glands, hormones, or metabolism. However, many disorders can be either genetic or acquired. For example, growth hormone deficiency can be related to mutations in one of three genes, but some individuals with this disorder do not have mutations in these genes. In a similar way, disorders related to the thyroid, including both Graves disease and Hashimoto disease, and the parathyroid, including both hypo- and hyperparathyroidism, have a genetic origin, but not all individuals who have these disorders have a family history of the disorder. In addition to genetics, many metabolic diseases result from environmental or autoimmune factors, and having one autoimmune disorder that leads to an alteration in metabolism increases the risk for having other autoimmune disorders.

Alterations and Therapies
Endocrine and Metabolic Disorders

ALTERATION	DESCRIPTION/ DEFINITION	MANIFESTATIONS	INTERVENTIONS AND THERAPIES

Changes in growth	Symptoms are caused by abnormal secretion of growth hormone from the pituitary gland.
	
	Examples:
	■ Hypothalamic disease
	■ Growth hormone deficiency
	■ Acromegaly
	■ Gigantism
		For alterations resulting from too much growth hormone, children will be larger than other individuals of the same age and gender. Adults may not have major signs or symptoms.
		    For alterations resulting from too little growth hormone, children will be smaller than other individuals of the same age and gender.
			Treatment of hypothalamic disease depends on the cause of the hypothalamic dysfunction. Tumors are treated with surgery or radiation. Hormonal deficiencies are treated with synthetic hormone administration.
			    Growth hormone deficiency is treated with synthetic growth hormone, administered by injection daily.
			    Acromegaly and gigantism treatment focuses on lowering the production of growth hormone along with reducing the negative effects of the tumor on the pituitary gland and surrounding tissues. Treatments include surgery, medication, and radiation.

Changes in thirst and urine output	Changes in the regulation of antidiuretic hormone or ions such as calcium, potassium, or sodium can lead to changes in thirst. *Example:* ■ Diabetes insipidus	Patients will complain of excessive thirst (polydipsia) or dry mouth, which is often accompanied by the excretion of large amounts of dilute urine (polyuria) if the thirst results in drinking excess fluids.	Treatment of diabetes insipidus includes the administration of the synthetic hormone, desmopressin, administered by nasal spray, oral tablets, or injection.

Changes in metabolism	Metabolic processes of the body increase or decrease as a result of too much or too little TH.
	
	Examples:
	■ Hyperthyroidism
	■ Hypothyroidism
	■ Graves disease
	■ Thyroid cancer
	■ Thyroid nodules
	■ Thyroiditis
		Increased metabolism results in excess energy and difficulty gaining weight. Decreased metabolism results in decreased energy, obesity, and difficulty losing weight.
		    Hypothyroidism may be accompanied by goiter formation, myxedema, or myxedema coma.
			Hyperthyroidism and Graves disease treatments include radioactive iodine (RAI), antithyroid medications, or a thyroidectomy.
			    Hypothyroidism treatment includes daily use of the synthetic TH levothyroxine, administered orally.
			    Thyroid cancer treatment includes surgery to remove the tumor or a thyroidectomy.
			    Thyroid nodules often require no treatment unless symptomatic. Treatment options range from medication to surgical removal.
			    Thyroiditis treatment depends on the clinical presentation.

Changes in calcium regulation	Alterations in hormones that regulate calcium levels (PTH, calcitonin) cause blood and bone calcium to be too high or too low.
	
	Examples:
	■ Hyperparathyroidism
	■ Hypoparathyroidism
		Increased calcium levels can lead to renal calculi.
		    Decreased calcium levels can lead to osteoporosis and severe muscle cramping.
		    Because calcium is important for neuronal signaling, muscle contraction, and many chemical reactions, abnormal calcium levels can cause manifestations in almost every body system.
			Hyperparathyroidism treatment includes surgical and pharmacologic intervention, including calcimimetics, hormone replacement therapy, and bisphosphonates.
			    Hypoparathyroidism treatment includes oral calcium carbonate tablets, vitamin D, and a diet rich in calcium and low in phosphorus.

(continued on next page)

Alterations and Therapies *(continued)*

ALTERATION	DESCRIPTION/ DEFINITION	MANIFESTATIONS	INTERVENTIONS AND THERAPIES

Changes in cortisol regulation	Symptoms result from excess or deficient secretion of cortisol from the adrenal glands.
	
	Examples:
	■ Addison disease
	■ Cushing syndrome
		Cortisol deficiency results in Addison disease, which is accompanied by muscle weakness, fatigue, weight loss, and other symptoms.
		    Excess cortisol results in Cushing syndrome, which is accompanied by a moon face and central obesity along with other symptoms.
			Addison disease is treated with oral or injected corticosteroids.
			    Cushing syndrome is treated with either decreasing corticosteroid dosage or surgery to remove a tumor, depending on the cause.

Changes in glucose regulation	Changes in insulin secretion, regulation, and response alter the body's ability to control blood glucose levels. *Examples:* ■ T1D ■ T2D	Clinical manifestations can include hypoglycemia or hyperglycemia, diabetic ketoacidosis, weight gain, thirst, frequent urination, increased susceptibility to infection, fatigue, and other symptoms.	Depending on the etiology, treatment may include insulin replacement therapy, changes to diet and exercise, blood glucose monitoring, and diabetes medications such as metformin or rosiglitazone.

Changes in sleep patterns	Alterations in melatonin homeostasis can interfere with circadian rhythms and sleep patterns.
	
	Examples:
	■ Jet lag
	■ Seasonal affective disorder
	■ Insomnia
		Clinical manifestations include difficulty falling asleep or staying asleep and fatigue.	Jet lag is generally temporary and does not require treatment. For patients who travel frequently, pharmacologic treatment may include benzodiazepine or nonbenzodiazepine sleeping pills, or the implementation of light therapy.
			    Seasonal affective disorder treatment includes light therapy, pharmacologic intervention with antidepressants, and psychotherapy.
			    Treatment for insomnia includes behavioral and lifestyle changes, prescription sleep aids, and complementary health approaches such as valerian or melatonin.

Disorders that are heavily influenced by environmental factors include obesity and T1D, although genetics may also play a role in these disorders in some individuals. One cause of obesity is consistently consuming more calories than what the body can expend each day, and obesity then contributes to the development of multiple conditions, including T2D and heart disease. Other factors that increase the risk for developing a metabolic disorder include the presence of a tumor in an endocrine gland or removal or damage of an endocrine gland during surgery for other conditions.

Clinical Reasoning Questions Level I

1. What risk factors are present (modifiable and unmodifiable) for osteoporosis and possible fracture?
2. Discuss safety risks that are present for Ms. Bell.
3. What further interview questions should the nurse ask?

Clinical Reasoning Questions Level II

4. What are two priority nursing diagnoses for Ms. Bell at this time?
5. What independent nursing interventions can you perform to help make Ms. Bell more comfortable and safe while in the clinic?
6. What tests do you anticipate will be done for Ms. Bell at this visit?

Case Study » Part 1

Mary Bell is a 65-year-old woman who comes to the clinic with back and hip pain. Her past medical history includes chronic obstructive pulmonary disease (COPD) with intermittent steroid use, hypertension, depression, gastroesophogeal reflux disease (GERD), and tobacco abuse. Ms. Bell lives alone, cooks for herself, has no family living nearby, and does not exercise. The nurse's observations are that Ms. Bell is a frail, elderly-looking woman who is in moderate pain and moves cautiously. Her gait is unstable.

Concepts Related to Metabolism

The hormones of the endocrine system are integral to homeostasis (see the Concepts Related to Metabolism feature on the next page). For example, the regulation of phosphates and other buffer systems by the endocrine system helps maintain acid–base balance in the body. In the kidney, hormones regulate the excretion and reabsorption of electrolytes and water. Hormones are also responsible for helping

Concepts Related to
Metabolism

CONCEPT	RELATIONSHIP TO METABOLISM	NURSING IMPLICATIONS
Collaboration	▪ Patients with endocrine or metabolic disorders may have comorbidities that require care by multiple healthcare providers. ▪ Many metabolic disorders are rare and may require working with a specialist; some may require surgery, which requires working with a surgical team and others.	▪ Advocate for patients with metabolic disorders to receive care by the appropriate specialist. ▪ Maintain adequate communication among all healthcare providers to develop a complete understanding of the patient's condition(s).
Fluids and Electrolytes	▪ ↑ Aldosterone production → ↑ sodium and water retention → fluid excess → edema ▪ Liver cirrhosis → ↓ albumin production → fluid excess → edema ▪ Dehydration and hypovolemia → ↑ antidiuretic hormone and ↑ aldosterone → sodium and water retention ▪ Metabolic disorders (e.g., Cushing syndrome, diabetes insipidus) → hypernatremia ▪ Adrenal insufficiency → hyponatremia and hyperkalemia ▪ Chronic kidney disease → ↑ metabolic waste products → ↑ uric acid (gout) and ↓ sensitivity to insulin (diabetes)	▪ Fluid deficit and fluid excess will cause changes in vital signs. ▪ Assess for skin turgor, urine output, urine specific gravity, and weight. ▪ Monitor children and older adults closely for dehydration if lab tests reveal that related hormones are abnormally high or low. ▪ For older adults, changes in fluid status related to hormone dysregulation may cause changes in mental status. ▪ Monitor patients for fluid and electrolyte levels.
Mobility	▪ ↓ Calcium → ↓ bone density → ↑ bone fractures → ↓ mobility	▪ Older adults with low calcium or low bone density should be monitored for risk for falls, which lead to bone fractures, especially hip fractures. ▪ Individuals with bone fractures should be encouraged to consume adequate levels of calcium to promote calcium deposition in bones.
Perfusion	▪ ↑ Aldosterone → ↑ sodium and water retention → ↑ preload → ↑ overstretching of heart muscle → ineffective heart contraction → heart failure ▪ ↑ Aldosterone → ↑ sodium and water retention → ↑ blood volume → ↑ blood pressure ▪ ↓ Aldosterone → ↓ sodium and water retention → fluid deficit → ↓ preload → ↓ cardiac output → ↑ heart rate and ↓ blood pressure ▪ Regulation of electrolytes by hormones → ion availability → heart muscle contraction ▪ Thyrotoxicosis/hyperthyroidism → ↑ myocardial oxygen demand → angina ▪ Hypothyroidism → ↑ vascular resistance → ↑ blood pressure ▪ Ischemia of heart vessels → electrolyte imbalances and hormone release → ↓ myocardial contractility → ↓ cardiac output, ↓ blood pressure, and ↓ tissue perfusion ▪ Insulin resistance → DM → ↑ blood pressure and obesity → ↑ risk of stroke	▪ Closely monitor patients with alterations in metabolism for changes in perfusion. ▪ Closely monitor heart rate and blood pressure, because changes to these vital signs are often early signs of problems. ▪ Monitor intake and output, water and electrolyte levels, and edema, as they can radically alter blood volume and heart workload.
Reproduction	▪ Pregnancy → ↑ thyroid size and activity → ↑ metabolic function and ↑ metabolic demand → allows use of both glucose and fats for energy source ▪ Pregnancy → ↑ steroid sex hormones → ↑ sodium and water retention → ↑ weight gain and blood volume ▪ Pregnancy → ↑ parathyroid gland size and activity → meet calcium demands of growing baby ▪ Hypothalamic stimulation of anterior pituitary gland → follicle-stimulating hormone and luteinizing hormone release → ovum growth and ovulation → woman ready for fertilization ▪ Anterior pituitary secretes prolactin → prepares for lactation	▪ Monitor pregnant patients for gestational diabetes and other metabolic or hormonal changes. ▪ Patients with uncontrolled hypothyroidism or hyperthyroidism are at increased risk for miscarriage and other complications such as preeclampsia and low birth weight. ▪ Encourage pregnant women to consume adequate iodine to support the development of the baby's thyroid.
Stress and Coping	▪ ↑ Stress → ↑ cortisol → ↓ inflammatory response and changes metabolism of carbohydrates and fats	▪ All assessments related to metabolic disorders should also include an assessment of the patient's stress level and coping ability.

maintain normal sleep–rest patterns. The inflammatory process that plays a role in the response to injury or infection is controlled in part by cortisol, an adrenal hormone. Cortisol also plays a role in the stress response. Mobility and the risk for bone fracture is related to calcium regulation, which is controlled by PTH and calcitonin. Perfusion by the cardiovascular system is controlled in part by the endocrine system; blood volume and pressure is regulated by sodium and water levels, which are under the control of several hormones, and heart rate and blood flow are regulated by epinephrine and norepinephrine, which are secreted from the adrenal medulla. The development of the reproductive system is regulated by hormones from the reproductive glands, which play a role in human sexuality and reproduction.

These examples are only a small glimpse of how the endocrine system controls metabolism and regulates the physiologic effects of the body to maintain health and wellness. The Concepts Related to Metabolism feature links additional concepts integral to metabolism, which are presented in alphabetical order.

Health Promotion

The nurse can promote health in patients with metabolic or endocrine disorders by routinely monitoring affected hormone levels, monitoring fluid and electrolyte levels, testing for related secondary disorders, and providing patient teaching about the importance of regularly taking hormone supplements if needed (see the Patient Teaching feature). Health promotion also involves reminding the patient to report worsening or additional signs and symptoms, providing information on appropriate nutritional support for the condition, and encouraging the patient to maintain a healthy weight and exercise routine.

Modifiable Risk Factors

Many metabolic disorders have nonmodifiable risk factors, and the patient cannot prevent the onset of disease. However, patients who consume a diet that is deficient in vitamins and other nutrients or who have a sedentary lifestyle are at increased risk for many metabolic disorders. For example, patients who consume more calories than they expend, especially if their diet is high in fats and refined sugars, are at increased risk for obesity and T1D.

Another risk factor for many metabolic diseases is taking medications that can affect hormone levels. For example, long-term use of glucocorticoids can increase a patient's risk of developing Cushing syndrome. Taking supplemental hormones can cause disorders that are opposite to the disorder they are being used to treat; for example, taking supplemental TH for hypothyroidism can result in hyperthyroidism if the hormone levels are not regulated appropriately. Nurses should discuss side effects of medications with patients to help them understand their risk for metabolic disorders and to help them identify signs and symptoms of metabolic disorders related to their medication.

Nursing Assessment

Because hormones affect all of the tissues and organs in the body, manifestations of dysfunction often are nonspecific,

Patient Teaching
Hormone Replacement Therapy

Patients who have had an endocrine gland removed or who have a hormone deficiency (e.g., hypothyroidism, hypoparathyroidism) must take hormone replacement therapy for life. Failure to take these medications can result in potentially life-threatening conditions. Therefore, nurses can promote patient health by teaching patients about the importance of regularly taking their hormone supplements.

- Failure to take supplemental TH can result in fatigue, dry skin, hoarseness, muscle weakness, depression, weight gain, and other symptoms. If the untreated hypothyroidism is severe, it could result in myxedema or myxedema coma.
- Failure to take vitamin D and calcium supplements to treat hypoparathyroidism can result in hypocalcemia, which causes muscle cramps, tetany, and convulsions, depending on severity. Hypocalcemia can also result in brittle bones that are at increased risk for fracture.
- Failure to take growth hormone supplements in pediatric patients can result in short stature and delayed puberty. Untreated growth hormone deficiency can also lead to high cholesterol and osteoporosis.
- Failure to take corticosteroids for adrenal insufficiency (Addison disease) can result in addisonian crisis, which is characterized by low blood pressure, low blood sugar, and high blood potassium. This is a life-threatening condition.
- Failure to take insulin in insulin-dependent (type 1) diabetes results in hyperglycemia, which can result in ketoacidosis and diabetic coma. Long-term hyperglycemia can lead to complications with the eyes, kidneys, nerves, and heart.

sometimes making assessment of endocrine function more difficult than assessment of other body systems.

Observation and Patient Interview

Although many metabolic disorders are not observable, the nurse should be aware of visible signs associated with metabolic disorders, including changes to fat distribution (e.g., central obesity, buffalo hump), changes to body weight (weight gain or weight loss), and changes to skin color or texture (see the Endocrine Assessments feature). Because many symptoms of metabolic disorders are not observable, the nurse should conduct a thorough health assessment interview and physical assessment if an endocrine disorder is suspected.

A health assessment interview to determine problems with the endocrine system may be part of a health screening or a total health assessment, or the interview may focus on a chief complaint (e.g., increased urination, changes in energy levels). When conducting a health assessment interview and a physical assessment, the nurse should consider genetic influences on the health of the adult. The nurse should ask if any immediate family members have or have had endocrine disorders and, if so, the family member's age at onset and gender.

If the patient has a problem with endocrine function, the nurse analyzes its onset, characteristics and course, severity, precipitating and relieving factors, and any associated symptoms, noting the timing and circumstances. The nurse should ask the patient about any changes in normal growth and development and in height and weight. The nurse can often detect changes in the size of extremities by asking whether the patient has had to have rings enlarged or to buy increasingly larger gloves and shoes. The nurse should also identify enlargement of the neck by asking whether the patient has difficulty finding shirts or blouses with a collar that fits.

Interview questions may include:

General
- Have you had any problems with an endocrine gland (pituitary, thyroid, parathyroid, adrenal, pancreas, ovaries, testes)?
- If you had a problem with any of these glands, how was it treated (medications, surgery, diet, hormone replacement)?
- Does anyone in your family have an endocrine disorder? If so, what family member is affected? At what age did the disorder begin? How does it affect that individual?
- Do you smoke, drink alcohol, or use recreational drugs? If so, how much, what kind, and how often?
- Have you ever been tested for high or low blood sugar?

Nutrition and Metabolism
- Describe what you eat as well as how much (and what type of) fluid you drink in a 24-hour period.
- Do you take any nutritional supplements, herbs, or vitamins?
- Have you noticed any change in your hunger or thirst?
- Has your weight changed? If so, by how many pounds (gain or loss) and over what time period?
- Have you noticed any change in your energy level? If so, explain.
- Have you noticed any change in your ability to tolerate heat or cold?
- Have you noticed any difficulty swallowing? If so, explain.
- Have you noticed any change in the texture of your skin? If so, what were they?
- Have you noticed any change in the color, odor, amount, or frequency of your urination? If so, describe it.
- Describe your physical activities in a usual day.
- Do some activities make you very tired? Explain how you feel.
- How many hours of sleep do you get each night?
- Do you feel nervous and unable to rest?
- Do you sweat at night?
- Have you noticed any change in the color or condition of your skin and hair (color, dryness, oiliness, bruises)?

Cognition and Sensory Perception
- Have you noticed any problem with your memory?
- Do you feel restless, anxious, or confused?

- Have you noticed any change in your voice?
- Have you had any headaches, memory loss, changes in sensation, or depression? If so, describe them.
- Have you noticed any change in your vision? If so, describe it.
- Have you had any heart palpitations?
- Have you had any abdominal pain? If so, what is it like, and where is it located?
- Have you had any pain or stiffness in your muscles and joints?

Stress and Coping
- How does this condition make you feel about yourself?
- How do you feel about taking medications?
- How does this condition affect your relationships with others? Your work?
- Does stress seem to make your condition worse? Explain.
- Describe what you do when you feel stressed.
- Describe any social or community pressures or activities that affect how you care for and feel about this condition.

Physical Examination
During the physical assessment, assess for any manifestations that might indicate a genetic disorder. If findings indicate genetic risk factors or alterations, ask whether the patient is willing to undergo genetic testing and, if so, refer for appropriate genetic counseling and evaluation.

The only endocrine organ that can be palpated is the thyroid gland; however, other assessments that provide information about endocrine problems include inspection of the skin, hair, nails, facial appearance, reflexes, and musculoskeletal system. Measuring and monitoring trends in height and weight and in vital signs also provide clues to altered function of the endocrine system.

The Endocrine Assessments feature describes the physical assessment, normal and abnormal findings, and lifespan and developmental considerations.

Diagnostic Tests
The results of diagnostic tests support the diagnosis of a specific disease, provide information to identify or modify the appropriate medication or therapy used to treat the disease, and help nurses monitor the patient's responses to treatment and nursing care interventions. Specific diagnostic tests to assess the structure and function of the glands of the endocrine system include:

- Hemoglobin A1C
- T_3, T_4, TSH
- Individual hormone levels—parathyroid, catecholamines, estrogen, progesterone, growth hormone, and so on
- Serum electrolytes
- Liver enzymes (AST, ALT, LDH)
- Bilirubin
- Serum albumin
- Serum calcium

Endocrine Assessment

ASSESSMENT/ METHOD	NORMAL FINDINGS	ABNORMAL FINDINGS	LIFESPAN OR DEVELOPMENTAL CONSIDERATIONS
Skin Assessment			
Inspect the skin color.	Skin color should be even and appropriate to the age and race of the patient.	■ Hyperpigmentation may be seen in patients with Addison disease or Cushing syndrome. ■ Hypopigmentation may be seen in patients with DM, hyperthyroidism, or hypothyroidism. ■ A yellowish cast to the skin might indicate hypothyroidism. ■ Purple striae over the abdomen and bruising may be present in patients with Cushing syndrome.	■ Older patients' skin becomes pale due to decreased melanin production and decreased dermal vascularity. ■ In general, children's skin is smoother than adults' skin because of lack of exposure to the elements and lack of coarse hair.
Palpate the skin, assessing texture, moisture, and the presence of lesions.	Skin should be appropriate to the patient's race, smooth, warm, dry, and intact, without abnormal lesions.	■ Rough, dry skin often is seen in patients with hypothyroidism, whereas smooth and flushed skin can be a sign of hyperthyroidism. ■ Lesions (e.g., ulcerations) on the lower extremities might indicate DM.	■ Older patients' skin is drier because of decreased production of sebum. Older patients perspire less because of decreased activity of sweat glands. Older patients may also have a variety of lesions because of aging of the skin, such as senile keratosis and senile lentigines (age or liver spots). ■ In early childhood, sebaceous glands are minimally active, and although exocrine glands function, they produce little sweat.
Nails and Hair Assessment			
Assess the texture, distribution, and condition of the nails and hair.	Hair should be of normal texture and appropriately distributed for gender and age; nail surfaces should be smooth, with even color.	■ Increased pigmentation of the nails often is seen in patients with Addison disease. ■ Dry, thick, brittle nails and hair may be apparent in patients with hypothyroidism; thin, brittle nails and thin, soft hair may be apparent in patients with hyperthyroidism. ■ Hirsutism (excessive facial, chest, or abdominal hair) may be seen in women with Cushing syndrome.	■ Older patients' nails may appear thickened and yellow because of decreased circulation to the extremities. Hair feels coarser and drier in older adults. Dark-skinned patients may have thicker nails. Individuals of Black African descent tend to have very dry scalps and dry, fragile hair. During toddlerhood, hair grows thicker and usually loses curliness. Fine hair becomes visible in distal portions of the upper and lower extremities. Nails are usually pink, convex, and smooth throughout childhood and adolescence.

Endocrine Assessment *(continued)*

ASSESSMENT/ METHOD	NORMAL FINDINGS	ABNORMAL FINDINGS	LIFESPAN OR DEVELOPMENTAL CONSIDERATIONS
Facial Assessments			
Inspect the symmetry and form of the face.	The face should be bilaterally symmetrical.	■ Variations of form and structure may indicate growth abnormalities, such as acromegaly.	■ Older patients may have shrinkage of the lower face and folding in of the mouth because of mandibular resorption of bone due to aging. ■ During toddlerhood, the nasal bridge is low and the mandible and maxilla are small, making the face seem small compared with the skull. In school-age children, the skull seems to grow disproportionately faster than the rest of the cranium.
Inspect the position of the eyes.	Eyes should be equal in position on both sides of the face. Eyelids should close over the eyes.	■ **Exophthalmos** (protruding eyes) may be seen in patients with hyperthyroidism.	■ Some Asians and other groups may have a common variation of epicanthic folds or narrowed palpebral fissures, giving an impression that the upper border of the iris is covered. The palpebral fissures of Asians typically have an upward slant. The eyes of some African Americans protrude more than those of other ethnicities, and both men and women may have eyes that protrude beyond the 21 mm standard.
Thyroid Gland Assessment			
Palpate the thyroid gland for size and consistency. Stand behind the patient, and place your fingers on either side of the trachea below the thyroid cartilage (see **Figure 12–3** ❯❯). Ask the patient to tilt the head to the right. Now ask the patient to swallow. As the patient swallows, displace the left lobe while palpating the right lobe. Repeat to palpate the left lobe.	The thyroid gland is not usually palpable. If it is, the lobes should feel smooth, rubbery, and free of nodules.	■ The thyroid may be enlarged in patients with Graves disease or a goiter. ■ Multiple nodules may be seen in patients with metabolic disorders, whereas the presence of only one nodule may indicate a cyst or a benign or malignant tumor. ■ One enlarged nodule suggests malignancy.	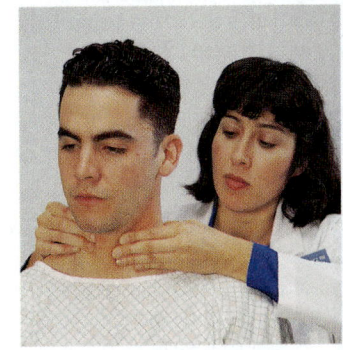 **Figure 12–3** ❯❯ Palpating the thyroid gland from behind the patient. ■ The older patient's thyroid may feel more nodular and irregular because of fibrotic changes that occur with aging. It may be palpated lower in the neck because of age-related changes. In children, the isthmus is the only portion of the thyroid that should be palpated. "Shotty" nodes (small, nontender, mobile) are commonly palpated in children between ages 3 and 12.

(continued on next page)

Endocrine Assessment *(continued)*

ASSESSMENT/ METHOD	NORMAL FINDINGS	ABNORMAL FINDINGS	LIFESPAN OR DEVELOPMENTAL CONSIDERATIONS
Motor Function Assessment			
Assess the deep tendon reflexes (DTRs). DTRs are assessed with the reflex hammer and include the biceps reflex, brachioradialis reflex, triceps reflex, patellar reflex, and Achilles reflex.	Normal values range from 1+ (present but decreased) to 2+ (normal) to 3+ (increased).	■ Increased reflexes may be seen in patients with hyperthyroidism; decreased reflexes may be seen in those with hypothyroidism.	■ Some older patients may have decreased DTRs because of a decrease in the number of nerve axons and increased demyelination of the nerve axons. There is also a decrease in transmission of impulses along with a delay in reaction time. ■ In children, the nervous system grows rapidly during the postnatal period, reaching 25% of adult capacity at birth, 50% by age 1, 80% by age 3, and 90% by age 7. Development takes place in an orderly fashion, but each child develops at his or her own pace.
Sensory Function Assessment			
Test the patient's sensitivity to pain, temperature, vibration, light touch, and stereognosis (the ability to identify an object merely by touch). Ask the patient to close his or her eyes. Then, compare symmetrical areas on both sides of the body, and compare the distal to the proximal regions of the extremities: ■ To test pain, use the blunt and sharp ends of a new safety pin. Discard the pin after use. ■ To test temperature, use cups or other containers of cold and hot (not scalding) water. ■ To test vibration, use a tuning fork over one of the patient's finger or toe joints. ■ To test light touch, use a cotton wisp. ■ To test stereognosis, place in the patient's hand a simple, familiar object, such as a rubber band, cotton ball, or button. Ask the patient to identify the object.	Sensory function should be bilaterally intact.	■ Peripheral neuropathy and paresthesias (altered sensations) may occur in patients with diabetes, hypothyroidism, or acromegaly.	■ In some older patients, light touch and pain sensations may be decreased. ■ In children, touch is well developed at birth. Sensitivity to touch and discriminations should be present. The thresholds of touch, pain, and temperature are higher in older children than in infants.

Endocrine Assessment (continued)

ASSESSMENT/ METHOD	NORMAL FINDINGS	ABNORMAL FINDINGS	LIFESPAN OR DEVELOPMENTAL CONSIDERATIONS
Musculoskeletal Assessment			
Inspect the size and proportions of the patient's body structure.	Size and proportion of the body structure should be bilaterally equal.	▪ Extremely short stature may indicate **dwarfism**, which is caused by insufficient growth hormone. ▪ Extremely large bones may indicate acromegaly, which is caused by excessive growth hormone.	▪ An exaggerated thoracic curve (kyphosis) is common with aging. ▪ Growth charts are used to detect deviation from the norm in children and are used from birth to prepubescent adolescence.
Assessing for Hypocalcemic Tetany			
Assess for **Trousseau sign** (spasmodic muscle contractions induced by pressure on the nerves going to those muscles; a test for hypocalcemia) with resulting tetany by inflating a blood pressure cuff above the antecubital space to a point greater than systolic blood pressure for 2–5 minutes.	A normal finding is no carpal spasm in response to compression of the arm by the blood pressure cuff.	▪ Decreased calcium levels cause the patient's hand and fingers to contract (**carpal spasm**).	▪ Older adults may experience tremors with movement including hands and head, which are not associated with disease. ▪ DTRs and superficial reflexes are the same for children and adults, although the triceps reflex is absent until age 6.
Assess for **Chvostek sign** (facial grimacing caused by repeated contractions of the facial muscle; a test for hypocalcemia) by tapping your finger in front of the patient's ear at the angle of the jaw.	A normal finding is no facial grimacing in response to tapping the patient's face in front of the ear.	▪ Decreased calcium levels cause the patient's lateral facial muscles to contract.	▪ Chvostek sign is an appropriate test for hypocalcemia in patients of any age.

Case Study » Part 2

Ms. Bell's T score is found to be –3.2 in the spine and –3 in the hip. She continues to have pain. Ms. Bell has been started on a bisphosphonate. Her COPD is also exacerbated, and she is started back on steroids. When she comes back to the clinic for a follow-up, she is coughing deeply.

Clinical Reasoning Questions Level I

1. What interview questions would be a priority to ask at today's visit?
2. What teaching can be done today to help Ms. Bell understand her diagnosis?

Clinical Reasoning Questions Level II

3. What added risks (related to fracture) are present with Ms. Bell's COPD exacerbation?
4. What type of medications can aggravate Ms. Bell's GERD and why?

Independent Interventions

Patients with metabolic diseases often require interprofessional care for multiple problems. They often face exhausting diagnostic tests, changes in physical appearance and emotional responses, and permanent alterations in lifestyle. Nursing care is directed toward meeting the patient's physiologic needs, providing education, and ensuring psychologic support for the patient and family. A holistic approach to the complex needs of patients with metabolic disorders is an essential component of nursing care.

Following assessment of an individual for metabolic disorders, the nurse can educate the patient regarding the diagnostic testing, disease state, and therapies. If medications are prescribed, the nurse should provide teaching about how and when to take the medications, what the side effects are, and when to report side effects or changes in their condition to the physician. The nurse should also provide patient teaching related to the complications that could result from the condition and from not taking medications or supplements as prescribed. Patient teaching related to the treatment plan includes medication teaching and providing education about any monitoring devices that the patient needs to use, such as a glucometer for individuals with DM.

The nurse can serve as educator, coach, and advocate to help the patient attain optimum health and prevent complications by teaching about proper nutrition for their disorder, referring the patient to a nutritionist, or encouraging the patient to maintain an exercise routine that is appropriate for their health status. The nurse can provide education about coping mechanisms the patient can use to cope with their disorder and the physical, mental, and emotional effects it may have. The nurse can aid the patient in finding community resources for patient support in the quest for health, especially for patients who have common health problems such as obesity, diabetes, or alcoholism.

Collaborative Therapies

Diagnostic testing can be confusing for patients. The health-care provider will most likely order blood tests, electrolytes and kidney function tests, thyroid and liver function tests, an electrocardiogram (ECG), and a full physical evaluation. In addition to testing for the disorder directly, the physician may order tests to rule out common comorbidities. The patient may not understand the need for these tests, so the nurse can help explain tests to the patient, including the expected procedure and the reason the test is needed.

In addition to diagnostic tests, continual monitoring of hormone and electrolyte levels and kidney, liver, and heart function will be needed throughout the patient's lifetime. This monitoring is required because each patient needs medication or hormone levels titrated individually due to individual differences in absorption, metabolism, and excretion of drugs.

Pharmacologic Therapy

The goals of hormone pharmacotherapy vary widely. In many cases, a hormone is administered as replacement therapy for patients who are unable to secrete sufficient quantities of their own endogenous hormones. However, it is important to note that hormone replacement is not the only pharmacologic intervention in endocrine disorders. Medications may also be modulators and inhibitors of endocrine activity when there is an interruption or increase in hormone activity.

An example of replacement therapy is administering TH after the thyroid gland has been surgically removed. Replacement therapy supplies the same low-level amounts of the hormone that would normally be present in the body. In contrast, in overactive thyroid disease, antithyroid agents may have to be used to inhibit TH synthesis and release. In T1D, the hormone insulin is a necessary lifetime replacement, but in T2D, it may not be started until later in the progression of the disease. Oral medications that improve insulin sensitivity, those that make the pancreas produce insulin, and those that block incretin degradation or replace the incretin hormone may be used. In osteoporosis, selective serum receptor modulators appear to prevent bone loss by imitating estrogen's effect on bone density. The inhibitory action of bisphosphonates slow bone resorption and preserve bone mass. The patient should be aware that treatment is ongoing and should not stop when hormone levels return to normal. The patient should also be aware that oral medication and monthly or yearly medications may require regularly scheduled appointments and are important to prevent interruption in therapy. For example, when thyroid replacement therapy is started, it is for life, and the patient's physician will monitor hormone levels and adjust medication as

needed. The nurse can be part of this team by ensuring that the patient knows how important it is to take the medicine regularly and separate it from other medications and food to optimize absorption.

Nonpharmacologic Therapy

Collaboration with a certified exercise physiologist and certified dietitian may be part of the collaborative team approach to care for patients with a metabolic disorder. A behavioral therapist may be helpful for patients who have difficulty making changes on their own. For example, behavioral therapy may be helpful for patients who abuse alcohol and for those who use food as a coping mechanism.

Complementary Health Approaches

Many patients are turning to complementary health approaches to help them manage lifelong endocrine disorders. Common therapies used to manage endocrine disorders include acupuncture, meditation, yoga, massage, and nutritional supplements. These therapies can help reduce stress and support optimal body functioning, including optimal functioning of the endocrine glands. Before pursing integrative health practices to manage metabolic disorders, nurses should encourage patients to talk to a professional who has experience both with the complementary health approach and with the patient's specific metabolic disorder.

Case Study ›› Part 3

Ms. Bell falls at the grocery store and is brought to the emergency department where she is diagnosed with a fracture of L3 and L4. She is admitted to the medical surgical floor for several days for conservative treatment focusing on alleviating her pain and preventing further injury.

Clinical Reasoning Questions Level I

1. What is the anticipated mortality outcome for a spine fracture versus a hip fracture?
2. In the hospital, what other team members may be called in to help with Ms. Bell's care?

Clinical Reasoning Questions Level II

3. Develop a discharge plan for Ms. Bell that includes safety and medication education.
4. While in the hospital, Ms. Bell is treated with heparin. Comment on the use of long-term heparin therapy for Ms. Bell.

Lifespan Considerations

Like most body systems, the endocrine system, and therefore metabolism, changes throughout the lifespan. Most endocrine glands provide a similar function from the time of birth to the time of death. However, specific hormones may play additional roles during childhood to support the normal growth and development of body systems. In a similar way, endocrine glands of pregnant and nursing women take on additional roles to support the growth and development of the baby. Older adults also see normal age-related changes to endocrine glands as they age.

An assessment of infants and children for alterations in metabolism must include a review of family history to determine if the child has any potential genetic causes for

Medications
Metabolic and Endocrine Disorders

CLASSIFICATION AND DRUG EXAMPLES	MECHANISMS OF ACTION	NURSING CONSIDERATIONS
Insulin *Drug examples:* Short-acting [Humalog(R)] Intermediate-acting (NPH) Long-acting (insulin detemir) forms	Insulin is a replacement therapy; it is an endogenous hormone secreted by the beta cells of the pancreas. It lowers the blood glucose level by stimulating the passage of glucose across cell membranes and uptake into the cells. It also promotes the conversion of glucose to glycogen and inhibits the production of hepatic glucose from glycogen.	▪ Date vials at first use and discard vials past the expiration date. ▪ Refrigerate, but do not freeze, insulin vials not currently in use. ▪ Store insulin in a cool place, and avoid exposure to temperature extremes or sunlight. ▪ Store compatible mixtures of insulin for no longer than 1 month at room temperature or 3 months at 2–8°C (36–46°F). ▪ Discard any vials with discoloration, clumping, granules, or solid deposits on the sides. ▪ Insulin pens not in use can be kept in the refrigerator but, while in use, can be kept out of the refrigerator. They should not be exposed to extreme temperatures and should be discarded 30 days after opening (always check package insert for discarding mixed insulin pens).
Oral Glucose Control Agents *Drug examples:* Biguanides Sulfonylureas Meglitinides Thiazolidinediones Alpha-glucosidase inhibitors Dipeptidyl peptidase-4 (DPP-4) inhibitors	These drugs increase insulin sensitivity and decrease glucose production.	▪ Administer one to three times each day, with meals. ▪ Assess for hypoglycemia. ▪ Use caution with biguanides for patients with renal failure. ▪ Monitor for diarrhea for patients prescribed biguanides and diarrhea and flatulence with alpha-glucosidase inhibitors. ▪ Certain sulfonylureas (chloropamide and tolbutamide) may interact with alcohol causing headache, flushing, and nausea. ▪ Thiazolidinediones may increase the risk for heart failure and cause liver toxicity.
Antithyroid Agents *Drug examples:* Potassium iodide (Thyro-Block) Methimazole (Tapazole) Propylthiouracil Radioactive iodine (I-131, Iodotope)	These drugs inhibit TH synthesis and release.	▪ Assess for hypersensitivity to iodine before giving medication (e.g., ask patients about allergies to shellfish). ▪ Dilute liquid iodine sources in water or orange juice to disguise bitter taste. ▪ Monitor for increased bleeding tendencies if the patient is also taking anticoagulants (iodine increases their effect). ▪ Administer drugs at the same time each day with meals to maintain stable blood levels.
Thyroid Agents *Drug examples:* Levothyroxine sodium (T_4; Levoxyl, Levothroid, Synthroid) Liothyronine sodium (T_3; Cytomel) Liotrix (T_3–T_4; Thyrolar)	Thyroid agents increase blood levels of TH, raising the metabolic rate.	▪ For best absorption give 1 hour before meals or 2 hours after meals. ▪ Thyroid preparations potentiate the effect of anticoagulant drugs. ▪ Thyroid medications potentiate the effect of digitalis. ▪ The effect of insulin may change as thyroid function increases. ▪ During dose adjustment, take the patient's pulse before administering the drug. Report a pulse greater than 100 bpm.
Calcium Regulation Agents *Drug examples:* Calcitonin: Calcitonin—human (Cibacalcin) Calcitonin—salmon (Calciman, Miacalcin)	The drugs oppose the effects of PTH, which acts to increase the blood level of calcium.	▪ Parenteral and nasal spray forms may cause an anaphylactic-type allergic response. ▪ Alternate nostrils daily when administering calcitonin nasal spray. ▪ Observe for side effects. ▪ Teach the patient the proper technique for handling and injecting the drug at home. ▪ Hot flashes are a common side effect.

(continued on next page)

Medications *(continued)*

CLASSIFICATION AND DRUG EXAMPLES	MECHANISMS OF ACTION	NURSING CONSIDERATIONS
Selective Estrogen-receptor Modulators (SERMs) *Drug example:* Raloxifene hydrochloride (Evista)	SERMs appear to prevent bone loss by mimicking estrogen's beneficial effects on bone density in postmenopausal women.	▪ Teach the patient clinical manifestations for blood clots in the legs (deep vein thrombosis) and in the lung (pulmonary embolism); report these immediately. ▪ Assess for a history of blood clots as this is a contraindication for this drug. ▪ Medication should be taken with calcium and vitamin D to prevent or treat osteoporosis. ▪ Hot flashes are a common side effect.
Synthetic Parathyroid Hormone (SERMs) *Drug examples:* Teriparatide (Forteo) Raloxifene (Evista)	SERMs bind with high affinity to the estrogen receptor; they have estrogen agonist and antagonist properties that vary depending on the target organ. This prevents bone loss, improves bone mineral density, and decreases the risk of vertebral fracture.	▪ Teach the patient to stop taking the medication if lightheadedness or a fast or pounding heartbeat occurs with each injection. ▪ The patient should avoid cigarettes and alcohol while taking this drug as they can affect bone mineral density. ▪ Patients may be at an increased risk for bone cancer when taking this drug. ▪ Impaired thinking or judgment may occur when taking this drug. Teach the patient to use caution. ▪ Monitor prescribed laboratory tests such as bone density, liver function, and plasma lipid tests. ▪ Assess for and immediately report any clinical manifestations associated with a thromboembolic event. ▪ Hot flashes are a common side effect. ▪ Teach the patient to notify the healthcare provider immediately if calf pain or tenderness occurs.
Bisphosphonates *Drug examples:* Alendronate sodium (Fosamax) Etidronate disodium (Didronel) Ibandronate (Boniva) Pamidronate disodium (Aredia) Risedronate sodium (Actonel) Tiludronate disodium (Skelid)	Bisphosphonates are potent inhibitors of bone resorption that may be used to prevent and treat osteoporosis. They inhibit bone breakdown, preserve bone mass, and increase bone density in the hip and vertebrae.	▪ Bisphosphonates should not be taken by a woman with a history of blood clots. ▪ They should be taken on an empty stomach, first thing in the morning, with water. ▪ The patient should remain upright for 30 minutes and should not eat or drink anything else for 30 minutes to avoid esophagitis. Hold calcium and vitamin D supplements for 60 minutes or longer after taking the medication. ▪ Monitor for pathologic fractures and bone pain. ▪ Monitor for gastrointestinal side effects. ▪ Monitor kidney function, especially creatinine level. ▪ Monitor BUN, calcium, vitamin D, urinalysis, and serum phosphate and magnesium levels. ▪ Monitor dietary habits for adequate intake of vitamin D, calcium, and phosphate.

Source: Data from Adams, M. P., Holland, L. N., & Urban, C. (2017). *Pharmacology for nurses: A pathophysiologic approach* (5th ed.). Hoboken, NJ: Pearson Education.

metabolic dysregulation. The parent or guardian will play a significant role in the patient interview for younger children with a metabolic disorder, but adolescents should be allowed to answer questions on their own as much as possible, as they may not share their symptoms with a parent present. For older adults, cognitive changes may require the nurse to address questions to an adult child, spouse, or other family member, but the older adult should be addressed directly unless cognitive problems require help.

In children and adolescents, the thyroid may not be palpable, or the thyroid isthmus may be the only palpable part of the thyroid. If the thyroid is palpable in children, it indicates an enlarged thyroid or goiter. In older adults, the thyroid may feel nodular and irregular. Older adults may have difficulty swallowing to allow proper assessment of the thyroid gland, and some may feel anxiety related to having hands on their throat. Speak to the patient in calm, reassuring tones, describing the expected movement so the patient feels more comfortable. For other lifespan considerations related to assessment of the endocrine system, see the Endocrine Assessments feature.

Interventions and therapies for metabolic disorders will depend on the age of the patient and the specific disorder. Disorders related to hormone deficiency will require treatment with exogenous hormones, and the dose prescribed will depend on the patient's age and the normal hormone level for that age group. Children and older adults may need higher or lower levels of hormone depending on the hormone and their stage of development, and the dosage will need to be carefully titrated to achieve the desired effect and reduce the risk of complications. Children with a metabolic disorder will need extensive teaching on how to live with and manage a lifelong disease, and this patient teaching should be age appropriate. Even young children can learn to manage their own disease if they are taught properly, and this teaching should continue as they develop and become more responsible and more able to comprehend the physiology of the disease.

The Endocrine System in Children

The endocrine system is responsible for sexual differentiation during fetal development and for stimulating growth and development during childhood and adolescence. Growth hormone, produced by the anterior pituitary gland, is secreted in pulses when the child is in Stage 4 sleep. Growth hormone stimulates the growth of muscles and improves bone mineralization. The level of growth hormone released increases progressively during childhood, with peak levels being secreted during the growth spurt associated with puberty. Multiple hormones in the endocrine system, including growth hormone, TH, adrenal and gonadal androgens, and estrogen, are responsible for skeletal growth and maturation, including the appearance of secondary ossification centers in the bones (Kini & Nandeesh, 2012). In addition to its role in skeletal growth and maturation, the thyroid gland also contributes to the development of the brain and nervous system in children.

The thymus is one endocrine gland that functions specifically in childhood and adolescence to stimulate the development of T cells. After puberty, the thymus is gradually replaced with fatty tissue and no longer contributes to T cell development. The function of the thymus is to prevent autoimmunity.

The role of the gonads in sexual development in children is detailed in the module on Sexuality.

The most common alterations in metabolism in children are usually genetic/congenital or autoimmune in nature or related to the presence of a tumor. For example, a pituitary tumor can result in too much or too little production of growth hormone, resulting in extremely tall or extremely short stature in children. In contrast to adults, solitary thyroid nodules are more likely to be malignant in children (Gerber, Reilly, & Bhayani, 2015). Autoimmune disorders common in children include T1D, hyperthyroidism (Graves disease), and hypothyroidism (Hashimoto disease). More information about these diseases in children will be presented in the exemplars associated with this module. Obesity in children will also be discussed in the exemplar on Obesity in the module on Nutrition.

Endocrine disorders that relate to the reproductive system in children include precocious puberty and congenital adrenal hyperplasia. Precocious puberty results in early puberty in children, typically before the age of 8 years in girls and before the age of 9 years in boys. In addition to early puberty, precocious puberty can result in early closure of epiphyseal plates in the bones and thus short stature. Precocious puberty is frequently caused by environmental factors such as exposure to certain chemicals. In contrast, congenital adrenal hyperplasia is an inherited disorder of the adrenal glands that results in decreased cortisol and aldosterone production and increased androgen production in children. This causes abnormal genitals in girls at birth, but boys often appear normal. Boys and girls with congenital adrenal hyperplasia have alterations in their reproductive systems that result in male-like characteristics in girls and early puberty in boys (U.S. National Library of Medicine, 2014). Adrenal insufficiency can also affect children, causing weakness, fatigue, nausea, dehydration, and other symptoms.

The Endocrine System in Pregnant Women

Pregnant women present a unique case with regard to the function of the endocrine system, because during pregnancy, the previously minor role of the uterus in the endocrine system becomes greatly enhanced as the uterus and placenta become endocrine glands to support the development of the fetus. When a woman is pregnant, the uterus becomes an endocrine gland secreting prolactin and relaxin, and the placenta becomes an endocrine gland secreting progesterone, estrogens, human chorionic gonadotropin, human placental lactogen, and inhibin. Each of these hormones has a specific function in pregnancy and reproduction.

Relaxin prepares the lining of the uterus for pregnancy, promotes implantation of the fertilized ovum, and stimulates growth of the placenta. During pregnancy, it relaxes the walls of the uterus to inhibit contractions. Outside the uterus, relaxin produces changes in the cardiovascular and renal systems to help prepare the pregnant woman's body for increased blood flow and volume and increased waste products. When the time for delivery of the baby comes, relaxin stimulates rupture of the membranes and softening and opening of the cervix and vagina to prepare for the birth (Society for Endocrinology, 2015a).

Human chorionic gonadotropin (hCG) is produced by the cells surrounding the embryo that will eventually form the placenta; it is the hormone that is detected by home pregnancy tests. hCG stimulates the corpus luteum to produce progesterone to help maintain the pregnancy during the first trimester until the placenta can take over production of progesterone. hCG also helps increase the blood supply to the uterus and helps prepare the uterus for the implanting embryo (Society for Endocrinology, 2015b).

Progesterone and estrogen play a vital role in stimulating uterine development and maintaining the pregnancy (see the module on Reproduction). Human placental lactogen plays a role in providing maternal nutrition to the growing fetus. Inhibin decreases follicle-stimulating hormone levels and regulates placental function. Prolactin is classically known for stimulating milk production in the female breast after delivery, among other roles.

In addition to hormones secreted by the uterus and placenta, other hormones have additional functions during and after pregnancy. For example, oxytocin, which is secreted from the posterior pituitary, stimulates uterine contractions during childbirth and stimulates the flow of milk from the breast during breastfeeding. Pregnancy also increases the demand on the thyroid gland to increase TH secretion because the mother's thyroid must produce TH for the fetus during the first weeks of development. hCG and estrogen are the primary hormones that increase thyroid gland stimulation during pregnancy. The HPA axis also contributes to pregnancy by providing additional nutrients to the fetus and helping clear fetal waste.

The pregnant woman's body undergoes many metabolic and endocrine changes during pregnancy, and most of these changes are considered normal. However, occasionally pregnancy will stimulate a metabolic or endocrine change that causes detrimental effects to the mother and/or fetus. One of the most common metabolic disorders of pregnancy is gestational diabetes. In gestational diabetes, hormones from the placenta produce insulin resistance in the mother, causing high blood glucose levels for both the mother and fetus. This usually begins around gestational week 24. Gestational diabetes can result in babies with macrosomia and breathing problems, and it increases the risk of requiring a cesarean delivery. The baby is also at higher risk for developing obesity and T2D later in life. Gestational diabetes usually resolves spontaneously after birth, but it requires careful glucose monitoring and a diet change for the pregnant woman.

Alterations in TH regulation are also common during pregnancy. Pregnant women are at increased risk of developing either hyperthyroidism or hypothyroidism, which can lead to adverse obstetric outcomes such as miscarriage, low infant birth weight, preterm delivery, placenta abruptio, and postpartum hemorrhage. In addition to common causes of hyper- and hypothyroidism, pregnancy provides unique etiologies for thyroid dysregulation. For example, pregnancy-specific conditions that can lead to hyperthyroidism include hyperemesis gravidarum (characterized by severe nausea, vomiting, weight loss, and electrolyte imbalances) and gestational trophoblastic disease (including both hydatidiform moles and choriocarcinomas). In addition, pregnant women with preexisting hypothyroidism may require a change in dosage of their thyroid replacement hormones.

The pituitary gland normally enlarges during pregnancy; however, if the pituitary gland enlarges too much, it can cause vision changes due to encroachment on the optic chiasm (Corenblum, 2015). Pregnancy can also cause diabetes insipidus and hypopituitarism. Pregnancy-specific conditions that can cause hypopituitarism include Sheehan syndrome and lymphocytic hypophysitis. Sheehan syndrome often develops in women who lost a significant amount of blood during childbirth, causing damage to the pituitary gland. This results in permanent hypopituitarism (Mayo Clinic, 2014a). Lymphocytic hypophysitis is an autoimmune disorder that affects the pituitary gland, especially the pituitary stalk, causing hypopituitarism. It is also often associated with diabetes insipidus.

In addition to metabolic and endocrine changes that occur as a result of pregnancy, women who have preexisting metabolic conditions will require additional monitoring during pregnancy. Pregnancy often either resolves or worsens preexisting metabolic conditions, necessitating a change in therapy during the duration of the pregnancy.

The Endocrine System in Older Adults

See **Table 12–2** » for normal age-related changes to the endocrine system in adults. Older age is a risk for the development of many metabolic disorders, including hypothyroidism and T2D. However, most metabolic disorders are also commonly found in younger individuals, so they are not specifically associated with older adults, and they do not have different manifestations in older adults as compared with younger adults. One metabolic disorder that is frequently associated with older age is osteoporosis, which will be discussed in Exemplar 12.D. In addition to the effect of age on the endocrine system directly, older age also increases the risk of metabolic disorders due to the presence of tumors, injuries, infection, and surgery.

TABLE 12–2 Age-Related Endocrine Changes

Age-Related Change	Significance
Pituitary: ↓ production of ACTH, TSH, FSH	Decreased secretion of glucocorticoids, 17-ketosteroids, progesterone, androgen, and estrogen (and thus lower levels on diagnostic tests)
Thyroid: ↑ in fibrosis and nodularity, ↓ in gland activity	Lower basal metabolic rate Increased incidence of hypothyroidism Palpable nodules
Adrenal medulla: ↑ secretion and level of norepinephrine, ↓ beta-adrenergic response to norepinephrine	Decreased response to beta-adrenergic and receptor-blocking medications Possible contribution to increased incidence of hypertension
Pancreas: calcification of blood vessels and distention and dilation of pancreatic ducts	Decreased production of lipase with reduced fat absorption and digestion, leading to intolerance of fatty foods and indigestion Decreased absorption of fat-soluble vitamins
Pancreas: delayed and decreased insulin release; believed to be accompanied by decreased sensitivity to circulating insulin	Decreased ability to metabolize glucose with higher and more prolonged blood glucose levels, possibly contributing to increased incidence of T2D with aging (however, higher-than-normal blood glucose levels are not unusual in older adults without diabetes)

REVIEW The Concept of Metabolism

RELATE Link the Concepts

Linking the concept of metabolism with the concept of fluids and electrolytes:

1. In T1D, the underlying problem of hyperglycemia leads to acidosis. Explain why the patient with severe hyperglycemia needs fluid replacement as well as insulin.
2. How would changes in aldosterone secretion affect the ability of a patient to maintain proper fluid and electrolyte balance?

Linking the concept of metabolism with the concept of safety:

3. How can the nurse help the patient with osteoporosis prevent falls at home?
4. List some of the mobilization aids that may be used by the patient with osteoporosis.

Linking the concept of metabolism with the concept of stress and coping:

5. A patient who has had a lifelong battle with obesity feels that everyone is looking at her when she goes to the gym, so she often skips her exercise sessions. What suggestions could you make to help her include exercise in her lifestyle?
6. A patient with obesity has given up trying to lose weight because she says that her whole family is large and there is always food around her. What advice can you give her regarding weight loss strategies at home?

READY Go to Volume 3: Clinical Nursing Skills

- SKILLS 1.1–1.4   General Assessment
- SKILLS 1.10–1.27   Physical Assessment
- SKILL 2.24   Oral Medication: Administering
- SKILL 2.31   Injection, Intramuscular: Administering
- SKILL 5.1   Intake and Output: Measuring
- SKILL 8.1   Endocrine Disorders: Assessing
- SKILL 8.2   Endocrine Disorders: Complementary Health Approaches
- SKILL 8.4   Capillary Blood Specimen for Glucose: Measuring
- SKILL 8.5   Diabetes: Managing

REFER Go to Pearson MyLab Nursing and eText

- Additional review materials
- Appendix B: Diagnostic Values and Laboratory Tests

REFLECT Apply Your Knowledge

Jenna Hubbard, 26, brought in her 8-month-old son, Trevor, because of a muscle spasm that appeared very painful. She also reports that he commonly has facial twitching. Jenna's obstetric history indicates that she developed gestational diabetes, and Trevor was born large for gestational age. Blood tests indicate that Trevor has hyperphosphatemia and hypocalcemia. He also has a positive Chvostek sign.

Clinical Reasoning Questions Level I

1. Which electrolyte imbalance is most likely the cause of Trevor's symptoms?
2. A deficiency in which endocrine hormone could cause this electrolyte imbalance?

Clinical Reasoning Questions Level II

3. How would you assess Trevor for pain?
4. What nursing diagnoses are appropriate for Trevor? For Jenna?
5. What patient teaching would you provide for Jenna?

>> Exemplar 12.A
Type 1 Diabetes Mellitus

Exemplar Learning Outcomes

12.A Analyze type 1 diabetes mellitus as it relates to metabolism.

- Describe the pathophysiology of type 1 diabetes.
- Describe the etiology of type 1 diabetes.
- Compare the risk factors and prevention of type 1 diabetes.
- Identify the clinical manifestations of type 1 diabetes.
- Outline the complications of type 1 diabetes.
- Summarize diagnostic tests and therapies used by interprofessional teams in the collaborative care of an individual with type 1 diabetes.
- Differentiate care of patients with type 1 diabetes across the lifespan.
- Apply the nursing process in providing culturally competent care to an individual with type 1 diabetes.

Exemplar Key Terms

Dawn phenomenon, *810*
Diabetes mellitus, *808*
Diabetic ketoacidosis (DKA), *810*
Diabetic nephropathy, *815*
Diabetic neuropathies, *815*
Diabetic retinopathy, *814*
Euglycemia, *824*
Exogenous insulin, *809*
Glucagon, *808*
Gluconeogenesis, *808*
Glucosuria, *809*
Glycogenolysis, *808*
Hyperglycemia, *809*
Hypoglycemia, *813*
Insulin, *808*
Insulin reaction, *813*
Ketosis, *809*
Microalbuminuria, *815*
Polydipsia, *809*
Polyphagia, *809*
Polyuria, *809*
Somatostatin, *808*
Somogyi phenomenon, *810*

Overview

Diabetes mellitus (often referred to more simply as *diabetes*) is a disorder of hyperglycemia resulting from defects in insulin secretion, insulin action, or both, leading to abnormalities in carbohydrate, protein, and fat metabolism (NIDDK, 2016a). According to the American Diabetes Association (ADA, 2015a), there are four major types of diabetes:

- T1D—5% of diagnosed cases
- T2D—95% of diagnosed cases
- Gestational diabetes—9.2% of all pregnancies
- Other specific types of diabetes—1–2% of diagnosed cases.

Role of Hormones

The pancreas produces hormones necessary for the metabolism and cellular utilization of carbohydrates, proteins, and fats. The cells that produce these hormones are clustered in groups called the islets of Langerhans. These islets have three different types of cells:

1. Alpha cells produce the hormone **glucagon**, which stimulates the breakdown of glycogen in the liver, the formation of carbohydrates in the liver, and the breakdown of lipids in both the liver and the adipose tissue. The primary function of glucagon is to decrease glucose oxidation and to increase blood glucose levels. Through **glycogenolysis** (the breakdown of liver glycogen) and **gluconeogenesis** (the formation of glucose from fats and proteins), glucagon prevents blood glucose from decreasing below a certain level when the body is fasting or between meals. The action of glucagon is initiated in most individuals when blood glucose falls below approximately 70 mg/dL.
2. Beta cells secrete the hormone **insulin**, which facilitates the movement of glucose across cell membranes into cells, thus decreasing blood glucose levels. Insulin prevents the excessive breakdown of glycogen in the liver and in muscle, facilitates the formation of lipid while inhibiting the breakdown of stored fats, and helps to move amino acids into cells for protein synthesis. After secretion by the beta cells, insulin enters the portal circulation, travels directly to the liver, and is then released into the general circulation. Circulating insulin is rapidly bound to receptor sites on peripheral tissues (especially muscle and fat cells) or is destroyed by the liver or kidneys. Insulin release is regulated by blood glucose: It increases when blood glucose levels increase, and it decreases when blood glucose levels decrease. When an individual eats food, insulin levels begin to rise in minutes, peak in 30–60 minutes, and return to baseline in 2–3 hours.
3. Delta cells produce **somatostatin**, which is believed to be a neurotransmitter that inhibits the production of both glucagon and insulin.

Blood Glucose Homeostasis

All body tissues and organs require a constant supply of glucose; however, not all tissues require insulin for glucose uptake. The brain, liver, intestines, and renal tubules do not require insulin to transfer glucose into their cells. Skeletal muscle, cardiac muscle, and adipose tissue require insulin for glucose movement into the cells.

Normal blood glucose is maintained in healthy individuals primarily through the actions of insulin and glucagon. Increased blood glucose levels, amino acids, and fatty acids stimulate pancreatic beta cells to produce insulin. As the cells of cardiac muscle, skeletal muscle, and adipose tissue take up glucose, the resulting decrease in plasma levels of nutrients suppresses the stimulus to produce insulin. If blood glucose falls, glucagon is released to raise hepatic glucose output, which raises glucose levels. Epinephrine, growth hormone, T_4, and glucocorticoids (often referred to as *glucose counterregulatory hormones*) also stimulate an increase in glucose in times of hypoglycemia, stress, growth, or other increased metabolic demand. The regulation of blood glucose levels by insulin and glucagon is illustrated in **Figure 12–4 »**.

Pathophysiology and Etiology

Pathophysiology

The destruction of the beta cells of the islets of Langerhans in the pancreas—the only cells in the body that make insulin—is the cause of T1D. When beta cells are destroyed, insulin is no longer produced. Although T1D may be classified as either an autoimmune or an idiopathic disorder, 90% of the cases are immune mediated. The disorder begins with insulinitis, a chronic inflammatory process that occurs in response to the autoimmune destruction of islet cells. This process, which slowly destroys beta cell production of insulin, usually occurs over a long preclinical period, with the onset of hyperglycemia occurring when 80–90% of beta cell function is lost. Researchers believe that both alpha cell and beta cell functions are abnormal, with a lack of insulin and a relative excess of glucagon resulting in hyperglycemia.

Etiology

The onset of T1D most often occurs in childhood and adolescence, but it may occur at any age, even in the 80s and 90s. The actual cause and exact sequence are not completely understood.

Genetic predisposition plays a role in the development of T1D (see the Focus on Diversity and Culture feature), and environmental factors are believed to trigger development of the disorder. The trigger can be a viral infection (e.g., mumps, rubella, coxsackievirus B4) or a chemical toxin (e.g., those found in smoked and cured meats). As a result of exposure to the virus or chemical, an abnormal autoimmune response occurs in which antibodies respond to normal islet beta cells as though they were foreign substances—in other words, by destroying them.

Risk Factors

Although the risk in the general population ranges from 1 in 400 to 1 in 1000, the child of an individual with diabetes has a risk of 1 in 20 to 1 in 50. Genetic markers that determine immune responses have been found in 95% of individuals diagnosed with T1D. The presence of these markers does

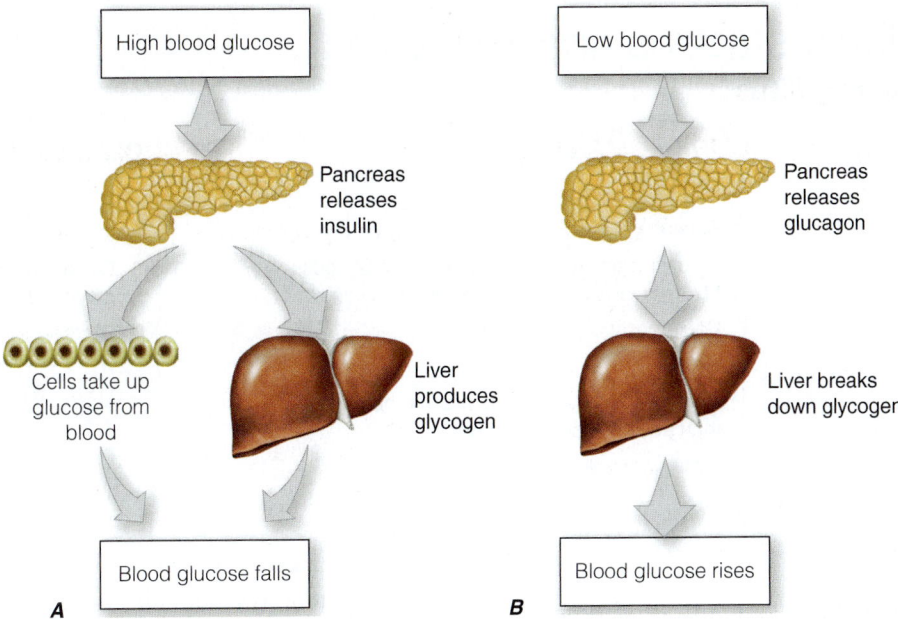

Figure 12–4 ❯❯ Regulation (homeostasis) of blood glucose levels by insulin and glucagon. **A,** High blood glucose is lowered by insulin release. **B,** Low blood glucose is raised by glucagon release.

not guarantee that the individual will develop T1D, but it does indicate increased susceptibility. These individuals may also develop other autoimmune disorders such as Graves disease, Addison disease, autoimmune hepatitis, myasthenia gravis, pernicious anemia, celiac disease, and vitiligo (ADA, 2016a).

Prevention

There is no way to prevent T1D (CDC, 2014b). Researchers, however, are working to fully understand what causes or triggers this type of DM. A better understanding of the pathophysiology and triggers of T1D could mean preventing it in the future. Individuals diagnosed with this type of diabetes are taught to prevent the short- and long-term complications of this disease process (Smith-Marsh, 2014).

Clinical Manifestations

T1D is characterized by **hyperglycemia** (elevated blood glucose levels), a breakdown of body fats and proteins, and development of **ketosis** (an accumulation of ketone bodies produced during oxidation of fatty acids). As was mentioned earlier, the manifestations of T1D appear when approximately 90% of the beta cells are destroyed. However,

manifestations may appear at any time during the loss of beta cells if an acute illness or stress increases the demand for insulin beyond the reserves of the damaged cells.

The clinical manifestations of T1D result from a lack of insulin to transport glucose across the cell membrane into the cells. The accumulation of glucose molecules in the circulating blood results in hyperglycemia. Hyperglycemia causes serum hyperosmolality, drawing water from the intracellular spaces into the general circulation. The increased blood volume increases renal blood flow, and the hyperglycemia acts as an osmotic diuretic. The resulting osmotic diuresis increases urine output (**polyuria**). When the blood glucose level exceeds the renal threshold for glucose—usually approximately 180 mg/dL—glucose is excreted in the urine (**glucosuria**). The decrease in intracellular volume and the increased urinary output cause dehydration. The mouth becomes dry, and the activation of thirst sensors causes the individual to drink increased amounts of fluid (**polydipsia**).

Because glucose cannot enter the cells without insulin, energy production decreases. This decrease in energy stimulates hunger, causing the individual to eat more food (**polyphagia**). Despite increased food intake, the individual loses weight as the body loses water and breaks down proteins and fats in an attempt to restore energy sources. Malaise and fatigue accompany the decrease in energy. Blurred vision also is common, resulting from osmotic effects that cause the lenses of the eyes to swell.

Thus, the classic manifestations of T1D are polyuria, polydipsia, and polyphagia, accompanied by weight loss, malaise, and fatigue. Depending on the degree of insulin deficiency, the manifestations vary from slight to severe. Individuals with T1D require **exogenous insulin** (insulin from a source outside the body) to maintain life. See the Clinical Manifestations and Therapies feature for an overview.

Focus on Diversity and Culture
Risk and Incidence of Type 1 Diabetes

Certain ethnicities have a higher rate of T1D. In the United States, Caucasians are more susceptible when compared to African Americans and Hispanic Americans. Individuals of Chinese and South American descent have a lower risk for developing T1D (Smith-Marsh, 2016a).

Clinical Manifestations and Therapies
Type 1 Diabetes Mellitus

ETIOLOGY	CLINICAL MANIFESTATIONS	CLINICAL THERAPIES
Immune-mediated insulin deficiency caused by pancreatic beta-cell destruction	▪ Polyuria, polydipsia ▪ Recent weight loss, but patient may be overweight ▪ Ketoacidosis on initial presentation in 30–40% of cases, and continued risk for ketoacidosis ▪ Rapid onset of symptoms ▪ Ketosis ▪ Initial period of decreased insulin requirement, then need of insulin for survival ▪ Hyperglycemia	▪ Blood glucose monitoring ▪ Insulin ▪ Dietary management, balancing carbohydrate intake to insulin ▪ Exercise

Complications

The individual with diabetes, regardless of type, is at increased risk for complications involving many body systems. Alterations in blood glucose levels, alterations in the cardiovascular system, neuropathies, increased susceptibility to infection, and periodontal disease are common. In addition, the interaction of several complications can cause problems in the feet. The Multisystem Effects feature shows the progression from cardinal signs to acute and late complications for the patient with diabetes. A discussion of each of these complications follows; nursing care and related collaborative care are discussed later in the exemplar.

Acute Complications

The following discussion provides additional information about hyperglycemia and hypoglycemia. **Table 12–3 ≫** compares DKA, hyperosmolar hyperglycemic state (HHS), and hypoglycemia. Note that DKA and hypoglycemia can occur in both T1D and T2D, but HHS occurs only in T2D. HHS will be discussed in detail in Exemplar 12.B.

Hyperglycemia

The major problems resulting from hyperglycemia in the individual with diabetes are DKA and HHS. Two other problems are the dawn phenomenon and the Somogyi phenomenon.

Dawn Phenomenon

The **dawn phenomenon** is a rise in blood glucose between 4 a.m. and 8 a.m. that is not a response to hypoglycemia. This condition occurs in individuals with both T1D and T2D. The exact cause is unknown, but it is believed to relate to nocturnal increases in growth hormone, which decrease peripheral uptake of glucose.

Somogyi Phenomenon

The **Somogyi phenomenon** is a combination of hypoglycemia during the night with a rebound morning rise in blood glucose to hyperglycemic levels. The hyperglycemia stimulates the counterregulatory hormones, which in turn stimulate gluconeogenesis and glycogenolysis and inhibit peripheral glucose use. This process may cause insulin resistance for 12–48 hours (ADA, 2014a).

Diabetic Ketoacidosis

As the pathophysiology of untreated T1D continues, the insulin deficit causes fat stores to break down; the result is continued hyperglycemia and mobilization of fatty acids with a subsequent ketosis. **Diabetic ketoacidosis (DKA)** develops when there is an absolute deficiency of insulin and an increase in the insulin counterregulatory hormones. Glucose production by the liver increases, peripheral glucose use decreases, fat mobilization increases, and ketogenesis (ketone formation) is stimulated. Increased glucagon levels activate the gluconeogenic and ketogenic pathways in the liver. In the presence of insulin deficiency, hepatic overproduction of beta-hydroxybutyrate and acetoacetic acids (ketone bodies) causes increased ketone concentrations and increased release of free fatty acids. Because of a loss of bicarbonate, which occurs when the ketone is formed, bicarbonate buffering does not occur, and a metabolic acidosis—namely, DKA—occurs. Depression of the central nervous system from the accumulation of ketones and the resulting acidosis may cause coma and death if left untreated (Kishore, 2014). For additional details, see **Figure 12–5 ≫**.

DKA also may occur in an individual with diagnosed diabetes when energy requirements increase during physical or emotional stress. Stress states initiate the release of gluconeogenic hormones, resulting in the formation of carbohydrates from protein or fat. The individual who is sick, who has an infection, or who decreases or omits insulin doses is at a greatly increased risk for developing DKA.

DKA involves four metabolic problems:

1. Hyperosmolarity from hyperglycemia and dehydration
2. Metabolic acidosis from an accumulation of ketoacids
3. Extracellular volume depletion from osmotic diuresis
4. Electrolyte imbalances (e.g., loss of potassium and sodium) from osmotic diuresis

Manifestations of DKA result from severe dehydration and acidosis, and DKA requires immediate medical attention. Admission to the hospital is appropriate when the individual has a blood glucose level greater than 250 mg/dL, a decreasing pH, and ketones in the urine. If the patient is alert and conscious, fluids may be replaced orally. In the first 12 hours of treatment, adults usually require 8–10 L of fluid to replace losses from polyuria and vomiting. However,

Multisystem Effects of
Diabetes

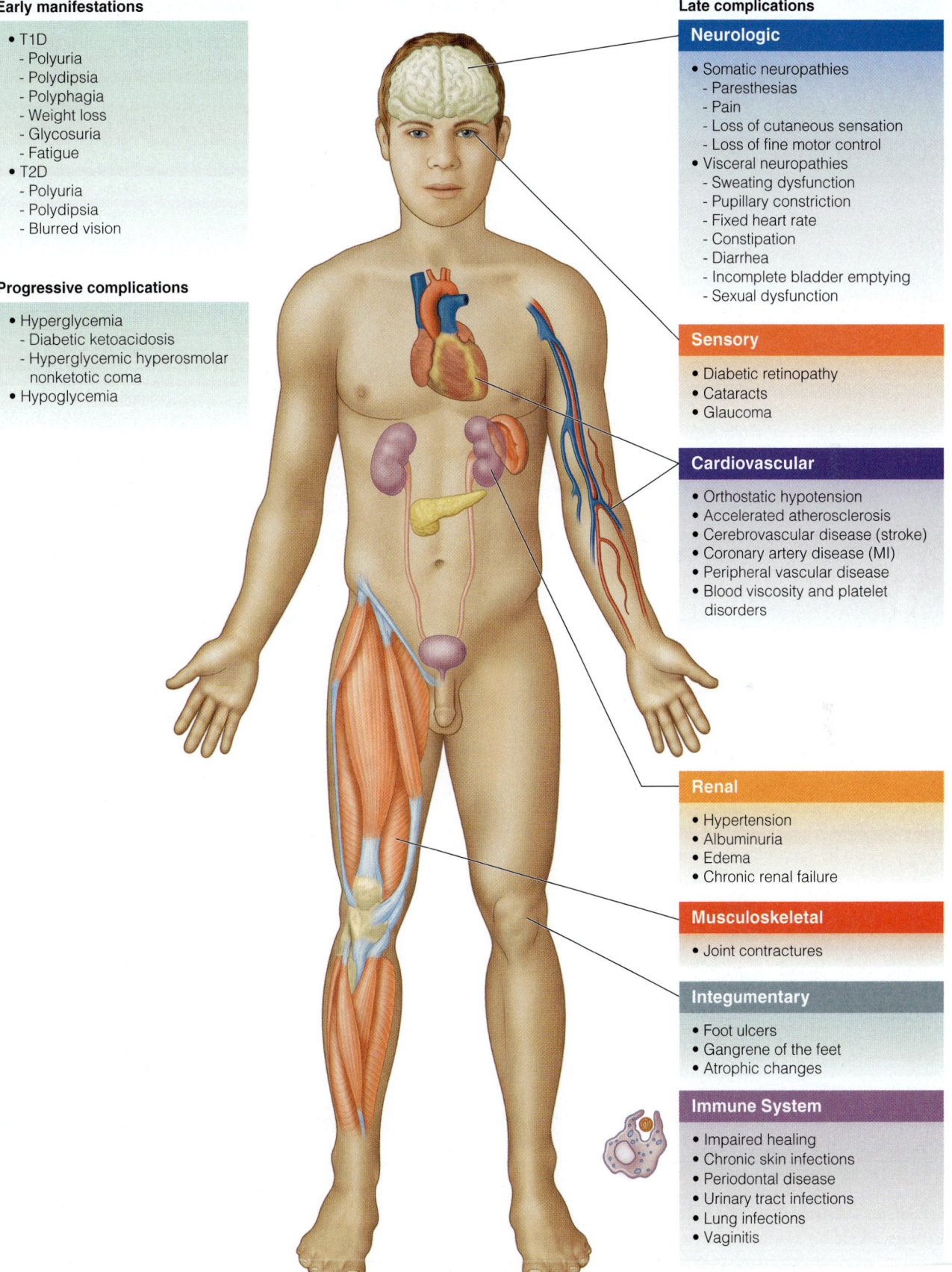

Early manifestations

- T1D
  - Polyuria
  - Polydipsia
  - Polyphagia
  - Weight loss
  - Glycosuria
  - Fatigue
- T2D
  - Polyuria
  - Polydipsia
  - Blurred vision

Progressive complications

- Hyperglycemia
  - Diabetic ketoacidosis
  - Hyperglycemic hyperosmolar nonketotic coma
- Hypoglycemia

Late complications

Neurologic

- Somatic neuropathies
  - Paresthesias
  - Pain
  - Loss of cutaneous sensation
  - Loss of fine motor control
- Visceral neuropathies
  - Sweating dysfunction
  - Pupillary constriction
  - Fixed heart rate
  - Constipation
  - Diarrhea
  - Incomplete bladder emptying
  - Sexual dysfunction

Sensory

- Diabetic retinopathy
- Cataracts
- Glaucoma

Cardiovascular

- Orthostatic hypotension
- Accelerated atherosclerosis
- Cerebrovascular disease (stroke)
- Coronary artery disease (MI)
- Peripheral vascular disease
- Blood viscosity and platelet disorders

Renal

- Hypertension
- Albuminuria
- Edema
- Chronic renal failure

Musculoskeletal

- Joint contractures

Integumentary

- Foot ulcers
- Gangrene of the feet
- Atrophic changes

Immune System

- Impaired healing
- Chronic skin infections
- Periodontal disease
- Urinary tract infections
- Lung infections
- Vaginitis

TABLE 12–3 Comparison of Diabetic Ketoacidosis, Hyperosmolar Hyperglycemic State, and Hypoglycemia

		DKA	HHS	Hypoglycemia
Diabetes type		Both	T2D	Both
Onset		Slow	Slow	Rapid
Cause		↓ Insulin	↓ Insulin	↑ Insulin
		Infection	Older age	Omitted meal/snack
				Error in insulin dose
Risk factors		Surgery	Surgery	Surgery
		Trauma	Trauma	Trauma
		Illness	Illness	Illness
		Omitted insulin	Dehydration	Exercise
		Stress	Medications	Medications
			Dialysis	Lipodystrophy
			Hyperalimentation	Renal failure
				Alcohol intake
Assessments	Skin	Flushed, dry, warm	Flushed, dry, warm	Pallid, moist, cool
	Perspiration	None	None	Profuse
	Breath	Fruity	Normal	Normal
	Vital signs	↓ BP	↓ BP	↓ BP
		↑ P	↑ P	↑ P
		R Kussmaul	R normal	R normal
	Mental status	Confused	Lethargic	Anxious; restless
	Fluid intake	Increased	Increased	Normal
	Gastrointestinal effects	Nausea/vomiting	Nausea/vomiting	Hunger
		Abdominal pain	Abdominal pain	
	Fluid loss	Moderate	Profound	Normal
	Level of consciousness	Decreasing	Decreasing	Decreasing
	Energy level	Weak	Weak	Fatigue
	Other	Weight loss	Weight loss	Headache
		Blurred vision	Malaise	Altered vision
			Extreme thirst	Mood changes
			Seizures	Seizures
Laboratory findings	Blood glucose	>300 mg/dL	>600 mg/dL	<50 mg/dL
	Plasma ketones	Increased	Normal	Normal
	Urine glucose	Increased	Increased	Normal
	Urine ketones	Increased	Normal	Normal
	Serum potassium	Abnormal	Abnormal	Normal
	Serum sodium	Abnormal	Abnormal	Normal
	Serum chloride	Abnormal	Abnormal	Normal
	Plasma pH	<7.3	Normal	Normal
	Osmolality	>340 mOsm/L	>340 mOsm/L	Normal
Treatment		Insulin	Insulin	Glucagon
		IV fluids	IV fluids	Rapid-acting carbohydrate
		Electrolytes	Electrolytes	IV solution of 50% glucose

Note: BP = blood pressure; IV = intravenous; P = pulse; R = respiration.

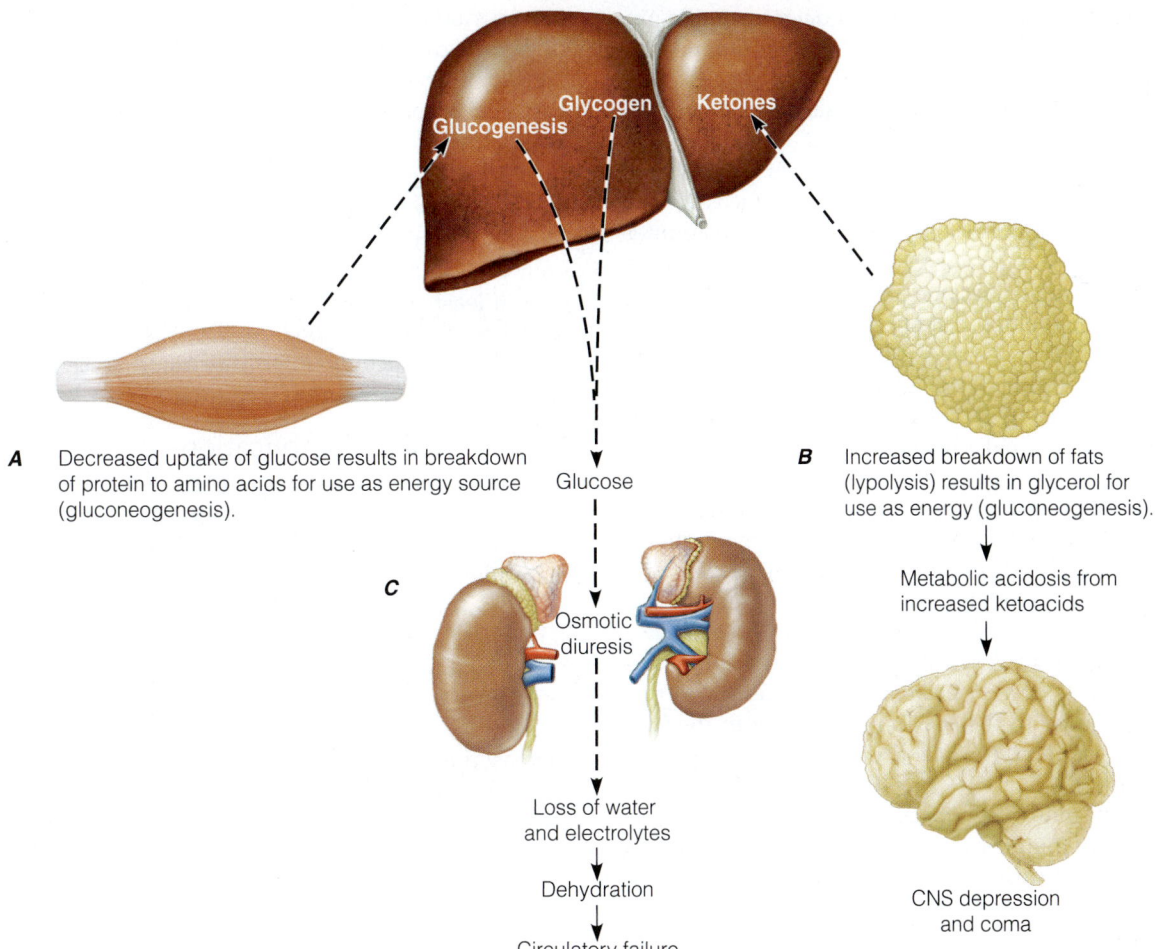

A   Decreased uptake of glucose results in breakdown of protein to amino acids for use as energy source (gluconeogenesis).

Glucogenesis   Glycogen   Ketones

Glucose

B   Increased breakdown of fats (lypolysis) results in glycerol for use as energy (gluconeogenesis).

Metabolic acidosis from increased ketoacids

C   Osmotic diuresis

Loss of water and electrolytes

Dehydration

Circulatory failure

CNS depression and coma

Figure 12–5 ❯❯ In type 1 diabetes mellitus, without adequate insulin, muscle **(A)**, and fat **(B)**, cells are metabolized to provide sources of energy. Amino acids from skeletal muscle are converted to glucose in the liver; glycerol from fat cells is converted to glucose and fatty acids (ketoacids), which cause central nervous system (CNS) depression and coma. Increased glucose **(C)** causes osmotic diuresis, leading to dehydration and decreased circulatory volume. These processes create the symptoms of diabetic ketoacidosis. The symptoms can be reversed with IV insulin to lower blood glucose. Administration of IV fluids raises blood volume to prevent circulatory failure; electrolytes are monitored and corrected.

alterations in level of consciousness, vomiting, and acidosis are common, necessitating intravenous (IV) fluid replacement. The initial fluid replacement may be accomplished by administering 0.9% saline solution at a rate of 500–1000 mL/hr. After 2–3 hours (or when blood pressure is returning to normal), administration of 0.45% saline at 200–500 mL/hr may continue for several more hours. When the blood glucose level reaches 250 mg/dL, dextrose is added to prevent rapid decreases; hypoglycemia could result in fatal cerebral edema.

Regular insulin is used in the treatment of DKA and may be given by various routes, depending on the severity of the condition. Mild ketosis may be treated with subcutaneous insulin, whereas severe ketosis requires an IV infusion of insulin.

The electrolyte imbalance of primary concern in patients with DKA is depleted body stores of potassium. At first, serum potassium levels may be normal, but they decrease during treatment. In DKA (and as a result of rehydration), the body loses potassium from increased urinary output, acidosis, catabolic state, and vomiting or diarrhea. Potassium

replacement is begun early in the treatment, usually by adding potassium to the rehydration fluids. Replacement is essential for preventing cardiac dysrhythmias secondary to hypokalemia. Cardiac rhythms and potassium levels must be monitored every 2–4 hours.

Hypoglycemia

Hypoglycemia (low blood glucose levels) is common in individuals with T1D, and it occasionally occurs in individuals with T2D who are treated with oral hypoglycemic agents. This condition often is called *insulin shock,* **insulin reaction,** or *the lows* in patients with T1D. Hypoglycemia results primarily from a mismatch between insulin intake (e.g., an error in insulin dose), physical activity, and carbohydrate availability (e.g., omitting a meal). The intake of alcohol and drugs, such as chloramphenicol (Chloromycetin), sodium warfarin (Coumadin), monoamine oxidase inhibitors, probenecid (Benemid), salicylates, and sulfonamides, also can cause hypoglycemia.

The manifestations of hypoglycemia result from a compensatory autonomic nervous system response and from impaired cerebral function caused by a decrease in the glucose available for use by the brain. The manifestations vary, particularly in older adults (see Table 12–3). The onset is sudden, and blood glucose usually is less than 45–60 mg/dL. Severe hypoglycemia may cause death.

Individuals who have T1D for 4 or 5 years fail to secrete glucagon in response to a decrease in blood glucose. These patients then depend on epinephrine to serve as a counter-regulatory response to hypoglycemia. However, this compensatory response can become absent or blunted, and the individual then develops a syndrome called *hypoglycemia unawareness*. In this syndrome, the individual does not experience symptoms of hypoglycemia, even though it is present. Because treatment is not initiated in the absence of symptoms, the individual is likely to have episodes of severe hypoglycemia.

When mild hypoglycemia occurs, immediate treatment is necessary. Individuals experiencing hypoglycemia should take approximately 15 g of a rapid-acting sugar. This amount of sugar is found, for example, in three glucose tablets, half a cup of fruit juice or regular soda, 8 oz of skim milk, five Life Savers candies, three large marshmallows, or 3 tsp of sugar or honey. Sugar should not be added to fruit juice. Adding sugar to the fruit sugar already in the juice could cause a rapid rise in blood glucose, with persistent hyperglycemia.

If the manifestations continue, the 15/15 rule should be followed: Wait 15 minutes, monitor blood glucose, and if the blood glucose is low, eat another 15 g of carbohydrate. This procedure can be repeated until blood glucose levels return to normal (Evert, 2014; Haire-Joshu, 1996). Individuals with diabetes should have some source of carbohydrate readily available at all times so that hypoglycemic symptoms can be quickly reversed. If hypoglycemia occurs more than two or three times a week, the individual's diabetes management plan should be adjusted.

Patients with diabetes who have severe hypoglycemia often are hospitalized. The criteria for hospitalization are one or more of the following:

- Blood glucose is less than 50 mg/dL, and the prompt treatment of hypoglycemia has not resulted in recovery of sensorium.
- The patient has coma, seizures, or altered behavior.
- The hypoglycemia has been treated, but a responsible adult cannot be with the patient for the following 12 hours.
- The hypoglycemia was caused by a sulfonylurea drug.

If the patient is conscious and alert, 10–15 g of an oral carbohydrate may be given. If the patient has an altered level of consciousness, administer parenteral glucose or glucagon. Give 20–50 mL of 35–50% glucose, usually at a rate of 10 mL over 1 min by IV push. This is the most rapid method of increasing blood glucose levels. Then, start a continuous IV infusion of glucose 10–20% at 50–200 mL/hr (Diabetes in Control, 2012).

Glucagon is an antihypoglycemic agent that raises blood glucose by promoting the conversion of hepatic glycogen to glucose. It is used in severe insulin-induced hypoglycemia and may be given in the recommended dose of 1 mg by the subcutaneous, intramuscular, or IV route. Glucagon has a short period of action; an oral (if the patient is conscious) or IV carbohydrate should be administered following the glucagon to prevent a recurrence of hypoglycemia. If the patient has been unconscious, glucagon may cause vomiting when consciousness returns.

Chronic Complications

Chronic complications of T1D and T2D occur as a result of poor blood glucose control. These complications develop over at least 10 or more years. Uncontrolled blood glucose damages the body's blood vessels. These complications are referred to as microvascular (tiny blood vessel) and macrovascular (large blood vessel) complications.

Microvascular Complications

Alterations in the microcirculation in the individual with diabetes involve structural defects in the basement membrane of smaller blood vessels and capillaries. (The basement membrane is the structure that supports and serves as the boundary around the space occupied by epithelial cells.) These defects cause the capillary basement membrane to thicken; the eventual result is decreased tissue perfusion. Changes in basement membranes are believed to be caused by one or more of the following: presence of increased amounts of sorbitol (a substance formed as an intermediate step in the conversion of glucose to fructose), formation of abnormal glycoproteins, or problems in the release of oxygen from hemoglobin. The effects of alterations in the microcirculation affect all body tissues but are seen primarily in the eyes and the kidneys (Smith-Marsh, 2016b).

Diabetic Retinopathy

Diabetic retinopathy refers to the changes in the retina that occur in the individual with diabetes. The retinal capillary structure undergoes alterations in blood flow, leading to retinal ischemia and breakdown in the blood–retinal barrier. Diabetic retinopathy is the leading cause of blindness in individuals between 20 and 74 years of age (CDC, 2015a). Retinopathy has three stages:

1. *Stage I: nonproliferative retinopathy.* Dilated veins, microaneurysms, edema of the macula, and presence of exudates characterize this stage.
2. *Stage II: preproliferative retinopathy.* Retinal ischemia causes infarcts of the nerve fiber layer, with characteristic "cotton wool" patches on the retina. Shunts form between occluded and patent vessels.
3. *Stage III: proliferative retinopathy.* As fibrous tissue and new vessels form in the retina or optic disc, traction on the vitreous humor may cause hemorrhage or retinal detachment.

The prevalence of retinopathy is strongly related to the duration of the diabetes (ADA, 2016a). If exudate, edema, hemorrhage, or ischemia occurs near the fovea, the individual experiences visual impairment at any stage. In addition, the individual with diabetes is at increased risk for developing cataracts (opacity of the lens) as a result of increased glucose levels within the lens itself. Screening for retinopathy is important, because laser photocoagulation surgery has proven to be beneficial in preventing loss of vision.

Diabetic Nephropathy

Diabetic nephropathy is a disease of the kidneys characterized by the presence of albumin in the urine, hypertension, edema, and progressive renal insufficiency. In the United States, this disorder accounts for 44% of new cases of end-stage renal disease requiring dialysis or transplantation. Nephropathy occurs in 20–40% of individuals with diabetes and is the single leading cause of end-stage renal disease (ADA, 2016a).

The exact pathologic origin of diabetic nephropathy is unknown. It has been established, however, that thickening of the basement membrane of the glomeruli eventually impairs renal function, and it has been suggested that an increased intracellular concentration of glucose supports the formation of abnormal glycoproteins in the basement membrane and mesangium. The accumulation of these large proteins stimulates glomerulosclerosis (fibrosis of the glomerular tissue). Glomerulosclerosis thickens the basement membrane and simultaneously makes it functionally leaky, allowing large molecules (e.g., proteins) to be lost in the urine. Kimmelstiel-Wilson syndrome is a type of glomerulosclerosis found only in individuals with diabetes. In advanced nephropathy, tubular atrophy occurs, and end-stage renal disease results. (See the module on Fluids and Electrolytes for a discussion of renal failure.)

The first indication of nephropathy is **microalbuminuria** (a low but abnormal level of albumin in the urine). Without specific interventions, individuals with T1D and sustained microalbuminuria develop overt nephropathy, accompanied by hypertension, over a period of 10–15 years (ADA, 2016a).

Because hypertension accelerates the progress of diabetic nephropathy, aggressive antihypertensive management should be instituted. Management includes control of hypertension with angiotensin-converting enzyme (ACE) inhibitors (e.g., captopril [Capoten]), weight loss, reduced salt intake, and exercise.

Diabetic Neuropathy

Peripheral and visceral neuropathies are disorders of the peripheral nerves and the autonomic nervous system. In individuals with diabetes, these disorders often are called **diabetic neuropathies**. The manifestations depend on the locations of the lesions.

The etiology of diabetic neuropathies involves thickening of the walls of the blood vessels that supply nerves, causing a decrease in nutrients; demyelinization of the Schwann cells that surround and insulate nerves, slowing nerve conduction; and formation and accumulation of sorbitol within the Schwann cells, impairing nerve conduction.

Note that manifestations depend on which nerve fibers are involves. As their names imply, polyneuropathies are bilateral sensory disorders involving multiple nerve fibers; mononeuropathies are isolated peripheral neuropathies that affect a single nerve. Visceral neuropathies, also called autonomic neuropathies because of their autonomic nervous system involvement, cause various manifestations depending on the area of the autonomic nervous system that is involved. **Table 12–4 >>** outlines various diabetic neuropathies.

TABLE 12–4 Types of Diabetic Neuropathies

Subtype of Diabetic Neuropathy	Manifestations
Peripheral Neuropathies	
Polyneuropathies	■ Manifestations first in the toes and feet, then progress upward ■ Fingers and hands involved only in later stages of diabetes ■ Distal paresthesias (e.g., numbness, tingling) ■ Pain (aching, burning, shooting) or impaired sensations of pain ■ Cold feet ■ Loss of temperature sense ■ Loss of two-point discrimination ■ Loss of vibration sense
Mononeuropathies	■ Palsy of the cranial nerve III accompanied by headache, eye pain, and inability to move the eye ■ Radiculopathy, most often in the chest ■ Diabetic femoral neuropathy with motor and sensory deficits (e.g., pain, weakness) in the anterior thigh and medial calf
Visceral Neuropathies	
Sweating dysfunction	■ Anhidrosis (absence of sweating) of the hands and feet ■ Increased sweating on face or trunk
Abnormal pupillary function	■ Constricted pupils that dilate slowly in the dark
Cardiovascular dysfunction	■ Fixed cardiac rate that does not change with exercise ■ Postural hypotension ■ Failure to increase cardiac output or vascular tone with exercise
Genitourinary dysfunction	■ Changes in bladder function (e.g., inability to empty the bladder completely, loss of sensation of bladder fullness, increased risk for urinary tract infection) ■ Sexual dysfunctions in men (e.g., ejaculatory changes, impotence) ■ Sexual dysfunctions in women (e.g., changes in arousal patterns, vaginal lubrication, and orgasm)

Macrovascular Complications

The macrocirculation (large blood vessels) in individuals with diabetes (T1D and T2D) undergoes changes as a result of atherosclerosis; abnormalities in platelets, red blood cells, and clotting factors; and changes in arterial walls. Atherosclerosis has an increased incidence and earlier age of onset in individuals with diabetes (although the reason is unknown). Other risk factors that contribute to the development of macrovascular disease of diabetes are hypertension, hyperlipidemia, cigarette smoking, and obesity. Alterations in the vascular system increase the risk of the long-term complications of coronary artery disease, cerebral vascular disease, and peripheral vascular disease.

Coronary Artery Disease

Coronary artery disease is a major risk factor for the development of myocardial infarction in individuals with diabetes, especially the middle-age to older adult with diabetes. Individuals with diabetes who have myocardial infarction are more prone to develop congestive heart failure as a complication of the infarction and also are less likely to survive in the period immediately following the infarction. Coronary artery disease is the most common cause of death in individuals with diabetes (NIDDK, 2014b).

Hypertension

Hypertension (blood pressure greater than or equal to 140/90 mmHg) is a common comorbidity of diabetes. It affects 20–60% of all individuals with diabetes and is a major risk factor for cardiovascular disease (CVD) and microvascular complications such as retinopathy and nephropathy. Hypertension may be reduced by weight loss, exercise, and decreased sodium intake and alcohol consumption. If these methods are not effective, treatment with antihypertensive medications is necessary.

Stroke (Cerebrovascular Accident)

Individuals with diabetes, especially older adults with T2D, are two to six times more likely to have a stroke. Although the exact relationship between diabetes and cerebral vascular disease is unknown, hypertension (a risk factor for stroke) is a common health problem in those who have diabetes. In addition, atherosclerosis of the cerebral vessels develops at an earlier age and is more extensive in individuals with T2D, possibly due to low level of vitamin D (ADA, 2012).

The manifestations of impaired cerebral circulation are similar to those of hypoglycemia or HHS, namely, blurred vision, slurred speech, weakness, and dizziness. Individuals with these manifestations have potentially life-threatening health problems and require constant medical attention.

Peripheral Vascular Disease

Peripheral vascular disease of the lower extremities accompanies both types of diabetes, but the incidence is greater in individuals with T2D. Atherosclerosis of vessels in the legs of individuals with diabetes begins at an earlier age, advances more rapidly, and is equally common in men and women. Impaired peripheral vascular circulation leads to peripheral vascular insufficiency with intermittent claudication (pain) in the lower legs and ulcerations of the feet. Occlusion and thrombosis of large vessels and small arteries and arterioles, as well as alterations in neurologic function and infection, result in gangrene (necrosis, or the death of tissue). Gangrene from diabetes is the most common cause of nontraumatic amputations of the lower leg. In individuals with diabetes, dry gangrene is most common; it is manifested by cold, dry, shriveled, and black tissues of the toes and feet. The gangrene usually begins in the toes and moves proximally into the foot.

Alterations in Mood

Depression affects approximately 20% of individuals with diabetes. Individuals with diabetes and co-occurring depressive symptoms report lower quality of life and greater difficulty managing self-care. They also have higher hemoglobin A1C levels, are less likely to adhere to the treatment regimen, and are less likely to maintain physical exercise and a healthy diet (van Dooren, Nefs, Schram, Verhey, Denollet, & Pouwer, 2013). Treating depression has been associated with better control of serum glucose, so screening for depression is an important part of assessing the individual's ability to manage the disease. Tests to identify the scope of depression are available (see the module on Mood and Affect).

Interventions to help patients with depression include antidepressant medications and psychotherapy focused on restoring logical thinking and problem-solving skills, but treating the depression alone does not improve self-management. Stress management programs and education in the self-management of diabetes are positively correlated with improved self-care. Nurses can assist patients who are depressed by correcting misconceptions about depression, identifying individual strengths in managing diabetes, acknowledging negative feelings that are expressed, suggesting problem-solving behaviors to better manage the disease, and referring to appropriate resources (National Institute of Mental Health, 2015).

Increased Susceptibility to Infection

The individual with diabetes has an increased risk of developing infections. The exact relationship between infection and diabetes is not clear, but many dysfunctions that result from diabetic complications predispose the individual to develop an infection. Vascular and neurologic impairments, hyperglycemia, and altered neutrophil function are believed to be responsible (Weintrob & Sexton, 2015).

The individual with diabetes may have sensory deficits that result in inattention to trauma and vascular deficits that decrease circulation to the injured area. In this situation, the normal inflammatory response is diminished, and healing is slowed.

Nephrosclerosis and inadequate bladder emptying with retention of urine predispose the individual with diabetes to pyelonephritis (inflammation of the kidney and the pelvis) and urinary tract infections. Bacterial and fungal infections of the skin, nails, and mucous membranes are common, and tuberculosis is more prevalent in individuals with diabetes than in the general population. Hospitalized patients with a blood glucose greater than 220 mg/dL have higher infection rates (ADA, 2016a).

Periodontal Disease

Although periodontal disease does not occur more often in individuals with diabetes, it does progress more rapidly, especially if the diabetes is poorly controlled. This more rapid progression is believed to be caused by microangiopathy, with changes in vascularization of the gums. As a result, gingivitis (inflammation of the gums) and periodontitis (inflammation of the bone underlying the gums) occur.

Complications Involving the Feet

The high incidence of problems with and amputations of the feet in individuals with diabetes is the result of angiopathy, neuropathy, and infection. Individuals with diabetes are at high risk for amputation of a lower extremity, with an even greater risk in those who have had diabetes for more than 10 years, are male, have poor glucose control, or have cardiovascular, retinal, or renal complications.

Vascular changes in the lower extremities of the individual with diabetes result in arteriosclerosis. Diabetes-induced arteriosclerosis tends to occur at an earlier age, has an equal incidence in men and women, is usually bilateral, and progresses more rapidly. The blood vessels most often affected are located below the knee. Blockages form in the large, medium, and small arteries of the lower legs and feet. Multiple occlusions with decreased blood flow result in the manifestations of peripheral vascular disease (see the exemplar on Peripheral Vascular Disease in the module on Perfusion for more details).

Diabetic neuropathy of the foot produces multiple problems. Because the sense of touch and perception of pain are absent, the individual with diabetes may have some type of foot trauma without being aware of it. This lack of awareness increases the risk for trauma to the tissues of the feet, leading to ulcer development. Infections commonly occur in traumatized or ulcerated tissue.

Despite the many potential sources of foot trauma in the individual with diabetes, the most common are cracks and fissures caused by dry skin or infections (e.g., athlete's foot), blisters caused by improperly fitting shoes, pressure from stockings or shoes, ingrown toenails, and direct trauma (e.g., cuts, bruises, burns). The individual with diabetic neuropathy who has lost the perception of pain may not be aware these injuries have occurred. In addition, when a part of the body loses sensation, the individual tends to dissociate from or ignore that part, so an injury may go unattended for days or weeks—or may even be forgotten entirely.

Foot lesions usually begin as a superficial skin ulcer. In time, the ulcer may extend deeper, into muscles and bone and lead to an abscess or osteomyelitis. Gangrene can develop on one or more toes; if untreated, the whole foot eventually becomes gangrenous. (Care of the feet, an essential part of patient and family education, is discussed later in this exemplar.)

Collaboration

The results of a 10-year DM Control and Complications Trial (DCCT), sponsored by the National Institutes of Health (NIH), have significant implications for the management of T1D. Individuals in the study who kept their blood glucose levels close to normal by frequent monitoring, several daily insulin injections, and lifestyle changes that included exercise and a healthier diet reduced by 60% their risk for the development and progression of complications involving the eyes, the kidneys, and the nervous system. Treatment of the patient with diabetes focuses on maintaining blood glucose at levels as nearly normal as possible through medications, dietary management, and exercise. In order to help the patient with diabetes reach the optimal glycemic goal, a team approach that includes collaboration among many sources yields the best outcome for the patient. Depending on the available resources and the patient's needs, the interprofessional team may include a certified diabetes educator, a nurse, a family physician, specialists, a dietitian, a podiatrist, and a psychologist and/or psychiatrist, as well as family and friends (Aschner et al., 2010; Tapp et al., 2012).

Diagnostic Tests

Laboratory tests are conducted for screening purposes to diagnose diabetes, and ongoing diagnostic tests are conducted to evaluate the effectiveness of diabetes management. Definitions of normal blood glucose levels vary in clinical practice, depending on the laboratory that performs the assay.

Diagnostic Screening

Four diagnostic tests may be used to diagnose diabetes, and each must be confirmed, on a subsequent day, with another of the four tests. The following diagnostic criteria are recommended by the ADA (2016a):

1. Hemoglobin A1C $\geq$6.5%. This test should be performed in a laboratory using a method that is certified and standardized to the DCCT assay.
2. Symptoms of diabetes plus casual plasma glucose (PG) concentration >200 mg/dL (11.1 mmol/L). *Casual* is defined as any time of day without regard to time since last meal.
3. Fasting plasma glucose (FPG) >126 mg/dL (7 mmol/L). *Fasting* is defined as no caloric intake for 8 hours.
4. Two-hour PG >200 mg/dL (11.1 mmol/L) during an oral glucose tolerance test (OGTT). The test should be performed with a glucose load containing the equivalent of 75 g anhydrous glucose dissolved in water.

When using these criteria, the following levels are used for the FPG:

- Normal fasting glucose = 100 mg/dL (6.1 mmol/L)
- Impaired fasting glucose (IFG) >100 mg/dL (6.1 mmol/L) and <126 mg/dL (7.0 mmol/L)
- Diagnosis of diabetes >126 mg/dL (7 mmol/L)

When these criteria are used, the following levels are used for the OGTT:

- Normal glucose tolerance = 2 hour PG <140 mg/dL (7.8 mmol/L).
- Impaired glucose tolerance (IGT) = 2 hour PG >140 (7.8 mmol/L) and <200 mg/dL (11.1 mmol/L).
- Diagnosis of diabetes = 2 hour PG >200 mg/dL (11.1 mmol/L).

Note that although either method may be used to diagnose diabetes, in a clinical setting the FPG is the recommended screening test for adults who are not pregnant (ADA, 2016a).

Diabetes Management Monitoring

The following diagnostic tests may be used to monitor diabetes management:

- **Fasting blood glucose (FBG).** This test is often ordered, especially if the patient is experiencing symptoms of hypoglycemia or hyperglycemia. In most individuals, the normal range is 70–110 mg/dL.

- **Hemoglobin A1C.** This test determines the average blood glucose level over approximately the previous 2–3 months. When glucose is elevated or control of glucose is erratic, glucose attaches to the hemoglobin molecule and remains attached for the life of the hemoglobin, which is about 120 days. The normal level depends on the type of assay done, but values above 6.5% are considered elevated (ADA, 2016a). The ADA recommends that hemoglobin A1C be performed at the initial assessment, and then at regular intervals, individualized to the medical regimen used.

- **Urine glucose and ketone levels.** These are not as accurate in monitoring changes in blood glucose as blood levels. The presence of glucose in the urine indicates hyperglycemia. Most individuals have a renal threshold for glucose of 160–180 mg/dL; that is, when the blood glucose exceeds 180 mg/dL, glucose is not reabsorbed by the kidney and spills over into the urine. This number varies greatly, however. Ketonuria (the presence of ketones in the urine) occurs with the breakdown of fats and is an indicator of DKA; however, fat breakdown and ketonuria also occur in states of malnutrition.

- **Urine test for the presence of albumin (albuminuria).** If albuminuria is present, a 24-hour urine test for creatinine clearance is used to detect the early onset of nephropathy.

- **Serum cholesterol and triglyceride levels.** These indicate atherosclerosis and an increased risk of cardiovascular impairments. The ADA (2016a) recommends treatment goals to lower low-density lipoprotein (LDL) cholesterol to less than 100 mg/dL, raise high-density lipoprotein (HDL) cholesterol to more than 40 mg/dL in men and more than 50 mg/dL in women, and lower triglycerides to less than 150 mg/dL.

- **Serum electrolytes.** Levels are measured in patients who have DKA or HHS (specific to T2D) to determine imbalances.

Monitoring Blood Glucose

Individuals with diabetes must monitor their condition daily or as directed by their provider by testing glucose levels. Two types of tests are available. The first type, long used before the development of devices to directly measure blood glucose, is urine testing for glucose and ketones. Urine testing is less commonly used today. The second type, direct measurement of blood glucose, is widely used in all types of healthcare settings and in the home.

Urine Testing for Ketones and Glucose

Urine testing for glucose and ketones was at one time the only available method for evaluating the management of diabetes. An inexpensive, noninvasive, and painless test, it has unpredictable results and cannot be used to detect or measure hypoglycemia. In the healthy state, glucose is not present in the urine because insulin maintains serum glucose below the renal threshold of 160–180 mg/dL. The accuracy of this measurement is not reliable in diabetes because the renal threshold may rise with aging or secondary to diabetes. Urine testing is recommended to monitor hyperglycemia and ketoacidosis in individuals with T1D who have unexplained hyperglycemia during illness or pregnancy. Ketones may be detected through urine testing and reflect the presence of DKA. Individuals who choose not to self-monitor blood glucose by other methods may use urine testing.

Self-Monitoring of Blood Glucose

Self-monitoring of blood glucose (SMBG) allows the individual with DM to monitor and achieve metabolic control and decrease the danger of hypoglycemia. The ADA recommends that all patients with diabetes be taught some method of monitoring glycemic control. The timing of SMBG is highly individualized, depending on the patient's diagnosis, general disease control, and physical state. SMBG is recommended three or more times a day for patients with T1D using multiple insulin injections or insulin pump therapy.

When adding or modifying therapy, patients with both T1D and T2D should test more often than usual. SMBG is also useful when the individual is ill or pregnant or has manifestations of hypoglycemia or hyperglycemia. Both hypoglycemia and hyperglycemia may contribute to complications and decrease quality of life. With the information assessed with SMBG, patients can alter their diet, their physical activity, and even their medication to reduce the postprandial increases, reduce their risk for complications, and feel better because they no longer experience wide swings in glucose levels (McCulloch, 2015).

The ADA annually publishes a comprehensive list of currently available blood glucose-monitoring machines and test strips with approximate prices in *Diabetes Forecast.* Most medical insurance policies cover the cost of these machines, known as *glucose meters,* and the test strips. Many companies provide the meter free of cost. Testing supplies are specific to each glucose meter, so the recipient is obligated to purchase supplies for that particular meter.

The following equipment is needed for SMBG:

- A lancet device to perform a finger-stick for obtaining a drop of blood (e.g., Autolet, Penlet, Soft Touch; see **Figure 12–6 ≫**).

- A blood glucose monitor (e.g., Glucometer, AccuChek, One Touch). If the most accurate measurement is desired or recommended, the manufacturer's instructions must be followed carefully. If the timing or amount of the blood on the strip is not exact, the test will not be accurate. Meters include a memory of previous glucose readings to show a pattern of control. Most of the meters no longer require coding and are simple to use by just placing the strip in the meter and applying a small drop of blood.

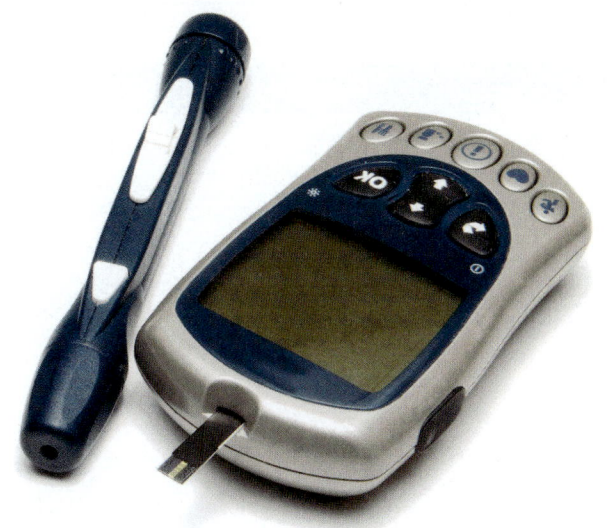

Source: Rob Byron/Shutterstock.

Figure 12–6 》 Lancet and blood glucose monitor for SMBG.

A technology for continuous blood glucose monitoring (CGM) has become available in recent years. The CGM has a sensor that is inserted under the skin. This sensor continuously sends data useful as a warning for high or low glucose levels. Finger-stick measurements are required before therapy adjustments are made. The CGM may be used for diagnostic evaluation; patients wear the pump for 3 days under the supervision of physicians and nurses. The data reveal patterns of glycemic control useful for treatment (McCulloch, 2015).

A CGM technology currently in development involves a bio-implant that would provide data wirelessly for 1–5 years after being inserted. Noninvasive CGM technologies that are being developed include infrared monitoring and ultrasound (McCulloch, 2015).

Factors that Affect Glucose Meter Performance

According to the U.S. Food and Drug Administration (FDA, 2015), several factors affect the accuracy of blood glucose test results. The quality of the meter and test strips and the patient's ability to use the meter correctly contribute to the degree of accuracy. Other factors can create false positive or false negative readings.

Hematocrit

Patients with higher hematocrit values usually test falsely low in blood glucose, and patients with lower hematocrit test falsely higher. Anemia and sickle cell anemia are two conditions that can affect hematocrit values.

Other Substances

Overdoses of many medications cause inaccurate results. Glucose meters and supplies vary in sensitivity to medications. Uric acid (a natural substance in the body that can be more concentrated in some individuals with DM), glutathione (an antioxidant also called *GSH*), and ascorbic acid (vitamin C) are known to interfere with accurate results.

Using Correct Supplies and Sample Volume

The test strips must be compatible with the glucose meter, must not be outdated, and must not have been exposed to air and humidity, which can alter strip sensitivity. The volume of blood required depends on the type of strip that is used. Please refer to product guidelines for this information.

Pharmacologic Therapy

The pharmacologic treatment for DM depends on the type of diabetes. Individuals with T1D must have insulin; those with T2D are usually able to control glucose levels with an oral hypoglycemic medication, but they may require insulin if control is inadequate.

Insulin

The individual with T1D requires a lifelong exogenous source of the insulin hormone to maintain life. Insulin is not a cure for diabetes; rather, it is a means of controlling hyperglycemia. Insulin is also necessary in other situations, such as these:

- An individual with diabetes is unable to control glucose levels with oral antidiabetic drugs and/or diet. The ADA (2016a) also states that if a newly diagnosed patient with diabetes has markedly symptomatic and/or increased blood glucose, insulin should be considered at the outset with or without additive agents.

- An individual with diabetes is experiencing physical stress (e.g., infection, surgery) or is taking corticosteroids.

- A woman with gestational diabetes is unable to control glucose with diet.

- An individual with diabetes has DKA or HHS.

- An individual with diabetes is receiving high-calorie tube feedings or parenteral nutrition.

Preparations of insulin are derived from animals (pork pancreas) or synthesized in the laboratory from either an alteration of pork insulin or recombinant DNA technology, using strains of *Escherichia coli* to form a biosynthetic human insulin. Insulin analogs have been developed by modification of the amino acid sequence of the insulin molecule. Although different types are prescribed on an individualized basis, it is standard practice to prescribe human insulin.

Insulins are available in rapid-acting, short-acting, intermediate-acting, and long-acting preparations. The trade names and times of onset, peak, and duration of action are listed in **Table 12–5 》**.

Insulin lispro (Humalog) is a human insulin analog that is derived from genetically altered *E. coli* that includes the gene for insulin lispro. It is classified as a rapid-acting or ultra-short-acting insulin. Compared to regular insulin, insulin lispro has a more rapid onset (less than 15 minutes), an earlier peak of glucose lowering (30–60 minutes), and a shorter duration of activity (3–4 hours). Thus, lispro should be administered 15 minutes before a meal, rather than 30–60 minutes before as recommended for regular insulin. Patients with T1D usually also require concurrent use of a longer acting insulin product. Lispro is much less likely than regular insulin to cause tissue changes and may lower the risk of nocturnal hypoglycemia in patients with T1D.

TABLE 12–5 Insulin Preparations

	Name	Onset (H)	Peak (H)	Duration (H)
Rapid acting	Lispro (Humalog)	0.25	1–1.5	3–4
	Aspart (NovoLog)	0.25	40–50 minutes	3–5
	Glulisine (Apidra)	0.25	1–1.5	3–5
Short acting	Regular (Novolin R, Humulin R)	0.5–1	2–3	4–6
Intermediate acting	NPH (Novolin N, Humulin N)	2	6–8	12–16
Long acting	Glargine (Lantus)	2 (onset and peak not defined)	16–20	24 +
	Detemir (Levemir)	1	6–23	24 +
Combinations	Humalog 50/50	0.5	3	6–12
	Humalog 75/25	0.25	2–4	6–12
	NovoLog 70/30	0.25	1–4	12–24
	Humulin 70/30	0.5	4–8	24
	Novolin 70/30	0.5	4–8	24

Regular insulin is unmodified crystalline insulin, classified as a short-acting insulin. Regular insulin is clear in appearance and is the only insulin preparation that can be given intravenously; the other types are suspensions and could be harmful if given by this route. Regular insulin is also used to treat DKA, to initiate treatment for newly diagnosed T1D, and in combination with intermediate-acting insulins to provide better glucose control.

The onset, peak, and duration of action of insulin can be changed with the addition of acetate buffers and protamine. Zinc and protamine are added to NPH insulins to prolong their action, and they are classified as intermediate- or long-acting insulins. These preparations appear cloudy when properly mixed prior to injection. Protamine and zinc are foreign substances and may cause hypersensitivity reactions. As of July 6, 2005, Lilly discontinued manufacture of pork insulins and Humulin U and Humulin Lente insulin.

Insulin glargine (Lantus) is a 24-hour, long-acting rDNA human insulin analog that is given subcutaneously once or twice a day, usually at bedtime, to treat patients with both T1D and T2D. It has a relatively constant effect (i.e., it does not have a peak time of effect). It is not recommended for use in pregnancy. Glargine should not be mixed with other insulins; the pH is incompatible (RxList, 2016). Glargine cannot be used in insulin pumps.

SAFETY ALERT Glargine (Lantus) and detemir (Levemir) are clear, unlike other intermediate- or long-acting insulins. Do not mistake these for regular insulin. Do not mix them with any other insulins. Do not inject them intravenously, only subcutaneously.

Insulin is dispensed as 100 units/mL (U-100) and 500 units/mL (U-500) in the United States. U-100 is the standard insulin concentration used. U-500 insulin is used only in rare cases of insulin resistance when patients require very large doses. U-500 and all the analog insulins require a prescription.

Nursing implications for administering insulin are outlined in Skill 2.35 in Volume 3 of this title, and instructions for the patient are provided in the Patient Teaching feature.

The considerations for administering insulin include routes of administration, syringe and needle selection, preparing the injection, sites of injection, mixing insulins, and insulin regimens.

>> Go to Volume 3, Clinical Nursing Skills, Skill 2.35, for steps to teach patients how to administer insulin.

All insulins are given parenterally, although current research is investigating the development of a nasal spray and an oral preparation of insulin. Only regular insulin is given by both subcutaneous and IV routes; all others are given only subcutaneously. If the IV route is not available, regular insulin may also be administered intramuscularly in an emergency situation.

Regular or rapid-acting insulins are used in continuous subcutaneous insulin infusion (CSII) devices, often called *insulin pumps* (e.g., MiniMed). CSII devices have a small pump that holds a syringe of insulin, connected to a subcutaneous needle by tubing. The pump is about the size of a pager and can be worn on a belt or tucked into a pocket. The needle is placed in the skin, usually in the abdomen, and is changed every 3 days. This device delivers a constant amount of programmed insulin throughout each 24-hour period. It also can be used to deliver a bolus of insulin manually (e.g., before meals).

Maintaining normal blood glucose during hospitalization decreases the risk of postoperative infections and shortens hospital stays. Healing is impaired when hemoglobin is glycosylated (hemoglobin A1C); glycosylated Hgb has increased affinity for oxygen, putting tissues at risk for ischemia (Humphers et al., 2014). Further, diabetes leads to small-vessel disease, which impairs circulation and oxygenation of tissue for healing.

IV insulin infusions are preferable for maintaining normal blood glucose during hospitalization, although their use depends on frequent blood glucose monitoring and intensive nursing care. Supplements of regular insulin following sliding-scale prescriptions (relative to monitored blood glucose levels) are ineffective management protocols, risking both hyperglycemia and hypoglycemia. These supplements treat hyperglycemia after it has occurred rather than pre-venting it. The current trend is to use a basal insulin along with a fixed dose for carbohydrate intake and a correction factor that is geared to the patient (ADA, 2016a).

Many individuals with diabetes believe the pump allows more normal regulation of blood glucose and pro-vides greater lifestyle flexibility. When recommended pro-cedures are followed, pumps are as safe as multiple-injection therapy. A potential complication is an undetected inter-ruption in insulin delivery, which may result in a rapid onset of DKA. The needle site must be kept clean and changed regularly (usually every 2–3 days) to prevent inflammation and infection.

Other special injection products are available for individ-uals with physical handicaps. These products include auto-matic injectors and jet spray injectors. Prefilled syringes are useful for individuals who are visually impaired or traveling. Prefilled syringes are stable for up to 30 days if stored in the refrigerator.

The vial of insulin in use may be kept at room temperature for up to 4 weeks. Stored vials should be kept in the refrigera-tor and brought to room temperature prior to administration.

Regular insulin does not require mixing. If the solution is cloudy or discolored, the vial should be discarded. The other types of insulin must be mixed to disperse the parti-cles evenly throughout the solution. Mix the vial by gently rolling it between the hands; vigorous shaking causes bub-ble formation and frothing, which make the dose inaccu-rate. It is critical that no air bubbles remain in the prepared dose, because even a small bubble can displace several units of insulin.

Although in theory any area of the body with subcutane-ous tissue can be used for injections of insulin, certain sites are recommended (see **Figure 12–7 》**). The rate of absorption

and peak of action of insulin differ according to the site. The site that allows the most rapid absorption is the abdomen, fol-lowed by the deltoid muscle, then the thigh, and then the hip. Because of the rapid absorption, the abdomen is the recom-mended site.

》 *Go to Volume 3, Clinical Nursing Skills, Chapter 2, for techniques to minimize discomfort of injections.*

Do not massage the site after administering the injection, because massaging may interfere with absorption; however, pressure may be applied for about 1 minute. Insulin should not be injected into an area to be exercised (e.g., the thigh before a vigorous walk) or to which heat will be applied; exercise or heat may increase the rate of absorption and cause a more rapid onset and peak of action.

Lipodystrophy (hypertrophy of subcutaneous tissue) or lipoatrophy (atrophy of subcutaneous tissue) may result if the same injection site is used repeatedly, especially with pork and beef insulins. The tissues become hardened and have an orange-peel appearance. The use of refrigerated insulin may trigger the development of tissue atrophy or hypertrophy. These problems rarely occur with the use of human insulins. Lipodystrophy and lipoatrophy alter insu-lin absorption, delaying its onset or retaining the insulin in the tissue for a period of time instead of allowing it to be absorbed into the body. Lipodystrophy usually resolves if the area is unused for a minimum of 6 months.

Aspirin Therapy

Individuals with diabetes are up to four times more likely to die from CVD. It is recommended that a once-daily dose of 81–325 mg enteric-coated aspirin be given to reduce athero-sclerosis in patients with vascular disease or increased car-diovascular risk factors. Aspirin therapy is contraindicated for patients with aspirin allergy, bleeding tendency, antico-agulant therapy, recent gastrointestinal bleeding, or active liver disease (ADA, 2016a).

Nutrition Management

The management of diabetes requires a careful balance between the intake of nutrients, the expenditure of energy, and the dose and timing of insulin. Although everyone has the same need for basic nutrition, the individual with diabe-tes must eat a more structured diet to prevent hyperglyce-mia. The goals for dietary management for individuals with diabetes, based on guidelines established by the ADA (2016a), are as follows:

- Maintain as near normal blood glucose levels as possible by balancing food intake with insulin or oral glucose.

- Achieve optimal serum lipid levels.

- Provide adequate calories to maintain or attain reason-able weights, and to recover from catabolic illness.

- Prevent and treat the acute complications of insulin-treated DM, short-term illnesses, and exercise-related problems, or the long-term complications of diabetes.

- Improve overall health through optimal nutrition, using Dietary Guidelines for Americans and ChooseMyPlate.

The ADA (2016a) recommends that carbohydrate intake be individualized to the patient's needs, with recommended

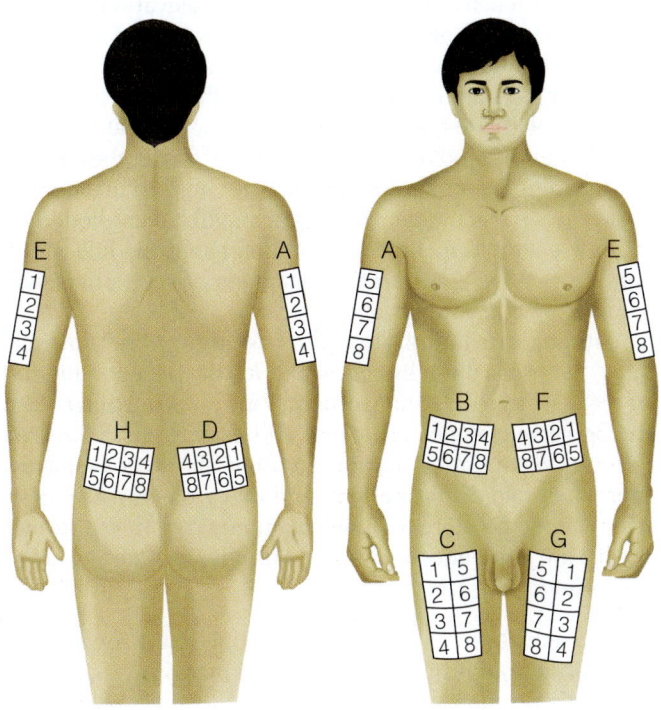

Figure 12–7 》 Sites of insulin injection.

allowances of 45–65% of the daily diet. Carbohydrates contain 4 kcal/g and intake should not be restricted to less than 130 g/day. This group of nutrients consists of plant foods (grains, fruits, vegetables), milk, and some dairy products. Carbohydrates can be divided into simple sugars and complex carbohydrates. Glycemic index is the rate at which a food raises blood glucose and, thus, insulin. Proponents of low-carbohydrate diets use glycemic index as the scientific foundation for decreasing intake of foods with a high glycemic index. However, many factors affect the digestion of carbohydrates; to date, research does not support using glycemic index as a basis for therapy. The ADA (2016a) does not recommend reliance on glycemic index as a method to treat or prevent diabetes.

The use of sucrose as part of the total carbohydrate content in the diet does not impair blood glucose control in individuals with diabetes. Sucrose and sucrose-containing foods must be substituted for other carbohydrates gram for gram. Dietary fructose (from fruits and vegetables or from fructose-sweetened foods) produces a smaller rise in PG than sucrose and most starches, so it may offer an advantage as a sweetening agent. However, large amounts of fructose have potentially adverse effects on serum cholesterol and LDL cholesterol, so amounts used should be controlled.

The recommended daily protein intake is 15–20% of total daily kilocalorie intake. Protein has 4 kcal/g. Sources of protein should be low in fat, low in saturated fat, and low in cholesterol. Although this amount of protein is much less than most individuals normally consume, it is recommended to help prevent or delay renal complications. To help the patient accept the decrease in the amount of protein, the nurse may suggest a less severe restriction at diagnosis with a gradual decrease to take place over a period of years.

Dietary fats should be low in saturated fat and cholesterol. Saturated fats should be no higher than 7% of the total kilocalories allowed per day, with dietary cholesterol less than 200 mg/day. Fat has 9 kcal/g. Sources of the different types of fat include:

- *Saturated fat.* Sources are animal meats (meat and butter fats, lard, bacon), cocoa butter, coconut oil, palm oil, and hydrogenated oils.

- *Polyunsaturated fat.* Sources are oils of corn, safflower, sunflower, soybean, sesame seed, and cottonseed.

- *Monosaturated fat.* Sources are peanut oil, olive oil, and canola oil.

Limiting fat and cholesterol intake may help prevent or delay the onset of atherosclerosis, a common complication of diabetes.

Dietary fiber may be helpful in treating or preventing constipation and other gastrointestinal disorders, including colon cancer. It also helps provide a feeling of fullness, and large amounts of soluble fiber may be beneficial to serum lipids. Soluble fiber is found in dried beans, oats, and barley, and in some vegetables and fruits (e.g., peas, corn, zucchini, cauliflower, broccoli, prunes, pears, apples, bananas, oranges). Insoluble fiber, which is found in wheat and corn, and in some vegetables and fruits (e.g., carrots, Brussels sprouts, eggplant, green beans, pears, apples, strawberries), does facilitate intestinal motility and give a feeling of fullness.

The ideal level of fiber has not been determined, but an intake of 20–35 g/day is recommended. An increase in fiber may cause nausea, diarrhea or constipation, and increased flatulence, especially if the individual does not also increase fluid intake. Fiber in the diet should therefore be increased gradually.

Although the body requires sodium, most individuals consume much more than is needed each day, especially in processed foods. The recommended daily intake is 1000 mg of sodium per 1000 kcal, not to exceed 3000 mg. The primary concern about sodium is its association with hypertension, a common health problem in individuals with diabetes. It is suggested that table salt (which is 40% sodium) and processed foods high in sodium be avoided in the diabetes meal plan. In normotensive and hypertensive individuals, reduced sodium intake of 2300 mg per day with a diet high in fruits and vegetables and low in fat lowers blood pressure (ADA, 2015d).

The diet plan for individuals with diabetes restricts the amount of refined sugars. As a result, many individuals use noncaloric sweeteners and foods or drinks made with noncaloric sweeteners. Commercially produced nonnutritive sweeteners are approved for use by the FDA. Although questions have been raised about the safety of these substances in laboratory animal studies, they are considered safe for use by humans. Included in this category of sweeteners are saccharin (Sweet'N Low), aspartame or neotame (Nutrasweet, Equal), sucralose (Splenda), acesulfame potassium (Sunett), and stevia (Truvia). The nonnutritive sweeteners have negligent amounts of or no kilocalories, do not produce dental caries, and produce very little or no change in blood glucose levels.

Individuals with diabetes also use nutritive sweeteners, including fructose, agave, honey, sorbitol, and xylitol. The kilocalorie content of these substances is similar to that of table sugar (sucrose), but they cause less elevation in blood glucose. They are often included in foods labeled as "sugar free." Sorbitol may cause flatulence and diarrhea.

Researchers are continuing to study the safety and effectiveness of the sweeteners. In addition, the FDA recommends that the food industry label products with the amount of each ingredient in milligrams per serving and the number of servings per container. When teaching patients about diet, the nurse should include information about the kilocalorie content of sweeteners and the meaning of such phrases as *sugar free* and *dietetic* on labels.

Although drinking alcoholic beverages is not encouraged, neither is it totally prohibited for the patient with diabetes. Alcohol consumption may potentiate the hypoglycemic effects of insulin and oral agents. The ADA (2016a) recommends that men with diabetes consume no more than two drinks per day and that women with diabetes consume no more than one drink per day. In the following list are guidelines for individuals who include alcohol in their diet plan:

- The signs of intoxication and hypoglycemia are similar; thus the individual with T1D is at increased risk for an insulin reaction.

- Liqueurs, sweet wines, wine coolers, and sweet mixes contain large amounts of carbohydrate.

- Light beer is the recommended alcoholic drink.
- Alcohol should be consumed with meals and included in the daily food intake. In most instances, the alcohol is substituted for fat in calculating the diet; a drink with 1.5 oz of alcohol is the equivalent of two fat exchanges (90 kcal).

Several systems for meal planning are available to the individual with diabetes. These systems include a consistent-carbohydrate diabetes meal plan, exchange lists, point systems, food groups, carbohydrate counting, and calorie counting. No matter what system is used, however, it must take into account the individual's eating habits, diet history, food values, and special needs. Altering foods and meal patterns is often one of the most difficult parts of diabetes management; careful consideration of individualized preferences enhances compliance with the diet. Although the ADA recommends that a registered dietitian provide the nutrition prescription, nurses must know what is prescribed and be able to reinforce teaching and answer questions.

Sick-Day Management

When the individual with diabetes is sick or has surgery, blood glucose levels increase, even though food intake decreases. The individual often mistakenly alters or omits the insulin dose, causing further problems. The guidelines for dietary management during illness focus on preventing dehydration and providing nutrition for promoting recovery. In general, sick-day management includes the following:

- Monitoring blood glucose at least four times a day throughout an illness
- Testing urine for ketones if blood glucose is greater than 240 mg/dL
- Continuing to take the usual insulin dose or oral hypoglycemic agent
- Sipping 8–12 oz of fluid each hour
- Substituting easily digested liquids or soft foods if solid foods are not tolerated (The substituted liquids and foods should be carbohydrate equivalents, for example, 1/2 cup sweetened gelatin, 1/2 cup fruit juice, one Popsicle, 1/4 cup sherbet, and 1/2 cup regular soft drink.)
- Calling the healthcare provider if unable to eat for more than 24 hours or if vomiting and diarrhea last for more than 6 hours.

Exercise

The third component of diabetes management is a regular exercise program. The benefits of exercise are the same for everyone, with or without diabetes: improved physical fitness, improved emotional state, weight control, and improved work capacity. In individuals with diabetes, exercise increases the uptake of glucose by muscle cells, potentially reducing the need for insulin. Exercise also decreases cholesterol and triglycerides, reducing the risk of cardiovascular disorders. Individuals with diabetes should consult their primary healthcare provider before beginning or changing an exercise program. The ability to maintain an exercise program is affected by many factors, including

fatigue and glucose levels. It is as important to assess the individual's usual lifestyle before establishing an exercise program as it is before planning a diet. Factors to consider include the patient's usual exercise habits and living environment, as well as community programs. The exercise that the individual enjoys most is probably the one that he or she will continue (throughout patients should be cautioned to use proper footwear, inspect the feet daily and after exercise, avoid exercise in extreme heat or cold, and avoid exercise during periods of poor glucose control).

In the individual with T1D, glycemic responses to exercise vary according to its type, intensity, and duration. Other factors that influence responses include the timing of exercise in relation to meals and insulin injections and the time of day of the activity. Unless these factors are integrated into the exercise program, the individual with T1D has an increased risk of hypoglycemia and hyperglycemia. Following are general guidelines for an exercise program:

- Individuals who have frequent hyperglycemia or hypoglycemia should avoid prolonged exercise until glucose control improves.
- The risk of exercise-induced hypoglycemia is lowest before breakfast, when free-insulin levels tend to be lower than they are before meals later in the day or at bedtime.
- Low-impact aerobic exercises are encouraged.
- Exercise should be moderate and regular; brief, intense exercise tends to cause mild hyperglycemia, and prolonged exercise can lead to hypoglycemia.
- Exercising at a peak insulin action time may lead to hypoglycemia.
- SMBG is essential both before and after exercise.
- Food intake may need to be increased to compensate for the activity.
- Fluid intake, especially water, is essential.

Young adults may continue participating in sports with some modifications in diet and insulin dosage. Blood sugar of less than 100 mg/dL should be treated with a carbohydrate source prior to beginning exercise (ADA, 2016a). Athletes should begin training slowly, extend activity over a prolonged period, take a carbohydrate source (e.g., drink consisting of 5–10% carbohydrate) after about 1 hour of exercise, and monitor blood glucose levels for possible adjustments. In addition, a snack should be available after the activity is completed. It may be necessary to omit the usual regular insulin dose prior to an athletic event; even if the athlete is hyperglycemic at the beginning of the event, blood glucose levels will fall to normal after the first 60–90 minutes of exercise. Individuals with T1D should avoid exercise in the presence of ketones in the urine.

Surgery

Surgical management of diabetes involves replacing or transplanting the pancreas, pancreatic cells, or beta cells. Although it is still in the investigative stage, many researchers believe that transplantation of the tail of the pancreas is the most promising technique for achieving long-term disease control. Islet cell transplantation has had moderate success, and research is continuing. Other research is being conducted in the use of an internally implanted artificial pancreas or closed-loop artificial beta cells.

Surgery is a stressor that often alters self-management and glycemic control in individuals with diabetes. In response to stress, levels of catecholamines, cortisol, glucagon, and growth hormone increase, as does insulin resistance. Hyperglycemia occurs, and protein stores are decreased. In addition, diet and activity patterns change, and medication types and dosages vary. As a result, surgical patients who have diabetes are at increased risk for postoperative infection, delayed wound healing, fluid and electrolyte imbalances, hypoglycemia, and DKA (Loh-Trivedi & Rothenberg, 2015).

The patient should be in the best possible metabolic state preoperatively. Screening for complications and regular monitoring of blood glucose are part of preoperative preparation. Oral hypoglycemic agents may be withheld for 1 or 2 days before surgery, and during the perioperative period, regular insulin is often administered to the patient with T2D and to those with hyperglycemia but not diagnosed with diabetes. All patients with hyperglycemia, whether diagnosed with diabetes or not, follow a carefully prescribed insulin regimen individualized to specific needs.

The insulin regimen in the perioperative period is individualized. When the patient is NPO, short-acting insulin should not be given without IV glucose. Patients with both types of diabetes and patients with hyperglycemia who are critically ill in the perioperative period should receive IV glucose and insulin infusion in an intensive care unit. The target blood glucose level during surgery is between 110 and 140 mg/dL. This level prevents hypoglycemia, which is difficult to detect under anesthesia, and prevents glycosuria, dehydration, and impaired wound healing. IV infusion of glucose, insulin, and added potassium is appropriate for all hyperglycemic patients undergoing surgery (ADA, 2016a).

The surgical procedure should be scheduled for as early as possible in the morning to minimize the length of fasting. If there is no food intake after surgery, IV dextrose should be administered, accompanied by subcutaneous regular insulin every 6 hours for the noncritically ill surgical patient. The dose can be adjusted to blood glucose levels. Although kilocalorie intake is decreased postoperatively, stress can increase insulin requirements. Glucose control is also affected postoperatively by nausea and vomiting, anorexia, and gastrointestinal suction.

During the postoperative period, the patient with T2D may continue to require insulin or may resume oral medications, depending on glucose control. The patient with T1D may require reduced insulin as healing progresses and stress diminishes. Regular blood glucose monitoring is essential, as are assessments for hypoglycemia.

Lifespan Considerations

Diabetes unfortunately can affect individuals of any age. The presence of diabetes complicates care for other acute illnesses and injuries, and it has wide-ranging complications for individuals who are pregnant. Care of individuals with diabetes is complex, for varying reasons, regardless of the individual's stage of life. However, the developmental stages of childhood and children's cognitive levels take on particular importance when assessing and caring for children with diabetes or any chronic illness. The nurse needs to carefully assess the child's readiness to handle self-care. The orientation to the present and rebelliousness that come with adolescence may affect treatment adherence. In collaboration with parents and caregivers, nurses assess the pediatric patient's ability to participate in treatment, provide self-care, and adhere to treatment regimens.

T1D in Children and Adolescents

Some 208,000 Americans children and adolescents have diabetes (T1D and T2D), with just under 20,000 new cases being diagnosed each year (ADA, 2016b). The clinical manifestations of all forms of diabetes in children are hyperglycemia, which includes increased thirst, hunger, urination, fatigue, and blurred vision (see **Figure 12–8 »**). Weight loss is an additional symptom in children with T1D. The clinical manifestations of T1D usually appear as an acute event that requires emergency intervention. Some 20–25% of all DKA cases are due to new-onset diabetes. DKA is caused by an absolute lack of insulin and, although research studies have found some measurable insulin concentrations, the levels are inadequate to meet the metabolic needs of the child. The clinical hallmarks of DKA are dehydration and electrolyte imbalance.

SAFETY ALERT Nurses should teach parents that extreme sleepiness and irritability can be signs of hypoglycemia or hyperglycemia in toddlers. They should check blood glucose levels if their toddler is demonstrating these behaviors.

Speedy diagnosis and treatment are required to prevent further deterioration. Therapy is aimed at correcting the metabolic acidosis, restoring fluid and electrolyte balance, and achieving **euglycemia** (a normal concentration of glucose in the blood). The frequent blood sugar monitoring, IV fluids, and insulin drips required for treatment mandate that the child be cared for in an intensive care environment until stabilized.

To achieve optimal glycemic control and prevent acute complications, children with diabetes require a dedicated and knowledgeable team of caregivers. The team consists of a primary care provider (who may be an endocrinologist or a family physician with training in childhood diabetes), a dietitian, a certified diabetes educator, a school nurse, and trained personnel who may be involved in the daily activities of the child in school or child care. The team may also include a social worker or psychologist with education in behavioral modification to address problems that may arise in dealing with a chronic disease in childhood. It is imperative that there be a team approach involving open communication within the group. A plan of care is developed by the primary care provider, the certified diabetes educator, and the parents and child (if appropriate) and is disseminated to the other team members.

Federal laws that protect children with diabetes include the Rehabilitation Act of 1973, the Individuals with Disabilities Education Act of 1990 (reauthorized most recently in 2004) and the Americans with Disabilities Act of 1990. Any

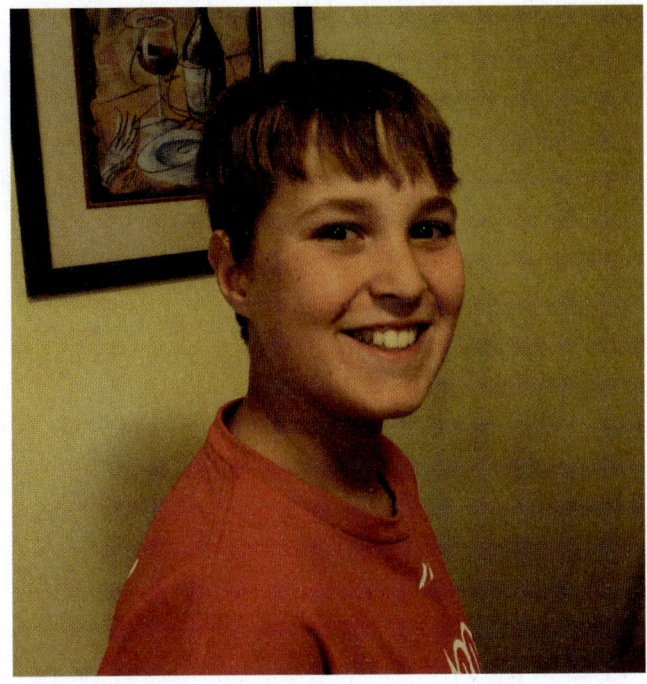 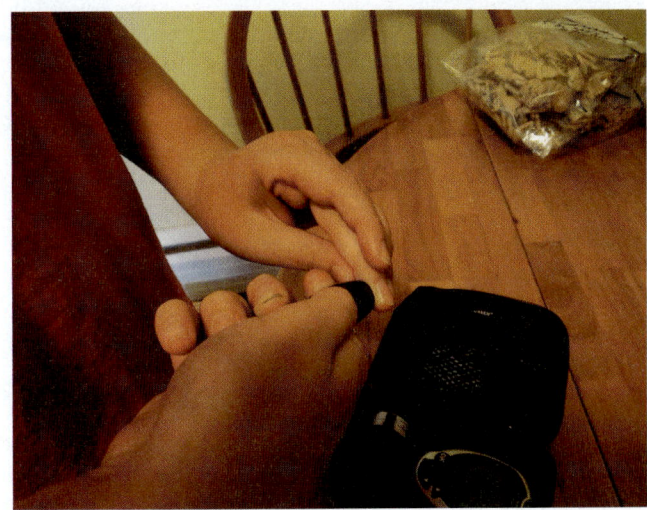

Source: Michael Grey.

Figure 12–8 》》 Six months ago, Ethan, 11 years old, was going for an annual physical, and his grandmother, a retired nurse, noted to his parents that Ethan was often tired and very thirsty; she suggested the family discuss these symptoms with Ethan's pediatrician. By that evening, Ethan was in the emergency department having his blood sugar regulated, and the family spent the next day at a specialized center learning how to manage his newly diagnosed type 1 diabetes mellitus. Today, Ethan is thriving. He tests his glucose level frequently, and injects himself with insulin four times a day: at breakfast, lunch, and dinner, and at bedtime. He is very careful with his diet and he maintains an active lifestyle. He knows that if his glucose level is high, he needs to drink water and let a responsible adult know.

school or child care that is open to the public must provide for the special needs of the child with diabetes by providing a written individualized education plan (IEP) that is developed in partnership with the child's parents and, if the child is old enough, the child.

The child must be allowed to participate in all sports and extracurricular activities that are available at the school or child care (see Section 504 of the Rehabilitation Act of 1973). It is important for parents, school personnel, and the child's treatment team to work together to ensure both the child's health and safety at school and the child's potential for success in the school environment, whether in the class or on the field. A child's success in school is greatly improved by development of a diabetes management plan for use by caregivers and school personnel. A thorough diabetes management plan ensures privacy for checking blood pressure, training of school personnel on diabetes management, and instructions for when to call the parents, the treating healthcare provider, or 9-1-1.

》》 **Stay Current:** For information on diabetes management plans and other strategies for helping children with diabetes succeed in school, see guidelines provided by the CDC at http://www.cdc.gov/features/diabetesinschool/

Diagnostic Tests

A hemoglobin (A1C) level of 6.5% or higher in combination with a random blood PG level of 200 mg/dL or higher or a fasting PG of 126 gm/dL or higher confirms the presence of diabetes. Fasting is defined as no caloric intake for at least 8 hours.

In children with T1D, the diagnosis may be confirmed by the presence of autoantibodies to glutamic acid decarboxylase, pancreatic islet beta cells (tyrosine phosphatase IA-2), and/or insulin. Some forms of T1D have no evidence of autoimmunity and are termed idiopathic. This type of diabetes can also occur in children who are obese, and documentation of C peptide levels (which indicate the activity of the pancreatic beta cells) and the presence or absence of immune markers along with a careful family history and evaluation of presenting symptoms may be useful to the physician in attaining the correct diagnosis. This will be helpful in distinguishing T1D from T2D in children when there is a need (American Association of Clinical Endocrinologists, 2015).

Glucose Monitoring

Children require more frequent glucose monitoring than adults and have different targets because of their erratic oral intake and activity (see **Table 12–6 》》**). By age 6–8, most children can take some responsibility for obtaining and reading a blood glucose sample or injecting insulin.

Insulin

For pediatric patients with T1D, exogenous insulin is a life-long requirement. However, children who are newly diagnosed may go through a partial remission phase when blood sugars are close to normal with smaller amounts of insulin. It is believed that this phenomenon results from activation of the remaining beta cells, and scientists now think that it is important for patients in this honeymoon phase to continue

TABLE 12–6 Plasma Blood Glucose and Hemoglobin A1C Goals for T1D by Age Group

Age Group	Plasma Blood Glucose Goal Range (mg/dL)		Hemoglobin A1C (%)	Rationale
	Before Meals	**Bedtime/ Overnight**		
Toddlers and preschoolers (0–6 years)	100–180	110–200	<8.5	Vulnerability to hypoglycemia
				Insulin sensitivity
				Unpredictability in dietary intake and physical activity
				A lower goal (< 8.0%) is reasonable if it can be achieved without excessive hypoglycemia.
School age (6–12 years)	90–180	100–180	<8	Vulnerability to hypoglycemia
				A lower goal (< 7.5 %) is reasonable if it can be achieved without excessive hypoglycemia.
Adolescents and young adults (13–19 years)	90–130	90–150	<7.5	A lower goal (< 7.0%) is reasonable if it can be achieved without excessive hypoglycemia.

Key concepts in setting glycemic goals:

- Goals should be individualized, and lower goals may be reasonable based on benefit–risk assessment.
- Blood glucose goals should be modified in children with frequent hypoglycemia or hypoglycemia unawareness.
- Postprandial blood glucose values should be measured when there is a discrepancy between preprandial blood glucose values and A1C levels and to help assess glycemia in those on basal/bolus regimens.

Glycemic goals may need to be modified to take into account the fact that most children younger than age 6 or 7 have a form of "hypoglycemic unawareness." They lack the cognitive capacity to recognize and respond to hypoglycemic symptoms and may be at greater risk for hypoglycemia. Children under 5 years of age may be at risk for permanent cognitive impairment after episodes of severe hypoglycemia.

Sources: Based on American Diabetes Association. (2016a). Standards of medical care in diabetes—2016. *Diabetes Care, 39* (Suppl. 1). Retrieved from http://care.diabetesjournals.org/content/suppl/2015/12/21/39.Supplement_1.DC2/2016-Standards-of-Care.pdf; International Diabetes Federation. (2013). *Pocketbook for management of diabetes in childhood and adolescence in under-resourced countries.* Retrieved from http://www.idf.org/sites/default/files/attachments/ISPAD-LFAC-Pocketbook-final-2.pdf; National Diabetes Education Program. (2014). *Overview of diabetes in children and adolescents.* Retrieved at https://www.niddk.nih.gov/health-information/health-communication-programs/ndep/living-with-diabetes/youth-teens/diabetes-children-adolescents/Documents/overview-of-diabetes-children_508_2016.pdf

Patient Teaching
Ten Tips for Better Glucose Control in Children

10. **Be persistent.** Parents need to stay involved in the day-to-day management of their child's blood sugar until the child is old enough and mature enough to self-manage responsibly.

9. **Provide structure.** Maintaining daily routines helps keep glucose in control. This step may be a challenge, but sticking as close as possible to a routine usually results in better glucose control.

8. **Support year-round exercise.** To maintain consistent insulin sensitivity, the child should participate in an activity during the week and on the weekends. Excessive activity at one time with extended periods of inactivity at other times can cause major glucose swings.

7. **Keep accurate, consistent records.** Although glucose meters have memories, the input of information is limited. There is also a psychologic effect to writing down blood sugars and food intake. Special notations also help identify a probable cause when blood sugar control is erratic.

6. **Think like a pancreas.** Understanding the underlying basic physiology of the pancreas assists in making correct decisions in relation to food intake and insulin administration. This understanding is not acquired overnight, but with time, experience, and education and support from a trained professional, a child with diabetes gets to know her or his own diabetes better than anyone else.

5. **Demand quality from your healthcare team.** Although the decisions regarding diabetes are made by the child and the parents, the diabetes care team has the expertise to support and guide the child through a life with diabetes.

4. **Network with other families.** Support groups and other children with diabetes can be a powerful system to enable the child and the parents.

3. **If it's broken, fix it.** For the child with diabetes, small things can become big things quickly. The child and the parents need to be vigilant for illness and stresses that may cause wide fluctuations in glucose control.

2. **Involve the child.** Children are more apt to follow rules if they have been involved in making the rules. Allowing children to make decisions gives them the confidence to feel some control over the disease. For example, young children can choose the finger that will be stuck for glucose measurement.

1. **Let kids be kids.** Sometimes the glucose police need to take a break. Constantly nagging a child to attain perfect numbers results in breakdowns in communication between the child and parent, and the child may give up on even trying to self-manage. The parent should take time for fun and relaxation with and without the child, just as they would if diabetes was not in the picture.

Source: Based on Scheiner, G. (2015). *Top ten tips for better glucose control.* Retrieved from http://www.diabetesselfmanagement.com/Articles/Kids-And-Diabetes/top-10-tips-for-better-blood-glucose-control/

TABLE 12–7 Recommended Insulin Doses for Children with T1D

During the partial remission phase (honeymoon)	Total daily dose <0.5 unit/kg/day
Prepubertal children (outside partial remission phase)	Total daily dose 0.7–1 unit/kg/day
Puberty (usually requires substantial increase)	Total daily dose 1–2 units/kg/day

Source: Data from Danne, T., Bangstad, H. J., Deeb, L., Jarosz-Chobot, P., Mungaie, L., Saboo, B., … International Society for Pediatric and Adolescent Diabetes. (2014). ISPAD Clinical Practice Consensus Guidelines 2014: Insulin treatment in children and adolescents with diabetes. *Pediatric Diabetes, 15*(Suppl. 20), 115–134. doi:10.1111/pedi.12184

taking insulin by injection to preserve the remaining beta cells for as long as possible (Joslin Diabetes Center, 2016).

Daily insulin dosage for children depends on many factors, including age, weight, stage of puberty, duration and phase of diabetes, state of injection sites, nutritional intake and distribution, exercise patterns, daily routine, results of glucose monitoring, and comorbid illness. See **Table 12–7 »** for recommended doses based on body weight.

The correct dose is the dose that achieves the best control for a child without causing hypoglycemia and that at the same time allows healthy progression and growth according to the weight and height charts. For information on how insulin is administered, please see Exemplar 12.B on T2D. Continuous subcutaneous insulin infusion (CSII) devices (insulin pumps) are fairly popular with young individuals and may be a good option for families with children who require intensive insulin therapy (see the Evidence-Based Practice feature).

In addition to the correct daily insulin dosage determined for the child, an additional amount of insulin may need to be administered with a meal based on the child's premeal blood glucose level. This additional amount of insulin is referred to as the *correction factor* and is given to reach the postmeal glucose target (Osborn et al., 2014). The healthcare team works with the child to determine the correction factor.

The child and parents also need to learn how to adjust the amount of rapid insulin necessary to cover carbohydrate (CHO) intake at a meal. The insulin-to-CHO ratio (I:C) may differ according to meal and activity level. The healthcare team or certified diabetes educator works with the child and family to determine appropriate ratios and to teach them how to calculate these ratios for different situations (McDermott, 2010; Osborn et al., 2014).

Nutrition Management

Dietary recommendations for children with diabetes are based on healthy eating guidelines that are also suitable for all children and adults. (See **Table 12–8 »** for age-specific nutrition recommendations for children with T1D.)

Managing Complications

Although the complications of diabetes for children are similar to those for adults, a few specific complications are more

Evidence-Based Practice

Intensive Insulin Therapy and Mealtime Behaviors

Intensive insulin therapy is designed to mimic the body's production of insulin by delivering multiple doses of insulin throughout the day via multiple injections or insulin pump. Intensive insulin therapy allows patients more flexibility in timing meals and snacks and in the quantity of carbohydrates consumed. Further, intensive insulin therapy is thought to prevent long-term complications of diabetes. These factors make intensive insulin therapy attractive to families with young children whose schedules are variable because of parents' work and child and family activities common among this age group.

Problem

Early childhood is a critical time for the development of healthy eating behaviors. Does the flexibility intensive insulin therapy provides result in more successful mealtime behaviors and healthy eating for young children who receive the therapy?

Evidence

In a one-sample, cross-sectional study of 39 young children, researchers found that a more healthful diet was related to fewer behavioral problems at mealtime. Using the Behavioral Pediatric Feeding Assessment Scale, researchers determined that greater adherence to a healthy diet at meals correlated to parent–child behaviors at mealtimes (Patton, Dolan, Cheng, & Powers, 2013). Challenging behaviors observed during meals included child time away from the table (an average of 2 minutes per child per meal) and time children spent talking (an average of 6 minutes per child per meal). These behaviors resulted in less time eating (Patton, Dolan, Smith, et al., 2013).

Implications

The results of the small study sample are supported by the body of knowledge of child development. Toddlers can be temperamental as they seek to expand their independence and may be less hungry because of their slower growth rate. They may also experience food jags, where they show interest in only one or two specific foods at a time. Young children are also easily distracted at mealtimes by television and other interruptions (Ball et al., 2017). Therefore, parents of young children with diabetes may find mealtimes especially challenging.

Nurses can help by assessing child dietary intake and mealtime quality and encouraging parents to share their successes and concerns—what works and what does not—as well as their frustrations related to feeding children with diabetes. Referrals to a professional who can provide behavioral strategies that target mealtime can help parents assess and improve their mealtime strategies.

Critical Thinking Application

1. What strategies would you suggest to improve parent–child interactions at mealtime for the parents of a 2-year-old with diabetes? For the parents of a 5-year-old?

2. What challenges related to dietary adherence do you think would be common for adolescents? What strategies would you suggest to adolescents and their parents?

TABLE 12–8 Age-Specific Nutritional Recommendations

Age	Nutritional Recommendations
Infants and toddlers	<ul><li>Encourage mothers to breastfeed their infants up to 12 months.</li><li>Frequent small meals (grazing) may promote better glycemic control. Care must be taken to match the feeding schedule and the insulin.</li><li>Insulin pump therapy has proven to be effective in infants and toddlers and reduces the trauma of frequent injections. Rapid-acting insulin as a bolus is usually given after the meal so a more accurate estimation of insulin dosing to match food intake can occur.</li><li>Encourage a variety of tastes, colors, and textures of foods while considering personal and cultural preferences.</li><li>Episodes of food refusal and sickness often cause parental distress. Support from the healthcare team is essential.</li></ul>
Schoolchildren	<ul><li>Focus on adapting the diabetes regimen to fit the active life of the school-age child. Give advice regarding carbohydrate intake to prevent hypoglycemia and how to adjust insulin and intake when sports activities are involved.</li><li>The team should discuss sleepover and party advice.</li><li>The team should discuss special occasions like birthdays and Halloween.</li><li>Frequent consults with a pediatric nutritionist help with problem solving in this age group.</li></ul>
Adolescents	<ul><li>Weight monitoring is recommended for early recognition of both weight loss and inappropriate weight gain, which may be associated with insulin omission for weight control or may be indicative of an eating disorder.</li><li>Teach adolescents how to read food labels to help plan carbohydrate intake.</li><li>Meals and snacks should be eaten at the same time each day. However, erratic eating behavior is not uncommon among adolescents. Parties, vacations, and peer pressure may all contribute.</li><li>Advise on how to make healthy choices in restaurants.</li><li>Advise on safe consumption of alcohol and the risk of prolonged hypoglycemia.</li></ul>

Sources: Data from Ayling, R. (2012). Nutritional management of diabetes mellitus in infants and children. In R. R. Watson, G. Grimble, V. R. Preedy, & S. Zibaldi (Eds.), *Nutrition in infancy*. New York, NY: Springer; Hess-Fischi, A. (2016). *Meal planning for children with type 1 diabetes: Understanding carbohydrates for optimal blood glucose management.* Retrieved from http://www.endocrineweb.com/guides/type-1-children/meal-planning-children-type-1-diabetes; KidsHealth. (2013). *Eating out when you have diabetes.* Retrieved from http://kidshealth.org/kid/diabetes_basics/diabetes-nutrition/eating_out_diabetes.html?tracking=K_RelatedArticle; Smart, C., Annan, F., Bruno, L., Higgins, L. A., & Acerini, C. L. (2014). Nutritional management in children and adolescents with diabetes. *Pediatric Diabetes, 15*(S20), 135–153.

prevalent in children with diabetes. Celiac disease, an immune-mediated disorder characterized by the inability to hydrolyze peptides contained in gluten, occurs with increased frequency in individuals with T1D (1–16% of individuals compared with 0.3–1% of the general population). Celiac disease (also called *nontropical sprue*) may be asymptomatic, but general symptoms include poor growth, delayed puberty, nutritional deficiencies, and hypoglycemia. A gluten-free diet is the only accepted treatment for celiac disease (ADA, 2016a).

Another autoimmune disorder that occurs with increased frequency in individuals with T1D is thyroid disease. It occurs in 17–30% of patients with T1D. The thyroid dysfunction is usually hypothyroidism, but the autoimmune disorder may be expressed as the less common hyperthyroidism.

Eating disorders are another possible complication of T1D in children. When hyperglycemia is present, calories are lost and weight loss occurs; therefore, diabetes is unique in that body weight and shape can be altered by stopping insulin. The risks are obvious, but it has been found that insulin omission for weight control occurs in 12–15% of adolescents. Recognition of this potential disorder by the nurse and reporting to the appropriate caregiver can prevent further deterioration in glycemic control for the adolescent with T1D (Rewers et al., 2014).

Another serious acute complication of diabetes in children is frequent and severe hypoglycemia. Children are at higher risk for hypoglycemia than adults because of children's erratic nutritional intake and increased activity levels and growth spurts. Insulin or oral medication error in dose administration is also implicated as a cause of frequent hypoglycemia. Postexercise hypoglycemia can occur several hours after the activity because of the continued uptake of glucose in the muscles in relation to the presence of circulating insulin from the injections. The child and parents must be aware that the adjustment of insulin doses and frequent glucose monitoring prevent profound and unpredictable hypoglycemic events.

Diabetic Ketoacidosis

As stated earlier, DKA is a life-threatening event that occurs when the body lacks sufficient insulin to promote glucose as a fuel source and begins to break down fat for fuel instead. Ketones, the by-products of fat breakdown, build up in the blood and urine. Often the first and acutely presenting sign of T1D, DKA can result from infection or serious illness, injury, surgery, missed doses of insulin, or overwhelming stress (Jeha & Haymond, 2016). Symptoms for children and adolescents are similar to those of adults: excessive thirst, nausea and vomiting, increased urination, anorexia, abdominal pain, shortness of breath, and fruity-scented breath are common symptoms of DKA. If left untreated, DKA can cause depression of the central nervous system, resulting in coma and even death.

Priority interventions for the child or adolescent with DKA include the following:

- Assessment of physiologic parameters such as vital signs, respiratory status, mental status, and blood sugar is ongoing.

- Cardiac monitoring is required because of potential hypokalemia, which can result in lethal dysrhythmias. Insulin in the presence of excess glucose moves potassium into the cells and thus causes serum hypokalemia. There is also loss of total body potassium due to the osmotic diuresis that occurs (Jeha & Haymond, 2015).

- Intake and output are monitored hourly.

- IV fluids are given in boluses of 10–20 mL/kg if hypovolemia is present.

- Insulin infusions are titrated to bring the blood sugar down slowly, as too rapid a decrease can lead to cerebral complications and neurologic changes.
- Once the acidosis is corrected and the blood sugar is improved, the insulin drip is tapered off, and subcutaneous insulin is initiated.
- Food is reintroduced when the patient is alert and the blood glucose has been stabilized.

Alcohol Use

In adolescents and young adults, alcohol use and diabetes present a special concern. Alcohol use in combination with oral hypoglycemic medication and/or insulin can result in profound hypoglycemia because of the following (ADA, 2014b):

- Even small amounts of alcohol may impair someone's ability to detect the onset of hypoglycemia and therefore take appropriate action to correct it.
- Other individuals may mistake hypoglycemia for intoxication.
- Alcohol has been shown to impair the hormonal counterregulatory responses to low blood glucose levels.
- Small amounts of alcohol can augment the cognitive deficits associated with hypoglycemia in individuals with T1D.

- Alcohol use may be associated with a delayed effect that increases the risk of next-day hypoglycemia.

This result may occur many hours after alcohol intake due to impaired mobilization of glycogen stores as the liver detoxifies the alcohol and to the impairment of counterregulatory hormones. Patients in these age groups should be cautioned against drinking alcohol, but if they choose to do so, they should make sure they eat food to accompany the alcohol.

Long-term Complications

The long-term complications of diabetes remain the same for children as for adults with this lifelong disease. Those living with diabetes are at increased risk for alterations in the cardiovascular system, including coronary artery disease, hypertension, stroke, and peripheral vascular disease. Diabetic retinopathy, diabetic nephropathy, peripheral and visceral neuropathies, and periodontal disease are also concerns. Individuals with diabetes are at increased risk for amputation of a lower extremity, and that risk increases for individuals who have lived with diabetes for more than 10 years.

Monitoring and Treatment

Monitoring blood pressure and lipid levels is essential to lowering long-term risks for children with diabetes. **Table 12–9 »** outlines screening and treatment recommendations.

TABLE 12–9 Screening and Treatment Recommendations for Children with T1D

	Screening Recommendations	Treatment Recommendations
Nephropathy	■ At age 10 with diabetes for 5 years: annual screening for microalbuminuria with a random spot sample for albumin-to-creatinine ratio (ACR)	■ Confirmed, persistently elevated ACR on two additional urine specimens from different days can be treated with an ACE inhibitor.
Hypertension	■ Hypertension is defined as an average systolic and diastolic blood pressure greater than the 90th percentile for age, sex, and height measured on at least three separate days. Normal blood pressure for age, sex, and height, with treatment options is available at http://www.nhlbi.nih.gov/	■ Treatment for high normal blood pressure (above the 90th percentile) should include dietary intervention and exercise. If target blood pressure is not reached within 3–6 months of lifestyle intervention, pharmacologic treatment with ACE inhibitors should be considered. ■ The goal of treatment is to have the blood pressure less than 130/80 or below the 90th percentile for age.
Dyslipidemia	■ Assess for family history of elevated total cholesterol or an early cardiac event. If present or if no family history is known, a fasting lipid profile should be done on children older than age 2. ■ If there is no family concern, the first screening can take place at puberty or approximately 10 years of age. ■ Abnormal lipid profiles should be monitored annually. ■ If lipids are normal, monitor every 5 years.	■ Initial treatment of elevated lipids is the optimization of glucose control. ■ After glucose control is achieved, initial treatment of elevated lipid profile includes medical nutrition therapy and following the diet and lifestyle recommendations approved by the American Heart Association. ■ If the introduction of lifestyle changes fails to correct the problem, statin therapy is reasonable in children over the age of 10 years. ■ The goal is an LDL of less than 100 mg/dL.
Retinopathy recommendations	■ The first ophthalmologic exam should occur once the child is 10 years of age and has had diabetes for 3–5 years.	■ Treatment depends on findings and recommendation by the ophthalmologist.
Thyroid disorders	■ Children with T1D should be screened for thyroid perioxidase and thyroglobulin antibodies at diagnosis. ■ TSH should be measured after metabolic control is established and then, if normal, rechecked every 1–2 years or if symptoms are present.	■ Treatment depends on findings and symptoms of thyroid disorder.
Celiac disease	■ Children with T1D should be screened for celiac disease by measuring transglutaminase or antiendomysial antibodies with documentation of normal serum IgE levels. ■ Testing should also be done in children with signs and symptoms of celiac disease or in children with frequent unexplained hypoglycemia or deterioration in glucose control.	■ Children with positive antibodies should be referred to a gastroenterologist. ■ Children with biopsy-confirmed celiac disease should be placed on a gluten-free diet, and a dietitian who is experienced in dealing with both celiac disease and diabetes should be consulted.
Psychosocial assessment and care	■ Assessment of psychologic and social situation, attitudes about the illness, affect, mood, and psychiatric history should be part of the ongoing care.	■ When glucose management is poor, screening for depression and diabetes-related stress, anxiety, and eating disorders is appropriate.

Source: Adapted from American Diabetes Association (2016a). *Standards of medical care for diabetes—2016.* Retrieved from http://care.diabetesjournals.org/content/suppl/2015/12/21/39.Supplement_1.DC2/2016-Standards-of-Care.pdf

As the child matures and approaches puberty, special circumstances may occur. The nurse must be ready to assess and implement education strategies to help the adolescent deal with these situations. It is not uncommon for children to go through a period of erratic glucose control as they approach puberty. The reasons may be physiologic as well as behavioral. The nurse should be aware of this possibility when a child with previously well-controlled T1D suddenly finds it harder to control her glucose levels.

Complementary Health Approaches

Regardless of the type of diabetes, the cornerstones for diabetes management in children are diet, exercise, medication (insulin and/or oral medications), and glucose monitoring. However, many individuals have chosen to use complementary health approaches to enhance their diabetes management. Use of complementary health approaches is often more prevalent in children whose parents used alternative therapies. Many complementary health approaches have no basis in scientific evidence. A key point to remember in using complementary health approaches in children is that, because of their age, children may react to therapies differently than adults. Parents of children who have chosen to use complementary health approaches must communicate this choice to the physician and diabetes educator to ensure safe and coordinated care. In turn, nurses and healthcare providers should assess the patient for use of complementary health approaches at each medical interaction (NIDDK, 2016b).

Some of the more prevalent therapies are dietary supplements such as alpha-lipoic acid, chromium, omega-3 fatty acids, polyphenols, garlic, magnesium, coenzyme Q10, ginseng, and vanadium. Some botanicals are used, such as prickly pear cactus, gurmar, *Coccinia indica*, aloe vera, fenugreek, and bitter melon, but as with other complementary health approaches, there is limited research on their effectiveness in adults and even less information on their use in children (National Center for Complementary and Alternative Medicine, 2013).

Pregnant Women with T1D

Women of childbearing age who are diagnosed with T1D require specific care. Family planning, along with effective contraception, should be prescribed and used until the woman is prepared and ready to become pregnant. These patients should also receive preconception counseling that addresses the importance of glycemic control. Glycemic control is essential to reduce the risk of spontaneous abortion, congenital anomalies, preeclampsia, intrauterine fetal demise, macrosomia, neonatal hypoglycemia, and neonatal hyperbilirubinemia (ADA, 2016a).

When providing care to a pregnant woman with T1D, the nurse should teach the importance of self-monitoring the fasting, preprandial, and postprandial glucose in order to achieve glycemic control. The nurse should also closely monitor the patient's A1C, as this laboratory value tends to be lower than normal during pregnancy because of increased red blood cell turnover. The target A1C during pregnancy is less than 6.5%. Pregnant women may require changes in their insulin dosages as a result of this phenomenon (ADA, 2016a).

Pregnant women with T1D are at an increased risk for diabetic retinopathy. It is essential for the nurse to counsel pregnant women regarding this risk. Women of childbearing age who are diagnosed with T1D and planning a pregnancy should have eye examinations before pregnancy. Pregnant women with T1D should have an eye examination during each trimester of the pregnancy and for 1-year postpartum to monitor for the development, or progression, of diabetic retinopathy (ADA, 2016a).

T1D in Older Adults

The prevalence of diabetes becomes greater with age, increasing from 11.3% with diagnosed diabetes in those age 20 years or older to 26.9% in those age 65 or older (ADA, 2015a). Although most older adults with diabetes have T2D, improved survival rates have resulted in an increased number of older adults with T1D.

The picture is further complicated by the fact that blood glucose levels increase with age, beginning in the 50s. The normal physiologic changes of aging may mask manifestations of the onset of diabetes. In addition, older adults may have misconceptions about the causes of diabetes (see the Focus on Diversity feature). For these reasons, it is more difficult to diagnose diabetes in older adults, because these patients may be mistakenly diagnosed with the disease simply because they exhibit essentially normal age-related changes in glucose and may not report behaviors or manifestations that signal that other processes are at work. The relationship between normal increases in glucose levels and the presence of diabetes is not yet understood.

Signs and symptoms of diabetes in older adults may not include the classic symptoms of polyuria and thirst. Conditions such as orthostatic hypotension, periodontal disease, infections, stroke, gastric hypotony, impotence, neuropathy, confusion, and glaucoma should be considered potential indicators of diabetes. These conditions also may increase the potential for complications from the disease or its treatment (ADA, 2016a).

The older adult with diabetes has multiple, complex healthcare problems and needs, including risks for polypharmacy, depression, cognitive impairment, urinary incontinence, injurious falls, and persistent pain (ADA, 2016a). The older adult with diabetes also has a longer recovery period after surgery or serious illness, often requiring insulin to maintain blood glucose levels. The benefits and risks of treatment to maintain glycemic control as well as blood pressure and lipid management must be carefully balanced.

Older adults diagnosed with T1D are at an increased risk for morbidity and mortality associated with CVD. Evidence suggests that this increased risk is due to poorly controlled A1C, elevated cholesterol and triglycerides, and hypertension that is poorly controlled with pharmacologic treatment. Older adults with T1D who smoke, have an elevated BMI, and participate in little physical activity have even more risk for CVD. Therefore, nurses should assess older adults' clinical risk factors for CVD with each encounter (Lee et al., 2015).

Strategies to manage CVD for older adults with T1D focus on tight control of blood glucose along with controlling modifiable risk factors. Strategies include HDL control along with a heart healthy diet and increased physical activity appropriate for age. More research is necessary in order to further enhance the plan of care for older adults with T1D to decrease the risk for CVD (Lee et al., 2015).

Focus on Diversity and Culture
Tailoring Patient Education for Individuals with Diabetes

A study of 593 adults 60 years old and older who had been diagnosed with diabetes for 2 or more years found that education level was a strong predictor of beliefs about diabetes. In particular, patients with low education levels had consistently different beliefs about the causes of diabetes (Grzywacz et al., 2012). This suggests that individuals with diabetes who have attained lower levels of education require more individualized patient teaching related to diabetes, even if they have been diagnosed and in treatment for some time. Nurses should carefully assess patients' level of understanding and provide follow-up education as needed.

NURSING PROCESS

The responses of patients with diabetes to their illness are often complex and individual, involving multiple body systems. Assessments, planning, and implementation differ for the patient with newly diagnosed diabetes, the patient with long-term diabetes, and the patient with acute complications of diabetes. The plan of care and the content of teaching also differ according to the type of diabetes and the patient's age, culture, and intellectual, psychologic, and social resources.

Teaching the patient (and family) to self-manage diabetes is a nursing responsibility. Even if a formal teaching plan is developed and implemented by an advanced practice nurse, each nurse who interacts with the patient must be able to reinforce this knowledge and answer questions. Teaching is necessary for both the individual who is newly diagnosed and for the individual who has had diabetes for years. In fact, the latter may need almost as much teaching as the newly diagnosed patient. Products for diabetes care, especially insulins, have changed dramatically, and knowledge about risk reduction to prevent complications has increased.

The ADA recommends that teaching be carried out on three levels. The first level focuses on survival skills; the individual learns basic knowledge and skills in diabetes management for the first week or two while adjusting to the idea of having the disease. The second level deals with home management, emphasizing self-reliance and independence in the daily management of diabetes. The third level aims at improving lifestyle and educating the patient to individualize self-management of the illness.

Health promotion activities primarily focus on preventing the complications of diabetes. The patient should prevent or decrease excess weight, follow a sensible and well-balanced diet, and maintain a regular physical exercise program. These same activities, when combined with medications and self-monitoring, also are beneficial in reducing the onset of complications.

Assessment

The following data is collected through the health history and physical examination:

- **Observation and patient interview.** Observe the patient for any pain when walking back to the examination room; this may be an indicator of diabetes. During the patient interview, ask questions regarding any family history of diabetes; history of hypertension or other cardiovascular problems; history of dizziness, numbness or tingling in hands or feet, and any change in vision (e.g., blurring) or speech; pain when walking; frequent voiding; change in weight, appetite, infections, and healing; problems with gastrointestinal function or urination; or altered sexual function.

- **Physical examination.** The physical assessment for a patient diagnosed with T1D includes monitoring the height–weight ratio and vital signs; monitoring visual acuity, cranial nerves, and the sensory ability in the extremities (e.g., touch, hot/cold, vibration); and palpating peripheral pulses and a close inspection of the skin and mucous membranes (e.g., hair loss, appearance, lesions, rash, itching, vaginal discharge).

Children generally are admitted to the hospital at the time of diagnosis. The nurse assesses the child's physiologic status, focusing on vital signs and level of consciousness. The nurse assesses hydration by checking mucous membranes, skin turgor, and urine output. Blood initially is collected hourly to monitor blood gases, glucose, and electrolytes. Once the child is stable, the nurse assesses dietary and caloric intake and the ability of the child or family to manage care.

If parents waited to seek care until the child began to experience symptoms of DKA, they may feel guilty at the time of diagnosis. The nurse should assess their coping mechanisms, family strengths and resources, and ability to manage the disease, as well as the educational needs of both the child and the parents. The nurse should identify family stressors that may cause challenges in the long-term management of diabetes, including access to health insurance and other financial considerations.

Diagnosis

The goals of care are to maintain function, prevent complications, and teach self-management. Although many NANDA-I nursing diagnoses are appropriate for the individual with diabetes, the following address some of the more common problems:

- *Knowledge, Deficient*
- *Skin Integrity, Risk for Impaired*
- *Infection, Risk for*
- *Injury, Risk for*
- *Fluid Volume: Deficient, Risk for*
- *Sexual Dysfunction*
- *Coping, Ineffective.*

(NANDA-I © 2014)

Planning

The nursing plan of care is focused on helping the patient learn to provide self-care and reduce the risk of complications. Goals of care include, but are not limited to, the following:

- The patient will describe how to administer medications and respond to side effects appropriately.
- The patient will demonstrate meal planning compliant with the ADA diet.

- The patient will demonstrate proper foot care and inspection.
- The patient will demonstrate the proper procedure for monitoring blood sugar levels.
- The patient will describe strategies for reducing the risk of infection.

Implementation

Nursing care for the patient with diabetes is individualized and focuses on teaching the patient and family about the disease and its management, planning dietary intake, providing emotional support, and creating strategies for daily management in the community. Some hospitals have developed clinical pathways to streamline and standardize diabetes care. The nurse should include the following when teaching the patient and family about care at home:

- Information about normal metabolism, diabetes, and how diabetes changes metabolism
- How diet helps keep blood glucose in the normal range; the number of kilocalories required and why; the amount of carbohydrates, meats, and fats allowed and why; and how to calculate the diet while integrating personal food preferences
- How exercise helps lower blood glucose, the importance of a regular exercise program, types of exercise, integrating personal exercise preferences, and how to handle increased activity
- SMBG, how to care for equipment, and what to do about a high or low blood glucose level
- Medications:
  a. *Insulin: subcutaneous agents.* Type, dosage, mixing instructions (if necessary), times of onset of insulin effect and of peak actions and duration of action, how to get and care for equipment, how and where to give injections
  b. *Hypoglycemic agents: oral delivery.* Type, dosage, side effects, and interaction with other drugs (T2D only)
- Manifestations of acute complications of hypoglycemia and hyperglycemia, and what to do when they occur
- Hygiene, including skin care, dental care, and foot care
- What to do about food, fluids, and medications when the patient is sick
- Helpful resources.

Teaching may have to be adapted to the special needs and developmental level of a child or older adult. However, because 40% of all individuals with diabetes are over the age of 65, considering the special needs of the older population is particularly essential. Uncontrolled diabetes in the older adult increases the potential for functional loss, social disengagement, and increased morbidity and mortality. Education for self-care allows the older adult to be more actively involved in diabetes management and decreases the potential for acute and chronic complications from the disease. Considerations for teaching the older adult with diabetes include the following:

- Changes in diet may be difficult to implement for many reasons. Favorite foods are difficult to give up. Balanced meals at regular intervals may not have been part of the patient's lifestyle. Purchasing, storing, and preparing foods may be a problem. Dentures may not fit well. Changes in taste sensation often cause the patient to increase the use of salt and sugar. (For more information on nutrition and the older adult, see the module on Nutrition.)
- Exercise of any type may not have been part of the activities of daily living. An exercise plan must be individualized for any physical limitations imposed by other chronic illnesses, such as arthritis, Parkinson disease, chronic respiratory diseases, and/or CVD.
- Diagnosis of a chronic illness threatens a patient's independence and feelings of self-worth. After years of taking care of themselves, older adults with diabetes may now have to depend on others for help in meeting self-care needs. This change of circumstance often leads to withdrawal from social interactions with others.
- Money to purchase medications and supplies often must be taken out of a fixed income.
- Visual deficits may make insulin administration difficult or impossible. Visual deficits also can interfere with blood glucose monitoring, food preparation, exercises, and foot care.

Caring interventions may also focus on the risks for impaired skin integrity, infection, and injury, as well as on sexual dysfunction and ineffective coping. Interventions for each diagnosis are discussed in the following section.

Maintain Skin Integrity

The patient with diabetes is at increased risk for altered skin integrity as a result of decreased tissue perfusion from cardiovascular complications, infection, and decreased or absent sensation from neuropathies. In addition, poor vision increases the risk of trauma, and an open lesion is more prone to infection and delayed healing.

Impaired skin and tissue integrity, with resultant gangrene, is especially common in the feet and lower extremities. In fact, individuals with diabetes are at significant risk for lower extremity gangrene. The nurse should conduct baseline and ongoing assessments of the patient's feet, including the following:

- Musculoskeletal assessment that includes foot and ankle joint range of motion, bone abnormalities (e.g., bunions, hammertoes, overlapping digits), gait patterns, use of assistive devices for walking, and abnormal wear patterns on shoes
- Neurologic assessment that includes sensations of touch and position, pain, and temperature
- Vascular examination that includes assessment of lower extremity pulses, capillary refill, color and temperature of skin, and edema
- Assessment of hydration status, including dryness or excessive perspiration
- Assessment for lesions, fissures between toes, corns, calluses, plantar warts, ingrown or overgrown toenails, redness over pressure points, blisters, cellulitis, or gangrene.

Peripheral neuropathies may result in altered perception of pain, loss of DTRs, loss of cutaneous pressure and position sensation, foot drop, changes in the shape of the foot, and changes in bones and joints. Peripheral vascular disease may cause intermittent claudication, absent pulses, delayed venous filling on elevation, dependent rubor, and gangrene. Injuries, lesions, and changes in skin hydration potentiate infections, resulting in delayed healing and tissue loss in the individual with diabetes.

- Teach foot hygiene. The patient should wash the feet daily with lukewarm water and mild hand soap; pat them dry and dry well between the toes; and apply a very thin coat of lubricating cream if dryness is present (but not between the toes). Proper hygiene decreases the chance of infection. The temperature receptors in the patient's feet may be impaired, so the water should always be tested before use.

- If the patient smokes, discuss the importance of not smoking. Nicotine in tobacco causes vasoconstriction, further decreasing the blood supply to the feet.

- Discuss the importance of maintaining blood glucose levels through prescribed diet, medication, and exercise. Hyperglycemia promotes the growth of microorganisms.

- Conduct foot care teaching sessions (see the Patient Teaching feature) as often as necessary. Foot care is a priority in diabetes management to prevent serious problems. Many individuals with diabetes are unaware of lesions or injury until infection and compromised circulation are far advanced. The hows and whys of each component must be included in teaching. A variety of methods may be used, including demonstration, return demonstration, audiovisual aids, and written lists. If the patient is wearing shoes and socks, ask him or her to remove them to practice foot care effectively.

Promote Healthy Behaviors

The individual with diabetes is at increased risk for infection. The risk of infection is believed to result from vascular insufficiency that limits the inflammatory response, neurologic abnormalities that limit the awareness of trauma, and a predisposition to bacterial and fungal infections. In addition to monitoring for signs of infection, the nurse should do the following:

- Use and teach meticulous hand hygiene. Hand hygiene is the single most effective method for preventing the spread of infection.

- Discuss the importance of skin care. Using lukewarm water and mild soap, keep the skin clean and dry. Individuals with diabetes are more prone to develop furuncles and carbuncles; the infection often increases the need for insulin. Clean, intact skin and mucous membranes are the first line of defense against infection.

- Teach dental health measures, such as the importance of regular dental examinations (every 4–6 months), brushing teeth using a soft toothbrush and fluoridated toothpaste twice daily, and flossing as recommended. Teach patients to make adjustments to insulin if dental surgery is needed.

Patient Teaching
Foot Care

General Information

- Never go barefoot. Wear slippers when leaving the bed during the night.
- Do not use commercial corn medicines or pads, chemicals (e.g., boric acid, iodine, hydrogen peroxide), or over-the-counter cortisone medications on the feet.
- Do not put heating pads, hot water bottles, or ice packs on the feet. If the feet become cold at night, wear socks or use extra blankets.
- Do not allow the feet to become sunburned.
- Do not put tape on the feet.
- Do not sit with the legs crossed at the knees or ankles.

Buying and Wearing Shoes and Stockings

- Shoes that allow 0.5–0.75 in. of toe room are best; there should be room for the toes to spread out and wiggle. The lining and inside stitching should be smooth, and the insole should be soft. The sole should be flexible and cushion the foot. The heel should fit snugly, and good arch support should be present.
- Do not wear open-toed shoes, sandals, high heels, or thongs; these increase the risk of trauma.
- Buy shoes late in the afternoon, when feet are at their largest; always buy shoes that feel comfortable and do not need to be "broken in."
- Shoes made of natural fibers (e.g., leather, canvas) allow perspiration to escape.

- Check the shoes before each wearing for foreign objects, wrinkled insoles, and cracks that might cause lesions.
- Socks or stockings made of wool or cotton allow perspiration to dry.
- Do not wear garters, knee stockings, or pantyhose; these may interfere with circulation.
- Wear insulated boots in the winter.

Inspecting the Feet

- Check the feet daily for red areas, cuts, blisters, corns, calluses, or cracks in the skin. Check between the toes for cracks or reddened areas.
- Check the skin of the feet for dry or damp areas.
- Use a mirror to check each sole and the back of each heel.
- If you are unable to inspect the feet daily, be sure that someone else does.

Care of Toenails

- Cut the toenails after washing, when they are softer and easier to trim.
- Cut the nails straight across with a clipper, and smooth edges and corners with an emery board.
- Do not use razor blades to trim the toenails.
- If you are unable to see your feet well or to reach them easily, have someone else trim the nails. If the nails are very thick or ingrown, if the toes overlap, or if circulation is poor, get professional care from a podiatrist.

- Teach women with diabetes the symptoms and preventive measures for vaginitis caused by *Candida albicans*. The symptoms are an odorless white or yellow cheese-like discharge and itching. Poor personal hygiene and clothing that keeps the vaginal area warm and moist increase the risk of vaginitis. The infection may spread to the urinary tract and result in urinary tract infections; preventing and treating vaginitis decrease this risk.

Maintain Safety

The patient with diabetes is at risk for injury from multiple factors. Neuropathies may alter sensation, gait, and muscle control. Cataracts or retinopathy may cause visual deficits. Hyperglycemia often causes osmotic changes in the lenses of the eye; the result is blurred vision. In addition, changes in blood glucose alter levels of consciousness and may cause seizures. The impaired mobility, sensory deficits, and neurologic effects of complications of diabetes increase the risk of accidents, burns, falls, and trauma. To help the patient decrease the risk of injury, the nurse can do the following:

- Assess for the presence of contributing or causative factors that increase the risk of injury: blurred vision, cataracts, decreased adaptation to dark, decreased tactile sensitivity, hypoglycemia, hyperglycemia, hypovolemia, joint immobility, and unstable gait. A knowledge base is necessary to develop an individualized plan of care. The risk of injury increases with the number of factors identified.

- Reduce environmental hazards in the healthcare facility, and teach the patient about safety in the home and in the community (see the module on Safety for more information).

- Monitor for and teach the patient and family to recognize and seek care for the manifestations of DKA in the patient with T1D: hyperglycemia, thirst, headaches, nausea and vomiting, increased urine output, ketonuria, dehydration, and decreasing level of consciousness.

- Monitor for and teach the patient and family to recognize and treat the manifestations of hypoglycemia: low blood glucose, anxiety, headache, uncoordinated movements, sweating, rapid pulse, drowsiness, and visual changes. Teach the patient and family to carry some form of rapid-acting sugar source at all times.

- Recommend that the patient wear a medical alert bracelet or necklace that identifies the patient as an individual with diabetes. In case of sudden severe illness or accident, a medical alert bracelet allows immediate medical attention for diabetes.

Maintain Sexual Health

Sexuality is a complex and inseparable part of every individual. It involves not only physical sexual activities but also an individual's self-perception as a man or woman, roles and relationships, and attractiveness and desirability. Changes in sexual function and sexuality have been identified in both men and women with diabetes.

To monitor the patient with diabetes for issues involving sexual dysfunction, the nurse should do the following:

- Include a sexual history as a part of the initial and ongoing assessment of the patient with diabetes. See the module on Sexuality for information on assessing a patient's sexual history and when to make referrals for counseling.

- Provide information about the actual and potential physical effects of diabetes on sexual function. Include the effect of poor control of blood glucose on sexual function as part of any teaching plan. Patients benefit from basic information about male and female anatomy, the sexual response cycle, and how diabetes can affect these parts of the body. Changes in blood glucose levels not only may cause changes in desire and physical response but also may alter sexual responses as a result of depression, anxiety, and fatigue.

Promote Effective Coping

Coping is the process of responding effectively to internal or environmental stressors or potential stressors. When coping responses are ineffective, the stressors exceed the individual's available resources for responding. The patient diagnosed with diabetes is faced with lifelong changes. New diet, exercise habits, and medications must be integrated into the lifestyle and carefully controlled. Daily injections may be a reality. Fear of potential complications and of negative effects on the future is common.

If the patient is unable to cope successfully with these changes or lacks a strong support system, emotional stress can interfere with glycemic control. In addition, unsuccessful coping often results in noncompliance with prescribed treatments, further impairing glycemic control and increasing the potential for acute and chronic complications.

Assess the patient's psychosocial and financial resources. Provide information about support groups and resources such as suppliers of products, journals, books, and cookbooks for individuals with diabetes. Patients who are living on limited incomes or are without health insurance may need assistance in accessing special programs offered by pharmaceutical companies or local clinics to help them pay for their prescriptions. Sharing with others who have similar problems provides opportunities for mutual support and problem solving. Using available resources improves the ability to cope.

For more information on strategies to promote coping, see the module on Stress and Coping.

Evaluation

Expected outcomes of nursing care of the patient with diabetes are individualized on the basis of the nursing care plan and the goals established during the planning phase. These outcomes may include the following:

- The patient demonstrates an age-appropriate understanding of diabetes self-management through medication, diet, exercise, and blood glucose self-monitoring activities.
- The patient's skin integrity remains intact.
- The patient remains free of infection.
- The patient remains free of injury.

If patient outcomes are not met, assess the patient's diet and medication adherence. Failure to adhere to treatment regimens can cause rapid changes in the patient's condition and necessitate admittance to the hospital. If the patient is not following dietary restrictions or taking medication properly, determine the cause for nonadherence and develop a care plan that addresses these causes.

Nursing Care Plan
A Patient with T1D

Jim Meligrito, age 24, is a third-year nursing student at a large Mid-western university. Mr. Meligrito also works 20 hours a week as a campus student security guard. His working hours are 8 p.m. to mid-night, five nights a week. He lives with his father, who also is a stu-dent. Neither of the men likes to cook, and they usually eat "whatever is handy." Mr. Meligrito has smoked 8–10 cigarettes a day for 5 years.

Mr. Meligrito was diagnosed with T1D at age 12. Although his insulin dosage has varied, he currently takes a total of 32 U of insulin each day, 10 U of NPH, and 6 U of regular insulin each morning and evening. He monitors his blood glucose about three times a week. He feels that he is too busy for a regular exercise program and that he gets enough exercise in clinicals and in weekend sports activi-ties. He has not seen a healthcare provider for over a year.

One day during a 6-hour clinical laboratory in pediatrics, Mr. Meligrito notices that he is urinating frequently, is thirsty, and has blurred vision. He also is very tired, but he blames all his symptoms on drinking a couple of beers and having had only 4 hours of sleep the night before while studying for an exam, and on the stress he has been under lately from school and work. When he remembers that he forgot to take his insulin that morning, he realizes he must have hyperglycemia but decides that he will be all right until he gets home in the afternoon. Around noon, he begins having abdominal pain, feels weak, has a rapid pulse, and vomits. When he reports his physical symptoms to his clinical instructor, she immediately sends him, accompanied by another student, to the hospital emergency department.

ASSESSMENT

As soon as Mr. Meligrito arrives at the emergency department, his blood glucose level is measured at 300 mg/dL. Urine sam-ples and additional blood samples are sent to the laboratory for analysis. Hemoglobin A1C is 9.5%, urine shows the pres-ence of ketones, electrolytes are normal, and pH is 7.1. His vital signs are as follows: T 37.2°C (99°F); P 140 bpm; R 28/min; BP 102/52 mmHg. An IV infusion of 1000 mL of normal (0.9%) saline with 40 mEq of KCl is started at a rate of 400 mL/hr. IV regular insulin at 5 U/hr (diluted in 0.9% saline) is begun. Hourly blood glucose monitoring also is initiated. Mr. Meligrito is nau-seated and lethargic but remains oriented. Three hours later, he has a blood glucose level of 160 mg/dL, and his pulse and blood pressure are normal. He is dismissed from the emer-gency department after making an appointment for the next morning with the hospital's diabetes nurse educator. When he meets with the diabetes educator, he says that he no longer feels in control of the diabetes or his future goal of becoming a nurse anesthetist.

DIAGNOSES

Nursing diagnoses that may be appropriate for Mr. Meligrito include the following:

- *Powerlessness* related to a perceived lack of control of diabetes because of present demands on time
- *Knowledge, Deficient* of self-management of diabetes
- *Role Performance, Ineffective* related to uncertainty about his capacity to achieve the desired role as a registered nurse.

(NANDA-I © 2014)

PLANNING

The expected outcomes for the plan of care specify that Mr. Meligrito will:

- Identify those aspects of diabetes that can be controlled and participate in making decisions about self-managing his care
- Demonstrate an understanding of diabetes self-management through planned medication, diet, exercise, and blood glucose self-monitoring activities
- Explore and clarify his perceptions of his role as a student nurse and verbalize his ability to meet his expectations.

IMPLEMENTATION

The following interventions may be appropriate for Mr. Meligrito:

- Mutually establish specific and individualized short-term and long-term goals for self-management to control blood glucose.
- Provide opportunities to express his feelings about himself and his illness.
- Explore perceptions of his own ability to control his illness and his future, and clarify these perceptions by providing information about resources and support groups.

- Facilitate his decision-making abilities in self-managing his prescribed treatment regimen.
- Provide positive reinforcement for increasing his involvement in self-care activities.
- Provide relevant learning activities about insulin administration, dietary management, exercise, SMBG, and healthy lifestyle.

EVALUATION

After taking an active part in the weekly educational meetings for 2 months, Mr. Meligrito has greatly enhanced his understanding of and compliance with self-management of his diabetes. He states that he finally understands how insulin, food, and exercise affect his body, having previously thought they were "just things I should do when I wanted to." He decides to perform self-management activities 1 week at a time rather than think too far into (and thereby feel overwhelmed by) the future. Both son and father have devel-oped a workable meal schedule and weekly grocery list, and they have begun eating breakfast and dinner together. Jim and a friend have arranged to walk 2–3 miles three times a week on a commu-nity hiking trail. To gain a sense of control over his illness, he has also worked out a schedule that allows time for school, health-care, and himself.

CRITICAL THINKING

1. What is the pathophysiologic basis for the changes in temperature, pulse, respiration, and blood pressure that were recorded on Mr. Meligrito's admission to the hospital emergency department?

2. How can smoking and poor self-management of diabetes increase the risk of long-term complications?

3. Is powerlessness a common response to a chronic illness? Why or why not?

4. What does the hemoglobin A1C of 9.5% suggest about Mr. Meligrito's control of his diabetes?

REVIEW Type 1 Diabetes Mellitus

RELATE Link the Concepts and Exemplars

Linking the exemplar of type 1 diabetes mellitus with the concept of development:

1. In consideration of development, how would you approach diabetes teaching for an 8-year-old?

2. Based on developmental level, how would your teaching of a 15-year-old about diabetes differ from your teaching of an adult?

Linking the exemplar of type 1 diabetes mellitus with the concept of sensory perception:

3. When caring for a patient with diabetic neuropathy, what teaching would you provide to reduce the risk of injury?

4. When caring for a patient with diabetic retinopathy, what strategies would you teach to facilitate a normal standard of living for the patient?

READY Go to Volume 3: Clinical Nursing Skills

REFER Go to Pearson MyLab Nursing and eText

- Additional review material

REFLECT Apply Your Knowledge

Emily Davis is a young adult who was diagnosed with T1D during adolescence. Ms. Davis and her husband, Brad, would like to start a family within the next year. They meet with a women's health nurse practitioner to discuss their options and any special precautions that they must take to ensure that Ms. Davis's health, along with the health of their baby, is maintained during this process.

Ms. Davis's T1D is treated with an insulin pump to maintain her blood glucose levels. Her last documented A1C was 6.7%, and her current BMI is 29. She denies alcohol consumption and the use of tobacco products. She exercises daily by taking a 45-minute walk with her husband in the evenings. Thus far, she has not experienced any long-term complications associated with her T1D diagnosis.

1. What pre-pregnancy testing should the nurse include in the plan of care for this patient?

2. What are some of the risks for Ms. Davis and her baby that are directly related to the T1D diagnosis?

3. What are Ms. Davis's teaching needs while she and her husband try to conceive? What will their teaching needs be during pregnancy and the postpartum period?

» Exemplar 12.B
Type 2 Diabetes Mellitus

Exemplar Learning Outcomes

12.B Analyze type 2 diabetes mellitus as it relates to metabolism.

- Describe the pathophysiology of type 2 diabetes.
- Describe the etiology of type 2 diabetes.
- Compare the risk factors and prevention of type 2 diabetes.
- Identify the clinical manifestations of type 2 diabetes.
- Summarize diagnostic tests and therapies used by interprofessional teams in the collaborative care of an individual with type 2 diabetes.

- Differentiate care of patients with type 2 diabetes across the lifespan.
- Apply the nursing process in providing culturally competent care to an individual with type 2 diabetes.

Exemplar Key Terms

Acanthosis nigricans, *839*
Endogenous insulin, *836*
Hyperosmolar hyperglycemic state (HHS), *837*
Prediabetes, *837*

Overview

T2D was formerly labeled *non-insulin-dependent diabetes mellitus* or *adult-onset diabetes*; however, a disturbingly large number of children are being diagnosed with T2D because of the increase in childhood obesity (Mayo Clinic, 2014b). This type of diabetes results from insulin resistance with a defect in compensatory insulin secretion. Over time, the body does not produce enough insulin to keep blood glucose levels within normal limits (ADA, 2015b).

Pathophysiology and Etiology

Pathophysiology

T2D is a condition of fasting hyperglycemia that occurs despite the availability of **endogenous insulin** (insulin that is produced by the individual's own body). The level of insulin produced varies in T2D, and despite the availability

of insulin, its functioning is impaired by insulin resistance. Insulin resistance exceeds the ability of the pancreas to compensate, and over time the pancreas fails to produce enough insulin to meet body needs (ADA, 2016b). Whatever the cause, there is insufficient production of insulin to prevent the breakdown of fats with resultant ketosis; thus, T2D is characterized as a nonketotic form of diabetes. However, the amount of insulin available is not sufficient to lower blood glucose levels through the uptake of glucose by muscle and fat cells.

Etiology

In the United States, the incidence of T2D has increased 33% since 2003. This type of diabetes can occur at any age, but it usually is seen in individuals who are of middle age and older. A major factor in the development of T2D is cellular resistance to the effect of insulin. This resistance is increased by obesity, inactivity, illnesses, medications, and increasing

Focus on Diversity and Culture
Risk and Incidence of Type 2 Diabetes

While most of the genetic risk for T2D results from complex polygenic risk factors, certain ethnicities are at an increased risk for developing this disease process. African Americans, Native Americans, and Hispanic Americans are 2–6 times more likely than Caucasians to be diagnosed with T2D (CDC, 2015b; McCulloch & Robertson, 2014).

age. In obesity, insulin has a decreased ability to influence glucose metabolism and uptake by the liver, skeletal muscles, and adipose tissue. The exact reason is not clear, but weight loss and exercise may improve the mechanism responsible for insulin receptor binding or postreceptor activity (McCulloch & Robertson, 2014).

Statistics related to the rates of diagnosed diabetes by race/ethnicity from the ADA (2016b) are as follows: Non-Hispanic Whites, 7.6%; Asian Americans, 9%; Hispanics, 12.8 %; Non-Hispanic Blacks, 13.2%; American Indians and Alaska Natives, 15.9%.

Risk Factors

The major risk factors for T2D are as follows:

- The patient has a history of diabetes in parents or siblings. Although no human leukocyte antigen linkage has been identified, the children of an individual with T2D have a 15% chance of developing this type of diabetes and a 30% risk of developing a glucose intolerance (the inability to metabolize carbohydrate normally).

- The patient is obese. Obesity is defined as being at least 20% over the desired body weight or having a BMI (the weight in kilograms divided by the square of the height in meters) of at least 27. Obesity, especially of the upper body, decreases the number of available insulin receptor sites in cells of skeletal muscles and adipose tissues, a process called *peripheral insulin resistance*. In addition, obesity impairs the ability of the beta cells to release insulin in response to increasing glucose levels.

- The patient is physically inactive or has an overall sedentary lifestyle. Individuals who are physically active fewer than 3 times per week are an increased risk for T2D (CDC, 2016a).

- The patient has a race/ethnicity more prone to T2D (see the Focus on Diversity and Culture feature).

- The woman has a history of gestational diabetes, polycystic ovary syndrome, or delivery of a baby weighing more than 9 lb.

- The patient has hypertension (140/90 mmHg or more in adults or on therapy for hypertension), HDL cholesterol of less than 35 mg/dL, and/or a triglyceride level of 250 mg/dL or more.

- The patient has a metabolic syndrome. The National Cholesterol Education Program's Adult Treatment Panel III (NCEP/ATP III) identified metabolic syndrome as a cluster of factors that increase an individual's risk for developing cardiovascular disease. Hypertension, abdominal obesity, dyslipidemia, elevated C-reactive protein, and a fasting blood glucose greater than 100 mg/dL increase the risk of T2D, coronary heart disease, and stroke. Studies have shown that metabolic syndrome is prevalent and increases with age and BMI. Studies also note that the prevalence varies by race and ethnicity, but the pattern is different for men and women (Meigs, 2015).

The term **prediabetes** describes individuals who are at increased risk of developing T2D. An estimated 86 million Americans have prediabetes (CDC, 2016a). Prediabetes is characterized by an A1C of 5.7% or higher; a fasting blood glucose between 100 and 125 mg/dL, which is high but not high enough to be classified as diabetes; or an oral glucose tolerance test (OGTT) 2-hour blood glucose of 140–199 mg/dL. These test results indicate a risk for progression to diabetes, but it is not inevitable (ADA, 2015c). Individuals with prediabetes are at increased risk for other adverse health outcomes, such as heart disease and stroke (CDC, 2016a).

Prevention

Many individuals diagnosed with prediabetes will develop T2D within 5 years if lifestyle changes are not implemented (CDC, 2016a). Studies suggest that weight loss (losing 7% of the current body weight) and increased physical activity (moderate exercise, such brisk walking 30 minutes 5 times per week) among individuals with prediabetes prevent or delay diabetes and may return blood glucose levels to within normal limits (ADA, 2015c).

The CDC recommends that individuals diagnosed with prediabetes participate in a CDC-approved diabetes prevention lifestyle change program.

>> **Stay Current:** Visit the website of the National Diabetes Prevention Program to learn more about Lifestyle Change Program details: http://www.cdc.gov/diabetes/prevention/lifestyle-program/experience/index.html

Clinical Manifestations

Clinical manifestations of T2D (insulin resistance and decreased insulin production that affects glucose processing) include fatigue, extreme thirst, frequent urination, extreme hunger, weight loss, infection, slow wound healing, and blurry vision. Because most individuals diagnosed with T2D are insulin resistant, these specific manifestations and therapies are explored here.

Complications of T2D

The individual with diabetes, regardless of type, is at increased risk for complications involving many body systems. Alterations in blood glucose levels, alterations in the cardiovascular system, neuropathies, increased susceptibility to infection, and periodontal disease are common. In addition, the interaction of several complications can cause problems in the feet. Because T2D may go undetected for years, individuals with T2D often have microalbuminuria and overt nephropathy shortly after diagnosis. Microalbuminuria is also a well-established marker of increased cardiovascular risk in those with diabetes (ADA, 2016a). A discussion of each of these complications can be found in Exemplar 12.A on T1D.

Hyperosmolar hyperglycemic state (HHS) occurs in individuals who have T2D and is characterized by a plasma

Clinical Manifestations and Therapies
Type 2 Diabetes Mellitus

ETIOLOGY	CLINICAL MANIFESTATIONS	CLINICAL THERAPIES
Insulin resistance with relative insulin secretory defect	■ Obesity, little or no weight loss, or possible significant recent weight loss ■ Acanthosis nigricans ■ Slow onset of symptoms ■ Polyuria, polydipsia ■ Glycosuria without ketonuria on initial presentation in 33% of cases ■ Ketoacidosis on initial presentation in 5–25% of cases ■ Lipid disorders ■ Hypertension ■ Androgen-mediated problems (e.g., acne, hirsutism, menstrual disturbances, polycystic ovary disease) ■ Excessive weight gain and fatigue caused by insulin resistance ■ Hyperglycemia	■ Diet with low-fat foods and decreased calories ■ Decreased sedentary activity time, or increased routine physical activity ■ Blood glucose monitoring ■ Oral medication (metformin) to improve insulin sensitivity

osmolarity of 340 mOsm/L or greater (the normal range is 280–300 mOsm/L), greatly elevated blood glucose levels (more than 600 mg/dL and often as high as 1000–2000 mg/dL), and altered levels of consciousness. HHS is a serious, life-threatening medical emergency. Mortality is high—even higher than for DKA—because the metabolic changes are serious and because individuals with diabetes usually are older and have other medical problems that either cause or are caused by HHS.

The precipitating factors associated with HHS include infection, therapeutic agents, therapeutic procedures, acute illness, and chronic illness. The most common precipitating factor is infection. The manifestations of this disorder may be slow to appear, with onset ranging from 24 hours to 2 weeks. The manifestations are initiated by hyperglycemia, which causes increased urine output, and with increased output, plasma volume decreases and glomerular filtration rate drops. As a result, glucose is retained, and water is lost. Glucose and sodium accumulate in the blood and increase serum osmolarity.

Serum hyperosmolarity results in severe dehydration, which reduces intracellular water in all tissues, including the brain. The individual with HHS has dry skin and mucous membranes, extreme thirst, and altered levels of consciousness (progressing from lethargy to coma). Neurologic deficits may include hyperthermia, motor and sensory impairment, positive Babinski sign, and seizures. Metabolic acidosis is not part of the pathology; despite elevated blood glucose, sufficient insulin is present to prevent metabolism of fats with the resulting fatty acids and ketones of DKA.

Treatment is similar to that of DKA: correcting fluid and electrolyte imbalances and providing insulin to lower hyperglycemia. In general, treatment modalities include the following:

■ Establish and maintain adequate ventilation.

■ Correct shock with adequate IV fluids.

■ If the patient is comatose, institute nasogastric suction to prevent aspiration.

■ Maintain fluid volume with IV isotonic or colloid solutions, administering potassium intravenously to replace losses.

■ Administer insulin to reduce blood glucose, usually until blood glucose levels reach 250 mg/dL (because ketosis is not present, there is no need to continue insulin, as with DKA).

Collaboration

Treatment of the patient with T2D focuses on maintaining blood glucose at levels as nearly normal as possible through medications, dietary management, and exercise. Primary care providers are able to care for the patient diagnosed with T2D. However, collaboration among many sources yields the best outcome for the patient. Depending on the available resources and the patient's needs, the interprofessional team may include a certified diabetes educator, a nurse, a family physician, specialists, a dietitian, a podiatrist, and a psychologist and/or psychiatrist, as well as family and friends (Tapp et al., 2012).

Studies of patients with T2D who have gastrointestinal surgery for morbid obesity show complete remission in over three quarters of the cases. Laparoscopic adjustable gastric banding (LAGB) and Roux-en-Y gastric bypass (RYGB) result in remarkable reductions in blood glucose levels and hemoglobin A1C. RYGB, which alters gastrointestinal anatomy, improves insulin sensitivity and is associated with total remission of T2D in a significant percentage of patients (Ikramuddin et al., 2013).

Diagnostic Tests

For many illnesses, there is a major distinction between screening and diagnostic testing. However, for diabetes the same tests are used for both screening and diagnosis (ADA, 2016a). Testing for T2D in patients who are asymptomatic should be considered for patients who are overweight or obese (BMI greater than 25) who have one or more other risk factors for T2D. All patients, however, should be tested at the age of 45 years. If testing is normal, repeat testing is completed at 3-year intervals.

Tests used to screen for T2D include measurement of FPG, a glycated hemoglobin (A1C), and a 2-hour PG during an OGTT. Because of its inconvenience, however, the OGTT is not commonly used for screening, except in pregnant women (McCulloch & Hayward, 2016). Refer to Exemplar 12.A on T1D for more information regarding diagnostic testing for diabetes.

Pharmacologic Therapy

Individuals with T2D are usually able to control glucose levels with an oral hypoglycemic medication, but they may require insulin if control is inadequate. This often occurs during hospitalization. Patients with T2D cannot be treated with oral medications during hospitalization because of the risk of hypoglycemia from not eating and the slow response of these medications to correct hyperglycemia.

There is growing acceptance of the need to achieve tighter control of blood sugar in individuals who are hospitalized with hyperglycemia, whether they are diagnosed with diabetes, have unrecognized diabetes, or have hospital-related diabetes. Although there is no clear evidence for specific goals for hospitalized patients who are not critically ill, the ADA (2016a) suggests that reasonable targets are less than 140 mg/dL premeal and less than 180 mg/dL random if these targets can be safely achieved.

Hypoglycemic Agents

Hypoglycemic agents are used to treat individuals with T2D. These medications lower blood sugar by stimulating or increasing insulin secretion, preventing breakdown of glycogen to glucose by the liver, and increasing peripheral uptake of glucose by making cells less resistant to insulin. Peripheral uptake is uptake by muscles and fat in the arms and legs rather than in the trunk. Some hypoglycemic agents keep blood sugar low by blocking absorption of carbohydrates in the intestines. The most recent pharmacologic therapy in treating T2D includes the incretin effect. Incretin hormones, which are hormones released from the gut endocrine cells during meals, play a significant role in insulin secretion. GLP-1 (glucagon-like peptide) and GIP (glucose-dependent insulinotropic polypeptide or gastric inhibitory polypeptide) may be responsible for as much as 70% of postprandial insulin secretion in healthy individuals. This secretion is greatly reduced or absent in individuals with T2D. Exenatide (Byetta) and liraglutide (Victoza) are considered GLP-1 agonists and are administered subcutaneously. They help to stimulate insulin and amylin secretion from the pancreatic beta cells, which leads to decreased hepatic gluconeogenesis, slowed gastric emptying, and increased satiety. Another drug related to the incretin effect is the oral preparation of dipeptidyl peptidase IV (DPP-IV) inhibitors. These medications work by inhibiting the DPP-IV enzyme and therefore preventing the inactivation of endogenous GLP-1. These medications are sitagliptin (Januvia) and linagliptin (Tradjenta). A potential side effect of GLP-1 or DPP-IV inhibitors is pancreatitis, and the patient must be monitored for this (Inzucchi, Berganstal, & Buse, 2012).

Exercise

An exercise program is especially important for the patient with T2D. The benefits of regular exercise include weight loss in individuals who are overweight, improved glycemic control, increased well-being, socialization with others, and a reduction of cardiovascular risk factors. A combination of diet, exercise, and weight loss often decreases the need for oral hypoglycemic agents. This decrease is due to an increased sensitivity to insulin, increased kilocalorie expenditure, and increased self-esteem. Regular exercise may prevent T2D in high-risk individuals (CDC, 2016a).

Following are general guidelines for an exercise program:

- Before beginning the program, have a medical screening for previously undiagnosed hypertension, neuropathy, retinopathy, and nephropathy.
- Begin the program with mild exercises, and gradually increase intensity and duration.
- Self-monitor blood glucose before and after exercise.
- At least 150 minutes a week of moderate-intensity physical activity is recommended (ADA, 2015c).

Lifespan Considerations

The increasing prevalence of T2D in both children and adults is linked to increasing rates of obesity. Environmental determinants of obesity in the United States include shifts in food consumption, changes in physical activity levels, and higher levels of television viewing with marketing of food, especially to children. The CDC (2015d) is focusing on using the best available evidence to implement intervention programs. The CDC states that for maximum population impact, the focus should be on strategies that alter food consumption and on physical activity environments where individuals live, learn, work, play, and pray. Examples of interventions include support for breastfeeding in the workplace and increasing safety in communities so that children can safely play and walk/bike to school.

T2D in Children

The incidence of T2D has increased in children and adolescents since the early 1990s and is attributed to the rise in childhood obesity. T2D, along with the comorbidities associated with T2D, are risk factors for vascular disease later in life. Therefore, it is essential to identify and treat children for T2D (Laffel & Svoren, 2016).

Clinical manifestations of T2D in children may be less acute than those of T1D, presenting with a range of symptoms that are related to hyperglycemia and that may vary in severity and may include weight gain. Another presenting symptom in children with T2D is the marker of insulin resistance typified by skin changes. **Acanthosis nigricans** is a condition in which the skin is velvety in texture and brownish black in color with hyperkeratotic plaques. Acanthosis nigricans usually appears in the folds of the skin, especially in the neck, thigh, axillae, and knuckles (see **Figure 12–9 ⟫**). It is believed to be related to direct and indirect activation of IGF-1 (insulin-like growth factor) receptors that results in proliferation of keratinocytes and fibroblasts. The skin appears dark and thick. There may also be darkening of the mucous membranes, eyelids, and nail beds (Nimblett, 2012).

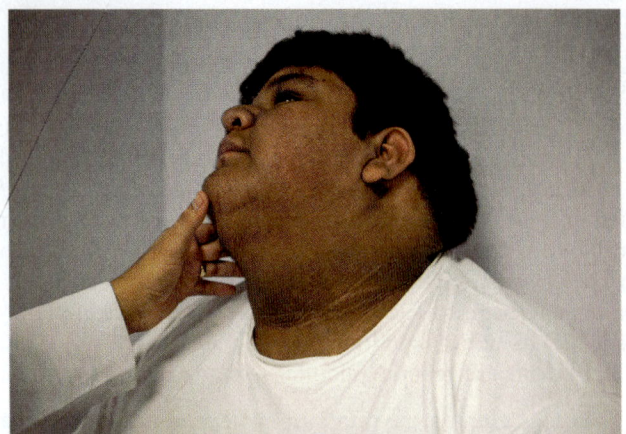

Source: Benedicte Desrus/Alamy Stock Photo.

Figure 12–9 ❯❯ Acanthosis nigricans.

Once a pediatric patient is diagnosed with T2D, the child must have healthcare visits at specific intervals. Assessments and other considerations for managing T2D in children and adolescents are outlined in **Table 12–10** ❯❯.

The child or adolescent newly diagnosed with either type of DM requires a nursing assessment of physiologic as well as psychosocial, environmental, and developmental needs. On the basis of the assessment findings, the nurse can develop a plan of care that involves the parents and the child at every stage of the nursing process. Ongoing evaluation of interventions will help the child with diabetes live a healthy and well-adjusted life.

Children and adolescents with T2D require the care of a collaborative team and careful communication among all adults caring for the child in any situation. Education in skills required to manage T2D can be initiated as early as the family and child feel it is acceptable. Nurses should always assess the child's developmental stage and take that into account when planning teaching and health promotion. For example, the preschool-age child who seeks greater control and autonomy may benefit from choosing which snacks to eat. Most school-age children are able to (and need to) learn how to recognize the symptoms of hypoglycemia and hyperglycemia and what to do in the event one of these occurs. Adolescents may exhibit resistance to complying with treatment, as they may find it embarrassing to be singled out as different from their peers or may feel resentful about their illness and the restrictions that it imposes.

The nurse should continually assess barriers to implementing the teaching plan. Health promotion and teaching topics to cover include diet; medication; exercise; glucose monitoring; and prevention, recognition, and intervention for acute complications. The family that has difficulty coping may need referral to a counselor who can help deal with the realities of managing diabetes in a child. The nurse should review with the family any action plans or instructions to be shared with school or child care personnel.

Nutrition and exercise are the keystones for clinical management of T2D in children and adolescents, even though there is little evidence regarding the nutritional treatment of T2D in children. Therefore, the recommendations from pediatric diabetologists are derived from a combination of recommendations for treatment of children who are overweight and obese, adults with T2D, and children with T1D. The overall goal of therapeutic intervention for children with T2D is to achieve and maintain an age-appropriate BMI. The increase in the number of overweight youth has been associated with increased caloric intake and a sedentary lifestyle. Children with a BMI greater than the 85th percentile for age

TABLE 12–10 Provider Schedule for Managing T2D in Youth

Time Frame	Tasks
At diagnosis	■ Establish a baseline hemoglobin A1C, lipid profile (repeat every 3–5 years); refer for eye exam. ■ Initiate diabetes education. ■ Administer psychosocial assessment. ■ Establish goals for care and discuss them with the child (if appropriate) and parents. ■ Evaluate for microalbuminuria. ■ Refer for nutrition therapy, behavioral therapy, and family and community support as needed.
Quarterly	■ Assess injection sites. ■ Assess psychosocial adjustment and self-management skills. ■ Assess dietary needs and physical activity levels. ■ Discuss tobacco, alcohol, and drug use. ■ Measure hemoglobin A1C and fasting glucose levels. ■ Review glucose records.
Annually	■ Administer the influenza vaccine. ■ Perform a physical assessment. ■ Evaluate for microalbuminuria. ■ Conduct a foot assessment. ■ Refer for an eye exam (ophthalmologist may recommend frequency).

Sources: Data from Copeland, K. C., Silverstein, J., Moore, K. R., Prazer, G. E., Raymer, T., ... Flinn, S. (2013) Management of newly diagnosed type 2 diabetes mellitus (T2DM) in children and adolescents. *Pediatrics, 131*(2), 364–382; Laffel, L., & Svoren, B. (2014). Management of type 2 diabetes mellitus in children and adolescents. *UpToDate.* Retrieved from https://www.uptodate.com/contents/management-of-type-2-diabetes-mellitus-in-children-and-adolescents?source=search_result&search=management+of+type+2+DM+in+children&selectedTitle=1~150#H18; Springer, S. C., Silverstein, J., Copeland, K., Moore, K. R., Prazar, G. E., Raymer, T., ... Flinn, S. K. (2013). Management of type 2 diabetes mellitus in children and adolescents. *Pediatrics, 131*(2), e648–e664.

TABLE 12–11 Nutritional and Activity Guidelines for Youth with T2D

Target Areas	Guidelines
Food modification	■ Individualize food intake based on age, sex, and physical activity (should include consultation with dietitian and/or a certified diet educator). ■ Limit snack intake (especially snacks with high sugar and fat content, such as potato chips, fast food, desserts). Consumption of sugar-free drinks in place of sweet drinks can be encouraged. ■ Provide a meal plan designed by a dietitian and/or certified diet educator to include high-fiber foods, low-fat foods, and low-concentrated sugar. To prevent or treat hypoglycemia, sweet drinks such as 100% juice with no sugar added can also be included in the diet. ■ Both the child and the family should be included in the teaching regarding blood glucose levels and carbohydrate intake.
Physical activity	■ Physical activity should be at least 30–60 minutes per day most days of the week. ■ Limit sedentary activities such as watching TV and playing video games.
Psychosocial support	■ Encourage peer support groups and family participation in the lifestyle change. Children are not generally worried about long-term complications, so the change in lifestyle must be made attractive to them with exercises and foods that they will accept.

and sex should be counseled to increase activity and decrease intake of high-calorie foods while adequately meeting the nutrition needs of the growing child. Other goals include optimization of blood glucose and lipid and blood pressure values to prevent the long-term complications of diabetes (CDC, 2016b). Nutritional and activity guidelines for children with T2D are found in **Table 12–11 》**.

Pharmacolgic Therapy

Hypoglycemic agents are not the first-line therapy for children with T2D. Instead, the focus is on decreased insulin sensitivity with advancing sexual maturity, physical growth, and the ability to provide self-management. However, diet and exercise alone are effective for metabolic control in less than 10% of those with T2D, and an oral medication usually is required. Metformin (Glucophage) is the only oral hypoglycemic agent approved for use in some children, and it is used as an adjunct to diet and exercise (Laffel & Svoren, 2014). Metformin therapy typically shows improvement in blood glucose control in 1–2 weeks; however, the full effect of blood glucose control may take up to 3 months (Mayo Clinic, 2015).

Glycemic control is defined as an A1C of less than 7% and a fasting PG of less than 130 mg/dL. It is important to note that providers might reasonably suggest more stringent A1C goals (less than 6.5%) or less stringent A1C goals (less than 7.5%) depending on individual circumstances (ADA, 2016a). If these goals are unrealistic in the short term for an individual patient, it is reasonable to set a higher target initially and then decrease the target as tolerated. Use of realistic goals may help to engage the patient and promote adherence to prescribed therapies (Laffel & Svoren, 2014).

SAFETY ALERT Successful maintenance of glycemic control depends in part on frequency of glucose monitoring. Be sure to assess for frequency of monitoring at each patient interaction.

If the pediatric patient experiences ketosis or severe hyperglycemia (random PG concentrations greater than or equal to 250 mg/dL or an A1C greater than 9%), insulin therapy may be initiated and metformin introduced after stability in glycemic control is achieved. Severe hyperglycemia is toxic to the pancreatic islet cells. Insulin is beneficial in these circumstances as it can help to restore endogenous insulin production (Laffel & Svoren, 2014).

Children with T2D are insulin resistant; therefore, they require relatively high doses of insulin to restore glycemic control. A starting dose of insulin ranges from 0.75 to 1.25 units/kg/day but can be as high as 2 units/kg/day. Glycemic control is monitored by finger-stick glucose testing, and the insulin dose is adjusted accordingly. Children who are prescribed insulin therapy for T2D should monitor their blood glucose three or more times each day. Once glycemic control is achieved, metformin can be added to the regimen. Some patients may be weaned off insulin, but others may require a combination to control blood glucose levels (Laffel & Svoren, 2014).

Managing Challenges

Those who care for children and adolescents with T2D face several potential challenges. Most diabetes training and education materials are designed for children and adolescents with T1D. The emphasis on insulin and glucose monitoring may not be appropriate for youth with T2D. Most medications used in T2D have been tested for safety and efficacy only in individuals older than 18. The American Academy of Pediatrics has recommendations regarding comorbidity screening and management of complications such as hypertension, dyslipidemia, retinopathy, microalbuminuria, and depression (Copeland et al., 2013).

The decision to recommend weight reduction versus weight maintenance depends on the age of the patient, the degree of obesity, and the presence of comorbidities. In children who are still growing, weight maintenance will lead to a reduction in BMI. Weight maintenance is a crucial component in the successful management of T2D in the pediatric population (Laffel & Svoren, 2014).

Glycemic control is a balance between food intake and physical activity. Teach the child and family the importance of providing small meals to avoid wide glycemic excursions. The diet should reduce caloric intake while providing adequate nutrition for normal health and growth. A dietitian can provide instruction on how to adjust dietary habits and behaviors in order to ensure adequate nutrition while reducing caloric intake (Laffel & Svoren, 2014).

Increased physical activity is also a necessary component of the plan of care for a child diagnosed with T2D. Increased physical activity improves insulin sensitivity and will assist in weight reduction or maintenance. Children and adolescents diagnosed with T2D should be encouraged to engage in moderate to vigorous physical activity for at least 1 hour per day. Non-academic screen time should also be limited. When planning care and teaching needs, the nurse should start with more modest goals and then generally reduce the allowed screen time (Laffel & Svoren, 2014).

Adolescents can be resistant to following therapeutic regimens. Nurses, diabetes educators, and other healthcare providers should assess adolescent patients' adherence to the treatment plan and to look for interventions that meet adolescents' preferences and interests. Peer support groups and technology-based interventions are two types of strategies that may be helpful in promoting adherence among adolescents (see the Evidence-Based Practice feature).

Other special situations include the adolescent driver, who needs education about the effects of hypoglycemia on safe driving. Drivers with diabetes should always check their blood glucose before driving and should have a source of carbohydrate with them at all times. Education regarding onset, peak, and duration of insulin may have to be reviewed before the youth takes on the new responsibility of driving.

Pregnant Women with T2D

Women with T2D who have been treated with diet and oral medications generally require insulin for blood glucose management during pregnancy. In some cases, glyburide or metformin can be continued. However, women who are taking these drugs when they become pregnant should speak with their healthcare provider in order to determine the best course of therapy (Barss & Repke, 2015).

Pregestational T2D is often associated with obesity; therefore, weight management during pregnancy is a priority when providing care. Recommended weight gain during pregnancy for an overweight woman is 15–25 lb, and 10–20 lb for a woman who is obese. Dietary planning and activity should be discussed early in pregnancy for these women (ADA, 2016a).

Glycemic control is often easier to achieve in women diagnosed with T2D during pregnancy when compared to those diagnosed with T1D. Much higher doses of insulin are often required for pregnant women diagnosed with T2D, which may necessitate concentrated insulin formations. Insulin requirements will dramatically drop after childbirth (ADA, 2016a).

Pregnant patients diagnosed with T2D often have comorbidities that place the pregnancy at higher risk when compared with T1D. For example, hypertension can be exacerbated during pregnancy. Women with T2D are at an increased risk for pregnancy loss during the third trimester, whereas individuals with T1D are at a greater risk for pregnancy loss during the first trimester (ADA, 2016a).

T2D in Older Adults

Older adults diagnosed with T2D are at risk for developing a similar spectrum of complications as compared with younger patients with T2D. In addition, older adults are at high risk for polypharmacy, functional disabilities, and common geriatric syndromes such as cognitive impairment, depression, urinary incontinence, falls, and persistent pain.

The goals of T2D management are similar to those in younger adults and include management of hyperglycemia and risk factors. Because of the heterogeneous population, management of T2D for the older adult must be

Evidence-Based Practice

Use of Technology to Promote Healthy Behaviors in Adolescents with T2D

Problem

Adolescents with diabetes face developmental and environmental challenges to treatment adherence. Can technology assist in promoting healthy behaviors in adolescents with T2D?

Evidence

For some time, researchers have been studying the use of technology, or eHealth, in health promotion and as part of an overall treatment plan for adolescents (Tercyak et al., 2009). Woolford and colleagues (2010) examined the use of tailored text messages as part of an overall weight-management program for adolescents with T2D. Using a library of 90 messages tailored to individual patients' characteristics, researchers found that participants were enthusiastic about the messages and reported them to be helpful, especially the messages that provided meal suggestions. In another study, researchers examined the effects of three different tech-based interventions with adolescents with T2D: website only; website with monthly group meetings and follow-up calls; and website with text message support. Over a 12-month period, the adolescents using the website in combination with group sessions and follow-up calls showed improvements in sedentary behavior and the use of behavior-change strategies (Patrick et al., 2013).

Implications

Nurses working with adolescents may want to work with the patient's diabetes care manager to incorporate the use of technology into the treatment plan targeting eHealth to the patient's specific needs and involving parents in both development of the treatment plan and oversight in the use of technology to promote adherence and safe patient use of the internet and social media.

Critical Thinking Application

1. How can technology be used to enhance dietary adherence for the adolescent diagnosed with T2D?

2. How should social media be incorporated into the adolescent's plan of care?

individualized and take into account current health status. This population is at an increased risk for hypoglycemia; therefore, this is an important consideration when establishing goals and choosing therapeutic agents for the older adult.

SAFETY ALERT Make frequent assessments to monitor for symptoms of HHS in the older adult who has had major surgery.

NURSING PROCESS

The plan of care for the patient with T2D is similar to that for T1D. Refer to Exemplar 12.A on T1D for further information. The differences in the nursing care provided to the patient with T2D are explored here.

Assessment

The following data are collected through the health history and physical examination:

- *Observation and patient interview.* Observe the patient for any outward signs of complications associated with T2D. During the interview, determine which medications are prescribed and review the glucose log, if the patient brings it to the visit. Inquire about diet (carbohydrate intake), weight gain/loss, exercise, and urine output (increased urine output could indicate osmotic diuresis secondary to hyperglycemia). For children and adolescents, assess mealtime patterns and behaviors.

- *Physical examination.* Assess the patient's vital signs (decreased blood pressure and increased heart rate may indicate fluid volume deficit related to hyperglycemia; elevated temperature could indicate infection). Assessment for microvascular and macrovascular complications is essential and should include capillary refill (decreased refill could indicate decreased perfusion due to microvascular changes). A thorough skin assessment is essential to determine risk for impaired integrity.

Diagnosis

The goals of care are to maintain function, prevent complications, and teach self-management. Although many NANDA-I nursing diagnoses are appropriate for the individual with T2D, the following address some of the more common problems:

- *Knowledge, Deficient*
- *Skin Integrity, Risk for Impaired*
- *Infection, Risk for*
- *Injury, Risk for*
- *Tissue Perfusion: Peripheral, Risk for Ineffective*
- *Fluid Volume: Deficient, Risk for*
- *Sexual Dysfunction*
- *Coping, Ineffective.*

(NANDA-I © 2014)

Planning

The nursing plan of care is focused on helping the patient learn to provide self-care and reduce the risk of complications. Goals of care include, but are not limited to, the following:

- The patient will describe how to administer medications and respond to side effects appropriately.
- The patient will demonstrate meal planning compliant with the ADA diet.
- The patient will demonstrate proper foot care and inspection.
- The patient will demonstrate the proper procedure for monitoring blood sugar levels.
- The patient will describe strategies for reducing risk of infection.

Implementation

Nursing interventions to treat a patient diagnosed with T2D are similar to those for patients diagnosed with T1D. Refer to Exemplar 12.A on T1D to review implementation for a patient with diabetes. The interventions explored here are specific to T2D.

SMBG by patients with T2D who are not using insulin should provide enough data to help them reach glucose goals. Postprandial blood glucose is often the most useful information for evaluating the level of glycemic control in patients with T2D (ADA, 2016a). Patients who check only their fasting glucose would be unaware of the postprandial results.

Monitor for and teach the patient and family to recognize and seek care for the manifestations of HHS in the patient with T2D. Manifestations include extreme hyperglycemia, increased urinary output, thirst, dehydration, hypotension, seizures, and decreasing level of consciousness. HHS is a life-threatening condition requiring recognition and treatment.

Evaluation

Expected outcomes of nursing care of the patient with T2D are individualized on the basis of the nursing care plan and the goals established during the planning phase. These outcomes may include the following:

- The patient demonstrates an age-appropriate understanding of diabetes self-management through medication, diet, exercise, and blood glucose self-monitoring activities.
- The patient's skin integrity remains intact.
- The patient remains free of infection.
- The patient remains free of injury.

If patient outcomes are not met, assess the patient's diet and medication adherence. Failure to adhere to the treatment regimen can cause rapid changes in the patient's condition and necessitate admittance to the hospital. If the patient is not following dietary restrictions or taking medication properly, determine the cause for nonadherence and develop a care plan that addresses these causes.

REVIEW Type 2 Diabetes Mellitus

RELATE Link the Concepts and Exemplars

Linking the exemplar of type 2 diabetes mellitus with the concept of stress and coping:

1. How might a diagnosis of T2D increase the stress or anxiety level of a child? An older adult?

2. What nursing interventions do you think would help reduce a child's stress level? An adolescent's? A parent's?

Linking the exemplar of type 2 diabetes mellitus with the concept of advocacy:

3. In what ways can the nurse in a pediatric office help parents learn to advocate for their child in the school or child care setting?

4. How can nurses advocate for patients with diabetes in their communities?

READY Go to Volume 3: Clinical Nursing Skills

REFER Go to Pearson MyLab Nursing and eText

- Additional review materials

REFLECT Apply Your Knowledge

Mary Wills is a 12-year-old girl whose mother brings her to her healthcare provider's office for symptoms related to a cold and sore throat. When the nurse weighs Mary, she notes that Mary is in the 90th percentile for her height and age. Blood work reveals an elevated blood glucose level of 250. Mary says she feels fine and is just a little tired because of her cold. Her mother says that Mary does not play outside very much, preferring to watch TV or read in bed at home. Mary has a few friends, but when they come over, they play computer games or look at books. Mary is not involved in any school activities.

A diet recall with Mary's mother reveals that the family eats takeout food almost every night because both parents work, get home late, and do not feel like cooking. Plenty of snacks are always on hand in case the kids get hungry while waiting for the parents to get home from work. Breakfast is usually a honey bun on the school bus. Mary eats a school lunch and also brings her own snacks. The only family event is going together to get ice cream. Both parents are also obese and sedentary.

Mary's mother has tried some herbs she has seen advertised on TV to help herself and the children lose weight.

1. What can the nurse tell Mary's mother about the risk factors for T2D in children?

2. Develop a teaching plan of care to help Mary and her mother cope with the new diagnosis of T2D (include skills for survival).

3. Mary's mother would like to start using some of the medications she has seen advertised in magazines to treat Mary. She feels that herbs and vitamins are better than prescription drugs. What could the nurse say to Mary's mother regarding the use of dietary supplements and complementary health approaches?

» Exemplar 12.C
Liver Disease

Exemplar Learning Outcomes

12.C Analyze liver disease as it relates to metabolism.

- Describe the pathophysiology of liver disease.
- Describe the etiology of liver disease.
- Compare the risk factors and prevention of liver disease.
- Identify the clinical manifestations of liver disease.
- Summarize diagnostic tests and therapies used by interprofessional teams in the collaborative care of an individual with liver disease.
- Differentiate care of patients with liver disease across the lifespan.
- Apply the nursing process in providing culturally competent care to an individual with liver disease.

Exemplar Key Terms

Alcoholic cirrhosis, *845*
Balloon tamponade, *853*
Cirrhosis, *845*
Gastric lavage, *853*
Hematochezia, *852*
Laënnec cirrhosis, *845*
Paracentesis, *852*
Transjugular intrahepatic portosystemic shunt (TIPS), *853*

Overview

The liver is a complex organ with multiple metabolic and regulatory functions. Optimal liver function is essential to health. Because of the significant amount of blood in the liver at all times, it is exposed to the effects of pathogens, drugs, toxins, and possibly malignant cells. As a result, liver cells may become inflamed or damaged, or cancerous tumors may develop.

The essential functions of the liver include the metabolism of proteins, carbohydrates, and fats. It also is responsible for the metabolism of steroid hormones and most drugs; it detoxifies alcohol and other substances. It synthesizes essential blood proteins—albumin and clotting factors, in particular. Ammonia, a toxic by-product of protein metabolism, is converted to urea in the liver for elimination by the kidneys. The liver produces bile, an essential substance for absorbing fats and eliminating bilirubin from the body. Minerals and fat-soluble vitamins are stored in the liver, as is glycogen (stored carbohydrate for energy reserves). The Kupffer cells that line the sinusoids phagocytize foreign cells and damaged blood cells.

The liver is vital to the digestion and metabolism of nutrients; the production of plasma proteins, including those involved in clotting; and the metabolism and excretion of compounds such as bilirubin, steroid hormones, and ammonia, as well as toxins (e.g., alcohol) and drugs. Impaired function of liver cells has multiple effects, including:

- Impaired protein metabolism with decreased production of albumin and clotting factors. Low albumin levels contribute to edema in peripheral tissues and *ascites* (accumulation of fluid in the abdomen) as plasma oncotic pressure is reduced. Impaired clotting-factor production increases the risk for bleeding.

- Disrupted glucose metabolism and storage with resulting alterations in blood glucose levels (either hyperglycemia or hypoglycemia).

- Reduced bile production that impairs the absorption of lipids and fat-soluble vitamins. Inadequate vitamin K, a fat-soluble vitamin, affects the production of clotting factors, leading to a bleeding tendency.

- Impaired metabolism of steroid hormones (including estrogen and testosterone) that leads to feminization in men and irregular menses in women.

Although many different disorders can disrupt liver function, their manifestations relate to three primary effects: disrupted liver cell function, impaired bilirubin conversion and excretion leading to jaundice, and disrupted blood flow through the liver, with resulting portal hypertension. Cirrhosis of the liver is examined here in more detail because it is the most common cause of liver disease in the United States and demonstrates most of the symptoms commonly found in chronic degenerative liver disease.

Cirrhosis is the end stage of chronic liver disease. It is a progressive, irreversible disorder, eventually leading to liver failure. Cirrhosis that results from chronic hepatitis C is the most common type of cirrhosis in North America, followed by **alcoholic cirrhosis** (or **Laënnec cirrhosis**) (NIDDK, 2014a). Cirrhosis also may result from chronic hepatitis B; prolonged obstruction of the biliary (bile drainage) system; long-term, severe right heart failure; and other, uncommon, liver diseases.

Pathophysiology and Etiology

Pathophysiology

In cirrhosis, functional liver tissue is gradually destroyed and replaced by fibrous scar tissue. As hepatocytes and liver lobules are destroyed, the metabolic functions of the liver are lost. Structurally abnormal nodules encircled by connective tissue form. This fibrous connective tissue forms constrictive bands that disrupt blood and bile flow within liver lobules. Blood no longer flows freely through the liver to the inferior vena cava. This restricted blood flow leads to portal hypertension (increased pressure in the portal venous system).

Etiology

The incidence and mortality attributable to cirrhosis and chronic liver disease vary significantly among populations.

Alcoholic Cirrhosis

Alcoholic (or Laënnec) cirrhosis is the end result of alcoholic liver disease. Its development is directly related to

alcohol consumption—specifically the total amount of alcohol consumed, the number of years of excessive alcohol consumption, and blood alcohol levels. Women develop cirrhosis at lower overall levels of alcohol use than men. The reason may be less effective metabolism of alcohol in women, resulting in higher blood alcohol levels (MedlinePlus, 2015).

Alcohol causes metabolic changes in the liver: Triglyceride and fatty acid synthesis increases, and a decrease in the formation and release of lipoproteins leads to fatty infiltration of hepatocytes (fatty liver). At this stage, abstinence from alcohol can allow the liver to heal. However, with continued alcohol abuse, the disease continues to progress. Inflammatory cells infiltrate the liver (alcoholic hepatitis), causing necrosis, fibrosis, and destruction of functional liver tissue. In the final stage of alcoholic cirrhosis, regenerative nodules form, and the liver shrinks and develops a nodular appearance. Malnutrition commonly accompanies alcoholic cirrhosis.

Biliary Cirrhosis

When bile flow is obstructed within the liver or in the biliary system, the retained bile damages and destroys liver cells close to the interlobular bile ducts. This activity leads to inflammation, fibrosis, and formation of regenerative nodules.

Posthepatic Cirrhosis

Advanced progressive liver disease resulting from chronic hepatitis B or C or from an unknown cause is called *posthepatic* or *postnecrotic cirrhosis*. Chronic viral hepatitis appears to be the leading cause of posthepatic cirrhosis in the United States (NIDDK, 2014a). In patients with this type of cirrhosis, the liver is shrunken and nodular, with fibrosis and extensive loss of liver cells.

Focus on Diversity and Culture
Cirrhosis

- Although cirrhosis/chronic liver disease is the 12th leading cause of death overall in the United States, it is the 7th leading cause of death for individuals of Hispanic (or Latino) origin (CDC, 2015c) and the 10th leading cause for White men (CDC, 2016c).

- Non-Hispanic Blacks and Mexican Americans have a higher prevalence of cirrhosis (Scaglione et al., 2015).

- Chronic liver disease is also a leading cause of death among Native Americans and Alaska Natives (Office of Minority Health, 2015).

- Although there is no clear explanation for these differences, contributory factors are thought to include:

  a. Socioeconomic and environmental factors that lead to greater stress and alcohol consumption among certain populations

  b. Patterns of alcohol consumption (e.g., consuming alcohol without food calories)

  c. Variations in alcohol metabolism among populations

See the exemplar on Alcohol Abuse in the module on Addiction for information on the prevalence and etiology of alcohol abuse.

Risk Factors

For most patients, high-risk behaviors are the risk factors for cirrhosis. While many patients tolerate alcohol use in moderation with no adverse effects on the liver, excess alcohol use is the leading cause of cirrhosis. Injection drug use also is a significant risk factor, increasing the risk for contracting bloodborne hepatitis (B, C, or D). These types of viral hepatitis can lead to chronic hepatitis and, ultimately, to cirrhosis.

Prevention

Patients diagnosed with liver disease are at an increased risk for cirrhosis. To prevent cirrhosis from occurring, it is essential for the patient to:

- See the healthcare provider on a regular basis. This is especially important for those diagnosed with hepatitis.
- Maintain a healthy weight
- Avoid alcoholic beverages and illegal drugs
- Take all medications as prescribed; this is especially important for those diagnosed with autoimmune hepatitis (NIDDK, 2013).

Clinical Manifestations

Early in the course of cirrhosis, few manifestations may be present. The liver usually is enlarged and may be tender. A dull, aching pain in the right upper abdominal quadrant may be present. Other early signs include weight loss, weakness, and anorexia. Bowel function is disrupted with diarrhea or constipation (NIDDK, 2014b).

As the disease progresses, manifestations related to liver cell failure and portal hypertension develop. Impaired metabolism causes such manifestations as bleeding, ascites, gynecomastia (breast enlargement) in men and infertility in women, jaundice, and neurologic changes. Portal hypertension accounts for such manifestations as ascites, peripheral edema, anemia, and low white blood cell (WBC) and platelet counts. See the Multisystem Effects of Cirrhosis feature.

Treatment of cirrhosis is supportive and directed at slowing the progression to liver failure and reducing complications. It can include medications to help regulate protein metabolism; maintenance of fluid and electrolyte balance; and supportive therapies, including treatment of underlying problems (e.g., malnutrition, anemia, bleeding, encephalopathy, renal failure, infections).

Portal Hypertension

Portal hypertension causes blood to be rerouted to adjoining, lower pressure vessels. This *shunting* of blood involves collateral vessels. Affected veins, which become engorged and congested, are located in the esophagus, rectum, and abdomen. Portal hypertension increases the hydrostatic pressure in vessels of the portal system. Increased hydrostatic pressure in the capillaries pushes fluid out, contributing to ascites formation.

Splenomegaly

Because portal hypertension causes blood to be shunted into the splenic vein, the spleen enlarges (splenomegaly). Splenomegaly increases the rate at which red blood cells (RBCs), WBCs, and platelets are removed from circulation and destroyed. This increased destruction of blood cells leads to anemia (low RBC count), leukopenia (low WBC count), and thrombocytopenia (low platelet count) (NIDDK, 2014b).

Ascites

Ascites is the accumulation of plasma-rich fluid in the abdominal cavity. Although portal hypertension is the primary cause of ascites, decreased serum proteins and increased aldosterone also contribute to the fluid accumulation. *Hypoalbuminemia* (low serum albumin) decreases the colloidal osmotic pressure of plasma. This pressure normally holds fluid in the intravascular compartment, but when the plasma colloidal osmotic pressure decreases, fluid escapes into extravascular compartments. *Hyperaldosteronism* (an increase in aldosterone) causes sodium and water retention, contributing to ascites and generalized edema.

Esophageal Varices

Esophageal varices are enlarged, thin-walled veins that form in the submucosa of the esophagus. These collateral vessels form when blood is shunted from the portal system because of portal hypertension. The thin-walled varices may rupture and cause massive hemorrhage; even eating high-roughage foods can precipitate bleeding in these patients. Thrombocytopenia, platelet deficiency, and impaired production of clotting factors by the liver contribute to the risk for hemorrhage.

Portal Systemic Encephalopathy

Portal systemic encephalopathy (also known as *hepatic encephalopathy*) results from cerebral edema and the accumulation of neurotoxins in the blood. Ammonia, a by-product of protein metabolism, contributes to hepatic encephalopathy. Ammonium ion is produced as proteins and amino acids are broken down by bacteria in the intestinal tract. The ammonia produced is normally converted by the liver to urea before entering the general circulation. However, as functional liver tissue is destroyed, ammonia can no longer be converted to urea, and it accumulates in the blood. Other nervous system depressants, such as narcotics and tranquilizers, also may contribute to hepatic encephalopathy. Accumulation of other metabolic toxins is thought to contribute as well. Additional factors are constipation, blood transfusions, gastrointestinal bleeding, hypoxia, high-protein diet, severe infection, and surgery.

Asterixis (also known as liver flap) is a muscle tremor that interferes with the ability to maintain a fixed position of the extremities and causes involuntary jerking movements. It also is an early sign of portal systemic encephalopathy. Asterixis primarily affects the upper extremities, but it may affect the tongue and feet. The nurse may elicit asterixis by instructing the patient to extend the arms and dorsiflex the wrists; if present, asterixis causes a downward flapping of the hands.

Individuals with portal systemic encephalopathy also develop changes in personality and mentation. Agitation, restlessness, impaired judgment, and slurred speech are early manifestations; as the condition progresses, confusion, disorientation, and incoherence develop. Cerebral edema that leads to increased intracranial pressure and cerebral hypoxia is the leading cause of death in individuals with portal systemic encephalopathy and liver failure.

Multisystem Effects of
Cirrhosis

Endocrine
- Gynecomastia in males

Potential complication
- Diabetes mellitus

Respiratory
- Dyspnea

Hepatic
- Atrophic, nodular liver
- Splenomegaly

Potential complication
- Liver cancer

Gastrointestinal

Esophageal
- Esophageal varices

Stomach/intestines
- Abdominal pain
- Anorexia
- Ascites
- Nausea
- Clay-colored stools
- Peptic ulcers
- GI bleeding
- Hemorrhoids

Immune System
- Leukocytopenia
- ↑ susceptibility
  to infections

Neurologic
- Portal system encephalopathy
  (agitation → lethargy → stupor → coma)
- Paresthesias
- Sensory disturbances
- Asterixis ("liver flap")

Cardiovascular
- Bounding pulse
- Pulmonary hypertension
- Portal hypertension
- Dysrhythmias

Hematologic
- ↓ clotting factors
- Thrombocytopenia
- Anemia

Potential complication
- Disseminated intravascular
  coagulation

Reproductive
- Oligomenorrhea (female)
- Testicular atrophy (male)

Integumentary
- Jaundice (skin, sclera of eyes)
- Erythema of palms
- Spider angioma
- ↓ body hair
- Pruritis
- Ecchymoses
- Caput medusae (dilated veins
  around the umbilicus)

Metabolic Processes
- Fluid and electrolyte imbalances
  - Hypoalbuminemia
  - Hypokalemia
  - Hypocalcemia
- Malnutrition
- Muscle wasting

Hepatorenal Syndrome

Although the cause is unclear, renal failure with azotemia (excess nitrogenous waste products in the blood), sodium retention, oliguria, and hypotension may develop in patients with advanced cirrhosis and ascites. Hepatorenal syndrome appears to be the result of imbalanced blood flow, resulting in constriction of vessels leading to and within the kidneys. The syndrome may be precipitated by gastrointestinal bleeding, aggressive diuretic therapy, or an unknown cause.

Spontaneous Bacterial Peritonitis

Patients with cirrhosis and ascites may develop bacterial peritonitis even in the absence of known contamination of the peritoneal cavity or other specific risk factors (e.g., paracentesis).

The inflammatory response to peritonitis worsens ascites by increasing the permeability of capillaries in the mesentery. The manifestations of spontaneous bacterial peritonitis may be subtle, with increased abdominal discomfort or pain, fever, increasing ascites, worsening encephalopathy, and an overall decline in condition.

Collaboration

Care for the patient with cirrhosis is holistic, addressing physiologic, psychosocial, and spiritual needs, and the nurse is responsible for coordinating care among providers. The importance of including the family in the plan of care cannot be overemphasized, particularly if alcohol abuse is identified as the cause. Counseling, job coaching, and

Clinical Manifestations and Therapies
Liver Disease

ETIOLOGY	CLINICAL MANIFESTATIONS	CLINICAL THERAPIES
Impaired plasma protein synthesis (hypoalbuminemia) Disrupted hormone balance and fluid retention Increased pressure in portal venous system	Edema, ascites	▪ Diuretics ▪ Sodium and fluid restrictions ▪ Paracentesis ▪ Transjugular intrahepatic portosystemic shunt (TIPS)
Decreased clotting factor synthesis Increased platelet destruction by enlarged spleen Impaired vitamin K absorption and storage	Bleeding, bruising	▪ Ferrous sulfate, folic acid to treat anemia ▪ Vitamin K to reduce risk of bleeding ▪ For acute bleeding, possible administration of packed RBCs, fresh frozen plasma, or platelets to promote hemostasis ▪ Institution of bleeding precautions
Increased pressure in portal venous system with collateral vessel development	Esophageal varices	▪ Beta-blocker nadolol with isosorbide mononitrate ▪ For bleeding esophageal varices, central line insertion; monitoring of central venous and pulmonary artery pressures ▪ Upper endoscopy with gastric lavage ▪ Balloon tamponade ▪ TIPS
Engorged veins in the gastrointestinal system Alcohol ingestion Impaired bile synthesis and fat absorption	Gastritis, anorexia, diarrhea	▪ Cessation of alcohol intake ▪ Nutrition therapy ▪ Supportive therapy
Impaired bilirubin metabolism and excretion	Jaundice	▪ Supportive therapy
Impaired nutrient metabolism Impaired fat absorption Impaired hormone metabolism	Malnutrition, muscle wasting	▪ Arranging for consultation with a dietitian for meal planning
Accumulated metabolic toxins Impaired ammonia metabolism and excretion	Asterixis, encephalopathy	▪ Medications to reduce nitrogenous load and lower serum ammonia levels ▪ Protein restrictions in acute encephalopathy ▪ Parenteral nutrition as needed

behavioral therapy may be helpful. Consultation with a nutritionist can help to reinforce any patient teaching the nurse has provided as well as give the patient an additional resource in this area.

Diagnostic Tests

Studies to confirm the diagnosis of cirrhosis and identify its cause and effects are performed. Diagnostic tests may include the following:

- *Liver function studies.* These include studies of *alanine aminotransferase, aspartate aminotransferase, alkaline phosphatase,* and *gamma-glutamyltransferase.* All four may be elevated in patients with cirrhosis, but usually not as severely as in patients with acute hepatitis. Elevations in these enzymes may not correlate well with the extent of liver damage in cirrhosis.
- *Complete blood count (CBC) with platelets.* A low RBC count, hemoglobin, and hematocrit demonstrate anemia related to bone marrow suppression, increased RBC destruction, bleeding, and deficiencies of folic acid and vitamin B_{12}. Platelet counts are low, related to increased destruction by the spleen. Leukopenia (low WBC count) also relates to splenomegaly.
- *Coagulation studies.* A prolonged prothrombin time results from impaired production of coagulation proteins and lack of vitamin K.
- *Serum electrolytes.* Hyponatremia is common, resulting from hemodilution. Hypokalemia, hypophosphatemia, and hypomagnesemia are also frequently seen, related to malnutrition and altered renal excretion of these electrolytes.
- *Bilirubin.* Both direct (conjugated) and indirect (unconjugated) bilirubin usually are elevated in patients with severe cirrhosis.
- *Serum albumin.* Hypoalbuminemia results from impaired liver production.
- *Serum ammonia.* Levels are elevated, because the liver fails to effectively convert ammonia to urea for renal excretion.
- *Serum glucose and cholesterol.* These levels frequently are abnormal in patients with cirrhosis.
- *Abdominal ultrasound.* This test is performed to evaluate liver size, detect ascites, and identify liver nodules. Ultrasound may be used in conjunction with *Doppler studies* to evaluate blood flow through the liver and spleen (Allan, Kerry, & Phillips, 2010).
- *Esophagoscopy.* Upper endoscopy may be done to determine the presence of esophageal varices.
- *Liver biopsy.* This test is not always necessary to diagnose cirrhosis, but it may be done to distinguish cirrhosis from other forms of liver disease. Biopsy may be deferred if the patient's bleeding time is prolonged (e.g., prothrombin time more than 3 seconds over the control).

Pharmacologic Therapy

Medications are used to treat the complications and effects of cirrhosis; they do not reverse or slow the process of cirrhosis itself. Known hepatotoxic drugs and alcohol are avoided, as are drugs metabolized by the liver (e.g., barbiturates, sedatives, hypnotics, acetaminophen). Several groups of drugs are commonly prescribed:

- Diuretics reduce fluid retention and ascites. Spironolactone (Aldactone) is frequently the drug of first choice, because it addresses increased aldosterone levels, one of the causes of ascites. If additional diuresis is necessary, a loop diuretic, such as furosemide (Lasix), may be added to the regimen.
- Medications to reduce the nitrogenous load and lower serum ammonia levels are added when manifestations of hepatic encephalopathy develop. Two commonly administered medications are lactulose and neomycin. Both exert their effects locally, in the bowel. Lactulose reduces the number of ammonia-forming organisms in the bowel and increases the acidity of colon contents, converting ammonia into ammonium ion. Ammonium ion is not absorbable and is excreted in the feces. Neomycin sulfate is a locally acting antibiotic that also reduces the number of ammonia-forming bacteria in the bowel.
- The beta-blocker nadolol (Corgard) may be given together with isosorbide mononitrate (Ismo, Imdur, Monoket) to prevent rebleeding of esophageal varices. This drug combination also lowers hepatic venous pressure.
- Ferrous sulfate and folic acid are given as indicated to treat anemia. Vitamin K may be ordered to reduce the risk of bleeding. When bleeding is acute, packed RBCs, fresh frozen plasma, or platelets may be administered to restore blood components and promote hemostasis.
- Antacids are prescribed as indicated. A drug regimen to treat *Helicobacter pylori* infection also may be effective.
- Oxazepam (Serax), a benzodiazepine antianxiety/sedative drug, is not metabolized by the liver and may be used to treat acute agitation.

Nutritional Therapy

Dietary support is an essential part of care for the patient with cirrhosis. Dietary needs change as hepatic function fluctuates. Nutritional therapy often involves the following:

- Sodium intake is restricted to less than 2 g/day, and fluids are restricted as necessary to reduce ascites and generalized edema. Fluids often are limited to 1500 mL/day. Fluid needs are calculated based on response to diuretic therapy, urine output, and serum electrolyte values.
- Unless serum ammonia levels are high, a palatable diet with adequate calories and protein is recommended. Most individuals with mild chronic encephalopathy can tolerate 60–80 g of protein daily. Protein restriction is rarely justified for patients with cirrhosis because they are already in a state of malnutrition. Plant protein is preferred to animal protein. When encephalopathy resolves and serum ammonia levels stabilize, protein intake is allowed as tolerated. The diet is high in calories and includes moderate fat intake to promote healing. Parenteral nutrition is used as needed to maintain nutritional status when food intake is limited (Wolf, 2017).

- Vitamin and mineral supplements are ordered based on laboratory values. Deficiencies in the B-complex vitamins, particularly thiamin, folate, and B_{12}, and in the fat-soluble vitamins A, D, and E, are common. These vitamins may need to be administered in a water-soluble form. Patients with alcohol-induced cirrhosis are at high risk for magnesium deficiency, which requires replacement therapy.

Surgery

Liver transplantation is indicated for some patients with irreversible, progressive cirrhosis. A decline in functional status, increasing bilirubin levels, falling albumin levels, and increasing problems with complications that respond poorly to treatment are indications for liver transplantation. Malignancy, active alcohol or drug abuse, and poor surgical risk are contraindications for the surgery.

Lifespan Considerations

There are two liver disorders that affect the pediatric population, biliary atresia and cirrhosis. Two other disease processes, viral hepatitis and hyperbilirubinemia, are discussed in-depth in the module on Digestion and the module on Reproduction.

Biliary Atresia

Biliary atresia is a condition in which the extrahepatic bile ducts fail to develop or are closed. This disorder leads to cholestasis, cirrhosis, portal hypertension, end-stage liver disease, and death by 2 years of age if not treated (Flanigan, 2013; Moreira et al., 2012; Sira, Taha, & Sira, 2014). Biliary atresia is the leading cause for pediatric liver transplantation (Moreira et al., 2012).

The specific cause of biliary atresia is not known. It is believed to be caused by the absence or blockage of the extrahepatic bile ducts. This results in blocked bile flow from the liver to the duodenum, causing inflammation and fibrotic changes in the liver. In addition to blockage, the disease can also be caused by hepatocellular dysfunction. The lack of bile acids also interferes with digestion of fat and absorption of fat-soluble vitamins A, D, E, and K, resulting in steatorrhea and nutritional deficiencies. Without treatment the disease is fatal.

Newborns and infants with biliary atresia are initially asymptomatic. Jaundice may not be detected until 2–3 weeks after birth. At that point, bilirubin levels increase and are often accompanied by both abdominal distention and hepatomegaly. As the disease progresses, splenomegaly occurs. The child experiences easy bruising, prolonged bleeding time, and intense itching. Stools have a putty-like consistency and are white or clay colored because of the absence of bile pigments. The child's urine is tea-colored because of the excretion of bilirubin and bile salts. Avoidant–restrictive food intake disorder (failure to thrive) and malnutrition occur as the disease progresses.

The child is diagnosed based on the history, physical examination, and laboratory evaluation. Laboratory findings reveal elevated bilirubin, serum aminotransferase, and alkaline phosphatase levels, along with prolonged prothrombin time, and an increased ammonia level

(Schwarz, 2014). A percutaneous liver biopsy suggests biliary atresia, and an exploratory laparotomy and intraoperative cholangiography confirms the diagnosis (Robie, Overfelt, & Xie, 2014).

Treatment for biliary atresia involves surgical intervention to correct the obstruction (hepatoportoenterostomy) along with supportive care. In a hepatoportoenterostomy (Kasai procedure), a segment of the intestine is anastomosed to the porta hepatis. This procedure promotes bile flow from the liver. IV antibiotics are administered in the postoperative period to prevent cholangitis. Prophylactic oral antibiotics are continued for 1–2 years after surgery (Flanigan, 2013).

Up to 80% of children who have the Kasai procedure will eventually need a liver transplant (Mieli-Vergani & Tizzard, 2012). Advances in transplantation surgery now make it possible to perform partial liver transplants from living donor resections. This enables transplantation to be performed before the child develops end-stage liver disease (Flanigan, 2013).

Supportive care includes the administration of intramuscular vitamin K prior to invasive procedures and surgery to decrease the risk of bleeding afterward and vitamins A, D, E, and K to provide supplementation since absorption of these vitamins is impaired. As the liver disease worsens, the child may need cholestyramine and antihistamines to help decrease itching. Ursodeoxycholic acid (Actigall) may be given to the child to promote bile flow (Schwarz, 2014). Enteral feedings may be needed as well (Flanigan, 2013).

Cirrhosis

Cirrhosis can occur in children of any age as the end stage of several disorders such as hepatitis and biliary atresia (Hassan & Balistreri, 2016; Squires & Balistreri, 2016). The diffuse destruction and regeneration of the hepatic parenchymal cells caused by these disease processes results in an increase in fibrous connective tissue and disorganization of the liver structure. Progressive scarring leads to altered blood flow to the liver, which causes further deterioration of liver function (Squires & Balistreri, 2016).

Clinical manifestations of cirrhosis in children vary. Hepatomegaly may be evident on examination along with jaundice as the disease progresses. Jaundice is sometimes the only sign of hepatic dysfunction, so its appearance must be investigated. Pruritus is common in children with cirrhosis, although it is not related to the degree of hyperbilirubinemia, as with adult patients. Other clinical manifestations include ascites, portal hypertension, encephalopathy, and variceal hemorrhage (Squires & Balistreri, 2016).

Diagnostic evaluation is based on the child's history of infection or disease with liver involvement. Physical examination often reveals jaundice, skin changes, ascites, and hemodynamic instability. Laboratory evaluation reveals abnormal liver function tests. A liver biopsy may help determine the extent of the parenchymal damage.

Medical management focuses on treating the child's symptoms and achieving optimal nutritional status and growth. Liver transplantation is the most common treatment for biliary atresia and is the only treatment for end-stage liver disease.

NURSING PROCESS

Nursing care of patients with cirrhosis is aimed at reducing further liver damage, teaching the patient to make healthier lifestyle choices, and minimizing the symptoms of the disease.

Assessment

Assessment data related to cirrhosis include the following:

- **Observation and patient interview.** Observe for current manifestations, including abdominal distention, bleeding, bruising, and jaundice. During the patient interview, ask about abdominal pain or discomfort, recent weight loss, weakness, and anorexia; altered bowel elimination; pruritus (itching); altered libido or erectile dysfunction; duration of symptoms; and history of liver or gallbladder disease. Assess for patterns and extent of alcohol or injection drug use and use of other prescription and nonprescription drugs.
- **Physical examination.** The physical examination for this patient includes monitoring vital signs; conducting a mental status exam; inspecting the color and condition of skin and mucous membranes; and palpating peripheral pulses for the presence of peripheral edema. Conduct a focused abdominal assessment, including appearance, shape and contour, bowel sounds, abdominal girth, percussion for liver borders, and palpation for tenderness and liver size.

Diagnosis

Nursing care of the patient with cirrhosis presents many challenges, because liver function affects all body systems. Many NANDA-I nursing diagnoses may apply. The diagnoses discussed in this section focus on problems with fluid and electrolyte balance, disturbed thought processes, risk for bleeding, skin integrity, and nutrition; they include the following:

- *Fluid Volume: Excess*
- *Confusion, Risk for Acute*
- *Protection, Ineffective*
- *Skin Integrity, Impaired*
- *Nutrition, Imbalanced: Less than Body Requirements.*

(NANDA-I © 2014)

Planning

Expected outcomes for a patient with cirrhosis may include any of the following:

- The patient will maintain liver function tests within normal limits.
- The patient will maintain proper hydration levels as indicated by urine specific gravity tests.
- The patient will maintain appropriate diet.
- The patient will report regular bowel elimination pattern.
- The patient will be oriented to surroundings, person, time, and place.
- The patient will maintain vital signs within normal limits.
- The patient will avoid alcohol and illicit drug use.

Implementation

With all patients (including children and young adults), the nurse should stress the relationship between alcohol and drug abuse and liver diseases. Specific interventions deal with excess fluid volume, acute confusion, ineffective protection, impaired skin integrity, and imbalanced nutrition.

Balance Fluid Volume

Cirrhosis affects water and salt regulation because of portal hypertension, hypoalbuminemia, and hyperaldosteronism. Signs of fluid volume overload and portal hypertension may develop, such as ascites, peripheral edema, internal hemorrhoids and varices, and prominent abdominal wall veins. Careful monitoring is necessary, because treatment measures can lead to further fluid and electrolyte imbalances. The nurse's responsibilities may include the following:

- Weigh the patient daily. Assess for jugular vein distention, measure abdominal girth daily, check for peripheral edema, and monitor intake and output. Careful assessment to detect fluid shifts is important.
- Assess the patient's urine specific gravity. Specific gravity measures the concentration of urine, an indicator of hydration.
- Provide a low-sodium diet (500–2000 mg/day), and restrict fluids as ordered. Excess sodium leads to water retention and can increase fluid volume, ascites, and portal hypertension.

SAFETY ALERT Monitor the patient with cirrhosis for signs of impaired renal function, such as oliguria, a fixed specific gravity of approximately 1.012, central edema (around the eyes and of the face), and increasing serum creatinine and BUN levels. These signs may indicate hepatorenal syndrome or acute renal failure from another cause.

Promote Mental Status

Accumulated nitrogenous waste products and other metabolites affect mental status and thought processes. Effects of hepatic encephalopathy can range from mild confusion to agitation to coma. The nurse's responsibilities include the following:

- Assess neurologic status, including level of consciousness and mental status. Observe for signs of early encephalopathy, such as asterixis and changes in handwriting and speech. Early identification of evidence of encephalopathy allows prompt intervention. Subtle changes in neurologic functioning are important.
- Avoid factors that may precipitate hepatic encephalopathy. Avoid hepatotoxic medications and drugs that depress the central nervous system. Cautious use of medications and close monitoring can eliminate iatrogenic causes of encephalopathy.
- Plan for consistent nursing care assignments if possible. Consistent care providers facilitate early identification of subtle neurologic changes that indicate hepatic encephalopathy.

- Provide a low-protein diet as prescribed; teach the family the importance of maintaining diet restrictions. Nitrogenous by-products from dietary protein increase serum ammonia levels.

- Administer medications or enemas as ordered to reduce nitrogenous products. Monitor bowel function, and provide measures to promote regular elimination and prevent constipation. Orally or rectally administered (per enema) medications are ordered to reduce intestinal bacteria and the ammonia they produce. Regular bowel elimination promotes protein and ammonia elimination in the feces.

- Orient the patient to surroundings, person, and place; provide simple explanations and reassurance. Modification of verbal interactions to the level of understanding and mental status of the patient may reduce anxiety and agitation.

SAFETY ALERT Closely monitor patients who have experienced gastrointestinal bleeding for signs of hepatic encephalopathy. Blood in the intestinal tract is digested as a protein, which increases serum ammonia levels and the risk for hepatic encephalopathy.

Minimize Bleeding

Impaired coagulation, esophageal varices, and possible acute gastritis place the patient with cirrhosis at significant risk for hemorrhage. Clotting is altered by vitamin K deficiency; by impaired manufacture of coagulation factors II, VII, IX, and X; and by increased platelet destruction because of splenomegaly. To prevent or minimize bleeding, the nurse does the following:

- Monitor vital signs, and report tachycardia or hypotension. Increased pulse and decreasing blood pressure may indicate hypovolemia caused by hemorrhage.

- Institute bleeding precautions. Preventive measures can decrease the risk for active bleeding.

- Monitor coagulation studies and platelet count, and report abnormal results. Coagulation studies help to determine the risk for bleeding and the need for treatment.

- Carefully monitor the patient who has had bleeding esophageal varices for evidence of rebleeding, such as hematemesis (blood in the vomit), **hematochezia** (bright blood in the stool) or tarry stools, and signs of hypovolemia or shock. Rebleeding is common following variceal hemorrhage, especially within the first week.

SAFETY ALERT Carefully monitor the respiratory status of the patient with a Sengstaken-Blakemore or Minnesota tube, which may be used in the treatment of esophageal varices. Displacement of the tube can obstruct the airway unless an endotracheal tube is in place. The esophageal balloon prevents the patient from swallowing oral secretions, increasing the risk for aspiration. Keep the head of the bed elevated 45 degrees to reduce the risk of aspiration and promote gas exchange.

Promote Skin Integrity

Severe jaundice with bile salt deposits on the skin may cause pruritus. Scratching related to the pruritus damages the skin and impairs its integrity. Malnutrition, particularly protein deficiency, and edema also increase the risk

for tissue breakdown and impaired skin integrity. To maintain the patient's skin integrity, the nurse should take the following actions:

- Use warm water rather than hot water when bathing the patient. Hot water increases pruritus.

- Use measures to prevent dry skin: Apply an emollient or lubricant as needed to keep skin moist, avoid soap or preparations with alcohol, and do not rub the skin. Dry skin contributes to pruritus.

- If indicated, apply mittens to the hands to prevent scratching. Patients with encephalopathy may not understand the need to refrain from scratching.

- Institute measures to prevent skin and tissue breakdown: Turn the patient at least every 2 hours, use an alternating-pressure mattress, and frequently assess skin condition. Frequent position changes relieve pressure and promote circulation and tissue oxygenation.

- Administer a prescribed antihistamine (to relieve pruritus) cautiously. Decreased liver function increases the risk for altered drug responses.

Promote Balanced Nutrition

The patient with cirrhosis is at risk for malnutrition for a number of reasons. These reasons include possible chronic alcohol use, anorexia, impaired vitamin and mineral absorption, and impaired protein metabolism. In addition, salt and protein restrictions may make the diet less palatable and appealing to the patient. To protect the patient against malnutrition, the nurse should do the following:

- Weigh the patient daily. Instruct the patient to weigh self at least weekly at home. Weight is a good indicator of both nutritional status and fluid balance. Short-term weight fluctuations tend to reflect fluid balance, while longer-term weight fluctuations are more reflective of nutritional status.

- Provide small meals with between-meal snacks. A small meal is more appealing for a patient with anorexia. Between-meal snacks help the patient to maintain adequate calorie and nutrient intake.

- Unless protein is restricted because of impending hepatic encephalopathy, promote protein and nutrient intake by providing nutritional supplements, such as Ensure or instant breakfasts. The sodium and protein content of all meals and snacks must be calculated when these nutrients are restricted.

- Arrange a consultation with a dietitian for diet planning while the patient is hospitalized and when at home. The dietitian can provide detailed instructions, sample menus, and suggestions for improving the palatability of the diet to promote intake.

Manage Complications

Paracentesis (aspiration of fluid from the peritoneal cavity) may be a diagnostic or a therapeutic procedure (to relieve severe ascites that does not respond to diuretic therapy). The goal of paracentesis is to relieve respiratory distress caused by excess fluid in the abdomen. Ascites fluid may be withdrawn in moderate amounts of 500 mL to 1 L daily to reduce the risk of fluid and electrolyte imbalances.

Large-volume paracentesis (withdrawal of 4–6 L of fluid at one time) may be used. Albumin often is administered intravenously during large-volume paracentesis to maintain intravascular volume as the pressure of the ascites fluid in the abdomen is relieved.

Bleeding esophageal varices are life-threatening and require intensive care management. Restoration of hemodynamic stability is the first priority. A central line is inserted, and central venous and pulmonary artery pressures are monitored. Blood is given to restore blood volume, and fresh frozen plasma may be administered to restore clotting factors. Somatostatin or octreotide, both of which constrict blood vessels in the gut, is given intravenously to reduce blood flow in the portal venous system. Vasopressin, which produces generalized vasoconstriction, also may be used.

When the patient's blood pressure and cardiac output have stabilized, upper endoscopy is performed to evaluate and treat the varices. A large nasogastric tube is inserted before endoscopy, and **gastric lavage** (irrigation of the stomach with large quantities of normal saline) is performed to improve visualization. During endoscopy, the varices may be banded or sclerosed to reduce the risk of recurrent bleeding. In *banding* (*variceal ligation*) small rubber bands are placed on varices to occlude blood flow. *Endoscopic sclerosis* involves injecting a sclerosing agent directly into the varices to induce inflammation and clotting.

Balloon tamponade of bleeding varices may be used if bleeding cannot be controlled through vasoconstriction or if endoscopy is unavailable. A multiple-lumen nasogastric tube (e.g., a Sengstaken-Blakemore or Minnesota tube) is inserted, and the gastric and esophageal balloons are inflated to apply direct pressure on the bleeding varices. Tension is applied to the tube to further compress the varices. Balloon tamponade carries a number of risks, including aspiration, airway obstruction, and tissue ischemia and necrosis. An endotracheal tube is inserted before nasogastric intubation to support the airway and reduce the risk of aspiration. This short-term measure is used only until more definitive treatment can be performed.

SAFETY ALERT When caring for a patient with a multiple-lumen nasogastric tube, always deflate the esophageal balloon before the gastric balloon. This practice prevents the balloon from becoming misplaced and occluding the airway. Always keep an appropriate syringe at the bedside to deflate the esophageal balloon should the patient develop respiratory distress.

A **transjugular intrahepatic portosystemic shunt (TIPS)** is used to relieve portal hypertension and its complications of esophageal varices and ascites. A channel is created through the liver tissue with a needle inserted transcutaneously. An expandable metal stent is inserted into this channel to allow blood to flow directly from the portal vein into the hepatic vein, bypassing the cirrhotic liver. The shunt relieves pressure in esophageal varices and allows better control of fluid retention with diuretic therapy. Stenosis and occlusion of the shunt are frequent complications. TIPS also increases the risk of developing hepatic encephalopathy (because of decreased perfusion of the liver and impaired ammonia metabolism), and it may reduce long-term survival. It generally is used as a short-term measure until a liver transplantation can be performed.

Patient Teaching
Home Care for the Patient with Cirrhosis

Cirrhosis is a chronic, progressive disease. Therefore, the patient and family assume major roles in managing the disease and its manifestations and in preventing complications. Teaching topics for home care include the following:

- The absolute necessity of avoiding alcohol and other hepatotoxic drugs. Suggest inpatient or community-based alcohol treatment programs and Alcoholics Anonymous as indicated.
- Diet and fluid intake restrictions and recommendations. Include suggestions to promote nutritional intake and increase the flavor of food when sodium is restricted.
- Prescribed medications. Include their timing, intended and adverse effects, and manifestations to report to the primary care provider.
- Bleeding precautions.
- Manifestations of potential complications to be reported to the primary care provider. Stress the importance of promptly reporting evidence of gastrointestinal bleeding for prompt intervention for potential hemorrhage.
- Skin care techniques to reduce pruritus and the risk of damage.
- Ways to manage fatigue and conserve energy.
- Referrals for home health services, dietary consultation, social services, and counseling as needed by the patient and family. Suggest local support groups where available. If appropriate, suggest hospice services for the patient with end-stage liver disease.

Evaluation

The evaluation of the patient with cirrhosis includes:

- Monitoring laboratory data such as liver function tests. Elevated liver enzymes indicate hepatocellular destruction. Liver function tests should remain stable during the treatment phase of the disease.
- Monitoring other lab tests including CBC, hematocrit (Hct) and hemoglobin (Hgb), coagulation studies, serum electrolytes, serum albumin, serum ammonia levels, and urine specific gravity tests. These values are expected to improve if therapy is successful.
- Assessing vital signs and level of consciousness for improvement.

Other data that indicate improvement include absence of bruising and bleeding, improved appetite, improved mobility, adequate urinary output and bowel elimination, decreasing ascites (as evidenced by decreasing girth measurements), restorative sleep patterns, and decreased discomfort.

If patient outcomes are not met, assess the patient's diet and medication adherence. Failure to adhere to treatment regimens can cause rapid changes in the patient's condition and necessitate admittance to the hospital. If the patient is not following dietary restrictions or taking medication properly, determine the cause for nonadherence and develop a care plan that addresses these causes.

>> Go to **Pearson MyLab Nursing and eText** to see a Nursing Care Plan for a patient with alcoholic liver disease.

REVIEW Liver Disease

RELATE Link the Concepts and Exemplars

Linking the exemplar of liver disease with the concept of addiction:

1. What nursing strategies might help the patient with alcohol addiction experiencing symptoms of liver disease find the motivation to abstain from alcohol?

2. The family of a patient who is addicted to alcohol and has liver disease informs the nurse that the patient has relapsed and returned to regular alcohol use after discharge from an alcohol treatment center. What assessment data would the nurse collect from the patient?

Linking the exemplar of liver disease with the concept of tissue integrity:

3. When caring for a patient with jaundice resulting from liver disease, what specific skin care measures might the nurse initiate to reduce the risk of altered skin integrity?

4. What factors increase the risk of altered skin integrity in the patient with chronic or acute liver disease?

READY Go to Volume 3: Clinical Nursing Skills

REFER Go to Pearson MyLab Nursing and eText

- Additional review materials
- Nursing Care Plan: A Patient with Alcoholic Liver Disease

REFLECT Apply Your Knowledge

Saul Mendato is a 60-year-old man with a history of alcohol-induced cirrhosis. His wife found him unconscious and called EMS to take him to the emergency department. The nurse evaluating his laboratory values notes the following: total bilirubin, 4.6 mg/dL; serum ammonia, 95 mcg/dL; platelets, 68,000/mm^3; and RBC, 4.2 million/mm^3.

1. Based on the laboratory reports, Mr. Mendato is at most risk for which complication of cirrhosis?

2. What are the priorities of nursing care?

3. What outcomes would be appropriate for this patient?

≫ Exemplar 12.D
Osteoporosis

Exemplar Learning Outcomes

12.D Analyze osteoporosis as it relates to metabolism.

- Describe the pathophysiology of osteoporosis.
- Describe the etiology of osteoporosis.
- Compare the risk factors and prevention of osteoporosis.
- Identify the clinical manifestations of osteoporosis.
- Summarize diagnostic tests and therapies used by interprofessional teams in the collaborative care of an individual with osteoporosis.

- Differentiate care of patients with osteoporosis across the lifespan.
- Apply the nursing process in providing culturally competent care to an individual with osteoporosis.

Exemplar Key Terms

Cancellous bone, *854*
Diaphysis, *854*
Metaphysis, *854*
Osteoporosis, *854*

Overview

Osteoporosis (literally defined as "porous bones") is a metabolic bone disorder characterized by loss of bone mass, increased bone fragility, and increased risk of fractures. The reduced bone mass is caused by an imbalance in the processes that influence bone growth and maintenance. Although osteoporosis may result from an endocrine disorder or malignancy, it most often is associated with aging and is a result of inadequate calcium intake. In children, osteoporosis can be related to imbalanced nutrition or other pathologic conditions.

Pathophysiology and Etiology

Pathophysiology

Although the exact pathophysiology of osteoporosis is unclear, it is known to involve an imbalance in the activity of osteoblasts that form new bone and osteoclasts that resorb bone. Until age 35, the time of peak bone mass, formation occurs more rapidly than resorption. After peak bone mass

has been achieved, slightly more bone is lost than is gained (about 0.7% per year); this loss is accelerated if the diet is deficient in vitamin D and calcium. In women, bone loss increases after menopause (with loss of estrogen), then slows but does not stop at about age 60. The decline of testosterone levels in men with aging is a more gradual process, and the associated bone loss occurs more slowly.

Osteoporosis affects the **diaphysis** (shaft of the bone) and the **metaphysis** (portion of the bone between the diaphysis and the epiphysis). The diameter of the bone increases, thinning the outer supporting cortex. As osteoporosis progresses, trabeculae are lost from **cancellous bone** (the spongy tissue of bone), and the outer cortex thins to the point where even minimal stress will fracture the bone (International Osteoporosis Foundation, 2015b).

Etiology

The National Osteoporosis Foundation (2016a) has found that osteoporosis is a health threat for an estimated 54 million Americans who have osteoporosis or low bone mass, increasing their risk for the disease. Although osteoporosis can occur at any age and in both men and women, 80% of those with osteoporosis are older women. One in three women and one in five men over age 50 will have an osteoporosis-related fracture in his or her remaining lifetime (International Osteoporosis Foundation, 2015a).

There are two types of osteoporosis: primary and secondary. Primary osteoporosis may be either type 1, which is associated with menopause, or type 2, which associated with decreasing bone formation that accompanies the aging process. Type 1 osteoporosis has been linked to estrogen deficiency resulting in increased calcium reabsorption from bone as the lack of estrogen renders the body more sensitive to PTH. Type 2 osteoporosis typically results as the kidneys lose their ability to process vitamin D, causing decreased calcium absorption, which in turn increases sensitivity to PTH and bone reabsorption (Bethel, 2016).

Secondary osteoporosis occurs as the result of a disease process or a deficiency or as an effect of a drug. Renal hypercalciuria is one of the more common causes of secondary osteoporosis and is treated with thiazide diuretics. Many patients with primary osteoporosis also have one or more secondary factors, such as Cushing syndrome, adrenal insufficiency, calcium deficiency, or DM (Bethel, 2016). Medications that increase risk for osteoporosis are outlined in **Box 12–1 »**.

Risk Factors

The risk for developing osteoporosis depends on how much bone mass is achieved between ages 25 and 35 and, afterward, on how much bone mass is lost. Certain diseases, lifestyle habits, and ethnic backgrounds increase the risk of developing osteoporosis. Different variables affect the risk of osteoporosis. Some of these variables can be modified, but others cannot.

Unmodifiable Risk Factors

Unmodifiable risk factors include being female, thin, and/or having a small frame. A personal history of fracture after age 50 also is a risk factor. Other unmodifiable risk factors include gender, family history, age, ethnicity, other chronic diseases, and current low bone mass.

Family History

Those with a family history of osteoporosis are at increased risk for developing osteoporosis themselves. Those with a history of fracture in a first-degree relative also are at higher risk.

Age and Gender

Both men and women are susceptible to osteoporosis as they age, because the osteoblasts and osteoclasts undergo alterations that diminish their activity. Women (especially White and Asian women), however, have a significantly higher risk for the manifestations and complications of osteoporosis, because their peak bone mass is 10–15% less than that of men. In addition, age-related bone loss begins earlier and proceeds more rapidly in women, beginning in their 30s and accelerating before menopause. Age-related bone loss in men occurs 15–20 years later than in women and at a slower rate. Estrogen in women and testosterone in men appear to help prevent osteoporosis; the decreasing levels of these hormones associated with aging contribute to bone loss.

Ethnicity

Osteoporosis is more common in Caucasian and Asian populations. The incidence of osteoporosis and fractures of the hip and spine are lower in African American patients (due to greater bone density) when compared to Caucasian patients (International Osteoporosis Foundation, 2015c).

Prevention

Modifiable Risk Factors

Modifiable risk factors are caused primarily by an unhealthy diet or lifestyle choices, which impact bone biology, resulting in decreased bone mineral density. Some of these risk factors increase the risk of fracture independently of their effect on the bone itself. These factors can be modified by preventive strategies.

Poor Nutrition

Dietary intake plays a role in the development of osteoporosis. Calcium is an essential mineral in the process of bone formation and other significant body functions. When the intake of calcium through the diet is insufficient, the body compensates by removing calcium from the skeleton, weakening the bone tissue. A high intake of diet soda with a high phosphate content also can deplete calcium stores.

Vitamin D is also essential as it facilitates calcium absorption from the intestines into the blood. For most individuals, casual exposure to the sun for at least 10–15 minutes per day is usually sufficient; however, some individuals may require food or supplemental sources of vitamin D (International Osteoporosis Foundation, 2015d).

Acidosis, which may result from a high protein diet, contributes to osteoporosis in two ways. First, acidosis may result in calcium being withdrawn from the bone as the kidneys attempt to buffer the excess acid. Second, acidosis may directly stimulate osteoclast function.

Box 12–1
Medications and Secondary Osteoporosis

Prolonged use of certain medications increases the risk of developing osteoporosis. Among the medications identified are (Bethel, 2016; Weinberg & Schambelan, 2016):

- Heparin therapy, which increases bone reabsorption
- Antiretroviral therapy
- Some psychotropic drugs, including selective serotonin reuptake inhibitors, lithium, and some antipsychotics
- Furosemide
- Some chemotherapeutics

Note that patients taking glucocorticoids for more than 3 months are at risk for glucocorticoid-induced osteoporosis. Glucocorticoids can slow the rate of bone formation and interfere with how the body uses calcium, leading to bone loss. These medications are often prescribed to control rheumatic diseases and include prednisone, prednisolone, dexamethasone, and cortisone. Patients with moderate to severe persistent asthma who take these medications for frequent exacerbations are also at risk.

Body Weight

Any individual with a BMI less than 20 regardless of age, sex, or weight loss is at a greater risk for both bone loss and subsequent risk for fracture. This is especially true for patients diagnosed with anorexia nervosa. Low body weight in female patients causes the body to stop producing estrogen. Low levels of estrogen negatively affect bone density (National Osteoporosis Foundation, 2016b). Underweight individuals have two-fold increased risk for fracture when compared to people with a BMI greater than 25 (International Osteoporosis Foundation, 2015a).

Substance Abuse

Both cigarette smoking and excess alcohol intake are risk factors for osteoporosis. Smoking decreases the blood supply to bones, and nicotine slows the production of osteoblasts and impairs the absorption of calcium, contributing to decreased bone density. Alcohol has a direct toxic effect on osteoblast activity, suppressing bone formation during periods of alcohol intoxication. In addition, heavy alcohol use may be associated with nutritional deficiencies that contribute to osteoporosis. Moderate alcohol consumption in postmenopausal women, however, may increase bone mineral content, possibly by increasing levels of estrogen and calcitonin.

Sedentary Lifestyle

Weight-bearing exercises, such as walking, influence bone metabolism in several ways. The stress of this type of exercise causes an increase in blood flow to bones, which brings growth-producing nutrients to the cells. Walking causes an increase in osteoblast growth and activity.

Individuals who lead a sedentary lifestyle are more likely to have a hip fracture than those who lead a more active lifestyle. For example, women who sit more than 9 hours per day are 50% more likely to experience a hip fracture when compared with women who sit less than 6 hours per day (International Osteoporosis Foundation, 2015a).

Clinical Manifestations

The most common manifestations of osteoporosis are loss of height; progressive curvature of the spine; low back pain; and fractures of the forearm, spine, or hip. Osteoporosis often is called the "silent disease," because bone loss occurs without symptoms; the problem may not become apparent until the patient has a fracture or radiologic studies reveal the condition.

The loss of height occurs as vertebral bodies collapse. Acute episodes generally are painful, with radiation of the pain around the flank into the abdomen. Vertebral collapse can occur with little or no stress; minimal movements, such as bending, lifting, or jumping, may precipitate the pain. In some patients, vertebral collapse may occur slowly, accompanied by little discomfort.

Along with loss of height, characteristic dorsal kyphosis and cervical lordosis develop, accounting for the buffalo hump (sometimes referred to as a "dowager's hump") often associated with aging. The abdomen tends to protrude and the knees and hips flex as the body attempts to maintain its center of gravity (see **Figure 12–10 ≫**).

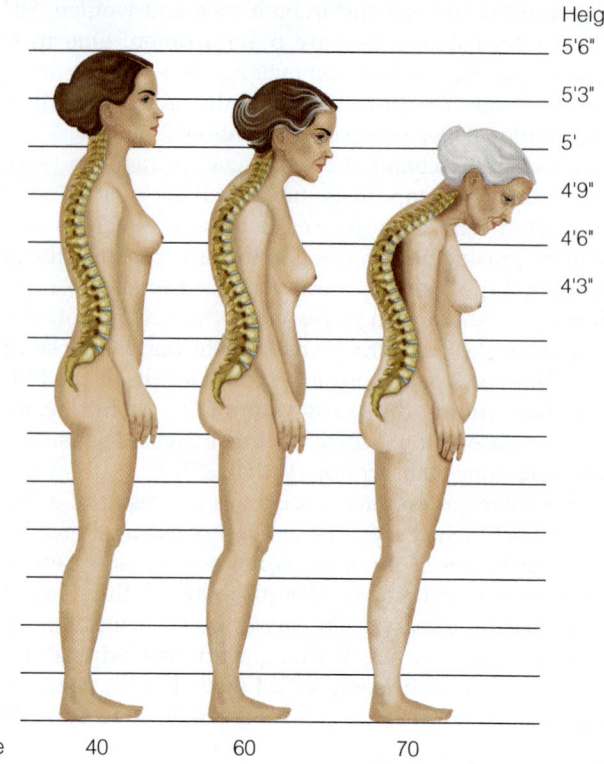

Figure 12–10 ≫ Spinal changes caused by osteoporosis. As the condition progresses, height can be reduced by as much as 7 in.

Fractures are the most common complication of osteoporosis, and the disease is responsible for more than 1.5 million fractures each year. These include more than 500,000 vertebral fractures, 300,000 hip fractures, 200,000 wrist fractures, and 300,000 fractures at other sites (Bethel, 2016). There may be no obvious manifestations of osteoporosis until fractures occur. Some fractures are spontaneous; others may result from everyday activities. Wrist and vertebral fractures have not been shown to increase patient disability or mortality, but the persistent pain and associated changes in posture may restrict the patient's activities or interfere with activities of daily living.

Pharmacotherapy is used for prevention and treatment of osteoporosis. Medications used include hormonal agents, bisphosphonates, and selective estrogen receptor modulators. Estrogen replacement therapy reduces bone loss, increases bone density in the spine and hip, and reduces the risk of fractures in postmenopausal women. It is particularly recommended for women who have undergone surgical menopause before age 50, and it often is prescribed for women with other risk factors. Estrogen therapy alone is associated with an increased risk of endometrial cancer, so it usually is prescribed in combination with progesterone; this is referred to as hormone replacement therapy (Camacho, 2014).

Collaboration

Care of the patient with osteoporosis focuses on stopping or slowing the process, alleviating the symptoms, and preventing complications. Proper nutrition and exercise are important components of the treatment program.

Diagnostic Tests

The manifestations of osteoporosis can mimic those of other bone disorders. Therefore, diagnostic tests are needed to differentiate osteoporosis from other problems.

Dual-energy x-ray absorptiometry (DEXA) measures bone density in the lumbar spine or hip and is considered highly accurate. Bone density tests are reported using T-scores. A T-score between −1.0 and −2.5 indicates low bone density, or osteopenia. A T-score of −2.5 or below indicates osteoporosis. Ultrasound transmits painless sound waves through the heel of the foot to measure bone density. This 1-minute test is not as sensitive as DEXA, but it is accurate enough for screening purposes.

Laboratory tests include alkaline phosphatase, which may be elevated following a fracture, and serum bone Gla protein (osteocalcin), which can be used as a marker of osteoclastic activity and is therefore an indicator of the rate of bone turnover. This test is most useful to evaluate the effects of treatment rather than to indicate the severity of the disease.

Physical Therapy

Nurses may collaborate with physical therapists to design appropriate exercises for patients with osteoporosis. This collaboration may be particularly helpful for patients who have a comorbid condition that limits exercise, such as COPD. Patients who have problems with balance may benefit from tai chi or yoga, both of which can benefit individuals with osteoporosis. If a nurse working with a female athlete suspects an eating disorder or amenorrhea, the nurse should discuss counseling and nutrition referrals with the patient.

Dietary Management

Patients who have osteoporosis or who are at risk for later development of the disease benefit from choosing healthy menu items, particularly those high in calcium and vitamin D. Calcium-rich foods include dairy, vegetables, and beans. Food supplemented with extra calcium includes orange juice, breakfast cereals, and breads. Foods rich in vitamin D include fish. Foods with vitamin D added include milk, cereal, and breads. If inadequate calcium and vitamin D are found in the diet, patients may take supplements to ensure that the body has an adequate supply of these nutrients.

Pharmacologic Therapy

Selected drugs for osteoporosis are listed in the Medications feature in the module on Metabolism. Calcium gluconate and other calcium compounds are used to treat and prevent osteoporosis. Oral calcium supplements are best taken with meals or within 1 hour following meals. It is recommended that adults 50 years of age and over should obtain at least 1000–1200 mg per day of elemental calcium. The most common adverse effect is hypercalcemia caused by taking too much of the supplement. Symptoms include lethargy, drowsiness, weakness, headache, anorexia, nausea and vomiting, increased urination, and thirst. Calcium

supplementation is contraindicated in patients with ventricular fibrillation, metastatic bone cancer, renal calculi, or hypercalcemia. Caution should be taken in administering calcium supplements with digoxin, tetracyclines, and calcium channel blockers. The recommended dose of vitamin D is 1000 international units for adults 50 and older. High-risk patients and older adults may need more (National Osteoporosis Foundation, 2015a).

The most common drug class for treating osteoporosis is the bisphosphonates. These drugs are structural analogs of pyrophosphate, a natural substance that inhibits bone resorption. Bisphosphonates inhibit bone resorption by suppressing osteoclast activity, thus increasing bone density and reducing the incidence of fractures by about 50%. Examples are etidronate (Didronel), alendronate (Fosamax), tiludronate (Skelid), and pamidronate (Aredia). Adverse effects include gastrointestinal problems such as nausea, vomiting, abdominal pain, and esophageal irritation. Oral bisphosphonates should be taken on an empty stomach, as tolerated by the patient, because they are poorly absorbed. Recent studies suggest that once-weekly dosing with bisphosphonates may give the same bone density benefits as daily dosing because of the extended duration of drug action.

Lifespan Considerations

Osteoporosis in Children

While osteoporosis is often associated with the aging process, children can also develop this disease process. When diagnosed in the pediatric patient, osteoporosis is often referred to as metabolic bone disease. Children at risk for developing osteoporosis include those with decreased mechanical loading (Szadek & Scharer, 2014). This tends to occur with diagnoses such as spina bifida or cerebral palsy as these disease processes interfere with ambulation, which causes limited pressure on the bones. As a result, bones in the affected extremities and the spine have lower mass. Some other conditions associated with lower bone mass include Turner syndrome, growth hormone deficiency, osteogenesis imperfecta, juvenile rheumatoid arthritis, and diabetes. Other risk factors for osteoporosis in the pediatric population include children who are immobilized as a result of casting or bracing for the treatment of a disorder or injury. Children who are treated for some types of cancer may also be at risk for osteoporosis.

≫ **Stay Current:** Visit the website of the Osteogenesis Imperfecta Foundation to learn more about this disorder: http://www.oif.org/

Adolescent athletes may also be at an increased risk for osteoporosis. This is especially true if the adolescent participates in a sport that emphasizes leanness, such as gymnastics or cross-country running. The leanness found in many adolescent female athletes increases the risk for female athlete triad. This health problem causes low bone mass, disordered eating, and amenorrhea.

≫ **Stay Current:** Visit the website of the Female Athlete Triad Coalition to learn more about this disorder: http://www.femaleathletetriad.org/

Osteoporosis in Pregnant Women

Pregnancy and breastfeeding cause changes in, and often place extra demands on, women's bones. Most women do not experience bone problems during pregnancy and breast-feeding. If problems do occur, they are often easily corrected.

During pregnancy, the growing fetus needs adequate amounts of calcium to develop the skeleton. If the mother does not eat a diet that is rich in calcium, the fetus draws what it needs from the mother's bones. Any bone mass that is lost during pregnancy, however, is typically restored within several months after childbirth.

Several studies indicate that breastfeeding also affects maternal bones. Evidence suggests that some women may lose up to 5% of their bone mass while breastfeeding. Restoration occurs within several months once the infant is weaned from the breast (NIH Osteoporosis and Related Bone Diseases National Resource Center, 2015).

Some studies suggest that pregnancy is good for women's overall bone health. Evidence suggests that the more times women are pregnant (for at least 28 weeks' gestation), the greater the bone density and the lower the risk for fracture (NIH Osteoporosis and Related Bone Diseases National Resource Center, 2015).

Osteoporosis in Older Adults

With menopause and decreasing estrogen levels, bone loss accelerates in women. Normal age-related changes of aging coupled with common conditions found with older adults (visual impairment, loss of balance, neuromuscular dysfunction, dementia, immobilization, and the use of sleeping pills) increase the risk for fracture (International Osteoporosis Foundation, 2015c). Nurses should encourage regular bone density monitoring in older adult women and provide education on fall prevention. See the module on Mobility for fall prevention strategies.

NURSING PROCESS

Osteoporosis is both preventable and treatable; therefore, nursing care focuses primarily on planning and implementing interventions to prevent the disease, its manifestations, and the resulting injuries. An important aspect of preventing osteoporosis is educating patients under age 35. Health promotion activities to prevent or slow osteoporosis focus on calcium intake, exercise, and health-related behaviors.

Assessment

The nurse should collect the following data through the health history and physical examination:

- **Observation and patient interview.** Observe the patient for any physical manifestations of osteoporosis. During the patient interview, ask questions regarding age; risk factors; history of fractures; smoking history; alcohol intake; medications; usual diet; menstrual history, including menopause; usual exercise/activity level; and low back pain.
- **Physical examination.** Measure the patient's height and assess spinal curves.

Diagnosis

While there may be some variance regarding appropriate NANDA-I nursing diagnoses among patients who are at

risk for or have osteoporosis, the following should be considered:

- *Injury, Risk for*
- *Nutrition, Imbalanced: Less than Body Requirements*
- *Pain, Acute.*

(NANDA-I © 2014)

Planning

Planning should be structured around self-care strategies that reduce patients' risk for developing osteoporosis and/or minimize its symptoms and effects. Appropriate goals for patients may include the following:

- The patient will participate in weight-bearing exercises for approximately 30 minutes a day at least 4 days per week.
- The patient's bone density will be evaluated at least every other year.
- The patient will get sufficient nutrition, particularly calcium and vitamin D, through diet or diet in combination with dietary supplements and sun exposure.
- The patient will be able to discuss risk factors for osteoporosis and how to prevent or minimize them.
- The patient with a high risk for injury will modify the home and work environments to minimize risk of falling.

Implementation

Nursing care of patients who have osteoporosis focuses on teaching about the disease process, helping to maintain physical mobility and nutrition, and solving problems associated with pain and injury.

Prevent Injury

Falls that would result in little or no injury in the healthy adult may cause fractures in the patient with osteoporosis. Even normal movements, such as twisting, bending, lifting, or rising from bed, can precipitate a vertebral fracture. The nurse should take care to do the following:

- Implement safety precautions as necessary for the patient who is hospitalized or in a long-term care facility. Maintain the bed in a low position; encourage patient to call for assistance to prevent the patient from getting up alone. Provide nighttime lighting in toilet facilities. Most falls are preventable, particularly in hospitals and long-term care facilities.
- Avoid using restraints on the patient who is hospitalized or a resident in a long-term care facility if at all possible. Restraints may actually increase the patient's risk of falling and the risk of injury associated with a fall.
- Encourage older adults to use assistive devices to maintain independence in activities of daily living. Walking sticks, canes, and other assistive devices encourage patient independence and support activities that promote bone growth.
- Teach older patients about safety and fall precautions. An assessment of the patient's home for safety and fall risks

may reduce the risk of fractures and, in turn, the cost of hospitalization and potential disability and/or death.

Promote Balanced Nutrition

Most Americans do not maintain their recommended daily intake of calcium. Patients therefore must be made aware of the relationship between an adequate calcium intake and maintaining strong bones. The following are steps the nurse can take to help patients ingest adequate calcium:

- Teach adolescents, pregnant or lactating women, and adults through age 35 to eat foods that are high in calcium and to maintain a daily calcium intake of 1200–1500 mg, as recommended by the National Institutes of Health.

- Encourage postmenopausal women to maintain a calcium intake of 1000–1500 mg daily, through either diet or a calcium supplement. Calcium needs for postmenopausal women vary depending on age.

- Teach patients who are taking calcium supplements about the importance of taking the medication at the proper time and about the possible side effects. Free hydrochloric acid is needed for calcium absorption. Calcium carbonate supplement (e.g., Tums) should be taken 30–60 minutes before meals to allow adequate absorption. Calcium citrate supplements should be taken with meals to prevent gastrointestinal distress. Calcium supplements should be taken in divided doses (two to three times daily) for improved distribution, because the body requires calcium 24 hours per day.

- Inform patients that calcium absorption requires sufficient levels of vitamin D. Patients who are at risk for insufficient levels of vitamin D may need to take a vitamin D supplement in combination with their calcium supplement. The National Institutes of Health recommends 400–800 IU of vitamin D daily for those under 50 years of age and 800–1000 IU for those age 50 and older.

Relieve Acute Pain

Pain and immobilization can occur in the advanced stages of osteoporosis. Acute pain usually results from a complicating fracture, especially a compression fracture of the vertebrae. For patients experiencing pain, the nurse can do the following:

- Suggest the application of heat to relieve pain. A heating pad may offer temporary pain relief. To avoid a rebound effect (when the muscles and joints become sore and stiff from too much heat), the heat should be removed every 20–30 minutes.

- Suggest that the patient take over-the-counter anti-inflammatory pain medications for treatment of both acute and chronic pain. Patients should be instructed in the dosage and frequency as noted on the manufacturer's label. Continuous administration of ibuprofen or other nonsteroidal anti-inflammatory drugs (NSAIDs) can be useful to provide relief from pain, but patients must be cautioned not to exceed dosage recommendations.

SAFETY ALERT Teach patient on long-term anti-inflammatory medications to watch for bright red bleeding from the stomach (in vomitus) or dark black bowel movements.

Encourage Exercise

Patients need to understand the role of physical activity and weight-bearing exercises in preventing and slowing bone loss. The nurse should inform patients that swimming and water aerobic exercises are not as beneficial for maintaining bone density because they are not weight-bearing activities. The nurse should also do the following:

- Before beginning teaching related to exercise, determine the patient's preexisting health problems and consult with the patient's primary provider to ensure safety in beginning an exercise regimen.

- Teach the patient who is able to participate in weight-bearing exercises to perform such exercises for a sustained period of 30–40 minutes at least three times a week. The mechanical force of weight-bearing exercises promotes bone growth. Bones weaken and demineralize without exercise. Walking is an easy, low-impact form of exercise. Swimming (including walking on the bottom of the pool) does not require the needed weight bearing.

- Determine the patient's interests and help the patient to plan an exercise regimen in keeping with the patient's preferences.

Promote Healthy Behaviors

Behaviors that help to prevent osteoporosis include not smoking, avoiding excessive alcohol intake, and limiting caffeine intake to two or three cups of coffee each day. The nurse should make sure the patient understands the importance of these behaviors.

Evaluation

The nurse should evaluate outcomes when planning with the patient at the patient's annual checkup. The nurse should ask the patient about any pharmacologic therapies at each healthcare visit to ensure that the patient is taking the prescribed medications and to provide the opportunity to discuss any possible side effects.

Expected outcomes for the patient with osteoporosis include the following:

- The patient identifies and implements strategies to change or modify lifestyle factors such as smoking cessation, weight-bearing exercise, and moderation in alcohol use.

- The patient achieves adequate calcium and vitamin D intake.

- The patient identifies and eliminates safety hazards.

- The patient experiences relief from acute pain.

If patient outcomes are not met, additional education about medication, diet, and activity adherence may be necessary. Failure to adhere to treatment regimens can heighten the bone density loss and increase the risk for injury, especially fractures. If the patient is not following the plan of care properly, determine the reasons for nonadherance and develop a care plan that addresses them.

Nursing Care Plan

A Patient with Osteoporosis

Nancy Bauer is a 53-year-old schoolteacher. She has been married for 36 years and has two children. Ms. Bauer is 65 inches tall. She has smoked one pack of cigarettes a day for 30 years and drinks one to two glasses of wine with dinner each evening. She does not exercise routinely. Ms. Bauer has had symptoms of menopause for 8 years, including hot flashes in the early years and mood swings more recently. She has never been on hormone replacement therapy.

Ms. Bauer is currently seeking medical advice for continuous low back pain. The pain is not relieved with an over-the-counter analgesic, and she frequently wakes up during the night because of the pain. She is diagnosed with osteoporosis.

ASSESSMENT

The nurse practitioner notes that Ms. Bauer's vital signs are within normal limits. She has full range of motion of all extremities and is able to stand and bend over, but she reports discomfort when returning to the upright position. Ms. Bauer has a slightly pronounced "hump" on her upper back and is 1 inch shorter than her stated height on admission. Her muscle strength is symmetrical and strong.

DIAGNOSES

Nursing diagnoses that may be appropriate for Ms. Bauer include the following:

- *Pain, Acute* of the lower spine related to vertebral compression
- *Knowledge, Deficient* related to osteoporosis and treatment to prevent further damage
- *Nutrition, Imbalanced: Less than Body Requirements* related to inadequate intake of calcium
- *Injury, Risk for* related to effects of change in bone structure secondary to osteoporosis.

(NANDA-I © 2014)

PLANNING

The goals for the plan of care specify that Ms. Bauer will:

- Verbalize a decrease in back pain
- Be able to describe ways to treat her osteoporosis and prevent further complications
- Verbalize an understanding of the current research and treatment regarding osteoporosis
- Verbalize how stopping smoking can help to prevent further progression of osteoporosis
- Seek consultation for supplements and medications to prevent further bone loss
- Design a program of physical activity to prevent complications of osteoporosis
- Verbalize safety precautions to prevent fractures resulting from falls.

IMPLEMENTATION

The following nursing interventions may be appropriate for Ms. Bauer:

- Teach back-strengthening exercises.
- Refer to an osteoporosis support group if available.
- Provide realistic, yet optimistic, feedback about loss of height and bone integrity and the potential outcomes of treatment.
- Assess the patient's current knowledge base, and correct any misconceptions regarding treatment of osteoporosis.
- Provide current educational literature regarding treatment of osteoporosis.
- Instruct the patient in dietary and calcium supplements that help to prevent the effects of osteoporosis.
- Discuss physical exercises that help to prevent complications resulting from osteoporosis.
- Review safety and fall precautions, and provide literature regarding how to create a safe home environment.

EVALUATION

On her return visit after 6 months, Ms. Bauer reports that she feels much better. She is no longer irritable and does not experience mood swings, because she has been taking her prescribed hormone replacement for 6 months. She is eating products rich in calcium and is taking a twice-daily supplement of calcium with vitamin D. Ms. Bauer has reduced her wine intake to one glass in the evening and now drinks decaffeinated coffee and tea. She also states that since she stopped smoking, she has been walking 30–45 minutes every day.

CRITICAL THINKING

1. What is the rationale for stopping smoking and limiting caffeine and alcohol intake in the treatment of osteoporosis?

2. What foods would you encourage for patients who are at high risk for osteoporosis and whose serum cholesterol and LDL/HDL ratios indicate a high risk for cardiovascular disease?

3. What physical activities would you consider beneficial in helping to prevent the effects of osteoporosis in a woman who uses a wheelchair or has limited mobility?

4. Develop a care plan for Ms. Bauer for the nursing diagnosis *Risk for Trauma*.

REVIEW Osteoporosis

RELATE Link the Concepts and Exemplars

Linking the exemplar of osteoporosis with the concept of fluids and electrolytes:

1. Create a flowchart diagramming the relationship between calcium and osteoporosis.

2. In addition to calcium, what other electrolytes are required for calcium to be properly metabolized and absorbed into the bone? Explain the physiology involved.

Linking the exemplar of osteoporosis with the concept of safety:

3. What safety issues will the nurse address in caring for a patient with osteoporosis? Why?

4. What strategies will the nurse recommend to reduce the risk of fractures for a patient with osteoporosis? Why?

READY Go to Volume 3: Clinical Nursing Skills

REFER: Go to Pearson MyLab Nursing and eText

- Additional review materials

REFLECT Apply Your Knowledge

Mary Martin is a 75-year-old woman who was recently widowed. She has a limited income because her husband's pension terminated when

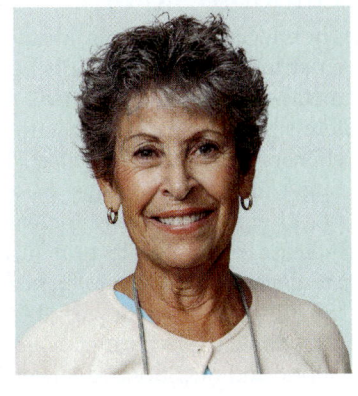

he died, and she has moved in with her son, his wife, and their three teenage children. Ms. Martin has cataracts and glaucoma, for which she sees an ophthalmologist regularly; otherwise, she is in good health.

Ms. Martin goes to the community health fair with her friend. While at the fair, she has a bone density screening and is told that she needs further evaluation for low bone density, a finding commonly associated with osteoporosis. In a follow-up visit with her primary care provider, Ms. Martin is told that her bone scan shows evidence of decreased bone mineral density consistent with osteoporosis. She is told to introduce weight-bearing exercise into her activities, to increase her calcium intake to 1500 mg/day, and to take vitamin D supplements. She also is given a prescription for alendronate (Fosamax).

1. What teaching will the nurse provide Ms. Martin?

2. What outcomes are appropriate for Ms. Martin?

3. What recommendations will the nurse make to reduce the risk of injury when assessing Ms. Martin's home?

» Exemplar 12.E Thyroid Disease

Exemplar Learning Outcomes

12.E Analyze thyroid disease as it relates to metabolism.

- Describe the pathophysiology of thyroid disease.
- Describe the etiology of thyroid disease.
- Compare the risk factors and prevention of thyroid disease.
- Identify the clinical manifestations of thyroid disease.
- Summarize diagnostic tests and therapies used by interprofessional teams in the collaborative care of an individual with thyroid disease.
- Differentiate care of patients with thyroid disease across the lifespan.
- Apply the nursing process in providing culturally competent care to an individual with thyroid disease.

Exemplar Key Terms

Euthyroid, *862*
Exophthalmos, *862*
Goiter, *862*
Graves disease, *862*
Hashimoto thyroiditis, *868*
Hyperthyroidism, *861*
Hypothyroidism, *868*
Myxedema, *868*
Myxedema coma, *870*
Proptosis, *862*
Thyroid crisis, *864*
Thyroid storm, *864*
Thyroidectomy, *865*
Thyroiditis, *864*
Thyrotoxicosis, *861*
Toxic multinodular goiter, *864*

Overview

The thyroid gland is a small saddle-shaped gland that wraps around the anterior portion of the trachea. Altered production or use of TH affects all major organ systems. In the adult, TH changes primarily affect metabolism and cardiovascular, gastrointestinal, and neuromuscular function. Thyroid disorders are among the most common endocrine disorders and, if left untreated, can result in cardiac disease and ultimately death.

HYPERTHYROIDISM

Hyperthyroidism (also called **thyrotoxicosis**) is a disorder caused by excessive delivery of TH to the peripheral tissues. Because the primary effect of TH is to increase metabolism and protein synthesis, hyperthyroidism affects all major organ systems.

Pathophysiology and Etiology

Pathophysiology

The effects of hyperthyroidism are the result of increased circulating levels of TH. This hormonal excess increases the metabolic rate and heightens the sympathetic nervous system's physiologic response to stimulation. The sensitizing effect of abnormally elevated TH levels increases the cardiac rate and stroke volume. As a result, cardiac output and peripheral blood flow increase. Elevated TH levels also increase carbohydrate, protein, and lipid metabolism. Lipids are depleted, glucose tolerance decreases, and protein degradation increases; the result is a negative nitrogen balance. Over time, the hypermetabolic effects of excess TH result in caloric and nutritional deficiencies.

Etiology

Hyperthyroidism results from many different factors, including autoimmune stimulation (as in Graves disease), excess secretion of TSH by the pituitary gland, thyroiditis, neoplasms (e.g., toxic multinodular goiter), and an excessive intake of thyroid medications. The most common etiologies of hyperthyroidism are Graves disease and toxic multinodular goiter.

Risk Factors

Women are at increased risk for hyperthyroidism, being 8 times more likely than men to develop the condition. Genetic factors, such as a family history of Graves disease, also contribute to increased risk. Other risk factors are increased iodine intake and being between 20 and 40 years in age (NIDDK, 2012a).

Prevention

Hyperthyroidism caused by Graves disease is a genetic condition that cannot be prevented. Individuals who smoke are more likely to develop hyperthyroidism. Based on these data, individuals with a family history of this disorder should be educated about their increased risk and encouraged not to smoke (Mount Sinai Hospital, 2016a).

Clinical Manifestations

The patient with hyperthyroidism typically has an increased appetite yet loses weight and may have hypermotile bowels (characterized by increased peristalsis, bloating, and pain) and diarrhea. Additional manifestations related to hypermetabolism include heat intolerance, insomnia, palpitations, and increased sweating. The skin is smooth and warm; the hair may become fine; and hair loss in the scalp, eyebrow, axillary, or pubic areas of the body is common. Emotional lability also is common. See the Multisystem Effects of Hyperthyroidism feature.

Treatment of hyperthyroidism focuses on reducing the production of TH by the thyroid gland, thus establishing a **euthyroid** (normal thyroid) state, and preventing or treating complications. Depending on the patient's age and physical status, medications, RAI therapy, or surgery may be used.

Graves Disease

Graves disease, the most common cause of hyperthyroidism, is an autoimmune disorder sometimes associated with the presence of other autoimmune disorders, such as T1D, rheumatoid arthritis, and virtiglio (NIDDK, 2012a). Patients with Graves disease have an antibody in their serum that binds to TSH receptors in the thyroid follicles and causes the thyroid cells to hyperfunction. When this antibody binds to the TSH receptors on the thyroid gland, it stimulates hormone synthesis and secretion, enlarging the gland. The cause is unknown, but there is a hereditary link.

Patients with Graves disease have an enlarged thyroid gland (**goiter**) and manifestations of hyperthyroidism. The goiter can result from excess TSH stimulation (when the amount of circulating TH is deficient), abnormal growth-stimulating immunoglobulins, or substances that inhibit TH synthesis. A goiter may be present in patients with hyperthyroidism or hypothyroidism.

The ophthalmopathy (disease of the eye) of Graves' disease is manifested as proptosis and visual dysfunction. **Proptosis** (forward displacement of the eye) occurs in about one third of cases (NIDDK, 2012a). This forward protrusion of the eyeballs (also known as **exophthalmos**) results from an accumulation of inflammation by-products in the retro-orbital tissues. Many times, the sclera is visible above the iris. The upper lids often are retracted, and the individual has a characteristic unblinking stare (see **Figure 12–11 >>**). Proptosis usually is bilateral, but it may involve only one eye. The patient may experience blurred vision, diplopia, eye pain, lacrimation, and photophobia. The inability to close the eyelids completely over the protruding eyeballs increases the risk of corneal dryness, irritation, infection, and ulceration. Infiltration of the muscles that move the eye and of the optic nerve leads to paralysis and vision loss. The treatment of Graves disease may stabilize these symptoms but generally does not reverse the changes in the eyes.

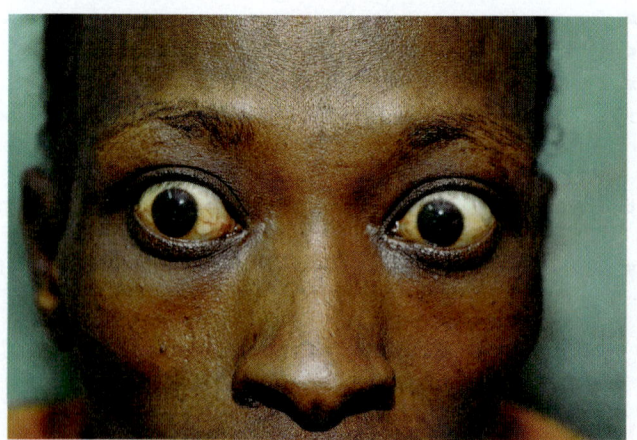

Source: Medicshots/Alamy Stock Photo.

Figure 12–11 >> Exophthalmos in a patient with Graves disease. The disease causes edema of fat deposits behind the eyes and inflammation of the extraocular muscles. The accumulating pressure forces the eyes outward from their orbits.

Multisystem Effects of
Hyperthyroidism

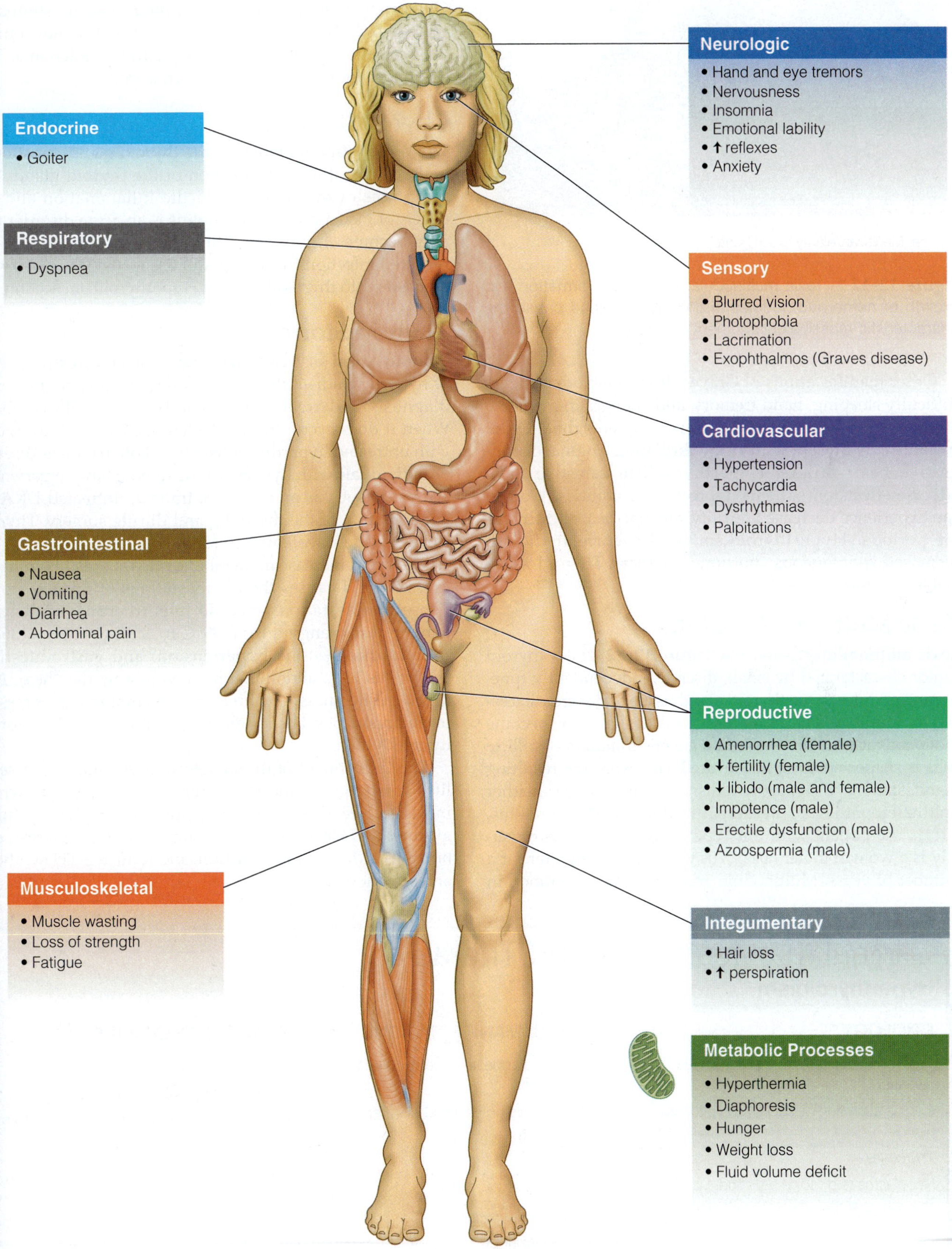

Neurologic
- Hand and eye tremors
- Nervousness
- Insomnia
- Emotional lability
- ↑ reflexes
- Anxiety

Endocrine
- Goiter

Respiratory
- Dyspnea

Sensory
- Blurred vision
- Photophobia
- Lacrimation
- Exophthalmos (Graves disease)

Cardiovascular
- Hypertension
- Tachycardia
- Dysrhythmias
- Palpitations

Gastrointestinal
- Nausea
- Vomiting
- Diarrhea
- Abdominal pain

Reproductive
- Amenorrhea (female)
- ↓ fertility (female)
- ↓ libido (male and female)
- Impotence (male)
- Erectile dysfunction (male)
- Azoospermia (male)

Musculoskeletal
- Muscle wasting
- Loss of strength
- Fatigue

Integumentary
- Hair loss
- ↑ perspiration

Metabolic Processes
- Hyperthermia
- Diaphoresis
- Hunger
- Weight loss
- Fluid volume deficit

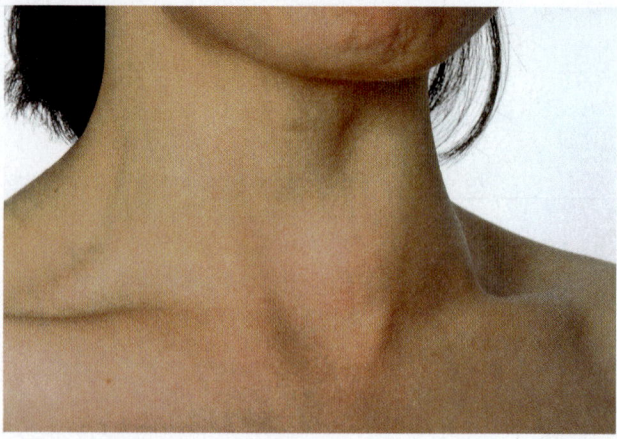

Source: Mediscan/Alamy Stock Photo.

Figure 12–12 》》 Toxic multinodular goiter. The formation and growth of numerous nodules in the thyroid gland cause the characteristic massive enlargement of the neck.

Other manifestations of Graves disease include fatigue, difficulty sleeping, hand tremors, and changes in menstruation ranging from decreased flow to amenorrhea. Older patients may present with atrial fibrillation, angina, or congestive heart failure. Hyperthyroidism can also have adverse effects on patients' reproductive abilities. Women can experience decreased fertility, amenorrhea, and irregular periods. Hyperthyroidism is also correlated with increased spontaneous abortion (American Thyroid Association, 2014a).

Toxic Multinodular Goiter

Toxic multinodular goiter (see **Figure 12–12 》》**) is a thyroid tumor characterized by small, discrete, independently functioning nodules in the thyroid gland tissue that secrete excessive amounts of TH. How these nodules grow or become independent is not known, but a genetic mutation of follicle cells is suspected. Despite elevated TH levels, the resulting manifestations of hyperthyroidism develop slowly; neither ophthalmopathy nor dermopathy develop (MedlinePlus, 2014). The patient with this type of hyperthyroidism usually is a woman in her 60s or 70s who has had a goiter for a number of years. Multinodule goiters are most common in

postmenopausal women and may present as both hypothyroidism and hyperthyroidism.

Excess TSH Stimulation

Overproduction of TSH by the pituitary usually stimulates the thyroid gland to produce excess TH. The elevation in TSH secretion often results from a pituitary adenoma. This secondary form of hyperthyroidism is rare.

Thyroiditis

Thyroiditis (inflammation of the thyroid gland) most often is the result of a viral infection of the thyroid gland. The symptoms of thyroiditis are acute inflammation and the effects of increased TH. Thyroiditis is an acute disorder that may become chronic, resulting in a hypothyroid state as repeated infections destroy gland tissue. (See the discussion of Hashimoto thyroiditis in the Hypothyroidism section.)

Thyroid Storm

Thyroid storm (also called **thyroid crisis**) is an extreme state of hyperthyroidism that is rare today because of improved diagnosis and treatment methods (MedlinePlus, 2014). When it does occur, those affected usually are individuals with untreated hyperthyroidism (most often Graves disease) or individuals with hyperthyroidism who have experienced a stressor, such as an infection, trauma, untreated DKA, or manipulation of the thyroid gland during surgery. Thyroid storm is a life-threatening condition.

The rapid increase in metabolic rate that results from the excessive TH causes the manifestations of thyroid storm. These manifestations include hyperthermia, with body temperatures ranging from 39°C to 41°C (102°F to 106°F); tachycardia; systolic hypertension; and gastrointestinal symptoms (e.g., abdominal pain, vomiting, diarrhea). Agitation, restlessness, and tremors are common, progressing to confusion, psychosis, delirium, and seizures. The mortality rate is high.

Rapid treatment of thyroid storm is essential to preserve life. Treatment includes cooling without aspirin (which increases free TH) or inducing shivering; replacing fluids, glucose, and electrolytes; relieving respiratory distress; stabilizing cardiovascular function; and reducing TH synthesis and secretion.

Clinical Manifestations and Therapies
Hyperthyroidism

ETIOLOGY	CLINICAL MANIFESTATIONS	CLINICAL THERAPIES
Autoimmune stimulation (as in Graves disease)	▪ Increased appetite accompanied by weight loss	▪ Pharmacotherapy
Excess secretion of TSH by the pituitary gland	▪ Hypermotile bowels and diarrhea	▪ Radioactive iodine (RAI) therapy
Thyroiditis	▪ Heat intolerance	▪ Surgery (subtotal or total thyroidectomy)
Neoplasms (e.g., toxic multinodular goiter)	▪ Insomnia	
Excessive intake of thyroid medications.	▪ Palpitations	
	▪ Increased sweating	
	▪ Emotional lability	

Collaboration

The focus of care of the patient with hyperthyroidism is on preventing complications until the TH levels can be brought into the normal range. Because hyperthyroidism is generally treated by destruction of all or part of the thyroid gland, thereby reducing or eliminating the production of TH, it is important for the patient to recognize the need for lifelong thyroid supplementation to replace the hormone that will no longer be produced by the thyroid gland following treatment. The patient should understand symptoms to report immediately to the healthcare provider and signs and symptoms of both hyperthyroidism and hypothyroidism.

Diagnostic Tests

Hyperthyroidism is diagnosed according to the manifestations of the specific disorders causing excessive TH and by diagnostic test results (see **Table 12–12 》**). Elevated levels of TH (both T_3 and T_4) and increased RAI uptake are diagnostic criteria of hyperthyroidism.

The following diagnostic tests may be ordered:

- **TA test.** Serum TA is measured to determine whether a thyroid autoimmune disease is causing the patient's symptoms. TA is elevated in Graves disease.

- **TSH test (sensitive assay).** Serum TSH levels are measured and compared with T_4 levels to differentiate pituitary from thyroid dysfunction. The best indicator of primary hyperthyroidism (e.g., in Graves disease) is suppression of TSH below 0.1 mcg/mL. When the sensitive TSH is not suppressed, the hyperthyroidism is caused by a TSH-secreting pituitary tumor.

- **T_4 test.** Serum T_4 levels are measured to determine TH concentration and to test thyroid gland function. T_4 levels are elevated in hyperthyroidism and in acute thyroiditis.

- **T_3 test.** Serum T_3 is measured by radioimmunoassay, which measures bound and free forms of this hormone. This test is effective for the diagnosis of hyperthyroidism. T_3 levels also may be elevated in thyroiditis.

- **T_3 uptake test.** T_3 uptake is measured by an in vitro test in which the patient's blood is mixed with radioactive T_3; the results are elevated in hyperthyroidism.

- **RAI uptake test.** An RAI uptake test (thyroid scan) measures the absorption of 131-I or 123-I by the thyroid gland.

A calculated dose of RAI is given orally or intravenously, and the thyroid is then scanned (often after 24 hours). The distribution of radioactivity in the gland is recorded (increased uptake of RAI is seen in Graves disease). In addition, the scan reveals the size and shape of the gland.

- **Thyroid suppression test.** RAI and T_4 levels are measured first. The patient then takes TH for 7–10 days, after which the tests are repeated. Failure of hormone therapy to suppress RAI and T_4 indicates hyperthyroidism.

Pharmacologic Therapy

Hyperthyroidism is treated by administering antithyroid medications that reduce TH production. Because these drugs do not affect the release or activity of hormone that is already formed, therapeutic effects may not be seen for several weeks. To rapidly decrease the cardiovascular symptoms associated with hyperthyroidism, a beta-blocker, such as propanolol (Inderal), is part of initial treatment.

Radioactive Iodine Therapy

Because the thyroid gland takes up iodine in any form, RAI (or 131-I) concentrates in the thyroid gland and damages or destroys thyroid cells so that they produce less TH. The RAI is given orally. Results typically occur in 6–8 weeks. In most instances, the patient is not hospitalized during treatment and does not require radiation precautions. This type of therapy is contraindicated for pregnant women, because RAI crosses the placenta and can have negative effects on the developing fetal thyroid gland. Because the amount of gland destroyed by RAI therapy is not readily controllable, the patient may develop hypothyroidism and require lifelong TH replacement. Adverse reactions include thyroiditis and cardiac instability caused by liberation of stored TH in the gland (American Thyroid Association, 2016a). Patients should be taught to measure their pulse rate and notify the provider if the rate exceeds 100 bpm following therapy until released stores of TH diminish.

Surgery

Some patients with hyperthyroidism have such enlarged thyroid glands that pressure on the esophagus or trachea causes problems with breathing or swallowing. In these patients, a **thyroidectomy** (removal of all or part of the gland) is indicated. A subtotal thyroidectomy usually is performed; this procedure leaves enough of the gland in place to produce an adequate amount of TH. A total thyroidectomy is performed to treat cancer of the thyroid; the patient then requires lifelong hormone replacement (Mount Sinai Hospital, 2016b).

Before surgery, the patient should be in as nearly a euthyroid state as possible. The patient may be given antithyroid drugs to reduce hormone levels and iodine preparations to decrease the vascularity and size of the gland (which also reduces the risk of hemorrhage during and after surgery).

Lifespan Considerations
Hyperthyroidism in Children

The clinical manifestations of hyperthyroidism in the pediatric population are similar to those seen in adults; however, hyperthyroidism may have unique effects on the child's

TABLE 12–12 Laboratory Findings in Hyperthyroidism

Test	Normal Values	Findings
Serum thyroid antibodies (TA)	Negative to 1:20	Increased
Serum TSH (sensitive assay)	0.35–5.5 mU/mL	Decreased in primary hyperthyroidism
Serum T_4	4.5–11.5 mcg/dL	Increased
Serum T_3	80–200 ng/dL	Increased
T_3 uptake	25–35 relative percentage	Increased
Thyroid suppression		Increased RAI uptake and T_4 levels

growth and development. Clinical manifestations of pediatric hyperthyroidism include modest acceleration of linear growth and epiphyseal maturation along with distractibility associated with unexplained poor school performance and emotional lability. The age at onset of puberty and the attainment of pubertal stages does not appear to be altered by hyperthyroidism. Female pediatric patients who have undergone menarche may develop oligomenorrhea or secondary amenorrhea along with anovulatory cycles. Hyperthyroidism is also associated with an increased aromatization of androgens to estrogens (LaFranchi, 2016a).

Hyperthyroidism in Pregnant Women

Hyperthyroidism in pregnancy occurs in 1 of every 500 pregnancies and is usually caused by Graves disease. Although Graves disease may first appear during pregnancy, a woman with preexisting disease may actually see improvement in symptoms during the second and third trimesters. This remission is the result of the general suppression of the immune system that occurs during pregnancy. The disease process is typically exacerbated during the first few months after birth. Pregnant women with Graves disease should be monitored monthly during gestation (NIDDK, 2012b).

Hyperthyroidism in pregnancy may be caused by hyperemesis gravidarum. The severe nausea and vomiting associated with this condition is triggered by high levels of hCG, which can cause temporary hyperthyroidism. This condition resolves during the second half of the pregnancy (NIDDK, 2012b).

Uncontrolled hyperthyroidism during pregnancy can lead to congestive heart failure, preeclampsia, thyroid storm, miscarriage, premature birth, and low birth weight. If the pregnant patient was treated for Graves disease in the past with surgery or RAI, the TSI antibodies may still be present in her blood and can travel across the placenta to the fetus' bloodstream stimulating the thyroid gland. If the mother is being treated with antithyroid medication, fetal hyperthyroidism is less likely because these drugs cross the placenta (NIDDK, 2012b).

Hyperthyroidism in a newborn can result in rapid heart rate, leading to heart failure; early closure of the fontanelles; poor weight gain; irritability; and breathing issues due to an enlarged thyroid gland that presses against the trachea. Because of these possible clinical manifestations, the newborn should be closely monitored by the healthcare team (NIDDK, 2012b).

Hyperthyroidism in Older Adults

While Graves disease is a common cause for hyperthyroidism for the older adult patient, toxic nodular goiter is seen more frequently in this population. Older adults who are diagnosed with hyperthyroidism often exhibit only one or two symptoms, while younger patients often have multiple symptoms. Treatment for hyperthyroidism includes antithyroid drugs and RAI. Surgery, however, is rarely recommended due to the older adult's increased operative risks (American Thyroid Association, 2014b).

Because of increased preexisting cardiac, central nervous system, and thyroid disease in older adults, these patients are closely monitored during therapy. This is especially true during the initial phase of treatment. Once thyroid function is within the normal range with oral medication, the health care provider makes a decision on definitive treatment with RAI. There is some controversy, however, about the normal level of TSH for this population (American Thyroid Association, 2014b).

NURSING PROCESS

Nursing care of the patient with hyperthyroidism is focused on providing patient education regarding the disease process, treatment options, and posttreatment self-care. In caring for the patient with hyperthyroidism, the nurse should recognize the impact that increased metabolism rates will have on the patient's ability to concentrate on information presented by the nurse.

Assessment

The following data are collected through the health history and physical examination:

- **Observation and patient interview.** Observe for clinical manifestations associated with hyperthyroidism. Ask the patient about other diseases, family history of thyroid disease, when symptoms began, severity of symptoms, intake of thyroid medications, menstrual history, changes in weight, and bowel elimination patterns.
- **Physical examination.** Evaluate muscle strength, tremors, vital signs, cardiovascular and peripheral vascular systems, integument, size of thyroid, presence of bruit over thyroid, eyes and vision.

Diagnosis

For the patient with hyperthyroidism, the nurse must consider the patient's responses to the systemic effects of the disorder. Although each patient may have different needs, the NANDA-I diagnoses discussed in this exemplar focus on the most common problems:

- *Cardiac Output, Decreased*
- *Comfort, Impaired*
- *Health Maintenance, Ineffective*
- *Infection, Risk for*
- *Nutrition, Imbalanced: Less than Body Requirements*
- *Body Image, Disturbed.*

(NANDA-I © 2014)

Planning

Nursing care is directed at symptom resolution and patient teaching related to self-care and the treatment plan. Goals appropriate for a patient with hyperthyroidism include the following:

- The patient will report improvement of clinical manifestations.
- The patient will describe situations necessitating intervention by the healthcare provider.
- The patient will explain how to take prescribed medications.

Implementation

Hyperthyroidism is often treated on an outpatient basis, so it is important that the patient understand how to provide self-care, what symptoms to monitor for, and when to call the provider. Emphasis should be on teaching patients about the importance of taking medications daily and not skipping a dose because symptoms are absent.

Monitor Cardiac Output

The patient with hyperthyroidism is at risk for alterations in cardiac output. Excess TH directly affects the heart, increasing heart rate and stroke volume. Increases in the metabolic demands and oxygen requirements of peripheral tissues increase the demands on the heart, and systolic hypertension, angina, arrhythmias, or cardiac failure may occur. The patient often has palpitations and shortness of breath and is easily fatigued. The risk of complications is greater in patients with preexisting cardiovascular disorders. To deal with this risk, the nurse should do the following:

- Monitor blood pressure, pulse rate and rhythm, respiratory rate, and breath sounds. Assess for peripheral edema, jugular vein distention, and increased activity intolerance. Higher TH level increases cardiac rate, stroke volume, and tissue demand for oxygen, causing stress on the heart. This stress may result in hypertension, arrhythmias, tachycardia, and congestive heart failure.

- Suggest keeping the environment as cool and free of distractions as possible. Decrease stress by explaining interventions and by teaching relaxation procedures. A physically comfortable and psychologically calm environment can reduce stimuli and stressors. Stress increases circulating catecholamines, which further increase cardiac workload.

- Encourage the patient to balance periods of activity with periods of rest. Rest periods decrease energy expenditure and tissue requirements for oxygen and thus decrease demands on the heart by lowering the cardiac workload.

Promote Visual Health

Visual changes that occur in patients with hyperthyroidism include difficulty in focusing, diplopia (double vision), and visual loss. If the patient is unable to close the eyelids because of exophthalmos, the risk of corneal dryness with resultant infection or injury increases. Visual deficits also may result from pressure on the optic nerve from retro-orbital edema and shortening of the eye muscles. Although treatment of hyperthyroidism may stop the progression of eye changes, not all symptoms are reversible. To address the possibility of visual changes, the nurse should do the following:

- Monitor visual acuity, photophobia, integrity of the cornea, and lid closure. The cornea is at risk for dryness, injury, conjunctivitis, and corneal infections. Injury and infection of the cornea can result in further loss of visual acuity.

- Teach measures for protecting the eye from injury and maintaining visual acuity:
  a. Use tinted glasses or shields as protection.
  b. Use artificial tears to moisten the eyes.
  c. Use cool, moist compresses to relieve irritation.
  d. Cover or tape the eyelids shut at night if they do not close.
  e. Elevate the head of the bed to 45 degrees to promote periorbital fluid decrease.
  f. Have the patient promptly report any pain or changes in vision.

These measures decrease the risk of injury, provide comfort, decrease periorbital edema that can compromise vision further, and ensure immediate care for problems, thereby minimizing the risk of further visual loss.

Promote Balanced Nutrition

The hypermetabolic state that occurs in hyperthyroidism causes gastrointestinal hypermotility, with nausea, vomiting, diarrhea, and abdominal pain. Although the patient may have an increased appetite and eat more than usual, weight loss continues. To help the patient maintain adequate nutrition, the nurse should do the following:

- Monitor nutritional status through results of laboratory tests. Serum albumin, transferrin, and total lymphocyte counts commonly are lower than normal in patients with nutritional deficits. A negative nitrogen balance signifies a catabolic state in which protein is lost and metabolic demands are not being met.

- Ask the patient to check weight daily (at the same time each day) and to keep a record of results. Regular monitoring detects continued weight loss, which can result from not meeting the body's metabolic demands.

- In collaboration with a dietitian, teach the patient about the need for a diet high in carbohydrates and protein that includes between-meal snacks. Six small meals a day may be more desirable than three large meals. Caloric intake may need to be increased to 4000 kcal/day if weight loss exceeds 10–17% for height and frame. Increased nutrients are necessary as part of a well-balanced diet and to meet metabolic demands. Patients often are better able to increase food intake by eating frequent, small meals. A 1 lb weight gain requires approximately 3500 extra kilocalories.

Improve Body Image

Physical changes that are common in hyperthyroidism include exophthalmos, goiter, tremors, hair loss, increased perspiration, loss of strength, fatigue, weight loss, and changes in reproductive and sexual function (amenorrhea in women leading to infertility, erectile dysfunction and azoospermia in men leading to infertility, and changes in libido in both genders). In addition, the patient often has mood changes and insomnia and is constantly nervous and anxious. There may even be periods of psychosis (Ross, 2016c). These changes are frightening not only for the patient but also for family members. To help the patient deal with the physical changes and their effects, the nurse should establish a trusting relationship, encourage the patient to verbalize feelings and ask questions, and provide reliable information.

Evaluation

Expected outcomes for the patient with hyperthyroidism include the following:

- The patient's cardiac status stabilizes.
- The patient regains or maintains visual acuity.

- The patient takes in an appropriate number of calories per day and exhibits no further weight loss.
- The patient communicates feelings about changes in body image and verbalizes coping mechanisms.
- The patient explains the importance of daily medications and proper self-administration.

If patient outcomes are not met, additional education about diet, medication adherence, and coping strategies may be necessary. Failure to adhere to the treatment regiments can cause rapid changes in the patient's condition necessitating hospital admission. If the patient is not following the prescribed diet and medication regimen, determine the cause for the nonadherence and develop a plan of care that addresses these causes.

HYPOTHYROIDISM

Hypothyroidism is a disorder that results when the thyroid gland produces an insufficient amount of TH.

Pathophysiology and Etiology

Pathophysiology

When TH production decreases, the thyroid gland enlarges in a compensatory attempt to produce more hormone. The goiter that results is usually a simple or nontoxic form.

The hypothyroid state in adults is sometimes called **myxedema**. The term reflects the characteristic accumulation of nonpitting edema in the connective tissues throughout the body. The edema is the result of water retention in mucoprotein (hydrophilic proteoglycans) deposits in the interstitial spaces. The face of a patient with myxedema appears puffy, the tongue is enlarged, and the voice is hoarse and husky (Surks, 2016).

Etiology

Hypothyroidism may be either primary or secondary. Primary hypothyroidism, which is more common, may be caused by congenital defects in the gland, loss of thyroid tissue following treatment of hyperthyroidism with surgery or radiation, antithyroid medications, thyroiditis, or endemic iodine deficiency. Secondary hypothyroidism may result from pituitary TSH deficiency or peripheral resistance to TH.

The cardiac drug amiodarone (Cordarone), which contains 75 mg of iodine per 200 mg tablet, is increasingly being implicated in causing thyroid problems (Ross, 2016b). Clofibrate, estrogens, methadone, amiodarone, and birth control pills increase T_4 measurement; anabolic steroids, androgens, lithium, phenytoin, propranolol, interferon alfa, and interleukin-2 decrease T_4 measurement in thyroid tests. Of course, the drugs propylthiouracil and methimazole, which are used to treat hyperthyroidism, decrease T_4 measurement as well (Ross, 2015b).

The disorder can occur at any stage of life, but it is common in women between the ages of 30 and 60. The incidence rises after age 50. Therefore, careful evaluation of symptoms is important in the older adult, because manifestations of hypothyroidism often are thought to be the result of aging instead of a pathologic process.

Risk Factors

Anyone can develop hypothyroidism; however, it is more common among women older than 50 years; individuals who have a close relative with an autoimmune condition and individuals who have had thyroid surgery, received radiation to the neck, or been treated with RAI or antithyroid medication. Other factors that result in decreased TH include iodine deficiency and Hashimoto thyroiditis.

Iodine Deficiency

Iodine is necessary for synthesis and secretion of TH. Iodine deficiency may result from certain goitrogenic drugs, which block TH synthesis; lithium carbonate, which is used to treat bipolar mental disorders; and antithyroid drugs. Goitrogenic compounds in foods such as turnips, rutabagas, and soybeans also may block TH synthesis if consumed in sufficient quantities.

In areas of the world where the soil is deficient in iodine, dietary intake of iodine may be inadequate. Individuals living in these areas are more prone to become hypothyroid and to develop simple goiter. In the United States, the use of iodized salt has reduced this risk.

Hashimoto Thyroiditis

Hashimoto thyroiditis is the most common cause of goiter and primary hypothyroidism in adults and children. In this autoimmune disorder, antibodies develop that destroy thyroid tissue. Functional thyroid tissue is replaced with fibrous tissue, and TH levels decrease. In addition, decreasing levels of TH during the early stages of the disease prompt the gland to enlarge in an attempt to compensate, causing a goiter. However, as the disease progresses, the thyroid gland becomes smaller. This disorder is more common in women than in men and has a familial link.

Prevention

For patients who live in a developed country, such as the United States, there is nothing that can be done to prevent hypothyroidism, as most diets contain adequate amounts of iodine. If the patient lives in a country where iodine deficiency is common, taking iodine supplements may help to prevent the development of this disease process. Therefore, there is no known way to prevent hypothyroidism if the patient consumes adequate amount of iodine (American Thyroid Association, 2016b).

Clinical Manifestations

Hypothyroidism has a slow onset, with manifestations occurring over months or even years. Patients with hypothyroidism characteristically have goiter, fluid retention and edema, decreased appetite, weight gain, constipation, dry skin, dyspnea, pallor, hoarseness, and muscle stiffness. Many patients have a decreased sense of taste and smell, menstrual disorders, anemias, and cardiac enlargement. The pulse typically is slow in patients with hypothyroidism, and sleep apnea is more common. See the Multisystem Effects of Hypothyroidism feature.

Deficient amounts of TH cause abnormalities in lipid metabolism, with elevated serum cholesterol and triglyceride levels. As a result, the patient is at increased risk for

Multisystem Effects of
Hypothyroidism

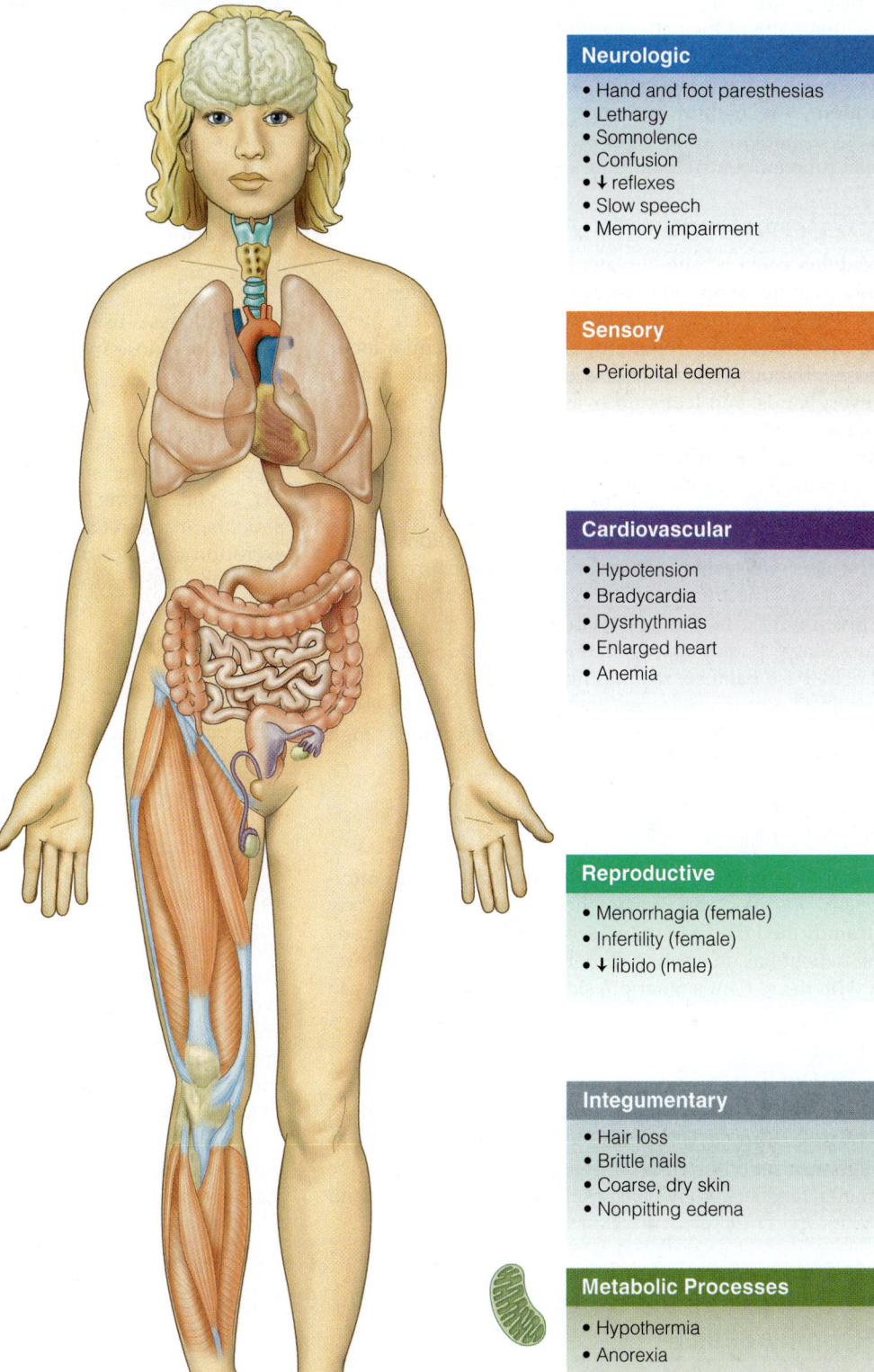

Neurologic
- Hand and foot paresthesias
- Lethargy
- Somnolence
- Confusion
- ↓ reflexes
- Slow speech
- Memory impairment

Sensory
- Periorbital edema

Cardiovascular
- Hypotension
- Bradycardia
- Dysrhythmias
- Enlarged heart
- Anemia

Reproductive
- Menorrhagia (female)
- Infertility (female)
- ↓ libido (male)

Integumentary
- Hair loss
- Brittle nails
- Coarse, dry skin
- Nonpitting edema

Metabolic Processes
- Hypothermia
- Anorexia
- Weight gain
- Systemic edema

Endocrine
- Goiter

Respiratory
- Pleural effusion

Gastrointestinal
- Constipation

Musculoskeletal
- Muscle stiffness
- Weakness
- Fatigue

atherosclerosis and cardiac disorders. Decreased renal blood flow and glomerular filtration rate reduce the kidney's ability to excrete water, which may cause hyponatremia.

Because a decrease in TH levels lowers metabolic rate and heat production, hypothyroidism affects all body systems. Treatment of the patient with hypothyroidism focuses on diagnosis, prevention or treatment of complications, and replacement of the deficient TH. With early and continued treatment, the mental and physical symptoms rapidly reverse in patients of all ages, and both appearance and mental function return to normal.

Myxedema Coma

Myxedema coma is a life-threatening complication of long-standing, untreated hypothyroidism usually triggered by an acute illness or trauma. It is characterized by severe metabolic disorders (e.g., hyponatremia, hypoglycemia, lactic acidosis); hypothermia; a shallow edema, especially around the eyes, hands, and feet; cardiovascular collapse; impaired mentation; and coma. Although rare, myxedema coma most commonly occurs during the winter months in older women with chronic hypothyroidism (Ross, 2015a).

Myxedema coma may be precipitated by trauma, infection, failure to take thyroid replacement medications, use of central nervous system depressants, and exposure to cold temperature. The treatment of myxedema coma addresses the precipitating factors and manifestations and involves maintaining a patent airway; maintaining fluid, electrolyte, and acid–base balance; maintaining cardiovascular status; increasing body temperature; and increasing TH levels. If myxedema coma is left untreated, the mortality rate is high (Ross, 2015a).

Collaboration

Collaboration with the patient's pharmacist will help minimize any side effects and ensure the patient is not taking any contraindicated medications prescribed by different doctors. If the patient has an existing comorbid condition, collaboration with the patient's other physicians may be necessary to ensure optimal care.

Diagnostic Tests

Hypothyroidism is diagnosed by the clinical manifestations and by a decrease in TH, especially T_4 (see **Table 12–13 》**). TSH concentration often is increased, because the negative hormonal feedback from TH is lost. The same laboratory and

TABLE 12–13 Laboratory Findings in Hypothyroidism

Test	Normal Values	Findings
Serum TA	None to 1:20	Normal
Serum TSH	0.35–5.5 mU/mL (mU = microunit)	Increased in primary hypothyroidism
Serum T_4	4.5–11.5 mcg/dL	Decreased
Serum T_3	80–200 ng/dL	Decreased
T_3 uptake	25–35 relative percentage	Decreased
Thyroid suppression		No change in RAI uptake or T_4 levels

diagnostic tests used to diagnose hyperthyroidism also are used to diagnose hypothyroidism, with opposite results in most cases.

Pharmacologic Therapy

Hypothyroidism is treated with medications that replace TH. Levothyroxine (LT_4) is the treatment of choice. In older patients, an age-related decrease in serum albumin and renal excretion can increase the amount of available drug and cause an exaggerated pharmacologic effect. Therefore, the older patient may require less thyroid medication than a younger patient.

Surgery

If the patient with hypothyroidism has a goiter large enough to cause respiratory difficulties or dysphagia, a subtotal thyroidectomy may be performed.

Lifespan Considerations

Hypothyroidism in Infants and Children

Congenital hypothyroidism occurs in approximately 1 in every 2000–4000 newborns. It is one of the most common and preventable causes of intellectual disability. The longer the condition goes undetected, the lower the individual's IQ later in life (LaFranchi, 2016a).

Most newborns with congenital hypothyroidism have few, if any, clinical manifestations of TH deficiency. Therefore, newborn screening programs have been developed to measure heel-stick blood specimens for T_4 and TSH. The

Clinical Manifestations and Therapies
Hypothyroidism

ETIOLOGY	CLINICAL MANIFESTATIONS	CLINICAL THERAPIES
Decrease in TH production	Hypothermia	■ Pharmacotherapy
Possibly primary or secondary	Decreased appetite accompanied by weight gain	■ Subtotal thyroidectomy if goiter is large enough to cause respiratory difficulties or dysphagia
	Systemic edema	

mplementation of these programs has been largely successful as the number of children with intellectual disability has decreased as result of diagnosis and intervention LaFranchi, 2015).

The overall goal of treatment is to ensure normal rowth and development by restoring the serum T_4 concentration rapidly to the normal range. Oral levothyroxine is the treatment of choice. Treatment is initiated to all ewborns/infants with a clearly positive screen test. In ases in which the test yields borderline results, a treatnent decision is made after results of the confirmatory ests return. Clinical evaluation should be performed very few months for the first 3 years of life. For those atients whose congenital hypothyroidism is permanent, nyroid replacement therapy is required throughout life LaFranchi, 2016b).

Hypothyroidism in Pregnant Women

Hypothyroidism in pregnancy is often caused by Hashimoto isease, but it also can occur as a result of existing hypothyidism that is inadequately treated and from the prior estruction, or removal, of the thyroid gland prior to pregancy. Hypothyroidism occurs in up to 5 of 1000 pregnanies (NIDDK, 2012b).

Uncontrolled hypothyroidism during pregnancy can ead to preeclampsia, anemia, miscarriage, low birth veight, stillbirth, or congestive heart failure (although this a rare occurrence). TH is crucial to fetal brain and nervous system development Therefore, uncontrolled hypoyroidism, especially in the first trimester of pregnancy, an affect the fetus's growth and brain development NIDDK, 2012b).

Clinical manifestations of hypothyroidism in pregnancy nclude extreme fatigue, cold intolerance, muscle cramps, onstipation, and problems with both concentration and nemory. High levels of TSH, or low levels of free T_4, confirm ne diagnosis. Note, however, that test results must be interreted with caution due to the normal pregnancy-related hanges in thyroid function (NIDDK, 2012b).

Hypothyroidism in pregnancy is treated with synthetic H, referred to as thyroxine. Women with preexisting hypoyroidism will often require an increased thyroxine dose in rder to maintain normal thyroid function. Synthetic thyroxie is safe, and necessary, for the well-being of the fetus NIDDK, 2012b).

Hypothyroidism in Older Adults

he thyroid gland undergoes some degree of atrophy, fibrois, and nodularity during the aging process. Therefore, lder adults are at risk for hypothyroidism. Symptoms aused by the aging process are often misdiagnosed as yperthyroidism, and include a decrease in hair growth; ails that are thick, brittle, and yellow; sagging facial skin; ones that become more prominent; decreased DTRs; and a ower response when answering questions. While these naifestations should not be ignored, it is important to iagnose the older adult patient based on laboratory data nd not symptomology alone.

Older adult patients should be treated conservatively as H increases myocardial oxygen demand, increasing the

patient's risk for cardiac arrhythmias, angina pectoris, and myocardial infarction. Pharmacologic treatment includes 50 mg of levothyroxine per day. This dose is often decreased by 25 mg/day for those patients with a history of coronary artery disease (Ross, 2016a).

NURSING PROCESS

Assessment

Collect the following data through the health history and physical examination. Further focused assessments are described in the Implementation section. When assessing the older adult, be aware of normal changes with aging as outlined in the Lifespan Considerations feature.

- *Observation and patient interview.* Observe the patient for clinical manifestations of hypothyroidism during the interview process. Ask questions related to pituitary diseases, when symptoms began, severity of symptoms, treatment of hyperthyroidism with medications or RAI, thyroid surgery, treatment of head or neck cancer with radiation, diet, use of iodized salt, bowel elimination, and respiratory difficulties
- *Physical examination.* Assess the patient's muscle strength, DTRs, vital signs, cardiovascular and peripheral vascular systems, integument, thyroid gland, and weight.

Diagnosis

In planning and implementing care for patients with hypothyroidism, the nurse takes into account that the disorder affects all organ systems. Although many nursing diagnoses might be valid, this section focuses on patient problems with cardiovascular function, elimination, and skin integrity.

Appropriate nursing diagnoses include:

- *Cardiac Output, Decreased*
- *Constipation*
- *Skin Integrity, Impaired*
- *Verbal Communication, Impaired*
- *Self-Esteem, Situational Low.*

(NANDA-I © 2014)

Planning

Goals for the patient with hypothyroidism include the following:

- The patient's pulse and blood pressure will remain within established limits.
- The patient will not exhibit arrhythmias.
- The patient's skin will remain warm and dry to touch.
- The patient will remain free of edema.
- The patient will maintain visual acuity.
- The patient will participate in activities without heart rate exceeding or falling below established limits.
- The patient's elimination pattern will return to normal.
- The patient's skin will remain intact.

Implementation

Care of the patient with hypothyroidism is always individualized on the basis of the specific manifestations the patient experiences as well as unique needs. When care is planned, interventions are indicated on the basis of the nursing diagnosis and goals of treatment.

Monitor Cardiac Output

A TH deficit causes a reduction in heart rate and stroke volume, resulting in decreased cardiac output. Fluid may also accumulate in the pericardial sac (from the edema characteristic of hypothyroidism), and coronary artery disease may be present, further compromising cardiac function. The nurse should take the following actions:

■ Monitor blood pressure, rate and rhythm of apical and peripheral pulses, respiratory rate, and breath sounds. Hypotension indicates decreasing peripheral blood. Fluid in the pericardial sac restricts cardiac function. Monopolysaccharide deposits in the respiratory system decrease vital capacity and cause hypoventilation.

■ Suggest that the patient avoid being chilled (e.g., increase room temperature, use additional bed covers, avoid drafts). Chilling increases metabolic rate and puts increased stress on the heart.

■ Explain the need to alternate periods of activity with periods of rest. Ask the patient to report any breathing difficulties, chest pain, heart palpitations, or dizziness. Activity increases demands on the heart and should be balanced with rest. Symptoms of cardiac stress include dyspnea, chest pain, palpitations, and dizziness.

Prevent Constipation

The patient with hypothyroidism is likely to have a reduced appetite and decreased food intake, a diminished activity level because of muscle aches and weakness, and reduced peristalsis, to the point where fecal impactions may occur. To prevent or minimize constipation, the nurse should do the following:

■ Encourage a fluid intake of up to 2000 mL/day. Discuss preferred liquids and the best times of day to drink fluids. If kilocalorie intake is restricted, ensure that liquids have no kilocalories or are low in kilocalories. Sufficient fluid intake is necessary to promote proper stool consistency.

■ Discuss ways to maintain a high-fiber diet. Diets high in fiber and fluid produce soft stools. Fiber that is not digested absorbs water, which adds bulk to the stool and assists in the movement of fecal material through the intestines.

■ Encourage activity as tolerated. Activity influences bowel elimination by improving muscle tone and stimulating peristalsis.

Maintain Skin Integrity

The patient with hypothyroidism is at risk for impaired skin integrity related to the accumulation of fluid in the interstitial spaces and to dry, rough skin. Decreased peripheral circulation, decreased activity levels, and slow wound healing further increase the risk. The following interventions are for the older patient who is hospitalized for surgery or severe hypothyroidism.

To help the patient maintain skin integrity, the nurse should do the following:

■ Monitor skin surfaces for redness or lesions, especially if the patient's activity is greatly reduced. Use a scale for pressure ulcer risk assessment to identify patients at risk. Hypothyroidism causes dry, rough, edematous skin, conditions that increase the risk of skin breakdown.

■ Provide measures to promote optimal circulation or teach them to the patient who is immobile:
   a. Use a turning schedule if the patient is on bedrest, or teach the patient to change position every 2 hours.
   b. Limit the time for sitting in one position; shift weight or lift the body using armrests every 20–30 minutes.
   c. Use pillows, pads, or sheepskin or foam cushions for bed and/or chair.

■ Prolonged pressure, especially in patients with edema and circulatory impairment, can occlude capillaries and cause hypoxic tissue damage.

■ Teach and implement a schedule of range-of-motion exercises.

■ Provide or teach the patient measures to maintain skin integrity:
   a. Take baths only as necessary; use warm (not hot) water.
   b. Use gentle motions when washing and drying skin.
   c. Use alcohol-free skin oils and lotions.

Dry skin and edema increase the risk of skin breakdown. Hot water, rough massage, and alcohol-based preparations may increase skin dryness, further impairing the body's ability to maintain skin integrity.

SAFETY ALERT Lift the patient up in bed to prevent tissue damage from shearing forces.

Evaluation

Expected outcomes for the patient with hyperthyroidism include the following:

■ The patient's vital signs remain, or return to, within established limits both at rest and with activity.

■ The patient exhibits a normal cardiac rhythm.

■ The patient's skin remains intact without edema.

■ The patient's visual acuity is maintained within established limits.

■ The patient's elimination pattern remains within normal limits.

Evaluation involves determining whether the patient has met expected outcomes and, in the event that outcomes have not been met, modifying outcomes or making changes to the nursing care plan. Any diagnostic tests should be repeated to ensure that medications are at appropriate levels.

Nursing Care Plan

A Patient with Hypothyroidism

Jane Lee is a 60-year-old retired nurse living with her husband and daughter on a farm that has been in the family for four generations. Ms. Lee has gained 4.5 kg (10 lb) in the past few months, even though she is rarely hungry and eats much less than normal. She is always tired and weak—so tired that she has not even been able to help with the chores on the farm or do housework. She is concerned about her appearance and the way she sounds when she talks. Her face is puffy, and her tongue always feels thick. Mr. Lee convinces his wife to make an appointment at a health center in a nearby town.

ASSESSMENT	DIAGNOSES	PLANNING
Brian Henning, RN, completes the health assessment for Ms. Lee at the health center. He finds that she now weighs 68 kg (150 lb), an increase of 4.5 kg (10 lb) over her weight at her last visit 6 months earlier. Ms. Lee states that she always feels cold, tired, and weak. She also states that she is constipated, has difficulty remembering things, and looks different. Physical assessment findings include a palpable and bilaterally enlarged thyroid; dry, yellowish skin; nonpitting edema of the face and lower legs; and slow, slurred speech. Diagnostic tests reveal the following abnormal findings: T_3, 56 ng/dL (normal range, 80–200 ng/dL); T_4, 3.1 mcg/dL (normal range, 4.5–11.5 mcg/dL); TSH increased. The medical diagnosis is hypothyroidism, and Ms. Lee is started on levothyroxine at 0.05 mg daily.	Nursing diagnoses that may be appropriate for Ms. Lee include the following: ■ *Constipation* related to decreased peristalsis, as evidenced by hard, formed stools every 4 days ■ *Verbal Communication, Impaired* related to changes in speech patterns and enlarged tongue ■ *Self-Esteem, Situational Low* related to changes in physical appearance and activity intolerance (NANDA-I © 2014)	The patient goals based on the plan of care for Ms. Lee include that she will: ■ Regain normal bowel elimination patterns, having a soft, formed stool at least every other day ■ Experience improvement in verbal communication ■ Regain positive self-esteem as medication reduces physical changes and fatigue.

IMPLEMENTATION

The following nursing interventions may be appropriate for Ms. Lee:

■ Teach the patient to increase fluids, bulk, and fiber in her diet to help regain a normal bowel elimination pattern of a soft, formed stool every other day.

■ Stress that the patient must take medication as prescribed and should not expect an immediate reversal of the symptoms affecting her speech.

■ Advise the patient to plan activities around rest periods. Encourage the patient's husband and daughter to help with housecleaning and cooking.

EVALUATION

On return to the health center 2 months later, Ms. Lee reports that she is no longer constipated but is continuing to drink six glasses of water and to eat oatmeal every day. She no longer feels cold, is regaining her normal energy, and even feels well enough to plant her garden. Her speech is clear and easy to understand. As she leaves the examining room, Ms. Lee says, "It's hard to believe that I have changed so much—now I look and feel like the 'old' me!"

CRITICAL THINKING

1. What physical changes that normally occur with aging are similar to the manifestations of hypothyroidism?

2. Describe the factors that put Ms. Lee's safety at risk. What alterations in her home environment would you suggest to promote safety until the prescribed medication takes effect?

3. The patient taking oral thyroid medications may become hyperthyroid. List the manifestations you would include in a teaching plan to signal this condition.

REVIEW Thyroid Disease

RELATE Link the Concepts and Exemplars

Linking the exemplar of thyroid disease with the concept of mood and affect:

What strategies might you employ when teaching a patient diagnosed with hypothyroidism and disturbed body image?

What impact might hypothyroidism have on the patient's mood and affect, and how would this impact alter the nursing plan of care?

Linking the exemplar of thyroid disease with the concept of stress and coping:

3. For what stressors would you assess the patient diagnosed with hypothyroidism?

4. The time between initial diagnosis of hyperthyroidism and symptom relief may be several weeks to months as additional diagnostic testing is performed and treatments are decided upon. What teaching might help the patient cope with the symptoms of hyperthyroidism?

READY Go to Volume 3: Clinical Nursing Skills

REFER Go to Pearson MyLab Nursing and eText

■ Additional review materials

REFLECT Apply Your Knowledge

Judy Smith is a 55-year-old woman who has recently returned to the United States after a lengthy missionary assignment in South Africa. She arrives at the provider's office today requesting a "head-to-toe" physical examination, including a Pap smear and mammogram. Ms. Smith has been reassigned to serve in the Fiji Islands, where healthcare is scarce, so she would like a full workup. Vital signs: T_O 99°F; P 112 bpm; R 22/min; BP 134/92 mmHg; weight: 101 lb; height: 5 ft 2 in.; overall physical appearance: thin, looks older than stated age, wispy gray hair in matted bun. You note that Ms. Smith has a visible goiter, and as you question her about it, she says, "Oh, I've had that

for a long time. My mother had one, too." She states that she has been going through "the change of life" (for the past 5 years) and is having frequent hot flashes. She has lost 10 lb over the past few years from what she describes as "self-imposed caution" when eating in South Africa.

As Ms. Smith is talking, you note she has slight tremors as she pushes her hair from her eyes. Her face is flushed, and she is fanning herself throughout the interview. She is anxious and fidgets a lot. Her hair is thin and shiny, and her goiter is palpable, which has caused an enlargement of her neck. She denies sleep apnea but states that she snores.

1. What focused health history would be appropriate to elicit from Ms. Smith?

2. What physical assessment will you perform to obtain a complete picture of Ms. Smith's status?

3. Based on physical assessment, what nursing diagnosis best describes Ms. Smith's health?

References

Adams, M. P., Holland, L. N., & Urban, C. (2017). *Pharmacology for nurses: A pathophysiologic approach* (5th ed.). Hoboken, NJ: Pearson Education.

Allan, R., Kerry, T., & Phillips, M. (2010). Accuracy of ultrasound to identify chronic liver disease. *World Journal of Gastroenterology, 28,* 3510–3520.

American Association of Clinical Endocrinologists. (2015). AACE/ACE diabetes guidelines. *Endocrine Practice, 21*(Suppl. 1), 1–87. Retrieved from https://www.aace.com/files/dm-guidelines-ccp.pdf

American Diabetes Association. (2012). *Vitamin D deficiency may contribute to clogged arteries in people with type 2 diabetes.* Retrieved from http://www.diabetes.org/research-and-practice/we-are-research-leaders/recent-advances/archive/vitamin-d-deficiency-may.html

American Diabetes Association. (2014a). *Common terms: S–Z.* Retrieved from http://www.diabetes.org/diabetes-basics/common-terms/common-terms-s-z.html?referrer= https://www.google.com/

American Diabetes Association. (2014b). *Alcohol.* Retrieved from http://www.diabetes.org/food-and-fitness/food/what-can-i-eat/alcohol.html

American Diabetes Association. (2015a). *Fast facts: Data and statistics about diabetes.* Retrieved from http://professional.diabetes.org/sites/professional.diabetes.org/files/media/fast_facts_12-2015a.pdf

American Diabetes Association. (2015b). *Facts about type 2.* Retrieved from http://www.diabetes.org/diabetes-basics/type-2/facts-about-type-2.html

American Diabetes Association. (2015c). *Fitness: Types of activity: What we recommend.* Retrieved from http://www.diabetes.org/food-and-fitness/fitness/types-of-activity/what-we-recommend.html

American Diabetes Association. (2015d). *Cutting back on sodium.* Retrieved from http://www.diabetes.org/food-and-fitness/food/what-can-i-eat/food-tips/cutting-back-on-sodium.html

American Diabetes Association. (2016a). Standards of medical care in diabetes—2016. *Diabetes Care, 39*(Suppl. 1). Retrieved from http://care.

diabetesjournals.org/content/suppl/2015/12/21/39.Supplement_1.DC2/2016-Standards-of-Care.pdf

American Diabetes Association. (2016b). *Statistics about diabetes.* Retrieved from http://www.diabetes.org/diabetes-basics/statistics/?referrer=https://www.google.com/

American Thyroid Association. (2014a). *Thyroid and pregnancy.* Retrieved from http://www.thyroid.org/wp-content/uploads/publications/ctfp/volume7/issue12/ct_public_v712_3.pdf

American Thyroid Association. (2014b). *Thyroid disease in the older patient.* Retrieved from http://www.thyroid.org/wp-content/uploads/patients/brochures/ThyroidDisorderOlder_broch.pdf

American Thyroid Association. (2016a). *Hypothyroidism.* Retrieved from http://www.thyroid.org/hypothyroidism/

American Thyroid Association. (2016b). *Radioactive iodine.* Retrieved from http://www.thyroid.org/radioactive-iodine/

Aschner, P., Horton, E., Leiter, L. A., Munro, N., & Skyler, J. S. (2010). Practical steps to improving the management of type 1 diabetes: Recommendations from the Global Partnership for Effective Diabetes Management. *International Journal of Clinical Practice, 64*(3), 305–315.

Ball, J. W., Bindler, R. C., Cowen, K., & Shaw, M. (2017). *Principles of pediatric nursing: Caring for children* (7th ed.). Hoboken, NJ: Pearson Education.

Barss, V. A., & Repke, J. T. (2015). Patient information: Care during pregnancy for women with type 1 and 2 diabetes mellitus (Beyond the basics). *UpToDate.* Retrieved from http://www.uptodate.com/contents/care-during-pregnancy-for-women-with-type-1-or-2-diabetes-mellitus-beyond-the-basics

Bethel, M. (2016). Osteoporosis. *Medscape.* Retrieved from http://emedicine.medscape.com/article/330598-overview

Camacho, P. M. (2014) Osteoporosis drugs and medications: Medications that help treat or prevent osteoporosis. *Endocrineweb.* Retrieved from https://www.endocrineweb.com/conditions/osteoporosis/osteoporosis-drugs-medications

Centers for Disease Control and Prevention (CDC). (2014a). *National Diabetes Statistics Report, 2014.* Retrieved from http://www.cdc.gov/diabetes/pdfs/data/2014-report-estimates-of-diabetes-and-its-burden-in-the-united-states.pdf

Centers for Disease Control and Prevention (CDC). (2014b). *Diabetes report card, 2014.* Retrieved from http://www.cdc.gov/diabetes/pdfs/library/diabetesreportcard2014.pdf

Centers for Disease Control and Prevention (CDC). (2015a). *Vision health initiative—Common eye disorders.* Retrieved from http://www.cdc.gov/visionhealth/basics/ced/index.html

Centers for Disease Control and Prevention (CDC). (2015b). *Hispanic health.* Retrieved from http://www.cdc.gov/vitalsigns/hispanic-health/

Centers for Disease Control and Prevention (CDC). (2015c). *2014 National diabetes statistic report.* Retrieved from http://www.cdc.gov/diabetes/data/statistics/2014statisticsreport.html

Centers for Disease Control and Prevention (CDC). (2015d). *Combating childhood obesity.* Retrieved from http://www.cdc.gov/features/PreventChildhoodObesity/index.html

Centers for Disease Control and Prevention (CDC). (2016a). *National diabetes prevention program.* Retrieved from http://www.cdc.gov/diabetes/prevention/prediabetes-type2/index.html

Centers for Disease Control and Prevention (CDC). (2016b). *Strategies to prevent obesity.* Retrieved from http://www.cdc.gov/obesity/strategies/minority-health-month.html

Centers for Disease Control and Prevention. (2016c). *Health, United States, 2016.* Retrieved from https://www.cdc.gov/nchs/data/hus/hus16.pdf#020

Copeland, K., Silverstein, J., Moore, K. R., Prazer, G. E., Raymer, T., … Flinn, S. (2013). Management of newly diagnosed Type 2 diabetes mellitus in children and adolescents. *Pediatrics,131*(2), 364–382. doi:10.1542/peds.2012-3494

Corenblum, B. (2015). Pituitary disease and pregnancy. *Medscape.* Retrieved from http://emedicine.medscape.com/article/127650-overview

Danne, T., Bangstad, H. J., Deeb, L., Jarosz-Chobot, P., Mungaie, L., Saboo, B., … International Society for Pediatric and Adolescent Diabetes. (2014).

ISPAD Clinical Practice Consensus Guidelines 2014: Insulin treatment in children and adolescents with diabetes. *Pediatric Diabetes, 15*(Suppl. 20), 115–134. doi:10.1111/pedi.12184

Diabetes in Control. (2012). *Diabetic emergencies: Hypoglycemia caused by insulin, part 3.* Retrieved from http://www.diabetesincontrol.com/diabetic-emergencies-hypoglycemia-caused-by-insulin-part-3/

Evert, A. B. (2014). Treatment of mild hypoglycemia. *Diabetes Spectrum, 27*(1), 58–62. Retrieved from http://www.ncbi.nlm.nih.gov/pmc/articles/PMC4522892/

Flanigan, L. M. (2013). Biliary atresia and choledochal cyst. In N. T. Browne, L. M. Flanigan, C. A. McComiskey, & P. Pieper (Eds.), *Nursing care of the pediatric surgical patient* (3rd ed., pp. 435–446). Burlington, MA: Jones & Bartlett.

Gerber, M. E., Reilly, B. K., & Bhayani, M. K. (2015). Pediatric thyroid cancer. *Medscape.* Retrieved from http://emedicine.medscape.com/article/853737-overview

Grzywacz, J. G., Arcury, T. A., Ip, E. H., Nguyen, H. T., Saldana, S., Reynolds, T., … Quandt, S. A. (2012). Cultural basis for diabetes-related beliefs among low- and high-education African American, American Indian, and white older adults. *Ethnicity & Disease, 22*(4). Retrieved from https://ethndis.org/edonline/index.php/ethndis/article/view/438

Guaraldi, F., & Salvatori, R. (2012). Cushing syndrome: Maybe not so uncommon of an endocrine disease. *Journal of the American Board of Family Medicine, 25*(2), 199–208.

Haire-Joshu, D. (Ed.). (1996). *Management of diabetes mellitus: Perspectives of care across the life span* (2nd ed.). St. Louis, MO: Mosby.

Hassan, H. H. A-K., & Balistreri, W. F. (2016). Neonatal cholestasis. In R. M. Kliegman, B. F. Stanton, J. W. St. Geme III, & N. F. Schor (Eds.), *Nelson textbook of pediatrics* (20th ed., pp. 1928–1932). Philadelphia, PA: Elsevier Saunders.

Herdman, T. H. & Kamitsuru, S. (Eds.). *Nursing Diagnoses—Definitions and Classification 2015–2017.* Copyright © 2014, 1994–2014 NANDA International. Used by arrangement with John Wiley & Sons, Inc. Companion website: www.wiley.com/go/nursingdiagnoses

Hess-Fischi, A. (2016). *Meal planning for children with type 1 diabetes: Understanding carbohydrates for optimal blood glucose management.* Retrieved from http://www.endocrineweb.com/guides/type-1-children/meal-planning-children-type-1-diabetes

Humphers, J. M., Shibuya, N., Fluhman, B. L., & Jupiter, D. (2014). The impact of glycosylated hemoglobin and diabetes mellitus on wound-healing complications and infection after foot and ankle surgery. *Journal of the American Podiatric Medical Association, 104*(4), 320–329. Retrieved from https://www.researchgate.net/publication/263432555_The_Impact_of_Glycosylated_Hemoglobin_and_Diabetes_Mellitus_on_Wound-Healing_Complications_and_Infection_After_Foot_and_Ankle_Surgery

Ikramuddin, S., Korner, J., Lee, W. J., Connett, J. E., Inabnet, W.B., Billington, C. J., … Bantle, J. P. (2013). Roux-en-Y gastric bypass vs. intensive medical management for the control of type 2 diabetes, hypertension, and hyperlipidemia: The Diabetes Surgery Study randomized clinical trial. *Journal of the American Medical Association, 309*(21), 2240–2249.

International Diabetes Federation. (2013). *Pocketbook for management of diabetes in childhood and adolescence in under-resourced countries.* Retrieved from http://www.idf.org/sites/default/files/attachments/ISPAD-LFAC-Pocketbook-final-2.pdf

International Osteoporosis Foundation. (2015a). *Pathophysiology: Biological causes of osteoporosis.* Retrieved from http://www.iofbonehealth.org/pathophysiology-biological-causes-osteoporosis

International Osteoporosis Foundation. (2015b). *What is osteoporosis.* Retrieved from http://www.iofbonehealth.org/what-is-osteoporosis

International Osteoporosis Foundation. (2015c). *Fixed risk factors.* Retrieved from http://www.iofbonehealth.org/fixed-risk-factors

International Osteoporosis Foundation. (2015d). *Modifiable risk factors.* Retrieved from http://www.iofbonehealth.org/modifiable-risk-factors

Inzucchi, S., Berganstal, R., & Buse, J. (2012). Management of hyperglycemia in type 2 diabetes: A patient centered approach. Position Statement of ADA and EASD. *Diabetes Care, 35*(6), 1364–1379.

Jeha, G. S., & Haymond, M. W. (2015). Treatment and complications of diabetic ketoacidosis in children. *UpToDate.* Retrieved from https://www.uptodate.com/contents/treatment-and-complications-of-diabetic-ketoacidosis-in-children?source=search_result&search=DKA&selectedTitle=3~150

Jeha, G. S., & Haymond, M. W. (2016). Clinical features and diagnosis of diabetic ketoacidosis in children. *UpToDate.* Retrieved from https://www.uptodate.com/contents/clinical-features-and-diagnosis-of-diabetic-ketoacidosis-in-children?source=search_result&search=DKA&selectedTitle=4~150

Joslin Diabetes Center. (2016). *Will diabetes go away?* Retrieved from http://www.joslin.org/info/will_diabetes_go_away.html

Kini, U., & Nandeesh, B. N. (2012). Physiology of bone formation, remodeling, and metabolism. In I. Fogelman, G. Gnanasegaran, & H. van der Wall (Eds.), *Radionuclide and hybrid bone imaging* (pp. 29–57). New York, NY: Springer.

Kishore, P. (2014). *Diabetic ketoacidosis.* Retrieved from http://www.merckmanuals.com/professional/endocrine-and-metabolic-disorders/diabetes-mellitus-and-disorders-of-carbohydrate-metabolism/diabetic-ketoacidosis-dka

Laffel, L., & Svoren, B. (2014). Management of type 2 diabetes in children and adolescents. *UpToDate.* Retrieved from https://www.uptodate.com/contents/management-of-type-2-diabetes-mellitus-in-children-and-adolescents?source=search_result&search=treating+DM+in+children&selectedTitle=6~150

Laffel, L., & Svoren, B. (2016). Epidemiology, presentation, diagnosis of type 2 diabetes mellitus in children and adolescents. *UpToDate.* Retrieved from https://www.uptodate.com/contents/epidemiology-presentation-and-diagnosis-of-type-2-diabetes-mellitus-in-children-and-adolescents?source=search_result&search=type+2+DM+in+children&selectedTitle=1~150

LaFranchi, S. (2015). Clinical features and detection of congenital hypothyroidism. *UpToDate.* Retrieved from http://www.uptodate.com/contents/clinical-features-and-detection-of-congenital-hypothyroidism

LaFranchi, S. (2016a). Clinical manifestations and diagnosis of hyperthyroidism in children and adolescents. *UpToDate.* Retrieved from https://www.uptodate.com/contents/clinical-manifestations-and-diagnosis-of-hyperthyroidism-in-children-and-adolescents

LaFranchi, S. (2016b). Treatment and prognosis of congenital hypothyroidism. *UpToDate.* Retrieve from http://www.uptodate.com/contents/treatment-and-prognosis-of-congenital-hypothyroidism

Lee, S. I., Patel, M., Jones, C. M., & Narendran, P. (2015). Cardiovascular disease and type 1 diabetes: Prevalence, prediction, and management in an aging population. *Therapeutic Advances in Chronic Disease 2015, 6*(6), 347–374. Retrieved from http://www.ncbi.nlm.nih.gov/pmc/articles/PMC4622313/pdf/10.1177_2040622315598502.pdf

Loh-Trivedi, M., & Rothenberg, D. M. (2015). *Perioperative management of the diabetic patient.* Retrieved from http://emedicine.medscape.com/article/284580-overview

Mayo Clinic. (2014a). *Sheehan's syndrome.* Retrieved from http://www.mayoclinic.org/diseases-conditions/sheehans-syndrome/basics/definition/con-20029870

Mayo Clinic. (2014b). *Type 2 diabetes in children.* Retrieved from http://www.mayoclinic.com/health/type-2-diabetes-in-children/DS00946

Mayo Clinic. (2015). *Metform—oral route.* Retrieved from http://www.mayoclinic.org/drugs-supplements/metformin-oral-route/proper-use/drg-20067074

McCulloch, D. K. (2015). Patient information: Self-blood glucose monitoring in diabetes mellitus (Beyond the basics). *UpToDate.* Retrieved from https://www.uptodate.com/contents/self-blood-glucose-monitoring-in-diabetes-mellitus-beyond-the-basics

McCulloch, D. K., & Hayward, R. A. (2016). Screening for type 2 diabetes mellitus. *UpToDate.* Retrieved from http://www.uptodate.com/contents/screening-for-type-2-diabetes-mellitus

McCulloch, D. K., & Robertson, R. P. (2014). Pathogenesis of type 2 diabetes mellitus. *UpToDate.* Retrieved from https://www.uptodate.com/contents/pathogenesis-of-type-2-diabetes-mellitus

McDermott, M. (2010). *Endocrine secrets: Questions you will be asked on rounds, in the clinic, on oral exams* (5th ed.). St. Louis, MO: Mosby.

MedlinePlus. (2014). *Thyroid storm.* Retrieved from https://www.nlm.nih.gov/medlineplus/ency/article/000400.htm

MedlinePlus. (2015). *Alcoholic liver disease.* Retrieved from https://www.nlm.nih.gov/medlineplus/ency/article/000281.htm

Meigs, J. B. (2015). The metabolic syndrome (insulin resistance syndrome or syndrome X). *UpToDate.* Retrieved from https://www.uptodate.com/contents/the-metabolic-syndrome-insulin-resistance-syndrome-or-syndrome-x?source=search_result&search=metabolic+syndrome&selectedTitle=1~150

Michels, A., & Michels, N. (2014). Addison disease: Early detection and treatment principles. *American Family Physician, 89*(7), 563–568.

Mieli-Vergani, G., & Tizzard, S. A. (2012). Biliary atresia and Kasai's surgery—When is it too late? *Pediatric OnCall Journal, 9*(9). Retrieved from http://www.pediatriconcall.com/Journal/Article/FullText.aspx?artid=511&type=J&tid=&imgid=&reportid=358&tbltype=

Moreira, R. K., Cabral, R., Cowles, R. A., & Lobritto, S. J. (2012). Biliary atresia: A multidisciplinary approach to diagnosis and management. *Archives* of Pathology and Laboratory Medicine, 136(7), 746–760.

Mount Sinai Hospital. (2016a). Hyperthyroidism. Retrieved from http://www.mountsinai.org/patient-care/health-library/diseases-and-conditions/hyperthyroidism#prevention

Mount Sinai Hospital. (2016b). Thyroidectomy. Retrieved from http://www.mountsinai.org/patient-care/health-library/treatments-and-procedures/thyroidectomy

National Center for Complementary and Alternative Medicine. (2013). Children and complementary health approaches. Retrieved from http://nccam.nih.gov/health/children/

National Diabetes Education Program. (2014). Overview of diabetes in children and adolescents. Retrieved at https://www.niddk.nih.gov/health-information/health-communication-programs/ndep/living-with-diabetes/youth-teens/diabetes-children-adolescents/Documents/overview-of-diabetes-children_508_2016.pdf

National Institute of Diabetes and Digestive and Kidney Disease (NIDDK). (2012a). Hyperthyroidism. Retrieved from http://www.niddk.nih.gov/health-information/health-topics/endocrine/hyperthyroidism/Pages/fact-sheet.aspx

National Institute of Diabetes and Digestive and Kidney Disease (NIDDK). (2012b). Pregnancy and thyroid disease. Retrieved from https://www.niddk.nih.gov/health-information/health-topics/endocrine/pregnancy-and-thyroid-disease/Pages/fact-sheet.aspx

National Institute of Diabetes and Digestive and Kidney Disease (NIDDK). (2013). Hypothyroidism. Retrieved from http://www.niddk.nih.gov/health-information/health-topics/endocrine/hypothyroidism/Pages/fact-sheet.aspx

National Institute of Diabetes and Digestive and Kidney Disease (NIDDK). (2014a). Cirrhosis. Retrieved from https://www.niddk.nih.gov/health-information/health-topics/liver-disease/cirrhosis/Pages/ez.aspx

National Institute of Diabetes and Digestion and Kidney Disease (NIDDK). (2014b). Diabetes, health disease, and stroke. Retrieved from https://www.niddk.nih.gov/health-information/diabetes/preventing-diabetes-problems/heart-disease-stroke

National Institute of Diabetes and Digestive and Kidney Disease (NIDDK). (2016a). What is diabetes? Retrieved from https://www.niddk.nih.gov/health-information/diabetes/overview/what-is-diabetes

National Institute of Diabetes and Digestive and Kidney Disease (NIDDK). (2016b). Complementary and alternative medical therapies for diabetes. Retrieved from https://www.niddk.nih.gov/health-information/diabetes/manage-monitoring-diabetes/complementary-alternative-medical-therapies-diabetes

NIH Osteoporosis and Related Bone Diseases National Resource Center. (2015). Pregnancy, breastfeeding, and bone health. Retrieved from https://www.niams.nih.gov/health_info/bone/Bone_Health/Pregnancy/default.asp

National Institute of Mental Health. (2015). Chronic illness and mental health. Retrieved from http://www.nimh.nih.gov/health/publications/chronic-illness-mental-health-2015/index.shtml#pub1

National Osteoporosis Foundation. (2014). Clinician's guide to prevention and treatment of osteoporosis.

Retrieved from https://www.nof.rg/2014/09/09/nofs-clinicians-guide-published-by-osteoporosis-international/

National Osteoporosis Foundation. (2016a). General facts. Retrieved from https://www.nof.org/prevention/general-facts/

National Osteoporosis Foundation. (2016b). What women need to know. Retrieved from https://www.nof.org/prevention/general-facts/what-women-need-to-know/

Nimblett, A. (2012) A telltale lesion: Acanthosis nigricans in children can be a precursor of type 2 diabetes. Advanced Healthcare Network for NPs & PAs. Retrieved from http://nurse-practitioners-and-physician-assistants.advanceweb.com/Features/Articles/A-Telltale-Lesion.aspx

Office of Minority Health. (2015). Chronic liver disease and American Indians/Alaska Natives. Retrieved from https://minorityhealth.hhs.gov/omh/browse.aspx?lvl=4&lvlid=32

Ogden, C. L., Carroll, M. D., Kit, B. K., & Flegal, K. M. (2014). Prevalence of childhood and adult obesity in the United States, 2011–2012. Journal of the American Medical Association, 311(8), 806–814.

Osborn, K. S., Wraa, C. E., Watson, A. B., & Holleran, R. (2014). Medical-surgical nursing: Preparation for practice (2nd ed.). Upper Saddle River, NJ: Pearson Education.

Patrick, K., Norman, G. J., Davila, E. P., Calfas, K. J., Raab, F., Gottschalk, M., … Colvin, J. R. (2013). Outcomes of a 12-month technology-based intervention to promote weight loss in adolescents at risk for type 2 diabetes. Journal of Diabetes Science and Technology, 7(3), 759–770.

Patton, S. R., Dolan, L. M., Cheng, M., & Powers, S. W. (2013). Dietary adherence and mealtime behaviors in young children with diabetes on type 1 intensive insulin therapy. Journal of the Academy of Nutrition and Dietetics, 113(2), 258–262.

Patton, S. R., Dolan, L. M., Smith, L. B., Brown, M. B., & Powers, S. W. (2013). Examining mealtime behaviors in families of young children with type 1 diabetes on intensive insulin therapy. Eating Behaviors, 14(4), 464–467.

Rewers, M., Pihoker, C., Donaghue, K., Hanas, R., Swift, P., & Klingensmith, G. (2014). Assessment and monitoring of glycemic control in children and adolescents with diabetes. Pediatric Diabetes, 15 (Suppl. 20), 102–114.

Robie, D. K., Overfelt, S. R., & Xie, L. (2014). Differentiating biliary atresia from other causes of cholestatic jaundice. American Surgeon, 80(9), 827–831.

Ross, D. S. (2015a). Myxedema coma. UpToDate. Retrieved from http://www.uptodate.com/contents/myxedema-coma?source=search_result&search=myxedema+coma&selectedTitle=1~22

Ross, D. S. (2015b). Patient information: Antithyroid drugs (Beyond the basics). UpToDate. Retrieved from http://www.uptodate.com/contents/antithyroid-drugs-beyond-the-basics

Ross, D. S. (2016a). Amiodarone and thyroid dysfunction. UpToDate. Retrieved from http://www.uptodate.com/contents/amiodarone-and-thyroid-dysfunction

Ross, D.S. (2016b). Treatment of hypothyroidism. UpToDate. Retrieved from http://www.uptodate.com/contents/treatment-of-hypothyroidism?source=search_result&search=treatment+of+hypothyroid+ism&selectedTitle=1%7E150

Ross, D. S. (2016c). Thyroid storm. UpToDate. Retrieved from http://www.uptodate.com/contents/thyroid-storm

RxList. (2016). Lantus. Retrieved from http://www.rxlist.com/lantus-drug/medication-guide.htm

Scaglione, S., Kliethermes, S., Cao, G., Shoham, D., Durazo, R., Luke, A., & Volk, M. L. (2015). The epidemiology of cirrhosis in the United States: A population-based study. Journal of Clinical Gastroenterology, 49(8), 690–696.

Scheiner, G. (2015). Top ten tips for better glucose control. Retrieved from http://www.diabetesselfmanagement.com/Articles/Kids-And-Diabetes/top-10-tips-for-better-blood-glucose-control/

Schwarz, S. M. (2014). Pediatric biliary atresia. Retrieved from http://emedicine.medscape.com/article/927029-overview

Sira, M. M., Taha, M., & Sira, A. M. (2014). Common misdiagnoses of biliary atresia. European Journal of Gastroenterology & Hepatology, 26(11), 1300–1305.

Smart, C., Annan, F., Bruno, L., Higgins, L. A., & Acerini, C. L. (2014). Nutritional management in children and adolescents with diabetes. Pediatric Diabetes, 15(S20), 135–153.

Smith-Marsh, D. E. (2014). Type 1 diabetes prevention. Retrieved from http://www.endocrineweb.com/conditions/type-1-diabetes/type-1-diabetes-prevention

Smith-Marsh, D. E. (2016a). Type 1 diabetes risk factors. Retrieved from http://www.endocrineweb.com/conditions/type-1-diabetes/type-1-diabetes-risk-factors

Smith-Mash, D. E. (2016b). Type 1 diabetes complications. Retrieved from http://www.endocrineweb.com/conditions/type-1-diabetes/type-1-diabetes-complications

Society for Endocrinology. (2015a). Relaxin. Retrieved from http://www.yourhormones.info/hormones/relaxin.aspx

Society for Endocrinology. (2015b). Human chorionic gonadotropin. Retrieved from http://www.yourhormones.info/hormones/human_chorionic_gonadotrophin.aspx

Squires, J. E., & Balistreri, W. F. (2016). Manifestations of liver disease. In R. M. Kliegman, B. F. Stanton, J. W. St. Geme III, & N. F. Schor (Eds.), Nelson textbook of pediatrics (20th ed., pp. 1922–1928). Philadelphia, PA: Elsevier Saunders.

Surks, M. I. (2016). Clinical manifestations of hypothyroidism. UpToDate. Retrieve from http://www.uptodate.com/contents/clinical-manifestations-of-hypothyroidism?source=search_result&search=hypothyroidism&selectedTitle=3~150

Szadek, L. L., & Scharer, K. (2014). Identification, prevention, and treatment of children with decreased bone mineral density. Journal of Pediatric Nursing, 29, e3–e14.

Tapp, H., Phillips, S. E., Waxman, D., Alexander, M., Brown, R., & Hall, M. (2012). Multidisciplinary team approach to improved chronic care management for diabetic patients in an urban safety net ambulatory care clinic. Journal of the American Board of Family Medicine, 25(2), 245–246. Retrieved from http://www.jabfm.org/content/25/2/245.full.pdf+html

Tercyak, K. P., Abraham, A. A., Graham, A. L., Wilson, L. D., & Walker, L. R. (2009). Association of multiple behavioral risk factors with adolescents' willingness to engage in ehealth promotion. Journal of Pediatric Psychology, 34(5), 457–469.

U.S. Food and Drug Administration. (2015). Blood glucose monitoring devices. Retrieved from http://www.fda.gov/medicaldevices/productsandmedicalprocedures/InVitroDiagnostics/Glucose-TestingDevices/default.htm

U.S. National Library of Medicine. (2014). *Congenital adrenal hyperplasia*. Retrieved from https://www.nlm.nih.gov/medlineplus/ency/article/000411.htm

van Dooren, F. E. P., Nefs, G., Schram, M. T., Verhey, F. R. J., Denollet, J., & Pouwer, F. (2013). Depression and risk of mortality in people with diabetes mellitus: A systemic review and meta-analysis. *PLoS One*. Retrieved from http://journals.plos.org/plosone/article?id=10.1371/journal.pone.0057058

Weinberg, M., & Schambelan, M. (2016). *Bone and calcium disorders in HIV-infected patients*. Retrieved from http://www.uptodate.com/contents/bone-and-calcium-disorders-in-hiv-infected-patients

Weintrob, A. C., & Sexton, D. J. (2015). Susceptibility to infections in persons with diabetes mellitus. *UpToDate*. Retrieved from https://www.uptodate.com/contents/susceptibility-to-infections-in-persons-with-diabetes-mellitus

Wolf, D. C. (2017). Cirrhosis. *Medscape*. Retrieved from http://emedicine.medscape.com/article/185856-overview

Woolford, S. C., Clark, S. C., Strecher, V. J., & Resnicow, K. (2010). Tailored mobile phone messages as an adjunct to obesity treatment for adolescents. *Journal of Telemedicine and Telecare, 16*(8), 458–461.

Wright, N. C., Looker, A. C., Saag, K. G., Curtis, J. R., Delzell, E. S., Randal, S., & Dawson-Hughes, B. (2014). The recent prevalence of osteoporosis and low bone mass in the United States based on bone mineral density at the femoral neck or lumbar spine. *Journal of Bone and Mineral Research, 29*(11), 2520–2526.

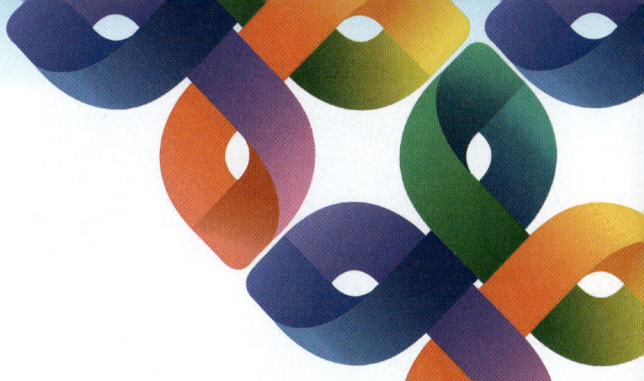

Module 13
Mobility

Module Outline and Learning Outcomes

The Concept of Mobility

Normal Mobility

13.1 Analyze the physiology of mobility in the body.

Alterations to Mobility

13.2 Differentiate alterations in mobility.

Concepts Related to Mobility

13.3 Outline the relationship between mobility and other concepts.

Health Promotion

13.4 Explain the promotion of healthy mobility.

Nursing Assessment

13.5 Differentiate among common assessment procedures and tests used to examine mobility.

Independent Interventions

13.6 Analyze independent interventions nurses can implement for patients with alterations in mobility.

Collaborative Therapies

13.7 Summarize collaborative therapies used by interprofessional teams for patients with alterations in mobility.

Lifespan Considerations

13.8 Differentiate considerations related to the care of patients with alterations in mobility throughout the lifespan.

Mobility Exemplars

Exemplar 13.A Back Problems

13.A Analyze back problems as they relate to mobility.

Exemplar 13.B Fractures

13.B Analyze fractures as they relate to mobility.

Exemplar 13.C Hip Fractures

13.C Analyze hip fractures as they relate to mobility.

Exemplar 13.D Multiple Sclerosis

13.D Analyze multiple sclerosis (MS) as it relates to mobility.

Exemplar 13.E Osteoarthritis

13.E Analyze osteoarthritis (OA) as it relates to mobility.

Exemplar 13.F Parkinson Disease

13.F Analyze Parkinson disease (PD) as it relates to mobility.

Exemplar 13.G Spinal Cord Injury

13.G Analyze spinal cord injury (SCI) as it relates to mobility.

 The Concept of Mobility

Concept Key Terms

5 *Ps* neurovascular assessment, **888**	Atrophy, **901**	Discs, **900**	Osteoblasts, **899**	Sarcomeres, **900**
Ambulation, **897**	Axial skeleton, **880**	Epiphyseal plate, **899**	Osteoclast, **900**	Sarcopenia, **901**
Appendicular skeleton, **880**	Bradykinesia, **882**	Kyphosis, **899**	Range of motion (ROM), **888**	Sprain, **883**
	Cartilage, **880**	Ligaments, **880**		Strain, **884**
	Crepitation, **881**	Lordosis, **899**	Resorption, **900**	Tendons, **880**

The musculoskeletal system is made of the bones and joints of the skeletal system and the muscles, ligaments, tendons, and cartilage of the muscular system. The skeletal and muscular systems work together to support body weight, control movements, and provide stability. Some musculoskeletal structures, such as the rib cage and skull, provide protection for other organs, including the heart, lungs, and brain. The musculoskeletal system allows the performance of gross movement, such as walking, and fine movement, such as writing.

The musculoskeletal system works in tandem with the circulatory and nervous systems. The bones store nutrients and produce white and red blood cells. The blood subsequently provides oxygen, calcium, and other nutrients to strengthen bones; it also transports electrolytes that are needed for muscle movement. Nerves innervate the

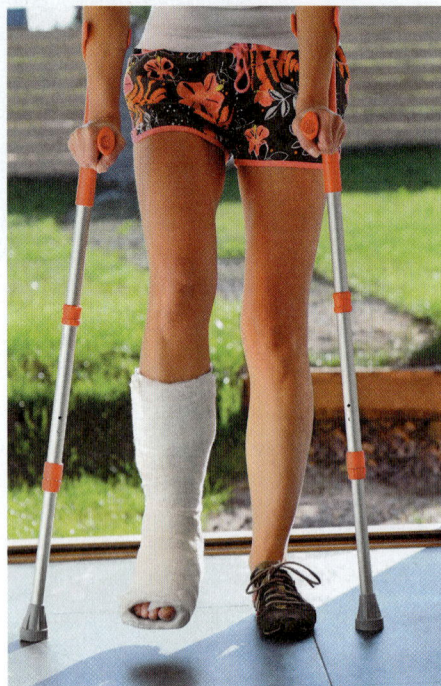

Source: Domin domin/E+/Getty Images.

Figure 13–1 ❯❯ What difficulties would you expect this college student to have trying to manage her schedule while navigating the campus on crutches with her ankle in a cast?

muscles to provide the electrical stimulus needed to initiate contraction.

Alterations in musculoskeletal integrity have a detrimental effect on the individual's ability to perform activities of daily living (ADLs), communicate, and participate in recreational activities. Impaired mobility is a common source of frustration and pain for patients with musculoskeletal dysfunction or injury (see **Figure 13–1** ❯❯).

Normal Mobility

Most individuals take mobility for granted until a disease or an injury restricts their freedom of movement. Because the musculoskeletal system is interconnected, injury to one structure can impair the function of other structures as well.

Physiology Review

The basic components of the musculoskeletal system include the bones, muscles, joints, tendons, ligaments, and cartilage. The bones provide the framework of the body. Joints are formed between bones, and muscular contraction stimulates movement of bones at the joints. Tendons, ligaments, and cartilage connect bones with either muscles or other bones and provide cushioning during movements.

Skeleton

The human skeleton consists of 206 bones that are divided into the **axial skeleton** (ribs, sternum, vertebral column, and skull) and the **appendicular skeleton** (pectoral girdles, upper limbs, pelvic girdle, and lower limbs). Bones have several functions, including forming the body structure, supporting soft tissues, protecting vital organs, providing a point of attachment for muscles, storing minerals, and forming blood cells.

Muscles

The three types of muscle are skeletal muscle, smooth muscle, and cardiac muscle. Skeletal muscle is critical for physical mobility. Skeletal muscles attach to bones via tendons; thus, muscle contraction causes movement of the skeletal bones. The human body contains more than 640 skeletal muscles that are under voluntary control by the nervous system.

Joints

Joints are formed where two bones meet; they hold the skeleton together while providing mobility. Structural and functional classifications of joints are generally interrelated. However, some joints, such as the epiphyseal plate in children (cartilaginous/synarthrosis), fall outside this general classification.

Ligaments, Tendons, and Cartilage

Ligaments, tendons, and cartilage are all connective tissues composed of differing amounts of collagen fibers, proteoglycan matrix, cells such as fibroblasts or chondroblasts, and other structural components. **Ligaments** connect bones to other bones to form a joint. They strengthen and stabilize the joint and may limit the mobility of some joints. **Tendons** connect bones to muscles and carry the contractile forces from the muscle to the bone to cause movement. **Cartilage** is a type of flexible connective tissue found throughout the body. For example, cartilage connects the ribs to the sternum, covers the epiphyses of long bones to cushion the joint, and provides structure for the nose. Cartilage is less flexible than muscle, but not as rigid as bones. Of these three types of connective tissue, cartilage is the only one that does not contain blood vessels.

❯❯ Go to **Pearson MyLab Nursing and eText** for a MiniModule that thoroughly reviews the physiology of mobility.

Alterations to Mobility

Changes in the function of the musculoskeletal system affect nearly every aspect of life. It does not matter whether the patient is healthy and wants to increase physical fitness or has a medical condition that limits mobility; most patients are distressed when mobility is less than optimal. Alterations in the muscles, bones, and joints are linked to a variety of health problems, including arthritis, fractures, neurologic disorders, and traumatic injuries. Regardless of its cause, impaired mobility or immobility can lead to a number of other health alterations (see the Safety Alert feature). The Concepts Related to Mobility section outlines some of the ways in which mobility is integrated with other concepts. The exemplars in this module describe some of the most common alterations in mobility, and present nursing considerations to keep in mind when caring for patients with limited mobility.

SAFETY ALERT Along with exacerbating existing musculoskeletal impairment, immobility can lead to a host of other problems, including atelectasis (collapse of one or more sections of the lungs) and pneumonia; decreased gastrointestinal motility and paralytic ileus; and impaired tissue perfusion, which can predispose the patient to developing pressure injuries. The nurse should encourage and facilitate patient activities that safely promote mobility, including frequent turning and repositioning as well as ambulation as ordered by the patient's primary care provider.

Alterations and Manifestations

Manifestations of musculoskeletal problems will differ depending on their etiology. For example, a patient with a fractured wrist may have trouble writing, whereas a patient with osteoarthritis (OA) of the knee will have limited walking ability. Common medical conditions that cause alterations in mobility include back problems (e.g., herniated discs, scoliosis), fractures, multiple sclerosis (MS), OA, Parkinson disease (PD), and spinal cord injuries (SCIs) (see the Alterations and Therapies feature).

Alterations and Therapies
Mobility

ALTERATION	DESCRIPTION	MANIFESTATIONS	INTERVENTIONS AND THERAPIES
Herniated disc	A spinal disc that slips out of place or ruptures	<ul><li>Back pain that spreads to the buttocks and legs (herniated disc in lower back) or to the shoulders and arms (herniated disc in upper back)</li><li>Tingling or numbness</li><li>Muscle spasms or weakness</li><li>Limited mobility</li></ul>	<ul><li>Rest</li><li>Pharmacologic therapy to manage pain and prevent muscle spasms</li><li>Physical therapy</li><li>Complementary health approaches</li><li>Surgery to remove or replace the disc</li></ul>
Scoliosis	A sideways or abnormal S- or C-shaped curve of the spine	<ul><li>Back pain</li><li>Uneven hips or shoulders</li><li>Obvious abnormal curve of the spine upon inspection</li><li>Leaning to one side</li><li>Exhaustion of the spine after sitting or standing</li><li>Difficulty breathing</li></ul>	<ul><li>Regular checkups</li><li>Exercises to improve back strength</li><li>Back brace to prevent further curving</li><li>Surgery to correct curve</li><li>Emotional support</li></ul>
Fractures	A break in the continuity of a bone	<ul><li>Pain from damage to surrounding tissues</li><li>Visible fracture on an x-ray</li><li>Protrusion of bone out of skin</li><li>Limited mobility</li></ul>	<ul><li>Ice packs to limit swelling</li><li>Pharmacologic therapy to reduce pain and swelling and prevent infection</li><li>Immobilization with a splint, brace, cast, or traction</li><li>Surgery to stabilize bone or replace fractured bone</li></ul>
Multiple sclerosis	An autoimmune disease that causes damage to the myelin sheath around nerves	<ul><li>Loss of balance, dizziness</li><li>Muscle spasms</li><li>Numbness or tingling</li><li>Problems moving arms or legs</li><li>Tremor or weakness in arms or legs</li><li>Bowel and bladder problems</li><li>Eye, hearing, and speech problems</li><li>Cognitive deficits</li></ul>	<ul><li>Pharmacologic therapy to slow the progression of disease and decrease severity of attacks</li><li>Physical therapy</li><li>Speech therapy</li><li>Assistive devices for mobility</li><li>Healthy lifestyle (nutrition, activity, rest)</li><li>Safety measures to prevent falls</li><li>Counseling</li></ul>
Osteoarthritis	Degeneration of cartilage and bone in a joint	<ul><li>Joint pain and swelling</li><li>Joint stiffness</li><li>Loss of joint flexibility</li><li>Bone spurs</li><li>Crackling sounds (**crepitation**) during joint movement</li><li>Joint tenderness</li></ul>	<ul><li>Pharmacologic therapy to reduce pain and swelling</li><li>Physical therapy</li><li>Reduction of stress on affected joints</li><li>Injections of corticosteroids or hyaluronic acid (HA)</li><li>Surgery to realign bones or replace joints</li><li>Gentle exercises</li><li>Weight loss</li><li>Application of warm or cold compresses</li></ul>

(continued on next page)

Alterations and Therapies *(continued)*

ALTERATION	DESCRIPTION	MANIFESTATIONS	INTERVENTIONS AND THERAPIES
Parkinson disease	A motor system disorder caused by the loss of dopamine neurons	• Tremor in the hands, arms, legs, jaw, and face • Rigidity and stiffness of the limbs and trunk	• Pharmacologic therapy to manage symptoms • Deep brain stimulation (DBS) • Healthy lifestyle
		• **Bradykinesia** (slowness of movement) • Impaired balance and coordination • Lack of affect • Slurred speech	• Walking carefully • Occupational therapy • T'ai chi and qigong to improve balance
Spinal cord injury	Direct damage to the spinal cord or indirect damage due to disease of surrounding tissues	• Weakness or numbness below the injury • Muscle spasticity • Loss of bladder and bowel control • Pain • Paralysis • Difficulty breathing	• Immobilization of the spine • Pharmacologic treatment to reduce pain and swelling and prevent further damage • Surgery to remove tissue, fluid, or objects pressing on the spinal cord • Bedrest • Spinal traction • Physical and occupational therapy

Back Problems

Back problems can arise from a variety of causes, including trauma, degenerative disorders, muscle irritation, and pregnancy. Strain over time, poor posture, and improper lifting are common causes of back pain. Being overweight or having poor physical fitness also contributes to back problems. Two common causes of back problems, herniated discs and scoliosis (see **Figure 13–2** »), are discussed in Exemplar 13.A.

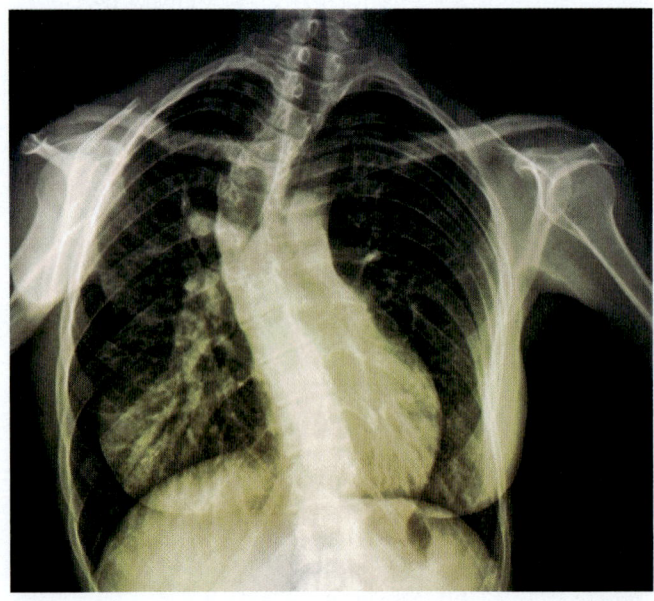

Figure 13–2 » Scoliosis.

Fractures

A fracture is a break in the continuity of a bone. Depending on the location, a fracture can greatly impair mobility and cause excessive pain for the patient. Two factors that affect the severity of the fracture are the nature of the event (e.g., a fall) and the strength of the bone. Falls, blunt trauma, motor vehicle crashes, child abuse, and repetitive forces are all common causes of fractures.

A hip fracture, in particular, occurs when the neck, head, or lesser or greater trochanter of the upper femur is fractured. Seventy percent of hip fractures occur in older female adults, and they are most likely to occur as the result of a fall (Mayo Clinic, 2015a). The incidence of hip fractures is increased in individuals with loss of bone density and muscle mass (Mayo Clinic, 2015a). In younger individuals, hip fractures are usually the result of sports injuries or motor vehicle crashes. Hip fractures are covered in detail in Exemplar 13.C.

Multiple Sclerosis

MS is an autoimmune disorder that destroys the myelin sheath around nerves, disrupting transmission of nerve impulses. This impairs the brain's ability to communicate with the rest of the body, resulting in a variety of symptoms, including sensory and motor disturbances and alterations in bowel and bladder control. Symptom attacks vary in location and severity, and they can last for days, weeks, or months. MS is given a differential diagnosis after other conditions are ruled out. There are no tests that are specific to MS (Mayo Clinic, 2015b). MS is explored in detail in Exemplar 13.D.

Osteoarthritis

OA is characterized by degeneration of cartilage and bone in a joint, sometimes accompanied by bone spurs, or bony growths on normal bone. OA is a normal process of aging due to wear and tear on a joint. The most commonly affected joints are the knees, hips, hands, and spine. Ankle and foot joints can also be involved, especially if the individual is overweight. OA is covered in detail in Exemplar 13.E.

Parkinson Disease

PD is a central nervous system (CNS) disorder caused by degeneration of neurons that produce the neurotransmitter dopamine. PD affects approximately 1% of individuals over the age of 60, and it is more common in men than women (Hauser, 2013). Because PD is a progressive disease, early symptoms may not be noticed for several months, and full expression of symptoms may not be seen for many years after diagnosis. PD is explored in detail in Exemplar 13.F.

Spinal Cord Injuries

SCIs are medical emergencies that may result in permanent disability or paralysis. Spinal cord trauma often results from motor vehicle crashes, assault, gunshot wounds, sports injuries, and falls. The location of the injury will determine the type and severity of symptoms. Cervical injuries may affect the arms, legs, and trunk of the body. One of the most serious possible effects of cervical injury is paralysis of breathing muscles. Thoracic and lumbar sacral injuries usually affect the legs and may cause loss of bowel and bladder control. SCIs are covered in Exemplar 13.G.

Other Alterations That Affect Mobility

Bruises occur when traumatic force ruptures blood vessels, causing localized pooling of blood. Common symptoms of bruises include skin discoloration ("black-and-blue") and tenderness. Bruises usually heal on their own without further treatment as the body clears away the pooled blood.

Joint disorders are a primary cause of decreased mobility; they can affect one or multiple joints. For example, joint disorders of the head include temporomandibular joint (TMJ) syndrome, which affects chewing and talking. Joint disorders of the elbows and knees may include *tendinitis* (inflammation of a tendon), *synovitis* (inflammation of the synovial membrane; see **Figure 13–3 »**), and *bursitis* (inflammation

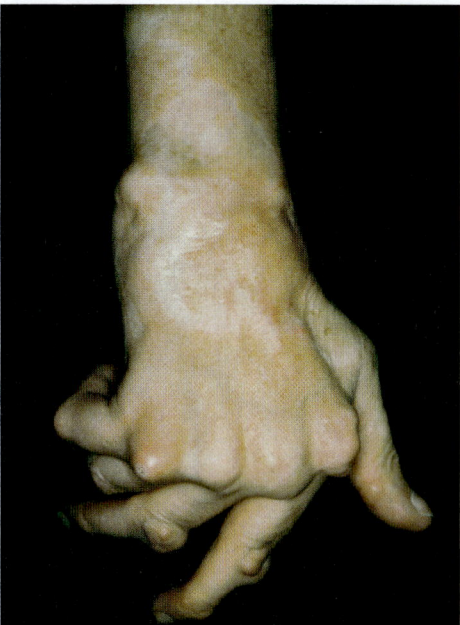

Figure 13–4 » Rheumatoid arthritis with rheumatoid nodules, ulnar deviation, and swan-neck deformity of fingers.

of a bursa). Joint disorders found in the hand and wrist include joint *effusion* (presence of excess fluid), rheumatoid arthritis (RA; see **Figure 13–4 »**), Dupuytren's contracture (thickening and contracture of the tissue beneath the skin of the palm and fingers), and carpal tunnel syndrome (see **Figure 13–5 »**). Joint disorders of the foot include *gout* (buildup of uric acid; see **Figure 13–6 »**), bunions (hallux valgus, a lateral deviation of the great toe; see **Figure 13–7 »**), club foot, and hammertoe.

Traumatic injuries are also a source of limited mobility, including sprains, strains, muscle injuries, and bruises. A **sprain** is a stretching or tearing of ligaments. The most common sprains are ankle and knee sprains. Sprains may also occur in the shoulder, elbow, wrist, and hip. Sprains

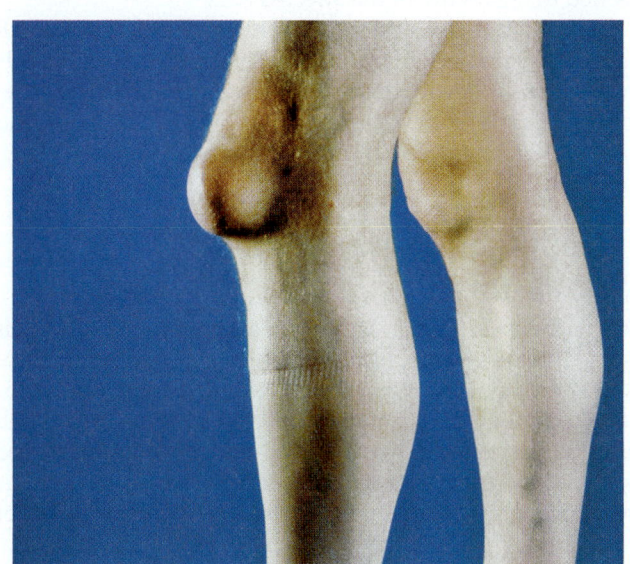

Figure 13–3 » Synovitis.

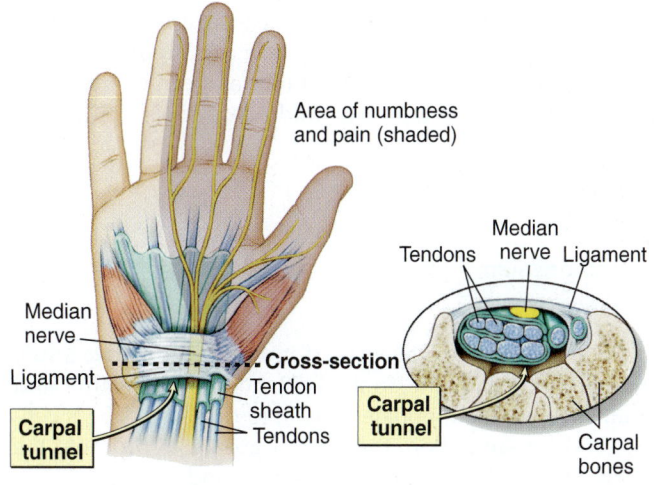

Area of numbness and pain (shaded)

Median nerve

Ligament

Carpal tunnel

Cross-section

Tendon sheath

Tendons

Tendons

Median nerve

Ligament

Carpal tunnel

Carpal bones

Figure 13–5 » Carpal tunnel syndrome.

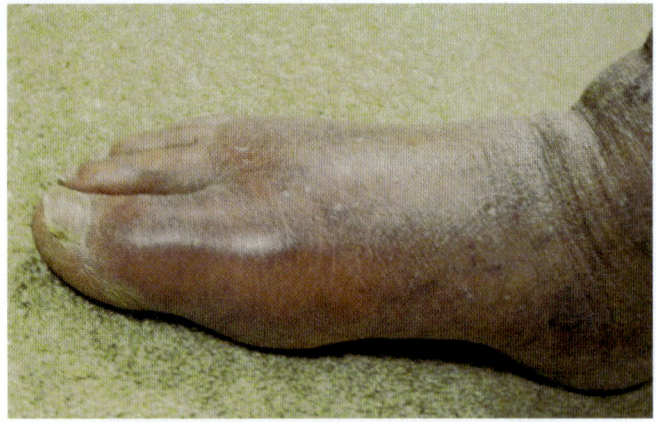

Source: David Cole/Alamy Stock Photo.

Figure 13–6 》 Gout.

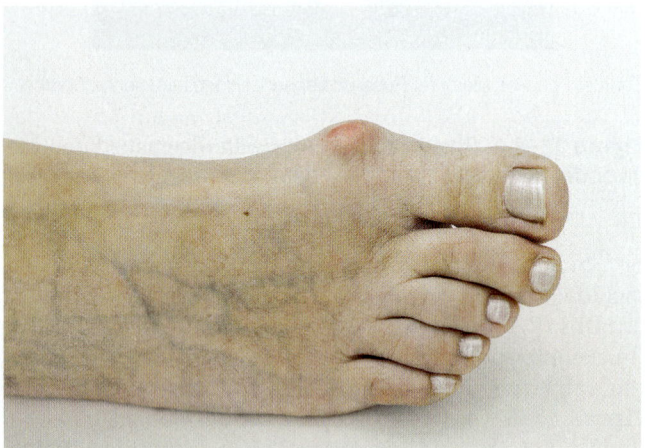

Source: Photographee.eu/Shutterstock.

Figure 13–7 》 Bunion (hallux valgus).

are often accompanied by pain, swelling, and bruising. A **strain** is a stretching or tearing of a muscle or tendon. Symptoms include pain, swelling, and muscle spasms. Strains often occur in the lower back muscles and hamstrings. Muscles strains that cause tearing are often simply called *tears,* such as a rotator cuff tear (see **Figure 13–8 》**). Sprains and strains are usually minor and can be treated at home with **RICE** therapy and mild pain relievers (Karim & Brukner, 2015):

Rest

Ice

Compression

Elevation.

RICE therapy has been used universally for the initial treatment (within the first 24–72 hours) of sprains and strains. While the rationale may be to decrease pain, swelling, and inflammation, the overall goal is to promote the healing process. The acronym has been updated to **POLICE** to include protection and optimal loading instead of rest (Karim & Brukner, 2015; Maffulli et al., 2013). Optimal load

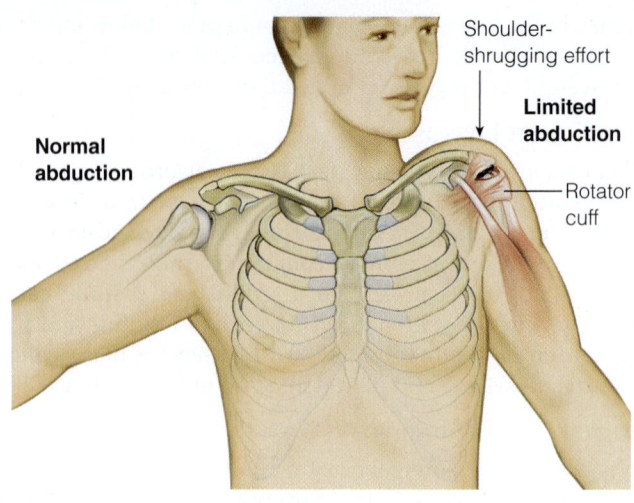

Figure 13–8 》 Rotator cuff tear.

(load applied to structures that maximizes physiologic adaptation) promotes optimal healing. These protocols are available best practice options that providers may decide to use with patients with suspected or confirmed muscle injuries.

Protection

Optimal

Load

Ice

Compression

Elevation.

Walker Gallego, Kerstman, and Shaw (2015) reported that, despite several recent studies, it has not been determined if cold therapy actually promotes healing, but it does dull the pain of inflammation. Severe sprains and strains may be treated with surgery, and physical therapy may be needed to regain use of the affected area.

Maffulli and colleagues (2013) reported the initial treatment (2–3 days after injury) for muscle injuries may include the use of heat or cold therapy. The goal of heat therapy is to reduce muscle contractions, reduce neural tension, and increase flexibility. Heat must not be applied until any structural injuries have been ruled out.

Genetic Considerations and Risk Factors

One of the primary risk factors for alterations in mobility is aging. Joint problems that decrease mobility, including OA, gout, kyphosis, lower back pain, and inflammatory disorders, become more common as individuals age. An increased risk of fractures, particularly hip fractures, is associated with osteoporosis in older adults. In addition, some diseases that limit mobility, such as PD, primarily affect the older generation.

Genetic factors are also linked to alterations in mobility. Genetic mutations that affect the musculoskeletal or nervous systems will likely affect the individual's mobility (see **Box 13–1 》**).

Box 13–1
Genetic Disorders That Affect Mobility

- Muscular dystrophy (MD) is characterized by progressive weakness and degeneration of skeletal muscles, leading to muscle dysfunction and causing difficulty with advanced motor skills (e.g., running, hopping) and progressive difficulty walking. Breathing difficulties and cognitive deficits are also common. Affected muscles eventually atrophy or undergo pseudohypertrophy. There are more than 30 types of MD, including Duchenne MD and myotonic MD. Duchenne MD is an X-linked disorder, so it primarily affects boys. However, girls can be carriers of the disease. Myotonic MD is the most common type of adult-onset MD.
- Marfan syndrome is a disorder of the connective tissues that affects the lungs, heart, blood vessels, eyes, and skeleton. It causes individuals to have long limbs and digits compared to the rest of the body. Deficiencies in the connective tissue lining the brain may cause pain, numbness, and weakness in the legs, and cardiovascular effects may be life-threatening.
- Amyotrophic lateral sclerosis (ALS) is a neurologic disorder that affects the neurons responsible for voluntary muscle movement. Symptoms include weakness or paralysis in the limbs, slurred speech, trouble swallowing, muscle cramps, and difficulty breathing.
- Ellis–van Creveld syndrome is a rare disorder that affects bone growth. It may cause cleft lip or palate, polydactyly (extra digits), short arms and legs, and tooth abnormalities.
- Other mobility disorders that may have a genetic component include rheumatoid arthritis, gout, developmental dysplasia of the hip, ankylosing spondylitis, and systemic lupus erythematosus.

Case Study » Part 1

Darrell Hayes is a 42-year-old man who is experiencing lower back pain. As the nurse at his primary care clinic, you are responsible for obtaining Mr. Hayes's medical history and conducting a preliminary assessment. Mr. Hayes's height is 71" and his weight is 225 lb (body mass index [BMI] is 31). Mr. Hayes states that his back pain has gradually increased during the past several years because his job on an assembly line requires him to repeatedly bend and twist. Within the past week, his pain has gotten worse, and it now radiates down his left leg into his knee. He rates his pain as a 6 on a scale of 0–10. He adds that his pain is relieved by rest, but gets worse when he bends. Mr. Hayes's vital signs include temperature 99.2°F oral; pulse 88 bpm; respirations 18/min; and BP 139/84 mmHg. During the straight-leg-raise test, Mr. Hayes can raise his left leg to approximately 45 degrees before he is in severe pain. He is able to extend and lift his right leg to nearly 90 degrees, but he still experiences moderate pain. After a physical exam by the healthcare provider, Mr. Hayes is diagnosed with sciatica and a suspected herniated lumbar disc. He is referred to an orthopedic surgeon for further evaluation.

Clinical Reasoning Questions Level I

1. What factors may contribute to Mr. Hayes's condition?
2. Describe at least three simple tests the physician may perform to identify a potential herniated disc.

Clinical Reasoning Questions Level II

3. What patient teaching points will help prevent exacerbation of Mr. Hayes's back injury?

4. What diagnostic tests can be used to determine the exact location of the herniated disc?
5. What nonpharmacologic nursing interventions might decrease Mr. Hayes's back pain?

Concepts Related to Mobility

Mobility is related to several concepts. Some conditions will limit mobility or cause immobility, whereas other conditions may be caused by immobility. Conditions that may limit mobility include pain, fatigue, respiratory disorders, cardiovascular disease, nervous system disorders, and musculoskeletal diseases or injuries. Immobility may cause or affect problems with constipation, decubitus ulcers, metabolic disorders, depression, coping, or spirituality.

Snook and Oliver (2015) studied the perceptions of wellness in patients age 22–72 years old with mobility impairments (without other disabilities). They identified six themes they considered most prevalent in regards to thoughts of wellness.

> These included overcoming barriers, pain management, psychological wellness, physical activity and nutrition, social connectedness and family support, and spirituality. The last four themes are common to models of wellness for individuals without mobility impairments, whereas the first two—overcoming barriers and pain management—are unique findings for adults with mobility impairments. (Snook & Oliver, 2015, p. 290)

Patients with alterations in mobility accompanied by chronic or poorly managed pain may have difficulty performing their ADLs. Ongoing pain may also affect mood and relationships. Pain management was identified as an important factor by the participants in the Snook and Oliver study (2015). Although some patients may experience chronic pain, others may have acute pain during the first few days following an injury or flare up of a chronic issue that requires short-term pain management.

Some patients may experience difficulty performing activities that were once considered simple, such as walking, talking, dressing, or eating. Physical activity and maintaining a nutritious diet are among the self-care interventions patients reported as helping them cope with stress (Snook & Oliver, 2015). Patients with chronic or progressive mobility impairments (e.g., paralysis, PD) may require increasing levels of assistance from family members and caregivers, which puts these individuals at risk for caregiver burnout.

Physically active people are more likely to have improved moods over people who are inactive or have low activity levels. Patients with mobility impairments are at a higher risk for developing mood and affect disorders. Rosenburg, Bombardier, Atherholt, Jensen, and Motl (2013) reported that in the general population, approximately 17% of people have a major depressive episode in their lifetime, whereas the lifetime prevalence of major depression may be as high as 50% in individuals with MS.

Assessing and fostering spirituality and/or religiosity of patients with mobility impairments should be part of the standard of care. For patients with chronic or progressive impairments, the nurse may need to reassess patients' spiritual needs and provide support on either an ongoing or an intermittent basis, depending on each patient's needs.

Patients with medical conditions related to alterations in mobility may benefit from interprofessional care that includes some combination of the nurse and/or case manager, a disease specialist, a physical therapist (PT) or an occupational therapist (OT), a personal trainer, or a nutritionist. Patients with a prolonged decrease in mobility who develop anxiety or depression may benefit from counseling.

Although communication is always important, accurate communication is especially important at the time of care transitions, including patient discharge from a clinic or other facility. The discharging nurse needs to ensure the patient understands discharge instructions that may include weight or activity limitations, medications that may include pain medications or anti-inflammatory medications, when and how to wear any splints or braces, cast care, or who to call about any problems. Dossa, Bokhour, and Hoenig (2012) reported that discharged patients were often dissatisfied because of the lack of communication among hospital staff, the primary physician and surgeon, the physician and patient, and the discharge nurse and the patient or family members and friends.

Patients with hip fractures, joint injuries, or other mobility impairments will require fall-prevention strategies. Some less-obvious mobility impairments will require prudent nursing assessments and clinical judgments. For example, Suttanon and colleagues (2012) identified balance and mobility impairments in patients with mild to moderately severe Alzheimer disease (AD). When considering safety factors for a patient with AD or another form of dementia, it will be necessary to assess the patient's activity level, balance, and mobility. The Concepts Related to Mobility feature links some, but not all, of the concepts integral to mobility. They are presented in alphabetical order.

Health Promotion

Good lifestyle habits are vital to preventing many bone, muscle, and joint problems. Good nutrition, especially adequate calcium intake, helps maintain strong bones and provide ions for muscle contraction and nerve transmission. In addition, a regular exercise routine stimulates the body to build muscle strength and deposit minerals in bones. Regular exercise also helps maintain flexibility in joints and prevent the development or worsening of some joint disorders, including OA and back pain.

Modifiable Risk Factors

Obesity is a major risk factor for mobility problems. Excess weight strains the joints and increases the rate at which cartilage and other protective materials are destroyed, leading to OA, back pain, and joint inflammation. Obesity also makes common movements, including climbing stairs, getting in and out of a car, and walking, more difficult. Encouraging patients who are overweight or obese to lose weight is an important nursing intervention to prevent alterations in mobility.

Promotion of mobility begins even before birth. Good maternal nutrition during pregnancy can prevent some disorders that impair mobility. For example, taking folic acid during pregnancy is known to reduce the risk of spina bifida (myelomeningocele), which can cause partial or complete loss of sensation and paralysis of the legs. A well-balanced diet also helps the fetus develop strong bones and muscles and make essential nerve connections.

Screenings

Screenings to prevent or detect musculoskeletal disorders are not routinely included in annual physicals for adults. However, some screening tools are available for patients who have risk factors for specific disorders. For example, older adults may have a bone density scan to detect osteoporosis. Treatment for osteoporosis can strengthen bones and help prevent fractures. Spinal screenings for school-age children can detect scoliosis so observation and treatment can begin early to prevent progression of the disease. Genetic testing can also be done for patients with a family history of MD, Marfan syndrome, PD, and others.

Nursing Assessment

Assessment of the patient for alterations in the musculoskeletal and nervous systems that affect mobility includes observation and patient interview, physical assessment, and diagnostic tests. The nursing assessment includes gathering information to determine whether the patient is experiencing musculoskeletal dysfunction; the primary manifestations of musculoskeletal disorders are pain and limited mobility. Pain assessments are described in Exemplar 13.A and elsewhere in this module. Other manifestations related to limited mobility include fatigue, weight changes, and inflammation.

Observation and Patient Interview

Observe patients as they ambulate across the room or to the examination room. Observe for balance, uneven gait, difficulty bearing weight, and use of assistive devices or furniture for balance or support. Observe for signs of pain, such as facial grimacing or guarding, or moaning or wincing with movement, bending, or weight bearing. Note any findings. Observation in the clinic or inpatient setting may be similar to that for the home setting.

For the patient with alterations in mobility, the nursing assessment should include questions about the patient's lifestyle, such as physical activity required at work, ability to perform ADLs, participation in sports or exercise programs, time spent in sedentary activities, and nutritional habits. Assess for pain, and ask patients who report pain about any medications or interventions they may be using to relieve pain. The patient history should also include information about the onset, severity, timing, and symptoms associated with the limitations in mobility as well as factors that increase or decrease mobility. In addition, information about past injuries, joint pain, or neurologic problems is beneficial when developing nursing diagnoses. Patient interview questions include:

History

- Have you ever experienced a bone or muscle injury or problem? If so, describe it.
- Have you ever taken medications to treat a bone or muscle injury or problem? If so, what were they?
- Have you ever received treatments for a bone or muscle injury or problem, such as surgery, physical therapy, or alternative treatments? If so, describe them.

Concepts Related to
Mobility

CONCEPT	RELATIONSHIP TO MOBILITY	NURSING IMPLICATIONS
Collaboration	Alterations in mobility require interaction among multiple clinicians to help the patient regain full mobility.	■ Refer patients to a personal trainer or nutritionist to help build strong muscles and bones. ■ Refer patients to PTs or OTs to increase both gross and fine motor movements. ■ Refer patients to counselors to help with stress and coping.
Comfort	↑ Pain → ↓ activity tolerance → ↑ muscle atrophy and bone resorption. ↑ Fatigue (especially muscle fatigue) → ↓ muscle control and ↓ balance. Patients at end of life often have ↓ mobility in general.	■ Advocate for adequate pain management, and give pain medications as prescribed. ■ Encourage mild exercise programs for patients with pain and fatigue to build muscle strength and prevent bone loss. ■ Teach patients the importance of alternating periods of activity with periods of rest. ■ Encourage adequate calcium intake. ■ Assist with mobility for patients in pain or at the end of life. ■ Provide palliative care for patients at the end of life who are immobile.
Health, Wellness, Illness, and Injury	↑ Physical activity → ↑ muscle mass/strength and bone density. ↓ Mobility → ↑ actual or perceived barrier.	■ Encourage physical activity for patients with decreased mobility to help them gain strength. ■ Teach patients the importance of physical activity for maintaining health and wellness. ■ Assess patients' perception of any barriers to healing or ADLs. ■ Refer patients to appropriate resources (social services, governmental agencies, or community resources).
Mood and Affect	↓ Sense of self-worth or perception of life → ↑ risk of depression. ↓ Immobility → ↓ mood or affect → ↑ risk of self-harm or suicide.	■ Assess mood and affect. ■ Discuss signs and symptoms with healthcare providers as appropriate. ■ Make appropriate referrals. ■ Stay with patients; institute safety/suicide precautions.
Safety	Infants' learning mobility → ↑ risk of injury (e.g., falls, drowning, head injury). Children and adolescents who are involved in sports or other activities are at ↑ risk of injury, causing ↓ mobility. ↓ Mobility → ↑ risk of falls and fractures, especially in older adults.	■ Teach parents safety precautions for children at different stages of life. ■ Teach children and adults the importance of using safety equipment such as helmets, pads, and seat belts. ■ Assess homes of older patients with decreased mobility for safety hazards to help prevent falls. ■ Teach the proper use of assistive mobility devices, such as canes, walkers, and crutches.
Stress and Coping	↓ Mobility → ↑ stress → difficulty coping.	■ Teach patients coping methods to counteract the stress of decreased mobility. ■ Encourage patients to adhere to the treatment plan to increase mobility. ■ Teach patients methods to reduce stress.

■ Has anyone in your family been diagnosed with a musculoskeletal or nervous disorder?

Current Problem

■ Describe the pain you are experiencing (onset, intensity, location, etiology, duration). What relieves the pain or makes it worse?

■ Do you have any symptoms accompanying your pain, such as swelling, muscle spasms, cognitive deficits, balance problems, numbness, stiffness, or muscle weakness?

■ Do your symptoms limit your ADLs, such as walking, bathing, cooking, or participating in social activities?

■ Are you currently taking any medications or other treatments to help decrease your symptoms?

- Do you need to use assistive devices for ambulation or ADLs?
- Does your condition affect your ability to sleep at night?
- Has your condition ever caused you to fall?
- Describe how this condition affects your relationships, your ability to work, or how you feel about yourself.
- Does your condition contribute to feelings of stress? How do you cope with that stress?
- If the patient is injured, ask the following questions:
  - Describe how the injury occurred.
  - How does it feel when you try to bend the joint (knee, ankle, shoulder) or use the affected area (hand/wrist, foot)?
  - How does it feel when you try to bear weight on the affected area (leg, foot)?

Lifestyle

- Describe your typical dietary intake in a 24-hour period, especially your calcium intake.
- Do you take vitamins or other supplements? If so, what type and how often?
- Describe your physical activity in a 24-hour period.
- Do you participate in a regular exercise program?
- Does your job require you to do any physical labor, including lifting, bending, or twisting?
- Do you smoke, drink, or use drugs? Do you feel this is contributing to your condition?
- Are there any responsibilities that you may require assistance with at home, such as grocery shopping, pet care, laundry, and so forth?
- Are there any barriers that you can think of that may make it difficult for you to return to your home? (For example, if the patient is non-weight-bearing, are there stairs in the home or leading into the home?)
- How would you describe yourself in regard to religiosity or spirituality?
  - If the patient reports being religious, consider assessing for any religious beliefs behind or practices related to the injury.
  - Consider exploring how the patient may find comfort in spirituality.

Physical Examination

Physical assessment of the patient with potential musculoskeletal or neurologic problems should include inspection and palpation of bones, muscles, and joints for deformities, tenderness, and pain (see the Mobility Assessment feature). **Range of motion (ROM)**, the measurement of movement around a joint, is a key component of mobility. A range-of-motion (ROM) assessment should test the patient's ability to move joints (see **Table 13–1 》** and the Mobility Assessment feature). A goniometer should be used to measure ROM (see **Figure 13–9 》**). The assessment may require the patient to perform actions while standing, sitting, and supine. Joints should be clearly visible during the assessment; the remainder of the patient's body should be draped for privacy. The exam should progress logically from head to toe and proximal to distal.

TABLE 13–1 Muscle Function Grading Scale

Score	Description
0	No muscle contraction; paralysis
1	Muscle contracts, but limb does not move
2	Muscle movement only in absence of gravity
3	Full ROM against gravity
4	Full ROM against mild resistance
5	Full ROM against full resistance

Physical assessment also includes assessing the patient's neurovascular status through use of the **5 Ps neurovascular assessment**:

1. **Pain.** Assess for pain using a 0–10 pain scale. Also assess for pain with movement if movement will not cause further damage. Determine the location, quality, and etiology of the patient's pain.
2. **Pulses.** Compare distal pulses between the injured or affected extremity and the unaffected extremity. Lack of distal pulse may indicate compartment syndrome or arterial compromise.
3. **Pallor.** Observe skin color in the injured or affected extremity and in the skin in general. General pallor may indicate severe loss of blood, whereas pallor and coolness of the injured extremity indicates decreased arterial supply. In contrast, warmth and cyanosis may indicate venous stasis.
4. **Paresthesia.** Ask the patient about changes in sensation, such as burning, tingling, or numbness. The presence of paresthesia indicates neural damage or involvement.
5. **Paralysis/paresis.** For the patient with a fracture, assess the patient's ability to move body parts distal to the fracture, such as fingers and toes. Inability to move indicates paralysis, whereas muscle weakness indicates paresis. Paralysis or paresis may indicate nerve or tendon damage.

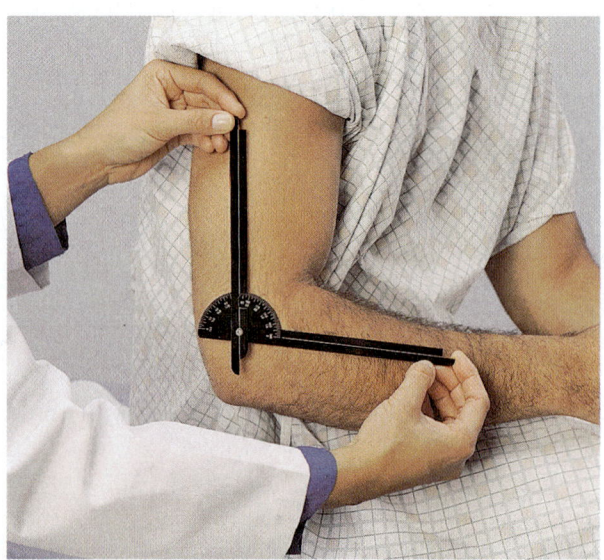

Figure 13–9 》 Using a goniometer to measure joint ROM.

Mobility Assessment

ASSESSMENT/METHOD	NORMAL FINDINGS	ABNORMAL FINDINGS	LIFESPAN OR DEVELOPMENTAL CONSIDERATIONS
Physical Assessment			
Inspect for deformities. Palpate for tenderness and pain. Measure extremities for length and circumference. Assess muscle mass and strength.	Patient should have no deformities, tenderness, or pain. Extremities should be bilaterally equal in length and circumference. Patient should have full ROM against resistance. Dominant side should be stronger than nondominant side.	■ Deformities such as scoliosis, bunions, nodules, Boutonnière, and swan-neck ■ Presence of inflammation, tenderness, or pain ■ Unequal bilateral strength, length, or circumference ■ Unable to move against resistance	■ Assessment of older patients, patients in pain, or patients who are weak may take extra time. ■ All procedures and tests should be fully described for patients before they are performed, especially for children who may be frightened.
Gait and Posture Assessment			
Inspect body posture and gait. Inspect the spine for curvature.	Body posture should be upright. Gait should be smooth and steady. Cervical and lumbar spine should be concave. Thoracic spine should be convex.	■ Joint problems or muscle weakness may cause changes in gait or posture. ■ Flattened lumbar curve and decreased spinal mobility may be evidence of herniated lumbar disc. ■ Scoliosis is a lateral S- or C-shaped curve of the spine.	■ Lordosis may be seen in patients with obesity or pregnant patients. ■ Kyphosis is common in older adults. ■ Scoliosis may be observed in children.
Joint Assessment			
Inspect joints for inflammation and deformities. Palpate joints for tenderness, warmth, pain, and crepitus. Observe for symmetry of use.	There should be no visible inflammation or deformities. Joints should have no tenderness, pain, warmth, or crepitation. Use of extremities should be symmetrical.	■ Deformities include tissue loss, tissue overgrowth, contractures, and shortening of the muscles and tendons. ■ Edema may cause bulging. ■ Inflammation (arthritis, bursitis, tendinitis, osteomyelitis) is indicated by redness, swelling, warmth, and pain. ■ Crepitation is evidence of lost cartilage.	■ Older adults often have some degree of cartilage loss (OA). ■ Athletes who overuse joints may have inflammation from chronic use (e.g., tennis elbow).
Range-of-Motion Assessment			
The nurse should provide resistance by pushing in the opposite direction (test both ROM and muscle strength).	Muscles should have full ROM against full resistance. Flexion to 45 degrees Extension to 55 degrees Lateral bending to 40 degrees Rotation to 70 degrees.	■ Clicking or popping noises ■ Decreased ROM ■ Pain ■ Swelling ■ Neck pain and limited ROM may indicate herniated cervical disc or cervical spondylosis. ■ Immobile neck with head and neck thrust forward may indicate ankylosing spondylitis.	■ Nonverbal infants and small children may need the nurse to physically perform motions. Individuals with cognitive impairment may need extra guidance or assistance from the nurse. ■ Older adults may naturally have less flexibility of joints compared to children and young adults.

(continued on next page)

Mobility Assessment *(continued)*

ASSESSMENT/METHOD	NORMAL FINDINGS	ABNORMAL FINDINGS	LIFESPAN OR DEVELOPMENTAL CONSIDERATIONS
Temporomandibular joint: Palpate the joint while the patient opens and closes the mouth (see **Figure 13–10** »). ***Cervical spine:*** Flexion: Touch chin to chest. Extension: Look at the ceiling. Lateral bending: Touch ear to shoulder on each side. Rotation: Touch chin to each shoulder.	Patient should open and close mouth smoothly with full ROM and no pain or sound. Left and right lateral bending, flexion and extension, and rotation should occur without pain or difficulty.	▪ Pain in jaw ▪ "Locking" of jaw ▪ Difficulty or discomfort with chewing ▪ Aching pain near ear or face ▪ Difficulty or pain may occur with left and right lateral bending, flexion and extension, and rotation. ▪ Juvenile rheumatoid arthritis may affect joints of the cervical spine. ▪ Instability of the cervical spine is not uncommon in pediatric orthopedics. (It does not always result in injury or problems.)	▪ Problems may occur at any age, but are most common in women ages 20–40. ▪ Children may complain of symptoms similar to those of an adult; however, they may complain of hearing cracking or popping in their jaw. ▪ Trauma: Children younger than 11 years are more likely to experience upper cervical spine ligamentous injuries or fractures. ▪ Adolescents are more likely to experience fractures and injuries to the lower cervical spine.
Lumbar spine: Flexion: Touch toes with fingers (see **Figure 13–11A** »). Extension: Bend backward. Lateral bending: Bend right and left (Figure 13–11B). Rotation: Twist shoulders right and left (Figure 13–11C).	Flexion to 90 degrees Extension to 30 degrees Lateral bending to 35 degrees Rotation to 30 degrees	▪ Decreased ROM or pain may indicate abnormal curvature, arthritis, herniated disc, or muscle spasm.	▪ Trauma: Male patients are more likely to sustain a spinal injury than female patients. ▪ Injury is more common between ages 16 and 30.

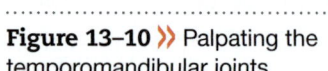

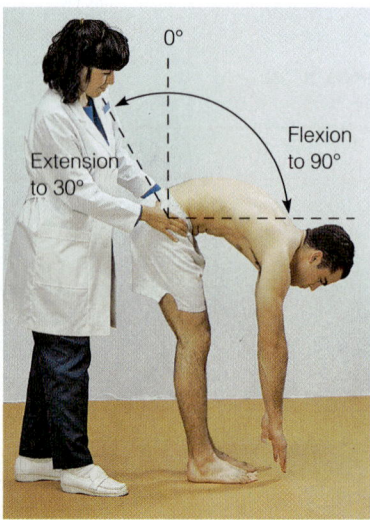

Figure 13–10 » Palpating the temporomandibular joints.

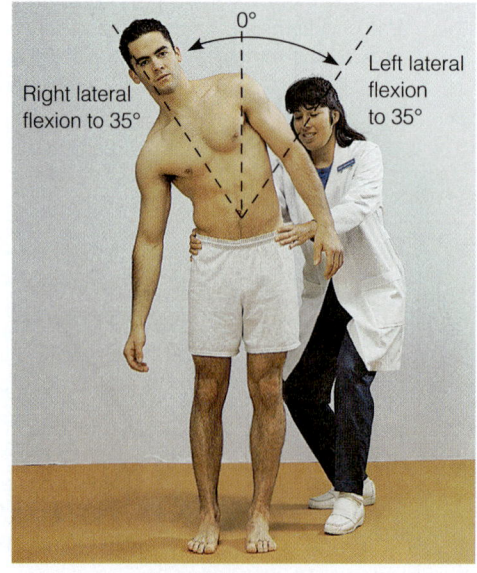

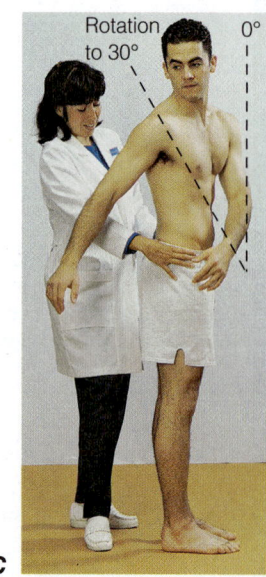

A   B   C

Figure 13–11 » ***A,*** Forward flexion of spine. ***B,*** Lateral flexion of spine. ***C,*** Rotation of spine.

Mobility Assessment *(continued)*

ASSESSMENT/METHOD	NORMAL FINDINGS	ABNORMAL FINDINGS	LIFESPAN OR DEVELOPMENTAL CONSIDERATIONS
Shoulders: Flexion: Slowly raise straight arms from at the side to over the head. Hyperextension: Put straight arms behind the back. Internal rotation: Put forearm behind the lower back. Abduction: Raise straight arm out to the side. Adduction: Put straight arm across the chest.	Flexion to 180 degrees Hyperextension to 50 degrees Internal rotation to 90 degrees Abduction to 180 degrees Adduction to 50 degrees	▪ Tendinitis is evidenced by pain of the biceps tendon. ▪ Rotator cuff tears often cause pain at rest, which worsens when lying on the affected side; pain with movement up or down; and pain with lifting. ▪ Ruptured supraspinatus tendon prevents full abduction. ▪ Bursitis and calcium deposits limit abduction and cause pain.	▪ Rotator cuff tears may be caused by normal wear and tear and are more common after the age of 40. In young people, they are more commonly caused by an injury.
Elbows: Flexion: Touch hands to shoulders. Extension: Straighten elbows. Supination: Bend elbow 90 degrees and turn palm up. Pronation: Bend elbow 90 degrees and turn palm down.	Flexion to 160 degrees Extension to 180 degrees Supination and pronation to 90 degrees	▪ Inflammation may indicate arthritis. ▪ Pain and tenderness of lateral epicondyle indicate tennis elbow. ▪ Dislocation of the elbow joint may be caused by a sudden pull on the extended forearm, such as by an adult tugging on an uncooperative child.	▪ Tennis elbow is most common between ages 30 and 50 years. ▪ Toddlers with "nursemaid's elbow" may not use one of their upper extremities.
Wrists: Flexion: Bend wrist down. Extension: Bend wrist up. Ulnar deviation: Bend wrist toward little finger. Radial deviation: Bend wrist toward thumb.	Flexion to 90 degrees Extension to 70 degrees Ulnar deviation to 55 degrees Radial deviation to 20 degrees	▪ Arthritis causes pain and swelling of the wrist. ▪ Fractures may cause pain, swelling, deformity, and possible decreased blood circulation to the hand. ▪ Carpel tunnel syndrome may cause gradual onset of tingling or burning in the thumb, index, and middle fingers. Pain may be worse at night.	▪ Wrist injuries are commonly caused by falls with hands extended to catch self. ▪ Snowboard and skateboard falls may result in injuries to young people. ▪ Carpal tunnel syndrome usually only occurs in adults.
Fingers: Flexion: Make a fist. Extension: Open hand. Abduction: Spread fingers. Adduction: Close fingers.	Patient should be able to complete all tasks with full ROM.	▪ Arthritis: Flexion and extension are decreased; finger joints become stiff, painful, and swollen. ▪ Swollen fingers with chalky discharge may indicate gout. ▪ Trigger finger will cause a popping or clicking sensation in the finger and a tender lump at the base of the finger; the finger will become fixed in a bent position.	▪ OA is more commonly seen in older adults; rheumatoid arthritis is much less common. It affects women more often than men, and onset is around 20 years of age. ▪ Gout is more common in men. ▪ Trigger finger is more common in women, and usual onset is after age 40.
Hips: (Patient should lie down.) Flexion: Bring bent knee up to chest. Hyperextension: Lie on abdomen, and lift each leg. Abduction: Move straight leg out to the side. Internal rotation: Bend knee, and swing it toward other leg. External rotation: Bend knee, and swing it to the side.	Flexion to 120 degrees Hyperextension to 30 degrees Abduction to 45 degrees Internal rotation to 40 degrees External rotation to 45 degrees	▪ Limited ROM or pain may indicate arthritis or fracture.	The risk of hip fractures increases 10 times in 20-year intervals beginning at the age of 40 (Reeve & Loveridge, 2014).

(continued on next page)

Mobility Assessment *(continued)*

ASSESSMENT/METHOD	NORMAL FINDINGS	ABNORMAL FINDINGS	LIFESPAN OR DEVELOPMENTAL CONSIDERATIONS
Knees: Flexion: Do a deep knee bend. Extension: Sit down, and hold the legs out straight.	Flexion to 130 degrees Extension to 180 degrees	▪ Synovitis is common with knee trauma. ▪ Swelling may indicate inflammation and excess fluid buildup in the articular capsule or bursitis.	Sports injuries are a common cause of mobility impairments in children and adolescents. Soccer, basketball, and skiing are common sports for knee injuries.
Ankles: Dorsiflexion: Point foot to ceiling. Plantar flexion: Point foot to floor. Inversion: Walk on the outside (lateral portion) of feet (see **Figure 13–12** ≫). Eversion: Walk on the inside (medial portion) of feet (see Figure 13–12).	Dorsiflexion to 20 degrees Plantar flexion to 45 degrees Inversion to 30 degrees Eversion to 20 degrees	▪ Contractures or injuries to the Achilles tendon may cause pain and decreased ROM. ▪ Arthritis may cause pain or contractures, especially after bedrest.	The most common ankle injuries occur in men between 15 and 24 years old. Women older than 30 years experience more ankle injuries than men. The ankle is most commonly injured during sports or walking on uneven ground. Risks of ankle injury increase with the use of high-heeled shoes, loose fitting shoes (clogs), twisting, falling, jumping and landing awkwardly, or sudden impact. Gout is one of the most painful types of arthritis. Gout often occurs in the great toe; it is more common in men.
Toes: Flexion: Curl toes down. Extension: Straighten toes. Abduction: Spread toes apart. Adduction: Bring toes together.	Flexion to 90 degrees Patient should be able to perform all tasks.	▪ Lateral deviation of the great toe is hallux valgus and causes bunions. ▪ Swollen, inflamed, and painful toes indicate arthritis or gout. ▪ Hyperextension of the metatarsophalangeal joint and flexion of the proximal interphalangeal joint indicate hammertoe.	Bunions: 9 out of 10 patients with bunions are women, often because they wear tight shoes and/or high heels. Morton's neuroma: Patients often report it "feels like walking on a marble"; 8 out of 10 patients with Morton's neuroma are women, often because they wear tight-fitting footwear (ski boots, skates, tight shoes).

Special Assessments

Phalen test. Hold wrists in acute flexion for 60 seconds (see **Figure 13–13** ≫).	Patient should feel no tingling, numbness, or pain.	▪ Numbness, tingling, or pain may indicate carpal tunnel syndrome.	N/A

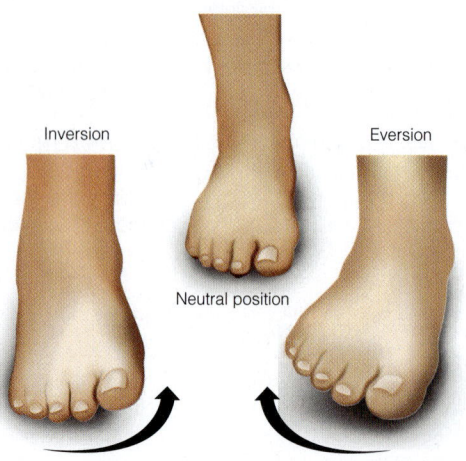

Figure 13–12 ≫ Inversion and eversion of the ankle and foot.

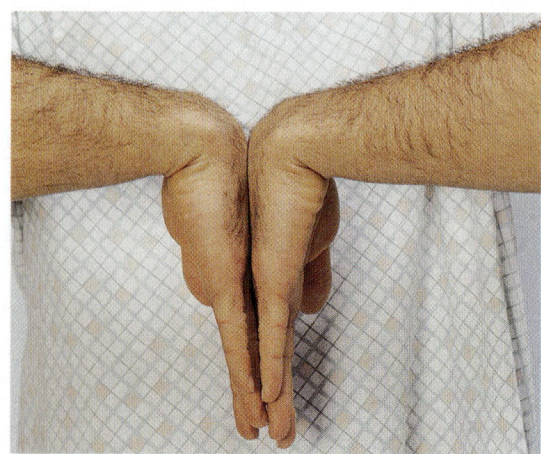

Figure 13–13 ≫ Phalen test.

Mobility Assessment *(continued)*

ASSESSMENT/METHOD	NORMAL FINDINGS	ABNORMAL FINDINGS	LIFESPAN OR DEVELOPMENTAL CONSIDERATIONS
Bulge test. Milk upward on the medial knee, and tap the lateral side of the patella (see **Figure 13–14 »**).	No bulge of fluid should appear on the medial knee.	■ Fluid bulge indicates effusion in the knee instead of swelling.	N/A
Ballottement test. Apply downward pressure on the knee while pushing the patella backward against femur (see **Figure 13–15 »**).	The patella should not move.	■ Increased fluid will cause a tapping sound as the patella displaces the fluid and hits the femur.	N/A
McMurray test. When the patient is lying down, ask the patient to turn the flexed knee toward the center of the body. Stabilize the knee, and apply pressure on the lower leg (see **Figure 13–16 »**).	No pain or clicking should be present.	■ Pain, locking, or popping may indicate meniscus injury.	N/A

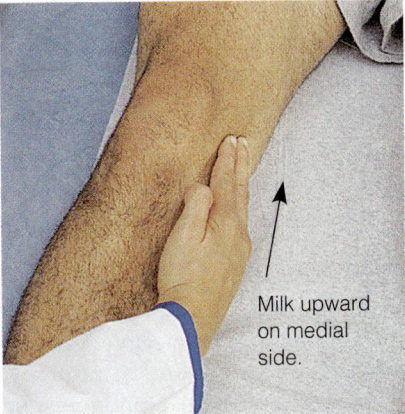

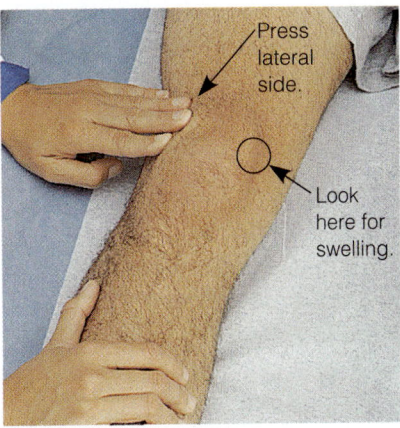

Press lateral side.

Look here for swelling.

Milk upward on medial side.

Figure 13–14 » Checking for the bulge sign.

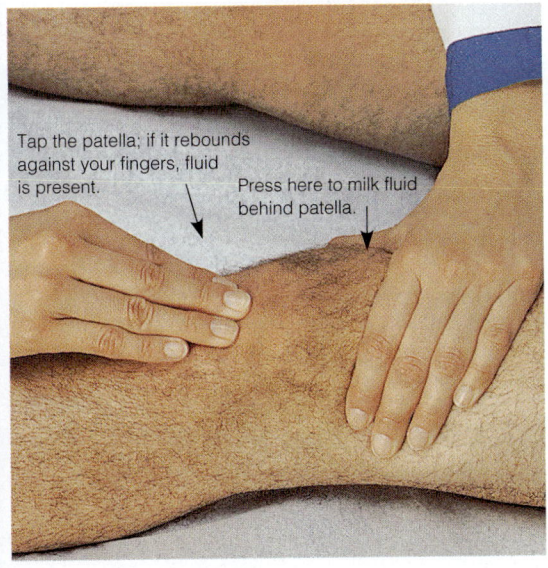

Tap the patella; if it rebounds against your fingers, fluid is present.

Press here to milk fluid behind patella.

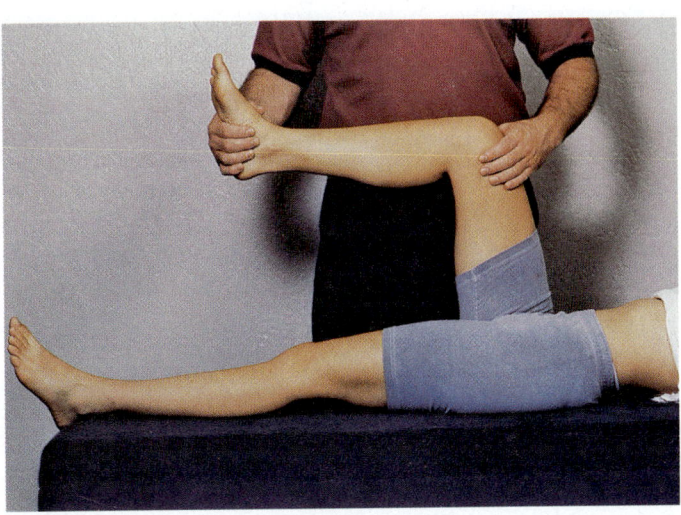

Figure 13–15 » Checking for ballottement.

Figure 13–16 » McMurray test.

(continued on next page)

Mobility Assessment (continued)

ASSESSMENT/METHOD	NORMAL FINDINGS	ABNORMAL FINDINGS	LIFESPAN OR DEVELOPMENTAL CONSIDERATIONS
Thomas test. While the patient is lying down, ask the patient to extend one leg while bringing the opposite leg to the chest (see **Figure 13–17** »).	Extended leg should not rise off the table.	A hip flexion contracture will cause the extended leg to rise off the table.	N/A

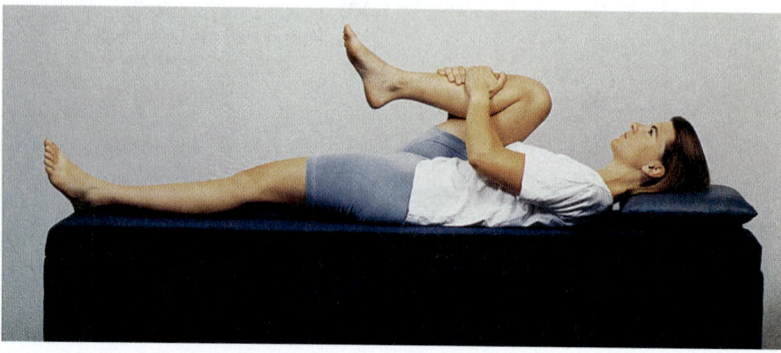

Figure 13–17 » Thomas test for hip contracture.

Diagnostic Tests

Tests used to detect musculoskeletal and neurologic problems that may alter mobility include blood tests (see **Table 13–2** »), imaging tests, and electrical tests. These tests can be used to support a diagnosis and identify the efficacy of current treatments.

» *Selected diagnostic tests are described in Appendix B at* **Pearson MyLab Nursing and eText**.

Imaging tests include bone density scans (e.g., dual-photon absorptiometry, dual-energy x-ray absorptiometry, technetium bone scan, peripheral bone density test), CT scans (e.g., classic CT, discography, quantitative CT), MRI, and x-rays (e.g., classic x-rays, arthrography). Many of these tests can be performed with or without specific dyes to detect alterations in bone or connective tissue structures, including joint structures; osteoporosis; unusual bone formation; bone fractures; spinal disc problems; spinal stenosis; and torn muscles, ligaments, and cartilage.

TABLE 13–2 Blood Tests for Musculoskeletal Disorders

Test	Function
Alkaline phosphatase (ALP)	ALP is produced by bone and other organs. Increased ALP may indicate bone disease, bone fracture, bone tumors, osteomalacia, Paget disease, or rickets. Decreased ALP may indicate Wilson disease.
Calcitonin/parathyroid hormone	Calcitonin and parathyroid hormone (PTH) have opposite actions in the regulation of blood calcium levels, which is vital for bone and muscle strength and function. Increased calcitonin may indicate a thyroid tumor. PTH may be increased in osteoporosis that does not respond to therapy. Increased PTH may suggest kidney disease, parathyroid gland tumors, lack of calcium, or vitamin D disorders.
Calcium (Ca)	Increased blood Ca levels could indicate the presence of metastatic bone tumors, Paget disease, bone fractures, or hyperparathyroidism. Decreased blood Ca levels could indicate hypoparathyroidism, osteomalacia, or vitamin D deficiency.
Creatine kinase (CK)	CK is used to detect muscle damage, muscle inflammation, rhabdomyolysis, polymyositis, and MD. CPK-MM is specific for skeletal muscle.
Growth hormone (GH)	High levels of GH may indicate acromegaly or gigantism. Low levels of GH may result in dwarfism.
Human leukocyte antigen-B27 (HLA-B27)	The presence of HLA-B27 indicates an increased risk for ankylosing spondylitis and arthritis.
Phosphorus (P)	Increased levels may indicate hypoparathyroidism. Decreased levels may indicate hyperparathyroidism or lack of vitamin D, which increases the risk of rickets and osteomalacia.
Rheumatoid factor (RF)	Elevated level may indicate rheumatoid arthritis, scleroderma, lupus erythematosus, and adult Still disease.
Uric acid	Increased uric acid levels may indicate gout, excessive exercise, and a variety of non–musculoskeletal-related disorders.

SAFETY ALERT Patients with metal implants such as pacemakers; heart valves; brain, eye, or ear implants; and infusion catheters should not undergo MRIs because the strong magnetic field may damage the implants and cause injury to the patient. Individuals with embedded shrapnel may also be at risk for injury. Most orthopedic and dental implants are safe for MRIs, but they may distort the image. Patients scheduled to undergo MRI scanning should be screened for potential contraindications.

Other tests include electrical tests such as electromyography (EMG), neurologic tests such as a nerve conduction study, and joint aspiration. EMG testing, which is used to analyze the electrical activity of the muscle, can be useful in determining whether nerve compression is present. In conjunction with EMG testing, nerve conduction studies are often administered to determine if nerves are functioning normally. Nerve conduction studies can be especially useful in the detection of carpal tunnel syndrome or ulnar nerve entrapment. Joint aspiration may be used to remove accumulated fluid from a joint. Through laboratory analysis, the aspirated fluid may be sent for laboratory analysis to detect infection, as well as blood or fat droplets, which may indicate a fracture.

Case Study » Part 2

Mr. Hayes is under the care of an orthopedic spine surgeon. After 6 weeks of implementing a regimen that includes ibuprofen, moist heat packs, and alternating periods of rest and mild activity, Mr. Hayes returns to his surgeon's office. He now complains of numbness and tingling in his left leg. He states that he constantly feels like his leg has "fallen asleep." He has been trying to limit his bending and twisting at work, but he has to move quickly to meet productivity standards on the assembly line. The ibuprofen seems to dull the pain, but the pain often returns before his next dose of medication is scheduled. On the basis of the severity of symptoms, the surgeon decides to refer Mr. Hayes to the pain clinic for an epidural cortisone injection. First, he needs to obtain a myelogram to confirm the exact location of the disc that is causing Mr. Hayes's pain. The myelogram results indicate that Mr. Hayes has a herniated disc at L4–L5. After Mr. Hayes is admitted to the pain clinic, an anesthesiologist administers an epidural cortisone injection in the L4–L5 region and also prescribes the muscle relaxant cyclobenzaprine.

Clinical Reasoning Questions Level I
1. What symptoms indicate that Mr. Hayes's condition is worsening?
2. What nursing interventions should be implemented for Mr. Hayes before, during, and after his myelogram and epidural cortisone injection?
3. Prior to his myelogram and epidural injection, what assessment questions should the nurse ask Mr. Hayes to ensure his safety?

Clinical Reasoning Questions Level II
4. What adverse reactions may occur during the myelogram? How can the nurse assess for adverse effects and complications related to this procedure?
5. What coping strategies might the nurse suggest for Mr. Hayes?
6. What instructions should be included in Mr. Hayes's discharge teaching?

Independent Interventions

Primary categories of independent nursing interventions for the patient with impaired mobility include education, comfort promotion, injury prevention, fostering independence, and

Patient Teaching
Proper Body Mechanics for Lifting

The nurse should teach proper body mechanics to all patients, from school-age children to older adults. Body mechanics are especially important for individuals, including nurses, who regularly perform physical labor such as lifting, bending, and twisting. Guidelines for proper body mechanics for lifting heavy objects include the following:

- Start with the feet apart, with one foot slightly forward to provide balance.
- Bend at the knees, not the back.
- Use the large muscles of the legs and arms rather than the weaker back muscles to lift heavy objects.
- Stand close to the object, and lift it straight up.
- Distribute weight evenly between both feet.
- Use the feet to pivot rather than twisting or turning with the back.
- Use a back brace to support the back for frequent heavy lifting.
- If possible, slide, roll, or push an object rather than lift it.
- If the object is too heavy to lift alone, ask for help.

reducing social isolation. While the specific nursing interventions are dependent on the patient and the nature of the impairment, certain considerations within these five categories are applicable to a majority of these patients.

Providing Education

For patients who are ambulatory or will resume ambulation, patient teaching should include instruction about body mechanics and proper posture (see the Patient Teaching feature). Even simple modifications in turning, lifting, and bending practices can significantly enhance the patient's healing and reduce the risk for further injury. In addition, because obesity is a risk factor for impaired mobility, patients should be educated as to the importance of regular exercise and good nutrition. Teaching should also incorporate discussion of any medications added to the patient's regimen, including safe administration, actions, side effects, and precautions associated with the drugs.

Promoting Comfort

During periods of immobility, patient positioning and proper padding of joints and bony prominences can prevent discomfort and help prevent skin breakdown. Braces and support devices, such as splints and wrist braces, also help promote comfort by stabilizing weak or injured musculoskeletal structures. The nurse should be knowledgeable in the application of these devices, as well as care of patients whose treatment plan includes their use. When a splint or brace is in place, the nurse should routinely assess the surrounding area for signs and symptoms of circulatory impairment, including skin pallor or blanching, weak or absent pulses, and impaired sensation.

Preventing Injury

Traumatic injury, certain neurologic conditions, and decreased mobility are associated with an increased risk for contractures. The patient should be encouraged to perform exercises and stretches, and to utilize braces and splints as prescribed by the patient's primary healthcare provider, PT, and OT (Ma, 2016a).

The patient's environment should be screened for potential hazards, including loose floor coverings, inadequate lighting, and obstructed walkways. In addition, the nurse should ensure that the patient is properly using any assistive devices and provide instruction as needed.

Fostering Independence

There are many ways for nurses to foster independence for patients with mobility impairments. The nurse may begin with helping the patient prioritize what is important to him or her. For example, in what aspects of life does the patient find it important to remain independent? This will vary significantly depending on the age of the patient. For example, the child may find it important to be able to use the toilet independently. An older adult may feel it is important to live independently.

Some common interventions for promoting independence for any age include:

- Be encouraging, as this promotes trying.
- Offer assistance in determining adjustments that may be needed.
- Avoid helping or doing something for a patient because it will get done faster.
- Encourage the patient to ease out of his or her comfort zone, as creating a challenge often provides an opportunity to learn something or see what is possible.
- Foster adjustments that might be necessary to allow the patient to go out independently, rather than in a group.
- Provide information about the proper screenings and healthcare necessary to maintain adequate health to promote independence in healthcare choices and decisions. Screenings and healthcare will vary depending on medical conditions. For example, screening for a patient with diabetes will include eye examinations to assess for retinopathy, which could make independence difficult.

Reducing Social Isolation

Social isolation is a concern for people with mobility impairments. This may be due to lack of transportation, inability to access the internet to find and maintain social opportunities, or inability to access facilities (older buildings that have not been updated to meet regulations). Some individuals with disabilities may fear going out because of the concern others will stare at them. Others may organize outings to avoid having to manage a visit to a public bathroom. The type of home setting (e.g., second floor apartment) can increase the risk of isolation. Although some people may want to live in a private home or their own apartment, this can increase the likelihood of social isolation. Strategies to help patients reduce social isolation include the following:

- Discuss with the patient and family members how relying too much on paid assistance may make it difficult for the patient to develop relationships with others. For example, family members may wish to hire a driver for

the patient, but the patient may be capable of taking the bus, which is a great social opportunity. A patient who does not need 24-hour care may feel uncomfortable inviting friends over.

- Help the patient explore social networks.
- Discuss living arrangements that may promote social interaction, such as assisted living, apartments with dining halls, or homes that have group living.

The nurse should promote involvement in community groups that align with the patient's personal interests.

Collaborative Therapies

Collaborative interventions include rehabilitative services designed to help the patient preserve or regain mobility, as well as pharmacologic interventions. Physical therapy may be prescribed by the patient's primary care provider, and therapeutic exercises are implemented by the PT and the physical therapy assistant (PTA). In some clinical settings, the nurse may also implement portions of the patient's physical therapy regimen.

For the patient with alterations in mobility, the primary care provider may also order occupational therapy. Exercises and activities implemented by the OT and occupational therapy assistant (OTA) are designed to help the patient maintain and optimize skills that are necessary to complete ADLs, such as bathing, housework, and meal preparation. The OT can also help identify necessary modifications to the patient's home environment that will allow the patient to function as independently as possible.

Preservative interventions are especially important for patients who must remain in bed for prolonged periods. The main types of rehabilitative services include exercise and assisted ambulation. Assisted ambulation includes the use of assistive devices such as crutches, canes, and walkers. These devices can be used during rehabilitation to help patients maintain mobility and prevent further injury. This rehabilitation should begin as early as possible in the patient's care.

Exercise

Exercise is vital to maintaining muscle strength. Muscles that are not used atrophy and become weak, especially during prolonged bedrest. Specific exercises can be performed to promote strength and ROM, reduce joint pain and stiffness, and increase flexibility and endurance. Exercise also promotes proper alignment of bones and joints; helps to prevent edema, thrombophlebitis, and pressure injuries; and stimulates circulation and lung expansion. Exercises can be either passive or active. Passive exercises are administered by the nurse, therapist, or therapy assistant. Active exercises are performed by the patient.

- ***Range-of-motion exercises*** are passive exercises that help the patient maintain joint mobility during periods of restricted physical activity. The therapist or nurse moves joints through their full ROM to maintain or increase strength and flexibility. Before beginning the therapy, the nurse should explain all exercises to the patient and determine the patient's baseline ROM. If the patient experiences pain, ROM exercises should be stopped. As the patient heals, he or she may begin active ROM exercises without the assistance of the healthcare provider.

- **Resistive exercises** are active exercises in which the patient works against resistance to increase muscle strength. Resistance can be provided by weights or by the therapist or nurse supplying resistive force.
- **Isometric exercises** are active exercises used to maintain strength when a joint is immobilized. The patient is instructed to contract a specific muscle group against another muscle group or immovable object. This prevents overall movement of the body part(s). Isometric exercises are most beneficial for patients who are immobilized while an injury is healing or who experience severe pain during movement.

Ambulation

Ambulation is the ability to walk from place to place independently with or without an assistive device. The patient who is unable to ambulate is at higher risk for thrombophlebitis, osteoporosis, muscle atrophy, constipation, and urinary incontinence and infection. The longer a patient is immobile, the harder it is to overcome these effects. In addition to reducing the risk of complications, early ambulation provides several benefits for the patient, including strengthening muscles, increasing joint flexibility, stimulating circulation and preventing thrombophlebitis, providing pressure relief, and improving self-esteem.

Safe, effective ambulation requires adequate leg muscle strength. For patients who are immobile, strengthening exercises should be performed several times daily. When patients are ready to ambulate, they first should sit at the edge of the bed to allow for assessment of vertigo or postural hypotension. Assessment of vital signs, especially blood pressure, may be appropriate. When patients are ready, the nurse should assist them to a standing position. During ambulation, assistance from a nurse or use of an assistive device also may be needed. The nurse should encourage patients to verbalize any physical complaints or concerns throughout the activity period. To avoid overexertion and potential injury, short, frequent periods of ambulation are preferable to extended periods of activity.

Assistive Devices

Assistive devices are used to provide support and balance for the patient and increase confidence in independent ambulation. They reduce the pressure exerted on an injured limb, help to prevent further injury, and assist in healing. Assistive devices include crutches, canes, and walkers.

Crutches commonly feature one of three designs: axillary, Lofstrand, or platform. Axillary crutches are most common for short-term use; body weight is typically supported by the wrists. Lofstrand crutches use a forearm piece for stability. Platform crutches are used for patients who are unable to bear weight on their wrists. Patients can use two crutches for non-weight-bearing ambulation or one crutch for stability and partial weight-bearing ambulation. Crutches must be fitted to the patient. If using axillary crutches, the axillary portion should be placed about 2 inches below the underarm, and the hand piece should allow a 20- to 30-degree elbow flexion. Rubber tips should be placed on the bottom

of all crutches for safety. Upper body and trunk strength are necessary for proper use of crutches.

Walkers have four legs to provide maximum stability for the patient. The patient's arms support the majority of the body weight to relieve pressure on the lower extremities. Walkers are generally used for patients with severe injuries, such as spinal cord surgery or hip replacement surgery, or for patients who are unsteady, such as older adults. Some walkers are available with wheels on the front legs to provide ease of walking while preventing further injury. Walkers without wheels should be used only for patients who are steady enough to stand on their own and bear their full weight for short times while they move the walker forward. All walker legs without wheels have rubber tips to ensure stability. Rubber tips should be replaced if excessive wear is evident. Some walkers have platforms for sitting, should the patient become weary. Like crutches, walkers should be adjusted to fit the patient's height.

Canes are often used by patients who can bear weight, but are unsteady or have one weak limb. Many types of canes are available; they can be wooden or metal, have a C-handle or functional grip handle, and have one or four rubber-cushioned feet at the base. Canes should be adjusted for the patient's height. Canes are available in a variety of styles to fit the personality of the patient if needed for long-term use. Collapsible canes are also available for ease of storage.

Selecting an assistive device may depend on the patient's age and preference. See examples in **Box 13–2 »**.

Pharmacologic Therapy

Pharmacologic treatment of musculoskeletal disorders incorporates a wide variety of medications, including pain relievers (see Exemplar 3.A, Acute and Chronic Pain), muscle relaxants, anti-inflammatory drugs, bone growth stimulators, and neurologic drugs (see the Medications feature). Medications used for specific disorders are discussed in more detail in the exemplars in this module.

Collaborative treatment of patients with musculoskeletal disorders may also include nutritional guidance, chiropractic care, support groups, spiritual care, and counseling. For patients with chronic mobility problems, collaborative care should incorporate family members and caregivers.

Box 13–2
Use of Assistive Devices Across the Lifespan

- Toddlers and preschool children may prefer to crawl or scoot, have a parent carry them, or have a walking cast rather than learn how to use an assistive device.
- Active school-age children, adolescents, and young adults will likely choose a walking cast or axillary crutches for ambulation assistance. Patients with long-term assistance needs may prefer Lofstrand crutches rather than axillary crutches.
- Middle-age adults will likely choose crutches or a cane for assistance, depending on the need for weight-bearing or non-weight-bearing assistance.
- Older adults may feel unstable on crutches, so they may instead choose a walker or cane depending on the amount of support needed. Patients who need to avoid putting weight on the injured limb may prefer a wheelchair for mobility.

Medications

Musculoskeletal Disorders

CLASSIFICATION AND DRUG EXAMPLES	MECHANISMS OF ACTION	NURSING CONSIDERATIONS
Anti-Inflammatory Drugs Nonsteroidal anti-inflammatory drugs (NSAIDs) *Drug examples:* Ibuprofen Aspirin Naproxen Diclofenac Indomethacin Celecoxib	These drugs block production of inflammatory mediators by inhibiting COX-1 and/or COX-2. *May also be used as an:* ■ Analgesic ■ Antipyretic ■ Antiplatelet	■ Aspirin therapy is not commonly recommended for children and should be avoided in children with an active virus or infection, particularly influenza. ■ These drugs may interfere with clinical tests such as pregnancy tests, urine tests, and liver function tests. ■ Patients should be monitored for GI distress, bleeding, and allergic reactions.
Antispasmodics Skeletal muscle relaxants *Drug examples:* Cyclobenzaprine Dantrolene Baclofen Chlorzoxazone Orphenadrine Methocarbamol Carisoprodol Tizanidine	These drugs may act in the CNS to decrease nerve transmission to skeletal muscles. They may interfere with calcium release during muscle stimulation. *May also be used as an:* ■ Analgesic	■ Patients should be observed carefully for CNS effects, including confusion, depression, and hallucinations (more common in people over age 65). ■ These drugs may cause orthostatic hypotension, loss of spasticity, or dizziness, increasing the risk of falls during ambulation. ■ Patients should not drive or participate in other hazardous activities until they know how these drugs affect them. ■ Effects may be additive with other CNS depressants such as alcohol. ■ Monitor patients for allergic response. ■ Cyclobenzaprine is not recommended for pediatric use. ■ Some drugs may discolor urine.
Direct-Acting Antispasmodic Drugs *Drug examples:* AbobotulinumtoxinA IncobotulinumtoxinA OnabotulinumtoxinA RimabotulinumtoxinB	These drugs block the release of acetylcholine (necessary for voluntary contraction of skeletal muscles) from cholinergic nerve terminals.	■ Because of the ability of these medications to spread to other parts of the body, serious effects include angina, difficulty breathing, extreme muscle weakness, dysrhythmias, difficulty swallowing, and loss of bladder control. ■ Instruct patients on gradual onset.
Bone Growth Stimulators Bisphosphonates *Drug examples:* Alendronate Risedronate Ibandronate Zoledronic acid	These drugs inhibit osteoclast-mediated bone resorption.	■ Use cautiously in patients with renal impairment or liver disease. ■ Hypocalcemia should be corrected before therapy begins; do not administer within 2 hours of consuming calcium.

Source: Data from Adams, M. P., Holland, L. N., & Urban, C. (2017). *Pharmacology for nurses: A pathophysiologic approach* (5th ed.). Hoboken, NJ: Pearson Education.

SAFETY ALERT Discussion about the safety of medications at home should include how to store medications so that children cannot access them. Nurses should remind grandparents to store medications out of reach of grandchildren. There have been numerous accounts of child deaths related to accidental ingestion of medications. In addition, nurses should explain safe disposal practices. For example, children have eaten Fentanyl patches found in waste baskets.

Lifespan Considerations

Bones and muscles adapt as an individual ages. Some bones fuse during infancy, and bones and muscles in children grow in length as the child ages. This growth ability is turned off in adults, so bones begin to undergo remodeling. In older adults, the musculoskeletal system undergoes physiologic changes that decrease strength and mobility.

Mobility Considerations in Children and Adolescents

A child's musculoskeletal system goes through many important changes as the child grows (see **Figure 13–18 »**). The bones of an infant's skull are not fused at birth, allowing the bones to shift as needed as the head passes through the birth canal. This also provides flexibility of the skull as the infant's head grows, preventing excess pressure on the brain. The spaces between the skull bones form membrane-covered fontanels, or "soft spots." The two largest fontanels are the anterior fontanel (between the frontal and parietal bones) and the posterior fontanel (between the parietal bones and occipital bone). The posterior fontanel usually closes between 1 and 2 months of age, whereas the anterior fontanel remains open until between 7 and 19 months of age (National Library of Medicine, 2015).

An infant's spine adapts as the child develops. At birth, the infant's spinal column is a C-shaped convex curve. As the infant learns to hold up his or her head, the cervical spine forms a concave curve. Likewise, as the infant starts to crawl and walk, the lumbar spine also forms a concave curve. This gives the spine its characteristic S-shape. This process usually takes about a year to complete. If the spine does not form these curves, the infant may have **kyphosis** (convex curvature) or **lordosis** (concave curvature), both of which can decrease mobility.

Long bones of children are also unique in that they contain cartilage between the epiphysis and diaphysis, called the **epiphyseal plate**. **Osteoblasts** (cells that produce the matrix for bone formation) at the epiphyseal plate work to produce new bone and deposit calcium to increase the length of the bone (secondary ossification), creating a bone that is more porous than adult bone. This is one reason calcium intake is vital for children and adolescents. Adequate calcium intake allows the body to form strong bones to prevent fractures and osteoporosis. The rapid bone growth in children allows fractures to heal more quickly, but it may also produce "growing pains" as the lengthening bones pull on the muscles. When individuals reach skeletal maturity between the ages of 18 and 25, the epiphyseal plates close and leave behind epiphyseal lines.

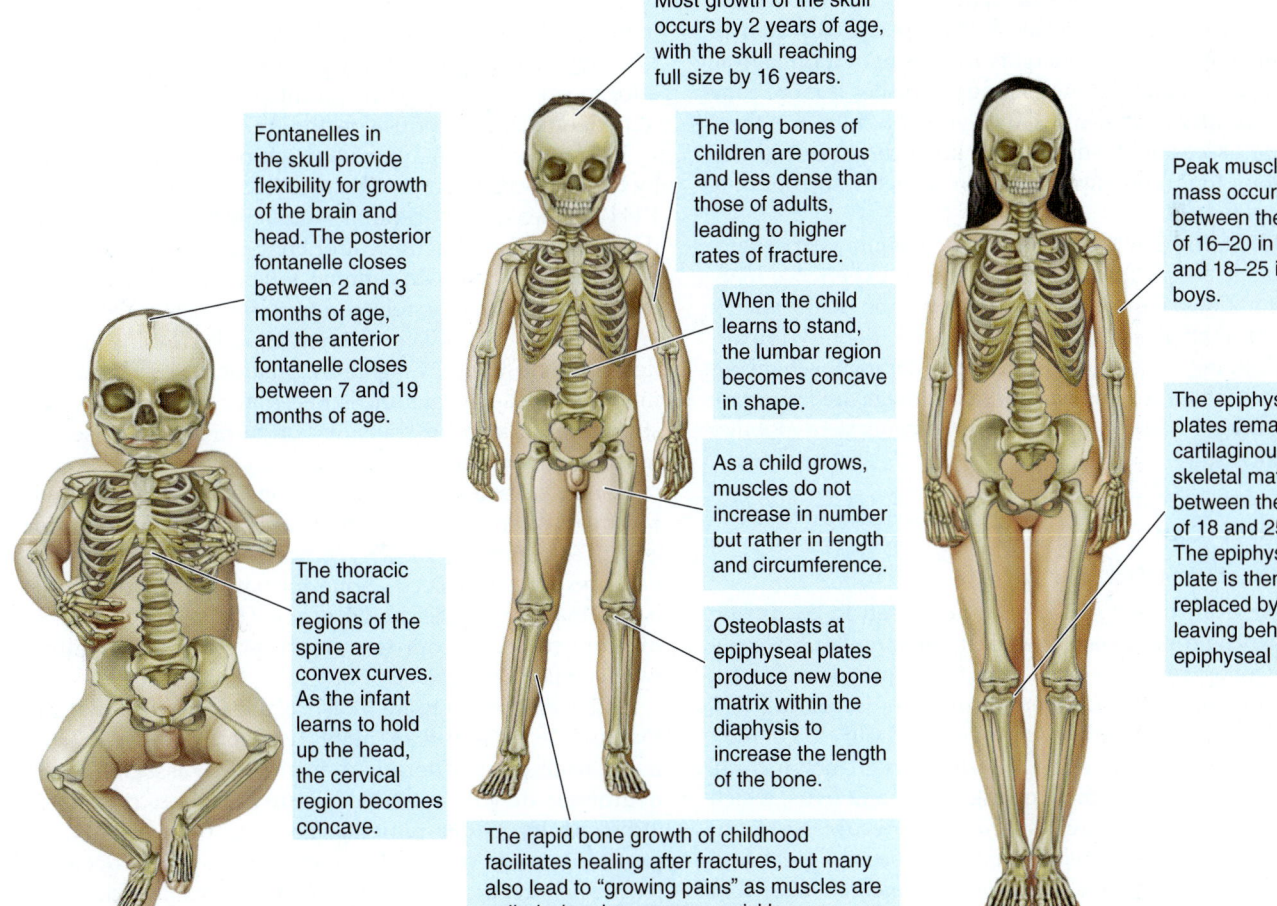

Most growth of the skull occurs by 2 years of age, with the skull reaching full size by 16 years.

Fontanelles in the skull provide flexibility for growth of the brain and head. The posterior fontanelle closes between 2 and 3 months of age, and the anterior fontanelle closes between 7 and 19 months of age.

The long bones of children are porous and less dense than those of adults, leading to higher rates of fracture.

When the child learns to stand, the lumbar region becomes concave in shape.

Peak muscle mass occurs between the ages of 16–20 in girls and 18–25 in boys.

The thoracic and sacral regions of the spine are convex curves. As the infant learns to hold up the head, the cervical region becomes concave.

As a child grows, muscles do not increase in number but rather in length and circumference.

The epiphyseal plates remain cartilaginous until skeletal maturity between the ages of 18 and 25. The epiphyseal plate is then replaced by bone, leaving behind an epiphyseal line.

Osteoblasts at epiphyseal plates produce new bone matrix within the diaphysis to increase the length of the bone.

The rapid bone growth of childhood facilitates healing after fractures, but many also lead to "growing pains" as muscles are pulled when bones grow quickly.

Figure 13–18 » Skeletal and muscle development throughout childhood.

An infant's spine also adapts as the child develops. At birth, the infant's spinal column is a C-shaped convex curve. As the infant learns to hold up his head, the cervical spine forms a concave curve. Similarly, as the infant starts to crawl and walk, the lumbar spine also forms a concave curve. This gives the spine its characteristic S-shape. This process usually takes about a year to complete. If the spine does not form these curves, the infant may suffer from kyphosis (convex curvature) or lordosis (concave curvature), both of which can decrease mobility.

Unlike the skeleton, muscles are almost completely formed at birth. Muscle growth occurs as **sarcomeres** (filaments made of actin or myosin) are added and lengthened in the muscle fibers; muscle fibers increase only in circumference and length, not in number. Skeletal muscle increases during childhood from about 25% of body weight at birth to 40–50% of body weight in adulthood, and boys and girls have equal amounts of muscle until around age 13–14. Muscle growth in girls continues until around age 16, with muscle mass peaking at ages 16–20. In contrast, muscles grow rapidly after age 13 and into late adolescence in boys, resulting in a growth period that is twice as long as that of girls, with muscle mass peaking at ages 18–25. Therefore, boys develop much more skeletal muscle than girls (Samour & King, 2013).

Certain alterations may be more prevalent among patients in specific age groups. For example, infants and children are most likely to have mobility alterations as a result of genetic disorders or congenital malformations. Assessment should be tailored to the specific disorder or malformation. Decreased mobility as a result of trauma from sports injuries, abuse, or motor vehicle crashes is more common in children, adolescents, and young adults. For these patients, assessment should focus on the specific area affected by the traumatic event, as well as the surrounding joints and tissues.

Children and adolescents in particular may experience body image and self-esteem issues if they experience long-term alterations of mobility, and these may be exacerbated if a physical malformation accompanies the mobility impairment. Ongoing assessment of stress and coping mechanisms as well as patient self-esteem and body image are important when working with children and adolescents with mobility impairments.

Mobility Considerations in Pregnant Women

Pregnant women will likely have decreased ROM during pregnancy, and back pain is a common complaint. Nearly 62% of women reporting back pain during pregnancy report the pain as moderately severe, with some reporting disabling back pain (Matthews, McConda, Lolli, & Daffner, 2015). Common causes of back pain in pregnancy include strain on the back from the growing uterus and fetus, which causes postural changes; abdominal weakness from stretched abdominal muscles, which may become weak and less able to support the spine; and hormonal changes that loosen the ligaments in the joints of the pelvis, causing instability and pain (American Congress of Obstetricians and Gynecologists, 2016). Back pain during pregnancy is managed

conservatively. The patient interview for pregnant women should include questions to determine if postural changes or other adaptations could increase mobility and decrease pain. The recommended pain medication is acetaminophen, as NSAIDS need to be avoided in pregnancy. Cauda equina syndrome (CES) is the only condition for which surgery is absolutely indicated for pregnant women (Matthews et al., 2015).

SAFETY ALERT Ultrasound and MRI are recommended during pregnancy, as they do not deliver ionizing radiation to the fetus.

Anticoagulation therapy may be needed for orthopedic injuries in pregnant women because of the hypercoagulable state of pregnancy and the potential immobility. Warfarin is contraindicated during pregnancy, as it may cause fetal hemorrhaging and/or abortion. Compression stockings and unfractionated heparin or low-molecular-weight heparin may be used during pregnancy (Matthews et al., 2015).

Mobility Considerations in Older Adults

After the skeleton has matured, bone remodeling continues throughout adulthood at a much slower rate. Bone **resorption** (the process by which bone is broken down and its minerals released into the blood) occurs when minerals stored in bones are needed for cellular processes, and bone formation (ossification) occurs when excess minerals are available. Bone stress also plays a role in the rate of bone remodeling; bones that are used frequently increase their rate of bone formation, whereas bones that are not used undergo a higher rate of bone resorption. These processes must remain in balance to preserve the structural integrity of the bone. Bone remodeling is also a critical factor in repair of bone injuries.

Hormones that regulate bone remodeling are controlled by blood calcium levels. When blood calcium levels are low, PTH is released to stimulate **osteoclast** (cell that breaks down bone tissue) activity and bone resorption to increase blood calcium levels. In contrast, when blood calcium levels are high, calcitonin is released to inhibit osteoclast activity and increase osteoblast activity, thus increasing mineral deposition in bones. Calcium regulation is a vital factor in mobility, because calcium is necessary not only for bone strength, but also for transmission of nerve impulses and muscle contraction.

Bones, muscles, joints, and connective tissue undergo many physiologic changes that decrease mobility in older adults (see **Figure 13–19** »). Bone density decreases as bone resorption exceeds bone formation, contributing to bones that are thinner and weaker. This increases the risk of bone fracture from trauma or overuse, especially in women after menopause.

Older adults are more likely to present with inflammatory and "wear-and-tear" mobility problems such as arthritis or back pain. Alterations in mobility associated with neurologic deficits, such as PD, are also more common in older adults. Older patients, patients with obesity, and patients who do not exercise regularly may have decreased ROM and strength or increased pain as a result of decreased muscle tone and stress on the joints.

Aging also produces changes in the spinal **discs**, which are located in between the vertebrae. Like ligaments, discs

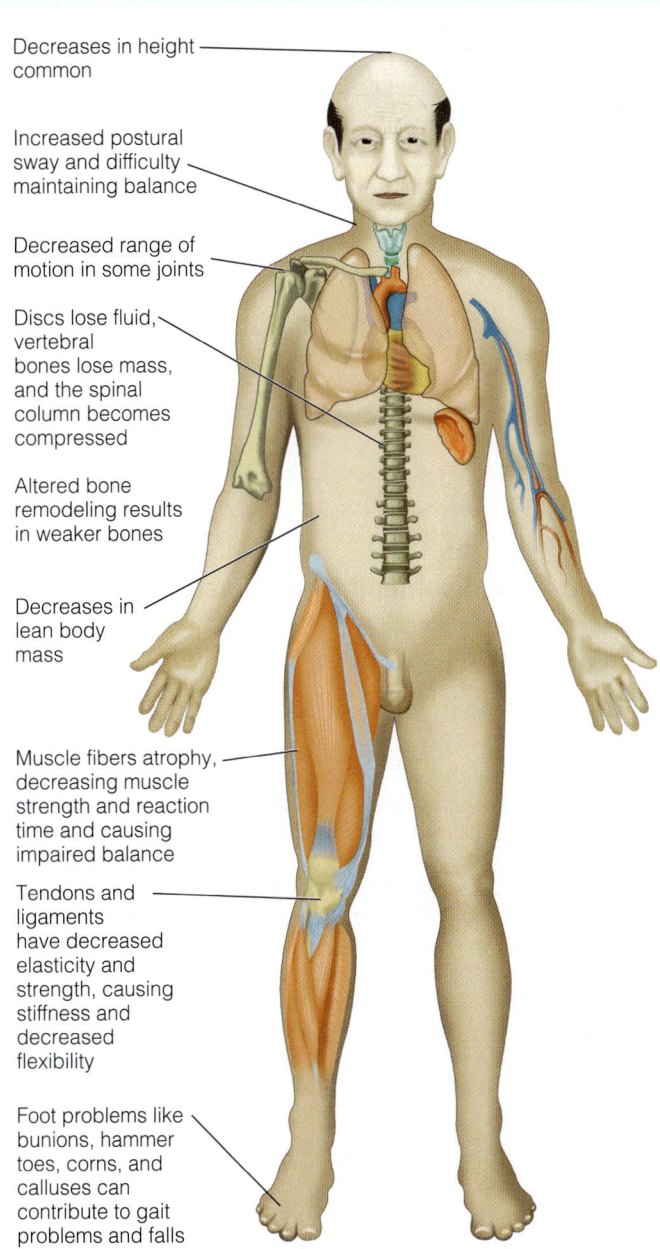

Decreases in height common

Increased postural sway and difficulty maintaining balance

Decreased range of motion in some joints

Discs lose fluid, vertebral bones lose mass, and the spinal column becomes compressed

Altered bone remodeling results in weaker bones

Decreases in lean body mass

Muscle fibers atrophy, decreasing muscle strength and reaction time and causing impaired balance

Tendons and ligaments have decreased elasticity and strength, causing stiffness and decreased flexibility

Foot problems like bunions, hammer toes, corns, and calluses can contribute to gait problems and falls

Figure 13–19 >> Normal changes of aging in the musculoskeletal system.

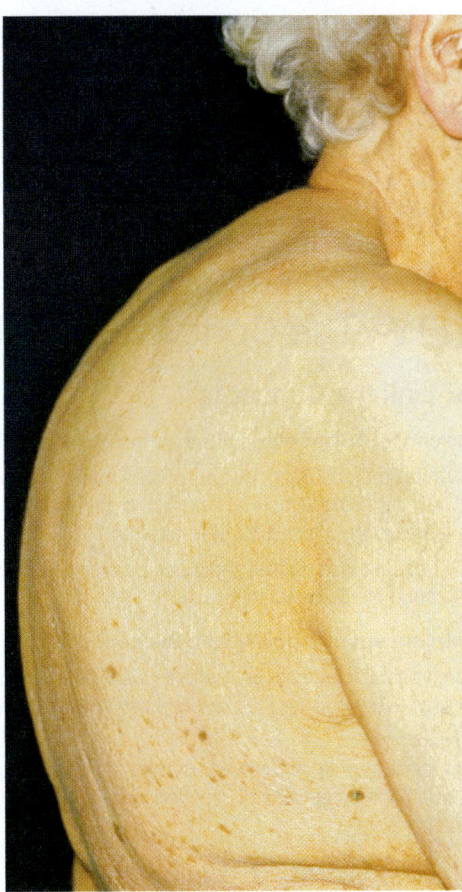

Source: Dr. P. Marazzi/Science Source.

Figure 13–20 >> Kyphosis (hunchback).

hold the vertebrae together. With their tough outer covering and fluid-filled center, discs serve as shock absorbers. Discs also allow the spine to be mobile. With aging, discs between the vertebrae lose fluid and become thinner. Combined with the decreased bone mass, disc changes lead to spinal column compression, resulting in shorter stature and stooped posture (see **Figure 13–20 >>**). Muscle fibers decrease, or **atrophy**, with age in a process called **sarcopenia**. This causes muscles to have less tone and decreased speed and power of contractions, partially as a result of changes in the nervous system, causing decreased muscle strength, slower reaction time, more rapid tiring, and impaired balance (Berman, Snyder, & Frandsen, 2016; Dugdale, 2012a).

Tendons and ligaments in joints have decreased elasticity, strength, and hydration, causing stiffness and decreased flexibility and ROM in the joints. Hips and knees may take

on a flexed position. Ligaments and tendons tear more easily and heal more slowly. Fluid in the joints may decrease, and cartilage may rub together and erode. This causes pain and inflammation and contributes to slow and unsteady movements, increasing the risk of falls (Berman et al., 2016; Dugdale, 2012a). These changes decrease activity tolerance in older adults, enhancing the effects of aging in the musculoskeletal system.

Case Study **>>** Part 3

The epidural cortisone injection that Mr. Hayes received for treatment of his herniated disc helped alleviate his numbness and tingling for approximately 3 weeks, but then the neurologic effects returned. Because of his severely limited mobility, Mr. Hayes has been unable to work. Within the past 2 days, he also has developed bowel and urinary incontinence. After an emergent office visit, Mr. Hayes's orthopedic spine surgeon diagnoses him with cauda equina syndrome (CES) and schedules him for an immediate discectomy, laminectomy, and spinal fusion. His surgery and anesthesia care are uneventful, with no reported complications. Twenty-four hours after the surgery, Mr. Hayes's vital signs include temperature 102.1°F oral; pulse 98 bpm; respirations 22/min; and BP 144/82 mmHg. He complains of moderate pain in his back, head, and left leg. His medications include codeine with ibuprofen for pain and inflammation.

Clinical Reasoning Questions Level I

1. What complication might Mr. Hayes's fever indicate? What priority nursing action should be implemented immediately?

2. Describe passive exercises that you can conduct with Mr. Hayes to help him maintain mobility while he is in the hospital.

3. What discharge instructions will you give Mr. Hayes when he is ready to return home?

Clinical Reasoning Questions Level II

4. Under what circumstances should you advocate for Mr. Hayes to receive additional pain medication?

5. What collaborative interventions will be beneficial in helping Mr. Hayes make a full recovery?

6. What independent nursing interventions can be implemented to promote comfort while Mr. Hayes is immobile?

REVIEW The Concept of Mobility

RELATE Link the Concepts

Linking the concept of mobility with the concept of development:

1. What exercise therapy might be appropriate for a 15-year-old male patient with a fractured tibia? How would the exercise regimen change if the patient were a 62-year-old man?

2. Describe patient teaching that should be provided to a 10-year-old female patient with juvenile arthritis.

Linking the concept of mobility with the concept of infection:

3. To which types of infections are patients with limited mobility more susceptible? What nursing interventions can help prevent infection in these patients?

4. Describe the elements of the nursing assessment that are used to identify signs and symptoms of infection for a patient with an open fracture.

READY Go to Volume 3: Clinical Nursing Skills

- SKILL 1.19 Musculoskeletal System: Assessing
- SKILL 1.22 Neurologic Status: Assessing
- SKILL 3.1 Pain in Newborn, Infant, Child, or Adult: Assessing
- SKILL 3.2 Pain Relief: Back Massage
- SKILL 3.3 Pain Relief: Complementary Health Approaches
- SKILL 9.1 Body Mechanics: Using
- SKILL 9.2 Range-of-Motion Exercises: Assisting
- SKILL 9.3 Ambulating Patient: Assisting
- SKILL 9.5 Logrolling Patient in Bed
- SKILL 9.13 Cane: Assisting
- SKILL 9.14 Crutches: Assisting
- SKILL 9.15 Walker: Assisting

- SKILL 15.1 Abuse: Newborn, Infant, Child, Older Adult: Assessing for
- SKILL 15.2 Fall Prevention: Assessing and Managing
- SKILL 15.5 Environmental Safety: Healthcare Facility, Community, Home

REFER Go to Pearson MyLab Nursing and eText

- Additional review materials
- MiniModule: Physiology of Mobility

REFLECT Apply Your Knowledge

Simone Addison, a 57-year-old woman, presents to an orthopedic clinic with complaints of pain with ambulation. As she is ambulating to the examination room, you notice that she has a steady gait without any assistive devices; however, she has a very notable limp as she ambulates. She tells you that she does not have insurance because she has a temporary job. She reports that she had started to run about 3 months ago in order to lose weight and become healthier. Over the past few weeks, she has experienced some pain in her left knee. She tells you that she has had an artificial left hip since she was a very young girl. Patient weight is 195 lb; height is 5'4".

The patient's left knee pain is reported to be from the introduction of running. The left knee image indicates normal findings. The orthopedist expresses surprise that Ms. Addison had a hip replacement at such a young age.

1. Discuss the issues that require collaboration with other healthcare professionals.

2. As a patient advocate, what actions may the nurse consider?

3. What are some appropriate nursing diagnoses for this patient?

4. What questions would you want to ask this patient to determine other potential nursing diagnoses?

» Exemplar 13.A Back Problems

Exemplar Learning Outcomes

13.A Analyze back problems as they relate to mobility.

- Describe the pathophysiology of back problems.
- Describe the etiology of back problems.
- Compare the risk factors for and prevention of back problems.
- Identify the clinical manifestations of back problems.
- Summarize diagnostic tests and therapies used by interprofessional teams in the collaborative care of an individual with back problems.

- Differentiate considerations for care of patients with back problems across the lifespan.
- Apply the nursing process in providing culturally competent care to an individual with back problems.

Exemplar Key Terms

Artificial disc surgery, *905*
Cauda equina syndrome (CES), *904*
Cobb angle, *910*
Discectomy, *905*

Exemplar Overview

Back pain is one of the most common medical problems in the United States. Approximately one out of four adults experiences at least 1 day of back pain within a 3-month period (National Institute of Arthritis and Musculoskeletal and Skin Diseases [NIAMSD], 2013). Back problems are associated with a decreased quality of life, including decreased mobility, increased pain and frustration, and loss of work hours. Although patients usually attribute back pain to a specific injury, back problems often result from years of improper bending, lifting, and standing, with one incident acting as "the straw that broke the camel's back."

Back problems are linked to certain lifestyle habits, including bad posture, low fitness level, smoking, athletic injuries, and occupational risk factors. Even children are susceptible to back pain as a result of carrying heavy backpacks. Diseases that contribute to back problems include degenerative disorders (spondylosis, spinal stenosis, osteoporosis), systemic disorders (osteomyelitis, osteoporosis, neoplasms), referred pain (gastrointestinal or genitourinary disorders, abdominal aortic aneurysms, hip pathology), and other disorders such as fibromyalgia and post–Lyme disease syndrome. Pregnancy is also a major cause of back pain based on changes in posture to compensate for increasing anterior weight. This exemplar focuses on two common causes of back problems: herniated discs and scoliosis.

HERNIATED DISC

A **herniated intervertebral disc** (also called a ruptured disc, slipped disc, or herniated nucleus pulposus) occurs when a spinal disc ruptures, allowing the fluid in the disc to leak out and irritate nearby nerves (see **Figure 13–21 》**). This also

causes a decrease in the ability of the disc to cushion the joints of the vertebrae, causing back pain and limiting mobility.

Pathophysiology and Etiology
Pathophysiology

Intervertebral discs lie between adjacent bones of the vertebral column. The outer annulus fibrosus is composed of strong fibrocartilage, whereas the inner nucleus pulposus contains loose fibers in a mucoprotein gel. These discs provide cushioning, shock absorption, and support for the vertebrae during movement. Herniation occurs when the nucleus pulposus protrudes through a compromised annulus fibrosus. This occurs most often in cervical and lumbar discs, but herniation of thoracic discs can occur as well. Herniation of a thoracic disc is a medical emergency that may result in paralysis.

Etiology

Loss of fluid content in the nucleus pulposus and increased susceptibility to tears in the annulus fibrosus occur with aging. This shrinks the disc, decreases its ability to absorb shock, and increases the risk of herniation. Because of the structure of the vertebral column and the pressure of body weight on the spine, herniation occurs most frequently at C5–C6, C6–C7, L4–L5, and L5–S1. Herniation may occur gradually because of degenerative changes such as OA or ankylosing spondylitis, or it may occur abruptly as a result of trauma such as lifting a heavy object or being in a motor vehicle crash. Abrupt herniation is associated with nerve root compression, severe pain, and muscle spasms. Gradual herniation usually results in a slow onset of pain and may be associated with neurologic symptoms such as weakness or tingling. If herniation occurs centrally rather than posterolaterally, it can put pressure on the spinal cord.

Risk Factors

Herniated discs are most common between the ages of 30 and 50, because discs naturally degenerate with age. Other risk factors for herniated discs include excess weight; regular heavy lifting, bending, and twisting; previous back problems; and smoking (NIAMSD, 2016). Genetic factors such as male gender, tall height, bone disorders, and degenerative disc disorders also contribute to increased risk of herniated discs.

Prevention

Prevention of herniated discs is primarily associated with good back care. This includes using good posture for sitting and standing, exercising regularly to keep back muscles strong, maintaining a healthy weight to decrease the pressure on the vertebral column, and using proper body mechanics (**Figure 13-22 》**). Weight-bearing exercises such as t'ai chi and yoga are a good place to start (NIAMSD,

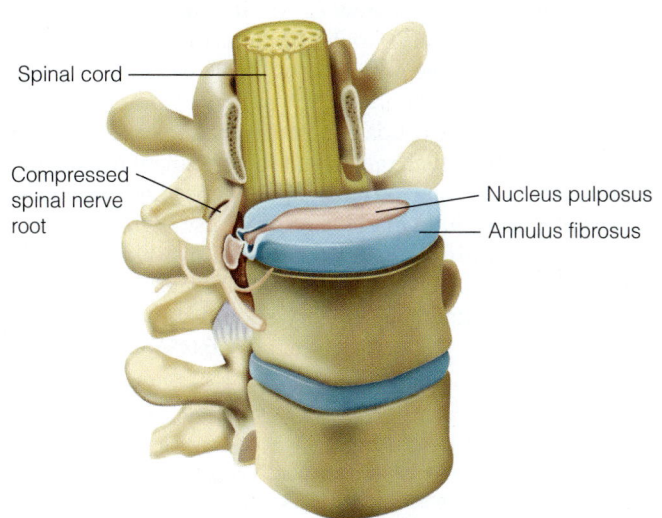

Figure 13–21 》 A herniated intervertebral disc. The herniated nucleus pulposus is applying pressure against the nerve root.

Spinal cord

Compressed spinal nerve root

Nucleus pulposus

Annulus fibrosus

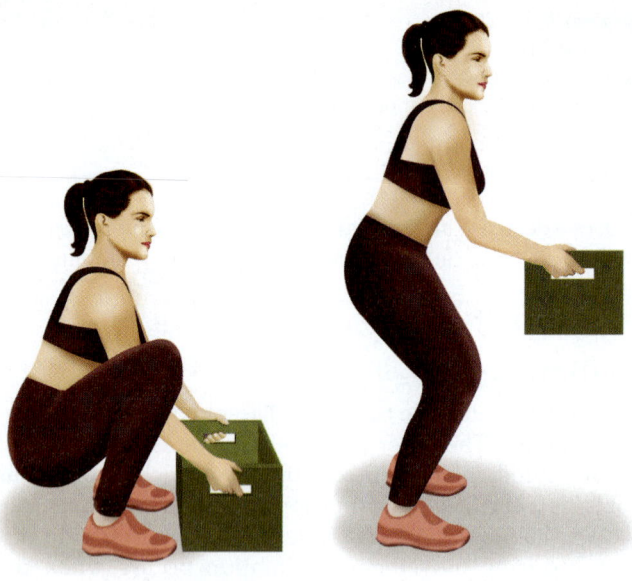

Source: Patricia Ladewig.

Figure 13–22 》 When picking up objects from floor level or lifting objects, it is important to use proper body mechanics.

2015). Use of proper body mechanics is especially important for pregnant women, who are highly susceptible to back pain because of the weight of the growing uterus and fetus.

Clinical Manifestations

Clinical manifestations of a herniated disc will depend on the severity and location of the herniation. The most common location of herniated discs is the lumbar region (L4–L5 and L5–S1), followed by the cervical region (C5–C6 and C6–C7).

If the herniated disc is not compressing a nerve, the patient may be asymptomatic. If nerve compression is present, clinical manifestations may include pain in the lower back, buttocks, thigh, and leg; numbness or tingling; and muscle weakness. The discs contain a jelly-like material; if a disc leaks, it may irritate the nerves and cause pain. The location of the symptoms depends on the area innervated by the compressed nerve (Mayo Clinic, 2014a).

Lumbar Discs

A herniated disc in the lumbar region may cause a condition called sciatica. **Sciatica** occurs when irritation or compression of all or part of the sciatic nerve, which originates in the lower back, produces pain and neurologic manifestations. The sciatic nerve is the longest nerve in the body and is made up of branches of the lumbar spinal nerve roots (see **Figure 13–23** 》). From its origin point in the lower back, the sciatic nerve divides into two main branches, each of which innervates one side of the lower portion of the body. On each side, one branch of the sciatic nerve travels through the pelvis, deep into the buttock, and then down the leg (Mayo Clinic, 2015c). Pressure on one or more of the lumbar nerve roots can also affect the sciatic nerve, leading to pain, burning, tingling, and numbness that radiates from the buttock into the leg and foot. Usually sciatica only affects one side of the body, and it may be more severe when standing, walking,

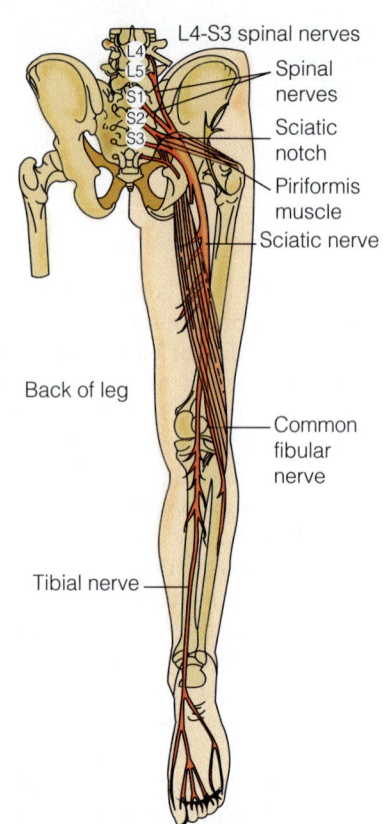

Figure 13–23 》 The sciatic nerve.

or sitting (Mayo Clinic, 2015c). Sciatica may also be aggravated by sneezing or coughing.

Other symptoms associated with lumbar disc herniation include a forward tilt to the trunk when standing and changes in mobility, motor function, and knee and ankle reflexes. Spinal changes may include an absence of normal lumbar lordosis or scoliosis of the lumbar spine. Some patients may experience muscle spasms and problems with sexual function.

The spinal cord does not extend through the entire spinal canal; rather, at approximately L1–L2, it branches into a bundle of free-flowing nerve roots. Because this portion of the spinal cord resembles a horse's tail, it is called the cauda equina, which means "horse's tail" in Latin. Compression of the nerve roots of the cauda equina can lead to **cauda equina syndrome (CES)**, which may result in permanent neurologic impairment, including urinary incontinence and paralysis. Causes of CES include massive lumbar disc herniation, spinal stenosis, epidural hematoma, epidural abscess, and trauma (Schiel, 2015). CES is a medical emergency (Mayo Clinic, 2014b). Immediate surgery should be performed to relieve pressure on the nerves (see the Safety Alert feature).

SAFETY ALERT Symptoms of CES include severe low back pain, bladder or bowel dysfunction, impaired sensation in the genital or saddle region, and sexual dysfunction. Although not always present, unilateral or bilateral sciatica may also occur. When the nerves are not completely compressed, any of the symptoms may be observed. When compression is complete, the presence of all of these symptoms is common (Schiel, 2015).

Cervical Discs

Similar to lumbar disc herniation, cervical disc herniation can result in numbness, tingling, muscle spasms, and weakness in the areas serviced by the affected nerves. A stiff neck is also a common feature of cervical disc herniation. In addition, neck and shoulder pain that shoots into the arm or fingers is likely present. The location and intensity of pain may depend on the movement of the neck and area of herniation (American Association of Neurological Surgeons [AANS], 2014). If a cervical disc compresses the spinal cord instead of a nerve root, symptoms in the lower body may be similar to those seen with lumbar disc herniation.

Collaboration

Care of a patient with a herniated disc includes identifying the herniated disc and determining a course of treatment. Nursing interventions are aimed at preparing the patient for diagnostic testing and teaching the patient about pharmacologic, nonpharmacologic, and surgical interventions. The nurse may need to collaborate with physicians, chiropractors, pharmacists, and PTs during care of a patient with a herniated disc.

Diagnostic Tests

In addition to a health history and physical exam, diagnosis of a herniated disc may include performing one or more diagnostic tests to rule out other causes of back pain. Tests may include mobility tests, imaging tests, and blood tests. Mobility tests include the straight-leg-raise test, gait tests, reflex tests, and muscle strength tests (Ogiela, 2012). These tests can help the physician determine the location, intensity, and cause of pain as well as the associated effects of the herniated disc or other back problems.

A CT scan is the most common imaging test that can conclusively identify a herniated disc, but an MRI may also be needed for more severe cases. A **myelogram**, during which dye is injected into the spinal fluid and visualized by x-ray, may be used to identify areas of pressure on the spinal cord or nerves due to herniated discs (Mayo Clinic, 2014a). Diagnostics may also include an **electromyogram**, which measures the electrical activity of the muscles at rest and during contraction. A nerve conduction study may be used to measure the speed of the electrical impulse through the nerve; this is helpful to identify damage and destruction (Johns Hopkins Medicine, n.d.a). Several blood tests can be used to test for inflammation, infection, and arthritis, including a complete blood count (CBC), erythrocyte sedimentation rate, C-reactive protein, and HLA-B27 (NIAMSD, 2016).

Surgery

Surgical treatment of a herniated disc is reserved for the most severe cases in which patients do not respond to other therapies. Other indications for spinal surgery include progressive leg weakness or numbness, loss of normal bowel and bladder functions, difficulty standing or walking, and back and leg pain that limits normal activity (AANS, 2014). The type of surgery chosen depends on the location of the disc and the integrity of the spinal column:

- A **laminectomy** is performed to remove the lamina, or the part of the vertebra that covers the spinal canal. This enlarges the spinal canal and relieves pressure on the associated nerves. During a **laminotomy**, which is a similar procedure, only a portion of the lamina is removed. A laminectomy or laminotomy is often performed in conjunction with other procedures, such as a discectomy or spinal fusion.

- A **discectomy** is performed to remove all or part of the herniated disc. Muscles and other tissues are dissected away from the spine to allow for surgical exposure of the ruptured disc. After removal of the disc, surrounding structures are returned to their natural positions. A microdiscectomy may be performed if there is no need for surgical intervention on bones, ligaments, or muscles. Compared to a discectomy, microdiscectomy requires a smaller incision and less disruption of tissues.

- **Spinal fusion** is performed to join two or more vertebrae together using bone grafts, screws, and rods. This prevents motion between the two vertebrae and reduces pain. Bone grafts are usually taken from the hip or pelvis. Tissue rejection may occur if donor bone is used. After spinal fusion, the fused area is immobile. Spinal fusion can be performed on the anterior spine by an incision in the patient's abdomen or on the posterior side by an incision in the patient's back.

- During an **artificial disc surgery**, a herniated disc is replaced with an artificial disc, similar to a traditional hip or knee replacement. This may be done as an alternative to spinal fusion to maintain flexibility of the spinal joint.

- Newer technology has allowed the use of laser surgery to treat herniated discs. During laser surgery, the surgeon inserts a needle into the disc and delivers laser energy to vaporize the tissue in the disc. This reduces the size of the disc and relieves pressure on the nerves. The usefulness of laser discectomy is still being debated (NIAMSD, 2013).

Pharmacologic Therapy

First-line therapy for a herniated disc includes NSAIDs to reduce pain and swelling. If the patient is experiencing neurologic problems such as numbness or sciatica, additional medications may include opioids for severe pain and antispasmodics to reduce muscle spasms (see the Medications feature and exemplar on Acute and Chronic Pain in the module on Comfort). Medications used to treat neuropathic pain, such as gabapentin (Neurontin), pregabalin (Lyrica), and duloxetine (Cymbalta), may also be useful for reducing pain related to nerve damage and have milder side effects compared to opioids. Tramadol (Ultram), which is a centrally acting opiate receptor agonist, may be used to treat moderate to severe pain. Epidural injection of cortisone/corticosteroids or anesthetics may also help reduce pain and inflammation (Mayo Clinic, 2014a). Nursing responsibilities include teaching the patient about dosing, side effects, and contraindications. If severe pain and neurologic symptoms are still present after 1–2 months, surgery may be considered.

Nonpharmacologic Therapy

There are many nonpharmacologic treatment options for individuals with herniated discs. Hot or cold packs can be used individually or alternately to dilate the blood vessels

Clinical Manifestations and Therapies
Herniated Disc

ETIOLOGY	CLINICAL MANIFESTATIONS	CLINICAL THERAPIES
Lumbar herniated disc	▪ The condition may have no symptoms if the disc is not pressing on a nerve. If the disc is pressing on a nerve root, manifestations may include pain in the hip, lower back, and lower extremities; sciatica; CES; limited mobility; muscle spasms; paresthesia of the lower extremities; foot drop; changes in knee and ankle reflexes; and inability to walk on the toes or sides of the feet.	▪ Application of heat or cold ▪ NSAIDs or other analgesics ▪ Antispasmodics ▪ Neuropathic pain medications ▪ Epidural cortisone injections ▪ Surgery ▪ Physical therapy ▪ Chiropractic therapy
Sciatica	▪ Manifestations include severe pain that radiates across the buttocks, down the leg, and into the knee or foot; and positive straight-leg-raise test.	▪ NSAIDs or other analgesics ▪ Antispasmodics ▪ Epidural cortisone injections ▪ Surgery ▪ Physical therapy
Cauda equina syndrome	▪ Manifestations include bowel and bladder incontinence associated with a herniated lumbar disc and paralysis of lower extremities.	▪ Emergency surgery to relieve pressure on the cauda equina
Cervical herniated disc	▪ The condition may have no symptoms if the disc is not pressing on a nerve. If the disc is pressing on a nerve root, manifestations may include pain in the neck, shoulders, and upper extremities; paresthesia in the upper extremities; decreased biceps and supinator reflexes; and hyperactive triceps reflex. If the disc is pressing on the spinal cord rather than nerve roots, the condition may cause neurologic deficits in the lower body.	▪ Application of heat or cold ▪ NSAIDs or other analgesics ▪ Antispasmodics ▪ Nerve pain medications ▪ Epidural cortisone injections ▪ Surgery ▪ Physical therapy ▪ Chiropractic therapy

and increase oxygen supply to the area (heat) or to reduce inflammation by decreasing blood flow to the area (cold). Patients with herniated discs should be encouraged to maintain their normal activities. Activity restrictions and strict bedrest are no longer recommended. Mild, low-impact exercise may be helpful to strengthen the back.

SAFETY ALERT Patients with herniated discs should consult a clinician before beginning an exercise regimen. Some exercises, especially those that require bending and twisting, may exacerbate symptoms.

Other forms of nonpharmacologic therapy may require collaboration with a healthcare professional, such as a PT or chiropractor. Patients may receive intradiscal electrothermal therapy, in which a needle is inserted into the disc and heated to thicken and seal the disc wall to prevent bulging. Chiropractic therapy uses spinal manipulation to adjust the spine and surrounding tissues, possibly reversing the protrusion of the nucleus pulposus. Massage therapy may benefit patients with herniated discs by relieving muscle tension, stiffness, and spasms and improving joint flexibility and ROM. The Clinical Manifestations and Therapies feature lists therapies that are used in treating herniated discs at different locations.

Lifespan Considerations
Herniated Discs in Children

Herniated discs are rare in children, although they have become more common and are often caused by trauma. Children with herniated discs may not experience back pain. Symptoms may include sciatica, numbness, tingling, or weakness in one or both legs. Treatment begins with physical therapy. If that is not effective, a discectomy may be necessary. Children often recover from this surgery better than adults, returning to school and activities quickly (Children's Healthcare of Atlanta, 2016).

Herniated Discs in Pregnant Women

Nearly half of women report back pain during pregnancy. Approximately 70% of the women with back pain during pregnancy reported the pain was severe, and about 9% reported complete disability related to the pain. A herniated disc is rare, however, occurring in about 1 in 10,000 pregnancies (Matthews et al., 2015). Most often the symptoms resolve after delivery.

Herniated Discs in Older Adults

Herniated discs are more common in younger adults. As people age, the jelly-like nucleus pulposus dries out and the space between the discs becomes smaller, making the discs unlikely to herniate (American Academy of Orthopaedic Surgeons [AAOS], 2012). Most older adults experience recovery similar to younger adults with nonsurgical interventions.

NURSING PROCESS

The primary goals of treatment for a patient with a herniated disc include relieving pain, healing the involved disc, and regaining mobility. The nurse's role in this process includes assessing the patient; providing information about procedures, medications, and therapies; encouraging and supporting the patient; and providing proficient nursing care before and after procedures.

Assessment

Nursing assessment begins with interviewing the patient regarding the primary complaint, then obtaining a health history. The health history should include the patient's description of the pain, previous back injuries or surgeries, current medications, risk factors for back pain, type of employment, and typical recreational activities. A physical assessment may include tests for muscle strength, coordination, gait and posture, sensation, and reflexes. The 5 *P*s neurovascular assessment may be used to determine neurovascular status. (See the 5 *P*s neurovascular assessment in the Concept of Mobility.)

Diagnosis

Nursing diagnoses for a patient with a herniated disc may include the following:

- *Injury, Risk for*
- *Mobility: Physical, Impaired*
- *Pain, Acute*
- *Pain, Chronic*
- *Sleep Pattern, Disturbed*
- *Knowledge, Deficient*
- *Role Performance, Ineffective.*

(NANDA-I © 2014)

Planning

Goals for a patient with a herniated disc may include the following:

- The patient will develop no motor deficits.
- The patient will develop no sensory deficits.
- The patient will remain free from infection.
- The patient will demonstrate normal bowel function, including the presence of bowel sounds in all quadrants.
- The patient will demonstrate normal urinary function, including urine production at a rate of at least 0.5 mL/kg/hr.
- The patient will report diminished pain to allow performance of ADLs.

- The patient will correctly verbalize proper use of medications for pain, inflammation, and muscle spasms.
- The patient will verbalize emotions and concerns related to all treatments, including invasive procedures.
- The patient will perform job responsibilities without work absences.

Implementation

Nursing interventions for patients with a herniated disc include promoting safety, preventing onset or exacerbation of neurologic deficits, providing adequate pain relief, and explaining treatment options. For patients who must undergo surgery, the general principles of nursing care of postsurgical patients apply, in addition to considerations that are specific to patients who undergo spinal surgery. (Also see the module on Perioperative Care.)

In outpatient settings, nurses will:

- Assess patients' neurologic and mobility status
- Assess patients' knowledge of diagnosis and understanding of the treatment regimen and provide patient teaching as necessary
- Assess patients' response to immobilization and other treatments and therapies, including stress and coping mechanisms.

In all settings, nurses will:

- Provide medication teaching
- Provide information about diagnostic procedures
- Teach patients about physical restrictions as ordered by the primary care provider.

In in-patient settings, nurses may perform additional interventions:

- Apply cervical collar as indicated
- Maintain spinal precautions as needed (do not twist or bend the spine until spinal injury has been ruled out)
- Administer pain medications as ordered
- Prepare patients for surgical procedures as appropriate
- Assess neurologic status following any procedures
- Provide postoperative assessments and instructions.

Prevent Injury

To prevent spinal injury and complications related to disruption of a surgical site, the nurse teaches patients to avoid bending and twisting. The nurse encourages patients to maintain body alignment that decreases stress on the vertebral column, such as flexing the hips when in the supine position; placing a small pillow under the knees (lumbar disc) or neck (cervical disc) to decrease pressure on the nerve roots; and using a firm mattress to support the spinal column. Patients with alterations in mobility should be assisted with positioning and ambulation.

Promote Comfort

For patients with pain related to a herniated disc, the nurse assesses pain on a 0–10 scale, with 0 representing no pain and 10 representing severe pain. The nurse reassesses pain following administration of pain medication. Adequate pain management may require a primary care provider's referral for physical therapy to develop a safe, but effective, exercise program. Exercise should strengthen muscles and increase mobility without increasing pain. For the patient with chronic back pain, counseling referrals may be necessary to treat frustration, depression, and anxiety. Because the patient with a herniated disc will receive care from multiple clinicians, adequate documentation is essential for maintaining continuity of care.

The nurse should also teach the patient about coping techniques for pain, including depending on others for help with ADLs, alternating rest and activity, and engaging in enjoyable activities. Adequate pain management and effective coping techniques are helpful in promoting adequate sleep–rest patterns. Inadequate sleep can amplify pain and increase frustration and irritability. See the exemplar on Acute and Chronic Pain in the module on Comfort for information on nonpharmacologic management of pain.

The nurse teaches patients about the purpose of medications, the expected response, possible side effects and adverse reactions, and safe administration. For example, steroids may be used to reduce inflammation. The nurse also teaches patients with diabetes how the medications may affect their blood glucose levels. The nurse provides information about complementary health approaches and assesses patients for use of herbal supplements that may be contraindicated with prescribed medications. During follow-up visits, the nurse evaluates patients' responses to medications and other methods used to minimize pain.

For patients in inpatient settings, the nurse will also:

- Monitor frequently for changes in symptoms that may indicate a worsening of the patient's condition, including alterations in mobility and sensation
- Administer pain medications as ordered around the clock or by a patient-controlled analgesic pump
- Reposition as indicated to promote comfort and reduce risk of skin breakdown
- Provide nonpharmacologic pain reduction measures.

Educate the Patient About Procedures and Treatments

Multiple procedures may be used to diagnose a herniated disc, including muscle, sensation, and reflex tests and imaging tests. In addition, multiple treatment options are available for herniated discs depending on the severity of symptoms and location of the herniation. All this information may be confusing to a patient and, coupled with moderate to severe pain, may increase the patient's anxiety. Therefore, a primary nursing responsibility when caring for a patient with a herniated disc is explaining diagnostic procedures and treatment options in a way that the patient will understand. This is especially important for invasive procedures that require injections (e.g., myelogram, cortisone injection) or surgery (e.g., discectomy, spinal fusion). Patients often feel increased anxiety about spinal procedures because of the risk of unintentional nerve damage and the fear of paralysis.

Interventions include:

- Assess for signs of anxiety, as heightened anxiety affects learning ability.
- Discuss the treatment plan as prescribed, and give the patient time to ask questions; provide information as indicated. (This may also help reduce anxiety.)
- Discuss the need for a ride home, as indicated for some outpatient procedures. For example, patients receiving epidural steroid injections require a driver, whereas patients receiving cortisone injections may be able to drive themselves home.

Provide Preoperative and Postoperative Care to the Surgical Patient

Nursing care of patients who require surgical treatment of a herniated disc includes both preoperative teaching and postoperative management of pain and care of the incision site. The nurse should demonstrate techniques that will be performed postoperatively and encourage the patient to practice the techniques. Logrolling, which maintains neutral alignment of the spine when turning, is performed by the nurse for the first day or two after surgery and then by the patient. This technique helps to prevent spinal injury and promotes proper healing of the spine. Deep breathing and an incentive spirometer are used to prevent respiratory complications, and leg exercises should be performed to prevent circulatory complications. A fracture bedpan is most comfortable for the patient who must remain flat in bed following surgery. Eating while lying flat is also a technique that the patient may want to practice, as this may be necessary postoperatively. The nurse should do the following:

- Promote wound healing by positioning and turning the patient appropriately and assessing the wound for hematomas, cerebrospinal fluid (CSF) leakage, and infection.
- Monitor the patient for nerve root compression or injury. Assess for hand, arm, and leg strength; the ability to move the fingers and toes and dorsiflex the foot; and the ability to detect touch, as appropriate.
- Monitor the patient for complications associated with surgery, including pain, urinary retention, respiratory and circulatory complications, and decreased mobility.

Evaluation

The patient should be evaluated frequently for progress toward identified outcomes. Satisfactory progress will include a reported decrease in the patient's pain, increased mobility, full ROM of joints, normal sensory perception, lack of neurologic deficits, and absence of infection and other complications from surgery.

SCOLIOSIS

Scoliosis is a lateral, or sideways, curve of the spine; it can be C-shaped or S-shaped. It is often noticed during the growth spurt just before puberty. Most cases of scoliosis are mild, but severe scoliosis can cause a rotation of the spine, leading to deformities and disability.

Pathophysiology and Etiology

Pathophysiology

A small degree of sideways curvature is found in many individuals. Scoliosis is diagnosed if the sideways curvature measures more than 10 degrees (see **Figure 13–24** ≫) (Mehlman, 2012). Mild scoliosis reflects a curve between 10 and 20 degrees, moderate scoliosis is a curve between 20 and 40 degrees, and severe scoliosis is a curve over 40 degrees. Scoliosis can be classified as either structural or nonstructural. *Nonstructural scoliosis* occurs as the spine bends to compensate for poor posture, differences in leg length, presence of tumors, adaptation to pain, or other physical conditions. Nonstructural scoliosis is usually corrected by alleviating the underlying cause of the curve. *Structural scoliosis* is a more severe form that involves deformities of the bones in the spinal column.

Etiology

Scoliosis of unknown etiology is called *idiopathic scoliosis*. Most often it is found between the age of 10 and the time of growth completion (AAOS, 2015a). Research suggests that idiopathic scoliosis may be the result of abnormal force exerted on the spine by surrounding connective tissues and muscles (Mehlman, 2012). *Congenital scoliosis* occurs when the individual is born with a curved spine. This usually results from incomplete formation or separation of the vertebrae, and it can be associated with other health issues such as heart and kidney problems. *Neuromuscular scoliosis* occurs when medical conditions that affect the nerves and muscles, such as cerebral palsy, MD, or SCI, lead to sideways curvature of the spine.

The most common curve pattern is a right thoracic curve (Mehlman, 2012). Left lumbar, right thoracolumbar, and double major curve patterns are also common. The lateral curvature of the spine causes several structural changes to the skeleton. As the curve worsens, the vertebrae rotate, causing a twisting of the spine. The ribs on the inside of the curve are forced closer together, and the ribs on the outside of the curve are spread farther apart (see Figure 13–24). This causes formation of the typical rib hump that is most obvious when the individual performs the Adam forward bend test. Likewise, the spinal disc spaces are narrowed on the inside curve and wider on the outside of the curve. This creates an asymmetric vertebral canal that may cause additional complications such as paresthesia.

Risk Factors

Adolescents are at greatest risk of developing scoliosis as they go through a growth spurt just before puberty, usually between the ages of 9 and 15. However, girls are more likely to progress to a greater curvature than boys (Mayo Clinic, 2016a). Of people with idiopathic scoliosis, about 30% are found to have a family history of scoliosis (AAOS, 2015a). Other risk factors for developing scoliosis include having a neuromuscular disorder such as cerebral palsy or MD and having a family history of scoliosis.

Clinical Manifestations

Common manifestations of scoliosis include a spinal curvature to one side, uneven hips or shoulders, differences in leg length, tiredness of the spine, a prominent shoulder blade, and a rib bump. Although not common, back pain may accompany scoliosis. Severe scoliosis may cause heart and lung problems such as difficulty breathing and pneumonia; compression of nerve roots may cause paralysis. Curvature of more than 100 degrees may increase mortality rates.

Mild curves of scoliosis (less than 20 degrees) often do not progress and do not need treatment. Moderate and severe curves (20 degrees to over 100 degrees) will require treatment, especially if the curve continues to progress. Scoliosis curves often worsen as the child grows; progression of curvature dramatically slows when the child stops growing. For girls, this is usually 2 years after the start of menstruation. For boys, growth usually stops in the late teens or early 20s. Curves usually progress only 0.5 to 1 degree per year or less in adults.

Types of Scoliosis

Congenital scoliosis is present at the time of birth. There is no known cause for congenital scoliosis; however, certain types of host and environmental factors have been identified (Zheng, Xin, & Jianxiong, 2015). Hypoxia and vitamin A deficiency are leading factors, and others that increase the risk include valproic acid, boric acid, hyperthermia, and alcohol use. Zheng and colleagues (2015) recommended further research to shed light on the epidemiology of congenital scoliosis.

Idiopathic scoliosis is classified as one of four types depending on the age of onset. Symptoms and risk factors may vary for each age group (Mehlman, 2012):

- *Infantile idiopathic scoliosis* occurs from birth to 3 years of age. It typically results in a left thoracic curve of the

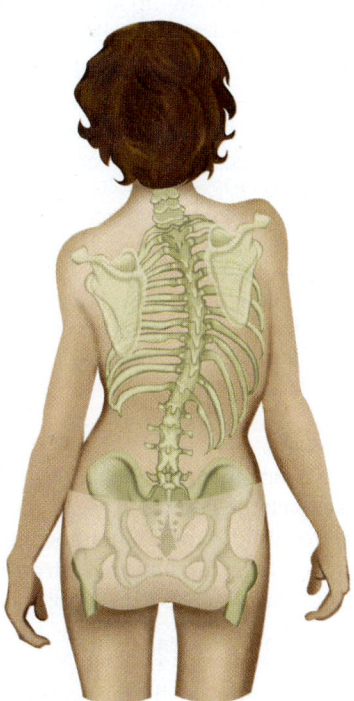

Figure 13–24 ≫ Scoliosis is diagnosed if the sideways curvature measures more than 10 degrees.

spine and is most commonly seen in boys of European descent. Infantile scoliosis may resolve as the child ages.

- *Juvenile idiopathic scoliosis* occurs in children between 3 and 9 years of age. Symptoms are similar to those of adolescent scoliosis. Children with juvenile idiopathic scoliosis are most likely to have progression of the curve and require surgery.

- *Adolescent idiopathic scoliosis* occurs in children between 10 and 19 years old. This is the most common type of scoliosis; progression of the curvature is seen more frequently in girls. Progression is more likely to occur in younger children with large curves than in older children with small curves.

- *Adult idiopathic scoliosis* may be present from childhood or may develop as a result of aging. Aging causes may be related to degenerative changes of the spine (often called adult degenerative scoliosis), osteoporosis, previous fractures, spondylolisthesis, infections, or tumors. Involvement of the entire spine, including the neck, is more common in adults than in children. Back pain and pain radiating down the legs is also more common in adults (Scoliosis Research Society, 2017).

Collaboration

Nursing care for patients with scoliosis ranges from periodic observation to surgical care. This is often achieved through collaboration with school nurses, physicians, surgeons, PTs, and the patient's family. The goal of treatment is to limit or stop the progression of the spinal curvature.

Diagnostic Tests

Most schools require scoliosis screenings for children between the ages of 10 and 15 years. One of the primary screening tests for scoliosis is the Adam forward bend test, in which the individual leans forward at the waist with the arms hanging straight down (see Figure 13–25). This allows the clinician to see the spine more clearly. In patients with scoliosis, the Adam test often causes an obvious rib hump, usually on the right side. However, the Adam test may be negative in some patients with scoliosis, so it should never be used as the only diagnostic test. A **scoliometer** can be used to measure the patient's rib hump when in the Adam position.

X-rays are the most common imaging test used to definitively diagnose scoliosis. Using an x-ray of the spine, physicians can determine the angle of the curve using the Cobb method (Cobb, 1948). The Cobb method uses lines drawn from the end vertebrae (the vertebrae at the upper and lower limits of the curve that tilt most dramatically toward the apex of the curve) to estimate the degree of curvature. The angle found at the intersection of the two lines is the **Cobb angle**. The degree of **vertical rotation** can be determined with the Nash-Moe method (Nash & Moe, 1969). In this method, a vertebra at the apex of the curve is divided into three equal segments on the half of the vertebra on the convex side of the curve. The location of the pedicle of the vertebra in relation to the segments determines the grade of rotation, with no rotation being the lowest and grade 4 rotation being the highest at over 90 degrees of rotation. Other imaging tests may include MRIs, CT scans, and bone scans.

Surgery

Surgical correction of scoliosis is available for patients with a Cobb angle of greater than 50 degrees. Surgery is usually performed only on patients whose curvature progression is not slowed by bracing and whose bones have stopped growing. If curve progression is severe (at least 45 degrees) before the child has stopped growing, surgeons may insert a rod that can be adjusted in length as the child grows; adjustments usually occur every 6 months (Mayo Clinic, 2016a). Scoliosis surgery involves spinal fusion combined with inserting metal rods on either side of the spine, which are held together by hooks, screws, and wires until the bone heals. Surgery can correct the lateral curvature of the spine, but it often does not correct the abnormal rotation of the spine.

After surgery, most patients will not require long-term therapy or postoperative casting. However, they will need to be on bedrest during the recovery period and may need to wear a brace such as a **thoracolumbar sacral orthosis (TLSO)**, also called the underarm brace or Boston brace, for several months to help support the spine. The TLSO is contoured to conform to the body and is almost invisible under the clothes. In severe cases, halo traction may be used to provide support for the spine. Complications of surgery may include bleeding, infection, nerve damage, and disc degeneration.

After spinal surgery, the patient will need to limit activities for 6–8 months. In addition, the patient will need to adapt to new body mechanics. Because spinal surgery involves fusion of the spine, the patient will need to learn to perform simple tasks without bending or twisting the torso. Nursing care should include teaching the patient how to move properly and confirming that the patient can independently perform ADLs. Collaboration with a PT is usually required. The nurse should emphasize the importance of following the treatment regimen, including wearing a supportive brace and attending follow-up appointments. The nurse should give written instructions to the patient and parents to promote adherence to the treatment plan.

SAFETY ALERT Infection related to spinal surgery that involves the spinal instrumentation and bone graft can compromise the outcome of the deformity correction and delay recovery. Clinical signs of deep wound infection include pain, persistent wound drainage, erythema, wound rupture, and a positive culture from a wound aspirate. The majority of postoperative wound infections occur between 3 days and 3 months (AANS, 2016). Deep wound infections can occur early or as late as 8 years after surgery. The most common spinal infections are Staphylococcus aureus and Escherichia coli (AANS, 2016).

Pharmacologic Therapy

Scoliosis usually is not treated with medication. If needed, patients can take over-the-counter (OTC) analgesics, such as acetaminophen, for mild pain. Pain associated with severe scoliosis or spinal surgery may require stronger pain medications, such as prescription NSAIDs or opioids.

Nonpharmacologic Therapy

Nonpharmacologic therapy will depend on the Cobb angle (angle of the spinal curvature viewed on frontal plane x-ray). Weiss, Turnbull, Tournavitis, and Borysov (2016) reported that, historically, patients with Cobb angles of 15–25 degrees were treated conservatively with physical therapy. For patients with Cobb angles between 20 and 40 degrees, medical management includes wearing a brace (Weiss et al., 2016). Patients with great than 40-degree angles were considered for spinal fusion surgery. Weiss and colleagues' review of the current literature found no evidence to support spinal fusion in the long term. Rather, the current evidence supports physical therapy and brace treatment.

The choice of brace will depend on the size and location of the curve. The two main types of braces are the TLSO and the Milwaukee brace (full torso brace). The TLSO is the most common type of brace worn both before and after surgery. The Milwaukee brace has a neck ring with rests for the chin and back of the head and wide bars in the front and back. This type of brace is more cumbersome than the TLSO, and compliance is a major problem. Therefore, it is used only when a TLSO is inadequate, such as for curvatures in the cervical spine (Mayo Clinic, 2016a). Braces should be worn between 12 and 23 hours per day; brace success increases with increasing time spent wearing the brace each day. This may be a difficult issue for some patients, because adoles-

cents who wear a brace for scoliosis may be at risk for altered self-image (see the Evidence-Based Practice feature).

Multiple studies have shown that alternative therapies such as chiropractic treatment, electrical stimulation, biofeedback, nutritional supplements, and exercise are ineffective in the treatment of scoliosis (Mayo Clinic, 2016a; Weiss et al., 2016).

Lifespan Considerations

Although scoliosis is most commonly found in childhood, it does have implications from the time it is found through adulthood.

Scoliosis in Children and Adolescents

Congenital scoliosis is a sideways curve that is present at birth. It is not often found until adolescence. Children born with congenital scoliosis may also have kidney or bladder problems. Congenital scoliosis is a rare type of scoliosis; however, it has a 75% chance of progressing without surgical intervention (Boston Children's Hospital, 2017).

Evidence-Based Practice
Adolescent Self-Image and Braces

Problem
Scoliosis is often diagnosed during middle and high school. Adolescents with moderate to severe curves that require surgery or bracing are at risk for disturbed body image.

Evidence
Carrasco and Ruiz (2016) completed a qualitative, phenomenologic, and hermeneutic study to explore the experience of young women, ages 15–22 years, living with a body deformity due to idiopathic adolescent scoliosis (IAS). Carrasco and Ruiz recognized that it is not uncommon for adolescents to be dissatisfied with their body image, even without scoliosis. Previous studies had shown that adolescents with scoliosis had difficulty with self-esteem, psychosocial aspects, and perceptions of health. A factor that may play an important piece in the aspect of self-esteem is the timing of deformity developments. During self-discovery, teenagers are learning about their bodies and experiencing growth and development; the development of a deformity is likely to affect self-esteem and mental health.

Twelve young women who were admitted to have surgical procedures for IAS volunteered for the phenomenologic study (Carrasco & Ruiz, 2016). During interviews, the women described dissatisfaction with their body appearance, voiced having social difficulties, and reported that the curvatures of scoliosis needed to be fixed. They described feeling different and trying to hide the deformity with clothing.

Because of feeling different, they reported experiencing anxiety, embarrassment, and guilt. Some personal comments included:

- [. . .] but I was ashamed or if I noticed it or if someone said anything . . . people who would see it . . . but no . . . luckily it wasn't that evident . . .
- My whole problem was aesthetic [. . .] I had a really bad time . . .
- It [was] very evident, because I'm very skinny so it showed a lot . . . so one of my bones was higher than the other and I couldn't wear some dresses

- Well . . . scoliosis in my life has been nothing but more problems . . . more inferiority complex, and that's it

Some women described their experiences with physical pain related to their curvatures as causing problems with their social lives. There were reports of not being able to participate in normal activities because of the pain. Some of their statements included:

- I [. . .] have had a hard time because of the pain [. . .] and the pain during the previous year . . . it was too much . . . no matter how much medicine I took
- I had a hard time, I would walk home for an hour and my ribs would hurt so much and sometimes I couldn't leave my house

Carrasco and Ruiz (2016) found that a significant concern for these women was the sense of inferiority and embarrassment due to their deformity. Living with scoliosis had a negative impact on the women's psychosocial domain and social relationships. The women saw surgery as a way to solve a problem and rid them of the deformity.

Implications
Adolescents, especially girls, are susceptible to poor self-image when faced with a visible deformity such as scoliosis and the treatment that goes with that diagnosis. Therefore, nurses and other healthcare professionals should create a comfortable atmosphere that encourages patients to share their fears and concerns. Emotional support should be a nursing priority when caring for an adolescent patient, and nurses should provide suggestions for ways in which the patient can build self-esteem and confidence.

Critical Thinking Application
Describe how a nurse can play a key role in providing support for patients with scoliosis after diagnosis. Consider ways in which a nurse can build self-esteem and confidence in a male patient versus a female patient. Identify signs or symptoms of low self-esteem that a nurse should look for in adolescent patients with scoliosis.

Clinical Manifestations and Therapies
Scoliosis

ETIOLOGY	CLINICAL MANIFESTATIONS	CLINICAL THERAPIES
Mild scoliosis	■ Spinal curvature with a Cobb angle 15–25 degrees	■ Observation every 3–6 months ■ Physical therapy
Moderate scoliosis	■ Spinal curvature with a Cobb angle between 20 and 40 degrees; uneven hips or shoulders; differences in leg length; tiredness of the spine	■ Bracing for 12–23 hours per day with a TLSO or Milwaukee brace ■ Counseling or support groups ■ Mild pain medications
Severe scoliosis	■ Spinal curvature with a Cobb angle of greater than 40 degrees; prominent shoulder blade and/or rib bump; back and leg pain; difficulty breathing; nerve root compression	■ Surgical correction of the curve ■ Bracing after surgery with a TLSO brace ■ Nonopioid or opioid analgesics ■ Counseling or support groups ■ Physical therapy

Scoliosis in Pregnant Women

Scoliosis in the mother does not increase risk factors for the fetus during pregnancy or the mother's pregnancy risk factors. The physician and other healthcare providers should know the mother's diagnosis of scoliosis, as it may affect procedures such as an epidural during the labor process. A surgically placed rod may make it impossible to have an epidural, as some physicians will refuse to place an epidural with the presence of a rod. However, the rod does not prevent pregnancy. Patients with or without spinal fusions may experience more back pain than patients without scoliosis.

Scoliosis in Adults and Older Adults

Although most types of scoliosis are diagnosed in childhood and adolescence, myopathic deformity and secondary scoliosis may develop in adulthood (see **Table 13–3** »).

TABLE 13–3 Types of Scoliosis in Adults

Type	Cause	Characteristics
Idiopathic curve	No known cause	Most common type
Congenital curve	Present at birth; patient born with it	May not be recognized during childhood May worsen with age because of wear and tear
Paralytic curve	Often caused by SCIs that result in paralysis	Develops over time because of muscles around the spine not working
Myopathic deformity	May result from muscular disease (MD, polio, cerebral palsy)	Similar to paralytic curve, as it develops over time because of muscles around the spine not working properly
Secondary scoliosis	Secondary, caused by another spinal condition (degeneration, osteoporosis, imbalance of spine)	Develops over time

Treatment of scoliosis in adults begins with conservative measures similar to those used for adolescents, including physical therapy, exercise, and braces. Surgery is considered as a last resort. As patients with IAS age, they are more likely to experience chronic or acute back pain than patients without IAS (Scoliosis Research Society, 2017).

NURSING PROCESS

Nursing care for a patient with scoliosis may include teaching the patient and family about scoliosis and its treatment options, monitoring curvature progression, providing emotional support, and caring for the patient before and after surgery.

Assessment

Assessment of a patient with scoliosis includes a health history and physical examination. The health history should include identifying any family history of scoliosis, because individuals with parents or siblings with scoliosis are at higher risk for developing the disorder. It should also include a history of past spinal problems and assessment of other symptoms such as back pain.

A physical examination should include scoliosis screening and referral for diagnostic tests. The initial scoliosis screening is often performed by a school nurse for children in middle and high school. Girls are often screened twice; boys are usually screened once. A scoliosis screening includes several visual examinations:

- When the patient is standing, determine whether the head is centered; whether the hips, shoulders, or rib cage appears uneven; whether one shoulder blade is more prominent; whether the legs are the same length; or whether the body leans to one side. Closely assess the spine to determine whether it appears to be straight.
- When the patient is in the Adam position, assess the spine for obvious curvature, a rib hump, or asymmetry of the back. The physical examination should include palpation

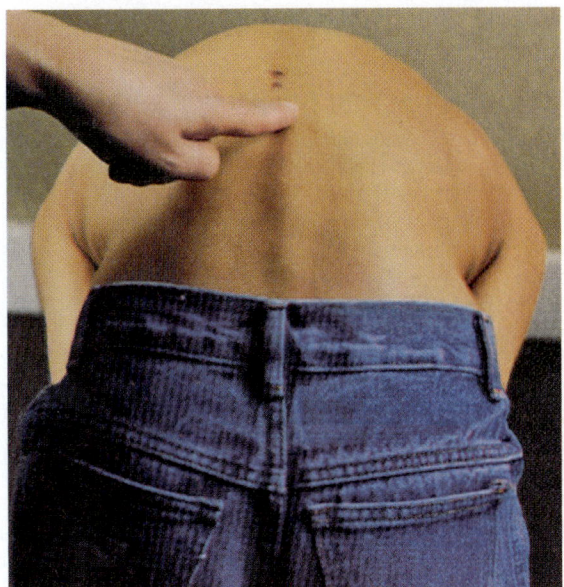

Source: George Dodson/Pearson Education, Inc.

Figure 13–25 ❯❯ Inspection of the spine for scoliosis. Ask the child to slowly bend forward at the waist, with arms extended toward the floor. Run your forefinger down the spinal processes, palpating each vertebra for a change in alignment. A lateral curve to the spine or a one-sided rib hump is an indication of scoliosis.

of each vertebra to detect abnormal alignment of the spine that may not be visible (see **Figure 13–25** ❯❯). If any abnormalities are detected, use a scoliometer to measure the deformity while the patient is in the Adam position.

Patients with a spine curvature greater than 10 degrees should be monitored every 6 months for curvature progression. If the curve appears to progress dramatically, the patient should be referred to a physician for follow-up.

Diagnosis

Nursing diagnoses related to patients with scoliosis may include the following:

- *Breathing Pattern, Ineffective*
- *Skin Integrity, Risk for Impaired*
- *Mobility: Physical, Impaired*
- *Activity Intolerance, Risk for*
- *Knowledge, Deficient*
- *Body Image, Disturbed*
- *Self-Esteem, Risk for Chronic Low*
- *Coping, Ineffective*
- *Social Isolation.*

(NANDA-I © 2014)

Planning

Expected outcomes for patients with scoliosis may include the following:

- The patient will demonstrate effective breathing patterns as evidenced by adequate oxygenation and activity tolerance.

- The patient and family will express understanding of treatment options appropriate for severity of spine curvature.
- The patient will report compliance with prescribed brace wear.
- The patient will state the importance of follow-up every 6 months.
- The patient will communicate fears and emotions about diagnosis and treatment.
- The patient's curvature will not progress during treatment with the brace.

Patients who undergo surgery for scoliosis will have additional outcomes related to surgical procedures:

- The patient will demonstrate proficiency with breathing exercises.
- The patient will demonstrate no manifestations of neurologic impairment.
- The patient will demonstrate no signs or symptoms of postoperative infection.
- The patient will accurately describe surgical procedure and postoperative expectations.
- The patient will verbalize understanding of the importance of limiting activities after surgery.

Implementation

Nursing interventions for patients with scoliosis will depend on the degree of curvature and the proposed treatment. For patients with mild scoliosis who require observation without medical treatment, nursing interventions may include emotional support, teaching about the importance of attending regular follow-up appointments, and teaching proper body mechanics. For patients with moderate scoliosis who require bracing, nursing care will additionally include teaching the patient about brace wear and care, emphasizing the importance of wearing the brace for the prescribed amount of time each day, encouraging the patient to maintain social interactions, and teaching the patient about clothing that can help disguise the presence of the brace. Care of patients who undergo surgery will likely incorporate the nursing interventions indicated in the care of patients with mild and moderate scoliosis, as well as nursing interventions related to preoperative and postoperative care. For all patients, referral to community support groups or to an individual who has had similar treatment for scoliosis may be beneficial.

Evaluation

Evaluation of the patient with scoliosis will include regular assessment of the curvature of the spine as well as assessment of the skin under the brace to confirm skin integrity. Evaluation should also include interviewing the patient about compliance with brace wear and self-image problems. During long-term care of the patient with scoliosis, the patient's needs will change significantly based on the patient's physiologic response to care, as well as his or her ability to cope with the challenges associated with this disorder. The nursing care plan should be revised and updated to reflect the patient's current needs, including those within the psychosocial realm.

❯❯ Go to **Pearson MyLab Nursing and eText** to see Chart 1: Nursing Care Plan: A Child Undergoing Scoliosis Surgery.

REVIEW Back Problems

RELATE Link the Concepts and Exemplars

Linking the exemplar of back problems with the concept of addiction:

1. What focused assessment should the nurse implement for a patient with chronic back problems who has been taking Percocet for pain?

2. A 46-year-old female patient diagnosed with back problems was admitted last evening with an alcohol overdose. What is the priority of nursing care for this patient?

Linking the exemplar of back problems with the concept of family:

3. Patients with reduced mobility related to back problems often require care from family members. Describe methods to relieve caregiver role strain for parents caring for a child, a partner caring for a partner, and adult daughters and sons caring for older parents.

4. How can the nurse advocate for a child with scoliosis whose parents do not agree with the treatment plan?

READY Go to Volume 3: Clinical Nursing Skills

REFER Go to Pearson MyLab Nursing and eText

- Additional review materials
- Chart 1: Nursing Care Plan: A Child Undergoing Scoliosis Surgery

REFLECT Apply Your Knowledge

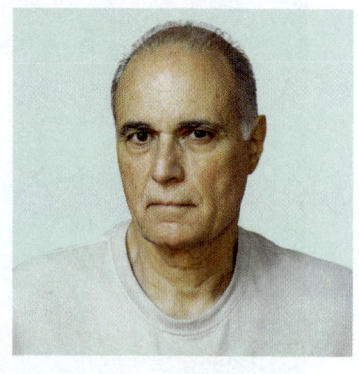

Gilbert Martin is a 53-year-old man who is married to Helen Martin. Mr. Martin has a son from a previous marriage and a stepdaughter whom he has raised since she was 3 years old. Mr. Martin's father recently passed away, so he has been helping his mother manage her affairs. Mr. Martin works as a delivery truck driver for a construction company. His job includes assisting with the loading and unloading of construction materials. Mr. Martin considers himself to be in good health, with the exception of chronic back pain. Mr. Martin also has hyperlipidemia, for which he takes atorvastatin (Lipitor) 20 mg/day. Mr. Martin sees his primary care provider once a year for triglyceride and liver function tests and has been encouraged to follow a low-fat diet.

1. What nonpharmacologic interventions may be implemented to help Mr. Martin reduce his chronic back pain?

2. What factors place Mr. Martin at risk for exacerbation of his back problems?

3. Describe how the stress in Mr. Martin's life may be affecting his chronic low back pain.

≫ Exemplar 13.B Fractures

Exemplar Learning Outcomes

13.B Analyze fractures as they relate to mobility.

- Describe the pathophysiology of fractures.
- Describe the etiology of fractures.
- Compare the risk factors for and prevention of fractures.
- Identify the clinical manifestations of fractures.
- Summarize diagnostic tests and therapies used by interprofessional teams in the collaborative care of an individual with a fracture.
- Differentiate considerations for care of patients with fractures across the lifespan.
- Apply the nursing process in providing culturally competent care to an individual with fractures.

Exemplar Key Terms

Cast, *921*
Compartment syndrome, *917*
Deep venous thrombosis (DVT), *917*
Delayed union, *916*
Fracture, *914*
Malunion, *916*
Nonunion, *916*
Open reduction and internal fixation (ORIF), *920*
Reduction, *920*
Splint, *921*
Traction, *921*

Overview

A bone **fracture** is a break in the continuity of a bone. Fractures are most common in patients who have experienced trauma and in older adults. Fractures vary in type, location, and severity.

Pathophysiology and Etiology

Pathophysiology

Humans are born with at least 270 bones, some of which fuse together to form the 206 bones found in an adult body. Any of these bones can be fractured. Fractures can be classified according to the break pattern of the bone (see **Figure 13–26 ≫**).

Etiology

Two main factors contribute to development of a fracture: the strength of the force acting against the bone and the strength of the bone. When the force acting on the bone is greater than the bone strength, the bone will fracture. The force acting on the bone may be a direct blow, compression, twisting, trauma such as a fall, or repetitive forces such as running. Single large forces are likely to cause bone fractures at the point of impact

Closed

- Bone breaks but skin remains intact.
- Also called a simple fracture.

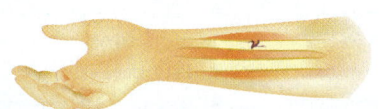

Open

- Bone breaks and protrudes through the skin; increased risk of osteomyelitis,
- Also called a compound fracture.

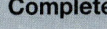
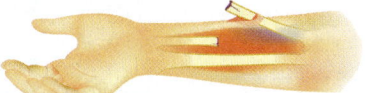

Complete

- Fracture involves the entire width of the bone.

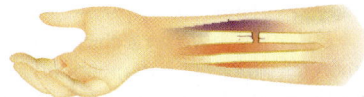

Greenstick

- Bone fragments are still partially joined.
- Also called an incomplete fracture.
- Occurs commonly in children.

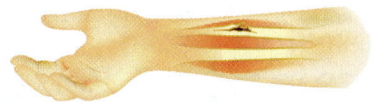

Comminuted

- Bone fragments into many pieces.
- Common in individuals with brittle bones, such as patients with osteogenesis imperfecta.

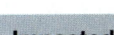

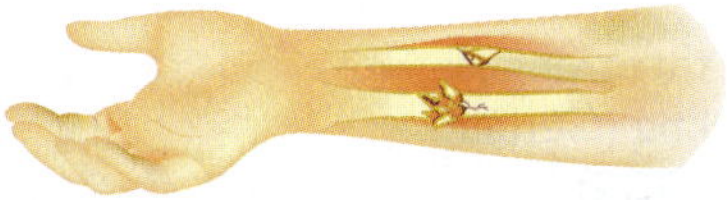

Impacted

- The two ends of the bone are forced together.
- Also called a buckle fracture.
- Often seen with children's arm and hip fractures.

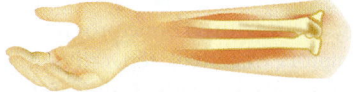

Oblique

- Fracture occurs diagonal to the bone's axis.

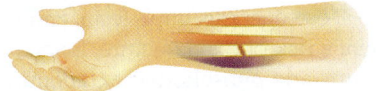

Transverse

- Fracture occurs at a right angle to the bone's axis.

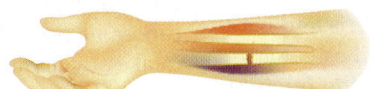

Linear

- Fracture occurs parallel to the bone's axis.

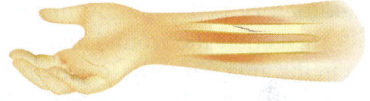

Displaced

- Broken ends of bones move out of correct anatomical alignment.
- Also called an unstable fracture.
- Requires immediate attention to prevent further damage.

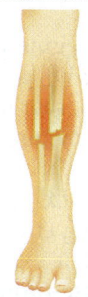

Nondisplaced

- Broken ends of bones remain aligned.
- Also called a stable fracture.

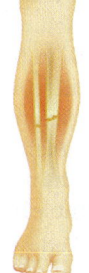

Avulsion

- A fragment of bone is separated from the rest of the bone.
- May also involve displacement of surrounding tissues.

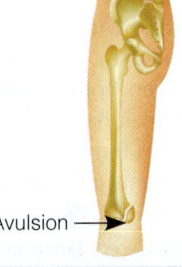

Avulsion →

Stress

- Caused by small repetitive forces on the bone.
- Often caused by participation in sports or exercise.

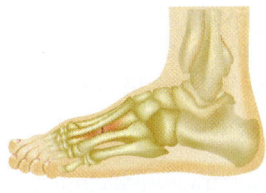

Spiral

- Fracture spirals around the bone.
- Occurs as the result of a twisting force, often during sports.
- Occurs commonly in children.

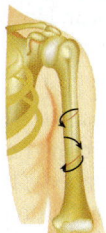

Depression

- Bone is forced inward.
- Occurs commonly in skull fractures.

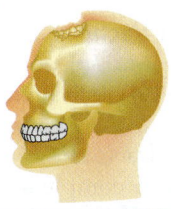

Pathologic

- Caused by a disease that weakens the bone such as osteoporosis, bone cancer, and osteogenesis imperfecta.

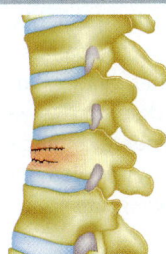

Compression

- Bone is crushed; occurs most commonly in vertebrae.
- Common in patients with osteoporosis.

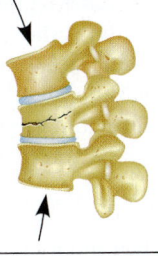

Compressed

Figure 13–26 》 Common fractures.

(direct force), whereas small repetitive forces are likely to cause fractures at the weakest point of the affected bone (indirect force). The strength of the bone is related to the individual's nutritional status as well as the presence of pathologic conditions such as osteoporosis, bone cancer, or Paget disease.

SAFETY ALERT When a child presents with a fracture that is uncommon for his or her age group, abuse should be suspected. However, because a fracture does not always imply abuse, the nurse should tactfully interview the patient and caregiver and follow institutional protocols for further investigation when abuse is suspected. During the interview, the nurse should consider this question: Does the story match the injury?

Fracture Healing

Healing of a fractured bone progresses through three stages: inflammatory (reactive), reparative, and remodeling (Gerber, 2015; Pountos, Georgouli, Calori, & Giannoudis, 2012).

- In the *inflammatory (reactive) phase,* damage to the bone, blood vessels, and surrounding tissues causes bleeding and the formation of a hematoma around the injury. Inflammatory cells, mainly macrophages and neutrophils, then enter the wound and degrade debris and bacteria in the area. This phase usually lasts until osteoblasts and endothelial cells begin to proliferate at the fracture site, usually a few days.

- In the *reparative phase,* fibroblasts, osteoblasts, and chondroblasts begin to secrete collagen to form fibrocartilage, which develops into a soft callus that joins the fractured bone. Endothelial cells begin to form blood vessels in the damaged area. Once the soft callus is formed, it is replaced by woven bone through endochondral ossification, which forms a hard callus. This woven bone is immature bone with a random collagen and bone structure. The reparative phase usually lasts 6–8 weeks for relatively simple fractures.

- In the *remodeling phase,* woven bone is replaced by highly organized lamellar bone. Lamellar bone is stronger and more compact, with better blood circulation compared to woven bone. Because bones are being continually remodeled, bone fractures usually heal without a scar. However, it may be several years before the bone returns to its original strength.

A bone that fractures and undergoes normal healing is called a union. Multiple factors can influence bone healing (see **Table 13–4 ⟩⟩**). If the bone does not heal properly, it may be classified as a delayed union, nonunion, or malunion. A **nonunion** is a fracture that shows no clinically significant progress toward complete healing for at least 3 months based on x-rays. This may occur at any point along the healing process. A **delayed union** occurs when the healing process takes significantly longer than expected. Healing time is related to the size of the bone. Phalanges typically heal in about 3 weeks, whereas femur fractures take about 12 weeks (Schubert, n.d.). A **malunion** occurs when the bone fragments join in a position that is not anatomically correct. Nonunions and malunions may need to be surgically corrected.

Risk Factors

The primary risk factors associated with bone fractures are age, presence of bone disease, and poor nutrition. Younger patients are more likely to sustain fractures related to sports injuries,

TABLE 13–4 Factors Influencing Bone Healing

Location	Positive Factors	Negative Factors
Local	■ Immobilization ■ Timely correction of displacement ■ Application of ice ■ Electrical stimulation	■ Open fracture ■ Delay in correction of displacement ■ Deep bone infection ■ Presence of foreign body in fracture
Systemic	■ Adequate growth hormone, vitamin D, and calcium ■ Adequate blood supply ■ Absence of infection or disease ■ Younger age ■ Moderate activity level prior to injury	■ Malnutrition ■ Immunocompromised status ■ Decreased circulation (as in diabetes and peripheral vascular disease) ■ Advanced age ■ Osteoporosis

whereas older patients are at higher risk of fractures related to falls and disease. Bone diseases that decrease the strength of the bone, such as osteoporosis, osteogenesis imperfecta, and bone cancer, increase the patient's risk of bone fracture. Inadequate intake of vitamin D, calcium, and phosphorus also contributes to poor bone strength. Lifestyle habits, such as participation in dangerous activities, can also increase the risk of fracture.

Prevention

Fracture prevention begins with education. Children and young adults should be taught the importance of using safety equipment (e.g., seat belts, helmets, knee and elbow pads) to help prevent fractures. Practicing good lifestyle habits (e.g., exercising regularly, maintaining a healthy weight) can also increase bone strength and prevent fractures.

Creating a safe living environment is also key to the prevention of fractures. For example, parents of toddlers and young children can use protective gates at stairways, and older adults in particular can remove rugs and clutter that increase the risk for falls. Older adults should also have regular screenings for osteoporosis and risk assessments for falls. Osteoporosis screenings are particularly important for women after menopause, because the loss of estrogen during menopause decreases calcium absorption and increases the risk for osteoporosis. For more teaching points to help older adults prevent falls and fractures, see the Patient Teaching feature.

Clinical Manifestations

Clinical manifestations of bone fracture include pain due to tissue trauma and a visible fracture on an x-ray. Pain is generally due to an interruption in the continuity of the bone; damage to ligaments, tendons, and other surrounding tissues; and muscle spasms. Depending on the severity of the fracture, other manifestations may include visible deformity if the bone is displaced, swelling from inflammation, and numbness due to nerve damage. Internal or external loss of blood may result in hypovolemic shock or ecchymosis. If the fractured pieces of bone grate against each other, crepitus may be heard.

Complications

Complications associated with fractures include compartment syndrome, deep venous thrombosis (DVT), fat emboli,

Patient Teaching

Fall Prevention in Older Adults

Several lifestyle changes can help older adults decrease their risk of fractures related to falls. If needed, a nurse can visit the patient's home to perform an environmental safety assessment.

- Start a mild or moderate exercise program to help improve balance and strength.
- Wear sensible shoes with nonslip soles and good support, both inside and outside the house.
- Walk slowly and carefully in areas that may be slippery, including icy or wet surfaces or polished floors. Use a walker or cane if needed for extra stability. Avoid walking in socks or slippers that lack traction.
- Ask a physician or pharmacist how medications may affect balance and alertness or change bone or muscle strength.
- Make sure hallways and stairways have adequate lighting, even at night. Make room lights, lamps, and flashlights easily accessible.
- Keep rooms free of clutter, including clothing, paper, electric cords, and throw rugs.
- Install handrails on stairs and around the toilet and bathtub. Also place a rubber mat in the tub or shower.
- Avoid using a stepstool if possible. If necessary, use a sturdy stepstool with a wide base and handrail for balance.
- Seek treatment for health conditions that may affect bone or muscle strength, neuronal control of muscles, balance, or vision loss.

infection, or loss of sensation. Development of complications depends on the type and severity of fracture and the patient's personal factors.

Compartment Syndrome

Individual muscles are surrounded by fascia, and the muscle tissue, nerves, and blood vessels within the fascia are part of a compartment. Fasciae are designed to hold the muscle in place; therefore, they do not expand, and pressure can build up within the compartment. **Compartment syndrome** occurs when edema and swelling cause increased pressure in a muscle compartment, leading to decreased blood flow and potential muscle and nerve damage (Ma, 2016b). Decreased blood flow leads to dilation of the blood vessels, causing more edema and stimulating a cycle of continually increasing pressure in the limb. If ischemia to the compartment continues for a significant length of time, the muscles and nerves may die, and the limb may need to be amputated.

Symptoms of compartment syndrome include severe pain and tenderness, swelling, paresthesia, pallor, numbness or paralysis, and decreased or absent pulse and poikilothermia (normalization to room temperature) in the distal portion of the affected limb. Compartment syndrome is most common in the lower leg and forearm, but it can also occur in the hand, foot, thigh, and upper arm. The nurse should suspect compartment syndrome if the patient's complaints of pain and swelling are disproportionate to negative x-ray findings. It can result from a fracture, muscle bruise, crush injury, or bandage that is too tight, such as a cast. Compartment syndrome is a medical emergency; the first step in treatment is to remove a tight cast. If internal pressure is causing the symptoms, it is generally treated by surgery (i.e., fasciotomy)

to relieve pressure (National Library of Medicine, 2014). Patients with a bone fracture in an extremity should be regularly evaluated for swelling, pain, discoloration, and neurovascular function in the fractured limb. Methods to prevent compartment syndrome include elevation and ice to reduce swelling and delaying casting until the swelling is gone.

Compartment syndrome can lead to many complications, including paralysis, the need for amputation, or a Volkmann contracture. A *Volkmann contracture* is a deformity of the wrist, hand, and fingers caused by ischemia to the forearm, usually as a result of compartment syndrome. Ischemia in the forearm causes the nerves and muscles to become scarred and shortened, forcing the joint to be permanently bent (Ma, 2016c). A Volkmann contracture is common after elbow injuries, especially in children.

Deep Venous Thrombosis

Deep venous thrombosis (DVT) occurs when a blood clot, or thrombus, forms in one of the deep veins, usually in the leg. Symptoms include redness and warmth of the skin, leg pain, cramping, and swelling. If DVT is suspected, the nurse should report the symptoms to a physician immediately. The physician may order a venogram or Doppler ultrasound to visualize the blood clot and confirm diagnosis. DVT is usually treated with bedrest to prevent dislodgement of the clot, anticoagulants such as heparin or warfarin to prevent further clotting, thrombolytics such as tissue plasminogen activator (tPA) to break down the clot, or surgery to insert a filter in the vena cava to prevent blood clots from traveling to vital organs. Measures to prevent DVT include early immobilization of the fracture, regular exercise, prophylactic anticoagulants, and use of compression stockings or boots (Mayo Clinic, 2014c).

If the blood clot dislodges from the leg, it can travel to the brain and cause a cerebrovascular accident (CVA, or stroke). In the lungs, a blood clot can cause a pulmonary embolism. In the coronary arteries, a blood clot can lead to myocardial infarction (MI) and other severe damage (Dugdale, 2012b). Risk factors for development of DVT include decreased blood flow, blood vessel injury, and altered blood coagulation (see **Table 13–5 >>**). Other risk factors include older age, obesity, poor circulation, inactivity or bedrest, smoking,

TABLE 13–5 Risk Factors for Deep Venous Thrombosis

Risk Factor	Nursing Implications for Patients with Fractures
Blood stasis in a vein	Immobility from casting and bedrest can decrease blood flow in the limb. Encourage early ambulation, active or passive exercises, and the use of compression stockings or boots to prevent blood stasis.
Blood vessel injury	Blood vessels may be injured by the force that caused the fracture, by movement of the fractured bone, or during surgical repair of the bone, causing clots to form at the site of injury. Target assessments to the location of suspected blood vessel injury.
Altered blood coagulation	Excess blood loss from injury or surgery may cause the body to increase production of platelets and clotting factors. The presence of tissue debris or fat in the vein may also promote clot formation. Assess the patient for coagulation disorders, and monitor use of medications that alter blood clotting.

and cancer. (For more information about DVT, pulmonary embolism, and stroke, see the module on Perfusion.)

Fat Embolism Syndrome

Fat embolism may occur in conjunction with closed long bone or pelvic fractures. Fat emboli released from the bone marrow enter the bloodstream and become trapped in the pulmonary and dermal capillaries. In most patients, release of fat from the bone marrow after a fracture produces no symptoms. Patients who experience release of large amounts of fat, as many as 90% of major trauma victims, may experience a fat embolism. While rare, if the condition progresses to fat embolism syndrome (FES), multiple systems may be affected, and there is a high morbidity and mortality rate (Bulauitan, 2015).

Respiratory consequences are typically the first symptom of FES to occur (Bulauitan, 2015). In severe cases, dyspnea may progress to respiratory failure with tachypnea and hypoxia. A syndrome similar to acute respiratory distress syndrome (ARDS) may develop (see the exemplar on ARDS in the module on Oxygenation). Neurologic symptoms may include confusion, restlessness, seizures, or coma. A transient petechial rash usually covers the upper anterior trunk, arms, and neck as well as the buccal mucosa and conjunctiva. Other symptoms may include Purtscher retinopathy (sudden loss of vision, most often associated with traumatic injury) and mild fever.

Treatment of FES is supportive and includes oxygen administration; approximately one half of patients will require mechanical ventilation. Neurologic symptoms usually resolve with adequate oxygenation, and the petechial rash disappears spontaneously within a week. Prophylactic treatment with corticosteroids and early immobilization of the injury may reduce the risk of FES. FES is rarely seen in children under the age of 10.

Infection

Impaired skin integrity as a result of an open fracture or surgical correction of a fracture increases the risk of bacterial contamination and development of an infection. Common infecting organisms include *Pseudomonas*, *Staphylococcus*, and *Clostridium*. Patients with greater soft tissue damage or with a compromised immune system are at higher risk of infection. Signs of infection include warmth, redness, pain, swelling, stiffness, fever, chills, and purulent drainage. Treatment includes administration of antibiotics according to the infecting agent and proper hygiene of the infection site. Hygiene care may include debridement, drainage, and culture for identification of the infecting organism. Infection due to fractures can cause cellulitis (see the exemplar on Cellulitis in the module on Infection), osteomyelitis, or gangrene. If the infection is severe or does not respond to antibiotics, tissue death may occur, necessitating amputation.

Collaboration

A bone fracture is an emergency situation that often requires the collaboration of multiple healthcare professionals, including nurses, physicians, surgeons, and PTs. The majority of bone fractures are treated with nonpharmacologic therapy, including casts, traction, and pain management. Electrical bone stimulation is an alternative therapy that may also be beneficial (see the Evidence-Based Practice feature).

Evidence-Based Practice
Smoking and Fractures

Problem

Bone fractures take extensive time to heal, and occasionally patients have delayed union or nonunion of fractures. Smoking increases the risk for nonunion, malunion, osteomyelitis, infections, and lower functional scores. Smoking has been shown to increase the risk of delayed bone healing (Truntzer, Vopat, Feldstein, & Matityahu, 2015).

Evidence

Previous studies had shown that smoking cessation 4 weeks prior to surgery reduced surgical risks to the level of nonsmokers when compared to individuals who smoked in the 4 weeks prior to surgery. A similar tendency is seen with individuals who smoke during the healing time of bone fractures (Truntzer et al., 2015). The 4000+ toxins found in cigarettes may lead to delayed healing. Nicotine affects bone density and the healing process by decreasing circulation through peripheral vasoconstriction (Miller, 2014). Studies found that there were increased numbers of nonunion rates in individuals who continued to smoke after lumbar fusion surgery than in the nonsmokers. The nonunion rates for those who quit smoking prior to surgery or after surgery were lower than the smokers who continued to smoke after surgery (Truntzer et al., 2015).

Implications

Nurses in all settings should incorporate the U.S. Public Health Service's 5 As of smoking into the patient interview and history taking. Although there are several reasons to incorporate the 5 As of smoking in general practice, it may be especially important to include them when working with individuals with fractures. The 5 As of smoking consist of:

- **Ask** all patients about their histories.
- **Advise** all patients to quit using personalized, but nonjudgmental language.
- **Assess** motivation to quit: "How do you feel about your smoking?" "Are you ready to give it up?"
- **Assist** by assessing readiness to quit and providing resources and referrals.
- **Arrange** support follow-up with the local smoking cessation service (Miller, 2014).

Critical Thinking Application

1. Determine your comfort level of discussing smoking cessation with patients. If you are a smoker, how does this create bias in your thoughts?
2. Develop a teaching plan for smoking cessation related to bone healing after a fracture. How do nonunions, malunions, infections, or other complications affect the patient? How could these facts be used to encourage smoking cessation and be built into the teaching plan?
3. Once you are working as a registered nurse, how could you promote the use of the U.S. Public Health Service's 5 As of smoking at your work setting?

Clinical Manifestations and Therapies
Fractures and Complications

ETIOLOGY	CLINICAL MANIFESTATIONS	CLINICAL THERAPIES
Bone fracture	■ Pain ■ Fracture on x-ray ■ Swelling, deformity, numbness ■ Loss of blood, crepitus	■ Immobilization (casts, traction) ■ Surgical repair ■ Analgesics for pain ■ RICE therapy (rest, ice, compression, elevation)
Compartment syndrome	■ Edema, swelling, ischemia ■ Severe pain, tenderness ■ Paresthesia, numbness, paralysis ■ Absent distal pulse ■ Poikilothermia ■ Skin discoloration (pallor, cyanosis) ■ Renal failure (late symptom)	■ Removal of tight cast ■ Fasciotomy ■ Ice ■ Elevation
Deep venous thrombosis	■ Redness, warmth ■ Leg pain, cramping, swelling ■ Dislodged clots (emboli) may cause stroke, pulmonary embolism, or MI.	Treatment: ■ Bedrest ■ Anticoagulants ■ Thrombolytics ■ Surgical insertion of filter Prevention: ■ Early immobilization of the fracture ■ Regular exercise ■ Early ambulation ■ Compression stockings or boots
Fat embolism syndrome	■ Dyspnea, respiratory failure ■ Petechial rash ■ Confusion, seizures, coma ■ Purtscher retinopathy ■ Fever	■ Administration of oxygen ■ Mechanical ventilation ■ Corticosteroids ■ Early immobilization of injury
Infection	■ Warmth, redness ■ Pain, swelling, stiffness ■ Fever, chills ■ Purulent drainage	■ Antibiotics ■ Analgesics ■ Antipyretics ■ Wound hygiene ■ Amputation

The nurse's primary roles include assessing the patient, maintaining patient comfort, assisting with procedures, providing patient education, and referring the patient to specialists as needed.

Emergency Care

The primary objectives of emergency care of a patient with a fracture include immobilizing the fracture and preventing infection. If emergency care is provided outside a medical facility, immobilization should not include trying to reset the bone if it is out of alignment. Instead, the nurse should apply splints above and below the joint to reduce mobility and prevent further damage to the area. Cervical immobilization is essential if a spinal fracture is suspected. If the patient is bleeding, the nurse should apply a pressure dressing, and sterile dressings should be applied to all open wounds. Once the patient is stabilized and the fracture immobilized, the nurse should assess the extremities for pulses, movement, and sensation. Ice packs may be applied to reduce swelling if needed. Patients may also need to be treated for shock (see the exemplar on Shock in the module on Perfusion).

Diagnostic Tests

The primary diagnostic test for a fractured bone is an x-ray (see **Figure 13–27** ❯❯). Other complementary methods used for diagnosis include patient history; physical assessment;

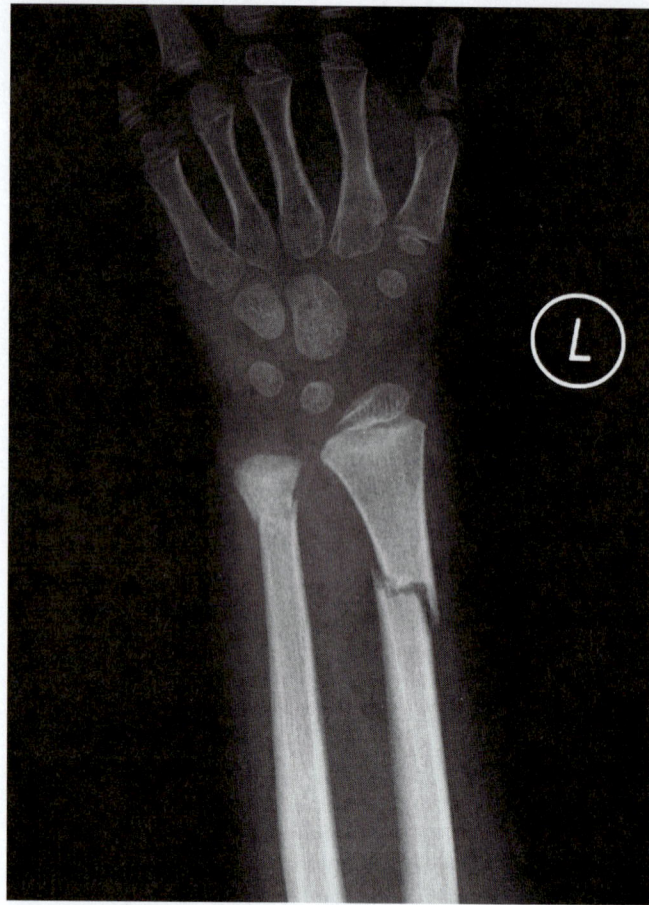

Source: *kuehdi/Shutterstock.*

Figure 13–27 ›› X-ray of fractured forearm.

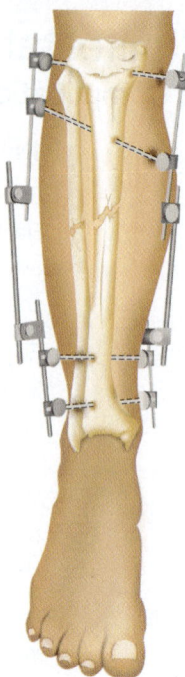

Figure 13–28 ›› In external fixation, pins are placed through the bone above and below the fracture site to immobilize the bone. External fixation rods hold the pins in place.

other imaging studies such as bone scans, MRIs, or CT scans; and blood tests such as blood chemistry studies, CBC, and coagulation studies.

Surgery

For severe fractures that require direct visualization to repair, such as open fractures and comminuted fractures, the patient will undergo surgery. The two main types of surgical repair for bone fractures are external fixation and internal fixation. With external fixation, metal pins and screws are placed into the bone above and below the fracture. The pins and screws are then attached to a metal bar outside the skin (see **Figure 13–28** ››). This is often performed if damage to soft tissues prevents internal fixation. The nurse is responsible for monitoring the patient for infection and neurovascular function.

Open reduction and internal fixation (ORIF) is the surgical procedure used to internally repair a bone fracture. During **reduction**, the bone is placed in correct alignment. Nails, screws, pins, wires, plates, or rods are then inserted into the bone to hold the bone in place (see **Figure 13–29** ››). Plates are attached on the outer surface of the bone, whereas rods may be inserted through the marrow space in the center of the bone. Fractures of the long bones are commonly repaired by ORIF; internal fixation allows shorter hospital stays, earlier return to full function, and fewer instances of

nonunion and malunion (AAOS, 2014a). Complications of fracture reduction may include infection, neurovascular or vascular injury, and leg length discrepancy.

Pharmacologic Therapy

Pharmacologic therapy for patients who sustain bone fractures primarily includes analgesics for pain. For severe fractures, opioids or patient-controlled analgesics are prescribed. In addition to opioids, NSAIDs may be administered for both pain and inflammation. See Exemplar 3.A, Acute and Chronic Pain, for a thorough discussion of opioid and nonopioid analgesics, including their side effects and nursing implications. Other common medications for patients with

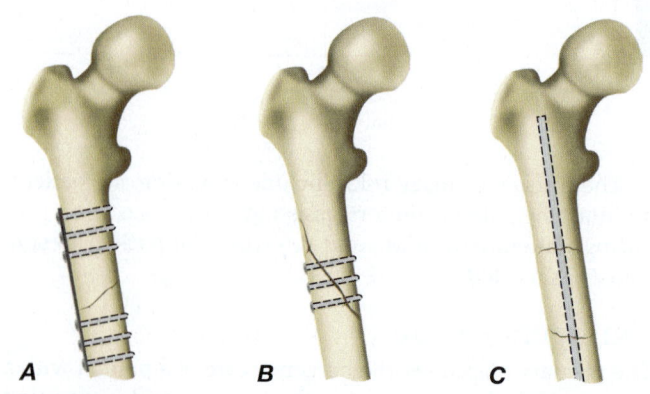

A   B   C

Figure 13–29 ›› Internal fixation hardware is entirely within the body. **A,** Fixation of a short oblique fracture using a plate and screws above and below the fracture. **B,** Fixation of a long oblique fracture using screws through the fracture site. **C,** Fixation of segmental fracture using a medullary nail.

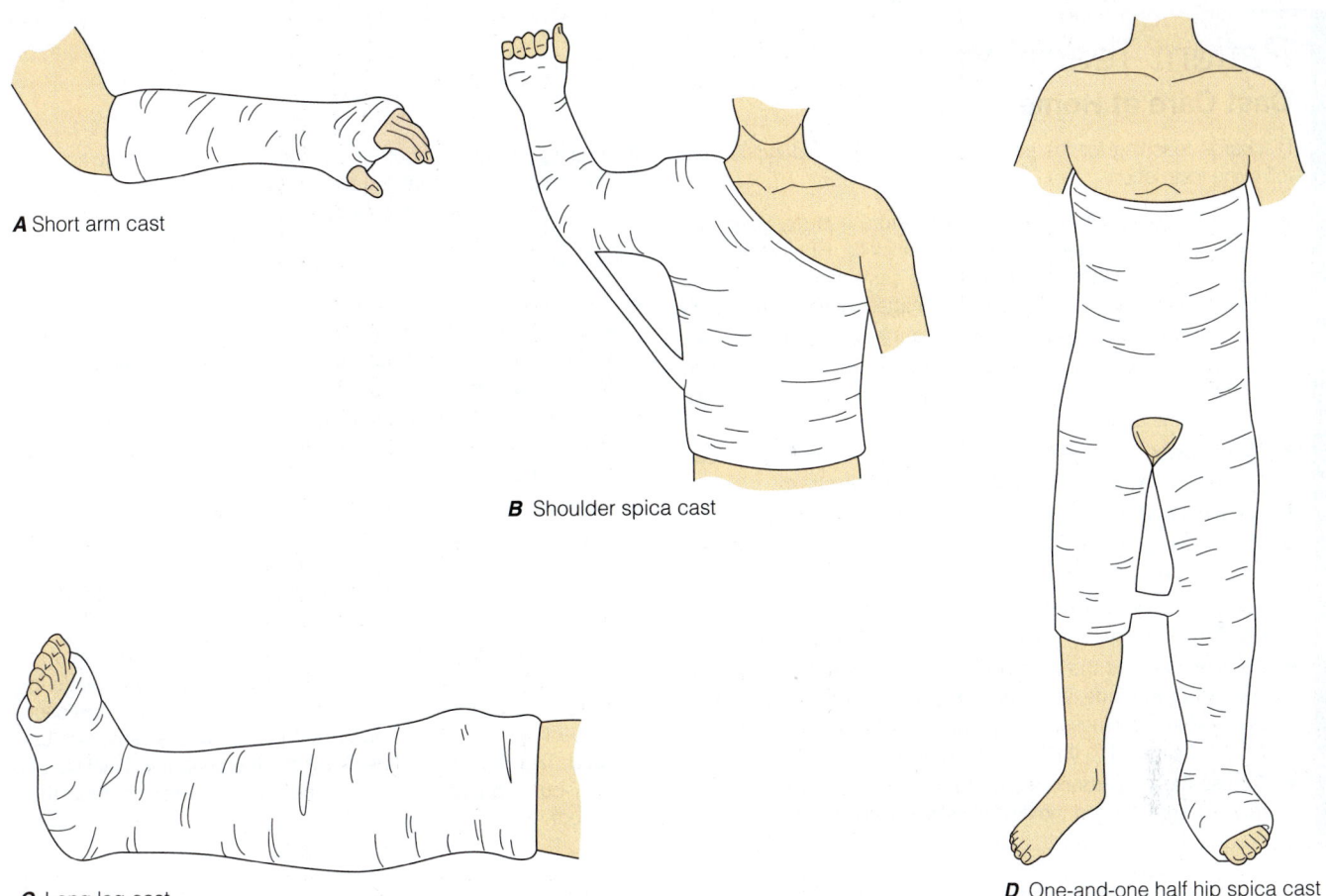

A Short arm cast

B Shoulder spica cast

C Long leg cast

D One-and-one half hip spica cast

Figure 13–30 ⟫ Examples of types of casts used to immobilize fractures.

bone fractures include antibiotics to prevent or treat infections and anticoagulants to prevent or treat DVT.

Casts and Splints

A **cast** is a rigid device used to immobilize, support, and protect fractured bones and the surrounding soft tissue (see **Figure 13–30** ⟫). A cast is usually applied to a stable fracture after it has been reduced. Casts are custom made from plaster or fiberglass to exactly fit the injured limb and cannot be easily removed by the patient. Fiberglass is lighter, "breathes" better, and is more compatible with x-rays than plaster, but plaster is less expensive and shapes better than fiberglass. Cotton padding is usually applied under the cast for patient comfort and to protect the skin. A cast should cover the joint above and below the fractured bone to prevent bone movement and facilitate healing. A functional cast may also be applied that allows limited movement of nearby joints; a functional cast works for some, but not all, fractures. Nursing care of the patient with a cast includes performing neurovascular assessments, palpating the cast for "hot spots" that may indicate infection, reporting drainage promptly, assessing the patient for compartment syndrome, and educating the patient about proper cast care at home (see the Patient Teaching feature).

A **splint** provides less support than a cast, but it can be easily adjusted to accommodate swelling and prevent compartment syndrome. Splints are usually ready made with Velcro straps that allow the splint to be easily removed. Splints may also be formed using fiberglass or plaster, then molded to fit the fractured region. Because of their ability to expand, splints are often used to stabilize fresh injuries before the swelling has subsided, as well as after the reparative phase of healing to allow some movement of the joints.

Traction

Traction is the use of weights, ropes, and pulleys to apply force to a fractured bone to maintain proper alignment of the bone for healing (see **Figure 13–31** ⟫). It may also help stretch muscles that have contracted or are producing muscle spasms. The two main types of traction are skin traction and skeletal traction.

SAFETY ALERT For the patient whose injury requires traction, do not let weights rest on the bed or the floor. This will cause inadequate force on the bone and may change the alignment of the fracture, causing a malunion.

During *skin traction*, equipment such as splints, bandages, and boots are placed on the injured limb, and a force is applied to soft tissues such as the skin, muscles, and tendons through the use of a weight and pulley system attached to the bed. Skin traction is used only when a small amount of weight (e.g., 5–7 lb) is needed for traction, because skin cannot tolerate larger weights. Skin traction is often used to

Patient Teaching

Cast Care at Home

Discharge teaching for the patient with a cast should include the following instructions:

- Do not apply pressure to the cast before it is dry, because dents in the cast may cause pressure injuries. Fiberglass casts dry in less than 1 hour, whereas plaster casts may take up to 48 hours to dry. If the cast becomes damaged, notify a physician.

- Do not get the cast wet, especially if it is a plaster cast. Use plastic or waterproof shields around the cast while showering or bathing. If a fiberglass cast becomes wet, dry it with a blow dryer on the cool setting.

- Do not place any objects in the cast. Itching under the cast can be relieved by using a blow dryer on the cool setting.

- Keep dirt and other irritants away from the inside of the cast.

- Do not remove any part of the cast, including padding and rough edges.

- Elevate the injured extremity above the heart as often as possible, and apply ice to the cast to prevent swelling under the cast.

- Regularly assess the injured extremity for symptoms of compartment syndrome, including increased pain and swelling, loss of sensation, coolness, and changes in color. If the cast feels as if it is becoming too tight, see a physician immediately.

- Assess the skin around the cast regularly. If the skin becomes raw or looks infected, notify a physician immediately.

- If using a sling, distribute the weight of the cast evenly around the neck. Ensure that the sling strap remains flat around the neck to prevent impaired circulation.

The nurse should also consider the following points:

- If the patient is using crutches, teach him or her proper crutch walking or refer the patient to a PT. Provide the patient with verbal and written instructions regarding the physician's orders for bearing weight on the injured leg.

- For leg fractures, refer the patient to a PT to teach crutch walking, limited weight bearing, and transferring and to conduct a home safety inspection.

- Refer the patient to home care agencies for ongoing monitoring of wound healing and local medical equipment sources for crutches, wheelchairs, slings, elevated toilet seats, and other equipment that may facilitate healing or prevent further injury.

- The provider may order x-rays at follow-up appointments to track the healing progress of the fracture. If the cast needs to be removed for skin or bone assessment or because the cast is too large after swelling is decreased, a cast saw will be used. The cast saw will be noisy and the patient will feel vibration, but a guard will prevent the cast saw from cutting the patient.

---

control muscle spasms, to maintain alignment of a fracture before or after internal fixation, or to provide traction if skeletal pins become infected and must be removed. Common methods of skin traction include Buck traction, Dunlop traction, Russell traction, and Bryant traction (see **Box 13–3 》》**).

SAFETY ALERT Skin traction is contraindicated in older adults with frail skin, because it may tear the skin and increase the risk for infection.

Skeletal traction is used when a greater force needs to be applied to the fracture or when skin traction is contraindicated. Skeletal traction may be used in conjunction with skin traction, depending on the location and severity of the fracture. For skeletal traction, pins, wires, or screws are surgically implanted into the bone under sterile conditions while the patient is under local or general anesthesia. Weights (usually around 25 lb) are then attached to the implanted hardware in one or more directions to maintain the fracture in correct

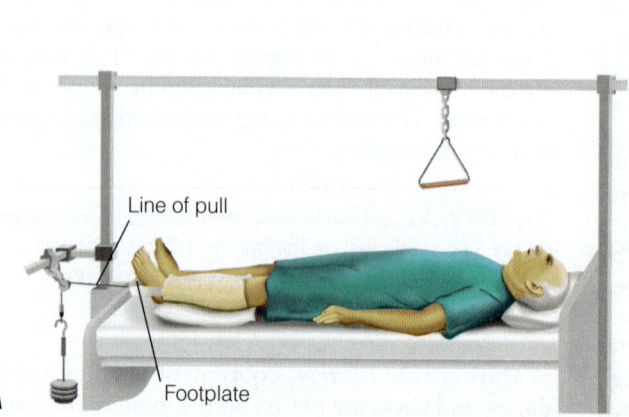
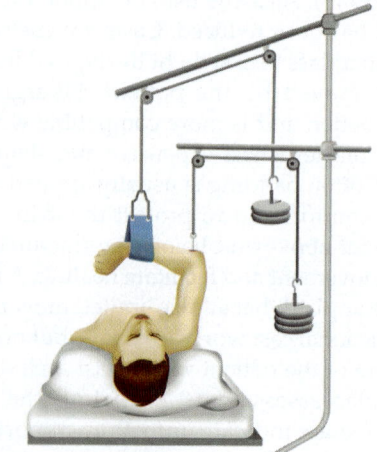

Figure 13–31 》》 Traction is the application of a pulling force to maintain bone alignment during fracture healing. Different fractures require different types of traction. **A,** Skin traction applies force to the soft tissues through a pulley system attached to the bed, such as Buck traction shown here for stabilization of the knee and hip. **B,** Skeletal traction applies force directly to the bone, such as the traction used here for a humerus fracture.

Box 13–3
Common Traction Methods

Skin Traction

- *Buck traction* (see **Figure 13–32** ≫) is the most common orthopedic traction procedure; it is used for fractured or dislocated hips and knee injuries. The foot on the injured side is placed in a foam boot with a small weight (usually 5 lb) attached with a rope and pulley system, and the knee and hip are kept straight. Buck's traction can be unilateral or bilateral.
- *Dunlop traction* (skin or skeletal traction) is used to immobilize a humeral supracondylar fracture in children. The elbow is maintained in a flexed position to prevent circulation and nerve problems.
- *Russell traction* (see **Figure 13–33** ≫) is used for fractured femurs, hip and knee contractures, and other hip and knee problems. The knee is suspended in a sling, and the knee and lower leg are attached to a series of three pulleys and weights. The angle between the thigh and the bed is approximately 20 degrees, and the hips and knees remain slightly flexed.
- *Bryant traction* (see **Figure 13–34** ≫) is used to immobilize both lower extremities to treat a fractured femur or developmental dysplasia of the hip in infants and toddlers. The legs are suspended vertically in the air with the hips at a 90-degree angle and the knees slightly flexed. The buttocks are raised slightly off the bed, and the position of the lower body is maintained by weights and pulleys.

Skeletal Traction

- *Skeletal cervical traction* uses Crutchfield, Gardner-Wells, or Vinke tongs inserted into the parietal area of the skull to immobilize the spine after cervical fracture. The tongs are then attached to a pulling device for stabilization.
- *Halo traction* (see **Figure 13–35** ≫) involves the use of a ring and skull pins attached to a sheepskin jacket and support rods designed to be worn by the patient. The screws may need to be tightened periodically to ensure correct alignment of the spine. A halo apparatus is used for fractures of the cervical spine or to correct the alignment of the spine in scoliosis.
- *90–90 traction* (see **Figure 13–36** ≫) is commonly used in children with a displaced fractured femur. A pin is inserted into the femur close to the knee and attached to a pulley and weight system so the hip and knee are both flexed at a 90-degree angle. The opposite leg may be unrestricted or may be placed in Buck or Russell traction for immobilization.
- *Balanced suspension traction* uses both skeletal traction and suspension to support the injured limb. One example is traction for a fractured femur. A Thomas leg splint is applied to the thigh, and a Pearson attachment is attached to the Thomas splint at the knee by clamps. A sling supports the lower leg and provides knee flexion. A footplate is used to support the foot. Weights are attached to both the Thomas splint and the Pearson attachment. The thigh is suspended at a 45-degree angle, while the lower leg is horizontal with the bed.

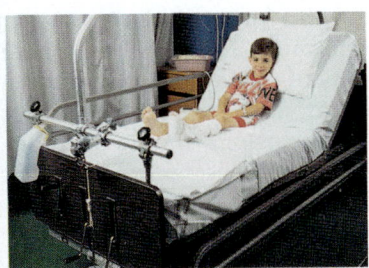

Figure 13–32 ≫ Buck traction.

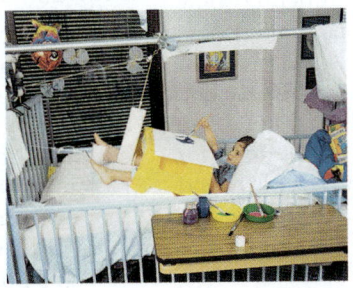

Figure 13–33 ≫ Russell traction.

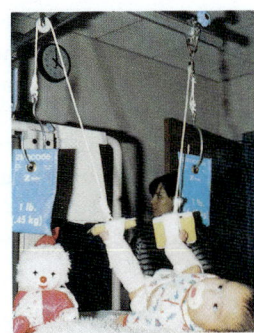

Figure 13–34 ≫ Bryant traction.

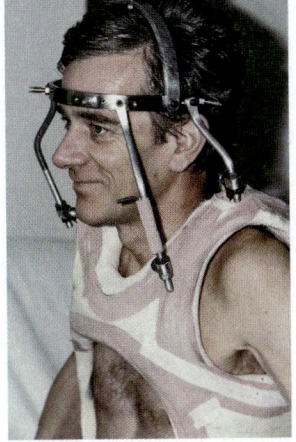

Source: Dr. P. Marazzi/Science Source.

Figure 13–35 ≫ Halo traction.

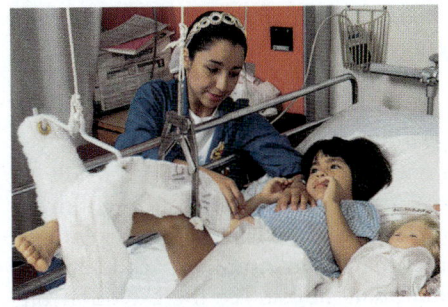

Figure 13–36 ≫ 90–90 traction.

alignment. The most common types of skeletal traction include Dunlop traction, skeletal cervical traction, halo traction, 90–90 traction, and balanced suspension traction (see Box 13–3). Skeletal pins and other hardware must be cleaned frequently to reduce the risk of infection. If a pin becomes infected, the nurse should notify the patient's physician. The pin may need to be removed and placed elsewhere, or the patient may need to use skin traction instead of skeletal traction. In addition, the patient with a pin infection should be treated with antibiotics.

Nonpharmacologic Pain Management

Nonpharmacologic management of pain for patients with bone fractures includes RICE therapy (rest, ice, compression, and elevation). Compression should be enough to provide support for the injured area, as is provided by a cast or splint, but it should not decrease blood flow to the area and cause compartment syndrome. For nonpharmacologic nursing interventions related to pain management, see the exemplar on Acute and Chronic Pain in the module on Comfort.

Lifespan Considerations

A patient's age plays a role in the type of fracture the patient is likely to experience.

Fractures in Infants

An infant's inability to communicate location or nature of pain makes discovering fractured bones difficult. Some signs of possible bone fractures include inconsolable crying, crying when an area around a broken bone is touched, limited movement of an extremity, swelling of an extremity, or a deformity of an area or extremity. Fractured collar bones are a frequent birth injury (Birth Injury Guide, 2016). Risks for long bone fractures include cesarean birth, breech birth, and low birth weight.

Fractures in Toddlers

Although not a fracture, "nursemaid's elbow" is a common childhood injury worth consideration. This injury often occurs when a caregiver pulls a child by the hand with a quick motion, as may occur when pulling the child from a dangerous situation (e.g., going into busy street) or to assist the child onto a step. The medical term is radial head subluxation when there is a partial separation of the radiocapitellar joint (AAOS, 2014b). The main symptoms include holding the arm stiffly and not wanting to use it. Treatment is reduction of the joint. Prevention includes education on avoiding swinging children by the hands or pulling by the hands and encouraging people to pick children up under their arms.

Fractures in Children

Children often experience long bone fractures as a result of sports and play. Spiral fractures are common in children because of the porous nature of their bones; unexplained midshaft spiral fractures may be an indicator of child abuse. (For more information about abuse, see the exemplar on Abuse in the module on Trauma.) Children often recover quickly from fractures because their bones have a rapid growth rate and the epiphyseal plates have not yet been sealed.

Fractures in Adolescents

Athletes, such as long-distance runners or gymnasts, often experience stress fractures related to repetitive force on specific bones. In addition to repeated stress, adolescents are likely to sustain stress fractures as a result of imbalanced nutrition.

Fractures in Adults and Older Adults

Adults may have a lengthened recovery time because their bones have a slower rate of tissue growth; this is especially true for women after menopause and older adults in general. Older adults with osteoporosis have increased risk of hip fractures and are more likely to develop complications such as DVT and infection. Alterations in mental status increase risk for injury in adults of all ages.

NURSING PROCESS

Nursing care for patients with a fracture includes pain management, patient teaching, assessment for complications, and emotional support. Each patient's needs will depend on the location and severity of the fracture and the emotional trauma of the situation that caused the fracture.

Assessment

Assessment of a patient with a fracture includes obtaining a health history and performing a physical examination. Depending on the severity of the fracture, physical examination may need to be performed frequently to assess for complications. The health history should include the patient's age; a history of chronic illnesses that may increase risk for complications; medications, especially anticoagulants; a history of previous musculoskeletal injuries; the patient's normal activity level; and the history of the event that caused the fracture.

Physical assessment should include an assessment of distal pulses in the injured extremity, edema and swelling, skin color and temperature, deformity, ROM, and sensation. A 5 *P*s neurovascular assessment should also be conducted, which includes assessment of pain, pulses, pallor, paresthesia, and paralysis/paresis. For further description of the 5 *P*s neurovascular assessment, see the Concept of Mobility section.

Diagnosis

Examples of nursing diagnoses for the patient with a fracture may include the following:

- *Risk for Peripheral Neurovascular Dysfunction* related to compression of nerves
- *Risk for Ineffective Tissue Perfusion: Peripheral* related to impaired circulation and potential thrombus formation
- *Risk for Infection* related to surgical incision and insertion of hardware

- *Impaired Skin Integrity* related to open bone fracture
- *Acute Pain* related to bone and soft tissue damage
- *Impaired Mobility: Physical* related to fractured femur
- *Risk for Disuse Syndrome* related to use of traction to stabilize fracture
- *Deficient Knowledge* related to cast care
- *Disturbed Body Image* related to halo traction
- *Anxiety* related to external fixation.

(NANDA-I © 2014)

Planning

Planning care for the patient with a bone fracture will depend on the location and severity of the injury and the prescribed treatment by the physician. For example, a patient with a tibia fracture who needs a cast will require very different care from a patient with arm, leg, and spine fractures that need traction or surgery. Common goals for patients with fractures may include the following:

- The patient will not demonstrate signs or symptoms of a wound infection from an open fracture, skeletal pins, or surgical incision.
- The patient will develop no neurovascular complications related to the fracture or treatment.
- The patient will regain full function in the injured extremity.
- The patient will describe pain as less than 3 on a scale of 0–10.

Implementation

The primary goals of nursing care for a patient with a fracture include managing pain, maintaining proper fracture alignment, promoting mobility, monitoring for neurovascular status, preventing infections, preventing complications, and providing discharge instructions. If surgical treatment is required, the nurse may also prepare the patient for hospital admission or transfer to the surgery department. In a community setting, nursing care may involve administering first aid and arranging for transport of the patient to an emergency department (ED).

Pain associated with a bone fracture is often severe and may slow the healing process or be an indication of a complication such as compartment syndrome or DVT. The location, duration, and etiology of pain should be determined before analgesics are given. After the cause of pain is identified, several nursing interventions may be implemented:

- Administer analgesics as prescribed. Analgesics should be given around the clock for the first 24–48 hours. If medications are given prn, remind the patient to request medication before the pain becomes severe. Addiction to opioids is not likely if taken as prescribed for the recommended duration.
- Elevate the injured area, and apply ice packs to decrease swelling.
- Drain fluids from drainage devices (e.g., Hemovac drain), and monitor the drainage for possible hematoma.

- Encourage the patient to move frequently, including changing positions to relieve pressure, wiggling fingers or toes to improve circulation, and ambulating to reduce complications.
- Teach the patient alternative methods of pain management, including relaxation, distraction, imagery, and social interaction.
- Notify the physician of unrelieved pain, and advocate for increased pharmacologic intervention or assessment for complications such as compartment syndrome.

Provide Effective Pain Management

The nurse should regularly assess the patient for pain and for muscle spasms and swelling, which may increase pain. The nurse should also monitor vital signs per protocol or as ordered. The nurse should administer pain medications as prescribed and monitor the effectiveness of pain medications to advocate for stronger pain relief if needed. Nursing interventions to reduce pain include elevating the injured extremity, providing ice to reduce swelling, and using non-pharmacologic methods to reduce pain, such as distraction, deep breathing, and relaxation techniques. When patients must be moved, movement should be performed gently and slowly to reduce pain and muscle spasms, and the injured extremity should be supported above and below the fracture site to prevent displacement of bony fragments and nerve damage.

Maintain Proper Alignment

Proper alignment of the fractured bones is essential to prevent malunion of the fracture. A splint, a cast, traction, or internal or external fixation will be applied to reduced fractures to immobilize the joints and hold the bones in place. The nurse is responsible for providing verbal and written instructions to the patient and family for splint or cast care. When caring for patients in traction, the nurse is responsible for helping the patient maintain proper body alignment with the weight and pulley systems as well as ensuring that the weights are always hanging freely. Patients with internal or external fixation will need instructions on weight bearing and care of external pins.

Promote Mobility

Fractures of the hips and lower extremities alter the patient's gait and mobility. The nurse is responsible for assisting with ambulation as soon as allowed by the provider. Early ambulation increases circulation and reduces the risk of complications, especially DVT. If ambulation is restricted, such as for patients in traction, the nurse should help the patient with passive and active exercises in the uninjured limbs to maintain blood flow and strengthen muscles. The patient should also be repositioned every 1–2 hours to prevent skin breakdown. Promoting mobility may also include teaching patients how to use assistive devices such as crutches or a walker or referring the patient to a physical therapist. Proper use of assistive devices increases patient safety and decreases risk of further injury. For patients with a hip or pelvis fracture, patient mobility may require a wheelchair or wheeled cart.

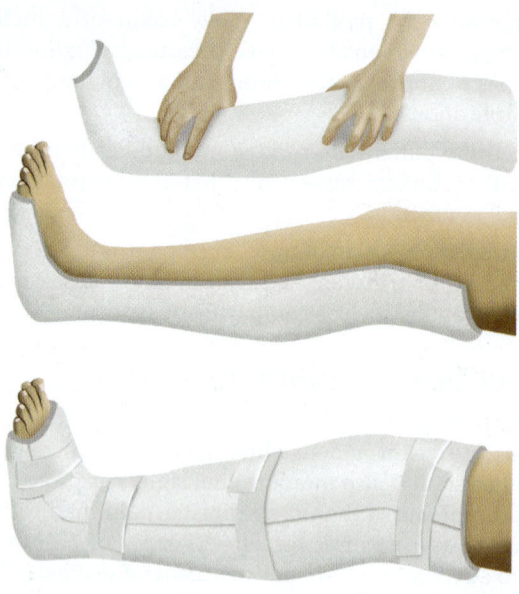

Figure 13–37 >> Bivalving is the process of splitting the cast down both sides to alleviate pressure on or allow visualization of the extremity.

Monitor Neurovascular Status

The patient's neurovascular status should be monitored using the 5 *P*s neurovascular assessment (see the Concept of Mobility section for review of the 5 *P*s neurovascular assessment). The injured limb should be assessed for swelling, cramping, temperature, hematoma, movement, capillary refill, and sensation to touch. The patient should be assessed every 15 minutes for the first 2 hours after a cast is applied and every 1–2 hours thereafter depending on facility policy and the patient's condition. The nurse should report abnormal findings immediately, because they could indicate a life- or limb-threatening complication such as compartment syndrome or DVT. A cast saw should be readily available for emergency cast removal or bivalving (see **Figure 13–37 >>**), which may become necessary in the event of emergent swelling. If compartment syndrome is suspected, the nurse should assist the provider in measuring compartment pressure. Pressure greater than 30 mmHg indicates compartment syndrome, and a fasciotomy may be needed. If DVT is suspected or diagnosed, the nurse should administer anticoagulants as prescribed.

Prevent Infection

Patients with open fractures, surgical repair, or skeletal pins are at increased risk of infection from the wound. Patients with a cast or skin traction and those on bedrest may also be at risk for infection if the skin develops pressure injuries. For general care of wounds, see the exemplar on Wound Healing in the module on Tissue Integrity. Nursing interventions related to monitoring fracture-related wounds for infection include providing skeletal pin care, drawing blood to monitor white blood cell counts, obtaining culture samples, checking vital signs,

using sterile technique to change dressings, and assessing the wound for signs of infection and drainage. Skeletal pin care will differ based on facility guidelines and physician preference, but may include gently cleansing the pin site daily to weekly with a cleansing solution such as sterile saline or chlorhexidine to remove crusts from the pins. The nurse should administer antibiotics as prescribed. Prophylactic antibiotics may be given for wounds with a high risk of infection, such as wounds related to a motor vehicle crash.

Provide Discharge Instructions

Most patients will receive emergency care for a fracture and return home the same day. Discharge instructions are an important aspect of nursing care for these patients. Teaching topics include cast care, activity restrictions, taking pain medications before pain becomes severe, signs of complications, and injury prevention. Patients with leg fractures who must use stairs may need special instructions for crutches, or they may need a referral to have a temporary or permanent ramp installed. A referral to home healthcare may be needed for older patients.

Evaluation

Evaluation of the patient depends on the location and severity of the fracture as well as the treatment received. Evaluation may include analysis of bone healing with x-rays, assessment of the patient's pain and neurovascular status, assessment of the patient's ROM and ability to ambulate independently, and assessment for other complications. Patient goals should include full function of the affected body part with no prolonged complications.

In the event the patient experiences complications or healing does not progress as expected, re-evaluation will be necessary, and nursing diagnoses and the care plan will need to be revised. Areas to consider include assessing for signs and symptoms of infection, assessing for neurovascular complications, assessing level of functioning of the injured limb or area, and pain assessment. In the event the patient reports significant pain during the follow-up call the day after casting, the nurse should assess for adherence to the treatment plan and assess for compartment syndrome. For example, questions to ask the patient with a cast on an upper extremity include:

■ On the hand with the cast, what color are the fingertips?

■ How do the fingers feel, warm or cold?

■ Is there feeling in the fingertips?

■ When you press down on the fingernail, how many seconds does it take for the nail to turn pink again?

■ Has the arm been elevated above the level of the heart?

If compartment syndrome is suspected, inform the patient that this is a medical emergency that requires immediate attention. If the patient lives far from the medical facility, the patient may need to call 9-1-1 or remove the cast. The patient should elevate the extremity, apply ice to decrease the swelling, and seek immediate medical attention.

Nursing Care Plan
A Patient with an Arm Fracture

Anthony Mandel, a 15-year-old boy, enjoys mountain biking with his friends on park trails. Today, in his attempt to jump a hill while cycling, Anthony lost control of his bike and flipped forward over the handlebars, landing on his extended left arm. He felt and heard a bone snap, and he could see bone through a wound in his left arm. His friends called Anthony's mother, who rushed to the scene and transported Anthony to the ED.

ASSESSMENT

Upon admission to the ED, the dorsal aspect of Anthony's left distal forearm reveals a 4-inch laceration with obvious deformity. Fractured bone is visible. He denies hitting his head, losing consciousness, or any other injuries. Anthony is pale, anxious, and complaining of pain. The digits on his left hand are warm and pink, and radial pulses are strong and equal bilaterally. Anthony denies numbness or tingling in his left arm or hand, but he continues to complain of pain, which he rates as 10 on a scale of 0–10, with 10 being the worst. Anthony's vital signs include temperature 98.9°F oral; pulse 102 bpm; respirations 20/min; and BP 119/68 mmHg. An x-ray reveals a fractured left distal radius. The ED nurse inserts an IV access device in Anthony's right hand, and he is sedated with midazolam (Versed) 1 mg IV and given fentanyl 50 mcg IV for analgesia. After requesting a consultation by the on-call orthopedic surgeon, the ED physician irrigates Anthony's wound and realigns the fractured bone. The ED physician then applies a sterile dressing to the wound. For stabilization and to prevent further injury to surrounding tissues, the ED physician places a splint on Anthony's left arm. After obtaining consent for surgery from Anthony's mother, the orthopedic physician orders that Anthony be scheduled for emergent ORIF of the left distal radius. Anthony's fracture is surgically repaired without incident, and the surgeon applies a splint to Anthony's left forearm. He is discharged to home that evening.

DIAGNOSES

- *Risk for Infection* related to compound fracture
- *Risk for Ineffective Peripheral Tissue Perfusion for* related to bone fracture and splint
- *Impaired Skin Integrity* related to open fracture of left distal radius
- *Acute Pain* related to left distal radius fracture
- *Fear* related to unknown diagnosis and treatment
- *Deficient Knowledge* related to manifestations of complications related to bone fracture

(NANDA-I © 2014)

PLANNING

- The patient will maintain normal distal pulse, capillary refill, and sensation in fingers.
- The patient's wound will demonstrate no signs or symptoms of infection.
- The patient will verbalize a pain intensity of less than 3 on a scale of 0–10.
- The patient and mother will demonstrate knowledge of signs and symptoms to report to the physician immediately.
- The patient and mother will verbalize understanding of cast care.
- The patient's fear will be diminished after diagnosis and treatment.
- The patient and mother will demonstrate knowledge of and practice good wound hygiene.

IMPLEMENTATION

- Routinely assess the patient for signs and symptoms of impaired circulation in the left arm, including pallor, diminished or absent pulses, and reports of numbness or tingling.
- Protect the patient's splint from contamination.
- Administer preoperative antibiotics as ordered.
- Elevate the patient's injured limb above the level of his heart.
- Administer pain medication as prescribed by the physician.
- Explain the surgical admission process to the patient and his mother and encourage them to ask questions.
- Teach the patient and mother signs and symptoms of complications related to bone fractures, including compartment syndrome and infection.

EVALUATION

Five days postoperatively, Anthony's mother transports him to the orthopedic surgeon's office for a follow-up visit. He denies complaints and reports that he is having "just a little bit of pain, maybe a 0 on a 0–10 scale." Anthony's left hand is warm, his fingers are pink and mobile, and his left radial pulse is strong. Anthony's mother reports that Anthony is taking his prophylactic antibiotic as prescribed. Anthony is scheduled for another follow-up visit in 2 weeks, at which time he remains free from complications and has no complaints. Four weeks following his injury, Anthony's cast is removed, and he begins a short course of physical therapy to regain full mobility in his injured arm.

CRITICAL THINKING

1. Why did the physicians apply a splint to Anthony's fractured arm instead of a cast?
2. Describe methods of wound cleansing that must be implemented to remove dirt and debris from the laceration on Anthony's left arm.
3. Develop a list of written discharge instructions the nurse would provide to Anthony and his mother.

REVIEW Fractures

....

RELATE Link the Concepts and Exemplars

Linking the exemplar on fractures with the concept of safety:

1. What safety principles can you teach children to decrease their risk for sustaining a bone fracture? Adolescents? Older adults?

2. What safety principles should you teach patients with a leg fracture? Arm fracture? Spine fracture?

Linking the exemplar on fractures with the concept of perfusion:

3. What nursing interventions will reduce the risk of DVT in the patient in traction with a broken femur?

4. What are the nursing priorities for patients with decreased perfusion to fingers or toes?

READY Go to Volume 3: Clinical Nursing Skills

REFER Go to Pearson MyLab Nursing and eText

- Additional review materials

REFLECT Apply Your Knowledge

Saul Genmar is a 21-year-old man who has recently graduated from college and is working as a car salesman. He is engaged to Joanne Bolit, who is a 19-year-old college sophomore. Ms. Bolit lives at home when she is not in school, and Mr. Genmar has an apartment with three friends. The previous night, Mr. Genmar and his friends met at a local tavern to watch a football game and drink beer. While traveling home, Mr. Genmar was involved in a one-car motor vehicle crash, during which he drove off the road in a residential area and struck a tree. Mr. Genmar's injuries were limited to his right leg, and no one else was injured. Mr. Genmar has a compound fracture of his right tibia and has returned from surgery with an external fixation device and is in traction. Ms. Bolit came to visit and is lying on the bed next to Mr. Genmar.

1. What is your priority of care for Mr. Genmar as you begin your shift?

2. How will you address the patient and his girlfriend when you enter the room to deliver care?

3. What teaching interventions will you initiate for both Mr. Genmar and Ms. Bolit?

›› Exemplar 13.C
Hip Fractures

Exemplar Learning Outcomes

13.C Analyze hip fractures as they relate to mobility.

- Describe the pathophysiology of hip fractures.
- Describe the etiology of hip fractures.
- Compare the risk factors for and prevention of hip fractures.
- Identify the clinical manifestations of hip fractures.
- Summarize diagnostic tests and therapies used by interprofessional teams in the collaborative care of an individual with a hip fracture.
- Differentiate considerations for care of patients with hip fractures across the lifespan.
- Apply the nursing process in providing culturally competent care to an individual with a hip fracture.

Exemplar Key Terms

Arthroplasty, *931*
Avascular necrosis, *928*
Extracapsular hip fractures, *928*
Hemiarthroplasty, *931*
Intracapsular hip fractures, *928*
Revision surgery, *931*

Overview

A hip fracture is a break in the neck, head, or trochanter region of the upper femur (see **Figure 13–38 ››**). Although hip fractures are most often associated with older adults, they can occur at any age as a result of trauma. Hip fractures often result in long-term functional impairment in older adults.

Pathophysiology and Etiology

Pathophysiology

There are two types of hip fractures: intracapsular and extracapsular. Extracapsular fractures can be further divided into intertrochanteric or subtrochanteric. **Intracapsular hip fractures** occur at the head or neck of the femur within the capsule of the hip joint. **Extracapsular hip fractures** occur within the trochanter region, which is between the neck and diaphysis of the femur. *Intertrochanteric fractures* take place between the neck and the lesser or greater trochanter, whereas *subtrochanteric fractures* occur immediately below the lesser trochanter (AAOS, 2009).

Hip fractures to the neck and intertrochanteric regions are the most common. Fractures of the neck are especially dangerous because the fracture often cuts off the blood supply to the head and neck of the femur, causing **avascular necrosis** (death of bone tissue due to lack of blood supply; also called osteonecrosis). This may also prevent cartilage and supporting bone from receiving adequate blood, leading to arthritis (AAOS, 2009). Extracapsular hip fractures are less likely to develop avascular necrosis because of a more diverse blood supply.

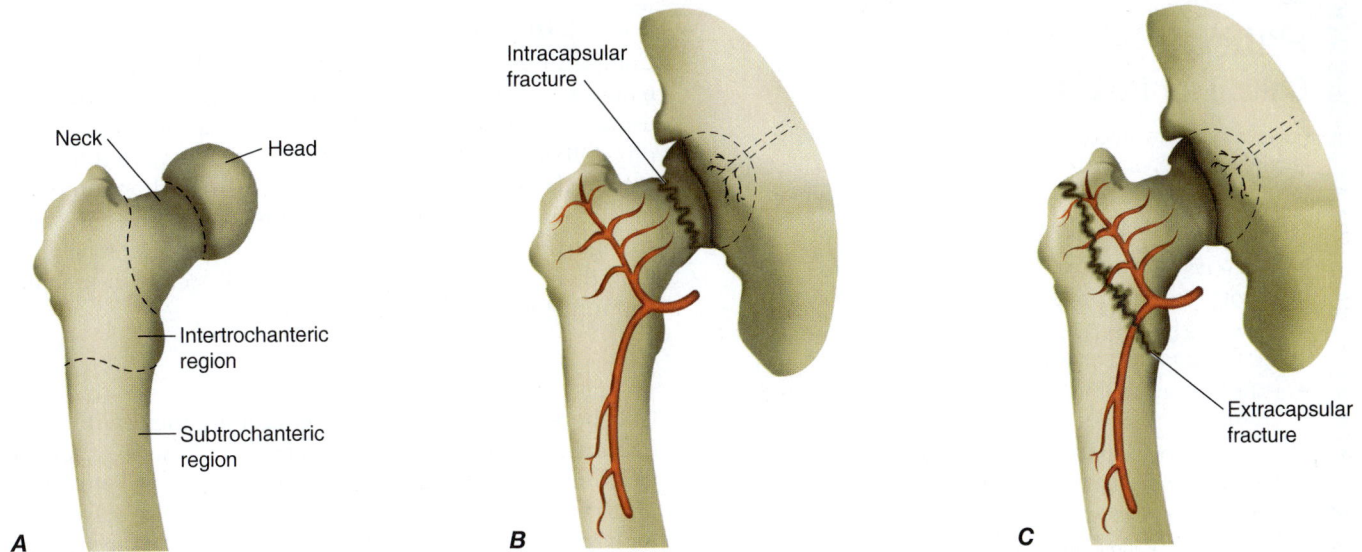

Figure 13–38 >> Regions where hip fractures may occur: **A,** The head of the femur, the neck of the femur, and the trochanteric regions of the femur. **B,** Intracapsular fractures occur across the head or neck of the femur. **C,** Extracapsular fractures occur across the trochanteric regions.

Etiology

Hip fractures are usually the result of trauma, such as a fall or motor vehicle crash. In older adults, a hip fracture is most often the result of falling sideways from a standing height onto the hip. Individuals with weak bones may sustain a hip fracture from simply standing on the leg and twisting (Mayo Clinic, 2015a). Common causes of hip fractures in children are motor vehicle and bike crashes, whereas teens are likely to sustain hip fractures due to sports injuries (Boston Children's Hospital, 2016a). Adults may fracture a hip as the result of a motor vehicle crash, a fall from a great height, or other severe trauma.

Risk Factors

The greatest risk factors for a hip fracture are old age and osteoporosis. Hip fracture rates increase exponentially with age; adults ages 85 and older are 10–15 times more likely to sustain a hip fracture than adults ages 60–65 (Mayo Clinic, 2015a). Older age is associated with osteoporosis, decreased muscle mass, vision and balance problems, and a slower reaction time. Osteoporosis occurs when new bone is not formed as quickly as the old bone is removed, causing bones to become brittle and less dense. Women after menopause are at an increased risk of developing osteoporosis. Women sustain approximately 70% of all hip fractures, and White women are more likely to sustain a hip fracture than Black or Asian women (Mayo Clinic, 2015a).

Other risk factors for hip fractures include chronic medical conditions that cause fragile bones, such as endocrine disorders, intestinal disorders, or cancer; some medications that weaken bone or cause dizziness; nutritional problems such as eating disorders or lack of calcium or vitamin D; physical inactivity, especially lack of weight-bearing exercise; and tobacco and alcohol use (Mayo Clinic, 2015d).

Prevention

Falls are the major cause of hip fractures, especially in older adults. One out of every three adults age 65 and older falls each year, and 20–30% of these individuals sustain severe injuries such as hip fractures (Centers for Disease Control and Prevention [CDC], 2012). Therefore, preventing falls is the best method of preventing hip fractures. Keys to fall prevention include performing weight-bearing exercises daily; assessing the home for fall hazards; asking a physician or pharmacist about medication side effects that may affect balance, bone density, or muscle strength; and getting vision checked yearly. Excessive alcohol use that may impair balance and vision should also be avoided. For more tips on preventing falls in older adults, see the Patient Teaching feature on fall prevention in Exemplar 13.B.

In addition to preventing falls, maintaining bone health and screening for bone disease are also methods to prevent hip fractures. Bone health can be maintained by exercise, a healthy diet, and adequate intake of calcium and vitamin D. Women past menopause who are not taking estrogen should consume 1500 mg of calcium daily; all other adults should consume 1000 mg of calcium daily. In 2011, the U.S. Preventive Services Task Force recommended osteoporosis screenings for all women ages 65 and older and for women younger than age 65 who are at high risk for osteoporosis. Tests to screen for osteoporosis include dual-energy x-ray absorptiometry of the hip and lumbar spine and quantitative ultrasonography of the calcaneus.

>> **Stay Current:** Visit https://www.uspreventiveservicestaskforce.org/ to see the U.S. Preventive Services Task Force 2017 recommendations for osteoporosis screening.

A mobility assessment is essential to measuring an older adult's risk of falls. This should include assessing the patient's gait, balance, and ability to change position. For example, the nurse should monitor the patient's ability to get up from a chair, turn while walking, raise the foot completely off the floor, and sit down. Difficulty with any of these tasks increases the patient's risk for falls. The World Health Organization provides the Fracture Risk Assessment (FRAX) tool to help estimate a patient's risk of fracture, including hip fracture, at http://www.shef.ac.uk/FRAX/index.aspx.

Patient Teaching
Calling for Help After a Fall

Patients with a fractured hip may be unable to move to get help after a fall. Patients at risk for falls and hip fractures should be taught how to notify emergency services in the event of a fall and injury. Options include the following:

- Turn on your stomach and crawl to a phone.
- Scoot to the phone on your bottom or uninjured side.
- Crawl to a stairway, and use the stairs to gradually lift yourself to a standing position.
- Participate in a 24-hour emergency alert service, such as Lifeline.
- Keep a bell or phone near the floor rather than on the wall or counter so it can be reached from a fallen position.
- Keep a cell phone with you at all times.
- Ask a friend or family member to check in daily.
- Cover up with a blanket to stay warm until help arrives.

Clinical Manifestations

Patients with a hip fracture will experience severe pain in the hip, upper thigh, groin, or lower back, especially when attempting to flex or rotate the hip. They may be unable to move, stand, or walk (see the Patient Teaching feature). The patient may feel stiffness as well as bruising and swelling in the hip area. The leg on the side of the injured hip may appear shorter than the uninjured leg and may turn outward. In severe injuries, bone may be visible through the skin.

Hip fractures are usually the result of trauma. Therefore, other injuries may also be present, such as additional bone fractures; head injuries; or damage to the intestines, bladder, or reproductive organs.

Complications

Complications associated with a hip fracture result from a major loss of mobility and include DVT, pressure injuries, urinary tract infections (UTIs), pneumonia, and muscle atrophy. Other complications include postoperative infection, mental deterioration, avascular necrosis, and nonunion or malunion of the bone. Most patients lose muscle mass and strength after sustaining a hip fracture. Even after rehabilitation, there is a likelihood of continued decline in mobility and function (PubMed Health, 2014).

Collaboration

Collaborative care team members for a patient with a hip fracture may include nurses, treating physicians (e.g., orthopedic surgeon, the patient's primary care physician), pharmacists, and PTs and OTs. The nurse should also collaborate with any specialists the patient may consult for specific conditions, especially respiratory and cardiac conditions. If the patient needs rehabilitative care after discharge from an acute care facility, the nurse may refer the patient to social services.

Diagnostic Tests

Diagnosis of a fractured hip is based on a physical exam and imaging tests. A fractured hip is usually evident based on the abnormal position of the leg and hip. X-rays are the primary imaging tool used to diagnose hip fractures and determine the location of the fracture. CT scans and MRIs can also be used to detect hairline fractures that are not visible by x-ray.

Surgery

The first-line treatment for a hip fracture is surgery. Surgery should take place as soon as possible after the fracture; ideally, the patient should be taken to a healthcare facility that offers

Clinical Manifestations and Therapies
Hip Fracture

ETIOLOGY	CLINICAL MANIFESTATIONS	CLINICAL THERAPIES
Intracapsular hip fracture	▪ Fracture to the head or neck of femur ▪ Pain in the hip region ▪ Inability to move or stand, outward turn of the leg, shorter leg on injured side	▪ Repaired with individual screws or compression hip screw with plate ▪ Repair of damaged cartilage ▪ Hemiarthroplasty or arthroplasty ▪ Analgesics ▪ Prophylactic antibiotics or anticoagulants ▪ Bisphosphonates ▪ Traction or casting ▪ Physical and occupational therapy
Extracapsular hip fracture	▪ Fracture to the trochanter region of the femur ▪ Pain in the hip region ▪ Inability to move or stand, outward turn of the leg, shorter leg on injured side	▪ Repaired with compression hip screw or intramedullary nail in marrow canal or plate on outside of bone ▪ Analgesics ▪ Prophylactic antibiotics or anticoagulants ▪ Bisphosphonates ▪ Traction or casting ▪ Physical or occupational therapy

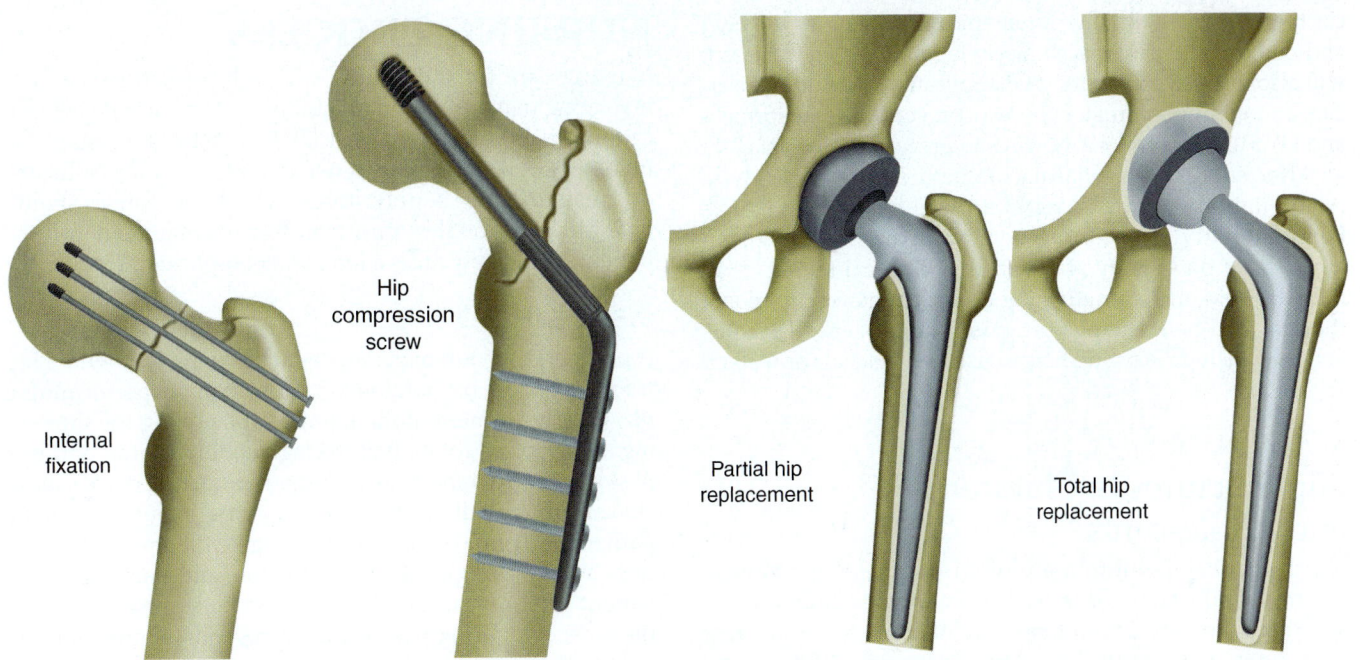

Figure 13–39 》 Repair of intracapsular and extracapsular hip fractures.

24-hour surgical care. The type of surgery will depend on the condition of the patient and the location and severity of the fracture. The goal of surgery is to reduce pain, stabilize the fracture, and return the patient to a normal activity level. The three basic types of surgery are repair with hardware, partial hip replacement, and total hip replacement (see **Figure 13–39 》**).

Repair of an intracapsular fracture often involves using individual screws (percutaneous pinning) for internal fixation or a single larger screw (hip compression screw,) that slides within the barrel of a plate. If the fracture is displaced, ORIF surgery will be conducted to realign the fracture. If damage is only to the head of the femur, the goal of surgery is to repair the cartilage that has been injured. If the acetabulum, or socket of the hip, is fractured, it may require surgical repair as well.

Repair of an extracapsular fracture involves the use of a compression hip screw similar to an intracapsular fracture or the insertion of an intramedullary nail into the marrow canal of the bone through an opening made in the greater trochanter. The nail is secured in place by screws at the top and bottom of the nail. As an alternative, a plate may be used on the outside of the bone to immobilize the fracture.

In older patients with avascular necrosis, severe fracture, or other underlying bone conditions, hip replacement may be the best treatment option. Hip replacement can involve replacement of the ball, or head, of the femur (partial hip replacement or **hemiarthroplasty**), or replacement of the ball and socket, or head and acetabulum (total hip replacement, or **arthroplasty**, see Figure 13–39). Total hip replacement is often the best option for patients with previous joint damage from arthritis (Mayo Clinic, 2015a).

Complications associated with hip replacement include dislocation of the prosthesis, infection, and delayed healing. Hip dislocation occurs because the artificial ball and socket are smaller than the original bone, allowing the ball to become dislodged in certain positions, such as when the knee is pulled up to the chest. In addition, failure of the prosthesis

may occur. Over time, particles wear off the joint surfaces, causing inflammation and loosening of the prosthesis. After 10 or more years of wear, this may create a need for **revision surgery**, or replacement of the artificial joint. Revision surgery carries greater risk than the original hip replacement surgery (NIAMSD, 2013). For this reason, internal fixation or casting of the fractured hip is traditionally preferred over hip replacement in younger patients. However, newer technology is increasing the longevity of hip prostheses, and hip replacement surgery is on the rise for younger, active patients.

SAFETY ALERT Because of potential complications associated with hip replacement surgery, hip replacement is contraindicated for patients with limited mobility prior to the fracture (e.g., patients who are bedridden or wheelchair bound), patients at high risk for infection (e.g., patients who are immunocompromised), and patients who are too ill to undergo any form of anesthesia.

Pharmacologic Therapy

Patients with a hip fracture will likely require pain medications, such as opioids or patient-controlled analgesia. Medications may also be given to high-risk patients to prevent complications, including antibiotics to prevent infection and anticoagulants to prevent DVT. Anti-inflammatory agents may be used for patients with a worn prosthesis in an attempt to avoid revision surgery. Patients may also receive bone density enhancers (e.g., bisphosphonates) to help stimulate bone growth, especially if a noncemented prosthesis is implanted or if the patient is at risk for a second hip fracture.

Nonpharmacologic Therapy

For patients who cannot undergo surgery or who have a stable hip fracture, the hip fracture will be managed by nonsurgical methods, including bedrest, traction, or casting. Traction will likely include either Buck or Russell traction (see Box 13–3). Traction may also be used briefly for patients awaiting surgery.

Casting will likely involve a hip spica cast, such as the one-and-one half hip spica cast shown in Figure 13–30D. Treatment will also involve prevention of complications, including exercise and compression stockings to prevent muscle stiffness and DVT and respiratory exercises to prevent pneumonia.

After surgery, nonpharmacologic therapy will include rehabilitation such as physical and occupational therapy. Early mobility is encouraged; many patients will begin ambulation on the day after surgery. Physical therapy will include ROM and strengthening exercises, and occupational therapy will help the patient gain independence in ADLs and may include learning how to use a wheelchair or walker.

Lifespan Considerations

Hip Fractures in Children and Adolescents

Hip fractures in children are often due to motor vehicle crashes. Children's bones heal more quickly than adults' and therefore need prompt medical attention to set the fracture and immobilize the joint. Hip fractures in children may involve the epiphyseal plate, which lies between the head and neck of the femur; physicians must account for epiphyseal plates in bones when performing treatment. Treatment for hip fractures in children often involves casting or repair surgery rather than hip replacement surgery. Adolescents are more likely to experience a hip fracture from a motor vehicle collision, bicycle collision, or sports injury. For both children and adolescents, time of healing in a cast is about 4–6 weeks (Boston Children's Hospital, 2016a).

Hip Fractures in Young Adults

Femoral neck fractures are uncommon in young adults and require a high-energy injury, such as a motor vehicle collision, a fall from a high area, and work injuries (Hakim & Volpin, 2015). Treatment emphasizes maintaining natural hip anatomy and mechanics.

Hip Fractures in Older Adults

Older adults may not be capable of returning to an independent lifestyle after a hip fracture (CDC, 2015). Approximately 20% of patients will have another hip fracture within 2 years (Mayo Clinic, 2015a). About 50% of patients will experience another fracture in about 3–5 years (Mitchell, as cited in Pollack, 2013).

Erika J. Mitchell, MD, spoke adamantly at the annual meeting of the Clinical Orthopaedic Society about the concerns of fragility fractures, especially hip fractures (Pollack, 2013). Mitchell reported that the mortality rate for hip fractures has changed little over the past 30 years. The 30-day mortality rate is approximately 9%; for patients with an acute medical condition, the mortality rate increases to 17%. For patients who develop pneumonia after hip fracture, the mortality rate increases to 43%; for patients who experience heart failure during treatment of the hip fracture, it increases to 65%. Emphasis is placed on getting the patient moving early, despite the patient's complaints of pain and feeling too tired. Additional emphasis is placed on nutrition, DVT prophylaxis, and avoiding sensory deprivation.

NURSING PROCESS

Nursing care for the patient with a hip fracture includes managing pain, promoting mobility, and preventing complications such as infection and DVT. Nursing care may also involve referring the patient to a PT or OT, home healthcare, or assistive device supply stores. In addition, nurses should provide emotional support and encouragement for the patient, who likely faces a long and complicated recovery.

Assessment

A preoperative nursing assessment of the patient with a hip fracture begins by obtaining vital signs and performing a physical assessment of the injured hip, looking for shortening and external rotation of the leg, mobility status, and loss of skin integrity related to a compound fracture or skin abrasions from the fall or accident. The nurse should assess the patient for degree of injury (including hematoma, inflammation, and swelling), cognitive function, and pain level. The patient's neurovascular status should be assessed by using the 5 *P*s, comparing neurovascular responses in the injured limb to the uninjured limb (see Exemplar 13.B).

SAFETY ALERT Paralysis is a sign of severe nerve damage and should be reported to the physician immediately.

The nurse should obtain a medical history, including a history of the current traumatic event and a past history of osteoporosis or other conditions that affect strength, mobility, balance, and coordination. Because hip fractures often occur in older patients and patients are at higher risk for developing complications as they age, obtaining the patient's age is a vital part of the nursing assessment. A history of other medical conditions or medications that may affect the patient's treatment should also be noted. To complete the nursing assessment, the nurse may be responsible for arranging and transporting the patient to imaging procedures such as an x-ray.

Postoperative assessment of the patient with a hip fracture involves many of the same assessments that were conducted preoperatively, including vital signs, pain intensity, cognitive dysfunction, and the 5 *P*s neurovascular assessment. (See the Concept of Mobility section for a review of the 5 *P*s neurovascular assessment.) In addition, assessment should include the patient's ability to ambulate, oxygenation status, presence of infection of the surgical incision, urinary or bowel complications associated with anesthesia and immobility, and signs of DVT.

Diagnosis

Examples of nursing diagnoses that may be appropriate for inclusion in the plan of care for the patient with a hip fracture may include the following:

- *Risk for Infection* related to surgical incision
- *Acute Pain* related to fractured hip
- *Impaired Physical Mobility* related to inability to move hip joint
- *Impaired Skin Integrity* related to skin abrasions
- *Risk for Falls* related to insufficient strength and balance
- *Acute Confusion* related to traumatic event

- *Anxiety* related to lengthy rehabilitation process
- *Deficient Knowledge* related to treatment options for fractured hip
- *Stress Overload* related to multiple severe injuries and their treatment
- *Caregiver Role Strain* related to caring for an individual with limited mobility.

(NANDA-I © 2014)

Planning

Goals for the patient with a hip fracture may include the following:

- The patient will achieve adequate pain control, as evidenced by reports of pain that rate no higher than 3 on a scale of 0–10.
- The patient will ambulate independently after surgery and rehabilitation.
- The patient will have adequate wound healing of skin abrasions.
- The patient will not develop an infection from wounds or surgical incisions.
- The patient will demonstrate increased muscle strength and balance.
- The patient will be oriented to time, location, and environment.
- The patient will verbalize decreased anxiety with understanding of the rehabilitation process.
- The patient will verbalize an understanding of treatment options for a hip fracture.
- The patient will implement nonpharmacologic methods to reduce stress.
- The patient's caregiver will ask for help when needed to provide relief from caregiver responsibilities.

Implementation

Nursing interventions begin at the community level with fall prevention programs. Nurses working in clinics or other community-based facilities can promote safety by assessing risk factors related to falls for patients of any age. Some potential risk factors include medications that may cause alterations in mentation, unsteady gait, orthostatic hypotension, or household items such as throw rugs.

Nursing interventions for patients with a hip fracture are similar to general recommendations for patients with other types of bone fractures, including managing pain, maintaining proper alignment, promoting mobility, monitoring the patient's neurovascular status, and monitoring for infection (see Exemplar 13.B). In the hospital setting, nursing interventions may include pre- and postoperative interventions, emotional care, and instructions for home care. Preoperatively, the nurse will assess the patient's understanding of the available treatment options for a hip fracture.

Plan Effective Preoperative and Postoperative Care

The majority of patients with a hip fracture will undergo surgery to repair or replace the injured hip. Preoperative

interventions include pain management, immobilization of the hip with traction or other restraints, and providing information about the treatment plan. Preoperative care may also include administering prescribed prophylactic antibiotics and transporting the patient to surgery.

Postoperative nursing interventions are aimed at managing pain, promoting mobility, and preventing complications. The nurse teaches the patient about correct positioning of the hip to prevent hip displacement after arthroplasty. The nurse also assists the patient with ambulation as soon as prescribed by the physician. The nurse should teach the patient about preventing DVTs as well as signs and symptoms of DVTs. Anticoagulants should be administered prophylactically. Patients who are bedridden should perform respiratory exercises to maintain lung function and should be monitored for signs of pneumonia and other respiratory complications. Patients who are bedridden are at high risk of deconditioning and should be assisted with ROM or receive passive ROM to prevent muscle atrophy. The nurse should turn patients who are bedridden or who have limited mobility frequently to prevent pressure injuries. The nurse should perform wound hygiene for the surgical incision and any other skin wounds; infections should be treated promptly with antibiotics.

Promote Psychosocial Wellness

Although physical care of the patient is important for recovery after a hip fracture, emotional and mental care of the patient is also a major nursing intervention needed for patients with a hip fracture. Whether the patient is younger and has experienced a traumatic motor vehicle crash or sports injury or is older and experienced a fall in the home, a hip fracture causes emotional distress related to the traumatic event. Most patients will experience anxiety or fear related to extreme pain, an unknown diagnosis and treatment plan, or a poor prognosis. Older patients may experience confusion as a result of the trauma or surgery, and they also may feel despair over their loss of independence.

Postoperative nursing interventions in the hospital setting may include the following:

- Orient the patient to the time, day, place, and situation.
- Assess the need for pain medication.
- Administer pain medications as ordered or needed.
- Assess the surgical wound for signs and symptoms of infection.
- Change the surgical dressing as ordered.
- Encourage the patient and family to share their feelings about the traumatic event, treatment, rehabilitation, and long-term care options.
- Provide information about the patient's condition, and explain the treatment plan.
- Provide verbal and written instructions for care.
- Refer the patient and family to a home health agency, rehabilitation center, or long-term care facility.
- Promote a trusting relationship so the patient can express concerns and ask questions about his or her condition or treatment plan.
- Support the use of coping mechanisms to decrease stress, including the use of family, friends, and support services.

Provide Thorough Discharge Instructions

The patient who has had surgery for a hip fracture will need extensive care after leaving the hospital. This may be provided at home or in a rehabilitation or long-term care facility. Patients who will be cared for at home and their caregivers will need proper training to ensure maximal healing. Topics for instruction may include the following:

- Proper use of an abduction pillow (if ordered) while resting or sleeping to maintain proper hip alignment
- Proper sitting and bending techniques, including sitting on a high chair and using a high toilet seat to prevent excess flexion of the hip
- Proper use of a walker or cane
- Explanation of weight-bearing limitations as prescribed by the physician
- Explanation of all medications, including dosage, schedule, and potential side effects
- Referral to PTs, home care agencies, or local medical equipment sources as needed.

Evaluation

The patient should be evaluated for return of mobility, absence of neurologic complications, a decrease in pain, and complications from the fracture and from surgery. Evaluation should also include assessment of the patient's emotional state throughout treatment. Participation in physical therapy and other rehabilitation programs should be evaluated to determine if the patient is benefiting from the exercise and returning to full function.

The nurse will evaluate the patient to determine whether the identified goals have been met after completion of intervention. Assessment of patients recovering at home should include adherence to all discharge instructions as well as the treatment regimen and assessment of patient and family/caregiver coping and functioning. Ongoing evaluation of postoperative patients is essential to promote healing, reduce the risk of mental and functional deterioration, and reduce the risk for complications leading to readmission.

Nursing Care Plan

Presurgical Care of a Patient with a Hip Fracture

Giorgina Mancini is a 68-year-old woman with a history of OA and osteoporosis. She has lived alone since her husband died 3 years ago, but she is well known in her neighborhood for providing delicious food made from scratch to anyone who stops by at mealtime. While carrying groceries up the front steps to her porch, Mrs. Mancini falls and lands on her right hip. Her neighbor, who witnesses the fall, calls 9-1-1, and Mrs. Mancini is transported by ambulance to the local ED.

ASSESSMENT	DIAGNOSES	PLANNING
The nurse conducting Mrs. Mancini's initial assessment finds that her right leg is externally rotated and shortened. Mrs. Mancini complains of severe pain with an intensity of 8 on a 0–10 pain scale. Her legs and feet are warm with strong pedal pulses bilaterally. She denies numbness or tingling. Mrs. Mancini is able to move the toes on her right foot, and she has full ROM in her left leg. Her vital signs include temperature 97.8°F oral; pulse 80 bpm; respirations 22/min; and BP 112/63 mmHg. Diagnostic tests include CBC, serum electrolytes, and x-ray studies of the right hip and pelvis. The CBC reveals a hemoglobin of 10.4 g/dL, which is slightly decreased from normal. The physician orders type and crossmatch for two units of blood. All other blood tests are within normal limits. The x-ray reveals a fracture in the right lesser trochanter region. Mrs. Mancini is admitted to the hospital with an order for 10 lb of straight leg traction. Surgery to repair the fracture with an intramedullary nail in the marrow canal is scheduled for the next morning.	■ *Risk for Ineffective Peripheral Tissue Perfusion* related to fractured right hip and soft tissue damage ■ *Acute Pain* related to fractured right hip and soft tissue damage ■ *Impaired Physical Mobility* related to fractured right femur and application of traction ■ *Impaired Skin Integrity* related to abrasions sustained during a fall ■ *Risk for Infection* related to contaminated skin wounds ■ *Impaired Social Interaction* related to not being home to provide food for visitors (NANDA-I © 2014)	■ The patient will develop no complications related to impaired peripheral circulation. ■ The patient will verbalize a decrease in pain to a 4 or less on a scale of 0–10. ■ The patient will participate in passive ROM exercises. ■ The patient will allow proper care of abrasions, including cleansing and application of a sterile bandage. ■ The patient will not develop an infection of the abrasions. ■ The patient will provide a phone number of a close friend or family member to be present in the hospital as needed during her recovery.

IMPLEMENTATION

- Administer pain medications and traction as prescribed by the physician.
- Turn the patient every 2 hours to prevent pressure injuries.
- Apply compression stockings to the patient's legs.
- Conduct passive ROM exercises on the patient's left leg and both arms every 4 hours while awake to enhance circulation.

- Assess the patient every 2–4 hours for neurovascular status of the right leg.
- Clean abrasions with sterile solution, and apply a sterile bandage.
- Provide patient teaching about traction and hip repair surgery.
- Call a close friend or family member to encourage visitation of the patient as tolerated.

Nursing Care Plan *(continued)*

EVALUATION

The patient expressed a decrease in pain from 8 to 5 after pain medication and a further reduction to 3 after traction. The patient's abrasions from the fall were cleaned and appeared minor. A sterile bandage and antibiotic ointment were applied to each abrasion. The nurse conducted passive ROM exercises for the patient twice in the evening and once in the morning before surgery.

Compression stockings were applied. Neurovascular checks revealed no complications. The patient was prepped for surgery, including receiving preoperative teaching and prophylactic antibiotics. Several friends have visited and waited at the hospital during the surgery. A new care plan reflecting postoperative interventions will be developed.

CRITICAL THINKING

1. Prepare a document explaining the process of traction and its necessity while waiting for surgery.

2. Why is it important for Mrs. Mancini to feel connected to friends and family members during her hospital stay?

3. Develop a postoperative care plan for Mrs. Mancini.

REVIEW   Hip Fractures

RELATE Link the Concepts and Exemplars

Linking the exemplar of hip fractures with the concept of health, wellness, and illness:

1. Describe the modifiable risk factors and teaching interventions for patients at risk for hip fractures.

2. In an older female patient, what findings from a nutritional screening would indicate an increased risk for hip fractures? What teaching could the nurse provide to lower this risk?

Linking the exemplar of hip fractures with the concept of elimination:

3. What nursing interventions can be implemented for a patient with a hip fracture who is taking opioids for pain management and has developed constipation?

4. Develop a care plan for a patient with urinary retention after hip replacement surgery.

READY Go to Volume 3: Clinical Nursing Skills

REFER Go to Pearson MyLab Nursing and eText

- Additional review materials

REFLECT Apply Your Knowledge

Maria Haley is 65 years old and lives alone in her two-story house. Her husband Del passed away 2 years ago, but left her financially comfortable if she is careful. Mrs. Haley has two grown children who are both married, but she has no grandchildren yet. Her children both live in another state. Mrs. Haley is active at the senior center in town, is an avid bridge player, and enjoys relatively good health. She is taking simvastatin 20 mg/day for a slightly elevated cholesterol level. Mrs. Haley also takes 10 mg of lisinopril once a day for borderline hypertension with good control. Because Mrs. Haley lives alone, she does not bother to cook much and fixes frozen dinners or soup for her meals at night. As active as Mrs. Haley is, she does not do much exercising and weighs 140 lb, which is a 10 lb increase over last year's weight. Mrs. Haley drives, but admits to the nurse that things seem blurry at night.

1. What factors put Mrs. Haley at risk for hip fracture?

2. During her annual checkup, what safety teaching regarding risks for hip fracture will you address with Mrs. Haley?

3. What nutritional suggestions might you implement to help with the prevention of hip fractures?

4. What recommendations regarding exercise will you make to Mrs. Haley?

›› Exemplar 13.D
Multiple Sclerosis

Exemplar Learning Outcomes

13.D Analyze multiple sclerosis (MS) as it relates to mobility.

- Describe the pathophysiology of MS.
- Describe the etiology of MS.
- Compare the risk factors for and prevention of MS.
- Identify the clinical manifestations of MS.
- Summarize diagnostic tests and therapies used by interprofessional teams in the collaborative care of an individual with MS.
- Differentiate considerations for care of patients with MS across the lifespan.
- Apply the nursing process in providing culturally competent care to an individual with MS.

Exemplar Key Terms

Axon, *936*
Demyelination, *936*
Exacerbation, *937*
Lesions, *936*
Multiple sclerosis (MS), *936*
Myelin, *936*
Oligodendrocytes, *936*
Plaques, *936*
Pseudoexacerbation, *937*
Remyelination, *936*

Overview

Multiple sclerosis (MS) is an immune-mediated disorder of the CNS in which immune cells attack the myelin sheath around nerve cells, causing decreased transmission of nervous signals. **Myelin** forms a fatty insulating layer around nerve cells to increase the speed of electrical transmission along the nerve. Symptoms of MS often go into remission after the initial manifestation of the disease, making MS difficult to diagnose. Each individual affected by MS will experience a different set of symptoms and a range of severity of symptoms depending on the nerves that are affected.

Pathophysiology and Etiology

Pathophysiology

The CNS consists of the brain, spinal cord, and optic nerves. Each **axon**, or nerve fiber, in the CNS is covered by a myelin sheath to protect the nerve and increase the efficiency of electrical impulses along the neuron membranes. In some individuals, cells of the immune system, such as lymphocytes and macrophages, cross the blood–brain barrier and attack and destroy the myelin sheath in a process called **demyelination**. This causes inflammation and leads to the formation of **lesions** (areas of inflammation and damage) in the surrounding area.

In addition to the myelin sheath, the underlying axon as well as **oligodendrocytes** (cells that produce myelin) may be damaged by the immune system. Unlike damage to the myelin sheath, which can be repaired by oligodendrocytes over time, damage to the axons is not reversible. However, repeated attacks on the myelin may stimulate the formation of scar tissue, or **plaques**, causing permanent damage. Axon damage and a lack of myelin disrupt nerve impulses in the CNS, causing neurologic symptoms such as muscle weakness, visual disturbances, and balance and coordination problems (Multiple Sclerosis Association of America [MSAA], 2013). The pattern of inflammation, damage, and repair causes MS to manifest in one of four patterns (see **Box 13–4 》**).

Etiology

MS is generally characterized as an autoimmune disease. However, because the exact antigen is unknown, many scientists prefer to call MS an immune-mediated process. The events that trigger the immune response against the myelin sheath are unknown, but links have been found to environmental, infectious, and genetic factors. Environmental factors may include geography, sunlight, and environmental toxins. Individuals who were born in an area with a high incidence of MS and move to an area of little or no incidence of MS prior to the age of 15 have been shown to lower their risk of developing MS to that of the new area. Individuals who live farther from the equator and are exposed to less sunlight are more likely to develop MS, causing some scientists to believe that vitamin D plays a protective role. Multiple studies have attempted to link viruses to the development of MS, including measles virus, herpes virus, rubella virus, HTLV-1, *Chlamydia pneumoniae*, and Epstein-Barr virus (NMSS, n.d.b.).

Box 13–4
Classifications of Multiple Sclerosis

The four main classifications of MS are relapsing-remitting MS, primary-progressive MS, secondary-progressive MS, and progressive-relapsing MS (MSAA, 2013; National Multiple Sclerosis Society [NMSS], n.d.a.).

- *Relapsing-remitting MS* is the most common form of MS at the time of diagnosis, affecting approximately 85% of patients with MS. Individuals with relapsing-remitting MS experience clearly defined flare-ups with worsening neurologic function followed by periods of partial or complete remission with few or no symptoms. Remission is thought to occur when oligodendrocytes repair the damaged myelin sheath (**remyelination**). Patients can experience periods of relapse that last for days or months and periods of remission that last from weeks, to months, to years.
- *Primary-progressive MS* affects approximately 10% of patients with MS. These individuals experience a slow, but nearly continuous, worsening of their disease from the time of onset with no distinct remissions. The rate of progression may vary over time, from temporary minor improvements, to plateaus, to obvious worsening of symptoms.
- *Secondary-progressive MS* develops within 10 years of diagnosis in about half of the patients with relapsing-remitting MS who are not receiving treatment. Individuals with secondary-progressive MS experience an initial period of relapsing-remitting MS, followed by a progressive form of the disease with or without occasional flare-ups and minor remissions. This form of MS may develop as a result of the eventual destruction of oligodendrocytes, preventing the body from repairing the myelin sheath.
- *Progressive-relapsing MS* is relatively rare, occurring in only 5% of individuals with MS. These individuals experience a steady worsening of disease with acute relapses. In contrast to relapsing-remitting MS, the periods between relapses are characterized by continued progression of the disease rather than remission of symptoms.

Genetic factors may also play a role in the development of MS. MS is not hereditary, but individuals with a first-degree relative such as a parent or sibling with MS have a significantly increased risk of developing MS. The risk of developing MS is approximately 0.1% for the general population. For first-degree relatives, this risk increases to 3–5%, whereas the risk is 31% for identical twins (MSAA, 2013).

Risk Factors and Prevention

Several other risk factors have been linked to the development of MS. MS is usually diagnosed in individuals between the ages of 20 and 40, although individuals as young as 2 and as old as 75 have been diagnosed with MS. Women are twice as likely as men to develop MS (Mayo Clinic, 2015b). Traditionally it was thought that individuals of European descent were more prone to MS, but recent research demonstrates that rates of MS are similar in African Americans, who have different, and often worse, symptoms that people of European descent (NMSS, n.d.c.). Smoking also increases the risk of developing MS, and individuals with MS who smoke are at greater risk for escalation of disease symptoms (MSAA, 2013). As the Focus on Diversity and Culture feature

Focus on Diversity and Culture
Parasites

Parasites tend to weaken the immune response. Therefore, individuals with an increased likelihood for parasitic infection, such as those who live in developing countries, are less likely to be diagnosed with MS, which is triggered by a strong immune response. With improved sanitation and decreased exposure to parasites, the diagnosis of MS is on the rise in these countries (MSAA, 2013).

explains, individuals in certain countries may also be at more risk.

There is currently no cure for MS and no absolute way to prevent it. Individuals may decrease their risk of developing MS by avoiding smoking and taking vitamin D supplements. Parents with children at a higher risk for developing MS should evaluate their living situation to determine if their family is living in an area of high risk for the development of MS.

Clinical Manifestations

Clinical manifestations of MS depend on the location and severity of damage in the CNS. No two patients will present with the same set of symptoms, and many manifestations are common to other diseases, making diagnosis difficult. Manifestations of MS may be persistent, may go into remission, or may become exacerbated depending on the immune process causing them. Individuals experiencing exacerbation may have one or more symptoms that last from days to months, and symptoms can be different during distinct exacerbations. A true **exacerbation** must last at least 24 hours and must be separated from the previous attack by at least 30 days. Symptoms that last for less than 24 hours are termed *paroxysmal attacks*.

Common signs and symptoms of MS include fatigue, paresthesia (numbness, tingling, burning), lack of coordination and balance, unsteady gait, tremor, bladder and bowel dysfunction, visual disturbances (unilateral loss of vision, optic neuritis, double vision, blurred vision, oscillopsia, red–green color distortion), dizziness, sexual dysfunction (impotence, dyspareunia, anorgasmia), pain (headache, Lhermitte sign, trigeminal neuralgia, allodynia), cognitive dysfunction (lack of concentration, memory loss, reasoning problems, poor judgment), depression, anxiety, and muscle spasticity or weakness in one or more limbs (see the Multisystem Effects feature). Less common symptoms include speech disorders, swallowing problems, hearing loss, seizures, breathing problems, itching, "MS hug" (a sensation of a tight band around the abdomen), and partial or complete paralysis.

Although there is no common trigger for relapse, several factors may influence a relapse. Many patients cite stress and fatigue as contributors to flare-ups. Some patients experience heat sensitivity, or a relapse of symptoms associated with increases in body temperature (e.g., fever caused by infection). Infection and increased body temperature may cause a **pseudoexacerbation**, or a temporary aggravation of symptoms that is directly related to a trigger and subsides as soon as the trigger is removed.

The primary symptoms of MS that result from demyelination may lead to secondary and tertiary symptoms as well. Secondary symptoms result from chronic primary symptoms. For example, individuals with urinary retention may develop UTIs, individuals with muscle weakness in the legs may develop muscle atrophy and pressure injuries from immobility, and individuals with balance problems and an unsteady gait may fall and fracture a bone. Tertiary symptoms relate to psychosocial problems, such as relationship difficulties, loss of a job because of decreased performance, or hopelessness. Tertiary symptoms often occur as a result of symptom exacerbation and lack of coping skills.

Cultural differences have also been observed in patients with MS. Although White patients are more susceptible to developing MS, Black patients with MS tend to be older and have more symptoms at the time of diagnosis. These symptoms are usually limited to the optic nerve and spinal cord, making Black patients more susceptible to vision and mobility problems. They also tend to have more progressive disease that is less responsive to current disease-modifying therapies. In contrast, Hispanic patients are usually younger than White patients at diagnosis, and they tend to have fewer mobility problems and bladder and bowel dysfunction than White patients. However, they may experience more depression and have less access to services needed to treat MS (MSAA, 2013).

Collaboration

The variety of symptoms associated with MS increases the need for collaboration among multiple clinicians, including nurses, neurologists, immunologists, urologists, ophthalmologists, obstetricians, pulmonologists, cardiologists, primary care providers, therapists (physical, occupational, speech, psychologic), nutritionists, and home health agencies. In particular, nursing care will focus on symptom management, patient teaching, emotional support, and referrals to other healthcare services, depending on the patient's disease manifestations.

Diagnostic Tests

No single test can be used to definitively diagnose MS. Instead, the medical history, physical examination, and several diagnostic tests are used to diagnose it. Diagnostic tests include an MRI, lumbar puncture, evoked potential test, and blood tests (Mayo Clinic, 2015b; MSAA, 2013; NMSS, n.d.a). Using these tests, the patient must meet three criteria to be diagnosed with MS: lesions in at least two separate areas of the CNS, evidence that the two areas of damage occurred at least 1 month apart, and the ability to rule out all other possible diagnoses.

- An *MRI* is used to detect the presence of lesions in the CNS that may indicate demyelination and MS. Gadolinium may also be injected to help detect areas of current disease activity.

- A *lumbar puncture*, or spinal tap, is used to obtain a sample of CSF. The CSF is then tested for the presence of elevated immunoglobulins (IgG), oligoclonal bands, and myelin breakdown products, all of which are indicative of MS.

Multisystem Effects of
Multiple Sclerosis

Respiratory
- Diminished cough reflex
Potential complication
- Respiratory infections

Urinary
- Hesitancy
- Frequency
- Retention
- Reflex bladder emptying
Potential complications
- Recurring UTIs
- Incontinence

Gastrointestinal
Oral/esophageal
- Difficulty chewing
- Dysphagia
Upper/lower GI
- ↓ or absent sphincter control
- Bowel incontinence
- Constipation

Musculoskeletal
- Fatigue
- Limb weakness
- Ataxic movements (shaky, irregular, uncoordinated)
- Intention tremors
- Spasticity
- Muscular atrophy
- Dragging of foot and foot drop
- Dysarthria with slurred speech

Neurologic
- Emotional lability (euphoria or depression)
- Forgetfulness
- Apathy
- Scanning speech
- Impaired judgment
- Irritability
Potential complications
- Convulsive seizures
- Dementia

Sensory
Visual
- Blurred vision
- Diplopia
- Nystagmus
- Visual field defects (blind spots)
- Eye pain
Auditory
- Vertigo
- Nausea
Tactile (especially hands or legs)
- Numbness
- Paresthesias (tingling, burning sensation)
- Diminished sense of temperature
- Pain with spasms
- Loss of proprioception
Potential complication
Visual
- Blindness

Reproductive
- Impotence (male)
- Loss of genital sensation
- Painfully heightened sensation (female)
- Vaginal dryness

Clinical Manifestations and Therapies
Multiple Sclerosis

ETIOLOGY	CLINICAL MANIFESTATIONS	CLINICAL THERAPIES
Primary symptoms (result from demyelination)	■ Sensory disturbances (visual, hearing, speech, balance, pain) ■ Motor disturbances (weakness, paresthesias, bowel and bladder dysfunction, unsteady gait, spasticity, breathing problems) ■ Cognitive dysfunction (concentration, memory, reasoning, judgment, depression)	■ Disease-modifying therapies ■ Symptom-specific medications ■ Corticosteroids to treat exacerbations ■ Assistive devices ■ Physical therapy or rehabilitation
Secondary symptoms (result from prolonged primary symptoms)	■ Pressure injuries ■ Osteoporosis ■ Aspiration pneumonia ■ UTIs ■ Back or hip pain ■ Muscle atrophy, poor postural alignment ■ Bone fractures	■ Antibiotics ■ Analgesics ■ Bisphosphonates ■ Physical therapy ■ Immobilization of fractures ■ Nutrition and fluids
Tertiary symptoms (psychosocial complications)	■ Social problems (partner, family, friends, social isolation) ■ Vocation problems (loss of job, loss of transportation) ■ Emotional problems (depression, irritability, hopelessness)	■ Psychologic counseling ■ Antidepressants ■ Referral to home care, transportation assistance ■ Encouragement to engage in social interaction ■ Patient teaching to minimize isolation ■ Caregiver support ■ Vocational rehabilitation

■ *Evoked potential tests* measure the electrical activity of the brain in response to stimulation of sensory nerve pathways, specifically visual evoked potentials, brainstem auditory evoked potentials, and sensory evoked potentials. These tests are able to detect the slowing of electrical conduction that is caused by demyelination of the nerves. Evoked potential tests are often useful for identifying a second demyelinating event that causes no clinical symptoms and does not create a lesion that is detectable by MRI.

■ *Blood tests* are used to rule out other infectious or inflammatory diseases that may mimic the symptoms of MS.

Surgery

Surgery is not a common treatment for patients with MS. However, patients with specific symptoms may require surgery. For example, patients with severe pain may undergo a rhizotomy, which selectively destroys problematic nerve roots in the spinal cord. Likewise, patients with spasticity may undergo musculoskeletal surgery to lengthen or transfer a tendon or muscle to reduce tension. Surgery may also be indicated to allow for placement of a pump that administers intrathecal baclofen therapy (ITB).

Pharmacologic Therapy

Pharmacologic therapy is the mainstay of treatment for patients with MS. Since 1993, 10 disease-modifying therapies have been approved for the treatment of relapsing-remitting MS; the primary result of taking these medications is a decrease in the number of relapses.

■ The beta interferons (Avonex, Betaseron, Extavia, Rebif) reduce the number of inflammatory cells that cross the blood–brain barrier, leading to a reduction of neuronal inflammation. Beta interferons can slow the progression of disease and decrease the severity of attacks. Side effects may include reactions at the injection area, liver damage, and mood changes. Nursing responsibilities include assessing liver function and CBC for baseline parameters and every 3 months to test side effects, assessing the injection site, and monitoring changes in the patient's condition and function to assess for efficacy.

■ Glatiramer acetate (Copaxone) blocks the immune system's attack on myelin. Side effects may include flushing, chest pain, or heart palpitations.

■ Fingolimod (Gilenya) traps immune cells in the lymph nodes, making them unable to access the CNS. Side effects include bradycardia, diarrhea, cough, and headache.

■ Natalizumab (Tysabri) interferes with the movement of immune cells across the blood–brain barrier; it is used only in patients who cannot tolerate other treatments because it increases the risk of developing a fatal brain infection (multifocal leukoencephalopathy).

- Mitoxantrone (Novantrone) is an immunosuppressant that is only used to treat advanced MS because of cardiovascular and other serious side effects.
- Teriflunomide (Aubagio) is a pyrimidine synthesis inhibitor that inhibits the function of lymphocytes. It may cause serious liver damage.
- Dimethyl fumarate (Tecfidera) is thought to inhibit immune cells and have antioxidant properties that protect the nerves from damage. Side effects may include flushing and gastrointestinal events.
- Baclofen (Lioresal) is administered to reduce spasticity in patients with a variety of disorders, including cerebral palsy, traumatic SCI, and MS. ITB may be considered when oral baclofen fails to adequately reduce spasticity in patients with certain conditions, including MS.

SAFETY ALERT Disease-modifying therapies may cause damage to a fetus. Therefore, they are not approved for women who are pregnant. Women who want to become pregnant should discontinue their MS medications before attempting to conceive. These drugs are also not recommended during breastfeeding.

Disease-modifying therapies are not approved for the treatment of progressive forms of MS. Therefore, patients with MS are often treated with medications that are specific for their symptoms (see **Table 13–6 »**). When a new medication is added to the regimen of a patient with MS, the nurse is responsible for reviewing with the patient the dosage and schedule for taking the medication and teaching the patient and family about side effects they should report to the physician.

Some medications may require tests for adverse side effects. For example, patients taking corticosteroid therapy for exacerbations should be monitored for glucose intolerance,

TABLE 13–6 Medications for Symptoms of Multiple Sclerosis

Symptom	Medication Examples
Acute exacerbations	Dexamethasone, methylprednisolone, adrenocorticotropic hormone (ACTH), prednisone
Fatigue	Amantadine, fluoxetine, modafinil
Spasticity	Baclofen, dantrolene, diazepam, tizanidine
Constipation	Bisacodyl, docusate, glycerin, magnesium hydroxide
Pain	Carbamazepine, clonazepam, gabapentin, phenytoin
Erectile dysfunction	Alprostadil, sildenafil, tadalafil, vardenafil
Depression	Bupropion, citalopram, duloxetine, paroxetine, sertraline
Urinary tract infection	Ciprofloxacin, methenamine, sulfamethoxazole + trimethoprim
Bladder dysfunction	Imipramine, desmopressin, oxybutynin, prazosin, tamsulosin
Tremor	Isoniazid, buspirone, propranolol
Walking	Dalfampridine

Source: Data from Adams, M. P., Holland, L. N., & Urban, C. (2017). *Pharmacology for nurses: A pathophysiologic approach* (5th ed.). Hoboken, NJ: Pearson Education.

osteoporosis, and cataract formation. Patients taking muscle relaxants for spasticity should be monitored for hepatotoxicity, dizziness, and skeletal muscle activity. Some muscle relaxants may produce withdrawal symptoms if not tapered during discontinuation. The nurse should be familiar with the potential adverse effects of each drug and conduct tests to monitor the patient's condition as prescribed by the physician.

Nonpharmacologic Therapy
The progressive, lifelong nature of MS requires that patients not only take medications as needed for symptoms, but also participate in nonpharmacologic therapies to reduce symptoms and regain functionality. This could include rehabilitation, proper nutrition and fluids, and good lifestyle habits. Rehabilitation includes the following (NMSS, n.d.d):

- Physical therapy emphasizes walking, strength, and balance by encouraging stretching, ROM exercises, strength training, gait training, and training in the use of assistive devices. The goal of physical therapy is to maintain optimal functioning and prevent complications.
- Occupational therapy is used to enhance independence, productivity, and safety for activities related to personal care, leisure, and employment.
- Speech-language therapy is used for patients with speech or swallowing problems related to MS to enhance clarity of speech and promote safe swallowing and overall health.
- Cognitive therapy is used to help treat changes in the patient's ability to think, reason, concentrate, and remember.
- Vocational rehabilitation offers job training, job placement assistance, mobility training, and assistive technology assessments in an effort to help patients maintain their current employment or find new employment that accepts their limitations.

Maintaining a healthy lifestyle is essential for patients with MS to reduce complications and exacerbations. In addition to rehabilitation, patients should participate in a regular mild exercise program such as walking, swimming, and weight training to increase muscle strength and balance. Fatigue is a common symptom of MS, so patients should get plenty of rest. Symptoms may be exacerbated by increased body temperature, so the patient should be encouraged to avoid excessive heat and to keep cool by staying in air-conditioned areas and drinking cold beverages. Eating a balanced diet and maintaining adequate hydration will help the patient maintain a healthy weight and maintain bone and muscle health. The patient's diet may need to be adapted to accommodate changes in the patient's ability to chew and swallow as well as movement limitations such as tremor and muscle weakness. The nurse may also teach patients methods to reduce stress, such as t'ai chi, massage, deep breathing, or distraction techniques (Mayo Clinic, 2015b).

Complementary Health Approaches
Complementary health approaches are commonly used by patients with MS. However, many of these therapies are unsubstantiated by clinical trials, so patients should be

cautioned in their use of complementary health approaches. Many therapies, such as acupuncture, aromatherapy, therapeutic horseback riding, electromagnetic therapy, massage, and prayer have low risk and may be beneficial for some symptoms. Other therapies, such as hyperbaric oxygen, marijuana, and bee venom therapy, carry more risk than benefit. Herbal remedies may benefit specific symptoms, such as valerian for insomnia or cranberry for prevention of UTIs, but others may irritate the urinary tract, interact with steroid medications, or stimulate the immune system (Reitman & Kalb, 2012). Low-dose naltrexone has also been suggested as an alternative therapy, and studies indicate that it improves the patient's quality of life, but has no impact on physical symptoms (NMSS, n.d.d.).

Lifespan Considerations

MS in Children and Adolescents

Studies suggest that 2–5% of individuals with MS experience symptoms before the age of 18. Diagnosis is more challenging in children than adults because of the multitude of other childhood disorders with symptoms similar to MS. In addition to symptoms experienced by adults, children with MS often experience seizures and mental status changes that are not common in adults, and children have a higher rate of relapse. Children with MS may have reduced academic performance, difficulty in family and peer relationships, and distorted self-image. MS usually progresses more slowly in children, but because of the early onset of symptoms, disability may accumulate at a younger age compared to patients with adult-onset MS (NMSS, n.d.e.).

MS in Pregnant Women

Because MS most commonly affects women of childbearing age, women with MS must decide whether they want to become pregnant. Evidence suggests that pregnancy does not influence the overall course of disease, and MS does not affect a woman's ability to become pregnant. However, pharmacologic treatment of MS involves drugs that may be harmful to a fetus. Pregnant women are usually protected from exacerbations during the second and third trimester, but they have a 20–40% risk of developing a flare-up in the first 6 months postpartum. Women who experience gait difficulties before pregnancy may experience an exacerbation of these symptoms, especially during the third trimester when the woman's center of gravity naturally shifts. Bladder problems and fatigue may also be intensified in pregnant women with MS compared to pregnant women without MS (NMSS, n.d.f). Pregnant women with MS may experience decreased pain during labor as a result of sensory deficits.

MS in Older Adults

The life expectancy and average age of individuals with MS has increased significantly over the past 20 years (Sanai et al., 2016). Older adults living with MS typically show more severe symptoms than younger people living with MS. This may be due to the progression of the disease and/or the aging process, which brings increasing weakness and loss of muscle mass. Caregivers, who are often aging spouses or partners, may increasingly require assistance. Older adults with MS may be more agreeable to using assistive devices now than when they were younger.

NURSING PROCESS

Individuals who are diagnosed with MS are often in their prime of life. The physical, emotional, and cognitive effects of MS can affect every area of the individual's life, including relationships, work, and self-image. In particular, the individual's relationship with a partner may become strained because the progressive course of the disease means increasing assistance with ADLs is required. Loss of independence and the strain on financial resources that a chronic illness creates can lead to social isolation, depression, feelings of helplessness, and a lack of desire to perform ADLs and self-care.

The nurse plays a major role in the healthcare of individuals with MS. Nurses have the most contact with the patient and therefore have the responsibility to follow and document the progression of the patient's disease course and treatment. Continued assessment of the timing and severity of exacerbations, effectiveness of medications, and the patient's functional status are integral to good nursing care. The nurse is in a unique position to listen to the patient, offer emotional and physical support, teach the patient about the disease and how to prevent exacerbations, and refer the patient to the needed services.

Assessment

- **Observation and patient interview.** Nursing assessment of the patient with diagnosed or suspected MS begins with observation and health history. Observe the patient's gait, posture, and degree of independence. The initial medical history includes onset, type, intensity, and pattern of symptoms; factors that affect symptoms; ongoing medical problems and medications; past history of surgery, trauma, or infection; health history of family members; and exposure to environmental hazards. The nurse should also assess how current symptoms affect the patient's everyday life. Following the initial assessment of the patient's health history, recurring assessments should evaluate the progression of signs and symptoms and the patient's coping responses to any changes.

- **Physical examination.** A physical examination begins by observing the patient's ability to move and walk, affect, balance and coordination, hygiene, and speech. The Expanded Disability Status Scale (EDSS; Kurtzke, 1983) is frequently used to assess neurologic impairment in patients with MS. This scale combines a general Disability Status Scale with a Functional System (FS) grade. The FS is divided into pyramidal, cerebellar, brainstem, sensory, bowel and bladder, visual, cerebral, and other. It is rated on 0–5, with 5 indicating a high level of problems. Using the 0–10 EDSS scale, patients with scores greater than 4 have some degree of gait disability. The tool is widely used by clinicians to determine the disability of the patient with MS (Tarver, 2015).

An MS Functional Composite (MSFC) scale can also be used to assess specific physical function using three tests. A nine-hole peg test is used to assess arm function, a timed 25 ft walk test assesses leg function, and the MS Symptom Checklist (MSSC) assesses the presence of 26 common MS symptoms in the areas of motor function, sensory disturbance, mental and emotional concerns, bowel and bladder elimination, and brainstem symptoms.

SAFETY ALERT Patients with chronic or progressive diseases such as MS are at increased risk for developing depression. Assess patients with MS for depression and suicidal ideation at each healthcare interaction.

Diagnosis

Patients with MS may have a variety of nursing diagnoses that could be related to any of the 12 domains depending on the location of myelin damage and resulting symptoms. A sample of relevant nursing diagnoses includes the following:

- *Mobility: Physical, Impaired*
- *Urinary Incontinence, Functional*
- *Constipation*
- *Fatigue*
- *Self-Care Deficit: Bathing*
- *Hopelessness*
- *Body Image, Disturbed*
- *Role Strain, Caregiver*
- *Role Performance, Ineffective*
- *Sexual Dysfunction*
- *Coping, Ineffective.*

(NANDA-I © 2014)

Planning

Just as a variety of nursing diagnoses may be appropriate for inclusion in the plan of care for a patient with MS, numerous patient goals are also relevant to these nursing diagnoses. For example, patient goals related to the previously described nursing diagnoses may include the following:

- The patient will participate in physical and occupational therapy and an exercise program to maintain independent physical mobility.
- The patient will state methods to reduce urinary incontinence and how to discreetly deal with urinary incontinence when outside the home.
- The patient will verbalize understanding of methods to prevent and treat constipation.
- The patient will receive 8 hours of sleep per night and rest as needed during the day to decrease fatigue.
- The patient will demonstrate maximum independence during ADLs, such as personal care and bathing.
- The patient will receive psychologic counseling as needed.
- The patient will accept and adapt to debilitating symptoms and participate in programs to regain maximal function.

- The patient's caregiver will receive help from home health agencies, family, and friends to provide relief from caregiver duties.
- The patient will participate in vocational rehabilitation and find a job that accommodates individuals with disabilities.

Implementation

Nursing interventions for many symptoms related to MS can be found in other exemplars throughout this textbook. See Table 13–6 for medications used to manage symptoms related to MS. This section discusses nursing interventions for symptoms specific to MS and mobility. In addition, one primary nursing intervention is patient teaching (see the Patient Teaching feature).

In outpatient settings, appropriate nursing interventions will include a combination of the following:

- Facilitate a home safety assessment to determine the patient's ability to function safely at home and evaluate the need for any assistance in the home, with the long-term goal being that the patient will be able to live at home as long as possible.
- Facilitate arrangements for home healthcare.
- Provide safety teaching related to safe body mechanics and fall prevention.
- Establish patient baseline to help identify exacerbations and subsequent return to baseline.
- Provide teaching or referral regarding a bladder training program to help the patient remain continent. Incontinence is linked to poor self-esteem and increased social isolation.

A recently developed survey, Assessing Relapse in Multiple Sclerosis (ARMS) Questionnaire, may serve as a helpful checklist for both patients and providers. Following treatment for the exacerbation, it may be helpful to ask patients to complete the corresponding posttreatment evaluation.

>> **Stay Current:** The ARMS Questionnaire can be found at: http://www.ncbi.nlm.nih.gov/pmc/articles/PMC3882990/figure/i1537-2073-14-3-148-f101/. The corresponding posttreatment questionnaire can be found at: http://www.ncbi.nlm.nih.gov/pmc/articles/PMC3882990/figure/i1537-2073-14-3-148-f102/.

Interventions for nurses working in the hospital setting might include:

- Encourage patient participation in decision making. Patients who participate in decision making regarding their treatment regimens have higher adherence rates and are more likely to report treatment challenges and symptom changes earlier.
- Teach intermittent urinary catheterization. Patient self-catheterization promotes independence.
- Administer medications as ordered to assist the patient's return to baseline.
- Administer antipyretics as ordered. Even small increases in body temperature can strongly affect conduction through partially demyelinated fibers.
- Teach the patient to use an incentive spirometer to promote respiratory function.

Patient Teaching

Multiple Sclerosis

MS is often diagnosed at a young age, and the patient will live with the disease for many years. Therefore, it is essential that the patient fully understand the disease and its implications. Teaching topics may include the following:

- The overall pathophysiology of the disease
- A projected disease course and disease classifications
- Symptoms commonly experienced by patients with MS
- Medications used to treat MS and its symptoms, including dosing, schedule, side effects, and drug–drug interactions
- Mechanisms to prevent exacerbations, such as managing fatigue and stress and avoiding cold and heat extremes, high humidity, physical overexertion, and infections
- Mechanisms to avoid complications, including pressure injuries, infections, and bone fractures
- Cautions for women who want to become pregnant or are pregnant or breastfeeding
- Safety modifications for the home
- Community resources, such as the National Multiple Sclerosis Society.

Promote Independent Mobility

The nurse should assess patients for ambulation ability at each appointment. Nursing interventions should aim to help patients remain independently mobile for as long as possible. The nurse should advocate for patients who may benefit from medications to reduce spasticity and increase walking ability. Patients experiencing difficulty with ambulation should be encouraged to begin an exercise program and physical therapy. The nurse may also need to assess patients' homes for safety to prevent falls in patients with an unsteady gait or muscle weakness.

Many patients resist using an assistive device for walking because of impaired self-image. The nurse plays an important role in teaching patients the advantages of assistive devices, including independence and increased safety. This may also include providing emotional support for patients to maintain a positive self-image while using assistive devices. Participation in physical therapy is essential for patients who need training in the use of ambulation devices. Patients may need multiple assistive devices depending on the activity. For example, a patient may use a cane at home for short distances, but a walker or wheelchair in public when longer distances are involved.

For patients who use a wheelchair, the nurse should provide information about motorized wheelchairs, handicap-accessible transportation services, and home modifications that will increase the patients' ability to move around the home or town. Methods to prevent complications such as pressure injuries and urinary retention should also be discussed.

Promote Self-Care

Patients with motor deficits such as tremor, walking difficulties, ataxia, muscle weakness, or spasticity may have trouble performing self-care, including bathing, eating, toileting, dressing, transferring, and hygiene care. The ability of patients to perform ADLs should be a guide to determine how much assistance the patients need in all areas of life. Patients who need assistance with ADLs are usually still able to make adequate decisions about self-care, even if they cannot physically perform the activities. Therefore, caregivers should be encouraged to consult patients about their preferences for self-care. Maintaining some control over basic activities is essential to patients' emotional well-being and should be incorporated into each nursing intervention.

Helping the patient maintain independence in ADLs is essential for promoting a positive self-image and encouraging participation in social activities. Nursing interventions could include encouraging the patient to wear arm or wrist braces to provide stability during self-care activities; teaching the patient to perform self-care activities when energy levels are high; using assistive devices while eating, such as plate guards and modified utensils; modifying the consistency of foods to make eating easier; and receiving assistance from others for meal preparation. The nurse can also teach patients techniques for bowel and bladder control, including adequate fluid intake, scheduling regular voiding, self-catheterization, bowel training, and exercise to maintain muscle strength. Patients with self-care deficits may also benefit from occupational therapy.

Facilitate Referrals for Collaborative Care

In addition to a neurologist, patients with MS will need integrated care from multiple healthcare workers. Specialty care is essential for these patients. For example, a patient with urinary incontinence or retention or chronic UTIs should be referred to a urologist. Patients who want to become pregnant should be referred to an obstetrician. Patients with motor deficits should be referred to a PT or an OT. Patients with depression or anxiety need to receive counseling and treatment from a psychologist or psychiatrist. Patients with swallowing difficulties should see a nutritionist to find a diet with adequate nutrition that is easy to swallow and a speech-language therapist to maintain swallowing function. Patients with visual disturbances should be referred to an ophthalmologist. All patients need an individualized healthcare team to help maintain optimal functioning.

Evaluation

MS is an ever-changing disease that requires constant evaluation and revision of the care plan to meet the current needs of the patient. Evaluation should include assessing for disease exacerbation as well as for progression from relapsing-remitting MS to secondary-progressive MS. The nurse should evaluate type and severity of symptoms and should re-evaluate medications related to each symptom for necessity and effectiveness. The nurse should continually evaluate the presence of complications such as infection, because complications may lead to an exacerbation. Other points of evaluation include mobility and the need for assistive devices, the emotional stability of the patient, and areas of deficient knowledge.

Nursing Care Plan
A Patient with Multiple Sclerosis

Holly West, a 42-year-old female patient who grew up in Canada, was diagnosed with MS approximately 7 years ago, although she has had mild symptoms for 12 years. She works as a grocery manager at a store near her home. She lives with her husband and two children, ages 14 and 17. Mrs. West has recently experienced worsening urinary incontinence, fatigue, weakness, and mobility issues due to spasticity in her leg muscles. She also has a fever, chest congestion, and a productive cough. After evaluation at her local hospital's ED, she is admitted to the hospital for evaluation and treatment of pneumonia and exacerbation of her MS.

ASSESSMENT

Carl Kartler, RN, is assigned to care for Mrs. West. Her primary complaint is congestion and the inability to cough up sputum. She also states, "I'm so tired of missing work. My husband has to take care of me like I'm a baby." Vital signs include temperature 101.0°F oral; pulse 92 bpm; respirations 28/min; and BP 112/62 mmHg. Auscultation of Mrs. West's lungs reveals scattered rhonchi throughout, and her oxygen saturation is 96% on room air. She is pale, but her skin is warm and dry. The physician orders a STAT respiratory treatment of aerosolized albuterol for Mrs. West, after which her breath sounds are improved; rhonchi are diminished. Her course of therapy also will include ACTH and IV antibiotics.

DIAGNOSES

- *Ineffective Airway Clearance* related to excessive mucus production
- *Ineffective Breathing Pattern* related to presence of sputum in the airways
- *Functional Urinary Incontinence* related to damaged nerves that control bladder function
- *Impaired Physical Mobility* related to weakness and spasticity of leg muscles
- *Fatigue* related to infection and MS
- *Ineffective Role Performance* related to inability to perform home and work roles
- *Bathing Self-Care Deficit* related to muscle weakness
- *Hyperthermia* related to infectious process

(NANDA-I © 2014)

PLANNING

- The patient will maintain a patent airway.
- The patient will freely expectorate sputum.
- The patient's lung sounds will be clear on auscultation.
- The patient's oxygen saturation will remain above 95% on room air.
- The patient will demonstrate knowledge of bladder training.
- The patient will be free from infection.
- The patient will participate in physical therapy to increase muscle strength and balance.
- The patient will rest as needed during the day to prevent fatigue.
- The patient will verbalize an ability to adapt work and self-care to her level of energy.

IMPLEMENTATION

- Encourage coughing, deep breathing, and expectoration of sputum.
- Administer respiratory treatments as ordered.
- Assess breath sounds every 4 hours and as needed.
- Assess oxygen saturation every 4 hours and as needed.
- Administer oxygen as needed per medical orders and hospital protocol.
- Administer antibiotic therapy as ordered.
- Administer ACTH as ordered.
- Teach the patient bladder training techniques, including Kegel exercises, delayed urination, and scheduled urination.

- Facilitate patient referral to a urologist as ordered for bladder incontinence and risk for UTI.
- Facilitate patient referral to a PT or an OT as ordered to increase muscle strength and the ability to perform ADLs as well as assistive device training if needed.
- Teach the patient the importance of performing activities during peak energy levels.
- Teach the patient the importance of resting throughout the day.
- Encourage independence with mobility and self-care. Assist with ADLs as needed based on the patient's fatigue levels.
- Offer and facilitate patient referral to an MS support group.

EVALUATION

After 5 days in the hospital, Mrs. West is ready for discharge. She denies dyspnea, and her lungs are clear to auscultation. Her oxygen saturation is 99% on room air. Mrs. West is given an additional 10-day prescription of antibiotics and verbalizes an understanding of the importance of completing the course of antibiotics. She demonstrates good pulmonary hygiene techniques and has been referred to a PT. After attending physical therapy and receiving instruction on cane use, Mrs. West has increased independence for ambulation. Occupational therapy has increased her ability to perform ADLs, and she understands the importance of performing strenuous activities during times of peak energy. Mrs. West still requires some help with eating in the evening when she is most fatigued. She has been referred to a urologist and has verbalized understanding of bladder training techniques.

CRITICAL THINKING

1. How would you change the care plan for Mrs. West if she used a wheelchair?

2. What teaching points should you provide for Mrs. West's husband about helping with self-care activities?

3. Develop a care plan for the nursing diagnosis Deficient Knowledge related to prevention of infection.

REVIEW Multiple Sclerosis

RELATE Link the Concepts and Exemplars

Linking the exemplar of MS with the concept of sensory perception:

1. What assessment findings would you anticipate for a patient with MS regarding alterations in visual acuity?

2. If the demyelination from MS is affecting the patient's brainstem, what physical assessment data are a priority for the nurse to gather related to sensory perception?

Linking the exemplar of MS with the concept of mood and affect:

3. How will the administration of interferon beta-1a put the patient at risk for alterations in mood and affect?

4. What mental health data are a priority for the nurse to assess before planning care for the patient with MS?

READY Go to Volume 3: Clinical Nursing Skills

REFER Go to Pearson MyLab Nursing and eText

- Additional review materials

REFLECT Apply Your Knowledge

Elena Jones is a 48-year-old charge nurse who works in a busy pediatric intensive care unit. She works 3 days a week doing 12-hour shifts and attends management and committee meetings on her days off. Mrs. Jones lives with her husband Brett and their three children: Debbie, 16; Jason, 11; and Ryan, 8. Brett is a remodeler who runs his business out of the home. Debbie is busy visiting colleges that are interested in recruiting her because she is a star soccer player. She has been sneaking out of the house at night to visit her boyfriend. Jason has been in trouble in school for sassing teachers and has mild attention-deficit/hyperactivity disorder. Ryan has just discovered an interest in playing football after school.

Mrs. Jones began having symptoms of neck pain and blurred vision. She has consulted a number of physicians, but did not receive a satisfactory diagnosis until she saw a neurologist who ordered an MRI and diagnosed her with MS. Following her initial treatment, she quickly entered a period of remission that lasted for a few weeks. From that time on, she has experienced three to four exacerbations per year. She has had to quit her job because she is unable to walk and has blurred vision that precludes driving. Her physician begins prednisone infusions five times a week for 1 week during flare-ups of MS.

1. What role might stress be playing in exacerbating her MS? What strategies can you promote to reduce stress?

2. How might you guide Mrs. Jones's family to contribute to improving her condition?

3. What are your expected outcomes for Mrs. Jones's care?

≫ Exemplar 13.E Osteoarthritis

Exemplar Learning Outcomes

13.E Analyze osteoarthritis (OA) as it relates to mobility.

- Describe the pathophysiology of OA.
- Describe the etiology of OA.
- Compare the risk factors for and prevention of OA.
- Identify the clinical manifestations of OA.
- Summarize diagnostic tests and therapies used by interprofessional teams in the collaborative care of an individual with OA.
- Differentiate considerations for care of patients with OA across the lifespan.
- Apply the nursing process in providing culturally competent care to an individual with OA.

Exemplar Key Terms

Arthroplasty, *949*
Arthroscopy, *948*
Debridement, *948*
Joint fusion, *949*
Joint irrigation, *948*
Joint resurfacing, *948*
Osteoarthritis (OA), *945*
Osteotomy, *949*
Viscosupplementation, *950*

Overview

Osteoarthritis (OA) is the most common form of arthritis, affecting 50% of the world's population ages 65 years and older (Musumeci, Szychlinska, & Mobasheri, 2015). OA develops as wear and tear on the joints breaks down the cartilage in the joint, causing bone to rub on bone. It is the most common cause of disability in older adults and can affect any joint in the body, especially the hands, knees, and hips. Treatment aims to reduce pain, improve function of the affected joint, and slow disease progression.

Pathophysiology and Etiology
Pathophysiology

In healthy joints, the slick surface of articular cartilage covers the ends of bones, allowing the bones to glide over each other without friction during movement of the joint. Cartilage also absorbs shock from physical movement. As an individual ages, the cartilage begins to break down, becoming rough and eventually wearing away, allowing the bones to rub against each other. Particles that break off the joint irritate the synovial tissue, causing the pain, stiffness,

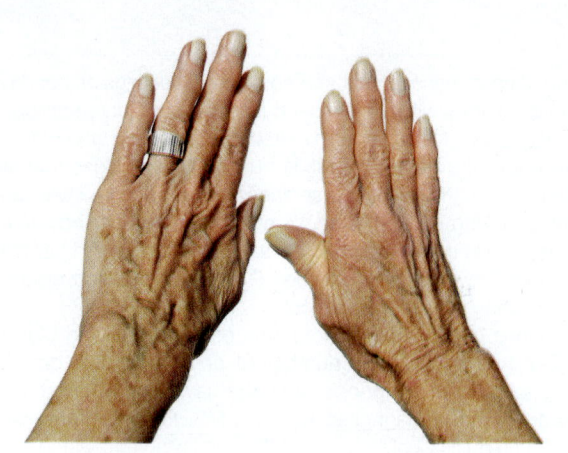

Figure 13–40 》》 Typical interphalangeal joint changes associated with osteoarthritis.

inflammation, and swelling characteristic of OA (see **Figure 13–40 》》**).

As OA progresses, slow-developing changes occur to the joint's synovium, subchondral bone, and cartilage. As changes to the joint occur, the joint no longer moves smoothly, causing mobility problems. OA typically involves the weight-bearing joints of the hips and knees, the digits of the hands and big toe, and the cervical and lumbar spine.

Etiology

OA can be classified as either idiopathic or secondary. Idiopathic OA has no identifiable cause, but most researchers believe it is caused by both mechanical and molecular factors. Idiopathic OA can be further divided into localized or generalized, with localized OA affecting one or two joints and generalized OA affecting three or more joints. Secondary OA is caused by an underlying condition, such as injury; congenital malformation; metabolic, endocrine, or neuropathic disease; or other medical cause.

Risk Factors

The greatest risk factor for OA is older age. OA rarely occurs in individuals under the age of 40, but at least 80% of individuals over age 55 have some x-ray evidence of the disorder. Sixty percent of individuals with arthritis are women (CDC, 2016). Men often develop OA in the hips, knees, and spine, whereas women usually develop OA in the hips, knees, and hands. Jobs that require hard labor, heavy lifting, bending, or repetitive motion are linked to increased rates of OA. Obesity also increases the risk of developing OA, because the added weight increases stress on weight-bearing joints, causing the joint to wear down more quickly.

Certain medical conditions may increase an individual's risk of developing OA. For example, individuals born with malformed joints (bow legs, unequal leg length) or defective cartilage have an increased risk of developing OA. In addition, diseases such as diabetes, hypothyroid, gout, and Paget disease increase the risk of developing OA. Joint injuries

from sports, accidents, or repetitive use also increase the risk of OA (CDC, 2016).

Prevention

Two of the most important guidelines for preventing OA are to maintain an ideal body weight and to participate regularly in a moderate exercise program. Weight-bearing joints endure three to six times the individual's body weight in force while walking. Therefore, being overweight magnifies the force on the joint and leads to rapid degeneration of the cartilage. Both inactivity and excessive exercise can lead to premature breakdown of the joint cartilage; a moderate exercise program that involves walking, jogging, cycling, or swimming provides the most benefit for keeping bones, muscles, and joints strong and functioning properly.

Other important guidelines for maintaining good joint health include using good posture and proper body mechanics, avoiding repetitive stress on joints, stopping an activity when the joint becomes painful, and avoiding injury to the joints. If an injury does occur, the patient should be encouraged to seek treatment immediately.

Clinical Manifestations

OA begins with mild symptoms and progressively worsens over time. Symptoms of OA vary depending on the joint affected and individual factors. Some patients with visible joint degeneration on x-ray have no associated symptoms in the affected joint. However, many patients with OA develop pain associated with joint degeneration; this pain is usually worsened by activity and relieved by rest. Pain and stiffness is also associated with prolonged inactivity, such as sleeping at night or taking a long car ride. Other symptoms include tenderness to the touch, swelling related to excess fluid in the joint (effusion), crackling or grating of the joint (crepitus) due to rough surfaces rubbing against each other, and bone spurs that contribute to joint swelling. This joint damage typically causes the joint to have a decreased ROM.

OA can lead to a host of complications as the severity of the condition worsens. Joint pain and degeneration, stiffness, unsteady gait, and certain medications increase the risk of falling, causing fractures and additional mobility limitations. As physical limitations increase, the patient may experience a decreased ability to perform ADLs. As the individual is less able to perform work responsibilities, he or she may develop financial difficulties related to the cost of treatment and lost wages. As the disability persists, the individual may develop anxiety, depression, and feelings of helplessness. Both the physical disability and the associated mood disorder may lead the individual to have difficulty participating in social and family activities.

Collaboration

Treatment of OA requires interprofessional care from nurses, primary care providers, rheumatologists, PTs and OTs, and many others. Because there is currently no cure for OA, treatment aims to relieve pain and maintain function of the joint. Helping patients learn how to cope with a chronic disease is also a vital part of nursing care for patients with OA. According to *Healthy People 2020* (U.S. Department of Health and Human Services, 2013), interventions that can reduce

Clinical Manifestations and Therapies
Osteoarthritis

ETIOLOGY	CLINICAL MANIFESTATIONS	CLINICAL THERAPIES
Knee	■ Pain, effusion ■ Crepitus ■ Instability ■ Deformity ■ Osteophytes ■ Stiffness, unsteady gait, limited movement	■ Rest, heat, ice ■ OTC analgesics ■ Assistive devices ■ Weight loss ■ Corticosteroid injections ■ Viscosupplementation ■ Osteotomy ■ Arthroplasty ■ Physical therapy, exercise
Hip	■ Referred pain to inguinal region, buttock, thigh, or knee ■ Limited ROM ■ Unsteady gait, stiffness	■ Rest, heat, ice ■ Physical therapy, exercise ■ Assistive devices ■ OTC analgesics ■ Weight loss ■ Corticosteroid injections ■ Joint resurfacing ■ Osteotomy ■ Arthroplasty
Shoulder	■ Pain ■ Stiffness ■ Thickened joint capsule ■ Loss of ROM ■ Crepitus	■ Physical therapy, exercise ■ OTC analgesics ■ Corticosteroid injections ■ Arthroscopic debridement ■ Joint resurfacing ■ Arthroplasty ■ Rest, heat, ice
Spine	■ Radiating pain ■ Stiffness, muscle spasm ■ Limited ROM ■ Nerve root compression, weakness, numbness	■ Rest, heat, ice ■ OTC analgesics ■ Weight loss ■ Spinal fusion ■ Back-strengthening exercises
Elbow	■ Pain ■ Loss of ROM ■ Grating or locking sensation ■ Swelling, numbness in fingers	■ OTC analgesics ■ Corticosteroid injections ■ Physical therapy, exercise ■ Arthroscopy ■ Osteotomy ■ Arthroplasty
Ankle	■ Pain, swelling, inflammation ■ Stiffness, difficulty walking ■ Limited ROM ■ Deformities	■ OTC analgesics ■ Orthotics ■ Physical therapy, exercise ■ Weight loss ■ Corticosteroid injections ■ Arthroscopic debridement ■ Joint fusion ■ Arthroscopy

(continued on next page)

Clinical Manifestations and Therapies (continued)

ETIOLOGY	CLINICAL MANIFESTATIONS	CLINICAL THERAPIES
Wrist	■ Pain, swelling ■ Stiffness, weakness ■ Limited ROM ■ Crepitus	■ Rest, heat, ice ■ OTC analgesics ■ Bracing ■ Corticosteroid injection ■ Joint fusion ■ Arthroplasty ■ Physical therapy, exercise
Fingers	■ Pain ■ Heberden nodes, Bouchard nodes ■ Crepitus ■ Swelling, tenderness ■ Decreased ROM ■ Cysts	■ Rest, heat, ice ■ OTC analgesics ■ Assistive devices ■ Splinting ■ Corticosteroid injection ■ Joint fusion ■ Arthroplasty
Toes	■ Pain ■ Heberden nodes, Bouchard nodes ■ Decreased ROM ■ Swelling	■ Rest, heat, ice ■ OTC analgesics ■ Corticosteroid injection ■ Joint fusion ■ Arthroplasty

arthritis pain and functional limitations include increased physical activity, self-management education, and weight loss among adults who are overweight or obese.

Diagnostic Tests

In addition to a medical history and physical examination, several tests can be used to help diagnose OA and track the disease's course. The most commonly used diagnostic test is an x-ray of the affected joint, but other tests may include an MRI, ultrasound, blood tests, and joint fluid analysis. An x-ray can reveal a narrowing of the space between bones in the joint, indicating a lack of cartilage. However, x-rays may not show signs of OA until significant cartilage loss has occurred. An x-ray may also show bone spurs or other bone damage. MRI and ultrasound produce more detailed images of the bone and soft tissues, including cartilage, ligaments, and tendons. This is a more sensitive way to determine the extent of joint damage.

Although there is no blood test available that can conclusively identify OA, blood tests can help rule out other causes of joint pain, such as rheumatoid arthritis. Joint fluid analysis is used to detect inflammation and the presence of bacteria (infection) or uric acid crystals (gout).

Surgery

Patients with severe arthritis that is not managed by medication and nonpharmacologic interventions may be good candidates for surgery. Depending on the joint and extent of damage, several options are available for surgery: arthroscopy, joint irrigation, joint resurfacing, osteotomy, joint fusion, and arthroplasty. The purpose of surgery is to remove damage, relieve pain, and restore function of the joint.

Arthroscopy and Joint Irrigation

In the procedure known as **arthroscopy**, a small arthroscope consisting of a small fiberoptic light source, magnifying lens, and camera is inserted into the joint to visualize the joint structures. Small surgical instruments may also be inserted into the joint to remove or trim structures that may be causing pain (**debridement**). Arthroscopy is often combined with **joint irrigation**, in which a fluid is injected into the joint to allow the surgeon to visualize joint structures more easily and to help remove debris and infection in the joint. Benefits of arthroscopic surgery for patients with OA are unpredictable, because the procedure is not designed to repair cartilage that is worn from the ends of bones. However, arthroscopic surgery does relieve pain in some patients with OA, and it can be used to treat OA in patients who have had little success with other treatments (Johns Hopkins Medicine, n.d.b). Arthroscopy can also be used to explore the extent of damage in the joint in preparation for future surgery.

Joint Resurfacing

In **joint resurfacing**, a small amount of bone is removed at the articulating surface of the joint, and a metal replacement is fitted over the end of the bone. Joint resurfacing is often performed instead of total joint replacement in younger patients in the early stages of arthritis. Artificial joints often wear out and need to be replaced within 15–20 years, and the amount of bone removed during arthroplasty makes revision complicated. Joint resurfacing removes less bone than arthroplasty, allowing younger patients to experience more successful total joint replacement later in life, when the metal component has become worn. Joint resurfacing is often performed for hip and shoulder joints.

Osteotomy

Osteotomy is a procedure that entails surgical removal of a wedge of bone above or below the joint to realign the joint and shift the weight away from the damaged portion of the joint. To further help redistribute weight, the tibia and femur are reshaped. Surgical staples or screws are inserted to stabilize the repositioned bones. This procedure is usually performed instead of joint replacement surgery if there is damage to only one side of the joint in healthy, younger adults. After an osteotomy, the patient should be able to participate in any physical activity enjoyed before the surgery, even high-impact exercise. Osteotomies are commonly performed on the knee and hip, but can be used for other joints as well.

Joint Fusion

Joint fusion, also known as arthrodesis, is used to permanently fuse two or more bones together at a joint using pins, plates, screws, and rods. A bone graft may also be used to stimulate bone growth at the site of fusion. Joint fusion is often recommended for badly damaged smaller joints, such as the spine, wrist, ankle, finger, or toe.

Arthroplasty

A total joint replacement is known as **arthroplasty**. In an arthroplasty, the surgeon removes the damaged joint surfaces and replaces them with plastic, metal, or ceramic prostheses. Prostheses may be joined to bone surfaces with cement, or they may contain porous surfaces that stimulate bone growth to hold the prosthesis in place.

Because of advances in technology, the surgeon can choose the type of prosthesis based on the patient's weight, sex, age, activity level, and general health. Artificial joints usually last about 15–20 years, so the best candidates for arthroplasty are older adults. Hip and knee arthroplasties (see **Figure 13–41 》**) are the most common, but other joints can also be replaced, including shoulders, elbows, ankles, wrists, fingers, and toes. Total recovery time after joint replacement of a major joint (hip, knee) is 4–6 weeks short term (independent function) and around 6 months long term (full function). The greatest risks after arthroplasty include infection, blood clots, and long-term breakdown of the artificial joint.

Pharmacologic Therapy

Many OTC medications are effective for treatment of mild to moderate OA pain. Acetaminophen (Tylenol) is usually suggested as a first-line therapy because most patients tolerate it well. However, acetaminophen can produce liver toxicity if taken in high doses or by patients with chronic liver disease or excess alcohol intake (see the Safety Alert feature). Ibuprofen (Advil, Motrin) and naproxen (Aleve) are NSAIDs that treat both pain and inflammation. Stronger NSAIDs are available by prescription, including the COX-2 inhibitor celecoxib (Celebrex). NSAIDs are generally well tolerated, but they can produce cardiovascular and gastrointestinal effects. For patients with severe OA pain, opioid analgesics

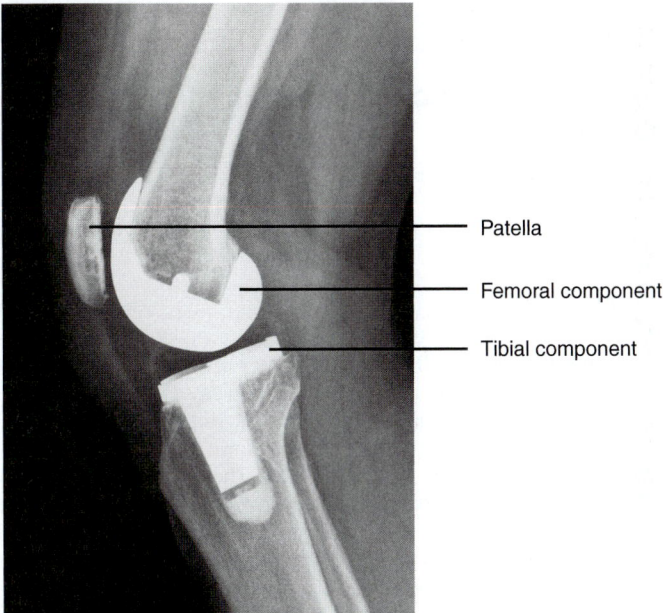

Source: Manx_in_the_world/iStock/Getty Images Plus/Getty Images.

Figure 13–41 》 Total knee replacement.

such as codeine, tramadol, or hydrocodone may be prescribed. However, opioids carry the risk of tolerance and addiction, so they should only be prescribed as a last resort. For more information about analgesics, see the exemplar on Acute and Chronic Pain in the module on Comfort.

SAFETY ALERT Since 2010, the U.S. Food and Drug Administration (FDA) has required manufacturers to provide specific language about the potential for liver damage on OTC medications that contain acetaminophen. The warning must include the information that exceeding a dosage of 4000 mg/day may result in severe liver damage. Manufacturers must also use language in regards to the maximum dosing. For example, acetaminophen 500 mg tablets would read: "Severe liver damage may occur if more than 8 tablets are taken in 24 hours, which is the maximum daily amount for this product" (U.S. FDA, 2015). Alternative language that may now be used states, **"Liver warning:** This product contains acetaminophen. Severe liver damage may occur if you take • more than 4000 mg of acetaminophen in 24 hours • with other drugs containing acetaminophen • 3 or more alcoholic drinks every day while using this product."

Source: From Notice to Industry: Final Guidance for Over-the-Counter Products that Contain Acetaminophen, U.S. Food and Drug Administration.

With any products containing acetaminophen, patients should be aware of the potential for unintentionally exceeding the maximum acetaminophen dosage due to simultaneously taking more than one medication that contains acetaminophen. Likewise, patients with impaired liver function may be at risk for toxicity-related injury, even when following the guidelines. Acetaminophen toxicity may cause severe liver damage, liver failure, and death.

Topical analgesic creams, rubs, and sprays may also be prescribed for patients with OA. These drugs are applied directly to the skin surrounding the joint. They work by stimulating nerve endings, depleting the neurotransmitter called substance P, or blocking prostaglandins to decrease

Evidence-Based Practice

Hyaluronic Acid Injections

Problem

Hyaluronic acid (HA) is a normal component of synovial fluid, where it acts as a lubricant and shock absorber. OA causes a reduced level of HA, leading to pain and reduced movement of the joint (AAOS, 2015b).

Evidence

Multiple studies have indicated that HA injections (**viscosupplementation**) are effective for the treatment of knee OA. HA works by restoring the elastic and viscous properties of the synovial fluid, theoretically improving joint movement and reducing pain (AAOS, 2015b). HA injections have not been shown to improve the condition of the cartilage (AAOS, 2015b). The number of injections administered is dependent on the product and patient response. Research has shown that corticosteroid injections and HA injections reduce joint pain; however, HA injections were found to last about a month longer than corticosteroid injections (Askari et al., 2016).

Implications

Viscosupplementation is a promising therapy for OA with few side effects. Therefore, it may be a preferred treatment for patients with severe OA who will not tolerate surgery. It appears to have fewer adverse effects compared to surgery and more long-term efficacy compared to corticosteroids. However, HA injections are more expensive and are currently approved only for knee OA. In addition, the most common adverse effect is infection, so patients with a compromised immune system should consider the risk versus benefit of such a treatment.

Critical Thinking Application

1. How would you describe the difference between cortisone and HA injections to an older patient with mild cognitive deficits (administration, mechanism of action, side effects, duration of effect, follow-up)?

2. Viscosupplementation is currently approved for knee injections. Some physicians have used it to treat OA in other joints. What would you say to a patient who is skeptical of the long-term side effects of this treatment?

3. If you were asked to develop a brochure stating the pros and cons of HA injections, what information would you include?

---

pain signals received by the brain. Examples include capsaicin cream (Capzasin, Zostrix), diclofenac gel (Voltaren), salicylates (Aspercreme, Bengay), and menthol (Icy Hot, Biofreeze). Nurses should teach patients to keep these topical medications away from the eyes, nose, and mouth and to discontinue use if irritation occurs.

Cortisone injections may also be administered for treatment of OA pain. The corticosteroid medication is injected directly into the joint to reduce inflammation and pain. Because frequent use of corticosteroids can cause joint damage, cortisone injections are limited to three to four injections per year for weight-bearing joints. A relatively new option for OA treatment by injection is HA (see the Evidence-Based Practice feature).

Nonpharmacologic Therapy

OA is a progressive disease, so early treatment can significantly improve outcomes and quality of life. In addition to treating pain with analgesics, nonpharmacologic treatment for OA includes heat and cold application, use of assistive technology, weight reduction, rest, and education about the disease, exercise, and coping techniques.

Heat can be applied to painful joints to decrease pain and improve flexibility. Heat application can include warm towels, hot packs, heating pads, or warm showers or baths. Cold in the form of ice packs or cold packs can be applied to reduce pain and swelling. Mild cold should be used for swelling, and deeper cold should be used for pain.

SAFETY ALERT To avoid skin injury, application of hot packs should not exceed 20 minutes, and cold packs should be applied for no more than 10–30 minutes.

Assistive technology can be used to help minimize stress placed on the affected joint. Canes, crutches, and walkers can be used to protect joints of the lower limbs, and devices such as grippers, reachers, dressing aids, and enlarged pens can reduce stress on the spine and upper limbs. Orthotics, such as braces or shoe inserts, may be beneficial to help maintain proper alignment of the joints. Many assistive devices can be bought commercially or custom made to meet the specific needs of the patient. The nurse may need to refer the patient to a PT or an OT for instruction about proper use of the assistive device.

Obesity is a major contributor to OA development, because excess weight dramatically increases the force on weight-bearing joints. Therefore, the nurse should encourage patients who are overweight or obese and who have OA of the knee, hip, or ankle to begin a weight-loss program. Weight-bearing joints withstand three to six times the force of the total body weight when the individual walks, so even a small reduction in weight can greatly reduce the force on the affected joint.

The nurse should encourage patients with OA to get adequate sleep and rest. Arthritis pain may interfere with nighttime sleep, so the nurse should teach the patient good sleep hygiene (see the exemplar on Sleep–Rest Disorders in the module on Comfort) and nonpharmacologic methods to reduce pain (see the exemplar on Acute and Chronic Pain in the module on Comfort). The nurse should encourage patients to get adequate rest throughout the day to prevent overstressing the affected joints. Rest should be done for short periods with the joint in correct alignment. In addition, the nurse should instruct the patient to stop an activity immediately and rest the joint for 12–24 hours if the arthritic joint is in use and develops increased pain. Resting the joint should result in decreased pain and swelling. If possible, the nurse should encourage the patient to find activities that do not require repetitive use of the injured joint. Assistive devices may be beneficial to promote rest of the injured joint.

Patient Teaching

Exercise Guidelines for Patients with OA

Exercise is an important aspect of nursing care for patients with OA. Exercise can increase flexibility, improve blood flow, help the patient lose weight, and improve mood. Types of exercises include the following:

- *Stretching* of all muscle groups for 10 minutes daily. Patients should avoid overstretching, because this can cause muscle damage.

- Active *range-of-motion* exercises daily for all joints. These exercises help keep joints limber.

- *Balance* and *agility* exercises can help maintain daily living skills.

- Low-intensity *isometric* exercises, or static exercises, can strengthen muscles without moving painful joints.

- *Isotonic*, or strengthening, exercises, in which a fixed weight is carried through the ROM, should start with small weights or a resistance band and a partial ROM. Resistance and range should be increased gradually.

- Low-impact *aerobic* exercises, such as walking, cycling, or swimming, are well tolerated by patients with OA. These exercises improve cardiovascular health, strengthen muscles, and improve balance and gait. Water exercises are especially beneficial for patients with OA of the weight-bearing joints, because water buoyancy helps decrease force on the joints.

Participating in a mild exercise program is an important treatment for OA. Exercises such as walking, biking, or swimming are best for patients with OA. The amount and type of exercise will depend on the joints involved and the extent of joint damage (see the Patient Teaching feature for exercise guidelines). The nurse should teach patients to stop exercising if they experience new pain. In addition, daily ROM exercises can strengthen muscles to provide support for the damaged joint. Physical therapy and other rehabilitation programs can help patients determine which exercises are best for their specific condition; rehabilitation is especially important after joint replacement surgery.

Some patients will not respond to traditional treatments for OA and will look for alternative ways to relieve pain. The Focus on Integrative Health feature provides further information on alternative treatments.

Complementary Health Approaches

Complementary health approaches for OA include acupuncture, massage, and gentle exercises (t'ai chi and yoga). The use of glucosamine and chondroitin for OA has shown mixed results in clinical trials, with most indicating that these nutritional supplements are no better than placebo, but may increase the risk of bleeding (Mayo Clinic, 2016b). Stem cell therapy using autologous mesenchymal stem cells (MSCs) is currently under investigation for use in patients with OA of the knee. Jo and colleagues (2014) found decreased pain and mobility following injection of MSCs in patients with OA of the knee and recommended further investigation.

Lifespan Considerations

OA in Children and Adolescents

Children can develop juvenile OA, which is usually secondary OA related to a congenital abnormality, genetic condition, or joint injury. Juvenile OA typically occurs only in the one or two joints affected by the abnormality or injury. Children with OA are less likely to become disabled and may outgrow the condition as they age. However, children and adolescents with joint abnormalities or injuries who do not develop OA during childhood are at increased risk of developing OA later in life.

OA in Pregnant Women

The increased weight due to pregnancy may cause increased pain related to OA. Pregnant and lactating women should be informed of the risks of any medications they are taking. Some medications, such as Celebrex, have unknown risk during pregnancy and lactation. Other medications, such as Cytoxan, are dangerous during pregnancy and lactation (Arthritis Foundation, n.d.).

OA in Older Adults

Acetaminophen is a first-line medication for older adults because of its efficacy and safety. Narcotics are considered safer than NSAIDS for older adults and are considered a second-line choice (Sholter & Lehman, 2012). Because of the risks of polypharmacy, a complete assessment of medication history and current medications and supplements is necessary before prescribing pain relievers for older adults. Mindfulness exercises and complementary health approaches such as yoga or t'ai chi may assist older adults in increasing mobility and reducing pain levels. Physical therapy is especially important in older adults to maintain or improve mobility of joint(s).

NURSING PROCESS

OA is a progressive and incurable disease. Nursing care for patients with OA focuses on reducing pain, maintaining mobility and function, and helping patients learn how to use assistive devices. If OA becomes severe, patients may also need pre- and postoperative nursing care. For patients who are overweight or obese, the nurse should encourage the patient to begin a weight-loss program to reduce force on weight-bearing joints.

Assessment

- ***Observation and patient interview.*** Observe how patient moves and ambulates. Does the patient require an assistive device or lean on furniture or a caregiver to move across a room? Observe for signs of pain such as grimacing or guarding or indications that the patient experiences difficulty with movement, such as shortness of breath. During the patient interview, assess for a family history of OA, description of symptoms (onset, location, intensity, modifying factors), physical activity (exercise, occupation, recreation), mobility, and ability to perform ADLs.

- ***Physical examination.*** A physical assessment should include height and weight and assessment of the affected joint, including appearance, temperature, pain, crepitus, ROM, deformities, and Heberden or Bouchard nodes.

Diagnosis

Nursing diagnoses related to OA may include the following:

- *Pain, Chronic*
- *Mobility: Physical, Impaired*
- *Lifestyle: Sedentary*
- *Self-Care Deficit: Dressing.*

(NANDA-I © 2014)

Planning

Patient goals for the individual with OA may include the following:

- The patient will verbalize understanding of the indications for and effects of analgesic medications.
- The patient will demonstrate knowledge of nonpharmacologic pain management techniques.
- The patient will verbalize an understanding of the need to rest when pain worsens during physical activity.
- The patient will perform ROM exercises daily.
- The patient will demonstrate increased ROM of the affected joint.
- The patient will begin a mild exercise program based on a PT's recommendations.
- The patient will enroll in nutritional counseling or a weight-loss program.
- The patient will independently perform dressing self-care with the use of assistive devices.

Implementation

Nursing interventions for patients with OA should aim to decrease pain, promote mobility through exercise, teach patients how to use assistive devices for ADLs and self-care, and encourage weight loss in patients who are overweight or obese. See the Patient Teaching feature.

Promote Comfort

Pain as a result of joint degeneration is the most common symptom of OA, and it influences the patient's ability to ambulate and perform ADLs. Therefore, pain management is the primary nursing intervention needed for patients with OA. The nurse should obtain a pain description and monitor pain levels with each patient interaction. Pain from OA is often managed by mild analgesics, which the patient should take on a regular schedule before pain becomes severe. The nurse should teach the patient nonpharmacologic pain management techniques, including good body mechanics, heat and ice, distraction techniques, guided imagery, and relaxation.

Pain associated with OA is cyclical: Joints stiffen with prolonged rest, causing pain when the patient begins movement. As movement warms and lubricates the joints, pain subsides. However, with excessive movement, the patient will begin to feel pain again, which is relieved by rest. Because of this cycle, the nurse should teach patients the importance of alternating rest and activity. Short periods of rest can help relieve joint stress while avoiding stiffness, and short periods of activity can prevent pain from overuse.

Patient Teaching
Home Care for Patients with OA

Patients with OA need to manage their condition while living at home. Several techniques can help patients cope with their disease and maintain function as the disease progresses. Modifications the patient can make include the following:

- Make home safety improvements, such as removing throw rugs and clutter, installing handrails, and placing commonly used items within easy reach.
- Learn about OA, including the disease process and treatments. (A resource such as the American Arthritis Society may be provided to patient.)
- Begin an exercise program to gain strength and ROM. If the patient is over the recommended weight, exercising may help in weight reduction.
- Avoid excessive or repetitive use of joints and overstretching of the muscles associated with the affected joint.
- Practice good posture, and avoid soft furniture that requires excessive effort to stand.
- Use pharmacologic and nonpharmacologic pain management techniques.
- Balance periods of activity with periods of rest.

Moderation of both rest and activity are key to maintaining mobility and reducing pain for patients with OA.

Optimize Physical Mobility

As previously mentioned, patients with OA benefit greatly from performing mild exercise. Exercise can increase the ROM of affected joints, strengthen muscles to provide support for the joint, and promote general health. Exercise can also help patients with OA in weight-bearing joints increase balance, coordination, and strength to promote independent ambulation. The nurse should assess patients with newly diagnosed OA for ROM of the affected joints as a baseline for future comparison, and ROM should be assessed with each subsequent nurse–patient interaction. The nurse should also perform a mobility assessment to determine whether patients have problems walking, sitting, rising, or climbing stairs. These assessments can help guide the nurse in suggesting appropriate exercises and assistive devices. The nurse should also teach patients a variety of exercises to promote mobility or should refer patients to PTs or OTs for teaching and rehabilitation.

Patients will need to learn how to perform ADLs while experiencing a progressive disorder that causes pain, stiffness, and decreased mobility of joints. Assistive devices play a key role in helping patients maintain independence in performing ADLs. Assistive devices can also help reduce stress on affected joints, which may help slow the progression of disease. The nurse should perform a functional assessment to determine which devices may provide the most benefit for patients; the assistive device needed will likely depend on the location of the OA. For example, patients with knee OA may benefit from the use of a cane or walker. Safety devices such as handrails and shower chairs may be beneficial for patients with hip OA. Patients with shoulder or spine

OA may benefit from the use of a reacher device, which can be used to grab objects over the head or on the floor. Patients with OA of the hand may need to use button or zipper hooks, toothbrushes or eating utensils with large handles, or electric can openers. The list of possible assistive devices is endless and can be tailored to the specific needs of patients. Once patients have chosen the appropriate assistive devices, the nurse should provide training or referrals for training in the proper use of each device.

Promote Balanced Nutrition

Patients who are overweight or obese will decrease their risk of disease progression if they begin a weight-loss program. Weight loss promotes general health and wellness and decreases the risk of a myriad of other chronic diseases. A weight-loss program should include both decreased caloric intake (balanced diet) and increased caloric expenditure (exercise). Many patients will benefit from a weight-loss support group or accountability program, such as

Weight Watchers, Curves, or one of the numerous other programs available.

Evaluation

The patient with OA should be evaluated in several areas with each follow-up appointment, including assessments for pain, ROM of the affected joint, ability to ambulate smoothly and independently, ability to independently perform ADLs, interference of the OA with the patient's preferred lifestyle, and adequate sleep and rest. Diagnostic tests such as x-rays should also be performed periodically to monitor joint space and osteophyte formation, especially if the patient reports increased pain or decreased ROM. Changes in the patient's condition necessitate a change in the nursing care plan.

>> Go to **Pearson MyLab Nursing and eText** to see Chart 2: Nursing Care Plan: A Patient with Osteoarthritis of the Knee

REVIEW   Osteoarthritis

RELATE Link the Concepts and Exemplars

Linking the exemplar of OA with the concept of comfort:

1. What assessment data will you gather to help plan for chronic pain relief in the patient with OA?

2. Compare and contrast the various complementary health approaches for pain relief for the patient with OA.

Linking the exemplar of OA with the concept of safety:

3. Create a safety plan for the patient with severe OA in both hands who lives alone.

4. What teaching interventions will you initiate for the patient with OA of the knees who is learning to use a walker?

READY Go to Volume 3: Clinical Nursing Skills

REFER Go to Pearson MyLab Nursing and eText

- Additional review materials
- Chart 2: Nursing Care Plan: A Patient with Osteoarthritis of the Knee

REFLECT Apply Your Knowledge

Maureen Murphy is a 68-year-old woman who has recently been diagnosed with OA in her right hip. Mrs. Murphy lives with her husband

Marty, who is 75 and has been diagnosed with early dementia. Mr. Murphy has a descending aortic aneurysm that required surgery 5 months ago. He has not recovered as well as expected and is frequently confused, forgetful, and weak. Mrs. Murphy is retired and carries good health insurance for herself and her husband. They both have modest retirement incomes and Social Security benefits. Mrs. Murphy is extremely well organized, pays attention to detail, and gets very agitated when her routine is interrupted. Mr. and Mrs. Murphy belong to a small community church and have many caring friends and neighbors.

Mrs. Murphy's healthcare provider recommends hip replacement, to which she readily agrees. She has been limping and in pain, which is causing problems as she attempts to care for her husband. The physician has told Mrs. Murphy that she will be in the hospital for 1 week after surgery and then 2 weeks at a rehabilitation hospital. Before surgery, Mrs. Murphy is trying to arrange for her husband's care as well as her own.

1. What priorities of care do you see for Mrs. Murphy prior to surgery?

2. What safety concerns do you anticipate for Mrs. Murphy and her husband when Mrs. Murphy is discharged from rehabilitation?

3. What resources will you recommend for Mrs. Murphy's home care after discharge from rehabilitation?

>> Exemplar 13.F
Parkinson Disease

Exemplar Learning Outcomes

13.F Analyze Parkinson disease (PD) as it relates to mobility.

- Describe the pathophysiology of PD.
- Describe the etiology of PD.
- Compare the risk factors for and prevention of PD.
- Identify the clinical manifestations of PD.
- Summarize diagnostic tests and therapies used by interprofessional teams in the collaborative care of an individual with a PD.

- Apply the nursing process in providing culturally competent care to an individual with PD.

Exemplar Key Terms

Bradykinesia, *954*
Cognitive deficits, *956*
Deep brain stimulation (DBS), *956*
Dopamine, *954*
Festination, *956*

Overview

Parkinson disease (PD) is a progressive neurologic disorder that primarily affects movement. It was first described in 1817 by James Parkinson, a British physician who called it the "shaking palsy." It is usually characterized initially by unilateral hand tremor, but progresses to include bilateral tremor, rigidity, **bradykinesia** (slow movements), and postural instability. These symptoms decrease the patient's quality of life and increase dependence on others. It is estimated that at least 500,000 individuals in the United States currently have PD, with approximately 50,000 new cases each year. The cost of care for these individuals is estimated at more than $6 billion annually (National Institute of Neurological Disorders and Stroke [NINDS], 2012).

Pathophysiology and Etiology

Pathophysiology

Dopamine is a brain neurotransmitter that regulates voluntary movement, reward-seeking behavior, memory and learning, attention, sleep, affect, and many other functions. Dopamine receptors are expressed throughout the brain, including the substantia nigra pars compacta (SNpc). The loss of dopaminergic neurons in the SNpc and decrease of striatal dopamine content characterize PD (Bassani, Vital, & Rauh, 2015). PD is also characterized by the presence of **Lewy bodies** in neurons. Lewy bodies are abnormal aggregates of proteins, including alpha-synuclein. The purpose of Lewy bodies, including whether they are helpful or harmful, is still under investigation.

Loss of dopaminergic neurons that connect the substantia nigra to the cholinergic neurons in the corpus striatum results in abnormal nerve-firing patterns that cause impaired movement (National Institutes of Health [NIH], 2012). Dopamine and acetylcholine must be balanced to produce smooth movement. When dopamine neurons are degenerated, acetylcholine signaling is increased, causing an imbalance that contributes to the clinical manifestations of PD.

Etiology

The cause of PD is unknown, but many researchers believe it results from a combination of genetic susceptibility and exposure to environmental factors or toxins, and some cases of PD appear to be hereditary. Most cases of PD are sporadic, which means the disease occurs randomly, with no apparent genetic link.

Risk Factors

Age is the primary risk factor for developing PD. The average age of onset is 60 years, and the risk increases with advancing age. Men are also at higher risk, with 50% more men than women developing PD. Some studies indicate that individuals who live in rural areas or work in certain professions are at higher risk, providing an environmental link for the development of PD. In a few individuals, PD is inherited; approximately 15–25% of individuals with PD have a relative with PD. Genetic mutation of several genes has been linked to PD, including *SNCA* (alpha-synuclein), *LRRK2*, and *PARK2* (NIH, 2012). Individuals with early-onset or juvenile PD are more likely to have a genetic mutation than individuals with late-onset PD.

Prevention

Because the cause of PD is unknown, there is no definitive way to prevent the development of the disease. However, several prevention techniques have been suggested by experts, including consuming a healthy diet that is high in fruits and vegetables, avoiding herbicides and pesticides, and consuming moderate amounts of caffeine and green tea. Consumption of nutritional supplements, including vitamins C, D, and E, coenzyme Q10, creatine, and stilbenes, may also help prevent PD (Chao, Leung, Wang, & Chang, 2012). Gao and colleagues (2012) reported that diets high in flavonoid-rich foods may lower PD risk in men. Foods high in flavonoids include berries, red wine, tea, and eggplant. The 20-year study of 130,000 men and women found that men who consumed high levels of flavonoid-rich foods were 40% less likely to develop PD than those who ate the least amount of flavonoid-rich foods. These findings were not found in women who participated in the study. Continued research is needed in the area of nutrition and prevention of PD.

Clinical Manifestations

Symptoms of PD are mild at the beginning of the disease and progressively worsen over time. The clinical manifestations of PD can be divided into motor and nonmotor symptoms. Motor symptoms include the four classic symptoms of PD: tremor, rigidity, bradykinesia, and postural instability. Nonmotor symptoms include cognitive deficits, emotional changes, and sleep problems. Patients with PD may experience these and many other symptoms during the progression of the disease. See the Multisystem Effects of Parkinson Disease feature.

Motor Symptoms

Motor symptoms associated with PD often begin unilaterally. With progression of the disease, motor symptoms begin to affect the patient bilaterally, but the side affected initially will continue to display more prominent deficits in motor function. Two of the three symptoms of tremor, rigidity, and bradykinesia are required for a diagnosis of PD. Postural instability generally develops later in the course of the disease.

Tremor, or trembling, of one hand is an early sign of PD; some individuals develop tremor in the foot or jaw before the hand. Tremor is most prominent when the individual is at rest, and it generally abates with movement. Tremor may be accompanied by a **"pill-rolling"** motion in which the thumb and fingers gently rub together. Trembling of both hands and the arms, legs, jaw, and face may occur as the disease progresses. Trembling may interfere with ADLs, including eating, dressing, bathing, walking, and talking. Tremor can be

Multisystem Effects of
Parkinson Disease

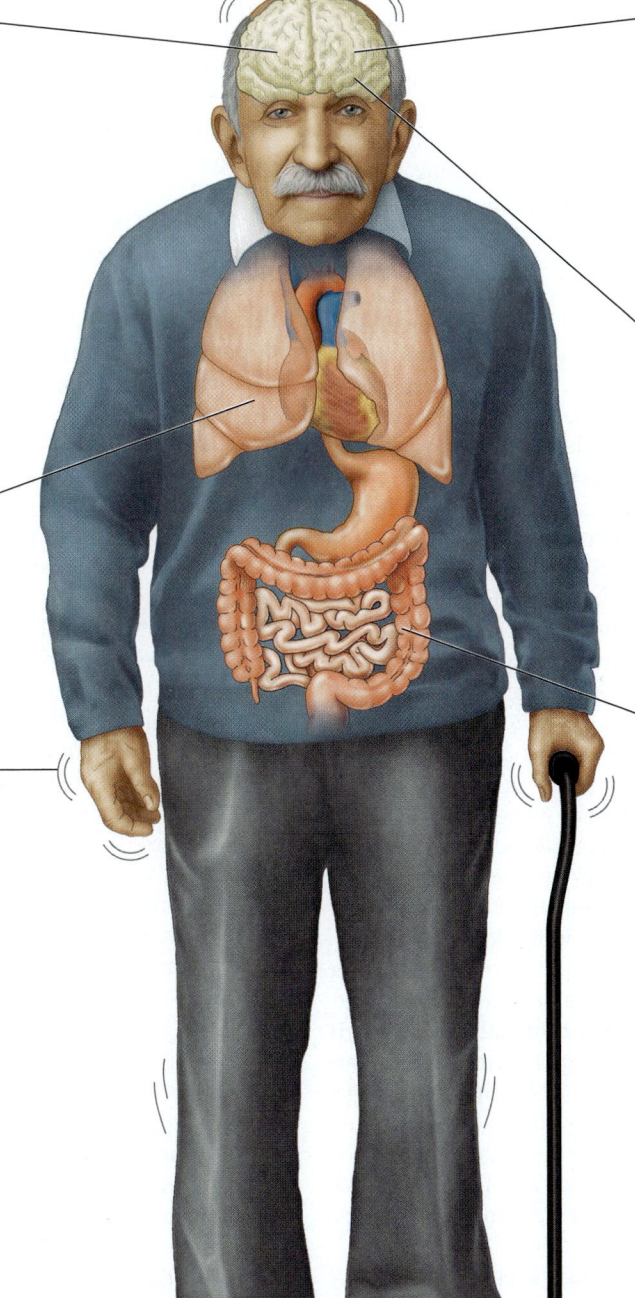

Neurologic

- Slowed thinking
- Confusion
- Memory loss
- Parkinson dementia
- Irritability
- Depression
- Fear
- Anxiety
- Panic attacks
- Social withdrawal
- Apathy

Respiratory

- Risk for aspiration with increasing oral motor impairment

Classic motor signs of PD

- Tremor
- Rigidity
- Bradykinesis
- Lack of affect
- Postural instability
- Parkinsonian gait

Sleep alterations

- Insomnia
- Daytime sleep attacks
- Restless leg syndrome
- Parasomnias
- Frequent awakening during the night
- REM sleep behavior disorders

Communication

- Speech deficits
- Slowed thinking
- Confusion
- Memory loss
- Apathy

Functional status/safety

- Progressive inability to perform ADLs
- Orthostatic hypotension
- Social withdrawal
- Bladder/bowel dysfunction
- Progressive immobility
- Difficulty chewing/swallowing
- Pain/numbness/weakness

exacerbated by stress or excitement. Tremor is generally the symptom that causes the individual to seek medical help.

Rigidity, or resistance to movement, occurs because of the involuntary contraction of all skeletal muscles. Muscles remain contracted when they should relax, upsetting the balance of opposing muscles and preventing movement.

This may lead to muscle aches or weakness. Muscle stiffness of the trunk and limbs can limit the ROM of joints and cause pain. For clinicians, rigidity is most obvious when another individual tries to move the patient's arm, which will move only in short, jerky movements known as "cogwheel" rigidity (NINDS, 2016a).

Bradykinesia, or slowed movement, affects both voluntary and automatic movements. Bradykinesia of voluntary movements causes the performance of ADLs, such as bathing and dressing, to take several hours. This can lead to frustration for the patient. Bradykinesia can also affect the ability of the patient to stand from a seated position. Steps may become shorter during walking, and the arms may not swing automatically. The patient may also have a decreased blink rate. Another common effect of bradykinesia is difficulty with speech, swallowing, and chewing. This manifests itself in excessive drooling, difficulty eating, slurred speech, lengthy pauses during speech, and a lower voice volume (**hypophonia**).

Postural instability may develop later in the course of the disease, along with a parkinsonian gait. **Postural instability** is characterized by a stooped posture that leads to balance problems and falls. It may lead to **retropulsion**, or the tendency to topple backward when bumped or when rising, standing, or turning. A **parkinsonian gait** is characterized by small, shuffling steps. The steps may be characterized by bradykinesia, or they may be rapid, as if the individual is trying to run (**festination**). When walking, the whole foot generally strikes the ground simultaneously, or the toe strikes first, which differs from the normal gait of the heel striking first. Individuals may also experience **freezing**, in which it feels as though their feet are stuck to the floor. This usually occurs on the first step or when pivoting, walking through a doorway, or crossing the street. Freezing may increase the risk of falling forward.

Nonmotor Symptoms

Some nonmotor symptoms appear early in the disease and include fatigue, irritability, and loss of sense of smell. Other nonmotor symptoms, such as dementia, occur later in the disease progression. These nonmotor symptoms can be just as debilitating to the individual as the motor symptoms.

Cognitive deficits usually begin with slowed thinking. Patients may also develop confusion and memory loss. Later in the course of disease, dementia may affect social interactions, language, reasoning, and other mental skills. This is normally referred to as *Parkinson dementia*; symptoms of Parkinson dementia are similar to those of Alzheimer dementia.

Emotional changes associated with PD may include depression, which can occur at any time throughout the course of the disease. Other forms of emotional changes include fear, anxiety, and panic attacks. An inability to cope may lead to social withdrawal and apathy.

Sleep problems are common among patients with PD and may be an early indicator of the disease. Fatigue may or may not be linked to sleep disturbances. Sleep disorders common to individuals with PD include insomnia, daytime sleep attacks, restless leg syndrome, parasomnias, and REM sleep behavior disorders. Frequent awakening during the night may be linked to lack of automatic muscle movement, forcing the individual to wake up to change positions during the night.

Parkinsonism

Individuals with the combination of motor symptoms typically seen in PD are said to have **parkinsonism**. Not everyone who has parkinsonism has PD. Parkinsonism can result from medications, head trauma, and other neurodegenerative disorders. Patients with tremor, bradykinesia, and rigidity that do not respond to dopaminergic drugs are usually classified as having parkinsonism rather than PD.

Collaboration

Care of the patient with PD often involves a neurologist, primary care provider, nurses, and therapists, among others. There is no cure for PD, so treatment is designed to help control symptoms and teach the patient how to live with the disease. Nursing care should also include support for the caregiver, especially as the disease progresses.

Diagnostic Tests

In 2011, the FDA approved an imaging technique called DaTscan for patients with symptoms of PD. DaTscan involves the injection of radioactive Ioflupane I-123, which binds to dopamine transporters (DaT) in the brain. This allows visualization of dopaminergic neurons using single photon emission computed tomographic scan (SPECT). Patients with degeneration of dopamine neurons will show less uptake of Ioflupane I-123, which can be evaluated by a trained neurologist. A DaTscan is helpful for differentiating between essential tremor and tremor due to parkinsonian syndromes, but it does not distinguish among PD and other dopamine degenerative disorders such as multiple system atrophy (MSA) or progressive supranuclear palsy (PSP) (Okun, 2014).

Patients should drink plenty of water the day of the test and 2 days after the test to promote excretion of the iodine. After the injection, the DaT agent takes about 3–6 hours to distribute throughout the body. The scan, once started, takes 30–45 minutes (Cedars-Sinai, 2016).

Other diagnostic tests for individuals with PD may include an MRI or blood tests to help rule out other causes of the patient's symptoms. A patient with PD will have normal results from an MRI or CT scan. In addition to ruling out other conditions, diagnosis of PD is based on the patient's medical history and a neurologic and physical examination.

Surgery

Surgical treatment of PD is reserved for patients with advanced disease. The most common surgical procedure is DBS. Pallidotomy or thalamotomy may also be used.

Deep brain stimulation (DBS) is a procedure in which a neurostimulator is implanted into the individual to send electrical signals to one of three brain regions: the subthalamic nucleus, the globus pallidus, or the thalamus. The subthalamic nucleus is the most common target and gives the best response. Stimulation of the globus pallidus or subthalamic nucleus reduces tremor, bradykinesia, and rigidity, whereas stimulation of the thalamus primarily reduces tremor. Patients may have DBS on one or both sides of the brain; stimulation will affect symptoms on the opposite side of the body (NINDS, 2016a). The DBS apparatus consists of three parts: the lead (electrode), which is placed in the brain; the neurostimulator, which is usually placed near the collarbone; and a thin, insulated wire, which connects the stimulator and the lead (Jasmin, 2012).

DBS often allows patients to decrease their dosage of levodopa, which can decrease side effects such as dyskinesias. Patients will need frequent follow-up for several months after surgery to adjust the neurostimulator settings and set a new medication dosage. Complications of DBS include

Clinical Manifestations and Therapies

Parkinson Disease

ETIOLOGY	CLINICAL MANIFESTATIONS	CLINICAL THERAPIES
Lower limb and trunk motor deficits	■ Tremor ■ Rigidity ■ Bradykinesia ■ Postural instability ■ Muscle cramps ■ Dystonia ■ Parkinsonian gait ■ Balance problems ■ Immobility, freezing ■ Stooped posture, retropulsion, festination	■ Levodopa ■ Dopamine- or levodopa-modifying drugs ■ Deep brain stimulation (DBS) ■ Walking and balance training ■ Exercise program ■ Physical therapy ■ Modification of the environment to reduce the risk of falls ■ Mobility devices
Upper limb motor deficits	■ Tremor (with pill-rolling) ■ Rigidity (especially cogwheel rigidity) ■ Bradykinesia ■ Micrographia ■ Muscle cramps ■ Dystonia ■ Uncoordinated hand movements ■ Inability to perform ADLs	■ Levodopa ■ Dopamine- or levodopa-modifying drugs ■ DBS ■ Allowing adequate time for ADLs ■ Exercise program ■ Occupational therapy ■ Assistive devices
Head and neck motor deficits	■ Tremor ■ Rigidity ■ Bradykinesia ■ Lack of affect ■ Dystonia ■ Oculogyric crisis ■ Difficulty chewing and swallowing, drooling ■ Speech deficits (slurred speech, lengthy pauses, hypophonia)	■ Levodopa ■ Dopamine- or levodopa-modifying drugs ■ DBS ■ Speech therapy ■ Providing soft foods
Cognitive effects	■ Confusion ■ Slowed thinking ■ Memory loss ■ Dementia	■ Rivastigmine ■ Promoting reorientation ■ Providing support to caregivers
Emotional effects	■ Anxiety ■ Fear, panic attacks ■ Depression, social withdrawal, apathy	■ Antidepressants ■ Anxiolytics ■ Support group
Sleep problems	■ Fatigue ■ Irritability ■ Restless leg syndrome ■ Sleep attacks, insomnia, parasomnias, REM sleep behavior disorders	■ Atypical antipsychotics ■ Good sleep hygiene
Bowel and bladder effects	■ Constipation ■ Urinary hesitancy or frequency	■ Oxybutynin ■ High-fiber diet ■ Laxatives, stool softeners ■ Adequate fluids ■ Bladder or bowel training
Other	■ Sexual dysfunction ■ Seborrhea ■ Hyperhidrosis ■ Anosmia ■ Orthostatic hypotension ■ Pain	■ Fludrocortisone ■ Sildenafil ■ Ketoconazole ■ Teaching the patient to change positions slowly

hemorrhage, infection, misplacement or dislodging of the leads, component failure, and stimulation-related adverse effects (Machado, Deogaonkar, & Cooper, 2012).

Pharmacologic Therapy

No pharmacologic cure is available for PD. However, many medications are effective at reducing the severity of symptoms. The goals of pharmacologic treatment for patients with PD are to improve the quality of life, reduce disability, and maintain the ability to work. The medications chosen by the physician will depend on the patient's age, symptoms, and response to the drug. Information about medications used to treat PD follows; also see the Medications feature.

Levodopa

The symptoms of PD result from a lack of dopamine in the brain. Therefore, the best way to treat PD is to increase brain dopamine levels. The primary drug used for this purpose is levodopa, which is the mainstay of PD treatment. Levodopa is effective at reducing tremor, bradykinesia, and rigidity, but problems with balance and nonmotor symptoms may not be relieved.

Levodopa is a natural chemical that can cross the blood–brain barrier and be converted directly to dopamine in the brain. Levodopa can also be converted to dopamine outside the brain, which leads to the most common side effects of nausea and orthostatic hypotension. Therefore, levodopa is almost always given in combination with carbidopa, which prevents levodopa from converting to dopamine until it reaches the brain.

As the patient continues to take levodopa, its effectiveness diminishes. This causes the patient to experience an **"on–off" effect** characterized by a sudden lack of symptom control and unexpected dyskinesias. With increasing doses and long-term exposure, levodopa usually causes dyskinesia, which may become less tolerable for the patient than the symptoms of PD. Therefore, many physicians hesitate to prescribe levodopa to patients too early in the course of the disease.

SAFETY ALERT Although the FDA requires generic drugs to show an "essential similarity" to the correlating brand name drug, generic substitutions may have different levels of efficacy and side effects in comparison to brand name counterparts. The patient should be cautioned to consult the primary care provider before switching to a generic drug. The patient should also report any differences in effectiveness and side effects after switching medications.

Dopamine Agonists

Dopamine agonists are not converted directly to dopamine; instead, they act similarly to dopamine in the brain by activating dopamine receptors. Dopamine agonists are not as effective as levodopa, so they are often used alone early in the course of disease when symptoms are minor. Dopamine agonists have a longer duration of action compared to levodopa, so they may also be used later in the disease with levodopa to prevent the "on–off" effect. In addition to the side effects seen with levodopa, dopamine agonists may also produce hallucinations, swelling, drowsiness, and compulsive behaviors such as gambling and overeating.

Dopamine Modifiers

Dopamine modifiers are used to extend the action of dopamine in the brain; they include the MAO-B (monoamine oxidase-B) inhibitors and the COMT (catechol-*O*-methyltransferase) inhibitors. MAO-B inhibitors may be given as monotherapy early in the course of disease to delay the need for levodopa therapy by a year or more. When given with levodopa, MAO-B inhibitors can enhance and prolong the response to levodopa and reduce wearing-off effects. COMT inhibitors reduce the breakdown of levodopa to an inactive intermediate product, thus increasing the availability of levodopa in the brain. When taken with levodopa, COMT inhibitors can decrease the duration of "off" periods and reduce the required dose of levodopa.

Other Medications

Anticholinergics were the first class of drugs used to treat PD. They reduce tremor and rigidity by decreasing acetylcholine and restoring the balance of acetylcholine and dopamine in the brain. Because of side effects in older adults and limited usefulness for most PD symptoms, anticholinergics are prescribed only to younger patients whose primary symptom is tremor.

Amantadine is an antiviral medication that can provide short-term relief of mild symptoms of PD. It may also be used in addition to levodopa to help control dyskinesia for patients in the later stages of PD.

Drugs for Nonmotor Symptoms

Patients with PD often experience many nonmotor symptoms. Classic medications for PD do not treat these symptoms, so additional medications are often prescribed, including antidepressants (amitriptyline, fluoxetine), anxiolytics (benzodiazepines), and atypical antipsychotics. The antipsychotics quetiapine and clozapine may be prescribed at bedtime to reduce frightening dreams or to treat psychosis; patients on clozapine should have their blood monitored frequently for agranulocytosis. Olanzapine and risperidone may be given to treat hallucinations, but like traditional antipsychotics, they may worsen PD motor symptoms.

Orthostatic hypotension may be treated with fludrocortisone, and sildenafil may be used to treat erectile dysfunction. Oxybutynin is often prescribed for patients with bladder dysfunction. Seborrheic dermatitis can be treated with ketoconazole. Rivastigmine can be used to treat dementia in PD.

Nonpharmacologic Therapy

Nonpharmacologic therapy is an essential aspect of treatment for patients with PD. In spite of regular medication usage, patients with PD still develop progressively worsening symptoms. Medications have limited effectiveness over time and frequently produce side effects. Therefore, nonpharmacologic therapies are used as an adjunct to help patients prolong the early, mild stage of disease and delay disability.

Exercise is the most important nonpharmacologic therapy for patients with PD (see the Evidence-Based Practice feature). The nurse should encourage patients to participate in an exercise program, especially a combination of walking and strength training. However, any type of exercise is beneficial for patients with PD; t'ai chi, yoga, and Alexander techniques may all provide some improvement in flexibility, balance, muscle strength, and posture.

Medications
Parkinson Disease Motor Symptoms

CLASSIFICATION AND DRUG EXAMPLES	MECHANISMS OF ACTION	NURSING CONSIDERATIONS
Levodopa *Drug examples:* ■ Levodopa ■ Levodopa/carbidopa	Metabolic precursor to dopamine; restores dopamine levels in the brain ***May also be used for:*** ■ Parkinsonism ■ Pain relief for shingles, bone pain	■ This drug is the cornerstone therapy for PD. ■ Effective dosage must be titrated, which may take several weeks to avoid adverse effects. ■ Long-term use of high doses causes dyskinesia. ■ Effectiveness may become less predictable over time; the drug may produce "wearing-off" or "on–off" effects. ■ A high-protein diet may interfere with levodopa absorption from the gastrointestinal tract; patients should avoid protein-rich meals when taking levodopa. ■ Do not take vitamin products containing vitamin B_6 if taking levodopa without carbidopa. ■ The drug should be used cautiously in patients with heart, kidney, liver, or endocrine disease. ■ Levodopa may interfere with several laboratory tests and other drugs; patients should be monitored for interactions. ■ A metabolite of levodopa may cause urine and sweat to be dark colored. ■ Psychologic side effects may be more common in older adults.
Dopamine Agonists *Drug examples:* ■ Pramipexole ■ Ropinirole ■ Apomorphine ■ Rotigotine ■ Bromocriptine	Mimic the role of dopamine in the brain ***May also be used for:*** ■ Restless leg syndrome ■ Reducing prolactin levels (bromocriptine)	■ These drugs may cause compulsive behaviors such as gambling, overeating, compulsive shopping, or hypersexuality; patients should be warned to report behaviors that are out of character to their physician. ■ Side effects are similar to levodopa and include nausea, hallucinations, sleep attacks, and orthostatic hypotension. ■ Apomorphine is an injectable, short-acting agonist used for quick relief of symptoms in patients who are experiencing "wearing-off" or "on–off" effects; it can be used up to five times daily. ■ Rotigotine is a transdermal patch that is replaced once per day; patients should rotate the placement of the patch. ■ Bromocriptine may produce fibrosis in the heart or chest cavity (pleuropulmonary fibrosis); it is rarely prescribed for PD.
MAO-B Inhibitors *Drug examples:* ■ Selegiline ■ Rasagiline	Prevents the breakdown of brain dopamine by inhibiting monoamine oxidase-B and interferes with dopamine reuptake in synapses ***May also be used for:*** ■ Depression ■ ADHD	■ These drugs can increase the risk of hallucinations if taken with levodopa and carbidopa. ■ Do not use in combination with most antidepressants and certain narcotics and decongestants. ■ Selegiline is available in an orally disintegrating formula for patients who have difficulty swallowing. ■ If levodopa-induced side effects occur when taking MAO-B inhibitors, the dose of levodopa should be reduced.
COMT Inhibitors *Drug examples:* ■ Entacapone ■ Tolcapone	Prolongs the actions of levodopa by blocking an enzyme that breaks down levodopa	■ Side effects are related to increased levodopa effect. ■ Tolcapone is rarely prescribed due to risk for liver failure; patients on tolcapone need regular monitoring of liver function. ■ COMT inhibitors are only effective in combination with levodopa. ■ Formulations of entacapone combined with levodopa and carbidopa are available in a single tablet. ■ Taper dose when discontinuing COMT inhibitors. ■ These drugs may cause urine to be brownish-orange. ■ These drugs should not be given with nonselective monoamine oxidase inhibitors.

(continued on next page)

Medications (continued)

CLASSIFICATION AND DRUG EXAMPLES	MECHANISMS OF ACTION	NURSING CONSIDERATIONS
Anticholinergics *Drug examples:* - Benztropine - Trihexyphenidyl	Decrease activity of acetylcholine *May also be used for:* - Drug-induced extrapyramidal symptoms	- These drugs are effective in only approximately half of patients for a brief period. - These drugs cause significant antimuscarinic effects, including confusion, dry mouth, urinary retention, blurred vision, and constipation, especially in older adults. - Intake and output should be monitored regularly. - These drugs may increase susceptibility to heat stroke if patient exercises vigorously in hot weather.
Other *Drug example:* - Amantadine	Exact mechanism unknown; may be related to an increased release of dopamine from neuronal storage sites *May also be used for:* - Treatment and prophylaxis of influenza A	- Patients should be taught to watch for side effects, including mottled skin (livedo reticularis), edema, agitation, and hallucinations. - Dosage should be reduced in patients with renal insufficiency. - Maximum effect occurs in 2 weeks to 3 months; effectiveness may wane after 6–8 weeks of treatment. Patients should be instructed to notify the physician when the drug is no longer effective. - Abrupt discontinuation of amantadine may produce parkinsonian crisis.

Source: Data from Adams, M. P., Holland, L. N., & Urban, C. (2017). *Pharmacology for nurses: A pathophysiologic approach* (5th ed.). Hoboken, NJ: Pearson Education.

Evidence-Based Practice
Exercise for Patients with PD

Problem

Patients with PD develop motor problems that cause changes in gait, muscle strength and coordination, and balance. These symptoms decrease the patient's mobility and ability to perform ADLs and increase the risk for falls and other complications.

Evidence

Exercise, including stretching, aerobic exercise, strength training, and dancing can help patients with PD increase their mobility and strength. A Cochrane review of eight trials (203 participants) indicated that treadmill training improved gait speed, stride length, and walking distance for individuals with PD in a variety of clinical trials. In addition, treadmill training was not significantly associated with adverse events or patient dropout (Mehrholz et al., 2010). Another study of 67 individuals with PD compared high-intensity treadmill exercise, low-intensity treadmill exercise, and stretching and resistance exercises for gait speed, cardiovascular fitness, and muscle strength. All three types of exercise improved distance on the 6-minute walk test, with the low-intensity treadmill group showing the most improvement. Both treadmill exercises improved cardiovascular fitness, whereas stretching and resistance improved muscle strength (Shulman et al., 2013). A third study of 121 individuals with PD indicated that individuals who participated in flexibility, balance, and function exercises had improved overall physical function and ADLs scores, whereas individuals who performed aerobic exercises showed improvement in walking economy (oxygen uptake) (Schenkman et al., 2012). Aerobic exercises have been found to promote cognitive and procedural functioning as well as motor functioning and physical fitness (Duchesne et al., 2015).

More recently, Dr. Karen Jaffe, a physician who has PD, started a program for patients with PD that includes everything from cycling to boxing to dancing (Michael J. Fox Foundation, 2016). A new study (IOS Press, 2017) demonstrated that exercising for 2.5 hours per week can significantly slow the progression of PD.

Implications

Patients should participate in both aerobic activity and strength training for maximum benefit. Exercises appear to slow disease progression, and they may improve body strength, so the individual is less disabled compared to patients who do not exercise. Exercise improves balance, minimizes gait problems, and strengthens muscles to increase physical functioning. Both structured exercise programs and general physical activity (walking, gardening, swimming, dancing) are beneficial for patients with PD (NINDS, 2016a). The nurse should help patients find exercise solutions that they enjoy in order to increase the likelihood of adherence to the exercise regimen. The Michael J. Fox Foundation (2015) reports swimming, yoga, and walking to be popular among patients with PD and recommends that patients discuss exercise programs with their treating provider before beginning any exercise regimen.

Critical Thinking Application

1. How would you explain the importance of exercise to a patient with mild PD who is skeptical of its beneficial effects?

2. What special considerations would you have when suggesting an exercise program for an older patient with severe bilateral tremor in his legs who requires a walker for ambulation?

3. Develop an exercise program for a 67-year-old male patient with a gait speed of 1.2 m/s, stride length of 0.79 m, cadence of 115 steps/min, and 6-minute walk distance of 472 m.

Focus on Integrative Health
Music and Motion Therapy

Dance therapy has been shown to be safe and effective at increasing health-related quality of life (HRQOL). It can affect HRQOL in as little as 2 weeks and improve HRQOL in individuals with severe or end-stage neurologic disorders, with participants reporting significant improvements in symptoms of anxiety, stress, and depression (Hackney & Bennett, 2014).

Some individuals with PD are finding a way to improve their HRQOL through the work of a nonprofit organization called InMotion. Cofounder Karen Jaffe, a physician and individual with PD, was looking for a way to decrease her symptoms of PD. InMotion empowers individuals with PD to take control of their lives. Participants engage with a variety of therapies, including Reiki, art, music, massage, and other therapies that provide energy and hope. At the same time, InMotion provides a circle of support and opportunity for social interactions in a place that allows individuals to leave the stigma of PD at the door (Michael J. Fox Foundation, 2016).

Participation in physical, occupational, and speech therapy can play an essential role in the ability of a patient with PD to remain mobile. *Physical therapy* often focuses on lower body strength and mobility to improve walking and prevent contractures and falls. Physical therapy may also help the patient become more proficient at transfers. *Occupational therapy* often focuses on the upper extremities, especially finger function, to improve the patient's ability to independently perform ADLs, such as cooking and grooming. Occupational therapy can also help a patient maintain the ability to perform work functions, allowing the patient to keep his or her job longer. *Speech therapists* help the patient with speech and swallowing, which can enhance the patient's daily functioning in the areas of communication and nutrition. Therapists are also responsible for helping patients learn how to use assistive devices that are within their area of expertise (PT: walkers, canes; OT: button hooks, electric razor; speech therapist: pen grips, "magic slate").

Lifespan Considerations

Approximately 5–10% of individuals with PD have "early-onset" or "young-onset" PD, which begins before the age of 50. Early-onset PD shares many clinical manifestations with older-onset PD. However, patients with early-onset PD generally have a slower disease progression and a lower rate of dementia. They are more likely to have dystonia at onset and dyskinesias (involuntary movements, such as a tic or spasm) in response to levodopa treatment. Early-onset PD is often inherited, although it may be idiopathic (National Parkinson Foundation [NPF], n.d.b).

Women with early-onset PD may be referred to a geneticist for any concerns prior to conception. When using contraceptives, women should be made aware that the effect of PD medication on the efficacy of birth control pills is not known. Many women with PD have successfully carried healthy babies to full term. Similar to any pregnant woman, women with PD should discuss all medications with their physicians.

NURSING PROCESS

Nurses are essential for evaluating the progression of the patient's PD, monitoring the patient's ability to perform ADLs and ambulate independently, and providing patient teaching and emotional support. Nurses also play a key role in performing patient assessments for changes in symptoms, effectiveness of medications, and new patient concerns. Documentation of this information is critical for current and future care of the patient.

Assessment

- **Observation and patient interview.** Observe the patient's gait and movements, assessing for the presence and degree of tremor and the need to rely on caregivers or assistive devices to ambulate. A general health history should include a history of brain disorders or trauma, exposure to environmental toxins, medication and drug use, and family history of PD. A PD-specific health history should include the patient's description of symptoms, including onset, duration, severity, aggravating or alleviating factors, response to medication, interference with mobility or ADLs, interference with work or relationships, "on–off" or "wearing-off" effects, and use of assistive devices. If needed, ask specifically about nonmotor symptoms, because many patients do not associate these symptoms with PD. Nonmotor symptoms include cognitive deficits, emotional changes, sleep problems, bladder and bowel changes, orthostatic hypotension, sexual dysfunction, and others.

- **Physical examination.** Physical assessment often follows the Unified Parkinson's Disease Rating Scale (UPDRS), which rates patients in 42 different areas in the categories of mentation, behavior, and mood; ADLs; motor examination; and complications of therapy (Fahn, Elton, & Members of the UPDRS Development Committee, 1987):
  - The mentation, behavior, and mood assessment includes intellectual impairment, thought disorder, depression, and motivation.
  - The ADL assessment includes speech, swallowing, handwriting, hygiene, walking, tremor, and others.
  - The motor examination assessment includes facial expression, tremor at rest, finger taps, hand movements, rapid alternating movement of hands, leg agility, ability to rise from a chair, posture, gait, bradykinesia, and others.
  - Complications included in the assessment are dyskinesias, "on–off" periods, sleep disturbances, and others.
  - The modified Hoehn and Yahr Staging Scale and Schwab and England Activities of Daily Living Scale are also included as part of the UPDRS.

In 2007, the Movement Disorder Society sponsored a revision of the UPDRS, called the MDS-UPDRS, which is divided into four parts: nonmotor experiences of daily living, motor experiences of daily living, motor examination, and motor complications. This revised scale was made available in 2008.

>> **Stay Current:** Visit the website of the Movement Disorder Society to see the latest rating scale.

Diagnosis

Nursing diagnoses related to PD may include, but are not limited to, the following:

- *Falls, Risk for*
- *Mobility: Physical, Impaired*
- *Self-Care Deficit: Feeding*
- *Fluid Volume: Deficient, Risk for*
- *Swallowing, Impaired*
- *Sleep Pattern, Disturbed*
- *Verbal Communication, Impaired*
- *Urinary Elimination, Impaired*
- *Constipation*
- *Fear*
- *Memory, Impaired*
- *Role Strain, Caregiver.*

(NANDA-I © 2014)

Planning

Patient goals for individuals with PD are specific to the nursing diagnoses included in the plan of care and will be tailored to the patient. Examples include the following:

- The patient will remain free from injury.
- The patient will demonstrate progressive improvement in scores for the 6-minute walk test.
- The patient will participate in a daily exercise program that includes walking and strength training.
- The patient will participate in occupational therapy to gain knowledge of assistive devices for feeding and will obtain kitchen utensils to aid in feeding self-care.
- The patient will maintain sufficient caloric intake necessary to meet increasing metabolic needs related to onset of tremor.
- The patient will participate in speech therapy for training in swallowing and enhanced verbal communication.
- The patient will verbalize an understanding of good sleep hygiene.
- The patient will participate in physical therapy to improve walking and balance.
- The patient will verbalize an understanding of bladder training techniques.
- The patient will demonstrate normal bowel elimination patterns, including one bowel movement daily.
- The patient will report episodes of freezing and demonstrate an understanding of techniques to overcome freezing.
- The patient will use techniques to augment memory, including writing down important information.
- The patient's caregiver will utilize help from friends, family, and healthcare agencies to provide relief from daily tasks.

Implementation

For most patients with PD, early implementation of strategies to maintain mobility and independently perform ADLs will provide the most benefit throughout the course of the disease.

These interventions may need to be adjusted as the disease progresses, but many therapies implemented early during the course of treatment will prolong the mild stage of the disease and provide muscle strength and coordination in the later stages of disease. Several techniques can be used by the patient to help minimize symptoms and prevent complications. The nurse plays a vital role in educating patients with PD about these preventive strategies (see the Patient Teaching feature).

Prevent Injury

Safety is a priority for patients with walking difficulties to maintain their mobility. Modifications such as using lift chairs, elevating the back legs of chairs, and installing a raised toilet seat can help patients with PD rise from a seated position more easily. Installing handrails for stability and removing floor hazards are all important safety modifications for patients with PD. These modifications can help patients be more confident while ambulating and may help prevent falls and other accidents.

Optimize Mobility

The best strategy for mobility that a nurse can provide for patients with PD is to encourage the patient to walk daily and participate in an exercise program. Aerobic exercise and strength training increase muscle strength, balance, and coordination to counteract the effects of tremor, rigidity, bradykinesia, and postural instability. ROM exercises can help with joint mobility and function and help prevent contractures. Treadmill walking can help increase stride length, gait, and cardiovascular health to help patients overcome the parkinsonian gait and maintain general physical fitness. For patients who cannot ambulate independently, a caregiver should be encouraged to help the patient ambulate several times daily.

Techniques for proper walking, including intentionally picking up the feet instead of shuffling and placing the heel on the floor first, can easily be provided to patients through oral and written instructions. The nurse can also teach tricks to overcome freezing, such as stepping over an imaginary line. Methods to maintain balance when walking, including standing upright and not carrying anything, are also beneficial for patients with PD. Understanding and implementing these techniques early in the course of disease will help patients naturally integrate these practices later in the disease when symptoms are more severe.

Participation in physical and occupational therapy is also vital for helping patients with PD maintain mobility as long as possible. The nurse is essential for referring patients to the proper therapy, providing patients with information about what to expect during therapy, and following up with patients to ensure that they are attending therapy sessions and that the therapy sessions are beneficial. Patients who require assistive devices for walking may receive training during physical therapy sessions, or the nurse may provide this training if needed.

When helping patients learn ambulation strategies, the nurse must also provide encouragement and emotional support. As the patient's disability increases, the patient will be more susceptible to fear, anxiety, and depression. The nurse can help the patient overcome these barriers by listening to the patient's fears, providing resources for support and mobility training, and helping the patient celebrate small victories related to the patient's mobility and physical functioning.

Patient Teaching
Strategies to Minimize Symptoms and Complications of PD

Strategies to minimize the effects of PD:

- Take medications on time, every time.
- Consume a varied and balanced diet; avoid high-protein meals because protein can decrease the transport of levodopa across the blood–brain barrier.
- Drink plenty of fluids, but avoid dehydrating fluids, such as coffee.
- Use a proper walking technique: Place the heel on the ground before the toe, stand up straight, look ahead instead of down, and do not move too quickly. Use an assistive device for balance if needed.
- Maintain a strong voice by taking a breath before speaking, expressing ideas in short sentences, speaking louder than necessary, reducing throat clearing and coughing, and resting the voice when it is tired.
- Stop smoking, and cut back on caffeine and alcohol consumption if they increase tremor or balance problems.
- Allow plenty of time for ADLs. Sit down to perform activities to conserve energy and use assistive devices such as items with large handles, footstools, and electric toothbrushes. See an OT for techniques to make ADLs easier.
- If bladder incontinence is a problem, try a regular schedule for going to the bathroom or use a protective pad for accidents. If pain is experienced during urination, a UTI may be present and should be treated by a physician.
- Practice good sleep hygiene.

Strategies to prevent complications associated with PD:

- See a speech-language pathologist to prevent or treat swallowing and speech problems.
- Discuss medications with a physician or pharmacist to prevent drug–drug and food–drug interactions.
- Increase fiber and fluid intake to prevent constipation.
- Maintain balance to prevent falls: Do not pivot the body before the feet, do not lean or reach, do not carry things while walking, avoid walking backward, remove obstacles and throw rugs, install handrails, and install adequate lighting that is easy to turn on and off.
- Participate in a support group to increase social interaction and prevent depression.
- Participate in an exercise program to maintain muscle strength and improve mobility, flexibility, balance, posture, and emotional well-being (see Evidence-Based Practice feature).
- Be cautious when driving. PD can affect the patient's ability to drive safely because of changes in perception, mental clarity, tremor, and medication side effects. Consider taking public transportation or arrange for a safety assessment through the local DMV.

》》 Stay Current: Additional tips are available at the website of the National Parkinson Foundation: http://www.parkinson.org/Parkinson-s-Disease/Living-Well.

Sources: Based on Mayo Clinic. (2015d). *Parkinson's disease.* Retrieved from http://www.mayoclinic.com/health/parkinsons-disease/DS00295; National Institutes of Health (NIH). (2012). Parkinson's disease. *NIHSeniorHealth.* Retrieved from https://nihseniorhealth.gov/parkinsonsdisease/whatisparkinsonsdisease/01.html; National Parkinson Foundation (NPF). (n.d.a). *Parkinson's disease: Living well.* Retrieved from http://www.parkinson.org/Parkinson-s-Disease/Living-Well; Stacy, M., Davis, T. L., Heath, S., Isaacson, S. H., Tarsy, D., Williams, M., & Moore, A. P. (2009). The clinicians' and nurses' guide to Parkinson's disease. *Medscape Education.* Retrieved from http://www.medscape.org/viewarticle/701955.

Promote Independence

In addition to difficulty ambulating, deficits in performing ADLs constitute a major burden for patients with PD and their caregivers. ADLs include cooking and eating, performing hygiene acts (bathing, dressing, grooming, brushing teeth, toileting), and maintaining a house (housework, laundry, driving, shopping, using the phone, managing finances). The nurse can promote independence in ADLs by encouraging the patient to take adequate time to perform each task. This takes planning on the part of the patient, especially if the patient is getting ready for an appointment or social activity, but it also requires patience from both the patient and caregiver.

The use of assistive devices is key to helping patients maintain their independence in performing ADLs. Assistive devices for cooking and eating include electric can openers, food processors, mixers, utensils with large handles, finger guards, sloped plates, and many others. Patients with severe hand tremor have difficulty transporting food from the plate to the mouth. The nurse can teach patients techniques to reduce tremor while eating, such as holding a piece of bread in the opposite hand or using purposeful movement. Swallowing is often a problem for patients with PD, so the nurse can encourage patients to prepare soft foods, to cut food into small pieces or puree food, and to eat smaller meals more

frequently. Speech therapy can help patients learn swallowing techniques to prevent choking and aspiration, and occupational therapy can help patients learn techniques to reduce tremor, grasp objects, and increase safety.

SAFETY ALERT Individuals with PD who have difficulty swallowing may aspirate foods that have a thin consistency, such as juice or broth. Products to thicken liquids to prevent aspiration should be used, and the nurse should stress the need for adequate hydration. Aspiration can lead to life-threatening complications, including pneumonia.

Assistive devices are often helpful for hygiene activities. Devices such as shower seats, retractable shower heads, button hooks, zipper pulls, long shoe horns, electric razors and toothbrushes, elevated toilet seats, and handrails can help patients maintain independence in performing personal hygiene. The nurse can provide suggestions for assistive devices, referrals for equipment suppliers, and training in the use of assistive devices. The nurse may also provide training to caregivers about assisting patients with hygiene care and helping patients overcome privacy or embarrassment issues when assistance is needed. An OT can also provide tools and techniques to aid patients in performing hygiene acts independently.

Patients with PD may also use assistive devices when maintaining a house. Magnifying glasses can enlarge small text. Phones with sound amplifiers and large buttons are easier for many patients to use. Apps or call services that provide reminders about upcoming appointments or when to take medications may be helpful. Patients can use public transportation, if available, to run errands or go to appointments. Reachers, grippers, and brushes and dusters with large or telescopic handles may be helpful in maintaining independence with housework. The nurse can provide suggestions, referrals, and training, and patients can participate in occupational therapy to learn more about maintaining independence in these activities. Patients with advanced disability may consider hiring a friend, family member, or company to provide assistance with housework or transportation.

Other ADLs that may be affected by PD are communication and sleep. The nurse can help the patient overcome these problems by providing oral and written information about vocal training and good sleep hygiene. Vocal training may include teaching patients to speak louder than they think is necessary, to take a deep breath before speaking, and to express their thoughts in short sentences. Referral to a speech therapist is also an essential aspect of treatment for patients with voice changes. If writing is a problem, the nurse can encourage patients to use writing tools with large handles or nonslip grips, to type messages, or to use a recording device to note important information. An OT can also provide training in writing techniques for the patient with PD. If sleep problems are severe and are not resolved by good sleep hygiene or a change in medication, the nurse may also recommend pharmacologic therapy.

Each patient with PD will have a unique set of difficulties in performing ADLs. The nurse should determine which ADLs are causing the most difficulty and provide insight into techniques, devices, and therapies that may help patients maintain independence in each area.

Evaluation

Evaluation of patients with PD includes regular assessment using the UPDRS to determine the patient's level of disability. Significant changes in the UPDRS score may indicate a need for a modification of pharmacologic, nonpharmacologic, or surgical therapy.

As mentioned previously, patients taking levodopa or carbidopa for long periods may experience changes in the efficacy of the medication over time or may experience increasing side effects as dosages are increased. The nurse should assess patient and caregiver knowledge of medications at each change in medication or dosage and provide additional education as needed. As the disease progresses, patients may experience hopelessness and depression. Evaluation should include an assessment of the patient's emotional status at each healthcare interaction. For all patients, the nurse should evaluate adherence to both pharmacologic and nonpharmacologic therapies and help patients find solutions to obstacles or barriers to adherence.

The physical and cognitive deterioration associated with the progression of PD puts the patient at risk for social isolation and neglect. The nurse should assess the patient's support system and resources at each stage of disease progression and make referrals to area resources as appropriate.

Nursing Care Plan
A Patient with Parkinson Disease

Benjamin Tinsley, age 86, was diagnosed with PD at age 74. Mr. Tinsley lives at home with his second wife, age 80, and he has a son who lives in the same city. Mr. Tinsley visited his primary care physician for routine follow-up.

ASSESSMENT	DIAGNOSES	PLANNING
Patient history indicates that Mr. Tinsley has had PD for 12 years. Initial pharmacologic therapy was pramipexole for 2 years, then levodopa/carbidopa for 7 years. Mr. Tinsley has been on levodopa/carbidopa plus entacapone for the past 3 years. Primary complaints include severe right-hand tremor, parkinsonian gait (requires assistive device when walking), low voice volume, difficulty rising from a seated position, and constipation. The right-hand tremor interferes with eating, hygiene care, and other ADLs, and Mr. Tinsley has lost 10 lb in the past 2 months. The parkinsonian gait and postural instability make walking and standing difficult, and Ms. Tinsley states that Mr. Tinsley falls at least once per day, which is often associated with freezing. The nurse completes Mr. Tinsley's physical assessment using the UPDRS and the Schwab and England ADL scale.	■ *Risk for Injury* related to altered mobility ■ *Impaired Walking* related to parkinsonian gait ■ *Impaired Transfer Ability* related to inability to rise from a seated position ■ *Imbalanced Nutrition: Less Than Body Requirements* related to right-hand tremor and difficulty self-feeding ■ *Self-Care Deficit: Bathing, Dressing, Feeding, Toileting* related to right-hand tremor and postural instability ■ *Constipation* related to inadequate physical activity and decreased food intake ■ *Impaired Verbal Communication* related to low voice volume (NANDA-I © 2014)	■ The patient will sustain no injuries. ■ The patient will participate in treadmill training during physical therapy. ■ The patient will acquire a chair lift and an elevated toilet seat with handrails and demonstrate understanding of how to use these assistive devices. ■ The patient will use purposeful movement to reduce tremor while eating. ■ The patient will purchase a shower chair and assistive devices for dressing. ■ The patient will ambulate at least four times daily and eat a diet high in fiber and fluids. ■ The patient will intentionally take a deep breath before speaking and speak louder than normal. ■ The patient will have handrails installed throughout his home.

Nursing Care Plan *(continued)*

IMPLEMENTATION

- Facilitate referral of the patient to physical therapy for the purpose of treadmill training and strength and balance training.
- Facilitate referral of the patient to occupational therapy for assistance with eating and hygiene care.
- Facilitate referral of the patient to speech therapy for vocal training.
- Refer the patient to equipment suppliers to purchase assistive and safety devices.
- Provide patient teaching in the use of assistive devices.

- Discuss the importance of consuming a balanced diet that is easy for the patient to eat.
- Provide training to the caregiver in the areas of hygiene care, assistance with standing and walking, removal of safety hazards, and proper meal preparation.
- Encourage the patient and caregiver to be patient when performing ADLs to help the patient maintain independence as long as possible.

EVALUATION

Mr. Tinsley returns to his primary care provider in 3 months for a follow-up appointment. He reports that he has been attending PT, OT, and speech therapy regularly, and with proper training on assistive devices, he is able to independently perform ADLs more frequently than before his previous appointment. He is still very slow in performing ADLs, but he is thankful that he can be independent. Mrs. Tinsley reports that this has helped lift some of her burden of caregiving as well. Mr. Tinsley has made slight improvement on his 6 min walk distance (302 m to 387 m), and he is better able to feed himself by using larger utensils and practicing purposeful movements. As a result, he has gained 3 lb since his last appointment. Mr. Tinsley reports that he still has difficulty rising from a seated position, and his constipation has not improved much.

CRITICAL THINKING

1. What additional nursing interventions can be implemented for improvement of Mr. Tinsley's constipation?
2. Describe the components of a focused nursing assessment to determine the severity of Mr. Tinsley's difficulty rising from a seated position.
3. Develop a nursing care plan for Mr. Tinsley that reflects the development of dysphagia (difficulty swallowing).

REVIEW   Parkinson Disease

RELATE Link the Concepts and Exemplars

Linking the exemplar of PD with the concept of cognition:

1. Describe the impact of PD on cognition.
2. What safety measures can the nurse initiate for the patient with PD who has alterations in cognition?

Linking the exemplar of PD with the concept of elimination:

3. What factors associated with PD put the patient at risk for constipation?
4. What nursing interventions might be appropriate for implementation when caring for the patient with PD who is at risk for developing urinary retention?

READY Go to Volume 3: Clinical Nursing Skills

REFER Go to Pearson MyLab Nursing and eText

- Additional review materials

REFLECT Apply Your Knowledge

Kody Manuel is a 65-year-old man who was diagnosed with PD 1 year ago. Mr. Manuel is retired from the railroad, where he worked in management. He lives with his daughter, Susan Ransone, and her husband, Val. They both work outside the home, and they have one infant daughter, Isabelle. Mr. Manuel has been able to care for himself at home while his daughter and son-in-law work. Isabelle is taken to a child care center in the morning by Mrs. Ransone, and Mr. Ransone picks her up in the evening.

Mr. Manuel was started on levodopa 1 month ago. He has been reading about PD online and is very disturbed by what he has learned. He does not think the levodopa is working for him, and he tells his daughter and son-in-law that he needs to move out in order to prevent disruption of their home as the disease progresses. While visiting the physician today, he tells the nurse about his plans to move.

1. What data should be obtained from Mr. Manuel before continuing the discussion about his decision to move out of his daughter's home?
2. What potential psychosocial concerns can the nurse identify based on Mr. Manuel's statements?
3. How should the nurse respond to Mr. Manuel's report that the levodopa is not working for him?

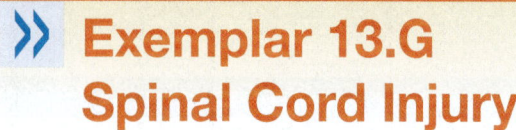

Exemplar 13.G
Spinal Cord Injury

Exemplar Learning Outcomes

13.G Analyze spinal cord injury (SCI) as it relates to mobility.

- Describe the pathophysiology of SCI.
- Describe the etiology of SCI.
- Compare the risk factors for and prevention of SCI.
- Identify the clinical manifestations of SCI.
- Summarize diagnostic tests and therapies used by inter-professional teams in the collaborative care of an individual with SCI.
- Differentiate considerations for care of patients with SCI across the lifespan.
- Apply the nursing process in providing culturally competent care to an individual with SCI.

Exemplar Key Terms

Autonomic dysreflexia, *971*
Complete SCIs, *969*
Compression, *967*
Hyperextension, *967*
Hyperflexion, *967*
Incomplete SCIs, *969*
Level of injury, *969*
Paraplegia, *970*
Rotational injuries, *967*
Spinal cord injury (SCI), *966*
Spinal shock, *969*
Tetraplegia, *970*
Transection, *967*

Overview

Spinal cord injury (SCI) is often the result of trauma from, for example, a motor vehicle crash, a fall, or a gunshot wound. SCI occurs when vertebrae or other objects are forced against the spinal cord, damaging nerve cells and preventing transmission of nerve impulses between the body and the brain. Depending on the extent and location of nerve damage, SCI can lead to anything from slight muscle weakness in a few muscles to complete loss of sensory and motor function. Approximately 17,000 new cases of SCI occur each year in the United States (National SCI Statistical Center [NSCISC], 2016).

Pathophysiology and Etiology

Pathophysiology

The brain and spinal cord are the two major components of the CNS. The spinal cord transports sensory signals from the body to the brain and motor signals from the brain to the body. The spinal cord consists of an H-shaped core of gray matter, which is made of neurons, support cells called glia, and blood vessels, and a surrounding area of white matter, which is made of myelin-coated axons (see **Figure 13–42 》》**). The gray matter is divided into four regions: interneurons of the dorsal horn that connect to visceral and somatic sensory neurons in the dorsal root, and visceral and somatic motor neurons of the ventral horn that combine to form the ventral root. The dorsal and ventral roots then join together on each side of the body to form the spinal nerve. The axons of the white matter make up the descending and ascending pathways. Descending pathways carry signals from the brain to control the motor neurons, and ascending pathways carry signals from the sensory neurons to the brain. Axons in the white matter travel from the brain along the entire length of the spinal cord until it connects with the desired spinal nerve.

The 33 bones of the vertebral column encase and protect the spinal cord. The vertebral column is divided into five

segments, and the spinal nerves protrude from each of these segments to innervate specific areas of the body (see **Figure 13–43 》》** and **Table 13–7 》》**) (NINDS, 2016a).

Between the bones of the vertebral column are spinal discs that provide cushioning during movement, and spinal nerves protrude from the spinal column between the vertebrae near the spinal discs. The spinal cord is more susceptible to direct injury by lesser or repetitive forces at the location of the spinal discs because of their soft nature, whereas damage to the portion of the spinal cord that is surrounded by hard vertebral bones requires greater force.

Most damage to the spinal cord occurs because of a sudden, traumatic force that distorts the normal structure of the vertebral column. When displaced bone fragments, disc material, or ligaments connecting the vertebrae come into contact with the spinal cord, the result is bruising or tearing of the nerves. The force may also cause damage to blood vessels in the gray matter, causing bleeding that can spread to the white matter and nearby segments of the spinal cord.

The initial physical trauma produces a series of events that kills neurons, demyelinates axons, and triggers an inflammatory response. Reduction in blood flow due to damage, swelling, and edema decreases oxygen and nutrient supply, causing many neurons to die; the cells in the gray matter are particularly susceptible. Swelling and edema can also cause direct compression of the nerves. Immune cells that are normally trapped in the blood vessels are able to leak into the spinal cord, where they cause an inflammatory response, scavenge debris, and fight infection. They may also secrete cytokines that cause damage to surrounding nerve cells and stimulate collagen production, forming scars. Release of neurotransmitters, especially glutamate, from damaged neurons causes a process called excitotoxicity that kills surrounding neurons and oligodendrocytes (cells that produce myelin) (NINDS, 2016b).

These and other cellular responses to traumatic SCI result in the destruction of nerves. When nerves are destroyed and can no longer transmit signals between the brain and the body, the individual experiences loss of motor and sensory

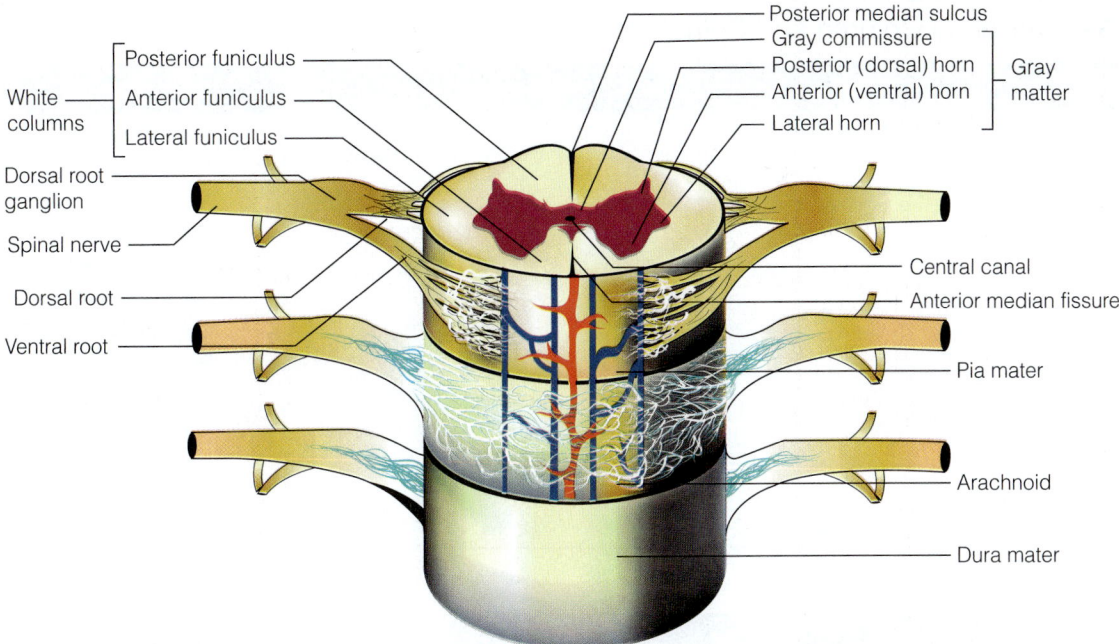

Figure 13–42 ❯❯ The structure of the spinal cord.

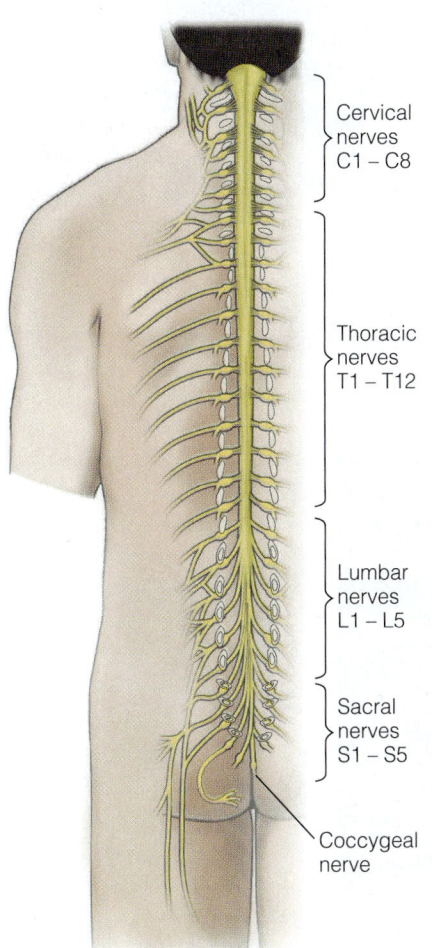

Figure 13–43 ❯❯ The vertebral column and spinal cord are divided into five segments, and spinal nerves protrude from each segment to innervate the body.

function. Sometimes, the spinal cord is only bruised or swollen, and the nerves begin to function again after the swelling goes down. However, many injuries result in neuronal damage that is not reversible.

Etiology

SCIs occur when excessive force causes hyperextension, hyperflexion, compression, rotation, or transection of the spinal cord (see **Figure 13–44 ❯❯**). **Hyperflexion** (forward bending beyond normal limits) and **hyperextension** (backward bending beyond normal limits) are usually caused by sudden acceleration–deceleration forces, such as occurs in a motor vehicle crash. During these rapid body movements, the most flexible portions of the spine, the cervical (C5–C7) and thoracolumbar (T12, L1) regions, are likely to sustain damage, including dislocated or fractured vertebrae, torn ligaments, and ruptured discs. These damaged structures can then cause injury to the spinal cord.

Compression of the spinal cord occurs when a vertical force is applied to the spinal column, such as occurs by falling and landing on the feet or buttocks or diving into shallow water. **Rotational injuries** are caused by lateral flexion or twisting of the head and neck. This can cause tearing of ligaments or dislocation or fracture of the vertebrae and an unstable spinal injury. **Transection** of the spinal cord occurs when the individual is injured by a gunshot, stabbing, or similar force that partially or completely severs the spinal cord.

The most common cause of SCI is vehicular crashes (35%), including those involving cars, motorcycles, bikes, and all-terrain vehicles (ATVs). Motor vehicle crashes can cause any one or a combination of the five types of forces and may involve both passengers and pedestrians. Falling is the second most common cause (approximately 25%), usually resulting in compression injuries. Violence (approximately 15%),

TABLE 13–7 Vertebral Column and Spinal Nerves

Segment	Label	Location	Innervation
Cervical	C1–C7 (vertebrae) C1–C8 (nerves)	Neck	Head and neck Diaphragm Upper limbs
Thoracic	T1–T12	Upper back; vertebrae attach to rib cage	Chest muscles Abdominal muscles Some back muscles
Lumbar	L1–L5	Lower back	Lower abdomen and back Parts of lower limbs
Sacral	S1–S5	Hip area	Bowels and bladder Buttocks (and anus) Parts of lower limbs Parts of external genital organs
Coccygeal	1–4 fused	Tailbone	Skin of the lower back

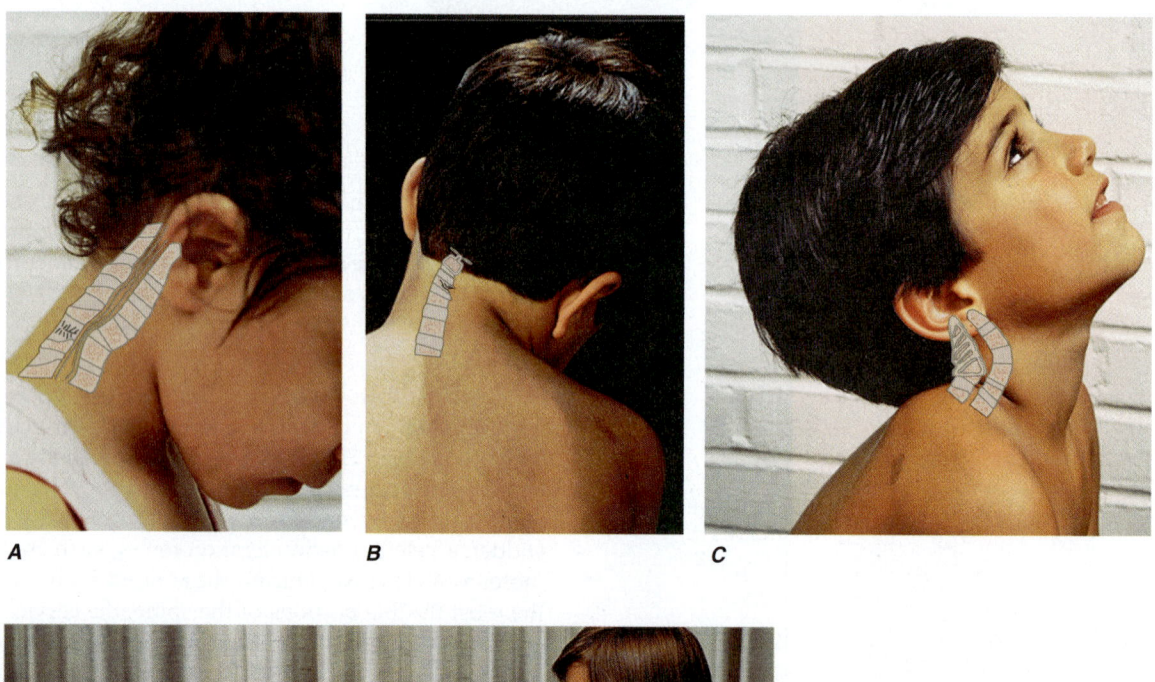

A B C

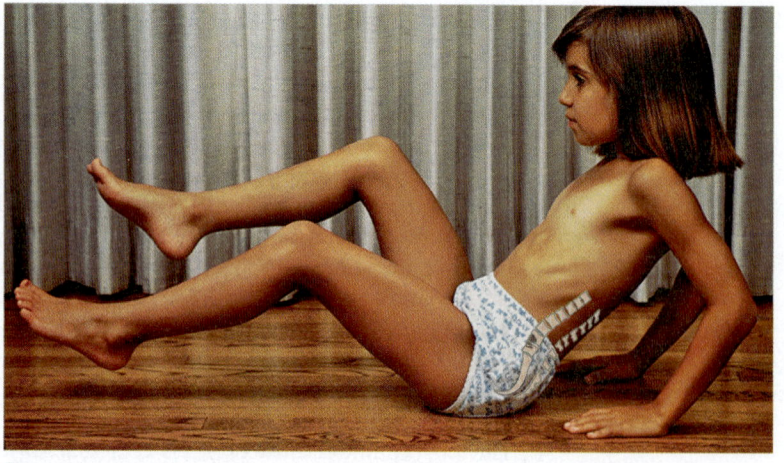

D

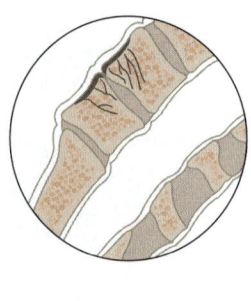

Figure 13–44 ≫ Mechanics of injury to the spinal cord: **A,** Hyperflexion, often due to diving and frontal motor vehicle crashes. **B,** Rotation, in which the head and neck are twisted. **C,** Hyperextension, often due to rear-end motor vehicle crashes and falls. **D,** Compression, due to falls that put vertical pressure on the spinal column. Infants and young children are at higher risk for injury to the brain and spinal cord because their bones and muscles are still developing.

especially gunshot wounds, typically results in transection of the spinal cord. SCIs associated with sports (9%) often result from football and diving. Diseases such as cancer, osteoporosis, and arthritis can also cause SCI (Mayo Clinic, 2014b).

Risk Factors

Eight out of ten new SCIs occur in male patients; the average age of injury is 42 years. Individuals who engage in risky behavior, such as diving into too-shallow pools, playing sports without protective gear, or driving ATVs or motorcycles at high speed over rough terrain, are also at higher risk for SCIs. Single young adult men are often the ones who engage in risky behavior, so it is not surprising that they have the highest risk for SCIs. Race and ethnicity can also contribute to the risk for SCIs: Among individuals who have sustained SCI since 2010, 63.5% are Non-Hispanic White, 22.0% are Non-Hispanic Black, 11.0% are Hispanic, 2.0% are Asian, 0.5% are Native American, and 1.0% are classified as Other (NSCISC, 2016). Older adults are more likely to sustain SCI from a fall, especially if the individual also has arthritis or osteoporosis.

Prevention

Prevention methods for SCI are similar to those for injury generally and include fall precautions for toddlers and older adults. Safe driving practices, use of vehicle restraint systems, use of a designated driver, and not driving under the influence of medications that affect mentation and awareness are practices that reduce the risk for SCI. Similar precautions related to sports and activities also reduce the risk for injury. Because diving into water that is too shallow is a common cause of compression injuries, individuals should always check water depth before diving and should never dive into above-ground pools. Individuals should wear appropriate safety gear for the type of sport or activity and avoid leading with the head (e.g., tackling in football, sliding headfirst in baseball).

Clinical Manifestations

Both the vertical location of the injury along the spinal column (called the **level of injury**) and the specific area of the spinal cord or spinal nerve that is damaged will determine the extent and type of physical manifestations the patient experiences after injury. All systems below the level of injury will be affected by damage to the spinal cord, so the higher the level of injury, the greater the extent of motor and sensory deficits. For example, a patient who experiences damage at the C3 level will experience more widespread effects than an individual with an injury at the T11 level.

Emergency signs and symptoms that may indicate SCI include extreme pain or pressure in the neck or back; weakness, paralysis, or lack of sensation in any part of the body; loss of bladder or bowel control; impaired breathing after injury; or an oddly positioned or twisted neck or back. Muscle spasms may also occur (Mayo Clinic, 2014b).

Approximately half of individuals with SCI develop **spinal shock**, which is characterized by spinal cord swelling; decreased blood flow and blood pressure; and complete loss of motor function, spinal reflexes, and autonomic function below the level of injury. During spinal shock, even undamaged nerves may have trouble communicating with the brain, causing paralysis and loss of reflexes and sensations in the limbs that are unrelated to the site of injury. Spinal shock usually occurs immediately after injury and can last from several hours to several weeks (NINDS, 2016b).

Classification of Spinal Cord Injury

SCIs can be classified as complete or incomplete using the American Spinal Injury Association (ASIA) Impairment Scale (see **Box 13–5** »). **Complete SCIs** involve a total loss of all sensory and motor function below the level of the injury. The diagnosis is usually determined by a loss of sensory function in the S4–S5 area, or anal area. Complete SCIs usually cause irreversible damage. **Incomplete SCIs** involve only a partial loss of sensory and motor function below the level of injury. Some individuals may detect sensation, but have little or no ability to move, whereas others may have movement with little or no sensation. The individual has a better chance of recovering sensory and motor function if the injury is incomplete (Chin, 2016).

Four main types of incomplete syndromes are associated with SCI (see **Table 13–8** »). CES, which is characterized by injury to the nerve roots emanating from the conus medullaris, is not a true SCI. It is characterized by bladder and bowel retention and should be treated by surgical decompression within 48 hours (Fehlings et al., 2013). (See Exemplar 13.A for further discussion of CES.)

Box 13–5
American Spinal Injury Association (ASIA) Impairment Scale (AIS)

*A = **Complete.*** No sensory or motor function is preserved in the sacral segments S4–S5.

*B = **Sensory incomplete.*** Sensory but not motor function is preserved below the neurologic level and includes the sacral segments S4–S5 (light touch, pin prick at S4–S5, or deep anal pressure), AND no motor function is preserved more than three levels below the motor level on either side of the body.

*C = **Motor incomplete.*** Motor function is preserved below the neurologic level, and more than half of key muscle functions below the single neurological level of injury (NLI) have a muscle grade of less than 3 (grades 0–2).

*D = **Motor incomplete.*** Motor function is preserved below the neurologic level, and at least half of key muscle functions below the NLI have a muscle grade ≥ 3.

*E = **Normal.*** If sensation and motor function as tested with the International Standards for Neurological Classification of Spinal Cord Injury (ISNCSCI) exam are graded as normal in all segments, and the patient had prior deficits, then the AIS grade is E. Someone without an initial SCI does not receive an AIS grade.

Source: American Spinal Injury Association: International Standards for Neurological Classification of Spinal Cord Injury, revised 2013; Atlanta, GA. Reprinted 2013.

TABLE 13–8 Syndromes Associated with Incomplete Spinal Cord Injury

Syndrome	Location and Cause of Injury	Symptoms	Prognosis
Central cord syndrome	Hyperextension of the neck, especially from falls and motor vehicle crashes; damage to the center of the spinal cord	More severe motor loss of the upper extremities than the lower extremities, bladder dysfunction (usually urinary retention), varying degrees of sensory loss below the level of injury	Almost all patients will have some degree of neurologic recovery, starting in the lower extremities and moving upward. However, some will have sustained functional loss. Younger patients have a higher recovery rate than older patients.
Anterior cord syndrome	Injury to the anterior two thirds of the spinal cord, especially the anterior spinal artery	Paraplegia below the level of injury (or tetraplegia for injuries higher than C7), bilateral loss of pain and temperature sensations with preservation of proprioception and vibratory senses below the level of injury	Patients with anterior cord syndrome have the worst prognosis for recovery of neurologic function and require long periods of rehabilitation. Only 10–20% of patients experience motor recovery.
Brown-Sequard syndrome	Hemisection of the spinal cord, usually caused by a penetrating trauma (gunshot, knife)	Ipsilateral (same side) motor paralysis and loss of proprioception and vibratory sense below the level of injury Contralateral (opposite side) loss of pain and temperature sensation below the level of injury	Patients have the best prognosis of all individuals with incomplete SCI syndromes; approximately 75–90% will recover functional motor strength and the ability to ambulate independently.
Conus medullaris syndrome	Injury to the conus medullaris, which is the tapered inferior end of the spinal cord; located at the L1 level	Symmetrical pattern of upper and lower motor neuron dysfunction, saddle anesthesia, variable degrees of lower extremity weakness, areflexic bladder and bowel	Prognosis for recovery of bowel and bladder function is poor.

Sources: Based on Chin, L. S. (2016). Spinal cord injuries. *Medscape Reference.* Retrieved from http://emedicine.medscape.com/article/793582-overview; Fehlings, M. G., Vaccaro, A. R., Boakye, M., Rossignol, S., Ditunno, J. F., Jr., & Burns, A. S. (2013). *Essentials of spinal cord injury: Basic research to clinical practice.* New York, NY: Thieme Medical.

Effects of Spinal Cord Injury Throughout the Body

SCI has many effects on the rest of the body. Individuals with SCI often experience paraplegia or tetraplegia depending on the level of injury (see **Figure 13–45**). **Tetraplegia** (also called *quadriplegia*) is paralysis of the upper and lower limbs and trunk; it is usually associated with a cervical injury. **Paraplegia** is paralysis of all or part of the trunk, legs, and pelvic organs; it is usually associated with spinal cord damage in the thoracic or lumbar regions. Incomplete tetraplegia (45.0%) is the most common neurologic category at

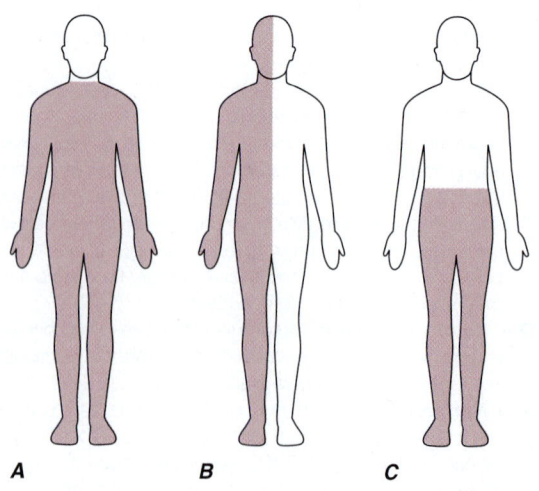

Figure 13–45 Types of paralysis. **A,** Complete quadriplegia or partial paralysis of the upper extremities and complete paralysis of the lower part of the body. **B,** Hemiplegia is paralysis of one half of the body when it is divided along the median sagittal plane. **C,** Paraplegia is paralysis of the lower part of the body.

discharge, followed by incomplete paraplegia (21.3%), complete paraplegia (20.0%), and complete tetraplegia (13.3%) (NSCISC, 2016). Hemiplegia can also occur, in which one half of the body is paralyzed when divided along the median sagittal plane.

Other common symptoms that are caused by SCI include pain, bladder and bowel problems, respiratory and cardiovascular problems, and reproductive problems. Pain can be due to either neurogenic pain resulting from damage to nerves in the spinal cord, or physiologic pain resulting from compensatory use of muscle groups (e.g., pain in shoulder muscles from pushing a wheelchair).

Urinary and bowel problems occur when nerves that innervate the muscles that control the urinary system or bowel no longer transmit signals properly. Muscles in the bladder, urethra, and sphincters no longer work together effectively, causing the bladder to empty without warning, become distended, or force urine back into the kidneys because of uncoordinated release of the bladder and urethral sphincter. Likewise, if the anal sphincter remains tight, bowel movements occur randomly when the bowel is full; however, if it is permanently relaxed ("flaccid bowel"), the individual is unable to have a bowel movement (NINDS, 2016b).

Individuals with complete thoracic or cervical injuries often lose control of respiratory muscles, including the diaphragm, intercostal muscles, neck muscles, and abdominal muscles. The higher the level of injury, the greater the loss of muscle control. For example, an individual with SCI at level C3 or higher loses control of all four muscle groups needed for breathing. These individuals require immediate ventilator support. The diaphragm is controlled by spinal nerves in the C3–C5 region, and nerves in the T1–T12 region control the intercostal and abdominal muscles; injuries in these regions will affect all muscles below the injury (Chin, 2016). Any injury below the C5 level conserves diaphragm function, but breathing tends to be rapid and shallow, and the individual cannot clear secretions from the lungs because of weak thoracic muscles (NINDS, 2016b).

Cardiovascular problems can occur for individuals with cervical injuries. Blood pressure instability, particularly hypotension, often occurs because of loss of tone in blood vessels and blood pooling in distal arteries. Damage to the cardiac accelerator nerves can cause bradycardia (slow heart rate) or arrhythmias in which the heart beats rapidly and irregularly. Arrhythmias usually appear in the first 2 weeks after injury (NINDS, 2016b).

SCIs can also cause reproductive problems for men and women. Many men with SCI are capable of having an erection, but the erection may not be hard enough or last long enough for intercourse. Men may also face fertility issues due to an inability to ejaculate or retrograde ejaculation, in which semen is deposited in the bladder instead of the urethra. Women often have no change in fertility, but they may have less satisfaction from intercourse. Women with an SCI who desire to become pregnant should discuss options with an obstetrician and other members of the healthcare team who are familiar with SCIs (Chin, 2016).

Complications

With each detrimental effect of SCI comes the potential for complications. The most common complications affect the cardiovascular system, respiratory system, integumentary system, and urinary system. In addition, patients may experience emotional changes due to the reality of their new situation.

Cardiovascular System

One of the most common and life-threatening complications of SCI is autonomic dysreflexia. **Autonomic dysreflexia** is the abrupt onset of excessively high blood pressure as the result of an overactive autonomic nervous system (ANS); it usually occurs in patients who have injuries above T5 (Chin, 2016). Autonomic dysreflexia is triggered by an irritation, pain, or other stimulus below the level of injury, such as an urge to urinate or defecate, pressure injuries, burns, or pressure from tight clothing. An overdistended bladder is the most common cause. When the irritated area tries to send a signal to the brain, the signal is blocked by the injury, causing a reflex action that stimulates the ANS to contract blood vessels, causing a rapid increase in blood pressure. Symptoms of autonomic dysreflexia include flushing, sweating, a pounding headache, bradycardia, sudden hypertension (less than 200/100 mmHg), vision changes, and goose bumps. Treatment should be immediate and may include changing positions, emptying the bladder or bowels, or removing tight clothing (NINDS, 2016b). If not treated immediately, autonomic dysreflexia can lead to seizures, stroke, MI, and death. Methods to avoid autonomic dysreflexia are outlined in the Patient Teaching feature.

Another common complication of SCI is DVT, especially for patients with little to no mobility. Individuals with SCI are at three times the risk for developing blood clots in comparison to other individuals with limited mobility. If blood clots become dislodged, they may travel throughout the body and cause stroke or pulmonary embolism, both of which are life-threatening complications. Anticoagulant therapy may be provided as a preventive measure.

Patient Teaching
Avoiding Autonomic Dysreflexia

Autonomic dysreflexia is caused by irritation or pain below the level of injury. Methods to avoid irritation include the following:

- Regularly empty the bladder and bowels.
- If using an indwelling catheter, keep the tubing free of kinks, and keep the drainage bag and tubes clean and empty.
- Treat UTIs promptly.
- Consume adequate fluid and fiber to prevent constipation.
- Change positions frequently.
- Regularly assess the skin for impaired integrity, including pressure injuries and ingrown toenails.
- Avoid burns, including sunburns.
- Do not wear clothing that is too tight.
- Take medications as prescribed to prevent pain and other complications that may initiate autonomic dysreflexia.
- Do not become overstimulated during sexual activity.

Respiratory System

If innervation of respiratory muscles is affected by SCI, multiple respiratory complications can occur in addition to difficulty breathing. Any loss of respiratory muscle control decreases lung capacity, increases respiratory congestion, and makes coughing difficult. If the patient is unable to draw enough air into the lungs, atelectasis (collapsed lung) may occur. An inability to clear secretions and use of mechanical ventilation increases the patient's risk for pneumonia. Individuals on mechanical ventilation increase their risk of developing complications by 1–3% per day of intubation. More than 25% of all deaths associated with SCI are related to ventilator-associated pneumonia (NINDS, 2016b). Symptoms of pneumonia include shortness of breath, pale skin, fever, a "heavy" chest, and increased congestion (Chin, 2016). Individuals with pneumonia should be treated immediately with antibiotics.

Integumentary System

SCIs are associated with a temporary or permanent loss of mobility. Many individuals must stay in bed for weeks while the spinal cord heals, or they may use a wheelchair for life. These individuals are at high risk for developing pressure sores if they are not turned or repositioned frequently. If pressure injuries do develop, decreased blood flow and nervous intervention inhibits the wound healing process, and it may also stimulate autonomic dysreflexia. Patients with SCI may also lose sensory perception to pain, touch, and temperature, putting these patients at high risk for burns and cuts. If not treated promptly, these injuries may cause infection or autonomic dysreflexia.

Urinary System

Every SCI has the potential to cause urinary problems. Many patients must undergo indwelling or intermittent catheterization, which dramatically increases their risk of developing a UTI. If urine backs up into the kidneys, it could cause a serious kidney infection. Kidney or bladder stones may also

Clinical Manifestations and Therapies
Spinal Cord Injury

ETIOLOGY	CLINICAL MANIFESTATIONS	CLINICAL THERAPIES
Spinal cord injury (general)	■ Pain ■ Loss of sensation ■ Loss of bladder or bowel control ■ Paralysis ■ Muscle spasms ■ Spinal shock ■ DVT ■ Reproductive problems	■ Immobilization ■ Spinal decompression surgery ■ Methylprednisolone ■ Analgesics ■ Antispasmodics ■ Catheterization ■ Skin care ■ ROM exercises ■ Rehabilitation
Cervical injury	*In addition to symptoms for general SCI:* ■ Tetraplegia ■ Oddly twisted neck ■ Weakness, loss of respiratory muscle control ■ Hypotension ■ Bradycardia, arrhythmias ■ Autonomic dysreflexia ■ Decreased peristalsis	*In addition to therapies for general SCI:* ■ Airway patency ■ External fixation or traction ■ Nasogastric decompression
Thoracic injury	*In addition to symptoms for general SCI:* ■ Paraplegia ■ Impaired breathing ■ Autonomic dysreflexia	*In addition to therapies for general SCI:* ■ Airway patency
Lumbar/sacral injury	*In addition to symptoms for general SCI:* ■ Paraplegia ■ CES	*In addition to therapies for general SCI:* ■ Surgery to relieve pressure on cauda equina

develop. For more information about UTIs, see the exemplar on UTIs in the module on Infection. For more information on other bladder and bowel problems, see the module on Elimination.

Emotional Changes

SCIs instantly cause a plethora of physical changes. Patients often go through a process of grief upon the loss of mobility and independence. Some patients will progress through the grief process and eventually accept their new condition. These patients have the best chance of having a good quality of life. Others, however, may be unable to accept their new condition and fight anger and depression for many years. These patients may need additional psychologic care, including medications and counseling.

Collaboration

Care of an individual with actual or suspected SCI begins with emergency care at the moment of injury and often continues throughout the remainder of the individual's life. Emergency care, surgical repair, and pharmacologic and nonpharmacologic therapies are all required for adequate treatment of an individual with SCI.

Emergency Care

SCI is not always obvious. All individuals who have trauma to the head or are unconscious should be treated as if they have SCI. Individuals with penetrating injuries near the spine and individuals who have experienced a fall or motor vehicle crash should also be suspected of having SCI. Initial care should focus on maintaining the patient's ability to breathe, preventing movement that could cause more damage, and preventing shock. About one third of patients will need respiratory support via intubation, particularly those with high cervical injuries. Immediate medical attention and transport to the hospital by emergency medical services are necessary. At the hospital, the patient should be transferred from the stretcher to the bed with the backboard still in place. The spine should be realigned using a rigid brace or axial traction as soon as possible after arrival at the hospital.

Diagnostic Tests

Diagnostic tests for SCI should include imaging tests such as x-rays, myelograms, CT scans, or MRIs. X-rays can reveal major vertebral fractures and other bone problems; x-rays must adequately show all regions of the spinal column so that no injuries, especially noncontiguous fractures (spinal fractures separated by at least one normal vertebra), are overlooked. Injecting a contrast dye during myelography allows the radiologist to directly view damage to the spinal cord and surrounding tissues. CT scans and MRIs are more sensitive than simple x-rays at detecting abnormalities, especially damage to soft tissue and small fractures. Imaging tests are useful for determining both the location of the injury and whether the spinal cord is being compressed.

Somatosensory evoked potentials or magnetic evoked potentials can be used to detect neural response to physiologic, electrical, or magnetic stimulation. Common sites for stimulation include the median nerve at the wrist, the common peroneal nerve at the knee, and the posterior tibial nerve (Chawla, 2012). Arterial blood gases (ABGs) should be monitored regularly to evaluate oxygenation and ventilation, and hemoglobin and hematocrit should be measured to detect major blood loss.

Surgery

The timing of surgical treatment for SCI is a controversial issue. Some studies indicate that early decompression (removal of debris that is compressing the spinal cord) results in a better recovery compared to late decompression, whereas other studies indicate that there is no difference in neurologic recovery between early and late decompression. A large study of six hospitals throughout North America compared outcomes between early decompression (less than 24 hours after injury) and late decompression (more than 24 hours after injury). This study found that the odds of at least a two-grade AIS improvement were 2.8 times higher in patients who underwent early decompression compared to late decompression (Fehlings et al., 2012). Spinal decompression surgery is most often performed in patients with progressive neurologic deterioration, facet dislocation (displacement of one vertebra on another), spinal nerve compression, and extradural lesions (Chin, 2016).

After SCI, surgery may also be needed to stabilize the spine. Spine stabilization may involve realigning the spine and using instrumentation such as rods and screws to internally immobilize the spine. A bone graft from the patient or bone bank is often added to promote fusion of the vertebrae. Surgery can also be performed to set up spinal traction using Gardner-Wells tongs or other traction devices (see **Figure 13–46 》**) or

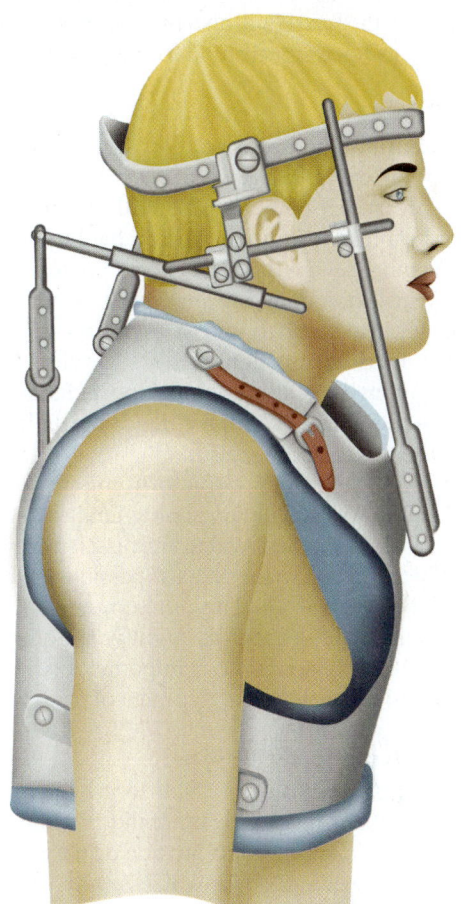

Figure 13–47 》 The halo external fixation device.

external fixation with a halo brace (see **Figure 13–47 》**). A halo brace is often used for patients with cervical fractures without major cord damage. The patient may be in traction or external fixation for several weeks or months.

Pharmacologic Therapy

Pharmacologic therapy for patients with SCI is primarily symptomatic. Symptoms that may require treatment include pain, constipation, infections, hypotension, and muscle spasticity. Medications to treat these symptoms are discussed elsewhere in this textbook. Most patients will receive high-dose methylprednisone within 8 hours after injury to improve neurologic recovery. Methylprednisolone appears to decrease inflammation and reduce damage to surrounding nerve cells. Adverse effects are usually minor. Prophylactic anticoagulation therapy (e.g., heparin, Coumadin) may be given to help prevent DVT and pulmonary embolism. Infections, especially pneumonia, should be treated promptly with appropriate antibiotics; pain can be treated with opioids, NSAIDs, and other analgesics as needed.

Nonpharmacologic Therapy

Patients with SCI will require extensive nursing care. Immediate nursing care involves maintaining an airway, assisting with ventilation, and immobilizing the patient. Nursing care also includes preventing complications such as urinary or bowel problems, pressure injuries, and infection. During the

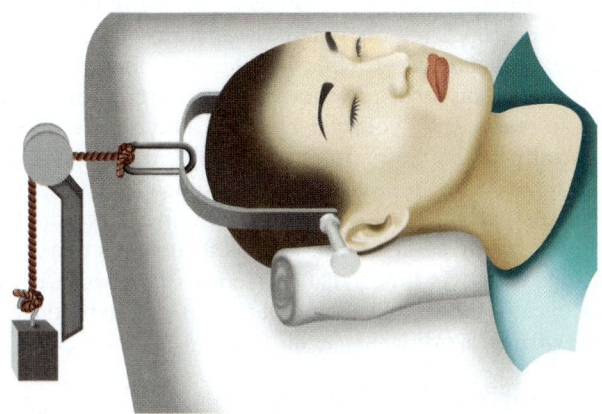

Figure 13–46 》 Cervical traction may be applied by any of several methods, including the Gardner-Wells method.

healing process, the nurse will also play a role in the patient's rehabilitation and patient teaching for home care.

Ventilation

The most important therapy for patients with SCI is to maintain a patent airway and assist with ventilation as needed. Patients with injuries above T12 will experience some decrease in respiratory muscle control; the higher the level of injury, the more severe the deficiencies. Some patients will require only insertion of an oropharyngeal airway, whereas others will require intubation and mechanical ventilation (Chin, 2016). During insertion of tubes, cervical alignment must be maintained at all times. Most individuals with a C4 injury and some with a C3 injury may eventually learn to breathe on their own (Chin, 2016).

Patients with decreased respiratory muscle control also have a hard time coughing and clearing lung secretions. The nurse should help the patient with cough assist treatments and encourage the patient to drink water if possible to keep secretions from becoming thick. The nurse may also teach the patient breathing exercises, such as incentive spirometry. Keeping the airway clear of secretions is important both for ease of breathing and to prevent the development of pneumonia.

Preventing Complications

Many primary complications related to the injury and secondary complications related to immobility can affect patients with SCI. Primary complications include urinary, bowel, and gastrointestinal problems. Most SCIs affect bladder and bowel control because of a disruption of nerve transmission to the muscles that control these organs. Individuals with bladder dysfunction often use intermittent or indwelling catheters to empty their bladders. Individuals with bowel dysfunction should implement a scheduled bowel program; if constipation is severe, the patient may need manual removal of stool to prevent fecal impaction. Gastrointestinal problems usually involve decreased peristalsis (ileus) and difficulty swallowing. Some patients will need a nasogastric tube to remove stomach contents (nasogastric decompression) to prevent aspiration pneumonia. Food or medicine can also be administered through the nasogastric tube as needed throughout recovery for patients with swallowing problems.

Secondary complications are often related to immobility. Patients with SCI may be on bedrest for an extended period, or they may use a wheelchair for the rest of their lives. Both the injury and immobility cause decreased blood flow, which can lead to complications such as pressure injuries, DVT, and infection. Nonpharmacologic interventions to prevent pressure injuries include turning the patient every 1–2 hours, providing good skin care, observing the patient's skin for damaged areas, padding hard surfaces (both exterior surfaces such as bedrailings and interior surfaces such as bony prominences), removing items that may cause compression of blood vessels (e.g., keys, belts, cell phones), performing passive and active ROM exercises, and ambulating if possible. For patients with severe pressure injuries, nonpharmacologic treatment may include covering the wound with a sterile dressing and eating foods high in protein to promote healing. In addition to many of these same interventions, compression stockings or boots can stimulate circulation in the legs to prevent DVT.

Individuals with SCI are at high risk for infection from additional bone fractures and skin wounds from the traumatic event, surgical incisions, traction or external fixation pins, pressure injuries, decreased airway clearance, and catheterization. Each of these types of infection requires different nonpharmacologic interventions. For example, skin wounds should be gently cleansed, covered with sterile gauze, and monitored for drainage and other signs of infection. Pneumonia can be prevented by keeping the airway clear of secretions, and UTIs can be prevented by keeping the bladder empty and using sterile technique during catheterization.

Rehabilitative and Home-Based Care

When the initial traumatic injuries have been treated and the patient is stabilized, the patient faces a long road to recovery to regain maximal function. Rehabilitation is a core component of this recovery. Rehabilitation team members may include a PT, OT, rehabilitation nurse, recreation therapist, and physiatrist. Therapists emphasize strengthening existing muscle function, redeveloping fine motor skills to perform ADLs, and learning new technology to increase independence (Mayo Clinic, 2014b). Rehabilitation will include learning how to use assistive devices such as a wheelchair, walker, or Lofstrand crutches as well as devices to aid with ADLs. Another vital component of rehabilitation is preparing patients to return home and live independently.

Rehabilitation for patients with partial lower limb function may include gait training. Gait training involves using mechanical or human assistance to help the patient walk on a treadmill. In addition to providing cardiovascular and respiratory benefits, gait training helps the patient gain joint stability, retrain the muscles to walk, increase walking speed, and gain independence. Secondary complications are also decreased. Gait training often uses a harness system to provide support and safety for the patient (Chin, 2016).

Lifespan Considerations

SCI in Children and Adolescents

Although SCI in the pediatric population accounts for only 5% of all new cases, it can have significant physiologic and psychologic consequences. Both the location and common mechanisms of injury are different for children than for adults. For cervical injuries, preteens are more likely to be injured in the C2 region, whereas teens sustain C4 injuries and adults sustain C4–C5 injuries (Boston Children's Hospital, 2016b). The most common causes of injury are motor vehicle crashes for younger children and sports injuries (especially football) for adolescents (NSCISC, 2016).

Children tend to have better neurologic recovery after SCI compared to adults. Incomplete injuries have the best prognosis, but even severe complete injuries can show improvement over time in children. However, there is a high incidence of neuromuscular scoliosis in children and preteens with SCIs (Mulcahey et al., 2013).

SCI in Pregnant Women

Pregnant women with SCI also need special care. Women with SCI are considered to be "high risk" during pregnancy, but that does not mean pregnancy should be avoided.

Instead, the woman will need to work closely with a team of healthcare professionals, including an obstetrician, neurologist, respiratory therapist, physiatrist, and nurse, to prevent complications and prepare for pregnancy, labor, and delivery. Pregnant women are at higher risk for autonomic dysreflexia (especially during labor and delivery), changes in bowel and bladder function, UTIs, pressure injuries, respiratory complications, muscle spasms, and swelling in the lower limbs. The woman may not be able to continue taking prescribed medications during pregnancy, so alternative therapies may be needed to manage symptoms.

Pregnant women with decreased sensation in the lower trunk may not feel the typical pains of labor, so they should be taught the common signs of labor such as changes in breathing, abdominal tightening, and backache. New mothers must also consider the effects of her SCI on breastfeeding; muscle spasticity may increase during breastfeeding, and women with limited sensation in their breasts may have reduced milk production (Chin, 2016).

SCI in Older Adults

As the general population increases, the number of individuals with SCI has increased. The older adult population has seen the highest increase in SCIs (Jain et al., 2015). Sixty percent of SCIs in the geriatric population are due to falls. The most common falls occur on the same level; from steps or stairs; and from slips, trips, or stumbling (Chen, Tang, Allen, & DeVivo, 2015).

NURSING PROCESS

SCI is a serious medical condition that requires collaboration between experts in a variety of fields. The nurse is an important part of this team. Nursing care of patients with SCI can be divided into emergency care, acute care of a stabilized patient, and rehabilitation. The nurse focuses on stabilizing the patient, preventing and treating complications, promoting self-care, and educating the patient and family. The nurse also plays a major role in the community to prevent SCI by promoting safety.

Assessment

Nursing assessment of the patient with SCI includes obtaining a health history and performing ongoing physical assessments. The health history should include questions about the patient's overall health before the traumatic event; an accounting of the traumatic event (time, location, and type of event); any medications the patient is taking; and any symptoms the patient is experiencing, including pain, numbness, and difficulty breathing.

The physical examination of a patient with SCI includes assessing vital signs regularly, assessing the patient's respiratory status, maintaining a patent airway, and assisting with breathing if needed. A neurologic examination should follow the ASIA International Standards for Neurological Classification of Spinal Cord Injury. This includes testing key muscles for strength using the muscle function grading scale (see Table 13–1), testing areas of innervation for each spinal nerve for sensation of light touch and pin prick, and scoring the patient on the ASIA Impairment Scale. The nurse should also assess the patient for reflexes, bowel sounds,

bladder distention, pain, ABGs, and other injuries from the event.

Diagnosis

Nursing diagnoses will vary with the level and extent of injury. Some nursing diagnoses that may apply to patients with a SCI include the following:

- *Ineffective Airway Clearance* related to impaired gag reflex
- *Risk for Aspiration* related to impaired gag reflex and gastrointestinal motility
- *Ineffective Breathing Pattern* related to impaired diaphragmatic innervation
- *Risk for Autonomic Dysreflexia* related to C7 SCI
- *Impaired Physical Mobility* related to T5 SCI
- *Acute Pain* related to injuries from motor vehicle crash
- *Urinary Retention* related to flaccid bladder
- *Bowel Incontinence* related to defecation reflex
- *Self-Care Deficit: Bathing, Dressing, Feeding, Toileting* related to upper limb paralysis
- *Risk for Post-Trauma Syndrome* related to traumatic event with life-changing injuries.

(NANDA-I © 2014)

Planning

Patient goals related to SCI may include the following:

- The patient will maintain a patent airway.
- The patient will participate in speech and occupational therapy as ordered to optimize control of muscles used for swallowing.
- The patient will maintain clear breath sounds and oxygen saturation of greater than 95% on room air.
- The patient will deny dyspnea.
- The patient will verbalize understanding of potential triggers of autonomic dysreflexia and will avoid these triggers.
- The patient will participate in physical and occupational therapy to regain as much mobility as possible.
- The patient will verbalize adequate pain control, as evidenced by reporting pain as tolerable and having pain no higher than 3 on a scale of 0–10.
- The patient will demonstrate safe, effective self-catheterization.
- The patient will develop techniques for using assistive devices to help with ADLs.
- The patient and caregiver will contact a home health agency to assist with ADLs.
- The patient will attend counseling sessions to overcome emotional trauma.

Implementation

The nursing interventions needed for patients with SCI will depend on the level, severity, and classification of the injury. Immediate care will include assistance with ventilation, immobilization, care of wounds, and bladder and bowel control. Interventions during the recovery phase will include assistance with mobility, exercise, and self-care activities and prevention of complications. Rehabilitation interventions will include assistance with ambulation, training for ADLs, and referral to rehabilitation therapy. Another vital component of rehabilitation is preparing patients to return home and live independently (see the Patient Teaching feature).

Interventions for a person suspected of having SCI (acute/emergent phase) in a community area include:

- Determine responsiveness.
- Call 9-1-1, and request assistance from others in the facility.
- Logroll the individual while maintaining spinal precautions. (If the patient walked into the healthcare facility, consider the need for a standing backboard and application of cervical collar.)
- Assess airway and breathing. Maintain a patent airway, and provide respirations as needed. Provide oxygen as available.
- Obtain patient history if the patient is alert and able to communicate prior to possible loss of consciousness. If the patient is unresponsive, determine if a friend or family member can provide history.

With the exception of calling 9-1-1, interventions will be similar in inpatient settings. Additional interventions will include:

- Establish IV access, and administer medications as ordered—possible use of IV methylprednisolone (Solu-Medrol, A-Methapred) (Mayo Clinic, 2014b).
- Complete a head-to-toe assessment that includes focused neurologic assessment and pain assessment.
- Prepare the patient for surgery as needed.
- Insert a Foley catheter as indicated.
- Assess the patient for anxiety.
- Turn the patient every 2 hours.
- Observe for and treat autonomic dysreflexia.
- Monitor respiratory status.
- Provide the patient and family education about SCI, interventions, and therapies.

Interventions following the postacute phase include patient teaching (see the Patient Teaching feature) and may include:

- Assess respiratory symptoms.
- Observe for signs and symptoms of autonomic dysreflexia, and provide teaching about it to the patient and family.
- Promote patient independence as appropriate.
- Teach self-catheterization as needed.
- Encourage and facilitate participation in physical, occupational, and speech therapy as needed.

Manage Emergent and Urgent Problems

Nursing interventions that need to be implemented immediately after injury will focus on immobilizing the spine and

providing an adequate airway. This may involve assisting the physician in applying a cervical brace and other immobilization devices and inserting an oropharyngeal airway, intubation tube, or nasogastric tube. This may also involve providing support to the patient while the patient is being moved from the transport bed to a hospital bed. The nurse will also be responsible for monitoring vital signs, ABGs, and machines used to stabilize the patient, such as a mechanical ventilator. Abnormal reports should be immediately reported to a physician, because they may indicate additional complications.

When the patient's status has stabilized, the nurse can begin to provide care for non–life-threatening injuries, such as skin wounds, bone fractures, and loss of bladder and bowel control. Nursing care involves cleansing skin wounds and applying an antibiotic ointment and sterile bandage. The patient may need an indwelling catheter and fecal incontinence pouch until the patient is able to perform self-catheterization, ambulate to the toilet, or participate in bowel and bladder training. If the patient is constipated, nursing care may include encouraging increased intake of fluids and fiber or manually removing impacted feces.

Provide Assistance with ADLs

Patients with SCI will be hospitalized, potentially for several weeks. During this time, nursing care includes assisting the patient with self-care activities (bathing, eating), monitoring vital signs every 4 hours, assessing the patient for complications (DVT, infection, pressure injuries, excess sputum, autonomic dysreflexia, distended bladder), and providing patient education and emotional support. The nurse should perform respiratory and neurologic assessments regularly, because worsening symptoms may require immediate intervention. Nursing interventions to help prevent complications include helping the patient perform ROM exercises, turning the patient every 2 hours, keeping the catheter and fecal pouch clean and empty, providing pin care for patients in traction or external fixation, helping the patient cough to clear sputum every 2 hours, and applying compression stockings or boots. The patient may also begin physical or occupational therapy during this time; the nurse may be responsible for providing referrals for therapy or transporting the patient to therapy sessions.

SAFETY ALERT Compression stockings or boots are necessary for patients who are immobile to help stimulate blood flow and to prevent DVT. However, they may also trigger autonomic dysreflexia in patients with SCI. If patients develop autonomic dysreflexia, compression stockings or boots should be immediately removed. In addition, compression stockings or boots can be removed for 30–60 minutes several times daily to provide relief for the patient.

Facilitate Rehabilitation

When the patient's injuries have healed as much as possible, the patient is ready to begin aggressive rehabilitation. The patient may be in the hospital, in an extended care facility, or at home during this time. Nursing care may include referring the patient to a rehabilitation facility, providing emotional support, performing periodic neurologic assessments, teaching the patient to use assistive devices, and training the patient or caregiver to perform catheterization. Providing bowel and bladder training for the patient may also be the responsibility of the nurse.

Evaluation

Evaluation of patients with SCI involves monitoring vital signs, performing neurologic assessments, and assessing the patient for signs and symptoms of complications that may range in severity from life-threatening to minor. The patient's emotional status should also be monitored; anger, frustration, anxiety, and depression are common emotions for patients with SCI. The goal of nursing care is to return the patient to as close to maximal physical health as possible. Areas to evaluate will include:

- **Airway and breathing.** The patient will maintain a patent airway, demonstrate no signs or symptoms of aspiration, and demonstrate effective ventilation. Effective ventilation is manifested by an oxygen saturation greater than 95%, absence of cyanosis, and ABGs within normal limits.

- **Complications.** The patient will remain free of complications, such as autonomic dysreflexia, DVT, UTI, and any alterations to skin integrity.

- **Elimination patterns.** The patient will demonstrate production of at least 0.5 mL/kg/hr of urine and will demonstrate adequate bowel elimination patterns, including passage of at least one stool daily.

Nursing Care Plan
A Patient with a Cervical Spinal Cord Injury

Caleb Peralta, a 20-year-old college junior, is admitted to the hospital by ambulance following a diving accident. He was socializing at a lake with friends, and on diving into the lake, he struck his head on a concealed rock formation.

ASSESSMENT	DIAGNOSES	PLANNING
When Mr. Peralta is admitted to the ED, he has flaccid paralysis involving all extremities. Below the clavicle, he has no sensation; he cannot feel or move his arms and legs. His bladder is distended, and bowel sounds are absent. Mr. Peralta was apneic at the scene; a friend performed rescue breathing for the patient until the ambulance crew arrived. Mr. Peralta was intubated by emergency medical personnel and manually ventilated while en route to the ED. Upon ED arrival, mechanical ventilation was initiated. Mr. Peralta's vital signs include temperature 96.8°F oral; pulse 57 bpm; respirations controlled at 16/min; and BP 92/61 mmHg. ABG results include pH 7.36, PaO$_2$ 54, PaCO$_2$ 41, and SaO$_2$ 96%. A CT scan indicates a fracture and SCI at the C5 level; halo traction is applied. A Foley catheter is inserted into his bladder, with immediate returns of 100 mL clear yellow urine. A nasogastric tube is inserted and attached to low-pressure continuous suction.	■ *Risk for Ineffective Airway Clearance* related to C5 SCI and tracheal intubation ■ *Risk for Aspiration* related to neurologic injury, tracheal intubation, and decreased peristalsis ■ *Impaired Swallowing* related to C5 SCI ■ *Ineffective Breathing Pattern* related to C5 SCI ■ *Impaired Gas Exchange* related to paralysis of respiratory muscles ■ *Impaired Physical Mobility* related to C5 SCI ■ *Urinary Retention* related to flaccid bladder ■ *Dysfunctional Gastrointestinal Motility* related to SCI ■ *Self-Care Deficit: Bathing, Dressing, Feeding, Toileting* related to upper extremity paralysis ■ *Risk for Impaired Skin Integrity,* related to immobility (NANDA-I © 2014)	■ The patient will maintain a patent airway. ■ The patient will demonstrate no signs or symptoms of aspiration. ■ The patient will demonstrate effective ventilation, as manifested by oxygen saturation of greater than 95%, absence of cyanosis, and ABGs within normal limits. ■ The patient will demonstrate no signs or symptoms of autonomic dysreflexia. ■ The patient will demonstrate no signs or symptoms of DVT. ■ The patient will demonstrate production of at least 0.5 mL/kg/hr of urine. ■ The patient will tolerate passive ROM. ■ The patient will demonstrate no signs or symptoms of UTI. ■ The patient will verbalize the time required for bathing and dressing. ■ The patient will demonstrate adequate bowel elimination patterns, including passage of at least one stool daily. ■ The patient's skin will remain intact and free from impairment, including skin breakdown or ulceration.

(continued on next page)

Nursing Care Plan (continued)

IMPLEMENTATION

- Monitor the patient's endotracheal tube placement and tube patency; administer tracheal suctioning as ordered and as needed to prevent obstruction.
- Routinely assess the patient's respiratory status, including breath sounds, continuous oxygen saturation monitoring, and ABG results as ordered.
- Avoid exposing the patient to triggers for autonomic dysreflexia, including bladder or bowel distention, constrictive garments, or development of pressure injuries.
- Monitor for signs and symptoms of autonomic dysreflexia, and immediately report any suspected manifestations to the physician.
- Administer IV fluid as ordered; monitor for signs and symptoms of fluid volume overload.
- Insert a Foley catheter per the physician's order, and monitor and record fluid intake and output.

- Report decreased or inadequate urine output to the patient's physician.
- Routinely assess the patient's halo pins, and clean the sites per the physician's orders.
- Monitor and document nasogastric output.
- Turn the patient every 2 hours. Inspect the skin for breakdown or injury, and report any alterations to the patient's physician.
- Provide urinary hygiene care and catheter care as needed to prevent infection.
- Place and monitor a fecal incontinence pouch; empty pouch as needed, and report abnormalities or decreased stool production to the physician.
- Apply compression stockings or boots as needed to prevent DVT. Remove stockings during ROM exercises.
- Perform passive ROM exercises on the patient's extremities every 4 hours.

EVALUATION

After 2 weeks, Mr. Peralta is moved from the intensive care unit to the neurosurgical unit for continuing care. Because he is hospitalized in the city where he attends college, several hundred miles from home, his family (father, mother, and sister) have been able to visit only one weekend a month. His parents have requested that he be transferred to a rehabilitation hospital in his hometown when he is able to travel.

His vital signs have stabilized and are within normal limits. Mr. Peralta is still receiving oxygen by nasal cannula, but he is able to breathe without assistance. He has not regained sensation below the neck. One night, as his nurse is repositioning him and inspecting his back for indications of skin breakdown, he states, "I wish I had died when I hit my head. I can't even scratch my own nose. I'm useless."

CRITICAL THINKING

1. How should Mr. Peralta's care plan be modified based on his statement to the nurse?
2. If Mr. Peralta continues to have tetraplegia with no control of his bowel or bladder, develop a training session to educate his parents about how to care for him.
3. What types of rehabilitation therapy will be most beneficial for Mr. Peralta?

REVIEW Spinal Cord Injury

RELATE Link the Concepts and Exemplars

Linking the exemplar of SCI with the concept of ethics:

1. What is the healthcare team's ethical responsibility to a patient with tetraplegia who wants to remove the ventilator and be allowed to die?
2. A patient with a drug abuse problem has sustained a gunshot wound to the spinal cord and is in severe pain. How should you respond if the physician will not prescribe opioids?

Linking the exemplar of SCI with the concept of acid–base balance:

3. An unconscious patient with a T5 SCI has just been intubated and is being manually ventilated at a rate of 28 respirations per minute. The ED physician orders an ABG analysis. Presuming the patient's ABG results reflect hyperventilation, would the nurse expect the patient's $PaCO_2$ to be increased or decreased? What effect would uncompensated hyperventilation have on the patient's blood pH?
4. What nursing interventions should be implemented for a patient with SCI who develops respiratory acidosis?

READY Go to Volume 3: Clinical Nursing Skills

REFER Go to Pearson MyLab Nursing and eText

- Additional review materials

REFLECT Apply Your Knowledge

Robert Morris is a 25-year-old man who is in rehabilitation following SCI that resulted from falling from his parents' roof while cleaning gutters. He lost his balance and fell two stories to the ground, fracturing his L1 vertebrae. Mr. Morris had a job in the marketing department of a large department store in a town 15 miles away, but he does not think he will be able to continue working at the job following his injury. He is currently taking a medical leave of absence.

Mr. Morris is engaged to Laura Knecht, 25 years old, who is a newly graduated OT employed by a local hospital. They have dated since high school and always planned to marry. Ms. Knecht has been very supportive of Mr. Morris during his convalescence, but he has been noticeably cool and withdrawn toward her. Mr. Morris plans to live with his parents when he is discharged. They are concerned about Mr. Morris's treatment of Ms. Knecht, whom they love very much. His 18-year-old sister has been giving Mr. Morris a hard time about how he is treating his fiancée.

Mr. Morris is paralyzed from the waist down, and the physicians are not sure whether the paralysis is permanent. Mr. Morris spent 4 weeks in a rehabilitation hospital and is planning for discharge, after which he will receive physical therapy in the home. You are the home health nurse visiting Mr. Morris in the rehabilitation center to obtain a current assessment and begin developing his plan of care.

1. How should you respond to Mr. Morris if he confides his concerns that he will never be able to hold a decent job or have a family?
2. Why might Mr. Morris be attempting to distance himself from his fiancée? How should you address this issue?
3. Design Mr. Morris's initial plan of care for his first week at home.

References

Adams, M. P., Holland, L. N., & Urban, C. (2017). *Pharmacology for nurses: A pathophysiologic approach* (5th ed.). Hoboken, NJ: Pearson Education.

American Academy of Orthopaedic Surgeons (AAOS). (2009). *Hip fractures.* Retrieved from http://orthoinfo.aaos.org/topic.cfm?topic=A00392

American Academy of Orthopaedic Surgeons (AAOS). (2012). *Herniated disc in lower back.* Retrieved from http://orthoinfo.aaos.org/topic.cfm?topic=a00534

American Academy of Orthopaedic Surgeons (AAOS). (2014a). *Internal fixation for fractures.* Retrieved from http://orthoinfo.aaos.org/topic.cfm?topic=a00534

American Academy of Orthopaedic Surgeons (AAOS). (2014b). *Nursemaid's elbow.* Retrieved from http://orthoinfo.aaos.org/topic.cfm?topic=A00717

American Academy of Orthopaedic Surgeons (AAOS). (2015a). *Idiopathic scoliosis in children and adolescents.* Retrieved from http://orthoinfo.aaos.org/topic.cfm?topic=A00353

American Academy of Orthopaedic Surgeons (AAOS). (2015b). *Tennis elbow (lateral epicondylitis).* Retrieved from http://orthoinfo.aaos.org/topic.cfm?topic=A00068

American Association of Neurological Surgeons (AANS). (2014). *Herniated disc.* Retrieved from http://orthoinfo.aaos.org/topic.cfm?topic=a00534

American Association of Neurological Surgeons (AANS). (2016). *Spinal infections.* Retrieved from http://www.aans.org/Patient%20Information/Conditions%20and%20Treatments/Spinal%20Infections.aspx

American Congress of Obstetricians and Gynecologists. (2016). *Back pain during pregnancy.* Retrieved from http://www.acog.org/Patients/FAQs/Back-Pain-During-Pregnancy

American Spinal Injury Association: International Standards for Neurological Classification of Spinal Cord Injury, revised 2013; Atlanta, GA. Reprinted 2013.

Arthritis Foundation. (n.d.). *Arthritis medications in pregnancy: What's safe, what's not?* Retrieved from http://www.arthritis.org/living-with-arthritis/life-stages/pregnancy-family/arthritis-medication-pregnant-safety.php

Askari, A., Gholami, T., NaghiZadeh, M. M., Farjam, M., Kouhpayeh, S. A., & Shahabfard, Z. (2016, April). *Hyaluronic acid compared with corticosteroid injections for the treatment of osteoarthritis of the knee: A randomized control trial.* doi:10.1186/s40064-016-2020-0

Bassani, T. B., Vital, M. A. B. F., & Rauh, L. K. (2015). Neuroinflammation in the pathophysiology of Parkinson's disease and therapeutic evidence of anti-inflammatory drugs. *Arquivos de Neuro-Psiquiatria, 73*(7), 616–623. Retrieved from http://orthoinfo.aaos.org/topic.cfm?topic=a00534

Berman, A., Snyder, S. J., & Frandsen, G. (2016). Pain management. In *Kozier and Erb's fundamentals of nursing: Concepts, process, and practice* (10th ed.). Hoboken, NJ: Pearson Education.

Birth Injury Guide. (2016). *Infant broken bones.* Retrieved from http://www.birthinjuryguide.org/birth-injury/types/infant-broken-bones/

Boston Children's Hospital. (2016a). *Hip fracture: Overview.* Retrieved from http://www.childrenshospital.org/conditions-and-treatments/conditions/h/hip-fracture/overview

Boston Children's Hospital. (2016b). *Spinal cord injury in children.* Retrieved from http://www.childrenshospital.org/conditions-and-treatments/conditions/spinal-cord-injury

Boston Children's Hospital. (2017). *Congenital scoliosis.* Retrieved from http://www.childrenshospital.org/conditions-and-treatments/conditions/congenital-scoliosis/overview

Bulauitan, C. S. (2015). *Fat embolism: Background.* Retrieved from http://emedicine.medscape.com/article/460524-overview

Carrasco, M. I. B., & Ruiz, M. C. S. (2016). Idiopathic adolescent scoliosis: Living with a physical deformity. *Texto & Contexto—Enfermagem, 25*(2), e3640014 [Epub June 07, 2016]. Retrieved from http://orthoinfo.aaos.org/topic.cfm?topic=a00534

Cedars-Sinai. (2016). *DaTscan procedure information.* Retrieved from https://www.cedars-sinai.edu/Patients/Programs-and-Services/Imaging-Center/For-Patients/Exams-by-Procedure/Nuclear-Medicine/DatScan/DaTscan-Procedure-Information.aspx

Centers for Disease Control and Prevention (CDC). (2012). *Older adult falls: Important facts about falls.* Retrieved http://www.cdc.gov/homeandrecreationalsafety/falls/adultfalls.html

Centers for Disease Control and Prevention (CDC). (2015). *Hip fractures among older adults.* Retrieved from http://www.cdc.gov/HomeandRecreationalSafety/Falls/adulthipfx.html

Centers for Disease Control and Prevention (CDC). (2016). *Arthritis.* Retrieved from http://www.cdc.gov/arthritis/index.htm

Chao, J., Leung, Y., Wang, M., & Chang, R. C. (2012). Nutraceuticals and their preventive or potential therapeutic value in Parkinson's disease. *Nutrition Reviews, 70*(7), 373–386. doi:10.1111/j.1753-4887.2012.00484.x

Chawla, J. (2012). Clinical applications of somatosensory evoked potentials. *Medscape Reference.* Retrieved from http://emedicine.medscape.com/article/1139393-overview#a1

Chen, Y., Tang, Y., Allen, V., & DeVivo, M. J. (2015). Aging and spinal cord injury: External causes of injury and implications for prevention. *Topics in Spinal Cord Injury Rehabilitation, 21*(3), 218–226. Retrieved from http://doi.org/10.1310/sci2103-218

Children's Healthcare of Atlanta. (2016). *Pediatric neuro spine care for kids.* Retrieved from http://www.choa.org/childrens-hospital-services/neurosciences/programs-and-services/neurosurgery/services-and-technology/spine-care

Chin, L.S. (2016). Spinal cord injuries. *Medscape.* Retrieved from http://emedicine.medscape.com/article/793582-overview

Cobb, J. R. (1948). Outline for the study of scoliosis. In J. W. Edwards (Ed.), *AAOS, instructional course lectures* (Vol. 5, pp. 261–275). Ann Arbor, MI: American Academy of Orthopaedic Surgeons.

Dossa, A., Bokhour, B., & Hoenig, H. (2012). Care transitions from the hospital to home for patients with mobility impairments: Patient and family caregiver experiences. *Rehabilitation Nursing, 37*(6), 277–285. doi:10.1002/rnj.047

Duchesne, C., Lungu, O., Nadeau, A., Robillard, M. E., Bore, A., Bobeuf, F., . . . Doyon, J. (2015). Enhancing both motor and cognitive functioning in Parkinson's disease: Aerobic exercise as a rehabilitative intervention. *Brain and Cognition, 99*(2015), 68–77.

Dugdale, D. C., III. (2012a). Aging changes in the bones—muscles—joints. *MedlinePlus.* Retrieved from http://www.nlm.nih.gov/medlineplus/ency/article/004015.htm

Dugdale, D. C., III. (2012b). Deep venous thrombosis. *MedlinePlus.* Retrieved from http://www.nlm.nih.gov/medlineplus/ency/article/000156.htm

Fahn, S., Elton, R., & Members of the UPDRS Development Committee. (1987). Unified Parkinson's Disease Rating Scale. In S. Fahn, C. D. Marsden, D. B. Calne, & M. Goldstein (Eds.), *Recent developments in Parkinson's disease* (Vol. 2, pp. 153–163, 293–304). Florham Park, NJ: Macmillan Healthcare Information.

Fehlings, M. G., Vaccaro, A. R., Boakye, M., Rossignol, S., Ditunno, J. F., Jr., & Burns, A. S. (2013). *Essentials of spinal cord injury: Basic research to clinical practice.* New York, NY: Thieme Medical.

Fehlings, M. G., Vaccaro, A. R., Wilson, J. R., Singh, A., Cadotte, D. W., Harrop, J. S., . . . Rampersaud, R. (2012). Early versus delayed decompression for traumatic cervical spinal cord injury: Results of the Surgical Timing in Acute Spinal Cord Injury Study (STASCIS). *PLoS One, 7*(2), e32037. doi:10.1371/journal.pone.0032037

Gao, X., Cassidy, A., Schwarzschild, M. A., Rimm, E. B., & Ascherio, A. (2012). Habitual intake of dietary flavonoids and risk of Parkinson disease. *Neurology, 78*(15), 1138–1145. doi:10.1212/WNL.0b013e31824f7fc4

Gerber, R. (2015). *Healing bone fractures: Your body's do-it-yourself remodeling process.* Retrieved from http://www.dignityhealth.org/cm/content/pages/healing-bone-fractures-your-bodys-do-it-yourself-remodeling-process.asp

Hackney, M. E., & Bennett, C. G. (2014). Dance therapy for individuals with Parkinson's disease: Improving quality of life. *Journal of Parkinsonism and Restless Leg Syndrome*. doi.org/10.2147/JPRLS. S40042

Hakim, G., & Volpin, G. (2015). Surgical treatment of femoral neck fractures in young adults. *Israel Medical Association Journal, 17*(6), 380–382.

Hauser, R. A. (2013). Parkinson disease. *Medscape Reference*. Retrieved from http://emedicine.medscape. com/article/1831191-overview

Herdman, T. H. & Kamitsuru, S. (Eds.). *Nursing Diagnoses—Definitions and Classification 2015–2017.* Copyright © 2014, 1994–2014 NANDA International. Used by arrangement with John Wiley & Sons, Inc. Companion website: www.wiley.com/ go/nursingdiagnoses

IOS Press. (2017). Exercising 2.5 hours per week associated with slow decline for Parkinson's patients. *Neuroscience News*. Retrieved from http://neuroscience news.com/parkinsons-exercise-neurology-6282/

Jain, N. B., Ayers, G. D., Peterson, E. N., Harris, M. B., Morse, L., O'Connor, K. C., & Garshick, E. (2015). Traumatic spinal cord injury in the United States, 1993–2012. *JAMA, 313*(22), 2236–2243. doi:10.1001/ jama.2015.6250

Jasmin, L. (2012). Deep brain stimulation. *MedlinePlus*. Retrieved from http://www.nlm.nih.gov/ medlineplus/ency/article/007453.htm

Jo, C. H., Lee, Y. G., Shin, W. H., Kim, H., Chai, J. W., Jeong, E. C., . . . Yoon, K. S. (2014). Intra-articular injection of mesenchymal stem cells for the treatment of osteoarthritis of the knee: A proof-of-concept clinical trial. *Stem Cells, 32*, 1254–1266. doi:10.1002/stem.1634

Johns Hopkins Medicine. (n.d.a). *Nerve conduction studies*. Retrieved from http://www.hopkinsmedicine. org/healthlibrary/test_procedures/neurological/ nerve_conduction_velocity_92,p07657/

Johns Hopkins Medicine. (n.d.b). *Johns Hopkins sports medicine patient guide to knee arthroscopy*. Retrieved from http://www.hopkinsortho.org/knee_ arthroscopy.html

Karim, K., & Brukner, P. D. (2015). Management of musculoskeletal injuries in the mature athlete. In G. Whyte, M. Loosemore, & C. Williams (Eds.), *ABC of sports and exercise medicine* (pp. 38–40). Hoboken, NJ: John Wiley & Sons. Retrieved from https://books.google.com/ books?hl=en&lr=&id=U_bzBgAAQBAJ&oi=fnd& pg=PA38&dq=ice,+musculoskeletal,+&ots=eO1p_ e0Dzk&sig=A71G-UPj42Tw5oYhF6bF9- WqpxQ#v=onepage&q=ice%2C%20 musculoskeletal&f=false

Kurtzke, J. F. (1983). Rating neurologic impairment in multiple sclerosis: An expanded disability status scale (EDSS). *Neurology, 33*(11), 1444–1452.

Ma, C. B. (2016a). Contracture deformity. *MedlinePlus*. Retrieved from https://medlineplus.gov/ency/ article/003185.htm

Ma, C. B. (2016b). Compartment syndrome. *MedlinePlus*. Retrieved from https://medlineplus.gov/ ency/article/001224.htm

Ma, C. B. (2016c). Volkmann ischemic contracture. *MedlinePlus*. Retrieved from https://medlineplus. gov/ency/article/001221.htm

Machado, A. G., Deogaonkar, M., & Cooper, S. (2012). Deep brain stimulation for movement disorders: Patient selection and technical options. *Cleveland Clinic Journal of Medicine, 79*(Suppl. 2), S19–S24. doi:10.3949/ccjm.79.s2a.04

Maffulli, N., Oliva, F., Frizziero, A., Nanni, G., Barazzuol, M., Via, A. G., . . . Del Buono, A. (2013).

ISMuLT guidelines for muscle injuries. *Muscles, Ligaments and Tendons Journal, 3*(4), 241–249.

Matthews, L. J., McConda, D. B., Lalli, T. A. J., & Daffner, S. D. (2015). Orthostetrics: Management of orthopedic conditions in the pregnant patient. *Orthopedics (Online), 38*(10), e874–880. doi:10.3928/01477447-20151002-53

Mayo Clinic. (2014a). *Herniated disk: Tests and diagnosis*. Retrieved from http://www.mayoclinic.org/ diseases-conditions/herniated-disk/basics/tests- diagnosis/con-20029957

Mayo Clinic. (2014b). *Spinal cord injury*. Retrieved from http://www.mayoclinic.org/diseases- conditions/spinal-cord-injury/basics/risk- factors/con-20023837

Mayo Clinic. (2014c). *Deep vein thrombosis (DVT)*. Retrieved from http://www.mayoclinic.org/ diseases-conditions/deep-vein-thrombosis/ basics/definition/con-20031922

Mayo Clinic. (2015a). *Hip fractures*. Retrieved from http://www.mayoclinic.org/diseases-conditions/ hip-fracture/basics/definition/con-20021033

Mayo Clinic. (2015b). *Multiple sclerosis*. Retrieved from http://www.mayoclinic.org/diseases-condi- tions/multiple-sclerosis/home/ovc-20131882

Mayo Clinic. (2015c). *Sciatica*. Retrieved from http:// www.mayoclinic.org/diseases-conditions/ sciatica/basics/definition/con-20026478

Mayo Clinic. (2015d). *Parkinson's disease*. Retrieved from http://www.mayoclinic.org/diseases- conditions/parkinsons-disease/basics/definition/ con-20028488

Mayo Clinic. (2016a). *Scoliosis*. Retrieved from http:// www.mayoclinic.org/diseases-conditions/scolio- sis/home/ovc-20193685

Mayo Clinic. (2016b). *Osteoarthritis*. Retrieved from http://www.mayoclinic.org/diseases-conditions/ osteoarthritis/home/ovc-20198248

Mehlman, C. T. (2012). Idiopathic scoliosis. *Medscape Reference*. Retrieved from http://emedicine.med- scape.com/article/1265794-overview

Mehrholz, J., Friis, R., Kugler, J., Twork, S., Storch, A., & Pohl, M. (2010). Treadmill training for patients with Parkinson's disease. *Cochrane Database of Systematic Reviews*, Issue 2. Art. No.: CD007830. doi:10.1002/14651858.CD007830.pub2.

Michael J. Fox Foundation. (2015). Getting started: Exercise and Parkinson's disease. *Foxfeed Blog*. Retrieved from https://www.michaeljfox.org/ foundation/news-detail.php?getting-started-exer- cise-and-parkinson-disease

Michael J. Fox Foundation. (2016). Keeping "InMotion" to combat Parkinson's disease. *Foxfeed*. Retrieved from https://www.michaeljfox.org/ foundation/news-detail.php?keeping-inmotion- to-combat-parkinson-disease

Miller, S. (2014). How smoking can hinder fracture healing. *Emergency Nurse, 22*(4), 28. http://dx.doi. org/10.7748/en.22.4.28.e1219

Mulcahey, M. J., Gaughan, J. P., Betz, R. R., Samdani, A. F., Barakat, N., & Hunter, L. N. (2013). Neuromuscular scoliosis in children with spinal cord injury. *Topics in Spinal Cord Injury Rehabilitation, 19*(2), 96–103. http://doi.org/10.1310/sci1902-96

Multiple Sclerosis Association of America (MSAA). (2013). *MS overview*. Retrieved from http:// mymsaa.org/ms-information/overview/

Musumeci, G., Szychlinska, M. A., & Mobasheri, A. (2015). Age-related degeneration of articular cartilage in the pathogenesis of osteoarthritis: Molecular markers of senescent chondrocytes. *Histology and Histopathology, 30*, 1–12. Retrieved from http:// www.hh.um.es/

Nash, C. L., Jr., & Moe, J. H. (1969). A study of vertebral rotation. *Journal of Bone & Joint Surgery, 51*(2), 223–229.

National Institute of Arthritis and Musculoskeletal and Skin Diseases (NIAMSD). (2013). *Questions and answers about hip replacement*. Retrieved from http://www.niams.nih.gov/Health_Info/Hip_ Replacement/default.asp

National Institute of Arthritis and Musculoskeletal and Skin Diseases (NIAMSD). (2016). *Handout on health: Back pain*. Retrieved from https://www.niams.nih. gov/Health_Info/Back_Pain/default.asp

National Institute of Neurological Disorders and Stroke (NINDS). (2016a). *Parkinson's disease: Hope through research*. Retrieved from http://www. ninds.nih.gov/disorders/parkinsons_disease/ detail_parkinsons_disease.htm

National Institute of Neurological Disorders and Stroke (NINDS). (2016b). *Spinal cord injury: Hope through research*. Retrieved from http://www.ninds. nih.gov/disorders/sci/detail_sci.htm#186383233

National Institutes of Health (NIH). (2012). Parkinson's disease. *NIHSeniorHealth*. Retrieved from https://nihseniorhealth.gov/parkinsons- disease/whatisparkinsonsdisease/01.html

National Library of Medicine, National Institutes of Health. (2014). Compartment syndrome. *MedlinePlus*. Retrieved from https://www.nlm.nih. gov/medlineplus/ency/article/001224.htm

National Library of Medicine, National Institutes of Health. (2015). Fontanelles—bulging. *MedlinePlus*. Retrieved from https://www.nlm.nih.gov/ medlineplus/ency/article/003310.htm

National Multiple Sclerosis Society (NMSS). (n.d.a). *Diagnosing MS*. Retrieved from http://www. nationalmssociety.org/about-multiple-sclerosis/ what-we-know-about-ms/diagnosing-ms/index. aspx

National Multiple Sclerosis Society (NMSS). (n.d.b). *Research news & progress*. Retrieved from http:// www.nationalmssociety.org/Research/Research- News-Progress

National Multiple Sclerosis Society (NMSS). (n.d.c.). African Americans. Retrieved from http://www. nationalmssociety.org/What-is-MS/Who-Gets- MS/African-American-Resources

National Multiple Sclerosis Society (NMSS). (n.d.d). Complementary & alternative medicines. Retrieved from http://www.nationalmssociety. org/Treating-MS/Complementary-Alternative- Medicines

National Multiple Sclerosis Society (NMSS). (n.d.e). *Pediatric (child) MS*. Retrieved from http://www. nationalmssociety.org/about-multiple-sclerosis/ pediatric-ms/index.aspx

National Multiple Sclerosis Society (NMSS). (n.d.f). *Pregnancy and reproductive issues*. Retrieved from http://www.nationalmssociety.org/living-with- multiple-sclerosis/healthy-living/pregnancy/ index.aspx

National Parkinson Foundation (NPF). (n.d.a). *Parkinson's disease: Living well*. Retrieved from http://www.parkinson.org/Parkinson-s-Disease/ Living-Well

National Parkinson Foundation (NPF). (n.d.b). *Parkinson's disease overview*. Retrieved from http:// www.parkinson.org/parkinson-s-disease.aspx

National SCI Statistical Center. (2016). *Spinal cord injury (SCI) facts and figures at a glance*. Retrieved from https://www.nscisc.uab.edu/Public/ Facts%202016.pdf

Ogiela, D. (2012). Herniated disc. *MedlinePlus*. Retrieved from http://www.nlm.nih.gov/ medlineplus/ency/article/000442.htm

Okun, M.S. (2014). *What's hot in PD? An update on DAT scanning for Parkinson's disease diagnosis.* Retrieved from http://www.parkinson.org/find-help/blogs/whats-hot/april-2014

Pollack, P. (2013, January). Don't let hip fractures kill. *AAOS Now.* Retrieved from http://www.aaos.org/aaosnowissue/?issue=AAOSNow/2013/Jan

Pountos, I., Georgouli, T., Calori, G. M., & Giannoudis, P. V. (2012). Do nonsteroidal anti-inflammatory drugs affect bone healing? A critical analysis. *Scientific World Journal, 2012,* 606404. http://doi.org/10.1100/2012/606404

PubMed Health. (2014). *Anabolic steroids for improving recovery after hip fracture in older people.* Retrieved from http://www.ncbi.nlm.nih.gov/pubmedhealth/PMH0068640

Reeve, J., & Loveridge, N. (2014). The fragile elderly hip: Mechanisms associated with age-related loss of strength and toughness. *Bone, 61,* 138–148. Retrieved from https://www.ncbi.nlm.nih.gov/pmc/articles/PMC3991856/

Reitman, N., & Kalb, R. (2012). *Multiple sclerosis: The nursing perspective* (6th ed.). New York, NY: National Multiple Sclerosis Society.

Rosenburg, D. E., Bombardier, C. H., Atherholt, S., Jensen, M. P., & Motl, R. W. (2013). Self-reported depression and physical activity in adults with mobility impairments. *Archives of Physical Medicine and Rehabilitation, 94,* 731–736. doi:10.1016/j.apmr.2012.11.014

Samour, P. Q., & King, K. (2013). *Essentials of pediatric nutrition.* Burlington, MA: Jones & Bartlett.

Sanai, S. A., Saini, V., Benedict, R. H. B., Zivadinov, R., Teter, B. E., Ramanathan, M., & Weistock-Guttman, B. (2016). Aging and multiple sclerosis. *Multiple Sclerosis Journal, 22*(6) 717–725. doi:10.1177/1352458516634871

Schenkman, M., Hall, D. A., Baron, A. E., Schwartz, R. S., Mettler, P., & Kohrt, W. M. (2012). Exercise for people in early- or mid-stage Parkinson disease: A 16-month randomized controlled trial. *Physical Therapy, 92*(11), 1395–1410. doi:10.2522/ptj.20110472

Schiel, W. C. (2015). *Cauda equina syndrome.* Retrieved from http://www.medicinenet.com/cauda_equina_syndrome/article.htm

Schubert, R. (n.d.). *Fracture healing.* Retrieved from http://radiopaedia.org/articles/fracture-healing

Scoliosis Research Society. (2017). *Scoliosis: Types of adult scoliosis.* . Retrieved from http://www.srs.org/patients-and-families/conditions-and-treatments/adults/scoliosis

Sholter, D., & Lehman, R. (2012, April). Treatment of osteoarthritis in the elderly. *Drug Use in the Elderly.* Retrieved from https://www.albertadoctors.org/Publications%20-%20DUE%20Q/publications_dueq_apr12_pub.pdf

Shulman, L. M., Katzel, L. I., Ivey, F. M., Sorkin, J. D., Favors, K., Anderson, K. E., . . . Macko, R. F. (2013). Randomized clinical trial of 3 types of physical exercise for patients with Parkinson disease. *JAMA Neurology, 70*(2), 183–190. doi:10.1001/jamaneurol.2013.646

Snook, J., & Oliver, M. (2015). Perceptions of wellness from adults with mobility impairments. *Journal of Counseling & Development, 93*(3), 289–298. doi:10.1002/jcad.12027. Published by American Counseling Association, © 2015.

Stacy, M., Davis, T. L., Heath, S., Isaacson, S. H., Tarsy, D., Williams, M., & Moore, A. P. (2009). The clinicians' and nurses' guide to Parkinson's disease. *Medscape Education.* Retrieved from http://www.medscape.org/viewarticle/701955

Suttanon, P., Hill, K. D., Said, C. M., LoGiudice, D., Lautenschlager, N. T., & Dodd, K. J. (2012). Balance and mobility dysfunction and falls risk in older people with mild to moderate Alzheimer disease. *American Journal of Physical Medicine & Rehabilitation, 91*(1), 12–23. doi:10.1097/PHM.0b013e31823caeea

Tarver, M. L. (2015, July). *Kurtzke expanded disability status scale.* Retrieved from http://www.va.gov/MS/Professionals/Diagnosis/Kurtzke_Expanded_Disability_Status_Scale.asp

Truntzer, J., Vopat, B., Feldstein, M., & Matityahu, A. (2015). Smoking cessation and bone healing: Optimal cessation timing. *European Journal of Orthopaedic Surgery & Traumatology, 25*(2), 211–215. doi:10.1007/s00590-014-1488-y

U.S. Department of Health and Human Services. (2013). *Healthy People 2020: Arthritis, osteoporosis, and chronic back conditions.* Retrieved from http://www.healthypeople.gov/2020/topicsobjectives2020/overview.aspx?topicId=3

U.S. Food and Drug Administration (FDA). (2015). *Notice to industry: Final guidance for over-the-counter products that contain acetaminophen.* Retrieved from http://www.fda.gov/Drugs/DrugSafety/ucm310469.htm

U.S. Preventive Services Task Force. (2016, July). *Topic update in progress: Osteoporotic fractures: Screening.* Retrieved from http://www.uspreventiveservicestaskforce.org/Page/Document/UpdateSummaryDraft/osteoporosis-screening1?ds=1&s=osteoporosis%20screening

Walker Gallego, E. R., Kerstman, E., & Shaw, R. V. (2015). *NASA human research program-exploration medical capability: Approach to musculoskeletal injuries.* Retrieved from http://ston.jsc.nasa.gov/collections/trs/_techrep/TM-2015-218581.pdf

Weiss, H-R., Turnbull, D., Tournavitis, N., & Borysov, M. (2016, April). Treatment of scoliosis—Evidence and management (Review of the literature). *Middle East Journal of Rehabilitation and Health.* doi:10.17795/mejrh-35377

Zheng, L., Xin, Y., & Jianxiong, S. (2015). Environmental aspects of congenital scoliosis. *Environmental Science and Pollution Research, 22*(8), 5751–5755. doi:10.1007/s11356-015-4144-0

Module 14
Nutrition

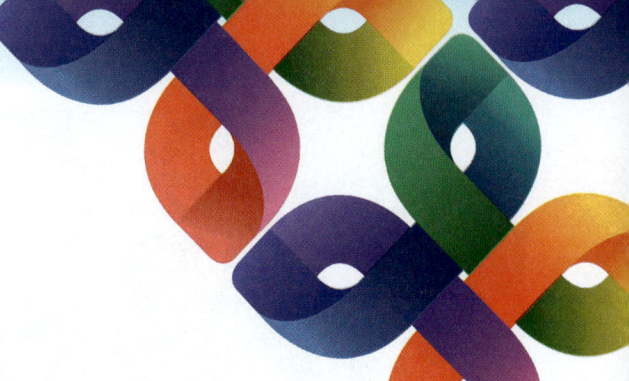

Module Outline and Learning Outcomes

The Concept of Nutrition

Normal Nutrition
14.1 Analyze the physiology of nutrition in the body.

Alterations to Nutrition
14.2 Differentiate among alterations in nutrition.

Concepts Related to Nutrition
14.3 Outline the relationship between nutrition and other concepts.

Health Promotion
14.4 Explain the promotion of healthy nutrition.

Nursing Assessment
14.5 Differentiate among common assessment procedures and tests used to evaluate nutritional status.

Independent Interventions
14.6 Analyze independent interventions nurses can implement for patients with alterations in nutrition.

Collaborative Therapies
14.7 Summarize collaborative therapies used by interprofessional teams for patients with alterations in nutrition.

Lifespan Considerations
14.8 Differentiate considerations related to the care of patients with alterations in nutrition throughout the lifespan.

Nutrition Exemplar

Exemplar 14.A Obesity
14.A Analyze obesity as it relates to nutrition.

» The Concept of Nutrition

Concept Key Terms

Absorption, **986**
Anthropometric
    measurements, **997**
Body mass index
    (BMI), **991**
Carbohydrates, **988**
Chyme, **990**
Dietary fiber, **988**
Dietary reference
    intakes (DRIs), **988**

Dietitian, **999**
Enteral nutrition, **1001**
Essential nutrient, **986**
Food choices, **983**
Food desert, **984**
Food insecurity, **984**
Food security, **984**
Hunger, **983**
Kilocalorie, **988**

Lactation consultant, **1003**
Lacto-ovo-vegetarian, **986**
Lacto-vegetarian, **986**
Lipids, **988**
Macronutrient, **986**
Micronutrient, **986**
Minerals, **989**
MyPlate, **988**
Nutrient density, **986**

Nutrients, **986**
Nutrition, **983**
Nutritionist, **999**
Overnutrition, **991**
Proteins, **988**
Satiety, **985**
Saturated fats, **988**
Sphincter, **990**

Total parenteral nutrition
    (TPN), **1002**
Undernutrition, **991**
Unsaturated fats, **988**
Vegan, **986**
Vitamins, **989**

Just as the body must have oxygen to sustain itself, nutritional intake is essential to ongoing health and physical well-being. Food intake is often considered enjoyable in itself and contributes to the emotional stability of individuals by providing opportunities for social interaction and communication. **Nutrition** is the science of the intake of nutrients and their actions in body functioning.

Normal Nutrition

One of the reasons individuals eat is because they are hungry (see **Figure 14–1** »). **Hunger** is a stimulus that encourages individuals to eliminate this feeling by eating. Theories suggest that hunger is a response to chemical mediators in the hypothalamus that promote food-seeking behaviors. However, the food choices that individuals make determine whether their nutritional intake is appropriate to meet their body's various needs and whether what they ingest may contribute to disease. Thus, food choice is a contributing factor to wellness and to illness.

Food Choice

Individuals base **food choices** on a number of factors (see **Table 14–1** »). The factor that most directly affects food choice is taste. Health-related diet changes also directly affect choice as individuals eliminate certain foods from the

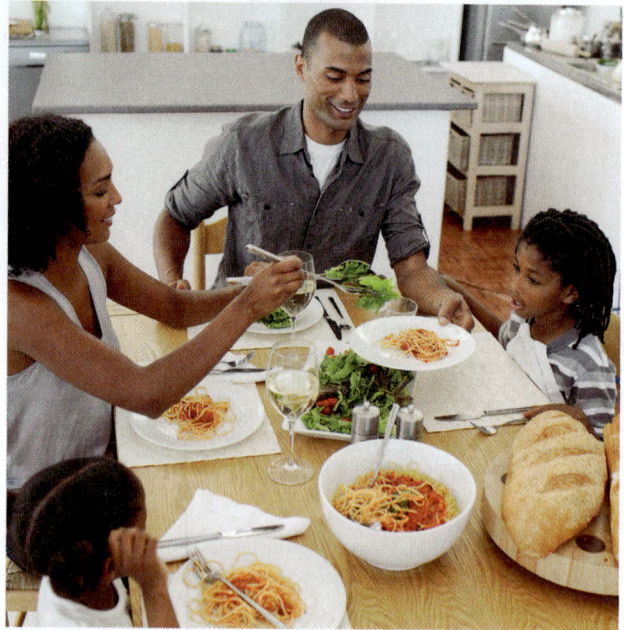

Source: ESB Professional/Shutterstock.

Figure 14–1 》 Individuals eat because they are hungry, but the food choices they make are contributing factors to wellness and illness.

TABLE 14–1 Factors Affecting Food Choice

Factor	Considerations
Taste	Preparation/cooking methods affect taste. Medication side effects can affect taste. Loss of taste buds in aging negatively affects taste. Illness may affect taste.
Smell	Pleasing aromas initiate the hunger reflex. Bad smells diminish interest. Appetizing smells may facilitate overeating.
Habits	People eat food that is familiar and may avoid unfamiliar foods. Toddlers often eat the same food item for several days in a row and refuse suggestions for alternatives. Adolescents are affected by what peers eat.
Convenience	Availability of prepared foods and takeout meals affects food choices. Convenient foods often are not nutritionally adequate. Supplement Nutrition Program (SNAP) and Meals on Wheels assist older adults in obtaining a healthier diet and maintaining a better weight status.
Packaging	Attractive packaging, including easy-to-read labels, motivates food selection. The appearance of food overall affects food choice.
Emotion	Eating with others affects food choice. Foods may be chosen unconsciously because of association with pleasure rather than nutritional value. Loneliness and depression may affect food choice and intake, especially among older adults.
Body image	Body image may affect choices that promote appropriate weight. Some individuals restrict food to lose weight. Body image is a significant factor in eating disorders.
Health	Some foods may meet specific health needs. Some foods may promote appropriate overall good health. Individuals may have hypersensitivity reactions or intolerances to some foods.
Cultural	Individuals may prefer foods from their country of origin, regardless of nutritional value. Some foods may play specific roles in traditional health practices.

diet to meet the recommendations of their healthcare provider. Other factors affecting food choice include food smell, food-related habits, convenience, packaging, and emotion. Body image, perceived health benefits, and cultural preferences also affect food choice.

Cost is another significant factor in food choice. Food prices have continued to increase, and a report on the state of hunger in the world from the Food and Agriculture Organization of the United Nations (2012) suggests that the price of food, rather than the availability of food, contributes to hunger in the United States and the rest of the world. The cost of a healthy diet is greater than that of a less healthy diet, and low- and average-income families may be unable to afford a healthy diet (Burns, Cook, & Mavoa, 2013). Zarnowiecki, Dollman, and Parlette (2014) suggest that socioeconomic status is associated with food availability and accessibility.

A **food desert** is any area of population where it is difficult to find good-quality, affordable fresh fruits, vegetables, and whole grains. In urban areas, a food desert is generally recognized as any populated area more than 1 mile from a grocery store that sells fresh fruits and vegetables. In rural areas, the distance is generally more than 10 miles. Distance and affordability greatly affect food choices for individuals and families, as does marketing. In one study of household food consumption among families living in food deserts, researchers concluded that a strategy of offering better prices for healthy foods than junk foods and changing marketing to promote healthy foods is needed to affect food selection among families living in these areas (Ghosh-Dastidar et al., 2014).

Income may affect food accessibility and food choices. According to an economic research report for the U.S. Department of Agriculture (USDA), 85.5% of American households

were food secure throughout the entire year of 2012. Of the remaining numbers, 5.7% had very minimal **food security**; that is, the members of the household had resources just sufficient to obtain appropriate quantities and variety of food. These numbers increased from previous years (Nguyen, Shuval, Bertmann, & Yaroch, 2015). **Food insecurity** means having no consistent access to sufficient nutritious food. Parents may go hungry to ensure that their children have adequate food to eat. According to Feeding America (2014), 15.3 million children experienced food insecurity in 2014. The percentage of children living in food-insecure households was 20% or more of the child population in 38 states and the District of Columbia (Coleman-Jensen, Nord Andrews, & Carlson, 2012). Food insecurity among children may be higher in the summer months, when children are unable to obtain meals at school (see **Figure 14–2 》**). Food insecurity is particularly prevalent among African Americans and aging veterans (Wang et al., 2015).

Portion size influences food choice. Many individuals are taught to eat what is placed before them without having a true understanding of the volume of food they consume.

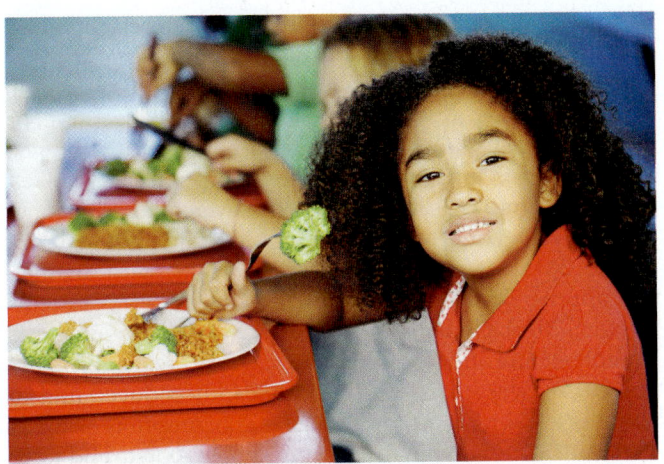

Source: Monkey business images/iStock/Getty Images.

Figure 14–2 ❯❯ For children living in poverty, their federally subsidized school lunches may be their only complete meals during the week, leaving them hungry on the weekend.

Americans have become accustomed to serving sizes that exceed recommended portion size. In many instances, these larger portions have become the norm. **Figure 14–3** ❯❯ illustrates the increases in food portions during the past 20 years. This increase in size contributes to overnutrition and resultant obesity. Many organizations provide aids that assist individuals to visualize and better identify appropriate portion sizes.

❯❯ **Stay Current:** The Centers for Disease Control and Prevention offers tips for how to avoid problems related to trends in portion size at http://www.cdc.gov/healthyweight/healthy_eating/portion_size.html.

Satiety is the feeling of fullness and satisfaction that should inhibit eating until the next meal. Results of studies suggest that satiety was significantly increased when protein replaced fat in meals containing the same number of calories. Whole grains may function in a similar manner. Food choices that increase satiety may be beneficial when considering the health risks associated with obesity and the importance of decreasing calorie intake (Pal, Radavelli-Bagatini, Hagger, & Ellis, 2014).

Food Safety

Each year in the United States over 48 million people succumb to foodborne illness. Many of these illnesses result in only minor discomforts of nausea, vomiting, and diarrhea. Some individuals require hospitalization, and figures from the Centers for Disease Control and Prevention (CDC) indicate that 3000 people in the United States die from foodborne illness each year. Over 31 known pathogens have been linked to these illnesses; the most common pathogens have been identified as norovirus, *Salmonella, Escherichia coli,* and *Campylobacter* (CDC, 2014a). Some foods, especially fish (e.g., shark, swordfish, king mackerel, tile fish), contain mercury that could be harmful, especially to pregnant women.

Nutritional Status

Nutritional health can be defined as the physical result of the balance between nutrient intake and nutritional

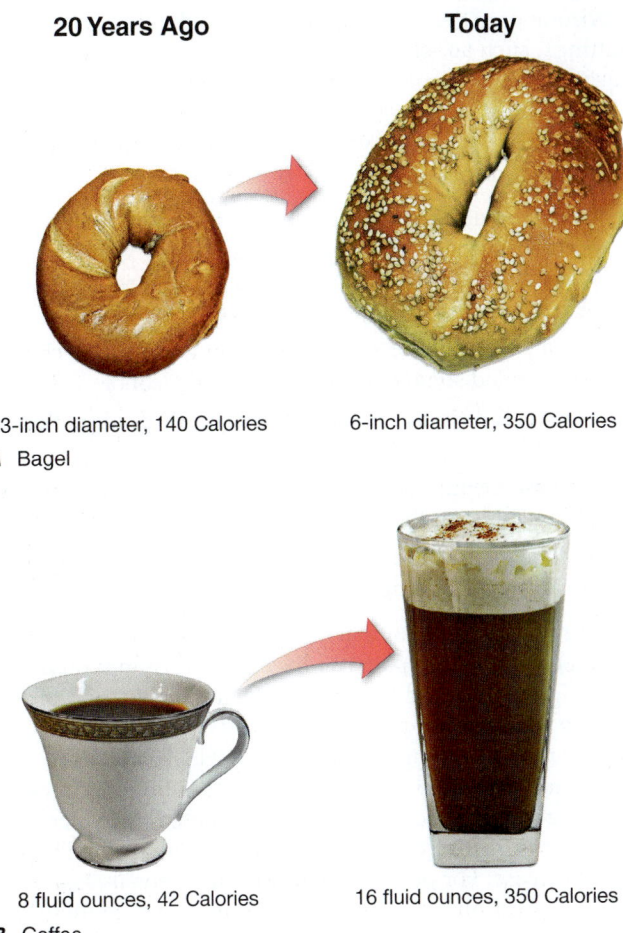

20 Years Ago   **Today**

3-inch diameter, 140 Calories   6-inch diameter, 350 Calories

A Bagel

8 fluid ounces, 42 Calories   16 fluid ounces, 350 Calories

B Coffee

Figure 14–3 ❯❯ Example of the increase in portion sizes over the past 20 years. *A,* A bagel has increased in diameter from 3 inches to 6 inches. *B,* A cup of coffee has increased from 8 fl oz to 16 fl oz and now commonly contains calorie-dense flavored syrup as well as steamed whole milk.

requirements. Patients who consume adequate nutrition to meet their individual needs and avoid habitual excesses and insufficiencies would be considered to be in good nutritional health. Any number of factors can impair nutritional health. For example, individuals who consume excess saturated fat may be at risk for elevated blood cholesterol and cardiovascular disease. They may be considered to have poor nutritional health due to overnutrition. There is also a predictable relationship between consuming sweets, snacks, and soft drinks during pregnancy and excessive weight gain (Renault et al., 2015). Poor nutritional health due to undernutrition is also possible: Women who consume less than the required amount of folic acid during pregnancy may place their unborn children at risk for certain birth defects, such as neural tube defects.

The objectives of the federal government's *Healthy People 2020* program address nutritional intake and include promotion of health and reduction of the risk of developing chronic diseases by encouraging Americans to consume healthful diets and to achieve and maintain healthy body weights. Emphasis is on modifying individual behavior patterns and habits and creating policies and environments that will support these behaviors in various settings, such as schools and local community-based organizations (U.S. Department of Health and Human Services [USDHHS], 2013).

Healthy People 2020's goals include the following key recommendations:

- Consume a variety of nutrient-dense foods within and across the food groups, especially whole grains, fruits, vegetables, low-fat or fat-free milk or milk products, and lean meats and other protein sources
- Limit the intake of saturated fat and trans fats, cholesterol, added sugars, sodium (salt), and alcohol
- Limit caloric intake to meet caloric needs as identified by the USDHHS
- Increase the number of fruits and the variety and number of vegetables in the diets of children 2 years and older
- Reduce obesity and increase the proportion of adults who are at a healthy weight.

The evidence is clear that many chronic diseases are linked to unhealthy dietary patterns. Excessive consumption of certain high-calorie and high-fat foods, in combination with a failure to consume plant-based foods, may contribute to higher rates of chronic diseases (USDHHS, 2013a).

A growing number of patients are adopting a vegetarian or vegan diet. For some, this choice is rooted in an increased awareness of the relationship between dietary intake and heart disease. For others, it is based on personal respect for animals and objection to the ways in which animals are raised for food and slaughtered in this country. In general, vegetarian diets are far lower in fat than diets that include meat. The **lacto-vegetarian** eats milk, cheese, and dairy foods but avoids meat, fish, poultry, and eggs. The **lacto-ovo-vegetarian** includes eggs, and the **vegan** eats only foods of plant origin. Some plans allow the inclusion of fish as well.

Vegan diet plans can lead to deficiencies in calcium, omega-3 fatty acids, iron, zinc, and vitamin B_{12}. The lack of vitamin B_{12} can lead to the development of pernicious anemia. These patients should include a daily source of vitamin B_{12} in their diets, such as a fortified breakfast cereal, fortified soy beverage, or meat substitute. All vegetarians should ensure that they get adequate amounts of calcium, iron, zinc, and vitamin D through foods such as tofu, lentils, and Swiss chard. To facilitate the **absorption** (intake) of iron into the body, patients should also consume sufficient quantities vitamin C.

Patients may experience food allergies or food intolerance. Food allergies can manifest as urticaria, angioedema, rhinoconjunctivitis, asthma, gastrointestinal disorders, and anaphylaxis. Researchers estimate that up to 15 million Americans have food allergies. This potentially deadly disease affects 1 in every 13 children (under 18 years of age) in the United States (Food Allergy Research and Education, 2016).

Examples of food intolerance include lactose and gluten intolerance. Lactose is a sugar found in milk and milk products. Lactose intolerance is caused by a deficiency of the enzyme lactase, which is produced by the cells lining the small intestine, and results in distressing gastrointestinal symptoms including nausea, abdominal pain, and diarrhea.

Lactose intolerance is discussed in detail in the exemplar on Malabsorption Disorders in the module on Digestion.

Gluten intolerance is often referred to as celiac disease. Gluten, a protein found in foods made with wheat, rye, or barley, can cause inflammation and edema in the bowel, which leads to interruption in the absorption of some key nutrients. Symptoms include diarrhea, weight loss, bloating, nausea, and vomiting (Rostami, Aldulaimi, & Rostami-Nejad, 2015). It can manifest systemically with anemia, osteoporosis, and rash (Ontvieros, Hardy, & Cabrera-Chavez, 2015). Gluten intolerance in children also manifests in short stature and iron deficiency anemia (Gokce & Arslantas, 2015). Symptoms can be significantly reduced and in some cases eliminated by reducing consumption of foods that contain gluten, such as processed flour, potato and tortilla chips, some soups, cereals, and breads, or eliminating them from the diet and following a gluten-free diet plan (Rostami, Rostami-Nejad, & Al Dulaimi, 2015).

Food security affects nutritional status. Adults with food insecurity report poor quality of life and conditions such as weight loss, compromised immune systems, and undiagnosed diabetes (Ding, Wilson, Garza, & Zizza, 2015). Children who lack food security often are underweight or experience wasting, growth effects, rickets, and tooth decay (Santin et al., 2014). Children who are hungry may also experience irritability and have difficulty paying attention in class.

Nutrients

Nutrients are substances found in food that the body needs for health and growth as well as for maintenance and repair. To eat a balanced and appropriate diet, experts suggest the inclusion of foods that are nutrient-dense. **Nutrient density** refers to the ratio of good nutrients to the calories a food contains. The most nutrient-dense foods contain an abundance of vitamins, minerals, fiber, and other key nutrients with a decreased amount of calories (http://www.nutrition-research.org). At the negative end of the nutrient density scale are foods such as candy, which is full of calories but has no essential nutrients.

The major nutrients are carbohydrates, proteins, lipids (fats), vitamins, minerals, and water. Nutrients are classified according to their work in the body. Carbohydrates, proteins, and fats supply energy and are termed **macronutrients** because the body needs them in large amounts to maintain health and well-being. Vitamins and minerals are considered **micronutrients** because they are needed in smaller amounts. This does not mean, however, that their role in the body is less important. Water is an **essential nutrient** needed for survival. Adequate water intake contributes to fluid balance. It also plays an important role in nerve and muscle functioning and in the transport of nutrients to all body systems. Nutrient use by the body is presented in **Figure 14–4 »**.

The USDA publishes the *Dietary Guidelines for Americans* every 3–5 years. They include recommended intake for sodium, moderation of alcohol use, safety in preparing meals, and age-specific nutrition needs.

»» Stay Current: The USDA's dietary guidelines for 2015–2020 are available at http://health.gov/dietaryguidelines/2015/guidelines

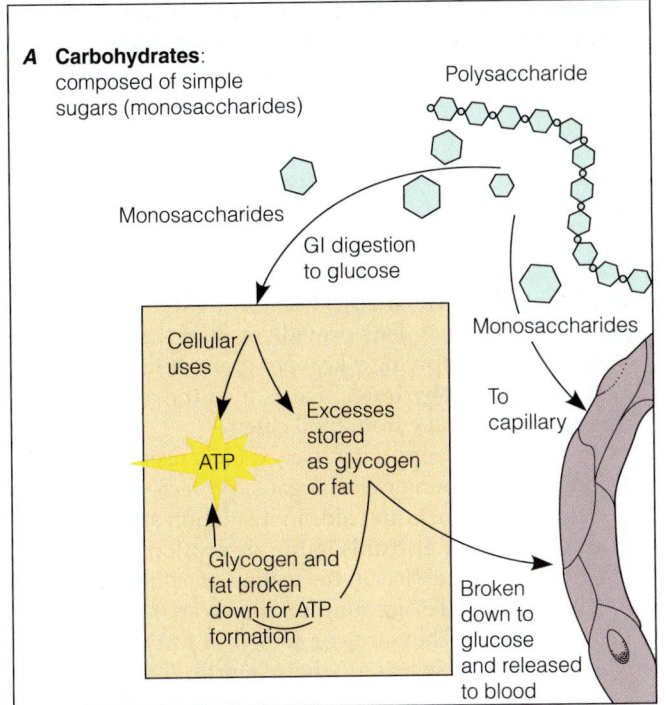

A **Carbohydrates**: composed of simple sugars (monosaccharides)

Polysaccharide

Monosaccharides

GI digestion to glucose

Cellular uses

ATP

Excesses stored as glycogen or fat

Glycogen and fat broken down for ATP formation

Monosaccharides

To capillary

Broken down to glucose and released to blood

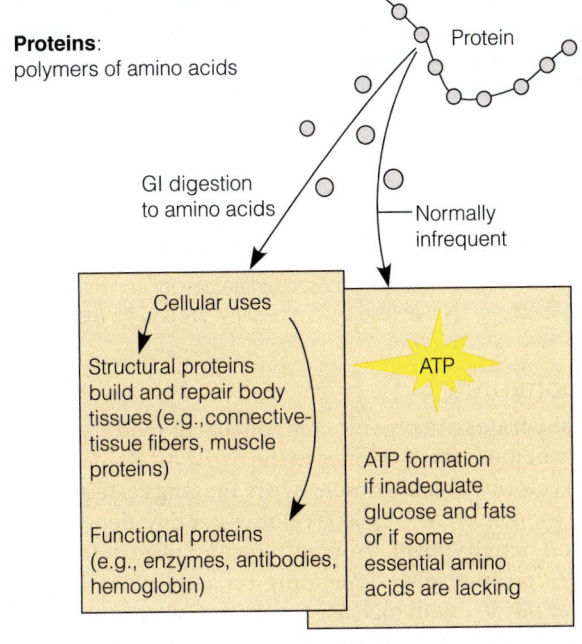

B **Proteins**: polymers of amino acids

Protein

GI digestion to amino acids

Normally infrequent

Cellular uses

Structural proteins build and repair body tissues (e.g.,connective-tissue fibers, muscle proteins)

Functional proteins (e.g., enzymes, antibodies, hemoglobin)

ATP

ATP formation if inadequate glucose and fats or if some essential amino acids are lacking

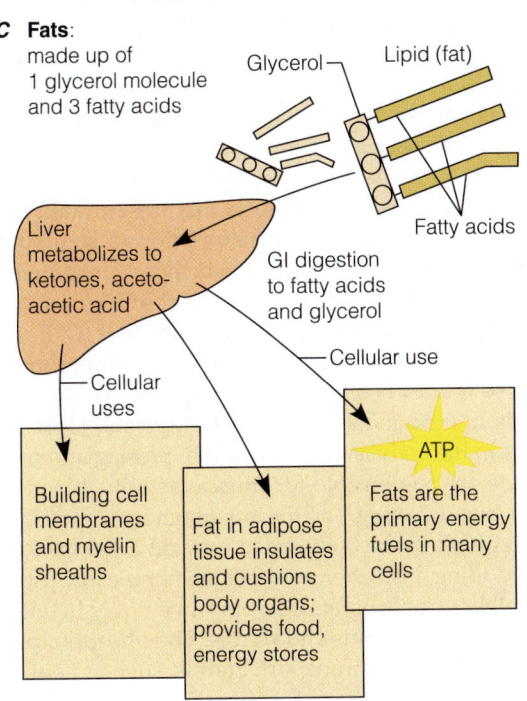

C **Fats**: made up of 1 glycerol molecule and 3 fatty acids

Glycerol

Lipid (fat)

Fatty acids

Liver metabolizes to ketones, aceto-acetic acid

GI digestion to fatty acids and glycerol

Cellular uses

Cellular use

ATP

Building cell membranes and myelin sheaths

Fat in adipose tissue insulates and cushions body organs; provides food, energy stores

Fats are the primary energy fuels in many cells

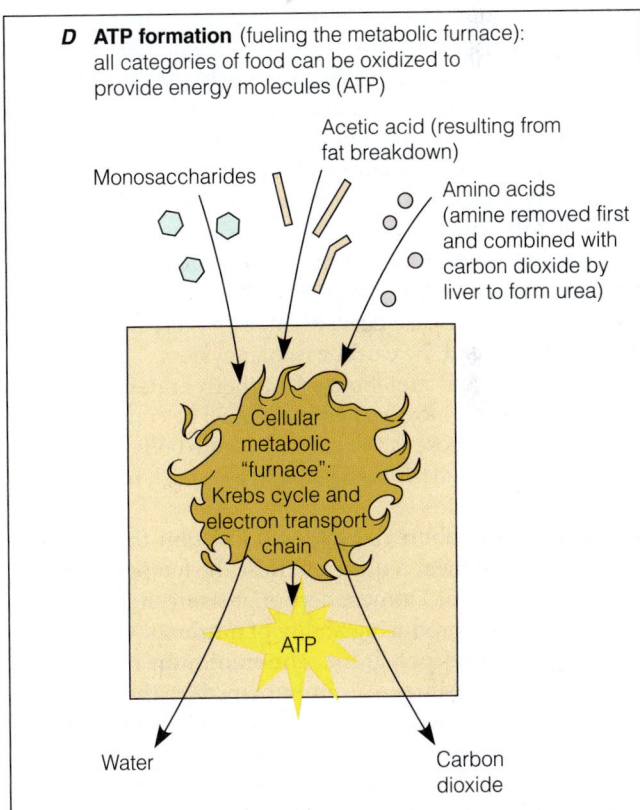

D **ATP formation** (fueling the metabolic furnace): all categories of food can be oxidized to provide energy molecules (ATP)

Monosaccharides

Acetic acid (resulting from fat breakdown)

Amino acids (amine removed first and combined with carbon dioxide by liver to form urea)

Cellular metabolic "furnace": Krebs cycle and electron transport chain

ATP

Water

Carbon dioxide

Figure 14–4 》 A schematic overview of nutrient use by body cells.

Many organizations provide information regarding suggested nutrient intake and supporting a healthy diet. **Dietary reference intakes (DRIs)**, developed by the Institute of Medicine (IOM), provide a standard for identifying needed amounts of each nutrient. The USDA's **MyPlate** plan outlines suggested food intake by food groups (e.g., bread and meat daily). The MyPlate plan illustrates the five food groups (fruits, vegetables, grains, protein, and dairy foods) that are the building blocks for a healthy diet using a place setting for a meal.

≫ **Stay Current:** Visit www.choosemyplate.gov for information about the five food groups that help build a healthy diet and for resources for families and professionals.

Carbohydrates

Carbohydrates are organic components of food that supply energy in the form of calories to the body. Adult men require more calories than women, with the suggested healthy range for men at 2400 to 3000 calories per day, depending on age and activity level. Women typically need 1600 to 2400 calories per day, also depending on activity, with greater calories needed with increased activity. Calorie needs generally decrease as a result of a decrease in the metabolic rate that occurs around the age of 50.

The primary sources of carbohydrates are plant foods. These foods contain sugars and starches. The simple sugars, called monosaccharides, are glucose, fructose, and galactose, which are quickly absorbed from the bloodstream. The disaccharides are sucrose, lactose, and maltose, which are found in milk, sugar cane, sugar beets, honey, and fruits. The polysaccharides are complex carbohydrates and are found in grains, legumes, and root vegetables. The polysaccharides break down more slowly than monosaccharides and disaccharides, and they supply energy for longer periods of time. **Dietary fiber** is a polysaccharide carbohydrate and contributes to disease prevention, especially in the gastrointestinal tract and the cardiovascular system.

Once ingested and metabolized, carbohydrates are converted primarily to glucose. All sugars must be converted to glucose because glucose is the only molecule body cells can use to make adenosine triphosphate (ATP), which transports energy in cells.

The **kilocalorie** (abbreviation: *kcal*) is a unit that represents the amount of heat required to raise the temperature of 1 kg of water by 1°C at 1 atmosphere of pressure. It is used to indicate the energy-producing ability of nutrients. Carbohydrates supply 4 kcal per gram. The minimum necessary daily carbohydrate intake is unknown, but the recommended daily intake is 125–175 g, most of which should be in the form of complex carbohydrates.

Because carbohydrates are not stored in the body in significant amounts, individuals must eat them throughout the day. When they are eaten in excess, the body converts the excess glucose to glycogen or fat. Glycogen is stored in the liver and muscles; fat is stored as adipose tissue. Excess intake of carbohydrates over time can result in obesity, dental caries, and elevated plasma triglycerides. Insufficient intake of carbohydrates over extended periods of time leads to tissue wasting from protein breakdown and metabolic acidosis from an excess of ketones as a by-product of fat breakdown.

Both the IOM and the USDA's *Dietary Guidelines for Americans* suggest that carbohydrates come from the consumption of foods high in fiber and low in added sugars. At least half of the grains consumed should be whole grains, and fruits and vegetables should complete the carbohydrate intake.

Lipids

Lipids, also known as fats, are substances that dissolve in alcohol but not in water. They contain carbon, hydrogen, and oxygen and serve as a secondary source of fuel for the body. Lipids are divided into three categories: triglycerides, phospholipids, and sterols. Most individuals use the term *fats* instead of *lipids*. Fats provide most of the energy for the body's work, supplying 9 kcal per gram of food eaten, twice that of the carbohydrates. Fat is also the storage form of excess energy intake from food eaten.

In addition to supplying energy, fat is useful in body protection. Fat surrounds vital organs, protects portions of the skeleton from shock, and aids in insulation and temperature management. Fat also aids in the absorption of the fat-soluble vitamins and assists in the feeling of satiety after a meal.

The triglycerides account for approximately 90%–95% of fats consumed. They are composed of fatty acids that are classified on the basis of their length. They are further defined according to the level of saturation and whether they are essential or nonessential. **Saturated fats** contain all the material they are capable of holding (i.e., they hold all the hydrogen ions they can). Fats that do not contain all of the material they are capable of holding and, thus, have a place where hydrogen ions are missing, are **unsaturated fats**. If only one set place is missing, the fat is termed *monounsaturated*. If two or more are missing, the fat is termed *polyunsaturated*. Research suggests that unsaturated fats are more heart-healthy and that consumption of some unsaturated fats such as olive oil can even be heart-protective.

Some fat is essential for the digestion, absorption, and transportation of the fat-soluble vitamins (vitamins A, D, E, and K). In this sense, *essential* means that the body cannot make the nutrient, so it must be ingested. Fat also contains the essential fatty acids, linoleic and linolenic acid. The primary role of these two acids in the body is the formation of prostaglandins. Prostaglandins are responsible for muscle activity, blood vessel response, blood clotting, and the inflammatory response. Other functions of fats in the body are to provide a storage form for energy, padding, insulation, and cell membrane integrity.

Two other groups of fats also play a vital role in body performance: phospholipids and sterols. The phospholipid lecithin plays a role in fat transport. Sterols, such as cholesterol, provide the bile necessary for digestion. Excessive cholesterol intake also plays a significant role in heart disease, as discussed in the module on Perfusion.

Proteins

Proteins are naturally occurring substances that consist of amino acids. They are essential components of all living organisms and vary from the other macronutrients in that they contain nitrogen, which fats and carbohydrates do not. Proteins are classified as essential or not essential and as either complete or incomplete. As with the fatty acids, essential amino acids are those that the body cannot supply, so they must be ingested.

Complete proteins contain all nine of the essential amino acids and are found in animal products such as meat, poultry, fish, milk, eggs, and cheese. Incomplete proteins do not contain all essential amino acids in the quantities necessary to support growth and development. Incomplete proteins are found in legumes, nuts, grains, cereals, and vegetables. Incomplete proteins can be combined in the diet or augmented by complementary food items to equal a complete protein. For example, rice contains small amounts of specific essential amino acids; however, these same essential amino acids are found in greater amounts in dry beans. Dry beans also contain smaller amounts of certain essential amino acids that can be found in larger amounts in rice. Together, these two foods can provide all of the essential amino acids the body needs.

Proteins perform many essential functions in the body. They continuously build new tissues, including muscles and red blood cells; they function as enzymes and antibodies; and they respond to injury to help prevent blood loss by clotting of the blood. In addition, they form hormones and help maintain fluid and electrolyte and acid–base balance. Proteins can also serve as an energy source, supplying 4 kcal per gram.

The recommended daily intake of protein is 56 g for men and 45 g for women. In healthy people with adequate caloric intake, the rates of protein synthesis and protein breakdown and loss are equal. If the breakdown and loss of proteins exceed intake, a negative nitrogen balance results, which can lead to metabolic complications. Excessive protein breakdown or loss may occur with burns, major illnesses, or altered emotional states. Protein deficits are manifested by weight loss, tissue wasting, edema, and anemia. Children with severe protein deficiency can develop marasmus and kwashiorkor. Marasmus is characterized by general malnutrition and is manifested by wasting of subcutaneous tissue and muscle and fat. Children with marasmus appear wrinkled. Kwashiorkor is due to protein deficiency with an adequate calorie intake. It is manifested by edema, primarily abdominal ascites, and dermatitis (Boyd, Andea, & Hughey, 2013).

When protein intake exceeds breakdown, a positive nitrogen balance occurs. This is normal during growth, tissue repair, and pregnancy. Excessive intake of proteins may affect the rate of protein use, as may taking anabolic steroids. Abnormal rates of protein use may also occur during times of stress, when the body releases adrenal corticosteroids to increase protein breakdown and conversion of amino acids to glucose. Excessive intake of proteins may lead to obesity and can have a significant impact on a number of body systems.

Vitamins

Vitamins are micronutrient compounds that are involved in regulating body functioning. With the exception of vitamins D and K, they must be consumed as a part of dietary intake. Vitamin D is manufactured by ultraviolet irradiation of cholesterol molecules in the skin, and vitamin K is synthesized by bacteria in the intestine. Vitamins are categorized as either fat- or water-soluble. The fat-soluble vitamins (A, D, E, and K) are found in the fats and oils of foods and require bile for absorption. These vitamins are stored in the liver and tissues until needed by the body. This storage ability also allows toxicities to develop if vitamins are

taken in excess. Any interruption in fat absorption can directly affect levels of fat-soluble vitamins. Vitamins have different roles and effects on the body. For example, the fat-soluble vitamin D plays a role in calcium absorption and transport.

The water-soluble vitamins, B complex and C, are absorbed with water in the gastrointestinal tract. However, vitamin B_{12} must become attached to intrinsic factor, a glycoprotein, to be absorbed. Water-soluble vitamins consumed in excess of body requirements are excreted in the urine. Each of the B vitamins plays a role in cellular functioning throughout the body. Vitamin C plays a significant role in tissue healing.

>> **Stay Current:** The most current information about the sources, functions, and minimum daily recommended intake levels for all of the vitamins is provided at https://fnic.nal.usda.gov/food-composition/vitamins-and-minerals.

Minerals

In the body, **minerals** are salts dissolved in water and, in this state, carry an electrical charge and are referred to as electrolytes. Minerals work with other nutrients to maintain fluid balance. The role of minerals in maintaining fluid and electrolyte balance is reviewed in detail in the module on Fluids and Electrolytes. In addition, minerals play a role in acid–base balance, which is further discussed in the module on Acid–Base Balance.

The most abundant mineral in the body is calcium, most of which exists in the bones and teeth. A very small amount of calcium exists in the blood, where it helps regulate metabolic functions. Calcium is constantly moving into and out of the bone as dictated by the body's demand for it. Phosphorus plays a role in energy production and participates in the buffer system. Like vitamins, each mineral has one or more health benefits.

The USDA dietary guidelines suggest that women of childbearing age consume foods that supply heme iron and add vitamin C–rich food to facilitate iron absorption. Women should also add 400 mcg per day of synthetic folic acid from fortified foods or supplements.

>> **Stay Current:** Information about the role of each mineral in the body and recommended intake can be found at http://ods.od.nih.gov/factsheets/list-VitaminsMinerals.

Water

Water comprises about 60% of an adult's body weight and about 75% of an infant's body weight. Obesity decreases the percentage of body weight from water.

Water serves the following functions in the body:

- Transports nutrient and wastes
- Regulates metabolic processes
- Serves as a solvent for vitamins, minerals, glucose, and amino acids
- Acts as a lubricant
- Acts as a cushion
- Regulates body temperature
- Maintains blood volume
- Assists in maintaining a healthy weight.

When adequate water is not ingested, the body will pull water from other sources, leading to increased blood viscosity, retention of toxicities and waste, and an increased risk for health interruption. Without water an individual can live only a few days. Dehydration, regardless of cause, accounts for multiple hospitalizations and even deaths, especially among infants and children (Jauregui et al., 2014).

Digestion and Metabolism

The Digestive Process

The digestive process begins in the mouth. Food is mechanically broken down by the teeth, and the salivary enzymes begin the chemical processes of digestion. The food bolus then moves down the esophagus, where no digestion takes place. The bolus moves through various **sphincters** (circular bands of muscle) that keep the bolus moving in one direction. The bolus then empties into the stomach, where food is stored and digestive enzymes further aid digestion and prepare the food to move into the small intestine. Minimal absorption occurs in the stomach, but the food bolus is further broken down by the chemical action of digestive enzymes. **Table 14–2 ≫** outlines the role of the various enzymes on nutrient digestion.

The bolus then becomes **chyme**, a mass composed of the food bolus, water, and digestive enzymes. It takes approximately 4 hours for the chyme to leave the stomach and enter the small intestine. The cells in the small intestine are individual and recognize the various nutrients needed for absorption. The cells are selective and can recognize and absorb all of the nutrients needed by the body. They are transported to cells via either the lymph system or small capillaries. Depending on their type, nutrients are absorbed all along the tract. Some, such as carbohydrates, are absorbed quickly; others, such as fats and proteins, are absorbed farther down the tract. The colon has the same type of action and is primarily responsible for the absorption of water and electrolytes. For more information, see the module on Digestion.

Metabolism

Metabolism is the chemical process that enables the body to use the energy extracted from ingested food. The type of metabolism that occurs is related to the type of cells undergoing metabolism. The liver is the organ primarily responsible for metabolic processes. Following digestion, the liver begins the metabolic processing of the various macronutrients. For carbohydrates, the liver converts complex sugars to glucose. It converts glucose to energy, and it converts glucose to fatty acids. For proteins, the liver removes ammonia from the blood and converts it to urea. It also makes plasma proteins such as the components of the coagulation cascade. For lipids, the liver manufactures bile and sends it to the gallbladder to aid in digestion. It also breaks down fatty acids for energy when needed. The liver also detoxifies alcohol and is responsible for the metabolism of all oral drugs. For more information, see the module on Metabolism.

Genetic Considerations

Genetic factors play a role in nutritional status, nutrient intake, and food choice. Genetically engineered crops such as soybeans, maize, canola, rice, and potatoes are readily available. The long-term effects of such crops on health and nutrition are not yet fully understood, prompting calls for increased research as well as federal regulations requiring mandated leveling and identification of genetically engineered foods (Tan & Epley, 2015).

Genetics plays a role in the nutritionally related disorders of lactose intolerance and hypercholesteremia. Additional information about these disorders can be found in the exemplar on Malabsorption Disorders in the module on Digestion and in the exemplar on Coronary Artery Disease in the module on Perfusion.

Studies are being conducted to identify the relationship among genetic variation, nutrient metabolism, and energy balance and their relationship to disease states such as heart disease (Petrosino & Matende, 2014). The researchers hope that data gained from these studies will explain why some patients respond to dietary intervention and others do not.

Alterations to Nutrition

Alterations to nutritional status take many forms. Overnutrition and undernutrition are major concerns throughout all populations and all ages and have direct effects on physical and emotional well-being (see the Alterations and Therapies feature). Appropriate food intake is essential to normal growth and development throughout the lifespan. Appropriate food choice is also a vital factor in disease management and intervention. Weight, which is affected by

TABLE 14–2 Selected Digestive Enzymes and Their Actions

Site of Production	Enzyme	Primary Action
Mouth	Salivary amylase	Digests carbohydrates in the mouth
Stomach	Gastric lipase	Digests lipids in the stomach
	Pepsin	Digests proteins in the stomach
Pancreas	Pancreatic amylase	Digests carbohydrates in the small intestine
	Pancreatic lipase	Digests lipids in the small intestine
	Proteases	Digests proteins in the small intestine
Small intestine	Lactase	Digests lactose in the small intestine
	Lipase	Digests lipids in the small intestine
	Maltase	Digests maltose in the small intestine
	Sucrase	Digests sucrose in the small intestine
	Various peptidases	Digest proteins in the small intestine

food choice and amount of intake, affects an individual's body image, self-concept, and overall self-efficacy (Olander et al., 2013).

Promotion of appropriate food intake is an essential part of nursing care. Food is often thought of as a form of comfort for patients, and when its intake is interrupted, their physiologic and psychologic well-being are affected. During times of acute illness or surgery of the gastrointestinal tract, traditional nutritional intake is often avoided because of impaired appetite, symptomatology, or postoperative care instructions. The inability to eat in a normal manner can produce psychologic discomfort, so nurses must be ready to assist patients in coping with these changes.

Alterations and Manifestations

Individuals who do not eat appropriate types and amounts of food may experience undernutrition or overnutrition. The Alterations and Therapies feature lists the most important excesses and deficiencies.

Undernutrition

According to the World Health Organization (WHO), undernutrition is the underlying cause of 3.1 million preventable maternal and child deaths worldwide each year, and it is associated with 45% of child deaths (WHO, 2016). In some discussions, the terms *malnutrition* and *undernutrition* are used interchangeably. Based on the most current literature review, **undernutrition** is the more accurate term and is representative of insufficient food intake and being hungry.

Children are the most visible victims of undernutrition. In 2014, approximately 15.3 million children under age 18 in the United States lived in households where there is food insecurity (Coleman-Jensen, Rabbit, Gregory, & Singh, 2015).

Undernutrition increases the risk of the development of infections in children due to a decrease in the immune response. It leads to slower bone development, and children experiencing undernutrition may be short for their developmental age. This is referred to as *stunting* and may be seen in nearly 24% of children worldwide (UNICEF, 2016). Hungry children may also experience learning disabilities due to lack of specific nutrients such as iodine.

One specific form of undernutrition in childhood is failure to thrive due to inadequate calorie intake and absorption or overexpenditure of calories. Failure to thrive occurs in 5%–10% of the children seen in primary care settings (Atalay & McCord, 2012). Data suggestive of failure to thrive include **body mass index (BMI)** at less than the 5th percentile, length for age less than the 5th percentile, and weight decline (Nangia & Tiwari, 2013). See the exemplar on Failure to Thrive in the module on Development for more information.

In adolescents and young adults, undernutrition can lead to growth failure, compromised immune status, poor wound healing, muscle loss, and physical and functional decline.

Individuals at risk for undernutrition include those who have a chronic illness or who are impoverished, older, or hospitalized; who impose self-enforced restrictive eating; or who have an alcohol abuse problem. See the Multisystem Effects of Undernutrition feature.

Overnutrition

The worldwide transition toward refined foods and the increased intake of animal protein and of fats are resulting in a significant increase in diseases directly linked to **overnutrition**, that is, the consumption of food such that the intake of nutrients exceeds that required for normal growth and metabolism. These diseases include obesity, diabetes, and cardiovascular diseases. Across the world, people are consuming increased levels of refined sugar; fat and sugar account for more than half of caloric intake, and refined grains have replaced whole grains. According to the Harvard Women's Health Watch (2014), many adults take in more sugar in a single day than their great-grandparents did in a week. There is also an established relationship between increasing BMIs in children and consumption of sugar-sweetened beverages and high-fat food (Millar et al., 2014, Purtell & Gershoff, 2015). Children under the age of 7 with existing diabetes increase their cardiovascular risk by increasing consumption of saturated fat and decreasing consumption of fruit and vegetables (Sundberg, Augustsson, Forsander, Cederholm & Axelsen, 2014).

In children and adults, overnutrition in the form of excess dietary intake of fat, especially saturated fat, has been associated with an increased risk of atherosclerosis. Being overweight and obese are linked to increased risk for hypertension, cardiovascular disease, type 2 diabetes, some cancers, degenerative joint disease, and other conditions. In addition, excess body weight has been shown to increase the risk of all-cause mortality in adults 30–74 years of age. In the United States, 63% of men and 55% of women 20–74 years of age are considered overweight or obese, a statistic that has increased by 25% during the past 30 years. In the United States, 31.8% of children from 2 to 19 years of age are overweight or obese (Ogden, Carroll, Kit, & Flegal, 2014). According to Catanese, Khan, Nelson, and Williams (2014), 30% of the world's population (2.1 billion people) are obese, and the number could rise to 50% by 2030. For additional information, see Exemplar 14.A on Obesity.

Prevalence

Obesity may be the most important manifestation of a nutritional imbalance. According to the CDC (2015a), more than one third of U.S. adults are obese. Obesity now affects 18% of all children and adolescents in the United States—triple the rate from just one generation ago. An estimated 3.5% of children and adolescents age 2–19 years are underweight (CDC, 2014b). An estimated 1.7% of adults are underweight, including 1.2% of older adults (CDC, 2012).

Genetic Considerations and Risk Factors

Many health alterations respond positively to changes in food intake. For example, in patients with elevated cholesterol,

Multisystem Effects of
Undernutrition

Endocrine
- ↓ thyroid hormones
- ↓ testosterone (male)
- ↓ estrogen (female)

Respiratory
- ↓ respiratory rate
- ↓ vital capacity

Hepatic
- Hepatomegaly
- ↓ bile synthesis

Gastrointestinal

Oral/esophageal
- Cheilosis
- Glossitis
- Gingivitis

Stomach/intestines
- Ascites
- Constipation
- Intestinal atrophy
- Steatorrhea
- ↓ gastric and pancreatic secretions

Potential complication
- Malabsorption syndrome

Musculoskeletal
- Muscle wasting
- Tenderness
- Impaired strength

Immune System
- ↓ cell-mediated and humoral immunity
- ↑ susceptibility to infections

Neurologic
- ↓ cognition
- ↓ consciousness (drowsiness, lethargy)
- Tremors
- Paresthesias
- Impaired coordination

Integumentary
- Hair: brittle, dull, dry, loss of color
- Nails: fragile, brittle, spoon-shaped
- Petechiae
- Poor wound healing

Cardiovascular
- Dysrthmias and conduction disturbances
- ↓ HR
- ↓ BP
- Enlarged heart

Potential complication
- Heart failure

Reproductive
- Amenorrhea

Metabolic Processes
- ↓ weight
- ↓ core body temperature
- Edema

Alterations and Therapies
Nutrition

ALTERATION	DESCRIPTION	MANIFESTATIONS	INTERVENTIONS AND THERAPIES
Carbohydrate excess	Excess occurs when carbohydrate intake exceeds the recommended intake.	▪ With excess carbohydrate intake, weight gain may be seen as well as elevated blood glucose and storage of excess intake as fat.	▪ Provide patients with the suggested intake for carbohydrates and provide education regarding weight management and appropriate exercise.
Carbohydrate deficiency	Deficiency occurs when carbohydrate intake is less than recommended.	▪ With deficiency, the body may use protein and fat for energy, leading to weight and muscle mass loss and ketonuria.	▪ Provide patients with the suggested intake for carbohydrates and provide education regarding weight management and appropriate exercise.
Protein excess	Excess occurs when protein intake exceeds the recommended intake.	▪ In the patient with normal kidney function, protein excess does not require nursing intervention. In the presence of both acute and chronic renal failure, limitations are placed on protein intake.	▪ Monitor blood urea nitrogen (BUN) and proteinuria. ▪ In the presence of hepatic failure, suggest further decreases in protein intake.
Protein deficiency	Deficiency occurs when protein intake is less than recommended.	▪ In the patient with normal kidney function, protein deficiency does not require nursing intervention. ▪ With illness, protein deficiency can lead to poor wound healing, lack of tissue integrity, and adverse effects on blood components.	▪ Patients who are vegetarians may need assistance in maintaining adequate protein intake. ▪ Individuals with critical illnesses who are receiving alternative nutrition may need protein-replacement therapy.
Mineral excess	Excessive levels occur when intake of minerals such as calcium exceeds the recommended amount.	▪ Excessive intake of calcium can lead to hypercalcemia and can place patients at risk for renal calculi.	▪ Provide patients with lists of foods high in calcium. Teach the relationship between vitamin D and calcium absorption.
Mineral deficiencies	Deficiency occurs when mineral intake is insufficient.	▪ Insufficient intake of calcium places patients at risk for osteoporosis.	▪ Provide patients with lists of foods high in calcium. Teach the relationship between vitamin D and calcium absorption.
Vitamin excess	Excessive levels occur when vitamin intake exceeds the recommended amount.	▪ Excessive intake of vitamin C can lead to diarrhea. ▪ Vitamin A toxicity is rare but can cause dry skin, headache, fatigue, and dizziness. Significant overdoses can lead to hepatotoxicity. ▪ Toxicity due to excess intake produces a flushing-like feeling; the patient becomes very red and hot.	▪ Teach patients about the risks for excessive vitamin intake.
Vitamin deficiencies	Deficiencies occur when intake of vitamins is insufficient.	▪ Deficiency of vitamin C can lead to scurvy. Vitamin C functions as an antioxidant. ▪ Deficiency of thiamine can lead to beriberi. ▪ Deficiency of niacin can lead to pellagra. ▪ Deficiency of vitamin B_6 can lead to convulsions and nerve damage. ▪ Deficiency of vitamin B_{12} can lead to pernicious anemia. ▪ Vitamin A deficiency is a worldwide concern and leads to increased risk for infections, night blindness, and keratinization. ▪ Vitamin D deficiency causes rickets in children and osteomalacia in older adults. ▪ Vitamin E deficiency is rare, except in premature infants, in whom it can lead to erythrocyte hemolysis. ▪ Vitamin K deficiency is rare except in newborns.	▪ Vitamin K is administered to newborns to help with their immature liver function and to aid in coagulation. ▪ Encourage intake of foods rich in each of the vitamins. ▪ Teach that exposure to sunlight assists in vitamin D formation.

dietary modifications affect total cholesterol and the amount of low-density lipoproteins. This leads to decreased risk of coronary artery disease. These choices are voluntary and are considered modifiable.

Some factors associated with food choice that patients cannot modify include allergies to specific food products, especially peanuts, eggs, and fruit; lactose intolerance and the need to avoid milk and milk products; and adjustment of carbohydrate intake in patients with diabetes. In many cases, these factors have a genetic link.

Some researchers consider age to be a nonmodifiable risk factor for obesity. According to researchers, as people age, hormone levels change, and when these changes are associated with a sedentary lifestyle, body fat begins to accumulate and muscle mass begins to decrease (Mayo Clinic, 2015). The loss in muscle tissue, accompanied by a declining metabolic rate, contributes to the increased risk of becoming overweight or obese.

Case Study » Part 1

Stacy Carpenter is a 9-year-old girl who is being seen in the pediatric clinic today for a well-child checkup because she wants to play softball in the fall. Stacy weighs 120 pounds, which places her at the 120th percentile for weight. She is 55 inches tall. Her blood pressure is 130/90 mmHg, and her heart rate is 90 bpm at rest. Stacy's mother is visibly overweight. She knows that obesity is a problem in many school-age children today and asks for help in changing Stacy's diet, lifestyle, and weight loss strategies. The nurse asks Stacy to do a quick 24-hour food recall. Stacy identifies the following:

- Breakfast: two Pop Tarts, glass of chocolate milk, and one glazed donut.

- Lunch: two slices of pepperoni pizza and two breadsticks, one serving of canned peaches, a bottle of fruit juice, and a sugar cookie for dessert.

- Supper: three chicken enchiladas, Mexican rice, refried beans, chips and salsa, and two sopapillas.

When the nurse asks about exercise, Stacy says that she really does not do any exercising except for recess at school.

Clinical Reasoning Questions Level I

1. In evaluating Stacy's diet, what findings would concern the nurse the most?
2. Why might Stacy's blood pressure be high?
3. What role, if any, does Stacy's ethnicity play in her weight problems?

Clinical Reasoning Questions Level II

4. What could be the cause of the elevation of Stacy's blood pressure?
5. What should the nurse teach Stacy's mother at this point?

Concepts Related to Nutrition

What individuals eat and why they eat it often involve complex factors. Some are related to their upbringing, some to likes and dislikes, some to convenience and costs, and some to the recommendations of healthcare providers. Treatment of many illnesses and disorders includes diets that limit intake of certain foods that place patients at risk for exacerbations of these health interruptions. Nurses need to be prepared to teach patients about foods that should be included or avoided in such diet plans. The Concepts Related to Nutrition feature links some, but not all, of the concepts

Concepts Related to
Nutrition

CONCEPT	RELATIONSHIP TO NUTRITION	NURSING IMPLICATIONS
Elimination	Decreased fiber intake → slowed peristalsis.	■ Fiber in the diet promotes bulk and draws fluid into the bowel, which aids in fecal elimination. Intake of fiber can reduce the need for laxatives in the treatment of constipation.
Fluids and Electrolytes	Normal levels of protein intake ↑ workload in poorly performing kidneys.	■ Protein-restricted diets are often implemented for patients with chronic renal failure.
Metabolism	Inadequate nutritional intake → hypoglycemia or diabetic ketoacidosis (DKA) in patients with diabetes.	■ Supply patients with diabetes with educational materials or guides about the management of their disease. Refer patients to specialized diabetes educators.
Mobility	Insufficient calcium and vitamin D → bone loss → osteoporosis and fractures.	■ Encourage patients to maintain their intake of calcium-rich and vitamin D–rich foods and to safely spend time in the sun for appropriate intervals.
Perfusion	Regular (in special populations) or increased sodium intake ↑ fluid retention.	■ Increased sodium intake, especially in salt-sensitive patients, can lead to increased blood pressure. Teach patients how to read labels and provide lists of low-sodium foods. Nurses must also be familiar with the DASH diet plan (http://dashdiet.org).
Tissue Integrity	Deficiency in protein intake → delayed wound healing.	■ Lack of protein intake leads to lack of cellular integrity that is manifested by edema. Patients recovering from major surgery, burns, or severe trauma may need additional protein intake to help provide for tissue healing.

related to nutrition. They are presented in alphabetical order.

Health Promotion

Health promotion and nutrition are often in the headlines. School lunch programs focus on good nutrition. Many restaurants provide nutritional information about meal items. Prevention and management of childhood obesity are the focus of several national and even international initiatives.

Modifiable Risk Factors

The primary modifiable risk factors for nutrition alterations are food choice, portion size, and nutritional intake. Because reducing the risk of alterations in nutrition can be difficult for patients with food sensitivities and patients living on limited incomes, nurses can help by providing information on local feeding programs and food resources, reliable websites that provide relevant dietary information and recipes, and health education programs that offer cooking classes and nutritional counseling.

Screenings

In many school systems, nutrition screening using BMI is considered a required screening in the same manner as scoliosis screening. Screening tools are discussed in the Nursing Assessment section.

Nursing Assessment

Nurses should know the common risk factors for poor nutritional status when they are gathering data for a nutritional assessment. Evaluation of nutritional status is an important part of total patient assessment and includes the following:

- Review of the nutritional history
- Food and fluid intake record
- Laboratory data
- Food–drug interactions
- Health history and physical assessment
- Anthropometric measurements
- Psychosocial assessment
- Access to food.

An initial nutrition screening provides an inexpensive, quick way of determining which patients need more extensive nutritional assessment by the healthcare team. The Joint Commission's patient care standards require that a nutritional screening occur within 24 hours of a patient's hospital admission, when the individual's condition meets the organization's criteria for such assessment (Joint Commission, 2012). When a patient is in the hospital for more than a week, nutritional assessment should be part of the daily plan of care.

Observation and Patient Interview

The initial assessment of nutritional status includes inspection of the body overall for signs of malnutrition, measurement

of height and weight with comparisons to identified norms, weight history (loss or gain), usual eating habits, ability to chew and swallow, and any recent changes in appetite or food intake. See the Nutrition Assessment feature for a summary of assessment methods.

One internationally recognized tool is the Mini Nutritional Assessment (MNA), a two-part tool that has been tested extensively. The MNA provides a reliable, rapid assessment for patients in the community or any healthcare setting. It is available in a number of languages. The first part of the screening asks about food intake, mobility, and BMI. It also screens for weight loss, acute illness, and psychologic health problems. The second part (G-R) of the MNA is completed if the patient scores 11 points or less. The entire assessment takes less than 15 minutes (Hsu, Ho, Kuo, Wang, & Tsai, 2014). A shorter version of the MNA with just six questions is also available. It provides initial information about risk that can be followed up by using the full MNA or other comprehensive tools.

>> **Stay Current:** The Mini Nutritional Assessment Short Form (MNA®-SF) is available as a free iPhone app through iTunes.

Assessment of nutritional status also involves a review of the patient's history, anthropometric data, and systems and laboratory results. The nurse also reviews socioeconomic factors with an emphasis on the patient's ability to purchase food, access to food sources, and food preparation abilities.

A major component of a patient's nutritional status is the foods the patient has eaten recently or foods (and portion sizes) the patient normally eats. Tools to collect this data include a 24-hour diet recall or a diet diary kept for 3 days, a week, or longer. To get as accurate a picture as possible, the patient should follow his or her standard typical intake. The healthcare team can then evaluate the patient's diet for nutrient intake and compare it to standard guidelines such as the DRIs. The healthcare team can use diet analysis software or evaluate items through nutrient food charts. This is a time-consuming procedure. However, when it is combined with other portions of the assessment, the healthcare team can determine adequacy of nutritional status and possible problem areas.

Questions to ask during the history include:

Current Nutritional Intake

- Do you follow a special diet? If so, why? Do you eat meat? Eggs?
- Have you noticed any weight gain or weight loss greater than 5 pounds during the past month?
- Have your eating habits changed during the past month? If so, how?
- Are you able to obtain food when you choose to do so? Where do you obtain your food?
- What is an example of a typical day of food intake?
- Do you modify your diet based on a disease or health interruption? If so, how?
- Do you take any nutritional supplements? If so, what and how often?

Nutrition Assessment

ASSESSMENT/ METHOD	NORMAL FINDINGS	ABNORMAL FINDINGS	LIFESPAN OR DEVELOPMENTAL CONSIDERATIONS
Height and Weight			
Weigh and measure the patient	Normal weights for adult men and women are available from several reference standards, including Health Check Systems (www.healthchecksystems.com/heightweightchart.htm) and the revised Metropolitan Life tables.	▪ Weight and/or height outside the outlined parameters can indicate under- or overnutrition.	▪ Muscle mass weighs more, so individuals with significant muscle mass and decreased body fat may need to use more refined methods such as dual-energy x-ray absorptiometry (DEXA) scanning to determine whether they are over- or underweight. DEXA uses a very low dose x-ray for measurement of body composition and body fat. ▪ Specific height and weight tables based on percentiles are useful for evaluating infants and children.
Body Mass Index (BMI)			
Use a formula to compare height to weight	Formula: **English BMI Formula** BMI = [Weight in Pounds/ (Height in inches × Height in inches)] × 703 **Metric BMI Formula** BMI = [Weight in kilograms/ (Height in meters × Height in meters)] (www.bmi-calculator.net/bmi-formula.php) Norms: 18.5–24.9	▪ Low BMI compared to the chart suggests being underweight or undernutrition; high BMI suggests being overweight or obese.	▪ BMI is calculated for individuals ages 20 and older. ▪ Growth percentile charts reflect height and weight more accurately in infants, children, and teens.
Waist-to-Height Ratio			
Measure waist circumference at a horizontal line 1 inch above the belly button	An online calculator will indicate whether a patient is underweight, at appropriate weight, or overweight.	▪ Waist-to-height ratio outside the outlined parameters indicates either under- or overnutrition.	▪ Those with a higher than normal range of upper-body fat are at risk for chronic diseases. ▪ This measurement may not be accurate in older adults.
Food Diary			
Have the patient write down everything eaten for 3 days or more	This method reviews specific nutrient intake over a designated period of time.	▪ The food diary documents lack of intake of specific nutrients and provides indications for over- or undernutrition.	▪ Foods should be recorded at the time eaten. This method is especially helpful in older adults who may eat the same food items every day, or who may eat simple meals such as cold cereal. ▪ This method is used as an adjunct to other nutritional screenings. ▪ It is especially helpful for mothers who question foods eaten by young children.
Food Frequency Questionnaires			
Conduct a 24-hour recall with the patient, completing a questionnaire, or using diet analysis software	The 24-hour recall evaluates the patient's diet for equivalency to recommended intake of various nutrients. Food frequency questionnaires ask the patient to report the frequency of consumption and portion size of approximately 125 line items over a defined period of time.	▪ These methods document deficits and excesses.	▪ The nurse can teach about replacements or changes in food choice. ▪ These methods identify deficiencies and excesses in the diet.
Six-Item Mini Nutritional Assessment			
Perform the Mini Nutritional Assessment with the patient	This six-item tool provides a general review of the nutritional status of older adults.	▪ This tool provides early problem identification.	▪ The assessment allows the nurse to teach about possible areas of deficiency.

- Do you have enough money to buy food?
- Do you use any special food preparation techniques?
- Do you count calories?
- Do you eat three meals per day?
- Describe a typical 24-hour diet.

Lifestyle

- Do you eat out often? If so, how many times a week?
- What type of restaurants do you frequent?

Physical

- Have you been diagnosed with a nutrition-related anemia?
- Do you have any physical problems that limit or affect your food intake, for example, dentition problems or trouble swallowing?
- Do you have any digestive problems, such as lactose intolerance, ulcers, constipation, or diarrhea?

Physical Examination

Anthropometric measurements are a set of quantitative measurements used to determine the size, shape, and composition of a human body. They include height and weight (length in babies), BMI, and waist-to-hip ratio. Data from these measures can help the nurse identify individuals who are at risk for undernutrition or overnutrition. Obtain height and weight first. Because individuals often report their height inaccurately, measure the patient's height using the measuring stick of a scale. Ask the patient to stand erect, look straight ahead, and position the heels together with the arms at the sides (Tipton et al., 2012). If the patient cannot stand, height estimates can be obtained using a knee height caliper. This device uses the distance between the patient's patella and heel to estimate height. Weight should be obtained at the same time each day, on the same scale, and with the patient wearing similar clothing. It is important for the scale to be calibrated. Findings are then compared with identified standards for gender and age.

Body mass index is calculated by dividing the weight (in kilograms or pounds) by the height (in centimeters or inches) squared. The formula for calculating BMI is the same for both adults and children. Many sources are available to assist patients in calculating their own BMIs.

>> **Stay Current:** Go to the CDC website to use the BMI calculators for adults (http://www.cdc.gov/healthyweight/assessing/bmi/adult_BMI/english_bmi_calculator/bmi_calculator.html) and for children and teens (https://nccd.cdc.gov/dnpabmi/Calculator.aspx).

Waist-to-height ratio also provides data about nutritional status and health risk. If the measurements indicate that the body has a higher than normal range of upper-body fat, the patient is at increased risk for chronic diseases, such as type 2 diabetes, heart disease, and high blood pressure.

>> **Stay Current:** Calculations for waist-to-height ratio can be obtained at https://www.healthstatus.com/calculate/waist-to-hip-ratio

Note that these data only serve as general indicators of nutritional status and do not provide any information regarding nutrient deficiency or excess, although some relationships have been found. For example, increased BMI and waist circumference values demonstrated significant correlations with elevated systolic and diastolic blood pressure in children and adults. All body systems are affected by nutritional intake (refer to the Multisystem Effects of Undernutrition feature above).

Cultural Considerations

Culture can affect food choices, and many cultures recognize both acceptable and prohibited food choices. These choices are based on food preparation, location, tradition, religious beliefs, and food availability in the culture of origin. For example, alligators exist in many parts of the world, but they are unacceptable as a food choice by many groups. Some practicing Muslim and Jewish individuals eat only meats that have been slaughtered, butchered, and/or stored and cooked according to their religion's traditional practices. Culture also affects food preparation and consumption. For example, some individuals will consume foods that contain a variety of meats while others are vegetarian.

Nurses who understand the relationships among culture, ethnicity, and food choices are better able to provide the education necessary in disease management. **Table 14–3 >>** outlines the dietary practices of selected religious groups. The Focus on Diversity and Culture feature outlines rates of under- and overnutrition in various populations along with rates of poverty and food insecurity.

>> **Stay Current:** Ethnic/cultural food pyramids are available for various populations from the USDA at https://fnic.nal.usda.gov/dietary-guidance/past-food-pyramid-materials/ethniccultural-food-pyramids.

Diagnostic Tests

Tests used to assist in the diagnosis of nutritional deficiencies include a lipid profile; a complete blood count; and serum glucose, serum albumin, and total protein levels. Low hematocrit levels may indicate anemia, such as iron deficiency anemia, or could indicate blood loss. A low serum albumin level may provide information as to the etiology of a patient's edema. Total protein level provides information about globulin as well. Elevated glucose levels could be an early indicator of prediabetes. Prealbumin (PAB), also called transthyretin (TTHY), is a hepatic protein found in the serum that provides a sensitive indication of protein deficiency because of its short half-life of 2 days. Depending on the laboratory test used, the normal PAB range is 15–36 mg/dL or 150–360 mg/L (SI units). PAB can also assess improvement in nutritional status with parenteral or enteral feeding; levels can increase by 1 mg/dL daily with adequate nutritional support.

Cholesterol levels normally range between 160 and 200 mg/dL in adult men and women. A cholesterol level below 160 mg/dL has been identified as a possible indicator of malnutrition. Serum levels of each of the vitamins and minerals can provide additional information about certain disease states, for example, in the diagnosis of anemias such as vitamin B_{12} or iron deficiency anemia.

TABLE 14–3 Dietary Practices of Selected Religious Groups

Religious Group	Dietary Practices*
Buddhist	Dietary customs vary depending on sect. Many are lacto-ovo-vegetarians because of restrictions on taking a life. Some eat fish, and most eat no beef or poultry. Monks fast at certain times of the month, avoid eating solid food after the noon hour, and are not allowed to store or cook their own food.
Hindu	All foods thought to interfere with physical and spiritual development are avoided. Many are lacto-vegetarians and/or avoid alcohol. The cow is considered sacred—an animal dear to the Lord Krishna. Beef is never consumed, and often pork is avoided.
Jewish	Kashrut is the body of Jewish law dealing with foods. The purpose of following the complex dietary laws is to conform to the Divine Will as expressed in the Torah. The term *kosher* denotes all foods that are permitted for consumption. To *keep kosher* means to follow dietary laws in the home. For some, this may require separate cooking and refrigeration areas. A lengthy list of prohibited foods, called *treyf*, includes pork and shellfish. The laws define how birds and mammals must be slaughtered and how foods must be eaten at the same meal. During Passover, special laws are observed, such as the elimination of leavened foods from the diet.
Mormon	Alcoholic beverages and coffee, tea, and other beverages containing caffeine are avoided. Mormons are encouraged to limit meat intake and emphasize grains in the diet.
Muslim	Overeating is discouraged, and consuming only two-thirds of capacity is suggested. Dietary laws are called *halal*. Prohibited foods are called *haram* and include pork and birds of prey. Laws define how animals must be slaughtered. Alcoholic drinks are not allowed. Fasting is required from sunup to sundown during the month of Ramadan.
Roman Catholic	Meat is not eaten on Fridays during Lent (40 days before Easter). No food or beverages (except water) are to be consumed for 1 hour before taking communion.
Seventh Day Adventist	Most are lacto-ovo-vegetarians. If meat is eaten, pork is avoided. Tea, coffee, and alcoholic beverages are not allowed. Water is not consumed with meals but is drunk before and after meals. Followers refrain from using seasonings and condiments. Overeating and snacking are discouraged.

Sources: Based on Boyle, M., & Long, S. L. (2015). *Personal nutrition* (8th ed., p. 19). Belmont, CA: Wadsworth; Diet Health, Inc. (n.d.). *Religion and dietary practices.* Retrieved from http://www.diet.com/g/religion-and-dietary-practices; Roth, R. A. (2014). *Nutrition and diet therapy* (11th ed., p. 48). Clifton Park, NJ: Cengage Learning.

*Many of the religious guidelines regarding food have practical applications for the society. For example, the Hindu prohibition against killing cattle respects the needs for Indian farmers to use cattle for power and cattle dung for fuel. Cows also supply milk to make dairy products. Some Christians forgo meat during Lent (the period before Easter), Jewish law includes an extensive set of dietary rules that govern the use of foods derived from animals, and Muslims fast between sunrise and sunset during Ramadan (the ninth month of the Islamic calendar).

Focus on Diversity and Culture
Nutrition

Overweight and Obesity

■ The prevalence of obesity has increased among Whites, Blacks, and Hispanics, especially among African American adolescents.

■ The prevalence of being overweight is highest among Mexican American men.

■ The prevalence of obesity is highest among Mexican American women.

■ Adults of low socioeconomic status have twice the rate of being overweight or obese in comparison to those of medium and high socioeconomic status.

Undernutrition

■ Undernutrition can contribute to growth retardation. By definition, 5% of children would be expected to be at the 5th percentile for height. However, up to 15% of Black children have growth retardation in the first year of life, and 11% of Asian and Pacific Islander children have growth retardation during the second year.

■ The number of older adults living at home who are malnourished is in the hundreds of thousands, with one expert estimating that over 1 million homebound older adults may be malnourished.

■ Between 35% and 50% of the older residents of long-term care facilities and as many as 65% of older adults in hospitals are malnourished.

■ Pregnant Mexican American women are more likely than those of other ethnic groups to have iron deficiency and low folic acid levels. Women of lower economic status and those with less education are also more likely to have inadequate folic acid or iron status.

■ Black women and adolescents under age 15 years are more likely to have insufficient gestational weight gain and deliver low-birth-weight babies than women of other populations.

Poverty and Food Insecurity

■ Poverty is a major risk factor for food insecurity and malnutrition. Public programs such as Women, Infants and Children (WIC) and the Supplemental Nutrition Assistance Program (SNAP; formerly the Food Stamp Program) help families in poverty obtain healthy food for their children (Nguyen et al., 2015).

■ In 2014, the U.S. official poverty rate was 14.8%. There were 46.7 million people living in poverty.

■ The poverty rate in 2014 for children under age 18 was 21.1%. The poverty rate for people age 18–64 was 13.5%, while the rate for people age 65 and older was 10.0%.

■ The prevalence of poverty is highest among Black and Hispanic populations.

Sources: Data from National Center for Children in Poverty. (2013). *Topics: Child poverty.* Retrieved from http://www.nccp.org/topics/childpoverty.html; U.S. Bureau of the Census. (n.d.). *Poverty.* Retrieved from https://www.census.gov/hhes/www/poverty/data/incpovhlth/2014/highlights.html; U.S. Department of Health and Human Services (USDHHS). (2013b). *Healthy People 2020: Nutrition and weight status—Overview.* Retrieved from http://www.healthypeople.gov/2020/topicsobjectives2020/overview.aspx?topicId=29

Case Study >> Part 2

Stacy Carpenter returns to the clinic 6 months later with complaints of feeling tired and having a sore throat. Stacy's weight remains at the 120th percentile, and her mother relates that Stacy is also being followed for elevated blood sugar. Her blood pressure is 136/92 mmHg. Stacy and her mom report that Stacy has not really changed her diet and that she is exercising some, but she really enjoys her video games and staying inside. She was not successful at her athletic events because she "could not run fast enough." A diet history is similar to that reported in her first visit.

Clinical Reasoning Questions Level I

1. What are the priorities for care for Stacy at this time?
2. What interventions might be appropriate for Stacy?

Clinical Reasoning Questions Level II

3. What risks, if any, does Stacy's blood pressure pose for her overall health?
4. What laboratory tests would you expect the practitioner to order?
5. What resources are available to help Stacy's mother with meal planning and food selection?

Independent Interventions

Nurses have daily opportunities for intervention in the area of nutrition, most often in the form of education about the relationship between food choices and health promotion and food choices and the management of illness and disease. Many of these interventions occur through the natural process of nurse–patient communication and should play a significant part in discharge teaching, especially in the area of food and medication interaction.

One of the goals of *Healthy People 2020* is for healthcare providers to give patients more comprehensive information regarding weight status and health outcomes. Nurses can assist with this by providing weekly opportunities for weight and diet evaluation. In addition, nurses can provide nutritional counseling for individuals who are over- or underweight and recommend various online resources or community programs that assist with weight management and healthy eating behavior.

Case Study >> Part 3

Stacy Carpenter comes to see the nurse in the clinic at her school. She tells the nurse about her feelings about her weight and her need to exercise. She has lost 7 pounds but says that she cannot seem to lose any more. She asks the nurse to help her develop a diet plan for 3 days considering that she eats breakfast and lunch at school.

Clinical Reasoning Questions Level I

1. How would you follow up with Stacy?
2. How would you encourage exercise?
3. What role should the school play in providing options for food choices?

Clinical Reasoning Questions Level II

4. What plan would you develop for Stacy?
5. What teaching would you perform at this time?
6. Would you include Stacy's peers? If so, how would you involve them?

Collaborative Therapies

Collaborative care for patients with alterations in nutrition can include consultation with or referral to a professional dietitian. **Dietitians** have advanced nutrition education, and their role is to provide expertise in the use of nutrition in a therapeutic fashion to treat disease. At times, the term *nutritionist* is used interchangeably with the term *dietitian*. **Nutritionists** advise individuals on the benefits of appropriate nutritional intake and diet planning. Most public health departments and long-term or assisted care facilities employ dietitians who can provide nutritional information, from weight loss management to weight gain, to intervention for constipation or eating disorders. Patients with diabetes should be referred to diabetes nurse educators, and patients with advanced cardiovascular risks should be referred to cardiac rehabilitation centers.

Weight loss clinics and personal trainers and other support personnel such as occupational and physical therapists can also be included as a part of healthcare teams to treat the problem of obesity. Primary care providers need to play a larger role in initiating and intervening in the prevention and treatment of childhood obesity.

Surgery

Collaborative interventions may include surgery and other invasive treatments. For people with morbid obesity, bariatric or lap band surgery is an option. Bariatric surgery may be considered in adolescents in severe cases of obesity resistant to previous weight loss attempts. Because of an absence of long-term follow-up, the overall physical and psychologic benefits of the surgery are not clear, and how long weight loss is maintained is not known (Lennerz et al., 2014). See Exemplar 14.A on Obesity for more information on pharmacologic therapy, behavior modification, and bariatric surgery for patients with obesity.

Many gastrointestinal surgeries will affect a patient's nutritional status. For example, patients with Crohn disease or ulcerative colitis may lose a portion of their bowel, affecting absorption (see the exemplar on Inflammatory Bowel Disease in the module of Inflammation for more information). Children can experience blockage of the outlet to the duodenum from the stomach and experience projectile vomiting due to pyloric stenosis. After surgery to repair the blockage, the infant is able to retain feedings. See the exemplar on Pyloric Stenosis in the module on Digestion for more information. Other pediatric disorders that affect nutritional intake are intussusception and megacolon.

Pharmacologic Therapy

Many of the pharmacologic agents specific to nutrition can be purchased over the counter. Protein drinks and protein powders to add to other foods are widely available. Vitamins can be purchased in the form of a multivitamin, which typically contains the recommended intakes of most vitamins and minerals needed on a daily basis. Vitamins and minerals can also be purchased individually.

Multiple claims are made about the health benefits of vitamin and mineral supplementation. Some of these are supported by research; many are not. Examples supported by research include folic acid supplementation during

Medications

Nutrition

CLASSIFICATION AND DRUG EXAMPLES	MECHANISMS OF ACTION	NURSING CONSIDERATIONS
Lipase Inhibitors *Drug examples:* Orlistat (Alli, Xenical)	Block absorption of dietary fats in the small bowel	■ Lipase inhibitors decrease absorption of fat-soluble vitamins and some medications such as warfarin (Coumadin). ■ Patients should restrict intake of fatty foods. ■ Individuals may experience flatus, diarrhea, stool urgency, and "greasy" stools.
Anorexiants *Drug examples:* Diethylpropion (Tenuate) Phentermine and topiramate (Qysmia) Locaserin (Belviq) Bupropion and naltrexone (Contrave) Liraglutide (Saxenda)	Suppress appetite by increasing the availability of norepinephrine in the brain; central nervous system stimulants 　Precise method of action of phentermine unknown but affects the hypothalamus, decreasing appetite 　Activates serotonin receptors, causing a feeling of fullness 　Reduces appetite by increasing dopamine activity and blocking opioid receptors 　Activates receptors for glucagon-like peptide, the appetite regulator for the brain, resulting in decreased calorie intake	■ Diethylpropion may produce nervous system effects such as confusion, insomnia, and tremors. ■ It has a risk for abuse. ■ Phentermine may produce paresthesia, dizziness, dysgeusia (alteration in taste), insomnia, constipation, and dry mouth. ■ Headache and upper respiratory tract infections can occur.
Vitamin Supplements *Drug examples:* Multiple vitamins Niacin Vitamin B_6 Vitamin B_{12} Vitamin C Vitamin D	Replace vitamins removed from food by cooking and/or correct deficiencies in food consumed in the diet 　Niacin—treats elevated cholesterol 　Vitamin B_6—supplements isoniazid (INH) therapy in the treatment of tuberculosis to prevent side effects of paresthesia and other neurologic discomforts 　Vitamin B_{12}—administered to patients with pernicious anemia who are unable to absorb vitamin B_{12} 　Vitamin C—assists with the absorption of iron in the treatment of anemia and aids in wound healing 　Vitamin D—assists with the absorption of calcium, administered to those who have insufficient intake as a component of osteoporosis treatment	■ Teach patients the importance of taking vitamins as recommended. Remind them that fat-soluble vitamins are stored in the body, and excess consumption can occur and can lead to toxicity. ■ In some preparations, niacin can lead to significant flushing. ■ Vitamin B_6 must be taken continuously during the treatment of INH. ■ Remind patients that vitamin B_{12} replacement will likely be lifelong. ■ Provide information relative to the role of vitamin C in promotion of wound healing. Note that vitamin C and iron should be taken at the same time to facilitate absorption. ■ Vitamin D is present in fortified cereals and included in the same formulation for treatment of osteoporosis or osteopenia (e.g., Fosamax D). It is also essential in the prevention of rickets.
Mineral Supplements *Drug examples:* Iron Calcium Folic acid	Iron is used to treat iron deficiency anemia and anemia due to blood loss 　Replacing lost calcium is especially important for postmenopausal women 　Folic acid is used in the prevention of open neural cords in the fetus	■ Provide information about foods high in iron and calcium. ■ Remind patients that iron may turn feces black and may lead to constipation; provide suggestions for increasing fiber in diet and encourage increased fluid intake. ■ If iron is prepared in a liquid format, patients need to use a straw because iron can stain teeth. For children, iron should be placed in the back of the mouth to avoid staining teeth. ■ Adolescents may often be deficient in iron because of blood loss during menses, the increased metabolic rate of growth, and poor nutrition intake.

Medications *(continued)*

CLASSIFICATION AND DRUG EXAMPLES	MECHANISMS OF ACTION	NURSING CONSIDERATIONS
		▪ Calcium is prepared in a variety of different forms, including tablets and gummies. It needs to be taken consistently. ▪ Calcium interferes with absorption of antibiotics such as tetracycline, so these medications must be taken several hours apart. ▪ Cereals and breads are often calcium fortified and could be added to the diet plan. ▪ Encourage intake of prenatal vitamins, especially folic acid. Folic acid levels are low in adolescents due to poor and inconsistent intake.
Protein and Nutrient Supplements *Drug examples:* Ensure Boost Nutrition bars	Provide needed protein and nutrient replacement for individuals who are unable to consume enough through traditional dietary intake	▪ Protein and nutrient supplements are helpful in the older adults who may have dentition or appetite problems and fail to consume adequate amounts of nutrients. ▪ Watch calorie intake, especially in patients with diabetes.
Intravenous administration of albumin, total parenteral nutrition (TPN)	Replace lost protein due to burns, major trauma, and significant surgical intervention or in situations in which the person cannot ingest oral nutrition.	▪ Follow dosage scheduling; a separate line or tubing may be needed. Monitor the infusion and timing of administration. ▪ Monitor serum albumin levels throughout administration.

Source: Data from Adams, M. P., Holland, L. N., & Urban, C. (2017). *Pharmacology for nurses: A pathophysiologic approach* (5th ed.). Hoboken, NJ: Pearson Education.

pregnancy and the prevention of open neural cords (American Academy of Pediatrics [AAP], 2013), vitamin C and facilitation of increased iron absorption (CDC, 2013), and increased tissue healing and calcium replacement in the prevention of osteoporosis (Ezzell & Castelow, 2014). Nurses must be familiar with the possible negative effects of misuse of these agents and be able to teach patients accordingly. See the Medications feature for more information on these supplements and other medications used in treating nutrition alterations.

SAFETY ALERT Excess consumption of some vitamins, especially the fat-soluble vitamins, can lead to significant toxicity. The disorder is referred to as hypervitaminosis. When taken in excess, vitamin D can cause bone destruction, rather than contributing to bone formation. Excess intake of vitamin C can lead to diarrhea, nausea, and stomach cramps (Manickavasagar et al., 2015).

Nonpharmacologic Therapy

Many individuals seek nutrition intervention for weight loss, dietary changes, health maintenance, and nutritional replacement or enhancement. Athletes who wish to add muscle mass may choose additional protein intake. Many patients take additional calcium for bone strength. Excess

intake of vitamins and other supplements may place patients at risk. Nurses must be able to provide patients with accurate and up-to-date information about these types of intervention and their strengths, weaknesses, and concerns.

Special Diets

Special diets are often suggested or prescribed to assist patients in managing their health and existing medical conditions. Disorders such as hypertension, hypercholesteremia, diabetes, irritable bowel disease, and celiac disease all respond favorably to the inclusion or omission of certain foods. See **Table 14–4 »** for some common special diets.

Some individuals are unable to consume food orally because of impairment of the gastrointestinal tract, temporary considerations following surgery, or other factors. These individuals may require nutrition therapy in the form of enteral or parenteral nutrition. **Enteral nutrition**, or tube feeding that provides nutrients directly to the stomach or small intestine, may be used to meet calorie and protein requirements in patients who are unable to consume enough food to meet the requirements. These patients may have impairment of the gastrointestinal tract, difficulty swallowing, unresponsiveness, oral or neck surgery or trauma,

TABLE 14–4 Selected Special Diets

Special Diet	Description and Use
Gluten-free	The gluten-free diets avoid the protein gluten, which is found in barley, rye and wheat. They are used as a medical treatment for celiac disease.
Dietary Approaches to Stop Hypertension (DASH)	This healthy eating plan is designed to lower blood pressure. It is low in saturated fat and sodium.
Ketogenic	This is a high-fat, low-carbohydrate diet in which dietary and body fat is converted into energy. It is used as a medical treatment for refractory epilepsy.
Low-fat/cholesterol	Low-fat/cholesterol diets include whole-grain products, fruits, and vegetables with a moderate amount of lean and low-fat animal-based food. Patients should choose lean meats, fish, and poultry.
Low-protein	Low-protein diets limit the intake of protein to 1–2 grams per day. They are used by patients experiencing kidney or liver disorders.
Low-sodium	Low-sodium diets limit the intake of sodium to less than 2 grams. Patients should avoid canned and processed foods and should not add salt to any meal.

anorexia, or serious illness. **Total parenteral nutrition (TPN)** is the intravenous administration of amino acids, often with added carbohydrates, fats, electrolytes, vitamins, and minerals. TPN is initiated when patients' nutritional requirements cannot be met through diet or enteral feedings and may be used concurrently with enteral nutrition. Patients who have undergone major surgery or trauma or who are seriously undernourished are often candidates for TPN. Enteral and parenteral nutrition are discussed further in the module on Digestion.

Lifespan Considerations

Although nutritional needs change throughout the lifespan, everyone needs vitamins, minerals, protein, fats, and carbohydrate intake. Nurses will meet individuals of all ages and needs, and for many patients, nutrition will be a primary area of intervention. Additional information about nutrition across the lifespan can be found in the Nutrition Assessment feature earlier in this module.

Nutrition for Infants

Infants and children have unique nutritional requirements due to the rapid physical and functional changes associated with growth and development. In their first year of life, children triple their birth weight. Adequate nutrient intake is essential for bone formation, teeth development, and the additional increase in metabolism that marks the years of rapid growth.

Nurses should encourage breastfeeding for all infants. The AAP (2012) recommends exclusive breastfeeding for the first 6 months, followed by continued breastfeeding as foods are introduced for the first full year of life. Not only does breastfeeding provide positive nutritional balance, but it also promotes gastrointestinal functioning, enhances immune function, and provides psychologic benefits (see **Figure 14–5 »**) (Ball, Bindler, Cowen, & Shaw, 2017). Exclusive breastfeeding reduced the incidence of otitis media by 50%, and any breastfeeding reduced the incidence of gastrointestinal disorders by 64%. Breastfeeding has also been associated with a reduction in the incidence of sudden infant death syndrome (AAP, 2012). For premature infants, breastfeeding may be even more important (Briere, McGrath, Cong, & Cusson, 2014). Support programs for breastfeeding

mothers are available from the AAP and other organizations. For mothers who are unable to breastfeed or choose not to, several ready-to-feed formulas are available that are nutritionally adequate to meet the needs of babies throughout the first year. Mothers who have difficulty breastfeeding may

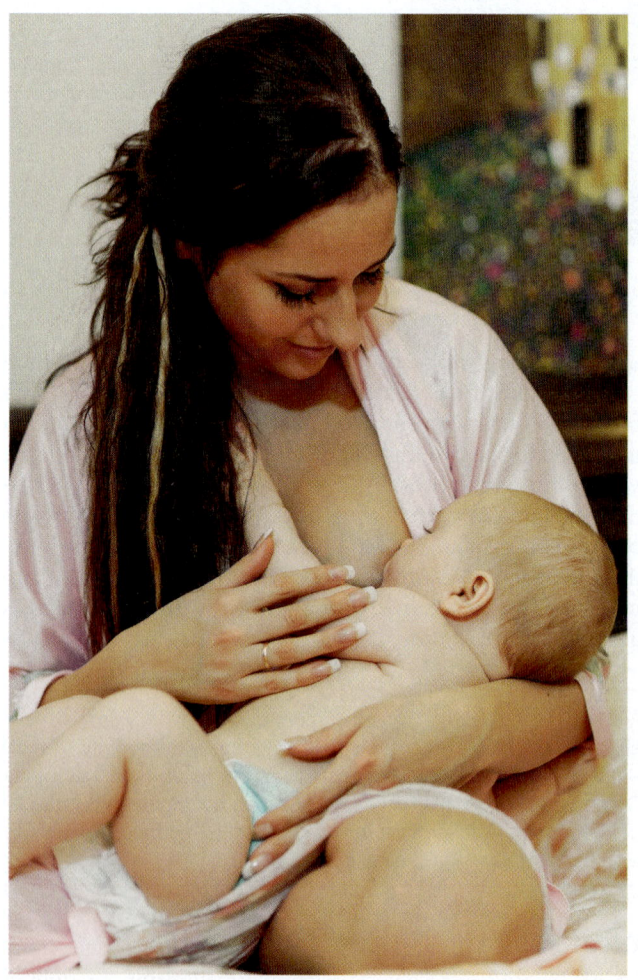

Source: Dmitry Melnikov/Shutterstock.

Figure 14–5 » Breastfeeding provides positive nutritional balance, promotes gastrointestinal functioning, enhances immune function, and provides psychological benefits.

benefit from a referral to a certified lactation consultant. The role of the **lactation consultant** is to provide breastfeeding support and care to mothers, infants, children, families, and communities. Lactation consultants may not be nurses but may have received training and certification, enabling them to provide necessary information and support to breastfeeding families. The presence of lactation consultants in obstetrician offices and hospitals leads to improved breastfeeding outcomes (Bass, Rodgers, & Baker, 2014; Torres, 2013).

>> **Stay Current:** Parents and healthcare providers can get information and view webinars on breastfeeding from the website of the American Academy of Pediatrics: http://www2.aap.org/breastfeeding

Nutrition for Children

The rapid rate of growth and development in children has a direct impact on their nutritional needs. Recommendations for adequate nutritional intake to meet these needs include the following:

- Make half of what is on the child's plate fruits and vegetables
- Choose healthy sources of protein, such as lean meat, nuts, and eggs
- Serve whole-grain breads and cereals because they are high in fiber. Reduce refined grains
- Broil, grill, or steam foods instead of frying them
- Limit fast food and junk food
- Offer water or milk instead of sugary fruit drinks and sodas (MedlinePlus, 2016).

>> **Stay Current:** The Mayo Clinic offers intake guidelines for calories, protein, fruits, vegetables, grains, and dairy for boys and girls in age groups ranging from 2–3 to 14–19. Go to http://www.mayoclinic.org/nutrition-for-kids/ART-20049335?p=1

Vlasak and Frisina (2015) confirm that knowledge about nutrition should begin at home. Parents play a key role in educating their children about healthy food choices, good nutrition, and healthy portion sizes. Parents can use everyday items to help children learn portion size and reduce unnecessary calorie intake (Small, Lane, Vaughn, Melnyk, & McBurnett, 2015). Children mimic what they see others doing; thus, children should see parents eating lean meats, complex carbohydrates, and vegetables (Wellard et al., 2014). Children can assist with shopping and purchasing healthy items. They should assist with cooking and learn how to prepare nutritious meals.

Because much of children's food intake occurs at school, teachers and school nurses have a part in shaping the views and behaviors that students will use in their futures. Weichselbaum and Buttriss (2014) confirmed the importance of a "whole school" approach to good nutrition, including education and the types of food and drink available at schools.

>> **Stay Current:** Information regarding children and fruit and vegetable intake, cutting back on sweet treats, healthy school lunches and snack tips for parents is available in both English and Spanish from http://www.nutrition.gov/life-stages/children/food-nutrition

Nutrition for Adolescents

Adolescence is a time of rapid physical, emotional, and social growth. Adolescents experience periods of "growth spurts" during which their nutritional and caloric needs increase significantly. Girls experience a change in fat disposition, and boys experience an increase in muscle mass and lean body tissue. Adolescent girls may have reached close to their adult height prior to adolescence, and boys may experience significant skeletal growth (Thompson, Manore, & Vaughan, 2014). Calcium intake is especially important, with one estimate suggesting that 26% of adult calcium deposition is established in early adolescence, with peak rates of calcium deposition occurring at 12.5 years for women and 14.0 years for men (Donaldson & Gordon, 2013). With inappropriate intake of calcium, precursors to osteoporosis may appear during adolescence.

Bone health in adulthood depends on bone density acquired during adolescence. The identification of risk factors associated with poor bone health early in adolescence and the provision of nutrition education, exercise, and lifestyle counseling can help teenagers maximize bone mass before their skeletal growth is completed, thus improving bone health into adulthood and beyond (Donaldson & Gordon, 2013).

Adolescence is also a time of increased independence in making decisions, including decisions about food choice. Adolescence is a time of identity formation, and adolescents align with peers in regard to food selection. One factor that continues to provide a strong impact on adolescents' food choices is parental food choices (Williams & Mummery, 2012). At times this factor is negative, when adolescents move away from family traditions; at other times, it is positive, with food choices being made based on a food's familiarity and comfort. Studies on food consumption suggest that caloric information or nutrient content is not a major consideration in choice among adolescents (Williams & Mummery, 2012).

During adolescence and young adulthood, young women experience social pressure to be thin, leading them to significantly limit dietary intake. Extreme dieting is particularly dangerous in the adolescent years because poor intake affects calcium and other nutrient levels and also causes a loss of estrogen. Eating disorders lead to complications such as cardiac dysrhythmias, electrolyte imbalances, and even death. In men, by contrast, there is pressure to gain muscle mass, which may lead to poor food choices.

Magee, Everts, and Jamison (2012) note that obesity prevention and management can be an important part of the practice of advanced practice nurses because their role enables them to take the time necessary to collaborate with patients and their families. Family functioning is an important factor in the success of nutrition programs (Van Ryzin & Nowicka, 2013).

Another *Healthy People 2020* goal is to reduce the proportion of children and adolescents who are considered obese (USDHHS, 2013). See Exemplar 14.A on Obesity for more information on obesity in children and adolescents.

Nutrition for Pregnant Women

Because the fetus is entirely dependent on the mother for its nutritional supply and ultimately quality of life, appropriate nutritional intake is critical for pregnant women. Nutrition for pregnant patients involves eating healthy foods that include more protein, iron, calcium, and folic acid. An increase in calories is also indicated (Wyness, 2015). Sensible weight gain goals are an increase of 2–4 pounds total during the first trimester and an increase of 3–4 pounds per month for the second and third trimesters. For more information refer to the exemplar on Antepartum Care in the module on Reproduction.

Nutrition for Older Adults

Older adults have unique nutritional requirements due to the physical and functional changes that occur with aging. Although many older adults experience a decline in physical activity level and have lower calorie needs, older adults need more vitamin D, calcium, vitamin B_{12}, and vitamin B_6. Obtaining a well-balanced diet while consuming fewer calories overall can present a challenge to many older adults.

Obesity is also a concern among the older adult population. Decreased metabolic rate, lack of exercise, high carbohydrate intake, hormonal changes in women, and polypharmacy, which can lead to undernutrition, can also result in overnutrition. Obesity places older adults at risk for cardiovascular disease, diabetes, and musculoskeletal disruption (Singh & Kaur, 2012).

A variety of factors place the nutritional well-being of older adults at risk. Physiologic changes can affect food choices and consumption and place older adults at risk for undernutrition. These changes include the following:

- Xerostomia (decreased salivation due to decreased function of salivary glands) decreases the taste of food, impairs chewing, and can lead to avoidance of certain foods (Daly & Smith, 2015).
- Loss of teeth, dental caries, and ill-fitting dentures often lead to decreased protein and fruit and vegetable intake due to chewing difficulties.
- Older adults may not realize they are thirsty and therefore may fail to consume adequate water throughout the day. This is a specific problem among older adults with dementia. Caregivers must be cognizant of the need to offer liquids repeatedly throughout the day.
- A decreased number of taste buds leads to decreased interest in foods, lack of desire to eat, and decreased intake leading to appetite dysregulation. Some sources classify this decreased intake as "anorexia of the elderly" (Donini et al., 2013). The loss of taste buds also results in increased use of additional amounts of spices, such as

---

Patient Teaching
Nutrition Across the Lifespan

Nutrition plays an important role throughout the lifespan, from prevention of birth defects to healthy growth and development and successful living into late adulthood. Nurses are at the direct point of contact with patients throughout the community, and education, especially nutrition education relative to food choice, is a distinct service that nurses are prepared to provide.

Infants

- Infant formulas are developed to meet the needs of specific age groups.
- In the first few weeks of life, feeding should occur on demand, especially for breastfed babies.
- The first week of life is critical in establishing breastfeeding. Lactation consultants can play a significant role in success.
- Breastfeeding is recommended for the first 6 months. Some sources suggest vitamin D supplementation in breastfed infants.

Children

- Toddlers often eat food in a repetitive format.
- Teach patients about choking hazards and the size of food.
- Children can be iron-deficient and may need supplements.
- School lunch programs may be the child's best option for appropriate food intake.

Adolescents

- Results of studies indicate adolescents need ongoing education and support to assist in making healthy food choices, avoid under- or overnutrition, and maintain health.
- Fast-food consumption is associated with higher total calorie intake and poorer diet quality (Powell & Nguyen, 2015).
- Body image may affect food choice.
- Peers significantly influence adolescent food intake.
- Adolescents who are obese are more likely to become adults who are obese.

Pregnant Women

- Teach pregnant women the importance of eating breakfast. If they experience early nausea, they can consider eating dry toast.
- Teach pregnant women to drink plenty of fluids throughout the day and avoid too much caffeine.
- Eating foods that are high in fiber helps with nausea and aids in the prevention of constipation.
- Pregnant women should remember to take prenatal vitamins. They are important for iron and for folic acid. Additional folic acid may be indicated to help prevent certain birth defects such as open neural cord.
- Increased calcium is also an essential part of the mother's diet to promote adequate skeletal development (Ezzell & Castelow, 2014).

Adults

- Food choice for adults is often set from earlier years. When health interruptions require alteration of food intake and moving to better food choices, adults will need education and support to transfer this knowledge to a lifestyle.
- Obesity continues to be a national health problem.

Older Adults

- Chewing and swallowing are frequent problems for older adults and are direct factors in food choice.
- Access to food and socioeconomic factors play a significant role in food choices.
- Loneliness and/or depression occur due to loss of a spouse and/or friends. Decreased appetite and social isolation may result.
- Polypharmacy may contribute to alterations in taste.
- Chronic disease may adversely affect meal planning and food choices.

salt, which may affect overall health, especially in older adults with hypertension.

- Cognitive impairment, particularly with dementia, leads to decreased nutrient and overall food intake. Individuals with dementia may hold food in their mouth, refuse to open their mouth, or turn their head away in a direct refusal to eat. Other behaviors such as wandering may affect mealtimes.

Constipation is a frequent complaint among older adults. Its etiology includes decreased fluid intake; lack of exercise; normal, age-related decreases in peristalsis; decreased fiber intake (related to lack of or ill-fitting dentition); decreased metabolism; and the misconception that a bowel movement needs to occur daily. Medications may also contribute to constipation in this population (Gallegos-Orozco, Foxx-Orenstein, Sterler, & Stoa, 2012).

Some medications can affect food taste, promote nausea and vomiting, cause dry mouth, and suppress appetite. Because older adults frequently take multiple medications,

the impact is even greater for them. In addition, interactions occur between nutrients and drugs that can affect expected pharmacokinetics and pharmacodynamics. The aging process may also lead to accidental overdose or omission of drugs due to forgetfulness or repeated dosing (Hanlon, Schmader, & Semla, 2013).

One of the goals of *Healthy People 2020* is to improve the health, function, and quality of life of older adults (USDHHS, 2013). The federal government acknowledges that nutritional intake among older adults remains a concern. The Older Americans Act (OAA) provides nutrition services that include meals served at group sites such as senior centers, schools, churches, or senior housing complexes; home-delivered nutrition services; and family caregiver support (Napili & Colello, 2013).

》 Stay Current: An excellent website that can assist older adults in understanding nutritional status and choice is MyPlate for Older Adults, created by Tufts University, found at http://hnrca.tufts.edu/myplate. The website, which provides printable material in English, Spanish, and Chinese, can also be used by nurses for nutritional guidance.

Nursing Care Plan
A Patient with Undernutrition

Joe Calhoun is a 72-year-old man who is being seen at the clinic today for his annual physical exam. Mr. Calhoun is 6 ft tall and weighs 155 pounds. In a quick review of his history, the nurse notes that since his last visit 6 months ago, Mr. Calhoun has lost 15 pounds.

ASSESSMENT	DIAGNOSES	PLANNING
After an initial head–to-toe exam that is within the expected norms for Mr. Calhoun's age, the nurse also notes that Mr. Calhoun's mucous membranes are pale and that his pulse is slightly elevated at 90 bpm. His blood pressure is 120/70 mmHg. Previous vital signs for Mr. Calhoun were a pulse of 70 bpm and a blood pressure of 140/80 mmHg. His current medications include losartan (Avapro) 150 mg for blood pressure, simvastatin for cholesterol, and aspirin 81 mg daily. He takes no other prescription or over-the-counter medications except ibuprofen (Advil) as needed for headache. The nurse questions Mr. Calhoun about changes in his life and nutritional intake during the past 6 months. The nurse also asks Mr. Calhoun to do a 24-hour dietary recall. Mr. Calhoun tells the nurse that his wife Irene died 6 months ago and that he has been sad and has difficulty cooking for himself. He is able to drive and goes to the grocery store each week. His daughter checks on him daily by phone because she lives in another state. His friends from church check on him, too. They used to bring him casseroles, but that has not happened recently. His dietary recall was as follows: "I eat cereal for breakfast and dinner and go to the senior citizens' center for lunch." He also states that the food he cooks does not taste like his wife's cooking and that "It's hard to cook for one." Mr. Calhoun denies having any difficulty chewing and has his own teeth. He denies constipation. He states he has no problem swallowing. The nurse calculates that at best Mr. Calhoun is consuming 900 calories each day, and many of these are empty calories. His complete blood count (CBC) report identifies a red blood cell (RBC) count of 3.9/mcL and a hemoglobin and hematocrit of 13 g/dL and 37%, respectively.	■ *Nutrition, Imbalanced: Less than Body Requirements* ■ *Cardiac Output, Decreased,* related to anemia ■ *Social Isolation* related to loneliness. (NANDA-I © 2014)	Goals for Mr. Calhoun's care include: ■ The patient will increase intake of protein to at least 3 ounces per day. ■ The patient will increase intake of fresh vegetables to at least one meal per day. ■ The patient will increase calorie intake by 300–500 calories per day. ■ The patient will gain 2 pounds by next visit (1 month). ■ The patient will socialize at least once a week with friends from church.

(continued on next page)

Nursing Care Plan *(continued)*

IMPLEMENTATION

- Instruct the patient to take one multivitamin daily.
- Refer the patient to a dietitian.
- Teach the patient to weigh himself first thing every Saturday and record the weights in a diary, noting any weight loss or gain.
- Encourage the patient to add one high-protein drink to his daily diet.

- In coordination with a dietitian, teach the patient how to perform a 3-day diet history for evaluation.
- Reinforce consumption of high-density foods.
- Encourage the patient to continue going to the senior citizens' center or to weekly lunch with church friends.
- Refer the patient for psychologic counseling.

EVALUATION

At his follow-up appointment 1 month later, Mr. Calhoun has gained 2 pounds. He continues to meet with the dietitian weekly and is consuming 200–300 more calories a day. He looks less pale, although his CBC demonstrates that he is still slightly anemic. His RBC count, hemoglobin, and hematocrit have increased some. He is taking his vitamins and protein drink daily. He relates that cooking for himself is still difficult and that at times he has to "make himself eat." He has been meeting with friends from church at least once a week and sometimes more often, and he says, "It has helped me a lot. They understand how much I miss Irene."

CRITICAL THINKING

1. What resources (e.g., congregate meal centers, senior citizen centers) are available in your community to help senior citizens who live alone? What is the nurse's role in assisting patients to find resources once patients have been discharged from care?

2. What intervention would you suggest if this patient demonstrated early stages of dementia?

3. With the expected increase in the senior citizen population and the likelihood that there will be many more men in Mr. Calhoun's situation, what proactive intervention can nurses implement to help prepare to care for these individuals?

REVIEW The Concept of Nutrition

RELATE Link the Concepts

Linking the concept of nutrition with the concept of metabolism:

1. Describe the relationship among calcium, vitamin D, and the treatment of osteoporosis.

2. What foods would provide additional calcium and vitamin D in a patient's diet?

Linking the concept of nutrition with the concept of development:

3. What are the symptoms of failure to thrive and what factors place a 1-year-old infant at greatest risk for the disorder?

4. What type of teaching plan should be developed to assist a mother with food choices to treat failure to thrive in a 1-year-old?

Linking the concept of nutrition with the concept of healthcare systems:

5. Develop at least four strategies to assist an 86-year-old woman who does not drive to gain access to her local food store on a weekly basis.

6. What normal physiologic changes of aging might affect this patient's nutritional well-being?

READY Go to Volume 3: Clinical Nursing Skills

- Skill 1.2   Height: Newborn, Child, and Adult, Measuring
- Skill 1.4   Weight: Newborn, Child, and Adult, Measuring
- Skill 10.1   Body Mass Index (BMI): Assessing
- Skill 10.2   Diet, Therapeutic: Managing
- Skill 10.5   Nutrition: Assessing

REFER Go to Pearson MyLab Nursing and eText

- Additional review materials

REFLECT Apply Your Knowledge

Valerie Athenopoulos is turning 40 years old in a few days. Over the past 6–8 months, she has been experiencing dyspepsia and chronic diarrhea, which at times changes to constipation. She also complains of bloating and belching. She states that at times her stools are loose and look greasy. The nurse practitioner asks Ms. Athenopoulos to do a diet history. Foods eaten include white bread, luncheon meats, oatmeal for breakfast, soup, and French fries. After reviewing the foods in the diary, the nurse practitioner suspects that Ms. Athenopoulos is experiencing gluten intolerance and, in consultation with the provider, makes a diagnosis of celiac disease with thoughts that the disorder is progressing in its intensity. The healthcare team suggests that Ms. Athenopoulos begin a diet that eliminates the majority of foods that contain gluten from her diet.

1. What is the relationship between gluten and celiac disease?

2. What is the relationship between obesity and celiac disease?

3. Are the manifestations of celiac disease different in children?

4. How might growth and development be affected in children and adolescents with celiac disease?

5. Develop a 48-hour diet plan for Ms. Athenopoulos that eliminates gluten from her diet

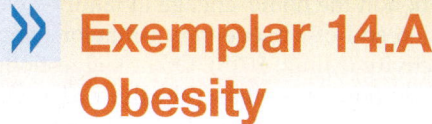

Exemplar 14.A
Obesity

Exemplar Learning Outcomes

14.A Analyze obesity as it relates to nutrition.

- Describe the pathophysiology of obesity.
- Describe the etiology of obesity.
- Compare the risk factors and prevention of obesity.
- Identify the clinical manifestations of obesity.
- Summarize diagnostic tests and therapies used by interprofessional teams in the collaborative care of an individual with obesity.
- Differentiate care of patients with obesity across the lifespan.
- Apply the nursing process in providing culturally competent care to an individual with obesity.

Exemplar Key Terms

Basal metabolic rate (BMR), *1007*
Body mass index (BMI), *1008*
Lower body obesity, *1008*
Metabolic syndrome, *1009*
Morbid obesity, *1009*
Obesity, *1007*
Triglycerides, *1007*
Upper body obesity, *1008*
Very-low-calorie diets, *1010*

Overview

Obesity (which is an excess of adipose tissue) is one of the most prevalent preventable health problems in the United States. It has serious physiologic and psychologic consequences and is associated with increased morbidity and mortality. Obesity contributes more to poor health-related quality of life than do smoking, excess alcohol use, and poverty. Obesity figures for children are controversial, with both decreases and increases being reported (Obesity Rate for Young Children Plummets 43% in a Decade, 2014; Skinner, Perrin, & Skelton, 2016). The most recent national data on obesity prevalence among adults, adolescents, and children shows that 35% of adults and 17% of children and adolescents were obese in 2011–2012 (Ogden et al., 2014). Between 4% and 6% of adolescents are severely obese (Kelly et al., 2013). A report by Marchiondo (2014) suggests that obesity among nurses equals that in the general population, suggesting that nutritional intake and food choices should be a focus for practitioners as well as patients.

Adults age 60 and over were more likely to be obese than younger adults. Among women, 42% of those age 60 and over were obese, compared to 31% of women age 20–39. There was no significant difference in obesity prevalence between men and women at any age. Non-Hispanic Blacks had the highest age-adjusted rates of obesity (47.8%); the rate among Mexican Americans was 42.5% (Ogden et al., 2014).

Pathophysiology and Etiology

Pathophysiology

All body activities, including activities of daily living and those necessary to maintain cell and tissue function, require the intake of nutrients and the production of energy. The body stores excess nutrients and energy to meet the body's needs when required nutrients are unavailable. This ability to store and release energy is important in maintaining body function. More than 70% of the energy expended each day goes to maintaining the **basal metabolic rate (BMR)**—essentially, the "cost" (in kilocalories) of being alive. Physical activity accounts for only 5%–10% of the energy spent daily.

Energy is stored primarily as fat in adipose tissue. Although mature fat cells (adipocytes) do not multiply, the immature cells in adipose tissue can multiply, particularly when exposed to estrogen during puberty, in late adolescence, during breastfeeding, and in middle-age adults who are overweight. Fat cells store excess energy as **triglycerides**, which are formed from dietary fats and carbohydrates. The body breaks down the triglycerides in fat cells when they are needed to provide energy (Porth & Matfin, 2015).

Etiology

Obesity occurs when excess calories are stored as fat. It can result from excess energy intake, decreased energy expenditure, or a combination of the two. The etiology of obesity is not, however, as simple as excess kilocalorie intake in relation to energy expenditure. The systems that regulate food intake, energy storage, and energy expenditure are complex and not fully understood.

Appetite, which affects food intake, is regulated by the central nervous system and by emotional factors. The hunger center in the hypothalamus stimulates appetite in response to stimuli such as hypoglycemia. As nutrient levels rise, the satiety center sends the message to stop eating, and gastrointestinal filling and hormonal factors assist in promoting satiety. However, appetite may have little relationship to hunger; some individuals eat to relieve depression or anxiety or to promote feelings of well-being.

Several hormones are involved in regulating obesity: thyroid hormone, insulin, and leptin (a peptide produced by fatty tissue that suppresses appetite and increases energy expenditure). Some studies suggest that leptin resistance is associated with obesity. Insulin is associated with body fat distribution.

Risk Factors

Heredity may contribute as much as 25%–40% of the risk for obesity. However, it is difficult to separate the role of environment from that of genetic factors. A strong correlation exists between the weight of adopted children and their biological parents, and identical twins tend to have similar BMIs regardless of whether they are raised together or apart, providing further evidence of a genetic link to obesity. Although several genes that contribute to appetite and fat deposition have been identified, obesity as a purely genetic condition is rare in all populations (Collins, Ryan, & Truby, 2013; Wang et al., 2015; Zegers et al., 2012).

Physical inactivity is probably the most important contributor to obesity. Even when inactive individuals consume fewer calories, they continue to gain weight because of a lack of energy expenditure. Cultural and environmental factors, such as labor-saving devices, reliance on the automobile for transportation, and an increasingly sedentary lifestyle, contribute to decreased energy expenditure among adults in the United States. Increased time spent watching television is seen as a major contributor to the increase in obesity among children, adolescents, and older adults (Hamer, Weiler, & Stamatakis, 2014).

Socioeconomic status also tends to correlate with the risk for being overweight or obese. In the United States, women with low incomes or low educational levels are more likely to be obese than are those with higher socioeconomic status (Ogden, Carroll, Kit, & Flegal, 2012). The association between socioeconomic status and obesity is less clear in men.

Prevention

Strategies for the prevention of obesity begin before birth. Prenatal education of parents should include content such as the positive effects of breastfeeding through the first 6 months of life, supporting places for safe exercise, and pursuing legislation that places limits on unhealthy food advertising (Mintz, 2015). Parents should be encouraged to promote good nutrition in the home, engage in family-style dining, limit television and other sedentary behaviors, and promote physical activity (Mintz, 2015). Other suggestions for prevention include population-based health programs through faith communities (Opalinski, Dyess, & Grooper, 2015); using technology (Schuman, 2015); patient education through all settings, including schools, clinics, and private providers, regarding healthy nutritional intakes and the important balance between nutrient consumption and expenditure, including programs such as the National Football League's Rush Play 60 (NFL, 2016); and partnership with public health organizations (Sommers & Heiser, 2013). Prevention should occur in all age groups and in all ethnicities. School nurses are at the forefront in prevention strategies (Quelly, 2015).

Clinical Manifestations

While obesity often is discussed as a matter of weight, it is more accurately defined by the **body mass index (BMI)**, which is an indirect measure of the amount of body fat, or adipose tissue (see **Table 14–5 »**). Adipose tissue is created when energy consumption exceeds energy expenditure. The terms *overweight* and *obese* are not mutually exclusive; a patient who is obese is also overweight.

The two major types of body fat distribution are upper body and lower body obesity. **Upper body obesity** (also called *central obesity*) is identified by a waist-to-hip ratio greater than 1 in men or 0.8 in women. Individuals with upper body obesity tend to have more intra-abdominal fat and higher levels of circulating free fatty acids (Porth & Matfin, 2015). As a result, upper body obesity is associated with a greater risk of complications such as hypertension, abnormal blood lipid levels, heart disease, stroke, and elevated insulin levels. Men tend to have more intra-abdominal fat than women, although women develop a central fat distribution pattern after menopause.

Lower body obesity (also known as *peripheral obesity*) is identified by a waist-to-hip ratio less than 0.8 and is more

TABLE 14–5 Classification of Overweight and Obesity by BMI, Waist Circumference, and Associated Disease Risks

	BMI	Obesity Class	Disease Risk Relative to Normal Weight and Waist Circumference[a]	
			Men 102 cm (40 in.) or Less, Women 88 cm (35 in.) or Less	Men >102 cm (40 in.), Women >88 cm (35 in.)
Underweight	<18.5		—	—
Normal	18.5–24.9		—	—
Overweight	25.0–29.9		Increased	High
Obese	30.0–34.9	I	High	Very high
	35.0–39.9	II	Very high	Very high
Extreme obesity	≥40.0	III	Extremely high	Extremely high

Source: From National Heart, Lung, and Blood Institute (2013). *Classification of overweight and obesity by BMI, waist circumference, and associated disease risks.* Retrieved from http://www.nhlbi.nih.gov/health/public/heart/obesity/lose_wt/bmi_dis.htm

[a]Disease risk for type 2 diabetes mellitus, hypertension, and cardiovascular disease. Increased waist circumference also can be a marker for increased risk even in individuals of normal weight.

Clinical Manifestations and Therapies
Obesity

CLINICAL MANIFESTATIONS	CLINICAL THERAPIES
BMI of 25–26.9 with two or more comorbidities	■ Diet, exercise, and behavior modification
BMI of 27–29.9 with two or more comorbidities	■ Diet, exercise, and behavior modification ■ Pharmacotherapy
BMI of 30–34.9 with two or more comorbidities (obesity class I)	■ Diet, exercise, and behavior modification ■ Pharmacotherapy ■ Surgery
BMI of 35–39.9 with two or more comorbidities (obesity class II)	■ Diet, exercise, and behavior modification ■ Pharmacotherapy ■ Surgery
BMI of ≥40 (obesity class III)	■ Diet, exercise, and behavior modification ■ Pharmacotherapy ■ Surgery

Note: Diet, exercise, and behavior modification can be appropriate for patients with hypertension, hyperlipidemia, diabetes, and other obesity-related complications.

TABLE 14–6 Problems Associated with Obesity

Body System	Related Problems
Cardiovascular	Atherosclerosis, hypercholesterolemia Coronary heart disease Heart failure Hypertension Stroke Varicosities Venous thrombosis
Endocrine	Endometrial cancer Type 2 diabetes mellitus
Gastrointestinal	Colon cancer Gallstones Hiatal hernia
Genitourinary	Cancers of the breast, uterus, and prostate Stress incontinence
Musculoskeletal	Low back pain Joint pain Muscle strains and sprains Osteoarthritis
Reproduction	Complications of pregnancy Decreased spermatogenesis Polycystic ovarian syndrome
Respiratory	Sleep apnea Other sleep disorders
Other	Depression Binge-eating disorder Postoperative complications

commonly seen in women. The risk for hyperinsulinemia, abnormal lipids, and heart disease is lower in individuals with lower body obesity than in those with upper body obesity. Lower body obesity may be more difficult to treat, however.

Because obesity has many contributing factors, its treatment is far more complex than just reducing the amount of food consumed. Most experts recommend an individualized program of exercise, diet, and behavior modification designed to meet the patient's specific needs. Pharmacotherapy usually is recommended only as an adjunct when traditional therapies have been unsuccessful. Surgical treatment (bariatric surgery) generally is limited to patients with **morbid obesity** (BMI ≥40, or >200% of ideal body weight) who are unable to lose weight through diet and exercise or have serious obesity-related problems, such as metabolic syndrome, hypertension, or heart disease. See the Clinical Manifestations and Therapies feature for more information.

Complications of Obesity

Obesity is a significant risk factor for cardiovascular disease. Approximately 60% of individuals with obesity have **metabolic syndrome**, a cluster of conditions that include three or more of the following symptoms: increased waist circumference, hypertension, elevated blood triglycerides and fasting blood glucose, and low high-density lipoprotein (HDL) cholesterol. Metabolic syndrome is an identified risk factor for atherosclerosis and coronary heart disease. Obesity-associated obstructive sleep apnea also contributes to the risk for heart failure (Bingolm, Pihtili, Cagatay, Okumus, & Kiyan, 2015; Qaseem et al., 2013). A more complete list of health-related problems associated with obesity is provided in **Table 14–6 》**.

Collaboration

Successful treatment of obesity—that is, sustained achievement of normal body weight without adverse consequences—is rarely achieved. Treatment typically focuses on reducing the health risks associated with obesity by changing both eating and exercise habits.

Diagnostic Tests

Diagnostic tests that may be part of the physical assessment include the following:

■ **Body mass index.** Used to identify excess adipose tissue. Calculations may not reflect as accurately the extent of adipose tissue in individuals who are highly muscular (e.g., body builders) or in those who have lost muscle mass (e.g., older adults).

- **Anthropometry.** Includes measurements of height, weight, waist circumference, and waist-to-hip ratio. Men with a waist measurement of 102 cm (40 in.) or greater and women with a waist measurement of 88 cm (35 in.) or greater have a higher risk for complications of obesity.

- **Underwater weighing (hydrodensitometry).** Considered the most accurate way to determine body fat, this technique involves submerging the whole body and then measuring the amount of displaced water.

- **Bioelectrical impedance.** Uses a low-energy electrical impulse to determine the percentage of body fat by measuring the electrical resistance of the body.

Other diagnostic tests may be done to help identify a physiologic cause or complications related to obesity. These tests include:

- **Thyroid profile.** Includes a total triiodothyronine (T_3) and T_3 uptake, free thyroxine (T_4) and total T_4, free T_4 index, and thyroid-stimulating hormone (TSH) profile and is done to rule out thyroid disease.

- **Serum glucose.** Measured to identify coexisting diabetes.

- **Serum cholesterol.** Measured to assess for elevated levels.

- **Lipid profile.** HDL levels may be reduced in patients with obesity, whereas low-density lipoprotein (LDL) levels are elevated.

- **Electrocardiography.** Performed to detect effects of obesity on the heart (e.g., rate or rhythm disruptions, myocardial infarction, heart enlargement).

Exercise

Exercise is a critical element in losing weight and keeping it off. Physical activity increases energy consumption and promotes weight loss while preserving lean body mass. Such activity improves physical fitness, decreases appetite, promotes self-esteem, and increases the BMR. Patients may benefit from consulting with a physical therapist or personal trainer who will help them develop an exercise plan that reflects their physical condition, interests, lifestyle, and abilities.

Patients with obesity may experience excess fatigue, tachycardia, and shortness of breath with activity. These symptoms result from the physiologic effects of excess weight as well as a sedentary lifestyle. Evaluation by a healthcare practitioner is important for any patient before beginning an exercise program. The practitioner instructs the patient to increase the duration and intensity of activity and to stop exercising and report symptoms if chest pain or shortness of breath occurs. An aerobic exercise program of 30–40 minutes of exercise five or more days a week promotes weight loss while reducing adipose tissue, increasing lean body mass, and promoting long-term weight control. (See the module on Health, Wellness, Illness, and Injury for more details.)

Nutrition Management

Collaboration with a nutritionist helps patients to identify nutritious foods that appeal to them and that can be included in a diet plan to create a daily 500- to 1000-kcal deficit. The recommended diet should be low in kilocalories and fat, contain adequate nutrients and minerals, and be high in dietary fiber. The patient should eat regular meals with small servings. A gradual, slow weight loss of no more than 1–2 lb/week is recommended. For most individuals, this means a diet of 1000–1200 kcal/day for most women and 1200–1600 kcal/day for men. Fewer than 1200 kcal each day may lead to loss of lean tissue and nutritional deficiencies. Excessive calorie restrictions also can lead to failure to follow the prescribed diet, feelings of guilt, and overeating.

"Yo-yo" dieting (repeated cycles of weight loss and gain) may lead to a metabolic deficiency that makes subsequent weight loss efforts increasingly difficult. Therefore, it is critical that dieters take any weight loss effort seriously and include plans for long-term maintenance. The best approach is to modify dietary intake without severe restrictions, eating a well-balanced, low-fat diet and developing improved eating habits.

Very-low-calorie diets generally are reserved for patients who have a BMI greater than 30 (Weight-Control Information Network ([WIN], 2013b). In a typical program, the patient, under close medical supervision, consumes 400–800 kcal/day or less, including 45–70 g of high-quality protein, 30–50 g of carbohydrate, and approximately 2 g of fat per day for 1–2 months. Exercise, nutrition, and behavior modification counseling should accompany the diet. The patient generally experiences a dramatic and rapid weight loss while maintaining lean body mass. Suppression of hunger brought on by ketone production associated with fat metabolism is an added benefit of the diet. Complications generally are minor, and benefits include decreased blood pressure and lower blood glucose, cholesterol, and triglyceride levels along with improved exercise tolerance. Very-low-calorie diets may not be appropriate for use in individuals over age 50 because of normal loss of lean body mass and adverse effects of the diet. Adverse effects generally are minor but can include fatigue, constipation, nausea, diarrhea, and gallstone formation (WIN, 2013b).

Behavior Modification

Behavior modification is a critical component of successful weight management. Strategies such as keeping food diaries, eliminating cues that precipitate eating, and changing the act of eating often are helpful.

Recording food intake, amount, location of eating, and situations that induce eating often helps the dieter to gain self-control. These strategies generally are most effective when used in combination with other behavior modification approaches.

Researchers have found that for most overweight individuals, eating is regulated by external cues, such as the proximity to food and the time of day. In contrast, in adults of normal weight, hunger and satiety are the cues that regulate

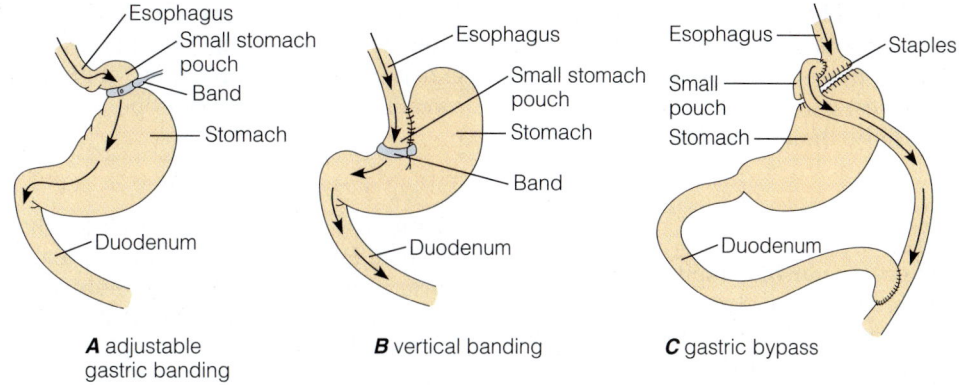

A adjustable gastric banding

B vertical banding

C gastric bypass

Figure 14–6 ⟫ Types of surgical procedures to treat obesity: **A,** adjustable gastric banding; **B,** vertical banded gastroplasty; and **C,** Roux-en-Y gastric bypass surgery.

eating. Strategies to control food cues include keeping food out of view, eliminating snack foods, and eating only in designated areas.

Other behavior modification approaches focus on helping patients to examine factors that affect eating behaviors. Examining their lifestyle, personality, and environment helps patients to understand eating behaviors and their consequences. The goal is to empower individuals who are stimulated to eat to choose instead to participate in activities that are not related to food.

Social support and group programs such as Weight Watchers, Overeaters Anonymous, and Take Off Pounds Sensibly promote weight loss success through peer support. Most organized programs require participants to pay a fee, which may improve compliance.

Surgery

Surgical treatment of obesity (bariatric surgery) generally is limited to patients who are morbidly obese and unable to lose weight through diet and exercise or have serious obesity-related problems, such as metabolic syndrome, hypertension, or heart disease (WIN, 2013a). Patients must be able to tolerate surgery and be free of addiction to alcohol or other drugs. A thorough psychologic evaluation is done before surgery. The benefits of surgery include major weight loss; improved blood pressure; and reduced risk of diabetes, sleep apnea, angina, heart failure, blood lipid levels, and venous disease. Bariatric surgery is not without risk, however, and the decision to undergo surgery is a significant one.

The most common bariatric surgical procedures in the United States are the gastric bypass; the sleeve gastrectomy, in which 80% of the stomach is removed; adjustable gastric band surgery; and combined restrictive/malabsorptive surgeries such as the Roux-en-Y.

Restrictive Procedures

Restrictive procedures limit food intake by restricting stomach capacity. They include adjustable gastric banding and the vertical banded gastroplasty. In adjustable gastric banding (see **Figure 14–6A ⟫**), a hollow band of silicone rubber is placed around the upper (proximal) portion of

the stomach. The band is inflated with saline solution to create a small stomach pouch with a narrow passage to the rest of the stomach. The amount of band inflation can be adjusted with a port implanted under the skin. The vertical banded gastroplasty (see Figure 14–6B) uses both a band and staples to create a small stomach pouch. Both procedures may be performed laparoscopically and can be reversed if necessary. Few nutritional deficiencies are associated with restrictive bariatric procedures. Vomiting is a common postoperative risk with restrictive procedures. The band may slip or break, necessitating a return to surgery. Approximately 15%–20% of patients who undergo vertical banded gastroplasty procedures require a second procedure. For this reason, and because of the increased complexity of the vertical banded procedure, it is performed less commonly than adjustable gastric banding (WIN, 2013a).

Restrictive procedures are safer but generally less effective in the long term than combined approaches. While patients typically lose approximately 50% of their excess body weight within the first year after restrictive procedures, fewer than one quarter of these patients maintain that weight loss over a 10-year period (WIN, 2013a).

Restrictive/Malabsorptive Procedures

Restrictive/malabsorptive surgeries both restrict stomach capacity, limiting food intake, and bypass a portion of the small intestine, restricting the absorption of calories and nutrients. In the Roux-en-Y gastric bypass (see Figure 14–6C), a small stomach pouch is created to restrict food intake. A Y-shaped section of the jejunum is then attached to the pouch to allow food to bypass the lower stomach and duodenum. This limits calorie and nutrient absorption. A more complex procedure, the biliopancreatic diversion, carries a higher risk of nutritional deficiencies and is used less frequently.

Restrictive/malabsorptive surgeries have the advantage of producing rapid weight loss that is maintained over time. Many patients maintain a 60%–70% weight loss for 10 years or more following Roux-en-Y gastric bypass surgery (WIN, 2013a). These surgeries also help to improve obesity-associated health problems, such as type 2 diabetes mellitus, hypertension, and sleep apnea. Because these procedures allow food to bypass the duodenum and jejunum, nutrient deficiencies, particularly of iron, calcium, vitamin B$_{12}$, and, possibly, the fat-soluble vitamins, are common.

Complications of Surgery

Although the risk for postoperative complications is high, the mortality rate for bariatric procedures is low (<1% for restrictive surgeries and up to 5% for combination procedures). Possible postoperative complications include anastomosis leakage with peritonitis, abdominal wall herniation, gallstones, wound infections, deep venous thrombosis, nutritional deficiencies, and gastrointestinal symptoms. Dumping syndrome, which can be precipitated by a meal that is high in simple carbohydrates, may develop following combined bariatric surgeries. In dumping syndrome, stomach contents move rapidly through the small intestine, drawing fluid into the intestine by osmosis. The patient experiences nausea, bloating, abdominal pain, weakness, sweating, and possibly syncope.

Lifespan Considerations

Obesity is a significant concern throughout all phases of the lifespan. Sullivan (2014) suggests that obesity prevention starts prenatally and that childbirth educators are in a unique position to lay a foundation of healthy eating that can last a lifetime.

Obesity in Children and Adolescents

According to the CDC, *overweight* is defined as a BMI at or above the 85th percentile and below the 95th percentile for children and teens of the same age and sex. *Obesity* is defined as a BMI at or above the 95th percentile for children and

Evidence-Based Practice
Intervention in Preventing Childhood Obesity

Problem

According to the most recent data (2011–2012), the prevalence of childhood obesity remains significant throughout the United States, with 1 out of 6 children identified as obese (CDC, 2015b). Data from the most recent National Health and Nutritional Examination Survey (NHANES) study indicates that over one third of children and adolescents consume fast food on a given day, accounting for 12.4% of their caloric intake (Vikraman, Fryar, & Ogden, 2015).

Obesity in childhood predisposes children to multiple physical and psychosocial problems and can be a contributing factor to early mortality. Major contributing factors were determined to be lack of exercise, intake of sugar-sweetened beverages, availability of high-carbohydrate food choices, and use of food as a reward. The highest risk factors for childhood obesity were parental obesity and unhealthy food choices in the home environment.

Evidence

Significant health and social consequences are associated with childhood obesity (Sundberg et al., 2014). Research suggests that genetic, home, school, and community factors all contribute to the problem (Mehta et al., 2014).

During the past decade, obesity among 2- to 5-year-olds decreased from 13.9% in 2003–2004 to 8.4% in 2011–2012 (CDC, 2015b). Research has identified relationships between breastfeeding (Lefebvre & John, 2014), eating breakfast daily (Chowdhury et al., 2016), and eating with family (Berge et al., 2014) and reductions in childhood obesity. One community in Massachusetts found that with total community support, the obesity rates dropped significantly and the results spread to the family as well, with parents' BMI decreasing by 0.5 points (Coffield et al., 2015). New York saw similar results from interventions such as eliminating sugary drinks from beverage vending machines, moving from whole to 1% fat and skim milk in school meals, increasing fiber in meals, and integrating physical movements into classroom activities.

Implications

Nutrition may directly or indirectly influence cognitive performance (Smith & Scholey, 2014). Given the fact that children who are obese are often the target of teasing and harassment and their self-esteem is adversely affected, nutrition can be said to affect social competence (Jackson & Cunningham, 2015). Nurses in the community, especially in local school systems, are strategically placed to provide education to children and their families about appropriate food choices and the factors that lead to childhood obesity. Most researchers suggest that the problem is not only food intake but also lack of exercise. Nurses can provide opportunities and suggestions for constructive play and share this information with teachers and parents (Rabbitt & Coyne, 2012). In 2011, through funding from the CDC, a 4-year Childhood Obesity Research Demonstration project (CORD) was developed, which aims to improve children's nutrition and physical activity behaviors in the places where they live, learn, and play. A summary report on the findings is still pending at the time of this writing. The project identifies three key interventions: increasing physical activity and consumption of fruits, vegetables, and healthier beverages; ensuring that children get enough sleep; and decreasing screen time and consumption of high-sugar drinks and high carbohydrate foods (CDC, 2015c).

Critical Thinking Application

Given the significant picture of childhood obesity, what role can the nurse play in its prevention? What role should parents play? What role should schools play? What role should primary care providers play? How can nurses encourage community involvement for increased outcome improvement across the country?

teens of the same age and sex (CDC, 2015b). Fractures, musculoskeletal pain, lower-extremity misalignment, and impaired mobility are more prevalent in children and adolescents who are obese than in those who are not obese (Kish, 2015). Hyperlipidemia, hypertension, and abnormal glucose tolerance occur with greater frequency in children and adolescents who are obese. Children with obesity have increased risks for cardiovascular disease, diabetes, and cancer in later life (Ning et al., 2014); hypertension; decreased self-esteem; depression; and an increase in total health care expenditures (Arai et al., 2015).

Obesity in Pregnant Women

Obesity in pregnancy is problematic for both the mother and the child. Maternal obesity is one of the most common high-risk maternal conditions (Poston & Patel, 2014). Women with obesity have higher rates of menstrual irregularities and higher incidences of infertility. Some obese women may not know they are pregnant, thus delaying prenatal care (Flick & Artal, 2013). For the mother, obesity can lead to gestational diabetes (Stadtlander, 2014), insulin resistance and dyslipidemia (Martin et al., 2014), gestational hypertension (Flick & Artal, 2013), anemia (Phillips et al., 2014), cardiovascular and respiratory complications (Gaillard, Felix, Duijts, & Jaddoe, 2014), risk of nonelective cesarean section, and significant incidences of preterm birth (Hancke et al., 2015). For the fetus, the risks associated with maternal obesity include macrosomia (Bautista-Castaño et al., 2013), congenital heart disease (Brite, Laughon, Troendle, & Mills, 2014), birth injury, and admission to a special care unit following delivery (Ahluwalla, 2015). These babies are more likely to be obese in later life (Balogh, 2015). Research suggests that women who are obese should begin a weight loss program prior to trying to conceive (Martin, Krishna, Ellis, Paccione, & Madell, 2014). Although opinions differ, some researchers suggest it is safe for pregnant women to be active, maintain their present weight, and even lose weight (Flick & Artal, 2013).

Obesity in Older Adults

Studies suggest that the population of individuals age 45–64 are more likely to be overweight than other age groups (Pruchno, Wilson-Genderson, & Gupta, 2014). Over the past 5 years, the obesity rate among people age 65 and older has increased by 4 percentage points, from 23.4% in 2008 to 27.4% in 2014 (Rettner, 2014). Obesity in older adulthood is related to higher risks for adverse brain changes and poor cognition due to reduced perfusion to the brain, with many individuals demonstrating markers for Alzheimer disease, especially patients with comorbidities such as heart failure (Alosco, Spitznagel, & Gunstad, 2014). Obesity can also lead to an increase in generalized inflammation in older adults (Ellis, Crowe, & Lawrence, 2013). Older adults who are obese typically have insufficient muscle strength to remain active, leading to increased adipose tissue and further loss of muscle mass and strength. The contribution of obesity to impaired function is progressive, as excessive adiposity and loss of muscle strength/mass are cyclically reinforcing.

NURSING PROCESS

Maintaining a healthy weight throughout the lifespan begins in childhood. Children and teenagers who are obese become adults who are obese. Nurses should promote healthy eating, including a diet rich in whole grains, fruits, and vegetables and low in fat. The USDA's MyPlate and Harvard's Healthy Eating Pyramid provide visual guidance for appropriate food choices to maintain a healthy, well-balanced diet. Encourage all children and adults to maintain an active lifestyle, engaging in at least 30 minutes of aerobic activity daily. Urge parents to limit the time that children spend watching television, using the computer, and playing video games. Discuss the effects of smoking and excess alcohol use on nutrition and activity.

Adults commonly gain approximately 20 pounds between early and middle adulthood. Educate patients to reduce the number of calories they consume as their energy needs change.

Assessment

Collect the following data through the health history and physical examination:

- **Observation and patient interview.** Observe the patient's general appearance, posture, and gait. Obesity often makes rising to a standing and ambulation position difficult due to pressure on joints and increased respiratory effort. Record the patient's current and usual weight and ask about any recent weight gains or losses. Review family history of obesity, and assess the patient's usual diet and food intake. A 24-hour diet recall is a useful tool to accomplish a quick review of the patient's food and resultant caloric intake. Assessment should also include a review of the patient's usual exercise and activity patterns, with a special focus on the identification of self-imposed restriction due to excesses in weight. For example, does the patient state it is painful to ambulate, or that shortness of breath impedes activity? Does the patient feel unsteady with gait? The assessment should include present comorbidities such as cardiovascular disease or diabetes. Gather data about all medications, prescription and other, taken by the patient, and assess the patient's body image and perception of his or her weight and its effect on the patient's health.

- **Physical examination.** Specific physical assessment data should include vital signs and weight and height, making certain to measure height and not depend on the patient's self reporting. Review skinfold measurements and waist-to-hip ratio. Assess skin integrity, including inspection of skin under the breasts and abdominal folds or any other areas where skin folds impede oxygenation or trap moisture and may lead to skin breakdown.

> **SAFETY ALERT** Use of an inappropriate size of sphygmomanometer is a common source of error in measuring blood pressure in patients with obesity. Choose a cuff on which the width of the bladder is 40% of the circumference of the arm and the length of the bladder is sufficient to cover at least 65% of the arm circumference.

Although body weight may be used to identify obesity, measures of body fat are more accurate. Men at ideal body weight have 10%–20% body fat, whereas women at ideal body weight have 20%–30% body fat.

Diagnosis

Nursing care for patients who are overweight or obese is community-based and holistic, focusing on both physiologic and psychologic responses to weight and appearance. Appropriate NANDA-I nursing diagnoses may include the following:

- *Overweight, Risk for*
- *Overweight*
- *Obesity*
- *Self-Esteem, Chronic Low*
- *Knowledge, Deficient*
- *Activity Intolerance*
- *Health Maintenance, Ineffective.*

(NANDA-I © 2014)

Planning

Although many factors contribute to obesity, it always involves an imbalance of kilocalorie consumption and energy expenditure. Patient education includes exercise, diet, and behavior modification. Goals are individualized based on classification of obesity, risk factors, and treatments and may include the following:

- The patient will make sensible dietary choices to plan meals within the caloric limitations chosen by the collaborative team.
- The patient will follow an exercise routine planned in collaboration with the healthcare team.
- The patient will relate strategies to deal with hunger and making unhealthy food choices.
- The patient will attend support group meetings to help meet weight loss goals.
- The patient will demonstrate appropriate weight loss, attending regular weigh-in appointments.

Implementation

Caring interventions focus on diet, exercise, and behavior modification. The nurse should do the following:

- Encourage the patient to identify the factors that contribute to excess food intake. Identification of cues for eating helps the patient to eliminate or reduce these cues.
- Establish realistic weight-loss goals and exercise/activity objectives. Small, reasonable goals, such as loss of 1–2 lb/week, increase the likelihood of success.
- Assess the patient's nutritional knowledge, and discuss well-balanced diet plans. Provide necessary teaching about diet. Knowledge empowers the patient to participate and make appropriate diet choices.
- Discuss behavior modification strategies, such as self-monitoring and environmental management. Behavior modification, diet, and exercise are critical to promoting successful long-term weight loss.
- Monitor weight loss, blood pressure, and laboratory data, including blood glucose and lipid levels. Continuing assessment is important, not only to evaluate the safety of weight loss strategies but also to reinforce the positive benefits of weight loss.

Encourage Exercise

The patient may need a medical evaluation before beginning an exercise program. The nurse can assist the patient in setting up an exercise program by doing the following:

- Assess the patient's current activity level and tolerance of that activity. Assess vital signs.
- After medical clearance, plan with the patient a program of regular, gradually increasing exercise. Consider a consultation with an exercise physiologist.

Promote Weight Loss

For a weight loss and maintenance program to be successful, patients who are overweight must modify their dietary intake in a world of daily temptations. Most patients who are overweight or obese experience some difficulty integrating all the components of a weight-loss program into a daily routine. Obstacles to exercise may include a busy schedule, activity intolerance, impaired physical mobility, lack of equipment, and the embarrassment of being fat. To assist the patient in formulating a successful weight loss program, the nurse can do the following:

- Discuss the patient's ability and willingness to incorporate changes into daily patterns of diet, exercise, and lifestyle. This discussion provides a basis on which to build realistic goals with the patient.
- Help the patient to identify behavior-modification strategies and support systems for weight loss and its maintenance. Weight loss and maintenance are most successful if the patient establishes lifestyle patterns that promote interest and motivation and, thus, exercise and diet management. Family and social support is critical for successful adherence to the therapeutic regime.
- Have the patient establish strategies for dealing with stress eating or interruptions in the therapeutic regime. A sense of failure associated with overeating or lack of exercise can lead to further overeating. Identifying positive strategies to

deal with these situations promotes self-acceptance and limits self-punishment through overeating.

Promote Self-Esteem

Although many patients with obesity have accepted their weight and body appearance on some level, most individuals who are overweight or obese have been subjected to ridicule, prejudice, and health problems attributed to being "fat." These experiences, coupled with day-to-day problems such as finding attractive clothing or a chair large enough to sit on, can affect self-esteem. Many patients report that "fat" jokes or comments contribute to their sense of negative self-worth. To help patients deal with these issues, the nurse should do the following:

- Encourage patients to verbalize the experience of being overweight, and validate their experience. This approach provides baseline data to use in developing individualized interventions to address self-esteem issues.

- Set small goals, and offer positive feedback and encouragement. Small goals provide more opportunities for success. Positive feedback and encouragement provide a comfortable environment in which to develop self-esteem.

- Refer patients for counseling as appropriate. Many patients benefit from counseling for issues related to self-esteem.

Evaluation

Expected outcomes of nursing care are individualized based on the nursing care plan. These outcomes may include the following:

- The patient identifies and understands factors contributing to weight gain.

- The patient understands and applies behavioral modification techniques to reduce weight.

- The patient accomplishes the desired weight loss at a rate of 1–2 lb/week.

- The patient incorporates physical activity into routines.

Nursing Care Plan

A Patient with Obesity

Sam Elliott, age 57, has gained 30 pounds since retiring 2 years ago. The most active things he does each day are "puttering around" and "walking to the end of the driveway to get the mail." His diet includes juice, oatmeal, a muffin, and coffee with cream for breakfast; donuts and coffee with friends midmorning; a bologna-and-cheese sandwich with chips and a root beer for lunch; and cheese, crackers, and wine before a dinner of meat, potatoes, vegetables, and dessert. He tells the nurse, "I have never had to diet. Now, I just don't know how to get this weight off."

ASSESSMENT	DIAGNOSES	PLANNING
Mr. Elliott is 173 cm (5 ft 8 in.) tall and weighs 91.2 kg (201 lb). His BMI is 30.1. His cholesterol is 240 mg/dL (normal, 150–200 mg/dL), with an HDL of 37 mg/dL (normal male value, >45 mg/dL) and an LDL of 180 mg/dL (normal, <130 mg/dL). His BP is 138/90 mmHg. His fasting blood glucose is normal at 103 mg/dL. His electrocardiogram shows normal sinus rhythm. He reports fatigue and shortness of breath with activity. His healthcare provider has advised a weight loss of 30 pounds and a regular exercise program.	Nursing diagnoses that may be appropriate to Mr. Elliot include the following: - *Obesity* related to food intake in excess of energy expenditure - *Health Maintenance, Ineffective,* related to knowledge deficit - *Activity Intolerance* related to sedentary lifestyle (NANDA-I © 2014)	The goals for the plan of care specify that Mr. Elliot will: - Lose 1 pound each week. - Walk 30 minutes 5 days each week. - Verbalize an understanding of the relationship between weight loss, weight control, and exercise. - Identify behavior-modification strategies to avoid overeating. - Identify support systems for behavior modification.

IMPLEMENTATION

The following nursing interventions may be appropriate for Mr. Elliot:

- Assess weight and blood pressure once or twice each week.

- Discuss current eating habits and strategies to reduce fat and calorie intake.

- Discuss cues that promote eating, and identify strategies to eliminate or reduce these cues.

- Teach how to keep a food diary to examine and change eating habits.

- Discuss the role of regular exercise in weight loss and weight control. Explain how to maintain an exercise record to track the intensity and duration of activity.

- Discuss lifestyle and behavior modification strategies to promote successful weight loss and control.

(continued on next page)

Nursing Care Plan (continued)

EVALUATION

Two weeks after changing his diet and beginning to exercise, Mr. Elliott has lost 2 pounds. He has maintained a food diary. He has identified boredom as a cue to eating. As a result, he has started volunteering at the local hospital, where he is working with children. He is walking for 30 minutes 5 days a week. He plans to increase his activity periods to 45 minutes. He verbalizes commitment to a lifelong plan of exercising and eating a low-fat diet. His BP has ranged from 132/76 to 136/84 mmHg. He plans to have the employee health nurse at the hospital check his weight and BP each week and to join Weight Watchers for ongoing support.

CRITICAL THINKING

1. What are some possible pathophysiologic bases for Mr. Elliott's abnormal cholesterol, HDL, and LDL levels?

2. Develop a teaching plan for a group of men and women who are overweight.

3. Identify potential barriers to losing weight and strategies to reduce or eliminate these barriers.

REVIEW Obesity

RELATE Link the Concepts and Exemplars

Linking the exemplar of obesity with the concept of culture and diversity:

1. Research perceptions about being obese and overweight in several cultures, and identify the cultural differences.

2. How would you teach a patient from a culture that values obesity as a sign of status to make healthier food choices?

Linking the exemplar of obesity with the concept of health, wellness, and illness:

3. What teaching would you provide an adolescent patient who is obese to promote health and reduce the risk of complications in later life?

4. Is it possible to be obese and still maintain optimal health? Explain your answer.

REFER Go to Pearson MyLab Nursing and eText

- Additional review material

REFLECT Apply Your Knowledge

Jenna Riley is a healthy but overweight 14-year-old girl who lives with her mother, Evelyn, and her brother, Jason. Her older sister, Jessica, lives a short distance away in her own apartment with her new infant son, Ryan. Jenna misses having her older sister around,

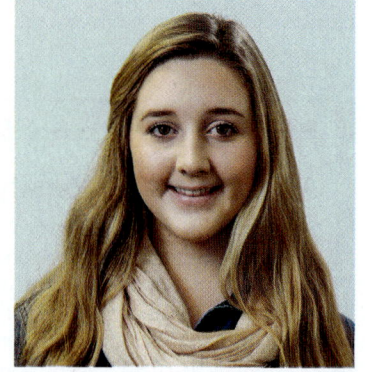

and she looks up to Jessica. Jenna has had minimal contact with her father during the past 10 years and does not really know him. Because her mother works a few evenings a week, Jenna is responsible for her younger brother. She gets along well enough with Jason, but she thinks he is a weirdo.

Jenna is a good student in the eighth grade at the local middle school. She has many friends and spends a great deal of time on the phone or in computer chat rooms talking with them each evening. Jenna is self-conscious about her weight, however. She knows she should try to lose weight, but she does not know how and does not have much discipline when it comes to resisting snacks. She finds it very hard to not join her friends when they eat.

1. What risk factors does Jenna face as a result of obesity?

2. What patient teaching will you provide Jenna?

3. What support groups might you recommend for Jenna?

4. Devise a 1-week meal plan for Jenna that reflects healthy eating and promotes sensible weight loss.

References

Adams, M. P., Holland, L. N., & Urban, C. (2017). *Pharmacology for nurses: A pathophysiologic approach* (5th ed.). Hoboken, NJ: Pearson Education.

Ahluwalla, M. (2015). Supporting the individual needs of obese pregnant women: Effects of risk-management processes. *British Journal of Midwifery, 23*(10), 702–708.

Alosco, M. L., Spitznagel, J. B., & Gunstad, J. (2014). Obesity as a risk factor for poor neurocognitive outcomes in older adults with heart failure. *Heart Failure Review, 19*, 403–411.

American Academy of Pediatrics (AAP). (2012). Policy statement: Breastfeeding and the use of human milk. *American Academy of Pediatrics, 129*(3), 600–603.

American Academy of Pediatrics (AAP). (2013). *Where we stand: Folic acid.* Retrieved from http://www.healthychildren.org/English/ages-stages/prenatal/pages/Where-We-Stand-Folic-Acid.aspx

Arai, L., Panca, M., Morris, A., Curtis-Tyler, K., Lucas, P. J., & Roberts, H. M. (2015, April 8). Time,

monetary and other costs of participation in family-based child weight management interventions: Qualitative and systematic review evidence. *PLOS Online*, 1–12.

Atalay, A., & McCord, M. (2012). Characteristics of failure to thrive in a referral population implications for treatment. *Clinical Pediatrics, 51*, 219–225.

Ball, J. W., Bindler, R. C., Cowen, K., & Shaw, M. (2017). *Principles of pediatric nursing: Caring for children* (7th ed.). Hoboken, NJ: Pearson Education.

Balogh, V. (2015). The consequences of maternal obesity. *International Journal of Childbirth Education, 30*(1), 54–58.

Bass, C. A., Rogers, M., & Baker, H. R. (2014). Can placing a lactation consultant in the obstetric office magically increase exclusive breastfeeding rates? *Journal of Obstetric, Gynecologic & Neonatal Nursing, 14*, S52.

Bautista-Castaño, I., Henriquez-Sanchez, P., Alemán-Perez, N., Garcia-Salvador, J. J., Gonzalez-Quesada, A., García-Hernández, J. A., & Serra-Majem, L. (2013). Maternal obesity in early pregnancy and risk of adverse outcomes. *PLoS One, 8*(11), e80410. Retreived from https://www.ncbi.nlm.nih.gov/pmc/articles/PMC3835325/

Berge, J. M., Wall, M., Hsueh, T.-F., Fulkerson, J. A., Larson, N., & Neumark-Sztainer, D. (2014). The protective role of family meals for youth obesity: 10-year longitudinal associations. *Journal of Pediatrics, 166*(2), 296–301.

Bingolm, Z., Pihtili, A., Cagatay, P., Okumus, G., & Kiyan, E. (2015). Clinical predictors of obesity hypoventilation syndrome in obese subjects with obstructive sleep apnea. *Respiratory Care, 1* (online journal).

Boyd, K. P., Andea, A., & Hughey, L. C. (2013). Acute inpatient presentation of kwashiorkor: Not just a diagnosis of the developing world. *Pediatric Dermatology, 30*(6), e240–e241.

Boyle, M., & Long, S. L. (2015). *Personal nutrition* (8th ed.). Belmont, CA: Wadsworth.

Briere, C.-E., McGrath, J., Cong, X., & Cusson, R. (2014). An integrative review of factors that influence breastfeeding duration of premature infants after NICU hospitalization. *Journal of Gynecological and Neonatal Nursing, 43*, 272–281.

Brite, J., Laughon, S. K., Troendle, J., & Mills, J. (2014). Maternal overweight and obesity and risk of congenital heart defects in offspring. *International Journal of Obesity, 38*(6), 878–892.

Burns, C., Cook, C., & Mavoa, H. (2013). Role of expendable income and price in food choice by low income families. *Appetite, 71*(1), 209–217.

Catanese, D., Khan, A., Nelson, S., & Williams, J. (2014). Global cost of obesity, *U. S. News Digest Weekly, 6*(48), 1–2.

Centers for Disease Control and Prevention (CDC). (2012). *Prevalence of underweight among adults aged 20 years and over: United States, 1960–1962 through 2007–2010.* Retrieved from http://www.cdc.gov/nchs/data/hestat/underweight_adult_07_10/underweight_adult_07_10.htm

Centers for Disease Control and Prevention (CDC). (2013). *Nutrition for everyone: Vitamins and minerals.* Retrieved from http://www.cdc.gov/nutrition/everyone/basics/vitamins

Centers for Disease Control and Prevention (CDC). (2014a). *Estimates of foodborne illness in the United States.* Retrieved from http://www.cdc.gov/foodborneburden

Centers for Disease Control and Prevention (CDC). (2014b). *Prevalence of underweight among children and adolescents aged 2–19 years: United States, 1963–1965 through 2011–2012.* Retrieved from http://www.cdc.gov/nchs/data/hestat/underweight_child_11_12/underweight_child_11_12.htm

Centers for Disease Control and Prevention (CDC). (2015a). *Adult obesity facts.* Retrieved from https://www.cdc.gov/obesity/data/adult.html

Centers for Disease Control and Prevention (CDC). (2015b). *Childhood obesity facts.* Retrieved from http://www.cdc.gov/obesity/data/childhood.html

Centers for Disease Control and Prevention (CDC). (2015c). *Childhood Obesity Research Demonstration Project (CORD).* Retrieved from http://www.cdc.gov/nccdphp/dnpao/division-information/programs/researchproject.html

Chowdhury, E. A., Richardson, J. D., Holman, G. D., Tsintzas, K., Thompson, D., & Betts, J. A. (2016). The causal role of breakfast in energy balance and health: A randomized controlled trial in obese adults. *American Journal of Clinical Nutrition, 103*(3), 747–756. doi:10.3945/ajcn.115.122044

Coffield, E., Nihlser, A. J., Sherry, B., & Economos, C. D. (2015). Shape up Somerville: Change in parent body mass indexes during a child-targeted, community-based environmental change intervention. *American Journal of Public Health, 105*(2), e83–e89.

Coleman-Jensen, A., Nord, M., Andrews, M., & Carlson, S. (2012, September). Household food security in the United States. *USDA Economic Research Report,* No. 141.

Coleman-Jenson, A., Rabbit, M., Gregory, C., & Singh, A. (2015). Household food security in the United States in 2014. *USDA Economic Research Report, 194.* Retrieved from http://www.ers.usda.gov/media/1896841/err194.pdf

Collins, J., Ryan, L., & Truby, H. (2014). A systematic review of the factors associated with interest in predictive genetic testing for obesity, type II diabetes and heart disease. *Journal of Human Nutrition and Dietetics, 27*(5), 479–488.

Daly, B., & Smith, K. (2015). Promoting good dental health in older people: Role of the community nurse. *British Journal of Community Nursing, 20*(9).

Diet Health, Inc. (n.d.). *Religion and dietary practices.* Retrieved from http://www.diet.com/g/religion-and-dietary-practices

Ding, M., Wilson, N. L., Garza, K. B., & Zizza, C. A. (2015). Undiagnosed prediabetes among food insecure adults. *American Journal of Health Behavior, 38*(2), 225–233.

Donaldson, A. B., & Gordon, C. M. (2013, April). Bone health in adolescents. *Contemporary Pediatrics, 14*–20.

Donini, L. M., Poggiogalle, E., Piredda, M., Pinto, A., Barbagallo, M., Cucinotta, D., & Sergi, G. (2013). Anorexia and eating patterns in the elderly. *PLoS One, 8*(5), e63539. doi:10.1371/journal.pone.0063539

Ellis, A., Crowe, K., & Lawrence, J. (2013). Obesity-related inflammation: Implications of older adults. *Journal of Nutrition in Gerontology and Geriatrics, 32,* 253–290.

Ezzell, D. A., & Castelow, C. (2014, July). Calcium and the developing other: Guidance for a healthy child and a healthy self. *International Journal of Childbirth Education.*

Feeding America. (2014). *Hunger in America.* Retrieved from http://feedingamerica.org/hunger-in-america/hunger-facts/hunger-and-poverty-statistics.aspx

Flick, A., & Artal, R. (2013, July). Obesity and weight gain in pregnancy. *Contemporary OB GYN,* 26–36.

Food Allergy Research and Education. (2016). *Food allergy basics: Facts and statistics.* Retrieved from http://www.foodallergy.org/facts-and-stats

Food and Agriculture Organization of the United Nations. (2012). *The state of food insecurity in the world 2012: Economic growth is necessary but not sufficient to accelerate reduction of hunger and malnutrition.* Retrieved from http://www.fao.org/docrep/016/i3027e/i3027e.pdf

Gaillard, R., Felix, J. F., Duijts, L., & Jaddoe, V. W. V. (2014). Childhood consequences of maternal obesity and excessive weight gain during pregnancy. *Obstetricia et Gynecologica, 93,* 1085–1089.

Gallegos-Orozco, J. F., Foxx-Orenstein, A. E., Sterler, S. M., & Stoa, J. M. (2012). Chronic constipation in the elderly. *American Journal of Gastroenterology, 107*(1), 18–25.

Ghosh-Dastidar, B., Cohen, D., Hunter, G., Zenk, S. N., Huang, C., Beckman, R., & Dubowitz, T. (2014). Distance to store, food prices, and obesity in urban food deserts. *American Journal of Preventive Medicine, 47*(5), 587–595.

Gokce, S., & Arslantas, E. (2015). Changing faces and clinical features of celiac disease in children. *Pediatrics International, 57*(1), 107–112.

Hamer, M., Weiler, R., & Stamatakis, E. (2014). Watching sport on television, physical activity, and risk of obesity in older adults. *BMC Public Health, 14*(10), 1–4.

Hancke, K., Gundelach, T., Hay, B., Sander, S., Reister, F., & Weiss, J. M. (2013). Pre-pregnancy obesity compromises obstetric and neonatal outcomes. *Journal of Perinatal Medicine, 43*(2), 141–146.

Hanlon, J. T., Schmader, K. E., & Semla, T. P. (2013). Update of studies on drug-related problems in older adults. *Journal of the American Geriatric Society, 61,* 1365–1368.

Harvard Women's Health Watch. (2014). *What too much sugar could do to your heart.* Retrieved from http://www.health.harvard.edu/staying-healthy/what-too-much-sugar-could-do-to-your-heart

Herdman, T. H. & Kamitsuru, S. (Eds.). *Nursing Diagnoses—Definitions and Classification 2015–2017.* Copyright © 2014, 1994–2014 NANDA International. Used by arrangement with John Wiley & Sons, Inc. Companion website: www.wiley.com/go/nursingdiagnoses

Hsu, M. F., Ho, S. C., Kuo, H., Wang, J., & Tsail, A. C. (2014). Mini-Nutritional Assessment (MNA) is use for assessing the nutritional status of patients with chronic obstructive pulmonary disease: A cross-sectional study. *COPD: Journal of Chronic Obstructive Pulmonary Disease, 11*(3), 325–332.

Jackson, S. L., & Cunningham, S. A. (2015). Social competence and obesity in elementary school. *American Journal of Public Health, 105*(1), 153–158.

Jauregui, J., Nelson, D., Choo, E., Stearns, B., Levine, A. C., Liebmann, O., & Shah, S. P. (2014, May 2). External validation and comparison of three pediatric clinical dehydration scales. *PLOS Open Access.*

Joint Commission. (2012). *Nutritional, functional, and pain assessments and screens.* Retrieved from http://www.jointcommission.org/mobile/standards_information/jcfaqdetails.aspx?StandardsFAQId=471&StandardsFAQChapterId=78

Kelly, A. S., Barlow, S. E., Rao, G., Inge, T. H., Hayman, L. L., Steinberger, J., . . . Daniels, S. R. (2013). Severe obesity in children and adolescents: Identification, associated health risks, and treatment approaches. A scientific statement from the American Heart Association. *Circulation, 128*(15), 1689–1712.

Kish, W. J. (2015). *Comorbidities and complications of obesity in children and adolescents.* Retrieved from http://www.uptodate.com/contents/comorbidities-and-complications-of-obesity-in-children-and-adolescents

Lefebvre, C. M., & John, R. M. (2014). The effect of breastfeeding on childhood overweight and obesity: A systematic review of the literature. *Journal of the American Association of Nurse Practitioners, 26*(7) 386–401.

Lennerz, B. S., Wabitsch, M., Lippert, H., Wolff, S., Knoll, C., Weiner, R., . . . Stroh, C. (2014). Bariatric surgery in adolescents and young adults—safety and effectiveness in a cohort of 345 patients. *International Journal of Obesity, 38,* 334–340.

Magee, S. D., Everts, C., & Jamison, M. (2012). Increased body mass index interventions: A provider comparison study. *Kansas Nurse, 87*(6), 15–18.

Manickavasagar, B., McArdle, A. J., Yadav, P., Shaw, V., Dixon, M., Blomhoff, R., . . . Shroff, R. (2015). Hypervitaminosis A is prevalent in children with CKD and contributes to hypercalcemia. *Pediatric Nephrology, 30*(2), 317–325.

Marchiondo, K. (2015). Stemming the obesity epidemic: are nurses credible coaches? *Medsurg Nursing, 23*(3), 155–158.

Martin, A., Krishna, I., Ellis, J., Paccione, R., & Madell, M. (2014). Super obesity in pregnancy: difficulties in clinical management. *Journal of Perinatology, 34,* 495–502.

Mayo Clinic. (2015). *Obesity: Risk factors.* Retrieved from http://www.mayoclinic.org/diseases-conditions/obesity/basics/risk-factors/con-20014834

MedlinePlus. (2016). *Child nutrition.* Retrieved from https://www.nlm.nih.gov/medlineplus/childnutrition.html

Mehta, T., Fontaine, K. R., Keith, S. W., Bangalore, S. S., de los Campos, G., Bartolucci, A., . . . Allison, D. B. (2014). Obesity and mortality: Are the risks declining? Evidence from multiple prospective studies in the United States. *Obesity Reviews, 15*(8), 619-629.

Millar, L., Rowland, B., Nichols, M., Swinburn, B., Bennett, C., Skouteris, H., & Allender, S. (2014). Relationship between raised BMI and sugar sweetened beverage and high fat food consumption among children. *Obesity, 22*(5), E96–E103.

Mintz, B. B. (2014, October). Childhood obesity: Parents have the power to foster change! *Eparent,* 8–12.

Nangia, S., & Tiwari, S. (2013). Failure to thrive. *Indian Journal of Pediatrics, 80*(7), 585–589.

Napili, A., & Colello, K. J. (2013). Funding for the Older Americans Act and other aging services programs. *Congressional Research Service.* Retrieved from http://www.fas.org/sgp/crs/misc/RL33880.pdf

National Center for Children in Poverty. (2013). *Topics: Child poverty.* Retrieved from http://www.nccp.org/topics/childpoverty.html

National Football League (NFL). (2016). *NFL rush.* Retrieved from http://www.nflrush.com

National Heart, Lung, and Blood Institute. (2013). *Classification of overweight and obesity by BMI, waist circumference, and associated disease risks.* Retrieved from http://www.nhlbi.nih.gov/health/public/heart/obesity/lose_wt/bmi_dis.htm

Nestlé Nutrition Institute. (2013). *Mini nutritional assessment.* Retrieved from http://www.mna-elderly.com/forms/mini/mna_mini_english.pdf

Nguyen, B. T., Shuval, K., Bertmann, F., & Yaroch, A. L. (2015). The Supplemental Nutrition Assistance Program, food insecurity, dietary quality, and obesity among U.S. adults. American Journal of Public Health, 105(7), 1453–1459.

Ning, Y., Yang, S., Evans, R. K., Stern, M., Sun, S., Francis, G. L., & Wickham, E. P. (2014). Changes in body anthropometry and composition in obese adolescents in a lifestyle intervention program. *European Journal of Nutrition, 53,* 1093–1102.

Obesity Rate for Young Children Plummets 43% in a Decade. (2014). *The New York Times.* Retrieved from http://www.nytimes.com/2014/02/26/

health/obesity-rate-for-young-children-plummets-43-in-a-decade.html

Ogden, C. L., Carroll, M. D., Kit, B. K., & Flegal, K. M. (2012, January). Prevalence of obesity in the United States, 2009–2010. *NCHS Data Brief, 82.* Retrieved from http://www.cdc.gov/nchs/data/databriefs/db82.pdf

Ogden, C. L., Carroll, M. D., Kit, B. K., & Flegal, K. M. (2014). Prevalence of childhood and adult obesity in the United States, 2011–2012. *Journal of the American Medical Association, 311*(8), 808–814.

Olander, E. K., Fletcher, H., Williams, S., Atkinson, L., Turner, A., & French, D. P. (2013). What are the most effective techniques in changing obese individuals' physical activity self-efficacy and behavior: A systematic review and meta-analysis. *International Journal of Behavioral Nutrition and Physical Activity, 10,* 29. doi:10.1186/1479-5868-10-29

Ontvieros, N., Hardy, M. Y., & Cabrera-Chavez, F. (2015). Assessing of Celiac disease and nonceliac gluten sensitivity. *Gastroenterology Research and Practice, 15*(4), 1–13.

Opalinski, A., Dyess, S., & Grooper, S. (2015). Do faith communities have a role in addressing childhood obesity? *Public Health Nursing, 32*(6), 721–730.

Pal, S., Radavelli-Bagatini, S., Hagger, M., & Ellis, V. (2014). Comparative effects of whey and casein proteins on satiety in overweight and obese individuals: A randomized controlled trial. *European Journal of Clinical Nutrition, 68*(9), 980–986.

Petrosino, S. P., & Matendo, B. N. (2014). Nutrition supplementation, diet and genetics and their impact on Parkinson Disease (PD), a review of studies. *Nutrition Health and Food Engineering, 1*(6), 1–12.

Phillips, A. K., Roy, S. C., Guilbert, T. W., Auger, A. P., Blohowiak, S. E., Coe, C. L., & Kling, P. J. (2014). Neonatal iron status is impaired by maternal obesity and excessive weight gain during pregnancy. *Journal of Perinatology, 34,* 513–518.

Porth, C., & Matfin, G. (2015). *Pathophysiology: Concepts of altered health states* (9th ed.). Philadelphia, PA: Lippincott.

Poston, L., & Patel, N. (2014). Dietary recommendations for obese pregnant women: Current questions and controversies. *Acta Obstetricia et Gynecologica Scandinavica, 92,* 1081–1084.

Powell, L. M., & Nguyen, B. T. (2015). Fast food and restaurant consumption among children and adolescents: Effect on energy, beverage and nutrient intake. *Pediatrics, 135*(2), 322–330.

Pruchno, R., Wilson-Genderson, M., & Gupta, A. K. (2014). Neighborhood food environment and obesity in community-dwelling older adults: Individual and neighborhood effects. *American Journal of Public Health, 104*(5), 924–929.

Purtell, K. M., & Gershoff, E. T. (2015). Fast food consumption and academic growth in late childhood. *Clinical Pediatrics, 54*(9), 871–877.

Qaseem, A., Holty, J. E. C., Owens, A. C., Dallas, P., Starkey, M., & Shekelle, P. (2013). Management of obstructive sleep apnea in adults: A clinical practice guidelines. *Annals of Internal Medicine, 159*(7), 471–483.

Quelly, S. B. (2015). Childhood obesity prevention: A review of school nurse perceptions and practices. *Pediatric Nursing, 19*(204), 198–209.

Rabbitt, A., & Coyne, I. (2012). Childhood obesity: Nurses' role in addressing the epidemic. *British Journal of Nursing, 21*(12), 731–735.

Renault, K. M., Carlsen, E. M., Norgaard, K., Nilas, L., Pryde, O., Secher, N. J., . . .Halidorsson, T. I. (2015). Intake of sweets, snacks and soft drinks

predicts weight gain in obese pregnant women: Detailed analysis of the results of a randomized controlled trial. *PLoS One, 10*(7), 1–15.

Rettner, R. (2014, January 27). US obesity rates have risen most in older adults. *Life Science.* Retrieved from http://www.livescience.com/49587-obesity-rates-older-adults.html

Rostami, K., Aldulaimi, D., & Rostami-Negad, M. (2015). Gluten free diet is a cure not a poison! *Gastroenterolgy and Hepatology, 8*(2), 93–94.

Rostami, K., Rostami-Negad, M., & Al Dulaimi, D. (2015). Post gastroenteritis gluten intolerance. *Gastroenterology Hepatology, From Bed to Bench, 8*(1), 66–70.

Roth, R. A. (2014). *Nutrition and diet therapy* (11th ed.). Clifton Park, NJ: Cengage Learning.

Santin, G. C., Martins, C. C., Pordeus, I. A., Calixto, F. F., & Ferreira, F. M. (2014). Food insecurity and oral health: A systematic review. *Brazilian Research in Pediatric Dentistry and Integrated Clinic, 14*(4), 335–346.

Schuman, A. J. (2015, April 1). Using tech to fight kids' obesity. *Contemporary Pediatrics.*

Singh, S., & Kaur, K. (2012). Association of age with obesity related variables and blood pressure among women. *Annals of Biological Research, 3*(7), 3633–3637.

Skinner, A. C., Perrin, E. M., & Skelton, J. A. (2016). Prevalence of obesity and severe obesity in U.S. children, 1999–2014. *Obesity, 24*(5), 1116–1123.

Small, L., Lane, H., Vaughn, L., Melnyk, B., & McBurnett, D. (2015). A systematic review of the evidence: The effects of portion size manipulation with children and portion education/training interventions on dietary intake with adults. *Worldviews on Evidence-Based Nursing, 10*(2), 69–81.

Smith, M. A., & Scholey, A. B. (2014). Nutritional influences on human neurocognitive functioning. *Frontiers in Human Neuroscience, 8,* 1–2.

Sommers, J. K., & Heiser, C. (2013, Winter). The role of community, state, territorial and tribal public health in obesity prevention. *Journal of Law, Medicine & Ethics,* 35–39.

Stadtlander, L. (2014). Maternal obesity and the development of child obesity. *International Journal of Childbirth Education, 29*(2), 21–25.

Sullivan, D. H. (2014). Obesity prevention starts prenatally. *International Journal of Childbirth Education, 29*(2), 12–15.

Sundberg, F., Augustsson, M., Forsander, G., Cederholm, U., & Axelsen, M. (2014). Children under the age of seven with diabetes are increasing their cardiovascular risk by their food choices. *Acta Paediatrica, 103,* 404–410.

Tan, S., & Epley, B. (2014). Much ado about something: The first amendment and mandatory labeling of genetically engineered foods. *Washington Law Review, 89*(3), 301–328.

Thompson, J., Manore, M., & Vaughan, L. (2014). *The science of nutrition* (3rd ed.). Glenview, IL: Pearson.

Tipton, P. H., Aigner, A. J., Finto, D., Haislet, J. A., Pehl, L., Sanford, P., & Williams, M. (2012). Consider the accuracy of height and weight measurements. *Nursing, 5,* 50–53.

Torres, J. M. C. (2013). Breast milk and labour support: Lactation consultants' and doulas' strategies of navigating the medical context of maternity care. *Sociology of Health & Illness, 55*(6), 924–938.

UNICEF. (2016). *Undernutrition contributes to nearly half of all deaths in children under 5 and is widespread in Asia and Africa.* Retrieved from http://data.unicef.org/nutrition/malnutrition.html

U.S. Bureau of the Census. (n.d.). *Poverty*. Retrieved from https://www.census.gov/hhes/www/poverty/data/incpovhlth/2014/highlights.html

U.S. Department of Health and Human Services (USDHHS). (2013a). *Healthy People 2020: Nutrition and Weight Status—Objectives*. Retrieved from http://www.healthypeople.gov/2020/topicsobjectives2020/objectiveslist.aspx?topicId=29.

U.S. Department of Health and Human Services (USDHHS). (2013b). *Healthy People 2020: Nutrition and weight status—Overview*. Retrieved from http://www.healthypeople.gov/2020/topicsobjectives2020/overview.aspx?topicId=29

Van Ryzin, M. J., & Nowicka, P. (2013). Direct and indirect effects of a family-based intervention in early adolescence on parent–youth relationship quality, late adolescent health, and early adult obesity. *Journal of Family Psychology, 27*(1), 106–116.

Vikraman, S., Fryar, C. D., & Ogden, C. L. (2015). Caloric intake from fast food among children and adolescents in the United States, 2011–2012. *NCHS Data Brief No. 213*. Retrieved from *National Center for Health Statistics* website: http://www.cdc.gov/nchs/data/databriefs/db213.htm

Vlasak, E., & Frisina, G. (2015). Good nutrition starts at home. *The Exceptional Parent, 45*(2).

Wang, E. A., McGinnis, K. A., Goulet, J., Bryant, K., Gibert, C., Leaf, D. A., . . . Fiellin, D. A. (2015, May–June). Food insecurity and health: Data from the Veterans aging cohort study. *Public Health Reports, 130*, 261–268.

Weichselbaum, E., & Buttress, J. L. (2014). Diet, nutrition and schoolchildren: An update. *British Nutrition Foundation Nutrition Bulletin, 19*, 9–73.

Wellard, L., Chapman, K., Woflenden, L., Dodds, P., Hughes, C., & Wiggers, J. (2014). Who is responsible for selecting children's fast food meals, and what impact does this have on energy content of the selected meals? *Nutrition and Dietetics, 78*, 172–177.

Williams, S. L., & Mummery, W. K. (2012). Associations between adolescent nutrition behaviours and adolescent and parent characteristics. *Nutrition & Dietetics, 69*, 85–101.

Weight-Control Information Network. (2013a). *Weight loss for life*. Retrieved from http://win.niddk.nih.gov/publications/for_life.htm

Weight-Control Information Network. (2013b). *Very-low-calorie diets*. Retrieved from http://win.niddk.nih.gov/publications/low_calorie.htm

World Health Organization (WHO). (2016). *Infant and young child feeding*. Retrieved from http://who.int/mediacentre/factsheets/fs342/en

Wyness, L. (2015). Vitamin supplementation and nutrition during pregnancy and breast-feeding. *British Journal of Midwifery, 23*(10), 695–701.

Zarnowiecki, D. M., Dollman, J., & Parietta, N. (2014). Associations between predictors of children's dietary intake and socioeconomic position: A systematic review of the literature. *Obesity Reviews, 15*, 375–391.

Zegers, D., Hendricks, D., Verrijken, A., Van Hoorenbeeck, K., Van Camp, J. K., deCraemer, V., . . . Beckers, S. (2012). Screening for genetic variants in BDNF that contribute to childhood obesity. *Pediatric Obesity, 9*, 36–42.

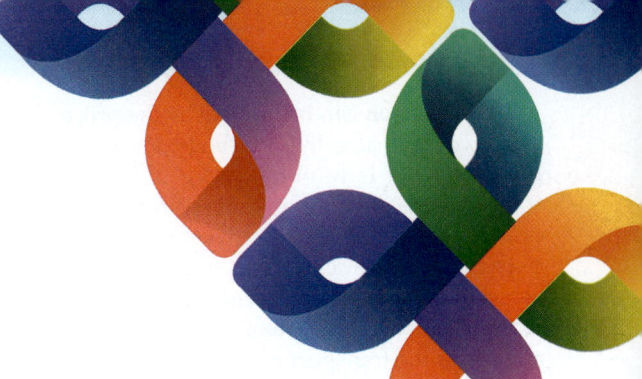

Module 15
Oxygenation

Module Outline and Learning Outcomes

The Concept of Oxygenation

Normal Oxygenation
15.1 Analyze the physiology of oxygenation in the body.

Alterations to Oxygenation
15.2 Differentiate among alterations in oxygenation.

Concepts Related to Oxygenation
15.3 Outline the relationship between oxygenation and other concepts.

Health Promotion
15.4 Explain the promotion of healthy oxygenation.

Nursing Assessment
15.5 Differentiate among common assessment procedures and tests used to examine oxygenation.

Independent Interventions
15.6 Analyze independent interventions nurses can implement for patients with alterations in oxygenation.

Collaborative Therapies
15.7 Summarize collaborative therapies used by interprofessional teams for patients with alterations in oxygenation.

Lifespan Considerations
15.8 Differentiate considerations related to the care of patients with alterations in oxygenation throughout the lifespan.

Oxygenation Exemplars

Exemplar 15.A Acute Respiratory Distress Syndrome
15.A Analyze acute respiratory distress syndrome (ARDS) as it relates to oxygenation.

Exemplar 15.B Asthma
15.B Analyze asthma as it relates to oxygenation.

Exemplar 15.C Chronic Obstructive Pulmonary Disease
15.C Analyze chronic obstructive pulmonary disease (COPD) as it relates to oxygenation.

Exemplar 15.D Cystic Fibrosis
15.D Analyze cystic fibrosis as it relates to oxygenation.

Exemplar 15.E Respiratory Syncytial Virus/Bronchiolitis
15.E Analyze RSV/bronchiolitis as it relates to oxygenation.

Exemplar 15.F Sudden Infant Death Syndrome
15.F Analyze sudden infant death syndrome (SIDS) as it relates to oxygenation.

The Concept of Oxygenation

Concept Key Terms

Alveoli, **1022**	Chronic obstructive pulmonary disease (COPD), **1025**	Hypocarbia, **1033**	Percussion, **1030**	Spirometry, **1033**
Apnea, **1026**		Hypoventilation, **1026**	Pleural friction rub, **1030**	Stridor, **1030**
Arterial blood gases (ABGs), **1033**		Hypoxemia, **1024**		Suctioning, **1036**
Atelectasis, **1030**	Crackles, **1030**	Hypoxia, **1024**	Pleural space, **1024**	Surfactant, **1022**
Auscultation, **1022**	Cyanosis, **1025**	Incentive spirometry, **1037**	Pneumothorax, **1026**	Symmetry, **1030**
Bradypnea, **1026**	Dyspnea, **1026**	Inspiration, **1022**	Pulmonary function tests (PFTs), **1033**	Tachypnea, **1026**
Bronchial sounds, **1024**	Eupnea, **1022**	Orthopnea, **1026**		Thoracentesis, **1034**
Bronchoscopy, **1034**	Expiration, **1022**	Oxygenation, **1022**	Pulse oximetry, **1033**	Ventilation, **1022**
Bronchovesicular sounds, **1024**	Homeostasis, **1033**	Palpation, **1030**	Respiration, **1022**	Ventilation-perfusion (V-Q), **1024**
	Hypercapnia, **1033**	Patent airway, **1024**	Respiratory depression, **1026**	
Chest x-ray (CXR), **1033**	Hypercarbia, **1033**	Peak expiratory flow rate (PEFR), **1033**	Retractions, **1025**	Vesicular sounds, **1024**
	Hyperventilation, **1026**		Rhonchi, **1030**	Wheezing, **1030**
	Hypocapnia, **1033**			

Oxygenation can be defined as the process of providing oxygen to all cells of the body. The function of the respiratory system is to obtain oxygen from atmospheric air, transport this air through the respiratory tract into the alveoli, and ultimately diffuse oxygen into the blood to carry oxygen to all the cells of the body. The respiratory system achieves all this through **ventilation**, which includes **inspiration** (inhaling) and **expiration** (exhaling). Inspiration allows for the transport of oxygen to the alveoli, where oxygen is exchanged for carbon dioxide. During expiration, carbon dioxide is expelled from the body. **Respiration** technically refers to the exchange of oxygen and carbon dioxide at the cellular level; however, this term is commonly used synonymously with ventilation.

Breathing, which typically is an automatic process, contributes to vital oxygenation of the cells and tissues. When oxygenation decreases, the respiratory system typically compensates by increasing the respiratory rate. Alterations in breathing patterns should be immediately addressed, as impaired oxygen delivery can be life-threatening.

Normal Oxygenation

Normal oxygenation depends on healthy development and function of the respiratory system, as well as intricate cellular and organic processes that allow for effective gas exchange. The following sections provide an overview of the physiologic process involved in normal oxygenation, as well as discussion of alterations to oxygenation.

Physiology Review

Adequate oxygenation depends on a healthy, intact respiratory system. The respiratory system obtains oxygen from the air and transports it into the alveoli, where oxygen diffuses into capillaries and is carried by the blood to all cells of the body. The respiratory system also allows for the removal of carbon dioxide from the body.

The upper respiratory system is the inlet for air into the body. The nose typically is the primary entry for air. The nose is divided into two nares, which are moist, pink, mucosa-lined passageways. Nares warm, humidify, and filter air as it is breathed into the nose. In the upper respiratory tract, two primary protective mechanisms prevent foreign matter from entering the lower respiratory tract: sneezing and cilia. Foreign matter that enters the nose irritates the nasal passages and induces sneezing, which is a reflexive action that clears foreign matter and debris from the upper airway. This reflexive action is active even in the neonatal period. Cilia are microscopic hairs within the posterior portion of the nares that trap small particles of foreign matter to prevent their entry into the lower respiratory tract. The cilia propel foreign matter into the pharynx to be coughed out or swallowed.

Breathing also occurs through the mouth, allowing air to enter the respiratory system through the pharyngeal cavity. The respiratory system shares this cavity with the gastrointestinal system, providing passage for air during breathing and for food or drink during swallowing. However, the epiglottis prevents food and fluids from passing through the glottis, which serves as the entryway into the lower respiratory tract. The epiglottis is pendulous tissue that covers the tracheal opening during swallowing or any time foreign matter contacts the glottis. The closure of the epiglottis is a reflexive response.

The lower respiratory tract is enclosed in the musculoskeletal structures of the neck and thoracic cavity. The trachea, which sits midline in the neck, is the entrance for air into the lungs. During normal breathing, the muscular structures of the neck are relaxed and the larynx easily rises and falls with each swallow. The chest wall effortlessly and symmetrically rises and falls with each equally spaced breath. Inspiration is half the rate of expiration. **Eupnea** describes breathing within the expected respiratory rates. **Auscultation**, listening to the body's sounds with a stethoscope, is an important assessment method. Effective respiratory assessment, including recognition of normal breath sounds by auscultation, requires an understanding of respiratory anatomy and physiology.

At the carina, the trachea bifurcates (divides in two) into bronchi to access the right and left lungs (see **Figures 15–1 》** and **15–2 》**). The right bronchus is shorter and wider than the left. The trachea and larger bronchi are supported by C-shaped cartilage rings, as well as by smooth muscle. Each bronchus further divides into yet smaller airway passages called bronchioles. The bronchioles, which are supported by smooth muscles only, dilate and constrict in response to autonomic nervous system regulation of the smooth muscles supporting them. Bronchioles give rise to the alveolar ducts, which branch into alveolar sacs that are made up of individual alveoli.

The **alveoli** compose the terminal (final) structures of the lower respiratory system. Alveoli serve as the sites of gas exchange, specifically carbon dioxide (CO_2) and oxygen. Alveoli are not directly connected to a specific bronchiole, but are interconnected to the terminal airways and to each other (see **Figure 15–3 》**). This structural design facilitates the filling of each alveolus with air. Specialized cells within the alveoli produce surfactant. **Surfactant** controls surface tension and, in turn, keeps the alveoli from collapsing and sticking to themselves. Alveolar macrophages keep the alveoli region free of microbes and are swept upward from the alveolar region by cilia in the airway passages. Macrophages are large cells of the immune system that remove waste and harmful microorganisms from the alveoli and from other areas of the body. Mast cells in the alveoli mediate the immune response within the airways.

Alveoli have a simple squamous epithelial lining and basement membrane that interface with the basement membrane and epithelial lining of pulmonary capillaries. This interface is where oxygen and carbon dioxide diffusion occurs. The concentration of oxygen is greater in the alveoli than in the blood in the capillaries, so oxygen diffuses across the membranes into the blood. The concentration of carbon dioxide is greater in the blood, so it diffuses into the alveoli.

The lungs are also described in terms of their lobes. The lobes lie obliquely in the thoracic cavity. The right lung has three lobes; the left lung has two lobes. The inferior lobes are the largest. Most of the inferior lobes lie in the posterior thoracic cavity. Each lung has a pleural lining to aid respiration and separate it from the other lung. The pleural lining has two layers; the visceral pleura covers the surface of each lung, and the parietal pleura lines the inside of the chest wall. A tiny amount of fluid between the visceral and parietal pleura allows these structures to glide across one

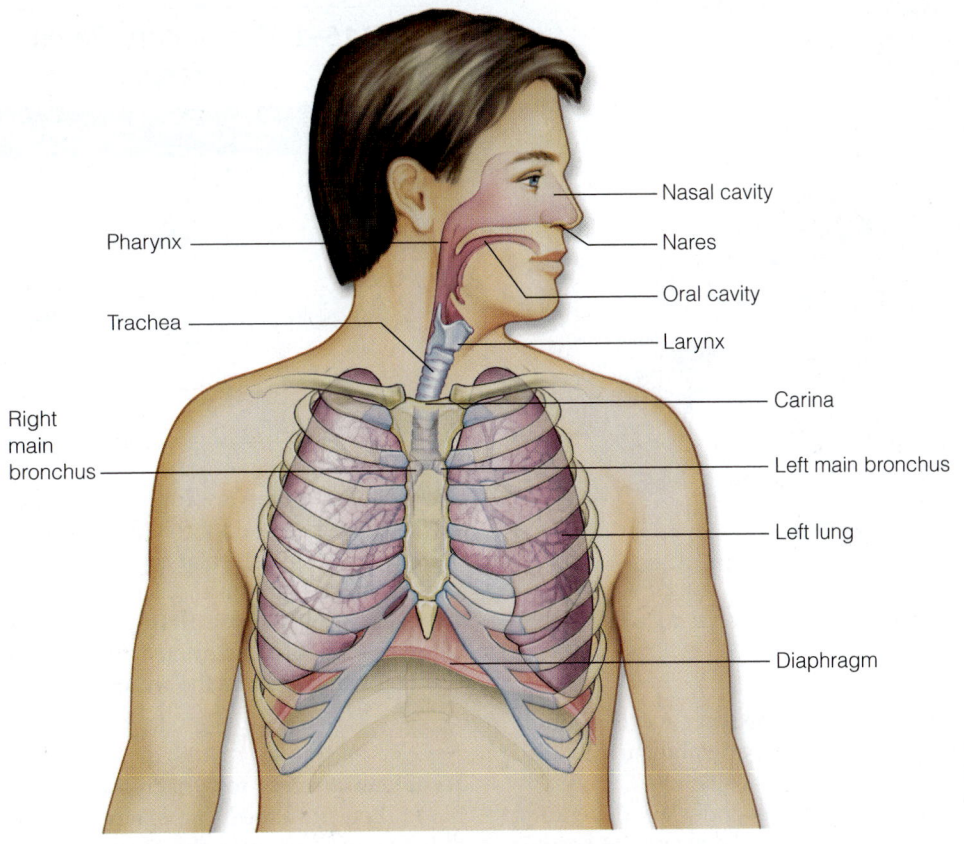

Figure 15–1 ≫ Anatomy of the respiratory system.

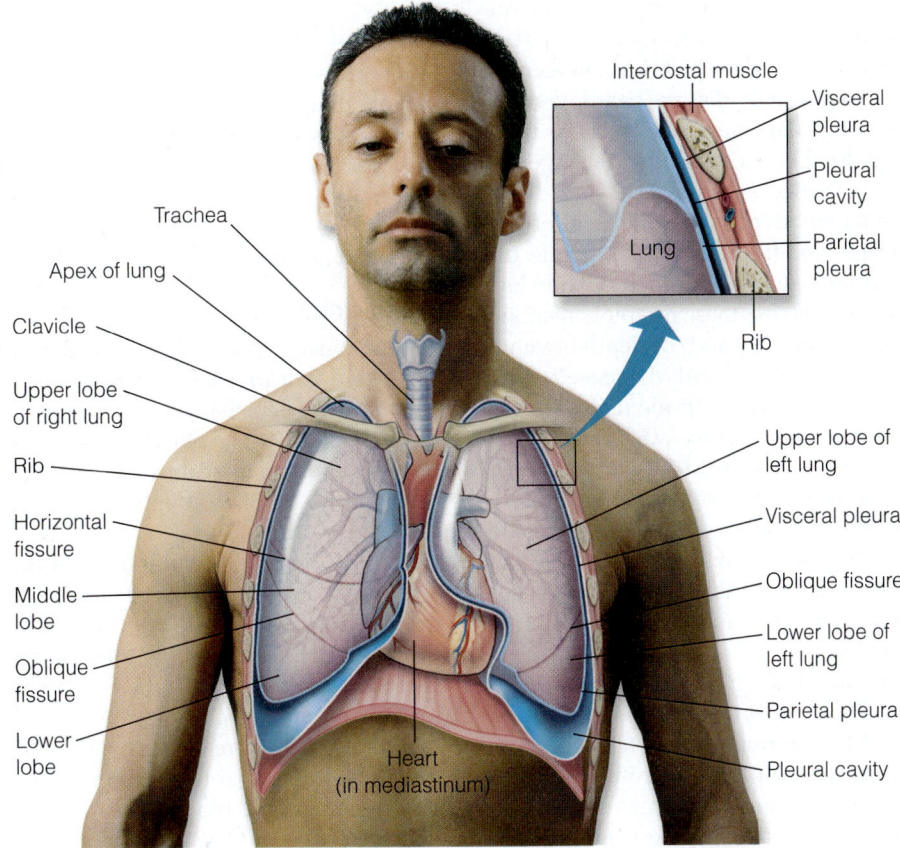

Figure 15–2 ≫ Anterior view of thorax and lungs.

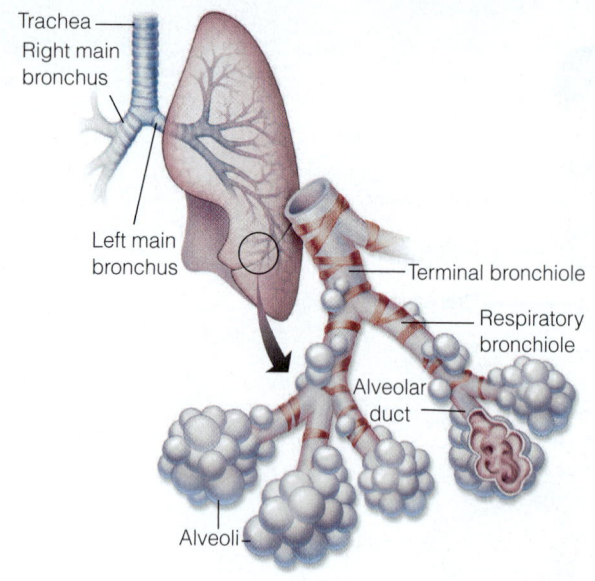

Figure 15–3 » Respiratory bronchioles, alveolar ducts, and alveoli.

TABLE 15–1 Respiratory Rates Throughout the Lifespan

Age Group	Rate (Breaths/Min)
Newborns	30–80
Infants	30–60
Toddlers	20–40
Preschoolers	22–34
School-age children	15–25
Adolescents	12–20
Adults	12–20
Older adults	15–20

The ability of the respiratory system to deliver oxygen to the blood depends on inflated and well-oxygenated alveoli and well-perfused alveolar capillaries. The movement of oxygen across the alveolar–capillary membrane into a capillary is represented by the **ventilation-perfusion (V-Q)** ratio. The concentrations of oxygen and carbon dioxide dictate the movement of each gas across the alveolar–capillary membrane.

Alterations to Oxygenation

Hypoxemia refers to a decreased level of oxygen in the blood. Left untreated, hypoxemia may result in decreased delivery of oxygen to the tissues, or **hypoxia**. Even mild impairments in oxygenation can cause fatigue, irritability, and discomfort. More severe alterations in oxygenation may be fatal if left untreated.

Alterations and Manifestations

Alterations in oxygenation can be described in the context of gas exchange, airway patency, and respiratory patterns. Damage to the supporting thoracic structures, either by injury or disease, can interfere with effective respiration. Irritation or inflammation of the respiratory mucosa also affects the ability of the respiratory system to obtain adequate oxygenation for the cells within the body.

Gas Exchange

As previously discussed, the level of carbon dioxide in arterial blood is a primary stimulus for ventilation. From the standpoint of acid–base balance, carbon dioxide levels fluctuate in response to the blood's hydrogen ion concentration. To be more specific, in healthy individuals the respiratory drive is primarily stimulated by the concentration of hydrogen ions $[H^+]$ in the arterial blood, which varies in direct response to the arterial blood concentration of carbon dioxide (CO_2).

An increase in the arterial blood's $[H^+]$ causes a corresponding increase in the arterial blood level of CO_2; in turn, the blood pH decreases (i.e., the blood becomes more acidic). By contrast, a decrease in $[H^+]$ causes the blood level of CO_2 to decrease and, as a result, the blood pH increases (i.e., the blood becomes more alkaline). However, a healthy respiratory system is capable of compensating for an increase or decrease in arterial blood CO_2.

An increase in CO_2 in the bloodstream typically triggers an increase in ventilation. Increasing the rate and/or depth of ventilations increases the release of CO_2, which in turn

another without friction during inspiration and expiration. The region between the visceral and parietal pleura is called the **pleural space**.

The nature and quality of breath sounds vary depending on the site of auscultation. For example, **bronchial sounds** are loud, high-pitched sounds heard over the trachea. Bronchial sounds are longer on exhalation than inhalation. **Bronchovesicular sounds**, which are medium in loudness and pitch, are heard on each side of the sternum and between the scapulae. Bronchovesicular sounds typically are equal in duration during inspiration and expiration. **Vesicular sounds** are soft, low-pitched sounds that are heard over the peripheral lung fields. Vesicular sounds, which are most prominently heard in the lung bases, typically are longer on inhalation than exhalation (Sarkar et al., 2015).

The drive to breathe largely depends on the level of carbon dioxide in the arterial blood. Receptor sites within the medulla and pons are sensitive to blood carbon dioxide levels. When carbon dioxide levels rise, these receptors respond by stimulating an increase in the rate and/or depth of ventilation. The typical breathing rate is regularly spaced, with inspiration half as long as expiration (I:E [ratio of inspiration to expiration] = 1:2). Normal respiratory rates range from 30–80 breaths per minute in newborns to 12–20 breaths per minute in an adult. **Table 15–1 »** shows normal respiratory ranges for various age groups. Quality of breathing refers to the effort involved in taking a breath and the sounds that may occur with inspiration or expiration. Effective breathing requires a **patent airway**, meaning an airway that is open and free of obstruction.

Receptor sites in the aortic arch and carotid arteries monitor oxygen levels. These receptors induce inspiration when oxygen levels fall below normal. Stretch receptors within the lungs control the volume of air inhaled with each breath. During relaxed states, the lungs will fill to approximately 500 mL. Strenuous exercise results in deeper breaths of increasing volume to meet the oxygen demands of skeletal muscles.

decreases the amount of CO_2 in the bloodstream. The opposite is also true. The respiratory system typically responds to a decrease in blood CO_2 by decreasing the rate and/or depth of ventilations, which allows for the buildup of CO_2 in the bloodstream. This manner of compensation allows for maintenance of the correct amount of arterial CO_2, which is necessary to maintain the proper acid–base balance in the bloodstream. As previously discussed, the exchange of oxygen and CO_2 occurs in the alveoli; thus, alveolar function is critical not only to oxygenation, but also to maintaining the body's delicate acid–base balance. Intact neural function also is essential to respiratory function.

Both impaired neural regulation and damaged alveoli can limit the respiratory system's ability to compensate for increases or decreases in blood CO_2. For example, **chronic obstructive pulmonary disease (COPD)** often is associated with an increased level of carbon dioxide in the blood. For individuals with emphysema, which is one form of COPD, alveolar damage limits the exchange of oxygen and carbon dioxide; as a result, these individuals retain carbon dioxide. (See the module on Acid–Base Balance for more detailed discussion of acid–base imbalances and the mechanisms by which the body compensates for these alterations.)

Along with CO_2 retention, individuals with COPD often experience a chronic decrease in blood oxygen levels. As previously discussed, hypoxemia refers to a decreased level of oxygen in the blood, while hypoxia refers to a decrease in delivery of oxygen to the tissues. **Retractions**, which manifest as a drawing in of the chest wall, are an early indicator of hypoxia. **Cyanosis**, a bluish discoloration of the skin and mucous membranes, is a late sign of hypoxia. In individuals

with darker pigmentation, cyanosis may present as gray discoloration of the skin. An indicator of chronic hypoxemia is clubbed nail beds. Clubbed nail beds have an angle of 180° or greater, depending on the duration of time an individual has had hypoxemia.

Abnormalities within the alveolar–capillary bed system alter V-Q ratios. Airflow in an alveolus blocked by sputum, inflammation with its complementary swelling, atelectasis, or fluid volume excesses can cause decreased ventilation. Blood clots, plaque buildup, and emphysemic alveoli interfere with capillary blood flow. Each of these V-Q mismatches results in inadequate oxygenation of body cells. Any and all of these types of V-Q mismatch may occur simultaneously (see **Figure 15–4 >>**).

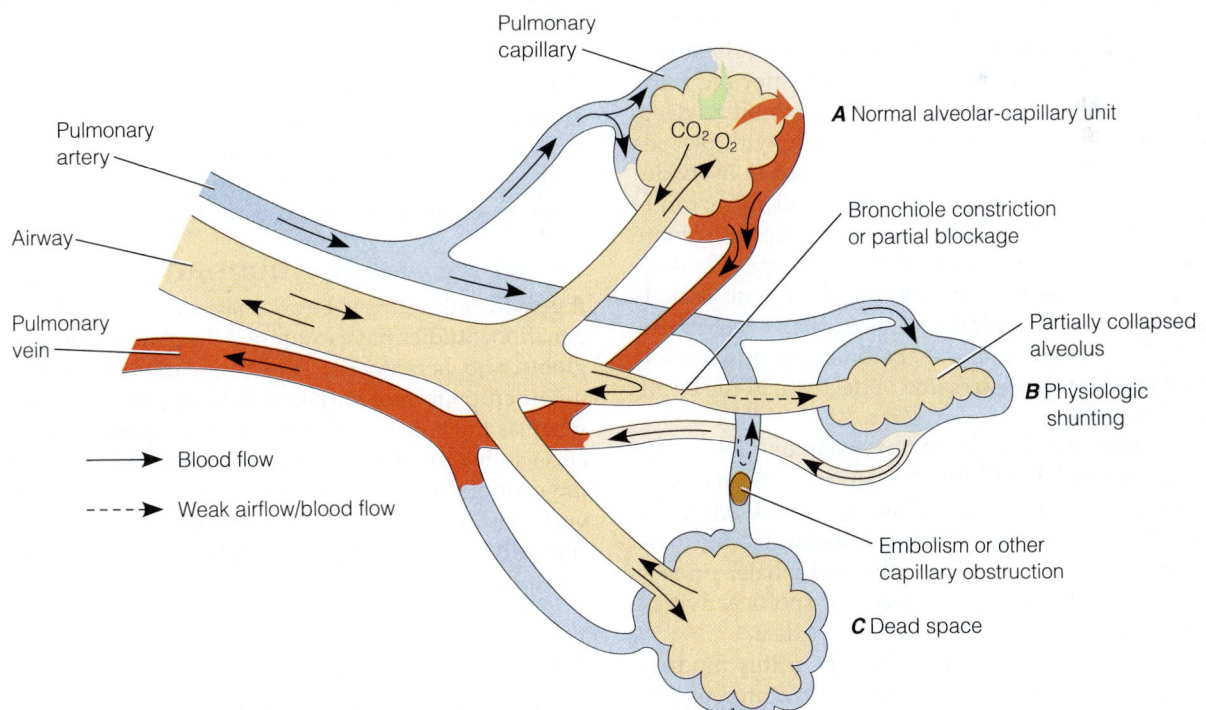

Figure 15–4 >> Ventilation–perfusion relationships. **A,** Normal alveolar–capillary unit with an ideal match of ventilation and blood flow. Maximum gas exchange occurs between alveolus and blood. **B,** Physiologic shunting: a unit with adequate perfusion but inadequate ventilation. **C,** Dead space: a unit with adequate ventilation but inadequate perfusion. In the latter two cases, gas exchange is impaired.

Airway Patency

Loss of airway patency can result from increased sputum production from upper and lower respiratory infection or irritation. Thick sputum secretions are of special concern in relation to blocking large and small airways. Inflammation of airways due to infections or irritants narrows airways, decreasing the movement of air through the respiratory system. Airway obstruction is the primary cause of atelectasis, which, as previously discussed, refers to the collapse of all or part of a lung, affecting the exchange of oxygen and carbon dioxide.

Respiratory Patterns

Respiratory rate, rhythm, depth, and quality determine adequate oxygenation to the cells. A respiratory rate greater than 20 breaths per minute in adults is called **tachypnea**. Anxiety or stress may cause an individual to breathe very rapidly, inhaling and exhaling deeply. **Hyperventilation** is rapid and deep inhalation and exhalation of air from the lungs. In **hypoventilation**, an abnormally slow respiratory rate leads to inadequate oxygen delivery to the lungs as well as an increase in retention of carbon dioxide. A respiratory rate of less than 10 breaths per minute in adults is called **bradypnea**. *Respiratory arrest* is characterized by **apnea**, which is the absence of breathing.

Dyspnea, labored breathing or shortness of breath that is uncomfortable or painful, also occurs when breathing is insufficient to meet oxygen demand. Exertional dyspnea occurs with activity. **Orthopnea** is difficulty breathing when in the supine position. Several breathing patterns with irregular rates, rhythms, depth, and quality indicate abnormalities within other body systems. Kussmaul breathing occurs in the presence of metabolic acidosis and results in very deep and rapid breaths. These deep, rapid exhalations increase the elimination of carbon dioxide, affecting acid–base balance. Cheyne-Stokes respirations exhibit as deep, rapid breathing and slow, shallow breathing with periods of apnea. Cheyne-Stokes respirations are seen in individuals with congestive heart failure, increased intracranial pressure (ICP), and drug overdoses. Biot respirations are seen in individuals with central nervous system disorders. Biot respirations present as shallow breathing with periods of apnea. As a result of central nervous system effects, medications such as benzodiazepines, barbiturates, and opioids may cause **respiratory depression**, a decrease in the depth and rate of breathing.

Any alteration that impairs the oxygenation process can be life-threatening. In addition to determining and then treating the presenting alteration, nurses should determine its cause. A mild case of exercise-induced asthma may require only administration of an albuterol inhaler prior to the individual participating in exercise or sports activities. By contrast, COPD is much more difficult to treat.

In addition to the exemplars detailed in this module, other diseases and some injuries, such as a fractured pleural rib, can cause impairment in oxygenation. Sickle cell disease, an inherited blood disorder, impairs the transport of oxygen through the blood and can cause a variety of complications, including organ failure (see the module on Cellular Regulation for more information).

Pneumothorax

Normal lung inflation occurs as a result of a vacuum effect. Expansion of the chest cavity during inspiration creates a negative pressure inside the pleural space, which causes expansion of the lungs. However, air entry into the pleural space—either through an opening in the chest wall or by way of an opening in the lung—causes a loss of the negative pressure that is needed to produce lung expansion. With the entry of air into the pleural space, the pressure between the pleural space and the outside of the body is equalized, leading to a loss of the vacuum effect and subsequent lung collapse. This condition is referred to as **pneumothorax**. Signs and symptoms of a pneumothorax include sudden sharp pleuritic pain, worsened by movement such as breathing and coughing; decreased or absent breath sounds over the affected side; asymmetrical chest wall movement; shortness of breath; and cyanosis.

A pneumothorax that occurs without any identifiable cause is termed a *spontaneous pneumothorax*. Risk factors for spontaneous pneumothorax also include respiratory disorders such as emphysema, cystic fibrosis, and tuberculosis. A *tension pneumothorax* typically results from a traumatic injury, such as a lung puncture caused by a fractured rib or a gunshot wound. Tension pneumothorax occurs when increasing intrapleural pressure causes compression and shifting of structures inside the mediastinum, such as the heart and the trachea. Tension pneumothorax is a life-threatening emergency that requires immediate decompression either through needle decompression or chest tube insertion.

Prevalence

The inability to oxygenate properly can occur at any point during the lifespan. Very young children (less than 1 year of age) and older adults (over the age of 65) are at increased risk for alterations in oxygenation. Very young children are more susceptible to respiratory disorders that affect oxygenation. Older adults carry an increased risk of developing a variety of health impairments (e.g., respiratory ailments, cardiovascular issues) that can affect oxygenation.

Genetic Considerations and Risk Factors

A genetic link seems to be associated with alterations in oxygenation. Studies have examined the genetic effect of hemoglobin and hematocrit. There appears to be a significant inherited pattern of variation in hemoglobin concentration, whereas the hematocrit shows a lower genetic effect. Differences in hemoglobin concentration and hematocrit between the genders add to the evidence of genetic control of these variables and, therefore, the ability to oxygenate. Women typically have lower concentrations of hemoglobin and hematocrit compared to men (Kravitz & Robergs, 2013).

Case Study >> Part 1

Melissa Dawson is a 30-year-old woman who was diagnosed with severe persistent asthma as a young child. She presents at her pulmonologist's office at 0900 on Thursday after calling and requesting to be worked in because she is not "getting enough air." As the nurse working with Ms. Dawson's pulmonologist, you conduct her patient interview and initial assessment when she comes to the clinic.

It takes a little time to get through the patient interview; Ms. Dawson can speak only a few words at a time and appears short of breath. Ms. Dawson reports that she came down with bronchitis over the holiday weekend and went to an urgent care clinic to get an antibiotic. The physician's assistant at the clinic prescribed a Z-pack (azithromycin). Ms. Dawson states she has been on 40 mg prednisone since Monday for asthma symptoms and has been using her rescue inhaler 4 times daily in addition to her Flovent Diskus (fluticasone) inhaler. Ms. Dawson tells you that she woke up in the middle of the night unable to get enough air and that her nail beds were blue. She used her rescue inhaler, and her symptoms improved enough that she decided not to go the emergency department but to wait and call the office first thing this morning.

You observe that Ms. Dawson is holding back tears. She is sitting on the exam table leaning forward with her hands on her knees. Her voice is hoarse. Her face is pale, and she has dark rings around her eyes. Ms. Dawson tells you her voice gets hoarse only when she is very, very sick. On taking her vitals, you note that Ms. Dawson's blood pressure is elevated and her respirations are 32. Her oxygen saturation (SaO_2) is 91% on room air. When you auscultate her lungs, you hear decreased breath sounds. The pulmonologist puts her on 4 L/min oxygen by nasal cannula.

Clinical Reasoning Questions Level I

1. Which of Ms. Dawson's signs and symptoms are consistent with altered oxygenation?
2. Why might Ms. Dawson's blood pressure be high?
3. Why might Ms. Dawson be close to tears?

Clinical Reasoning Questions Level II

4. What is the priority nursing diagnosis for Ms. Dawson at this time?
5. What independent nursing interventions can you perform to help make Ms. Dawson more comfortable while she waits for the specialist?
6. *Refer to Exemplar 15.B on Asthma:* What additional interventions should the nurse anticipate implementing as part of Ms. Dawson's immediate care?

Concepts Related to Oxygenation

Inadequate levels of oxygenation can affect acid–base balance. Decreased levels of oxygen can lead to a condition known as respiratory acidosis, in which levels of CO_2 increase, resulting in vasodilation of the vessels. The patient experiences increased ICP and an increased heart rate.

A decrease in oxygen levels in the blood can also affect cellular regulation. When oxygenation is decreased, as seen with anemia or blood loss, the systemic workload increases, and blood is shunted from the periphery to the vital organs.

Patients with impaired oxygenation may also experience cognitive impairment. Patients may exhibit memory loss, may have slurred speech, or may appear incoherent. Nurses must carefully assess patients with signs of impaired cognition in order to rule out acute brain injury.

Alterations and Therapies
Oxygenation

ALTERATION	DESCRIPTION	MANIFESTATIONS	INTERVENTIONS AND THERAPIES
Hypoxemia	Decreased level of oxygen	▪ Chest wall in-drawing (early manifestation) ▪ Cyanosis (late manifestation)	▪ Identify and treat the underlying cause. ▪ Administer oxygen if O_2 saturation level falls below 90%.
Dyspnea	Labored breathing or shortness of breath	▪ Clearly audible, labored breathing; anxiety ▪ Distressed facial expression ▪ Nasal flaring	▪ Identify and treat the underlying cause. ▪ Administer oxygen if O_2 saturation level falls below 90%.
Apnea	Absence of breathing	▪ Lack of respiratory effort that can lead to respiratory arrest	▪ Identify and treat the underlying cause. ▪ Administer respiratory stimulants, as appropriate.
Tachypnea	A respiratory rate greater than 20 breaths per minute for children and adults, 60 breaths per minute for an infant	▪ Excessive rapid breathing ▪ Rapid breathing at rest ▪ Shallow breathing	▪ Identify and treat the underlying cause.
Orthopnea	Difficulty breathing when lying down	▪ Dyspnea while lying down	▪ Identify and treat the underlying cause. ▪ Elevate the head, neck, and chest while sleeping.
Pneumothorax	Lung collapse caused by the collection of free air within the pleural space	▪ Chest pain ▪ Shortness of breath	▪ Identify and treat the underlying cause. ▪ Observe the patient. ▪ Use needle decompression or chest tube insertion. ▪ Surgery

Concepts Related to
Oxygenation

CONCEPT	RELATIONSHIP TO OXYGENATION	NURSING IMPLICATIONS
Acid–Base Balance	$\uparrow CO_2 \rightarrow$ vasodilation $\rightarrow \uparrow$ ICP and pulse rate.	■ Patient may have headache, irritability, $\downarrow$ LOC, and flushed skin. ■ May be seen in patients with chest trauma, aspiration, pneumonia, or overdose. ■ Be alert to patients with problems related to airway clearance, limited ambulation, anxiety, or signs/symptoms of $\downarrow O_2$.
Cellular Regulation	$\downarrow O_2$ increases systemic workload and shunts blood from periphery to vital organs.	■ Be alert to signs/symptoms of fatigue, pallor, jaundice, and tachycardia. ■ Anticipate the need for vitamin supplements, blood transfusions, and dietary changes. ■ Consider activity intolerance.
Cognition	$\downarrow O_2$ to brain can cause changes in cognition.	■ Assess mentation. Rule out acute brain trauma before considering other causes.
Comfort	$\downarrow O_2$ to tissues manifests as pain.	■ Assess related symptoms such as $\uparrow$ pulse, respirations, BP, restlessness, anxiety, diaphoresis, and patient reports of discomfort. ■ Anticipate need for additional assessments, medications for pain relief, and diversional therapies.
Perfusion	$\downarrow$ Tissue perfusion creates oxygen deficit to organs.	■ Assess perfusion, including pulses, nail beds, color, and body position for comfort and orientation. ■ Administer oxygen. ■ Anticipate the need for pharmacotherapy to improve cardiac output. ■ Anticipate surgery to correct a defect. ■ Monitor arterial blood gases.
Stress and Coping	$\uparrow$ Difficulty breathing $\rightarrow$ anxiety, fear, fatigue, and difficulty with activities of daily living.	■ Ensure adequate oxygenation. ■ Promote balance between activity and rest. ■ Limit all unnecessary environmental stressors (e.g., harsh lighting, loud noises). ■ Explain expected outcomes of treatments/procedures. ■ Acknowledge the patient's fear/anxiety and provide reassurance.

Perfusion can also be affected by inadequate amounts of oxygen in the blood. Decreased tissue perfusion creates oxygen deficit to organs. The patient may exhibit changes in pulse rate and blood pressure due to an increased workload on the heart. Color, capillary refill, and orientation may be affected because of decreased oxygenation to the tissues. The Concepts Related to Oxygenation feature links some, but not all, of the concepts integral to oxygenation. They are presented in alphabetical order.

Health Promotion

A number of factors can affect a healthy respiratory system. Exposure to airborne irritants (e.g., cigarette smoke, pollen, chemicals, pollution) may produce an inflammatory response within the airways. Infectious illnesses of the respiratory tract and hemoglobin disorders such as sickle cell disease interfere with effective respiratory function. Lifestyle behaviors may affect respiratory health. Some medications affect respiratory rate and depth. Inflammation, infection, sputum production, and compromised airflow generally contribute to alterations in respiratory health. *Healthy People 2020* has several directives related to promoting respiratory health (Centers for Disease Control and Prevention [CDC], 2016). These include directives to manage environmental air quality to decrease the concentration of respiratory irritants affecting asthma and COPD in the United States, and programs to encourage the use of vaccination to decrease the transmission of preventable diseases, many of which are transmitted by respiratory secretions.

Modifiable Risk Factors

Several modifiable risk factors are associated with alterations in oxygenation. Any alteration that affects the heart's ability to pump and circulate blood throughout the body, such as hypertension or atherosclerosis, can cause alterations in oxygenation as the blood carries and circulates oxygen. Other modifiable risk factors that affect the body's ability to oxygenate properly include obesity, type 2 diabetes, smoking, and stress and anxiety. Taking control of these variables can promote oxygenation and respiratory health.

Smoking and Tobacco Cessation

Tobacco smoke exposure causes increased mucus production and reduced cilia action within the airway passages. Individuals who smoke present with a chronic cough due to airway irritation and excessive mucus production. Prolonged exposure to tobacco smoke yields a decline in pulmonary function due to damage to pulmonary structures. Because the capacity of the respiratory system to compensate is great, the sense of pulmonary decline occurs well after irreversible damage has occurred. All healthcare providers should encourage smoking cessation and advise nonsmoking individuals to avoid secondary smoke.

Tobacco use is more than a habit; it is an addiction. If the patient opts to continue smoking or using tobacco, the nurse should show respect for the patient's decision and the right to choose. Nicotine replacement therapy (NRT) may be appropriate for some patients, particularly during extended periods of hospitalization. Among smokers who are admitted to the intensive care unit (ICU) or a general medical unit, research suggests that NRT in combination with behavioral counseling increases the likelihood of abstinence (Goldwire, Lehano, & Ostenson, 2015). Forms of NRT include patches, lozenges, gum, oral inhalers, and nasal spray (Goldwire et al., 2015). The nurse should help the patient who expresses an interest in quitting in developing a plan and provide a referral to a support group or to a counselor or other professional as needed. Counselors or other people trained to assist with smoking cessation can help with decision making. For more information, see the exemplar on Nicotine Use in the module on Addiction. **Table 15–2 »** lists strategies to decrease tobacco use.

Nursing Assessment

Assessment of a patient's respiratory system includes both subjective and objective data obtained through physical assessment and taking the patient's health history. Note that the following signs and symptoms signal hypoxia:

- Increasing restlessness, irritability, or unexplained sudden confusion
- Rapid heart rate accompanied by a rapid respiratory rate.

Observation and Patient Interview

During the health history, the nurse elicits information on lifestyle behaviors, any current trouble breathing, presence of cough or sputum, and any risk factors (e.g., occupational exposure to chemicals, allergies, recent illness, cigarette smoking).

Current Respiratory Problems

- Have you noticed any changes in your breathing pattern (e.g., shortness of breath, difficulty breathing, need to be in upright position to breathe, rapid and shallow breathing)?
- If so, which of your activities might cause these symptoms to occur?
- How many pillows do you use to sleep at night?

History of Respiratory Disease

- Have you had colds, allergies, asthma, tuberculosis, bronchitis, pneumonia, or emphysema?
- How frequently have these occurred? How long did they last? And how were they treated?
- Have you been exposed to any pollutants?

Lifestyle

- Do you smoke? If so, how much? If not, did you smoke previously, and when did you stop?
- Does any member of your family smoke?
- Is there cigarette smoke or are there other pollutants (e.g., fumes, dust, coal, asbestos) in your workplace?
- Do you drink alcohol? If so, how many drinks (mixed drinks, glasses of wine, or beers) do you usually have per day or per week?
- Describe your exercise patterns. How often do you exercise and for how long?

Presence of Cough

- How often and how much do you cough?
- Is it productive (i.e., accompanied by sputum) or nonproductive (i.e., dry)?
- Does the cough occur during a certain activity or at certain times of the day?

TABLE 15–2 Interventions for Tobacco Cessation

	Hospital	Community
ASSESS	■ Assess and document tobacco use on admission. ■ Assess history of attempts to quit, including what was helpful and what was not. ■ Assess willingness to quit at this time.	■ Assess and document tobacco use, history of attempts to quit, and willingness to quit at every healthcare interaction.
ASSIST	■ Seek NRT during hospitalizations and suggest to individuals who have had NRT during hospitalization that they are on their way to quitting. ■ Provide tobacco cessation publications and teach about physiologic consequences of tobacco use with daily care interactions such as taking vital signs.	■ Request a tobacco cessation medication order from the primary care provider. ■ Provide resources for counseling and support groups for the individual willing to attempt to quit tobacco use.
ARRANGE	■ Collaborate with individuals who desire to quit to arrange tobacco cessation support group contacts and request in-hospital tobacco cessation teaching.	■ Establish a plan for follow-up contact for the individual willing to attempt to quit tobacco use within 1 week of the quit date. ■ Continue to ask tobacco users about quitting tobacco use at each visit.

Source: Based on the Tobacco Cessation Clinical Practice Guidelines as established by the U.S. Department of Health and Human Services, https://www.ahrq.gov/professionals/clinicians-providers/guidelines-recommendations/tobacco/clinicians/references/quickref/index.html

Description of Sputum

- When is the sputum produced?
- What is the amount, color, thickness, and odor of the sputum?
- Is it ever tinged with blood?

Presence of Chest Pain

- How does going outside in the heat or the cold affect you?
- Do you experience any pain with breathing or activity?
- Where is the pain located?
- Describe the pain. How does it feel?
- Does it occur when you breathe in or out?
- How long does it last, and how does it affect your breathing?
- Do you experience any other symptoms when the pain occurs (e.g., nausea, shortness of breath or difficulty breathing, light-headedness, palpitations)?
- What activities precede your pain?
- What do you do to relieve the pain?

Presence of Risk Factors

- Do you have a family history of lung cancer, cardiovascular disease (including strokes), or tuberculosis?
- The nurse should also note the patient's weight, activity pattern, and dietary assessment. Risk factors include obesity, sedentary lifestyle, and diet high in saturated fats.

Medication History

- Have you taken or do you take any over-the-counter or prescription medications for breathing (e.g., bronchodilator, inhalant, narcotic)?
- If so, which ones? And what are the dosages, times taken, and results, including side effects? Are you taking them exactly as directed?

Physical Examination

Physical assessment begins with simple observation during the initial interaction with the patient. The assessment of any body system requires a systematic approach using all five senses to ensure that nothing is missed. The nurse uses his or her eyes to observe expected and unexpected findings, a process called *inspection*. The nurse uses **palpation** to feel the areas related to the body system for **symmetry**, equality of the size, shape, or condition of opposite sides of the body. Next, the nurse uses **percussion**, a method of tapping the chest or back to assess underlying structures; tones heard during percussion determine solid-filled or air-filled spaces at the area percussed. Finally, the nurse uses auscultation to hear the sounds within the respiratory system. Use of a stethoscope facilitates the hearing of sounds within the body. Any assessment is best supported by obtaining a full set of vital sign measurements with pulse oximetry.

Adventitious Breath Sounds

Adventitious breath sounds are abnormal breath sounds that may be heard on lung auscultation. Examples of adventitious breath sounds include the following:

- **Stridor** is a high-pitched sound within the trachea and larynx that suggests narrowing of the tracheal passage.

- **Crackles** are high-pitched popping sounds, much like when milk pours over crisped rice cereal. Crackles are heard on inspiration and are caused by fluid associated with or resulting from inflammation or exudates within the lung fields or localized atelectasis. **Atelectasis** is the collapse of all or part of a lung affecting the exchange of oxygen and carbon dioxide. Obstruction is the primary cause of atelectasis. Causes of obstructive atelectasis include mucus plugs, foreign objects, and airway stenosis (narrowing) due to disease (Mayo Clinic, 2015a). Atelectasis also may be the result of nonobstructive factors. For example, shallow respirations can lead to the development of nonobstructive atelectasis. Conditions such as pneumonia, pneumothorax, and pleural effusion also may cause nonobstructive atelectasis (Mayo Clinic, 2015a).

- **Rhonchi** are coarse, low-pitched sounds that continue throughout inspiration. Rhonchi may indicate blockage of large airway passages, which can sometimes be cleared with coughing.

- **Wheezing** is a high-pitched whistling sound most often heard on expiration and caused by the narrowing of bronchi, but wheezes can also be heard on inspiration. Unlike rhonchi, wheezes typically do not disappear after coughing (Bohadana, Izbicki, & Kraman, 2014).

- **Pleural friction rub** is associated with pleural inflammation and occurs when inflamed pleural surfaces slide across one another. This low-pitched, crackling sound typically is present during both inspiration and expiration (Bohadana et al., 2014).

Patient Presentation

The patient who presents with breathing problems may provide a number of objective and subjective indicators that confirm the report. Self-posturing (leaning forward or against a table or wall to breathe) may be evident. A patient may have difficulty speaking, taking breaths in the middle of sentences. The individual's voice may be raspy. In the absence of a productive cough, repeated throat clearing may indicate the presence of phlegm. Individuals who cannot breathe well often become frustrated when answering questions because the effort to answer further impairs breathing, and the effort to breathe quickly brings on fatigue. A pulse oximetry reading that is within normal limits does not always mean the patient is breathing effectively. For example, a pulse oximetry reading above 90% may not be a true indicator of the level of respiratory distress if the patient has used an albuterol inhaler within the past 30–60 minutes of presenting at the clinic or emergency department. Increased frequency of use of albuterol inhalers or nebulizer treatments indicates a severe respiratory episode. See the Oxygenation Assessment for an outline of the assessment procedure.

Patients who present with impairment at or near respiratory failure will not be able to respond to questions. Assessment questions should be tailored and asked of any family member or friend accompanying the patient to the emergency department. The patient's regular healthcare provider should be notified immediately on the patient's arrival at the hospital. The immediate concern is to return the patient's respiratory status as near to normal as possible.

Oxygenation Assessment

ASSESSMENT/ METHOD	NORMAL FINDINGS	ABNORMAL FINDINGS	LIFESPAN OR DEVELOPMENTAL CONSIDERATIONS
Nasal Assessment			
Inspect the nose symmetry.	The nose should be midline and symmetrical.	■ Asymmetry indicates trauma or surgery.	■ Nasal flaring in the neonate may be indicative of respiratory compromise.
Inspect nasal cavity using a flashlight.	The septum should fall midline and be intact. The mucosa of the nares should be pink and moist without drainage. Both nares should be patent.	■ Redness and/or swelling is observed. ■ Deviated septum narrows or occludes one naris. ■ Foreign bodies may be found in the nares, especially of infants, toddlers, and preschoolers. ■ Purulent or watery nasal drainage is present. ■ Pale turbinates are seen.	■ Nasal passages of neonates and small children are smaller than those of adults. Ensuring a clear nasal cavity may decrease the risk for respiratory compromise, as neonates and infants are nasal breathers.
Respiratory Rate Assessment			
Count respiratory rate for one full minute, counting one inspiration and one expiration as one breath.	Normal respiratory rate is eupnea (see Table 15–1 for developmental impact on rate).	■ Bradypnea ■ Tachypnea ■ Apnea ■ Cheyne-Stokes respirations	■ A child's respiratory rate is higher than that of an adult's. Rely on both sight and touch to obtain an accurate respiratory rate. Neonates are sporadic breathers so short periods of apnea (less than 15 seconds) are expected.
Assess quality of breathing: determine regularity in timing. Assess depth of inspiration. Observe effort to breathe.	The I:E ratio is normally 1:2. The cycle of inspiration and expiration should be followed by a resting period in which the sensors of the respiratory system will initiate the next cycle. Normal breathing is referred to as eupnea.	■ Shortness of breath ■ Dyspnea ■ Orthopnea	■ Infants and children have softer chest walls and depend more heavily on the diaphragm to breathe. Therefore, they exhibit what is known as "seesaw" breathing, an indicator of severe distress. ■ In older adults, lifestyle choices such as smoking can affect the quality of breathing, as can the development of respiratory diseases.
Inspection of Thoracic Cavity			
Anteroposterior diameter is half the transverse diameter.	Normal ratio is 1:2. (See **Figures 15–5 》** and **15–6 》**.)	■ Anteroposterior equals transverse thoracic diameter measurements, called a barrel chest.	■ Rapid growth early in life, the plateau in young adulthood, and decline in later life can affect normal ratios.
Inspection of the Muscles of Breathing			
Observe muscles of breathing.	The chest wall gently rises and falls with each breath. The muscles in the neck are relaxed. The trachea is midline. The intercostal muscles raise the chest upward and outward with inhalation, then calmly relax with exhalation.	■ Retraction of the intercostals occurs. ■ Sternocleidomastoid muscles of the neck contract. ■ Posturing occurs.	■ Infants and children are more likely than adults to experience retractions and posturing with respiratory ailments. The adult patient is more likely to compensate in other ways.

(continued on next page)

Oxygenation Assessment (continued)

ASSESSMENT/METHOD	NORMAL FINDINGS	ABNORMAL FINDINGS	LIFESPAN OR DEVELOPMENTAL CONSIDERATIONS
Inspection and Palpation of the Thoracic Wall for Symmetry			
Assess thoracic wall.	Symmetrical movement of the hands is observed with symmetrical hand placement on the chest wall. The trachea is midline.	■ Asymmetry of movement occurs. ■ Decreased expansion occurs. ■ The trachea shifts from midline.	■ Rapid growth early in life, the plateau in young adulthood, and decline in later life can affect normal symmetry. Respiratory ailments can also affect thoracic wall symmetry.
Skin Assessment in Relation to the Respiratory System			
Assess color of skin.	Skin color should be normal for race or ethnicity.	Cyanosis is a blue tinge to the skin in fair individuals and gray coloration of the skin in darker pigmented individuals.	■ Acrocyanosis is a normal finding for neonates/newborns. Cyanosis at any other stage of development is considered an abnormal finding.
Assess nail beds.	Nail beds are an extension of the finger and are normally curved with a 160° angle of the nail bed to the finger.	Clubbed nail beds have an angle of 180° or greater, depending on the duration of time an individual has had hypoxemia.	■ Clubbing of the nails can occur with chronic cardiovascular or respiratory disease. Knowledge of the patient's baseline is essential to the assessment process.

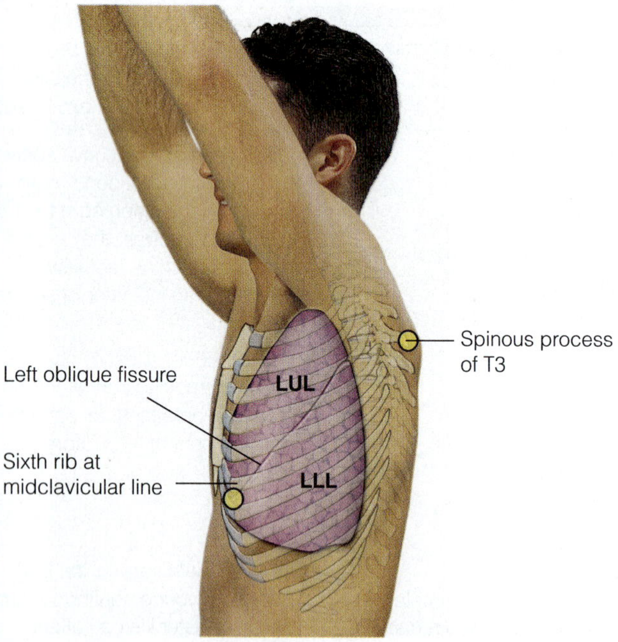

Figure 15–5 》 Lateral view of lobes of the left lung.

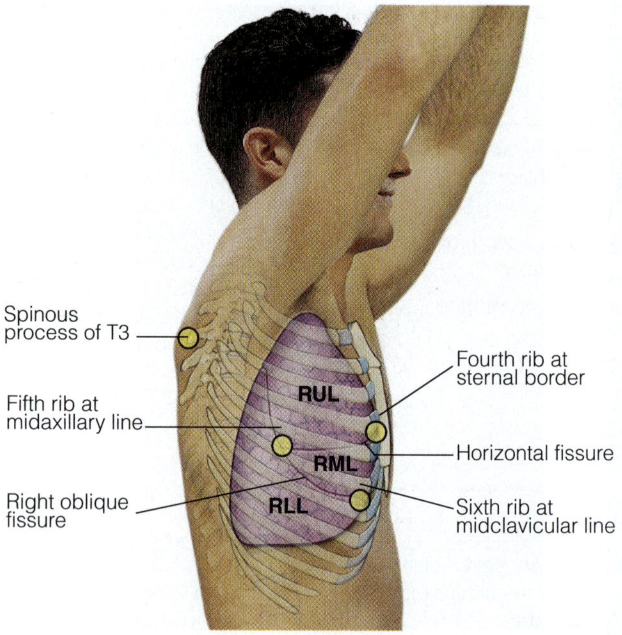

Figure 15–6 》 Lateral view of lobes of the right lung.

Diagnostic Tests

Specific diagnostic tests are used to assess for abnormalities of the respiratory system and to monitor for changes in individuals with chronic oxygenation impairment. Tests are used to determine the presence of inflammation or infection, detect changes in acid–base balance, and view thoracic structures.

A sputum specimen may be taken to identify the presence of microbes, metabolites of inflammation, and immunoglobulins. Sputum is expectorant matter that may contain mucus, cellular debris, blood, microorganisms, and/or purulent matter from the respiratory tract. Nurses should ensure that the liquid obtained from an individual is from the lung fields and not from spit from the mouth. Proper identification of

TABLE 15–3 Arterial Blood Gas Values

pH	7.35–7.45
$PaCO_2$	35–45 mmHg
PaO_2	75–100 mmHg
HCO_3^-	24–28 mEq/L

the microbe facilitates the selection of the appropriate antibiotic, antiviral, or antifungal agents to treat the inflammation. **Arterial blood gases (ABGs)** provide a direct indication of oxygen and carbon dioxide exchange and the acid–base balance within the blood. The major chemical components monitored by ABG are hydrogen ions (pH), carbon dioxide (CO_2), oxygen (O_2), and bicarbonate (HCO_3^-). See **Table 15–3** ≫ for normal ABG laboratory values. Each ABG component is reviewed in turn.

Initial assessment focuses on the oxygen-related values of the ABGs, including the arterial blood oxygen saturation (SaO_2) and the partial pressure of oxygen in the arterial blood (PaO_2). More specifically, the SaO_2 is a measure of the percentage of hemoglobin that is carrying oxygen. The PaO_2 is a measure of the amount of oxygen dissolved in the arterial blood. SaO_2 in a healthy individual without any respiratory abnormalities is greater than 95%. PaO_2 must be interpreted in the context of whether or not the patient is receiving oxygen therapy, as supplemental oxygen administration typically causes a significant increase in PaO_2. For the patient who is breathing room air, normal PaO_2 ranges from 75 to 100 mmHg (Kee, 2018).

Carbon dioxide values also are assessed. In the blood, normal carbon dioxide values range from 35 to 45 mmHg. An increase in blood levels of carbon dioxide to above 45 mmHg is referred to as **hypercarbia** (or **hypercapnia**). By contrast, **hypocarbia** (also known as **hypocapnia)** refers to a decrease in blood levels of carbon dioxide to below 35 mmHg. See the module on Acid–Base Balance for an in-depth discussion of ABGs.

The kidneys help maintain the body's acid–base balance by excreting or reabsorbing acids and bases. For example, the kidneys respond to an increase in the blood's acidity (which corresponds with a decrease in blood pH) by increasing renal reabsorption of bicarbonate (HCO_3^-), which is a base. In response to an increase in the blood's alkalinity (which corresponds with an increase in blood pH), the renal system increases bicarbonate excretion. Bicarbonate values range from 24 to 28 mEq/L.

The body naturally tends toward maintenance of **homeostasis**, a state of balance even in the presence of changing conditions, or *dynamic equilibrium*. Maintenance of blood pH is essential to promoting homeostasis. In relation to ABGs or acid–base balance, maintenance of homeostasis requires the body to alter carbon dioxide and bicarbonate levels in order to keep the blood pH level within a normal range of 7.35–7.45. A blood pH of less than 7.35 indicates acidosis, while a blood pH of greater than 7.45 indicates alkalosis (Kee, 2018). When one component of the acid–base balance equation changes in response to an alteration in the other component, this process is reflective of the body's attempt at *compensation*. For example, the individual who experiences kidney failure may also experience an increase

in respiratory rate. Increased ventilation allows for an increase in the removal of carbon dioxide from the body by way of expiration. See the module on Acid–Base Balance for a detailed discussion of the mechanisms involved in the physiologic regulation of serum pH.

Pulse oximetry is a noninvasive method of assessing arterial blood oxygenation. A clip or adhesive device with an infrared probe analyzes blood as it perfuses past the view of the two opposing sensors of the probe. Expected SaO_2 values in a healthy individual (one who has no alterations in pulmonary function) are greater than 95%.

Individuals who respond poorly to bronchodilators or who have poor oxygenation may benefit from assessment of their pulmonary function. Diagnosis and differentiation of reactive airway diseases necessitate the use of **pulmonary function tests (PFTs)**. PFTs demonstrate changes in pulmonary health related to ventilation airflow, lung volume and capacity, and the diffusion of gas. They also incorporate spirometry, peak flow meters, and the body plethysmograph. PFTs include measurement of inspired and expired air as well as the diffusion ability of the alveolar–capillary membrane. A spirometer is used to measure airflow and lung volumes. **Spirometry** measures inhalation and exhalation, although the key measurements are forced expiratory volume over 1 second (FEV_1) and the ratio of FEV_1 to forced vital capacity (FEV_1/FVC). In other words, how much and how quickly an individual exhales air as measured by spirometry is an indicator of the degree of pulmonary function deficit. **Box 15–1** ≫ diagrams all the PFTs. Results outside the anticipated range for the individual's age, gender, height, and weight may indicate the need to alter care interventions.

Peak expiratory flow rate (PEFR) is used to monitor the ability of an individual to exhale a specific volume of air related to the individual's age, gender, height, and weight. PEFR allows individuals with asthma to monitor the reactivity of their lungs and adjust asthma treatments according to the plan developed by the primary care or specialty provider and the individual. PEFR is not diagnostic for reactive airway diseases such as asthma and COPD.

An anterior–posterior **chest x-ray (CXR)** allows for two-dimensional visualization of the contents of the thoracic cavity. CXRs reveal the presence of fluids, exudates, or masses within the thoracic cavity. CT scans and MRIs provide more information about the structures within the thoracic cavity.

Thoracic CT produces cross-sectional images of the contents of the chest. It may be used with dye to determine the presence of pulmonary embolism. MRI allows for assessment of pulmonary embolism without the use of dye and is best for visualizing soft tissue and vascular structures. MRI is contraindicated in the individual who has implanted metal devices.

Pulmonary angiography and pulmonary V-Q scans demonstrate the ventilation and perfusion activities of the respiratory system. A pulmonary angiogram is used to identify structural changes in the pulmonary vasculature. Structural changes that cause occlusions may include blood clots, tumors, aneurysms, and overinflated alveoli. A pulmonary ventilation-perfusion scan (V-Q scan) uses radioactive isotopes to identify defects of ventilation and perfusion. Injected radioactive albumin helps identify defects of perfusion, whereas inhaled radioactive gas identifies defects of ventilation.

Box 15–1
Pulmonary Function Tests

Pulmonary function tests (PFTs) are performed in a pulmonary function laboratory. After preparing the patient, the nurse applies a nose clip, and the alert patient breathes into a spirometer or body plethysmograph, a device for measuring and recording lung volume in liters versus time in seconds. The nurse instructs the patient on how to breathe for specific tests; for example, to inhale as deeply as possible and then exhale to the maximal extent possible. Respiratory capacities are calculated using measured lung volumes to assess pulmonary status. The specific values determined by PFT and illustrated in **Figure 15–7 »** include the following:

- *Total lung capacity (TLC)* is the total volume of the lungs at their maximum inflation. Four values are used to calculate TLC:
  a. *Total volume (TV),* the volume inhaled and exhaled with normal quiet breathing (also called tidal volume)
  b. *Inspiratory reserve volume (IRV),* the maximum amount that can be inhaled over and above a normal inspiration
  c. *Expiratory reserve volume (ERV),* the maximum amount that can be exhaled following a normal exhalation
  d. *Residual volume (RV),* the amount of air remaining in the lungs after maximal exhalation.
- *Vital capacity (VC)* is the total amount of air that can be exhaled after a maximal inspiration. It is calculated by adding together the TV, IRV, and ERV.

- *Inspiratory capacity (IC)* is the total amount of air that can be inhaled following a normal quiet exhalation. It is calculated by adding the TV and IRV.
- *Functional residual capacity (FRC)* is the volume of air left in the lungs after a normal exhalation. The ERV and RV are added to determine the FRC.
- *Forced expiratory volume (FEV_1)* is the amount of air that can be exhaled in 1 second.
- *Forced vital capacity (FVC)* is the amount of air that can be exhaled forcefully and rapidly after maximum air intake.
- *Minute volume (MV)* is the total amount or volume of air breathed in 1 minute.

In older patients, residual capacity is increased and vital capacity is decreased. These age-related changes result from the following:

- Calcification of the costal cartilage and weakening of the intercostal muscles, which reduce movement of the chest wall
- Vertebral osteoporosis, which decreases spinal flexibility and increases the degree of kyphosis, further increasing the anterior–posterior diameter of the chest
- Diaphragmatic flattening and loss of elasticity.

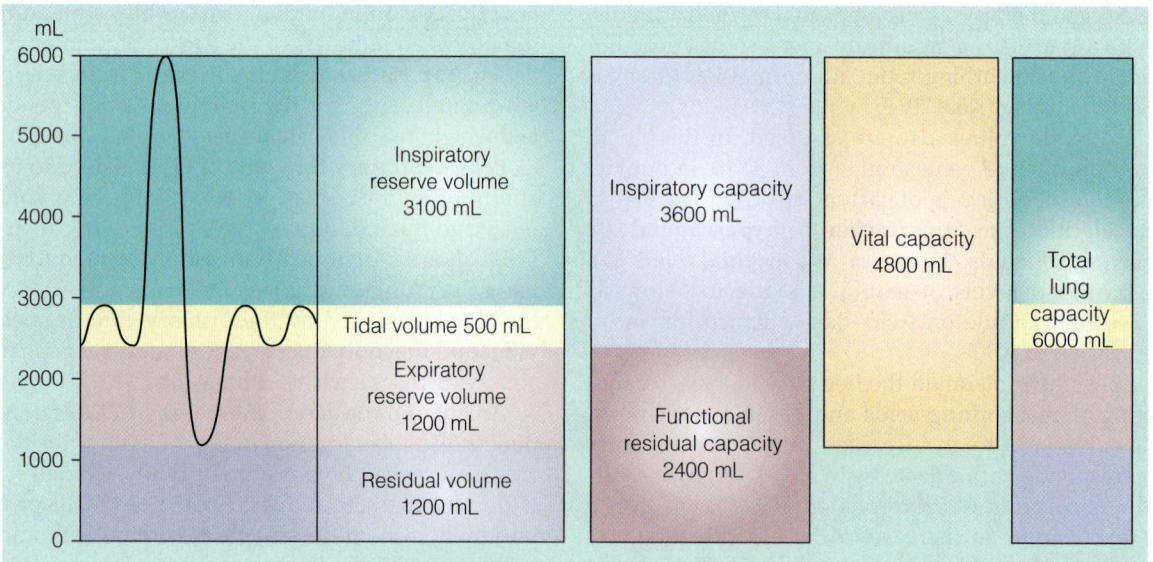

Figure 15–7 » The relationship of lung volumes and capacities. Volumes (in milliliters) shown are for an average adult man.

Bronchoscopy, a procedure that allows direct visualization of the lungs, is usually performed by a pulmonologist but may be performed by a primary care or emergency care physician. A bronchoscope is inserted orally into the trachea and advanced to the bronchi bifurcation. Bronchoscopy may be used for direct visualization and photography of pulmonary structures, suctioning of mucous plugs from larger bronchioles, and collection of lung tissue biopsy specimens. Sedation is necessary for patient comfort.

Thoracentesis is both an intervention and a diagnostic test. Thoracentesis is performed to drain excessive pleural fluid from between the pleural linings. The fluid drained is often analyzed for blood, fiber, and microbe content.

Case Study » Part 2

Ms. Dawson is prescribed Advair Diskus (fluticasone and salmeterol) to replace her Flovent Diskus and has a follow-up appointment in 7 days. She fills her prescription for Advair and begins using it later that evening. Upon trying to go to sleep, Ms. Dawson experiences difficulty breathing when lying down. She takes two puffs of her rescue inhaler and props herself up with three pillows and feels more comfortable. She falls asleep without difficulty.

At 0400 the next morning, Ms. Dawson awakens coughing. She gets up for a drink of water and continues to cough and has trouble catching her breath. She is sweating profusely and begins to feel dizzy. Ms. Dawson is able to make it back to her bed and calls her mother, but she is unable to explain her symptoms before passing out. Ms. Dawson's mother is concerned when her daughter does not respond. Aware of Ms. Dawson's recent exacerbation, she calls 911.

Ms. Dawson is transported to the emergency department. You are the admitting nurse in the emergency department. The paramedics give you their field report: 30-year-old woman found unconscious in her home. Vital signs upon initial assessment include temperature within normal limits; heart rate 100 bpm; respirations 28/min; and BP 140/92 mmHg. Paramedics report that initial pulse oximeter readings were 85%, but they improved to 90% with oxygen administration—8 L/min by face mask. Ms. Dawson is continued on 8 L/min oxygen by face mask in the emergency department. She is now alert and oriented but says she still feels like she cannot catch her breath. The current pulse oximeter reading is 93%. The physician on call orders a blood gas analysis, which is drawn per protocol.

Blood gas results reveal severe respiratory acidosis. You perform a follow-up respiratory assessment and note that breath sounds are significantly decreased and the patient appears cyanotic. Pulse oximeter readings have fallen to 90% despite increasing her oxygen to 10 L/min by face mask. Ms. Dawson is admitted to the hospital for further treatment.

Clinical Reasoning Questions Level I

1. Why would Ms. Dawson experience easier breathing with the use of pillows at bedtime?
2. Why does Ms. Dawson feel dizzy and pass out?
3. What does a pulse oximeter measure? Is this an accurate way to measure oxygenation?
4. Ms. Dawson's blood gas results reveal severe respiratory acidosis. What would you expect her ABG results to be?

Clinical Reasoning Questions Level II

5. Why did the pulmonologist add Advair to the current treatment regimen?
6. Why is the finding of significantly decreased breath sounds important?
7. *Refer to Exemplar 15.A on Acute Respiratory Distress Syndrome.* What independent interventions can you perform to help Ms. Dawson reduce her anxiety while she is on mechanical ventilation?

Independent Interventions

Independent nursing interventions for patients with alterations in oxygenation focus on improving gas exchange and enhancing breathing patterns. Examples of appropriate interventions include deep breathing exercises, positioning, encouraging smoking cessation, monitoring activity intolerance, promoting secretion clearance, suctioning, and assisting with activities of daily living (ADLs).

For all patients exhibiting signs of respiratory difficulty, nurses monitor vital signs, fluid status, and laboratory results. Tachypnea, tachycardia, an elevated blood pressure, and increasing hypoxemia and hypercapnia are signs of compromised respiratory status. Hypoxia and dyspnea can cause anxiety, which compounds the problem by increasing the respiratory rate. As always, administer medications, such as bronchodilators and anti-inflammatory drugs, as ordered and monitor for desired and adverse effects.

Deep Breathing Exercises

Individuals who experience alterations in oxygenation may benefit from deep breathing exercises. These exercises work on the body's sympathetic nervous system to influence the body's respiratory system. Controlling the effort of respiration can ultimately improve oxygenation.

Deep breathing exercises are also known as diaphragmatic, or abdominal, breathing. The diaphragm is forced down when it contracts, which in turn causes the abdomen to expand. The negative pressure this expansion causes within the chest forces air into the lungs while also pulling blood into the chest, thereby improving venous return to the heart.

Individuals perform deep breathing exercises in two steps:

1. Place one hand on the chest and the other hand on the abdomen and then take a deep breath. To ensure that the diaphragm is pulling air into the base of each lung, the hand on the abdomen should rise higher than the hand on the chest.
2. Depress the abdomen while exhaling through the mouth to ensure that all air is expelled.

It takes time and repetition to train the body in the technique of deep breathing, so the activity should be repeated several times a day.

Positioning

Positioning affects oxygenation. Fowler position may benefit individuals experiencing alterations in oxygenation (see **Figure 15–8 »**). Fowler position decreases the compression of the chest due to gravity to improve breathing.

Fowler position has several variations based on the elevation of the patient's head. In high-Fowler position, the patient's head is elevated 80–90 degrees; in standard Fowler position, 45–60 degrees; and in semi-Fowler position, 30–45 degrees. High-Fowler position may be used to feed a patient on feeding precautions or to deliver a breathing treatment. Fowler position may be used to increase comfort during eating and other activities. Semi-Fowler may be used for patients receiving tube feedings to decrease the risk for aspiration.

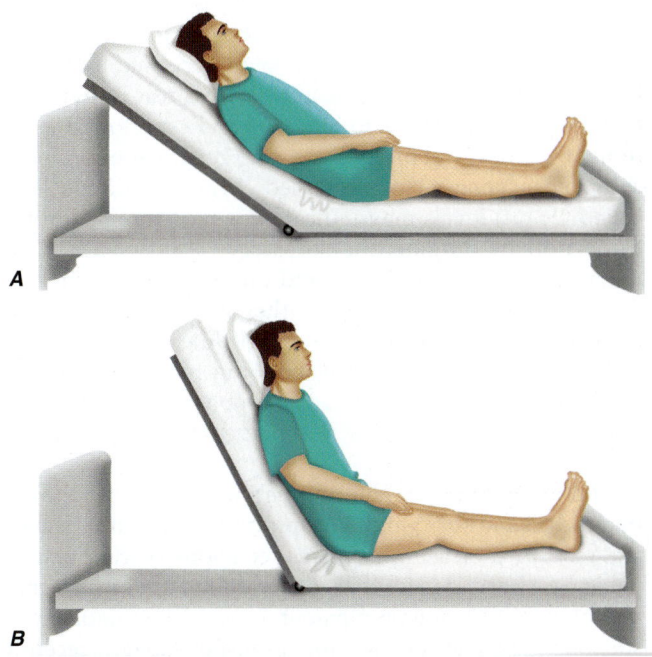

Figure 15–8 » *A,* Fowler position. *B,* High-Fowler position.

Monitor Activity Tolerance

Alterations in the respiratory system can affect activity levels. An individual may not have sufficient physiologic or psychologic energy to endure or complete required or desired daily activities. For the patient with poor oxygenation, fatigue or weakness can occur from participating in too many activities too close together. Dyspnea or shortness of breath occurs at varying points in an exercise program, depending on the individual's endurance level. Nurses may need to adapt schedules for patients who are hospitalized and alternate periods of activity with periods of rest. For patients who manage their treatment at home, the nurse may need to provide education related to activity tolerance.

Individuals who are too weak to provide their own care may need assistance with ADLs. The family and the healthcare team must collaborate to provide sufficient support to the individual with compromised oxygenation, while encouraging the individual to do as much as possible to maintain appropriate physical strength and prevent deteriorating physical or mental condition.

Promote Secretion Clearance

Lung sounds that indicate the presence of fluids or exudates will benefit from deep breaths and coughing to clear pulmonary secretions. Patients unable to clear their own secretions will require suction. Individuals who are producing sputum with a cough may require the collection of a sputum specimen. They may benefit from postural drainage to clear secretions from various lung fields. (See Volume 3: Clinical Nursing Skills for these skills.)

Suctioning

When patients have difficulty handling their secretions or an airway is in place, suctioning may be necessary to clear air passages. **Suctioning** is the aspiration of secretions through a catheter connected to a suction machine or wall suction outlet. Even though the upper airways (the oropharynx and nasopharynx) are not sterile, sterile technique is recommended for all suctioning to avoid introducing pathogens into the airways.

The nurse decides when suctioning is needed by assessing the patient for signs of respiratory distress or evidence that the patient is unable to cough up and expectorate secretions. Dyspnea, bubbling or rattling breath sounds, poor skin color (cyanosis), or decreased oxygen saturation (also called O_2 sat) levels may indicate the need for suctioning. Good nursing judgment is necessary, because suctioning irritates mucous membranes and can increase secretions if performed too frequently. In other words, suctioning is based on clinical need, not a fixed schedule.

Oral and oropharyngeal suctioning remove secretions from the upper respiratory tract. Nasopharyngeal and nasotracheal suctioning provide closer access to the trachea and requires sterile technique.

Following endotracheal intubation or a tracheostomy, the trachea and surrounding respiratory tissues are irritated and react by producing excessive secretions. Sterile suctioning is necessary to remove these secretions from the trachea and bronchi to maintain a patent airway. The frequency of suctioning depends on the patient's health and how recently the intubation was done. Suctioning may also be necessary in patients who have increased secretions because of pneumonia or inability to clear secretions because of altered level of consciousness (LOC).

Collaborative Therapies

An intervention or therapy that requires a medical order or that is implemented by other healthcare professionals is called a collaborative intervention. Improved nutrition, pharmacologic therapies, administration of oxygen, and use of a chest tube are all examples of collaborative interventions to improve oxygenation.

Nutrition Management

Individuals with respiratory alterations often need an increased calorie intake but lack the endurance to consume adequate nutrition. Increased calories are necessary because the increased work of breathing burns more calories. A nutritionist is able to assist the individual to select foods and supplements to meet daily caloric and nutritional needs. A nutritionist can guide the individual in developing menus consisting of frequent, small, nutritious meals.

Pharmacologic Therapy

Therapeutic management related to promoting and maintaining effective respiratory system function focuses on the individual's ability to maintain a patent airway through the automatic protective mechanisms in the upper and lower respiratory tracts. The ability of the individual to maintain breathing patterns within the acceptable rates and quality for the individual's age group is also assessed. Inspiration and expiration must provide adequate ventilation of the lung fields (see **Figure 15–9 》**). Individuals also must demonstrate an ability to breathe easily without the use of positioning or accessory muscles. Adequate alveolar gas exchange requires effective ventilation.

Bronchodilators may be administered to treat symptoms consistent with bronchoconstriction caused by disorders such as asthma and chronic bronchitis. Bronchodilators relax the smooth muscles of the airway, improving airflow. Common bronchodilators of short duration (short-acting beta-agonists, or SABAs) include levalbuterol (Xopenex) and albuterol (Proventil, Ventolin). Inflammation of the airways also contributes to impaired oxygenation.

The administration of oral or inhaled corticosteroids to reduce inflammation also may be ordered by the primary care or specialty care provider. Because oral steroids have a number of side effects, they are usually administered for a short period of time. Exogenous (i.e., obtained from a source outside the body) steroid administration can cause suppression of natural corticosteroid production by the adrenal glands. The degree of adrenal suppression that occurs is dependent on the length of medication therapy. Because of this, discontinuation of corticosteroid medications requires a progressive, step-wise reduction (tapering) of the medication. Abrupt discontinuation can cause adrenal crisis, which is characterized by manifestations associated with insufficient glucocorticoid production, such as profound hypotension, tachycardia, and cardiovascular collapse. For discussion of the effects of corticosteroids, see the module on Inflammation.

Inhalation

Exhalation

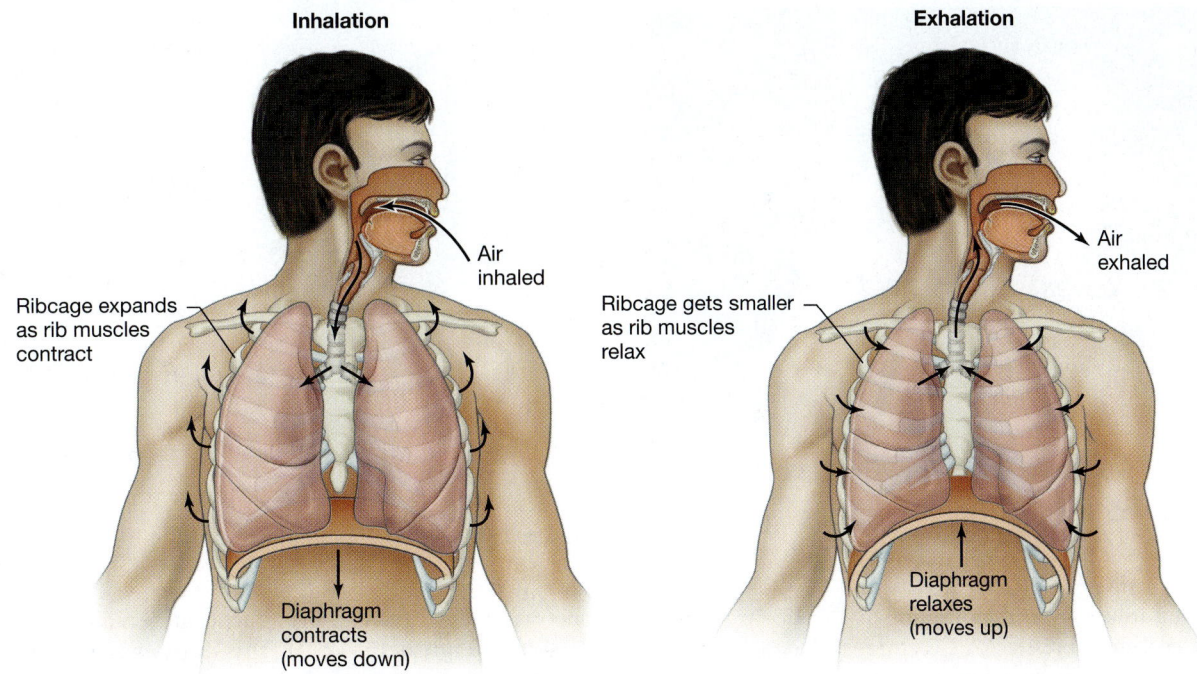

Figure 15–9 >> Respiratory inspiration: lateral and anterior views. Note the volume expansion of the thorax as the diaphragm flattens.

Individuals with chronic respiratory problems such as COPD and asthma usually benefit from use of a long-acting beta-agonist (LABA) in combination with an inhaled corticosteroid (ICS). Commonly prescribed preparations include Symbicort, Dulera, and Advair. Because LABAs may be contraindicated in some individuals, inhaled corticosteroids are available without the addition of the LABA; common examples are budesonide (Pulmicort) and mometasone furoate (Asmanex).

SABAs and corticosteroids can be administered through a nebulizer. Nebulizers aerosolize a solution of medication so that it can be directly inhaled by the patient via a mouthpiece or mask.

Anticholinergic medications relax the smooth muscles of the airways and decrease mucous secretions by blocking the parasympathetic effect. The most commonly prescribed anticholinergic agent for impaired respiratory function is an ipratropium bromide inhaler (e.g., Atrovent). Inhaled anticholinergics are a good alternative for patients who cannot tolerate beta-agonists and can be effective in relieving bronchospasm resulting from the use of beta-blocker medications.

Xanthines, such a theophylline (Slo-Bid) also are used to treat asthma, chronic bronchitis, and emphysema. Xanthines cause small airway dilation and increase heart rate and renal blood flow. Because of the narrow therapeutic range of this type of medication and the potential for serious side effects, patients taking xanthines should have periodic blood tests to ensure they are maintaining optimal therapeutic levels and to guard against the risk of toxicity.

Additional medications may be prescribed. These can vary depending on the nature of the respiratory impairment. Allergic asthmatic individuals, for example, may take immunotherapy (allergy shots) or other medications for allergies to prevent attacks.

Medication adherence in individuals with chronic or recurrent respiratory impairment is critical. Some medications used for treating respiratory diseases are fairly expensive and may carry higher copayments. For individuals who require multiple prescription medications to maintain respiratory health, the combined costs of these medications may be overwhelming. Most pharmaceutical companies have programs to assist patients who lack health insurance or whose standard of living is at or close to the poverty level.

Incentive Spirometry

Incentive spirometry is a breathing exercise using an incentive spirometer that helps patients breathe deeply to expand the lungs. This process can help patients clear mucus secretions and increase the amount of oxygen delivered to the bronchi and alveoli. Incentive spirometry is often prescribed for postoperative patients as well as for some patients with pulmonary alterations. The nurse or respiratory therapist usually provides an initial demonstration with return demonstration by the patient, after which most patients are able to use the incentive spirometer independently.

Oxygen Administration

Decreases in oxygen saturation in arterial blood indicate a need for supplemental oxygen. A variety of devices can be used to administer oxygen to an individual. The selection of a device depends on the amount of oxygen needed to relieve hypoxemia. When administering oxygen, an increase in flow rate yields an increase in the concentration of oxygen that is delivered. However, the maximum concentration of oxygen that is delivered varies by device. Noninvasive devices require patent airways to be effective.

The most common and comfortable device is the nasal cannula (see **Figure 15–10** >>). The nasal cannula delivers flow

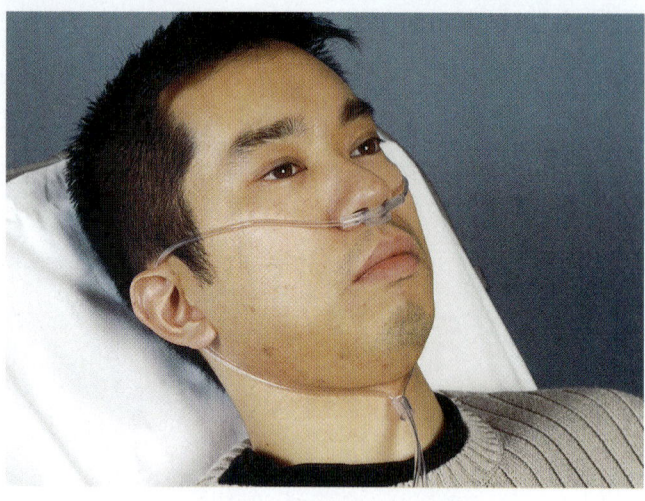

Figure 15–10 ›› A nasal cannula.

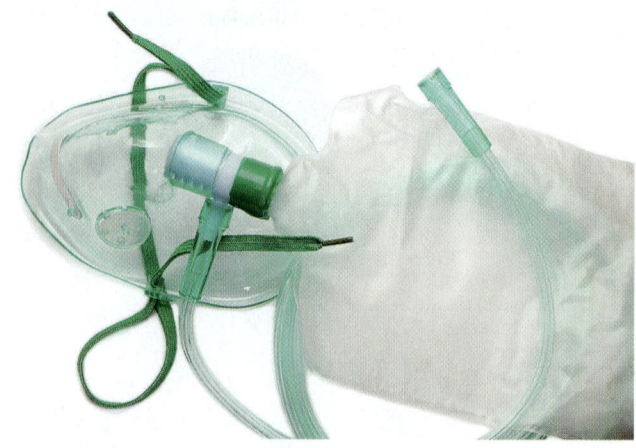

Figure 15–12 ›› A nonrebreather mask.

rates from 2 to 6 L/min that administer 24–45% fraction of inspired oxygen (FiO_2). An Oxymizer also delivers air through the nasal passage, but it has an added reservoir for oxygen. This additional reservoir increases the amount of oxygen inhaled with each breath. A Vapotherm delivers oxygen via a nasal cannula, but it warms and filters oxygen and increases the positive end-expiratory pressure of oxygen delivery via the cannula. Vapotherms are used in neonatal ICUs. Another common device is a simple mask that covers the mouth and nose. It is fitted to the individual's face size. The mask itself provides an additional gas reservoir to that provided by the nasopharynx alone (see **Figure 15–11** ››). Flow rates may be set from 5 L/min to 8 L/min. The FiO_2 delivered is from 40–50%. To attain FiO_2 levels of 60% or more, masks that have an attached reservoir are necessary to provide adequate oxygen. The nonrebreather mask has a

one-way valve between the attached reservoir and the face mask (see **Figure 15–12** ››). This ensures that appropriate levels of oxygen are inhaled, with no carbon dioxide from exhaled gases. Oxygen delivery at a specified flow rate requires the use of a venturi mask (see **Figure 15–13** ››).

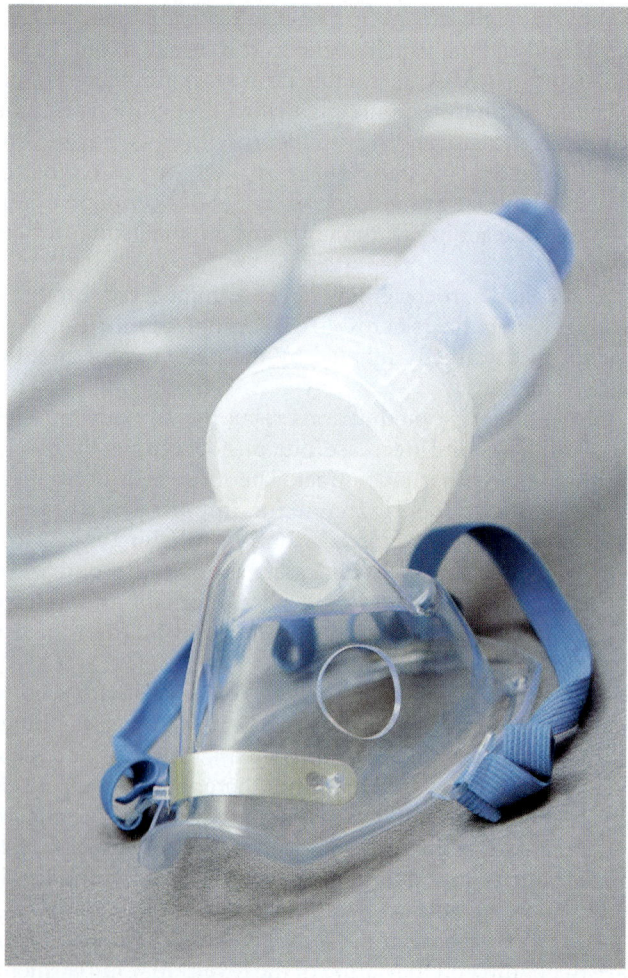

Figure 15–13 ›› A venturi mask.

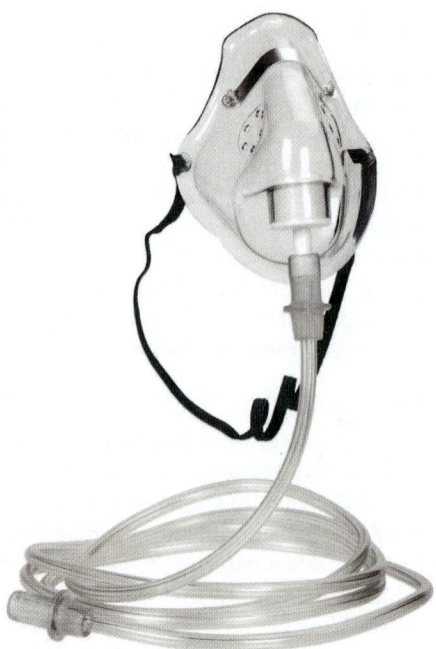

Figure 15–11 ›› A simple face mask.

Venturi masks are set with a specific oxygen flow rate and specific jet adapter device. Flow rates of 24–50% may be set with the venturi mask.

Nursing care for the patient receiving supplemental oxygen includes ensuring that flow is sufficient as required, that the patient is reasonably comfortable with the manner of oxygen administration, and that indwelling catheters (lines) remain clear. For the patient being discharged to home with supplemental oxygen, both the nurse and the respiratory therapist delivering the oxygen to the home must teach the patient how to use the devices properly, the importance of checking oxygen levels in tanks, the need for a portable device for trips outside of the house, and the need to maintain the lines and keep them clear of obstruction.

SAFETY ALERT Because oxygen supports combustion, no one should smoke in a room where supplemental oxygen is being used. The recommendation is to put a warning sign against smoking due to the risk of fire or explosion in every room where supplemental oxygen is used.

Patients who are prescribed supplemental oxygen may feel they have lost their quality of life. The nurse can explain that supplemental oxygen will help the patients maintain their quality of life and that the patients can still participate in any number of activities. The nurse should be alert to any possible signs of depression in patients whose oxygen impairment is sufficient to warrant supplemental oxygen. Frustration, rising medical costs, and other issues can contribute to depression in patients with respiratory impairment.

Chest Tube Management

A chest tube (also called a chest drain or thoracic catheter) is used to treat conditions in which air or fluid enters the pleural cavity, causing lung collapse. Inserted under emergency conditions and treated as a surgical procedure, a chest tube will typically remain in place for 2–5 days until the patient's x-rays indicate that all fluid has been drained from the pleural cavity.

Case Study » Part 3

Ms. Dawson has been hospitalized for 10 days. During the course of her care, she required tracheal intubation and mechanical ventilation. Further examination of her symptoms, including CXRs and blood cultures, revealed that pneumonia was the culprit for her sudden asthma exacerbation. Within 24 hours of beginning intravenous (IV) antibiotics, Ms. Dawson was weaned from the ventilator and extubated. She has completed a 10-day course of IV antibiotics and no longer requires supplemental oxygenation to maintain oxygen saturations above 93%.

You are preparing Ms. Dawson for discharge to her home. Discharge instructions include self-administration of nebulizer treatments 3–4 times per day as needed, as well as chest percussion, vibration, and postural drainage (PVD) for persistent congestion. Because she lives alone, Ms. Dawson will need assistance with her self-care. Fortunately, her mother will be staying with her. The respiratory therapist has completed teaching sessions with Ms. Dawson and her mother that include how to perform chest PVD, as well as how to use the nebulizer. Her admission medications are continued, with the addition of the nebulizer treatments, which include albuterol and acetylcysteine (Mucomyst). You have completed Ms. Dawson's teaching about the

safe administration and effects of her newly added medications. Ms. Dawson's continued care includes a follow-up appointment with her pulmonologist in 3 days, as well as instructions to return to the emergency department immediately should she experience difficulty breathing or any other problems.

Clinical Reasoning Questions Level I

1. What additional patient education do you anticipate Ms. Dawson will need at her follow-up appointment?
2. When Ms. Dawson goes to the pulmonologist's office for her follow-up, what will the nurse's assessment include?
3. For healthy patients without respiratory disorders, what is the normal oxygen saturation level (SaO_2)?

Clinical Reasoning Questions Level II

4. What are the priorities for Ms. Dawson's care in order to decrease her risk of developing pneumonia in the future?
5. How does chest physical therapy help to decrease chest congestion?
6. What education would Ms. Dawson require when prescribed two forms of rescue medications for asthma (albuterol by both inhaler and nebulizer treatment)?
7. Where would you look for the most recent research on nursing care of patients receiving mechanical ventilation?

Lifespan Considerations

Normal oxygenation across the lifespan depends on both the structure and function of the respiratory system. Coexisting health alterations also may influence oxygenation. In addition, age-related variations affect ventilation and oxygenation. The following sections provide an overview of lifespan considerations related to oxygenation.

Oxygenation in Infants and Children

Age-related physiologic differences in respiratory system structures significantly affect oxygenation. For example, a child's airway is shorter and narrower than an adult's. The infant's airway is approximately 4 mm in diameter, about the width of a drinking straw, in contrast to the adult's airway diameter of 20 mm. The child's little finger is a good estimate for the child's tracheal diameter and can be used for a quick assessment of airway size. The trachea primarily increases in length rather than diameter during the first 5 years of life. Also, the tracheal division of the right and left bronchi is higher in a child's airway and at a different angle than in an adult's (see **Figure 15–14 »**). The cartilage that supports the trachea is more flexible and has the potential to compress the airway if the head and neck are not appropriately positioned.

At birth, the lung tissue contains an estimated 50 million alveoli, which are not fully developed, and the distal bronchioles that extend to the alveoli are narrow and fewer in number than in an adult. After 8 years of age, the alveoli begin increasing in size and complexity. The number of alveoli increases to more than 300 million by adulthood (Brashers, 2010; Chan et al., 2013). Although alveoli are fewer in number in children, oxygen consumption is higher than in adults because of the child's high metabolic rate.

Because their intercostal muscles are immature, children under 6 years of age primarily breathe with their diaphragm. However, once the intercostal muscles develop and the child

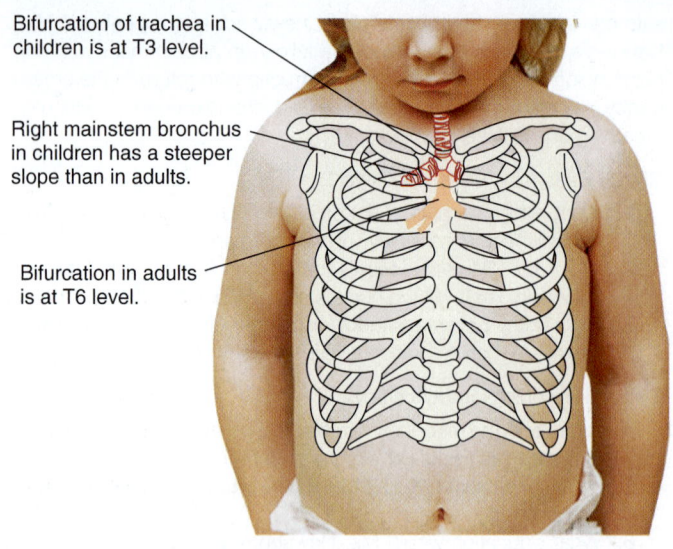

Bifurcation of trachea in children is at T3 level.

Right mainstem bronchus in children has a steeper slope than in adults.

Bifurcation in adults is at T6 level.

Figure 15–14 》》 In children, the trachea is shorter and the angle of the right bronchus at bifurcation is more acute than in the adult. The nurse must allow for these differences when resuscitating or suctioning.

can use them more effectively, diaphragm breathing decreases. In addition to immature muscles, young children have flexible ribs made primarily from cartilage rather than bone.

Because of their narrower airways, infants and preschoolers are at risk for airway obstruction by foreign objects, such as coins and small toys (see **Figure 15–15 》》**). Airway obstruction may also be caused by infection. Upper respiratory infections are common but usually not serious in infants and children. Any condition that causes edema of the airway or accumulation of secretions increases the airway resistance in children because of their narrower airways (see **Figure 15–16 》》**).

Airway resistance is measured by the force required to move oxygen through the trachea to the lungs. As oxygen flows to the alveoli, it passes through small areas, generating friction and increasing resistance. If edema and swelling are present, such as when the child has a respiratory infection, the child must increase the breathing rate in order to maintain adequate oxygenation. This causes negative pressure in the airways, further narrowing the airway.

Likewise, because infants and young children have a decreased number of alveoli, disease processes affecting a small number of alveoli can have a much larger impact on a child's clinical condition because of the increased proportion of lung involvement. For example, involvement of 1 million alveoli secondary to pneumonia would be 4% of the lung for a pediatric patient but only 0.33% for an adult. This causes the child's oxygenation status to deteriorate faster than an adult's. If a child experiences respiratory distress, oxygen consumption increases, and negative pressure in the lungs may cause retractions, seen as sunken areas of skin around the ribs during inspiration (see **Figure 15–17 》》**). As the child works harder to breathe, muscle fatigue develops rapidly because fewer glycogen stores are present in the

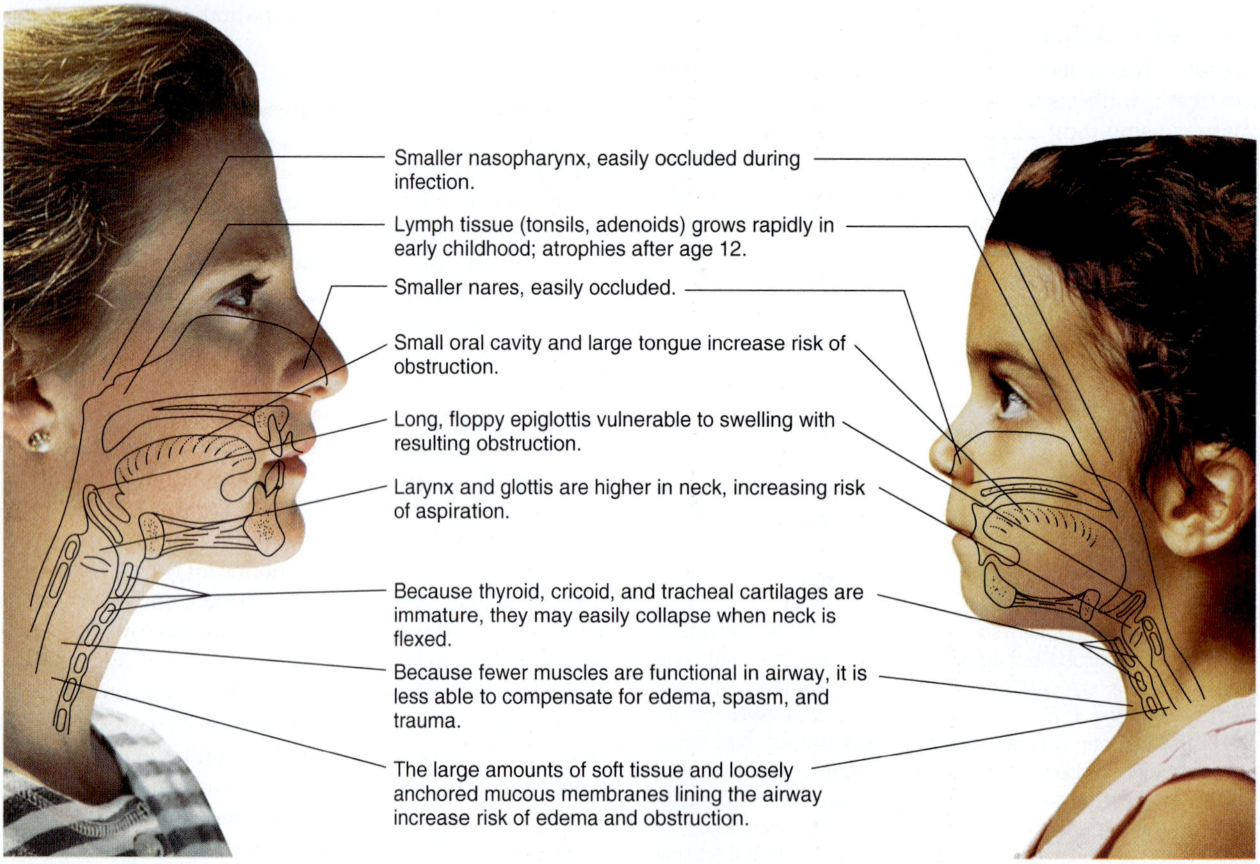

Smaller nasopharynx, easily occluded during infection.

Lymph tissue (tonsils, adenoids) grows rapidly in early childhood; atrophies after age 12.

Smaller nares, easily occluded.

Small oral cavity and large tongue increase risk of obstruction.

Long, floppy epiglottis vulnerable to swelling with resulting obstruction.

Larynx and glottis are higher in neck, increasing risk of aspiration.

Because thyroid, cricoid, and tracheal cartilages are immature, they may easily collapse when neck is flexed.

Because fewer muscles are functional in airway, it is less able to compensate for edema, spasm, and trauma.

The large amounts of soft tissue and loosely anchored mucous membranes lining the airway increase risk of edema and obstruction.

Figure 15–15 》》 Children's airways are smaller and less developed than adults' airways. An upper respiratory tract infection, allergic reaction, positioning of the head and neck during sleep, and the small objects children play with can have serious consequences in children.

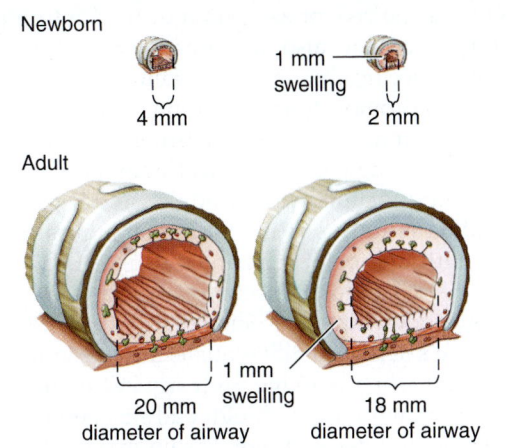

Newborn

1 mm
swelling

4 mm

2 mm

Adult

1 mm
swelling

20 mm
diameter of airway

18 mm
diameter of airway

Figure 15–16 》 The diameter of an infant's airway is approximately 4 mm, in contrast to an adult's airway diameter of 20 mm. An inflammatory process in the airway causes swelling that narrows the airway, and airway resistance increases. Note that swelling of 1 mm reduces the infant's airway diameter to 2 mm, but the adult's airway diameter is only narrowed to 18 mm. Air must move more quickly in the infant's narrowed airway to get the same amount of air to the lungs. The friction of the quickly moving air against the side of the airway increases airway resistance. The infant must use more effort to breathe and breathe faster to get adequate oxygen.

muscles. See the Oxygenation Assessment feature for additional discussion of lifespan and developmental considerations related to pediatric patients.

Nurses can promote lung health and oxygenation in children by encouraging their parents to quit smoking. Secondhand smoke causes the child's lungs to develop more slowly, and it increases the risk of developing respiratory infections. Secondhand smoke can also trigger asthma in children, and it can increase their incidence of wheezing and coughing (CDC, 2014c). Health promotion for children also includes encouraging immunization against influenza and pneumonia.

Many aspects of the lung and respiratory exam for children are similar to those for adults. The following section will

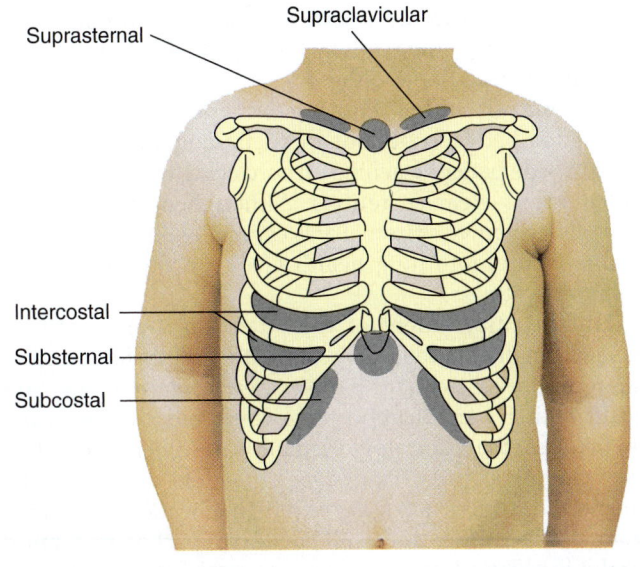

Supraclavicular

Suprasternal

Intercostal

Substernal

Subcostal

Figure 15–17 》 Retraction sites.

highlight only the differences between children and adults that the nurse might encounter. When assessing the infant, start with inspection of the chest. Infants typically have a barrel-shaped chest, with the lateral diameter increasing as the child grows. Check the infant for pectus carinatum and pectus excavatum. Pectus carinatum occurs when the sternum protrudes and increases the anteroposterior diameter of the chest; pectus excavatum occurs when the sternum is depressed, which decreases the anteroposterior diameter of the chest. During breathing, flaring of the lower costal margins and movement of the abdomen rather than the chest is normal for infants because they breathe through the nose and use the diaphragm when breathing. The normal respiratory rate for newborns is 30–80 breaths/min and for infants is 30–60 breaths/min. During palpation, note the infant's facial expression or presence of crying to detect areas of pain or tenderness. In newborns, palpate the area near the clavicle for crepitus, especially if the clavicle was injured during delivery. Assess infants for tactile fremitus; infants with asthma may have decreased tactile fremitus, and infants with pneumonia may have increased tactile fremitus. When auscultating the lungs, use a pediatric stethoscope and avoid listening through clothing. In infants, the areas over which bronchovesicular breath sounds are heard are small and may be hard to find.

For toddlers through elementary-age children, in addition to inspection for pectus carinatum and pectus excavatum, assess the vertebral column for kyphosis or scoliosis, which can make breathing more difficult. The barrel chest found in infants should not be present in children over 6 years old. Retractions should also not be present in this age group. The normal respiratory rate for toddlers is 20–40 breaths/min, for preschoolers 22–34 breaths/min, and for school age children 15–25 breaths/min. A respiratory rate higher than 60 breaths per minute indicates respiratory distress and requires immediate treatment. When palpating this age group, ask the child about the presence of pain in addition to observing facial expressions. Children in this age group should also be able to voluntarily repeat words or numbers to assess for tactile fremitus. If percussion is performed, toddlers and preschoolers will usually have hyperresonance because of the thin chest wall, but school-age children will have resonance more similar to that of an adult. Percussion in children requires a lighter touch than percussion in adults, and the nurse may need to feel the percussion rather than hear an audible sound. During auscultation, ask the child to breathe deeply. Children of this age group should be able to follow the nurse's directions. Use a pediatric stethoscope for younger children. If the child crosses the arms in front of the chest during auscultation of posterior lung sounds, more lung tissue will be exposed, allowing for better assessment. The nurse may hear stridor in children with croup.

If a child in respiratory distress does not respond to standard medications or treatments, the nurse may recommend an x-ray to determine if a foreign object is present. If the child is in severe respiratory distress because of total airway obstruction by a foreign object, the nurse should attempt to clear the obstruction using back blows and chest thrusts in infants or abdominal thrusts in older children. If possible, the foreign body should be visualized with a laryngoscope and removed with a Magill forceps. This is often done in an operating room if time permits to help protect and maintain the child's airway.

Oxygenation in Pregnant Women

Pregnancy increases metabolic demands, which creates an increased need for oxygen. The pregnant woman's growing uterus raises the diaphragm, and the ability to expand the lungs decreases. As such, respiratory rate increases with pregnancy to keep up with the increased oxygen needs of the baby. The chest circumference of the pregnant woman also increases to accommodate body changes. In addition, changes to the upper respiratory mucosa increase the pregnant woman's likelihood of developing nasal stuffiness and epistaxis (nosebleeds), even in the absence of other underlying pathology.

Assessment of lungs and respiration should be similar for pregnant women as for other adults of a similar age. However, in addition to the pregnant woman's respiratory rate increasing slightly, residual capacity decreases, and minute ventilation, alveolar ventilation, and tidal volume all increase. Blood pH may become more alkaline because of changes in respiration and blood gases. Pregnant women should also be assessed for rhinitis of pregnancy and epistaxis due to nasal changes in pregnancy. During active labor, pregnant women may experience hyperventilation and tachypnea, causing hypocapnia and respiratory alkalosis. The laboring woman's oxygenation status should be monitored closely to prevent adverse effects on the baby's oxygenation status before birth (Madappa & Sharma, 2015).

For pregnant women, many interventions can remain the same for alterations in oxygenation, taking into consideration positioning that may be harmful to the fetus, including avoiding prolonged supine positioning to prevent restricting blood flow through the vena cava. Prompt resolution of underlying conditions affecting oxygenation in the pregnant woman is essential to ensure that both mother and baby maintain adequate oxygen levels and distribution. Treatment of pregnant women with chronic respiratory conditions should be made in consultation with both a pulmonologist and the woman's treating obstetrician. Check the pregnancy category for all medications before administering to a pregnant patient because many medications can harm the fetus. In addition, metabolism, blood volume, and albumin level are all altered in pregnant women, so dosing of safe medications may need to be altered.

Oxygenation in Older Adults

As adults age, their ribcage may change shape, causing the ribcage to not expand and contract as well as it used to. The diaphragm also weakens with age. Tissues that support the structure of the airways also weaken, allowing the airways to collapse more easily. In addition, the nervous system becomes less efficient, decreasing the older adult's ability to control breathing and decreasing the cough reflex. Together, these changes reduce the older adult's lung function (Martin, 2014).

Normal changes to the lungs of older adults increase their risk of developing infections such as pneumonia and bronchitis. They also have an increased risk of developing breathing disorders such as sleep apnea. Changes to the cough reflex also increase the older adult's risk of choking on food, and the increased incidence of gastroesophageal reflux with age increases the risk of aspiration of food into the lower respiratory tract. This also increases the risk of developing pneumonia, specifically aspiration pneumonia.

Nurses can promote lung health and oxygenation in older adults by encouraging them to stop smoking and by encouraging them to engage in physical activity. Exercise can improve lung function in older adults, and it prevents the accumulation of mucus in the lungs that occurs with lying down or sitting for long periods. Mucus accumulation increases the risk of lung infections, especially after surgery or in conjunction with other illnesses (Martin, 2014).

The nurse's ability to differentiate changes in respiratory rate is critical when working with any individual but particularly when working with older adults, because pulmonary function declines with age. The normal respiratory rate for older adults is 15–20 breaths/min. Nurses should expect to hear decreased breath sounds on assessment, and inspiratory crackles are commonly heard as well. In addition, nurses should assess older adults for scoliosis and kyphosis, which are common in this population and often contribute to difficulty breathing.

Older adults are at increased risk for acute respiratory diseases such as pneumonia and chronic diseases such as emphysema and chronic bronchitis. Nursing assessment of older adults with difficulty breathing includes assessing for possible infection. Vesicular breath sounds with a longer expiratory phase may be reflective of respiratory alterations with an obstructive component, such as COPD and asthma (Sarkar et al., 2015). Pneumonia may not present with the usual symptom of a fever, but may present with atypical symptoms, such as confusion, weakness, loss of appetite, and increased heart rate and respiration. In assessing adults with chronic illness, nurses should assess for any changes in medication (including compliance with the therapeutic regimen), fluid and nutrition status, and cognition. Nurses should remember that older patients who are too ill to sit up for a respiratory examination may have artifacts upon examination due to positioning.

Older adults also need special considerations when treating alterations in oxygenation. Older adults are susceptible to aspiration of secretions because of a decreased gag reflex and cough reflex. Therefore, they frequently need suctioning. Nurses should use a lower suction pressure for older adults than for younger adults because of older adults' fragile oral mucosa. Some older adults may be susceptible to hypoxemia related to suctioning, so hyperoxygenation may be needed between periods of suctioning. Nurses should also provide patient teaching on enhancing coughing to help older adults clear secretions. Although useful for most patients, incentive spirometry is especially helpful for older adults to promote lung health after surgery or during a respiratory illness.

Nursing assessment of the older adult also includes assessment of adherence to treatment regimens for any alterations and assessment of barriers to adherence. Is the older adult taking a medication for a comorbid condition that might affect the respiratory system? Is the older adult taking medications as prescribed? Does the older adult have the financial resources necessary to refill medications in a timely manner? These factors can all have an impact on respiratory health in older adults.

REVIEW The Concept of Oxygenation

RELATE Link the Concepts

Linking the concept of oxygenation with the concept of infection:

1. Why would alterations in oxygenation lead to an increased risk of certain infections?
2. What are some ways to decrease the risk of infections caused by alterations in oxygenation?

Linking the concept of oxygenation with the concept of mobility:

3. How might alterations in oxygenation affect mobility?
4. What are some nursing interventions that can decrease the risk of altered mobility for patients with alterations in oxygenation?

Linking the concept of oxygenation with the concept of perfusion:

5. How are the concepts of oxygenation and perfusion related?
6. What disease processes related to oxygenation can affect the body's ability to perfuse adequately?

Linking the concept of oxygenation with the concept of cognition:

7. How might an alteration in oxygenation affect an individual's orientation?
8. How might lack of oxygenation to the brain be detected?

READY Go to Volume 3: Clinical Nursing Skills

- SKILL 1.7   Pulse Oximeter: Using
- SKILL 1.8   Respirations: Newborn, Infant, Child, Adult, Obtaining
- SKILL 1.23   Nose and Sinuses: Assessing
- SKILL 1.27   Thorax and Lungs: Assessing
- SKILL 2.21   Inhaler, Metered-Dose: Administering
- SKILL 2.22   Nasal Medication: Administering
- SKILL 11.14 Suctioning, Oropharyngeal and Nasopharyngeal: Newborn, Infant, Child, Adult

REFER Go to Pearson MyLab Nursing and eText

- Additional review materials

REFLECT Apply Your Knowledge

Grayson Garrett, a 67-year-old man, has been admitted to the hospital for treatment of complications related to chronic kidney disease (CKD). Mr. Garrett's medical history also includes hypertension. Mr. Garrett's vital signs include temperature 99.1°F; pulse 91 bpm; respirations 30/min; BP 139/82 mmHg; and pulse oximetry 97%. Mr. Garrett's diagnostic tests include a complete blood count (CBC), serum electrolyte panel, CXR, and ABGs. Mr. Garrett's ABG results include the following values: pH = 7.36, $PaCO_2$ = 32 mmHg, PaO_2 = 86 mmHg, and HCO_3^- = 21 mEq/L.

1. Which acid–base imbalance is commonly associated with renal failure?
2. Do Mr. Garrett's ABG results reflect the presence of an acid–base imbalance? Explain your answer.
3. Why is Mr. Garrett's respiratory rate increased?
4. What interventions can the nurse implement to help decrease Mr. Garrett's respiratory rate?

» Exemplar 15.A
Acute Respiratory Distress Syndrome

Exemplar Learning Outcomes

15.A Analyze acute respiratory distress syndrome (ARDS) as it relates to oxygenation.

- Describe the pathophysiology of ARDS.
- Describe the etiology of ARDS.
- Summarize risk factors for ARDS.
- Compare methods for preventing ARDS.
- Identify the clinical manifestations of ARDS.
- Summarize diagnostic tests and therapies used by interprofessional teams in the collaborative care of an individual with ARDS.
- Differentiate care of patients with ARDS across the lifespan.
- Apply the nursing process in providing culturally competent care to an individual with ARDS.

Exemplar Key Terms

Acute respiratory distress syndrome (ARDS), *1043*
Barotrauma, *1050*
Bilevel ventilator (BiPAP), *1048*
Continuous positive airway pressure (CPAP), *1048*
Negative pressure ventilator, *1048*
Noninvasive positive pressure ventilation (NIPPV), *1048*
Pneumomediastinum, *1050*
Pneumopericardium, *1050*
Positive end-expiratory pressure (PEEP), *1048*
Positive pressure ventilators, *1048*
Refractory hypoxemia, *1043*
Terminal weaning, *1050*
Weaning, *1050*

Overview

Acute respiratory distress syndrome (ARDS) is a disorder with rapid onset characterized by noncardiac pulmonary edema and progressive **refractory hypoxemia** (the decrease of arterial oxygen despite administration of oxygen at high flow rates). ARDS is widely recognized as a severe form of acute

respiratory failure. Among hospitalized patients with ARDS, the estimated mortality rate is 32% (Radbel et al., 2014).

Extensive lung tissue inflammation and small blood vessel injury occur, with malfunction of other organs following. The onset of ARDS is rapid, with an ABG showing respiratory failure. The initial admitting diagnoses of individuals who develop ARDS are varied, with most individuals presenting to the hospital with another critical event, such as a drug overdose or exposure to a toxic inhalant, and being admitted to intensive care. Both direct and indirect injuries to the body can result in ARDS.

Pathophysiology and Etiology
Pathophysiology

The underlying pathology in ARDS is acute lung injury resulting from an unregulated systemic inflammatory response to acute injury or inflammation. Inflammatory cellular responses and biochemical mediators damage the alveolar–capillary membrane. This damage develops rapidly, often within 90 minutes of the systemic inflammatory response and within 24 hours of the initial insult.

Damaged capillary membranes allow plasma and blood cells to escape into the interstitial space. Increased interstitial pressure and damage to the alveolar membrane allow fluid to enter the alveoli. Within the alveoli, the fluid dilutes and inactivates surfactant. The inflammatory process damages surfactant-producing cells, leading to a deficit of surfactant, increased alveolar surface tension, and alveolar collapse with atelectasis. The lungs become less compliant, and gas exchange is impaired. As the syndrome progresses, hyaline membranes form, further reducing gas exchange and compliance. Finally, fibrotic changes occur in the lungs. Intra-alveolar septa thicken, and alveolar surface area for gas exchange is reduced. Hypoxemia becomes refractory or resistant to improvement with supplemental oxygen, and the $PaCO_2$ rises as diffusion is further impaired.

Figures 15–18 » and **15–19 »** illustrate the pathogenesis and pathophysiology of ARDS. As ARDS progresses, tissue hypoxia becomes significant, and metabolic acidosis develops. Both carbon dioxide exchange and oxygen exchange become impaired, leading to combined respiratory and metabolic acidosis. Sepsis and multiple organ system dysfunction of the kidneys, liver, gastrointestinal tract, central nervous system, and cardiovascular system are the leading causes of death in ARDS. If the process is halted before sepsis or organ system dysfunction occurs, the long-term prognosis for recovery is good.

Etiology

ARDS develops in nearly 200,000 Americans each year (American Lung Association [ALA], n.d.) and affects all ages (ALA, 2013; National Heart, Lung, and Blood Institute [NHLBI], 2012a) with a mortality rate ranging from 25% to 45%. The risk of mortality from ARDS is greater for men than women and greater for African Americans than people of other races. Compared to patients who develop ARDS from pulmonary infections or trauma, patients who develop ARDS from sepsis have poorer outcomes. Therefore, the prognosis for patients with ARDS depends on a number of factors, including the underlying cause of ARDS and any health alterations that may coexist with this cause (NHLBI, 2012a).

Risk Factors

As stated earlier, direct and indirect insults to the lungs may result in ARDS. Pulmonary infections are a direct insult to

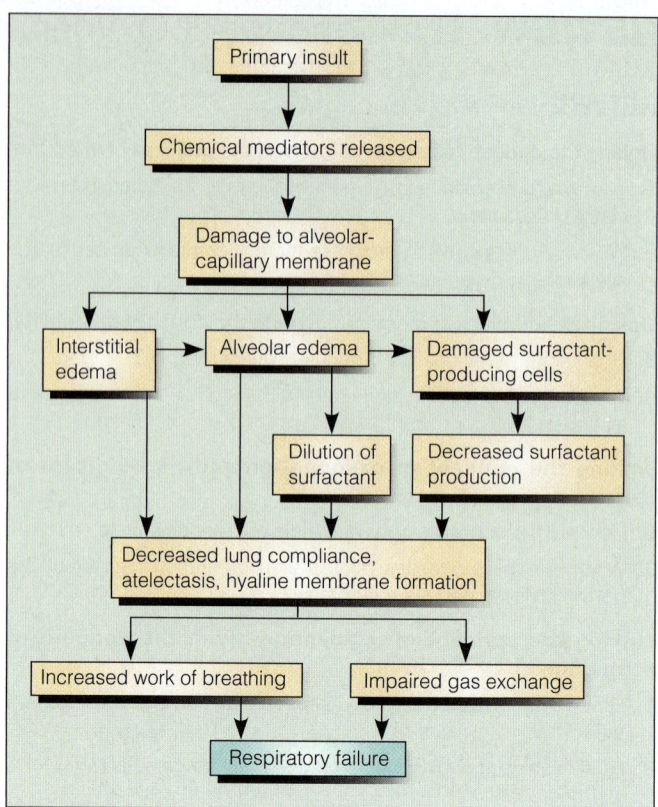

Figure 15–18 » Pathogenesis of acute respiratory distress syndrome.

lung tissue. Aspiration of gastric contents and inhalation injuries, such as smoke inhalation and saltwater inhalation from near-drowning in saltwater, can result in ARDS. Indirect insults, including overall body sepsis, trauma, and gastrointestinal infections such as pancreatitis, also may result in ARDS. Drug overdoses, especially with tricyclic antidepressants, are associated with ARDS. Multiple blood transfusions have caused the development of ARDS, as has cardiopulmonary bypass. Sepsis is the most common cause of ARDS. Mortality is highest in individuals who are older than 70 years, who are immunocompromised, and who have chronic liver failure. Smoking may increase the risk for ARDS. Current research suggests that exposure to high levels of air pollution is a risk factor for ARDS, as well (Ware et al., 2015).

Prevention

Much of ARDS prevention involves identifying and preventing the risk factors for ARDS and initiating timely interventions. For example, to decrease the risk of aspiration, one of the most significant risk factors for ARDS, elevate the head of the bed for patients in respiratory distress, particularly when the patients ingest food, whether they do that by mouth or through a nasogastric tube.

Clinical Manifestations

The initial manifestations of ARDS will typically develop a full day or two following the initial insult. To identify the change in pulmonary status, rely on baseline laboratory data as well as diagnostic tests. Dyspnea and tachypnea manifest early, and the laboratory results will be consistent with the presenting illness. With the exception of direct pulmonary illness, a CXR will often show the lungs to be clear of infiltrates, and ABG values may be within the normal range.

As progressive respiratory distress develops, the patient's respiratory rate, intercostal retractions, and use of accessory muscles of respiration will all increase. As the demand for oxygen to the cells of the body increases, tachycardia occurs. At first, breath sounds are clear, but rales, also called crackles, and rhonchi will develop later. Cyanosis develops and may not improve with oxygen administration. CXR will show interstitial changes with patchy infiltrates, and the pulse oximetry and ABG levels may demonstrate hypoxemia refractory to oxygen administration. Changes in mental status, including such changes as increased agitation, confusion, and lethargy, will occur as respiratory failure progresses.

Collaboration

Patients with ARDS are seriously ill and require contributions from many members of the healthcare team. In addition to nurses, respiratory therapists, dietitians, physical therapists, and physicians may play a significant role in the provision of healthcare services to the patient. The role of the nurse is to constantly monitor the patient's condition, respond to subtle cues indicating a change, and intervene

appropriately. The focus of nursing care is discussed in more detail in the Nursing Process section.

Diagnostic Tests

Several diagnostic tests can be used to diagnose ARDS. These tests include:

- ABG analysis to determine low levels of oxygen in the blood
- Chest radiography (CXR or chest CT) to determine fluid in the lungs
- Blood tests such as a CBC, blood chemistries, and blood cultures to help find the cause of ARDS (e.g., infection)
- Sputum culture to determine the exact cause of infection (National Institutes of Health, 2012).

Pharmacologic Therapy

Although no definitive drug therapy currently exists for ARDS, a number of medications may be used. Inhaled nitric oxide reduces intrapulmonary shunting and improves oxygenation by dilating blood vessels in better ventilated areas of the lungs. Surfactant therapy may be prescribed because of the decrease in surfactant production that is often associated with ARDS.

Interventions to block the inflammatory response, such as using nonsteroidal anti-inflammatory agents (NSAIDs) and corticosteroids, are under investigation. Corticosteroids may be used late in the course of ARDS to improve oxygenation and lung mechanics when fibrotic changes occur.

Clinical Manifestations and Therapies
Acute Respiratory Distress Syndrome

ETIOLOGY	CLINICAL MANIFESTATIONS	CLINICAL THERAPIES
Hypoxia	■ Dyspnea ■ Tachypnea ■ Intercostal retractions ■ Tachycardia ■ Cyanosis ■ Atelectasis	■ Bronchodilators, beta-agonists, corticosteroids ■ Oxygen administration ■ Monitoring of pulmonary artery pressures and cardiac output ■ Mechanical ventilation ■ Continuous positive airway pressure (CPAP), bilevel ventilator (BiPAP), or positive end-expiratory pressure (PEEP) as necessary ■ Prone positioning ■ Surfactant therapy
Nutritional imbalance	■ Confusion ■ Fluid–electrolyte imbalance ■ Weakness or fatigue	■ Fluid replacement ■ Total parenteral/enteral nutrition or enteral feedings ■ Nutritional analysis ■ Monitoring of serum electrolytes
Activity intolerance	■ Irritability ■ Fatigue ■ Confusion ■ Lethargy ■ Inability to maintain ADLs	■ Splitting of care as needed to prevent overtaxing the patient ■ Assessing LOC as indicated ■ Assessing vital signs and respiratory status before, during, and after any physical activity

Acute respiratory distress syndrome (ARDS) is a severe form of acute respiratory failure that occurs in response to pulmonary or systemic insults. ARDS is characterized by noncardiogenic pulmonary edema resulting from inflammatory damage to alveolar and capillary walls. Many disorders may precipitate ARDS, although sepsis is the most common.

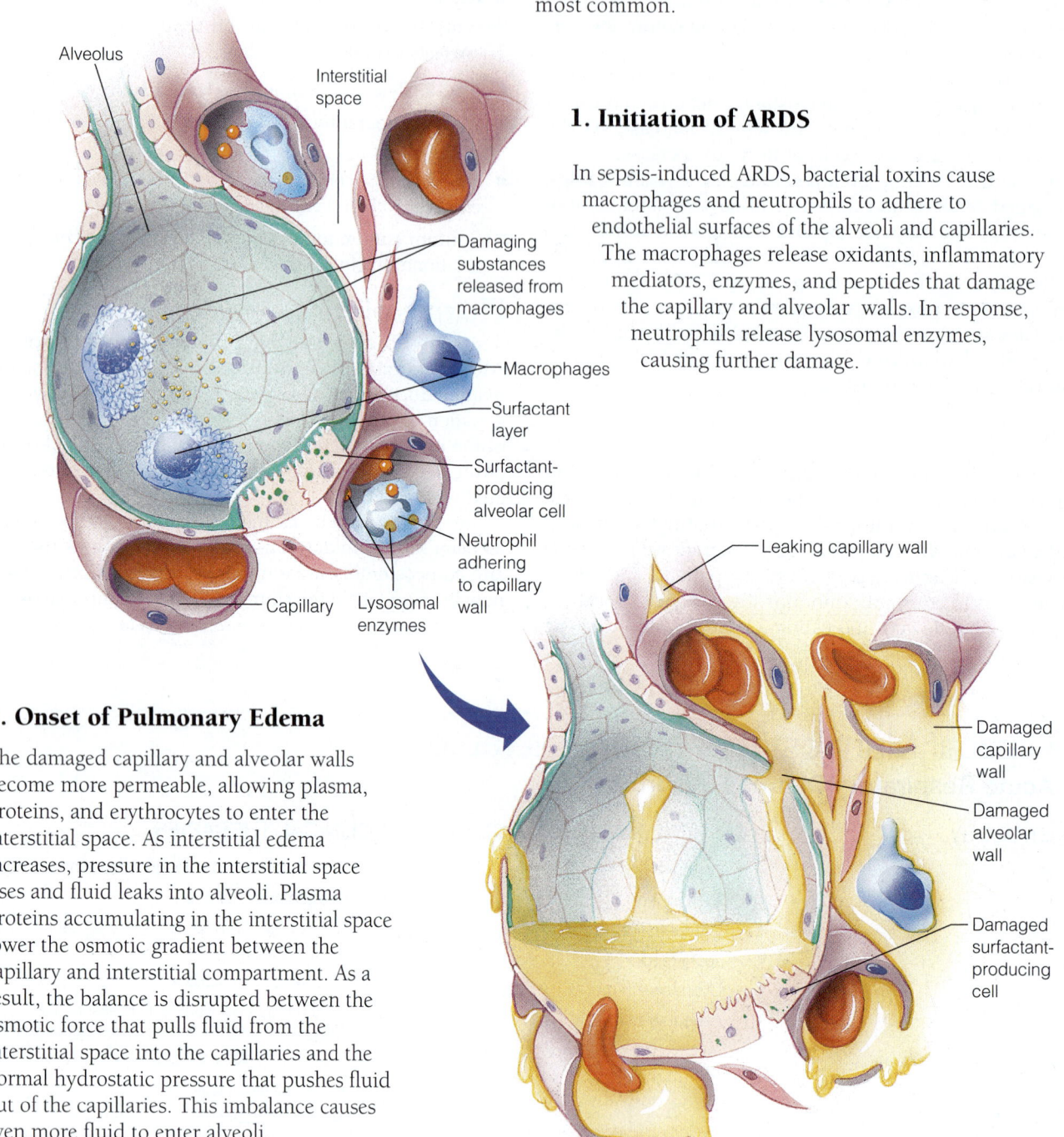

1. Initiation of ARDS

In sepsis-induced ARDS, bacterial toxins cause macrophages and neutrophils to adhere to endothelial surfaces of the alveoli and capillaries. The macrophages release oxidants, inflammatory mediators, enzymes, and peptides that damage the capillary and alveolar walls. In response, neutrophils release lysosomal enzymes, causing further damage.

2. Onset of Pulmonary Edema

The damaged capillary and alveolar walls become more permeable, allowing plasma, proteins, and erythrocytes to enter the interstitial space. As interstitial edema increases, pressure in the interstitial space rises and fluid leaks into alveoli. Plasma proteins accumulating in the interstitial space lower the osmotic gradient between the capillary and interstitial compartment. As a result, the balance is disrupted between the osmotic force that pulls fluid from the interstitial space into the capillaries and the normal hydrostatic pressure that pushes fluid out of the capillaries. This imbalance causes even more fluid to enter alveoli.

Figure 15–19 » Pathophysiology of acute respiratory distress syndrome.

4. End-Stage ARDS

Fibrin and cell debris from necrotic cells combine to form hyaline membranes, which line the interior of the alveoli and further reduce alveolar compliance and gas exchange. Because CO_2 cannot diffuse across hyaline membranes, $PaCO_2$ levels now begin to rise while PaO_2 levels continue to fall. Rising $PaCO_2$ levels can lead to respiratory acidosis. Without respiratory support, respiratory failure will develop.
Even with aggressive treatment, almost 50% of patients with ARDS die.

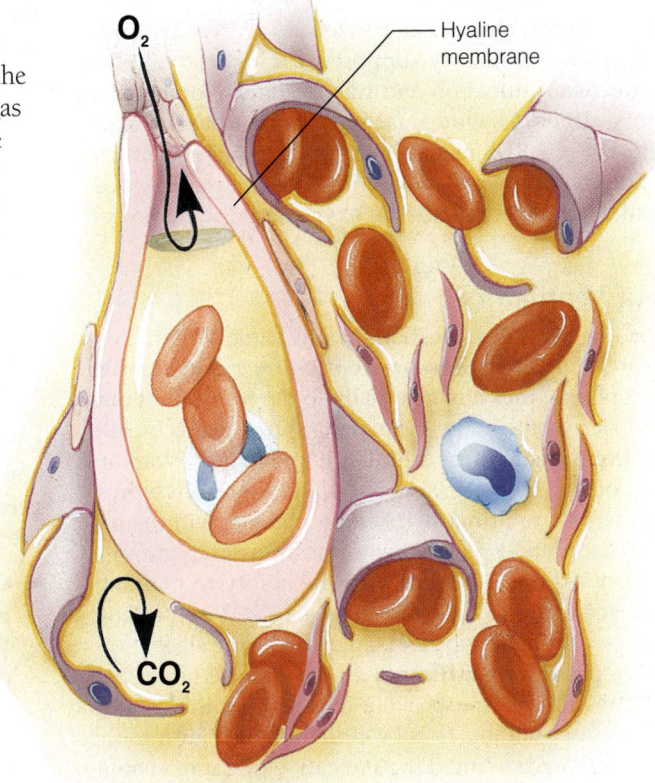

3. Alveolar Collapse

Protein-rich fluid accumulates in the alveoli, inactivating surfactant and damaging type II alveolar cells that produce surfactant. (Surfactant is important in maintaining alveolar compliance—the ability of tissue to stretch or distend.) As active surfactant is lost, the alveoli stiffen and collapse, leading to atelectasis, which increases breathing effort.

Decreased alveolar compliance, atelectasis, and fluid-filled alveoli interfere with gas exchange across the alveolar-capillary membrane. Blood oxygen (PaO_2) levels fall. Because carbon dioxide diffuses more readily than oxygen, however, blood carbon dioxide ($PaCO_2$) levels also fall initially as tachypnea causes more CO_2 to be expired.

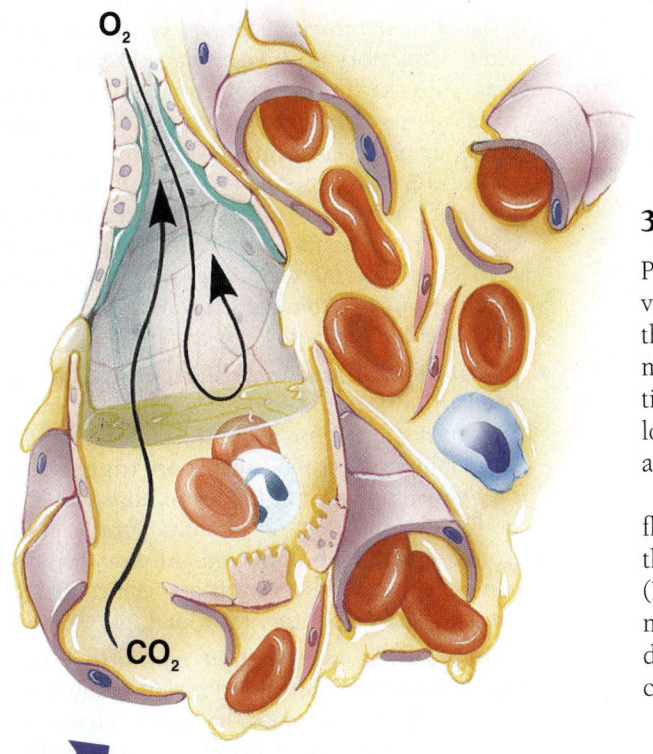

Figure 15–19 》 Pathophysiology of acute respiratory distress syndrome. (*continued*)

Ventilatory Support

Ventilatory support may be categorized as invasive or noninvasive. Invasive ventilatory support includes interventions such as tracheal intubation and tracheotomy. Noninvasive ventilatory support includes face masks and nasal masks. The mainstay of ARDS management is endotracheal intubation and mechanical ventilation. With ARDS, it is rarely possible to maintain adequate tissue oxygenation with oxygen therapy alone.

Types of Ventilators

Two broad, general classifications of mechanical ventilators are available. **Negative pressure ventilators** create negative (subatmospheric) pressure externally to draw the chest outward and air into the lungs, mimicking spontaneous breathing. The iron lung, cuirass ventilator, and PulmoWrap are examples of negative pressure ventilators. Negative pressure ventilators are primarily used by patients with neuromuscular disorders (e.g., postpolio syndrome, amyotrophic lateral sclerosis) that interfere with the ability to maintain adequate ventilation. They also may be used by patients who require ventilator support primarily during sleep.

Positive pressure ventilators are used more often than negative pressure ones, especially in treating patients with acute respiratory failure. These ventilators push air into the lungs rather than drawing it in as negative pressure ventilators do. The amount of air delivered with each breath can be delivered in milliliters (volume ventilator) or until a specific pressure is reached (pressure ventilators). Either invasive ventilation using an endotracheal tube or tracheostomy or noninvasive modalities can be used.

Noninvasive positive pressure ventilation (NIPPV) provides respiratory support by way of a tight-fitting full face mask, nasal mask, nasal shield, or nasal pillows. If effective, NIPPV may prevent the need for tracheal intubation. Primary goals of NIPPV center on providing ventilatory support to patients with obstructive sleep apnea, neuromuscular disease, or impending respiratory failure (e.g., advanced COPD). NIPPV also may be used for patients in respiratory failure who refuse intubation. The degree of success varies and is primarily limited by patient intolerance as a result of the physical and psychologic discomfort of wearing a mask when dyspneic (Jones & Park, 2014). NIPPV tends to be more successful in patients without significant underlying lung disease (e.g., respiratory failure related to neuromuscular disease). NIPPV is not appropriate for use in treating patients whose condition warrants immediate tracheal intubation. Likewise, NIPPV is contraindicated for use in patients who demonstrate a significant decrease in LOC. The patient's underlying condition also must be considered, as certain conditions are more responsive to NIPPV; for example, hypercapnic respiratory failure and exacerbation of COPD tend to be more responsive to this form of ventilatory assistance (Jones & Park, 2014).

Several variables are used to trigger, cycle, and limit airflow with positive pressure ventilators. The trigger prompts the ventilator to deliver a breath. The patient's inspiratory effort triggers ventilator-assisted breaths. Ventilator-controlled breaths usually are triggered by a preset time interval (e.g., a breath is delivered every 5 sec for a rate of 12 breaths/min). The ventilator cycle, or duration of inspiration, can be limited by volume, pressure, flow, or time. Volume-cycled ventilators deliver air until a preset volume is delivered. Pressure-cycled ventilators cycle off when a preset pressure is achieved within the airways. Flow-cycled ventilators are cycled by a preset inspiratory flow rate, and time-cycled ventilators deliver air for a set time interval. Airflow delivered by the ventilator also can be limited by factors such as airway pressure (e.g., a volume-cycled ventilator can be set to immediately stop inspiratory flow if airway pressure exceeds a preset value).

Modes of Ventilation

A number of different modes or patterns of ventilation may be used with positive pressure ventilators. The mode determines whether a breath is initiated by the patient or the ventilator and the pattern of airway support provided by the ventilator. CPAP, BiPAP, assist-control mode ventilation (ACMV), synchronized intermittent mandatory ventilation (SIMV), PEEP, pressure-support ventilation, and pressure-control ventilation are common modes of ventilation in use today.

- ***Continuous positive airway pressure.*** **Continuous positive airway pressure (CPAP)** applies positive pressure to the airways of a patient who is breathing spontaneously. CPAP may be used with either endotracheal intubation or a tight-fitting face mask. All breathing is spontaneous (patient triggered) and pressure controlled. CPAP is used to help maintain open airways and alveoli, decreasing the work of breathing.

- ***Bilevel ventilators.*** A **bilevel ventilator (BiPAP)** provides inspiratory positive airway pressure as well as airway support during expiration. Bilevel ventilation is primarily used at night with a tight-fitting mask (nasal, facial, or oral). Three modes of ventilation can be used with BiPAP: (a) spontaneous breathing (S); (b) timed mode (T), in which pressure-supported breaths are delivered at a predetermined rate; and (c) spontaneous/timed (S/T), in which the ventilator switches to timed mode if spontaneous breathing falls below a preset rate (International Ventilator Users Network, [IVUN], 2015).

- ***Assist-control mode ventilation.*** ACMV is frequently used to initiate mechanical ventilation and when the patient is at risk for respiratory arrest (e.g., overdose, head injury). Assisted breaths are triggered by inspiratory effort; however, if the respiratory rate falls below a preset number (e.g., 14 breaths/min), ventilator-controlled breaths are delivered. All breaths, assisted and controlled, are delivered at a specific tidal volume or pressure and inspiratory flow rate.

- ***Synchronized intermittent mandatory ventilation.*** SIMV allows the patient to breathe spontaneously, without ventilator assistance, between delivered ventilator breaths. Mandatory or ventilator-controlled breaths are delivered at a preset rate, volume, and/or pressure, coordinated with the patient's inspiratory efforts. This mode of ventilation is used to support ventilation, to exercise respiratory muscles between ventilator-assisted breaths, and during the weaning process (Society of Critical Care Anesthesiologists [SOCCA], 2013).

- ***Positive end-expiratory pressure.*** **Positive end-expiratory pressure (PEEP)** requires intubation and can be applied to any of the previously described ventilator

TABLE 15–4 Ventilator Settings

Parameter	Description
Rate (*f*)	Number of ventilator breaths per minute; usually 12–15 in adults using ACMV; may be lower in SIMV
Tidal volume (V_t)	Amount of gas delivered with each ventilator breath; usually 8–10 mL/kg body weight
Oxygen concentration (FiO_2)	Percentage of oxygen delivered with ventilator breaths; can be set between 21% (room air) and 100%
I:E ratio	Duration of inspiration to expiration; usually 1:2–1:1.5
Flow rate	Speed at which air is delivered
Sensitivity	Effort required by patient to initiate ventilator-assisted breath
Pressure limit	Maximal pressure within airways that will terminate a ventilator breath

modes. With PEEP, a positive pressure is maintained in the airways during exhalation and between breaths. Keeping alveoli open between breaths improves V-Q relationships and diffusion across the alveolar–capillary membrane. This reduces hypoxemia and allows use of lower percentages of inspired oxygen. PEEP is particularly useful for treating patients with ARDS.

- *Pressure-support ventilation.* Pressure-support ventilation (PSV) delivers ventilator-assisted breaths when the patient initiates an inspiratory effort. The cycle is flow limited; inspiration is terminated when inspiratory airflow falls below a preset rate. This mode decreases the work of breathing. It can be used in combination with SIMV when the respiratory drive is depressed. Ventilator support can be gradually withdrawn during weaning.

- *Pressure-control ventilation.* Pressure-control ventilation controls pressure within the airways to reduce the risk of airway trauma (e.g., following thoracic surgery). Ventilation is time triggered and time cycled, but pressure is limited. The ventilator maintains a preset airway pressure throughout inspiration. Because all breaths are controlled by the ventilator, heavy sedation may be required to prevent competition between inspiratory effort and ventilator control.

With mechanical ventilation, the FiO_2 (fraction of inspired oxygen—the percentage of oxygen administered) is set at the lowest possible level to maintain a PaO_2 higher than 60 mmHg and oxygen saturation of approximately 90%. When the PaO_2 cannot be maintained with less than 50% inspired oxygen, oxygen toxicity may accentuate ARDS. Adding positive end-expiratory pressure (PEEP) to mechanical ventilator settings is often necessary in order to prevent collapse of alveoli and promote oxygenation. The patient who does not require intubation but needs additional respiratory support may receive bilevel ventilation (BiPAP) or continuous positive airway pressure (CPAP). Maintaining open airways and alveoli enhances gas diffusion and reduces V-Q mismatch. PEEP increases intrathoracic pressure resulting in a decrease in cardiac output while increasing the risk of barotrauma, which can result in long-term pulmonary complications. Either assist-control or synchronized intermittent mandatory ventilation may be used along with PEEP in treating the patient with ARDS. It is important to remember that mechanical ventilation does not cure ARDS; it simply supports respiratory function while the underlying problem is identified and treated.

Ventilator Settings

In addition to choosing the mode of ventilation, other parameters are set to meet individual patient needs when positive pressure ventilation is used (see **Table 15–4 »**). The most important of these parameters are rate, tidal volume, and oxygen concentration.

For most adult patients, the rate is initially set between 12 and 15 ventilator breaths per minute. With ACMV or SIMV, the patient's respiratory rate often is higher than the ventilator setting because of spontaneous breathing. Exhaled carbon dioxide ($ETCO_2$) or the $PaCO_2$ may be used to determine the rate. A $PaCO_2$ of less than 35 mmHg indicates hyperventilation and respiratory alkalosis and the need to reduce the set rate. A $PaCO_2$ above 45 mmHg or an $ETCO_2$ greater than 45 mmHg indicates hypoventilation and the need to increase the rate.

The tidal volume setting controls the amount of gas delivered with each ventilator breath. The normal adult tidal volume at rest is approximately 7 mL/kg body weight, or 400–550 mL. The tidal volume delivered by mechanical ventilation is slightly higher (500–750 mL) to compensate for tubing dead space. Higher tidal volumes can cause lung tissue trauma.

The percentage of oxygen delivered with ventilator breaths is adjusted to maintain the oxygen saturation and PaO_2 within acceptable ranges. Because prolonged delivery of high oxygen concentrations increases the risk of oxygen toxicity and pulmonary fibrosis, the FiO_2 is set at the lowest possible level for adequate tissue oxygenation. For most patients, the goal is to maintain an oxygen saturation of greater than 90%. Lower oxygen saturation levels may be appropriate for patients with long-standing COPD.

Complications

Although endotracheal intubation and mechanical ventilation can be lifesaving in respiratory failure, they are not without risk. Improper endotracheal tube placement or advancement of the tube into a mainstem bronchus can result in ventilation of one lung only. The inflated lung becomes overdistended and traumatized, and the uninflated lung develops atelectasis. Complications associated with NIPPV include gastric dilation, aspiration, facial skin necrosis, drying of the eyes and mucous membranes, stress, and claustrophobia (Mahmoodpoor & Golzari, 2015).

- *Ventilator-associated pneumonia (VAP).* Infection is a significant risk associated with intubation and mechanical ventilation. Normal upper respiratory tract defense mechanisms are bypassed, and often the cough reflex is inhibited or impaired. Oral secretions and gastric contents can enter the respiratory system via the open epiglottis, necessitating frequent, meticulous oral hygiene. Secretions may become thick and tenacious, increasing the risk of atelectasis.

- **Barotrauma. Barotrauma** (also called volutrauma) is lung injury caused by alveolar overdistention. Both the volume of delivered gas and the pressures under which it is delivered can contribute to barotraumas. As a result, overdistended alveoli rupture, allowing air to escape into the pulmonary interstitial spaces and the mediastinum, pleural space, and other tissues. Subcutaneous emphysema, pneumothorax, and pneumomediastinum are possible results of barotrauma. Subcutaneous emphysema, or air in the subcutaneous tissue, causes tissue swelling of the chest, neck, and face. A "crackling" or air bubble popping sensation is felt on palpation of subcutaneous emphysema. Swelling may be massive. Once the cause is corrected, the air is gradually reabsorbed.

- **Pneumothorax.** Pneumothorax is identified by signs of unequal chest expansion, a sudden loss of or significant decrease in breath sounds on the affected side, and a hyperresonant percussion tone. Rapid chest tube insertion is necessary to prevent tension pneumothorax and cardiovascular compromise. **Pneumomediastinum** is the presence of air in the mediastinum (the space between the lungs that contains the heart, great vessels, trachea, and esophagus). Air in the mediastinal space can interfere with the function of all of these organs and lead to such complications as **pneumopericardium** (air in the pericardial sac). Pneumomediastinum may have few manifestations, but the CXR shows widening of the mediastinal space.

- **Cardiovascular effects.** Positive pressure ventilation increases intrathoracic pressure, which can interfere with venous return to the heart and ventricular filling. As a result, cardiac output falls. Use of PEEP increases the effects of mechanical ventilation on cardiac output. The decreased cardiac output can affect liver and kidney function secondarily.

- **Gastrointestinal effects.** Gastrointestinal complications are commonly associated with prolonged mechanical ventilation. Stress ulcers (erosive gastritis) may develop, leading to painless gastrointestinal hemorrhage. Histamine H_2-receptor blockers or sucralfate are often used to prevent stress ulcers. Air leaks around the endotracheal tube can cause gastric distention; a nasogastric tube often is inserted to prevent vomiting. Sedation and other medications used during mechanical ventilation can slow intestinal motility, leading to constipation.

Weaning from Ventilator Support

The process of removing ventilator support and reestablishing spontaneous, independent respirations is called **weaning**. Weaning begins only after the underlying process causing respiratory failure has been corrected or stabilized. The process and time required for weaning depend on factors such as preexisting lung condition, duration of mechanical ventilation, and the patient's general condition, both physical and psychologic. In all cases, the vital signs, respiratory rate, extent of dyspnea, blood gases, and clinical status are used to evaluate weaning and its progress.

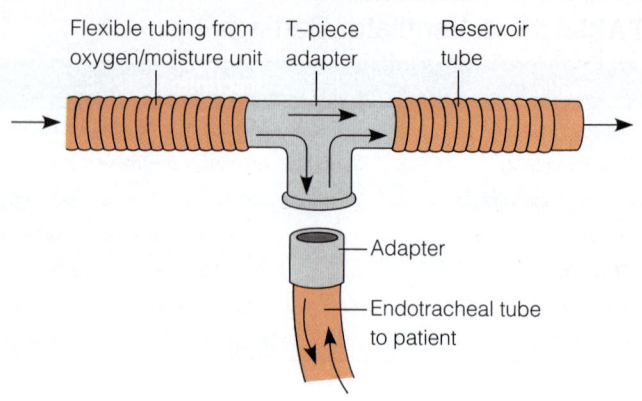

Figure 15–20 》 A T-piece, or "blow-by," unit for weaning from mechanical ventilation.

Following a brief period of mechanical ventilation, a T-piece unit or CPAP may be used for weaning. In T-piece weaning, the ventilator is removed for brief periods during which oxygen is delivered using a T-piece (see **Figure 15–20 》**). The duration of periods off the ventilator is gradually increased until the patient can maintain adequate independent respirations for several hours. Vital signs, oxygen saturation, $ETCO_2$, and PaO_2 are carefully monitored during the process. If signs of respiratory distress develop, the patient is placed back on the ventilator at the previous settings. When mechanical ventilation is no longer needed, the endotracheal tube is removed. CPAP weaning follows a similar process, with trials of spontaneous breathing supported by the ventilator in CPAP mode.

Both SIMV and PSV are used for weaning when the duration of mechanical ventilation has been longer and reconditioning of respiratory muscles is needed. When SIMV is used, the number of mandatory ventilator-assisted breaths is gradually decreased as ABG, $ETCO_2$, and respiratory rate are monitored. When the patient is able to tolerate SIMV at 4 breaths/min without rest periods or greater ventilatory support, CPAP or T-piece weaning is attempted before extubation (SOCCA, 2013).

Weaning is a primary use for PSV. At first, PSV is set slightly below the peak inspiratory pressures required during volume-cycled ventilation. Pressure support levels are gradually decreased, often in a cyclic pattern of periods of minimal support alternating with periods of higher support to recondition respiratory muscles. When the PSV level reaches 8–10 cm H_2O, extubation is considered (SOCCA, 2013).

When an illness is terminal or irreversible with a poor prognosis, terminal weaning may be requested by the patient or family. **Terminal weaning** is the gradual withdrawal of mechanical ventilation when survival without assisted ventilation is not expected. Unlike weaning when recovery is expected, which usually occurs in an ICU, the patient is moved to a quiet medical–surgical room, a hospice room, or even the patient's home before terminal weaning is initiated. Family members are encouraged to remain with the patient throughout the process. If possible, decisions about sedation and analgesia before and during weaning are made with the patient, as are decisions about hydration and nutritional support following weaning. Ventilator support is gradually withdrawn using the same modes described earlier (SIMV or PSV). Analgesia and sedation are given to promote comfort during weaning.

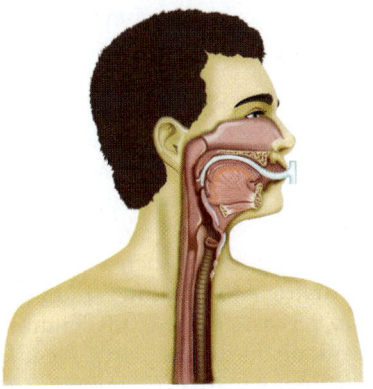

Figure 15–21 》 An oropharyngeal airway in place.

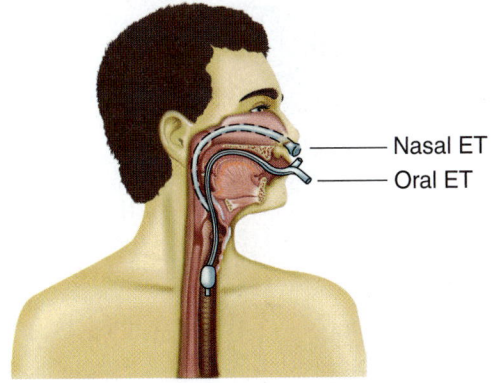

Nasal ET
Oral ET

Figure 15–23 》 An endotracheal tube in place.

Artificial Airways

Artificial airways are inserted to maintain a patent air passage for a patient whose airway has become or may become obstructed. A patent airway is necessary so that air can flow to and from the lungs. Four of the more common types of airways are oropharyngeal, nasopharyngeal, endotracheal, and tracheostomies.

Oropharyngeal and Nasopharyngeal Airways

Oropharyngeal and nasopharyngeal airways are used to keep the upper air passages open when they may become obstructed by secretions or by the tongue. These airway devices are easy to insert and have a low risk of complications. Sizes vary and should be appropriate to the size and age of the patient.

Oropharyngeal airways (see **Figure 15–21** 》) can stimulate the gag reflex and are used only for semiconscious or unconscious patients (e.g., because of general anesthesia or opioid overdose). Careful insertion of the oropharyngeal airway device is essential to preventing damage of the oral structures or accidental dislodgement of loose teeth, which could result in airway obstruction or aspiration. Note that oral airway insertion is contraindicated for patients with an intact gag reflex, as it can cause complications such as vomiting and laryngospasm in these patients.

Nasopharyngeal airways are generally well tolerated by alert patients and are inserted through the naris, terminating in the oropharynx (see **Figure 15–22** 》). When caring for a patient with a nasopharyngeal airway, provide frequent oral

and nares care, repositioning the airway in the other naris every 8 hours or as ordered to prevent necrosis of the mucosa. Prior to insertion, coat the nasopharyngeal airway device with a water-soluble lubricant.

SAFETY ALERT Nasopharyngeal airway insertion is contraindicated in patients who have bleeding disorders or who are receiving anticoagulant therapy, as damage to the nasal mucosa may cause uncontrollable bleeding. Insertion of a nasopharyngeal airway also is contraindicated in patients with a known or suspected facial fracture, including patients who demonstrate nasal bleeding following a traumatic head injury. Cranial vault fractures may allow for passage of the nasopharyngeal airway into the brain.

Endotracheal Tubes

Endotracheal tubes are most commonly inserted in patients who have had general anesthesia or who are in emergency situations in which mechanical ventilation is required. An endotracheal tube is inserted by the primary care provider, nurse, or respiratory therapist with specialized education. It is inserted through the mouth or the nose and into the trachea with the guide of a laryngoscope (see **Figure 15–23** 》). The tube terminates just superior to the bifurcation of the trachea into the bronchi. The tube may have an air-filled cuff to prevent air leakage around it. Because an endotracheal tube passes through the epiglottis and glottis, the patient is unable to speak while the tube is in place.

Tracheostomies

Patients who need long-term airway support may have a tracheostomy. A tracheostomy is an opening into the trachea through the neck. A tube is usually inserted through this opening, and an artificial airway is created. Tracheostomy is done using one of two techniques: the traditional open surgical method or a percutaneous insertion. The percutaneous method can be done at the bedside in a critical care unit. The open technique is done in the operating room: A surgical incision is made in the trachea just below the larynx, and a curved tracheostomy tube is inserted to extend through the stoma into the trachea (see **Figure 15–24** 》).

The nurse provides tracheostomy care for the patient with a new or recent tracheostomy to maintain patency of the tube and reduce the risk of infection. A tracheostomy may initially need to be suctioned and cleaned as often as every 1–2 hours. After the initial inflammatory response

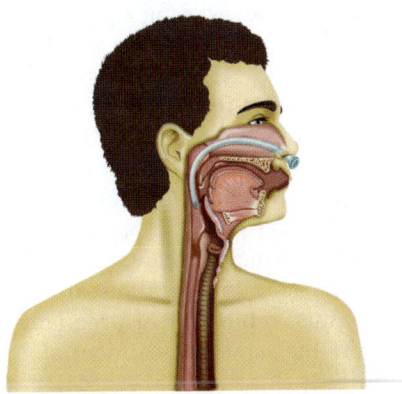

Figure 15–22 》 A nasopharyngeal airway in place.

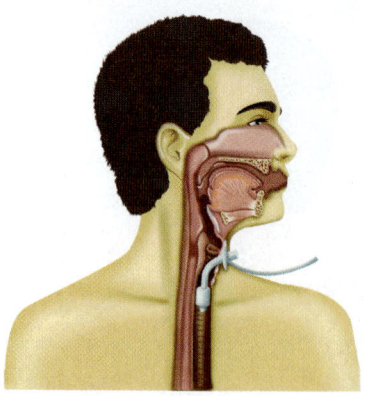

Figure 15–24 >> A tracheostomy tube in place.

subsides, tracheostomy care may only need to be done once or twice a day, depending on the patient's condition.

When the patient breathes through a tracheostomy, air is no longer filtered and humidified as it is when passing through the upper airways; therefore, special precautions are necessary. Humidity may be provided with a mist collar. Patients with long-term tracheostomies may wear a light scarf or a 4-in. × 4-in. gauze held in place with a cotton tie over the stoma to filter air as it enters the tracheostomy.

Nutrition and Fluids

The patient on mechanical ventilation requires close monitoring of fluid and electrolyte status as well as adequate nutrition. Mechanical ventilation promotes sodium and water retention as a result of its effects on cardiac output. Renal perfusion is decreased, stimulating the renin–angiotensin–aldosterone system to retain sodium and water. A Swan-Ganz catheter is often inserted to monitor pulmonary artery pressures and cardiac output. An arterial line allows repeated blood gas analysis and continuous arterial pressure monitoring. Serum electrolytes are drawn frequently; and intake, output, and daily weight are carefully monitored. Enteral or parenteral nutrition is provided during mechanical ventilation because the endotracheal tube prohibits eating. A nasogastric, gastrostomy, or jejunostomy feeding tube is placed for enteral nutrition. A jejunostomy tube may be used to reduce the risk of regurgitation and aspiration.

Other Clinical Therapies

Atelectasis frequently occurs in dependent lung regions in patients with ARDS. Prone positioning in conjunction with mechanical ventilation reduces the pressure of surrounding tissue on dependent regions and improves oxygenation.

Other management strategies include treatment of any infection and correction of the underlying condition. Infections are treated with IV antibiotic therapy tailored to the causative organism. Low molecular weight heparin may be ordered to prevent thrombophlebitis and possible pulmonary embolus or disseminated intravascular coagulation, a possible complication of ARDS.

Lifespan Considerations

ARDS can affect patients in any age group. However, common causes of ARDS, appropriate treatments and nursing interventions, and possible outcomes may differ depending on whether the patient is a child, pregnant woman, or older adult.

ARDS in Children

As in adult patients, the most common causes of ARDS in pediatric patients are pneumonia, aspiration, major trauma, near-drowning, and systemic infection. Children who are immunocompromised are at increased risk. Overall, the incidence of pediatric ARDS is low; studies estimate a rate between 2.9 and 9.5 cases per 100,000 children per year. The mortality rate among this population is somewhere between 22% and 35% (Cheifetz, 2011; Cornfield, 2013). The exact validity of these statistics is unclear, because it is widely believed that ARDS is underdiagnosed in the pediatric population. Likely reasons for underdiagnosis include hesitance to obtain invasive measures of arterial blood oxygenation in children, as well as difficulty identifying ARDS in children with lower respiratory tract infections (Rotta et al., 2015).

Because of the relatively low incidence of ARDS among pediatric patients, clinical guidelines related to the management of care for these patients were developed only recently (Pediatric Acute Lung Injury Consensus Conference Group [PALLIC], 2015). These guidelines reflect a variety of inherent differences between adult and pediatric patients, including the fact that children (especially infants and young children) have more compliant chest walls; higher sedation requirements and baseline airway resistance; and lower hematocrit and functional residual capacity. Because their lungs are not yet fully developed, children are also at higher risk for ventilator-related lung damage (Cheifetz, 2011).

The new pediatric ARDS guidelines include recommended ventilator settings and advise against routine use of inhaled nitric oxide, exogenous surfactant, corticosteroids, and prone positioning in children. They also recommend that intubation be used only in patients who do not respond to other measures or who have signs and symptoms of worsening ARDS, in an attempt to limit the risk of acquired infection and avoid complications from pain. However, the majority of the current recommendations highlight the need for additional research to determine ideal care modalities for pediatric patients with ARDS (PALLIC, 2015).

ARDS in Pregnant Women

ARDS is rarely seen in pregnant patients; various studies put the incidence somewhere between 1 in 3000 and 1 in 6000 deliveries. Despite low rates in this population, the condition often has devastating results, with a maternal mortality rate as high as 44% (Philip & Sharma, 2011). Common obstetric causes of ARDS in pregnant women include preeclampsia; amniotic fluid embolism; obstetric hemorrhage; and sepsis due to infection of the uterus, fetal membranes, or kidneys. Other common causes include pneumonia, aspiration, blood transfusion, and trauma (Duarte, 2014). ARDS has also been linked to influenza (H1N1) during pregnancy (Samanta et al., 2014).

Ethical concerns limit medical research involving pregnant women; thus, treatment of pregnant patients with ARDS is largely the same as treatment of any other adult patient (Philip & Sharma, 2011). Major goals include ensuring adequate ventilation and providing nutritional support. Administration of nitric oxide and corticosteroids may be appropriate (Duarte, 2014). Prone positioning can help patients maintain oxygen levels, although care must be taken in the third trimester of pregnancy to ensure there is adequate maternal blood flow to the placenta (Samanta et al., 2014). Close fetal monitoring is also critical and can help determine when the infant should be delivered. There is no research indicating that maternal outcomes improve on delivery, although immediate delivery is obviously beneficial to the fetus when the mother's ARDS has led to compromised placental oxygen transfer (Philip & Sharma, 2011), especially if the fetus is at least 20–24 weeks of gestational age.

ARDS in Older Adults

Older adults, especially those over age 70, are at greater risk for ARDS than the rest of the adult population. This heightened risk is at least partially due to age-related changes in respiratory physiology, including loss of elastic tissue, increased chest diameter, and decreased muscle strength. Mortality rates are also higher among older adults, especially those who have ARDS accompanied by multisystem organ failure (Lorente & Artigas, 2012).

As compared to their younger counterparts, older adults with ARDS are less likely to be admitted to the ICU. Even when placed in a critical care unit, older adults are still less likely to receive the same intensity of care as other patients with ARDS, including use of mechanical ventilation (Lorente & Artigas, 2012). Thus, while older adults are able to recover from the acute phase of ARDS in about the same time as younger patients, they are significantly more likely to die from multiple organ failure and other complications (Brock & Jablonski, 2010). Older adults may also be at increased risk for injuries from mechanical ventilation (Lorente & Artigas, 2012). Together, these factors help explain the increased mortality rate among older adults.

There is little evidence as to whether various therapies for ARDS itself are more or less successful in the older adult population (Lorente & Artigas, 2012). However, research suggests that treatments aimed at prevention of nonpulmonary organ complications help improve overall outcomes (Brock & Jablonski, 2010). Adequate nutrition, including a diet high in omega-3 and -6 fatty acids, also appears to contribute to improved oxygen levels and lung function in older adults (Cohen et al., 2014).

NURSING PROCESS

Caring for the patient with ARDS requires careful and continuous monitoring of airway, breathing, and circulation. Changes in LOC, oxygenation, or perfusion require rapid nursing interventions to maintain life. The focus of nursing care is on meeting these essential patient needs.

Assessment

Collect assessment data through the health history and physical assessment:

- **Observation and patient interview.** Previous respiratory alterations, previous illnesses and surgeries, and any illness or direct or indirect injury in the previous 3–4 days

- **Physical examination.** Respiratory rate and rhythm; auscultation of the lungs; LOC, including orientation; baseline vital signs; peripheral perfusion.

Confusion, agitation, and anxiety are early signs of hypoxemia, especially in older adults. Changes from baseline vital signs alert the nurse to subtle changes in cardiac or respiratory status. Individuals developing ARDS may express desperate anxiety because of the inability to get enough air to relieve their shortness of breath.

Diagnosis

Any combination of the following NANDA-I diagnoses may be appropriate for the individual with ARDS:

- *Confusion, Risk for Acute*
- *Airway Clearance, Ineffective*
- *Breathing Pattern, Ineffective*
- *Ventilation: Spontaneous, Impaired*
- *Impaired Gas Exchange*
- *Cardiac Output, Decreased*
- *Ventilatory Weaning Response, Dysfunctional*
- *Fluid Volume: Imbalanced, Risk for*
- *Imbalanced Nutrition: Less Than Body Requirements*
- *Infection, Risk for*
- *Pain, Acute*
- *Anxiety.*

   (NANDA-I © 2014)

Additional NANDA-I diagnoses may be appropriate depending on the underlying condition causing the acute respiratory distress.

Planning

The goal of care for individuals with ARDS is to protect the lungs from fibrotic damage while providing adequate oxygenation to the body systems. Expected outcomes may include the following:

- The patient will be oriented to name, place, and time with each healthcare personnel interaction.
- The patient will receive adequate ventilatory support to maintain oxygenation of body cells.
- The patient will maintain a patent airway.
- The patient will maintain cardiac output adequate to perfuse all body systems.
- The patient will receive adequate nutrition to maintain body processes.
- The patient will be free of any sign or symptom of infection.
- The patient will remain free of thrombosis.
- The patient will manage pain successfully.
- The patient will cope with or be free from anxiety.

Implementation

All body systems are at risk of failure caused by poor oxygenation and alterations in perfusion. The healthcare team will identify and treat the causative agent, as this is critical to returning the patient to normal health. Common interventions for the patient with ARDS include the following:

- Conduct CBC, chemistry panel, ABGs, blood cultures, sputum cultures, and gastric and stool cultures as indicated by symptoms.
- Monitor vital signs at least hourly. Continual monitoring may be required.
- Monitor oxygenation status with ABGs and pulse oximetry.
- Monitor neurologic status, including orientation and LOC.
- Auscultate lung and heart sounds.
- Provide analgesia, anxiolytics, and sedation medications as ordered.
- Provide beta-agonist to maintain patent airways as ordered.
- Maintain head of bed at 30° or higher.
- Position the individual prone for 30 minutes to an hour as tolerated three or four times a day. This position may facilitate oxygenation of the posterior alveoli and posterior drainage.
- Suction airway as needed.
- Monitor hemodynamic status with central venous catheters or pulmonary artery catheter as ordered.
- Monitor renal function by intake and output as well as blood urea nitrogen and creatinine levels.
- Place Foley catheter.
- Administer IV fluids as needed, but avoid fluid overload.
- Monitor glucose level, and maintain levels within normal limits.
- Assess peripheral pulses.

Maintain a Patent Airway

Ineffective airway clearance may either cause respiratory failure or occur as a result of interventions. Impaired ventilation frequently leads to acute respiratory failure. Although intubation and mechanical ventilation can be lifesaving measures, they also increase the risk of respiratory infection and ineffective secretion management.

- Perform PVD as ordered. These techniques help loosen secretions and move them into larger airways for removal by coughing or suctioning.
- Assess fluid balance and maintain adequate hydration. Adequate hydration helps liquefy secretions.
- Suction as needed to maintain a patent airway. Indicators for suctioning include crackles and rhonchi on auscultation, frequent coughing or setting off of the high-pressure alarm, and increasing restlessness or anxiety. Although patients with a tracheostomy can usually cough up secretions, the length and diameter of endotracheal tubes makes this extremely difficult. Even with humidification, secretions often become thick and tenacious, further inhibiting their removal.
- Obtain sputum for culture if it appears purulent or is odorous. Culture is necessary to identify pathogens and guide antibiotic therapy.

- Firmly secure the endotracheal or tracheostomy tube. Provide adequate slack on ventilator tubing to prevent tension on the tube when turning, positioning, or transferring the patient to a chair or stretcher. If prescribed, loosely restrain the patient's hands. These measures are important to ensure proper airway placement and prevent inadvertent removal of the tube.

Promote Spontaneous Ventilation

The ability of the patient with ARDS to maintain adequate ventilation is impaired. This is a concern both before initiation of mechanical ventilation and during the weaning process.

- Place the patient in Fowler or high-Fowler position. Sitting positions decrease pressure on the diaphragm and chest, improving lung ventilation and decreasing the work of breathing.
- Minimize activities and energy expenditures by assisting with ADLs, spacing procedures and activities, and allowing uninterrupted periods of rest. Rest is vital to reduce oxygen and energy demands.
- Promptly report worsening ABG and oxygen saturation levels. Close assessment of these values allows timely intervention as needed.
- Administer oxygen as ordered, monitoring response. Observe closely for respiratory depression, especially in the patient with COPD. Oxygen administration reduces the hypoxemic respiratory drive. Chronically high $PaCO_2$ levels depress the respiratory center; hypoxemia may provide the only respiratory drive.

SAFETY ALERT Promptly report signs of respiratory distress, including tachypnea, tachycardia, nasal flaring, use of accessory muscles, intercostal retractions, cyanosis, increasing restlessness, anxiety, or decreased LOC. These may be early manifestations of respiratory failure and inability to maintain ventilatory effort.

Enhance Cardiac Output

With positive pressure ventilation, increased intrathoracic pressure decreases cardiac output. When PEEP is applied, intrathoracic pressure increases further; this can significantly decrease venous return, ventricular filling, stroke volume, and cardiac output. Manifestations of decreased cardiac output include hypotension and compensatory tachycardia as the heart attempts to maintain cardiac output despite decreased stroke volume. In the patient who is already hypoxic because of ARDS, this drop in cardiac output can increase tissue damage. Urine output falls, and dysrhythmias may develop. A fall in urine output to less than 30 mL/hour is often the first sign of decreased cardiac output; therefore, urine output should be recorded hourly.

- Assess LOC at least every 4 hours. Altered LOC, confusion, and restlessness are early signs of cerebral hypoxia resulting from decreased cardiac output.
- Monitor pulmonary artery pressures, central venous pressure, and cardiac output readings every 1–4 hours. Changes in these measurements may indicate worsening cardiac status.

- Assess heart and lung sounds frequently. Increasing crackles or abnormal heart sounds may indicate heart failure.
- Weigh daily at the same time. Accurate daily weights are the best indicator of fluid volume status.
- Provide frequent skin care, keeping skin clean and dry and protecting pressure points. Tissue hypoxia increases the risk of skin breakdown, which in turn increases the risk of infection and sepsis.
- Administer analgesics, sedatives, and neuromuscular blockers as needed. These medications may be prescribed to decrease cardiac workload.

Monitor for Dysfunctional Ventilatory Weaning Response

Assessment findings indicative of dysfunctional weaning include the following:

- Dyspnea, apprehension, or agitation
- Decreasing oxygen saturation level
- Cyanosis or pallor, diaphoresis
- Increased blood pressure, pulse, and respiratory rate
- Diminished or adventitious breath sounds, use of accessory muscles
- Decreased LOC
- Deteriorating ABG values
- Shallow, gasping breaths or paradoxical abdominal breathing.

The patient with dysfunctional ventilatory weaning response has difficulty adjusting to reduced mechanical ventilator support, prolonging the weaning process. Airway congestion, inadequate rest or nutrition, pain, anxiety, and a nonsupportive environment are factors that can contribute to difficulty weaning. With ARDS, the pathologic processes of the disease and its effects on gas exchange may be responsible for a prolonged or ineffective weaning process.

- Assess vital signs every 15–30 minutes following changes in ventilator settings and during T-piece trials. Vital signs (heart and respiratory rates in particular) can provide early signs of hypoxemia and poor tolerance of the weaning process.
- Place in Fowler or high-Fowler position.
- Fully explain all weaning procedures, along with expected changes in breathing. Adequate explanations help reduce anxiety and improve cooperation.
- Remain with the patient during initial periods following changes of ventilator settings or T-piece trials. This provides reassurance and allows close monitoring of the response.
- Limit procedures and activities during weaning periods. Reducing energy expenditures and cardiac work facilitates the weaning process.
- Provide diversion, such as television or radio. Diversion helps distract the focus from breathing.
- Begin weaning procedures in the morning, when the patient is well rested and alert; weaning may be discontinued overnight to provide rest. The work of breathing increases during the weaning process; adequate rest is important.
- When SIMV is used for weaning, decrease the SIMV rate by increments of two breaths per minute. Slow reduction of ventilator support allows respiratory muscle reconditioning and gradual resumption of the work of breathing.
- Avoid administering drugs that may depress respirations during the weaning process (except as ordered at night to facilitate rest when ventilator support is provided). Sedatives or analgesics that depress respirations can impair the weaning process.
- Keep oxygen at the bedside following weaning and extubation. Supplemental oxygen may be necessary to maintain adequate blood and tissue oxygenation.
- Provide pulmonary hygiene with percussion and postural drainage. Maintaining patent airways and adequate alveolar ventilation is vital during the weaning process.

SAFETY ALERT Frequently assess respiratory status following weaning and extubation. Keep an intubation kit readily available following extubation; be prepared to provide emergency reintubation. Laryngeal spasm or laryngeal edema may develop following extubation, necessitating reintubation to maintain respirations.

Relieve Anxiety

Critical illness creates anxiety for any patient. In ARDS, this anxiety is compounded by the presence of an endotracheal tube or tracheostomy, mechanical ventilator, numerous monitors and equipment, and potentially, neuromuscular blockade and paralysis of voluntary muscles. Fear of continued dependence on the mechanical ventilator and inability to return to a normal life may compound this anxiety.

- Explain all monitors, procedures, unusual sounds, and machinery. Understanding the environment and the various sounds and alarms reduces anxiety.
- Provide a simple means of communication, such as a whiteboard or iPad, or use methods such as looking to the right for "yes" and to the left for "no." Reassure the patient that endotracheal tube removal restores the ability to speak. The inability to speak and call out for help is frightening for the patient. Providing an alternative means of communication helps reduce anxiety.
- Encourage frequent family visits, especially if the time of visitations is being limited. Encourage family participation in care. Family visits help reduce anxiety and feelings of abandonment. Allowing family members to participate in care helps reduce their anxiety as well.
- Explain to the family that the patient can hear and understand. Emphasize the importance of talking to the patient, not over or about the patient. Talking to the patient about everyday things reduces the patient's sense of isolation and fear.
- Attend to physical needs promptly and completely. This provides reassurance that needs will be met even though the patient is unable to ask for assistance.
- Reassure the patient that intubation and mechanical ventilation are temporary measures to allow the lungs to rest

and heal. Reinforce that the patient will be able to breathe independently again. The patient may fear continued dependence on mechanical ventilation.

SAFETY ALERT Frequently monitor the patient's anxiety level. High levels of anxiety increase oxygen use and often interfere with the ability to work with the respirator. This can increase hypoxemia and further increase anxiety; intervention is necessary to break this cycle.

Prepare for Discharge

Provide referrals to home health and respiratory care services as indicated, as well as for occupational therapy and counseling as needed. When preparing the patient who has recovered from ARDS and the family for home care, provide patient teaching about ARDS itself and the need to tailor activities until maximal respiratory function returns, to avoid smoking and exposure to smoke and other pollutants, and to obtain immunizations for pneumonia and influenza.

Evaluation

The patient's response to nursing care is evaluated often, and nursing care is adjusted accordingly. Expected outcomes for the patient with ARDS often include:

- The patient attained and maintained an effective airway throughout the hospitalization.

- The patient's oxygen saturation remained greater than 90% throughout the hospitalization.
- The patient's cardiac output remained stable throughout the hospitalization.
- The patient was successfully weaned off the mechanical ventilator before discharge.
- The patient demonstrated no signs or symptoms of aspiration of gastric contents throughout the hospitalization.
- The patient's ABG results were within normal limits prior to hospital discharge.
- The patient was able to successfully use coping mechanisms to manage anxiety.
- Following completion of discharge teaching, the patient verbalized understanding of the importance of avoiding secondhand smoke and pollutants.

Successful treatment of ARDS requires continual monitoring of the patient and application of the nursing process. If one type of intervention is not successful, the nurse should continue to consult with the physician and others on the care team, implement appropriate nursing interventions, and assist in any needed procedures. The nurse may need to implement physician orders for different types of ventilation, continually adjust ventilator pressure, monitor the patient for exacerbations, and report changes to the care team.

REVIEW Acute Respiratory Distress Syndrome

RELATE Link the Concepts and Exemplars

Linking the exemplar of acute respiratory distress syndrome with the concept of acid–base balance:

1. What impact will ARDS likely have on acid–base balance, and how can the nurse intervene to promote normal balance?
2. Are the symptoms of ARDS entirely the result of acid–base imbalance, or are other factors involved? Explain your answer.

Linking the exemplar of acute respiratory distress syndrome with the concept of grief and loss:

3. When caring for a patient with ARDS who is not responding to treatments as anticipated, what nursing care might the family require as it deals with the possibility of the patient's death?
4. How might you, as the nurse, help to support the family in this process?

Linking the exemplar of acute respiratory distress syndrome with the concept of comfort:

5. When caring for a patient with ARDS, what symptoms might the patient exhibit that may signal the patient is in discomfort?
6. What treatments or diversional activities may be appropriate for this patient?

READY Go to Volume 3: Clinical Nursing Skills

REFER Go to Pearson MyLab Nursing and eText

- Additional review material
- Nursing Care Plan: A Patient with Acute Respiratory Distress Syndrome

REFLECT Apply Your Knowledge

Mr. Robert Michaels is a 75-year-old man with emphysema, asthma, high blood pressure, and almost complete hearing loss. A lifelong smoker, he quit smoking a few years ago when he was diagnosed with emphysema. For some time, he has been on oxygen therapy at night. He takes several medications daily, including 10 mg of prednisone, a corticosteroid inhaler, albuterol by nebulizer, and high blood pressure medication with a diuretic.

Two days ago, Mr. Michaels felt sick and was running a fever. His wife took him to his primary care provider's office, where he was diagnosed with an upper respiratory infection and sent home with an oral antibiotic. Mr. Michaels woke up in the middle of the night in respiratory distress. Ms. Michaels called 911, and her husband was transported by ambulance to the emergency department, where he was diagnosed with pneumonia and ARDS. Mr. Michaels was placed on mechanical ventilation and admitted to the critical care unit.

1. What are the nursing priorities for Mr. Michaels?
2. What considerations need to be given to Mr. Michaels' hearing loss?
3. What factors are likely to exacerbate his respiratory function?
4. How can you promote oxygenation for this patient?

Exemplar 15.B
Asthma

Exemplar Learning Outcomes

15.B Analyze asthma as it relates to oxygenation.

- Describe the pathophysiology of asthma.
- Describe the etiology of asthma.
- Summarize risk factors for asthma.
- Compare methods for preventing asthma.
- Identify the clinical manifestations of asthma.
- Summarize diagnostic tests and therapies used by interprofessional teams in the collaborative care of an individual with asthma.
- Differentiate care of patients with asthma across the lifespan.
- Apply the nursing process in providing culturally competent care to an individual with asthma.

Exemplar Key Terms

Airway remodeling, *1057*
Asthma, *1057*
Edema, *1057*
Hyperresponsiveness, *1057*
Hyperventilation, *1058*
Orthopneic position, *1068*
Status asthmaticus, *1058*

Overview

Asthma is the persistent inflammation of the lungs characterized by recurrent episodes of shortness of breath, difficulty breathing, chest tightness or pressure, coughing (especially at night), and wheezing. While most episodes or asthma "attacks" are relatively brief, some patients may experience longer episodes with some degree of airway impairment daily. Mild, brief episodes may resolve spontaneously, but most asthma attacks require treatment. Asthma in early life may lead to an irreversible decline of pulmonary function in adulthood as a result of permanent, structural changes called **airway remodeling**. These changes can lead to progressive or permanent loss of lung function.

Pathophysiology and Etiology

Pathophysiology

In asthma, the airways are in a persistent state of inflammation. During symptom-free periods, airway inflammation in asthma is subacute or quiet. Even during these periods, however, inflammatory cells, such as eosinophils, neutrophils, and lymphocytes, may be found in airway tissues, and **edema** (swelling caused by excess fluid in bodily tissue) may be present.

A variety of triggers may initiate an acute inflammatory response, during which resident inflammatory cells interact with inflammatory mediators, cytokines, and additional infiltrating inflammatory cells (see the Etiology section). The inflammatory response resulting from exposure to one of these triggers leads to bronchoconstriction, airway edema, and impaired clearance of secretions. Airway narrowing impedes airflow and increases the work of breathing; trapped air mixes with inhaled air, impairing gas exchange.

In an individual with asthma, any combination of these stimuli may result in airway **hyperresponsiveness** (an exaggerated bronchoconstrictor response) and airway obstruction from overproduction of mucus and edema of the airway mucosa (see **Figure 15–25 »**). Sensitized mast cells in the bronchial mucosa release inflammatory mediators, such as histamine, prostaglandins, and leukotrienes. Resident and

infiltrating inflammatory cells also produce inflammatory mediators, such as cytokines, bradykinin, and growth factors. These mediators stimulate parasympathetic receptors and bronchial smooth muscle to produce bronchoconstriction. They also increase capillary permeability, which allows

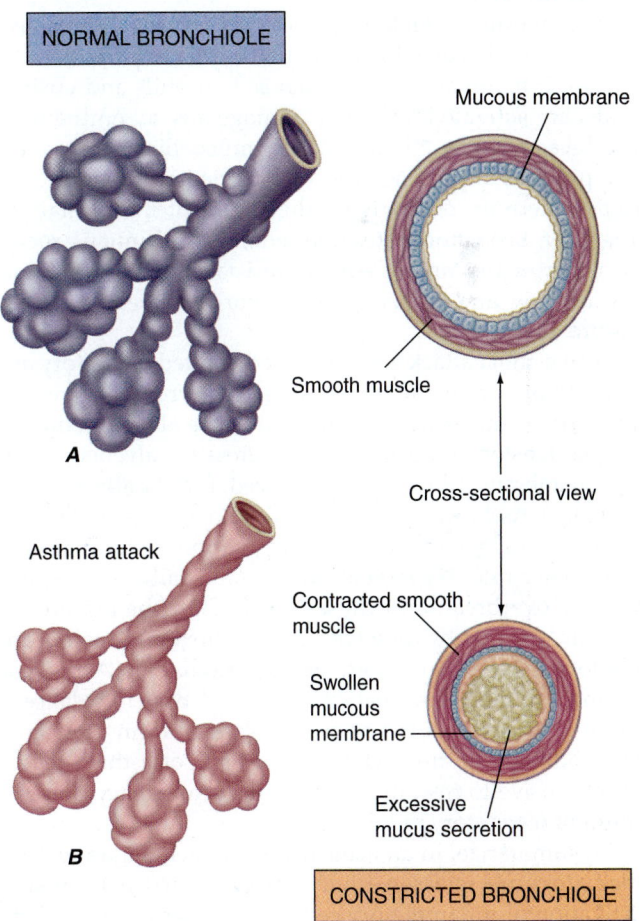

Figure 15–25 » Changes in bronchioles during an asthma attack. **A,** Normal bronchiole. **B,** Bronchiole during asthma attack.

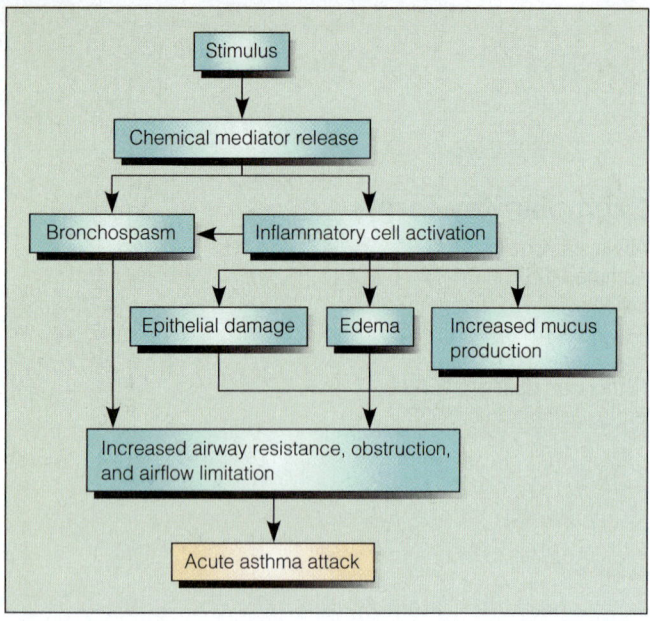

```
                    ┌──────────┐
                    │ Stimulus │
                    └──────────┘
                         │
                         ▼
            ┌─────────────────────────┐
            │ Chemical mediator release │
            └─────────────────────────┘
              │                    │
              ▼                    ▼
     ┌──────────────┐   ┌─────────────────────────┐
     │ Bronchospasm │◄──│ Inflammatory cell activation │
     └──────────────┘   └─────────────────────────┘
              │          │        │          │
              │          ▼        ▼          ▼
              │  ┌──────────┐ ┌──────┐ ┌─────────────┐
              │  │ Epithelial│ │ Edema│ │Increased mucus│
              │  │  damage  │ │      │ │  production  │
              │  └──────────┘ └──────┘ └─────────────┘
              │        │        │          │
              ▼        ▼        ▼          ▼
     ┌────────────────────────────────────────────┐
     │ Increased airway resistance, obstruction,    │
     │ and airflow limitation                       │
     └────────────────────────────────────────────┘
                         │
                         ▼
                ┌──────────────────┐
                │ Acute asthma attack │
                └──────────────────┘
```

Figure 15–26 》 Pathogenesis of an acute episode of asthma.

plasma to escape and leads to mucosal edema. Production of mucus is stimulated; excess mucus collects in the narrowed airways.

The asthma attack is prolonged by the late-phase response, which develops 4–12 hours after exposure to the trigger. Inflammatory cells, such as basophils and eosinophils, are activated, and they damage airway epithelium, produce mucosal edema, impair mucociliary clearance, and produce or prolong bronchoconstriction. The degree of hyperreactivity depends on the extent of inflammation. Together, bronchoconstriction, edema, and mucus secretion narrow the airway. Airway resistance increases, limiting airflow and increasing the work of breathing (see **Figure 15–26 》**).

If an asthma attack goes untreated, limited expiratory airflow traps air distal to the spastic, narrowed airways. Trapped air mixes with inspired air in the alveoli, reducing oxygen tension and gas exchange across the alveolar–capillary membrane. Blood flow is reduced, further affecting gas exchange. As a result, hypoxemia develops. Hypoxemia and increased lung volume caused by trapping stimulate the respiratory rate. **Hyperventilation** (unusually fast respiration, or overbreathing) causes the $PaCO_2$ (the amount of pressure exerted by dissolved carbon dioxide) to fall, leading to respiratory alkalosis. (See the module on Acid–Base Balance for more information about acid–base imbalances.) **Status asthmaticus** is a severe, prolonged form of asthma that is difficult to treat. Untreated asthma or asthma that is unresponsive to treatment is a medical emergency that can result in respiratory failure.

To summarize, in an acute asthma attack, inflammatory mediators are released from sensitized airways, causing activation of inflammatory cells. This progression leads to bronchoconstriction, airway edema, and impaired mucociliary clearance. Airway narrowing limits airflow and increases the work of breathing; trapped air mixes with inhaled air, impairing gas exchange.

Etiology

Common allergens that can cause airway inflammation include pollens, weeds, molds, dust mites, and animal dander. Allergic asthma is an alteration of type I hypersensitivity, which is explained in more detail in the module on Immunity.

Asthma also may occur from exposure to aspirin and other nonsteroidal drugs. It may result from exercise, cold or hot air, viral infections, and even stress. Genetic involvement seems to be a component, but the role played by genetics in asthma is not clear. Occupational asthma arises from exposure to respiratory irritants in the workplace.

According to the Centers for Disease Control and Prevention (CDC, 2015a), asthma affects more than 9% of children in the United States, making it the most common serious chronic childhood illness. Overall, asthma affects some 25 million Americans (CDC, 2015a), resulting in both direct and indirect costs, such as lost workdays each year, either for adult patients with asthma or for caregivers staying home with children with asthma (Rappaport & Bonthapally, 2012).

Risk Factors

Risk factors include genetic factors, exposure to certain infections early in life, air pollution, and allergies. Early childhood exposure to respiratory syncytial virus (RSV), parainfluenza virus, adenovirus, mycoplasma, and chlamydia has been associated with the development of asthma. Atmospheric air can be polluted by ozone, industrial gaseous wastes, and particulate matter, such as pollens or tobacco smoke. Obesity, maternal smoking, and premature birth also increase the risk for asthma.

Prevention

Asthma attacks often can be prevented by avoiding allergens and environmental triggers. Modifying the home environment by controlling dust, removing carpets, covering mattresses and pillows to reduce dust mite populations, and installing air-filtering systems may be useful. Pets may need to be removed from the household. Stuffed animals provide wonderful living spaces for dust mites and should be removed from bedrooms. Eliminating all tobacco smoke in the house is vital. Wearing a mask that retains humidity and warm air while exercising in cold weather may help prevent attacks of exercise-induced or cold-triggered asthma. Early treatment of respiratory infections is vital to prevent exacerbations.

The patient with moderate or severe asthma who is prescribed controller medications (e.g., long-acting bronchodilators and inhaled corticosteroids) to prevent asthma attacks must take these daily in order for the medicine to be effective. Adherence to medication regimens varies greatly among those with asthma, as some will stop taking the medication once symptoms improve, which only increases the likelihood of another asthma attack. Patient teaching about prevention must include the issue of adherence to medication regimens.

Cultural and language barriers have an effect on the management of asthma (see the Focus on Diversity and Culture feature).

Focus on Diversity and Culture
Asthma Management

Although asthma is a general concern that crosses all racial and ethnic lines, people in different racial and ethnic groups differ in how they use preventive medications for asthma. Research points to differences in communication practices and health beliefs as possible factors (Seeleman et al., 2012). Overcoming communication barriers is crucial when cultural or language barriers exist. Therefore, when patients have little or no English proficiency, the use of formal interpreters is necessary to effectively and accurately transfer health-related information. To effectively promote proper self-management of care among all patients regardless of culture or ethnicity, the active development of cultural competence is also critical to increase awareness of how different cultural beliefs influence health-related perceptions (Seeleman et al., 2012).

Poverty also plays a role in asthma management. The prevalence of asthma is higher among groups whose income-to-poverty levels are lower (CDC, 2015a; Federal Interagency Forum on Child and Family Statistics, 2016). A National Center for Health Statistics study found that the percentage of children ages 0–17 years who currently have asthma and have received an asthma management plan increased between 2002 and 2013 from 41% to 51%. During the same time span, there were no changes in the percentages of children with asthma who received an asthma management plan and who lived in families with incomes less than 100% of the poverty level. This lack of difference held true among children in families with incomes 100–199% of the poverty level (Federal Interagency Forum on Child and Family Statistics, 2015). Although the incidence of asthma is higher among children in lower income families, asthma management has not increased or improved for those children in recent years, though it has for children in general.

Clinical Manifestations

Clinical manifestations of asthma include coughing, wheezing, shortness of breath, chest tightness, tachypnea and tachycardia, and anxiety and apprehension. Asthma is defined by severity and control as well as by the frequency of exacerbations. Asthma that is not well controlled is evident by daytime symptoms, nocturnal awakenings because of symptoms, frequent use of a SABA, and inability to perform or difficulty performing normal activities, including exercise.

The onset of symptoms may be either abrupt or insidious, and an attack may subside rapidly or persist for hours or days. With more severe attacks, use of accessory muscles for respirations, retractions, loud wheezing, and distant breaths sounds may be noted. Activity intolerance and fatigue are common, especially if an episode lasts for more than a few minutes. Fatigue, anxiety, apprehension, and severe dyspnea that allows only one or two words to be spoken between breaths may occur with persistent severe episodes. The onset of respiratory failure is marked by inaudible breath sounds with reduced wheezing and an ineffective cough. Without careful assessment, this apparent relief of symptoms can be misinterpreted as improvement.

The frequency of attacks and the severity of symptoms vary greatly from person to person. Although some people have infrequent, mild episodes, or flares, others have nearly continuous manifestations. See the Clinical Manifestations and Therapies feature for a summary of the categories of asthma severity.

Severity of asthma symptoms can be difficult for the patient to describe and for the nurse to assess. A PEFR measurement provides an objective assessment of lung function that allows patients to monitor symptoms and communicate their severity to others. Using small, inexpensive PEFR meters, patients take readings at varying times of day over several weeks to establish their personal best or normal PEFR. This value is then used to evaluate the severity of the airway obstruction. Traffic colors are used for simplicity: Green (80–100% of personal best) indicates asthma that is under control; yellow (50–80%) means caution, indicating a need for medication or treatment; and red (50% or less) signals an immediate need for a bronchodilator and further medical treatment if the level does not return to the yellow range immediately following administration of the bronchodilator.

Collaboration

Patients with asthma may benefit from a collaborative effort that includes a number of healthcare providers, including a respiratory therapist. The role of the nurse is discussed in more detail in the Nursing Process section.

Diagnostic Tests

An important diagnostic tool for a patient with persistent asthma is the PEFR. Nurses should encourage all patients to use their peak flow meters daily and to keep a record of their readings, even on days when they are in the green zone (80–100% of personal best). At each healthcare interaction, nurses should remind patients with persistent asthma of the importance of using their peak flow meters.

For patients who are suspected of having allergic asthma, scratch or patch testing and immunoglobulin E (IgE) testing can be used to determine the severity of the patient's allergies as well as specific triggers to which the patient reacts. Allergy testing normally is available only through an allergist or immunologist and is described in more detail in the module on Immunity.

Other diagnostic tests that may be useful for the patient with asthma include the following:

- CBC with differential if infection is suspected
- ABGs to monitor acid–base balance
- Pulmonary function studies
- CXR
- Oxygen saturation monitoring
- Transcutaneous oxygen and carbon dioxide monitoring.

≫ Go to **Pearson MyLab Nursing and eText** to see Appendix B for information on diagnostic tests that may be useful for the patient with asthma.

Pharmacologic Therapy

Medications are used to prevent and control asthma symptoms, reduce the frequency and severity of exacerbations, and reverse airway obstruction. Drugs used for long-term control of asthma are taken daily to maintain control of the disease. The primary drugs in this group

Clinical Manifestations and Therapies
Asthma

SEVERITY	CLINICAL MANIFESTATIONS	CLINICAL THERAPIES
Mild intermittent	■ Daytime symptoms occur no more than twice a week. ■ Nighttime symptoms occur no more than twice per month. ■ Peak flow rates between attacks are normal. ■ Attacks (or flares) last hours to a few days. ■ Typical symptoms include shortness of breath, labored breathing, and fatigue.	■ Medications include bronchodilators or beta-agonists, usually via inhaler or nebulizer. A beta-agonist is usually prescribed for use before anticipated exposure (e.g., exercise). ■ A short course of oral corticosteroids may be prescribed if the attack lasts beyond 1 day or is related to an infection or other disease process that may extend recovery time. Inhaled corticosteroids usually take a few days to work and may not be prescribed for intermittent asthma except during periods of exposure to known triggers (e.g., ragweed). ■ If triggers include allergens, oral antihistamine may be prescribed.
Mild persistent	■ Daytime symptoms occur more than twice a week but less than once per day. ■ Nighttime symptoms occur more than twice a month. ■ Exacerbations may affect activity. ■ Typical symptoms include shortness of breath, labored breathing, and fatigue.	■ Medications include bronchodilators or beta-agonists. A LABA may be prescribed for daily use regardless of whether the patient is symptomatic. ■ Inhaled corticosteroids are prescribed for daily use to prevent symptoms during likely periods of exacerbation. ■ If triggers include allergens, antileukotrienes may be prescribed.
Moderate persistent	■ Symptoms occur daily. ■ A short-acting bronchodilator (e.g., albuterol inhaler) is used daily. ■ Nighttime symptoms occur more than once a week. ■ Exacerbations may last for days. ■ Exacerbations affect activity. ■ Symptoms of exacerbations include shortness of breath, labored and painful breathing, and chest tightness; symptoms may include coughing, wheezing, tachypnea, tachycardia, and fatigue.	■ Medications include LABAs, inhaled corticosteroids, and antileukotrienes (if allergens are triggers). ■ Immunotherapy may be tried if triggers include allergens. ■ Cromolyn sodium or theophylline (long-acting bronchodilators) may be prescribed. ■ A nebulizer may be prescribed for use during exacerbations. ■ Oral corticosteroids may be prescribed for use during exacerbations lasting more than 1–2 days.
Severe persistent	■ Continuous symptoms occur with frequent exacerbations. ■ Physical activity is limited. ■ Symptoms include shortness of breath, labored and painful breathing, chest tightness, coughing, wheezing, tachypnea, tachycardia, difficulty speaking without pausing for breathing, and extreme fatigue.	■ Medications include LABA inhalers, inhaled corticosteroids, and antileukotrienes (if allergens are triggers). ■ Immunotherapy may be tried if triggers include allergens. ■ Cromolyn sodium or theophylline may be prescribed. ■ Oral corticosteroids may be prescribed for use during exacerbations lasting more than 1–2 days. ■ Steroids and beta-agonists delivered via nebulizer may be prescribed and used daily or as needed during exacerbations.

are anti-inflammatory agents, long-acting bronchodilators, and leukotriene modifiers. Quick-relief medications provide prompt relief of bronchoconstriction and airflow obstruction with associated wheezing, cough, and chest tightness. Short-acting adrenergic stimulants (rapid-acting bronchodilators), anticholinergic drugs, and methylxanthines fall into this category.

A stepwise approach for managing asthma is recommended. This approach is based on the severity of disease (see **Table 15–5** 》). For all patients, an inhaled SABA is recommended for quick relief of acute symptoms. Strategies for long-term control may need to be modified if a short-acting bronchodilator is needed more than twice a week (NHLBI, 2014).

TABLE 15–5 Stepwise Approach to Asthma Management for Adults

Step/Disease Severity	Preferred Treatment	Alternative or as-Needed Treatment
Step 1: Intermittent	Inhaled SABAs as needed	
Step 2: Mild persistent	Low-dose inhaled corticosteroids	Use cromolyn, leukotriene receptor antagonist, or theophylline; administer inhaled SABAs as needed.
Step 3: Mild-moderate persistent	Low-dose inhaled corticosteroids *and* long-acting inhaled β_2-agonist OR medium-dose inhaled corticosteroids	Combine low-dose inhaled corticosteroid with leukotriene receptor antagonist, theophylline, or zileuton; administer inhaled SABAs as needed.
Step 4: Moderate persistent	Medium-dose inhaled corticosteroids *and* long-acting inhaled β_2-agonist	Combine medium-dose inhaled corticosteroid with leukotriene receptor antagonist, theophylline, or zileuton; administer inhaled SABAs as needed.
Step 5: Moderate-severe persistent	High-dose inhaled corticosteroid *and* long-acting inhaled β_2-agonist	Consider adding omalizumab for patients with allergies; administer inhaled SABAs as needed. Ipatroprium, or tiotropium bromide inhaler may be added.
Step 6: Severe persistent	High-dose inhaled corticosteroid *and* long-acting inhaled β_2-agonist *and* oral corticosteroid	Consider adding omalizumab for patients with allergies; administer inhaled SABAs as needed. Ipatroprium or tiotropium bromide inhaler may be added.

Source: From National Heart, Lung, and Blood Institute (NHLBI). (2012b). *Asthma care quick reference.* Retrieved from https://www.nhlbi.nih.gov/files/docs/guidelines/asthma_qrg.pdf

Many of the drugs used for continued asthma management and relief of an acute attack can be administered by a metered-dose inhaler (MDI), dry powder inhaler (DPI), or nebulizer. The advantages of administering medications locally by inhalation include rapid onset and reduced systemic effects. In an MDI, a chemical propellant is used to deliver the medication when the canister is depressed. In contrast, a DPI contains no propellant. Instead, the medication is released by inhaling rapidly through the mouthpiece.

Bronchodilators

Most patients with asthma need bronchodilator therapy to relieve bronchoconstriction by relaxing the smooth muscles of the airway. Inhalation of nebulized medication is the preferred means of administration.

The primary bronchodilators used include adrenergic stimulants, methylxanthines, and anticholinergic agents. These drugs often are administered in combination with an anti-inflammatory agent. Adrenergic stimulants (beta$_2$-agonists) affect receptors on smooth muscle cells of the respiratory tract, causing smooth muscle relaxation and bronchodilation. Long-acting adrenergic stimulants, such as inhaled salmeterol and oral sustained-release albuterol, are used in conjunction with anti-inflammatory drugs to control symptoms but are not appropriate to treat an acute episode of asthma. Inhaled SABAs, such as albuterol and levalbuterol, administered by MDI or DPI are the treatment of choice for quick relief. They act within minutes, but their duration generally is short, lasting only 4–6 hours. Tachycardia and muscle tremors (common side effects of adrenergic agonists) are minimal with inhalation therapy.

Anticholinergic medications prevent bronchoconstriction by blocking parasympathetic input to bronchial smooth muscle. Ipratropium bromide, an anticholinergic drug administered by MDI, is useful when asthma symptoms are poorly controlled by adrenergic stimulants alone. In September 2015, the Food and Drug Administration approved the use of tiotropium bromide (Spiriva inhaler) for the treatment of asthma in patients ages 12 and older who continued to struggle despite daily administration of a LABA with an inhaled corticosteroid. Adding an anticholinergic to daily treatment has been shown to help improve outcomes in

these patients (Medscape, 2015). Note that anticholinergic drugs act more slowly than adrenergic stimulants, requiring as much as 60–90 minutes to achieve maximal effect.

Theophylline is a methylxanthine sometimes used as adjunctive treatment for asthma. It relaxes bronchial smooth muscle and may also inhibit the release of chemical mediators of the inflammatory response. Regular monitoring of serum theophylline levels is necessary because of wide individual variations in metabolism and elimination of the drug and its toxic effects. The therapeutic serum level of theophylline is 10–20 mcg/mL. Signs and symptoms of theophylline toxicity include hypotension, tachycardia, dysrhythmias, seizures, circulatory failure, and respiratory arrest (Adams, Holland, & Urban, 2017).

Theophylline may be used as a long-term bronchodilator, given once or twice daily. A related drug, aminophylline, may be administered intravenously to treat an acute, severe exacerbation of the disease.

Corticosteroids and NSAIDs

Corticosteroids and two NSAIDs, cromolyn sodium and nedocromil, are used to suppress airway inflammation and reduce asthma symptoms. Corticosteroids block the late response to inhaled allergens and reduce edema and bronchial hyperresponsiveness. The preferred route of administration is by MDI or DPI to minimize systemic absorption and reduce the many adverse effects of prolonged steroid use (cushingoid effects). For a severe acute attack, corticosteroids may be given systemically to alleviate symptoms and induce remission.

Cromolyn sodium and nedocromil are anti-inflammatory agents used to prevent acute episodes of asthma. They reduce airway hyperreactivity and inhibit the release of mediator substances. These drugs are used for long-term control of asthma, not quick relief. Cromolyn sodium and nedocromil have a wide margin of safety and few side effects.

Leukotriene Modifiers

The leukotriene modifiers montelukast (Singulair), zafirlukast (Accolate), and zileuton (Zyflo Filmtab) are oral medications that reduce the inflammatory response in some patients with asthma. They appear to improve lung function, diminish

Patient Teaching
Using a Metered-Dose or Dry Powder Inhaler

For all inhalers, patients should follow the manufacturer's directions to insert the inhaler canister into the mouthpiece or spacer and prime the inhaler.

Metered-Dose Inhaler

- Remove the mouthpiece cap. Shake the canister vigorously for 3–5 seconds.
- Exhale slowly and completely.
- Holding the inhaler with the mouthpiece down and the canister up, place the mouthpiece in your mouth, closing your lips around it if a spacer is being used. When no spacer is used, hold the mouthpiece directly in front of your mouth.
- Press and hold the canister down while inhaling deeply and slowly for 3–5 seconds (see **Figure 15–27 》》**).
- Hold your breath for 10 seconds, release pressure on the container, remove the spacer from your mouth, and exhale. Wait 20–30 seconds before repeating the procedure for a second puff.
- Rinse your mouth after using the inhaler to minimize systemic absorption and drying of the mucous membranes.
- Rinse the inhaler mouthpiece and spacer after use; store in a clean location.

Dry Powder Inhaler

- Keep the inhaler and medication in a clean, dry location. Do not refrigerate it or store it in a humid place (e.g., bathroom).
- Remove the cap and hold the inhaler upright or level as indicated by the manufacturer's insert. Inspect to be sure that the mechanism is clean and the mouthpiece is clear.
- If necessary, load the dose into the inhaler, following manufacturer's directions. For some inhalers, removing the cap from the mouthpiece is sufficient to load the dose.
- Hold the inhaler level with the mouthpiece end facing toward you.
- Breathe out slowly and completely. Tilt your head back slightly.

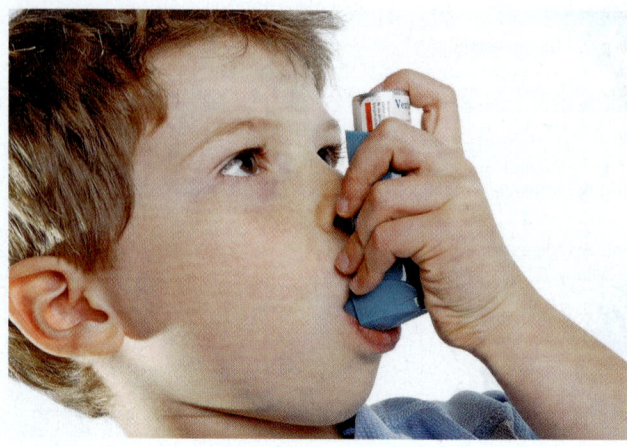

Source: Jacopin/BSIP SA/Alamy Stock Photo.

Figure 15–27 》》 Proper use of a metered-dose inhaler.

- Place the mouthpiece in your mouth with your teeth over the mouthpiece. Seal your lips around the mouthpiece. Do not block the inhaler with your tongue.
- Breathe in rapidly and deeply through your mouth over 2–3 seconds to activate the flow of medication.
- Remove the inhaler from your mouth and hold your breath for 10 seconds.
- Exhale slowly through pursed lips to allow the medication to enter distal airways. To prevent clogging never exhale into the inhaler mouthpiece.
- Rinse your mouth or brush your teeth after using the inhaler to avoid a bad taste from the medication and to prevent a yeast infection (if a corticosteroid medication is being used).
- Store the inhaler in a clean, sealed plastic bag; do not wash the inhaler unless directed to do so by the manufacturer. Clean the mouthpiece weekly using a dry cloth.

symptoms, and reduce the need for short-acting bronchodilators. These drugs affect the metabolism and excretion of other medications, such as warfarin and theophylline, and they may cause liver toxicity. Nursing implications for medications used to treat asthma are outlined in the Medications feature.

Lifespan Considerations

Asthma can occur in patients of all ages, and the number of people affected by asthma is increasing. Asthma is typically managed by patients and families outside of the hospital setting, making age-appropriate education and interventions essential for preventing asthma exacerbations.

Asthma in Children and Adolescents

Asthma interferes with a child's ability to sleep, concentrate in school, and play and causes multiple frustrations for both the child and the family. In addition, asthma attacks can be frightening for both the child and parents. The nurse plays

an essential role by assessing the parents' understanding of their child's asthma management at each healthcare interaction and by providing important patient teaching regarding use of asthma medications and avoidance of triggers. For example, if someone in the family smokes, the nurse provides education on the danger that secondhand smoke poses to those with asthma. The nurse also provides parents and caregivers with information about smoking cessation programs and therapies available in their area.

Inappropriate use of medication can increase a child's risk for another attack. Therefore, parents and other caregivers must understand how, when, and why to give medications. Children with asthma should have written asthma action plans that both parents and caregivers (including classroom teachers, coaches, and others who care for or supervise the child) can follow (see the Evidence-Based Practice feature). Action plans ensure that medications are given in a timely manner without risk of overdose, and they ensure successful outcomes for the child and family.

Medications
Asthma

CLASSIFICATION AND DRUG EXAMPLES	MECHANISMS OF ACTION	NURSING CONSIDERATIONS
Beta-Adrenergic Agonists *Drug examples:* Albuterol (ProAir, Proventil, Ventolin) Levalbuterol (Xopenex) Salmeterol (Serevent) Formoterol (Foradil) *Combination products:* Albuterol/ipratropium (Combivent) Salmeterol/fluticasone (Advair) Formorterol/mometasone (Dulera) Formorterol/budesonide (Symbicort)	Beta-adrenergic agonists affect sympathetic receptors in the respiratory tract. Administered by MDI or DPI, these drugs are the treatment of choice for acute bronchial asthma. Nearly all of the drugs in this class (epinephrine and isoproterenol being the exceptions) selectively activate β_2-receptors at the doses typically used to treat asthma. β_2-Receptor activation results in smooth muscle relaxation and bronchodilation. Formoterol and salmeterol are highly selective to β_2-receptors, resulting in fewer adverse effects. Formoterol and salmeterol have been shown to increase the risk of serious asthma exacerbations and death, however. These drugs should only be used when the disease cannot be adequately controlled with other medications. Oral forms of adrenergic agonists are not effective in treating an acute attack because of their slow onset. When administered orally or parenterally, their effect on sympathetic nervous system receptors can produce undesirable side effects such as nervousness, irritability, tachycardia, and cardiac dysrhythmias.	▪ Use with caution in patients with hypertension, cardiovascular disease or dysrhythmias, hyperthyroidism, or diabetes. ▪ These drugs may cause potentially dangerous cardiac stimulation in patients with hypoxemia and acidosis. ▪ When given by inhaler, wait 1–2 minutes between puffs to allow airways to dilate, permitting the second dose to reach distal airways. ▪ Observe for the desired effect of reduced dyspnea and wheezing. Central nervous system stimulation (anxiety, irritability, and insomnia) and tremor are common side effects. Health Education for the Patient and Family ▪ Use the prescribed inhaler or nebulizer as directed. ▪ If you are taking a bronchodilator along with another medication by inhalation, use the bronchodilator first to open your airways and enhance the effectiveness of the second medication. ▪ Rinse your mouth after using inhalers to reduce systemic absorption of the medication. ▪ Report palpitations, irregular pulse, and other side effects to the physician.
Methylxanthines *Drug examples:* Theophylline (Bronkotabs, Quibron, Slo-Phyllin Theolair, Theo-Dur, others) Aminophylline (Somophyllin)	The methylxanthines are central nervous system stimulants that are chemically related to caffeine. These drugs produce bronchodilation through relaxation of bronchial smooth muscle. As central nervous system stimulants, they produce adverse effects such as nervousness, insomnia, and tremors. When administered in large doses, convulsions may result. Once the drugs of choice for preventing and treating asthma attacks, they are now used primarily to prevent nocturnal asthma in adults. Theophylline has a narrow margin of safety and high potential for toxicity. Because the metabolism and excretion of theophylline vary significantly from person to person—affected by such factors as age, smoking, genetic factors, alcoholism, and other chronic diseases—monitoring of serum levels is vital.	▪ The therapeutic blood level for theophylline is *adult: 5–20 mcg/mL, older adult: 5–18 mcg/mL.* ▪ Monitor for manifestations of toxicity. Anorexia, nausea, vomiting, restlessness, insomnia, cardiac dysrhythmias, and seizures are early manifestations. Other manifestations include epigastric pain, hematemesis, diarrhea, headache, irritability, muscle twitching, palpitations, tachycardia, flushing, and circulatory failure. ▪ Administer with meals or a full glass of water or milk to minimize gastric irritation. ▪ Monitor the effect closely when administering concurrently with other medications such as barbiturates, anticonvulsants, thyroid hormone, beta-blockers, bronchodilators, and others. ▪ Aminophylline is incompatible with many other IV drugs. Use a separate line or flush the line with normal saline before and after administering any other preparation. Health Education for the Patient and Family ▪ Oral methylxanthines are ineffective to treat an acute asthma attack; do not delay other treatment by using these drugs. ▪ Check with the physician before taking any over-the-counter medications or other prescription drugs while on theophylline. ▪ Do not smoke while using this drug. ▪ Report adverse effects to the physician.

(continued on next page)

Medications *(continued)*

CLASSIFICATION AND DRUG EXAMPLES	MECHANISMS OF ACTION	NURSING CONSIDERATIONS
Anticholinergics *Drug examples:* Atropine Ipratropium bromide (Atrovent) Tiotropium bromide (Spiriva) *Combination products:* Albuterol/ipratropium (Combivent)	Anticholinergics are potent bronchodilators, blocking muscarinic receptors of the parasympathetic nervous system. Activation of muscarinic receptors produces smooth muscle contraction and bronchoconstriction; blockade of these receptors facilitates smooth muscle relaxation and bronchodilation. Atropine is used infrequently because of its tendency to dry secretions of the mucous membranes and other side effects. Ipratropium and tiotropium bromide are available as inhalers and have fewer side effects than atropine.	▪ Assess for possible contraindications to the drug, including hypersensitivity, glaucoma, prostatic hypertrophy, or bladder–neck obstruction. ▪ Assess for desired and/or adverse effects: improving or worsening symptoms; nausea, vomiting, or abdominal cramping; anxiety; dizziness; and headache. ▪ Provide ice chips, fluids, or hard candy to relieve dry mouth. Health Education for the Patient and Family ▪ To prevent overdose, take no more than the prescribed number of doses per day. ▪ If the drug becomes less effective over time, notify the physician.
Corticosteroids *Drug examples:* Mometasone (Asmanex) Ciclesonide (Alvesco) *Combination products:* Salmeterol/fluticasone (Advair) Formoterol/mometasone (Dulera) Formoterol/budesonide (Symbicort)	The anti-inflammatory effect of corticosteroids helps both prevent and treat acute episodes. Corticosteroids are used to reduce the frequency and severity of asthma attacks and allow reduced dosages of other drugs. The beneficial effects of corticosteroids for asthma result from their ability to decrease the synthesis and release of inflammatory mediators (e.g., histamine, leukotrienes), reduce inflammatory cell activation and infiltration, and decrease airway edema. Corticosteroids also decrease mucus production in the airways and increase the number and receptivity of β_2-receptors. The cushingoid side effects of corticosteroids, always a major concern with their use, are minimized when they are inhaled. Note that the combination product salmeterol/fluticasone is associated with an increased risk of serious asthma exacerbations and death. It is recommended for use only when asthma is inadequately controlled using other medications or for patients who clearly require both a bronchodilator and an inhaled corticosteroid for managing their asthma (Adams et al., 2017).	▪ Administer inhaler doses after bronchodilators to facilitate transport of the medication to distal airways. ▪ Assess for common side effects: sore throat, hoarseness, and oropharyngeal or laryngeal *Candida albicans* infection. ▪ Administer antifungal medications or gargles as ordered. Health Education for the Patient and Family ▪ Rinse your mouth after using the inhaler, and maintain good oral hygiene to reduce the risk of fungal infections. ▪ Do not use these medications to alleviate the symptoms of an acute attack. ▪ You may require several weeks of continued therapy before you notice a beneficial effect. ▪ Notify the physician if you develop weight gain, fluid retention, muscle weakness, redistribution of fat, or mood changes.
Mast Cell Stabilizers *Drug examples:* Cromolyn sodium (Intal) Nedocromil	Cromolyn sodium and nedocromil inhibit inflammatory cells in the airway, blocking early and late responses to inhaled antigens. Both drugs also prevent bronchoconstriction in response to inhaling cold air. These drugs act primarily by stabilizing the cytoplasmic membrane of mast cells, preventing the cells from releasing inflammatory mediators such as histamine. These drugs are used only for preventing asthma attacks, not to treat an acute attack. They are administered by MDI and have a wide margin of safety. Patients using nedocromil may complain of an unpleasant taste.	▪ Evaluate for potential adverse effects of wheezing and bronchoconstriction. Health Education for the Patient and Family ▪ Gargling or sipping water can decrease the throat irritation associated with nebulizer treatment. ▪ Use the appropriate technique. Inhale deeply with your head tipped back to open your airways, hold your breath, and then exhale. Repeat until all of the drug has been inhaled. ▪ These drugs are used only to prevent asthma attacks; they are not effective in treating an acute attack. ▪ You may require several weeks before you notice a beneficial effect.

Medications *(continued)*

CLASSIFICATION AND DRUG EXAMPLES	MECHANISMS OF ACTION	NURSING CONSIDERATIONS
Leukotriene Modifiers *Drug examples:* Montelukast (Singulair) Roflumilast (Daliresp) Zafirlukast (Accolate) Zileuton (Zyflo)	Leukotriene modifiers interfere with the inflammatory process in the airways by suppressing the effects of leukotrienes, a group of inflammatory mediators. Leukotrienes are powerful bronchoconstrictors and vasodilators; blocking their synthesis or their receptors improves airflow, decreases symptoms, and reduces the need for short-acting bronchodilators. They are used for maintenance therapy in adults and children over the age of 12 as an alternative to inhaled corticosteroid therapy. They are not used to treat an acute attack.	▪ Administer at least 1 hour before or 2 hours after meals. ▪ These drugs inhibit some liver enzymes, affecting the metabolism of warfarin and possibly terfenadine and theophylline. Monitor prothrombin times and theophylline blood levels. ▪ Monitor liver enzymes, because these drugs may be toxic to the liver. Health Education for the Patient and Family ▪ Take the drugs as prescribed on an empty stomach. ▪ Notify the physician if you note a change in color of your stools or urine or if you are jaundiced.

Source: Data from Adams, M. P., Holland, L. N., & Urban, C. (2017). *Pharmacology for nurses: A pathophysiologic approach* (5th ed.). Hoboken, NJ: Pearson Education.

Inhalers, typically the preferred method of asthma medication administration, are relatively inefficient and present special challenges for infants and young children. Many devices require cooperation, coordination, and appropriate technique for the child to receive the appropriate dose.

Children ages 7 and older are usually able to use MDIs and coordinate medication release and inspiration; children ages 4–7 may prefer to use a holding chamber or spacer with a valve. Spacers enhance the amount of the drug that reaches the lungs, and valves prevent the escape of medication during

Evidence-Based Practice
Asthma Management in Adolescence

Problem

Adolescent failure to follow medication regimens for asthma is well documented. Given the challenges inherent in working with this age group, nurses should know what barriers adolescents face in following asthma protocols as well as what interventions and supports promote adherence with asthma treatment regimens.

Evidence

Asthma control often relies more on lifestyle management than on medication management. Blaakman and colleagues (2014) found that forgetfulness, hurrying, and competing demands of school and social obligations impede the ability of adolescents with asthma to follow their treatment regimens. Equally as important, the researchers discovered school-based barriers, which included adolescents' concerns of how others' perceive their need to leave class to take medication, the need to obtain hall passes, and the interruption of school routines. The researchers found that routines played an important role in medication adherence and that many teens reported that fewer asthma symptoms were an incentive to take their medications. They also reported that independence in managing their own medications reduced parental stressors associated with taking medications. Perceptions of normalcy are also important. Mammen and colleagues (2016) found that adolescents based their decision to use their rescue medications in part on their individual perceptions of normal, and that teens with more severe asthma tolerated a more severe acuity of symptoms as "normal."

Interventions that have shown promise in increasing adolescent adherence to medication regimens include peer-led interventions, both in-person and using social media (Rhee, McQuillian, & Belyea,

2012; Rhee, Pesis-Katz, & Xing, 2012), and text medication reminders (Bhatti et al., 2015). Rhee et al. (2012) found that adolescents involved in peer-led groups were four to five times more likely to visit school clinics for their asthma symptoms than adolescents in similar adult-led groups.

Implications

Adolescents face a number of barriers to medication adherence. The evidence suggests that adolescents with asthma can successfully manage their own medications when they implement routines and participate in interventions that are conducive to their developmental level and preferences for using technology. This suggests the need to include questions that target what adolescent patients perceive as hindering their adherence as well as what they would find helpful in managing their treatment plans. Collaboration with school personnel (e.g., school nurses, coaches, teachers) may be necessary to inform the assessment and provide additional support in the school setting.

Critical Thinking Application

Consider the possible perceptions and beliefs of adolescents with asthma in your practice setting.

1. How would you assess adolescents' perceptions of and barriers to medication adherence?

2. How would you assess the role that peers play in an adolescent's lifestyle choices and asthma management?

3. Develop an education program for adolescents that explains asthma and discusses how adolescents can help their friends who have asthma stay healthy and safe.

use. In children younger than 4, a spacer with a mask attachment is more appropriate because children in this age range tend to be nasal breathers. The mask should fit the child's face and have a flexible seal to prevent air from leaking around the facial features. Many manufacturers now offer child-friendly masks that resemble cartoon characters or super heroes to make the masks more appealing. Play or distraction may also improve cooperation for medication delivery (van Aalderen et al., 2015).

Nebulizers do not require coordination of breathing, making them easier for young children to use. They include a mask or a mouth piece and provide humidification during treatment that may be beneficial. While nebulizers are not more effective than MDIs with a spacer, they may lead to better outcomes because the child only needs to breathe in and out normally. Nebulizers require a power source and take time to complete treatment. Infants and young children may have difficulty cooperating for the duration of the treatment (Smith & Goldman, 2012).

DPIs activate when the patient takes a breath, so puffs do not need to be coordinated with inhalation. DPIs do not require a spacer, and they do not use propellant. DPIs can be used by children ages 5 and older; however, children with severe asthma may not be able to produce enough airflow to get an adequate dose of medication (van Aalderen et al., 2015).

The nurse should also teach the child and parent when and how to use the PEFR meter. Growing children will have gradually increasing peak flow readings as their lungs grow and they exhale larger volumes of air with each breath. Daily use of peak flow monitors is particularly important in pediatric patients in order to track baseline or "normal" expiratory flow. Baseline should be reestablished as recommended by the physician.

>> **Stay Current:** Additional resources for parents can be found at the following websites:

- American Academy of Allergy, Asthma, and Immunology: http://www.aaaai.org
- Allergy and Asthma Network Mothers of Asthmatics: http://www.allergyhome.org/blogger/allergy-asthma-network-mothers-of-asthmatics-aanma-and-our-community/

Asthma in Pregnant Women

Pregnancy has significant effects on the respiratory physiology of all women because of elevation of the diaphragm. In general, tidal volume and ventilations per minute are increased during pregnancy while functional residual capacity and residual volume are decreased. As a result, changes in respiratory status in pregnant patients can be rapid. This is especially true of patients with asthma (Little & Sinert, 2014).

Asthma is the most common respiratory disease in pregnancy and affects 8% of all women in their childbearing years (American College of Allergy, Asthma, and Immunology [ACAAI], n.d.). One third of patients with asthma experience improvement in their asthma during pregnancy, one third experience little or no change, and the remaining third of patients experience worsening of their asthma during pregnancy. The highest incidence of asthma exacerbation in patients who are pregnant occurs between 24 and 36 weeks of gestation. Asthma is often dormant during labor and birth, but PEFR should be monitored to detect changes in maternal respiratory status (ACAAI, n.d.).

Asthma has been linked with higher rates of hyperemesis gravidarum, preeclampsia, and uterine hemorrhage in expectant mothers. Asthma can also have an impact on fetal health. Prematurity and low birth weight are more common among infants of women who have asthma (ACAAI, n.d.). These infants are also at increased risk of congenital malformations such as cleft lip and cleft palate.

SAFETY ALERT Perinatal mortality is higher in infants born to women with asthma (Murphy & Schatz, 2014). The goal of therapy is to prevent maternal exacerbations, because even a mild exacerbation can cause severe hypoxia-related complications in the fetus.

Caring for a woman who is pregnant and has asthma calls for an interprofessional effort. If the patient is not already in the care of a pulmonologist, the nurse should make a referral. Encourage the patient to talk with the pulmonologist about a stepwise action plan so that the patient knows what to do in the event of an exacerbation. Encourage the patient to use her peak flow meter daily as a method of monitoring her condition and to use standard precautions to reduce the risk of acquiring respiratory viruses. If an exacerbation occurs, it should be managed in the same way as for a woman who is not pregnant because the asthma drugs used are less of a threat to the fetus than a serious asthma attack (ACAAI, n.d.). However, use of epinephrine should be avoided in severe exacerbations because of its effects on the fetus (Little & Sinert, 2014).

Asthma in Older Adults

Prevalence of asthma among older adults is similar to that of other age groups, although the condition is often underdiagnosed and undertreated. This is due in part to difficulty differentiating symptoms of asthma from those of other common, age-related respiratory conditions. Cough is one of the most common symptoms of asthma in older adults; it can also be indicative of COPD, congestive heart disease, and pulmonary fibrosis. In addition, respiratory comorbidities in older adults differ from those in other age groups. Sinus issues such as nasal obstruction, loss of smell, and headache often occur in older adults with asthma, while younger adults typically experience allergic rhinitis (Yáñez et al., 2014).

Allergic factors appear to play less of a role in asthma in older adults than in other age groups. The development of asthma in older adults appears to be primarily the result of age-related lung and immune changes, environmental exposure, and other health conditions. In addition, older adults have higher morbidity from asthma than other age groups. This increased rate is believed to be related to muscular, cellular, and physiologic changes that occur in the respiratory system with age (Yáñez et al., 2014).

Among the older adult population, coexisting health alterations are a primary concern for management of asthma. Depending upon the type of condition and the medications prescribed to manage it, these conditions may negatively affect the patient's ability to control asthma and increase the risk of drug interactions (Melani, 2013). Memory problems and socioeconomic conditions also present challenges for disease management, as do improper use of inhaled medications.

For older adults, effective patient teaching and evaluation of self-management protocols are essential to promoting effective asthma control. Adherence to treatment regimens in older adults with asthma is often poor, and frequent follow-up and monitoring are important. In addition, some inhalation devices are difficult for older adults to use because of dexterity and inspiratory flow issues; as a result, spacers or nebulizers may be more appropriate for patients than MDIs or DPIs (Yáñez et al., 2014).

NURSING PROCESS

The immediate priority for nursing care is to help the patient maintain oxygenation and a patent airway. The long-term goal of care is to improve an individual's ability to function and ability to participate in ADLs and exercise, with the ultimate goal of improving the patient's quality of life.

Assessment

Assessment of the patient experiencing an acute asthma attack must be very focused and timely. For patients with persistent asthma, assessment should focus on concerns and symptoms at each healthcare interaction, but also on the patient's overall quality of life. Cool clammy skin, changes in LOC (e.g., agitation, lethargy, confusion), and cyanosis indicate worsening hypoxia and the need for emergency treatment.

- *Observation and patient interview.* During the patient interview, inquire about current symptoms, including chest tightness, shortness of breath, and dyspnea; duration of current attack; measures used to relieve symptoms and their effect; identified precipitating factors for the attack; frequency of attacks; current medications; and known allergies. Observe the position or posturing of the individual. Self-posturing (e.g., a tripod stance) may indicate respiratory distress.

  During the health history, the nurse also assesses how effectively asthma is being controlled. This includes assessment of how often symptoms require use of SABAs, how often the patient wakes with symptoms, and how often the patient requires primary or emergency care to address asthma management. A history of symptom and control issues for the previous few weeks may help the nurse understand how asthma affects the patient. Encourage the patient to monitor PEFR and keep a daily log to help the patient recognize and respond to changes in oxygenation status earlier, as this may help reduce the extent of exacerbations. A daily log may also help identify triggers or exposures that aggravate asthma symptoms.

- *Physical examination.* During the physical examination, note the apparent level of distress and LOC; skin color; vital signs; respiratory rate and excursion; breath sounds throughout lung fields; and apical pulse. Auscultate lung sounds, inspect and palpate the chest for symmetry, and assess for use of accessory muscles, which indicates an increased need for oxygen at the alveolar level. In addition, assess for the presence and nature of pulmonary secretions (thinned secretions are easier to expectorate than thick mucus) and for tobacco use.

Diagnosis

The age and developmental level of the patient, the severity of the patient's asthma and its etiology, and the presence of comorbid conditions (if any) will affect the nursing diagnosis of the patient. The following diagnoses may be appropriate for patients with asthma:

- *Breathing Pattern, Ineffective*
- *Airway Clearance, Ineffective*
- *Gas Exchange, Impaired*
- *Activity Intolerance*
- *Anxiety*
- *Health Management, Ineffective.*

  (NANDA-I © 2014)

Planning

The planning process is informed by the assessment of the patient's current condition and the patient's goals for the future. Together, the nurse and patient will develop a plan of care that may include the following goals:

- The patient will experience improved asthma control as evidenced by fewer and less severe exacerbations.
- The patient will require fewer healthcare interactions to maintain asthma control.
- The patient will reduce exposure to irritants that aggravate asthma symptoms.
- The patient will experience improved quality of life (as evidenced by fewer days missed from school or work, greater ease and comfort, and ability to participate in health promotion activities).

Implementation

Patients with asthma require careful monitoring and rapid intervention during exacerbations in order to prevent hypoxia and promote oxygenation. Because of the chronic nature of the disorder, patients are often the best source of information regarding the implementations that work best for them, and they should be consulted when planning and implementing care.

Promote Effective Gas Exchange

For patients in all settings, the nurse administers nebulizer treatments and provides humidification as ordered. Nebulizer treatments are used to administer bronchodilators and other medications; humidity helps loosen secretions. The nurse also promotes increase in the patient's fluid intake to help keep secretions thin. Prior to discharge, the nurse provides any additional patient teaching related to environmental, behavior, or pharmacologic management.

In hospital or residential settings (e.g., rehabilitation centers, nursing centers), additional interventions to promote effective gas exchange will include:

- Assess ABG results and pulse oximetry readings; notify the physician of abnormal values or changes in status. These values provide information about gas exchange and the adequacy of alveolar ventilation. A fall in oxygen saturation levels is an early indicator of impaired gas exchange.

- Place in Fowler, high-Fowler, or **orthopneic position** (with head and arms supported on the overbed table) to facilitate breathing and lung expansion. These positions reduce the work of breathing and increase lung expansion, especially of basilar areas.
- Administer oxygen as ordered. If a mask is used, monitor closely for feelings of claustrophobia or suffocation. Supplemental oxygen reduces hypoxemia. Small children may require use of a pediatric tent. Oxygen therapy via mask or tent can be frightening; monitor the patient for anxiety during administration.

SAFETY ALERT Frequently assess respiratory status (at least every 1–2 hours): respiratory rate and depth, chest movement or excursion, breath sounds, and PEFR. Note manifestations of ineffective breathing, including rapid rate, shallow respirations, nasal flaring, use of accessory muscles, and intercostal retractions. Respiratory status can change rapidly during an acute asthma attack and its treatment. Decreasing PEFR readings indicate worsening airflow restriction. Slowed, shallow respirations with significantly diminished breath sounds and decreased wheezing may indicate exhaustion and impending respiratory failure. Immediate intervention is necessary.

Help Relieve Anxiety

Acute exacerbations of asthma can produce significant anxiety. Fear of being unable to breathe and feelings of suffocation associated with acute asthma are significant. Financial or other concerns may cause the patient to want to avoid hospitalization. Increasingly frequent and severe episodes may cause fear for the future. Hypoxia contributes to anxiety as well, stimulating the sympathetic nervous system and the fight-or-flight response. Nursing interventions for the patient presenting with an acute exacerbation of asthma in any setting include assessing the patient's anxiety level, helping the patient identify coping skills that have been successful in the past, and including the patient in care and planning decisions without making excessive demands. Additional interventions include reducing excessive environmental stimuli, allowing supportive family members to remain with the patient, and assisting the patient to use relaxation techniques.

Promote Adherence to Therapeutic Regimen

Once acute asthma is under control and effective respirations have been reestablished, the nurse should ensure the patient understands the importance of adhering to the treatment plan in order to prevent recurring attacks.

- Assess the patient's level of understanding about asthma and the prescribed treatment regimen. Provide additional information and teaching as indicated.
- Discuss the patient's perception of the illness and its effect on his or her lifestyle. Open discussion can help identify conflicts between lifestyle and the treatment regimen.
- Assist the patient and significant others to identify problems or difficulties integrating the treatment regimen into their lifestyle. Asthma and its management may necessitate lifestyle modifications to prevent acute exacerbations, which can significantly affect family members.
- Assess knowledge and understanding of prescribed medications, use of over-the-counter preparations, and use of

integrative therapies. This is important to determine misperceptions or possible misuse of medications.
- Provide verbal and written instructions at the patient's level of understanding.
- Refer to counseling, support groups, or self-help organizations to help the patient and family adapt to living with asthma and the treatment regimen.

Provide Education Regarding Activity Intolerance

Patients with mild asthma may not experience any activity intolerance except during and immediately following a flare. For patients with moderate to severe asthma, however, activity intolerance can greatly limit quality of life.

- Teach the patient how to monitor cardiopulmonary response to activity by taking his or her own pulse and blood pressure.
- Teach the patient how to monitor and record peak flow rates before and after activities.
- Help the patient assess his or her capacity to sustain activities and determine activities and exercises in which the patient can participate.
- Assess the need for short-acting bronchodilators before activity or exercise.
- Teach the patient to alternate periods of activity with periods of rest.
- Assist the patient with ADLs as needed.

Evaluation

The nurse evaluates the patient's response to treatment, which may be compared to the following common expected outcomes:

- The patient maintains oxygen saturation greater than 90%.
- The patient demonstrates proper use of medications.
- The patient lists common triggers for asthmatic exacerbation and strategies to avoid triggers.
- The patient and family members list symptoms requiring immediate notification of the primary provider.
- The patient responds appropriately to asthma flare-up.
- The patient maintains optimal nutrition to promote health.
- The patient describes appropriate follow-up care to control the condition.

If the patient or the patient's family does not understand the prescribed treatment regimen, assess barriers to adherence and continue to work with them to promote understanding. If the patient's asthma exacerbation continues, provide information about additional medications that the patient can take, using the stepwise approach for asthma management that is appropriate for the patient's age. If the patient continues to experience exacerbations despite following the treatment regimen, advocate for the prescribing provider to re-evaluate the treatment regimen with the patient. Continue patient teaching about methods to prevent asthma attacks and how to remain calm and reduce anxiety during an attack.

Nursing Care Plan
A Patient with Asthma

Sarah Mitchell is a 35-year-old working mother with moderate persistent asthma. Her known triggers are allergies to dust mites, cockroach feces, grass and tree pollens, and some molds. She takes immunotherapy once a week and takes maintenance medications daily. She works as a full-time preschool teacher.

Ms. Mitchell calls her allergist's office asking to be seen because she is having a bad asthma flare. She reports having to use her rescue inhaler every 3–4 hours, that her chest is very tight, and that she is having trouble breathing. She has used her home peak flow meter three times since late yesterday and has been in the yellow zone each time. She did not sleep last night because of her asthma symptoms.

ASSESSMENT

The nurse, Clancy O'Hara, admits Ms. Mitchell when she arrives at the allergist's office. During the health history Ms. Mitchell confirms she is compliant with her medication regimen. She takes a LABA in combination with a low-dose corticosteroid, a daily antihistamine, and montelukast. In checking Ms. Mitchell's medical record, Nurse O'Hara notes that the patient is maintaining her scheduled immunotherapy appointments. Ms. Mitchell reports that she is not aware of any unusual allergy exposure but says that several of her students have a cold this week.

On physical examination, Nurse O'Hara notes that Ms. Mitchell's vital signs are as follows: T 37°C (98.6°F); P 96 bpm; R 36/min; BP 128/86 mmHg. Other assessment data include needing to pause frequently while speaking, use of accessory muscles for respirations, and scattered wheezes audible over both lung fields with stethoscope. ABG results are pH 7.32, PaO_2 88 mmHg, $PaCO_2$ 47 mmHg, and HCO_3 38 mEq/L. Pulses are strong and equal bilaterally, and the patient expectorates a small amount of white mucus into a tissue.

DIAGNOSES

- *Ineffective Breathing Pattern* related to exacerbation of asthma
- *Impaired Gas Exchange* related to bronchoconstriction and mucus in airways
- *Fatigue* related to ineffective sleep pattern
- *Activity Intolerance* related to inadequate oxygenation

(NANDA-I © 2014)

PLANNING

Together Nurse O'Hare and Ms. Mitchell agree on the following outcomes:

- The patient's breathing will return to the green zone within 24 hours.
- The patient's need for her rescue inhaler will decline within 3 days and return to baseline within 1 week.
- The patient will maintain baseline respiratory rate and pattern sufficient to meet her ADLs within 72 hours.

IMPLEMENTATION

Ms. Mitchell's provider prescribes a higher-dose inhaled steroid to use 10–15 minutes after she uses her LABA. The provider also gives Ms. Mitchell a short, tapered course of prednisone. Ms. O'Hare initiates the following implementations:

- Teaches Ms. Mitchell how to properly self-administer medications and about possible side effects associated with steroid use, including those that should be reported immediately
- Explains the importance of taking the steroid as ordered and not stopping the medication suddenly
- Provides strategies for managing fatigue, including a handout with written instructions

- Teaches Ms. Mitchell the importance of proper nutrition and hydration in asthma management
- Observes Ms. Mitchell's technique when measuring peak flow
- Reviews signs and symptoms indicating worsening condition and instructs Ms. Mitchell to call the provider if these occur
- Schedules Ms. Mitchell to return in 6 weeks for a further evaluation but tells her to call the office if her symptoms worsen or if she sees no meaningful improvement in 3–4 days.

EVALUATION

Ms. Mitchell returns in 6 weeks for her follow-up appointment and reports improvement of symptoms and no further recurrence. She expresses a desire to continue on the higher-dose steroid until school is out. Ms. O'Hare assesses that Ms. Mitchell's breathing rate and pattern have returned to baseline. Peak flow measurements indicate Ms. Mitchell's breathing is within her green zone, and breath sounds are clear and equal bilaterally.

CRITICAL THINKING

1. Why is the prescription of the short, tapered course of oral prednisone appropriate for Ms. Mitchell? Why is the continued use of the higher-dose inhaled corticosteroid appropriate? What special teaching will the patient taking steroids require?

2. What should the nurse teach Ms. Mitchell about the importance of nutrition and hydration to asthma management?

3. What signs and symptoms would you want Ms. Mitchell to report to the provider immediately?

REVIEW Asthma

RELATE Link the Concepts and Exemplars

The patient has a history of severe persistent asthma, taking a daily LABA in combination with an inhaled corticosteroid, montelukast, and albuterol in both oral, inhaler, and nebulizer form for emergencies. Oral prednisone is prescribed approximately twice a year for severe flare-ups.

Linking the exemplar of asthma with the concept of metabolism:

1. What risk factors does this patient have for osteoporosis? Explain the rationale for your answer.

2. What risk factors does this patient have for diabetes and obesity? Explain the rationale for your answer.

Linking the exemplar of asthma with the concept of acid–base balance:

3. When caring for a patient in status asthmaticus, what would you anticipate finding when analyzing ABG results? Explain the pathophysiology resulting in these findings.

4. What nursing interventions could be initiated to promote acid–base balance?

Linking the exemplar of asthma with the concept of cognition:

5. How could asthma affect an individual's ability to comprehend? Explain your answer with appropriate rationales.

6. What nursing interventions could be initiated to promote cognition?

READY Go to Volume 3: Clinical Nursing Skills

REFER Go to Pearson MyLab Nursing and eText

- Additional review materials

REFLECT Apply Your Knowledge

Hannah McGregor, a 9-year-old with asthma, lives at home with her parents and two brothers, who are 6 and 4 years old. Hannah developed asthma at approximately 5 years of age and has had wheezing episodes that were generally controlled by rescue medications. Two weeks ago, Hannah had a severe episode of asthma that started at school and was possibly associated with the paint or glue used on a project. She did not have any quick-relief medications at school, and she delayed going to the school nurse so that she could finish her project. By the time her mother arrived to pick her up, Hannah was in respiratory distress. After receiving treatment in the emergency department, Hannah was admitted to the pediatric ICU.

Hannah and her mother are in the health center to meet with the provider to learn more about asthma management. At today's visit, Hannah's lungs are clear to auscultation, and her PEFR is in the green zone. Ms. McGregor reports that she has given all prescribed medications since the hospitalization. Both Hannah and her mother are motivated to prevent a future hospital admission if possible. The nurse uses a model to show Hannah how asthma narrows her airway and makes it difficult to breathe. The nurse then works with Ms. McGregor and Hannah to develop a plan for asthma control with daily medications.

1. What are the current recommendations for managing Hannah's asthma and to help prevent asthma episodes?

2. How should Hannah handle future episodes that start at school?

3. What arrangements are needed for Hannah to have access to her medications at school?

›› Exemplar 15.C
Chronic Obstructive Pulmonary Disease

Exemplar Learning Outcomes

15.C Analyze chronic obstructive pulmonary disease (COPD) as it relates to oxygenation.

- Describe the pathophysiology of COPD.
- Describe the etiology of COPD.
- Summarize the risk factors for COPD.
- Compare methods for preventing COPD.
- Identify the clinical manifestations of COPD.
- Summarize diagnostic tests and therapies used by interprofessional teams in the collaborative care of an individual with COPD.
- Differentiate care of patients with COPD across the lifespan.
- Apply the nursing process in providing culturally competent care to an individual with COPD.

Exemplar Key Terms

Air trapping, *1071*
Barrel chest, *1073*
Bronchitis, *1071*
Chronic bronchitis, *1071*
Chronic obstructive pulmonary disease (COPD), *1070*
Emphysema, *1071*
Expectorate, *1078*
Forced expiratory volume in 1 second (FEV$_1$), *1073*
Percussion, *1075*
Postural drainage, *1075*
Pursed-lip breathing, *1073*
Sputum, *1070*
Tripod position, *1073*
Vibration, *1075*

Overview

Obstructive pulmonary diseases are those that cause obstruction of the airways, usually through a combination of bronchoconstriction and inflammation. These include bronchitis (chronic or acute) and emphysema (NHLBI, 2013a).

The term **chronic obstructive pulmonary disease (COPD)** is used to describe a specific progressive disorder that slowly alters the structures of the respiratory system over time, irreversibly affecting lung function. The disease is one of periodic exacerbations, often related to respiratory infection, with increased symptoms of dyspnea and **sputum**

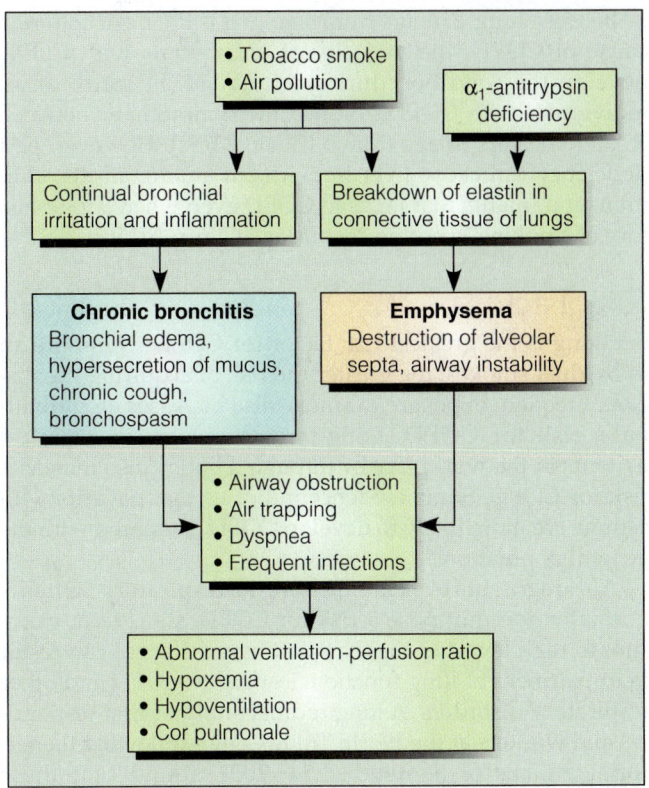

Figure 15–28 》 Pathogenesis of chronic obstructive pulmonary disease.

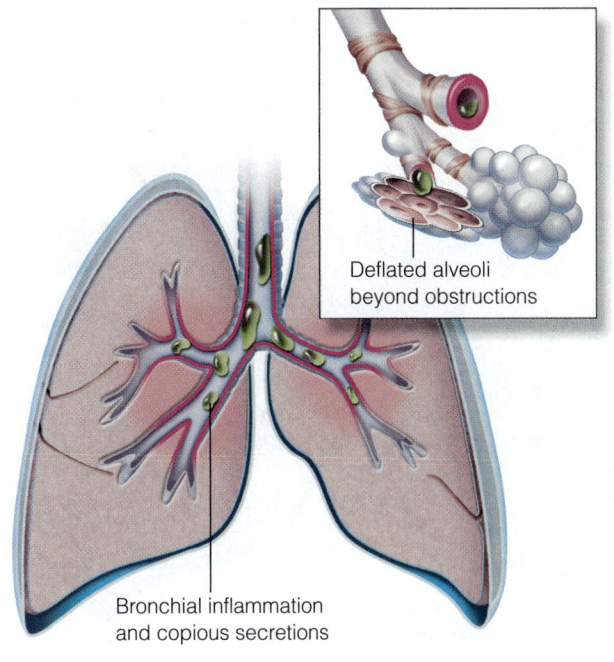

Figure 15–29 》 Chronic bronchitis.

(mucus or mucopurulent matter expectorated from the lungs) production. Unlike acute processes in which lung tissues recover, airways and lung parenchyma do not return to normal following an exacerbation; instead, they demonstrate progressive destructive changes. COPD is not curable, but it can be managed (and sometimes prevented) with appropriate medical interventions and lifestyle choices.

Although one or the other may dominate, COPD typically includes components of both chronic bronchitis and emphysema, two distinctly different processes. Small airways disease, narrowing of small bronchioles, is also part of the COPD complex. Through different mechanisms, these processes cause airways to narrow, resistance to airflow to increase, and expiration to become slow or difficult (see **Figure 15–28** 》). The result is a mismatch between alveolar ventilation and blood flow or perfusion, leading to impaired gas exchange.

Pathophysiology and Etiology

Pathophysiology

COPD results from repeated exposure to respiratory irritants that begin to damage the structures of the respiratory system. Damage to the large and small airway passages causes increased mucus production, causing arrest in cilia action. Excessive amounts of fluid accumulate with the lung mucosal cells, causing edema. In turn, edema causes narrowing of airway passages, resulting in airflow limitation, **air trapping** (decreased airflow with exhalation), and ultimately, hyperinflation of the lungs. This process leads to **bronchitis** (best defined as inflammation of the mucous membranes of the bronchial tubes).

Chronic bronchitis is a disorder of excessive bronchial mucus secretion (see **Figure 15–29** 》). It is characterized by a productive cough lasting 3 or more months in 2 consecutive years (Mayo Clinic, 2014). Cigarette smoke is the major factor implicated in the development of chronic bronchitis. Inhaled irritants lead to a chronic inflammatory process with vasodilation, congestion, and edema of the bronchial mucosa. Goblet cells increase in size and number, and mucous glands enlarge. Thick, tenacious mucus is produced in increased amounts. Changes in bronchial squamous cells impair the ability to clear mucus (Herfs et al., 2012). Narrowed airways and excess secretions obstruct airflow; expiration is affected first, then inspiration. Because ciliary function is impaired, normal defense mechanisms are unable to clear the mucus and any inhaled pathogens. Recurrent infection is common in chronic bronchitis.

Emphysema is characterized by destruction of the walls of the alveoli, with resulting enlargement of abnormal air spaces (see **Figure 15–30** 》). Deficiency of α_1-antitrypsin, an enzyme that normally inhibits the activity of proteolytic enzymes and tissue destruction in the lungs, contributes to the development of emphysema in some individuals, especially when combined with exposure to cigarette smoke. Inflammatory cells that collect in distal airway tissues appear to lead to destruction of elastic fibers in the respiratory bronchioles and alveolar ducts. Alveolar wall destruction causes alveoli and air spaces to enlarge, with loss of corresponding portions of the pulmonary capillary bed. As a result, the surface area for alveolar–capillary diffusion is reduced, affecting gas exchange. Elastic recoil is lost, reducing the volume of air that is passively expired. The loss of support tissue also affects airways, increasing the risk of expiratory collapse and further air trapping. Either respiratory bronchioles or alveoli may be the primary tissue involved anatomically. As in chronic bronchitis, cigarette smoking is strongly implicated as a causative factor in most cases of emphysema.

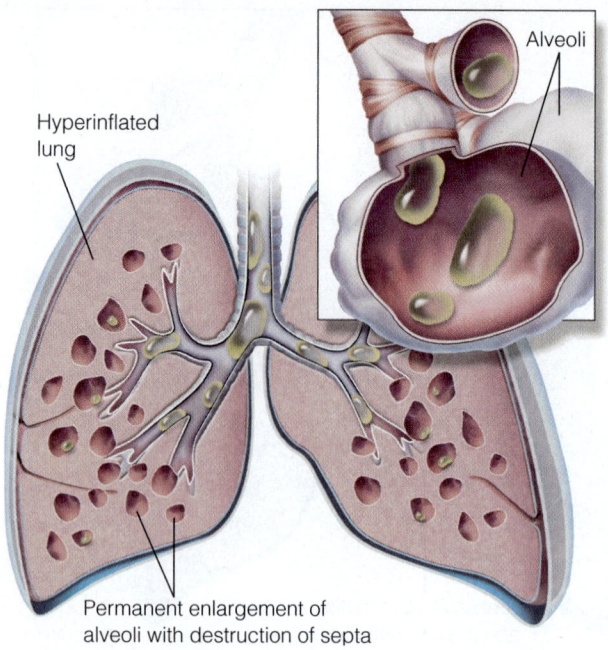

Labels on figure: Hyperinflated lung; Alveoli; Permanent enlargement of alveoli with destruction of septa

Figure 15–30 ≫ Emphysema.

Asthma often exists as a comorbid disease in the patient with COPD. Patients who have lived with moderate to severe persistent asthma for most of their lives may develop COPD as a result of airway remodeling and damage to alveoli over time (see Exemplar 15.B on Asthma).

Etiology

COPD is included among the leading causes of death, disability, and illness in the United States. In most cases, the individual with COPD is over age 50, is a current or former smoker, and has a 20 pack-per-year smoking history. With aging, the individual with COPD experiences worsening lung function (University of Maryland Medical Center [UMMC], 2012). Mortality rates are nearly equal for women and men, though rates for women have significantly increased since 1970. By 2020, the estimated costs of care for individuals with COPD are expected to reach $90 billion annually (CDC, 2014a). Although COPD is not curable, the symptoms of the disease can be managed.

Cigarette smoking accounts for approximately 80% of cases. Other causes that have contributory effects of COPD on the lungs include exposures to occupational respiratory irritants and air pollution (both indoors and outdoors) in industrialized nations. The use of wood, coal, or animal dung for cooking fires in close quarters in less-developed nations increases the risk of COPD in women from those countries.

Among individuals with COPD, approximately 1% of cases are linked to a deficiency of alpha-1 antitrypsin (AAt), which is an inherited genetic abnormality (Mayo Clinic, 2015b). Also referred to as *genetic COPD* (Alpha-1 Foundation, n.d.), this disorder is caused by a deficiency of the protein AAt, which is produced by the liver. AAt is necessary for normal lung development and function; therefore, lack of this protein causes pulmonary complications.

Because lung damage from smoking is the most common cause of COPD, the majority of individuals with COPD develop the condition during adulthood. In many cases, individuals with COPD first become symptomatic between 35 and 40 years of age (Mayo Clinic, 2015c). However, AAt deficiency can cause liver impairment among adults, children, and infants that leads to COPD even when a long history of smoking is not present (Mayo Clinic, 2015b).

Risk Factors

Smoking is the greatest risk factor for COPD: The more an individual smokes, the greater the risk of acquiring the disease. Frequent exposure to smoke also increases an individual's risk for COPD. Long-term exposure to chemical irritants in the workplace or through a hobby also increases risk for COPD. Some evidence indicates that patients with asthma are more likely to develop COPD compared with the general population.

Although short-term exposure to respiratory irritants normally does not pose a risk for COPD, short-term exposure to high levels of highly irritating substances can result in impairment of lung function, leading to COPD and other respiratory disorders. A longitudinal study of first responders and workers at the World Trade Center following the terrorist attacks of September 11, 2001, found that these individuals experienced significantly decreased lung function within the first year following the attacks. The exposure-related decrease in lung function of the study participants within that year was equivalent to 12 years of aging-related decline in lung function (Banauch et al., 2006). Current research suggests a persistent increased risk for the development of numerous chronic illnesses among these individuals, including asthma, sinusitis, obstructive airway disease, and spirometric abnormalities (Glaser et al., 2014; Wisnivesky et al., 2011).

Prevention

The key to preventing COPD is to refrain from behaviors that have been linked with the etiology of the disease. Patients should not smoke or should quit smoking, if possible. They should also decrease their exposure to secondhand smoke, occupational respiratory irritants, and air pollutants. This is especially important for Hispanic patients because they have an increased risk of developing COPD, and because tobacco use is the leading preventable cause of death among Hispanics living in the United States. Issues associated with this high rate of tobacco use appear to include acculturation, education levels, and alcohol and substance abuse (Rodríguez-Esquivel et al., 2009). A 2007 study found that Hispanic patients with COPD do not receive referral to smoking cessation classes as frequently as patients of other ethnicities (Adams et al., 2008). A 2015 study subsequently suggested that culturally specific education materials provided in the patient's preferred language promoted increased utilization of smoking cessation strategies (Rodríguez-Esquivel et al., 2015). Nurses working with Hispanic patients who exhibit chronic cough and sputum or who are diagnosed with COPD should inquire about nicotine and alcohol use and provide patient teaching and appropriate referrals in these areas.

Box 15–2
Classification of COPD by Severity

GOLD 1: Mild. Usually, but not always, chronic cough and sputum production; mild airflow limitation; FEV_1/forced vital capacity (FVC) less than 0.70; FEV_1 predicted to be greater than 80%

GOLD 2: Moderate. Usually worse symptoms, with shortness of breath typically developing on exertion; FEV_1/FVC less than 0.70; FEV_1 predicted to be 50–80%

GOLD 3: Severe. Worse symptoms, with noticeable shortness of breath; FEV_1/FVC less than 0.70; FEV_1 predicted to be 30–50%

GOLD 4: Very severe. Severe symptoms; FEV_1/FVC less than 0.70; FEV_1 predicted to be less than 30%

Source: From Global Initiative for Chronic Obstructive Lung Disease (GOLD). (2017). *Global strategy for the diagnosis, management and prevention of COPD.* Retrieved from http://goldcopd.org/gold-2017-global-strategy-diagnosis-management-prevention-copd/

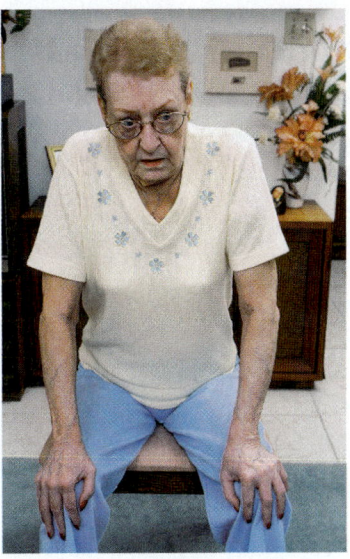

Figure 15–31 》 Typical appearance of a patient with emphysema. Note the patient's anxious expression and assumption of the tripod position, leaning forward with the hands on the knees.

Clinical Manifestations

The clinical presentation of COPD varies from simple chronic bronchitis without disability to chronic respiratory failure and severe disability. **Forced expiratory volume in 1 second (FEV_1)** is the amount of air that can be exhaled in 1 second as measured by a spirometer. A patient's FEV_1 reading, combined with symptom manifestations, determines the patient's level of COPD severity. **Box 15–2 》** outlines the classifications of COPD severity.

Manifestations are typically absent or minor early in the disease. Initial symptoms are chronic cough and sputum production, which tend to begin long before changes in pulmonary function. No incidence of shortness of breath occurs in the early stages of pulmonary decline as a result of COPD. When the patient finally seeks care, chronic productive cough, dyspnea, and exercise intolerance often have been present for as long as 10 years. The cough typically occurs in the mornings and often is attributed to "smoker's cough." Dyspnea initially occurs only on extreme exertion; as the disease progresses, dyspnea becomes more severe and accompanies mild activity. Manifestations characteristic of chronic bronchitis and emphysema develop. Manifestations of chronic bronchitis include a cough that produces copious amounts of thick, tenacious sputum; cyanosis; and evidence of right-sided heart failure, including distended neck veins, edema, liver engorgement, and an enlarged heart. Adventitious lung sounds, including loud rhonchi, and possible wheezes are prominent on auscultation.

SAFETY ALERT Chronic cough and sputum are not normal occurrences. An individual experiencing chronic cough and sputum beyond 3–4 days should consult with a healthcare professional. Individuals with a smoking history as well as chronic cough and sputum production should have PFTs to determine lung function.

Emphysema is insidious in onset. Dyspnea is the first symptom. It initially occurs only with exertion but may progress to become severe, even at rest. Cough is minimal or absent. Air trapping and hyperinflation increase the anteroposterior chest diameter, a condition called **barrel chest**. The patient often is thin, is tachypneic, uses accessory muscles of

respiration, and often assumes a **tripod position** (a position of sitting and leaning forward) (see **Figure 15–31 》**). On auscultation, breath sounds are diminished, and the percussion tone is hyperresonant. The patient may utilize **pursed-lip breathing**. Pursed-lip breathing involves exhaling through a narrow opening between the lips to prolong the expiratory phase in an effort to promote more alveolar emptying while maintaining open alveoli. Prolonged impairment of gas exchange as a result of COPD eventually results in cardiac dysfunction. Chest pain and hypertension may be the earliest manifestations, indicating that the heart is having to work harder to provide oxygen through the bloodstream. Congestive heart failure eventually may result. Patients with COPD should be seen by their specialist or primary care provider at least every 6 months in order for their disease progression to be evaluated and therapies to be modified or added.

The work of breathing requires calories. Caloric demand increases as the effort to breathe increases. Tachypnea makes eating more difficult. Increased caloric demand with decreased caloric intake often occurs in the latter stages of COPD, often resulting in weight loss and possibly anemia.

Anxiety related to increasing periods of dyspnea occurs with exacerbations in moderate and severe COPD. Severe COPD can result in impairment of other body systems because of insufficient airflow, further restricting quality of life.

Collaboration

Nurses will find it helpful to collaborate with physical therapists, nutritionists, pharmacists, family members, and sometimes counselors to help patients achieve outcomes and improve their quality of life. In particular, nurses should be aware of who is caring for the patient with COPD who continues to live at home and should discuss with the patient and family the need for those individuals to have sufficient information and training so they can provide care that meets best practice guidelines.

Clinical Manifestations and Therapies
Chronic Obstructive Pulmonary Disease

ETIOLOGY	CLINICAL MANIFESTATIONS	CLINICAL THERAPIES
Bronchitis	■ Chronic cough with mucus production ■ Dyspnea ■ Tachycardia ■ Narrowed airway passages ■ Wheezing ■ Air trapping	■ Smoking cessation ■ Bronchodilators ■ Corticosteroids ■ Fluids to thin secretions ■ Elevating the head of the bed ■ Low-flow oxygen ■ Monitoring of ABGs and oxygen ■ Mechanical ventilation if patient cannot meet oxygen demands
Emphysema	■ Air trapping ■ Possible wheezing ■ Dyspnea ■ Barrel chest ■ Pursed-lip breathing ■ Posturing	■ Oxygen administration as needed ■ Pursed-lip breathing technique ■ Patient education of posture changes to improve ventilation ■ Low-flow oxygen ■ Monitoring of ABGs and oxygen ■ Mechanical ventilation if patient cannot meet oxygen demands ■ Nutritional assessment and increased calorie intake

Cardiac dysfunction	■ Chest pain
	■ Poor perfusion
	■ Arrhythmias, particularly premature ventricular contractions
	■ Hypertension
	■ Cardiac hypertrophy
	■ Congestive heart failure
		■ Medications:
		  a. Positive inotropics
		  b. Calcium blockers
		  c. Antiarrhythmic medications
		  d. Diuretics
		  e. Nitrites
		  f. Antihypertensives
		■ Monitoring of exercise tolerance
		■ Holter monitoring
		■ Antiembolism stockings to improve venous return
		■ Fluid restrictions if cardiac dysfunction not medically managed

Diagnostic Tests

Diagnostic tests are used to help establish the diagnosis of COPD and identify the predominant component: emphysema or chronic bronchitis. These procedures also are used to assess respiratory status and monitor treatment effectiveness.

- PFT to diagnose and evaluate the extent and progression of COPD
- Ventilation and perfusion scanning to determine the extent of V-Q mismatch (i.e., the extent to which the lung tissue is ventilated but not perfused [dead space] or perfused but inadequately ventilated [physiologic shunting])
- Serum α_1-antitrypsin levels to assist in determining etiology
- ABGs to evaluate gas exchange and acid–base balance
- Pulse oximetry to monitor oxygen saturation of the blood
- Capnography (ETCO$_2$) to evaluate alveolar ventilation (ETCO$_2$ levels above 45 mmHg indicate inadequate ventilation; levels below 35 mmHg indicate impaired perfusion.)
- CBC with differential to monitor RBCs and hematocrit and to check for the presence of bacterial infection
- CXR to monitor the extent of secretions in the alveolar sacs and to assess for the presence of pulmonary infection.

≫ Go to **Pearson MyLab Nursing and eText** to see Appendix B for more detailed information about related diagnostic tests.

SAFETY ALERT Hypercapnia (elevated PaCO$_2$ levels) often is chronic in patients with COPD (CO$_2$ retainers). In these patients, administering oxygen can further increase the PaCO$_2$, which contributes to worsening of V-Q mismatch. While oxygen is a mainstay of treatment for many patients with COPD, careful titration of oxygen is recommended (Abdo & Heunks, 2012).

Surgery

When medical therapy is no longer effective, lung transplantation may be an option. Both single and bilateral transplantations have been performed successfully. Among recipients of lung transplants, the 1-year survival rate is nearly 80%, and the 5-year survival rate is over 50% (Healthline, 2016). Lung reduction surgery is an experimental surgical intervention for advanced diffuse emphysema and lung hyperinflation. The procedure reduces the overall volume of the lung, reshapes it, and improves elastic recoil. As a result, pulmonary function and exercise tolerance improve, and dyspnea is reduced.

Pharmacologic Therapy

Immunization against pneumococcal pneumonia and a yearly influenza vaccine are recommended to reduce the risk of respiratory infections. A broad-spectrum antibiotic may be prescribed if infection is suspected. Recent studies indicate that patients with purulent sputum and increased dyspnea will likely benefit from antibiotic therapy, even if no other signs of infection are present. Current recommendations are to prescribe antibiotics only if known infection is present (GOLD, 2017).

Bronchodilators improve airflow and reduce air trapping in patients with COPD, resulting in improved dyspnea and exercise tolerance. By relaxing bronchial smooth muscle, bronchodilators widen the airway and allow for improved ventilation; they have no anti-inflammatory properties. An anticholinergic agent administered by MDI, such as ipratropium or titropium bromide, is frequently prescribed. It has a longer duration of action than the short-acting beta$_2$-adrenergic stimulant bronchodilators and few side effects. A LABA may be used in combination therapy. Oral theophylline, a methylxanthine, is a weak bronchodilator and has a narrow therapeutic range, but it may be prescribed for its other effects. Theophylline stimulates the respiratory drive, strengthens diaphragmatic contractions, and improves cardiac output. As a result, dyspnea, exercise tolerance, and quality of life improve for the patient with COPD. Bronchodilators are discussed in further detail, including their nursing implications, in Exemplar 15.B on Asthma.

Corticosteroid therapy may be used when asthma is a major component of COPD. It also improves symptoms and exercise tolerance and may reduce the severity of exacerbations and the need for hospitalization. Oral corticosteroids, such as prednisone, are used initially. If a beneficial response occurs, the amount is reduced to the lowest effective dose. Every-other-day dosing or administration by inhaler is preferred to minimize steroid side effects, such as cushingoid effects, mood swings, and increased risk for osteoporosis and vertebral fractures.

Retrospective studies indicate that the use of statins results in significant improvement for the patient with COPD. Statins are associated with a decrease in all-cause mortality (Horita et al., 2014) as well as a reduction in the rate of myocardial infarction (Cao et al., 2015). Statins may also target airway inflammation; however, this mechanism may be more pronounced among individuals with coexisting cardiovascular disease (Ingebrigtsen et al., 2015). In contrast to the retrospective studies, however, current prospective studies conducted by the NHLBI indicate that statins have no effect on COPD exacerbations (Criner et al., 2014).

Oxygen Therapy

Long-term oxygen therapy is used for severe and progressive hypoxemia. Oxygen therapy improves exercise tolerance, mental functioning, and quality of life in patients with advanced COPD. It also reduces the rate of hospitalization and increases the length of survival. Oxygen may be used intermittently, at night, or continuously. Patients with severe hypoxemia see the greatest benefit with continuous oxygen administration. Home oxygen may be supplied as liquid oxygen, compressed gas cylinders, or oxygen concentrators.

An acute exacerbation of COPD may necessitate oxygenation and inspiratory positive pressure assistance with a face mask or intubation and mechanical ventilation.

According to the *hypoxic drive theory*, patients whose blood carbon dioxide levels remain chronically elevated, such as individuals who have COPD, develop a decreased response to hypercarbia. Therefore, hypercarbia is no longer a stimulus for breathing. Instead, individuals who experience chronic hypercarbia become dependent on a low level of oxygen in the blood as a stimulus for breathing. In keeping with this theory, among patients with chronic hypercarbia, the alleviation of hypoxia by way of supplemental oxygen administration may lead to respiratory depression or even respiratory failure (Jerath et al., 2015). Despite research to suggest that patients with chronic hypercarbia do not depend on hypoxia as a stimulus for breathing (Kim et al., 2008), fear of blunting the hypoxic drive remains a potential barrier to the administration of supplemental oxygen to patients with COPD. Rather than withholding oxygen therapy from patients with COPD, current recommendations include judiciously titrating the concentration of oxygen to maintain the patients' oxygen saturation between 88% and 92% (Abdo & Heunks, 2012; Austin et al., 2010).

Percussion, Vibration, and Postural Drainage

Percussion, vibration, and postural drainage are dependent nursing functions performed according to a primary care provider's order. **Percussion**, sometimes called *clapping*, is forceful striking of the skin with cupped hands. Mechanical percussion cups and vibrators are also available. When the hands are used, the fingers and thumb are held together and flexed slightly to form a cup, as one would to scoop up water. Percussion over congested lung areas can mechanically dislodge tenacious secretions from the bronchial walls. Cupped hands trap the air against the chest, and the trapped air sets up vibrations through the chest wall to the secretions. When done correctly, the percussion action should produce a hollow, popping sound. Percussion is avoided over the breasts, sternum, spinal column, and kidneys.

Vibration is a series of vigorous quiverings produced by hands that are placed flat against the patient's chest wall. Vibration is used after percussion to increase the turbulence of the exhaled air and thus loosen thick secretions. It is often done alternately with percussion.

Postural drainage is the drainage by gravity of secretions from various lung segments. Secretions that remain in the lungs or respiratory airways promote bacterial growth and subsequent infection. They also can obstruct the smaller airways and cause atelectasis. Secretions in the major airways, such as the trachea and the right and left main bronchi, are usually coughed into the pharynx, where they can be expectorated, swallowed, or effectively removed by suctioning.

A wide variety of positions is necessary to drain all segments of the lungs, but not all positions are required for every patient. The nurse will use only those positions that drain specific affected areas. The lower lobes require drainage most frequently, because the upper lobes drain by gravity. Before postural drainage, the nurse may give the patient a bronchodilator medication or nebulization therapy to loosen secretions. Postural drainage treatments are scheduled two or three times daily, depending on the degree of lung congestion. The best times include before breakfast, before lunch, in the late afternoon, and before bedtime. The nurse should avoid hours shortly after meals, because postural drainage at these times can be tiring and may induce vomiting.

The nurse needs to evaluate the patient's tolerance of postural drainage by assessing the stability of the patient's vital signs, particularly the pulse and respiratory rates, and by noting signs of intolerance, such as pallor, diaphoresis, dyspnea, nausea, and fatigue. Some patients do not react well to certain drainage positions, and the nurse must make appropriate adjustments. For example, some patients become dyspneic in Trendelenburg's position and require only a moderate tilt or a shorter time in that position.

The sequence for postural drainage treatment is usually as follows: positioning, percussion, vibration, and removal of secretions by coughing or suction. Each position is usually assumed for 10–15 minutes, although beginning treatments may start with shorter times and gradually increase.

Following postural drainage treatments, the nurse should auscultate the patient's lungs; compare the findings to the baseline data; and document the amount, color, and character of expectorated secretions.

Other Interventions

Smoking cessation not only can prevent COPD from developing but also can improve lung function once the disease has been diagnosed. With smoking cessation, FEV_1 improves, and survival is prolonged, largely because of lower rates of lung cancer and heart disease. More information about nicotine abuse can be found in the exemplar on Nicotine Use in the module on Addiction.

In addition to refraining from smoking, the patient should avoid exposure to other airway irritants and allergens. The patient should remain indoors during periods of significant air pollution to prevent exacerbations of the disease. Air-filtering systems or air conditioning may be useful.

Pulmonary hygiene measures, including hydration, effective coughing, percussion, and postural drainage, are used to improve clearance of airway secretions. Cough suppressants are usually ineffective, and the patient should generally avoid sedatives because they may cause retention of secretions.

Exercise

Unless disabling cardiac disease is present, a regular exercise program is beneficial for improving exercise tolerance, enhancing the ability to perform ADLs, and preventing deterioration of physical condition.

Regular exercise improves exercise tolerance, muscle strength, and quality of life in patients with COPD and also reduces dyspnea and fatigue (Gloeckl, Marinov, & Pitta, 2013). Exercise may be conducted independently or in the context of a pulmonary rehabilitation program. Regardless of setting, exercise programs should be tailored to the individual to increase adherence. Breathing exercises are used to slow the respiratory rate and relieve accessory muscle fatigue. Pursed-lip breathing slows the respiratory rate and helps maintain open airways during exhalation by keeping positive pressure in the airways. Abdominal breathing relieves the work of accessory muscles of respiration.

Focus on Integrative Health
Chronic Obstructive Pulmonary Disease

Complementary health approaches may be useful to help manage symptoms of COPD. Dietary measures, such as minimizing intake of dairy products and salt, may help reduce mucus production and keep mucus more liquefied. Be sure to recommend measures to replace the protein and calcium in dairy products to help maintain nutritional balance. Hot herbal teas made with peppermint may act as expectorants to help relieve chest congestion.

Patients may be interested in trying complementary health approaches to assist them in quitting smoking. While additional studies are needed to evaluate the effectiveness of complementary health approaches for use in quitting smoking, current research suggests that acupuncture and hypnotherapy may be effective in promoting smoking cessation (Tahiri et al., 2012). Likewise, Hasan et al. (2014) found that hypnotherapy may be more effective than NRT for promotion of smoking cessation.

Hydration

Adequate fluid intake is essential to help thin and expectorate respiratory secretions, as well as to ensure overall fluid volume balance. A low-sodium diet is recommended to prevent water retention (DeBellis & Fetterman, 2012). Recommended fluid volume intake must take into consideration coexisting conditions, especially those that require restriction of fluid intake, such as heart failure or renal disease.

Humidifiers are devices that add water vapor to inspired air. Room humidifiers provide cool mist to room air. Nebulizers are used to deliver humidity and medications. They may be used with oxygen delivery systems to provide moistened air directly to the patient. Humidifiers prevent mucous membranes from drying and becoming irritated and loosen secretions for easier expectoration.

NURSING PROCESS

Nursing care is focused on promoting oxygenation. Health promotion activities include smoking cessation, reducing the risk of infection, and maintaining patient safety. Because of the chronic nature of this disease process, teaching the patient how to maximize self-care while knowing when to notify the healthcare team is another important role of the nurse.

Assessment

Focused assessment for the patient with COPD includes collecting the following data:

- ***Observation and patient interview.*** Current symptoms, including cough, sputum production, shortness of breath or dyspnea, and activity tolerance; frequency of respiratory infections and most recent episode; previous diagnosis of emphysema, chronic bronchitis, or asthma; current medications; smoking history in pack-years (packs per day times number of years smoked); and history of exposure to secondhand smoke and to occupational or other pollutants
- ***Physical examination.*** General appearance, weight for height, and mental status; vital signs, including temperature; skin color and temperature; anteroposterior:lateral

chest diameter; use of accessory muscles, nasal flaring, or pursed-lip breathing; respiratory excursion and diaphragmatic excursion; percussion tone; breath sounds throughout; neck veins, apical pulse and heart sounds, peripheral pulses, and edema.

Auscultation of the chest may yield very little information to aid in establishing the diagnosis of COPD. Often, lung sounds are distant or reduced, although occasionally wheezes or inspiratory crackles may be heard. These sounds, however, are also associated with other diagnoses. Heart sounds may be difficult to hear if the patient has a barrel chest. Auscultation over the xiphoid process (the lowest portion of the sternum) makes it easier to hear heart tones.

The nurse should inspect and palpate the chest for symmetry. Increased anteroposterior diameter indicates chronic respiratory effort. The nurse should also assess the use of accessory muscles during breathing and observe the position of the individual. Upright posturing is an effective aid for ease of breathing. Self-posturing may indicate respiratory distress. An individual with COPD may sit upright with support of an overbed table.

Because COPD is a progressive and deteriorating illness, many patients with COPD reach the point at which they can no longer continue to live successfully at home. The nurse working with the patient with COPD at home may want to use a home care assessment for oxygenation for patients with COPD (see **Box 15–3 »**).

Diagnosis

Patients with COPD have multiple nursing care needs. Because of the obstructive nature of the disease, airway clearance is a high priority. Nutritional deficit is common,

particularly when emphysema is predominant. Because this chronic disease affects all functional health patterns, psychosocial issues are also of concern in planning nursing care. NANDA-I diagnoses appropriate for the patient with COPD include the following:

- *Breathing Pattern, Ineffective*
- *Airway Clearance, Ineffective*
- *Activity Intolerance*
- *Imbalanced Nutrition: Less Than Body Requirements*
- *Coping: Family, Compromised*
- *Decisional Conflict: Smoking.*

(NANDA-I © 2014)

Planning

Nursing care of the patient with COPD, especially in later stages, requires careful planning in order to meet the patient's oxygenation demands. Possible outcomes for this patient may include the following:

- The patient will adapt breathing patterns to meet oxygenation demands adequately.
- The patient will experience ease of respirations with the use of positioning and pursed-lip breathing.
- The patient will maintain a patent airway, allowing adequate oxygenation.
- The patient will maintain oxygen saturation levels above 90%.
- The patient will tolerate activity levels, allowing completion of ADLs.

Box 15–3
Home Care Assessment: Oxygenation

Patient

- *Self-care abilities.* Ability to ambulate and perform ADLs independently
- *Exercise and activity pattern.* Type and regularity of usual exercise, perceived and actual energy for desired and required leisure activities
- *Assistive devices required.* Supplemental oxygen, humidifier, nebulizer treatments, or inhalers; walker, cane, or wheelchair; grab bars, shower chair, and other devices to promote safety and minimize energy expenditure; scale to monitor weight on a regular basis
- *Home environment.* Factors that impair airway clearance, gas exchange, or activity tolerance; indoor pollutants, such as cigarette smoke, dust, and allergens (e.g., pets); lack of humidity in the air; barriers, such as stairs
- *Current level of knowledge.* Importance of avoiding smoking and other pollutants; dietary salt and other restrictions if appropriate; recommended activities; medications; need to limit exposure to respiratory infections; use of prescribed nebulizer, multidose inhaler, powdered dose inhaler, or home oxygen; activity level.

Family

- *Caregiver availability, skills, and responses.* Ability and willingness to provide care as needed (help with ADLs, providing meals, assisting with transportation and shopping, caring for dependents, and performing treatments, such as percussion and postural drainage)
- *Family role changes and coping.* Effect on financial status, parenting and spousal roles, sexuality, and social roles
- *Alternate potential primary or respite caregivers.* Other family members, volunteers, church members, paid caregivers or housekeeping services, and available community respite care

Community

- *Environment.* Usual temperature and humidity; presence of air pollutants, such as automobile exhaust, industrial smoke and pollutants, and smoke from field burning
- *Current knowledge of and experience with community resources.* Medical and assistive equipment and supply companies, respiratory and physical therapy services, home health agencies, local pharmacies, available financial assistance, and support and educational organizations, such as the local lung association and COPD support groups.

Implementation

The highest priorities of nursing implementation are aimed at promoting oxygenation, which includes monitoring and promoting airway clearance and effective breathing patterns. Ongoing reassessment to determine effectiveness of interventions will help guide the nursing plan of care. For patients in the hospital, the nurse should assist with ADLs as necessary to help the patients conserve energy and reduce fatigue. Regardless of setting, the nurse should teach and assist with techniques to control and improve breathing pattern: pursed-lip breathing, abdominal breathing, and relaxation techniques.

Promote Airway Clearance

Both chronic bronchitis and emphysema affect the ability to maintain open airways. In chronic bronchitis, copious amounts of thick, tenacious mucus impair ciliary action, making it difficult to clear mucus from the airways. The loss of supporting tissue caused by emphysema increases the risk for airway collapse. In both cases, air is trapped distally, and less oxygen is available to the alveoli for diffusion. Normal respiratory defense mechanisms are impaired, and mucus-plugged airways provide an ideal environment for bacterial growth. Respiratory infection further impairs airway clearance and is often the cause of an acute exacerbation.

- Encourage a fluid intake of at least 2000–2500 mL/day unless contraindicated to help keep mucus thin.
- Place in Fowler, high-Fowler, or orthopneic position; encourage movement and activity to tolerance.
- Assess respiratory status every 1–2 hours or as indicated. Adventitious sounds should decrease with effective intervention. Diminished or absent breath sounds may indicate increasing airway obstruction and possible atelectasis.
- Monitor ABG results. Increasing hypoxemia, hypercapnia, and respiratory acidosis may indicate increasing airway obstruction.
- Weigh daily, monitor intake and output, and assess mucous membranes and skin turgor. Dehydration causes respiratory secretions to become thicker, more tenacious, and difficult to **expectorate** (expel or spit out); fluid overload can further compromise respiratory status.
- Assist with coughing and deep breathing at least every 2 hours while the patient is awake (see the Patient Teaching feature).
- Provide tissues and a paper bag to dispose of expectorated sputum. This important infection control measure reduces the spread of respiratory organisms to other people.
- Refer to a respiratory therapist, and assist with or perform percussion and postural drainage as needed. Percussion helps loosen secretions in airways; postural drainage facilitates movement of these secretions out of the respiratory tract.
- Administer expectorant and bronchodilator medications as ordered. Coordinate timing with respiratory treatments.

Patient Teaching
Effective Coughing Techniques

Several coughing techniques may be useful. For controlled cough technique, teach the patient as follows:

1. Following prescribed bronchodilator treatment, inhale deeply and hold breath briefly.
2. Cough twice, the first time to loosen mucus and the second to expel secretions.
3. Inhale by sniffing to prevent mucus from moving back into deep airways.
4. Rest. Avoid prolonged coughing to prevent fatigue and hypoxemia.

For huff coughing, teach the patient to:

1. Inhale deeply while leaning forward.
2. Exhale sharply with a "huff" sound to help keep airways open while mobilizing secretions.

Using expectorants and bronchodilators before coughing, percussion, and postural drainage increases their effectiveness in clearing airways.

- Provide supplemental oxygen as ordered. Supplemental oxygen helps maintain adequate blood and tissue oxygenation.

SAFETY ALERT Prepare for intubation and mechanical ventilation if respiratory status deteriorates (increasing hypoxemia and hypercapnia, decreased LOC, cyanosis, or worsening airway obstruction). Respiratory failure is a possible complication of an acute exacerbation of COPD and requires immediate intervention to preserve life.

Promote Balanced Nutrition

With advanced COPD, minimal activity, including eating, can cause fatigue and dyspnea. The patient may be unable to consume a full meal without resting. At the same time, the increased work of breathing increases metabolic demands, and more calories are required. The patient may appear cachectic (thin and wasted). Poor nutritional status further impairs immune function and increases the risk of a complicating infection.

- Assess nutritional status, including diet history, appropriate weight for height, and anthropometric (skinfold) measurements. It is important to differentiate nutritional status from body type rather than assume a nutritional impairment.
- Observe and document food intake, including types, amounts, and caloric intake. This information can provide direction for supplementation if needed.
- Monitor laboratory values, including serum albumin and electrolyte levels. These values provide information about the adequacy of nutritional intake, including protein.
- Consult with a dietitian to plan meals and nutritional supplements that meet caloric needs. More concentrated

sources of high-energy foods may be required to maintain caloric intake without excess fatigue. A diet high in proteins and fats without excess carbohydrates is recommended to minimize carbon dioxide production during metabolism.

- Provide frequent, small feedings with between-meal supplements to maintain intake and reduce fatigue associated with eating.
- Place the patient in a seated or high-Fowler position for meals to promote lung expansion and reduce dyspnea.
- Assist the patient with choosing preferred foods from the menu; encourage family members to bring food from home if allowed.
- Keep snacks at the bedside to provide additional caloric intake.
- Provide mouth care before meals to enhance the appetite.
- If the patient is unable to maintain oral intake, consult with the primary care provider about enteral or parenteral feedings. Maintenance of caloric and nutrient intake is vital to prevent catabolism.

Promote Family Coping

Chronic illness affects the entire family structure. Roles and relationships change; additional demands are placed on the family. Family members may blame the patient for causing the illness or may have distorted perceptions about it, even denying its existence. They may refuse to assist or participate in care. The patient may develop an attitude of helplessness or dependence or may demonstrate anger, hostility, or aggression.

- Assess the effect of the illness on the family to assist in planning appropriate interventions.
- Provide information and teaching about COPD to help the family gain an understanding of the patient's condition and needs.
- Help family members recognize behaviors and attitudes that may hinder effective treatment, such as continuing to smoke in the house.
- Initiate a care conference involving the patient, family, and healthcare team members from a variety of disciplines. A wide range of perspectives and areas of expertise aids in problem solving and facilitates communication.
- Refer the patient and family to support groups and pulmonary rehabilitation programs as available.

Evaluation

Observe and record the patient's breathing and vital signs, focusing on trends and patterns. Compare the patient's actual respiration and breathing patterns to the outcome goal established. Some interventions may require time before progress is observed. For example, improving the ease of breathing may occur readily with a change in medications, but quitting smoking may take months or years.

Potential outcomes to evaluate the effectiveness of care may include:

- The patient consistently maintains oxygen saturation greater than 90%.

Patient Teaching
Home Care for Patients with COPD

When preparing for home care for a patient with COPD, the nurse must teach both the patient and the patient's family and caregivers the following:

- Maintain adequate fluid intake (at least 2.0–2.5 quarts of fluid daily).
- Avoid respiratory irritants, including cigarette smoke (both primary and secondary), other smoke sources, dust, aerosol sprays, air pollution, and very cold, dry air.
- Prevent exposure to infection, especially upper respiratory infections.
- Receive a pneumococcal vaccine and annual influenza immunization.
- Follow the prescribed exercise program, maintain ADLs, and balance rest and exercise.
- Maintain nutrient intake (e.g., eating small, frequent meals and using nutritional supplements to provide adequate calories).
- Identify early signs of an infection or exacerbation, and seek medical attention for the following: fever, increased sputum production, purulent (green or yellow) sputum, upper respiratory infection, increased shortness of breath or difficulty breathing, decreased activity tolerance or appetite, and increased need for oxygen.
- Understand prescribed medications, including purpose, proper use, and expected effects.
- Avoid use of over-the-counter medications unless approved by the physician.
- Understand other prescribed therapies, such as use of home oxygen, percussion, postural drainage, and nebulizer treatments.
- Wear an identification band and carry a list of medications at all times in case of an emergency.

The nurse should also provide referrals to home care services, such as home health, assistance with ADLs (as needed), home maintenance services, respiratory therapy and home oxygen services, and other agencies such as Meals on Wheels and senior services as indicated.

- The patient modifies ADLs to reduce fatigue related to activity intolerance.
- The patient demonstrates appropriate use of medications (e.g., inhalers).

Because COPD is a chronic condition, patients with COPD will need continual re-evaluation to ensure that medications are providing relief, the patient is maintaining appropriate activity levels, and the patient is adhering to the treatment plan, including any smoking cessation program. Patients with a history of smoking usually require multiple attempts before they successfully quit smoking for the long term, so the nurse should evaluate the patient's success and provide encouragement to the patient at each interaction.

Nursing Care Plan
A Patient with COPD

Anna Mercurio, known as "Happy" to all her friends, is an 83-year-old widow who lives with her two adult sons. During the past 15 years, Mrs. Mercurio has become increasingly short of breath while gardening and walking, two of her favorite activities. She also has developed a chronic cough that is particularly bad in the mornings. Ten years ago, her family physician told her that she had emphysema. She is admitted to the hospital with possible pneumonia and acute exacerbation of COPD.

ASSESSMENT

Jeff Harris, RN, admits Mrs. Mercurio to the medical unit. In the nursing history, Nurse Harris notes that she denies ever smoking but says that her husband and two sons have been smokers "for practically their whole lives." She says she lived an active life before developing lung disease, but her breathing and coughing have progressed so that she now must rest after just a few minutes of housework or other activity. Her cough is productive of moderate to large amounts of sputum, particularly in the mornings. She developed increasing shortness of breath and sputum 2 days ago. This morning, she could not complete her morning activities without resting, so she contacted her doctor.

On physical examination, Nurse Harris notes the following: The skin is very warm, dry, and dusky colored. The patient pauses frequently while speaking to breathe. Respirations are 36/minute and fairly shallow; the patient coughs frequently, producing large amounts of thick, tenacious green sputum. Other vital signs: temperature 39°C (102.4°F); pulse 115 bpm and irregular; BP 186/60 mmHg. The patient appears very thin: weight 43.6 kg (96 lb), height 160 cm (63 in.). Anteroposterior:lateral chest diameter approximately 1:1; moderate kyphosis noted. Chest is hyperresonant to percussion. Auscultation reveals distant breath sounds with scattered wheezes and rhonchi throughout lung fields. CXR shows flattening of the diaphragm, slight cardiac enlargement, prominent vascular and bronchial markings, and patchy infiltrates. Initial laboratory work reveals moderate erythrocytosis, leukocytosis, and low serum albumin. ABG results: pH 7.19, PaO_2 54 mmHg, $PaCO_2$ 59 mmHg, HCO_3, 30 mg/dL, and oxygen saturation 88%. Admitting orders include sputum specimen for culture; IV penicillin G, 2 million units every 4 hours; albuterol/ipratropium (Combivent) inhaler, two puffs every 6 hours; salmeterol/fluticasone (Advair) DPI, twice a day; bedrest with bathroom privileges; oxygen per nasal cannula at 2 L/min continuously; and regular diet.

DIAGNOSES

- *Ineffective Airway Clearance* related to pneumonia and COPD
- *Impaired Gas Exchange* related to acute and chronic lung disease
- *Impaired Spontaneous Ventilation* related to loss of hypoxemic respiratory drive and respiratory muscle fatigue
- *Impaired Home Maintenance* related to activity intolerance

(NANDA-I © 2014)

PLANNING

- The patient will expectorate secretions effectively.
- The patient will return to the level of pulmonary function prior to acute exacerbation.
- The patient will demonstrate improved ABG and oxygen saturation values.
- The patient will maintain spontaneous respirations without excess fatigue.
- The patient will verbalize a willingness to allow her sons or a housekeeper to assist with daily household tasks.

IMPLEMENTATION

- Assess respiratory status and LOC every 1–2 hours until stable, then at least every 4 hours.
- Closely monitor the response to oxygen therapy, including skin color, oxygen saturation, sputum consistency, and respiratory drive.
- Ensure adequate fluid intake as ordered and provide a bedside humidifier.
- Monitor the patient for signs and symptoms of fluid volume overload, including adventitious breath sounds, bounding pulses, and increased blood pressure.
- Elevate the head of the bed to at least 30° at all times.
- Teach the "huff" coughing technique.

- Administer medications as ordered, providing the ipratropium inhaler before the fluticasone inhaler. Provide mouth care after inhalers.
- Contact respiratory therapy for percussion and postural drainage following inhaler treatments.
- Provide uninterrupted rest periods following treatments and procedures.
- Meet with Mrs. Mercurio and her sons to develop a postdischarge care plan.
- Refer to the home health department for nursing follow-up.
- Refer Mrs. Mercurio to social services for possible assistance with home maintenance.

Nursing Care Plan *(continued)*

EVALUATION

After the first day in the hospital, Mrs. Mercurio's condition begins to improve slowly. On discharge 6 days later, she is able to provide self-care with less fatigue and dyspnea. She is using oxygen at night only, admitting that it is just for security. Although a few scattered wheezes and rhonchi are still present in her lungs, Mrs. Mercurio's sputum is thinner, white, and easily expectorated. She will take oral penicillin V for an additional 10 days at home. She will also continue using the Advair and Combivent inhalers as prescribed at home. Although Mrs. Mercurio's sons admit they will probably never be able to quit smoking, they have agreed to smoke only in the garage or outside. A home health nurse will initially evaluate Mrs. Mercurio's progress three times weekly. Arrangements have been made for a housekeeper to come twice a week for cleaning and laundry. Mrs. Mercurio is glad to be returning home and grateful for the arrangements that have been made.

CRITICAL THINKING

1. Mrs. Mercurio has never been a smoker but has had long-term exposure to secondhand smoke. How does secondhand smoke contribute to lung diseases in adults and children?

2. The patient with an acute exacerbation of COPD is at risk for respiratory failure. What changes in Mrs. Mercurio's assessment findings could indicate this complication may be developing?

3. Develop a nursing care plan for Mrs. Mercurio for the nursing diagnosis *Risk for Infection* related to secondhand smoke exposure.

REVIEW   Chronic Obstructive Pulmonary Disease

RELATE Link the Concepts and Exemplars

Linking the exemplar of chronic obstructive pulmonary disease with the concept of fluids and electrolytes:

1. Why is it important for the patient with COPD to drink sufficient fluids?

2. Why might a patient with COPD who is confined to bed choose to drink less, and how can the nurse promote hydration in this patient?

Linking the exemplar of chronic obstructive pulmonary disease with the concept of safety:

3. Why is it important for the nurse to assess the patient with COPD for risk for injury related to the use of oxygen?

4. What teaching should the nurse provide to a patient who will be discharged with home oxygen therapy for the first time?

Linking the exemplar of chronic obstructive pulmonary disease with the concept of infection:

5. Why is the patient with COPD at a greater risk for developing respiratory infections?

6. What therapies could be used to decrease the risk of infection in the patient with COPD?

READY Go to Volume 3: Clinical Nursing Skills

REFER Go to Pearson MyLab Nursing and eText

- Additional review materials

REFLECT Apply Your Knowledge

James Winston is a 58-year-old man living in North Carolina. Before retiring this past fall, he worked on a heavy-machinery production line most of his adult life. He served in the Marines during the Vietnam War. Throughout his work years, he was a weekend gardener. He has smoked a pack of cigarettes every day since high school, and he has increased to two packs a day since retirement. "I have been lying around the house waiting for spring so I can garden," he says.

Now that spring has arrived, trees are blooming, grass is again in need of mowing, and Mr. Winston is admitted to the medical unit with shortness of breath. The initial assessment demonstrates an afebrile man with vital signs as follows: temperature 98.9°F, pulse 88 bpm, respirations 32/min, BP 164/96 mmHg, and pulse oximetry reading 89%. Mr. Winston is tachypneic, sitting upright and forward with his hands on his knees. He has removed his oxygen face mask because he says, "It smothers me."

1. What other assessment data are needed before providing care for this patient?

2. What are the priority interventions for Mr. Winston? Why do these take priority?

3. What diagnostic examination would confirm the patient has COPD?

4. What interventions may be necessary for Mr. Winston to resume the healthy behaviors in his life?

» Exemplar 15.D
Cystic Fibrosis

Exemplar Learning Outcomes

15.D Analyze cystic fibrosis as it relates to oxygenation.

- Describe the pathophysiology of cystic fibrosis.
- Describe the etiology of cystic fibrosis.
- Summarize the risk factors for cystic fibrosis.
- Describe methods for preventing cystic fibrosis.
- Identify the clinical manifestations of cystic fibrosis.
- Summarize diagnostic tests and therapies used by interprofessional teams in the collaborative care of an individual with cystic fibrosis.

- Differentiate care of patients with cystic fibrosis across the lifespan.
- Apply the nursing process in providing culturally competent care to an individual with cystic fibrosis.

Exemplar Key Terms

Overview

Cystic fibrosis (CF) is an inherited disorder that affects the secretory glands, particularly the glands that are responsible for secreting mucus, digestive enzymes, and sweat. In turn, CF affects the lungs and sinuses as well as the digestive organs, including the pancreas, intestines, and liver. CF also affects the reproductive organs (NHLBI, 2013b).

Among Caucasians, CF is relatively common, occurring in 1 in 2500 to 3500 infants. CF is less common among people of color. For example, it is found in approximately 1 in 17,000 African Americans and in approximately 1 in 31,000 Asian Americans (U.S. National Library of Medicine, 2012).

In the United States, CF affects approximately 30,000 individuals. Worldwide, an estimated 70,000 people are diagnosed with this disorder. Nearly 1000 new cases of CF are diagnosed annually. Almost 50% of individuals with CF are 18 years of age or older; however, in more than 75% of cases, diagnosis of CF occurs before 2 years of age (Cystic Fibrosis Foundation, n.d.a).

Pathophysiology and Etiology

Pathophysiology

CF stems from a mutation of the *CFTR* gene, which causes absence or dysfunction of the **cystic fibrosis transmembrane conductance regulator (CFTR) protein**. The CFTR protein is central to the movement of chloride into and out of the body cells (Haack, Aragão, & Novaes, 2013). The mutation associated with the CF gene affects not only chloride but also the movement of salt (as sodium chloride) and water into and out of the cells (Mayo Clinic, 2015d). To be more specific, CF involves cellular entry of too much salt and not enough water. Mucus secretions are typically relatively thin and watery and serve as natural lubricants. However, the genetic defect associated with CF causes the production of thick, sticky mucus that obstructs ducts and passageways within the body, including the airways (see **Figure 15–32 》**) and pancreatic ducts.

This viscous mucus not only accumulates in respiratory passages and causes airway occlusion, but it also creates an environment that supports bacterial growth (Osborn et al., 2014). As part of the immune response, white blood cells react to the localized infection, releasing sticky chemical substances into the mucus and worsening the degree of obstruction, as well as exacerbating the existing inflammation and infection (Osborn et al., 2014). Although CF is most often diagnosed before 2 years of age (Cystic Fibrosis Foundation, n.d.a), manifestations of the disorder are variable and may emerge later in the individual's life. In some cases, patients may remain completely asymptomatic for several years before developing signs or symptoms of CF (Haack et al., 2013).

Etiology

The genetic mutation associated with CF causes either absence or dysfunction of the CFTR protein, which is responsible for regulating the movement of chloride across cellular membranes (see **Figure 15–33 》**). Chloride is essential to cellular function, including regulating water balance within the tissues. This water balance is needed to ensure adequate production of mucus (U.S. National Library of Medicine, 2012). This genetic abnormality allows an excess of salt (sodium chloride) to enter the cells; at the same time, not enough water is allowed to enter the cells. Because of this imbalance, cells in the lungs and pancreas, as well as other in organs, secrete abnormally viscous, sticky mucus that occludes respiratory passageways (U.S. National Library of Medicine, 2012) as well as ducts within the digestive and reproductive systems (NHLBI, 2013b). The characteristic manifestations of CF occur as a result of the mucus-clogged passageways and ducts.

Risk Factors

As an **autosomal recessive disorder**, development of CF requires that the affected individual receive two abnormal *CFTR* genes in order to express the disease. In the case of autosomal recessive disorders, each of the affected individual's parents carries one copy of the abnormal gene. However, as carriers of the defective gene, neither parent typically demonstrates signs or symptoms of CF (U.S. National Library of Medicine, 2012).

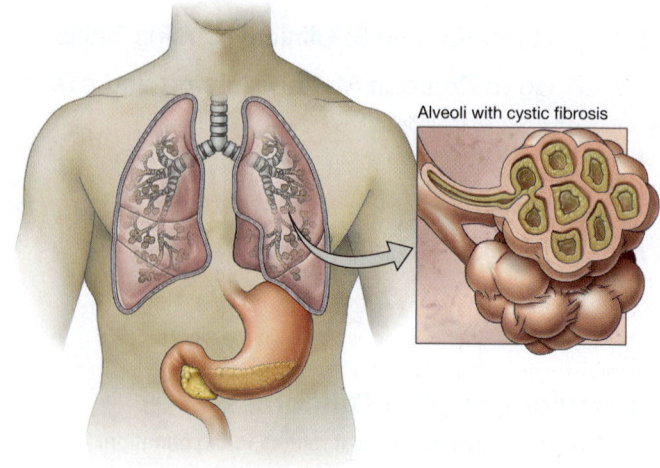

Alveoli with cystic fibrosis

Figure 15–32 》 Cystic fibrosis.

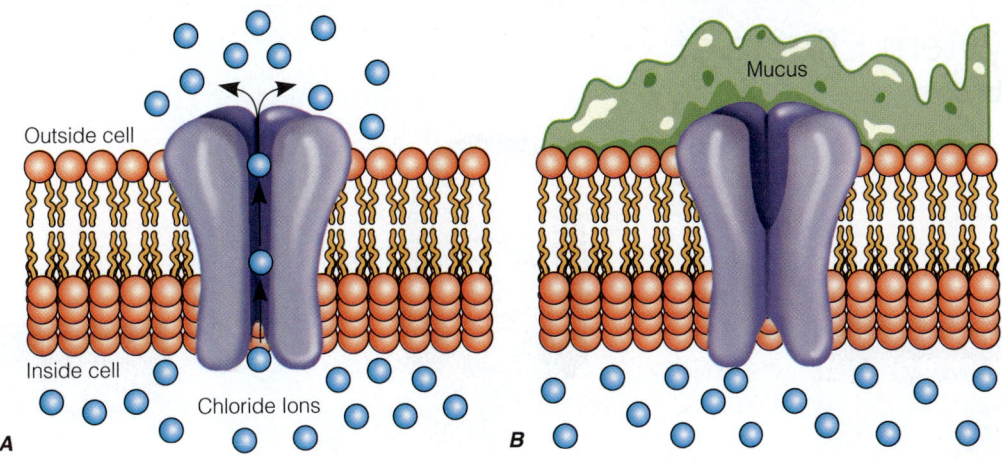

Figure 15–33 ❯❯ Gene mutations in cystic fibrosis. ***A,*** A normal CTFR channel moves chloride ions to the outside of the cell. ***B,*** A mutant CTFR channel does not move chloride ions, causing a sticky mucus to build up on the outside of the cell.

Because development of CF requires the inheritance of two *CFTR* genes (one from each parent), the offspring of parents who carry the *CFTR* gene are not guaranteed to develop the disorder. For example, when both parents are carriers of the *CFTR* gene, each conception allows for a 25% possibility that two abnormal genes will be passed to the child, along with a 50% possibility that the child will be a carrier of one *CFTR* gene. Each conception also allows for a 25% possibility that the child will not carry the *CFTR* gene.

Prevention

Genetic screening can be done using blood or a saliva sample to assess an individual's carrier status. Genetic screening is recommended for individuals who have a personal or family history of CF. In addition, genetic screening is advised for the individual whose partner either has CF or has a family history of CF (NHLBI, 2013b). Although not 100% accurate, genetic screening allows for detection of faulty *CFTR* genes in approximately 90% of cases (NHLBI, 2013b).

Clinical Manifestations

An increased level of chloride in the sweat is a hallmark manifestation and is one basis for diagnosis of CF. As a result of increased mucus viscosity, clinical manifestations of CF also commonly include respiratory problems, such as a chronic cough and susceptibility to infection. Chronic sinusitis may occur as a result of accumulation of viscous nasal secretions that become infected and produce inflammation (Johns Hopkins Cystic Fibrosis Center, n.d.a). Gastrointestinal alterations, such as chronic diarrhea and nutritional deficiencies, are common. However, because CF affects multiple organs and body systems, specific manifestations vary among individuals (Haack et al., 2013). Likewise, the effects of CF range in terms of severity. (See Multisystem Effects of Cystic Fibrosis.)

In many cases, common manifestations associated with CF include chronic, recurrent episodes of respiratory infections, including bronchiectasis and pneumonia (Mayo

Clinic, 2015d). Subsequent damage to the structures of the respiratory system can cause the development of scar tissue (fibrosis) and cyst formation in the lungs (U.S. National Library of Medicine, 2012). Pneumothorax also may develop during later stages of the disease (Kioumis et al., 2014). Pulmonary damage caused by persistent infections may ultimately lead to respiratory failure and death.

Obstruction of pancreatic ducts by viscous mucus secretions may impair the production of pancreatic enzymes, which are necessary for food digestion. As a result, malnutrition and delays in growth and development may occur (Osborn et al., 2014). Pancreatic duct obstruction also may interfere with insulin production, causing impaired blood glucose control (U.S. National Library of Medicine, 2012). Approximately 20% of patients with CF develop diabetes by 30 years of age (Mayo Clinic, 2015d). Additional gastrointestinal sequelae of CF may include blockage and inflammation of the bile duct, which transports bile from the liver and gallbladder to the small intestine. Impairment of the bile duct may cause hepatic dysfunction and gallstone formation (Mayo Clinic, 2015d).

The majority of men who have CF will demonstrate congenital bilateral absence of the vas deferens (CBAVD). This complication comprises obstruction and impaired development of the vas deferens (the tube that connects the testes and the prostate gland, allowing for sperm transport) (U.S. National Library of Medicine, 2012). The vas deferens may also be absent (Mayo Clinic, 2015d). Men who have CBAVD typically experience infertility and, for those who desire to parent a child, necessary interventions may include fertility treatment or surgical procedures (Mayo Clinic, 2015d; U.S. National Library of Medicine, 2012). Women with CF also are subject to reproductive complications, including decreased fertility. While successful conception and pregnancy are possible, the physiologic changes associated with pregnancy may exacerbate the effects of CF (Mayo Clinic, 2015d).

In the past, CF was considered to be a fatal childhood disease. However, as a result of improved therapies and disease management strategies, the survival rate among individuals with CF has greatly improved.

Multisystem Effects of
Cystic Fibrosis

Respiratory

- Viscous, sticky mucus
- Respiratory infections
- Chronic cough
- Chronic sinusitis
- Bronchiectasis
- Pneumonia
- Cysts
- Fibrosis
- Pneumothorax

Gastrointestinal

- Chronic diarrhea
- Nutritional deficiencies
- Obstructed pancreatic ducts
- Blocked bile ducts
- Gallstones
- Abdominal pain
- Bowel obstruction/
  intussusception

Musculoskeletal

- Delayed growth and
  development
- Osteopenia
- Osteoporosis
- Fractures

Neurologic

- Depression
- Anxiety

Cardiovascular

- Clubbing of fingers and toes
- Cyanosis

Reproductive

- Delayed puberty
- Blockage or absence of
  vas deferens
- Decreased fertility
  (men and women)
- Pregnancy complications

Integumentary

- Salty skin

Metabolic Processes

- Diabetes

Clinical Manifestations and Therapies
Cystic Fibrosis

ETIOLOGY	CLINICAL MANIFESTATIONS	CLINICAL THERAPIES
Viscous respiratory secretions	<ul><li>Airway obstruction</li><li>Hypoxia</li><li>Hypoxemia</li><li>Dyspnea</li><li>Infection</li></ul>	<ul><li>Monitoring airway patency</li><li>Oral suctioning</li><li>Oxygen therapy</li><li>Frequent auscultation of breath sounds</li><li>Chest physiotherapy</li><li>Maintaining current immunizations</li><li>Pathogen-specific antibiotics</li><li>Pharmacologic treatments</li><li>Surgical treatments as warranted (e.g., endoscopy and lavage, excision of nasal polyps)</li><li>Psychosocial support</li></ul>
Viscous gastrointestinal and digestive system secretions	<ul><li>Impaired nutrition</li><li>Impaired insulin production and glucose control</li><li>Chronic diarrhea; typically loose, oily stools</li><li>Delayed growth and development</li><li>Intestinal and bile duct blockages</li><li>Abdominal pain</li><li>Gallstone formation</li></ul>	<ul><li>Early diagnosis and treatment of disease</li><li>Nutritional supplementation</li><li>Nutritional supervision by a dietitian</li><li>Enteral feeding</li><li>Pharmacologic treatments</li><li>Surgical treatments as warranted (e.g., feeding tube placement, bowel surgery)</li><li>Monitoring weight and height/length</li><li>Monitoring achievement of developmental milestones</li><li>Psychosocial support</li></ul>
Viscous reproductive system secretions	<ul><li>Decreased fertility (men and women)</li><li>Increased pregnancy-related complications (women)</li></ul>	<ul><li>Genetic counseling</li><li>Fertility treatment</li><li>Psychosocial support</li></ul>

Collaboration

Because CF affects multiple target organs and body systems, collaboration among several healthcare providers will likely be necessary and will depend on the organs and systems affected and the severity of symptoms. Collaboration may include the patient's primary healthcare provider, respiratory specialists, gastrointestinal and nutritional specialists, and reproductive specialists and obstetricians, among others.

Diagnostic Tests

Prenatal screening for CF involves taking a blood sample from the mother to determine whether she carries normal *CFTR* genes. If both of the mother's *CFTR* genes are normal, the infant will not have CF. However, if the mother does carry an abnormal gene, then the father will also receive a blood test. If both parents carry the abnormal gene, the infant has a 25% chance of having CF and a 50% chance of being a carrier only (Johns Hopkins Cystic Fibrosis Center, n.d.b).

If both of the parents are carriers of an abnormal *CFTR* gene, then they can choose to perform prenatal testing on the fetus (Johns Hopkins Cystic Fibrosis Center, n.d.b). Genetic testing using either **amniocentesis** or **chorionic vil-**

lus sampling (CVS) can determine whether the fetus has CF (NHLBI, 2013b). CVS typically occurs between weeks 10 and 13 of the pregnancy, earlier than amniocentesis is typically performed (Mayo Clinic, 2015e), usually around weeks 15–18 (Johns Hopkins Cystic Fibrosis Center, n.d.b). The American College of Obstetricians and Gynecologists recommends that all couples considering having a child be tested to determine if they are carriers for CF (Cystic Fibrosis Foundation, n.d.b).

Newborns across all 50 states and Washington, DC, are tested for CF (Mayo Clinic, 2015d; NHLBI, 2013b), and most children born in the United States are screened at birth, with the majority of CF diagnoses occurring by the age of 2 (Cystic Fibrosis Foundation, n.d.c). Parents who forgo prenatal testing should have their newborn baby screened for CF (Johns Hopkins Cystic Fibrosis Center, n.d.b). This testing involves a blood test to determine how much immunoreactive trypsinogen, or IRT, the newborn's pancreas is releasing (Mayo Clinic, 2015d). If this test shows high enough levels of IRT to be of concern, then a sweat test is administered at a center accredited by the Cystic Fibrosis Foundation (Cystic Fibrosis Foundation, n.d.c), typically at the age of 1 month (Mayo Clinic, 2015d). The **sweat test**, which is typically administered twice, measures the amount of salt in the baby's sweat and is most effective for a CF diagnosis; a high level of salt confirms the diagnosis (NHLBI, 2013b). Genetic testing, which is done via a blood test, confirms the specific defects on the gene responsible for the condition (Mayo Clinic, 2015d).

Older children or adults who were not screened at birth for CF may be tested for the condition if they show warning signs, such as bronchiectasis, chronic lung or sinus infections, nasal polyps, pancreatitis, or male infertility (Mayo Clinic, 2015d). In 2013, 20.8% of diagnoses were in children ages 2–15, and 6.8% were in patients ages 16 years or older (Cystic Fibrosis Foundation, n.d.c). Testing for older children or adults is the same as for newborns in whom CF is suspected: sweat testing and genetic testing through blood samples (Mayo Clinic, 2015d).

Surgery

Many surgical and other medical procedures exist to help individuals with CF manage the effects of the disease. However, their use depends on each patient's presentation and management needs. Examples of surgical and medical procedures used for the treatment of CF include:

- Nasal polyps may be removed to improve breathing.
- Mucus may be removed through endoscopic lavage to improve breathing (Mayo Clinic, 2015d).
- Oxygen therapy may be used for advanced lung disease; this typically involves providing pure oxygen through nasal prongs or a mask (NHLBI, 2013b). Oxygen therapy is recommended when the blood–oxygen level declines severely; breathing pure oxygen helps prevent pulmonary hypertension (Mayo Clinic, 2015d).
- Digestive treatments may involve using a feeding tube at night to receive additional nutrients or having bowel surgery if a bowel blockage or intussusception (i.e., a section of bowel folds in on itself) occurs (Mayo Clinic, 2015d).

Pharmacologic Therapy

Pharmacologic therapy is essential for patients with CF to help open the airways, break up mucus, and treat infections and inflammation. These medications are necessary to maintain adequate oxygenation and nutrition and prevent complications.

Bronchodilators

The Cystic Fibrosis Foundation recommends the use of bronchodilators such as albuterol (Proventil, Ventolin) before chest physical therapy or before administration of other inhaled medications to improve mucus clearance and delivery of medications (Cystic Fibrosis Foundation, n.d.d; Osborn et al., 2014). Depending on the needs of the patient and the formulations available, bronchodilators can be administered orally or by inhalation. Bronchodilators are typically used only in patients with milder disease for specific purposes. For patients with significant airflow obstruction, bronchodilators may produce a paradoxical decrease in airflow, so they should be used with caution.

Mucolytics

Mucolytics are medications that help break up thick mucus secretions in the airways of patients with CF. The two primary mucolytics recommended for patients with CF are dornase alfa (Pulmozyme) and hypertonic saline (Mogayzel et al., 2013). Dornase alfa is a DNase I endonuclease that cleaves DNA strands. White blood cells that get trapped in the thick mucus secretions release denatured DNA, contributing to mucus thickening. By cleaving these DNA strands, dornase alfa helps decrease the viscosity of the mucus. Dornase alfa is generally used daily, although similar results have been obtained from alternate day dosing. Because of cost constraints associated with dornase alfa, many clinics prefer to recommend alternate day dosing.

Inhalation of 7% hypertonic saline helps hydrate and thin mucus so it is more easily expelled. This helps improve lung function and decrease the number of pulmonary exacerbations (Sharma, 2015). Bronchodilators should be administered before hypertonic saline to limit bronchospasm often associated with inhalation of hypertonic saline. Hypertonic saline is generally less expensive than dornase alfa, but it is associated with lower tolerability due to irritation of the airways. In addition, hypertonic saline and dornase alfa should never be mixed in the same nebulizer because the saline will inactivate the dornase alfa.

Antibiotics

The accumulation of thick mucus in the airways provides an ideal environment for the growth of bacteria, so patients with CF are at high risk for infection with bacteria such as *Pseudomonas aeruginosa*, *Staphylococcus aureus*, *Haemophilus influenzae*, and *Burkholderia cepacia* complex (Bhatt, 2013). In addition, infection increases mucus production, which further inhibits oxygenation. Therefore, prompt treatment with organism-specific antibiotics is essential for patients with CF. Patients should be encouraged to finish their full course of antibiotics as prescribed to decrease the risk of developing resistant strains of bacteria.

Oral antibiotics are frequently used for mild infections, IV antibiotics are for more severe infections, and inhaled antibiotics are specifically for patients with *P. aeruginosa* infections. *P. aeruginosa* is the most common infectious agent in patients with CF. Inhaled antibiotics include tobramycin solution (TOBI, Bethkis), tobramycin powder (TOBI Podhaler), and aztreonam solution (Cayston) (Cystic Fibrosis Foundation, n.d.e). Other antibiotics used include gentamicin, piperacillin, cephalosporins, and fluoroquinolones (Sharma, 2015).

Because patients with CF have altered distribution and metabolism of drugs, they should be given higher doses of antibiotics than other patients with the same infection (Osborn et al., 2014). Depending on the patient's needs, antibiotics can be administered continuously or intermittently, and the patient may take one or more antibiotics simultaneously (Sharma, 2015).

CFTR Modulators

CFTR modulators are a major revolution in the treatment of CF, because they target the cause of the problem rather than just the clinical manifestations. The first CFTR modulator, ivacaftor (Kalydeco), is approved for treatment of patients age 2 and over with one of the following mutations: R117H, G178R, S549N, S549R, G551D, G551S, G1244E, S1251N, S1255P, and G1349D. Ivacaftor works by helping the CFTR protein work correctly and by helping salt and fluid move into the airways. The second CFTR modulator is a combination of ivacaftor and lumacaftor (Orkambi). The combination drug is targeted to patients age 12 and over who have two copies of the F508del mutation, which is the most common mutation. This drug works by moving the defective CFTR protein to the cell surface and helping increase its activity once it is in place (Cystic Fibrosis Foundation, n.d.f). CFTR modulators should be taken orally twice daily with fat-containing foods (Pettit & Fellner, 2014). Because CFTR modulators are relatively new drugs, they may be prohibitively expensive for most patients unless they receive help with payment. Nurses should be aware of this cost for qualifying patients and help them find resources to decrease the out-of-pocket cost.

Vaccination

Because the risk for respiratory infection is high in patients with CF, most guidelines recommend that they stay up to date on their immunizations, including annual influenza vaccines. Other vaccines that are recommended include measles and pertussis, both of which have elements of respiratory involvement. Because of the increased risk of infection, patients with CF should receive the inactivated version of vaccines rather than the live version if this option is available.

Anti-inflammatory Drugs

Airway inflammation is a hallmark of CF. Inflammation contributes to the accumulation of neutrophils in the airways, which then contributes to the thickening of mucus. The most common anti-inflammatory medication prescribed for patients with CF is ibuprofen (Lands & Stanojevic, 2013). However, toxicity with chronic use is a concern. Long-term use of corticosteroids is not recommended for patients with CF. Several other anti-inflammatory drugs are undergoing clinical trials for use in patients with CF.

Digestive Drugs

The pancreas secretes digestive enzymes that enter the small intestine through a duct. However, in patients with CF, this small duct is clogged with thick mucus, and the digestive enzymes cannot reach the intestines. Therefore, almost 90% of patients with CF take oral pancreatic enzymes (pancrelipase; Creon, Pancreaze) to help aid in digestion and absorption of nutrients (Cystic Fibrosis Foundation, n.d.g). These enzymes contain lipase, amylase, and protease and are given as a capsule. Capsules should be taken before every meal or snack and are effective for about 1 hour after taking them. The number of capsules taken depends on the individual and the type of meal being consumed. The beads in the capsules are designed to dissolve in the small intestine to release the enzymes; because of this design, the capsules can be opened and the beads mixed with soft foods for administration to infants and small children who cannot swallow the capsules. Pancreatic enzymes help digest carbohydrates, proteins, and fats; absorb vitamins and minerals; and maintain a healthy weight (Cystic Fibrosis Foundation, n.d.g).

Many patients with CF also take vitamin and mineral supplements in addition to pancreatic enzymes to help maintain a healthy nutritional status. Supplemental vitamins needed include vitamins A, D, E, and K—the fat-soluble vitamins. Supplementation of water-soluble vitamins is unnecessary for most patients with CF. Supplemental minerals needed include calcium, iron, zinc, and sodium chloride. The amount of vitamins or minerals needed depends on the patient's weight, height, and nutritional status.

Nonpharmacologic Therapy

Because CF has no cure, the goals of CF therapy involve alleviating the complications associated with CF. Nonpharmacologic therapy for CF attempts to address the physical ailments and complications that arise from CF. Nonpharmacologic therapies can assist in loosening and removing mucus from the lungs to keep airways clear, preventing or treating intestinal blockages, maintaining healthy nutrition and hydration, and ensuring appropriate hygiene (NHLBI, 2013b).

Coughing is the most basic of the **airway clearance techniques**, or ACTs, because it is an involuntary reflex. An individual with CF should not attempt to suppress coughs, because these can clear the larger airways of mucus (Cystic Fibrosis Foundation, n.d.h). As an involuntary reflex, coughing is a hardwired physiologic response to obstructions of the airway, but huffing is a more controlled and potentially less exhausting alternative to coughing. Huffing involves holding a breath and then actively exhaling it to move the mucus out of the lungs (Cystic Fibrosis Foundation, n.d.h). Although all ACTs involve coughing or huffing (Cystic Fibrosis Foundation, n.d.d), coughing and huffing ideally should be used in conjunction with other ACTs to move mucus out of the smaller airways as well (Cystic Fibrosis Foundation, n.d.h).

Chest physical therapy (CPT) is an ACT that involves **percussion** (clapping or pounding on the chest) as well as vibration and deep breathing (Cystic Fibrosis Foundation, n.d.i). CPT aims to loosen mucus from the lungs so that it can be expelled (NHLBI, 2013b). Posture can improve drainage by raising the parts of the lungs to be drained as high as possible (Cystic Fibrosis Foundation, n.d.i); individuals might sit or lie on their stomachs with their heads down while engaging in CPT (NHLBI, 2013b). While the individual is in a good posture for drainage so that gravity is at work on the mucus (Cystic Fibrosis Foundation, n.d.i), clapping on the chest or using vibration creates force that helps with drainage (NHLBI, 2013b). The clapping involves drumming cupped hands against the front and back of the chest in a rhythmic motion (see **Figure 15–34** ≫) (Mayo Clinic, 2015c). The frequency of CPT is typically one to four times a

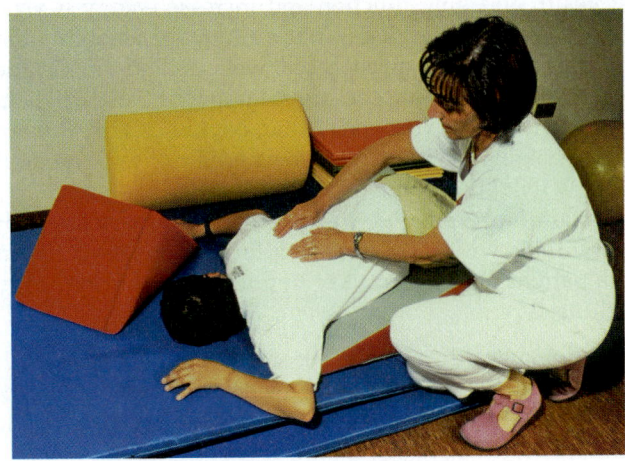

Source: Mauro Fermariello/Science Source.

Figure 15–34 ≫ Therapist performing chest physical therapy on a boy with cystic fibrosis.

Focus on Diversity and Culture
Cystic Fibrosis

In both developed and developing nations, research has demonstrated the impact of poverty on patients with CF (Kerem & Cohen-Cymberknoh, 2016). Compared to children who are from affluent socioeconomic backgrounds, children with CF who are from socioeconomically disadvantaged populations demonstrate greater lung dysfunction, more significant growth-related alterations, and higher mortality rates (Kerem & Cohen-Cymberknoh, 2016).

Socioeconomic status (SES) does not appear to significantly influence treatment of complications in the healthcare setting. Research suggests that pulmonary exacerbations tend to be treated aggressively among individuals with low SES (Kerem & Cohen-Cymberknoh, 2016). However, adherence to maintenance regimens may represent an area of weakness for patients with low SES; in particular, nonadherence with ACT has been identified as a challenge among this population (Oates et al., 2015).

Among individuals of lower SES, cultural, ethnic, and spiritual factors may influence caregivers' compliance with home maintenance regimens for CF, which are complex and time-consuming (Kerem & Cohen-Cymberknoh, 2016). Assessment of barriers to adherence to home maintenance regimens, as well as collaboration with the pediatric patient's caregiver to identify needs related to education and resources, are necessary to promote adherence to maintenance regimens and, in turn, ensure optimal patient health.

day (Mayo Clinic, 2015d), although frequency varies with individual need, and CPT is typically performed either before meals or at least 1.5 hours after meals. The duration of each session is usually 20–40 minutes (Cystic Fibrosis Foundation, n.d.i).

The treatment plan for patients with CF may include pulmonary rehabilitation to improve the quality of life for those who have chronic breathing problems. Activities include exercise training, nutritional counseling, techniques for conserving physical energy, education on the management of lung disease, and breathing strategies (Mayo Clinic, 2015c; NHLBI, 2013b). Increased physical fitness can improve overall health and lung function and increase energy (Cystic Fibrosis Foundation, n.d.j), but pulmonary rehabilitation includes attention to all aspects of wellness and can include psychologic counseling and group support if those will help the individual (Mayo Clinic, 2015d; NHLBI, 2013b). Pulmonary rehabilitation is intended to be used alongside medical therapy (NHLBI, 2013b).

Attention to positive lifestyle choices is essential for individuals with CF. Lifestyle interventions essential in this patient population vary by individual but typically include:

- Eating a healthy, well-balanced diet that is high in both fat and calories and includes a variety of fruits and vegetables as well as whole grains (Johns Hopkins Cystic Fibrosis Center, n.d.c; NHLBI, 2013b)

- Maintaining a high fluid intake and following provider recommendations regarding vitamins, nutritional supplements, and extra fiber or salt (Mayo Clinic, 2015d)

- Participating in regular exercise and fitness-related activities to improve lung function and mood, maintain bone strength, and manage problems such as diabetes and heart disease

- Refraining from smoking and actively avoiding second-hand smoke

- Practicing good hygiene, including proper and frequent hand cleansing (Mayo Clinic, 2015d)

- Coughing into a tissue, disposing of the tissue immediately, and cleansing hands with an alcohol-based gel to avoid spreading infections (Cystic Fibrosis Foundation, n.d.h)

- Seeking emotional support and counseling as needed to help cope with anxiety, stress, or depression related to management of a chronic illness (NHLBI, 2013b)

Lifespan Considerations

Thanks to better screening and treatment options, more and more individuals with CF are living well into their 30s, 40s, and beyond. This trend highlights the need for interventions specific to each stage of the human lifespan, from the prenatal period to adulthood.

Cystic Fibrosis in Infants and Children

Today, genetic testing means that many parents are aware of their child's CF diagnosis before the child is born. Some parents decide to undergo prenatal testing because of a family history of CF or because they are members of a group at elevated risk for the condition. Other parents seek testing because of a prenatal ultrasound finding known as *hyperechoic* or *echogenic bowel*, in which abnormally thick meconium appears to obstruct the fetus's intestinal tract. Although echogenic bowel often resolves itself before birth, about 10% of fetuses with this condition are affected by CF (Johns Hopkins Cystic Fibrosis Center, 2015a). Still other parents discover their child has CF as a result of routine neonatal screening. This screening is not 100% accurate, however, which means that some cases of CF are not detected until a child is anywhere from several weeks to several years old (Johns Hopkins Cystic Fibrosis Center, 2015a). In such cases, the first sign of CF may be that the parents discern a salty taste when kissing their infant's skin (NHLBI, 2013b).

Another early indicator of CF is meconium ileus (MI). As with echogenic bowel, this condition occurs when abnormal meconium blocks the lower digestive tract and prevents the passage of stool. Symptoms of MI are typical of those of bowel obstruction, including vomiting and abdominal distention. Immediate treatment is critical to prevent bowel twisting, perforation, and other complications; enemas are usually effective in removing the blockage, although surgery is sometimes necessary. MI affects roughly 18% of babies with CF, and 98% of full-term infants who are born with MI are ultimately diagnosed with CF (Johns Hopkins Cystic Fibrosis Center, n.d.b).

In addition to MI and other types of bowel obstruction that can develop at any age, children with CF demonstrate a greater risk for *intussusception*, a condition in which a portion of the intestine slides into itself in a telescoping manner (Mayo Clinic, 2015d). Risk of intussusception is highest after age 4. Other digestion-related problems often observed in children with CF include unusually bulky, fatty, and/or smelly stools and constipation. About 20% of children with CF experience rectal prolapse because of the amount of exertion required to pass a bowel movement combined with the stress of frequent coughing. Pancreatic and liver dysfunction are also common because of blockage of the ducts that carry secreted substances from these organs to the intestines. Over time, these blockages lead to the development of diabetes, cirrhosis, and/or portal hypertension in a small percentage of pediatric patients (Children's Hospital of Pittsburgh, 2015).

CF-related digestive issues mean that many children with this disease have a hard time obtaining adequate nutrients from the food they eat. This, in turn, can result in poor weight gain, delayed growth and development, and in some cases, failure to thrive (Johns Hopkins Cystic Fibrosis Center, 2015a). To help counter these problems, parents may be instructed to provide their children with vitamin supplements, extra calories via nutritional supplementation, and pancreatic enzyme replacements. Administration of extra salt may be recommended because many children with CF lose salt in their sweat. For some pediatric patients, tube feedings and/or administration of exogenous insulin may also be required (Cystic Fibrosis Center of North Shore–Long Island Jewish Health System, 2015a).

Respiratory difficulties are the other typical indicator of CF in children. Airway obstruction is a primary concern among pediatric patients because even a tiny amount of mucus can result in significant or complete airway obstruction. Immediate symptoms of airway obstruction include shortness of breath, persistent coughing, wheezing, and exercise intolerance. Possible longer-term effects include recurrent chest, sinus, and bronchial infections; pneumonia; nasal polyps; and clubbing of the fingers and toes due to impaired oxygenation (Children's Hospital of Pittsburgh, 2015).

Vigilant assessment and monitoring of airway patency and respiratory status is required to protect the safety of neonatal and pediatric patients. To prevent respiratory problems, parents are taught to perform postural drainage and percussion (PD&P) and other forms of CPT. In some cases, infants may benefit from other airway clearance techniques, including use of positive expiratory pressure (PEP) masks and assisted autogenic drainage (Cystic Fibrosis Trust, 2013). Vibration can be effected through the use of a mask designed for that purpose, as well as by way of other devices, such as an exhalation device that uses vibrations. In addition, an inflatable vest that uses high-frequency airwaves (high frequency chest wall oscillation, or HFCWO) to mobilize mucus may be used (NHLBI, 2013b). Parents should also encourage their child to engage in regular physical activity to help keep the chest clear and build muscle strength.

Based on multiple long-term studies that evaluated the effectiveness of airway clearance techniques—including postural drainage, PEP, and HFCWO—no superior method was identified (McIlwaine, Son, & Richmond, 2014). However, McIlwaine et al. (2012) reported that PEP was more effective than HFCWO for maintenance of respiratory health among patients with CF. For pediatric patients, selection of the appropriate technique should take patient preference into consideration (Main, 2013).

Staying up to date on childhood immunizations, especially the influenza and pneumococcal vaccines, is critical to preventing further respiratory complications (Children's Hospital of Pittsburgh, 2015). Children over age 6 may also benefit from administration of inhaled hypertonic saline. Note, however, that in patients younger than age 6, administration of inhaled hypertonic saline has been shown to be no more effective than administration of inhaled isotonic saline (Rosenfeld et al., 2012).

Cystic Fibrosis in Adolescents

During adolescence, patients will continue to require CPT and administration of appropriate enzymes, vaccines, and other drugs. Nutritional supplementation also remains necessary for proper growth and development. Because teenagers with CF are at elevated risk for osteoporosis, osteopenia, and broken bones, both weight-bearing exercise and administration of extra calcium and vitamin D are particularly important (Cystic Fibrosis Center of North Shore–Long Island Jewish Health System, 2015b).

Because of delayed growth and development, many adolescents with CF begin puberty 18–24 months later than their peers without CF (Cystic Fibrosis Center of North Shore–Long Island Jewish Health System, 2015b). Some girls, however, do not experience menstruation because of disease-related nutritional deficiencies. Even with delayed onset of puberty, more than 90% of patients with CF achieve normal adult height (Johns Hopkins Cystic Fibrosis Center, n.d.d).

Teenagers with CF are generally able to go to school, work, date, and do nearly everything their peers without CF can do—as long as they engage in appropriate self-care. Thus, around the ages of 12–14, adolescents should be taught about the various ways CF affects their body, as well as specific actions they can take to promote and maintain good health. Appropriate self-care includes not just getting adequate nutrition and sleep, but also scheduling provider appointments, managing daily medication regimens, and making important healthcare decisions. Parents should be encouraged to give their children greater independence and autonomy while ensuring they continue to adhere to their therapeutic plan. Providing adequate emotional and social support is critical, because teenagers with CF are at increased risk for depression, stress, poor self-esteem, and related issues. Adolescents with CF should also be encouraged to think about their future education and career plans, because many of these patients will live well into their adult years (Cystic Fibrosis Center of North Shore–Long Island Jewish Health System, 2015b).

Cystic Fibrosis in Adults

For patients with CF, nutritional supplementation, CPT, and various pharmacologic treatments remain important throughout the adult years. Adulthood also brings several unique concerns. For example, long-term damage to the lungs, pancreas, and liver mean that organ transplantation may be necessary. Surgery may also be performed to promote normal bowel function and proper draining of the sinuses (Mayo Clinic, 2015d). Women with CF frequently have weak pelvic floor muscles, so Kegel exercises are important to help prevent and decrease urinary incontinence (Johns Hopkins Cystic Fibrosis Center, 2015b).

Fertility is an area of concern for an increasing number of adult patients with CF. Women with CF who receive adequate nutrition and have good lung function have fertility rates similar to those of the general population; however, because of blockage or absence of the vas deferens, only about 2–3% of men with CF are fertile (Johns Hopkins Cystic Fibrosis Center, n.d.d). Thus, men with CF are increasingly turning to a technique known as *intracytoplasmic sperm injection (ICSI)* to help their partners conceive. With this technique, the physician inserts a needle into the epididymis to extract sperm. The sperm are then used for in vitro fertilization, with a success rate of about 50% (Johns Hopkins Cystic Fibrosis Center, n.d.c).

Cystic Fibrosis in Pregnant Women

Women with CF are typically able to conceive, although the outcome of their pregnancy depends heavily on their respiratory health. In general, mothers with good lung function are less likely to experience preterm delivery and thus more likely to have healthier babies. Still, overall fetal outcomes are good for mothers with CF. Between 70% and 90% of pregnancies end in live birth, and the rate of spontaneous miscarriage is about the same as in the general population. Many women can deliver naturally, although cesarean section is necessary in up to one third of cases (Goddard & Bourke, 2009), especially when the stress of pushing puts too much strain on the mother's lungs (Cystic Fibrosis Trust, n.d.).

Not surprisingly, women with CF tend to have lower than average weight gain during pregnancy. Therefore, nutritional supplementation is often necessary to promote maternal and fetal well-being. CF also places pregnant women at higher than average risk of gestational diabetes, with up to 33% of pregnant women with CF requiring administration of exogenous insulin (Thorpe-Beeston & Madge, 2016).

For some women, pregnancy necessitates a change in their normal therapeutic regimen for CF. Although most drugs used in the treatment of CF are considered safe for the fetus, others—including certain antibiotics—may need to be discontinued until the postpartum period (Cystic Fibrosis Center of North Shore–Long Island Jewish Health System, 2015c).

NURSING PROCESS

Because of the chronic nature of CF, the nurse plays an essential role in the continuity of care for patients with CF. Thorough assessment at each encounter is necessary to help the patient maintain adequate oxygenation and nutritional status.

Assessment

With each interaction, the nurse should perform a thorough assessment related to oxygenation and nutrition.

- ■ ***Observation and patient interview.*** Observe the patient for difficulty breathing, coughing, mucus expectoration, cyanosis, and overall appearance. Note patient positioning that may indicate difficulty breathing, such as the tripod position. Ask about periods of dyspnea, effort required to breathe, fatigue, changes in sputum production or color, effective use of coughing and huffing, effective use of CPT, current medications and supplements, and nutritional intake. Because chronic illness is a risk factor for depression, ask about any psychosocial problems the patient may be having, including depression and anxiety related to illness or aspects of the treatment regimen. Ask about pain in the chest or abdomen.

- ■ ***Physical examination.*** The physical examination should begin by taking vital signs, including temperature, pulse, respiratory rate, and blood pressure. The patient should also be weighed at every examination to help monitor nutritional status. In addition, the physical examination should include respiratory and gastrointestinal assessments. Respiratory assessments include determining respiratory rate and depth, SpO_2, and FEV_1; using auscultation to listen for grunting, wheezing, crackles, and other abnormal lung sounds; and inspecting the patient for rib retraction, nasal flaring, and clubbing. The nurse may be asked to collect sputum samples to determine the presence of pathogens in the lungs. If the patient complains of chest or abdominal pain, refer him or her for a chest or abdominal x-ray to identify pneumothorax, effusion, or bowel obstruction.

Diagnosis

The age and development of the patient, the presence of infection, and the patient's success at maintaining the strict regimen of therapies required for treating CF will influence the nurse's diagnosis. The following diagnoses may be appropriate for patients with CF:

- ■ *Breathing Pattern, Ineffective*
- ■ *Airway Clearance, Ineffective*
- ■ *Fluid Volume, Deficient*
- ■ *Imbalanced Nutrition: Less than Body Requirements*
- ■ *Activity Intolerance, Risk for*
- ■ *Caregiver Role Strain, Risk for.*

(NANDA-I © 2014)

Planning

The planning process depends on the patient's oxygenation and nutritional status. The planning process should include the patient and family members as appropriate as well as all the healthcare professionals involved in the patient's care. Specific plans for care may include:

- ■ The patient will report that less effort is required to maintain adequate oxygenation.
- ■ The patient will demonstrate proper airway clearance techniques.
- ■ The patient's fluid intake will equal fluid output.
- ■ The patient will demonstrate knowledge of proper nutritional requirements.
- ■ The patient will maintain a healthy weight.
- ■ The patient will report an ability to participate in physical activities.
- ■ The patient's caregiver will report the use of appropriate coping techniques and identify sources of support.

Implementation

Many nursing interventions for patients with CF will focus on helping keep the airways patent by clearing them of mucus and preventing respiratory infections. This is a daily intervention for most patients with CF, and airway clearance techniques are frequently performed multiple times each day. Therefore, the nurse plays a primary role in providing teaching for the patient and the patient's caregiver to follow at home. The nurse must also provide patient teaching related to maintaining adequate nutritional and fluid intake.

Promote Effective Breathing

Patients with CF are at high risk for ineffective breathing patterns related to mucus in the airways. The nurse can promote effective breathing using several methods:

- Teach patients when to call their primary care provider if a pulmonary exacerbation happens at home. Patients should call their provider or the CF center if they experience increased coughing, chest congestion, or sputum production. In addition, a decrease in appetite or weight or an increase in fatigue should prompt patients to call their provider.

- Administer bronchodilators as prescribed before beginning airway clearance techniques or administering inhaled mucolytics. This helps open the airways to allow more medication to penetrate the smaller airways, making airway clearance techniques more effective.

- Teach patients how to use incentive spirometry to promote oxygenation (see **Figure 15–35 》**). Incentive spirometry encourages patients to take slow, deep breaths. Two goals for patients during incentive spirometry are to keep the air flow within a certain range, measured by a floating marker on the side of the spirometer, and to reach a specific lung volume, measured by reaching a stationary goal marker. For patients with CF, incentive spirometry can improve FVC and FEV1, resulting in improved lung function (Sokol et al., 2015). See Skill 11.5 in Volume 3 on using an incentive spirometer.

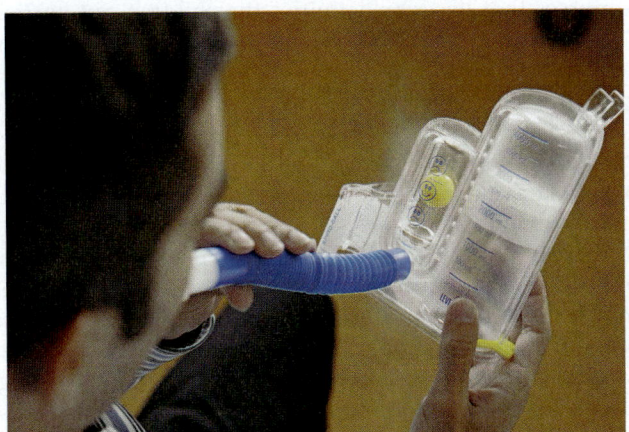

Source: Javier Larrea/age fotostock/Alamy Stock Photo.

Figure 15–35 》 Incentive spirometer.

- Administer pure oxygen to patients as prescribed to promote oxygenation. Continually monitor patients' SpO_2 and report to the healthcare provider any problems that may require changes to the oxygen administration.

SAFETY ALERT Do not administer cough suppressants to patients with CF. Coughing is an essential method of clearing mucus from the airways, and if the cough is suppressed, patients will be at higher risk for airway obstruction due to mucus in the airways.

Promote Airway Clearance

Airway clearance techniques are an essential part of everyday therapy for patients with CF.

- Teach patients about airway clearance techniques such as huffing and coughing.

- Administer mucolytics as prescribed before beginning CPT. This helps loosen sticky secretions so they can more easily be expelled.

- Assist patients with CPT, or teach patients or caregivers how to perform CPT (see the Patient Teaching feature).

- During pulmonary exacerbations, CPT should be administered more frequently than normal. Patients may require CPT up to four times daily for 1 hour per session during severe exacerbations.

Control and Prevent Infection

Because respiratory infections can cause pulmonary exacerbations for patients with CF, the nurse is essential in helping control the spread of infection for patients with CF in the hospital as well as teaching patients and caregivers how to prevent infection in the community.

- Teach the patient how to self-administer inhaled antibiotics, including how to use an inhaler or nebulizer.

- Teach the patient about the importance of receiving vaccinations, including the annual influenza vaccine.

- Teach the patient and caregiver hand hygiene techniques to prevent the spread of infection. This includes teaching about the importance of using alcohol-based hand cleansers after coughing.

- Teach the patient proper respiratory hygiene, including expectorating into a clean tissue and immediately disposing of the tissue; avoiding sharing eating utensils and cups; and properly cleansing any device that enters the mouth, including spirometers, inhalers, and nebulizers.

- Teach the patient to avoid close contact with other individuals with CF. Individuals with CF should stand no closer than 3 feet apart from other individuals with CF to prevent the spread of infectious agents. Drug-resistant and virulent pathogens can pass more easily between two individuals with CF than between an individual with CF and someone without CF.

- Use proper infection control procedures when caring for patients with CF to reduce the risk of transferring healthcare-associated infections.

Patient Teaching

Percussion and Postural Drainage

CPT uses gravity (through postural drainage) and percussion (through clapping or vibration on the chest or back) to loosen mucus in the lungs preparatory to coughing it up. Teach patients to do the following:

- Perform clapping forcefully with the steady beat of a cupped hand and wrist. Properly done, a popping sound should be produced (not a slapping sound), and although forceful, the clapping should not hurt. Another person may need to perform the clapping for hard-to-reach areas or for young children. As an alternative, a special cup designed for this purpose can be used rather than cupped hands.

- Perform vibration by gently shaking the ribs with a flattened hand while holding in a deep breath. Another person may need to do the vibration while the individual concentrates on breathing.

- Use soft supports during postural drainage. Pillows, sofa cushions, cribs with adjustable mattresses or tilts, foam wedges, bean bag chairs, and other soft items can be used to help position the patient comfortably.

- Use devices to aid in percussion therapy, such as an electric chest clapper, also called a mechanical percussor; an inflatable therapy vest; a small handheld vibratory breathing device; or a mask that creates vibrations.

- Perform percussion and postural drainage when the stomach is empty. The ideal time is before a meal. If the patient performs CPT after a meal, wait at least 1.5 hours after eating.

- Use appropriate positions for postural drainage. Postural drainage can be performed while sitting, lying down flat on the back or on either side, and with the head held in different positions.

- Hold the chosen postural position for at least 5 minutes while percussing the chest in the prescribed manner.

- Percuss or vibrate only on the upper ribs and never over the spine, breastbone, stomach, and lower ribs or back. Percussing these areas may cause trauma to the spleen on the left, the liver on the right, or the kidneys in the lower back. Never percuss or vibrate on bare skin.

- Stop CPT if the patient experiences difficulty breathing, vomiting, or severe discomfort such as nausea or pain. The patient should call the primary care provider immediately if these events occur.

Sources: Data from Cystic Fibrosis Foundation. (n.d.i). *Chest physical therapy.* Retrieved from https://www.cff.org/Living-with-CF/Treatments-and-Therapies/Airway-Clearance/Chest-Physical-Therapy/; Mayo Clinic. (2015d). *Cystic fibrosis.* Retrieved from http://www.mayoclinic.org/diseases-conditions/cystic-fibrosis/basics/definition/con-20013731; National Heart, Lung, and Blood Institute (NHLBI). (2013b). *What is cystic fibrosis?* Retrieved from http://www.nhlbi.nih.gov/health/health-topics/topics/cf

Monitor Nutrition Status

In addition to maintaining respiratory health, patients with CF must maintain an adequate nutritional status. This is made more difficult by the inadequate digestion and absorption of nutrients that is common for patients with CF. If patients are unable to maintain adequate nutrition through normal oral consumption of foods, advocate for the patients to receive nutrition through nasogastric or gastronomy tube feedings. Teach patients with feeding tubes (and their caregivers) how to administer feedings each night and how to help care for the feeding equipment. Assess for patient adherence to the nutrition plan, and make referrals or schedule follow-ups with a nutritionist or dietitian as necessary. Provide patient teaching about appropriate nutrition intake (see the Patient Teaching feature). Caloric intake may need to be increased even more than normal during pulmonary exacerbations. Monitor patients for signs of electrolyte or fluid imbalance, especially hyponatremia, hypochloremia, and dehydration.

Encourage Physical Activity

Participating in an exercise program is essential for patients with CF to maintain overall health and wellness. Physical activity helps loosen mucus in airways and strengthen respiratory muscles. This helps patients produce stronger coughs to expel mucus more efficiently. Physical activity also improves nutrition and helps patients with CF maintain body weight, and it improves gastrointestinal motility to promote better digestion. Therefore, nurses should strongly encourage patients with CF to participate in regular physical activity.

- Because physical activity increases sweat production, patients who engage in physical activity are at high risk for hyponatremia and dehydration. Therefore, patients with CF should be encouraged to drink adequate fluids (e.g., sports drinks, tomato juice) and eat salty snacks during exercise even if they do not feel thirsty or hungry.

- Teach patients the signs of dehydration, including headache, weakness, fatigue, dark urine, and vomiting. Patients who are dehydrated should rehydrate immediately with fluids that contain high amounts of salt. As an alternative, fluids with low salt could be consumed in addition to a salty snack.

- Advocate for children with CF to be able to participate in physical activities at school. This may involve providing instructions for the school teachers, administrators, or nurses that describe activities the children can participate in and precautions that need to be taken to prevent dehydration.

Provide Patient and Caregiver Support

When an infant or child is diagnosed with CF, the nurse plays a key role in providing emotional support for parents as they accept the diagnosis and learn about the disease. As the patient with CF ages, the nurse also plays a major role in providing support to the patient as the patient becomes more independent and learns how to manage the disease without help from caregivers. One major way that nurses can provide emotional support is through patient teaching. Understanding the disease process and how to treat the disease will help patients and caregivers to better cope with the disease. Another important intervention is to offer voluntary annual screening with a mental health specialist to assess for and treat depression and anxiety. Individuals

Patient Teaching

Dietary Recommendations

- A high-calorie, high-fat diet is typically recommended for individuals with CF because they may need as much as 50% more daily calories than people without CF.

- A high-fat diet for a person with CF means a diet that is 35–40% fat.

- Individuals with CF must monitor their nutritional status, paying close attention to nutritional indicators such as their body mass index, to prevent malnutrition. Children may need to be shown how to maintain proper nutritional habits.

- Although a high-calorie, high-fat diet is not typically associated with health, it can be healthy for individuals with CF if it is well-rounded and contains a good quantity and variety of fruits, vegetables, and grains.

- Individuals with CF should eat whenever they are hungry and may need to take several meals per day, in addition to snacking as often as once an hour. Eating should be regular even if the individual with CF is not hungry, although eating times should also be flexible to cater to fluctuations in appetite and need.

- To increase caloric intake, add dairy products such as grated cheese, whole milk, half and half, cream, enriched milk, or butter to whatever these can go with. Add fruits, nuts, or brown sugar to cereal or eat these as snacks.

- Increase protein intake with meat, chicken, and fish (breaded or battered to add more calories) and boiled eggs.

- Have easily transportable snacks on hand such as graham crackers, granola bars, protein shakes, muffins, pretzels, chips, or dried fruits.

- Take supplements for fat-soluble vitamins and select minerals.

- Take oral pancreatic enzymes before each meal or snack to aid in digestion and absorption and reduce gas and bloating.

- During the summer or during intense exercise, increase salt intake to replace salt lost in the sweat.

Sources: Data from Cystic Fibrosis Foundation. (n.d.). *Healthy eating.* Retrieved from https://www.cff.org/Living-with-CF/Treatments-and-Therapies/Nutrition/Healthy-Eating/; Johns Hopkins Cystic Fibrosis Center. (2015b). *Treatments.* Retrieved from http://www.hopkinscf.org/what-is-cf/treatments/; Kaneshiro, N. K. (2014). Cystic fibrosis—nutritional considerations. *MedlinePlus.* Retrieved from https://www.nlm.nih.gov/medlineplus/ency/article/002437.htm; Mayo Clinic. (2015c). *Cystic fibrosis.* Retrieved from http://www.mayoclinic.org/diseases-conditions/cystic-fibrosis/basics/definition/con-20013731; National Heart, Lung, and Blood Institute (NHLBI). (2013b). *What is cystic fibrosis?* Retrieved from http://www.nhlbi.nih.gov/health/health-topics/topics/cf.

with CF and their parent caregivers are at an increased risk for depression and anxiety (Cystic Fibrosis Foundation, n.d.k.). Nurses can also provide emotional support by providing information about support groups for both patients and caregivers and information about financial resources. Encourage patients to ask for help when they need it, and provide referrals for counseling as appropriate.

Evaluation

The patient with CF must be continually evaluated to ensure adequate oxygenation and nutrition. Expected outcomes may include:

- The patient successfully expectorated large amounts of mucus to enhance breathing.

- The patient has followed physician orders for prescribed antibiotics.

- The patient demonstrated proper use of a nebulizer.

- The patient's caregiver demonstrated proper techniques to enhance airway clearance.

- The patient has verbalized an understanding of the importance of participating in physical activities.

- The patient has verbalized knowledge of appropriate nutritional habits.

- The patient's caregiver has indicated an interest in joining a support group for parents of children with CF.

The chronic nature of CF means that the patient may frequently not meet expected outcomes, especially during a pulmonary exacerbation. The nurse should adjust treatments as necessary, including recommending increased nutritional intake, increased CPT, and appropriate physical activity as tolerated by the patient. The nurse should also advocate with the physician if any medications need to be altered, including increasing medication dosages or administering oxygen.

Nursing Care Plan

A Patient with Cystic Fibrosis

Matthew Bauer is a 14-year-old boy who was diagnosed with CF shortly after birth. For most of his life, Matthew's CF has been well controlled thanks to a combination of pharmacologic and nonpharmacologic therapies. Although Matthew has experienced moderate delays in physical growth and development typical of individuals with CF, he has always engaged in the same basic activities as other members of his peer group. He is a freshman at a local public high school.

Last week, Matthew's mother called the CF specialist's office to request an appointment as soon as possible. Mrs. Bauer reported that Matthew's respiratory symptoms seemed to be worsening despite his normal course of CPT, supplemental vitamins, Pancreaze, Ventolin, and 7% hypertonic saline. She expressed concern that Matthew might have a respiratory infection or that it might be time to consider adding a CFTR modulator to his regular treatment regimen.

(continued on next page)

Nursing Care Plan *(continued)*

ASSESSMENT

The nurse, Juanita Suarez, greets the Bauers when they arrive at the specialist's office. During the health history, Mrs. Bauer reiterates that Matthew is compliant with his therapeutic regimen. She also mentions how proud she is that Matthew has assumed responsibility for many of his self-care tasks, including drug administration. Mrs. Bauer confirms that her son eats a well-balanced diet high in fat and calories, drinks plenty of water, and engages in regular exercise. In checking Matthew's chart, Nurse Suarez notes that he is up to date on all recommended vaccinations, including the seasonal flu vaccine. Neither Matthew nor Mrs. Bauer recall being exposed to anyone who has a respiratory infection more severe than the common cold.

On physical examination, Nurse Suarez records Matthew's vital signs as follows: T 37°C (98.6°F); P 86 bpm; R 30/min; BP 115/64 mmHg. Nurse Suarez notes that Matthew has lost 10 lb since his last visit; has lung sounds including wheezes and crackles; demonstrates rib retraction, nasal flaring, and other difficulty when breathing; and is coughing up copious amounts of mucus.

Nurse Suarez asks to speak with Matthew alone. After Mrs. Bauer leaves the room, Matthew explains that he is not actually as compliant with his therapeutic regimen as he has led his mother to believe. In reality, he is performing his breathing exercises and using his PEP device only once per day, rather than the recommended two or more times. Matthew also mentions that he forgets to take his vitamin supplements and medications at least 2–3 days per week. When he does remember, he sometimes neglects to follow the doctor's instructions; for example, he often takes his Ventolin after his inhaled hypertonic saline, rather than before. Matthew further states that he tends to eat junk food when his mother's not around, especially during school lunch period.

When Nurse Suarez asks Matthew why he is not following his treatment regimen, he says, "I'm going to die young anyway, so why bother punishing myself with all these stupid therapies? It's not like they make a difference." Matthew also says he does not see the point in doing his schoolwork because he doubts he will ever go to college or have a job, and he is tired of his mother nagging him about his health.

DIAGNOSES

- *Ineffective Airway Clearance* related to increased presence and stasis of respiratory secretions caused by noncompliance with medication and CPT regimen
- *Ineffective Breathing Pattern* related to exacerbation of CF symptoms
- *Imbalanced Nutrition: Less than Body Requirements* related to failure to take supplements as prescribed and maintain adequate dietary intake
- *Ineffective Health Management* related to feelings of powerlessness and desire to rebel against parents
- *Hopelessness* related to perceived inability to alter the course and rapidity of the disease process

(NANDA-I © 2014)

PLANNING

Together Matthew, Mrs. Bauer, and Nurse Suarez agree on the following outcomes:

- The patient will resume taking all medications and supplements on a daily basis, as prescribed by the physician.
- The patient will perform breathing exercises and use his PEP device as instructed at least two times per day.
- The patient will eat three complete and well-balanced meals per day, to be supplemented with healthy snacks as desired.
- The patient will verbalize his concerns to his mother and agree to fully comply with his therapeutic regimen. In return, the patient's mother will grant the patient additional independence and inquire less frequently about his health status, provided there is demonstrable evidence that the patient is in compliance with the therapeutic regimen.
- The patient will verbalize understanding of the fact that proper medical and self-care can extend the length and quality of life for patients with CF.

IMPLEMENTATION

The CF specialist opts against prescribing a CFTR modulator until Matthew resumes his full therapeutic regimen and sees what results it yields. She orders a sputum culture to rule out the possibility of an ongoing respiratory infection. In addition, she recommends that Matthew enroll in a pulmonary rehabilitation program, as well as "jump start" the clearing of his respiratory tract by having his mother percuss his chest at least twice per day for the next 7 days. After speaking with the physician, Nurse Suarez initiates the following interventions:

- Obtains a sputum sample from Matthew and sends it to the lab for culture and sensitivity (C&S).
- Explains that a course of antibiotics may be prescribed at a later date, depending on the results of the C&S. Emphasizes that if an antibiotic is prescribed, it must be taken directly as ordered until the full prescription is completed.
- Reviews instructions for successful chest percussion with Matthew and his mother.
- Demonstrates proper CPT techniques for Matthew, including breathing exercises and use of the PEP device. Observes Matthew perform each of these techniques before leaving the office.
- Instructs Matthew regarding proper dosing and administration of all prescribed medications.

- Suggests strategies for obtaining adequate nutrition, and provides Matthew and his mother with a handout showing a sample diet for teenagers with CF.
- Recommends that Matthew download a smartphone app that can be used by both the patient and his mother; the app reminds Matthew to complete his maintenance therapies and also allows Matthew's mother to confirm his adherence to treatment protocols.
- Encourages Matthew and his mother to engage in open dialogue about their feelings and concerns.
- Offers to speak with the primary care provider to obtain a referral to a mental health professional for general assessment and enhancement of coping skills.
- Teaches Matthew that therapeutic advances have greatly expanded the average lifespan of patients with CF, thus potentially allowing them to pursue higher education, hold a job, and even have a family.
- Refers Matthew to a pulmonary rehabilitation program to foster both physical and psychologic wellness.
- Schedules Matthew to return in 4 weeks for a further evaluation but tells him to call the office if his symptoms worsen or if he sees no meaningful improvement in 1–2 weeks.

Nursing Care Plan (continued)

EVALUATION

At the 4-week evaluation, Matthew has regained 5 of the 10 pounds he lost. Matthew reports improvement of his respiratory symptoms, as well as increased (but still not perfect) compliance with his pharmacologic and nonpharmacologic therapeutic regimens. Matthew also reports that he has been using the recommended cell phone app, which has been helpful with reminding him to follow his treat-ment regimen. Mrs. Bauer indicates that she and Matthew have been getting along better and says her son's attitude has begun to improve. Nurse Suarez notes that Matthew's respirations are easier and less frequent, his lung sounds have decreased, and the sputum that he is expelling seems thinner and less sticky.

CRITICAL THINKING

1. At the initial office visit, what specific teaching should the nurse provide Matthew with regard to medication dosing and administration? Why?

2. In addition to reduced respiratory rate, what other changes (if any) would you expect to observe in Matthew's vital signs at his 4-week evaluation?

3. At the evaluation visit, what nursing interventions might the nurse consider to help Matthew more fully comply with his therapeutic regimen?

REVIEW Cystic Fibrosis

RELATE Link the Concepts and Exemplars

Linking the exemplar of cystic fibrosis with the concept of nutrition:

1. What actions might you suggest to the parents of a pediatric patient with CF to help their child meet his or her daily nutritional requirements?

2. How might inadequate nutritional intake accelerate the course of disease in adult patients with CF?

Linking the exemplar of cystic fibrosis with the concept of development:

3. What strategies might be useful in helping an 8-year-old patient with CF better understand the nature of his or her disease, as well as the required therapies and treatments?

4. Prepare a patient teaching plan for a 14-year-old girl with CF who is beginning to perform age-appropriate self-care tasks.

Linking the exemplar of cystic fibrosis with the concept of family:

5. How might you incorporate elements of family-centered care into your nursing practice when caring for a newborn with CF? Provide specific examples.

6. How might a diagnosis of CF have an impact on the relationship between a child with CF and his or her parents? Between the child and his or her siblings?

READY Go to Volume 3: Clinical Nursing Skills

REFER Go to Pearson MyLab Nursing and eText

- Additional review materials

REFLECT Apply Your Knowledge

Jeremy and Leah Hansen are parents of a 3-month-old boy named Henry, who is their only child. Several weeks ago, the Hansens brought Henry to the pediatrician's office because they were concerned about his persistent coughing, wheezing, and large amounts of respiratory mucus. Although the Hansens suspected Henry merely has a cold, they felt a doctor's appointment was warranted given his age.

After observing Henry's symptoms and noting that his growth was not proceeding along the expected curve, the pediatrician asked the Hansens about Henry's intake and output patterns. Ms. Hansen explained that Henry was breastfed, so she was not sure exactly how much he was consuming. However, she did report that Henry was eating at roughly 3-hour intervals, staying at the breast for approximately 20–30 minutes per feed, and appeared to be latching well, despite his breathing problems. Ms. Hansen also mentioned that Henry typically had at least 8 or 9 bowel movements each day, often accompanied by a great deal of straining and gas. In addition, she reported surprise at how large, bulky, and foul-smelling each bowel movement was, because they had been told that the feces of breast-fed babies were usually liquid and had little to no smell.

On the basis of Henry's symptoms and history, the pediatrician decided to administer a sweat test to screen for CF. After Henry's first and second sweat tests came back positive, a blood sample was taken and sent for genetic testing to confirm the diagnosis of CF. While they wait for genetic confirmation, the Hansens are referred to a pediatric CF specialist so they can learn more about the condition and begin to put together a plan of care.

1. During their first meeting with the specialist and her nursing staff, the Hansens mention that Henry passed the routine CF screen administered by the hospital at the time of his birth. They ask how it is possible for their son to have the disease given the results of this initial screening. How should the nurse reply?

2. Which pharmacologic therapies may be appropriate for Henry, assuming the diagnosis of CF is confirmed via genetic testing? What, if any, drugs are contraindicated?

3. What instruction should the nurse provide to the Hansens with regard to various nonpharmacologic therapies that may benefit their son? In what ways do these therapies differ for pediatric patients as compared to adult patients?

4. The Hansens tell the specialist that they had planned on having more children but are no longer sure whether this is a wise choice. What information can the nurse offer the Hansens regarding the heritability of CF, as well as the potential burden of caring for one or more children with this condition?

Exemplar 15.E
Respiratory Syncytial Virus/Bronchiolitis

Exemplar Learning Outcomes

15.E Analyze RSV/bronchiolitis as it relates to oxygenation.

- Describe the pathophysiology of RSV/bronchiolitis.
- Describe the etiology of RSV/bronchiolitis.
- Summarize the risk factors for RSV/bronchiolitis.
- Identify the clinical manifestations of RSV/bronchiolitis.
- Compare methods for preventing RSV/bronchiolitis.
- Summarize diagnostic tests and therapies used by interprofessional teams in the collaborative care of an individual with RSV/bronchiolitis.
- Differentiate care of patients with RSV/bronchiolitis across the lifespan.
- Apply the nursing process in providing culturally competent care to an individual with RSV/bronchiolitis.

Exemplar Key Terms

Apnea, *1096*
Atelectasis, *1096*
Bronchiolitis, *1096*
Comorbidity, *1097*
Play therapist, *1098*
Respiratory syncytial virus (RSV), *1096*
Rhinorrhea, *1097*

Overview

Respiratory syncytial virus (RSV) is a highly contagious respiratory infection that affects almost all children before 2 years of age. While individuals of any age can contract the disease, it is likely to present as a simple cold or be asymptomatic in children older than 2 years. Only children age 2 years and younger will normally experience the more severe form of the disease. Older adults who are already at risk for impaired oxygenation may also be at risk for acquiring the more severe form of RSV, although they are at lower risk than young children. Because acquired immunity to the virus is weak, individuals may have repeated infections of RSV throughout their lifespan, although the symptoms tend to be less severe with repeated exposure.

Bronchiolitis is a lower respiratory tract illness that occurs when an infecting agent (virus or bacterium) causes inflammation and obstruction of the small airways (the bronchioles). Among children 12 months of age and younger, bronchiolitis is the most common cause of hospital admissions (Ralston et al., 2014). Children with bronchiolitis have an increased risk for wheezing and asthma later in childhood (Kusel et al., 2012).

Pathophysiology and Etiology

RSV is a highly contagious viral infection that is spread by direct physical contact with respiratory secretions or an infected individual. Virus droplets have also been detected in air as many as 22 feet from the infected individual. Bronchiolitis is most often caused by RSV (CDC, 2013a).

Pathophysiology

RSV infects the squamous epithelial cells of the bronchioles and alveoli. Large masses of cells called syncytia develop when infected cells merge with adjacent cells, which subsequently burst and die. The resulting debris clogs the minute airways of the lower respiratory tract, irritating the airway and resulting in edema and mucosal secretions. Partial airway obstruction and bronchospasms follow. As the virus spreads through the airway cells, this cycle repeats. Although the airways are only partially obstructed and do allow air in, mucus and airway swelling prevent the expulsion of air, causing wheezing and crackles in the airways and the manifestation of acute rhinorrhea. Air trapping and hyperinflation occur in some areas; in other areas, **atelectasis** (collapse of one or more portions of the lungs, including at least parts of the alveoli) occurs. Hypoxemia results from the mismatch between the air and the blood reaching the alveoli. Therefore, the patient with RSV is at risk for respiratory failure as the carbon dioxide level increases and the oxygen level decreases. **Apnea**, or the absence of respirations, and pulmonary edema may also occur.

Etiology

RSV is a primary cause of respiratory infections among both children and older adults. By the age of 2, nearly all children in the United States have been infected with RSV. RSV leads to the hospitalization of more than 50,000 children under 5 years of age each year (CDC, 2015b). The rate of hospitalization is three to five times higher for Alaskan Native infants than for other U.S. infants. Factors such as household crowding, increased indoor cohabitation during the winter season, lack of running water, and use of woodstoves all contribute to an increased risk of RSV hospitalization in Native Alaskan infants (Bruden et al., 2015).

RSV infections claim the lives of approximately 14,000 older adults out of more than 170,000 adults infected by the virus each year (CDC, 2015b). In the Western hemisphere, RSV is associated with up to 63% of all acute respiratory infections in children and up to 81% of infections in children who require hospitalization (Bont, Checchia, Fauroux et al., 2016).

Infection with RSV is the most common cause of bronchiolitis, although other potential causes are adenovirus, parainfluenza virus, influenza virus, and human meta pneumovirus. RSV occurs in epidemics from October to March every year. Transmission occurs directly, through contact with respiratory secretions, or indirectly, through contaminated surfaces. The infected child sheds the virus for 3–8 days, and the incubation period is between 2 and 8 days. It is common for reinfection to occur throughout life through siblings or other close family contacts. Infants younger than 24 months with chronic lung disease who have required medical therapy within 6 months of the onset of RSV season are at risk for RSV, as well as infants with significant congenital heart disease and preterm infants under 35 weeks of gestation. RSV is a common cause of lower respiratory tract infections in infants and children (American Academy of Pediatrics [AAP], 2015).

Risk Factors

The risk of infection with RSV is higher for infants and toddlers who are not breastfed or who live in homes with secondary cigarette exposure, attend child care, live in crowded conditions, or are socioeconomically disadvantaged (CDC, 2014b).

Risk of infection is higher when the parent or caregiver smokes. Tobacco smoke increases mucus production and reduces the action of cilia within the airway passages. Exposure to secondhand smoke is thought to alter maturation of the respiratory epithelium.

Infants and toddlers who have a history of prematurity, chronic lung disease, acyanotic congenital heart disease, or reduced immunity are at greater risk for complications from RSV and may require hospitalization. As mentioned, all children under the age of 2 have smaller airways, so they are at risk for serious complications from RSV/bronchiolitis as compared with older children and adults. In adults, high-risk populations include older adults, those with chronic pulmonary disease, and those with congestive heart failure.

Prevention

The best way to prevent RSV is through good hand hygiene and infection control measures. This can be accomplished through frequent hand cleansing with soap and water and avoiding sharing items such as food, cups, or utensils with infected individuals. RSV can survive on hard surfaces (e.g., crib rails, tables) for several hours. Soft surfaces such as tissues also allow for the survival of RSV, though to a lesser extent than hard surfaces (CDC, 2014b).

Infants who are at a high risk for serious RSV infections and associated complications may be given the medication palivizumab (Synagis) (CDC, 2014b). Palivizumab is not effective in the treatment of acute RSV infection, nor is this medication recommended by the American Academy of Pediatrics (AAP) for use in the general prevention of healthcare-associated RSV infection (Committee on Infectious Diseases and Bronchiolitis Guidelines Committee, 2014).

Clinical Manifestations

The typical clinical presentation in otherwise healthy children begins 3–5 days after exposure to the virus. The early signs of a mild infection include **rhinorrhea** (drainage of mucus from the nose), cough, irritability, and a low-grade fever for 1–3 days. Copious mucus secretions occur in the lung fields and nasal passages and are usually green in color. The fever can lead to dehydration.

Signs and symptoms of a more serious infection may occur even in infants and toddlers with no history of **comorbidity** (the presence of one or more additional disease processes). These signs and symptoms, which call for medical care, include increased irritability, excessive coughing, and wheezing. Of even more concern are marked retractions of the ribcage, nasal flaring, rapid respiratory rate, blue skin, listlessness, and, most important, periods without breathing. Call 911 to provide transport to the hospital when a child presents with these symptoms.

Clinical Manifestations and Therapies
RSV/Bronchiolitis

ETIOLOGY	CLINICAL MANIFESTATIONS	CLINICAL THERAPIES
Increased airway secretions	<ul><li>Rhinorrhea</li><li>Cough</li><li>Shortness of breath</li></ul>	Treatment at home may include:<ul><li>Fluids</li><li>Rest</li><li>Antipyretics</li><li>Nasal suctioning using bulb syringe in children too young to clear their own airway.</li></ul>
Partial airway obstruction caused by increased secretions and resulting edema	<ul><li>Wheezing and crackles</li><li>Fever</li><li>Irritability</li><li>Anorexia</li><li>Poor fluid intake</li><li>Tachypnea</li><li>Grunting</li><li>Retractions</li></ul>	Treatment by the primary care provider may include:<ul><li>Increased fluid intake</li><li>Antipyretics</li><li>Airway suctioning to relieve obstructions</li><li>Positioning to optimize oxygenation</li><li>Administration of oxygen via tent or hood.</li></ul>
Hypoxia	<ul><li>Apnea</li><li>Tachypnea</li><li>Marked retractions of the ribcage</li><li>Use of accessory muscles</li><li>Listlessness</li><li>Cyanosis</li><li>Respiratory acidosis</li></ul>	Treatment at the emergency department may include:<ul><li>Hydration with IV or oral fluids to prevent insensible fluid loss</li><li>Humidified oxygen therapy</li><li>Bronchodilators, steroids, and beta-agonists</li><li>Suctioning to remove excess secretions if the child cannot cough or swallow</li><li>Cardiopulmonary monitoring and pulse oximetry</li><li>Intubation and mechanical ventilation.</li></ul>

Collaboration

Newborns and infants who demonstrate signs of respiratory distress while infected with RSV will require hospitalization. The plan of care includes monitoring breathing patterns, maintaining patent airways, promoting adequate fluid and caloric intake, and supporting appropriate developmental behaviors. The respiratory therapist and nurse collaborate to monitor breathing patterns and keep airways clear of secretions. Infants who need endotracheal intubation will be closely cared for by the respiratory therapist.

Rapid breathing rates may require delivery of fluids and nutrition via an IV line. A nutritionist collaborates with the healthcare team to ensure that caloric intake meets the needs of the infant with RSV. A **play therapist** (a therapist educated in recreational activities related to the various age groups of people) is available in larger healthcare facilities to encourage age-appropriate activities for children's play needs.

Diagnostic Tests

Laboratory tests that are used to identify RSV include rapid diagnostic assays, which may be used for analysis of respiratory specimens. At present, most laboratories use antigen detection tests, which may be supplemented with cell culture. Compared with culture, the sensitivity of antigen detection tests generally ranges from 80% to 90%. Real-time polymerase chain reaction (RT-PCR) assays are now commercially available for RSV as well. In comparison to antigen detection, RT-PCR assays are more sensitive (CDC, 2015d). CXRs show hyperinflation, patchy atelectasis, and other signs of inflammation. ABGs may be indicated to assess the effectiveness of gas exchange.

Pharmacologic Therapy

Few medications are prescribed for RSV infection and bronchiolitis. Moreover, certain medications that were previously recommended for use in treating bronchiolitis are no longer recommended.

Although past recommendations for treatment of bronchiolitis included bronchodilators and nebulized epinephrine (Selden & Scarfone, 2009), the AAP currently does not recommend including these medications in the treatment plan (Ralston et al., 2015). While some studies suggest bronchodilators produce temporary benefits, the majority of infants with bronchiolitis do not benefit from bronchodilator administration. In addition, bronchodilators produce undesirable side effects, including tachycardia and tremors (Ralston et al., 2015). While nebulized epinephrine may be of some benefit when used as a rescue treatment for patients with severe bronchiolitis, the AAP does not recommend epinephrine for general use in treating infants and children (Ralston et al., 2015). However, some evidence suggests epinephrine may be useful as a rescue agent for patients whose bronchiolitis is severe (Ralston et al., 2015).

Corticosteroids are not recommended for treatment of bronchiolitis, as these medications demonstrate questionable effectiveness and are associated with potential negative side effects (Ralston et al., 2015). Likewise, antibacterial medications are not indicated for the treatment of bronchiolitis unless the presence of a concurrent bacterial infection has been confirmed or is strongly suspected (Ralston et al., 2015).

Current recommendations for treating bronchiolitis (Ralston et al., 2015) do include nebulized hypertonic saline, which may be useful in promoting mucociliary clearance and increasing the expectoration of respiratory secretions. However, the benefits of nebulized hypertonic saline require repeated treatments. As such, this intervention is recommended for use only in patients who have been admitted to the hospital and not as an acute intervention in emergency settings (Ralston et al., 2015).

Nonpharmacologic Therapy

As no effective therapy for RSV infection and bronchiolitis currently exists, recommended interventions emphasize preventing the spread of infection. To prevent the spread of the virus to other children in the hospital, children with RSV are roomed together, placed on the same unit, or isolated completely. Quarantined children receive humidified oxygen to maintain their pulse oximetry oxygen saturation readings at 90% or greater (Ralston et al., 2015). Which delivery method for the humidified oxygen is used—a hood, face tent, mask, or nasal cannula—is based on the child's response and the degree of humidity and desired concentration of oxygen. Additional supportive care includes oral or IV hydration and facilitation of breathing through nasal suctioning. The critical care unit provides care to children with apnea or respiratory failures; usually these children are intubated and ventilated when they become too fatigued to breathe effectively on their own.

SAFETY ALERT For the first several months of life, infants are obligate nose breathers (Gnagi & Schraff, 2013), meaning the infant's nose is the preferential route for air exchange. In infants, always perform oral suctioning prior to nasal suctioning, as suctioning the infant's nose may stimulate the infant to gasp, leading to aspiration of oral secretions.

Lifespan Considerations

RSV in Adults

RSV infection is usually asymptomatic in individuals over age 2. However, some groups of adults are at higher risk of symptomatic infection, including individuals who work in healthcare or with small children. Typical symptoms in this population correspond to those of upper respiratory tract infection and include rhinorrhea, cough, headache, pharyngitis, fever, and fatigue. In most cases, symptoms resolve within 5 days (CDC, 2015c).

Emerging evidence also suggests that RSV is a significant cause of morbidity and mortality in older adults, as well as in individuals who are immunosuppressed or have underlying medical conditions. Older adults who live in long-term care facilities are particularly at risk, with studies estimating that between 5% and 10% of nursing home residents experience symptomatic infection each year (Falsey et al., 2014). Among older adults and individuals with chronic disease, symptoms of RSV infection tend to be more severe and consistent with those of pneumonia and other lower respiratory tract infections (CDC, 2015d).

For young children, antigen detection tests are generally considered reliable tools for diagnosing RSV. However, among older children and adults, RSV antigen detection tests are less reliable because of the lower viral loads in these individuals' respiratory specimens. Thus, for older children and adults, RT-PCR assays are more useful in the diagnosis of RSV (CDC, 2015d).

As with pediatric patients, there is no specific treatment available for adult adults with RSV. If provided, therapeutic measures focus on maintaining adequate hydration and oxygenation and promoting airway clearance. Limiting the spread of infection is also a major goal. Methods for prevention and care of RSV are currently limited. Researchers hope to develop more effective antiviral therapies and/or an RSV vaccine in the years ahead (Lee et al., 2013).

Bronchiolitis in Adults

Among adults, bronchiolitis is rare and has not been thoroughly studied (King, 2015; Vasudevan et al., 2012). Despite the relative shortage of research, numerous known etiologies are linked to the development of adult bronchiolitis. For example, in addition to infectious causes, inhalation of mineral or organic dust may lead to the development of bronchiolitis in adults. Bronchiolitis is also increasingly observed in veterans who served in Iraq or Afghanistan, most likely due to inhalation of sand, dust, and various substances released by burn pits, sulfur fires, combat smoke, and human waste (Colella, Cook, & Graziani, 2014).

For diagnosis of adult bronchiolitis, high-resolution CT scanning is a more effective diagnostic test than CXR (King, 2015). No specific treatment is available for adult bronchiolitis. Therapies vary depending on the severity of the disease and may include administration of oxygen and/or mechanical ventilation; however, evidence suggests that mechanical ventilation may worsen the condition in the long run. When adult bronchiolitis occurs because of inhalational injuries, the disease is usually progressive and has a poor prognosis. Although some patients stabilize after a period of decline, many experience respiratory failure within months or years (Colella et al., 2014).

NURSING PROCESS

Nursing management focuses on alleviating symptoms and preventing further distress by maintaining airway patency, promoting effective respiratory function, and supporting overall physiologic function and hydration while also reducing anxiety for the child and the family and preparing the family for the rigors of home care. Another focus of care should be to prevent the further spread of RSV and other organisms through the use of airborne and standard precautions.

Assessment

Assessment allows the nurse to determine the severity of symptoms. The nurse should collect assessment data through the health history and physical assessment:

- *Observation and patient interview.* Symptoms and behaviors for the previous 2 weeks, eating habits, fluid intake, any previous breathing problems or illnesses, birth history, and a list of those who provide care for the child other than the parents (e.g., grandparents, child care providers, and babysitters)

- *Physical examination.* Breathing pattern, including rate, rhythm, and quality; inspection and palpation of the chest; use of accessory muscles when breathing, which indicates an increased need for oxygen; and self-posturing.

Most children continue to play despite illness. Increased fatigue levels will interfere with play. Lack of play is an indication of severe illness in children.

Infants who are premature, have cardiac or respiratory disorders, or are immunocompromised have the greatest risk of severe RSV requiring hospital care. The nurse should assess for a more pronounced cough, wheezing, fevers to 102°F, and poor feeding. They should also assess for signs of increased respiratory effort: marked retractions with nasal flaring, rapid respiratory rate, cyanosis, listlessness, and apnea.

SAFETY ALERT In an infant with bronchiolitis, watch for these signs of life-threatening illness: central cyanosis, respiratory rate greater than 70 breaths per minute, listlessness, and apneic episodes. The infant's chest will be hyperinflated, and because air exchange is so diminished, breath sounds will be greatly reduced during auscultation.

Diagnosis

Likely NANDA-I diagnoses for the infant or child with RSV infection include the following:

- *Breathing Pattern, Ineffective*
- *Airway Clearance, Ineffective*
- *Gas Exchange, Impaired*
- *Electrolyte Imbalance, Risk for*
- *Fluid Volume: Imbalanced, Risk for*
- *Imbalanced Nutrition: Less Than Body Requirements*
- *Activity Intolerance.*

(NANDA-I © 2014)

Planning

Care of the infant with RSV infection requires collaboration between the parents and the healthcare team. Goals often include the following:

- The patient's breathing patterns will remain at or return to regular rate, rhythm, and quality for the individual's age group.
- The patient's airways will remain clear of secretions; swelling of mucosal linings will decrease to normal for the individual's age group.
- The patient's fluid intake will meet daily requirements for the individual's age group.
- The patient's daily nutritional needs will be met as required for the individual's age group.
- The pediatric patient will return to play activities as expected for the child's developmental level.

Implementation

The priority of nursing care is maintaining a clear airway and promoting oxygenation. Parents of children requiring hospitalization are normally very anxious and protective.

Including them in providing care and teaching the importance of interventions may help reduce that anxiety and allow them a measure of control in their child's life.

Promote Airway Clearance

The nurse working with a patient who cannot clear the airway effectively should:

- Monitor temperature, pulse, respiration, blood pressure, and pulse oximetry.
- Auscultate lung sounds.
- Encourage oral fluids to maintain thinned pulmonary secretions. Thinned secretions are easier to expectorate than thick, tenacious mucus. IV fluids may be needed for the child with respiratory rates too great to safely feed orally or for the child who is too weak to consume adequate fluid volumes.
- Suction the mouth and nose to maintain a patent airway.
- Provide patient teaching to the parents related to airway clearance and when to return to the primary care provider or the hospital (see the Patient Teaching feature).
- Administer medications as ordered.

Promote Effective Breathing Pattern

The nurse working with a patient with an ineffective breathing pattern should:

- Teach the parents or caregiver how to observe breathing patterns. Observable retractions of the ribcage indicate respiratory distress. If these are observed, the child should be taken to the hospital.
- Continue to monitor breathing pattern, including rate, rhythm, and quality.
- Inspect and palpate chest for use of accessory muscles. Use of accessory muscles may indicate an increased need for oxygen.
- Assess for self-posturing. A tripod stance indicates respiratory distress.
- Administer bronchodilators and oxygen therapy as ordered.

Patient Teaching
Caring for the Child with RSV/Bronchiolitis

Parents of a child with RSV/bronchiolitis require some specific instructions in order to care for their child at home and prevent the need for hospitalization. Teaching points include the following:

- Clearing oral and nasal passages with a bulb syringe.
- When to return the child to the primary care provider or hospital. Signs and symptoms that indicate additional care is required include increasing irritability, wheezing, coughing, and visible retractions of the ribcage.
- When to call 911. Manifestations that require emergency care include rapid respiratory rate, blue coloring of the skin, listlessness, marked retractions with nasal flaring, and apnea.
- Not smoking around infants and children.

Promote Adequate Nutrition

Children with RSV and bronchiolitis are at risk for impaired nutrition and require additional interventions:

- Monitor dietary intake. Adequate calories support healing.
- Offer foods that the patient prefers in small, frequent feedings.
- Encourage parents to continue to feed the child and provide liquids as normal. The child should not be forced to eat. If the child is not eating or drinking as much as normal, he or she may need more frequent feedings.
- Take daily weight measurements, if in hospital setting.

Monitor Fluid Balance

Nursing interventions related to the child's risk for fluid volume deficit due to fever and poor oral intake include the following:

- Teach parents to count diapers per day.
- Encourage oral intake.
- Record intake and output. Weigh each diaper for accurate output.
- Assess for poor skin elasticity, dry mucous membranes, and decreased urinary output.
- Monitor IV fluid rate if IV fluids are ordered.

Reduce Fatigue

Nursing interventions to reduce fatigue associated with activity intolerance include the following:

- Organize care to allow for rest periods.
- Assess the capacity to play. Even children who are ill play. Children who do not exert themselves to play may be experiencing increased fatigue levels, which may indicate the disease is more severe. Follow-up with the primary care provider may be necessary.

Evaluation

When caring for a child with RSV or bronchiolitis, the child must be evaluated after treatment. Successful recovery will result in the following outcomes:

- The patient's breathing patterns returned to a rate, rhythm, and quality that is appropriate for the patient's age.
- The patient's airway remained clear through suctioning and coughing.
- The patient had appropriate fluid, electrolyte, and caloric intake to meet nutritional needs.
- The patient returned to appropriate play based on developmental age.

Most patients will recover from RSV or bronchiolitis over time. The nurse's role is to continually monitor the patient's breathing and nutritional status, provide patient teaching to the patient and parents, and promote play. Exacerbations may require additional interventions and collaborations based on the severity and type of symptoms.

REVIEW Respiratory Syncytial Virus/Bronchiolitis

RELATE Link the Concepts and Exemplars

Linking the exemplar of respiratory syncytial virus/bronchiolitis with the concept of comfort:

1. What can you do to help a 3-month-old baby with RSV infection feel more comfortable?

2. What would you do differently to provide comfort to a 2-year-old with RSV infection?

Linking the exemplar of respiratory syncytial virus/bronchiolitis with the concept of stress and coping:

3. How can you help parents to cope with the fear and anxiety related to hospitalization of their child?

Linking the exemplar of respiratory syncytial virus/bronchiolitis with the concept of infection:

4. What treatment methods are most effective for an infant who is experiencing complications associated with RSV?

5. How can the spread of RSV be reduced?

READY Go to Volume 3: Clinical Nursing Skills

REFER Go to Pearson MyLab Nursing and eText

- Nursing Care Plan: A Patient with RSV
- Additional review materials

REFLECT Apply Your Knowledge

Ryan Riley is 9 months old. He has been sick off and on for the past week with a cold. He is not interested in eating or playing and has

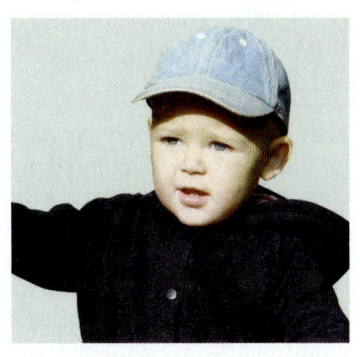

no energy. Ryan's mother, Jessica, leaves him in the care of her boyfriend, Casey Holmes, while she goes to work. Mr. Holmes puts Ryan in his crib and leaves him alone all evening. During the course of the evening, Ryan gets worse and has nothing to drink. When Ms. Riley comes home later that evening, Ryan feels very sick and is having problems breathing. She immediately takes him to the hospital.

At the emergency department, Dr. Gordon asks Ms. Riley how long Ryan has been sick, how many wet diapers he had in the past day, and when he last ate. Ms. Riley tells Dr. Gordon that Ryan has had a cold for a week or so but just got sick today. She admits that she does not know when he last ate or the number of wet diapers he has had. She tells Dr. Gordon that she has been working a lot of hours during the past several days. Dr. Gordon diagnoses Ryan with RSV infection and dehydration.

1. What signs and symptoms are priorities for the nursing assessment?

2. What are likely NANDA-I diagnoses for Ryan?

3. What are the priority nursing interventions for Ryan?

4. What tests or therapies is Dr. Gordon likely to order for Ryan?

» Exemplar 15.F
Sudden Infant Death Syndrome

Exemplar Learning Outcomes

15.F Analyze sudden infant death syndrome (SIDS) as it relates to oxygenation.

- Describe the pathophysiology of SIDS.
- Describe the etiology of SIDS.
- Summarize the risk factors for SIDS.
- Compare methods for preventing SIDS.
- Summarize diagnostic tests and therapies used by interprofessional teams in the collaborative care of a family experiencing SIDS.
- Apply the nursing process in providing culturally competent care for a family experiencing SIDS.

Exemplar Key Terms

Prone, *1102*
Sudden infant death syndrome (SIDS), *1101*
Sudden unexpected infant deaths (SUIDs), *1101*
Supine, *1102*

Overview

Each year in the United States approximately 3500 sudden, unexpected infant deaths occur (AAP, 2016). Among these fatalities, which are collectively referred to as **sudden unexpected infant deaths (SUIDs)**, the most common causes include sudden infant death syndrome (SIDS), unknown causes, and accidental suffocation and strangulation in bed (ASSB). Of the three classifications of SUIDs, SIDS is the most prevalent, comprising approximately half of SUIDs

(CDC, 2015d). Further, SIDS is the leading cause of death among infants between the ages of 1 and 12 months (U.S. National Library of Medicine, 2015).

Sudden infant death syndrome (SIDS) is the sudden death of an apparently healthy infant that remains unexplained after other possible causes have been ruled out through autopsy, death scene investigation, and review of the medical history. At present, SIDS is unpredictable, and it is impossible to prevent in some cases. Because many infants whose lives are claimed by SIDS are found inside their cribs,

SIDS is also sometimes referred to as "crib death" (U.S. National Library of Medicine, 2015).

Pathophysiology and Etiology

Pathophysiology

There is no confirmed causative factor or pathophysiology for SIDS; it can be diagnosed only after a review of the child's clinical history, examination of the scene of death, and an autopsy that fails to find a cause of death. Sudden and unexplained infant deaths are investigated for cause. The CDC tabulates data to determine trends and similarities in relation to infant deaths. Nurses must be aware that data related to infant deaths are gathered and reported for research purposes and must know the procedures for gathering and reporting such data in the clinic or hospital where they work.

Etiology

SIDS is called a syndrome because the autopsy and clinical findings characteristic of most deaths of children from SIDS are varied and do not identify a disease process as the cause of death.

Three factors that occur simultaneously lead to SIDS. First, the infant must have a vulnerability, an abnormality in the brainstem, which controls respiratory and autonomic responses to stressors during sleep. Second, significant stressors that contribute to SIDS must be present, such as prone or side sleeping, face-down sleeping, and bed sharing. When infants are in the prone or side-lying positions, the brainstem abnormality compromises their protective reflexes, such as arousal and head turning, against asphyxia. Third, infants must be in a critical developmental period within the first 6 months of life. Although the question has been raised (Miller et al., 2015), researchers have identified no significant causal relationship between vaccinations and SIDS (CDC, 2015d; McCarthy et al., 2013; Stratton et al., 2003; Venneman et al., 2007).

Risk Factors

In addition to age, infant and maternal risk factors associated with an increased incidence of SIDS include the following (CDC, 2013b, 2015e; U. S. National Library of Medicine, 2015):

- Preterm and low birth weight
- Race: most common in American Indians and Alaska Natives, followed by non-Hispanic Blacks, non-Hispanic Whites, Hispanics, and Asian or Pacific Islanders
- Gender: more common in boys than in girls
- Sleeping in a prone or side-lying position
- Exposure to environmental tobacco smoke or mother who smoked during pregnancy
- Overheating (e.g., overdressing, too many bed covers)
- Bed sharing, especially with people who smoke or are under the influence of alcohol or drugs
- Loose bedding: use of pillows, comforters, quilts, and blankets
- Sleeping on soft surfaces: waterbeds, sofas, pillows, with stuffed toys

Infants placed **prone** (face-down) to sleep are at greatest risk. Infants should always be placed **supine** (on the back). The side-lying position also increases risk. Risk increases if a baby who has consistently been placed supine is placed prone for a nap or nighttime sleep. This often occurs when a caregiver other than a parent cares for the child. Grandparents, child care workers, and healthcare workers should be told to consistently place infants supine.

Maternal smoking during pregnancy and exposure to secondhand smoke during infancy have been correlated with an increased incidence of SIDS. Smoking outside, away from babies, does not decrease the risk because smoky hair and clothes also affect babies' respiratory status. While co-sleeping is associated with an increased risk of SIDS among all infants, the risk for SIDS is even greater among infants who co-sleep with mothers who smoke cigarettes (Zhang & Wang, 2013). Nurses should advise mothers to abstain from smoking during pregnancy, as well as in the postpartum period.

A previous case of SIDS in the family increases the risk for SIDS recurrence. Other risk factors associated with SIDS involve infant sleeping environments. Babies placed on soft sleeping surfaces with loose bedding are at increased risk, as are babies who are overheated or who share a bed with adults or other children. Sleeping with a baby on the couch, a recliner chair, or soft bedding places the baby at risk.

In an effort to educate parents and caregivers about strategies for decreasing infants' risk for SIDS, the Back to Sleep campaign was launched in 1994. This campaign was founded as a partnership between the National Institute of Child Health and Human Development (NICHD), the AAP, the Maternal and Child Health Bureau of the Health Resources and Services Administration, the SIDS Alliance (now known as First Candle), and the Association of SIDS and Infant Mortality Programs (USDHHS, 2015). Now known as the Safe to Sleep campaign, this program offers educational resources and safety guides aimed at reducing the incidence of SIDS.

» **Stay Current:** Visit the Safe to Sleep website at https://www. nichd.nih.gov/sts/Pages/default.aspx.

Prevention

In 2016, the American Academy of Pediatrics published a policy statement related to safe sleep recommendations (AAP, 2016). A brief summary is shown below. Read the full report as listed in the Stay Current feature.

The AAP recommends the following for safe infant sleeping:

- Infants should always be placed on their back for sleeping until 1 year of age. Side sleeping is not safe.
- Breastfeeding is recommended because it is associated with a reduced risk of SIDS.
- Infants should sleep in the same bedroom as their parents, close to the parents' bed, but not in the bed, for at least their first 6 months, and preferably for their first year. They should sleep on a separate surface designed for infants.
- There should be no soft objects in the infant's sleep area— no pillows, soft toys, quilts, comforters, sheepskins, crib bumpers, or loose bedding such as blankets.
- Offer a pacifier at naptime and bedtime, but there is no need to replace it if it falls out.
- Avoid exposure to smoke, alcohol, and illicit drugs during pregnancy and after birth.
- Dress infants appropriately for the environment—avoid overheating, and especially avoid covering the face and head of the infant.

» Stay Current: Read the full report on SIDS from the AAP's Task Force on Sudden Infant Death Syndrome at http://pediatrics.aappublications. org/content/138/5/e20162938

SAFETY ALERT Even when room-sharing without co-sleeping, Carpenter et al. (2013) found that maternal use of cannabis or any illegal drugs increased an infant's risk for SIDS 11 times. To effectively educate parents who smoke about reducing the risks for SIDS, assessment should include tactful exploration of all parental smoking habits, including asking about which substances are being smoked, as well as sensitively exploring the issue of drug use.

Clinical Manifestations

There are no warning signs or early clinical manifestations to indicate that a baby will die of SIDS. Cardiopulmonary arrest is the first and only symptom, and deaths are rarely observed. Parents typically discover the infant dead in the crib after having heard no cries or other disturbances. Clinical evidence of SIDS after death includes frothy, blood-tinged secretions from the mouth and nares and evidence that the infant struggled or changed position.

Collaboration

All members of the healthcare team must work together to promote safety for infants in order to reduce the occurrence of SIDS. All new parents should be taught the importance of safe sleep recommendations for their infants as outlined in the Prevention section. Patients who purchase used older cribs and linens need to be taught how to assess them for safety because guidelines at the time of manufacture were different than those for bedding designed today. Infants at increased risk should be identified as early as possible to initiate precautions.

Modeling Protective Behaviors

Members of the healthcare team are in a perfect position to teach new families to care for their baby. Protective behaviors should be modeled as well as taught. All members of the healthcare team need to place newborns on their backs for sleep. Because many nurses and physicians were educated that the appropriate sleep position for babies was prone, some healthcare providers may find it difficult to alter behaviors from what they learned to the positioning that is now supported by research. Supine positioning for sleeping has been found to be even more protective of SIDS for the premature infant. Neonatal healthcare workers, nursery, and pediatric healthcare personnel need to be conscious of their positioning behaviors, particularly because parents observe positioning behaviors of healthcare workers and then copy those behaviors.

Addressing the Psychosocial Needs of the Family

Even if a family follows all the precautions, sudden infant death may occur. The emergency department confirms the nature of the infant's death. The nurse's role, along with the rest of the interprofessional team, is to be empathetic and support the family in the acute phase of their grief.

The range of services for the support of families experiencing SIDS should include religious support such as baptism services, grief counseling, assistance with funeral arrangements, and, when appropriate, counseling on the cessation of breastfeeding. If the family is religious, a spiritual leader of the family's particular belief system should come to the family's aid at this time. Other healthcare providers who were involved with the infant's care may also provide emotional support to the family, and some healthcare providers even attend the funeral.

Reassure the parents that they are not responsible for the infant's death. It may also be necessary to reassure older children that they are not in danger of SIDS and that they also are not in any way responsible. Counsel the parents about the potential reactions of siblings to help them respond to the needs of their other children. Assist the parents in contacting other family members to mobilize their support.

Evidence-Based Practice

Compliance with Safe to Sleep Recommendations

Problem

Compared to previous recommendations for preventing SIDS, current recommendations are more complex. For example, the Safe to Sleep guidelines address not only infant positioning but also maintaining a safe sleep environment and abstaining from co-sleeping (bed sharing). The increased complexity of the recommendations may lead to decreased parental compliance with current guidelines for the prevention of SIDS (Goodstein, Bell, & Krugman, 2015).

Evidence

The Safe to Sleep recommendations include supine positioning during sleep, using a firm sleep surface, breastfeeding, room sharing without co-sleeping, routine immunizations, and the use of a pacifier. Items that should be avoided include soft bedding, toys, layered clothing, and crib bumpers (USDHHS, 2015). Research suggests that parental adherence to current recommendations for the prevention of SIDS is significantly increased when nurses model the behaviors that are reflective of all current guidelines for preventing SIDS and obtain parental signatures on a document acknowledging receipt of education related to current guidelines (Goodstein et al., 2015).

Implications

Nurses should demonstrate endorsement of all current recommendations for reducing SIDS-related deaths, including modeling and implementing all recommendations as soon as the infant is clinically stable and up to discharge. Nurses working with parents of newborns must provide additional patient teaching and follow-up, as well as ensuring that parents understand the teaching. All parents should receive documented education on safe infant sleep practices, including voluntary acknowledgement forms indicating that education has been provided with regard to the specific current guidelines (Goodstein et al., 2015).

Critical Thinking Application

1. Identify barriers to educating parents and caregivers about current recommendations for preventing sleep-associated deaths.

2. Describe methods for evaluating parental understanding of the current guidelines for prevention of SIDS.

Support groups for those who have experienced the death of a child can help parents, siblings, and other family members express their fears and work through their feelings about the infant's death. Nurses in perinatal or pediatric care as well as social workers may direct the family to such a group. It may also be possible for local hospice organizations to provide support to families grieving the loss of a child. Remember that the parents may also need extra support at a later time with the birth of a subsequent newborn.

Refer to the module on Grief and Loss for more information.

>> **Stay Current:** The First Candle organization at http://www. firstcandle.org can help families locate a support group in their geographic area.

When a Death Occurs

The assessment carried out after the death of an infant in the home is completed by a medical examiner and law enforcement agents. Other potential causes have to be ruled out. Sudden, unexplained infant deaths may be the result of homicide, undiagnosed genetic disorders, accidents, or other cardiopulmonary pathologies. Investigative questions are utilized to establish the cause and manner of the death or to support the investigator's findings in court.

Families who have suddenly lost a baby are interviewed. The purpose of the interview is to determine any cause, clinical or accidental, and to rule out homicide. The CDC stresses balancing investigation with supporting the grieving family. Often, the investigation has the positive effect of demonstrating the family's innocence to friends and neighbors.

The physical address of the location where the death occurred is recorded. An assessment of the scene, including orientation of fixtures and body placement as well as body appearance, is completed. A health history of the infant, including diet, metabolic disorders, birth defects, and maternal pregnancy history, is recorded. A pathologist summarizes the findings from the autopsy and investigation reports to determine the cause of death.

This process can be intimidating to family members, who may resent these intrusions during the time of grief and who may reject findings that they do not understand or with which they do not agree. Collaborative care for these families may include grief counselors, chaplains and religious leaders, nurses (including school nurses working with older children who lose a sibling), and psychotherapists. In particular, the parents' grief will be acute, and they should receive a psychosocial assessment at each healthcare interaction.

NURSING PROCESS

Nursing care is focused on prevention. When caring for the family who lost an infant to SIDS, the priority of care is to support the parents in the grieving process, reduce feelings of guilt, provide referrals to support groups, and help the parents cope with their loss.

Assessment

Nurses who provide care during pregnancy and early infancy should assess for risk for SIDS and not hesitate to ask appropriate questions. They should collect assessment data through the health history and physical assessment:

- **Observation and patient interview.** Does the mother or any other member of the household smoke? How and where does the mother put the child to sleep? What other caregivers put the child to sleep? What are the child's breathing patterns? Will the mother breastfeed or use formula? Has there been a previous death of an infant within the family?
- **Physical examination.** Note respiratory rate and patterns of the infant.

Diagnosis

The following NANDA-I diagnoses are appropriate for the infant at risk for SIDS and immediate family members:

- *Sudden Infant Death Syndrome, Risk for*
- *Knowledge, Deficient*
- *Parenting, Readiness for Enhanced.*

    (NANDA-I © 2014)

The following NANDA-I diagnoses may be appropriate for those families who have just lost a baby to SIDS:

- *Grieving*
- *Family Coping, Compromised*
- *Spiritual Distress, Risk for.*

    (NANDA-I © 2014)

Planning

Nurses collaborate with families to design appropriate outcomes with the goal of decreasing an infant's risk for SIDS. These outcomes may include the following:

- Parents and other adults living in the household will describe appropriate habits to lower the risk for SIDS, including putting the infant on his back to sleep.
- Any adult in the household who smokes will participate in a smoking cessation program.
- Parents who lose a baby to SIDS will participate in grief counseling or a support group if ready and comfortable doing so.

The nurse on duty when the baby is brought to the emergency department should determine if the family has spiritual support and notify the hospital chaplain or offer to call the family's spiritual leader.

Implementation

Patient teaching is an important nursing intervention. By educating parents of newborns on preventive strategies, nurses can continue to reduce the number of SIDS deaths occurring annually.

Reduce Risk for SIDS

Nursing interventions focus on teaching parents how to reduce risks. For nursing interventions related to helping parents and caregivers cope with the profound effects of infant death, see the module on Grief and Loss.

Patient Teaching
SIDS

Preventive measures emphasize teaching parents the principles outlined in the U.S. Department of Health and Human Services (2015) Safe to Sleep campaign, which include the following:

- Ensure that the infant is placed on his or her back (supine position) for any sleep period, including at night and during naps.
- Keep the sleep area free from potential hazards. No pillows, toys, soft objects, or loose bedding should be near the infant.
- Eliminate the use of blankets during sleep time; instead, dress the infant in one-piece sleep clothing to promote warmth and comfort (USDHHS, 2015).

>> **Stay Current:** Visit the Safe to Sleep website at https://www.nichd.nih.gov/sts/Pages/default.aspxto learn more about SIDS prevention.

Evaluation

Expected outcomes for families at risk for an infant dying of SIDS include:

- The infant's parents were able to explain the importance of supine sleeping.
- The infant's parents and family were able to explain the importance of protecting the infant from breathing secondhand cigarette smoke.
- The infant's parents were able to explain the importance of avoiding co-sleeping behaviors.
- The infant's parents were able to explain the importance of avoiding the use of loose clothing or blankets when the infant is sleeping.

Expected outcomes for families who have recently lost an infant to SIDS include:

- The parents have expressed their feelings of grief and loss.
- The parents have started attending a support group for individuals who have lost a child.
- The parents are demonstrating appropriate coping mechanisms for their grief.

REVIEW Sudden Infant Death Syndrome

RELATE Link the Concepts and Exemplars

The parents of an infant who has died of SIDS ask the emergency department nurse for ideas on how they can tell the 2-year-old sibling that the baby has died.

Linking the exemplar of sudden infant death syndrome with the concept of development:

1. What suggestions might the nurse make based on the language developmental of a typical 2-year-old?
2. How would the nurse's suggestions differ if the family asks for ideas for how to tell a 10-year-old sibling what has happened?

Linking the exemplar of sudden infant death syndrome with the concept of family:

3. What resources could you recommend to the family of an infant who died of SIDS in your community?
4. What strategies might you suggest to family members of an infant who died from SIDS who are displaying unhealthy coping methods?

Linking the exemplar of sudden infant death syndrome with the concept of grief and loss:

5. What interventions can the nurse implement to help the family who has lost an infant due to SIDS?

6. How can the nurse help the family respond to a sibling's response to loss?

READY Go to Volume 3: Clinical Nursing Skills

REFER Go to Pearson MyLab Nursing and eText

- Additional review materials

REFLECT Apply Your Knowledge

Susan Miller is a 24-year-old, gravida 2 para 2 woman in the postpartum unit. Her son died at the age of 4 months because of SIDS. Ms. Miller expresses fear that her newborn daughter, Grace, could also die from SIDS. She has heard that if SIDS occurs in a family, the likelihood of recurrence is great.

1. What are possible nursing diagnoses for Ms. Miller? For Grace?
2. Create a teaching plan that includes typical infant care, stressing behaviors that can reduce the risk of SIDS for this mother and child.
3. What coping strategies might you suggest to Ms. Miller to help her reduce her anxiety related to a reoccurrence of SIDS with her new daughter?

References

Abdo, W. F., & Heunks, L. M. (2012). Oxygen-induced hypercapnia in COPD: Myths and facts. *Journal of Critical Care, 16*(5), 323.

Adams, S. G., Hospenthal, A. C., Baillargeon, G. M., Kazis, L. E., Pugh, J. A., & Anzueto, A. (2008). Hispanic patients with COPD did not receive referral to smoking cessation courses as commonly as patients of other ethnicities. *American*

Journal of Respiratory and Critical Care Medicine, 177(5), 473–478.

Alpha-1 Foundation. (n.d.). *Lung disease.* Retrieved from http://www.alpha1.org/Newly-Diagnosed/Learning-about-Alpha-1/Lung-Disease

American Academy of Pediatrics (AAP). (2015). *Respiratory syncytial virus (RSV).* Retrieved from

https://www.healthychildren.org/English/health-issues/conditions/chest-lungs/Pages/Respiratory-Syncytial-Virus-RSV.aspx

American Academy of Pediatrics (AAP). (2016). *SIDS and other sleep-related infant deaths: Updated 2016 recommendations for sale infant sleeping environment.* Retrieved from http://pediatrics.aappublications.org/content/138/5/e20162938

American College of Allergy, Asthma, and Immunology (ACAAI). (n.d.). *Pregnancy and asthma: Overview*. Retrieved from http://acaai.org/asthma/who-has-asthma/pregnancy

American Lung Association (ALA). (n.d.). *Learn about ARDS*. Retrieved from http://www.lung.org/lung-health-and-diseases/lung-disease-lookup/ards/learn-about-ards.html

American Lung Association (ALA). (2013). Acute respiratory distress syndrome (ARDS). *Lung Disease Data: 2012*. Retrieved from http://www.lungusa.org

Austin, M. A., Wills, K. E., Blizzard, L., Walters, E. H., & Wood-Baker, R. (2010). Effect of high flow oxygen on mortality in chronic obstructive pulmonary disease patients in prehospital setting: Randomised controlled trial. *BMJ, 341*, c5462.

Banauch, G. I., Hall, C., Weiden, M., Cohen, H. W., Aldrich, T. K., Christodoulou, V. ... Prezant, D. J. (2006). Pulmonary function after exposure to the World Trade Center collapse in the New York City Fire Department. *American Journal of Respiratory Care and Critical Care Medicine, 174*, 312–319.

Bhatt, J. M. (2013). Treatment of pulmonary exacerbations in cystic fibrosis. *European Respiratory Review, 22*(129), 205–216.

Bhatti, H. M., Alame W., Adams, J., Montego, J. M., Pansare, M. V., Poowuittikal, P., & Secord, E. A. (2015). Texting medication reminders for better control in children and teens: An update. *Journal of Clinical Allergy & Immunology* (Suppl. 135.2), AB 50.

Blaakman, S. W., Cohen, A., Fagnano, M., & Halterman, J. S. (2014). Asthma medication adherence among urban teens: A qualitative analysis of barriers, facilitators and experiences with school-based care. *Journal of Asthma, 51*(5), 522–529.

Bohadana, A., Izbicki, G., & Kraman, S. S. (2014). Fundamentals of lung auscultation. *New England Journal of Medicine, 370*(8), 744–751.

Bont, L., Checchia, P. A., Fauroux, B., Figueras-Aloy, J., Manzoni, P., Paes, B., . . . Carbonell-Estrany, X. (2016). Defining the epidemiology and burden of severe respiratory syncytial virus infection among infants and children in Western countries. *Infectious Diseases and Therapy, 5*(3), 271–298. http://doi.org/10.1007/s40121-016-0123-0

Brashers, V. L. (2010). Alterations in pulmonary function. In K. L. McCance, S. E. Heuther, V. L. Brashers, & N. R. Rote, *Pathophysiology: The biological basis for disease in adults and children* (6th ed., pp. 1266–1304). St. Louis, MO: Mosby Elsevier.

Brock, A. J., & Jablonski, R. A. (2010). Physiology of aging: Impact on critical illness and treatment. In M. D. Foreman, T. T. Fulmer, & K. Milisen (Eds.), *Critical care nursing of older adults* (p. 245). New York, NY: Springer.

Bruden, D. J. T., Singleton, R., Hawk, C. S., Bulkow, L. R., Bentley, S., Anderson, L. J., ... Hennessy, T. W. (2015). Eighteen years of respiratory syncytial virus surveillance. *Pediatric Infectious Disease, 34*(9), 945–950.

Cao, C., Wu, Y., Xu, Z., Lv, D., Zhang, C., Lai, T., ... Shen, H. (2015). The effect of statins on chronic obstructive pulmonary disease exacerbation and mortality: A systematic review and meta-analysis of observational research. *Scientific Reports, 5*, 16461. Retrieved from http://www.nature.com/articles/srep16461

Carpenter, R., McGarvey, C., Mitchell, E. A., Tappin, D. M., Vennemann, M. M., Smuk, M., & Carpenter, J. R. (2013). Bed sharing when parents do not smoke: Is there a risk of SIDS? An individual level analysis of five major case–control studies. *BMJ Open, 3*(5), e002299.

Centers for Disease Control and Prevention (CDC). (2013a). *Bronchiolitis: Causes*. Retrieved from http://www.mayoclinic.org/diseases-conditions/bronchiolitis/basics/causes/con-20019488

Centers for Disease Control and Prevention (CDC). (2013b). *SIDS (sudden infant death syndrome)*. Retrieved from http://www.cdc.gov/sids

Centers for Disease Control and Prevention (CDC). (2014a). *Increase expected in medical care costs for COPD*. Retrieved from http://www.cdc.gov/features/ds-copd-costs/

Centers for Disease Control and Prevention (CDC). (2014b). *Respiratory syncytial virus: Transmission and prevention*. Retrieved from http://www.cdc.gov/rsv/about/transmission.html

Centers for Disease Control and Prevention (CDC). (2014c). *Health effects of secondhand smoke*. Retrieved from http://www.cdc.gov/tobacco/data_statistics/fact_sheets/secondhand_smoke/health_effects/index.htm#children

Centers for Disease Control and Prevention (CDC). (2015a). *Asthma*. Retrieved from http://www.cdc.gov/nchs/fastats/asthma.htm

Centers for Disease Control and Prevention (CDC). (2015b). *Respiratory syncytial virus infection (RSV): Trends and surveillance*. Retrieved from http://www.cdc.gov/rsv/research/us-surveillance.html

Centers for Disease Control and Prevention (CDC). (2015c). *Respiratory syncytial virus infection (RSV): For healthcare professionals*. Retrieved from http://www.cdc.gov/rsv/clinical/

Centers for Disease Control and Prevention (CDC). (2015d). *Sudden infant death syndrome (SIDS)*. Retrieved from http://www.cdc.gov/vaccinesafety/concerns/sids.html

Centers for Disease Control and Prevention (CDC). (2015e). *Sudden unexpected infant death and sudden infant death syndrome*. Retrieved from http://www.cdc.gov/sids/data.htm

Centers for Disease Control and Prevention (CDC). (2016). Respiratory diseases. *Healthy People 2020*. Retrieved from https://www.healthypeople.gov/2020/topics-objectives/topic/respiratory-diseases

Chan, J. K., Charrier, J. G., Kodani, S. D., Vogel, C. F., Kado, S. Y., Anderson, D. S., ... Van Winkle, L. S. (2013). Combustion-derived flame generated ultrafine soot generates reactive oxygen species and activates Nrf2 antioxidants differently in neonatal and adult rat lungs. *Particle and Fibre Toxicology, 10*(34), 1–18.

Cheifetz, I. M. (2011). Pediatric acute respiratory distress syndrome. *Respiratory Care, 56*(10), 1589–1599. doi:10.4187/respcare.01515

Children's Hospital of Pittsburgh. (2015). *Cystic fibrosis*. Retrieved from http://www.chp.edu/our-services/transplant/liver/education/liver-disease-states/cystic-fibrosis

Cohen, J., Tehilla, M., Anbar, R., & Singer, P. (2014). Food for thought: The effects of nutritional support on outcomes in hospitalized elderly patients and the critically ill. *Advances in Critical Care, 2014*, 1–7. doi:10.1155/2014/871328

Colella, C., Cook, C., & Graziani, J. (2014). Constrictive bronchiolitis: Consider this diagnosis when assessing Iraq and Afghan veterans with respiratory symptoms. *Advance for NPs and PAs*. Retrieved from http://nurse-practitioners-and-physician-assistants.advanceweb.com/Features/Articles/Constrictive-Bronchiolitis.aspx

Committee on Infectious Diseases and Bronchiolitis Guidelines Committee. (2014). Updated guidance for palivizumab prophylaxis among infants and young children at increased risk of hospitalization for respiratory syncytial virus infection. *Pediatrics, 134*(2), 415–420.

Cornfield, D. (2013). Acute respiratory distress syndrome in children: Physiology and management. *Current Opinion in Pediatrics, 25*(3), 338–343. doi:10.1097/MOP.0b013e328360bbe7

Criner, G. J., Connett, J. E., Aaron, S. D., Albert, R. K., Bailey, W. C., Casaburi, R., ... Lazarus, S. C. (2014). Simvastatin for the prevention of exacerbations in moderate-to-severe COPD. *New England Journal of Medicine, 370*, 2201–2210.

Cystic Fibrosis Center of North Shore–Long Island Jewish Health System. (2015a). *Living with CF: Newborns and infants*. Retrieved from http://www.cfcareli.com/livingwithcf_infants.php

Cystic Fibrosis Center of North Shore–Long Island Jewish Health System. (2015b). *Living with CF: Tweens and teens*. Retrieved from http://www.cfcareli.com/livingwithcf_tweensteens.php

Cystic Fibrosis Center of North Shore–Long Island Jewish Health System. (2015c). *Living with CF: Adults*. Retrieved from http://www.cfcareli.com/livingwithcf_adults.php

Cystic Fibrosis Foundation. (n.d.a). *About cystic fibrosis*. Retrieved from https://www.cff.org/What-is-CF/About-Cystic-Fibrosis/

Cystic Fibrosis Foundation. (n.d.b). *Carrier testing for CF*. Retrieved from https://www.cff.org/What-is-CF/Testing/Carrier-Testing-for-CF/

Cystic Fibrosis Foundation. (n.d.c). *Diagnosed with cystic fibrosis*. Retrieved from https://www.cff.org/What-is-CF/Diagnosed-with-Cystic-Fibrosis/

Cystic Fibrosis Foundation. (n.d.d). *Airway clearance techniques (ACTs)*. Retrieved from https://www.cff.org/Living-with-CF/Treatments-and-Therapies/Airway-Clearance/Airway-Clearance-Techniques/

Cystic Fibrosis Foundation. (n.d.e). *Antibiotics*. Retrieved from https://www.cff.org/Living-with-CF/Treatments-and-Therapies/Inhaled-Medications/Antibiotics/

Cystic Fibrosis Foundation. (n.d.f). *CFTR modulator basics*. Retrieved from https://www.cff.org/Living-with-CF/Treatments-and-Therapies/CFTR-Modulators/CFTR-Modulator-Basics/

Cystic Fibrosis Foundation. (n.d.g). *Enzymes*. Retrieved from https://www.cff.org/Living-with-CF/Treatments-and-Therapies/Nutrition/Enzymes/

Cystic Fibrosis Foundation. (n.d.h). *Coughing and huffing*. Retrieved from https://www.cff.org/Living-with-CF/Treatments-and-Therapies/Airway-Clearance/Coughing-and-Huffing/

Cystic Fibrosis Foundation. (n.d.i). *Chest physical therapy*. Retrieved from https://www.cff.org/Living-with-CF/Treatments-and-Therapies/Airway-Clearance/Chest-Physical-Therapy/

Cystic Fibrosis Foundation. (n.d.j). *Why fitness matters*. Retrieved from https://www.cff.org/Living-with-CF/Treatments-and-Therapies/Fitness/Why-Fitness-Matters/

Cystic Fibrosis Foundation. (n.d.k). *Anxiety and CF*. Retrieved from https://www.cff.org/Life-With-CF/Daily-Life/Emotional-Wellness/Anxiety-and-CF/

Cystic Fibrosis Trust. (2013). *Factsheet: Physiotherapy treatment for babies and toddlers with cystic fibrosis*. Retrieved from https://www.cysticfibrosis.org.uk/life-with-cystic-fibrosis/cystic-fibrosis-care/staying-active/exercise-and-physiotherapy#whatiscfphysiotherapy

Cystic Fibrosis Trust. (n.d.). *Fertility and pregnancy*. Retrieved from http://cysticfibrosis.org.uk/fertility#na

DeBellis, H. F., & Fetterman, J. W. (2012). Enteral nutrition in the chronic obstructive pulmonary disease (COPD) patient. *Journal of Pharmacy Practice, 25*(6), 583–585.

Duarte, A. G. (2014). ARDS in pregnancy. *Clinical Obstetrics and Gynecology, 57*(4), 862–870.

Falsey, A. R., McElhaney, J. E., Beran, J., van Essen, G. A., Duval, X., Esen, M., … Taylor, S. (2014). Respiratory syncytial virus and other respiratory viral infections in older adults with moderate to severe influenza-like illness. *Journal of Infectious Diseases, 209*(12), 1873–1881. doi:10.1093/infdis/jit839

Federal Interagency Forum on Child and Family Statistics. (2015). *Asthma management plan.* Retrieved from https://www.childstats.gov/americaschildren15/special4.asp

Federal Interagency Forum on Child and Family Statistics. (2016). *America's children in brief: Key national indicators of well-being, 2016.* Retrieved from https://www.childstats.gov/americaschildren

Glaser, M. S., Webber, M. P., Zeig-Owens, R., Weakley, J., Liu, X., Ye, F., … Hall, C. B. (2014). Estimating the time interval between exposure to the World Trade Center disaster and incident diagnoses of obstructive airway disease. *American Journal of Epidemiology, 180*(3), 272–279.

Gloeckl, R., Marinov, B., & Pitta, F. (2013). Practical recommendations for exercise training in patients with COPD. *European Respiratory Review, 22*(128), 178–186.

Gnagi, S. H., & Schraff, S. A. (2013). Nasal obstruction in newborns. *Pediatric Clinics of North America, 60*(4), 903–922.

Goddard, J., & Bourke, S. J. (2009). Review: Cystic fibrosis and pregnancy. *The Obstetrician and Gynaecologist, 11,* 19–24.

Goldwire, M., Lehano, C., & Ostenson, A. (2015). Nicotine replacement therapy in the hospitalized patient. *US Pharmacist, 40*(8), HS20–HS24.

Goodstein, M. H., Bell, T., & Krugman, S. D. (2015). Improving infant sleep safety through a comprehensive hospital-based program. *Clinical Pediatrics, 54*(3), 212–221.

Haack, A., Aragão, G. G., & Novaes, M. R. C. G. (2013). Pathophysiology of cystic fibrosis and drugs used in associated digestive tract diseases. *World Journal of Gastroenterology: WJG, 19*(46), 8552–8561.

Hasan, F. M., Zagarins, S. E., Pischke, K. M., Saiyed, S., Bettencourt, A. M., Beal, L., … McCleary, N. (2014). Hypnotherapy is more effective than nicotine replacement therapy for smoking cessation: Results of a randomized controlled trial. *Complementary Therapies in Medicine, 22*(1), 1–8.

Healthline. (2016). *Lung transplant.* Retrieved from http://www.healthline.com/health/lung-transplant#Overview1

Herdman, T. H. & Kamitsuru, S. (Eds.). *Nursing Diagnoses—Definitions and Classification 2015–2017.* Copyright © 2014, 1994–2014 NANDA International. Used by arrangement with John Wiley & Sons, Inc. Companion website: www.wiley.com/go/nursingdiagnoses

Herfs, M., Hubert, P., Poirrier, A. L., Vandevenne, P., Renoux, V., Habraken, Y., … Delvenne, P. (2012). Proinflammatory cytokines induce bronchial hyperplasia and squamous metaplasia in smokers: Implications for chronic obstructive pulmonary disease therapy. *American Journal of Respiratory Cell and Molecular Biology, 47*(1), 67–79.

Horita, N., Miyazawa, N., Kojima, R., Inoue, M., Ishigatsubo, Y., Ueda, A., & Kaneko, T. (2014). Statins reduce all-cause mortality in chronic obstructive pulmonary disease: A systematic review and meta-analysis of observational studies. *Respiratory Research, 15,* 80.

Ingebrigtsen, T. S., Marott, J. L., Nordestgaard, B. G., Lange, P., Hallas, J., & Vestbo, J. (2015). Statin use and exacerbations in individuals with chronic obstructive pulmonary disease. *Thorax, 70*(1), 33–40.

International Ventilator Users Network (IVUN). (2015). *Home ventilator guide.* Saint Louis, MO: Author. Retrieved from http://www.ventusers.org/edu/index.html

Jerath, R., Crawford, M. W., Barnes, V. A., & Harden, K. (2015). Widespread depolarization during expiration: A source of respiratory drive? *Medical Hypotheses, 84*(1), 31–37.

Johns Hopkins Cystic Fibrosis Center. (n.d.a). *Effects of CF: Sinus.* Retrieved from http://www.hopkinscf.org/what-is-cf/effects-of-cf/sinus/

Johns Hopkins Cystic Fibrosis Center. (n.d.b). *Diagnosis.* Retrieved from http://www.hopkinscf.org/what-is-cf/diagnosis/

Johns Hopkins Cystic Fibrosis Center. (n.d.c). *Treatments.* Retrieved from http://www.hopkinscf.org/what-is-cf/treatments/

Johns Hopkins Cystic Fibrosis Center. (n.d.d). *Effects of CF: Reproduction.* Retrieved from http://www.hopkinscf.org/what-is-cf/effects-of-cf/reproduction/

Johns Hopkins Cystic Fibrosis Center. (2015a). *Diagnosis: presentations: echogenic bowel.* Retrieved from http://www.hopkinscf.org/what-is-cf/diagnosis/presentations/echogenic-bowel/

Johns Hopkins Cystic Fibrosis Center. (2015b). *Treatments.* Retrieved from http://www.hopkinscf.org/what-is-cf/treatments/

Jones, L. D., & Park, J. G. (2014). Noninvasive positive pressure ventilation. *Hospital Medicine Clinics, 3*(2), e149–e161.

Kaneshiro, N. K. (2014). Cystic fibrosis—nutritional considerations. *MedlinePlus.* Retrieved from https://www.nlm.nih.gov/medlineplus/ency/article/002437.htm

Kee, J. L. (2018). *Laboratory and diagnostic tests with nursing implications* (10th ed.). Upper Saddle River, NJ: Pearson Education.

Kerem, E., & Cohen-Cymberknoh, M. (2016). Disparities in cystic fibrosis care and outcome: Socioeconomic status and beyond. *CHEST, 149*(2), 298–300.

Kim, V., Benditt, J. O., Wise, R. A., & Sharafkhaneh, A. (2008). Oxygen therapy in chronic obstructive pulmonary disease. *Proceedings of the American Thoracic Society, 5*(4), 513–518.

King, T. E. (2015). Chronic bronchiolitis in adults. In V. Cottin, J. Codrier, & L. Richeldi (Eds.), *Orphan lung diseases: A clinical guide to rare lung disease* (pp. 17–27). London, England: Springer-Verlag.

Kioumis, I. P., Zarogoulidis, K., Huang, H., Li, Q., Dryllis, G., Pitsiou, G., … Zarogoulidis, P. (2014). Pneumothorax in cystic fibrosis. *Journal of Thoracic Disease, 6*(Suppl. 4), S480–S487. http://doi.org/10.3978/j.issn.2072-1439.2014.09.27

Kravitz, L., & Robergs, R. (2013). *Is it genetic?* Retrieved from http://www.unm.edu/~lkravitz/Article%20folder/genetics.html

Kusel, M. M., Kebadze, T., Johnston, S. L., Holt, P. G., & Sly, P. D. (2012). Febrile respiratory illnesses in infancy and atopy are risk factors for persistent asthma and wheeze. *European Respiratory Journal, 39*(4), 876–882.

Lands, L. C., & Stanojevic, S. (2013). Oral non-steroidal anti-inflammatory drug therapy for lung disease in cystic fibrosis. *Cochrane Database of Systematic Reviews, 6,* CD001505.

Lee, N., Lui, G. C. Y., Wong, K. T., Li, T. C. M., Tse, E. C. M., Chan, J. Y. C., … Chan, P. K. S. (2013). High morbidity and mortality in adults hospitalized for respiratory syncytial virus infections. *Clinical Infectious Diseases, 57*(8), 1069–1077. doi:10.1093/cid/cit471

Little, M., & Sinert, R. (2014). *Asthma in pregnancy.* Retrieved from http://emedicine.medscape.com/article/796274-overview#a11

Lorente, J. A., & Artigas, A. (2012). Acute respiratory failure in the elderly. In B. Guidet (Ed.), *Personnes âgées et reanimation* (pp. 243–244). Paris, France: Springer-Verlag France.

Madappa, T., & Sharma, S. (2015). Pulmonary disease and pregnancy. *Medscape.* Retrieved from http://emedicine.medscape.com/article/303852-overview

Mahmoodpoor, A., & Golzari, S. E. (2015). Noninvasive positive-pressure ventilation. *New England Journal of Medicine, 373*(13), 1279–1279.

Main, E. (2013). What is the best airway clearance technique in cystic fibrosis? *Paediatric Respiratory Reviews, 14S,* 10–12.

Mammen, J. R., Rhee, H., Norton, S. A., & Butz, A. M. (2016). Perceptions and experiences underlying self-management and reporting of symptoms in teens with asthma. *Journal of Asthma* [Epub ahead of print].

Martin, L. J. (2014). Aging changes in the lungs. *MedlinePlus.* Retrieved from https://www.nlm.nih.gov/medlineplus/ency/article/004011.htm

Mayo Clinic. (2014). *Bronchitis: Symptoms.* Retrieved from http://www.mayoclinic.org/diseases-conditions/bronchitis/basics/symptoms/con-20014956

Mayo Clinic. (2015a). *Atelectasis: Causes.* Retrieved from http://www.mayoclinic.org/diseases-conditions/atelectasis/basics/causes/con-20034847

Mayo Clinic. (2015b). *COPD: Causes.* Retrieved from http://www.mayoclinic.org/diseases-conditions/copd/basics/causes/con-20032017

Mayo Clinic. (2015c). *COPD: Risk factors.* Retrieved from http://www.mayoclinic.org/diseases-conditions/copd/basics/risk-factors/con-20032017

Mayo Clinic. (2015d). *Cystic fibrosis.* Retrieved from http://www.mayoclinic.org/diseases-conditions/cystic-fibrosis/basics/definition/con-20013731

Mayo Clinic. (2015e). *Chorionic villus sampling.* Retrieved from http://www.mayoclinic.org/tests-procedures/chorionic-villus-sampling/basics/definition/prc-20013566

McCarthy, N. L., Weintraub, E., Vellozzi, C., Duffy, J., Gee, J., Donahue, J. G., … DeStefano, F. (2013). Mortality rates and cause-of-death patterns in a vaccinated population. *American Journal of Preventive Medicine, 45*(1), 91–97.

McIlwaine, M., Agnew, J. L., Alarie, N., Lands, L., Ratjen, F., Milner, R., & Davidson, A. G. F. (2012). Canadian national airway clearance study: Positive expiratory pressure mask versus high frequency chest wall oscillation. *Journal of Cystic Fibrosis, 11*(Suppl. 1), S23.

McIlwaine, M. P., Son, N. M. L., & Richmond, M. L. (2014). Physiotherapy and cystic fibrosis: What is the evidence base? *Current Opinion in Pulmonary Medicine, 20*(6), 613–617.

Medscape. (2015). *Tiotropium (spiriva respimat) gets asthma indication in US.* Retrieved from http://www.medscape.com/viewarticle/851102

Melani, A. S. (2013). Management of asthma in the elderly patient. *Clinical Interventions in Aging, 8,* 913–922.

Miller, E. R., Shimabukuro, T. T., Hibbs, B. F., Moro, P. L., Broder, K. R., & Vellozzi, C. (2015). Vaccine safety resources for nurses—The CDC supports nurses in promoting vaccination. *American Journal of Nursing, 115*(8), 55–58.

Mogayzel, P. J. Jr., Naureckas, E. T., Robinson, K. A., Mueller, G., Hadjiliadis, D., Hoag, J. B. … Pulmonary Clinical Practice Guidelines Committee.

(2013). Cystic fibrosis pulmonary guidelines: Chronic medications for maintenance of lung health. *American Journal of Respiratory and Critical Care Medicine, 187*(7), 680–689.

Murphy, V. E., & Schatz, M. (2014). Asthma in pregnancy: A hit for two. *European Respiratory Review, 23*(131), 64–68.

National Heart, Lung, and Blood Institute (NHLBI). (2012a). *What is ARDS?* Retrieved from http://www.nhlbi.nih.gov/health/health-topics/topics/ards

National Heart, Lung, and Blood Institute (NHLBI). (2012b). *Asthma care quick reference.* Retrieved from https://www.nhlbi.nih.gov/files/docs/guidelines/asthma_qrg.pdf

National Heart, Lung, and Blood Institute (NHLBI). (2013a). *What is COPD?* Retrieved from http://www.nhlbi.nih.gov/health/health-topics/topics/copd

National Heart, Lung, and Blood Institute (NHLBI). (2013b). *What is cystic fibrosis?* Retrieved from http://www.nhlbi.nih.gov/health/health-topics/topics/cf

National Heart, Lung, and Blood Institute (NHLBI). (2014). *How is asthma treated and controlled?* Retrieved from http://www.nhlbi.nih.gov/health/health-topics/topics/asthma/treatment

National Institutes of Health. (2012). *Acute respiratory distress syndrome (ARDS).* Retrieved fromhttp://www.nhlbi.nih.gov/health/health-topics/topics/ards

Oates, G. R., Stepanikova, I., Gamble, S., Gutierrez, H. H., & Harris, W. T. (2015). Adherence to airway clearance therapy in pediatric cystic fibrosis: Socioeconomic factors and respiratory outcomes. *Pediatric Pulmonology, 50*(12), 1244–1252.

Osborn, K. S., Wraa, C. E., Watson, A. B., & Holleran, R. (2014). *Medical-surgical nursing: Preparation for practice* (2nd ed.). Upper Saddle River, NJ: Pearson.

Pediatric Acute Lung Injury Consensus Conference Group (PALLIC). (2015). Pediatric acute respiratory distress syndrome: Consensus recommendations from the pediatric acute lung injury consensus conference. *Pediatric Critical Care Medicine, 16*(5), 428–439.

Pettit, R. S., & Fellner, C. (2014). CFTR modulators for the treatment of cystic fibrosis. *Pharmacy & Therapeutics, 39*(7), 500–511.

Philip, J., & Sharma, S. K. (2011). Respiratory disorders in pregnancy. In D. R. Gambling, M. J. Douglas, & R. S. F. McKay (Eds.), *Obstetric anesthesia and uncommon disorders* (pp. 75–77). Cambridge, England: Cambridge University Press.

Radbel, J., Mehta, K., Shah, N., Soni, R., & Singh, J. (2014). The sharp decline in ARDS mortality: Analysis of 856,293 national inpatient sample admissions. *Chest, 146*(4_MeetingAbstracts), 210A–210A.

Ralston, S. L., Lieberthal, A. S., Meissner, H. C., Alverson, B. K., Baley, J. E., Gadomski, A. M., ... Hernandez-Cancio, S. (2014). Clinical practice guideline: The diagnosis, management, and prevention of bronchiolitis. *Pediatrics, 134*(5), e1474–e1502.

Ralston, S. L., Lieberthal, A. S., Meissner, H. C., Alverson, B. K., Baley, J. E., Gadomski, A. M., ... Hernandez-Cancio, S. (2015). Clinical practice guideline: The diagnosis, management, and prevention of bronchiolitis. *Pediatrics, 134*(5), e1474–e1502.

Rappaport, H., & Bonthapally, V. (2012). The direct expenditures and indirect costs associated with

treating asthma in the United States. *Journal of Allergy & Therapy, 3*(2), 1–8.

Rhee, H., McQuillan, B. E., & Belyea, M. J. (2012). Evaluation of a peer-led asthma self-management program and benefits of the program for adolescent peer leaders. *Respiratory Care, 57*(12), 2082–2089. doi:10.4187/respcare.01488

Rhee, H., Pessis-Katz, I., & Xing, J. (2012). Cost benefits of a peer-led asthma self-management program for adolescents. *Journal of Asthma, 49*(6), 303-613. doi:10.3109/02770903.2012.694540

Rodríguez-Esquivel, D., Cooper, T. V., Blow, J., & Resor, M. (2009). Characteristics associated with smoking in a Hispanic sample. *Addictive Behaviors, 34,* 593–598.

Rodríguez-Esquivel, D., Webb-Hooper, M., Baker, E. A., & McNutt, M. D. (2015). Culturally specific versus standard smoking cessation messages targeting Hispanics: An experiment. *Psychology of Addictive Behaviors, 29*(2), 283–289.

Rosenfeld, M., Ratjen, F., Brumback, L., Daniel, S., Rowbotham, R., McNamara, S., ... ISIS Study Group. (2012). Inhaled hypertonic saline in infants and children younger than 6 years with cystic fibrosis: The ISIS randomized controlled trial. *Journal of the American Medical Association, 307*(21), 2269–2277.

Rotta, A. T., Piva, J. P., Andreolio, C., Brunow de Carvalho, W., & Garcia, P. C. R. (2015). Progress and perspectives in pediatric acute respiratory distress syndrome. *Revista Brasileira de Terapia Intensiva, 27*(3), 266–273. doi:10.5935/0103-507X.20150035

Samanta, S., Samanta, S., Wig, J., & Baronia, A. K. (2014). How safe is the prone position in acute respiratory distress syndrome at late pregnancy? *American Journal of Emergency Medicine, 32*(6). Retrieved from https://www.ncbi.nlm.nih.gov/pubmed/24412021

Sarkar, M., Madabhavi, I., Niranjan, N., & Dogra, M. (2015). Auscultation of the respiratory system. *Annals of Thoracic Medicine, 10*(3), 158.

Selden, J. A., & Scarfone, R. J. (2009). Bronchiolitis: An evidence-based approach to management. *Clinical Pediatric Emergency Medicine, 10,* 75–81.

Seeleman, C., Stronks, K., van Aalderen, W., & Bot, M. L. E. (2012). Deficiencies in culturally competent asthma care for ethnic minority children: A qualitative assessment among care providers. *BMC Pediatrics, 12*(1), 47.

Sharma, G. D. (2015). Cystic fibrosis treatment and management. *Medscape.* Retrieved from http://emedicine.medscape.com/article/1001602-treatment#d1

Smith, C., & Goldman, R. (2012). Nebulizers versus pressurized metered-dose inhalers in preschool children with wheezing. *Canadian Family Physician, 58*(5), 528–530.

Society of Critical Care Anesthesiologists (SOCCA). (2013). *Residents' guide to learning in the intensive care unit* (4th ed.). Park Ridge, IL: Author.

Sokol, G., Vilozni, D., Hakimi, R., Lavie, M., Sarouk, I., Bar, B. E. ... Efrati, O. (2015). The short-term effect of breathing tasks via an incentive spirometer on lung function compared with autogenic drainage in subjects with cystic fibrosis. *Respiratory Care, 60*(12), 1819–1825.

Sommers, M. S. (2011). Color awareness: A must for patient assessment. *American Nurse Today, 6*(1), 6.

Stratton, K., Almario, D. A., Wizemann, T. M., & McCormick, M. C. (2003). *Immunization safety review: Vaccinations and sudden unexpected death in infancy.* Washington, DC: The National Academies Press.

Tahiri, M., Mottillo, S., Joseph, L., Pilote, L., & Eisenberg, M. J. (2012). Alternative smoking cessation aids: A meta-analysis of randomized controlled trials. *The American Journal of Medicine, 125*(6), 576–584.

Thorpe-Beeston, J. G., & Madge, S. (2016). Sexual and reproductive issues. In A. Bush, D. Bilton, & M. Hodson (Eds.), *Hodson and Geddes' cystic fibrosis* (4th ed., pp. 386–396). Boca Raton, FL: CRC Press/Taylor & Francis.

University of Maryland Medical Center (UMMC). (2012). *Chronic obstructive pulmonary disease.* Retrieved from https://umm.edu/health/medical/reports/articles/chronic-obstructive-pulmonary-disease

U.S. Department of Health and Human Resources (USDHHS). (2015). *Safe to sleep—Public education campaign.* Retrieved from https://www.nichd.nih.gov/sts/Pages/default.aspx

U.S. National Library of Medicine. (2012). *Cystic fibrosis: What is cystic fibrosis?* Retrieved from http://ghr.nlm.nih.gov/condition/cystic-fibrosis

U.S. National Library of Medicine. (2015). *Sudden infant death syndrome.* Retrieved from https://www.nlm.nih.gov/medlineplus/suddeninfantdeathsyndrome.html

van Aalderen, W., Garcia-Marcos, L., Gappa, M., Lenney, W., Pedersen, S., Dekhuijzen, R., & Price, D. (2015). How to match the optimal currently available inhaler device to an individual child with asthma or recurrent wheeze. *Primary Care Respiratory Medicine, 25.* doi:10.1038/npjpcrm.2014.88

Vasudevan, V. P., Suryanarayanan, M., Shahzad, S., & Megjhani, M. (2012). Mycoplasma pneumoniae bronchiolitis mimicking asthma in an adult. *Respiratory Care, 57*(11), 1974–1976.

Vennemann, M. M., Butterfass-Bahloul, T., Jorch, G., Brinkmann, B., Findeisen, M., Sauerland, C., ... Mitchell, E. A. (2007). Sudden infant death syndrome: No increased risk after immunisation. *Vaccine, 25*(2), 336–340.

Ware, L. B., Zhao, Z., Koyama, T., May, A. K., Matthay, M. A., Lurmann, F. W., ... Calfee, C. S. (2015). Long-term ozone exposure increases the risk of developing the acute respiratory distress syndrome. *American Journal of Respiratory and Critical Care Medicine* [Advance online publication]. doi:10.1164/rccm.201507-1418OC

Wisnivesky, J. P., Teitelbaum, S. L., Todd, A. C., Boffetta, P., Crane, M., Crowley, L., ... Landrigan, P. J. (2011). Persistence of multiple illnesses in World Trade Center rescue and recovery workers: A cohort study. *The Lancet, 378*(9794), 888–897.

Yáñez, A., Cho, S., Soriano, J., Rosenwasser, L., Rodrigo, G., Rabe, K., ...WAO Special Committee on Asthma. (2014). Asthma in the elderly: What we know and what we have yet to know. *WAO Journal, 7*(16). Retrieved from http://www.waojournal.org/content/7/1/8

Zhang, K., & Wang, X. (2013). Maternal smoking and increased risk of sudden infant death syndrome: A meta-analysis. *Legal Medicine, 15*(3), 115–121.

Module 16
Perfusion

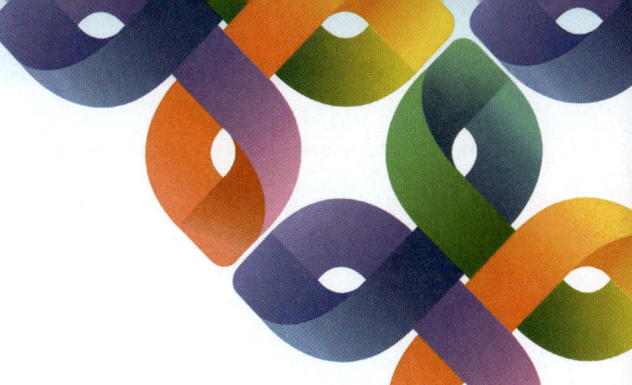

Module Outline and Learning Outcomes

The Concept of Perfusion

Normal Perfusion

16.1 Analyze the physiology of perfusion in the body.

Alterations to Perfusion

16.2 Differentiate alterations in perfusion.

Concepts Related to Perfusion

16.3 Outline the relationship between perfusion and other concepts.

Health Promotion

16.4 Explain the promotion of healthy perfusion.

Nursing Assessment

16.5 Differentiate common assessment procedures and tests used to examine perfusion.

Independent Interventions

16.6 Analyze independent interventions nurses can implement for patients with alterations in perfusion.

Collaborative Therapies

16.7 Summarize collaborative therapies used by inter-professional teams for patients with alterations in perfusion.

Lifespan Considerations

16.8 Differentiate considerations related to the assessment and care of patients with alterations in perfusion throughout the lifespan.

Perfusion Exemplars

Exemplar 16.A Cardiomyopathy

16.A Analyze cardiomyopathy as it relates to perfusion.

Exemplar 16.B Congenital Heart Defects

16.B Analyze congenital heart defects as they relate to perfusion.

Exemplar 16.C Coronary Artery Disease

16.C Analyze coronary artery disease (CAD) as it relates to perfusion.

Exemplar 16.D Deep Venous Thrombosis

16.D Analyze deep venous thrombosis (DVT) as it relates to perfusion.

Exemplar 16.E Disseminated Intravascular Coagulation

16.E Analyze disseminated intravascular coagulation (DIC) as it relates to perfusion.

Exemplar 16.F Heart Failure

16.F Analyze heart failure as it relates to perfusion.

Exemplar 16.G Hypertension

16.G Analyze hypertension as it relates to perfusion.

Exemplar 16.H Hypertensive Disorders of Pregnancy

16.H Analyze hypertensive disorders of pregnancy as they relate to perfusion.

Exemplar 16.I Life-Threatening Dysrhythmias

16.I Analyze life-threatening dysrhythmias as they relate to perfusion.

Exemplar 16.J Peripheral Vascular Disease

16.J Analyze peripheral vascular disease (PVD) as it relates to perfusion.

Exemplar 16.K Pulmonary Embolism

16.K Analyze pulmonary embolism (PE) as it relates to perfusion.

Exemplar 16.L Shock

16.L Analyze shock as it relates to perfusion.

Exemplar 16.M Stroke

16.M Analyze stroke as it relates to perfusion.

» The Concept of Perfusion

Concept Key Terms

The essential function of the cardiovascular and pulmonary systems is to provide a continuous supply of oxygenated blood to every cell in the body. The physiologic process of perfusion requires the heart to transport and distribute blood throughout the body. Changes in perfusion affect all human functions, including self-care, comfort, mobility, fluid volume status, respiration, and tissue integrity. Impaired perfusion may also affect self-concept and role performance.

Normal Perfusion

The heart is a hollow, cone-shaped organ, approximately the size of an adult's fist and weighing less than 1 lb. It is located in the mediastinum of the thoracic cavity, between the vertebral column and the sternum, and is flanked laterally by the lungs. Two thirds of the heart mass lies to the left of the sternum; the upper base lies beneath the second rib, and the pointed apex is approximate with the fifth intercostal space (ICS), midpoint to the clavicle (see **Figure 16–1** »).

The Pericardium

The heart is covered by the **pericardium**, a double layer of fibroserous membrane (see **Figure 16–2** »). The pericardium encases the heart and anchors it to surrounding structures, forming the pericardial sac. The snug fit of the pericardium prevents the heart from overfilling with blood. The pericardium consists of two layers—the visceral and parietal layers.

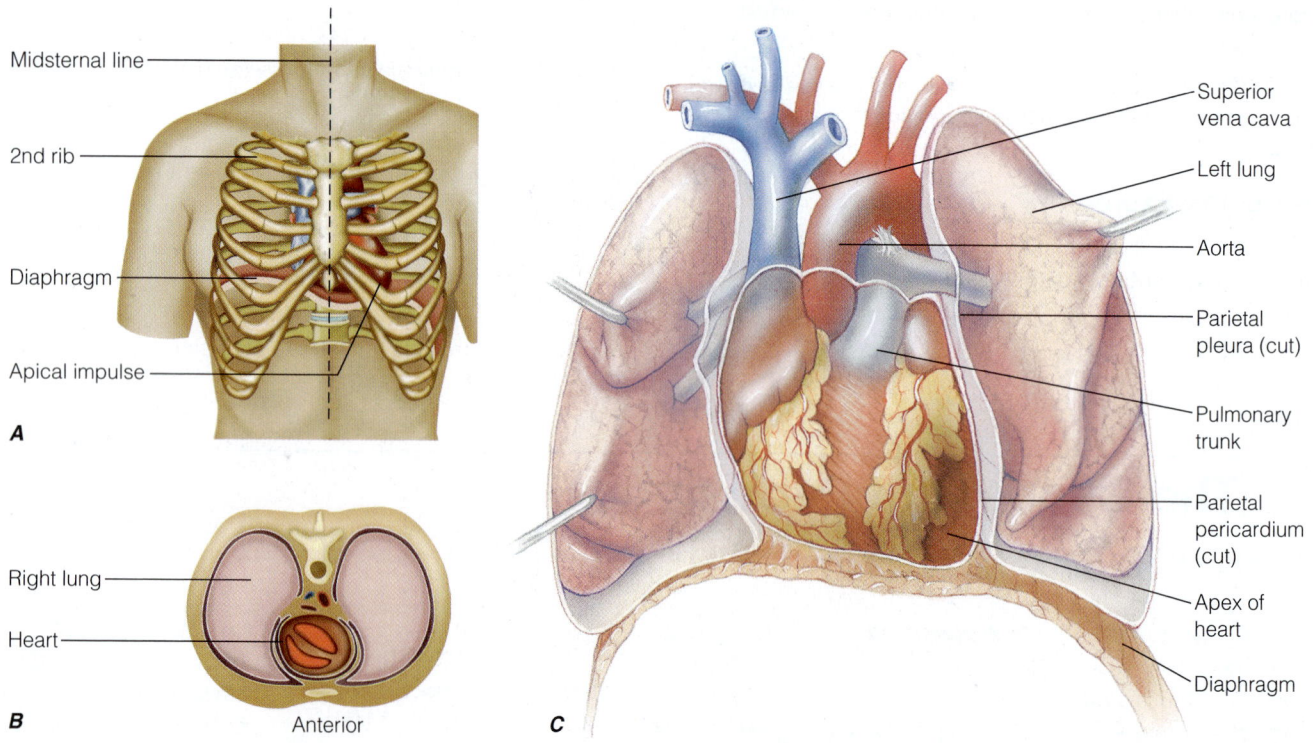

Figure 16–1 » Location of the heart in the mediastinum of the thorax. **A,** Relationship of the heart to the sternum, ribs, and diaphragm. **B,** Cross-sectional view showing relative position of the heart in the thorax. **C,** Relationship of the heart and great vessels to the lungs.

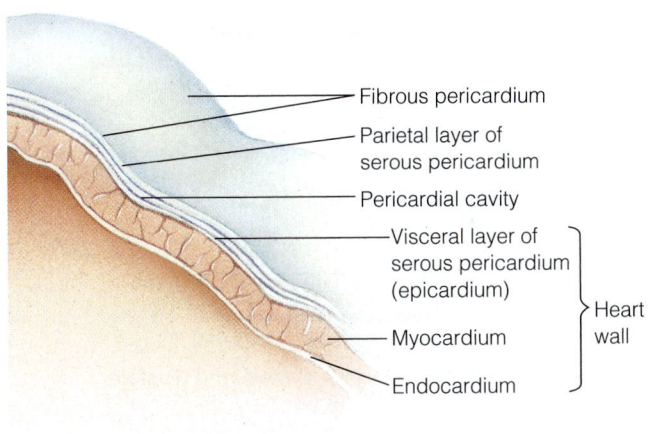

Fibrous pericardium
Parietal layer of serous pericardium
Pericardial cavity
Visceral layer of serous pericardium (epicardium)
Myocardium
Endocardium
} Heart wall

Figure 16–2 》 Coverings and layers of the heart.

The small space between these layers is called the pericardial cavity. A serous lubricating fluid produced in this space cushions the heart as it contracts.

Layers of the Heart Wall

The heart wall consists of three layers of tissue: the epicardium, the myocardium, and the endocardium (see Figure 16–2). The epicardium covers the entire heart and great vessels, then folds over to form the parietal layer lining the pericardium. The myocardium, the middle layer of the heart wall, consists of specialized cardiac muscle cells (myofibrils). These cells provide the bulk of the contractile heart muscle.

The endocardium, which is the innermost layer, is a thin membrane composed of three layers; the innermost layer is made up of smooth endothelial cells that line the inside of the heart's chambers and great vessels.

Chambers and Valves of the Heart

The heart has four hollow chambers: two atria (left and right) and two ventricles (left and right). They are separated longitudinally by the interventricular septum (see **Figure 16–3 》**). The right atrium receives deoxygenated blood from the body. Specifically, the superior vena cava returns blood from the head, neck, arm, and chest; the inferior vena cava returns blood from the lower body; and the coronary sinus drains blood from the heart. The deoxygenated blood then travels to the right ventricle, from which it is pumped through the pulmonary artery to the pulmonary capillary bed for oxygenation. Oxygenated blood then travels through the pulmonary veins to the left atrium and then to the left ventricle. The blood is then pumped out of the left ventricle through the aorta, at which point it enters the arterial circulation.

Each chamber of the heart is separated by a valve that allows unidirectional blood flow to the next chamber or great vessel (see Figure 16–3). The atria are separated from the ventricles by the two atrioventricular (AV) valves: the tricuspid valve on the right side, and the bicuspid (or mitral) valve on the left. The chordae tendineae anchor the flaps of the valves to the papillary muscles. These structures control the movement of the AV valves to prevent backflow of blood. The ventricles are connected to their great vessels by the semilunar valves. On the right, the pulmonary

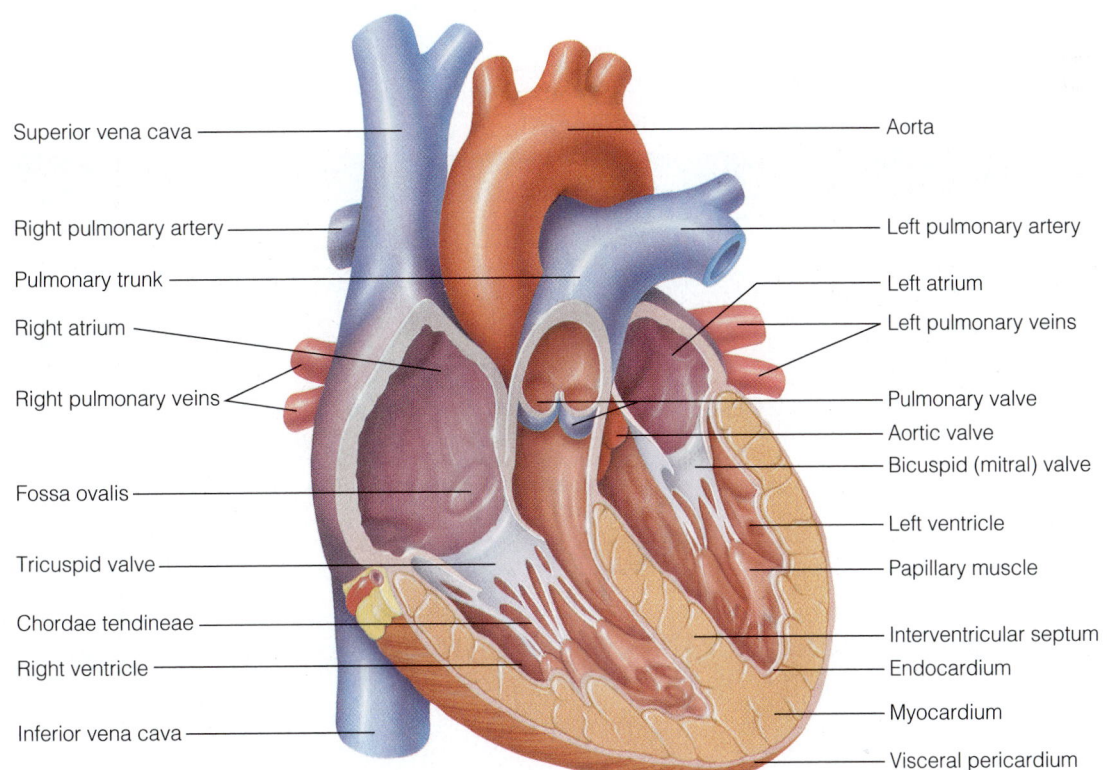

Superior vena cava
Right pulmonary artery
Pulmonary trunk
Right atrium
Right pulmonary veins
Fossa ovalis
Tricuspid valve
Chordae tendineae
Right ventricle
Inferior vena cava

Aorta
Left pulmonary artery
Left atrium
Left pulmonary veins
Pulmonary valve
Aortic valve
Bicuspid (mitral) valve
Left ventricle
Papillary muscle
Interventricular septum
Endocardium
Myocardium
Visceral pericardium

Figure 16–3 》 The internal anatomy of the heart, frontal section.

(pulmonic) valve joins the right ventricle with the pulmonary artery. On the left, the aortic valve joins the left ventricle to the aorta.

Normal Heart Sounds

Closure of the heart valves causes the "lub dub" sounds that can be heard through auscultation over the precordium, which is the part of the anterior chest wall over the heart. The syllable "lub" characterizes the **first heart sound (S_1)**, which is produced by closure of the AV valves when the ventricles fill. The syllable "dub" characterizes the **second heart sound (S_2)**, which is produced by closure of the semilunar valves when the ventricles empty blood into the aorta and pulmonary arteries.

The two heart sounds relate to the contraction and relaxation phases of the heart's activity. The phase of ventricular contraction is called **systole**. The ventricles fill and then contract in the systolic phase to expel blood into the aorta and pulmonary arteries. When the AV valves close (S_1), the systolic phase begins, and when the aortic and pulmonic valves close, the systolic phase ends. The phase of ventricular relaxation is called **diastole**. The ventricles relax and then fill during atrial contraction in the diastolic phase, which begins as the aortic and pulmonic valves (S_2) close and ends as the AV valves (S_1) close (see **Figure 16–4 》**).

Toward the end of inspiration, splitting of S_2 may occur because of a slight difference in how long the semilunar valves take to close. This is considered normal when the splitting is from an increase in intrathoracic pressure during inspiration. A split sound ("t-dub" instead of "dub") results during inspiration because the aortic valve closes just slightly earlier than the pulmonic valve, but during expiration, the S_2 is not split ("dub") because the valves close at the same time.

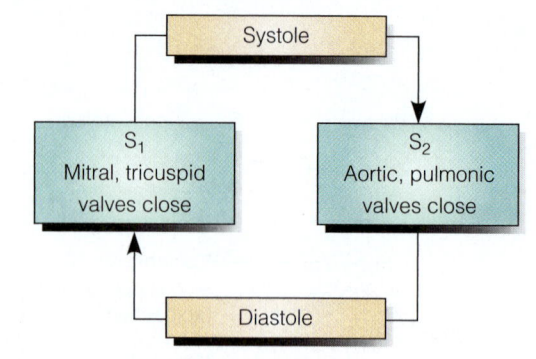

Figure 16–4 》 Heart sounds in systole and diastole.

In some healthy individuals, two other heart sounds may occur. The **third heart sound (S_3)**, also called a **ventricular gallop**, follows S_2 and happens when blood flow into the ventricles as the AV valves open causes vibrations during diastole. The S_3 sound may be heard in children, in young adults, or in pregnant women during the third trimester. Atrial contraction and ejection of blood into the ventricles in late diastole together cause the **fourth heart sound (S_4)**, also called an **atrial gallop**. The S_4 sound may be heard in children, in well-conditioned athletes, and in healthy older adults without cardiac disease. Although often normal, both the S_3 and S_4 sounds may be associated with pathologic conditions such as myocardial infarction (MI) or heart failure.

Interpretation of heart sounds is based on pitch, duration, intensity, phase, and location on the precordium. **Table 16–1 》** provides information about the characteristics of heart sounds.

TABLE 16–1 Characteristics of Heart Sounds

Heart Sounds			Cardiac Cycle Timing	Auscultation Site	Position	Pitch
S_1 S_1 — S_2 LUB — dub			Start of systole	Apex with diaphragm	Position does not affect the sound	High
S_2 S_1 — S_2 lub — DUB			End of systole	Both at second ICS; pulmonary component best at left sternal border (LSB); aortic component best at right sternal border (RSB) with diaphragm	Sitting or supine	High
Split S_1 S_1 — S_2 T			Beginning of systole	If normal, at second ICS, LSB; abnormal if heard at apex	Best heard in the supine position	High

TABLE 16–1 Characteristics of Heart Sounds *(continued)*

Heart Sounds	Cardiac Cycle Timing	Auscultation Site	Position	Pitch
S_3 	Early diastole right after S_2	Apex with the bell	Auscultated best in left lateral position or supine	Low
S_4 	Late diastole right before S_1	Apex with the bell	Auscultated best in left lateral position or supine	Low

Additional Heart Sounds

The valves of the heart typically open silently, but tissue damage may cause additional heart sounds. Valvular disease causes clicks and snaps. Mitral stenosis may cause an opening snap. Damage to the pulmonic and aortic valves may cause ejection clicks, and prolapse of the mitral valve may cause nonejection clicks. Inflammation of the pericardial sac causes friction rubs, in which the surfaces of the parietal and visceral layers of the pericardium produce a rubbing or grating sound because they cannot slide smoothly. **Table 16–2 »** provides information regarding interpretation of additional heart sounds.

Disruption of blood flow into the heart, between the chambers of the heart, or from the heart into the pulmonary or aortic systems causes harsh, blowing sounds commonly known as **heart murmurs**. Murmurs are graded in terms of audibility on a scale of 1 to 6, with grade 1 being the quietest and barely audible with a stethoscope, and grade 6 being the

TABLE 16–2 Additional Heart Sounds

Clicks		Heart Sounds	Cardiac Cycle Timing	Auscultation Site	Position	Pitch
		Aortic click	Early systole	Second ICS, RSB for aortic click and apex with diaphragm	Sitting or supine position may increase sound	High
		Pulmonic click	Early systole	Second ICS, LSB for pulmonic click with diaphragm	Sitting	High
		Opening snap	Early diastole	Third to fourth ICS, LSB with diaphragm	Sitting or supine position may increase sound	High
		Friction rub	Can occur at any time	Best heard with the diaphragm; location variable	May be heard in any position, but heard best when the patient sits forward	High, harsh in sound, grating

loudest with visible thrill and thrust. Heart murmurs may vary in quality (blowing, harsh, musical, rasping, or rumbling) and pitch (high, medium, or low) and can occur in systole, diastole, or both.

Pulmonary, Systemic, and Coronary Circulation

Because each side of the heart receives and ejects blood, the heart is often described as a double pump. Blood enters the right atrium and moves to the pulmonary bed at almost the exact same time that blood is entering the left atrium. The circulatory system has two main parts: the pulmonary circulation and the systemic circulation. The pulmonary circulation moves blood through the capillary bed surrounding the lungs to link with the gas exchange system of the lungs. The systemic circulation supplies blood to all other body tissues. In addition, the heart muscle is supplied with blood via the coronary circulation.

Pulmonary Circulation

The **pulmonary circulation** consists of the right side of the heart, the pulmonary artery, the pulmonary capillaries, and the pulmonary vein. Deoxygenated blood from the venous system enters the right atrium through the superior and inferior vena cava and is transported to the lungs via the pulmonary artery and its branches (see **Figure 16–5 》**). After oxygen and carbon dioxide are exchanged in the pulmonary capillaries, oxygen-rich blood returns to the left atrium through several pulmonary veins. Blood is then pumped out of the left ventricle through the aorta and its major branches to supply all body tissues. This second circuit of blood flow is called the systemic circulation.

Systemic Circulation

The **systemic circulation** is a high-pressure system responsible for moving blood to peripheral areas of the body. It consists of the left side of the heart, the aorta and its branches, the systemic arterial system, the capillaries that supply the brain and peripheral tissues, the systemic venous system, and the venae cavae.

Coronary Circulation

The **coronary circulation** is a network of vessels that supply the heart muscle. The left and right coronary arteries originate at the base of the aorta and branch out to encircle the myocardium (see **Figure 16–6A 》**). These arteries supply blood, oxygen, and nutrients to the myocardium. The left main coronary artery divides to form the anterior descending and circumflex arteries. The anterior descending artery supplies the anterior interventricular septum and the left ventricle. The circumflex branch supplies the left lateral wall of the left ventricle. The right coronary artery supplies the right ventricle and forms the posterior descending artery. The posterior descending artery supplies the posterior portion of the heart.

Ventricular contraction delivers blood through the pulmonary circulation and the systemic circulation. However, during ventricular relaxation, the coronary arteries fill with oxygen-rich blood. After the blood perfuses the heart muscle, the cardiac veins drain the blood into the coronary sinus, which empties into the right atrium of the heart (see Figure 16–6B).

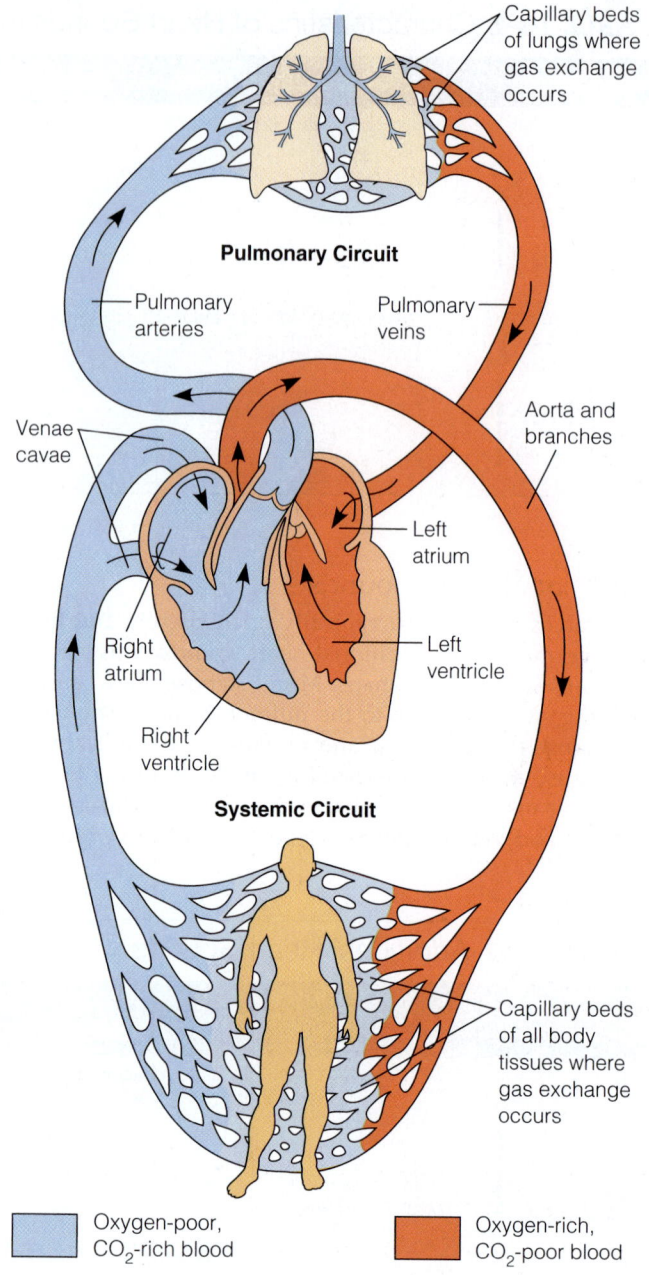

■ Oxygen-poor, CO_2-rich blood	■ Oxygen-rich, CO_2-poor blood

Figure 16–5 》 Pulmonary and systemic circulations.

The Cardiac Cycle and Cardiac Output

The contraction and subsequent relaxation of the heart constitute one heartbeat; this process is called the **cardiac cycle** (see **Figure 16–7 》**). Ventricular filling is followed by ventricular systole, during which the ventricles contract and eject blood into the pulmonary and systemic circuits. Systole is followed by a relaxation phase known as diastole. During diastole, the atria contract, the ventricles refill, and the myocardium is perfused. The complete cardiac cycle normally occurs about 70–80 times per minute. This is recorded as the heart rate.

During diastole, the volume in the ventricles increases to approximately 120 mL (the end-diastolic volume). At the end of systole, approximately 50 mL of blood remains in the

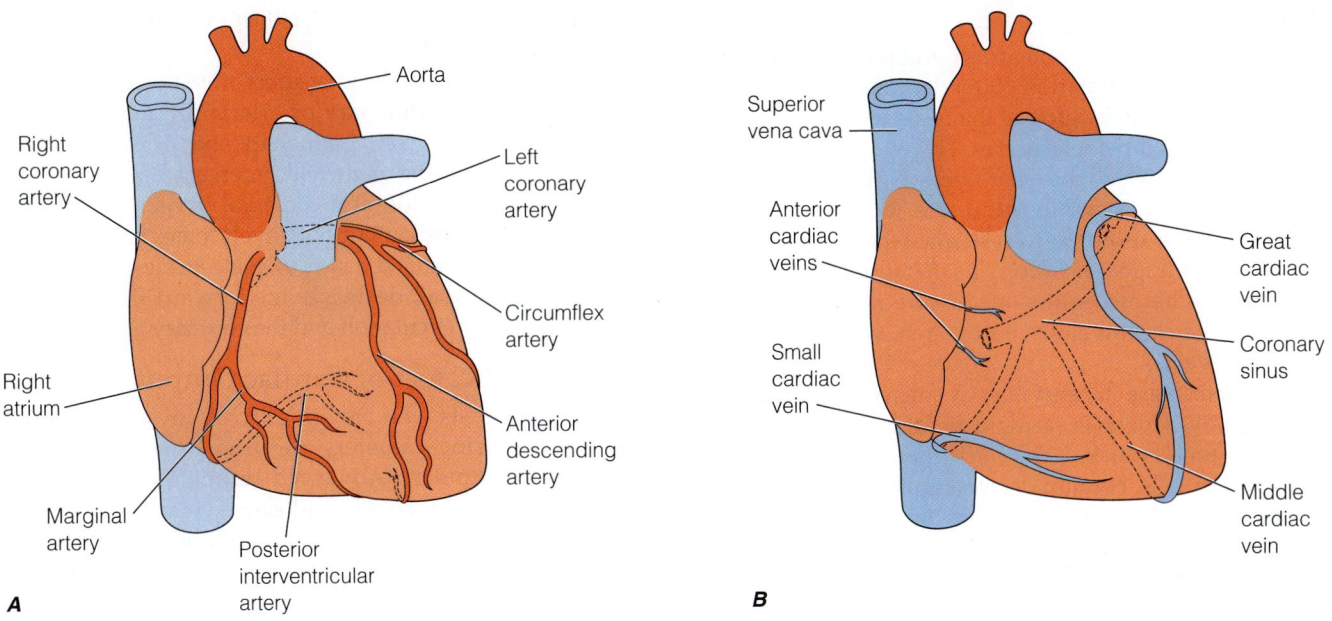

Figure 16–6 ›› Coronary circulation. **A,** Coronary arteries. **B,** Coronary veins.

ventricles (the end-systolic volume). The difference between the end-diastolic volume and the end-systolic volume is called the **stroke volume (SV)**. SV ranges from 60 to 100 mL/beat and averages approximately 70 mL/beat in an adult. **Cardiac output (CO)** is the amount of blood pumped by the ventricles into the pulmonary and systemic circulations in 1 minute. Multiplying the SV by the heart rate (HR) determines the CO:

$$HR \times SV = CO$$

The **ejection fraction** is the SV divided by the end-diastolic volume; it represents the fraction or percent of the diastolic volume that is ejected from the heart during systole. For example, an end-diastolic volume of 120 mL divided by an SV of 80 mL equals an ejection fraction of 66%. The normal ejection fraction ranges from 50 to 70%.

The average adult CO ranges from 4 to 8 L/min CO is an indicator of the heart's ability to function as a pump. If the heart cannot pump effectively, CO and tissue perfusion are decreased. In turn, body tissues that do not receive enough blood and oxygen (carried in the blood via hemoglobin) become **ischemic** (deprived of oxygen). If these tissues do not receive enough blood flow to maintain cellular function, the cells within them will die (resulting in necrosis or infarction).

Activity level, metabolic rate, physiologic and psychologic stress responses, age, and body size all influence CO. In addition, CO is determined by the interaction of four major factors: heart rate, contractility, preload, and afterload. Changes in each of these variables influence CO intrinsically, and each variable can be manipulated to affect CO. The heart's ability to respond to an increase in strenuous activity and adjust its CO is called **cardiac reserve**.

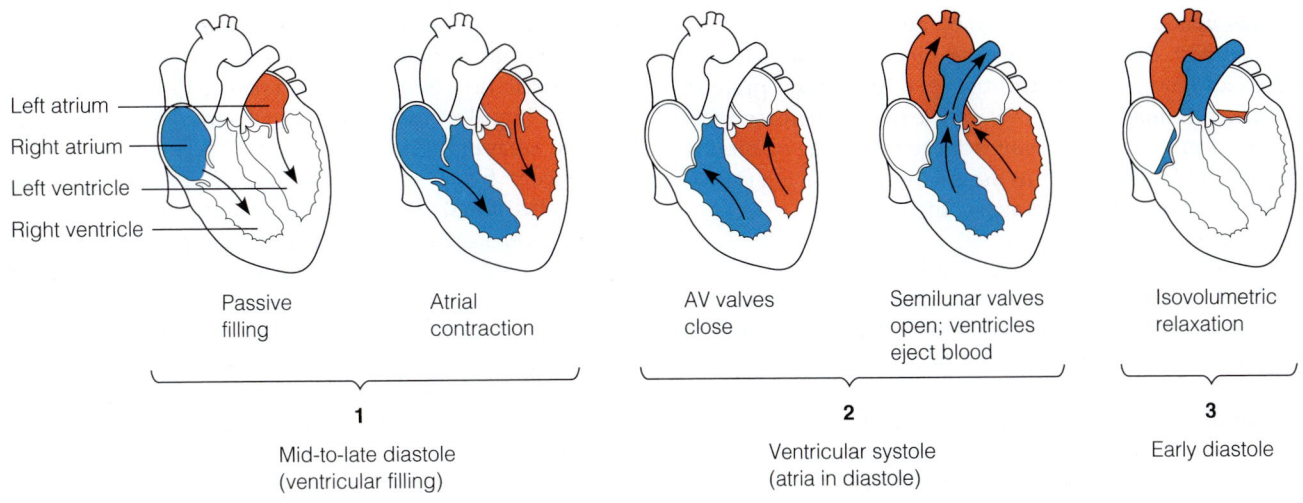

Figure 16–7 ›› The cardiac cycle has three events: (1) ventricular filling in mid-to-late diastole, (2) ventricular systole, and (3) isovolumetric relaxation in early diastole.

Heart Rate

Heart rate is affected by both direct and indirect autonomic nervous system stimulation. Direct stimulation is accomplished through innervation of the heart muscle by sympathetic and parasympathetic nerves. The sympathetic nervous system (SNS) increases the heart rate, whereas the parasympathetic vagal tone slows the heart rate. Reflex regulation of the heart rate in response to systemic blood pressure (BP) also occurs through activation of sensory receptors. These are known as baroreceptors or pressure receptors and are located in the carotid sinus, aortic arch, venae cavae, and pulmonary veins.

With an increase in heart rate, CO increases if there is no change in SV. However, a rapid heart rate decreases the amount of time available for ventricular filling during diastole. CO then falls, because decreased filling time decreases SV. Coronary artery perfusion also decreases, because the coronary arteries fill primarily during diastole. Because the number of cardiac cycles is decreased, CO decreases during bradycardia if SV stays the same.

Contractility

Contractility is the inherent capability of the cardiac muscle fibers to shorten. Poor contractility of the heart muscle reduces the forward flow of blood from the heart, increases the ventricular pressures from accumulation of blood volume, and reduces CO. Increased contractility may stress the heart.

Preload

Preload is the amount of cardiac muscle fiber tension or "stretch" that exists at the end of diastole. Preload is influenced by venous return and the compliance of the ventricles. The relationship between cardiac muscle fiber length and the force with which the fibers contract to accomplish ventricle emptying is referred to as Starling's law of the heart.

Cardiac muscle fiber stretch has a physiologic limit. Just as continuous overstretching of a rubber band causes the band to relax and lose its ability to recoil, overstretching of the cardiac muscle fibers eventually results in ineffective contraction. For example, disorders such as renal disease and congestive heart failure (CHF) result in sodium and water retention and increased preload. Likewise, vasoconstriction increases venous return and thereby increases preload.

In contrast, too little circulating blood volume results in decreased venous return and therefore decreased preload. Decreased preload reduces SV and leads to decreased CO. Decreased preload may result from hemorrhage or maldistribution of blood volume, as occurs in third spacing (movement of fluid into the interstitial compartment).

Afterload

Afterload is the force the ventricles must overcome to eject their blood volume. The right ventricle must generate enough tension to open the pulmonary valve and eject its volume into the low-pressure pulmonary arteries. Right ventricle afterload is measured as pulmonary vascular resistance. In contrast, the left ventricle ejects its load by overcoming the pressure behind the aortic valve. Afterload of the left ventricle is measured as **systemic vascular resistance (SVR)**. Arterial pressures are much higher than pulmonary pressures; thus, the left ventricle has to work much harder than the right ventricle.

Alterations in vascular tone affect afterload and ventricular work. As the pulmonary or arterial BP increases (e.g., through vasoconstriction), pulmonary and/or SVR increases, and the work of the ventricles increases. As workload increases, consumption of myocardial oxygen increases. A compromised heart cannot effectively meet this increased demand for oxygen, and a vicious cycle ensues. By contrast, a very low afterload decreases the forward flow of blood into the systemic circulation and the coronary arteries.

Clinical Indicators of Cardiac Output

For many patients who are critically ill, invasive hemodynamic monitoring catheters are used to measure CO in quantifiable numbers. Advanced technology, however, is not the only way to identify and assess compromised blood flow. Because CO perfuses the body's tissues, clinical indicators of low CO may manifest through changes in organ function resulting from compromised blood flow. For example, a change in level of consciousness (LOC) may indicate decreased blood flow to the brain.

The **cardiac index** is a patient's CO adjusted for his or her body size or body surface area (BSA). Because it takes into account the patient's BSA, the cardiac index provides useful data regarding the heart's ability to perfuse the tissues. A patient's BSA is expressed in square meters (m^2), and the cardiac index is calculated by dividing the patient's CO by his or her BSA. Cardiac measurements are considered adequate if they fall within the range of 2.5 to 4.2 L/min/m^2. For example, two patients are determined to have a CO of 4 L/min. This parameter is within normal limits. However, one patient is 157 cm (5'2") tall and weighs 54.5 kg (120 lb), with a BSA of 1.54 m^2. This patient's cardiac index is $4 \div 1.54$, or 2.6 L/min/m^2, which is within the acceptable range. The second patient is 188 cm (6'2") tall and weighs 81.7 kg (280 lb), with a BSA of 2.52 m^2. This patient's cardiac index is $4 \div 2.52$, or 1.6 L/min/m^2, which is outside the acceptable range.

The Conduction System of the Heart

The cardiac cycle, perpetuated by a complex electrical circuit, is commonly known as the intrinsic conduction system of the heart. Cardiac muscle cells possess an inherent characteristic of self-excitation. Self-excitation enables them to initiate and transmit impulses independent of a stimulus. However, specialized areas of myocardial cells typically exert a controlling influence in this electrical pathway. One of these specialized areas is the sinoatrial (SA) node, located at the junction of the superior vena cava and right atrium (see **Figure 16–8** »). The SA node acts as the normal "pacemaker" of the heart and typically generates an impulse 60–100 times per minute. This impulse travels across the atria via internodal pathways to the AV node, in the floor of the interatrial septum. The very small junctional fibers of the AV node slow the impulse, slightly delaying its transmission to the ventricles. The impulse then passes through the bundle of His at the AV junction and continues down the interventricular septum, through the right and left bundle branches, and out to the Purkinje fibers in the ventricular muscle walls.

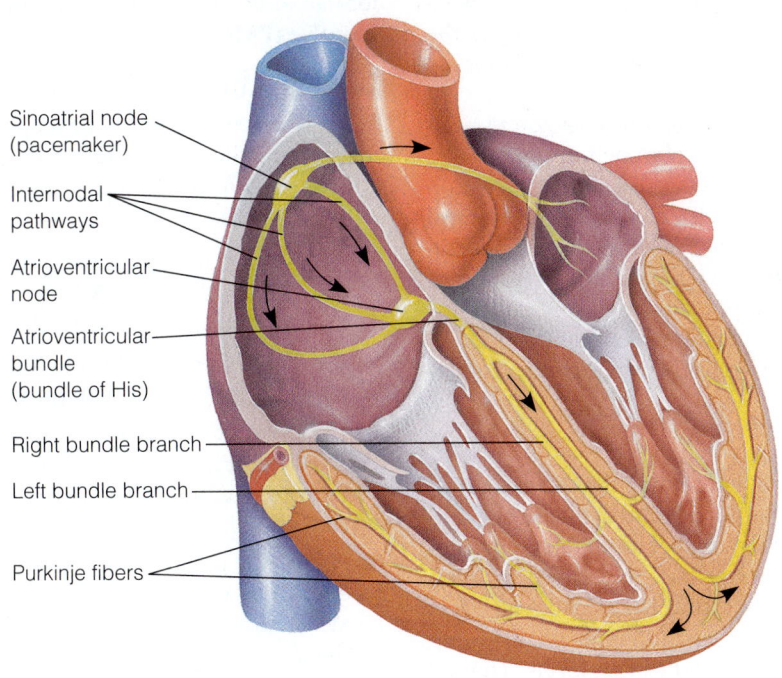

Figure 16–8 》 The intrinsic conduction system of the heart.

Sinoatrial node (pacemaker)
Internodal pathways
Atrioventricular node
Atrioventricular bundle (bundle of His)
Right bundle branch
Left bundle branch
Purkinje fibers

The Action Potential

The impulses from the SA and AV nodes stimulate a series of changes in ion concentration across the membrane of each cardiac muscle cell. This movement of sodium, potassium, and calcium ions causes an electrical impulse that stimulates muscle contraction. This electrical activity, called the **action potential**, produces the waveforms recorded by an **electrocardiography** (a diagnostic test of cardiac function).

In the resting state, positive and negative ions align on either side of the cell membrane, producing a relatively negative charge within the cell and a positive extracellular charge (see **Figure 16–9** 》). At this point, the cell is said to be polarized. The negative resting membrane potential is maintained at approximately –90 mV by the sodium–potassium pump in the cell membrane.

Depolarization

Depolarization is the phase when the heart contracts. Two types of ion channels function to produce the electrical changes that occur during depolarization: the fast sodium channels and the slow calcium channels. A fast action potential occurs in atrial and ventricular muscle cells and the Purkinje conduction system using the fast sodium channels. A slow action potential occurs in the SA and AV nodes using the slow calcium channels. The action potential for contraction of the heart is initiated in the SA node. When a resting cell is stimulated by an electrical charge from a neighboring cell or a spontaneous event, its cell membrane permeability changes. Sodium ions enter the cell, and the membrane

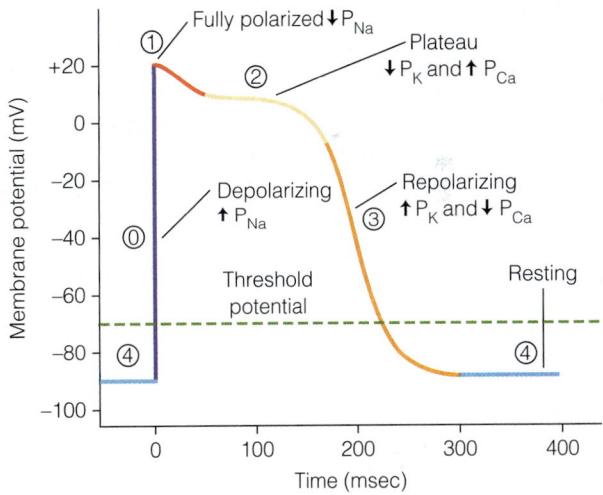

Figure 16–9 》 Action potential of a cardiac muscle cell. In the resting state (phase 4), the cell membrane is polarized; the cell's interior has a negative charge compared to that of extracellular fluid. On depolarization (phase 0), sodium ions diffuse rapidly across the cell membrane into the cell, and calcium channels open. In the fully depolarized state (phase 1), the cell's interior has a net positive charge compared to its exterior. During the plateau period (phase 2), calcium moves into the cell and potassium diffusion slows, prolonging the action potential. In phase 3, calcium channels close, the sodium–potassium pump removes sodium from the cell, and the cell membrane again becomes polarized, with a net negative charge.

becomes less permeable to potassium ions. Addition of positively charged ions to the intracellular fluid changes the membrane potential from negative to slightly positive, at +20 to +30 mV.

As the cell becomes more positive, it reaches the **threshold potential**, or the point at which an action potential is capable of being generated. The response to the action potential in the myocardial muscle cells causes a chemical reaction of calcium within the cell. This in turn causes actin and myosin filaments to slide together, producing cardiac muscle contraction. The action potential then spreads to surrounding cells, causing coordinated muscle contraction. As soon as the myocardium is completely depolarized, repolarization begins.

Repolarization

Repolarization is the process that returns the cell to its resting, polarized state. During repolarization, fast sodium channels close abruptly, and the cell begins to regain its negative charge. During the plateau phase, muscle contraction is prolonged as slow calcium–sodium channels remain open. When these channels close, the sodium–potassium pump restores ion concentrations to normal resting levels. The cell membrane is then ready for the next cycle. Each heartbeat represents one cardiac cycle, with one depolarization and repolarization cycle and one complete cardiac muscle contraction and relaxation (systole and diastole).

Only pacemaker cells normally demonstrate **automaticity** (the ability to generate an electrical impulse). Pacemaker cells have a resting potential that is much less negative (−70 to −50 mV) than other cardiac muscle cells. Their threshold potential is also lower than other myocardial cells. These differences result from constant leakage of sodium and potassium ions into the cell.

Myocardial cells have a unique protective property known as the **refractory period**. During the refractory period, cardiac cells resist stimulation. This protects cardiac muscle from spasm and tetany. During the absolute refractory period, depolarization will not occur, regardless of cell stimulation. The absolute refractory period is followed by the relative refractory period. During the relative refractory period, a greater-than-normal stimulus is required to generate an action potential. During the supernormal period that follows, a mild stimulus will cause depolarization. Many cardiac dysrhythmias are triggered during the relative refractory and supernormal periods.

Pulse

The **pulse** is a wave of blood created by contraction of the left ventricle of the heart. The pulse wave generally represents the SV output or the amount of blood that enters the arteries with each ventricular contraction. In a healthy individual, the pulse reflects the heartbeat. The pulse rate is the same as the rate of the heart's ventricular contractions. However, in some types of cardiovascular disease, the heartbeat and pulse rates can differ. For example, a patient's heart may produce weak pulse waves that are not detectable far from the heart. In these instances, the nurse should assess both the heartbeat and the peripheral pulse. A **peripheral pulse** is a pulse located away from the heart (e.g., in the foot or wrist). In contrast, the apical pulse is a central pulse. It is

located at the apex of the heart and is the **point of maximal impulse (PMI)**.

Factors Affecting the Pulse

Pulse rate is expressed in beats per minute (bpm). This rate varies according to a number of factors. The nurse should consider each of the following factors when assessing a patient's pulse:

- **Age.** As age increases, the pulse rate gradually decreases overall. See **Table 16–3** ≫ for specific variations in pulse rates from birth to adulthood.
- **Gender.** After puberty, the average male patient's pulse rate is slightly lower than the average female patient's.
- **Exercise.** The pulse rate normally increases with activity. The rate of increase in professional athletes is often less than in average individuals because of greater cardiac size, strength, and efficiency.
- **Fever.** The pulse rate increases (a) in response to the lowered BP that results from peripheral vasodilation associated with elevated body temperature and (b) because of the increased metabolic rate.
- **Medications.** Some medications decrease the pulse rate, and others increase it. For example, cardiotonics (e.g., digitalis preparations) lower the heart rate, whereas epinephrine raises it.
- **Hypovolemia.** Loss of blood from the vascular system normally increases pulse rate. In adults, the loss of circulating volume results in an adjustment of the heart rate to increase BP as the body compensates for the lost blood volume. Adults can usually lose up to 10% of their normal circulating volume without adverse effects.
- **Stress.** In response to stress, sympathetic nervous stimulation increases the overall activity of the heart. Stress increases the rate as well as the force of the heartbeat. Fear and anxiety as well as the perception of severe pain stimulate the sympathetic system.

TABLE 16–3 Variations in Pulse and Respirations by Age

Age	Pulse (per Minute)	Respirations (per Minute)
Newborn	100–205 (awake) 90–160 (asleep)	30–80
Infant	100–180 (awake) 80–160 (asleep)	30–60
Toddler	98–140 (awake) 80–120 (asleep)	20–40
Preschooler	98–140 (awake) 80–120 (asleep)	22–34
School age	70–120 (awake) 50–90 (asleep)	15–25
Adolescent	50–90	12–20
Adult	60–100	12–20
Older adult	60–100	15–20

- *Position changes.* When an individual is sitting or standing, blood usually pools in dependent vessels of the venous system. Pooling results in a transient decrease in venous blood return to the heart and a subsequent reduction in BP and increase in heart rate.
- *Pathology.* Certain diseases, such as some heart conditions or conditions that impair oxygenation, can alter the resting pulse rate.

Blood Pressure

Arterial blood pressure is a measure of the pressure exerted by the blood as it flows through the arteries. Because the blood moves in waves, two types of BP are measured. The **systolic blood pressure** is the pressure of the blood as a result of contraction of the ventricles, that is, the pressure of the height of the blood wave. The **diastolic blood pressure** is the pressure when the ventricles are at rest. Diastolic pressure is the lower pressure and is present at all times within the arteries. The difference between the diastolic and the systolic pressures is called the **pulse pressure**. A normal pulse pressure is about 40 mmHg but can be as high as 100 mmHg during exercise. A consistently elevated pulse pressure occurs in arteriosclerosis. A low pulse pressure (e.g., less than 25 mmHg) occurs in conditions such as severe heart failure.

BP is measured in millimeters of mercury (mmHg) and recorded as a fraction: systolic pressure over the diastolic pressure. A typical BP for a healthy adult is just below 120/80 mmHg (pulse pressure of 40). A number of conditions are reflected by changes in BP. Because BP can vary considerably among individuals, the nurse must know a specific patient's baseline BP. For example, if a patient's usual BP is 180/100 mmHg and it is assessed following surgery to be 120/80 mmHg, this significant drop may indicate complications and must be reported to the primary care provider.

Determinants of Blood Pressure

Arterial BP is the result of several factors: the pumping action of the heart, the peripheral vascular resistance (PVR; the resistance supplied by the vessels through which the blood flows), and the blood volume and viscosity.

Pumping Action of the Heart

When the heart pumps weakly, less blood is pumped into arteries (lower CO), and the BP decreases. When the heart pumps strongly, the volume of blood pumped into circulation increases (higher CO), and the BP increases.

Peripheral Vascular Resistance

Peripheral resistance can increase BP, especially the diastolic pressure. Factors that create resistance in the arterial system are the capacity of the arterioles and capillaries, the compliance of the arteries, and the viscosity of the blood.

The internal diameter or capacity of the arterioles and the capillaries determines in great part the PVR. The smaller the space within a vessel, the greater the resistance. Arterioles normally are in a state of partial constriction. Increased vasoconstriction raises the BP, whereas decreased vasoconstriction lowers the BP. If the elastic and muscular tissues of the arteries are replaced with fibrous tissue, the arteries lose much of their ability to constrict and dilate. This condition is known as **arteriosclerosis**.

Compliance of the arteries refers to their ability to contract and expand. When an individual's arteries become less compliant, as can happen during the process of aging, greater pressure is required to pump blood into the arteries, thus increasing the BP.

Blood Volume

When the blood volume decreases (e.g., as a result of a hemorrhage or dehydration), the BP decreases because of decreased fluid in the arteries. On the contrary, when the volume increases (e.g., as a result of a rapid intravenous [IV] infusion), the BP increases because of the greater fluid volume within the circulatory system.

Blood Viscosity

BP is higher when the blood is highly **viscous** (thick), that is, when the proportion of red blood cells (RBCs) to blood plasma is high. This proportion is referred to as the **hematocrit**. Viscosity increases markedly when the hematocrit is more than 60–65%.

Factors Affecting Blood Pressure

Factors that affect BP are age, exercise, stress, race, gender, medications, obesity, diurnal variations, and disease processes.

- *Age.* At day 10, the average systolic pressure of newborns is 90 mmHg. This pressure rises with age, reaching a peak at the onset of puberty, and then tends to decline somewhat. In older adults, elasticity of the arteries is decreased—the arteries are more rigid and less yielding to the pressure of the blood. This produces an elevated systolic pressure. Because the walls no longer retract as flexibly with decreased pressure, the diastolic pressure may also be high.
- *Exercise.* Physical activity increases the CO and BP; thus 20–30 minutes of rest following exercise is indicated before resting BP can be reliably assessed.
- *Stress.* Stimulation of the SNS increases CO and vasoconstriction of the arterioles, thus increasing the BP. However, severe pain can decrease BP greatly by inhibiting the vasomotor center and producing vasodilation.
- *Race.* African American men over 35 years of age have higher BPs than Caucasian men of the same age.
- *Gender.* After puberty, women usually have lower BPs than men of the same age; this difference is thought to be due to hormonal variations. After menopause, women generally have higher BPs than before.
- *Medications.* Many medications, including caffeine, increase or decrease the BP.
- *Obesity.* Both childhood and adult obesity predispose individuals to hypertension.
- *Diurnal variations.* Pressure is usually lowest early in the morning, when the metabolic rate is lowest, then rises throughout the day and peaks in the late afternoon or early evening.
- *Disease process.* Any condition affecting CO, blood volume, blood viscosity, and/or compliance of the arteries has a direct effect on BP.

Hemostasis

Hemostasis is the process by which the body slows and stops the flow of blood. Careful regulation of hemostasis is essential to perfusion. Without adequate mechanisms of hemostasis, even minor injuries could result in shock, tissue damage, and death due to uncontrolled bleeding. However, too much hemostatic activity can also be problematic, because unwanted clot formation in the absence of injury could lead to blocked blood vessels and other health problems.

Hemostasis is a complicated process that involves multiple chemical mediators and interactions. For the sake of simplicity, researchers divide the overall process into three basic steps: vasoconstriction, formation of a platelet plug, and the coagulation cascade. Once tissue repair begins and the clot is no longer necessary, it is gradually broken down via fibrinolysis.

Vasoconstriction

The first major step in hemostasis is vasoconstriction, or narrowing of the injured blood vessel due to contraction of smooth muscle in the vessel wall. Vasoconstriction is triggered by substances released at the site of injury and by nerve impulses from nearby pain receptors. However, this effect is only temporary (Kumar, Abbas, & Aster, 2013).

Platelet Plug Formation

Exposed collagen fibers at the injury site bind with von Willebrand factor (vWF), a plasma protein. One end of each vWF molecule attaches to the collagen in the vessel wall, while the other end attracts and binds platelets. This binding activates the platelets, causing them to change from smooth disks to spherical shapes with long arms. The binding also causes the platelets to release chemical mediators that attract even more platelets to the area. Within a few minutes, the aggregated, activated platelets stick to each other and to the vessel wall well enough to form a small plug that closes the hole in the vessel.

The Coagulation Cascade

Platelet plugs are temporary, and they cannot patch large holes. To fully stop the bleeding, the body requires a stronger, larger, longer-lasting patch. The process by which this patch is formed is called **coagulation**, or **clotting**, and it involves a complex series of events called the **coagulation cascade** (see **Figure 16–10 »**).

The coagulation cascade involves multiple plasma proteins called **clotting factors**. Thirteen clotting factors have been identified thus far; each is denoted by a Roman numeral. Under normal circumstances, inactive clotting factors circulate in the blood. Initiation of the coagulation cascade converts the clotting factors to their active form. The exact sequence of activation depends upon whether coagulation proceeds via the intrinsic or the extrinsic pathway.

- In the **intrinsic pathway**, exposed collagen in the wall of the damaged blood vessel triggers a series of reactions that culminate in activation of Factor X.

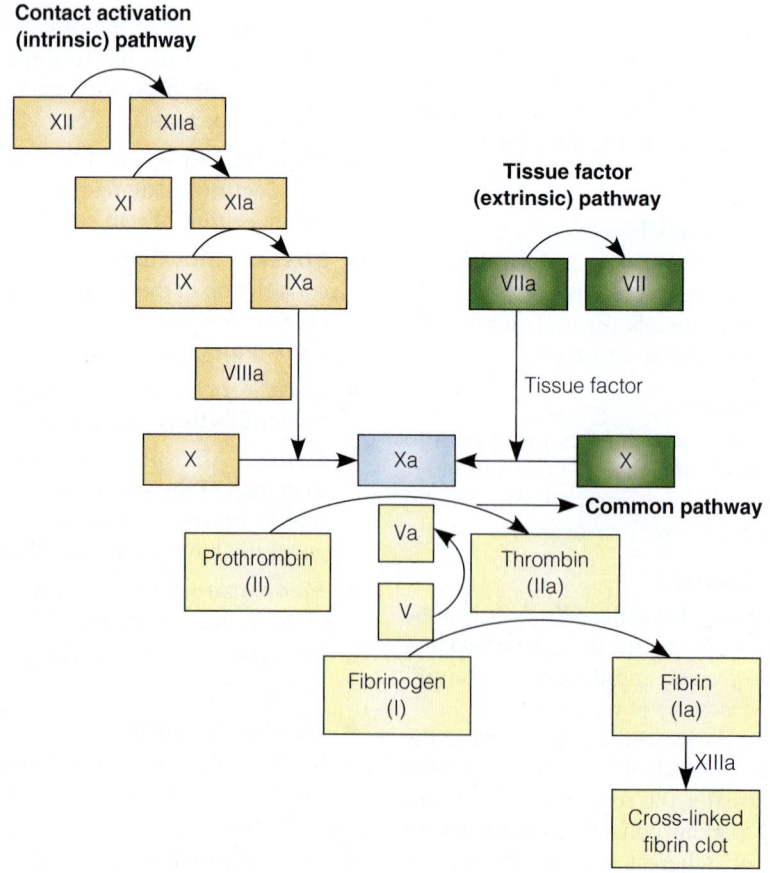

Figure 16–10 » Coagulation cascade.

- The **extrinsic pathway** is initiated when blood leaks out of a vessel and into the tissue spaces. Factor VII within the leaked blood binds with **tissue factor (TF)**, a protein found on the surface of some body cells. This binding starts a series of reactions that leads to Factor X activation. Although both pathways result in activation of Factor X, the reaction sequence in the extrinsic pathway is shorter and more rapid than that in the intrinsic pathway.

From this point, the two pathways converge in the common pathway. In the common pathway, Factor X combines with Factor V to form a complex called prothrombin activator or prothrombinase. This complex then converts **prothrombin** (or Factor II) in the blood to **thrombin** (Factor IIa). Finally, thrombin converts **fibrinogen** (or Factor I) in the blood into **fibrin** (Factor Ia). The fibrin strands intertwine with each other and bind with platelets in the area to form a stable, insoluble clot.

Fibrinolysis

About 24–48 hours after clot formation, the injured blood vessel is usually healed to the point that the clot is no longer needed. At this point, the body starts to break down the clot through the process of **fibrinolysis**. Fibrinolysis begins when new, healthy tissue at the site of injury secretes an enzyme called tissue plasminogen activator (tPA). The tPA then acts on **plasminogen**, an inactive protein incorporated into the clot, converting it to active **plasmin**. Slowly but steadily, the plasmin digests the fibrin strands and dissolves the clot.

Genetic Considerations

Various genetic factors have been shown to influence perfusion. One such factor is gender. For example, the risk for heart disease in women increases after menopause because of the drop in estrogen production. Women who experience menopause early double their risk of developing heart disease. Age typically becomes a risk factor for women at 55 years old. In addition, women are more likely to experience angina than men.

Research also reveals that heart disease tends to run in families. If a person's father or brother had a heart attack before age 55, or if the person's mother or sister had a heart attack before age 65, that person is more likely to develop heart disease. Men are more likely to have heart attacks earlier in life than women.

Alterations to Perfusion

Nurses care for many patients with alterations in perfusion secondary to the prevalence of cardiac disease. Patients may present with cardiac disease as a primary diagnosis, or they may be seen for a variety of other problems complicated by a secondary diagnosis of cardiac disease. Patients with alterations to perfusion will likely have alterations to other concepts as well, especially acid–base balance. Acute respiratory acidosis exists when an acute ventilation failure occurs. Common causes include drug-induced respiratory depression, inadequate ventilation due to neuromuscular disease or paralysis, and airway obstruction. Chronic respiratory acidosis is usually secondary to other medical conditions, such as chronic obstructive pulmonary disease (COPD),

neuromuscular disorders, severe restrictive ventilator defects, and thoracic skeletal deformities. Likewise, patients with metabolic acidosis have pulmonary vasoconstriction and increased pulmonary vascular pressures, leading to right ventricular failure and generalized myocardial depression.

Alterations and Manifestations

Clotting Disorders

Disorders of clotting can result in excessive bleeding (as discussed in Exemplar 16.E on Disseminated Intravascular Coagulation) or excessive clotting (as discussed in Exemplar 16.D on Deep Venous Thrombosis). Clotting can occur only if the body has sufficient platelets and clotting factors. Bleeding disorders result when either platelets or one or more clotting factors do not work properly or when the supply of platelets and clotting factors is insufficient. Von Willebrand disease is the most common of these disorders (Office on Women's Health, 2012). It results from a defect or deficiency in vWF and can cause bleeding to be unusually excessive. This condition is usually hereditary (Mayo Clinic, 2014a). Another well-known but rare disorder, hemophilia, is caused by a genetic mutation that results in uncontrolled bleeding due to a lack of clotting factors in men who inherit the mutation. Women who inherit the mutation become carriers (Office on Women's Health, 2012). Although small cuts typically do not present a problem, internal bleeding can be life-threatening for people with hemophilia (Mayo Clinic, 2014b). Excessive blood clotting, or hypercoagulation, results when clots fail to dissolve properly and subsequently limit or obstruct blood flow, potentially causing heart attacks, strokes, organ damage, or death. Excessive clotting disorders can be genetic or acquired through other conditions (American Heart Association [AHA], 2015a).

Alterations to Pediatric Cardiology

Most pediatric perfusion disorders are related to congenital cardiac defects. With recent advances in pediatric cardiology, children who would not have survived to their first birthday are now entering adolescence. As a result, nurses may care for patients with profound alterations in cardiac anatomy requiring special considerations when planning care. Cardiac congenital anomalies are discussed in more detail in Exemplar 16.B. See the Lifespan Considerations section for more information on issues related to perfusion in children.

Common Cardiovascular Illnesses of Adulthood

Coronary artery disease (CAD) is the leading cause of death in the United States. CAD occurs when the arteries supplying the heart muscle harden and become narrow. The buildup, called atherosclerosis, is made up of cholesterol and other materials. As the arteries become narrower, the heart muscle does not receive a sufficient amount of blood or oxygen. Patients with CAD may experience angina (chest pain), MI (heart attack), dysrhythmias, or heart failure.

MIs occur when the flow of oxygenated blood to a section of heart muscle is blocked. Blockages need immediate treatment or the heart muscle begins to die. Necrotic tissue is replaced with scar tissue, which may result in long-term cardiac disease. Another cause of MI is severe spasms of a

TABLE 16–4 Age-Related Cardiac Changes

Age-Related Change	Significance
Myocardium: ↓ efficiency and contractility. **Sinoatrial (SA) node:** ↑ in thickness of shell surrounding the node and ↓ in number of pacemaker cells.	Decreased CO when under physiologic stress, with resulting tachycardia that lasts longer than in younger people. The individual may require rest time between physical activities.
Left ventricle: Slight hypertrophy, prolonged isovolumetric contraction phase and relaxation time; ↑ time for diastolic filling and systolic emptying cycle.	SV may increase to compensate for tachycardia, leading to increased BP.
Valves and blood vessels: Aorta is elongated and dilated, valves are thicker and more rigid, and resistance to peripheral blood flow increases by 1% per year.	BP increases to compensate for increased peripheral resistance and decreased CO.

coronary artery, resulting in interrupted blood supply to a section of the heart. These spasms may occur without the presence of atherosclerosis. Prompt, rapid medical treatment significantly improves the patient's outcome. Approximately 50% of those who die from an MI do so within 60 minutes of the first symptom.

Common Cardiovascular Illnesses of Aging

Cardiovascular disease can have a slow onset with progressive deterioration of other organ systems, such as the kidneys and lungs. Some conditions, such as hypertension or hyperlipidemia, are risk factors for more serious conditions. These conditions require ongoing assessment and treatment (see **Table 16–4 》**).

Prevalence

High BP affects 29% (70 million) of American adults. More than 360,000 deaths in 2013 were attributed to high BP. Of people who have a first heart attack, 69% have high BP, as do 77% of people who have a first stroke and 74% of people with chronic heart failure. Only about half of people who have high BP (52%) have it under control (Centers for Disease Control and Prevention [CDC], 2015a).

Heart disease is the leading cause of death for both men and women. One of every four deaths in the United States is attributed to heart disease, amounting to 610,000 deaths annually. Coronary heart disease is most common, killing 370,000 people annually. Every year, about 525,000 Americans have a first heart attack, and 210,000 have a repeat attack (CDC, 2015b).

About 5.1 million people in the United States have heart failure, which is the primary cause of death in 55,000 people each year, and a contributing cause of death in 280,000 people. About half of people with heart failure die within 5 years of diagnosis (CDC, 2015c).

Every year, more than 795,000 Americans have a stroke, and about 610,000 of these strokes are first strokes. Stroke kills almost 130,000 Americans each year, which is 1 in every 20 deaths. Stroke is the leading cause of long-term disability.

Box 16–1
Genetic Considerations for Cardiac Disorders

- Familial hypercholesterolemia is a single-gene disorder that results in atherosclerosis and CAD at an earlier age than in the general population (i.e., before age 55 in men and age 65 in women). However, increased cholesterol levels may also be inherited and are a risk factor for CAD in both men and women.
- Marfan syndrome is an autosomal dominant inherited disorder that affects the skeleton, eyes, and cardiovascular system. Cardiovascular effects include dilation of the proximal aorta and aortic dissection associated with degeneration of the elastic fibers in the tunica media of the aorta. Thoracic aortic aneurysms may also be present.
- Supraventricular aortic stenosis is a genetic vascular disorder resulting in hourglass-shaped stenosis of the ascending aorta. It may also affect other major arteries, including the pulmonary, carotid, cerebral, renal, and coronary arteries.
- Hypertrophic cardiomyopathy, a disease of sarcomere proteins, has a genetic transmission.
- Williams syndrome is a rare genetic disorder characterized by characteristic "elfin-like" features and heart and blood vessel problems (as well as other physical problems).
- Long QT syndrome is an inherited genetic disorder that results from structural abnormalities of the potassium channels in the heart, leading to dysrhythmias. This can result in unconsciousness and may cause sudden cardiac death (SCD) in teenagers and young adults when exposed to stressors ranging from exercise to loud sounds.

Genetic Considerations and Risk Factors

Risk factors for perfusion abnormalities may be identified as nonmodifiable or modifiable. Nonmodifiable risk factors are not affected by changes in patient behavior. They include age, gender, race, family history, and personal health history. The nurse should consider genetic influences on the health of the adult. During the patient interview, the nurse should ask about family members with health problems affecting cardiac function or a family history of high cholesterol levels or early-onset CAD. During the physical assessment, the nurse should assess for manifestations that might indicate a genetic disorder (see **Box 16–1 》**). If data are found to indicate genetic risk factors or alterations, the nurse should ask about genetic testing and refer for appropriate genetic counseling and evaluation.

Case Study 》 Part 1

During your shift, Mr. Bill Evans, a 64-year-old man, presents to the emergency department after collapsing at home. His wife states that just before losing consciousness, Mr. Evans seemed confused and complained of numbness and tingling in his left arm and of double vision. She also states that her husband's speech was slurred and the left side of his face drooped. He has a history of CAD, hypertension, CHF, atrial fibrillation, and diabetes. Current vitals are T 98.9°F; P 91 bpm; R 24/min; and BP 182/98 mmHg. Mr. Evans has regained consciousness and is aware of his surroundings but demonstrates right-sided weakness, slurred speech, and difficulty forming words.

Clinical Reasoning Questions Level I

1. What symptoms of alterations in perfusion does Mr. Evans demonstrate?

Alterations and Therapies
Perfusion

ALTERATION	DESCRIPTION	MANIFESTATIONS	INTERVENTIONS AND THERAPIES
Coronary artery disease (CAD)	As plaque builds within the coronary artery, the diameter of the artery decreases. This reduces blood flow to the cardiac muscle until an MI occurs. Necrosis of the heart muscle may occur as a result of decreased perfusion.	■ Pain or discomfort in chest; may also include atypical locations such as arm, left shoulder, back, neck, or jaw ■ Shortness of breath ■ Cold, clammy skin ■ Feeling of indigestion or fullness ■ Dizziness, anxiety ■ Rapid, irregular heart rate	■ Administer oxygen. ■ Administer nitrates for vasodilatory effects. ■ Conduct telemetry monitoring. ■ Administer tissue plasminogen activator, streptokinase, or other medication to eliminate clots preventing perfusion of cardiac muscle. ■ Administer antiarrhythmic medications. ■ Implement bedrest. ■ Implement anxiety reduction measures. ■ The patient may be prepped for coronary artery bypass grafting (CABG).
Cardiomyopathy	Inflammation of the cardiac muscle results in an increase in heart size and reduced cardiac function. Cardiomyopathy may be classified as primary (no known cause) or secondary (results from hypertension, valvular disease, artery disease, congenital heart defects, or another known cause) and as dilated, hypertrophic, or restrictive.	■ Signs and symptoms may not present until later in the disease ■ Shortness of breath, especially with physical exertion; may include cor pulmonale ■ Fatigue ■ Lower-extremity edema ■ Arrhythmias ■ Heart murmur	■ Administer medications (calcium channel blockers [CCBs], beta-blockers, antidysrhythmics). ■ Monitor vital signs, including pulse ox. ■ Conduct focused cardiac/respiratory assessment for detection of crackles, dry cough, murmurs, or extra heart sounds. ■ Monitor intake and output. ■ Assess capillary refill time. ■ Instruct patient to avoid nitrates (because they lower BP) and digoxin (because it increases the force of contractions). ■ Administer antibiotics to reduce the risk for bacterial endocarditis. ■ Treatment may include septal myectomy, ethanol ablation, or implantable cardioverter–defibrillator (ICD). ■ Heart failure management ■ Fluid and sodium restriction
Dysrhythmia	Dysrhythmia is irregular electrical pattern seen on an ECG. It may result from new or existing CAD, serum electrolyte imbalances, injury, congenital defect, MI, or malfunction of conduction system.	■ Irregular heart rate	■ Conduct cardiac monitoring. (Notify healthcare provider of changes in heart rate or rhythm.) ■ Administer antidysrhythmic medications as ordered. ■ Administer supplemental O_2 as needed. ■ Structure activities of daily living (ADLs) to provide for adequate rest periods. ■ Monitor lab values.
Valvular heart disease	Valvular heart disease may be acquired or congenital. It may be caused by valvular stenosis or valvular insufficiency.	■ Shortness of breath ■ Weakness or lightheadedness ■ Chest discomfort ■ Edema of lower extremities ■ Palpitations ■ Rapid weight gain (2–3 lb per day)	■ Provide patient teaching to include diet, lifestyle changes, and signs and symptoms of heart failure. ■ Medications may include diuretics, antidysrhythmics, vasodilators, angiotensin-converting–enzyme (ACE) inhibitors, beta-blockers, and/or anticoagulants; they may also include antibiotics to prevent bacterial endocarditis.

(continued on next page)

Alterations and Therapies (continued)

ALTERATION	DESCRIPTION	MANIFESTATIONS	INTERVENTIONS AND THERAPIES
Cardiogenic shock	Cardiogenic shock is inadequate perfusion of the tissues as a result of blood loss, infection, destruction of or inadequate production of blood cells, reduced CO caused by cardiac disease, or systemic vasodilation.	■ Confusion ■ Loss of consciousness ■ Sudden, rapid heartbeat ■ Diaphoresis ■ Tachypnea ■ Decreased urine output ■ Extremities cool to touch	■ Administer fluids and, depending on cause, blood transfusions or volume expanders. ■ Medications may include vasoconstrictors and other drugs needed to treat the underlying cause. ■ Monitor and assess cardiorespiratory function and oxygen saturation. ■ Administer oxygen as indicated. ■ Assess LOC, and report significant deviations from baseline. ■ Patients in acute shock may require mechanical ventilation.
Hypertension	Pressure in the arterial blood vessels is elevated, causing the heart to pump with much more force in order to overcome higher pressures. Causes may be primary (no known cause) or secondary (result of another disease process).	■ Often asymptomatic until hypertension becomes significant ■ May present with headaches (particularly in the a.m.), dizziness, nausea, nosebleeds, fatigue, and difficulty sleeping	■ Assess cardiovascular risk status. ■ Encourage lifestyle changes. ■ Conduct a nutritional assessment. ■ Encourage smoking cessation. ■ Obtain detailed family history.
Hypertensive disorders of pregnancy	BP elevates, causing damage to nephrons with leakage of protein into the urine. As BP continues to rise, it can result in fetal demise, seizures, stroke, and death.	■ Proteinuria, headache, edema of hands and lower extremities	■ Instruct patient to reduce sodium intake. ■ Monitor BP. ■ Elevate extremities. ■ If BP exceeds acceptable limits, patient will be admitted and IV magnesium sulfate administered. ■ If unable to control BP with magnesium sulfate, the only option is to deliver the baby, which will resolve the problem and gradually return BP to normal limits.

2. Identify three nonmodifiable risk factors related to alterations in perfusion.
3. Describe the pathophysiology of a cerebrovascular accident (CVA).

Clinical Reasoning Questions Level II

4. Would you expect that Mr. Evans experienced a hemorrhagic or ischemic CVA? Why?
5. What issues can you identify as priorities in caring for this patient?
6. What are some potential complications that the nurse needs to be aware of?

Concepts Related to Perfusion

In addition to acid–base balance, a number of concepts and systems affect and are affected by adequate (or impaired) perfusion, including, but not limited to, cognition, comfort, fluids and electrolytes, intracranial regulation, and oxygenation.

Because of autoregulation, the brain has the ability to maintain relatively constant blood flow despite changes in perfusion pressure, and therefore is able to maintain cognition. Clinical signs or symptoms of ischemia can be seen when cerebral perfusion pressure drops below the lower limit of autoregulation. Altered mental status is an early symptom of decreased cerebral blood flow. Without adequate cerebral blood flow, energy-dependent brain processes cease, leading to irreversible brain injury. Adequate cerebral blood flow or intracranial regulation must be maintained to ensure adequate cerebral perfusion pressure.

The heart generates sufficient CO to transport and distribute blood to the body's tissues. Impaired tissue perfusion results when the blood supply available to a site of injury is present but decreased. Comfort can be a concern, as pain is a common symptom.

Inadequate fluid resuscitation may lead to multiple-organ failure and death due to fluid and electrolyte imbalances. Hypovolemia causes a decrease in extracellular

Concepts Related to
Perfusion

CONCEPT	RELATIONSHIP TO PERFUSION	NURSING IMPLICATIONS
Acid–Base Balance	Retention of CO_2 Low pH, low or normal $PaCO_2$	▪ Evaluate patient's respiratory drive and function. Treat underlying problem. Reestablish effective ventilation. ▪ Assess for lactic acidosis and acute renal failure.
Assessment	Impaired perfusion can be evident by changes in vital signs and physical signs and symptoms.	▪ Monitor hypotension, changes in respiration and heart rate signaling either compensation or decompensation, decrease in oxygen saturation, increase in capnography, and lack of temperature regulation. ▪ Assess physical signs and symptoms such as retractions, skin pallor and turgor, perspiration, decreased mental status, and capillary refill.
Cellular Regulation	Internal respiration is impaired by an insufficient amount of hemoglobin in the blood, thereby impairing oxygenation.	▪ Patient may require a blood transfusion. Evaluate mental status, noting development of confusion and labs such as blood type and screen. Monitor vital signs and respiratory status related to possible fluid volume overload or allergic reaction. Supply supplemental O_2 as needed.
Cognition	Hypoxemia can cause altered mental state.	▪ Assess mental status. Rule out acute brain injury.
Comfort	↓ Perfusion of tissues may manifest as pain.	▪ Note abdominal pain, chest pain, changes in extremity temperature, pain in extremities, ↑ BP, ↑ respirations, restlessness, and anxiety. ▪ Monitor vital signs, pain scale, redness, and swelling in extremities. Administer O_2 as needed. Administer meds as ordered.
Fluids and Electrolytes	Fluid volume excess may result in hypervolemia, impaired gas exchange, and other life-threatening alterations. Fluid volume deficit may result in hypovolemia, impaired gas exchange related to anemia, fluid and electrolyte imbalances, and other life-threatening alterations.	▪ Decrease work of breathing. Administer supplemental O_2 as needed. Maintain perfusion pressure pharmacologically with vasopressors or by the infusing of crystalloid and or colloid fluids. Monitor pulse ox and arterial blood gases (ABGs). ▪ Balance fluids. Ensure bedrest. Conduct a focused pulmonary assessment. Assess for jugular venous distention (JVD). Assess for chest pain, nausea and vomiting, and shortness of breath.
Intracranial Regulation	Cerebral blood flow (CBF)	▪ Regulate to meet brain's metabolic needs. ↑ CBF can ↑ intracranial pressure (ICP). ↓ CBF may result in cerebral ischemia. ▪ Monitor vital signs. Observe pupils and level of consciousness. Assess using the Glasgow Coma Scale. Maintain correct body positioning. Observe for signs and symptoms of ↑ ICP.
Oxygenation	Factors affecting transport of respiratory gases to the tissues	▪ Patient may experience ↓ energy, restlessness, tachypnea, tachycardia, hypertension, and confusion. ▪ Monitor vital signs. Use high-Fowler positioning, if able. Encourage deep breathing. Administer O_2. Provide for periods of rest between activities.

fluid. In severe cases, inadequate tissue perfusion may occur. A loss of blood volume causes an inappropriate redistribution of body fluids and electrolytes via passive transport.

Respiratory gases are transported by RBCs, resulting in oxygenation by means of internal respiration. Ventilation, diffusion, and perfusion are essential for gas exchange to occur. The process of perfusion pumps bloods from the cardiovascular system to the lungs. The Concepts Related to Perfusion feature links some, but not all, of the concepts integral to perfusion. They are presented in alphabetical order.

Health Promotion

Modifiable risk factors usually stem from an individual's lifestyle, and primary prevention methods require lifestyle modifications before the individual has been diagnosed with an alteration in perfusion. Secondary prevention methods require immediate changes after diagnosis to help prevent a worsening of the disease. *Healthy People 2020* has identified 25 objectives for health promotion related to heart disease and stroke (Office of Disease Prevention and Health Promotion [ODPHP], 2016).

Modifiable Risk Factors

Modifiable risk factors increase an individual's risk of developing alterations in perfusion. Health promotion related to these risk factors is aimed at altering the individual's lifestyle by encouraging healthy habits. Most interventions that focus on the primary prevention of cardiovascular injury include quitting smoking, encouraging a normal BMI by eating a healthy diet, and starting a daily regimen of physical activity.

Secondary Risk Factors

Secondary risk factors are those that contribute to an individual's risk for developing heart disease. Examples of methods used to reduce secondary risk factors include controlling high BP, decreasing high blood cholesterol and stress, and abstaining from alcohol or consuming only small amounts of alcohol. A lower stress level has been associated with lowering BP and slowing intrinsic heart rate by reducing the production of stress hormones such as cortisol, adrenaline, and norepinephrine, which increases perfusion to muscular tissues. A lower stress level then contributes to a decrease in the myocardial oxygen demand. Stress reduction strategies are discussed in detail in the module on Stress and Coping.

Screenings

A patient's first symptom of impaired perfusion may present as MI or sudden death. Patients may not experience preceding chest pain or other signs and symptoms associated with impaired perfusion. Because of this, screening tests may be performed for individuals with risk factors for CAD to detect signs of CAD before serious events occur.

BP screenings are an easy way to identify a substantial risk factor for altered perfusion. Most screening activities are covered by insurance providers related to the decreased cost of wellness measures compared to hospitalization and chronic care. This is why the Affordable Care Act mandates that preventive care be provided for free (U.S. Centers for Medicare & Medicaid Services, n.d.). BP screenings are recommended for all individuals of adult age. An optimal BP is below 120 mmHg systolic and below 80 mmHg diastolic.

Monitoring serum lipids is another screening that can identify a risk for altered perfusion. The U.S. Preventive Services Task Force (USPSTF) recommends all men over 35 years old and women over 45 years old have a screening for lipid disorders. It is also strongly recommended that those who are 20 years of age and older who have an increased risk of coronary heart disease have a serum lipid screening (USPSTF, 2015).

An ECG may be ordered to detect electrical changes, such as ST depressions or Q waves that suggest CAD or signs of a previous MI. Results of the ECG may indicate the need for further testing. Another type of screening is a stress test. These screenings place the heart under controlled stress to detect the presence of blockages that may limit flow. There are two types of basic stress testing. Exercise cardiac stress testing involves exercising the patient under controlled conditions to stress the heart. The second basic type of stress testing is physiologic stress testing, which involves chemically stressing the heart to mimic the effects of exercise. This type of testing may be considered for patients with limited mobility.

The physician may order that a radionuclide be used in conjunction with the stress test to assess the perfusion of coronary arteries. This involves injecting a radioactive isotope (usually thallium, technetium, or Cardiolite) into the patient's vein. Once the isotope has been absorbed by normal heart muscle, an image of the heart's cross-section becomes visible. The nuclear images are viewed with the patient at rest and then again after exercise. The two sets of images are then compared. If present, blockages will be evident as "cold spots" on the images taken after exercise.

Stress echocardiography may be used to supplement screenings for CAD. Echocardiography produces sound waves that are used to produce images of the heart at rest and at the peak of exercise. In hearts with normal blood flow, the left ventricle demonstrates stronger contractions of the heart muscle during peak exercise. In patients with CAD, a left ventricle segment not receiving adequate blood flow will exhibit reduced contractions. Stress echocardiography may be used in patients with false-positive stress tests. Contrast agents such as perflutren (Definity) may be injected into the venous system to help view the left ventricular wall motility during an echocardiogram, especially in those who are obese and those who retain a certain amount of carbon dioxide in their lungs, such as patients with COPD or those who have a history of smoking.

Electron beam CT offers new technology for CAD screening. This test can identify calcium blockages as mild as 10–20%. With mild blockages, the recommended treatment is risk factor modification. Calcium scoring may be used to persuade those at risk to engage in lifestyle modifications. Scores range from zero (no evidence of CAD) to over 400 (extensive evidence of CAD). Not all insurance plans cover calcium scoring at this time.

Lifestyle Modifications

Lifestyle modifications, such as proper nutrition and exercise, are important to health promotion in patients at risk for alterations in perfusion. Keeping a patient's body mass index (BMI) below 25 helps reduce the risk of CAD (National Heart, Lung, Blood Institute [NHLBI], 2012a). Serum lipids are also altered by a proper diet and normal BMI. Obesity is also associated with diabetes, which can damage blood vessels through its disease process, which impairs perfusion. Loss of as little as 4.5 kg (10 lb) reduces BP in many individuals (AHA, 2016a). Weight loss also reduces risk for stroke and other cardiovascular diseases. A balanced diet, such as the DASH (Dietary Approaches to Stop Hypertension) diet, is recommended for weight loss.

Regular exercise (e.g., walking, cycling, jogging, swimming) reduces BP and contributes to weight loss, stress reduction, and feelings of well-being. Previously sedentary patients are encouraged to engage in aerobic exercise for 30–45 minutes per day 5–6 days per week.

A definitive link exists between cigarette smoking and cardiovascular disease. Patients who smoke are strongly urged to quit. Smoking also reduces the effect of some antihypertensive medications, such as propranolol (Inderal). Smoking

Box 16–2
Heart-Healthy Lifestyle Modifications

- Maintain normal body weight; lose weight if overweight.
- Dietary modifications: Eat a diet rich in fruits, vegetables, and low-fat dairy products; reduce sodium intake; reduce intake of cholesterol and of total and saturated fat.
- Limit alcohol intake to no more than 1 oz of ethanol (1/2 oz for women and lighter-weight individuals) per day.
- Engage in aerobic exercise for 30 minutes most days of the week (5–6 days/week).
- Stop smoking.
- Use stress management techniques, such as relaxation therapy.

cessation aids, such as nicotine patches and gum, contain lower amounts of nicotine and usually do not raise BP. Nurses should encourage patients to talk with their healthcare provider before choosing a smoking cessation strategy.

Stress stimulates the SNS, increasing vasoconstriction, SVR, CO, and BP. Regular, moderate exercise is the treatment of choice for reducing stress in patients with cardiovascular disease. Relaxation techniques, such as biofeedback, therapeutic touch, yoga, and meditation, to relax both mind and body may also lower BP, although their effect has not been proven in hypertension management. **Box 16–2 》** outlines health promotion strategies to reduce risks for hypertension and cardiovascular disease.

Nursing Assessment

Nursing assessment (including assessment of pulse and BP) and collection of subjective data are essential to designing the nursing plan of care. Symptoms such as pain, fatigue, and shortness of breath are assessed by the careful questioning of the patient.

Observation and Patient Interview

Signs and symptoms associated with altered perfusion may appear on observation. Observation starts with direct assessment of the patient's actions and appearance as the nurse is interviewing the patient. The nurse should particularly pay attention to the patient's breathing, coughing, skin color and temperature, edema, pregnancy, mental status, and neck vein distension.

Dyspnea and Edema

Dyspnea, or difficulty breathing, may be observed when a patient is experiencing a decrease in oxygenated blood in the circulatory system. This may be attributed to a failure in the body's internal or external respiration by mechanical or chemical means. External respiration provides oxygen to internal respiration when the patient breathes air through the mouth and nose, down the trachea, through the bronchi, and into the bronchioles. Internal respiration is accomplished chemically by alveoli in the lungs when they exchange carbon dioxide from the patient's oxygen-poor venous blood for oxygen inhaled through external respiration. Internal respiration is also accomplished by the cellular and chemical transfer of oxygen for carbon dioxide in the body's tissues.

The myocardial muscle may be unable to adequately move blood from either side of the heart, causing CHF. In this case, the patient may lose his or her breath quickly while talking and/or have a wet sounding cough. In severe exacerbations, the patient may have pulmonary edema, and the wet cough will be accompanied by frothy, pink sputum. The nurse may observe edema in the patient's extremities, especially the legs and feet, because they are the areas farthest from the heart.

Cyanosis and Pallor

The nurse may observe bluish coloration of the skin or cyanosis when perfusion is inadequate, as with hypoxia. Peripheral cyanosis typically is observed in the extremities such as the finger and toenails, but it can also be evident in the patient's lips and mucous membranes. This condition is caused by an increase in unoxygenated hemoglobin in the capillaries. Central cyanosis, which is observed on the patient's trunk and abdomen, is associated with the failure of external respiration and the inability of the lungs to receive oxygen.

Pallor or paleness of the skin can also be observed in those with decreased perfusion. As decreased perfusion progresses, the body shunts blood centrally to the vital organs and brain. This diversion of blood is accomplished by vasoconstriction, which manifests by whiteness or paleness of capillaries secondary to impaired tissue perfusion. Vasoconstriction can also yield cool and dry skin, while vasodilation may cause the patient's skin to feel clammy.

Mental Status

As oxygen becomes unavailable to the brain, the patient's mental status may become altered. The patient may also show signs and symptoms of dizziness and fatigue. This may be apparent by the patient's gait and inability to ambulate as usual. In these situations, the nurse should assess the patient's LOC and orientation to person, place, time, and situation.

Jugular Vein Distention

If the venous blood supply becomes too congested, central venous pressure (CVP) will increase and cause distention of the blood vessels in the neck. As the heart loses its ability to pump blood efficiently, blood vessels that branch off of it directly become engorged with blood. JVD is an abnormal finding that indicates functional or structural deficiency of the circulatory system. It is best assessed when the patient is in semi-Fowler's position.

Patient Interview

An assessment interview to determine problems with cardiac structure and function may be conducted during a health screening or total health assessment or may focus on a chief complaint (e.g., chest pain). If the patient has a problem with cardiac function, the nurse should analyze its onset, characteristics, course, severity, precipitating and relieving factors, and any associated symptoms, noting the timing and circumstances. For example, the nurse should ask the patient with chest pain (also see **Table 16–5 》**):

- What is the location of the chest pain you experienced? Did it move into other areas of your chest, back, neck, jaw, or arm?

TABLE 16–5 Assessing Chest Pain

Characteristic	Examples
Location	Substernal, precordial, jaw, back
	Localized or diffuse
	Radiation to neck, jaw, shoulder, arm
Character/quality	Pressure; tightness; crushing, burning, or aching quality; heaviness; dullness; "heartburn" or indigestion
Timing	Onset: Sudden or gradual?
	Duration: How many minutes does the pain last?
	Frequency: Is the pain continuous or periodic?
Setting/precipitating factors	Awake, at rest, sleep interrupted?
	With activity? With eating, exertion, exercise, elimination, emotional upset?
Intensity/severity	Can range from 0 (*no pain*) to 10 (*worst pain ever felt*)
Aggravating factors	Activity, breathing, temperature
Relieving factors	Medication (nitroglycerin, antacid), rest; there may be no relieving factors
Associated symptoms	Fatigue, shortness of breath, palpitations, nausea and vomiting, sweating, anxiety, lightheadedness, dizziness

- Describe the type of activity that brings on your chest pain.
- Have you felt lightheaded during the times your heart is racing?

The nurse should explore the patient's history for heart disorders, such as angina, heart attack, CHF, hypertension, and valvular disease. The nurse should ask the patient about previous heart surgery or illnesses, such as rheumatic fever, scarlet fever, or recurrent streptococcal throat infections. Also ask about the presence and treatment of other chronic illnesses, such as diabetes mellitus, bleeding disorders, or endocrine disorders. The nurse should then review the patient's family history for CAD, hypertension, stroke, hyperlipidemia, diabetes, congenital heart disease, or sudden death. Questions to ask relate to the patient's medical history, lifestyle, signs and symptoms, sleep and rest, sense of self, and stress and coping ability. Some examples include the following:

Current and Past Medical History

- Have you ever had any problems with your heart, such as angina (pain), heart attack, or disease of the valves? If so, describe. How were these problems treated?
- Have you been diagnosed with high BP? If so, how is it treated?
- Have you had your cholesterol checked recently? If so, what is it? If you have high cholesterol, how is it treated?
- Have you ever had tests to check the function of your heart? If so, describe them.
- Do you take any medications to make your heart function more effectively, such as aspirin, medications to control heart rate, anticoagulants, or diuretics? If so, how often do you take them?
- Do you have a pacemaker? If so, at what age did you receive it, and for what problem? How do you check the batteries?

Lifestyle

- Do you smoke, chew tobacco, or use snuff or e-cigarettes? If so, how often and how much?
- Do you drink alcohol? If so, what type, how much, and for how long?
- Describe your food and liquid intake during a 24-hour period. How often do you eat fried foods, fast foods, or meat?
- How much salt do you use on food?
- Do you eat high-fiber foods? If so, what are they, and how often do you eat them?
- Do you consume energy drinks? If so, what type and how often?

Signs and Symptoms

- Have you had a recent weight gain or loss? Explain.
- Have you noticed any change in the color of your skin (e.g., pale, dusky, flushed)? If so, do you know what causes this?
- Have you had any swelling in your feet or legs? If so, where and how much? What do you do to relieve it?
- Describe any chest pain you have experienced. When did it occur? Where was it located? On a scale of 0–10, with 10 being the worst pain you have ever had, rate the pain and describe it (e.g., burning, crushing, stabbing, squeezing, heavy, tight).
- What were you doing when the pain began (e.g., were you working or resting)? Did it begin suddenly or gradually? How long did it last?
- Did you have any other symptoms with the pain, such as nausea or vomiting, sweating, racing heart, pale skin, or palpitations?
- What made the pain worse? What did you do to try to relieve the pain? Did that work?
- Have you experienced any numbness or tingling, dizziness or lightheadedness, or palpitations? If so, describe.
- Have you ever used oxygen?

Sleep and Rest

- How long do you sleep each night? Do you feel rested after you sleep?
- Does your heart problem interfere with your ability to sleep and rest? Explain.
- How many pillows do you use at night?
- Where do you sleep at night (e.g., in a recliner to breathe more easily)?
- Do you ever feel short of breath while you are resting or sleeping? If so, does this wake you up? Explain.

Self

- How does having this condition make you feel about yourself?
- How does this condition affect your relationships with others?
- Has having this condition interfered with your ability to work? Explain.
- Has this condition interfered with your usual sexual activity?
- Have you ever had chest pain during sexual activity? What do you do for it?

- Has having this condition created stress for you?
- Have you experienced any kind of stress that makes this condition worse? Explain.
- Describe what you do when you feel stressed.
- Describe how specific relationships or activities help you cope with this problem.
- Describe specific cultural beliefs or practices that affect how you care for and feel about this problem.
- Are there any specific treatments that you would not use to treat this problem?

Physical Examination

Four procedures are necessary to perform a complete physical assessment of the cardiovascular system: inspection, palpation, percussion, and auscultation. The nurse gathers objective data during these procedures related to heart function as measured in terms of heart rate and the quality and characteristics of the heart sounds. The nurse also assesses skin color and temperature, abnormal pulsations, and the characteristics of the patient's respiratory effort to observe for signs of appropriate cardiac function related to oxygen perfusion. To know what data gathered during a physical health assessment means, it is necessary to know what is normal and expected in terms of functional parameters and observational findings.

Anatomical Landmarks for Cardiovascular Assessment

The sternum, clavicles, and ribs are examples of anatomical landmarks that assist the assessment of the cardiovascular system. The nurse can make critical observations concerning underlying pathologic mechanisms by correlating assessment findings with the overlying body landmarks. A cardiac assessment uses many of the landmarks identified during the respiratory assessment, including but not limited to the sternum and the second through fifth ICS.

The flat, narrow center bone of the upper anterior chest is the sternum (see **Figure 16–11 》**), which in adults has three parts: upper, or the manubrium; middle, or the body; and inferior, or the xiphoid process. In adults, the average length

of the sternum is 7 in., or 18 cm. The sternum serves as a vertical landmark during cardiovascular assessment. The angle of Louis assists in locating the second ICS. The clavicles attach to the sternum at the top of the manubrium above the first rib. The midclavicular line serves as a landmark for cardiovascular assessment.

The flat, arched bones that form the thoracic cage are the ribs. Ribs form pairs, and there is an ICS between each of 12 pairs of ribs. Each ICS is numbered successively; the first ICS lies between the first and second ribs (see Figure 16–11). The ICS are horizontal landmarks for cardiac assessment that serve to locate the base of the heart and the apex of the heart as well as to auscultate valvular sounds. To locate the second ICS, feel for the angle of Louis, then slide the finger laterally to the second rib, and finally slide the finger down below the rib until reaching the ICS. Locate each succeeding ICS by sliding the finger over the rib into the ICS.

Inspection

A typical adult will exhibit the following characteristics in a visual inspection:

- Skin color should be even and homogeneous over the entire aspect of the body.
- Eye function and appearance should be symmetrical in nature, with pink, moist conjunctiva; white sclera; and clear cornea. The region surrounding the eye, also called the periorbital area, should be level, and the eyes should display no signs of exophthalmos.
- Lips should be smooth in texture with no evidence of cyanosis.
- The head should be fixed and remain upright when unsupported. The skull should be proportionate to the face.
- The skin of the earlobe should be flat with no creases.
- The jugular veins should be flat and not visible unless the patient is sitting at an angle lower than 45 degrees.
- Carotid pulsations can be palpated and auscultated bilaterally with symmetrical appearance.
- The fingernails should be slightly curved or flat with no evidence of cyanosis; the fingers should be round, even, and proportionate.
- Respirations should be regular, even, and unlabored.
- ICS and clavicles should be visible.
- Vasculature of the trunk should be flat and uniform with no visible bulges or masses.
- There should be no pulsations over the pericardium, with only aortic pulsations visible in the suprasternal notch in patients who are thin.
- The temperature and color of the lower extremities should be homogeneous, with uniform and symmetrical hair distribution.
- The skeleton should display no malformations, and the neck and extremities should be in proportion to the torso.
- A slight vibration should be palpable at the apical aspect of the pericardium.

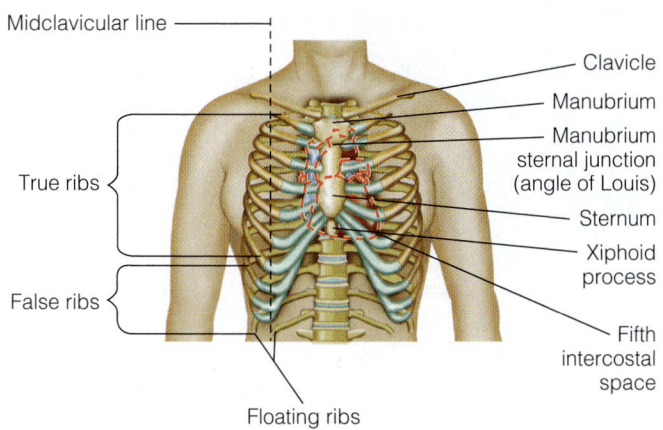

Labels: Midclavicular line, True ribs, False ribs, Floating ribs, Clavicle, Manubrium, Manubrium sternal junction (angle of Louis), Sternum, Xiphoid process, Fifth intercostal space

Figure 16–11 》 Landmarks for cardiovascular assessment.

- There should be a dull percussion over the torso until the midclavicular line intersects at the fifth ICS.
- S_1 and S_2 heart sounds should be equal and audible at the intersection of the third ICS and the LSB or Erb's point.
- No murmurs should be present upon auscultation.

Physical assessment of the cardiovascular system follows an organized pattern:

1. Inspect the patient's head and neck, including the eyes, ears, lips, face, skull, and neck vessels, noting symmetry.
2. Inspect the upper extremities, chest, abdomen, and lower extremities for swelling, masses, tenderness, and excessive warmth.
3. Palpate the precordium and carotid pulses for abnormalities such as crepitus, swelling, masses, tenderness, and excess warmth. Pulsation that correlates with the patient's peripheral pulses should be observed at the PMI or the fourth or fifth ICS at the midclavicular line; this may be difficult in patients who are obese and more prevalent in patients who are thin or have anxiety, hyperthyroidism, or stress.
4. Percuss the chest to determine the cardiac borders.
5. Auscultate the heart in five areas with the diaphragm and the bell of the stethoscope.
   - **Aortic Valve:** Second ICS at RSB
   - **Pulmoic Valve:** Second ICS at LSB

   - **Erb's Point:** Third ICS at LSB
   - **Tricuspid Valve:** Forth or Fifth ICS at LSB
   - **Mitral Valve:** Fifth ICS at midclavicular line.
6. Auscultate the carotid and the apical pulses, noting the presence of bruits at the carotid pulses.

Helpful hints for the physical assessment are listed in **Box 16–3 》**.

Perfusion Assessment

ASSESSMENT/METHOD	NORMAL FINDINGS	ABNORMAL FINDINGS	LIFESPAN OR DEVELOPMENTAL CONSIDERATIONS
Apical Impulse Assessment			
First using the palmar surface and then repeating with finger pads, palpate the precordium for symmetry of movement and the apical impulse for location, size, amplitude, and duration. The sequence for palpation is shown in **Figure 16–12 》**. To locate the apical impulse, ask the patient to assume a left lateral recumbent position. Simultaneous palpation of the carotid pulse may also be helpful.	The apical impulse is not palpable in all patients but may be palpated in the mitral area and has only a brief, small amplitude.	■ An enlarged or displaced heart is associated with an apical impulse lateral to the midclavicular line or below the fifth left ICS.	■ The apical impulse is often not visible in older and pediatric patients. Assessment remains the same as in the adult population.

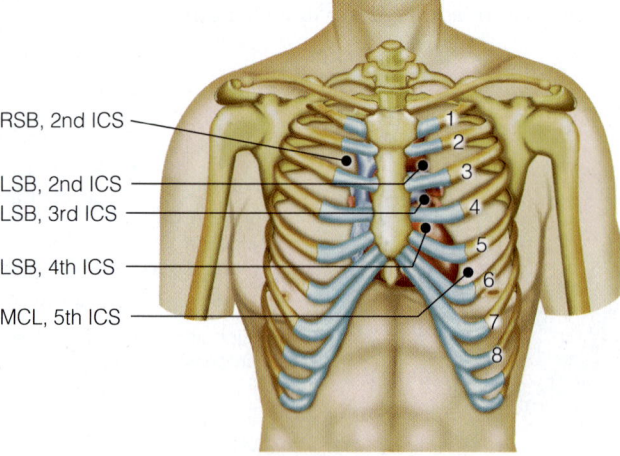

RSB, 2nd ICS
LSB, 2nd ICS
LSB, 3rd ICS
LSB, 4th ICS
MCL, 5th ICS

Figure 16–12 》 Areas for inspection and palpation of the precordium, indicating the sequence for palpation.

Perfusion Assessment *(continued)*

ASSESSMENT/METHOD	NORMAL FINDINGS	ABNORMAL FINDINGS	LIFESPAN OR DEVELOPMENTAL CONSIDERATIONS
		■ Increased size, amplitude, and duration of the apical impulse are associated with left ventricular volume overload (increased afterload) in conditions such as hypertension and aortic stenosis and with pressure overload (increased preload) in conditions such as aortic or mitral regurgitation.	■ When assessing a pediatric patient, it may be more beneficial to auscultate the apical pulse in the area of the left nipple at the fourth ICS.
		■ Increased amplitude alone may occur with hyperkinetic states, such as anxiety, hyperthyroidism, and anemia.	
		■ Decreased amplitude is associated with a dilated heart in cardiomyopathy.	
		■ Displacement alone may also occur with dextrocardia, diaphragmatic hernia, gastric distention, or chronic lung disease.	
		■ A **thrill** (a palpable vibration over the precordium or an artery) may accompany severe valve stenosis.	
		■ A marked increase in amplitude of the apical impulse at the right ventricular area occurs with right ventricular volume overload in atrial septal defect.	
		■ An increase in amplitude and duration occurs with right ventricular pressure overload in pulmonic stenosis and pulmonary hypertension. A lift or heave may also be seen in these conditions and in chronic lung disease.	
		■ A palpable thrill in this area occurs with ventricular septal defect (VSD).	
		■ Right ventricular enlargement may produce a downward pulsation against the fingertips.	
		■ An accentuated pulsation at the pulmonary area may be present in hyperkinetic states.	
		■ A prominent pulsation reflects increased flow or dilation of the pulmonary artery.	
		■ A thrill may be associated with aortic or pulmonary stenosis, aortic stenosis, pulmonary hypertension, or atrial septal defect.	
		■ Increased pulsation at the aortic area may suggest aortic aneurysm.	
		■ A palpable S_2 may be noted with systemic hypertension.	

(continued on next page)

Perfusion Assessment *(continued)*

ASSESSMENT/METHOD	NORMAL FINDINGS	ABNORMAL FINDINGS	LIFESPAN OR DEVELOPMENTAL CONSIDERATIONS
Palpate the subxiphoid area with the index and middle finger.	Diastolic movements of S_3 and S_4 may be felt.	■ Right ventricular enlargement may produce a downward pulsation against the fingertips. ■ An accentuated pulsation at the pulmonary area may be present in hyperkinetic states. ■ A prominent pulsation reflects increased flow or dilation of the pulmonary artery. ■ A thrill may be associated with aortic or pulmonary stenosis, aortic stenosis, pulmonary hypertension, or atrial septal defect. ■ Increased pulsation at the aortic area may suggest aortic aneurysm. ■ A palpable S_2 may be noted with systemic hypertension.	■ This method is useful in patients with an increased anterior-posterior diameter. ■ It is useful in infants because respiratory excursions may interfere with parasternal palpation.

Cardiac Rate and Rhythm Assessment

ASSESSMENT/METHOD	NORMAL FINDINGS	ABNORMAL FINDINGS	LIFESPAN OR DEVELOPMENTAL CONSIDERATIONS
Auscultate heart rate.	The heart rate should be 60–100 bpm, with regular rhythm.	■ A heart rate of more than 100 bpm is tachycardia. A heart rate of less than 60 bpm is bradycardia.	■ Consider using a pediatric chest piece when auscultating heart sounds on a pediatric patient or very thin adult.
Simultaneously palpate the radial pulse while listening to the apical pulse.	The radial and apical pulses should be equal.	■ If the radial pulse falls behind the apical rate, the patient has a **pulse deficit**, indicating weak, ineffective contractions of the left ventricle.	■ Digitalis toxicity may be associated with pulse deficit, especially in older adults. ■ Atrial fibrillation, which is more prevalent in older adults, may cause inefficient left ventricle filling and ejection. This, in turn, can decrease the strength of the peripheral pulses, making them difficult to palpate.
Auscultate heart rhythm.	The heart rhythm should be regular.	■ Dysrhythmias (abnormal heart rate or rhythms) may be regular or irregular in rhythm; their rates may be slow or fast. Irregular rhythms may occur in a pattern (e.g., an early beat every second beat, called bigeminy), sporadically, or with frequency and disorganization (e.g., atrial fibrillation). A pattern of gradual increase and decrease in heart rate that is within the normal range and that correlates with inspiration and expiration is called sinus arrhythmia.	■ Sinus arrhythmia can be a normal variant caused by respirations in pediatric patients.

Perfusion Assessment *(continued)*

ASSESSMENT/METHOD	NORMAL FINDINGS	ABNORMAL FINDINGS	LIFESPAN OR DEVELOPMENTAL CONSIDERATIONS
Heart Sounds Assessment			
See guidelines for cardiac auscultation in **Box 16–4 »**. Identify S_1, and note its intensity. At each auscultatory area, listen for several cardiac cycles. See Figure 16–13 for auscultation areas.	S_1 is loudest at the apex of the heart.	▪ An accentuated S_1 occurs with tachycardia, states in which CO is high (e.g., fever, anxiety, exercise, anemia, stress, hyperthyroidism), complete heart block, and mitral stenosis. ▪ A diminished S_1 occurs with first-degree heart block, mitral regurgitation, CHF, CAD, and pulmonary or systemic hypertension. The intensity is also decreased with obesity, emphysema, and pericardial effusion. Varying intensity of S_1 occurs with complete heart block and grossly irregular rhythms.	▪ Review history for presence of pacemaker. ▪ Presence of asymptomatic bradycardia may not be of importance in older adults.
Listen for splitting of S_1.	Splitting of S_1 may occur during inspiration.	▪ Abnormal splitting of S_1 may be heard with right bundle branch block and premature ventricular contractions (PVCs).	▪ PVCs, which are usually benign in adults, can cause splitting of S_1 heart sound.
Identify S_2, and note its intensity.	S_2 immediately follows S_1 and is loudest at the base of the heart.	▪ An accentuated S_2 may be heard with hypertension, exercise, excitement, and conditions of pulmonary hypertension, such as CHF and cor pulmonale. ▪ A diminished S_2 occurs with aortic stenosis, a fall in systolic BP (shock), and increased anteroposterior chest diameter.	▪ S_2 heart sounds can be more intense in patients who are thin.
Listen for splitting of S_2.	No splitting of S_2 should be heard.	▪ Wide splitting of S_2 is associated with delayed emptying of the right ventricle, resulting in delayed pulmonary valve closure (e.g., mitral regurgitation, pulmonary stenosis, right bundle branch block). ▪ Fixed splitting occurs when right ventricular output is greater than left ventricular output and pulmonary valve closure is delayed (e.g., with atrial septal defect and right ventricular failure). ▪ Paradoxic splitting occurs when closure of the aortic valve is delayed (e.g., left bundle branch block).	▪ Splitting of S_2 heart sounds can be auscultated as a normal variant in older adults who require left ventricle (LV) pacing.
Identify extra heart sounds in systole.	No extra heart sounds should be heard.	▪ Ejection sounds (or clicks) result from the opening of deformed semilunar valves (e.g., aortic and pulmonary stenosis). ▪ A midsystolic click is heard with mitral valve prolapse.	▪ A fourth heart sound is commonly present in older adults without evidence of a cardiovascular event.

(continued on next page)

Perfusion Assessment *(continued)*

ASSESSMENT/METHOD	NORMAL FINDINGS	ABNORMAL FINDINGS	LIFESPAN OR DEVELOPMENTAL CONSIDERATIONS
Identify the presence of extra heart sounds in diastole.	No extra heart sounds should be heard.	▪ An opening snap results from the opening sound of a stenotic mitral valve. ▪ A pathologic S_3 (a third heart sound that immediately follows S_2, called a ventricular gallop) results from myocardial failure and ventricular volume overload (e.g., CHF and mitral or tricuspid regurgitation). ▪ An S_4 (a fourth heart sound that immediately precedes S_1, called an atrial gallop) results from increased resistance to ventricular filling after atrial contraction (e.g., hypertension, CAD, aortic stenosis, cardiomyopathy). ▪ A combined S_3 and S_4 is called a summation gallop and occurs with severe CHF.	▪ Extra heart sounds are considered abnormal in patients of any age.
Identify extra heart sounds in both systole and diastole.	No extra heart sounds should be heard during systole and diastole.	▪ A pericardial friction rub results from inflammation of the pericardial sac, as with pericarditis.	▪ Heart sounds such as murmurs can be audible during both systole and diastole in pediatric patients who are nonpathologic.

Murmur Assessment

Identify any murmurs. Note location, timing, presence during systole or diastole, and intensity.	No murmurs should be heard.	▪ Midsystolic murmurs are heard with semilunar valve disease (e.g., aortic and pulmonary stenosis) and with hypertrophic cardiomyopathy (HCM).	▪ Innocent murmurs do not require treatment.
Use the following scale to grade murmurs: I = Barely heard II = Quietly heard III = Clearly heard IV = Loud V = Very loud VI = Loudest; may be heard with stethoscope off the chest. (A thrill may accompany murmurs of grade IV to grade VI.) Note pitch (low, medium, or high), and quality (harsh, blowing, or musical). Note pattern/shape, crescendo, decrescendo, and radiation/transmission (to axilla or neck).		▪ Pansystolic (holosystolic) murmurs are heard with AV valve disease (e.g., mitral and tricuspid regurgitation, ventricular septal defect). ▪ A late systolic murmur is heard with mitral valve prolapse. ▪ Early diastolic murmurs occur with regurgitant flow across incompetent semilunar valves (e.g., aortic regurgitation). ▪ Mid-diastolic and presystolic murmurs, such as with mitral stenosis, occur with turbulent flow across the AV valves. ▪ Continuous murmurs throughout systole and all or part of diastole occur with patent ductus arteriosus (PDA).	▪ Pulmonary flow murmurs, still murmurs, and venous hums are often seen in children as a normal part of development. They do not require treatment.

Box 16–4

Guidelines for Cardiac Auscultation

1. Locate the major auscultatory areas on the precordium (see **Figure 16–13 》**).
2. Choose a sequence of listening. Either begin from the apex and move upward along the sternal border to the base, or begin at the base and move downward to the apex. One suggested sequence is shown in Figure 16–13.
3. Listen first with the patient in the sitting or supine position. Then, ask the patient to lie on his or her left side, and focus on the apex. Finally, ask the patient to sit up and lean forward. These position changes bring the heart closer to the chest wall and enhance auscultation. Carry out the following steps when the patient assumes each of these positions:
   a. First, auscultate each area with the diaphragm of the stethoscope to listen for high-pitched sounds (S_1, S_2, murmurs, and pericardial friction rubs).
   b. Next, auscultate each area with the bell of the stethoscope to listen for lower-pitched sounds (S_3, S_4, and murmurs).
   c. Listen for the effect of respirations on each sound. While the patient is sitting up and leaning forward, ask the patient to exhale and hold the breath while you listen to heart sounds.

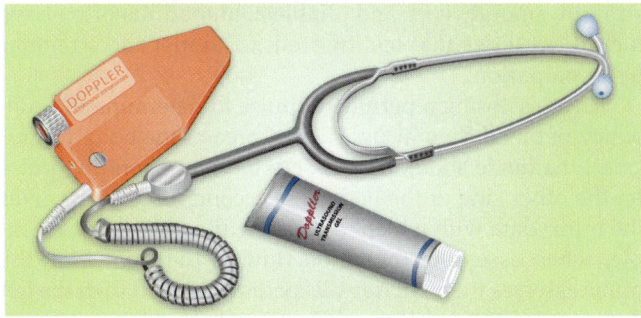

Source: Rick Brady/Pearson Education, Inc.

Figure 16–14 》 A Doppler ultrasound stethoscope (DUS).

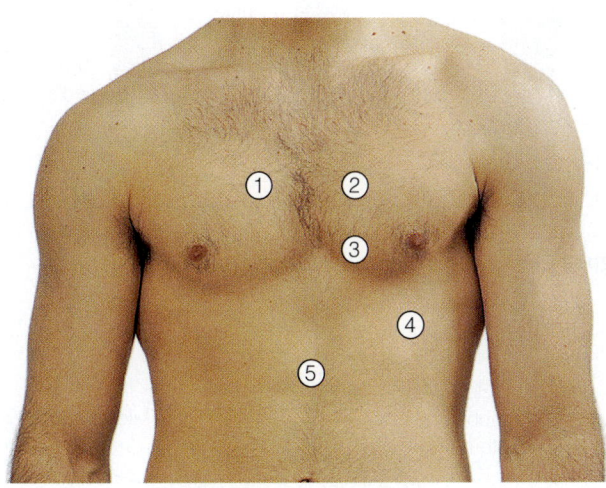

Figure 16–13 》 Areas for auscultation of the heart.

Assessing the Pulse

A pulse is commonly assessed by palpation (feeling) or auscultation (hearing). The middle three fingertips are used for palpating all pulse sites except the apex of the heart, which requires a stethoscope. A Doppler ultrasound stethoscope (DUS; see **Figure 16–14 》**) is used for pulses that are difficult to assess. The DUS has earpieces similar to standard stethoscope earpieces, but it has a long cord attached to a volume-controlled audio unit and an ultrasound transducer. The DUS detects movement of RBCs through a blood vessel. In contrast to conventional stethoscopes, it excludes environmental sounds.

A pulse is normally palpated by applying moderate pressure with the three middle fingers of the hand. The pads on the most distal aspects of the finger are the most sensitive areas for detecting a pulse. Using excessive pressure can obliterate a pulse, whereas too little pressure may fail to detect it. Before the nurse assesses the resting pulse, the patient should assume a comfortable position. The nurse should also be aware of the following:

- Any medication that could affect the heart rate.
- Whether the patient has been physically active. If so, wait 10–15 minutes until the patient has rested and the pulse has slowed to its usual rate.
- Any baseline data about the normal heart rate for the patient. For example, a physically fit athlete may have a heart rate below 60 bpm.
- Whether the patient should assume a particular position (e.g., sitting). In some patients, the rate changes with the position because of changes in blood flow volume and autonomic nervous system activity.

When assessing the pulse, the nurse collects the following data: the rate, rhythm, volume, arterial wall elasticity, and bilateral equality. An excessively fast heart rate (e.g., over 100 bpm in an adult) is referred to as **tachycardia**. A heart rate in an adult of less than 60 bpm is called **bradycardia**. If a patient has either tachycardia or bradycardia, the apical pulse should be assessed.

The **pulse rhythm** is the pattern of the beats and the intervals between the beats. Equal time elapses between beats of a normal pulse. A pulse with an irregular rhythm is referred to as a **dysrhythmia** or **arrhythmia**. It may consist of random, irregular beats or a predictable pattern of irregular beats (documented as "regularly irregular"). When a dysrhythmia is detected, the apical pulse should be assessed. An ECG is necessary to define the dysrhythmia further.

Pulse volume, also called the pulse strength or amplitude, refers to the force of blood with each beat. The pulse volume is usually the same with each beat. It can range from absent to bounding. A normal pulse can be felt with moderate pressure of the fingers and can be obliterated with greater pressure. A forceful or full blood volume that is obliterated only with difficulty is called a full or bounding pulse. A pulse that is readily obliterated with pressure from the fingers is referred to as weak, feeble, or thready.

The elasticity of the arterial wall reflects its expansibility or its deformities. A healthy, normal artery feels straight, smooth, soft, and pliable. Older adults often have inelastic arteries that feel twisted (tortuous) and irregular upon palpation.

When assessing a peripheral pulse to determine the adequacy of blood flow to a particular area of the body (perfusion), the nurse should also assess the corresponding pulse on the other side of the body. The second assessment gives the nurse data with which to compare the pulses. For example, when assessing the blood flow to the right foot, the nurse assesses the right dorsalis pedis pulse and then the left dorsalis pedis pulse. If the patient's right and left pulses are the same, the patient's dorsalis pedis pulses are bilaterally equal. The pulse rate does not need to be counted when assessing for perfusion and equality.

When a peripheral pulse is located, it indicates that pulses more proximal to that location will also be present. For example, if the dorsalis pedis, the most distal pulse of the lower extremity, cannot be felt, the nurse next palpates for the posterior tibial pulse. If it is not felt, the popliteal pulse must be assessed. If the popliteal pulse is found, it is not necessary to assess the femoral pulse since it must also be present in order for the more distal pulse to exist.

Pulse Sites

A pulse may be measured in nine sites (see **Figure 16–15** »).

1. **Temporal**, where the temporal artery passes over the temporal bone of the head. The site is superior (above) and lateral to (away from the midline of) the eye.
2. **Carotid**, at the side of the neck where the carotid artery runs between the trachea and the sternocleidomastoid muscle.

SAFETY ALERT Never press both carotids at the same time because this can cause a reflex drop in BP or pulse rate.

---

3. **Apical**, at the apex of the heart. In an adult, this is located on the left side of the chest, about 8 cm (3 in.) to the left of the sternum (breastbone) and at the fourth, fifth, or sixth ICS. In older adults, the apex may be further left if any health conditions have resulted in an enlarged heart. Before 4 years of age, the apex is left of the midclavicular line (MCL); between 4 and 6 years, it is at the MCL (see **Figure 16–16** »). For a child 7–9 years of age, the apical pulse is located at the fourth or fifth ICS.
4. **Brachial**, at the inner aspect of the biceps muscle of the arm or medially in the antecubital space.
5. **Radial**, where the radial artery runs along the radial bone, on the thumb side of the inner aspect of the wrist.
6. **Femoral**, where the femoral artery passes alongside the inguinal ligament.
7. **Popliteal**, where the popliteal artery passes behind the knee.
8. **Posterior tibial**, on the medial surface of the ankle where the posterior tibial artery passes behind the medial malleolus.
9. **Pedal (dorsalis pedis)**, where the dorsalis pedis artery passes over the bones of the foot, on an imaginary line drawn from the middle of the ankle to the

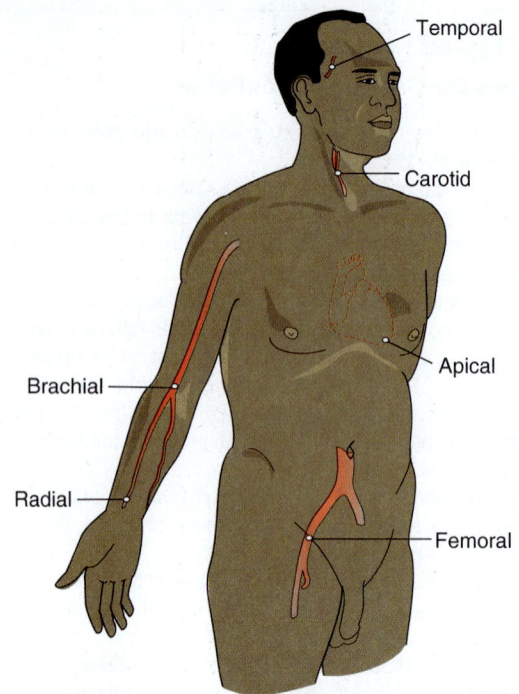

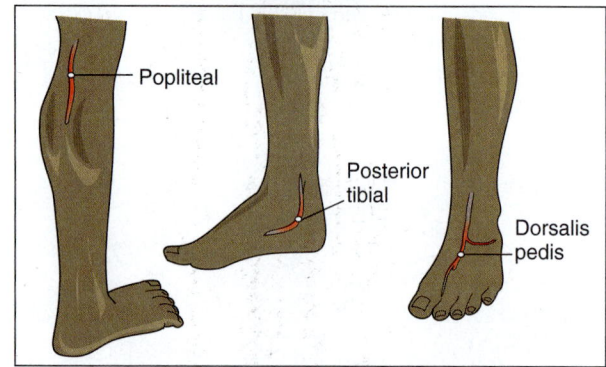

Figure 16–15 » Nine sites for assessing pulse.

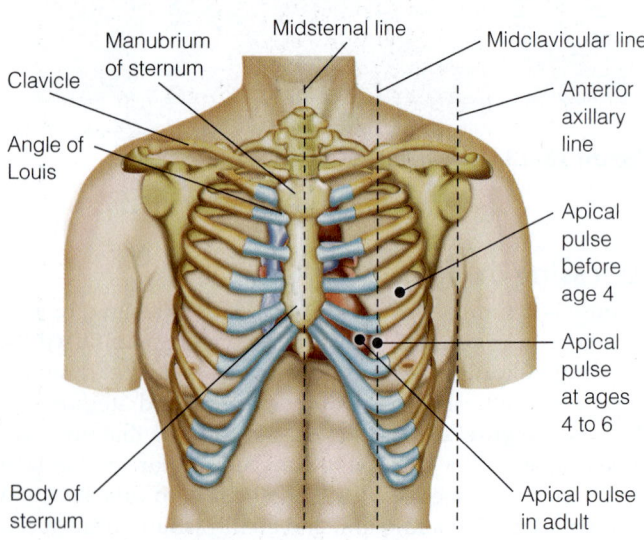

Figure 16–16 » Location of the apical pulse for a child under 4 years old, a child 4–6 years old, and an adult.

TABLE 16–6 Reasons for Using Specific Pulse Site

Pulse Site	Reasons for Use
Radial	Readily accessible
Temporal	Used when radial pulse is not accessible
Carotid	Used during cardiac arrest/shock in adults
	Used to determine circulation to the brain
Apical	Routinely used for infants and children up to 3 years of age
	Used to determine discrepancies with radial pulse
	Used in conjunction with some medications
Brachial	Used to measure BP
	Used during cardiac arrest for infants
Femoral	Used in cases of cardiac arrest/shock
	Used to determine circulation to the leg
Popliteal	Used to determine circulation to the lower leg
Posterior tibial	Used to determine circulation to the foot
Pedal	Used to determine circulation to the foot

space between the big and second toes. The radial site is most commonly used in adults. It is easily found in most people and readily accessible. Some reasons for use of each site are given in **Table 16–6 》**.

Apical Pulse Assessment

The nurse should assess the apical pulse in patients whose peripheral pulse is irregular or unavailable as well as in patients with known cardiovascular, pulmonary, and renal diseases. It is commonly assessed prior to administering medications that affect heart rate. The apical site is also used to assess the pulse for newborns, infants, and children 2–3 years old.

Apical-Radial Pulse Assessment

An **apical-radial pulse** may need to be assessed for patients with certain cardiovascular disorders. The apical and radial rates are normally identical. An apical pulse rate greater than a radial pulse rate can indicate that the thrust of the blood from the heart is too weak for the wave to be felt at the peripheral pulse site, or it can indicate that vascular disease is preventing impulses from being transmitted. Any discrepancy between the two pulse rates is called a pulse deficit and needs to be reported promptly. In no instance is the radial pulse greater than the apical pulse.

Patients who need to monitor their pulse at home should be provided patient teaching related to taking and recording a pulse. The nurse may need to assist the patient in obtaining and using an electronic pulse device or taking a pulse manually (see Patient Teaching feature).

Assessing Blood Pressure

BP is measured with a BP cuff and a sphygmomanometer. The BP cuff consists of a rubber bag (a bladder) that can be inflated with air. It is covered with cloth and has two tubes attached to it. One tube connects to a rubber bulb that inflates the bladder. A small valve on the side of this bulb traps and releases the air in the bladder. The other tube is

Patient Teaching
Monitoring Pulse in the Home

- Teach patients to monitor their pulse manually prior to taking medications that affect the heart rate. Tell patients to report any notable changes in heart rate or rhythm (regularity) to the healthcare provider.
- Using an index and middle finger, palpate the radial artery on the ventral side of the wrist toward the same side as the thumb.
- Using a clock with a second hand, count the number of palpations in 60 seconds.
- Keep a log of the intensity, regularity, and rate of your pulse, including the date and time the pulse was taken.

attached to a sphygmomanometer. The sphygmomanometer indicates the pressure of the air within the bladder.

The two types of sphygmomanometers are aneroid and digital. The aneroid sphygmomanometer is a calibrated dial with a needle that points to the calibrations (see **Figure 16–17A 》**), and the sounds of the patient's systolic and diastolic BPs are heard through a stethoscope. Digital (electronic) sphygmomanometers (see Figure 16–17B), which eliminate the need for a stethoscope, are used in many agencies. Electronic BP devices should be calibrated periodically to check accuracy. All healthcare facilities should have manual BP equipment available as backup.

DUSs are also used to assess BP (see Figure 16–14). These are of particular value when BP sounds are difficult to hear, such as in infants, patients with obesity, and patients in

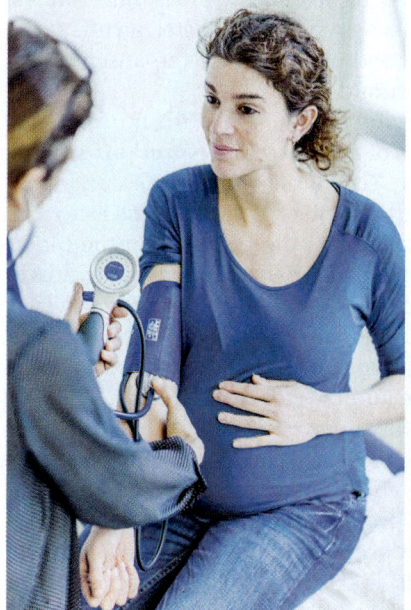
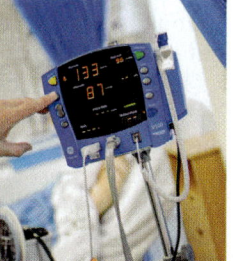

A   *B*

Sources: A, Phanie/Alamy Stock Photo; *B,* Wunkley/Alamy Stock Photo.

Figure 16–17 》 A, An aneroid sphygmomanometer and cuff. **B,** An electronic blood pressure monitor registers systolic and diastolic blood pressures and often other vital signs.

shock. Systolic pressure may be the only BP obtainable with some ultrasound models.

Blood Pressure Sites

The BP is typically assessed in the patient's upper arm using the brachial artery and a standard stethoscope. Assessing the BP on a patient's thigh may be indicated in these situations:

- The BP cannot be measured on either arm (e.g., because of burns or other trauma).
- The BP in one thigh is to be compared with the BP in the other thigh.

BP is not measured on a particular patient's limb in the following situations:

- The shoulder, arm, or hand (or the hip, knee, or ankle) is injured or diseased.
- A cast or bulky bandage is on any part of the limb.
- The patient has had surgical removal of axilla (or hip) lymph nodes on that side, such as for cancer.
- The patient has an IV infusion in that limb.
- The patient has an arteriovenous fistula (e.g., for renal dialysis) in that limb.

Methods

BP can be assessed directly or indirectly. Direct (invasive monitoring) measurement involves the insertion of a catheter into the brachial, radial, or femoral artery. Arterial pressure is represented as wavelike forms displayed on a monitor. With correct placement, this pressure reading is highly accurate.

Two noninvasive methods of measuring BP are the auscultatory and palpatory methods. The auscultatory method is most commonly used in hospitals, clinics, and homes. Required equipment is a sphygmomanometer, a cuff, and a stethoscope. When carried out correctly, the auscultatory method is relatively accurate.

When taking a BP using a stethoscope, the nurse identifies phases in the series of sounds called **Korotkoff sounds** (see **Figure 16–18 »**). The nurse pumps the cuff up to about 30 mmHg above the point where the pulse is no longer felt, which is identified as the point when the blood flow in the artery is stopped. The pressure is then slowly released (2–3 mmHg per second) while the nurse observes the readings on the manometer and relates them to the sounds heard through the stethoscope. Five phases occur but may not always be audible (see **Box 16–5 »**).

The palpatory method may be used if the Korotkoff sounds cannot be heard and electronic equipment to amplify the sounds is not available. It may also be used to prevent misdirection from the presence of an auscultatory gap. An *auscultatory gap,* which occurs particularly in patients who have hypertension, is the temporary disappearance of sounds normally heard over the brachial artery when the cuff pressure is high followed by the reappearance of the sounds at a lower level. This temporary disappearance of sounds occurs in the latter part of phase 1 and phase 2 and may cover a range of 40 mmHg. If a palpated estimation of the systolic pressure is not made prior to auscultation, the nurse may begin listening in the middle of this range and

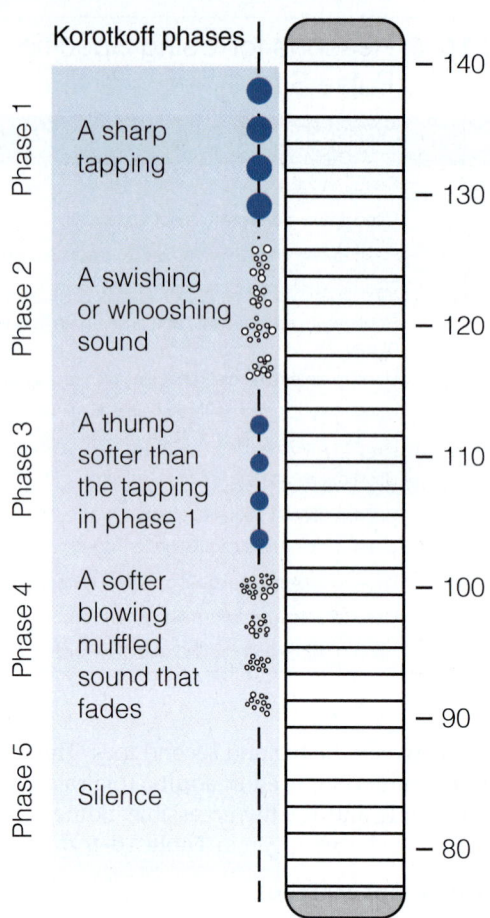

Figure 16–18 » Korotkoff sounds can be differentiated into five phases. In the illustration, the blood pressure is 138/90 or 138/102/90 mmHg.

Box 16–5
Korotkoff Sounds

- **Phase 1.** The pressure level at which the first faint, clear tapping or thumping sounds are heard. These sounds gradually become more intense. To ensure that they are not extraneous sounds, the nurse should identify at least two consecutive tapping sounds. The first tapping sound heard during deflation of the cuff is the systolic BP.
- **Phase 2.** The period during deflation when the sounds have a muffled, whooshing, or swishing quality.
- **Phase 3.** The period during which the blood flows freely through an increasingly open artery and the sounds become crisper and more intense and again assume a thumping quality but softer than in phase 1.
- **Phase 4.** The time when the sounds become muffled and have a soft, blowing quality.
- **Phase 5.** The pressure level when the last sound is heard. This is followed by a period of silence. The pressure at which the last sound is heard is the diastolic BP in adults.*

*In agencies where the fourth phase is considered the diastolic pressure, three measures are recommended (systolic pressure, diastolic pressure, and phase 5). These may be referred to as systolic, first diastolic, and second diastolic pressures. The phase 5 (second diastolic pressure) reading may be zero; that is, the muffled sounds are heard even when there is no air pressure in the BP cuff. In some instances, muffled sounds may not be heard. In this case, a dash is inserted where the reading would normally be recorded (e.g., –/–/110 mmHg).

underestimate the systolic pressure. In the palpatory method of BP determination, instead of listening for the blood flow sounds, the nurse uses light to moderate pressure to palpate the pulsations of the artery as the pressure in the cuff is released. The pressure is read from the sphygmomanometer when the first pulsation is felt.

Common Errors in Assessing Blood Pressure

The importance of the accuracy of BP assessments cannot be overemphasized. Many assessments of a patient's health are made on the basis of BP, which is an important indicator of the patient's condition and is used as a basis for identifying nursing interventions. Two possible reasons for BP errors are haste on the part of the nurse and subconscious bias. For example, a nurse may be influenced by the patient's previous BP measurements or diagnosis and "hear" a value consistent with the practitioner's expectations. Some reasons for erroneous BP readings are given in **Table 16–7 》》**.

SAFETY ALERT Electronic/automatic BP cuffs can be left in place for many hours. Remove the cuff and check skin condition periodically.

Hypotension

Hypotension is a below normal BP reading—one that is consistently between 85 and 110 mmHg in an individual whose baseline BP is typically higher. **Orthostatic hypotension** is a BP that falls when the patient sits or stands. It usually results from peripheral vasodilation in which blood leaves the central body organs, especially the brain, and moves to the periphery, often causing the individual to feel lightheaded or faint. Causes of hypotension include dehydration, bleeding, severe burns, and use of certain

TABLE 16–7 Selected Sources of Error in Blood Pressure Assessment

Error	Effect
Bladder cuff too narrow	Erroneously high
Bladder cuff too wide	Erroneously low
Arm unsupported	Erroneously high
Insufficient rest before the assessment	Erroneously high
Repeating assessment too quickly	Erroneously high systolic or low diastolic readings
Cuff wrapped too loosely or unevenly	Erroneously high
Deflating cuff too quickly	Erroneously low systolic and high diastolic readings
Deflating cuff too slowly	Erroneously high diastolic reading
Failure to use the same arm consistently	Inconsistent measurements
Arm above level of the heart	Erroneously low
Assessing immediately after a meal or while patient smokes or has pain	Erroneously high
Failure to identify ausculatory gap	Erroneously low systolic pressure and erroneously low diastolic pressure

Patient Teaching
Taking Blood Pressure Readings in the Home

- Rest for at least 5 minutes before taking a BP measurement. Wait 30 minutes after drinking any caffeinated beverage, using tobacco, or exercising before taking a measurement. Do not take BP measurements when under stress.

- Sit still in a chair, feet flat on the floor and legs uncrossed, with the upper arm bare and supported so that it is at heart level.

- Wrap the BP cuff around the arm so that it fits snugly with the lower edge about an inch above the bend of the elbow. The middle of the cuff must be directly above the eye of the elbow. It may be necessary to show the patient exactly how to do this.

- Inflate the cuff quickly, either by pumping the squeeze bulb or pushing a button, to the point that it feels tight around the arm. It will feel slightly uncomfortable.

- Open the valve slightly to allow the pressure to fall slowly.

- As the pressure falls, record the systolic pressure by noting the reading at the point that the sound of blood pulsing is first audible.

- As the pressure continues to fall, record the diastolic pressure by noting the reading at the point that the sound of blood pulsing ceases to be audible.

- Measure at the same times daily, such as morning and evening. For each measurement session, take several readings a minute apart.

- Accurately record all results. BP is optimal when it is less than 120/80 mmHg most of the time. If several high readings are recorded, not just one, the patient should contact a healthcare professional. A reading of more than 180/110 mmHg, if accurate, is indicative of hypertensive crisis, and emergency medical treatment is required.

Sources: Data from American Heart Association (AHA). (2016a). *Monitoring your blood pressure at home*. Retrieved from http://www.heart.org/HEARTORG/Conditions/HighBloodPressure/KnowYourNumbers/Monitoring-Your-Blood-Pressure-at-Home_UCM_301874_Article.jsp#.WOTqKPnyuUk; Cleveland Clinic. (2014). *Checking your blood pressure at home*. Retrieved from https://my.clevelandclinic.org/health/diseases_conditions/hic_Hypertension_High_Blood_Pressure/hic_Checking_Your_Blood_Pressure_at_Home; U.S. National Library of Medicine. (2014a). *Blood pressure measurement*. Retrieved from https://www.nlm.nih.gov/medlineplus/ency/article/007490.htm

analgesics. Patients with hypotension should be carefully monitored for fall risks.

Patients at risk for hypo- or hypertension may need to take BP readings at home. If this is the case, the nurse should ensure that the equipment the patient uses is calibrated against a system known to be accurate and ensure the patient knows how to take accurate and useful BP measurements (see the Patient Teaching feature).

Diagnostic Tests

The results of diagnostic tests of cardiac function are used to support the diagnosis of a specific disease, to provide information to identify or modify the appropriate medications or therapy used to treat the disease, and to help nurses monitor the patient's responses to treatment and nursing interventions. Diagnostic tests appropriate for determining cardiac function may include:

- Serum cholesterol, triglycerides, and lipids
- Stress/exercise tests
- X-ray, MRI, CT, or positron-emission tomography
- Echocardiogram
- Transesophageal echocardiography

- Cardiac catheterization with either coronary angiography or coronary arteriography
- Pericardiocentesis
- Electrocardiography (see **Boxes 16–6** ›› and **16–7** ››)
- Troponin, MB isoenzyme of creatine kinase (CK).

Regardless of the type of diagnostic test, the nurse is responsible for explaining the procedure and any special preparation needed, assessing for medication use that may

Box 16–6
The Electrocardiogram

The **electrocardiogram (ECG)** is a graphic record of the heart's activity. Electrodes applied to the body surface are used to obtain a graphic representation of cardiac electrical activity. These electrodes detect the magnitude and direction of electrical currents produced in the heart. They attach to the ECG by an insulated wire called a **lead**. The electrocardiograph converts the electrical impulses it receives into a series of waveforms that represent cardiac depolarization and repolarization. Placement of electrodes on different parts of the body allows different views of this electrical activity, much like turning the head while holding a camera provides different views of the scenery. ECG waveforms and patterns are examined to detect dysrhythmias as well as myocardial damage, effects of drugs, and electrolyte imbalances.

The ECG waveforms reflect the direction of electrical flow in relation to a positive electrode. Current flowing toward the positive electrode produces an upward (positive) waveform; current flowing away from the positive electrode produces a downward (negative) waveform. Current flowing perpendicular to the positive pole produces a biphasic (both positive and negative) waveform. Absence of electrical activity is represented by a straight line, the **isoelectric line**.

The ECG waveforms are recorded by a heated stylus and reproduced on heat-sensitive paper. The paper is marked at standard intervals representing time and voltage or amplitude (see **Figure 16–19** ››). Each small box is 1 mm². The recording speed of the standard ECG is 25 mm/second, so each small box represents 0.04 second. Five small boxes horizontally and vertically make one large box, equivalent to 0.20 second. Five large boxes represent 1 full second. Measured vertically, each small box represents 0.1 mV.

Both bipolar and unipolar leads are used in recording the ECG. A bipolar lead uses two electrodes of opposite polarity (negative and positive). A unipolar lead uses one positive electrode and a negative reference point at the center of the heart. The electrical potential between the two monitoring points is graphically recorded as the ECG waveform.

The heart can be viewed from both the frontal plane and the horizontal plane (see **Figure 16–20** ››). The frontal plane is an imaginary cut through the body that views the heart from top to bottom (superior to inferior) and side to side (right to left). This perspective of the heart is analogous to a paper doll cutout. It provides information about the inferior and lateral walls of the heart. The horizontal plane is a cross-sectional view of the heart

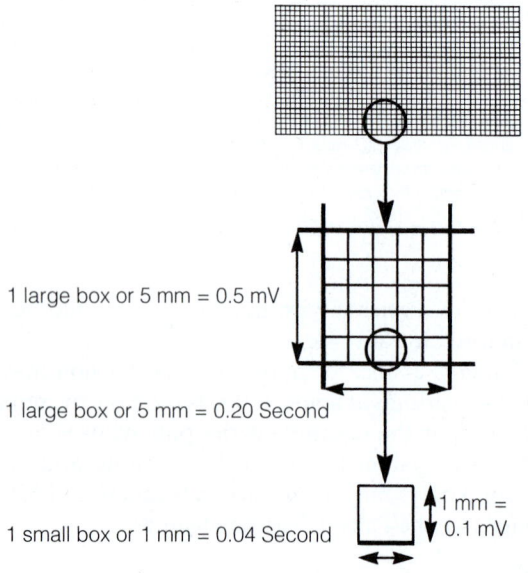

1 large box or 5 mm = 0.5 mV

1 large box or 5 mm = 0.20 Second

1 small box or 1 mm = 0.04 Second   1 mm = 0.1 mV

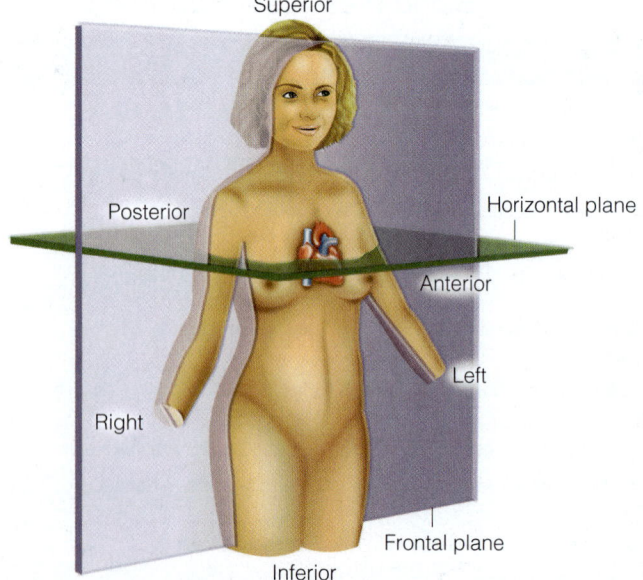

Superior

Posterior

Horizontal plane

Anterior

Right

Left

Frontal plane

Inferior

Figure 16–19 ›› Time and voltage measurements on ECG paper at a recording speed of 25 mm/second.

Figure 16–20 ›› Planes of the heart. Frontal plane, Horizontal plane.

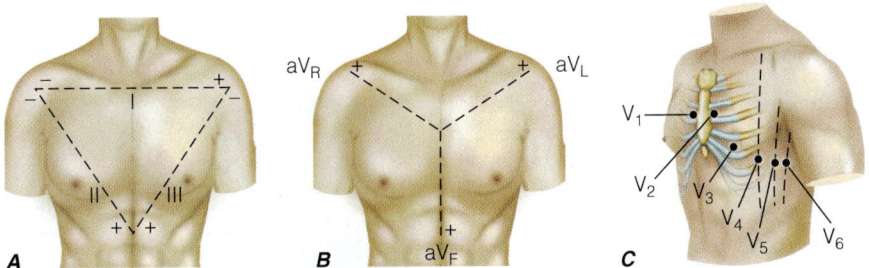

Figure 16–21 ❯❯ Leads of the 12-lead ECG. **A,** Bipolar limb leads I, II, III. **B,** Unipolar limb leads aV$_R$, aV$_L$, aV$_F$. **C,** Unipolar precordial leads V$_1$–V$_6$.

from front to back (anterior to posterior) and side to side (right to left). Information regarding the anterior, septal, and lateral walls of the heart, as well as the posterior wall, is obtained from this view.

A standard 12-lead ECG provides a simultaneous recording of six limb leads and six precordial leads (see **Figure 16–21** ❯❯). The limb leads provide information about the heart in the frontal plane and include three bipolar leads (I, II, and III) and three unipolar leads (aV$_R$, aV$_L$, and aV$_F$). The bipolar limb leads measure electrical activity between a negative lead on one extremity and a positive lead on another. The unipolar limb leads (called augmented leads) measure the electrical activity between a single positive electrode on a limb (right arm [R], left arm [L], or left leg [F for foot]), and the center of the heart.

The precordial leads, also known as chest leads or V leads, view the heart in the horizontal plane. They include six unipolar leads (V$_1$, V$_2$, V$_3$, V$_4$, V$_5$, and V$_6$) that measure electrical activity between the center of the heart and a positive electrode on the chest wall.

The cardiac cycle is depicted as a series of waveforms, the P, Q, R, S, T, and U waves (see **Figure 16–22** ❯❯):

- The *P wave* represents atrial depolarization and contraction. The impulse is from the SA node. The P wave precedes the QRS complex and is normally smooth, round, and upright. P waves may be absent when the SA node is not acting as the pacemaker. Atrial repolarization occurs during ventricular depolarization and usually is not seen on the ECG.
- The *PR interval* represents the time required for the sinus impulse to travel to the AV node and into the Purkinje fibers. This interval is measured from the beginning of the P wave to the beginning of the QRS complex. If no Q wave is seen, the beginning of the R wave is used. The PR interval is normally 0.12–0.20 second (up to 0.24 second is considered normal in patients over age 65). PR intervals greater than 0.20 second indicate a delay in conduction from the SA node to the ventricles.
- The *QRS complex* represents ventricular depolarization and contraction. The QRS complex includes three separate waves: The Q wave is the first negative deflection, the R wave is the positive or upright deflection, and the S wave is the first negative deflection after the R wave. All three waves may not be present in every QRS, but the name remains unchanged. The normal duration of a QRS complex is less than 0.12 second. QRS complexes of greater than 0.12 second indicate delays in transmitting the impulse through the ventricular conduction system.

- The *ST segment* signifies the beginning of ventricular repolarization. The ST segment, which is the period from the end of the QRS complex to the beginning of the T wave, should be isoelectric. An abnormal ST segment is displaced (elevated or depressed) from the isoelectric line.
- The *T wave* represents ventricular repolarization. It normally has a smooth, rounded shape that is usually less than 10 mm tall. It usually points in the same direction as the QRS complex. Abnormalities of the T wave may indicate myocardial ischemia or injury or electrolyte imbalances.
- The *QT interval* is measured from the beginning of the QRS complex to the end of the T wave. It represents the total time of ventricular depolarization and repolarization. Its duration varies with gender, age, and heart rate; it is usually 0.32–0.44 second long. Prolonged QT intervals indicate a prolonged relative refractory period and a greater risk of dysrhythmias. Shortened QT intervals may result from medications or electrolyte imbalances.
- The *U wave* is not normally seen. It is thought to signify repolarization of the terminal Purkinje fibers. If present, the U wave follows the same direction as the T wave. It is most commonly seen in hypokalemia.

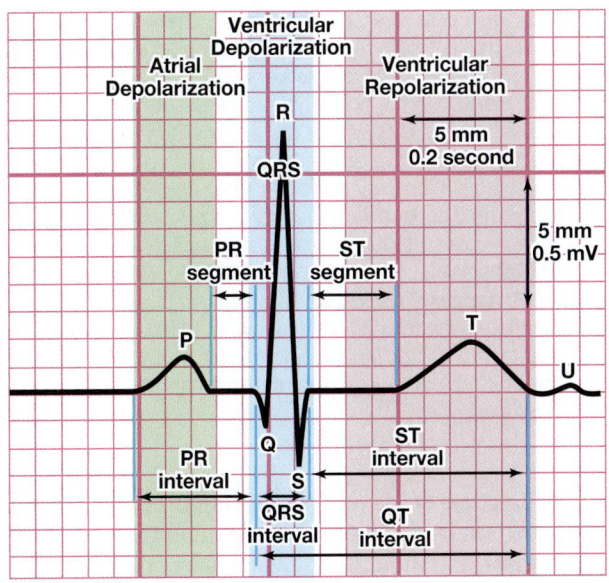

Figure 16–22 ❯❯ Normal ECG waveform and intervals.

Box 16–7
Interpreting an Electrocardiogram

Interpreting an ECG strip to determine the cardiac rhythm is a skill that takes practice to learn and master. Many methods are used to analyze ECGs, and it is important to use a consistent method for such analysis. Identifying and interpreting complex dysrhythmias require advanced skills and knowledge obtained through further training. One method for analyzing an ECG strip is the following:

- **Step 1: Determine rate.** Assess heart rate. Use P waves to determine the atrial rate and R waves for the ventricular rate. Several approaches can determine the heart rate:
  a. Count the number of complexes in a 6-second rhythm strip (the top margin of ECG paper is marked at 3-second intervals), and multiply by 10. This provides an estimate of the rate and is particularly valuable if rhythms are irregular.
  b. Count the number of large boxes between two consecutive complexes, and divide 300 (the number of large boxes in 1 min) by this number. For example, there are 6 large boxes between two R waves; 300 divided by 6 equals a ventricular rate of 50 bpm. Memorize the following sequence for rapid rate determination: 300, 150, 100, 75, 60, 50, 43. One large box between complexes equals a rate of 300; two large boxes, a rate of 150; three, a rate of 100; and so forth.
  c. Count the number of small boxes between two consecutive complexes, and divide 1500 (the number of small boxes in 1 min) by this number. For example, there are 19 small boxes between two R waves; 1500 divided by 19 equals a ventricular rate of 79 bpm. This is the most precise measurement of heart rate.
- **Step 2: Determine regularity.** Regularity is the consistency with which the P waves or QRS complexes occur. In a regular rhythm, all waves occur at a consistent rate. Rhythm regularity is determined by measuring the interval between consecutive waves. Place one point of an ECG caliper (a measuring device) on the peak of the P wave (for atrial rhythm) or the R wave (for ventricular rhythm). Adjust the other point to the peak of the next wave, P to P or R to R (see **Figure 16–23** 》). Keeping the calipers set at this distance, evaluate the intervals between consecutive waves. The rhythm is regular if all caliper points fall on succeeding wave peaks. As an alternative, use a strip of blank paper on top of the ECG strip, and mark the peaks of two or three consecutive waves. Then, move the paper along the strip to consecutive waves. Wave peaks that vary by more than one to three small boxes (depending on the rate) are irregular. Irregular rhythms may be irregularly irregular (if the intervals have no pattern) or regularly irregular (if a consistent pattern to the irregularity can be identified).
- **Step 3: Assess P waves.** The presence or absence of P waves helps determine the origin of the rhythm. All the P waves should be alike in size and shape (morphology). If P waves are not seen or if they differ in shape, the rhythm may not originate in the SA node.

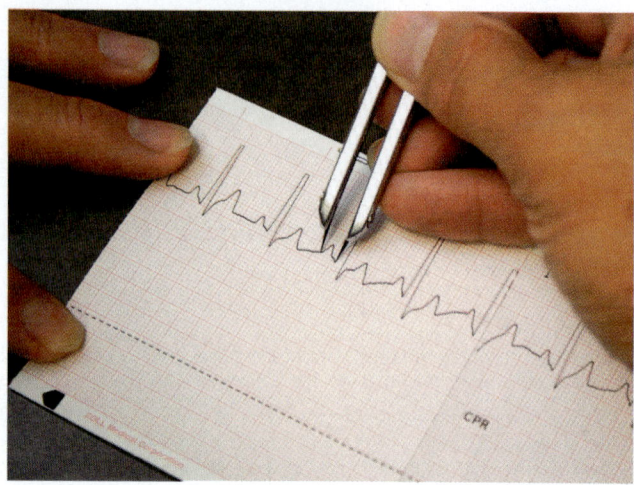

Source: London Robert/Pearson Education, Inc.

Figure 16–23 》 Using calipers to evaluate intervals between consecutive waves.

- **Step 4: Assess the P to QRS relationship.** Determine the relationship between P waves and QRS complexes. There should be one—and only one—P wave for every QRS complex, because the normal stimulus for ventricular contraction originates in the SA node.
- **Step 5: Determine interval durations.** To evaluate impulse transmission through the cardiac conduction system, measure the PR interval, QRS duration, and QT interval. To measure, count the number of small boxes from the beginning of the interval to the end, and multiply by 0.04 second. Then, determine whether the interval duration is within its normal limits. For example, assume the PR interval is 3.5 small boxes wide, or 0.14 second. This is within the normal limits of 0.12–0.20 second. This interval should be consistent, not varying from beat to beat. A PR interval of greater than 0.20 second or one that varies from beat to beat is abnormal.

The QRS complex duration is normally between 0.06 and 0.10 second. A QRS complex of greater than 0.12 second indicates delayed ventricular conduction.

The QT interval is normally 0.32–0.44 second. It varies inversely with the heart rate: The faster the heart rate, the shorter the QT interval. As a general rule, the QT interval should be no more than half the previous R–R interval. A prolonged QT interval indicates a prolonged relative refractory period of the heart.

- **Step 6: Identify abnormalities.** Note the presence and frequency of **ectopic** (extra) beats, deviation of the ST segment above or below the baseline, and abnormalities in waveform shape and duration.

---

affect the outcome of the test, supporting the patient during the examination as necessary, documenting the procedures as appropriate, and monitoring the results of the test.

Case Study 》 Part 2

Mr. Evans is transferred to the intensive care unit (ICU) and placed on cardiac monitoring. A CVA care path is initiated. A CT scan confirms an ischemic stroke of the right parietal/temporal region, and he continues to have trouble managing his secretions. His work of breathing is increasing. Supplemental O_2 is now being delivered via nonrebreather mask. His O_2 sats are in the high 80s. Vitals are now T 99.8°F; P 94 bpm; R 26/min; and BP 120/76 mmHg.

Shortly after Mr. Evans' arrival in the ICU, you notice bilateral crackles in his lungs. On auscultation, you note they are worse on the right side. Mr. Evans has pitting edema in his lower extremities, and his urine output has decreased significantly. He is difficult to arouse and is oriented to person only. Physician and respiratory therapy have been called to assess the need for possible mechanical ventilation.

Independent Interventions

Nursing interventions are aimed at supporting, improving, and promoting perfusion adequate to meet the patient's oxygenation needs and prevent tissue damage. Depending on the disease process involved, this may include caring interventions to reduce stress on the heart, decrease cardiac workload, increase the efficacy of cardiac contractions, and meet fluid needs.

Nurses also provide teaching at a primary level to reduce the risk of cardiac disease in later life. Lifestyle modifications, such as reducing fat intake, participating in regular aerobic exercise, and eating a well-balanced diet, are influential in reducing the risk of CAD.

Promoting Circulation and Cardiopulmonary Function

Interventions for circulatory problems usually fall into three broad categories: inputs, outputs, and pressure supports. Inputs include arterial lines, venous lines, fluids, drug regimens, transfusions, and blood component therapies. Outputs include suctioning with specialized equipment such as a Hemovac and chest tubes and procedures such as thoracentesis. Pressure supports include dressings, direct compression, tourniquets, and cardiopulmonary resuscitation (CPR). An evaluation of the planned actions should be continuous and modified as the patient's condition dictates.

In coping with alterations in perfusion, care should be directed toward promoting, maintaining, or regaining cardiopulmonary function. The nurse observes, interviews, and examines the patient to identify actual and/or potential circulatory problems. The nurse evaluates the patient's responses as appropriate, deficient, or excessive and plans interventions accordingly. The nurse attempts to reduce patient stress, support adaptive behaviors, replace deficiencies, modify or remove excessive responses, and prevent injury and complications. The nurse should evaluate planned actions, report patient responses, and assist in modifying the interventions as indicated.

Continuous Monitoring

With patients who report or display the symptomology of impaired perfusion, continuous cardiopulmonary monitoring is required. Vital signs such as pulse, heart rate and rhythm displayed by ECG, oxygen saturation, respirations, and BP are particularly important. Other invasive measurements may also be warranted, such as CVP or arterial BP. CVP measures the amount of venous blood return to the heart, which reflects preload, whereas arterial BP gives a more accurate and continuous assessment of mean arterial pressure (MAP) and left ventricular ejection. Caring for patients with invasive lines requires frequent assessment of the catheter insertion site for infection, air embolism, occlusion from tube kinking or clotting, and bleeding from the use of heparinized saline or other anticoagulation medications. Radial arterial catheterization sites specifically should be assessed for signs and symptoms of compartment syndrome and damage to the median or radial nerve.

CO and SV may need to be monitored as well. There are three main methods for calculating SV, which is then used to determine CO. One method is obtained by subtracting the end systolic volume from the end diastolic blood volume (SV = EDV – ESV). The second method for calculating SV is to divide CO by heart rate (SV = CO/HR). The third method for figuring SV is through thermodilution equations that are usually performed by computer programs during cardiac catheterization.

Pulmonary capillary wedge pressure (PCWP), as well as right atrial and right ventricular pressures, can also be obtained during cardiac catheterization by a Swan-Ganz catheter. While right atrial and right ventricular pressures are measured in their respective chambers, the PCWP is obtained when the cardiac catheter is guided out of the right atrial, past the tricuspid valve, then out of the right ventricular through the pulmonic valve, and into the pulmonary artery. This measurement allows an indirect determination of left atrial pressure, which may be altered by mitral valve stenosis, aortic stenosis, left ventricular infarct, ischemia, or injury.

Fetal monitoring for patients who are pregnant is also warranted in most situations to assess fetal perfusion and oxygenation. Fetal heart rate (FHR) can be monitored externally of the mother's uterus or, in cases in which the fetal membranes have been artificially or naturally ruptured, a small electrode can be inserted into the scalp of the presenting fetus's head by needle and removed after birth. FHR accelerations and decelerations need to be assessed along with uterine contractions via tocodynametery in order to assess for possible fetal hypoxia. See the module on Reproduction for more information on monitoring FHR.

Recording and interpreting ECGs is a vital skill when assessing patients for altered perfusion. Identifying the segments of the ECG for regularity, size, shape, and relationship to the isoelectric line serve as the basis for this skill. For example, a depressed T wave may demonstrate ischemia or decreased perfusion to the myocardial muscle. If ischemia continues and sufficient blood flow is not restored to the tissue, injury or infarction may be indicated by ST segment elevation and or depression depending on the lead that is assessed. If circulation is not restored expediently during infarction, necrosis of the heart muscle will occur, leading to possible heart failure and death.

Cardiopulmonary Resuscitation

CPR may be required for patients who have perfusion-related problems. Providing oxygenated blood to the cerebral and myocardial tissues by physically compressing the heart is essential when the heart is not providing adequate blood flow. The coronary arteries are located directly off the ascending aorta and depend exclusively on the ejection of blood from the left ventricle to supply the myocardial muscle tissue with oxygenated blood. Therefore, CPR is vital to patient survival in the event of asystole or ineffective ventricular filling and ejection that is caused by lethal arrhythmias such as ventricular tachycardia (VT) and fibrillation. Electrical defibrillation may be required by the nurse during these lethal arrhythmias to restore the normal electrical conduction of the heart and return the patient to a life-sustaining rhythm.

Assessing Application of Compression Devices

Proper fitting and application of compression devices such as stockings or sequential compression devices (SCDs) are important interventions for patients who are at increased risk of developing deep venous thrombosis (DVT) related to poor venous return (see the Patient Teaching feature). If compression stockings place uneven pressure on the patient's skin, decubitus ulcers may result. If the patient does not receive the proper size of stocking, ineffective venous return may occur, leading to a greater incidence of DVT. If stockings are too tight, arterial circulation can be impeded, which decreases perfusion to lower extremities, such as the toes.

Patient Teaching
Compression Stockings

Compression stockings are used to control edema in the lower extremities, which may cause pain, prevent venous return and wound healing, and aid in the causation of DVT. Proper application and care of compression stockings is required to ensure patient safety and treatment efficacy.

Application
- Apply compression stockings before getting out of bed. If applied before legs are dependent, edema and pain can be decreased.
- When slipping on the stockings, make sure there are no wrinkles or creases that may create increased pressure to specific parts of the skin.
  - Roll and gather fabric so that the stocking can be worked from toes, over the heel, and then up the leg.
- Remove stockings only when taking a shower or at bedtime. A good idea is to schedule both at the same time.
- After removing the stockings, elevate legs and feet to at or above heart level.

Care Instructions
- Follow manufacture instructions for washing. Most stockings are machine washable.
- Dry stockings by laying them out flat. Stockings may shrink or become damaged if placed in the dryer.
- Petroleum products have been noted to damage the elastic in the stocking's fabric.

Contact Provider
- If pain or numbness increases from baseline
- If new wounds appear after the application and use of stockings
- If cyanosis or pallor is assessed through opening at toes and feet.

Providing Psychosocial Support

Underlying serious illness results in an uncertain prognosis, which is often accompanied by fear and which can bring distress to both patients and family members. In addition, patients and their families often must adjust to dramatic changes in lifestyle. Nurses can help patients with alterations in perfusion and their families by engaging in the following:

- Encourage the patient and family to verbalize concerns and ask questions.
- Answer questions truthfully. Providing honest answers is vital to developing a therapeutic nurse–patient relationship. Accurate responses allow the patient and family to set priorities as they plan for an uncertain future.
- Help the patient and family identify coping strategies to manage this significant situational stressor. Implementing previously effective coping methods may provide the skills to manage the current crisis.
- Provide emotional support. The presence of a caring nurse helps reduce the fear and anxiety associated with a crisis.
- Maintain a calm environment. A calm environment provides reassurance that the situation is under control, reduces anxiety, and promotes rest.
- Teach relaxation techniques. Relaxation techniques can reduce muscle tension and other signs of anxiety. Gaining control over physical responses can help the patient gain a sense of control over the situation.
- Respond promptly when the patient calls for help. Prompt response to expressed needs helps develop a trusting relationship and a sense of security that assistance is readily available.

The nurse should provide information about community resources, including support groups for patients with heart disease and their family members and educational programs and classes. Community hospitals and organizations such as the American Heart Association [AHA] offer myriad educational and support offerings.

Collaborative Therapies

The primary goal of collaborative therapies related to alterations in perfusion is reducing risk and disease progression. This may include increasing physical activity, stress management, and smoking cessation. Nutrition is also important to heart health and may help control some CAD risk factors. Treatment is dependent on the patient's symptoms and severity of underlying disease.

Surgery

When a patient requires heart surgery, the heart must be stilled for the procedure. A perfusionist uses a heart-lung machine (a type of artificial pump) to propel oxygenated blood to the patient's tissues during the operation. This sustains the patient's circulatory and respiratory function until the operation is complete and the heart can resume its normal function. Perfusionists are also responsible for controlling the temperature of the patient during surgery and administering various types of blood products and medications (Mayo Clinic, 2014c).

If decreased perfusion is noted during ECG, serial cardiac enzymes blood draws, or stress test, the patient may require percutaneous transluminal coronary intervention (PTCA) to open blocked coronary arteries and restore perfusion to cardiac muscle and tissue. A nurse performs a preprocedure checklist and assessment on the patient in a holding area, including shaving the surgical site such as the groin or the anterior wrists in order to access the femoral and radial arteries, respectively. Patients are placed under conscious sedation during the procedure. Patients typically do not require ventilation, but they do require supplemental oxygenation by nasal cannula or nonrebreather mask. A circulating nurse monitors vital signs and provides the cardiologist and scrub technician with drugs and equipment. Angioplasty or inflation of a balloon to compress plaque against the coronary artery walls may be employed along with bare metal or drug-coated stents to create a patent lumen in the blood vessel, thus restoring perfusion. The patient may need to take an anticoagulant to prevent restenosis related to thrombus.

Cardiac Rehabilitation

Cardiac rehabilitation is a medically supervised program designed to aid patients who are recovering from acute myocardial infarction (AMI), heart surgeries, and percutaneous coronary interventions. Cardiac rehabilitation begins with admission for a cardiac event such as an AMI or a revascularization procedure. It consists of three phases:

- Phase 1 of the program is the inpatient phase. A thorough assessment of the patient's history, current status, risk factors, and motivation is obtained. During this phase, activity progresses from bedrest to independent performance of ADLs and ambulation. Both subjective and objective responses to increasing activity levels are evaluated. Excess fatigue, shortness of breath, chest pain, tachypnea, tachycardia, and cool, clammy skin indicate activity intolerance.

- Phase 2, immediate outpatient cardiac rehabilitation, begins within 3 weeks of the cardiac event. The goals for the outpatient program are to increase the patient's activity level, participation, and capacity; improve psychosocial status and treat anxiety or depression; and provide education and support for risk factor reduction.

- Phase 3, a continuation program, helps transition the patient to independent exercise and exercise maintenance. The time between visits may be increased as the patient is provided with opportunities to implement modifications discussed in the rehabilitation program.

Cardiac rehabilitation programs offer a combination of physical activity and exercise, risk factor management, medication administration and education, nutrition counseling, and smoking cessation programs. Cardiac rehabilitation education may range from weight management to CPR to sexual dysfunction. Psychosocial health will also be addressed. At all stages, nurses working with patients in cardiac rehabilitation (whether in a primary care setting or at a rehabilitation facility) focus on listening to the patient and family and addressing their concerns and reinforcing patient education and adherence to the treatment regimen.

Pharmacologic Therapy

Many of the medications administered by nurses have an impact on perfusion. Beta-blockers, antihypertensives, cardiac glycosides, and even some narcotics have a profound impact on cardiac functioning and perfusion. The Medications feature describes some of the more commonly prescribed medications. More specific Medications charts for cholesterol-lowering drugs, antiplatelet drugs, anticoagulants, heart failure drugs, antihypertensives, antidysrhythmic drugs, and shock can be found in the relevant exemplars.

Nonpharmacologic Therapy

To guard against atherosclerosis, patients should follow a heart-healthy diet based on fruits, vegetables, legumes (beans and peas), and whole grains. This kind of diet includes consuming fat-free or low-fat dairy products as well as eating fish twice a week, especially salmon, tuna, and trout that are high in omega-3 fatty acids. A heart-healthy diet avoids large amounts of red meat and sugary foods and beverages, and it is low in saturated fats, trans fats, cholesterol, and sodium. A heart-healthy diet can help patients control their weight, BP, cholesterol, and blood glucose (Mayo Clinic, 2015a; NHLBI, 2016).

In conjunction with a heart-healthy diet, some patients may be interested in using nutritional and/or herbal supplements. Evidence regarding the value of these supplements is mixed. For example, while dietary intake of omega-3 fatty acids has been shown to contribute to cardiovascular health, research suggests that consumption of fish oil and other omega-3 supplements has minimal, if any, benefits (Kwak et al., 2012; Mohebi-Nejad & Bikdeli, 2014; Rizos et al., 2012). Likewise, even though foods rich in vitamin E and beta carotene are part of a heart-healthy diet, high supplemental doses of these antioxidants are not recommended and may actually be harmful (Cleveland Clinic, 2016a; National Center for Complementary and Integrative Health [NCCIH], 2016a). Experts also warn against use of herbal supplements such as ephedra, garlic, ginkgo, goldenseal, licorice root, black cohosh, ginger, ginseng, and feverfew, as these can either interact with prescribed cardiac medications or produce unwanted cardiac side effects on their own (Cleveland Clinic, 2016b; Rabito & Kaye, 2013).

Patients who are overweight can reduce two major risk factors for atherosclerosis—high BP and high cholesterol—by losing just 5–10 pounds. Losing weight reduces the risk of patients developing diabetes, or it can help patients who already have diabetes control their condition (Mayo Clinic, 2015a). To screen patients for weight-related health risks, the nurse should measure waist circumference. If most of the patient's fat is around the waist instead of at the hips, the risk for heart disease and type 2 diabetes is higher. A waist size that is greater than 35 inches for women or greater than 40 inches for men represents a heightened risk (NHLBI, 2016).

Patients can condition their muscles to use oxygen more efficiently through regular exercise, which also may improve circulation and promote the development of new blood vessels, called collateral vessels, that form a natural bypass around obstructions. Exercise also helps lower BP and reduces the risk of diabetes (Mayo Clinic, 2015a). Patients should speak with their primary care provider before they start a new exercise plan and ask how much and what kinds of physical activity

Medications
Perfusion

CLASSIFICATION AND DRUG EXAMPLES	MECHANISMS OF ACTION	NURSING CONSIDERATIONS
Statins *Drug examples:* Atorvastatin (Lipitor) Fluvastatin (Lescol) Lovastatin (Mevacor) Pravastatin (Pravachol) Simvastatin (Zocor)	These drugs inhibit 3-hydroxy-3-methylglutaryl coenzyme (HMG-CoA), a reductase, which results in less cholesterol biosynthesis.	▪ Assess triglyceride, total cholesterol, low-density lipoprotein (LDL), and high-density lipoprotein (HDL) levels. ▪ Avoid use in patients who are or may become pregnant or are nursing. ▪ Monitor liver function tests. ▪ Avoid use in patients with liver disease or heavy alcohol consumption. ▪ Teach the patient to avoid alcohol while taking. ▪ Assess for muscle pain, tenderness, or weakness.
Antihypertensive Drugs **Diuretics** *Drug examples:* Furosemide (Lasix) Hydrochlorothiazide (Microzide) Bumetanide (Bumex) Triamterene (Dyrenium) Spironolactone (Aldactone) Metolazone (Mykrox)	These drugs reduce fluid volume in the vessels.	▪ Monitor serum electrolyte levels. ▪ Obtain the patient's weight daily. ▪ Teach the patient the importance of complying with the medication regimen. ▪ Assess hydration status. ▪ Monitor breath sounds for fluid volume excess.
ACE inhibitors and angiotensin II receptor blockers (ARBs) *Drug examples:* Benazepril (Lotensin) Captopril (Capoten) Lisinopril (Prinivil) Losartan (Cozaar) Valsartan (Diovan)	Angiotensin II is a potent natural vasoconstrictor; its actions are blocked by ACE inhibitors and angiotensin inhibitors.	▪ Follow vital sign changes. ▪ First dose may cause severe hypotension, so monitor BP carefully. ▪ The first dose is best administered at bedtime. ▪ Monitor BP carefully if given intravenously and with subsequent alteration in LOC if this occurs. ▪ Teach the patient to report the development of a persistent dry cough if taking an ACE inhibitor. ▪ Assess for angioedema, which can be life-threatening. ▪ Monitor complete blood count for neutropenia or agranulocytosis.
Combination Drugs *Drug examples:* Combines hydrochlorothiazide with propranolol, metoprolol, timolol, or bisoprolol	These drugs contain a diuretic, usually a potassium-sparing diuretic, and another class of drugs, such as adrenergic agents or ACE inhibitors.	▪ Monitor serum electrolyte levels. ▪ Obtain the patient's weight daily. ▪ Teach the patient the importance of complying with the medication regimen. ▪ Assess hydration status. ▪ Monitor breath sounds for fluid volume excess.
Direct Vasodilators *Drug examples:* Hydralazine (Apresoline) Minoxidil (Loniten) Nitroprusside (Nipride)	These drugs cause dilation of blood vessels.	▪ These may produce reflex tachycardia. ▪ These may produce angina in patients with CAD. ▪ Monitor for sodium and water retention. ▪ IV nitroprusside is the drug of choice for treating hypertensive emergency, but care must be taken not to drop BP too quickly. The drugs metabolize to cyanide, so careful monitoring is required.

Medications *(continued)*

CLASSIFICATION AND DRUG EXAMPLES	MECHANISMS OF ACTION	NURSING CONSIDERATIONS
Adrenergic Antagonists *Drug examples:* Beta-adrenergic blockers (atenolol [Tenormin], metoprolol [Lopressor]) Alpha$_1$-adrenergic antagonists (doxazosin [Cardura], prazosin [Minipress]) Alpha$_2$-adrenergic agonists (clonidine [Catapress], methyldopa [Aldomet]) Alpha$_1$- and beta-blocker (labetalol [Trandate]) Adrenergic neuron blockers (reserpine)	These drugs reduce autonomic nervous system effects by blocking beta$_1$-adrenergic receptor sites in the heart, blocking alpha$_1$-adrenergic receptors in arterioles, stimulating alpha$_2$ receptors in the brainstem, and/or blocking peripheral adrenergic neurons.	▪ Monitor vital signs. ▪ Hold medication if heart rate is less than 60 bpm or if BP is less than 90/60 mmHg. ▪ Use care when ambulating, monitoring for potential orthostatic hypotension. ▪ Monitor patients with diabetes for hypoglycemia.
Calcium Channel Blockers (CCBs) *Drug examples:* Nifedipine (Procardia) Verapamil (Calan) Diltiazem (Cardizem)	These drugs treat angina, dysrhythmias, and hypertension, reducing available calcium, muscular contractility, PVR, and BP.	▪ Obtain baseline ECG, heart rate, and BP before beginning therapy. ▪ Teach the patient to maintain a daily BP log and about the need for complying with the medication regimen. ▪ Use is contraindicated in patients with third-degree block of sick sinus syndrome (SSS). ▪ Monitor for tachycardia and hypotension if administered by IV. ▪ Teach the patient to avoid grapefruit juice.
Cardiac Glycosides *Drug example:* Digoxin (Cardoxin)	These drugs cause the heart to beat more forcefully and more slowly, improving CO (positive inotropic affect).	▪ Monitor serum potassium. ▪ Administer with caution to older adults and to those post-MI or with incomplete heart block or renal insufficiency. ▪ Side effects such as drowsiness, fatigue, dizziness, visual disturbances, anorexia, nausea, or vomiting may indicate toxic levels. ▪ Follow serum drug levels in order to maintain therapeutic levels.
Phosphodiesterase Inhibitors *Drug example:* Milrinone (Primacor)	These drugs block the enzyme phosphodiesterase in cardiac and smooth muscle, increasing the amount of calcium available for myocardial contraction, which results in positive inotropic actions and vasodilation.	▪ Assess serum potassium levels. ▪ Monitor for dysrhythmia. ▪ During IV administration, monitor for ventricular dysrhythmias.
Organic Nitrates *Drug examples:* Isosorbide dinitrate (Dilatrate) Nitroglycerin (Nitrostat)	These drugs are potent vasodilators that dilate both arterial and venous smooth muscle. Dilation of veins reduces preload.	▪ Monitor BP frequently for hypotension. ▪ To prevent falls, reduce dizziness, and reduce the oxygen demands on the heart, have the patient lie down when taking this medication for chest pain. ▪ Teach the patient how to take medication when having chest pain and how often it may be repeated before calling 9-1-1. ▪ Use is contraindicated in patients with cardiac tamponade and pericarditis or patients with head injury, shock, or increased ICP. ▪ Teach the patient to avoid alcohol consumption, which can lead to severe hypotension and cardiovascular collapse.

(continued on next page)

Medications (continued)

CLASSIFICATION AND DRUG EXAMPLES	MECHANISMS OF ACTION	NURSING CONSIDERATIONS
Thrombolytics *Drug examples:* Reteplase (Retavase) Alteplase (Activase) Streptokinase (Streptase)	These drugs are administered to dissolve clots resulting in MI or stroke, with quick restoration of circulation.	▪ The drugs must be administered within 12 hours after symptom onset; they are best if given within 3 hours after ischemic stroke. ▪ Research suggests patients older than 75 years do not experience reduced mortality from these drugs. ▪ Monitor patients carefully for bleeding, because all clots, even those formed as the result of venipuncture, are dissolved. ▪ In patients who may be receiving thrombolytics, attempt to minimize invasive procedures in order to avoid future bleeding sites. ▪ Do not administer to patients who have recently (within the past 2 weeks) fallen, been involved in a motor vehicle crash, or experienced any form of trauma. ▪ Closely monitor cardiac rhythm, because return of perfusion to the blocked vessel often results in reperfusion arrhythmias that may include VT.
Anticoagulants* *Drug examples:* Heparin Low-molecular-weight heparins (LMWH) Oral anticoagulants (e.g., warfarin [Coumadin]) *More detailed information on anticoagulants can be found in Exemplar 16.D on Deep Venous Thrombosis	Anticoagulants are used to prevent clot extension and lower the risk for DVT and pulmonary embolism (PE).	▪ Assess for history of unexplained or active bleeding. Assess laboratory results for abnormal clotting profile or evidence of active bleeding. ▪ Monitor for unusual or masked bleeding. Promptly report any evidence of bleeding such as hematemesis, hematuria, bleeding gums, or unexplained abdominal or back pain. ▪ Teach patient not to take aspirin, nonsteroidal anti-inflammatory drugs (NSAIDs), or other over-the-counter drugs unless cleared by their healthcare provider. ▪ For patients taking warfarin, keep vitamin K available to reverse effects of warfarin in the event of excessive bleeding or hemorrhage.

Source: Based on Adams, M. P., Holland, L. N., & Urban, C. (2017). *Pharmacology for nurses: A pathophysiologic approach* (5th ed.). Hoboken, NJ: Pearson Education.

are safe (NHLBI, 2016). Most patients will need to exercise at least a half hour if not an hour most days, breaking up this activity into 10-minute stretches if needed. Exercise can also be incorporated into everyday activities: taking the stairs instead of the elevator, walking during lunch breaks, and doing exercises while watching TV (Mayo Clinic, 2015a).

Patients should never smoke or use tobacco in any way. Smoking, even secondhand smoke and use of e-cigarettes, damages the arteries. If patients do use tobacco, quitting as soon as possible is the best way to halt the progression of atherosclerosis and reduce the risk of complications (Mayo Clinic, 2015a). Patients should talk with their primary care physicians about which programs and products might best help them quit. Patients who have trouble quitting smoking on their own should consider joining a support group or taking classes in how to quit, which many hospitals, workplaces, and community groups offer (NHLBI, 2016).

Stress reduction can help patients control the progress of atherosclerosis. Techniques include muscle relaxation and deep breathing (Mayo Clinic, 2015a). Other possibilities are

meditation, physical activity such as exercise, relaxation therapy, having constructive discussions with friends or family, and stress management programs (NHLBI, 2016).

Patients with hypotension should drink more water and less alcohol, eat smaller portions at meals that are low in carbs, and change body positions slowly (Mayo Clinic, 2015a). They also might try using compression stockings. Doctors may prescribe the use of compression stockings for patients with varicose veins or spider veins or for those who have just had surgery (U.S. National Library of Medicine, 2014b).

Avoiding hypertension involves the same activities and lifestyle choices that guard against atherosclerosis: eating a healthy diet, exercising regularly, avoiding smoking or other tobacco use, maintaining a healthy body weight, and avoiding or reducing stress (Mayo Clinic, 2015b; NHLBI, 2015a). Patients should also reduce their salt intake, following the DASH diet (Mayo Clinic, 2015a), and limit their alcohol intake as well (Mayo Clinic, 2015b; NHLBI, 2015a).

Finally, there is limited clinical evidence that chelation therapy, which involves injection of a substance called EDTA (ethylenediaminetetraacetic acid) into the blood, may reduce the risk of cardiac events, especially in older patients with diabetes. EDTA binds with heavy metals in the bloodstream, making it easier for the body to remove these substances. Although chelation is a proven treatment for heavy metal poisoning, further research is needed before it can be routinely recommended as a method for preventing heart disease, especially since chelation therapy presents a high risk of side effects (NCCIH, 2016b).

Lifespan Considerations

Although perfusion must be maintained throughout the lifespan, patients of different ages have different needs related to perfusion. This is particularly true for children, as differences in pediatric cardiology affect not only how children respond to cardiac alterations but also how they respond to therapy.

Transition from Fetal to Pulmonary Circulation

Before birth, blood flows from the placenta to the fetus through the umbilical vein to the ductus venosus (the fetal vascular channel between the umbilical vein and the inferior vena cava) and into the right atrium of the heart. The **foramen ovale** (an opening between the atria of the fetal heart) allows blood to flow from the right atrium to the left atrium and then into the left ventricle. Blood is then pumped into the aorta and systemic circulation. Some blood returns from the head and upper extremities to the superior vena cava and right atrium, and some blood travels to the right ventricle, where it is pumped into the pulmonary artery. The majority of the blood from the pulmonary artery passes through the ductus arteriosus, the vascular channel between

the pulmonary artery and the aorta, and into the systemic circulation. A small amount of the blood from the pulmonary artery goes to the lungs. Blood eventually returns to the placenta by way of the umbilical arteries.

After the umbilical cord has been cut, the newborn must quickly adapt to receiving oxygen from the lungs. The transition from fetal to pulmonary circulation occurs in just a few hours. The first breath expands the lungs. Blood that previously flowed through the ductus arteriosus to the aorta begins flowing to the lungs. Increased pulmonary blood flow and decreased **pulmonary vascular resistance** (pressure within the pulmonary blood vessels that must be overcome in order for blood to flow through the vessel) result. Pressure in the left atrium increases as increased blood flow is returned from the lungs through the pulmonary veins.

The force or resistance of the blood in the body's blood vessels that helps return blood to the heart is called **systemic vascular resistance (SVR)**. After the umbilical cord is cut, SVR increases, and right atrial pressure falls. Increased pressure in the left atrium stimulates closure of the foramen ovale. The flaps of the foramen ovale close, and fibrin deposits permanently seal the opening, unless there is excess pressure on the right side of the heart. In response to higher oxygen saturation, the ductus arteriosus normally constricts and closes within 18 hours after birth. Permanent closure occurs 2–3 weeks after birth, unless oxygen saturation remains low. Because fetal tissues have adapted to low oxygen saturation, newborns with cyanotic heart disease may appear relatively comfortable even when the arterial partial pressure of oxygen (PaO_2) is between 20 and 25 mmHg. In contrast, healthy newborns typically have a PaO_2 of between 50 and 70 mmHg. Older children and adults would rapidly develop acidosis and cerebral anoxia with such a low PaO_2. **Figure 16–24 》** compares fetal and postnatal circulation.

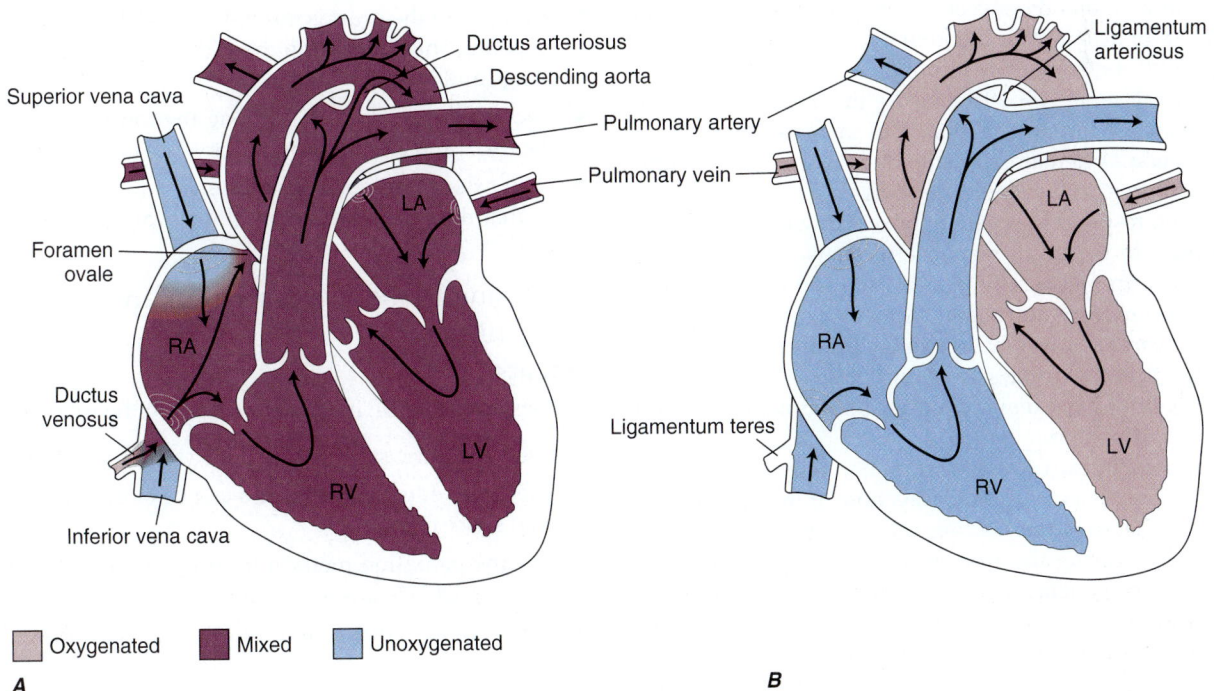

Oxygenated　Mixed　Unoxygenated

A　**B**

Figure 16–24 》 The arrows indicate the flow of blood through the heart while the color indicates level of oxygen saturation in the blood. **A,** Fetal circulation. **B,** Pulmonary circulation. LA, left atrium; LV, left ventricle; RA, right atrium; RV, right ventricle.

Perfusion in Infants and Children

Cardiac Development

Cardiac Functioning

Infants have a greater risk of heart failure because the immature heart is more sensitive to volume or pressure overload. During infancy, the heart's muscle fibers are less developed and less organized, resulting in limited functional capacity. SV does not increase substantially until the heart muscle is fully developed at 5 years of age. As the child's heart grows and develops, the systolic BP rises, reaching adult levels by puberty. The infant's metabolic rate and oxygen requirements double at birth. This results in a higher neonatal heart rate—one that can maintain a high CO and adequate oxygen transport. A newborn's heart rate is about 100–205 beats per minute while awake because of the demand for oxygen-rich blood. The heart rate gradually slows throughout childhood and settles between 50–90 beats per minute by the late teen years. Factors influencing neonatal heart rate include physical and emotional stress, exercise, fever, and respiratory distress. As infants experience tachycardia, CO is increased. There is little cardiac reserve capacity until oxygen demands begin to decrease.

Oxygenation

Hematocrit and hemoglobin concentrations appropriate for the child's age are necessary for adequate oxygen transport. The oxygen arterial saturation is the amount of oxygen that can potentially be delivered to the tissues. **Desaturated blood** results when oxygenated and deoxygenated blood mix because of a congenital heart defect. Cyanosis, which indicates **hypoxemia** (lower-than-normal amounts of oxygen in the blood), results from a concentration of 5 or more grams of deoxygenated hemoglobin per 100 mL of blood or from arterial saturations of less than 85%. Infants who display cyanosis while feeding or crying may have an abnormal shunting of blood between heart chambers, resulting in an increase of desaturated blood in the arterial circulation.

The child's bone marrow responds to chronic hypoxemia by producing more RBCs to increase the amount of hemoglobin available for oxygenation. This increase is known as **polycythemia**. A hematocrit value of 50% or higher is common in children with cyanotic heart defects.

Children respond to severe hypoxemia with bradycardia as opposed to the adult response of tachycardia. Cardiac arrest in children generally results from prolonged hypoxemia related to respiratory failure or shock rather than from a primary cardiac insult (as in adults). Bradycardia is therefore a significant warning sign of cardiac arrest. Appropriate management of hypoxemia often reverses bradycardia and prevents cardiac arrest.

Alterations in cardiovascular function may be the result of a congenital defect, acquired infection, or injury. Congenital heart disease is the leading cause of death, excluding prematurity, during the first year of life. Although heart defects may be genetic or part of a chromosome syndrome, many children do not have other types of birth defects. Rapid advances in the treatment of congenital heart defects have allowed children to undergo surgery at younger ages. As a result, nursing care required to identify and manage infants and children with heart disease has become more challenging.

Assessing Pulse in Infants and Children

Infants and Young Children

Nurses assessing pulse in infants and young children should do the following:

- Use the apical pulse for the heart rate of newborns, infants, and children 2–3 years old.
- Place a baby in the supine position, and offer a pacifier if the baby is crying or restless. Crying and physical activity will increase the pulse rate. For this reason, take the apical pulse rate of infants and small children before assessing body temperatures.
- Locate the apical pulse in the fourth ICS, lateral to the MCL during infancy.
- Brachial, popliteal, and femoral pulses may be palpated. Because of a normally low BP and rapid heart rate, infants' other distal pulses may be hard to feel.
- Newborn infants may have heart murmurs that are not pathologic but reflect functional incomplete closure of fetal heart structures (ductus arteriosus or foramen ovale).

Preschoolers and Older Children

Nurses assessing pulse in preschoolers and older children should do the following:

- To take a peripheral pulse, position the child comfortably in the adult's arms, or have the adult remain close by. This may decrease anxiety and yield more accurate results.
- To assess the apical pulse, assist younger children to a comfortable supine or sitting position.
- Demonstrate the procedure to the child using a stuffed animal or doll, and allow the child to handle the stethoscope before beginning the procedure. This will decrease anxiety and promote cooperation.
- The apex of the heart is normally located in the fourth ICS in young children and in the fifth ICS in children 7 years of age and over.
- Locate the apical impulse along the fourth ICS, between the MCL and the anterior axillary line (see Figure 16–16).
- Count the pulse prior to other uncomfortable procedures so that the rate is not artificially elevated by the discomfort.

Assessing Blood Pressure in Infants and Children

Infants

Nurses assessing BP in infants should do the following:

- Use a pediatric stethoscope with a small diaphragm.
- The lower edge of the BP cuff can be closer to the antecubital space of an infant.
- Use the palpation method if auscultation with a stethoscope or DUS is unsuccessful.
- Arm and thigh pressures are equivalent in children under 1 year of age.
- One quick way to determine the normal systolic BP of a child is to use the following formula:

Normal systolic BP = 80 + (2 × child's age in years)

Children

Nurses assessing BP in children should do the following:

- BP should be measured in all children over 3 years of age and in children under 3 years of age with certain medical conditions (e.g., congenital heart disease, renal malformation, medications that affect BP).

- Explain each step of the process and what it will feel like. Demonstrate on a doll.

- Use the palpation technique for children under 3 years old.

- Cuff bladder width should be 40%, and length should be 80–100% of the arm circumference.

- Take the BP prior to other uncomfortable procedures so that the BP is not artificially elevated by the discomfort.

- In children, the diastolic pressure is considered to be the onset of phase 4, where the sounds become muffled.

- In children, the thigh pressure is about 10 mmHg higher than the arm pressure.

Perfusion in Pregnant Women

Blood flow increases to some organ systems during pregnancy—the uterus, placenta, and breast—without changes to blood flow to the liver and brain, causing increased workload. Early in pregnancy, CO begins to increase, with a peak at 30–50% above prepregnancy levels after 25–30 weeks of gestation. CO generally remains elevated during the third trimester.

At term, the pulse rate may increase by as many as 10–15 bpm. BP decreases slightly, falling to its lowest point during the second trimester, and then gradually rebounds, increasing to near-prepregnancy levels by the end of the third trimester.

The uterus interferes with the return of blood flow and causes blood stasis in the lower extremities as it enlarges, exerting pressure on pelvic and femoral vessels. During late pregnancy, this interference may produce effects such as dependent edema and varicosity of the veins in the legs, vulva, and rectum (hemorrhoids). Increased blood volume in the lower legs may also lead to postural hypotension.

Pressure on the vena cava from the enlarging uterus when the woman lies supine may reduce blood flow to the right atrium; lower BP; and cause dizziness, pallor, and clamminess. Research indicates that there may also be pressure on the aorta and its collateral circulation as the uterus enlarges (Cunningham et al., 2014). This condition goes by various names, including supine hypotensive syndrome, vena caval syndrome, and aortocaval compression (see **Figure 16–25 ≫**). The woman may correct this problem by lying on her left side or by placing a pillow or wedge under her right hip as she lies in a supine position.

Blood volume progressively and rapidly increases from the first trimester until roughly 30–34 weeks of gestation, at which point it plateaus at approximately 40–50% above prepregnancy levels until birth. Increases in both erythrocytes and plasma cause this increase (Gordon, 2012).

In women who receive an iron supplement, the erythrocyte volume increases by approximately 30% total, but this number is less than 18% in women who receive no iron supplement. The increase in erythrocytes enables the transport of the additional oxygen that pregnancy requires. Plasma volume increases during pregnancy by an average

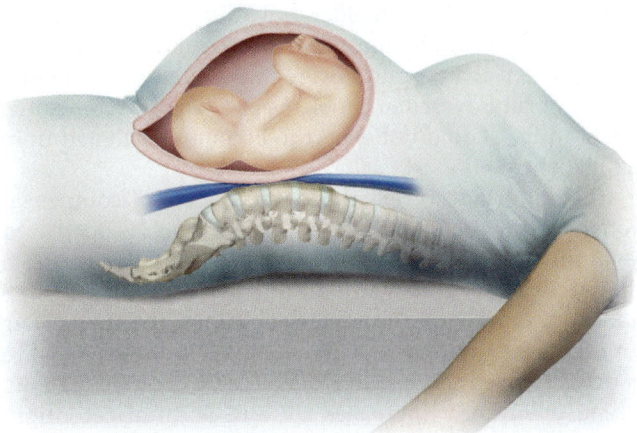

Source: Ladewig, P. W., London, M. L., & Davidson, M. C. (2013). *Contemporary maternal-newborn nursing care* (8th ed.). Reprinted and electronically reproduced by permission of Pearson Education, Inc. New York, NY.

Figure 16–25 ≫ Vena caval syndrome. The gravid uterus compresses the vena cava when the woman is supine. This reduces the blood flow returning to the heart and may cause maternal hypotension.

of approximately 50%. Because the increase in plasma volume is 20% greater than the erythrocyte increase, the hematocrit decreases slightly (Gordon, 2012), a decrease known as **physiologic anemia of pregnancy** (pseudoanemia).

Because iron is necessary for hemoglobin formation and hemoglobin is the oxygen-carrying component of erythrocytes, an increase in erythrocyte levels results in the pregnant woman needing a corresponding increase in iron. The gastrointestinal absorption of iron moderately increases during pregnancy, but even so it is usually necessary to supplement the diet with extra iron to meet the needs of the fetus and the RBCs.

Leukocyte production increases slightly to an average of $8500/mm^3$, with a range of 5600 to $12,200/mm^3$, reaching $20,000–30,000/mm^3$ during labor and the early postpartum period. This increase in white blood cells (WBCs) is normal and does not indicate the presence of infection for a clinical diagnosis (Gordon, 2012).

Fibrin and plasma fibrinogen levels increase during pregnancy, and clotting factors VII, VIII, IX, and X increase for pregnant women even though blood-clotting time for pregnant women does not differ significantly from that of nonpregnant women. Pregnancy, therefore, is a somewhat hypercoagulable state. Together with venous stasis in late pregnancy, these changes increase the risk that the pregnant woman will develop venous thrombosis during pregnancy.

Perfusion in Older Adults

Normal Changes of Aging

Because a wide range of changes occurs with aging, it is often difficult to distinguish between disease processes and the natural consequences of aging. A decrease in cardiovascular reserve or in CO may be the result of deconditioning or disease and not the result of the natural aging processes. Differences in cardiovascular functioning also exist from one individual to another. An older individual with a good family history and healthy lifestyle can enjoy much greater cardiac function than a middle-age individual with a family history of cardiovascular problems or a history of smoking. Older adults should not expect to become debilitated from aging alone.

It is important to remember the concept of compensation in cardiovascular function. Changes such as decreased renal functioning may occur with aging, and this causes a change in other systems in an attempt to improve functioning. Sometimes these compensatory changes cause problems of their own. For example, kidneys that are poorly perfused as a result of decreased CO produce renin, which eventually increases BP and sodium retention. These gradual compensatory changes are initially benign but can lead to decreased cardiac and renal function and to fluid overload. See **Figure 16–26** ›› for normal cardiovascular changes of aging.

Another feature of aging is the atypical presentation of disease in the older adult. For example, a middle-age individual experiencing an MI will most likely complain of the typical substernal chest pain with radiation down the left arm; however, the older adult may complain of heartburn, nausea and vomiting, or excessive fatigue. Complaints of fatigue, decreased activity, sleep disturbance, or pain are not normal and should be investigated. The older adult has a decreased capacity to adapt to stress to the cardiovascular system and may need medical or nursing interventions. Therefore, nurses should be alert to possible problems and include a wide range of diagnostic possibilities in any given situation. Mental status changes should not be assumed to be the result of dementia. Mental status changes, in addition to agitation and falls, may be the first sign of cardiac problems in the older adult. The nurse should conduct a thorough assessment of any older adult patient complaining of or exhibiting changes in mental status.

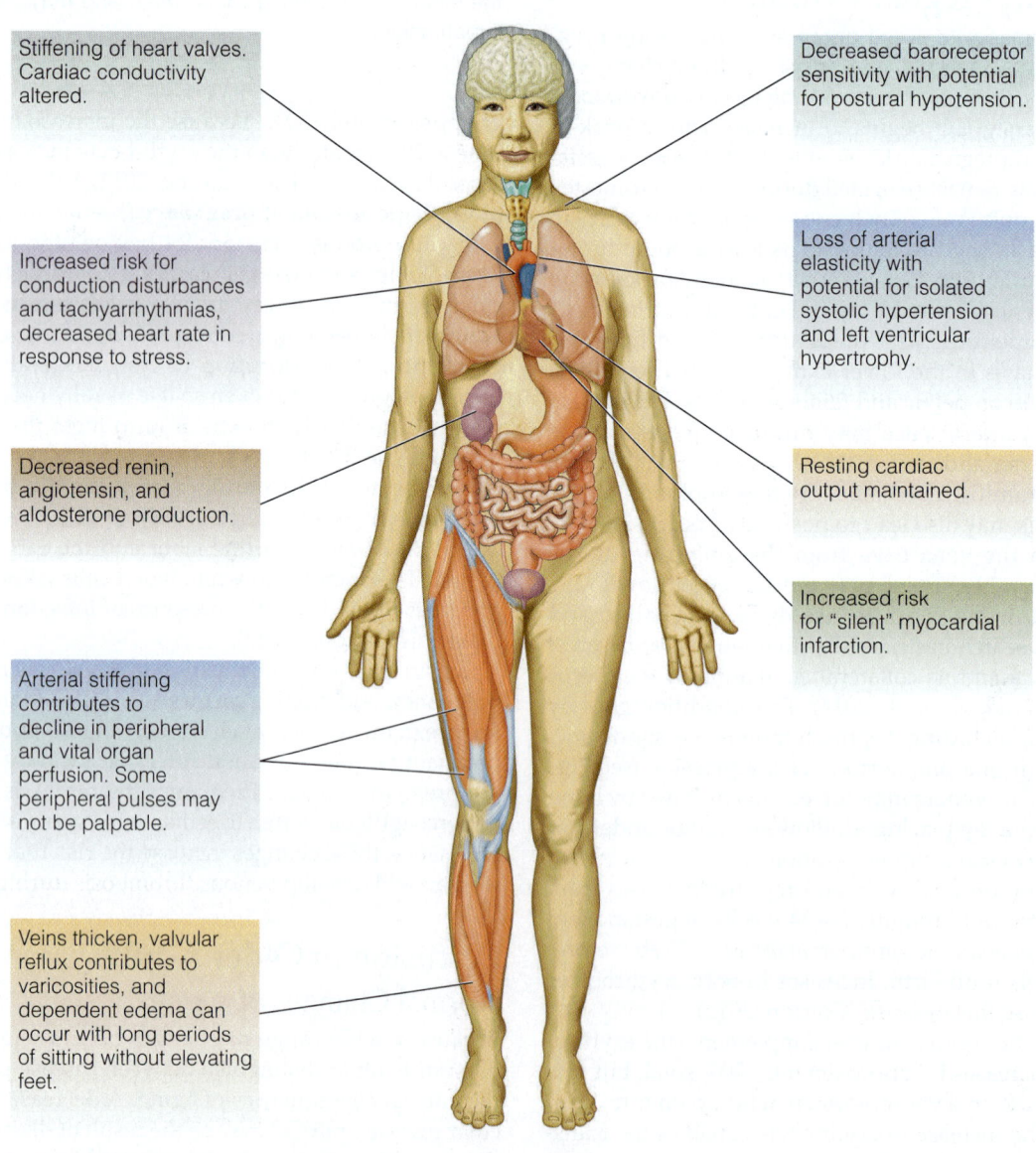

Stiffening of heart valves. Cardiac conductivity altered.

Increased risk for conduction disturbances and tachyarrhythmias, decreased heart rate in response to stress.

Decreased renin, angiotensin, and aldosterone production.

Arterial stiffening contributes to decline in peripheral and vital organ perfusion. Some peripheral pulses may not be palpable.

Veins thicken, valvular reflux contributes to varicosities, and dependent edema can occur with long periods of sitting without elevating feet.

Decreased baroreceptor sensitivity with potential for postural hypotension.

Loss of arterial elasticity with potential for isolated systolic hypertension and left ventricular hypertrophy.

Resting cardiac output maintained.

Increased risk for "silent" myocardial infarction.

Figure 16–26 ›› Normal changes of aging in the cardiovascular system.

Cardiovascular System

Specific changes in the cardiovascular system with aging include **myocardial hypertrophy** (an increase in the size of muscle cells of the myocardium). This will change the function of the left ventricular wall and the ventricular septum. The left ventricular wall thickens after the age of 60. Heart valves become stiff with aging as the result of fibrosis and calcification (Strait & Lakatta, 2012). In addition, changes in the valve rings can contribute to stenosis or incompetence, resulting in changes in the heart muscle and its chambers.

Resting heart rate is relatively unchanged with normal aging, and in the absence of disease, CO is not much changed. However, a slight decline in CO does occur after age 20. The average man with a CO of 5.0 L/min at age 20 will likely have a CO of 3.5 L/min at age 75. This CO is sufficient to maintain normal adult functioning. The heart has the ability to increase its rate in response to stress.

Electrical activity of the heart is affected in aging, with a decrease in the number of normal pacemaker cells in the SA node. By age 75, only 10% of the original pacemaker cells are still functional. Under normal circumstances, this number still supports cardiac function. Likewise, the number of cells in the AV node, left and right bundle branches, and bundle of His is lower for the older adult. Fat and collagen deposition may also be increased in these regions. Fibrosis of the AV node can lead to AV block with no other cardiac pathology. The AV node refractory period is also increased with aging. The ECG shows no specific changes with age, although some lengthening of the PR, QRS, and QT intervals has been described. In some patients, the stress of acute or chronic illness may precipitate conduction abnormalities.

Vascular System

The vascular system undergoes myriad changes with aging. The layers of the vascular system change, with a thickening of the intimal and medial layers. For arteries, the endothelial layer becomes irregular with more connective tissue. Lipid deposits and calcification occur. Calcification can extend to the medial layer with increased collagen deposits. These changes can all lead to decreased elasticity or "hardening" of the arterial walls. BP elevation frequently occurs with aging, although it is not considered a normal variant. Isolated systolic hypertension (systolic BP greater than 140 mmHg) is frequently seen in the older individual. The arterial wall diameter normally is controlled by a balance of systems, including the autonomic nervous system and beta-adrenergic stimulation. However, decreased responsiveness to beta-adrenergic stimulation may be noted in older patients.

Pulmonary System

Pulmonary changes that occur with aging can affect cardiovascular function. Decreased chest wall compliance is the result of decreased elasticity of lung tissue and stiffness of thoracic and spinal joints. An increase in anteroposterior diameter seen with aging can lead to higher residual volumes. Airway closure in dependent lung areas can occur at higher volumes. This removes portions of the lung from exchange functions. A combination of early airway closure, decreased diffusing capacity, increased lung volumes, and changes in alveolar structure can lead to lower arterial oxygen tension (PaO_2). Because carbon dioxide is diffused more readily, no change in $PaCO_2$ (arterial carbon dioxide tension) is noted with aging. Elevated $PaCO_2$ indicates pathology. Age-related changes that increase susceptibility to pneumonia and other infections include decreased ciliary functioning and suppression of the immune system.

Renal System

Renal function declines with age, and the kidneys decrease in size and weight. Functional decline is the result of decreased renal blood flow and decreased glomerular filtration. By age 80, the glomerular filtration rate is reduced 30–50% compared with that of the 30-year-old. Because of a concomitant decrease in muscle mass, serum creatinine levels are not elevated. However, the clearance rate for creatinine and other chemicals, including many medications, is reduced. This results in a longer half-life for drugs administered to the older adult. With aging, decreased levels of renin and aldosterone are found in the plasma. This leads to an increased sensitivity to dietary sodium consumption. Decreased ability to clear sodium from the blood can lead to body water overload. This increased preload can tax the myocardium. In addition, an antidiuretic hormone (ADH) is less able to be suppressed when serum osmolality is low, and this results in further retention of body water. A decreased ability to concentrate urine can result in dehydration. In addition to monitoring for fluid volume depletion, older patients should be monitored for fluid volume excess because they have a decreased ability to adapt to sudden increases in intravascular volume.

Assessing Pulse in Older Adults

Nurses assessing pulse in older adults should understand the following:

- If the patient has severe hand or arm tremors, the radial pulse may be difficult to count.
- Cardiac changes in older adults (e.g., decrease in CO, sclerotic changes to heart valves, dysrhythmias) often indicate that obtaining an apical pulse will be more accurate.
- Older adults often have decreased peripheral circulation, so pedal pulses should also be checked for regularity, volume, and symmetry.
- The pulse returns to baseline after exercise more slowly than with other age groups.

Assessing Blood Pressure in Older Adults

Nurses assessing BP in older adults should do the following:

- Skin may be very fragile. Do not allow cuff pressure to remain high any longer than necessary.
- If the patient has arm contractures, assess the BP by palpation, with the arm in a relaxed position. If this is not possible, take a thigh BP.
- Determine if the patient is taking antihypertensives and, if so, when the last dose was taken.

Medications that cause vasodilation (e.g., antihypertensive medications) along with the loss of baroreceptor efficiency in older adults place them at increased risk for having orthostatic hypotension. Dehydration, bleeding, severe burns, and some analgesics can also cause hypotension in older adults. Measuring BP while the patient is in the lying, sitting, and standing positions and noting any changes can determine this. To assess for orthostatic hypotension, the nurse should:

- Place the patient in a supine position for 10 minutes.

- Record the patient's pulse and BP.

- Assist the patient to slowly sit or stand. Support the patient in case of faintness.

- Immediately recheck the pulse and BP in the same sites as previously.

- Repeat the pulse and BP after 3 minutes.

- Record the results. A rise in pulse of 15–30 beats per minute or a drop in BP of 20 mmHg systolic or 10 mmHg diastolic indicates orthostatic hypotension (Mayo Clinic, 2014d).

Case Study » Part 3

On day 4 of admission, you go into Mr. Evans's room to perform the morning assessment and find that his BP is 258/128 mmHg and pulse is 112 bpm. He was placed on mechanical ventilation 2 days ago. During the prescribed sedation vacation, you note that he is minimally responsive and grimaces as if in pain. Upon auscultation, you note that his lungs have crackles throughout, and you are suctioning pink frothy sputum via the closed suctioning system.

Clinical Reasoning Questions Level I
1. What do you think may have caused this complication?
2. What additional assessments are needed?
3. What lab or diagnostic test do you expect the physician to order?

Clinical Reasoning Questions Level II
4. Utilize the SBAR format to provide this new information to the physician.
5. What medications do you expect to be found on the patient's medication administration record?
6. What is the priority nursing intervention at this time?

REVIEW The Concept of Perfusion

RELATE Link the Concepts

Linking the concept of perfusion with the concept of inflammation:

1. Why does tissue become swollen and red around the site of injury?

2. How is the process of tissue repair affected by alterations in perfusion?

Linking the concept of perfusion with the concept of cognition:

3. Describe the cognitive impairments a nurse might observe in a patient with elevated ICP.

4. Describe the pathophysiology of hypoxia as it relates to perfusion and cognitive impairments.

Linking the concept of perfusion with the concept of elimination:

5. Describe the link between CO and renal failure.

6. Define renal autoregulation.

7. What class of drugs may be administered to improve renal perfusion pressure?

READY Go to Volume 3: Clinical Nursing Skills

- SKILL 1.1   Appearance and Mental Status: Assessing
- SKILLS 1.5–1.9 Vital Signs
- SKILL 1.17   Heart and Central Vessels: Assessing
- SKILL 1.22   Neurologic Status: Assessing
- SKILL 1.24   Peripheral Vascular System: Assessing
- SKILL 1.25   Skin: Assessing
- SKILL 1.27   Thorax and Lungs: Assessing
- SKILL 2.4   Feet: Caring for
- SKILL 2.11   Medications: Preparing and Administering
- SKILL 2.24   Oral Medication: Administering
- SKILL 2.36   Intravenous Medications: Adding to Fluid Containers
- SKILL 3.1   Pain in Newborn, Infant, Child, or Adult: Assessing

- SKILL 3.13   Physiological Needs of the Dying Patient: Managing
- SKILL 4.9   Commode: Assisting
- SKILL 5.1   Intake and Output: Measuring
- SKILL 5.9   Infusion: Initiating
- SKILL 5.10   Infusion: Maintaining
- SKILL 9.2   Range-of-Motion Exercises: Assisting
- SKILL 9.3   Ambulating Patient: Assisting
- SKILL 9.7   Positioning Patient in Bed
- SKILL 9.12   Turning Patient: Lateral or Prone Position in Bed
- SKILL 10.2   Diet, Therapeutic: Managing
- SKILL 10.5   Nutrition: Assessing
- SKILL 11.4   Chest Physiotherapy: Preparing Patient
- SKILL 11.8   Oxygen Delivery Systems: Using
- SKILL 11.22   Cardiac Compressions, External: Performing
- SKILL 12.5   Antiemboli Stockings: Applying
- SKILL 12.6   Pneumatic Compression Device: Applying
- SKILL 12.7   Sequential Compression Devices: Applying
- SKILL 12.9   ECG, 12-Lead: Recording
- SKILL 12.10   ECG, Leads: Applying
- SKILL 12.11   ECG, Strip: Interpreting
- SKILL 14.22   Newborn: Assessing

REFER Go to Pearson MyLab Nursing and eText

- Additional review materials

REFLECT Apply Your Knowledge

Nathan is a very athletic and active 15-year-old boy who presents to the emergency department for sudden syncope and collapse during a soccer game. Nathan and his parents deny any pertinent medical history, serious diseases, or cardiac disorders. After triaging Nathan, further questioning yields that Nathan has experienced periodic chest pain/pressure, shortness of breath, and palpitations during conditioning, but he attributed the signs and symptoms to being out of shape from not playing in any leagues during summer. Nathan denies any illegal drug use or tobacco smoking.

Clinical Reasoning Questions Level I

1. What tests, orders, and medications would you expect the provider to order?

2. Because Nathan has no pertinent cardiac history or risk factors such as obesity or lack of exercise, what pathophysiology

of altered perfusion could be causing Nathan's signs and symptoms?

3. How might you phrase your questions for Nathan according to his stage of development?

Clinical Reasoning Questions Level II

4. What priorities would you highlight in particular for patient teaching in adolescents?

5. After Nathan is discharged from care or hospitalization, what medications might you expect a cardiologist to prescribe during follow-up?

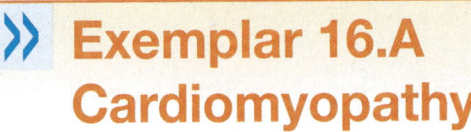

» Exemplar 16.A
Cardiomyopathy

Exemplar Learning Outcomes

16.A Analyze cardiomyopathy as it relates to perfusion.

- Describe the pathophysiology of cardiomyopathy.
- Describe the etiology of cardiomyopathy.
- Compare the risk factors and prevention of cardiomyopathy.
- Identify the clinical manifestations of cardiomyopathy.
- Summarize diagnostic tests and therapies used by interprofessional teams in the collaborative care of an individual with cardiomyopathy.
- Differentiate care of patients with cardiomyopathy across the lifespan.
- Apply the nursing process in providing culturally competent care to an individual with cardiomyopathy.

Exemplar Key Terms

Arrhythmogenic right ventricular dysplasia (ARVD), *1157*
Cardiomyopathy, *1155*
Dilated cardiomyopathy (DCM), *1155*
Hypertrophic cardiomyopathy (HCM), *1155*
Peripartum cardiomyopathy (PPCM), *1159*
Restrictive cardiomyopathy (RCM), *1157*
Syncope, *1157*

Overview

The term **cardiomyopathy** refers to diseases that affect the heart muscle and its ability to pump effectively. In patients with cardiomyopathy, the heart becomes enlarged, thick, or rigid (AHA, 2015b). In rare instances, sections of heart muscle are replaced with scar tissue. The heart eventually becomes weaker and less able to pump blood throughout the body. This inability to function normally can lead to heart failure, dysrhythmias, and disorders of the heart valves.

The AHA (2015b) classifies cardiomyopathies as either acquired or inherited. Acquired cardiomyopathies develop as a result of other diseases, conditions, or factors. Inherited cardiomyopathies are the result of genetic conditions passed from parent to child. In some cases, it is unclear whether cardiomyopathy is acquired or inherited.

Pathophysiology and Etiology

Cardiomyopathies are categorized by their pathophysiology and presentation into five types: dilated, hypertrophic, restrictive, arrhythmogenic right ventricular dysplasia (ARVD), and unclassified (AHA, 2015c). **Table 16–8** » compares the causes, pathophysiology, manifestations, and management of each type.

Dilated Cardiomyopathy

Dilated cardiomyopathy (DCM) is the most common type of cardiomyopathy and a common cause of heart failure. As

many as one third of individuals with DCM inherit the disease from their parents. DCM most commonly occurs between the ages of 20 and 60. Men are more likely than women to be diagnosed (AHA, 2015b).

With DCM, both the heart's ventricles and its atria can lose the ability to pump efficiently. End-diastolic and end-systolic volumes increase, reducing the left ventricular ejection fraction and decreasing cardiac output (CO) (Goswarmi et al., 2014). As the heart muscle begins to dilate and become thinner, the left ventricular chamber enlarges, eventually progressing to enlargement of the right ventricle and atria. Over time, the muscle becomes weaker, and heart failure can occur (AHA, 2015d). Clinical manifestations of DCM include shortness of breath, fatigue, swelling of the lower extremities and abdomen, and jugular venous distention (JVD). Disorders of the heart valves, dysrhythmias, and blood clots may occur with disease progression (Goswarmi et al., 2014).

The cause of DCM is unknown, although it is commonly associated with exposure to toxins, metabolic conditions, and infections. Reversible DCM may develop as a result of alcohol or cocaine abuse, chemotherapeutic drugs, pregnancy, or systemic hypertension. Up to one third of cases are as a result of inherited mutations (AHA, 2015d). Several different gene and chromosome aberrations are associated with DCM.

Hypertrophic Cardiomyopathy

Hypertrophic cardiomyopathy (HCM) is characterized by decreased compliance of the left ventricle and hypertrophy

TABLE 16-8 Classifications of Cardiomyopathy

	Dilated	Hypertrophic	Restrictive	Arrhythmogenic Right Ventricular Dysplasia	Unclassified
Causes	Usually idiopathic; may be inherited or acquired as a result of chronic alcoholism or myocarditis	Inherited; may be acquired as a result of chronic hypertension	Usually acquired as a result of amyloidosis, radiation, or myocardial fibrosis	Inherited cause of sudden death in young people and athletes; rare in individuals younger than 10 and older than 40	Inherited
Pathophysiology	Scarring and atrophy of myocardial cells Thickening of ventricular wall Dilation of heart chambers Impaired ventricular pumping Increased end-diastolic and end-systolic volumes Mural thrombi common	Hypertrophy of ventricular muscle mass Small left ventricular volume Septal hypertrophy may obstruct left ventricular outflow Left atrial dilation	Excess rigidity of ventricular walls restricts filling. Myocardial contractility remains relatively normal.	Genetically determined myocardial dystrophy Evidence of fibrofatty replacement of right ventricle and subepicardial regions of left ventricle	May progress to dilated or restrictive cardiomyopathies (RCMs)
Manifestations	Heart failure Cardiomegaly Dysrhythmias, S_3 and S_4 gallop; murmur of mitral regurgitation	Left ventricular hypertrophy Dysrhythmias Loud S_4 Sudden death Dyspnea, anginal pain, syncope	Dyspnea, fatigue Right-sided heart failure Mild to moderate cardiomegaly S_3 and S_4 gallop Mitral regurgitation murmur	Ventricular tachyarrhythmias High risk of sudden death	Symptoms of heart failure, chest pain, dysrhythmias, progression to heart failure and/or death Patients may be asymptomatic with detection during routine screenings or postmortem.
Management	Management of heart failure Implantable cardioverter–defibrillator (ICD) as needed Cardiac transplantation	Beta-adrenergic blockers Antidysrhythmic drugs Calcium channel blockers (CCBs) ICD, dual-chamber pacing Surgical excision of part of the ventricular septum	Management of heart failure Exercise restriction	Antiarrhythmics and implantation of defibrillators Prescreening for sport eligibility can detect asymptomatic patients	Treatment specific to type of cardiomyopathy Treatment may mirror that for heart failure. Monitor lab values as predictors of poor outcomes.

of the ventricular muscle mass. In HCM, the heart muscle becomes abnormally thick, which decreases the heart's ability to pump blood. Ventricular filling is impaired, leading to small end-diastolic volumes and low CO (Shah, 2016). The heart's conduction system may also be affected, leading to increased risk for life-threatening dysrhythmias.

The pattern of left ventricular hypertrophy is unique in that the muscle may not hypertrophy equally. This is known as *asymmetric septal hypertrophy*. In a majority of patients, the interventricular septal mass, especially the upper portion, increases to a greater extent than the free wall of the ventricle. The enlarged upper septum narrows the passage through which blood enters the aorta, impairing ventricular outflow (Shah, 2016).

HCM is usually inherited. Approximately half of individuals with this condition inherited the genetic mutation for the disease (Shah, 2016).

Restrictive Cardiomyopathy

Restrictive cardiomyopathy (RCM) is characterized by rigid ventricular walls that restrict the heart's ability to stretch and fill with blood. Decreased ventricular compliance reduces blood flow and may result in diastolic dysfunction and heart failure (Vainrib, William, & Goswarmi, 2014). Contractility is unaffected, and the ejection fraction is normal. Limited therapies are available for RCM; they consist of symptomatic, supportive, and pharmaceutical interventions.

Causes of RCM include scarring of the heart or amyloidosis. RCM may occur after heart transplantation. Fibrosis of the myocardium and endocardium causes excessive stiffness and rigidity of either or both ventricles.

Arrhythmogenic Right Ventricular Dysplasia

Patients with **arrhythmogenic right ventricular dysplasia (ARVD)** are at high risk for ventricular tachyarrhythmias and sudden death due to thickening of the heart muscle. ARVD results when the body progressively replaces the muscle of the right ventricle with fatty and fibrous tissue. ARVD may range in classification from mild to severe. Both men and women are affected, and the condition accounts for up to one fifth of sudden cardiac deaths (SCDs) in individuals under age 35 (Framingham Heart Study, 2015). ARVD is commonly associated with SCD in athletes. Treatment options range from no treatment to medications and surgery.

Most cases of ARVD are hereditary. Family studies suggest that the condition is the result of a genetic mutation of the desmosomal proteins (Burke & Butany, 2015). Family members of patients with ARVD should be closely screened for signs and symptoms of the illness.

Unclassified Cardiomyopathy

Cardiomyopathies that do not fit under the dilated, hypertrophic, restrictive, or arrhythmogenic types are referred to as unclassified cardiomyopathy. One example is left ventricular noncompaction, which occurs when there are muscle projections inside the right ventricle. Takotsubo cardiomyopathy, sometimes called "broken heart syndrome," is another example. It occurs when extreme stress leads to failure of the heart muscle (NHLBI, 2015b). Causes of unclassified cardiomyopathy vary depending upon the particular condition.

Risk Factors and Prevention

Risk factors for cardiomyopathies include a family history of cardiomyopathy, heart failure, sudden cardiac arrest, endocrine and metabolic diseases, alcoholism, and hypertension. Many forms of cardiomyopathy are idiopathic and often result in death. Although cardiomyopathies cannot be prevented, patients may reduce the risk of developing conditions that can lead to or complicate cardiomyopathies by living a heart-healthy lifestyle. This includes avoiding alcohol and drug use,

getting enough sleep, eating a heart-healthy diet, getting regular exercise, reducing stress, and avoiding smoking (Mayo Clinic, 2015c; NHLBI, 2015b). See the Health Promotion section in the module on Perfusion for more information.

Clinical Manifestations

All cardiomyopathies cause progressive weakening of the heart and decreased ability to pump blood and maintain regular rhythm. There are, however, subtle differences in the symptoms associated with each type of cardiomyopathy:

- **Dilated cardiomyopathy (DCM).** Manifestations of DCM develop gradually. Some patients may be asymptomatic or have minor symptoms with little impact on activities of daily living (ADLs). Heart failure often presents years after the onset of dilation and pump failure. Both right- and left-sided failure may be accompanied by dyspnea on exertion, orthopnea, paroxysmal nocturnal dyspnea, weakness, fatigue, peripheral edema, and ascites. Both S_3 and S_4 are commonly heard, as well as an AV regurgitation murmur (Goswarmi et al., 2014). As DCM progresses, patients begin to experience dysrhythmias. Patients with ventricular dysrhythmias are high risk for sudden death.

- **Hypertrophic cardiomyopathy.** Individuals with HCM may experience angina that results from ischemia caused by overgrowth of the ventricular muscle, coronary artery abnormalities, or decreased coronary artery perfusion. **Syncope**, or temporary loss of consciousness, results when outflow tract obstruction severely decreases CO and cerebral blood flow. Ventricular dysrhythmias and atrial fibrillation are common. Other manifestations of HCM include dyspnea, fatigue, dizziness, and palpitations. Symptoms develop as physical activity and oxygen demand increase, commonly during and after exercise (AHA, 2015b). A harsh systolic ejection murmur of variable intensity, heard best at the lower left sternal border (LSB) and apex, is characteristic in HCM. An S_4 murmur may also be noted (Shah, 2016).

- **Restrictive cardiomyopathy.** Patients with RCM may live a normal life and present as asymptomatic or with very few symptoms of illness. Others develop symptoms that worsen as heart function decreases. Less common are fainting and chest pain or pressure occurring during exercise or during periods of rest (exercise intolerance). Jugular venous pressure is elevated, and S_3 and S_4 are common (Vainrib et al., 2014).

- **Arrhythmogenic right ventricular dysplasia.** ARVD is usually diagnosed in patients younger than age 40. In many cases, ARVD is asymptomatic; the first manifestation is often sudden death. When symptoms do occur, they typically include dysrhythmias and conduction disturbances. These symptoms are relatively nonspecific, as are the results of blood and imaging tests (Burke & Butany, 2015).

- **Unclassified cardiomyopathy.** Unclassified cardiomyopathies do not fit into a specific category and include a variety of primary diseases of the heart muscle that result in cardiac dysfunction. Manifestations differ from disease to disease within this category.

Clinical Manifestations and Therapies
Cardiomyopathy

ETIOLOGY	CLINICAL MANIFESTATIONS	CLINICAL THERAPIES
Heart failure (left and right sided) often develops as the result of reduced CO.	■ Dyspnea on exertion, orthopnea, paroxysmal nocturnal dyspnea ■ Weakness, fatigue ■ Peripheral edema ■ Ascites	■ Treatment of underlying cause ■ Medications, including diuretics, vasodilators, beta-adrenergic blockers, and CCBs ■ Daily monitoring of patient's weight, intake, and output ■ Elastic stockings to improve venous return ■ Abdominocentesis to reduce ascites ■ Sleeping in semi-Fowler position ■ Periods of activity followed by periods of rest
Dysrhythmias are common because dilation of the heart muscle damages conduction pathways and leads to the formation of alternate paths.	■ ECG may show supraventricular tachycardias (SVTs), atrial fibrillation, and complex ventricular tachycardias (VTs).	■ Treatment of underlying cause ■ Medications, including antidysrhythmics, nitrates, and beta-adrenergic blockers ■ May require an implanted cardiac defibrillator (ICD) ■ Patient teaching regarding awareness of pulse rate and rhythm and when to interact with healthcare team
Angina may result from ischemia caused by overgrowth of the ventricular muscle, coronary artery abnormalities, or decreased coronary artery perfusion.	■ Chest pain radiating to the jaw, back, or left arm ■ Shortness of breath ■ Activity intolerance ■ Intermittent claudication ■ Nausea or vomiting	■ Treatment of underlying cause ■ Medications, including nitrates and beta-adrenergic blockers ■ Patient teaching regarding how to respond to symptoms and when to call 9-1-1 ■ Surgery may be required to repair damaged coronary arteries
Syncope may occur when outflow tract obstruction severely decreases CO and blood flow to the brain.	■ Dizziness, lightheadedness, fainting ■ Nausea	■ Treatment of underlying cause ■ Medications, including beta-adrenergic blockers ■ Patient teaching about the importance of sitting down as soon as symptoms start in order to prevent injuries from falls

Collaboration

The overall goals of treatment of cardiomyopathies are to manage the signs and symptoms, delay disease progression, and reduce the risk for complications. The treatment plan may include pharmacologic interventions, surgically implanted devices, or both. Treatment of HCM and ARVD focuses on reducing contractility and preventing SCD. Strenuous physical exertion is restricted. Dietary and sodium restrictions may help diminish manifestations.

Diagnostic Tests

Diagnosis begins with a thorough history and physical assessment, including exploration of signs and symptoms of illness and family history of cardiomyopathy, heart failure, or sudden cardiac arrest. Other diagnostic tests include:

■ Echocardiography
■ Electrocardiography and ambulatory ECG monitoring
■ Chest x-ray
■ Hemodynamic studies
■ Cardiac stress testing
■ Radionuclear scans
■ Cardiac catheterization and coronary angiography

■ Myocardial biopsy
■ Genetic testing.

Pharmacologic Therapy

Angiotensin-converting–enzyme (ACE) inhibitors, angiotensin II receptor blockers (ARBs), and CCBs may be prescribed to lower BP. Beta-blockers, CCBs, and digoxin are commonly used to slow the heart rate (although digoxin is avoided in HCM because of the hypercontractile pump). Beta-blockers may also be prescribed to relax the heart, stabilize the rhythm, and slow the heart's pumping action in patients with HCM. These drugs should be used with caution in patients with DCM. Diuretics may be added to aid in the treatment of heart failure. Anticoagulants are given to reduce the risk of thrombus formation and embolization. Electrolyte imbalances should be corrected because they may be a sign of dehydration, heart failure, high BP, or other illnesses. Aldosterone blockers may be used to correct imbalances. Antidysrhythmics may be administered to help prevent abnormal heart rhythms but are used with caution due to significant side effects.

Surgery

Cardiac transplantation is the definitive treatment for DCM, although organ rejection is a lifelong risk for the recipient.

With RCM, transplantation is not a viable option because the underlying process causing fibrosis is not eliminated, and eventually, the transplanted organ is affected as well. (See Exemplar 16.F for more information about cardiac transplantation.) Left ventricular assist devices (LVADs) may be used to support CO until a donor heart is available. The LVAD is an electronic pump surgically implanted into the abdominal cavity that aids in the perfusion of blood throughout the body.

Surgical ventricular remodeling is an alternative to transplantation. During the procedure, the size of the left ventricle is reduced to improve heart function and reduce the overall size of the muscle. The surgeon either removes a section or makes a tuck in the existing muscle.

An ICD or pacemaker may be inserted to control life-threatening dysrhythmias or help maintain a stable heart rhythm. When needed, these devices send an electrical impulse to stimulate cardiac contraction. The most common type of pacemaker attaches to the heart in two places, allowing healthcare providers to alter the sequence of contractions within the heart muscle.

Lifespan Considerations

Although individuals of all ages can have cardiomyopathy, certain forms are more prevalent in certain groups. Also, cardiomyopathies may affect members of different groups in different ways.

Cardiomyopathy in Infants and Children

Cardiomyopathy is one of the leading causes of cardiac death in children (Children's Cardiomyopathy Council, 2015). According to the Pediatric Cardiomyopathy Registry, 1 out of every 100,000 children in the United States under 18 is diagnosed with cardiomyopathy. The majority are under 12 months, with children ages 12–18 comprising the next largest group (AHA, 2015e).

DCM in pediatric patients appears along a spectrum of symptoms, ranging from no symptoms to congestive heart failure (CHF). In cases involving subtle symptoms, infants and young children are sometimes wrongly diagnosed with a viral upper respiratory tract infection or recurrent "pneumonia." Older children and adolescents are more likely to present with decreased capacity for exercise or susceptibility to fatigue; hence, they are less likely than younger children to be misdiagnosed with viral syndromes. In patients with DCM caused by viral myocarditis, the number and severity of CHF symptoms can increase so rapidly that the child can require emergency hospitalization and advanced life support within 1–2 days (AHA, n.d.a).

HCM is most often diagnosed during infancy or adolescence and is the second most common form of heart muscle disease. An estimated 35–40% of cardiomyopathies in children are hypertrophic. Like DCM, HCM presents along a spectrum, with some children having no symptoms while others have severe symptoms that include dysrhythmias and heart failure. Symptoms of CHF are often present in children less than 1 year old, while older children may be asymptomatic. Onset of symptoms often coincides with rapid growth and development in late childhood and early adolescence and with the rigorous activity of competitive sports (AHA, n.d.b).

RCM is the least common cardiomyopathy among children; it accounts for only 2.5–5% of diagnosed cardiomyopathies, or less than one per million children. Diagnosis of RCM usually occurs around age 5 or 6. RCM is slightly more prevalent among girls than boys, and family history of cardiomyopathy is present in about 30% of cases. Genetics are believed to play a role in most cases, even though the condition is usually idiopathic in the pediatric population. Initial symptoms in children often appear to be lung-related rather than heart-related. A history of chronic lung infection or asthma is common in children with RCM; cardiac involvement may be apparent only after chest x-ray reveals an enlarged heart or when a physical exam reveals abnormal findings. Other symptoms include abnormal heart sounds, fainting, fluid in the abdomen, liver enlargement, and edema of the face or extremities. In some patients, sudden death may be the first indication of RCM (AHA, n.d.c).

SAFETY ALERT Children with cardiomyopathy should not play competitive sports because of the possibility of collapse or increased heart failure. Low-impact activities may be appropriate based on a child's clinical status and should be discussed with the child's healthcare provider.

Cardiomyopathy in Pregnant Women

Peripartum cardiomyopathy (PPCM) is a relatively rare but serious form of DCM that leads to dysfunction of the left ventricle during the last month of pregnancy or the first 5 months postpartum. It typically occurs in women with no history of heart disease. As heart function decreases, the lungs, liver, and other body systems are affected. Heart dysfunction is usually reversible but may progress and necessitate heart transplantation. A heart biopsy may be indicated to determine the underlying cause. Subsequent pregnancy poses a high risk for complications, especially for patients who experience permanent enlargement of the heart (MedlinePlus, 2014a).

PPCM is most common in pregnant women over 30, although it may occur in childbearing women of any age. Risk factors include multiple pregnancies, obesity, poor nourishment, smoking, alcoholism, hypertension, and African American descent. Certain medications may also increase the risk (MedlinePlus, 2014a). See the Focus on Culture and Diversity feature for more information about risk factors for PPCM.

The cause of PPCM is unknown. However, systolic dysfunction and pulmonary edema should be ruled out. Nutritional disorders have been suggested but not validated (Carson, 2014). The left ventricle may not demonstrate dilation but the ejection fraction is typically reduced below 45% (Givertz, 2013). PPCM usually presents with anemia and infection. As a consequence, treatment focuses on underlying abnormalities. PPCM may resolve with bedrest as the heart gradually returns to normal size.

Cardiomyopathy in Older Adults

Cardiomyopathies are less common in older adults than in young adults and children. Only 10% of individuals

Focus on Diversity and Culture
Peripartum Cardiomyopathy in African American Women

Evidence suggests there is a correlation between PPCM and African ancestry. Rates of PPCM tend to be highest in African countries and countries where the population is predominantly of African descent (Gentry et al., 2010). In the United States, prevalence of PPCM is much higher among African American women than women of other racial backgrounds. An estimated 1 in 1421 African American mothers will develop this condition, as compared to 1 in 2675 Asian mothers, 1 in 4075 Caucasian mothers, and 1 in 9861 Hispanic mothers (Sliwa & Böhm, 2014).

Research further suggests that African American mothers with PPCM are less likely to see improved ventricular functioning upon recovery. An estimated 61% of Caucasian patients experienced improved functioning, but only 40% of African American patients saw improvement, even though members of both groups received therapy at similar rates (Sliwa & Böhm, 2014; Sliwa et al., 2014). Mortality rates due to PPCM are also higher among African Americans (Sharma & Russel, 2015).

In the United States, African American race is a risk factor for PPCM. Other risk factors include hypertension and two or more previous pregnancies. Because these risk factors frequently occur together, it is difficult to determine if race alone is a primary predictor or whether risk is based on a combination of factors (Gentry et al., 2010). Nurses should be prepared to counsel African American patients about their risk, particularly if other risk factors are present.

diagnosed with DCM are 65 or older (Arnold, 2015). HCM is also less common in the older population, though the number of patients over 60 diagnosed with this condition has been increasing (Maron et al., 2013). HCM in older adults tends to be benign and is less likely to lead to progressive heart failure and death than in children or younger adults (Cardiomyopathy UK, 2015). This may be because patients living past age 60 have milder forms of the condition. Treatment guidelines for older patients with HCM are not well established; however, the low morbidity and mortality rates among older patients do not support use of the defibrillator devices frequently implanted in younger patients (Maron et al., 2013).

RCM is the most common cardiomyopathy in older adults (Mayo Clinic, 2015c). Age-related decreases in the heart's contractile function and progressive stiffness of the ventricles can precipitate the condition, particularly in the presence of coronary artery disease (CAD), hypertension, or valvular calcification. RCM may also be the result of senile systemic amyloidosis (SSA), a nonhereditary, progressive disease that typically affects men in their 70s or 80s. SSA occurs when amyloid deposition in the heart leads to increased stiffening and deterioration of cardiac function. No specific treatment for SSA exists, and care is primarily focused on treating symptoms (Quarta, Kruger, & Falk, 2012).

Older patients may also be diagnosed with cardiomyopathy of aging. This is a blanket term used to describe heart failure or dysrhythmias that do not have a well-defined cause or cannot be attributed to a specific cardiomyopathy. Treatment of these conditions depends on the symptoms and health of individual patients.

NURSING PROCESS

Nursing assessment and care for patients with cardiomyopathies are similar to those for patients with heart failure. Because understanding and recognizing the symptoms are keys to learning how to manage the illness, patient and family education is vital. Some degree of activity restriction is often necessary. The nurse should teach patients to conserve energy while performing ADLs and encourage them to alternate periods of activity with periods of rest. Strong support systems are beneficial as the patient adapts to required lifestyle changes. Important lifestyle modifications include limiting salt, fat, and fluids in the diet; regular exercise; maintaining an appropriate weight; smoking cessation; limiting or eliminating alcohol; and stress reduction.

The patient with HCM requires care similar to that provided for the patient with myocardial ischemia. Nitrates and other vasodilators are avoided. If surgery is performed, nursing care is similar to that for any patient undergoing open heart surgery. Genetic counseling should be initiated to identify those at familial risk.

Assessment

The nurse should obtain both subjective and objective data when assessing the patient with cardiomyopathy:

- **Observation and patient interview.** Review health history, and note hypertension, diabetes, cardiac disease, and previous episodes of heart failure. Review family history, and note cardiomyopathy in close relatives. Record information about increased shortness of breath, dyspnea with exertion, and decreased activity tolerance. Assess sleep patterns for evidence of paroxysmal nocturnal dyspnea, and note whether additional pillows are used for sleeping. Ask about recent weight gain, episodes of coughing, chest or abdominal pain, anorexia, or nausea. Review current medications, typical diet and activity, and any recent changes in health.

- **Physical examination.** Assess vital signs, including apical and peripheral pulses. Observe general appearance, and note work of breathing, ease of conversation, position changes, and apparent anxiety. Examine skin and mucous membranes for color. Assess JVD and capillary refill. Note presence and degree of edema. Auscultate heart and breath sounds. Palpate the chest to assess heart size. Examine the abdomen, and note contour, tenderness in the right upper quadrant, and liver enlargement. Auscultate bowel sounds. Draw blood for testing as necessary.

Diagnosis

Appropriate nursing diagnoses for patients with cardiomyopathy include the following:

- *Cardiac Output, Decreased*
- *Fatigue*
- *Fluid Volume, Excess*
- *Activity Intolerance*
- *Knowledge, Deficient*
- *Grieving.*

(NANDA-I © 2014)

Planning

The plan of care is based on the type and severity of cardiomyopathy. Goals may include:

- The patient will maintain BP within specified limits.
- The patient will alter lifestyle to demonstrate adjustment to alterations in activity level caused by the disease process.
- The patient will modify diet to support long-term management of the condition.

Implementation

When providing care, the nurse must monitor for subtle changes in vital signs and LOC. Alterations in peripheral capillary refill time, pulse rate or volume, and LOC may be early warning signs of decreased perfusion. In many cases, the patient and family manage the condition in the home. For more information about preparing patients to manage their cardiomyopathies, see the Patient Teaching feature.

Monitor Cardiac Output

As the heart fails as a pump, stroke volume (SV) and tissue perfusion decrease. Nursing interventions that address these issues include the following:

- Encourage periods of rest throughout the day. Elevate the head of the bed to reduce the work of breathing. Provide a bedside commode, and assist with ADLs. Instruct the patient to avoid the Valsalva maneuver (i.e., trying to exhale against a closed airway, as when straining to lift an object or have a bowel movement). These interventions reduce cardiac workload.
- Administer prescribed medications as ordered. Medications are used to decrease cardiac workload and increase the effectiveness of contractions.
- Administer supplemental oxygen as needed. This decreases the effects of hypoxia and ischemia and results in increased oxygenation and perfusion.
- Monitor vital signs and oxygen saturation as indicated. Decreased CO stimulates the sympathetic nervous system (SNS) to increase the heart rate in an attempt to restore CO. Tachycardia at rest is common. Diastolic BP may initially be elevated because of vasoconstriction. In late stages, compensatory mechanisms fail, and BP falls. Oxygen saturation levels provide a measure of gas exchange and tissue perfusion.
- Monitor BNP (brain natriuretic peptide) levels, and report trends. BNP levels indicate the severity of heart failure: As the cardiac index decreases and left ventricular pressures increase, BNP levels increase.
- Auscultate heart and breath sounds regularly. S_1 and S_2 sounds may be diminished if cardiac function is poor. A ventricular gallop (S_3) is an early sign of heart failure; an atrial gallop (S_4) may also be present. Crackles are often heard in the lung bases; increasing crackles, dyspnea, and shortness of breath indicate worsening heart failure.

Monitor Fluid Volume

As CO falls, compensatory mechanisms cause salt and water retention, thereby increasing blood volume. Increased fluid volume places additional stress on the failing ventricles, making them work harder to shift the fluid load. Interventions for patients experiencing fluid volume excess include the following:

- Restrict fluids as ordered. Allow choices of fluid type and timing of intake, scheduling most fluid intake during morning and afternoon hours. Offer ice chips and frequent mouth care; provide hard candies if allowed. Providing choices increases the patient's sense of control. Ice chips, hard candies, and mouth care help relieve dry mouth and thirst.
- Monitor intake and output. Notify the healthcare provider if urine output is less than 30 mL/hr. Diuretics may reduce circulating volume, producing hypovolemia despite persistent peripheral edema. A fall in urine output may indicate reduced CO and renal ischemia.
- Weigh the patient at the same time each day, ideally after the patient has voided but before breakfast. Weight is an objective measure of fluid status: 1 L of fluid is equal to 2.2 lb of weight. Significant weight gain may indicate worsening heart failure.
- Record abdominal girth every shift. Note complaints of loss of appetite, abdominal discomfort, or nausea. Venous congestion can lead to ascites and may affect gastrointestinal function and nutritional status.
- Assess respiratory status and lung sounds at least every 4 hours. Notify the provider of significant changes. Declining respiratory status indicates worsening left heart failure.
- Monitor hemodynamic measurements. Report significant changes and trends. Hemodynamic measurements provide a means of monitoring condition and response to treatment.

Monitor Activity

Patients with heart failure have little or no cardiac reserve to meet increased oxygen demands. As the disease progresses, activity intolerance increases, which may impede self-care. Nursing interventions to help the patient minimize activity intolerance include:

- Provide written and verbal information regarding expected activity level. Written information provides a reference. Verbal information allows clarification and validation of the material.
- Plan and implement progressive activities. Use passive and active range-of-motion (ROM) exercises as appropriate. Consult with a physical therapist on an activity plan. Progressive activity slowly increases exercise capacity by strengthening and improving cardiac function without strain. Activity also helps prevent skeletal muscle atrophy. ROM exercises prevent complications of immobility.
- Assist with ADLs as needed, but encourage independence when possible. Assisting with ADLs helps ensure that care needs are met while reducing cardiac workload. Involving the patient promotes a sense of control and reduces a sense of helplessness.
- Organize care to allow rest periods for the patient.

Implement a Low-Sodium Diet

Diet is an important part of long-term management of heart failure. It also helps reduce fluid retention. When implementing a low-sodium diet, the nurse should do the following:

- Discuss the rationale for sodium restrictions to foster adherence with the prescribed diet.
- Consult with a dietitian to plan and review a low-sodium and, if necessary for weight control, low-calorie diet. Give the patient a list of high-sodium, high-fat, and high-cholesterol foods to avoid. Dietary planning and teaching increase the patient's sense of control and participation in disease management.

Evaluation

The effectiveness of nursing care and collaborative treatment is evaluated using nursing diagnoses and anticipated outcomes or goals. These may include the following:

- The patient verbalizes symptoms that must be immediately reported to the healthcare provider.
- The patient maintains BP within acceptable range as a means of demonstrating adequate tissue perfusion.
- The patient identifies activity tolerance strategies important for maintaining as normal a lifestyle as possible.
- The patient articulates the need for a low-sodium diet.

If patient outcomes are not met or the patient's condition worsens, referral to a healthcare provider who specializes in cardiomyopathies may be appropriate, and further assessment and testing may be required. ECG, chest x-rays, and cardiac catheterization may be appropriate means of

Patient Teaching
Cardiomyopathy

Cardiomyopathies are chronic, progressive disorders generally managed in the home and community care settings, unless surgery or transplant is planned or end-stage heart failure develops. When educating the patient and family about home care, include the following topics:

- Availability of community resources regarding support groups and respite care
- Activity restrictions and dietary changes to reduce manifestations and prevent complications
- Prescribed drug regimen, its rationale, and its intended and possible adverse effects
- Disease process, the expected outcomes, and treatment options
- Symptoms to report to the healthcare provider or for which immediate care is needed
- Cardiopulmonary resuscitation (CPR) procedures and available training sites
- Referrals to home and social services and counseling as indicated
- Cardiac transplantation, including the procedure, the need for lifetime immunosuppression to prevent organ rejection, and the risks of postoperative infection and immunosuppression.

assessing the patient. In some cases, defibrillator or pacemaker implantation, ventricular reconstruction, or heart transplantation may be indicated.

REVIEW Cardiomyopathy

RELATE Link the Concepts and Exemplars

Linking the exemplar of cardiomyopathy with the concept of oxygenation:

1. What physical assessment findings related to oxygenation would you anticipate for the patient with cardiomyopathy?
2. What are the priority interventions for a patient who presents to the emergency department with dyspnea and a history of cardiomyopathy?

Linking the exemplar of cardiomyopathy with the concept of comfort:

3. A patient with cardiomyopathy reports fatigue that is interfering with ADLs. What strategies might you recommend to help this patient improve independence in performing ADLs?
4. What techniques would be beneficial for the patient with cardiomyopathy to improve sleep and rest at home?

READY Go to Volume 3: Clinical Nursing Skills

REFER Go to Pearson MyLab Nursing and eText

- Additional review materials

REFLECT Apply Your Knowledge

Tyler Jones is a 28-year-old man who plays professional tennis. He is 6 feet 2 inches tall and weighs 180 pounds. Mr. Jones's wife, Sylvia, owns a popular local restaurant. Mr. and Ms. Jones have a 2-year-old son, Brandon. Mr. Jones is away much of the year for out-of-town matches. The Joneses have a strong family support system nearby to assist with Brandon's care.

Mr. Jones's father died suddenly at the age of 30 while running track. After an autopsy, he was diagnosed with HCM. Mr. Jones's mother is alive and healthy, helps Ms. Jones at the restaurant, and cares for Brandon when needed.

Mr. Jones has had occasional twinges of chest pain when practicing tennis. He has decided to see his regular healthcare provider for a full physical.

1. What factor in Mr. Jones's history puts him at greater risk for cardiomyopathy?
2. What assessment data will you obtain when examining Mr. Jones?
3. How will you respond to Mr. Jones when he tells you that he is afraid he will die suddenly at a young age, like his father?

» Exemplar 16.B
Congenital Heart Defects

Exemplar Learning Outcomes

16.B Analyze congenital heart defects as they relate to perfusion.

- Describe the pathophysiology of congenital heart defects.
- Describe the etiology of congenital heart defects.
- Compare the risk factors and prevention of congenital heart defects.
- Identify the clinical manifestations of congenital heart defects.
- Summarize diagnostic tests and therapies used by interprofessional teams in the collaborative care of an individual with a congenital heart defect.
- Differentiate care of patients with congenital heart defects across the lifespan.
- Apply the nursing process in providing culturally competent care to an individual with congenital heart defects.

Exemplar Key Terms

Aortic stenosis, *1168*
Atrial septal defect (ASD), *1164*
Atrioventricular (AV) canal, *1165*
Coarctation of the aorta (COA), *1168*
Congenital heart defect, *1163*
Endocardial cushion defect, *1165*
Heaving, *1179*
Holosystolic, *1165*
Hypercyanotic episode, *1166*
Hypoplastic left heart syndrome (HLHS), *1169*
Patent ductus arteriosus (PDA), *1163*
Pulmonary atresia, *1167*
Septal defect, *1163*
Shunt, *1172*
Tetralogy of Fallot (TOF), *1167*
Total anomalous pulmonary venous return, *1171*
Transposition of the great arteries (TGA), *1170*
Tricuspid atresia, *1167*
Truncus arteriosus, *1170*
Ventricular septal defect (VSD), *1165*

Overview

The term **congenital heart defect** refers to a defect in the heart or great vessels that results from an alteration in normal fetal development or the persistence of a fetal structure that does not convert to extrauterine anatomy after birth. In the United States, an estimated 8 infants per 1000 live births are born with a congenital heart defect (AHA, 2013a). Many of these defects have no known cause; others may be hereditary or a result of maternal medication use while pregnant. The majority of children with congenital heart defects survive to adulthood and live active, productive lives.

Pathophysiology and Etiology

Congenital heart defects were previously categorized as cyanotic or acyanotic. Current standards of practice categorize them by pathophysiology and hemodynamics. The resulting categories include the following:

- Heart defects that increase pulmonary blood flow
- Heart defects that decrease pulmonary blood flow
- Heart defects that result in obstructed systemic blood flow
- Mixed defects.

The following sections explore each category of defect in greater detail.

» **Stay Current:** The National Heart, Lung, and Blood Institute is an excellent source of information about conditions that affect perfusion. Information about congenital heart defects can be found on their website at http://www.nhlbi.nih.gov/health/health-topics/topics/chd.

Defects that Increase Pulmonary Blood Flow

The most common congenital heart defects involve an opening between the left and right sides of the heart (**septal defect**) or an opening in the aorta (**patent ductus arteriosus [PDA]**). These openings occur normally during fetal development and typically close on their own before or shortly after birth; failure to close allows blood to flow between the left and right sides of the heart. The pressures on the left side of the heart are higher than the pressures on the right side. This results in blood shunting from the left side to the right side of the heart and increases the amount of blood pumped to the lungs. In turn, increased blood flow to the lungs causes increased pulmonary vascular resistance (constriction of the pulmonary vascular bed, in an effort to reduce the blood flow) and pulmonary artery hypertension. Over time, right ventricular hypertrophy develops to compensate for increasing pulmonary vascular resistance. The size of the opening and volume of blood passing through it determine how quickly the child becomes symptomatic.

Table 16–9 » describes the pathophysiology, clinical manifestations, and clinical therapy for heart defects that increase pulmonary blood flow.

Defects that Decrease Pulmonary Blood Flow

Defects that obstruct pulmonary blood flow result in little or no blood reaching the lungs to be oxygenated. If an atrial or ventricular septal opening exists between the left and right side of the heart, the right-sided pressures exceed those on

TABLE 16–9 Pathophysiology, Clinical Manifestations, and Clinical Therapy for Heart Defects that Increase Pulmonary Blood Flow

Defect Pathophysiology, Clinical Manifestations, and Clinical Therapy	Anatomy

Patent Ductus Arteriosus (PDA)

PDA is a common congenital defect. When pulmonary circulation is established and systemic vascular resistance (SVR) increases at birth, pressures in the aorta become greater than pressures in the pulmonary arteries. Blood is shunted from the aorta to the pulmonary arteries, increasing circulation to the pulmonary system. In cases in which the passageway between the blood vessels does not close, some blood returns to the lungs. PDA is often seen in premature infants. The ductus arteriosus in the preterm newborn is not as responsive to the increased oxygen content with the conversion to pulmonary circulation, and it is less likely to close.

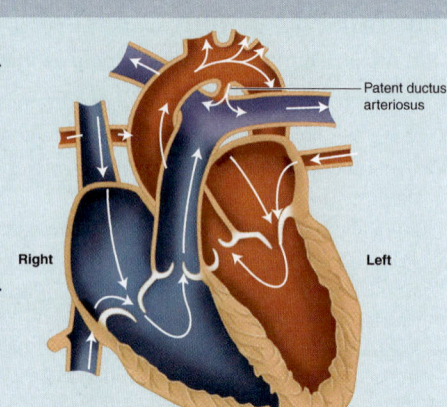

Clinical Manifestations
Manifestations include dyspnea; tachypnea; tachycardia; full, bounding pulses; and widened pulse pressure; hypotension may be noted when CO is low.
CHF, intercostal retractions, hepatomegaly, and growth failure with a large PDA may be seen.
A continuous "machinery" murmur during systole and diastole and a thrill in the pulmonic area may be present. The patient has high risk for respiratory infections, pneumonia, and infective endocarditis.

Diagnostic Procedures
Chest x-ray and ECG demonstrate left ventricular hypertrophy.
On echocardiogram, PDA is visible and a left-to-right shunt can be measured.

Clinical Therapy
IV indomethacin often stimulates closure of the PDA and may be given to some newborns.
Transcatheter occlusion is the least invasive surgical option and has become the treatment of choice.
  Surgical ligation of the ductus arteriosus is another option. Prophylaxis for infective endocarditis may be necessary until the PDA is closed.

Prognosis
No long-term sequelae occur if the PDA is treated before pulmonary vascular disease develops. If it is not treated, the child's lifespan is shortened as pulmonary hypertension and pulmonary vascular obstructive disease develop. Patients undergoing treatment should live healthy lives after appetite, growth, and activity levels return to normal.

Atrial Septal Defect (ASD)

An **atrial septal defect (ASD)** occurs when there is an opening in the atrial septum permitting left-to-right shunting of blood. ASD is commonly recognized in adulthood. Subtle physical examination findings and minimal symptoms during the first two to three decades of life often contribute to a delay in diagnosis. Approximately 70% of ASDs are detected in the fifth decade of life (Adler & Ellis, 2015). The disease sequelae depend on the size of the defect, size of the shunt, and associated abnormalities.

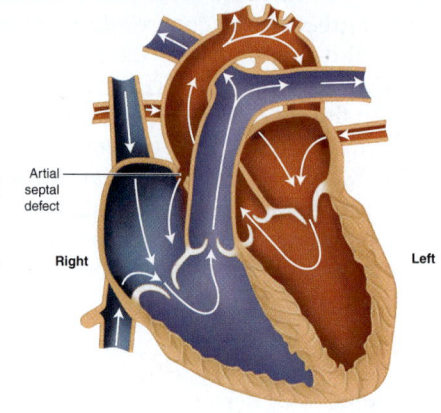

Clinical Manifestations
Infants and young children usually have no symptoms. Small and moderate-size ASDs may not be diagnosed until the preschool years or later. They are often considered after a heart murmur is detected on routine examination.
Abnormal findings may be found on chest x-ray or ECG.
Presenting symptoms include pulmonary arterial hypertension, atrial dysrhythmias, exercise intolerance, and CHF.
Heart sound S_1 may be split, reflecting forceful right ventricular contraction and delayed closure of the tricuspid leaflets (Adler & Ellis, 2015).
A soft systolic ejection murmur occurs in the pulmonic area with wide splitting of the second heart sound (S_2). The split S_2 is fixed because of reduced respiratory variation. It occurs only if pulmonary artery pressure is normal and pulmonary vascular resistance is low.
Mid-systolic murmur may be heard at lower LSB, due to increased blood flow across the tricuspid valve.
Mitral valve regurgitation may be present in patients with an ostium primum defect and an associated cleft of the mitral valve.

Diagnostic Procedures
Transthoracic echocardiography may clarify an uncertain diagnosis by providing direct visualization of most ASDs.
Chest x-ray often demonstrates cardiomegaly in patients presenting with a clinically significant left-to-right shunt.
MRI has been used successfully to identify the size and position of larger ASDs but is of limited value in visualizing small defects.
ECG reveals little information unless the ASD is large or has excessive shunting or right ventricular hypertrophy is present.

Clinical Therapy
Spontaneous closure of some ASDs occurs within the first 4 years of life. No activity limitations are needed.
Surgery to close or patch the ASD is performed when increased pulmonary blood flow causes CHF or when spontaneous closure has not occurred by 4 years of age. Minimally invasive approaches have increased in recent years.

Prognosis
The mortality rate for surgical repair is less than 1% for patients younger than age 45 who are not experiencing heart failure and have systolic pulmonary artery pressure less than 60 mmHg (Adler & Ellis, 2015). Many patients with uncorrected small and moderate-size ASDs live to middle age without symptoms. CHF, pulmonary hypertension, and atrial dysrhythmias are likely to develop by the sixth decade in untreated adults.

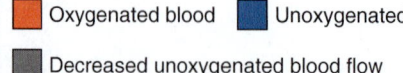

TABLE 16–9 Pathophysiology, Clinical Manifestations, and Clinical Therapy for Heart Defects that Increase Pulmonary Blood Flow *(continued)*

Defect Pathophysiology, Clinical Manifestations, and Clinical Therapy	Anatomy

Ventricular Septal Defect (VSD)

A **ventricular septal defect (VSD)** consists of one or more holes in the septum and results in increased pulmonary blood flow. Blood is shunted from the left ventricle to the right ventricle, where it enters the pulmonary artery. A VSD occurs in approximately 2–6 of every 1000 live births. VSDs may be primary anomalies or single components of intracardiac anomalies, including tetralogy of Fallot (TOF), complete AV canal defects, transposition of the great arteries (TGA), and correct transpositions (Ramaswamy & Srinivasan, 2015). Second to bicuspid aortic valves, VSDs are the most common congenital heart defect.

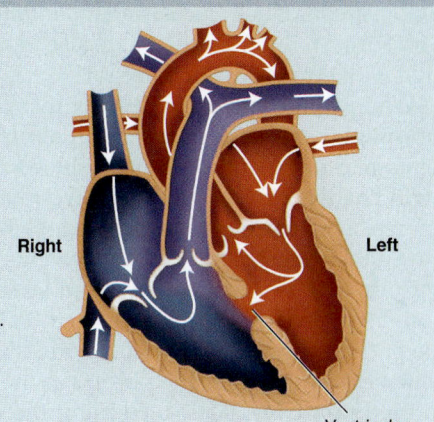

Right   Left

Ventricular septal defect

Clinical Manifestations

Symptoms depend on the size of the defect and degree of left-to-right shunt. Adults usually present with small to moderate defects because larger ones would have been identified earlier in life.
A murmur may be detected on routine examination in infants with small defects.
Excessive sweating during feedings may be observed in infants with moderate defects as a result of increased sympathetic tone.
Fatigue with feedings may occur due to increased CO. The presentation is similar to that for exercise intolerance.
Lack of adequate growth is due to increased caloric need.
Patients experience frequent respiratory infections.
A systolic murmur is auscultated at the third or fourth left ICS at the sternal border.
Patients experience signs of CHF with moderate to large defects.
Tachypnea is experienced only with exercise and not at rest (Eisenmenger syndrome).

Diagnostic Procedures

Chest x-ray, MRI, and ECG may provide useful but inconclusive information with small to moderate defects. An enlarged heart and pulmonary vascular markings may be seen on a chest x-ray when a large VSD causes shunting. Right and left ventricular hypertrophy may be seen on ECG.
Echocardiography establishes the diagnosis when shunting is present.
Cardiac catheterization may be beneficial prior to surgery. Findings usually reveal increased oxygen in the right ventricle and increased systolic pressure in the right ventricle and pulmonary artery.

Clinical Therapy

Most small VSDs close spontaneously within the first 6 months of life. Treatment is conservative when no signs of CHF or pulmonary artery hypertension are present.
Surgical patching of VSD during infancy is typically performed when poor growth is noted.
Closure of VSD by transcatheter device during cardiac catheterization may be used to repair some defects.
Prophylaxis for infective endocarditis may be required.

Prognosis

Highest risk associated with surgical repair is in the first few months of life. Children typically respond well to surgery and experience substantial catch-up growth. Tachyarrhythmias and right bundle branch block are possible complications.

Atrioventricular (AV) Canal (Endocardial Cushion Defect)

Atrioventricular (AV) canal, also known as **endocardial cushion defect**, refers to a combination of defects in the atrial and ventricular septa and portions of the tricuspid and mitral valves. As a result of these defects, blood moves freely among the four heart chambers, mixing oxygen-rich and oxygen-poor blood. The amount of blood flowing from the heart to the lungs increases, commonly causing symptoms in children. AV canal is estimated to occur in 3–5% of live births. This defect is also seen in approximately 9 out of every 10,000 children with Down syndrome (Pettersen & Seib, 2016). Most complex AV canal defects result in AV valve and large septal defects between both atria and ventricles.

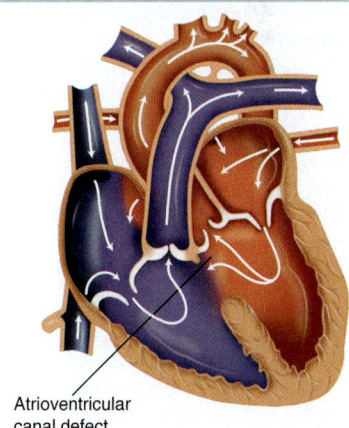

Atrioventricular canal defect

Clinical Manifestations

Severity of symptoms depends on the amount of mitral regurgitation and left-to-right shunting of blood across the septum.
Infants may present with CHF, tachypnea, tachycardia, failure to gain weight and grow, frequent pneumonia, pallor, sweating, cyanosis, and trouble breathing, especially during feedings.
A **holosystolic** (heard during the entire phase of systole) murmur is loudest at the left lower sternal border, and the intensity reflects the amount of mitral regurgitation. The S$_1$ heart sound is accentuated, and the S$_2$ is split.

Diagnostic Procedures

Chest x-ray shows cardiomegaly and pulmonary vascular markings.
ECG reveals atrial enlargement, right ventricular hypertrophy, and an incomplete right bundle branch block.
Echocardiography reveals dilation of the ventricles, septal defects, and details of valve malformation.
Cardiac catheterization reveals increased oxygen in the right atrium and increased right ventricle and/or pulmonary artery pressure.

Clinical Therapy

Surgery is performed during infancy to prevent pulmonary vascular disease.
Palliative pulmonary artery banding may be used to reduce blood flow to the lungs and alleviate CHF so the infant can grow before corrective surgery.
Oxygen may be required until surgery, but it may increase pulmonary blood flow and worsen CHF.
Patches are placed over septal defects, and valve tissue is used to form functioning valves. The mitral valve may be replaced.
Prophylaxis for infective endocarditis is required.

Prognosis

Long-term survival following surgery is good, although follow-up operations are necessary for 10–20% of patients (Ginde et al., 2015). Dysrhythmias and mitral valve insufficiency may occur postoperatively. There is no difference in short-term survival rates between infants with and without Down syndrome.

the left, resulting in right-to-left shunting. In this case, cyanosis often results.

The bone marrow is stimulated to produce more RBCs to increase the hemoglobin available to carry oxygen. Polycythemia may result and place the child at risk for thromboembolism. Over time, platelet survival is reduced and clotting factors are impaired, increasing the infant's risk of bleeding with surgery. Brain abscesses are also more common in children with cyanotic heart defects.

When infants and children with cyanosis rise in the morning, they may experience an abrupt decrease in systemic resistance and pulmonary blood flow. This physiologic change can trigger a **hypercyanotic episode** (also known as a hypoxic or "tet" episode) when combined with the sudden increase in CO and venous return associated with crying, feeding, exercise, and straining with defecation. The partial pressure of oxygen (PO_2) is lowered, and the partial pressure of carbon dioxide (PCO_2) rises. Hypoxemia becomes progressively worse as the respiratory center in the brain overreacts, increasing the respiratory effort. The extra respiratory effort further increases CO and

contributes to a life-threatening decline unless rapid intervention is successful.

Table 16–10 》 describes the pathophysiology, clinical manifestations, and clinical therapy for heart defects that decrease pulmonary blood flow.

Defects that Obstruct Systemic Blood Flow

Defects that obstruct systemic blood flow prevent sufficient blood from traveling to the body. For example, an anatomical stenosis of the aorta obstructs blood flow, causing a pressure load on the left ventricle and decreased CO. The greater the narrowing, the more obstructed the systemic blood flow. This results in higher pressure in the ventricle and decreased CO. Neonates with severe left outflow obstruction or left ventricular dysfunction may develop decreased CO and shock.

The pathophysiology, clinical manifestations, and clinical therapy for heart defects that obstruct the systemic blood flow are shown in **Table 16–11 》**.

TABLE 16–10 Pathophysiology, Clinical Manifestations, and Clinical Therapy for Heart Defects that Decrease Pulmonary Blood Flow

Defect Pathophysiology, Clinical Manifestations, and Clinical Therapy	Anatomy
Pulmonary Stenosis Pulmonary stenosis (PS), or abnormal narrowing of the valve allowing blood flow into the pulmonary artery, increases preload and results in right ventricular hypertrophy. PS accounts for 8–12% of congenital heart defects and can sometimes be seen to progress during the last 12 weeks of pregnancy (Lowenthal, 2014). It is often observed in children with Noonan syndrome, an autosomal dominant congenital disorder that affects both male and female patients. Children with Noonan syndrome typically present with distinct facial characteristics, including a webbed neck and flat-bridged nose. **Clinical Manifestations** PS is often present without symptoms. Dyspnea and fatigue may occur on exertion. Signs of heart failure and hepatosplenomegaly are rare but may result from chronic pressure overload. Chest pain on exertion may occur in severe cases. A loud systolic ejection murmur with a widely split S_2 and a thrill may be found with maximal intensity at the left upper sternal border. A pulmonic ejection click usually denotes a mild to moderate degree of stenosis. With severe stenosis, it may become buried in the first heart sound. **Diagnostic Procedures** Chest x-ray may show an enlarged pulmonary artery with normal heart size and normal pulmonary vascularity. ECG may show right atrial enlargement and right ventricular hypertrophy. Echocardiography provides information about the pressure gradient across the valve and size of valve ring. Cardiac catheterization findings include increased right ventricular pressure and a normal to slightly lowered pulmonary artery pressure. **Clinical Therapy** Dilation by balloon valvuloplasty, performed during cardiac catheterization, treats simple PS. Surgical valvotomy may be used when other defects such as VSD are present. Surgical resection may be needed for narrowing above the valve area. Pulmonary regurgitation may result but typically does not present as a significant problem. **Prognosis** PS does not typically increase in severity. Lifelong infective endocarditis prophylaxis is recommended.	Right Left Pulmonary stenosis

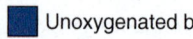

□ Oxygenated blood   ■ Unoxygenated blood   ■ Mixed oxygenated blood and unoxygenated blood
■ Decreased unoxygenated blood flow

TABLE 16–10 Pathophysiology, Clinical Manifestations, and Clinical Therapy for Heart Defects that Decrease Pulmonary Blood Flow *(continued)*

Defect Pathophysiology, Clinical Manifestations, and Clinical Therapy	Anatomy

Tetralogy of Fallot

Tetralogy of Fallot (TOF) consists of four defects—pulmonary stenosis, right ventricular hypertrophy, VSD, and an overriding aorta (aorta positioned directly over a VSD). Some children have a fifth defect, an open foramen ovale or ASD. TOF affects 3–6 of every 10,000 infants born (Bhimji & Mancini, 2015). With TOF, elevated pressures in the right side of the heart cause a right-to-left shunt.

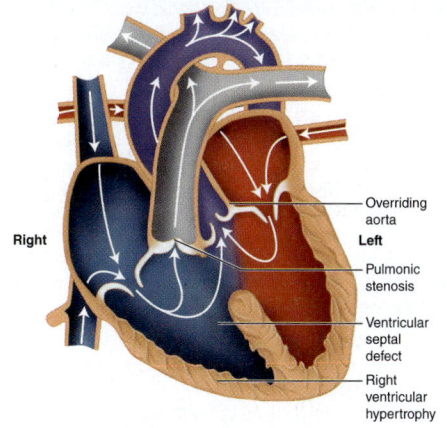

Clinical Manifestations
The infant develops hypoxia and cyanosis as the ductus arteriosus closes. The degree of PS determines the severity of symptoms.
A systolic murmur is heard in the pulmonic area and is transmitted to the suprasternal notch. A thrill may be palpated in the pulmonic area.
Polycythemia, hypoxic episodes, metabolic acidosis, poor growth, clubbing of the fingers, and exercise intolerance may develop.
Toddlers with uncorrected defects instinctively squat (assume a knee–chest position) to decrease the return of systemic venous blood to the heart.

Diagnostic Procedures
Chest x-ray shows a boot-shaped heart, resulting from the large right ventricle, decreased pulmonary vascular markings, and a prominent aorta.
ECG shows right ventricular hypertrophy.
Echocardiography shows the VSD, obstruction of pulmonary outflow, an overriding aorta, and the size of the pulmonary arteries.
Cardiac catheterization reveals the severity of the anatomical defects.
Blood tests demonstrate an elevated hematocrit and hemoglobin and increased clotting time.

Clinical Therapy
Management of hypercyanotic episodes includes placing the infant in the knee–chest position, calming the child, giving oxygen, and administering IV morphine and propranolol. Monitoring for metabolic acidosis or prolonged unconsciousness is critical.
A total repair is often performed at or around 12 months of age. A palliative shunt procedure (e.g., Blalock–Taussig) may be performed.

Prognosis
Not all children benefit from surgery, but most have improved longevity and quality of life.

Pulmonary Atresia and Tricuspid Atresia

Pulmonary atresia is the absence of a connection between the right ventricle and the pulmonary artery at the site of the pulmonary valve or in the main pulmonary artery. It occurs in about 1 out of every 10,000 babies (CDC, 2014a). In **tricuspid atresia**, the tricuspid valve is absent. Blood flows to the left side of the heart through the foramen ovale. A PDA provides the only flow of blood to the pulmonary arteries. A VSD or TGA is often present.

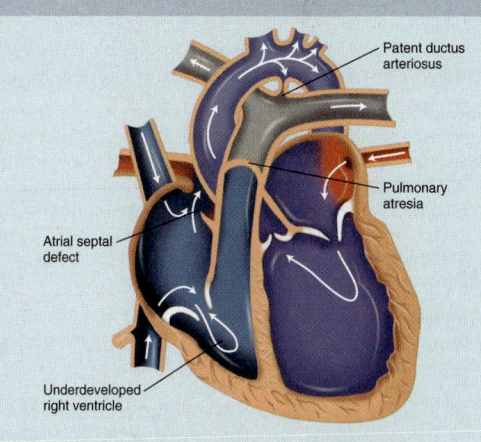

Clinical Manifestations
Cyanosis is present at birth.
Tachypnea, CHF, pulmonary edema, hepatomegaly, acidosis, hypoxic episodes, clubbing, polycythemia, and growth delays occur.
A continuous murmur from the PDA is heard in the pulmonic area. A single S_2 is heard in the aortic area, and a harsh systolic murmur may be heard in the tricuspid area.

Diagnostic Procedures
Chest x-ray may reveal a normal sized or slightly enlarged heart.
ECG may reveal right atrial hypertrophy.
Echocardiography shows a small hypoplastic right ventricular cavity and tricuspid valve, an absent right ventricular outflow tract, a dilated right atrium, and right-to-left shunting across the atrial septum.

Clinical Therapy
Prostaglandin E_1 is given immediately to maintain a PDA. Digoxin and diuretics are also used.
Rastelli balloon atrial septostomy is performed to increase the atrial opening (refer to Table 16–14).
Rastelli or modified Fontan procedure results in improved survival.

Prognosis
Outcome depends on the size of the pulmonary outflow tract developed by surgery and the fibrosis in the right ventricle. The child has increased risk for dysrhythmia and right ventricular dysfunction.

TABLE 16–11 Pathophysiology, Clinical Manifestations, and Clinical Therapy for Heart Defects that Obstruct the Systemic Blood Flow

Defect Pathophysiology, Clinical Manifestations, and Clinical Therapy	Anatomy

Aortic Stenosis

In **aortic stenosis (AS)**, narrowing of the aortic valve obstructs blood flow to systemic circulation. The valve is often bicuspid rather than tricuspid. The pressure gradient across the valve usually increases as the child grows and CO increases.

Clinical Manifestations

Most infants and children are asymptomatic, with normal growth and development. Life-threatening AS is detected in some newborns. CHF develops in infants with significant stenosis.

BP is normal, but a narrow pulse pressure may be noted. Peripheral pulses may be weak. The child may complain of chest pain after exercise, but exercise intolerance is uncommon. Syncope and dizziness are serious signs that require intervention.

A systolic heart murmur and thrill occur in the aortic or pulmonic areas with transmission to the neck. An ejection click may be heard. Splitting of the S_2 heart sound may be noted with severe AS.

Diagnostic Procedures

Chest x-ray is usually normal but may reveal a slight prominence of the left ventricle and aorta with increased severity.

ECG is usually normal in mild cases but with increased severity may show mild left ventricular hypertrophy and inverted T waves.

Echocardiography reveals the number of the valve cusps, pressure gradient across the valve, and size of the aorta.

Stress testing may be used in asymptomatic children to determine the amount of obstruction present with exercise.

Clinical Therapy

Newborns with life-threatening AS need prostaglandin E_1 to maintain a PDA until the aortic valve can be dilated.

The aortic valve may be successfully dilated by balloon valvuloplasty during cardiac catheterization. Surgical valvuloplasty may also be performed. Surgical treatment is palliative rather than curative.

Aortic valve replacement is performed when stenosis is severe or if significant regurgitation results from other interventions.

Prognosis

Chest pain, syncope, and sudden death can occur in symptomatic children, particularly during vigorous exercise. Stenosis is usually progressive during childhood as the valve calcifies. Valve replacement may be necessary once the child reaches adulthood, requiring lifelong anticoagulant therapy. Lifelong infective endocarditis prophylaxis is required.

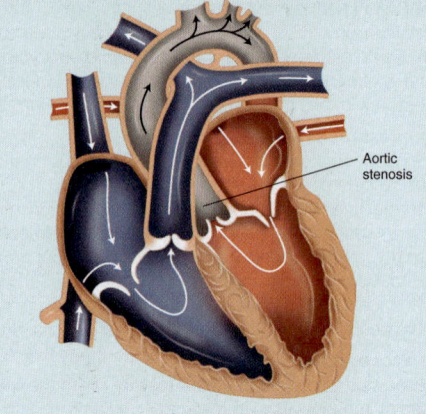

Aortic stenosis

Coarctation of the Aorta

In **coarctation of the aorta (COA)**, narrowing or constriction in the descending aorta, often near the ductus arteriosus or left subclavian artery, obstructs the systemic blood outflow. When this occurs, the heart must pump harder to force blood through the narrow part of the aorta.

COA may range from mild to severe; in some cases, it may not be diagnosed until adulthood. It often occurs with other heart defects and requires careful follow-up. COA is commonly seen in patients with certain genetic disorders, such as Turner syndrome (a chromosomal abnormality occurring only in female patients).

Clinical Manifestations

Symptoms are dependent on the rate of blood flow through the artery, but constriction is progressive. Infants may present with symptoms during the first few days of life; others may not present until adolescence.

Back pressure of blood and congestion of the lungs progresses to heart failure. Symptoms include dyspnea, coughing, fatigue, and swelling of feet and legs.

One distinguishing clinical feature is a difference between the femoral and carotid pulses.

A distinctive harsh murmur may be heard when a stethoscope is placed over the patient's back.

Diagnostic Procedures

Chest x-ray may reveal cardiomegaly, pulmonary venous congestion, and indentation of the descending aorta. Rib notching may be seen but is rare in patients younger than 10 years of age. MRI shows the site of coarctation.

ECG shows left ventricular hypertrophy; right ventricular hypertrophy may be seen in severe cases.

Echocardiography shows the size of the aorta, the actual coarctation, and the function of the aortic valve and left ventricle.

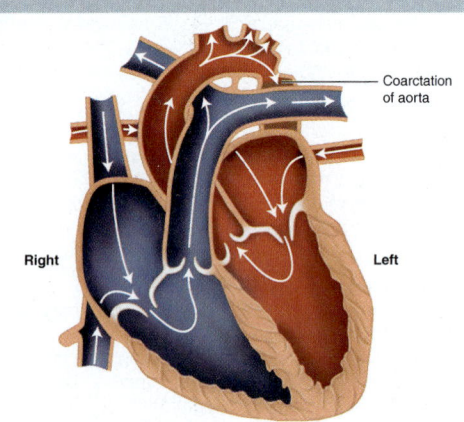

Coarctation of aorta

Right   **Left**

🟥 Oxygenated blood	🟦 Unoxygenated blood	🟪 Mixed oxygenated blood and unoxygenated blood
⬛ Decreased unoxygenated blood flow		

TABLE 16–11 Pathophysiology, Clinical Manifestations, and Clinical Therapy for Heart Defects that Obstruct the Systemic Blood Flow *(continued)*

Defect Pathophysiology, Clinical Manifestations, and Clinical Therapy	Anatomy

Clinical Therapy

Angioplasty occurs during cardiac catheterization for initial relief and recurrence.
   A catheter, with a balloon on the end is threaded into the aorta through the groin and into the blood vessels. Once the catheter reaches the coarctation, the physician inflates the balloon to expand the aorta. When the aorta is fully expanded, the balloon and catheter are removed.

Surgical resection with end-to-end anastomosis or with patching using the subclavian artery may be performed. Repair in the first year of life is recommended to decrease exposure to hypertension.

Prognosis

Prognosis depends on the severity of the defect and success of treatment.

Hypoplastic Left Heart Syndrome

Hypoplastic left heart syndrome (HLHS) is one of the most severe congenital heart defects. In HLHS, the left side of the heart does not form correctly during fetal growth, resulting in underdeveloped heart structures (CDC, 2015d). In patients with an absence of stenosis of the mitral and aortic valves, an abnormally small left ventricle, a small aorta, and aortic or mitral stenosis or atresia develops. HLHS accounts for roughly 1.5% of congenital heart defects (Syamasundar Rao, Turner, & Gessner, 2015).

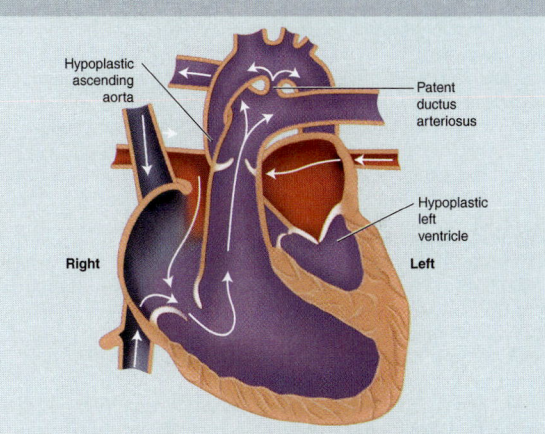

Clinical Manifestations

Once closure of the ductus arteriosus occurs, the newborn may have progressive cyanosis, tachycardia, tachypnea, dyspnea, retractions, and decreased peripheral pulses.

A systolic murmur may be present or absent.

Poor peripheral perfusion, pulmonary edema, and CHF can lead to shock, acidosis, and death.

Diagnostic Procedures

Chest x-ray shows cardiomegaly and increased pulmonary vascularity.

Echocardiography shows the small left ventricle. Diagnosis may occur prenatally during routine ultrasound scans.

Cardiac catheterization may be performed in preparation for surgical intervention. An atrial septostomy may be considered to promote homogeneity of the blood.

Clinical Therapy

An infusion of prostaglandin E_1 is usually begun to promote an open pathway for the blood to enter circulation from the right ventricle. The medication prevents closure of the PDA.

Supplemental oxygen is avoided because it tends to promote blood flow to the lungs, which may decrease blood flow to the body and place excessive demands on the stressed right ventricle.

Treatment options include comfort or palliative care; the Norwood, Glenn, or Fontan procedures (depending upon the child's age); and heart transplantation.

Surgery is performed in three stages. The Norwood procedure is performed in the first week of life, followed by the Glenn procedure at approximately 3–8 months of age, and then the Fontan procedure (see Table 16–14) at between 18 months and 3 years of age.

Heart transplantation is limited by the scarcity of newborn organs and a lifelong need for antirejection therapy. However, the lifetime incidence of rejection is lower in patients who receive transplants as newborns.

Prognosis

Once considered fatal within the first month of life, HLHS now has a 5-year survival rate around 65% (Marshall, 2015). Treatment decisions may be difficult because the parents must consider the potential for distress associated with multiples surgeries and the high medical costs. Children are restricted from competitive sports and very demanding physical activities but otherwise have a good quality of life. If failure of the single ventricle occurs, the child may require a heart transplant during adolescence or adulthood.

Mixed Defects

Many complex congenital heart conditions involve a combination of defects that make the newborn dependent on mixing pulmonary and systemic circulations for survival. This mixing of oxygen-rich and oxygen-poor blood results in a general, desaturated systemic blood flow and cyanosis. Pulmonary congestion may occur because of increased pulmonary blood flow and obstruction of systemic flow. The pathophysiology, clinical manifestations, and clinical therapy for mixed heart defects are shown in **Table 16–12** ⟩⟩.

TABLE 16–12 Pathophysiology, Clinical Manifestations, and Clinical Therapy for Mixed Heart Defects

Defect Pathophysiology, Clinical Manifestations, and Clinical Therapy	Anatomy

Transposition of the Great Arteries

In **transposition of the great arteries (TGA)**, the pulmonary artery and the aorta are transposed. TGA is life-threatening at birth, with initial survival depending on an open ductus arteriosus and foramen ovale. TGA is estimated to occur in approximately 5 out of every 10,000 babies born (CDC, 2014b). An ASD or VSD may also be present.

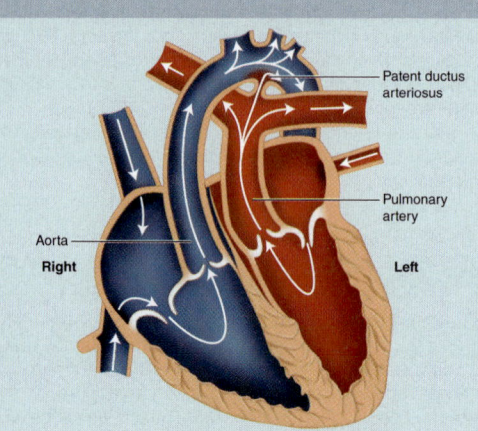

Clinical Manifestations

Cyanosis, apparent soon after birth, progresses to hypoxia and acidosis. Cyanosis does not improve with oxygen administration. Cyanosis may be less prevalent when a large VSD is present.

CHF may develop immediately or over days or weeks. Tachypnea (60 breaths/min) is often present without retractions or other signs of dyspnea.

A systolic murmur is present if a VSD is present; no other murmur is generally heard. The S_2 heart sound is loud.

Infants take a long time to feed and need frequent rest periods because of rapid respiratory rate and increasing fatigue.

Growth failure may be evident as early as 2 weeks of age if corrective surgery is not performed.

Diagnostic Procedures

Chest x-ray may reveal a classic egg-shaped heart on a string (narrow superior mediastinum) with enlarged ventricles and increased pulmonary vascular markings.

ECG reveals right ventricular hypertrophy.

Echocardiography often shows the abnormal position of the great arteries rising from ventricles.

Hyperoxia test confirms a cyanotic congenital heart defect.

Cardiac catheterization shows increased right ventricular pressure, and the catheter can enter the aorta through the right ventricle.

Blood tests reveal an increased hematocrit and hemoglobin or polycythemia.

Clinical Therapy

Prostaglandin E_1 is ordered to maintain a PDA until a palliative procedure can be performed. Oxygen is administered for severe hypoxemia.

Balloon atrial septostomy may be performed during cardiac catheterization in newborns as a first stage. The defect may also be corrected surgically. Other defects may be repaired in stages as the infant grows.

Corrective surgery (arterial switch or atrial switch) is usually performed before 1 week of age.

Prognosis

Survival without surgery is impossible. The overall survival rate following an arterial switch is greater than 90% (Charpie, Maher, & Berul, 2015). Dysrhythmias, decreased right ventricular function, pulmonary vascular disease, and sudden death are long-term complications after the Mustard and Senning atrial switch procedures. Follow-up every 6–12 months is recommended. Other complications of surgical repair include pulmonary artery or aortic stenosis, coronary artery obstruction, and mitral regurgitation. Infective endocarditis prophylaxis may be necessary.

Truncus Arteriosus

In **truncus arteriosus**, a single large vessel empties both ventricles and provides circulation for the pulmonary, systemic, and coronary circulations. A VSD is usually present. Truncus arteriosus is an uncommon congenital heart defect characterized by a single semilunar valve. In addition, the pulmonary arteries originate from the common arterial trunk distal to the coronary arteries and proximal to the first brachiocephalic branch of the aortic arch (McElhinney, Wernovsky, & Alejos, 2015).

■ Oxygenated blood	■ Unoxygenated blood	■ Mixed oxygenated blood and unoxygenated blood
■ Decreased unoxygenated blood flow		

TABLE 16–12 Pathophysiology, Clinical Manifestations, and Clinical Therapy for Mixed Heart Defects *(continued)*

Defect Pathophysiology, Clinical Manifestations, and Clinical Therapy	Anatomy

Clinical Manifestations

Cyanosis develops soon after birth, although this is also a condition of increased pulmonary blood flow. Severe CHF, dyspnea, retractions, fatigue, poor feeding, poor growth, polycythemia, clubbing, increased pulse pressure, bounding peripheral pulses, widened pulse pressure, frequent respiratory infections, and cardiomegaly occur.

The VSD produces a harsh systolic murmur in the lower sternal border. A systolic click may be heard in the apex and pulmonic area.

Diagnostic Procedures

Chest x-ray shows cardiomegaly, a large aorta, and increased pulmonary vascular markings.

ECG reveals right and left ventricular hypertrophy.

Echocardiography shows the absence of two semilunar valves.

Cardiac catheterization documents a left-to-right shunt at the level of the ventricle and pressure that is equal in the ventricles, the truncus, and pulmonary arteries.

Clinical Therapy

The Rastelli procedure is performed to close the VSD and create a passage to pulmonary arteries. Repeated surgery is necessary to enlarge the pulmonary artery conduit.

Digoxin and diuretics are given.

Prognosis

Survival is improved, but truncal valve stenosis and regurgitation result. The long-term prognosis is unknown. The child should not participate in competitive sports.

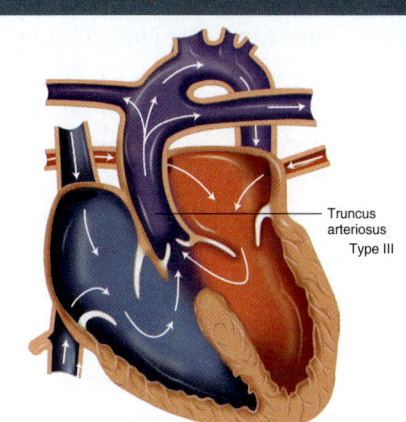

Truncus arteriosus Type III

Total Anomalous Pulmonary Venous Return

In **total anomalous pulmonary venous return**, the pulmonary veins empty into the right atrium, or into veins leading to the right atrium, rather than into the left atrium. The foramen ovale must remain patent for mixed blood from the right atrium to pass to the systemic circulation. Any obstruction of the pulmonary veins increases the condition's severity. Total anomalous pulmonary venous return is rare, occurring in approximately 1 out of every 10,000 births (CDC, 2014c).

Clinical Manifestations

Mild cyanosis and frequent respiratory infections occur. Increased cyanosis may occur with feedings as the filled esophagus compresses the common pulmonary vein.

If the pulmonary veins are obstructed in any way, cyanosis will be increased. Increased pulmonary blood flow will result in signs of CHF.

A precordial bulge may be palpated. The S_2 heart sound has a wide, fixed split when there is no pulmonary vein obstruction. An ejection murmur and gallop rhythm may be heard in the pulmonic area.

Diagnostic Procedures

Chest x-ray shows cardiac enlargement, a large pulmonary artery, and increased pulmonary blood flow.

ECG reveals hypertrophy of the right atrium and ventricle.

Echocardiography shows enlargement of the right atrium, a patent foramen ovale, and lack of connection between the pulmonary veins and left atrium.

Cardiac catheterization shows a higher oxygen level in the right atrium and the abnormal circulation.

Clinical Therapy

Prostaglandin E_1 is given to maintain a PDA.

Hypoxemia and CHF are treated.

Balloon atrial septostomy may be performed to promote better mixing of blood so surgery can be delayed until the infant is stabilized.

Surgery to reconnect or baffle the pulmonary veins to the left atrium is performed.

Prognosis

Prognosis is good when the defect is caught and repaired early and if there is no obstruction of the pulmonary veins at the new connection to the heart. Left untreated, the heart will continue to enlarge, resulting in heart failure.

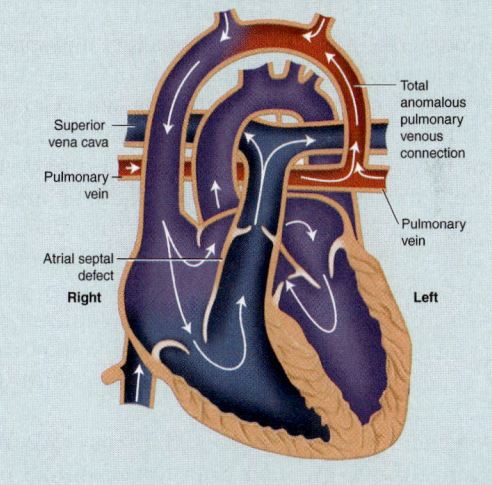

Superior vena cava

Pulmonary vein

Atrial septal defect

Right

Total anomalous pulmonary venous connection

Pulmonary vein

Left

Etiology

Most congenital heart defects develop during the first 8 weeks of gestation. They are usually the result of combined genetic and environmental factors. These may include the following:

- Fetal exposure to drugs (e.g., phenytoin, lithium, warfarin, valproic acid)
- Maternal viral infections (e.g., rubella, Coxsackie B5)
- Maternal metabolic disorders (e.g., phenylketonuria, diabetes mellitus, hypercalcemia)
- Maternal complications of pregnancy (e.g., increased age, antepartal bleeding)
- Genetic factors (family recurrence patterns)
- Chromosomal abnormalities (e.g., Turner syndrome, Noonan syndrome, DiGeorge syndrome, *cri du chat* syndrome, Down syndrome, trisomy syndromes 13, 18, and 21).

Deletion of chromosome 22q11 is associated with congenital heart disease, particularly TOF, interrupted aortic arch, VSD, and truncus arteriosus (McDonald-McGinn, Emanuel, & Zacai, 2013). Knowledge about other chromosome deletions or mutations associated with cardiovascular defects is emerging. Because of the genetic component, the incidence of congenital heart defects is expected to slowly increase as patients live longer and begin families of their own.

Risk Factors and Prevention

Specific environmental and genetic risk factors may play a role in the development of congenital heart defects. Maternal diabetes (type 1 or type 2) or infection with German measles (rubella) during pregnancy can impair fetal heart development. Medications such as isotretinoin (marketed under the brand names Amnesteem and Claravis, among others) and lithium (used to treat bipolar disorder) can increase the risk of congenital heart defects when taken during pregnancy. Consumption of alcohol and cigarettes while pregnant also increases risk. Heredity plays a significant role as well; congenital heart disease runs in families and is associated with genetic conditions such as Down syndrome (Mayo Clinic, 2016a).

Women considering pregnancy should discuss their risk factors with a healthcare provider prior to becoming pregnant. Genetic counseling is beneficial to women with congenital heart defects because there is a risk of passing these conditions to offspring. Some people with congenital heart defects may also have other genetic conditions of which they are unaware. These conditions may include a number of health problems with a wide range of severity, and affected individuals may have as much as a 50% likelihood of passing these conditions to their children (AHA, 2015f).

Prevention of congenital heart disease may not be possible because the causes of most congenital heart defects are unknown. It is possible, however, for women who are pregnant or who plan to become pregnant to control various risk factors. Risk reduction strategies include being vaccinated for rubella, managing chronic medical conditions such as diabetes, and discussing the risks associated with any medications with a physician. Other important measures include avoiding harmful substances like alcohol and cigarettes and taking a daily multivitamin that contains 400 micrograms of folic acid (Mayo Clinic, 2016b).

Some fetal heart abnormalities can be detected before birth through fetal echocardiography. This enables more timely medical or surgical intervention at birth and improves postdelivery survival. Some fetal heart problems involve tachycardia; mothers may have to take medication to help control this condition in their unborn child. This medication can affect fetal well-being, and maternal admission to a labor and delivery unit for monitoring may be required. Knowing that a heart problem exists during the prenatal stage gives the family an opportunity to learn about the problem and prepare psychologically and practically for the child's needs (AHA, 2015g).

Clinical Manifestations

The presence of a heart murmur is often the first indication of a congenital heart defect. A murmur indicates blood is flowing with higher-than-normal pressure to get through a narrowed valve or vessel, or is flowing through a **shunt** (an abnormal anatomical opening that allows movement of blood between the systemic and pulmonary circulation). Other clinical manifestations and the timing of their appearance vary by the pathophysiology and severity of the defect. Some infants and children, such as those with a small ASD, may be asymptomatic except for a heart murmur. Older children may have additional symptoms, such as exercise intolerance, chest pain, dysrhythmias, and syncope.

Defects that Increase Pulmonary Blood Flow

An infant's heart rate, respiratory rate, and metabolic rate are increased when pulmonary blood flow increases. Sucking breast milk or formula takes energy, and diaphoresis often occurs with feeding. The infant may be unable to take in enough calories to support metabolic rate and growth, resulting in poor weight gain. Dyspnea, tachypnea, intercostal retractions, and periorbital edema may occur if CHF develops. Frequent respiratory infections occur as the moist environment in the lungs supports bacterial growth. See Table 16–9 for the pathophysiology, clinical manifestations, and clinical therapy for specific congenital heart defects with increased pulmonary blood flow.

Defects that Decrease Pulmonary Blood Flow

Initial clinical manifestations in infants include cyanosis shortly after birth, dyspnea, and a loud murmur. The skin may be ruddy or mottled before cyanosis is observed. Cyanosis that does not respond as expected to oxygen is a classic sign (see **Figure 16–27 »**). Signs and symptoms of chronic hypoxemia include fatigue, clubbing of the fingers and toes, exertional dyspnea, and delayed developmental milestones. The infant may need to stop sucking periodically during feedings to breathe, and diaphoresis may be seen with the increased work of feeding. These infants have a higher metabolic rate, and inadequate calories may be consumed, resulting in poor weight gain. See Table 16–10

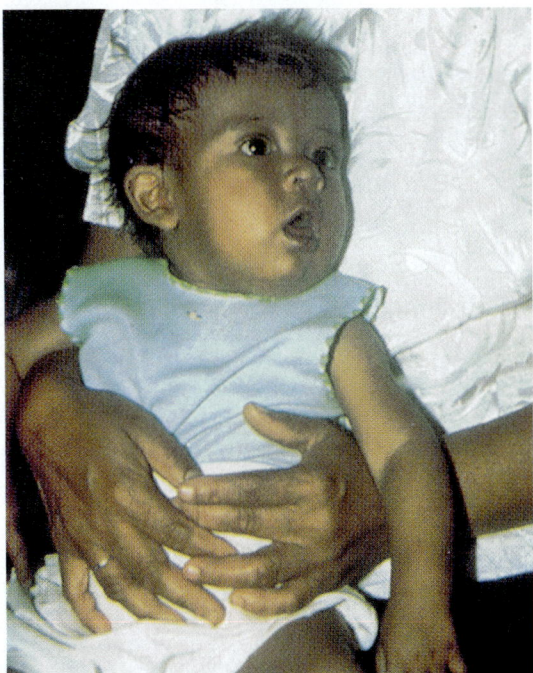

Figure 16–27 ›› The infant is cyanotic because of a heart defect that reduces pulmonary blood flow.

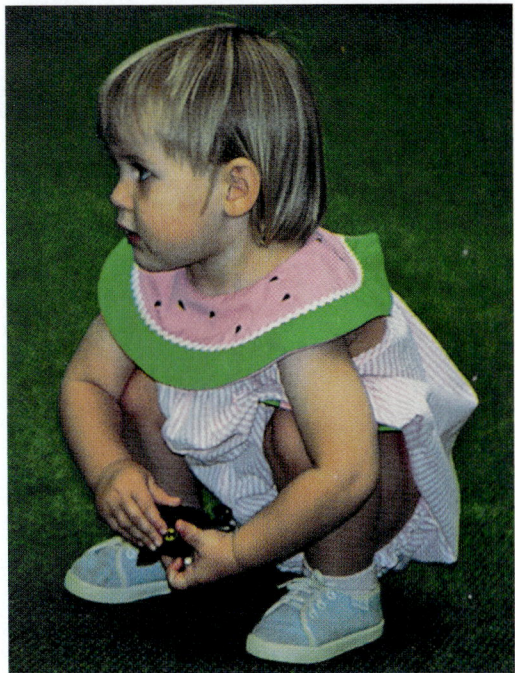

Figure 16–28 ›› A young child with an uncorrected or partially corrected defect that reduces pulmonary blood flow may squat (assume a knee–chest position) to reduce systemic blood flow return to the heart.

for the pathophysiology, clinical manifestations, and clinical therapy for these defects.

When the infant or child has severe obstruction to pulmonary blood flow, hypercyanotic episodes can develop suddenly. These episodes usually appear between 2 months and 2 years of age. Signs include increased rate and depth of respirations; increased heart rate; increased cyanosis, pallor, and poor tissue perfusion; diaphoresis; irritability and crying; and seizures and loss of consciousness. Toddlers with uncorrected cyanotic heart disease often squat to relieve dyspnea (see **Figure 16–28** ››). The knee–chest position reduces CO by decreasing venous return from the lower extremities and by increasing SVR. Older children may have additional symptoms, such as exercise-induced dizziness and syncope. These are serious signs indicating a need for medical evaluation.

Defects that Obstruct Systemic Blood Flow

Low CO is responsible for diminished pulses, poor color, delayed capillary refill time, and decreased urinary output. The blood cannot move past the obstruction, so it backs up into the left atrium and then the lungs, causing CHF and pulmonary edema. Children with mild obstruction may have leg cramps, cooler feet than hands, and stronger pulses and higher BP in the upper extremities than in the lower extremities. Decreased blood supply to the gastrointestinal tract may lead to necrotizing enterocolitis (see Table 16–11).

Mixed Defects

These complex congenital heart defects demonstrate varying degrees of cyanosis and CHF. When the pulmonary vascular resistance is lower than systemic resistance,

pulmonary congestion develops, followed by CHF. With decreased pulmonary blood flow, the infant will most likely present with severe cyanosis and polycythemia. See Table 16–12 for the pathophysiology and clinical manifestations of mixed defects.

Collaboration

Regular, ongoing follow-up with a primary healthcare provider and cardiologist is important for patients diagnosed with a congenital heart defect. Even with advances in medical treatment, not all patients are cured. Further surgeries may be needed after initial childhood surgeries. Diet and nutrition are important for those with feeding and weight gain issues. Many patients may also be placed on lifelong medications to improve heart function and help lower BP. Activity level should be discussed with the healthcare provider prior to beginning any exercise program.

Diagnostic Tests

Diagnostic procedures and laboratory tests used in the evaluation of congenital cardiac conditions are described in **Table 16–13** ››.

Pharmacologic Therapy

Medications administered to children with congenital heart defects may include any of those discussed in the Pharmacologic Therapy section in the Concept of Perfusion. In addition, prostaglandin may be administered to maintain fetal circulation, specifically to maintain a PDA, which allows blood to pass through the ductus and perfuse the rest

TABLE 16–13 Diagnostic Procedures and Laboratory Tests Used to Evaluate Cardiac Conditions

Diagnostic Procedure	Purpose	Nursing Implications
Cardiac catheterization	This invasive medical procedure is used in the diagnosis and treatment of various conditions. A flexible tube or catheter is inserted into a blood vessel in the arm, groin, or neck and threaded until it reaches the heart. Practitioners may place dye in the catheter to assist in the visualization of blood flow. They may perform ultrasound or heart muscle biopsies during catheterization. The practitioner can also use cardiac catheterization to view the overall flow of blood between the heart chambers and arteries.	■ Patient should be NPO 6–8 hours prior to procedure. ■ Check orders related to administration of routine and scheduled medications. Blood thinners and antiplatelet medications will most likely be placed on hold. ■ Ensure any lab work specific to the procedure has been reviewed and placed on the medical record. ■ Prep patient for procedure, as ordered. ***Postprocedure:*** ■ After sheath removal, apply consistent pressure to the access site for 20–30 minutes. Monitor vital signs per order. ■ Assess the access site frequently. Palpate and assess temperature, color, pulses, and patient discomfort. ■ Document access site assessment, including hematoma size and characteristics; skin color and temperature; and presence of pedal pulses, bruits, or both. ■ After stabilization of access site, elevate head of bed to 30 degrees. ■ Provide parent with education regarding common complications and methods to prevent bleeding. Clear instructions should emphasize when to seek medical assistance.
Chest x-ray	This radiographic exam of the chest, lungs, heart, large arteries, ribs, and diaphragm reveals the size and contour of the heart and characteristics of pulmonary vascular markings.	■ Explain the procedure to parent and child to alleviate stress and anxiety. Two images are usually taken from different angles. ■ Explain to the parent that the equipment limits radiation as much as possible. ■ Explain to the child that the tech may ask him or her to inhale and exhale deep breaths.
Echocardiography	This noninvasive test uses sound waves to create a moving picture of the heart. It is important for diagnosing congenital heart defect and its progression over time.	■ Decrease anxiety by reassuring the child that the exam is painless.
Electrocardiography (ECG)	This noninvasive test records the electrical activity of the heart. It demonstrates the heart's rate and rhythm and records the strength and timing of electrical signals as they pass through the heart.	■ Document current medications. ■ Reassure the child that the procedure is painless. ■ Explain to the parent and child the need to remain still during the recording.
Exercise testing	This test is typically performed on a treadmill or stationary bicycle to evaluate controlled increases in activity. The child is usually connected to ECG leads, a BP cuff, and a pulse oximetry monitor. Once the test begins, the machine's acceleration and pitch are increased in intervals. The test concludes when the child demonstrates noticeable fatigue or a predetermined stopping point is reached. The test is beneficial for identifying cardiac compensation or inadequate CO.	■ Educate the child and parents about the procedure. ■ Reassure the child that the test can be stopped at any point. ■ Instruct the child (in age appropriate terms) to report dizziness, shortness of breath, chest pain, and excessive fatigue. ■ Assess vital signs prior to, during, and after the exam.
Holter monitor (ambulatory ECG)	This procedure is used when a 24- to 48-hour recording of the heart's electrical activity is ordered. An ECG demonstrates the rate and rhythm of the heart and also records the strength and timing of electrical signals as they pass through the heart.	■ Normal daily activity is typically not limited. ■ Remind the parent and child to avoid submersing the electrodes in water. Swimming and bathing are not allowed until the test is completed. ■ Ask the parent to keep a daily log of activities and sleeping and eating habits.
Hyperoxitest	This is the most sensitive tool for differentiating primary pulmonary and cyanotic congenital heart disease. If cyanosis is respiratory in nature, PCO_2 should greatly improve with 100% O_2 supplementation.	■ Administer oxygen through a plastic hood for at least 10 minutes to replace all alveolar air with oxygen.
Magnetic resonance imaging (MRI)	This imaging test uses powerful magnets and radio waves to create images of the heart's myocardium, structure, valve function, blood vessels, and other soft tissues.	■ Verify that the child has no metal implants. ■ Reduce anxiety by discussing the shape, size, and sounds of the machine. ■ Administer sedation as ordered. ■ Monitor vital signs and LOC as appropriate.

TABLE 16–13 Diagnostic Procedures and Laboratory Tests Used to Evaluate Cardiac Conditions *(continued)*

Laboratory Test	Purpose	Nursing Implications
Arterial blood gas (ABG)	A sample of arterial blood is analyzed to help determine the status of pulmonary gas exchange and acid–base balance. Blood is drawn from either a direct arterial |puncture or an arterial line.	■ If ordered, a topical agent may be used to decrease pain associated with the needlestick. ■ After collecting the sample, place pressure on the puncture site for 5–10 minutes to decrease chances of hematoma.
Complete blood count (CBC)	Venous blood is collected and analyzed to assess the status of RBCs, WBCs, hemoglobin, hematocrit, and platelets.	■ Educate the parent and child about the procedure. ■ Follow hospital policy regarding skin preparation. ■ Apply light pressure and bandage to site after puncture.
Serum digoxin level	A venous blood sample is drawn to assess serum digoxin levels of patients receiving this medication.	■ Collect amount of blood recommended for procedure. ■ Educate the parent and child about the procedure. ■ Document last dosage and time of medication.
Antistreptolysin O antibody titer	This test detects previous infection by group A *Streptococcus*.	■ Educate the parent and child about the procedure. ■ Follow hospital policy regarding skin preparation.
Erythrocyte sedimentation rate (ESR)	This test detects the rate at which RBCs coagulate. The ESR increases with inflammation and assists in detecting acute illness.	■ Educate the parent and child about the procedure. ■ Follow hospital policy regarding skin preparation.
C-reactive protein (CRP)	This test detects the level of CRP produced by the liver. The CRP rises when there is inflammation in the body.	■ Educate the parent and child about the procedure. ■ Follow hospital policy regarding skin preparation.
Serum lipid panel	This test is used to measure total cholesterol, HDL, LDL, and triglycerides.	■ Follow orders regarding the need to fast.

Sources: Data from American Heart Association (AHA). (2015h). *Common tests for congenital heart defects.* Retrieved from http://www.heart.org/HEARTORG/Conditions/CongenitalHeartDefects/SymptomsDiagnosisofCongenitalHeartDefects/Common-Tests-for-Congenital-Heart-Defects_UCM_307412_Article.jsp; Morton, P. G., & Fontaine, D. K. (2013). *Critical care nursing: A holistic approach.* New York, NY: Wolters Kluwer/Lippincott Williams & Wilkins; National Heart, Lung, and Blood Institute (NHLBI). (2012b). *What is cardiac catheterization?* Retrieved from http://www.nhlbi.nih.gov/health/health-topics/topics/cath

of the body. Prostaglandin is used only for defects that rely on the PDA.

Surgery

One third of infants born with congenital heart defects develop life-threatening symptoms in the first few days of life. Treatment depends on the severity of symptoms and whether the condition is imminently life-threatening.

Interventional catheterization or surgical correction is the treatment of choice for many heart defects. Many defects can be completely repaired. For complex heart defects, however, treatment may be only a palliative procedure, meaning it does not create normal anatomical or hemodynamic results but allows adequate blood flow to oxygenate the tissues. A palliative procedure may be used for a child with a potentially fatal condition or as an initial procedure while the infant is small and before definitive corrective surgery can be performed. **Table 16–14** ❯❯ lists the types of cardiac catheterization and surgical interventions performed on children with congenital heart defects.

Lifespan Considerations

Congenital heart disease is a concern for patients across the lifespan. An estimated 2 million people in the United States are affected, including infants, children, adolescents, and adults (CDC, 2015e). Considerations tend to focus on infants and children because these conditions are present from birth, but many patients born with congenital heart defects survive into adulthood.

Congenital Heart Defects in Infants

Although critical congenital heart defects may present with severe or life-threatening symptoms in the immediate postnatal period, more simple conditions may present no symptoms (MedlinePlus, 2014b). Symptoms of critical defects in infants include cyanosis, rapid breathing and grunting while breathing, flared nostrils, shortness of breath during feedings, and edema around the eyes or in the legs and abdomen (Mayo Clinic, 2016b). An estimated 4.2% of all neonatal deaths are due to congenital heart disease, and these deaths tend to occur within 28 days of birth (CDC, 2015e). About 40,000 infants are born with congenital heart defects each year in the United States. Roughly one quarter of these children have a critical condition that requires intervention prior to the first birthday. Survival is dependent upon the timing of diagnosis, the severity of the condition, and the way in which the condition is treated. Approximately 95% of babies with noncritical conditions and 69% of babies with critical conditions are expected to survive to age 18. Infants with congenital heart defects have an increased risk for neurodevelopmental delays (see the Evidence-Based Practice feature).

Congenital Heart Defects in Children and Adolescents

Critical congenital heart defects are typically diagnosed in infancy, but conditions that are less severe may not manifest until childhood or adolescence. As the child grows and circulation requirements increase, the heart struggles to meet

TABLE 16–14 Clinical Interventions for Congenital Heart Defects

Heart Catheterization Procedure	Description of Intervention	Therapeutic Use and Defect Treated
Balloon angioplasty and valvuloplasty	A deflated balloon is threaded up to the coronary arteries to widen blocked areas where blood flow is reduced or completely obstructed.	Used as a primary or adjunctive treatment for PS, AS, and COA.
Patent ductus arteriosus (PDA) closure	Catheters are inserted in the groin and advanced to the aorta. A coil or plug may be placed, via the catheter, to occlude the defect.	Used to correct PDA.
Rashkind balloon atrial septostomy	A balloon catheter is used to increase oxygen saturation and enlarge a defect.	Used in the treatment of TGA.
Transcatheter closure	An umbrella- or clamshell-shaped device is inserted to plug a septum defect.	Used to correct atrial and ventral septal defects.

Surgical Procedure	Description of Intervention	Therapeutic Use and Defect Treated
Aorta resection with end-to-end anastomosis	Aortic isthmus and ductal tissues are resected, along with the inferior and lower lateral side of the aorta.	Used to correct COA.
Blalock–Taussig shunt	A Gore-Tex tube is placed from the innominate artery to the pulmonary artery.	Used as a palliative treatment for TOF, pulmonary atresia, tricuspid atresia, and other defects affecting blood supply to the lungs; in most cases, final repair will need to be done at a later time.
Brock procedure	This operation involves excision of fibromuscular obstruction in the right ventricle. The excision is completed using a surgical instrument inserted through the right ventricle.	Used as a palliative procedure to increase pulmonary blood flow and reduce right-to-left shunting in TOF.
Damus–Kaye–Stansel procedure	Aorta and pulmonary artery are joined using a patch.	Used as a corrective procedure for TGA and complex single-ventricle defects.
Fontan procedure	This operation results in the flow of systemic venous blood to the lungs without passing through a ventricle.	Performed to treat some complex congenital heart defects, including tricuspid atresia, pulmonary atresia, HLHS, and a double-inlet ventricle.
Glenn procedure	This operation involves connecting the superior vena cava to the right pulmonary artery and detaching it from the right atrium.	Used in patients with HLHS and other conditions requiring the redirection of blood flow.
Jatene procedure	This operation involves switching the main pulmonary artery and the aorta and relocating the ostia of the coronary arteries to the new aorta.	Used as a corrective procedure for TGA.
Mustard or Senning procedure	This operation restores circulation but reverses the direction of blood flow in the heart. Blood is pumped to the lungs via the left ventricle and pumped throughout the body via the right ventricle.	Used in patients diagnosed with TGA.
Norwood procedure	This procedure reroutes blood flow around some of the defective areas of the heart by creating new pathways for blood circulation to and from the lungs.	Used in patients with HLHS; variations for the procedure may be used to treat conditions in which one of both of the lower chambers of the heart are defective.
Norwood procedure with Sano modification	A Gore-Tex tube graft connects the right ventricle and pulmonary arteries, provides pulmonary blood flow, and replaces the Blalock–Taussig shunt used in the Norwood procedure.	Used to treat HLHS.
Patch aortoplasty	This surgery widens the narrowing section of the descending aorta. A synthetic patch is used.	Used to correct COA.
Pulmonary artery banding	This procedure creates a narrowing of the main pulmonary artery that decreases blood flow to the branch pulmonary arteries and reduces pulmonary blood flow.	Used in patients with pulmonary overcirculation and left-to-right shunting who require pulmonary blood flow reduction and those diagnosed with TGA.
Rastelli procedure	This operation involves excision of right ventricular muscle with large intraventricular baffle sutured into place. This results in closure of the VSD and redirection of left ventricular outflow to the aortic valve. A conduit is used to achieve right ventricular to pulmonary artery continuity.	Used to repair TGA with VSD and pulmonary stenosis.
Ross procedure	Patient's diseased aortic valve is replaced with his or her own pulmonary valve, or the pulmonary valve is replaced with a cadaver pulmonary valve.	Used as a treatment for AS.
Subclavian flap aortoplasty	Lengthwise incision is made along coarctation to create a flap that enlarges the constricted area. One benefit of this procedure is the possibility that the anastomosis may grow as the child ages.	Used as a corrective treatment for COA.
Transplantation	Patient's diseased heart is replaced with viable donor heart.	Used in cases of severe heart failure or when a badly damaged or defective heart cannot be made to function adequately through medical or surgical treatment.

Sources: Data from American Heart Association (AHA). (n.d.d). *Therapeutic cardiac catheterizations for children with congenital heart disease.* Retrieved from http://www.heart.org/idc/groups/heart-public/@wcm/@hcm/documents/downloadable/ucm_307680.pdf; Mayo Clinic. (2016b). *Disease and conditions: Congenital heart defects in children.* Retrieved from http://www.mayoclinic.org/diseasesconditions/congenital-heart-defects/basics/definition/con-20034017; MedlinePlus. (2015). *Congenital heart defect—corrective surgery.* Retrieved from https://www.nlm.nih.gov/medlineplus/ency/article/002948.htm

Evidence-Based Practice
Neurodevelopmental Outcomes in Children with Complex Congenital Heart Disease

Problem

Infants with congenital heart disease are at increased risk of neurodevelopmental delays for a variety of reasons. Infants born with these conditions are more likely to be born at younger gestational age and more likely to experience preoperative acidosis or hypoxia, all of which affect neurodevelopmental outcomes. Patients with congenital heart disease typically undergo early heart surgery, which also affects neurodevelopmental outcomes. As a result, patients may experience problems with cognitive and neurologic skills.

Evidence

A study of children born with congenital heart disease at the Arkansas Children's Hospital from 1998 through 2003 examined academic achievement. When assessed during third and fourth grade (9–10 years old), these children were 8 times more likely to receive special education services than their peers, and their achievement test scores were 7–13% below average. Surgery outside of the neonatal period was a significant predictor of decreased reading proficiency, with children who had surgery during the first 28 days after birth scoring higher than those who had surgery after this period (Mulkey et al., 2014).

Another study examined executive function in children ages 10–19 with congenital heart defects. Executive function is defined as neurologic skills involved in mental control and self-regulation; it includes mental flexibility, problem solving, verbal skills, and visual/spatial skills. The study found that children with congenital heart defects were twice as likely to struggle with executive function as those in the control group. The researchers also noted that individuals with more severe congenital heart defects experienced more problems with executive function than individuals whose manifestations were less severe (Cassidy et al., 2015).

Motor development may also be impaired in individuals with congenital heart disease. A study of adolescents with congenital heart defects revealed greater problems with fine and gross motor functioning than adolescents in a control group. These discrepancies were similar to those found in studies of younger children with congenital heart disease (Schaefer et al., 2013).

Implications

Together, these studies suggest that children with congenital heart disease are at greater risk for neurodevelopmental problems. Evidence-based interventions that address certain areas of neurodevelopment—including executive function and motor skills—have shown promising results in other populations, although little research exists on the efficacy of these interventions for patients with congenital heart disease (Calderon & Bellinger, 2015). Nurses who work with children with congenital heart defects should be sure to include neurologic assessment as part of the child's holistic assessment at each healthcare interaction. In addition, nurses should include assessment of parent coping and the need for education related to both their child's heart condition and any neurodevelopmental deficits.

Critical Thinking Application

1. What implications does this information have for nurses working with children in primary care clinics?

2. What implications does this information have for nurses working in early childhood intervention and school settings?

3. What resources are available in your community for children younger than 5 years old who have cognitive impairments? Motor problems? For children 5 years old and older?

---

demand. When this occurs, symptoms develop. These symptoms may include tiring easily, becoming short of breath during physical activity, and swelling in the extremities (Mayo Clinic, 2016b).

When congenital heart disease is suspected, the child may be referred to a pediatric cardiologist for evaluation and diagnosis. Chest x-rays may be used to detect heart enlargement, and ECG or echocardiography may be used to evaluate heart rhythm, structure, and function. In older children, an exercise stress test may also be ordered. Treatment depends on the particular defect and its overall impact on health and quality of life. Corrective surgery is necessary for many patients diagnosed in childhood or adolescence, and pharmacologic and dietary maintenance may be necessary both before and after surgical procedures (AHA, 2015h).

Regardless of whether congenital heart disease is diagnosed in infancy, childhood, or adolescence, children and adolescents may struggle to cope with their condition. Research suggests that lifelong medical monitoring and medication use, along with recurrent hospital stays, may negatively affect self-esteem (Bertoletti et al., 2014). This is especially true of adolescent patients who face bullying or social exclusion because of their physical limitations that prevent participation in sports or other activities. Adolescents may also struggle with issues of independence and acquisition of healthy behaviors.

Teaching older children and adolescents about their condition can lead to improved coping strategies. The nurse must provide age-appropriate education directly to these patients in addition to providing parent teaching about congenital heart disease (Ahn, Lee, & Choi, 2014).

Congenital Heart Defects in Pregnant Women

Pregnancy presents special concerns for patients with congenital heart disease because of the strain it places on the heart and circulation. Pregnancy may exacerbate symptoms in patients previously diagnosed with congenital heart disease; it may also cause symptoms to manifest for the first time in previously undiagnosed patients. Despite these issues, with proper medical care most women with congenital heart disease can carry an infant to term (Pereira & Warnes, 2014).

During pregnancy, the volume of blood in the mother's body increases by about 50%. This increase begins during the first trimester and peaks during the second trimester. The increase in volume increases the pressure load on the heart. Some congenital heart defects tolerate this increase better than others (Pereira & Warnes, 2014). Medical management of pregnancy focuses on these issues of cardiac load. Patients may also require teaching about anxiety reduction, as many pregnant women with congenital heart disease experience increased anxiety about their condition (Ramaswamy & Srinivasan, 2015).

Vaginal delivery is preferable to cesarean section for most patients with congenital heart disease because they will likely lose less blood with vaginal birth. Risk of wound infection and thrombophlebitis are also concerns with cesarean birth (Ramaswamy & Srinivasan, 2015). Women with complex congenital heart disease may need to deliver prior to term; when possible, they should undergo induction of vaginal delivery. Shorter labors (less than 24 hours) are preferred, and cesarean may be necessary if labor is slow. Dilated aorta, pulmonary hypertension, and aortic stenosis are contraindications for vaginal delivery (Pereira & Warnes, 2014).

Prepregnancy counseling is important for any woman with congenital heart disease who wishes to become pregnant. Counseling helps the patient understand the personal risk posed by her condition as well as the risk to the fetus. Counseling also helps determine what type of medical management will be required during gestation as well as whether there are any contraindications for pregnancy. Maternal medications should be reviewed during these sessions, and any medications that pose a fetal risk should be discussed. Genetic counseling related to the heritability of the mother's condition may also be discussed at this time. When necessary, the patient should be referred to a cardiologist who specializes in pregnancy management (Pereira & Warnes, 2014).

Congenital Heart Defects in Adults

Many individuals with congenital heart disease do not continue to receive proper follow-up care into adulthood. These patients may experience recurrence of symptoms such as activity intolerance, cyanosis, or shortness of breath years after initial treatment for their condition. There are several common reasons for symptom recurrence. In some cases, conditions that were surgically corrected may worsen over time. Corrective surgery may also cause scarring in the heart tissue that gives rise to other heart problems. Conditions that were treated medically rather than surgically may worsen, necessitating surgical repair in adulthood (Mayo Clinic, 2016a).

Numerous complications of congenital heart disease may develop during adulthood. Common complications include dysrhythmias, endocarditis, stroke, heart failure, pulmonary hypertension, and heart valve problems. Severity of complications may be associated with the severity of the specific defect. Some complications can lead to sudden death if not treated properly or in a timely manner (Mayo Clinic, 2016a). Diagnostic procedures may include cardiac imaging and catheterization. Treatments range from medication to implantable devices to open heart surgery, depending upon the type and severity of complications.

In addition to complications directly related to congenital heart disease, patients are at risk of developing other common diseases of adulthood. In some cases, these conditions may affect patients with congenital heart disease differently than the rest of the population (CDC, 2015f). Thus, patients with congenital heart disease must regularly see a physician for assessment and treatment appropriate to their history and current conditions.

Congenital Heart Defects in Older Adults

Prior to the inception of effective surgical interventions, patients who survived infancy were treated medically. Corrective surgeries for congenital heart disease were first performed in the 1950s as staged procedures for older children. Infant surgeries began in the 1970s and were limited to one or two common procedures. Thus, older patients with congenital heart disease include individuals who received only medical treatment, individuals who had multiple surgeries later in life, and individuals who had single surgeries in infancy (Bhatt et al., 2015).

Disease management in older adults must take into consideration the specific treatment modalities previously used to treat or correct patients' defects. It should also consider acquired heart disease, which may present with symptoms similar to those of congenital heart disease. The likelihood of developing cardiovascular disease or CAD increases with age, with mortality rates for these conditions being substantially higher in individuals age 65 and older. Prevention measures and risk management for acquired diseases are essential in patients with congenital heart disease, as is regular assessment by a cardiologist (Bhatt et al., 2015).

NURSING PROCESS

Nursing care of pediatric patients with congenital heart defects should address the family's needs as well as the child's. Parents and other caregivers are often overwhelmed by the complexity of the child's condition, worried the child will die, and confused by the decisions they are asked to make. Siblings are often frightened as a result of the anxiety they sense from the adults in their life and also need support.

Assessment

The first assessment finding in a child with a congenital heart defect is frequently a heart murmur. The location and sound of the murmur can provide significant detail regarding the type of defect the child has. The nurse gathers other objective and subjective information useful for patient assessment through interview and examination:

- **Observation and patient interview.** Review family history of heart defects or other congenital anomalies. Review the mother's history of prenatal and antenatal care. Record information related to breathing problems and shortness of breath. Observe the child's current respiratory pattern, and note rapid breathing and gasping breaths. Discuss feeding issues and problems with weight gain, and assess length and head circumference. Review sleeping and activity patterns, and observe the child for signs of fatigue. Note the color and temperature of the child's skin, the color of the mucous membranes, and any clubbing of the fingers. Assess parental coping and understanding of the child's condition.

- **Physical examination.** Assess various body systems for signs and symptoms of a cardiac condition. Use the

TABLE 16–15 Assessment Guidelines for the Child with a Cardiac Condition

Assessment Focus	Assessment Guidelines
Respirations	■ Inspect rate, depth, and respiratory effort. ■ Determine whether a cough is present. ■ Identify signs of increased respiratory effort: tachypnea, dyspnea, retractions, nasal flaring, and expiratory grunting. ■ Auscultate for adventitious sounds (wheezes, crackles).
Pulses	■ Assess pulse rate, rhythm, and quality. ■ Compare apical, brachial, and radial pulse rates. ■ Compare brachial and femoral pulses for strength.
Blood pressure	■ Compare BP to expected value for age, sex, and height percentiles. ■ Compare BP values between upper and lower extremities.
Color	■ Observe overall color; note pallor, dusky color, or cyanosis. ■ Contrast color in peripheral and central locations (e.g., nail beds to mucous membranes). Note whether crying improves or worsens color.
Heart	■ Inspect the anterior chest for bulging or **heaving** (lifting of the chest wall during contraction). ■ Palpate the chest wall for pulsations, heaves, or vibrations. ■ Locate the point of maximum intensity. ■ Auscultate the heart sounds and their quality (loud versus weak, distinct versus muffled). Muffled or indistinct sounds are associated with CHF or a heart defect. ■ Note presence of extra heart sounds or murmurs. Describe murmurs by intensity, location, radiation, timing, and quality. ■ Auscultate the heart with the child in sitting and reclining positions to detect differences in heart sounds.
Fluid status	■ Observe for signs of periorbital, facial, or peripheral edema. ■ Observe for abdominal distention. ■ Palpate the liver to detect hepatomegaly. ■ Observe for signs of dehydration with acute illnesses.
Activity and behavior	■ Determine whether exercise intolerance is present. ■ Assess whether the child tires with feeding. ■ Identify changes in activity level or behavior.
General	■ Assess growth. ■ Note presence of diaphoresis and when it occurs.

guidelines in **Table 16–15 》** to perform a comprehensive physical assessment of the cardiovascular system.

Diagnosis

Potential nursing diagnoses for the child with a congenital heart defect that increases pulmonary blood flow include the following:

- *Fluid Volume, Excess*
- *Infant Feeding Pattern, Ineffective*
- *Infection, Risk for*
- *Family Processes, Interrupted.*

    (NANDA-I © 2014)

Examples of nursing diagnoses that may apply to a child with a congenital heart defect that decreases pulmonary blood flow include the following:

- *Cardiac Output, Decreased*
- *Infection, Risk for*
- *Caregiver Role Strain*
- *Activity Intolerance.*

    (NANDA-I © 2014)

Examples of nursing diagnoses for a child following cardiac surgery include the following:

- *Breathing Pattern, Ineffective*
- *Pain, Acute*
- *Imbalanced Fluid Volume, Risk for*
- *Infection, Risk for.*

    (NANDA-I © 2014)

Planning

The goal when caring for children with congenital heart defects is to ensure long, healthy lives. The treatment plan should include interventions aimed at supporting perfusion throughout the body. Other treatment goals include the following:

- The child will maintain heart rate and oxygenation levels consistent with CO specific to the heart defect.
- The child will maintain adequate energy levels by engaging in activities appropriate to capabilities.
- The parents and family will verbalize concerns and fears related to the child's diagnosis.

- The parents and family will articulate resources available in the community, such as support groups and financial assistance agencies.
- The parents will articulate an understanding of the child's diagnosis and participate in the treatment plan.

Implementation

The nurse should participate with members of the cardiology team to educate the family about the child's condition. Appropriate information may include the following:

- General information about the congenital heart defect, including a description of the heart's anatomy and physiology and of the defect itself
- Information about genetic and environmental influences associated with the defect
- Overview of the child's prognosis and timing of medical and surgical interventions
- Interventions for CHF if it develops.

Provide Psychosocial Support

Parents often need support for anxiety about uncertain surgical outcomes. In addition, some parents may be concerned that signing consent for surgery places the child in more danger of illness or even death. When working with parents who are anxious about their child's condition, the nurse should do the following:

- Determine whether the parents have a support system as they learn about the child's diagnosis and make difficult decisions about surgery.
- Identify resources for support, such as social services, spiritual care, or a parent of a child with a similar heart defect, if adequate support systems are not already in place.
- Encourage parents to seek genetic counseling when planning future pregnancies.

Teach Presurgical Home Care

Children with congenital heart defects are often managed at home prior to surgery. The nurse should prepare parents to manage their child's condition by doing the following:

- Teach parents to encourage feeding and remind them that infants with congenital heart disease may take longer to eat than other infants.
- Encourage breastfeeding because of its beneficial effects for the infant.
- Suggest switching the infant to high-calorie formula if weight gain is an issue.
- Explain that feedings through a nasogastric or gastrostomy tube may be given at night or 24 hours a day to ensure that adequate calories are ingested, but encourage parents to continue offering formula orally to provide positive oral stimulation.
- Discuss the importance of reducing the child's exposure to infectious diseases, as well as the necessity of frequent hand hygiene by caregivers. Respiratory infections make hypoxemia worse in children with cyanosis, and fever increases metabolic rates and oxygen demands.
- Explain that disturbances in electrolyte balance may lead to vomiting, diarrhea, and certain drug toxicities. Instruct

parents to contact the healthcare provider if the child experiences fever, poor feeding, vomiting, or diarrhea.
- Emphasize the importance of routine health maintenance and promotion visits. Immunizations should be given according to the recommended schedule, and prophylaxis for respiratory syncytial virus should be provided during the peak season.

SAFETY ALERT Babies with congenital heart defects typically do best when fed on demand, because these children tend to tire easily during longer feedings.

Prepare for Surgery

When the child is preschool age or older, preparation for hospitalization and scheduled surgeries is essential to help alleviate the child's fear and anxiety. Interventions may include:

- After carefully assessing the child's developmental level, explain the procedure in simple, age-appropriate language that will help the child understand what will be happening. Be mindful of the language you use, and avoid technical terms and detailed descriptions that may frighten the child.
- Describe the surgical preparation procedures to the child and, if possible, take the child on a tour of the preoperative area to familiarize him or her with the environment.
- Encourage the child to ask any questions he or she may have.
- Help parents manage their anxiety during the preoperative period. The child will exhibit more anxiety if he or she senses anxiety in the parents.
- Provide parents with information about how the child will look postoperatively and the equipment that will be used in the child's care.
- Explain to parents the type of care that will be provided in the hospital during the immediate postoperative period and the type of care that must be provided at home following discharge.
- If available, connect the patient and family with the hospital's child life specialists. These specially trained professionals can provide emotional and other support before, during, and after the procedure.

Provide Postoperative Care

In the immediate postoperative period, the child will be cared for in the intensive care unit (ICU). When the child returns to the general nursing unit, nurses should be prepared to do the following:

- Assess for signs of surgical complications, such as infection, dysrhythmias, and impaired tissue perfusion.
- Monitor vital signs, including BP and pain.
- Auscultate the apical pulse to detect irregular heart rate or bradycardia, both of which are signs of reduced CO that require immediate intervention.
- Assess the respiratory system for breath sounds, respiratory effort, and signs of distress that may indicate pneumonia or fluid in the pleural space.
- Check pulse oximetry, capillary refill, extremity warmth, pedal pulses, LOC, and urine output to assess impaired tissue perfusion.

- Monitor the child's temperature, and inspect the incision site. Fever, excessive incisional pain, spreading erythema around the incision, and wound drainage beginning 3–4 days postoperatively may be signs of infection.

Manage Pain

Pain management is an important component of postoperative care and will likely include the following:

- Twenty four–hour IV opioids provided for several days postoperatively until the child is taking fluids.
- Round-the-clock oral analgesics may be given once the child is taking oral fluids and foods.
- Lifting and moving techniques that avoid stress on the incision and reduce potential pain should be used. The nurse will need to teach parents appropriate techniques.

Promote Respiratory Function

Pain in the chest following surgery can make breathing difficult or uncomfortable for the child. The nurse should promote respiratory function by doing the following:

- Encourage the child to take deep breaths and cough or perform spirometry exercises regularly to promote full lung expansion.
- Provide a pillow or new stuffed animal for the child to hold against the chest to help reduce pain from coughing and deep breathing.
- Prepare the patient for chest physiotherapy treatments with a physical or respiratory therapist for children under 3 years of age.

Manage Fluids and Nutrition

The nurse should encourage the infant or child to begin oral fluids and nutrition when permitted. When beginning oral food and fluids, the nurse should do the following:

- Assess intake and output carefully.
- Encourage parents to bring in favorite foods for the child when they can be tolerated.
- Administer antibiotics as ordered.
- Convert the line to a heparin or saline lock if IV antibiotics are continued after the child's oral intake is normal.

Promote Activity

Returning to normal activity is an important step in the recovery process. In helping the child resume normal activities, the nurse should do the following:

- Encourage the child to increase activity gradually, with longer periods out of bed every day and adequate rest periods to promote healing.
- Provide opportunities for therapeutic play and fun activities so the child can better manage the stresses associated with pain and frightening procedures.

SAFETY ALERT Be mindful for signs and symptoms of posttraumatic stress disorder (PTSD) in the child as well as the parents. Both parents and children experience heart surgery as a traumatic event, and nurses must include psychosocial assessment as part of the ongoing assessment process for these children and their families.

Plan Discharge and Postsurgical Home Care

Infants and children may be discharged from the hospital within a few days of surgery. The nurse should prepare parents for discharge by doing the following:

- Provide information to parents over the course of several days to allow them adequate time to prepare for care of the child at home. Walk parents through basic care routines, and answer any questions they may have.
- Encourage a nutritious diet and snacks so the infant or child has an opportunity to catch up from previous growth deficits. Coordinate with a nutritionist or dietitian if necessary.
- Discuss pain management, and encourage use of acetaminophen or ibuprofen for pain management after discharge.
- Explain the need for slow but steady return to normal activity. Discuss appropriate activities for the child as well as the need for adequate rest.
- Discuss the risk for infective endocarditis, especially in the first 6 months after surgery. Explain the need for prophylactic antibiotics for invasive procedures.

See the Patient Teaching feature for additional information about social and emotional considerations following surgery.

Patient Teaching
Social and Emotional Considerations Following Congenital Heart Defect Repair

Parents of a child with congenital heart disease may be anxious about their child's health, even after corrective surgery. The nurse should reassure parents of children with a complete correction of the cardiac defect that there should be no further cardiovascular problems. They should provide parents with full information about the child's defect and the surgery performed to share with the child's current and future healthcare providers. The nurse should encourage parents to allow the child to live a normal, active life and promote independence wherever possible.

The nurse should also prepare parents for potential behavior problems that may result from the stress of hospitalization. Examples of common problems include nightmares, separation anxiety, and overdependence on parents. The nurse should encourage parents to reassure children about their security and to promote play and other means to deal with their feelings. If the child's symptoms continue for several weeks, a referral for psychologic evaluation and care may be needed.

Focus on Integrative Health
Congenital Heart Defects

The nurse should caution parents of children with congenital heart defects against using integrative therapies, such as herbal products, that may interfere with prescribed medications. Products containing ginkgo are known to interact with warfarin, which is of particular concern for any child on anticoagulant therapy. The adverse effects of herbal remedies have not been fully identified.

Evaluation

Examples of expected outcomes of nursing care include the following:

- The child's pain is managed effectively.
- Full lung expansion is maintained with incentive spirometry exercises or chest physiotherapy.
- The child's incision heals without infection.

If patient outcomes are not met, the child should be evaluated by a pediatric cardiologist. Further tests may be necessary, including chest x-rays, ECG, and echocardiography. Additional treatment may also be needed and may include cardiac catheterization or further surgical interventions.

Nursing Care Plan
A Patient with VSD

Gwen Polasani is a newborn girl. She is the third child of Theresa and Jason Polasani, who also have a 4-year-old girl and a 6-year-old boy at home. Gwen was born earlier today via uncomplicated vaginal delivery.

ASSESSMENT

Upon admission to the newborn nursery, Gwen is weighed (4000 g), measured (chest, 33 cm; length, 53.34 cm), and found by exam to be at 39 weeks of gestation. Vital signs are T 98.0°F; P 148 bpm; R 52/min; BP 68/44 mmHg. When performing a complete assessment, you find nothing abnormal until assessing heart sounds, when you hear a loud systolic murmur. An echocardiogram is ordered, which demonstrates a large VSD.

The pediatrician recommends monitoring Gwen's condition and allowing her to remain in the normal nursery and spend time with her mother as long as she is stable. Two days later, Gwen's weight has increased to 4400 g, she is edematous, and she has course crackles throughout the lung fields. She is tachypneic, and her oxygen saturation is 88% on room air. She is lethargic, and vital signs are T 98°F; P 188 bpm; R 76/min; BP 54/36 mmHg. The pediatrician diagnoses Gwen with CHF secondary to her VSD, and she is transferred to the neonatal intensive care unit (NICU).

DIAGNOSES

- *Decreased Cardiac Output* related to cardiac anomaly (VSD)
- *Excess Fluid Volume* related to heart failure
- *Impaired Skin Integrity, Risk for* related to altered fluid status
- *Imbalanced Nutrition, Less than Body Requirements* related to increased metabolic needs and rapid tiring during feedings
- *Compromised Family Coping* related to situational crisis with child's health problems

(NANDA-I © 2014)

PLANNING

Goals of care include the following:

- Gwen's CO will be sufficient to meet the body's metabolic demands.
- Gwen will manifest adequate oxygenation.
- Gwen's peripheral and central edema will decrease.
- Gwen's intake and output will be balanced once excess fluid is excreted.
- Gwen will demonstrate expected weight gain for age.

IMPLEMENTATION

- Administer digoxin as ordered.
- Take apical pulse, and listen to heart sounds regularly, especially before each dose of digoxin. Record apical pulse with each recorded dose of digoxin.
- Place newborn on a cardiorespiratory monitor.
- Prevent injury by monitoring for digoxin side effects and serum potassium level.
- Stagger care to provide for rest periods.
- Place newborn in semi-Fowler position.
- Evaluate respiratory rate and sounds.
- Take pulse oximetry readings to determine oxygen saturation.
- Provide oxygen and humidification if ordered. Observe for diaphoresis, a sign of increased respiratory effort.
- Administer diuretics as ordered.
- Weigh and measure abdominal girth daily. Observe for peripheral edema.
- Measure intake and output carefully by weighing diapers.
- Maintain fluid restrictions as ordered.
- Monitor electrolytes.

- Provide skin care for edematous body parts, and elevate extremities.
- Change newborn's position frequently.
- Inspect skin frequently for redness and skin breakdown over pressure points.
- Hold newborn at a 45-degree angle for feeding.
- Give frequent small feedings with rest periods between, or insert a feeding tube per order.
- Use high-calorie formula.
- Transition to supplemental nasogastric feeding if the newborn is not able to gain weight.
- Involve parents in care as much as possible, encourage them to room in or visit the newborn frequently, and have them hold the baby often.
- At discharge, provide clear instructions and information about what to do in an emergency as well as whom and where to call with questions.
- Allow parents to verbalize questions, concerns, and feelings.
- Refer parents to support groups or other resources as needed.

Nursing Care Plan *(continued)*

EVALUATION

Expected outcomes used to evaluate Gwen's response to care include the following:

- The child's CO is sufficient, as indicated by increased energy, adequate feeding intake, and decreased edema.
- The child maintains normal serum levels of potassium and therapeutic levels of digoxin.
- The child has adequate energy to eat.
- The child has normal respiratory rate for age, with no evidence of adventitious sounds or diaphoresis.

- The child's intake and output are proportional, and electrolyte levels remain within normal ranges.
- The child has no skin breakdown after edema resolves.
- The child gains recommended weight according to growth grids, with all dietary requirements met.
- The parents participate in developing and implementing the treatment plan and in providing care to the child.

CRITICAL THINKING

1. How would you explain Gwen's congenital defect and a rationale for why she developed CHF?
2. Why would Gwen have an increased metabolic rate and need for increased calories?
3. How will Gwen's care needs change as she grows if surgery is delayed until she is older?

REVIEW Congenital Heart Defects

RELATE Link the Concepts and Exemplars

Linking the exemplar of congenital heart defects with the concept of family:

1. What is the priority of care for the family of a newborn diagnosed with a congenital heart defect that decreases pulmonary blood flow?
2. How might you support the family of a child who requires extensive and numerous open heart surgeries?

Linking the exemplar of congenital heart defects with the concept of development:

3. Why might the child with a significant unrepaired congenital defect fail to meet developmental milestones?
4. What interventions would the nurse initiate for the family whose infant is not meeting developmental milestones due to a congenital heart defect?

READY Go to Volume 3: Clinical Nursing Skills

REFER Go to Pearson MyLab Nursing and eText

- Additional review materials

REFLECT Apply Your Knowledge

Caleb Sexton, a male infant, is just a few hours old; he was born at 32 weeks' gestation to Mr. and Mrs. Sexton. Mr. Sexton, age 26, is in law school, and Mrs. Sexton, age 25, teaches first grade at the local elementary school. Caleb is their first child. He is taken to the NICU, where he is examined and diagnosed with TOF following a cardiac echocardiogram.

Mr. and Mrs. Sexton leave the NICU in a state of shock and do not even know what questions to ask the neonatologist. The practitioner has told them that Caleb will require open heart surgery when he is older and has adequate weight gain. Until that time, Caleb will be treated medically. The idea of taking him home with such a serious heart problem is truly frightening to both parents. Mr. Sexton finds himself wondering whether his son will survive and, if he does, whether he will ever be able to act like a normal child.

1. How will you help the parents understand the pathophysiology of Caleb's heart defect?
2. What is your priority nursing diagnosis for Caleb?
3. Create a teaching plan for the family to prepare them for Caleb's discharge from the hospital.

>> Exemplar 16.C
Coronary Artery Disease

Exemplar Learning Outcomes

16.C Analyze coronary artery disease (CAD) as it relates to perfusion.

- Describe the pathophysiology of CAD.
- Describe the etiology of CAD.
- Compare the risk factors and prevention of CAD.

- Identify the clinical manifestations of CAD.
- Summarize diagnostic tests and therapies used by interprofessional teams in the collaborative care of an individual with CAD.
- Differentiate care of patients with CAD across the lifespan.
- Apply the nursing process in providing culturally competent care to an individual with CAD.

Exemplar Key Terms

Overview

Coronary artery disease (CAD) is a leading cause of death for men and women in the United States, claiming the lives of about 370,000 Americans each year (NHLBI, 2015a). CAD is caused by impaired blood flow to the myocardium, usually due to accumulation of atherosclerotic plaque in the coronary arteries. CAD may be asymptomatic, or it may lead to angina pectoris, acute coronary syndrome (ACS), myocardial infarction (MI; heart attack), dysrhythmias, heart failure, and even sudden death.

Angina pectoris (or angina) is chest pain resulting from reduced coronary blood flow, which causes a temporary imbalance between myocardial blood supply and demand. The imbalance may be caused by CAD, atherosclerosis, or vessel constriction that impairs the myocardial blood supply. Hypermetabolic conditions, such as exercise, thyrotoxicosis, stimulant abuse, hyperthyroidism, and emotional stress, can also increase myocardial oxygen demand and precipitate angina. Other conditions that affect blood and oxygen supplies and trigger angina include anemia, heart failure, ventricular hypertrophy, and pulmonary diseases.

Acute coronary syndrome (ACS) refers to any condition that develops as a result of sudden, reduced blood flow to the heart. ACS includes unstable angina and acute myocardial ischemia.

An **acute myocardial infarction (AMI)**, which involves the necrosis (death) of myocardial cells, is a life-threatening event. AMI occurs when blood flow to a portion of the cardiac muscle is blocked. If circulation to the affected myocardium is not promptly restored, loss of functional myocardium will occur, affecting the heart's ability to maintain effective CO. This, in turn, may ultimately lead to cardiogenic shock and death.

Heart disease—including CAD—remains the leading cause of death in the United States. Of the major heart diseases, MI and other forms of ischemic heart disease cause the majority of deaths. Approximately 735,000 cases of MI occur in the United States each year (CDC, 2015g), although only a fraction of cases are fatal. The majority of deaths from MI occur during the initial period after symptoms begin: approximately 60% within the first hour and 40% before hospitalization. Heightening public awareness of the manifestations of MI, the importance of immediate medical assistance, and the value of training in CPR techniques is vital to decreasing the number of MI-related deaths.

Pathophysiology and Etiology

The most common cause of CAD is buildup of atherosclerotic plaque in the coronary arteries. Plaque accumulation causes reduced blood supply to the heart muscle, which eventually leads to ischemia, angina, and ACS, among other problems.

Pathophysiology

A thorough understanding of CAD begins with a review of the basic mechanisms of coronary circulation. The two main coronary arteries—left and right—supply blood, oxygen, and nutrients to the myocardium. They originate in the root of the aorta, just outside the aortic valve. The left main coronary artery divides to form the anterior descending and circumflex arteries. The anterior descending artery supplies the anterior interventricular septum and the left ventricle, including the apex of the heart. The circumflex branch supplies the lateral wall of the left ventricle. The right coronary artery supplies the right ventricle and forms the posterior descending artery. Also known as the posterior interventricular artery, this vessel supplies blood to the posterior portion of the heart. (For more information, see Figure 16–7 in the Concept of Perfusion.)

Blood flow through the coronary arteries is regulated by several factors. Aortic pressure is the primary factor. Other factors include heart rate (most of the flow occurs during diastole, when the muscle is relaxed), metabolic activity of the heart, blood vessel tone (constriction), and collateral circulation. Although no connections exist between the large coronary arteries, smaller arteries are joined by **collateral channels**. Sometimes referred to as collateral circulation, these are small blood vessels that develop to connect small coronary arteries. Should larger vessels become occluded, collateral channels provide alternative routes for blood flow.

Coronary atherosclerosis is the most common cause of reduced coronary blood flow. **Atherosclerosis** is a progressive disease characterized by plaque formation that affects the intimal and medial layers of large and midsized arteries. Atherosclerosis is initiated by unknown factors that cause lipoproteins and fibrous tissue to accumulate in the arterial wall. Although the precise mechanisms of atherosclerosis are unknown, abnormal lipid metabolism and injury to, or inflammation of, endothelial cells lining the arteries appear to be key to its development.

In the bloodstream, most lipids are transported while attached to proteins called apoproteins, forming assemblies known as lipoproteins. High levels of certain lipoproteins increase the risk of atherosclerosis. For example, low-density lipoproteins (LDLs), which are high in cholesterol, carry cholesterol to peripheral tissues, where some of it is released to be taken up and incorporated into cells for use in producing energy. Likewise, very low-density lipoproteins (VLDLs), which are large molecules composed primarily of triglycerides and cholesterol, carry triglycerides to muscle and fat cells. When the triglycerides are released into these tissues, the remainder of the molecule becomes an LDL. Because the fats they carry can accumulate in the arteries, both LDLs and VLDLs contribute to atherosclerosis. High-density lipoproteins (HDLs), in contrast, attract cholesterol, returning it from peripheral tissues to the liver. This, in turn, reduces the risk of atherosclerosis.

The atherosclerotic process typically begins when accumulated fats and cholesterol cause damage to the arterial endothelium. Other potential mechanisms of vessel injury include hypertension, environmental toxins, infections, and inflammatory processes. Regardless of cause, after such vessel injury occurs, materials begin to collect in the intimal lining of the artery. First, atherogenic (atherosclerosis-promoting) lipoproteins gather and appear to bind with the extracellular portion of the vessel endothelium. WBCs called macrophages then migrate to the injured site as part of the inflammatory process. Next, contact with platelets, cholesterol, and other blood components stimulates smooth muscle cells and connective tissue within the vessel wall to proliferate abnormally. Although blood flow is not affected at this stage, the early atherosclerotic lesion appears as a yellowish, fatty streak on the inner arterial lining.

As time passes, the early lesion transforms into a fibrous plaque because of the enlargement of smooth muscle cells, proliferation of collagen fibers, and further accumulation of blood lipids. The lesion now protrudes into the arterial lumen and is fixed to the inner wall of the intima. It may invade the muscular media layer of the vessel as well. The developing plaque not only gradually occludes the vessel lumen, but it also impairs the vessel's ability to dilate in response to increased oxygen demands. As the plaque expands, it can produce severe stenosis or total occlusion of the artery.

The final stage of the atherosclerotic process is the development of **atheromas**, which are complex lesions consisting of lipids, fibrous tissue, collagen, calcium, cellular debris, and capillaries. These calcified lesions can ulcerate or rupture, stimulating thrombosis. The vessel lumen may be rapidly occluded by the thrombus (clot), or the clot may embolize to occlude a distal vessel.

Plaque formation involved in atherosclerosis may be eccentric (located in a specific, asymmetric region of the vessel wall) or concentric (involving the entire vessel circumference). Plaques tend to develop in locations where arteries bifurcate, curve, or narrow. Certain vessels have a higher likelihood of being affected, including the coronary arteries (especially the left anterior descending artery), the renal arteries, the bifurcation of the carotid arteries, and the branching sections of peripheral arteries. Manifestations of the atherosclerotic process usually do not appear until approximately 75% of the arterial lumen has been occluded. In addition to occluding blood flow, atherosclerosis weakens arterial walls and is a major cause of aneurysm in vessels such as the aorta and iliac arteries.

Myocardial Ischemia

As CAD advances and the circumference of the coronary arteries declines, blood supply to the cardiac tissue is reduced. The imbalance between myocardial blood supply and demand eventually causes temporary and reversible myocardial ischemia. **Ischemia** results when a tissue's oxygen supply is inadequate to meet its metabolic demands.

The ability of cardiac tissue to satisfy its metabolic demands largely depends on two key factors: coronary perfusion and myocardial workload. Coronary perfusion can be affected by several mechanisms. For example:

- One or more vessels may be partially occluded by large, stable areas of plaque.
- Platelets may aggregate in narrowed vessels, forming a thrombus.
- Normal or already narrowed vessels may spasm.
- A drop in BP may lead to inadequate flow through coronary vessels.
- Normal coronary autoregulation mechanisms may be interrupted as coronary blood flow becomes pressure-dependent.

Myocardial workload may similarly be affected by heart rate, myocardial contractility, preload, and afterload. The blood's oxygen content and hematocrit levels are also contributing factors to myocardial ischemia. For more information on possible causes of myocardial ischemia, see **Table 16–16 》**.

When myocardial ischemia occurs, cellular processes in the affected tissue are compromised as adenosine triphosphate (ATP) stores are depleted. Reduced oxygen causes the affected cells to switch from aerobic metabolism to anaerobic metabolism. Anaerobic metabolism leads to lactic acid buildup in the cells. It also affects cell membrane permeability, releasing substances such as histamine, kinins, and specific enzymes that stimulate terminal nerve fibers in the cardiac muscle and send pain impulses to the central nervous system. This pain radiates to the upper body because

TABLE 16–16 Selected Causes of Myocardial Ischemia

Condition	Effect on Myocardial Workload
Atherosclerosis	Restricts blood flow
Thrombosis	Causes sudden, severe myocardial ischemia and possible heart attack
Coronary artery spasm	Decreases or prevents blood flow to part of the heart muscle
Bleeding, infection, or severe illness	Increases the metabolic demands of the heart and may cause a decrease in BP

the heart shares the same **dermatome** (an area supplied with afferent nerve fibers by a single posterior spinal root) as this region.

Therapeutic strategies to reduce ischemia-related cardiac injury include reestablishment of myocardial perfusion before irreversible damage occurs. Researchers estimate that each 30-minute delay from onset of symptoms to primary intervention results in an 8% increase in the relative risk of 1-year mortality.

Angina

Angina is chest pain that results from ischemia. It can be a one-time event or a chronic condition. Angina is categorized into three types:

1. **Stable angina** is the most common and predictable form of angina. It occurs with a predictable amount of activity or stress and is a common manifestation of CAD. Stable angina usually occurs when the work of the heart is increased by physical exertion, exposure to cold, or stress. Stable angina is relieved by rest and nitrates.
2. **Prinzmetal (variant) angina** is atypical angina that occurs unpredictably (unrelated to activity) and often at night. It is caused by coronary artery spasm with or without an atherosclerotic lesion. The exact mechanism of coronary artery spasm is unknown. It may result from hyperactive SNS responses, altered calcium flow in smooth muscle, or reduced prostaglandins that promote vasodilation.
3. **Unstable angina** is angina that occurs with increasing frequency, severity, and duration. Pain is unpredictable, occurs with decreasing levels of activity or stress, and may even occur at rest. Patients with unstable angina are at risk for MI. (Unstable angina is discussed in more detail in the section on ACS.)

Not all myocardial ischemia produces angina. Many patients with ischemic heart disease experience what is known as asymptomatic or silent myocardial ischemia. Patients at risk for silent ischemia include those already affected by stable angina, unstable angina, postinfarction angina, or variant angina. Other risk factors include diabetes and history of cardiac arrest, heart transplant, percutaneous coronary intervention, or cardiac bypass surgery. Silent ischemia often occurs with exercise and is associated with a higher relative risk of serious cardiac events.

Acute Coronary Syndrome

ACS is a dynamic state in which coronary blood flow is acutely reduced but not fully occluded. The resulting ischemia causes injury to myocardial cells. ACS may be precipitated by one or more of the following events: rupture or erosion of atherosclerotic plaque, formation of a thrombosis, coronary artery spasm (e.g., Prinzmetal angina), progressive vessel obstruction by atherosclerotic plaque or restenosis following a percutaneous revascularization procedure, inflammation of a coronary artery, or an increase in myocardial oxygen demand and/or a decrease in supply (i.e., acute blood loss or anemia).

Most people who are affected by ACS have significant atherosclerotic occlusion of one or more coronary arteries.

Atherosclerotic plaque may form stable or unstable lesions. Whereas stable lesions progress by gradually narrowing the vessel lumen (often causing angina), unstable (or complicated) lesions are prone to rupture and thrombus formation. When this occurs, ACS or another acute ischemic heart disease results.

With ACS, plaque rupture is often triggered by hemodynamic factors, such as increases in heart rate, blood flow, and BP in response to a surge of SNS activity. In fact, sympathetic hyperactivity has been shown to impair autonomic nervous system control of the cardiovascular system (Mancia & Grassi, 2014), and acute mental stress has been found to be a risk factor for atherosclerosis (Steptoe & Kivimaki, 2013).

After the unstable plaque ruptures or erodes, the exposed lipid core of the plaque stimulates platelet aggregation and the extrinsic clotting pathway. Thrombin is generated, and fibrin is deposited, forming a clot that severely impairs or obstructs blood flow to the heart tissue distal to the area of plaque rupture. As a result, the cells in that tissue become ischemic. Injured myocardial cells contract less effectively, potentially reducing CO if a large area of myocardium is affected. The ischemic myocardial cells also release lactic acid, which stimulates pain receptors and causes chest pain. In addition, ischemia and injury affect electrical impulse conduction, producing inverted T waves and possibly elevated ST segments on an ECG.

Acute Myocardial Infarction

MI occurs when blood flow to a portion of the cardiac muscle is completely blocked, resulting in prolonged tissue ischemia and irreversible cell damage. The coronary occlusion involved in MI is usually caused by ulceration or rupture of a complicated atherosclerotic lesion. When the lesion ruptures or ulcerates, substances are released that stimulate platelet aggregation, thrombin generation, and local vasomotor tone. As a result, the vessel constricts, and a thrombus forms, occluding the vessel and interrupting blood flow to the myocardium distal to the obstruction.

During an MI, lack of adequate oxygen and nutrients causes injury to the myocardial cells. The cells' oxygen, glycogen, and ATP stores are rapidly depleted. Cellular metabolism shifts to an anaerobic process, producing hydrogen ions and lactic acid. Cellular acidosis increases the cells' vulnerability to further damage, and intracellular enzymes are released through damaged cell membranes into interstitial spaces. If ischemia lasts more than 20–45 minutes, irreversible hypoxemic damage leads to cellular death and tissue necrosis.

The lack of adequate blood flow associated with MI causes alterations in the heart's pumping ability. Cellular acidosis, electrolyte imbalances, and hormones released in response to cellular ischemia affect impulse conduction. As a result, the risk for dysrhythmias increases and myocardial contractility decreases, reducing SV, CO, BP, and tissue perfusion.

The subendocardium is the first portion of the heart to experience damage during AMI, within 20 minutes of injury, because this area is the most susceptible to changes in coronary blood flow. If blood flow is restored at this point, the infarction is limited to subendocardial tissue, and the event is categorized as a subendocardial or non-Q-wave infarction. If blood flow is not restored, the damage progresses to the epicardium within 1–6 hours. When all layers of the myocardium are affected, the event is known as a transmural infarction. A significant Q wave develops with a transmural infarction, indicating the patient sustained a Q-wave MI. Complications such as heart failure are more frequently associated with Q-wave MIs. In comparison, patients with non-Q-wave MIs may experience favorable early prognosis, but late complications include recurrent angina, transmural myocardial infarction, and sudden death.

Following an MI, the necrotic or infarcted cardiac muscle is surrounded by regions of injured and ischemic tissues. Tissue in the ischemic area is potentially viable; restoration of blood flow minimizes the amount of tissue that is lost. The surrounding tissue also undergoes metabolic changes. It may be stunned (meaning its contractility is impaired for hours or even days following reperfusion) or hibernating (a process that protects myocytes until perfusion is restored). In some cases, myocardial remodeling may occur, with cellular hypertrophy and loss of contractility in regions distant from the infarction. These changes are dependent on the rate at which blood flow is restored to the site of injury.

When a larger artery is compromised during an MI, the collateral vessels that connect smaller arteries in the coronary system dilate to maintain blood flow to the cardiac muscle. The degree of collateral circulation helps determine the extent of myocardial damage from ischemia. Acute occlusion of a coronary artery without any collateral flow results in massive tissue damage and may cause death. In contrast, progressive narrowing of larger coronary arteries allows collateral vessels to develop and enlarge, meeting the demand for blood flow. Thus, good collateral circulation can limit the size of an MI.

MIs are described by reference to the damaged area of the heart, and the coronary artery that is occluded determines the area of damage. MI usually affects the left ventricle, because it is the major "workhorse" of the heart; its muscle mass is greater, as are its oxygen demands. Occlusion of the left anterior descending artery affects blood flow to the anterior wall of the left ventricle and part of the interventricular septum, causing an *anterior* MI. Occlusion of the left circumflex artery causes a *lateral* MI. Right ventricular, inferior, and posterior infarcts involve occlusions of the right coronary artery and posterior descending artery. Occlusion of the left main coronary artery is the most devastating, causing ischemia of the entire left ventricle and a grave prognosis. Identifying the infarct site helps predict possible complications and determine appropriate therapy.

Although rupture or ulceration of atherosclerotic plaque is the most common cause of AMI, it may also develop as a result of cocaine intoxication. Cocaine increases SNS activity by both increasing the release of catecholamines from central and peripheral stores and interfering with their reuptake. The resulting increase in catecholamine concentration increases heart rate and contractility, increases the automaticity of cardiac tissues and the risk of dysrhythmias, and causes vasoconstriction and hypertension. The patient with cocaine-induced MI may present with an altered LOC, confusion, restlessness, seizure activity, tachycardia, hypotension, increased respiratory rate, and respiratory crackles.

(Additional information about the effects of cocaine can be found in the module on Addiction.)

Etiology

The underlying causes of atherosclerosis, CAD, and their resulting conditions are unknown. An individual's tendency to develop cardiovascular disease may be inherited. Lifestyle habits such as diet, smoking, and physical activity also play a role.

Risk Factors

Although the exact causes of atherosclerosis have not yet been determined, certain risk factors are linked to the development of atherosclerotic plaques. The Framingham Heart Study (FHS) in particular has provided vital research into the relationship between risk factors and the development of heart disease. (See the Evidence-Based Practice feature for more information on the FHS.) Research into CAD continues, with investigators looking at potential causative factors, manifestations, and protective measures across many populations.

Broadly speaking, a number of risk factors have been identified, many of which are listed in **Table 16–17 》**. The following sections discuss these and other risk factors in greater depth.

Nonmodifiable Risk Factors

As shown in Table 16–17, age is a prominent nonmodifiable risk factor for CAD. For men, the risk of developing CAD rises around age 45, whereas for women, it increases around age 55. More than 50% of individuals who experience a heart attack are age 65 or older, and just over 80% of deaths caused by MI occur in this age group (Griffin, Kapadia, & Rimmerman, 2013).

Gender is another nonmodifiable risk factor for CAD, although the link between gender and CAD risk varies by age, as mentioned. Premenopausal women are less likely to be diagnosed with CAD than their same-age male counterparts. However, once women go through menopause, their risk of CAD is roughly equal to that of men (World Heart Federation, 2016a). Additional CAD risk factors that are unique to women are described in detail later in this exemplar.

Beyond age and gender, race and ethnicity also affect a person's likelihood of CAD. Various studies indicate that

TABLE 16–17 Risk Factors for CAD

Nonmodifiable Risk Factors	Modifiable Risk Factors	
	Pathophysiologic	**Lifestyle**
Age	Hyperlipidemia	Cigarette smoking
Men: 45 years or older	Elevated LDL	Obesity
Women: 55 years or older	Reduced HDL	Physical inactivity
Gender	High BP	Atherogenic diet
Race and ethnicity	Diabetes mellitus	Use of oral contraceptives (women only)
Family history of CAD	Stress	Hormone replacement therapy (women only)
	Kidney disease	

African Americans, Mexican Americans, American Indians, Alaska Natives, and some Asian Americans are at elevated risk for this condition (U.S. National Library of Medicine, 2014b). Risk may be genetic, but also appears to be related to socioeconomic factors such as diet and access to healthcare.

Finally, individuals with a family history of CAD are more likely to develop it. The risk is particularly elevated among individuals with a father or brother who was diagnosed by age 55 or a mother or sister who was diagnosed by age 65. Furthermore, if both of a person's parents were diagnosed by age 55, then that person's risk of CAD may be boosted by as much as 50% (World Heart Federation, 2016b).

Focus on Diversity and Culture
Risk for CAD

The kidney converts inactive 25-hydroxyvitamin D obtained from sun exposure and nutritional intake to active vitamin D. Vitamin D then helps regulate calcium and phosphate levels in the blood (Starkebaum, 2014). Studies indicate that low amounts of 25-hydroxyvitamin D are associated with an increased risk of CAD in White and Chinese populations, but not in Black or Hispanic populations (Robinson-Cohen et al., 2013). Therefore, studies indicating that low 25-hydroxyvitamin D concentrations in the serum increases the risk for CAD need to be assessed for cultural variability. Studies performed primarily on White populations will likely provide different results than studies that are racially and ethnically diverse.

Emerging Risk Factors

As researchers learn more about the possible mechanisms of CAD, the list of potential risk factors continues to grow. For example, studies demonstrate a link between elevated serum levels of **homocysteine** (an amino acid that is a homologue of cysteine) and CAD. Until menopause, women have lower homocysteine levels than men, which may partially explain premenopausal women's lower risk for CAD. Research also reveals that homocysteine levels are negatively correlated with serum folate and dietary folate levels; that is, increasing folate intake lowers homocysteine levels.

Based on evidence that aspirin and antiplatelet therapies reduce the risk for MI, clot-promoting factors have been recognized as another emerging risk factor for CAD. Inflammation has also been identified as a risk factor. Inflammatory processes may increase the development of atherosclerotic plaque, and they are implicated in plaque rupture. Inflammation also promotes clot formation at the site of ruptured plaque. However, because the exact role of inflammatory and clot-promoting factors remains unclear, routine screening for these factors is not currently recommended (Pothineni, Karathanasis, & Mehta, 2016).

Still other evidence indicates that a group of risk factors collectively known as metabolic syndrome greatly elevates the likelihood of CAD. In fact, metabolic syndrome has emerged as a risk factor for premature CAD equal to cigarette smoking. Patients are said to have metabolic syndrome if they exhibit three or more of the conditions listed in **Box 16–8 》**. These conditions are themselves the result of obesity, physical

Evidence-Based Practice
The Framingham Heart Study

Problem
What role do genetics and lifestyle play in cardiovascular disease?

Evidence
Since 1948, the FHS has been committed to identifying common factors or characteristics that contribute to cardiovascular disease. The first cohort of the study included 5209 participants from the town of Framingham, Massachusetts, who had not yet developed obvious symptoms of cardiovascular disease or sustained a heart attack or stroke (FHS, 2015). Careful monitoring of this and subsequent study cohorts has resulted in valuable information about multiple risk factors associated with cardiovascular disease.

Over the years, one topic of particular interest to the FHS researchers has been identifying which components of the American lifestyle are linked to high rates of cardiovascular disease and disability. The researchers ultimately determined that the most significant lifestyle risk factors are an unhealthy diet, physical inactivity, obesity, and cigarette smoking. A major implication of these findings is the value of practicing primary preventive education. In fact, in the years since the launch of the FHS, many national awareness campaigns have been formed to better educate the American public about these risk factors. It is especially important to provide young children with information about the effects of lifestyle on the cardiovascular system and then to reinforce this knowledge throughout childhood and into the teen and young adult years.

Such efforts will help ensure that healthy choices become habits, thereby reducing cardiac disease rates in the years ahead.

More recent, the FHS has been beneficial in lending insight into genetic influences and their role in assessing cardiovascular risk. In addition, the study has helped link certain genes to congenital heart defects and other structural abnormalities. Going forward, the researchers involved in the FHS hope to learn more about the genetics of CAD and other forms of cardiovascular disease, including possible multifactorial patterns of inheritance.

Implications
Findings from the FHS support the need for nurses to be vigilant in providing education related to lifestyle modifications for patients at risk for or diagnosed with coronary heart disease, and in particular for patients with a family history of cardiovascular illness.

Critical Thinking Application
1. What kinds of strategies can be used in elementary school settings to teach about cardiovascular health in a fun, informative manner?

2. Identify three possible health implications related to the role of genetics and increased cardiovascular risk.

3. What changes do you need to make in your lifestyle to role model heart-healthy living?

Box 16–8
Conditions Associated with Metabolic Syndrome

- Large waistline (40 in. or greater for men; 35 in. or greater for women)
- High triglyceride levels (150 mg/dL or greater)
- Low HDL levels (less than 40 mg/dL for men and 50 mg/dL for women)
- Hypertension (130/85 mmHg or greater)
- Elevated fasting blood glucose (100 mg/dL or greater)

Sources: Data from American Academy of Family Physicians. (2014). *Metabolic syndrome: Diagnosis and tests.* Retrieved from http://familydoctor.org/familydoctor/en/diseases-conditions/metabolic-syndrome/diagnosis-tests.html; Cleveland Clinic. (2015a). *Metabolic syndrome.* Retrieved from https://my.clevelandclinic.org/health/diseases_conditions/hic_Metabolic_Syndrome; Mayo Clinic. (2014e). *Metabolic syndrome: Tests and diagnosis.* Retrieved from http://www.mayoclinic.org/diseases-conditions/metabolic-syndrome/basics/tests-diagnosis/con-20027243

inactivity, and genetics. In addition to increasing the likelihood of CAD, metabolic syndrome elevates a person's risk of insulin resistance and type 2 diabetes (Cleveland Clinic, 2015a; International Diabetes Federation, 2015).

Risk Factors Unique to Women

Although gender is itself a nonmodifiable risk factor for CAD, there are several additional risk factors that are unique to women. Each of these factors—including early menopause and use of certain contraceptives—involves fluctuations in hormone levels.

At menopause, a woman's risk for CAD rises because changes in hormone levels cause her serum HDL levels to drop and her LDL levels to rise. Thus, the earlier a woman enters menopause, the more likely she is to develop CAD and experience MI. This is true whether early menopause occurs naturally or as a result of surgery. For example, women who undergo a bilateral oophorectomy without hormone replacement before age 35 are 8 times more likely to have an MI than women who experience natural menopause during the typical age range.

As mentioned previously, estrogen replacement therapy reduces the risk for CAD and MI in women who experience early menopause. Oral contraceptives, by contrast, have been demonstrated to elevate the risk for CAD, especially in women who smoke, are obese, have hypertension, and/or are genetically predisposed toward CAD. This increased risk is due to the tendency of oral contraceptives to raise LDL levels while lowering HDL levels. Risk of CAD and MI is greatest among oral contraceptive users who smoke and are older than age 35.

Prevention

Prevention of CAD focuses on modifiable risk factors, including both lifestyle factors and pathologic conditions that predispose the patient to developing CAD. Behavioral or lifestyle factors—such as diet, activity level, obesity, and smoking—can be controlled or completely eliminated with significant commitment by the patient, although ongoing support from the healthcare team is vital for success. Pathologic conditions that contribute to CAD include hypertension, diabetes mellitus, and hyperlipidemia. Although these conditions are not a matter of choice, they are modifiable risk factors that can often be controlled through medication, weight control, diet, and exercise.

Diet

An atherogenic diet is one that promotes the formation of atheromas and thereby contributes to CAD. Most Americans are aware that diets high in saturated and trans fats, cholesterol, and salt are strongly atherogenic; however, fewer people are aware that diet is a risk factor for CAD independent of such intake. In particular, diets low in fruits, vegetables, whole grains, and unsaturated fatty acids appear to promote CAD, whereas diets high in these foods appear to have a protective effect.

Activity Level

Physical inactivity is associated with a higher risk for CAD. Research data indicate that people who maintain a regular program of physical activity are less prone to developing CAD than sedentary people. The cardiovascular benefits of exercise include increased availability of oxygen to the heart muscle, decreased oxygen demand and cardiac workload, and increased myocardial function and electrical stability. Other positive effects of regular physical activity include decreases in BP, blood lipids, insulin levels, platelet aggregation, and weight.

Obesity

Obesity, or the presence of excess adipose tissue, is generally defined as a BMI of 30 (calculated as the weight in kilograms divided by the square of the height in meters) or greater. Obesity is a significant risk factor for CAD in that people who are obese have higher rates of hypertension, diabetes, and hyperlipidemia. In fact, in the FHS, men over age 50 who were obese had twice the incidence of CAD and AMI of men who were within 10% of their ideal weight.

Fat distribution also affects the risk for CAD. In particular, central obesity, or a large amount of intra-abdominal fat, is associated with increased risk. The best indicator of central obesity is an individual's waist circumference. A waist-to-hip ratio of greater than 0.8 (women) or 0.9 (men) increases the risk for CAD.

Cigarette Smoking

Cigarette smoking contributes to a range of health problems, not the least of which is CAD. The effects of smoking on the cardiovascular system are dose-dependent, but generally speaking, male cigarette smokers have 2–3 times the risk for developing heart disease compared with nonsmokers, whereas female smokers have up to 4 times the risk. For both men and women who stop smoking, however, the risk of CAD may be reduced by up to 50% within 1 year of tobacco cessation (World Health Organization [WHO], 2016).

Tobacco smoke promotes CAD in several ways. Carbon monoxide damages the vascular endothelium, promoting cholesterol deposition. Nicotine stimulates catecholamine release, which causes an increase in BP, heart rate, and myocardial oxygen use. Nicotine also constricts arteries, limiting tissue perfusion. Furthermore, nicotine reduces HDL levels and increases platelet aggregation, thereby increasing the risk of thrombus formation.

Hypertension

Hypertension is a condition characterized by consistent systolic BP readings of greater than 140 mmHg and/or consistent diastolic BP readings of greater than 90 mmHg. Hypertension is common, affecting more than one third of people over age 50 in the United States. Its prevalence is higher in African American individuals than in Hispanic individuals, and higher in Hispanic individuals than in White individuals. Hypertension damages the endothelial cells of the arteries, possibly due to excess pressure and altered characteristics of blood flow. This damage can stimulate the development of atherosclerotic plaque, thus leading to increased risk of CAD.

Diabetes Mellitus

Diabetes mellitus contributes to CAD in several ways. For example, diabetes is associated with higher blood lipid levels, a higher incidence of hypertension, and obesity—all of which are CAD risk factors in their own right. In addition, diabetes affects the endothelium of blood vessels, thereby contributing to the atherosclerotic process. Hyperglycemia and hyperinsulinemia, altered platelet function, elevated fibrinogen levels, and inflammation also are thought to play a role in the development of atherosclerosis in people with diabetes.

Hyperlipidemia

Hyperlipidemia is defined as an abnormally high level of blood lipids and lipoproteins. Lipoproteins carry cholesterol in the blood. As previously described, LDLs are the primary carriers of cholesterol. High LDL levels (memory cue: LDLs = less desirable lipoproteins) promote atherosclerosis, because LDL deposits cholesterol on artery walls. In contrast, HDLs (memory cue: HDLs = highly desirable lipoproteins) help clear cholesterol from the arteries, transporting it to the liver for excretion. HDL levels of 60 mg/dL or greater have a protective effect, reducing the risk of CAD, whereas HDL levels below 40 mg/dL for men and 50 mg/dL for women are associated with an increased risk for CAD (Cleveland Clinic, 2013; Mayo Clinic, 2016c).

In addition to LDL and HDL levels, triglyceride levels are another important risk factor for CAD. Triglycerides are compounds of fatty acids bound to glycerol and used for fat storage by the body. Recall that triglycerides are carried on VLDL molecules, which transform into LDL molecules when the triglycerides are released into the tissues. As with LDL levels, elevated triglycerides contribute to the risk for CAD. **Table 16–18 »** lists desirable and high-risk levels for total cholesterol, LDL cholesterol, and triglycerides.

Clinical Manifestations

CAD is often asymptomatic. When clinical manifestations of CAD do occur, the most common indications are angina and MI. Although angina and MI have a similar initial presentation, important differences exist. Differentiating between ischemic causes of chest pain and other causes can be subtle and complex; for this reason, chest pain should be assessed by an experienced healthcare professional.

TABLE 16–18 Classification of Serum Cholesterol and Triglyceride Values

	Total Cholesterol (mg/dL)	Low-Density Lipoprotein Cholesterol (mg/dL)	Triglycerides (mg/dL)
Optimal		< 100	
Desirable	< 200	100–129	< 150
Borderline high	200–239	130–159	150–199
High	≥ 240	160–189	200–499
Very high		≥ 190	≥ 500

Sources: Data from Cleveland Clinic. (2013). *What do cholesterol numbers mean?* Retrieved from https://my.clevelandclinic.org/health/diseases_conditions/hic_Cholesterol/hic_what_do_cholesterol_numbers_mean; Mayo Clinic. (2016c). *High cholesterol: Diagnosis.* Retrieved from http://www.mayoclinic.org/diseases-conditions/high-blood-cholesterol/diagnosis-treatment/diagnosis/dxc-20181913; National Heart, Lung, and Blood Institute (NHLBI). (2014). *How is high blood cholesterol diagnosed?* Retrieved from https://www.nhlbi.nih.gov/health/healthtopics/ topics/hbc/diagnosis

Angina

The cardinal manifestation of angina is chest pain. The pain typically is precipitated by an identifiable event, such as physical activity, strong emotion, stress, eating a heavy meal, or exposure to cold. The classic sequence of angina is activity–pain, rest–relief. The patient may describe the pain as a tight, squeezing, heavy pressure or a constricting sensation. It characteristically begins beneath the sternum and may radiate to the jaw, neck, shoulder, or arm. Less characteristically, the pain may be felt in the jaw, epigastric region, or back. Anginal pain usually occurs in a crescendo–decrescendo pattern (increasing to a peak, then gradually decreasing) and typically lasts 2–5 minutes. It generally is relieved by rest.

Additional manifestations of angina include dyspnea, pallor, tachycardia, and anxiety and fear. Women frequently present with atypical symptoms, including indigestion, nausea, vomiting, fatigue, and upper back pain. Manifestations of angina are summarized in **Box 16–9 »**.

The severity of angina can be graded by the degree to which it limits the patient's activities. Class I angina does not

Box 16–9
Manifestations of Angina

- **Chest pain.** Substernal or precordial (across the chest wall); may radiate to neck, arms, shoulders, or jaw
- **Quality of pain.** Tight, squeezing, constricting, or heavy sensation; may also be described as burning, aching, choking, dull, or constant
- **Associated manifestations.** Dyspnea, pallor, tachycardia, anxiety, or fear
- **Atypical manifestations.** Indigestion, nausea, vomiting, or upper back pain
- **Precipitating factors.** Exercise or activity, strong emotion, stress, cold, or heavy meal
- **Relieving factors.** Rest, position change, or nitroglycerin

occur with ordinary physical activity. It is prompted by strenuous, rapid, or prolonged physical exertion. Class II angina may develop with rapid or prolonged walking or stair climbing, whereas Class III angina significantly limits ordinary physical activities. The patient with Class IV angina may have angina with any level of exertion, primarily at rest.

Acute Coronary Syndrome

The cardinal manifestation of ACS is chest pain, usually substernal or epigastric. The pain often radiates to the neck, left shoulder, and/or left arm. The pain may occur at rest, and it typically lasts longer than 10–20 minutes. In ACS, the chest pain is more severe and prolonged than that previously experienced by the patient. It may be a new onset of pain, or it may represent a pattern of increasing frequency and severity of anginal pain. Dyspnea, diaphoresis, pallor, and cool skin may be present. Tachycardia and hypotension may occur. The patient may be nauseated or feel lightheaded.

Acute Myocardial Infarction

Pain is a classic manifestation of MI. The chest pain that results from MI is more severe than anginal pain. However, it is not the intensity of the chest pain that distinguishes MI from angina or ACS, but rather its duration and continuous nature. During MI, the onset of pain is sudden and usually not associated with activity. In fact, most MIs occur in the early morning. Patients with a history of angina may have more frequent anginal attacks in the days or weeks before an MI (unstable angina or ACS). The chest pain associated with MI may be described as crushing and severe; as pressure, heaviness, or a squeezing sensation; or as chest tightness or burning. The pain often begins in the center of the chest (substernal) and may radiate to the shoulders, neck, jaw, or arms. It lasts more than 15–20 minutes and is not relieved by rest or nitroglycerin.

Compensatory mechanisms cause many other symptoms of MI. SNS stimulation causes anxiety, tachycardia, and vasoconstriction. This results in cool, clammy, mottled skin. Pain and blood chemistry changes stimulate the respiratory center, causing tachypnea. The patient often has a sense of impending doom and death. Tissue necrosis triggers an inflammatory reaction that increases WBC count and elevates body temperature. Serum cardiac enzyme levels rise as enzymes are released from necrotic cardiac cells.

Other manifestations of MI vary depending on the location and amount of infarcted tissue. Hypertension, hypotension, or signs of heart failure may develop. Vagal stimulation may cause nausea and vomiting, bradycardia, and hypotension. Hiccupping may develop as a result of diaphragmatic irritation. If a large vessel is occluded, the first sign of MI may be sudden death. Typical manifestations of MI are listed in **Box 16–10 »**.

It is not uncommon for someone experiencing chest pain for the first time to attribute it to indigestion. Healthcare providers should ensure that patients understand the possible implications of such pain in order to promote calling 9-1-1, because the first hour following the beginning of chest pain is a time of increased risk for sudden death. Also, if thrombolytic medications (also called fibrinolytics) are considered for treatment (discussed in the Collaboration section), it is vitally important for the patient to be seen in the

emergency department as soon as possible after ischemia occurs.

The risk for complications associated with MI is related to the size and location of the MI. Possible complications include dysrhythmias, pump failure, cardiogenic shock, infarct extension, structural defects, pericarditis, and Dressler syndrome.

Dysrhythmias

Infarcted tissue is **arrhythmogenic**—that is, it alters the generation and conduction of electrical impulses in the heart. This increases the risk for disturbances or irregularities of heart rhythm (**dysrhythmias**), which are the most frequent complication of MI.

Premature ventricular contractions (PVCs) are especially common following AMI, developing in more than 90% of patients. PVCs may be predictive of more dangerous dysrhythmias, such as ventricular tachycardia (VT) or ventricular fibrillation (VF). The risk of VF is greatest the first hour after MI. In fact, VF is a frequent cause of SCD associated with AMI, but its incidence declines with time.

If the infarcted tissue is part of a conduction pathway, electrical conduction within the heart may be affected. Any degree of AV block may occur following MI, especially when the anterior wall is infarcted. First-degree and Mobitz I (Wenckebach) blocks are most common, although complete heart block may develop. **Bradydysrhythmia** (abnormal slow rhythms) also may occur, particularly when the inferior wall of the ventricle is affected.

Pump Failure

MI reduces myocardial contractility, ventricular wall motion, and compliance. Impaired contractility and filling may produce pump failure. The risk of heart failure is greatest when large portions of the left ventricle are infarcted. Heart failure may also be more severe with an anterior infarction. Loss of 20–30% of the left ventricular muscle mass may cause manifestations of left-sided heart failure, including dyspnea, fatigue, weakness, and respiratory crackles on auscultation. Inferior or right ventricular MI may lead to right-sided heart failure, with manifestations such as neck vein distention and peripheral edema. Hemodynamic monitoring is often initiated for patients with evidence of heart failure.

Box 16–10
Manifestations of AMI

- Substernal or precordial chest pain that may radiate to the neck, jaw, shoulder(s), or left arm
- Tachycardia and tachypnea
- Dyspnea and shortness of breath
- Nausea and vomiting
- Anxiety and a sense of impending doom
- Diaphoresis or sweating
- Cool, mottled skin; diminished peripheral pulses
- Hypotension or hypertension
- Palpitations and dysrhythmias
- Signs of left-sided heart failure
- Decreased LOC.

Cardiogenic Shock

Cardiogenic shock, or impaired tissue perfusion resulting from pump failure, results when functioning myocardial muscle mass decreases by more than 40%. In this situation, the heart is unable to pump enough blood to meet the needs of the body and maintain organ function. Low CO resulting from cardiogenic shock also impairs perfusion of the coronary arteries and myocardium, further increasing tissue damage. Mortality from cardiogenic shock is greater than 70%, although this can be reduced by prompt intervention with revascularization procedures.

Infarct Extension

During the first 10–14 days after an MI, approximately 10% of patients experience extension or reinfarction in the area of the original infarction. Extension of the MI is characterized by increased myocardial necrosis from continued impairment of blood flow and ongoing injury. Expansion of the MI is described as a permanent expansion of the infarcted area from muscle thinning and dilation. Infarct extension and expansion may cause continuing chest pain, hemodynamic compromise, and worsening heart failure.

Structural Defects

Following MI, necrotic muscle is replaced by scar tissue that is thinner than the ventricular muscle mass. This can lead to such complications as ventricular aneurysm, rupture of the interventricular septum or papillary muscle, and myocardial rupture:

- A **ventricular aneurysm** is an outpouching of the ventricular wall. It may develop when a large section of the ventricle is replaced by scar tissue. Because the aneurysm does not contract during systole, SV decreases. Also, blood may pool within the aneurysm, causing clots to form.

- Ischemia of the papillary muscle or chordae tendineae may cause structural damage leading to papillary muscle dysfunction or rupture. This affects AV valve function (usually the mitral valve), causing **regurgitation**, or the backflow of blood into the atria during systole. The interventricular septum may perforate or rupture due to ischemia and infarction.

- Myocardial rupture is a risk between days 4 and 7 after MI, when the injured tissue is soft and weak. This potential complication of MI is often fatal.

Pericarditis

Tissue necrosis—including that associated with MI—prompts an inflammatory response. One potential result of that response is **pericarditis**, or inflammation of the pericardial tissue surrounding the heart. Pericarditis is a complication of AMI that usually occurs within 2–3 days of the event, causing chest pain that may be aching or sharp and stabbing. This pain is often aggravated by movement or deep breathing. When pericarditis is present, a pericardial friction rub may be heard on auscultation of the patient's heart sounds.

Dressler Syndrome

Dressler syndrome, which is thought to be a hypersensitivity response to necrotic tissue or an autoimmune disorder, may develop days to weeks after AMI. Dressler syndrome is a symptom complex characterized by fever, chest pain, and dyspnea. It may spontaneously resolve or recur over several months, causing significant discomfort and distress to affected individuals.

Clinical Manifestations and Therapies
Coronary Artery Disease

ETIOLOGY	CLINICAL MANIFESTATIONS	CLINICAL THERAPIES
Damage to the cardiac cells is accompanied by anaerobic metabolism, increasing the risk of dysrhythmias.	■ Manifestations include PVCs, tachycardia, heart block, and increased risk for VF. ■ Patient may experience pulse rate irregularities and possible weak pulse.	■ Antidysrhythmic medications ■ Oxygen administration ■ Nitrates to restore cardiac perfusion ■ Placement of stent in coronary artery to restore cardiac perfusion ■ Continuous cardiac monitoring
Increased quantities of lactic acid accumulate in the cardiac tissue, causing pain.	■ Manifestations include a feeling of pressure or banding around the chest, with reports of acute and severe pain that may be stabbing or burning. ■ Patient may experience radiation of pain to the left arm, jaw, back, or neck.	■ Administration of an analgesic (often morphine sulfate), which causes both coronary vasodilation and pain control ■ Administration of nitrates and oxygen to reduce ischemia ■ Continuous cardiac monitoring
CO and SNS stimulation are reduced, causing tachypnea.	■ Skin color may be gray or pale. ■ Capillary refill time may be delayed if cardiac output is significantly reduced. ■ Patient may experience possible hypotension, symptoms of shock, and/or altered LOC.	■ Reduction of the cardiac workload ■ Administration of oxygen ■ Administration of vasoconstricting medications to improve BP as indicated

Collaboration

Care of patients with CAD focuses on management of risk factors to slow the atherosclerotic process and maintain myocardial perfusion. Until manifestations of chronic or acute ischemia are experienced, the diagnosis is often presumptive based on the patient's history and presence of risk factors. Specific therapeutic measures may be initiated once patients experience angina or MI.

Management of stable angina focuses on maintaining coronary blood flow and cardiac function, and it may require medical therapy. As for patients with CAD, risk factor management is a vital component of care for patients with angina.

Patients who are experiencing MI require rapid, more aggressive care. Immediate treatment goals for these patients include:

- Relieving chest pain
- Reducing the extent of myocardial damage
- Maintaining cardiovascular stability
- Decreasing cardiac workload
- Preventing complications.

Long-term care focuses on slowing the process of CAD and reducing the risk of future MI.

Rapid assessment and diagnosis are critical in treating AMI because for these patients, "Time is muscle." The evolution of AMI is dynamic: The quicker an artery is reopened (whether medically, surgically, or spontaneously), the more myocardium can be salvaged. Survival and long-term outcomes following AMI improve according to the rate at which circulation is restored to the infarcted heart muscle. Also, reestablishing blood flow reduces myocardial oxygen demand.

One major problem interfering with timely reperfusion is delay in receiving medical care following symptom onset. Delays may arise during transport to the hospital or during evaluation in the emergency department, although most frequently they occur because patients are slow to recognize the symptoms of AMI and/or to seek medical assistance. Many factors are cited as reasons for treatment delay, including advanced age, gender (with women often waiting longer than men to seek help), denial, limited access to medical care, solitary living arrangements, and the perception that symptoms are not serious (AHA, 2015i). Again, once patients do have contact with medical personnel, immediate evaluation is essential to early diagnosis and treatment.

Diagnostic Tests

A variety of tests may be appropriate for patients with known or suspected CAD. Prior to diagnosis, laboratory testing can be used to assess for risk factors, such as an abnormal blood lipid profile. A blood lipid profile includes measurement of a patient's total serum cholesterol, as well as HDL, LDL, and triglyceride levels. Patients with hyperlipidemia, or an elevated total cholesterol, are at greater risk for atherosclerosis (see Table 16–18). Elevated LDL and triglyceride levels and decreased HDL levels are also risk factors. Conducting a blood lipid profile further enables calculation of the patient's ratio of HDL to total cholesterol.

This ratio should be at least 1:5, with 1:3 being ideal. In patients with a strong family history of premature CAD or familial hyperlipidemia, lipoprotein(a) levels may be measured, because elevated levels of lipoprotein(a) may independently increase the risk of CAD. Still other subsets of blood lipids may be measured in selected patients.

Diagnostic tests to identify subclinical (asymptomatic) CAD may be indicated when multiple risk factors are present. Relevant diagnostic tests include the following:

- **C-reactive protein (CRP)** is a serum protein associated with inflammatory processes. Elevated blood levels of this protein may be predictive of CAD.

- **Ankle-brachial blood pressure index (ABI)** is an inexpensive, noninvasive test for peripheral vascular disease (PVD) that may be predictive of CAD. With this test, the systolic BP in the patient's brachial, posterior tibial, and dorsalis pedis arteries is measured by Doppler. An ABI of less than 0.9 in either leg indicates the presence of peripheral arterial disease and a significant risk for CAD.

- **Exercise electrocardiograph (ECG) testing** may be performed. ECGs are used to assess the patient's response to increased cardiac workload induced by exercise. The test is considered positive for CAD if myocardial ischemia is detected on the ECG (indicated by depression of the ST segment by more than 3 mm; see **Figure 16–29 »**), the patient develops chest pain, or the test is stopped because of excess fatigue, dysrhythmias, or other symptoms before the predicted maximal heart rate is achieved.

- **Electron beam CT** creates a three-dimensional image of the heart and coronary arteries that can reveal plaque and

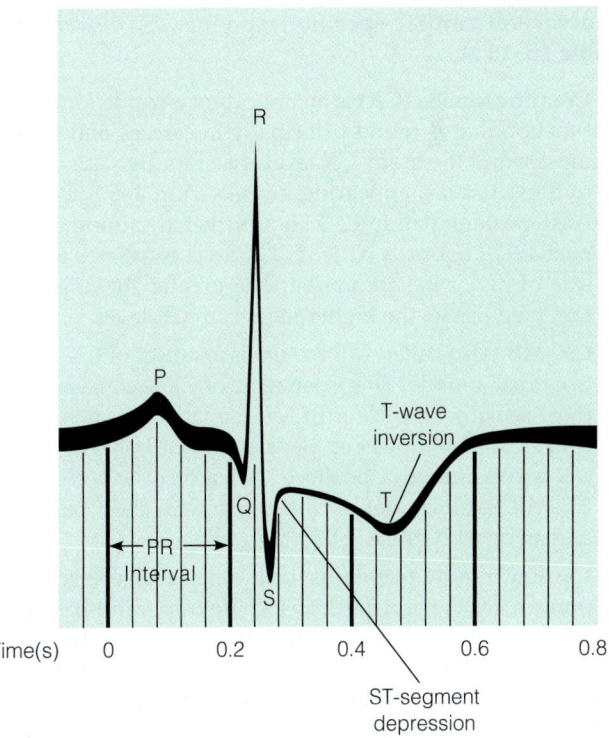

Figure 16–29 » ECG changes during an episode of angina. Note characteristic T-wave inversion and ST-segment depression of myocardial ischemia.

TABLE 16–19 Cardiac Markers

Marker	Normal Level	Primary Tissue Location	Significance of Elevation	Changes Occurring with MI		
				Appears	Peaks	Duration
CK (CPK)	Men: 55–170 units/L	Cardiac muscle, skeletal muscle, brain	Indicates injury to muscle cells	4–6 hr	12–24 hr	3–4 days
	Women: 30–135 units/L					
CK-MB	0–6% of total CK	Cardiac muscle	Indicates MI, cardiac ischemia, myocarditis, cardiac contusion, and/or defibrillation	4–6 hr	18–24 hr	3–4 days
cT_nT	< 0.2 ng/mL	Cardiac muscle	Indicates acute MI and/or unstable angina	1–3 hr	12–16 hr	10–14 days
cT_nI	0.1–0.5 ng/mL	Cardiac muscle	Indicates acute MI and/or unstable angina	1–3 hr	12–16 hr	5–9 days

other abnormalities. This noninvasive test requires no special preparation and can identify patients at risk for developing myocardial ischemia.

- *Myocardial perfusion imaging* may be used to evaluate myocardial blood flow and perfusion, both at rest and during stress testing (exercise or mental stress). Perfusion imaging studies are costly; therefore, they are not recommended for routine CAD risk assessment.

Diagnostic testing to establish the diagnosis of AMI involves assessing serum levels of various **cardiac markers**, or proteins released from necrotic heart muscle. Cardiac marker tests are ordered on admission and for three succeeding determined time frames. Serial blood levels help establish the diagnosis and determine the extent of myocardial damage. The proteins most specific for diagnosis of MI are CK (also called creatine phosphokinase [CPK]), CK-MB, and several cardiac-specific troponins, as described in **Table 16–19 >>**.

- **Creatine kinase (CK)** is an important enzyme for cellular function that is found principally in cardiac and skeletal muscle and the brain. CK levels rise rapidly with damage to these tissues, appearing in the serum 4–6 hours after AMI, peaking within 12–24 hours, then declining over the next 48–72 hours. A patient's CK level correlates with the size of his or her infarction: The greater the amount of infarcted tissue, the higher the serum CK level.

- **CK-MB** (also called MB bands) is a subset of CK specific to cardiac muscle. This isoenzyme of CK is considered the most sensitive indicator of MI. Elevated CK alone is not specific for MI; however, elevated CK-MB of greater than 6% is considered a positive indicator of MI. Note that CK-MB levels do not normally rise with chest pain from angina or with causes other than MI.

- **Cardiac muscle troponins**, including cardiac-specific troponin T (cT_nT) and cardiac-specific troponin I (cT_nI), are proteins released during MI that are sensitive indicators of myocardial damage. These proteins are part of the actin–myosin unit in cardiac muscle and normally are not detectable in the blood. With necrosis of cardiac muscle, however, troponins are released and blood levels rise. The specificity of cT_nT and cT_nI to cardiac muscle necrosis makes these markers particularly useful when skeletal muscle trauma contributes to elevated CK levels (e.g.,

when CPR has been performed or traumatic injury occurred at the time of the MI). Furthermore, tests for these troponins are sensitive enough to detect very small infarctions that do not cause significant CK elevation. cT_nI remains elevated for 5–9 days, and cT_nT remains elevated for 7–10 days after MI, which makes them useful for diagnosing MI when medical treatment is delayed.

Beyond the aforementioned tests, other laboratory tests used in the diagnosis of AMI include the following:

- *Myoglobin* is one of the first cardiac markers to be detectable in the blood after an MI, because it is released within a few hours after symptom onset. Measurement of myoglobin levels can be helpful in assessing reperfusion after thrombolysis.

- *Complete blood counts* in patients who have experienced MI will show elevated WBCs resulting from inflammation of the injured myocardium. The ESR will also be elevated because of inflammation.

- *Arterial blood gas (ABG) testing* may be ordered to assess patients' blood oxygen levels and acid–base balance.

Electrocardiography, echocardiography, and myocardial nuclear scans are the most common nonlaboratory diagnostic tests performed when AMI is suspected. With the exception of electrocardiography, the timing of these tests depends on the patient's immediate condition. Hemodynamic monitoring may also be initiated in the unstable patient following MI. General information regarding these tests is as follows:

- *An electrocardiogram* reflects changes in conduction resulting from myocardial ischemia and necrosis. Classic ECG changes seen in AMI include T-wave inversion, ST-segment elevation, and formation of a Q wave. Ischemic changes in the heart are indicated by depression of the ST segment or inversion of the T wave (see Figure 16–29). With myocardial injury, elevation of the ST segment occurs (see **Figure 16–30A >>**). Significant Q-wave development (see Figure 16–30B) indicates a transmural, or full-thickness, infarction. Myocardial damage can be localized using a 12-lead ECG.

- *Echocardiography* is the use of ultrasound technology to create images of the heart. It is performed to evaluate

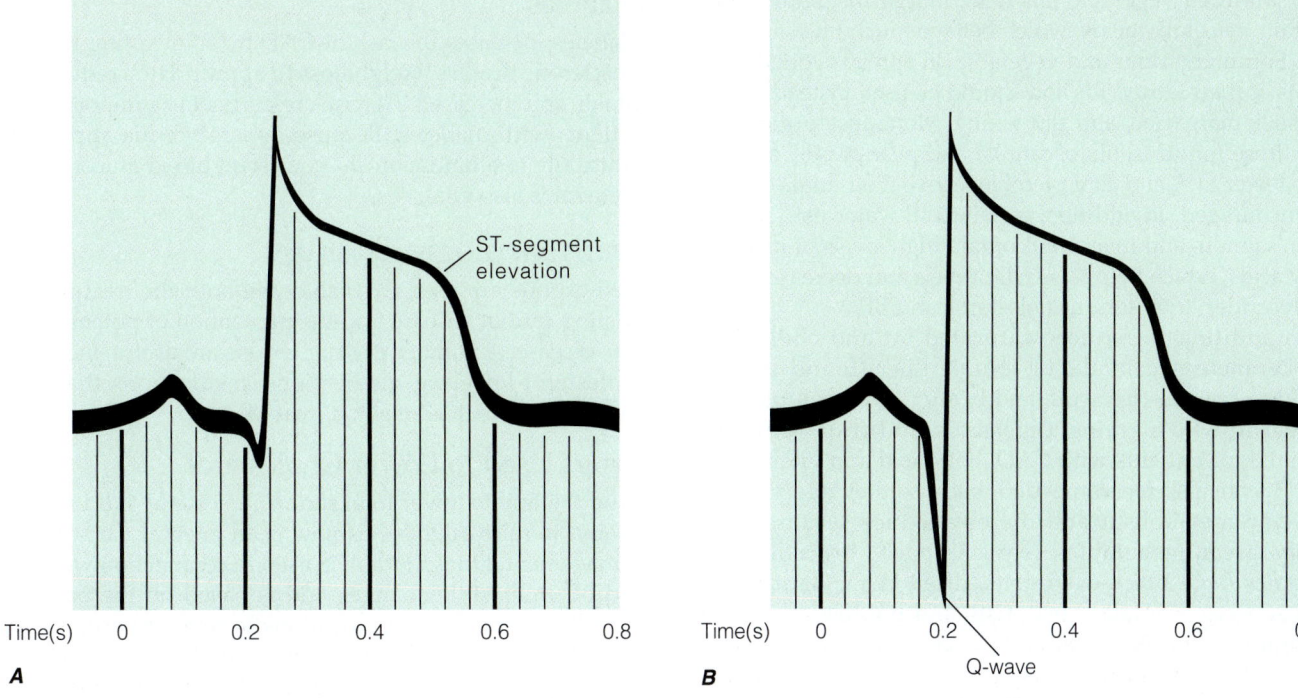

Figure 16–30 》 ECG changes characteristic of MI. **A,** ST-segment elevation characteristic of myocardial injury. **B,** Clinically significant Q-wave characteristic of a transmural infarction.

cardiac wall motion and left ventricular function. Stunned and infarcted tissue does not contract as effectively (if at all) as healthy myocardium.

- ***Radionuclide imaging*** may be performed to evaluate myocardial perfusion. These studies cannot differentiate between AMI and old scar tissue, but they do help identify specific areas of myocardial ischemia and damage.

- ***Hemodynamic monitoring*** may be initiated when AMI significantly affects CO and hemodynamic status.

Conservative Management

Conservative management of CAD focuses on risk factor modification, including smoking, diet, exercise, and management of contributing conditions, such as hypertension and diabetes.

Smoking

Smoking cessation reduces the risk for CAD within months after quitting and improves cardiovascular status. Individuals who quit reduce their risk of CAD by up to 50% within 1 year of cessation, regardless of how long they smoked before quitting (WHO, 2016). In addition, smoking cessation improves HDL levels, lowers LDL levels, and reduces blood viscosity. For these and other reasons, patients who have CAD should be advised to stop smoking and referred for support as appropriate. Nurses should also engage in health promotion activities that focus on preventing children, teenagers, and adults from starting to smoke. See Table 15–2 in the module on Oxygenation for interventions for tobacco cessation.

TABLE 16–20 Dietary Recommendations for Patients with CAD

Nutrient	Recommendation
Calories	Adjusted to attain or maintain desirable body weight
Total fat	25–35% of total calories
▪ Saturated fat	▪ Less than 7% of total calories
▪ Polyunsaturated fat	▪ Up to 10% of total calories
▪ Monounsaturated fat	▪ Up to 20% of total calories
Cholesterol	▪ Less than 200 mg/day
Carbohydrates (primarily complex carbohydrates [e.g., whole grains, fruits, vegetables])	50–60% of total calories
Dietary fiber	20–30 g/day
Protein	About 15% of total calories

Sources: Data from Lehne, R. A. (2013). *Pharmacology for nursing care* (8th ed.). St. Louis, MO: Elsevier Saunders; National Heart, Lung, and Blood Institute (NHLBI). (2005). *Your guide to lowering your cholesterol with TLC.* Retrieved from http://www.nhlbi.nih.gov/files/docs/public/heart/chol_tlc.pdf; Patton, K. (2013). Hypertension/hyperlipidemia/hyperhomocysteinemia and nutrition approaches. In M. L. Corrigan, A. A. Escuro, & D. F. Kirby (Eds.), *Handbook of clinical nutrition and stroke.* New York, NY: Humana Press.

Diet

Dietary recommendations for patients with CAD include reducing the consumption of saturated fat and cholesterol, as well as developing strategies to lower LDL levels (see **Table 16–20 》**). Most fats are a mixture of saturated and unsaturated fatty acids. The highest proportions of saturated fat are found in whole-milk products, red meats, and coconut oil. Therefore, nonfat dairy products, fish, and poultry are recommended as primary protein sources. Note also that solidified vegetable fats (e.g., margarine, shortening) contain *trans* fatty acids, which behave much like saturated fats. Soft margarines and vegetable oil spreads contain low levels of *trans* fatty acids and should be used instead of butter, stick margarine, and shortening. Monounsaturated fats, like those found in olive, canola, and peanut oils, actually help lower LDL and cholesterol levels, so their intake should be encouraged. In addition, certain cold-water fish, such as tuna, salmon, and mackerel, contain high levels of omega-3 fatty acids, which help raise HDL levels and decrease serum triglycerides, total serum cholesterol, and BP.

In addition to reduced saturated fat and cholesterol intake, increased intake of soluble fiber (found in oats, psyllium, pectin-rich fruit, and beans) and insoluble fiber (found in whole grains, vegetables, and fruit) is recommended for patients with CAD. Folic acid and vitamins B_6 and B_{12} are also recommended, because they affect homocysteine metabolism and thereby reduce serum levels. Leafy green vegetables (e.g., spinach, broccoli) and legumes (e.g., black-eyed peas, dried beans, lentils) are rich sources of folate. Meat, fish, and poultry are rich in vitamins B_6 and B_{12}. Vitamin B_6 is also found in soy products, while vitamin B_{12} is found in fortified cereals. Increased intake of antioxidant nutrients (vitamin E, in particular) and foods rich in antioxidants (fruits and vegetables) further appears to increase HDL levels and have a protective effect against CAD.

Moderate alcohol consumption may provide some health benefits for patients with CAD, particularly middle-age and older adults. Alcohol consumption should be limited to no more than two drinks per day for men or one drink per day for women. The health benefits for individuals who drink versus those who abstain have not been fully investigated, however.

Patients being treated for CAD who are overweight or obese are encouraged to lose weight via a combination of healthy eating and increased exercise. Patients should be informed that high-protein, high-fat weight-loss programs are not recommended for weight reduction.

Exercise

Regular physical exercise reduces the risk for CAD in several ways. It lowers VLDL, LDL, and triglyceride levels, and it raises HDL levels. Regular exercise also reduces BP and insulin resistance. Unless contraindicated, all patients are encouraged to participate in at least 30 minutes of moderate-intensity physical activity 5–6 days each week. To achieve weight loss and prevent weight gain, experts recommend 60–90 minutes of moderate intensity exercise daily. Exact physical activity requirements vary from person to person and may need to be increased to obtain maximum weight-loss goals (CDC, 2015h).

Hypertension

Although hypertension often cannot be prevented or cured, it can be controlled. Hypertension control (i.e., maintaining a BP of less than 130/80 mmHg) is vital to reduce its atherosclerosis-promoting effects and the workload of the heart. Management strategies include reduced sodium intake, increased calcium intake, regular exercise, stress management, and pharmacologic therapy.

Diabetes

Diabetes increases the risk of CAD by accelerating the atherosclerotic process. Weight loss (if appropriate), reduced fat intake, and increased exercise are particularly important for patients with diabetes. Because hyperglycemia appears to contribute to atherosclerosis, consistent blood glucose management is also vital.

Pharmacologic Therapy

Medications are used extensively in both the treatment of existing cardiac disease and the prevention of potential cardiac disease. A number of drug groups are useful, including cholesterol-lowering medications, medications that treat angina, and medications that treat MI.

Drugs Used to Lower Cholesterol

Drug therapy to lower total serum cholesterol and LDL levels and to raise HDL levels now is an integral part of CAD management. Drug therapy is used in conjunction with diet and other lifestyle changes and is based on the patient's overall risk for CAD. Medications to treat hyperlipidemia are expensive; thus, the cost–benefit ratio needs to be considered, because long-term treatment may be required. The four major classes of cholesterol-lowering drugs are statins, bile acid sequestrants, niacin (also called nicotinic acid), and fibric acid agents. The statins, including lovastatin (Mevacor), pravastatin (Pravachol), simvastatin (Zocor), and others, are first-line drugs for treating hyperlipidemia. They effectively lower LDL levels and may also increase HDL levels. All are taken by mouth.

SAFETY ALERT In rare cases, statins can cause myopathy, so all patients should be instructed to report muscle pain and weakness or brown urine. Liver function tests should also be monitored during therapy, because statins may increase liver enzyme levels.

The other classes of cholesterol-lowering drugs—bile acid sequestrants, niacin, and fibric acid agents—are primarily used when combination therapy is required to effectively reduce serum cholesterol levels. These drugs may also be used for selected patients, such as younger adults and women who wish to become pregnant, or to specifically lower triglyceride levels.

For more information on the various classes of cholesterol-lowering drugs, refer to the Medications feature.

Drugs Used to Treat Angina

Various drugs may be used for both acute and long-term relief of angina. The goal of drug treatment is to reduce oxygen demand and increase oxygen supply to the myocardium. The three main classes of drugs used to treat angina are organic nitrates, beta-adrenergic blockers, and CCBs. Patients with angina are also frequently placed on daily aspirin therapy.

Organic Nitrates

Organic nitrates, which come in both short- and long-acting forms, are used to treat acute anginal attacks and prevent angina. Short-acting sublingual nitroglycerin is the drug of choice for treating acute angina. It takes effect

Medications
Cholesterol-Lowering Drugs

CLASSIFICATION AND DRUG EXAMPLES	MECHANISMS OF ACTION	NURSING CONSIDERATIONS
Statins *Drug examples:* Lovastatin (Mevacor) Pravastatin (Pravachol) Simvastatin (Zocor) Fluvastatin (Lescol) Atorvastatin (Lipitor)	Statins inhibit the enzyme 3-hydroxy-3-methyl-glutaryl coenzyme A (HMG-CoA) reductase in the liver, reducing LDL synthesis and lowering serum levels. Statins are first-line treatment for elevated LDL and are used in conjunction with diet and lifestyle changes. Although their side effects are minimal, in rare cases, they may cause serious adverse effects, including increased serum liver enzyme levels, rhabdomyolysis, and myopathy.	▪ Monitor serum cholesterol and liver enzyme levels before and during therapy. Report elevated liver enzyme levels. ▪ Assess for muscle pain and tenderness. Monitor the patient's CK level if present. ▪ If the patient is taking digoxin concurrently, monitor for and report digoxin toxicity. Health Education for the Patient and Family ▪ The patient should promptly report muscle pain, tenderness, or weakness; skin rash, hives, or changes in skin color; and abdominal pain, nausea, or vomiting. ▪ The patient should not use these drugs if pregnant or planning to become pregnant. ▪ The patient should inform the healthcare provider if taking any other medications concurrently.
Bile Acid Sequestrants *Drug examples:* Cholestyramine (Questran) Colestipol (Colestid) Colesevelam (Welchol)	Bile acid sequestrants lower LDL levels by binding bile acids in the intestine, thus reducing the reabsorption of cholesterol and increasing its excretion in the stool. These drugs also reduce cholesterol production in the liver. Bile acid sequestrants are used in combination therapy regimens and for women who are considering pregnancy. Their primary disadvantages are inconvenience of administration (because of bulk), potential drug interactions, and possible gastrointestinal side effects (e.g., bloating, constipation, reduced absorption of vitamins and minerals).	▪ Mix cholestyramine and colestipol powders with 60–180 mL of water or juice; administer once or twice a day as ordered with meals. ▪ Store in a tightly closed container. Health Education for the Patient and Family ▪ The patient should promptly report constipation, severe gastric distress with nausea and vomiting, unexplained weight loss, black or bloody stools, or sudden back pain. ▪ Drinking ample amounts of fluid while taking these drugs reduces the problems of constipation and bloating. ▪ The patient should not omit doses, because this may affect the absorption of other drugs the patient is taking.
Niacin *Drug examples:* Nicobid Nicolar Niaspan	Niacin, in both prescription and nonprescription forms, lowers total and LDL cholesterol and triglyceride levels. The crystalline form and Niaspan, a prescription extended-release tablet, also raise HDL levels. Because the doses required to achieve significant cholesterol-lowering effects are associated with multiple side effects, niacin is generally used in combination therapy, particularly with the statin drugs.	▪ Give oral preparations with meals accompanied by a cold beverage to minimize gastrointestinal effects. ▪ Administer with caution to patients who have active liver disease, peptic ulcer disease, gout, or diabetes. ▪ Monitor blood glucose, uric acid levels, and liver function tests during treatment. Health Education for the Patient and Family ▪ Flushing of the face, neck, and ears may occur within 2 hours following dose; these effects generally subside as treatment continues. Alcohol use during niacin therapy may worsen this effect. ▪ The patient should report weakness or dizziness with changes in posture (lying to sitting; sitting to standing). The patient should also change positions slowly to reduce the risk of injury.

(continued on next page)

Medications *(continued)*

CLASSIFICATION AND DRUG EXAMPLES	MECHANISMS OF ACTION	NURSING CONSIDERATIONS
Fibric Acid Agents *Drug examples:* Gemfibrozil (Lopid) Fenofibrate (Tricor) Fenofibric acid (Fibricor)	Fibric acid agents (also called fibrates) are used to lower serum triglyceride levels; they have only a slight to modest effect on LDL. These drugs affect lipid regulation by blocking triglyceride synthesis. They are used to treat very high triglyceride levels and may be used in combination with statins.	■ Monitor serum LDL and VLDL levels, electrolytes, glucose, liver enzymes, renal function tests, and complete blood count during therapy. Report abnormal values. ■ Up to 2 months of treatment may be required to achieve a therapeutic effect; rebound, with decreasing benefit, may occur in the second or third month of treatment. Health Education for the Patient and Family ■ The patient should take with meals if the drug causes gastric distress. ■ The patient should promptly report flulike symptoms (e.g., fatigue, muscle aching, soreness, weakness). ■ The patient should not use this drug if pregnant or planning to become pregnant. The patient should use reliable birth control measures while taking this drug. ■ The patient should contact the healthcare provider before stopping this drug or taking any over-the-counter preparations.

within 1–2 minutes, decreasing myocardial work and oxygen demand through venous and arterial dilation, which in turn reduces preload and afterload. It may also improve myocardial oxygen supply by dilating collateral blood vessels and reducing stenosis. Rapid-acting nitroglycerin is also available as a buccal spray in a metered system. For some patients, the spray form may be easier to handle than small nitroglycerin tablets.

Longer-acting nitroglycerin preparations (oral tablets, ointment, or transdermal patches) are used to prevent attacks of angina, not to treat acute attacks. The main problem with long-term nitrate use is development of tolerance (i.e., a decreasing effect from the same dose of medication). Tolerance can be limited by a dosing schedule that allows a nitrate-free period of at least 8–10 hours per day. This is usually scheduled at night, when angina is less likely to occur.

Headache is a common side effect of both short- and long-acting nitrates and may limit the usefulness of these medications. Nausea, dizziness, and hypotension are also common effects of nitrate therapy.

Beta-Adrenergic Blockers

Beta-adrenergic blockers, including propranolol, metoprolol, nadolol, and atenolol, are considered first-line drugs for treating stable angina. These medications block the cardiac-stimulating effects of norepinephrine and epinephrine, thus preventing anginal attacks by reducing heart rate, myocardial contractility, and BP; this in turn reduces myocardial oxygen demand. Beta-adrenergic blockers may be used alone or with other medications to prevent angina.

SAFETY ALERT Beta-adrenergic blockers are contraindicated for patients with asthma or severe chronic obstructive pulmonary disease (COPD), because they may cause severe bronchospasm. They are not used in patients with significant bradycardia or AV conduction blocks, and they are used cautiously in patients with heart failure. In addition, beta-adrenergic blockers should not be used to treat Prinzmetal angina, because they may make it worse.

Calcium Channel Blockers

CCBs reduce myocardial oxygen demand and increase myocardial blood and oxygen supply. These drugs (which include verapamil, diltiazem, and nifedipine) lower BP, reduce myocardial contractility, and in some cases, lower heart rate, thus decreasing myocardial oxygen demand. They are also potent coronary vasodilators, effectively increasing oxygen supply.

Like beta-adrenergic blockers, CCBs are used for long-term prophylaxis because they act too slowly to effectively treat acute attacks of angina. However, because these drugs may actually increase ischemia and mortality in patients with heart failure or left ventricular dysfunction, they are not usually prescribed in the initial treatment of angina. CCBs are also used cautiously in patients with dysrhythmias, heart failure, or hypotension.

Drugs Used to Treat Myocardial Infarction

Analgesic, thrombolytic, and antidysrhythmic agents are among the principal classes of drugs used in treating AMI. Additional drugs frequently used in patients with MI include beta-adrenergic blockers, ACE inhibitors, and anticoagulant and antiplatelet medications, among others.

Analgesics

Pain stimulates the SNS, increasing heart rate and BP and, in turn, myocardial workload. For this reason, pain relief is a vital element of treatment for patients who are experiencing AMI.

Several types of medications are used to alleviate pain associated with AMI, with organic nitrates—specifically, nitroglycerin—being a common choice. Patients may receive up to three 0.4-mg doses of sublingual nitroglycerin at 5-minute intervals. IV nitroglycerin may then be continued for the first 24–48 hours after AMI to reduce myocardial work. As previously mentioned, nitroglycerin does not just relieve pain; it also decreases myocardial oxygen demand and may increase the supply of oxygen to the myocardium. In addition, nitroglycerin is a peripheral and arterial vasodilator that reduces afterload. It dilates coronary arteries and collateral channels in the heart, increasing coronary blood flow to save myocardial tissue at risk. Nitroglycerin may, however, cause reflex tachycardia or excessive hypotension, so close monitoring by the nurse is necessary during administration.

SAFETY ALERT Ask male patients about use of sildenafil (Viagra) within the prior 24 hours, because combining sildenafil and nitroglycerin can precipitate a significant drop in BP.

Morphine sulfate is the drug of choice for MI-related pain that is unrelieved by nitroglycerin and for sedation. Following an initial IV dose of 4–8 mg, small doses (2–4 mg) of morphine may be repeated intravenously every 5 minutes until pain is relieved. When administering morphine, the nurse must assess the patient frequently for pain relief and possible adverse effects of analgesia, such as excessive sedation. Pain that is unrelieved by expected or usual doses of morphine should be reported to the healthcare provider, because it may indicate a complication such as extension of the infarct. Antianxiety agents such as lorazepam (Ativan) may also be administered to promote rest.

Thrombolytics

Thrombolytic agents, which are drugs that dissolve or break up blood clots, are first-line drugs used to treat acute MI when access to a cardiac catheterization lab for revascularization procedures is not immediately available. Thrombolytic drugs activate the fibrinolytic system to lyse (destroy) clots, thereby restoring blood flow to obstructed arteries. Early thrombolytic administration (within 6 hours of MI onset) limits infarct size, reduces heart damage, and improves outcomes. However, activation of the fibrinolytic system can cause multiple complications; in fact, approximately 0.5–5% of patients who receive thrombolytic drugs experience serious bleeding complications. Furthermore, not every patient is a candidate for thrombolytic therapy. For example, these drugs are contraindicated in patients with known bleeding disorders, active peptic ulcer disease, hemorrhagic ophthalmic conditions, or history of severe hypertension; patients who are concurrently on anticoagulant therapy; patients who have had a recent invasive or surgical procedure; and patients who are pregnant.

Several thrombolytic agents are commonly used today. Among these, there are few demonstrated differences in effectiveness but big differences in cost. Streptokinase, a biological agent derived from group C *Streptococcus* organisms, is the least expensive thrombolytic drug. Its primary drawback is the risk for a severe hypersensitivity reaction, including anaphylaxis. Streptokinase is administered by IV infusion. Anisoylated plasminogen streptokinase activator complex (APSAC) is a related drug that can be administered by bolus over a period of 2–5 minutes. It has many of the same effects as streptokinase but is considerably more expensive. Tissue plasminogen activator, tenecteplase, and reteplase are more effective than streptokinase and APSAC in reestablishing myocardial perfusion (especially when the patient's pain developed more than 3 hours earlier), but these drugs are the most expensive thrombolytics.

Antidysrhythmics

Dysrhythmias are a common complication of AMI, particularly in the first 12–24 hours. Antidysrhythmic medications are therefore used as needed to treat dysrhythmias, and they may also be given prophylactically to prevent dysrhythmias. Ventricular dysrhythmias are treated with a class I or class III antidysrhythmic. Symptomatic bradycardia (i.e., bradycardia with associated hypotension and other signs of low CO) is treated with IV atropine, 0.5–1 mg. IV metoprolol, amirodorone, or diltiazem may be ordered to treat atrial fibrillation or other SVTs.

Beta-Adrenergic Blockers

Following AMI, beta-adrenergic blockers such as propranolol (Inderal), atenolol (Tenormin), and metoprolol (Lopressor) reduce pain, limit infarct size, and decrease the incidence of serious ventricular dysrhythmias. These drugs also decrease the patient's heart rate, thus reducing cardiac work and myocardial oxygen demand. Initial doses are given intravenously. However, oral beta-adrenergic blocker therapy has been shown to suggest lower mortality and reinfarction rates. For more information on beta-adrenergic blockers, refer to the section on drugs used in the treatment of angina.

Angiotensin-Converting–Enzyme Inhibitors

ACE inhibitors are useful in reducing mortality associated with AMI. These drugs decrease ventricular remodeling following MI, thereby reducing the risk for subsequent heart failure. Furthermore, although it is not known whether ACE inhibitors will prevent ischemic events, they have been demonstrated to decrease the risk of stroke or heart attack. For this reason, ACE inhibitors are sometimes also prescribed for patients at high risk of CAD and/or MI, including those with diabetes or those with other risk factors.

Anticoagulant and Antiplatelet Medications

Anticoagulant and antiplatelet medications are often prescribed to maintain coronary artery patency following thrombolysis or a revascularization procedure. For example, abciximab (ReoPro) suppresses platelet aggregation and reduces the risk of reocclusion following angioplasty. It also improves vessel opening with thrombolytic therapy, permitting lower doses of thrombolytic drugs to be used. Likewise, standard or low-molecular-weight heparin (LMWH) preparations often are given to patients with AMI. Heparin helps establish and maintain patency of the affected coronary artery. It also is used, along with long-term warfarin, to prevent systemic or pulmonary embolism in patients with significant left ventricular impairment or atrial fibrillation after AMI.

Beyond these medications, aspirin is now considered an essential part of both preventing and treating AMI. Aspirin inhibits the aggregation of platelets and decreases the risk of blood clots. Thus, patients with angina and other risk factors for MI are often started on prophylactic low-dose aspirin therapy (80–325 mg/day). Likewise, patients who are experiencing AMI may be given a 160- to 325-mg aspirin tablet by emergency personnel, with the instruction that the tablet is to be chewed (for buccal absorption). This initial dose is followed by a daily oral dose of 160–325 mg. Aspirin is contraindicated for patients with a history of aspirin sensitivity, bleeding disorders, or active peptic ulcer disease. Also, patients on long-term aspirin therapy should be screened for aspirin resistance. See the Medications feature for additional information on the nursing implications of aspirin and other antiplatelet drugs.

Medications
Antiplatelet Drugs

CLASSIFICATION AND DRUG EXAMPLES	MECHANISMS OF ACTION	NURSING CONSIDERATIONS
Oral Antiplatelet Drugs *Drug examples:* Aspirin Clopidogrel (Plavix)	Antiplatelet drugs suppress platelet aggregation in the arteries, preventing development of an arterial thrombus. Aspirin and clopidogrel block different platelet activation pathways to inhibit aggregation and clot formation. The dose of aspirin given to achieve antiplatelet effects is low, typically 80 mg/day.	■ Inquire about history of intracranial hemorrhage, upper gastrointestinal bleeding, peptic ulcer disease, or known bleeding tendency. ■ Observe for and report increased bruising, petechiae, purpura, and apparent or occult bleeding (e.g., melena, hematemesis). ■ Do not administer concurrently with warfarin (Coumadin). Health Education for the Patient and Family ■ Take as directed. Aspirin should be taken with food or milk; clopidogrel may be taken at any time of day. ■ Do not use NSAIDs or other over-the-counter drugs that may contain aspirin or NSAIDs unless prescribed by your healthcare provider. ■ Check with your healthcare provider before using any herbal remedies (e.g., evening primrose oil, feverfew, garlic, ginkgo biloba, grapeseed extract) while taking these medications. ■ Report unusual bruising or excessive bleeding. ■ Inform all care providers (including dental professionals) about use of these drugs.
Intravenous Antiplatelet Drugs *Drug examples:* Abciximab (ReoPro) Eptifibatide (Integrilin) Tirofiban (Aggrastat)	The intravenously administered antiplatelet drugs abciximab, eptifibatide, and tirofiban block the final common pathway of platelet activation and thus are more effective than orally administered antiplatelet drugs. However, the risk of bleeding is greater with these medications than with the orally administered antiplatelet drugs.	■ Determine history of bleeding disorders, intracranial hemorrhage, or recent trauma or surgery. ■ Inquire about recent use of oral antiplatelet or anticoagulant drugs. ■ Monitor complete blood count, including hemoglobin, hematocrit, and platelet count; clotting studies, including prothrombin time (PT), international normalized ratio (INR), and partial thromboplastin time (PTT); vital signs; and ECG during therapy. ■ Maintain separate IV lines for blood draws and for administration of other drugs during infusion. ■ Closely observe for and immediately report anaphylaxis or bleeding uncontrolled by pressure. Keep resuscitation equipment readily available. ■ Maintain bedrest during infusion. Health Education for the Patient and Family ■ These drugs are given to reduce the risk of clotting and MI. They help maintain blood flow through the affected vessel following angioplasty and stent placement. ■ Immediately report any chest tightness, difficulty breathing, shortness of breath, or itching that develops during the infusion. ■ Your risk of bleeding should return to normal within about 2 days following the infusion. ■ Immediately report any unusual bruising or bleeding.

Other Medications

Patients with pump failure and hypotension may receive IV dopamine, a vasopressor. At low doses (less than 5 mg/kg/min), dopamine improves blood flow to the kidneys, preventing renal ischemia and possible acute renal failure. With increasing doses, dopamine increases myocardial contractility and causes vasoconstriction, thereby improving BP and CO.

Patients affected by both MI and hyperlipidemia may be prescribed cholesterol-lowering agents. Also, a stool softener, such as docusate sodium, may be given following MI to maintain normal bowel function and reduce straining.

Nonpharmacologic Therapy

In patients with CAD, clinical therapy is employed primarily in cases of suspected or confirmed MI. Continuous monitoring and care are provided in the intensive coronary care unit for the first 24–48 hours, after which time less intensive monitoring (e.g., telemetry) may be appropriate.

Bedrest is prescribed for the first 12 hours after MI to reduce the cardiac workload, and an IV line is established to allow rapid administration of emergency medications. A bedside commode is allowed, because it generally provides a less stressful experience than using a bedpan. If the patient's condition is stable, sitting in a chair at the bedside is permitted after 12 hours. Activities are gradually increased as tolerated. A quiet, calm environment with limited outside stimuli is preferred. Visitors are limited to promote rest. Oxygen is administered by nasal cannula at 2–5 L/min to improve oxygenation of the myocardium and other tissues.

A liquid diet may be prescribed for the first 4–12 hours following MI to reduce gastric distention and myocardial work. After that, a low-fat, low-cholesterol, reduced-sodium diet is allowed. Sodium restrictions may be lifted after 2–3 days if no evidence of heart failure is present. Small, frequent feedings are often recommended. Drinks containing caffeine, as well as very hot and cold foods, may also be limited.

In addition to these measures and administration of appropriate medications, patients who have experienced MI often benefit from various revascularization procedures and/or other invasive therapeutic techniques, as described in the following sections.

Revascularization Procedures

Several procedures may be used to restore blood flow and oxygen to ischemic tissue. Nonsurgical percutaneous techniques include transluminal coronary angioplasty, placement of intracoronary stents, and coronary atherectomy, while the primary surgical technique is coronary artery bypass grafting (CABG). Other current and emerging options include minimally invasive coronary artery surgery and transmyocardial laser revascularization. Factors that influence the choice of revascularization strategy may include any of the following: diabetes mellitus, chronic kidney disease, systolic dysfunction, previous history of CABG, and type of MI.

Percutaneous Coronary Revascularization

Percutaneous coronary revascularization (PCR) procedures are used to restore blood flow to the ischemic myocardium in patients with CAD. Each year, approximately 600,000 PCR procedures are performed in the United States.

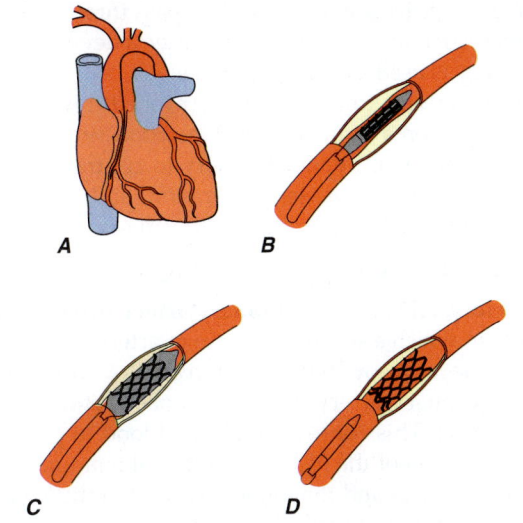

Figure 16–31 》 Percutaneous coronary revascularization. **A,** The balloon catheter with the stent is threaded into the affected coronary artery. The stent is positioned across the blockage **(B)** and expanded **(C)**. **D,** The balloon is deflated and removed, leaving the stent in place.

PCR procedures are similar to the procedure used for coronary angiography. First, a catheter is introduced into the arterial circulation and guided into the opening of the narrowed coronary artery. A flexible guidewire is inserted through the catheter lumen into the affected vessel. The guidewire is then used to thread an angioplasty balloon, arterial stent, or other therapeutic device into the narrowed segment of the artery. The procedure is performed in the cardiac catheterization laboratory using local anesthesia. The hospital stay following the procedure is short (1–2 days), minimizing costs.

Several types of PCR procedures exist. In a **percutaneous transluminal coronary angioplasty (PTCA)**, a balloon-tipped catheter is threaded over the guidewire, with the balloon positioned across the area of narrowing (see **Figure 16–31 》**). The balloon is inflated in a step-by-step fashion for approximately 30 seconds to 2 minutes to compress the plaque against the arterial wall, with the goal of reducing the vessel obstruction to less than 50% of the arterial lumen. PTCA is typically accompanied by placement of a **stent**. Intracoronary stents are metallic scaffolds used to maintain an open arterial lumen. Stents have been shown to reduce the rate of restenosis by approximately one third. During angioplasty, the stent is placed over a balloon catheter, guided into position, and expanded as the balloon is inflated. It then remains in the artery as a prop after the balloon is removed. Over time, endothelial cells will completely line the inner wall of the stent to produce a smooth inner lining. Antiplatelet medications (aspirin and ticlopidine) are given following stent insertion to reduce the risk of thrombus formation at the site.

In contrast to stent procedures, which enlarge the artery by displacing plaque, **atherectomy** procedures remove plaque from the identified lesion. Several types of atherectomy exist. In *directional atherectomy*, the catheter shaves plaque off the vessel walls using a rotary cutting head, retaining the fragments in its housing and removing them from the vessel. In *rotational atherectomy*, the catheter pulverizes plaque into particles small enough to pass through the coronary microcirculation. In *laser atherectomy,* a device that emits laser energy is used to remove plaque.

Complications following PCR procedures vary and include hematoma at the catheter insertion site, pseudoaneurysm, embolism, hypersensitivity to contrast dye, dysrhythmias, bleeding, vessel perforation, and restenosis or reocclusion of the treated vessel.

Coronary Artery Bypass Grafting

Surgery for CAD involves **coronary artery bypass grafting (CABG)**, in which a section of a vein or artery is used to create a connection, or bypass, between the aorta and the blocked coronary artery beyond the obstruction (see **Figure 16–32** »). This connection allows blood to perfuse the ischemic portion of the heart. The internal mammary artery (IMA) in the chest and the saphenous vein in the leg are the vessels most commonly used for CABG.

Bypass grafts are safe and effective. Although anginal pain may recur after surgery, angina is totally relieved or significantly reduced in 90% of patients who undergo complete revascularization. CABG is a viable option for blockages that cannot be treated with angioplasty. Many people remain symptom-free for as long as 10–15 years.

During CABG surgery, a median sternotomy commonly is used to access the heart. The heart is usually stopped during surgery, so a cardiopulmonary bypass (CPB) pump is used to maintain perfusion to the rest of the organs. In this scenario, venous blood is removed from the body through a cannula

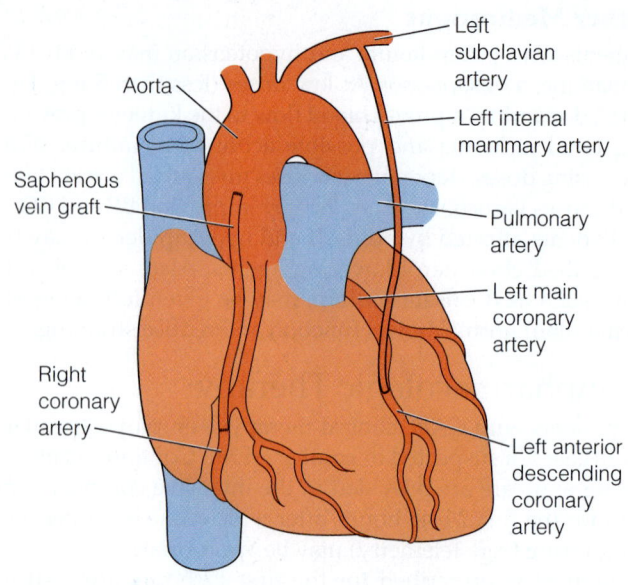

Figure 16–32 » Coronary artery bypass grafting using the internal mammary artery and a saphenous vein graft.

placed in the right atrium or the superior and inferior venae cavae. Blood then circulates through the CPB pump, where it is oxygenated, has its temperature regulated, and is filtered. Oxygenated blood is returned to the body through a cannula in the ascending aorta (see **Figure 16–33** »). CPB enables

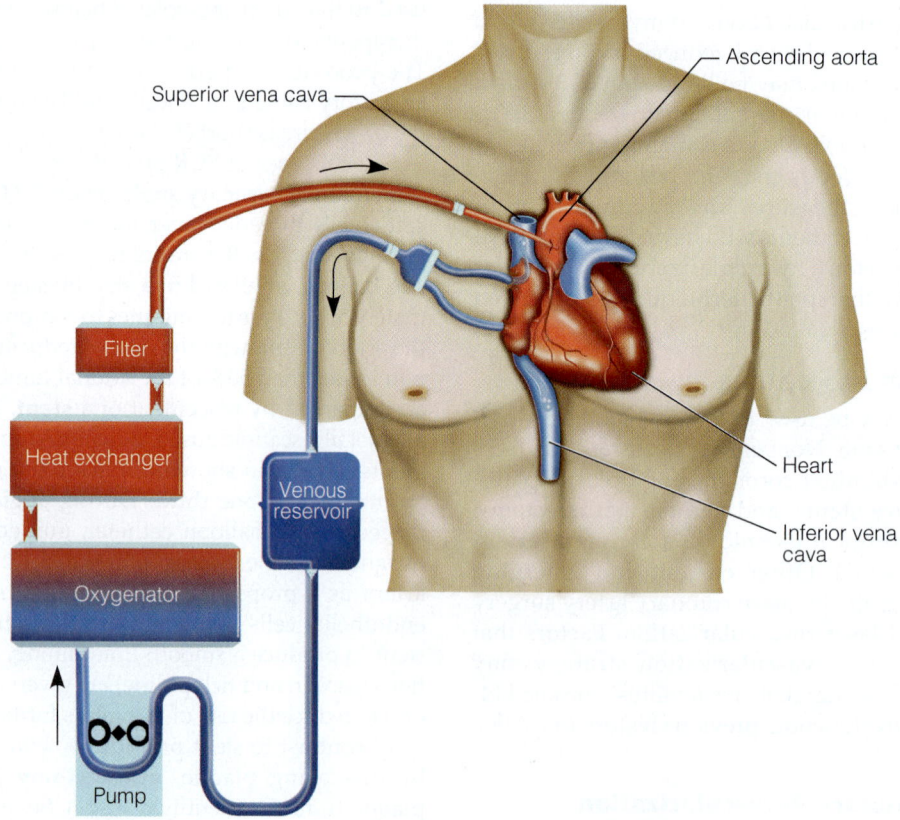

Figure 16–33 » A diagrammatic representation of cardiopulmonary bypass. A cannula in the superior and inferior venae cavae removes venous blood, which is then pumped through an oxygenator and heat exchanger. After filtering, oxygenated blood is returned to the ascending aorta.

surgeons to operate on a quiet heart and a relatively blood-less field. Hypothermia can be maintained to reduce the patient's metabolic rate and decrease oxygen demand during surgery.

When the saphenous vein is used for the bypass graft, it is excised from its normal attachments in the leg, flushed with a cold heparinized saline solution, and then reversed so that its valves do not interfere with blood flow. When appropriate, a laparoscopic approach may be used to remove the vein. The vein is then anastomosed (grafted) to the aorta and the coronary artery, distal to the occlusion (see Figure 16–32). This provides a bridge, or conduit, for blood flow past the obstruction. If the IMA is used instead of the saphenous vein, its distal end is excised and anastomosed to the coronary artery distal to the obstruction. The IMA often is used to revascularize the left coronary artery because of the greater oxygen demand of the left ventricle.

Once grafting is completed, CPB is discontinued, and the patient is rewarmed. Rewarming stimulates the heart to resume beating. Temporary pacing wires are sutured in place and passed through the chest wall in case temporary pacing is necessary. Chest tubes are placed in the pleural space and mediastinum to drain blood and reestablish negative pressure in the thoracic cavity. The sternum is closed using heavy wires and bone wax. The skin is closed with sutures or staples, and sterile dressings are applied over sternal and leg incisions.

Newer techniques have been developed that allow surgeons to perform CABG without cardioplegia (stopping the heart) and use of a CPB. Off-pump coronary artery bypass (OPCAB) also permits use of a smaller incision for access. Although CPB is employed for the majority of coronary artery bypass procedures, OPCAB is a promising alternative. Lower mortality and morbidity rates as well as faster recovery rates have been demonstrated for patients undergoing OPCAB as compared to CABG.

Minimally Invasive Coronary Artery Surgery

Minimally invasive coronary artery surgery is a potential future alternative to CABG. Two approaches may be used: *Port-access coronary artery bypass* uses several small holes, or "ports," in the chest wall to access vessels for connection to the CPB pump and the surgical site. The femoral artery and femoral vein may also be used. With the *minimally invasive direct coronary artery bypass (MIDCAB)* approach, CPB is avoided altogether. Instead, a small surgical incision and several chest wall ports are used to graft a chest wall artery to the affected coronary vessel while the heart continues to beat.

Transmyocardial Laser Revascularization

Transmyocardial laser revascularization is a procedure in which a laser is used to drill tiny holes into the myocardial muscle itself to provide collateral blood flow to ischemic muscle. Patients whose coronary artery obstructions are too diffuse to bypass are candidates for this more advanced surgical treatment.

Other Invasive Procedures

For patients with large MIs and evidence of pump failure, invasive devices may be used to temporarily take over the function of the heart, allowing the injured myocardium to heal. For example, the intra-aortic balloon pump (IABP) is widely used to augment CO. Ventricular assist devices are indicated for patients requiring more or longer-term artificial support than the IABP provides.

Intra-Aortic Balloon Pump

The **intra-aortic balloon pump (IABP)**, also called intra-aortic balloon counterpulsation, is a mechanical circulatory support device that may be used after cardiac surgery or to treat cardiogenic shock following AMI. The IABP temporarily supports cardiac function, allowing the heart to recover gradually by decreasing myocardial workload and oxygen demand and increasing perfusion of the coronary arteries.

With the IABP procedure, a catheter with a 30- to 40-mL balloon is introduced into the aorta, usually via the femoral artery. The balloon catheter is connected to a console that regulates the inflation and deflation of the balloon. The IABP catheter inflates during diastole, increasing perfusion of the coronary and renal arteries, and deflates just before systole, decreasing afterload and cardiac workload (see **Figure 16–34 》**). The inflation–deflation sequence is triggered by the ECG pattern. During the most acute period, the balloon inflates and deflates with each heartbeat (1:1 ratio), providing maximal assistance to the heart. As the patient's condition improves, the IABP is weaned to inflate–deflate at varying intervals (e.g., 1:2, 1:4, and 1:8). This provides a continually decreasing amount of support as the heart muscle recovers. When mechanical assistance is no longer required, the IABP catheter is removed.

Ventricular Assist Devices

Use of a **ventricular assist device (VAD)** to aid the failing heart is becoming more common as technology advances. Whereas an IABP can supplement cardiac output by approximately 10–15%, a VAD temporarily takes partial or complete control of cardiac function, depending on the type of device used. VADs may be used for patients with AMI and/or cardiogenic shock when there is a chance for recovery of normal

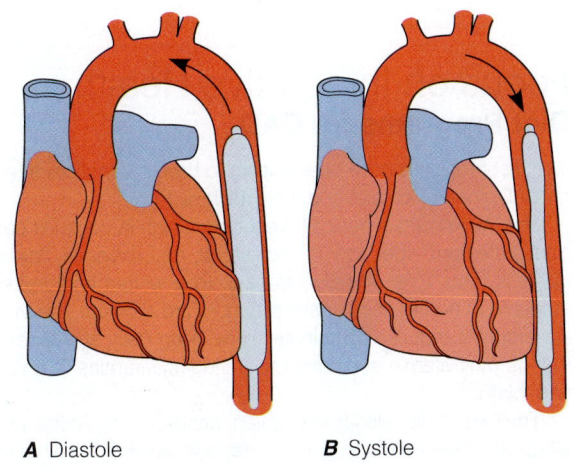

A Diastole   *B* Systole

Figure 16–34 》 The intra-aortic balloon pump. **A,** When inflated during diastole, the balloon supports cerebral, renal, and coronary artery perfusion. **B,** The balloon deflates during systole, so cardiac output is unimpeded.

heart function after a period of cardiac rest. These devices may also be used as a bridge to heart transplantation.

Nursing care for the patient with a VAD is supportive and includes assessing hemodynamic status and monitoring for complications associated with the device. Patients with a VAD are at considerable risk for infection, so strict aseptic technique must be used with all invasive catheters and dressing changes. Pneumonia is also a risk because of immobility and ventilatory support. Mechanical failure of the VAD is life-threatening and requires immediate medical attention.

Cardiac Rehabilitation

Cardiac rehabilitation is a medically supervised program designed to aid people with recovery from MI, heart attacks, heart surgeries, and percutaneous coronary interventions. See the Collaborative Therapies section in the module on Perfusion for a description of the phases of cardiac rehabilitation.

Complementary Health Approaches

Diet and exercise programs that emphasize physical conditioning and a low-fat diet rich in antioxidants have been shown to be effective in managing CAD (see the Focus on Integrative Health feature). Supplements of vitamins C, E, B_6, and B_{12}, as well as folic acid, may also be beneficial. Other potentially helpful complementary health approaches include consumption of red wine or grape juice, foods containing bioflavonoids, green tea, nuts, and herbal supplements and garlic (effective only for hypertension). The nurse should emphasize the need for patients to talk to their healthcare providers before taking any herbal preparations, because interactions with prescribed drugs are common. Behavioral therapies of benefit for patients with CAD include relaxation and stress management, guided imagery, treatment of depression, anger and hostility management, meditation, tai chi, and yoga.

Lifespan Considerations

Women and older adults often present with manifestations of MI different from those of younger and middle-age men.

Focus on Integrative Health
Diet Programs for CAD

Two diet programs have been shown to have a beneficial effect on CAD: the Pritikin diet and the Ornish diet.

The Pritikin diet is basically vegetarian, high in complex carbohydrates and fiber, low in cholesterol, and extremely low in fat (less than 10% of daily calories). Egg whites and limited amounts of nonfat dairy or soy products are allowed. The Pritikin program requires 45 minutes of walking daily and recommends multivitamin supplements, including vitamins C and E and folate.

The Ornish diet also is vegetarian, although egg whites and a cup of nonfat milk or yogurt per day are allowed. No oil or fat is permitted, even for cooking. Two ounces of alcohol are allowed each day. The Ornish program also calls for stress reduction, emotional-social support systems, daily stretching, and walking for 1 hour three times a week.

However, heart disease is the number one cause of death in both groups, making early recognition and aggressive treatment vital.

MI in Women

As compared to men, women are more likely to have a "silent" or unrecognized heart attack or to present in cardiac arrest or with cardiogenic shock. One reason for this situation is that women often experience atypical chest pain. For example, many women have epigastric pain, indigestion, nausea, and vomiting, causing them to blame their discomfort on heartburn or gastroenteritis. Shortness of breath is another common symptom in women, as are fatigue and weakness of the shoulders and upper arms. These atypical symptoms mean that many women do not immediately realize the true nature of their condition and delay seeking care as a result. Yet another factor contributing to treatment delay is that many women tend to ignore chest pain as they have historically been the caregivers and not the recipients of care.

Because of these and other factors, women who experience MI traditionally have worse diagnosis and treatment outcomes than their male counterparts. It is therefore important for healthcare providers to stress the importance of quickly seeking medical help for atypical manifestations of MI. Prompt diagnosis and intervention reduce the mortality and morbidity of MI in women, just as they do in men. Educational initiatives should be directed toward all age groups, because the increasing incidence of heart disease in younger women indicates a clear need for support across the lifespan.

MI in Older Adults

Like women, older adults commonly have atypical symptoms of MI. For instance, older people often seek treatment for vague complaints of difficulty breathing, confusion, fainting, dizziness, abdominal pain, or cough. They frequently attribute their symptoms to a stroke. The prevalence of silent ischemia is also greater in older adults.

The atypical nature of their pain means that many older adults neither seek nor receive prompt treatment, putting them at greater risk for widespread cardiac damage, complications, and death. Thus, both patient education about atypical manifestations of MI and prompt diagnosis and intervention are critical to reducing mortality and morbidity in older adults.

NURSING PROCESS

Nursing care for the patient with known or suspected CAD varies depending on the exact nature of the patient's condition. For example, the focus of care for patients with angina is on reducing myocardial oxygen demand and improving oxygen supply, whereas the focus of care for the patient with AMI is on reducing cardiac work, identifying and treating complications in a timely manner, and preparing the patient for rehabilitation.

Despite such differences, education is a critical element of nursing care for all patients. Nurses are instrumental in educating adults about their risk for CAD, promoting participation in screening programs to identify that risk, and teaching all patients measures to reduce their risk for CAD. For example, nurses may present information about healthy lifestyle habits to community and religious groups, to schoolchildren (grades K–12), and through the print media. In promoting healthy lifestyle habits, nurses can help reduce the incidence, morbidity, and mortality of CAD.

With regard to health promotion, nurses must provide patient education regarding avoiding or stopping all forms of tobacco use and should emphasize both the adverse effects of smoking and the benefits of quitting. Nurses also need to provide information about dietary recommendations to maintain optimal cholesterol levels and a healthy weight. Nurses also must teach patients the benefits of regular exercise. For patients with cardiovascular risk factors, nurses should encourage regular screening for hypertension, diabetes, and abnormal blood lipids.

In addition to undertaking these health promotion measures, the nurse should emphasize the importance of actively managing CAD risk factors to slow progression of the disease by following treatment regimens and making important lifestyle modifications. More specific nursing actions related to assessment, diagnosis, planning, implementation, and evaluation of patients with CAD and/or AMI are described in the following sections.

Assessment

Nursing assessment for CAD, AMI, and angina must be both timely and ongoing. Assessment strategies include the following:

- **Observation and patient interview.** Observe the patient for obvious signs of distress, including signs of fear or anxiety, panic, wide eyes that dart between objects or people, grasping the area of the body that is in pain, and decreased consciousness. Observe manifestations such as shortness of breath, loss of consciousness, grimacing, grasping of the chest, and other signs that may indicate that the patient is experiencing chest pain or a loss of perfusion. Record complaints of chest pain, including its location, intensity, character, radiation, and timing, and associated symptoms, such as nausea, heartburn, shortness of breath, and anxiety. Assess the patient's current diet, exercise patterns, and medications; smoking history and pattern of alcohol intake; history of heart disease, hypertension, or diabetes; and family history of CAD or other cardiac problems.
- **Physical examination.** Record the patient's vital signs and heart sounds; strength and equality of peripheral pulses; and skin color and temperature (central and peripheral); current weight and its appropriateness for height; BMI; waist-to-hip ratio; skin color, temperature, and moisture; LOC; cardiac rhythm (on bedside monitor); and bowel sounds and abdominal tenderness.

Diagnosis

A variety of nursing diagnoses may be appropriate, depending on the exact nature of the patient's condition. For example, nursing diagnoses that may apply to the patient with suspected or known CAD include the following:

- *Health Maintenance, Ineffective*
- *Obesity*

- *Enhanced Knowledge, Readiness for*
- *Activity Intolerance, Risk for*
- *Impaired Cardiovascular Function, Risk for*
- *Sedentary Lifestyle.*

(NANDA-I © 2014)

Along the same lines, nursing diagnoses that may be appropriate for a patient with angina include:

- *Activity Intolerance*
- *Pain, Acute*
- *Anxiety*
- *Health Management, Ineffective*
- *Decreased Cardiac Tissue Perfusion, Risk for.*

(NANDA-I © 2014)

Nursing diagnoses for patients with AMI frequently mirror those for patients with angina. Additional appropriate diagnoses may be as follows:

- *Knowledge, Deficient*
- *Fear*
- *Coping, Ineffective*
- *Peripheral Tissue Perfusion, Ineffective*
- *Decreased Cardiac Output, Risk for*
- *Fluid Volume, Risk for Imbalanced.*

(NANDA-I © 2014)

Planning

Planning for patients with known or suspected CAD varies depending on individual symptoms and diagnoses. The plan of care for a patient at risk for CAD may include the following goals, among others:

- The patient will verbalize modifiable risk factors.
- The patient will describe dietary changes to reduce the risk for CAD.
- The patient will make appropriate lifestyle modifications, such as increasing activity level or quitting smoking.

Planning for patients with symptomatic CAD focuses not only on education, but also on symptom reduction and/or control. Typical goals include such things as:

- The patient will describe lifestyle choices that may worsen CAD.
- The patient will prevent cardiac muscle damage by adhering to the treatment regimen.
- The patient will control her BP by taking medications as prescribed, making appropriate dietary changes, and exercising as tolerated.

As previously described, problems with tissue perfusion are common among patients with CAD, especially those who have also experienced MI. Care planning for patients with ineffective perfusion may include the following goals:

- The patient will understand how to take all prescribed medications and what symptoms to report to the healthcare provider.

- The patient will reduce activity level as needed to maintain optimal tissue perfusion.
- The patient will describe emergency actions to take when experiencing chest pain.

Implementation

The focus of nursing care for patients with CAD, angina, and/or MI is on improving CO, reducing cardiac workload, maximizing function, and teaching the patient how to care for her- or himself at home while reducing the risk of further cardiac damage. It is important to treat the patient holistically, dealing with psychosocial, spiritual, and cultural needs in addition to physical needs. Learning of a diagnosis that affects the heart is very frightening for most patients, and they often require assistance in coping with fear and anxiety. Although patients requiring cardiac rehabilitation will work with specially trained nurses and therapists, nurses in both hospital and primary care settings will be in the position to provide both direct interventions and important health education for patients and their families. Some specific nursing interventions that may be beneficial to patients with CAD are described next.

Promote Balanced Nutrition

Interventions that promote balanced nutrition may be appropriate for patients who are obese, who have a waist-to-hip ratio of greater than 0.8 (women) or 0.9 (men), or whose diet history or serum cholesterol levels indicate a need to reduce fat and cholesterol intake. When working with these patients, the nurse should consider taking the following actions:

- Encourage assessment of food intake and eating patterns to help identify areas that can be improved. Patients often are unaware of their fat and cholesterol intake, particularly when they eat many meals away from home. Careful assessment increases awareness and allows the patient to make conscious changes.
- Discuss American Heart Association (AHA) and Therapeutic Lifestyle Change (TLC) dietary recommendations, emphasizing the role of diet in heart disease. Provide guidance regarding specific food choices, including healthy alternatives. Specific diet information and suggestions will help the patient make better food choices.
- Refer the patient to a clinical dietitian for diet planning and further teaching. Suggest cookbooks that offer low-fat recipes to encourage healthier eating, and distribute AHA and American Cancer Society (ACS) recipe pamphlets and information on low-fat eating. These resources provide tools for the patient to use as eating patterns change.
- Encourage gradual but progressive dietary changes. Drastic changes in eating patterns may cause frustration and discourage the patient from maintaining a healthy diet over the long term.
- Discourage the use of high-fat, low-carbohydrate, or other fad diets for weight loss. These diets may adversely affect serum cholesterol and triglyceride levels, and they often are too drastic to maintain over the long term.
- Encourage reasonable goals for weight loss (e.g., 1.0–1.5 lb per week and a 10% weight loss over 6 months).

Provide information about weight loss programs and support groups, such as Weight Watchers and Take Off Pounds Sensibly (TOPS). Gradual but steady weight loss is more likely to be sustained. Recognized programs that emphasize healthy eating provide support and incentive for making lifetime dietary changes.

Promote Effective Health Maintenance

Patients with risk factors for CAD may be unable to identify or independently manage those risk factors. To promote more effective health maintenance in these patients, the nurse should do the following:

- Discuss risk factors for CAD, stressing how changing or managing those factors that can be modified reduces the patient's overall risk for the disease. Patients with significant nonmodifiable risk factors may be discouraged, which can affect their ability to eliminate or control modifiable risk factors unless the nurse offers support.
- Discuss the immediate benefits of smoking cessation. Provide resource materials from the AHA, the ACS, and the American Lung Association. Refer to a structured smoking cessation program to increase the likelihood of success in quitting. Long-time smokers may assume that the damage from smoking has already been done and that quitting would not be "worth the price." In such cases, provide evidence indicating otherwise.
- Help the patient identify specific sources of psychosocial and physical support for smoking cessation, dietary modification, and lifestyle change. Supportive individuals, support groups, and aids such as nicotine patches help the patient achieve success and provide encouragement during difficult times (e.g., during withdrawal symptoms).
- Discuss the benefits of regular exercise for cardiovascular health and weight loss. Help the patient identify favorite forms of exercise or physical activity. Encourage 30 minutes of continuous aerobic activity (e.g., walking, running, bicycling, swimming) four to five times a week. Recommend identification of an "exercise buddy" to help maintain motivation. Engaging in preferred activities with a partner maintains motivation and increases the likelihood of remaining on an exercise program. Encourage continuation of the exercise plan, even when days are missed. Remind the patient that exercise is cumulative, so increasing the duration of exercise on subsequent days can "make up" for a lost day.
- Provide information and teaching about prescribed medications, such as cholesterol-lowering drugs. Discuss the relationship between hypertension, diabetes, and CAD. Teaching is important to promote understanding of and adherence with the prescribed drug regimen.

Manage Acute Pain

Chest pain occurs when the oxygen supply to the heart muscle does not meet the demand. Myocardial ischemia and infarction cause pain, as does reperfusion of an ischemic area following thrombolytic therapy or emergent PTCA. Because pain stimulates the SNS and increases cardiac work, pain relief is a priority of care for the patient with AMI. Appropriate nursing interventions include the following:

- Assess the patient for verbal and nonverbal signs of pain. Document the characteristics and intensity of the pain, using a standard pain scale. Verify nonverbal indicators of pain with the patient. Frequent, careful pain assessment allows early intervention to reduce the risk of further damage. Pain is a subjective experience; its expression may vary with location and intensity, previous experiences, and cultural and social background. Pain scales provide an objective tool for measuring pain and a way to assess pain relief or reduction.

- If the patient is hypoxic, administer oxygen at 2–5 L/min via nasal cannula. Supplemental oxygen increases oxygen supply to the myocardium, decreasing ischemia and pain. Note that recent research suggests that oxygen administration may increase the risk of myocardial damage in patients who do not have hypoxia (Stub et al., 2015).

- Promote physical and psychologic rest, and provide information and emotional support. Rest decreases cardiac workload and SNS stimulation, promoting comfort. Information and emotional support help decrease anxiety and provide psychologic rest.

- Titrate IV nitroglycerin as ordered to relieve chest pain, maintaining a systolic BP of greater than 100 mmHg. Nitroglycerin decreases chest pain by dilating peripheral vessels, reducing cardiac work, and dilating coronary vessels, including collateral channels, thus improving blood flow to ischemic tissue.

- Administer 2–4 mg of morphine by IV push for chest pain as needed. Morphine is an effective narcotic analgesic for chest pain. It decreases pain and anxiety, acts as a venodilator, and decreases the patient's respiratory rate. The resulting reduction in preload and SNS stimulation reduces cardiac work and oxygen consumption.

Monitor Tissue Perfusion

Cardiac muscle damage affects compliance, contractility, and CO. The extent of the effect on tissue perfusion depends on the location and amount of damage. Anterior wall infarcts have a greater effect on CO than do right ventricular infarcts. Infarcted muscle also increases the risk for cardiac dysrhythmias, which can further affect the delivery of blood and oxygen to the tissues. Interventions to promote adequate tissue perfusion include the following:

- Assess and document the patient's vital signs. Report increases in heart rate and changes in rhythm, BP, and respiratory rate. Decreased CO activates compensatory mechanisms that may cause tachycardia and vasoconstriction, increasing cardiac work.

- Assess the patient for changes in LOC; decreased urine output; moist, cool, pale, mottled, or cyanotic skin; dusky or cyanotic mucous membranes and nail beds; diminished to absent peripheral pulses; and delayed capillary refill. These are manifestations of impaired tissue perfusion. A change in LOC is often the first manifestation of altered perfusion, because cerebral function depends on a continuous supply of oxygen.

- Auscultate heart and breath sounds. Note any abnormal heart sounds (e.g., an S_3 or S_4 gallop, a murmur) or adventitious lung sounds. These sounds may indicate impaired cardiac filling or output, increasing the risk for decreased tissue perfusion.

- Monitor the patient's ECG rhythm continuously. Dysrhythmias can further impair CO and tissue perfusion.

- Monitor the patient's oxygen saturation levels, and administer oxygen as ordered. Also obtain and assess ABG levels as indicated. Oxygen saturation is an indicator of gas exchange, tissue perfusion, and the effectiveness of oxygen administration. ABG levels provide a more precise measurement of blood oxygen levels and acid–base balance.

- Administer antidysrhythmic medications as needed. Dysrhythmias affect tissue perfusion by altering CO.

- Obtain serial CK, isoenzyme, and troponin levels as ordered. Levels of various cardiac markers (CK isoenzymes in particular) correlate with the extent of myocardial damage.

- Plan for invasive hemodynamic monitoring. Hemodynamic monitoring facilitates AMI management and treatment evaluation by providing a means of assessing pressures in the systemic and pulmonary arteries, the relationship between oxygen supply and demand, CO, and cardiac index.

Promote Effective Coping

Coping mechanisms help an individual deal with a life-threatening event or with acute changes in health. However, certain coping mechanisms may be detrimental to restoring health, particularly if the patient relies on them for a prolonged period. Denial, for example, is a common coping mechanism among patients after an MI. During the initial stages, denial can reduce anxiety, but continued denial can interfere with learning and treatment adherence. Nursing interventions to promote effective coping include the following:

- Establish an environment of caring and trust. Encourage patients to express their feelings. A trusting nurse–patient relationship provides a safe environment for the patient to discuss feelings of helplessness, powerlessness, anxiety, and hopelessness.

- Accept denial as a coping mechanism, but do not reinforce it. Denial may initially help by diminishing the psychologic threat to health and decreasing anxiety. However, its prolonged use can interfere with cooperation and acceptance of reality, possibly delaying treatment and hindering recovery.

- Note aggressive behaviors, hostility, or anger. These signs can indicate anxiety. Anxiety and depression, if not addressed, can lead to poor cardiac outcomes. Assess the reasons behind the behaviors, and provide additional support or information. Patients who continue to exhibit anxious, angry, or depressive behaviors may require a referral to a mental health specialist.

- Help the patient identify positive coping skills used in the past (e.g., problem-solving skills, verbalization of feelings, asking for help, prayer). Reinforce use of these positive coping behaviors. Coping behaviors that have been successful in the past can help the patient deal with the current situation. These familiar methods can also decrease feelings of powerlessness.

- Provide opportunities, as possible, for the patient to make decisions about the plan of care. This promotes self-confidence and independence. Participating in care planning gives the patient a sense of control and the opportunity to use positive coping skills.

- Provide privacy for the patient and family members to share their questions and concerns. Privacy offers an opportunity for the patient and family members to share their feelings and fears, give support and encouragement to one another, relieve anxiety, and establish effective coping methods.

Manage Fear

Fear of death and disability can be a paralyzing emotion that adversely affects the patient's recovery from AMI. To help the patient manage such fear, the nurse should do the following:

- Identify the patient's level of fear, noting verbal and nonverbal signs. This information enables the nurse to plan appropriate interventions. Because patients may not voice their concerns, attention to nonverbal indicators is especially important. Controlling fear helps decrease SNS responses and catecholamine release that may foster further feelings of fear and anxiety.

- Acknowledge the patient's perception of the situation, and allow the patient to verbalize concerns. A sudden change in health status causes anxiety and fear of the unknown. Verbalizing these fears may help the patient cope with change while also permitting the healthcare team to provide information and correct misconceptions.

- Encourage questions, and provide consistent, factual answers. Repeat information as needed. Accurate, consistent information can reduce fear. Honest explanations help strengthen the patient–nurse relationship and help the patient develop realistic expectations. Anxiety and fear decrease the ability to concentrate and retain data, so information may need to be repeated.

- Encourage self-care. Allow the patient to make decisions regarding the plan of care. This promotes personal responsibility for health and allows some control over the situation. Patients' confidence increases as their dependence decreases.

- Administer antianxiety medications as ordered. These medications promote rest and relaxation and decrease feelings of anxiety, which may act as barriers to health restoration.

- Teach nonpharmacologic methods of stress reduction (e.g., relaxation techniques, mental imagery, music therapy, breathing exercises, meditation, massage). Stress management techniques can help reduce tension and anxiety, provide a sense of control, and enhance coping skills.

Promote Effective Cardiac Perfusion

The pain of angina results from impaired oxygen supply to the myocardium. Nursing interventions that may promote effective cardiac perfusion, prevent ischemia, and shorten the duration of pain include the following:

- Instruct the patient to keep prescribed nitroglycerin tablets always on hand so one can be taken at the onset of pain. Anginal pain indicates myocardial ischemia. Nitroglycerin reduces cardiac work and may improve myocardial blood flow, relieving ischemia and pain.

- Teach the patient about prescribed medications to maintain myocardial perfusion and reduce cardiac work. Emphasize that long-acting organic nitrates, beta-adrenergic blockers, and CCBs are used to *prevent* anginal attacks, not to *treat* acute attacks. It is important for the patient to understand the purpose and use of prescribed drugs to maintain optimal myocardial perfusion.

- Instruct the patient to take sublingual nitroglycerin before engaging in activities that precipitate angina (e.g., climbing stairs, sexual intercourse). This prophylactic dose of nitroglycerin helps maintain cardiac perfusion when increased work is anticipated, thereby preventing ischemia and chest pain.

- Encourage the patient to implement and maintain a progressive exercise program under the supervision of his or her primary care provider or cardiac rehabilitation professional. Exercise slows the atherosclerotic process and helps develop collateral circulation to the heart muscle.

- Refer the patient to a smoking cessation program as indicated. Nicotine causes vasoconstriction and increases the heart rate, decreasing myocardial perfusion and increasing cardiac workload.

- Space activities to allow rest between them. Activity increases cardiac work and may precipitate angina. Spacing of activities allows the heart to recover.

Promote Adherence to the Therapeutic Regimen

Patients with CAD, angina, and/or MI may exhibit strong denial. Because many people think of the heart as the locus of life itself, problems such as angina remind people of their mortality, an uncomfortable fact. Denial may lead to "forgetting" to take prescribed medications or attempting activities that will precipitate angina. Some patients, by contrast, may become afraid to engage in activities because of anticipated chest pain. Their inactivity may actually hasten the atherosclerotic process and inhibit collateral circulation development, thus worsening their angina. The nurse can help avoid outcomes like this by promoting more effective therapeutic regimen management. Appropriate nursing interventions include the following:

- Assess the patient's knowledge and understanding of CAD and angina. Assessment allows tailoring of teaching and interventions to the needs of the patient.

- Teach about angina and atherosclerosis as needed, building on the patient's current knowledge base. This can help the patient understand that angina is a manageable disease and that pain can usually be controlled and progression of the disease slowed.

- Provide written and verbal instructions about prescribed medications and their use. Written instructions

Patient Teaching

Cardiac Rehabilitation and Home Care

Cardiac rehabilitation begins with admission to the health-care facility and continues through the inpatient stay and after discharge into the rehabilitative period. The emphasis is on realistic application of information to maintain lifestyle changes.

Assessing the patient's readiness to learn is an important first step in preparing for home care. The patient in strong denial may not identify any relevance to the information being taught. Evaluate the patient's ability to learn, assessing physiologic and psychologic health, beliefs regarding personal responsibility for health, and expectations of the healthcare system. Also assess the patient's developmental level, ability to perform psychomotor tasks, cognitive function, learning disabilities, and existing knowledge base, as well as the influence of previous learning experiences. Provide written material to supplement teaching and encourage questions.

Be sure to include the following topics in teaching for home care:

- The normal anatomy and physiology of the heart, and the specific area of heart damage
- The process of CAD and implications of MI
- Purposes and side effects of prescribed medications
- The importance of adhering with the medical regimen and cardiac rehabilitation program and of keeping follow-up appointments
- Information about community resources, such as the local chapter of the AHA

After discharge, follow up by telephone within 1 week and periodically thereafter during the recovery period. Provide telephone numbers of resource personnel who are available to respond to questions and concerns after discharge. Motivational and social support may be helpful to patients in adopting healthier behaviors after AMI.

Because the patient who has had an MI is at high risk for SCD, encourage family members to learn CPR and provide information about community resources for CPR training.

reinforce teaching and are available to the patient for future reference.

- Stress the importance of taking chest pain seriously while maintaining a positive attitude. Although it is vital for the patient to recognize the significance of chest pain and deal with it appropriately, it is also important to maintain a positive outlook.
- Refer the patient to a cardiac rehabilitation program or other organized activities and support groups for patients with CAD. Programs such as these help the patient develop risk factor management strategies, maintain a program of supervised activity, and gain coping skills. See the Patient Teaching feature for more information.

Evaluation

Care is evaluated on the basis of the patient's progress toward identified goals. For example, it may be based on achievement of the following expected outcomes:

- The patient demonstrates adequate circulation as evidenced by PaO_2 and $PaCO_2$ values within normal limits.
- The patient maintains systolic BP, pulse pressure, mean BP, central venous pressure (CVP), and/or pulmonary wedge pressures within the normal range.
- The patient reduces anginal events and demonstrates proper actions when angina begins.
- The patient shows an absence of complications resulting from CAD.

Depending on the patient's progress toward the nursing goals, additional interventions may be needed, including administration of additional medications as ordered or preparing the patient for surgery. This may involve providing additional patient teaching related to the medications or surgical procedures, providing emotional support to the patient and family, and prepping the surgical site. If surgery is necessary, the patient will need postoperative care that is appropriate for the type of surgery that was performed.

Nursing Care Plan

A Patient with AMI

Betty Williams, a 62-year-old woman who works as a psychologist, is admitted to the emergency department with complaints of severe substernal chest pain. Mrs. Williams states that the pain began after lunch, about 4 hours ago. She initially attributed it to indigestion. She describes the pain, which now radiates to her jaw and left arm, as "really severe heartburn." It is accompanied by a "choking feeling," severe shortness of breath, and diaphoresis. The pain is unrelieved by rest, antacids, or three sublingual nitroglycerin tablets (0.4 mg).

Mrs. Williams' SaO_2 is only 91%, so oxygen is started via nasal cannula at 2 L/min. Central and peripheral IV lines are inserted. A 12-lead ECG and the following lab work are obtained: cardiac troponins, CK and CK isoenzymes, ABG levels, complete blood count,

and a chemistry panel. Morphine sulfate is administered, and it relieves Mrs. Williams's pain.

Mrs. Williams's medical history includes type 2 diabetes, angina, and hypertension. She has a 45-year history of cigarette smoking, averaging 1.5–2 packs per day. Family history reveals that Mrs. Williams's father died at age 42 of AMI, and her paternal grandfather died at age 65 of AMI. Mrs. Williams is taking the following medications: tolbutamide (Orinase), hydrochlorothiazide, and isosorbide (Isordil).

Based on ECG changes and cardiac markers, an acute anterior MI is diagnosed. Mrs. Williams has no contraindications to thrombolytic therapy and is deemed a good candidate. IV alteplase (Activase) is given by bolus, followed by IV infusions of alteplase and heparin. She is transferred to the coronary care unit.

(continued on next page)

Nursing Care Plan (continued)

ASSESSMENT

Dan Morales, RN, is Mrs. Williams's primary care nurse. Mrs. Williams is alert and oriented to person, place, and time. Vital signs are as follows: temperature 99.6°F (37.5°C) oral; pulse 118 bpm; respirations 24/min with adequate depth; and BP 172/92 mmHg. Auscultation reveals a fourth heart sound (S_4) and fine crackles in the bases of both lungs. The ECG shows sinus tachycardia with occasional PVCs. Mrs. Williams's skin is cool and slightly diaphoretic. Her capillary refill is less than 3 seconds, and her peripheral pulses are strong and equal. Her nail beds are pink.

A triple-lumen central line is in place. Nitroglycerin is infusing at 200 mcg/min in the distal lumen. The alteplase infusion is in the middle lumen, and a heparin infusion is in the proximal lumen. The peripheral IV line has a saline lock.

Mrs. Williams states, "The pain is better since the nurse in the ER gave me a shot, but it has been coming and going. I would rate it a four right now, but it was terrible before. The physician told me that this drug I'm getting will quickly open up the artery that is blocked. I hope it works! Do many people get this drug?"

DIAGNOSES

- *Acute Pain* related to ischemic myocardial tissue
- *Anxiety* related to change in health status
- *Fear* related to health status
- *Ineffective Protection* related to the risk of bleeding secondary to thrombolytic therapy
- *Risk for Decreased Cardiac Output* related to altered cardiac rate and rhythm

(NANDA-I © 2014)

PLANNING

Goals of care include the following:

- The patient will rate chest pain as 2 or lower on a pain scale of 0–10.
- The patient will verbalize reduced anxiety and fear.
- The patient will demonstrate no signs of internal or external bleeding.
- The patient will maintain adequate cardiac output during and following reperfusion therapy.

IMPLEMENTATION

- Instruct the patient to report all chest pain. Monitor and evaluate pain using a scale of 0–10. Titrate IV nitroglycerin infusion for chest pain; stop infusion if systolic BP is below 100 mmHg. Administer 2–4 mg of morphine intravenously for chest pain unrelieved by nitroglycerin infusion.
- Encourage the patient to verbalize fears and concerns. Respond honestly, and correct misconceptions about the disease, therapeutic interventions, or prognosis.
- Assess the patient's knowledge of CAD. Explain the purpose of thrombolytic therapy to dissolve the fresh clot and reperfuse the heart muscle, limiting heart damage.
- Explain the need for frequent monitoring of vital signs and potential bleeding.

- Assess the patient for manifestations of internal or intracranial bleeding, such as complaints of back or abdominal pain, headache, decreased LOC, dizziness, bloody secretions or excretions, or pallor. Test all stools, urine, and vomitus for occult blood. Notify the healthcare provider immediately of any abnormal findings.
- Monitor the patient for signs of reperfusion, including decreased chest pain, return of ST segment to baseline, and reperfusion dysrhythmias (e.g., PVCs, bradycardia, heart block).
- Continuously monitor the ECG for changes in cardiac rate, rhythm, and conduction. Assess vital signs.
- Treat dangerous dysrhythmias or other cardiac events per protocol. Notify the healthcare provider when such events occur.
- Discuss continuing cardiac care and rehabilitation with the patient.

EVALUATION

The initial morphine dose reduced Mrs. Williams's chest pain from a rating of 8 to 4. The nitroglycerin infusion and thrombolytic therapy further reduce her pain to 2. The nitroglycerin infusion is gradually discontinued after 24 hours. As her pain subsides, Mrs. Williams states that she feels "much better now that the pain is gone. I was afraid it would just get worse." She verbalizes an understanding of thrombolytic therapy to limit myocardial damage. No indications of bleeding problems are noted. Reperfusion is indicated by relief of chest pain, return of the ST segment to baseline on the ECG, early peaking of CK levels, and increased frequency of PVCs but no significant dysrhythmias. Mrs. Williams remains in the coronary care unit for 36 hours and is then transferred to the floor.

CRITICAL THINKING

1. How would the initial plan of care have changed if Mrs. Williams were not a candidate for thrombolytic therapy?

2. Two days after her initial therapy, Mrs. Williams complains of palpitations. You notice frequent PVCs on the ECG monitor. What do you do?

3. What health promotion topics would you teach Mrs. Williams before discharge?

4. Mrs. Williams states, "I've been smoking for over 45 years, and I'm not going to stop now! Besides, it calms me down when I'm anxious." How would you respond to this statement?

REVIEW Coronary Artery Disease

RELATE Link the Concepts and Exemplars

Linking the exemplar of CAD with the concept of health, wellness, and illness:

1. What nutritional recommendations will you teach the patient with, or at risk for, CAD?

2. What will you teach the patient about physical fitness and exercise in regard to reducing the risk of CAD?

Linking the exemplar of CAD with the concept of metabolism:

3. What role does obesity play with regard to risk for CAD? Explain the physiology of this impact.

4. What teaching would you provide a patient with type 2 diabetes mellitus to reduce the risk of CAD?

READY Go to Volume 3: Clinical Nursing Skills

REFER Go to Pearson MyLab Nursing and eText

- Additional review materials.

REFLECT Apply Your Knowledge

Norma James is a 65-year-old widow who lives alone. Although Mrs. James has lived in the neighborhood for years, she is somewhat socially isolated. She has two adult sons with whom she has limited contact; they live out of the state and rarely call. She has only a few individuals whom she considers friends; she does not particularly like people and prefers the company of her six cats.

Mrs. James has a long history of type 2 diabetes mellitus and hypertension. In recent years, she has been diagnosed with atrial fibrillation. She has several healthcare providers and takes multiple medications, including:

- Glucotrol, 10 mg, twice a day

- Captopril, 50 mg, twice a day

- Digoxin, 125 mcg, once a day

- Coumadin, 5 mg, once a day.

Mrs. James has a known drug allergy to penicillin.

Mrs. James does not work outside the home and has very limited savings, so she relies on Social Security benefits for income. She smokes about 1/2 pack of cigarettes a day and has been a smoker since she was in her 20s. She reports that she drinks alcohol "a couple times a year, usually a glass of wine at a special dinner."

Mrs. James does not drive but relies on her friends, neighbors, or the city bus for transportation. She lives near a grocery store and prides herself on being able to get most things she needs without any assistance. She spends most of her time alone at home and occupies herself by watching television, reading, and doing crossword and jigsaw puzzles.

1. According to Mrs. James's history, what are her risks for developing CAD?

2. What lifestyle changes would you discuss with Mrs. James to reduce this risk?

3. Create a teaching plan to help Mrs. James understand her lifestyle behaviors that are increasing her risk of developing CAD.

≫ Exemplar 16.D
Deep Venous Thrombosis

Exemplar Learning Outcomes

16.D Analyze deep venous thrombosis (DVT) as it relates to perfusion.

- Describe the pathophysiology of DVT.
- Describe the etiology of DVT.
- Compare the risk factors and prevention of DVT.
- Identify the clinical manifestations of DVT.
- Summarize diagnostic tests and therapies used by interprofessional teams in the collaborative care of an individual with DVT.
- Differentiate care of patients with DVT across the lifespan.
- Apply the nursing process in providing culturally competent care to an individual with DVT.

Exemplar Key Terms

Deep venous thrombosis (DVT), *1211*
Superficial thrombophlebitis, *1211*
Thrombophlebitis, *1211*
Venous thrombectomy, *1217*
Venous thrombosis, *1211*
Virchow's triad, *1212*

Overview

Thrombophlebitis—sometimes called phlebitis—is a condition in which a blood clot forms and blocks one or more veins. Clots typically form in the legs but can form in the arms and neck in rare instances. When the blockage occurs near the skin's surface, it is known as **superficial thrombophlebitis**; when it occurs deep in a muscle, it is known as a **deep venous thrombosis (DVT)** (Mayo Clinic, 2014f). DVT typically occurs in the large veins of the lower leg and thigh.

Pathophysiology and Etiology

A thrombus is a clot that forms in a vein or artery. The formation of such a clot is referred to as thrombosis, and when the formation occurs in a vein, it is known as a **venous thrombosis**. DVT is the result of venous thrombosis deep in the muscle tissue. The blood clots involved in DVT may travel to the lungs; when this occurs, patients develop a life-threatening PE. Because these two conditions often occur together, they are collectively referred to as a venous thromboembolism (VTE) (Mayo Clinic, 2015d).

Pathophysiology

Three pathologic factors, called **Virchow's triad**, are associated with the formation of a thrombus (Hull & Harris, 2013):

1. Circulatory stasis
2. Vascular damage
3. Hypercoagulability.

Vascular damage stimulates the clotting cascade. Platelets aggregate at the site of the trauma, particularly when circulatory stasis is present. Platelets and fibrin form the initial clot. RBCs become trapped in the fibrin meshwork, and the thrombus propagates (grows) in the direction of blood flow. This triggers the inflammatory response, causing tenderness, swelling, and erythema in the area of the thrombus.

The thrombus initially floats within the vein. Pieces of the thrombus may break loose and travel through the circulation as emboli. Fibroblasts eventually invade the thrombus, scarring the vein wall and destroying venous valves. Permanent valve damage may occur because of thrombosis, even if valve patency is restored. Valve damage will most likely affect directional flow.

Deep venous thrombi occur in the deep veins of the body that lead to the vena cava. The deep veins of the legs—primarily in the calves—and of the pelvis provide the most hospitable environment for venous thrombosis (see **Figure 16–35** 》). There are also deep veins in the arms, chest, and neck, but thrombi typically do not form in these locations. Approximately one half of DVTs are asymptomatic. If symptoms are present, they depend on the clot's location and size.

SAFETY ALERT When a thrombus damages the vein or its valves, postthrombotic syndrome may develop. This condition occurs when damaged valves allow blood to backflow and pool and may result in pain, edema, discoloration of the skin, and skin lesions. Postthrombotic syndrome may occur at any time following DVT.

Etiology

Thrombi can be either venous or arterial. Venous thrombi tend to occur at sites where the vein is normal but blood flow is low. Arterial thrombi tend to occur at sites of arterial plaque rupture. DVT is a common complication of hospitalization, surgery, and immobilization. Other factors associated with venous thrombosis include venous injury, cancer, pregnancy, oral contraceptive or hormone replacement use,

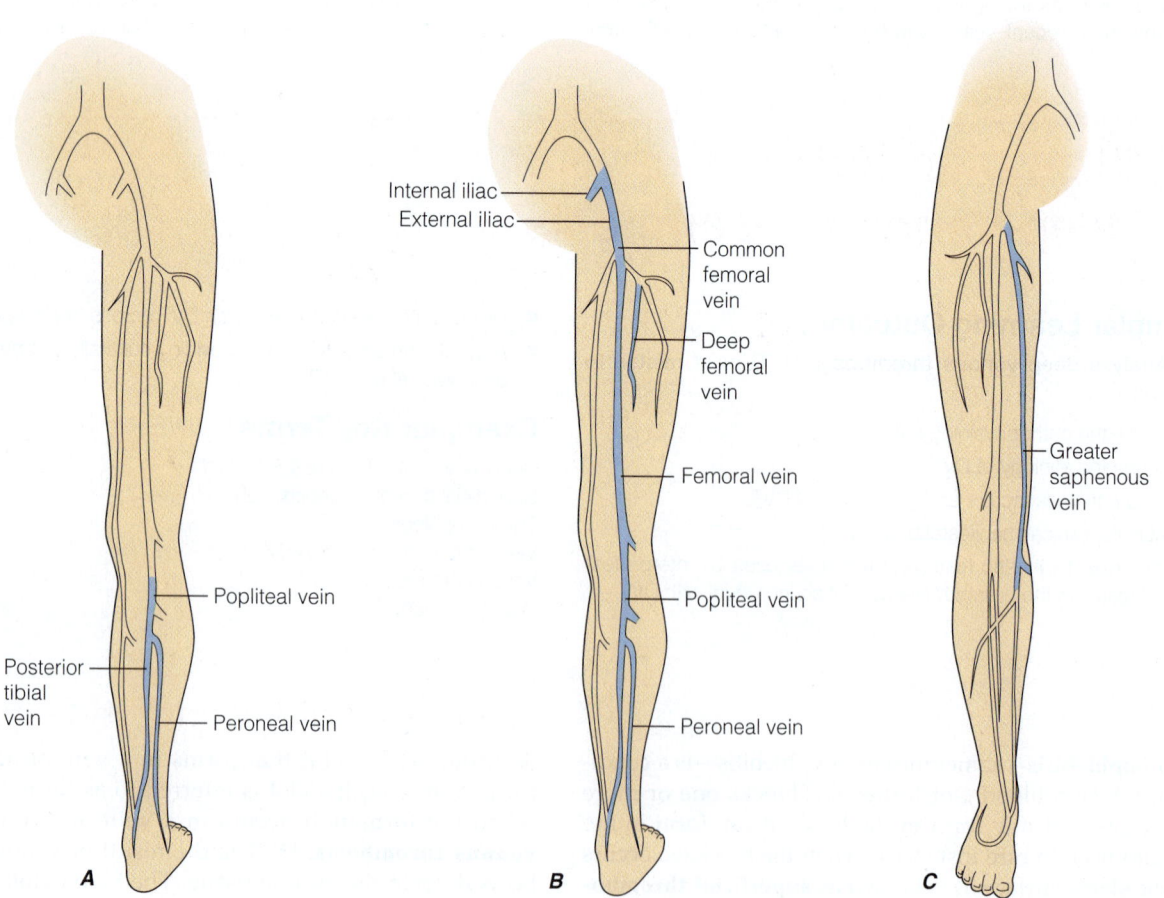

Figure 16–35 》 Common locations of venous thrombosis. **A,** The most common sites of DVT. **B,** DVT extending from the calf to the iliac veins. **C,** Superficial venous thrombosis.

Box 16–11
Factors Associated with Venous Thrombosis

- Immobilization: MI, heart failure, stroke, postoperative
- Surgery: orthopedic, thoracic, abdominal, genitourinary
- Cancer: pancreatic, lung, ovary, testes, urinary tract, breast, stomach
- Trauma: fractures of the spine, pelvis, femur, tibia; spinal cord injury
- Pregnancy and delivery
- Hormone therapy: oral contraceptives, hormone replacement therapy
- Coagulation disorders

Box 16–12
Manifestations of DVT

- Often asymptomatic
- Dull, aching pain in affected extremity, especially when walking
- Possible tenderness, warmth, and erythema along affected vein
- Edema of affected extremity
- Cyanosis of affected extremity

clotting disorders, obesity, and a personal or family history of DVT (CDC, 2015i) (see **Box 16–11** »).

Risk Factors and Prevention

Individual preventive approaches minimize the risk factors that can predispose individuals to DVT. Specific conditions warranting prevention include the following:

- *Orthopedic procedures.* Orthopedic surgery is associated with a high risk of DVT. Major procedures include total hip replacement, with an estimated DVT incidence of 40–60%; traumatic hip fracture repair, with an incidence of 45–60%; and total knee replacement, with an incidence of 40–85% (Kakkar & Rushton-Smith, 2013).

- *Atrial fibrillation.* Individuals with atrial fibrillation can form thrombi within the atria that can enter the general circulation and cause stroke. The risk of DVT is increased during the first 6 months following diagnosis of atrial fibrillation (Enga et al., 2014).

- *Acute myocardial infarction.* Patients who have had an AMI have a high incidence of DVT (Dobromirski & Cohen, 2012). Older patients with heart failure, recurrent angina, or ventricular dysrhythmias are most at risk.

- *Ischemic stroke.* Estimates of DVT incidence following ischemic stroke vary greatly. The majority of studies suggest that DVT occurs in about 20% of patients, though some research suggests that incidence may be as high as 80% in Western countries (Liu et al., 2014).

In many cases, prophylactic anticoagulant therapy is prescribed to lower the risk of DVT. LMWHs prevent DVT in patients who are undergoing general or orthopedic surgery, are experiencing acute medical illness, or are on prolonged bedrest. Oral anticoagulation may be used as a prophylactic measure in patients with fractures or those undergoing orthopedic surgery.

Elevating the foot of the bed with the knees slightly flexed promotes venous return. It is also important for patients to get up and start moving as soon as possible after surgery, injury, or illness, provided that they are physically capable and that doing so does not pose other risks to their health. Early mobilization and leg exercises such as ankle flexion and extension assist venous flow by muscle compression. Medical compression stockings or intermittent pneumatic compression devices may be used on patients with limited mobility, with a high risk of bleeding, or for whom prophylactic medications are contraindicated (CDC, 2015h).

Clinical Manifestations

Many patients with DVT experience no symptoms. When symptoms are present, they may differ greatly in severity (Patel & Chun, 2015). Manifestations of DVT are primarily caused by the inflammatory process that accompanies the thrombus. Aching pain in the affected extremity, particularly upon walking, is the most common symptom; a dull or tight feeling in the calf is also common. Tenderness, swelling, warmth, and erythema may be noted along the course of involved veins. The affected extremity is often edematous and may be cyanotic. In rare cases, a cord may be palpated over the affected vein. See **Box 16–12** » for a summary of the manifestations of DVT.

The major complications of DVT are recurrent DVT and PE. PE occurs when the clot or clot fragments break loose from the vein wall. As the clot travels, it moves through progressively larger veins and into the right side of the heart. From there, it enters the pulmonary circulation, where it eventually occludes arterial flow to a portion of the lungs. This results in a mismatch between ventilation and perfusion in a portion of the lungs. The effect on gas exchange depends on the size of the embolism and the vessel it occludes.

Collaboration

Venous thrombosis must be differentiated from other causes of extremity pain, such as cellulitis, muscle strain, contusion, and lymphedema. Patient history, physical examination, and diagnostic tests are used to establish the diagnosis. Treatment focuses on preventing further clotting or extension of the clot and addressing underlying causes.

Diagnostic Tests

Laboratory studies that may be ordered include D-dimer, PT (measured as an INR), PTT, activated partial prothrombin time (aPTT), bleeding time, and platelet count. Information about these studies can be found in Appendix B. Diagnostic tests for DVT include the following:

- *Duplex venous ultrasonography* is a noninvasive test used to visualize the vein and measure the velocity of blood flow in the veins. Although the clot often cannot be visualized directly, its presence can be inferred by an inability to compress the vein during the examination.

- *Plethysmography* is a noninvasive test that measures changes in blood flow through the veins. It is often used in conjunction with Doppler ultrasonography. Plethysmography is most valuable in diagnosing thromboses of larger or more superficial veins.
- *MRI* is another noninvasive means of detecting DVT. It is particularly useful when thrombosis of the vena cava or pelvic veins is suspected.
- *Ascending contrast venography* uses an injected contrast medium to assess the location and extent of venous thrombosis. Although invasive, expensive, and uncomfortable, contrast venography is the most accurate diagnostic tool for venous thrombosis. It is used when the results of less invasive tests leave the diagnosis unclear (University of Rochester Medical Center, 2016).

Pharmacologic Therapy

Anticoagulants that prevent clot propagation and enable the body's own lytic system to dissolve clots are the mainstay of treatment for venous thrombosis. Thrombolytic drugs such as streptokinase or tissue plasminogen activator (tPA) may accelerate the process of clot lysis and prevent damage to venous valves. Thrombolytic therapy may be recommended to dissolve a blood clot. This therapy is most likely to be used in patients who have serious complications related to DVT and who have low risk of serious bleeding. Thrombolytic outcomes are best in cases with a short time frame between diagnosis and start of therapy.

NSAIDs such as indomethacin (Indocin) or naproxen (Naprosyn) may be ordered to reduce inflammation in the veins and provide symptomatic relief, particularly for patients with superficial venous thrombosis.

Anticoagulants

Anticoagulants are given to prevent clot extension and reduce the risk of subsequent PE. These drugs act by inhibiting the action of one or more clotting factors, thereby disrupting the coagulation cascade, prolonging bleeding time, and stopping clots from forming and/or growing larger. Major categories of anticoagulant medications include heparin, warfarin, LMWHs, direct thrombin inhibitors, and Factor Xa inhibitors (Adams, Holland, & Urban, 2017). Each type of anticoagulant is described in greater detail in the Medications feature, as well as in the following sections.

Heparin and Warfarin

For most patients with DVT, anticoagulation is initiated with unfractionated heparin, although LMWHs may also be used. Following an initial IV bolus of unfractionated heparin, additional units are infused over a 24-hour period. The dosage is calculated to maintain the aPTT at approximately twice the control or normal value. An infusion pump is used to deliver the prescribed dosage. Frequent monitoring of the infusion is an important nursing responsibility. Subcutaneous heparin injections may be used as an alternative to IV infusion in some instances.

Oral anticoagulation with warfarin may be initiated concurrently with heparin therapy. Overlapping heparin and warfarin therapy for 4–5 days is important because the full anticoagulant effect of warfarin is delayed. Warfarin

doses are adjusted to maintain an INR greater than 2.0 (Medscape, 2015).

Once this level has been achieved, the heparin is discontinued, and a maintenance dose of warfarin is prescribed to prevent recurrent thrombosis. Anticoagulation generally is continued for at least 3 months. When DVT recurs or risk factors such as altered coagulability or cancer are present, anticoagulant therapy may be prolonged. Regular follow-up is necessary to be sure INR remains within the desirable range for anticoagulation.

Low-Molecular-Weight Heparins

LMWHs are increasingly used to prevent and treat venous thrombosis. These medications are more effective and carry lower risks for bleeding and thrombocytopenia than conventional unfractionated heparins. In addition, they do not require the close laboratory monitoring of unfractionated heparins. LMWHs are administered subcutaneously in fixed doses once or twice daily, which makes them appropriate for both inpatient and outpatient treatment. See the Focus on Diversity and Culture feature for information about potential patient concerns regarding heparin and LMWHs.

SAFETY ALERT Some foods and supplements can increase the risk of a bleeding episode for patients on anticoagulant therapy. Patients should avoid ginger, garlic, green tea, and ginkgo while taking heparin or warfarin.

Direct Thrombin Inhibitors

Direct thrombin inhibitors are advantageous in that they inactivate both free and bound thrombin. However, the FDA currently limits use of these drugs to a few specific situations. In particular, bivalirudin and argatroban are given to patients undergoing percutaneous coronary intervention, as well as patients at risk for thrombocytopenia related to heparin therapy; desirudin is used to prevent DVT in patients undergoing hip replacement surgery; and dabigatran is given to patients with atrial fibrillation and/or patients who have received parenteral anticoagulants for 5–10 days (Adams et al., 2017).

Factor Xa Inhibitors

Factor Xa inhibitors are a newer category of anticoagulants. Whereas heparin and LMWHs indirectly inhibit Factor Xa, these medications disrupt the coagulation cascade by directly impairing the function of Factor Xa. Factor Xa inhibitors may be used on an outpatient basis to prevent and treat DVT, as well as to reduce the risk of clots and stroke in patients with atrial fibrillation.

Factor Xa inhibitors are as effective as warfarin yet offer several advantages over older anticoagulants. For example, they are administered by mouth, present a lower risk of interaction with food or other drugs, and do not necessitate frequent INR monitoring. Factor Xa inhibitors are not risk-free, however. Rapid discontinuation without substitution of another anticoagulant may lead to serious ischemic events. Also, these drugs should not be used in patients who are undergoing neuraxial anesthesia or spinal puncture, because they increase the risk of long-term paralysis due to epidural or spinal hematoma (Adams et al., 2017).

Medications

Anticoagulants

CLASSIFICATION AND DRUG EXAMPLES	MECHANISMS OF ACTION	NURSING CONSIDERATIONS
Heparin	Heparin disrupts the clotting cascade by enhancing the action of antithrombin III, a normally occurring plasma protein that inhibits the effects of thrombin. Inhibited thrombin function prevents the conversion of fibrinogen to fibrin, thus interfering with formation of a stable fibrin clot. At therapeutic levels, heparin prolongs the thrombin time, clotting time, and aPTT. When given intravenously, its effect is immediate. Given subcutaneously, its onset of action is within 1 hour. Heparin has a short biological half-life and should be given frequently or via continuous infusion. *Heparin-induced thrombocytopenia (HIT)* is a potential complication of therapy with unfractionated heparin.	■ Assess for history of unexplained or active bleeding. Assess laboratory results for abnormal clotting profile or evidence of active bleeding. ■ Give a test dose as indicated to patients with a history of multiple allergies and/or asthma. ■ Administer by deep subcutaneous injection; abdominal sites are preferred. Avoid injecting within 2 in. of the umbilicus. Rotate sites. Do not aspirate prior to injecting or massage after the injection. ■ IV solutions may be diluted with dextrose, normal saline, or Ringer's solution. Use an infusion pump. ■ Keep protamine sulfate, a heparin antagonist, available to treat excessive bleeding. ■ Monitor and report abnormal laboratory results and aPTT values outside the desired range. ■ Promptly report evidence of bleeding, such as hematemesis, hematuria, bleeding gums, or unexplained abdominal or back pain. Health Education for the Patient and Family ■ Report unusual bleeding or excessive menstrual flow. ■ Use an electric razor and a soft-bristle toothbrush; prevent injury by clearing pathways, using a night-light, and other measures. Do not consume alcohol. ■ Avoid contact sports while on anticoagulant therapy. ■ Do not consume large amounts of food rich in vitamin K (yellow and dark green vegetables). ■ Do not use aspirin or NSAIDs while on heparin therapy unless advised to do so by your healthcare provider. ■ Wear a medical alert tag, and advise all healthcare providers (including dentists and podiatrists) of therapy.
Warfarin (Coumadin)	Warfarin interferes with synthesis of vitamin K–dependent clotting factors by the liver (specifically, Factors II, VII, IX, and X), leading to depletion of these factors. Warfarin has no effect on already circulating clotting factors or on existing clots. Rather, it inhibits extension of existing thrombi and formation of new clots. Its action is cumulative and more prolonged than that of heparin.	■ Assess laboratory results and history for evidence of abnormal bleeding. ■ Multiple drugs affect the metabolism and protein binding of warfarin; note all medications, and assess for interactions with warfarin. ■ Do not give during pregnancy because warfarin may cause congenital malformations. ■ Oral tablets may be crushed and given without regard to meals. ■ Dilute IV warfarin with supplied diluent; administer within 4 hours by direct IV injection at a rate of 25 mg/min. ■ Keep vitamin K available to reverse effects of warfarin in the event of excessive bleeding or hemorrhage. ■ Monitor PT or INR; report values outside the desired range. Health Education for the Patient and Family ■ If bleeding occurs (e.g., hematemesis, bright red or black tarry feces, hematuria, bleeding gums, excessive bruising), do not take the prescribed dose, and notify the healthcare provider immediately. Report rash or manifestations of hepatitis (dark urine, malaise, yellow skin or sclera). ■ Take warfarin at the same time every day; do not change brands, because their effects may differ. ■ Menstrual bleeding may be slightly increased; contact the healthcare provider if it increases significantly. Use reliable birth control to prevent pregnancy while taking warfarin. Immediately contact the healthcare provider if you think you may be pregnant.

(continued on next page)

Medications *(continued)*

CLASSIFICATION AND DRUG EXAMPLES	MECHANISMS OF ACTION	NURSING CONSIDERATIONS
		▪ Take precautions to prevent injury and bleeding: Use a soft-bristle toothbrush and electric razor, wear shoes, and use a night-light. Avoid participating in contact sports.
		▪ Do not smoke, use alcohol, or take over-the-counter drugs unless specifically recommended by the healthcare provider. Notify all healthcare providers, including dentists and podiatrists, of therapy. Wear a medical alert tag.
		▪ Obtain lab tests as scheduled, and keep all scheduled follow-up appointments.
Low-Molecular-Weight Heparins (LMWHs) **Drug examples:** Dalteparin (Fragmin) Enoxaparin (Lovenox) Tinzaparin (Innohep)	LMWHs are the most bioavailable fraction of heparin. They provide a more precise and predictable anticoagulant effect than unfractionated heparin because they act primarily by inhibiting active Factor X. Like unfractionated heparin, LMWHs prevent conversion of prothrombin to thrombin, liberation of thromboplastin from platelets, and formation of a stable clot. LMWHs cannot be used interchangeably with each other or with unfractionated heparin. Although the risk of HIT is significantly lower with LMWHs, patients who were previously treated with unfractionated heparin may develop HIT when treated with LMWHs.	▪ Assess for evidence of active bleeding; a history of bleeding disorders or thrombocytopenia; or sensitivity to heparin, sulfites, or pork products. ▪ Monitor for unusual or masked bleeding. PT and aPTT levels may be within normal levels even in the presence of hemorrhage. ▪ Administer by deep subcutaneous injection into abdominal wall, thigh, or buttocks. Rotate sites. Do not aspirate or massage. Health Education for the Patient and Family ▪ Pay close attention to subcutaneous self-administration technique, timing of doses, and site rotation. Do not rub site after administering to minimize bruising. ▪ Do not take aspirin, NSAIDs, or other over-the-counter drugs unless recommended by your healthcare provider. ▪ Promptly report excessive bruising or bleeding, chest pain, difficulty breathing, itching, rash, or swelling to your healthcare provider. ▪ Keep follow-up appointments as scheduled.
Direct Thrombin Inhibitors **Drug examples:** Argatroban (Acova, Novastan) Bivalirudin (Angiomax) Dabigatran (Pradaxa) Desirudin (Iprivask)	Direct thrombin inhibitors bind with thrombin's active site, inactivating the thrombin and preventing formation of fibrin clots. They act on both circulating thrombin and thrombin that is attached to clots. Patients typically receive these drugs until they obtain an appropriate aPTT value. Use of direct thrombin inhibitors is limited to a few specific situations. Dabigatran is the only oral medication in this class.	▪ Assess for evidence of active bleeding or history of bleeding disorders. ▪ Obtain baseline aPTT prior to starting drug therapy. ▪ Patients with moderate kidney disease may require adjusted dosing. Patients with severe kidney disease should not receive these medications. ▪ Monitor patients for excessive or unusual bleeding. ▪ Note that bivalirudin and argatroban are meant to be administered in conjunction with aspirin therapy. Health Education for the Patient and Family ▪ Promptly report excessive bruising or bleeding, chest pain, or difficulty breathing to your healthcare provider. ▪ Take dabigatran with food to reduce risk of gastrointestinal side effects, including diarrhea, nausea, vomiting, and gastrointestinal bleeding.
Factor Xa Inhibitors **Drug examples:** Apixaban (Eliquis) Edoxaban (Savaysa) Rivaroxaban (Xarelto)	Unlike older classes of anticoagulants, Factor Xa inhibitors work by directly impairing the function of Factor Xa in the coagulation cascade. Factor Xa inhibitors are administered by the oral route. They are used to prevent and treat DVT and to reduce the risk of clots and stroke in patients with atrial fibrillation. These medications work as well as warfarin but with lower risk of drug interactions and no need for frequent INR monitoring.	▪ Assess for evidence of active bleeding or history of bleeding disorders. ▪ Monitor patients for excessive or unusual bleeding. ▪ Do not rapidly discontinue these drugs unless another anticoagulant has been substituted, or serious ischemic events may result. ▪ Do not use in patients undergoing neuraxial anesthesia or spinal puncture because there is a risk of epidural or spinal hematoma, which may result in long-term paralysis. ▪ Specific antidotes to these drugs are not yet available. Health Education for the Patient and Family ▪ Promptly report excessive bruising or bleeding to your healthcare provider. ▪ Take all doses exactly as prescribed. ▪ Do not discontinue these medications without healthcare provider notification and close supervision.

Focus on Diversity and Culture
Pork-Derived Heparin

Heparin is the drug of choice for initiating anticoagulant therapy. It has been used as an anticoagulant since the 1930s and is one of the oldest drugs still in use. In the United States, heparin is derived from material extracted from the intestinal mucosa of pigs. Other countries may use material extracted from the lung or intestine of cows, sheep, turkeys, or other meat animals (Science Board to the Food and Drug Administration, 2014).

When administering heparin, the nurse should be aware of any restrictions patients may have related to pork products. Some religions forbid the use or consumption of pork, and administering heparin to these patients may violate their beliefs. The prohibition on pork primarily affects Muslim patients, but it may also have an impact on Hindu or Jewish patients (Queensland Department of Health, 2013). In addition, patients who are vegetarian or vegan may also be opposed to the use of heparin.

For some adherents of faiths with a pork prohibition, medical use of porcine-derived products is a gray area. For example, while many Muslim patients are forbidden to consume pork under normal circumstances, some make exceptions in emergency situations or cases of extreme necessity. For these individuals, if no suitable, equally effective alternative is available, use of porcine heparin may be permissible (Zarif, Murad, & Yusof, 2013). IV or subcutaneous administration of pork-derived medications may also be acceptable to some groups, as may be medicines with a chemically modified pork component. The nurse should encourage patients who are in doubt about the acceptability of heparin to speak with their religious leader.

Chemically derived alternatives to heparin do exist, but sufficient research about their effectiveness has yet to be completed (Szummer et al., 2015). If these drugs are available, the nurse should present them as an alternative to heparin and explain the differences and potential risks. The nurse should also secure informed consent from patients with potential objections to heparin prior to administration (Sadat-Ali & Al-Turki, 2013).

The U.S. Food and Drug Administration (FDA) is considering reintroducing bovine heparin into the United States after having removed it in the 1990s over concerns about bovine spongiform encephalopathy (commonly called mad-cow disease) (Science Board to the Food and Drug Administration, 2014). If these medications become available, they may represent an acceptable alternative for some patients.

Surgery

DVT is typically treated with conservative measures and anticoagulation. In some cases, however, surgery is required to remove the thrombus, prevent its extension into deep veins, or prevent the effects of embolization.

Venous thrombectomy is done when thrombi lodge in the femoral vein and their removal is necessary to prevent PE or gangrene. Successful thrombus removal rapidly improves venous circulation. The duration of this effect varies from patient to patient.

When DVT is recurrent and anticoagulant therapy is contraindicated, a filter may be inserted into the vena cava to capture emboli from the pelvis and lower extremities, preventing PE. Several different filters are available (see **Figure 16–36** »). The Greenfield filter is widely used for its ability to trap emboli within its apex while maintaining patency of the vena cava. The filter can be inserted under fluoroscopy with local anesthesia. Mortality and morbidity associated with the filter are very low.

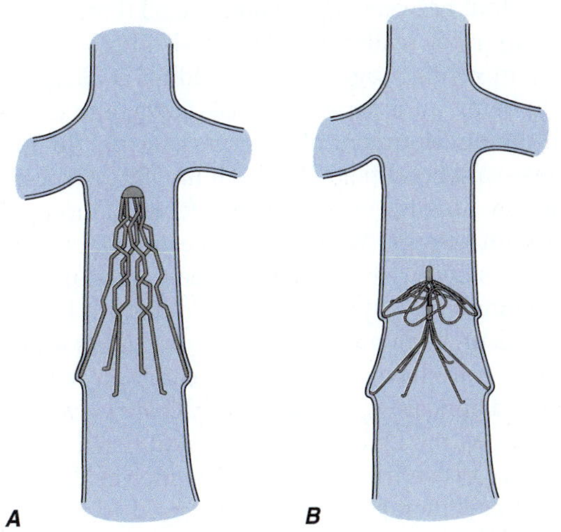

Superficial thrombophlebitis of the great saphenous vein can progress to DVT. It may be treated by ligating and dividing the vein where it joins the femoral vein to prevent clot extension into the deep venous system. Superficial thrombophlebitis that involves infection can lead to septic venous thrombosis. When this occurs, the affected vein is excised to control infection. Antibiotic therapy is also initiated (Rosh & Khait, 2015).

Nonpharmacologic Therapy

Treatment of venous thrombosis also includes measures to relieve symptoms and reduce inflammation. With superficial venous thrombosis, applying warm, moist compresses over the affected vein, resting the extremity, and using anti-inflammatory agents typically provide relief of symptoms.

Bedrest may be ordered for patients with DVT. The duration of bedrest typically is determined by the extent of leg edema. The legs are elevated 15–20 degrees, with the knees slightly flexed, above the level of the heart to promote venous return and discourage venous pooling. When permitted, walking is encouraged, as is avoiding prolonged standing or sitting. Crossing the legs also is avoided, as are tight-fitting garments or stockings that bind.

SAFETY ALERT Elastic antiembolism stockings or pneumatic compression devices are contraindicated in patients with known DVT, but they are frequently ordered by physicians for use in the prevention of DVTs. These devices stimulate the muscle-pumping mechanism that promotes the return of blood to the heart; therefore, they may dislodge a thrombus and cause PE.

A   *B*

Figure 16–36 » Venal caval filters. **A,** Greenfield filter. **B,** Nitinol filter.

Lifespan Considerations

DVT can occur in patients of all ages, and some factors associated with this condition are common across age groups. These include immobility, trauma, surgery, and cancer. In addition, patients of all ages with more than one co-occurring risk factor are increasingly likely to develop a DVT. Certain populations are more likely to develop DVT than others, and diagnosis and treatment methods may be different for patients in different groups.

DVT in Infants and Children

DVT is rare in children, with a 0.05% incidence (Aabideen et al., 2013). Prematurity and sepsis predispose newborns to DVT. Risk factors for older infants and children include congenital heart disease, cardiac catheterization, and nephrotic syndrome. DVT is often asymptomatic in children; when symptoms occur, they are nonspecific and include acute pain and swelling of the extremities. Initial treatment typically includes unfractionated or LMWH; over time, the patient is transitioned to oral warfarin (Howard, 2015).

DVT in Adolescents and Young Adults

Risk for DVT in adolescents and young adults is 8 times greater than in infants and young children, although the risk for this group is still lower than that of the general population (Johns Hopkins, 2013). During adolescence and young adulthood, thrombosis is twice as likely to occur in female patients as in male patients, whereas in the general population male patients have a slightly higher risk (Indiana Hemophilia & Thrombosis Center [IHTC], 2012; Patel & Chun, 2015). One factor that places young women at increased risk is use of contraceptives containing estrogen and progestin, often called combined hormonal contraception. Use of combined oral contraception (birth control pills) increases the risk of thrombosis 3–4 times, although other combined contraceptive methods can increase risk as well. Women with clotting disorders or a history of thrombosis who use combined hormonal contraception are at greatest risk of developing DVT. Progestin-only contraceptive methods and nonhormonal methods do not appear to increase risk of thrombosis (James, n.d.).

Symptoms of DVT in adolescents and young adults include swelling, pain, warmth, and tenderness of the extremity. Diagnosis and treatment methods are similar to those for other populations and typically include anticoagulant therapy. Young women on anticoagulant therapy may experience heavy menstrual bleeding. When this occurs, patients should continue with therapy and receive counseling about managing menstrual flow (James, n.d.). Sexually active young women taking warfarin should use birth control because of the teratogenic effects of the drug, but it is important that these patients avoid combined hormonal contraceptives (Howard, 2015).

DVT in Pregnant Women

During pregnancy and the first few weeks of the postnatal period, a woman's risk of DVT and PE are 4–5 times higher than that of a woman of the same age who is not pregnant. Inherited clotting disorders further increase this risk (Mayo Clinic, 2014f; Springel & Peng, 2014), as do pregnancy-related changes to the body. Blood volume and pressure in the leg veins and pelvis are increased during pregnancy. Hormonal changes also increase the stress on blood vessels and may increase clotting factors in the blood (James, n.d.). Venous stasis is typically increased in the lower body, and mobility may be somewhat decreased. Risk of developing DVT during pregnancy is greatest before 20 weeks of gestation, peaking at 11–15 weeks. Evidence also suggests that risk of thrombosis is greater during the postpartum period than during pregnancy (Springel & Peng, 2014). Depending upon a patient's health history, DVT prophylaxis may be indicated.

DVT during pregnancy is more likely to occur in the left leg than the right leg; this is believed to be due to compression of the left iliac vein by the right iliac artery. In addition, 12% of DVT in pregnancy occurs in the pelvic veins, while pelvic vein DVT is seen in only 1% of the general population (Springel & Peng, 2014). The symptoms of DVT during pregnancy are similar to those of pregnancy in general and include pain and swelling of the legs, dyspnea, tachycardia, and tachypnea. Diagnosis of DVT in pregnancy relies heavily on the D-dimer test and ultrasonography. When pelvic DVT is suspected, MRI may also be used.

Heparin is the preferred anticoagulant in pregnant women because it does not cross the placenta. Warfarin can cross the placenta and has teratogenic effects on the fetus. Patients should be monitored for progressive VTE and heparin allergies for the duration of anticoagulant therapy. Anticoagulant therapy does not increase the risk of delivery bleeding, but it may be temporarily discontinued if the patient needs regional anesthesia. In patients with planned deliveries, therapy may be discontinued or altered several days prior to delivery. Therapy is typically restarted within several hours after delivery. Patients may also be gradually transitioned from heparin to warfarin during the postpartum period. Both heparin and warfarin are considered safe for lactating mothers (Springel & Peng, 2014).

DVT in Older Adults

Age is a risk factor for DVT, and the risk for thrombosis increases 30-fold between age 30 and age 80 (Patel & Chun, 2015). Fatality rates related to VTE are also higher in older adults than in younger age groups (Geldhof et al., 2014). In addition to being an independent risk factor, age is associated with the development of other risk factors, including venous stasis and conditions that limit mobility. Cancer and cancer therapy are also important risk factors among older adults. As with younger women, use of estrogen-containing drugs increases DVT risk in older women (James, n.d.).

DVT is commonly asymptomatic in older adults. When symptoms occur, they are nonspecific. A patient's known comorbidities may have symptoms in common with DVT, complicating diagnosis. Age-related body changes can lead to false positives on the D-dimer test, and additional testing is often necessary to confirm diagnosis (Schouten et al., 2012).

Anticoagulant therapy is commonly used to treat older adults with DVT, but older adults are at higher risk of bleeding complications (Geldhof et al., 2014). Multiple comorbidities, decreased kidney function, decreased body weight, dementia, and increased risk of falls complicate the use of anticoagulant therapy in older adults (Thaler, Pabinger, & Ay, 2015). Most drugs are administered in a similar fashion and at comparable doses in older and younger patients, but monitoring may occur more frequently in older adults.

The use of anticoagulant prophylaxis in older adults is typically based on the co-occurrence of multiple risk factors. This is of special concern to patients with chronic immobility living in long-term care settings, because age and immobility alone are not typically considered sufficient risk factors to justify prophylaxis (Robinson, 2013).

NURSING PROCESS

Prevention of venous thrombosis is an important component of nursing care for all at-risk patients. To promote venous blood flow from the lower extremities, the nurse should position patients with the feet elevated and the knees slightly bent. Avoid placing pillows under the knees and positioning patients with hips and knees sharply flexed. Use a recliner chair or footstool when patients are sitting. Ambulate patients as soon as possible, and maintain a regular schedule of ambulation throughout the day. Teach ankle flexion and extension exercises, and frequently remind patients to perform these exercises. Apply compression stockings and pneumatic compression devices when appropriate. Instruct patients to avoid crossing their legs when in bed or sitting. Inquire about possible prophylactic heparin or warfarin therapy for patients undergoing orthopedic surgery or other high-risk procedures. Frequently assess IV sites. Change the site and catheter as dictated by agency protocol and if evidence of local inflammation is noted.

Assessment

The nurse should assess patients at risk for venous thrombosis for manifestations and risk factors and obtain objective and subjective data:

- **Observation and patient interview.** Review personal and family history of DVT, PE, and clotting disorders. Discuss any recent surgical procedures or traumatic injuries. Note complaints of leg or calf pain, duration and characteristics of pain, and the effect of the pain on the patient's ability to walk. Review current medications. Discuss exercise and regular physical activities. Observe for shortness of breath, cough, or chest pain, as these may be signs that an embolus has moved to the lungs.

- **Physical examination.** Assess vital signs, including temperature. Examine the affected extremity for redness and warmth. Assess for tenderness, particularly in the calf and the medial thigh. Palpate the extremity, and note any cordlike structures. Note the presence of edema and whether it is unilateral or bilateral. Measure the diameter of the affected extremity.

Diagnosis

Nursing diagnoses that apply to the patient with DVT include the following:

- *Pain, Acute*
- *Protection, Ineffective*
- *Physical Mobility, Impaired*
- *Ineffective Peripheral Tissue Perfusion, Risk for.*

(NANDA-I © 2014)

Planning

Goals of nursing care may include the following:

- The patient will experience pain control sufficient to allow rest and comfort.
- The patient will not experience complications resulting from embolization of the thrombus.
- The patient will have adequate tissue perfusion to prevent cellular damage.

Implementation

In addition to preventive measures, priority nursing diagnoses for the patient with venous thrombosis relate to managing pain, maintaining tissue perfusion and integrity, and addressing potential adverse effects of prescribed treatments.

Manage Pain

The pain associated with venous thrombosis results from inflammation of the involved vein. It may be aggravated by use of the involved extremity. Edema and swelling may contribute to discomfort. Measures to reduce the inflammation often help relieve the pain. The nurse should do the following:

- Regularly assess pain location, characteristics, and level using a standardized pain scale. Report increasing pain or changes in pain location or characteristics. Tissue substances released during the inflammatory process can stimulate pain receptors. In addition, localized swelling presses on pain-sensitive structures in the area of the inflammation, contributing to discomfort. As inflammation and swelling are reduced, pain should abate. Continued or increasing pain may indicate extension of the thrombosis. Sudden chest pain may indicate a PE, necessitating immediate intervention.

- Measure calf and thigh diameter of the affected extremity on admission and daily thereafter. Report increases promptly. The inflammatory process causes vasodilation and increases vessel permeability, in turn causing edema of the affected extremity. Baseline and subsequent measurements provide a measure of treatment effectiveness.

- Apply warm, moist heat to the affected extremity at least four times daily using compresses or an aqua-K pad. Moist heat penetrates tissues to a greater depth. Warmth promotes vasodilation, allowing reabsorption of excess fluid into the circulation. Vasodilation also reduces resistance within the affected vessel, reducing pain. As edema subsides, pressure on the surrounding tissues is relieved, thereby reducing pain.

- Maintain bedrest as ordered. Using leg muscles during walking exacerbates the inflammatory process and increases edema. This, in turn, increases venous compression and pain.

Promote Effective Peripheral Perfusion

As thrombi develop, they occlude the lumen of the vein and obstruct blood flow. In addition, the accompanying inflammatory response may precipitate vessel spasms, further impairing arterial and venous blood flow as well as tissue perfusion. Impaired tissue perfusion in turn deprives tissues of nutrients and oxygen. As a result, distal tissues of the affected extremity are at risk for ulceration and infection. Nursing interventions include the following:

■ Assess the skin of the affected lower leg and foot at least every 8 hours, or more often as indicated. Frequent assessment is important to detect early signs of tissue breakdown and implement measures to protect vulnerable tissues. Early intervention allows healing and restoration of tissue integrity; if allowed to continue, the process can lead to necrosis and potential gangrene.

■ Elevate the patient's extremities at all times, keeping knees slightly flexed and legs above the level of the heart. Elevation of the extremities promotes venous return and reduces peripheral edema. Knee flexion promotes muscle relaxation.

■ Use mild soaps, solutions, and lotions to clean the affected leg and foot daily. Pat dry after washing, and apply a non–alcohol-based lotion or moisturizing cream. Daily hygiene with nondrying soaps and solutions removes potential pathogens from the skin surface, maintains skin integrity, and is the first line of defense against infection. Caustic or harsh soaps or solutions can dry and crack the skin, increasing the risk for infection.

■ Use an egg-crate mattress or sheepskin on the bed as needed. Egg-crate mattresses and sheepskins distribute weight more evenly, preventing excess pressure on affected tissues.

■ Encourage frequent position changes (at least every 2 hours) while awake. Frequent position changes reduce pressure on bony prominences and edematous tissue, reducing the risk of tissue breakdown.

Reduce Risk for Injury

Anticoagulant therapy interferes with the body's normal clotting mechanisms, increasing the risk for bleeding and hemorrhage. Interventions to reduce the patient's risk for adverse effects from anticoagulant therapy include the following:

■ Monitor laboratory results, including the INR, aPTT, hemoglobin, and hematocrit as indicated.

■ Report values outside the normal or desired range. Coagulation studies are used to monitor the effect of anticoagulant medications. Values within the desired range prevent further clot development while carrying a low risk for bleeding and hemorrhage. A fall in the hemoglobin and hematocrit may indicate undetected bleeding.

Encourage Mobility

Prolonged bedrest rarely is required, and it is associated with many problems, including constipation, joint contractures, muscle atrophy, and boredom. Nursing care goals include maintaining joint ROM, minimizing muscle atrophy, and reducing boredom. Interventions appropriate to assist patients in meeting these goals include the following:

■ Encourage active ROM (performed by the patient) exercises at least every 8 hours (see Patient Teaching feature in Exemplar 16.M on Stroke). Provide passive ROM (performed by the nurse) as needed. ROM exercises maintain joint mobility and prevent contractures. Active ROM also helps prevent muscle atrophy and preserve function. While passive ROM exercises do not prevent muscle atrophy, they do maintain joint mobility.

■ Encourage frequent position changes, deep breathing, and coughing. Prolonged immobility can lead to impaired airway clearance and respiratory complications, such as atelectasis or pneumonia. Turning, coughing, and deep breathing facilitate expulsion of secretions from the respiratory tract, airway clearance, and alveolar ventilation.

■ Encourage increased fluid and dietary fiber intake. Constipation is a frequent complication of immobility that results from decreased gastrointestinal motility and loss of abdominal muscle strength. Increasing fluid and fiber intake helps maintain soft, easily expelled stools.

■ Assist the patient with and encourage ambulation as allowed. Ambulation promotes venous blood flow, helps maintain muscle tone and joint mobility, and increases sense of well-being.

■ Encourage diversional activities, such as reading, television or video games, and socializing. Boredom may lead to dozing and inertia, with little physical movement or mental stimulation, increasing the risk for complications of immobility.

Promote Effective Cardiopulmonary Perfusion

A thrombus that forms in the deep veins of the legs or pelvis may break loose or fragment, becoming an embolism. Emboli that originate in the venous system usually become trapped in the pulmonary circulation (i.e., PE). Gas exchange in the affected area is impaired as blood flow ceases or is reduced to an area of the lungs that is well ventilated. Interventions to promote effective gas exchange include the following:

■ Frequently assess the patient's respiratory status, including rate, depth, ease, and oxygen saturation levels. A mismatch of ventilation and perfusion can significantly affect gas exchange, leading to rapid and shallow respirations, dyspnea and air hunger, and a fall in oxygen saturation levels.

■ Initiate oxygen therapy, elevate the head of the bed, and reassure the patient who is experiencing manifestations of PE. Oxygen therapy and elevating the head of the bed promote ventilation and gas exchange in those alveoli that are well perfused, helping maintain tissue oxygenation. Reassurance helps reduce anxiety and slow the respiratory rate, promoting greater respiratory depth and alveolar ventilation.

Patient Teaching
Home Care for DVT

Treatment measures for DVT may be initiated and carried out on an outpatient basis or continued for an extended period of time following hospital discharge. The nurse should include the following topics when teaching for home care:

- Explanation of the disease process
- Treatment measures, including laboratory tests and their purposes as well as medications and adverse effects that should be reported
- Appropriate methods of heat application
- Prescribed activity restrictions
- Measures to prevent future episodes of DVT
- The importance of follow-up visits and laboratory tests as scheduled.

The nurse should refer patients to community nursing services for continued assessment and reinforcement of teaching. The nurse can also provide referrals for assistance with ADLs and home maintenance services as indicated. The nurse should consider referral for physical therapy if needed.

SAFETY ALERT Sudden increases in heart rate, stabbing chest pain, shortness of breath, and bloody cough may indicate that a DVT has moved through the bloodstream to the lungs, causing a PE. Patients with a PE may require emergency care.

Evaluation

Patient outcomes are evaluated based on their progress in meeting established goals and may include the following:

- The patient identifies warning signs of DVT.
- The patient vocalizes the risks associated with decreased mobility.
- The patient maintains an anticoagulant therapy regimen without complications.
- The patient and nurse collaborate with the interprofessional team to identify DVT recurrence strategies.
- The patient is free of long-term complications.

If patient outcomes are not met, recurrent DVT or other complications may develop. Depending upon the extent and severity of complications, the patient may require hospitalization and surgical intervention.

Nursing Care Plan
A Patient with DVT

Mrs. Opal Hipps, age 75, lives alone with her dog, Sunny, in her family home in the suburbs. Mrs. Hipps retired from her job as a postal clerk 10 years ago and now spends a lot of time reading and watching television. During the past week, she has developed a vague, aching pain in her right leg. She ignored the pain until last night, when it developed into a much more severe pain in her right calf. She noticed that her right lower leg seemed larger than the left, and it was very tender to the touch. After seeing her healthcare provider and undergoing Doppler ultrasound studies, Mrs. Hipps is admitted to the hospital with the diagnosis of DVT in the right leg. She is placed on bedrest and IV heparin. You are assigned to admit and care for Mrs. Hipps.

ASSESSMENT	DIAGNOSES	PLANNING
You notice that Mrs. Hipps was admitted 14 months ago for repair of a fractured femur. Mrs. Hipps says, "This business about a blood clot really has me worried." She also tells you that she is worried about who will care for her dog while she is in the hospital. Physical findings include the following: height, 157 cm (62 in.); weight, 68 kg (149 lb); temperature, 37.3°C (99.2°F); vital signs within normal limits otherwise. Her left leg is warm and pink, with strong peripheral pulses and good capillary refill. Her right calf is dark red, very warm, and dry to the touch. It is tender to palpation. The right femoral and popliteal pulses are strong, but the pedal and posterior tibial pulses are difficult to locate. The right calf diameter is 1.27 cm (0.5 in.) larger than the left.	• *Acute Pain* related to inflammatory response in the affected vein • *Anxiety* related to unexpected hospitalization and uncertainty about the seriousness of her illness • *Ineffective Peripheral Tissue Perfusion* related to decreased venous circulation in the right leg • *Risk for Impaired Skin Integrity* related to pooling of venous blood in the right leg (NANDA-I © 2014)	Goals of care include the following: • The patient will verbalize relief of right leg pain by the day of discharge. • The patient will verbalize reduced anxiety by the second day of hospitalization. • The patient will demonstrate reduction in right leg diameter by 0.25 in. (0.64 cm) by the fifth day of hospitalization.

IMPLEMENTATION

- Elevate legs, maintaining slight knee flexion, while in bed.
- Apply warm, moist compresses to right leg using a 2-hours-on, 2-hours-off schedule around the clock.
- Administer prescribed analgesics and evaluate their effectiveness.
- Spend time with Mrs. Hipps to explain venous thrombosis and its treatment.
- Arrange for a friend or neighbor to care for Mrs. Hipps' dog.
- Monitor laboratory values to assess effect of anticoagulant therapy; report values outside the desired range.
- Assist with progressive ambulation when allowed.
- Inspect legs and feet, and record findings every 8 hours.

(continued on next page)

Nursing Care Plan *(continued)*

EVALUATION

Seven days after admission, the pain in Mrs. Hipps's right leg has subsided and the diameter of her right calf is equal to that of her left calf. Mrs. Hipps admits that her fears relate to a cousin who was hospitalized for a similar problem and had his leg amputated. After you talk with her about her condition and the steps she can take to prevent its recurrence, Mrs. Hipps is much less anxious. Before discharge, you review instructions for antiembolism stockings, daily walking, warfarin schedule, and scheduled follow-up appointment. Mrs. Hipps' neighbor, Kate Kent, comes to pick her up. As you are helping Mrs. Hipps into the car, Ms. Kent hands her a small brown dog and says, "I took good care of Sunny for you, but he's missed you." Mrs. Hipps smiles, and assures you that she will call the number you provided if she has any questions.

CRITICAL THINKING

1. Describe the pathophysiologic reasons for the pain in Mrs. Hipps' right leg.

2. How would you respond if Mrs. Hipps tells you she does not have the money to buy the prescribed anticoagulant when she goes home?

3. How would you change your teaching and discharge planning if Mrs. Hipps had difficulty caring for herself?

4. Design a plan of care for Mrs. Hipps for the nursing diagnosis of *Activity Intolerance*.

REVIEW Deep Venous Thrombosis

RELATE Link the Concepts and Exemplars

Linking the exemplar of DVT with the concept of mobility:

1. What strategies can you implement to reduce the risk of DVT in the patient who is confined to bed?

2. Develop a teaching plan aimed at reducing the risk of DVT in an older patient who has limited mobility.

Linking the exemplar of DVT with the concept of reproduction:

3. Why is the pregnant patient at increased risk for DVT?

4. Explain the specific factors that increase the risk for DVT at each stage of pregnancy (prenatal, antenatal, and postpartum).

READY Go to Volume 3: Clinical Nursing Skills

REFER Go to Pearson MyLab Nursing and eText

- Additional review materials

REFLECT Apply Your Knowledge

Jennifer Walker, age 20, is a college student who is majoring in business. She lives with her boyfriend, Sam Hough, age 21, in an off-campus apartment. They enjoy walking around the campus with their dog, Shelby, and playing tennis and golf. Mr. Hough's parents are both physicians, and Ms. Walker's mother is a nurse.

At her examination several months ago, Ms. Walker obtained a prescription for oral contraceptives. She has been taking them daily. She recently began to notice pain in her left leg when she walks. She ignored it for several days, thinking she had just pulled a muscle while playing tennis, but the pain got worse. Today she is unable to put any pressure on the leg. She also notes a red area on the calf of her leg that is hot to the touch and very tender. She calls the campus clinic and makes an appointment to be seen today.

1. What factors in Ms. Walker's history put her at risk for developing a DVT?

2. What is your priority nursing diagnosis for Ms. Walker?

3. What teaching will you provide Ms. Walker during her visit to the campus clinic?

≫ Exemplar 16.E
Disseminated Intravascular Coagulation

Exemplar Learning Outcomes

16.E Analyze disseminated intravascular coagulation (DIC) as it relates to perfusion.

- Describe the pathophysiology of DIC.
- Describe the etiology of DIC.
- Compare the risk factors and prevention of DIC.
- Identify the clinical manifestations of DIC.
- Summarize diagnostic tests and therapies used by interprofessional teams in the collaborative care of an individual with DIC.

- Differentiate care of patients with DIC across the lifespan.
- Apply the nursing process in providing culturally competent care to an individual with DIC.

Exemplar Key Terms

Disseminated intravascular coagulation (DIC), *1223*
Fibrin degradation products, *1223*
Schistocytes, *1225*

Overview

Disseminated intravascular coagulation (DIC) is a disruption of hemostasis characterized by widespread intravascular clotting and bleeding. DIC may be acute and life-threatening, or it may be relatively mild.

Pathophysiology and Etiology

Pathophysiology

In DIC, a traumatic injury or causative agent activates the clotting cascade. Both the intrinsic and extrinsic cascades may be activated, with activation of the extrinsic cascade being more common. Cascade activation causes the proteins that control clotting to become overactive and causes small clots to form in blood vessels. These clots restrict blood flow to the brain, liver, or other organs (MedlinePlus, 2013). In time, widespread clotting in the microvasculature depletes clotting factors and activates anticoagulant production, causing hemorrhage (see **Figure 16–37** »). Thus, patients may experience both clotting and bleeding with DIC. Organ dysfunction may also result from damage to the microvasculature.

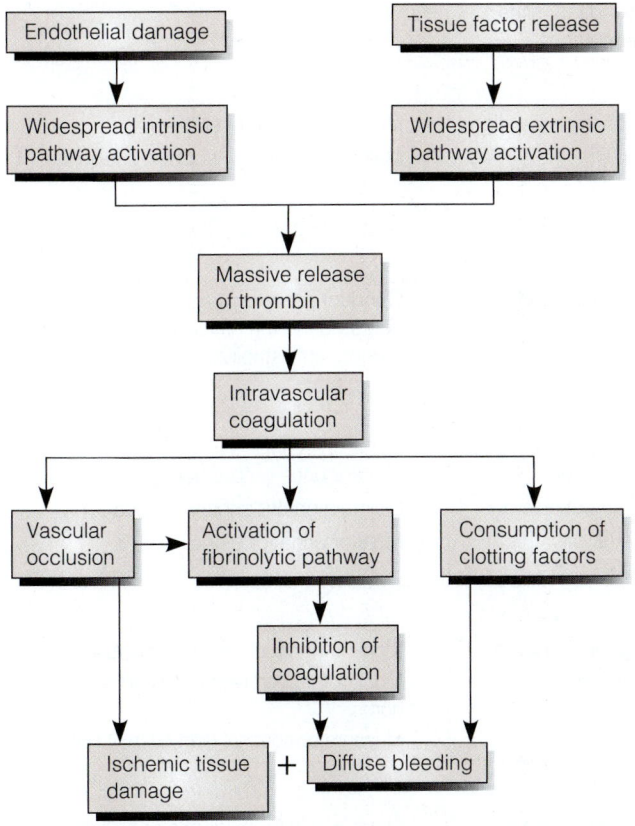

Figure 16–37 » Disseminated intravascular coagulation (DIC). Endothelial cell injury or release of TFs activates the intrinsic or extrinsic clotting pathway (or both). As a result, numerous microthrombi form throughout the vasculature, causing ischemic tissue damage. Simultaneously, rapid consumption of clotting factors and activation of fibrinolytic mechanisms trigger widespread bleeding.

The sequence of DIC is as follows:

1. Endothelial damage, TFs, or toxins stimulate the clotting cascade.
2. Excess thrombin within the circulation overwhelms naturally occurring anticoagulants.
3. Widespread clotting occurs within the microvasculature.
4. Thrombi and emboli impair tissue perfusion, leading to ischemia, infarction, and necrosis.
5. Clotting factors and platelets are consumed faster than they can be replaced.
6. Clotting activates fibrinolytic processes, which begin to break down clots.
7. **Fibrin degradation products** (potent anticoagulants) are released, contributing to bleeding.
8. Clotting factors are depleted, the ability to form clots is lost, and hemorrhage occurs.

Etiology

DIC is triggered by endothelial damage, release of tissue factors (TFs) into the circulation, or inappropriate activation of the clotting cascade by an endotoxin or products of microorganisms. Although DIC can occur as a complication of any condition that causes endothelial damage or the release of TFs, it most commonly presents in severe sepsis and septic shock. Gram-negative and gram-positive bacteria are most commonly associated with DIC, but viruses, fungi, and parasitic infections may also cause this condition (Levi & Schmaier, 2015).

It is estimated that DIC occurs in as many as 1% of all hospitalized patients (Levi & Schmaier, 2015). DIC is a complication or an effect of the progression of an illness, not a specific illness itself. It occurs secondary to an underlying condition and is typically associated with other clinical conditions (see **Box 16–13** »).

Risk Factors and Prevention

Risk factors for DIC include hemolytic reactions to blood transfusions, blood infections by bacteria or fungi, and

---

Box 16–13
Conditions That May Precipitate Disseminated Intravascular Coagulation

Tissue Damage
- Trauma: burns, gunshot wounds, frostbite, head injury
- Obstetric complications: septic abortion, abruptio placentae, amniotic fluid embolus, retained dead fetus
- Neoplasms: acute leukemia, adenocarcinomas
- Hemolysis
- Fat embolism

Vessel Damage
- Aortic aneurysm
- Acute glomerulonephritis
- Hemolytic uremic syndrome

Infections
- Bacterial infection or sepsis
- Viral or mycotic infections
- Malaria

improperly formed blood vessels (large hemangioma). Certain types of leukemia, pancreatitis, and liver diseases are also risk factors. Recent surgery or anesthesia and severe tissue damage such as burns or head injuries also increase the risk of developing DIC. Pregnancy complications are a risk factor as well; these will be discussed further in the Lifespan Considerations section. To prevent DIC, patients should seek treatment for the disorders, impairments, and conditions that can lead to DIC (MedlinePlus, 2013).

SAFETY ALERT Patients with liver disease are more likely to experience severe thrombotic complications of chronic DIC than other patients.

Clinical Manifestations

The manifestations of DIC are the result of both clotting and bleeding, although bleeding is more obvious. Bleeding may be internal or external and range from oozing at injection sites to frank hemorrhage from bodily orifices. DIC may be either acute or chronic. Acute DIC develops rapidly over hours or days and requires immediate treatment. Chronic DIC develops slowly, over weeks or months. It lasts longer and is not typically diagnosed as quickly as acute DIC. Chronic DIC causes excessive blood clotting but usually does not lead to bleeding. Patients with cancerous tumors and aortic aneurysms are commonly affected by chronic DIC (Levi & Schmaier, 2015). See the Clinical Manifestations and Therapies feature.

Clinical Manifestations and Therapies
Disseminated Intravascular Coagulation

ETIOLOGY	CLINICAL MANIFESTATIONS	CLINICAL THERAPIES
Cardiovascular System		
Tachycardia Hypotension Circulatory collapse Major vessel thrombosis	▪ Decreased perfusion ▪ Shock ▪ Inappropriate clotting ▪ Tissue necrosis and gangrene ▪ Oozing from wounds, IV sites, and mucous membranes	▪ Administer fluids as ordered. ▪ Monitor intake and output. ▪ Monitor vital signs. ▪ Maintain bedrest.
Respiratory System		
Tachypnea Decreased breath sounds Pleural friction rub Acute respiratory distress syndrome (ARDS)	▪ Impaired gas exchange resulting from microclots in the pulmonary vasculature	▪ Monitor respiratory status. ▪ Maintain ventilatory support if required.
Central Nervous System		
Confusion Coma Seizures Focal deficits	▪ Impaired cerebral perfusion	▪ Conduct neurologic assessment every 2 hours during the critical period, then every 4 hours until stabilized.
Urinary System		
Oliguria Anuria Renal failure Hematuria	▪ Impaired renal perfusion ▪ Impaired clotting mechanism leading to bleeding	▪ Monitor urine output hourly. ▪ Maintain patent urinary catheter. ▪ Monitor urine for blood.
Gastrointestinal System		
Gastrointestinal bleeding Abdominal distention Bleeding from mucous membranes Occult blood in stool or emesis	▪ Impaired clotting mechanisms leading to bleeding	▪ Monitor for occult blood in stools and emesis. ▪ Monitor for overt signs of bleeding from gums. ▪ Measure abdominal girth every 4 hours.
Integumentary System		
Petechiae Purpura Ecchymosis Bleeding or oozing from wounds or IV access site Pallor Cool extremities Cyanosis of extremities	▪ Impaired clotting mechanism leading to bleeding ▪ Impaired tissue perfusion	▪ Monitor skin for evidence of bleeding. ▪ Protect from injury. ▪ Monitor distal pulses, temperature, and capillary refill.

Collaboration

Treatment of DIC is directed toward treating the underlying disorder and preventing further bleeding or massive thrombosis. Supportive measures are essential as resuscitation of the patient's circulatory system is primary to enhance perfusion.

Diagnostic Tests

Diagnostic tests are used to confirm the diagnosis of DIC and evaluate the risk for hemorrhage. Relevant diagnostic tests include the following:

- *Complete blood count and platelet count* are used to evaluate the hemoglobin, hematocrit, and number of circulating platelets. **Schistocytes** (fragmented RBCs) may be noted as a result of cell trapping and damage within fibrin thrombi. The platelet count is decreased.
- *Coagulation studies* show prolonged PT, PTT, and thrombin time as well as a low fibrinogen level caused by depletion of clotting factors. A declining fibrinogen level on two consecutive readings can help make the diagnosis of DIC.
- *Fibrin degradation products or fibrin split products* are increased as a result of the fibrinolysis that occurs with DIC.
- *Fibrinogen* levels may be decreased or normal in circumstances where elevated levels are expected.
- *D-dimer* is elevated in both acute and chronic DIC.

Nonpharmacologic Therapy

When bleeding is the major manifestation of DIC, fresh frozen plasma, cryoprecipitate, and platelet concentrates are given to restore clotting factors and platelets. Heparin, although controversial because it may exacerbate bleeding in addition to preventing further clotting, may be administered. Heparin interferes with the clotting cascade and may prevent further clotting factor consumption as a result of uncontrolled thrombosis. It is used when bleeding is not controlled by plasma and platelets, as well as when the patient has manifestations of thrombotic problems, such as acrocyanosis (cyanotic, or blue, color in the hands and/or feet) and possible gangrene. Long-term heparin therapy (administered by injection or continuous infusion using a portable pump) may be necessary for patients with chronic DIC.

In severe cases of DIC, supportive care is essential to maintain life. Intracranial bleeding may result in altered LOCs, damage to the respiratory center, and increased ICP. Supportive care may include mechanical ventilation and control of organ damage caused by reduced perfusion.

SAFETY ALERT LMWH is associated with lower risk of bleeding and organ failure than unfractionated heparin when used to treat patients with DIC.

Lifespan Considerations

DIC can occur in patients of any age, but children and pregnant women are populations of particular interest. In both groups, the conditions underlying DIC differ from those of the general population, though the pathophysiology of the condition remains the same.

DIC in Infants and Children

Newborns are at increased risk of bleeding disorders due to their natural deficiencies in the quality and quantity of coagulation factors compared to older children and adults. In addition, birth trauma, asphyxia, necrotizing enterocolitis, and sepsis predispose infants to DIC (Victoria State Government, 2012). In older children, as with adults, DIC may be caused by endothelial damage. It may also be associated with pathologic processes, including hypoxia, acidosis, or shock. Systemic disease states such as congenital heart disease and rickettsial infection may lead to DIC as well (Hockenberry & Wilson, 2014).

Manifestations of DIC in infants and children are similar to those in the general population and include integumentary issues, hypotension, and infarction or ischemia (Hockenberry & Wilson, 2014). In neonates, blood may ooze from the umbilicus or circumcision, and the child may exhibit more birth-related bruising than is normal (Victoria State Government, 2012). Older children may experience headaches or lightheadedness, nosebleeds or bleeding gums, and blood in the urine or stool (Children's Hospital Nashville, 2016). Diagnosis is based on repeated laboratory testing of the blood and clinical observation (Soundar et al., 2013). Treatment regimens are similar to those for the general population and include blood products and anticoagulants.

DIC in Pregnant Women

Pregnant patients are at increased risk of acute DIC due in part to changes in hemostatic mechanisms as a result of pregnancy. These include an increase in coagulation factors and a decrease in natural anticoagulants (Sahin et al., 2014). The risk of developing DIC increases if patients have experienced preeclampsia, fetal death, amniotic fluid embolism, or septic abortion. Placental abruption also increases the risk of DIC, and the degree of placental separation appears to be correlated with the severity of DIC. This is likely due to the leakage of fluid similar to a coagulation factor from the placenta. DIC also occurs in some patients affected by hemolysis, elevated liver enzymes, and low platelet counts—a condition commonly referred to as HELLP (hemolysis, elevated liver enzymes, low platelet count; see Exemplar 16.H on Hypertensive Disorders of Pregnancy for more information). HELLP is thought to be a variant of preeclampsia (Levi & Schmaier, 2015).

Bleeding is the most common manifestation of DIC in pregnant patients. Ecchymosis, mucosal oozing, and bleeding of the gastrointestinal tract or incision sites are common. Loss of blood may lead to altered mental state and hypoxia. If blood loss is severe, renal failure or hypovolemic shock may occur. Some patients may develop abdominal compartment syndrome, characterized by increased pressure in the abdominal cavity that disrupts the circulation (Sahin et al., 2014).

Diagnosis is based on a combination of laboratory tests and observation. Blood testing for DIC is typically less reliable in pregnant women than other women because of changes in circulating levels of coagulation factors. As a result, blood tests are typically conducted sequentially.

Treatment involves replacement of blood and blood products, use of anticoagulants, and supportive care. For patients with acute DIC, management of major obstetric bleeding episodes may be necessary and is similar to that of trauma patients (Sahin et al., 2014).

NURSING PROCESS

DIC is a complex disorder that is managed by a critical care team. Nursing care focuses on assessing the bleeding, preventing further injury, and administering prescribed therapies.

Because all body systems can be involved, careful assessment of all systems is needed on a continuous basis. The nurse should observe for petechiae, ecchymoses, and oozing every 1–2 hours. The nurse should also check dependent areas because blood will pool there. IV sites are particularly prone to oozing and should be assessed every 15 minutes. The nurse should examine stool for the presence of blood and measure blood loss as accurately as possible. The nurse should also assess extremities for capillary refill, warmth, and pulses and frequently assess vital signs and LOC. In addition, the nurse should measure intake and output and monitor urine for the presence of blood. Blood urea nitrogen (BUN) and creatinine should be monitored to assess renal function.

The nurse should institute bleeding-control precautions, monitor prescribed therapy (transfusion or anticoagulant therapy), and report any signs of complications. In addition, the nurse should monitor oxygen saturation and ABGs. If the patient requires mechanical ventilation, the nurse should maintain patency of the airway and ensure correct endotracheal tube position.

The nurse should implement measures to maintain skin integrity, such as gentle repositioning. A nutritional plan of tube feedings or total parenteral nutrition should be implemented. The nurse should identify family members' coping strategies and support system to facilitate their ability to manage this life-threatening crisis.

Assessment

Focused nursing assessment for DIC includes the following objective and subjective data:

- *Observation and patient interview.* Review recent medical history, and note any blood transfusions or trauma. If the patient is female, inquire about current pregnancy and recent spontaneous or therapeutic abortion. Discuss the presence of any known malignancies. Note any history of abnormal bleeding episodes or hematologic disorders. Ask about exposure to infectious diseases, and observe for symptoms of those diseases. Inquire about blood in emesis, stool, or urine. Observe for nosebleeds, bleeding gums, and bruising or ecchymosis.
- *Physical examination.* Assess vital signs, and auscultate heart and breath sounds. Examine the hands, feet, and digits, and note the color, temperature, and condition of the skin. Assess the girth and contour of the abdomen, and auscultate bowel sounds. Palpate the abdomen, and note any tenderness or guarding. Examine skin and mucous membranes for petechiae or purpura. Note any

bleeding from puncture wounds or injections, IV sites, or incisions. Note any abnormal bleeding from the nose, mouth, or mucous membranes.

Diagnosis

Patients with acute DIC are often critically ill, with multiple nursing care needs. Septic shock may precipitate DIC, and hemorrhagic shock may occur as a complication of DIC. (See Exemplar 16.L on Shock for more information on the types of shock.) Priority nursing diagnoses discussed in this section include the following:

- *Peripheral Tissue Perfusion, Ineffective*
- *Gas Exchange, Impaired*
- *Pain, Acute*
- *Fear.*

(NANDA-I © 2014)

Planning

Goals of nursing care may include the following:

- The patient will have increased vascular volume as evidenced by hemodynamic stability and adequate urine output.
- The patient will maintain adequate gas exchange, related to mechanical ventilation, as evidenced by ABG results and oxygen saturation monitoring within normal limits.
- The patient will experience adequate pain control, as evidenced by ability to rest comfortably.
- The patient will show early recognition of illness progression by frequently monitoring vital signs after discharge and reporting abnormal results to the healthcare provider.

Implementation

Care of the patient diagnosed with acute DIC often requires specialized nursing in critical care. Continuous monitoring for inadequate oxygenation, altered perfusion, and bleeding are priorities of nursing care. Patients with DIC also require psychosocial support to help manage fear related to diagnosis and consequences of serious illness (see the Independent Interventions section in the Concept of Perfusion).

Promote Effective Tissue Perfusion

Thrombi and emboli forming throughout the microcirculation affect the perfusion of multiple organs and tissues. In addition, bleeding as a result of clotting factor consumption affects CO and blood flow to these tissues. Appropriate interventions include the following:

- Assess extremity pulses, warmth, and capillary refill. Monitoring central and peripheral tissue perfusion facilitates early treatment of impaired perfusion.
- Monitor the patient's LOC and mental status.
- Carefully reposition the patient at least every 2 hours. Position changes facilitate circulation and tissue perfusion and provide an opportunity to assess for purpura, pallor, and bleeding.
- Discourage the patient from crossing the legs, and do not elevate the knees on the bed or with a pillow. These

positions may impair arterial and venous flow to the lower legs and feet, increasing vascular stasis and the risk for thrombosis.

- Minimize use of tape on the skin; use binders, nonadhesive dressings, and other devices as needed. Preventing skin trauma reduces the risk for bleeding and potential infection.

Monitor Gas Exchange

Microclots in the pulmonary vasculature are likely to interfere with gas exchange in the patient with DIC. Nursing interventions to promote gas exchange include the following:

- Monitor the patient's oxygen saturation continuously. Administer oxygen as ordered. Oxygen saturation levels are a noninvasive means of assessing gas exchange. Supplemental oxygen promotes gas exchange and reduces cardiac work, relieving dyspnea.

- Place the patient in the Fowler or high-Fowler position as tolerated. Elevating the head of the bed improves diaphragmatic excursion and alveolar ventilation.

- Maintain bedrest. Bedrest reduces oxygen demands and cardiac work.

- Encourage deep breathing and effective coughing. Increased respiratory depth and clearance of secretions from airways improves alveolar ventilation and oxygenation.

- Institute cautious nasotracheal suctioning if cough is ineffective or an endotracheal tube is in place. Removal of secretions facilitates ventilation and oxygenation. However, care must be used to minimize suction-induced hypoxia and airway trauma.

- Administer analgesics and antianxiety drugs as needed to control pain and anxiety. Provide reassurance and comfort measures. Pain and anxiety increase the respiratory rate and decrease the depth of respirations, reducing effective ventilation and gas exchange.

Manage Pain

Both the underlying cause of DIC and the tissue ischemia from microvascular clots can cause pain. Identifying the etiology of pain is important for recognizing potential

Patient Teaching
Disseminated Intravascular Coagulation

Although the immediate crisis of acute DIC is resolved before discharge, the patient may have some continuing effects of the disorder, such as impaired tissue integrity of distal extremities. Teach the patient and family about specific care needs, such as foot care or dressing changes. Provide instruction about any continuing medications and follow-up care.

Patients with chronic DIC may require continuing heparin therapy, using either intermittent subcutaneous injections or a portable infusion pump. Teach the patient and family members how to administer the injection or manage the infusion pump. Provide a referral to home healthcare or a home IV management service for assistance. Discuss the manifestations of excessive bleeding or recurrent clotting that need to be reported to the healthcare provider.

complications or harmful effects of DIC and instituting effective treatment. Nursing interventions to minimize pain include the following:

- Handle extremities gently. Gentle handling reduces the risk of further injury to and pain in ischemic tissues.

- Apply cool compresses to painful joints. Application of cold decreases pain through the gate-control mechanism.

Evaluation

The patient's response to nursing care may be evaluated using the following expected outcomes:

- The patient experiences no long-term complications from DIC.

- The family demonstrates effective coping techniques to deal with severity of patient's illness.

- The patient's bleeding is controlled.

- The patient's body systems are capable of meeting needs of oxygenation and perfusion to prevent tissue destruction.

If patient outcomes are not met, the patient may require additional hospitalization until both DIC and the underlying condition can be managed appropriately.

REVIEW Disseminated Intravascular Coagulation

RELATE Link the Concepts and Exemplars

Linking the exemplar of DIC with the concept of elimination:

1. What pathophysiology places the patient with DIC at increased risk for renal failure?

2. Prioritize care for the patient diagnosed with DIC who experiences acute renal failure as a result.

Linking the exemplar of DIC with the concept of intracranial regulation:

3. What assessment findings would indicate possible increased intracranial pressure (ICP) in the patient diagnosed with DIC?

4. What is your priority nursing intervention if signs of increased ICP are found in the patient with DIC?

READY Go to Volume 3: Clinical Nursing Skills

REFER Go to Pearson MyLab Nursing and eText

- Additional review materials
- Nursing Care Plan: A Patient with DIC

REFLECT Apply Your Knowledge

Rhonda Fischer, age 29, has just delivered her fourth child at 39 weeks' gestation. The baby was delivered by emergency cesarean section due to fetal intolerance of labor. This occurred after attempted induction of labor for prolonged rupture of membranes and chorioamnionitis.

Ms. Fischer was placed on IV antibiotics prior to surgery and is now on the postpartum unit. During a focused assessment, the nurse notes that Ms. Fischer is having frank bleeding from her incision and is oozing blood from around her IV site. Her vital signs include T_O 99.7°F; P 96 bpm; R 28/min; BP 100/65 mmHg.

1. What laboratory data would you want to review first on Ms. Fischer's medical record?

2. What nursing diagnosis would you add to Ms. Fischer's plan of care based on these assessment findings?

3. What nursing interventions would you initiate for Ms. Fischer?

4. What patient teaching would you provide Mr. and Ms. Fischer to explain the diagnosis of DIC made by the obstetrician?

≫ Exemplar 16.F Heart Failure

Exemplar Learning Outcomes

16.F Analyze heart failure as it relates to perfusion.

- Describe the pathophysiology of heart failure.
- Describe the etiology of heart failure.
- Compare the risk factors for and prevention of heart failure.
- Identify the clinical manifestations of heart failure.
- Summarize diagnostic tests and therapies used by interprofessional teams in the collaborative care of an individual with heart failure.
- Differentiate care of patients with heart failure across the lifespan.
- Apply the nursing process in providing culturally competent care to an individual with heart failure.

Exemplar Key Terms

Cardiac tamponade, *1241*
Decompensation, *1228*
Frank–Starling mechanism, *1229*
Heart failure, *1228*
Hemodynamics, *1235*
Mean arterial pressure (MAP), *1235*
Nocturia, *1232*
Orthopnea, *1232*
Paroxysmal nocturnal dyspnea, *1232*

Overview

Heart failure is a condition in which the heart is unable to pump enough blood into circulation to meet the body's needs (NHLBI, 2015c). Heart failure occurs when the heart muscle is damaged or stressed. The damage or extra workload affects the heart's ability to contract (pump) blood to the periphery or to relax enough for blood from the periphery to return to the heart. Heart failure is often caused by a combination of ineffective contraction and relaxation. As a result of the heart's inability to meet the body's demands, CO falls, leading to decreased tissue perfusion. The body initially adjusts to the reduced CO by activating compensatory mechanisms to restore tissue perfusion. These compensatory mechanisms may result in vascular congestion, hence the term *congestive heart failure*. As these mechanisms are exhausted, heart failure ensues, with increased morbidity and mortality.

Heart failure is a progressive condition, developing over time as the heart muscle becomes weaker. It is frequently a long-term effect of coronary heart disease and MI when left ventricular damage is extensive enough to impair CO. It may also be the result of a primary cardiac muscle disorder, such as cardiomyopathy or myocarditis.

Structural disorders, inflammatory disorders, and hypertension may also lead to heart failure when the heart muscle is damaged by the long-standing excessive workload associated with these conditions. Patients with no history of abnormal myocardial function may present with manifestations of heart failure as a result of acute excessive demands placed on the heart by conditions such as volume overload, hyperthyroidism, and massive pulmonary embolus (see **Table 16–21 ≫**).

Pulmonary edema is a common consequence of heart failure. It is an abnormal accumulation of fluid in the interstitial tissue and alveoli of the lungs. Cardiogenic pulmonary edema, which will be discussed in this exemplar, is a sign of severe cardiac **decompensation** (failure of compensatory mechanisms to restore tissue perfusion). Pulmonary edema is a medical emergency. Its onset may be acute or gradual, progressing to severe respiratory distress. Immediate treatment is necessary.

Pathophysiology and Etiology

Pathophysiology

The mechanical pumping action of cardiac muscle propels blood into the pulmonary and systemic vascular systems for

TABLE 16–21 Selected Causes of Heart Failure

Impaired Myocardial Function	Increased Cardiac Workload	Acute Noncardiac Conditions
Coronary heart disease	Hypertension	Volume overload
Cardiomyopathies	Valve disorders	Hyperthyroidism
Rheumatic fever	Anemias	Fever, infection
Infective endocarditis	Congenital heart defects	Massive pulmonary embolus

TABLE 16–22 Compensatory Mechanisms Activated in Heart Failure

Mechanism	Physiology	Effect on Body Systems	Complications
Frank–Starling mechanism	The greater the stretch of cardiac muscle fibers, the greater the force of contraction.	■ Increased contractile force leading to increased CO	■ Increased myocardial oxygen demand ■ Limited by overstretching
Neuroendocrine response	Decreased CO stimulates the SNS and catecholamine release.	■ Increased heart rate, BP, and contractility ■ Increased vascular resistance ■ Increased venous return	■ Increased vascular resistance ■ Tachycardia, with decreased filling time and decreased CO ■ Increased myocardial work and oxygen demand
Neuroendocrine response	Decreased CO and decreased renal perfusion stimulate the renin-angiotensin system. Angiotensin stimulates aldosterone release from the adrenal cortex. Antidiuretic hormone (ADH) is released from the posterior pituitary. Atrial natriuretic peptide (ANP) and brain natriuretic peptide (BNP) are released. Blood flow is redistributed to vital organs (heart and brain).	■ Vasoconstriction and increased BP ■ Salt and water retention by the kidneys ■ Increased vascular volume ■ Water excretion inhibited ■ Increased sodium excretion ■ Diuresis ■ Vasodilation ■ Decreased perfusion of other organ systems ■ Decreased perfusion of skin and muscles	■ Increased myocardial work ■ Renal vasoconstriction and decreased renal perfusion ■ Increased preload and afterload ■ Pulmonary congestion ■ Fluid retention and increased preload and afterload ■ Pulmonary congestion ■ Renal failure ■ Anaerobic metabolism and lactic acidosis
Ventricular hypertrophy	Increased cardiac workload causes myocardial muscle to hypertrophy and ventricles to dilate.	■ Increased contractile force to maintain CO	■ Increased myocardial oxygen demand ■ Cellular enlargement

reoxygenation and delivery to the tissues. The performance of cardiac muscle is measured by the amount of blood pumped from the ventricles in 1 minute, referred to as CO. Effective CO depends on adequate functional muscle mass and the ability of the ventricles to work together. CO is normally regulated by the oxygen needs of the body: as oxygen use increases, CO increases to maintain cellular function. The ability of the heart to increase CO under these circumstances is known as cardiac reserve. Ventricular damage reduces cardiac reserve.

CO is a product of heart rate and SV. Heart rate affects CO by controlling the number of ventricular contractions per minute. It is influenced by the autonomic nervous system, catecholamines, and thyroid hormones. Activation of a stress response (e.g., hypovolemia, fear) stimulates the SNS, increasing heart rate and the heart's contractility. Elevated heart rate increases CO. Very rapid heart rate, however, shortens ventricular filling time (diastole), reducing SV and CO. On the other hand, a slow heart rate reduces CO simply because of fewer cardiac cycles.

SV is the volume of blood ejected with each heartbeat. It is determined by preload, afterload, and myocardial contractility, all of which are described in the Concept of Perfusion section. In addition to CO and SV, ejection fraction is another important measurement of the heart's effectiveness. As described in the Concept of Perfusion, a normal ejection fraction is 50–70%.

When the heart begins to fail, CO, SV, and ejection fraction all decrease. When this occurs, mechanisms compensate for impaired function and maintain CO. The primary compensatory mechanisms include the following: (1) the Frank–Starling mechanism; (2) neuroendocrine responses, including activation of the SNS and the renin-angiotensin

system; and (3) myocardial hypertrophy. These mechanisms and their effects are summarized in **Table 16–22**.

Decreased CO initially stimulates aortic baroreceptors, which in turn stimulate the SNS. Stimulation of the SNS produces both cardiac and vascular responses through the release of norepinephrine. Norepinephrine increases heart rate and contractility by stimulating cardiac beta-receptors. CO improves as both heart rate and SV increase. Norepinephrine also causes arterial and venous vasoconstriction, increasing venous return to the heart. Increased venous return increases ventricular filling and myocardial stretch, increasing the force of contraction (the **Frank–Starling mechanism**). Overstretching the muscle fibers past their physiologic limit results in ineffective contractions.

Blood flow is redistributed to the brain and the heart to maintain perfusion of these vital organs. Decreased renal perfusion causes renin to be released from the kidneys. Activation of the renin angiotensin system produces additional vasoconstriction and stimulates the adrenal cortex to produce aldosterone and the posterior pituitary to release ADH. Aldosterone stimulates sodium reabsorption in renal tubules, promoting water retention. ADH acts on the distal tubule to inhibit water excretion, and it also causes vasoconstriction. The effect of these hormones is significant vasoconstriction as well as salt and water retention, with a resulting increase in vascular volume. Increased ventricular filling increases the force of contraction, improving CO.

The effects of the renin-angiotensin system and ADH release are counterbalanced to a certain extent by two additional hormones. The increased vascular volume and venous return prompted by vasoconstriction and sodium and water retention increase the volume and pressures in the heart. Stimulation of stretch receptors in the atria and ventricles leads to the release of ANP and BNP from stores in the atria (ANP and BNP) and ventricles (BNP). These hormones promote sodium and water excretion and inhibit the release of norepinephrine, renin, and ADH, with resulting vasodilation. Although beneficial, the effects of these hormones are too weak to completely counteract the vasoconstriction and the sodium and water retention that occurs in heart failure.

Ventricular remodeling occurs as the heart chambers and myocardium adapt to fluid volume and pressure increases. The chambers dilate to accommodate excess fluid resulting from increased vascular volume and incomplete emptying. This additional stretch initially causes more effective contractions. Ventricular hypertrophy occurs as existing cardiac muscle cells enlarge, increasing their contractile elements (actin and myosin) and force of contraction.

Although these responses may help in the short-term regulation of CO, it is now recognized that they also hasten the deterioration of cardiac function. The onset of heart failure is heralded by decompensation. Heart failure progresses as a result of the very mechanisms that initially maintain circulatory stability.

A rapid heart rate shortens diastolic filling time, compromises coronary artery perfusion, and increases myocardial oxygen demand. Resulting ischemia further impairs CO. Beta-receptors in the heart become less sensitive to continued SNS stimulation, thus decreasing heart rate and contractility. As the beta-receptors become less sensitive, norepinephrine stores in the cardiac muscle become depleted. In contrast, alpha-receptors on peripheral blood vessels become increasingly sensitive to persistent stimulation, promoting vasoconstriction and increasing afterload and cardiac work.

As mentioned, ventricular hypertrophy and dilation initially increase CO, but chronic distention eventually causes the ventricular wall to thin and degenerate. The purpose of hypertrophy is thus defeated. In addition, chronic overloading of the dilated ventricle eventually stretches the fibers beyond the optimal point for effective contraction. The ventricles continue to dilate to accommodate the excess fluid, but the heart loses the ability to contract forcefully. The heart muscle may eventually become so large that the coronary blood supply is inadequate, causing ischemia.

Chronic distention exhausts stores of ANP and BNP. The effects of norepinephrine, renin, and ADH prevail, and the renin-angiotensin pathway is continually stimulated. This mechanism ultimately raises the hemodynamic stress on the heart by increasing both preload and afterload. As heart function deteriorates, less blood is delivered to the tissues and the heart itself. Ischemia and necrosis of the myocardium further weaken the already failing heart, and the cycle repeats.

In normal hearts, the cardiac reserve allows the heart to adjust its output to meet the metabolic needs of the body, increasing the CO by up to 5 times the basal level during exercise. Patients with heart failure have minimal to no cardiac reserve. At rest, they may be unaffected; however, any stressor (e.g., exercise, illness) taxes their ability to meet the demand for oxygen and nutrients. Manifestations of activity intolerance when the individual is at rest indicate a critical level of cardiac decompensation.

Classifications

Heart failure is classified in several ways, depending on the underlying pathology. Classifications include systolic versus diastolic failure, left-sided versus right-sided failure, low-output versus high-output failure, and acute versus chronic failure. Although not a class of heart failure, pulmonary edema is an important consequence of the various classes of heart failure.

Systolic Versus Diastolic Failure

Systolic failure occurs when the ventricle fails to contract adequately to eject a sufficient volume of blood into the arterial system. Systolic function is affected by loss of myocardial cells due to ischemia and infarction, cardiomyopathy, or inflammation.

Diastolic failure occurs when the heart cannot completely relax in diastole, disrupting normal filling. Passive diastolic filling decreases, increasing the importance of atrial contraction to preload. Diastolic dysfunction results from decreased ventricular compliance caused by hypertrophic and cellular changes and impaired relaxation of the heart muscle.

Left-Sided Versus Right-Sided Failure

Depending on the pathophysiology involved, either the left or the right ventricle may be primarily affected. In chronic heart failure, however, both ventricles typically are impaired to some degree.

Coronary heart disease and hypertension are common causes of left-sided heart failure, whereas right-sided heart failure often is caused by conditions that restrict blood flow to the lungs, such as acute or chronic pulmonary disease. Left-sided heart failure also can lead to right-sided failure, as pressures in the pulmonary vascular system increase with congestion behind the failing left ventricle.

As left ventricular function fails, CO falls. Pressures in the left ventricle and atrium increase as the amount of blood remaining in the ventricle after systole increases. These increased pressures impair filling, causing congestion and increased pressures in the pulmonary vascular system. Increased pressures in this normally low-pressure system increase fluid movement from the blood vessels into interstitial tissues and the alveoli (see **Figure 16–38 »**). The manifestations of left-sided heart failure result from pulmonary congestion (backward effects) and decreased CO (forward effects).

In right-sided heart failure, increased pressures in the pulmonary vasculature or right ventricular muscle damage impair the right ventricle's ability to pump blood into the pulmonary circulation. The right ventricle and atrium become distended, and blood accumulates in the systemic venous system. Increased venous pressures cause abdominal organs to become congested and peripheral tissue edema to develop (see **Figure 16–39 »**). Dependent tissues tend to be affected because of the effects of gravity.

Low-Output Versus High-Output Failure

Patients with heart failure resulting from coronary heart disease, hypertension, cardiomyopathy, and other primary cardiac disorders develop low-output failure and manifestations such as those previously described. Patients in hypermetabolic states (e.g., hyperthyroidism, infection, anemia,

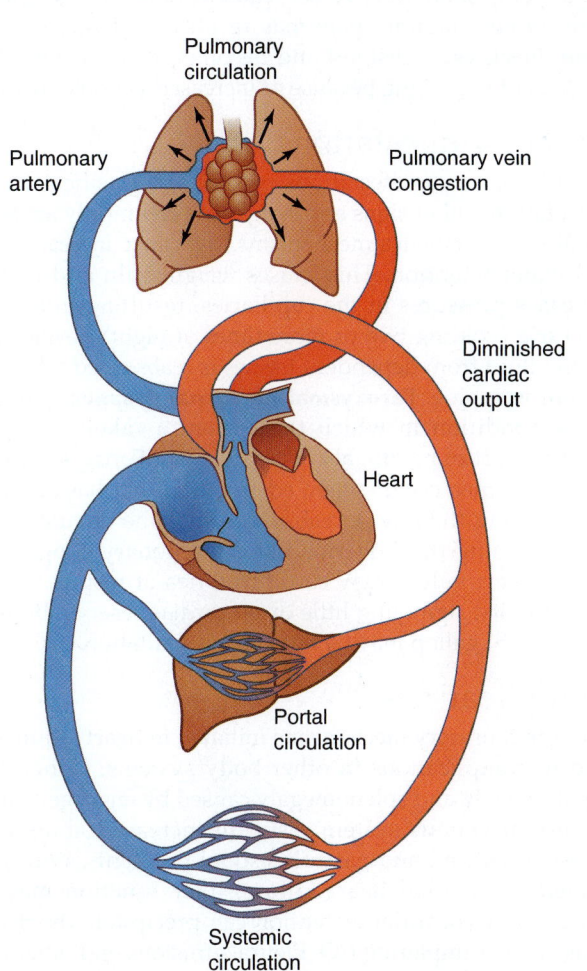

Figure 16–38 ≫ The hemodynamic effects of left-sided heart failure.

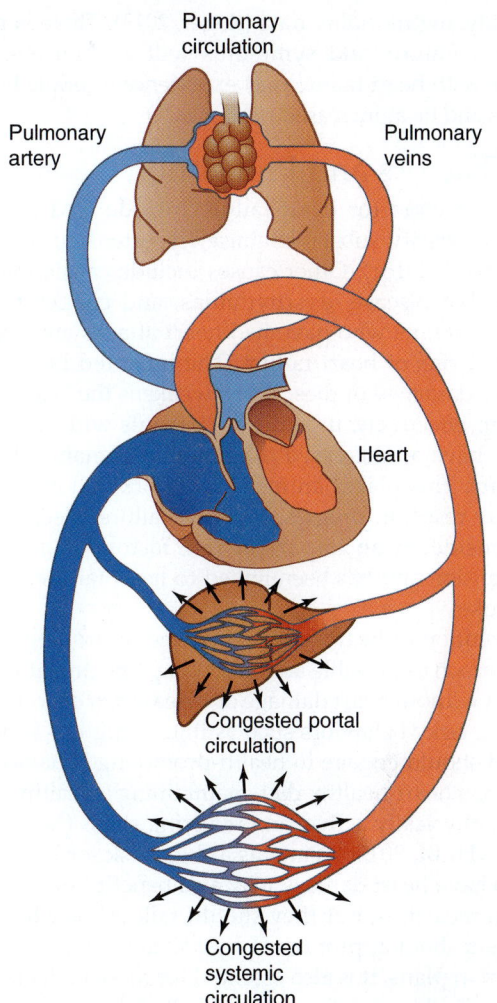

Figure 16–39 ≫ The hemodynamic effects of right-sided heart failure.

pregnancy) require increased CO to maintain blood flow and oxygen to the tissues. If the increased blood flow cannot meet the oxygen demands of the tissues, compensatory mechanisms are activated to further increase CO, which in turn further increases oxygen demand. Thus, even though CO is high, the heart is unable to meet increased oxygen demands. This condition is known as high-output failure.

Acute Versus Chronic Failure

Acute failure is the abrupt onset of a myocardial injury (e.g., massive MI) resulting in suddenly decreased cardiac function and signs of decreased CO. Chronic failure is a progressive deterioration of the heart muscle as a result of cardiomyopathies, valvular disease, or coronary heart disease.

Pulmonary Edema

In cardiogenic pulmonary edema, the contractility of the left ventricle is severely impaired. The ejection fraction falls because the ventricle is unable to eject the blood that enters it, causing a sharp rise in end-diastolic volume and pressure. Pulmonary hydrostatic pressures rise, ultimately exceeding the osmotic pressure of the blood. As a result, fluid leaking from the pulmonary capillaries congests interstitial spaces in the tissues, decreasing lung compliance and interfering with

gas exchange. As capillary and interstitial pressures increase further, the tight junctions of the alveolar walls are disrupted, and the fluid enters the alveoli, along with large RBCs and protein molecules. Ventilation and gas exchange become severely disrupted, and hypoxia worsens.

Etiology

The National Heart, Lung, and Blood Institute (NHLBI, 2015c) estimates that 5.7 million people in the United States have heart failure. At-risk populations include those 65 years of age and older, African Americans, patients who are overweight, and patients with a history of MI (NHLBI, 2015a). Children diagnosed with congenital heart defects can also develop heart failure. Congenital heart defects cause the heart to work harder, weakening the heart muscle, which can lead to heart failure.

The prognosis for a patient with heart failure depends on the underlying cause of the heart failure and how effectively the precipitating factors can be treated. Estimates of the 5-year survival rate for patients with heart failure are roughly 50%; estimates of 10-year survival fall between 10 and 26% (CDC, 2015c; Dumitru & Baker, 2016; Roger, 2013; Taylor et al., 2012). It is worth noting that survival rate estimates are a source of some debate, due in part to the methods used for collecting and analyzing mortality data (Roger, 2013). There is no cure for heart failure, and symptoms will worsen over time. Patients with heart failure may experience multiple hospitalizations and be at increased risk for SCD.

Risk Factors and Prevention

Key risk factors for heart failure include CAD, cigarette smoking, obesity, substance abuse, hypertension, and diabetes (NHLBI, 2015c). Other causes include cardiomyopathy, heart valve disease, dysrhythmias, and congenital heart defects. Patients who have had heart attacks are also at an increased risk of heart failure. The infarcted heart muscle becomes damaged or dies, which weakens the heart's ability to pump effectively. In addition, patients with severe lung disease have an increased oxygenation demand placed on the heart. This places an increased workload on the heart and may result in progressive heart failure. Sleep apnea is also considered an important risk factor for developing hypertension and has been linked to heart failure, diabetes, and stroke.

Prevention of heart failure involves controlling risk factors as much as possible and following a treatment regimen. Patients without heart damage or disease can concentrate on avoiding risky behaviors such as illicit drug use and smoking and should engage in health-promoting behaviors such as eating a heart-healthy diet, maintaining a healthy weight, staying physically active, and reducing stress (Mayo Clinic, 2015e; NHLBI, 2015c). Patients at high risk for heart failure or who have heart damage may also benefit from these prevention measures, but they should talk to their healthcare providers about appropriate physical activities and specific prevention plans. It is also essential for these patients to take all prescribed medications (NHLBI, 2015c).

Clinical Manifestations

The manifestations of systolic failure are those of decreased CO: weakness, fatigue, and decreased exercise tolerance. The manifestations of diastolic failure include shortness of breath, tachypnea, and respiratory crackles if the left ventricle is affected; they include distended neck veins, liver enlargement, anorexia, and nausea if the right ventricle is affected. Many patients have components of both systolic and diastolic failure. See Multisystem Effects of Heart Failure.

Left-Sided Failure

Fatigue and activity intolerance are common early manifestations of left-sided heart failure. Dizziness and syncope also may result from decreased CO. Pulmonary congestion causes dyspnea, shortness of breath, and cough. The patient may develop **orthopnea** (difficulty breathing when supine), prompting use of two or three pillows or a recliner for sleeping. Cyanosis from impaired gas exchange may be noted. On auscultation of the lungs, inspiratory crackles (rales) and wheezes may be heard in lung bases. An S_3 gallop may be present, reflecting the heart's attempts to fill an already distended ventricle.

Right-Sided Failure

In right-sided heart failure, edema develops in the feet and legs or, if the patient is bedridden, in the sacrum. Congestion of gastrointestinal tract vessels causes anorexia and nausea. Right upper quadrant pain may result from liver engorgement. Neck veins distend and become visible, even when the patient is upright, because of increased venous pressure.

Other Manifestations

In addition to manifestations of specific classifications of heart failure, other signs and symptoms commonly are seen. A fall in CO activates mechanisms that cause increased salt and water retention. This causes weight gain and further increases pressures in the capillaries, resulting in edema. **Nocturia** (voiding two or more times at night) develops as edema fluid from dependent tissues is reabsorbed while the patient is supine. **Paroxysmal nocturnal dyspnea**, a frightening condition in which the patient awakens at night acutely short of breath, also may develop. Paroxysmal nocturnal dyspnea occurs when edema fluid that has accumulated during the day is reabsorbed into the circulation at night, causing fluid overload and pulmonary congestion. Severe heart failure may cause dyspnea at rest as well as with activity, signifying little or no cardiac reserve. Both an S_3 and an S_4 gallop may be heard on auscultation.

Complications

The compensatory mechanisms initiated in heart failure can lead to complications in other body systems. Congestive hepatomegaly and splenomegaly caused by engorgement of the portal venous system result in increased abdominal pressure, ascites, and gastrointestinal problems. With prolonged right-sided heart failure, liver function may be impaired. Myocardial distention can precipitate dysrhythmias, further impairing CO. Pleural effusions and other pulmonary problems may develop.

The patient with acute pulmonary edema presents with classic manifestations (see **Box 16–14** »). Dyspnea, shortness of breath, and labored respirations are acute and severe,

---

Box 16–14
Manifestations of Pulmonary Edema

Respiratory
- Tachypnea
- Paroxysmal nocturnal dyspnea
- Labored respirations
- Cough productive of frothy, pink sputum
- Dyspnea
- Crackles, wheezes
- Orthopnea

Cardiovascular
- Tachycardia
- Cool, clammy skin
- Hypotension
- Hypoxemia
- Cyanosis
- Ventricular gallop

Neurologic
- Restlessness
- Feeling of impending doom
- Anxiety

Multisystem Effects of
Heart Failure

Respiratory

- Dyspnea on exertion
- Shortness of breath
- Tachypnea
- Orthopnea
- Dry cough
- Crackles (rales) in lung bases

Potential complications
- Pulmonary edema
- Pneumonia
- Cardiac asthma
- Pleural effusion
- Cheyne-Stokes respirations
- Respiratory acidosis

Gastrointestinal

- Anorexia, nausea
- Abdominal distention
- Liver enlargement
- Right upper quadrant pain

Potential complications
- Malnutrition
- Ascites
- Liver dysfunction

Musculoskeletal

- Fatigue
- Weakness

Neurologic

- Confusion
- Impaired memory
- Anxiety, restlessness
- Insomnia

Cardiovascular

- Activity intolerance
- Tachycardia
- Palpitations
- S_3, S_4 heart sounds
- Elevated central venous pressure
- Neck vein distention
- Hepatojugular reflux
- Splenomegaly

Potential complications
- Angina
- Dysrhythmias
- Sudden cardiac death
- Cardiogenic shock

Genitourinary

- Decreased urine output
- Nocturia

Integumentary

- Pallor or cyanosis
- Cool, clammy skin
- Diaphoresis

Potential complication
- Increased risk for tissue breakdown

Metabolic Processes

- Peripheral edema
- Weight gain

Potential complication
- Metabolic acidosis

accompanied by orthopnea. Cyanosis is present, and the skin is cool, clammy, and diaphoretic. A productive cough with pink, frothy sputum develops as a result of fluid, RBCs, and plasma proteins in the alveoli and airways. Crackles are heard throughout the lung fields on auscultation. As the condition worsens, lung sounds become harsher. The patient often is restless and highly anxious, although severe hypoxia may cause confusion or lethargy.

SAFETY ALERT Pulmonary edema is a medical emergency. Without rapid and effective intervention, severe tissue hypoxia and acidosis will lead to organ system failure and death.

Collaboration

The main goals for care of the patient with heart failure are to slow its progression, reduce cardiac workload, improve cardiac function, and control fluid retention. Treatment strategies are based on the evolution and progression of heart failure (see **Table 16–23 》**).

Diagnostic Tests

Diagnosis of heart failure is based on patient history, physical examination, and diagnostic findings. Relevant diagnostic tests include the following:

- *Atrial natriuretic peptide (ANP), also called atrial natriuretic hormone, and brain natriuretic peptide (BNP)* are hormones released by the heart muscle in response to changes in blood volume. Blood levels of these hormones increase in heart failure. BNP levels, in particular, have been shown to positively correlate with pressures in the left ventricle and the pulmonary vascular system. The level of BNP in the blood increases as the symptoms of heart failure worsen and decreases when the heart failure stabilizes. BNP levels may be elevated in women and patients over age 60 who do not have a diagnosis of heart failure. Therefore, they should not be considered as the primary diagnostic tool.

- *Serum electrolytes* are measured to evaluate fluid and electrolyte status. Serum osmolarity may be low because of fluid retention. Sodium, potassium, and chloride levels provide a baseline for evaluating the effects of treatment; serum calcium and magnesium are measured as well.

- *Urinalysis, blood urea nitrogen (BUN), and serum creatinine* are obtained to evaluate renal function.

- *Liver function tests,* including alanine aminotransferase, aspartate aminotransferase, lactate dehydrogenase, serum bilirubin, and total protein and albumin levels, are obtained to evaluate possible effects of heart failure on liver function.

- *Thyroid function tests* can indicate hyperthyroidism and hypothyroidism, which can produce symptoms resembling those of heart failure.

- *Arterial blood gas (ABG)* levels are determined to evaluate gas exchange in the lungs and tissues in the patient with acute heart failure.

TABLE 16–23 Stages of Heart Failure

Stage	Description	Recommended Interventions
I (mild)	Patient has no limitation of physical activity. Patient has no shortness of breath noted with normal physical activity.	Regular exercise Smoking cessation Treatment of hypertension Treatment of hyperlipidemia Discontinuation of alcohol or illegal drug use Low-sodium diet Possible addition of ACE inhibitor, ARB, or beta-adrenergic blocker to medication regimen
II (mild)	Patient has some physical limitations due to fatigue, shortness of breath, or palpitations. Patient is comfortable at rest.	Class I interventions ACE inhibitor or ARB, and beta-adrenergic blocker as indicated Surgical options: coronary artery repair, valve repair or replacement
III (moderate)	Patient has increased physical limitations. Less than normal physical activity results in fatigue, shortness of breath, or palpitations. Patient is comfortable at rest.	Class I interventions Addition of diuretic, ACE inhibitor, ARB, and/or beta-adrenergic blocker to medication regimen Possible addition of aldosterone inhibitor, digitalis, hydralazine, or nitrates Further restriction of dietary sodium Weight monitoring Fluid restriction, as needed Discontinuation of drugs that worsen condition Surgical options: biventricular pacing, implantable cardioverter–defibrillator (ICD)
IV (severe)	Any degree of physical activity results in increased discomfort. Patient exhibits symptoms of cardiac insufficiency at rest.	Interventions for Stages I, II, and III Evaluation for available options Possible interventions: heart transplant, VADs, surgery, research therapies, continuous infusion of IV heart pump medication, palliative or hospice care

Sources: Data from American Heart Association (AHA). (2015j). *Classes of heart failure.* Retrieved from http://www.heart.org/HEARTORG/Conditions/HeartFailure/AboutHeartFailure/Classes-of-Heart-Failure_UCM_306328_Article.jsp; Dumitru, I., & Baker, M. M. (2016). *Heart failure.* Retrieved from http://emedicine.medscape.com/article/163062-overview; Yancy, C. W., Jessup, M., Bozkurt, B., Butler, J., Casey, D. E., Drazner, M. H., . . . Wilkoff, B. L. (2013). 2013 ACCF/AHA guideline for the management of heart failure. *Journal of the American College of Cardiology, 62*(16), e147–e239. doi:10.1016/j.jacc.2013.05.019

- **Chest x-ray** may show pulmonary vascular congestion and cardiomegaly in heart failure.
- **Electrocardiography** is used to identify ECG changes associated with ventricular enlargement and to detect dysrhythmias, myocardial ischemia, or infarction.
- **Echocardiography with Doppler flow studies** are performed to evaluate left ventricular function. Either transthoracic echocardiography or transesophageal echocardiography may be used.

Hemodynamic Monitoring

Hemodynamics is the study of forces involved in blood circulation. Hemodynamic monitoring is used to assess cardiovascular function in the patient who is critically ill or unstable. The main goals of invasive hemodynamic monitoring are to evaluate cardiac and circulatory function and the response to interventions. Hemodynamic parameters include heart rate, arterial BP, central venous or right atrial pressure, pulmonary pressures, and CO. Direct hemodynamic parameters are obtained straight from the monitoring device (e.g., heart rate, arterial and venous pressures). Indirect or derived measurements are calculated using the direct data (e.g., cardiac index, MAP, SV). Invasive hemodynamic monitoring is routinely used in critical care units.

Hemodynamic monitoring systems measure the pressure within a vessel and convert it into an electrical waveform that is amplified and displayed. Key system components include an invasive catheter threaded into an artery or vein connected to a transducer by stiff, high-pressure tubing. Additional components include stopcocks and a continuous flushing system with normal saline or heparinized saline and an infusion pressure bag to prevent clots from forming in the catheter. **Figure 16–40** ≫

illustrates a pressure transducer and typical hemodynamic monitoring system.

Hemodynamic pressure monitoring may be used to measure peripheral artery pressures or central pressures. Although the information it provides is valuable, the procedure is not without risk. Some of the potential complications of central pressure monitoring include bleeding, hematoma, pneumothorax, hemothorax, arterial puncture, dysrhythmias, venospasm, infection, air embolism, thromboembolism, brachial nerve injury, and thoracic nerve injury.

Intra-Arterial Pressure Monitoring

With intra-arterial pressure monitoring, an indwelling arterial line allows for direct and continuous monitoring of systolic, diastolic, and MAPs and provides easy access for arterial blood sampling. Arterial lines are used to assess blood volume, to monitor the effects of vasoactive drugs, and to obtain frequent ABG determinations. Because the invasive catheter is inserted directly into the artery, it offers immediate access for blood gas measurements and blood testing.

The arterial BP reflects the CO and the resistance to blood flow created by the elastic arterial walls (SVR). The systolic BP, normally approximately 120 mmHg in healthy adults, reflects the pressure generated during ventricular systole. During diastole, elastic arterial walls keep a minimum pressure within the vessel (diastolic BP) to maintain blood flow through the capillary beds. The average diastolic pressure in a healthy adult is 80 mmHg. The **mean arterial pressure (MAP)** is the average pressure in the arterial circulation throughout the cardiac cycle. It reflects the driving pressure, or perfusion pressure, an indicator of tissue perfusion. The formula MAP = CO × SVR often is used to show the relationships between factors determining the BP. MAP can also be calculated by adding

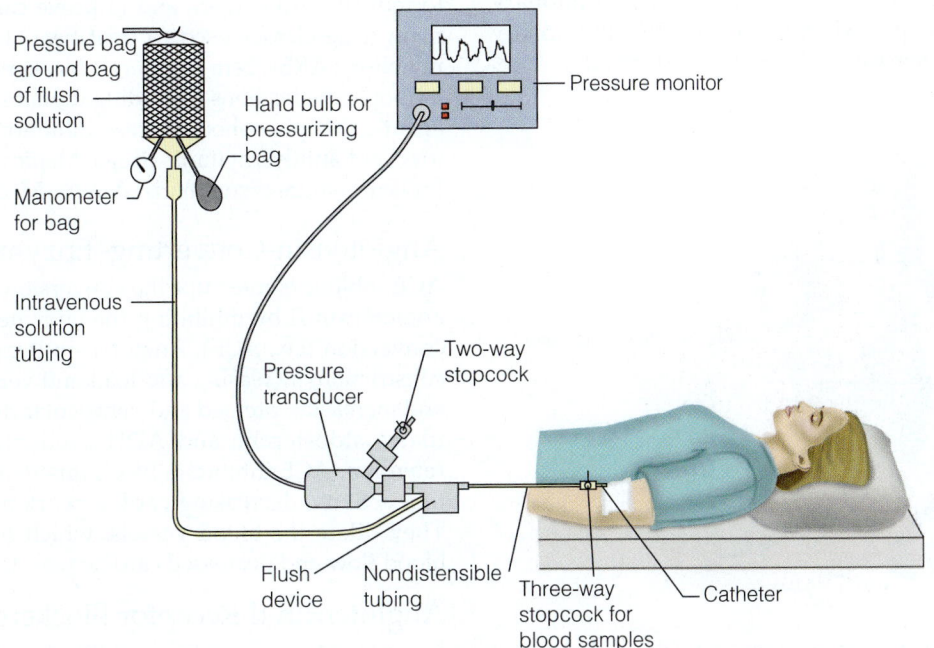

Figure 16–40 ≫ A hemodynamic monitoring setup.

one-third of the pulse pressure (PP) to the diastolic BP (DBP)—that is, MAP = DBP + PP/3. For example, a BP of 120/80 results in a MAP of 93. MAPs of 70 to 90 mmHg are desirable. Perfusion to vital organs is severely jeopardized at MAPs of 50 or less; MAPs of greater than 105 mmHg may indicate hypertension or vasoconstriction.

Venous Pressure Monitoring

CVP and right atrial pressure are measures of blood volume and venous return. They also reflect right-heart filling pressures. Pressures are elevated in right-sided heart failure. CVP and right atrial pressure are primarily used to monitor fluid volume status. To measure venous and atrial pressures, a catheter is inserted in the internal jugular or subclavian vein. The distal tip of the catheter is positioned in the superior vena cava just above or just inside the right atrium. CVP may be measured in either centimeters of water (cm H_2O) or millimeters of mercury (mmHg). The normal range for CVP is 2–8 cm H_2O or 2–6 mmHg, but CVP varies in individual patients. Hypovolemia and shock decrease CVP; fluid overload, vasoconstriction, and cardiac tamponade increase CVP.

Pulmonary Artery Pressure Monitoring

A pulmonary artery catheter is a flow-directed, balloon-tipped catheter first used in the 1970s to evaluate left ventricular and overall cardiac function. The pulmonary artery catheter is often called a Swan–Ganz catheter, after the physicians who developed it. It is inserted into a central vein and threaded into the right atrium. A small balloon at the tip allows the catheter to be drawn into the right ventricle and, from there, into the pulmonary artery (see **Figure 16–41 》**). The inflated balloon carries the catheter forward until the balloon wedges in a small branch of pulmonary vasculature. Once in place, the balloon is deflated, and multiple lumens of the catheter allow measurement of pressures in the right atrium, pulmonary artery, and left ventricle (see **Figure 16–42 》**). The normal pulmonary artery pressure is approximately 25/10 mmHg; normal mean pulmonary artery pressure is approximately 15 mmHg. Pulmonary artery pressure is increased in left-sided heart failure.

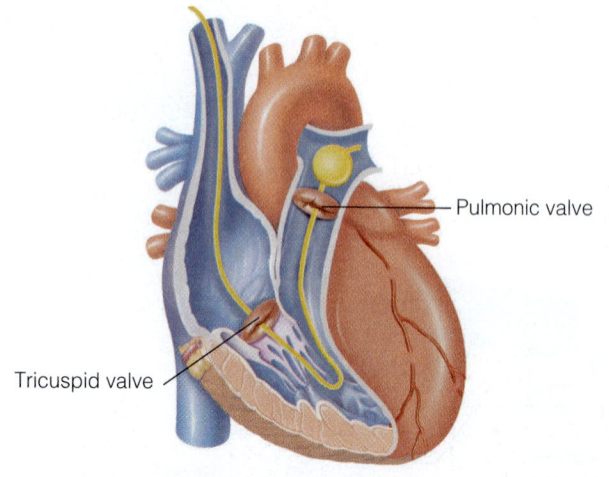

Figure 16–41 》 Inflation of the balloon on the flow-directed catheter allows it to be carried through the pulmonic valve into the pulmonary artery.

Pulmonic valve

Tricuspid valve

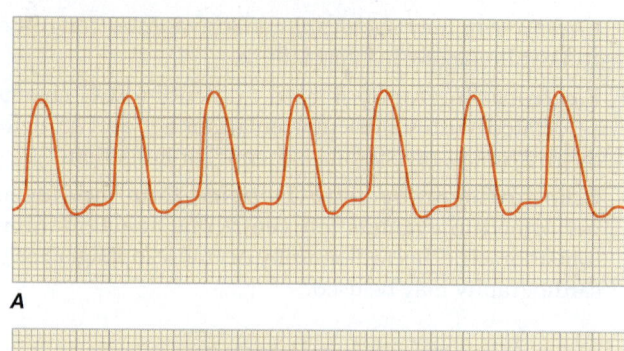

A

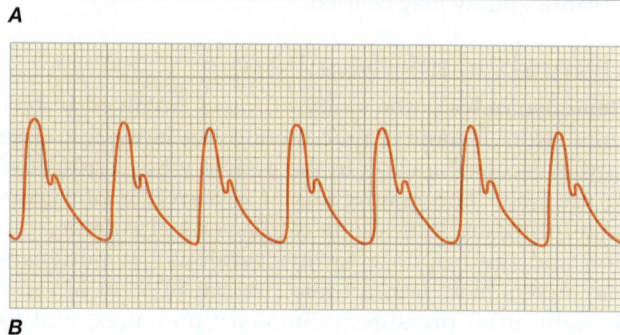

B

Figure 16–42 》 Typical waveforms seen when measuring, **A,** right ventricular (RV) pressure and, **B,** pulmonary artery pressure (PAP).

Inflation of the balloon effectively blocks pressure from behind the balloon and allows measurement of pressures generated by the left ventricle. This is known as the pulmonary artery wedge pressure (PAWP) and is used to assess left ventricular function. The normal PAWP is 8–12 mmHg. PAWP is increased in left ventricular failure and pericardial tamponade, and decreased in hypovolemia.

Pharmacologic Therapy

Patients with heart failure often receive multiple medications to reduce cardiac work and improve cardiac function. The main drug classes used to treat heart failure are the ACE inhibitors, ARBs, beta-adrenergic blockers, diuretics, positive inotropic medications (including digitalis, sympathomimetic agents, and phosphodiesterase inhibitors), direct vasodilators, and antidysrhythmic drugs. Medication administration for heart failure is summarized in the Medications feature.

Angiotensin-Converting–Enzyme Inhibitors

ACE inhibitors interrupt the conversion of angiotensin I to angiotensin II by inhibiting the enzyme that mediates the conversion (i.e., ACE). Angiotensin II causes intense vasoconstriction, increasing afterload and ventricular wall stress and increasing preload and ventricular dilation. It also stimulates aldosterone and ADH production, causing fluid retention. ACE inhibitors block this renin-angiotensin system activity, decreasing cardiac work and increasing CO. They dilate the blood vessels, which results in increased blood flow and decreased cardiac workload.

Angiotensin II Receptor Blockers

In contrast to ACE inhibitors, ARBs do not block the production of angiotensin II; instead, they block its action. The pharmacologic effect is similar, and they also are used in

Medications
Heart Failure

CLASSIFICATION AND DRUG EXAMPLES	MECHANISMS OF ACTION	NURSING CONSIDERATIONS
Angiotensin-Converting–Enzyme (ACE) Inhibitors *Drug examples:* Enalapril (Vasotec) Lisinopril (Prinivil, Zestril) Captopril (Capoten) Fosinopril (Monopril) Quinapril (Accupril) Ramipril (Altace) **Angiotensin II Receptor Blockers (ARBs)** *Drug examples:* Candesartan (Atacand) Valsartan (Diovan)	ACE inhibitors and ARBs prevent acute coronary events and reduce mortality in heart failure. ACE inhibitors interfere with production of angiotensin II, resulting in vasodilation, reduced blood volume, and prevention of its effects in the heart and blood vessels. In heart failure, ACE inhibitors reduce afterload and improve CO and renal blood flow. They also reduce pulmonary congestion and peripheral edema. ACE inhibitors suppress myocyte growth and reduce ventricular remodeling in heart failure. Although the pharmacologic effect of ARBs is similar, they block the action of angiotensin II at the receptor rather than interfering with its production.	■ Do not give these drugs in the second and third trimesters of pregnancy. ■ Carefully monitor patients who are volume-depleted or have impaired renal function. ■ Use an infusion pump when administering ACE inhibitors intravenously. ■ Monitor BP closely for 2 hours following the first dose and as indicated thereafter. ■ Monitor serum potassium levels; ACE inhibitors can cause hyperkalemia. ■ Monitor WBC count for potential neutropenia. Health Education for the Patient and Family ■ Take the drug at the same time every day to ensure a stable blood level. ■ Monitor BP and weight weekly. Report significant changes to your healthcare provider. ■ Avoid making sudden position changes. Lie down if you become dizzy or lightheaded, particularly after the first dose. ■ Report any signs of easy bruising and bleeding, sore throat, fever, edema, or skin rash. Immediately report swelling of the face, lips, or eyelids and any itching or breathing problems. ■ A persistent, dry cough may develop if you are taking an ACE inhibitor. Contact your healthcare provider if this becomes a problem. ■ Take captopril 1 hour before meals.
Diuretics *Drug examples:* Spironolactone (Aldactone) Furosemide (Lasix) Bumetanide (Bumex) Hydrochlorothiazide (HydroDIURIL)	Diuretics act on different portions of the kidney tubule to inhibit reabsorption of sodium and water and promote their excretion. With the exception of the potassium-sparing diuretics (spironolactone, triamterene, and amiloride), diuretics also promote potassium excretion, increasing the risk of hypokalemia. Spironolactone, an aldosterone receptor blocker, reduces symptoms and slows progression of heart failure. Aldosterone receptors in the heart and blood vessels promote myocardial remodeling and fibrosis, activate the SNS, and promote vascular fibrosis (which decreases compliance) and baroreceptor dysfunction.	■ Obtain baseline weight and vital signs. ■ Monitor BP, intake and output, weight, skin turgor, and edema as indicators of fluid volume status. ■ Assess for volume depletion, particularly with loop diuretics (furosemide, ethacrynic acid, and bumetanide): dizziness, orthostatic hypotension, tachycardia, and muscle cramping. ■ Report abnormal serum electrolyte levels to the healthcare provider. Replace electrolytes as indicated. ■ Do not administer potassium replacements to patients receiving a potassium-sparing diuretic. ■ Evaluate renal function by assessing urine output, BUN, and serum creatinine. ■ Administer IV furosemide slowly, no faster than 20 mg/min. Evaluate for signs of ototoxicity. Do not administer this drug or ethacrynic acid concurrently with aminoglycoside antibiotics (e.g., gentamicin), which are also ototoxic.

(continued on next page)

Medications (continued)

CLASSIFICATION AND DRUG EXAMPLES	MECHANISMS OF ACTION	NURSING CONSIDERATIONS
		Health Education for the Patient and Family ■ Drink at least 6–8 glasses of water per day. ■ Take the diuretic at times that will be least disruptive to your lifestyle, usually in the morning and early afternoon if a second dose is ordered. Take with meals to decrease gastric upset. ■ Monitor BP, pulse, and weight weekly. Report significant weight changes to your healthcare provider. ■ Report any of the following to your healthcare provider: severe abdominal pain; jaundice; dark urine; abnormal bleeding or bruising; flulike symptoms; and signs of hypokalemia, hyponatremia, or dehydration (e.g., thirst, salt craving, dizziness, weakness, rapid pulse). ■ Avoid sudden position changes because they may cause dizziness or feelings of faintness. ■ Unless you are taking a potassium-sparing diuretic, integrate potassium-rich foods into your diet. Limit sodium use.
Cardiac Glycoside *Drug example:* Digoxin (Lanoxin)	Digitalis improves myocardial contractility by interfering with ATP in the myocardial cell membrane and increasing the amount of calcium available for contraction. The increased force of contraction causes the heart to empty more completely, increasing SV and CO. Improved CO improves renal perfusion, decreasing renin secretion. This decreases preload and afterload, reducing cardiac work. Digitalis also has electrophysiologic effects, slowing conduction through the AV node. This decreases heart rate and reduces oxygen consumption.	■ Assess apical pulse before administering. Withhold digitalis, and notify the healthcare provider if heart rate is below 60 bpm and/or manifestations of decreased CO are noted. Record apical rate on medication record. ■ Evaluate the ECG for scooped (spoon-shaped) ST segment, AV block, bradycardia, and other dysrhythmias (especially PVCs and atrial tachycardias). ■ Report manifestations of digitalis toxicity: anorexia, nausea and vomiting, abdominal pain, weakness, vision changes (e.g., diplopia, blurred vision, yellow-green or white halos seen around objects), and new-onset dysrhythmias. ■ Assess potassium, magnesium, calcium, and serum digoxin levels before giving digitalis. Hypokalemia can precipitate toxicity even when the serum digitalis level is in the "normal" range (*adult:* 0.5–2 ng/mL, 0.5–2 nmol/L [SI units]; *infants:* 1–3 ng/mL). ■ Monitor patients with renal insufficiency or renal failure and older adults for digitalis toxicity. ■ Prepare to administer digoxin immune Fab (Digibind) for digoxin toxicity. Health Education for the Patient and Family ■ Take your pulse daily before taking your digoxin. Do not take digoxin if your pulse is below 60 bpm or if you are weak, fatigued, lightheaded, dizzy, short of breath, or having chest pain. Instead, notify your healthcare provider immediately. ■ Contact your healthcare provider if you develop manifestations of digitalis toxicity: palpitations, weakness, loss of appetite, nausea, vomiting, abdominal pain, blurred or colored vision, or double vision. ■ Avoid using antacids and laxatives, which decrease digoxin absorption.

Medications *(continued)*

CLASSIFICATION AND DRUG EXAMPLES	MECHANISMS OF ACTION	NURSING CONSIDERATIONS
		■ Notify your healthcare provider immediately if you develop manifestations of potassium deficiency: weakness, lethargy, thirst, depression, muscle cramps, or vomiting. ■ Incorporate potassium-rich foods into your diet: fresh orange or tomato juice, bananas, raisins, dates, figs, prunes, apricots, spinach, cauliflower, and potatoes.
Phosphodiesterase Inhibitors *Drug examples:* Inamrinone (Inocor) Milrinone (Primacor)	Phosphodiesterase inhibitors are used in treating acute heart failure to increase myocardial contractility and cause vasodilation. The net effects are an increase in CO and a decrease in afterload.	■ Use an infusion pump to administer these agents. Monitor hemodynamic parameters carefully. ■ Avoid discontinuing these drugs abruptly. ■ Change solutions and tubing every 24 hours. ■ Inamrinone is given as an IV bolus over 2–3 minutes, followed by an infusion of 5–10 mg · kg^{-1} · min^{-1}. ■ Inamrinone may be infused full strength or diluted in normal or half-strength saline. Do not mix this drug with dextrose solutions. After dilution, inamrinone can be piggybacked into a line containing a dextrose solution. ■ Monitor liver function and platelet counts; inamrinone may cause hepatotoxicity and thrombocytopenia. Health Education for the Patient and Family ■ Notify the healthcare provider if you experience abdominal pain or notice a skin rash or bruising.
Beta-Adrenergic Blockers (Antagonists) Carvedilol (Coreg) Metropolol (Toprol-XL)	These drugs block the cardiac actions of the sympathetic nervous system to slow the heart rate and reduce blood pressure.	■ Abrupt withdrawal is not advised. ■ Monitor BP and pulses.
Vasodilators *Drug examples:* Hydralazine with isosorbide dinitrate (BiDil) Nesiritide (Natrecor) Sacubitril/valsartan (Entresto)	Hydralazine with isosorbide dinitrate relaxes blood vessels and lowers blood pressure. Nesiritide causes vasodilation which contributes to reduced preload. Sacubitril/valsartan inhibits the renin-angiotensin-aldosterone system (RAAS) and increases levels of atrial natriuretic peptides.	■ Monitor BP, peripheral pulses, and urinary output. These drugs may cause severe hypotension. ■ Nesiritide is administered intravenously. ■ Monitor for dysrhythmias. Nesiritide may cause dysrhythmias. ■ Do not use sacubitril/valsartan in pregnant women.

heart failure to slow its progression, reduce manifestations, and prevent cardiac complications.

Beta-Adrenergic Blockers

Beta-adrenergic blockers improve cardiac function in heart failure by inhibiting SNS activity. This prevents the long-term deleterious effects of sympathetic stimulation. Because beta-adrenergic blockers reduce the force of myocardial contraction and may actually worsen symptoms, they are used in low doses. The combination of ACE inhibitors and beta-adrenergic blockers improves patient outcomes.

Diuretics

Patients with symptomatic heart failure often are treated with diuretics, which relieve symptoms related to fluid retention. Diuretics may, however, cause significant electrolyte imbalances and rapid fluid loss. Patients with severe heart failure are often treated with a loop, or high-ceiling, diuretic, such as furosemide (Lasix), bumetanide (Bumex), or torsemide (Demadex). These drugs have rapid onset of action, inhibiting chloride reabsorption in the ascending loop of Henle and thus prompting sodium and water excretion. Their major drawback is their efficacy in promoting diuresis; loss of vascular volume can stimulate the SNS. Thiazide diuretics may be used for patients with less severe manifestations of heart failure. These agents promote fluid excretion by blocking sodium reabsorption in the terminal loop of Henle and the distal tubule.

Vasodilators

Vasodilators relax smooth muscle in blood vessels, causing dilation. Arterial dilation reduces PVR and afterload, reducing myocardial work. Venous dilation reduces venous return and preload. Pulmonary vascular relaxation reduces pulmonary capillary pressure, allowing reabsorption of fluid from interstitial tissues and the alveoli. Vasodilators include nitrates and hydralazine.

Nitrates produce both arterial and venous vasodilation. They may be given by nasal spray or by the sublingual, oral, or IV route. Sodium nitroprusside is a potent vasodilator that may be used to treat acute heart failure. It can cause excessive hypotension, however, so it is often given along with dopamine or dobutamine to maintain the BP. Isosorbide or nitroglycerin ointment may be used in long-term management of heart failure.

In 2005, the FDA approved a new drug for treatment of heart failure in African Americans. This drug, known as BiDil, is a combination of two vasodilators, hydralazine and isosorbide, in fixed doses. BiDil has proven beneficial in extending life, improving heart failure symptoms, and decreasing hospital readmissions related to heart failure. See the Diversity and Culture Feature for more information about heart failure in African American patients.

Cardiac (Digitalis) Glycosides

Cardiac glycosides, sometimes called digitalis glycosides, are used judiciously in symptomatic heart failure. These drugs contain digitalis, which has a positive inotropic effect on the heart, increasing the strength of myocardial contraction by increasing the intracellular calcium concentrations. Digitalis also decreases SA node automaticity and slows conduction through the AV node, increasing ventricular filling time.

Digitalis has a narrow therapeutic index, which means that therapeutic levels are very close to toxic levels. Early manifestations of digitalis toxicity include anorexia, nausea and vomiting, headache, altered vision, and confusion. A number of cardiac dysrhythmias are also associated with digitalis toxicity, including sinus arrest, SVTs and VTs, and high levels of AV block. Low serum potassium levels increase the risk of digitalis toxicity, as do low magnesium and high calcium levels. Older adults are at particular risk for digitalis toxicity.

Digitalis levels may be affected by a number of other drugs. The nurse should check for potential interactions.

Antidysrhythmics

Dysrhythmias are common in patients with heart failure. Although PVCs may be frequent, they are often not associated with an increased risk of VT and fibrillation. Because many antidysrhythmic medications depress left ventricular function, PVCs are frequently left untreated in heart failure. Amiodarone is the drug of choice to treat nonsustained VT, which is associated with a poor prognosis. See the Medication feature on page 1281.

SAFETY ALERT NSAIDs can interfere with the effectiveness of heart failure medications. Nurses should teach patients to avoid NSAIDs whenever possible and to check for NSAIDs in any over-the-counter medications they may use.

Nutrition and Activity

A sodium-restricted diet is recommended to minimize sodium and water retention. Intake is generally limited to 1.5–2 g of sodium per day, a moderate restriction. See the exemplar on

Focus on Diversity and Culture
African American Patients and Heart Failure

African American patients are more likely to experience symptoms of heart failure than patients of other races. In addition, they tend to have more hospital stays related to heart failure and are more likely to die from heart failure than other patients (NHLBI, 2015c). The increased likelihood of heart failure among African Americans is thought to be associated with atherosclerotic risk factors (Roger, 2013). High BP, obesity, and diabetes are other risk factors for heart failure that disproportionately affect African Americans (AHA, 2015k).

African American patients tend to develop heart failure at younger ages, are more likely to have renal insufficiency, and are more likely to have poorly controlled hypertension than other patients with heart failure. In addition, African Americans tend to have lower ejection fractions at diagnosis than other patients. As with the general population, African American patients may present with vascular congestion and pulmonary edema and are often treated with diuretics. They may be treated with other typical heart failure medications as well, but have been shown to respond more favorably to treatment with the vasodilators isosorbide dinitrate and hydralazine than patients of other racial backgrounds (Cuyjet & Akinboboye, 2014). These two drugs are often administered in combination; the medication BiDil is a combination of these medications that is marketed specifically to African American patients.

Discharge planning is especially important. The nurse should teach patients about the importance of diet, exercise, and medication as well as recognition of symptoms and the importance of seeking care in a timely manner (Cuyjet & Akinboboye, 2014).

Fluid and Electrolyte Imbalance in the module on Fluids and Electrolytes for a list of high-sodium foods to avoid and for patient teaching regarding a sodium-restricted diet.

Exercise intolerance is a common early manifestation of heart failure. Activity may be restricted to bedrest during acute episodes of heart failure to reduce cardiac workload and allow the heart to recompensate. Prolonged bedrest and continued activity limitations, however, are not recommended. A moderate, progressive activity program is prescribed to improve myocardial function. Aerobic exercise should be performed 3–7 days per week; each session should include a 10- to 15-minute warm-up period, 20–30 minutes of exercise at the recommended intensity, and a cool-down period. It is important for patients to listen to their bodies by working with the cardiac rehab team in order to develop an awareness of the target heart rate. Flexibility exercises and weight training should be part of the exercise routine.

Surgery

In end-stage heart failure, devices to provide circulatory assistance or surgery may be required. Surgery may be used to treat the underlying cause of failure (e.g., replacement of diseased valves) or improve quality of life. Heart transplantation is currently the only clearly effective surgical treatment for end-stage heart failure; however, its use is limited by availability of donor hearts.

Circulatory Assistance

Devices such as the intra-aortic balloon pump (IABP) or a left-ventricular assist device (LVAD) may be used when the patient is expected to recover or as a bridge to transplantation. Newer devices that will allow longer term support outside the hospital are in the developmental stages. These devices will either serve as a bridge to transplantation or allow the myocardium to heal over an extended period of time.

Cardiac Transplantation

Heart transplantation is the treatment of choice for end-stage heart disease. Approximately 88% of cardiac transplantation patients are living 1-year posttransplantation, and 75% are living 5-years posttransplantation (Mayo Clinic, 2015f).

The most frequently used transplantation procedure leaves the posterior walls of the atria, the superior and inferior venae cavae, and the pulmonary veins of the recipient intact (see **Figure 16–43A** ≫). The atrial walls of the donor heart are then anastomosed to the recipient's atria (see Figure 16–43B), and the donor pulmonary artery and aorta are anastomosed to the recipient vessels (see Figure 16–43C). Care is taken to avoid damaging the sinus node of the donor heart and to ensure integrity of the suture line to prevent postoperative bleeding. Donor organs typically are obtained from young accident victims with no evidence of cardiac trauma.

Nursing care of the patient with a heart transplant is similar to care of the patient with any cardiac surgery. Bleeding is a major concern during the early postoperative period. Chest tube drainage is frequently monitored (initially every 15 minutes), as are the CO, pulmonary artery pressures, and CVP. **Cardiac tamponade** (compression of the heart) can develop, presenting as either a sudden event or a gradual process. Chest tubes are gently milked (not stripped) as needed to maintain patency. Atrial dysrhythmias are relatively common following cardiac transplantation. Temporary pacing wires are placed during surgery because the conduction system may be disrupted by surgical manipula-tion or postoperative swelling. Hypothermia is induced during surgery; postoperatively, the patient is gradually rewarmed over a 1- to 2-hour period. Prevention of rapid rewarming and shivering are important to maintain hemodynamic stability and reduce oxygen consumption. Cardiac function is impaired in up to 50% of transplanted hearts during the early postoperative period. After the transplant procedure, recipients may be placed on a combination of inotropic agents while the donor heart regains energy stores and is able to maintain adequate CO.

Infection and rejection are major postoperative concerns; these are the chief causes of mortality in patients with a transplantation. Rejection may develop immediately after transplantation (a rare occurrence), within weeks to months, or years after the transplantation. Acute rejection usually presents within weeks of the transplantation, developing when the transplanted organ is recognized by the immune system as foreign. Lymphocytes infiltrate the organ, and myocardial cell necrosis can be detected on biopsy. Patients are started on immunosuppression therapy soon after surgery and are maintained on a regimen that typically includes one to three drugs. Although immunosuppressive medications help prevent organ rejection, they impair the patient's defenses against infection. Early postoperative infections commonly are bacterial or fungal. Multiple invasive lines, prolonged ventilator support, and immunosuppressive therapy contribute to the transplant recipient's risk for infection. Infection control interventions are required to prevent healthcare-associated infections. Nursing care should be aimed at reducing exposure to exogenous pathogens, maintaining strict hand hygiene procedures, and instituting neutropenic precautions for those with weakened immune systems.

The donor heart is denervated during the transplant procedure. Lack of innervation by the autonomic nervous system affects the heart rate (usually 90–110 bpm in transplanted hearts) and its response to position changes, stress, exercise, and certain drugs.

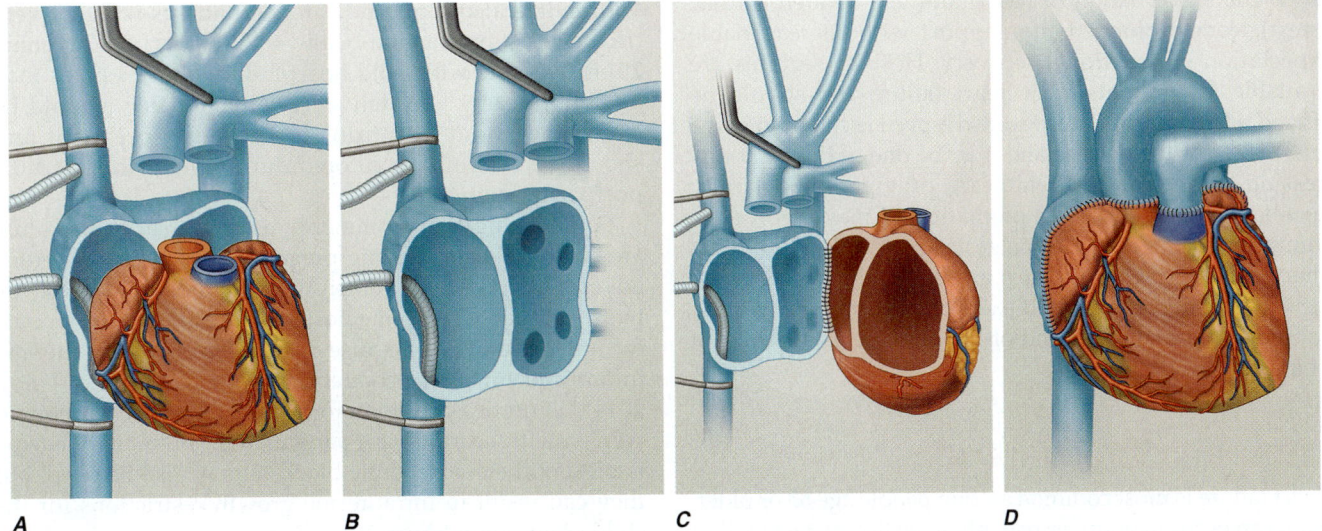

A   **B**   **C**   **D**

Figure 16–43 ≫ Cardiac transplantation. **A,** The heart is removed, leaving the posterior walls of the atria intact. **B,** The donor heart is anastomosed to the atria, **C,** and, **D,** the great vessels.

Other Procedures

Other surgical procedures, such as cardiomyoplasty and ventricular reduction surgery, do not improve the prognosis or quality of life in patients with end-stage heart failure. Cardiomyoplasty involves wrapping the latissimus dorsi muscle around the heart to support the failing myocardium. The muscle is stimulated in synchrony with the heart, providing a more forceful contraction and increasing CO. In ventricular reduction surgery (or partial ventriculectomy), the size of the damaged heart is reduced by excising a portion of the left ventricular wall. This procedure increases the ventricular diameter to a more optimal size. The efficiency of the remaining left ventricle improves, and the failing heart pumps more effectively.

Complementary Health Approaches

Strong evidence supports the use of several complementary health approaches for heart failure. Hawthorn, a shrubby tree, contains natural cardiotonic ingredients in its blossoms, leaves, and fruit. It increases the force of myocardial contraction, dilates blood vessels, and has a natural ACE inhibitor. Studies have shown that adding extract of hawthorn to standard heart failure medications might worsen early disease progression. Hawthorn should not be used without consultation with the primary care provider and experienced herb practitioner. Nutritional supplements of coenzyme Q10, magnesium, and thiamine may be used in conjunction with other treatments. Coenzyme Q10 improves mitochondria function and energy production.

End-of-Life Care

Unless the patient receives a cardiac transplant, chronic heart failure is ultimately a terminal disease. The patient and family need honest discussions about the anticipated course of the disease and treatment options. The nurse should discuss advance directives, such as the living will and healthcare power of attorney, and differentiating potential acute events from which recovery would be anticipated (e.g., a reversible exacerbation of heart failure, a sudden cardiac arrest) from prolonged life support without reasonable expectation of functional recovery. Hospice services are available for patients with heart failure and should be offered when appropriate. Severe dyspnea is common in the final stages of the disease and may be one of the most distressing symptoms for healthcare providers and family members. Treatment is symptomatic and may involve the administration of narcotic analgesic and/or diuretics. Nonpharmacologic measures, such as positioning and decreasing the patient's anxiety and exertion, may also be helpful. For more information on end-of-life care, see the module on Comfort.

Lifespan Considerations

Heart failure is most common among people age 65 or older, but it can occur in younger patients as well. Risk factors that increase the likelihood of heart failure at any age include being overweight, having had a heart attack, and being

African American. Treatment of heart failure depends upon the type and the cause of the condition.

Heart Failure in Children

Children with congenital heart defects may develop heart failure because defects cause the heart to work harder and weaken the muscle. Heart failure in children is typically the result of overcirculation failure or pump failure. In overcirculation failure, an overload blood flow pattern occurs in one or more of the sections of the heart, leading to an interruption in the normal blood flow. As a result, the heart becomes an inefficient pump. Pump failure occurs when one of the heart valves does not function properly, causing pressure to build up inside the heart chambers (AHA, 2015l). In rare circumstances, severe chest trauma may result in pump failure.

Children typically do not have the same symptoms of heart failure or receive the same treatments as adults (NHLBI, 2015c). Symptoms in children include difficulty breathing, excessive sweating, low BP, and poor feeding or growth. If heart failure is the result of overcirculation, surgery may be necessary to repair the defect causing the condition. If heart failure is related to pump failure, valve replacement surgery may be necessary. A pacemaker or mechanical pump may be implanted. Pharmacologic treatments for both causes of heart failure may include diuretics and afterload reducers. Following treatment, the child may experience an improvement in symptoms; this is known as compensated heart failure. Even when a child enters compensated heart failure, the underlying causes may still exist (AHA, 2015l).

Heart Failure in Pregnant Women

During pregnancy, women experience a 30–50% increase in CO and a 40–50% increase in blood volume. Heart rate and SV also increase during pregnancy. For women with heart failure, these increases can lead to decompensation and worsening heart failure. As a result, pregnancy is contraindicated in patients with stage III or stage IV heart failure. It is also contraindicated in patients with left ventricular ejection fraction below 40% (Naderi & Raymond, 2014). Patients with mild heart failure (stage I or II) may be able to carry and deliver a baby, but they should be counseled about risk prior to becoming pregnant and should be carefully monitored during pregnancy and the postpartum period.

Some medications commonly used to treat heart failure are contraindicated during pregnancy because of potential adverse effects on the fetus; ACE inhibitors and ARBs are two examples. Certain medications are also not appropriate for nursing mothers because of their effects on the nursing infant and on milk production (DeCara, Lang, & Foley, 2014). Diuretics are commonly prescribed for pregnant women with heart failure, particularly if pulmonary edema is present. Beta-adrenergic blockers may also be used, but they can result in intrauterine growth restrictions for the child (Anthony & Sliwa, 2015)

Women without a history of heart failure may develop the condition during pregnancy. One common cause of heart failure in pregnancy is peripartum cardiomyopathy (PPCM), discussed in Exemplar 16.A on Cardiomyopathy (DeCara et al., 2014). Preeclampsia, chronic hypertension, and pulmonary hypertension may also lead to heart failure in pregnant patients (Anthony & Sliwa, 2015).

Heart Failure in Older Adults

The diseases that tend to occur in old age can lead to heart failure, and the prevalence of heart failure increases with age. In the United States, heart failure is a leading cause of hospital stays among individuals on Medicare, and older patients with heart failure are more likely to have poor treatment outcomes (Lazzarini et al., 2013; NHLBI, 2015c).

As the heart ages, the number of cardiac cells and the functional capacity of these cells decreases. The remaining cells compensate through hypertrophy. Cardiac function is decreased as a result of these changes. At the same time, older patients tend to experience myocardial fibrosis as a result of changes in the rennin-angiotensin system, enhanced inflammation, and oxidative stress. These changes exacerbate existing cardiac conditions; they can also create problems in patients with no history of cardiac issues (Lazzarini et al., 2015).

Older adults with heart failure typically present with hypertension and pulmonary edema. Symptoms tend to have a gradual onset and are often accompanied by decreased appetite and weight loss. Common symptoms in the general population, such as shortness of breath, may occur but are often attributed to other conditions associated with aging. As a result, older patients with heart failure are less likely than younger patients to be referred to a cardiologist or other specialist for treatment (Lazzarini et al., 2013).

Pharmacologic treatment of older adults with heart failure is similar to that of the general population. There is concern about the efficacy of these treatments because of underrepresentation of older adults in clinical trials for heart failure medications. Drug interactions and nonadherence are also areas of concern with older adults (Lazzarini et al., 2013).

NURSING PROCESS

Health promotion activities to reduce the risk for and incidence of heart failure are directed at lifestyle changes. Offer information about and assistance with smoking cessation and substance abuse recovery. Teach patients about coronary heart disease, the primary underlying cause of heart failure. Discuss risk factors for coronary heart disease and ways to reduce those risk factors with both patients and caregivers.

Hypertension also is a major cause of heart failure. Screen and refer patients with elevated BP to a primary care provider as indicated. Discuss the importance of effectively managing hypertension to reduce the future risk for heart failure. For patients with diabetes, stress the relationship between effective diabetes management and reduced risk for heart failure.

Heart failure affects the patient's quality of life, interfering with such daily activities as self-care and role performance. Reducing the oxygen demand of the heart is a major nursing care goal for the patient in acute heart failure. This includes providing rest and carrying out prescribed treatment measures to reduce cardiac work, improve contractility, and manage symptoms.

Assessment

The nurse should obtain the following subjective and objective data when assessing the patient with heart failure:

- **Observation and patient interview.** Review history of cardiac disease or previous episodes of heart failure. Discuss other risk factors, including hypertension or diabetes. Discuss diet and activity levels, and note activity tolerance and dyspnea with exertion. Note episodes of paroxysmal nocturnal dyspnea and the number of pillows used for sleeping. Discuss recent weight gain or loss, anorexia, or nausea. Review current medications. Observe for shortness of breath, presence of cough, and chest or abdominal pain. Note ease of breathing, conversing, and changing positions.

- **Physical examination.** Assess vital signs, including apical pulse and peripheral pulses. Assess general appearance, note the color of skin and mucous membranes, and observe for neck vein distention. Assess capillary refill. Note the presence and degree of edema. Auscultate heart sounds, breath sounds, and bowel sounds. Palpate the abdomen, noting contour, tenderness, and liver enlargement. Note signs of apparent anxiety.

Diagnosis

Nursing diagnoses appropriate for the patient diagnosed with heart failure may include the following:

- *Cardiac Output, Decreased*
- *Fluid Volume, Excess*
- *Activity, Intolerance*
- *Knowledge, Deficient.*

(NANDA-I © 2014)

Planning

Goals of care for the patient with heart failure often include the following:

- The patient will describe the purpose of each medication prescribed.

- The patient will describe which symptoms to report to the healthcare provider.

- The patient will maintain adequate oxygenation, as demonstrated by respiratory status, breath sounds, oxygen saturation, and vital signs.

- The patient will maintain adequate tissue perfusion and myocardial function, as demonstrated by capillary refill, hemodynamic monitoring, assessment of pulses, and vital signs.

- The patient will meet the body's energy needs through adequate and appropriate nutrition.

Implementation

Nursing care is focused on promoting perfusion, improving oxygenation, and reducing fear and anxiety. A diagnosis of a disorder related to the heart often produces great fear of death and disability in the patient because the heart is vital to life. Helping the patient and family to cope with this fear is an important component of nursing care. Anxiety secondary to hypoxia is also anticipated and requires nursing intervention.

Maintain Cardiac Output

As the heart fails as a pump, SV and tissue perfusion decrease. Nursing interventions to assist patients in maintaining CO include the following:

- Encourage rest, explaining the rationale. Elevate the head of the bed to reduce the work of breathing. Provide a bedside commode, and assist with ADLs. Instruct to avoid the Valsalva maneuver. These measures reduce cardiac workload.

- Monitor the patient's vital signs and oxygen saturation as indicated. Decreased CO stimulates the SNS to increase the heart rate in an attempt to restore output. Tachycardia at rest is common. Diastolic BP may initially be elevated because of vasoconstriction; in late stages, compensatory mechanisms fail and BP falls. Oxygen saturation levels provide a measure of gas exchange and tissue perfusion.

- Monitor the patient's BNP levels, reporting trends. BNP levels indicate the severity of heart failure: As the cardiac index decreases and left ventricular pressures increase, BNP levels increase. Noting trends provides additional information about CO and effectiveness of the cardiac pump.

- Auscultate the patient's heart and breath sounds according to unit policy and clinical indications. The S_1 and S_2 heart sounds may be diminished if cardiac function is poor. A ventricular gallop (S_3) is an early sign of heart failure; an atrial gallop (S_4) may also be present. Crackles are often heard in the lung bases; increasing crackles, dyspnea, and shortness of breath indicate worsening failure.

- Administer supplemental oxygen as ordered. This improves oxygenation of the blood, decreasing the effects of hypoxia and ischemia.

- Administer prescribed medications as ordered. Drugs are used to decrease the cardiac workload and increase the effectiveness of contractions.

Monitor Fluid Volume

As CO falls, compensatory mechanisms cause salt and water retention, increasing blood volume. This increased fluid volume places additional stress on the already failing ventricles, making them work harder to move the fluid load. The nurse should do the following:

- Assess the patient's respiratory status and auscultate lung sounds at least every 4 hours. Notify the healthcare provider of significant changes in condition.

Declining respiratory status indicates worsening left heart failure.

- Monitor the patient's intake and output. Notify the healthcare provider if urine output is less than 30 mL/hr. Weigh the patient around the same time each day. Careful monitoring of fluid volume is important during treatment of heart failure. Diuretics may reduce circulating volume, producing hypovolemia despite persistent peripheral edema. A fall in urine output may indicate significantly reduced CO and renal ischemia. Weight is an objective measure of fluid status: 1 L of fluid is equal to 2.2 lb of weight.

- Record the patient's abdominal girth every shift. Note complaints of a loss of appetite, abdominal discomfort, or nausea. Venous congestion can lead to ascites and may affect gastrointestinal function and nutritional status.

- Monitor and record the patient's hemodynamic measurements. Report significant changes and negative trends. Hemodynamic measurements provide a means of monitoring condition and response to treatment.

- Restrict fluids as ordered. Allow choices of fluid type and timing of intake, scheduling most fluid intake during morning and afternoon hours. Offer ice chips and frequent mouth care; provide hard candies if allowed. Providing choices increases the patient's sense of control. Ice chips, hard candies, and mouth care relieve dry mouth and thirst and promote comfort.

Patient Teaching
Home Care for a Patient with Heart Failure

Heart failure may be a chronic condition requiring active participation by the patient and family for effective management. In preparation for home care, the nurse should discuss the following topics with the patient and the patient's family:

- The disease process and its effects on the patient's life
- Warning signals of cardiac decompensation that require treatment
- Desired and adverse effects of prescribed drugs, monitoring for those effects, and the importance of compliance with drug regimen to prevent acute and long-term complications of heart failure
- Prescribed diet and sodium restrictions, practical suggestions for reducing salt intake, and AHA materials and recipes
- Exercise recommendations to strengthen the heart muscle and improve aerobic capacity (see **Box 16–15 »**)
- The importance of keeping scheduled follow-up appointments to monitor disease progression and effects of therapy.

The nurse should provide referrals for home healthcare and household assistance (shopping, transportation, personal needs, and housekeeping) as indicated. Referrals to community agencies, such as local cardiac rehabilitation programs, heart support groups, or the AHA, can provide the patient and family with additional materials and psychosocial support.

Box 16–15
Home Activity Guidelines for the Patient with Heart Failure

- Perform as many activities as independently as you can.
- Space your meals and activities.
  a. Eat six small meals a day.
  b. Allow time during the day for periods of rest and relaxation.
- Perform all activities at a comfortable pace.
  a. If you get tired during any activity, stop what you are doing and rest for 15 minutes.
  b. Resume activity only if you feel up to it.
- Stop any activity that causes chest pain, shortness of breath, dizziness, faintness, excessive weakness, or sweating. Rest. Notify your healthcare provider if your activity tolerance changes and if symptoms continue after rest.
- Avoid straining. Do not lift heavy objects. To prevent constipation, eat a high-fiber diet and drink plenty of water. Use laxatives or stool softeners, as approved by your healthcare provider, to avoid constipation and straining during bowel movements.
- Begin a graded exercise program. Walking is good exercise that does not require any special equipment (except a good pair of walking shoes). Plan to walk twice a day at a comfortable, slow pace for the first couple of weeks at home, and then gradually increase the distance and pace. Below is a suggested schedule—but progress at your own speed. Take your time. Aim for walking at least three times per week (every other day).

Week 1	200–400 feet	Twice a day, slow and leisurely pace
Week 2	1/4 mile	15 minutes, minimum of three times per week
Weeks 2–3	1/2 mile	30 minutes, minimum of three times per week
Weeks 3–4	1 mile	30 minutes, minimum of three times per week
Weeks 4–5	1 1/2 mile	30 minutes, minimum of three times per week
Weeks 5–6	2 miles	40 minutes, minimum of three times per week

Monitor Activity

Patients with heart failure have little or no cardiac reserve to meet increased oxygen demands. As the disease progresses and cardiac function is further compromised, activity intolerance increases. The low CO and inability to participate in activities may hinder self-care. The nurse should do the following:

- Organize nursing care to allow rest periods. Grouping activities together allows adequate time to "recharge."
- Assist the patient with ADLs as needed. Encourage independence within prescribed limits. Assisting with ADLs helps ensure that care needs are met while reducing cardiac workload. Involving the patient promotes a sense of control and reduces helplessness.

- Plan and implement progressive activities. Use passive and active ROM exercises as appropriate. Consult with the physical therapist on an activity plan. Progressive activity slowly increases exercise capacity by strengthening and improving cardiac function without strain. Activity also helps prevent skeletal muscle atrophy. ROM exercises prevent complications of immobility in patients who are severely compromised.
- Provide written and verbal information about activity after discharge. Written information provides a reference for important information. Verbal information allows clarification and validation of the material. See the Patient Teaching feature for more information.

SAFETY ALERT Patients with unstable stage III or stage IV decompensated heart failure should abstain from sexual activity until their condition is stabilized and well managed.

Provide a Low-Sodium Diet

Diet is an important part of long-term management of heart failure to manage fluid retention. The nurse should do the following:

- Discuss with the patient the rationale for sodium restrictions. Understanding fosters compliance with the prescribed diet.
- Consult with a dietitian to plan and teach a low-sodium and, if necessary for weight control, low-kilocalorie diet. Provide a list of high-sodium, high-fat, high-cholesterol foods to avoid. Provide AHA materials. Dietary planning and teaching increase the patient's sense of control and participation in disease management. Food lists are useful memory aids.

Evaluation

Patient progress toward goals is evaluated on the basis of the following suggested expected outcomes:

- The patient describes each medication prescribed along with the symptoms that should be reported to the provider immediately.
- The patient explains the importance of daily weights and keeping a log, along with the importance of reporting significant weight gain.
- The patient chooses appropriate foods from a menu reflecting a low-sodium diet.
- The patient modifies the daily routine to allow adequate periods of rest and activity.

If patient outcomes are not met, additional education about diet and medication compliance may be necessary. Failure to adhere to treatment regimens can cause rapid changes in the patient's condition and necessitate admittance to the hospital. If the patient is not following dietary restrictions or taking medication properly, the nurse should determine the cause for noncompliance and develop a care plan that addresses these causes.

Nursing Care Plan
A Patient with Heart Failure

Arthur Jackson is a 67-year-old man. One year ago, he had a large anterior wall MI and underwent subsequent coronary artery bypass surgery. On discharge, he was started on a regimen of enalapril (Vasotec), digoxin, furosemide (Lasix), and a potassium chloride supplement. He is now in the cardiac unit complaining of severe shortness of breath, hemoptysis, and poor appetite for 1 week. He is diagnosed with acute heart failure.

ASSESSMENT

Mr. Jackson refuses to settle in bed, preferring to sit in the bedside recliner in the high-Fowler position. He states, "Lately, this is the only way I can breathe." Mr. Jackson states that he has not been able to work in his garden without getting short of breath. He complains of his shoes and belt being too tight.

When you obtain his nursing history, Mr. Jackson insists that he takes his medications regularly. He states that he normally works in his garden for light exercise. In his diet history, he reports eating bacon daily and takeout Chinese food twice this week. He states that he has stopped salting his food but admits he does not know how to track sodium intake.

Mr. Jackson's vital signs are as follows: temperature 97.5°F (36.5°C); pulse 124 bpm and irregular; respirations 28/min and labored; and BP 95/72 mmHg. The cardiac monitor shows atrial fibrillation. An S_3 is noted on auscultation; the cardiac impulse is left of the midclavicular line. Mr. Jackson has crackles and diminished breath sounds in the bases of both lungs. Significant JVD, 3+ pitting edema of feet and ankles, and abdominal distention are noted. Liver size is within normal limits by percussion. Skin is cool and diaphoretic. Chest x-ray shows cardiomegaly and pulmonary infiltrates.

DIAGNOSES

- *Excess Fluid Volume* related to impaired cardiac pump and salt and water retention
- *Activity Intolerance* related to impaired CO
- *Ineffective Health Maintenance* related to lack of knowledge about diet restrictions

(NANDA-I © 2014)

PLANNING

Goals of care include the following:

- The patient will demonstrate loss of excess fluid by weight loss and decreases in edema, JVD, and abdominal distention.
- The patient will demonstrate improved activity tolerance.
- The patient will verbalize understanding of diet restrictions.

IMPLEMENTATION

- Take hourly vital signs and hemodynamic pressure measurements.
- Administer and monitor the effects of prescribed diuretics and vasodilators.
- Weigh the patient daily; strictly monitor the patient's intake and output.
- Monitor the patient for edema.
- Enforce fluid restriction of 1500 mL/24 hr (600 mL day shift, 600 mL evening shift, and 300 mL at night).
- Auscultate heart and breath sounds every 4 hours and as indicated.
- Administer oxygen via nasal cannula at 2 L/min. Monitor oxygen saturation continuously; notify the healthcare provider if it falls below 94%.

- Place the patient in a high-Fowler or other position of comfort.
- Notify the healthcare provider of significant changes in laboratory values or vital signs.
- Teach the patient about all medications and how to take and record pulse.
- Design an activity plan that incorporates preferred activities and scheduled rest periods.
- Instruct the patient about sodium-restricted diet. Let patient select meal choices within allowed limits.
- Consult a dietitian for planning and teaching the patient about a low-sodium diet.

EVALUATION

Mr. Jackson is discharged after 3 days in the cardiac unit. He has lost 8 lb during his stay, and he states that it is much easier to breathe and his shoes fit better. He is able to sleep in the semi-Fowler position with only one pillow. His peripheral edema has resolved. While Mr. Jackson was in the cardiac unit, he and his wife met with a dietitian, who helped them develop a realistic eating plan to limit sodium, sugar, and fats. The dietitian also provided a list of high-sodium foods to avoid. Mr. Jackson is relieved to know that he can still enjoy Chinese food prepared without monosodium glutamate (MSG) or added salt. You and the physical therapist worked together to design a progressive activity plan with Mr. Jackson that he will continue at home. He remains in atrial fibrillation, a chronic condition. His knowledge of digoxin and Coumadin has been assessed and reinforced. You confirm that he is able to accurately check his pulse and can list signs of digoxin toxicity.

CRITICAL THINKING

1. Mr. Jackson's medication regimen remains the same after discharge. What specific teaching does he need related to potential interactions of these drugs?

2. Mr. Jackson tells you, "Talk to my wife about my medications. She's the one in charge now." How would you respond?

3. Design an exercise plan for Mr. Jackson to prevent deconditioning and conserve energy.

4. Mr. Jackson tells you, "Sometimes I forget whether I have taken my aspirin, so I'll take another just to be sure. After all, they are only baby aspirin. One or two extra a day shouldn't hurt, right?" What is your response?

5. Mr. Jackson is admitted to the neuro unit 6 months later with a CVA. What is the probable cause of his stroke?

REVIEW Heart Failure

RELATE Link the Concepts and Exemplars

Linking the exemplar of heart failure with the concept of oxygenation:

1. What is the nursing priority of care for a patient with heart failure and pulmonary edema? Explain your answer.

2. What impact does heart failure have on a patient's oxygenation status if pulmonary edema is not found?

Linking the exemplar of heart failure with the concept of cognition:

3. Why might heart failure induce confusion in the older patient?

4. What teaching would you provide the family of an older patient diagnosed with heart failure who becomes suddenly confused and disoriented?

READY Go to Volume 3: Clinical Nursing Skills

REFER Go to Pearson MyLab Nursing and eText

- Additional review materials

REFLECT Apply Your Knowledge

Dr. Danilo Ocampo is a 74-year-old retired pathologist. He lives in his home with Lydia, his wife of 51 years. Their only child was killed some years ago in a motor vehicle crash. Dr. Ocampo was born and raised in the Philippines and came to the United States when he was 23. He has a few nephews and nieces in the Philippines, but no relatives live nearby.

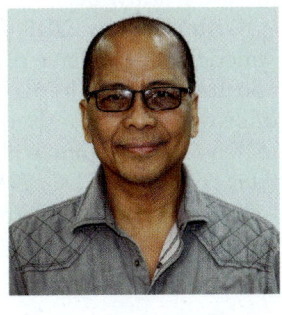

Dr. Ocampo's health has been declining for the past few years. He has a medical history that includes hypertension, MI, angina, and class II heart failure. Because of these cardiovascular disorders, he takes multiple medications, including metoprolol, lisinopril, spironolactone, furosemide (intermittently as needed), potassium supplements (when taking furosemide), aspirin, isosorbide dinitrate, and nitroglycerin. He is concerned his current treatment plan may not be effective; he experiences a number of side effects from his medications and has been admitted multiple times to the hospital. He usually feels better after a few days in the hospital but typically checks himself out of the hospital before his physicians are ready to discharge him.

Dr. Ocampo spends most of his time and energy managing the household and caring for his wife, who has dementia.

1. What interventions can you initiate to help Dr. Ocampo minimize the side effects of the multiple medications he is taking?

2. What nutritional assessment would be appropriate for Dr. Ocampo? Why?

3. Should you intervene to help Dr. Ocampo accept help with the care of his wife to decrease his own stress and improve his health? Explain your answer.

» Exemplar 16.G
Hypertension

Exemplar Learning Outcomes

16.G Analyze hypertension as it relates to perfusion.

- Describe the pathophysiology of hypertension.
- Describe the etiology of hypertension.
- Compare the risk factors and prevention of hypertension.
- Identify the clinical manifestations of hypertension.
- Summarize diagnostic tests and therapies used by interprofessional teams in the collaborative care of an individual with hypertension.

- Differentiate care of patients with hypertension across the lifespan.
- Apply the nursing process in providing culturally competent care to an individual with hypertension.

Exemplar Key Terms

Hypertensive emergency, *1250*
Hypertensive encephalopathy, *1252*
Peripheral vascular resistance (PVR), *1248*
Primary hypertension, *1249*
Secondary hypertension, *1250*
Step-down therapy, *1257*

Overview

In November of 2017, the American College of Cardiology in conjunction with the American Heart Association presented new guidelines for hypertension. The definition of normal blood pressure has been lowered to **less than** 120/80 mmHg. Elevated BP begins when systolic BP rises above 120 mmHg while diastolic is still below 80 mmHg (ACC, 2017). **Table 16–24 »** identifies classifications of BP for adults ages 18 and older.

Hypertension is an important public health issue. Although it rarely causes symptoms or noticeably limits the patient's functional health, hypertension is a major risk factor for coronary heart disease, heart failure, stroke, and renal failure. Hypertension and its consequences are not unique to the United States. The World Health Organization (2013)

TABLE 16–24 Classification of Blood Pressure for Adults (ACC, 2017)

Category	Definition (mmHg)	Examples (mmHg)
Normal	Less than 120/80	112/75
		119/79
Elevated	Systolic from 120–129 *and* diastolic less than 80	125/72
		129/79
Stage 1 hypertension	Systolic from 130–139 *or* diastolic from 80–89	130/79
		129/80
Stage 2 hypertension	Systolic at least 140 *or* diastolic at least 90	135/90
		140/85
Hypertensive crisis	Systolic over 180 *and/or* diastolic over 120	180/90
		165/120

states that hypertension is responsible for approximately 51% of cerebrovascular disease (stroke) and 45% of heart disease worldwide.

With the new 2017 guidelines, well over 80 million American adults have high BP. Although the identification and treatment of hypertension in the United States have improved significantly during the past 18 years, approximately 20% of adults with hypertension remain unaware of their condition (CDC, 2015a). Although 77% of adults with hypertension are being treated for the disorder, effective BP control is achieved in only about 54% (AHA, 2016b).

Pathophysiology and Etiology
Pathophysiology

The factors that affect arterial circulation are blood flow, PVR, and BP. BP is the force exerted against the walls of the arteries by the blood as it is pumped from the heart. It is most accurately referred to as mean arterial pressure (MAP), which denotes the average pressure in the arterial circulation throughout the cardiac cycle. MAP is regulated mainly by CO and PVR, as represented by the formula MAP = CO × PVR. For clinical use, MAP may be estimated by calculating the diastolic BP plus one third of the pulse pressure, or one third of the systolic pressure plus two thirds of the diastolic pressure.

Blood flow refers to the volume of blood transported in a vessel, in an organ, or throughout the entire circulation over a given period. It is commonly expressed as liters or milliliters per minute or as cubic centimeters per second. Blood flow through the circulatory system requires sufficient blood volume to fill the blood vessels and pressure differences within the system to allow blood to move forward. The arterial, or supply, side of the circulation has relatively high pressures created by the thick elastic walls of the arteries and arterioles. The venous, or return, side of the system is a low-pressure system of thin-walled, distensible veins. Blood flows through the capillaries, linking these two systems from the higher pressure arterial side to the lower pressure venous side.

The arterial BP is created by the ejection of blood from the heart during systole (CO) and the tension (resistance to blood flow) created by the elastic arterial walls (SVR). BP rises as the heart contracts during systole, ejecting its blood. This pressure wave is felt as the peripheral pulse and is heard as Korotkoff sounds during BP measurement. In healthy adults, average systolic pressure is less than 120 mmHg. During diastole, elastic arterial walls maintain a minimum pressure to maintain blood flow through the capillary beds. Average diastolic pressure in a healthy adult is less than 80 mmHg.

CO is determined by blood volume and the ability of the ventricles to fill and effectively pump blood. Factors contributing to SVR include vessel length, blood viscosity, and vessel diameter and distensibility (compliance). While vessel length and blood viscosity remain relatively constant, vessel diameter and compliance are subject to normal regulatory activities and disease. These factors also affect **peripheral vascular resistance (PVR)**, which refers to the opposing forces or impedance to blood flow as the arterial channels become more and more distant from the heart. PVR is determined by three factors:

1. **Blood viscosity.** The greater the viscosity, or thickness, of the blood, the greater its resistance to moving and flowing.
2. **Length of the vessel.** The longer the vessel, the greater the resistance to blood flow.
3. **Diameter of the vessel.** The smaller the diameter of a vessel, the greater the friction against the walls of the vessel, leading to greater impedance of blood flow.

Factors Influencing Arterial Blood Pressure

The arterioles normally determine the SVR as their diameter changes in response to a variety of stimuli. These stimuli include the following:

- **Sympathetic nervous system (SNS) stimulation** occurs when baroreceptors in the aortic arch and carotid sinus signal the SNS via the cardiovascular control center in the medulla when MAP changes. A drop in MAP stimulates the SNS, increasing the heart rate and CO and constricting arterioles (except in skeletal muscle). As a result, BP rises. A rise in MAP has the opposite effect, decreasing heart rate and CO and causing arteriolar vasodilation.

- **Circulating epinephrine and norepinephrine** from the adrenal cortex (e.g., the fight-or-flight response) have the same effect as SNS stimulation.

- **Renin-angiotensin-aldosterone system** responds to renal perfusion. A drop in renal perfusion stimulates renin release. Renin converts angiotensinogen to angiotensin I, which is subsequently converted to angiotensin II in the lungs by ACE. Angiotensin II is a potent vasoconstrictor. It also promotes sodium and water retention, both directly and by stimulating the adrenal medulla to release aldosterone. Both SVR and CO increase, raising BP.

- **Atrial natriuretic peptide (ANP) and brain natriuretic peptide (BNP)** are released from atrial cells in response to stretching by excess blood volume. These hormones promote vasodilation and sodium and water excretion, lowering BP.

- **Adrenomedullin** is a peptide synthesized and released by endothelial and smooth muscle cells in blood vessels. It is a potent vasodilator.

- **Vasopressin or antidiuretic hormone (ADH),** from the posterior pituitary gland, promotes water retention and vasoconstriction, raising BP.

- **Local factors,** such as inflammatory mediators and various metabolites, can promote vasodilation, affecting BP.

Other factors that can affect vessel compliance are the extent of arteriosclerosis (hardening of the arteries) and the extent of atherosclerosis (plaque accumulation). **Figure 16–44 ≫** summarizes the interrelationships of major factors regulating BP. The cardiovascular system adapts to increased blood volume by increasing CO. Autoregulatory mechanisms in the systemic arteries react to the increased volume, causing vasoconstriction. The increased SVR causes hypertension.

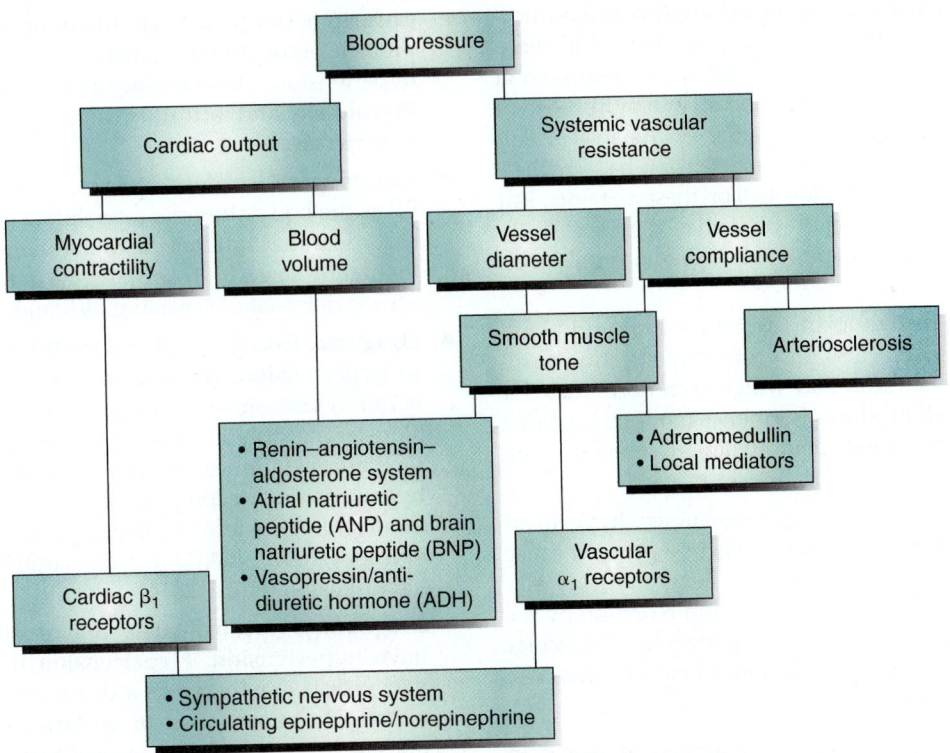

Figure 16–44 ≫ Factors affecting blood pressure.

Blood flow, PVR, and BP, which influence arterial circulation, are in turn influenced by various factors. These factors include the following:

- The sympathetic and parasympathetic nervous systems are the primary mechanisms that regulate BP. Stimulation of the SNS exerts a major effect on peripheral resistance by causing vasoconstriction of the arterioles, thereby increasing BP. Parasympathetic stimulation causes vasodilation of the arterioles, lowering BP.

- Baroreceptors and chemoreceptors in the aortic arch, carotid sinus, and other large vessels are sensitive to pressure and chemical changes and cause reflex sympathetic stimulation, resulting in vasoconstriction, increased heart rate, and increased BP.

- The kidneys help maintain BP by excreting or conserving sodium and water. When BP decreases, the kidneys initiate the renin-angiotensin mechanism. This stimulates vasoconstriction, resulting in the release of the hormone aldosterone from the adrenal cortex, increasing sodium ion reabsorption and water retention. In addition, pituitary release of ADH promotes renal reabsorption of water. The net result is an increase in blood volume and a consequent increase in CO and BP.

- Temperatures may also affect peripheral resistance: Cold causes vasoconstriction, whereas warmth produces vasodilation. Many chemicals, hormones, and drugs influence BP by affecting CO and/or PVR. For example, epinephrine causes vasoconstriction and increased heart rate; prostaglandins dilate blood vessel diameter (by relaxing vascular smooth muscle); endothelin, a chemical released by the inner lining of vessels, is a potent vasoconstrictor;

nicotine causes vasoconstriction; and alcohol and histamine cause vasodilation.

- Dietary factors, such as intake of salt, saturated fats, and cholesterol, elevate BP by affecting blood volume and vessel diameter.

- Race, gender, age, weight, time of day, position, exercise, and emotional state may also affect BP. These factors influence the arterial pressure. Systemic venous pressure, though it is much lower, is also influenced by such factors as blood volume, venous tone, and right atrial pressure.

Primary Hypertension

Primary hypertension, formerly known as essential hypertension, is a persistently elevated systemic BP. Approximately 70 million individuals in the United States have hypertension (CDC, 2015a). More than 90% of these individuals have primary hypertension, which has no identified cause (Madhur et al., 2014).

Primary hypertension is thought to develop from complex interactions among factors that regulate CO and SVR. These interactions may include:

- Excess SNS with overstimulation of alpha- and beta-adrenergic receptors, resulting in vasoconstriction and increased CO.

- Altered function of the renin-angiotensin-aldosterone system and its responsiveness to factors such as sodium intake and overall fluid volume. The renin-angiotensin-aldosterone system affects vasomotor tone as well as salt and water excretion. Chronically high levels of angiotensin II lead to arteriolar remodeling, which permanently increases SVR. In approximately 25% of individuals with primary hypertension, renin levels are lower than normal. Increased sodium intake increases the BP in these patients. Low plasma renin levels are more often seen in people of Sub-Saharan African ancestry than in those of European, North African, or Southwest Asian descent. Another 15% of patients with hypertension have higher-than-normal plasma renin levels. For these patients, salt intake has less of an effect on BP (Sahay & Sahay, 2012). Most individuals with hypertension have normal levels of renin activity.

- Other chemical mediators of vasomotor tone and blood volume, such as ANP, also play a role by affecting vasomotor tone and sodium and water excretion. Vascular endothelium itself produces hormones (endothelins) that also affect vasomotor tone. Endothelin-1 is a potent vasoconstrictor (Weil et al., 2012).

- The interaction between insulin resistance, hyperinsulinemia, and endothelial function may be a primary cause of hypertension. Excess insulin has several effects that may contribute to hypertension: sodium retention by the kidneys, increased SNS activity, hypertrophy of vascular smooth muscle, and changes in ion transport across cell membranes (Park et al., 2013).

The result of these interactions is sustained increases in blood volume and peripheral resistance. The cardiovascular system adapts to increased blood volume by increasing CO. Autoregulatory mechanisms in the systemic arteries react to the increased volume, causing vasoconstriction. The increased SVR causes hypertension.

It is unlikely that one single cause and pathologic process accounts for essential hypertension. Increasing evidence points to hypertension as a group of pathophysiologic mechanisms resulting in the common manifestation of elevated BP.

Secondary Hypertension

Secondary hypertension is elevated BP resulting from an identifiable underlying process. It accounts for only 5–10% of identified cases of hypertension. The pathophysiology of selected causes of secondary high BP can be summarized as follows:

- *Kidney disease.* Any disease that affects renal blood flow (e.g., renal artery stenosis) or renal function (e.g., glomerulonephritis, renal failure) can lead to hypertension. Disruption of the blood supply stimulates the renin-angiotensin-aldosterone system, with resulting vasoconstriction as well as sodium and water retention. Altered kidney function affects the elimination of water and electrolytes, leading to hypertension.

- *Coarctation of the aorta.* Coarctation of the aorta is narrowing of the aorta, usually just distal to the subclavian arteries. Reduced renal and peripheral blood flow stimulates the renin-angiotensin-aldosterone system and local vasoconstrictive responses, raising the BP. A marked difference between pressures in the upper and lower extremities is common, with weak pulses and poor capillary refill in the lower extremities.

- *Endocrine disorders.* Adrenal gland disorders, such as Cushing syndrome and primary aldosteronism, can cause hypertension. A rare tumor of the adrenal medulla, pheochromocytoma, causes persistent or intermittent hypertension. Other endocrine disorders, such as hyperthyroidism and pituitary disorders, also can lead to hypertension.

- *Neurologic disorders.* Increased ICP causes an elevated BP as the body attempts to maintain cerebral blood flow. Disorders that interfere with autonomic nervous system regulation (e.g., high spinal cord injury) may allow the SNS to dominate, increasing SVR and BP.

- *Drug use.* Estrogen and oral contraceptive use may lead to hypertension, possibly by prompting sodium and water retention and affecting the renin-angiotensin-aldosterone system. Stimulant drugs, such as cocaine and methamphetamines, increase SVR and CO, resulting in hypertension. Decongestants, estrogen and other hormones, corticosteroids, cyclosporine, antidepressants, and long-term NSAID use also contribute to secondary hypertension (Hurd, 2014).

- *Pregnancy.* Approximately 10% of all pregnant women have hypertension. Hypertension may predate pregnancy, or it may occur as a direct response to the pregnancy. The mechanism of gestational hypertension is unclear. It is a significant cause of maternal and fetal morbidity and mortality, and it requires careful perinatal management. (See Exemplar 16.H on Hypertensive Disorders of Pregnancy for more information.)

- *Hypothyroidism.* Twenty to forty percent of patients with hypothyroidism have hypertension. Thyroid hormone is a smooth muscle relaxant; therefore, hypothyroidism may lead to increased vascular resistance as well as increases in serum norepinephrine and aldosterone and decreases in endothelial relaxation factor production. Hypothyroidism is also associated with CAD.

- *Obstructive sleep apnea.* Sleep apnea has an adverse effect on the autonomic nervous system, as shown by increased levels of plasma catecholamines. The incidence and degree of hypertension is directly proportional to the frequency and severity of apneic episodes. Sleep apnea also interrupts the normal pattern of BP reduction during sleep.

The pattern of secondary hypertension varies depending on its cause. Pheochromocytoma may cause attacks of hypertension that last for minutes to hours, accompanied by anxiety, palpitations, diaphoresis, pallor, and nausea and vomiting. Primary aldosteronism may cause hypertension, weakness, paresthesias, polyuria, and nocturia. Symptoms of kidney disease accompany hypertension when a renal disorder is the cause.

Hypertensive Crisis

Some patients with hypertension may develop rapid, significant elevations in systolic and/or diastolic pressures. The reasons for this are not clearly understood. In a **hypertensive crisis** (also called *malignant hypertension* or *hypertensive emergency*), systolic pressure is greater than 180 mmHg, and/or diastolic pressure is higher than 120 mmHg. Immediate treatment (within 1 hour) is vital to prevent cardiac, renal, and vascular damage and reduce morbidity and mortality. Intense cerebral artery spasms help protect the brain from excess pressure; however, cerebral edema often develops. Prolonged severe hypertension damages walls of the arterioles and renal blood vessels and may lead to intravascular coagulation and acute renal failure.

Etiology

Hypertension primarily affects middle-age and older adults: More than 65% of individuals ages 65–74 and over 70% of those age 75 and older have hypertension (CDC, 2015a). An age-related increase in the systolic BP is the primary factor leading to the high incidence of hypertension in older adults. Unlike the diastolic BP, which tends to rise until approximately age 50 and then decline, the systolic BP continues to rise with age (Vishram et al., 2012).

The prevalence of hypertension is significantly higher in Black patients than in White and Hispanic patients. Over 43% of Black adults have hypertension, whereas fewer than 34% of adult White and Hispanic individuals are affected. More White men than White women have hypertension; in Black and Hispanic patients, more women than men are affected (CDC, 2015a). Native Americans and Alaska Natives are also at high risk for hypertension-related illnesses. This population is 1.3 times as likely as White adults to have high BP (Office of Minority Health, 2015). Essential hypertension affects individuals of all income groups, having great financial effects because of its effects on other body systems.

Risk Factors

A number of risk factors have been identified for primary hypertension (see **Box 16–16**). Genes play a role, as do environmental factors. In addition, men, African Americans, smokers, older adults, pregnant women with preeclampsia, and individuals with collagen or renal disease are at higher risk for a hypertensive emergency. Most hypertensive emergencies occur when patients suddenly stop taking their medications or their hypertension is poorly controlled.

Box 16–16
Factors Contributing to Hypertension

Modifiable Factors
- High sodium intake
- Low potassium, calcium, and magnesium intake
- Obesity
- Excess alcohol consumption
- Insulin resistance
- Low activity level
- Hypothyroidism
- Low vitamin D levels
- Depression
- Tobacco use

Nonmodifiable Factors
- Genetic factors
- Age
- Family history
- Race

Specific risk factors for hypertension include the following:

- **Family history.** Studies show a genetic link in approximately one third of individuals diagnosed with primary hypertension. Genes involved in the renin-angiotensin-aldosterone system and other genes that affect vascular tone, salt and water transportation in the kidney, obesity, and insulin resistance likely are involved in the development of hypertension, although no consistent genetic linkages have been found.

- **Age.** The incidence of hypertension rises with increasing age. Aging affects baroreceptors involved in BP regulation as well as arterial compliance. As the arteries become less compliant, pressure within the vessels increases. This is often most apparent as a gradual increase in the systolic pressure with aging.

- **Race.** Primary hypertension is more common and more severe in African Americans than in individuals of other ethnic backgrounds (AHA, 2015k; 2015m). It also tends to develop at an earlier age and is associated with more cardiovascular and renal damage. More African Americans with hypertension have low renin levels and altered renal excretion of sodium at normal BP levels. This genetic tendency to conserve salt may have developed as an adaptation to harsh environmental conditions, where salt and water conservation are beneficial (Williams et al., 2014).

- **Mineral intake.** High sodium intake often is associated with fluid retention. Hypertension related to sodium intake involves a number of different physiologic mechanisms, including the renin-angiotensin-aldosterone system, nitric oxide, catecholamines, endothelin, and ANP (Copstead & Banasik, 2013). Low potassium, calcium, and magnesium intakes also contribute to hypertension by unknown mechanisms. The ratio of sodium to potassium intake appears to play a role, possibly through the effects of increased potassium intake on sodium excretion. Potassium also promotes vasodilation by reducing responses to catecholamines and angiotensin II. Calcium has a vasodilator effect as well. Although magnesium has been shown to reduce the BP, its mechanism of action is unclear.

- **Obesity.** Central obesity (fat cell deposits in the abdomen), as determined by an increased waist-to-hip ratio, has a stronger correlation with hypertension than does BMI or skinfold thickness. Although a clear correlation exists between obesity and hypertension, the relationship may be one of common cause. Genetic factors appear to play a role in the common triad of obesity, hypertension, and insulin resistance.

- **Insulin resistance.** Insulin resistance with resulting hyperinsulinemia is linked with hypertension through its effects of excess circulating insulin on the SNS, vascular smooth muscle, renal regulation of sodium and water, and ion transport across cell membranes. Insulin resistance may be a genetic or acquired trait. Although more commonly seen in individuals who are obese, insulin resistance also has been found in individuals of normal weight.

- **Excess alcohol consumption.** Regular consumption of three or more drinks a day increases the risk of hypertension. Decreasing or discontinuing alcohol consumption reduces the BP, particularly systolic readings. Lifestyle factors associated with excessive alcohol intake (obesity and lack of exercise) may contribute to hypertension as well.

- **Stress.** Physical and emotional stress cause transient elevations of BP, but the role of stress in primary hypertension is less clear. BP normally fluctuates throughout the day, increasing with activity, discomfort, or emotional responses such as anger. Stress activates angiotensin II, part of the renin-angiotensin system; angiotensin II then contributes to vasoconstriction and vascular smooth muscle hypertrophy (Girouard, 2016).
- **Physical inactivity.** Regular exercise is proven to reduce BP.
- **Vitamin D deficiency.** Current research demonstrates an association between decreased vitamin D levels and hypertension (Vitamin D Council, 2014).
- **Depression.** Hypertension is more common in individuals with depression and other personality traits such as impatience and hostility.

Prevention

Prevention of hypertension involves healthy lifestyle choices and habits (see Box 16–2). Patients with prehypertension should take steps to avoid progressing to high BP and to follow their treatment regimens. Strategies include maintaining a healthy weight and a healthy diet with reduced salt intake, engaging in regular physical activity, using stress management techniques, following medication regimens, and avoiding baths that are too hot (AHA, 2015n; NHLBI, 2015c).

Patients diagnosed with high BP should obtain regular medical care and follow their prescribed treatment plan. Healthy lifestyle habits can prevent high BP from occurring, can reverse prehypertension and help control existing hypertension, or can prevent the complications and long-term problems associated with this hypertension (NHLBI, 2015c).

Clinical Manifestations

The early stages of primary hypertension typically are asymptomatic, marked only by elevated BP. BP elevations initially are transient but eventually become permanent. When symptoms do appear, they are usually vague. Headache, generally in the back of the head and neck, may be present on awakening, subsiding during the day. Other symptoms result from target organ damage and may include nocturia, confusion, nausea and vomiting, and visual disturbances. Examination of the retina of the eye may reveal narrowed arterioles, hemorrhages, exudates, and papilledema (swelling of the optic nerve). The Clinical Manifestations and Therapies feature lists the etiology and clinical manifestations of life-threatening hypertension along with recommended treatments.

Sustained hypertension affects the cardiovascular, neurologic, and renal systems. The rate of atherosclerosis accelerates, increasing the risk for coronary heart disease and stroke. The workload of the left ventricle increases, leading to ventricular hypertrophy, which then increases the risk for coronary heart disease, dysrhythmias, and heart failure. Diastolic BP is a significant cardiovascular risk factor until age 50; systolic pressure then becomes the more important factor contributing to cardiovascular risk (AHA, 2015o). More than 360,000 American deaths in 2013 included hypertension as a primary or contributing cause (CDC, 2015j).

Accelerated atherosclerosis associated with hypertension increases the risk for cerebral infarction (stroke). Increased pressure in the cerebral vessels can lead to development of microaneurysms and an increased risk for cerebral hemorrhage. **Hypertensive encephalopathy**, a syndrome characterized by extremely high BP, altered LOC, increased ICP, papilledema, and seizures, may develop. Its etiology is unclear.

Clinical Manifestations and Therapies
Hypertension

ETIOLOGY	CLINICAL MANIFESTATIONS	CLINICAL THERAPIES
Hypertensive crisis	- Rapid onset - Blurred vision - Papilledema - Systolic pressure greater than 180 mmHg and/or diastolic pressure greater than 120 mmHg - Headache, confusion, motor or sensory deficits	- Administer medications: vasodilators, CCBs, ACE inhibitors, or adrenergic blockers. - BP should be lowered gradually to prevent shock. - Monitor patient's BP continuously. - Reduce patient anxiety, which can cause BP to rise. - Teach the importance of maintaining treatment for hypertension.
Stroke	- Sudden onset of loss of sensation and/or movement; may be hemiplegia, hemiparesis, flaccidity, spasticity, or sensory loss of vision, hearing, taste, touch, proprioception, or smell	- Monitor patient's LOC. - Administer medications: anticoagulants, thrombolytics, corticosteroids, or antihypertensives. - Prepare for surgery: carotid endarterectomy, extracranial–intracranial bypass, or carotid angioplasty. - Reduce patient's ICP to prevent further damage.

Hypertension also can lead to nephrosclerosis and renal insufficiency. Proteinuria and microscopic hematuria develop, as do signs of chronic renal failure. African Americans experience hypertensive kidney disease more frequently than Caucasians. Hypertension is a major contributor to end-stage renal disease.

Patients presenting with a hypertensive emergency may have manifestations such as headache, confusion, swelling of the optic nerve (papilledema), blurred vision, restlessness, and motor and sensory deficits. Manifestations of hypertensive emergencies are listed the Clinical Manifestations and Therapies feature.

Collaboration

Although primary hypertension cannot be cured, it can be controlled. Management focuses on reducing BP to less than 130 mmHg systolic and 80 mmHg diastolic. The ultimate goal of hypertension management is to reduce cardiovascular and renal morbidity and mortality. The risk of cardiovascular complications (coronary heart disease, heart failure, and stroke) decreases when the average BP is less than 130/80 mmHg; when the patient also has diabetes or renal disease, the treatment goal is a BP of less than 129/79 mmHg. Most individuals with hypertension require a combination of two or more drugs along with lifestyle changes to achieve recommended BP levels (Mayo Clinic, 2015b). **Figure 16–45** ≫ illustrates collaborative care for patients with hypertension.

SAFETY ALERT Isometric exercise (e.g., weight training) may not be appropriate for individuals with hypertension, because it can raise the systolic BP.

Diagnostic Tests

The patient with hypertension is evaluated for the presence of identifiable causes of hypertension, cardiovascular risk factors, and the presence or absence of target organ damage. Before treatment is started, the following diagnostic tests are performed: ECG, urinalysis, blood glucose, hematocrit, serum creatinine, vitamin D, calcium, and cholesterol and lipoprotein profile, including HDL, LDL, and triglycerides.

Additional tests may include urinary albumin excretion, evaluation of the glomerular filtration rate (e.g., creatinine clearance), and tests for emerging cardiovascular risk factors, such as C-reactive protein and homocysteine levels. Also, the following diagnostic tests may be ordered to differentiate primary from secondary hypertension:

- ***Renal function studies and urinalysis*** can identify renal causes of hypertension. Elevated serum creatinine and BUN; reduced creatinine clearance; and hematuria, proteinuria, and casts often indicate kidney disease.

- ***The serum potassium level*** is decreased in hyperaldosteronism.

- ***Blood chemistries,*** including serum electrolytes, glucose, and lipid studies, can detect abnormalities indicative of endocrine or cardiovascular disease.

- ***IV pyelography, renal ultrasonography, renal arteriography, and CT or MRI*** tests are conducted when secondary hypertension is suspected.

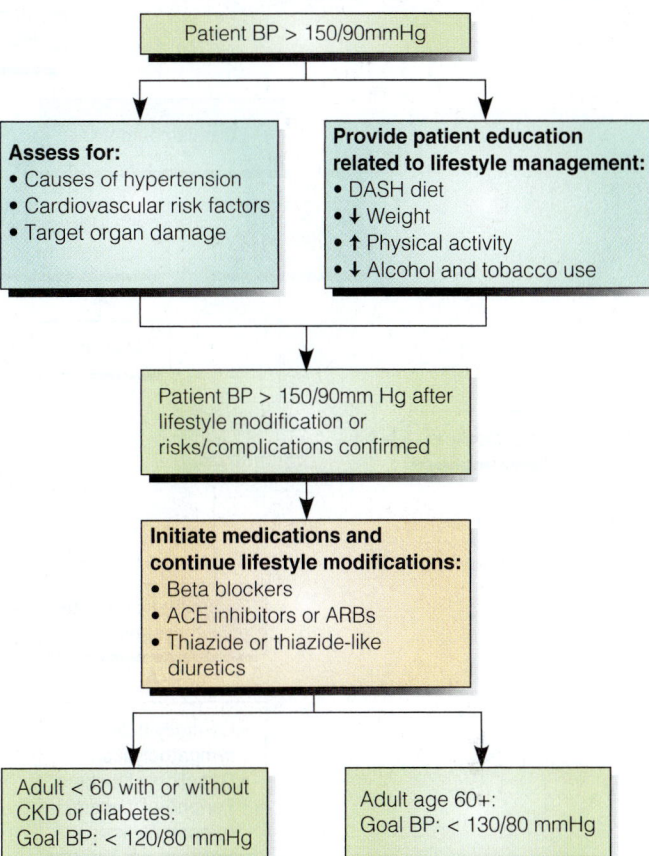

Sources: Based on American Heart Association. (2016). *Changes you can make to lower your blood pressure.* Retrieved from: http://www.heart.org/HEARTORG/Conditions/HighBloodPressure/Prevention-TreatmentofHighBloodPressure/Prevention-Treatment-of-High-Blood-Pressure_UCM_002054_Article.jsp# ; James, P. A., Oparil, S., Carter, B. L., Cushman, W. C., Dennison-Himmelfarb, C., Handler, J., . . . Ortiz, E. (2014). 2014 Evidence-based guideline for the management of high blood pressure in adults: Report from the panel members appointed to the Eighth Joint National Committee (JNC 8). *JAMA*, 311(5), 507–520.

Figure 16–45 ≫ Collaborative treatment of hypertension in adults.

Pharmacologic Therapy

Current pharmacologic treatment of hypertension involves using one or more of the following drug classes: diuretics, alpha-adrenergic blockers, beta-adrenergic blockers, alpha-2 adrenergic agonists, direct vasodilators, ACE inhibitors, ARBs, and CCBs (see the Medications feature). For most patients, two or more antihypertensive drugs selected from different drug classes are necessary to achieve effective control. These drug classes have different sites of action (see **Figure 16–46** ≫).

Drug Classes

Diuretics are the preferred treatment for systolic hypertension in older adults. Diuretics are relatively safe and well tolerated, and most are relatively inexpensive. Thiazide diuretics, such as hydrochlorothiazide (HydroDIURIL), are widely used. In major clinical studies, treatment with diuretics alone or in combination with other antihypertensives reduced systolic BP by 10–15 mmHg and diastolic BP by

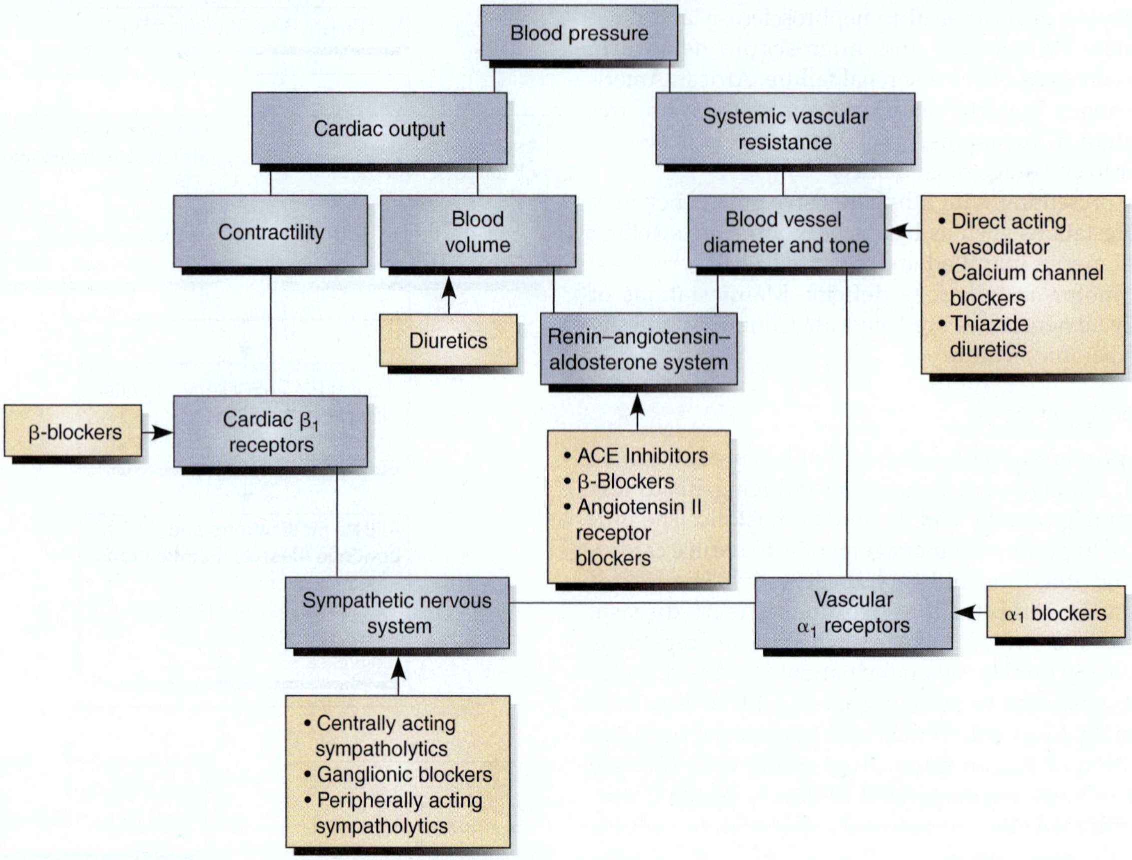

Figure 16–46 》 Sites of antihypertensive drug action.

5–10 mmHg; diuretics also reduced hypertension-linked morbidity and mortality related to coronary heart disease and stroke (Tamargo, Segura, & Ruilope, 2014). Diuretics control hypertension primarily by preventing tubular reabsorption of sodium, thus promoting sodium and water excretion and reducing blood volume. Thiazide diuretics also reduce SVR through an unknown mechanism. Diuretics are particularly effective in African Americans and in patients who are obese, are older, or have increased plasma volume or low renin activity. The adverse effects of diuretics generally are dose related. In addition to hypokalemia, diuretics may affect serum levels of glucose, triglycerides, uric acid, LDLs, and insulin.

SAFETY ALERT Patients who are prescribed potassium-sparing diuretics or ACE inhibitors for hypertension should not use salt substitutes. These substitutes often substitute potassium for sodium, which could result in hyperkalemia.

Patients with heart failure, coronary heart disease, or diabetes may initially be treated with a beta-blocker. These drugs lower BP, apparently by reducing PVR. They may also reduce the amount of renin released by the kidneys by blocking beta$_1$-receptors in the kidney. Beta-adrenergic blockers reduce the risk of complications such as heart failure and stroke.

SAFETY ALERT Beta blockers are contraindicated for patients with asthma or COPD because they promote bronchial constriction.

The ACE inhibitors and ARBs also are commonly used in the initial treatment of hypertension, particularly for patients with diabetes or heart failure, a history of MI, or chronic kidney disease. ACE inhibitors block formation of angiotensin II by inhibiting the action of ACE. Angiotensin II is a potent vasoconstrictor that also stimulates aldosterone release from the adrenal gland; blocking its action prevents vasoconstriction and sodium and water retention resulting from aldosterone release. ARBs have a very similar effect, although their action is to block angiotensin II receptors, thus preventing its vasoconstrictive and volume expansion effects.

Several drug classes work through their ability to promote vasodilation and reduce peripheral vascular resistance (PVR). Alpha$_1$-adrenergic blockers, such as prazosin and terazosin, block stimulation of alpha$_1$-receptors on arterioles and veins, preventing vasoconstriction. Because of their ability to dilate both arterioles and veins, alpha$_1$-adrenergic blockers can cause significant orthostatic hypotension, particularly following the initial dose. Calcium channel blocker (CCBs) promote dilation of arterioles, the primary regulators of PVR. These drugs can cause reflex tachycardia. Some CCBs (verapamil and diltiazem in particular) also suppress heart function, reducing SV and CO. Reflex tachycardia is minimal with these CCBs. Direct vasodilators, such as hydralazine and minoxidil, also directly affect the arterioles, reducing PVR. These drugs have little effect on veins, so the risk of orthostatic hypotension is minimal. They are, however, associated with reflex tachycardia and fluid retention, so they are rarely administered in single-drug treatment regimens.

Medications
Hypertension

CLASSIFICATION AND DRUG EXAMPLES	MECHANISMS OF ACTION	NURSING CONSIDERATIONS

Alpha-Adrenergic Blockers
 	
Drug examples:
Doxazosin (Cardura)
Prazosin (Minipress)
Terazosin (Hytrin)
	These drugs block alpha-receptors in vascular smooth muscle.
	    They decrease vasomotor tone and vasoconstriction.
	    These drugs reduce serum levels of LDLs and VLDLs.
		▪ Monitor patient for orthostatic hypotension, tachycardia, and palpitations.
		▪ Give first dose at bedtime to minimize "first-dose" syncope.
		▪ Encourage patient to change positions slowly.
		▪ Instruct patient to notify care provider if nasal congestion or impotence develops.
		▪ Notify primary care provider before discontinuing medication.

Angiotensin-Converting–Enzyme (ACE) Inhibitors *Drug examples:* Benazepril (Lotensin) Captopril (Capoten) Enalapril (Vasotec) Fosinopril (Monopril) Lisinopril (Prinivil, Zestril) Ramipril (Altace) Perindopril (Aceon)	These drugs lower BP by preventing conversion of angiotensin I to angiotensin II. They prevent vasoconstriction and sodium and water retention.	▪ Monitor patient for "first-dose" syncope, persistent cough, hyperkalemia. ▪ These drugs are less effective in African American patients. ▪ Report changes in WBC count, differential, serum potassium, BUN, or serum creatinine. ▪ These drugs are contraindicated in renal artery stenosis and pregnancy. ▪ Monitor patient for angioedema. ▪ Encourage patient to change positions slowly. ▪ Administer orally 1 hour before meals.
Angiotensin Receptor Blockers (ARBs) *Drug examples:* Losartan (Cozaar) Valsartan (Diovan)	These drugs block vasoconstriction and promote relaxation of blood vessels, thereby lowering BP.	▪ Monitor patient for headache, dizziness, orthostatic hypotension, rash, and diarrhea. ▪ Monitor patient for angioedema. ▪ Encourage patient to change positions slowly. ▪ These drugs are contraindicated in pregnancy.
Beta-Adrenergic Blocking Agents *Drug examples:* Acebutolol (Sectral) Atenolol (Tenormin) Metoprolol (Lopressor) Nadolol (Corgard) Propranolol (Inderal) *May be combined with alpha-adrenergic blocking agent:* Carvedilol (Corgard) Labetalol (Trandate)	These drugs reduce BP by preventing beta-receptor stimulation in the heart, resulting in decreased heart rate and CO. They interfere with renin release by kidneys, decreasing the effects of angiotensin and aldosterone.	▪ Monitor patient for bronchospasm, fatigue, sleep disturbances, nightmares, bradycardia, heart block, worsening heart failure, gastrointestinal disturbances, impotence, and increased triglyceride levels. ▪ These drugs are contraindicated in asthma, chronic lung disease, bradycardia, or heart block. ▪ Assess BP and apical pulse prior to administration. ▪ Report vital signs outside of parameters prior to administration. ▪ Encourage patient to change positions slowly. ▪ Notify physician of shortness of breath, cough, or extremity swelling. ▪ Do not discontinue without discussing with physician.
Calcium Channel Blockers (CCBs) *Drug examples:* Amlodipine (Norvasc) Diltiazem (Cardizem) Felodipine (Plendil) Isradipine (DynaCirc) Nicardipine (Cardene) Nifedipine (Procardia) Nisoldipine (Sular) Verapamil (Isoptin)	These drugs inhibit flow of calcium ions across the cell membrane of vascular tissue and cardiac cells. They relax arterial smooth muscle, lowering peripheral resistance through vasodilation.	▪ Monitor patient for impaired cardiac function and worsening heart failure. ▪ Prior to administration, assess BP, apical pulse, and liver and renal function. ▪ Do not administer verapamil or diltiazem to patients with severe hypotension or sinus or AV blocks. ▪ Administer with caution in patients also taking digoxin or a beta-blocker. ▪ Monitor vital signs and report bradycardia, AV block, or heart failure to primary care provider. ▪ These drugs may cause constipation. Patient should adjust diet as needed. ▪ Encourage patient to report shortness of breath, weight gain, or extremity swelling to primary care provider.

(continued on next page)

Medications *(continued)*

CLASSIFICATION AND DRUG EXAMPLES	MECHANISMS OF ACTION	NURSING CONSIDERATIONS
Alpha-2 Adrenergic Agonists *Drug examples:* Clonidine (Catapres) Guanfacine (Tenex) Methyldopa (Aldomet)	These drugs stimulate the alpha$_2$-receptors in the central nervous system to suppress sympathetic outflow to the heart and blood vessels. They decrease CO and vasodilation, reducing BP.	■ Severe reflex hypertension may occur if medication is abruptly discontinued. ■ Dry mouth and sedation are common adverse effects. ■ Clonidine is contraindicated in pregnancy. ■ Methyldopa is contraindicated for patients with active liver disease. ■ Obtain baseline vital signs, CBC, Coombs test, and liver function studies. ■ Administer oral doses at bedtime to minimize effects of sedation. ■ Promptly report lab value changes to physician. ■ Discontinue methyldopa if manifestations of liver dysfunction develop. ■ Take with meals to avoid gastrointestinal upset. ■ Do not discontinue or skip doses. ■ Report signs of depression or decreased mental acuity. ■ Encourage the patient to avoid driving if medication causes drowsiness.
Direct Vasodilators *Drug examples:* Hydralazine (Apresoline) Minoxidil (Loniten)	These drugs reduce BP by relaxing vascular smooth muscle and decreasing PVR. They are often prescribed in combination with a diuretic or beta-blocker because they can cause reflex tachycardia and fluid retention.	■ Monitor vital signs prior to administration. ■ Report peripheral edema and symptoms of volume overload and heart failure. ■ Immediately report muffled heart sounds or paradoxic pulse. Pericardial effusion and possible cardiac tamponade may develop with minoxidil therapy. ■ Discontinue hydralazine if lupus-like manifestations occur. ■ Encourage patient to change positions slowly. ■ Headache, palpitations, and rapid pulse may develop but should subside within 10 days. ■ Minoxidil may cause excess hair growth.
Thiazide Diuretics *Drug example:* Hydrochlorothiazide	These drugs prevent tubular reabsorption of sodium, promoting sodium and water excretion and reducing blood volume. They reduce SVR.	■ These drugs are the preferred treatment for systolic hypertension in older adults. ■ They are effective in African American patients. ■ Adverse effects tend to be dose related. ■ Monitor patient for hypokalemia.

Loop Diuretics
 	
Drug example:
Furosemide (Lasix)
	These drugs inhibit sodium and chloride reabsorption from the loop of Henle.
	    They act on kidneys to increase urine flow.
	    They may be used alone or in conjunction with other antihypertensives.
		■ Monitor patient for hyponatremia, hypokalemia, or hypomagnesemia.
		■ Encourage patient to change positions slowly.

Potassium-Sparing Diuretics *Drug example:* Spironolactone (Aldactone)	These receptor antagonists cause water and sodium excretion by the kidneys.	■ Monitor patient for skin rash, headache, dizziness, and gastrointestinal upset.

Other factors considered in selecting drugs for treating hypertension include demographic characteristics, concurrent conditions, quality of life, cost, and possible drug interactions. In general, diuretics and CCBs are more effective for treating hypertension in African Americans than beta-adrenergic blockers or ACE inhibitors. Beta-adrenergic blockers are preferred to treat hypertension with concurrent coronary heart disease and angina but are contraindicated for patients who have asthma or depression. Beta-adrenergic blockers also reduce exercise tolerance and may adversely affect lifestyle for some patients.

Drug Regimens

Treatment usually is initiated by using a single antihypertensive drug at a low dose. Unless otherwise indicated, a diuretic is recommended as the initial drug of choice. The dose is slowly increased until optimal BP control is achieved. If the drug does not effectively lower the BP or has troubling side effects, a different drug from another class of antihypertensive medications is substituted. If, on the other hand, the drug is tolerated well but does not lower BP to the desired level, a second drug from another class may be added to the treatment regimen.

Treatment of patients with stage 2 hypertension generally is more aggressive to minimize the risk of MI, heart failure, or stroke. When the patient's systolic BP is over 160 or diastolic BP is over 100, immediate therapy (and possible hospitalization) is vital.

After a year of effective hypertension control, an effort may be made to reduce the dosage and number of drugs. This is known as **step-down therapy**. It is more successful in patients who have made lifestyle modifications (see the Focus on Integrative Health feature). Careful BP monitoring is necessary during and after step-down therapy because BP often rises again to hypertensive levels.

Lifestyle Modifications

Lifestyle modifications are recommended for all patients whose BP falls within the elevated range (120–129/ <80 mmHg) and for everyone with intermittent or sustained hypertension. These modifications include weight loss, dietary changes, restricted alcohol use and cigarette smok-

---

Box 16–17
DASH Diet Recommendations

- Grains: 6–8 servings per day
- Vegetables: 4–5 servings per day
- Fruits: 4–5 servings per day
- Fat-free or low-fat milk and milk products: 2–3 servings per day
- Meats, poultry, and fish: 6 or fewer servings (1 oz each) per day
- Nuts, seeds, and legumes: 4–5 servings per week
- Fats and oils: 2–3 servings per day
- Sweets and added sugars: 5 or fewer servings per week (should be low in fat)

---

ing, increased physical activity, and stress reduction (see Box 16–2 in the Concept of Perfusion section).

Dietary approaches to managing hypertension focus on reducing sodium intake, maintaining adequate potassium and calcium intakes, and reducing total and saturated fat intake. A mild to moderate sodium restriction (no added salt) lowers BP and potentiates the effect of antihypertensive drugs for most patients. The DASH (Dietary Approaches to Stop Hypertension) diet has proven beneficial in lowering BP. This diet (see **Box 16–17**) focuses on whole foods rather than individual nutrients. It is rich in fruits and vegetables (up to 10 servings per day) and is low in total and saturated fats.

Complementary health approaches that assist individuals in reducing feelings of distress or anxiety may have some benefit in lowering BP. The nurse should encourage patients to notify their primary care providers before adding any new complementary health approaches. See the Focus on Integrative Health feature for additional information.

Lifespan Considerations

Hypertension is found in patients of all ages, especially as the U.S. population continues to become more obese. Age can play a significant role in the development and management of hypertension. Pregnancy also has several risk factors for the development of hypertension, and these factors are discussed in Exemplar 16.H.

Hypertension in Children and Adolescents

A child's normal BP changes during development (see **Table 16–25**). The risk for developing prehypertension and hypertension has been on the rise for children and adolescents, possibly due to a corresponding increase in obesity in this population (NHLBI, 2015d). Prehypertension is defined as having a BP that is between the 90th and 95th percentiles for the child's age, height, and sex. Hypertension is then defined as having a BP above the 95th percentile. Any child with a BP reading higher than 120/80 mmHg is also given a diagnosis of high BP, even if the BP is below the 90th percentile (Rodriguez-Cruz, 2015).

Physicians often overlook the problem of hypertension in children and adolescents even though hypertension in this

---

Focus on Integrative Health
Complementary Health Approaches for Lowering Blood Pressure

Behavioral and mind–body therapies may be helpful for some patients in lowering BP. BP increases in response to physiologic and psychologic stress and anxiety. Mind–body therapies, such as yoga and tai chi, meditation, and guided imagery, are designed to modify both physiologic and cognitive aspects of the stress response. In a study of older African American men and women with moderate hypertension, transcendental meditation was shown to reduce BP. Eastern exercises such as yoga and tai chi are gaining popularity as a means to reduce SNS activity. These treatments have not been fully explored but do not appear to be harmful. However, they should not replace a healthcare provider's advice regarding medication and aerobic exercise.

TABLE 16–25 Normal Blood Pressure in Children and Adolescents

Age	Systolic Blood Pressure (mmHg)	Diastolic Blood Pressure (mmHg)
Newborn (at birth)	50–70	30–45
Newborn (at day 10)	90	50
Infant (age 1)	Boys: 80–89 Girls: 83–90	Boys: 34–39 Girls: 38–42
Toddler (age 2)	Boys: 84–92 Girls: 85–91	Boys: 39–44 Girls: 43–47
Preschooler (age 4)	Boys: 88–97 Girls: 88–94	Boys: 47–52 Girls: 50–54
School age (age 9)	Boys: 95–104 Girls: 96–103	Boys: 57–62 Girls: 58–61
Adolescent (age 15)	Boys: 109–117 Girls: 107–113	Boys: 61–66 Girls: 64–67

population is increasing (Riley & Bluhm, 2012). Children should have their BP checked on a regular basis beginning at age 3 (NHLBI, 2015d). Regular BP readings in children are essential because hypertension in individuals in this group typically has no symptoms, although it can cause subtle changes in behavior and school performance (International Pediatric Hypertension Association [IPHA], 2016). When taking a BP reading in children, the nurse should use an appropriately sized cuff. The width of the rubber bladder should cover at least 40% of the child's upper arm from the olecranon to the acromion, and the length of the bladder should cover 80–100% of the circumference of the child's arm (Rodriguez-Cruz, 2015).

Hypertension in children can be either primary or secondary. Primary hypertension is often associated with obesity, a family history of hypertension, or diabetes mellitus. Secondary hypertension is often associated with kidney, heart, or endocrine abnormalities. Primary hypertension is often found in older children and adolescents, whereas secondary hypertension is often found in younger children. In contrast to adults, children have a lower risk of heart attack and stroke associated with hypertension, although if hypertension persists into adulthood, these risks increase. Childhood hypertension is often treated with lifestyle modifications, although children with stage 2 hypertension or hypertension that is not controlled by lifestyle changes may be prescribed medication (Mayo Clinic, 2015g). Clinical support for use of ACE inhibitors, ARBs, and CCBs is most prevalent (Rodriguez-Cruz, 2015).

Hypertension in Older Adults

BP tends to rise with age, so the risk for developing hypertension increases with age, with high BP affecting approximately 65% of Americans age 60 or older (NHLBI, 2015d). This increase in BP is typically caused by blood vessels losing flexibility with age (AHA, 2014a). Until age 45, a greater percentage of men have hypertension than women, but these percentages even out between the genders from age 45 to 64, after which point a greater percentage of women expe-

rience hypertension than men (AHA, 2014a; Mayo Clinic, 2015b). Because systolic BP continues to increase with age but diastolic BP does not, many older adults develop isolated systolic hypertension, in which the systolic BP is in the hypertensive range but the diastolic blood is normal (National Institute on Aging [NIA], 2015).

Treatment of older adults with antihypertensive medications should be closely monitored. Taking the wrong dose of medication at this age increases the risk of fainting or falling due to orthostatic hypotension. Falling can have devastating consequences in older adults. Complications related to polypharmacy may also occur in older adults, including an increased risk of kidney failure and death in patients who take a combination of an ACE inhibitor and an ARB. Therefore, treatment must be carefully adjusted to avoid any adverse effects in older adults, especially in patients with isolated systolic hypertension. Diuretics are the preferred treatment for older adults with hypertension; CCBs may also be beneficial.

NURSING PROCESS

Health promotion teaching and activities focus on modifiable risk factors for hypertension. The nurse should advise all patients (as well as children and adolescents) to stop smoking or never start. The nurse should discuss the risks of obesity, excess alcohol intake, and a sedentary lifestyle with patients. In addition, the nurse should encourage all patients to eat a diet rich in fruits and vegetables and low in total and saturated fat. The nurse can discuss the potential benefits of following the DASH diet or a similar eating plan. The nurse should advise all patients to remain active and engage in aerobic exercise 5 days or more each week and discuss the stress-reducing benefits of exercise. The nurse should also offer BP screening and refer patients for follow-up. The Patient Teaching feature lists topics for the nurse to cover in discussions about controlling a patient's hypertension.

Assessment

The nurse should obtain the following information during focused assessment of the patient with hypertension:

- **Observation and patient interview.** Individuals with hypertension often have no observable signs or symptoms. Therefore, the assessment of hypertension should focus on the patient interview and physical examination. Assess patients for complaints of morning headache or cervical pain; cardiovascular or central nervous system manifestations; history of hypertension, renal disease, or diabetes; family history of high BP, heart failure, or kidney disease; and current medications.

- **Physical examination.** The physical examination should start with a measure of vital signs, including BP in both arms as well as apical and peripheral pulses. The physical exam may also include an ophthalmologic exam of the retinal fundus as appropriate.

Diagnosis

Nursing diagnoses that may apply to the patient with primary hypertension include the following:

- *Health Maintenance, Ineffective*
- *Noncompliance*

Patient Teaching
Control of Hypertension

Effective control of hypertension requires the patient not only to participate in the plan of care but also to take an active role in managing the disease. Include the following topics when teaching the patient and family about hypertension:

- Specific lifestyle changes recommended for the patient and suggestions for implementing them, such as the following:
  a. Increase activity gradually. Develop a realistic exercise program that is enjoyable and fits into the individual's lifestyle.
  b. Adopt healthy eating patterns, following a low-fat, low-cholesterol, moderate-sodium diet that also is rich in fruits and vegetables and includes at least two servings of low-fat milk or milk products daily.
  c. Stop smoking. Participating in organized smoking cessation programs or using aids such as nicotine patches can help.
  d. Use alcohol in moderation, if at all, consuming no more than 1.5 oz of hard liquor, 5–10 oz of wine, or 12–20 oz of beer per day.

- e. Use stress-reducing techniques, such as meditation, relaxation, deep breathing, and exercise, to manage stress.
- Prescribed medications, their intended effect, dose and timing, interactions, and possible adverse effects. Discuss effects that should be reported to the healthcare provider and those that can be managed by the patient or that will diminish over time.
- The importance of monitoring BP and regular visits to the healthcare provider or hypertension clinic to monitor treatment. During follow-up visits, assess the patient's BP and specific laboratory work (e.g., serum creatinine, BUN, serum electrolytes) to evaluate the disease and the effects of antihypertensive medications.

Refer the patient to a dietitian or an organized weight loss program as indicated for further teaching and weight loss support.

- *Nutrition, Readiness for Enhanced*
- *Fluid Volume: Excess.*

(NANDA-I © 2014)

Planning

Goals of nursing care for the patient with primary hypertension include the following:

- The patient will describe lifestyle choices that can prevent, reduce, or resolve hypertension.
- The patient's BP will remain within the acceptable range for age and condition.
- The patient will reduce sodium consumption.
- The patient will maintain fluid balance.
- The patient will verbalize understanding of medication regimen and potential side effects.

Implementation

Primary nursing interventions for the patient with primary hypertension are aimed at preventing hypertension through patient teaching. Secondary interventions are aimed at controlling BP to prevent complications.

Promote Health Maintenance

When hypertension has been identified in a patient, knowledge about the disease and its management is vital for the patient. The patient's willingness to take responsibility for hypertension management is central to effective BP control. Adopting healthy lifestyle changes enhances drug therapy; in some cases, the need for medications may be eliminated or reduced. Because hypertension is often an asymptomatic disease and many antihypertensive drugs have unpleasant side effects, it is vital that the patient understand the chronic progressive nature of the

disease and its long-term consequences. The nurse's role in this process includes the following:

- Assist the patient in identifying current behaviors that contribute to hypertension. Using knowledge of hypertension risk factors, the nurse can help identify behaviors and factors contributing to hypertension that can be changed. Including the family in this process is important to reduce potential sabotage of the patient's efforts to adopt healthier behaviors.
- Assist the patient in developing a realistic health maintenance plan. Guide the patient in developing realistic goals and expectations for the treatment plan and for modifying risk factors such as smoking, exercise, diet, and stress.
- Help the patient and family identify strengths and weaknesses in maintaining health. Discussing areas of the health maintenance plan that are working well and those that present difficulties can help identify necessary changes in the plan and additional strategies for implementing it.

Promote Adherence

Failure to follow the identified treatment plan is a continuing risk for any patient with a chronic disease. Recommended lifestyle changes, such as diet, exercise, restricted alcohol intake, stress reduction, and smoking cessation, often are difficult to maintain on a continuing basis. In addition, prescribed medications may have undesirable effects, whereas hypertension itself often has no symptoms or noticeable effects. If a patient is not following the treatment plan, the nurse can take the following steps:

- Inquire about reasons for not adhering to the recommended treatment plan. Listen openly and without judging. Nonthreatening discussion of factors contributing to nonadherence validates the patient's self-esteem and partnership in the treatment plan.

■ Evaluate knowledge regarding hypertension, its long-term effects, and treatment. Provide additional information, and reinforce teaching as needed.

■ Assist the patient to develop realistic short-term goals for lifestyle changes. Smaller, gradual changes are more easily incorporated into lifestyle and daily activities, improving compliance.

■ Help the patient identify cues and develop reminders (e.g., written notes, medication box filled weekly) to assist with maintaining a schedule for exercise and medications.

■ Reassure the patient that relapse into old habits and behaviors is common. Encourage the patient to avoid feelings of guilt associated with relapse and to use the circumstance to renew efforts to comply with treatment.

Promote Balanced Nutrition

The relationship between obesity, excess alcohol intake, and hypertension is well documented. Hypertension is particularly associated with central obesity, identified by waist circumference greater than hip circumference. Although weight loss is difficult and takes commitment to changing both eating and exercise habits, most patients can achieve it. The nurse can assist in this effort by doing the following:

■ Assess the patient's usual daily food intake, and discuss with the patient possible contributing factors to excess weight, such as a sedentary lifestyle or using food as a reward or stress reliever. Inquire about diversional activities, exercise patterns, and previous weight reduction efforts (e.g., participation in weight reduction programs, using fad or crash diets). This provides direction for further teaching and for developing a realistic weight reduction plan.

■ Help the patient determine a realistic target weight (e.g., loss of 10% of current body weight over a 6-month period). Regularly monitor the patient's weight. Encourage a system of nonfood rewards for achieving small, incremental goals. Continuous incremental weight loss provides reassurance that the goal can be achieved and promotes permanent weight reduction.

■ Refer the patient to a dietitian for information about low-fat, low-calorie foods and eating plans. Focus on changing eating habits rather than "following a diet," as this promotes the sense that low-fat, low-calorie eating patterns should become a part of the patient's lifestyle rather than a short-term measure to be endured until the weight loss goal is achieved.

■ Recommend that the patient participate in an approved weight loss program such as Weight Watchers, Overeaters Anonymous, or Take Off Pounds Sensibly (TOPS). Organized programs provide structure for balanced weight reduction as well as mutual support.

Maintain Fluid Volume

Excess fluid volume often contributes to hypertension by increasing CO. A number of factors associated with hypertension can cause excess fluid volume, including sodium retention and disruption of the renin-angiotensin-aldosterone system. In addition, some antihypertensive drugs, such as CCBs and vasodilators, can contribute to excess fluid in the interstitial spaces and peripheral edema. The nurse should do the following:

■ Monitor the patient's intake and output, and weigh the patient daily (if in an acute or long-term care facility) or weekly (in the community). Rapid weight changes (over days) more accurately reflect fluid balance than intake and output records do. Weight changes and intake and output records help in monitoring the effects of therapy.

■ Monitor the patient for peripheral edema (sacral edema in the patient who is bedridden). Drugs such as vasodilators can cause fluid accumulation in interstitial tissues, leading to peripheral or dependent edema. Adding a diuretic to the treatment plan may be necessary.

■ Discuss the relationship between sodium intake and fluid retention. Refer the patient to a dietitian for teaching about a restricted sodium diet. Support the patient's efforts, and reassure the patient that lifestyle changes, such as consuming less sodium, take time.

■ Discuss the importance of adhering to treatment plans, such as dietary restrictions and medication schedules. Understanding the rationale for treatment measures promotes the patient's sense of control and encourages compliance with the treatment regimen.

Evaluation

Evaluation of the effectiveness of patient care may be based on the following expected outcomes:

■ The patient describes strategies for maintaining normal BP, including exercising, quitting smoking, losing weight, and managing stress.

■ The patient describes expected actions of medications, side effects to report to the healthcare provider, and the importance of taking medication every day.

■ The patient demonstrates accurate performance of BP monitoring and maintains a log of readings to share with the healthcare provider.

■ The patient demonstrates the ability to choose foods that are low in sodium.

If initial nursing interventions, lifestyle modifications, and medications do not decrease BP, the nurse can advocate for a change in medication, a combination of medications, and additional nonpharmacologic strategies. Many patients with uncontrolled hypertension fail to adhere to diet and exercise changes, so the nurse can provide additional patient teaching and recommend support groups that will help the patient remain accountable for making dietary and activity changes.

Nursing Care Plan
A Patient with Hypertension

Margaret Spezia is a married, 49-year-old woman with eight children whose ages range from 7 to 18 years. For the past 2 months, Mrs. Spezia has had frequent morning headaches as well as occasional dizziness and blurred vision. At her annual physical examination 1 month ago, her BP was 168/104 and 156/94 mmHg. She was instructed to reduce her fat and cholesterol intake, to avoid using salt at the table, and to start walking for 30–45 minutes daily. Mrs. Spezia returns to the clinic for follow-up.

ASSESSMENT

While escorting Mrs. Spezia to the exam room and obtaining her weight, BP, and history, Lisa Christos, RN, notices that Mrs. Spezia seems restless and upset. Nurse Christos says, "You look upset about something. Is everything OK?" Mrs. Spezia responds, "Well, my head is throbbing, and I'm sort of dizzy. I think I'm just overdoing it and not getting enough rest. You know, raising eight children is a lot of work and expense. I just started working part-time so we wouldn't get behind in our bills. I thought the extra money might relieve some of my stress, but I'm not so sure that's really happening. I'm not getting any better, and I'm worried that I'll lose my job or become disabled and that my husband won't be able to manage the children by himself. I really need to go home, but first, I want to get rid of this awful headache. Would you please get me a couple of aspirin or something?"

Mrs. Spezia's history shows a steady weight gain during the past 18 years. She has no known family history of hypertension. Physical findings include the following: height 63 in. (160 cm); weight 225 lb (102 kg); temperature 99°F (37.2°C); pulse 100 bpm and regular; respirations 16/min; and BP 180/115 mmHg (lying), 170/110 mmHg (sitting), and 165/105 mmHg (standing). Her skin is cool and dry, with capillary refill of 4 seconds in the right hand and 3 seconds in the left hand. Mrs. Spezia's total serum cholesterol is 245 mg/dL (normal: less than 200 mg/dL). All other blood and urine studies are within normal limits. Based on analysis of the data, Mrs. Spezia is started on amlodipine, 20 mg, and benazepril, 5 mg and is placed on a low-fat, low-cholesterol, no-added-salt diet.

DIAGNOSES

- *Fatigue* related to effects of hypertension and stresses of daily life
- *Obesity* related to excessive food intake
- *Ineffective Health Maintenance* related to inability to modify lifestyle
- *Deficient Knowledge* related to effects of prescribed treatment

(NANDA-I © 2014)

PLANNING

Goals of care include the following:

- The patient will reduce her BP readings to less than 140 mmHg systolic and 90 mmHg diastolic by the return visit next week.
- The patient will incorporate into her diet low-sodium and low-fat foods from a list provided.
- The patient will develop a plan for regular exercise.
- The patient will verbalize understanding of the effects of the prescribed drug, dietary restrictions, exercise, and follow-up visits to help control hypertension.

IMPLEMENTATION

- Teach the patient to take her own BP daily and record it, bringing the record to scheduled clinic visits.
- Teach the patient the name, dose, action, and side effects of her antihypertensive medication.
- Instruct the patient to walk for 15 minutes each day this week and to investigate swimming classes at the local pool.
- Discuss strategies for achieving a realistic weight loss goal.
- Refer the patient to a dietary consultation for further teaching about fat and sodium restrictions.
- Discuss stress-reducing techniques, helping identify possible choices.

EVALUATION

Mrs. Spezia returns to the clinic 1 week later. Her average BP is now 148/88 mmHg. She has lost 0.7 kg (1.5 lb) and states that her oldest daughter has suggested they join a weight reduction program together. Mrs. Spezia is walking for an average of 20 minutes at a local mall each day. She verbalizes an understanding of her medication and is taking it before dinner each day. She met with the dietitian and discussed ways to reduce the sodium and fat in her diet.

The dietitian provided a list of low-fat, low-sodium foods and recommended cookbooks to help Mrs. Spezia modify her cooking. Mrs. Spezia tells Ms. Christos, "I just can't believe how much better I feel already. My headaches are gone, and I've actually lost some weight—and I feel motivated to keep going. If I had only known how much better I could feel! I don't expect I'll ever go back to my old habits again; it's just not worth it!"

CRITICAL THINKING

1. Identify the factors that contributed to Mrs. Spezia's hypertension. Which were modifiable, and which were not?

2. What is the rationale for reducing sodium and fat in Mrs. Spezia's diet?

3. Suppose your patient with hypertension is homeless and has no source of income. How could you help ensure your patient would follow the treatment plan? What would you do if the patient did not follow it?

4. Discuss the role of stress in hypertension. What factors in Mrs. Spezia's life contribute to her stress level?

5. Develop a plan of care for the nursing diagnosis Situational Low-Self Esteem related to obesity.

REVIEW Hypertension

RELATE Link the Concepts and Exemplars

Linking the exemplar of hypertension with the concept of metabolism:

1. Create a plan of care, including nutrition, for the patient diagnosed with both hypertension and type 2 diabetes mellitus.

2. You receive a call from a patient who has been diagnosed with hypertension and diabetes mellitus. He is asking what over-the-counter medications would be safe to take to treat a mild upper respiratory infection (a cold). How will you respond to this question?

Linking the exemplar of hypertension with the concept of fluid and electrolytes:

3. Explain the impact hypertension has on urinary elimination.

4. What teaching will you provide the patient diagnosed with hypertension to reduce this impact on the renal system?

READY Go to Volume 3: Clinical Nursing Skills

REFER Go to Pearson MyLab Nursing and eText

- Additional review materials

REFLECT Apply Your Knowledge

Melinda Genmar is a 42-year-old woman with primary hypertension. She is married to Tom, who has a 17-year-old son, Paul, from a previous marriage. The Genmars have two children together, Sabrina, 14, and Charlie, 3. Mr. Genmar runs his own business installing sprinkler systems, and Mrs. Genmar is a real estate agent and home inspector. She spends a great deal of time in her car showing houses and taking the kids to their various after-school activities.

Mrs. Genmar's mother has type 2 diabetes; her father is fairly healthy. Mrs. Genmar has been prescribed several different antihypertensives, but her BP remains elevated. She recently was placed on captopril 50 mg twice a day, which seems to be maintaining her BP within acceptable limits.

1. What precautions would you teach Mrs. Genmar regarding captopril in conjunction with her lifestyle?

2. If you admitted Mrs. Genmar to the provider's office before captopril was prescribed, what interview questions would you want to explore in order to determine lifestyle factors that may be contributing to her continued hypertension?

3. What nutritional recommendations will you make to Mrs. Genmar to help her control her hypertension?

≫ Exemplar 16.H
Hypertensive Disorders of Pregnancy

Exemplar Learning Outcomes

16.H Analyze hypertensive disorders of pregnancy as they relate to perfusion.

- Describe the pathophysiology of hypertensive disorders of pregnancy.
- Describe the etiology of hypertensive disorders of pregnancy.
- Compare the risk factors and prevention of hypertensive disorders of pregnancy.
- Identify the clinical manifestations of hypertensive disorders of pregnancy.
- Summarize diagnostic tests and therapies used by interprofessional teams in the collaborative care of an individual with a hypertensive disorder of pregnancy.
- Differentiate care of patients with hypertensive disorders of pregnancy across the lifespan.
- Apply the nursing process in providing culturally competent care to an individual with a hypertensive disorder of pregnancy.

Exemplar Key Terms

Chronic hypertension, *1262*
Eclampsia, *1262*
Gestational hypertension, *1262*
HELLP syndrome, *1263*
Preeclampsia, *1262*
Superimposed preeclampsia, *1263*

Overview

Hypertension is the most common medical disorder among pregnant women and one of the major causes of pregnancy-related maternal deaths in the United States. Hypertension is said to complicate up to 1 in 10 pregnancies and affects an estimated 240,000 women in the United States each year (Mustafa et al., 2012). Elevated BPs and the results of the disease process in pregnancy can cause harm to both the mother and fetus and range in severity from minor complications to death.

The National High Blood Pressure Education Program (NHBPEP) classifies hypertensive disorders of pregnancy as follows: chronic hypertension, gestational hypertension, preeclampsia-eclampsia, and preeclampsia superimposed on chronic hypertension (NHBPEP, 2000). The diagnosis of **chronic hypertension** is based on a known history of hypertension prior to pregnancy, hypertension that is discovered during the pregnancy prior to 20 weeks' gestation, or hypertension that persists for more than 12 weeks postpartum. **Gestational hypertension** occurs in the second half of pregnancy in a previously normotensive mother. The diagnosis is made when the patient has a BP greater than or equal to 140/90 mmHg on at least two occasions that are at least 6 hours apart, after 20 weeks' gestation (King et al., 2015). **Preeclampsia** is defined according to the same criteria as gestational hypertension, accompanied by signs of end organ damage (see the Clinical Manifestations feature). **Eclampsia** is preeclampsia with the presence of seizures. Preeclampsia superimposed onto chronic hypertension (**superimposed preeclampsia**) occurs when a woman previously diagnosed with chronic hypertension develops hypertension-related end organ dysfunction in pregnancy or worsening hypertension that is resistant to treatment (August & Sibai, 2015).

Preeclampsia occurs in 3–7% of all pregnancies (U.S. National Library of Medicine, 2014c). Preeclampsia continues to be a major cause of maternal mortality, preterm births, perinatal death, and intrauterine growth restriction (Mayo Clinic, 2014g).

Pathophysiology and Etiology

Pathophysiology

Hypertension affects roughly 10% of pregnancies and may be either chronic (preexisting) or gestational. Gestational hypertension develops after 20 weeks' gestation and may persist through the 6-week postpartum period. Women who experience gestational hypertension are at greater risk for developing chronic hypertension later in life.

Hypertension may progress to preeclampsia in 3–7% of pregnancies. Early signs of preeclampsia include high BP and evidence of protein in the urine. Additional symptoms include swelling of the face, eyes, or hands and sudden weight gain of more than 0.9 kg (2 lb) per week. As preeclampsia progresses, more severe symptoms become evident. These include persistent headache, right-sided abdominal or shoulder pain, irritability, decreased urine output, nausea and vomiting, and vision changes. Preeclampsia is potentially fatal. Eclampsia, a serious complication of preeclampsia, is characterized by one or more seizures during pregnancy or the postpartum period. Accompanying severe epigastric pain may indicate hepatic involvement, which is commonly associated with **HELLP syndrome**. The characteristics of HELLP are hemolysis (H), elevated liver enzymes (EL), and low platelet count (LP). The most common reasons for critical illness and death related to eclampsia are stroke or rupture of the mother's liver.

The cure for preeclampsia is to deliver the baby by either induction or cesarean section. If the baby has not reached a safe gestational age, the mother may be monitored in the hospital and given medications to control her BP. When the mother has severe preeclampsia or eclampsia, the baby's well-being is threatened, and the baby must be delivered.

Etiology

The exact cause of preeclampsia is unknown. However, it has been identified as a disorder of placental dysfunction leading to a syndrome of endothelial dysfunction with associated vasospasm. Research has demonstrated abnormal placental development or placental damage from diffuse microthrombosis as playing a role in the development of maternal hypertension. An altered maternal immune response to fetal/placental tissue may also contribute to preeclampsia (Carson, 2014).

The vasculature of normal pregnant women typically demonstrates a decreased response to vasoactive peptides, such as angiotensin II and epinephrine, whereas women with preeclampsia demonstrate hyperresponsiveness to the same hormones. BPs may be labile in preeclampsia.

Research suggests that inadequate trophoblast invasion during formation of the placenta leads to incomplete remodeling of the uterine spiral arteries and placental hypoxia. The poorly perfused placenta then releases increased amounts of vasoactive factors, leading to a widespread activation of the maternal endothelium that, ultimately, results in elevated maternal BP, increased vascular permeability, vasospasm, and coagulopathies. The clinical manifestations and sequelae of preeclampsia are a result of vasospasm and increased permeability of the blood vessels (August & Sibai, 2015).

HELLP Syndrome

HELLP syndrome is most often related to severe preeclampsia and usually occurs as a complication of preeclampsia. However, in some documented cases, HELLP syndrome has occurred without a diagnosis of preeclampsia. Differential diagnoses include hepatitis, gallbladder disease, or idiopathic/thrombocytopenic purpura (ITP). HELLP syndrome is a multisystem disorder that is resolved only with delivery of the baby and placenta.

The hemolysis that occurs in HELLP syndrome is a microangiopathic hemolytic anemia. As RBCs pass through small, damaged blood vessels, they become distorted, resulting in vascular damage. Vasospasm occurs, and platelets begin to aggregate at the sites of injury, resulting in low platelet counts. Hepatic blood flow is impeded, causing an elevation in liver enzymes. The hepatic obstruction may then lead to periportal necrosis or intrahepatic hemorrhage. The patient may present with hyperbilirubinemia and jaundice. Signs of impending hepatic rupture include severe epigastric pain, liver distention, nausea, and vomiting. It is suspected that DIC is the primary process in HELLP syndrome. The risk factors for HELLP syndrome vary from those associated with preeclampsia. HELLP usually presents in the third trimester but has also been seen in the second trimester and in postpartum patients. Symptoms of HELLP in the postpartum period typically present within the first 48 hours but may be seen as long as 7 days after delivery.

Prompt diagnosis and initiation of therapy will ensure the best outcomes for the mother and fetus. Laboratory values typically worsen after delivery and peak within 24–48 hours after delivery. The peak lactate dehydrogenase level signals the beginning of recovery. The platelet count and coagulation studies may be used as predictive indicators for hemorrhagic complications. Complaints of severe right upper quadrant pain, neck pain, or shoulder pain should be considered for prompt evaluation.

Preeclampsia and HELLP syndrome are progressive and never resolve until after delivery of the placenta. In spite of this, about 5% of cases are atypical and are first recognized in the postpartum period (August & Sibai, 2015).

Risk Factors

The risk of preeclampsia is greater in pregnant women with a personal or family history of the illness. Other risk factors include a medical history of chronic hypertension or kidney disease, nulliparity, diabetes, coagulation disorders, lupus, obesity, age 40 years or older, and pregnancy characteristics such as twins or new paternity (Mayo Clinic, 2014g). Pregnancy-induced hypertension is most common in women of African descent and least common in Hispanics

(Nakimuli et al., 2014). Women without any identifiable risk factors may develop hypertensive disorders in pregnancy; thus, routine screening for all pregnant women is imperative. Pregnant women with high BP should discuss how to control their BP with their physicians (Mayo Clinic, 2015b).

Prevention

Prevention of hypertension for pregnant women involves the same actions as preventing hypertension for the general population, with a heavy emphasis on lifestyle choices such as eating a heart-healthy diet, engaging in regular physical activity, avoiding smoking, and managing stress. There is currently no known way to prevent preeclampsia. Women with known risks for hypertension or cardiovascular disease may benefit from making lifestyle modifications prior to becoming pregnant.

Clinical Manifestations

Preeclampsia is distinguished from chronic or gestational hypertension by the presence of abnormal proteinuria, defined as 2+ or greater on a urine dipstick, random urine protein/creatinine ratio of 0.3 or greater, or 0.3 gram of protein or greater in a 24-hour urine collection.

Severe features of preeclampsia include any or all of the following:

- BP greater than or equal to 160/110 mmHg
- Persistent or debilitating headache
- Persistent right upper quadrant or epigastric pain
- Serum creatinine greater than 1.1 mg/dL or double the patient's baseline
- Platelet count less than 100,000/microliter
- Liver enzymes elevated to at least twice the upper limit of normal
- Pulmonary edema
- Visual disturbances (scotomata, blurry vision, and rarely, blindness)
- Altered mental status or seizure.

Eclampsia, or eclamptic seizure, is a serious complication of preeclampsia, which manifests with convulsions, as in a grand mal seizure (August & Sibai, 2015).

Although they are not diagnostic criteria, edema and rapid weight gain may increase suspicion for preeclampsia because they are found in the presence of increased capillary permeability that causes leakage of intravascular fluid into interstitial space, where it is retained instead of being excreted by the kidneys. The Clinical Manifestations and Therapies feature provides more information about the signs and symptoms of preeclampsia and their treatment.

Fetal complications related to preeclampsia and eclampsia have a direct correlation with gestational age and the severity of maternal disease. Onset of preeclampsia prior to 34 weeks' gestation and preeclampsia with severe features place the fetus at a higher risk for perinatal morbidity and death (August & Sibai, 2015). Infant prematurity is a major complication.

Collaboration

The goal of medical management of the patient diagnosed with hypertension in pregnancy depends on gestational age

and severity of disease. The primary objective of treatment is to maintain the safety of the mother with delivery of a healthy baby. Prior to 34 weeks, corticosteroids may be administered to the mother to accelerate fetal lung maturity and reduce morbidity in the preterm infant. The severity of maternal disease should be weighed against the risks of infant prematurity.

Ongoing care of all pregnant patients requires providing care within the patient's own culture and belief systems. This is particularly important when caring for pregnant patients who are experiencing hypertension or another potential health crisis. The nurse should assess patients for use of any traditional healthcare practices or remedies popular within the patient's culture that may be contraindicated with the patient's current health status or treatment regimen. Different cultures may have different beliefs or attitudes regarding activity, sexual intercourse, and diet during pregnancy (Lauderdale, 2012). Some Chinese and Islamic patients may be hesitant to participate in invasive diagnostic techniques, so the nurse should always assess patients' understanding of recommended techniques and procedures (Spector, 2017). Other patients may be concerned about the use of medications during pregnancy. The nurse can help alleviate these concerns by providing patient teaching regarding the reasons a medication is prescribed, the benefits, and the possible side effects and risks.

Antepartum Management

Women with chronic hypertension who become pregnant are at a higher risk for the maternal and fetal complications associated with hypertension in pregnancy in addition to stroke and left ventricular hypertrophy. Many antihypertensive medications are contraindicated in pregnancy, so patients who require medication may be switched to methyldopa or labetalol. Women with chronic hypertension or a history of preeclampsia in prior pregnancies should be placed on a low-dose aspirin regimen (August, 2015). The pregnant woman should be instructed to take BP medications as directed and to not take any other medication or supplement unless her healthcare provider has approved it.

The normal, physiologic changes in the cardiovascular system related to pregnancy may cause a reduction in maternal BP and decreased medication requirements in the first 20 weeks. If the patient was on a sodium-restricted diet prior to pregnancy, she should continue this. Baseline laboratory studies should be done early in pregnancy and at regular intervals determined by the healthcare provider. Bi-weekly nonstress tests or biophysical profiles and ultrasound to evaluate fetal growth should be done in the third trimester (Norwitz & Repke, 2015).

Antepartum management for preeclampsia may include hospitalization to evaluate new-onset maternal and fetal conditions. Preeclampsia with severe features requires continued hospitalization for medical management of hypertension, seizure prophylaxis with IV magnesium sulfate, steroid administration, fetal surveillance, and ongoing assessment of the need for prompt delivery. There is no evidence in favor of antihypertensive medication unless maternal BP is in the severe range. Management at home may be considered for stable patients. If she remains at home, the patient will need to assess her BP daily. She will also need to log daily fetal movement. Activity restriction and dietary modifications do not alter the

Clinical Manifestations and Therapies
Hypertensive Disorders in Pregnancy

ETIOLOGY	CLINICAL MANIFESTATIONS	CLINICAL THERAPIES
Cerebral edema and cerebral vasospasm	▪ Hyperreflexia ▪ Headache ▪ Seizures ▪ Visual disturbances ▪ Presence of clonus ▪ Stroke ▪ Hypertensive encephalopathy	▪ Reduce external stimuli. ▪ Administer anticonvulsant: magnesium sulfate. ▪ Consider prompt delivery.
Increased vascular permeability	▪ Pulmonary edema ▪ Edema of the face, hands, and lower extremities ▪ Hemoconcentration	▪ Monitor breath sounds and oxygen saturation. ▪ Elevate extremities to reduce edema. ▪ Administer IV fluid to maintain intravascular volume and circulation. ▪ Monitor intake and output.
Loss of normal vasodilation of uterine arterioles	▪ Decreased placental perfusion ▪ Fetal growth restriction ▪ Decreased fetal movement ▪ Fetal hypoxia	▪ Provide regular antenatal fetal surveillance and continuous intrapartum fetal monitoring. ▪ Teach the patient to report decreased fetal movement. ▪ Nonreassuring fetal status may require prompt delivery.
Vasospasm	▪ Elevated serum creatinine, BUN, uric acid ▪ Decreased serum albumin ▪ Oliguria ▪ Proteinuria ▪ Elevated serum transaminases (liver enzymes) ▪ HELLP syndrome or coagulopathies ▪ Right upper quadrant or epigastric pain ▪ Palpable liver enlargement ▪ Hypertension ▪ Abruptio placentae	▪ Frequently monitor BP. ▪ Elevate extremities to reduce edema. ▪ Monitor laboratory values.

course or outcome of preeclampsia. When at rest, the patient may be encouraged to lie on her left side in order to maximize uterine and renal perfusion. She should avoid lying supine. Resting with her knees and hips bent with a pillow between her knees will help reduce the stress on her back. Nonstress tests and biophysical profiles are ordered bi-weekly by the attending provider. The patient will be weighed, her BP taken, and her home BP log reviewed at these visits. Weekly laboratory studies and monthly ultrasounds for growth may also be ordered (Norwitz & Repke, 2015).

The patient and family members should be educated to report worsening signs and symptoms of preeclampsia (see Patient Teaching feature).

Intrapartum Management

Induction of labor is initiated at term (at least 37 weeks) or if the risks to the mother and fetus outweigh the benefits of avoiding preterm delivery. Induction of labor is always preferable to cesarean delivery unless there is a category III fetal heart tracing.

Assessment for signs and symptoms of worsening preeclampsia should be ongoing. If the patient is on magnesium

sulfate to prevent seizures, the nurse is responsible for monitoring for symptoms of magnesium toxicity.

Laboratory values do not correlate well with adverse patient responses, so the diagnosis of magnesium toxicity is based on clinical observations. The first sign is usually loss of deep tendon reflexes. Other signs are shortness of breath, adventitious lung sounds, and decreased oxygen saturation. Magnesium is excreted by the kidneys, so the nurse should promptly report oliguria to the attending provider (Norwitz & Repke, 2015). The patient may also feel flushed, weak, or nauseated, but these are not signs of toxicity. Severe-range BPs may be treated with IV labetalol or hydralazine.

SAFETY ALERT Fetal status should be assessed continuously via electronic fetal monitoring. Magnesium easily crosses the placenta, and the fetal heart tracing may show a slightly decreased baseline rate and minimal variability. Toxicity can be reversed in the mother and infant with the administration of calcium gluconate (Norwitz & Repke, 2015). A pediatric team should be present at the delivery, and the nurse should anticipate that the baby may have difficulty breathing immediately after birth.

Patient Teaching
Progression of Preeclampsia

Preeclampsia can progress to preeclampsia with severe features, eclampsia, or HELLP syndrome. If the patient is on home monitoring for preeclampsia, the nurse should provide patient teaching about monitoring techniques and signs and symptoms of progression. The patient should be encouraged to schedule appointments to see her provider one to two times per week, depending on the provider's preference. If any signs or symptoms of disease progression are noted by the patient, she should notify her healthcare provider immediately.

Home monitoring techniques:

- Teach the patient to record fetal movements, including frequency, duration, type of movement, and factors that increase or decrease fetal movement.
- Teach the patient how to monitor BP at home and track BP readings over time.
- Teach the patient to monitor urine output and weight gain to assess for fluid retention and edema.

Signs and symptoms of complications:

- Edema of the hands, face, or eyes
- Severe, persistent headache
- Nausea and vomiting
- Vision changes, including sensitivity to light and blurry vision
- Abdominal pain, especially in the upper right abdomen
- Sudden, rapid weight gain
- Shoulder pain, especially the right shoulder
- Difficulty breathing
- Decreased urine production
- Seizures

Epidural and spinal anesthesia may be contraindicated in the presence of a low platelet count. Pain management options include IV medication, pudendal block, labor support, and maternal position changes.

Postpartum Management

The patient with preeclampsia usually improves rapidly after giving birth, although seizures can still occur up to 48 hours postpartum. The nurse will need to monitor the patient for the same signs of toxicity discussed previously.

Magnesium is a tocolytic and smooth muscle relaxer, so the risk for uterine atony and postpartum hemorrhage is high. The mother still requires vigilant monitoring of maternal vital signs, deep tendon reflexes, and respiratory and neurologic status. Magnesium infusion will continue for 24 hours after delivery in severe cases (American Congress of Obstetricians and Gynecologists [ACOG], 2013a).

Strict monitoring of input and output (I & O) is important because diuresis should occur with the return of normal kidney function, as the disease process starts to reverse itself. Monitoring of lab values will also confirm the progression of improvement. Many factors influence whether preeclampsia will recur. Illness severity, underlying illness, and the patient's genetic tendencies are all contributing risk factors. In addition, the patient with preeclampsia during pregnancy may have hypertension or be at risk for kidney disease later in life. Patients who have undergone long hospitalization, induction of labor, and continuous magnesium infusion may have difficulty breastfeeding. Delayed initiation of breastfeeding and separation of mother and baby are known to have a negative effect on breastfeeding success (King et al., 2015). The infant may be unable to leave the special care nursery due to the effects of prematurity and magnesium toxicity, and the mother's condition may not be stable for transport to the nursery for several days.

NURSING PROCESS

When caring for the pregnant woman with preeclampsia, it is important to remember that the nurse is caring for two patients, mother and baby. The needs of both individuals must be identified and met for a successful outcome.

Assessment

- ***Observation and patient interview.*** Note the presence of visible edema in the upper extremities and face of the patient with preeclampsia as well as obvious weight gain. Edema may be present in the lower extremities as well. Observe the patient's LOC during each interaction. For patients on bedrest in the hospital, observe for signs of uterine bleeding during each assessment. During the patient interview, begin by asking the patient about the presence of preeclampsia complications, including headache, changes in vision, presence of nausea or vomiting, and dizziness. Assess the patient's most common body positions during rest, dietary and fluid intake habits, and urinary output. Also ask the patient about the presence of pain, including severity, onset, duration, location, and triggers. The patient interview should also include the patient's history of seizures, especially seizures during pregnancy that may be related to eclampsia.

- ***Physical examination.*** Take and record BP during each antepartum visit. Report abnormal readings to the healthcare provider or midwife. Monitor respiratory status for respiratory rate, rhythm, signs of respiratory distress, and abnormal or absent lung sounds at every visit. Urine is also monitored for protein at each visit, and serum labs may be repeated weekly.

Diagnosis

Possible nursing diagnoses for the patient with preeclampsia include the following:

- *Fluid Volume: Excess*
- *Injury, Risk for*
- *Breastfeeding, Interrupted.*

(NANDA-I © 2014)

Planning

Goals of nursing care for the patient with preeclampsia may include the following:

- The patient will participate in monitoring fetal perfusion, including observing and tracking fetal movement.
- The patient will be encouraged to maintain a position on her left side when lying in bed and to avoid lying supine.
- The patient will maintain safety of herself and the fetus.
- The patient will have adequate fluid intake.
- The patient will have adequate urine output.

Implementation

In caring for a patient with preeclampsia, the focus of nursing care is to reduce the effects of the disease process while supporting the pregnancy. However, if BP continues to rise or remains elevated, delivery of the premature fetus may be unavoidable. In that case, nursing care is focused on optimizing outcomes for both the patient and the newborn.

Community-Based Nursing Care

The patient with preeclampsia must cope with several concerns. She may fear losing her unborn child, and she may be preoccupied with her spouse and other children. If placed on limited activity, she may experience concerns regarding finances and other aspects of family life. The nurse should help the patient identify and discuss these concerns. The nurse can offer information regarding the patient's condition and treatment plan as well as community resources and support groups.

The patient needs to know how to monitor her symptoms and immediately report signs of a worsening condition. She should be prepared to make frequent visits to the provider if requested.

Hospital-Based Nursing Care

Severe preeclampsia is cause for increased concern for the patient and her family. Immediate concerns are usually aimed at providing positive outcomes for the mother and infant. If the patient is admitted to the hospital, nursing interventions will include:

- **Maternal vital signs.** Monitor maternal vital signs every 5 minutes until they are stable. Assess lung sounds and pulse oximetry frequently. Assess BP at least every 1–4 hours. More frequent monitoring is needed with changes in patient status. Monitor temperature at least every 4 hours. Monitor pulse rate and respirations every 4 hours or hourly if the patient is on magnesium.
- **Fetal heart rate.** Check the fetal heart rate with maternal vital signs or continuously intrapartum or if the patient is on magnesium. Increase frequency of monitoring if changes are noted.
- **Urinary output.** Monitor and record intake and output every shift or more frequently per physician's order. Output should be at least 30 mL/hr.
- **Urine protein.** Monitor the patient's urine for protein after each void. A high level of protein in the urine is indicated by 300 mg/24 hr urine, greater than 1+ on urine

dip, or urine protein/creatinine ratio of greater than or equal to 0.3.

- **Urine specific gravity.** Monitor specific gravity of the urine with each voiding. Findings over 1.040 correlate with oliguria and proteinuria.
- **Edema.** Report periorbital swelling and swelling of the face even though they are not considered diagnostic criteria.
- **Weight.** Weigh the patient daily at the same time.
- **Pulmonary edema.** Monitor the patient for signs and symptoms of pulmonary edema.
- **Deep tendon reflexes.** Assess for evidence of hyperreflexia. The patellar reflex is the easiest to assess. Clonus should also be assessed by dorsiflexing the foot while the knee is held in a fixed position. Normally, no clonus is present.
- **Placental separation.** Monitor the patient for vaginal bleeding, or educate the patient to report the signs and symptoms of placental abruption if at home.
- **Headache.** Assess the patient for and report headaches, including their location, duration, and intensity.
- **Visual disturbance.** Assess for and report visual changes.
- **Epigastric pain.** Report complaints of epigastric pain for further examination. It is important to differentiate epigastric pain from simple heartburn, which tends to be less intense.
- **Laboratory blood tests.** Laboratory tests include hematocrit, BUN, creatinine, and uric acid levels to assess kidney function; clotting studies for any indication of thrombocytopenia or DIC; liver enzymes; and electrolyte levels.
- **Level of consciousness (LOC).** Report any changes in LOC or mental status.
- **Emotional well-being and level of understanding.** Be sure to consider the emotional needs of the patient who is experiencing the illness and facing possible premature delivery of her infant.

The occurrence of a convulsion is frightening to observers. It is important for the nurse to inform significant others of the possibility that a seizure may occur. A grand mal seizure has both a tonic phase, marked by pronounced muscular contraction and rigidity, and a clonic phase, marked by alternate contraction and relaxation of the muscles. During the tonic phase of the seizure, the patient should be turned on her side to aid circulation to the placenta. The nurse should monitor the patient's airway clearance in case the patient experiences vomiting. In an attempt to prevent injury, the side rails should be padded.

Nursing Management During Labor and Birth

During labor, the nurse should continuously monitor deep tendon reflexes, breath sounds, LOC, and intake and output. Monitoring activities at this stage include, but are not limited to the following: continuous assessment of the central nervous system, because changes could progress to eclamptic seizures; observing for signs of placental abruptions; monitoring laboratory values for changes or abnormal values; and assessing fetal heart rate for variability and accelerations. Late decelerations or a decrease or absence of variability indicates fetal distress.

A nonstimulating, quiet environment is recommended. The patient and her partner should be educated on the disease process and how care of a patient with preeclampsia may differ from that of a patient experiencing a normal pregnancy. The nurse should position the patient on her left side as much as possible to promote improved circulation to the heart, fetus, uterus, and kidneys. If the patient is unable to push while lying on her left side, encourage her to move into a semisitting position. If able, she can rest in the left lateral position during contractions.

A spouse, partner, or other supportive person is encouraged to remain with the patient during hospitalization to offer support. For continuity of care, the patient should be cared for by the same nurses throughout her stay.

Nursing Management During the Postpartum Period

The nurse must assess vaginal bleeding and observe the patient for signs of hypovolemic shock. Vital signs are monitored every 4 hours for 48 hours or hourly for 24 hours if the patient is on magnesium. Pertinent labs are checked daily. Intake and output are measured. Normal postpartum diuresis helps eliminate edema and is a favorable sign. However, the nurse continues to monitor the patient for signs of worsening preeclampsia in the postpartum period.

The patient should be monitored for signs and symptoms of postpartum depression (see the exemplar on Postpartum Depression in the module on Mood and Affect). The nurse will provide opportunities for frequent maternal–infant contact, provide breastfeeding support, and encourage family members to visit. The patient and significant other may have many questions, and the nurse should be available for discussion. The nurse should give family planning information. Oral contraceptives may be used if the woman's BP has returned to normal by the time they are prescribed (usually 4–6 weeks after birth).

Evaluation

Expected outcomes of nursing care include the following:

- The patient is able to verbalize the signs and symptoms of preeclampsia, the treatment plan, and the implications as they specifically relate to her pregnancy.
- The patient remains seizure free through the pregnancy and into the postpartum period.
- The patient and significant other can verbalize and report the signs and symptoms of worsening preeclampsia.
- The delivery has a positive outcome for both mother and newborn.

Regardless of the level of nursing care received, some patients will progress from hypertension to preeclampsia to eclampsia. The nurse's role when treating these patients is to provide continual assessment of the patient's condition and to collaborate with the patient's physician and other healthcare providers to implement changes to treatment as necessary, up to and including helping with labor and delivery. The nurse should provide supportive and emotional care to the patient, especially for patients who give birth to premature neonates. The nurse can provide patient teaching related to cesarean sections, premature birth, and recovery. The nurse also needs to provide continued evaluation of both the mother and neonate after delivery to identify any potential complications.

Nursing Care Plan
A Patient with Preeclampsia

Dianne Hardison, a 35-year-old primigravida, is 34 weeks pregnant. Three days ago, during a routine prenatal visit, her BP was 138/90 mmHg. Ms. Hardison's last in-office BP reading was 118/74 mmHg. She has also gained 2.3 kg (5 lb) since her visit last month. A trace level of protein was found in her urine. Ms. Hardison also reported experiencing some headaches during the past week.

They were not relieved by acetaminophen. The certified nurse midwife explained the signs and symptoms of preeclampsia and encouraged the patient to call the clinic if her condition worsened during the next few days. Ms. Hardison was sent home and scheduled to return to the office in 3 days.

ASSESSMENT	DIAGNOSES	PLANNING
Ms. Hardison returned to the clinic today with a BP of 144/92 mmHg and has been admitted to the hospital with worsening preeclampsia. She is placed on her left side when lying in bed. The nurse monitors her closely for worsening hypertension, proteinuria, oliguria, cerebral or visual disturbances, pulmonary edema, epigastric pain, and sudden onset of severe edema. She is also placed on seizure precautions. The fetus is assessed by biophysical profile and monitoring. The nurse reassures Ms. Hardison that everything will be done to make her comfortable and ensure the well-being of her baby. Ms. Hardison later reports headache, scotomata, and irritability. Other findings are as follows: BP of 146/92 mmHg; deep tendon reflexes are 3+; 600 mL of urine collected during the past 24 hours with a protein level of 5 g/L; weight gain of 1.8 kg (4 lb) during past 4 days; and 2+ pitting edema on lower extremities.	■ *Deficient Fluid Volume* related to fluid shift from intravascular to extravascular space secondary to vasospasm ■ *Risk for Injury* to fetus related to uteroplacental insufficiency secondary to vasospasm (NANDA-I © 2014)	Goals of care include the following: ■ The patient's BP will remain below the severe range. Signs and symptoms of preeclampsia will remain stable or decrease. ■ Adequate oxygenation and perfusion to the fetus will be maintained. Supplemental oxygen will be provided, if necessary. ■ The patient will maintain adequate urine output.

Nursing Care Plan (continued)

IMPLEMENTATION

- Avoid placing the patient in a supine position.
- Increase frequency of vital signs monitoring, as ordered.
- Monitor strict intake and output, and monitor each urine specimen for protein.
- Assess deep tendon reflexes and clonus.
- Assess for worsening edema.
- Administer magnesium sulfate per infusion pump as ordered.

- Monitor for signs of magnesium sulfate toxicity.
- Consult with a dietitian to provide a nutritionally sound meal plan.
- Educate the patient on how to monitor and record fetal movement throughout the day.
- Inform the patient of various tests that may be performed for fetal monitoring. Assure her that a nurse will be there to offer support during testing.

EVALUATION

Ms. Hardison's BP remains below the severe range. Her urine protein levels remain stable. Her deep tendon reflexes remain at 2+.

Tests measuring fetal status are within normal limits, indicating that uteroplacental sufficiency is maintained.

CRITICAL THINKING

1. A woman gives birth at 36 weeks of gestation after induction of labor for preeclampsia with severe features. The birth weight is graphed in the fifth percentile. What is the most likely reason for the low birth weight? How does preeclampsia affect the fetus as it grows and develops?

2. You are interviewing a patient diagnosed with preeclampsia without severe features at a follow-up outpatient visit. Upon questioning, the patient admits to having a headache most of the time for the past 5 days. What counseling would you provide for this patient on reporting new symptoms? Why?

3. Three women are being admitted to the antepartum unit. Two rooms are available: one private room and one double occupancy room. One woman being admitted is in preterm labor, the second has preeclampsia with severe features, and the third has third-trimester bleeding. Which room assignment would be most appropriate for the woman with preeclampsia? Why?

4. After performing your initial assessment on a patient with preeclampsia on a magnesium drip, you report the following findings: nausea and vomiting, blurred vision, absent deep tendon reflexes (previously deep tendon reflexes were 3+), and 70 mL of total urine output over 4 hours. Are these findings normal? What actions would you take, if any?

REVIEW   Hypertensive Disorders in Pregnancy

RELATE Link the Concepts and Exemplars

Linking the exemplar of hypertensive disorders in pregnancy with the concept of intracranial regulation:

1. What independent nursing interventions might you initiate to reduce the risk of seizures in the patient with preeclampsia who is 28 weeks pregnant?

2. When caring for a woman with preeclampsia who does not have severe features, what teaching would you provide to reduce disease advancement?

Linking the exemplar of hypertensive disorders in pregnancy with the concept of oxygenation:

3. What impact might preeclampsia have on fetal oxygenation?

4. List short- and long-term goals for the patient with preeclampsia aimed at optimizing patient and fetal oxygenation.

READY Go to Volume 3: Clinical Nursing Skills

REFER Go to Pearson MyLab Nursing and eText

- Additional review materials

REFLECT Apply Your Knowledge

Ginny Sims is a 36-year-old primigravida at 34 weeks' gestation. She is married to Paul, whose job as a buyer for a major department store chain requires a great deal of travel. The Simses had plans to have children when they first married, but they had trouble conceiving. Ms. Sims is the manager of a coffee shop. When she began feeling very tired and nauseated in the mornings, she decided that she was in early menopause because her period was late. As fatigue continued to impede her ability to concentrate at work, Ms. Sims finally made an appointment with her OB/GYN and found out she was pregnant. She and her husband are thrilled and cannot wait to greet their newborn. Mr. Sims is investigating the possibility of taking a job that does not involve so much travel so he can spend more time with his family.

Ms. Sims is seeing the nurse practitioner today for her routine prenatal examination. The nurse takes Ms. Sims's BP, and it is 140/92 mmHg, increased from her baseline of 110/70 mmHg. Ms. Sims's ankles are slightly swollen, and she admits to an occasional recurrent nagging headache. Her urine dip shows 2+ protein.

1. What further physical assessments would you perform to support the diagnosis of preeclampsia?

2. What teaching will you provide before sending Ms. Sims home from the office?

3. What assessment findings would indicate worsening preeclampsia in this patient?

»» Exemplar 16.I
Life-Threatening Dysrhythmias

Exemplar Learning Outcomes

16.I Analyze life-threatening dysrhythmias as they relate to perfusion.

- Describe the pathophysiology of life-threatening dysrhythmias.
- Describe the etiology of life-threatening dysrhythmias.
- Compare the risk factors and prevention of life-threatening dysrhythmias.
- Identify the clinical manifestations of life-threatening dysrhythmias.
- Summarize diagnostic tests and therapies used by interprofessional teams in the collaborative care of an individual with a life-threatening dysrhythmia.
- Differentiate care of patients with life-threatening dysrhythmias across the lifespan.
- Apply the nursing process in providing culturally competent care to an individual with a life-threatening dysrhythmia.

Exemplar Key Terms

Atrial kick, *1271*
Cardiac arrest, *1285*

DYSRHYTHMIAS

Overview

Heart muscle contracts in response to electrical stimulation. In the normal heart, electrical stimulation produces a synchronized, rhythmic heart muscle contraction that propels blood into the vascular system. Changes in cardiac rhythm affect this synchronized activity and the heart's ability to effectively pump blood to body tissues.

A cardiac **dysrhythmia** is an abnormal heart rate or rhythm; more specifically, it is a disturbance or irregularity in the electrical system of the heart. Cardiac dysrhythmias may be benign or have lethal consequences. Prompt recognition of a lethal dysrhythmia and quick action can truly be lifesaving.

Dysrhythmias develop for many reasons. Not all are pathologic; some alterations in cardiac rhythm occur in response to events such as exercise or fear. For example, a rapid heart rate as a result of exercise, fever, or excitement is a normal response to the body's demand for oxygen or to stimulation of the SNS. Slow heart rates also may be normal. Athletic heart syndrome, which results from long-term training of the heart muscle, allows the heart to beat more slowly and forcefully while maintaining adequate CO and tissue perfusion at a slower rate. Many athletes have a heart rate of less than 60 beats per minute (bpm), and the heart rate in a very-well-conditioned athlete may be as low as 44–48 bpm.

Aging also affects cardiac rhythm. The natural pacemaker of the heart loses some of its cells, resulting in a slightly slower heart rate. In older adults, the left ventricle tends to increase in size. This leads to an increase in

overall heart size but a decrease in the heart's filling capacity. The ECG of a normal, healthy older adult may appear slightly different from that of a younger individual. Dysrhythmias are seen more often and may be caused by heart disease. Heart murmurs may result from valve stiffness caused by the degeneration of muscle cells or calcification.

Regardless of cause, a dysrhythmia can significantly affect cardiac performance, depending on the health of the heart muscle. The patient's response to the dysrhythmia is key in determining the urgency and type of treatment needed.

Pathophysiology and Etiology

Pathophysiology

Five unique properties of cardiac cells allow effective heart function. Four of these properties are electrical; the fifth is cardiac muscle's mechanical response to electrical stimulation. These five properties include the following:

1. **Automaticity** is the ability of pacemaker cells to spontaneously initiate an electrical impulse (action potential). The SA node is the dominant pacemaker, generating impulses at 60–100 times a minute. Myocardial muscle cells do not possess this ability under normal circumstances.
2. **Excitability** is the ability of myocardial cells to respond to stimuli generated by pacemaker cells.
3. **Conductivity** is the ability to transmit an impulse from cell to cell. When one cell is stimulated, the impulse spreads rapidly throughout the heart muscle.

4. ***Refractoriness*** is the inability of cardiac cells to respond to additional stimuli immediately following depolarization. In the absolute refractory period, depolarization will not occur in response to any stimulus. A stronger-than-normal stimulus is required to initiate depolarization during the relative refractory period. This is followed by the supernormal period, during which a mild stimulus will cause depolarization.

5. ***Contractility*** is the ability of myocardial fibers to shorten in response to a stimulus. Heart muscle responds in an all-or-nothing manner: Stimulation of one muscle fiber causes the entire muscle mass to contract to its fullest extent as one unit.

Electrical activity of the heart is normally controlled by the cardiac conduction system (see Figure 16–10 earlier in this module). The impulse spreads through the atria, is briefly delayed at the AV node, then spreads through conduction pathways of the ventricles and to ventricular muscle. The AV nodal delay allows the atria to contract, delivering an extra bolus of blood to the ventricles before they contract (the **atrial kick**). The AV node also controls the number of impulses that reach the ventricles, preventing extremely rapid heart rates.

Dysrhythmias arise through disruption of the very properties that stimulate and control the heartbeat: automaticity, excitability, conductivity, and refractoriness. Dysrhythmias that result from altered impulse formation include changes in rate and rhythm and the development of ectopic beats. This category includes tachydysrhythmia (rapid heart rates), bradydysrhythmia (slow heart rates), and ectopic rhythms. These dysrhythmias result from a change in the automaticity of cardiac cells. The rate of impulse formation may abnormally increase or decrease. Aberrant (abnormal) impulses may originate outside normal conduction pathways, causing ectopic beats. **Ectopic beats** interrupt the normal conduction sequence and may not initiate a normal muscle contraction. Depending on the site and timing of abnormal impulses, they may have little effect on the patient or pose a significant threat.

Etiology

Ischemia, injury, and infarction of myocardial tissue affect its excitability and ability to conduct and respond to an electrical stimulus. Conduction abnormalities cause varying degrees of **heart block** (a block in the normal conduction pathways). Myocardial injury or MI can obstruct or delay impulse conduction. Bundle branch blocks are common in acute MI.

The reentry phenomenon, a phenomenon of normal and slow conduction, is a major cause of tachydysrhythmia. A stimulus such as an ectopic beat triggers the reentry phenomenon. The impulse is delayed in one area of the heart (e.g., an area of ischemia or injury), but is conducted normally through the rest. Muscle that has been depolarized by the normally conducted impulse is repolarized by the time the impulse traveling through the area of slow conduction reaches it, thus initiating another cycle of depolarization (Huether & McCance, 2012). The result is a dysrhythmia that propagates itself.

Several forms of reentry may occur. The impulse may travel through a set pathway to reenter repolarized tissue. Many atrial dysrhythmias follow this pattern, including atrial flutter. In functional reentry, local differences in the conduction of an impulse interrupt the normal wave of depolarization, sending it back upon itself in a spiral pattern and setting up a permanent rotation. This type of pattern suppresses normal pacemaker activity and can lead to atrial fibrillation (Huether & McCance, 2012).

Cardiac rhythms are classified according to the site of impulse formation or the site and degree of conduction block. Supraventricular rhythms arise above the ventricles. These rhythms usually produce a QRS complex within the normal range. Sinus rhythms, atrial rhythms, and junctional (arising from the AV junction) rhythms are all supraventricular rhythms. Ventricular rhythms originate in the ventricles and may prove fatal if left untreated. AV conduction blocks result from a defect in impulse transmission from the atria to the ventricles. The major normal and abnormal cardiac rhythms are summarized in **Table 16–26** ⟫.

Risk Factors

Individuals who have a history of heart disease, including CAD, prior heart surgery, high BP, congenital heart disease, heart attack, and other heart damage, are at high risk of developing a dysrhythmia. Alterations related to the endocrine system (including thyroid problems, diabetes mellitus, and electrolyte imbalances) can also increase an individual's risk. Sleep apnea is an additional risk factor. Alcohol, stimulants such as caffeine and nicotine, and some medications can also contribute to dysrhythmia development (Mayo Clinic, 2014h).

Prevention

Because a major risk factor for dysrhythmias is heart disease, methods used to increase heart health can help prevent dysrhythmias. These include maintaining a heart-healthy diet, participating in moderate physical exercise, maintaining a healthy weight, following treatment recommendations, limiting alcohol and caffeine consumptions, refraining from tobacco use of any kind, and avoiding medications that can cause dysrhythmias (Mayo Clinic, 2014h).

Clinical Manifestations

Cardiac dysrhythmias occur when the NSR of the heart is disturbed. **Normal sinus rhythm (NSR)** is the normal heart rhythm, in which impulses originate in the SA (sinus) node and travel through all normal conduction pathways without delay. All waveforms are of normal configuration, look alike, and have consistent (fixed) durations. The rate is 60–100 bpm.

The signs and symptoms associated with cardiac dysrhythmias often range from none to SCD (AHA, 2014b). More severe symptoms tend to occur in patients who have evidence of structural disease. Common symptoms include lightheadedness, dizziness, fluttering, a racing or slow heartbeat, shortness of breath, chest discomfort or pain, and syncope (Mayo Clinic, 2014h).

To improve understanding, rhythms are categorized according to the site of origination. Sinus node dysrhythmias

TABLE 16–26 Characteristics of Selected Cardiac Rhythms and Dysrhythmias

Rhythm/ECG Appearance	ECG Characteristics	Management
Supraventricular Rhythms		
Normal sinus rhythm (NSR) 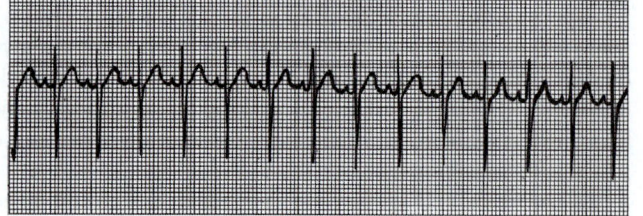	Rate: 60–100 bpm Rhythm: regular P:QRS: 1:1 PR interval: 0.12–0.20 sec QRS complex: 0.6–0.10 sec	None; normal heart rhythm
Sinus arrhythmia	Rate: 60–100 bpm Rhythm: irregular, varying with respirations P:QRS: 1:1 PR interval: 0.12–0.20 sec QRS complex: 0.6–0.10 sec	Generally none; considered a normal rhythm in the very young and very old
Sinus tachycardia	Rate: 101–150 bpm Rhythm: regular P:QRS: 1:1 (with very fast rates, P wave may be hidden in preceding T wave) PR interval: 0.12–0.20 sec QRS complex: 0.6–0.10 sec	Treated only if symptomatic or patient is at risk for myocardial damage Treatment of underlying cause (e.g., hypovolemia, fever, pain) Possible administration of beta-adrenergic blockers or verapamil
Sinus bradycardia	Rate: less than 60 bpm Rhythm: regular P:QRS: 1:1 PR interval: 0.12–0.20 sec QRS complex: 0.6–0.10 sec	Treated only if symptomatic Possible administration of IV atropine or isoproterenol, and/or pacemaker therapy
Premature atrial contractions (PACs)	Rate: variable Rhythm: irregular, with normal rhythm interrupted by early beats arising in the atria P:QRS: 1:1 PR interval: 0.12–0.20 sec, but may be prolonged QRS complex: 0.6–0.10 sec	Usually require no treatment Reduction of alcohol and caffeine intake, reduction of stress, and smoking cessation Possible administration of beta-adrenergic blockers
Paroxysmal supraventricular tachycardia (PSVT)	Rate: 100–280 bpm (usually 150–200 bpm) Rhythm: regular P:QRS: P waves often not identifiable PR interval: not measured QRS complex: 0.6–0.10 sec	Treatment if symptomatic Possible administration of vagal maneuvers (Valsalva, carotid sinus massage), oxygen therapy, adenosine or a beta-adrenergic blocker, temporary pacing, or synchronized cardioversion

TABLE 16–26 Characteristics of Selected Cardiac Rhythms and Dysrhythmias *(continued)*

Rhythm/ECG Appearance	ECG Characteristics	Management
Supraventricular Rhythms		
Atrial flutter	Rate: atrial, 240–360 bpm; ventricular rate depends on degree of AV block and usually is less than 150 bpm Rhythm: atrial, regular; ventricular, usually regular P:QRS: 2:1, 4:1, 6:1; may vary PR interval: not measured QRS complex: 0.6–0.10 sec	Medications to slow ventricular response, such as a beta-adrenergic blocker or CCB, followed by a class I antidysrhythmic agent or amiodarone; synchronized cardioversion
Atrial fibrillation	Rate: atrial, 300–600 bpm (too rapid to count); ventricular, 100–180 bpm in untreated patients Rhythm: irregularly irregular P:QRS: variable PR interval: not measured QRS complex: 0.06–0.10 sec	Synchronized cardioversion; medications to reduce ventricular response rate: metoprolol, diltiazem, or digoxin; anticoagulant therapy to reduce risk of clot formation and stroke
Junctional escape rhythm	Rate: 40–60 bpm; junctional tachycardia, 60–140 bpm Rhythm: regular P:QRS: P waves may be absent, inverted and immediately preceding or succeeding QRS complex, or hidden in QRS complex PR interval: less than 0.10 sec QRS complex: 0.06–0.10 sec	Treatment of cause if symptomatic
Ventricular Rhythms		
Premature ventricular contractions (PVCs)	Rate: variable Rhythm: irregular, with PVC interrupting underlying rhythm and followed by a compensatory pause P:QRS: no P wave noted before PVC PR interval: absent with PVC QRS complex: wide (greater than 0.12 sec) and bizarre in appearance; differs from normal QRS complex	Treatment if symptomatic or in presence of severe heart disease Avoiding stimulant use (caffeine, nicotine) Possible administration of beta-adrenergic blockers or class I or III antidysrhythmic agents in patients with severe heart disease who are symptomatic
Ventricular tachycardia (VT, V tach)	Rate: 100–250 bpm Rhythm: regular P:QRS: P waves usually not identifiable PR interval: not measured QRS complex: 0.12 sec or greater; bizarre shape	Treatment if VT is sustained, symptomatic, or associated with organic heart disease Possible administration of DC cardioversion or IV procainamide, lidocaine, or a class III antidysrhythmic agent if hemodynamic instability accompanies; surgical ablation or antitachycardia pacing with an ICD for repeated episodes If no pulse, treated as VF; CPR, if needed, followed by advanced cardiac life support algorithm

(continued on next page)

TABLE 16–26 Characteristics of Selected Cardiac Rhythms and Dysrhythmias *(continued)*

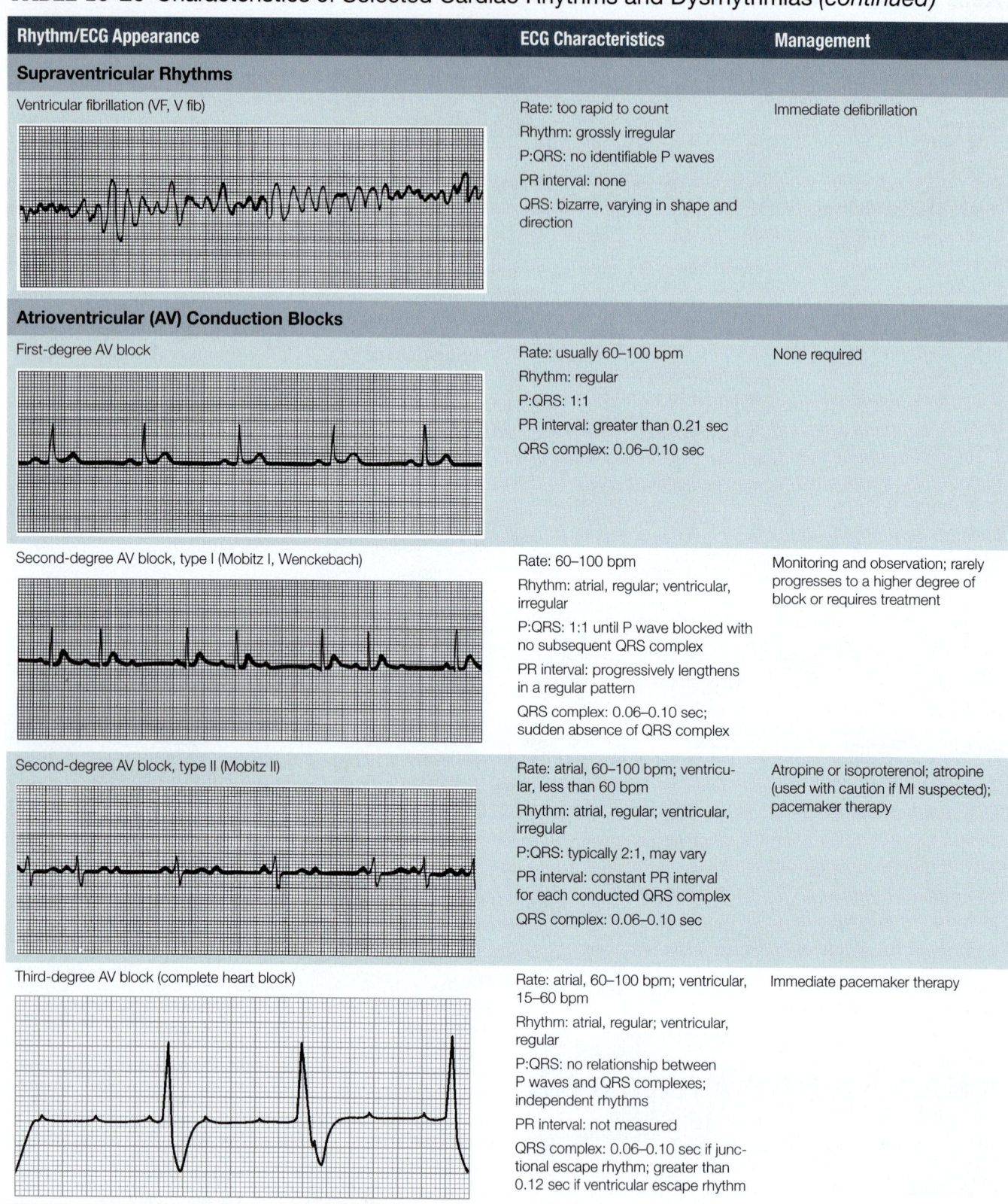

Rhythm/ECG Appearance	ECG Characteristics	Management
Supraventricular Rhythms		
Ventricular fibrillation (VF, V fib)	Rate: too rapid to count Rhythm: grossly irregular P:QRS: no identifiable P waves PR interval: none QRS: bizarre, varying in shape and direction	Immediate defibrillation
Atrioventricular (AV) Conduction Blocks		
First-degree AV block	Rate: usually 60–100 bpm Rhythm: regular P:QRS: 1:1 PR interval: greater than 0.21 sec QRS complex: 0.06–0.10 sec	None required
Second-degree AV block, type I (Mobitz I, Wenckebach)	Rate: 60–100 bpm Rhythm: atrial, regular; ventricular, irregular P:QRS: 1:1 until P wave blocked with no subsequent QRS complex PR interval: progressively lengthens in a regular pattern QRS complex: 0.06–0.10 sec; sudden absence of QRS complex	Monitoring and observation; rarely progresses to a higher degree of block or requires treatment
Second-degree AV block, type II (Mobitz II)	Rate: atrial, 60–100 bpm; ventricular, less than 60 bpm Rhythm: atrial, regular; ventricular, irregular P:QRS: typically 2:1, may vary PR interval: constant PR interval for each conducted QRS complex QRS complex: 0.06–0.10 sec	Atropine or isoproterenol; atropine (used with caution if MI suspected); pacemaker therapy
Third-degree AV block (complete heart block)	Rate: atrial, 60–100 bpm; ventricular, 15–60 bpm Rhythm: atrial, regular; ventricular, regular P:QRS: no relationship between P waves and QRS complexes; independent rhythms PR interval: not measured QRS complex: 0.06–0.10 sec if junctional escape rhythm; greater than 0.12 sec if ventricular escape rhythm	Immediate pacemaker therapy

originate in the sinus node. Supraventricular rhythms are those that originate above the ventricle. Junctional rhythms originate at the AV node. Ventricular rhythms originate below the AV node and are the most life threatening because of their impact on CO.

Sinus Node Dysrhythmias

Sinus node, also called SA node, dysrhythmias may occur as a normal compensatory response (e.g., to exercise) or because of altered automaticity. In these rhythms, as in NSR, the initiating impulse is from the SA node. They differ from

NSRs in rate or regularity of the rhythm. Sinus dysrhythmias include sinus arrhythmia, sinus tachycardia, and sinus bradycardia.

Sinus Arrhythmia

Sinus arrhythmia is a sinus rhythm in which the rate varies with respirations, causing an irregular rhythm. The rate increases during inspiration and decreases with expiration. Sinus arrhythmia is common in the very young and the very old. It can be caused by an increase in vagal tone, by digitalis toxicity, or by morphine administration.

Sinus Tachycardia

Sinus tachycardia has all of the characteristics of NSR, except that the rate is greater than 100 bpm. Tachycardia arises from enhanced automaticity in response to changes in the internal environment. SNS stimulation or blocked vagal (parasympathetic) activity increases the heart rate. Tachycardia is a normal response to any condition or event that increases the body's demand for oxygen and nutrients, such as exercise or hypoxia. In the patient on bedrest, tachycardia is an ominous sign. Sinus tachycardia may be an early sign of cardiac dysfunction, such as heart failure. Tachycardia is detrimental in patients with cardiac disease because it increases cardiac work and oxygen use.

Common causes of sinus tachycardia include exercise, excitement, anxiety, pain, fever, hypoxia, hypovolemia, anemia, hyperthyroidism, MI, heart failure, cardiogenic shock, PE, caffeine intake, and certain drugs, such as atropine, epinephrine (Adrenalin), or isoproterenol (Isuprel).

Manifestations of sinus tachycardia include a rapid pulse rate. The patient may complain of feeling that the heart is "racing," shortness of breath, and dizziness. In the presence of heart disease, sinus tachycardia may precipitate chest pain.

Sinus Bradycardia

Sinus bradycardia has all of the characteristics of NSR, but the rate is less than 60 bpm. Sinus bradycardia may result from increased vagal (parasympathetic) activity or from depressed automaticity due to injury or ischemia to the sinus node. Sinus bradycardia may be normal (e.g., in patients with athletic heart syndrome). The heart rate also normally slows during sleep because the parasympathetic nervous system is dominant at this time. Other causes of sinus bradycardia include pain, increased ICP, sinus node disease, AMI (especially with inferior wall damage), hypothermia, acidosis, and certain drugs.

Sinus bradycardia may be asymptomatic; it is important to assess the patient before treating the rhythm. Manifestations of decreased CO, such as decreased LOC, syncope (fainting), or hypotension, indicate a need for intervention.

Sick Sinus Syndrome

SSS results from sinus node disease or dysfunction that causes problems with impulse formation, transmission, and conduction. SSS is often found in older adults. It may be caused by direct injury to sinus tissue; fibrosis of conduction fibers associated with aging; and such drugs as digitalis, beta-adrenergic blockers, and CCBs.

ECG characteristics of SSS include sinus bradycardia; sinus arrhythmia; sinus pauses or arrest; and atrial tachydysrhythmias such as atrial fibrillation, atrial flutter, or atrial tachycardia. Bradycardia-tachycardia syndrome, characterized either by **paroxysmal** (occurring in bursts with an abrupt onset and termination) atrial tachycardia followed by prolonged sinus pauses or alternating periods of bradycardia and tachycardia, also may indicate sinus node dysfunction.

Manifestations of sinus node dysfunction often are intermittent, related to a drop in CO caused by the irregular rhythm. Fatigue, dizziness, lightheadedness, and syncope are common. The heart rate may not increase in response to stressors such as exercise or fever.

Supraventricular Dysrhythmias

When an action potential originates in atrial tissue outside the SA node, the resulting rhythm is classified as a supraventricular rhythm. In these dysrhythmias, an ectopic pacemaker takes over, or overrides, the SA node. They may also occur when the SA node fails; an escape rhythm develops as a failsafe mechanism to maintain the heart rate. The most common supraventricular dysrhythmias are PACs, SVT, atrial flutter, and atrial fibrillation. These rhythms may be paroxysmal.

Premature Atrial Contractions

PAC is an ectopic atrial beat that occurs earlier than the next expected sinus beat. PACs can arise anywhere in the atria. They are usually asymptomatic and benign, but they may initiate PSVT in susceptible individuals. PACs are common in older adults, often occurring without an obvious cause. Strong emotions, excessive alcohol intake, tobacco, and stimulants such as caffeine can precipitate PACs. They also may be associated with MI, heart failure and other cardiac disorders, hypoxemia, PE, digitalis toxicity, and electrolyte or acid–base imbalances. In patients with underlying heart disease, PACs may precede a more serious dysrhythmia.

The ECG tracing shows interruption of the underlying rhythm by a premature complex that looks similar to the underlying beats. The ectopic impulse of the PAC is usually conducted normally, leading to depolarization of cardiac muscle and a normal QRS complex. Because the impulse arises above the ventricles, it follows normal conduction pathways through the ventricles. The QRS complex is narrow or matches those of the underlying rhythm. The shape of the P wave of a PAC differs from normal P waves because its impulse arises outside the sinus node. A noncompensatory pause usually follows, as the PAC resets the SA node rhythm. The ectopic impulse occasionally may not be conducted through the heart, resulting in a lone P wave without a QRS, or a nonconducted PAC.

PACs cause few manifestations. If frequent, they may cause palpitations or a fluttering sensation in the chest. Early beats may be noted on auscultating or palpating the pulse.

Paroxysmal Supraventricular Tachycardia

PSVT is tachycardia of sudden onset and termination. PSVT is usually initiated by a reentry loop in or around the AV node; that is, an impulse reenters the same section of tissue over and over, causing repeated depolarizations.

PSVT occurs more frequently in women than men. SNS stimulation and stressors such as fever, sepsis, and hyperthyroidism may precipitate PSVT. It also may be associated with heart diseases such as coronary heart disease, MI, rheumatic heart disease, myocarditis, or acute pericarditis. Abnormal conduction pathways associated with Wolff–Parkinson–White (WPW) syndrome may account for PSVT.

PSVT affects ventricular filling and CO and decreases coronary artery perfusion. Its manifestations include palpitations and a "racing" heart, anxiety, dizziness, dyspnea, anginal pain, diaphoresis, extreme fatigue, and polyuria (urine output may reach up to 3 L in the first few hours after PSVT onset).

Atrial Flutter

Atrial flutter is a rapid and regular atrial rhythm thought to result from an intra-atrial reentry mechanism. Causes include SNS stimulation due to anxiety or caffeine and alcohol intake; thyrotoxicosis; coronary heart disease or MI; PE; and abnormal conduction syndromes, such as WPW syndrome. Older adults with rheumatic heart disease or valvular disease are especially vulnerable.

Two types of atrial flutter have been identified. Type I atrial flutter has an atrial rate of 240–340 bpm. It develops because of a reentry mechanism in the right atrium. The mechanism leading to type II atrial flutter has not been identified. In this type of flutter, the atrial rate is faster, up to 350 bpm.

Patients with atrial flutter may complain of palpitations or a fluttering sensation in the chest or throat. If the ventricular rate is rapid, manifestations of decreased CO, such as decreased LOC; hypotension; decreased urinary output; and cool, clammy skin, may be noted. The atrial kick (additional ventricular filling with atrial contraction) is lost because of inadequate atrial filling.

ECG characteristics include a "sawtooth" or "picket fence" appearance of P waves, which are labeled flutter (F) waves. The atrial rate is rapid, often around 300 bpm. As a protective mechanism, many impulses are blocked at the AV node, and the ventricular rate is rarely greater than 150–170 bpm. Atrial impulses usually are evenly conducted through the AV node, for example, two impulses to one QRS complex (2:1), four impulses to one QRS complex (4:1), or six impulses to one QRS complex (6:1). A constant conduction ratio results in a regular ventricular rhythm; the ventricular rhythm is irregular if the conduction ratio varies. The ventricular rate usually ranges from 150 to 170 bpm in 2:1 conduction and 60 to 75 bpm for lower conduction ratios. The T wave is usually hidden by overriding F waves; some F waves may be hidden in the QRS complex.

Atrial Fibrillation

Atrial fibrillation is a common dysrhythmia characterized by disorganized atrial activity without discrete atrial contractions. Extremely rapid atrial impulses bombard the AV node, resulting in an irregular ventricular response. Atrial fibrillation may occur suddenly and recur, or it may persist as a chronic dysrhythmia. Atrial fibrillation is commonly associated with heart failure, rheumatic heart disease, coronary heart disease, hypertension, and hyperthyroidism.

Manifestations of atrial fibrillation relate to the rate of the ventricular response. With rapid response rates, manifestations of decreased CO such as hypotension, shortness of breath, fatigue, and angina may develop. Patients with extensive heart disease may develop syncope or heart failure. Peripheral pulses are irregular and of variable amplitude (strength).

The specific ECG characteristics of atrial fibrillation include an irregular rhythm and the absence of identifiable P waves. The atrial rate is so rapid that it is not measurable. The ventricular rate varies.

Atrial fibrillation increases the risk for formation of thromboemboli. Organ infarction may occur as a result; the incidence of stroke is high.

Junctional Dysrhythmias

Rhythms that originate in AV nodal tissue are termed *junctional*. The AV junction includes the AV node and the bundle of His, which branches into the right and left bundle branches. An impulse arising from the AV junction may occur in response to failure of higher pacemakers, as in a junctional escape rhythm, or it may result from an abnormal mechanism, such as altered automaticity. An impulse arising from the AV junction may or may not be conducted back up to the atria. This conduction against the normal flow or pattern is called **retrograde conduction**. The resulting atrial wave, called a P′ wave, may be found before, during, or after the QRS complex, depending on the speed of conduction. The P′ wave is inverted in some ECG leads because the impulse moves from the AV node up to the atria instead of from the SA node down toward the AV node. In addition, the P′R interval is shorter than normal (less than 0.12 sec). The QRS complex is typically narrow.

A junctional rhythm may be due to drug toxicity (e.g., digitalis, beta-adrenergic blockers, CCBs) or other causes such as hypoxemia, hyperkalemia, increased vagal tone or damage to the AV node, MI, and heart failure. Loss of synchronized atrial contraction and the atrial kick may affect CO, leading to manifestations of decreased CO and impaired myocardial tissue perfusion. Heart failure may develop.

Premature junctional contractions occur before the next expected beat of the underlying rhythm. Isolated premature junctional contractions may occur in healthy individuals and are insignificant. Junctional tachycardia is a junctional rhythm with a rate greater than 60 bpm. It is caused by increased automaticity of AV nodal tissue. The ventricular rate is usually less than 140 bpm. Both rhythms are most commonly associated with digitalis toxicity, hypoxia, ischemia, or electrolyte imbalances.

Ventricular Dysrhythmias

Ventricular dysrhythmias originate in the ventricles. Because the ventricles pump blood into the pulmonary and systemic vasculature, any disruption of their rhythm can affect CO and tissue perfusion. A wide and bizarre QRS complex (greater than 0.12 sec) is a characteristic feature of ventricular dysrhythmias. This occurs because ventricular ectopic impulses begin and travel outside normal conduction pathways. Other characteristics include no relationship between the QRS complex and a P wave, increased amplitude of the QRS complex, an abnormal ST segment, and a T wave deflected in the opposite direction from the QRS complex.

Premature Ventricular Contractions

PVCs are ectopic ventricular beats that occur before the next expected beat of the underlying rhythm. They usually do not reset the atrial rhythm and are followed by a full compensatory pause. PVCs often have no significance in individuals without heart disease. Frequent, recurrent, or multifocal PVCs may be associated with an increased risk for lethal dysrhythmias. PVCs result from either enhanced automaticity or a reentry phenomenon. They may be triggered by anxiety or stress; tobacco, alcohol, or caffeine use; hypoxia, acidosis, and electrolyte imbalances; sympathomimetic drugs; coronary heart disease; heart failure; mechanical stimulation of the heart (e.g., the insertion of a cardiac catheter); or reperfusion after fibrinolytic therapy. The incidence and significance of PVCs is greatest after MI.

PVCs may be isolated or may occur in a specific pattern. Two PVCs in a row are called a **couplet**, or paired PVCs. Three consecutive PVCs (a **triplet**, or salvo) are a short run of VT. **Ventricular bigeminy** is characterized by a PVC following each normal beat; a PVC noted every third beat is called **ventricular trigeminy**. When the ventricular impulse arises from one ectopic site, all PVCs look the same (monomorphic) and are called **unifocal** PVCs. **Multifocal** PVCs arise from different ectopic sites and appear different from one another on the ECG (polymorphic).

The frequency and patterns of PVCs can be indicative of myocardial irritability and the risk for a lethal dysrhythmia. The following are considered warning signs in the patient with acute heart disease (e.g., an acute MI):

- PVCs that develop within the first 4 hours of an MI
- Frequent PVCs (six or more per minute)
- Couplets or triplets
- Multifocal PVCs
- R-on-T phenomenon (PVCs falling on the T wave)

In individuals without heart disease, isolated PVCs usually are insignificant and do not require treatment. In patients with preexisting heart disease, PVCs may indicate drug toxicity or an increased risk for lethal dysrhythmias and cardiac arrest. The risk is greatest following AMI.

Ventricular Tachycardia

VT is a rapid ventricular rhythm defined as three or more consecutive PVCs. VT may occur in short bursts, or "runs," or it may persist for more than 30 seconds (sustained VT). The rate is greater than 100 bpm, and the rhythm is usually regular. Reentry is the usual electrophysiologic mechanism responsible for VT. Myocardial ischemia and infarction are the most common predisposing factors for VT. VT also is associated with cardiac structural disorders such as valvular disease, rheumatic heart disease, or cardiomyopathy. It may occur in the absence of heart disease and with anorexia nervosa, metabolic disorders, or drug toxicity.

Nonsustained VT may occur paroxysmally and convert back to an effective rhythm spontaneously. The patient may experience a fluttering sensation in the chest or complain of palpitations and brief shortness of breath. Patients in sustained VT generally develop signs and symptoms of decreased CO and hemodynamic instability, including severe hypotension, a weak or nonpalpable pulse, and loss of consciousness. Allowed to continue, VT can deteriorate into VF. Sustained VT is a medical emergency that requires immediate intervention, particularly in patients with cardiac disease.

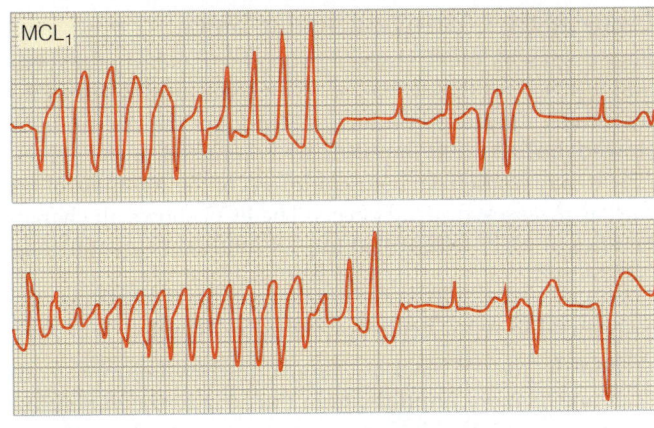

Figure 16–47 》 *Torsades de pointes.* Note the wide and bizarre QRS complexes of varying size, shape (morphology), and amplitude.

Torsades de pointes is a type of VT associated with long-QT syndrome (a prolongation of the QT interval). Long-QT syndrome may be genetic or acquired, occurring secondarily to electrolyte disruptions, MI, cocaine use, liquid protein diets, medications, or other conditions. In *torsades de pointes*, the QRS complexes vary in size, shape, and amplitude (see **Figure 16–47 》**). Patients with *torsades de pointes* typically present with recurrent episodes of palpitations, dizziness, and syncope. SCD can occur with the first episode.

Ventricular Fibrillation

VF is extremely rapid, chaotic ventricular depolarization that causes the ventricles to quiver and cease contracting; the heart does not pump. This is known as cardiac arrest; it is a medical emergency requiring immediate intervention with CPR. Death will follow the onset of VF within 4 minutes if the rhythm is not recognized and terminated and an effective perfusing rhythm reestablished.

VF is usually triggered by severe myocardial ischemia or infarction. It occurs without warning 50% of the time. It is the terminal event in many disease processes or traumatic conditions. VF may be precipitated by a single PVC or may follow VT. Other causes of VF include digitalis toxicity, reperfusion therapy, use of antidysrhythmic drugs, hypokalemia and hyperkalemia, hypothermia, metabolic acidosis, mechanical stimulation (as with the insertion of cardiac catheters or pacing wires), and electric shock.

Clinically, loss of ventricular contractions results in the absence of a palpable or audible pulse. The patient loses consciousness and stops breathing as perfusion ceases. The ECG shows grossly irregular, bizarre complexes with no discernible rate or rhythm.

Atrioventricular Conduction Blocks

Conduction defects that delay or block transmission of the sinus impulse through the AV node are called AV conduction blocks. Impaired conduction may result from tissue injury or disease, increased vagal (parasympathetic) tone, drug effects, or a congenital defect. AV conduction blocks vary in severity from benign to severe.

First-Degree Atrioventricular Block

First-degree AV block is a benign conduction delay that generally poses no threat, has no symptoms, and requires no treatment. Impulse conduction through the AV node is slowed, but all atrial impulses are conducted to the ventricles. It may result from injury or infarct of the AV node, other cardiac diseases, or drug effects. The ECG shows all characteristics of NSR, except that the PR interval is greater than 0.20 second.

Second-Degree Atrioventricular Block

Second-degree AV block is characterized by failure to conduct one or more impulses from the atria to the ventricles. Second-degree AV block presents as one of two patterns: type I and type II.

Second-Degree Atrioventricular Block—Type I

Type I second-degree AV block (also known as Mobitz type I or Wenckebach phenomenon) is characterized by a repeating pattern of increasing AV conduction delays until an impulse fails to conduct to the ventricles. On the ECG, PR intervals progressively lengthen until one QRS complex is not conducted (or dropped). The ventricular rate remains adequate to maintain CO, and the patient usually is asymptomatic. Mobitz type I AV block usually is transient, associated with acute MI or drug intoxication (e.g., digitalis, beta-blockers, CCBs). It rarely progresses to complete heart block.

Second-Degree Atrioventricular Block—Type II

Type II second-degree AV block (Mobitz type II) involves intermittent failure of the AV node to conduct an impulse to the ventricles without preceding delays in conduction. The PR interval remains constant, but not all P waves are followed by QRS complexes (e.g., there may be two P waves for every QRS). With second-degree AV block, the bundle of His and/or lower regions of the conduction system are blocked. Mobitz type II block is frequently associated with acute anterior wall MI and a high rate of mortality (Sovari et al., 2014). Manifestations of Mobitz type II block depend on the ventricular rate. Pacemaker therapy may be required to maintain CO.

Third-Degree Atrioventricular Block

Third-degree AV block (complete heart block) occurs when atrial impulses are completely blocked at the AV node and fail to reach the ventricles. As a result, the atria and ventricles are controlled by different and independent pacemakers, with separate rates and rhythms. The ventricular impulse arises from either junctional fibers (with a rate of 40–60 bpm) or a ventricular pacemaker at a rate of less than 40 bpm. The width of the QRS complex depends on the location of the escape pacemaker. The QRS is wide and the rate is slow when the rhythm arises distal to the bundle of His.

Third-degree AV block is frequently associated with an inferior or anteroseptal MI. Other causes include congenital conditions, acute or degenerative cardiac disease or damage, drug effects, and electrolyte imbalances. The slow escape rhythm significantly affects CO, causing manifestations such as syncope (known as a Stokes-Adams attack), dizziness, fatigue, exercise intolerance, and heart failure. Third-degree

AV block is life threatening and requires immediate intervention to maintain adequate CO.

Atrioventricular Dissociation

Complete dissociation of atrial and ventricular rhythms can occur in conditions other than third-degree AV block. The two primary factors leading to AV dissociation are severe sinus bradycardia and a slower pacemaker (junctional or ventricular) that competes with or exceeds the NSR. AV dissociation may result from acute myocardial ischemia or infarction, cardiac surgery, or drug effects. The ECG shows separate and competing atrial (P waves) and ventricular (QRS complexes) rhythms.

Intraventricular Conduction Blocks

Once the impulse enters the ventricles, its conduction through the right and left bundle branches may be impaired (bundle branch block). As a result, the impulse is conducted more slowly than normal through the ventricles. On the ECG, the QRS complex is prolonged. Its appearance varies, depending on the affected bundle (right or left). No clinical manifestations are typically associated with bundle branch block unless it occurs in conjunction with an AV block.

The Clinical Manifestations and Therapies feature lists the etiology and clinical manifestations of life-threatening dysrhythmias along with recommended treatments.

Collaboration

Cardiac dysrhythmias may be benign or critical. Recognizing lethal dysrhythmias is a matter of life and death. Major goals of care include identifying the dysrhythmia, evaluating its effect on patient well-being, and treating the underlying causes. This may involve correcting fluid and electrolyte or acid–base imbalances; treating hypoxia, pain, or anxiety; administering antidysrhythmic medications; or performing mechanical and surgical interventions.

Diagnostic Tests

Diagnostic tests for dysrhythmias include ECG, cardiac monitoring, and electrophysiology studies. Laboratory tests, such as serum electrolytes, drug levels, and ABGs, may be done to help identify the cause of the dysrhythmia.

Electrocardiogram

The 12-lead ECG may be required to accurately diagnose a dysrhythmia. It also provides information about underlying disease processes, such as MI or other cardiac disease. The ECG may also be used to monitor the effects of treatment.

Cardiac Monitoring

Cardiac monitoring allows continuous observation of the cardiac rhythm. It is used in many different circumstances (see **Box 16–18** 》). Different types of ECG monitoring are employed for different situations.

Continuous Cardiac Monitoring

Continuous monitoring of the cardiac rhythm is provided by bedside and central monitoring stations. Electrodes placed on the patient's chest attach to cables connected to a monitor. The heart rate and rhythm are visually displayed on a bedside monitor connected to a central monitoring

Clinical Manifestations and Therapies
Life-Threatening Dysrhythmias

ETIOLOGY	CLINICAL MANIFESTATIONS	CLINICAL THERAPIES
Decreased CO	■ Changes in LOC ranging from dizziness to complete loss of consciousness ■ Ischemia ■ Reduced tissue perfusion ■ Hypotension	■ Administer antidysrhythmic medications. ■ Perform defibrillation or cardioversion (external or implanted). ■ Install pacemaker (external or implanted). ■ Reduce cardiac workload.
Alterations in oxygenation	■ Cyanosis ■ Shortness of breath ■ Hypoxemia ■ Hypercapnia ■ Altered LOC ■ Death	■ Administer oxygen. ■ Provide mechanical ventilation. ■ Reduce activity to decrease oxygen demands on the body.
Stasis of blood in the heart	■ Increased risk of emboli formation that manifests differently depending on where the thrombus occurs ■ May result in MI, stroke, or DVT	■ Administer anticoagulants. ■ Treat the underlying dysrhythmia to promote movement of blood through the chambers of the heart.
Sudden cardiac death (SCD)	■ Pulselessness ■ Absence of respirations ■ Death	■ Perform CPR. ■ Administer antidysrhythmic medications. ■ Administer oxygen. ■ Conduct cardiorespiratory monitoring after successful resuscitation.

Box 16–18
Indications for Cardiac Monitoring

■ Perioperative monitoring of heart rate and rhythm
■ Detecting and identifying dysrhythmias
■ Monitoring the effects of cardiac and noncardiac diseases on the heart
■ Monitoring patients with potentially life-threatening conditions: major trauma (especially cardiac trauma), dissecting aneurysm, acute MI, heart failure, shock, and other emergency conditions
■ Evaluating responses to procedures and interventions such as drug therapies, diagnostic procedures, ablative techniques, angioplasty, cardiac catheterization, cardiac surgery, pacemaker function, and automated ICD function

station. The central station allows simultaneous monitoring of multiple patients within a nursing unit. Alarms on both bedside and central monitors warn of potential problems, such as very rapid or very slow heart rates. Alarm limits are preset by the nurse for the individual patient.

Telemetry may be used in acute care settings when the patient is ambulatory. Chest electrodes are connected to a portable transmitter worn around the neck or waist, and the ECG is transmitted electronically to a central monitoring station for continuous monitoring.

Home Monitoring
Patients often complain of palpitations or other heart symptoms but are asymptomatic during evaluation in a hospital or community-based setting. Ambulatory or Holter monitoring may be used to identify intermittent dysrhythmias, to detect silent ischemia, to monitor the effects of treatment, and to assess pacemaker or automatic cardioverter–defibrillator function. Electrodes are applied and the leads attached to the portable telemetry monitor that records and stores all electrical activity. Patients are instructed to leave the electrode pads in place during monitoring and record any cardiac symptoms or events (e.g., chest pain, palpitations, syncope) in a journal. After the prescribed period, usually 48–72 hours, the patient returns to the clinic, and the monitor is removed. Diary entries are compared to the recorded heart rhythms to identify the effects of dysrhythmias.

Electrophysiology Studies
Diagnostic cardiac electrophysiology procedures are performed to identify dysrhythmias and their causes. Electrophysiology studies are used to analyze components of the conduction system, identify sites of ectopic stimulation, and evaluate the effectiveness of treatment. Electrophysiology procedures can be employed for both diagnosis and therapeutic intervention.

In the electrophysiology laboratory, electrode catheters are guided by fluoroscopy into the heart through the femoral or brachial vein. The timing and sequence of electrical activation during normal and abnormal (aberrant) rhythms are observed and measured. Providers may use electrical stimulation to induce dysrhythmia similar to what the patient is experiencing. Following diagnosis, an electrophysiology procedure may be used to treat the dysrhythmia—for example, by overdrive pacing (stimulating the patient's heart to a rate faster than that of the tachydysrhythmia) to break the dysrhythmia cycle or ablative therapy to destroy the ectopic site. (For further information, see the Cardiac Mapping and Catheter Ablation section later in this exemplar.)

Nursing care for the patient undergoing an electrophysiology procedure is similar to that for the patient undergoing PCR. (See the discussion in the Revascularization Procedures section in Exemplar 16.C on Coronary Artery Disease for more details.) The nurse explains the procedure and expected sensations. The patient remains awake during the procedure; antianxiety medications or sedatives are given to reduce apprehension. IV heparin may be given during the procedure to reduce the risk of thromboembolism.

Pharmacologic Therapy

The goal of drug therapy is to suppress dysrhythmia formation. No drug has been found to be completely safe and effective. Antidysrhythmic drugs are primarily used for treatment of acute dysrhythmias, although they may also be used to manage chronic conditions. The overall goal of therapy is to maintain an effective CO by stabilizing cardiac rhythm. See the Medications feature.

Many antidysrhythmic drugs also have prodysrhythmic effects; that is, they can worsen existing dysrhythmias and precipitate new ones. Prior to administering antidysrhythmic medications, the nurse will want to obtain a thorough drug and medical history and measure baseline vital signs and cardiac rhythm. Labs should also be reviewed prior to initiating antidysrhythmic therapy.

Most antidysrhythmic drugs are classified by their effects on the cardiac action potential. Most are class I drugs, or fast sodium channel blockers. By blocking sodium channels, these drugs slow impulse conduction in the atria and ventricles. This class is further divided into subclasses A, B, and C. Class II drugs are beta-adrenergic blockers, which decrease SA node automaticity, AV conduction velocity, and myocardial contractility. Class III agents block potassium channels, delaying repolarization and prolonging the relative refractory period. Class IV drugs are CCBs. Their effect is similar to that of beta-blockers. Adenosine and digoxin do not fit within the major classes. Both drugs reduce SA node automaticity and slow AV conduction. Ibutilide and magnesium also fall outside the major classes but are used to treat dysrhythmias. The Medications feature identifies common antidysrhythmic drugs within each class and the nursing implications in caring for patients receiving these drugs.

Drugs that affect the autonomic nervous system may also be used to treat dysrhythmias. Sympathomimetics, such as epinephrine, stimulate the heart, increasing both heart rate and contractility. Anticholinergic agents, such as atropine, are used to decrease vagal tone and increase heart rate. Magnesium sulfate is an unclassified drug that has been shown to be safe and effective in treating VTs.

Countershock

Countershock is used to interrupt cardiac rhythms that compromise CO. Delivery of a direct current charge depolarizes all cardiac cells at the same time. This simultaneous depolarization may stop a tachydysrhythmia and allow the SA node to recover control of impulse formation. The two types of countershock are synchronized cardioversion and defibrillation.

Synchronized Cardioversion

Synchronized cardioversion delivers direct electrical current synchronized with the patient's heart rhythm. Synchronization of the shock with the QRS complex prevents VF by avoiding current delivery during the vulnerable period of repolarization. Cardioversion is usually done as an elective procedure to treat SVT, atrial fibrillation, atrial flutter, or hemodynamically stable VTs.

The nurse assists with cardioversion by preparing the patient before the procedure; obtaining any laboratory tests ordered; obtaining and documenting ECG strips before, during, and after treatment; setting up the equipment; and monitoring the patient's response.

Patients in atrial fibrillation are at high risk for thromboembolism following cardioversion. Loss of atrial contractions with atrial fibrillation leads to blood pooling in the atria, increasing the risk of clot formation. When the atria begin to contract following successful cardioversion, clots may be dislodged, embolizing to the pulmonary or systemic circulation. If possible, anticoagulants are given for several weeks before cardioversion is attempted.

Defibrillation

Unlike carefully synchronized cardioversion, **defibrillation** is an emergency procedure that delivers direct current without regard to the cardiac cycle. VF is immediately treated as soon as the dysrhythmia is recognized. Early defibrillation has been shown to improve survival in patients experiencing VF.

Defibrillation can be delivered by external paddles or pads or internal paddles. Conductive gel pads or paste are applied, and external paddles or pads are placed on the chest wall at the apex and base of the heart (see **Figure 16–48 »**). Internal paddles are applied directly on the heart and may be used in surgery, the emergency department, or critical care. Internal defibrillation is done only by a physician; external defibrillation may be performed by any healthcare provider who has been trained in the procedure. Automatic external defibrillators are available on most hospital units to allow early defibrillation for cardiac arrest.

Pacemaker Therapy

A **pacemaker** is a pulse generator used to provide an electrical stimulus to the heart when the heart fails to generate or conduct its own stimulus at a rate that maintains the CO. The pulse generator is connected to leads (insulated wires) passed intravenously into the heart or sutured directly to the epicardium. The leads sense intrinsic electrical activity of the heart and provide an electrical stimulus to the heart when necessary (pacing).

Pacemakers are used to treat both acute and chronic conduction defects, such as third-degree AV block. They also may be used to treat bradydysrhythmias and tachydysrhythmias.

Temporary pacemakers use an external pulse generator attached to a lead threaded intravenously into the right ventricle, to temporary pacing wires implanted during cardiac

Medications
Antidysrhythmic Drugs

CLASSIFICATION AND DRUG EXAMPLES	MECHANISMS OF ACTION	NURSING CONSIDERATIONS

Class I Drugs: Sodium Channel Blockers
 	
Class IA
Drug examples:
Quinidine (Cardioquin, Quinidex, Quinaglute)
Procainamide (Pronestyl, Procan SR)
Disopyramide (Norpace, Norpace CR)
	Decrease the flow of sodium into the cell and prolong the action potential
	Decrease automaticity, slow the rate of impulse conduction, and prolong refractoriness
	Used to treat both SVT and VT
		■ Obtain baseline data, including vital signs, cardiac rhythm (including rate, PR and QT intervals, and QRS duration), and physical assessment (especially cardiac, neurologic, and respiratory status).
		■ Assess medication regimen to identify drugs that may interfere with antidysrhythmic therapy.
		■ Monitor ECG to evaluate the effectiveness of therapy and assess for possible dysrhythmias precipitated by treatment.
		■ Immediately report to the physician any manifestations of drug toxicity:
		  • Procainamide: signs of heart failure; conduction delays or ventricular dysrhythmias; skin rash, myalgias or arthralgias, flu-like symptoms
		  • Disopyramide: urinary retention, heart failure, eye pain
		  • Lidocaine: changes in neurologic status, such as agitation, confusion, dizziness, nervousness
		  • Amiodarone: pulmonary fibrosis (increasing dyspnea, cough, hepatic dysfunction—changes in liver function tests, jaundice); vision changes, photosensitivity
		  • Digoxin: anorexia, nausea, vomiting; blurred or double vision; yellow-green halos; new-onset dysrhythmias.
		■ Use an infusion pump to administer IV infusions. Monitor the dose, and assess its appropriateness (in mg/min or mcg/kg/min).
		
		Heath education for the patient and family:
		■ Take the drug exactly as prescribed. Do not skip or double doses. Check with your physician if a dose is missed.
		■ Take your pulse, and record the rate daily before rising. Count the pulse for a full minute. Bring the record with you to each office or clinic visit.
		■ Report the following to the physician: irregular pulse rate or rhythm, dizziness, eye pain, changes in vision, skin rashes or color changes, wheezing or other respiratory problems, and changes in behavior.

Class IB *Drug examples:* Lidocaine (Xylocaine) Mexiletine (Mexitil) Phenytoin (Dilantin)	Decrease the refractory period but have little effect on automaticity Used primarily to treat ventricular dysrhythmias, including PVCs and VTs	
Class IC *Drug examples:* Flecainide (Tambocor) Propafenone (Rythmol)	Slow impulse conduction velocity Have little effect on refractoriness Used to reduce or eliminate tachy-dysrhythmias associated with reentry May be used to treat SVT	
Class II Drugs: Beta-Adrenergic Blockers *Drug examples:* Esmolol (Brevibloc) Propranolol (Inderal) Metoprolol (Toprol)	Decrease automaticity through the AV node Reduce the heart rate and myocardial contractility Used to treat SVT and to slow the ventricular response rate to atrial fibrillation May cause bronchospasm and are contraindicated for patients with asthma, COPD, or other restrictive or obstructive	
Class III Drugs: Potassium Channel Blockers *Drug examples:* Sotalol (Betapace) Amiodarone (Cordarone) Ibutilide (Corvert) Dofetilide (Tikosyn)	Block potassium channels, prolonging repolarization and the refractory period Primarily used to treat VT and VF Amiodarone: may be used to treat SVTs	
Class IV Drugs: Calcium Channel Blockers (CCBs) *Drug examples:* Verapamil (Calan, Verelan) Diltiazem (Cardizem, Dilacor XR)	Decrease automaticity and AV nodal conduction Used to manage SVTs Reduce myocardial contractility	
Other Drugs *Drug examples:* Adenosine (Adenocard) Digoxin	Decrease conduction through the AV node Used to treat SVTs	

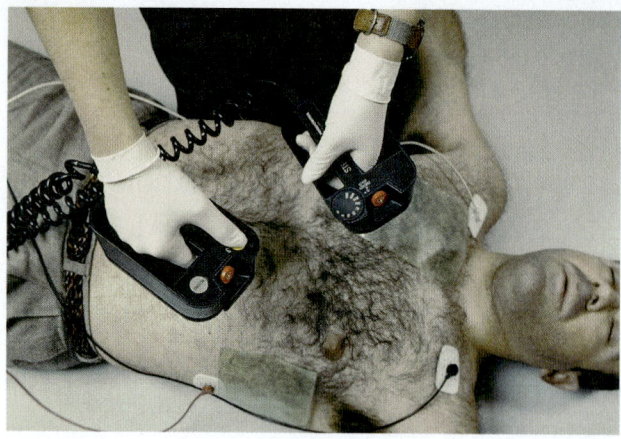

Figure 16–48 ❯❯ Placement of paddles for defibrillation.

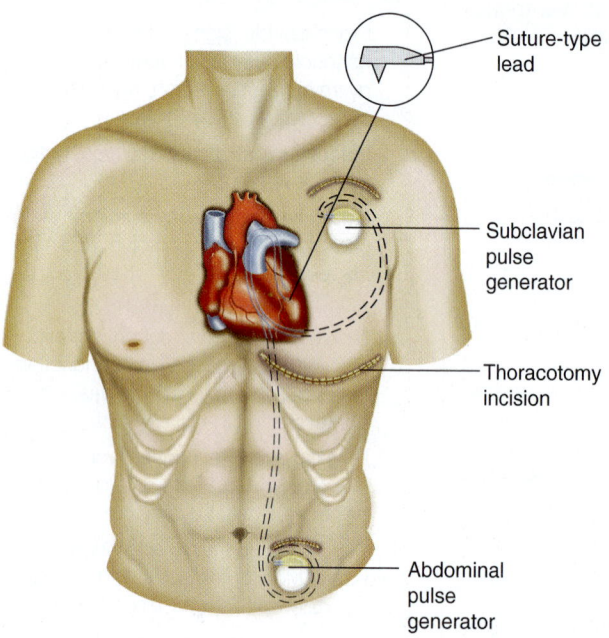

Figure 16–49 ❯❯ A permanent epicardial pacemaker. The pulse generator may be placed in subcutaneous pockets in the sub-clavian or abdominal regions.

Labels: Suture-type lead; Subclavian pulse generator; Thoracotomy incision; Abdominal pulse generator

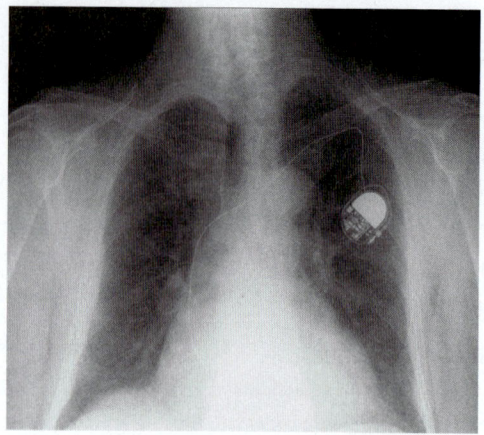

Source: Living Art Enterprises/Science Source.

Figure 16–50 ❯❯ A permanent transvenous (endocardial) pace-maker with the lead placed in the right ventricle via the subcla-vian vein.

TABLE 16–27 Terms Used to Describe Pacemaker Functions

Term	Definition
Asynchronous pacing	Pacemaker delivers a pacing stimulus at a set rate regardless of intrinsic cardiac activity
Base rate	Rate at which the pacemaker paces when no cardiac activity is sensed
Capture	The ability of the pacing stimulus to generate a car-diac depolarization
Demand pacing	Pacemaker delivers a pacing stimulus only when the intrinsic rate falls below the pacemaker's base rate
Dual-chamber pacing	Allows both the atria and the ventricles to be paced; most frequently used permanent pacing mode
Output	The electrical stimulus delivered by the pulse generator
Pacing spike	A small vertical spike noted on the ECG with every pacemaker stimulus
Rate-responsive pacing	Pacemaker has sensors that detect changes in the patient's physical activity and adjust the pacing rate accordingly
Sensing	The pacemaker's ability to identify and respond to intrinsic cardiac activity
Single-chamber pacing	Pacing of only the atria or the ventricles, not both; most commonly used temporary pacing mode

surgery, or to external conductive pads placed on the chest wall for emergency pacing. Permanent pacemakers use an internal pulse generator placed in a subcutaneous pocket in the subclavian space or abdominal wall. The generator connects to leads sewn directly onto the heart (epicardial) or passed transvenously into the heart (endocardial). Epicardial pacemakers (see **Figure 16–49** ❯❯) require surgical exposure of the heart. Leads may be placed during cardiac surgery or by using a small subxiphoid incision to expose the heart. Transvenous pacemaker leads are positioned in the right heart via the cephalic, subclavian, or jugular vein (see **Figure 16–50** ❯❯). Local anesthesia can be used for permanent pacemaker insertion.

Pacemakers are programmed to stimulate the atria or the ventricles (single-chamber pacing) or both (dual-chamber

pacing). **Table 16–27** ❯❯ defines terms used to describe pacemaker modes and functions. The most commonly used pacemakers either sense activity in and pace the ventricles only or sense activity in and pace both the atria and the ventricles. Dual-chamber or AV sequential pacing stimulates both chambers of the heart in sequence. AV pacing imitates the normal sequence of atrial contraction followed by ventricular contraction, improving CO.

Pacing is detected on the ECG strip by the presence of a pacing artifact (see **Figure 16–51** ❯❯). A sharp spike is noted before the P wave with atrial pacing and before the QRS

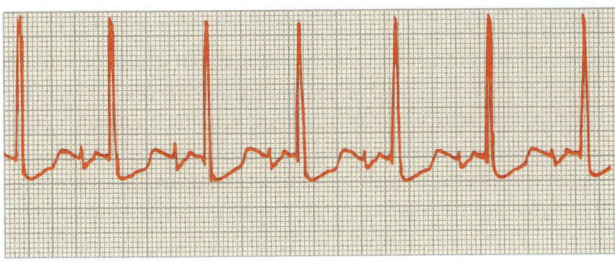

A

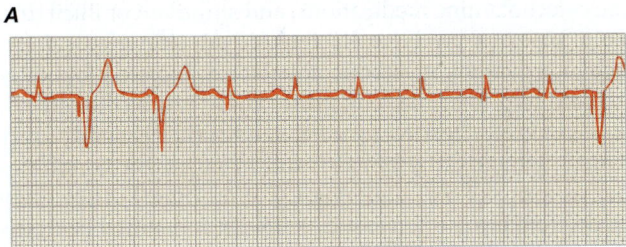

B

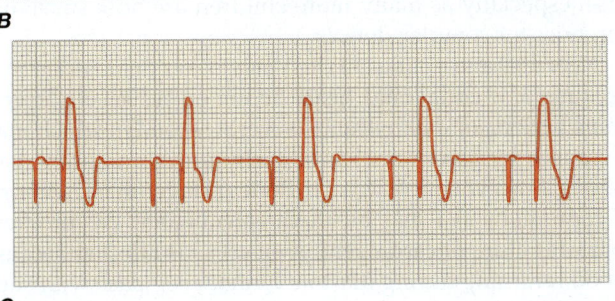

C

Figure 16–51 ⟫ Pacing artifacts. **A,** Atrial pacing and ventricular sensing. Note the pacer spike preceding the P wave. **B,** Ventricular demand pacing. Note the absence of pacer spikes when the patient's natural rhythm dominates. **C,** Atrioventricular pacing. Note the pacer spikes preceding both P waves and QRS complexes.

complex with ventricular pacing. Pacing spikes are seen before both the P wave and QRS complex in AV sequential pacing. Capture is noted if a contraction of the chamber occurs immediately following the pacer spike. Problems in sensing, pacing, and capture are noted in **Table 16–28** ⟫.

Box 16–19
Safety for Patients with a Temporary Pacemaker

- Ensure that all electrical equipment in use has a grounded plug; do not use adapters or extension cords.
- Encourage use of battery-powered equipment (e.g., electric razor).
- Remove any damaged electrical equipment from the unit, including equipment that has been abused (e.g., has been dropped in liquid, has had liquid spilled on it); has given anyone a shock; has frayed, worn, or otherwise damaged electrical cords or plugs; or has other evidence of impaired function, such as a hot smell during use or control knobs that are loose or do not consistently produce the expected response.
- Wear gloves when handling the pacemaker electrodes or wires.
- Insulate pacemaker terminals and pacing wires with nonconductive, moisture-proof material (e.g., a rubber glove).
- Test the pacemaker battery before use.
- Keep a spare pacemaker, cable, batteries, and battery tester available at all times.
- Immediately report any apparent deviation from expected pacemaker function.

Care of the patient with a temporary or permanent pacemaker focuses on monitoring for pacemaker malfunctioning, maintaining safety (see **Box 16–19** ⟫), and preventing infection and postoperative complications.

Implantable Cardioverter–Defibrillator

The ICD detects life-threatening changes in the cardiac rhythm and automatically delivers an electric shock to convert the dysrhythmia back into a normal rhythm. ICDs are used for survivors of sudden cardiac death (SCD), patients with recurrent VT, and patients with demonstrated risk factors for SCD. ICDs can deliver a shock as needed, provide pacing on demand, and store ECG records of tachycardic episodes.

TABLE 16–28 Potential Pacemaker Problems and Considerations for Preventing Complications

Device Complication	Considerations for Preventing Complications
Lead dislodgement	Examine active and passive fixation mechanisms.
Pneumothorax, hemothorax, or air embolism	Use fluoroscopic guidance of the subclavian puncture with careful technique. Use introducers with hemostatic valves.
Myocardial perforation during lead placement	Consider lead design prior to implantation. Ensure physician experience. Examine the patient's condition.
Extracardiac stimulation	Decrease voltage output or pulse width. The pacemaker may need to be reprogrammed or the leads repositioned.
Venous thrombosis and superior vena cava syndrome	Asymptomatic patients are usually not treated. Specific treatment for thrombosis or fibrosis is causative. Treatment varies from heparin therapy to percutaneous angioplasty or open surgical procedure. Surgery is the last resort.
Twiddler syndrome (leads become displaced due to the pacemaker box)	The size of the pacemaker pocket should be limited, with the device sutured to the fascia. Patients should be instructed not to manipulate device pockets.
Postpacemaker implant pericarditis	Use anti-inflammatory medications. Consider repositioning pacemaker leads and/or removing them.

A pulse generator connected to lead electrodes for rhythm detection and current delivery is implanted in the left pectoral region. The lead is threaded transvenously to the apex of the right ventricle. The ICD is programmed to sense a change in heart rate or rhythm. When it detects a potentially lethal rhythm, it shocks the heart to convert the rhythm. The device can be programmed or reprogrammed at the bedside as necessary. The ICD may be tested before discharge.

Local or general anesthesia is used, and the patient may be discharged within 24 hours. The lithium-powered battery must be surgically replaced every 5 years. Complications and nursing care are similar to those for a patient having a permanent pacemaker implant.

The patient may briefly lose consciousness before the device discharges but typically regains consciousness quickly after the episode. Some patients report significant discomfort with ICD discharge (like a "blow to the chest"). Anyone in direct contact with the patient when the device discharges may experience a tingling sensation.

Cardiac Mapping and Catheter Ablation

Cardiac mapping and catheter ablation are used to locate and destroy an ectopic focus. An ectopic focus is a cardiac stimulus, or pacemaker, that is located somewhere other than the SA node. Cardiac mapping and catheter ablation use electrophysiology techniques and can be performed in a cardiac catheterization laboratory. Cardiac mapping is used to identify the site of earliest impulse formation in the atria or ventricles. Intracardiac and extracardiac catheter electrodes and computer technology are used to pinpoint the ectopic site on a map of the heart. These same catheters can be used to deliver the ablative intervention.

Ablation destroys, removes, or isolates an ectopic focus. In most instances, radio-frequency energy produced by high-frequency alternating current is used to create heat as it passes through tissue. Catheter ablation is used to treat SVTs, atrial fibrillation and flutter, and in some cases, paroxysmal VT. Anticoagulant therapy may be started after catheter ablation to reduce the risk of clot formation at the ablation site.

Other Therapies

In addition to medications and interventional techniques, other measures may be used to treat selected dysrhythmias. Vagal maneuvers that stimulate the parasympathetic nervous system may be used to slow the heart rate in SVTs; these include carotid sinus massage and the Valsalva maneuver. Excessive slowing of the heart rate may result from carotid sinus massage, and it is performed only by a physician during continuous cardiac monitoring. The Valsalva maneuver increases intrathoracic pressure and vagal tone, slowing the pulse rate.

Lifespan Considerations

Some types of dysrhythmias are more frequent in children than in adults, whereas others are more frequent in older adults than younger individuals. The following sections detail these differences and provide additional information regarding dysrhythmias in pregnant women.

Dysrhythmias in Infants and Children

Cardiac dysrhythmias occur frequently in children but less commonly than in adults. Dysrhythmias can cause decreased CO and heart failure or can progress further to an even more serious dysrhythmia that could result in sudden death.

Tachydysrhythmias (e.g., sinus tachycardia) often occur with acute conditions, such as hypoxia, anemia, hypovolemia, shock, hyperkalemia or hypokalemia, hyperthyroidism, catecholamine medications, and stimulant or illicit drug use. Causes of bradycardia include specific medications, vagal stimulation, metabolic imbalances, hypoxia, hypothyroidism, hypothermia, and AMI. These types of dysrhythmias generally resolve once the underlying condition is treated. Some dysrhythmias result from genetic conditions, such as forms of SVT and long-QT syndrome. Less common dysrhythmias are often associated with congenital heart disease, especially as many more children are now surviving surgeries for complex defects.

Neonates and young children may be predisposed to SVT because of a congenital heart defect or WPW syndrome. Short periods of dysrhythmia (several seconds), which may be caused by paroxysmal atrial tachycardia, are rarely dangerous; however, prolonged episodes (longer than 24 hours) of continuous SVT may be life threatening and can progress to heart failure or cardiogenic shock. CO is affected because blood returning during diastole cannot keep pace with such a rapid heart rate.

Symptoms of dysrhythmias in children depend on age and development. Infants and toddlers may experience irritability, paleness, and difficulty feeding or eating. Older children may be able to state that they feel lightheaded or that their heart is fluttering. Other symptoms may include weakness, tiredness, fainting, chest pain, sweating, and shortness of breath.

Children suspected of having a dysrhythmia should be monitored for LOC, heart rate, and other vital signs. A cardiorespiratory monitor and pulse oximetry should be used to identify deterioration of the child's condition. An early indicator of cardiopulmonary compromise is a change in the child's mental status or LOC. Changes in color, weakness, irritability, and feeding patterns may indicate the development of hypoxia. Any child found to have an abnormal ECG finding, unusual heart rhythm, syncope (especially with exercise), or dizziness with palpitations should be referred to a pediatric cardiologist for evaluation.

Episodes of dysrhythmia are frightening for both children and parents, as are the unpredictability of recurrent episodes and the risk for SCD with some dysrhythmias. The nurse should provide support, encourage the parents to promote the child's normal development between episodes, and emphasize that medications help prevent or reduce episode frequency. Other nursing interventions include the following:

- Carefully explain the treatment plan and home care.
- Teach parents to take the child's apical pulse. Make sure parents are trained in CPR and use of the Valsalva maneuver.
- Provide telephone numbers of emergency medical facilities, and help parents plan how to seek emergency care.

- Make sure the parents and child with SVT understand the need to avoid using cardiac stimulant drugs, such as decongestants, because these drugs might trigger an episode.
- Describe and provide written instructions about the danger signs indicating a recurrence of the acute condition and how to seek emergency care.
- Prepare the child and family for procedures such as radio-frequency ablation or implantation of a pacemaker or ICD.

Dysrhythmias in Pregnant Women

In roughly half of women during pregnancy, premature atrial beats occur. In most cases, these are harmless and do not last. Although sustained dysrhythmia in pregnant women is relatively rare, for those pregnant women who have SVT or PSVT, symptoms such as shortness of breath, palpitations, and dizziness worsen in 20% of cases. Hormonal changes; changes in associated hemodynamic, hormonal, and autonomic changes; and changes in circulating blood volume, sleep, and emotion during pregnancy all may cause dysrhythmias to occur more frequently during pregnancy. Women with repaired congenital heart defects are at increased risk of dysrhythmias during pregnancy. Dysrhythmias in pregnancy are treated conservatively, with antidysrhythmic medications being used when the dysrhythmia causes symptoms or a drop in BP (Cleveland Clinic, 2015b).

Dysrhythmias in Older Adults

Aging affects the heart and the cardiac conduction system, increasing the incidence of dysrhythmias and conduction defects. Older adults may experience dysrhythmias even when no evidence of heart disease is found.

Older adults have a higher incidence of both ventricular and supraventricular dysrhythmias without detrimental effects compared with younger individuals. Ectopic beats, including short runs of VT, occur more commonly during exercise in older adults. These dysrhythmias do not affect cardiac morbidity or mortality. Fibrosis of the bundle branches can lead to AV blocks; a prolonged PR interval is common in patients over the age of 65. Older adults also have a higher incidence of diseases that may affect heart rhythm. An older patient with hyperthyroidism, for example, may present with atrial fibrillation, syncope, and confusion instead of the usual manifestations of goiter, tremor, and exophthalmos.

Assessment of the older adult for problems related to cardiac dysrhythmias focuses on the effect of the dysrhythmia on functional health status. In assessing the older adult, the nurse should do the following:

- Ask about a history of cardiovascular disease and current medications.
- Inquire about symptoms such as episodes of dizziness, lightheadedness, fainting, palpitations, chest pain, or shortness of breath.
- Ask about the relationship between symptoms such as palpitations and intake of certain foods and caffeine-containing beverages.
- Evaluate for other contributing factors, such as smoking or alcohol intake.
- Inquire about a history of falls, particularly any that occurred without apparent reason.

Older adults with a dysrhythmia will require patient teaching to reduce the risk of cardiac dysrhythmias and potential adverse consequences of dysrhythmias. The nurse should do the following:

- Emphasize the importance of taking medications as prescribed. Discuss possible effects of over-the-counter medications on the heart.
- Encourage the patient to reduce or eliminate caffeine intake. Caffeine increases the risk of ectopic beats and rapid heart rates.
- Encourage the patient to participate in a smoking cessation program and reduction or elimination of alcohol intake if appropriate.
- Encourage the patient to engage in regular exercise. Discuss the beneficial effects of exercise to maintain muscle mass, including cardiac muscle, and cardiovascular health.
- Instruct the patient to contact the primary care provider for evaluation of symptoms such as dizziness, fainting, frequent palpitations, shortness of breath, unexplained falls, or chest pain.

SUDDEN CARDIAC DEATH

Overview

Sudden cardiac death (SCD) is defined as unexpected death occurring within 1 hour of the onset of cardiovascular symptoms. It usually is caused by VF and cardiac arrest. **Cardiac arrest** is the cessation of heart function that precedes biological death. Worldwide, fewer than 6% of out-of-hospital victims of cardiac arrest survive. In communities of North America that have organized lay rescuer and automated external defibrillator (AED) programs, the survival rate is significantly better, ranging from 49 to 74% when a witnessed arrest caused by VF occurs (AHA, 2015p).

More than 50% of all deaths from coronary heart disease are attributed to SCD (Deo & Albert, 2012). Risk factors for SCD are those associated with coronary heart disease. SCD occurs most frequently in adults in their mid-30s to mid-40s (Cleveland Clinic, 2015c). Men are affected twice as often as women. Patients with dysrhythmias such as recurrent VT may have a higher risk of SCD. SCD is rare in children.

Pathophysiology and Etiology

Pathophysiology

Evidence of coronary heart disease with significant atherosclerosis and narrowing of two or more major coronary arteries is found in 75% of patients who experience SCD. Although most have had a previous MI, only 20–30% have had a recent AMI. An acute change in cardiovascular status precedes cardiac arrest by up to 1 hour; however, the onset often is instantaneous or abrupt. Tachycardia develops, and the number of PVCs increases. VT occurs, progressing to VF (Perrin & MacLeod, 2012). This causes blood flow to the brain to be reduced. Death follows unless emergency treatment occurs immediately.

Abnormalities of myocardial structure or function also contribute. Structural abnormalities include infarction, hypertrophy, myopathy, and electrical anomalies. Functional deviations are caused by such factors as ischemia followed by reperfusion, altered homeostasis, autonomic nervous system and hormone interactions, and toxic effects. The interactions of the two cause myocardial instability and may precipitate fatal dysrhythmias.

Etiology

More than 50% of all deaths due to coronary heart disease are attributed to SCD, and coronary heart disease increases the risk of SCD up to five times (Deo & Albert, 2012). Other cardiac pathologies, such as cardiomyopathy and valvular disorders, also may lead to SCD. Noncardiac causes of sudden death include electrocution, PE, and rapid blood loss from a ruptured aortic aneurysm.

VF is the most common dysrhythmia associated with SCD, accounting for 65–80% of cardiac arrests. Survival in these cases largely depends on potentially controllable or reversible electrophysiologic disturbances. Selected cardiac and noncardiac causes of SCD are listed in **Box 16–20 ≫**.

Risk Factors and Prevention

Risk factors for SCD are similar to those that cause CAD or any cardiac dysfunction. Smoking, obesity, hypertension, diabetes mellitus, sedentary lifestyle, and high-fat diets can result in cardiac disease (see the Focus on Diversity and Culture feature). Alterations in cardiac function can affect the electrical activity, resulting in dysrhythmias. Prevention of conditions such as hypertension and atherosclerosis can help prevent dysrhythmias as well; such prevention measures largely involve lifestyle choices such as eating a

Focus on Diversity and Culture
Risk for Sudden Cardiac Death

Multiple studies related to racial differences and SCD have indicated that African Americans are at much higher risk of SCD than individuals of other races, including Caucasians, Hispanics, and Asians (Fender, Henrikson, & Tereshchenko, 2014; Okin et al., 2012). African Americans are less likely to receive more advanced levels of treatment, such as an ICD, than Caucasians. African Americans also have a higher incidence of many risk factors related to SCD, including obesity, smoking, hypertension, and previously diagnosed heart disease. African Americans are also more likely to have genetic variants that predispose them to SCD, particularly mutations in cardiac potassium and sodium channels (Deo & Albert, 2012).

heart-healthy diet, not smoking, engaging in regular physical activity, and managing stress (see Box 16–2).

Clinical Manifestations

SCD may be preceded by typical manifestations of ACS or MI, including severe chest pain, dyspnea or orthopnea, and palpitations or lightheadedness. The event itself is abrupt, with complete loss of consciousness and death within minutes. If VT precedes cardiac arrest, consciousness and mentation may be impaired prior to collapse and loss of consciousness.

Collaboration

The goal of care for the patient with SCD is to restore CO and tissue perfusion. Treatment measures are initiated as soon as clinical cardiac arrest is verified by the absence of respirations and carotid or femoral pulses. Basic and advanced cardiac life support measures must be instituted within 2–4 minutes of cardiac arrest to prevent permanent neurologic damage and ischemic injury to other organs.

Basic Life Support

Basic life support begins with identification of the cardiac arrest and initiation of an emergency response. Providers trained in use of an AED should immediately defibrillate the patient who is in VF. Self-adhesive conductive pads attached to connecting cables are positioned on the chest (see **Figure 16–52 ≫**). The AED analyzes the rhythm and advises the provider to charge the device if VF is detected. After all personnel have been warned to stand clear, the shock button is depressed to deliver a shock. Following the shock, CPR is immediately initiated. After approximately 2 minutes, or five cycles of CPR, the rhythm is evaluated and circulation checked. The sequence of analysis, shock, CPR is continued, and advanced cardiac life support protocols are initiated (AHA, 2015p).

Cardiopulmonary resuscitation (CPR) is a mechanical attempt to maintain tissue perfusion and oxygenation using oral resuscitation and external cardiac compressions. All healthcare providers need to be proficient in CPR. The technique should be performed according to AHA guidelines and hospital protocol. Research demonstrates a clear

Box 16–20
Selected Causes of Sudden Cardiac Death

Cardiac Causes
- Coronary heart disease
- Reperfusion following ischemia
- Myocardial hypertrophy
- Cardiomyopathy
- Inflammatory myocardial disorders
- Valve disorders
- Primary electrical disorders
- Dissecting or ruptured aortic or ventricular aneurysm
- Cardiac drug toxicity

Noncardiac Causes
- Pulmonary embolism (PE)
- Cerebral hemorrhage
- Autonomic dysfunction
- Choking
- Electrical shock
- Electrolyte and acid–base imbalances

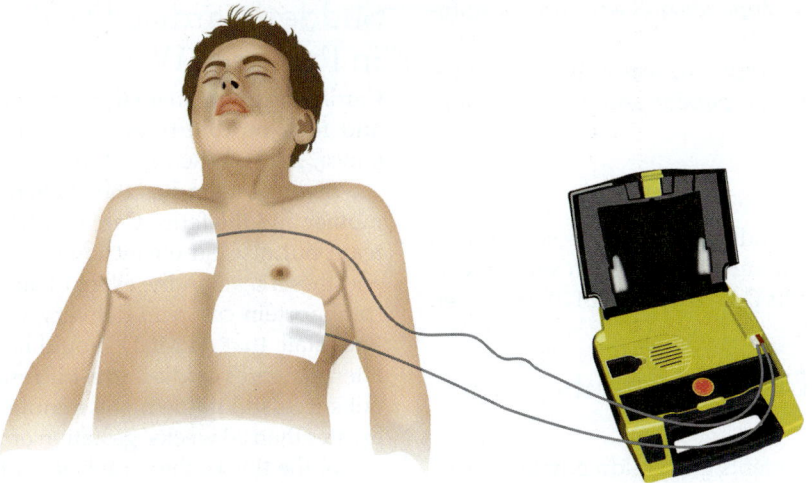

Figure 16–52 》 Schematic of an automated external defibrillator (AED) attached to a patient.

benefit from sustained, effective chest compressions, yet compressions often are interrupted for ventilation, assessment of pulses, and other measures. The 2015 AHA CPR guidelines reflect changes that align with current research findings (AHA, 2015c).

CPR carries a high risk for both cardiac and noncardiac trauma. CPR-related complications include injuries to the skin, thorax, upper airway, abdomen, lungs, heart, and great vessels. These complications can be minimized by adhering to accepted CPR techniques.

》 Stay Current: Visit the website of the AHA at http://www.heart.org to stay abreast of their latest recommendations. Note the new hands-only CPR that is recommended for use outside of hospital settings: http://www.heart.org/HEARTORG/CPRAndECC/HandsOnlyCPR/LearnMore/Learn-More_UCM_440810_FAQ.jsp.

Advanced Life Support

Advanced life support, provided by specially trained healthcare personnel, includes advanced airway support (insertion of a laryngeal mask airway, esophageal–tracheal Combitube, or endotracheal intubation) to maintain the airway and oxygenation, use of IV drugs following specific protocols, and additional interventions, such as repeated defibrillation procedures and cardiac pacing. Epinephrine, vasopressin, sodium bicarbonate, and antidysrhythmic drugs, such as amiodarone, lidocaine, procainamide, magnesium sulfate, and atropine are used to attempt to restore and maintain an effective cardiac rhythm.

Postresuscitation Care

Patients experiencing sudden cardiac arrest continue to have a poor prognosis, even with advances in the treatment of heart disease. Treatment depends on the underlying diagnosis. Specific considerations for patient care are found in **Box 16–21 》**.

After successful resuscitation, the nurse provides care specific to the patient's underlying disease processes and needs. IV infusions, such as lidocaine, or dopamine, may be ordered to prevent further dysrhythmias and maintain hemodynamic stability.

Box 16–21
Nursing Care of Patients Experiencing Sudden Cardiac Arrest

Nursing care of the patient experiencing sudden cardiac arrest requires prompt recognition of the event and immediate initiation of basic and advanced life support protocols. Fast and effective cardiac compressions and early defibrillation of unstable VT and fibrillation are the most important keys to the survival of a cardiac arrest event. Important concepts of emergency cardiac care include the following:

- Treat the patient, not the monitor. Recognize signs and symptoms of cardiac compromise early.
- Activate the emergency medical services system (call a code or 9-1-1).
- Begin and continue basic cardiac life support principles throughout the resuscitation effort.
- Continually assess the effectiveness of emergency interventions.
- Defibrillate pulseless VT or fibrillation as soon as possible.
- Initiate advanced life support protocols early.

Care for the Family

Nursing care of the patient experiencing sudden cardiac arrest includes providing care to the family. The nurse provides honest information about the patient's condition to the family in a supportive manner and assesses the family's coping abilities and resources.

If family members are present, they are usually offered a private consultation room in which to await the outcome. If the family members are not present, they are notified that their family member is not doing well and are asked to come to the hospital as soon as possible. The situation is presented in a careful manner to prevent the family from racing to the hospital, possibly precipitating an automobile crash. The nurse offers pastoral care or the family's choice of spiritual support during this difficult time. Attendance of family members during resuscitation efforts is controversial and depends on institutional protocols and family desires.

If the patient does not survive the arrest, the nurse provides postmortem care to the patient and emotional and spiritual support to the family.

Lifespan Considerations

As people age, the risk of sudden cardiac arrest increases (NHLBI, 2015e). As a result, most deaths from sudden cardiac arrest are in older adults (Mayo Clinic, 2014i). However, SCD can occur at any age.

Sudden Cardiac Death in Infants and Children

SCD most often occurs in infants and children with a structural defect in the heart. Cardiac arrest in infants and children can be the result of either progressive respiratory failure, shock, or both. It is less common but still possible for pediatric cardiac arrest to occur without warning as a sudden collapse following an arrhythmia—either a VF or VT.

Compressions and ventilations in CPR have shown improved survival results for children over using only compressions, even though compressions alone are preferable to no CPR for any victim of cardiac arrest (AHA, 2014c). This is in part because of the high rate of respiratory arrest in children. However, if the rescuer is not willing to perform mouth-to-mouth breaths, then compression-only CPR should be initiated (AHA, 2015c).

Infants and children require special considerations when CPR is needed. When performing CPR on neonates, thumbs should be placed side by side, or overlapping in very small neonates, and compressions should be performed below the nipple line. For infants, two fingers placed in the upright position should be used for compressions. For children, the provider should use two fingers plus the heel of the other hand to perform compressions (O'Connor, 2013). Although compressions without ventilation is now recommended for adults, this same recommendation has not been made for children because of the high rate of respiratory arrest in children.

Sudden Cardiac Death in Young People

Although it is rare, when sudden death occurs in people under age 35, the cause is often hidden heart defects or overlooked heart abnormalities, particularly hypertrophic cardiomyopathy. The context of these sudden deaths is frequently physical activity, such as participating in a sporting event. SCD among young adults, including athletes, is rare, with incidence rates increasing from 1 in 100,000 to 300,000 for athletes younger than 35 to 1 in 15,000 for joggers and 1 in 50,000 for marathon runners age 35 and older (Cleveland Clinic, 2015c; Mayo Clinic, 2014i). Individuals who experience syncope or seizures (both indicators of risk for SCD) during exercise should be encouraged to have a full physical performed to identify any cardiac abnormalities. Another risk factor for SCD is having a relative with an unexpected and unexplained sudden death before the age of 50. Children and young adults with these risks should be screened for cardiac abnormalities (American Academy of Pediatrics [AAP], 2012).

Sudden Cardiac Death in Pregnant Women

Cardiac arrest in pregnancy is associated with high maternal and fetal morbidity and mortality (Rodrigues, Clode, & Graca, 2014). When a pregnant woman is in cardiac arrest, the medical team has the challenge of caring for both the mother and the fetus. Care involves not only the emergency team but also an obstetric team, a neonatal team, and an anesthesia team in the event of an emergency cesarean birth (perimortem cesarean delivery, or PMCD). Current guidelines state that a PMCD should be performed by 5 minutes after maternal cardiac arrest if resuscitation measures were not successful in the first 4 minutes, especially if the fetus is greater than 20 weeks' gestation or if the uterus extends to or above the line of the umbilicus. If the gravid uterus is large enough to cause aortocaval compression, the fetus should be delivered by PMCD regardless of viability, but delivery of a fetus less than 20 weeks' gestation should not be performed if it does not interfere with maternal circulation (Jeejeebhoy et al., 2015).

The pregnant woman in cardiac arrest requires aggressive treatment within the first 4 minutes. The team should perform manual left uterine displacement to prevent aortocaval compression (Jeejeebhoy et al., 2015). The most experienced provider should manage the airway, and IV access should be placed above the diaphragm. If the mother has not responded within 4 minutes, the highest priority is delivery of the neonate (Jeejeebhoy & Morrison, 2013).

NURSING PROCESS

Caring for the patient with cardiac dysrhythmias requires the ability to recognize, identify, and in some cases, promptly treat the dysrhythmia. The urgency of intervention is determined by the effects of the dysrhythmia on the patient. Nursing care focuses on maintaining CO, monitoring the response to therapy, and teaching. Nurses working in critical care areas are likely to care for patients with dysrhythmias on a regular basis and should be certified in advanced cardiac life support.

Health promotion measures to prevent coronary heart disease also reduce the risk for dysrhythmias. In most cases, dysrhythmias develop as a result of ischemic or structural changes in the heart rather than develop in isolation. The nurse should advise patients who are at risk or who complain of occasional palpitations or "flutters" in their chest to reduce their intake of caffeine and other SNS stimulants, such as excess chocolate.

Assessment

Assessment is vital before treating any suspected dysrhythmia. What appears to be VT on the monitor may be the result of the patient scratching or even brushing teeth. Apparent asystole on the monitor may be the result of a loose electrode patch. Likewise, a heart rate of 52 bpm may not affect the overall CO in some patients.

The nurse obtains the following data when assessing the patient with a dysrhythmia:

- **Observation and patient interview.** Most symptoms of a dysrhythmia are not visible on observation. However, dysrhythmia is often accompanied by shortness of breath, which may cause breathing changes that are noticeable. For patients who are conscious, the patient interview may include the patient, the patient's family, or bystanders who were present during the episode of dysrhythmia or cardiac arrest. During the interview, assess for complaints of palpitations (the nurse should ask for further definition of palpitations), "fluttering" sensations, or a sensation of the heart racing; episodes of dizziness, lightheadedness, or syncope (fainting); timing (duration, time of day); correlation with food or beverage intake or activity; presence of chest pain, shortness of breath, or other associated symptoms; history of heart or endocrine disease (e.g., hyperthyroidism); and current medications.

■ *Physical examination.* Assess LOC; vital signs, including apical pulse for a full minute; regularity and amplitude of peripheral pulses; color; presence of dyspnea or adventitious lung sounds; ECG rhythm analysis; and oxygen saturation levels.

Diagnosis

Potential diagnoses for the patient experiencing a cardiac dysrhythmia include the following:

■ *Ineffective Tissue Perfusion: Cerebral, Risk for*
■ *Cardiac Output, Decreased*
■ *Activity Intolerance*
■ *Spontaneous Ventilation, Impaired*
■ *Spiritual Distress*
■ *Fear.*

(NANDA-I © 2014)

Planning

Goals for patient care of the patient with cardiac dysrhythmia may include the following:

■ The patient will receive supplemental oxygen to maintain or improve oxygenation; the patient may be intubated and mechanically ventilated.
■ The patient's oxygen demands will be minimized with bedrest and limited activity.
■ The patient will be monitored for dysrhythmias related to anemia, hypovolemia, electrolyte imbalances, and acidosis.
■ The patient will adhere to the medication regimen.
■ The patient will demonstrate knowledge of the disease process by verbalizing treatment goals.

Implementation

Addressing the effect of the dysrhythmia on CO is the priority of nursing care.

SAFETY ALERT Before treating any dysrhythmia, assess the patient, not just the monitor. Loose electrode pads, disconnected leads or cables, and muscle movement can simulate critical dysrhythmias. The patient's condition is the best indicator of the need for treatment.

Assess and Monitor Cardiac Output

Dysrhythmias can affect CO. Bradycardias decrease CO if the SV does not increase to compensate for the slow heart rate. Tachycardia reduces diastolic filling time, affecting SV and coronary artery perfusion. Loss of the atrial kick in junctional rhythms, atrial fibrillation, and AV blocks also decreases ventricular filling and CO. In VF, loss of ventricular contractions causes cardiac arrest and no CO. Nursing interventions related to decreased CO include the following:

■ Assess the patient for decreased CO: decreased LOC; tachycardia; tachypnea; hypotension; low oxygen saturation; diaphoresis; low urine output; cool, clammy, mottled skin; pallor or cyanosis; and diminished peripheral pulses. Initial signs of decreased CO may be subtle, such as decreased LOC. Early recognition of the dysrhythmia's effect on CO facilitates appropriate treatment and may prevent further adverse effects.
■ Monitor the patient's ECG; post the ECG strip every shift and when rhythm changes occur. Documenting cardiac rhythm provides a record of disease progression and treatment effectiveness.

SAFETY ALERT Assess the patient's vital signs, ECG, and oxygen saturation every 5–15 minutes during acute dysrhythmic episodes and during antidysrhythmic drug infusions. These data provide a record of CO during the dysrhythmia. Antidysrhythmic drugs can adversely affect heart rate, rhythm, and BP, further decreasing CO.

■ Assess the patient for underlying causes of dysrhythmias, such as hypovolemia, hypoxia, anemia, vagal stimulation, or medications. Sinus tachycardia often develops in response to tissue hypoxia. Vagal stimulation (e.g., the Valsalva maneuver) can precipitate bradycardia.
■ Assess the patient's serum electrolytes (especially potassium, calcium, and magnesium) and digitalis and antidysrhythmic drug levels as indicated. Report abnormal values. Electrolyte imbalances affect cardiac depolarization and repolarization and may cause dysrhythmias. Toxic levels of digitalis and antidysrhythmic drugs can precipitate further dysrhythmias. Impaired renal or hepatic function increases the risk for toxicity, as does aging.
■ Be prepared to administer antidysrhythmic medications as indicated. Implement advanced cardiac life support protocols as needed. Emergency drugs should be readily available, especially on units with high-risk patients. See the Medications feature for drugs used to treat common dysrhythmias that may affect CO.
■ If appropriate, instruct the patient to perform the Valsalva maneuver (bear down as if straining or coughing) for SVT or VT without angina. Vagal maneuvers stimulate the parasympathetic system and may terminate some dysrhythmias. The Valsalva maneuver is contraindicated if chest pain occurs with the dysrhythmia.
■ Prepare to assist the patient with cardioversion. Prepare the patient per orders or hospital protocol. Explain the procedure to reduce anxiety. Have emergency equipment readily available. Elective or emergency cardioversion is a treatment of choice for certain dysrhythmias.

On recognizing VF and cardiac arrest, begin emergency procedures. Call for help. Obtain a defibrillator, and immediately defibrillate the patient. If the defibrillator will be brought by another healthcare provider, begin CPR. Initiate advanced cardiovascular life support (ACLS) protocols, and assist with resuscitation measures as directed. CO ceases with VF. Immediate or early defibrillation has been shown to have the greatest positive impact on survival following cardiac arrest.

- After cardiac arrest, transfer the patient to critical care. Perform and document head-to-toe assessment; obtain laboratory tests, 12-lead ECG, and chest x-ray as ordered. Monitor and maintain oxygenation and IV infusions, and monitor vital signs and cardiac rhythm. The period following resuscitation is critical, necessitating careful monitoring. Postarrest assessment allows comparison of the patient's condition with prearrest status and may identify CPR-related injuries. Correcting electrolyte disturbances, hypoxia, and acid–base imbalances is important to prevent further dysrhythmias and potential adverse effects on CO. IV access is crucial to maintain drug infusions. Hemodynamic monitoring may be instituted. The 12-lead ECG documents myocardial status, and the chest x-ray provides information about pulmonary status and possible thoracic injury resulting from CPR.

- Notify the patient's family of significant changes in the patient's condition or cardiac arrest, providing up-to-date information. Prepare family members before visits by explaining interventions (e.g., invasive tubes, a ventilator, additional equipment) implemented since the last visit. Concern for the family and significant others is part of holistic nursing. Patients and families need and appreciate honest communication, information about their loved one's condition, and compassionate care. Preparing the family for critical changes in the patient's condition and plan of care helps them to cope with a situational crisis.

Plan for Discharge

Discharge planning for the patient diagnosed with a dysrhythmia includes patient education directed toward following the prescribed treatment plan and managing risk factors. The nurse should instruct the patient to take all medications as prescribed and to report any side effects to the healthcare provider when they first appear. The nurse should teach the patient how to monitor pulse daily and keep a diary of the recordings. The nurse should also explain that substances containing caffeine, tobacco, and alcohol should be avoided because they can contribute to an irregular heartbeat. Specific risk factors the patient can control include reducing high BP, monitoring cholesterol levels, losing weight, following a heart-healthy diet, stopping smoking, and engaging in regular physical activity as tolerated. The Patient Teaching features list topics that are particularly relevant for the patient with dysrhythmia and the patient at risk for sudden cardiac arrest.

Patient Teaching
Home Care for Patients with Dysrhythmias

Dysrhythmias have a significant physical and psychologic impact on the patient and all family members. Many of these patients and their families are under a great deal of stress from frequent hospitalizations, various treatment modalities, frustration, and the fear of SCD. It is important for the nurse to introduce coping strategies addressing these fears. The nurse should review the following topics when educating the patient and family for home care:

- Function, maintenance, precautions, and signs of malfunction or complications of any implanted device, such as a pacemaker or ICD
- Monitoring of pulse rate and rhythm
- Activity or dietary restrictions, and any potential effects of the dysrhythmia or its treatment on lifestyle

- Medication management to reduce the risk of dysrhythmias, including the desired and potential adverse effects of antidysrhythmic drugs
- Specific instructions related to planned diagnostic tests or procedures
- The importance of follow-up visits with the cardiologist
- The importance of and where to obtain training in CPR for the patient and family members.
- If the patient has an ICD implanted, discharge instructions should address fears, interference from magnets, carrying proper identification, and when to notify the healthcare provider.

Patient Teaching
Home Care for Patients at Risk for Sudden Cardiac Arrest

The risk for a future episode of sudden cardiac arrest requires careful, effective teaching for home care before discharge. The nurse should discuss the following topics with the patient and family:

- Risk factor reduction for coronary heart disease
- Planned diagnostic studies to identify the cause of sudden cardiac arrest and possible interventions

- The risks and benefits of an ICD if appropriate
- The importance of carrying a card at all times listing all current medications and the healthcare provider
- Early manifestations or warning signs of cardiac arrest
- The importance of training and maintaining proficiency in performing CPR (provide referral to local training providers or scheduled classes through the AHA or American Red Cross).

Evaluation

Nursing care should produce the following expected outcomes:

- By properly adhering to the prescribed medication regimen, the patient experiences a reduction in the frequency of dysrhythmic episodes.
- The patient and family both know how to respond appropriately should an episode of dysrhythmia occur.

The nurse should frequently monitor patients with a dysrhythmia to identify and respond to changes in heart rhythm as soon as possible to prevent complications and death. For patients whose dysrhythmia is not controlled by medication or a change in behaviors, the nurse should advocate for further treatment, including installation of a permanent pacemaker or other device if the patient would benefit from such a device. The nurse should provide patient teaching related to the device and warning signs related to increased risk of cardiac arrest.

Nursing Care Plan
A Patient with SVT

Elisa Vasquez, age 53, is admitted to the cardiac unit with complaints of palpitations, lightheadedness, and shortness of breath. Her history reveals rheumatic fever at age 12, with subsequent rheumatic heart disease and mitral stenosis. An IV line is in place, and she is receiving oxygen. Marcia Lewin, RN, is assigned to Ms. Vasquez.

ASSESSMENT	DIAGNOSES	PLANNING
Nurse Lewin's assessment reveals that Ms. Vasquez is moderately anxious. Her ECG shows SVT with a rate of 154 bpm. Vital signs are as follows: temperature 37.1°C (98.8°F) oral; respirations 26/min; and BP 95/60 mmHg. Peripheral pulses are weak but equal. Mucous membranes are pale pink, and skin is cool and dry. Fine crackles are noted in both lung bases. A loud S_3 gallop and a diastolic murmur are noted. Ms. Vasquez is still complaining of palpitations and tells Nurse Lewin, "I feel so nervous and weak and dizzy." Ms. Vasquez's cardiologist orders 6 mg of adenosine to be given via IV push and tells Nurse Lewin to prepare for additional adenosine administration if necessary. The cardiologist also tells Nurse Lewin to be ready to assist with synchronized cardioversion if drug therapy does not control the ventricular rate.	■ *Decreased Cardiac Output* related to inadequate ventricular filling associated with rapid tachycardia ■ *Ineffective Peripheral Tissue Perfusion* related to decreased CO ■ *Anxiety* related to unknown outcome of altered health state (NANDA-I © 2014)	Goals of care include the following: ■ The patient will maintain adequate CO and tissue perfusion. ■ The patient will demonstrate a ventricular rate within normal limits and stable vital signs. ■ The patient will verbalize reduced anxiety. ■ The patient will verbalize an understanding of the rationale for the treatment measures to control the heart rate.

IMPLEMENTATION

- Provide oxygen per nasal cannula at 4 L/min.
- Continuously monitor the patient's ECG for rate, rhythm, and conduction. Assess vital signs and associated symptoms with changes in ECG. Report findings to the physician.
- Explain the importance of rapidly reducing the heart rate. Explain the cardioversion procedure, and encourage questions.
- Encourage the patient to verbalize fears and concerns. Answer questions honestly, correcting misconceptions about the disease process, treatment, or prognosis.
- Administer IV diazepam as ordered before cardioversion.
- Document pretreatment vital signs, LOC, and peripheral pulses.
- Place an emergency cart with drugs and airway management supplies in the patient's unit.
- Assist with cardioversion as indicated.
- Assess the patient's LOC, level of sedation, cardiovascular and respiratory status, and skin condition following cardioversion.
- Document the procedure and postcardioversion rhythm and the patient's response to intervention.

EVALUATION

IV adenosine lowers Ms. Vasquez's heart rate to 138 bpm for a short time, after which it increases to 164 bpm, with a BP of 82/64 mmHg. Her cardiologist, Dr. Mullins, performs carotid sinus massage. The ventricular rate slows to 126 bpm for 2 minutes, revealing atrial flutter waves, then returns to 150 bpm. Dr. Mullins explains the treatment options, including synchronized cardioversion. Ms. Vasquez agrees to the procedure.

Ms. Vasquez is lightly sedated, and synchronized cardioversion is performed. One countershock converts Ms. Vasquez to regular sinus rhythm at 96 bpm, with a BP of 112/60 mmHg.

Ms. Vasquez is sleepy from the sedation but recovers without incident. She states that she feels "much better," and her vital signs return to her normal levels. She remains in NSR, with a rate of 86–92 bpm for the remainder of her hospital stay. Dr. Mullins places Ms. Vasquez on furosemide to treat manifestations of mild heart failure.

CRITICAL THINKING

1. What is the scientific basis for using carotid massage to treat SVTs? Was this an appropriate maneuver in the case of Ms. Vasquez?
2. What other treatment options might the physician have used to treat Ms. Vasquez's SVT if she had been asymptomatic with stable vital signs?
3. Develop a teaching plan for Ms. Vasquez related to her prescription for furosemide.

REVIEW Life-Threatening Dysrhythmias

RELATE Link the Concepts and Exemplars

Linking the exemplar of life-threatening dysrhythmias with the concept of safety:

1. What safety teaching will you provide the patient with atrial fibrillation?

2. Your patient has an internal pacemaker in place secondary to third-degree heart block. When you are providing safety instructions, the patient asks why battery-powered equipment is used rather than electrically powered equipment. How will you respond?

Linking the exemplar of life-threatening dysrhythmias with the concept of addiction:

3. What information will you provide the patient with SVT who plans to continue smoking cigarettes?

4. What alterations will you make to your plan of care for the patient with a dysrhythmia who abuses cocaine?

READY Go to Volume 3: Clinical Nursing Skills

REFER Go to Pearson MyLab Nursing and eText

- Additional review materials

REFLECT Apply Your Knowledge

Regina Moss, age 24, is 6 weeks postpartum after delivering her first baby, Mickey. The delivery was uncomplicated; Mickey weighed 8 pounds at birth. Mickey has adapted well to the home environment, eating and sleeping well. Ms. Moss lives with Greg Mackinnon, a foreman for a construction crew. Ms. Moss has taken 3 months leave from her job as a legal secretary. She is enjoying her time at home with Mickey and is not sure she wants to return to work full time when her leave is up. Both her parents and Mr. Mackinnon's live in town, and they have all offered to care for Mickey when Ms. Moss goes back to work.

This morning Mickey is pale and seems to be lethargic and is having trouble eating. Ms. Moss calls Mr. Mackinnon, and they go to the hospital, where they are told that Mickey has SVT. The emergency department physicians have given Mickey propranolol (Inderal) and are planning to admit him to the pediatric ICU.

1. What is your priority nursing diagnosis for Mickey?

2. What teaching will you provide Ms. Moss and Mr. Mackinnon?

3. How will you respond to Ms. Moss when she states that she must have done something wrong because Mickey had been so healthy?

» Exemplar 16.J
Peripheral Vascular Disease

Exemplar Learning Outcomes

16.J Analyze peripheral vascular disease (PVD) as it relates to perfusion.

- Describe the pathophysiology of PVD.
- Describe the etiology of PVD.
- Compare the risk factors and prevention of PVD.
- Identify the clinical manifestations of PVD.
- Summarize diagnostic tests and therapies used by interprofessional teams in the collaborative care of an individual with PVD.
- Differentiate care of patients with PVD across the lifespan.
- Apply the nursing process in providing culturally competent care to an individual with PVD.

Exemplar Key Terms

Arteriosclerosis, *1292*
Atherosclerosis, *1292*
Chronic venous insufficiency (CVI), *1292*
Intermittent claudication, *1293*
Peripheral vascular disease (PVD), *1292*
Rest pain, *1293*
Venous stasis, *1293*

Overview

Peripheral vascular disease (PVD), also called peripheral artery disease, refers to a category of circulation disorders that may occur when pathologic changes (arteriosclerosis and atherosclerosis) impair blood supply to peripheral tissues, particularly the lower extremities. **Arteriosclerosis**, which is characterized by thickening, loss of elasticity, and calcification of arterial walls, is the most common chronic arterial disorder. **Atherosclerosis** is a form of arteriosclerosis in which deposits of fat and fibrin obstruct and harden the arteries.

Chronic venous insufficiency (CVI) is a disorder of inadequate venous return over a prolonged period. It is a long-term condition that occurs because of a vein blockage or valve leakage in the leg veins, making it difficult for blood to return to the heart. Blood pools in the veins, causing stasis. DVT is the most common cause of CVI.

Pathophysiology and Etiology
Pathophysiology

Atherosclerotic lesions involve both the intima and the media of the involved arteries. Thromboses occur in the lower extremities more often than in the upper extremities. Arteriosclerosis in the abdominal aorta leads to the development of aneurysms as plaque erodes the vessel wall.

Plaque tends to form at arterial bifurcations. The vessel lumen is progressively obstructed, decreasing blood flow to the lower extremities. Tissue hypoxia or anoxia results. With gradual obstruction of the vessel, collateral circulation often develops. However, the collateral circulation is usually not adequate to supply tissue needs, especially when metabolic demand increases. Manifestations typically develop only when the vessel is occluded by 60% or more.

CVI results when venous blood collects and stagnates in the lower leg (**venous stasis**). Venous pressures in the calf and lower leg increase, particularly during ambulation. This increased pressure impairs arterial circulation to the lower extremities as well. The body's ability to provide sufficient oxygen and nutrients to the cells and remove metabolic waste products diminishes. Eventually, there is so little oxygen and nutrients that cells begin to die. The skin atrophies, and subcutaneous fat deposits necrose. Breakdown of RBCs in the congested tissues causes brown skin pigmentation. Venous stasis ulcers develop. Congested tissues impair the body's ability to increase the supply of oxygen, nutrients, and metabolic energy to heal the ulcer. As a result, the condition worsens and, over time, the ulcers enlarge. Congested venous circulation also prevents the blood from mounting effective inflammatory and immune responses, significantly increasing the risk for infection in the ulcerated tissue (Flugman & Clark, 2016).

Etiology

PVD primarily affects older adults, with greater prevalence rates seen in adults over age 80. Men are more often affected than women. African American patients are at increased risk, whereas those of Hispanic origin seem to have similar to slightly higher rates of peripheral artery disease when compared to non-Hispanic Whites. Overall, approximately 8 million people in the United States are estimated to have PVD (CDC, 2014d).

Risk Factors

Risk factors for PVD are similar to those for atherosclerosis and coronary heart disease; they include smoking, hypertension, high cholesterol, diabetes, family history of vascular disease, being overweight, and physical inactivity. Patients over the age of 50 also have an increased risk.

Several risk factors predispose a patient to the development of venous insufficiency. Thrombophlebitis sometimes results in damage to the valves of the deep veins. Obesity and occupations that require prolonged standing or sitting can also lead to venous insufficiency.

Prevention

Because PVD arises primarily from atherosclerosis and other disorders that impair cardiovascular function, prevention focuses on preventing these processes and includes maintaining a healthy lifestyle (e.g., maintaining a healthy weight and healthy diet with regular exercise) and following treatment regimens for chronic illnesses. Individuals who are at risk may be screened for PVD by their healthcare providers using an ankle-brachial index, or ABI (NHLBI, 2015f). Claudication medications in addition to lifestyle choices may also help slow or even reverse the progress of PVD symptoms; these include prescribed high BP medications and cholesterol-lowering medications and may also include drugs to prevent blood clots. All medications should only be taken as advised by a healthcare provider (AHA, 2014d).

Clinical Manifestations

Pain is the primary symptom of peripheral atherosclerosis. **Intermittent claudication** (a cramping or aching pain in the calves of the legs, the thighs, and the buttocks that occurs with a predictable level of activity) is characteristic of PVD. The pain is often accompanied by weakness and is relieved by rest.

Rest pain, in contrast, occurs during periods of inactivity. It is often described as a burning sensation in the lower legs. Rest pain increases when the legs are elevated and decreases when the legs are dependent (e.g., hanging over the side of the bed). The legs also may feel cold or numb along with the pain. Sensation is diminished, and the muscles may atrophy.

Peripheral pulses may be decreased or absent. A bruit (unusual sound made by blood rushing past an obstruction) may be heard over large affected arteries, such as the femoral artery and the abdominal aorta. The legs are pale when elevated but often are dark red (dependent rubor) when dependent. The skin often is thin, shiny, and hairless, with discolored areas. Toenails may be thickened. Areas of skin breakdown and ulceration may be evident. Edema may develop with severe PVD.

SAFETY ALERT The decreased sensation and skin breakdown that is common during PVD increases the risk for gangrene and amputation of an extremity. Teach patients with PVD how to assess their skin for breakdown and other injuries and how to perform proper foot and leg care.

Manifestations of peripheral atherosclerosis include intermittent claudication; rest pain; paresthesias; diminished or absent peripheral pulses; pallor with extremity elevation (redness of skin or rubor when dependent); thin, hairless skin; thickened toenails; and areas of discoloration or skin breakdown. Peripheral atherosclerosis may also induce rupture of abdominal aortic aneurysms and possible infection and sepsis.

Manifestations of CVI include lower extremity edema that worsens with standing; itching, dull leg discomfort or pain that increases with standing; thin, shiny, atrophic skin; cyanosis and brown skin pigmentation of lower leg and foot; possible weeping dermatitis; thick, fibrous (hard) subcutaneous tissue; and recurrent ulcerations of medial or anterior ankle.

The extremity is cyanotic. Recurrent stasis ulcers develop (see **Figure 16–53 ≫**), usually forming just above the ankle,

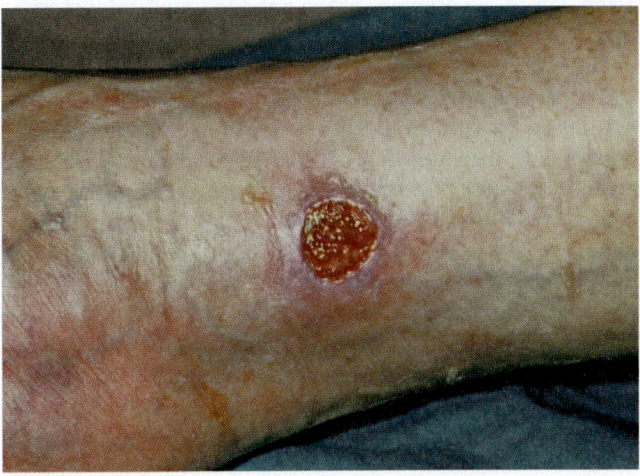

Source: Dr. P. Marazzi/Science Source.

Figure 16–53 ≫ Chronic venous insufficiency (CVI). Note the discoloration of the ankle and the stasis ulcer.

TABLE 16–29 Comparison of Arterial and Venous Leg Ulcers

Factor	Arterial Ulcers	Venous Ulcers
Location	Toes, feet, shin	Over medial or anterior ankle
Ulcer appearance	Deep, pale	Superficial, pink
Skin appearance	Normal to atrophic	Brown discoloration
	Pallor on elevation	Stasis dermatitis
	Rubor on dependency	Cyanosis on dependency
Skin temperature	Cool	Normal
Edema	Absent or mild	May be significant
Pain	Usually severe	Usually mild
	Intermittent claudication	Aching pain
	Rest pain	
Gangrene	May occur	Does not occur
Pulses	Decreased or absent	Normal

on the medial or anterior aspect of the leg. They heal poorly, forming scar tissue that breaks down easily. Tissue surrounding the ulcer is shiny, atrophic, and cyanotic, and there is a brownish pigmentation to the skin. Other skin changes, such as eczema or stasis dermatitis, also may develop. Necrosis and fibrosis of subcutaneous tissue cause the affected area of the leg to feel hard and somewhat leathery, but even the slightest trauma to the area can produce serious tissue breakdown. **Table 16–29** ≫ compares venous and arterial ulcers.

Collaboration

Management of PVD focuses on slowing the atherosclerotic process and maintaining tissue perfusion. Collaborative care for the patient with venous insufficiency focuses on relieving symptoms, promoting adequate circulation, and healing and preventing tissue damage.

The history and physical examination often establish the diagnosis of CVI. Because a history of DVT is a major risk factor, careful assessment of the patient's medical history is important. There are no specific diagnostic tests to confirm the diagnosis of CVI.

Conservative management of venous insufficiency focuses on reducing edema and treating ulcerations. Prolonged standing or sitting is discouraged. Graduated compression hosiery is ordered for daytime use, and frequent elevation of the legs and feet during the day is recommended. At night, the legs and feet should be elevated above the level of the heart by raising the foot of the mattress.

Treatment of associated stasis dermatitis varies based on the duration of the condition. Wet compresses of boric acid, buffered aluminum acetate (Burow solution), or isotonic saline solution are applied to acute weeping dermatitis four times a day for 1-hour periods. Following the compress, a topical corticosteroid (e.g., 0.5% hydrocortisone cream) is applied. Bedrest is prescribed during the acute period.

Stasis pigmentation is very difficult to treat, even when the underlying stasis dermatitis is well controlled with topical therapy. Some researchers have reported benefits from

treatment with a noncoherent intense pulsed light (IPL) source (Flugman & Clark, 2016).

The ulcer may be treated by using a semirigid boot applied to the foot and lower leg. This device may be made of Unna paste or Gauzetex bandage. Bony prominences must be well padded. The boot must be changed every 1–2 weeks, depending on the amount of drainage from the ulcer. This device often allows ambulatory treatment. A very large, chronic ulcer may require surgery. In this case, the incompetent veins are ligated, the ulcer is excised, and the area is covered with a skin graft.

Diagnostic Tests

Although PVD often can be diagnosed on the basis of the history and physical examination, diagnostic tests may be ordered to evaluate its extent. Noninvasive studies often are sufficient. Diagnostic tests for PVD include the following:

- **Segmental pressure measurements** use sphygmomanometer cuffs and a Doppler device to compare BPs between the upper and lower extremities (normally similar) and within different segments of the affected extremity. In PVD, the BP may be lower in the legs than in the arms.

- **Stress testing** using a treadmill provides functional assessment of limitations. In PVD, pressure at the ankle may decline even further with exercise, confirming the diagnosis. This may be done simultaneously for testing related to cardiovascular illness.

- **Doppler ultrasound** uses sound waves reflected off moving RBCs within a vessel to evaluate blood flow. The impulses may be translated into an audible signal or a graphic waveform. With significant PVD, the waveform becomes progressively flatter as the transducer is moved distally along the affected vessel. Segmental pressures may be used to locate the site of obstruction.

- **Duplex Doppler ultrasound** combines the audible or graphic Doppler ultrasound with ultrasound imaging to identify arterial or venous abnormalities. Ultrasonic imaging provides views of the affected vessel while Doppler ultrasound evaluates blood flow. *Color-flow Doppler ultrasound* provides color images of the vessel and blood flow.

- **Transcutaneous oximetry** evaluates oxygenation of tissues.

- **Angiography or magnetic resonance angiography** is done before revascularization procedures to locate and evaluate the extent of arterial obstruction. For angiography, a contrast medium is injected, and vessels are visualized using fluoroscopy and x-rays. Magnetic resonance angiography does not require injection of a contrast medium and may replace angiography.

Pharmacologic Therapy

Drug treatment of peripheral atherosclerosis is less effective than that for coronary heart disease. Medications to inhibit platelet aggregation, such as aspirin or clopidogrel (Plavix), are ordered to reduce the risk of arterial thrombosis. Cilostazol (Pletal), a platelet inhibitor with vasodilator properties, increases blood flow to the extremities, thereby improving claudication. Pentoxifylline (Trental) decreases blood viscosity and increases RBC flexibility, increasing blood flow to the microcirculation and tissues of the extremities.

Nonpharmacologic Therapy

Smoking cessation is vital for the treatment of PVD. Nicotine not only promotes atherosclerosis, but it also causes vasospasm, further reducing blood flow to the extremities.

Meticulous foot care is vital to prevent ulceration and infection. Elastic support hose, which reduce circulation to the skin, are avoided. Elevating the head of the bed on blocks may help relieve rest pain. Regular, progressively strenuous exercise, such as 30–45 minutes of walking daily, is important. The nurse should teach the patient to rest at the onset of claudication, resuming activity when the pain resolves.

Other measures to slow the process of atherosclerosis, such as controlling diabetes and hypertension, lowering cholesterol levels, and weight loss, also are recommended.

Surgery

Revascularization may be performed if symptoms are progressive, severe, or disabling. Other indications for surgery include symptoms that significantly interfere with ADLs, rest pain, and pregangrenous or gangrenous lesions. Either nonsurgical revascularization procedures or surgery may be performed.

Nonsurgical procedures include PTCA, stent placement, or atherectomy. Techniques may include balloon angioplasty to dilate the narrowed lumen, mechanical atherectomy to remove plaque, or laser or thermal angioplasty to vaporize the occluding material. In either case, a stent typically is placed at the time of angioplasty to maintain vessel patency. Iliac and femoral–popliteal PTCA initially reestablish good blood flow and relieve symptoms in more than 80% of patients. Practitioners may also insert a mesh framework, or stent, to help keep the artery open.

Surgical options include endarterectomy (to remove occlusive plaque from the artery) and bypass grafts. Knitted Dacron bypass grafts are commonly used. Both immediate graft patency and long-term graft patency are better with bypass grafting than with nonsurgical revascularization procedures. However, the risks for operative complications must be considered.

Complementary Health Approaches

Integrative therapies for PVD include interventions to improve circulation and reduce stress. A number of complementary health approaches may improve peripheral circulation: aromatherapy with rosemary or vetiver; biofeedback; healing or therapeutic touch and massage; herbals, such as ginkgo, garlic, cayenne, hawthorn, and bilberry; and exercise, including yoga. Aromatherapy and yoga also may reduce stress, as can breathing exercises, meditation, and counseling. In addition, complementary health approaches to reduce atherosclerosis and lower cholesterol levels may slow the progress of PVD. Measures such as a very-low-fat or vegetarian diet, including antioxidant nutrients or using vitamin C, vitamin E, or garlic supplements, and traditional Chinese medicine may be useful.

NURSING PROCESS

The nurse can help reduce the incidence and slow the progression of atherosclerosis by discussing healthy lifestyle habits with community and religious groups, with schoolchildren (grades K–12), and through the print media. The nurse should strongly encourage all patients to refrain from or stop using any tobacco products. The nurse should discuss the adverse effects of smoking and the benefits of quitting. The nurse should also provide information about dietary recommendations to maintain a healthy weight and optimal cholesterol levels. The nurse should discuss the benefits and importance of regular exercise. Finally, the nurse should encourage patients with cardiovascular risk factors to undergo regular screening for hypertension, diabetes, and hyperlipidemia.

Nursing care for the patient with CVI is primarily educative and supportive. Patient teaching includes the following recommendations:

- Elevate the legs while resting and during sleep.
- Walk as much as possible, but avoid sitting or standing for long periods of time.
- When sitting, do not cross the legs or allow pressure on the back of the knees (e.g., sitting on the side of the bed).
- Do not wear anything that pinches the legs (e.g., knee-high hose, garters, girdles).
- Wear elastic hose as prescribed. The elastic hose should be tighter over the feet than at the top of the leg. Put on the hose after the legs have been elevated.

SAFETY ALERT Teach patients who wear elastic hose or compression stockings to be sure the tops of the hose do not cut into their legs. This can cut off the circulation to the lower extremities, compounding the damage from PVD.

- Keep the skin on the feet and legs clean, soft, and dry.
- Follow guidelines in the Patient Teaching feature for care of the legs and feet.

Assessment

Focused assessment related to peripheral atherosclerosis includes the following:

- ***Observation and patient interview.*** Observe for signs of pain associated with PVD, such as limping or guarding. Observe for edema, skin discoloration, shiny skin, and other related signs of PVD or venous ulcers. During the patient interview, assess for complaints of pain, its relationship to exercise or rest, timing, associated symptoms, and relief measures; history of coronary heart disease, PVD, hyperlipidemia, hypertension, or diabetes; current medications; smoking history; and usual diet and activity patterns.
- ***Physical examination.*** During the physical examination, assess the patient's vital signs; strength and equality of peripheral pulses of all extremities; capillary refill; skin color, temperature, hair distribution, and presence of any discolorations or lesions; and movement and sensation of lower extremities.

Patient Teaching
Foot and Leg Care for the Patient with Peripheral Atherosclerosis

1. Keep legs and feet clean, dry, and comfortable.
   - Wash legs and feet daily in warm water, using mild soap.
   - Pat dry using a soft towel; be sure to dry between the toes.
   - Apply moisturizing cream to prevent drying.
   - Use powder on the feet and between the toes.
   - Buy shoes in the afternoon (when feet are largest); never buy shoes that are uncomfortable. Toes should not touch the tip of the shoe.
   - Wear a clean pair of cotton socks each day.
2. Prevent accidents and injuries to the feet.
   - Always wear shoes or slippers when getting out of bed.
   - Walk on level ground and avoid crowds, if possible.
   - Do not go barefoot.
   - Inspect legs and feet daily; use a mirror to examine backs of legs and bottoms of feet.
   - Have a professional foot care provider trim toenails and care for corns, calluses, ingrown toenails, or athlete's foot.
   - Always check the temperature of the water before stepping into a tub.
   - Do not let the legs or tops of the feet get sunburned.
   - Report leg or foot problems (increased pain, cuts, bruises, blistering, redness, or open areas) to the healthcare provider.
3. Improve blood supply to the legs and feet.
   - Do not cross legs.
   - Do not wear garters or knee stockings.
   - Do not swim or wade in cold water.

Diagnosis

Nursing diagnoses that may be useful for the patient with PVD include the following:

- *Peripheral Tissue Perfusion, Ineffective*
- *Pain, Chronic*
- *Skin Integrity, Impaired*
- *Activity Intolerance.*

(NANDA-I © 2014)

Nursing diagnoses that may apply to the patient with CVI include the following:

- *Body Image, Disturbed*
- *Health Maintenance, Ineffective*
- *Infection, Risk for*
- *Physical Mobility, Impaired*
- *Skin Integrity, Impaired*
- *Peripheral Tissue Perfusion, Ineffective.*

(NANDA-I © 2014)

Planning

Goals of nursing care for the patient with CVI may include the following:

- The patient will stop smoking.
- The patient will learn appropriate foot and wound care.
- The patient will maintain adherence with medications and wound care.
- The patient will maintain activity and exercise as tolerated.

Implementation

Nursing care for the patient with CVI is focused on improving tissue perfusion and preventing tissue damage. Any time tissues receive inadequate blood supply, the patient will experience very severe pain. As a result, pain management until perfusion can be improved is also a primary nursing focus.

Promote Tissue Perfusion

Impaired blood flow to the lower extremities affects gas, nutrient, and waste product exchange between the capillaries and cells. Oxygen and nutrient deprivation impairs cell function and tissue integrity, causing pain and impaired healing. Pain develops with exercise and when extremities are elevated. Interventions to promote tissue perfusion include the following:

- Position the patient with extremities elevated. Elevation promotes venous return from the extremity, increasing circulation and relieving pain.
- Discuss the benefits of regular exercise. Exercise promotes the development of collateral circulation to ischemic tissues and slows the process of atherosclerosis.
- Use a foot cradle and lightweight blankets, socks, and slippers to keep extremities warm. Avoid electric heating pads or hot water bottles. Keeping extremities warm conserves heat, prevents vasospasm, and promotes arterial flow. External heating devices are avoided to reduce the risk of burns in the patient with impaired sensation. The foot cradle protects tissues from compression by linens.
- Encourage frequent position changes. Instruct the patient to avoid crossing the legs or using a pillow under the knees. Position changes promote blood flow and reduce damage caused by pressure. Leg crossing and excessive flexion of the hip or knee joints can compress partially obstructed arteries and impair blood flow to distal tissues.
- Assess peripheral pulses, pain, color, temperature, and capillary refill every 4 hours and as needed. Use a Doppler device if pulses are not palpable. Mark pulse locations with a marker. Assessment data provide a baseline for evaluating the effectiveness of interventions and identifying changes in arterial blood flow.

Patient Teaching
Home Care for Patients with PVD

Discuss the following topics when preparing the patient and family for home and community-based care:

- Smoking cessation strategies and ways to avoid second-hand smoke
- Prescribed medications and anticoagulants, their purpose, doses, and desired and adverse effects
- Signs of excess bleeding to report to the practitioner
- Skin surveillance and foot care
- Recommended diet and exercise
- Weight loss strategies if appropriate

If revascularization or surgery has been performed, include the following topics as appropriate:

- Incision care
- Manifestations of complications (e.g., infection, graft leakage, thrombosis) to be reported to the practitioner
- Activity limitations

Provide referrals to home health services, physical or occupational therapy, and home maintenance assistance services as indicated. Consider resources such as Meals on Wheels for patients who have severe limitations from their disease.

Manage Pain

Impaired blood flow results in tissue ischemia. Metabolism shifts from an efficient aerobic process to an anaerobic process. Lactic acid and metabolic waste products accumulate in tissues, causing pain. Severe and cramping pain generally occurs with exercise early in the disease. Rest initially produces relief, similar to the process of angina. As the disease progresses, pain develops with less exercise and often occurs even at rest. Rest pain disrupts sleep and the patient's sense of well-being and has significant disruptive effects on life roles. The following nursing interventions may help to control the patient's pain:

- Keep the extremities warm. Cooling leads to vasoconstriction, increasing pain. Warming the extremities promotes vasodilation and improves arterial flow, reducing pain.
- Teach pain relief and stress reduction techniques, such as relaxation, meditation, and guided imagery. Pain increases stress. The stress response leads to vasoconstriction, increasing pain. Stress reduction techniques, when combined with other measures to promote blood flow, can help reduce pain.
- Assess pain at least every 4 hours using a standard pain scale. Pain is a subjective experience. Using a standard pain scale allows evaluation of treatment measures in relieving pain and restoring blood flow. Examples of pain scales can be found in the exemplar on Acute and Chronic Pain in the module on Comfort.

Promote Skin Integrity

Patients with PVD are at risk for impaired skin integrity as a result of oxygen and nutrient deprivation. Chronic tissue ischemia leads to dry, scaly, and atrophied skin. Pruritus can lead to scratching; minor injuries may go unnoticed because of impaired sensation. Impaired tissue healing can lead to ulceration, infection, and potential gangrene. The following are appropriate nursing interventions to promote skin integrity in these patients:

- Provide meticulous daily skin care, keeping the skin clean and dry. Apply a moisturizing cream to dry or scaly areas. Intact skin is the body's first defense against bacterial

invasion. Ischemic tissues of the injured extremity provide an excellent medium for microorganism growth. Keeping the skin clean, dry, and supple decreases the risk of breakdown.

- Apply a bed cradle. The bed cradle suspends bed linens over the legs, preventing them from placing pressure on extremities and injured tissues. Minimizing pressure on the tissues promotes capillary blood flow.
- Provide an egg-crate mattress, flotation pad, sheepskin, or heel protectors. Ischemic tissues may be damaged by minor trauma, such as that created by the shearing forces of skin against bed linens.

Encourage Activity

Pain and impaired perfusion of peripheral tissues may limit the patient's ability to engage in desired activities, even impairing self-care. The nurse can take the following actions to encourage the patient to be active:

- Unless contraindicated, encourage gradual increases in duration and intensity of exercise. Teach the patient to rest with the extremities dependent when claudication develops, resuming activity after pain has abated. Gradual increases in the duration and intensity of exercise promote development of collateral circulation, improve exercise tolerance, provide a sense of well-being, and support self-esteem.
- Encourage frequent position changes and active ROM exercises. Encourage self-care to the extent possible. Position changes relieve pressure on tissues, improving capillary circulation and reducing tissue ischemia. ROM exercises help prevent muscle atrophy and joint contractures. Self-care supports self-esteem.
- Assist with care activities as needed. Severe claudication or rest pain may limit activities. Muscle atrophy of affected extremities is common, leading to fatigue and weakness.
- Provide diversional activities during periods of prescribed bedrest. Encourage relaxation techniques to reduce muscle tension. Diversional activities help prevent the boredom and stress associated with enforced rest. Relaxation techniques reduce vasoconstriction induced by stress, improving peripheral circulation.

Evaluation

The patient's progress toward goals may be evaluated on the basis of the following expected outcomes:

- The patient provides a return demonstration of proper positioning of the affected extremity.
- The patient begins a smoking cessation program.
- The patient verbalizes proper wound care techniques to the nurse.
- The patient verbalizes signs and symptoms of infection prior to discharge.

PVD is a slow-healing, chronic disease that may require years of therapy. Patients are rarely successful at implementing all the beneficial lifestyle changes immediately. Therefore, the nurse can continue to encourage the patient to implement all the changes required for healing, including using proper skin and wound care techniques, implementing dietary changes, participating in regular physical activity, taking medications as prescribed, and using compression and elevation techniques as ordered. Because of the length of therapy required, the nurse should provide emotional support and encouragement for the patient to continue making positive changes. The nurse should document the patient's progress and share this progress with the patient to help encourage the patient to maintain the therapeutic regimen. If the patient is following all recommendations and healing still has not occurred, the nurse should advocate for further evaluation of the treatment plan.

REVIEW Peripheral Vascular Disease

RELATE Link the Concepts and Exemplars

Linking the exemplar of PVD with the concept of infection:

1. What factors related to PVD would increase the risk for infection in wounds to the lower extremities?
2. What patient teaching will you provide the patient with PVD to reduce the risk of infection?

Linking the exemplar of PVD with the concept of comfort:

3. Explain the relationship between physical exercise and pain in the patient with PVD.
4. Compare the pain experienced during exercise by a patient with PVD to that of a patient with angina.

READY Go to Volume 3: Clinical Nursing Skills

REFER Go to Pearson MyLab Nursing and eText

- Additional review materials

REFLECT Apply Your Knowledge

Vincent D'Angelo is a 69-year-old man who retired recently from Ford Motor Company, where he worked on the assembly line in a truck factory. He and his wife Pat are enjoying retirement and spending time together. Mr. and Ms. D'Angelo own their own home. Their children, Laurie and Peter, live nearby. Mr. D'Angelo has not had any major health issues until recently, when he started experiencing pain during evening walks with his wife.

Mr. D'Angelo drinks an occasional glass of wine at special functions. Ten years ago, he quit a two-pack-a-day smoking habit. The D'Angelos eat relatively healthy meals, mostly cooked by Ms. D'Angelo. She has finally convinced Mr. D'Angelo to see his primary care provider to find out why he is having leg pain.

1. Describe the noninvasive diagnostic tests that the physician might order to confirm Mr. D'Angelo's diagnosis of PVD.
2. What nursing assessments will you perform to support the diagnosis of PVD?
3. Create a teaching plan to reduce the risk of complications associated with PVD for Mr. D'Angelo.

➤➤ Exemplar 16.K
Pulmonary Embolism

Exemplar Learning Outcomes

16.K Analyze pulmonary embolism (PE) as it relates to perfusion.

- Describe the pathophysiology of PE.
- Describe the etiology of PE.
- Compare the risk factors and prevention of PE.
- Identify the clinical manifestations of PE.
- Summarize diagnostic tests and therapies used by interprofessional teams in the collaborative care of an individual with PE.

- Differentiate care of patients with PE across the lifespan.
- Apply the nursing process in providing culturally competent care to an individual with PE.

Exemplar Key Terms

Dead space, *1300*
Embolus, *1298*
Lyse, *1302*
Pulmonary embolism (PE), *1298*
Thromboemboli, *1298*

Overview

Pulmonary embolism (PE), or pulmonary thromboembolism, is the obstruction of blood flow in part of the pulmonary vascular system by an **embolus** (a particle or aggregate of blood, fat, or pathogens or a bubble of air) traveling from one area of the body to another. **Thromboemboli** (emboli created by a blood clot) that develop in the venous system or the right side of the heart are the most frequent cause of PE. Other sources of emboli include tumors that have invaded the venous circulation; fat or bone marrow entering the circulation as a result of fracture or other trauma; amniotic fluid released into the circulation during childbirth; and IV injection of air or other foreign substances.

PE is a medical emergency. Fifty percent of deaths from PE occur within the first 2 hours following embolization. In many cases, DVT has not been recognized or treated; often, embolization also goes undetected. Prompt treatment can help save lives and prevent complications associated with PE.

Pathophysiology and Etiology

Pathophysiology

The right side of the heart receives deoxygenated blood from the systemic venous circulation. The entire output of the right ventricle enters the pulmonary circulation via the pulmonary artery. This artery branches into successively smaller arteries, arterioles, and capillaries of the pulmonary vascular system. Each alveolus of the lungs is surrounded by a meshwork of capillaries. Oxygen and carbon dioxide readily diffuse across the alveolar–capillary membrane, driven by a concentration gradient. The partial pressure of oxygen in the alveolus is greater than that in the capillary; therefore, oxygen diffuses into the blood. Carbon dioxide diffuses from the capillaries into the alveoli, driven by the higher pressure of dissolved carbon dioxide in venous blood.

A match between blood flow through the pulmonary vascular system (perfusion) and lung ventilation is necessary for effective respiration (gas exchange) (see **Figure 16–54 »**). Local factors regulate ventilation and perfusion to maintain this match. A low alveolar PO_2 constricts alveolar capillaries,

directing blood flow to better ventilated areas of the lung. A high alveolar PCO_2 causes local bronchodilation, increasing airflow and eliminating excess carbon dioxide.

Thrombi that affect only the deep veins of the calf rarely embolize to the pulmonary circulation. However, thrombi often propagate proximally to the popliteal and ileofemoral veins. There, they may break loose to become an embolus. As vessels of the venous system become progressively larger, the embolus moves freely until it enters the pulmonary arterial system, with its progressively smaller vessels leading to the pulmonary capillary beds (see **Figure 16–55 »**).

The impact of a pulmonary embolus depends on the extent to which pulmonary blood flow is obstructed, the size of the embolus, its nature, and any secondary effects of the obstruction. The effects can range widely:

- Occlusion of a large pulmonary artery with sudden death. Gas exchange is significantly reduced or prevented, and CO falls dramatically as blood fails to move through the pulmonary vascular system and return to the left side of the heart.

- Lung tissue infarction caused by occlusion of a significant portion of pulmonary blood flow. Fewer than 10% of pulmonary emboli result in pulmonary infarction.

- Obstruction of a small segment of the pulmonary circulation with no permanent lung injury.

- Chronic or recurrent, possibly multiple, small emboli with recurring symptoms.

Obstruction of pulmonary blood flow by an embolus affects both perfusion and ventilation. Neurohumoral

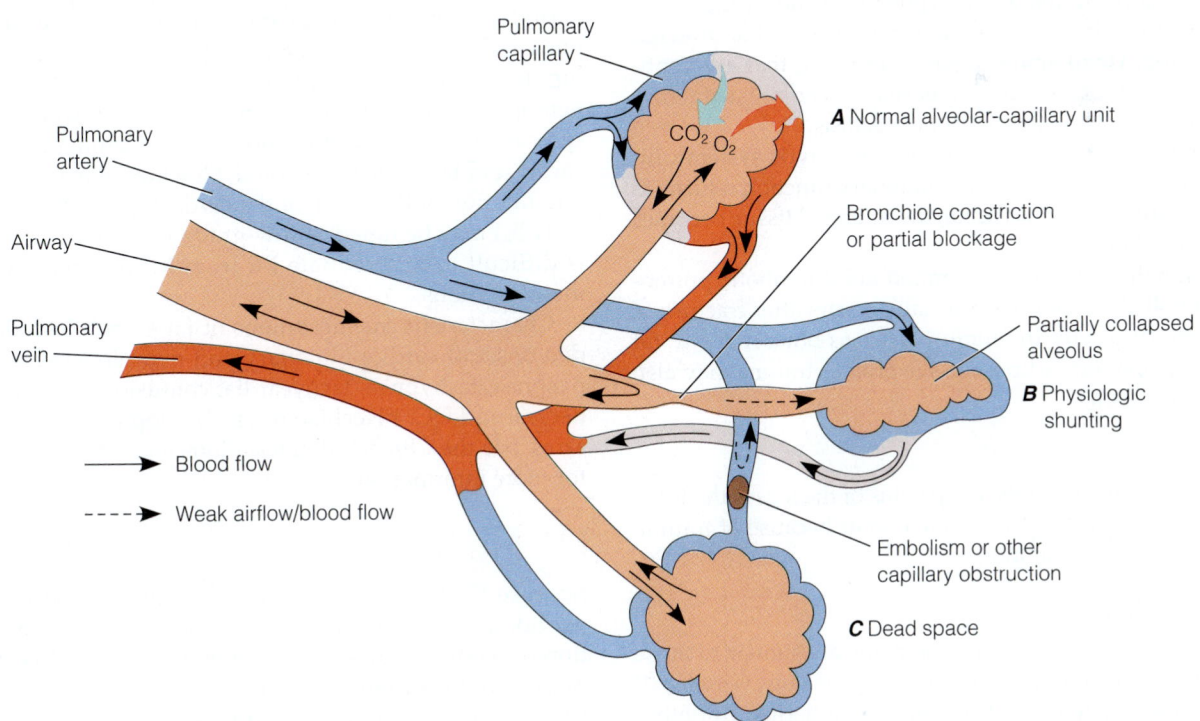

Figure 16–54 » Ventilation-perfusion relationships. **A,** Normal alveolar–capillary unit with an ideal match of ventilation and blood flow. Maximum gas exchange occurs between alveolus and blood. **B,** Physiologic shunting: a unit with adequate perfusion but inadequate ventilation. **C,** Dead space: a unit with adequate ventilation but inadequate perfusion. In the latter two cases, gas exchange is impaired.

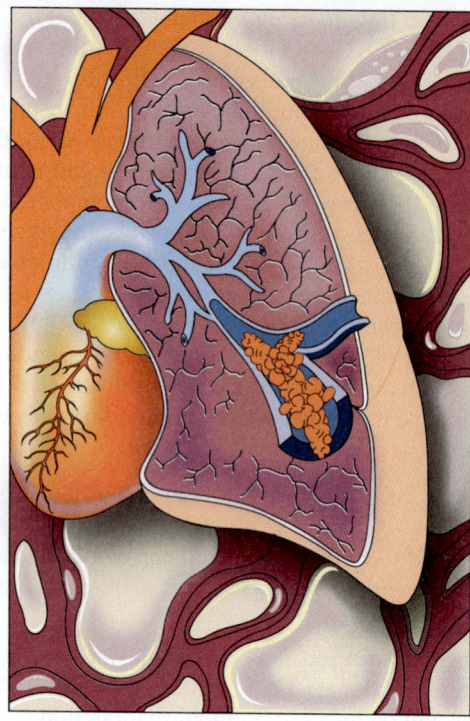

Figure 16–55 » A thromboembolism lodged in a pulmonary vessel.

reflexes triggered by obstruction cause vasoconstriction, increasing pulmonary vascular resistance. In severe cases, this can lead to pulmonary hypertension and right ventricular heart failure. Systemically, hypotension and a drop in CO may develop. Bronchoconstriction occurs in the affected area of lung. **Dead space** (areas of the lung that are ventilated but not perfused) increases. Alveolar surfactant decreases, increasing the risk for atelectasis.

If infarction does not occur, the fibrinolytic system ultimately dissolves the clot, and pulmonary function returns to normal. If infarction does occur, the infarcted tissue becomes scarred and fibrotic.

Fat emboli are the most common nonthrombotic pulmonary emboli. A fat embolism usually occurs after fracture of long bone (typically the femur) releases bone marrow fat into the circulation. Adipose tissue or liver trauma may also lead to fat emboli.

Etiology

Thrombus arising from the deep veins of the legs is the leading cause of PE. Fat emboli, which occur because of trauma or surgery, are less common.

Risk Factors

The risk factors for pulmonary embolus are similar to those for DVT and include stasis of venous blood flow, vessel wall damage, and altered blood coagulation. Inherited thrombophilias and certain cancers that produce coagulation factors make clot formation more likely (Mayo Clinic, 2014j). Risk factors for DVT include prolonged immobility; trauma, including hip and femur fractures; surgery (orthopedic, pelvic, and gynecologic surgery in particular); MI and heart

failure; obesity; and advanced age. A family history of DVT or PE may also indicate risk for the condition (CDC, 2015k). Women who use oral contraceptives or estrogen therapy are at risk, as are women during pregnancy and childbirth. Smoking cigarettes also increases the risk of pulmonary emboli. The incidence of PE is higher in Black patients than White patients, although procoagulant disorders such as factor V Leiden and prothrombin gene disorders are more prominent in White patients than in Black patients (Buckner & Key, 2012).

Prevention

To begin preventing PE, it is crucial to prevent the clots caused by DVT. Hospitals commonly take aggressive measures to prevent such clots, including administering anticoagulants before or after an operation for individuals who are at risk for clots (or for those who were admitted with a heart attack, stroke, or cancer complications); using compression stockings to keep blood from stagnating during surgery and/or pneumatic compression to squeeze the leg veins with air to improve blood flow; encouraging physical activity in patients as soon as possible following surgery; and elevating legs during bedrest. Patients may help prevent PE while traveling by taking breaks from sitting, flexing their ankles while seated, drinking plenty of fluids, and wearing support stockings (Mayo Clinic, 2015h).

Clinical Manifestations

The clinical manifestations of PE depend on the size and location of the emboli. Small emboli may be asymptomatic. Manifestations usually develop abruptly, over a period of minutes. The most common symptoms are dyspnea and pleuritic chest pain. Anxiety, a sense of impending doom, and cough are also common. Diaphoresis and hemoptysis may develop. A massive pulmonary embolus can cause syncope and cyanosis. On examination, tachycardia and tachypnea are noted. Crackles may be heard on auscultation of the chest, and a cardiac gallop (S_3 and possibly S_4) may be noted. A low-grade fever may develop. It is difficult to differentiate PE from MI or pneumonia by manifestations.

Characteristic manifestations of fat emboli include sudden onset of cardiopulmonary and neurologic symptoms: dyspnea, tachypnea, tachycardia, confusion, delirium, and decreased LOC. Petechiae often develop on the chest and arms. See the Clinical Manifestations and Therapies feature for more information.

Collaboration

Because DVT may not be identified until PE occurs, prevention is the primary goal in treating PE. Early ambulation of medical and surgical patients is an effective means of preventing venous stasis and reducing the incidence of PE. External pneumatic compression of the legs is also effective for patients undergoing neurosurgery, urologic surgery, or major surgery of the hip or knee, or when anticoagulant therapy is contraindicated. Other preventive measures include elevating the legs and active and passive leg exercises.

Clinical Manifestations and Therapies
Pulmonary Embolism

ETIOLOGY	CLINICAL MANIFESTATIONS	CLINICAL THERAPIES
Hypoxia due to blockage of alveoli by thrombus	<ul><li>Restlessness</li><li>Chest pain</li><li>Dyspnea</li><li>Cyanosis</li><li>Use of accessory muscles when breathing</li><li>Respiratory acidosis</li><li>Tachycardia</li><li>Tachypnea</li><li>Feeling of impending doom</li></ul>	<ul><li>Administer oxygen.</li><li>Reposition the patient to decrease the work of breathing.</li><li>Prepare the patient for the possibility of intubation and mechanical ventilation.</li><li>Begin anticoagulant therapy as ordered.</li><li>Monitor lab values.</li><li>Maintain a low-stimulus environment to decrease oxygen demands.</li></ul>
Rupture of small arterioles due to arterial congestion	<ul><li>Auscultation of coarse crackles in the affected lobe</li><li>Cough with or without the presence of blood</li><li>Dyspnea</li></ul>	<ul><li>Explain hemoptysis to help alleviate patient and family member concerns.</li><li>Administer oxygen as ordered.</li><li>Maintain patent airway. Suction prn.</li></ul>
Alveolar collapse related to tissue necrosis and inflammatory process	<ul><li>Hypoxia</li><li>Dyspnea</li><li>Productive cough</li><li>Chest pain</li></ul>	<ul><li>Administer oxygen.</li><li>Reposition the patient to facilitate adequate air exchange.</li><li>Promote use of an incentive spirometer to facilitate postural drainage.</li></ul>
Inflammatory process	<ul><li>Elevated temperature</li><li>Tachycardia</li><li>Tachypnea</li><li>Dehydration</li><li>Cough</li></ul>	<ul><li>Administer antipyretics.</li><li>Conduct laboratory testing to aid in diagnosis of causative agent.</li><li>Administer antibiotics and IV fluids as ordered.</li></ul>

SAFETY ALERT When applying external pneumatic compression boots, be sure to apply the correct size boots. Compression boots that are too small or too large will be ineffective at preventing DVT and PE. Ensure that boots of all sizes, including extra-large boots, are on hand.

When PE occurs, treatment is supportive. Oxygen therapy is initiated, and analgesics may be ordered to relieve severe pleuritic pain and anxiety. Pulmonary artery and wedge pressures are monitored with a balloon (Swan-Ganz) catheter. COs also may be assessed. Cardiac rhythm is monitored to detect dysrhythmias.

Diagnostic Tests

Before performing clinical tests, patients with suspected PE should undergo criteria testing with the Pulmonary Embolism Rule-out Criteria (PERC), Modified Wells Criteria, or Geneva Criteria. Patients who have a low probability of having a PE on the basis of these criteria will probably not need to undergo further testing, but they should continue to be monitored, because a small percentage of patients with a low score eventually have a PE. Criteria that indicate risk for

PE include the following (BMJ Best Practice, 2015; Kline et al., 2004; Weber, 2014):

- Pulse rate greater than 99 bpm
- Pulse oximetry less than 95% on room air
- History of DVT or PE
- Hemoptysis
- Recent surgery or trauma requiring hospitalization; cancer
- Unilateral leg swelling or limb pain.

If the criteria testing indicates that the patient is at risk for a PE, then the patient should undergo further testing. The studies performed to diagnose pulmonary emboli differ from those used to diagnose DVT and include the following:

- *Plasma D-dimer levels* are highly specific to the presence of a thrombus. *D-dimer* is a fragment of fibrin formed during lysis of a blood clot; elevated blood levels indicate thrombus formation and lysis (e.g., DVT and PE).
- *Chest CT with contrast* is the principal test used to diagnose PE. Chest CT effectively shows large, central

pulmonary emboli; newer-generation scanners also can detect peripheral emboli.

- *Lung scans,* including perfusion and ventilation scans (V/Q scans), may be used. In a perfusion lung scan, radiotagged albumin is injected intravenously and distributed in the lungs by the pulmonary blood flow. The lungs are then scanned for distribution of the isotope. An area of lung in which the isotope cannot be detected is suggestive of occluded blood flow and PE. For a ventilation scan, a radiotagged gas is inhaled, and the lungs are scanned for gas distribution. Combined perfusion and ventilation scans allow identification of areas of the lungs that are ventilated but not perfused, a characteristic of PE.

SAFETY ALERT Radioisotopes used in lung scans may cause allergic reactions in some individuals. Before a lung scan is performed, the nurse should ask the patient about any previous allergic reactions to radioisotopes. In addition, because of the potential harm to the fetus due to radiation, female patients should be asked if they are pregnant or may be pregnant before beginning the tests. Breastfeeding mothers should be cautioned to refrain from breastfeeding for 24–48 hours.

- *CT pulmonary angiography* is the definitive test for PE when other, less invasive tests are inconclusive. It is possible to detect very small emboli with angiography. A contrast medium injected into the pulmonary arteries illustrates the pulmonary vascular system on x-ray.
- *Chest x-ray* often shows pulmonary infiltration and occasionally pleural effusion.
- *Electrocardiography* is ordered to rule out AMI as the cause of symptoms. Electrocardiographic findings commonly associated with PE include tachycardia and nonspecific T-wave changes.
- *Arterial blood gas (ABG)* measurements usually show hypoxemia (PaO_2 less than 80 mmHg) and often respiratory alkalosis (pH greater than 7.45, $PaCO_2$ less than 35 mmHg) caused by tachypnea and hyperventilation.
- *$ETCO_2$* (end-tidal carbon dioxide, a measurement of carbon dioxide exhaled) may be measured to evaluate alveolar perfusion. The normal $ETCO_2$ reading is 35–45 mmHg; it is decreased when pulmonary perfusion is impaired.
- *Coagulation studies* are ordered to monitor the response to therapy. The aPTT (also called PTT) is used to assess the intrinsic clotting pathway and the response to heparin therapy. Desired levels with anticoagulant therapy are 1.5–2 times the control value. The risk of recurrent thromboembolism is high at lower levels; the risk of bleeding increases at higher levels. The INR is used to assess the extrinsic clotting system and oral anticoagulation with warfarin (Coumadin). The goal of anticoagulant therapy is to achieve a therapeutic INR range of 2.0–3.0.

Pharmacologic Therapy

Anticoagulant therapy is the standard treatment for preventing pulmonary emboli. It is often initiated in high-risk patients who have no evidence of PE to prevent possible devastating effects. In the patient with DVT or a pulmonary embolus, anticoagulants are administered to prevent further clotting and embolization.

For the patient with a pulmonary embolus, heparin therapy is initiated with an IV bolus of 5000–10,000 units, followed by continuous infusion at the rate of 1000–1500 units/hr. The aPTT or PTT is monitored frequently until stabilized. Heparin therapy is typically continued for approximately 5 days, or until oral anticoagulant therapy has become fully effective.

Oral anticoagulant therapy with warfarin sodium (Coumadin) is initiated at the same time as heparin. Warfarin sodium alters the synthesis of vitamin K–dependent clotting factors and requires 5–7 days to be fully effective. Anticoagulant therapy is continued for 2–3 months when few risk factors for thromboemboli exist; long-term therapy is used when chronic disorders that increase the risk of thromboemboli are present.

Bleeding is a risk associated with anticoagulant therapy. Although major hemorrhage is uncommon, it occurs in approximately 5% of patients receiving IV heparin. Cardiac, hepatic, and renal disease all increase the risk of significant bleeding, as does age over 60 years. The use of fractionated and low molecular weight heparin is associated with fewer adverse effects and may be considered. Current research suggests that Factor X inhibitors are also effective and result in fewer side effects and drug interactions (Ouellette, Kamangar, & Harrington, 2015). Protamine, a protein that combines with heparin to inactivate it, is used to stop its anticoagulant effect if major bleeding occurs. Vitamin K is given to treat bleeding associated with warfarin therapy.

Fibrinolytic therapy may be used to treat a massive pulmonary embolus and hypotension. Streptokinase, urokinase, or tissue plasminogen activators are used to **lyse** (disintegrate) the embolus, restore pulmonary blood flow, and reduce pulmonary artery and right heart pressures. Although fibrinolytic therapy may not reduce the mortality associated with pulmonary embolus, it may reduce the incidence of pulmonary hypertension, which can develop 3–5 years after an embolism. Fibrinolysis significantly increases the risk of bleeding, particularly cerebral bleeding. Contraindications to fibrinolysis include intracranial disease, recent stroke, active bleeding or a bleeding disorder, pregnancy, severe hypertension, and recent surgery or trauma. Because of the increased risk of hemorrhage, invasive procedures are avoided after fibrinolysis.

Surgery

When anticoagulant therapy fails to prevent recurrent emboli or is contraindicated, an umbrella-like filter may be inserted into the inferior vena cava to trap large emboli while allowing continued blood flow (see Figure 16–36). The filter usually is inserted percutaneously, via either the femoral or jugular vein.

SAFETY ALERT If a patient has a vena cava filter inserted and still has many emboli in the legs, the filter may become clogged, causing severe edema in the lower extremities. Monitor the patient for edema, and implement preventive measures to reduce or prevent edema.

Lifespan Considerations

PE in children is rare and presents with ambiguous symptoms, so it is underrecognized and underdiagnosed in this population. PE may be more common in pregnant women, as it is the sixth leading cause of maternal death (Schwartz, Malhotra, & Weinberger, 2016). Considerations for diagnosing and treating PE in older adults are similar to those for the general adult population.

Pulmonary Embolism in Children

Risk factors for PE in children include obesity (BMI of 25 or greater), immobilization, indwelling central line, malignancy, prior PE or DVT, a hypercoagulable state, and excessive estrogen state (use of oral contraceptives or peripartum state) (Agha et al., 2013; Lee et al., 2012). Presenting symptoms typically include tachypnea, tachycardia, chest pain, shortness of breath, and cough. Very few children present with hemoptysis, which is more common in adults with PE (Agha et al., 2013).

Tools to diagnose PE, such as the PERC or Wells Criteria, have not been validated in children. Although some adult predictive tools may be beneficial for use in children, others may not accurately predict the risk of PE in children (Agha et al., 2013). V/Q scans, CT pulmonary angiography, and magnetic resonance pulmonary angiography are useful in diagnosing children with PE, but the D-dimer test (useful in diagnosing adults) is not (Dijk et al., 2012; Lee et al., 2012). Treatment generally includes unfractionated heparin or low-molecular-weight heparin. The mortality rate for children with a PE is around 10%, but the cause of death is usually related to the underlying condition rather than the PE (Dijk et al., 2012).

Pulmonary Embolism in Pregnant Women

Symptoms of PE in pregnant women are similar to other adults. However, identification of PE in pregnant women is complicated by the fact that many symptoms of PE, including shortness of breath, leg edema, and tachycardia, are common in normal pregnancies (ACOG, 2013b).

If a pregnant women is suspected of having PE and DVT, a bilateral venous compression ultrasound of the lower extremities should be performed. If PE without DVT is suspected, the first diagnostic test should be a chest x-ray. If the chest x-ray is normal, a V/Q scan should be performed, followed by CT pulmonary angiography if the V/Q scan is inconclusive. If the chest x-ray is abnormal, the CT pulmonary angiography should be performed first rather than the V/Q scan (ACOG, 2013b). When attempting to diagnose pregnant women with PE, the Wells Criteria and D-dimer test should be used with caution. The Wells Criteria have not been validated in pregnant women, and D-dimer naturally increases in the second trimester (Emergency Care Institute New South Wales, 2016).

Pregnant women with suspected PE or DVT should be treated with unfractionated heparin or low-molecular-weight heparin. Warfarin should not be used, because it may harm the fetus. Thrombolytic therapy and more invasive procedures have not been tested for safety in pregnant women, and therefore should be used with caution. However, insertion of a vena cava filter appears to be safe if heparin use is contraindicated. If the woman is close to delivery, IV heparin should be used because of its short half-life. If needed, the woman can be switched to IV heparin when she is close to delivery, and then she can be returned to her previous therapeutic regimen after the risk of bleeding has passed. While the pregnant woman is being treated with anticoagulants, her anticoagulant status should be monitored carefully, and the dose required to maintain the desired anticoagulant state may increase as the woman gains weight during pregnancy. Anticoagulant therapy should be continued for at least 6 weeks postpartum, with a total of 6 months of therapy. Both heparin and warfarin have been shown to be safe for breastfeeding (ACOG, 2013b).

NURSING PROCESS

The nurse plays a primary role in preventing PE. Encouraging patients to ambulate after surgery or illness, applying compression stockings or pneumatic compression devices, teaching and encouraging leg exercises, and discouraging the use of pillows under the knees all help prevent DVT and subsequent pulmonary emboli.

The nurse can teach patients to reduce the risks associated with long periods of immobility. For example, to prevent venous stasis and pooling, the patient should stop every 1–2 hours during long automobile trips for a brief stretch and walk, get up every hour or so and do leg exercises while seated during long flights, avoid sitting for long periods of time during work or leisure time, and avoid crossing the legs. Regular exercise, such as walking, also reduces the risk for DVT. The nurse should instruct patients who stand for long periods to use well-fitted elastic stockings, being careful to avoid hose that bind around the knee or thigh. The nurse can also assist patients with smoking cessation and identifying alternatives to oral contraceptives and hormone replacement therapies.

Assessment

Because PE can be a medical emergency, assessment may be focused. In other instances, when emboli are small and not life-threatening, a more extensive nursing assessment may be done. The nurse should obtain the following data when assessing the patient with, or at risk for, a pulmonary embolus:

- *Observation and patient interview.* Most patients with a PE have no observable signs at onset. However, some patients may show signs of chest pain or shortness of breath. Note these signs, and interview the patient related to the potential presence of PE. In particular, assess for chest pain, shortness of breath, and other symptoms, including onset, severity, and precipitating factors; history of recent surgery, venous thrombosis, or other risk factor, such as childbirth or malignancy; and current medications. The patient interview may include using one or more of the criteria tools such as PERC or Wells criteria to assess the patient's relative risk of PE.

- *Physical examination.* Assess the patient for LOC, presence of respirations, and pulse; skin color, temperature, and moisture; vital signs, including apical pulse and temperature; breath sounds and heart sounds; oxygen saturation level; neck vein distention; and peripheral edema.

Diagnosis

Nursing diagnoses appropriate for a patient with PE may include the following:

- *Gas Exchange, Impaired*
- *Cardiac Output, Decreased*
- *Protection, Ineffective*
- *Pain, Acute*
- *Anxiety.*

(NANDA-I © 2014)

Planning

Goals of nursing care for the patient with PE are individualized on the basis of the patient's specific needs and may include the following:

- The patient will demonstrate an oxygen saturation that remains greater than 94%.
- The patient will verbalize fears resulting from respiratory distress.
- The patient will obtain relief from pain to allow for adequate rest and comfort.
- The patient will demonstrate adequate tissue perfusion.
- The patient's vital signs will remain within normal limits.

Implementation

The primary and most emergent focus of nursing care for the patient with PE is to promote oxygenation and gas exchange. Other considerations include pain management and reduction of the anxiety that often results from hypoxia.

Compensate for Impaired Gas Exchange

PE results in areas of the lung that are ventilated but not perfused; these areas receive no capillary blood flow. If the embolus is large and a major segment of the lung is not perfused, gas exchange is significantly affected. Nursing interventions are directed toward compensating for impaired gas exchange and include the following:

- Place the patient in the Fowler or high-Fowler position with the lower extremities dependent (e.g., hanging over the side of the bed). This position facilitates maximal lung expansion and reduces venous return to the right side of the heart, lowering pressures in the pulmonary vascular system.
- Maintain the patient on bedrest. Bedrest reduces metabolic demands and tissue needs for oxygen.
- Frequently assess the patient's respiratory status, including rate, depth, effort, lung sounds, and oxygen saturation. Impaired ventilation will further compromise gas exchange and worsen hypoxemia. Oxygen saturation can be monitored continuously and noninvasively to evaluate gas exchange.
- Monitor the patient's ABG results, reporting abnormal findings as indicated. ABG results are used to assess gas exchange and tissue oxygenation. An arterial line may be inserted for monitoring arterial pressure and for arterial blood sampling.

Preserve Cardiac Output

The impact of a large pulmonary embolus on hemodynamic status can be significant. Pressures in the pulmonary vascular system and right side of the heart increase; blood return to the left side of the heart, and CO may significantly decrease. A central line for hemodynamic monitoring may be instituted. Nursing interventions focus on preserving adequate BP and organ function until cardiopulmonary status stabilizes and may include the following:

- Instruct the patient to report chest pain or other symptoms. Decreased CO and an increased workload resulting from pulmonary hypertension may cause anginal pain.
- Assess the patient's skin color and temperature. These assessments monitor tissue perfusion.
- Auscultate the patient's heart sounds every 2–4 hours, and report any abnormalities. Sounds such as an S_3 or S_4 gallop may indicate cardiac compromise.
- Monitor the patient's cardiac rhythm. A drop in CO and other hemodynamic alterations resulting from PE can precipitate dysrhythmias, which in turn can further impair CO.
- Administer vasopressors and other medications as ordered. Carefully monitor the response to prescribed medications. Drugs may be prescribed to maintain adequate arterial pressure and tissue perfusion. The use of potent drugs, such as vasopressors, require careful monitoring for desired and adverse effects.
- Monitor the patient's pulmonary arterial pressures, neck vein distention, and peripheral edema. Report findings as indicated. Right-sided heart failure is a potential complication of PE because of increased pulmonary arterial pressures.
- Maintain IV and arterial access sites as well as central lines. The patient may be in unstable and critical condition, potentially needing immediate interventions to maintain life.

Promote Safety

Fibrinolytics and anticoagulant therapy impair normal clotting mechanisms, increasing the risk for bleeding and hemorrhage. This risk is particularly acute during the first 24–48 hours following fibrinolytic drug administration. Nursing interventions that promote safety include the following:

- Assess the patient's medication regimen for possible drug interactions that could potentiate or inhibit anticoagulant effects. Drug interactions can increase the risk for hemorrhage or further embolus formation.
- Maintain adequate fluid intake. Administer stool softeners as ordered. These measures help prevent constipation and straining, which may precipitate bleeding of hemorrhoids.
- Assess the patient frequently for overt and covert signs of bleeding: bleeding gums; hematuria; obvious or occult blood in stool or vomitus; incisional bleeding, or bleeding or bruising of injection sites or with minor trauma; joint pain or immobility; and abdominal or flank pain. Careful

monitoring is necessary to identify early signs of abnormal bleeding and prevent potential hemorrhage.

- Report coagulation study results outside the desired range for anticoagulant therapy. Levels less than the target range may indicate an increased risk for further clot development and pulmonary emboli; levels above the target range indicate an increased risk for bleeding.

- Keep protamine sulfate available for heparin therapy and vitamin K available for warfarin (Coumadin) therapy. Bleeding or hemorrhage resulting from excess anticoagulant may require antidote administration to rapidly reverse the anticoagulant effects.

- Avoid invasive procedures, injections, and venous punctures when possible, particularly during and following fibrinolytic therapy. Invasive procedures increase the risk of tissue trauma and bleeding.

- Maintain firm pressure on injection and venipuncture sites. Maintain pressure for 30 minutes following arterial puncture. Firm pressure reduces the risk for bleeding into the tissues.

Maintaining safety following discharge is essential. See the Patient Teaching feature on topics to address with the patient and family prior to discharge.

Relieve Anxiety

PE is a physiologic and psychologic threat to safety and integrity. It is a major physiologic stressor, eliciting a strong neuroendocrine stress response. The feeling of suffocation and inability to catch one's breath that accompanies a pulmonary embolus is also a strong psychologic stressor. Fear, anxiety, and apprehension are common responses. The following nursing interventions will help relieve the patient's anxiety:

- Assess the patient's anxiety. Appropriate interventions are determined by the level of anxiety.

- Explain procedures and treatments, using short, simple sentences. Providing clearly understood, simple instructions reduces fear of the unknown.

- Reduce environmental stimuli, and use a calm, reassuring manner. These measures help reduce anxiety for both the nurse and the patient.

- Allow supportive family members to remain with the patient as much as possible. Calm, supportive family members provide further reassurance.

Patient Teaching
Pulmonary Embolism

Discuss the following topics when preparing the patient with PE and family members for home care:

- Use of prescribed anticoagulant, including drug interactions, scheduled laboratory testing, and manifestations of bleeding to report to the primary care provider
- Use of a soft toothbrush and electric razor to reduce the risk of bleeding
- Avoiding aspirin (unless prescribed) and other over-the-counter medications unless approved by the healthcare provider
- Importance of wearing a medic alert tag for anticoagulant use
- Health promotion measures to reduce the risk of recurrent PE
- Symptoms of recurrent PE, such as sudden chest pain, shortness of breath, and possibly bloody sputum
- Strategies for smoking cessation.

- Remain with the patient as much as possible. The presence of a caring nurse helps reduce fear.
- Administer morphine sulfate as ordered. Morphine is given to reduce pain and anxiety.

Evaluation

The patient's progress toward meeting the goals set during the planning stage of care is evaluated on the basis of the following expected outcomes:

- The patient maintains adequate tissue perfusion to promote oxygenation and healing.
- The patient's pain is controlled to facilitate rest and recovery.
- The patient maintains effective airway clearance.

The nurse should provide continuous assessment and evaluation of the patient with a PE. Even if the patient is currently stable, the status can change at any moment, especially if additional thromboses dislodge and travel to the lungs. The nurse should have assessment tools and treatments readily available to care for the patient at risk for a PE.

Nursing Care Plan
A Patient with Pulmonary Embolism

Frank Marlin, a 52-year-old man, is traveling home with his wife from their 3-week vacation in Australia. The flight is 14 1/2 hours long. As they approach their destination, Mr. Marlin experiences a sharp, stabbing pain in his right chest, which he assumes is a pulled muscle that resulted from a sudden cough he developed a few hours ago. When the plane lands, Mr. and Ms. Marlin gather their carry-on luggage and walk through the concourse toward the baggage area.

As they walk, Mr. Marlin notices that he feels short of breath. He tells his wife he needs to sit down for a minute, secretly worried that he might be having a heart attack, but the pain remains on the right side of his chest. He begins to feel increasingly anxious, and Ms. Marlin notices that her husband is breathing rapidly and perspiring. She asks for help from a customer service clerk, who calls the paramedics. They transport Mr. Marlin to the local emergency department.

(continued on next page)

Nursing Care Plan (continued)

ASSESSMENT	DIAGNOSES	PLANNING
On admission to the emergency department, the nurse collects the following data: temperature 99.2°F tympanic; pulse 98 bpm; respirations 26/min; and BP 142/84 mmHg. Mr. Marlin's oxygen saturation is 87%. His breath sounds clear and equal, with fine rales in the upper right base. His lips and fingernails are mildly cyanotic. Mr. Marlin is alert, oriented, and anxious, asking the nurses, "Am I going to die?" His chest x-ray is normal; however, CT with contrast shows obstructed pulmonary circulation in the right upper lobe. His D-dimer level is elevated. Mr. Marlin is diagnosed with right lobe pulmonary emboli.	▪ *Impaired Gas Exchange* related to decreased perfusion to lungs ▪ *Acute Pain* related to decreased cardiac tissue oxygenation ▪ *Anxiety* related to feeling suffocated (NANDA-I © 2014)	Goals of care include the following: ▪ The patient's gas exchange will improve, as evidenced by an oxygen saturation of greater than 90%. ▪ The patient will have his pain controlled to improve his comfort, as evidenced by a reported pain level of 3 or less. ▪ The patient will experience reduced anxiety, as evidenced by his ability to sleep and to express less fear.

IMPLEMENTATION

- Apply oxygen via face mask.
- Place cardiorespiratory monitor and oxygen saturation monitor on the patient to allow for continuous monitoring of vital signs and oxygen saturation.
- Administer analgesics, per orders, and evaluate the patient's response to medication.
- Teach the patient and family about risk factors contributing to development of pulmonary emboli.
- Answer patient and family questions about the diagnosis of pulmonary emboli.

- Promote deep breathing.
- Position the patient in the semi-Fowler position to maximize expansion of healthy lungs.
- Remain with the patient until vital signs normalize and oxygen saturation improves.
- Administer anticoagulants, and teach the patient how to reduce bleeding risk.

EVALUATION

Mr. Marlin remains hospitalized for 5 days and is discharged on oral warfarin. Follow-up CT with contrast shows resolution of the emboli without permanent scarring or damage to lung tissue.

CRITICAL THINKING

1. On the basis of Mr. Marlin's symptoms, rate the severity of his pulmonary emboli.
2. What measures might you implement to reduce the patient's anxiety?
3. Could Mr. Marlin's vital signs have been monitored manually instead of with placement of a cardiorespiratory monitor? Why is the monitor placed?

REVIEW Pulmonary Embolism

RELATE Link the Concepts and Exemplars

Linking the exemplar of PE with the concept of acid–base balance:

1. What impact on acid–base balance would you anticipate finding when reviewing the results of an ABG drawn from a patient with a significant PE?
2. What assessment findings would you anticipate when examining a patient with a significant PE?

Linking the exemplar of PE with the concept of comfort:

3. Contrast the effectiveness of pharmacologic and nonpharmacologic therapies to control the pain associated with PE.
4. What risk is associated with administration of narcotics to a patient with pulmonary emboli? How would you reduce these risks?

READY Go to Volume 3: Clinical Nursing Skills

REFER Go to Pearson MyLab Nursing and eText

- Additional review materials

REFLECT Apply Your Knowledge

Jennifer Walker is a 20-year-old woman who is attending college in the Midwest. She is majoring in business and lives with her boyfriend, Sam Hough, age 21, in an off-campus apartment. Ms. Walker had an annual physical with a physician on campus at the beginning of the school year and obtained a prescription for oral contraceptives. Ms. Walker and Mr. Hough enjoy walking around the campus with their dog, Shelby, and are very active playing tennis and golf. Mr. Hough's parents are both physicians, and Ms. Walker's mother is a nurse.

Ms. Walker begins to notice that she has pain in her left leg when she walks Shelby and when she is playing tennis. Mr. Hough suggests that she return to the physician for a checkup.

Ms. Walker's physician admits her to the hospital with a diagnosis of thrombophlebitis and places her on heparin and bedrest.

Ms. Walker is on her third day in the hospital, and she and Mr. Hough are studying together in her room when she develops dyspnea and chest pain and becomes very apprehensive. Mr. Hough goes to the nurse's station to inform the staff of Ms. Walker's new symptoms.

1. What is the priority intervention for Ms. Walker at this time?
2. What is the physiologic rationale for pain control for Ms. Walker?
3. Create a plan of care for Ms. Walker and Mr. Hough regarding teaching interventions needed for discharge.

» Exemplar 16.L
Shock

Exemplar Learning Outcomes

16.L Analyze shock as it relates to perfusion.

- Describe the pathophysiology of shock.
- Describe the etiology of shock.
- Compare the risk factors and prevention of shock.
- Identify the clinical manifestations of shock.
- Summarize diagnostic tests and therapies used by interprofessional teams in the collaborative care of an individual with shock.
- Differentiate care of patients with shock across the lifespan.
- Apply the nursing process in providing culturally competent care to an individual with shock.

Exemplar Key Terms

Anaphylactic shock, *1313*
Cardiogenic shock, *1311*
Distributive shock, *1312*
Hypovolemic shock, *1311*
Neurogenic shock, *1312*
Obstructive shock, *1312*
Septic shock, *1312*
Shock, *1307*
Tone, *1307*
Vasogenic shock, *1312*

Overview

Shock is a clinical syndrome characterized by a decrease in blood flow to body organs and tissues, resulting in inadequate oxygenation and life-threatening cellular dysfunction.

To maintain cellular metabolism, the cells of all body organs and tissues require a regular and consistent supply of oxygen and removal of metabolic wastes. This homeostatic regulation is maintained primarily by the cardiovascular system and depends on four physiologic components:

1. CO sufficient to meet bodily requirements
2. An uncompromised vascular system, in which the vessels have a diameter sufficient to allow unimpeded blood flow and have good **tone** (ability to constrict or dilate to maintain normal pressure)
3. A volume of blood sufficient to fill the circulatory system, and a BP adequate to maintain blood flow
4. Tissues that are able to extract and use the oxygen delivered through the capillaries.

In a healthy individual, these components function as a system to maintain tissue perfusion. During shock, however, one or more of the components is disrupted.

Pathophysiology and Etiology

Pathophysiology

When one or more cardiovascular components do not function properly, the body's hemodynamic properties are altered. As a consequence, tissue perfusion may be inadequate to sustain normal cellular metabolism. The result is the clinical syndrome known as shock.

The manifestations of shock result from the body's attempts to maintain vital organs (in particular, the heart and brain) and to preserve life following a drop in cellular perfusion. However, if the injury or condition triggering shock is severe enough or of long enough duration, then cellular hypoxia and cellular death occur.

Shock is triggered by a sustained drop in MAP. This drop can occur after a decrease in CO, a decrease in the circulating blood volume, or an increase in the size of the vascular bed as a result of peripheral vasodilation. If intervention is timely and effective, the physiologic events that characterize shock may be stopped; if not, shock may lead to death.

Classes of Shock

Shock is frequently classified in terms of severity using the system outlined in **Table 16–30 »** and described in more detail in the following sections.

Class I: Early Shock

The initial stage of shock, known as class I or early shock, begins when baroreceptors in the aortic arch and carotid sinus detect a sustained drop in MAP of less than 10 mmHg from normal levels. The circulating blood volume may decrease (usually to less than 500 mL), but not enough to cause serious effects in an adult patient. (See the Lifespan Considerations section for information regarding blood volume changes in children.)

The body reacts to the decrease in arterial pressure as it would to any physical stressor. The cerebral integration center initiates the body's response systems, causing the SNS to increase the heart rate and force of cardiac contraction, thus increasing CO. Sympathetic stimulation also causes peripheral vasoconstriction, resulting in increased SVR and a rise in arterial pressure. The net result is that the perfusion of cells, tissues, and organs is maintained.

TABLE 16–30 Classification of Hemorrhagic Shock and Patient Presentation

	Early/Class I	Compensatory/Class II	Decompensated/Class III	Refractory/Class IV
Blood loss	< 750 mL	750–1500 mL	1500–2000 mL	> 2000 mL
% of blood volume loss	< 15%	15–30%	30–40%	> 40%
Heart rate	< 100	100–120	120–140	> 140
Blood pressure	Normal	Normal	Decreased	Decreased
Pulse pressure	Normal or increased	Decreased	Decreased	Decreased
Capillary refill	Normal	Mildly increased	Usually delayed	Delayed
Respiratory rate	Normal	Mildly increased	Moderate tachypnea	Marked tachypnea
Urine output	> 30 mL/hr	20–30 mL/hr	5–15 mL/hr	Anuria
Mental status	Normal to slightly anxious	Mildly anxious to agitated	Anxious to confused	Lethargic to obtunded

Source: Data from American College of Surgeons Committee on Trauma. (2017). *Advanced trauma life support* (10th ed.). Chicago, IL: American College of Surgeons.

Symptoms are almost imperceptible during the early stage of shock. The pulse rate may be slightly elevated. If the injury is minor or of short duration, arterial pressure is usually maintained, and no further symptoms occur.

Class II: Compensatory Shock

Class II or compensatory shock in adults begins after the MAP falls 10–15 mmHg below normal levels. The circulating blood volume is reduced by 15–30% (1000 mL or more), but compensatory mechanisms are able to maintain BP and tissue perfusion to vital organs, thereby preventing cell damage. Compensatory mechanisms of shock include the following:

- Stimulation of the SNS results in the release of epinephrine from the adrenal medulla and the release of norepinephrine from the adrenal medulla and the sympathetic fibers. Both hormones rapidly stimulate the alpha- and beta-adrenergic fibers. Stimulated alpha-adrenergic fibers cause vasoconstriction in the blood vessels that supply the skin and most of the abdominal viscera. Perfusion of these areas decreases. Stimulated beta-adrenergic fibers cause vasodilation in vessels supplying the heart and skeletal muscles (beta$_1$ response) and increase the heart rate and force of cardiac contraction (beta$_2$ response). Furthermore, blood vessels in the respiratory system dilate, and the respiratory rate increases (beta$_2$ response). Thus, stimulation of the SNS results in increased CO and oxygenation of these tissues.

- The renin-angiotensin response occurs as blood flow to the kidneys decreases. Renin released from the kidneys converts a plasma protein to angiotensin II, which causes vasoconstriction and stimulates the adrenal cortex to release aldosterone. Aldosterone causes the kidneys to reabsorb water and sodium and to lose potassium. The absorption of water maintains circulating blood volume while increased vasoconstriction increases SVR, maintaining central vascular volume and raising BP.

- The hypothalamus releases adrenocorticotropic hormone, causing the adrenal glands to secrete aldosterone. Aldosterone promotes the reabsorption of water and sodium by the kidneys, preserving blood volume and pressure.

- The posterior pituitary gland releases ADH, which increases renal reabsorption of water to increase intravascular volume. The combined effects of hormones released by the hypothalamus and posterior pituitary glands work to conserve central vascular volume.

- As MAP falls in the compensatory stage of shock, decreased capillary hydrostatic pressure causes a fluid shift from the interstitial space into the capillaries. The net gain of fluid raises the blood volume.

Working together, these compensatory mechanisms can maintain MAP for only a short period of time. During this period, perfusion and oxygenation of the heart and brain are adequate. If effective treatment is provided, the process is arrested and no permanent damage occurs. However, unless the underlying cause of shock is reversed, these compensatory mechanisms soon become harmful, and shock perpetuates shock.

Class III: Decompensated Shock

Class III shock, also called decompensated or progressive shock, occurs after a sustained decrease in MAP of 20 mmHg or more below normal levels and a blood volume loss of 30–40%. Although the compensatory mechanisms in the previous stage remain activated, they are no longer able to maintain MAP at a level sufficient to ensure perfusion of vital organs.

During decompensated shock, the vasoconstriction response that first helped sustain MAP eventually limits blood flow to the point at which cells become oxygen deficient. To remain alive, the affected cells switch from aerobic to anaerobic metabolism. The lactic acid formed as a by-product of anaerobic metabolism contributes to an acidotic state at the cellular level. As a result, production of ATP, the source of cellular energy, is inefficient. Lacking energy, the sodium–potassium pump fails. Potassium moves out of the cell, while sodium and water move inward. As this process continues, the cell swells, cell membrane integrity is lost, and cell organelles are damaged. Lysosomes within the cell spill out their digestive enzymes, which disintegrate any remaining organelles. Some enzymes spread to adjacent cells, where they erode and rupture cell membranes.

The acid by-products of anaerobic metabolism dilate the precapillary arterioles and constrict the postcapillary venules. This causes increased hydrostatic pressure within the capillary, and fluid shifts back into the interstitial space.

The capillaries also become increasingly permeable, allowing serum proteins to shift from the vascular space into the interstitium. The buildup of plasma proteins increases the osmotic pressure in the interstitium, further accelerating the fluid shift out of the capillaries.

Throughout this period, heart rate and vasoconstriction increase, but perfusion of the skin, skeletal muscles, kidneys, and gastrointestinal organs is greatly diminished. Cells in the heart and brain become hypoxic, while other body cells and tissues become ischemic and anoxic. A generalized state of acidosis and hyperkalemia ensues. Unless this stage of shock is treated rapidly, the patient's chances of survival are poor.

Class IV: Refractory Shock

If shock progresses to class IV, also known as refractory or irreversible shock, tissue anoxia becomes so generalized and cellular death so widespread that no treatment can reverse the damage. Even if MAP is temporarily restored, too much cellular damage has occurred to maintain life. Death of cells is followed by death of tissues, which results in death of organs. Death of vital organs contributes to subsequent death of the body.

Effects of Shock on Body Systems

Whatever its causes, shock produces predictable effects on the body's organ systems, as described in the following sections and shown in Multisystem Effects of Shock.

Cardiovascular System

Perfusion and oxygenation of the heart are adequate in the early stages of shock. As shock progresses, myocardial cells become hypoxic, and myocardial muscle function diminishes. At first, the BP may be normal or even slightly elevated (as a result of compensatory mechanisms), and the heart rate may increase only slightly. Sympathetic stimulation increases the heart rate (a sinus tachycardia of 120 bpm is common) in an effort to increase CO. As a result of vasoconstriction and decreased blood volume, the palpated pulse is rapid, weak, and thready; as shock progresses, peripheral pulses are usually not palpable.

Tachycardia reduces the time available for left ventricular filling and coronary artery perfusion, further reducing CO. With progressive shock, altered acid–base balance, hypoxia, and hyperkalemia damage the heart's electrical systems and contractility. As a consequence, cardiac dysrhythmias may develop. Decreased blood volume with decreased venous return also decreases CO, and BP falls.

The BP changes produced by shock are characterized by a progressive decrease in both systolic and diastolic pressures and a narrowing pulse pressure. Auscultation of BP is often difficult or impossible and is an inaccurate reflection of BP status. For this reason, hemodynamic monitoring is usually required to follow the patient's cardiovascular status accurately.

Respiratory System

During shock, oxygen delivery to cells may be impaired by a drop in circulating blood volume or, in the case of blood loss, by an insufficient number of RBCs that carry oxygen. Although the respiratory rate increases because of compensatory mechanisms that promote oxygenation, the number of alveoli that are perfused decreases, and gas exchange is impaired. As a result, blood oxygen levels decrease, and carbon dioxide levels increase. As perfusion of the lungs diminishes, carbon dioxide is retained, and respiratory acidosis occurs.

A complication of decreased perfusion of the lungs is ARDS, or "shock lung" (see the exemplar in the module on Oxygenation). The exact mechanism that produces ARDS is unknown, but some contributing factors have been identified. The pulmonary capillaries become increasingly permeable to proteins and water, resulting in noncardiogenic pulmonary edema. Production of surfactant, which controls surface tension within alveoli, is impaired, and the alveoli collapse or fill with fluid. This potentially lethal form of respiratory failure may result from any condition that causes hypoperfusion of the lungs, but it is most common in shock caused by hemorrhage, severe allergic responses, trauma, and infection.

Gastrointestinal System

The gastrointestinal organs normally receive 25% of the CO through the splanchnic circulation. Shock constricts the splanchnic arterioles and redirects arterial blood flow to the heart and brain. Gastrointestinal organs consequently become ischemic and may be irreversibly damaged.

Gastric mucosa tend to ulcerate when ischemic. Lesions of the gastric and duodenal mucosa (stress ulcers) can develop within hours of severe trauma, sepsis, or burns (Clarke et al., 2015). Gastrointestinal ulcers may hemorrhage within 2–10 days following the original cause of shock. In addition, the permeability of damaged mucosa increases, allowing enteric bacteria or their toxins to enter the abdominal cavity and then progress to the circulation, resulting in sepsis.

Gastric and intestinal motility is impaired during shock, and paralytic ileus may result. If the episode of shock is prolonged, necrosis of the bowel may occur. In many cases, alterations in the structure and function of the gastrointestinal tract impair absorption of nutrients.

Shock also alters the metabolic functions of the liver. Gluconeogenesis (the process of forming glucose from noncarbohydrate sources) and glycogenolysis (the breakdown of glycogen into glucose) initially increase. This process allows blood glucose levels to increase as the body attempts to respond to the stressor; however, as shock progresses, liver function becomes impaired, and hypoglycemia develops. Metabolism of fats and protein is impaired, and the liver can no longer effectively remove lactic acid, contributing to the development of metabolic acidosis.

The destruction of the liver's Kupffer cells (phagocytes that destroy bacteria) causes a further problem. Bacteria may proliferate within the circulatory system, causing overwhelming bacterial infection and toxicity.

Neurologic System

The primary effects of shock on the neurologic system involve changes in mental status and orientation. Cerebral hypoxia produces altered LOCs, beginning with apathy and lethargy and progressing to coma. A common early symptom of cerebral hypoxia is restlessness. Continued ischemia

Multisystem Effects of
Shock

Respiratory

- ↑ respiratory rate
- Respiratory acidosis

Potential complication
- ARDS

Urinary

- ↓ renal perfusion
- ↓ GFR

Late
- Oliguria

Potential complications
- Acute tubular necrosis
- Kidney failure

Hepatic

Early
- ↑ glucose production

Progressive
- ↓ glucose production = hypoglycemia
- ↓ lactic acid conversion = metabolic acidosis

Potential complication
- Destroyed Kupffer cells = systemic bacterial infections

Gastrointestinal

Early
- ↓ GI motility

Late
- Paralytic ileus
- Ulceration of GI mucosa

Potential complication
- Bowel necrosis

Neurologic

- ↓ cognition
- ↓ sympathetic activity
- ↓ consciousness

Early
- Restlessness, apathy

Progressive
- Lethargy

Late
- Coma

Cardiovascular

Early
- No change

Progressive
- Slightly ↑ BP
- Slowly ↑ HR
- Sinus tachycardia
- Thready pulse

Late
- MAP <60 mmHg
- Steadily ↓ BP
- Steadily ↓ CO
- Imperceptible pulses

Integumentary

- Pallor (skin, lips, oral mucosa, nail beds, conjunctiva)
- Cool, moist skin

Late
- Edema

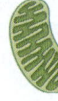

Metabolic Processes

- ↓ temperature
- Thirst
- Acidosis (metabolic and respiratory)

of brain cells eventually causes swelling, resulting in cerebral edema, neurotransmitter failure, and irreversible brain damage.

As cerebral ischemia worsens, the sympathetic activity and vasomotor centers are depressed. This leads to a loss of sympathetic tone, causing systemic vasodilation and pooling of blood in the periphery. As a result, venous return and CO decrease further.

SAFETY ALERT An early sign of shock is a change in LOC. Late signs of shock include mental status changes, hypotension, and marked tachycardia.

Renal System

During the progressive stage of shock, blood that normally perfuses the kidneys is shunted to the heart and brain, resulting in renal hypoperfusion. The drop in renal perfusion is reflected in a corresponding decrease in the glomerular filtration rate. Urine output is reduced, and the urine that is produced is highly concentrated. Oliguria of less than 20 mL/hr indicates progressive shock.

Healthy kidneys can tolerate a drop in perfusion for only approximately 30 minutes; thereafter, acute tubular necrosis develops (Silberberg, 2013). As tubular necrosis occurs, epithelial cells slough off and block the tubules, disrupting nephron function. The accumulating loss of functional nephrons eventually causes renal failure. Without normal renal function, metabolic waste products are retained in the plasma.

If treatment restores renal perfusion, the kidneys can regenerate the lost epithelial cells in the tubules, and renal function usually returns to normal. However, in patients who are older, chronically ill, or in sustained shock, loss of renal function may become permanent.

Effects on Skin, Temperature, and Thirst

In most types of shock, blood vessels supplying the skin are vasoconstricted, and the sweat glands are activated. As a result, changes in skin color occur. The skin of Caucasian patients becomes pale. In individuals with darker skin (e.g., those of African, Hispanic, or Mediterranean descent), shock-related skin color changes may be assessed as paleness of the lips, oral mucous membranes, nail beds, and conjunctiva. The skin is usually cool and moist and, in the later stages of shock, often edematous.

Body temperature decreases as shock progresses, the result of a decrease in overall body metabolism. Some individuals with shock become thirsty, probably a response to decreased blood volume and increased serum osmolality.

Etiology

Shock is identified according to its underlying cause. All types of shock progress through the same stages and exert similar effects on body systems. Any differences are noted in the following discussion.

Hypovolemic Shock

Hypovolemic shock is caused by a decrease in intravascular volume of 15% or more (Kolecki & Menckhoff, 2014). In hypovolemic shock, the amount of venous blood returning

to the heart decreases, and ventricular filling drops. As a result, SV, CO, and BP decrease. Hypovolemic shock is the most common type of shock, and it often occurs simultaneously with other forms of shock.

The decrease in circulating blood volume that triggers hypovolemic shock may result from any of the following:

- Loss of blood volume from hemorrhage (e.g., from surgery, trauma, gastrointestinal bleeding, blood coagulation disorders, or ruptured esophageal varices)
- Loss of intravascular fluid from the skin because of injuries such as burns
- Loss of blood volume from severe dehydration
- Loss of body fluid from the gastrointestinal system because of persistent and severe vomiting or diarrhea or continuous nasogastric suctioning
- Renal losses of fluid because of diuretic use or endocrine disorders, such as diabetes insipidus
- Conditions causing fluid shifts from the intravascular compartment to the interstitial space
- Third spacing because of disorders such as liver diseases with ascites, pleural effusion, or intestinal obstruction.

Hypovolemic shock affects all body systems. Its effects vary depending on the patient's age, the patient's general state of health, the extent of injury or severity of illness, the length of time before treatment is provided, and the rate of volume loss.

Manifestations of hypovolemic shock result directly from the decrease in circulating blood volume and the initiation of compensatory mechanisms (see **Figure 16–56** »»). The loss of circulating blood volume reduces CO by decreasing venous return to the heart. As a result, BP drops, and the body induces the sympathetic compensatory responses. If the fluid loss is less than 500 mL in adults, the sympathetic response is generally adequate to restore CO and BP to near normal, although the heart rate may remain elevated.

With a sustained loss of blood volume (1000 mL or more in adults), the shock stage progresses. Heart rate and vasoconstriction increase, and blood flow to the skin, skeletal muscles, kidneys, and abdominal organs decreases. Several renal mechanisms and a decline in capillary pressure help conserve blood volume. The amount of blood flowing to cells eventually is too low to oxygenate them and sustain production of cellular energy. Anaerobic metabolism begins, and cells lose their physical integrity. If untreated, shock causes multiple organ failure and death.

SAFETY ALERT Underlying conditions can affect the body's response to hypovolemic shock. For example, atherosclerosis affects many vital organs' sensitivity to even the slightest reduction in blood flow. In addition, patients who take beta-blockers may not present with tachycardia as an early indicator of shock. This important sign can be masked because of beta-adrenergic blockade. These patients will require early invasive monitoring in order to avoid excessive or inadequate volume restoration.

Cardiogenic Shock

Cardiogenic shock occurs when the heart's pumping ability is compromised to the point that it cannot maintain CO and

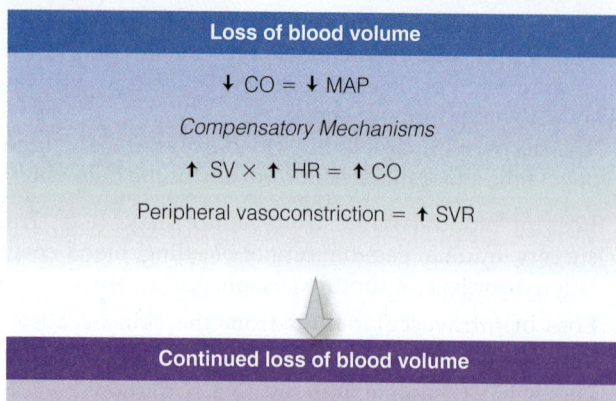

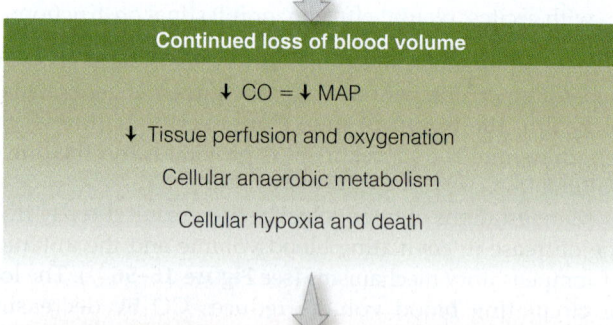

Key CO: Cardiac output
     HR: Heart rate
     MAP: Mean arterial pressure
     SV: Stroke volume
     SVR: Systemic vascular resistance

Figure 16–56 》 Stages of hypovolemic shock.

adequate tissue perfusion. The loss of pumping action may be caused by any of the following conditions:

- MI
- Cardiac tamponade
- Restrictive pericarditis
- Cardiac arrest
- Dysrhythmias, such as VF or VT
- Pathologic changes in the valves
- Cardiomyopathies from hypertension, alcohol, bacterial or viral infections, or ischemia
- Complications of cardiac surgery

- Electrolyte imbalances, especially changes in normal potassium and calcium levels
- Drugs affecting cardiac muscle contractility
- Head injuries causing damage to the cardioregulatory center.

MI is the most common cause of cardiogenic shock. Patients admitted to the hospital for treatment of MI or cardiac surgery are at risk for cardiogenic shock. The severity and progression of shock are related to the amount of myocardial damage.

Whatever the exact cause of cardiogenic shock, the decrease in CO leads to a decrease in MAP. Heart rate may increase due to compensatory mechanisms. However, tachycardia increases myocardial oxygen consumption and decreases coronary perfusion. The myocardium becomes progressively depleted of oxygen, causing further myocardial ischemia and necrosis. The typical sequence of shock is essentially unchanged in cardiogenic shock.

Cyanosis is more common in cardiogenic shock because stagnating blood increases extraction of oxygen from the hemoglobin at the capillary beds. As a result, the skin, lips, and nail beds may appear cyanotic. As cardiac failure and cardiogenic shock progress, left ventricular end-diastolic pressure increases. The increase is transmitted to the pulmonary capillary bed, and pulmonary edema may occur. Also, retention of blood in the right side of the heart increases right atrial pressure, which leads to JVD as a result of backflow through the vena cava.

Obstructive Shock

Obstructive shock is caused by an obstruction in the heart or great vessels that either impedes venous return or prevents effective cardiac pumping action. The causes of obstructive shock are impaired diastolic filling (e.g., pericardial tamponade, pneumothorax), increased right ventricular afterload (e.g., pulmonary emboli), and increased left ventricular afterload (e.g., aortic stenosis, abdominal distention). The manifestations are the result of decreased CO and BP, with reduced tissue perfusion and cellular metabolism.

Distributive Shock

Distributive shock, also called **vasogenic shock**, includes several types of shock that result from widespread vasodilation and decreased peripheral resistance. Because the blood volume does not change, relative hypovolemia results.

Septic Shock

Septic shock, also known as septicemia, is the leading cause of death for patients in ICUs. It is one part of a progressive syndrome called systemic inflammatory response syndrome. This condition is most often the result of gram-negative bacterial infections (e.g., *Pseudomonas, Escherichia coli, Klebsiella*) but may also follow gram-positive infections from *Staphylococcus* and *Streptococcus* bacteria. Septic shock is discussed in more detail in the exemplar on Sepsis in the module on Infection.

Neurogenic Shock

Neurogenic shock is the result of an imbalance between parasympathetic and sympathetic stimulation of vascular smooth muscle. If parasympathetic overstimulation or sympathetic understimulation persists, sustained vasodilation occurs, and blood pools in the venous and capillary beds.

Neurogenic shock causes a dramatic reduction in SVR as the size of the vascular compartment increases. As SVR decreases, pressure in the blood vessels becomes too low to drive nutrients across capillary membranes, and cellular metabolism is impaired.

A variety of conditions can cause neurogenic shock by increasing parasympathetic stimulation or inhibiting sympathetic stimulation of the smooth muscle of blood vessels. Examples include head injury, trauma to the spinal cord, insulin reactions (which cause hypoglycemia, decreasing glucose to the medulla), use of central nervous system depressant drugs, anesthesia, severe pain, and prolonged exposure to heat.

Bradycardia occurs early in neurogenic shock, but tachycardia begins as compensatory mechanisms are initiated. CVP drops as veins dilate, venous return to the heart decreases, SV decreases, and MAP falls. In early stages, the extremities are warm and pink (from the pooling of blood), but as shock progresses, the skin becomes pale and cool.

Anaphylactic Shock

Anaphylactic shock is the result of a widespread hypersensitivity reaction (called *anaphylaxis*). The pathophysiology in this type of shock includes vasodilation, pooling of blood in the periphery, and hypovolemia with altered cellular metabolism. These alterations occur when a sensitized individual comes in contact with an allergen (a foreign substance to which an individual is hypersensitive). Many different allergens can cause anaphylactic shock, including medications, blood administration, latex, foods, snake venom, and insect stings. Anaphylactic shock is discussed in more detail in the exemplar on Hypersensitivity in the module on Immunity.

Risk Factors and Prevention

Risk factors and prevention strategies vary for different types of shock. For example, advancing cardiac disease increases the risk for cardiogenic shock. Thus, prevention of cardiogenic shock involves taking the same steps as for preventing heart disease: controlling BP to avoid hypertension, not smoking, exercising regularly, maintaining a healthy weight, and reducing the intake of cholesterol and saturated fats. Individuals who practice high-risk behaviors, ranging from driving while under the influence of a mind-altering substance to participating in dangerous sports, are at increased risk for trauma and shock that results from bleeding or multisystem injury, while patients with diseases that slow the body's ability to clot (e.g., hemophilia) are at increased risk for hemorrhagic shock. Because shock often results from trauma or infection, safety measures aimed at preventing trauma, such as use of helmets, seatbelts, and other protective gear, and preventing infection, such as good hand hygiene and infection control measures, should be used consistently. Nurses are responsible for teaching patients safety measures that can prevent injury and infection.

Clinical Manifestations

The onset of shock may be rapid or slow, depending on its cause and severity. Signs of early shock may be nonspecific. As the body compensates for hypotension or hypovolemia, signs of shock include tachycardia, increased respiratory effort, and decreased urine output. The patient may also be diaphoretic (perspire excessively). Specific manifestations for different forms of shock are listed in the Clinical Manifestations and Therapies feature.

If treatment is not begun in the early stages of shock, the condition may progress until the patient can no longer compensate. At that time, the systolic BP drops, and the pulse pressure narrows. Reduced cerebral blood flow ultimately results in a decreased LOC. If shock is not reversed, it progresses to cardiopulmonary failure and death.

Collaboration

Medical care for the patient in shock focuses on treating the underlying cause, increasing arterial oxygenation, and improving tissue perfusion. Depending on the cause and type of shock, interventions include emergency care measures, oxygen therapy, fluid replacement, and medications. Emergency care is often the first course of collaborative action.

Diagnostic Tests

The following tests can help identify the type of shock and assess the patient's physical status:

- **Blood hemoglobin and hematocrit.** Changes in hemoglobin and hematocrit concentrations usually occur in hypovolemic shock. These changes reflect the underlying etiology. In hypovolemic shock resulting from hemorrhage, hemoglobin and hematocrit concentrations are lower than normal. In hypovolemic shock resulting from intravascular fluid loss, hemoglobin and hematocrit concentrations are higher than normal.

- **Arterial blood gases (ABGs).** ABGs are used to determine oxygen and carbon dioxide levels and blood pH. The effects of shock and of the body's compensatory mechanisms often cause a decrease in pH, a decrease in PaO_2 and total oxygen saturation, and an increase in $PaCO_2$.

- **Serum electrolytes.** Measurement of serum electrolytes helps determine the severity and progression of shock. As shock progresses, glucose and sodium levels decrease, and potassium levels increase.

- **Blood urea nitrogen (BUN), serum creatinine levels, urine specific gravity, and osmolality.** These measurements are used to check renal function. As perfusion of the kidneys is decreased and renal function is reduced, BUN and creatinine levels increase, as does urine specific gravity and osmolality.

- **Blood cultures.** In cases of septic shock, blood cultures are critical to identifying the causative organism and choosing appropriate antibiotic therapy.

- **White blood cell (WBC) count and differential.** These measurements are important for patients with septic or anaphylactic shock. The total WBC count is increased in

Clinical Manifestations and Therapies
Shock

ETIOLOGY	CLINICAL MANIFESTATIONS	CLINICAL THERAPIES
Hypovolemic shock	**Early Stage** ■ BP: Normal to slightly decreased ■ Pulse: Slightly increased from baseline ■ Respirations: Normal (baseline) ■ Skin: cool, pale (in periphery), moist ■ Mental status: Alert and oriented ■ Urine output: Slight decrease ■ Other: Thirst, decreased capillary refill time **Compensatory and Decompensated Stages** ■ BP: Hypotension ■ Pulse: Rapid, thready ■ Respirations: Increased ■ Skin: Cool, pale (includes trunk); poor turgor with fluid loss, edematous with fluid shift ■ Mental status: Restless, anxious, confused, or agitated ■ Urine output: Oliguria (less than 30 mL/hr) ■ Other: Marked thirst, acidosis, hyperkalemia, decreased capillary refill time, decreased or absent peripheral pulses **Refractory Stage** ■ BP: Severe hypotension (systolic pressure often is less than 80 mmHg) ■ Pulse: Very rapid, weak ■ Respirations: Rapid, shallow; crackles and wheezes ■ Skin: Cool, pale, mottled with cyanosis ■ Mental status: Disoriented, lethargic, comatose ■ Urine output: Anuria ■ Other: Loss of reflexes, decreased or absent peripheral pulses	■ Take action to control further blood loss. ■ Administer IV fluid and volume expanders. ■ Administer blood (in severe cases). ■ Administer oxygen. ■ Monitor effectiveness of respiratory effort; mechanical ventilation may be required to meet the body's oxygen demands. ■ Support vital functions until perfusion is restored. ■ Assess LOC. ■ Monitor lab data, including hemoglobin, hematocrit, ABGs, serum electrolytes, and BUN. ■ Administer medications as ordered (e.g., diuretics, sodium bicarbonate, antidysrhythmic agents, cardiac glycosides). ■ Keep patient NPO until gastrointestinal function returns to normal.
Cardiogenic shock	■ BP: Hypotension ■ Pulse: Rapid, thready; distention of veins of hands and neck ■ Respirations: Increased, labored; crackles and wheezes; pulmonary edema ■ Skin: Pale, cyanotic, cold, moist ■ Mental status: Restless, anxious, lethargic progressing to comatose ■ Urine output: Oliguria to anuria ■ Other: Dependent edema, elevated CVP, elevated pulmonary capillary wedge pressure, dysrhythmias	■ Administer IV fluid cautiously to avoid fluid overload, which places more stress on the heart. ■ Treat underlying cause. ■ Administer medications as ordered (e.g., diuretics, sodium bicarbonate, antidysrhythmic agents, cardiac glycosides). ■ Administer oxygen. ■ Monitor effectiveness of respiratory effort; mechanical ventilation may be required to meet the body's oxygen demands. ■ Support vital functions until perfusion is restored. ■ Assess LOC. ■ Monitor lab data, including ABGs, serum electrolytes, BUN, creatinine, cardiac enzymes, CVP, pulmonary wedge pressure, and CO. ■ Keep patient NPO until gastrointestinal function returns to normal.

Clinical Manifestations and Therapies *(continued)*

ETIOLOGY	CLINICAL MANIFESTATIONS	CLINICAL THERAPIES
Obstructive shock	■ Pulse: Tachycardia ■ Respirations: Tachypnea ■ BP: Hypotension ■ Urine output: Decreased ■ Other: Delayed capillary refill in extremities, peripheral edema	■ Treat underlying cause. ■ Reduce cardiac workload. ■ Administer oxygen. ■ Monitor effectiveness of respiratory effort; mechanical ventilation may be required to meet the body's oxygen demands. ■ Support vital functions until perfusion is restored. ■ Assess LOC.
Distributive (vasogenic) shock	■ Pulse: Tachycardia ■ Respirations: Tachypnea ■ BP: Hypotension ■ Urine output: Decreased ■ Other: Delayed capillary refill in extremities, peripheral edema, absent or weak peripheral pulses	■ Treat underlying cause. ■ Administer IV fluids. ■ Administer oxygen. ■ Monitor effectiveness of respiratory effort; mechanical ventilation may be required to meet the body's oxygen demands. ■ Administer vasoconstricting medications as ordered to increase PVR and restore perfusion.
Septic shock	***Early (Warm) Septic Shock*** ■ BP: Normal to hypotension ■ Pulse: Increased, thready ■ Respirations: Rapid and deep ■ Skin: Warm, flushed ■ Mental status: Alert, oriented, anxious ■ Urine output: Normal ■ Other: Increased body temperature; chills; weakness; nausea, vomiting, and diarrhea; decreased CVP ***Late (Cold) Septic Shock*** ■ BP: Hypotension ■ Pulse: Tachycardia, arrhythmias ■ Respirations: Rapid, shallow, dyspneic ■ Skin: Cool, pale, edematous ■ Mental status: Lethargic to comatose ■ Urine output: Oliguria to anuria ■ Other: Normal to decreased body temperature, decreased CVP	■ Treat underlying cause. ■ Administer antibiotics and IV fluids. ■ Administer oxygen. ■ Monitor effectiveness of respiratory effort; mechanical ventilation may be required to meet the body's oxygen demands. ■ Assess for potential DIC. ■ Support vital functions until perfusion is restored. ■ Assess LOC. ■ Obtain cultures prior to administration of antibiotics to determine source of infection and pathogen involved.
Neurogenic shock	■ BP: Hypotension ■ Pulse: Slow and bounding ■ Respirations: Vary ■ Skin: Warm, dry ■ Mental status: Anxious, restless, lethargic progressing to comatose ■ Urine output: Oliguria to anuria ■ Other: Lowered body temperature	■ Treat underlying cause. ■ Administer IV fluids. ■ Reduce parasympathetic stimulation or sympathetic understimulation. ■ Administer medications as ordered (e.g., corticosteroids, vasoconstrictors/ vasopressors).

(continued on next page)

Clinical Manifestations and Therapies (continued)

ETIOLOGY	CLINICAL MANIFESTATIONS	CLINICAL THERAPIES
Anaphylactic shock	■ BP: Hypotension ■ Pulse: Increased, dysrhythmias ■ Respirations: Dyspnea, stridor, wheezes, laryngospasm, bronchospasm, pulmonary edema ■ Skin: Warm, edematous (lips, eyelids, tongue, hands, feet, genitals) ■ Mental status: Restless, anxious, lethargic to comatose ■ Urine output: Oliguria to anuria ■ Other: Paresthesias, pruritus, abdominal cramps, vomiting, diarrhea	■ Remove allergen (if still present). ■ Treat underlying cause. ■ Administer medications as ordered (e.g., corticosteroids, albuterol and intramuscular epinephrine to treat histamine-induced bronchospasm). ■ Administer oxygen. ■ Monitor BP and respirations. ■ Insertion of an artificial airway may be required to maintain a functional airway if tracheal edema occurs.

septic shock. Elevated neutrophils indicate acute infection, increased monocytes indicate a bacterial infection, and increased eosinophils indicate an allergic response.

■ **Serum cardiac enzymes.** Levels of several enzymes are elevated in cardiogenic shock: lactate dehydrogenase, creatine kinase, and serum glutamic-oxaloacetic transaminase.

■ **Central venous catheterization.** This procedure can aid in the differential diagnosis of shock and provide information about the heart's preload. A pulmonary artery catheter may be inserted to monitor cardiac dynamics, fluid balance, and the effects of vasoconstrictors and vasopressors.

Depending on the patient's condition, other diagnostic tests may be ordered to determine the extent of injury or damage or to locate the site of internal hemorrhage. These tests might include x-ray studies, CT scans, MRI, endoscopic examinations, and echocardiograms. Newer diagnostic methods for hypoperfusion include gastric tonometry (which measures $PaCO_2$ in the gastric lumen) and sublingual $PaCO_2$ measurement. With either method, an increase in $PaCO_2$ may be indicative of a decrease in MAP.

Pharmacologic Therapy

When fluid replacement alone is not sufficient to reverse shock, vasopressors (drugs causing vasoconstriction) and inotropic drugs (drugs improving cardiac contractility) may be administered. These drugs increase venous return through vasoconstriction of peripheral vessels; they also improve the heart's pumping ability by facilitating myocardial contractility and by dilating coronary arteries to increase perfusion of the myocardium.

The primary drugs used in the treatment of shock are listed in the Medications feature. Other drugs that may be administered to patients with shock include the following:

■ Diuretics to increase urine output after fluid replacement has been initiated

■ Sodium bicarbonate to treat acidosis

■ Calcium to replace calcium lost as a result of blood transfusions

■ Antidysrhythmic agents to stabilize heart rhythm

■ Broad-spectrum antibiotics to suppress organisms responsible for septic shock

■ Epinephrine, antihistamines, and inhaled beta$_2$-agonists to treat anaphylactic shock

■ Morphine to dilate veins and decrease anxiety.

Oxygen Therapy

Establishing and maintaining a patent airway and ensuring adequate oxygenation are critical nursing interventions in reversing shock. All patients in shock (even those with adequate respirations) should receive oxygen therapy (usually by mask or nasal cannula) to maintain the PaO_2 at greater than 80 mmHg during the first 4–6 hours of care. If a patient cannot maintain the PaO_2 at this level with unassisted respiration, ventilatory assistance may be necessary.

Fluid Replacement Therapy

The most effective treatment for the patient with hypovolemic shock is to administer IV fluids or blood. Fluids are also used to treat septic, neurogenic, and anaphylactic shock. However, the patient with cardiogenic shock may require either fluid replacement or restriction, depending on pulmonary artery pressure.

Various fluids may be administered alone or in combination as part of fluid replacement therapy in treating shock. Whole blood or blood products increase the oxygen-carrying capacity of the blood and thus increase oxygenation of cells. Fluid replacements, such as crystalloid and colloid solutions, increase circulating blood volume and tissue perfusion. Fluid replacements are administered in massive amounts through two large-bore peripheral lines or a central line.

Crystalloid Solutions

Crystalloid solutions contain dextrose or electrolytes dissolved in water; they are hypertonic, isotonic, or hypotonic.

Medications
Shock

CLASSIFICATION AND DRUG EXAMPLES	MECHANISMS OF ACTION	NURSING CONSIDERATIONS
Sympathomimetics **Vasoconstrictors (drugs causing vasoconstriction)** *Drug examples:* Norepinephrine (Levophed) Phenylephrine (Neo-Synephrine) Epinephrine **Inotropes (also called cardiotonics)** *Drug examples:* Dopamine (Intropin) (receptors are dose dependent) Dobutamine (Dobutrex) Isoproterenol (Isuprel)	Sympathomimetics mimic the fight-or-flight response of the SNS, selectively stimulating alpha-adrenergic and beta-adrenergic receptors. Many of these drugs have both vasopressor (vaso-constricting) effects and positive inotropic effects. Stimulation of alpha-adrenergic receptors results in vasoconstriction and increased systemic BP. Stimulation of beta-adrenergic receptors increases the force and rate of myocardial contraction. The physiologic effects of these drugs include improved perfusion and oxygenation of the heart, with increased SV and heart rate, and increased CO. In turn, increased CO increases tissue perfusion and oxygenation. The major disadvantage is that increases in SV and heart rate also increase the oxygen requirements of the myocardium. These drugs may be used during the early stages of shock, especially in types of shock characterized by vasodilation. Note that epinephrine is used primarily to treat anaphylactic shock.	■ Carefully monitor responses in the older adult, who may be especially sensitive to sympathomimetics and require lower doses. ■ Use the IV route only with continuous-infusion pumps. Carefully adjust the dose to accommodate the patient's cardiovascular status (as ordered by the physician or by written protocol). ■ Document lung sounds, vital signs, and hemodynamic parameters before starting the medication and then according to institutional policy (usually every 5–15 minutes). ■ Monitor for signs of dysrhythmias and hypertension. ■ Record and monitor urine output. Report output of less than 30 mL/hr. ■ Be aware that the sympathomimetics are incompatible with sodium bicarbonate or alkaline solutions. ■ When administering drugs that cause vasoconstriction, such as norepinephrine (Levophed), monitor the IV insertion site for infiltration. If infiltration does occur, stop the infusion, and notify the physician immediately. (Infiltration may cause ischemia and necrosis of tissue.) Health education for the patient and family: ■ Because these drugs mimic a physiologic reaction to stress, they may cause feelings of anxiety. ■ Close monitoring to adjust the dose will be carried out by qualified nurses using written protocols. ■ Report heart palpitations or chest pain immediately.
Vasodilators *Drug example:* Nitroglycerin (Nitrostat) Nitroprusside (Nipride)	Drugs that cause vasodilation act directly on smooth muscle, affecting both arterioles and veins. Peripheral resistance, CO, and pulmonary wedge pressure are all reduced as a result of the vasodilation. These effects decrease both the heart's oxygen need and pulmonary congestion. Vasodilators are used primarily in the treatment of cardiogenic shock and may be combined with a sympathomimetic (e.g., dopamine).	■ Protect these drugs from light by wrapping the IV bag in the package that is provided. ■ Mix only with 5% dextrose in water. ■ Infuse with an infusion pump, and use within 4 hours of reconstitution. ■ Do not add other medications to the solution. ■ Assess mental status, BP, and pulse before initiating medication. Thereafter, assess BP and pulse according to institutional policy (usually every 5 minutes initially, then every 15 minutes until stable, and then every hour). ■ Monitor the patient for confusion, dizziness, tachycardia, dysrhythmias, hypotension, and adventitious breath sounds. If they occur, report them immediately, and slow the infusion to a keep-open rate. ■ Monitor the patient receiving nitroprusside for signs of thiocyanate poisoning (nausea, disorientation, muscle spasms, and decreased or absent reflexes) if infusion lasts longer than 72 hours. ■ Keep the patient in bed with side rails up. Health education for the patient and family: ■ It is important to stay in bed and change positions slowly to avoid dizziness. ■ BP and pulse are taken frequently to assist in adjusting the dose of medication. ■ Headache is a common side effect.

(continued on next page)

Medications *(continued)*

CLASSIFICATION AND DRUG EXAMPLES	MECHANISMS OF ACTION	NURSING CONSIDERATIONS
Colloid Solutions (Plasma Expanders) *Drug examples:* Albumin 5% (Albuminar-5, Buminate 5%) Albumin 25% (Albuminar-25, Buminate 25%) Dextran 40 (Gentran 40) Dextran 70 (Gentran 70, Macrodex) Dextran 75 (Gentran 75) Hetastarch (Hespan [HES]) Plasma protein fraction (Plasmanate, Plasma-Plex, Plasmatein, Protenate)	These solutions are blood volume expanders and are used to treat hypovolemic shock caused by surgery, hemorrhage, burns, or other trauma. Albumin and plasma protein fraction are prepared from healthy blood donors. Dextran and hetastarch are synthetically prepared large molecules. The solutions promote circulatory volume and tissue perfusion by rapidly expanding plasma volume. Dextran solutions are used infrequently.	▪ Before infusion begins, establish a baseline of vital signs, lung sounds, heart sounds, and (if possible) CVP and pulmonary artery wedge pressure. ▪ Start administration of ordered IV fluids, using a large-gauge (18- or 19-gauge) infusion needle. ▪ Take and record vital signs as required by institutional policy (usually every 15–60 minutes) and patient status. ▪ Take and record intake and output every 1–2 hours. ▪ Monitor the patient for manifestations of CHF or pulmonary edema (dyspnea, cyanosis, cough, crackles, or wheezes). If these manifestations appear, stop the fluids, and notify the physician immediately. ▪ Monitor the patient for bleeding from new sites; an increase in BP may cause bleeding in severed vessels that did not bleed with decreased BP. ▪ Monitor the patient for manifestations of dehydration (dry lips; scant, dark-colored urine; loss of skin turgor). Increased IV fluids are usually ordered if the patient becomes dehydrated. ▪ Monitor the patient for manifestations of circulatory overload (JVD, increase in CVP, or increase in pulmonary artery wedge pressure). If these manifestations occur, slow the rate of infusion, and notify the physician. ▪ Monitor PT, partial thromboplastin time, and platelet counts. ▪ If administering dextran or plasma protein fraction, have epinephrine and antihistamines readily available for any manifestations of a hypersensitivity reaction (fever, chills, rash, headache, wheezing, or flushing). ▪ Maintain the patient on bedrest with side rails elevated. Health Education for the Patient and Family ▪ The solutions are given to replace lost serum protein, which helps maintain the volume of blood. ▪ Vital signs are taken frequently to ensure the patient's safety.

Hypertonic solutions include 3% saline. Isotonic solutions include normal saline (0.9%), lactated Ringer's solution, and Ringer's solution. Hypotonic solutions include one half normal saline (0.45%) and 5% dextrose in water.

Hypertonic crystalloid solutions pull fluid into the vascular space to promote excretion. Isotonic and hypotonic crystalloid solutions increase fluid volume in both the intravascular and the interstitial space. Of the total amount infused, only approximately 25% remains in the intravascular system; the remaining 75% moves into the interstitial space. As a consequence, fluid volume is only minimally expanded by infusion of crystalloid solutions, and the potential for peripheral edema is increased when they are used. However, lactated Ringer's solution (an electrolyte solution) and 0.9% saline are the fluids of choice in treating hypovolemic shock, especially during the emergency phase of care while blood is being typed and cross-matched. Large amounts of these solutions may be infused rapidly, increasing blood volume and tissue perfusion.

Colloid Solutions

Colloid solutions contain substances (colloids) that should not diffuse through capillary walls. Hence, colloids tend to remain in the vascular system and increase the osmotic pressure of the serum, causing fluid to move into the vascular compartment from the interstitial space. As a result, plasma volume expands. Colloid solutions used to treat shock include 5% albumin, 25% albumin, hetastarch, plasma protein fraction, and dextran (see the Medications feature).

Colloid products reduce platelet adhesiveness and have been associated with reductions in blood coagulation. Therefore, the patient's PT, INR, platelet count, and aPTT should be monitored when these solutions are administered.

Blood and Blood Products

If hypovolemic shock is caused by hemorrhage, infusion of blood and blood products may be indicated. The goal of blood administration is to keep the hematocrit at 30–35% and the hemoglobin level between 12.5 and 14.5 g/100 mL for adults. Available blood and blood products include packed RBCs, platelet concentrate, fresh-frozen plasma, and cryoprecipitate. Often, packed RBCs are given to provide hemoglobin concentration and are supplemented with crystalloids to maintain an adequate circulatory volume.

Lifespan Considerations

Regardless of age, shock occurs when circulation fails and tissue and organ perfusion is inadequate. However, special considerations must be taken for individuals in specific age groups.

Shock in Neonates and Infants

Shock is often the result of hypotension and hypovolemia. In neonates and infants, the total blood volume is very small (see **Box 16–22**)). Therefore, even a small amount of blood loss can be devastating. This effect is even more pronounced for low-birth-weight and very-low-birth-weight neonates. Monitoring BP in neonates, especially preterm neonates, is difficult because reference ranges for BP are not well studied (Gupta & Sinha, 2014). Although an accurate BP during shock is often obtained through invasive methods using an arterial catheter, this method may not be useful in preterm infants with very tiny arteries. Use of automated Doppler may be more useful in these infants.

Adequate perfusion depends on CO. In the neonate, heart rate contributes to CO to a greater degree than SV. Therefore, a prolonged very high (greater than 180 bpm) or very low (less than 80 bpm) heart rate can compromise CO, contributing to shock (Gupta & Sinha, 2014). In premature infants, presence of PDA or patent foramen ovale can disrupt blood flow and lead to hypotension and cardiac failure. Because oxygen delivery in neonates depends more on CO than BP, hypotension (which normally signals an early stage of shock in the adult) usually indicates a later stage of shock in neonates.

Risk factors for neonatal shock include umbilical cord accident, fetal or neonatal hemolysis or hemorrhage, maternal problems such as infection or hypotension, asphyxia, neonatal sepsis, and other complications. Shock is a major cause of neonatal morbidity and mortality. The prognosis depends on the cause of the shock and amount of damage done during the period of inadequate perfusion. Treatment depends on the type of shock, ranging from vasopressor administration to blood volume expansion. Supportive measures include securing the airway, providing oxygen, achieving IV access, and infusing colloid or crystalloid solutions or whole blood as appropriate. A fluid bolus of 20 mL/kg should be given, with additional fluids being administered as needed. Delayed treatment can lead to cerebral palsy, epilepsy, and mental retardation. Nurses should prepare parents of infants with shock for the potential for neurodevelopmental problems and the need for extensive follow-up care for complications (Gupta & Sinha, 2014).

Shock in Children

Over 35% of children seen in pediatric emergency departments are in shock, which increases their risk of mortality. Early use of pediatric advanced life support (PALS) decreases the likelihood of mortality in these children (see **Box 16–23**)). Children are at risk of the same types of shock as adults. Some common causes of hypovolemic shock in

---

Box 16–22
Blood Volume in Children

A child's total blood volume varies by weight. A child has approximately 80 mL of blood for every kilogram of body weight.

- **Newborn:** 3 kg × 80 mL = 240 mL (1 cup)
- **5-year-old:** 25 kg × 80 mL = 2000 mL (2 quarts)
- **13-year-old:** 50 kg × 80 mL = 4000 mL (1 gallon)

Box 16–23
Pediatric Advanced Life Support (PALS)

The AHA has developed guidelines for CPR and emergency cardiovascular care for pediatric patients, including patients in shock. Guidelines that may be appropriate for children in shock include the following (De Caen et al., 2015):

- One healthcare provider should immediately begin chest compressions. This requires only hands, which avoids the delay that occurs when equipment is needed. The rate should be at least 100 compressions per minute, and compression depth should be approximately 1.5 inches in infants and 2 inches in children. Allow complete recoil between each compression.
- One or two healthcare providers should begin ventilations with a bag and mask. The time needed for gathering equipment may delay the start of assisted ventilation compared to the time needed to start chest compressions. Be sure to select a mask of the correct size, providing a tight seal between the mask and face. Avoid delivering excessive ventilation, which may increase intrathoracic pressure and decrease venous return.
- One healthcare provider should obtain a monitor and defibrillator. If defibrillation is needed, it should be given with minimal interruption to chest compressions. Infant-sized paddles should be used for infants under 10 kg. Children should receive an initial dose of 2–4 J/kg.
- One healthcare provider should establish vascular access. Vascular access is needed for administration of fluids and medications. Access at multiple points may be needed depending on the solutions to be administered. For infants and children, intraosseous access may be more appropriate than IV access.
- One healthcare provider should calculate and prepare anticipated medications based on the child's weight. If weight is not known, the child's length may be an appropriate substitute. A body length measured with a tape that provides precalculated doses should be available for emergency situations. Special precautions should be taken for children who are obese; dosages based on body weight may be too high, but dosages based on height may be insufficient.

children include gastroenteritis, burns, diabetes insipidus, heat stroke, trauma, surgery, and intestinal obstruction. Children with gastroenteritis can lose up to 20% of their circulating volume within 1–2 hours, and clinical deterioration may be rapid if rehydration efforts are hindered by continued vomiting. Common causes of distributive shock in children include anaphylaxis, head injury, and sepsis. Cardiogenic shock may be caused by dysrhythmias, congenital heart disease, and cardiomyopathies. Obstructive shock may be caused by tension pneumothorax, PE, and acute cardiac tamponade (Pasman & Watson, 2015).

In children, the definition of septic shock is slightly different from that for adults. Septic shock in children involves sepsis plus cardiovascular dysfunction, but it does *not* have to include hypotension as it does in adults. The signs of cardiovascular dysfunction will depend on age-specific values for vital signs and WBC counts (Biban et al., 2012). Signs and symptoms of shock in children include altered mental status, tachypnea, tachycardia, reduced urine output, delayed capillary refill (less than 2 sec), temperature instability, and metabolic acidosis (Pasman & Watson, 2015). Hypotension is a late sign of shock in children, and it is correlated with a poor prognosis.

Treatment of shock in children involves aggressive fluid replacement, which can prevent the child from progressing to uncompensated or irreversible shock. Early fluid replacement, even in the absence of hypotension, provides the best chance for recovery for many pediatric patients. For septic shock, early treatment with antibiotics also reduces mortality in children (Biban et al., 2012). Supportive measures should be the same as for neonates and infants.

Shock in Pregnant Women

Causes of shock in pregnant women include trauma, antepartum hemorrhage (e.g., related to placenta previa, placental abruption, or uterine rupture), septic abortion, chorioamniotic and postpartum infection, valvular disease, PPCM, amniotic fluid embolism, and many others (Baldisseri & Sharma, 2014). Shock in a pregnant woman differs from shock in other adults because of the normal physiologic changes that take place during pregnancy and the concern during treatment for both the mother and fetus. Normal cardiovascular changes of pregnancy include an increase in blood volume, heart rate, SV, and CO and a decrease in peripheral resistance and BP. Shock can affect all of these measures, and because fetal perfusion and oxygenation depend on the mother's circulation, the fetus is also at risk for circulatory failure if the mother's circulation fails during shock.

Pregnant women in shock should be ventilated to maintain their oxygenation status; respiratory alkalosis should be avoided because it decreases uterine blood flow. If CPR is needed, the pregnant woman should be placed in a left lateral tilt position to avoid pressure on the vena cava.

The first-line vasoactive drug for pregnant women in shock is ephedrine. If the cause of shock is postpartum hemorrhage, oxytocin should be administered (Baldisseri & Sharma, 2014). If the cause of shock is sepsis, the nurse should monitor the patient for complications. Complications of severe sepsis and septic shock are associated with increased rates of preterm labor, fetal infection, and preterm

delivery. Onset of sepsis can be precipitous, with patients transitioning suddenly from an apparently healthy state to a state of septic shock, multiple organ dysfunction syndrome, or even death. Early detection improves the outcome and survivability in severe sepsis and septic shock in pregnancy, and it allows for prompt recognition of the source of infection and targeted therapy (Barton & Sibai, 2012).

While the mother is being treated for shock, the fetus should undergo continuous heart rate monitoring. Fetal bradycardia may be an indication of hypoxia. In addition, an ultrasound may be needed to assess fetal movement and reactivity as well as amniotic fluid volume. Fetal distress may necessitate delivery of the neonate. Therefore, emergency equipment should be available for cesarean section and neonatal care.

Shock in Older Adults

Older adults are more likely to progress to shock, have poorer outcomes from shock, and have a higher risk of mortality due to shock as compared to younger adults. With aging comes a relative decrease in sympathetic activity in relation to the cardiovascular system. Cardiac compliance also decreases with age. Older adults who have a heart attack, especially those with a history of heart failure, diabetes, or hypertension, have an increased risk of cardiogenic shock (Mayo Clinic, 2014k). In addition, many older adults experience secondary volume depletion because of chronic diuretic use or malnutrition. Older adults have a lower tolerance for hypovolemia than younger adults, so they should be aggressively treated with fluids during hypovolemic shock (Kolecki & Menckhoff, 2014). Older adults are also highly susceptible to septic shock, in part because they are at higher risk for infections such as pneumonia and urinary tract infections (Mayo Clinic, 2016d). This is especially true for older adults who are immunocompromised, such as patients undergoing radiation and chemotherapy treatments, and for older adults with multiple comorbidities (Englert & Ross, 2015).

The nurse should assess the older adult with shock for preshock functional status, including identifying any difficulties with ADLs and instrumental ADLs. Preshock functional status is often a predictor of the outcome for the older adult. In addition, a sudden decrease in the ability to perform ADLs may be an older adult's only sign of sepsis (Englert & Ross, 2015).

Aggressive fluid administration can cause problems in older adults with diastolic dysfunction, which is common in this age group (Nasa, Juneja, & Singh, 2012). Although aggressive fluid administration is often necessary, the nurse should carefully monitor the older patient for signs of fluid overload. In addition, common treatments such as dobutamine administration may have a lesser effect on an older patient or cause a dysrhythmia, especially if the patient has a history of CAD (Englert & Ross, 2015; Nasa et al., 2012). For patients with sepsis, antibiotic dosing should be based on age-related differences in pharmacokinetics and the patient's ability to metabolize and excrete the drug. However, an initial bolus dose and aggressive dosing should still be maintained, because inadequate antibiotic therapy is associated with poor outcomes in the older adult population (Nasa et al., 2012).

Mechanical ventilation of older adults during shock is associated with increased mortality. If mechanical ventilation is needed, a low tidal volume is preferred over traditional tidal volume. Mechanical ventilation is a life-sustaining treatment that may be against the patient's wishes, especially if the patient has a do-not-resuscitate (DNR) order or advance directive. The medical staff should talk to the patient or patient's family to determine the patient's wishes for potential end-of-life care, because the rate of mortality due to shock is relatively high in older adults. If the older adult does survive, he or she will most likely be discharged to a nursing home or other care facility (Nasa et al., 2012).

NURSING PROCESS

Nursing care for the patient with shock often requires rapid assessment and reaction to subtle symptoms in order to prevent a downward cascade of events. Anticipating the potential for shock can promote rapid intervention when symptoms are caught early.

Assessment

Nursing assessments are critical in preventing shock. The exact nature of the assessment depends on the type of shock the patient is experiencing:

- *Hypovolemic shock.* Patients who have undergone surgery, have sustained multiple traumatic injuries, or have been seriously burned are most likely to develop hypovolemic shock. Monitoring fluid status is essential to prevent shock in these patients and includes daily assessments of weight, fluid intake by all routes, measurable fluid loss (e.g., urine, vomitus, wound drainage, gastric drainage, chest tube drainage), and fluid loss that must be estimated, such as fluid lost via profuse perspiration and wound drainage. Assessment for the critically ill patient is ongoing and includes fluid balance, hemodynamic values, and vital signs.
- *Cardiogenic shock.* Patients with left anterior wall MIs are at risk for developing cardiogenic shock. Nursing care to prevent development of cardiogenic shock focuses on maintaining or improving myocardial oxygen supply by providing immediate pain relief, maintaining rest, and administering supplemental oxygen.
- *Neurogenic shock.* The risk of neurogenic shock is increased in patients who have spinal cord injuries and those who have received spinal anesthesia. Preventive nursing care includes maintaining immobility of the patient with spinal cord trauma and elevating the head of the bed 15–20 degrees following spinal anesthesia. Elevations of more than 20 degrees, however, can potentiate headaches following spinal anesthesia and should be avoided.
- *Anaphylactic shock.* The nurse can prevent anaphylactic shock by collecting information about the patient's allergies and drug reactions during the health history, noting these allergies clearly on all documents, and placing a special armband on the patient. Careful and frequent assessments during blood administration may prevent serious reactions to blood or blood products.
- *Septic shock.* Patients who are hospitalized, debilitated, or chronically ill, and those who have undergone invasive procedures or tube insertions are at high risk for septic shock. Nursing care to prevent septic shock includes careful and consistent hand hygiene, use of aseptic techniques for procedures (e.g., catheterization, suctioning, changing dressings, starting and maintaining IV fluids or medications), and monitoring for local and systemic manifestations (e.g., WBC, differential counts) of infection. Reduction of unnecessary catheter and central line use, along with early removal of these devices, also decreases the likelihood of septic shock and reflects recommendations made in the Joint Commission's 2016 National Patient Safety Goals for Hospitals (see the module on Safety).

Diagnosis

Different types and causes of shock will determine which nursing diagnoses are most appropriate. Priority nursing diagnoses that may be appropriate for patients with any type of shock include the following:

- *Cardiac Output, Decreased*
- *Tissue Perfusion, Risk for Ineffective Cerebral*
- *Tissue Perfusion, Risk for Decreased Cardiac*
- *Anxiety.*

(NANDA-I © 2014)

Planning

Goals of nursing care for patients with shock may include the following:

- The patient's airway, breathing, and circulation will be maintained.
- The patient's perfusion will be maintained adequately to meet the body's needs.
- The patient will understand all procedures.
- The patient will verbalize feelings to reduce anxiety.
- The patient's cardiac workload will be reduced.

Implementation

Because nurses in the emergency department and ICU actively help resuscitate patients in hypovolemic shock, they frequently have guidelines or protocols for nursing actions such as:

- Assisting in assessing and establishing IV access for the patient
- Calculating the correct amount of and preparing IV fluid to be administered
- Employing IV push or a pressure bag to ensure rapid fluid administration
- Monitoring the patient's physiologic response to the fluid bolus over the course of 5 minutes
- Preparing a second and third fluid bolus.

Because hypothermia may hinder the effectiveness of treatment, the nurse should use warmed IV fluids for resuscitation.

When administering packed RBCs, the nurse should verify that the correct blood has been obtained for the patient.

To prevent clotting during blood administration, the nurse must change the IV fluid to normal saline. The nurse should also carefully assess the patient for a transfusion reaction during administration, monitoring the patient's physiologic circulatory responses for signs of improvement or deterioration in status. If any deterioration occurs, the nurse must notify the physician immediately.

Preserve Cardiac Output

Decreased CO is the primary problem for patients with shock. Although much of the care related to this diagnosis is collaborative, many independent nursing interventions are critical in the care of patients with shock. These include the following:

- Assess and monitor cardiovascular function via BP, heart rate and rhythm, pulse oximetry, peripheral pulses, and hemodynamic monitoring of arterial pressures, pulmonary artery pressures, and CVPs.

- Conduct a baseline assessment to establish the stage of shock. If palpable peripheral pulses and audible (to auscultation) BP are lost, it is essential to insert central arterial, venous, and pulmonary artery catheters to accurately establish progression of shock and evaluate the patient's response to therapy.

- Measure and record the patient's intake and output (total output and urinary output) hourly. A decrease in circulating blood volume with hypotension and the effect of the compensatory mechanisms associated with shock can cause renal failure. Urinary output of less than 30 mL/hr in an acutely ill adult indicates reduced renal blood flow.

- Monitor the patient's bowel sounds, abdominal distention, and abdominal pain. Decreased splanchnic blood flow reduces bowel motility and peristalsis; paralytic ileus may result.

- Monitor the patient for sudden, sharp chest pain and for dyspnea, cyanosis, anxiety, and restlessness. Hemoconcentration and increased platelet aggregation may result in pulmonary emboli.

- Maintain bedrest, and provide (to the extent possible) a calm, quiet environment. Place the patient in a supine position with the legs elevated approximately 20 degrees, trunk flat, and head and shoulders elevated higher than the chest (approximately 10 degrees) (see **Figure 16–57 »**). Limiting activity and ensuring rest decrease the heart's

workload. The supine position with legs elevated increases venous return; however, this position should not be used for patients with cardiogenic shock. The Trendelenburg position is no longer recommended, because it causes the abdominal organs to press against the diaphragm (limiting respirations), decreases filling of the coronary arteries, and initiates aortic and carotid sinus reflexes.

Promote Tissue Perfusion

As shock progresses, diminished tissue perfusion causes ischemia and hypoxia of major organ systems. As shock worsens, blood flow and oxygenation of the lungs, heart, and brain are also impaired. Hypoxia and ischemia result from decreased tissue perfusion in the kidneys, brain, heart, lungs, and gastrointestinal tract and the periphery. The following nursing interventions address tissue perfusion:

- Monitor the patient's skin color, temperature, turgor, and moisture. Decreased tissue perfusion is evidenced by the skin becoming pale, cool, and moist; as hemoglobin concentrations decrease, cyanosis occurs.

- Monitor the patient's cardiopulmonary function by regularly assessing BP (by auscultation or hemodynamic monitoring), rate and depth of respirations, lung sounds, pulse oximetry, JVD, CVP measurements, and peripheral pulses (brachial, radial, dorsalis pedis, and posterior tibial), including presence, equality, rate, rhythm, and quality. (If unable to palpate pulses, use a device such as a Doppler ultrasound flowmeter to assess peripheral arterial blood flow.) Baseline vital signs are necessary to determine trends in subsequent findings. As shock progresses, BP decreases, and the pulse becomes rapid, weak, and thready. As perfusion of the lungs decreases, crackles, wheezes, and dyspnea are commonly assessed. Capillary refill is prolonged, and peripheral pulses are weak or nonpalpable. Neck veins that cannot be seen when the patient is in the supine position indicate decreased intravascular volume. CVP is an accurate means of determining fluid status in the patient with shock; the findings will be low (5–15 cm H_2O or 2–6 mm Hg is normal) in hypovolemic shock because of the decreased blood volume.

- Monitor the patient's body temperature. An elevated body temperature increases metabolic demands, depleting energy reserves. It also increases myocardial oxygen demand and may place the patient with previous cardiac problems at even greater risk for hypoperfusion.

- Monitor the patient's urinary output per indwelling urinary catheter hourly, using a urometer. Urine output is a reliable indicator of renal perfusion.

- Assess the patient's mental status and LOC. The appropriateness of the patient's behavior and responses reflects the adequacy of cerebral circulation. Restlessness and anxiety are common in early shock; during later stages, the patient may become lethargic and progress to a comatose state. Altered LOCs are the result of both cerebral hypoxia and the effects of acidosis on brain cells.

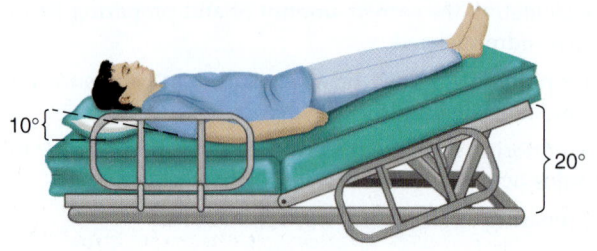

Figure 16–57 » The patient in shock should be positioned with the lower extremities elevated approximately 20 degrees (knees straight), and the head elevated about 10 degrees.

Relieve Anxiety

Many patients with hypovolemic shock have experienced some form of major trauma and may have multiple life-threatening injuries. Following on-the-scene treatment, the patient is usually admitted to the healthcare setting through the emergency department. Surgery may be required to treat injuries, followed by care in a critical care unit. Throughout this sequence of events, treatment is invasive, and contact with family is minimal. Common patient and family responses to these situations of uncertainty, instability, and change include anxiety, fear, and powerlessness. These responses are affected by age, developmental level, cultural and ethnic background, experience with illness and the healthcare system, and availability of support systems. The nurse can help relieve the patient's anxiety by doing the following:

- Assess the cause(s) of the anxiety, and manipulate the environment to provide periods of rest. Reducing stimuli that cause anxiety is calming and facilitates rest, which is necessary for the patient at risk for bleeding.
- Administer pain medications as prescribed. Pain precipitates and/or aggravates anxiety.
- Provide interventions to increase the patient's comfort and reduce restlessness. Examples of such interventions include:
  - Maintain a clean environment. Unfamiliar sounds, sights, and odors can increase anxiety.
  - Provide skin and oral care. Damp skin or a dry mouth increases discomfort.
  - Monitor the effectiveness of ventilation or oxygen therapy. Inadequate gas exchange with a decrease in oxygen or an increase in carbon dioxide in the blood may cause the patient to experience a "feeling of doom."
  - Eliminate all nonessential activities. Activity increases the body's need for oxygen.
  - Remain with the patient during procedures. Listening and touch provide support in an environment in which the patient often feels alone and abandoned.
  - Speak slowly and calmly, using short sentences and touch as appropriate. Severe anxiety interferes with the ability to understand others and to respond appropriately.
- Provide support for the patient and family:
  - Provide time, space, and privacy for family members.
  - Allow family members access to the patient when feasible.
  - Encourage the patient to express feelings and concerns. Provide anticipatory guidance to prepare for recovery or death and to support realistic hope.
  - Acknowledge the beliefs, values, and expectations of the patient and family.

Allowing the family access to the patient reduces anxiety and gives both the patient and the family some feeling of control. If the patient's prognosis is poor, access and involvement allow the family to begin the grieving process.

Patient Teaching
Care of the Family of a Patient in Shock

Both the patient and patient's family may experience significant anxiety throughout the process of treating the patient for shock. This is a life-threatening condition that occurs unexpectedly, and the patient and family are often unprepared to cope with the situation. Therefore, the nurse should provide teaching about the patient's situation and condition, as well as provide information about resources the patient and family can use. For example, the nurse can:

- Provide information about pastoral care that is available to the patient and family. Spiritual support is especially important if the patient's condition deteriorates and death is imminent.
- Provide information about temporary housing and meals that may be available to the family while their loved one is in the hospital for an extended period.
- Teach the family how to reduce stimulation so the patient can get adequate rest and reduce energy consumption. This may include asking only one or two family members to be present with the patient at any one time. The nurse should teach the visiting family to remain quiet during the visit.
- Teach the family how to provide simple care for the patient, including appropriate and timely position changes, administration of ice chips, and skin care.
- Teach the family signs and symptoms that require notification of the nursing staff, including changes in LOC, shortness of breath, increase in pain, and other visible signs of distress.

If recovery is expected, contact provides the patient and family with a feeling of hope. Supporting the patient and family facilitates concrete problem solving, promotes acceptance of the illness and its implications, and helps them begin to establish ways of managing the illness experience.

Evaluation

Expected nursing care outcomes for patients with shock may include the following:

- The patient maintains adequate airway and oxygenation.
- The patient maintains adequate urinary output.
- The patient does not progress to uncompensated shock.
- The family adequately copes with the stress of the patient's condition.

If evaluation indicates that the patient's condition has worsened, the nurse will need to review the care plan and implement additional nursing interventions to ensure that the patient maintains adequate oxygenation and perfusion. This may involve placing the patient on mechanical ventilation per the provider's orders, administering prescribed medications or blood components, reviewing laboratory results, and providing supportive care for both the patient and family.

Nursing Care Plan
A Patient with Shock

Huang Mei Lan is a 43-year-old unmarried woman who lives alone in a major West Coast city. Ms. Huang came to America 15 years ago from China, and she speaks English well. Her family still lives in China. She worked in a neighborhood sewing shop until 3 years ago, when she was diagnosed with breast cancer. Her treatment included mastectomy of the affected breast and follow-up chemotherapy.

ASSESSMENT

Last month, Ms. Huang experienced a recurrence of cancer in the liver. Surgery to remove the tumor and a lobe of the liver was performed, and chemotherapy is planned. Ms. Huang has a central line, a urinary catheter, and a midline abdominal surgical incision. She is underweight, weak, and depressed.

Ms. Huang's primary nurse enters her room early in the morning to make an initial assessment and finds Ms. Huang huddled in the middle of the bed. Ms. Huang reports that she feels cold. The nurse finds Ms. Huang's dressing saturated with bright red blood. She rolls Ms. Huang onto her side and finds the bed filled with blood. The nurse measures the size of the blood stain and records it (18 × 38 in). Her vital signs are T 99.2°F; P 110 bpm; R 30/min; BP 106/66 mmHg. Her pulse is weak and regular. Her skin is cool, dry, and pale with poor turgor. She is alert and oriented but restless and appears anxious. Ms. Huang states she is nauseated and suddenly begins vomiting and is incontinent of liquid stool. Laboratory data indicate leukocytosis; respiratory alkalosis; and reduced respirations, hemoglobin, and hematocrit.

Plasma expanders in the form of albumin are administered while a type and crossmatch for 4 units of blood are performed. The IV fluid rate is increased, and the patient's vital signs are monitored. Ms. Huang is taken back to surgery to repair the source of the bleeding and loses an additional 2 pints of blood. She receives 3 units of blood in the operative suite and returns to the unit with the fourth unit running. The physician's orders indicate that dopamine is to be started if Ms. Huang's BP falls below 90/60 mmHg following administration of the fourth unit.

Despite treatment, Ms. Huang's condition worsens. Her BP continues to drop, her skin becomes cool and cyanotic, and she begins to have periods of disorientation. She is transferred to the critical care unit. As she is being prepared for transfer, she begins to cry and asks, "Am I going to die?"

DIAGNOSES

- *Deficient Fluid Volume* related to bleeding, vomiting, diarrhea, and shift of intravascular volume to interstitial spaces
- *Ineffective Breathing Pattern* related to rapid respirations and progression of hypovolemic shock
- *Risk for Ineffective Cerebral Tissue Perfusion* related to progression of hypovolemic shock with decreased CO, hypotension, and massive vasodilation
- *Anxiety* related to hypoxia, serious health status, and transfer to critical care unit
- *Fear* related to worsening of health status and possible death

(NANDA-I © 2014)

PLANNING

Goals of care include the following:
- Maintain adequate oxygenation.
- Maintain adequate circulating blood volume.
- Promote breathing to maintain acid–base within acceptable parameters.
- Promote stable hemodynamic status.
- Assist the patient to verbalize increased ability to cope with stressors.

IMPLEMENTATION

- Continuously monitor oxygenation status, including pulse oximetry, skin color, and breathing pattern, and respiratory status, including respiratory rate, rhythm, and breath sounds.
- Monitor neurologic status, including mental status and LOC.
- Continuously monitor cardiovascular status, including arterial BP; rate, rhythm, and quality of pulses; central venous pressure; pulmonary artery pressure; and CO.
- Monitor results of ABGs, blood counts, clotting times, and platelet counts.
- Monitor urinary output hourly, reporting any output of less than 30 mL/hr.
- Administer blood and IV fluids as ordered.
- Explain procedures, and provide comfort measures (e.g., oral care, skin care, turning, positioning).
- Maintain a calm, supportive manner when interacting with the patient, and respond to her call signal as soon as possible.

EVALUATION

After administration of the fourth unit of blood, Ms. Huang's BP has stabilized above the defined parameters. Her urine output is less than 30 mL/hr for 3 hours, and fluid administration is increased until her urine output improves and hemodynamic status stabilizes. She remains in the critical care area for 2 days and is then transferred back to the oncology unit.

CRITICAL THINKING

1. Vasopressors may be used in the treatment of shock. Explain the rationale for their use.
2. While monitoring Ms. Huang's ABGs, the nurse notes that her PaO_2 is less than 60 mmHg and her $PaCO_2$ is greater than 50 mmHg. What do these findings indicate, and why have they occurred?
3. Ms. Huang has been given large amounts of colloids intravenously. Hemodynamic monitoring indicates higher-than-normal central venous pressure and pulmonary artery pressure. What do these findings indicate? What physical assessments would you make to confirm the changes?

REVIEW Shock

RELATE Link the Concepts and Exemplars

Linking the exemplar of shock with the concept of spirituality:

1. You are caring for a pediatric patient in hypovolemic shock following a bicycle crash. The family members refuse blood, explaining that it is against their religious beliefs. How will you respond?

2. What options for treatment might be considered for this child that do not conflict with the family's religious beliefs?

Linking the exemplar of shock with the concept of fluids and electrolytes:

3. Contrast administration of IV fluids for the patient in hypovolemic shock versus the patient in cardiogenic shock.

4. Contrast administration of colloids versus crystalloids in treating the patient with hypovolemic shock.

READY Go to Volume 3: Clinical Nursing Skills

REFER Go to Pearson MyLab Nursing and eText

- Additional review materials

REFLECT Apply Your Knowledge

Stacie Horton is a 15-year-old patient who required a heart transplant 5 years ago to repair damage done by a viral illness. She is compliant with her medication regimen and adheres to the prescribed diet. She lives with her parents and older brother. Although she appreciates the watchfulness of her parents, Stacie sometimes wishes her family would not hover over her as much as they do. Stacie is captain of the cheerleading squad at her school, where she is also an honor student.

Stacie is in class and begins to feel faint and nauseated. Her skin is cold and clammy, and her color is slightly cyanotic. Her respirations are 30/min, and her pulse is weak and thready at a rate of 124 bpm. Knowing her history, the teacher alerts the school nurse, who immediately calls 9-1-1 and Stacie's family.

1. As the school nurse, what interventions will you initiate for Stacie until the paramedics arrive?

2. If you were the nurse admitting Stacie in the emergency department, what would your priority assessment include?

3. When Stacie's parents arrive, what family teaching will you initiate?

» Exemplar 16.M
Stroke

Exemplar Learning Outcomes

16.M Analyze stroke as it relates to perfusion.

- Differentiate types of stroke.
- Describe the pathophysiology of each type of stroke.
- Describe the etiology of each type of stroke.
- Compare the risk factors and prevention of stroke.
- Identify the clinical manifestations of stroke.
- Summarize diagnostic tests and therapies used by interprofessional teams in the collaborative care of an individual with stroke.
- Differentiate care of patients with stroke across the lifespan.
- Apply the nursing process in providing culturally competent care to an individual with stroke.

Exemplar Key Terms

Agnosia, *1329*
Aneurysm, *1327*
Aphasia, *1330*
Apraxia, *1329*
Arterial ischemic stroke, *1334*
Contralateral deficit, *1326*
Dysphagia, *1338*
Flaccidity, *1330*
Hemianopia, *1329*
Hemiparesis, *1330*
Hemiplegia, *1330*
Neglect syndrome, *1329*
Penumbra, *1326*
Proprioception, *1328*
Sinovenous thrombosis, *1334*
Spasticity, *1330*
Stroke, *1325*
Transient ischemic attack (TIA), *1326*

Overview

A **stroke** (also known as a *cerebrovascular accident* or *brain attack*) is a condition in which neurologic deficits result from a sudden decrease in blood flow to a localized area of the brain. Strokes may be *ischemic,* occurring when the blood supply to a part of the brain is suddenly interrupted by a thrombus (blood clot), embolus (foreign matter traveling through the circulation), or stenosis (narrowing); or they may be *hemorrhagic,* occurring when a blood vessel breaks open and spills blood into spaces surrounding neurons. The neurologic deficits caused by ischemia and the resultant necrosis of brain cells vary according to the area of the brain involved, the size of the affected area, and the length of time blood flow is decreased or stopped. A major loss of blood supply to the brain can cause severe disability or death. When the duration of decreased blood flow is short and the anatomical area involved is small, the individual may not be aware that any damage has occurred.

On average, someone in the United States has a stroke every 40 seconds, and someone dies of a stroke every 4 minutes. Stroke is the fourth leading cause of death and disability in North America, where approximately 795,000 individuals experience a new or recurrent stroke each year. Of those,

160,000 die, and many who survive are left with some type of functional impairment. Although strokes occur in every age group, the highest incidence occurs in individuals over 65 years of age; indeed, only 28% of strokes occur in individuals under age 65. Strokes occur more frequently in men than in women, although the risk of stroke may be greater in women during pregnancy and for the first 6 weeks postpartum (American Stroke Association, 2015).

Pathophysiology and Etiology

The brain, which makes up only 2% of an adult's total body weight, receives approximately 20% of the CO each minute (approximately 750 mL) and accounts for 20% of the body's oxygen consumption. Cerebral blood flow, especially in the deep cerebral vessels, is largely self-regulated by the brain to meet metabolic needs. This self-regulation (also called autoregulation) allows the brain to maintain a constant blood flow despite changes in systemic BP. However, autoregulation is not effective when systemic BP falls below 50 mmHg or rises above 160 mmHg. In the latter case, the increased systemic pressure (as occurs in hypertension) causes an increase in cerebral blood flow with resultant overdistention of cerebral vessels. Cerebral blood flow also increases in response to increased carbon dioxide concentrations, increased hydrogen ion concentrations, and decreased oxygen concentrations.

When blood flow and oxygenation to cerebral neurons are decreased or interrupted, pathophysiologic changes at the cellular level take place within 4–5 minutes. Cellular metabolism ceases as glucose, glycogen, and ATP are depleted and the sodium–potassium pump fails. Cells swell as sodium draws water into them. Cerebral blood vessel walls also swell, further decreasing blood flow. Even if circulation is restored, vasospasm and increased blood viscosity can continue to impede blood flow. Severe or prolonged ischemia leads to cellular death. A central core of dead or dying cells is surrounded by a band of minimally perfused cells, called the **penumbra**. Although cells in the penumbra have impaired metabolic activity, their structural integrity is maintained. The survival of these cells depends on the timely return of adequate circulation, the volume of toxic products released by adjacent dying cells, the degree of cerebral edema, and alterations in local blood flow (Jauch & Stettler, 2015).

A stroke is characterized by gradual or rapid onset of neurologic deficits caused by compromised cerebral blood flow. The neurologic deficits that occur as a result of stroke can often be used to identify the affected region of the brain. Because the motor pathways cross at the junction of the medulla and spinal cord (decussation), strokes lead to loss or impairment of sensorimotor functions on the side of the body opposite the side of the brain that is damaged. Because of this effect, known as a **contralateral deficit**, a stroke in the right hemisphere of the brain is manifested by deficits in the left side of the body, and a stroke in the left hemisphere is manifested by deficits in the right side of the body.

Ischemic Stroke

As previously mentioned, ischemic strokes result from blockage and/or stenosis of a cerebral artery, decreasing or stopping blood flow and ultimately causing a brain infarction. The blockage may result from a blood clot (either as a thrombus or an embolus) or from stenosis of a vessel caused by plaque buildup. Plaque may cause stenosis in large blood vessels (called large vessel disease) or small blood vessels (called small vessel disease). Large vessel disease usually is the result of thrombi. Small vessel strokes, called *lacunar infarcts,* are small to very small infarcts in the deep, noncortical areas of the brain or the brainstem. Ischemic strokes are classified as transient, thrombotic, or embolic.

Transient Ischemic Attack

A **transient ischemic attack (TIA)**, sometimes called a *ministroke*, is a brief period of localized cerebral ischemia that causes neurologic deficits lasting for less than 24 hours (Hickey, 2013). The deficits may be present for only minutes or may last for hours. TIAs are often warning signals of an ischemic thrombotic stroke. One or many TIAs may precede a stroke, with the time between the TIA and a stroke ranging from hours to months. Of the 50,000 Americans who have a TIA each year, approximately one third will have an acute stroke sometime in the future (National Institute of Neurological Disorders and Stroke [NINDS], 2015).

The etiology of TIA includes inflammatory artery disorders, sickle cell disease, atherosclerotic changes in cerebral blood vessels, thrombosis, and emboli. Neurologic manifestations of a TIA vary according to the location and size of the cerebral vessel involved. Manifestations have sudden onset and often disappear within minutes or hours. Commonly occurring deficits include contralateral numbness or weakness of the leg, hand, forearm, and corner of the mouth (because of middle cerebral artery involvement); aphasia (because of ischemia of the left hemisphere); and visual disturbances, such as blurring (because of involvement of the posterior cerebral artery). The patient may also experience a visual disturbance called amaurosis fugax (a fleeting blindness of one eye, described as a shade coming down over vision with the affected eye).

Thrombotic Stroke

A thrombotic stroke is caused by occlusion of a large cerebral vessel by a thrombus (blood clot). Thrombotic strokes most often occur in older individuals who are resting or sleeping. The BP is lower during sleep, so there is less pressure to push the blood through an already narrowed arterial lumen, and ischemia may result.

Thrombi tend to form in large arteries that bifurcate and have narrowed lumens as a result of atherosclerotic plaque. The plaque involves the intima of the arteries, causing the internal elastic lamina to become thin and frayed with exposure of underlying connective tissue. This structural change causes platelets to adhere to the rough surface and release the molecule adenosine diphosphate (ADP). ADP initiates the clotting sequence, and the thrombus forms. A thrombus may remain in place and continue to enlarge, completely occluding the lumen of the vessel, or part of it may break off and become an embolus.

The most common locations for thrombi are the internal carotid artery, the vertebral arteries, and the junction of the vertebral and basilar arteries. Thrombotic strokes affecting the smaller cerebral vessels are called lacunar strokes, because the infarcted areas slough off, leaving a small cavity or "lake" in the brain tissue. A thrombotic stroke usually affects only one region of the brain, supplied by a single cerebral artery.

A thrombotic stroke occurs rapidly but progresses slowly. It often begins with a TIA and continues to worsen over 1–2 days; the condition is called a stroke-in-evolution. When maximum neurologic deficit has been reached, usually in 3 days, the condition is called a completed stroke. At that time, the damaged area of brain tissue is edematous and necrotic.

Embolic Stroke

An embolic stroke occurs when a blood clot or clump of matter traveling through the cerebral blood vessels becomes lodged in a vessel that is too narrow to permit further movement. The area of the brain supplied by the blocked vessel becomes ischemic. The most frequent sites of cerebral emboli are at bifurcations of vessels, particularly those of the carotid and middle cerebral arteries. This type of stroke is typically seen in patients who are younger than those who experience thrombotic strokes. Embolic stroke occurs when the patient is awake and active.

Many embolic strokes originate from a thrombus in the left chambers of the heart, formed during atrial fibrillation. These are referred to as cardiogenic embolic strokes. Emboli result when parts of the thrombus break off and are carried through the arterial system to the brain. Cerebral emboli may also be the result of carotid artery atherosclerotic plaque, bacterial endocarditis, recent MI, rheumatic heart disease, and ventricular aneurysm.

An embolic stroke has sudden onset and causes immediate deficits. If the embolus breaks into smaller fragments and is absorbed by the body, manifestations will disappear in a few hours to a few days. If the embolus is not absorbed, manifestations will persist. Even if the embolus is absorbed, the vessel wall where the embolus lodges may be weakened, increasing the potential for cerebral hemorrhage.

Hemorrhagic Stroke

A hemorrhagic stroke, or intracranial hemorrhage, occurs when a cerebral blood vessel ruptures. It occurs most often in individuals with a sustained increase in systolic–diastolic BP. It can also occur due to an **aneurysm** (a bulging weak area in the wall of an artery) that ruptures, releasing blood into the brain.

There are two types of hemorrhagic strokes: intracerebral hemorrhage and subarachnoid hemorrhage. Intracerebral hemorrhage results from bleeding within the brain. Subarachnoid hemorrhage results from bleeding into the spaces around the brain. As a result of the blood vessel rupture, blood enters the brain tissue, the cerebral ventricles, or the subarachnoid space, compressing adjacent tissues and causing blood vessel spasm and cerebral edema. Blood in the ventricles or subarachnoid space irritates the meninges and brain tissue, causing an inflammatory reaction and impairing absorption and circulation of cerebrospinal fluid (CSF).

A hemorrhagic stroke usually occurs suddenly, often when the affected individual is engaged in activity. Although hypertension is the most common cause, a variety of factors may contribute to a hemorrhagic stroke, including rupture of a plaque-encrusted artery wall; a ruptured intracranial aneurysm; trauma; erosion of blood vessels by tumors; arteriovenous malformations; anticoagulant therapy; and blood disorders. Hemorrhagic stroke is most commonly linked with poor outcomes.

The onset of manifestations from a hemorrhagic stroke is rapid. Manifestations depend on the location of the hemorrhage but may include vomiting, headache, seizures, hemiplegia, and loss of consciousness. Pressure on the brain tissue from increased ICP may cause coma and death.

Risk Factors

Specific stroke risk factors include the following:

- **Hypertension.** Hypertension is the leading cause of stroke (AHA, 2015q). Increased systolic and diastolic BP are associated with damage to all blood vessels, including the cerebral vessels. Individuals with hypertension have a 4–6 times greater risk for stroke than individuals without hypertension.

- **Heart disease.** Atrial fibrillation increases the risk for stroke, because when the heart's upper chambers do not beat effectively, pooling or clotting of the blood may result. If a clot dislodges into the bloodstream and travels to the brain, a stroke can occur. Heart failure, dilated cardiomyopathy, heart valve disease, and some types of congenital heart defects also increase the risk of stroke.

- **Diabetes mellitus.** Diabetes leads to vascular changes in both the systemic and cerebral circulation. Patients with diabetes often have high BP and high blood cholesterol and are overweight, all factors that raise the risk for stroke.

- **Sleep apnea.** Considered a major risk for stroke, sleep apnea increases BP and causes decreased oxygen and increased carbon dioxide in the blood.

- **Blood cholesterol levels.** Increased blood cholesterol levels contribute to the risk of atherosclerosis, including in arteries in the cerebral circulation.

- **Smoking.** Cigarette smoking doubles an individual's risk for ischemic stroke and increases the risk for cerebral hemorrhage. The use of hormonal contraceptives combined with smoking greatly increases the risk for stroke.

- **Sickle cell disease.** Changes in the shape of the RBCs increase blood viscosity and produce erythrocyte clumps that may occlude small cerebral vessels.

- **Substance abuse.** The injection of unpurified substances increases the risk for a stroke, and abuse of certain drugs can decrease cerebral blood flow and increase the risk for intracranial hemorrhage. Substances associated with strokes include marijuana, anabolic steroids, heroin, amphetamines, and cocaine.

- **Living in the "stroke belt."** Individuals who live in the Southeastern United States have the highest stroke mortality rate in the country. The reason for this has not been identified.

- **Ethnicity.** African Americans have almost twice the number of first-ever strokes compared to Caucasians. Hispanic Americans have an increased incidence of intracerebral hemorrhage, subarachnoid hemorrhage, ischemic stroke, TIA, and TIA at a younger age as compared to non-Hispanic Whites (CDC, 2015l).

Other risk factors are family history of stroke, obesity, sedentary lifestyle, recent viral and bacterial infections, and previous TIAs. Risk factors specific to women include hormonal contraceptive use, pregnancy, childbirth, menopause, migraine headaches with aura, autoimmune disorders (e.g., diabetes, lupus), and clotting disorders.

The risk for a recurrent stroke is 25–35% within the individual's lifetime (National Stroke Association, 2016). The risk is highest immediately after a stroke, then decreases with time.

Prevention

Preventing stroke involves the same measures as preventing or managing heart disease: controlling BP to prevent or reduce hypertension, lowering dietary intake of cholesterol and saturated fats, not smoking, controlling diabetes, maintaining a healthy weight, and exercising regularly. Health promotion activities focus on stroke prevention, especially for individuals with known risk factors. Eating a fruit- and vegetable-rich diet also helps. Patients who have already had an ischemic stroke may be prescribed antiplatelet drugs and anticoagulants to help prevent another stroke (Mayo Clinic, 2015i). Patients should take medicine exactly as prescribed for all conditions that increase the risk of stroke, such as heart disease, high cholesterol, hypertension, or diabetes (CDC, 2014e).

The National Stroke Association recommends the following three-step guidelines for preventing a stroke (National Stroke Association, n.d.a):

1. Review the risk factors to identify personal risk for stroke.
2. Reduce these risk factors through lifestyle changes and medication.
3. Recognize the signs and symptoms of stroke by memorizing **FAST.**
   Face: Is there facial drooping?
   Arm: Is there arm weakness?
   Speech: Is speech slurred?
   Time: Call 9-1-1 if these are present.

It is also vital to increase public awareness of the signs of TIA and stroke, as well as the need to call 9-1-1 or seek care immediately if any of the following warning signs occur:

- Sudden weakness or numbness of the face, arm, or leg, especially on one side of the body
- Sudden confusion, difficulty speaking, or difficulty understanding speech
- Sudden trouble walking, dizziness, or loss of coordination
- Sudden difficulty with vision in one or both eyes
- Sudden severe headache without a cause.

Clinical Manifestations

Manifestations of stroke vary according to the cerebral artery involved and the area of the brain affected. Women with stroke are more likely to report nontraditional manifestations (e.g., disorientation, confusion, loss of consciousness) than men. Manifestations are sudden in onset, focal, and

---

Box 16–24
Manifestations of Stroke by Involved Cerebral Vessel

Internal Carotid Artery
- Contralateral paralysis of the arm, leg, and face
- Contralateral sensory deficits of the arm, leg, and face
- Aphasia (if the dominant hemisphere is involved)
- Apraxia, agnosia, and/or unilateral neglect (if the nondominant hemisphere is involved)
- Homonymous hemianopia

Middle Cerebral Artery
- Drowsiness, stupor, coma
- Contralateral hemiplegia of the arm and face
- Contralateral sensory deficits of the arm and face
- Global aphasia (if the dominant hemisphere is involved)
- Homonymous hemianopia

Anterior Cerebral Artery
- Contralateral weakness or paralysis of the foot and leg
- Contralateral sensory loss of the toes, foot, and leg
- Loss of ability to make decisions or act voluntarily
- Urinary incontinence

Vertebral Artery
- Pain in the face, nose, or eye
- Numbness and weakness of the face on the involved side
- Problems with gait
- Dysphagia

---

usually one sided. The most common manifestation is weakness of the face and arm and sometimes the leg. Other common manifestations include numbness on one side, loss of vision, speech difficulties, sudden severe headache, and difficulties with balance. The various deficits associated with involvement of a specific cerebral artery are collectively referred to as *stroke syndromes*, although the deficits often overlap, as shown in **Box 16–24 》**.

Complications

Typical complications of stroke include sensory–perceptual deficits, cognitive and behavioral changes, communication deficits, motor deficits, and elimination disorders. These may be transient or permanent, depending on the degree of ischemia and necrosis as well as time of treatment. As a result of these neurologic deficits, the patient with a stroke may also have complications that involve many different body systems (see **Box 16–25 》**). These complications often cause serious alterations in the patient's functional health status.

Sensory–Perceptual Changes

Strokes often involve pathologic changes in neurologic pathways that alter the ability to integrate, interpret, and attend to sensory data. The patient may experience deficits in vision, hearing, equilibrium, taste, and smell. The ability to perceive vibration, pain, warmth, cold, and pressure may be impaired, as may **proprioception** (the body's sense of its position). The loss of these sensory abilities increases the risk for injury.

Box 16–25
Complications of Stroke

Integument
- Pressure injuries

Neurologic
- Hyperthermia
- Neglect syndrome
- Seizures
- Agnosias
- Communication deficits: expressive aphasia, receptive aphasia, global aphasia, agraphia
- Visual deficits: homonymous hemianopia, diplopia, decreased acuity
- Cognitive changes: memory loss, short attention span, distractibility, poor judgment, poor problem-solving ability, disorientation
- Behavioral changes: emotional lability, loss of social inhibitions, fear, hostility, anger, depression
- Increased ICP
- Alterations in consciousness
- Sensory loss to touch, pain, heat, cold, pressure

Respiratory
- Respiratory center damage

- Airway obstruction
- Decreased ability to cough

Gastrointestinal
- Dysphagia
- Constipation
- Stool impaction

Genitourinary
- Incontinence
- Frequency
- Urgency
- Urinary retention
- Renal calculi

Musculoskeletal
- Hemiplegia
- Contractures
- Bony ankylosis
- Disuse atrophy
- Dysarthria

Specific sensory–perceptual deficits may include the following:

- **Hemianopia** is the loss of half of the visual field of one or both eyes. When the same half is missing in each eye, the condition is called homonymous hemianopia (see **Figure 16–58** »).

- **Agnosia** is the inability to recognize one or more subjects that were previously familiar; agnosia may be visual, tactile, or auditory.

- **Apraxia** is the inability to carry out some motor pattern (e.g., drawing a figure, getting dressed) even when strength and coordination are adequate.

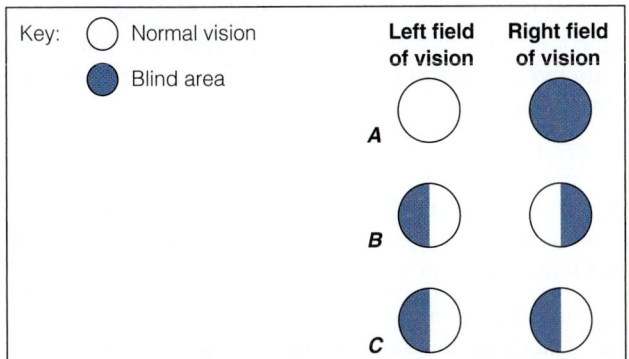

Figure 16–58 » Abnormal visual fields. **A,** Normal left field of vision with loss of vision in right field. **B,** Loss of vision in temporal half of both fields (bitemporal hemianopia). **C,** Loss of vision in nasal field of right eye and temporal field of left eye (homonymous hemianopia).

Another form of sensory–perceptual deficit is the **neglect syndrome** (or unilateral neglect), in which the patient has a disorder of attention. In this syndrome, the patient cannot integrate and use perceptions from the affected side of the body or from the environment on the affected side and therefore ignores that part. In severe cases, the patient may even deny the paralysis. This deficit is more common following a stroke of the right hemisphere, where damage to the parietal lobe (a center for mediation of directed attention) results in perceptual deficits.

Pain and discomfort may accompany a stroke, with the patient experiencing acute pain, numbness, or strange sensations. Although not common, damage to the thalamus may cause central stroke pain or central pain syndrome. The pain in this syndrome includes hot and cold, burning, tingling, and sharp, stabbing pain, most often in the extremities. It is worsened by movement and temperature changes. The painful sensations are not relieved by pain medications, nor are there any specific treatments.

Cognitive and Behavioral Changes

A change in consciousness, ranging from mild confusion to coma, is a common manifestation of stroke. This change may result from tissue damage following ischemia or hemorrhage involving either the carotid or vertebral arteries. Altered consciousness may also be the result of cerebral edema or increased ICP.

Behavioral changes associated with stroke include emotional lability (in which the patient may laugh or cry inappropriately), loss of self-control (manifested by behavior such as swearing or refusing to wear clothing), and decreased tolerance for stress (resulting in anger or depression). Intellectual changes may include memory loss, decreased attention span, poor judgment, and inability to think abstractly.

Communication Disorders

Communication is a complex process involving motor function, speech, language, memory, reasoning, and emotions. Communication disorders are usually the result of a stroke affecting the dominant hemisphere. The left hemisphere is dominant for language in approximately 88% of individuals who are right-handed and 78% of individuals who are left-handed. The remaining individuals are either ambilateral (no dominant hemisphere; 12% of right-handed and 15% of left-handed individuals) or right hemisphere dominant (7% of left-handed individuals) (Mazoyer et al., 2014).

Many different communication impairments may occur following stroke, and most are partial. Disorders of communication affect both speech (the mechanical act of articulating language through the spoken word) and language (the vocal or written formulation of ideas to communicate thoughts and feelings). Language involves oral and written expression as well as auditory and reading comprehension. Among these disorders are the following:

- **Aphasia** is the inability to use or understand language. It may be expressive, receptive, or mixed (global):
  - *Expressive aphasia.* A motor speech problem in which the individual can understand what is being said but can respond verbally only in short phrases; also called Broca aphasia.
  - *Receptive aphasia.* A sensory speech problem in which the individual cannot understand the spoken (and often written) word. Speech may be fluent but with inappropriate content; also called Wernicke aphasia.
  - *Mixed or global aphasia.* Language dysfunction in both understanding and expression.
- *Dysarthria* is any disturbance in muscular control of speech.

Motor Deficits

Body movement results from a complex interaction between the brain, spinal cord, and peripheral nerves. The motor areas of the cerebral cortex, basal ganglia, and cerebellum initiate voluntary movement by sending messages to the spinal cord, which then transmits the messages to the peripheral nerves. A stroke may interrupt the central nervous system component of this relay system and produce effects in the contralateral side ranging from mild weakness to severe limitation of any kind of movement.

Depending on the area of the brain involved, a stroke may cause weakness, paralysis, and/or spasticity. Specific motor deficits include the following:

- **Hemiplegia** is paralysis of the left or right half of the body (see **Figure 16–59** 》).
- **Hemiparesis** is weakness of the left or right half of the body.
- **Flaccidity** is absence of muscle tone (hypotonia).
- **Spasticity** is increased muscle tone (hypertonia), usually with some degree of weakness. The flexor muscles are usually more strongly affected in the upper extremities, and the extensor muscles are more strongly affected in the lower extremities.

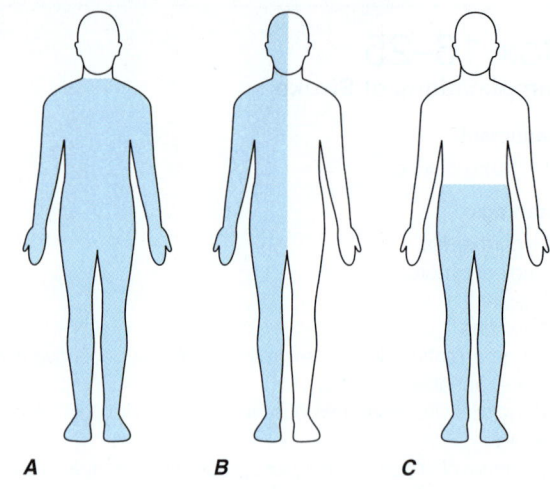

Figure 16–59 》 Types of paralysis. **A,** Quadriplegia is complete or partial paralysis of the upper extremities and complete paralysis of the lower part of the body. **B,** Hemiplegia is paralysis of one-half of the body when it is divided along the median sagittal plane. **C,** Paraplegia is paralysis of the lower part of the body.

When the corticospinal tract is involved, the affected arm and leg almost always are initially flaccid and then become spastic within 6–8 weeks. Spasticity often causes characteristic body positioning: adduction of the shoulder, pronation of the forearm, flexion of the fingers, and extension of the hip and knee. There is often foot drop, outward rotation of the leg, and dependent edema in the involved extremities.

Motor deficits resulting from stroke may result in altered mobility, further impairing body function. Complications of immobility involve multiple body systems and include orthostatic hypotension, increased thrombus formation, decreased CO, impaired respiratory function, osteoporosis, renal calculi, contractures, and decubitus ulcers.

Elimination Disorders

Disorders of bladder and bowel elimination are common. A stroke may cause partial loss of the sensations that trigger bladder elimination, resulting in urinary frequency, urgency, or incontinence. Bowel habits and control of urination may be altered as a result of cognitive deficits, immobility, and dehydration.

Collaboration

The type of treatment received by a patient with stroke depends on the stage of the disease. In general, there are three treatment stages:

1. Stroke prevention
2. Acute care immediately after a stroke
3. Rehabilitation after a stroke

The patient with an acute stroke may receive medical and/or surgical treatment. Treatment during the acute care phase focuses on diagnosing the type and cause of the stroke, supporting cerebral circulation, and controlling or preventing further deficits. The overall goals of stroke care, as defined

Clinical Manifestations and Therapies
Stroke

ETIOLOGY	CLINICAL MANIFESTATIONS	CLINICAL THERAPIES
Damage to neurons, depending on number and location, often results in loss of sensory and/or motor function.	■ Hemiplegia ■ Hemiparesis ■ Flaccidity ■ Paresthesias ■ Spasticity ■ Weakness ■ Paralysis	Initial therapy aimed at reducing the amount of brain injury includes: ■ Medications: Anticoagulant, thrombolytic, corticosteroids ■ BP control ■ Maintaining fluid, oxygen, and nutritional status. Following the initial insult, therapy is aimed at rehabilitation focused on restoring any function lost because of cellular damage: ■ Physical therapy ■ Occupational therapy ■ Home health assessment.
Alterations in the ability to communicate often result when cellular damage occurs on the dominant side of the brain.	■ Aphasia (expressive aphasia, receptive aphasia, mixed or global aphasia) ■ Dysarthria	■ Develop alternative means of communicating (e.g., use of hand signals). ■ Refer the patient for speech therapy. ■ Allow the patient time to express thoughts.
Sensory–perceptual deficits may occur if neurologic pathways are affected.	■ Vision, hearing, equilibrium, taste, or smell deficits ■ Altered ability to perceive vibration, pain, warmth, cold, and pressure ■ Altered proprioception ■ Hemianopia ■ Agnosia ■ Apraxia ■ Neglect syndrome	■ Provide reassurance and support. ■ Provide physical and occupational therapy when the patient's condition stabilizes. ■ Maintain patient safety.
Pain or strange sensations may result from damage to the thalamus.	■ Pain that may be hot, cold, burning, tingling, or sharp and stabbing in the extremities, worsened by movement or temperature changes, and not relieved by analgesics	No treatment has been identified.
Cognitive and behavioral changes can result from ischemia or hemorrhage involving either the carotid or vertebral arteries, cerebral edema, or increased ICP.	■ Emotional lability ■ Loss of self-control ■ Decreased tolerance for stress ■ Memory loss, decreased attention span ■ Poor judgment, lack of ability for abstract thought	■ Provide behavioral and cognitive therapy when condition stabilizes.

by the AHA (2013b), are to minimize brain injury and maximize patient recovery by way of the following measures:

- Rapid recognition and reaction to stroke warning signs
- Rapid emergency medical services (EMS) dispatch
- Rapid EMS system transport and hospital prenotification
- Rapid diagnosis and treatment in the hospital.

Note that in recent years, the focus of care has shifted from the nearest hospital to certified stroke centers (when available). Certified stroke centers offer immediate, appropriate care from entrance to the emergency department to discharge following rehabilitation.

Diagnostic Tests

Diagnosis of stroke begins with a complete history and careful physical assessment, including a thorough neurologic examination. The time of onset of stroke manifestations is a critical part of assessment. The National Institutes of Health Stroke Scale is a clinical evaluation tool widely used to assess neurologic outcome and degree of recovery. A portion of the scale is illustrated in **Table 16–31 》**. The full scale measures LOC, vision, facial paralysis, motor abilities, ataxia, sensation, language, and attention.

Imaging tests are used to identify an increased risk for stroke or to identify pathophysiologic changes after a stroke has occurred. CT is the first imaging technique used to

TABLE 16–31 National Institutes of Health Stroke Scale: Assessment of Level of Consciousness

Instructions	Scale Definition	Score
1a. Level of Consciousness (LOC): The investigator must choose a response, even if a full evaluation is prevented by such obstacles as an endotracheal tube, language barrier, or orotracheal trauma/bandages. A 3 is scored only if the patient makes no movement (other than reflexive posturing) in response to noxious stimulation.	0 = Alert, keenly responsive 1 = Not alert, but arousable by minor stimulation to obey, answer, or respond 2 = Not alert, requires repeated stimulation to attend, or is obtunded and requires strong or painful stimulation to make movements (not stereotyped) 3 = Responds only with reflex motor or autonomic effects or totally unresponsive, flaccid, areflexic	_____
1b. LOC Questions: The patient is asked the month and his or her age. The answer must be correct. There is no partial credit for being close. Aphasic and stuporous patients who do not comprehend the questions will score a 2. Patients unable to speak because of endotracheal intubation, orotracheal trauma, severe dysarthria from any cause, language barrier, or any other problem not secondary to aphasia are given a 1. It is important that only the initial answer be graded and that the examiner not "help" the patient with verbal or nonverbal cues.	0 = Answers both questions correctly 1 = Answers one question correctly 2 = Answers neither question correctly	_____
1c. LOC Commands: The patient is asked to open and close the eyes, then to grip and release the nonparetic hand. Substitute another one-step command if the hands cannot be used. Credit is given if an unequivocal attempt is made but not completed because of weakness. If the patient does not respond to the command, the task should be demonstrated (pantomime) and the results scored (i.e., follows none, one, or two commands). Patients with trauma, amputation, or other physical impediments should be given suitable one-step commands. Only the first attempt is scored.	0 = Performs both tasks correctly 1 = Performs one task correctly 2 = Performs neither task correctly	_____

Source: From Stroke Scale. Published by National Institutes of Health.

Note: This is a sample of only one part of the National Institutes of Health Stroke Scale. The entire scale may be viewed as a PDF file at https://stroke.nih.gov/resources/scale.htm.

demonstrate the presence of hemorrhage, tumors, aneurysm, ischemia, edema, and tissue necrosis. A CT scan also can demonstrate a shift in intracranial contents and is useful in distinguishing the type of stroke (e.g., a hemorrhagic stroke results in an increase in density). Cerebral infarctions usually are visible with a CT scan 6–8 hours poststroke; hemorrhage is visible immediately. Other imaging tests that may be used for diagnosis include cerebral arteriography, transcranial Doppler ultrasound, MRI, magnetic resonance angiography, positron emission tomography (PET), and single-photon emission CT. A perfusion- and diffusion-weighted imaging (DWI) test can be used to identify cerebral ischemia immediately after stroke onset and also to identify areas of possible reversible damage (the penumbra).

In addition to imaging tests, a blood test has recently been approved to screen for recurrent stroke risk. The PLAC test scans the blood for high levels of lipoprotein-associated phospholipase A_2, which is more common in individuals who have had strokes. For some patients, a lumbar puncture may be performed to obtain CSF for examination if there is no danger of increased ICP. A thrombotic stroke may elevate CSF pressure; after a hemorrhagic stroke, frank blood may be seen in the CSF.

SAFETY ALERT Removal of CSF when ICP is increased can result in herniation of the brainstem. Therefore, lumbar puncture should not be performed in patients with increased ICP.

Pharmacologic Therapy

Medications may be administered to prevent stroke in patients with TIAs or a previous stroke, as well as to treat patients during the acute phase of a stroke. Refer to Medications features throughout the module.

Stroke Prevention

Use of medications to prevent stroke is based on the patient's history of TIA or previous stroke and on other factors in the patient's medical history. Among the most frequently prescribed medications are antiplatelet and anticoagulant drugs, antihypertensives, and cholesterol-lowering drugs.

Antiplatelet agents are often used to reduce the risk of stroke in patients with TIAs or previous stroke history. Antiplatelet drugs commonly used to prevent clot formation and blood vessel occlusion include aspirin, clopidogrel (Plavix), dipyridamole (Persantine), and ticlopidine (Ticlid). Daily low-dose aspirin reduces TIA occurrence and stroke risk by interfering with platelet aggregation. Ticlopidine (Ticlid) is a platelet-aggregation inhibitor that reduces thrombotic stroke risk. In patients with atrial fibrillation, use of anticoagulants like warfarin (Coumadin), rivaroxaban (Xarelto), apixaban (Eliquis), dabigatran (Pradaxa), and edoxaban (Savaysa) can help reduce stroke risk by preventing clots from forming in the heart, from which they could travel to the brain (Adams et al., 2017).

Given that high BP is the leading cause of stroke, antihypertensive therapy is another common preventive measure. Of the various classes of antihypertensives, research indicates that thiazide diuretics, CCBs, ACE inhibitors, and ARBs are most useful in reducing stroke risk. Even though beta blockers are useful in lowering BP, they are of only limited effectiveness in the prevention of stroke (Silver, 2016). For more information on these medications, refer to Exemplar 16.G on Hypertension.

Like high BP, elevated cholesterol levels also increase a person's likelihood of stroke. Thus, cholesterol-lowering drugs are frequently included in stroke prevention efforts.

Statins such as atorvastatin (Lipitor), simvastatin (Zocor), and lovastatin (Mevacor) are most frequently prescribed and considered the standard of treatment. Fibric acid agents like fenofibrate (Tricor) and fenofibric acid (Fibricor) may also be prescribed, although evidence supporting the use of these drugs is less compelling than the evidence supporting statin use (Wang et al., 2015). Additional information on these drug classes can be found in Exemplar 16.C on Coronary Artery Disease.

Acute Stroke

During the acute phase of an ischemic stroke, medications are given to break up existing clots, prevent further thrombosis formation, increase cerebral blood flow, and protect cerebral neurons. The type of medication used depends on the type of stroke and other patient characteristics.

Fibrinolytic therapy using the recombinant tissue plasminogen activator alteplase (rt-PA, tPA) is the gold standard for the treatment of acute ischemic stroke. This drug converts plasminogen to plasmin, resulting in fibrinolysis of the clot. According to American Stroke Association guidelines, tPA is most effective when given intravenously within 3 hours after the onset of manifestations. However, in patients age 80 and under without a history of both diabetes mellitus and prior stroke, IV tPA can be administered up to 4.5 hours after onset of manifestations (Demaerschalk et al., 2016). To prevent stroke recurrence, patients who receive tPA typically begin anticoagulant or antiplatelet therapy no sooner than 24 hours after tPA administration (Zinkstok & Roos, 2012). The Evidence-Based Practice feature further discusses the use of tPA in treating stroke.

In patients for whom tPA is contraindicated (e.g., those over age 80, those with a history of diabetes and stroke), pharmacologic treatment of acute ischemic stroke is usually limited to administration of aspirin (Anderson et al., 2012). Otherwise, antiplatelet and/or anticoagulant drug therapy is not routinely recommended, although there are a few specific clinical situations in which it may be useful (e.g., in patients with atrial fibrillation who are experiencing stroke caused by an embolism that originated in the heart). In such cases, the most commonly used medications are heparin, LMWH, warfarin (Coumadin), and enoxaparin (Lovenox) (Shahpouri et al., 2012). These medications do not dissolve an existing clot; rather, they prevent further extension of the clot and formation of new clots. Sodium heparin may be given subcutaneously or by continuous IV drip, while warfarin sodium may be given orally.

SAFETY ALERT Anticoagulant and antiplatelet medications are *never* administered to a patient with a hemorrhagic stroke. Because hemorrhagic stroke involves bleeding in the brain, administration of these drugs would perpetuate the bleeding and worsen the patient's condition.

Management of hypertension during the acute phase of stroke is controversial, but if the patient is eligible for fibrinolytic therapy, BP control is necessary to decrease the risk for bleeding. If the BP is sustained at systolic levels greater than 185 mmHg or diastolic levels greater than 110 mmHg, the patient cannot be treated with IV tPA.

Corticosteroids, such as prednisone or dexamethasone, have been used to treat cerebral edema related to stroke, but

Evidence-Based Practice
Treating Stroke with tPA

Problem

Stroke is a leading cause of severe, long-term disability in the United States (American Stroke Association, 2015). The risk of disability and death can be reduced in individuals who experience a sudden ischemic stroke by administering thrombolytics to dissolve blood clots.

Evidence

tPA is the most commonly administered drug used in thrombolytic therapy (U.S. National Library of Medicine, 2015). In ideal situations, patients receive tPA within 90 minutes after arriving in the emergency department, but positive outcomes have been seen when tPA is administered as long as 12 hours after initial symptom onset. To be most effective, tPA should be administered within 3 hours of the warning signs of a stroke to increase the chances of recovery (National Stroke Association, n.d.b). tPA restores the brain's blood flow by dissolving the blood clot that caused the stroke.

tPA is the only drug treatment for acute ischemic stroke approved by the U.S. Food and Drug Administration (National Stroke Association, n.d.b). An enzyme found naturally in the body, tPA converts plasminogen to plasmin, an enzyme that dissolves blood clots. Physicians administer additional tPA intravenously to speed up this process. The most common complication of tPA therapy is brain hemorrhage. Early identification of stroke warning signs and prompt thrombolytic therapy are instrumental in helping patients achieve full recovery.

Implications

Nurses must frequently monitor patients' vital signs following administration of tPA. Patients are at increased risk for bleeding and should not be given anticoagulants or antiplatelet agents for 24 hours after administration of tPA. It is also important for the patient to avoid foods that influence the body's clotting mechanism, including spinach, lettuce, broccoli, cabbage, cauliflower, and vegetable oil. Acute care may be delivered via a specialized team of nurses and other interprofessional members. LOC and neurologic status are important indicators of further brain hemorrhage and should be monitored continuously during the hospitalization.

Critical Thinking Application

1. A patient arrives in the emergency department with an ischemic stroke and receives tPA. What is the priority nursing assessment?

2. Prior to administering tPA to a patient admitted with a diagnosis of stroke, what serum lab value should the nurse check? Why?

3. Think of a slogan that increases public awareness of the 3-hour window recommended for treatment with tPA.

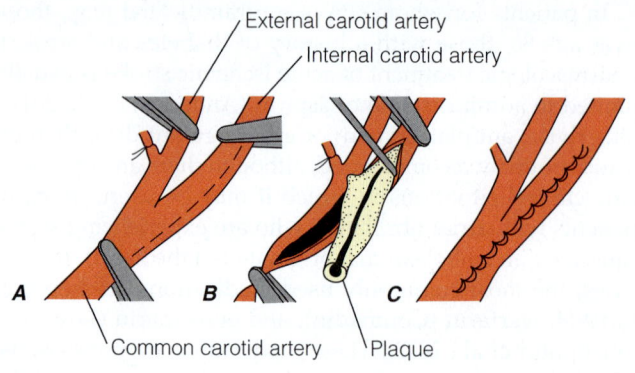

External carotid artery
Internal carotid artery

A   B   C

Common carotid artery   Plaque

Figure 16–60 》 Carotid endarterectomy. **A,** The occluded area is clamped off and an incision is made in the artery. **B,** Plaque is removed from the inner layer of the artery. **C,** To restore blood flow through the artery, the artery is sutured, or a graft is completed.

the results are not always positive. If the patient has increased ICP, hyperosmolar solutions (e.g., mannitol) or diuretics (e.g., furosemide) may be administered. Anticonvulsants, such as phenytoin (Dilantin), and barbiturates may be prescribed if increased ICP causes seizures.

Surgery

Surgery may be performed to prevent the occurrence of a stroke, to restore blood flow when a stroke has already occurred, or to repair vascular damage or malformations. In individuals who have had TIAs or are in danger of having another stroke, a carotid endarterectomy at the carotid artery bifurcation may be performed to remove atherosclerotic plaque (see **Figure 16–60 》**).

When an occluded or stenotic vessel is not directly accessible, an extracranial–intracranial bypass may be performed. Bypass of the internal carotid, middle cerebral, or vertebral arteries may be required. The indications for the bypass are manifestations of ischemia caused by TIAs or a mild completed stroke. The procedure reestablishes blood flow to the affected area of the brain.

A carotid angioplasty with stenting is an option for treating cerebral stenosis. During the procedure, a balloon catheter is inserted through an artery in the patient's arm or leg. Under fluoroscopy, the catheter is advanced to the area of carotid artery stenosis, and a small filter is inserted to catch any clots or pieces of debris that might break loose. The balloon is inflated to widen the artery, and a permanent stent is inserted.

Rehabilitation

Various types of therapy are necessary for poststroke rehabilitation. Types and goals of therapy are as follows:

- **Physical therapy** may help prevent contractures and improve muscle strength and coordination. Physical therapists teach exercises that help patients relearn how to walk, sit, lie down, and change from one type of movement to another.
- **Occupational therapy** provides assistive devices and a plan for regaining motor skills lost as a result of stroke.

These skills include eating, drinking, bathing, cooking, reading, writing, and toileting.

- **Speech and language therapy** is provided to help the patient relearn language and communication skills as well as improve swallowing.

Lifespan Considerations

Strokes can affect people of any age, from infants through older adults. Special considerations for patients at various stages throughout the lifespan are as follows.

Stroke in Neonates

The greatest risk for stroke in neonates is the time extending from immediately before birth to 30 days after birth. Stroke occurs in approximately 1 in 4000 live births. Risk factors for stroke in neonates include chorioamnionitis, premature rupture of membranes during pregnancy, and maternal pre-eclampsia (National Stroke Association, n.d.c). In addition, neonates are in a hypercoagulable state because of clotting factors that cross the placenta and an increased percentage of RBCs. Labor and delivery can also increase stress on the arteries and the veins in the head, potentially leading to clot formation.

Many times, stroke is missed in neonates because the signs are vague and the diagnosis is uncommon. Signs of stroke are often not noticed until the infant is several months old. Stroke warning signs in infants include seizures, extreme sleepiness, and favoring the use of only one side of the body (early handedness) (National Stroke Association, n.d.c). Signs of seizure in neonates include repetitive facial movements, staring, apnea, and jerking of the muscles of the face, arms, or legs.

The two most common types of ischemic stroke that occur in newborns are **sinovenous thrombosis**, which involves a clot in one of the veins of the brain, and **arterial ischemic stroke**, which involves a clot in one of the arteries of the brain. Neonates may also experience hemorrhagic stroke. Stroke in the fetus is generally diagnosed by fetal MRI or ultrasound. Stroke in neonates is diagnosed with ultrasound, a head CT, or an MRI. Treatment only can occur after birth, and it generally involves anticoagulant administration for ischemic stroke.

Because of the plasticity of the newborn brain, damage done to the neonatal brain can be minimized because healthy areas of the brain compensate for the damaged area. Therefore, a newborn may be developmentally normal, even after a stroke. However, many neonates develop permanent deficiencies such as cerebral palsy; epilepsy; or language, cognitive, or behavioral problems (International Alliance for Pediatric Stroke [IAPS], 2014).

Stroke in Children and Adolescents

Each year, approximately 5 in 100,000 children between 1 month and 19 years of age have a stroke. Between 20 and 40% of children die after stroke, ranking stroke among the top 12 causes of death in children (AHA, 2014e). Strokes are more common in children under age 2 than in older children, and among children, boys and African Americans are at a higher risk for stroke than other groups. Common causes of adult strokes such as hypertension, irregular heartbeat, and hardening arteries are rare in children, whose risk factors for stroke include congenital heart defects, sickle cell disease, immune disorders, arterial diseases, abnormal blood clotting, trauma to the head or neck, and maternal history of infertility.

Symptoms of stroke in children and teens include severe headaches, vomiting, sleepiness, dizziness, seizures, language problems, and loss of balance or coordination (IAPS, 2014; National Stroke Association, n.d.c). As in neonates, the most common types of stroke in children are arterial ischemic stroke and sinovenous thrombosis. The effects of stroke in a child are generally the same as in an adult—most commonly, hemiparesis or hemiplegia, unilateral neglect, aphasia, dysphagia, decreased field of vision and visual perception problems, mood changes and loss of emotional control, cognitive changes or impairment, and behavior or personality changes. Younger people generally are more resilient than older people in recovering lost abilities from stroke, and children frequently recover their ability to speak and use their arms and legs following a stroke (AHA, 2015r). However, 60% of children with stroke have permanent complications, including seizures, weakness, vision problems, hemiparesis, and hemiplegia (AHA, 2014e; National Stroke Association, n.d.c). In addition, children who have one stroke have a 15–18% risk for recurrent stroke (IAPS, 2014).

Although treatment with tPA is common in adults, use of tPA is controversial in children, because safety studies have not been performed in this population. Current treatment includes supportive care; controlling high BP, increased ICP, and seizures; antithrombotic therapy; and surgery to relieve ICP if needed (National Stroke Association, n.d.c).

Stroke in Pregnant Women

Pregnancy increases the risk of stroke because of the effect that increased hormone levels have on blood vessel walls and clotting. The increase in BP associated with pregnancy, especially in patients with preeclampsia, also increases stroke risk. In one study, 0.16% of patients with a hypertensive disorder of pregnancy had a stroke, whereas only 0.03% of patients without a hypertensive disorder of pregnancy had a stroke (Leffert et al., 2015). Stroke risk increases during the third trimester and in the first 6 weeks after birth (Stroke Association, 2012). Strokes during pregnancy are treated the same way as any other stroke in adults, although use of tPA is limited to eligible women only (Selim & Molina, 2013).

NURSING PROCESS

Even though many individuals who have a stroke experience full recovery, a substantial number are left with disabilities that affect their physical, emotional, interpersonal, family, and professional status. The nursing care they need is often complex and multidimensional, and continuity of care is vital as patients move between acute care settings, long-term care settings, rehabilitation centers, and the home.

The nurse caring for a patient who has had a stroke requires knowledge and skill to meet the patient's needs during both the acute and rehabilitative phases of care. The patient may have losses in multiple areas: mobility, ability to provide self-care, communications, concept of self, and interpersonal or intimate relationships with others. Holistic,

individualized nursing care is essential in all settings and focuses on promoting the achievement of maximum potential and quality of life.

The patient's family often faces many changes. A young to middle-age adult with a family member who has had a stroke may face economic difficulties and social isolation. A middle-age adult family member may become the caretaker for an older parent, in essence switching roles with the parent. An older adult may not be able to care for a spouse and may have to accept nursing home placement. In addition, an older adult who has no family may have to struggle alone to regain the ability to function independently. Although not all of these problems are amenable to nursing solutions, the nurse is most often the healthcare provider who assesses and identifies the needs of each individual and who provides information and referrals to patients and families to help meet those needs.

Because a stroke has the potential to cause many different health problems, a wide variety of nursing diagnoses may be appropriate. Each patient will be affected differently, depending on the degree of ischemia and area of the brain involved. Nursing diagnoses discussed in this section focus on problems with cerebral tissue perfusion (specific to nursing care during the acute phase), physical mobility, self-care, communication, sensory–perceptual deficits, bowel and urine elimination, and swallowing (specific to prevention of complications and rehabilitation).

Assessment

During the assessment phase, the nurse should collect the following data through the health history and physical examination:

- *Observation and patient interview.* Observation of the patient includes noting visible signs of stroke, including paralysis or weakness of one side of the body, facial drooping, and difficulty speaking or understanding speech. Ask the patient or patient's family member about risk factors, previous stroke history, drug use (including prescribed, over-the-counter, and street drugs), smoking history, when manifestations began, severity of manifestations, presence of incontinence, LOC, and family support systems.
- *Physical examination.* The physical examination of a patient with a suspected stroke should include assessment of LOC, motor strength, coordination, communication, cranial nerve function, sensory function, stroke scale, vital signs, skin integrity, and mobility status.

If the patient is a woman, her risks for stroke are different than those of a man, and she should be asked questions specific to her gender. Questions relating to the uniqueness of women's symptoms include inquiries regarding sudden face and limb pain, sudden nausea, sudden hiccups, sudden shortness of breath, palpitations, and generalized weakness.

Diagnosis

Nursing diagnoses that may apply to the patient with stroke include the following:

- *Tissue Perfusion: Risk for Ineffective Cerebral*
- *Physical Mobility, Impaired*

- *Self-Care Deficit, Dressing*
- *Verbal Communication, Impaired*
- *Urinary Elimination, Impaired*
- *Constipation, Risk for*
- *Swallowing, Impaired.*

(NANDA-I © 2014)

Planning

Goals of care for the patient who has had a stroke include the following:

- The patient's BP will be maintained within prescribed limits.
- The patient will understand the importance of cardiac rehabilitation.
- The patient will ambulate and increase activity as tolerated.
- The patient will participate in therapies that maximize communication techniques.

Implementation

The focus of care for the patient who has had a stroke is determined by the severity of the stroke, the neurologic deficits that result, and whether the patient is in the acute or rehabilitative stage. In the acute phase, ensuring airway, breathing, and circulation are the priority focus. Once the ABCs of care are met, the nurse's priority shifts to reducing loss of neurologic function. Providing psychosocial support for the patient and family also is an important nursing role.

Maintain Cerebral Perfusion

Initial assessment and care focus on identifying changes that may indicate altered cerebral perfusion. The nurse monitors the patient's airway, breathing, circulation, and neurologic status and provides interventions to maintain cerebral perfusion. Nursing interventions related to maintaining cerebral perfusion in the acute care setting are as follows:

- Monitor the patient's respiratory status and airway patency. Auscultate pulmonary sounds, and monitor respiratory rate and results of studies of ABGs. The patient is often unconscious, and breathing may be impaired. Respiratory complications develop rapidly, as manifested by crackles, wheezes, rapid respirations, and respiratory acidosis.
- Suction as necessary, using care to avoid prolonged suctioning, which can increase ICP.
- Place the patient in a side-lying position.
- Administer oxygen as prescribed. Oxygen decreases the risk for hypoxia and hypercapnia, which can increase cerebral ischemia and ICP.
- Monitor the patient's mental status and LOC, watching for restlessness, drowsiness, lethargy, inability to follow commands, and unresponsiveness. Frequent monitoring of neurologic status is necessary to detect changes. Alterations in mental status, LOC, and movement indicate increased ICP, the major cause of death in the acute phase of a stroke.

- Monitor the patient's strength and reflexes, and assess for pain, headache, decreased strength, sluggish pupillary reflexes, absent gag or swallowing reflexes, hemiplegia, Babinski sign, and decerebrate or decorticate posturing. Alterations in strength and reflexes indicate increased ICP.
- Continuously monitor the patient's cardiac status. A stroke may cause cardiac dysrhythmias, including bradycardia, PVCs, tachycardia, and AV block. Characteristic ECG changes include a shortened PR interval, peaked T waves, and a depressed ST segment.
- Monitor the patient's body temperature. Hyperthermia may develop if the hypothalamus is affected.
- Maintain accurate intake and output records, and measure urinary output via an indwelling catheter. A stroke may damage the pituitary gland, resulting in diabetes insipidus and possible dehydration from greatly increased urinary output.
- Monitor the patient for seizures. Pad the side rails, and administer prescribed anticonvulsants. Seizures may be the result of cerebral tissue damage or increased ICP. Padded side rails prevent injury if seizure occurs, while anticonvulsants prevent or treat seizures.

Promote Physical Mobility

The goals of care for patients with impaired mobility are to maintain and improve functional abilities (by maintaining normal function and alignment, preventing edema of extremities, and reducing spasticity) and to prevent complications. Nursing interventions related to physical mobility include the following:

- Encourage active ROM exercises for unaffected extremities (see the Patient Teaching feature), and perform passive ROM exercises for affected extremities every 4 hours during the day and evening shifts and once during the night shift. Support the joint during passive ROM exercises. Active ROM exercises maintain or improve muscle strength and endurance and help maintain cardiopulmonary function. Passive ROM exercises do not strengthen muscles but do help maintain joint flexibility.
- Turn the patient every 2 hours around the clock, following a posted schedule for side-to-side and supine-to-prone position changes (verify prone positioning with the healthcare provider first). Maintain body alignment, and support the extremities in the proper position with pillows. Elevate the head of the bed 30 degrees. Turning on a regular basis, accompanied by proper positioning, maintains joint function, alleviates pressure on bony prominences that can lead to skin breakdown, decreases dependent edema in hands and feet, reduces ICP, and reduces the risk of complications resulting from immobility (see **Figure 16–61 》》**).
- Monitor the patient's lower extremities each shift for symptoms of thrombophlebitis. Assess for increased warmth and redness in calves; measure the circumference of the calves and thighs. Patients on bedrest (especially those with loss of muscle strength and tone) are particularly prone to development of DVT. Promptly report manifestations of thrombophlebitis.

Patient Teaching

Active Range-of-Motion Exercises

Patients who have had a stroke can help build their strength by performing active ROM exercises. These exercises are performed by the patient with no help from the nurse or family. Patients should perform the exercises at the same time each day and in the same order each time, preferably from head to toe. Exercises should be performed first on the unaffected side of the body, then the affected side of the body. The patient can use the unaffected side to help move the affected side through the exercises if needed. Performing active ROM exercises on the affected side helps the patient learn to use muscles that have lost functionality because of the stroke. Teach the patient to use slow movements and to stop if pain occurs. Appropriate active ROM exercises may include the following:

- **Neck.** Perform lateral flexion, rotation, flexion, extension, and hyperextension
- **Shoulder.** Perform flexion, extension, hyperextension, internal rotation, external rotation, abduction, adduction, and circumduction
- **Elbow.** Perform flexion, extension, and hyperextension
- **Wrist.** Perform adduction, abduction, flexion, extension, and hyperextension
- **Fingers.** Perform adduction, abduction, flexion, extension, and hyperextension; also perform opposition with the thumb
- **Back.** Perform lumbar rotation, lateral flexion, flexion, and extension
- **Hips.** Perform flexion, extension, hyperextension, abduction, adduction, internal rotation, external rotation, and circumduction
- **Knee.** Perform flexion and extension
- **Ankle.** Perform dorsiflexion and plantar flexion
- **Foot.** Perform inversion, eversion, flexion, extension, abduction, and adduction
- **Toes.** Perform adduction, abduction, flexion, extension, and hyperextension

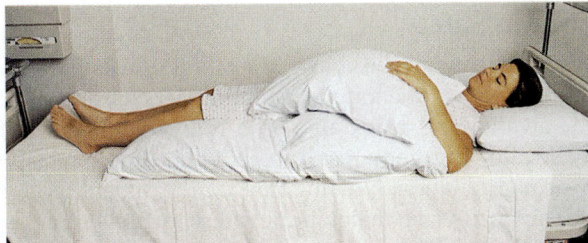

A

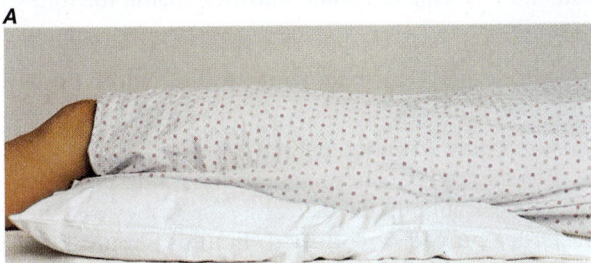

B

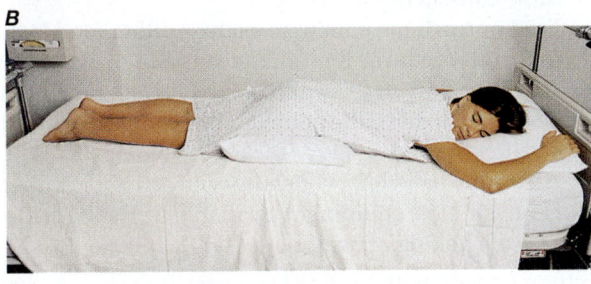

C

Source: George Dodson/Pearson Education, Inc.

Figure 16–61 ❯❯ Positioning the patient with hemiplegia is important in preventing deformity of the affected extremities. **A,** With the patient in a supine position, place a pillow in the axilla (to prevent adduction) and under the hand and arm, with the hand higher than the elbow (to prevent flexion and edema). **B,** When the patient is lying supine, use a pillow from the iliac crest to the middle of the thigh to prevent external rotation of the hip. **C,** When the patient is in the prone position, place a pillow under the pelvis to promote hip hyperextension.

- Collaborate with the physical therapist as the patient gains mobility, using consistent techniques to move the patient from the bed to the wheelchair and to help the patient ambulate. Use of consistent techniques facilitates rehabilitation.

Promote Self-Care

The patient who has had a stroke may have self-care deficits due to impaired mobility or mental confusion. It is important for patients to perform as much of their own physical care and grooming as possible to promote functional ability, increase independence, decrease feelings of powerlessness, and improve self-esteem. Nursing interventions to promote self-care include:

- Encourage the patient to use the unaffected arm to bathe, brush teeth, comb hair, dress, and eat. Use of the unaffected arm promotes functional ability and independence.
- Teach the patient to put on clothing by first dressing the affected extremities and then dressing the unaffected extremities. This technique facilitates self-dressing with minimal assistance.
- Collaborate with the occupational therapist in scheduling times for training to promote the upper extremity functioning necessary for ADLs. Encourage the use of assistive devices (if required) for eating, physical hygiene, and dressing. Following a regular schedule in daily routines promotes learning. Use of assistive devices promotes independence and decreases feelings of powerlessness. Optimal grooming facilitates positive self-concept.

Before establishing a plan to increase self-care, determine which hand was dominant before the stroke. If the patient's dominant side is affected, self-care will be more difficult.

Promote Verbal Communication

The patient who loses communication abilities requires intensive speech therapy and emotional support. It is important for the nurse to determine the exact nature of the impairment when planning interventions and helping family members understand specific problems. Although the speech therapist is usually most involved with speech rehabilitation, nurses must plan interventions to meet communication needs during all phases of care. These interventions may include the following:

- Communicate with the patient using the following guidelines:
  a. Approach and treat the patient as an adult.
  b. Do not assume that the patient who does not respond verbally cannot hear. Do not use a raised voice when addressing the patient.
  c. Allow adequate time for the patient to respond.
  d. Face the patient, and speak slowly.
  e. When you do not understand the patient's speech, be honest and say so.
  f. Use short, simple statements and questions.
- Accepting the patient and providing dignity and respect enhances the nurse–patient relationship. Allowing adequate response time and using short verbal statements or questions while facing the patient motivates the patient to communicate and decreases frustration.
- Accept the patient's frustration and anger as a normal reaction to the loss of function. Anger represents the patient's frustration at the inability to control the loss of function.
- Try alternative methods of communication, including writing tablets, flash cards, and computerized talking boards. Patients who are unable to communicate verbally may be able to use other methods effectively.

Promote Urinary and Bowel Elimination

Both urinary and bowel elimination may be altered because of neurologic deficits, impaired mobility, cognitive impairment, communication deficits, or preexisting problems (especially if the patient is an older adult). Other causes can include changes in food and fluid intake and side effects of medications. Urinary incontinence or retention, constipation, and fecal impaction are the usual manifestations. Nursing interventions to promote normal elimination include the following:

- Encourage bladder training by having the patient void on schedule (e.g., every 2 hours, rather than in response to the urge to void). Voiding on schedule promotes bladder tone and urine storage.
- Teach Kegel exercises. To perform Kegel exercises, the patient contracts the perineal muscles as though stopping urination, holds the contraction for 5 seconds, and then releases. Kegel exercises increase pubococcygeal muscle tone and bladder control, decreasing incontinence.
- Use positive reinforcement (verbal praise) for successful management of urinary elimination. Positive reinforcement can be a useful part of the teaching program.
- Discuss prestroke bowel habits as well as patterns of bowel elimination since the stroke.
- If the patient is able to swallow without difficulty, encourage fluids (up to 2000 mL/day) and a high-fiber diet. Increased fluids and fiber stimulate intestinal motility.
- Increase physical activity as tolerated. Increased activity stimulates intestinal motility.

Additional interventions appropriate in hospital settings may include the following:

- Assess for urinary frequency, urgency, incontinence, nocturia, and voiding in small amounts. In addition, assess the patient's ability to respond to the need to void, ability to use the call light, and ability to use toileting equipment.
- Assist in using the toilet facilities at the same time each day (based on usual patterns of bowel elimination), ensuring privacy and having the patient sit in an upright position if possible. Establishing a regular daily time for bowel movements in the upright position and in privacy promotes normal bowel elimination.
- Administer prescribed stool softeners if the patient is following a bowel elimination routine or is not drinking sufficient fluids. Stool softeners help prevent formation of hard stool that is more difficult to expel.

Maintain Safety

A stroke may impair the ability to swallow. Weakness or lack of coordination of the tongue, attention deficits, and deficits in the swallowing reflex all play a role. **Dysphagia** (difficulty swallowing) may result in choking, drooling, aspiration, or regurgitation. Nursing care for the patient receiving acute care focuses on maintaining safety by preventing aspiration and ensuring adequate nutrition, using the following interventions:

- Monitor results of swallowing studies before providing oral food and fluids.
- Ensure safety when the patient is eating.
  a. Position the patient in an upright sitting position with the neck slightly flexed.
  b. Order puréed or soft food. Liquids should be of the same consistency as honey.
  c. Feed or teach the patient to eat by putting food behind the front teeth on the unaffected side of the mouth. Teach the patient to swallow one bite at a time. It may be helpful to have the patient tuck his or her chin while swallowing.
  d. Assess the patient for coughing with eating or drinking.
  e. Have suction equipment available at the bedside in case of choking or aspiration.
- Sitting upright with the head and neck first slightly flexed and then the chin tilted forward helps the patient swallow. The patient can usually swallow puréed or soft foods more easily than liquid or solid foods. Using the unaffected side of the mouth helps prevent food from collecting in the mouth and makes swallowing safer; in addition, food is less likely to fall out of the mouth. Coughing may be indicative of dysphagia.
- Monitor the patient's lung sounds. Coarse lung sounds heard in the right upper and/or lower lobes may indicate aspiration, because the right bronchus is the first division of the bronchi and where most aspirations occur.

- Minimize distractions and, if necessary, give the patient step-by-step instructions for eating. Distractions increase the risk of aspiration. Complex activities are easier to perform when broken down into small steps.

Evaluation

Patient outcomes may be evaluated based on the following expected outcomes:

- The patient participates in assigned therapies.
- The patient communicates effectively.
- The patient's significant other and family members participate in the patient's care.
- The patient experiences minimal complications resulting from immobility, dysphagia, and reduced motor or sensory function.

During acute care after a stroke, the patient's status may change often, so frequent evaluation is important. With every change in status, the nurse will need to revise the nursing care plan to best meet the patient's needs. This may involve administration of prescribed medications, helping the patient change positions, assisting the patient with urination or defecation, analyzing laboratory results and vital signs, and providing supportive care for the patient and family. During rehabilitation, the nurse will need to evaluate the patient's progress in regaining strength, movement, and verbal skills. Changes in the patient's status may indicate a worsening of the patient's condition, necessitating additional nursing interventions, or it may indicate recovery and readiness for discharge.

Nursing Care Plan

A Patient with Stroke

Orville Boren is a 63-year-old man who had a stroke caused by right cerebral thrombosis 3 days ago. He is a history instructor at the local community college. His hobbies are wood carving and gardening. Mr. Boren is also an active member of his church. For the past 2 years, Mr. Boren has been taking medication for hypertension, but his wife Emily reports that he often forgets to take it and that his BP was high at his last physical examination.

Mrs. Boren tells the staff that she has never had to worry about her husband's health before and that she wants to learn everything she can to care for him at home. However, she says that her husband was always the one to make the decisions and pay the bills. Mrs. Boren adds that the children, grandchildren, neighbors, and family pastor all want to see Mr. Boren back at home as soon as possible.

ASSESSMENT	DIAGNOSES	PLANNING
Carol Merck, RN, the nurse assigned to Mr. Boren, completes a health history and physical assessment, with Mrs. Boren providing information for the history. Mrs. Boren reports that her husband did have several spells of dizziness and blurred vision the week before his stroke, but they lasted only a few minutes and he believed them to be caused by "old age and working out in the sun." On the morning of admission, Mr. Boren woke up and could not move his left arm or leg; he also could not speak sensibly. Mrs. Boren called 9-1-1, and an ambulance took her husband to the hospital.	*Feeding Self-Care Deficit* related to loss of the ability to use the left hand and arm	Goals of care include the following:
	Impaired Swallowing related to cerebral injury	■ The patient will learn to use his right hand to feed himself.
	Risk for Aspiration due to impaired swallowing	■ The patient will learn techniques for and engage in exercises that promote proper swallowing.
Physical assessment findings include the following: Mr. Boren is drowsy but responds to verbal stimuli. Although he does not respond verbally, he can nod his head to indicate "yes." Flaccid paralysis is present in his left arm and left leg, with no response noted to touch in those extremities. (He is left-handed.) Visual fields are decreased in a pattern consistent with homonymous hemianopia. A CT scan, negative on admission, is repeated the day after admission and confirms the medical diagnosis of a right-brain stroke caused by a thrombus of the middle cerebral artery.	*Impaired Physical Mobility* related to neurologic deficits causing left hemiplegia	■ The patient will learn and demonstrate techniques for reducing the risk of aspiration when eating.
	Risk for Impaired Skin Integrity related to inability to change position	■ The patient will participate in exercises necessary to maintain muscle strength and tone.
	Impaired Verbal Communication related to cerebral injury	■ The patient will maintain skin integrity.
Mr. Boren's medical treatment includes oral aspirin, 300 mg/day, as well as continuation of his prior antihypertensive therapy.	*Deficient Knowledge* related to the medication regimen and need for BP control	■ The patient will practice and implement speech therapy activities while at the same time using alternative methods of communication.
	Ineffective Role Performance related to impaired verbal communication and physical mobility	■ The patient will demonstrate an understanding of the medication regimen, as well as the need for proper BP control.
	(NANDA-I © 2014)	■ The patient will formulate realistic goals and plans for the future.

(continued on next page)

Nursing Care Plan *(continued)*

IMPLEMENTATION

- Arrange mealtimes so that Mr. Boren is sitting up by the window in a clean, semi-private environment.
- Provide adaptive devices (silverware with thick handles and nonslip plates).
- Encourage Mrs. Boren to visit at mealtimes, to assist with meals, and periodically to bring a favorite food from home.
- Teach Mr. and Mrs. Boren about appropriate foods and feeding techniques to facilitate swallowing and reduce the risk of aspiration.
- Arrange for Mr. Boren to work with a speech therapist, physical therapist, and occupational therapist.
- Conduct passive ROM exercises on the left arm and leg; schedule active ROM exercises for the right extremities as well as quadriceps and gluteal sets every 4 hours during waking hours.

- Keep the skin clean and dry at all times.
- Establish and maintain a regular schedule for turning when Mr. Boren is in bed.
- Place objects (e.g., call bell, tissues) on the unaffected side, and approach Mr. Boren from that side.
- Support attempts to communicate verbally, but provide Mr. Boren with a large marker and tablet when needed for communication purposes.
- Teach Mr. Boren about the risks and benefits of his medication regimen.
- Encourage Mr. and Mrs. Boren to formulate realistic goals and plans for the future.

EVALUATION

Mr. Boren is discharged to his home after being in the hospital for 5 days. During the first 2 months after discharge, Martha Grimes, RN, the home health nurse, visits Mr. and Mrs. Boren at home. At the end of 2 months, Mr. Boren is using his right hand to feed himself. He has regained partial use of his left arm and leg and is using a walker to move around the house and yard; he is even able to work in his flower garden. His skin has remained intact, and his vision is back to normal. He is slowly relearning speech; this has been the most difficult change for him to accept. Once he writes on his tablet, "I think God has forgotten me."

CRITICAL THINKING

1. Hypertension is sometimes referred to as the "silent killer." Provide justifications for this statement.
2. The functional changes Mr. Boren has experienced may make a return to teaching difficult. What other uses of his knowledge and abilities might you suggest?
3. What would be your reply if, after you had completed passive ROM on Mr. Boren's left arm, he wrote: "I just ignore that part of my body—it doesn't work anyway"?

REVIEW Stroke

RELATE Link the Concepts and Exemplars

Linking the exemplar of stroke with the concept of thermoregulation:

1. What impact related to thermoregulation might be seen in the patient who has had a massive stroke?
2. You are caring for a patient who had a stroke. The patient requires mechanical ventilation because of inadequate breathing patterns. The patient's temperature is 106.2°F axillary. What are your priorities of care? Will over-the-counter antipyretics be effective? Explain your answer.

Linking the exemplar of stroke with the concept of safety:

3. You are caring for a 56-year-old male patient in the rehabilitation facility who experienced a stroke 6 months ago, resulting in hemiplegia of the left side. What risks to safety do you anticipate for this patient?
4. What interventions, including patient teaching, will you provide to reduce this patient's risk of injury?

READY Go to Volume 3: Clinical Nursing Skills

REFER Go to Pearson MyLab Nursing and eText

- Additional review materials

REFLECT Apply Your Knowledge

Ted Marist is a 68-year-old man who lives with his wife Maggie in a condominium on the sixth floor of a high-rise building. Mr. Marist is recently retired from the police force. Mr. Marist smoked two packs a day until 1 year ago, when his physician discovered a bruit in his right carotid artery. The physician placed Mr. Marist on Coumadin (1.5 mg/day), and his wife insisted that he quit smoking. He still smokes an occasional cigarette when he is out with friends, but he no longer smokes regularly. The Marists have three grown children and five grandchildren.

Mrs. Marist attempts to regulate her husband's diet and encourages him to take a walk with her every night after dinner. The Marists have come to the physician's office today to have Mr. Marist's clotting times checked. Mrs. Marist says she is very concerned because her husband has had two episodes of staring off into space and not responding to her questions. She says his eyes were open but he looked like "there was nobody home behind his eyes" and even when she screamed he did not respond. When the episode stopped, he complained of a headache and insisted on taking a nap, saying he felt much better when he awoke.

1. What do you suspect is causing Mr. Marist's symptoms?
2. How will you respond to Mrs. Marist's concerns when she tells you about these events?
3. What orders do you anticipate receiving from the provider related to these symptoms?
4. Considering Mr. Marist's history, for what type of stroke is he most at risk?

References

Aabideen, K., Ogendele, M., Ahmad, I., & Amegavie, L. (2013). Deep vein thrombosis in children. *Pediatric Reports, 5*(2), 48–49. doi:10.4081/pr.2013.e13

Adams, M. P., Holland, L. N., & Urban, C. (2017). *Pharmacology for nurses: A pathophysiologic approach* (5th ed.). Hoboken, NJ: Pearson Education.

Adler, D. H., & Ellis, A. R. (2015). *Atrial septal defect.* Retrieved from http://emedicine.medscape.com/article/162914-overview

Agha, B. S., Sturm, J. J., Simon, H. K., & Hirsh, D. A. (2013). Pulmonary embolism in the pediatric emergency department. *Pediatrics, 132*(4), 663–667.

Ahn, J. A., Lee, S., & Choi, J. Y. (2014). Comparison of coping strategy and disease knowledge in dyads of parents and their adolescent with congenital heart disease. *Journal of Cardiovascular Nursing, 29*(6), 508–516. doi:10.1079/JCN.0000000000000090

American Academy of Family Physicians. (2014). *Metabolic syndrome: Diagnosis and tests.* Retrieved from http://familydoctor.org/familydoctor/en/diseases-conditions/metabolic-syndrome/diagnosis-tests.html

American Academy of Pediatrics (AAP). (2012). Pediatric sudden cardiac arrest: Section on cardiology and cardiac surgery. *Pediatrics, 129*(4), e1094–e1102.

American College of Cardiology. (2017). New ACC/AHA high blood pressure guidelines lower definition of hypertension. Retrieved from http://www.acc.org/latest-in-cardiology/articles/2017/11/08/11/47/mon-5pm-bp-guideline-aha-2017

American College of Surgeons Committee on Trauma. (2017). *Advanced trauma life support* (10th ed.). Chicago, IL: American College of Surgeons.

American Congress of Obstetricians and Gynecologists (ACOG). (2013a). *Committee opinion. Emergent therapy for acute-onset, severe hypertension with pre-eclampsia or eclampsia.* Retrieved from http://www.acog.org/~/media/Districts/District%20II/PDFs/Optimizing_Protocols_In_OB_HTN_Series_3-%20Version%201.pdf?dmc=1

American Congress of Obstetricians and Gynecologists (ACOG). (2013b). *Pulmonary embolism in pregnancy: Diagnosis and treatment.* Retrieved from http://www.acog.org/~/media/Districts/District%20VIII/PulmonaryEmbolismPregnancy.pdf?dmc=1&ts=20140525T0200225053

American Heart Association (AHA). (n.d.a). *Dilated cardiomyopathy.* Retrieved from http://www.heart.org/idc/groups/heart-public/@wcm/@hcm/documents/downloadable/ucm_312224.pdf

American Heart Association (AHA). (n.d.b). *Hypertrophic cardiomyopathy.* Retrieved from http://www.heart.org/idc/groups/heart-public/@wcm/@hcm/documents/downloadable/ucm_312225.pdf

American Heart Association (AHA). (n.d.c). *Restrictive cardiomyopathy.* Retrieved from http://www.heart.org/idc/groups/heart-public/@wcm/@hcm/documents/downloadable/ucm_312227.pdf

American Heart Association (AHA). (n.d.d). *Therapeutic cardiac catheterizations for children with congenital heart disease.* Retrieved from http://www.heart.org/idc/groups/heart-public/@wcm/@hcm/documents/downloadable/ucm_307680.pdf

American Heart Association (AHA). (2013a). *Statistical fact sheet: Congenital cardiovascular defects.* Retrieved from https://www.heart.org/idc/groups/heart-public/@wcm/@sop/@smd/documents/downloadable/ucm_319830.pdf

American Heart Association (AHA). (2013b). *Stroke treatments.* Retrieved from http://strokeassociation.org/STROKEORG/AboutStroke/Treatment/Stroke-Treatments_UCM_310892_Article.jsp

American Heart Association (AHA). (2014a). *Know your risk factors for high blood pressure.* Retrieved from http://www.heart.org/HEARTORG/Conditions/HighBloodPressure/UnderstandYourRiskforHighBloodPressure/Understand-Your-Risk-for-High-Blood-Pressure_UCM_002052_Article.jsp#.Vnf5Xr_2uzQ

American Heart Association (AHA). (2014b). *Symptoms, diagnosis, and monitoring of arrhythmia.* Retrieved from http://www.heart.org/HEARTORG/Conditions/Arrhythmia/SymptomsDiagnosisMonitoringofArrhythmia/Symptoms-Diagnosis-Monitoring-of-Arrhythmia_UCM_002025_Article.jsp#.VumM-uZQuzR

American Heart Association (AHA). (2014c). *Understand your risk for cardiac arrest.* Retrieved from http://www.heart.org/HEARTORG/Conditions/More/CardiacArrest/Understand-Your-Risk-for-Cardiac-Arrest_UCM_307909_Article.jsp#.VumRPOZQuzR

American Heart Association (AHA). (2014d). *Prevention and treatment of PAD.* Retrieved from http://www.heart.org/HEARTORG/Conditions/More/PeripheralArteryDisease/Prevention-and-Treatment-of-PAD_UCM_301308_Article.jsp#

American Heart Association (AHA). (2014e). *Knowing no bounds: Stroke in infants, children, and youth.* Retrieved from https://www.heart.org/idc/groups/heart-public/@wcm/@adv/documents/downloadable/ucm_462442.pdf

American Heart Association (AHA). (2015a). *What is excessive blood clotting (hypercoagulation)?* Retrieved from http://www.heart.org/HEARTORG/Conditions/More/What-Is-Excessive-Blood-Clotting-Hypercoagulation_UCM_448768_Article.jsp#

American Heart Association (AHA). (2015b). *Cardiomyopathy in adults.* Retrieved from http://www.heart.org/HEARTORG/Conditions/More/Cardiomyopathy/Cardiomyopathy_UCM_444459_SubHomePage.jsp

American Heart Association (AHA). (2015c). *Highlights of the 2015 American Heart Association guidelines update for CPR and ECC.* Retrieved from https://eccguidelines.heart.org/wp-content/uploads/2015/10/2015-AHA-Guidelines-Highlights-English.pdf

American Heart Association (AHA). (2015d). *Dilated cardiomyopathy (DCM).* Retrieved from http://www.heart.org/HEARTORG/Conditions/More/Cardiomyopathy/Dilated-Cardiomyopathy-DCM_UCM_444187_Article.jsp

American Heart Association (AHA). (2015e). *Pediatric cardiomyopathies.* Retrieved from http://www.heart.org/HEARTORG/Conditions/More/CardiovascularConditionsofChildhood/Pediatric-Cardiomyopathies_UCM_312219_Article.jsp#

American Heart Association (AHA). (2015f). *Understand your risk for congenital heart defects.* Retrieved from http://www.heart.org/HEARTORG/Conditions/CongenitalHeartDefects/UnderstandYourRiskforCongenitalHeartDefects/Understand-Your-Risk-for-Congenital-Heart-Defects_UCM_001219_Article.jsp#.Vmhsbr_2v3s

American Heart Association (AHA). (2015g). *Detection of a heart defect in the fetus.* Retrieved from http://www.heart.org/HEARTORG/Conditions/CongenitalHeartDefects/SymptomsDiagnosisofCongenitalHeartDefects/Detection-of-a-Heart-Defect-in-the-Fetus_UCM_315673_Article.jsp#.VnB0m7_2uzR

American Heart Association (AHA). (2015h). *Common tests for congenital heart defects.* Retrieved from http://www.heart.org/HEARTORG/Conditions/CongenitalHeartDefects/SymptomsDiagnosis ofCongenitalHeartDefects/Common-Tests-for-Congenital-Heart-Defects_UCM_307412_Article.jsp

American Heart Association (AHA). (2015i). Part 9: Acute coronary syndromes. In *2015 American Heart Association Guidelines for CPR and ECC.* Retrieved from https://eccguidelines.heart.org/index.php/circulation/cpr-ecc-guidelines-2/part-9-acute-coronary-syndromes/

American Heart Association (AHA). (2015j). *Classes of heart failure.* Retrieved from http://www.heart.org/HEARTORG/Conditions/HeartFailure/AboutHeartFailure/Classes-of-Heart-Failure_UCM_306328_Article.jsp

American Heart Association (AHA). (2015k). *African-Americans and heart disease, stroke.* Retrieved from http://www.heart.org/HEARTORG/Conditions/More/MyHeartandStrokeNews/African-Americans-and-Heart-Disease_UCM_444863_Article.jsp

American Heart Association (AHA). (2015l). *Heart failure in children and adolescents.* Retrieved from http://www.heart.org/HEARTORG/Conditions/HeartFailure/AboutHeartFailure/Heart-Failure-in-Children-and-Adolescents_UCM_311919_Article.jsp#

American Heart Association (AHA). (2015m). *African Americans and cardiovascular diseases: Statistical fact sheet, 2013 update.* Retrieved from http://www.heart.org/idc/groups/heart-public/@wcm/@sop/@smd/documents/downloadable/ucm_319568.pdf

American Heart Association (AHA). (2015n). *Changes you can make to manage high blood pressure.* Retrieved from http://www.heart.org/HEARTORG/Conditions/HighBloodPressure/PreventionTreatmentofHighBloodPressure/Prevention-Treatment-of-High-Blood-Pressure_UCM_002054_Article.jsp#

American Heart Association (AHA). (2015o). *Understanding blood pressure readings.* Retrieved from http://www.heart.org/HEARTORG/Conditions/HighBloodPressure/AboutHighBloodPressure/Understanding-Blood-Pressure-Readings_UCM_301764_Article.jsp#.VruLMfkrLIV

American Heart Association (AHA). (2015p). *2010 American Heart Association guidelines for cardiopulmonary resuscitation and emergency cardiovascular care science.* Retrieved from https://circ.ahajournals.org/content/122/18_suppl_3/S639.full

American Heart Association (AHA). (2015q). *How high blood pressure can lead to stroke.* Retrieved from http://www.heart.org/HEARTORG/Conditions/HighBloodPressure/WhyBloodPressureMatters/Stroke-and-High-Blood-Pressure_UCM_301824_Article.jsp

American Heart Association (AHA). (2015r). *Pediatric stroke.* Retrieved from http://www.strokeassociation.org/STROKEORG/AboutStroke/StrokeInChildren/Stroke-In-Children_UCM_308543_SubHomePage.jsp

American Heart Association (AHA). (2016a). *Monitoring your blood pressure at home.* Retrieved from http://www.heart.org/HEARTORG/Conditions/HighBloodPressure/SymptomsDiagnosisMonitoringofHighBloodPressure/How-to-Monitor-and-Record-Your-Blood-Pressure_UCM_303323_Article.jsp#

American Heart Association (AHA). (2016b). *Heart disease, stroke, and research statistics at-a-glance.* Retrieved from http://www.heart.org/idc/groups/ahamah-public/@wcm/@sop/@smd/documents/downloadable/ucm_480086.pdf

American Heart Association (AHA). (2016c). *Changes you can make to lower your blood pressure.* Retrieved from: http://www.heart.org/HEARTORG/Conditions/HighBloodPressure/PreventionTreatmentofHighBloodPressure/Prevention-Treatment-of-High-Blood-Pressure_UCM_002054_Article.jsp#

American Stroke Association. (2015). *What is stroke?* Retrieved from http://www.strokeassociation.org/STROKEORG/AboutStroke/About-Stroke_UCM_308529_SubHomePage.jsp

Anderson, D., Larson, D., Bluhm, J., Charipar, R., Fiscus, L., Hanson, M., . . . Zinkel, A. (2012). *Institute for Clinical Systems Improvement: Diagnosis and initial treatment of ischemic stroke.* Retrieved from https://www.icsi.org/_asset/xql3xv/Stroke.pdf

Anthony, J., & Sliwa, K. (2015). Decompensated heart failure in pregnancy. *Cardiac Failure Review, 2*(1). Retrieved from https://www.radcliffecardiology.com/articles/decompensated-heart-failure-pregnancy

Arnold, J. M. O. (2015). *Dilated cardiomyopathy.* Retrieved from http://www.merckmanuals.com/home/heart-and-blood-vessel-disorders/cardiomyopathy/dilated-cardiomyopathy

August, P. (2015). Management of hypertension in pregnant and postpartum women. *UpToDate.* Retrieved from http://www.uptodate.com/contents/management-of-hypertension-in-pregnant-and-postpartum-women?source=machineLearning&search=hypertension +in +pregnancy&selectedTitle=1%7E150&sectionRank=1&anchor=H53704432#H53704432

August, P., & Sibai, B. M. (2015). Preeclampsia: Clinical features and diagnosis. *UpToDate.* Retrieved from http://www.uptodate.com/contents/preeclampsia-clinicalfeaturesanddiagnosis?source=machineLearning&search=preeclampsia&selectedTitle=1%7E150&sectionRank=1&anchor=H6#H6

Baldisseri, M. R., & Sharma, S. (2014). *Shock and pregnancy.* Retrieved from http://emedicine.medscape.com/article/169450-overview#showall

Barton, J. R., & Sibai, B. M. (2012). Severe sepsis and septic shock in pregnancy. *Obstetrics and Gynecology, 120*(3), 689–706.

Bertoletti, J., Marx, G. C., Hattge, S. P., & Pellanda, L. C. (2014). Quality of life and congenital heart disease in childhood and adolescence. *Arquivos Brasileiros de Cardiologia, 102*(2), 192–198. doi:10.5935/abc.20130244

Bhatt, A. B., Foster, E., Kuehl, K., Alpert, J., Brabeck, S., Crumb, S., . . . Tseng, Z. H. (2015). Congenital heart disease in the older adult: A scientific statement from the American Heart Association. *Circulation, 131,* 1884–1931. doi:10.1161/CIR.0000000000000204

Bhimji, S., & Mancini, M. C. (2015). *Tetralogy of Fallot.* Retrieved from http://emedicine.medscape.com/article/2035949-overview

Biban, P., Gaffuri, M., Spaggiari, S., Zaglia, F., Serra, A., & Santuz, P. (2012). Early recognition and management of septic shock in children. *Pediatric Reports, 4*(1), e13.

BMJ Best Practice. (2015). Revised Geneva Criteria for pulmonary embolism. Retrieved from http://bestpractice.bmj.com/best-practice/monograph/116/diagnosis/criteria.html

Buckner, T. W., & Key, N. S. (2012). Clinical update: Venous thrombosis in blacks. *Circulation, 125,* 837–839.

Burke, A. P., & Butany, J. (2015). *Arrhythmogenic right ventricular cardiomyopathy pathology.* Retrieved from http://emedicine.medscape.com/article/2017949-overview#a1

Calderon, J., & Bellinger, D. C. (2015). Executive function deficits in congenital heart disease: Why is intervention important? *Cardiology in the Young, 25*(7), 1238–1246. doi:10.1017/S1047951115001134

Cardiomyopathy UK. (2015). *Study of older people with hypertrophic cardiomyopathy.* Retrieved from http://www.cardiomyopathy.org/news--media/latest-news/post/82-study-of-older-people-with-hypertrophic-cardiomyopathy

Carson, M. (2014). *Peripartum cardiomyopathy.* Retrieved from http://emedicine.medscape.com/article/153153-overview

Cassidy, A. R., White, M. T., DeMaso, D. R., Newburger, J. W., & Bellinger, D. C. (2015). Executive function in children and adolescents with critical cyanotic congenital heart disease. *Journal of the International Neuropsychological Society, 21*(1), 34–49. doi:10.1017/S1355617714001027

Centers for Disease Control and Prevention (CDC). (2014a). *Facts about pulmonary atresia.* Retrieved from http://www.cdc.gov/ncbddd/heartdefects/pulmonaryatresia.html

Centers for Disease Control and Prevention (CDC). (2014b). *Facts about transposition of the great arteries.* Retrieved from http://www.cdc.gov/ncbddd/heartdefects/tga.html.

Centers for Disease Control and Prevention (CDC). (2014c). *Facts about total anomalous pulmonary venous return or TAPVR.* Retrieved from http://www.cdc.gov/ncbddd/heartdefects/tapvr.html

Centers for Disease Control and Prevention (CDC). (2014d). *Peripheral arterial disease (PAD) fact sheet.* Retrieved from http://www.cdc.gov/dhdsp/data_statistics/fact_sheets/fs_pad.htm

Centers for Disease Control and Prevention (CDC). (2014e). *Preventing stroke: Control medical conditions.* Retrieved from http://www.cdc.gov/stroke/medical_conditions.htm

Centers for Disease Control and Prevention (CDC). (2015a). *High blood pressure facts.* Retrieved from http://www.cdc.gov/bloodpressure/facts.htm

Centers for Disease Control and Prevention (CDC). (2015b). *Heart disease facts.* Retrieved from http://www.cdc.gov/heartdisease/facts.htm

Centers for Disease Control and Prevention (CDC). (2015c). *Heart failure fact sheet.* Retrieved from http://www.cdc.gov/dhdsp/data_statistics/fact_sheets/fs_heart_failure.htm

Centers for Disease Control and Prevention (CDC). (2015d). *Facts about hypoplastic left heart syndrome.* Retrieved from http://www.cdc.gov/ncbddd/heartdefects/hlhs.html

Centers for Disease Control and Prevention (CDC). (2015e). *Congenital heart defects (CHDs).* Retrieved from http://www.cdc.gov/ncbddd/heartdefects/data.html

Centers for Disease Control and Prevention (CDC). (2015f). *Living with a congenital heart defect.* Retrieved from http://www.cdc.gov/ncbddd/heartdefects/living.html

Centers for Disease Control and Prevention (CDC). (2015g). *Heart attack.* Retrieved from http://www.cdc.gov/heartdisease/heart_attack.htm

Centers for Disease Control and Prevention (CDC). (2015h). *Physical activity for a healthy weight: Why is physical activity important?* Retrieved from http://www.cdc.gov/healthyweight/physical_activity/index.html

Centers for Disease Control and Prevention (CDC). (2015i). *Venous thromboembolism (blood clots).* Retrieved from http://www.cdc.gov/ncbddd/dvt/facts.html

Centers for Disease Control and Prevention (CDC). (2015j). *Understanding blood pressure readings.* Retrieved from http://www.heart.org/HEARTORG/Conditions/HighBloodPressure/AboutHighBloodPressure/Understanding-Blood-Pressure-Readings_UCM_301764_Article.jsp#.VruLMfkrLIV

Centers for Disease Control and Prevention (CDC). (2015k). *Venous thromboembolism (blood clots).* Retrieved from http://www.cdc.gov/ncbddd/dvt/facts.html

Centers for Disease Control and Prevention (CDC). (2015l). *Stroke facts.* Retrieved from http://www.cdc.gov/stroke/facts.htm

Charpie, J. R., Maher, K. O., & Berul, C. I. (2015). *Transposition of the great arteries.* Retrieved from http://emedicine.medscape.com/article/900574-overview

Children's Cardiomyopathy Council. (2015). *About the disease.* Retrieved from http://www.childrenscardiomyopathy.org/site/causes.php

Children's Hospital Nashville. (2016). *Disseminated intravascular coagulation.* Retrieved from http://thechildrenshospitalnashville.com/hl/?/96584/Disseminated-Intravascular-Coagulation

Clarke, R. H., Gbadehan, E., Dim, U. R., & Ferraro, R. M. (2015). *Stress-induced gastritis.* Retrieved from http://emedicine.medscape.com/article/176319-overview#showall

Cleveland Clinic. (2013). *What do cholesterol numbers mean?* Retrieved from https://my.clevelandclinic.org/health/diseases_conditions/hic_Cholesterol/hic_what_do_cholesterol_numbers_mean

Cleveland Clinic. (2014). *Checking your blood pressure at home.* Retrieved from https://my.clevelandclinic.org/health/diseases_conditions/hic_Hypertension_High_Blood_Pressure/hic_Checking_Your_Blood_Pressure_at_Home

Cleveland Clinic. (2015a). *Metabolic syndrome.* Retrieved from https://my.clevelandclinic.org/health/diseases_conditions/hic_Metabolic_Syndrome

Cleveland Clinic. (2015b). *Women and abnormal heart beats.* Retrieved from http://my.clevelandclinic.org/services/heart/disorders/arrhythmia/women-abnormal-heart-beats

Cleveland Clinic. (2015c). *Sudden cardiac death (sudden cardiac arrest).* Retrieved from http://my.clevelandclinic.org/services/heart/disorders/arrhythmia/sudden-cardiac-death

Cleveland Clinic. (2016a). *Treatments and procedures: Antioxidants, vitamin E, beta carotene, and cardiovascular disease.* Retrieved from http://my.clevelandclinic.org/services/heart/services/vitamin_e

Cleveland Clinic. (2016b). *Drugs, devices and supplements: Herbal supplement safety.* Retrieved from http://my.clevelandclinic.org/health/drugs_devices_supplements/hic-herbal-supplements/hic-herbal-supplement-safety

Copstead, L. C., & Banasik, J. L. (2013). *Pathophysiology* (5th ed.). St. Louis, MO: Saunders.

Cunningham, F. G., Leveno, K. J., Bloom, S. L., Spong, C. Y., Dashe, J., Hoffman, B. L., . . . Sheffield, J. S. (2014). *Williams obstetrics* (23rd ed.). New York, NY: McGraw-Hill.

Cuyjet, A. B., & Akinboboye, O. (2014). Acute heart failure in the African American patient. *Journal of Cardiac Failure, 20*(7), 533–540. doi:10.1016/j.cardfail.2014.04.018

De Caen, A. R., Berg, M. D., Chameides, L., Gooden, C. K., Hickey, R. W., Scott, H. F., . . . Samson, R. A. (2015). Part 12: Pediatric advanced life support: 2015 American Heart Association Guidelines Update for Cardiopulmonary Resuscitation and Emergency Cardiovascular Care. *Circulation, 132,* 5526–5542.

DeCara, J. M., Lang, R. M., & Foley, M. R. (2014). *Management of heart failure during pregnancy.* Retrieved from http://www.uptodate.com/contents/management-of-heart-failure-during-pregnancy

Demaerschalk, B. M., Kleindorfer, D. O., Adeoye, O. M., Demchuk, A. M., Fugate, J. E., Grotta, J. C., . . . Smith, E. E. (2016). Scientific rationale for the inclusion and exclusion criteria for intravenous alteplase in acute ischemic stroke. *Stroke, 47,* 581–641.

Deo, R., & Albert, C. M. (2012). *Sudden cardiac death: Epidemiology and genetics of sudden cardiac death. Circulation, 125,* 620–637. doi:10.1161/CIRCULATIONAHA.111.023383

Dijk, F. N., Curtin, J., Lord, D., & Fitzgerald, D. A. (2012). Pulmonary embolism in children. *Paediatric Respiratory Reviews, 13*(2), 112–122.

Dobromirski, M., & Cohen, A. T. (2012). How I manage venous thromboembolism risk in hospitalized medical patients. *Blood, 120*(8), 1562–1569. doi:10.1182/blood-2012-03-0378901

Dumitru, I., & Baker, M. M. (2016). *Heart failure.* Retrieved from http://emedicine.medscape.com/article/163062-overview

Emergency Care Institute New South Wales. (2016). *Pulmonary thromboembolism (PE)—Evaluation in the pregnant patient.* Retrieved from http://www.ecinsw.com.au/PE-pregnant

Enga, K. F., Rye-Holmboe, I., Hald, E. M., Løchen, M. L., Mathiesen, E. B., Njølstad, I., . . . Hansen, J. B. (2014). Atrial fibrillation and future risk of venous thromboembolism: The Tromsø study. *Journal of Thrombosis and Haemostasis, 31,* 10–16. doi:10.1111/jth.12762

Englert, N. C., & Ross, C. (2015). The older adult experiencing sepsis. *Critical Care Nursing Quarterly, 38*(2), 175–181.

Fender, E. A., Henrikson, C. A., & Tereshchenko, L. (2014). Racial differences in sudden cardiac death. *Journal of Electrocardiology, 47*(6), 815–818.

Flugman, S. L., & Clark, R. A. (2016). *Statis dermatitis.* Retrieved from http://emedicine.medscape.com/article/1084813-overview

Framingham Heart Study (FHS). (2015). *Welcome to the Framingham Heart Study.* Retrieved from http://www.framinghamheartstudy.org

Geldhof, V., Vandenbriele, C., Verhamme, P., & Vanassche, T. (2014). Venous thromboembolism in the elderly: Efficacy and safety of non-VKA oral anticoagulants. *Thrombosis Journal, 12*(21). doi:10.1186/1477-9560-12-21

Gentry, M. S., Dias, J. K., Luis, A., Patel, R., Thornton, J., & Reed, G. L. (2010). African-American women have a higher risk for developing peripartum cardiomyopathy. *Journal of the American College of Cardiology, 55*(7), 654–659. doi:10.1016/j.jacc.2009.09.043

Ginde, S., Lam, J., Hill, G. D., Cohen, S., Woods, R. K., Mitchell, M. E., . . . Earing, M. G. (2015). Long-term outcomes after surgical repair of complete atrioventricular septal defect. *Journal of Thoracic and Cardiovascular Surgery, 150*(2), 369–374.

Girouard, H. (Ed.). (2016). *Hypertension and the brain as an end-organ target.* Basel, Switzerland: Springer International Publishing.

Givertz, M. M. (2013). Peripartum cardiomyopathy. *Circulation, 127,* 622–626. doi:10.1161/CIRCULATIONAHA.113.001851

Gordon, M. C. (2012). Maternal physiology. In S. G. Gabbe, J. R. Niebyl, & J. L. Simpson (Eds.), *Obstetrics: Normal and problem pregnancies* (6th ed.). Philadelphia, PA: Saunders.

Goswarmi, V. J., Suleman, A., Sander, G. E., Celebi, M. N., & Wilklow, F. E. (2014). *Dilated cardiomyopathy.* Retrieved from http://emedicine.medscape.com/article/152696-overview

Griffin, B. P., Kapadia, S. R., & Rimmerman, C. M. (2013). *The Cleveland Clinic cardiology board review* (2nd ed.). Philadelphia, PA: Lippincott Williams & Wilkins.

Gupta, S., & Sinha, S. K. (2014). *Shock and hypotension in the newborn.* Retrieved from http://emedicine.medscape.com/article/979128-overview

Herdman, T. H. & Kamitsuru, S. (Eds.). *Nursing Diagnoses—Definitions and Classification 2015–2017.* Copyright © 2014, 1994–2014 NANDA International. Used by arrangement with John Wiley & Sons, Inc. Companion website: www.wiley.com/go/nursingdiagnoses.

Hickey, J. V. (2013). *The clinical practice of neurological and neurosurgical nursing* (7th ed.). Philadelphia, PA: Lippincott Williams & Wilkins.

Hockenberry, M. J., & Wilson, D. (2014). *Wong's nursing care of infants and children.* St. Louis, MO: Mosby.

Howard, S. C. (2015). *Pediatric thromboembolism.* Retrieved from http://emedicine.medscape.com/article/959501-overview#a5

Huether, S. E., & McCance, K. L. (2012). *Understanding pathophysiology* (5th ed.). St. Louis, MO: Mosby Elsevier.

Hull, C. M., & Harris, J. A. (2013). Venous thromboembolism and marathon athletes. *Circulation, 128,* 469–471. doi:10.1161/CIRCULATIONAHA.113.004586

Hurd, R. (2014). *Drug-induced hypertension.* Retrieved from https://www.nlm.nih.gov/medlineplus/ency/article/000155.htm

Indiana Hemophilia & Thrombosis Center (IHTC). (2012). *Blood clot formation (thrombosis).* Retrieved from http://www.ihtc.org/patient/blood-disorders/clotting-disorders/thrombosis/

International Alliance for Pediatric Stroke (IAPS). (2014). *Get the facts about pediatric stroke.* Retrieved from http://iapediatricstroke.org/about_pediatric_stroke.aspx

International Diabetes Federation. (2015). *IDF definition of the metabolic syndrome: Frequently asked questions.* Retrieved from http://www.idf.org/metabolic-syndrome/faqs

International Pediatric Hypertension Association (IPHA). (2016). *Welcome to IPHA!* Retrieved from http://www.iphapediatrichypertension.org/

James, A. (n.d.). *Women's health.* Retrieved from https://www.stoptheclot.org/learn_more/womens_health_faq.htm

James, P. A., Oparil, S., Carter, B. L., Cushman, W. C., Dennison-Himmelfarb, C., Handler, J., . . . Ortiz, E. (2014). 2014 Evidence-based guideline for the management of high blood pressure in adults report from the panel members appointed to the Eighth Joint National Committee (JNC 8). *JAMA, 311*(5), 507–520.

Jauch, E. C., & Stettler, B. (2015). *Ischemic stroke.* Retrieved from http://emedicine.medscape.com/article/1916852-overview

Jeejeebhoy, F. M., & Morrison, L. J. (2013). Maternal cardiac arrest: A practical and comprehensive review. *Emergency Medical International, 2013,* 274814.

Jeejeebhoy, F. M., Zelop, C. M., Lipman, S., Carvalho, B., Joglar, J., Mhyre, J. M., . . . Callaway, C. W. (2015). Cardiac arrest in pregnancy: A scientific statement from the American Heart Association. *Circulation, 132,* 1747–1773.

Johns Hopkins. (2013). *Study sheds light on risk of life-threatening blood clots in hospitalized children.* Retrieved from http://www.hopkinsmedicine.org/news/media/releases/study_sheds_light_on_risk_of_life_threatening_blood_clots_in_hospitalized_children

Kakkar, A. K., & Rushton-Smith, S. K. (2013). Incidence of venous thromboembolism in orthopedic surgery. In J. V. Llau (Ed.), *Thromboembolism in orthopedic surgery* (pp. 11–17). London, United Kingdom: Springer-Verlag.

King, T., Brucker, M. C., Kriebs, J. M., Ofahey, J. O., Gegor, C. L., & Varney, H. (2015). *Varney's midwifery* (5th ed.). Burlington, MA: Jones & Bartlett.

Kline, J. A., Mitchell, A. M., Kabrhel, C., Richman, P. B., & Courtney, D. M. (2004). Clinical criteria to prevent unnecessary diagnostic testing in emergency department patients with suspected pulmonary embolism. *Journal of Thrombosis and Haemostasis, 2*(8), 1247–1255.

Kolecki, P., & Menckhoff, C. R. (2014). *Hypovolemic shock clinical presentation.* Retrieved from http://emedicine.medscape.com/article/760145-clinical#showall

Kumar, V., Abbas, A. K., & Aster, J. C. (2013). *Robbins basic pathology* (9th ed.). Philadelphia, PA: Elsevier Saunders.

Kwak, S. M., Myung, S. K., Lee, Y. J., & Seo, H. G. (2012). Efficacy of omega-3 fatty acid supplements (eicosapentaenoic acid and docosahexaenoic acid) in the secondary prevention of cardiovascular disease: A meta-analysis of randomized, double-blind, placebo-controlled trials. *Archives of Internal Medicine, 172*(9), 686–694.

Ladewig, P. W., London, M. L., & Davidson, M. C. (2013). *Contemporary maternal-newborn nursing care* (8th ed.). Reprinted and electronically reproduced by permission of Pearson Education, Inc., New York, NY.

Lauderdale, J. (2012). Transcultural perspectives in childbearing. In M. M. Andrews & J. C. Boyle (Eds.), *Transcultural concepts in nursing care* (6th ed., pp. 91–122). Philadelphia, PA: Lippincott, Williams, & Wilkins.

Lazzarini, V., Mentz, R. J., Fiuzat, M., Metra, M., & O'Connor, C. M. (2013). Heart failure in elderly patients. *European Journal of Heart Failure, 15*(7), 717–723.

Lee, E. Y., Tse, S. K. S., Zurakowski, D., Johnson, V. M., Lee, N. J., Tracy, D. A., & Boiselle, P. M. (2012). Children suspected of having pulmonary embolism: Multidetector CT pulmonary angiography—thromboembolic risk factors and implications for appropriate use. *Radiology, 262*(1). Retrieved from http://pubs.rsna.org/doi/full/10.1148/radiol.11111056

Leffert, L. R., Clancy, C. R., Bateman, B. T., Bryant, A. S., & Kuklina, E. V. (2015). Hypertensive disorders and pregnancy-related stroke: Frequency, trends, risk factors, and outcomes. *Obstetrics and Gynecology, 125*(1), 124–131.

Lehne, R. A. (2013). *Pharmacology for nursing care* (8th ed.). St. Louis, MO: Elsevier Saunders.

Levi, M. M., & Schmaier, A. H. (2015). *Disseminated intravascular coagulation.* Retrieved from http://emedicine.medscape.com/article/199627-overview

Liu, L., Zheng, H., Wang, D. Z., Wang, Y., Hussain, M., Sun, H., . . . Wang, Y. (2014). Risk assessment of deep-vein thrombosis after acute stroke: A prospective study using clinical factors. *CNS Neuroscience & Therapeutics, 20*(5), 403–410. doi:10.1111/cns.12227

Lowenthal, M. A. (2014). *Pulmonic valvular stenosis*. Retrieved from http://emedicine.medscape.com/article/759890-overview

Madhur, M. S., Riaz, K., Dreisbach, A. W., & Harrison, D. G. (2014). *Hypertension*. Retrieved from http://emedicine.medscape.com/article/241381-overview

Mancia, G., & Grassi, G. (2014). The autonomic nervous system and hypertension. *Circulation Research, 114*, 1804–1814. doi:10.1161/CIRCRESAHA.114.302524

Maron, B. J., Rowin, E. J., Casey, S. A., Haas, T. S., Chan, R. H. M., . . . Maron, M. S. (2013). Risk stratification and outcome of patients with hypertrophic cardiomyopathy ≥ 60 years of age. *Circulation, 127*, 585–593. doi:10.1161/CIRCULATIONAHA.112.136085

Marshall, A. (2015). *Hypoplastic left heart syndrome*. Retrieved from http://www.uptodate.com/contents/hypoplastic-left-heart-syndrome

Mayo Clinic. (2014a). *Von Willebrand disease*. Retrieved from http://www.mayoclinic.org/diseases-conditions/von-willebrand-disease/basics/definition/con-20030195

Mayo Clinic. (2014b). *Hemophilia*. Retrieved from http://www.mayoclinic.org/diseases-conditions/hemophilia/basics/definition/con-20029824

Mayo Clinic. (2014c). *Cardiovascular perfusionist*. Retrieved from http://www.mayo.edu/mshs/careers/cardiovascular-perfusionist

Mayo Clinic. (2014d). *Orthostatic hypotension (postural hypotension): Definition. Try these steps to reduce stress*. Retrieved from http://www.mayoclinic.org/diseases-conditions/orthostatic-hypotension/basics/definition/con-20031255

Mayo Clinic. (2014e). *Metabolic syndrome: Tests and diagnosis*. Retrieved from http://www.mayoclinic.org/diseases-conditions/metabolic-syndrome/basics/tests-diagnosis/con-20027243

Mayo Clinic. (2014f). *Disease and conditions: Deep vein thrombosis (DVT)*. Retrieved from http://www.mayoclinic.org/diseases-conditions/deep-vein-thrombosis/basics/definition/con-20031922

Mayo Clinic. (2014g). *Preeclampsia: Definition*. Retrieved from http://www.mayoclinic.org/diseases-conditions/preeclampsia/basics/definition/con-20031644

Mayo Clinic. (2014h). *Heart arrhythmia: Overview*. Retrieved from http://www.mayoclinic.org/diseases-conditions/heart-arrhythmia/home/ovc-20188123

Mayo Clinic. (2014i). *Sudden death in young people: Heart problems often blamed*. Retrieved from http://www.mayoclinic.org/sudden-death/art-20047571

Mayo Clinic. (2014j). *Deep vein thrombosis (DVT): Risk factors*. Retrieved from http://www.mayoclinic.org/diseases-conditions/deep-vein-thrombosis/basics/risk-factors/con-20031922

Mayo Clinic. (2014k). *Cardiogenic shock: Prevention*. Retrieved from http://www.mayoclinic.org/diseases-conditions/cardiogenic-shock/basics/prevention/con-20034247

Mayo Clinic. (2015a). *Arteriosclerosis/atherosclerosis*. Retrieved from http://www.mayoclinic.org/diseases-conditions/arteriosclerosis-atherosclerosis/manage/ptc-20167079

Mayo Clinic. (2015b). *High blood pressure (hypertension)*. Retrieved from http://www.mayoclinic.org/diseases-conditions/high-blood-pressure/basics/definition/con-20019580

Mayo Clinic. (2015c). *Cardiomyopathy: Definition*. Retrieved from http://www.mayoclinic.org/diseases-conditions/cardiomyopathy/basics/definition/con-20026819

Mayo Clinic. (2015d). *Diseases and conditions: Pulmonary embolism*. Retrieved from http://www.mayoclinic.org/diseases-conditions/pulmonary-embolism/basics/definition/con-20022849

Mayo Clinic. (2015e). *Diseases and conditions: Heart failure*. Retrieved from http://www.mayoclinic.org/diseases-conditions/heart-failure/basics/definition/con-20029801

Mayo Clinic. (2015f). *Tests and procedures: Heart transplant*. Retrieved from http://www.mayoclinic.org/tests-procedures/heart-transplant/basics/results/prc-20014050

Mayo Clinic. (2015g). *High blood pressure in children*. Retrieved from http://www.mayoclinic.org/diseases-conditions/high-blood-pressure-in-children/basics/definition/con-20033799

Mayo Clinic. (2015h). *Pulmonary embolism: Prevention*. Retrieved from http://www.mayoclinic.org/diseases-conditions/pulmonary-embolism/basics/prevention/con-20022849

Mayo Clinic. (2015i). *Stroke: Self-management*. Retrieved from http://www.mayoclinic.org/diseases-conditions/stroke/manage/ptc-20117267

Mayo Clinic. (2016a). *Disease and conditions: Congenital heart defects in adults*. Retrieved from http://www.mayoclinic.org/diseases-conditions/congenital-heart-disease/basics/definition/con-20034800

Mayo Clinic. (2016b). *Disease and conditions: Congenital heart defects in children*. Retrieved from http://www.mayoclinic.org/diseases-conditions/congenital-heart-defects/basics/definition/con-20034017

Mayo Clinic. (2016c). *High cholesterol: Diagnosis*. Retrieved from http://www.mayoclinic.org/diseases-conditions/high-blood-cholesterol/diagnosis-treatment/diagnosis/dxc-20181913

Mayo Clinic. (2016d). *Sepsis: Symptoms and causes*. Retrieved from http://www.mayoclinic.org/diseases-conditions/sepsis/symptoms-causes/dxc-20169787

Mazoyer, B., Zago, L., Jobard, G., Crivello, F., Joliot, M., Perchey, G., . . . Tzourio-Mazoyer, N. (2014). Gaussian mixture modeling of hemispheric lateralization for language in a large sample of healthy individuals balanced for handedness. *PLoS ONE, 9*(6), e101165.

McDonald-McGinn, D. M., Emanuel, B. S., & Zacai, E. H. (2013). *22q11.2 deletion syndrome*. Retrieved from http://www.ncbi.nlm.nih.gov/books/NBK1523

McElhinney, D. B., Wernovsky, G., & Alejos, J. C. (2015). *Transposition of the great arteries*. Retrieved from http://emedicine.medscape.com/article/900574-overview

MedlinePlus. (2013). *Disseminated intravascular coagulation (DIC)*. Retrieved from https://www.nlm.nih.gov/medlineplus/ency/article/000573.htm

MedlinePlus. (2014a). *Peripartum cardiomyopathy*. Retrieved from http://www.nlm.nih.gov/medlineplus/ency/article/000188.htm

MedlinePlus. (2014b). *Congenital heart defects*. Retrieved from https://www.nlm.nih.gov/medlineplus/congenitalheartdefects.html#cat8

MedlinePlus. (2015). *Congenital heart defect—corrective surgery*. Retrieved from https://www.nlm.nih.gov/medlineplus/ency/article/002948.htm

Medscape. (2015). *Drugs & diseases: Warfarin (Rx)*. Retrieved from http://reference.medscape.com/drug/coumadin-jantoven-warfarin-342182#0

Mohebi-Nejad, A., & Bikdeli, B. (2014). Omega-3 supplements and cardiovascular diseases. *Tanaffos, 13*(1), 6–14.

Morton, P. G., & Fontaine, D. K. (2013). *Critical care nursing: A holistic approach*. New York, NY: Wolters Kluwer/Lippincott Williams & Wilkins.

Mulkey, S. B., Swearingen, C. J., Melguizo, M. S., Reeves, R. N., Rowell, J. A., Gibson, N., . . . Kaiser, J. R. (2014). Academic proficiency in children following early congenital heart disease surgery. *Pediatric Cardiology, 35*(2), 344–352. doi:10.1007/s00246-013-0781-6

Mustafa, R., Ahmed, S., Gupta, A., & Venuto, R. (2012). A comprehensive review of hypertension in pregnancy. *Journal of Pregnancy, 2012*, 105918.

Naderi, S., & Raymond, R. (2014). *Pregnancy and heart disease*. Retrieved from http://www.clevelandclinicmeded.com/medicalpubs/diseasemanagement/cardiology/pregnancy-and-heart-disease/

Nakimuli, A., Chazara, O., Byamugisha, J., Elliott, A. M., Kaleebu, P., Mirembe, F., & Moffett, A. (2014). Pregnancy, parturition and preeclampsia in women of African ancestry. *American Journal of Obstetrics and Gynecology, 210*(6), 510–520.

Nasa, P., Juneja, D., & Singh, O. (2012). Severe sepsis and septic shock in the elderly: An overview. *World Journal of Critical Care Medicine, 1*(1), 23–30.

National Center for Complementary and Integrative Health (NCCIH). (2016a). *Antioxidants: In depth*. Retrieved from https://nccih.nih.gov/health/antioxidants/introduction.htm

National Center for Complementary and Integrative Health (NCCIH). (2016b). *Chelation for coronary heart disease*. Retrieved from https://nccih.nih.gov/health/chelation

National Heart, Lung, and Blood Institute (NHLBI). (2005). *Your guide to lowering your cholesterol with TLC*. Retrieved from http://www.nhlbi.nih.gov/files/docs/public/heart/chol_tlc.pdf

National Heart, Lung, and Blood Institute (NHLBI). (2012a). *Overweight and obesity*. Retrieved from http://www.nhlbi.nih.gov/health/health-topics/topics/obe/

National Heart, Lung, and Blood Institute (NHLBI). (2012b). *What is cardiac catheterization?* Retrieved from http://www.nhlbi.nih.gov/health/health-topics/topics/cath

National Heart, Lung, and Blood Institute (NHLBI). (2014). *How is high blood cholesterol diagnosed?* Retrieved from https://www.nhlbi.nih.gov/health/health-topics/topics/hbc/diagnosis

National Heart, Lung, and Blood Institute (NHLBI). (2015a). *Who is at risk for coronary heart disease?* Retrieved from http://www.nhlbi.nih.gov/health/health-topics/topics/cad/atrisk

National Heart, Lung, and Blood Institute (NHLBI). (2015b). *What is cardiomyopathy?* Retrieved from http://www.nhlbi.nih.gov/health/health-topics/topics/cm

National Heart, Lung, and Blood Institute (NHLBI). (2015c). *What is heart failure?* Retrieved from https://www.nhlbi.nih.gov/health/health-topics/topics/hf

National Heart, Lung, and Blood Institute (NHLBI). (2015d). *Description of high blood pressure*. Retrieved from http://www.nhlbi.nih.gov/health/health-topics/topics/hbp

National Heart, Lung, and Blood Institute (NHLBI). (2015e). *What is sudden cardiac arrest?* Retrieved from http://www.nhlbi.nih.gov/health/health-topics/topics/scda

National Heart, Lung, and Blood Institute (NHLBI). (2015f). *What is peripheral artery disease?* Retrieved from https://www.nhlbi.nih.gov/health/health-topics/topics/pad

National Heart, Lung, and Blood Institute (NHLBI). (2016). *How is atherosclerosis treated?* Retrieved from http://www.nhlbi.nih.gov/health/health-topics/topics/atherosclerosis/treatment

National High Blood Pressure Education Program. (2000). *Working group report on high blood pressure in pregnancy.* Retrieved from https://www.nhlbi.nih.gov/files/docs/guidelines/hbp_preg_archive.pdf

National Institute of Neurological Disorders and Stroke (NINDS). (2015). *Transient ischemic attack information page.* Retrieved from http://www.ninds.nih.gov/disorders/tia/tia.htm

National Institute on Aging (NIA). (2015). *High blood pressure.* Retrieved from https://www.nia.nih.gov/health/publication/high-blood-pressure

National Stroke Association. (n.d.a). *Preventing a stroke.* Retrieved from http://www.stroke.org/understand-stroke/preventing-stroke

National Stroke Association. (n.d.b). *Stroke treatments.* Retrieved from http://www.stroke.org/we-can-help/survivors/just-experienced-stroke/stroke-treatments

National Stroke Association. (n.d.c). *Pediatric stroke.* Retrieved from http://www.stroke.org/understand-stroke/impact-stroke/pediatric-stroke

National Stroke Association. (2016). *Steps against recurrent stroke (STARS).* Retrieved from http://www.stroke.org/sites/default/files/resources/STARSbrochure_0.pdf

Norwitz, E., & Repke, J. T. (2015). Preeclampsia: Management and prognosis. *UpToDate.* Retrieved from http://www.uptodate.com/contents/preeclampsia-management-and-prognosis?source=search_result&search=magnesium +sulfate&selectedTitle=3%7E118

O'Connor, R. E. (2013). *Cardiopulmonary resuscitation in infants and children.* Retrieved from https://www.merckmanuals.com/professional/critical-care-medicine/cardiac-arrest/cardiopulmonary-resuscitation-in-infants-and-children

Office of Disease Prevention and Health Promotion (ODPHP). (2016). *Healthy People 2020: Heart disease and stroke.* Retrieved from http://www.healthypeople.gov/2020/topics-objectives/topic/heart-disease-and-stroke/objectives

Office of Minority Health. (2015). *Heart disease and American Indians/Alaskan natives.* Retrieved from http://minorityhealth.hhs.gov/omh/browse.aspx?lvl=4&lvlid=34

Office on Women's Health. (2012). *Bleeding disorders fact sheet.* Retrieved from http://womenshealth.gov/publications/our-publications/fact-sheet/bleeding-disorders.html

Okin, P. M., Kieldsen, S. E., Julius, S., Dahlof, B., & Devereux, R. B. (2012). Racial differences in sudden cardiac death among hypertensive patients during antihypertensive therapy: The LIFE study. *Heart Rhythm, 9*(4), 531–537.

Ouellette, D. R., Kamangar, N., & Harrington, A. (2015). *Pulmonary embolism.* Retrieved from http://emedicine.medscape.com/article/300901-overview

Park, S. E., Rhee, E., Park, C., Oh, K. W., Park, S., Kim, S., & Lee, W. (2013). Impact of hyperinsulinemia on the development of hypertension in normotensive, nondiabetic adults: A 4-year follow-up study. *Metabolism Clinical and Experimental, 62*(4), 532–538.

Pasman, E. A., & Watson, C. M. (2015). *Shock in pediatrics.* Retrieved from http://emedicine.medscape.com/article/1833578-overview#showall

Patel, K., & Chun, L. J. (2015). *Deep venous thrombosis.* Retrieved from http://emedicine.medscape.com/article/1911303-overview

Patton, K. (2013). Hypertension/hyperlipidemia/hyperhomocysteinemia and nutrition approaches.

In M. L. Corrigan, A. A. Escuro, & D. F. Kirby (Eds.), *Handbook of clinical nutrition and stroke.* New York, NY: Humana Press.

Pereira, N. L., & Warnes, C. A. (2014). *Mayo Clinic talks: Pregnancy in women with congenital heart disease.* Retrieved from http://www.medscape.com/viewarticle/819157

Perrin, K. O., & MacLeod, C. E. (2012). *Understanding the essentials of critical care nursing* (2nd ed.). Upper Saddle River, NJ: Pearson Prentice Hall.

Pettersen, M. D., & Seib, P. M. (2016). *Pediatric complete atrioventricular septal defects.* Retrieved from http://emedicine.medscape.com/article/893914-overview#a6

Pothineni, N. V., Karathanasis, S. K., & Mehta, J. L. (2016). Immuno-inflammatory basis of atherosclerotic coronary artery disease. In W. S. Aronow & J. A. McClung (Eds.), *Translational research in coronary artery disease: Pathophysiology to treatment.* London, United Kingdom: Elsevier.

Quarta, C. C., Kruger, J. L., & Falk, R. H. (2012). Cardiac amyloidosis. *Circulation, 126*, 178–182. doi:10.1161/CIRCULATIONAHA.111.069195.

Queensland Department of Health. (2013). Guideline: *Medicines/pharmaceuticals of animal origin* (Document Number #QH-GDL-954). Retrieved from https://www.health.qld.gov.au/qhpolicy/docs/gdl/qh-gdl-954.pdf

Rabito, M. J., & Kaye, A. D. (2013). Complementary and alternative medicine and cardiovascular disease: An evidence-based review. *Evidence-Based Complementary and Alternative Medicine, 672097.* doi:10.1155/2013/672097

Ramaswamy, P., & Srinivasan, K. (2015). *Ventricular septal defects.* Retrieved from http://emedicine.medscape.com/article/892980-overview

Riley, M., & Bluhm, B. (2012). High blood pressure in children and adults. *American Family Physician, 85*(7), 693–700.

Rizos, E. C., Ntzani, E. E., Bika, E., Kostapanos, M. S., & Elisaf, M. S. (2012). Association between omega-3 fatty acid supplementation and risk of major cardiovascular disease events: A systematic review and meta-analysis. *JAMA, 308*(10), 1024–1033.

Robinson, A. M. (2013). Venous thromboembolism prophylaxis for chronically immobilized long-term care residents. *Annals of Long-Term Care, 21*(9). Retrieved from http://www.annalsoflongtermcare.com/article/venous-thromboembolism-prophylaxis-chronically-immobilized-long-term-care-residents

Robinson-Cohen, C., Hoofnagle, A. N., Ix, J. H., Sachs, M. C., Tracy, R. P., Siscovick, D. S., . . . de Boer, I. H. (2013). Racial differences in the association of serum 25-hydroxyvitamin D concentration with coronary heart disease events. *Journal of the American Medical Association, 310*(2), 179–188.

Rodrigues, A., Clode, N., & Graca, L. M. (2014). Cardiac arrest in pregnancy: Best practices are needed. *Acta Obstetrica e Ginecologica Portuguesa, 8*(2), 164–168.

Rodriguez-Cruz, E. (2015). *Pediatric hypertension.* Retrieved from http://emedicine.medscape.com/article/889877-overview#showall

Roger, V. L. (2013). Epidemiology of heart failure. *Circulation Research, 113*, 646–659. doi:10.1161/CIRCRESAHA.113.300268

Rosh, A. J., & Khait, L. (2015). *Superficial thrombophlebitis.* Retrieved from http://emedicine.medscape.com/article/463256-overview

Sadat-Ali, M., & Al-Turki, H. A. (2013). The use of porcine derived low molecular weight heparins in Muslims. *Saudi Medical Journal, 34*(8), 865.

Sahay, M., & Sahay, R. K. (2012). Low renin hypertension. *Indian Journal of Endocrinology and Metabolism, 15*(5), 728–739.

Sahin, S., Eroglu, M., Tetik, S., & Gazin, K. (2014). Disseminated intravascular coagulation in obstetrics: Etiopathogenesis and up to date management strategies. *Journal of Turkish Society of Obstetrics and Gynecology, 11*(1), 42–51.

Schaefer, C., von Rhein, M., Knirsch, W., Huber, R., Natalucci, G., Caflisch, J., . . . Latal, B. (2013). Neurodevelopmental outcome, psychological adjustment, and quality of life in adolescents with congenital heart disease. *Developmental Medicine & Child Neurology, 55*(12), 1143–1149. doi:10.1111/dmcn.12242

Schouten, H. J., Koek, H. L., Oudega, R., Geersing, G., Janssen, K. J. M., van Delden, J. J. M., & Moons, K. G. M. (2012). Validation of two age dependent D-dimer cut-off values for exclusion of deep vein thrombosis in suspected elderly patients in primary care: Retrospective, cross sectional, diagnostic analysis. *BMJ, 344*, e2985. doi:10.1136/bmj.e2985

Schwartz, D. R., Malhotra, A., & Weinberger, S. E. (2016). Pulmonary embolism in pregnancy: Epidemiology, pathogenesis, and diagnosis. *UpToDate.* Retrieved from http://www.uptodate.com/contents/pulmonary-embolism-in-pregnancy-epidemiology-pathogenesis-and-diagnosis

Science Board to the Food and Drug Administration. (2014). *Proposal to encourage the reintroduction of bovine heparin to the U.S. Market.* Retrieved from http://www.fda.gov/AdvisoryCommittees/CommitteesMeetingMaterials/ScienceBoardtotheFoodandDrugAdministration/ucm399395.htm

Selim, M. H., & Molina, C. A. (2013). The use of tissue plasminogen-activator in pregnancy: A taboo treatment or a time to think out of the box. *Stroke, 44*, 868–869.

Shah, S. N. (2016). *Hypertrophic cardiomyopathy.* Retrieved from http://emedicine.medscape.com/article/152913-overview

Shahpouri, M. M., Mousavi, S., Khorvash, F., Mousavi, S. M., & Hoseini, T. (2012). Anticoagulant therapy for ischemic stroke: A review of literature. *Journal of Research in Medical Sciences, 17*(4), 396–401.

Sharma, K., & Russel, S. D. (2015). An update on peripartum cardiomyopathy in the 21st century. *International Journal of Clinical Cardiology, 2*(3). Retrieved from http://clinmedjournals.org/articles/ijcc/ijcc-2-034.pdf

Silberberg, C. (2013). *Acute tubular necrosis.* Retrieved from https://www.nlm.nih.gov/medlineplus/ency/article/000512.htm

Silver, B. (2016). *Stroke prevention.* Retrieved from http://emedicine.medscape.com/article/323662-overview#a4

Sliwa, K., & Böhm, M. (2014). Incidence and prevalence of pregnancy-related heart disease. *Cardiovascular Research, 109*(2), 554–560. doi:10.1093/cvr/cvu012

Sliwa, K., Hilfiker-Kleiner, D., Mebazaa, A., Petrie, M. C., Maggioni, A. P., Regitz-Zagrosek, V., . . . Pieske, B. (2014). EURObservational research programme: A worldwide registry on peripartum cardiomyopathy (PPCM) in conjunction with the Heart Failure Association of the European Society of Cardiology Working Group on PPCM. *European Journal of Heart Failure, 16*, 583–591. doi:10.1002/ejhf.68

Soundar, E. P., Jariwala, P., Nguyen, T. C., Eldin, K. W., & Teruya, J. (2013). Evaluation of the International Society on Thrombosis and Haemostasis and Institutional Diagnostic Criteria of

Disseminated Intravascular Coagulation in pediatric patients. *American Journal of Clinical Pathology, 139,* 812–816. doi:10.1309?AJCPO64IWNLYCVVB

Sovari, A. A., Gaeta, T. J., Kocheril, A. G., & Levine, M. D. (2014). Second-degree atrioventricular block. Retrieved from http://emedicine.medscape.com/article/161919-overview

Spector, R. E. (2017). *Cultural diversity in health and illness* (9th ed.). Hoboken, NJ: Pearson Education.

Springel, E. H., & Peng, T. C. C. (2014). *Thromboembolism in pregnancy.* Retrieved from http://emedicine.medscape.com/article/2056380-overview

Starkebaum, G. A. (2014). 25-hydroxy vitamin D test. *MedlinePlus.* Retrieved from https://www.nlm.nih.gov/medlineplus/ency/article/003569.htm

Strait, J. B., & Lakatta, E. G. (2012). Aging-associated cardiovascular changes and their relationship to heart failure. *Heart Failure Clinics, 8*(1), 143–164.

Steptoe, A., & Kivimaki, M. (2013). Stress and cardiovascular disease: An update on current knowledge. *Annual Review of Public Health, 34,* 337–354. doi:10.1146/annurev-publhealth-031912-114452

Stroke Association. (2012). *Women and stroke.* Retrieved from https://www.stroke.org.uk/sites/default/files/women_and_stroke.pdf

Stroke Scale. Published by National Institutes of Health. Stub, D., Smith, K., Bernard, S., Nehme, Z., Stephenson, M., Bray, J. E., . . . Kaye, D. M. (2015). Air versus oxygen in ST-segment elevation myocardial infarction. *Circulation, 131*(24), 2143–2150.

Syamasundar Rao, P., Turner, D. R., & Gessner, I. H. (2015). *Pediatric hypoplastic left heart syndrome.* Retrieved from http://emedicine.medscape.com/article/890196-overview#a6

Szummer, K., Oldren, J., Lindhagen, L., Carrero, J. J., Evans, M., Spaak, J., . . . Jernberg, T. (2015). Association between the use of fondarparinux vs low-molecular-weight heparin and clinical outcomes in patients with non-ST-segment elevation myocardial infarction. *Journal of the American Medical Association, 313*(7), 707–716. doi:10.1001/jama.2015.517

Taylor, C., Roalfe, A. K., Iles, R., & Hobbs, F. D. R. (2012). Ten-year prognosis of heart failure in the community: Follow-up data from the Echocardiography Heart of England Screening (ECHOES) Study. *European Journal of Heart Failure, 14*(2), 176–184.

Tamargo, J., Segura, J., & Ruilope, L. M. (2014). Diuretics in the treatment of hypertension. Part 1: Thiazide and thiazide-like diuretics. *Expert Opinions in Pharmacotherapy, 15*(4), 527–547. Retrieved from http://www.redheracles.net/media/upload/research/pdf//244442541415009695.pdf

Thaler, J., Pabinger, I., & Ay, C. (2015). Anticoagulant treatment of deep vein thrombosis and pulmonary embolism: The present state of the art. *Frontiers in Cardiovascular Medicine, 2*(30). doi:10.3389/fcvm.2015.00030

University of Rochester Medical Center. (2016). *Health encyclopedia: Venogram.* Retrieved from https://www.urmc.rochester.edu/encyclopedia/content.aspx?ContentTypeID=92&ContentID=P08295

U.S. Centers for Medicare & Medicaid Services. (n.d.). *Health coverage rights and protections.* Retrieved from https://www.healthcare.gov/health-care-law-protections/

U.S. National Library of Medicine. (2014a). *Blood pressure measurement.* Retrieved from https://www.nlm.nih.gov/medlineplus/ency/article/007490.htm

U.S. National Library of Medicine. (2014b). *Heart disease—risk factors.* Retrieved from https://www.nlm.nih.gov/medlineplus/ency/patientinstructions/000106.htm

U.S. National Library of Medicine. (2014c). *Preeclampsia.* Retrieved from https://www.nlm.nih.gov/medlineplus/ency/article/000898.htm

U.S. National Library of Medicine. (2015). *Stroke.* Retrieved from http://www.nlm.nih.gov/medlineplus/stroke.html

U.S. Preventive Services Task Force. (2015). *Lipid disorders in adults (cholesterol, dyslipidemia): Screening.* Retrieved from http://www.uspreventiveservicestaskforce.org/Page/Document/UpdateSummaryFinal/lipid-disorders-in-adults-cholesterol-dyslipidemia-screening

Vainrib, A., William, A., & Goswarmi, V. J. (2014). *Restrictive cardiomyopathy.* Retrieved from http://emedicine.medscape.com/article/153062-overview

Victoria State Government. (2012). *Neonatal ehandbook: Bleeding conditions in neonates.* Retrieved from http://www.health.vic.gov.au/neonatalhandbook/conditions/bleeding-conditions.htm

Vishram, J. K. K., Borglykke, A., Andreasen, A. H., Jeppesen, J., Ibsen, H., Jorgensen, T., . . . Olsen, M. H. (2012). Impact of age on the importance of systolic and diastolic blood pressures for stroke risk. *Hypertension, 60,* 1117–1123.

Vitamin D Council. (2014). *Hypertension.* Retrieved from https://www.vitamindcouncil.org/health-conditions/hypertension/

Wang, D., Liu, B., Tao, W., Hao, Z., & Liu, M. (2015). Fibrates for secondary prevention of cardiovascular disease and stroke. *Cochrane Database of Systematic Reviews, 10* (Art. no. CD009580). doi:10.1002/14651858.CD009580.pub2

Weber, J. (2014). Venous thromboembolic disease. *Journal of the American Osteopathic College of Radiology, 3*(3), 2–7.

Weil, B. R., Westby, C. M., Greiner, J. J., Stauffer, B. L., & DeSouza, C. A. (2012). Elevated endothelin-1 vasoconstrictor tone in prehypertensive adults. *Canadian Journal of Cardiology, 28*(3), 347–353.

Williams, S. F., Nicholas, S. B., Vaziri, N. D., & Norris, K. C. (2014). African Americans, hypertension, and the renin angiotensin system. *World Journal of Cardiology, 6*(9), 878–889.

World Health Organization (WHO). (2013). *A global brief on hypertension: Silent killer, global public health crisis.* Retrieved from http://apps.who.int/iris/bitstream/10665/79059/1/WHO_DCO_WHD_2013.2_eng.pdf?ua=1

World Health Organization (WHO). (2016). *Fact sheet about health benefits of smoking cessation.* Retrieved from http://www.who.int/tobacco/quitting/benefits/en/

World Heart Federation. (2016a). *Cardiovascular disease risk factors.* Retrieved from http://www.world-heart-federation.org/cardiovascular-health/cardiovascular-disease-risk-factors/

World Heart Federation. (2016b). *Family history.* Retrieved from http://www.world-heart-federation.org/cardiovascular-health/cardiovascular-disease-risk-factors/family-history/

Yancy, C. W., Jessup, M., Bozkurt, B., Butler, J., Casey, D. E., Drazner, M. H., . . . Wilkoff, B. L. (2013). 2013 ACCF/AHA guideline for the management of heart failure. *Journal of the American College of Cardiology, 62*(16), e147–e239. doi:10.1016/j.jacc.2013.05.019

Zarif, M. M. M., Murad, A. H. A., & Yusof, A. F. (2013). The use of forbidden materials in medicinal products: An Islamic perspective. *Middle-East Journal of Scientific Research, 13,* 5–10. doi:10.5829.idosi.mejsr.2013.16.s.10022

Zinkstok, S. M., & Roos, Y. B. (2012). Early administration of aspirin in patients treated with alteplase for acute ischaemic stroke: A randomised control trial. *Lancet, 380*(9843), 731–7.

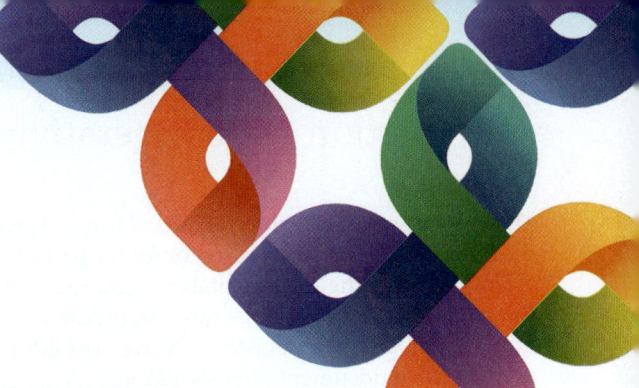

Module 17
Perioperative Care

Module Outline and Learning Outcomes

The Concept of Perioperative Care

Introduction to Perioperative Nursing

17.1 Summarize the scope of perioperative nursing.

Concepts Related to Perioperative Care

17.2 Outline the relationship between perioperative care and other concepts.

Preoperative Nursing

17.3 Explain the process of preoperative nursing.

Intraoperative Nursing

17.4 Explain the process of intraoperative nursing.

Postoperative Nursing

17.5 Explain the process of postoperative nursing.

Lifespan Considerations

17.6 Differentiate perioperative considerations throughout the lifespan.

» The Concept of Perioperative Care

Concept Key Terms

Adhesions, **1356**
Allogeneic blood
  transfusion, **1368**
ASA Physical Status
  Classification
  System, **1364**

Autologous blood
  transfusion, **1368**
Extubation, **1347**
Handoff report, **1349**
Hyperthermic, **1375**
Hypothermic, **1375**

Intraoperative, **1347**
Intubation, **1347**
Massive
  transfusion, **1350**
Malignant
  hyperthermia, **1356**

Normothermia, **1359**
Perioperative, **1347**
Postanesthesia care unit
  (PACU), **1370**
Postoperative, **1347**
Preoperative, **1347**

Preprocedure verification
  process, **1349**
Time-out, **1349**
Universal
  Protocol, **1347**

Perioperative is the term used to describe the three phases of surgical procedures: the preoperative phase, the intraoperative phase, and the postoperative phase. The **preoperative** phase is the phase preceding surgery in which the patient is identified as a candidate for surgical or procedural intervention. During the preoperative phase, the patient is assessed and prepared for surgery. Preoperative interventions include, but are not limited to, lab tests, medication administration, and physical assessment. The **intraoperative** phase is the actual surgical intervention phase. During the intraoperative phase, patients are often anesthetized, prepped, and draped, and the surgical procedure takes place. If necessary, a tracheal tube is inserted (**intubation**). On completion of the surgery or procedure, after the patient is stable and breathing effectively, the patient is prepared for the postoperative phase. At this point, the tracheal tube maybe removed (**extubation**). The **postoperative** phase is the recovery phase. It begins when the patient leaves the surgical suite and continues until the patient meets all discharge criteria. Postoperative nursing care is tailored to meet the patient's specific needs. Considerations that shape

postoperative care include the specific procedure performed and the patient's response to the procedure, the type of anesthetic administered and the patient's response to anesthesia, the patient's medical history, and any complications that develop during the postoperative period.

With the growth of surgery in outpatient facilities and other changes in the healthcare industry, nurses working in a variety of settings must be knowledgeable about perioperative care. For example, nurses working in dermatology offices are likely to assist with the removal of basal cell carcinomas using surgical procedures that generally involve local anesthesia. In pediatric offices, nurses may be required to provide nursing care for patients with minor wounds that require sutures. In medical–surgical units, nurses provide postoperative care to patients following a variety of procedures. Labor and delivery nurses provide postoperative care for women who deliver via cesarean section. Because of its applicability across settings and across the lifespan and because of the risks involved, surgical nursing care is related to a wide variety of concepts in nursing, some of which will be covered in the Concepts Related to Perioperative Care section.

Introduction to Perioperative Nursing

This module covers the three phases of surgical procedures in the order in which the phases occur for the patient. It includes a discussion of the documentation required in each of the three phases of perioperative care. According to the Association of periOperative Registered Nurses (AORN) (2013), the perioperative documentation should include all steps of the nursing process, including assessment, diagnosis, identified outcome, planning, implementation, and evaluation.

The Interprofessional Team

The surgical patient is cared for by an interprofessional team (see **Figure 17–1** »). The team's objectives are to assist the patient back to health and to maintain patient safety. For patients receiving anesthesia, the core perioperative team typically includes the following members:

- **Surgeon.** Performs the surgical procedure.
- **Anesthesia personnel.** Delivers anesthesia during the procedure and continually monitors the patient's physiologic status. This individual may be an anesthesiologist (medical doctor), certified registered nurse anesthetist (CRNA), or anesthesia assistant (AA).
- **Preoperative nurse.** Cares for the patient before the surgical event.
- **Circulating nurse.** Cares for the patient during the surgical event.
- **Surgical technician.** Chooses and passes surgical instruments and supplies to the surgeon during the procedure.
- **First assistant.** Assists the surgeon with the techniques of surgery.
- **Postoperative nurse.** Cares for the patient after the surgical procedures.

Support personnel may include:

- **Interpreter.** When the patient's primary language is not English, an interpreter gathers pertinent information in the preoperative phase and interprets information that must be exchanged between the patient and the nurse in the postoperative care phase.
- **Hospital liaison.** Advocates for the patient from the start of the admission process to the patient's release. The liaison may be a volunteer.
- **Nurse navigator.** Offers individualized assistance to patients, families, and caregivers to help overcome barriers in the healthcare system.
- **Radiology personnel.** Takes or evaluates radiologic films or tests during operative or invasive procedures.
- **Referral or specialty physician.** Plays a role in the patient's surgical care according to the physician's specialty in the patient's overall healthcare. A specialist might monitor the patient during the postoperative period in order to assist in attaining improved patient outcomes.
- **Respiratory therapist.** Assists in maintaining the patient's airway and oxygen status as needed during the postoperative period.
- **Social worker.** Assists in accessing resources for additional care of the patient as an inpatient and/or outpatient. For example, if the patient requires a walker to assist with mobility upon postoperative discharge, the social worker will work with the patient's insurance company and the walker manufacturer to obtain the walker for the patient.
- **Wound, ostomy, and continence nurse (WOCN).** Provides direct care and patient teaching related to wound healing, ostomy, and continence.
- **Additional disciplines.** Others contribute according to specialty to a positive patient outcome. Healthcare staff from another area of the facility, such as cardiology, may

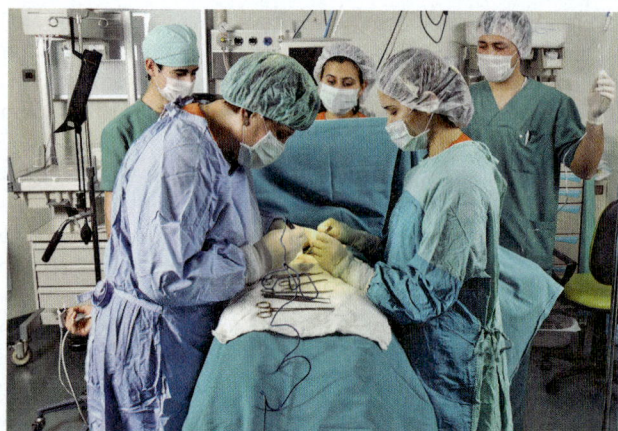

Source: Levent Konuk/Shutterstock.

Figure 17–1 » Surgical team in the operating room.

Focus on Diversity and Culture
Diversity in the Surgical Workforce

Cultural competency is the ability of the healthcare team to work effectively with patients from a variety of cultural, linguistic, social, and economic backgrounds. Cultivating cultural competency is essential in perioperative teams: numerous reports have shown evidence that people of color in the United States receive worse care and have worse health status indicators than do White populations (Rangrass, Ghaferi, & Dimick, 2014; Williams, Priest, & Anderson, 2016). Racial differences in health outcomes exist even when insurance status, income, age, and severity of conditions are similar. Ensuring optimal health outcomes in the preoperative, intraoperative, and postoperative phases depends heavily on the team's ability to communicate in culturally sensitive ways.

One challenge facing hospitals and surgical teams is that the American surgical workforce is lacking in diversity. While medical school graduates are almost equally split between men and women, there are twice as many men as women in surgical specialties (Data USA, 2017). And in 2015, 71.7% of surgeons were White, 20.1% were Asian, and the remaining 8.2% were Black, American Indian, and other people of color. In nursing schools in 2016, only 29% of students were people of color (National League of Nursing, 2017).

complete additional testing throughout the perioperative phase. For example, the patient may need an echocardiogram or an ultrasound of the cardiac system. Clergy may also provide spiritual/religious support to the patient and the patient's family.

Perioperative Diagnostic Tests

Lab work is done in the preoperative, intraoperative, and postoperative phases as needed (see **Table 17–1 >>**). In all phases, the results of the blood work are analyzed by the nurse as well as the anesthesiologist and surgeon. Once results have been analyzed, the interprofessional team communicates any concerns about abnormalities in the patient's lab results. Interpretation of the results of serum tests will take into account whether the patient is female or male or a pediatric, adult, or older patient.

Additional diagnostic tests, such as a pregnancy test, chest x-ray, or electrocardiogram (ECG), may be ordered depending on the surgical procedure and patient history.

>> *Go to* **Pearson MyLab Nursing and eText** *to see Appendix B for additional information about diagnostic tests, including lab values.*

Perioperative Safety Protocols and Precautions

Nurses, along with the rest of the interprofessional team, engage in a variety of interventions to ensure the safety of patients throughout the perioperative phases. AORN, the American Society of PeriAnesthesia Nurses (ASPAN), and the World Health Organization (WHO) created guidelines and safe practice recommendations for perioperative staff to utilize during the care of perioperative patients. In addition, The Joint Commission established a **Universal Protocol**— guidelines for healthcare professionals that are designed to prevent errors during surgical procedures. Each of these organizations emphasizes the need for preprocedure verification processes, time-outs, and handoff reports to ensure the safety of patients and prevent "never events" from occurring. Never events are surgical errors that should never occur, such as amputation of the incorrect limb. A **preprocedure verification process** is a standardized process used to verify that the correct procedure is being implemented on the correct patient at the correct site, and that all items necessary for the procedure are available. A **time-out** is a momentary pause and accuracy check taken by all members of the procedure team before an invasive procedure begins. A **handoff report** is a standardized communication process that captures all essential patient information for healthcare providers exchanging responsibility for patient care. To ensure accuracy, handoff reports frequently follow standardized formats such as SBAR (Situation, Background, Assessment, Recommendation) (The Joint Commission, n.d.). Healthcare facilities take these national guidelines and recommendations into account when creating protocols and policies for the perioperative staff to follow.

Preprocedure Verification Process

A preprocedure verification process is performed in all three perioperative phases (see **Table 17–2 >>**). The length of the verification process is based on the history of the patient and the content that needs to be covered. Preprocedure verification is designed to prevent errors, including surgery on the wrong patient or at the wrong site.

Medications

Medication errors and adverse drug events are common in perioperative care. According to a recent study, one in every two surgical procedures is accompanied by a medication error, and 5% of all medication administrations involve a medication error (Nanji, Patel, Shaikh, Seger, & Bates, 2015). Almost 80% of these errors were deemed preventable. Medication errors are costly. Andel, Davidow, Hollander, and Moreno (2015) reported that in 2008, medication errors in the United States cost $19.5 billion. The most common types of medication errors include labeling errors, wrong-dose errors, and omitted medication or failure to act (Nanji et al., 2016). To prevent medication errors, all staff should follow the rights of safe medication practices, which vary across states and agencies, but may include:

1. Right assessment
2. Right drug
3. Right dose
4. Right patient
5. Right route
6. Right time
7. Right documentation.

AORN (2013) and ASPAN (2012) created recommended practices and position statements for perioperative nurses to follow to assist with patient safety practices during medication preparation and administration. AORN focuses on six phases of medication use: procuring, prescribing, dispensing, transcribing, administering, and monitoring. AORN recommendations include, but are not limited to, the perioperative nurse being mindful of the seven rights of medication administration, following clear and concise medication orders, and continually assessing the therapeutic and adverse effects of the medication being administered. According to ASPAN, additional guidelines the perioperative nurse should follow to ensure safe medication practices include adopting the two-patient-identifier method during the preparation of the medication and before the administration of the medication, utilizing standard abbreviations used by the healthcare facility, and restricting unnecessary noise or distractions during patient care. The perioperative nurse should follow these recommendations and guidelines in all three perioperative phases.

SAFETY ALERT The two-patient-identifier method requires nurses and clinicians to identify the patient and match the treatment to the patient using two methods of identification. For example, the nurse may identify a patient by asking the patient to verbally identify him- or herself by name and birthdate and by comparing the name and birthdate given with the patient's wristband. These two identifiers are compared to the medical order, which should match *both* identifiers.

Medications are ordered for patients on the basis of the patient's health history, including medication history, physical assessment, the systems involved in the surgical procedure, and ongoing assessment of the patient's needs throughout perioperative care. Common medications administered to patients receiving surgical procedures include antiemetics, analgesics, anxiolytics, general anesthetics, and antibacterial drugs (see the Medications feature).

TABLE 17–1 Perioperative Diagnostic Tests

Diagnostic Test	Implication
Prothrombin time (PT) Time required for the patient's plasma to clot **Partial thromboplastin time (PTT)** Time required for the patient's blood to clot **Bleeding time** Time required for platelets to effectively stop bleeding; requires creation of a superficial skin wound	■ Due to bleeding risk, this can be the factor determining whether the surgical procedure occurs.
Capnography Comprehensive measurement and display of CO_2 levels in exhaled breath. Capnography depicts respiration, including metabolism, transport, and ventilation, which gives a picture of the respiratory process.	■ Capnography is performed in surgery to assist in determining adequate ventilation. Without adequate ventilation, appropriate levels of oxygenation cannot be maintained. Patients with inadequate oxygen levels can sustain irreversible brain damage. Capnography can also help the healthcare team determine whether the patient is experiencing a heart attack or hyperventilating.
Hematocrit (Hct) Measurement of the percentage of red blood cells in whole blood **Hemoglobin (Hgb)** Measurement of hemoglobin, which is a protein found in red blood cells that binds and carries oxygen **Red blood cells (RBC)** Measurement of the red blood cells in the blood; red blood cells contain hemoglobin, which transports oxygen throughout the body **Platelets** Assist in the formation of blood clots	■ Indications for transfusion of blood or blood products include substantial blood loss that causes a significant decrease in hemoglobin, hematocrit, and/or platelet count. In severe cases, a **massive transfusion** may be needed, which involves administration of a large volume of blood or blood products over a relatively short period of time.

Sodium (Na⁺)
Regulates blood and body fluids, nerve impulses, muscle activity and metabolic functions in the body
See Table 17–10 for potential intraoperative complications.
	■ **Hyponatremia:**
	   Nausea
	   Vomiting
	   Cramping
	   Edema
	   Muscle twitching
	   Signs of hypovolemia
	   Headache
	
	■ **Hypernatremia:**
	   Thirst
	   Orthostatic hypotension
	   Dry mouth and mucous membranes
	   Concentrated urine
	   Lethargy
	   Irritability
	   Fatigue

Potassium (K⁺)
Plays an important role in muscle and nerve activity. Potassium also assists in the transfer of nutrients and waste in the cells.
See Table 17–10 for potential intraoperative complications.
	■ **Hypokalemia:**
	   Abdominal distention
	   Loss of bowel sounds
	   Weakness
	   Severe arrhythmias
	
	■ **Hyperkalemia:**
	   Weakness
	   Nausea
	   Intestinal cramps
	   Diarrhea
	   Arrhythmias

pH Test of the acidity or alkalinity of cells	■ The normal range of blood pH is 7.35–7.45.

pCO₂
Measure of arterial CO_2 level
■ Decreased CO_2 = respiratory alkalosis.
   Note: Releasing too much CO_2 (hyperventilation), patient is releasing too much CO_2; breathing too fast.
■ Increased CO_2 = respiratory acidosis.
   Note: Retaining too much CO_2 (hypoventilation), patient is not expelling sufficient CO_2.
	■ When the body attempts to compensate for a primary acid–base alteration, a secondary imbalance may occur. For example, respiratory acidosis (which is caused by an excess of CO_2) may lead to increased retention of bicarbonate (HCO_3^-) by the kidneys as the body attempts to bring the pH to a more alkaline state and restore homeostasis.

HCO₃
■ Decreased HCO_3 = metabolic acidosis
■ Increased HCO_3 = metabolic alkalosis
	■ **Metabolic acidosis:**
	   Kussmaul respirations
	   Coma
	   Hypotension
	   Xerosis (dry skin)
	   Drowsiness
	   Fetor (strong offensive smell)
	   Asterixis (rapid tremor of the hand when the wrist is extended)
	   Pericardial rub during renal failure
	   Reduced skin turgor
	   Dry mucous membranes
	
	■ **Metabolic alkalosis:**
	   Weakness
	   Myalgia
	   Polyuria
	   Cardiac arrhythmias
	   Hypokalemia
	   Hypocalcemia
	   Jitteriness
	   Perioral tingling
	   Muscle spasms

TABLE 17–1 Perioperative Diagnostic Tests (*continued*)

Diagnostic Test	Implication
Human chorionic gonadotropin (HCG) or pregnancy test	▪ A pregnancy test is usually performed in the preoperative setting on all women of childbearing age. Medications administered during the perioperative phases can be harmful to an unborn fetus because the effects on the mother are transmitted to the fetus. Certain anesthetic medications may negatively affect fetal development. If a patient is scheduled for an elective procedure and the patient is determined to be pregnant, the procedure may be canceled. If the patient is scheduled for an emergent procedure, the procedure typically will proceed; however, special precautions will be taken to decrease any effects on the fetus and may include the patient's undergoing the procedure with an anesthetic block instead of general anesthesia.
Chest x-ray	▪ A chest x-ray is performed to assess for any respiratory problems, such as pneumonia. Respiratory infection could cause complications during anesthesia as well as the postoperative recovery period. A patient with such an infection who undergoes surgery may ultimately experience a longer hospital stay and unnecessary complications, such as a surgical site infection.
Electrocardiogram (ECG) Diagnostic test that evaluates the patient's cardiac rhythm	▪ A baseline ECG is conducted in the preoperative phase. If an abnormal rhythm is detected, consultation with a cardiology specialist, as well as medical treatment, may be required before the patient can proceed with surgery.
Total protein Tests for albumin and globulin levels	▪ Albumin levels are reflective of liver and kidney function. This is important because many medications are metabolized by the liver and excreted by the kidneys. ▪ Globulins or antibodies determine whether the patient is at a higher risk of acquiring an infection. One of globulin's primary functions is to transport in the blood nutrients that fight infection.
Blood glucose A measurement of the blood glucose (sugar) level in the patient's blood	▪ Increased blood glucose may indicate diabetes. Patients with diabetes are at greater risk for poor wound healing.

TABLE 17–2 Preprocedure Verification Process

Phase	Participating Surgical Team Members	Procedure (Content Covered During Preprocedure Verification Process)
Preoperative	Preoperative nurse Circulating nurse Anesthesia team Interpretation services if applicable	▪ Correct patient ▪ Correct surgical procedure ▪ Correct surgical site ▪ Surgical site marked by surgeon ▪ Review of pertinent patient history, including medications, allergies, health history, and abnormal labs
Intraoperative	Entire surgical team	Prior to initial surgical incision, change in surgeon, and/or change in position: ▪ Name of patient ▪ Consented procedure ▪ Allergies ▪ Antibiotic administered ▪ Any applicable implants ▪ Radiology records present and in the room ▪ Surgical prep is dry On conclusion of surgical procedure: ▪ Name of patient ▪ Consented procedure and actual procedure completed match ▪ All specimens acknowledged and approved by surgeon ▪ Surgical instrument and sponge counts correct
Postoperative	Postoperative (PACU) nurse Circulating nurse Anesthesia team Interpretation services if applicable	▪ Name of patient ▪ Surgical procedure completed ▪ Surgical side (if applicable) ▪ Review of pertinent patient history, including medications, allergies, health history, and abnormal labs ▪ Drains ▪ Implants placed ▪ Inform surgeon of any complications during intraoperative phase

Medications
Perioperative

CLASSIFICATION AND DRUG EXAMPLES	MECHANISMS OF ACTION	NURSING CONSIDERATIONS
Antiemetic *Drug examples:* Metoclopramide hydrochloride (Reglan) Dolasetron (Anzemet) Ondansetron (Zofran) Dexamethasone (Decadron) Aprepitant (Emend)	These drugs can be administered in the preoperative or postoperative phase. Most work in the brain to alter neural stimulation of the gut. ***May also be used for:*** ■ Treating nausea and vomiting associated with antineoplastic drugs	■ Monitor fluid and electrolytes. ■ Diarrhea and constipation are adverse effects. ■ Monitor patient cardiovascular status (for tachycardia and angina). ■ Extrapyramidal symptoms are possible. Administered in 1. Preoperative phase 2. Postoperative phase
Nonopioid Analgesics *Drug example:* Intravenous acetaminophen	These drugs provide temporary analgesia for mild to moderate pain. They decrease the patient's pain level in the postoperative phase.	■ Monitor for signs and symptoms of hepatotoxicity. Administered in 1. Preoperative phase 2. Postoperative phase
Anxiolytics *Drug examples:* Midazolam (Versed) Diazepam (Valium)	Benzodiazepines produce central nervous system (CNS) depression, resulting in sedation, musculoskeletal relaxation, and anticonvulsant activity. Sedatives relax the patient, but they do not relieve pain.	■ Monitor for adverse CNS effects (e.g., sedation). ■ Flumazenil (Romazicon) is used to reverse the adverse effects of sedatives. ■ Complete baseline and periodic liver function tests. Administered in 1. Preoperative phase 2. Intraoperative phase
Opioid Analgesics *Drug examples:* Morphine sulfate Fentanyl (Sublimaze) Hydromorphone (Dilaudid)	These drugs control moderate to severe pain but do not alter pain threshold. They may be used for sedation and/or pain relief.	■ These drugs can cause respiratory depression. ■ Naloxone hydrochloride (Narcan) reverses the effects of opiates, including respiratory depression, sedation, and hypotension (Wilson, Shannon, & Shields, 2013). Administered in 1. Intraoperative phase 2. Postoperative phase
General Anesthetics *Drug example:* Propofol (Diprivan)	These drugs are short-acting. They are commonly used during induction and maintenance of anesthesia.	■ Propofol should be inspected before use for particulate matter, discoloration, or evidence of separation of the emulsion. ■ Unused propofol should be discarded within 6 hours after filling the syringe or 12 hours after spiking a large volume for infusion. ■ These drugs have no reversal agent. Administered in 1. Intraoperative phase
Antibacterial Drugs Aminoglycosides Macrolides Tetracyclines Cephalosporins Penicillins Sulfonamides Fluoroquinolones *Drug examples:* Penicillin Vancomycin Levofloxacin (Levaquin)	These drugs decrease the risk for surgical site infections (SSIs).	■ Monitor for signs of allergic reaction. ■ Assess renal and hepatic function and vital signs. Administered in 1. Preoperative phase 2. Intraoperative phase 3. Postoperative phase

Source: Data from Adams, M. P., Holland, L.N., & Urban, C. (2017). *Pharmacology for nurses: A pathophysiologic approach* (5th ed.). Hoboken, NJ: Pearson Education.

Concepts Related to Perioperative Care

Assessment is the most significant concept during the perioperative process and encompasses most of the other concepts. It focuses on monitoring the patient's vital signs, including cardiac rhythm, oxygenation, acid–base balance, lab tests, pain, and input and output. Assessment also includes spiritual, cultural, and emotional aspects such as the patient's psychologic status, religion, sexual and cultural identification, and current and baseline developmental stage. Assessment may also include a nurse's communication with the healthcare and surgical team. Assessing what other team members gather from a nurse's communication is vital to a patient's safety.

All surgical procedures require patients to provide informed consent. Children and adolescents require informed parental consent for most procedures and in all but emergent life-threatening situations. Although the healthcare provider who will be conducting the procedure is responsible for providing the information and obtaining informed consent, nurses are responsible for ensuring that consent has been obtained, witnessing the appropriate individual signing the consent, and making sure all questions have been answered by appropriate personnel. Nurses also ensure that patients who do not speak English have the services of an interpreter

and that these patients fully understand all aspects of the procedure, including their right to decline.

Perfusion is particularly important during the perioperative process. Patients are at risk for overt blood loss and anemia related to surgical intervention. In addition, they may experience decreased tissue perfusion secondary to pressure on or over bony prominences such as the sacrum and the heels. The nurse should always assess intravenous (IV) patency before the patient enters the intraoperative stage. If the patient were to require a rapid fluid bolus, blood transfusion, or administration of medication, a lack of IV access could potentially prove to be fatal.

Stress and how the patient copes with it can alter the patient's experience during any stage of the perioperative process. In this area, the nurse can best meet the patient's needs by assessing the patient's preoperative developmental stage and consistently reassessing during the intraoperative and postoperative stages. Stress may cause regression to an earlier developmental stage, which may require the nurse to change the interventions and treatment modality for this patient.

Culture and diversity are essential considerations during the perioperative process. Cultural and religious considerations may affect the perioperative process. The patient's culture and/or religious practice may affect the patient's preferences on aspects such as blood transfusions, end-of-life

Concepts Related to
Perioperative Care

CONCEPT	RELATIONSHIP TO PERIOPERATIVE CARE	NURSING IMPLICATIONS
Assessment	Inadequate assessment → ↑ patient morbidity → ↑ recovery time → ↑ mortality	▪ Nursing care during the perioperative period begins and ends with assessment augmented by consistent and constant reassessment.
Comfort	↓ Mobility and ↑ hard surfaces (operating tables) → ↑ risk of pressure ulcers Perioperative process → ↑ anxiety, depression, physical, and emotional distress	▪ Premedication such as anxiolytics and antihistamines may aid in subduing a patient's anxiety. ▪ Nurses routinely administer analgesics during the perioperative process to aid in the patient's comfort or to decrease the signs and symptoms associated with the patient's disease process. ▪ Assessment of the patient's developmental stage during preadmission may help the nurse identify comfort needs.
Infection	↑ Infection-control measures and wound care → ↓ risk of infection	▪ Nurses must follow infection-control protocols. ▪ Nurses providing postoperative care must provide excellent wound care. Discharge teaching must include wound care and return demonstrations confirming the patient's ability to care for the wound.
Oxygenation	↑ Sedation → ↓ respiratory status ↑ Hypoxia → respiratory acidosis	▪ Nurses need to monitor the patient's respiratory status according to their facility's guidelines, especially with older adults and children because of the possibility for rapid deterioration.
Perfusion	↑ Perfusion → ↑ wound healing and recovery	▪ Perioperative nurses must be aware of blood transfusion policies and patient preferences. ▪ Nurses must be aware of the patient's hemodynamic status and understand the guidelines for transfusion. ▪ Nurses must assess IV access and patency perioperatively. ▪ Nurses must assess a patient's skin and tissue conditions, especially over bony prominences.
Stress and Coping	↓ Coping mechanisms and stress control → ↓ healing → ↑ time of recovery → ↓ prognosis	▪ Perioperative nurses must assess the patient's stress and coping mechanisms during the preoperative phase and reassess after the procedure.

decisions, and who is providing care during the perioperative period. The nurse must assess the patient's attitudes during the perioperative process and then advocate on the patient's behalf to provide complete and holistic care.

For surgical and healthcare teams, safety is of the utmost concern during the perioperative process. All ancillary staff must have productive and organized communication to coordinate safe and timely care during the perioperative period. Nursing care of the patient undergoing a surgical procedure begins with communication, which is critical throughout the perioperative phases. The feature lists some, but not all, of the concepts related to perioperative care. They are presented in alphabetical order.

Preoperative Nursing

Preoperative nursing care begins immediately when a patient is notified of the need for surgery. Nurses employ therapeutic communication to educate the patient about the upcoming procedure (see the Patient Teaching feature) and to assess the patient's health history and current physical status.

Preparing the Patient

Patients preparing for surgery often need to participate in preparations that are specific to the surgery being performed, the

site of the surgery, and the postoperative recovery. For example, abdominal or pelvic surgical procedures may require bowel preps, which patients complete the day before surgery. Bowel cleansing allows the surgeon to have a better view of the intestines in procedures such as a colonoscopy. This allows for better visualization of the inner lining of the intestines, which assists in diagnosing abnormalities, such as a polyp. The nurse should provide appropriate education to ensure that patients comply with necessary preparations. If patients have any questions, the nurse should provide informative answers.

The preoperative nurse reviews all surgical documents, such as the surgical consent form, with the patient in preparation for surgery. If the patient has questions about the scheduled surgical procedure, the nurse should notify the surgeon that the patient needs additional information. The preoperative phase also provides time for the preoperative nurse to establish a level of trust and confidence with the patient, which will help ease anxiety and facilitate patient care throughout the other perioperative phases. See the module on Tissue Integrity for more information on wound care and healing.

Nursing Assessment

Accurate and complete preoperative assessment is critical to ensuring that the patient achieves a good outcome during and after the surgical procedure.

Patient Teaching
Preparing the Patient for Surgery

Preparing the patient begins when the patient is identified as needing surgery and includes a variety of nursing interventions, from patient teaching to discharge planning. Nurses provide early patient teaching and reinforce preoperative instructions related to the following:

- The nature and anticipated length of the procedure, including expectations related to recovery time. For example, a single mother who will need to be hospitalized overnight will need to make arrangements for her children to be cared for until she returns home.
- Whether or not the patient should stop taking current medications in advance of the procedure, such as the following:
  - Anticoagulants
    - Nonsteroidal anti-inflammatory drugs (NSAIDs) such as aspirin and ibuprofen
    - P2Y12 platelet inhibitors such as clopidogrel (Plavix), prasugrel (Effient), and ticagrelor (Brilinta)
    - Warfarin (Coumadin)
    - Heparin
  - Tricyclic antidepressants
  - Herbal supplements
    - Ginkgo
    - St. John's wort
- Deep breathing and coughing exercises, which include the following:
  1. Cough twice, the first time to loosen mucus and the second to expel secretions.
  2. Inhale by sniffing to prevent mucus from moving back into the deep airways.

  3. Rest. Avoid prolonged coughing to prevent fatigue and hypoxemia.
- Surgical incision care (see the Patient Teaching feature on surgical wound care). This is especially important for outpatient surgical patients.
- Prevention of postoperative constipation, which may include the following:
  - Encouraging early postoperative ambulation
  - Advising the use of laxatives and stool softeners
  - Providing nutritional information such as guidelines for a diet high in fiber
- Pain control information such as the following:
  - Early ambulation decreases the risk of pain related to pulmonary complications and deep vein thrombosis.
  - Opioids increase drowsiness and may cause dizziness, nausea, itchiness, and constipation.
  - NSAIDs can increase the chance of bleeding and ulcers.
- Prevention of clot formation, with the application of thromboembolism-deterrent (TED) hose if appropriate. The patient should be given the following instructions:
  - Apply compression stocking early in the morning when first waking to decrease swelling.
  - Hand-wash stockings to increase their flexibility.
  - Line-dry compression stockings to maintain the correct size.

Education continues through discharge. Some healthcare facilities offer patients classes on preparing for surgery.

>> **Stay Current:** The Mayo Clinic offers a 45-minute class called Preparing for Surgery for their patients: www.mayoclinic.org/patienteducation-rst/surgeryadults.html.

Data Collection

During the preoperative phase, the nurse gathers important data about the patient's health history and current physical status (see **Table 17–3 »**). Assessment information gathered during the preoperative phase informs the plan of care that is implemented in the preoperative area and continues to inform the care plan through the intraoperative and postoperative phases. Vital signs, including blood pressure, pulse, respiration, and oxygen saturation, should be taken throughout the perioperative period, with the baseline vital signs being obtained during the preoperative phase.

Physical Examination

The surgeon is responsible for completing a full physical examination on the patient in the immediate preoperative period. The baseline assessment data provide a background that will enable nurses to discern physiologic changes during the perioperative period. The procedure team reassesses any component of a physical assessment when there is an apparent change from the patient's baseline. Depending on the surgical procedure, a focused assessment (and reassessments as necessary) is completed on the specific body system(s) involved in the procedure. Additional focused diagnostic testing may include tests such as a capillary blood glucose test for patients who have been previously diagnosed with diabetes (see Table 17–1).

Psychosocial Assessment

Psychosocial assessment of patients includes gathering information about their current level of stress and coping mechanisms. For patients who will need assistance with postoperative care after discharge, the nurse will assess the presence of competent help and the degree to which the caregiver is able to provide support to the patients. The nurse ensures that the cognitive function of older adult patients is sufficient for them to participate in informed consent. During the perioperative phases, the nurse has multiple opportunities to assess and determine whether patients are being abused. Patients often do not want to verbalize or admit to abuse, but the nurse is required to follow the healthcare organization's protocol on abuse when the nurse determines that it may be present. Questions to ask patients as part of the psychosocial assessment that directly relate to surgery include the following:

- I have some questions I will need to review with you as part of our perioperative assessment. Would you like for us to go through the questions by ourselves or would you like your family member present?

- How are you feeling about the surgical procedure?

- Do you feel safe in your home environment?

- Do you have any concerns you would like to address? For example, financial?

- Do you have any cultural or religious practices that the healthcare team needs to take into account while creating your perioperative plan of care?

- Do you have anyone who can assist you with daily routine care, such as bathing and preparation of food, upon discharge?

Many patients preparing to undergo surgery are concerned about their appearance. Older patients are often reluctant to part with wigs or hairpieces. Patients with limited mobility may be anxious about parting with prostheses or assistive devices. Reassure these patients by giving these important items to a family member who will return the item to the patient after surgery.

Nutritional Assessment

The preoperative nurse often performs the patient's nutritional assessment, which determines certain outcomes during and after surgery, including postoperative healing of the surgical wound. For example, patients with a high body mass index (BMI) are at increased risk for poor wound healing and surgical site infection. Perioperative nutritional assessment includes weight, BMI, food preferences, and total protein serum levels.

Pain Assessment

The nurse's assessment of the patient's pain begins in the preoperative phase and continues throughout all perioperative phases. The pain assessment scale is based on the patient's age, maturity level, and basic understanding of the question being asked. For example, a mature 12-year-old patient could use the numeric pain scale (0–10, with 0 = little to no pain and 10 = the maximum pain intensity) instead of the Wong-Baker FACES Pain Rating Scale. (See the module on Comfort for a full discussion of pain rating scales.) A patient with a primary language other than English may find it easier to understand the facial pain scale.

Patient Medication Review

Prescription medications are any medications that are prescribed by a licensed healthcare provider and dispensed by a pharmacy. The preoperative nurse documents the prescription medications the patient is taking, including the last dose and time the medication was administered. Examples of high-alert drugs for perioperative patients include beta-blockers, which affect blood pressure, and anticoagulant medications such as

Focus on Integrative Health
Over-the-Counter (OTC) Medications and Herbal Supplements

Herbal supplements can be a cause of concern during the perioperative process. The use of herbal supplements remains common in the United States (Wu, Wang, Tsai, Huang, & Kennedy, 2014). Herbal products, which include teas, dietary supplements, and some cosmetics, can cause serious complications during surgery. Herbal supplements can interfere with prescribed medications and may have properties such as anticoagulation of which the patient may not be aware. Ginkgo, garlic, ginger, ginseng, and St. John's wort are known to increase bleeding. Ephedra, golden seal, and licorice have been observed to increase blood pressure. Echinacea can cause immunosuppression, thus increasing the risk of infection. Kava, St. John's wort, and valerian root have been known to increase or interfere with the effects of anesthesia (Ehrlich, 2014).

Over-the-counter (OTC) medications are any medication (e.g., vitamin E, ibuprofen, aspirin) that the patient can obtain without a prescription. The perioperative nurse evaluates OTC medications to assess whether the patient is at risk for any complications during surgery. The nurse instructs the patient, if indicated, to stop taking, before surgery, any medication or supplement that can place the patient at an increased risk of bleeding.

TABLE 17–3 Essential Preoperative Assessment Data Collection

Assessment Data	Nursing Implications
Allergies	■ Before the patient is transported to surgery, the preoperative nurse confirms all patient allergies with the patient and updates the preoperative documentation accordingly, including adding any allergies not listed or deleting incorrect allergy information.
Previous surgeries: any invasive procedure for the patient	The nurse reviews all previous surgeries with the patient to determine the following: ■ The presence of any metal implants in the patient, which is important information when electrocautery is to be used ■ The presence of **adhesions** (scar tissue) from previous surgeries ■ Helpful information, such as patient history of being combative or nauseated when waking up from anesthesia
Personal or family history with anesthesia	■ The nurse assesses personal and family history regarding anesthesia to determine the patient's risk of presenting with **malignant hyperthermia**—a genetic disorder caused by exposure to certain anesthetic agents—as well as allergies or any other adverse events.
Hearing aids, glasses, and contact lenses	■ The patient removes contact lenses to prevent any potential damage to the eyes during surgery. ■ The patient removes glasses. The nurse can store them with the patient's belongings or give them to a family member to prevent the glasses from being damaged or lost. ■ The patient takes off removable hearing aids. If the patient has an implanted hearing aid such as a cochlear implant, the circulating nurse needs to be alerted. Electrosurgical units can deactivate hearing aids.
Loose teeth, crowns, caps, dentures, and other dental issues	■ For liability reasons as well as patient safety, the nurse notifies the surgical team if the patient has any loose teeth, cracks, crowns, and/or caps.
Pacemakers, prostheses, artificial joints, and other implanted devices	■ For patient safety and legal reasons, the patient must alert the surgical team of any previously implanted medical device.
NPO status	■ The patient must be NPO (have nothing to eat or drink by mouth) for 8 hours before surgery. These instructions vary for infants and very young children. ■ Eating or drinking anything other than clear liquids within the 8 hours before surgery increases the patient's risk of aspiration. ■ If the patient has had anything to eat or drink within 8 hours before surgery, the surgical procedure may be canceled, especially if the surgery is elective. ■ If the procedure is an emergency case, appropriate steps are taken to prevent complications such as aspiration.
Retained hardware or metal	■ To prevent patient injury, including burns, the patient removes any metal, including all jewelry, in the preoperative setting. ■ The nurse conducting the assessment also alerts the intraoperative team to the presence of any metal implants inside the patient, such as a metal rod or pin placed as part of orthopedic repair of a bone. ■ The nurse assesses older adult men for an implanted penile prosthesis, which increases the risk for injury during urinary catheterization.
Venous thromboembolism (VTE) assessment/ prophylaxis	■ The preoperative nurse assesses the patient for a history of VTEs. Certain factors may place the patient at higher risk for VTEs, such as a surgical procedure that lasts 30 minutes or longer. ■ Longer procedures can cause stasis or slowing of the blood, which can cause one or more VTEs to form. For this reason, the patient falls into the high-risk category. The physician can order pharmacologic and/or mechanical prophylaxis. ■ Pharmacologic prophylaxis, such as heparin or enoxaparin (Lovenox), interferes with coagulation and helps to prevent stasis and formation of emboli. ■ Mechanical prophylaxes, such as sequential compression devices, intermittently squeeze the leg, enhancing circulation.
Cultural assessment	■ Perioperative nurses should be aware of cultural differences among patients at their healthcare facility. This awareness includes assessment of cultural beliefs and practices that may affect the patient postoperatively. (See the module on Culture and Diversity for more information.) ■ Cultural conflicts between generations can arise. For example, some older adult patients may follow the instructions given by the surgical staff whether or not the patients understand the procedure or agree with the surgical staff. ■ In patriarchal cultures, the husband may speak for the wife even if she is the patient. In this scenario, the surgical team needs to be aware of the patient's culture in order to distinguish whether the husband is speaking because of his cultural role in the family or because the relationship is abusive and the husband is trying to exert control over his wife's decisions.
Communication assessment	■ The patient must understand the questions being asked and answer to the best of his or her ability. If English is not the patient's primary language, the perioperative nurse must ask for assistance from a trained interpreter who speaks the patient's primary language. If an interpreter is not available, the hospital should provide interpretation via telephone or the Internet. ■ If any members of the patient's family are present and do not speak English, the nurse must obtain assistance to communicate with them. This is required for all age groups. ■ The perioperative nurse should not allow a family member to interpret for the patient because of the risk of incorrect or incomplete translation. This could lead to the patient's not having all of the required information necessary for surgery or the surgical team's having incorrect or incomplete information about the patient. ■ Age and developmental characteristics also influence communication with the patient and family (see the modules on Communication and Development).
Drug and alcohol assessment	■ Drug and alcohol use can result in the patient's needing an increased amount of anesthetic medication to be utilized. ■ Patients who abuse drugs and alcohol may present with signs and symptoms of withdrawal in the postoperative setting. The postoperative nurse must be able to identify and assess for signs and symptoms of withdrawal.

warfarin (Coumadin), which place the patient at increased risk for bleeding. Medication delivered by skin patches, such as nicotine, estrogen, or fentanyl, must also be documented.

Informed Consent

A patient must give informed consent before any surgical procedure. The nurse's role in obtaining informed consent is to verify the patient's signature on the informed consent form. Informed consent is required not only for the procedure itself but also for administration of anesthesia and blood products. In addition, the patient must consent to financial responsibility for the procedure, to any photos or video taken, and to additional activities such as extra personnel present in the room during the procedure. See the module on Legal Issues for more information about informed consent.

Preoperative Nursing Diagnoses

Once the preoperative assessment is complete, the nurse begins creating the preoperative care plan. Some preoperative diagnoses include, but are not limited to, the following:

- *Fear*
- *Anxiety*
- *Knowledge, Deficient.*

(NANDA-I © 2014)

Focus on Diversity and Culture
Overcoming Language Barriers for Pediatric Surgical Patients

Nurses and other members of the healthcare team will frequently be faced with situations in which cultural and linguistic barriers make communicating with pediatric patients and their families difficult. A wide variety of tools are available to help the healthcare team interface with speakers of other languages. A good first step when working with a family that speaks a language other than English is to complete a communication assessment plan (CAP) to determine which resources will be most appropriate for a particular patient and family's needs. Once the CAP is complete, the nurse and patient's family can communicate about the nursing care plan through interpretation services, which will provide an interpreter who can facilitate both verbal and nonverbal understanding. If a particular healthcare facility does not have interpretive staff available, nurses may use telephonic interpretation services to communicate with patients. The operators of these services are available day and night and provide a telephone handset to both the nurse and patient while the interpreter translates on the other end of the line (Weldon et al., 2014).

Members of cultural and religious support teams can also provide translation services. These personnel may include chaplains or volunteers, who may be able to provide comfort and communication for the family. Visual aids can provide an easy translation technique. Educational texts are commonly available in multiple languages, including picture books for the pediatric patient. Creating a language board on which the healthcare provider can visually illustrate concepts can also be a helpful augmentation of translation services. Finally, the hospital should make an effort to employ multicultural personnel who speak a wide variety of languages to make the communication effort as seamless as possible.

TABLE 17–4 Preoperative Surgical Site Preparation

Type of Preparation	Explanation
Clipping of patient's hair	■ Whenever possible, hair at the surgical site should not be removed. However, if removal is necessary, clip the patient's hair in the preoperative setting to decrease the amount of hair contaminating the field. In some circumstances (e.g., gynecologic procedures), the patient's surgical site area is clipped during the intraoperative phase. ■ Clip hair with electric clippers (not a razor) immediately before the procedure.
Cast removal	■ If the patient has a cast, remove it in the preoperative setting to decrease the amount of dust contaminating the surgical arena.
Showers the day before surgery	■ Patients undergoing open class I surgical procedures below the chin should complete two preoperative showers with chlorhexidine gluconate (CHG) before surgery. When appropriate, the surgeon will instruct the patient accordingly in the physician's office. ■ Preoperative showers help to remove microorganisms from the skin. ■ Cleaning with a special soap before surgery can assist in the prevention of SSIs.

Sources: Based on Association of periOperative Registered Nurses (2013). *Perioperative standards and recommended practices.* Denver, CO: Author; Centers for Disease Control and Prevention (CDC). (2013). *Patient safety: Ten things you can do to be a safe patient.* Retrieved from http://www.cdc.gov/Features/PatientSafety/; Kamel, C., McGahan, L., Polisena, J., Mierzwinski, M., & Embil, J. M. (2012). Preoperative skin antiseptic preparations for preventing surgical site infections. *Infection Control and Hospital Epidemiology, 33*(6), 608–617.

The nursing care plan is based on the nursing assessment and diagnoses and will incorporate orders from the surgeon as well as care considerations for the patient's family.

Preparing the Surgical Site

The preoperative nurse either oversees or assists with preparation of the surgical site. According to AORN (2013) and the Centers for Disease Control and Prevention (CDC) (n.d.), site preparation is time-sensitive. For example, clipping a patient's hair around the surgical site the morning of surgery, rather than the day before, has been shown to result in fewer surgical site infections (SSIs). See **Table 17–4 »** for an overview of surgical site preparation.

Preoperative Interventions

Preoperative nursing interventions assist in preparing the patient for surgery and can save valuable time and improve patient outcomes after surgery. While the patient is waiting for surgery, the nurse can provide essential patient teaching related to postoperative care and expectations.

Preoperative Documentation

Information gathered during the preoperative assessment is documented according to agency protocol and is used as the baseline for care of the patient (see **Box 17–1 »**).

Patient Teaching
Postoperative Care and Incentive Spirometers

Deep breathing may be uncomfortable for the patient in the postoperative period, depending on the surgical procedure. An incentive spirometer is a device that the patient uses to breathe slowly and deeply after surgery or in the event of a disease process like pneumonia (Hadjiliadis, 2014). To teach a patient to use an incentive spirometer, the postoperative nurse should instruct the patient to do the following:

1. Sit upright while holding the device and seal lips around the mouthpiece.
2. Exhale a normal breath and then inhale slowly while watching the marker rise. The point is to get the marker as high as possible. The nurse may designate a desired height for the marker as a goal.
3. In another area, a ball or disc should be held floating in the middle of the chamber.
4. Sessions are usually 10–15 breaths every 1–2 hours.

See the modules on Infection and Oxygenation for more information about incentive spirometers.

Focus on Integrative Health
Music

As healthcare expenditures become an ever-increasing factor in patient care, noninvasive interventions such as music are being utilized as a way to decrease anxiety and pain and increase overall patient satisfaction (Stern, 2013). Systematic review has shown that music improves patients' outcomes in the perioperative arena as well as other areas of healthcare (Li, Wang, Chou, & Chen, 2015). While exactly which type of music to use and when it should be used in the perioperative process depend on the clinical situation and the preferences of the patient, overall use of music during the perioperative process demonstrates a positive correlation with a better patient experience (Hole, Hirsch, Ball, & Meads, 2015).

Box 17–1
Preoperative Documentation

Preoperative documentation includes, but is not limited to, the following:

1. History and physical assessment
2. Social assessment
3. Nutritional assessment
4. Systems assessment
   a. Integumentary
   b. Neurologic
   c. Cardiovascular
   d. Respiratory
   e. Gastrointestinal/abdominal
   f. Musculoskeletal
5. Pain assessment
6. Medication review
7. Medications administered in the preoperative setting
8. Perioperative care plan.

Case Study » Part 1

Rachel Poole is a 20-year-old woman in her junior year of nursing school. She was recently diagnosed with stage II breast cancer and is scheduled to have a bilateral total mastectomy with a free transverse rectus abdominis myocutaneous (TRAM) breast reconstruction. Ms. Poole is healthy except for her recent diagnosis and has been given an ASA II classification. Her vital signs in the preoperative area are: T_O 98.6°F, P 72 bpm, R 14/min, BP 110/70 mmHg. She is 5 ft 4 in. tall and weighs 125 lb. A type and screen has been ordered. Ms. Poole has signed all of her consent forms and is now slightly anxious, as she will be going to the operating room shortly. The preoperative nurse administers midazolam (Versed) 2 mg IV. Ms. Poole is monitored until she is transported to the intraoperative suite.

Clinical Reasoning Questions Level I

1. What are your next steps?
2. What additional assessment data would be helpful to have at this time? Why?

Clinical Reasoning Questions Level II

3. Would your next steps change if Ms. Poole's respirations change to 10/min? If so, how?
4. Referring to the module on Development, how would you explain the surgery to Ms. Poole? How would your strategies differ for a 60- to 70-year-old?

Intraoperative Nursing

Intraoperative nursing includes all aspects of a surgical or invasive procedure within the operating or procedure room. Constant monitoring of both the surgical environment and the patient is necessary to ensure patient safety. The intraoperative environment is a high-risk area, where there are increased risks for infection, surgical errors, wrong-site surgery, retained instruments, burns, and incorrect specimen labeling.

Intraoperative Nursing Diagnoses

The intraoperative nursing diagnoses are created after the intraoperative assessment but before the intraoperative planning. The intraoperative diagnoses may include, but are not limited to, the following:

- *Infection, Risk for*
- *Anxiety*
- *Fluid Volume, Deficient, Risk for*
- *Injury, Risk for*
- *Electrolyte Imbalance, Risk for*
- *Breathing Pattern, Ineffective.*

(NANDA-I © 2014)

Types of Surgical Procedures

Surgical procedures may be open, such as an abdominal hysterectomy, or laparoscopic, such as a laparoscopic hysterectomy. Closed procedures, such as closed reduction of a bone fracture, require no incision. Surgical procedures ending in "-ectomy" indicate the removal of an organ; examples include appendectomy and hysterectomy. Procedures that end in "-oscopy" indicate that a part of the body is being viewed; examples include colonoscopy and arthroscopy.

There are several types of surgical procedures, which may be performed for a variety of reasons.

- *Reconstructive surgery* may be performed to restore lost or reduced appearance or function. Facial reconstruction after a motor vehicle crash is an example of reconstructive surgery.
- *Diagnostic procedures* are conducted to determine or confirm a diagnosis. A biopsy of a mass is an example of a diagnostic procedure.
- *Elective surgery* is a procedure that is the recommended treatment for a condition that is not life-threatening. Knee-replacement surgery is an example of an elective surgery.
- *Emergency surgery* is a procedure that is performed when a condition creates the risk of loss of life or limb. Surgery to control internal hemorrhage is an example of emergency surgery.
- *Palliative surgery* may be performed to alleviate pain or symptoms associated with a disease. Palliative surgery does not cure or stop the course of the disease. Surgery intended to remove but not eradicate tumors is an example of palliative surgery.
- *Transplant surgery* replaces malfunctioning organs or other structures. A liver transplantation is an example of transplant surgery.

Laparoscopic procedures usually involve three small incisions approximately 1 cm in size to allow for insertion of thin surgical instruments into the patient's body. A laparoscope allows for visualization of internal body structures through use of a tiny video camera that transmits images to a monitor. Other instruments may be inserted for various purposes, such as manipulating organs for exploration of the site, removing tissue, or cauterizing blood vessels. Laparoscopic surgeries are less invasive than open surgeries and usually require a shorter hospital stay and recovery. Also, because the incision sites are small, the patient is at a lower risk for acquiring SSIs and experiences less blood loss. Surgeons have the option to convert from a laparoscopic procedure to an open procedure depending on the initial findings from the laparoscope. For example, an extensive amount of scar tissue and adhesions can impair laparoscopic visualization of the surgical site, making it necessary to convert to an open procedure.

Open surgical cases are procedures for which a surgical incision is required. Open procedures usually require a longer hospital stay and a longer recovery period. Open procedures also place the patient at a higher risk for blood loss. Larger incisions place the patient at a higher risk for complications, such as hypothermia and SSIs.

Length of Surgical Procedure

The length of the surgery will vary depending on the type of surgical procedure. Longer procedure times are associated with an increased risk for complications. Shorter procedures benefit patients of all ages; less exposure time means less risk for physiologic complications and reduction in the time required for healing. Generally speaking, the following statements hold true:

- The longer the procedure, the longer the patient is exposed to anesthesia, which may lengthen recovery time and increase the risk for complications.
- The longer the procedure, the greater the patient's risk of hypothermia, which can increase the time required for healing and the risk for VTE. The patient must maintain **normothermia**, a normal body temperature.
- Procedures that last 30 minutes or longer may require patients to wear sequential compression devices to prevent VTE. Review your healthcare facility's VTE prophylaxis guidelines or parameters, including pharmacologic and mechanical prophylaxis.
- The longer the procedure, the greater the risk for blood loss that may necessitate a blood transfusion, either intraoperatively or on admission to the medical unit.

Sterile Field and Hand Hygiene

The sterile field consists of the area utilized for the procedure and is handled only by intraoperative personnel who have completed the required hand scrub according to their healthcare facility's surgical hand scrub guidelines or policy. Many facilities follow the Recommended Practices for Sterile Technique, which is outlined in the AORN (2013) guidelines. AORN recommends a 3- to 5-minute surgical hand scrub before donning sterile gloves to reduce the microorganisms on the skin of personnel involved in the procedure. Hand hygiene should also be performed on completion of the surgery and whenever surgical gloves are removed. Hands must be scrubbed before and after eating and using the restroom, when hands are visibly soiled, and before and after caring for patients (AORN, 2013). See the module on Infection for more information on hand hygiene and preventing infection in the clinical setting.

Focus on Diversity and Culture
Jehovah's Witnesses and Blood Transfusion

Jehovah's Witnesses are one of the more notable religious groups whose beliefs complicate perioperative care. Members of this sect generally refuse transfusion of specific blood components. Their decision not to accept certain kinds of transfusions is related to a scriptural injunction against consuming blood. However, individuals vary in their interpretation of this scripture, so nurses should clearly determine the preference of individual patients. Nearly all Jehovah's Witnesses refuse transfusions of whole blood and the primary blood components, but many Witnesses accept the transfusion of derivative blood products such as albumin solutions, cryoprecipitate, clotting factor concentrates, and immunoglobulins (JPAC, 2016). Witnesses frequently carry a signed advance decision document listing the products and procedures that they do not find acceptable. Nurses should add a copy of this document to the patient's record and make the limitations of treatment clear to the perioperative team before the procedure begins. A member of the healthcare team should have a confidential discussion with the patient about the risks of his or her decision, but in the end the team must respect the patient's decision.

During Surgery

The nurse's responsibilities during surgery will vary according to the nature of the procedure and the composition of the surgical team. At all times, nurses act to promote the physiologic health of the patient by guarding against infection and preventing potential complications, including but not limited to complications during positioning of the patient, SSIs, and hypothermia.

Continuous Surveillance

The perioperative nurse must maintain continuous surveillance within the intraoperative setting. The nurse acts as the substitute for the senses temporarily lost by the patient during surgery, such as sight and hearing. Nurses are taught that they are patient advocates. In the operating room, the patient is unconscious, and the circulating nurse becomes the protector of that patient. To be comfortable being the spokesperson for the patient, the perioperative nurse needs to have self-confidence, which comes with experience. Also with experience, the nurse will learn the sounds of the operating room, for example, the anesthesia monitors and the conversations between the anesthesia team and the surgeon. Nurses learn by experience to recognize changes in the patient's heart rhythm, a change in blood pressure, or even a drop in oxygen saturation. The circulating nurse vigilantly monitors intraoperative events, including the patient's volume of blood loss, and other safety-related concerns. The nurse begins to learn these skills in nursing school and builds on them through gaining experience.

Intraoperative Safety Precautions

The intraoperative phase includes many dangerous combinations for both the patient and the healthcare team. For example, if a combustible skin cleansing solution comes into contact with a spark from an electrosurgical unit and high-flowing oxygen, a surgical fire may be ignited; this could result in burns, possibly severe ones, to the patient or to the surgical team. See **Table 17–5 》》** for specific safety precautions that must be followed during the intraoperative phase.

Positioning

Patients are positioned intraoperatively for access to the surgical site (see **Table 17–6 》》**). Joints, nerves, and skin must be protected during movement and final positioning. Padding is typically used under pressure points to prevent nerve injuries and protect the skin. Positioning the patient correctly is extremely important for the safety of the patient. For example, the brachial plexus can be damaged if the arm is not positioned correctly.

- When positioning the patient in the prone position, the intraoperative nurse has to rotate the patient's arm with the natural flow of the arm, or the patient's shoulder can be dislocated.

- In placing a patient in the lithotomy position, both legs need to be lifted and positioned in the stirrups at the same time or the patient's hips can potentially be dislocated.

- Depending on the procedure, the surgical bed may have to be placed in a specific position. For example, for a gynecology procedure, the patient is placed in the lithotomy position, but the bed is placed in the gynecologic position. This allows the patient's buttocks to be specifically placed at an opening in the bed and the bottom section of the surgical bed to be lowered or removed once the patient's legs have been placed in the stirrups, for easier access to the operative site.

Anesthesia

Generally speaking, patients undergoing surgical procedures require anesthesia. The type of anesthesia varies and depends on many variables, such as the type of surgical procedure and the level of systemic illness. For example, high blood pressure and obesity increase the risk level of anesthesia; conscious sedation (also known as monitored anesthesia care [MAC]) may be preferred over general anesthesia for patients with these conditions. See **Table 17–7 》》** for an overview of types of anesthesia.

The perioperative nurse's role is consistent regardless of the particular type of anesthesia being used in the procedure. In the preoperative phase, the nurse completes the preoperative assessment, confirms that the informed consent form has been completed, and prepares the patient for anesthesia (see **Box 17–2 》》**). In the intraoperative phase, the nurse assists with the application of monitors and assists with airway management as well as adjusting patient position as necessary and monitoring patient safety. In the postoperative phase, the nurse assists in placing the dressing, protects the patient during the return of reflexes, and prepares the patient to move into the postanesthesia care unit (Lewis, Dirksen, Heitkemper, & Bucher, 2014).

TABLE 17–5 Intraoperative Safety Precautions

Procedure	Nursing Implications
Electrosurgery An electrical method used to cut and cauterize tissue ■ There are two types of electrosurgery handpieces: *Bipolar:* The electrical current flows between the two points on the handpiece. *Monopolar:* The current flows through the patient. ■ If the patient has a pacemaker, the surgical team should use a bipolar handpiece if possible and refer to the facility's pacemaker guidelines during surgical procedures if applicable.	■ Always follow manufacturer guidelines. ■ The combination of alcohol-based preps, oxygen, and electrosurgery creates an ideal environment for surgical fires, increasing the risk for patient burns. The surgical team must ensure that the surgical prep is dry before draping. ■ Obtain the appropriate electrosurgery pad size (e.g., pediatric, adult) for the patient. ■ The preferred site for the electrosurgery pad is an area of large muscle or fat tissue. ■ Place the pad as close to the surgical site as possible. ■ Inspect and document the condition of the skin at the site of pad placement; remove hair if needed. ■ Never place the pad in the following locations: a. Over metal implants b. Over tattoos or scars c. Over skin that is not intact (e.g., abrasions, burns). ■ Remove any metal on the patient, including all jewelry, hearing aids, and eyeglasses, in the preoperative setting. ■ Alert the circulating nurse if the patient is wearing a hearing aid or has an implanted hearing aid such as a cochlear implant. Electrosurgical units can deactivate hearing aids. Depending on the regulations of your healthcare facility, external hearing aids may be removed before surgery. ■ When the pad is removed, the circulating nurse must assess the site for any changes from the patient's baseline skin assessment (e.g., burns, abrasions).
Light amplification by stimulated emission of electromagnetic radiation (LASER) A method used to cut body structures (e.g., tissue, kidney stones). Healthcare lasers are defined according to their relative hazard and the appropriate controls. Class 3 and 4 lasers are primarily used in healthcare organizations. Class 4 lasers are hazardous to the eyes and skin and can also cause fires; Class 3 lasers are hazardous under direct contact or exposure through reflection of a beam off of a reflective source, such as a mirror (AORN, 2013).	■ Always follow manufacturer guidelines. ■ Wear laser-approved protective goggles. ■ Place laser-approved protective goggles on the patient. ■ Cover all windows and reflective surfaces with a towel. ■ Lasers can damage the lens of the eye and cause sight damage. ■ Laser beams can go through windows and injure staff outside the operative room. Laser beams can also bounce off of reflective surfaces, causing fires and/or damage to staff's eyesight. ■ A laser safety officer (LSO) should be appointed as part of a laser safety program implemented by the healthcare organization administrators to monitor and oversee the control of laser hazards (AORN, 2013).
Pneumatic tourniquet A method used to obliterate circulation to an extremity (e.g., circulation to the knee during a total knee replacement)	■ Always follow manufacturer guidelines. ■ Complete a baseline skin assessment on the site before placing the tourniquet. ■ Always pad under the tourniquet before securing. ■ Use an appropriately sized tourniquet. ■ Follow the guidelines for the length of time the tourniquet should be inflated. ■ Document the times when the tourniquet is inflated and deflated.
Radiology A method used to take intraoperative photos or accomplish surgical placement of radiation for oncology patients	■ Always follow manufacturer guidelines. ■ Perioperative staff must make sure lead shields cover their bodies, including women's ovaries and men's testicles, because radiation can cause sterility. Staff should also wear a neck shield to protect the thyroid gland. ■ Staff should request a radiometer from their facility to measure their dose of radiation exposure.
Chemicals *Preps*—specific chemicals that are applied to a surgical site before incision to decrease the amount of pathogens on the skin surface and to decrease the chance of an SSI *Chemotherapy agents*—chemicals used in intraoperative oncology cases (e.g., hyperthermic intraperitoneal chemotherapy)	■ Always follow manufacturer guidelines because procedures may vary.

Sources: Based on Association of periOperative Registered Nurses (2013). *Perioperative standards and recommended practices.* Denver, CO: Author; Association of Surgical Technologists. (2012). *AST standards of practice for use of electrosurgery.* Retrieved from http://www.ast.org/uploadedFiles/Main_Site/Content/About_Us/Standard%20Electrosurgery.pdf; Board of Laser Safety. (2014). *Certified medical laser safety officer: Policies & procedures manual.* Retrieved from https://www.lasersafety.org/uploads/pdf/cmlso_pp_manual.pdf

TABLE 17–6 Surgical Positions

Patient Position	Steps to Safely Position the Patient
Supine The circulating nurse places the patient on his or her back and ensures that the accompanying steps are completed. 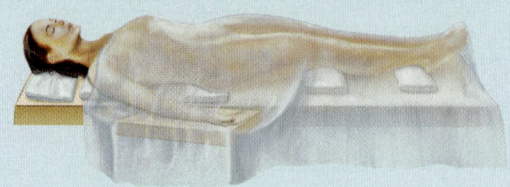	1. Gently secure arms on padded arm boards at less than a 90-degree angle with palms up. 2. As an alternative, and only if necessary, secure tucked arms at the patient's side with palms of hands facing in toward the thighs, elbows and hands protected and padded, and hands and wrists anatomically aligned. 3. Place pillows under the patient's knees. 4. Elevate bony prominences (e.g., heels) from the surface of the bed using pillows and a padded foot board for leg positioning. 5. Place a wedge under a pregnant patient's right hip/flanks to displace the uterus to the left.
Semi-Fowler (sitting) The circulating nurse places the patient in the sitting position and ensures that the accompanying steps are completed. 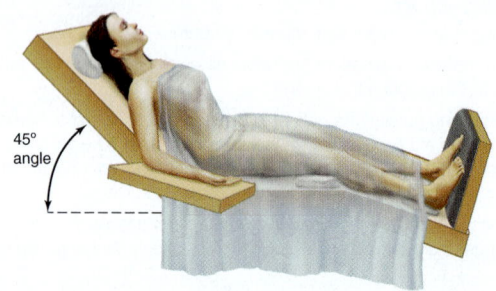	1. Gently secure arms on padded arm boards at less than a 90-degree angle with palms up. 2. Protect pressure points by properly positioning and padding the buttocks/sacrum and other bony prominences. 3. Elevate bony prominences (e.g., heels) from the surface of the bed using pillows and a padded foot board for leg positioning. 4. Lower the foot of the bed slightly to allow the knees to flex. 5. Support the patient's feet on a padded foot board to prevent plantar flexion and stretching of the tibial nerve. 6. Raise the back of the operating room bed to become the back rest, supporting the shoulders and torso with safety restraints.
Prone and Jackknife The circulating nurse places the patient on his or her stomach and ensures that the accompanying steps are completed. 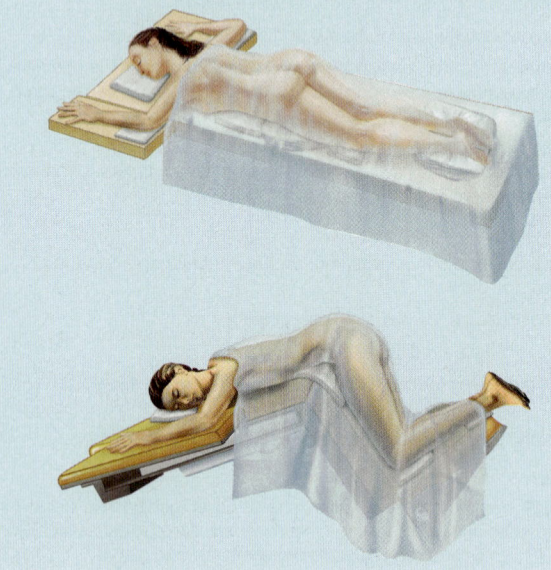	1. Maintain alignment of the cervical neck. 2. Elevate toes from the surface of bed. 3. Protect eyes to prevent ocular injury (e.g., pressure, corneal abrasion). 4. Ensure female breasts and male genitalia are not compressed.
Lateral The circulating nurse places the patient on his or her side (left or right) and ensures that the accompanying steps are completed. 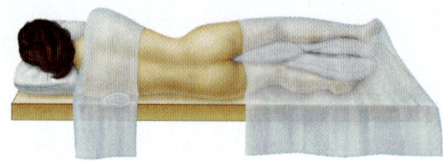	1. Initial the correct surgical side before the patient is transferred to the operating room. The initials must be visible after positioning, prepping, and draping. 2. Position the patient on the nonoperative side. 3. Pad pressure points on the dependent side (e.g., ear, acromion process, iliac crest, greater trochanter, lateral knee, malleolus). 4. Maintain correct spinal alignment when the patient is turned and stabilized in position. 5. Use axillary rolls or other devices to safely position arms and prevent brachial plexus injury.

TABLE 17–6 Surgical Positions (*continued*)

Patient Position	Steps to Safely Position the Patient
Trendelenburg or Reverse Trendelenburg The circulating nurse places the patient on his or her back with padded shoulder braces in place and ensures that the accompanying steps are completed. This position displaces the intestines into the upper abdomen. 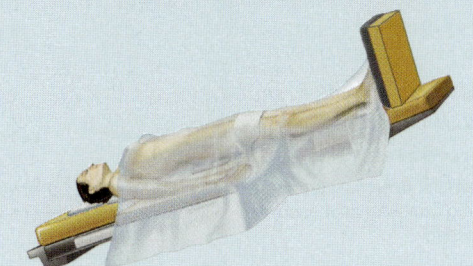	1. Monitor time in the head-down position to identify physiologic shifts. 2. Prevent the patient from sliding and shearing injuries. 3. Prevent injury to the patient's shoulders. 4. Support the feet on a padded foot board to prevent plantar flexion and stretching of the tibial nerve. 5. Prevent injury to the patient's brachial plexus. 6. Prevent injury to the patient's feet.
Lithotomy This is a gynecologic position. The circulating nurse places the patient on her back with both legs elevated in stirrups and ensures that the accompanying steps are completed. 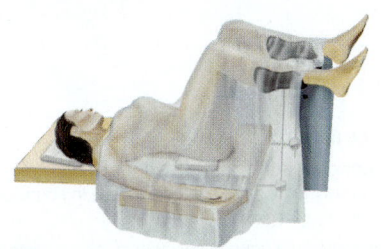	1. Pad ankles and heels. 2. Prevent stretching of the perineal nerve by ensuring that the hip and knee joints are not overextended. 3. Pad arms and gently secure on arm boards at less than a 90-degree angle with palms up. 4. Remove the patient's legs from stirrups slowly and bring them together simultaneously to prevent lumbosacral strain. 5. Raise and lower the patient's legs slowly and simultaneously to maintain hemodynamic status.
For all procedures: Before draping the patient, the circulating nurse must complete the accompanying steps for all surgical positions.	1. Evenly distribute pressure over bony prominences. 2. Assess the patient's body alignment to prevent musculoskeletal compromise. 3. Assess placement of safety straps. 4. Assess tissue perfusion. 5. Assess skin integrity and ensure that there is no pooling of solutions or wet surfaces. 6. Ensure the patient's circulatory, neurologic, and respiratory systems are not compromised.
For each surgical procedure, the circulating nurse must evaluate the patient postoperatively for injuries, covering all of the accompanying steps and documenting per agency requirements.	1. Check for skin injuries (e.g., reddened, bruised, tears). 2. Check for musculoskeletal and nerve injuries (e.g., aberrations in circulation, movement, and sensation). 3. Check for pressure ulcer development (e.g., identify the stages of pressure ulcer development). 4. Check for eye injuries.

Sources: Based on Association of periOperative Registered Nurses (2012). *Perioperative job descriptions and competency evaluation tools.* Denver, CO: Author; Gerken, S. (2013). Lateral and prone positioning risks in orthopaedic surgery. *AAOS Now, 7*(2); Osborn, K. S., Wraa, C. E., Watson, A. B., & Holleran, R. (2014). Intraoperative nursing. In *Medical-surgical nursing: Preparation for practice* (2nd ed., Ch. 18). Upper Saddle River, NJ: Pearson Education.

Box 17–2
Preparing the Patient for Anesthesia

The periods immediately before and after the patient is anesthetized can cause anxiety for the patient. Part of the perioperative nurse's role is to provide a comforting and calm atmosphere (Lewis et al., 2014). Consider using some of the following therapies to decrease the patient's anxiety, promote relaxation, reduce pain, and accelerate the healing process in the perioperative period:

- Use integrative therapies such as aromatherapy, music therapy, guided imagery, and even movies to calm the patient.
- Implement integrative health therapies before the patient's admission to the operating room or after the patient's arrival in the holding area.

- Ask if the patient has any last-minute questions to clarify remaining confusion.
- Validate that the correct preoperative medications were given as ordered.
- Ask whether the patient has any comfort needs and provide a pillow or position adjustment if he or she is uncomfortable.
- Ask the patient about valuables, prostheses, and last intake of food and fluid to ensure perioperative success.
- Cover the patient's hair before transfer to the operating room suite to prevent shedding.

TABLE 17–7 Types of Anesthesia

Type of Anesthesia	Definition
Local Anesthesia Localized specifically to surgical site *Used for:* ■ Invasive procedures that can be completed in the surgeon's office but instead are completed in a procedural setting for various reasons, such as presence of comorbidities or need for additional monitoring.	■ The patient is awake during the entire procedure. ■ A circulating nurse monitors the patient's vital signs and oxygen saturation. Anesthesia personnel may or may not provide patient care. ■ The patient's surgical area receives local anesthetics.
Conscious Sedation/Monitored Anesthesia Care (MAC) *Used for:* ■ Older adults, who are more prone to decreased renal function ■ Carpal tunnel syndrome ■ Stapedectomy	■ The patient is not intubated. ■ Small amounts of propofol are administered. ■ Anesthesia personnel monitor the patient. ■ Anesthesia personnel must be prepared to provide advanced airway management (e.g., tracheal intubation) and to convert to using general anesthesia if needed.
General Anesthesia A medically induced coma A paralytic agent is commonly administered in conjunction with the anesthetic agent. *Used for:* ■ Total abdominal hysterectomy ■ Craniotomy ■ Nephrectomy	■ The patient is intubated, utilizing intubation tubes such as an endotracheal tube or laryngeal mask airway. ■ The patient is unaware of what is happening and does not feel pain because of the anesthetic medications administered through the IV line. ■ The patient is monitored by anesthesia personnel.
Regional Anesthesia (e.g., spinal anesthesia, epidural anesthesia, femoral nerve block) A specific region of the patient is anesthetized *Used for:* ■ Cesarean birth ■ Toe/partial foot amputation ■ Hip replacements	■ The patient may be awake or sedated. ■ An anesthetic medication is injected into a specific body region to bathe targeted nerves, producing loss of sensation (and, in some cases, loss of mobility) in selected body regions. ■ It can be used in addition to general anesthesia. This assists with pain control in the postanesthesia care unit.

ASA Physical Classification Category

The American Society of Anesthesiologists (ASA) (2014) created the **ASA Physical Status Classification System**,* a physical risk classification category that helps to describe the patient's present state of physical illness before surgery. The ASA class is used as a predictor of the patient's risk for surgical complications. The ASA level is not used to estimate the possibility of anesthetic complications, nor does it dictate the type of anesthetic that will be administered. The ASA classifications are as follows:

ASA I: The patient is healthy, that is, free of health conditions or systemic disease.

ASA II: The patient demonstrates mild systemic disease, such as obesity, uncomplicated diabetes, or controlled hypertension.

ASA III: The patient has one severe systemic illness, such as coronary artery disease, angina, or poorly controlled hypertension.

ASA IV: The patient has a life-threatening severe illness such as pulmonary dysfunction.

ASA V: The patient is not expected to survive for more than 24 hours unless surgery occurs.

ASA VI: The patient is brain-dead but may be an organ donor.

*Republished with permission of American Society of Anesthesiologists, from ASA Physical Status Classification System, 2014; permission conveyed through Copyright Clearance Center, Inc.

Laryngeal Mask Airways and Endotracheal Tubes

The anesthesia provider will choose the type of airway management device used during general anesthesia. In certain instances, the anesthesia provider may opt to insert a laryngeal mask airway (LMA) (see **Figure 17–2 》**). An LMA is inserted blindly into the pharynx, forming a seal

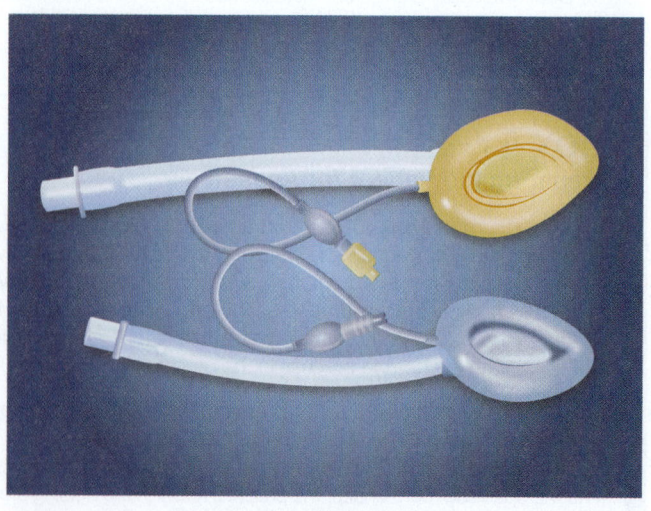

Figure 17–2 》 Laryngeal mask airway.

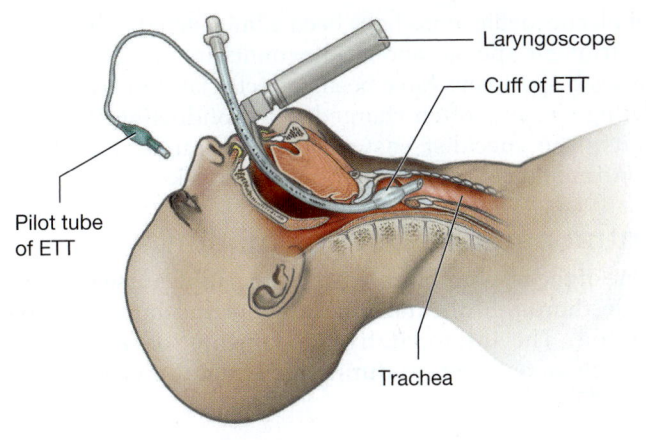

Pilot tube
of ETT

Laryngoscope

Cuff of ETT

Trachea

Figure 17–3 ⟩⟩ Using a laryngoscope to insert an endotracheal tube (ETT).

around the laryngeal inlet and creating positive-pressure ventilation. As an alternative to an LMA, an endotracheal tube (ET) may be used to manage the patient's airway. An ET is inserted through the vocal cords into the trachea with the use of a laryngoscope (see **Figure 17–3** ⟩⟩).

Surgical Site Preparation

Preparation of the surgical site occurs in the intraoperative setting, just before sterile draping of the patient. The purpose of a surgical prep is to help prevent SSIs. The circulating nurse always starts the prep at the surgical incision site and moves outward. Surgical preparation solutions are given an opportunity to completely dry before draping in order to prevent serious consequences, such as a surgical fire, which can burn the patient. Completing the surgical preparation just before draping decreases the chance of the surgical site being contaminated, which decreases the risk of acquiring an SSI. See **Table 17–8** ⟩⟩ for a list of commonly used surgical prep solutions and **Figure 17–4** ⟩⟩ for skin preparation for common surgical sites.

Head surgery

Unilateral chest surgery

Thoracoabdominal surgery

Abdominal surgery

Forearm, elbow, or hand surgery

Gynecologic surgery

Genitourinary surgery

Hip surgery

Thigh and leg surgery

Foot/lower leg surgery

Ankle, foot, or toe surgery

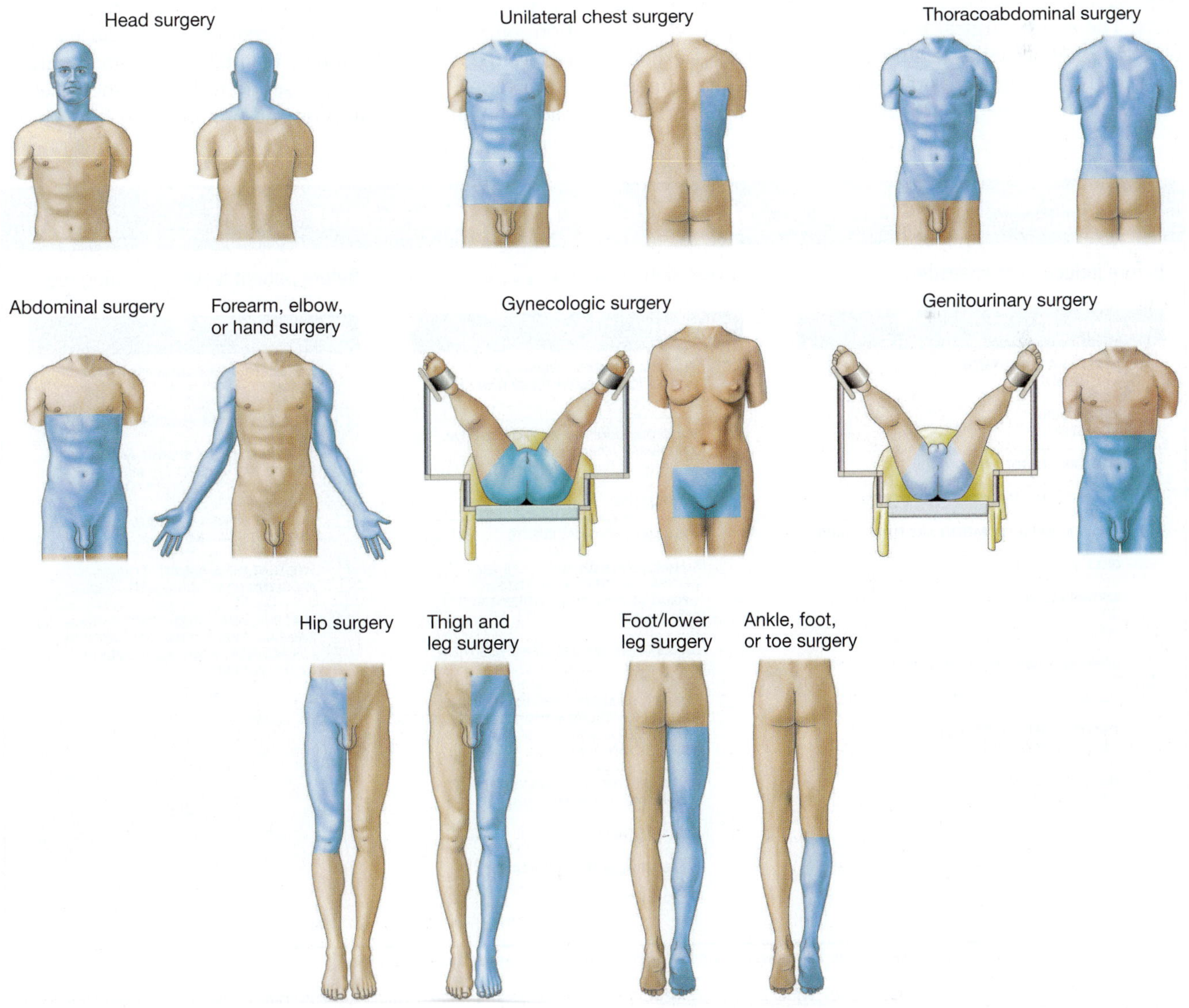

Figure 17–4 ⟩⟩ Skin preparation for common surgical sites.

TABLE 17–8 Commonly Used Surgical Prep Solutions

Surgical Prep Solutions	Uses and Precautions
Betadine scrub	■ Used for the initial wash or prep of surgical area ■ Cannot be used on mucous membranes
Betadine paint	■ Used for the final Betadine prep of the surgical area ■ Can be used on mucous membranes
ChloraPrep, DuraPrep	■ Alcohol-based; must be completely dry before patient is draped ■ Not for use on mucous membranes; avoid contact with ears and eyes
Ultradex scrub	■ Used when the patient has iodine and latex allergies

Surgical Safety Checklist

In 2009, the World Health Organization (WHO) created a Surgical Safety Checklist to assist perioperative staff in achieving best practice and maintaining the safety of the patient (Walker, Reshamwalla, & Wilson, 2012) (see **Figure 17–5 »**). Many hospitals use the checklist to ensure patient safety. The entire surgical team is required to periodically cease all other activities (a surgical time-out) and verbally verify such information as the patient's name; the surgery to be performed; the side or site of surgery; whether pro-

phylactic medications have been administered; whether all instrument, sponge, and needle counts are correct; and that any lab specimens have been correctly labeled. The circulating nurse is often charged with conducting the timeouts. The checklist ensures that the nurse documents confirmation of essential perioperative tasks.

Intraoperative Documentation

One of the responsibilities of the circulating nurse is to provide thorough documentation about the intraoperative period. The intraoperative documentation records all aspects of occurrences during the surgical procedure (see **Box 17–3 »**).

Infection

Many factors influence a patient's healing process, especially the patient's age, nutrition, and physical health. Pediatric patients and older adult patients are at higher risk of surgical complications for various reasons, including decreased immune status. Patients with poor health or poor nutrition status also are at greater risk for infection. Patients who have diabetes, take immunosuppressants, or have an increased BMI have an increased risk of acquiring an infection. Nurses and other members of the surgical team can reduce the risk of infection by maintaining aseptic technique at all times. Any break in aseptic technique increases the patient's chance for infection and prolonged healing period.

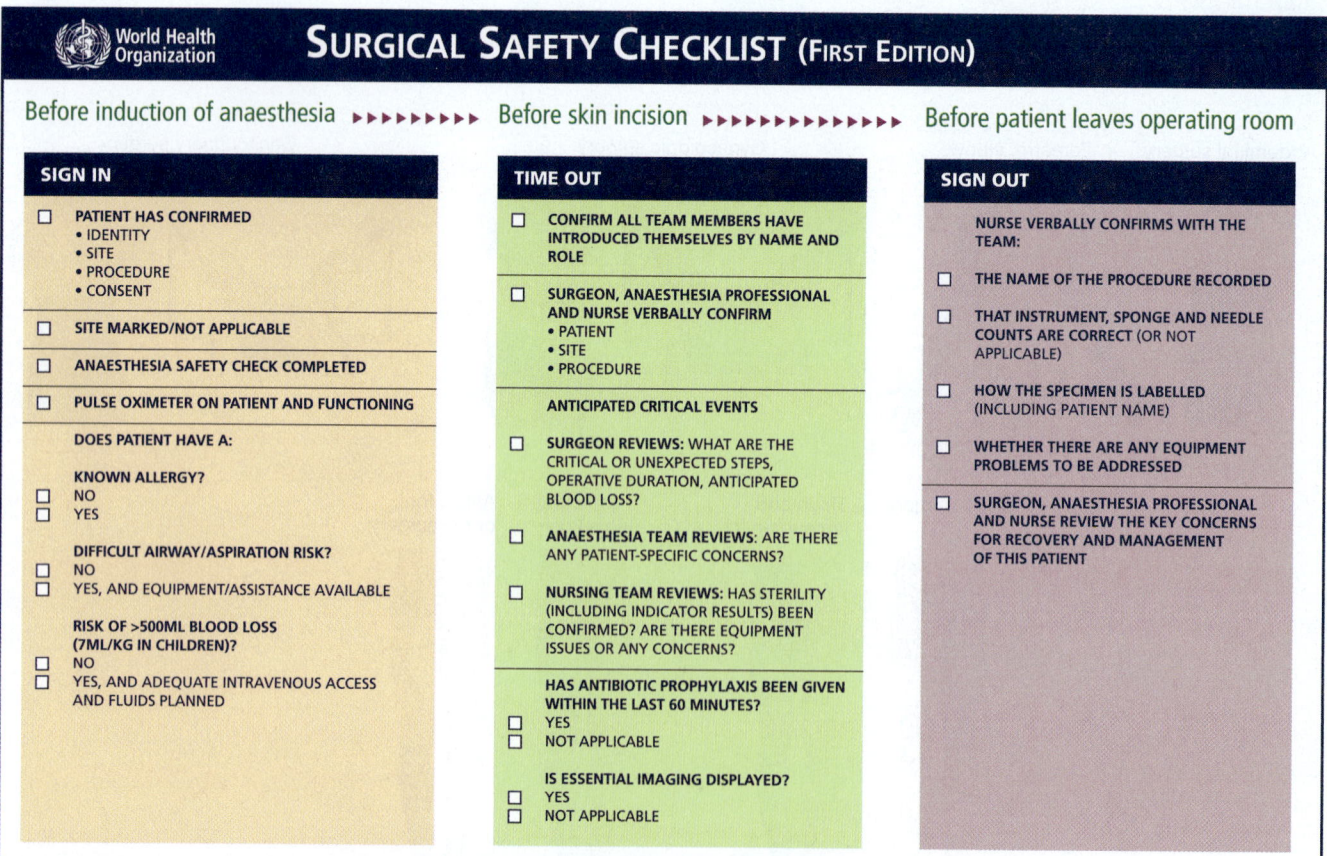

Source: World Alliance for Patient Safety (2008). *WHO surgical safety checklist and implementation.* Retrieved from http://www.who.int/patientsafety/safesurgery/tools_resources/SSSL_Checklist_finalJun08.pdf

Figure 17–5 » WHO Surgical Safety Checklist.

Evidence-Based Practice

Surgical Safety Checklist

Problem

Each year, millions of patients require surgical intervention and procedures, which account for approximately 13% of the world's total disability-adjusted life years (DALYs) (WHO, 2015b). It is no secret that while the purpose of doing surgery is to achieve a therapeutic outcome, the surgery itself is intentional and organized trauma to the patient's body. The overall crude mortality rate associated with surgery is 0.5–5%; complications account for an estimated 25% of cases of surgery-related mortality. Industrialized countries report that nearly half of their medical adverse events are attributed to surgical complications. What is most worrisome is that half of the complications and adverse events were deemed preventable (WHO, 2015b).

Evidence

The WHO decided to create a surgical safety checklist that could be implemented in operating rooms all over the world in all situations. Because the goal in creating the Surgical Safety Checklist (see Figure 17–5) was to improve patient safety by decreasing unnecessary surgical deaths and complications during the perioperative process, the WHO consulted nurses, physicians, anesthesiologists, and patients during development of the checklist (WHO, 2015a).

During the final stages of the checklist's development, the WHO reported that the overall death rate had been reduced from 1.5% to 0.8%, with a decrease in inpatient complications from 11% to 7%. Of the patients who were questioned about the checklist, 93.4% stated that they would like the checklist used if they were to have a surgical procedure (Walker et al., 2012). The checklist has also improved the

administration of prophylactic antibiotics before surgical procedures from 57% in 2007 to 79% in 2010 (Walker et al., 2012).

Implications

The WHO Surgical Safety Checklist has improved patient outcomes and will continue to change the landscape of the perioperative arena. As technology and surgical procedures change, so will the criteria of the checklist. To err may be human, as the saying goes, but prevention of complications during surgical procedures can help to decrease the mortality of surgical procedures, while also lessening the financial burden of extraneous healthcare costs not only to patients, but also to healthcare providers.

Critical Thinking Application

1. How might you as a nurse improve the quality of the WHO's Surgical Safety Checklist? If you have any suggestions or additions to the checklist, how would you share your ideas or results?

2. Why do you think it took until 2009 for a universal surgical checklist to be created and adopted? How might we keep such oversights from occurring with future healthcare modalities?

3. You are about to start a surgical procedure when you begin to implement the WHO Surgical Safety Checklist. It appears that no one on the surgical team is being attentive; instead, they are treating the checklist as an obstacle rather than a necessary part of the perioperative process. How do you change your milieu in this situation?

Box 17–3

Intraoperative Documentation

Intraoperative documentation includes, but is not limited to, the following:

1. Recognition that the handoff from the preoperative nurse to the intraoperative nurse is complete
2. Preoperative medical diagnosis
3. Postoperative medical diagnosis
4. Completion of consented surgical procedure
5. Type of anesthesia administered (e.g., general anesthesia)
6. ASA level
7. Intraoperative team members. Names of all individuals present for the surgical procedure must be documented. This should include medical sales representatives. All individuals should be listed on the intraoperative nurse's notes in case an unexpected event occurs. The individuals in the nurse's notes can be questioned as references for each individual's recognition of the specific outline of events. Observing students will also be entered in the operating room records and can be called as witnesses if necessary.
8. Times
   a. Start and stop times of anesthesia
   b. Start and stop times of procedure
   c. Antibiotic infusion times
9. Surgical preparation site
   a. Prep used
10. Skin assessment
    a. Initial
    b. Postoperative
11. Position or positions of patient
12. Positioning aids utilized

13. Foley insertion
14. Surgical instrument count, documenting correct or incorrect count. If an incorrect count occurs, documentation should include the steps taken to ensure that the missing instrument or sponge does not remain in the patient's body. For example, an x-ray can be taken to locate the item within the patient.
    a. Initial
    b. Ongoing
    c. Closing
    d. Shift change
15. Time-out(s)
    a. Name of individual completing the time-out
    b. Time the time-out is completed
16. Equipment used during procedure
17. Specimens collected
    a. Pathology (e.g., appendix)
    b. Laboratory (e.g., blood for diagnostic testing)
18. Tubes or drains placed
    a. Location
    b. Type
    c. Number
19. Dressing placed
    a. Location
    b. Type
20. Total fluid intake and output that occurred intraoperatively
    a. Intake
    b. Output
21. Medications used on the surgical field or given by the circulating nurse
22. Additional notes if necessary.

TABLE 17–9 Surgical Wound Classifications

Wound Classification Level	Definition
Class I—clean	The surgical wound is not infected and has no inflammation present. The alimentary, respiratory, genital, and urinary tract are not entered.
Class II—clean contaminated	There is no sign of infection, but the alimentary, respiratory, genital, or urinary tract is entered under controlled conditions. There is no break in sterile technique.
Class III—contaminated	Gross spillage from the gastrointestinal tract occurs. A major break in sterile technique will also cause a wound to be placed in this category.
Class IV—dirty, infected	Pus or evidence of bacterial inflammation is found. Tissue necrosis may be present.

1. If there is a minor break in sterility, the wound class level increases to the next level.
2. A major break in sterility automatically increases the wound class level to a Class III.
3. An open drain left in place increases the wound class one level.

Sources: Data from Chard, R. (2012). Wound classifications. *Issues, 88*(1), 108–109; Fry, D. E. (n.d.). *Surgical site infection: Pathogenesis and prevention.* Retrieved from http://www.medscape.org/viewarticle/448981; Zinn, J., & Swofford, V. (2014). Quality-improvement initiative: Classifying and documenting surgical wounds. *American Nurse Today, 9*(1).

Surgical Wound Classification

A circulating registered nurse typically determines surgical wound classification for all surgical procedures (see **Table 17–9**). The healthcare team uses classification of surgical wounds, including incisions, in predicting the risk of surgical site infection (Zinn, 2012). The surgeon and nurse determine the wound classification at the end of the surgical procedure to capture any events that may have occurred that would affect the wound classification (Zinn, 2012). As shown in Table 17–9, if there is a minor break in sterile technique, the wound class increases one level. The more breaks in sterile technique, the higher the wound class, which correlates with a higher risk of an SSI.

Potential Intraoperative Complications

For all patients undergoing a surgical procedure, the nurse must pay close attention to possible physiologic changes occurring within the patient. The nurse cannot assume that another team member is monitoring the patient. In the intraoperative setting, the nurse truly becomes the spokesperson for the patient and is the patient's advocate.

The circulating nurse must pay attention to the whole intraoperative environment, including changes in the sounds of the monitor and changes in the color and amount of the patient's urine. If the circulating nurse notices any change during the intraoperative phase from the patient's preoperative baseline assessment, the nurse notifies the entire intraoperative team. Communicating any patient issues to the entire intraoperative team ensures a better surgical outcome for the patient. A list of potential intraoperative complications is shown in **Table 17–10**.

Rapid Response Teams

Surgery and anesthesia are associated with serious risks for all patients. In the event of a cardiopulmonary arrest during the preoperative period, the nurse should follow hospital protocols to call a "code blue" for a rapid response team, in which a team of specially trained care providers responds immediately to begin resuscitative efforts. If a patient deteriorates during the intraoperative period, the surgical and anesthesia team members work together as needed to implement appropriate interventions.

Within the intraoperative and postoperative phases, a member of the healthcare team runs the code blue, and the rest of the interprofessional team members assist, including drawing up medications and recording rapid response documentation.

Blood Transfusions

Blood transfusions are administered primarily in the intraoperative and postoperative phases. Blood for transfusion can be obtained from two sources: the patient can donate his or her own blood; this type of transfusion is known as an **autologous blood transfusion**. The patient can also receive blood that has been donated by the community; this type of transfusion is known as **allogeneic blood transfusion**.

The three methods of autologous blood transfusion include preoperative blood donation, normovolemic hemodilution, and perioperative salvage of autologous blood, such as blood recovered during the intraoperative phase (Kumar, Chen, Nath, & Liu, 2012). In preoperative blood donation, the surgical patient donates his or her own blood before the surgical procedure for use during upcoming surgery. Preoperative blood donation was once promoted to decrease the need for allogeneic blood transfusions (Shander et al., 2012). However, donation of blood before surgery is labor-intensive, is more costly than using allogeneic blood, and presents an increased risk for bacterial contamination and ABO incompatibility error. In addition, a high percentage of preoperative blood goes to waste when the patient is hemodynamically stable (Su et al., 2015). Normovolemic hemodilution is a method of conserving blood during surgical procedures in which a patient's blood is collected and then infused back to the patient with either a colloid or crystalloid fluid; this process tends to dilute the blood (Society for the Advancement of Blood Management, n.d.). At the end of the procedure, the red blood cells that were withdrawn before the procedure are replaced, along with platelets and plasma, which assist in coagulation. Perioperative blood recovery is done through the use of blood recovery equipment in the intraoperative suite during surgery (American Society of Anesthesiologists Task Force on Perioperative Blood Management, 2015).

TABLE 17–10 Potential Intraoperative Complications

Potential Complications	Nursing Implications
Hypovolemia - Decreased fluid volume (e.g., blood volume) - Decreased blood pressure - Decreased urine output - Increased heart rate - Increased respiratory rate	- Assess the patient to determine any underlying cause. - Replenish fluid volume (e.g., crystalloids, colloids, blood transfusion). See the module on Fluids and Electrolytes for discussion of IV fluid therapy.
Hypervolemia - Increased fluid volume (e.g., excessive amounts of IV fluids) - Increased blood pressure - Increased heart rate - Increased respiratory rate - Decreased urine output	- Assess the patient to determine any underlying cause. - Administer medications as ordered to decrease volume (e.g., diuretics).
Hyponatremia - Decreased sodium - Edema (swelling) - Muscle twitching - Signs of hypovolemia	- Assess the patient to determine any underlying cause. - If the cause of hyponatremia is fluid volume overload, IV fluids may be restricted to allow for concentration effect. Severe hyponatremia may require administration of hypertonic saline. See the module on Fluids and Electrolytes for discussion of IV fluid therapy.
Hypernatremia - Increased sodium - Concentrated urine - Dry mucous membranes	- Assess the patient to determine any underlying cause. - If the cause of hypernatremia is dehydration, IV fluids may be administered to create a dilutional effect.
Hypokalemia - Decreased potassium - Abdominal distention - Severe arrhythmias	- Assess the patient to determine any underlying cause. - Administer medications as ordered to increase potassium level (e.g., IV potassium).
Hyperkalemia - Increased potassium - Arrhythmias	- Assess the patient to determine any underlying cause. - Administer medications as ordered to decrease potassium level (e.g., kayexalate or IV glucose and insulin).
Increased intracranial pressure (ICP) - Increased blood pressure - Decreased heart rate - Hyperthermia may increase ICP.	- Administer medications as ordered to decrease ICP (e.g., diuretics). - Use methods to decrease temperature if patient has an increased temperature.
Hypothermia - Decreased body temperature - Decreased heart rate - Decreased circulation	- Assess the patient to determine any underlying cause. - Utilize warming methods (e.g., body warmer). - Administer warmed IV fluid.
Hyperthermia - Increased body temperature - Increased heart rate - Increased blood flow	- Monitor patient's temperature in all perioperative phases. - Identify cause of hyperthermia and implement appropriate interventions.
Malignant hyperthermia - Genetic disorder that produces a life-threatening hypermetabolic state; manifestations include hypercarbia (increased CO_2), tachycardia, muscle rigidity, rhabdomyolysis (breakdown of skeletal muscle fibers), and hyperthermia. - Primary cause is patient's exposure to certain anesthetic agents, including succinylcholine and anesthetic gases. - Triggered by inhalation of anesthetic gases and IV use of depolarizing muscle relaxants.	- Review the patient's history as well as the patient's familial history regarding any complications with anesthesia during previous procedures. - Administer dantrolene. - Recognize the early signs of malignant hyperthermia (e.g., hypercarbia, tachycardia). - Be familiar with your institution's protocols for treatment of patients with suspected malignant hyperthermia.

Evidence-Based Practice

Capnography Respiratory Assessment During Intraoperative Procedures

Problem

Monitoring only a patient's respiratory status during anesthesia and conscious sedation has come under scrutiny. Prior methods of respiratory assessment have been limited to peripheral capillary oxygen saturation (SpO_2) and observation of quality, rate, and labor of respirations, all of which may show change only after extended periods of distress or lack of proper oxygenation. End-tidal carbon dioxide ($etCO_2$), or capnography monitoring, offers a more accurate and rapid measurement of a patient's oxygenation (Spiegel, 2013).

Evidence

Capnography measures the concentration of carbon dioxide in a patient's expired breath. Changes in $etCO_2$ can be tracked almost instantaneously, whereas SpO_2 levels may take an extended amount of time to show any change in ventilation or respiratory status (Press, Macario, Desai, & Tanaka, 2013). Capnography measures the amount of carbon dioxide in the airway, which provides a breath-to-breath measure of ventilation. $EtCO_2$ is measured by waveform on a capnography-capable monitor using either a special nasal cannula or a bag valve mask. The normal range of $etCO_2$ is 35–45 mmHg.

Implications

The ability to detect acute changes in a patient's respiratory status during sedation and/or anesthesia is imperative to maintaining the patient's life and health. As the technology advances, capnography equipment is quickly becoming more portable and easier to use (Kodali, 2013). This will make measuring $etCO_2$ the standard of care in monitoring patients' respiratory status during procedures (Spiegel, 2013). As this modality becomes more prevalent in the inpatient and outpatient surgical arenas, nurses will need to become more familiar with its setup, use, and monitoring during procedures. Capnography has also improved the quality of compressions used during cardiopulmonary resuscitation (CPR), greatly improving its use and efficacy (Press et al., 2013). Some of the other implications of capnography include adequacy of mechanical ventilation for patients with chronic obstructive pulmonary disease (COPD); diagnosing mechanical problems such as kinked tubes, circuit leak, or blocked tubes; and detection of proper feeding tube insertion, metabolic acidosis, and shunts in cyanotic heart diseases (Spiegel, 2013).

Critical Thinking Application

1. How might you as a nurse better implement new advances in technology, such as capnography monitoring, in your unit? How would you tackle biases toward reliance on older modalities to which other nurses might be accustomed?

2. As you begin setting up the equipment for monitoring capnography, your 78-year-old patient, who reports that she was a nurse for over 50 years, asks why you are using this during sedation for surgery to correct her right shoulder subluxation. How do you describe the new standard of care to your patient and how might you best teach her?

3. You are preparing a patient for sedation during a surgical procedure. You are setting up capnography and getting ready to apply it to the patient when the surgeon exclaims, "Stop setting that stuff up! I don't use it and never have! We have to get moving! I have three more cases left today." Your hospital and unit manager have just recently set capnography as the standard of care for monitoring a patient's respiratory and ventilation status during surgical procedures. How do you approach and handle this situation with the surgeon and the others involved in this patient's care?

Case Study » Part 2

Rachel Poole is a 20-year-old woman recently diagnosed with stage II breast cancer who is undergoing a bilateral total mastectomy with a free TRAM breast reconstruction. She is healthy except for her recent diagnosis and has been given an ASA II classification. To prepare for surgery, the circulating nurse transfers Ms. Poole to the operating room and assists her onto the operating room bed. She places Ms. Poole in the supine position with her arms laterally abducted less than 90 degrees and pressure points padded. The nurse places a safety strap over Ms. Poole's upper thighs. The anesthesia team medicates and intubates Ms. Poole. Then, the nurse places a Foley catheter. She places a pillow under Ms. Poole's knees and soft gel pads under her ankles. The nurse completes the intraoperative skin prep for the breast and reconstruction surgery because the breast surgeon and plastic surgeon will be performing surgery concurrently. The surgeons and surgical technologists drape the patient, and the nurse completes the preprocedure verification process for both procedures. During the procedure, Ms. Poole loses 2500 mL of blood.

Clinical Reasoning Questions Level I

1. Why are safety straps being used to secure Ms. Poole's legs and thighs?
2. What purpose do the pillow under Ms. Poole's knees and the gel pads under her ankles serve?

Clinical Reasoning Questions Level II

3. What vital signs would you expect with Ms. Poole's blood loss? How would you intervene?
4. What considerations would you need to address with a patient who has religious objections to blood transfusions?

Postoperative Nursing

The postoperative phase begins with admission to the designated postsurgical recovery area and concludes upon the patient's transfer to a hospital unit or discharge to home. Patients receiving general anesthesia typically are transferred to a **postanesthesia care unit (PACU)**. Patients who emerge from surgery in a more critical state may be transferred to the intensive care unit (ICU). Ensuring airway patency is a priority of care while the patient recuperates from anesthesia. The nurse places the patient on an ECG monitor and pulse oximeter, checks vital signs on a regular basis, and administers medications to control pain and to assist the patient through the recovery period. After recovery, the patient may be transferred to a medical-surgical floor or, depending on the nature of the procedure, discharged home.

Postoperative Nursing Care

Surgery and anesthesia produce numerous physiologic effects. A detailed, thorough handoff during the postoperative phase is imperative and occurs between the postoperative nurse, the intraoperative circulating nurse, and the anesthesia provider. After receiving the report, the postoperative nurse assesses the patient, revises goals in the patient's care plan as needed, and then continues with implementation of the care plan. If a patient experiences cardiopulmonary arrest during the postoperative period, a member of the healthcare team should call a code team to attempt to resuscitate the patient.

Immediate postoperative assessment of the patient postanesthesia includes the following:

- Airway patency, ability to protect airway, oxygen saturation, ventilation, and pulmonary hygiene
- Emergence from anesthesia, ability to move limbs, return of sensation, and mobility
- Cardiovascular status: blood pressure, heart rate and rhythm
- Protective reflexes (e.g., gag reflex, cough reflex)
- Skin assessment
- Fluid status
- Operative site: dressing, drainage (amount, type, color)
- Pain, nausea, vomiting
- Safety
- Bowel sounds and postoperative diuresis
- Advancing diet.

SAFETY ALERT Significant findings that must be reported immediately to the surgeon or anesthesiologist include prolonged unresponsiveness, decrease in level of consciousness, oxygen saturation 92% or lower, respiratory rate less than 10 per minute, tachycardia or bradycardia, hypertension or hypotension, weak or absent pulses, urine output less than 30 mL per hour, and bleeding more than expected at the incision site.

The postoperative diagnoses include, but are not limited to, the following:

- *Pain, Acute*
- *Gas Exchange, Impaired*
- *Anxiety*
- *Cardiac Output, Decreased, Risk for*
- *Fluid Volume, Deficient, Risk for.*

(NANDA-I © 2014)

Nursing interventions in the postoperative phase will vary according to the patient, the procedure, and the patient's evolving postoperative status. At all times, the nurse acts to ensure airway management, reduce the potential for postoperative complications (e.g., infection), and address patient pain and anxiety.

Risk Monitoring

Patients who undergo certain surgical procedures, such as colorectal surgery, are at a high risk for acquiring a urinary tract infection or urinary retention (Kang et al., 2012). Urinary tract infection is the leading cause of healthcare-associated infections in the United States and increases mortality rates and healthcare costs (Kang et al., 2012). When applicable, the postoperative nurse should complete a thorough assessment of the indwelling urinary (e.g., Foley) catheter, including maintaining strict intake and output calculations and documentation. For example, if the patient has received 1000 mL of fluid but has excreted only 30 mL into the Foley bag and the patient's abdomen is starting to distend, the postoperative nurse uses critical thinking skills to assess the source of the problem. The problem could be as simple as a bend in the Foley tubing that needs to be straightened, or it may be that the patient is retaining fluid and the surgeon and anesthesia personnel need to be notified. The postoperative nurse should also be alert to changes in the appearance of the patient's urine, such as cloudiness or the presence of blood. The nurse should report all abnormalities to the patient's attending physician. Before the patient is discharged home, the postoperative nurse removes the catheter and ensures that the patient is able to excrete an acceptable amount of urine without straining. The patient's urine flow must be normal for the patient. For example, if the patient states, "I really did not pass as much urine as I usually do at home," the postoperative nurse continues to assess the patient.

SAFETY ALERT The postoperative nurse must maintain IVs as ordered to replace body fluids lost as a result of the surgical procedure. Once oral intake is permitted, the nurse should offer only small sips of water. Anesthetics and narcotic analgesics impair mobility of the stomach, and large amounts of water may induce vomiting. If the patient cannot yet drink water, the surgeon may permit the patient to suck on ice chips.

Cultural Considerations

Cultural influences can affect every aspect of the patient's response to care. The postanesthesia care unit nurse should incorporate the patient's cultural needs and preferences into the plan of care whenever possible. For example, suppose that a patient arrives during the postoperative phase after a dilation and curettage because her fetus was unexpectedly found to be lifeless at 13 weeks' gestational age. Because of her religious beliefs, the patient requests to take the products of conception home with her, as she does not want to send her unborn child's remains to a funeral home. With regard to miscarriage, most healthcare facilities have protocols in place to guide the process of care when a patient chooses to take home the remains for the purpose of burial. The nurse should follow organizational policy while seeking to safely incorporate the patient's cultural preferences into the plan of care.

Postoperative Medications

During the postoperative phase, the patient recovers from anesthesia. Two types of medications typically are administered in the postanesthesia phase: pain medications and antiemetic medications. Pain medications include, but are not limited to, hydromorphone (Dilaudid), morphine, and sometimes fentanyl (Sublimaze) (see the Medications feature). Pain medications assist in lowering the patient's pain level and, in turn, decrease elevated blood pressure and pulse rate.

Antiemetic medications assist in decreasing nausea and vomiting (see Medications: Perioperative feature).

Airway

On completion of the intraoperative phase, most patients are extubated before transport to the postoperative phase. If the patient is not stable enough to be extubated and the plan is to place the patient on a ventilator, the patient often remains intubated and is transferred to the unit, usually the ICU, to be placed on a ventilator. If the patient is extubated during the intraoperative phase and is stable, he or she is transferred to the postoperative care unit. On arrival in the postoperative care unit, the drowsy patient is placed in a sitting position—if the surgeon's orders allow—to decrease the work of breathing. At times, the patient may need to be stimulated to independently maintain the airway. Stimulation may include various interventions to assist the patient to wake up postoperatively; for example, the nurse may rigorously rub the patient's sternum. The postoperative nurse may have to perform a chin lift maneuver to open the airway or administer Narcan to reverse respiratory depression caused by narcotics previously administered to the patient.

Cardiac Rhythms

Patients receiving general anesthesia are monitored with an ECG upon arrival in the postoperative care unit. Postoperative nurses all have Advanced Cardiovascular Life Support (ACLS) certification. ACLS prepares the postoperative nurse to recognize the various heart rhythms, causes for the specific heart rhythms, and the course of action needed to return the patient to a normal rhythm or the patient's baseline rhythm before surgery. Depending on the patient's heart rhythm, postanesthesia care nurses are trained to complete algorithms, including the administration of medications. For example, the patient arrives during the postoperative phase and is placed on an ECG monitor. The ECG monitor shows the patient presents with a pulse of 45 beats per minute and demonstrates labored breathing. On the basis of the assessment data, the nurse follows the bradycardia algorithm, including identifying and treating any underlying causes. The primary care provider who is directing the PACU should be immediately notified of any changes in the patient's condition.

If the patient goes into cardiac or respiratory arrest, a code blue is called and followed according to the healthcare facility's set guidelines.

Wound Management

The surgeon may write orders for a dressing change to be completed before the patient is discharged. Depending on the surgeon's preferences, the order may specifically state that the surgeon or the surgeon's assistant (e.g., physician assistant, nurse practitioner) will complete the first dressing change and the patient's nurse will only reinforce the dressing if necessary before discharge. This may occur when the initial dressing that was placed at the completion of surgery creates a pressure pack to the wound, which assists in decreasing bleeding from the incision. If given the order to change the dressing, the postoperative nurse will use clean technique to change the patient's surgical dressing to decrease the chance of the patient having a surgical site infection. See the module on Tissue Integrity for a discussion of wound care and healing.

Line and Drain Management

Postoperative patients typically have infusion lines and may have surgical drains that need to be managed by postoperative nurses. All tubing is labeled with the name of the line or drain, the date and time the line or drain was placed, and the initials of the individual who initiated the line and/or drain. Lines and drains are labeled to prevent serious errors, such as attaching suction to an IV line. Lines and drains can include, but are not limited to, IV lines, chest tubes, urinary catheters, and closed wound drainage systems. Drains are inserted to allow excessive fluid and purulent material to drain and to promote healing of underlying tissues. Without a drain, a wound may heal on the outside but trap discharge and purulent material internally, increasing the risk for abscess formation.

Proper maintenance of all lines and drains is imperative and is the responsibility of the nurse. For example, consider the IV line used to administer medications, fluids, and blood products. The nurse must make sure the IV line does not infiltrate, causing fluids to enter surrounding tissue, which can cause excessive pain for the patient and tissue damage around the IV site, depending on the medication being administered. When drains are used, the nurse is responsible for maintaining wound suction, which helps to drain excess discharge. This, in turn, assists in the formation of granulation tissue. In closed wound drainage systems, the drain is connected to electric suction or a portable suction device such as a Jackson-Pratt drain or a Hemovac drainage system (see **Figure 17–6 》》**). Directions for use are printed on the container and must be followed carefully to ensure that the container is emptied and the drainage plug replaced correctly in order to restore the vacuum function that is required for the closed drainage system to work.

SAFETY ALERT Note that the presence of blood in drainage tubes or more than the expected amount of drainage in chest tubes or drainage sites requires a report to the surgeon or anesthesia provider.

Sutures and Staples

Sutures can be absorbable or nonabsorbable; the human body considers both types of sutures to be foreign bodies. The choice of suture material depends on the type of body tissue being sutured. For example, absorbable synthetic sutures are used in cardiovascular or ophthalmic procedures because of their low affinity with microorganisms, whereas surgical gut sutures are used for soft tissues that heal quickly (MacKay-Wiggin, Ratner, & Sambandan, 2014).

Staples are utilized mainly to close the skin. Staples decrease the length of time in the operating room because they allow faster closure of the surgical incision than is possible with sutures (Galli & Constantinides, 2013). Staples offer a uniform tension and less distortion along the closure line (Galli & Constantinides, 2013). Another benefit to using staples rather than sutures to close the skin is that the skin heals better and is cosmetically more appealing. On the other hand, staples are more expensive and call for more attention to placement, especially when considering eversion of wound edges. Injury to the skin from using staples is comparable to that from using sutures.

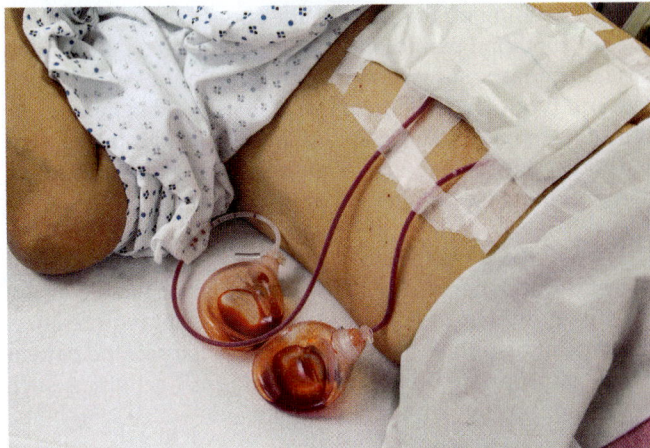

A

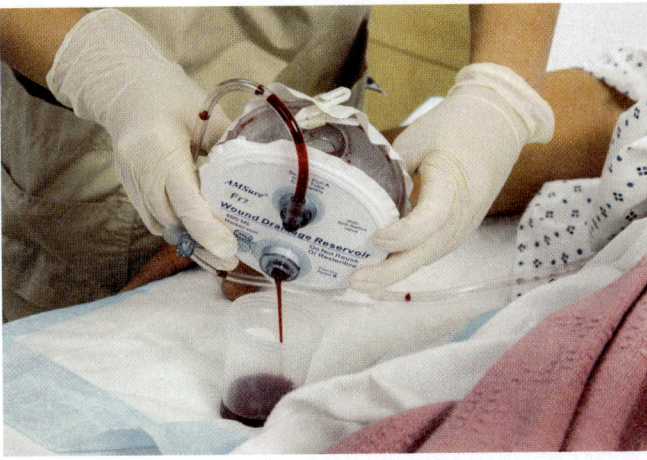

B

Figure 17–6 ⟫ Closed wound drainage systems. *A,* Jackson-Pratt drains. *B,* Hemovac drainage system.

Postoperative Documentation

A thorough postoperative assessment is imperative to minimize disruption to the patient's physiologic processes (see **Box 17–4 ⟫**).

Patient Recovery and Discharge

According to ASPAN (2012), each healthcare organization should create discharge criteria using the discharge assessment parameters created by ASPAN while also consulting with the anesthesia department and medical staff. Many healthcare facilities utilize a discharge scoring record, which assists in the objective determination of whether the patient is physically able to be discharged. One common scoring method is the Aldrete scoring system, which measures the patient's circulation, respiration, activity level, and oxygen saturation (see **Box 17–5 ⟫**). The Aldrete scoring system identifies two recovery phases:

- Phase 1 occurs with the discontinuation of anesthesia.
- Phase 2 begins when the patient's protective reflexes and motor functioning return, indicating that the patient is effectively recovering from anesthesia.

Box 17–4
Postoperative Documentation

Postoperative assessment and management include, but are not limited to, the review and documentation of the following (ASPAN, 2012):

1. Review of history and physical assessment
2. Systems assessment
   a. Respiratory
   b. Cardiovascular
   c. Neurologic
   d. Gastrointestinal/abdominal
   e. Urinary
   f. Musculoskeletal
   g. Integumentary
3. Pain assessment
4. Sedation assessment
5. Psychosocial assessment
6. Medication review and administration
7. Care of postoperative lines and drains (e.g., a Foley catheter)
8. Intake and output of fluids
9. Laboratory testing
10. Blood administration
11. Dressing changes
12. Discharge education.

Box 17–5
The Aldrete Score

The Aldrete scoring system is designed to assess a patient's transition from Phase 1 recovery to Phase 2 recovery, from discontinuation of anesthesia to return of protective reflexes and motor function.

Respiration	2 = Able to take deep breath and cough
	1 = Dyspnea/shallow breathing
	0 = Apnea
O₂ saturation	2 = Maintains >92% on room air
	1 = Needs O_2 inhalation to maintain O_2 saturation >90%
	0 = Saturation <90% even with supplemental oxygen
Consciousness	2 = Fully awake
	1 = Arousable on calling
	0 = Not responding
Circulation	2 = BP ±20% preop
	1 = BP ±20–49% preop
	0 = BP ±50% preop
Activity	2 = Able to move four extremities
	1 = Able to move two extremities
	0 = Able to move no extremities

The total score is 10. Patients scoring 8 or above (and/or patients who are returned to a similar preop status) are considered fit for transition to Phase 2 recovery.

If the patient does not meet the discharge criteria, he or she is transferred to a specified unit, such as an extended recovery or medical–surgical unit, for further monitoring until meeting the discharge criteria. The postoperative nurse and anesthesia personnel determine the team and equipment necessary for transport of the patient according to the patient's postoperative stability (ASPAN, 2012). For example, if the patient is having difficulty breathing and maintaining the desired oxygen saturation level and needs to be transported while on oxygen, a licensed professional would transport the patient. Once the patient meets the discharge criteria, the surgeon writes discharge orders, which include specific information on medications, wound care, nutrition, and physical activity. Before discharge, the postoperative or unit nurse educates the patient and the individual who will be driving the patient home (see the Patient Teaching feature).

Wound Care

The postoperative nurse instructs the patient to allow surgical dressings to fall off naturally, which may take up to about 1 week. The patient is usually allowed to have a shower 24 hours after surgery, but the patient may not soak in a bath until the surgical dressings have fallen off, as a precaution against the possible occurrence of a surgical site infection. The nurse instructs the patient on suture or staple care to prevent a surgical site infection. The nurse also teaches the patient to report the signs and symptoms of infection to the surgeon and gives the patient specific instructions on when to return to the surgeon's office for a postoperative appointment. During the postoperative appointment, the surgeon or nurse will remove the sutures or staples and complete a dressing change.

Nutrition

To help prevent nausea and vomiting, patients should start by eating bland foods and gradually advance to a normal diet. Depending on the surgery, the surgeon may prescribe a specific diet for a period of time. For example, a patient who has had bariatric surgery will be prescribed a specific serving size and type of food. Patients typically should increase their fluid intake on discharge. Increasing the fluid intake assists the body systems to return to normal, maintaining hydration and providing electrolytes necessary for homeostasis.

Physical Activity

The surgical patient is not allowed to drive or handle heavy machinery within 24 hours of procedures that require anesthesia administration. The surgeon also instructs the patient on the appropriate time to resume physical activities, such as running, cycling, or sexual activity.

Case Study >> Part 3

Rachel Poole, a 20-year-old woman diagnosed with stage II breast cancer, underwent a bilateral total mastectomy with a free TRAM breast reconstruction. The surgery was completed with no complications. Now that the procedure has been completed, the anesthesia provider extubates Ms. Poole before her transport to the PACU. Upon extubation, Ms. Poole's blood pressure drops to 70/30 mmHg, her pulse drops to 45 bpm, her respiratory rate drops to 8/min, and her oxygen saturation drops to 70% on 2 L oxygen through a nasal cannula.

Clinical Reasoning Questions Level I

1. What factors could be contributing to Ms. Poole's changes in vital signs?
2. Would calling a code be appropriate in this situation? Why or why not?

Clinical Reasoning Questions Level II

3. How would you intervene in this situation? Why?
4. What medications would you expect to use in this situation?

Lifespan Considerations

Perioperative care requires that nurses assess patients' needs related to lifespan and developmental considerations. For example, the nurse assesses the patient's ability to understand the surgery and provides education according to the patient's developmental level that takes into consideration differences in learning style and abilities. Priorities for care of patients in all stages of the lifespan include maintaining airway patency and tissue perfusion, monitoring the patient's temperature and vital signs, and ensuring safe administration of medications.

Perioperative Care of Infants

Preoperative nursing for infants focuses on aiding the patient in his or her development for adaption to the outside world. Parents can help to prepare the patient for surgery by adjusting care of the infant in a manner that will support their child's already established feeding and bonding routine. Soothing the infant with proper oral means such as pacifiers and breastfeeding can aid in helping the infant during preoperative procedures such as labs, physical assessments, and IV access. Nurses should assess whether the infant was born preterm (less than 37 weeks) or post-term (more than 42 weeks). Preterm infants may be small for ges-

---

Patient Teaching
Postoperative Discharge Instructions

Patients should adhere to the following instructions when they are discharged in the postoperative phase.

- Use pain medications as ordered; do not allow pain to become severe before taking the prescribed dose. Pain inhibits healing.
- Avoid using alcohol while taking opioids or other narcotic analgesics.
- Contact your primary care provider if you experience an increase in pain after increasing discomfort.
- Change dressings and perform wound care as instructed to promote healing and reduce the risk of infection.
- Promptly report any increase in redness, swelling, pain, or discharge from the incision or drain site to the surgical specialist's office.
- Gradually increase activities as ordered by the surgeon or primary care provider.
- Adequate rest, nutrition, and hydration are important to promote healing and immune function.

tational age (SGA), which makes them more prone to respiratory complications such as infection related to meconium aspiration and necrotizing enterocolitis (NEC) (Garg, Garg, & Lal, 2015). The family of a preterm infant is likely to be confused and emotionally unstable in any case, but especially if the infant requires surgery. Nurses working with families of preterm infants requiring perioperative care can work in a nurse navigator capacity to provide emotional outlets for the family and help overcome impediments in the healthcare system.

As nurses help the infant patient make the transition into the intraoperative stage, they give special care to the patient's respiratory status related to the immature status of the respiratory system and the possible lack of surfactant, which helps to generate negative pressure within the thoracic cavity, thus aiding in lung inflation. Glucose regulation is important during the perioperative process related to the neonate's lack of brown fat reserves along with concomitant NPO (nothing by mouth) or clear liquid diet during the preoperative period. Fluid and electrolyte balance is also of great concern related to the infant's large surface area of immature skin and relatively high fluid volume to weight ratio. Fluid overload during repair of such conditions such as patent ductus arteriosus (PDA) can cause pulmonary edema quite easily.

The postoperative infant patient will most often be transferred to and cared for in the neonatal intensive care unit (NICU) at the facility at which the infant had the procedure. At this stage, the nurse should focus largely on support for the parents. Assessment of parents' grief, guilt, anxiety, and coping mechanisms are necessary so that the nurse may better assist the infant in receiving necessary care required from the parents, such as bonding activities and breastfeeding. The nurse should keep in mind that surgery on the infant patient can be exhausting and demanding for the parents, who play a large part in comforting and caring for the neonate. Assessment of the infant's developmental stages and the needs of the infant's parents is important for consistent and thorough care of the postoperative neonate patient.

Perioperative Care of Children

During the preoperative stage, nurses preparing children for surgery should always assess and consider the child's developmental level when communicating information and explanations of the surgical procedure. Nurses should educate the patient according to the patient's developmental level and preferred learning style. Depending on the patient's developmental level and age, nurses should include the family as much as possible in the perioperative care plan. Whenever possible, preparation for the child's procedure should start at least 1 month before intervention, including assessment of the patient for language, hearing, or visual services. Sometimes, scheduling a tour of the facility is beneficial in easing fears in the pediatric patient and the patient's family. Nurses should educate the parents to assess the patient for sickness, including rash, fever, and blisters, one day before surgery (Children's National Health System, n.d.).

Surgical procedures create stress for both the pediatric patient and family members. Preoperative assessment includes assessing the patient and family's stress and coping skills. Nurses should be honest with the patient and family, especially regarding expectations about postoperative pain and how the care team is ready to respond and treat pain. To help younger patients cope with stress, nurses should promote comfort by offering choices whenever possible, such as by allowing younger patients to bring a comfort item, such as a stuffed animal or blanket. The nurse should ensure safe care of the comfort item by the family while the child is in the intraoperative phase. If the patient is unable to get comfortable in any of the perioperative phases, including before induction in the intraoperative phase, the nurse may allow the patient's parent or caregiver to sit with the patient, especially if the patient becomes agitated and disruptive. The patient's hospital room needs to be a nonthreatening place; therefore, procedures such as drawing blood or starting an IV may be performed in a treatment or procedure room rather than in the patient's hospital room. To promote safety, pediatric patients may also be assigned a one-to-one perioperative nurse ratio.

SAFETY ALERT Children who undergo surgery can become very emotional and confused when anesthesia wears off. For the child's well-being, provide comfort and allow the parents to provide comfort when it is safe to do so.

» Stay Current: Many pediatric hospitals have information on their websites, including lists of books that can help families prepare for a child's surgery. For example, see the website of The Children's National Health System: http://childrensnational.org/specialty-care-patients/preparing-for-your-visit/having-surgery-what-to-expect/countdown-checklists

During the intraoperative stage, nurses are the child's chief advocate and are placed in charge of a range of different tasks. For example, maintaining normothermia can be difficult for all patients under the age of 18, so the nurse acts to monitor and maintain the patient's temperature to determine which actions will be taken if the patient becomes **hyperthermic** (temperature above 37.8°C [100°F]) or **hypothermic** (temperature below 36.1°C [97°F]). For surgeries that will require electrocauterization, the nurse should identify the proper electrocautery pad size for the patient before the patient is transported to surgery. In the intraoperative phase, the nurse continuously monitors airway patency and is alert to signs and symptoms of respiratory distress, including distress that occurs after extubation (withdrawal of the breathing tube on completion of anesthesia and the surgical case). When performing surgery on children, the perioperative team must be prepared to implement additional safety measures as needed to protect the patient from injury, including falls or dislodged IV devices, and to promote safe emergence from anesthesia.

The nurse should promote the postoperative child's comfort and safety. The nurse needs to assess whether or not the parents have medications such as children's acetaminophen at home to treat the patient's pain. It may also be pertinent for a nurse to discuss care at home such as having plenty of clear liquids available in forms such as water, sugar water, Pedialyte, Jell-O, juices, and Popsicles (Children's National Health System, n.d.). The nurse should also discuss transportation concerns for the infant patient, specifically whether the parents have a properly sized car seat or booster seat. The nurse also should assess whether the parents have scheduled a follow-up appointment, have guidelines for contacting the healthcare provider if the patient displays worsening signs and symptoms, can fill and give prescription medications properly, and have information on when the school-age patient can return to school. Also, because of the need for constant care after a procedure, the nurse should ask the parents what arrangements they have made to have another adult present while the parents themselves recover.

Perioperative Care of Pregnant Women

Pregnant women constitute a unique population of patients when it comes to perioperative care. While cesarean birth, elective or emergent, can understandably be the most apparent surgical intervention for pregnant women, other emergencies such as acute appendicitis, cholecystitis, and intestinal obstruction may necessitate surgery. Nurses should be aware of special perioperative concerns for pregnant women.

During the preoperative period, the pregnant woman may require radiologic testing, an ultrasound, CT, or MRI. While radiation exposure during normal diagnostic testing usually does not harm the fetus, ionizing radiation can contribute to serious health consequences such as growth retardation, malformations, impaired brain function, and cancer (CDC, 2014). The risk for abnormal fetal brain development related to radiation exposure is at its most significant from 16 to 25 weeks' gestation (CDC, 2014). Ultrasound and MRI without radiologic intervention are both considered safe for mother and fetus. The pregnant women undergoing a surgical intervention or procedure warrants the same preoperative lab work and antibiotic prophylaxis as any other demographic with the specific addition of Group B Streptococcus (GBS) and newborn prophylaxis.

During the intraoperative phase, nurses should place the pregnant woman in the left lateral recumbent position so that the uterus is shifted off the vena cava, thus improving cardiac output and venous return. Pregnant women are also in a state of hypercoagulability, which places them at an increased risk for deep venous thrombosis (DVT) and pulmonary embolism (PE); as a consequence, pneumatic compression stockings or sequential compression devices (SCDs) are recommended during the intraoperative and postoperative periods. Fetal monitoring is indicated during the entire perioperative process. Abnormal organogenesis related to anesthesia is usually not a concern during surgery in pregnant women, but anesthesia has been associated with fetal death and spontaneous abortion (International Anesthesia Research Society, 2015).

During the postoperative period, nurses should continue fetal monitoring if the procedure is nonobstetric. If the procedure was a cesarean section, nurses must test the neonate's Apgar status at 1 and 5 minutes. Nurses should support the respiratory function of the neonate by suctioning the infant's mouth and then nose after the delivery procedure. Bleeding should be monitored postdelivery for signs and symptomatology of retained placenta or boggy uterus.

Focus on Diversity and Culture
Gaining Cultural Competence

Addressing ageist, racial, cultural, and economic disparities in healthcare is a key issue in attaining equal health outcomes for people of all backgrounds and ages. One of the most important efforts that nurses and other members of the healthcare team can make to address this disparity is engaging in culturally competent care education (CCCE) and working CCCE into nursing education and perioperative practice. There are several approaches to CCCE, and various learning tools are available to members of the healthcare team (Khoury et al., 2012):

- Cultural sensitivity focuses on biases and attitudes within the healthcare team. This approach rests on the fact that cultural competence is achieved when the key components of professionalism—empathy, humility, respect, and sensitivity—are met.
- Cultural adaptability emphasizes the importance of gaining general knowledge about health attitudes and habits specific to the members of different cultural groups. Nurses who frequently work with members of particular populations may benefit from the cultural adaptability approach.
- Cross-cultural skills are bolstered by focusing on the social, cultural, and health issues of various groups while always emphasizing the tenets of professionalism.
- The U.S. Department of Health and Human Services provides a variety of assessments for healthcare institutions to identify ways in which nurses can best serve diverse patient populations. These tools include self-assessment modules, a cultural competency curriculum, training modules, and resources crafted to improve deficiencies in culturally competent care.

In the event of fetal death during the surgical procedure, the nurse should focus special attention on the family's spiritual and cultural beliefs and practices. Activities such as grief counseling, assembling a memory kit, and parental interaction with the fetus or baby can play an important role in achieving closure.

Perioperative Care of Older Adults

Perioperative care of older adults requires the nurse to be aware of nuances related to aging. Preexisting conditions related to the normal aging process can result in perioperative complications in the older surgical patient (Bashaw & Scott, 2012). The nurse should pay specific attention to the patient's hearing status to evaluate whether the patient is understanding the procedure's possible risks and benefits so that the patient may make a proper informed decision. Older adults may have a lower speed of comprehension than younger adults, so nurses should check with the patient to ensure that information is being delivered at an understandable rate. If the patient cannot hear or understand the information being presented, provide information through alternative means. Dementia, confusion, risk for falls, and depression need to be considered during the perioperative period for all surgical patients ages 65 and older (Hilsgen, 2013). Because deep breathing and coughing assist in the prevention of pneumonia and other respiratory conditions related to surgery, nurses should teach these techniques in the preoperative phase. (See the module on Oxygenation for a discussion of deep breathing exercises and a patient-teaching feature on effective coughing techniques.)

As the older adult enters the intraoperative stage, maintaining normothermia becomes challenging because the aging process decreases the body's ability to maintain a normal body temperature. See the module on Thermoregulation for more information about maintaining normothermia in older adults. A skin assessment is essential because older adults have a predisposition to dry skin, loss of subcutaneous fat, and fragility of blood vessels (Hurd, 2014). The perioperative team must take special precautions when removing adhesives from the older adult patient's skin to prevent tearing of the skin. They must make sure to prevent the formation of pressure sores during the intraoperative period. The geriatric patient is also at higher risk for developing a VTE.

SAFETY ALERT Older adults are more vulnerable to postoperative infection than younger adults. Do not rely on the presence of fever to indicate infection in older adults. Patients in this population may have lower core body temperatures and decreased immune responses. Signs of infection in older adults often relate to cognitive changes such as confusion or agitation.

The postoperative older adult is at a higher risk for acquiring a surgical site infection, pneumonia, and other postoperative complications. Reinforce teaching related to moving, deep breathing, and coughing exercises. The nurse should assess the patient for risks for pressure ulcers, for example, poor nutritional status, diabetes or cardiovascular illness, and history of steroid use (which increases bruising and skin breakdown). The postoperative nurse will also assess and initiate plans for care after discharge. This includes arranging for necessary medical equipment (e.g., walkers, chair-height toilet seats). The nurse should help with organization and implementation of transportation and extended postsurgical care as needed. Communication with ancillary staff, family members, and community resources such as social or case workers may be needed at this time.

REVIEW The Concept of Perioperative Care

RELATE Link the Concepts

Linking the concept of perioperative care with the concept of development:

1. What strategies could you use to explain a diagnostic surgical procedure to a 5-year-old patient?

2. Prepare a patient teaching plan for a 10-year-old patient who must refrain from sports-related activities for 2 weeks after surgery.

Linking the concept of perioperative care with the concept of nutrition:

3. Why is it necessary to provide patient teaching related to withholding food before surgery?

4. How does altered nutrition status or malnutrition increase the risks associated with surgery?

Linking the concept of perioperative care with the concept of informatics:

5. What are the advantages of a surgical team using uniform language?

6. How might telehealth be used to assist patients to prepare for surgery before the day of the procedure?

READY Go to Volume 3: Clinical Nursing Skills

- SKILL 13.1   Preoperative Patient Teaching
- SKILL 13.2   Surgical Hand Antisepsis and Scrubs
- SKILL 13.3   Surgical Site: Preparing
- SKILL 13.4   Sterile Field: Maintaining
- SKILL 13.5   Sterile Gown and Gloves: Donning (Closed Method)
- SKILL 13.6   Surgical Patient: Preparing
- SKILL 16.3   Closed Wound Drains: Maintaining
- SKILL 16.4   Dressing, Dry: Changing
- SKILL 16.8   Elastic Bandage: Applying
- SKILL 16.9   Surgical Wound: Caring for

REFER Go to Pearson MyLab Nursing and eText

- Additional review materials

REFLECT Apply Your Knowledge

Mary Caruso, a 42-year-old woman, arrives in the postoperative anesthesia care unit (PACU). Ms. Caruso's mother died of colon cancer, and Ms. Caruso had a colonoscopy that revealed three precancerous polyps and one malignant polyp. She has just had a partial colectomy to remove the malignant section of her colon. The physician placed a closed drain system in her abdominal incision. The abdominal drain has drained 20 mL of blood-tinged fluid. Ms. Caruso has a urinary catheter in place that is draining 30 mL of clear urine every hour. During intubation, Ms. Caruso sustained a 3-mm laceration to her upper lip. Bleeding is controlled. Her heart rate is 48 bpm, indicating bradycardia. Ms. Caruso remains drowsy from the anesthesia, but she appears to be comfortable, with a limited amount of pain. The postanesthesia nurse raises Ms. Caruso's head and places her in the sitting position. The nurse supports her with pillows and provides a pillow for her to place on her stomach when she takes deep breaths.

Ms. Caruso sits up for 1 hour. Her vital signs include: T_O 98.6°F, P 65 bpm, R 14/min, BP 117/72 mmHg. Her respirations are regular and nonlabored. She is transferred to the medical–surgical unit for further observation for 24 hours before being discharged home.

1. What procedure could the nurse perform to assist in Ms. Caruso's prognosis? Explain why.

2. List some topics for discharge instructions that the postoperative nurse should anticipate.

References

American Society of Anesthesiologists. (2014). *ASA physical status classification system.* Retrieved from https://www.asahq.org/resources/clinical-information/asa-physical-status-classification-system

American Society of Anesthesiologists Task Force on Perioperative Blood Management. (2015). Practice guidelines for perioperative blood management. *Anesthesiology, 122*(2), 241–275. doi:10.1097/aln.0000000000000463

American Society of PeriAnesthesia Nurses (ASPAN). (2012). *2012–2014 Perianesthesia nursing standards, practice recommendations and interpretive statements.* Cherry Hill, NJ: Author.

Andel, C., Davidlow, S. L., Hollander, M., & Moreno, D. A. (2012). The economics of health care quality and medical errors. *Journal of Health Care Finance, 39*(1), 39–50.

Association of periOperative Registered Nurses (AORN). (2012). *Perioperative job descriptions and competency evaluation tools.* Denver, CO: Author.

Association of periOperative Registered Nurses (AORN). (2013). *Perioperative standards and recommended practices.* Denver, CO: Author.

Bashaw, M., & Scott, D. (2012). Surgical risk factors in geriatric perioperative patients. *AORN Journal, 96*(1), 58–74. doi:10.1016/j.aorn.2011.05.025

Centers for Disease Control and Prevention (CDC). (n.d.). *Frequently asked questions about surgical site infections.* Retrieved from http://www.cdc.gov/HAI/pdfs/ssi/SSI_tagged.pdf

Centers for Disease Control and Prevention (CDC). (2013). *Patient safety: Ten things you can do to be a safe patient.* Retrieved from http://www.cdc.gov/Features/PatientSafety/

Centers for Disease Control and Prevention (CDC). (2014). *Radiation and pregnancy: A fact sheet for clinicians.* Retrieved from http://emergency.cdc.gov/radiation/prenatalphysician.asp

Children's National Health System. (n.d.). *Countdown to surgery: Checklists for parents.* Retrieved from http://childrensnational.org/specialty-care-patients/preparing-for-your-visit/having-surgery-what-to-expect/countdown-checklists

Data USA. (2017). *Physicians and surgeons: Diversity.* Retrieved from https://datausa.io/profile/soc/291060/#demographics

Ehrlich, S. (2014). *Valerian: University of Maryland Medical Center.* Retrieved from http://umm.edu/health/medical/altmed/herb/valerian

Galli, S., & Constantinides, M. (2013). *Wound closure technique.* Retrieved from http://emedicine.medscape.com/article/1836438-overview#a1

Garg, P. M., Garg, P. P., & Lal, C. V. (2015). Necrotizing enterocolitis (NEC): A devastating disease of prematurity. *Journal of Neonatal Biology, 4,* 202. Retrieved from http://www.omicsgroup.org/journals/necrotizing-enterocolitis-nec-a-devastating-disease-of-prematurity-2167-0897-1000202.php?aid=62557

Hadjiliadis, D. (2014). Using an incentive spirometer. *MedlinePlus Medical Encyclopedia.* Retrieved from https://www.nlm.nih.gov/medlineplus/ency/patientinstructions/000451.htm

Herdman, T. H. & Kamitsuru, S. (Eds). *Nursing Diagnoses—Definitions and Classification 2015–2017.* Copyright © 2014, 1994–2014 NANDA International. Used by arrangement with John Wiley & Sons, Inc. Companion website: www.wiley.com/go/nursingdiagnoses.

Hilsgen, J. (2013). Gerioperative nursing care: Principles and practices of surgical care for the older adult. *AORN Journal, 97*(1), 154–155. doi:http://dx.doi.org/10.1016/j.aorn.2012.10.002

Hole, J., Hirsch, M., Ball, E., & Meads, C. (2015). Music as an aid for postoperative recovery in adults: A systematic review and meta-analysis. *The Lancet.* doi:10.1016/s0140-6736(15)60169-6

Hurd, R. (2014). Aging changes in skin. *MedlinePlus Medical Encyclopedia.* Retrieved from https://www.nlm.nih.gov/medlineplus/ency/article/004014.htm

Ibrahim, M. H., Azab, A., Kamal, N. M., Salama, M. A., Elshorbagy, H. H., Abdallah, E. A., Hammad, A., & Sherief, L. M. (2015). Outcomes of early ligation of patent ductus arteriosus in preterms, multicenter experience. *Medicine* (Baltimore), *94*(28):1.

International Anesthesia Research Society. (2015). *Surgery risk during pregnancy.* Retrieved from https://www.openanesthesia.org/surgery_risk_during_pregnancy/

Joint Commission, The. (n.d.). *The universal protocol for preventing wrong site, wrong procedure, and wrong person surgery.* Retrieved from http://www.jointcommission.org/assets/1/18/up_poster.pdf

JPAC. (2016). *Jehovah's witnesses and blood transfusion.* Retrieved from http://www.transfusion-guidelines.org/transfusion-handbook/12-management-of-patients-who-do-not-accept-transfusion/12-2-jehovah-s-witnesses-and-blood-transfusion

Kang, C., Chaudhry, O., Halabi, W., Nguyen, V., Carmichael, J., Mills, S., & Stamos, M. (2012). Risk factors for postoperative urinary tract infection and urinary retention in patients undergoing surgery for colorectal cancer. *American Surgeon, 78*(10), 1100–1104.

Kodali, B. S. (2013). Capnography outside the operating rooms. *Anesthesiology, 118*(1), 192–201. doi:10.1097/aln.0b013e318278c8b6

Kumar, N., Chen, Y., Nath, C., & Liu, E. (2012). What is the role of autologous blood transfusion in major spine surgery? *The American Journal of Orthopedics, 41*(6), E89–E95.

Lewis, S. L., Dirksen, S. R., Heitkemper, M. M., & Bucher, L. (2014). *Medical-surgical nursing: Assessment and management of clinical problems* (9th ed.). St. Louis, MO: Elsevier Mosby.

Li, H., Wang, H., Chou, F., & Chen, K. (2015). The effect of music therapy on cognitive functioning among older adults: A systematic review and meta-analysis. *Journal of the American Medical Directors Association, 16*(1), 71–77.

MacKay-Wiggin, J., Ratner, D., & Sambandan, D. (2014). *Suturing techniques periprocedural care.* Retrieved from http://emedicine.medscape.com/article/1824895-periprocedure

Nanji, K. C., Patel, A., Shaikh, S., Seger, D. L., & Bates, D. W. (2016). Evaluation of perioperative medication errors and adverse drug events. *Anesthesiology, 124,* 25–34.

National League of Nursing. (2017). Biennial survey of schools of nursing, academic year 2015–2016. Retrieved from http://www.nln.org/newsroom/nursing-education-statistics/biennial-survey-of-schools-of-nursing-academic-year-2015-2016

Press, C. D., Macario, A., Desai, A. M., & Tanaka, P. P. (2013). *End-tidal capnography.* Retrieved from http://emedicine.medscape.com/article/2116444-overview#a4

Rangrass, G., Ghaferi, A. A., & Dimick, J. B. (2014). Explaining racial disparities in outcomes after cardiac surgery: The role of hospital quality. *JAMA Surgery, 149*(3):223–227. doi: 10.1001/jamasurg.2013.4041

Shander, A., Van Aken, H., Colomina, M. J., Gombotz, H., Hofmann, A., Krauspe, R., ... Spahn, D. R. (2012). Patient blood management in Europe. *British Journal of Anaesthesia, 109*(1), 55–68.

Society for the Advancement of Blood Management. (n.d.). *Acute normovolemic hemodilution.* Retrieved from http://www.sabm.org/glossary/acute-normovolemic-hemodilution-anh

Spiegel, J. (2013). End tidal carbon dioxide: The most vital of vital signs. *Anesthesiology News, 39*(10), 21–27.

Stern, C. (2013). Music interventions for preoperative anxiety. *International Journal of Evidence-Based Healthcare, 11*(3), 208–209.

Su, L. L., Adamski, J., Gilman, E. A., Cusick, R., & Hernandez, J. S. (2015). Decreasing preoperative autologous blood donation: Collaboration between a hospital and a blood center to prompt change in physician ordering behavior. *Lab Medicine, 46,* 74–78.

Walker, I. A., Reshamwalla, S., & Wilson, I. H. (2012). Surgical safety checklists: Do they improve outcomes? *British Journal of Anaesthesia, 109*(1), 47–54.

Weldon, J. M., Miedema, F., Oakie, A., Langan, K., Myers, J., & Walter, E. (2014). Special needs populations: Overcoming language barriers for pediatric surgical patients and their family members. *AORN Journal.* Retrieved from https://www.aorn.org/websitedata/ceararticle/pdf_file/CEA14512-0001.pdf

Williams, D. R., Priest, N., & Anderson, N. (2016). Understanding associations between race, socioeconomic status and health: Patterns and prospects. *Health Psychology, 35*(4): 407–411. doi.org/10.1037/hea0000242

Wilson, B., Shannon, M., & Shields, K. (2013). *Pearson nurse's drug guide, 2013.* Upper Saddle River, NJ: Pearson Education.

World Alliance for Patient Safety (2008). *WHO surgical safety checklist and implementation.*

Retrieved from http://www.who.int/patientsafety/safesurgery/tools_resources/SSSL_Checklist_finalJun08.pdf

World Health Organization (WHO). (2015a). *World Health Organization (WHO) surgical safety checklist and getting started kit*. Retrieved from http://www.ihi.org/resources/Pages/Tools/WHOSurgicalSafetyChecklistGettingStartedKit.aspx

World Health Organization (WHO). (2015b). *Safe surgery*. Retrieved from http://www.who.int/patientsafety/safesurgery/en/

Wu, C., Wang, C., Tsai, M., Huang, W., & Kennedy, J. (2014). Trend and pattern of herb and supplement use in the United States: Results from the 2002, 2007, and 2012 National Health Interview Surveys. *Evidence-Based Complementary and Alternative Medicine*, 1–7.

Zinn, J. (2012). Surgical wound classification: Communication is needed for accuracy. *AORN Journal*, *95*(2), 274–278.

Zinn, J., & Swofford, V. (2014). Quality-improvement initiative: Classifying and documenting surgical wounds. *American Nurse Today*. Retrieved from http://www.americannursetoday.com/quality-improvement-initiative-classifying-and-documenting-surgical-wounds/

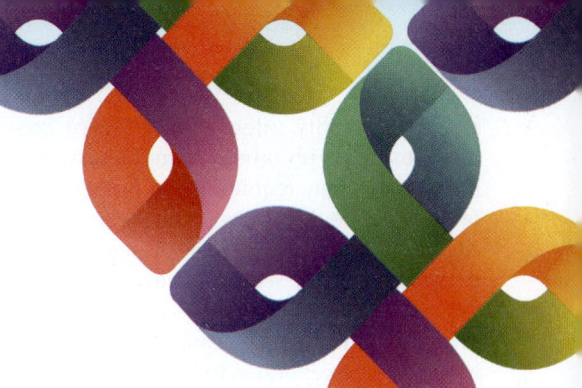

Module 18
Sensory Perception

Module Outline and Learning Outcomes

» The Concept of Sensory Perception

Concept Key Terms

The sensory organs provide pathways for stimuli to reach the brain, allowing individuals to experience the world in which they live. Sensory stimuli give meaning to events in the environment. The five senses—vision, hearing, touch, smell, and taste—are essential for growth, development, and survival. Normal sensory function enables or affects nearly every human activity, from reading a book to alerting someone to smoke from a fire. **Sensory perception** is protective, such as a mother sensing that the bath water is too hot as she sees the steam rise from the water. It is also complex, allowing individuals to master activities that require the use of multiple senses at once, such as driving a car.

Alterations in sensory functions can affect an individual's ability to experience the world; these alterations may limit self-care, mobility, safety, independence, communication, and relationships with others. Some deficits, such as mild vision impairment, may require only simple compensatory behaviors or assistive devices to overcome (e.g., eyeglasses). Other deficits, such as full hearing loss, present greater challenges. Some patients may experience impairments that put them at risk in institutional settings such as schools or assisted living facilities. The role of the nurse working with a patient with an alteration in sensory perception is to help the patient find ways to function safely in what are often confusing environments.

Normal Sensory Perception

The sensory process involves two components: reception and perception. **Sensory reception** is the process of receiving stimuli or data. These stimuli are either external or internal to the body. External stimuli are **visual** (sight), **auditory** (hearing), **olfactory** (smell), **tactile** (touch), and **gustatory** (taste). Gustatory stimuli can be internal as well. Other types of internal stimuli are kinesthetic and visceral. **Kinesthesia** refers to awareness of the position and movement of body parts. For example, an individual walking is normally aware of which leg is forward. A related sense is **stereognosis**, the ability to perceive and understand an object through touch by its size, shape, and texture. An individual holding a tennis ball is normally aware of its size, round shape, and soft surface without seeing it. **Visceral** means of, or relating to, any large organ within the body. Visceral organs may produce stimuli that make an individual aware of them (e.g., a full stomach). Sensory perception involves the conscious organization and translation of the data or stimuli into meaningful information.

For an individual to be aware of the surroundings, four aspects of the sensory process must be present:

- **Stimulus.** This is an agent or act that stimulates a nerve receptor.
- **Receptor.** A nerve cell acts as a receptor by converting the stimulus to a nerve impulse. Most receptors are specific, that is, sensitive to only one type of stimulus, such as visual, auditory, or touch.
- **Impulse conduction.** The impulse travels along nerve pathways to the spinal cord or directly to the brain. The cranial nerves (listed in **Table 18–1** ≫ along with their functions) are important nerves that control many actions required for sensory perception (see **Figure 18–1** ≫). For example, auditory impulses travel to the organ of Corti in the inner ear. From there, the impulses travel along the eighth cranial nerve to the temporal lobe of the brain.
- **Perception.** Perception, or awareness and interpretation of stimuli, takes place in the brain. Specialized brain cells interpret the nature and the quality of the sensory stimuli. The level of consciousness affects the perception of the stimuli.

The brain has the capacity to adapt to sensory stimuli. For example, an individual living in a city may not notice traffic noise that someone from a rural area finds loud and disturbing. The brain does not act on all stimuli immediately; some stimuli are stored in the memory to be used at a later date. Sensory processing is not the same as cognition or awareness. Cognition is the process by which an individual learns, stores, retrieves, and uses information. **Awareness** is the

TABLE 18–1 Cranial Nerves and Their Functions

Name	Function
I Olfactory	Sense of smell
II Optic	Vision
III Oculomotor	Eyeball movement: Moves eye medially, elevates eye or rolls it superiorly, depresses eye or rolls it inferiorly, elevates eye and turns it laterally
	Raising of upper eyelid
	Constriction of pupil
	Proprioception
IV Trochlear	Eyeball movement: depresses eye and turns it laterally
V Trigeminal	Sensation of the upper scalp, upper eyelid, nose, nasal cavity, cornea, and lacrimal gland
	Sensation of the palate, upper teeth, cheek, top lip, lower eyelid, and scalp; sensation of the tongue, lower teeth, chin, and temporal scalp
	Chewing
VI Abducens	Eyeball movement: Moves eye laterally
VII Facial	Movement of facial muscles
	Secretions of lacrimal, nasal, submandibular, and sublingual glands
	Sensation of taste
VIII Acoustic/Vestibulocochlear	Sense of balance
	Sense of hearing
IX Glossopharyngeal	Swallowing
	Gag reflex
	Secretions of parotid salivary gland
	Sense of taste
	Touch, pressure, and pain from pharynx and posterior tongue
	Pressure from carotid arteries
	Receptors to regulate blood pressure
X Vagus	Swallowing
	Regulation of cardiac rate
	Regulation of respirations
	Digestion
	Sensation from thoracic and abdominal organs
	Proprioception
	Sense of taste
XI Accessory	Movement of head and neck
	Proprioception
XII Hypoglossal	Movement of tongue for speech and swallowing

ability to perceive environmental stimuli and body reactions and to respond appropriately through thought and action. The normal, alert individual can assimilate many kinds of information at one time.

Understanding of sensory function and of alterations in sensory perception requires familiarity with the normal anatomic structure and physiologic function of each system involved in sensory perception. Knowledge of related structures and functions, and how they may differ along the lifespan, helps the nurse to provide timely and accurate assessment to reduce the individual's risk for injury or complications when alterations occur.

≫ Go to **Pearson MyLab Nursing and eText** for a Module on the review of the physiology of sensory perception.

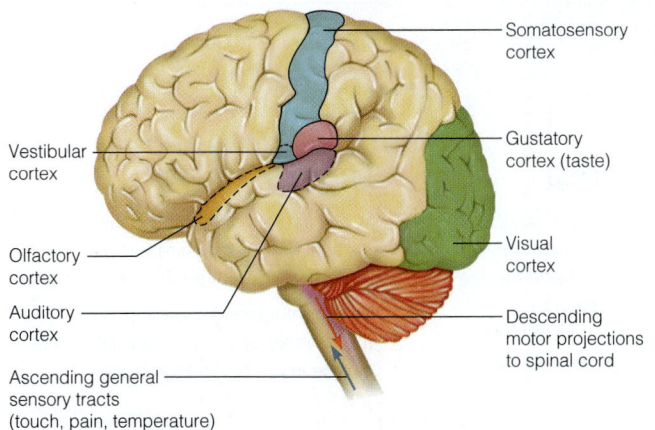

Vestibular cortex

Olfactory cortex

Auditory cortex

Ascending general sensory tracts
(touch, pain, temperature)

Somatosensory cortex

Gustatory cortex (taste)

Visual cortex

Descending motor projections to spinal cord

Source: From Marieb, E. N., & Hoehn, K. (2007). *Human anatomy & physiology* (7th ed., p. 455). Benjamin Cummings Publishing Company. Reprinted by permission of Pearson Education, Inc.

Figure 18–1 » The nerve impulses run along the ascending sensory tracts to reach the reticular activating system (RAS) and then the cerebral cortex where they are perceived.

Alterations of Sensory Perception

Alterations in sensory perception are common. Nurses work with patients with a variety of alterations from color blindness to eye injury to altered sense of taste. Alterations in sensory perception can affect patients and patient care in a number of ways. Specific alterations that are offered as exemplars of this concept are hearing impairment, diseases of the eye (cataracts, glaucoma, and macular degeneration), eye injuries, and peripheral neuropathy. An overview of some nonspecific alterations, such as vertigo, is provided here.

Alterations and Manifestations

A number of nonspecific alterations may result from aging, genetic factors, or underlying illness. Lifestyle factors, such as tobacco use, can also affect sensory perception. In all cases, identification of the cause begins with a thorough patient assessment. Some common nonspecific alterations in sensory perception are vertigo, color blindness, impaired olfaction (sense of smell), and taste disturbances.

Vertigo is a feeling of rotation or imbalance. It can be acute or chronic and can range from being merely distracting to being completely debilitating. It may or may not be accompanied by nausea. A patient with vertigo may have difficulty with balance and/or **nystagmus** (involuntary rapid eye movements). Vertigo is difficult to diagnose; it can be caused by strokes, brain tumors, head trauma, or viruses, or it can be idiopathic with no identifiable cause. A common cause of vertigo is vestibular neuritis, an infection of the vestibular nerve. In about 50% of cases of vestibular neuritis, the patient will report a prior upper respiratory infection. One common type of vertigo is benign paroxysmal positional vertigo (BPPV), which is caused by a disruption of the orientation of ear otoliths. Up to 42% of cases of vertigo will be diagnosed as BPPV. Treatment and prognosis for the resolution of vertigo depend on the etiology. Most patients will experience resolution within a few days, but some will experience recurring symptoms throughout their lifetime.

Color blindness affects approximately 1 in 10 men but very few women. It occurs when one or more pigments are missing within the cones in the retina. The most common variant of color blindness is the inability to distinguish between red and green. Less common is the inability to distinguish between blue and yellow. Many people with the blue–yellow variant also have problems distinguishing between green and red. *Achromatopsia* is a rare form of color blindness in which the individual cannot distinguish any color at all and sees only shades of gray.

Impaired sense of smell can occur for a number of reasons. It is commonly associated with respiratory illnesses such as the common cold. A decreased sense of smell is part of the normal aging process. Some medications, such as cholesterol-lowering medications and antibiotics, may alter the sense of smell temporarily. Patients who smoke tobacco or have undergone radiation treatment for head and neck cancers will have a decreased sense of smell. Because serious conditions such as brain tumors, Parkinson disease, or multiple sclerosis also may result in loss of smell, patients reporting a prolonged alteration in their sense of smell require further assessment.

Taste disturbances are an often-overlooked abnormality. Although a decrease in sense of taste is a normal part of aging, it is also associated with medication use, smoking, and infection. Gum disease can also affect taste. Because taste and smell are closely related, they may share an etiology when both are impaired. Patients reporting prolonged taste impairment require further assessment. In older adults, decreased taste sensation can lead to weight loss, requiring intervention. Impairment of vision and hearing and peripheral neuropathies are discussed in more detail in the exemplars in this module.

Prevalence

The prevalence of sensory perception disorders varies widely depending on the disorder. In 2012, 15% of adults age 18 and over reported having some difficulty hearing, and men were more likely to have trouble hearing than women (Centers for Disease Control and Prevention [CDC], 2014). Of individuals age 45–54, approximately 2% have disabling hearing loss; this increases to 8.5% in individuals age 55–64, 25% in individuals age 65–74, and 50% in individuals age 75 and older (National Institute on Deafness and Other Communication Disorders [NIDCD], 2015).

In a study of adults age 40 and over, the prevalence of myopia (i.e., nearsightedness) was 23.9%, and the prevalence of hyperopia (i.e., farsightedness) was 10.0%. In this same population, the prevalence for blindness (i.e., 20/200 visual acuity or worse) was 0.9%, that of cataracts was 17.1%, that of diabetic retinopathy was 5.4%, that of age-related macular degeneration was 2.1%, and that of open-angle glaucoma was 1.9% (National Eye Institute [NEI], 2010). For most alterations in vision except myopia, the prevalence increases significantly with age.

The prevalence of self-reported smell and taste disorders is estimated to be 10.6% and 5.3%, respectively (Bhattacharyya & Kepnes, 2015). However, this estimate may be low, as many individuals do not realize that they have impaired taste or smell or do not report their impairment. Taste and smell disturbances are associated with age but not gender.

Alterations and Therapies
Sensory Perception

ALTERATION	DESCRIPTION	MANIFESTATIONS	INTERVENTIONS AND THERAPIES
Eye injuries	Eye injuries are damage to the structure of the eye. They are a common cause of vision loss in children. Common causes include sports injuries and chemical exposure.	■ Manifestations vary based on type of injury but can range from redness and edema due to corneal abrasion to complete loss of vision (and/or eye) due to penetrating injury.	■ All eye injuries should be considered medical emergencies requiring immediate evaluation and intervention. ■ Treatment varies according to the type and severity of injury; treatments may include irrigation, foreign body removal, and surgery.
Cataracts	A breakdown of proteins within the lens results in the lens no longer being able to change shape to focus.	■ Opacification of the eye prevents **refraction** of light rays onto the retina. Cataracts may be congenital or acquired.	■ If vision is not affected, the patient will be monitored. If vision becomes impaired, the lens may be surgically removed and a new lens implanted.
Glaucoma	Glaucoma is optic neuropathy with gradual loss of peripheral vision. The two main types are open-angle and angle-closure glaucoma. Both types are associated with an increase in intraocular pressure.	■ Open-angle glaucoma may cause the gradual loss of peripheral vision, or "tunnel" vision, in both eyes. ■ Closed-angle glaucoma may cause severe eye pain, sudden onset of visual disturbances, and blurred vision.	■ Treatment includes medications to control intraocular pressure and preserve vision in open-angle glaucoma. ■ Surgical procedures include: Laser trabeculoplasty Photocoagulation Gonioplasty Laser iridotomy
Age-related macular degeneration (AMD)	This progressive disorder involves loss of central vision due to damage to the retina. The two types are nonexudative and exudative.	■ Symptoms usually develop gradually and include needing more light to read, blurriness of print, or a blurred or blind spot in central vision.	■ High-dose antioxidants and zinc are used to treat early-to-intermediate dry AMD. ■ Laser surgery or photodynamic therapy is used to treat wet AMD.
Hearing impairment	Hearing impairment is a defect in the ability of the ear structures to transmit sound signals to the brain. It may be congenital or noise-induced.	■ Impairment may range from a slight decrease in the ability to detect sounds to a complete inability to detect sound. Decreases in hearing may be associated with high or low frequencies.	■ Interventions and therapies include use of hearing aids or cochlear implants. ■ Some individuals who are deaf or hard of hearing may opt for use of sign language to communicate and not seek treatment to improve hearing.
Peripheral neuropathy	This condition occurs when trauma or disease processes interfere with innervation of peripheral nerves. Peripheral blood vessels constrict, peripheral nerve endings in the affected area experience decreased blood flow, and neuropathy develops.	■ Manifestations depend on the affected nerve(s) and the amount of damage. ■ Manifestations may include aching, shooting, or burning pain; weakness; or imbalance.	■ Interventions and therapies focus on treating the underlying cause and promoting safety and comfort.

Genetic Considerations and Risk Factors

Although lifestyle choices—such as wearing vision protection while woodworking, limiting the use of ear buds, or refraining from smoking—can reduce the risk for sensory impairment, genetic predisposition to illness and the pathology of certain coexisting disorders can lead to alterations in sensory perception.

Congenital and Hereditary Conditions

Many conditions lead to temporary or permanent impairment of sensory perception. Infants who are premature; whose mothers were infected prenatally with rubella, toxoplasmosis, or other viruses; or who have certain congenital and hereditary conditions are at a high risk for visual and/or hearing problems. More than 50% of all cases of hearing loss at birth can be linked to genetic abnormalities. Some occur in the absence of other problems. Others occur in conjunction with other genetic syndromes such as Treacher Collins syndrome and Down syndrome. Retinopathy of prematurity, low birth weight, and congenital cataracts are common causes of blindness or visual impairment in children. Fetal alcohol syndrome (FAS) is a major cause of prenatal visual and hearing disturbances.

Focus on Diversity and Culture
Cultural Background and the Prevalence of Blindness

Blindness affects African Americans more often than Caucasians and Hispanics. Glaucoma and cataracts are serious problems within the African American community and can lead to blindness. Beginning at age 40, African Americans should have a comprehensive dilated eye exam at least every 2 years. If an African American patient also has a diagnosis of diabetes, exams should be scheduled at least once a year (Varma, Bressler, & Doan, 2014). Nurses working with African American patients should inquire about the frequency of eye examinations at each healthcare interaction and teach patients about the risks associated with race, diabetes, and lack of regular eye care.

Auditory processing disorder, a condition in which the individual has difficulty differentiating individual sounds in words, is one of several hearing disorders with which a child may be born. It creates difficulty for individuals in some environments, especially school. Its cause is unknown.

In older adults, prevalence of some visual disorders may have a cultural or genetic component. African Americans and people of Hispanic origin have the highest prevalence of open-angle glaucoma. Visual impairment due to refractive error occurs two to three times more often in American Indian/Alaskan Natives than in Caucasians or African Americans (Mansberger et al., 2005).

Illness

Diseases such as atherosclerosis restrict blood flow to the receptor organs and the brain, thereby decreasing awareness and slowing responses. Hypertension, especially uncontrolled, can contribute to vision loss. Cerebrovascular accidents (strokes) can cause blindness, hearing loss, changes in taste or smell, or other sensory disturbances based on the location of damaged brain tissue. Uncontrolled diabetes mellitus can impair vision and is a leading cause of blindness in the United States. Maternal diabetes can also cause hearing loss in infants. Some central nervous system diseases cause varying degrees of paralysis and sensory loss. Repeated bouts of otitis media can cause permanent hearing loss in children.

Case Study » Part 1

Simon Thompson is a 10-year-old boy who is currently in the fifth grade. He has always been a good student, but this year his grades have not been very good. During a parent–teacher conference, Simon's teacher reported that Simon seemed to be squinting a lot. His parents scheduled an appointment with their primary care provider's office.

The nurse practitioner performs an ophthalmoscope exam and tests Simon's vision using a Snellen chart. On the basis of her findings, she advises Simon's parents to take him to see an ophthalmologist. The ophthalmologist determines that Simon's visual acuity is 20/100 and that he needs glasses to correct his vision. When he starts wearing his glasses, his 13-year-old sister and her friends tease

Simon every chance they get, and he becomes embarrassed at having to wear his glasses.

Clinical Reasoning Questions Level I
1. This scenario features a nurse practitioner. What is the role of the registered nurse in assessing sensory perception?
2. What are some possible nursing diagnoses for Simon at this time?

Clinical Reasoning Questions Level II
3. What patient teaching can the nurse provide to explain to Simon the connection between his eyesight and his grades?
4. What nursing interventions could help Simon cope with his embarrassment over wearing glasses?

Concepts Related to Sensory Perception

The loss or dysfunction of a sense can sometimes be difficult to diagnose and treat, especially in older adults who may accept loss of function as a normal part of the aging process even when pathology is present. In any stage of development, the loss of one or more senses can affect daily functioning and increase patients' risk for injury. For example, hearing loss that affects the inner ear's ability to maintain a sense of balance may result in vertigo or dizziness, which increases patients' risk for a fall. Falls, in turn, have the potential to decrease patients' mobility. Even minor impairments can cause overload of other senses, creating stress and anxiety for patients. Long-term impairment can lead to loss of independence and dignity or to depression, especially in patients who are not able to return to a normal level of functioning or who experience a change in their ability to perform familiar tasks or roles. Alterations in sensory perception can increase the risk for confusion, especially when patients find themselves in unfamiliar settings. Disorientation may result from either sensory deprivation or sensory overload. Infection may also play a role: Untreated or chronic ear infections may lead to structural changes in the ear and permanent hearing impairment. Infection also is one of many potential causes of peripheral neuropathy.

The role of the nurse is to provide thorough assessment, aid in an accurate diagnosis, support a safe environment, and assist the patient in achieving optimal functioning. While providing these services, the nurse must also recognize the patient's alterations in sensory perception and provide information and caring interventions in a way that is most beneficial to the patient. For example, a patient with a hearing impairment may benefit from the presence of a sign language interpreter during the assessment and when patient teaching is given.

The Concepts Related to Sensory Perception feature links some, but not all, of the concepts integral to sensory perception. They are presented in alphabetical order.

Health Promotion

Healthy sensory function can be promoted by incorporating environmental stimuli that provide appropriate sensory input that varies and is neither excessive nor too limited. Various colors, sounds, textures, smells, and body positions can provide multisensory stimulation. Nurses can teach parents to stimulate infants and children and teach family members to stimulate an older adult and others in the home who have sensory deficits. Nurses should explain that some trial and

Concepts Related to
Sensory Perception

CONCEPT	RELATIONSHIP TO SENSORY PERCEPTION	NURSING IMPLICATIONS
Cognition	Alterations in sensory perception → ↑ confusion. Sensory deprivation or overload → disorientation	■ Assess for sensory function by obtaining a complete patient history and performing a physical examination. ■ Pay close attention to mental status; loss or decrease in one or more senses can mimic senility in older adults. ■ Provide reorientation as needed. ■ Involve other members of the healthcare team if deficits are noted.
Communication	↓ Sight → ↓ ability to read written instructions and information → ↑ need for verbal communication ↓ Hearing → ↓ ability to hear verbal instructions and information → ↑ need for alternative communication methods (e.g., sign language interpreter, written communication)	■ For patients who are blind or have impaired vision, provide thorough verbal instructions. Verbally describe all parts of the assessment, especially assessments that require touch. If written instructions are required, provide instructions to a spouse, parent, or other family member or friend who is with the patient. ■ For patients who are deaf or have impaired hearing, provide thorough written instructions. Engage the involvement of a sign language interpreter during assessments to provide translation of questions, answers, and other information. ■ For patients who do not speak English and have impaired vision or hearing, advocate for the use of an interpreter who will be able to communicate with the patient in the patient's own language.
Infection	Eye infections can lead to a decrease in vision, especially chronic infections or severe infections. Ear infections that increase exudate in the inner ear can dampen hearing, causing the individual to hear muffled sounds rather than clear sounds. Individuals with diabetic neuropathy who injure their feet have an increased risk of infection, potentially leading to amputation in severe cases.	■ Provide patient education about the need to take antibiotics as prescribed. ■ Provide patient teaching related to preventing infection, for example, hand hygiene. ■ Treatment of illnesses that increase the risk for sensory deprivation is one of the best methods of prevention.
Safety	Sensory deficits → ↑ risk for injury (falls, burns) ↓ Sight or hearing → ↓ ability to read or listen to instructions → ↑ Risk for inadequate knowledge of treatments, side effects, warning signs	■ Assess the extent to which the deficit affects function, particularly safe movement. ■ Assist the patient to determine what coping mechanisms or assistive devices may promote safety. ■ Educate the patient and caregivers about increased risk for injury, and provide patient teaching related to safety. Schedule an in-home safety assessment as necessary.
Self	Alterations in senses → ↓ independence and dignity	■ Encourage verbalization of positive and negative feelings related to loss. ■ Teach the patient how to adapt to sensory deficit. ■ Provide for patient safety. ■ Encourage involvement with social and community groups to increase feelings of self-worth and contribution. ■ Provide referrals to organizations that may assist with involvement and interaction; assess for the need for referral related to lack of transportation.
Stress and Coping	Loss of one or more senses → sensory overload → sensory compensation → ↑ stress and anxiety Unresolved anger over loss of senses → ↓ quality of relationships, especially with immediate family members	■ Note whether the patient looks bored or confused because the patient may not communicate feeling overwhelmed or uninterested. ■ Eliminate extra noise and stimulus as needed. ■ Provide meaningful interaction and stimulation to reduce emotional or physical isolation. ■ Encourage verbalization of positive and negative feelings related to loss.

error may be necessary at first because it takes time to learn what materials and activities stimulate the patient and which activities the patient enjoys. Exercise and social activities often help to stimulate the mind and the senses.

Some loss of sensory function is inevitable as part of the normal aging process. However, nurses can promote patient health related to sensory perception by providing information about risk factors and encouraging patients to engage in activities that would slow or halt the loss of sensory perception such as minimizing exposure to loud noise to avoid hearing loss and wearing sunglasses or safety goggles when appropriate to protect the eyes.

Modifiable Risk Factors

For certain alterations in sensory perception, individual choices can significantly influence the development of a disorder or impairment. Nurses should teach patients who are at risk of sensory loss how to prevent or minimize the loss. Teaching topics include general health measures, such as getting regular eye examinations and controlling chronic diseases such as diabetes. Avoiding known risk factors, such as hot temperatures for the individual with impaired tactile senses, is also critical.

Smoking

Tobacco use can cause impairment in the senses of taste and smell. It can also cause problems with vision because it constricts the blood vessels that supply the eyes and optic nerve. For these and other reasons, nurses should encourage all patients who smoke to stop. See the Patient Teaching feature for the detrimental effects of smoking on the senses.

Ultraviolet Light Exposure

Although often overlooked, unprotected exposure to ultraviolet (UV) light can cause serious eye problems. In the short term, minor symptoms such as irritation or photokeratitis (corneal burn) may occur. Long-term effects of UV exposure can include serious visual disturbances (some of which will be discussed further in Exemplar 18.B on Diseases of the Eye and Exemplar 18.C on Eye Injuries). Several types of cancers, such as melanoma, basal cell, and squamous cell, can occur on the skin near the eye or on the eye itself. Long-term UV exposure also increases rates of cataracts and AMD. Advise patients to wear UVA/UVB blocking sunglasses and hats, minimize sun exposure, and avoid tanning beds.

Medication

Certain medications can alter an individual's awareness of environmental stimuli. Narcotics and sedatives, for example, can decrease awareness of stimuli. Some antidepressants can alter perceptions of stimuli. Anyone taking several medications concurrently may show alterations in sensory function. Older adults are especially at risk and need to be monitored carefully, particularly if they are simultaneously taking multiple medications for a variety of conditions.

Stress

During times of increased stress, individuals may find their senses overloaded and seek to decrease sensory stimulation. For example, a patient dealing with physical illness, pain, hospitalization, and diagnostic tests may wish to have only

Patient Teaching
Effects of Smoking on the Senses

- **Sight.** Smokers have an increased risk of developing cataracts and AMD as compared with nonsmokers (CDC, 2015a). Other potential eye problems related to smoking include uveitis, diabetic retinopathy, glaucoma, retinal detachment, conjunctivitis, and dry eyes. Smoking during pregnancy can lead to eye-related disorders in the infant, including blindness. Patients who smoke should be encouraged to eat foods that promote eye health, control their blood pressure and cholesterol, and visit their eye care professional regularly.

- **Smell.** Smoking causes nerve damage along the nerves in the nose that transmit signals to the brain. When these olfactory nerves are damaged, the sense of smell is impaired. If patients stop smoking, their sense of smell often recovers at least partially. However, if smoking continues long term, their nerves could be permanently damaged, and the loss of the ability to smell could be permanent.

- **Taste.** Smokers frequently lose the ability to taste as intensely as they did before smoking. The loss of the sense of taste is closely intertwined with the loss of the sense of smell in smokers. Taste often depends on smell, so when smokers' sense of smell is impaired, their sense of taste is impaired as well (Malaty & Malaty, 2013). However, patients who stop smoking often report a remarkable recovery in their sense of taste.

- **Hearing.** Current smokers are more likely to report a hearing loss than nonsmokers, and individuals who are regularly exposed to smoking (passive smokers) are also more likely to report a hearing loss (Dawes et al., 2014). The degree of hearing loss is correlated with the number of packs smoked daily and the number of years of smoking. Past smokers have a slightly improved sense of hearing over their counterparts who continue to smoke.

- **Touch.** Smoking can decrease the sense of touch and may lead to numbness and tingling in some sensitive individuals, especially when they smoke recreational drugs such as marijuana (Morris, 2014).

close support people visit. The patient may also need the nurse's help in reducing unnecessary stimuli (e.g., noise) as much as possible. Some patients, however, may seek sensory stimulation during times of low stress.

Isolation

Much research has been done to document the importance of touch in early life. Infants in incubators who are not touched will stop eating and fail to thrive. The same may be true for older adults, especially those with cognitive or sensory impairments. Institutionalized older adults who are deprived of caring touch and nurturing physical contact experience a diminishing quality of life, a lessening of their desire to relate to others, and a weakening of what may already be a fragile relationship with physical reality (Prieto-Flores et al., 2011).

Injuries

Injuries that may damage sensory organs can occur anywhere—at home, in the workplace, or at school. Each year more than 60 million children participate in organized sports. Of these, more than 2.6 million will end up with an injury that requires a visit to the emergency department, with the greatest number of injuries resulting from participation in football and basketball (Safe Kids Worldwide, 2015).

Many eye injuries are minor, but without timely and appropriate intervention, even a minor injury can threaten vision. For this reason, all eye injuries should be considered medical emergencies requiring immediate evaluation and intervention. Eye injuries will be explored in more detail in Exemplar 18.C on Eye Injuries.

Ear injuries of many types are common in children. Lacerations, infections, and hematomas may occur in the external ear structures, especially the pinna. Children may place foreign objects in the ear, and insects may enter the ear canal. Rupture of the tympanic membrane may result from head injuries, blows to the ear, or insertion of objects into the ear canal. Serous drainage from the ear can indicate a basilar skull fracture. Ruptured tympanic membranes in combination with conjunctival and retinal hemorrhage are indicative of shaken baby syndrome; retinal hemorrhage rarely occurs with any other type of injury. A nurse who suspects child abuse should follow agency protocol for reporting to Child Protective Services.

Regardless of age, any injury that results in earache, decreased hearing, persistent bleeding, or other discharge should be evaluated by a physician.

Screenings

Often, changes that occur in the domain of sensory perception happen very slowly or without the patient noticing any symptoms. By promoting routine screening, nurses can help to detect changes in sensory perception early, resulting in improved outcomes for the patient.

Hearing

Most newborns are routinely screened for hearing loss before leaving the hospital. Preschoolers and school-age children typically undergo periodic screening at their schools or healthcare provider's office; guidelines vary by state. Early detection of hearing problems is critical for children's everyday functioning and school performance. Adults should be screened at least every 10 years until the age of 50 and then every 3 years. Any patient who experiences an abnormal hearing screening or feels that there has been a change in hearing should be referred to a certified audiologist for a comprehensive evaluation (American Speech-Language-Hearing Association [ASHA], 2015b).

Vision

Current guidelines recommend that all children between the ages of 3 and 5 receive a vision screening at least once. Many states establish their own guidelines and periodically offer vision screening at school or as part of routine well-child visits. Any child suspected of having visual difficulties should be referred for a comprehensive ophthalmologic evaluation (U.S. Preventive Services Task Force, 2011). Beyond the age of 40, 7.5% of adults in the United States have visual impairment (Chou et al., 2013). Adults should receive a comprehensive eye exam at the age of 40. For individuals without comorbidities, eye exams should be repeated every 2–4 years for ages 40–54, every 1–3 years for ages 55–64, and every 1–2 years for ages 65 and above. For individuals at high risk, such as individuals with diabetes, eye exams should be given annually (American Academy of Ophthalmology [AAO], 2015a).

Taste, Smell, and Touch

There are currently no recommended screening guidelines for taste, smell, or touch. Most abnormalities in these senses are found when patients present to their healthcare providers with complaints of alterations.

Nursing Assessment

Nursing assessment of sensory-perceptual functioning includes six components: (1) observation and patient interview, (2) mental status examination, (3) identification of patients at risk, (4) the patient's environment, (5) the patient's social support network, and (6) physical examination.

Observation and Patient Interview

Nurses can obtain limited information about a patient's sensory impairments by careful observation. For example, a patient with visual impairment may wear glasses, squint when reading, carry and use a white cane, or run into objects when walking in an unfamiliar setting. Examination of the eyes may reveal a cloudy cornea that suggests blindness or other visual impairments. Likewise, a patient with hearing impairment may wear hearing aids, fail to respond when addressed, or use sign language or writing to communicate.

The nursing assessment begins with obtaining a thorough history from the patient. Inquire about the patient's current sensory functioning, sensory deficits, and any recent changes. Include questions designed to obtain information related to noise exposure—loud, constant sounds from any type of equipment, for example—as well as hobbies or work that can cause burns or injuries. Assess for chronic diseases or illness as well as medications taken by the patient, regardless of the type of impairment suspected. The following list provides examples of interview questions to elicit data about the patient's sensory-perceptual functioning.

Visual

- How would you rate your vision (excellent, good, fair, or poor)? Describe any recent changes in your vision.
- Do you wear eyeglasses or contact lenses?
- Do you have any difficulty seeing near or far objects or difficulty seeing at night?
- When did you last visit an eye doctor?

Auditory

- How would you rate your hearing (excellent, good, fair, or poor)? Describe any recent changes in your hearing.
- Do you wear a hearing aid?
- Can you locate the direction of sounds and distinguish various voices?
- Do you experience any dizziness or vertigo? Do you experience any ringing, buzzing, humming, crackling noises, or fullness in the ears?
- Are you exposed to any loud noises at work? If so, what are they? How much or how often?

Gustatory

- Have you experienced any changes in taste?
- Do you enjoy the taste of foods as you did previously?

Olfactory

- Have you experienced any changes in smell?
- Can you distinguish foods by their odors and tell when something is burning?
- Have you experienced any changes in appetite?

Tactile

- Are you experiencing any pain or discomfort?
- Have you experienced any decrease in your ability to perceive heat, cold, or pain in your limbs?
- Do you have any numbness or tingling in your extremities?

Kinesthetic

- Have you noticed any difficulty in perceiving the position of parts of your body?
- Do you need any assistance standing or sitting down?

In some instances, significant others or family members can provide data the patient cannot. For example, family members may discuss recent changes in the patient's hearing ability, such as inattention to others, recent mood swings, difficulty following clear instructions, frequent requests to have something repeated, and unusually loud radio or television volumes.

Mental Status Examination

Sensory alterations can cause changes in mental status, and an altered mental status can cause changes in sensory perception (Treas & Wilkinson, 2014). Assessment of mental status includes inquiring about any recent history of mood alterations or delirium. Assess for problems with cognitive function, including level of consciousness, orientation, memory, and attention span.

Identification of Patients at Risk

The patient may be at higher risk of developing sensory alterations if he or she has altered mobility, has multiple comorbidities, is older, is involved in contact sports, or smokes. Comorbidities associated with vision impairment include diabetes mellitus, heart problems, breathing problems, hypertension, joint problems, and stroke (Court et al., 2014). Comorbidities associated with hearing loss include diabetes, dizziness, and arthritis (Stam et al., 2014).

Patient's Environment

Nurses assess the patient's environment for quantity, quality, and type of stimuli. Inadequate environmental stimulation may place the patient at risk for sensory deprivation; excessive stimulation may increase the risk for sensory overload. Nonstimulating environments include those that severely restrict physical activity and limit social contact with family and friends. Because appropriate or meaningful stimuli decrease the incidence of sensory deprivation, nurses must consider the patient's healthcare environment for the presence of stimuli such as reading materials, visual and auditory devices (e.g., television, MP3 player, smartphone, iPad), number and compatibility of roommates (which may affect level of overall noise), and number of visitors. To assess a healthcare environment that produces excessive stimuli, the nurse also considers factors such as bright lights, noise, therapeutic measures, and frequency of assessments and procedures.

Patient's Social Support Network

The degree of isolation an individual feels is significantly influenced by the quality and quantity of support from family members and friends. Nurses assess whether the patient lives alone, who visits and when, and any signs indicating social deprivation. Signs of social deprivation may include withdrawal from contact with others to avoid embarrassment or to avoid dependence on others, negative self-image, reports of lack of meaningful communication with others, and absence of opportunities to discuss fears or concerns that facilitate coping mechanisms.

Physical Examination

Physical examination determines whether the senses are impaired. During the physical examination, nurses assess vision (including color vision); hearing; and the olfactory, gustatory, tactile, and kinesthetic senses. The examination should include assessment of the patient's visual and hearing abilities; perception of heat, cold, light touch, and pain; and awareness of the position of the body parts (proprioception). Specific sensory tests include the following:

- Visual acuity, using a Snellen chart or other reading material such as a newspaper, and visual fields, using picture charts for those with limited reading or language proficiency
- Hearing acuity, by observing the patient's conversation with others and by performing the whisper test and the Weber and Rinne tuning fork tests
- Olfactory sense, by identifying specific aromas
- Gustatory sense, by identifying three tastes such as lemon, salt, and sugar
- Tactile sense, by testing light touch, sharp and dull sensation, two-point discrimination, hot and cold sensation, vibration sense, position sense, and stereognosis.

If the patient uses sensory adaptive devices such as eyeglasses or a hearing aid, nurses should determine whether or not these function properly and whether the patient is compliant in using them.

Eye and Vision Assessment

Visual acuity is assessed with an eye chart, such as the Snellen chart or the E chart for testing distance vision (see **Figure 18–2 »**) and the Rosenbaum chart for testing near vision (see **Figure 18–3 »**). If the patient wears corrective lenses, test the patient's vision with and without the lenses. Nurses

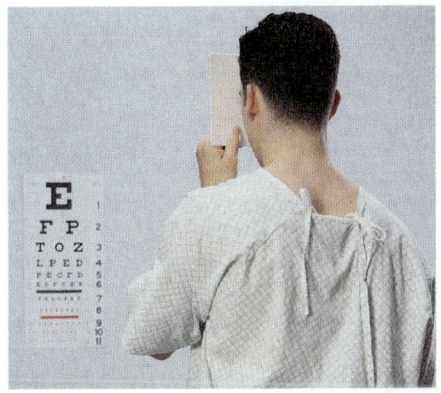

Figure 18–2 » Testing distant vision using the Snellen eye chart.

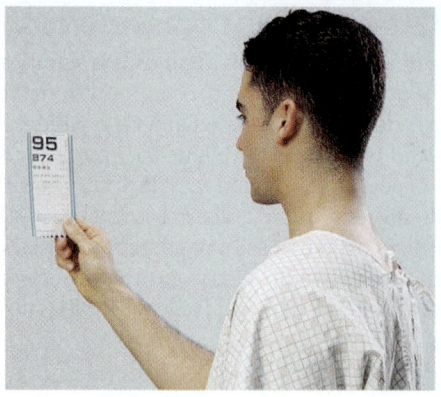

Figure 18–3 >> Testing near vision using Rosenbaum eye chart.

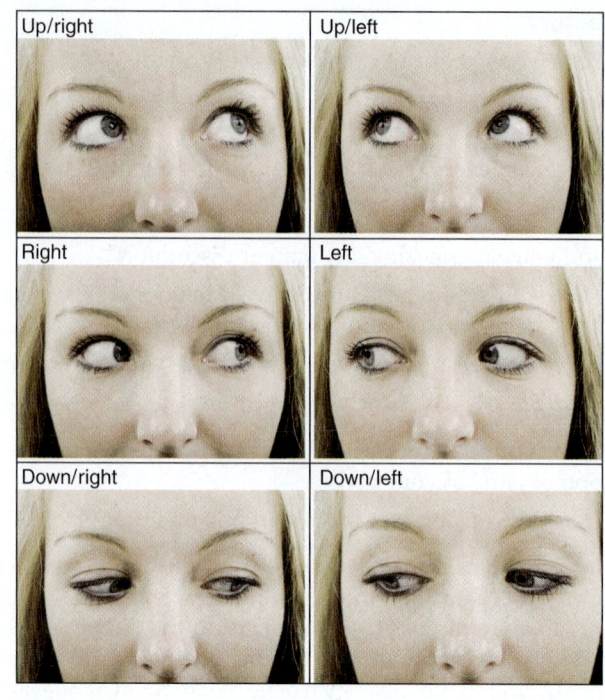

Figure 18–4 >> The six cardinal fields of vision.

can also assess a gross estimate of near vision by asking the patient to read from a magazine or newspaper.

The cardinal fields of vision are assessed to gain information about extraocular eye movements. Nurses should ask the patient to follow a pen or their finger while keeping the head stationary. Nurses move the pen or their finger through the six fields one at a time, returning to the central starting point before proceeding to the next field (see **Figure 18–4** >>).

The internal structures of the eye are assessed by using the ophthalmoscope, an instrument that allows visualization of the lens, the vitreous humor, and the retina. However, this assessment is usually performed by a physician or eye specialist.

See the Eye and Vision Assessment feature for assessment methods, normal and abnormal findings, and lifespan and development considerations.

Eye and Vision Assessment

ASSESSMENT/METHOD	NORMAL FINDINGS	ABNORMAL FINDINGS	LIFESPAN OR DEVELOPMENTAL CONSIDERATIONS
Vision Assessment			
Assess distance vision using the Snellen or E chart. The number at the end of the row indicates the visual acuity of a patient who can read that row at a distance of 20 feet. Ask the patient to cover one eye with an opaque cover. Then, ask the patient to read each row of letters, moving from largest letters to the smallest ones that the patient can see. Measure visual acuity in the other eye in the same way, and then assess visual acuity while the patient has both eyes uncovered.	When standing 20 feet from the chart, the patient can read the smallest line of letters with or without corrective lenses (recorded as 20/20).	■ Changes in distance vision are most commonly the result of **myopia** (nearsightedness). For example, a reading of 20/100 indicates impaired distance vision. An individual has to stand 20 feet from the chart to read a line that an individual with normal vision could read 100 feet from the chart.	■ For patients with limited English proficiency or whose developmental level makes using the Snellen chart a challenge, the E chart may be a more appropriate tool.
Assess near vision using a Rosenbaum chart or a card with newsprint held 12–14 inches from the patient's eyes. Visual acuity is measured in the same manner as with the Snellen chart.	Normal near visual acuity is 14/14 with or without corrective lenses.	■ The patient can read only lines larger than the 14/14 line with one or both eyes. ■ Tilting the head, squinting, or moving the card around may indicate that the patient has difficulty reading print.	■ Changes in near vision, especially in patients over age 45, can indicate **presbyopia**, an impairment in near vision resulting from a loss of elasticity of the lens related to aging. In younger patients, this condition is referred to as **hyperopia** (farsightedness). ■ Patients with low literacy levels may be embarrassed to admit that they do not know the letters on the card.

Eye and Vision Assessment *(continued)*

ASSESSMENT/METHOD	NORMAL FINDINGS	ABNORMAL FINDINGS	LIFESPAN OR DEVELOPMENTAL CONSIDERATIONS
Eye Movement Assessment			
Assess the cardinal fields of vision (see Figure 18–4).	The eyes should move through each field without involuntary movements.	■ Failure of one or both eyes to follow the object in any given direction may indicate extraocular muscle weakness or cranial nerve dysfunction. ■ Nystagmus is associated with neurologic disorders and the use of some medications.	■ In infants or toddlers, use a brightly colored object or toy to capture the child's attention.
Assess for **strabismus** (misalignment of the eyes) using the cover–uncover test: Hold a pen or your finger about 1 foot from the eyes and ask the individual to focus on that object. Cover one of the patient's eyes and note any movement in the uncovered eye; as you remove the cover, assess for movement in the eye that was just uncovered. Repeat the procedure with the other eye.	The uncovered eye should remain fixed straight ahead. The covered eye should remain fixed straight ahead after being uncovered.	■ One eye will deviate from the other when the individual is focusing on an object.	■ Strabismus can occur at any point in the lifespan, based on the underlying pathology. It may be considered a normal finding in newborns, but if it persists past 3 months it should be assessed by an ophthalmologist.
Assess **convergence** (ability of the eyes to turn inward together). Ask the patient to follow an object as you move it toward the patient's eyes.	Normally both eyes converge toward the center.	■ Failure of the eyes to converge equally on an approaching object may indicate a neuromuscular disorder or improper eye alignment.	■ Problems with convergence are usually diagnosed in school-age children when they have difficulty reading and may be interpreted as a learning disability rather than a visual problem.
Assess the corneal light reflex. Direct a light source onto the bridge of the nose from 12–15 inches away.	Observe for equal reflection of the light from each eye.	■ Reflections of the light from different sites on the eyes reveal improper alignment.	■ It may be difficult to assess this reflex in children because looking straight ahead requires cooperation.
Pupillary Assessment			
Observe pupil size and equality.	Pupils should be of equal size, 3–5 mm.	■ Pupils that are unequal in size (anisocoria) may indicate a severe neurologic problem, such as increased intracranial pressure.	■ Pupils that are unequal in size may be a normal finding in newborns. ■ One in five healthy patients will have a difference in pupil size up to 1 mm at some point in the lifespan. In older adults, the use of eyedrops to treat various eye disorders may cause pupil size to be unequal.
Assess direct and consensual pupil response. Ask the patient to look straight ahead. Shine a light obliquely into one eye at a time. Observe for constriction of the pupil in the illuminated eye (direct response).	The normal direct and consensual pupillary response is constriction.	■ Failure of the pupils to respond to light may indicate degeneration of the retina or destruction of the optic nerve.	■ This test requires cooperation, which may be difficult to obtain in newborns and small children or in individuals with mental disabilities.

(continued on next page)

Eye and Vision Assessment (continued)

ASSESSMENT/METHOD	NORMAL FINDINGS	ABNORMAL FINDINGS	LIFESPAN OR DEVELOPMENTAL CONSIDERATIONS
Test both eyes. To test consensual pupil response, again shine a light obliquely into one eye at a time as the patient looks straight ahead. Observe constriction of the pupil in the opposite eye (consensual response).		▪ A patient who has one dilated and unresponsive pupil may have paralysis of the oculomotor nerve. ▪ Some eye medications may cause unequal dilation, constriction, or inequality of pupil size. Morphine and narcotic drugs may cause small, unresponsive pupils, and anticholinergic drugs such as atropine may cause dilated, unresponsive pupils.	
Test for **accommodation** (the ability of the eye to adjust focal length). Hold an object at a distance of a few feet from the patient. The pupils should dilate. Ask the patient to follow the object as you bring it to within a few inches of the patient's nose.	The pupils should constrict and converge as they change focus to follow the object.	▪ Failure of accommodation along with lack of pupil response to light may signal a neurologic problem. ▪ Lack of response to light with appropriate response to accommodation is often seen in patients with diabetes.	▪ Consider using a brightly colored object or toy to get the attention and cooperation of a young child.

External Eye Assessment

Inspect the eyelids. *Source:* Mediscan/Alamy Stock Photo. **Figure 18–5 》** Ptosis.	Eyelids should be the color of the patient's facial skin, without redness, discharge, or drooping. The sclera should not be visible.	▪ Unusual redness or discharge may indicate an inflammatory state. ▪ Drooping of one eyelid, called **ptosis**, may be the result of a stroke, indicate a neuromuscular disorder, or may be congenital (see **Figure 18–5 》**). ▪ Unusual widening of the lids may be due to **exophthalmos**, protrusion of the eyeball, which is often associated with hyperthyroid conditions. ▪ Hordeolum (sty) is generally caused by staphylococcal organisms. ▪ A chalazion is an infection or retention cyst of the meibomian glands.	▪ Yellow plaques noted on or near the lid margins are referred to as xanthelasma and may indicate high lipid levels. This can occur between the ages of 15 and 73 but most commonly occurs during the 40s and 50s.

Eye and Vision Assessment *(continued)*

ASSESSMENT/METHOD	NORMAL FINDINGS	ABNORMAL FINDINGS	LIFESPAN OR DEVELOPMENTAL CONSIDERATIONS
Inspect the lacrimal puncta (orifice where tears are produced and secreted).	The puncta should be free of redness or discharge.	■ Unusual redness or discharge from the puncta may indicate an inflammation due to trauma, infection, or allergies.	■ Babies are occasionally born without one or more of their puncta or with partially opened puncta. ■ Puncta can become blocked or narrowed due to aging.
Inspect the bulbar and palpebral conjunctiva.	The conjunctiva should be clear, moist, and smooth. The upper and lower palpebral conjunctiva should be clear, without redness or swelling.	■ Increased erythema or the presence of exudate may indicate acute conjunctivitis. ■ A cobblestone appearance is often associated with allergies.	■ A fold in the conjunctiva, called a pterygium, is an abnormal growth that may be seen as a clouded area that extends over the cornea. It may interfere with vision if it covers the pupil. This occurs most often in patients ages 20–40.
Inspect the sclera.	The sclera is white in Caucasians; people with darker skin normally have yellow sclera.	■ Unusual redness may indicate an inflammatory state as a result of trauma, allergies, or infection. ■ Yellow discoloration of the sclera in patients with fair skin may be seen in conditions involving the liver, such as hepatitis. ■ Bright red areas in the sclera are often subconjunctival hemorrhages and may indicate trauma or bleeding disorders. They may also occur spontaneously.	■ Newborns with jaundice may have yellow sclera. ■ School-age children are more likely to develop "pink eye" (conjunctivitis), in which the conjunctiva becomes swollen and the sclera becomes pinkish or red. ■ Some children and older adults develop a blue sclera, which may indicate a thinning of the sclera. ■ Brown or gray spots in the sclera may be a result of Axenfeld loops (loops of posterior ciliary nerves); this is occasionally seen in children and is normal. ■ Pregnancy may increase the redness of the sclera. ■ Older adults often have a yellow tinge to their sclera due to UV light exposure over time.
Inspect the cornea.	The cornea is normally transparent.	■ Dullness, opacities, or irregularities of the cornea may be abnormal.	■ Corneal arcus is a thin, grayish-white arc seen toward the edge of the cornea. It is normal in older patients.
Assess corneal sensitivity. Lightly touch a wisp of cotton to the patient's cornea.	This action should cause a **corneal reflex** (blinking of the eye).	■ Failure of the corneal reflex may indicate a neurologic disorder.	■ Corneal sensitivity decreases with age.
Inspect the iris.	The iris is normally round, flat, and evenly colored.	■ Lack of clarity of the iris may indicate cloudiness of the cornea. ■ Constriction of the pupil accompanied by pain and circumcorneal redness indicates acute iritis.	■ The color of the iris may change as the patient ages, especially for patients with lighter-colored eyes.

(continued on next page)

Eye and Vision Assessment *(continued)*

ASSESSMENT/METHOD	NORMAL FINDINGS	ABNORMAL FINDINGS	LIFESPAN OR DEVELOPMENTAL CONSIDERATIONS
Palpate over the lacrimal glands, puncta, and nasolacrimal duct.	There should be no tenderness, drainage, or excessive tearing.	▪ Tenderness over any of these areas or drainage from the puncta may indicate an infectious process. (Wear gloves if you see any drainage.) ▪ Excessive tearing may indicate a blockage of the nasolacrimal duct.	▪ Infants are often born with a blocked nasolacrimal duct. This may resolve spontaneously, or it may require a procedure to open the ducts. Blocked tear ducts can lead to infection if not treated. ▪ Older adults are at increased risk for dry eye because of decreased production of tears by the lacrimal gland.

Ear and Hearing Assessment

Assessment of the ear and hearing usually starts with inspection of the external ear. The ears are usually equal in size and of the same skin color as the face and without palpable lesions. The otoscope is used to inspect both the external auditory canal and the tympanic membrane. The external ear canal should be smooth and without lesions and similar in color to the facial skin. The presence of **cerumen** (ear wax) is expected, but the amount present should not interfere with the exam or have a foul smell. The tympanic membrane should be shiny and translucent and pearly gray in color. A well-defined cone of light (light reflex) should be visible on the surface of the tympanic membrane. Any distortion or dullness of the cone of light may signal an infection or the presence of fluid behind the tympanic membrane.

The whisper test can be used to evaluate the patient's level of hearing. If hearing loss is noted, either unilaterally or bilaterally, a further evaluation can be performed with a tuning fork (see **Figures 18–6 》** and **18–7 》**). Nurses should hold the tuning fork at the base and make it ring softly by stroking the prongs or by lightly tapping them on the heel of the opposite hand. The vibrating tuning fork emits sound waves of a particular frequency, measured in hertz (Hz). Tuning forks with a frequency of 512–1024 Hz are preferred for auditory evaluation, because that range corresponds to the range of normal speech.

Many of the hearing tests performed in a general practitioner's office are difficult to do with infants and young children because they require a degree of cooperation. Nurses can perform some tests of basic hearing by clapping or using another means to create a noise and seeing whether the child looks for the source. Further evaluation typically is performed by an audiologist and/or an otolaryngologist (ear, nose, and throat physician).

The Ear and Hearing Assessment feature lists the techniques and methods used for assessing hearing, gives the

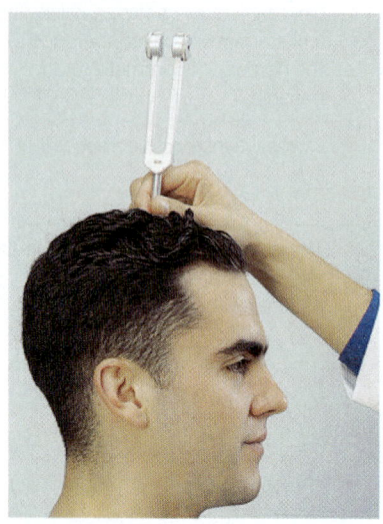

Figure 18–6 》 Performing the Weber test with a tuning fork.

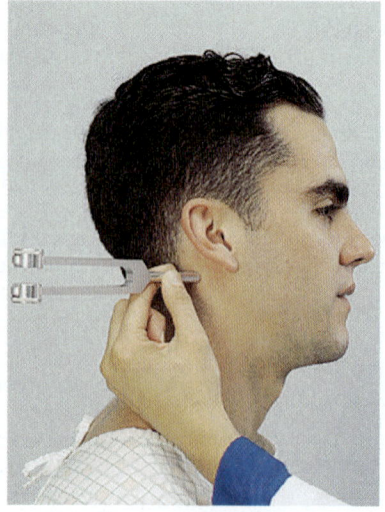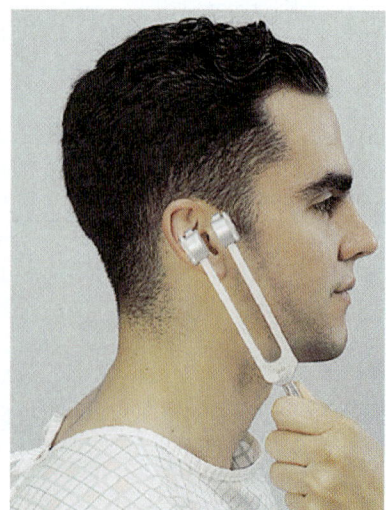

Figure 18–7 》 Performing the Rinne test with a tuning fork.

Ear and Hearing Assessment

ASSESSMENT/METHOD	NORMAL FINDINGS	ABNORMAL FINDINGS	LIFESPAN OR DEVELOPMENTAL CONSIDERATIONS
Hearing Assessment			
Perform the Weber test. Place the base of a vibrating tuning fork on the midline vertex of the patient's head (see Figure 18–6). Ask whether the patient hears the sound equally in both ears or better in one ear than the other.	Sound is normally heard equally in both ears.	■ Sound heard in, or lateralized to, one ear indicates either a conductive loss in that ear or a sensorineural loss in the other ear. With a conductive hearing loss, the sound will be louder on the impaired side. With a sensorineural hearing loss, the sound will be softer on the impaired side. ■ Conductive losses may be due to a buildup of cerumen, an infection such as otitis media, or perforation of the eardrum.	■ This test requires cooperation, so it probably cannot be performed in infants and toddlers. ■ Consider clapping or using an item that makes a noise to see whether the child will look to find the source. In some patients with autism, sudden loud noises are perceived as painful and may elicit a strong response.
Perform the Rinne test. Place the base of a vibrating tuning fork on the patient's mastoid bone. Ask the patient to indicate when the sound is no longer heard. When the patient does so, quickly reposition the tuning fork in front of the patient's ear, close to the ear canal. Ask whether the patient can hear the sound. If so, ask the patient to indicate when the sound is no longer heard. Repeat over the opposite mastoid bone (see Figure 18–7).	The patient with no conductive hearing loss will hear the sound twice as long by air conduction as by bone conduction.	■ Bone conduction is greater than air conduction in the ear with a conductive loss. The normal pattern is AC > BC (air conduction greater than bone conduction).	■ This test requires cooperation, so it probably cannot be performed in infants and toddlers. ■ Consider clapping or using an item that makes a noise to see whether the child will look to find the source. In some patients with autism, sudden loud noises are perceived as painful and may elicit a strong response.
Perform the whisper test. Ask the patient to occlude one ear with a finger. Stand 1–2 feet away from the patient, on the side of the unoccluded ear. Softly whisper numbers, and ask the patient to repeat them. Repeat the procedure, having the patient occlude the other ear. Note whether you need to raise your voice or to stand closer for the patient to hear you.	The patient should be able to repeat the numbers or words whispered by the nurse without difficulty. Note whether the nurse has to speak more loudly or if there is difficulty with one or both ears.	■ This test provides a rough estimate of hearing loss.	■ This test may be difficult to perform in young children because it requires cooperation and understanding of the words being spoken.
Perform the otoacoustic emissions test. This test uses an earphone and microphone to play sounds into the ear.	If the individual hears normally, the microphone will detect an echo.	■ Failure to detect an echo indicates hearing loss.	■ This test is performed almost exclusively on infants as part of the routine hearing screening.

(continued on next page)

Ear and Hearing Assessment *(continued)*

ASSESSMENT/METHOD	NORMAL FINDINGS	ABNORMAL FINDINGS	LIFESPAN OR DEVELOPMENTAL CONSIDERATIONS
External Ear Assessment			
Inspect the auricle (also called the pinna).	External ears are normally bilateral, equal in size, of equal color with the patient's face, and without redness or lesions.	▪ Unusual redness or drainage may indicate an inflammatory response to infection or trauma. ▪ Scales or skin lesions around the rim of the auricle may indicate skin cancer. ▪ Small, raised lesions on the rim of the ear are known as tophi and indicate gout. ▪ Ears that "stick out," are normal and do not require treatment.	▪ In children, abnormalities of the auricle may indicate disorders such as Down syndrome or Turner syndrome. ▪ Auricles may change in size and shape over the lifespan, especially in older adults. ▪ Older men may have longer ear hairs visible when inspecting the auricle.
Inspect the external auditory canal with an otoscope.	Canal walls should be skin-colored and smooth without lesions. Cerumen is normally present in small, odorless amounts.	▪ Unusual redness, lesions, or purulent drainage may indicate an infection. ▪ Cerumen varies in color and texture, but hardened, dry, or foul-smelling cerumen may indicate an infection or an impaction of cerumen that requires removal. People with darker skin tend to have darker cerumen. Cerumen buildup in children can lead to hearing impairment.	▪ When examining an infant or young child, have parents hold the child's head in their lap or against their chest to prevent sudden movements and to provide comfort. ▪ Allow older children to inspect the equipment before the exam. ▪ When inspecting the ear canal, pull the auricle down and back in children younger than 3 years of age, and up and back in children 3 years of age and older. ▪ Older adults may have a buildup of cerumen in the auditory canal.
Inspect the tympanic membrane with an otoscope.	The tympanic membrane should be pearly gray, shiny, and translucent without bulging or retraction.	▪ White, opaque areas or an inconsistent texture and color on the tympanic membrane may be scars from previous perforations due to infection, allergies, or trauma. ▪ Bulging membranes are indicated by a loss of bony landmarks and a distorted light reflex. Such bulges may be the result of otitis media or malfunctioning auditory tubes. ▪ Retracted tympanic membranes are indicated by accentuated bony landmarks and a distorted light reflex. Such retraction is often due to an obstructed auditory tube.	▪ Infants and young children are susceptible to otitis media, which results in a bulging of the tympanic membrane. ▪ Older adults may experience changes in the thickness and elasticity of the tympanic membrane.

Ear and Hearing Assessment (continued)

ASSESSMENT/METHOD	NORMAL FINDINGS	ABNORMAL FINDINGS	LIFESPAN OR DEVELOPMENTAL CONSIDERATIONS
Palpate the auricles and over each mastoid process.	There should be no pain or swelling on palpation.	■ Tenderness, swelling, or nodules may indicate inflammation of the external auditory canal or mastoiditis. ■ Stiffness of the auricles and other outer ear structures may indicate an endocrine abnormality.	■ Children and young adults with swimmer's ear may find manipulation of the auricles to be painful. ■ Older adults may have a loss of cartilage in the auricles.

normal and abnormal findings, and presents lifespan and developmental considerations. More information about lifespan considerations is presented in the section on lifespan considerations.

Taste, Smell, and Tactile Assessment

One reason decreased sense of smell often goes undetected is that it is not adequately tested. Most physical examination records state "cranial nerves II–XII intact," completely omitting cranial nerve I. Nurses can examine the mucous membranes of the nares using a penlight or an otoscope and speculum, taking care not to touch the septum. The mucous membranes of the nares should be free from polyps, slightly red in color, and without ulceration or copious exudates. Nurses can then ask the patient to occlude one side of the nose, close the eyes, and identify a familiar smell such as vanilla, coffee, or an alcohol swab. This maneuver is repeated on the opposite side using a different odor. Using familiar odors enhances the validity of the test. Commercially prepared scratch-and-sniff tests are available in some smell assessment clinics. These tests contain over 40 odorants and provide more complete information regarding deficits in smell. The patient with obvious deficits in smell should be referred to the primary care provider, an otolaryngologist, and a neurologist.

There are many different ways to test for tactile function using sharp, dull, warm, and cold objects. Regardless of the chosen assessment method, the key component of the exam is establishing the presence or absence of symmetry. Graphesthesia is the ability to recognize a letter that is "written" on the skin through touch. Two-point discrimination is performed by asking a patient to close the eyes and report whether one or two points of contact are felt on the skin. Other tests can be used to assess kinesthesia and stereognosis. An inability to identify superficial touch and pain sensation may indicate sensory loss. Nurses should identify the extent of sensory loss, such as all areas below the knee. Other sensory function tests (temperature, vibratory, deep pressure pain, and position sense) are performed when sensory loss is found. Assessment of taste is not usually done as part of a normal sensory examination. Most alterations of taste are found when the patient presents to the healthcare provider with a complaint of decrease in taste. If this occurs, the patient should be referred to a specialist.

The Cranial Nerve Assessment feature lists the testing methods and techniques, the normal and abnormal findings, and lifespan and development considerations for testing smell, taste, and tactile impairments. For specific considerations related to assessment of tactile function in infants and children, see the section on Lifespan Considerations.

Other Diagnostic Tests

Additional diagnostic tests may be necessary to diagnose a specific injury or disease process, to provide information to inform selection of medications or assistive devices, and to help nurses monitor the patient's responses to treatment and nursing interventions. Examples include the use of retinoscopy or refractometry to diagnose refractive errors of the eye that require corrective lenses or audiometry to evaluate the extent of hearing impairment. These more advanced exams are usually performed by a physician or eye specialist.

Case Study » Part 2

Simon Thompson has been trying to ignore the teasing from his sister and her friends. His grades are improving, and he is happy that he can see better. All of his friends have started to skateboard. For his 11th birthday, Simon asks his parents for a skateboard and is excited when he gets one.

Simon has been hanging out with his friends and skateboarding on the playground after school. He is afraid of breaking his glasses, so he takes them off and sets them by the slide. He has learned a new trick and is eager to show his friends. While he is showing them, he falls off of his skateboard and lands in a pile of sand. He feels as though he has sand in his left eye, so he rubs it hard. This makes his eye hurt, and his friends point out that his eye is now all red and watery. Simon gathers his glasses and his skateboard and heads home. By that evening, he is crying because his eye hurts so badly and the lights are bothering it. His parents note that his left eyelid is swollen and crusty. His mother takes him to the urgent care clinic, where he is diagnosed with a left corneal abrasion. Simon is given antibiotic drops, and his mother is instructed on how to apply an eye patch to protect the eye because Simon will not stop rubbing it.

Clinical Reasoning Questions Level I

1. What nursing diagnoses would be appropriate for Simon at this time?
2. What independent nursing interventions can the nurse do with Simon and his mother?

Cranial Nerve Assessment

ASSESSMENT/METHOD	NORMAL FINDINGS	ABNORMAL FINDINGS	LIFESPAN OR DEVELOPMENTAL CONSIDERATIONS
Assess Smell			
Test cranial nerve (CN) I. Note the patient's ability to smell scents (e.g., soap, coffee) with each nostril. This test is usually done only if a problem with the ability to smell is reported.	Sense of smell should be equal in both nostrils.	▪ Anosmia (an inability to smell) may be seen with lesions of the frontal lobe and may also occur with impaired blood flow to the middle cerebral artery.	▪ Smell decreases as part of the normal aging process. ▪ Tobacco use can alter the sense of smell.
Assess Tactile Sensation			
Assess the patient's ability to perceive sensations. Touch both sides of the body (the chest, abdomen, arms, and legs) with one or more of the following: ▪ Cotton wisp ▪ Sharp object ▪ Dull object ▪ Warm object ▪ Cold object ▪ Vibrating tuning fork placed on bony prominences.	The patient should be able to differentiate between soft and sharp and feel vibrations appropriately.	▪ Decreased sensation of pain occurs with injury to the spinothalamic tract. ▪ Decreased vibratory sensations are seen with injuries to the posterior column tract. ▪ Transient numbness of face, arm, or hand is seen with transient ischemic attacks. ▪ Sensory loss on one side of the body is seen with lesions of higher pathways to the spinal cord. ▪ Bilateral sensory loss is seen in polyneuropathy (a disease such as Guillain-Barré syndrome or diabetes mellitus). Sensations are impaired with strokes, brain tumors, and spinal cord trauma or compression.	▪ Withdrawal from noxious stimulation is assessed in newborns. ▪ Identification of specific stimuli requires understanding and cooperation and may not be able to be assessed in young children or those with developmental delays. ▪ Patients diagnosed with autism spectrum disorder may have unexpected responses ranging from little or no response to exaggerated reactions that are disproportionate to the amount of stimulation.
Assess Kinesthesia			
Assess sense of position (kinesthesia). Move the patient's finger or big toe up or down. Ask the patient to describe the movement.	The patient should be able to accurately describe the position of a finger or toe when it is moved up or down.	▪ Lesions of the posterior column of the spinal cord may affect sense of position.	▪ This test requires understanding and cooperation and may be difficult to assess on younger patients or those with developmental delays.
Assess Ability to Discriminate Fine Touch			
Ask the patient to identify the following: ▪ Object in hand with eyes closed, such as a coin or key (tests stereognosis) ▪ Number written on hand (tests graphesthesia) ▪ Two points of simultaneous pinpricks on the hand (tests two-point discrimination) ▪ Where the patient is being touched (tests localization) ▪ How many sensations are felt when the patient is touched simultaneously on both sides of the body (tests extinction).	The patient should be able to identify and discriminate fine touch.	▪ Inability to discriminate fine touch (stereognosis, graphesthesia, two points, point localization, and extinction) may occur with injury to the posterior columns or sensory cortex.	▪ This test requires understanding and cooperation and may be difficult to assess on younger patients or those with developmental delays.

Cranial Nerve Assessment (continued)

ASSESSMENT/METHOD	NORMAL FINDINGS	ABNORMAL FINDINGS	LIFESPAN OR DEVELOPMENTAL CONSIDERATIONS
Assess Taste			
Assessment of taste is usually not performed as part of a routine physical assessment but can be assessed through a questionnaire.	The patient should be able to distinguish between sweet, salty, bitter, sour, and umami.	▪ The patient is not able to distinguish among tastes, which is related closely to the sense of smell.	▪ A decrease in taste is a common part of the aging process. ▪ Tobacco use and certain medications can alter this sense.

Clinical Reasoning Questions Level II

3. *Refer to the module on Comfort.* Other than the eye patch, what strategies can the nurse implement to help Simon stop rubbing his eye?
4. *Refer to the module on Infection.* In addition to instilling the antibiotic eyedrops, what other patient teaching can the nurse provide to decrease the risk of developing an eye infection?
5. What additional patient education could the nurse provide to Simon and his mother before discharge?

Independent Interventions

Care of the patient with impaired sensory perception includes both independent and collaborative interventions. Independent interventions focus on education, injury prevention, and wellness promotion. Collaborative interventions include facilitating medical management of the patient's condition as well as interacting with other members of the healthcare team to optimize the patient's outcomes.

Many of the independent therapies relevant to care for the patient with alterations in sensory perception involve assessing the individual's understanding of both the alteration and the appropriate treatment. Patient teaching is essential, especially with regard to promoting safety.

Patient education includes teaching patients about appropriate use of any prescribed medications. If the plan of care calls for use of assistive devices, the nurse may provide instruction and verify the patients' effective use of the device. Common goals of care for patients with an alteration in sensory perception include preventing injury, restoring or maintaining function, promoting comfort, and preventing sensory overload or deprivation.

Preventing Sensory Overload

For patients who are at risk of overstimulation, nurses should assist with reducing the number and type of environmental stimuli. Nurses can counteract sensory overload by blocking stimuli and by helping the patients organize the stimuli and alter responses to the stimuli.

Dark glasses with UVA and UVB light protection can partially block light rays, and a window shade or curtain can reduce visual stimulation. Earplugs reduce auditory stimuli, as do soft background music and earphones. To further reduce sensory overload, nurses may need to schedule a

quiet period after implementation of several nursing measures together. By explaining the significance of environmental sounds, such as an intravenous (IV) pump alarm, nurses can help patients to organize them mentally. Nurses can encourage patients to employ relaxation techniques to reduce anxiety and stress despite continual sensory stimulation.

Preventing Sensory Deprivation

For patients at risk for sensory deprivation, newspapers, books, music, and television can be provided to stimulate the visual and auditory senses. Objects that are pleasant to touch, including soft fabrics, can provide tactile stimulation. Clocks that use color to differentiate night from day can help orient patients to time. Fresh flowers or a fragrant plant can also stimulate the olfactory sense.

Arrangements should also be made for people to visit and talk with the patients regularly. Many church and community groups provide people who will visit individuals who are confined to their homes or who reside in nursing homes.

Managing Acute Sensory Deficits

Nursing care of patients who have a sensory deficit includes encouraging the use of sensory aids to support residual sensory function, promoting the use of other senses, communicating effectively, and ensuring patient safety. Nurses also teach patients and families how to find freedom within the limitations imposed by the patients' sensory loss. For example, patients with visual impairments may find comfort and joy in attending live music performances, listening to podcasts and audiobooks, and downloading other reading material that has been converted into spoken word via the internet. Patients with hearing impairments may experience frustration when talking on the phone, even if they have a hearing aid that works well. These patients may increase use of communication via e-mail and text messages to minimize frustration with audio communications.

Sensory Aids

Sensory aids can be used in the healthcare setting as well as in the home. Many sensory aids are available for patients who have visual and hearing deficits. Examples are listed in **Box 18–1 ⟩⟩**. Service dogs are a popular but expensive example. Service dogs protect individuals with sensory impairments from risk and assist them with activities of daily

Box 18–1
Sensory Aids for Visual and Hearing Deficits

Visual
- Eyeglasses of the correct prescription, clean and in good repair
- Adequate room lighting, including night-lights
- Sunglasses or shades on windows to reduce glare
- Bright contrasting colors in the environment
- Magnifying glass
- Phone dialer with large numbers
- Clock with large numbers or auditory device
- Color code or texture code on stoves, washer, medicine containers, and so on
- Colored or raised rims on dishes
- Reading material with large print
- Braille or recorded books; podcasts
- Seeing-eye dog.

Hearing
- Hearing aid in good order
- Lip reading
- Sign language
- Amplified telephones
- Telecommunication device for the deaf (TDD)
- Amplified telephone ringers and doorbells
- Flashing alarm clock
- Flashing smoke detectors.

Box 18–2
Communicating with Patients Who Have a Visual or Hearing Deficit

Visual Deficit
- Always announce your presence when entering the patient's room and identify yourself by name.
- Stay in the patient's field of vision if the patient has a partial vision loss.
- Speak in a warm and pleasant tone of voice. Some people tend to speak louder than necessary when talking to someone who is blind.
- Always explain what you are about to do before touching the individual.
- Explain the sounds in the environment.
- Indicate when the conversation has ended and when you are leaving the room.

Hearing Deficit
- Before initiating conversation, convey your presence by moving to a position where the patient can see you or by gently touching the patient.
- Decrease background noises (e.g., television) before speaking.
- Talk at a moderate rate and in a normal tone of voice. Shouting does not make your voice more distinct and can make it more difficult for some patients to understand you.
- Address the individual directly. Do not turn away in the middle of a remark or story. Make sure the individual can see your face easily and that it is well lighted.
- Avoid talking when you have something in your mouth, such as chewing gum. Avoid covering your mouth with your hand.
- Keep your voice at about the same volume throughout each sentence without dropping the voice at the end of each sentence.
- Always speak as clearly and accurately as possible. Articulate consonants with particular care. Do not "overarticulate"; mouthing or overdoing articulation is just as troublesome as mumbling. Pantomime or write ideas, or use sign language or finger-spelling as appropriate.
- Use longer phrases, which tend to be easier to understand than short ones. For example, "Would you like a drink of water?" presents much less difficulty than "Would you like a drink?" Word choice is important: "Fifteen cents" and "fifty cents" may be confused, but "half a dollar" is clear.
- Pronounce every name with care. Make a reference to the name for easier understanding, for example, "Joan, the girl from the office" or "Sears, the big downtown store."
- Change to a new subject at a slower rate, making sure that the individual follows the change to the new subject. A key word or two at the beginning of a new topic is a good indicator.

living (ADLs), such as opening doors and fetching objects. Raising and training service dogs can cost upwards of $40,000 before the dog is ready to go into active service. The cost along with the shortage of trainers sometimes results in long waiting lists for service dogs. Some training programs provide dogs to individuals with sensory impairments free of charge.

Promoting the Use of Other Senses

For some individuals, when one sense is lost, one or more of the intact senses may be heightened to compensate for the impairment. To promote compensation, sensory stimulation techniques are used that are similar to those used to prevent sensory deprivation, as discussed previously. However, the type of stimulation needs to be adapted in accordance with the patient's specific deficit. For example, for a patient with a visual impairment, stimulation of hearing, taste, smell, and touch can be encouraged. A radio, recordings of music or books, clocks that chime, music boxes, and wind chimes can be used for auditory stimulation. Diets that include a variety of flavors, temperatures, and textures stimulate the taste buds. Taking sips of water between foods and eating foods separately can enhance the taste sensation. Fresh flowers, scented candles (safely used), room fragrances, brewing coffee, and baking can stimulate the sense of smell. Massage, hair brushing, grooming, different textures in clothing and upholstery fabrics, and pets can stimulate touch receptors.

Communicating Effectively

Communication with the patient who has sensory deficits should convey respect, enhance the individual's self-esteem, and ensure the exchange of correct information. For the patient with a hearing impairment, communication often requires concentrated effort. Fatigue compounded by an illness can further reduce the individual's ability to hear. An individual with impaired vision is unable to observe most nonverbal cues during communication and relies largely on the spoken word and tone of voice. Guidelines for communicating with individuals who have visual or hearing impairments are shown in **Box 18–2 »**.

Promoting Effective Coping

Moderate to acute sensory deficits affect the patient's quality of life. Mobility, ability to perform ADLs, and independence may all be affected by sensory deficits. A patient who develops successful coping mechanisms is less likely to experience injury and more likely to experience greater quality of life. Depending on the extent of the individual's limitations, eliciting the help of the patient's family or an outside source such as social workers and physical therapists may be helpful.

Impaired Vision

Research has established an association between vision impairment and greater disability in ADLs (e.g., bathing, dressing, eating) and instrumental tasks (e.g., shopping, housekeeping). Studies have also shown that visual impairment increases the risk of depression among older adults living in the community; some studies indicate that the rate of depression in older adults with visual disturbances is as high as 30% in North America (Margrain et al., 2012). Explanations for this relationship vary. One explanation is that vision loss leads to increased disability, which leads to depression. Another explanation is that loss of vision causes fear of losing one's autonomy and becoming dependent on another or others. Visual loss also affects how an individual obtains information (e.g., reading the newspaper). In addition, reading is often a leisure activity, and its loss can affect an individual's quality of life. It is important for the nurse to be aware of and assess for signs of depression and to intervene as appropriate if an older adult is experiencing depression as a result of a visual impairment.

In the healthcare setting, nursing interventions for patients with visual impairments should include optimizing safety through environmental organization. For individuals outside the healthcare setting, the nurse should teach patients and their families the importance of organizing the patient's living environment. Organizing the environment reduces the risk for injury and increases opportunities for independence. Features of a safe environment for the patient with a visual impairment include the following:

- An uncluttered environment with plenty of lighting
- Clear pathways (chairs pushed under tables, things put away); furniture should not be rearranged without orienting the patient
- Organized self-care articles within the patient's reach
- Call lights and assistive devices within easy reach.

SAFETY ALERT When assisting with ambulation, stand at the patient's side, walk about 1 foot ahead and allow the individual to grasp your arm. Confirm whether the patient prefers grasping your arm with the dominant or nondominant hand.

Impaired Hearing

For home safety, patients with impaired hearing should obtain devices that either amplify sounds or respond to sounds with flashing lights. These devices can be obtained from hearing aid dealers, telephone companies, and appliance stores. In most areas, providers of television programming offer closed captioning in their broadcasts, and most online streaming services also provide closed captioning. This can allow individuals with a hearing impairment to continue to enjoy television programs and movies and to access important news and weather updates.

Impaired Olfactory Sense

Patients with an impaired sense of smell should be taught about the dangers of cleaning with chemicals such as ammonia. Strong chemicals such as ammonia used in confined spaces such as a bathroom may affect patients before they smell the chemical. Because a gas leak can go undetected, patients should keep gas stoves and heaters in good working order. Food poisoning is a concern with patients who have difficulty detecting spoiled meat or dairy products. Patients need to carefully inspect food for freshness (check its color and texture) and check expiration dates on food packages.

Impaired Tactile Sense

Patients with an impaired sense of touch may not be aware of hot temperatures, which can cause burns, or pressure on bony prominences, which can produce pressure ulcers. Patients with impaired temperature perception should have the temperature adjusted on their hot water heater and test water temperature with a thermometer before bathing. Patients with decreased sensation to pressure must change their position frequently.

Collaborative Therapies

Treatment of altered sensory perception is based on the cause and severity of the problem. For many disorders, treatment will require collaboration with physicians and others who have been specially trained to evaluate and treat vision, hearing, and other sensory disorders.

For vision disorders, patients may be referred to an optometrist or ophthalmologist. An optometrist is trained to perform eye exams and prescribe corrective lenses to correct ordinary problems with visual acuity. However, if a more severe disorder is discovered that requires surgery or more advanced treatments, the patient should be referred to an ophthalmologist. Optometrists and ophthalmologists may work closely with an optician, who is trained to help fit glasses and frames, or with a physical or occupational therapist who is specifically trained to provide vision therapy.

For hearing disorders, patients may be referred to an audiologist or an otolaryngologist. An audiologist is trained to provide hearing exams and to provide prescriptions for hearing aids. Audiologists may also be able to diagnose and treat balance disorders or provide hearing or speech rehabilitation. Otolaryngologists are physicians who are trained to diagnose and treat ear, nose, and throat disorders, including performing surgery if needed. Otolaryngologists also can be consulted for patients who develop smell or taste disorders. Audiologists and otolaryngologists may also work closely with a hearing instrument specialist, who is trained to fit patients with hearing aids, or with a physical or occupational therapist who is trained in sound therapy (commonly used to help patients with tinnitus) or vestibular rehabilitation therapy (commonly used to help patients with balance disorders). Patients with new and permanent hearing loss may also be referred to a class to learn American Sign Language or lip reading.

If sight or hearing disorders or loss of feeling is related to loss of nerve conductance, the patient may be referred to a neurologist. Other specialists may also be used as needed, depending on the exact condition and type of sensory loss.

Surgery

Surgery is used to correct many types of sensory disorders, particularly sight and vision disorders. Surgeries to treat sight disorders include cataract surgery; glaucoma surgery; laser eye surgery to correct myopia, hyperopia, astigmatism, and other disorders; corneal transplant surgery; surgery to repair detached retinas; eye muscle surgery to correct strabismus; and many other types of surgery. Eye surgery is also often performed after a direct major injury to the eye.

Surgeries to treat hearing or ear disorders include surgery to remove tumors or polyps, surgery to correct congenital atresia of the ear canal, surgery to restore hearing loss (e.g., cochlear implant surgery), and surgery to reconstruct the tympanic membrane. Cosmetic surgery to reconstruct the outer ear may also be needed after trauma. Children with frequent otitis media may require surgery to insert ear tubes. Many other ear surgeries are available as well, depending on the disorder or alteration.

Individuals with alterations in smell and taste may also require surgery, particularly if the alteration is due to the presence of polyps, a deviated septum, or other treatable disorders.

Pharmacologic Therapy

The eye is vulnerable to a variety of conditions, many of which can be prevented, controlled, or reversed with proper treatment. Medicated eyedrops are often used to treat various eye disorders, including dry eye, allergies, and eye infections. Pharmacotherapy is of particular importance in the treatment of glaucoma and macular degeneration. Medications used to treat these alterations are discussed in the respective exemplars.

If hearing loss is the result of an infection, the infection can be treated with antibiotics in the form of medicated eardrops. If the infection is severe and persistent, qualified healthcare providers may consider perfusion of the inner ear with antibiotics. This treatment may restore hearing loss for some individuals. If hearing loss is due to impacted cerumen, gentle treatment with an ear wax softener and warm water should restore hearing when the cerumen is removed.

Treatment of olfactory impairment generally may be resolved by treating the underlying cause of the impairment. However, olfactory impairment sometimes presents with the onset of serious illnesses, such as diabetes, hypertension, and Parkinson disease. Treatment of the underlying disease does not always restore olfactory function.

Unfortunately, no medications are available to help patients who experience permanent hearing loss or permanent alterations of taste or smell.

Lifespan Considerations

Most individuals will not experience significant permanent sensory alterations over the span of their life. However, temporary sensory alterations are very common across the lifespan. For example, an upper respiratory infection may cause temporary loss of the ability to smell and taste. Patients with an ear infection may temporarily experience some hearing loss. To appropriately treat patients throughout the lifespan, nurses should be aware of several lifespan considerations. See the Eye and Vision Assessment, Ear and Hearing Assessment, and Cranial Nerve Assessment features for more on developmental considerations in assessment of sensory perception.

Sensory Perception in Infants

Healthy individuals are born with the ability to see, hear, taste, touch, and smell, and they have those same abilities throughout the lifespan. However, some normal changes do occur across the lifespan, particularly to infants' vision. Newborns are unable to focus on objects that are more than 8–10 inches away, and they cannot easily distinguish between images or move their eyes between two images. During the first 3 months of life, infants' eyes start to work together, and infants are more easily able to see and track objects. As their vision matures, infants develop depth perception and color vision. By 2 years of age, children's vision should be similar to adults' vision (American Optometric Association [AOA], 2015). During these early years, infants will also begin to develop taste preferences. Other senses should be well developed at birth.

Parents should be taught how to help develop their children's senses and to observe their babies for signs of vision or hearing problems (AOA, 2015). Infants with vision or hearing problems can have developmental and learning delays if deficits in vision and hearing are not detected early and treated.

Potential problems with vision involve strabismus; excessive tearing, which is a sign of blocked eye ducts; and encrusted eyelids, which is a sign of infection. Infants may also have **amblyopia** (lazy eye; one eye has reduced vision even with no identifiable cause, and the reduced vision is not correctable by corrective lenses), nystagmus, myopia, hyperopia, and cancer. Premature babies may develop retinopathy of prematurity, which results from replacement of retinal tissue with fibrous tissue (AOA, 2015). The AOA recommends that infants receive a comprehensive eye exam by 6 months of age. Optometrists participating in InfantSEE, managed by the AOA Foundation, provide free eye assessments for infants between the ages of 6 and 12 months. Nurses should be aware of this service and recommend participating optometrists to all parents of infants.

Treatment of amblyopia should occur in the first 2–4 years of life. The treatment for amblyopia commonly involves putting a patch over the healthy eye to encourage the "lazy" eye to process images, thus strengthening the eye and building nerve connections between that eye and the brain. Treatment of strabismus also often occurs early in life. Strabismus is treated with corrective lenses and an eye patch. If this does not correct the problem, surgery may be needed to alter the way the eye muscles work.

Newborns are routinely screened for hearing by using two different tests. The otoacoustic emissions test uses an earphone and microphone to play sounds in the baby's ear. If the baby hears normally, the microphone will detect an echo. If the baby has hearing loss, the echo will not be detected. The auditory brainstem response test uses electrodes to detect nerve responses after sounds are played for the infant through small earphones. Neither of these hearing tests require an observable response by the infant. The otoacoustic emissions test can be performed by the nurse, and if the infant fails the test, the infant can be referred to a specialist for the more complete auditory brainstem response test.

An infant's sense of touch is not routinely assessed. However, the nurse can often assess an infant's ability to detect touch using simple observation. For example, withdrawal responses to painful stimuli indicate normal sensory function.

Sensory Perception in Children and Adolescents

Children of all ages who have recurrent, severe otitis media or other problems that cause fluid buildup in the inner or middle ear may be at risk for developing hearing loss. Infants and children are also at increased risk of damage to the eye or ear due to injury. For example, allowing an infant or toddler to play with a sharp object increases the risk of severe injury to the child's eye, which may result in loss of vision or loss of the eye. Toddlers may stick small objects such as marbles in their ears, causing temporary hearing loss and potential damage to ear structures.

Children and adolescents in high-contact sports or extreme sports are at risk of losing sensory perception due to head injuries that alter nerve conduction of sensory signals or due to injuries directly to the sensory structure. Nurses can promote sensory health in children, adolescents, and young adults by teaching them to use helmets and other safety equipment when participating in sports and other athletic activities that may result in head injury and a subsequent loss of sensory perception.

Parents can protect their child's hearing by not exposing them to loud noises and by monitoring them for ear infection, cerumen buildup, and other conditions that might damage hearing. Nurses should encourage parents to immunize their children at the appropriate times, as preventable diseases such as mumps may contribute to hearing loss in children.

Vision screenings of toddlers and young children should include inspection of the eye for overall shape, structure, pupil shape, and red reflex. Vision screening may also involve photoscreening (uses the red reflex to detect eye problems), corneal light reflex testing (uses a penlight to detect the light reflection off the corneal surface), and cover testing (tests the misalignment of the eyes). Visual acuity tests can also be used. Eye charts for young children should feature pictures or shapes rather than letters (American Association for Pediatric Ophthalmology and Strabismus [AAPOS], 2014a). Vision screenings are not comprehensive eye exams, but they can detect problems that would be cause for referral to an optometrist or ophthalmologist.

Children should also have their hearing tested periodically at school or at their healthcare provider's office. Young children with hearing loss often receive early treatment with hearing aids, cochlear implants, or bone-anchored hearing aids. Some of these devices require surgery to implant the device into the child's ear.

For older children, specific tests can be used to assess for response to touch. To test superficial tactile sensation, the nurse can stroke the skin on the lower leg or arm with a cotton ball or a finger while the child's eyes are closed. Cooperative children over 2 years of age can normally point to the location touched. To test superficial pain sensation, the nurse can break a tongue blade to get a sharp point. After asking the child to close his or her eyes, the nurse can touch the child gently in various places on each arm and leg, alternating the sharp and dull ends of the tongue blade. A paper clip may also be used. Children over 4 years of age can normally distinguish between a sharp and dull sensation each time.

As with adults, a child's senses of taste and smell are not part of a normal physical assessment. Any alteration reported by the patient or patient's parent or guardian is cause for referral to a specialist.

Sensory Perception in Pregnant Women

Alterations related to hearing and balance that are more common in pregnancy are tinnitus and vertigo. Unless the alteration is unrelated to the pregnancy, most symptoms revert back to normal after delivery. If treatment is needed, many treatments, such as the use of hearing aids or corrective lenses, are safe for pregnant women. However, if medication is needed, the medication should be assessed for risks versus benefits in pregnant women.

Whereas many adults do not notice or report changes in smell and taste, pregnant women often report a heightened sense of smell, which may cause nausea and vomiting, or they may report cravings for odd combinations of food or very specific foods. These changes in smell and taste are temporary and will be relieved when the woman delivers her baby. However, the pregnant woman may be prescribed antiemetic medications to relieve nausea and vomiting.

Sensory Perception in Older Adults

Unless significant alterations occur, patients' senses, especially taste, smell, and touch, should remain relatively stable throughout life. However, older adults often lose some sensitivity in their hearing and vision as they age. As an individual ages, the structures inside the ears change, causing functional decline. This decreases the patient's ability to detect sound. The structures of the eyes also change, causing a decrease in sensitivity and reactivity to light. Visual acuity decreases, and eye muscle movement declines, resulting in a smaller visual field. Some changes in the ability to distinguish between colors may also occur. Older adults have fewer taste buds, and sensitivity to taste may decrease over time. Loss of nerve endings in the nose may also cause the sense of smell to diminish over time. Older adults may also have a reduced ability to detect touch, making them more susceptible to injury (Martin, 2014).

In addition to the normal loss of sensory perception due to aging, older adults are at higher risk of developing hearing disorders such as presbycusis (age-related loss of hearing, particularly of high-frequency sounds) and tinnitus and vision disorders such as glaucoma, AMD, and cataracts.

When assessing the senses of older adults, nurses should take into consideration declining vision and hearing. For example, assessment of vision should be done using high-contrast colors (e.g., black on white rather than gray on white), and the assessment should be done in a room with good lighting but minimal glare. Older adults have a harder time hearing consonants than vowels, so nurses should emphasize consonant sounds when talking and assessing hearing in older adults.

Case Study » Part 3

Simon Thompson has been instructed to keep his eye patch on for 3 days for comfort and to prevent him from rubbing his eye. His friends have been doing a new jump trick on their skateboards that Simon really wants to try. He borrows his friend's skateboard at the playground after school. He is having a hard time focusing with just one eye but does not want to look timid in front of his friends. Simon is able to do the jump trick but loses control and crashes into a metal bike rack on the playground. His friends rush over and notice that Simon's right eye is puffy and swollen and his nose has begun to bleed.

Simon's friends help him to get home, and his mother takes him to the emergency department, where Simon is diagnosed with a right maxillary fracture. He is continuing to experience epistaxis. He is scheduled for a surgical repair tomorrow.

Clinical Reasoning Questions Level I

1. What are some appropriate nursing diagnoses for Simon at this time?
2. What are some appropriate nursing diagnoses for Simon's mother at this time?

Clinical Reasoning Questions Level II

3. What diagnostic studies might have been ordered to diagnose Simon's maxillary fracture?
4. How could the nurse check to make sure that Simon does not have a basilar skull fracture?
5. What independent nursing interventions can be done to decrease swelling and maintain Simon's safety until surgery?
6. What additional patient education do you anticipate Simon will need at his postoperative follow-up appointment?

REVIEW The Concept of Sensory Perception

RELATE Link the Concepts

Linking the concept of sensory perception with the concept of development:

1. How might an alteration in sensory perception interfere with an infant or toddler's ability to meet developmental milestones?
2. How would your assessment of hearing for a 40-year-old man be different from your assessment of hearing for a 6-year-old girl?

Linking the concept of sensory perception with the concept of safety:

3. Discuss how different alterations in sensory perception might affect the safety of a 76-year-old woman.
4. Discuss how different alterations in sensory perception might affect the safety of a 4-year-old boy.

READY Go to Volume 3: Clinical Nursing Skills

- SKILL 1.13 Ears: Hearing Acuity, Assessing
- SKILL 1.14 Eyes: Visual Acuity, Assessing
- SKILL 1.22 Neurologic Status: Assessing
- SKILL 1.24 Peripheral Vascular System: Assessing
- SKILL 2.3 Eyes and Contact Lenses: Caring for
- SKILL 2.4 Feet: Caring for
- SKILL 2.6 Hearing Aid: Removing, Cleaning, and Inserting
- SKILL 2.17 Ear Medication: Administering
- SKILL 2.19 Eye Medication: Administering
- SKILL 3.3 Pain Relief: Complementary Health Approaches
- SKILL 15.5 Environmental Safety: Health Care Facility, Community, Home

REFER Go to Pearson MyLab Nursing and eText

- Additional review materials
- MiniModule: Physiology of Sensory Perception

REFLECT Apply Your Knowledge

Paul Holcomb is a 68-year-old man. While family members were visiting him and his wife over the holidays, their old oven caught on fire. The smoke detectors were activated, and everyone except Mr. Holcomb heard the alarms and evacuated the house. As the family gathered outside, they realized that he was missing. He was eventually rescued from the house by firefighters and sustained only minor injuries. However, after this incident, Mr. Holcomb's wife Elinor insisted that he get a hearing examination. During the nursing assessment before the audiologist performed the hearing exam, Mr. Holcomb told the nurse that he often has trouble hearing if there is noise in the background, that he cannot hear high-frequency sounds, and that everyone he talks to seems to mumble. His wife always tells him that he has the TV turned up too loud, but he still has trouble hearing it.

1. What additional assessment questions should the nurse ask Mr. Holcomb? What questions should the nurse ask Mrs. Holcomb?
2. What nursing diagnoses are appropriate for Mr. Holcomb at this time? For Mrs. Holcomb?
3. What independent interventions and patient teaching could the nurse implement for Mr. and Mrs. Holcomb during this appointment?
4. What are possible reasons for Mr. Holcomb's hearing impairment, and what are some treatments that the audiologist might suggest?

>> Exemplar 18.A Hearing Impairment

Exemplar Learning Outcomes

18.A Analyze hearing impairment as it relates to sensory perception:

- Describe the pathophysiology of hearing impairment.
- Describe the etiology of hearing impairment.
- Compare the risk factors for and prevention of hearing impairment.
- Identify the clinical manifestations of hearing impairment.
- Summarize diagnostic tests and therapies used by interprofessional teams in the collaborative care of an individual with hearing impairment.

- Differentiate considerations for care of patients with hearing impairment across the lifespan.
- Apply the nursing process in providing culturally competent care to an individual with hearing impairment.

Exemplar Key Terms

Decibels (dB), *1405*
Noise-induced hearing loss (NIHL), *1406*
Presbycusis, *1406*
Tinnitus, *1407*

Overview

Approximately 1 million children in the United States have some form of hearing impairment. Hearing loss is present in 2–3 out of every 1000 newborns (NIDCD, 2015). Hearing loss is a significant problem for adults as well, affecting an estimated 37.5 million adults (15%) in the United States. The problem of hearing loss is particularly significant in older adults, with about 25% of adults between the ages of 65 and 74 and 50% of those over age 75 experiencing a disabling hearing loss (NIDCD, 2015). As many as 70% of nursing home residents have impaired hearing.

Hearing impairments are expressed in terms of **decibels (dB)**, which are units of loudness, and rated according to severity (see **Table 18–2 >>**). Children who have only a mild hearing loss (35–40 dB) may miss as much as 50% of everyday conversation and are considered at high risk for difficulty in school. Anyone with a hearing loss of more than 90 dB is considered legally deaf.

Hearing loss impairs the ability to communicate in a world filled with sound and hearing individuals. A hearing deficit can be partial or total, congenital or acquired. It may affect one or both ears. In some types of hearing loss, the ability to perceive sound at specific frequencies is lost. In others, hearing is diminished across all frequencies.

Pathophysiology and Etiology

Pathophysiology

Many factors can be involved in alterations in hearing. For example, lesions in the outer ear, middle ear, inner ear, or central auditory pathways can result in hearing loss. The process of aging also can affect the structures of the ear and hearing.

Etiology

Hearing loss is classified as conductive, sensorineural, or mixed, depending on what portion of the auditory system is affected. Profound deafness is often a congenital condition.

Conductive Hearing Loss

Anything that disrupts the transmission of sound from the external auditory meatus to the inner ear results in a conductive hearing loss. The most common cause of conductive hearing loss is obstruction of the external ear canal. Impacted cerumen, edema of the canal lining, stenosis, and neoplasms may lead to canal obstruction. Other causes of conductive loss include a perforated tympanic membrane, disruption or fixation of the ossicles of the middle ear, fluid, scarring, and tumors of the middle ear. Conductive loss also occurs if the tympanic membrane does not fully vibrate, as in otitis media. In these cases, loss may be restored after the infection clears. Chronic and untreated ear infections may lead to ear structural changes and permanent hearing impairment. The loss of acuity may be gradual or rapid and results in diminished hearing in all ranges.

Sensorineural Hearing Loss

Disorders that affect the inner ear, the auditory nerve, or the auditory pathways of the brain may lead to a sensorineural hearing loss. In this type of hearing loss, sound waves are

TABLE 18–2 Severity of Hearing Loss

Type of Loss	Decibel Level (DB)	Hearing Ability
Slight/mild	16–40	Some speech sounds are difficult to perceive, particularly unvoiced consonant sounds.
Moderate	41–70	Most normal conversational speech sounds are missed.
Severe	71–90	Speech sounds cannot be heard at a normal conversational level.
Profound/deaf	91+	No sounds at all can be heard.

Sources: American Speech-Language-Hearing Association (ASHA). (n.d.b). *Degree of hearing loss.* Retrieved from http://www.asha.org/public/hearing/Degree-of-Hearing-Loss/; Royal National Institute for Deaf People. (n.d.). *Levels of hearing loss.* Retrieved from https://www.actiononhearingloss.org.uk/your-hearing/about-deafness-and-hearing-loss/glossary/levels-of-hearing-loss.aspx; Seattle Children's Hospital. (n.d.). *Degree of hearing loss.* Retrieved from https://www.seattlechildrens.org/pdf/degree-hearingloss-chart.pdf

effectively transmitted to the inner ear. In the inner ear, however, lost or damaged receptor cells, changes in the cochlear apparatus, or auditory nerve abnormalities decrease or distort the ability to receive and interpret stimuli. Conditions leading to sensorineural hearing loss may be congenital, genetic, or acquired. In sensorineural hearing loss, high-frequency sounds are most affected.

A significant cause of sensorineural hearing deficit is damage to the hair cells of the organ of Corti. In the United States, noise exposure is the major cause. Damage may result from either loud impulse noise (e.g., an explosion) or loud continuous noise (e.g., machinery). Exposure to a high level of noise (e.g., standing close to the stage or speakers at a rock concert) on an intermittent or continuing basis damages the hair and supporting cells of the organ of Corti. Other sources of potential damage to hearing include certain types of work (first responders, construction workers) and play (fireworks, concerts, firearms, ear buds, loud toys). Ototoxic drugs also damage the hair cells of the organ of Corti; when combined with high noise levels, the damage is greater and the resultant hearing loss is more profound.

Other causes of sensory hearing loss include prenatal exposure to rubella, viral infections, meningitis, trauma, Ménière disease, and aging. Tumors such as acoustic neuromas (vestibular schwannomas), vascular disorders, demyelinating or degenerative diseases, infections (bacterial meningitis in particular), or trauma may affect the central auditory pathways and produce a neural hearing loss.

Presbycusis

With aging, the hair cells of the cochlea degenerate, producing a progressive sensorineural hearing loss. In age-related hearing loss, or **presbycusis**, hearing acuity begins to decrease in early adulthood and progresses as long as the individual lives. Higher pitched tones and conversational speech are lost initially.

Risk Factors

Several risk factors are associated with hearing impairment. Individuals who are consistently exposed to loud noises on their job are at greater risk of developing hearing impairment. Likewise, individuals who are exposed to loud noises due to recreational activities, such as firearms, snowmobile engines, or loud music, have a higher risk of hearing impairment. Some medications and illnesses can also damage the inner ear, increasing the risk of hearing loss. Age is one of the greatest risk factors associated with hearing impairment (Mayo Clinic, 2017d).

Caucasians are twice as likely as African Americans to have hearing loss. Hispanics are less likely than non-Hispanics to experience difficulty with hearing. Very little research, however, has examined ethnic diversity and hearing impairment.

Prevention

Both the loudness of the noise and the length of exposure contribute to hearing damage. The level of noise is measured in decibels (dB). The louder the noise, the higher the decibel

Focus on Diversity and Culture
Deaf Culture

Deaf culture is a community that is shared by individuals who are deaf or hard of hearing, their family members, and others who self-identify with the Deaf community. It is usually based off a shared proficiency in a common sign language. Members of Deaf culture consider deafness to be a matter of difference rather than disability. Some people who have severe hearing impairments identify with Deaf culture because of its shared history and values, a unique language, and strong artistic and literary traditions. Deaf culture is increasingly gaining recognition in the mainstream. Indeed, the most recent statement from the United Nations Convention on the Rights of Persons with Disabilities states that individuals with disabilities, including those who are deaf, are entitled to be recognized and supported in their cultural and linguistic identities, specifically sign languages and Deaf culture (United Nations, 2006, Article 30, Para. 4).

level. Some examples of decibel levels of everyday sounds are shown in **Table 18–3 »**.

Although young children may be at higher risk, hearing impairment associated with the use of ear buds and headphones can affect individuals of any age group. In part because of the popular practice of listening to portable media devices (e.g., MP3 players and cell phones) through ear buds and headphones, **noise-induced hearing loss (NIHL)** continues to be a serious public health concern. This condition is associated with prolonged exposure to sounds of greater than or equal to 85 dB over an extended time period, including listening to loud music. NIHL may also be caused by a single exposure to an intense impulse sound at a volume of 120 dB or more, such as an explosive

TABLE 18–3 Decibel Levels of Everyday Sounds

Category	Decibel Level	Examples
Faint	20–30	Leaves rustling in a breeze, quiet library, whisper
Moderate	50	Moderate rainfall
	60	Dishwasher, clothes dryer, normal conversation
Very loud	70	Alarm clock, vacuum cleaner
	80–90	Hair dryer, food processor
Extremely loud	90	Passing motorcycle
	106	Snowblower, gas-powered lawn mower, sporting event
Painful	120	Siren
	124	Maximum volume of MP3 ear buds, MRI scanner
	140	Jet engine, firearms

Sources: Based on American Speech-Language-Hearing Association. (2015a). *Noise.* Retrieved from http://www.asha.org/public/hearing/Noise; Centers for Disease Control and Prevention (CDC). (2017). *Noise and hearing loss prevention.* Retrieved from http://www.cdc.gov/niosh/topics/noise/default.html; Center for Hearing, Speech and Language. (2014). *How loud is it?* Retrieved from http://www.chsl.org/soundchart.php

blast (CDC, 2015b). Prevention of NIHL includes avoiding situations that pose known risks and wearing ear protection when in environments that may involve exposure to known risks.

Warning signs that may suggest auditory damage include the inability to hear another individual's voice from a distance of 3 feet away, muffled sound perception, ringing in the ears (tinnitus), and ear pain.

Some medications can cause hearing disorders (see **Table 18–4 ≫**). The decision to discontinue a medication based on potential to damage hearing (ototoxicity) should be made in collaboration with the prescribing physician. Some drugs cannot be discontinued despite their potential for ototoxicity. The nurse should be aware of medication groups that can cause hearing damage and teach patients to monitor their hearing while they are taking these medications. One group requires special mention: platinum coordination complexes (cisplatin). These drugs are used in the treatment of many solid cancerous tumors and are among the most ototoxic drugs prescribed in clinical practice.

TABLE 18–4 Ototoxic Medications

Medication Category and Drug Examples	Uses
Aminoglycosides **Drug examples:** –Tobramycin –Gentamicin –Amikacin –Kanamycin –Neomycin –Streptomycin	These drugs are used in the treatment of advanced bacterial infections and tuberculosis. Hearing loss is more likely to occur in patients with renal disease or previous hearing difficulty. Hearing loss may result from either cochlear or vestibular complications.
Alkylating Agents **Drug examples:** –Cisplatin –Carboplatin	These drugs are used as chemotherapy for many solid tumors. Hearing loss starts with tinnitus, but changes can be profound and permanent. Hearing loss may start as soon as the first dose of treatment, but hearing loss may also be delayed until well after chemotherapeutic treatment is over.
Loop Diuretics **Drug examples:** –Bumetanide (Bumex) –Furosemide (Lasix) -Ethacrynic acid (Edecrin)	These drugs are diuretics that affect the ascending limb of the loop of Henle in the kidney. Hearing loss is most common in patients with renal failure who have also received aminoglycosides.
Others **Drug examples:** –Salicylates (aspirin) –Quinine –Chloroquine –Quinidine	Aspirin is commonly used as an antipyretic, anti-inflammatory agent, and anti-platelet agent. Quinine, chloroquine, and quinidine are anti-protozoan drugs commonly used to treat malaria. Ototoxicity with these drugs generally causes tinnitus, and effects are usually temporary. Hearing loss usually resolves once the drug is stopped. Ototoxicity is most common when the drug is given in high doses.

Source: Data from Adams, M. P., Holland, L. N., & Urban, C. (2017). *Pharmacology for nurses: A pathophysiologic approach* (5th ed.). Hoboken, NJ: Pearson Education.

Clinical Manifestations

Conductive hearing loss involves an equal loss of hearing at all sound frequencies. If the level of sound is greater than the threshold for hearing, speech discrimination is good. Because of this, the patient with a conductive hearing loss benefits from amplification by a hearing aid.

Sensorineural hearing losses typically affect the ability to hear high-frequency tones. This loss makes speech discrimination difficult, especially in a noisy environment. Hearing aids are often not useful in sensorineural hearing loss because they amplify both speech and background noise. The increased sound intensity may actually cause discomfort for the patient.

Tinnitus

Tinnitus is the perception of sound or noise in the ears without stimulus from the environment. The sound may be steady, intermittent, or pulsatile and is often described as a buzzing, roaring, or ringing. Tinnitus is usually associated with hearing loss (conductive or sensorineural); however, the mechanism that produces the sound is poorly understood. Tinnitus is often an early symptom of noise-induced hearing damage and drug-related ototoxicity. Tinnitus is especially associated with salicylate, quinine, or quinidine toxicity. Other etiologies include obstruction of the auditory meatus, presbycusis, middle or inner ear inflammations and infections, otosclerosis, and Ménière disease. Most tinnitus, however, is chronic and has no pathologic importance. Tinnitus can be very stressful and cause anxiety and/or depression for the individual experiencing it. Nurses should not minimize the distress that individuals with chronic tinnitus experience.

≫ **Stay Current:** You can hear some of the sounds that someone with tinnitus might experience by visiting the American Tinnitus Association at http://www.ata.org/understanding-facts/symptoms.

Collaboration

For proper treatment of an alteration in hearing, patients need to be diagnosed with the correct type of hearing loss. Nurses can help patients with explanations about the types of tests that will be performed and by providing the relevant education if an alteration is found.

Diagnostic Tests

Assessment protocols that can be performed for initial screening include the whisper test, otoscope examination, tympanogram, and use of a tuning fork to perform the Rinne and Weber tests. (See the Ear and Hearing Assessment feature in the Concept of Sensory Perception section.)

Surgery

For patients with a conductive hearing loss, reconstructive surgeries of the middle ear, such as a stapedectomy or tympanoplasty, may help to restore hearing. Stapedectomy, the removal and replacement of the stapes, is used to treat hearing loss related to otosclerosis. In a tympanoplasty, the structures of the middle ear are reconstructed to improve conductive hearing deficits. Chronic otitis media with necrosis and scarring of the middle ear is a common indication for this type of surgery.

Clinical Manifestations and Therapies
Hearing Impairment

ETIOLOGY	CLINICAL MANIFESTATIONS	CLINICAL THERAPIES
Conductive hearing loss	▪ Equal loss of hearing at all sound frequencies	▪ Hearing aids ▪ Treatment of underlying conditions such as otitis media ▪ Steroids and/or decongestants to reduce inflammation ▪ Surgery
Sensorineural hearing loss	▪ Decreased ability to hear high-frequency tones more than low-frequency tones ▪ Difficulty discriminating speech	▪ Cochlear implant
Presbycusis	▪ Cognitive and affective manifestations such as confusion, forgetfulness, and depression; poor health, reduced mobility; withdrawal; signs of impaired hearing, such as cupping a hand around the ear	▪ Hearing aids ▪ Steroids or decongestants to reduce inflammation
Tinnitus (mechanism not fully understood; etiology varies to include noise, ototoxicity, infection or inflammation, underlying conditions such as Ménière disease)	▪ Buzzing, roaring, or ringing in the ears	▪ Treatment of underlying cause ▪ Tinnitus maskers such as ambient noise

In myringotomy, a small hole is made in the tympanic membrane and then tympanostomy tubes are placed. This procedure is common in young children with repeated episodes of otitis media but can also be performed on older adults for chronic presence of middle ear fluid (effusion). The tubes allow equalization of air within the middle ear and prevent fluid accumulation.

For the patient with a sensorineural hearing loss, a cochlear implant may be the only hope for restoring sound perception. The cochlear implant consists of a microphone, speech processor, transmitter, receiver/stimulator, and electrodes (see **Figure 18–8 »**). Its function is more similar to the way the ear normally receives and processes sounds than it is to that of a hearing aid. The microphone picks up sounds and sends them to the speech processor, which selects and processes those that are useful. The receiver/stimulator and transmitter receive signals from the speech processor, convert them to electrical impulses, and send these impulses to the electrodes for transmission to the brain.

Cochlear implants provide sound perception but not normal hearing. The patient is able to recognize warning sounds such as automobiles, sirens, telephones, and doors opening or closing. Patients also receive stimuli to alert them to incoming communication so they can focus on the individual speaking. Many patients learn to interpret perceived sounds as words, especially when they have acquired the hearing loss as an adult.

Pharmacologic Therapy

For hearing loss that is caused by upper respiratory infections or seasonal allergies, decongestants may be helpful.

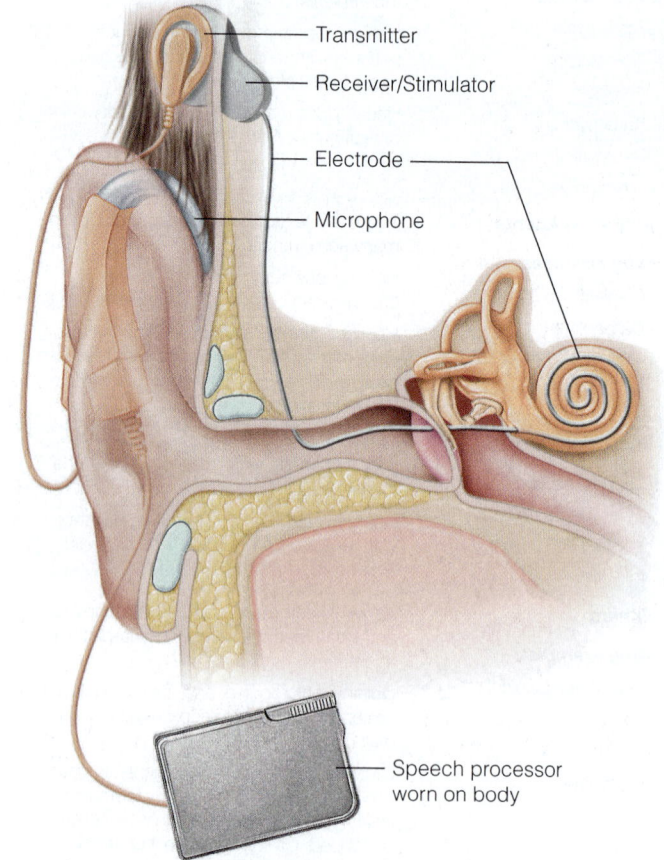

Transmitter
Receiver/Stimulator
Electrode
Microphone
Speech processor worn on body

Source: Courtesy of National Eye Institute, Published by National Institutes of Health.

Figure 18–8 » A cochlear implant for sensorineural hearing loss.

Medications

Temporary Hearing Loss

CLASSIFICATION AND DRUG EXAMPLES	MECHANISMS OF ACTION	NURSING CONSIDERATIONS
Adrenergic Drugs *Drug example:* Pseudoephedrine	These drugs enhance norepinephrine and epinephrine activity by stimulating alpha-adrenergic receptors. This causes vasoconstriction and reduces inflammation.	▪ Use with caution in patients with hyperthyroidism, hypertension, or heart disease. ▪ Instruct the patient to limit caffeine use because it can lead to hypertension and tachycardia.
Corticosteroids *Drug examples:* Prednisone Methylprednisolone	These drugs mimic hormones produced by the adrenal gland. They reduce inflammation and the immune response system.	▪ Warn the patient that grapefruit or grapefruit juice may alter the drug's uptake. ▪ Barbiturates may decrease effectiveness. ▪ Live vaccines should be avoided while taking corticosteroids.
Antibiotics *Drug examples:* Cephalosporins Penicillins Macrolides Tetracyclines Fluoroquinolones Sulfonamides	These drugs are used to treat bacterial infections. The choice of antibiotic is based on the bacteria causing the infection.	▪ Teach the importance of finishing the full course of antibiotics. ▪ Observe for signs of allergic reaction. ▪ Encourage adequate fluid intake. ▪ Monitor renal and/or hepatic function in long-term use. ▪ Monitor for ototoxicity. ▪ Warn patients taking macrolides that grapefruit or grapefruit juice may alter the drug's uptake.

Source: Data from Adams, M. P., Holland, L. N., & Urban, C. (2017). *Pharmacology for nurses: A pathophysiologic approach* (5th ed.). Hoboken, NJ: Pearson Education.

Sudden sensorineural hearing loss may initially be treated with steroids. For cases of otitis media, antibiotics may be prescribed. There are currently no medications available to treat permanent hearing loss.

Medications used for temporary hearing loss are presented in the Medications feature.

Nonpharmacologic Therapy

If hearing loss in a patient is permanent, a multiprofessional team is formed to assist the patient and family with adaptation to the disability. Team members may include any of the following: physician; nurse; speech/language, occupational, or physical therapist; audiologist; teacher; social worker; and family members and caregivers. For a patient whose hearing loss is correctable, the team may provide strategies and accommodations until surgery is completed or other treatments take effect. Therapists and social workers can often assist patients in obtaining assistive technology devices at relatively low cost, especially if these are not covered by insurance, and can help the patient learn how to use these tools.

Amplification

A hearing aid or other amplification device can help many patients with hearing deficits. These assistive devices do nothing to prevent, minimize, or treat the hearing loss itself. They amplify the sound that is presented to the hearing apparatus of the ear, which may bring the level of sound above the hearing threshold, allowing more accurate perception and interpretation of its meaning. When sound perception is distorted, a hearing aid may be less helpful because it simply amplifies the distorted sound. Hearing aids must be individually prescribed by an audiologist. Proper design, proper fit, and regular maintenance are necessary to maintain their effectiveness.

All hearing aids include a microphone, amplifier, speaker, earpiece, and volume control. Many include an option to turn off the microphone when using the telephone; others can be adjusted for the patient's pattern of hearing loss. Hearing aids are available in a variety of styles, each with advantages and disadvantages:

- Canal hearing aids (in-canal and completely-in-canal) are the least noticeable style, fitting in the ear canal. They are appropriate for mild to moderately severe hearing loss. These small and unobtrusive devices allow use of the telephone and can be worn during exercise. Because of their small size, the patient must have good manual dexterity to insert, clean, and change the batteries in canal hearing aids. For this reason, older patients or patients with impaired dexterity may be unable to use them.

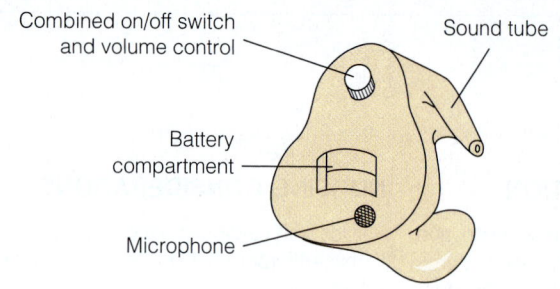

Figure 18–9 ⟩⟩ An in-ear hearing aid.

- The in-ear style of hearing aid fits into the external ear and is used for mild to severe hearing loss (see **Figure 18–9** ⟩⟩). Its larger size makes manipulation somewhat easier, although it still may be difficult for individuals who are less dexterous. A greater degree of amplification is possible with the in-ear aid. Many have a toggle switch for telephone usage.

- The behind-ear hearing aid allows finer adjustment of the level of amplification and is easier for the patient to manipulate (see **Figure 18–10** ⟩⟩). This device can be used by patients with mild to profound hearing loss. For the patient who wears glasses, this style can be modified, with all components fitting into the temple of the eyeglasses.

With both the in-canal and in-ear styles, cleaning is important. Small portals may become plugged with cerumen, interfering with sound transmission.

For the patient who does not have a hearing aid, an assistive listening device, or "pocket talker," with a microphone and earpieces is useful. Pocket talkers are available over the counter or through an audiologist and are relatively inexpensive. The earpiece requires no special fitting, and the external microphone allows the patient to focus on the desired sound rather than simply amplifying all sounds. Assistive listening devices may also be used in conjunction with a hearing aid.

Patients with tinnitus may find a white or pink noise–masking device helpful to promote concentration and rest.

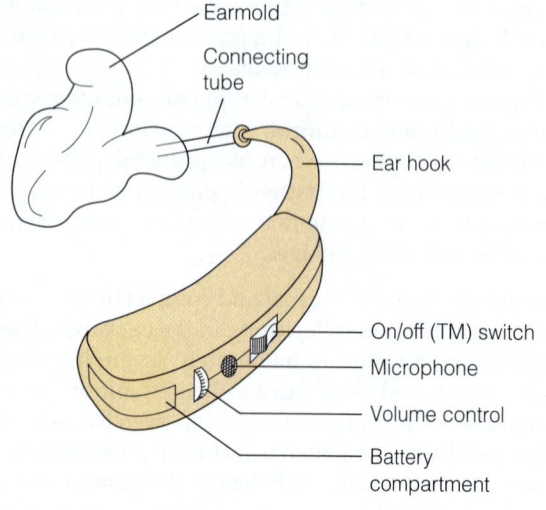

Figure 18–10 ⟩⟩ A behind-ear hearing aid.

These devices conduct a pleasant sound to the affected ear, allowing patients to block out the abnormal sound. White noise provides equal power per hertz, regardless of the frequency, whereas pink noise has decreasing power per hertz with increasing frequency. This allows pink noise to sound even or flat because each octave has equal power.

TTD/TTY telephones and phones with amplifiers are available to assist patients who are deaf or hearing impaired in communicating with the outside world. Being able to access the internet can make an extraordinary difference in the quality of life to an individual with a hearing impairment, who can thus communicate by e-mail, participate in online forums, make restaurant and airplane reservations online, and find comprehensive product information about items they may be considering purchasing.

Additional Therapies

For uncorrectable hearing loss, several approaches are used to enhance communication (see **Table 18–5** ⟩⟩). Patients with hearing impairment may receive speech therapy and instructions in lip reading, signing, cuing, and finger-spelling.

SAFETY ALERT Patients who have a hearing impairment may not be able to hear conventional alarms such as smoke detectors, intruder alerts, or carbon monoxide detectors. Additional therapies may need to include recommendations that the patient install alarms that flash lights or vibrate the bed rather than use a loud noise to alert the patient in case of emergency.

Lifespan Considerations

Hearing impairments occur throughout life, and the etiology behind the hearing loss is often different during different stages of the lifespan. These etiologies require specific considerations in management of the hearing loss.

TABLE 18–5 Communication Techniques for Patients Who Have a Hearing Impairment

Technique	Description
Cued speech	This supplement to lip reading uses eight hand shapes that represent groups of consonant sounds and four positions about the face that represent groups of vowel sounds. Cued speech is based on the sounds the letters make, not the letters themselves. The patient can "see-hear" every spoken syllable a hearing individual hears.
Oral approach	This approach uses only spoken language for face-to-face communication. It avoids the use of formal signs and uses hearing aids and residual hearing.
Total communication	Total communication uses speech and sign, finger-spelling, lip reading, and residual hearing simultaneously. The patient selects the communication technique depending on the situation.
Sign language	This separate language allows the user to communicate quickly and accurately with others who understand signs. The signs or hand movements represent words, concepts, feelings, and emotions. When a sign is not available, the word can be spelled out using signs. American Sign Language (ASL) is most often used; however, British Sign Language (BSL) is common in Europe.

Hearing Impairment in Infants and Children

More than 50% of hearing loss in children is genetic. Congenital hearing loss can be associated with dominant, recessive, or X-linked genes. The remainder is associated with complications during pregnancy or at the time of birth or with unknown causes. Although many infants with hearing loss have no known risk factors, identified risks include the following (Joint Committee on Infant Hearing, 2007):

- Family history of congenital hearing loss
- Neonatal intensive care stay of more than 5 days
- Exposure to assisted ventilation, ototoxic medications, loop diuretics, or chemotherapy for any amount of time
- In utero infections with TORCH (toxoplasmosis, rubella, cytomegalovirus, syphilis, herpes) pathogens
- Craniofacial abnormalities (e.g., cleft palate) and head trauma
- Presence of syndromes or diseases associated with hearing loss (neurofibromatosis; osteopetrosis; Usher, Waardenburg, Alport, Pendred, Jervell, Lange-Nielson, and Hunter syndromes; or Charcot-Marie-Tooth disease).

Another common cause of hearing loss in children is otitis media. Over 75% of children will experience otitis media within the first 3 years of life, and many of them will have multiple bouts of the disease. Depending on the severity and frequency of otitis media, hearing loss associated with this condition ranges from mild, temporary hearing impairment to permanent hearing loss (ASHA, n.d.a). For more about otitis media, see the exemplar on Otitis Media in the module on Infection.

All children should be screened for hearing impairment within the first month after birth. Infants who fail the hearing test should undergo additional testing and be diagnosed with hearing loss by 3 months of age. They should be fitted for amplification devices within 1 month of diagnosis. By the age of 6 months, infants with hearing loss should be enrolled in a program to help them develop communication skills to prevent a delay in development. Older children should receive a hearing evaluation if the caregiver or teacher indicates that the child may have hearing loss. Signs of hearing loss in older children include speech and language delays, difficulty understanding speech when background noise is present, not startling to loud sounds, attention or behavior problems, difficulty hearing TV or radio compared to other family members, and other similar signs (Cleveland Clinic, 2017).

To minimize the impact of hearing loss or deafness, early detection and intervention are critical. Screening by the child's healthcare provider as well as school screenings can help with early detection. Speech-language therapists can work closely with the child, parents, and school to maximize the child's educational success. Families of children with hearing loss should be given the opportunity to learn sign language with their child. Hearing aids (if appropriate), development of lip-reading skills, learning sign language, and use of printed text can help the child be successful in school (World Health Organization, 2017).

Hearing Impairment in Older Adults

Hearing loss in older adults is due to damage to the ear structures over a lifetime of listening to loud sounds as well as presbycusis. Because the hearing loss of presbycusis is gradual, the patient and family may not realize the extent of the deficit. The individual with a hearing impairment may be described as unsociable or paranoid. The family may worry that the individual is becoming increasingly forgetful, absentminded, or perhaps "senile." Depression, confusion, inattentiveness, tension, and negativism have been noted in older adults with hearing impairments. Functional problems such as poor general health, reduced mobility, and impaired interpersonal communication are also associated with hearing loss. Nurses need to be alert for signs of impaired hearing such as cupping an ear, difficulty understanding verbal communication when the individual cannot see the speaker's face, difficulty following conversation in a large group, and withdrawal from social activities. Hearing aids and other amplification devices are useful for most patients with presbycusis.

Fewer than one fifth of older patients with a hearing deficit have or use a hearing aid. Denial of the deficit, other health problems, poor visual acuity, and decreased manual dexterity all contribute to this low usage. Cost is another factor. Hearing aids can be expensive, and health insurance plans typically cover only one pair of hearing aids within a certain time frame. In most states, Medicare does not pay for hearing aids. Some patients therefore choose not to purchase hearing aids. Nurses can help older patients navigate their insurance as well as recommend other ways in which older patients can get help paying for hearing aids.

Because most older adults have some level of hearing loss, nurses should evaluate each patient for hearing impairment at every encounter. Nurses should encourage patients with significant hearing loss to get a thorough hearing examination from an otolaryngologist or other hearing specialist. They should advocate for patients to receive hearing aids or other hearing devices as appropriate. Nurses should provide patient teaching on proper use and care of any hearing devices (see SKILL 2.6, Hearing Aid: Removing, Cleaning, and Inserting in Volume 3) and provide emotional support and teaching to both the patient and family related to living with hearing loss.

NURSING PROCESS

Early identification of hearing loss is a key element in successful treatment. In planning and implementing nursing care for the patient with a hearing deficit, the type and extent of hearing loss, the patient's adaptation to the loss, and the availability of assistive hearing devices are considered, as well as the patient's ability and willingness to use assistive devices.

Assessment

- ***Observation and patient interview.*** A patient's level of hearing impairment can be observed by noting the patient's ability to respond to verbal cues or other noises. Ear problems that cause alterations in balance can be observed if the patient is unsteady or imbalanced. The patient interview should include questions about the patient's perceived ability to hear; the effect of hearing loss on the patient's function and lifestyle; and risk factors such as use of ototoxic medications, upper respiratory tract or frequent ear infection, and noise exposure. The patient should also be asked about the presence of vertigo and tinnitus.

- **Physical examination.** The physical examination should include inspection of the external ear and tympanic membrane to identify obstructions or infections. The physical examination should also include whisper, Rinne, and Weber tests and tests of balance and cranial nerve function.

Diagnosis

Possible nursing diagnoses for the patient with hearing impairment may include the following:

- *Injury, Risk for*
- *Verbal Communication, Impaired*
- *Social Isolation.*

(NANDA-I © 2014)

Planning

Appropriate outcomes for the patient with hearing impairment are based on the extent of the deficit and may include the following:

- The patient will remain free from injury.
- The patient will wear hearing protection and have no further loss of hearing.
- The patient will find the best method of communication with others, including sign language, hearing aids, writing, and lip reading.
- The patient will remain involved in the community, maintain social contacts, and have positive feelings of self-worth.

Implementation

All hearing loss can cause safety concerns for the patient and contribute to feelings of isolation and lowered self-esteem. Therefore, the goals of nursing care are to promote patient safety, encourage social interaction, and promote feelings of self-worth.

Promote Optimal Wellness

Whether the patient's hearing deficit is partial or total, impaired sound perception is the primary problem. The patient needs to understand what causes the deficit and what to expect for the future. Nursing interventions focus on maximizing available hearing and preventing further deterioration to the extent possible:

- Encourage the patient to talk about the hearing loss and its effect on ADLs. The patient may be denying the extent of the deficit or grieving the loss.

- Talk with the family members about techniques they can use to make communication with the patient easier. Family members can use the same techniques the nurse employs, as listed in Box 18–2.
- Provide information about the type of hearing loss. Refer to an audiologist for evaluation of the hearing loss and possible exploration of amplification devices.
- Remind the patient to replace batteries in hearing aids regularly and as needed. Hearing aid batteries usually last between 3 days and 3 weeks, depending on amount of use and type of battery. If a battery is old or has been improperly stored, its life may be reduced further.

Facilitate Communication

A hearing deficit impairs the patient's ability to receive and interpret verbal communication. A hearing loss affects the patient's ability to follow conversations, use the telephone, and enjoy TV or other forms of entertainment. Use the techniques outlined in Box 18–2 to improve communication.

Encourage Socialization

Patients with impaired hearing often become socially isolated. This isolation may be self-imposed because of difficulty communicating, especially in a group. Often, however, the isolation comes about gradually and without intention. Patients find social settings such as family dinners or community gatherings increasingly difficult. Friends and family become frustrated trying to communicate with patients who have a hearing impairment, and invitations to participate in social activities may dwindle. In addition, many adults with hearing loss are not employed, and many of those who are employed work in low-skilled jobs, which may not offer opportunities for social interaction.

The loss of the ability to communicate with other people can have a profound impact on everyday life and may create feelings of frustration and loneliness. This is especially prevalent in patients with congenital hearing loss if they have not been given the ability to learn sign language. Therefore, teaching for home and community-based care for the patient with hearing loss focuses on managing the deficit and developing coping strategies.

- Identify the extent and cause of the social isolation. Help to differentiate the reality of the isolation and its cause from the patient's perception of isolation. Identifying factors that contribute to isolation may provide the needed impetus to remedy the hearing loss.
- Encourage the patient to interact with friends and family on a one-to-one basis in quiet settings. The patient with impaired hearing is more successful in understanding conversations that take place in small groups and quiet settings.
- Involve the patient in activities that do not require acute hearing, such as checkers and chess. This provides the patient with an opportunity to interact socially without the stress of straining to hear.
- Refer the patient to resources such as support groups and senior citizen centers. These groups provide new social outlets.

Evaluation

Expected outcomes of nursing care for a patient with hearing impairment may include the following:

- The patient demonstrates successful establishment of a communication method.
- The patient manifests growth and developmental milestones to maximum potential.

- The patient and family demonstrate positive methods of coping.

For patients with permanent hearing impairment, the nurse will need to continually evaluate the patient for signs of isolation and depression with each interaction. Each interaction is an opportunity for the nurse to encourage the patient to connect with others, develop coping strategies, and learn multiple methods of communication.

REVIEW Hearing Impairment

RELATE Link the Concepts and Exemplars

Linking the exemplar of hearing impairment with the concept of development:

1. You are caring for a young child who receives a cochlear implant after being deaf from birth to age 5. How will the child's speech patterns differ from those of a normal 5-year-old?
2. What strategies can you use to help this patient improve speech patterns?

Linking the exemplar of hearing impairment with the concept of cognition:

3. How might hearing loss affect an older patient's cognition?
4. What measures would you implement to promote cognition in an older adult who has a hearing impairment?

READY Go to Volume 3: Clinical Nursing Skills

REFER Go to Pearson MyLab Nursing and eText

- Additional review materials

REFLECT Apply Your Knowledge

Corrine Matusiak is an 87-year-old woman who recently moved into an assisted living home after hospitalization for uncontrolled diabetes. She enjoyed reading, but for a long time she has not been able to read because of poor vision acuity. During the admission assessment, the nurse also documents a hearing loss.

1. Discuss the importance of a thorough sensory assessment in this patient.
2. Describe the benefits of improving Mrs. Matusiak's sensory deficits.
3. What recommendations will the nurse make to Mrs. Matusiak to improve her hearing?
4. How does diabetes mellitus affect Mrs. Matusiak's sense of hearing?

≫ Exemplar 18.B
Diseases of the Eye

Exemplar Learning Outcomes

18.B Analyze diseases of the eye as they relate to sensory perception.

- Describe the pathophysiology of the most common diseases of the eye.
- Describe the etiology of selected diseases of the eye.
- Compare the risk factors for and prevention of selected diseases of the eye.
- Identify the clinical manifestations of selected diseases of the eye.
- Summarize diagnostic tests and therapies used by interprofessional teams in the collaborative care of an individual with the most common diseases of the eye.
- Differentiate considerations for care of patients with the most common diseases of the eye across the lifespan.
- Apply the nursing process in providing culturally competent care to individuals with the most common diseases of the eye.

Exemplar Key Terms

Age-related macular degeneration (AMD), *1414*
Angle-closure glaucoma, *1414*

Blepharospasm, *1422*
Buphthalmos, *1422*
Cataract, *1414*
Congenital cataracts, *1414*
Congenital glaucoma, *1422*
Epiphora, *1422*
Extracapsular extraction, *1420*
Exudative macular degeneration, *1415*
Glaucoma, *1414*
Infantile glaucoma, *1422*
Intraocular pressure, *1414*
Juvenile glaucoma, *1422*
Juvenile macular degeneration, *1422*
Mydriasis, *1415*
Nonexudative macular degeneration, *1415*
Open-angle glaucoma, *1414*
Photophobia, *1416*
Radiation cataracts, *1414*
Secondary cataracts, *1414*
Traumatic cataracts, *1414*

Overview

There are many diseases that affect the eyes. The most common ones are cataracts, glaucoma, and macular degeneration. A **cataract** is an opacification (clouding) of the lens of the eye that can significantly interfere with light transmission to the retina and the ability to perceive images clearly. **Glaucoma** is characterized by optic neuropathy with gradual loss of peripheral vision and (usually) increased **intraocular pressure** (force within the eye causing tissue damage). **Age-related macular degeneration (AMD)** is the gradual process of degeneration in the macular area of the retina.

Cataracts

The incidence of cataracts is so common that even if it is not the primary diagnosis, most nurses will at some time take care of patients who either have cataracts or have had them surgically removed. Nurses should recognize that not all cataracts need to be removed in the early stages, but many patients will eventually have them surgically corrected.

Pathophysiology and Etiology

Most cataracts form as a result of the aging process. As the lens ages, its fibers and proteins change and degenerate. The proteins clump, clouding the lens and reducing light transmission to the retina. This process generally begins at the periphery of the lens; it gradually spreads to involve the central portion. The entire lens may eventually become opaque. The lens may also discolor over time, affecting the ability to accurately discriminate colors.

Four types of cataracts may occur independently of the aging process. **Secondary cataracts** can form after surgery performed to treat another eye disorder, such as glaucoma, or as an effect of medication or another primary disorder. Patients who require regular or recurring doses of corticosteroids, for example, are at risk for secondary cataracts. **Traumatic cataracts** may result from an injury to the eye. **Radiation cataracts** may result from long-term exposure to radiation. **Congenital cataracts** may appear in a child at birth or in childhood, usually in both eyes (NEI, 2015a).

The prevalence of cataracts increases rapidly with aging. Approximately 50% of individuals in the United States between the ages of 65 and 74 will develop a cataract; that increases to 70% of individuals over the age of 75. Men are affected less frequently than women. African Americans with cataracts lose their vision at a rate twice that of Caucasians, as a result of lack of or delay in treatment (Health Communities, 2015).

Risk Factors and Prevention

Age is the greatest single risk factor for cataracts. Genetics may contribute to the risk, although the link is unclear. Environmental and lifestyle factors play a role. Long-term exposure to sunlight (UVB rays) increases the risk for cataracts. Cigarette smoking and heavy alcohol consumption are associated with earlier cataract development. Eye trauma can precipitate cataract formation. Diabetes mellitus is associated with earlier development of cataracts. Certain drugs, such as systemic or inhaled corticosteroids, lovastatin (Mevacor),

phenytoin (Dilantin), chlorpromazine (Thorazine), and busulfan (Myleran) also prompt the formation of cataracts.

Although there are no known methods to prevent the development of cataracts, patients can reduce their risk of developing cataracts by not smoking, by refraining from heavy alcohol consumption, and by protecting their eyes from UVB rays. Maintaining a healthy weight and managing other health problems can also help reduce the risk of developing cataracts (Mayo Clinic, 2017a). A diet that includes adequate consumption or supplementation of vitamins C and E as well as lutein and zeaxanthin also reduces the risk of developing cataracts and slows the progression of cataracts (AOA, n.d.a).

Glaucoma

Glaucoma is a silent thief of vision. The patient typically experiences no manifestations other than narrowing of the visual field, which occurs so gradually that it often goes unnoticed until late in the disease process.

Pathophysiology and Etiology

Primary glaucoma, which has no identified cause, has two major forms in adults: open-angle glaucoma and angle-closure glaucoma. Open-angle glaucoma is the more common type. Both terms refer to the angle formed at the point where the iris meets the cornea in the eye's anterior chamber (see **Figure 18–11** »).

In **open-angle glaucoma**, the anterior chamber angle between the iris and cornea is normal (thus the term *open-angle*). However, the flow of aqueous humor through the trabecular meshwork and into the canal of Schlemm is relatively obstructed; the cause of this obstruction is unknown. The trabecular meshwork increasingly inhibits the outflow of aqueous humor, and the intraocular pressure gradually increases. The results are neuronal ischemia and optic nerve degeneration, leading to gradual loss of vision. Open-angle glaucoma tends to be a chronic and gradually progressive disease. It typically affects both eyes, although the pressures and progression may not be symmetric. Open-angle glaucoma is the most common form in adults, accounting for approximately 90% of all glaucomas. Open-angle glaucoma occurs more frequently in Latinos and African Americans than in Caucasians (Glaucoma Research Foundation, 2014).

In **angle-closure glaucoma** (also called closed-angle glaucoma), narrowing of the anterior chamber angle occurs because of corneal flattening or bulging of the iris into the anterior chamber (see Figure 18–11A for an illustration of the normal anterior chamber angle). When the lens thickens during accommodation or the iris thickens during pupil dilation, this angle can close completely. Closure of the angle blocks the outflow of aqueous humor through the trabecular meshwork and canal of Schlemm, and the intraocular pressure rises abruptly (see Figure 18–11B). This increase in intraocular pressure damages the neurons of the retina and the optic nerve, leading to a rapid and permanent loss of vision if not treated promptly. Patients may have intermittent episodes lasting several hours before they have a more typical prolonged attack of angle-closure glaucoma.

Because of the effect of pupil dilation on aqueous outflow in angle-closure glaucoma, episodes often occur in association

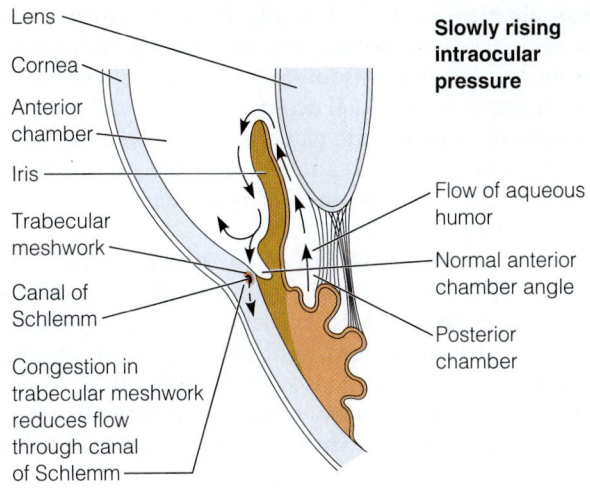

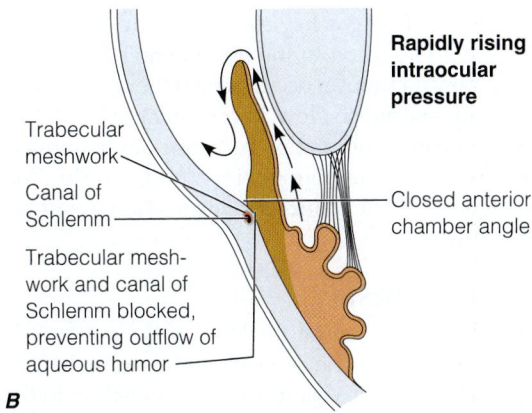

Source: Courtesy of National Eye Institute, Published by National Institutes of Health.

Figure 18–11 ≫ Forms of primary adult glaucoma. **A,** In chronic open-angle glaucoma, the anterior chamber angle remains open, but drainage of aqueous humor through the canal of Schlemm is impaired. **B,** In acute angle-closure glaucoma, the angle of the iris and anterior chamber narrows, obstructing the outflow of aqueous humor.

with darkness, emotional upset, or other factors that cause the pupil to dilate. Patients with a history of the condition must avoid medications, such as atropine and other anticholinergics, that can cause **mydriasis**, or dilation of the pupil. Angle-closure glaucoma is typically unilateral and occurs between 1 and 40 times for every 1000 Americans, with a higher incidence among certain ethnic groups such as Inuits and Asians (Freedman, Sinert, & Aherne, 2015).

The cause of glaucoma is unknown. It is thought to have a hereditary component, but no clear inheritance pattern has been identified. Cardiovascular disease or diabetes may contribute to its formation. In the United States, glaucoma affects over 3 million people over the age of 40; it remains undetected in approximately 50% of these cases (Glaucoma Research Foundation, 2015b).

Risk Factors and Prevention

Glaucoma is a leading cause of blindness worldwide. Age and race are the primary identified risk factors. Patients with

an immediate family member with glaucoma have a nine times higher chance of developing the disease. Long-term steroid use may be a contributing factor. Prior eye injuries, especially blunt trauma or penetrating injuries, may cause secondary glaucoma, called angle recession glaucoma, years later (Glaucoma Research Foundation, 2013).

For individuals with a high risk of glaucoma, prescription eyedrops are available that can help to reduce the risk of developing glaucoma. Regular comprehensive eye exams can also help to identify problems early so that they can be treated promptly to prevent further damage (BrightFocus Foundation, n.d.a; Stamper, 2012).

Exercise helps to lower intraocular pressure, which can help to reduce the risk of developing glaucoma. However, the benefit occurs only as long as exercise is done regularly. In addition, exercises that require the individual to place the head lower than the heart, such as certain yoga poses, can increase intraocular pressure, thus negating the beneficial effect of exercise (Stamper, 2012). Other methods to help prevent the development of glaucoma include eating a healthy diet that is high in vitamins, carotenoids, zinc, and omega-3 fatty acids; maintaining a healthy weight; preventing overexposure to sunlight; and refraining from smoking.

Macular Degeneration

The leading cause of legal blindness and impaired vision in people over the age of 60 is AMD, a gradual process of degeneration in the macular area of the retina. Among individuals ages 75 years or older, nearly one third are affected by AMD (BrightFocus Foundation, 2015a).

Pathophysiology and Etiology

Nonexudative, or dry, macular degeneration is the more common form of AMD. It is the early or intermediate stage of AMD and accounts for 90% of all cases. **Nonexudative macular degeneration** begins with the accumulation of deposits called drusen beneath the pigment epithelium of the retina. Over time, these deposits enlarge and increase in number. The pigment epithelium detaches in small areas and becomes atrophic, interfering with sensory function of the macula. Vision loss is typically not significant, and the disorder progresses slowly. However, there is a risk that the disorder will progress to an exudative stage of the disease.

In **exudative macular degeneration** (wet macular degeneration), vascular endothelial growth factor (VEGF) causes growth of abnormal blood vessels in the potential space between the choroid (vascular layer of the eye) and the retina (neurosensory layer). These new vessels are prone to leak, elevating the retina from the choroid and distorting vision. Although exudative macular degeneration typically is a gradual process, bleeding can lead to acute vision loss in some cases. All patients with exudative macular degeneration had the intermediate stage of the dry form first. With significant or repeated bleeding episodes, scar tissue forms, and central vision is permanently lost. This form accounts for only about 10% of all cases of AMD (BrightFocus Foundation, 2015a).

Approximately 15 million Americans have AMD, with 200,000 new diagnoses occurring each year. AMD is the number one cause of severe vision loss and legal blindness in Americans over the age of 60 (NEI, 2014). Although previous studies indicated that AMD was more prevalent in White populations than in Asian populations, more recent studies have found that the prevalence is the same in these populations (Cheung et al., 2012).

Risk Factors and Prevention

The most significant risk factor for developing AMD is aging. Other nonmodifiable risk factors include race, eye color, and family history (Fisher et al., 2016). AMD is seen more frequently in women, likely because women tend to live longer (BrightFocus Foundation, n.d.b). Modifiable risk factors include smoking, obesity, poor cardiovascular health, and excessive UV exposure. Alcohol consumption of more than 20 g per day is also associated with a higher risk of developing AMD (Adams et al., 2012).

Because smoking is a significant risk factor for developing AMD, patients can decrease their risk of developing AMD by not smoking. Individuals can also decrease their risk by reducing UV exposure, eating a healthy diet that is high in antioxidants and healthy fats, and maintaining a low BMI (see the Focus on Integrative Health feature). Managing other conditions, especially heart disease, can also lower the patient's risk of developing AMD (BrightFocus Foundation, n.d.b; Mayo Clinic, 2017e).

Clinical Manifestations

As a cataract interferes with light transmission through the lens, visual acuity decreases, affecting close and distance vision and causing glare. Glare affects the individual's ability to adjust between light and dark environments. Color discrimination is impaired, particularly in the blue to purple range. When the cataract is mature, the pupil may appear cloudy gray or white rather than black. Cataracts tend to occur bilaterally unless they are related to eye trauma; however, the cataract in one eye usually matures more rapidly than that in the other.

Open-angle glaucoma has no symptoms in many cases, and vision will remain normal for a while. Then, as the nerve becomes more damaged, blank spots will start to appear in the visual field. Although angle-closure glaucoma is also typically free of symptoms, it can cause intermittent pain or

Focus on Integrative Health
Antioxidants for Patients with Age-Related Macular Degeneration

Because antioxidants may help to slow vision loss in patients with AMD, patient teaching should include recommendations for eating foods that are high in antioxidants such as berries (cranberries, blueberries, blackberries, raspberries, strawberries); other fruits (purple or red grapes, apples with peels, pears, citrus fruits, stone fruits); nuts (pecans, walnuts, hazelnuts, pistachios, almonds); beans (red, kidney, pinto, black); green vegetables (broccoli, spinach, kale, collard greens, artichokes, okra, asparagus); white and red potatoes; orange vegetables (sweet potatoes, carrots, winter squash); and fish (sardines, salmon, oysters, mackerel, tuna, rainbow trout, herring).

photophobia (sensitivity to light). Symptoms such as severe eye and face pain, general malaise, nausea and vomiting, seeing colored halos around lights, and experiencing an abrupt decrease in visual acuity are associated with acute episodes of angle-closure glaucoma. The conjunctiva of the affected eye may be reddened, and the cornea may be clouded with corneal edema. The pupil may be fixed (nonreactive to light) at midpoint.

Patients with AMD will often report blurred vision, blind or blurry spots within their central visual field, and colors appearing less bright. They have difficulty adjusting when going from bright light to lower light situations. Patients with AMD will also report difficulty in recognizing people's faces. Because central visual fields are affected, the individual must learn to rely on peripheral fields in order to function.

Collaboration

Ophthalmologists play a key role in the care of patients with eye disease. In addition to the ophthalmologist, the healthcare team may include an occupational therapist, orientation and mobility specialists, low vision therapists, and a social worker. A vision rehabilitation program can help the patient find assistive and adaptive devices (NEI, 2015b). The ophthalmologist or other trained eye professional will perform diagnostic tests.

Diagnostic Tests

Cataracts are diagnosed on the basis of the patient's history and eye examination. The Snellen and Rosenbaum charts are used. (See the Eye and Vision Assessment feature in the Concept of Sensory Perception section.) A dilated eye exam with either an ophthalmoscope or slit-lamp examination provides a magnified view of the structures of the eye. Ophthalmoscope examination confirms the diagnosis by identifying the location and extent of a cataract. As the cataract matures, ophthalmoscopy reveals a dark area instead of the red reflex.

Although glaucoma cannot be predicted, prevented, or cured, in most cases it can be controlled, and vision can be preserved if glaucoma is diagnosed early. Because the most prevalent type of glaucoma, open-angle glaucoma, has few symptoms, routine eye examinations are recommended for early detection. Measurement of intraocular pressure, funduscopy to assess the optic disc, and visual field testing are used to diagnose glaucoma and monitor the effectiveness of treatment.

Almost 50% of patients with glaucoma will not have high intraocular pressure on examination, so a single pressure reading may miss the diagnosis. Regular pressure readings over time and an optic nerve examination are essential parts of a comprehensive eye examination. The following diagnostic studies are performed by an ophthalmologist or other eye specialist to detect and evaluate the presence, severity, type, and effects of glaucoma:

- *Tonometry* indirectly measures intraocular pressure. Contact or noncontact tonometry may be used. Routine tonometry screening is recommended for everyone over the age of 60. A single elevated pressure reading does not warrant a diagnosis of glaucoma, as variations in intraocular pressure occur throughout the day.

Clinical Manifestations and Therapies
Diseases of the Eye

DISEASES OF THE EYE	CLINICAL MANIFESTATIONS	CLINICAL THERAPIES
Congenital cataracts ■ These cataracts are rare. ■ The cause is usually unknown. ■ Congenital cataracts may occur with other birth defects such as congenital rubella, trisomy 21 (Down syndrome), Pierre Robin syndrome, trisomy 13 (Patau syndrome).	■ May be different from those of age-onset cataracts ■ Gray or white cloudy pupils ■ May have nystagmus ■ May not have "red eye" glow in photos	■ Treatment depends on severity. ■ If cataracts are mild, they may just be monitored, especially if they are bilateral. ■ If they are moderate to severe and seem to affect vision or if they are unilateral, surgical removal is usually recommended; an intraocular lens is usually implanted.
Age-related cataracts ■ Aging causes proteins in the lens to deteriorate and become cloudy. ■ By age 75, most people will have cataracts that affect vision. ■ Factors that speed formation include diabetes, UVA/UVB exposure, smoking, and family history.	■ Cloudy/opaque lens ■ May cause cloudy vision, halos, diplopia, or photophobia	■ Early cataracts or those with minimal effect on vision may require no surgical intervention. ■ UVA/UVB protection should be encouraged. ■ Safety measures should be utilized for decreased visual acuity. ■ Surgery is recommended if cataracts interfere with ADLs.
Open-angle glaucoma	■ No initial manifestations ■ Frequent lens changes in glasses ■ Impaired dark adaptation ■ Halos around lights ■ Gradual reduction of visual fields with preservation of central vision until late in the disease ■ Mild to severe increased intraocular pressure	■ Topical medications such as miotics, beta-blockers, and prostaglandin analogs may be prescribed. ■ Treatment may include carbonic anhydrase inhibitors. ■ Laser trabeculoplasty and trabeculectomy may be used.
Angle-closure glaucoma	■ Abrupt onset of eye pain, headache ■ Decreased visual acuity ■ Nausea and vomiting ■ Reddened conjunctiva ■ Cloudy cornea ■ Fixed pupil ■ Rapid, significant increase in intraocular pressure	■ Topical miotics or beta-blockers may be prescribed. ■ Treatment may include systemic osmotic agents and carbonic anhydrase inhibitors. ■ Laser iridotomy or peripheral iridectomy may also be used.
Nonexudative macular degeneration (dry)	■ Slow progression ■ Need for increasingly brighter light when reading ■ Possible blurriness of printed words ■ Difficulty recognizing faces ■ Overall haziness in vision ■ Blurred or blind spot in center of visual field; affects activities, such as reading and sewing	■ Treatment includes high-dose antioxidants and zinc.
Exudative macular degeneration (wet)	■ Possible abrupt onset ■ Visual distortions ■ Visual hallucinations ■ Impaired color vision ■ Blurred spot in center of visual field	■ Treatment may include laser surgery. ■ Photodynamic therapy may also be used.

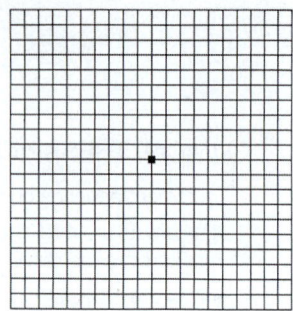

Figure 18–12 ⟩⟩ The Amsler grid.

- *Funduscopy* (visual inspection of the optic fundus using an ophthalmoscope; also called ophthalmoscopy) identifies pallor and an increase in the size and depth of the optic cup on the optic disc. These changes are significant for a diagnosis of glaucoma.
- *Gonioscopy* uses a gonioscope to measure the depth of the anterior chamber. This test differentiates open-angle from angle-closure glaucoma.
- *Visual field testing* identifies the degree of central visual field narrowing and peripheral vision loss. The patient with glaucoma may retain 20/20 central vision even when there is severe peripheral vision loss.

AMD is diagnosed through vision and retinal examinations. The Amsler grid was developed as a diagnostic tool for AMD (see **Figure 18–12 ⟩⟩**). Patients with wet AMD will report the same symptoms as those with dry AMD with the addition of visual distortions. Lines that are straight will appear crooked, bent, or irregular. Also, there may be a difference in the appearance of the size of objects between eyes (AAO, 2016a).

Diagnostic tests for AMD usually involve pupillary dilation, which can be an unsettling experience the first time the examination is performed. The nurse can instruct the patient on how the exam is performed, what to expect, and that the dilation is temporary.

SAFETY ALERT Visual distortions increase the risk of falls and other injuries. Warn patients with wet AMD to walk carefully and to test each step to ensure solid footing.

If treatment for wet AMD is planned, fluorescein angiography may be done. Pictures are taken as the dye passes through the blood vessels of the retina, allowing detection of leaks.

Optical coherence tomography (OCT) is relatively new. It is noninvasive and involves taking cross-sectional images of the retina to measure its thickness. Areas with thinning are noted in patients with advanced AMD (BrightFocus Foundation, 2015b).

Pharmacologic Therapy

No medications are available for treating cataracts. For glaucoma, topical medications are effective for many patients (Glaucoma Research Foundation, 2015a). The principal categories of medications used to treat glaucoma are beta-adrenergic blockers, prostaglandin analogs,

alpha₂-adrenergic agonists, and carbonic anhydrase inhibitors. Which therapy is prescribed depends on a number of factors, including patient health history. Topical beta-adrenergic blocking agents reduce intraocular pressure by decreasing the production of aqueous humor in the ciliary body. Because beta-blockers do not affect pupil size and lens accommodation, they do not have the adverse effects on visual acuity that adrenergic agonists do.

Prostaglandin analogs are a newer class of ophthalmics used to increase aqueous outflow. They are similar to beta-blockers in that their longer duration of action means that they require only a daily dose.

Alpha₂-adrenergic agonists dilate the pupil, reduce the production of aqueous humor, and increase its absorption, effectively reducing intraocular pressure in open-angle glaucoma. Brimonidine may be prescribed along with a beta-blocker or when beta-blockers are contraindicated. Apraclonidine may be prescribed when other drugs do not sufficiently reduce intraocular pressure, but adverse effects make it inappropriate for long-term use (Mayo Clinic, 2015).

The carbonic anhydrase inhibitors decrease production of aqueous humor and are used primarily as adjunctive therapy. Dorzolamide and brinzolamide are administered as eyedrops; acetazolamide may be given orally, intramuscularly, or intravenously.

In acute angle-closure glaucoma, diuretics may be administered intravenously to achieve a rapid decrease in intraocular pressure prior to surgical intervention. Both the acetazolamide and osmotic diuretics such as mannitol are used. Fast-acting miotic drops, such as acetylcholine, also are administered to constrict the pupil and draw the iris away from the angle and from the canal of Schlemm.

Angiogenesis inhibitors are the primary pharmacologic therapy used in the treatment of wet AMD. These drugs block the production of VEGF, thus slowing the progression of the disease (BrightFocus Foundation, 2015c; Mayo Clinic, 2017f). See the Medications feature for nursing considerations.

To help doctors, pharmacists, and patients identify their glaucoma eyedrops, the U.S. Food and Drug Administration has mandated that the tops of the eyedrop bottles be color coded. Some generic eyedrops and all brand-name drops adhere to the guidelines (AAO, 2015c).

⟩⟩ **Stay Current:** The color coding system development by the American Academy of Ophthalmology (AAO) can be seen at http://www.aao.org/about/policies/color-codes-topical-ocular-medications.

The role of the nurse in teaching patients to recognize side effects of these medications is critical. The nurse should ensure that the patient has been instructed on and understands how to properly instill eyedrops (refer to the Patient Teaching feature in Exemplar 18.C on Eye Injuries).

Surgery

Cataracts

Surgical removal is the only treatment used at this time for cataracts. It is performed when the cataract has developed to the point at which vision and ADLs are affected. A mature

Medications

Glaucoma and Macular Degeneration

CLASSIFICATION AND DRUG EXAMPLES	MECHANISMS OF ACTION	NURSING CONSIDERATIONS
Beta-adrenergic Blockers *Drug examples:* Timolol (Timoptic) Levobunolol (Betagan) Carteolol (Ocupress) Metipranolol (OptiPranolol)	These drugs decrease the production of aqueous humor in the eye, thus decreasing intraocular pressure.	▪ These drugs are prescribed for use once or twice a day depending on the specific drug and dosage form. ▪ Systemic absorption may occur; assess the patient for hypotension, bradycardia, and shortness of breath. ▪ Systemic effects may limit usefulness for certain patients. Assess the patient for contraindications (asthma, chronic obstructive pulmonary disease [COPD], heart block, or heart failure). ▪ Teach the patient to close the eye and occlude the lacrimal duct after administration to help reduce systemic absorption.
Prostaglandin Analogs *Drug examples:* Latanoprost (Xalatan) Bimatoprost (Lumigan) Travoprost (Travatan)	These drugs increase drainage of aqueous humor through the uveoscleral pathway. They reduce intraocular pressure by about 30%.	▪ The patient may experience change in iris color. ▪ The patient may notice blurred vision, eye pain (itching, burning, stinging), and eye redness.
Alpha$_2$-adrenergic Agonists *Drug examples:* Brimonidine tartrate (Alphagan) Apraclonidine (Iopidine)	These drugs decrease production of aqueous humor in the eye and increase drainage of aqueous humor through the uveoscleral pathway.	▪ Assess the patient for contraindications such as acute angle-closure glaucoma, hypertension, coronary artery disease, and dysrhythmias. ▪ Assess for central nervous system (CNS) side effects such as anxiety, nervousness, and muscle tremors. ▪ Allergic reactions are common with this class of drug; assess the patient for eye and eyelid erythema, itching and tearing of the eye, dry mouth and nose, and eye discomfort. ▪ Assess the patient for serious side effects such as chest pain, dizziness, trouble breathing, and swelling of the eye or extremities.
Carbonic Anhydrase Inhibitors *Drug examples:* Acetazolamide (Diamox): oral medication Methazolamide (Neptazane): oral medication Brinzolamide (Azopt) Dorzolamide (Trusopt)	These drugs decrease the production of aqueous humor into the eye. They are related to sulfa drugs.	▪ These drugs are used with other drugs to control pressures and in patients for whom beta-blockers are contraindicated because of heart failure or reactive airway disease. ▪ Oral medications may cause periorbital numbness and tingling in the fingers and toes, blurred vision, memory problems, frequent urination, nausea and vomiting, and keratopathy. ▪ These drugs may cause loss of potassium; assess daily weight and electrolytes. ▪ Allergy to sulfa is a contraindication. ▪ Use with caution in patients with renal or hepatic disease.
Combination Medications *Drug examples:* Cosopt (beta-blocker plus carbonic anhydrase inhibitor) Combigan (beta-blocker with alpha$_2$-adrenergic agonist)	The mechanism of action depends on the medication combination.	▪ The same nursing implications apply as for individual medications. ▪ These drugs may be beneficial to patients to have only one eye medication instead of two and may be available at a reduced cost.
Cholinergic Agonists (Miotics) *Drug examples:* Pilocarpine (Isopto Carpine, Pilopine, Pilostat) Carbachol (Isopto Carbachol)	These drugs increase drainage of aqueous humor through the trabecular meshwork via pupillary constriction.	▪ These drugs are rarely used routinely owing to their side effects. ▪ They may be beneficial in narrow-angle glaucoma. ▪ Myopic patients have increased risk of retinal detachment. ▪ Assess the patient for headaches, eye pain, and dim vision, especially in low light.

(continued on next page)

Medications (continued)

CLASSIFICATION AND DRUG EXAMPLES	MECHANISMS OF ACTION	NURSING CONSIDERATIONS
Angiogenesis Inhibitors *Drug examples:* Aflibercept (Eylea) Pegaptanib (Macugen) Ranibizumab (Lucentis)	These drugs block VEGF. VEGF stimulates angiogenesis and vasculogenesis and causes blood vessels to grow in the retina, which causes damage. These drugs are useful in treating the wet form of AMD.	▪ These drugs must be given by injection into the eye. ▪ Teach patients to be aware of and seek treatment for serious side effects: eye pain, erythema, edema, photophobia, headache, confusion, weakness or numbness.

Source: Data from Adams, M. P., Holland, L. N., & Urban, C. (2017). *Pharmacology for nurses: A pathophysiologic approach* (5th ed.). Hoboken, NJ: Pearson Education.

cataract also may be removed when it causes a secondary condition such as glaucoma or uveitis.

If an intraocular lens (an artificial lens to replace the diseased lens of the eye) is to be implanted during surgery, the corneal curvature will be measured via keratometry, and the anteroposterior diameter of the eye will be measured before surgery. This allows the healthcare team to determine the proper type of lens needed for the intraocular lens implant. The surgeon must make more careful measurements for a patient who has previously undergone LASIK surgery (AAO, 2016b).

Cataract surgery typically is done on an outpatient basis using local anesthesia. **Extracapsular extraction**, in which the anterior capsule, nucleus, and cortex of the lens are removed, leaving the posterior capsule intact, is the most common surgery (see **Figure 18–13** ≫). Using an operating microscope, the surgeon makes a small incision at the edge of the cornea and extracts the lens intact or via emulsification and aspiration (AAO, 2016b). After removal of the lens, the eye can no longer focus light on the retina, and vision is seriously affected. A plastic, acrylic, or silicone intraocular

lens that is implanted at the time of surgery rapidly restores binocular vision and depth perception. If the patient presents with bilateral cataracts, surgery is typically performed on only one eye at a time, with an interval of days to several weeks before surgery is performed on the second eye.

Between 10% and 50% of patients who undergo extracapsular extraction may develop opacification of the remaining posterior capsule 3–5 years after surgery (secondary cataract). Vision can be restored with another procedure (AAO, 2016b; Mayo Clinic, 2017b).

To decrease the risk of infection and aid in healing, the physician or surgeon will likely prescribe antibiotic eyedrops and anti-inflammatory eyedrops after surgery. Anti-inflammatory eyedrops can include either steroids or nonsteroidal anti-inflammatory drugs (NSAIDs), and they are sometimes prescribed together.

SAFETY ALERT Steroid anti-inflammatory ophthalmic drugs may increase intraocular eye pressure, so they are usually given for only 2–3 weeks rather than 4–6 weeks like the NSAIDs.

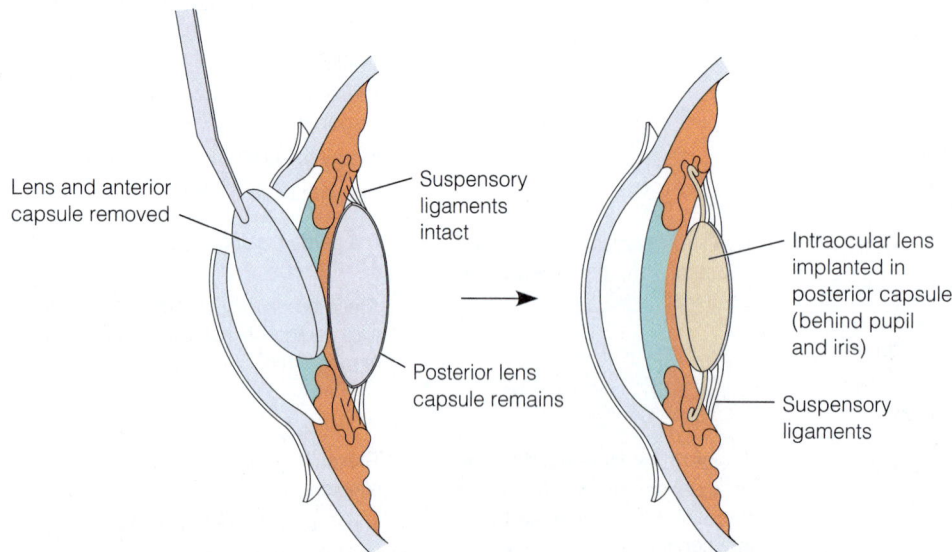

Source: Courtesy of National Eye Institute, Published by National Institutes of Health.

Figure 18–13 ≫ Extracapsular cataract extraction with removal of the lens and anterior capsule, leaving the posterior capsule intact. The intraocular lens is implanted within the posterior capsule.

Focus on Diversity and Culture
Cataract Surgery

National Health and Nutrition Examination Survey (NHANES) studies over the past several years have found a racial disparity among the number of individuals having cataract surgery. The studies found that non-Hispanic Whites have a higher prevalence of cataract surgery than non-Hispanic Blacks (Zhang et al., 2012). This is both because Blacks are less likely to have cataracts than Whites and because Blacks who require cataract surgery are less likely to undergo surgery as compared with Whites (Shahbazi, Studnicki, & Warner-Hillard, 2015). Blacks are more likely to develop cortical opacity, and Whites are more likely to develop nuclear opacity (Storey et al., 2013).

Glaucoma

Surgical management of glaucoma involves improving the drainage of aqueous humor from the anterior chamber of the eye or decreasing aqueous humor production. Trabeculoplasty and trabeculectomy filtration surgery are the most commonly used procedures. In a laser trabeculoplasty, an argon laser creates multiple burns spaced evenly around the trabecular meshwork. As they heal, tension on the resulting scars stretches and opens the meshwork. This noninvasive technique requires no incision and can be performed as an outpatient procedure, making it the treatment of choice. In trabeculectomy, a permanent fistula is created to drain aqueous humor from the anterior chamber of the eye into the space under the conjunctiva, where it can be absorbed into the systemic circulation. A trabeculectomy is usually performed under general anesthesia and requires hospitalization.

If these procedures are not effective, an argon laser or cyclocryotherapy may be employed to destroy portions of the ciliary body. This reduces the production of aqueous humor. Another surgical procedure involves inserting a glaucoma drainage device that regulates the outflow of aqueous humor.

Acute angle-closure glaucoma may be treated surgically with gonioplasty (also known as iridoplasty), laser iridotomy, or peripheral iridectomy. In gonioplasty, the healing and scarring of microscopic lesions created at the periphery of the iris draw the iris away from the cornea, widening the anterior chamber; this increases the angle and opens drainage channels for aqueous humor. In laser iridotomy, a laser is used to create multiple small perforations in the iris, which allow aqueous humor to drain from the posterior chamber to the anterior chamber. Iridectomy involves removal of a small segment of the iris to facilitate the flow of aqueous humor between the posterior and anterior chambers and to open the anterior chamber angle. Because of the high risk for a future attack of angle-closure glaucoma in the unaffected eye, these procedures are often performed prophylactically.

Age-related Macular Degeneration

Wet AMD is treated with laser surgery or photodynamic therapy. Although these treatments do not cure the disease, they may slow the rate of vision loss. In laser surgery, fragile blood vessels are destroyed, preventing bleeding. In photodynamic therapy, verteporfin, a drug that tends to adhere to the surface of new blood vessels, is injected systemically. Shining a light into the affected eye activates the drug and destroys new blood vessels. Risks include damage to surrounding healthy tissue, some vision loss, and continued growth of new vessels. Since the introduction of antiangiogenic drug therapy, surgical therapy has become less common for treating AMD.

Nonpharmacologic Therapy

If a cataract does not interfere with the ability to perform ADLs or is not associated with other eye pathology, then surgical removal is not necessary. Early cataracts can be managed with magnifying glasses, stronger prescription lenses, brighter lighting, or antiglare sunglasses (Mayo Clinic, 2017a).

For patients with glaucoma, relaxation and regular exercise may lower intraocular pressure and positively affect other risk factors, such as diabetes. Physical exercise, such as riding a stationary bicycle or walking briskly for 40 minutes several times a week, has been shown to have beneficial effects. Participants in one study have been able to lower their intraocular pressure enough that they no longer need to take beta blockers. Note that angle-closure glaucoma does not appear to be responsive to exercise (Glaucoma Research Foundation, 2016).

In its early or intermediate stages, the progress of dry AMD can be slowed through the use of high-dose antioxidants and zinc. Research has demonstrated a benefit when vitamin C, vitamin E, zinc, and copper are administered daily (NEI, 2013). Assistive devices that may be helpful to patients with AMD include magnifiers, large-print books and magazines, and high-intensity lighting to help the patient cope with the reduced vision of macular degeneration. Computers and handheld electronic devices, such as tablets and e-readers, allow users to increase text size and change brightness and contrast for easier reading. They also provide audio functionality, which enables use of audiobooks and podcasts.

Lifespan Considerations
Diseases of the Eyes in Infants and Children
Congenital Cataracts

Some children have congenital cataracts or develop cataracts during childhood. In earlier times, congenital cataracts in infants were often associated with the pregnant mother's infection with rubella during gestation; but since the advent of the rubella vaccine, very few cases of congenital cataracts are now related to rubella. Instead, common causes of cataracts in children are maternal infection during gestation, galactosemia and other metabolic disorders, genetic mutations (e.g., trisomy 21), and trauma (AAO, 2015b).

Infants and children with cataracts are often asymptomatic, however some will have an obviously opaque lens. Signs that a child may have a cataract include a lack of reaction to bright light, failure to notice toys or faces, and unexpected developmental delays. Testing for cataracts in children is similar to testing in adults, including a full ophthalmologic exam with a red reflex test and slit-lamp examination. If vision impairment is significant, the infant should undergo surgical removal of the cataract within the first 2 months of life. This is because the connections between the eye and the brain are still developing, and impairment or lack of light signals from the eye may cause the brain never to develop signaling paths for vision; the resulting amblyopia could lead to blindness if not treated promptly (AAPOS, 2015). For children older than 2 months, cataract surgery should be performed at the discretion of the physician. Many infants and children have an intraocular lens implanted at the same time.

Pediatric Glaucoma

Primary congenital glaucoma, which occurs in about 1 in every 10,000 births in the United States, is caused by an abnormal development in the ocular drainage system. Approximately 10% of cases are diagnosed at birth (**congenital glaucoma**); the majority (80%) are diagnosed by age 1 (**infantile glaucoma**). Childhood glaucoma diagnosed after the age of 3 is called **juvenile glaucoma**. Secondary congenital glaucoma results from disorders of the eye or the body, including Sturge-Weber syndrome, Axenfeld-Rieger syndrome, aniridia, and neurofibromatosis (Huang, 2014).

Glaucoma in young children can be difficult to diagnose. Parents and healthcare professionals should be alert for photophobia, excessive tearing (**epiphora**), and larger than normal eyes (**buphthalmos**). **Blepharospasm** (involuntary tight closure of the eyelids, corneal clouding, and Haab's striae) may also be present. Diagnosis requires a thorough eye exam. If necessary, anesthesia may be used to obtain an accurate exam with intraocular pressure readings.

The treatment of choice for pediatric glaucoma is trabeculotomy or goniotomy. Most pediatric patients also receive eyedrops and/or oral medications to control intraocular pressure. Many of the medications used in adults are also used in children. However, brimonidine is contraindicated in children because of its side effect profile, and miotic agents and adrenergic agents are not as effective in children as in adults (AAO, 2017). Although approximately 80–90% of pediatric patients with glaucoma who receive prompt diagnosis and treatment have near normal vision throughout their lifetime, some will sustain complications such as myopia, amblyopia, and strabismus (AAPOS, 2014b). Approximately 12–15% will develop blindness.

Juvenile Macular Degeneration

Juvenile macular degeneration, also called *macular dystrophy*, is the pediatric equivalent of AMD, although the pathophysiology is different in that juvenile macular degeneration is an inherited disorder. The most common type of juvenile macular degeneration is Stargardt disease; other types include Best disease and juvenile retinoschisis. Stargardt disease has a recessive inheritance pattern, whereas Best disease is a dominant disorder, and juvenile retinoschisis is X-linked.

All three forms of juvenile macular degeneration cause central vision loss. Symptoms can begin anytime in childhood or adolescence, and one eye may be affected more than the other. Stargardt disease is typically characterized by yellowish flecks, which are deposits of lipofuscin, in the macula. Patients with Best disease usually develop a yellow cyst under the macula that eventually ruptures, potentially harming the macula. The retina splits into two layers in patients with juvenile retinoschisis, harming the macula. Vision loss associated with juvenile macular degeneration is not treatable or preventable (AAO, 2015d).

Diseases of the Eyes in Pregnant Women

Glaucoma is very rare in women of child-bearing age. Most instances of glaucoma in this population are due to congenital glaucoma or diseases that cause early glaucoma, such as diabetes.

Many of the medications used to treat glaucoma have potential adverse effects on the fetus (Jindal, Salim, & Boonyaleephan, 2014; Salim, 2014). A relatively safe treatment option for a pregnant woman with glaucoma is argon laser trabeculoplasty. It has only short-term benefits, but this may be enough to provide relief of symptoms and prevent worsening of the glaucoma until the woman delivers the baby (Jindal et al., 2014).

Diseases of the Eyes in Older Adults

With the increasing number of older adults in the overall population, the prevalence of eye diseases will continue to increase. Two common conditions in older adults that may affect treatment of these diseases are tremors and cognitive decline. Hand tremors may make it difficult for the older adult to adequately apply eyedrops, and cognitive decline may cause older adults to forget to take their medications (Franks, 2013). Therefore, older adults with these conditions may need a family member or friend who can help them remember to take their medications and potentially apply eyedrops for them.

NURSING PROCESS

Providing a safe environment is a priority nursing intervention for any patient with an eye disease, whether or not it is the patient's primary diagnosis. The nurse should be alert to the potential for an eye disease in all patients.

Assessment

- *Observation and patient interview.* The nurse can observe general difficulties with vision based on the patient's ability to see objects and read text. The patient interview should include assessing the effect of vision changes on lifestyle and activities (e.g., ability to read, watch television, participate in work and recreational activities) and the patient's history of smoking, diabetes, and use of prescription drugs associated with increased risk of eye diseases.

The nurse may be able to observe the presence of cataracts if they are advanced enough to cloud the pupil. The patient interview should assess the patient's family history of eye diseases. The nurse should be alert for signs and symptoms that indicate a patient may have new and rapid onset of macular degeneration. If so, the patient should be referred for ophthalmologic evaluation. Early intervention may preserve a greater degree of vision and slow the progress of the disease.

- *Physical examination.* Physical examination for diseases of the eye should include testing the patient's distant and near vision, testing peripheral fields, and testing on an Amsler grid. Examination for specific eye disorders will depend on the signs and symptoms of the patient.

Diagnosis

Patients with diseases of the eyes have few physical care nursing needs. Patient advocacy, psychologic and emotional support, and teaching/learning needs are typically of high priority for these patients.

Nursing diagnoses for the patient with eye diseases may include the following:

- *Anxiety*
- *Fear*
- *Health Management, Ineffective*
- *Health Maintenance, Ineffective*
- *Injury, Risk for.*

(NANDA-I © 2014)

Planning

Appropriate outcomes for the patient diagnosed with an eye disease may include the following:

- The patient will remain free from injury.
- The patient will be able to articulate an understanding of the reasons for and risks involved with treatment.
- The patient will express feelings related to diagnosis and reduced vision.
- The patient will participate in self-care activities to protect the eyes from further damage and to maximize safety.
- The patient will follow self-care instructions.

Implementation

With the initial diagnosis of an eye disease, teaching focuses on the particular disorder and teaching adaptive strategies to deal with the effects of vision loss and upcoming treatments.

Prevent Injury

The following measures help to ensure the patient's safety while enhancing mobility and independence:

- Discuss possible adaptations in the home to prevent falls or other injuries. Often minor changes in the home environment, such as removing scatter rugs and small items of furniture and improving lighting, allow the patient to navigate safely in this already familiar environment.
- If applicable, provide instructions related to unilateral vision loss and change in depth perception such as reaching slowly for objects and using visual cues as to distance, especially when driving. Teach the patient to scan, turning the head fully toward the affected side to identify potential hazards and looking up and down to compensate for the loss of depth perception.
- For the patient in a hospital or other care facility, notify housekeeping and place a sign on the patient's door to alert all personnel not to change the arrangement of the patient's room. The patient with impaired vision is at high risk for falling in an unfamiliar environment. It is important to maintain a safe, familiar room.

SAFETY ALERT Raise two or three side rails on the patient's bed. Raised rails remind the patient to ask for assistance before ambulating in an unfamiliar environment.

Promote Wellness and Teach Principles of Self-Care

Conduct an eye and vision assessment at each healthcare interaction with the patient age 65 years and older; inquire about any problems with vision and the date of the patient's most recent appointment with an ophthalmologist or optometrist. Encourage the patient with diabetes, previous history of visual problems, or disorders that require frequent use of corticosteroids to see an ophthalmologist at least every 2 years. Assess for factors that may interfere with the patient's ability to provide self-care. A chronic condition that may affect the ability to administer eyedrops, such as arthritis, may indicate the need to include a family member in teaching.

- Assess the patient's ability to perform ADLs. The patient may be reluctant to request assistance, believing that he or she should be able to perform these familiar tasks.
- Discuss lifestyle adaptations that may be necessary if the patient must limit or discontinue nighttime driving or perhaps discontinue driving altogether (see the Patient Teaching feature).

Facilitate Orientation and Environmental Modifications

The patient with impaired vision requires orientation to the individual speaking and the environment in order to reduce anxiety.

- Address the patient by name and identify yourself with each interaction. Orient the patient to time, place, person, and situation. State the purpose of your visit. The patient with impaired vision must rely on input from the other senses. A lack of visual cues increases the importance of verbal ones.
- Provide any visual aids that are routinely used. Keep them close to the patient, making sure the patient knows where they are and can reach them easily. Easy access encourages the patient to use these items and enhances the ability to provide self-care.
- Provide or suggest other tools or items that can help to compensate for diminished vision, such as bright, nonglare lighting; books, magazines, and instructions in large print; an electronic tablet, which will allow the

Patient Teaching
Managing Glaucoma at Home

The patient with glaucoma must be provided with strategies for managing the disease at home. The patient needs to understand the importance of lifetime therapy to control the disease and prevent blindness. The patient with a permanent visual impairment needs information on achieving maximum independence while maintaining safety. The following topics should be discussed with the patient and family:

- Review the patient's prescribed medications, including the proper way to administer eyedrops. Stress the importance of reading the labels of all prescription and over-the-counter medications and consulting a physician if the patient is uncertain whether a medication is safe for individuals with glaucoma.
- Recommend that the patient wear sunglasses with UVA/UVB protection when outdoors, wear eye protection when using tools, and use reading or prescription glasses or contact lenses as necessary.
- Refer to community resources such as the National Association for Local Societies of Visually Impaired People, local libraries, and transportation services. Suggest helpful resources such as the Glaucoma Foundation.

patient to enlarge print and images; audiobooks; telephones with oversize push buttons; and a clock with numbers and hands that can be felt.

- If appropriate to the setting, assist with meals by reading menu selections and marking choices, describing the position of foods on a meal tray according to the clock system, placing the utensils in a readily accessible position, removing lids from containers, buttering bread, cutting meat, feeding the patient, or providing assistance as needed during the meal if the patient's visual impairment is new or temporary.

SAFETY ALERT Have the patient hold your arm or elbow and walk slightly ahead as a guide. Do not hold the patient's arm or elbow. Maintain the pace that is most comfortable for the patient. Describe the surroundings and progress as you proceed. Warn in advance of potential hazards, turns, and steps. There is no need to speak loudly unless the patient also has a hearing impairment. Teach the patient to feel the chair, bed, or commode with the hands and the back of the legs before sitting.

Promote Psychosocial Wellness

The actual or potential loss of sight threatens the patient's self-concept, role functioning, patterns of interaction, and, potentially, environment. The patient with impaired vision who functions well in a familiar environment will feel anxious in the unfamiliar setting of a hospital or care facility.

- Assess for verbal and nonverbal indications of anxiety level and for normal coping mechanisms. Repeated expressions of concern indicate anxiety, as does denial that the vision change will affect the patient's life. Nonverbal indicators include tension, difficulty concentrating or thinking, restlessness, and changes in vocalization (rapid speech, quivering voice). Physical indicators include tachycardia, dilated pupils, cool and clammy skin, and tremors. The patient may not recognize this feeling as anxiety. Identifying and acknowledging the anxiety can help the patient recognize and deal with it.
- Encourage the patient to verbalize fears, anger, and feelings of anxiety. Verbalizing helps to externalize the anxiety and allows fears to be addressed.
- Identify coping strategies that have been useful in the past, and adapt these strategies to the present situation. Previously successful coping strategies may be employed to increase the patient's sense of control.

Evaluation

Criteria that may reflect attainment of identified outcomes and successful resolution of nursing diagnoses include the following:

- The patient remains free from injury.
- The patient makes an informed decision regarding treatment.
- The patient verbalizes concerns and identifies appropriate resources.
- The patient verbalizes appropriate home care activities.
- The patient demonstrates correct medication administration.
- The patient lists resources available within the community.

Many patients with eye diseases will need continuous monitoring over several years and will require accommodations for impaired vision. The nurse may need to advocate for surgery or provide additional patient teaching on self-administration of eyedrops and the benefits of exercise.

Nursing Care Plan
A Patient with Glaucoma and Cataracts

Lila Rainey is an 80-year-old widow who lives alone in the house she and her late husband built 50 years ago. She has worn glasses for nearsightedness since she was a young girl; she now wears bifocals to correct her near vision as well. She was diagnosed 4 years ago with chronic open-angle glaucoma, for which she takes timolol maleate (Timoptic) 0.5%. Mrs. Rainey has recently noticed difficulty reading and watching television despite a new lens prescription. Because she is unable to see clearly, she has stopped reading or watching television; instead, she listens to the radio. She also has stopped driving at night because the glare of oncoming headlights makes it difficult for her to see. Although her glaucoma is still controlled with timolol maleate 0.5%, one drop in each eye twice a day, her intraocular pressure measurements have been gradually increasing. Mrs. Rainey has taken 325 mg of aspirin daily since a transient ischemic attack 8 years ago. She is being admitted to the outpatient surgery unit for cataract removal and intraocular lens implant in her right eye.

Nursing Care Plan *(continued)*

ASSESSMENT

Mrs. Rainey is admitted to the eye surgery unit by Susan Schafer, RN. In her assessment, Ms. Schafer finds Mrs. Rainey to be alert and oriented, though apprehensive about her upcoming surgery. Assessment findings include temperature 97.8°F oral; pulse 86 bpm; respirations 18/min; and BP 134/72 mmHg. Mrs. Rainey's neurologic, respiratory, cardiovascular, and abdominal assessments are essentially normal. However, she reports that she experiences occasional constipation. Her pupils are round and equal and react briskly to light and accommodation. Her conjunctivae are pink; her sclera and corneas are clear. Using the ophthalmoscope, Ms. Schafer notes that the red reflex in Mrs. Rainey's right eye is diminished. Ophthalmic examination shows visual acuity of 20/150 OD (right eye) and 20/50 OS (left eye) with corrective lenses. Her intraocular pressures are 21 mmHg OD and 17 mmHg OS. On funduscopic exam, no disease of the blood vessels, retina, macula, or disc is found. Ms. Schafer reviews the operative procedure with Mrs. Rainey, answering her questions and telling her what to expect after surgery. Following preoperative protocols, Mrs. Rainey is prepared and transported to surgery.

DIAGNOSES

- *Injury, Risk for,* related to myopia and lens extraction
- *Anxiety* related to anticipated surgery
- *Deficient Knowledge* related to lack of information regarding postoperative care
- *Home Maintenance, Impaired,* related to activity restrictions and impaired vision.

(NANDA-I © 2014)

PLANNING

Goals of nursing care may include:

- The patient will avoid injury.
- The patient will regain sufficient visual acuity to maintain ADLs, including reading and watching television for enjoyment.
- The patient will demonstrate a reduced level of anxiety.
- The patient will demonstrate the procedure for instilling eyedrops postoperatively.
- The patient will demonstrate knowledge of the home care she will require after surgery, signs of complications, and actions to take if complications occur.
- The patient will use appropriate resources to assist with home maintenance until vision stabilizes and activity restrictions are lifted.

IMPLEMENTATION

- Provide a safe environment, placing the call light and personal care items within easy reach.
- Encourage Mrs. Rainey to express her fears about surgery and its potential effect on vision.
- Explain all procedures related to surgery and recovery.
- Instruct Mrs. Rainey to avoid shutting her eyelids tightly, sneezing, coughing, laughing, bending over, lifting, or straining to have a bowel movement. Activities that may increase intraocular pressure must be avoided during the immediate postoperative period.

- Teach Mrs. Rainey to wear sunglasses during the day and a protective eye shield at night.
- Explain and demonstrate the procedure for administering eyedrops.
- Provide verbal and written instructions about postoperative care, including a schedule of follow-up examinations, potential complications, and actions to take in response to complications.
- Refer Mrs. Rainey to a discharge planner or social worker to help establish a plan for home maintenance.

EVALUATION

Mrs. Rainey is preparing for discharge 2 hours after her surgery. She is able to relate the recommended activity restrictions. She administers her own eyedrops before discharge and relates an understanding of the prescribed postoperative care and safety precautions. She verbalizes understanding of the need to wear a protective eye shield on the operative eye for 24 hours. Mrs. Rainey's daughter, Janice Dunne, will be transporting her home.

Ms. Dunne states that she plans to visit her mother two or three times a week to help with laundry and vacuuming until Mrs. Rainey can resume all of her household activities. Mrs. Rainey says that she "won't be so scared when I need my other eye done." She understands the chronic nature of her glaucoma and says that her vision is too important for her to neglect her timolol drops and routine eye exams.

CRITICAL THINKING

1. How has Mrs. Rainey's impaired vision affected her ADLs? Should she expect a full return to normal activities once her eye is healed? Why or why not?

2. Aside from books, television, and radio, what form of media entertainment might Mrs. Rainey enjoy?

3. Explain why constipation could be a source of complications following Mrs. Rainey's surgery. Describe dietary modifications

that could be implemented to ensure that Mrs. Rainey avoids complications related to bowel elimination.

4. Describe the purpose of a plan for home maintenance. What safety-related concerns should the discharge planner or social worker prioritize when creating a home maintenance plan for Mrs. Rainey?

REVIEW Diseases of the Eyes

RELATE Link the Concepts and Exemplars

You are caring for a patient who is scheduled to undergo surgery for cataracts. The patient is 78 years old and lives alone on a third-floor walk-up with no elevator.

Linking the exemplar of diseases of the eye with the concept of safety:

1. What safety issues will you address when teaching this patient?

2. What issues place this patient at increased risk for injury?

Sarah Schulman is a 40-year-old woman with severe, persistent asthma. In addition to receiving bimonthly immunotherapy, she takes an inhaled corticosteroid with a long-acting beta-agonist and an anti-histamine daily. Each year she has four or five acute exacerbations of asthma that usually require a taper of oral prednisone.

Linking the exemplar of diseases of the eye with the concept of oxygenation:

3. What are Ms. Schulman's risk factors for glaucoma?

4. What patient teaching should you provide Ms. Schulman to reduce her risk of developing glaucoma?

Linking the exemplar of diseases of the eye with the concept of cognition:

5. What effect might advancing macular degeneration have on a patient's cognition?

6. What strategies can you implement to promote cognitive functioning in a patient with macular degeneration?

READY Go to Volume 3: Clinical Nursing Skills

REFER Go to Pearson MyLab Nursing and eText

REFLECT Apply Your Knowledge

Celeste Martin, a 75-year-old widow with osteoporosis, has an appointment with her ophthalmologist this week. The ophthalmologist notes that Mrs. Martin's cataracts have continued to worsen and recommends that she consider surgery. Mrs. Martin does not admit that she is afraid to have surgery on her eyes. She tells the physician that she might have the surgery at some point but that she is too busy to do it right now. The physician gives Mrs. Martin a new prescription for her eyeglasses, knowing that this will help her vision at least for a little while. Mrs. Martin is told to increase the amount of light and to use reading glasses or a magnifying glass for reading.

1. What nursing diagnosis would be appropriate for Mrs. Martin?

2. How will the nurse address Mrs. Martin's concerns about surgery?

3. What factors may affect Mrs. Martin's home care?

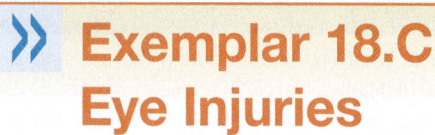

Exemplar 18.C
Eye Injuries

Exemplar Learning Outcomes

18.C Analyze eye injuries as they relate to sensory perception.

- Describe the pathophysiology of eye injuries.
- Describe the etiology of eye injuries.
- Compare the risk factors for and prevention of eye injuries.
- Identify the clinical manifestations of eye injuries.
- Summarize diagnostic tests and therapies used by interprofessional teams in the collaborative care of an individual with eye injuries.
- Differentiate considerations for care of patients with eye injuries across the lifespan.
- Apply the nursing process in providing culturally competent care to an individual with eye injuries.

Exemplar Key Terms

Aphakia, *1428*
Blepharism, *1432*
Corneal abrasion, *1427*
Enophthalmos, *1428*
Hyphema, *1428*
Penetrating injury, *1427*
Perforating injury, *1428*
Retinal detachment, *1428*

Overview

Any part of the eye may be affected by trauma, the exposed parts being particularly vulnerable. Abrasions, lacerations, and foreign bodies in the eye are the most common types of eye injuries. Traumatic injury also may be caused by a penetrating object, blunt force, or burns. The majority of eye injuries are preventable. Nurses can take the opportunity to teach eye safety to patients throughout their entire lifespan during well visits as well as when discussing alterations in patient's vision.

Pathophysiology and Etiology

The pathophysiology of a given eye injury depends on the nature of the injury. Later in this exemplar, the pathophysiology of selected injuries is discussed in conjunction with their clinical manifestations.

Eye injuries affect more than 2.5 million Americans every year. Each year 50,000 people will permanently lose all or part of their vision as a result of injury. Recreational sports, workplace injuries, fireworks, automobile accidents, and home accidents are all settings where eye injuries can occur (Aghadoost, 2014).

In the United States, approximately 2000 workers each day sustain a work-related eye injury that requires medical treatment (CDC, 2015c). Adults who are at greatest risk of eye injuries include contractors, woodworkers, welders, and electricians. Sources of eye trauma in the workplace include chemicals, projectiles, steam, radiation, and bloodborne pathogens (AOA, n.d.b).

Risk Factors

Around 73% of eye injuries occur in men. Almost half of all eye injuries happen to individuals ages 18–45. Occupational eye injuries are often associated with being distracted, tools that malfunction, performing an unfamiliar task, being rushed, and feeling fatigued (Blackburn et al., 2012). Individuals who perform at-home construction or maintenance projects are also at higher risk, even while performing simple tasks such as mowing the lawn or hammering nails (AAO, 2016e).

Certain sports are associated with eye injuries. The most common sports in which eye injuries occur are boxing and other full-contact martial arts, baseball, lacrosse, basketball, hockey, football, soccer, and racquet sports (AAO, 2016c).

Prevention

Protective eyewear is estimated to prevent more than 90% of all injuries (AAO, 2016f). Yet more than 78% of individuals presenting with eye injuries report not wearing eyewear at the time of injury. The type of eye protection that is required depends on the type of activity the individual is doing. Each home should have at least one pair of eyewear (glasses or goggles, depending on the activity) that is certified by the American National Standards Institute (ANSI). For home use, look for eyewear labeled "ANSI Z87." Standards for eye protection for sports and recreation are set by the American Society for Testing and Materials. Various types of protection are available based on the sport being played. Proper UV protection is recommended to shield eyes from glare while water skiing or snow skiing. The Occupational Safety and Health Administration determines what type of eye protection is required in the workplace. This information

---

Focus on Diversity and Culture
Eye Injuries in Migrant Workers

Eye injuries among migrant farm workers are underreported. These individuals are exposed to a variety of risks such as chemicals, machinery, tools, and airborne soil and particulates. Most migrant workers do not have jobs that provide workers' compensation coverage. They are also faced with tremendous pressure to support families in the United States or their country of origin. Because a limited number of clinics serve this population, many injuries go both unreported and untreated, or treatment may be delayed. In one study, most reported eye injuries among migrant farm workers were penetrating wounds or open wounds, typically caused by foreign objects (Quandt et al., 2012).

---

should be readily available through an individual's employer (AAO, 2016d).

Clinical Manifestations

Eye injuries can range from minor, with no loss of vision, to catastrophic, with complete loss of vision in one or both eyes. People are very dependent on their sense of sight, so the nurse should be cognizant of how impairments in vision can affect functioning, safety, and patient self-image.

Corneal Abrasion

Corneal abrasion is disruption of the superficial epithelium of the cornea. Objects that commonly cause corneal abrasion include contact lenses, eyelashes, small foreign bodies such as dust and dirt, and fingernails. Drying of the eye surface and chemical irritants also may result in a corneal abrasion.

Superficial abrasions of the cornea are extremely painful but generally heal rapidly without complication or scarring. Photophobia (sensitivity to light) and tearing are commonly present. When the stroma is damaged by a deep abrasion or laceration, there is an increased risk of infection, slowed healing, and scar formation.

Burns

The outer surface of the eye may be subjected to burns caused by heat, radiation, or explosion, but chemical burns are most common. Both acid and alkaline substances can burn the eye. Ammonia, products that contain lye (e.g., oven and drain cleaners), acids from car batteries, and other sources are often implicated in eye injuries. Burns caused by alkaline substances are particularly serious because tiny particles of the chemical may remain in the conjunctival sac, causing progressive damage. Acid causes rapid damage to the eye but generally causes less serious burns than alkaline substances.

Explosions and flash burn injuries pose the greatest risk for thermal burns of the eye. UV rays also can cause corneal damage ranging in severity from mild to extensive. Depending on the source of the UV light, these burns may be referred to as snowblindness, welder's arc burn, or flash burn.

The patient who experiences a burn to the eye will have a history of face and eye contact with a caustic substance or another burning agent and will complain of eye pain and decreased vision. The patient's eyelids may be swollen, and the face and lips may be affected. The appearance of the patient's eye may vary depending on the type of burn. The conjunctiva is typically reddened and edematous. Sloughing may be seen, particularly with chemical burns. The cornea often appears cloudy or hazy, and ulcerations may be evident.

Penetrating Trauma

Perforation of the eye has a variety of causes. Metal flakes or other particles produced by high-speed drilling or grinding, glass shards, or other substances may penetrate the eye. Bullets (including BBs), arrows, and knives can penetrate the eye. In a **penetrating injury**, the layers of the eye spontaneously reapproximate (join together) after entry of a sharp-pointed object or small missile (e.g., a BB) into the globe. Penetrating eye injuries are those that have a single entrance wound from the injury. There can be multiple such wounds, but they would have been caused by multiple sources. In a **perforating injury**, the layers of the eye do not spontaneously reapproximate, resulting in rupture of the globe and potential loss of ocular contents. A perforating eye injury involves an entrance and exit wound, both of which are caused by the same object (Yonekawa, Chodosh, & Eliott, 2013).

Penetrating injuries may not be readily apparent when the eye is inspected. They may be hidden because of tissue swelling, or they may be missed when the patient has other significant injuries that command attention. When the eyelid is lacerated or has a puncture wound, it is vital to inspect the underlying eye tissue for possible damage. Eye perforations cause pain, partial or complete loss of vision, and possibly bleeding.

Blunt Trauma

Sports injuries are a common cause of blunt trauma to the eye, which may be struck with a ball (baseballs, tennis balls, racquet balls, and handballs are frequently implicated) or injured during contact sports such as basketball, football, boxing, and wrestling. Motor vehicle crashes, falls, and physical assault are examples of other causes of blunt eye trauma.

Blunt trauma may lead to a minor eye injury such as lid ecchymosis (black eye) or subconjunctival hemorrhage, which is caused by rupture of a blood vessel in the conjunctiva. With subconjunctival hemorrhage, a well-defined bright area of erythema appears under the conjunctiva. No pain or discomfort is associated with the hemorrhage, and no treatment is necessary. The blood typically reabsorbs within 2–3 weeks.

Hyphema, bleeding into the anterior chamber of the eye, is a potential result of blunt eye trauma. When the highly vascular uveal tract of the eye is disrupted by blunt force, hemorrhage may result, filling the anterior chamber. The patient complains of feeling eye pain, experiencing decreased visual acuity, and seeing a reddish tint. Blood is visible in the anterior chamber.

An orbital blowout fracture is another potential result of blunt eye trauma. Although any part of the eye orbit may be fractured, the ethmoid bone on the orbital floor is the most likely site. Orbital contents, including fat, muscles, and the eye itself, may herniate through the fracture into the underlying maxillary sinus. The patient complains of diplopia (double vision), pain with upward movement of the affected eye, and decreased sensation on the affected cheek. The eye appears sunken (**enophthalmos**) and has limited movement on examination.

Detached Retina

Separation of the retina, or sensory portion of the eye, from the choroid, the pigmented vascular layer, is known as a **retinal detachment**. Although retinal detachment may be precipitated by trauma, it usually occurs spontaneously. The vitreous humor normally adheres to the retina at the optic disc, the macula, and the periphery of the eye. With aging, the vitreous humor shrinks and may pull the retina away

from the choroid. Therefore, aging is a common risk factor, as are myopia, glaucoma, trauma, previous retinal detachment, and **aphakia**, or absence of the lens (e.g., following lens removal for cataracts) (University of Michigan Kellogg Eye Center, n.d.; Wu & Pakalnis, 2014).

The retina may tear and fold back on itself, or it may remain intact but no longer adhere to the choroid. A break or tear in the retina allows fluid from the vitreous cavity to enter the defect. This, along with fluid that escapes from choroid vessels, the pull of gravity, and traction exerted by the vitreous humor, separates the retina from the choroid. The detached area may rapidly increase in size, escalating loss of vision. Unless contact between the retina and choroid is reestablished, the neurons of the retina become ischemic and die, causing permanent vision loss. For that reason, retinal detachment is a true medical emergency, requiring prompt ophthalmologic referral and treatment.

When the retina detaches, the patient experiences floaters, or spots, and lines or flashes of light in the visual field. Often the patient describes the sensation of having a curtain drawn across the vision, much like a curtain being drawn over a window. The area of the visual field affected is directly related to the area of detachment. For example, because light rays cross as they pass through the lens, a retinal tear in the superior portion of the eye results in a deficit in the lower part of the visual field. The patient feels no pain, and the eye appears normal to visual inspection.

Collaboration

Diagnostic tests and nursing and medical interventions vary widely depending on the extent of the eye injury. The nurse can reinforce the importance of protective eyewear, especially in the occurrence of minor injuries.

Diagnostic Tests

Diagnostic testing for eye injuries should begin with tests of visual acuity. Extraocular movements should be evaluated. The pupil should be tested for reactivity and size with a flashlight or ophthalmoscope. The ophthalmoscope should also be used to examine the fundus to check for presence of the red reflex (Family Practice Notebook, n.d.). A slit lamp is a high-intensity light source combined with a low-power microscope. It can be focused to shine a blue light in a thin beam and is often used in conjunction with fluorescein stain. Fluorescein is orange/yellow in color. When applied to the eye, it fills in any defect on the cornea. The defect will fluoresce under the cobalt blue light of the slit lamp. For eye injuries, it can be useful in identifying corneal injuries and retinal detachment (National Library of Medicine, 2015). Facial x-rays and CT scans are used to identify orbital fractures or foreign bodies in the globe. Ultrasonography may be employed to detect a detached retina or vitreous hemorrhage.

Surgery

Surgery is usually not necessary in the treatment of corneal abrasion, subconjunctival hemorrhage, or periorbital ecchymosis. For eye injuries caused by severe chemical burns, surgery may include debridement, tissue grafting, or even

Clinical Manifestations and Therapies
Eye Injuries

ETIOLOGY	CLINICAL MANIFESTATIONS	CLINICAL THERAPIES
Corneal abrasion	■ Intense pain and redness ■ Photophobia ■ Tearing	■ Identify the site of abrasion by touching a sterile fluorescein strip to the eye; the dye will adhere to the damaged epithelial cells. ■ Corneal abrasions often heal with no treatment. For patients with a high risk of infection, antibiotic ointment may be used. For patients with severe injury or risk of rubbing the eyes, such as small children, an eye patch may be used.
Burns (Alkaline burns, which readily penetrate the cornea, are more serious than acid burns.)	■ Pain and/or complaints of "blindness" or vision loss ■ Edematous, red conjunctiva ■ Swollen eyelids ■ Hazy or cloudy conjunctiva ■ Possible presence of ulcerations	■ For chemical burns, irrigate eyes with normal saline. ■ Pupils are dilated to reduce pain and prevent adhesions. ■ After irrigation is complete, patch the eyes and administer antibiotics as prescribed. ■ Apply topical anesthetic as prescribed.
Penetrating and perforating injuries	■ Pain ■ Bleeding ■ Extrusion of eye contents ■ Partial or complete vision loss	■ If a penetrating object is embedded in or sticking out of eye, do not remove it. Immobilize the object and protect the eye until the ophthalmologist arrives. ■ Manage pain. ■ Irrigate. ■ Assist the ophthalmologist as needed in removing the object. The object should be removed using a sterile cotton-tipped applicator or a sterile needle or other equipment. ■ Apply antibiotic ointment after removal. ■ Apply eye patch. ■ Surgery may be necessary.
Blunt trauma	■ Pain and redness ■ Ecchymosis ■ Subconjunctival hemorrhage ■ Hyphema ■ Possible diplopia, enophthalmos ■ *Note:* Be aware that retinal hemorrhage is a common presentation of shaken-baby syndrome.	■ Place the patient in semi-Fowler position. ■ Protect the injured eye with an eye shield; patch the unaffected eye to minimize eye movement. ■ Administer carbonic anhydrase inhibitor as prescribed.
Subconjunctival hemorrhage (caused by coughing, mild trauma, or increased physical activity)	■ Reddened area in conjunctiva	■ This injury usually heals spontaneously. ■ The patient should see an ophthalmologist if most of sclera is covered or if the condition does not clear up in 1–2 weeks.
Periorbital ecchymosis	■ Black eye or bruising of the skin around the eye	■ Apply ice to the eye area (both eyes) for 5–15 minutes every hour for the first 1–2 days after injury. (Even if only one eye is affected, both eyes may discolor.) ■ Apply warm compresses the second day after injury.
Foreign body on conjunctiva	■ Intense pain or feeling of something in the eye	■ The patient must not rub the eye. ■ Material on the surface of the eye is removed by closing the upper lid over the lower lid, irrigating or everting the upper lid, visualizing the material, and removing it with a slightly damp handkerchief. ■ If the foreign body cannot be removed, the eye is patched and the patient is transported to the emergency department.

(continued on next page)

Clinical Manifestations and Therapies *(continued)*

ETIOLOGY	CLINICAL MANIFESTATIONS	CLINICAL THERAPIES
Detached retina	▪ Floaters: irregular dark lines or spots in the field of vision ▪ Flashes of light ▪ Blurred vision ▪ Progressive deterioration of vision ▪ Sensation of a curtain or veil being drawn across the field of vision ▪ If the macula is involved, loss of central vision	▪ Prompt treatment is needed to preserve vision. ▪ Proper positioning is important. ▪ Cryotherapy, laser photocoagulation, or laser therapy may be needed. ▪ Scleral buckle may be needed to close the retinal break.

corneal transplant (Allina Health System, 2015). Penetrating wounds of the eye generally require surgical intervention by an ophthalmic surgeon. Surgical management of blunt trauma depends on the extent and type of injury, which may include corneal abrasions, globe rupture, retinal detachment, and lens dislocation (Colby, 2014). Conjunctival foreign bodies do not usually lead to injuries that require surgical treatment. However, nonsurgical removal of the foreign body, which is often performed in the emergency department, may be required.

Retinal detachment is a medical emergency; early diagnosis and treatment are essential in order to preserve vision. The manifestations and examination of the ocular fundus by ophthalmoscopy establish the diagnosis of retinal detachment. If the condition is left untreated, the detached portion will become necrotic because of separation from the vascular supply of the choroid. Permanent blindness in that portion of the eye results. Interventions are directed toward bringing the retina and choroid back into contact and reestablishing the blood and nutrient supply to the retina. Either cryotherapy, using a supercooled probe, or laser photocoagulation may be used to create an area of inflammation and adhesion to "weld" the layers together. Scleral buckling, during which an indentation or fold is surgically created in the sclera, may be performed to restore contact between the choroid and retina. Contact is maintained with a local

Medications
Eye Injuries

CLASSIFICATION AND DRUG EXAMPLES	MECHANISMS OF ACTION	NURSING CONSIDERATIONS
Topical Antibiotics *Drug examples:* Gentamicin Neomycin Tobramycin Erythromycin	These drugs are used to treat or prevent bacterial infection. The choice of antibiotic depends on the bacteria suspected.	▪ Instruct the patient on the proper use of eyedrops or ointments.
Cycloplegic Drugs *Drug examples:* Atropine Tropicamide Cyclopentolate	These drugs block the responses of the sphincter muscles of the iris and the muscles of the ciliary body to cholinergic stimulation. They cause pupillary dilation.	▪ Instruct the patient on the proper use of eyedrops. ▪ These drugs should not be used in patients with narrow-angle glaucoma.
Carbonic Anhydrase Inhibitors *Drug examples:* Acetazolamide (Diamox): oral medication Methazolamide (Neptazane): oral medication Brinzolamide (Azopt) Dorzolamide (Trusopt)	These drugs decrease the production of aqueous humor into the eye. They are related to sulfa drugs.	▪ Oral medications may cause periorbital numbness and tingling in the fingers and toes. ▪ These drugs may cause loss of potassium; assess daily weight and electrolytes. ▪ Allergy to sulfa is a contraindication. ▪ Use with caution in patients with renal or hepatic disease.

Source: Data from Adams, M. P., Holland, L. N., & Urban, C. (2017). *Pharmacology for nurses: A pathophysiologic approach* (5th ed.). Hoboken, NJ: Pearson Education.

implant on the sclera or an encircling strap or "buckle." In a procedure called pneumatic retinopexy, air is injected into the vitreous cavity. The patient is positioned so that the air bubble pushes the detached portion of the retina into contact with the choroid.

Pharmacologic Therapy

For treatment of corneal abrasion and following removal of a conjunctival foreign body, antibiotic ointment, such as erythromycin or sulfacetamide sodium, may be applied. Pharmacologic treatment of burns may include pain medications (oral or eyedrops), steroids (to decrease inflammation), and cycloplegic drops, such as atropine, tropicamide, or cyclopentolate, to cause pupillary dilation to decrease pain (Allina Health System, 2015). Following irrigation, a topical antibiotic ointment, such as gentamicin ophthalmic, is applied.

For penetrating and perforating injuries, pain is managed by using narcotic analgesics (e.g., morphine). The patient also may require sedation (e.g., diazepam) and antiemetic medications to prevent vomiting. Antibiotics such as IV cefazolin (Ancef) and gentamicin (Garamycin) are prescribed to prevent infection. Blunt trauma to the eye may require reduction of intraocular pressure with a carbonic anhydrase inhibitor, such as acetazolamide (Diamox) or dichlorphenamide (Daranide). Following surgical repair of retinal detachment, steroid medications may be used to reduce inflammation (Koerner, Koerner-Stiefbold, & Garwig, 2012). Treatment of subconjunctival hemorrhage and periorbital ecchymosis does not usually include medication.

Patient Teaching

Administering Eyedrops and Eye Ointments

To ensure safe, effective delivery of eye medication, patient teaching should include the following:

- Wash hands with soap and water. Rinse and dry hands.
- Read directions to determine whether drops need to be gently shaken.
- Check applicator/dropper tip for cracks or chips.
- Avoid touching the applicator tip to your eye or hands. It must be kept clean.
- Tilt your head back slightly, and pull down the lower eyelid with your index finger to form a pocket.
- Hold the applicator with the other hand, tip facing down, as close to the eye as possible without touching it.
- Use the other fingers on that hand as a brace against your face to stabilize your hand.
- Look up and gently squeeze medication into the lower eyelid pocket. Instill the prescribed amount of medication.
- Tip your head slightly down and close your eyes for 2–3 minutes. Try not to squint or blink.
- Apply gentle pressure to the lacrimal duct.
- Wipe any excess medication from your face with a tissue.
- Replace and tighten the applicator lid.
- To remove any medication, wash your hands.

Lifespan Considerations

Eye Injuries in Children

Pediatric eye injuries are often the result of play. Common causes of eye injuries in children include blunt trauma from a ball or fist, sharp trauma from projectiles such as sticks, chemical trauma from household chemicals, and burns from fireworks. Injuries can be to the eyelid, the bones surrounding the eye, or the eye itself. Corneal scratches, lacerations, and internal bleeding can all result from eye injuries. Depending on the severity of the injury, prompt treatment is often required. Treatment of eye injuries is similar for all ages, including eye irrigation and surgery as appropriate.

Nurses can help to prevent eye injuries in children by providing patient teaching, especially to parents, about how to keep children safe from injury. Nurses should promote the use of eye safety equipment during sports and other activities that could result in eye injury. Safety equipment for young children in the home may include safety gates for stairs and cushions or pads for sharp corners. Nurses should also teach parents to keep caustic chemicals out of the reach of children, to buy age-appropriate toys for their children, and not to allow children or other adults to handle fireworks. Teaching children how to safely use tools such as scissors and paper clips is also an important task for parents and nurses.

External eye injuries are very common in children and, by themselves, rarely indicate some form of abuse or nonaccidental trauma. However, two black eyes rarely occur by accident, and raccoon eyes accompanied by swelling and skin injury are likely to accompany nonaccidental fracture at the base of the skull (Becker & Dutelle, 2013). In these cases, nurses should assess the patient for potential abuse.

Eye Injuries in Older Adults

The number one cause of eye injury is falling, and most of the eye injuries related to falling occur in older adults (AAO, 2015e). Primary causes of eye injuries in older adults include slipping on wet surfaces and falling down stairs (Chupkov, 2016). Older adults are more at risk for falling than younger populations because of poor eyesight, getting used to bifocals that may cause altered depth perception, decreased sense of balance, and decreased cognition. Nurses should teach older adults methods to prevent falling in order to reduce the risk of eye injury in this population.

NURSING PROCESS

The nursing role involves educating people about the prevention of eye injuries and providing direct care to patients with eye injuries.

Assessment

Ocular injuries require immediate interventions simultaneously with assessment and collection of an accurate history. Determine the time, type, and extent of injury and the circumstances under which it occurred. In addition, ask about preexisting visual problems.

If the patient normally wears corrective lenses, perform a vision assessment while the patient is wearing lenses. Evaluate eye movement unless a penetrating object is present, and inspect the lid and eye for lacerations. Perform inspection using strong light and magnification with a headband loupe or slit lamp. **Blepharism** (spasms that cause the eye to blink continuously) and eye pain may prevent assessment of the injured eye. If eye pain and photophobia make opening the eye difficult, topical anesthesia may be applied before inspection. Fluorescein staining can help identify foreign bodies and abrasions. Note any conjunctival or anterior chamber hemorrhage as well as the presence or absence of the red reflex.

For the patient with a detached retina, the nursing focus is on early identification and treatment. Because early intervention is vital to preserve the patient's sight, recognizing early manifestations of retinal detachment and intervening appropriately to obtain definitive treatment for the patient is essential. Retinal detachment can be successfully treated on an outpatient basis, often in an ophthalmologist's office. If an ophthalmologist is not readily available, position the patient's head so that gravity pulls the detached portion of the retina into closer contact with the choroid. Keep in mind that patients with certain cardiorespiratory diseases may not tolerate this position.

Diagnosis

Nursing diagnoses for the patient with an eye injury may include the following:

- *Tissue Integrity, Impaired*
- *Pain, Acute*
- *Anxiety*
- *Tissue Perfusion, Ineffective.*

(NANDA-I © 2014)

Planning

Planning with the patient with an eye injury is based on the nature and extent of the injury. Typical outcomes may include the following:

- The patient will be free of pain associated with the injury.
- The patient will articulate and follow instructions regarding eye protection and the healing process.
- The patient will describe when to call the primary care provider in the event of worsening symptoms or condition.
- The patient will experience healing and restoration of vision to the maximum extent possible.

Implementation

All types of eye trauma pose the risk of violating the integrity of the eye, threatening vision. Therefore, the goals of nursing care are preserving vision and the integrity of the eye and preventing further damage.

Reduce Risk for Impaired Vision

- Assess vision in each eye and both eyes, with and without corrective lenses, upon the patient's entry to the emergency department or primary care setting. An initial assessment provides valuable information about the effect of the injury on the patient's vision and a baseline for future comparisons.

- Inspect the eye(s) carefully for evidence of foreign bodies, burns, penetrating injury, or blunt trauma. Note whether lacerations, burns, or other trauma are evident in tissues surrounding the eye. Eye trauma may be hidden by other injuries and thus remain untreated.

- If a burn or foreign body is present, consider administering anesthetic drops and irrigating the eye before or after the physician evaluates the patient. Irrigation to remove the chemical is a higher priority than assessment of the eye (see **Box 18–3** »).

- Remove any loose foreign bodies using a moist, sterile cotton-tipped applicator. Prompt removal of foreign bodies may prevent corneal abrasion.

- For a severe or penetrating injury, promote rest and stabilize the injured eye by applying an eye pad or gauze dressing loosely over both the affected and unaffected eye. Stabilize any penetrating object if possible. These measures reduce eye movement and can help preserve the patient's vision.

- Following treatment, apply eyedrops or ointment as prescribed, and apply an eye pad or shield if ordered. Apply an eye pad to the affected eye to reduce pain and photophobia and to promote healing.

Box 18–3
Eye Irrigation

Eye irrigation is a critical procedure for flushing chemicals and other small debris from the eye. Steps for eye irrigation include the following:

- Obtain normal saline for irrigation. If saline is not available, water may be used.
- If needed, apply a topical anesthetic, such as tetracaine drops, to relieve pain and make inspection and irrigation easier.
- Direct fluid from the inner to the outer canthus of the eye.
- Have the patient move the eyeball in all directions to properly irrigate.
- When irrigating, evert the eyelid to identify and remove material from the conjunctival sac.
- The eye should be rinsed thoroughly for at least 30 minutes. A special contact lens irrigating unit (Morgan lens) or a bottle of irrigant with IV tubing held to flush all eye surfaces may be useful.
- Slightly tip the patient's head to the affected side to prevent contamination of the unaffected eye.
- Irrigate until the pH of the eye is normal (in the range of 7.2–7.4).
- Following irrigation, apply a topical antibiotic ointment, such as gentamicin ophthalmic.

Patient Teaching

Eye Injuries: Prevention and First Aid

Teaching individuals and groups how to prevent eye injuries is an important nursing role, especially for patients involved in hazardous occupations and activities. Children in particular are at risk for eye injuries.

Although sports injuries readily come to mind, many eye injuries in children happen at home. All chemicals should be kept in a childproof area. Toys that can cause eye injury such as bows and arrows, darts, and BB guns should be used under careful adult supervision or avoided. Common items around the house such as scissors, paper clips, pencils, and rubber bands can also cause serious eye injury. It is important for parents to teach children the safe use of these items.

Protective eyewear should be used by participants in all sports that pose a risk of eye injury. Stress the importance of using seat belts to prevent eye injury in automobile crashes. Small children should not be left alone with dogs. When a dog bites a child age 4 or younger, eye injuries occur in about 15% of cases. Most often, it is a dog that the child is familiar with.

Instruct patients and their families about steps to take for a variety of eye injuries. If a chemical splash occurs, they should immediately flush the eye with copious amounts of water. Loose objects can sometimes be flushed from the eye with rapid blinking and tears. The patient or family should not try to remove objects from the eye on their own. If an abrasion, penetrating, or blunt injury is suspected, they should cover the eye loosely with sterile gauze and seek immediate medical attention. Instruct patients and their families not to remove objects that penetrate the eye (AAO, 2016g). Whenever the extent of injury is not clear, recommend that the child be evaluated in an emergency care facility.

- After an injury, discuss the following topics with the patient and family: prescribed medications and possible adverse effects, strategies to prevent further trauma, application of the eye pad or shield, avoidance of activities that increase intraocular pressure, and the importance of activity restrictions.

Interventions for Retinal Detachment

Restoring contact between the retina and choroid is a priority of nursing and medical care for the patient with retinal detachment. Vitreous humor may leak through a retinal tear, and fluid exudate may collect behind the tear, causing further detachment. If the macula is detached, central vision is lost, and the likelihood of restoring full vision decreases.

- Notify the patient's healthcare provider and ophthalmologist immediately. To preserve vision, immediate medical intervention is required in patients with retinal detachment.

- Position the patient so the area of detachment is inferior. For instance, for a superior temporal retinal detachment of the right eye (with corresponding vision loss in the inferior medial visual field of that eye), place the patient supine with head turned to the right. Correct positioning allows the contents of the posterior portion of the eye to place pressure on the detached area, bringing the retina in closer contact with the choroid.

- Maintain a confident attitude while carrying out priority interventions. Administering care in a calm though urgent manner helps to reassure the patient that the problem is treatable and that appropriate measures are being taken.

- Reassure the patient that most retinal detachments are successfully treated, usually on an outpatient basis. Reassurance can help allay the patient's fear of permanent vision loss.

- Explain all procedures fully, including the reason for positioning. Explanations facilitate understanding and help relieve anxiety in unfamiliar settings.

- Allow supportive family members or friends to remain with the patient as much as possible. Additional support helps to lower the patient's anxiety level.

Teaching for the patient undergoing surgical repair of retinal detachment is similar to that for patients experiencing other types of eye surgery. If the retina remains detached, provide instructions about the change in peripheral vision or other visual fields and changes in depth perception.

>> Go to **Pearson MyLab Nursing and eText** to see Chart 1, Nursing Care of the Patient Having Eye Surgery.

Discuss the following topics with the patient and family to prepare for home care:

- Limitations on positioning the head before or following repair

- Activity restrictions such as no bending or straining during bowel movements

- Use of an eye shield

- Early manifestations and the importance of seeking immediate treatment

- Follow-up treatment with the ophthalmologist.

Evaluation

Criteria that reflect the patient's achievement of identified outcomes and successful resolution of nursing diagnoses may include the following:

- The patient maintains optimal vision following injury.

- The patient experiences no loss of vision as the result of preventable complications.

- The patient reports pain management to acceptable levels.

If the expected outcomes are not met, the patient may need further evaluation for eye infections and treatment with topical antibiotics or referral for surgery, depending on the complication.

REVIEW Eye Injuries

RELATE Link the Concepts and Exemplars

Patrick Callahan is 75 years old and married. He was admitted to the medical surgical unit with a retinal detachment and is scheduled for a scleral buckling procedure in the morning.

Linking the exemplar of eye injuries with the concept of safety:

1. What is Mr. Callahan's priority nursing diagnosis?
2. What postoperative teaching would you include for Mr. Callahan and his wife before discharge to reduce his risk of injury?

Linking the exemplar of eye injuries with the concept of cognition:

3. You are caring for an older adult patient with an eye injury. How might her cognition be affected?
4. What nursing interventions might you initiate to reduce the impact of reduced vision on an adult patient's cognition?

READY Go to Volume 3: Clinical Nursing Skills

REFER Go to Pearson MyLab Nursing and eText

- Additional review materials
- Chart 1: Nursing Care of the Patient Having Eye Surgery

REFLECT Apply Your Knowledge

Seth Iyengar, age 17, presents to the emergency department with his parents after he was hit in the eye with a paintball. Seth was running through an outdoor course with his friends when his right eye was struck. At the time of his injury, Seth was not wearing the eye protection provided to him at the course. Seth reports eye pain and decreased visual acuity. Examination reveals visible blood in the right eye.

1. What are the potential nursing diagnoses?
2. What are the immediate nursing interventions?
3. What teaching might help Seth avoid injury in the future?

›› Exemplar 18.D
Peripheral Neuropathy

Exemplar Learning Outcomes

18.D Analyze peripheral neuropathy as it relates to sensory perception.

- Describe the pathophysiology of peripheral neuropathy.
- Describe the etiology of peripheral neuropathy.
- Compare the risk factors for and prevention of peripheral neuropathy.
- Identify the clinical manifestations of peripheral neuropathy.
- Summarize diagnostic tests and therapies used by interprofessional teams in the collaborative care of an individual with peripheral neuropathy.
- Differentiate considerations for care of patients with peripheral neuropathy across the lifespan.
- Apply the nursing process in providing culturally competent care to an individual with peripheral neuropathy.

Exemplar Key Terms

Charcot-Marie-Tooth (CMT) disease, *1436*
Guillain-Barré syndrome (GBS), *1435*
Mononeuropathies, *1435*
Paresthesias, *1435*
Peripheral neuropathy, *1434*
Polyneuropathies, *1435*

Overview

Peripheral neuropathy results when trauma or a disease process interferes with innervation of peripheral nerves. The overall effectiveness of blood vessels decreases, and superficial blood vessels constrict to divert blood to larger vessels. With the constriction of peripheral blood vessels, peripheral nerve endings in the constricted area experience decreased blood flow, and neuropathy develops. Although most peripheral neuropathies progress slowly over time, the symptoms, including pain and muscle weakness, can significantly affect quality of life. An estimated 20 million Americans have some form of peripheral neuropathy (National Institute of Neurological Disorders and Stroke [NINDS], 2015).

Pathophysiology and Etiology

The peripheral nervous system (PNS) links the CNS with the rest of the body. The PNS is responsible for receiving and transmitting information from and about the external environment. It consists of nerves, ganglia (groups of nerve cells), and sensory receptors located outside—or peripheral to—the brain and spinal cord. The PNS is divided into a sensory (afferent) division and a motor (efferent) division. Most nerves of the PNS contain fibers for both divisions, and all nerves are classified regionally as either spinal nerves or cranial nerves.

Pathophysiology

The main components of peripheral nerves are the axon and myelin. Peripheral neuropathy can be classified according to the predominant pathology: axonal degeneration or segmental demyelination. Damage to peripheral nerves can interrupt communication between the brain and the body, affecting normal muscle movement and sensory perception and causing pain.

The peripheral neuropathies (also called somatic neuropathies) include polyneuropathies and mononeuropathies.

Polyneuropathies, the most common types of neuropathy associated with diabetes, are bilateral sensory disorders. The manifestations appear first in the toes and feet and progress upward. The fingers and hands also may be involved, but usually only in later stages of diabetes. The manifestations of polyneuropathies depend on the nerve fibers involved.

Mononeuropathies are isolated peripheral neuropathies that affect a single nerve. Injury or trauma is the most common cause, although repetitive motions, such as those resulting in carpal tunnel syndrome, also can cause mononeuropathies.

Etiology

Neuropathies are classified according to cause: acquired, hereditary, or idiopathic. Acquired neuropathies include those caused by disease or illness, nutritional deficits, infection, trauma, and toxins. Hereditary, or inherited, neuropathies include Charcot-Marie-Tooth (CMT) disease. Idiopathic neuropathies are from an unknown cause and account for up to 30% of neuropathies.

The etiology of polyneuropathy is varied; it often is caused by systemic diseases, exposure to toxins, and poor nutrition (in particular, vitamin B deficiency). Damage from disease processes such as metabolic and endocrine disorders affects the body's ability to process waste products and utilize nutrients. Approximately 70% of individuals with diabetes develop some type of neuropathy (Foundation for Peripheral Neuropathy, 2015). Conditions that decrease oxygen supply may cause a thickening of the walls of blood vessels that supply nerves, resulting in a reduced blood flow. Autoimmune disorders and infections also can cause peripheral neuropathy. Viruses and bacteria can attack nerve tissues (or cause the body to attack nerve tissues), resulting in the destruction of nerve axons or the myelin sheath.

One of the most serious polyneuropathies is **Guillain-Barré syndrome (GBS)**, a demyelinating disorder of the peripheral nervous system that results from both a humoral- and cell-mediated immunologic response. GBS is one of the most common peripheral nervous system disorders, affecting approximately 3000–6000 people annually in the United States (CDC, 2015d). The cause is unknown, but precipitating events include a respiratory or gastrointestinal viral or bacterial infection 1–3 weeks before the onset of manifestations, surgery, viral immunizations, and other viral illnesses. In 60% of cases, *Campylobacter jejuni* is identified as the cause of the preceding infection.

GBS is characterized by progressive ascending flaccid paralysis, accompanied by **paresthesias** (subjective feelings of a change in sensation, such as numbness or tingling). About 20% of patients have respiratory involvement to the point that ventilatory assistance is required. GBS is often a medical emergency. In spite of this, approximately 80–90% of patients with GBS have a spontaneous recovery with little or no residual disabilities.

Sensory neuropathies with manifestations of numbness, tingling, and pain in the lower extremities affect about 30% of patients with AIDS. A GBS-type of inflammatory demyelinating polyneuropathy also can occur, resulting in progressive weakness and paralysis. In addition, untreated Lyme disease can cause extensive peripheral nerve damage.

Other disease processes that can result in peripheral neuropathy include the following:

- Alcoholic neuropathy is damage to the nerves that results from long-term excessive use of alcohol. Malnutrition is a serious complication of chronic alcoholism; thiamin (B_1) deficiency that may be associated with chronic alcoholism is characterized by progressive cognitive deterioration, confabulation, myopathy, and peripheral neuropathy.

- Inflammation, cancer, and toxins, including some types of chemotherapy, other medications, and environmental chemicals, such as lead, can damage nerve tissue and fibers, resulting in peripheral neuropathy.

- Inflammation and swelling in tendon sheaths can lead to peripheral neuropathy. The carpal tunnel is a canal through which flexor tendons and the median nerve pass from the wrist to the hand. Carpal tunnel syndrome develops from narrowing of the tunnel and compression of the median nerve as a result of inflammation and swelling of the synovial lining of the tendon sheaths.

The prognosis for patients with peripheral neuropathy ranges from the neuropathy resolving (e.g., the underlying cause is successfully treated) to cases in which the patient does not respond to treatment or the cause is not identified and the condition persists indefinitely.

Risk Factors and Prevention

Risk factors for acquired peripheral neuropathies include diabetes; alcohol use; vitamin deficiencies (particularly B vitamins); immune system suppression; autoimmune diseases; exposures to toxins; and kidney, liver, or thyroid disorders.

Age also appears to have a role in risk for peripheral neuropathy. Studies show that the incidence of peripheral neuropathy increases significantly in older adults. Although some changes in the peripheral system are due to the normal aging process, they are not usually associated with changes in functional status.

Height has been identified as a risk factor for the development of peripheral neuropathy, independent of gender or presence of diabetes mellitus. Men who are taller than 167 cm (5'6") and women who are taller than 159 cm (5'3") are at higher risk for developing peripheral neuropathy than individuals of shorter height, and they are at higher risk of amputation if they do develop peripheral neuropathy (Kote et al., 2013). This may be because the longer axon length increases the surface area available for exposure to toxins and the length of time needed for repair. This relationship between height and peripheral neuropathy may also be because of the increased hydrostatic pressure in the feet of taller individuals when they are standing. Nurses should be aware of this risk factor and use it to identify individuals who are at higher risk for peripheral neuropathy, especially if patients also have other risk factors, such as diabetes mellitus or excessive alcohol use.

Controlling medical conditions that increase the risk for peripheral neuropathy is one of the best prevention methods. A healthy diet of vegetables, fruits, and whole grains can help improve nerve health. Intake of vitamin B_{12} can be helpful as well. Avoiding triggers that contribute to nerve damage, such as repetitive motions, smoking, excessive alcohol consumption, toxic chemicals, and cramped positions, will also help in prevention of neuropathies (Mayo Clinic, 2017c).

Clinical Manifestations

Clinical manifestations of peripheral neuropathy depend on the affected nerve or nerves and the amount of damage. The patient with polyneuropathy commonly has distal paresthesias; pain described as aching, burning, or shooting; and feelings of cold feet. Other manifestations may include impaired sensations of pain, temperature, light touch, two-point discrimination, and vibration. With GBS, there is frequently a "stocking–glove" pattern—feeling as though stockings and gloves are being worn when they are not—with pain in the hands, feet, and legs.

Weakness in the arms or legs is often caused by damage to motor nerves; patients may report difficulty walking or running, stumbling, dropping things, and tiring easily. A general feeling of lack of coordination or clumsiness may be reported, and the patient may compensate by changing the walking pattern to maintain balance.

SAFETY ALERT Symptoms of numbness or weakness in the legs and feet increase the patient's risk for falls, which in turn increases the risk for injury and infection. Teach patients with peripheral neuropathy to be aware of obstacles that may cause tripping. Also teach patients how to call for help if they fall and cannot move.

The most common inherited peripheral neuropathy is **Charcot-Marie-Tooth (CMT) disease**, which is characterized by a slowly progressive degeneration of the muscles of the foot, lower leg, hand, and forearm. Symptoms usually present between adolescence and young adulthood.

Clinical Manifestations and Therapies
Peripheral Neuropathy

ETIOLOGY	CLINICAL MANIFESTATIONS	CLINICAL THERAPIES
Motor nerve damage	■ Muscle weakness ■ Cramps ■ Fasciculations ■ Muscle loss	■ Treatment of underlying cause ■ Physical therapy ■ Surgery if necessary (e.g., to remove tumor causing compression)
Sensory nerve damage	■ Numbness ■ Pain ■ Burning or shooting pain ■ Impaired touch, temperature, and pain sensation	■ Treatment of underlying cause ■ Medication ■ Physical therapy

Collaboration

Because peripheral neuropathy can involve multiple systems, collaboration is likely to include specialists (e.g., a neurologist or an endocrinologist, physical or occupational therapists, pain specialists). The primary goal of treatment is to correct or manage the underlying cause so that symptoms are controlled and further nerve damage is minimized.

Diagnostic Tests

Diagnostic tests for peripheral neuropathy may include the following:

- Electromyography
- Complete blood count (CBC)
- Thyroid function tests
- Serum levels for B_{12} and thiamin
- Metabolic panel
- Urine screening
- Nerve biopsy.

Lyme disease and HIV tests also may be indicated.

Surgery

Surgical intervention may be appropriate when peripheral neuropathies are caused by compression, as in the case of nerve tumors, carpal tunnel syndrome, and peripheral nerve injuries. Patients with CMT disease may also be good candidates for surgery, especially for foot reconstruction to straighten clawed toes, flatten high arches, and stabilize ankles. Neuropathies caused by medical pathologies such as diabetes cannot be treated with surgery.

SAFETY ALERT If an individual with peripheral neuropathy has an injury that gets infected and develops gangrene, surgery may be required to amputate the infected extremity. Therefore, nurses should encourage patients to regularly check their extremities for injury and infection to avoid progression to gangrene and amputation.

Pharmacologic Therapy

There is no single drug to treat pain resulting from peripheral neuropathy because drug therapy is individualized and based on comorbidities, extent of nerve damage, and nerve affected. Medications used include pain relievers, anticonvulsants, and antidepressants.

- ***Pain relievers.*** For mild symptoms, over-the-counter medications such as acetaminophen or ibuprofen may be helpful. More severe symptoms may require the use of an opiate.
- ***Antiseizure drugs.*** In recent years, the use of antiseizure drugs to treat nerve pain has increased. The mechanism of action related to nerve pain is poorly understood, but it is thought that antiseizure drugs may block pain receptors in the CNS. Some examples of antiseizure drugs used in treating nerve pain include carbamazepine (Carbatrol, Tegretol), gabapentin (Neurontin), pregabalin (Lyrica), and topiramate (Topamax).
- ***Antidepressants.*** Tricyclic antidepressants are thought to activate a descending serotonergic (5-HT1) antinociceptive pathway that creates an endogenous pain modulation

Medications
Peripheral Neuropathy

CLASSIFICATION AND DRUG EXAMPLES	MECHANISMS OF ACTION	NURSING CONSIDERATIONS
Antiseizure Drugs *Drug examples:* Carbamazepine (Carbatrol, Tegretol) Gabapentin (Neurontin) Pregabalin (Lyrica) Topiramate (Topamax)	The mechanism of action in controlling nerve pain is poorly understood. These drugs may block pain receptors in the CNS. *May also be used for:* Treatment of epilepsy	▪ Teach patients about the side effects of dizziness and drowsiness. ▪ Teach patients to avoid grapefruit and grapefruit juice. ▪ Teach patients to avoid antacids. ▪ Women who are breastfeeding or may become pregnant should avoid using these drugs.
Tricyclic Antidepressants *Drug examples:* Amitriptyline (Elavil) Nortriptyline (Pamelor)	These drugs are thought to activate a descending serotonergic (5-HT1) antinociceptive pathway, which creates an endogenous pain modulation system. *May also be used for:* Treatment of depression	▪ Teach patients about the side effects of dizziness and drowsiness, nausea, and decreased appetite. ▪ It may take 4–6 weeks for therapeutic plasma levels to be achieved. ▪ Take at bedtime to avoid drowsiness.
Serotonin-norepinephrine Reuptake Inhibitors *Drug examples:* Duloxetine (Cymbalta)	These drugs block the depletion of serotonin and norepinephrine in the CNS, which may help to modulate pain. *May also be used for:* Treatment of depression	▪ Teach patients about the side effects of dizziness and drowsiness, nausea, and decreased appetite. ▪ It may take 4–6 weeks for therapeutic plasma levels to be achieved. ▪ Administer with food.

Source: Data from Adams, M. P., Holland, L. N., & Urban, C. (2017). *Pharmacology for nurses: A pathophysiologic approach* (5th ed.). Hoboken, NJ: Pearson Education.

system. This action is different from how tricyclic antidepressants work in the treatment of depression. Some examples of tricyclic antidepressants are amitriptyline (Elavil) and nortriptyline (Pamelor). The serotonin-norepinephrine reuptake inhibitor (SNRI) duloxetine (Cymbalta) blocks the depletion of serotonin and norepinephrine in the CNS, which may help modulate pain receptors. They have side effects that include dizziness, drowsiness, nausea, and decreased appetite.

▪ *Lidocaine patch.* A lidocaine patch is a local anesthetic that is absorbed through the skin. Serious side effects can occur, including hives, confusion, weakness, fainting, and swelling of the lips, face, tongue, or throat (National Library of Medicine, 2013).

Nonpharmacologic Therapy

There is no specific treatment for polyneuropathy, because it is a symptom with many potential causes. The primary goals of treatment are to care for and manage the underlying cause. However, a combination of medication, lifestyle modifications, and physical therapy can be effective in treating symptoms and increasing quality of life. Physical or occupational therapy may help the patient maintain mobility and avoid further changes in functional status.

Changes in daily life may be required to maintain or restore health. Adherence with the therapeutic regimen for the primary condition (e.g., maintain blood glucose control) is important. Eating a healthy, well-balanced diet (vitamin supplements may be necessary), maintaining optimal weight, avoiding smoking, and limiting alcohol will promote overall health. Regular exercise will help to increase/maintain muscle strength. Daily foot care, as described in the Patient Teaching feature on Foot Care in the exemplar on Type 1 Diabetes Mellitus in the module on Metabolism, is imperative.

Complementary health approaches include acupuncture, biofeedback, massage, and transcutaneous electrical nerve stimulation (TENS) (see Focus on Integrative Health feature).

Lifespan Considerations

There are several etiologies of peripheral neuropathy that are seen throughout the lifespan, including GBS, CMT disease, and diabetic peripheral neuropathy. A discussion of each of these is included in the following sections.

Lifespan Considerations for Patients with Guillain-Barré Syndrome

Children rarely develop GBS. However, now that polio has been eradicated, GBS is the leading cause of acute motor paralysis in children (DiFazio et al., 2014). The average age range of children who have GBS is 4–8 years, but infants as young as 3 weeks old can be affected (DiFazio et al., 2014). In infants, floppy baby syndrome, which is characterized by hypotonia with no identifiable cause, should be considered a candidate for GBS diagnosis. Infants may also present with respiratory distress and difficulty feeding. Children younger

Focus on Integrative Health
Transcutaneous Electrical Nerve Stimulation (TENS)

TENS uses pulses of electrical current to generate nonpainful mild muscle twitches at the site of the pain. This inhibits transmission of pain signals to the brain, helping to decrease pain. TENS can be either conventional (low intensity, high frequency) or acupuncture-like (high intensity, low frequency) (Johnson, 2012). TENS can be self-administered and is relatively inexpensive, making it a good choice for pain treatment for many patients. In a small study, TENS was found to significantly decrease pain associated with peripheral neuropathy (Kilinc et al., 2014). Additional clinical trials are currently underway to further investigate the usefulness of TENS to treat peripheral neuropathy (National Institutes of Health, 2016).

than 6 years old may present with a refusal to walk and pain in the legs, whereas older children present with symptoms more similar to adults. GBS usually manifests in children as progressive, symmetrical, ascending muscle weakness with hyporeflexia or areflexia (Rosen, 2012). The most effective treatment in children is IV immunoglobulin. Plasmapheresis is not recommended for small children. Children are more likely to recover from GBS than adults, with a 90–95% rate of complete recovery within 3–12 months. The remaining 5–10% may have lifelong effects of the disease.

GBS also may affect pregnant women, although diagnosis is often complicated in pregnant women because symptoms of GBS mimic common complaints from women in the third trimester, when GBS is most likely to occur. GBS is often more severe in pregnant women, with severe disability affecting 20% of women after 1 year (Zafar et al., 2013), and symptoms worsen in the postpartum period due to a reversal of the decrease in cellular-mediated immunity that occurs during pregnancy (Vasudev & Raina, 2014). GBS should not affect the pregnant woman's ability to deliver vaginally, but she may have a decreased ability to bear down during labor, so vacuum extraction of the neonate may be required (Paul et al., 2012).

Clinical manifestations and treatment of GBS is the same for older adults as for other patients with GBS. However, older adults have increased risk of developing GBS, and mortality rates are higher in this population. The use of mechanical ventilation greatly increases the risk of death in older adults; this increased risk is often related to ventilator-associated pneumonia (Andary et al., 2015).

Lifespan Considerations for Patients with Charcot-Marie-Tooth Syndrome

CMT disease is a genetic disorder that can be evident at birth, but it more commonly appears in childhood, adolescence, or early adulthood. Although CMT is a genetic disorder, many forms of the disease are autosomal recessive, so parents often do not realize they are carriers of the disease until their child is diagnosed. For this reason, and in combination with the fact that symptoms are very mild early in the course of the disease, patients may not be diagnosed with CMT until years after symptoms begin.

Early in the course of the disease, symptoms may manifest as clumsiness due to foot drop and muscle weakness in the feet, ankles, and legs. As the patient ages, symptoms become more pronounced because of muscle wasting and lack of sensation in the extremities. This may lead to problems in dexterity and hand strength, making ADLs more difficult in older adults. In addition, the consistent alterations in posture to compensate for muscle problems can cause muscle and joint pain. Most older adults with CMT require walking aids such as a walker or cane (NHS, 2014).

Lifespan Considerations for Patients with Diabetic Peripheral Neuropathy

Diabetic peripheral neuropathy is rarely seen in children, although subclinical neuropathy is occasionally seen in adolescents (Louraki et al., 2012). Children and adolescents who are at higher risk for developing peripheral neuropathy include patients with poor glycemic control and longer duration of diabetes. Children with diabetes should be screened annually for peripheral neuropathy. Like other patients with diabetic peripheral neuropathy, children and adolescents should be taught how to properly control blood glucose levels and how to provide adequate foot care to prevent injury and infection.

NURSING PROCESS

Application of the nursing process to care of the patient with known or suspected peripheral neuropathy requires significant collaboration with the patient. Because the assessment interview may reveal aspects of the patient's condition that are not made evident through physical assessment, it is essential for the nurse to establish effective communication with the patient.

Assessment

A health assessment to determine problems with the peripheral nervous system may be conducted during a health screening, may focus on a chief complaint (e.g., tingling), or may be part of a total health assessment. Analyze onset, characteristics, course, severity, precipitating and relieving factors, and any associated symptoms, noting the time and circumstances.

- **Observation and patient interview.** Observation of a patient with peripheral neuropathy includes watching as the patient walks to notice drop foot, shuffling steps, or lack of coordinated movement that may indicate lack of feeling in the feet. The patient may also have trouble with coordination if peripheral neuropathy affects the hands. Questions about the patient's present health status include information about numbness, tingling sensations, tremors, problems with coordination or balance, and loss of movement in any part of the body. Carefully assess older adults for impaired balance and fall risk. Ask the patient about difficulty with other senses, including detecting odors. In addition, assess for mood and anxiety, changes in sleep patterns, and ability to perform self-care and ADLs, sexual activity, and weight. Inquire about use of medications, including over-the-counter products and herbal supplements. Ask about past history of seizures; fainting; dizziness; headaches; infection and any trauma; tumors; and surgery of the brain, spinal cord, or nerves. Discuss illnesses that may cause neurologic manifestations, including cardiac disease, strokes, pernicious anemia, sinus infections, liver disease, and/or renal failure. Also ask the patient about family history of neurologic health problems, diabetes mellitus, hypertension, seizures, or mental health problems. Question the patient about occupational hazards, such as exposure to toxic chemicals or materials, and the amount of time spent performing repetitive motions (e.g., data entry, assembly). Information about the patient's diet; use of tobacco, alcohol, or drugs; and use of safety and protective equipment also may be helpful.

- **Physical examination.** A physical examination should include testing peripheral pulses based on the affected extremities. A gait assessment should be performed to test the patient for gait, balance, and risk of falls. The gait assessment should include walking for a minimum of 10 ft. A vibration test can also be used to test sensation at each affected joint. A pressure test can be done by touching random points with a monofilament to detect sensation. Deep tendon reflexes should be tested. A physical exam should also include cranial nerve assessments.

Diagnosis

Nursing diagnoses for the patient with peripheral neuropathy will differ based on the type of neuropathy and comorbidities. They may include the following:

- *Injury, Risk for*
- *Tissue Perfusion: Peripheral, Ineffective*
- *Pain, Chronic.*
- *Anxiety.*

(NANDA-I © 2014)

Planning

Identified outcomes relevant to the plan of care for the patient with peripheral neuropathy may include the following:

- The patient will remain free from injury.
- The patient will report effective pain management through use of a predetermined pain rating scale.
- The patient will verbalize feelings and concerns related to sensory loss.

Implementation

Nursing care of the patient with peripheral neuropathy is focused on promoting patient safety and comfort. While the nursing plan of care is tailored to meet the needs of each patient, general interventions relevant to the plan of care for the patient with peripheral neuropathy target injury prevention and comfort promotion in both the physiologic and psychosocial realms.

Prevent Injury

Ensure patient safety. Patients with compromised feeling in the extremities may be unaware that they have sustained an injury. Teaching topics, depending on the type of peripheral neuropathy and the extent of nerve damage, may include the following:

- Foot care, as the patient may not feel injuries to the feet (see the Patient Teaching feature on Foot Care in the exemplar on Type 1 Diabetes Mellitus)

- Exercise
- Smoking cessation (see Table 15–2 in the module on Oxygenation)
- Avoidance of toxic chemicals
- Nutrition, stressing its importance and identifying sources of B_{12}
- Avoidance of repetitive motion and/or prolonged pressure
- Massage to improve circulation, stimulate nerves, and reduce pain.

Promote Comfort

Pain experienced with peripheral neuropathy varies. Pain and tenderness in muscles can be severe; interventions must be individualized to patient needs. The intense pain combined with altered sensations leads to anxiety. Nursing interventions can make a difference in breaking the cycle of increasing pain that leads to increased anxiety, which can cause more pain.

- Listen to the description of pain; determine the presence of triggers or a pattern. Acknowledging the patient's perception of pain is a basis for treatment; listening establishes trust.
- Use a pain scale for determining the extent of pain. Consistent measurement is essential to evaluate the degree of pain and the effectiveness of intervention.
- Provide analgesics as indicated; administer them on a regular schedule rather than waiting until pain becomes severe. Anticipating and managing pain before it becomes severe will decrease anxiety and avert the cycle of increased anxiety leading to increased pain.
- For patients with GBS, monitor for side effects of analgesics, particularly respiratory depression; assess respirations and lung sounds. Perform routine pulmonary care measures, and monitor for aspiration. Frequent respiratory monitoring is indicated.
- The following complementary health approaches may be used to help manage pain: application of heat/cold, guided imagery, relaxation techniques, and massage.

Evaluation

Nursing care is evaluated on the basis of patient progress in meeting expected outcomes, which may include the following:

- The patient experiences pain control to allow for rest and comfort.
- The patient lists strategies to reduce the risk of injury and promote safety.
- The patient describes a treatment plan to reduce further deterioration of sensation.

Neuropathic pain is usually a chronic condition that will require continual reevaluation by the nurse. Worsening symptoms should be remedied by advocating for stronger pain medications, advocating for surgery if appropriate, referring for appropriate therapy, and teaching additional coping mechanisms.

REVIEW Peripheral Neuropathy

RELATE Link the Concepts and Exemplars

Linking the exemplar of peripheral neuropathy with the concept of comfort:

1. How would nursing interventions for pain differ for a patient with GBS and a patient with carpal tunnel syndrome?

2. What patient teaching would you provide each patient to prevent and/or manage pain?

Linking the exemplar of peripheral neuropathy with the concept of metabolism:

3. What patient teaching would you provide the patient newly diagnosed with diabetes to reduce the risk of later development of peripheral neuropathy?

4. Describe the pathophysiology of diabetes that contributes to the development of peripheral neuropathy.

READY Go to Volume 3: Clinical Nursing Skills

REFER Go to Pearson MyLab Nursing and eText

- Additional review materials

REFLECT Apply Your Knowledge

Ramon Bandera is an assembly line worker who started to feel numbness in his feet at work, where he stands 8–10 hours a day. Of late, he has noticed that he tires more easily, but he has been ignoring it "for a while" because he fears losing his job if he complains. He called in sick today; he explained, "I feel like my feet are freezing and on fire at the same time." Mr. Bandera is 55 years old and lives alone on the second floor of an apartment complex. He is 6 ft tall and weighs 195 lbs. He eats "mostly junk," drinks four or five beers a night, and has smoked a pack of cigarettes a day for 30 years. Despite this, he reports "good health." Mr. Bandera was adopted and has no knowledge of his family's health history. His vital signs are temperature 98.9°F oral; pulse 80 bpm; respirations 20/min; and BP 130/80 mmHg.

1. What laboratory and diagnostic tests would you expect to be performed?

2. What nursing diagnosis would be appropriate for Mr. Bandera?

3. What interventions would you initiate for Mr. Bandera?

4. What teaching will Mr. Bandera need before discharge?

References

Adams, M. K., Chong, E. W., Williamson, E., Aung, K. Z., Makeyeva, G. A., Giles, G. G., . . . Simpson, J. A. (2012). 20/20—Alcohol and age-related macular degeneration: The Melbourne Collaborative Cohort Study. *American Journal of Epidemiology, 176*(4), 289–298.

Adams, M. P., Holland, L. N., & Urban, C. (2017). *Pharmacology for nurses: A pathophysiologic approach* (5th ed.). Hoboken, NJ: Pearson Education.

Aghadoost, D. (2014). Ocular trauma: An overview. *Archives of Trauma Research, 3*(2), e21639.

Allina Health System. (2015). *Chemical eye burns.* Retrieved from http://www.allinahealth.org/mdex/ND1420G.HTM

Andary, M. T., Oleszek, J. L., Maurelus, K., & White-McCrimmon, R. Y. (2015). *Guillain-Barre syndrome.* Retrieved from http://emedicine.medscape.com/article/315632-overview

American Academy of Ophthalmology (AAO). (2015a). *Policy statement: Frequency of ocular examinations.* San Francisco, CA: Author.

American Academy of Ophthalmology (AAO). (2015b). *Cataracts in children, congenital and acquired.* Retrieved from http://eyewiki.aao.org/Cataracts_in_Children,_Congenital_and_Acquired

American Academy of Ophthalmology (AAO). (2015c). *Color codes for topical ocular medications.* Retrieved from http://www.aao.org/about/policies/color-codes-topical-ocular-medications

American Academy of Ophthalmology (AAO). (2015d). *What is juvenile macular degeneration?* Retrieved from http://www.geteyesmart.org/eyesmart/diseases/juvenile-macular-degeneration.cfm

American Academy of Ophthalmology (AAO). (2015e). *Falls and brawls top list of causes for eye injuries in United States.* Retrieved from http://www.

aao.org/newsroom/news-releases/detail/falls-brawls-top-list-of-causes-eye-injuries-in-un

American Academy of Ophthalmology (AAO). (2016a). *What is macular degeneration?* Retrieved from https://www.aao.org/eye-health/diseases/amd-macular-degeneration

American Academy of Ophthalmology (AAO). (2016b). *Cataract treatment.* Retrieved from https://www.aao.org/eye-health/diseases/cataracts-treatment

American Academy of Ophthalmology (AAO). (2016c). *Eye health in sports and recreation.* Retrieved from https://www.aao.org/eye-health/diseases/injuries-sports

American Academy of Ophthalmology (AAO). (2016d). *Protective eyewear.* Retrieved from https://www.aao.org/eye-health/tips-prevention/injuries-protective-eyewear

American Academy of Ophthalmology (AAO). (2016e). *Eye injuries at home.* Retrieved from https://www.aao.org/eye-health/tips-prevention/injuries-in-home

American Academy of Ophthalmology (AAO). (2016f). *Preventing eye injuries.* Retrieved from https://www.aao.org/eye-health/diseases/preventing-injuries

American Academy of Ophthalmology (AAO). (2016g). *Children's eye injuries: Prevention and care.* Retrieved from https://www.aao.org/eye-health/tips-prevention/injuries-children

American Academy of Ophthalmology (AAO). (2017). *Glaucoma, congenital or infantile.* Retrieved from http://eyewiki.aao.org/Glaucoma,_Congenital_Or_Infantile

American Association for Pediatric Ophthalmology and Strabismus (AAPOS). (2014a). *Vision screening.* Retrieved from http://www.aapos.org/terms/conditions/107

American Association for Pediatric Ophthalmology and Strabismus (AAPOS). (2014b). *Glaucoma for children.* Retrieved from http://www.aapos.org/terms/conditions/55

American Association for Pediatric Ophthalmology and Strabismus (AAPOS). (2015). *Cataract.* Retrieved from http://www.aapos.org/terms/conditions/31

American Optometric Association (AOA). (2015). *Infant vision: Birth to 24 months of age.* Retrieved from http://www.aoa.org/patients-and-public/good-vision-throughout-life/childrens-vision/infant-vision-birth-to-24-months-of-age?sso=y

American Optometric Association (AOA). (n.d.a). *Nutrition and cataracts.* Retrieved from http://www.aoa.org/patients-and-public/caring-for-your-vision/nutrition/nutrition-and-cataracts?sso=y

American Optometric Association (AOA). (n.d.b). *Caring for your vision: Protecting your eyes at work.* Retrieved from http://www.aoa.org/patients-and-public/caring-for-your-vision/protecting-your-vision?sso=y#4

American Speech-Language-Hearing Association (ASHA). (2015a). *Noise.* Retrieved from http://www.asha.org/public/hearing/Noise

American Speech-Language-Hearing Association (ASHA). (2015b). *Who should be screened for hearing loss?* Retrieved from http://www.asha.org/public/hearing/Who-Should-be-Screened/

American Speech-Language-Hearing Association (ASHA). (n.d.a). *Causes of hearing loss in children.* Retrieved from http://www.asha.org/public/hearing/disorders/causes.htm

American Speech-Language-Hearing Association (ASHA). (n.d.b). *Degree of hearing loss.* Retrieved from http://www.asha.org/public/hearing/Degree-of-Hearing-Loss/

Becker, R. F., & Dutelle, A. W. (2013). *Criminal investigation*. Burlington, MA: Jones & Bartlett.

Bhattacharyya, N., & Kepnes, L. J. (2015). Contemporary assessment of the prevalence of smell and taste problems in adults. *The Laryngoscope, 125*(5), 1102–1106.

Blackburn, J., Levitan, E. B., MacLennan, P. A., Owsley, C., & McGwin, G. Jr. (2012). A case-crossover study of risk factors for occupational eye injuries. *Journal of Occupational and Environmental Medicine, 54*(1), 42–47.

BrightFocus Foundation. (2015a). *Age-related macular degeneration: Facts & figures*. Retrieved from http://www.brightfocus.org/macular/article/age-related-macular-facts-figures

BrightFocus Foundation. (2015b). *Screening & diagnosis*. Retrieved from http://www.brightfocus.org/macular/diagnosis-and-screening-tests

BrightFocus Foundation. (2015c). *Treatments for age-related macular degeneration*. Retrieved from http://www.brightfocus.org/macular/article/treatments-age-related-macular

BrightFocus Foundation. (n.d.a). *Prevention & risk factors*. Retrieved from http://www.brightfocus.org/glaucoma/prevention-and-risk-factors

BrightFocus Foundation. (n.d.b). *Prevention & risk factors*. Retrieved from http://www.brightfocus.org/macular/prevention-and-risk-factors

Center for Hearing, Speech and Language. (2014). *How loud is it?* Retrieved from http://www.chsl.org/soundchart.php

Centers for Disease Control and Prevention (CDC). (2014). *Summary health statistics for U.S. adults: National health interview survey, 2012*. Retrieved from http://www.cdc.gov/nchs/data/series/sr_10/sr10_260.pdf

Centers for Disease Control and Prevention (CDC). (2015a). *The new smoking story: Going blind*. Retrieved from http://www.cdc.gov/features/smoking-eyesight/

Centers for Disease Control and Prevention (CDC). (2015b). *Promoting hearing health in schools*. Retrieved from http://www.cdc.gov/healthy-schools/noise/promoting.htm

Centers for Disease Control and Prevention (CDC). (2015c). *Eye safety*. Retrieved from http://www.cdc.gov/niosh/topics/eye/

Centers for Disease Control and Prevention (CDC). (2015d). *Guillain-Barre syndrome*. Retrieved from http://www.cdc.gov/vaccinesafety/concerns/guillain-barre-syndrome.html

Centers for Disease Control and Prevention. (CDC). (2017). *Noise and hearing loss prevention*. Retrieved from http://www.cdc.gov/niosh/topics/noise/default.html

Cheung, C. M. G., Tai, E. S., Kawasaki, R., Tay, W. T., Lee, J. L., Hamzah, H., & Wong, T. Y. (2012). Prevalence of and risk factors for age-related macular degeneration in a multiethnic Asian cohort. *Archives of Ophthalmology, 130*(4), 480–486.

Chou, C-F., Cotch, M. F., Vitale, S., Zhang, X., Klein, R., Friedman, D. S., . . . Saaddine, J. B. (2013). Age-related eye diseases and visual impairment among U.S. adults. *American Journal of Preventive Medicine, 45*(1), 29–35.

Chupkov, M. (2016). *Falls top list of causes for eye injuries in United States*. Retrieved from http://www.aao.org/eye-health/news/falls-are-leading-cause-of-eye-injuries-in-us

Cleveland Clinic. (2017). *Hearing loss in children*. Retrieved from http://my.clevelandclinic.org/services/head-neck/diseases-conditions/hearing-loss-children

Colby, K. (2014). Eye contusions and lacerations. *Merck Manuals*. Retrieved from https://www.merckmanuals.com/professional/injuries;-poisoning/eye-trauma/eye-contusions-and-lacerations

Court, H., McLean, G., Guthrie, B., Mercer, S. W., & Smith, D. J. (2014). Visual impairment is associated with physical and mental comorbidities in older adults: A cross-sectional study. *BMC Medicine, 12*, 181.

Dawes, P., Cruickshanks, K. J., Moore, D. R., Edmondson-Jones, M., McCormack, A., Fortnum, H., & Munro, K. J. (2014). Cigarette smoking, passive smoking, alcohol consumption, and hearing loss. *Journal of the Association for Research in Otolaryngology, 15*(4), 663–674.

DiFazio, M. P., Patel, N. C., Tseng, B. S., Chhibber, S., & Patel, M. N. (2014). *Pediatric Guillain-Barré syndrome*. Retrieved from http://emedicine.medscape.com/article/1180594-overview

Family Practice Notebook. (n.d.). *Eye injury*. Retrieved from http://www.fpnotebook.com/eye/exam/Eyinjry.htm

Fisher, D. E., Klein, B. E. K., Wong, T. Y., Rotter, J. I., Li, X., Shrager, S., . . . Cotch, M. F. (2016). Incidence of age-related macular degeneration in a multi-ethnic United States population. *Ophthalmology 123*(6): 1297-1308.doi: 10.1016/j.ophtha.2015.12.026.

Foundation for Peripheral Neuropathy. (2015). *Home page*. Retrieved from https://www.foundationforpn.org/index.cfm

Franks, J. (2013). *Glaucoma in seniors: Symptoms & care*. Retrieved from http://www.aplaceformom.com/senior-care-resources/articles/glaucoma-in-seniors

Freedman, J., Sinert, R. H., & Aherne, A. (2015). *Acute-angle closure glaucoma: Epidemiology*. Retrieved from http://emedicine.medscape.com/article/798811-overview#a6

Glaucoma Research Foundation. (2013). *Traumatic glaucoma*. Retrieved from http://www.glaucoma.org/glaucoma/traumatic-glaucoma.php

Glaucoma Research Foundation. (2014). *Glaucoma facts and stats*. Retrieved from http://www.glaucoma.org/glaucoma/glaucoma-facts-and-stats.php

Glaucoma Research Foundation. (2015a). *Medication guide*. Retrieved from http://www.glaucoma.org/treatment/medication-guide.php

Glaucoma Research Foundation. (2015b). *Glaucoma facts and stats*. Retrieved from http://www.glaucoma.org/glaucoma/glaucoma-facts-and-stats.php

Glaucoma Research Foundation. (2016). *Alternative medicine*. Retrieved from http://www.glaucoma.org/treatment/alternative-medicine.php

Health Communities. (2015). *Cataracts*. Retrieved from http://www.healthcommunities.com/cataracts/overview-of-cataracts.shtml

Herdman, T. H. & Kamitsuru, S. (Eds.). *Nursing Diagnoses—Definitions and Classification 2015–2017* . Copyright © 2014, 1994–2014 NANDA International. Used by arrangement with John Wiley & Sons, Inc. Companion website: www.wiley.com/go/nursingdiagnoses

Huang, W. (2014). Pediatric glaucoma: A review of the basics. *Review of Ophthalmology*. Retrieved from http://www.reviewofophthalmology.com/content/d/pediatric_patient/c/47468/

Jindal, A. P., Salim, S., & Boonyaleephan, S. (2014). Glaucoma management in pregnancy and post-partum. Retrieved from the American Academy of Ophthalmology website: http://eyewiki.aao.org/Glaucoma_management_in_pregnancy_and_post-partum

Johnson, M. I. (2012). *Transcutaneous electrical nerve stimulation (TENS)*. eLS. doi:10.1002/9780470015902.a0024044

Joint Committee on Infant Hearing. (2007). Year 2007 position statement: Principles and guidelines for early hearing detection and intervention programs. *Pediatrics, 120*(4), 898–921.

Kilinc, M., Livanelioglu, A., Yildirim, S. A., & Tan, E. (2014). Effects of transcutaneous electrical nerve stimulation in patients with peripheral and central neuropathic pain. *Journal of Rehabilitation Medicine, 46*(5), 454–460.

Koerner, F., Koerner-Stiefbold, U., & Garwig, J. (2012). Systemic corticosteroids reduce the risk of cellophane membranes after retinal detachment surgery: A prospective randomized placebo-controlled double-blind clinical trial. *Graefe's Archive for Clinical and Experimental Ophthalmology, 250*(7), 981–987.

Kote, G. S. S., Bhat, A. N., K, T., Ismail, M. H., & Gupta, A. (2013). Peripheral insensate neuropathy—Is height a risk factor? *Journal of Clinical & Diagnostic Research, 7*(2), 296–301.

Louraki, M., Karayianni, C., Kanaka-Gantenbein, C., Katsalouli, M., & Karavanaki, K. (2012). Peripheral neuropathy in children with type 1 diabetes. *Diabetes & Metabolism, 38*(4), 281–289.

Malaty, J., & Malaty, I. A. (2013). Smell and taste disorders in primary care. *American Family Physician, 88*(12), 852–859.

Mansberger, S. L., Romero, F. C., Smith, N. H., Johnson, C. A., Cioffi, G. A., Edmunds, B., . . . Becher, T. M. (2005). Causes of visual impairment and common eye problems in northwest American Indians and Alaska Natives. *American Journal of Public Health, 95*(5), 881–886.

Margrain, T., Nollett, C., Shearn, J., Stanford, M., Edwards, R., Ryan, B., . . . Smith, D. (2012). The Depression in Visual Impairment Trial (DEPVIT): Trial design and protocol. *BMC Psychiatry, 12*(57). doi:10.1186/1471-22X-12-57

Marieb, E. N., & Hoehn, K. (2007). *Human anatomy & physiology* (7th ed., p. 455). Hoboken, NJ: Benjamin Cummings.

Martin, L. J. (2014). Aging changes in the senses. *Medline Plus*. Retrieved from https://www.nlm.nih.gov/medlineplus/ency/article/004013.htm

Mayo Clinic. (2015). *Apraclonidine (ophthalmic route): Side effects*. Retrieved from http://www.mayo-clinic.org/drugs-supplements/apraclonidine-ophthalmic-route/side-effects/drg-20062024

Mayo Clinic. (2017a). *Cataracts: Overview*. Retrieved from http://www.mayoclinic.org/diseases-conditions/cataracts/home/ovc-20215123

Mayo Clinic. (2017b). *Cataracts: Treatment*. Retrieved from http://www.mayoclinic.org/diseases-conditions/cataracts/diagnosis-treatment/txc-20215217

Mayo Clinic. (2017c). *Peripheral neuropathy: Overview*. Retrieved from http://www.mayoclinic.org/diseases-conditions/peripheral-neuropathy/home/ovc-20204944

Mayo Clinic. (2017d). *Hearing loss*. Retrieved from http://www.mayoclinic.org/diseases-conditions/hearing-loss/basics/definition/con-20027684

Mayo Clinic. (2017e). *Dry macular degeneration: Overview*. Retrieved from http://www.mayoclinic.org/diseases-conditions/dry-macular-degeneration/home/ovc-20164874

Mayo Clinic. (2017f). *Wet macular degeneration: Overview*. Retrieved from http://www.mayoclinic.org/diseases-conditions/wet-macular-degeneration/home/ovc-20164274

Morris, C. A. (2014). *Side effects of weed*. Retrieved from http://floridamarijuanainfo.org/medical-marijuana-in-florida/side-effects-of-weed/

National Eye Institute (NEI). (2010). *Statistics and data*. Retrieved from https://nei.nih.gov/eyedata

National Eye Institute (NEI). (2013). *NIH study provides clarity on supplements for protection against blinding eye disease*. Retrieved from https://nei.nih.gov/news/pressreleases/050513

National Eye Institute (NEI). (2014). *Age-related macular degeneration: What you should know*. Retrieved from https://nei.nih.gov/catalog/age-related-macular-degeneration-what-you-should-know

National Eye Institute (NEI). (2015a). *Facts about cataract*. Retrieved from https://nei.nih.gov/health/cataract/cataract_facts

National Eye Institute (NEI). (2015b). *Facts about age-related macular degeneration*. Retrieved from https://nei.nih.gov/health/maculardegen/armd_facts

National Institute of Neurological Disorders and Stroke (NINDS). (2015). *Peripheral neuropathy fact sheet*. Retrieved from http://www.ninds.nih.gov/disorders/peripheralneuropathy/detail_peripheralneuropathy.htm

National Institute on Deafness and Other Communication Disorders (NIDCD). (2015). *Quick statistics*. Retrieved from http://www.nidcd.nih.gov/health/statistics/pages/quick.aspx

National Institutes of Health (NIH). (2016). *Study of TENS in reducing symptoms of peripheral neuropathy induced by chemotherapy (CIPN)*. Retrieved from https://clinicaltrials.gov/ct2/show/NCT02107417

National Library of Medicine. (2013). *Lidocaine transdermal patch*. Retrieved from https://www.nlm.nih.gov/medlineplus/druginfo/meds/a603026.html

National Library of Medicine. (2015). *Slit-lamp exam*. Retrieved from http://www.nlm.nih.gov/medlineplus/ency/article/003880.htm

NHS. (2014). *Charcot-Marie-Tooth disease: Symptoms*. Retrieved from http://www.nhs.uk/Conditions/Charcot-Marie-Tooth-disease/Pages/Symptoms.aspx

Paul, A., Bandyopadhyay, K. H., & Patro, V. (2012). Anesthetic management of a parturient with Guillain-Barre syndrome posted for emergency caesarian section. *Journal of Obstetric Anaesthesia and Critical Care, 2*(1), 40–43.

Prieto-Flores, M., Forjaz, M., Fernandez-Mayoralas, G., Rojo-Perez, F., & Martinez-Martin, P. (2011). Factors associated with loneliness of noninstitutionalized and institutionalized older adults. *Journal of Aging and Health, 23*(1), 177–194.

Quandt, S., Schulz, M., Talton, J., Verma, A., & Arcury, T. (2012). Occupational eye injuries experienced by migrant farmworkers. *Journal of Agromedicine, 17*(1), 63–69.

Rosen, B. A. (2012). Guillain-Barre syndrome. *Pediatrics in Review, 33*(4), 164–171.

Royal National Institute for Deaf People. (n.d.). *Levels of hearing loss*. Retrieved from https://www.actiononhearingloss.org.uk/your-hearing/about-deafness-and-hearing-loss/glossary/levels-of-hearing-loss.aspx

Safe Kids Worldwide. (2015). *Sports and recreation safety fact sheet*. Retrieved from http://www.safekids.org/sites/default/files/documents/skw_sports_fact_sheet_feb_2015.pdf

Salim, S. (2014). Glaucoma in pregnancy. *Current Opinions in Ophthalmology, 25*(2), 93–97.

Seattle Children's Hospital. (n.d.). *Degree of hearing loss*. Retrieved from https://www.seattlechildrens.org/pdf/degree-hearingloss-chart.pdf

Shahbazi, S., Studnicki, J., & Warner-Hillard, C. W. (2015). A cross-sectional retrospective analysis of the racial and geographic variations in cataract surgery. *PLoS One, 10*(11), e0142459.

Stam, M., Kostense, P. J., Lemke, U., Merkus, P., Smit, J. H., Festen, J. M., & Kramer, S. E. (2014). Comorbidity in adults with hearing difficulties: Which chronic medical conditions are related to hearing impairment? *International Journal of Audiology, 53*(6), 392–401.

Stamper, R. L. (2012). *What can I do to prevent glaucoma?* Retrieved from http://www.glaucoma.org/gleams/what-can-i-do-to-prevent-glaucoma.php

Storey, P., Munoz, B., Friedman, D., & West, S. (2013). Racial differences in lens opacity incidence and progression: The Salisbury Eye Evaluation (SEE) study. *Investigative Ophthalmology & Visual Science, 54*(4), 3010–3018.

Treas, L. S., & Wilkinson, J. M. (2014). *Basic nursing: Concepts, skills, & reasoning*. Philadelphia, PA: F.A. Davis Company.

United Nations. (2006). *Convention on the rights of persons with disabilities*. Retrieved from http://www.un.org/disabilities/convention/conventionfull.shtml

University of Michigan Kellogg Eye Center. (n.d.). *Detached retina*. Retrieved from http://www.kellogg.umich.edu/patientcare/conditions/detached.retina.html#risk

U.S. Preventive Services Task Force. (2011). Vision screening for children one to five years of age: Recommendation statement. *American Family Physician, 84*(2), 221–222.

Varma, R., Bressler, N. M., & Doan, Q. V. (2014). Prevalence of and risk factors for diabetic macular edema in the United States. *JAMA Ophthalmology, 132*(11): 1334–1340. doi:10.1001/jamaophthalmol.2014.2854

Vasudev, R., & Raina, T. R. (2014). A rare case of Guillain-Barre syndrome in pregnancy treated with plasma exchange. *Asian Journal of Transfusion Science, 8*(1), 59–60.

World Health Organization. (2017). *Deafness and hearing loss*. Retrieved from http://www.who.int/mediacentre/factsheets/fs300/en/

Wu, L., & Pakalnis, V. A. (2014). *Postoperative retinal detachment*. Retrieved from http://emedicine.medscape.com/article/1224609-overview#showall

Yonekawa, Y., Chodosh, J., & Eliott, D. (2013). Surgical techniques in the management of perforating injuries of the globe. *International Ophthalmology Clinics, 53*(4), 127–137.

Zafar, M. S. H., Naqash, M. M., Bhat, T. A., & Malik, G. M. (2013). Guillain-Barre syndrome in pregnancy: An unusual case. *Journal of Family Medicine and Primary Care, 2*(1), 90–91.

Zhang, X., Cotch, M. F., Ryskulova, A., Primo, S. A., Nair, P., Chou, C-F., . . . Saaddine, J. B. (2012). Vision health disparities in the United States by race/ethnicity, education, and economic status: Findings from two nationally representative surveys. *American Journal of Ophthalmology, 154*, S53–S62.

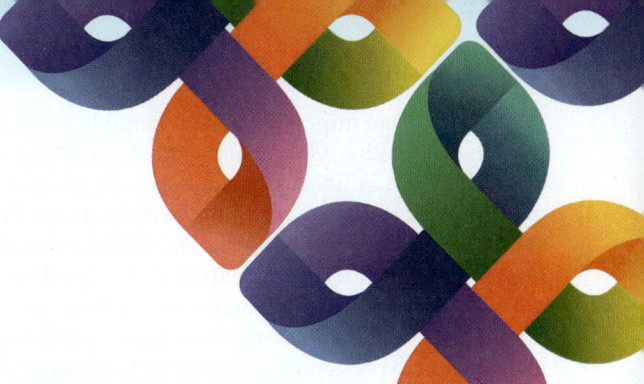

Module 19
Sexuality

Module Outline and Learning Outcomes

The Concept of Sexuality

Development of Sexuality
19.1 Outline the development of sexuality.

Sexual Health
19.2 Define and analyze the components of sexual health.

Alterations in Sexual Function
19.3 Differentiate alterations in sexuality.

Concepts Related to Sexuality
19.4 Outline the relationship between sexuality and other concepts.

Health Promotion
19.5 Explain the promotion of healthy sexuality.

Nursing Assessment
19.6 Differentiate among common assessment procedures and tests used to examine sexuality.

Independent Interventions
19.7 Analyze independent interventions nurses can implement for patients with alterations in sexuality.

Collaborative Therapies
19.8 Summarize collaborative therapies used by interprofessional teams for patients with alterations in sexuality.

Lifespan Considerations
19.9 Differentiate considerations related to the care of patients with alterations in sexuality throughout the lifespan.

Sexuality Exemplars

Exemplar 19.A Family Planning
19.A Analyze family planning as it relates to sexuality.

Exemplar 19.B Menopause
19.B Analyze menopause as it relates to sexuality.

Exemplar 19.C Menstrual Dysfunction
19.C Analyze menstrual dysfunction as it relates to sexuality.

Exemplar 19.D Sexual Dysfunctions
19.D Analyze sexual dysfunctions as they relate to sexuality.

Exemplar 19.E Sexually Transmitted Infections
19.E Analyze sexually transmitted infections as they relate to sexuality.

 ## The Concept of Sexuality

Concept Key Terms

Anal stimulation, 1450	Excitement phase, 1450	Intimacy, 1446	Phimosis, 1458	Sexual orientation, 1448
Anorgasmia, 1457	Galactorrhea, 1462	Masturbation, 1449	Plateau phase, 1450	Sexual response cycle, 1450
Balanitis, 1458	Gender dysphoria, 1449	Meatal stenosis, 1459	Primary sex characteristics, 1444	Sexual self-concept, 1446
Body image, 1446	Gender identity, 1447	Menarche, 1445	Prostatectomy, 1456	Spermarche, 1470
Climacteric, 1445	Gender-role behavior, 1447	Menopause, 1446	Puberty, 1444	Tanner stages, 1444
Colostrum, 1462	Genital intercourse, 1450	Menstruation, 1445	Rectocele, 1463	Testicular torsion, 1459
Cryptorchidism, 1459	Gynecomastia, 1452	Nabothian cysts, 1465	Resolution phase, 1451	Testosterone, 1444
Cystocele, 1463	Hydrocele, 1459	Nocturnal emissions, 1444	Secondary sex characteristics, 1444	Thelarche, 1444
Dissatisfaction problems, 1452	Hypospadias, 1459	Oral–genital sex, 1450	Semen, 1451	Transgender, 1449
Dyspareunia, 1457	Impotence, 1456	Orgasmic phase, 1450	Sensate focus, 1469	Transsexual, 1449
Epispadias, 1459	Intersex, 1449	Paraphimosis, 1458	Sexual health, 1446	Varicocele, 1459
Estrogen, 1444		Perimenopause, 1446		

Sexuality is an important part of being human. It contributes to healthy relationships and a sense of well-being. Sexuality is an individually expressed and highly personal phenomenon, and its meaning evolves from life experiences. Physiologic, psychosocial, religious, and cultural factors influence individual sexuality and lead to the wide range of attitudes and behaviors seen in humans. There are no normal, universal sexual behaviors. Satisfying or "normal" sexual expression can generally be described as whatever behaviors give mutual pleasure and satisfaction to the adults involved, without threat of coercion or injury to self or others.

Development of Sexuality

The development of sexuality begins at conception and continues throughout the lifespan. Although this section discusses development in terms of sexuality, nurses need to consider sexuality within the larger context of the development of the individual and the family and environmental contexts.

Birth to 12 Years

Several months after birth, when babies find their fingers and toes, they also find their genitals. They seem to experience a pleasurable sensation from the touch, but this is not a sexual experience. By the age of 3 years, more purposeful masturbation begins, and the orgasmic response is quite common, although boys do not ejaculate until after puberty. By age 2½ or 3, children know what gender they are and have beginning awareness of genital differences between boys and girls.

Around age 9 or 10, the first physical changes of **puberty**, or the process of sexual maturation, begin: the development of breast buds (**thelarche**) in girls and the growth of pubic hair in both boys and girls. As the adrenal glands mature, they produce more **testosterone** (the primary male sex hormone) and **estrogen** (the primary female sex hormone), which contribute to the first experiences of sexual attraction to another individual. Sexual maturity ratings based on **Tanner stages** may be assigned; these stages are defined by physical growth of the breasts and pubic hair in girls and the genitalia and pubic hair in boys. **Figure 19–1 》** depicts Tanner stages for breasts. **Figure 19–2 》** depicts Tanner stages for pubic hair changes in girls, and **Figure 19–3 》** shows Tanner stages for genital growth and pubic hair changes in boys.

Adolescence

During early adolescence (ages 12–13), primary and secondary sex characteristics continue to develop. **Primary sex characteristics** involve the reproductive organs themselves, whereas **secondary sex characteristics** involve bodily traits that develop over time and are influenced by a person's sex but not directly involved in reproduction.

For boys, the testes and scrotum increase in size, the skin over the scrotum becomes darker, pubic hair continues to grow, and axillary sweating begins. Development of the genitals to adult size takes approximately 5–6 years. At about ages 13–15, boys start to experience **nocturnal emissions** (spontaneous orgasm), or "wet dreams." The boy's voice

changes as his genitals grow, and he experiences a dramatic growth in height as puberty continues.

Boys mature about 2 years later than girls. Boys are often awkward, self-conscious, and concerned about body changes during this period. Because the onset of puberty for boys is not marked by an event as apparent as menses in girls, parents are less likely to talk with boys about sex and the sexual changes occurring in their body (Ball et al., 2017).

For girls, adolescence is marked by broadening of the pelvis and hips, continued development of breast tissue, ongoing pubic hair growth, and onset of axillary sweating. Also during this period, a girl's vaginal secretions become milky and

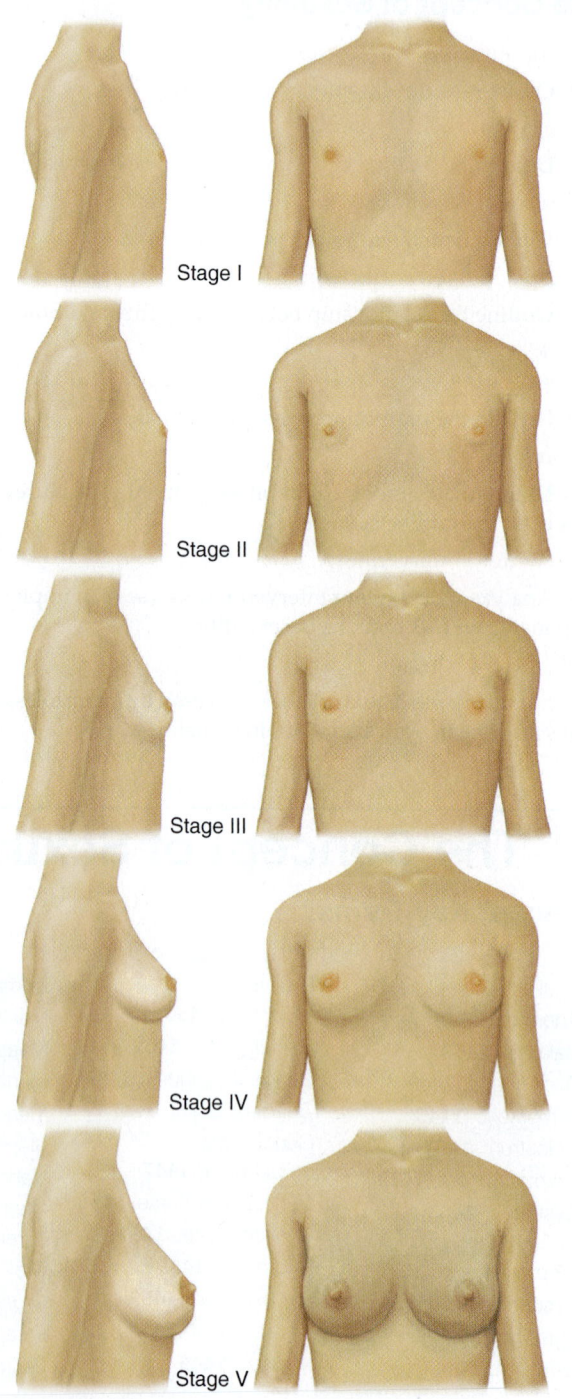

Stage I

Stage II

Stage III

Stage IV

Stage V

Figure 19–1 》 Tanner stages for the breasts.

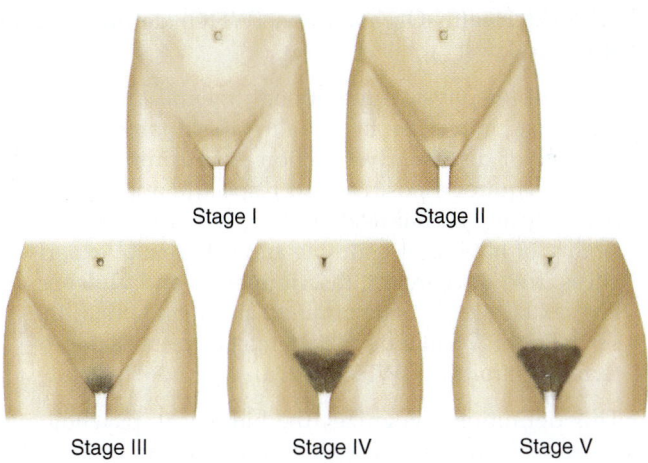

Stage I   Stage II

Stage III   Stage IV   Stage V

Figure 19–2 》 Tanner stages for pubic hair changes in girls.

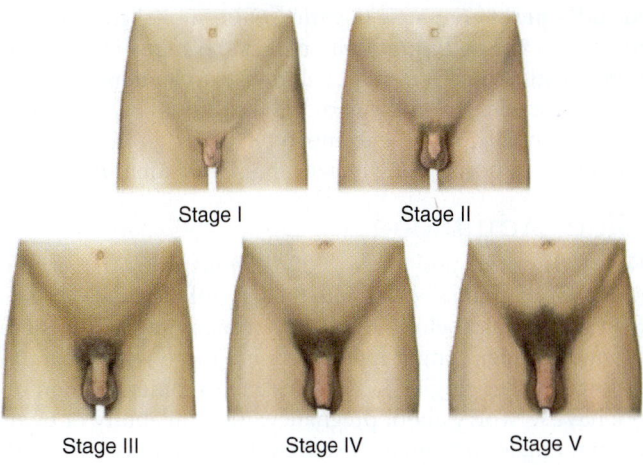

Stage I   Stage II

Stage III   Stage IV   Stage V

Figure 19–3 》 Tanner stages for genital and pubic hair changes in boys.

change from an alkaline to an acid pH. **Menarche** (first menses) usually occurs within 2 years of the start of breast and pubic hair changes. In the United States, the average age of menarche is 12 years old (Office on Women's Health, 2014a).

During their first few months or years of **menstruation**, girls may not have regular monthly periods, which can lead to embarrassment from unexpected bleeding and the stained clothing that results. Girls should therefore be taught to recognize subtle signs of impending menstruation, such as tender breasts and water retention or bloating. They should also be counseled regarding the use of feminine hygiene products so they can make intelligent choices about use of these products. In particular, parents and nurses should advise teenage girls to cleanse their hands thoroughly before inserting a tampon, to change tampons frequently, to alternate tampons with pads, and to use pads at night. These measures help decrease the risk of infection, including the risk of toxic shock syndrome, a particular type of *Staphylococcus aureus* infection (see the Patient Teaching feature). Thorough cleaning of the genital area and wiping from front to back also decrease the risk of infection and help prevent odors.

Patient Teaching
Preventing and Recognizing Toxic Shock Syndrome

Although menstruation-related staphylococcal toxic shock syndrome (TSS) is rare today, proper teaching is a critical component in its prevention, especially among women ages 15–25, who represent the group at greatest risk. Nurses should advise patients to change tampons every 4–8 hours, alternate tampons with pads, and use tampons with the lowest absorbency necessary for their menstrual flow.

Both patients and nurses should also be familiar with the symptoms of TSS, including nausea, vomiting, sudden high fever, chills, dizziness, diarrhea, headaches, hypotension, conjunctivitis, sunburn-like rash, and peeling skin on the hands and feet. When staphylococcal TSS is suspected, immediate hospitalization is necessary to prevent shock, organ damage, and/or death (Cleveland Clinic, 2014a).

When working with adolescents, nurses must also be aware that sexual experimentation frequently occurs at younger ages than it did in previous decades. Of 13,000 high school students surveyed in 2013, 5.6% had experienced sexual intercourse before age 13; 46.8% of the students in the survey sample had engaged in sexual intercourse at least one time; and 15.0% had engaged in intercourse with four or more partners during their life (Centers for Disease Control and Prevention [CDC], 2014a). The high incidence of sexual intercourse puts teenagers at risk for sexually transmitted infections (STIs) and unintended pregnancies. In 2013, about half of the 20 million new STIs in the United States were among individuals ages 15–24, and about 273,000 girls ages 15–19 gave birth (CDC, 2015a).

All adolescents want to know about sexual behaviors, but they are often uneasy discussing these concerns with their parents. Therefore, nurses and schools must be prepared to provide adolescents with accurate information about sexuality and sexual development. Also, during the nursing assessment, nurses should ask teenagers directly what they know about sex, contraception, and reproduction. They should provide factual information about sex, sexual actions and their consequences, an individual's right to make decisions regarding personal sexual expression, and the responsibilities of each individual with respect to sexual activity.

Young and Middle Adulthood

In young adulthood, many (but not all) individuals begin to form intimate relationships with long-term implications. Young adults are often concerned about normal sexual response for both themselves and their partners. Couples need to communicate their needs to one another early in their courtship so that a successful intimate relationship can develop and grow. Young adults should also be aware that sexual needs and responses may change, so each partner should listen and respond to the needs of the other.

During middle adulthood, both men and women experience decreased hormone production, causing the **climacteric** (transitional period in reproductive life). In men, this transition involves a reduction in Leydig cells and androgen with continued spermatogenesis. In women, the climacteric includes **perimenopause** (a period of hormonal change during which the body gradually makes the transition toward permanent infertility), and it culminates in **menopause** (cessation of menses) and the end of the ability to bear children (Blackburn, 2013). These events often affect an individual's sexual self-concept, body image, and sexual identity.

Older Adulthood

Research performed since 2000 demonstrates that many older adults enjoy sex well into their eighth decade. Reasons for this finding include the fact that many individuals are living healthier, longer lives; there are more widowed and divorced older singles looking for mates; older women do not have to worry about pregnancy; the availability of treatment for male and female sexual dysfunctions has increased; and society is increasingly accepting of sexual activity among older adults (Foster et al., 2012; Poynten, Grulich, & Templeton, 2013; Stewart & Graham, 2013).

Even with these changes, older adults may experience significant changes in sexual response. For men, more time may be needed to achieve an erection and to ejaculate, more direct genital stimulation is required to achieve an erection, erections may be less firm, the volume of ejaculated fluid decreases, and the intensity of contractions with orgasm may decrease. The time to the next erection will also be longer. In addition, erectile dysfunction (ED) becomes more common (Mayo Clinic, 2014a, 2014b). Older women remain capable of multiple orgasms and may, in fact, experience an increase in sexual desire after menopause. However, vaginal lubrication and elasticity decrease with menopause and the accompanying decline in estrogen, and the phases of the sexual response cycle may take longer to occur.

Older adults continue to need **intimacy**—chosen emotional interconnectedness between two individuals that includes mutual caring and responsibility. Intimacy may entail close body contact, hand holding, kissing, eye contact, closeness, companionship, verbal expressions of affection, social support, and meaningful activity (Kaplan & Berkman, 2013). Close friendships, sexual relationships, strong ties to family members, and beloved pets can all contribute to meeting an older adult's need for intimacy. However, these are not always available.

Age-related changes in sexual response in both men and women do not preclude a satisfying sex life. Because arousal takes longer for both partners, foreplay is even more important for older adults than for younger adults. Hugging, kissing, and caressing are sexual activities that both men and women enjoy. These activities can be preludes to sexual intercourse or satisfying activities in themselves. In general, older adults are open minded and knowledgeable about sexual matters, but the loss of a partner or problems with health status are common barriers to sexual expression in this population (DeLemater, 2012).

Sexual Health

Sexual health is an individual and constantly changing phenomenon that falls within the wide range of human sexual thoughts, feelings, needs, and desires. An individual's degree of sexual health is best determined by that individual, sometimes with the assistance of qualified professionals.

The World Health Organization (WHO) defines **sexual health** as follows:

[A] state of physical, emotional, mental and social well-being in relation to sexuality; it is not merely the absence of disease, dysfunction or infirmity. Sexual health requires a positive and respectful approach to sexuality and sexual relationships, as well as the possibility of having pleasurable and safe sexual experiences, free of coercion, discrimination and violence. For sexual health to be attained and maintained, the sexual rights of all individuals must be respected, protected and fulfilled (WHO, 2013a).

This definition recognizes the biological, psychologic, and sociocultural dimensions of sexuality, as well as the existence of certain sexual rights. Some of the rights identified by such groups as the WHO (2013b) and the World Association for Sexual Health (2013) include:

- The right to sexual freedom, including the right to decide to be sexually active or not and the right to choose sexual partners
- The right to sexual autonomy, integrity, privacy, and equity
- The right to sexual and reproductive healthcare services for the prevention and treatment of all sexual concerns, problems, and disorders
- The right to sexual education to seek, receive, and impart information in relation to sexuality
- The right to make free and responsible reproductive choices, including the decision of whether and when to have children.

Components of Sexual Health

Sexual health is a key element of personal well-being and is important for individuals of varying degrees of physical ability (see the Focus on Diversity and Culture feature). Five critical components of sexual health are sexual self-concept, body image, gender identity, gender-role behavior, and freedoms and responsibilities. Although each component is unique, they all work in concert to determine a person's sexual well-being.

Sexual Self-Concept

An individual's **sexual self-concept** (or how the individual values him- or herself as a sexual being) determines the gender and kinds of individuals to whom the person is attracted; the individual's values about when, where, how, and with whom he or she expresses his or her sexuality; and the individual's ability to freely choose sexual partners. A positive sexual self-concept enables individuals to form intimate relationships throughout life, whereas a negative sexual self-concept may impede the formation of relationships.

Body Image

Body image is a central part of a person's sense of self, and it is constantly changing. Pregnancy, aging, trauma, disease, and therapies can all alter an individual's appearance and function, thereby affecting the person's body image. In turn, how an individual feels about his or her body influences his or her sexuality. Individuals who feel good about their bodies

Focus on Diversity and Culture
Sexual Health in Individuals with Physical Disability, Disfigurement, and Other Alterations

Sexuality is a critical part of life for all people—including people with physical disabilities, disfigurements, and other alterations such as those that arise from paralysis, amputation, ostomies, and mastectomy. Individuals with these conditions unfortunately often face numerous social, psychologic, and physical roadblocks to sexual behavior and expression. When working with these patients, nurses should take special care to address issues related to sexual health. Some helpful actions may include the following:

- Reassure patients that the onset of physical disability, disfigurement, or another alteration need not mean discontinuation of sexual thoughts, desires, or behaviors.
- Take steps to cultivate positive body image in patients with disabilities and other alterations, including referral to psychologic services and support groups as appropriate.
- Remind patients that intimacy and sexual expression can take many forms other than penetrative sex, including kissing, caressing, and manual and oral stimulation.
- Encourage patients to consider adaptive positioning and use of assistive devices (e.g., specialized cushions, harnesses, and chairs; personal massagers/vibrators) when engaging in sexual activity.

Nurses should remain nonjudgmental when discussing issues of sexuality with patients who have disabilities and other physical alterations so as not to discourage or impede these individuals' interest in intimacy, romance, and sexual activity (Early, 2013; Lundy & James, 2016).

are likely to be comfortable with and enjoy sexual activity. In contrast, individuals who have a poor body image may respond negatively to sexual arousal.

Gender Identity

Gender identity refers to an individual's self-image as a female, male, or transgender person. Gender identity involves not only a biological component but also social and cultural norms. Gender identity is the result of a long series of developmental events that may or may not conform to an individual's apparent biological sex. Once a person's gender identity has been established, it cannot be easily changed. Additional information on variations in gender identity is provided later in the Sexuality and Gender section.

Gender-Role Behavior

Gender-role behavior is the outward expression of an individual's sense of maleness or femaleness, as well as the expression of what is perceived as gender-appropriate behavior. Each society defines its roles for men and women, and these roles are passed to subsequent generations as boys receive reinforcement for behaving in a "masculine" way and girls receive reinforcement for exhibiting "feminine" behaviors. Physical structure, variations in the internal sense of what is male or female, family values, and cultural values also influence gender-role behavior. The extent to which

gender-role behavior is defined by family values and roles varies both among families and among different cultures.

Freedoms and Responsibilities

Finally, sexual health includes both freedoms and responsibilities. Sexually healthy individuals engage in activities that are freely chosen, including both self-pleasuring and shared-pleasuring activities. Individuals also have freedom of their sexual thoughts, feelings, and fantasies, but they are likewise ethically motivated to exercise behavioral, emotional, and social responsibility for themselves. This includes taking steps to prevent unwanted pregnancy and STIs (Lamanna, Riedmann, & Stewart, 2014), knowing how to identify the warnings signs of and protect themselves from dating violence and date rape, and refraining from coercing or forcing sexual experiences on others. (Refer to the module on Trauma for more information.) In addition, all individuals have a responsibility to respect the sexual rights and freedoms of their partners.

Cultural Considerations

Many factors influence an individual's sexuality. Some of the most important include culture, religion, and personal expectations and ethics.

Culture

An individual's sexuality is regulated to some degree by culture. For example, culture influences the sexual nature of dress, rules about marriage, expectations of role behavior and social responsibilities, and specific sex practices. Societal attitudes vary widely. Depending on an individual's culture, premarital and extramarital sex and homosexuality may be unacceptable or tolerated. Polygamy (having several marriage partners) or monogamy (having only one marriage partner) may be the norm. As previously mentioned, gender-role behavior also varies from culture to culture.

Cultures further differ in terms of their attitude toward various aspects of the human body, including, for example, weight as a cultural determinant of attractiveness. Another practice that is often culturally determined is related to dress and nudity. In some Islamic cultures, women cover their entire bodies and faces; some cultures in New Guinea and Australia find complete nudity acceptable.

A culture's sexual attitudes and practices are sometimes controversial. Female circumcision, also known as female genital mutilation (FGM) or female ritual cutting, is a dangerous custom that is common in parts of Africa, Asia, and the Middle East. FGM involves removal of the clitoris, which may be accompanied by removal of the labia and closure of the vaginal entrance except for a small opening. Although FGM is illegal in Canada, the United States, and several African and European countries, female emigrants from countries where FGM is practiced often need medical care.

Male circumcision, or removal of the foreskin of the penis, is legal, less physically damaging, and far more common in Western culture; however, it also is the subject of much discussion. In 1971, the American Academy of Pediatrics (AAP) stated that there were no valid medical indications for circumcising newborns. Since then, research has revealed several benefits of male circumcision, including reduced likelihood of urinary tract infections (UTIs), STIs, HIV infection, and penile cancer. Today, the AAP's official position is that while the benefits of circumcision outweigh the risks, there is not sufficient data to recommend routine circumcision of all male infants and recommends that parents make the decision to circumcise in consultation with their pediatrician and base their decision on the child's best interests and medical needs as informed by religious, cultural, and ethnic traditions (AAP, 2015a).

As described previously, culture influences many aspects of sexuality, and it is so much a part of everyday life that it is often taken for granted. Healthcare providers tend to assume that others, including patients, share their own perspectives. For example, nurses may not realize that cultural prohibitions forbid certain patients from discussing sexual activity or from being physically examined by a healthcare provider of another gender. To provide sensitive nursing care in the realm of sexuality, nurses must avoid projecting their own cultural beliefs and preferences onto others. Furthermore, they must be careful to avoid believing that their own culture is more important than, and preferable to, any other culture (Spector, 2017).

Religion

Like culture, an individual's religion may influence sexual expression. Religious beliefs provide guidelines for acceptable and prohibited sexual behaviors, as well as the consequences of engaging in these behaviors. These guidelines may be detailed and rigid or broad and flexible. For example, some religions view forms of sexual expression other than male–female intercourse as unnatural and hold virginity before marriage to be the rule. Other religions mandate certain practices related to sexuality, such as male circumcision or avoidance of sexual activity while menstruating.

In some cases, a religion's values may conflict with the more flexible societal values that have developed in the United States. Areas of conflict can vary but often include societal acceptance of premarital sex, unwed parenthood, homosexuality, and abortion. These conflicts can create marked anxiety and potential sexual dysfunction in some individuals. Religious and cultural norms can also create conflicts within families. For example, family rejection of an adolescent's sexual orientation or gender identity is the most frequently cited factor for homelessness among lesbian, gay, bisexual, and transgender (LGBT) young people (Durso & Gates, 2012).

Personal Expectations and Ethics

Although ethics is integral to religion, ethical thought and ethical approaches to sexuality can be viewed separately from religion. For centuries, cultures have developed written or unwritten codes of conduct based on ethical principles. Personal expectations concerning sexual behavior come from these cultural norms. Thus, what one individual or culture views as bizarre, perverted, or wrong may be completely natural and right to another. Examples include masturbation, oral or anal intercourse, and cross-dressing. Moreover, many individuals accept a variety of sexual expressions provided they are performed by consenting adults, are practiced in private, and are not harmful. Couples need to explore and communicate clearly about various types of acceptable sexual expression to prevent domination of sexual decision making by one member of the pair.

Sexuality and Gender

Individuals experience and express their sexuality across a continuum; there is no distinct or specific "normal" for all individuals. Further, some people experience and express their gender outside the *gender binary*—the traditional female and male genders. There are also many differences in the priority individuals place on sexuality in their lives. Human expressions of sexuality and gender include sexual orientation, gender identity, erotic preferences, and sexual lifestyle.

Sexual Orientation

An individual's attraction to people of the same sex, the other sex, or both sexes is referred to as **sexual orientation**. Sexual orientation lies along a continuum with a wide range between the two extremes of exclusively heterosexual attraction and exclusively homosexual attraction. Individuals who are attracted to individuals of both genders are referred to as *bisexual*.

The origins of sexual orientation are not well understood. Biological theories describe sexual orientation in terms of the genetic composition of the individual, while psychologic theories stress the role of early learning experiences and cognitive processes. Other theories acknowledge the confluence of genetics and environment in the development of sexual orientation.

Whatever its source, an individual's sexual orientation is enduring and unlikely to change over the course of his or her lifetime. In fact, all major mental health organizations in the United States, including the American Psychological Association, the American Psychiatric Association, and the U.S. Substance Abuse and Mental Health Services Administration, have officially adopted the position that so-called conversion therapy aimed at changing an individual's sexual orientation is not just scientifically unfounded but also more likely to cause psychologic harm than to bring about lasting change in a person's sexual orientation (Drescher, 2015; Human Rights Campaign, 2015).

》 Stay Current: As of October 2015, four U.S. states and the District of Columbia have passed laws prohibiting licensed mental health providers from offering conversion therapy to minors, and 18 other states are considering similar measures. For an up-to-date list of states in which these laws apply, visit http://www.lgbtmap.org/equality-maps/conversion_therapy.

Data from the 2013 National Health Interview Survey indicate that roughly 1.6% of American adults identify as homosexual, 0.7% identify as bisexual, and 1.1% are either unsure of or unwilling to describe their orientation (CDC, 2013a). As these figures suggest, many individuals are uncomfortable disclosing their sexual orientation, in part because they are acutely aware of the discrimination they face in U.S. society. Actual percentages of homosexual, bisexual, and questioning Americans may be somewhat higher; for example, Gallup surveys estimate that 3.6% of American adults identify as LGBT (Cook, 2015). Nurses and other providers should be aware that individuals in these populations are at increased risk for disparities in healthcare access as well as certain health conditions and behaviors—again, partly due to discriminatory forces in American society (Ward et al., 2014).

Gender Identity

Gender identity is both a component of sexual health and one way in which individuals express their sexuality. Western culture is deeply committed to the idea that there are two sexes. Biologically speaking, however, there are many gradations running from female to male. Gender may be clear, a blending of both genders within the same individual, or unclear.

Intersex Individuals

About 1 in every 2000 babies is born with an **intersex** condition, in which contradictions are seen among chromosomal gender, gonadal gender, internal sex organs, and external genital appearance. What this means is that an intersex individual has some parts usually associated with males and some parts usually associated with females. Intersex anatomy may not be apparent at birth, although the gender of some intersex infants is ambiguous. In other cases, an intersex condition is not detected until puberty, until the individual is identified as an infertile adult, or until the individual dies and is autopsied.

》 **Stay Current:** For more information on intersex conditions and other disorders of sexual development, visit the Accord Alliance website at http://www.accordalliance.org.

Transgender and Transsexual Individuals

For some people, their gender identity is not consistent with their sexual anatomy. Today, the term **transgender** is used to describe those individuals whose gender identity and/or gender expression differs from the gender they were assigned at birth. Generally speaking, a *transgender man* is someone who was assigned the female gender at birth but now emotionally and psychologically identifies as a man; a *transgender woman* is someone who was assigned the male gender at birth but now emotionally and psychologically identifies as a woman. In years past, these individuals were often referred to as **transsexual**, although use of this term is now typically limited to those people who have changed or who seek to change their sexual anatomy through medical interventions (GLAAD, 2015a; Planned Parenthood of the Heartland, 2015). Transgender individuals' sexual orientation may be heterosexual, homosexual, or bisexual.

The terms *transgender* and *transsexual* are best used as adjectives, not nouns. Because people in the transgender community differ in how they describe themselves, it is best to ask which term an individual prefers.

》 **Stay Current:** For more information on respectful communication with transgender individuals, visit http://www.glaad.org/transgender/transfaq.

Members of the medical and psychologic professions often consider transgender individuals to be affected by a condition called **gender dysphoria**, which involves the individuals having strong and persistent feelings of discomfort with their assigned genders. The diagnosis of *gender dysphoria*, introduced in the fifth edition of the American Psychiatric Association's *Diagnostic and Statistical Manual of Mental Disorders* (DSM-5), replaces the now-outdated diagnosis of *gender identity disorder*. According to the American Psychiatric Association (2013a, 2013b), although not all transgender individuals will experience distress related to gender incongruence, many will become distressed if a supportive environment and physical interventions such as hormone therapy and/or surgery are not made available to them. Thus, the focus of the DSM-5 diagnosis is on the dysphoria rather than the issue of gender expression. Some advocacy groups reject any formal psychiatric diagnosis related to gender expression, because in their opinion, transgender identity is one of many normal variations on the spectrum of human sexual identity (GLAAD, 2015a).

Transgender individuals face increased risks to their personal safety. More than 50% of transgender individuals report experiencing sexual violence. Experiences of harassment and violence explain, in part, the increased risk for suicide among transgender individuals (FORGE, 2015; GLAAD, 2015b; Haas, Rodgers, & Herman, 2014; National Coalition of Anti-Violence Programs, 2014).

In addition, being transgendered puts women and men at extreme risk of ridicule and humiliation; hate violence; discrimination in hiring, housing, and employment practice; eviction without cause from restaurants and stores; limited access to healthcare and medical treatment; and poverty (Bradford et al., 2012; GLAAD, 2015a).

As outlined in the American Nurses Association Code of Ethics for Nurses (ANA, 2015), nurses have the responsibility to treat all individuals with respect and dignity. This is particularly important when working with transgender individuals, because these patients often face discrimination in healthcare settings. Disrespectful treatment by even a single healthcare provider increases the likelihood that a transgender patient will delay seeking medical care (Zunner & Grace, 2012).

As self-understanding and acceptance increase, many transgender people live part- or full-time as members of the gender with which they identify. Dressing in the clothing typically associated with that gender not only makes their outward appearance consistent with their inner identity and gender role but also increases their comfort with themselves.

Erotic Preferences and Sexual Lifestyle

Over a lifetime, sexual fantasies and single-partner sex are the most common sexual outlets for women and men; single and coupled individuals; and heterosexual, gay, lesbian, and bisexual individuals. Sexual activity may take a variety of forms, including masturbation, oral–genital sex, anal stimulation, and/or genital intercourse.

Masturbation

Masturbation is self-stimulation of the genitals for sexual pleasure. It may be an expression of the ongoing love affair that individuals have with themselves throughout their lifetime. Masturbation is the way individuals discover their erotic feelings and learn about their sexual response. *Mutual masturbation,* or masturbation shared with a partner, can provide sexual pleasuring and intimacy without hurrying to genital interaction before both partners are ready. It is also a safe alternative to unprotected genital sex.

1450 Module 19 Sexuality

Oral–Genital Sex

Oral–genital sex is use of the mouth to stimulate the genitals of a partner. Male-to-female or female-to-female oral–genital sex is called *cunnilingus*. This involves kissing, licking, or sucking of the female genitals, including the mons pubis, vulva, clitoris, labia, and vagina. *Fellatio* is female-to-male or male-to-male oral stimulation of the penis by licking and sucking. *Sixty-nine* is simultaneous oral–genital stimulation by two individuals. Like most sexual activity, oral–genital sex is not completely free of the potential for disease transmission, so safe sex practices should be used.

Anal Stimulation

Anal stimulation can be a source of sexual pleasure because the anus has a rich nerve supply. Stimulation may be applied by the fingers, mouth, or sex toys such as vibrators. The anus is surrounded by strong muscles, and the rectum contains no natural lubrication. Therefore, inserting a finger or penis into the rectum requires relaxation of the muscles and use of water-soluble lubricant.

Genital Intercourse

Genital intercourse is a common form of sexual activity. Among heterosexual couples, *penile–vaginal intercourse* (coitus) is common. During penile–vaginal intercourse, the man moves his penis back and forth along the woman's vaginal walls by rhythmic thrusting movements of his hips. At the same time, the woman may move her own body to match the partner's hip movements. Movements usually continue until orgasm is achieved by one or both partners. Simultaneous orgasm can be difficult to achieve. After coitus, caressing, hugging, and kissing can increase the shared intimacy.

The other form of genital intercourse is *anal intercourse,* during which the penis is inserted into the anus and rectum of the partner. Positions for anal intercourse are similar to those for penile–vaginal intercourse, with minor differences due to the position of the anus.

Current practice dictates the use of a condom in both forms of genital intercourse to prevent disease transmission. Because anorectal tissue is not self-lubricating, a lubricant must be used on the condom during anal sex. Also, because normal bacterial flora from the bowel can produce infection in other parts of the body, the used condom should be removed and another applied before inserting the penis into other body orifices.

There are many other varieties of sexuality that are beyond the scope of this module. These include several or many partners, nudism, swinging, group sex, fetishism, sexual sadism, and sexual masochism. Note that DSM-5 defines some of these sexual interests as disorders, but only if they involve some element of nonconsensual behavior (American Psychiatric Association, 2013a).

The Sexual Response Cycle

The human **sexual response cycle** follows a similar sequence of phases in women and men. This is true regardless of an individual's sexual orientation and regardless of whether the motive for sexual activity is true love or passionate lust. The most common model of the sexual response cycle was proposed by Masters and Johnson in 1966, and it involves four phases: excitement, plateau, orgasm, and resolution (Mark, 2012).

The sexual response cycle starts in the brain with conscious sexual desires. Sexually arousing stimuli, often called *erotic stimuli,* may be real or symbolic. Sight, hearing, smell, touch, and imagination can all invoke arousal. Sexual desire fluctuates within each individual and varies from individual to individual. Someone who suppresses or blocks conscious sexual desires may not experience any physiologic response. Although psychologic issues are the most common causes of lack of sexual desire, medications, drugs, and hormone imbalances can also interfere.

The **excitement phase** of the sexual response cycle involves two primary physiologic changes. *Vasocongestion* is an increase in blood flow to various parts of the body, resulting in erection of the penis and clitoris and swelling of the labia, testes, and breasts. Vasocongestion stimulates sensory receptors within these body parts, which in turn transmit messages to the conscious brain, where they are usually interpreted as pleasurable sensations. When stimulation is continued, vasocongestion increases until it either is released by orgasm or fades away. Likewise, *myotonia*, or an increase in muscle tension, may build until released by orgasm, or it may simply fade away.

Both vasocongestion and myotonia intensify in the next phase of the sexual response cycle, called the **plateau phase**. During this phase, individuals experience strong, prolonged sexual arousal. The plateau phase is typically maintained by physical stimulation. This stimulation can take many forms, from simple touch to full-on intercourse. There is no set period of time for the plateau phase; it can be as long or as brief as the participants wish (Planned Parenthood, 2014).

The **orgasmic phase** is the involuntary climax of sexual tension, accompanied by physiologic and psychologic release. This phase is considered the measurable peak of the sexual experience (see **Figure 19–4** »). Although the entire

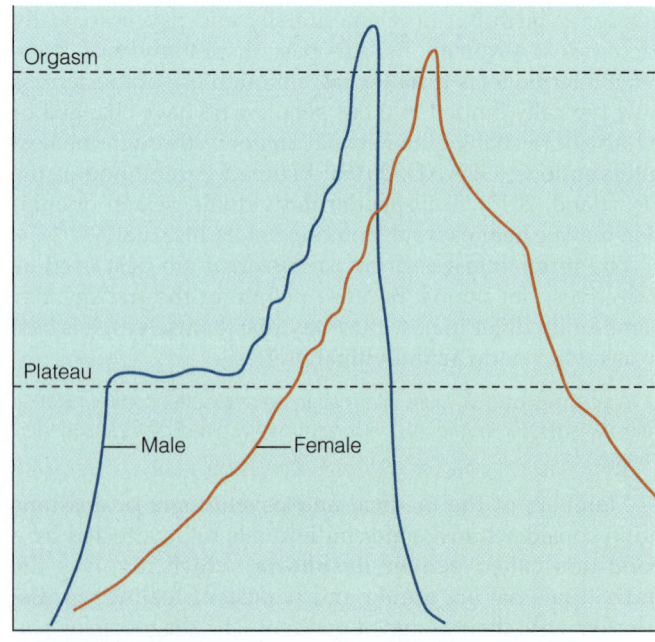

Figure 19–4 » Phases of the sexual response cycle.

body is involved, the major focus of the orgasm is the pelvic region. Male orgasms usually last 10–30 seconds, whereas female orgasms last 10–50 seconds. Men usually experience ejaculation and expel **semen** (a mixture of sperm and bodily secretions) as part of their orgasm. Before puberty and in later years, men may experience orgasms without ejaculation, however.

The **resolution phase**, or period of return to the unaroused state, may last 10–15 minutes after orgasm (or longer if there is no orgasm). This phase is quite varied in women; some women are capable of multiple successive orgasms followed by a longer period of resolution.

Since the 1960s, researchers have proposed several alternatives to Masters and Johnson's four-phase model. Some of these models acknowledge that the human sexual response does not always proceed in a linear series of steps, others reflect the fact that orgasm is not always achieved, and still others include nonphysiologic factors than can influence the sexual response. Despite its shortcomings, the Masters and Johnson model remains the best known and most common model in use today (Carroll, 2013; Mark, 2012).

Alterations in Sexual Function

The ability to engage in sexual behavior is of great importance to most people, but many individuals experience transient problems with their ability to respond to sexual stimulation. A small percentage of individuals will experience lifelong problems. These problems may be generalized to all sexual interactions and settings, or they may be situational, occurring only in specific settings or with specific types of sexual activity.

It is often difficult to sort out the many factors contributing to an individual's or couple's sexual problems. A number of past and current factors are generally involved. These problems can take a variety of forms, and some may even have a genetic component. All of these topics are described in greater detail in the following subsections.

Past and Current Factors

Sociocultural factors that interfere with an individual's sexual function often include a restrictive upbringing accompanied by inadequate sex education. Rigid gender-role socialization may inhibit exploration of sexual activities, positions, toys, and other lovemaking behaviors. If the religion with which an individual is affiliated believes that sex is only for procreation, the individual may have great difficulty celebrating the pleasure and fun of a loving sexual relationship. Another contributing factor for many sexual problems may be parental punishment for normal exploration of the genitals or normal childhood sex play. Also, the pressures of family and work may leave couples with too little time and not enough energy to enjoy sex.

Psychologic factors associated with impaired sexual function may include negative feelings that interfere with the ability to experience pleasure and joy. Some individuals experience guilt when they simply enjoy sex or when they participate in what they label "unusual" sexual activities; they may also have guilt regarding their choice of partner. Adults who have been sexually abused at any time in their lives may experience overwhelming anxiety when faced

with the decision to engage in sex. Common fears associated with sex include fear of pregnancy, STIs, or pain. Because vulnerability and intimacy are inherent in most sexual relationships, fear of these may lead to avoidance of sex. Fear of failure in sexual performance is also common and can become a vicious cycle; that is, fear of failure creates actual failure, which in turn produces more fear. *Spectatoring* is the detached appraisal of sexual performance or the body during a sexual act: "Am I going to lose my erection?" "Am I going to have an orgasm this time?" "My stomach is too flabby." "When did his thighs get that fat?" Such appraisal can limit sexual performance or inhibit feelings of pleasure. Finally, individuals with depression frequently lose interest in sexual activity and may experience a complete loss of sexual desire and fulfillment.

Cognitive factors that impede a person's sexual health may include internalization of negative expectations and beliefs. Individuals with low self-esteem may not understand how another person could value and love them and also find them sexually attractive. For individuals who have not yet accepted their sexual orientation or gender identity, this cognitive conflict may interfere with sexual relationships.

Sexual problems may also be symptomatic of relationship problems. Being in conflict with or angry with a partner is not conducive to positive sexual interaction. In some cases, individuals may lose their physical attraction to their partner or feel more attracted to someone else. Communication is an important part of the sexual relationship, and lack of it can lead to issues for any couple. Failure to communicate may result in one or both partners not knowing how to please the other. Disagreements about sexual frequency and/or activities may lead to further conflict.

Alterations and Manifestations

Numerous physical health factors can interfere with individuals' expressions of sexuality. For example, conditions such as heart disease, diabetes mellitus, joint disease, cancer, and some psychiatric disorders can affect sexual health and expression. Surgeries such as hysterectomy, prostate surgery, and radical surgeries can alter an individual's body image. Spinal cord injuries, traumatic amputations, or disfiguring accidents can negatively affect sexual functioning. In addition, the presence of an STI in one partner induces fear of transmission in the other, often resulting in abstinence from sexual contact. In some situations, however, the presence of an STI is unknown, and transmission occurs.

Many prescription medications beyond those intended to affect sexual functioning have side effects that alter sexual functioning. For example, antidepressants may slow ejaculation. Some street drugs, such as marijuana, amphetamines, and cocaine, enhance sexual functioning. Others, such as opioids and anabolic steroids, interfere with sexual functioning. **Table 19–1 》** provides an overview of the effects of several major classes of drugs on sexual function.

Specific alterations in sexual function are often placed into four broad categories: sexual desire disorders, sexual arousal disorders, orgasmic disorders, and sexual pain disorders (Cleveland Clinic, 2015b). Within each category, some disorders are specific to men, others are specific to women, and still others can affect either men or women. For more

TABLE 19–1 Effects of Various Drugs on Sexual Function

Drug Class	Possible Effects*
Alcohol	Increased risk for unsafe sexual behavior, decreased sexual desire, orgasmic dysfunction, ED, and reduction of male secondary sex characteristics
Alpha-adrenergic blockers (e.g., prazosin [Minipress], terazosin [Hytrin])	Ejaculatory dysfunction (ED)
Amphetamines	Increased risk for unsafe sexual behaviors, reduced erectile rigidity, enhanced and/or delayed orgasm, and prolonged time to ejaculation
Anabolic steroids	Testicular atrophy, reduced sperm count and possible infertility, **gynecomastia** (abnormal enlargement of the breasts), and increased risk of prostate cancer in men; growth of facial hair, menstrual changes or cessation, and enlargement of the clitoris in women
Angiotensin-converting enzyme (ACE) inhibitors	ED (although lower risk than with alpha- and beta-adrenergic blockers)
Antidepressants (e.g., tricyclics, monoamine oxidase inhibitors [MAOIs], selective serotonin reuptake inhibitors [SSRIs])	Decreased sexual desire, orgasmic dysfunction, ED, and delayed or failed ejaculation
Antihistamines	Decreased sexual desire, erectile and ejaculatory problems in men, and decreased lubrication in women
Antipsychotics	Decreased sexual desire, orgasmic dysfunction, ED, delayed or failed ejaculation
Antiseizure agents (e.g., carbamazepine [Tegretol], phenytoin [Dilantin])	Decreased sexual desire, diminished orgasm, ED in men, and decreased lubrication in women
Anxiolytic agents (benzodiazepines)	Decreased sexual desire, diminished orgasms, pain during intercourse, ED, and delayed ejaculation
Barbiturates	Decreased sexual desire, orgasmic dysfunction, and ED
Beta-adrenergic blockers (e.g., metoprolol [Toprol])	Decreased sexual desire and ED
Cocaine	Increased risk for unsafe sexual behavior, decreased sexual desire, and ED (typically with chronic use)
Diuretics	Decreased sexual desire, ED in men, and decreased lubrication in women
Fibrates	Decreased sexual desire and ED
H_2-receptor antagonists (e.g., cimetidine [Tagamet], ranitidine [Zantac])	Decreased sexual desire, ED, gynecomastia, and reduced sperm count
Marijuana	ED and reduced sperm count (with chronic use)
Narcotics	Increased risk for unsafe sexual behavior, decreased sexual desire, and erectile and ejaculatory dysfunction

*The nurse and patient must familiarize themselves with the specific medication prescribed or used because effects vary in each category of drug.

Sources: Data from CDC. (2014b). *Fact sheets: Excessive alcohol use and risk to men's health.* Retrieved from http://www.cdc.gov/alcohol/fact-sheets/mens-health.htm; Cleveland Clinic. (2013). *Medications that affect sexual function.* Retrieved from https://my.clevelandclinic.org/health/diseases_conditions/hic_An_Overview_of_Sexual_Dysfunction/hic_Medications_that_Affect_Sexual_Function; Cleveland Clinic. (2015a). *Medications that may cause erectile dysfunction.* Retrieved from https://my.clevelandclinic.org/health/diseases_conditions/hic_Erectile_Dysfunction_Overview/hic_Medications_That_May_Cause_Erectile_Dysfunction; Conaglen, H. M., & Conaglen, J. V. (2013). Drug-induced sexual dysfunction in men and women. *Australian Prescriber, 36,* 42–45; Koslov, D. S., & Andersson, K. E. (2013). Physiological and pharmacological aspects of the vas deferens—An update. *Frontiers in Pharmacology, 4,* 101; National Institute on Drug Abuse. (2012). *Drug facts: Anabolic steroids.* Retrieved from http://www.drugabuse.gov/publications/drugfacts/anabolic-steroids; Neel, A. B. (2012). *Seven meds that can wreck your sex life.* Retrieved from http://www.aarp.org/health/drugs-supplements/info-04-2012/medications-that-can-cause-sexual-dysfunction.html

information on each category and its associated disorders, see Exemplar 19.D on Sexual Dysfunction.

It is important to note that some individuals experience sexual desire, arousal, and orgasm yet still feel dissatisfied with their sexual relationships. These **dissatisfaction problems** are more commonly related to issues in the relationship than to the physiologic response. Because giving and receiving pleasure in a mutually intimate relationship are the primary goals of sex for most individuals, dissatisfaction problems may be more disturbing than other types of sexual dysfunctions.

At times, satisfaction problems may be situational. For example, one partner may choose an inconvenient time, or a partner may feel anxious and therefore cannot experience pleasure or joy. Situational problems may also arise during times of family stress, such as acute illness or personal or environmental trauma (e.g., assault and robbery, natural disaster, loss of home).

As previously mentioned, satisfaction problems are often related to relationship difficulties. The inability to communicate effectively in other relationship areas frequently results

in sexual frustration. Partners who are angry with each other and make love without resolving the conflict may feel unhappy about the relationship despite having experienced arousal and orgasm. Couples who define their relationship in terms of rigid, unequal power and gender roles may have difficulty negotiating and compromising about sexual issues. The individual with the lesser amount of power may feel helpless and dissatisfied with the sexual interchanges.

In addition, lack of intimacy and lack of feelings of connectedness are understandably related to satisfaction problems. Even couples in a committed relationship may complain of lack of intimacy. Dissatisfaction issues include lack of romance, love, tenderness, and nurturance. Fulfillment of sexuality, then, depends on the ability to relate to a partner in an intimate and mutually pleasing manner that is compatible with the individual's values and chosen lifestyle.

Prevalence

Numerous studies have sought to determine the prevalence of sexual dysfunction in specific populations. The general agreement in these studies is that sexual dysfunction is more prevalent in women than in men (Dahir, 2013; Faught, 2015). Most research has focused on the prevalence of female sexual dysfunction. For instance, Shifren and colleagues (2008) conducted a landmark national survey of 31,581 adult female respondents and determined that the prevalence rate for any sexual problem, including desire, arousal, and orgasm problems, was 43.1%. Note, however, that female sexual dysfunction is difficult to measure because of the variation in definitions and the varying degrees of perceived severity of dysfunction that women may experience (Burri et al., 2012).

Among women, the most common sexual dysfunction is low or absent sexual desire. Although many women occasionally deal with desire issues, some are affected to such a great degree that they are diagnosed with what the DSM-5 calls female sexual interest/arousal disorder. Previously known as hypoactive sexual desire disorder, this condition is believed to have a prevalence rate around 8% (Kingsberg & Woodard, 2015). In men, the most prevalent problem is ED. Overall, about 52% of men report at least occasional ED, with older men affected at higher rates. Complete ED follows a similar pattern. According to one study, the prevalence of complete ED rises from 5% at age 40 to 15% at age 70 (Lakin & Wood, 2012).

Regardless of gender, a variety of factors can increase a person's risk for altered sexual function. Common risk factors include the following:

- Altered body structure or function due to trauma, pregnancy, recent childbirth, anatomical abnormalities of the genitals, or a variety of diseases
- Physical, psychosocial, emotional, or sexual abuse
- Sexual assault
- Disfiguring conditions (e.g., burns, scars, ostomies)
- Specific medication therapy (see Table 19–1)
- Value conflicts between personal beliefs and religious doctrine
- Loss of a partner
- Lack of knowledge or misinformation about sexual functioning and expression.

Genetic Considerations

Researchers continue to investigate the connection between human genetics and altered sexual functioning. So far, the results are limited but promising. For instance, Burri and associates (2012) conducted a genome-wide association study involving more than 1400 adult female twins. Although not conclusive, this study suggests that there are at least two genetic factors related to the symptoms associated with female sexual dysfunction. Likewise, a number of studies have revealed genetic markers that appear to be associated with ED in men, as well as with the effectiveness of pharmacologic treatment for ED (Lippi et al., 2012; Lopushnyan & Chitaley, 2012).

Case Study » Part 1

The Jarvis family lives in a comfortable home in the suburb of a large city. Ralph Jarvis, 45, has his own construction business and has prospered, particularly in the past 5 years. His wife, Betty, 42, is a homemaker and hospital volunteer. They have two children. Matthew, 15, is into sports at school and is very popular. Jolene, 12½, is doing well in school and is friendly and outgoing. Eileen, Ralph's mother, came to live with the Jarvises when her husband, Tom, was killed in a car crash 2 years ago.

Today, Betty Jarvis has brought Jolene to the pediatrician's office for a check-up and her immunizations. In the interview with the nurse before seeing the nurse practitioner, Mrs. Jarvis explains that she is concerned because Jolene has not yet started her period. Mrs. Jarvis tells the nurse, "My sister and I started when we were 11."

Clinical Reasoning Questions Level I

1. What is the first physical sign that Jolene is beginning puberty?
2. What Tanner stage evidence would be seen if Jolene is nearing menarche?
3. What is the average age for menarche in the United States?

Clinical Reasoning Questions Level II

4. What is the priority nursing diagnosis for Jolene and her mother? Why?
5. *Refer to Exemplar 19.C on Menstrual Dysfunction:* At what age would a girl with secondary sex characteristics who has not yet started her period be diagnosed as having primary amenorrhea?
6. *Refer to Exemplar 19.E on STIs:* The immunization to prevent cervical cancer related to a sexually transmitted virus could be administered to Jolene today. What is the virus and the immunization?

Concepts Related to Sexuality

Sexuality is intricately related to many aspects of physical and psychologic health. For some patients, sexuality is a source of physical and mental pleasure and well-being, whereas for others, it is a source of psychologic and/or physical problems or distress. In addition, poor health or psychologic problems can result in sexual difficulties.

Psychologic factors linked to sexuality are vast and varied. For example, patients may experience stress, anxiety, anger, lowered self-esteem, and even mood disorders when their sexual practices or preferences vary from those typical of their culture. Alterations in sexual function, including any number of sexual desire, arousal, orgasm, or pain disorders, can contribute to feelings of anxiety, sadness, and depression. Likewise, certain psychologic conditions—especially mood disorders—may result in sexual dysfunction. Many times, the medications used to treat these disorders have side effects that can further impair sexual function. Conflict or poor communication with a partner, an inability to express personal needs, a lack of knowledge about sexual arousal and stimulation, and/or a history of trauma are still other contributors to alterations in sexuality.

Physical factors that may have an impact on sexuality include aging, chronic disease, poor perfusion, STI, and inflammation. Individuals with mobility issues related to musculoskeletal or neurologic disabilities may have difficulty with sexual relations and responses. The proximity and interrelatedness of the sexual organs and the organs of elimination may lead to difficulties such as UTIs, urinary retention, ejaculatory issues, or anal/rectal problems and constipation. In some cases, patients who have urinary or bowel problems may experience alterations in sexual function because of anxiety, embarrassment, or physical limitations related to these problems.

Because sexuality affects so many aspects of human health, nurses must be well versed in the possible causes, signs, symptoms, and results of alterations in sexual function. Good communication skills are essential, as sexuality is a difficult or taboo topic for many patients to discuss. Nurses can strengthen the therapeutic relationship by remaining sensitive to and nonjudgmental of patients' sexuality, while at the same time providing education and support, especially for individuals who are at elevated risk for sexual dysfunction, trauma, violence, and related problems.

The Concepts Related to Sexuality feature links some, but not all, of the concepts integral to sexuality. They are presented in alphabetical order.

Concepts Related to
Sexuality

CONCEPT	RELATIONSHIP TO SEXUALITY	NURSING IMPLICATIONS
Culture and Diversity	Different cultures vary with regard to what they consider "acceptable" sexual and gender-role behavior. Patients whose preferences vary from those of the larger culture are at elevated risk for stress, psychologic distress, and (in some cases) physical harm. Patients from some cultures may be uncomfortable discussing issues of sexuality and/or may prefer a care provider of the same gender.	■ Remain nonjudgmental when working with patients whose culture differs from your own. ■ Honor patients' cultural preferences when possible. ■ Use culturally sensitive language and terminology (e.g., when caring for a transgender patient). ■ Assess for signs of physical and psychologic trauma in patients from high-risk populations. ■ Refer patients to community resources as appropriate (e.g., support groups, counseling services, advocacy organizations).
Infection	Infection acquired via sexual relations may affect the genitals, anus, and/or mouth in men and women. HIV/AIDS may be acquired via sexual relations and cause immunodeficiency.	■ Be alert to signs and symptoms of STI, such as penile or vaginal discharge, fever, or genital lesions. ■ Provide education regarding safe sex practices. ■ Recommend regular testing for patients at elevated risk of STI. ■ Consider sexual activity as a possible contributor to urinary complaints (e.g., increased frequency, pain on urination).
Perfusion	↓ Perfusion → ↑ risk for ED due to alterations in arterial and/or venous flow	■ Assess for signs of vascular disease in patients who report ED. ■ Educate patients that some cardiac and antihypertensive medications can contribute to ED (see Table 19–1).
Reproduction	Patients who are experiencing alterations in sexual function may have difficulty conceiving. Postpartum women → ↑ risk of altered sexual function due to a combination of physical and psychologic causes (e.g., fluctuating hormones, ↑ stress, ↓ sleep)	■ Educate new and breastfeeding mothers about alterations in sexual function that commonly occur in the postpartum period. ■ Advise that patients abstain from penetrative sex for at least 6 weeks immediately postpartum. ■ When postpartum patients report pain during sex, suggest gradually building toward penetration and use of personal lubricants. ■ Encourage postpartum patients to engage in Kegel exercises, which can lead to increased pleasure during sex. ■ Refer patients to psychologic services as appropriate.
Safety	Transgender patients (especially women and people of color) → ↑ risk for violence	■ Assess transgender and other high-risk patients for signs of physical, emotional, and sexual violence. ■ Educate patients about strategies and resources for establishing and maintaining personal safety. ■ Refer patients to social services and/or law enforcement, as appropriate.
Trauma	↑ Trauma → ↑ risk for sexual dysfunction	■ Be aware that past sexual abuse and trauma can contribute to alterations in sexual function. ■ Use care and demonstrate compassion when asking patients about known or suspected trauma. ■ Note that patients who have experienced trauma may be uncomfortable during the physical assessment and/or may request a provider of a specific gender. ■ Conduct STI and pregnancy testing in patients who report recent sexual trauma. ■ Refer patients to psychologic counseling, social services, and/or law enforcement, as appropriate.

Health Promotion

A wide variety of practices can help preserve and promote patients' sexual health. At the most basic level, nurses should encourage patients to make healthy lifestyle choices similar to those that enhance cardiovascular health. By adopting a healthy lifestyle, patients significantly reduce their risk of sexual dysfunction related to acute or chronic illness. A healthy lifestyle also reduces the likelihood that patients will require antihypertensives and other medications that can impair sexual functioning.

Cancer Screenings

Regular screenings are another essential element in promoting sexual health. All patients can benefit from regular physical checkups and screening for hypercholesterolemia and hypertension, because these measures help prevent sexual dysfunction related to alterations in perfusion. Other useful screenings include regular cervical cancer screening for women of reproductive age and mammograms for women over age 40. Men should consider screenings for prostate cancer beginning at age 50, or earlier if they are at elevated risk (American Cancer Society, 2015a, 2015b). STI screenings should be offered to sexually active women and men.

>> **Stay Current:** Cancer screening guidelines for breast, cervical, prostate, and other cancers can be found on the American Cancer Society's website: http://www.cancer.org/healthy/findcancerearly/cancerscreeningguidelines/american-cancer-society-guidelines-for-the-early-detection-of-cancer.

Vaccinations

Vaccination is another action that helps promote sexual health. In particular, three vaccines (Gardasil, Gardasil 9, and Cervarix) to protect against human papilloma virus (HPV) infection are now available. These vaccines are all administered via three intramuscular injections delivered over a 6-month period, and they are most effective when received before patients become sexually active. Although all three vaccines protect against new cases of HPV, none of them are useful in the treatment of existing HPV infection (National Cancer Institute, 2015a).

- Gardasil protects against the types of HPV associated with cervical cancer; genital warts; and cancer of the anus, vagina, and vulva. It is approved for use in male and female patients ages 9–26. The vaccine lasts at least 8 years and is nearly 100% effective.

- Gardasil 9 offers the same protection as the original Gardasil, plus protection against five additional types of high-risk HPV. It is approved for use in male patients ages 9–15 and female patients ages 9–26. Like the original Gardasil, Gardasil 9 is nearly 100% effective, although its duration of efficacy is currently unknown.

- Cervarix protects against only the types of HPV that cause cervical cancer. It is approved for use solely in female patients ages 9–25. Protection from Cervarix lasts at least 9 years and is nearly 100% effective.

Regardless of which vaccine is chosen, the CDC recommends that routine immunization occur at age 11 or 12—meaning nearly all children would receive the vaccine prior

to engaging in sexual activity. However, patients will still benefit from vaccination after age 12, provided they have not yet been exposed to HPV (National Cancer Institute, 2015a).

Safer Sex Practices

For optimal health promotion, patients who engage in sexual activity need to know about and practice safer sex. Safer sex encompasses a variety of practices and precautions, as described in the Patient Teaching feature. For example, reducing the number of sexual partners—such as by entering into a long-term mutually monogamous relationship with an uninfected partner—reduces the risk of contracting an STI. Nurses should discourage patients who are not in a long-term monogamous relationship from engaging in unprotected sex, especially if the HIV status of their partner(s) is unknown. In terms of protection, latex condoms have been shown to reduce the risk of transmitting HIV and other infections. To be effective, condoms must be used with every sexual encounter involving vaginal, oral, or anal intercourse.

Patient Teaching
Guidelines for Safer Sex

- Practice mutual monogamy. If you are not in a mutually monogamous relationship, limit your number of sexual partners.

- Do not engage in unprotected sex, especially if you do not know your partner's HIV status. Remember that an individual may be infected, and infective, for up to 6 months before converting to seropositive status.

- When entering into a new monogamous relationship, both you and your partner should undergo HIV testing. If both tests are negative, practice abstinence or safer sex for 6 months, then get retested. If the results still indicate that both you and your partner are negative, sexual activity can probably be considered safe.

- Use latex condoms for oral, vaginal, or anal intercourse. Avoid natural or animal skin condoms, which allow the passage of HIV.

- Pre-exposure prophylaxis (PrEP) reduces the risk of getting HIV by 90% (CDC, 2017).

- For vaginal or anal sex, lubricate condoms with the spermicidal agent nonoxynol-9 for additional protection.

- Do not use an oil-based lubricant such as petroleum jelly, which can result in condom damage. Water-based lubricants are acceptable.

- To further decrease the risk of disease, engage in safer sexual practices that are less damaging to sensitive tissues (e.g., mutual masturbation, avoiding anal or oral sex).

- Do not use drugs or alcohol.

- Do not share needles, razors, toothbrushes, sex toys, or other items that may be contaminated with blood or body fluids.

- If you are HIV positive: Do not engage in unprotected sexual activity. Inform all current and former sexual partners and all healthcare providers (including dentists) of your HIV status. Do not donate blood, plasma, blood products, sperm, organs, or tissue. Women who are HIV positive should take steps to prevent pregnancy and should consult with their healthcare providers if they seek to become pregnant.

They also need to be applied and removed properly. Condoms' effectiveness is further improved when nonoxynol-9 (a spermicide) is used for lubrication; however, nonoxynol-9 may cause genital ulcers, which can facilitate transmission of bloodborne diseases, such as HIV and hepatitis. Pre-exposure prophylaxis (PrEP) is highly effective for preventing HIV if used as prescribed (CDC, 2017).

Nursing Assessment

Assessing a patient's sexual health can be a challenging task because it may be complicated by physiologic as well as social, cultural, and psychologic factors. For example, some patients may be hesitant or unwilling to discuss sexual issues because of embarrassment, self-consciousness, privacy concerns, fear of judgment, or cultural taboos. Other patients may be uncomfortable having their bodies—especially their reproductive and related structures—examined by a nurse or other healthcare provider who is not of the same gender as them. Still other patients might fail to share important details with the nurse because of lack of education about issues related to sexuality. For these and other reasons, assessment of a patient's sexuality requires deep clinical knowledge and strong interpersonal skills throughout all stages of the process.

Patient Interview

The interview stage of the assessment process must be tailored to the patient's gender. If the nurse does not understand certain words or phrases the patient uses, the nurse must clarify these terms to reduce barriers to successful communication. Some patients may be embarrassed to discuss health problems or concerns involving their reproductive organs. To help patients feel more comfortable, the nurse should ask questions in a nonthreatening, matter-of-fact manner, making sure to consider the psychologic, social, and cultural factors that affect sexuality and sexual activity. The nurse should use words that the patient can understand and should not be embarrassed or offended by the words the patient uses.

Interviewing Men

During the history or interview portion of the nursing assessment, the patient shares information about his sexual concerns or problems with his reproductive system. The interview may be conducted during a health screening, may focus on a chief complaint (e.g., discharge from the penis), or may be part of a total health assessment. The health assessment interview ideally precedes the physical examination.

Questions about the current problem:

- When did you first notice difficulty having an erection?
- Describe the changes in your ability to have an erection after you started taking medicine for high blood pressure.
- Have you tried any medications or remedies to help achieve or maintain an erection?

Questions about medical history:

- Do you have any chronic diseases, such as diabetes, cardiovascular disease, or thyroid disease?
- Have you ever had surgery of the penis or prostate?

Questions about psychosocial history:

- Do you use tobacco, alcohol, or drugs? If so, how much and how often?
- Is there anyone at home who is hurting you?

If the patient has a health problem, analyze its onset, characteristics and course, severity, precipitating and relieving factors, and any associated symptoms, noting the timing and circumstances. Also ask about any medications, over-the-counter drugs, herbal supplements, or vitamins the patient is taking in order to determine whether these substances may be affecting the reproductive system (see Table 19–1). In addition, this is a good time to assess what the patient may be using in an effort to relieve his symptoms. Men may be reluctant to discuss the use of sildenafil (Viagra), for instance, but it is important to ask because of potential drug interactions that may occur. Also, it is good practice to ask patients about their allergies in anticipation of any medications that may be ordered. If a procedure is planned, determine whether the patient has a latex allergy.

When questioning a male patient about his medical history, ask about chronic illnesses such as diabetes, cardiovascular disease, and thyroid disease. The effects of these illnesses and the treatments prescribed may cause **impotence**, or the inability to achieve or maintain an erection. Inquire about past illnesses and surgical procedures involving the genitoreproductive system, because these too can affect the patient's sexuality. For example, childhood mumps infections may result in sterility, and **prostatectomy** (surgical removal of the prostate) may lead to impotence. As with nearly any type of health problem, explore potentially relevant aspects of the patient's ethnic background and family history, because some conditions are more common among people from certain backgrounds. For example, the risk for testicular cancer is greatest in Caucasian men between the ages of 20 and 34 who were born in the United States or Europe. Another family-related risk factor is having a brother who was diagnosed with testicular cancer (American Cancer Society, 2015c).

Last but certainly not least, explore the patient's lifestyle, stressors, and social history. Ask about the frequency and nature of the patient's sexual activity, because frequent intercourse (especially if unprotected) increases the potential for STIs, including HIV infection. In addition, asking about sexual orientation may be appropriate, because intercourse with same-sex partners further increases the risk for HIV. Other questions related to the patient's sexuality may include number of sexual partners; history of premature ejaculation, impotence, or other sexual problems; history of sexual trauma; use of condoms or other contraceptives; and current level of sexual satisfaction.

Interviewing Women

The interview portion of the nursing assessment is the time when female patients share information about their sexual or reproductive concerns. As with male patients, the interview may be conducted during a health screening, may focus on a chief complaint (e.g., vaginal discharge), or may be part of a total health assessment. The interview ideally precedes the physical examination.

During the interview, the nurse begins to establish a professional, nonthreatening relationship with the patient. The woman may perceive the interview as less threatening if the discussion begins with more general questions and progresses to specific questions. Questions should be asked in a way that gives the patient permission to describe behaviors and manifestations. For example, the nurse should ask the patient about her menstrual and childbirth history before asking questions about STIs or sexual dysfunctions. Sample interview questions related to a female patient's current problem (in this case, painful intercourse), medical history, and psychosocial history include:

Questions about the current problem:

- When did you first experience painful intercourse?
- Is the pain occurring just as the penis enters the vagina, or does it occur with deep thrusting?
- Have you tried any medications or remedies for the pain? Have these things helped?
- When was your last menstrual period?

Questions about medical history:

- Do you have or have you had endometriosis?
- Have you ever had gynecologic surgery?

Questions about psychosocial history:

- Do you use tobacco, alcohol, or drugs? If so, how much and how often?
- Is there anyone at home who is hurting you?

The focused interview should be tailored to the patient's specific health problem. As with the assessment of other body systems, analyze and document the onset of the problem, its duration, its frequency, its precipitating and relieving factors, and any associated symptoms, as well as any treatment and self-care measures and their outcomes. Inquire about any medications, over-the-counter drugs, herbal supplements, or vitamins the woman is taking to determine whether these substances may be affecting the reproductive system (see Table 19–1). Ask specifically about use of birth control pills or other hormonal methods of pregnancy prevention, because many women forget to mention they are taking the pill or using a progestin intrauterine device. Furthermore, it is good practice to ask patients about allergies in anticipation of any medications that may be ordered. If a procedure is planned, determine if the patient has a latex allergy.

Taking a female patient's medical history includes asking questions about chronic illnesses, gynecologic surgery, menstrual history, and obstetrical history. Chronic illnesses may affect the function of the female reproductive system. For instance, diabetes increases the risk of vaginal infections and dryness, both of which interfere with sexual pleasure. Chronic heavy menstrual flow may result in anemia, and thyroid and adrenal disorders may affect secondary sex characteristics, the menstrual cycle, and the ability to become pregnant.

Obtaining information about the patient's family history is important because the risk for endometrial, ovarian, and breast cancers is higher in women with family histories of these disorders. Other aspects of a patient's family history may be important, too. For example, women who were exposed to diethylstilbestrol (DES) in utero have an increased risk of cancer of the cervix and vagina (American Cancer Society, 2015d).

Gather pertinent psychosocial information during the patient interview. This includes asking about the use of condoms to reduce risk for STIs. Ask whether the patient smokes, because a history of smoking increases the risk of cervical cancer in all women, as well as the risk of circulatory problems in women who use hormonal contraceptives. In some cases, inquiring about exposure to other carcinogenic substances may be useful; exposure to asbestos, for example, poses a risk of ovarian cancer.

Finally, ask questions related to the patient's sexual choices and behaviors. These include questions about number of partners; history of **anorgasmia** (absence of orgasm), **dyspareunia** (painful intercourse), or other problems with intercourse; history of sexual trauma; use of contraceptives or condoms; and current level of sexual satisfaction (Mayo Clinic, 2015a).

Physical Examination

When performing a physical assessment of the reproductive system and related parts of the body, the nurse should maintain a professional approach in order to reduce the patient's anxiety. Most patients consider their genitals, breasts, and rectum to be personal and private, which means the nurse must be nonjudgmental, gentle, and empathetic. The nurse must also use caution to avoid misperception by the patient of sexual harassment or abuse. This can be accomplished by touching in a non-intimate fashion, obtaining consent from the patient before performing any assessment or procedure, and explaining what will happen before proceeding. In addition, it is best to have another healthcare provider in the room during physical examination of the genitalia.

For more information on examining specific areas of a patient's body, refer to the Male and Female Sexual Health Assessment features.

Diagnostic Tests

Diagnostic tests related to sexuality and disorders of the reproductive system include both laboratory tests and imaging studies. For male patients, appropriate lab tests may include (but are not limited to) complete blood count (CBC) with differential; urinalysis; sperm analysis; culture and sensitivity (C&S) to identify causative organisms in infection; blood tests for syphilis, HIV, or herpes; serum hormone studies; and prostate-specific antigen (PSA) tests to screen for prostate cancer. Lab tests related to sexual and/or reproductive function in female patients may include CBC with differential, urinalysis, C&S, blood tests for STIs, and serum hormone studies. Other laboratory tests specific to women include pregnancy tests (urine or blood) and the Papanicolaou (Pap) test. Because the Pap test involves a pelvic examination, teaching about the procedure and the test is required. Neither pregnancy tests nor the Pap test require a woman to fast.

As previously mentioned, imaging studies are an important element in diagnosing many sexual and reproductive disorders. For example, both men and women may require

Male Sexual Health Assessment

ASSESSMENT/ METHOD	NORMAL FINDINGS	ABNORMAL FINDINGS	LIFESPAN OR DEVELOPMENTAL CONSIDERATIONS
Breast and Lymph Node Assessment			
Inspect and palpate the breasts and lymph nodes.	In men, the breasts should be flat with an erect nipple and an areola that is darker than the surrounding skin. The axillary area should be free of lesions and masses. The axillary and infraclavicular lymph nodes are usually nonpalpable.	■ An enlarged, smooth, firm, mobile, tender disk of breast tissue behind the areola indicates gynecomastia. ■ A hard, irregular nodule in or near the nipple area suggests carcinoma. ■ Enlarged axillary nodes are common with infections of the hands or arms but may be caused by cancer of the breast. ■ Enlarged supraclavicular nodes may indicate breast cancer metastasis.	■ Infant and adolescent boys may have gynecomastia related to changes in hormones. Most cases will resolve without treatment. ■ About 25% of men between the ages of 50 and 80 are affected by gynecomastia, often as a result of age-related hormonal fluctuations but also due to certain disease processes and medications.
External Genitalia Assessment			
Inspect the inguinal and femoral area for hernias. Ask the man to bear down or cough as you palpate (see **Figure 19–5** ❯❯). Inspect and palpate the inguinal lymph nodes.	There should be no bulging in the inguinal and femoral areas. The inguinal lymph nodes are normally nonpalpable. 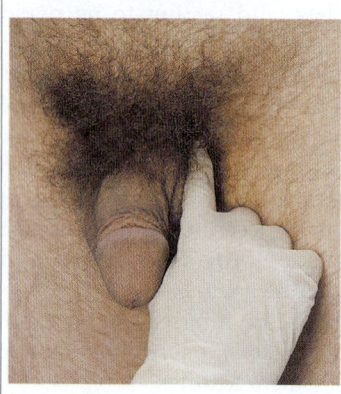 **Figure 19–5** ❯❯ Palpating the male inguinal area for bulges.	■ A bulge that increases with coughing or straining suggests a hernia. ■ Palpable or tender inguinal lymph nodes suggest infection of the lower abdomen, external genitalia, perianal area, leg, or foot.	■ Indirect inguinal hernia (resulting from incomplete closure of the inguinal ring after testicular descent) is the most common type of hernia in men of all ages. ■ Direct inguinal hernias (resulting from weakness in the abdominal wall) are more common in men over age 40.
Inspect the glans of the penis. If the man is uncircumcised, ask him to retract his foreskin.	When nonerect, the penis should be soft, flaccid, nontender, and without lesions. Note that some men have small, pearly papules around the edge of the glans; these are a normal and harmless anatomical variation.	■ **Phimosis** (tightness of the foreskin that prevents retraction) may be congenital or occur because of recurrent inflammation. ■ Narrow or inflamed foreskin may cause **paraphimosis**, in which the retracted foreskin becomes trapped over the glans and tightens on the penis, causing painful swelling. ■ **Balanitis** (inflammation of the glans) is associated with infection, irritation, or trauma. ■ Ulcers, vesicles, or warts suggest the presence of an STI. ■ In uncircumcised men, nodules or sores on the glans may be cancerous.	■ Phimosis is normal in newborn boys, but the foreskin should loosen over time. ■ Although more common in children, both phimosis and paraphimosis can occur at any age. ■ Balanitis is more common among uncircumcised male patients, especially young boys (due to poor personal hygiene and inability to fully retract the foreskin) and the older adults (due to hygiene issues and the presence of predisposing conditions like diabetes).

Male Sexual Health Assessment *(continued)*

ASSESSMENT/ METHOD	NORMAL FINDINGS	ABNORMAL FINDINGS	LIFESPAN OR DEVELOPMENTAL CONSIDERATIONS
Inspect the external urinary meatus. Press the glans between the thumb and forefinger to inspect inside (see **Figure 19–6 »**). Replace foreskin if appropriate.	The external urinary meatus is in the center of the glans. The opening should appear as a vertical slit. There should be no lesions, redness, or discharge. 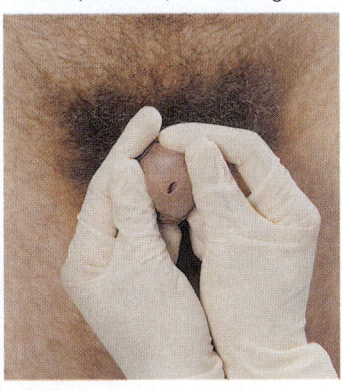 **Figure 19–6 »** Inspecting the external urinary meatus of men.	■ Erythema or discharge indicates inflammatory disease. Further assessment is required. ■ Abnormal narrowing of the external urinary meatus, called **meatal stenosis**, can cause pain or other difficulties with urination. Meatal stenosis may be a result of circumcision, surgery, infection, injury, or prolonged catheter use.	■ Inspection of the external urinary meatus may be difficult in young children because of inability to retract the foreskin. ■ Two congenital abnormalities sometimes observed in male newborns include **hypospadias** (in which the meatus is located on the underside of the glans) and **epispadias** (in which the meatus is located on the upper side of the glans). Both conditions usually require corrective surgery.
Inspect and palpate the shaft of the penis.	The skin on the shaft should not have any lesions or redness. The shaft should be free of masses and nontender.	■ Excoriation or inflammation suggests lice, scabies, or fungal infection. ■ Vesicles or chancres suggest herpes or syphilis. ■ Warts suggest HPV infection. ■ Fibrous plaques may be palpable in Peyronie disease.	■ During puberty, the penis first grows longer, then wider. It may reach full adult size as early as age 13 or as late as age 18. ■ The penis decreases in size from middle adulthood through old age.
Inspect the scrotum. If swollen, use transillumination: Darken the room and place a lighted flashlight behind and against the scrotum.	The scrotum should hang freely from the perineum. It is usually covered with hair. The testes and epididymis should not transilluminate.	■ A unilateral or bilateral poorly developed scrotum suggests **cryptorchidism** (failure of one or both testes to descend into the scrotum). ■ Swelling of the scrotum may indicate hernia, **hydrocele** (accumulation of fluid), or edema. Serous swelling will transilluminate; blood or tissue will not. ■ A scrotal mass may occur in cases of hernia where bowel loops have descended into the scrotum. ■ A unilateral scrotal mass that feels like a "bag of worms" is a **varicocele** (varicosity of the spermatic cord).	■ Cryptorchidism is usually detected in infant boys. ■ Hydrocele is more common in newborn boys. ■ As puberty begins, the testicles and scrotum nearly double in size. The scrotal skin thins and darkens, and hair follicles appear. ■ Adult men with varicocele may have fertility problems because of increased heat in the scrotum. ■ In older men, the scrotum sags, and the testicles are smaller and located lower in the scrotum.
Palpate each testis and epididymis.	The testes should be smooth, firm, and slightly tender. The epididymis is a comma-shaped organ on the posterior of each testis.	■ Tender, painful scrotal swelling occurs in acute inflammation of the testicles, inflammation of the epididymis, **testicular torsion** (twisting of the spermatic cord), and strangulated hernia. ■ A painless nodule in the testis may be associated with testicular cancer and needs to be further investigated.	■ Testicular torsion is more common in adolescents and is a surgical emergency. ■ Testicular cancer occurs infrequently and is more likely to affect men between the ages of 20 and 34.

(continued on next page)

Male Sexual Health Assessment (continued)

ASSESSMENT/METHOD	NORMAL FINDINGS	ABNORMAL FINDINGS	LIFESPAN OR DEVELOPMENTAL CONSIDERATIONS
Prostate Assessment			
Assess the prostate via digital rectal examination (DRE). Before conducting the DRE, have the patient lean over the exam table or lie on his left side with his right knee drawn up so you can inspect the anal area. Begin the DRE by inserting a gloved, well-lubricated index finger. Palpate the anterior rectal wall for the rounded, two-lobed posterior prostate. (The single anterior lobe is nonpalpable.)	The anal area should be free of lesions and excoriation. The prostate should be nontender, smooth, and about 2.5 cm long with a palpable median sulcus between the lobes.	■ Inflammation or skin damage in the anal area indicates infection, excoriation, or trauma. ■ Prostate enlargement with obliteration of the median sulcus suggests benign prostatic hyperplasia (BPH). ■ Painful enlargement with asymmetry and tenderness suggests prostatitis. ■ A hard, irregular nodule is suspicious for carcinoma.	■ The prostate grows slowly throughout a man's entire life. ■ In men in their 20s, the prostate is the size of a walnut; by age 40, it is about the size of an apricot; and by age 60, it is roughly lemon sized. ■ After age 50, symptoms related to BPH are common. By age 85, nearly all men are affected by this condition.

Sources: Data from American Academy of Pediatrics. (2015b). *Physical development in boys: What to expect.* Retrieved from https://www.healthychildren.org/English/ages-stages/gradeschool/puberty/Pages/Physical-Development-Boys-What-to-Expect.aspx; American Cancer Society. (2015e). *Do I have testicular cancer?* Retrieved from http://www.cancer.org/cancer/testicularcancer/moreinformation/doihavetesticularcancer/do-i-have-testicular-cancer-facts-and-risk-factors; Bickley, L., & Szilagyi, P. (2013). *Bates' guide to physical examination and history taking* (11th ed.). Philadelphia, PA: Wolters Kluwer/Lippincott Williams & Wilkins; Mayo Clinic. (2014c). *Enlarged breasts in men (gynecomastia).* Retrieved from http://www.mayoclinic.org/diseases-conditions/gynecomastia/basics/causes/con-20028710; Mayo Clinic. (2013a). *Inguinal hernia: Causes.* Retrieved from http://www.mayoclinic.org/diseases-conditions/inguinal-hernia/basics/causes/con-20021456. National Cancer Institute. (n.d.). *Understanding prostate changes: A health guide for men.* Retrieved from http://www.cancer.gov/types/prostate/understanding-prostate-changes; University of Rochester Medical Center. (2015). *Phimosis and paraphimosis.* Retrieved from https://www.urmc.rochester.edu/Encyclopedia/Content.aspx?ContentTypeID=90&ContentID=P03104

imaging via ultrasound, CT scan, or laparoscope. Most studies are done on an outpatient basis, and nurses are involved with patient teaching and assisting other healthcare providers with the procedure. Female patients may also require additional types of visualization, including hysteroscopic examinations and mammograms. In a hysteroscopic examination, an endoscope is used to visually inspect the uterine lining. In a mammogram, x-rays are used to generate an image of the breast tissue. For women with dense breast tissue, MRI and/or ultrasound imaging may be more useful than mammography in screening for cancer (Mayo Clinic, 2015b). Finally, both male and female patients may require biopsies of the breasts or genitals that necessitate special procedures and education.

Case Study » Part 2

Ralph Jarvis, age 45, has "not been himself" lately, and his wife is worried. Mr. Jarvis smokes about 10 cigarettes per day and has smoked since age 19. Over the past few weeks, he has gained a little weight and does not seem to have much energy. The only exercise he gets is walking around the construction site. His wife convinces him to go to Ms. Walker, the family's nurse practitioner, for a checkup. He is reluctant but agrees to go if his wife will go with him.

During the patient interview, Ms. Walker determines that Mr. Jarvis is healthy, but there is something he is unwilling to discuss. Ms. Walker says, "Mr. Jarvis, some of my male patients who are your age and smoke tell me they have sexual difficulties. Is this a concern for you?" Mr. Jarvis looks at his wife, who reaches for his hand and says, "Tell her, Ralph." This helps Mr. Jarvis admit that he was unable to attain an erection a couple of times and this has him worried.

Clinical Reasoning Questions Level I

1. What model of intervention is Ms. Walker using?
2. What further assessment questions might Ms. Walker ask Mr. and Ms. Jarvis?
3. In thinking about male gender and culture, is Mr. Jarvis's reluctance to talk about sex expected? Explain.

Clinical Reasoning Questions Level II

4. What is the priority nursing diagnosis for Mr. Jarvis at this time?
5. *Refer to Exemplar 19.D on Sexual Dysfunction:* How will Ms. Walker determine whether Mr. Jarvis's sexual problem is a matter of sexual desire or the physical ability to attain and maintain an erection? Give two examples of history questions Ms. Walker could ask.
6. *Refer to Exemplar 19.D on Sexual Dysfunction:* What are some lifestyle changes that Mr. Jarvis can make that will improve his health and likely enhance his sexual performance?

Female Sexual Health Assessment

ASSESSMENT/ METHOD	NORMAL FINDINGS	ABNORMAL FINDINGS	LIFESPAN OR DEVELOPMENTAL CONSIDERATIONS
Breast Assessment			
Inspect both breasts, first with the woman sitting with arms at her sides, then with her arms overhead, and again with her hands pressed on her hips and leaning forward. Be sure to lift the breasts and inspect underneath.	Breasts vary in size and shape. It is normal for one breast to be somewhat larger than the other. The color of the breasts should be the same as the woman's other skin. The tone should be firm and the texture smooth.	■ Retractions, dimpling (*peau d'orange*, or orange skin), erythema, and prominent venous patterns suggest underlying lesions and should be further investigated.	■ Newborns may have swollen breast tissue and/or leak a milky substance from their nipples. This is due to residual maternal hormones and should resolve within the first weeks of life. ■ Thelarche (beginning of breast development) occurs around ages 9–11. From that point on, the rate of breast growth varies. ■ During menstruation, a woman's breasts may become slightly larger. ■ During pregnancy and lactation, a woman's breasts enlarge and the blood vessels become more prominent. ■ After menopause, a woman's breasts often lose fat and begin to sag.
Inspect the areolae and nipples.	The nipples and areolae should be slightly darker than the surrounding skin (dark pink to dark brown). Montgomery tubercles (sebaceous glands) may be present. The nipples are usually equal in size and bilateral position. Most women's nipples are everted, although some women's nipples are normally inverted or flat.	■ Lesions, excoriation, or discharge may denote skin infection, mechanical injury, or lactation. ■ *Peau d'orange* may appear first on the areola. ■ Recent unilateral inversion of the nipple or asymmetry in pointing direction suggests underlying malignancy.	■ During pregnancy and lactation, the areolas become larger and darker. Montgomery tubercles may also be more pronounced. ■ Sore, cracked, and/or bleeding nipples are not unusual in lactating mothers, especially during the early weeks of breastfeeding. In some cases, however, they may be indicative of thrush.
Palpate both breasts. Examine all four quadrants of the breast, including the axillary tail (tail of Spence) (see **Figure 19–7 »**). The breasts should be palpated with the woman in a supine position, one at a time, with a small pillow under her shoulder. They should also be palpated when the woman has her arm extended over her head.	Breasts should feel smooth, firm, and elastic. Many women have nodularity or lumpiness that is uniform in both breasts. It is normal and caused by fibrocystic changes related to cyclic hormones.	■ Tenderness may be related to premenstrual fullness, fibrocystic changes, or inflammation. Tenderness has also been associated with cancer. ■ Nodules in the tail of the breast may be enlarged lymph nodes. ■ Hard, irregular, fixed unilateral masses that are poorly delineated suggest carcinoma. ■ Bilateral, single or multiple, round, mobile, well-delineated masses are consistent with fibrocystic breast changes or fibroadenoma. ■ Swelling, tenderness, erythema, and heat may be seen with mastitis or inflammatory breast cancer.	■ During menstruation, some women's breasts become more lumpy than usual. ■ Breast swelling and tenderness are early signs of pregnancy and may continue through childbirth and lactation. ■ In lactating women, painful lumps are typically indicative of mastitis and not breast cancer. ■ Premenopausal women typically have denser breast tissue than older women. ■ Breast cancer occurs more often among older women.

(continued on next page)

Female Sexual Health Assessment *(continued)*

ASSESSMENT/ METHOD	NORMAL FINDINGS	ABNORMAL FINDINGS	LIFESPAN OR DEVELOPMENTAL CONSIDERATIONS
Palpate the nipple and areola of each breast.	Nipples should be firm and elastic. There should be no discharge.	▪ Loss of nipple elasticity is seen in cancer. ▪ Bloody or serous discharge is associated with intraductal papilloma. ▪ Bilateral milky discharge not due to pregnancy or lactation is known as **galactorrhea**. It may be associated with pituitary tumors or certain drugs. ▪ Unilateral discharge from one or two ducts may be seen in fibrocystic breast changes, intraductal papilloma, or carcinoma.	▪ Pregnant women may begin to leak straw-colored **colostrum** (the precursor to milk) as early as week 16 of gestation. ▪ The nipple ducts of middle-age and older women are more palpable than those of younger women.

Axillary and Clavicular Lymph Node Assessment

With the patient sitting, inspect the axilla and clavicular areas. Palpate the axillary nodes in the central, lateral, pectoral, and subscapular areas (see **Figure 19–8** »). Palpate the supraclavicular (above the clavicle) lymph nodes.	The axillary areas are covered in hair unless shaved. The skin should be the color of the surrounding skin and free of lesions. The axillary and supraclavicular lymph nodes are usually nonpalpable.	▪ Redness, rash, irritation, or lesions may be due to allergy, shaving, or infection of the sweat glands or hair follicles. ▪ Enlarged axillary nodes may be due to infection in the hand or arm or caused by breast malignancy. ▪ Enlarged supraclavicular nodes are associated with metastasis from abdominal or thoracic carcinoma or generalized lymph swelling from systemic disease.	▪ Prior to age 70, the probability that breast cancer will metastasize to a woman's axillary lymph nodes decreases with age; after age 70, the probability increases with age.

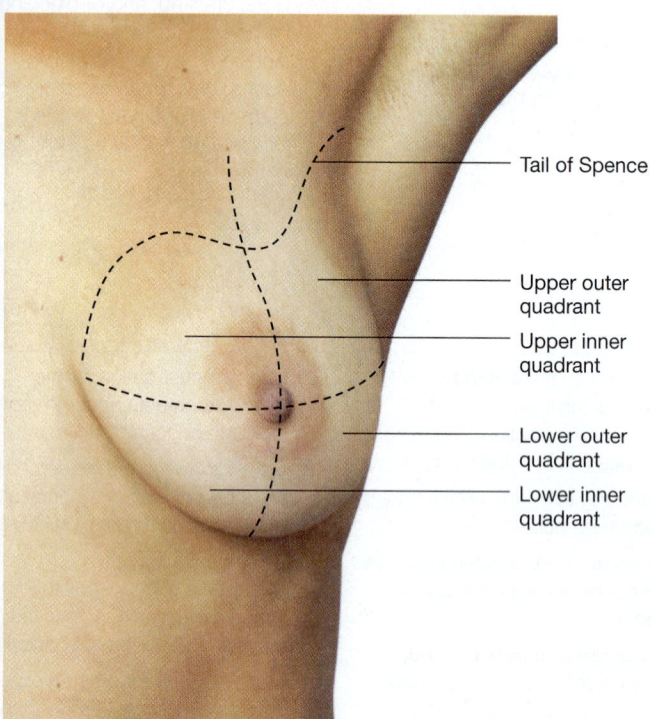

Tail of Spence

Upper outer quadrant

Upper inner quadrant

Lower outer quadrant

Lower inner quadrant

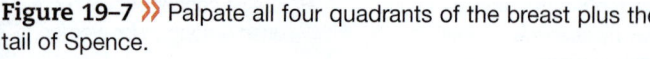

Figure 19–7 » Palpate all four quadrants of the breast plus the tail of Spence.

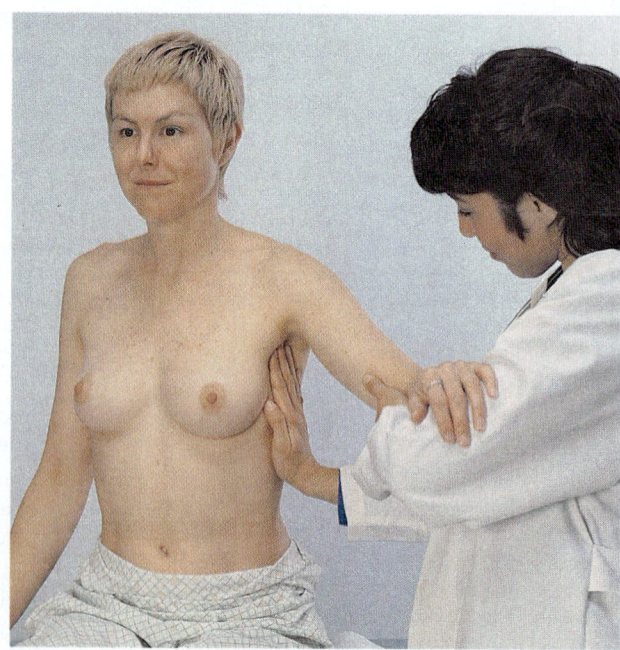

Figure 19–8 » Palpating the axillary lymph nodes.

Female Sexual Health Assessment *(continued)*

ASSESSMENT/ METHOD	NORMAL FINDINGS	ABNORMAL FINDINGS	LIFESPAN OR DEVELOPMENTAL CONSIDERATIONS
Hernia and Inguinal Lymph Node Assessment			
With the woman standing, inspect the inguinal and femoral areas. Palpate for inguinal lymph nodes.	The inguinal and femoral areas should be free of bulging masses. The inguinal lymph nodes are normally nonpalpable.	■ A bulge above the inguinal ligament denotes indirect inguinal hernia. ■ Femoral hernia occurs medially to the femoral artery and may feel like an enlarged lymph node. ■ Palpable or tender inguinal lymph nodes suggest infection in the lower vagina, external genitalia, lower abdomen, anal area, or perineum.	■ Indirect hernia is the most common hernia type in female patients of all ages. ■ Pregnancy sometimes contributes to development of an inguinal hernia. However, in some cases, pregnancy-associated varicosities of the round ligament mimic inguinal hernia.
External Genitalia Assessment			
Help the woman into the lithotomy position with knees flexed and separated. Vaginal examinations can also be done with the woman in a side-lying position with one leg drawn up. Inspect and palpate the labia majora and labia minora.	The labia majora are equal in size and covered with pubic hair. The labia minora are smooth, symmetric, and hairless.	■ Excoriation, rashes, vesicles, nodules, or other lesions suggest inflammatory or infective processes. ■ Varicosities may be present on the labia majora, especially during pregnancy. ■ Caking of discharge or smegma in tissue folds suggests vaginal infection or poor hygiene. ■ Chancres, ulcers, and vesicles may be signs of an STI. ■ Small, firm, cystic nodules suggest sebaceous cysts. ■ Wartlike lesions suggest HPV infection. ■ Ulcerated or red, raised lesions suggest vulvar carcinoma.	■ Older women or women with mobility issues may have difficulty assuming the lithotomy position. ■ During puberty, the pubic hair begins to change from fine, vellus hair to coarse, curly hair. At menopause, the pubic hair becomes more sparse and gray. ■ In postmenopausal women, the labia majora loses fat, and the labia and clitoris become thin, pale, and dry. ■ Vulvar carcinoma is a disease of older women.
Inspect the clitoris and vaginal opening (introitus).	The clitoris is small, sensitive, and made up of erectile tissue. The vaginal opening varies in size depending on age and parity.	■ Clitoral enlargement may be a sign of hormone imbalance. ■ Swelling, discoloration, and lacerations of the introitus may be due to trauma. ■ Bulging of the anterior vaginal wall at the introitus, with or without urinary incontinence, suggests **cystocele** (prolapsed bladder). ■ Bulging of the posterior wall of the vagina at the introitus suggests **rectocele** (rectal prolapse). ■ Yellowish discharge or lesions at the vaginal opening are signs of infection.	■ Newborn girls may have white or blood-tinged vaginal discharge due to residual maternal hormones. ■ Prior to ovulation, a woman's vaginal secretions become thicker, clearer, and more elastic. ■ Increased amounts of clear or white vaginal discharge are typical during pregnancy. ■ Pregnant women are at elevated risk of yeast infection. ■ After menopause, a woman's vaginal secretions decrease significantly.

(continued on next page)

Female Sexual Health Assessment *(continued)*

ASSESSMENT/ METHOD	NORMAL FINDINGS	ABNORMAL FINDINGS	LIFESPAN OR DEVELOPMENTAL CONSIDERATIONS
Palpate the urethra, Skene glands, and Bartholin glands. Place a gloved index finger under the urinary meatus and press up and toward the examiner to inspect the urethral opening and Skene ducts (see **Figure 19–9** »). Palpate the Bartholin glands by pressing with the thumb and index finger at 5 o'clock and 7 o'clock to the introitus (see **Figure 19–10** »).	The urinary meatus opens just over the vagina. The Skene ducts open at the posterior portion of meatus and are usually not visible. The Bartholin glands are on either side of the posterior introitus and are usually not palpable or visible.	■ Unilateral swelling, redness, and severe tenderness at 5 or 7 o'clock to the introitus indicates an abscess of a Bartholin gland. ■ Obstruction of the Skene ducts may lead to cyst formation. Most cysts are asymptomatic, but they can form abscesses and/or cause urethral obstruction and UTI. ■ Redness, swelling, or bulging tissue in or around the urethral opening may indicate infection or, in rare cases, urethral prolapse. ■ Any discharge from the urethra or Skene or Bartholin glands should be cultured to check for infection.	■ Bartholin gland cysts are most common in women of childbearing age. ■ Urethral prolapse is most common in prepubertal African American girls and postmenopausal Caucasian women.

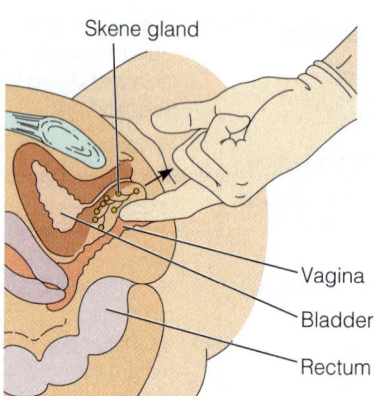
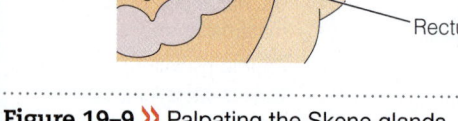

Figure 19–9 » Palpating the Skene glands.

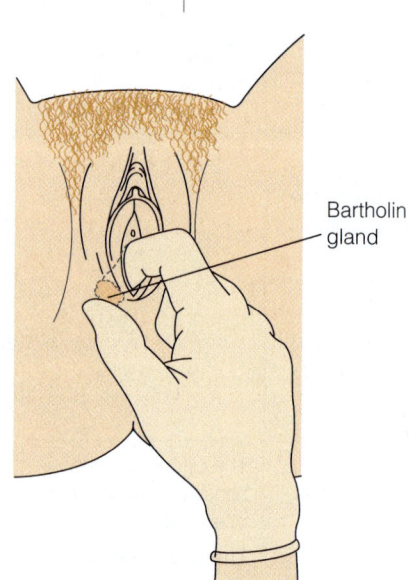

Figure 19–10 » Palpating the Bartholin glands.

Inspect and palpate the perineum.	The area between the vaginal opening and the anus should be the same color as the surrounding skin. Scars from episiotomy or laceration during childbirth are a normal finding.	■ Inflammation, excoriations, lesions, or growths may be seen with infection or cancer. ■ Fistulas or fissures may be the result of injury, trauma, infection, or spreading cancer.	■ Perineal swelling is normal during the last few weeks of pregnancy because of pressure from the fetus. ■ Perineal swelling, bruising, and tearing are common complications of vaginal birth. ■ In older women, perineal irritation often occurs as a result of urinary and/or fecal incontinence.

Female Sexual Health Assessment *(continued)*

ASSESSMENT/ METHOD	NORMAL FINDINGS	ABNORMAL FINDINGS	LIFESPAN OR DEVELOPMENTAL CONSIDERATIONS
Vaginal and Cervical Assessment			
Use a vaginal speculum to inspect the vagina and cervix. Select the size of speculum most appropriate for the size of the patient's introitus.	The vaginal wall and fornices should be pink and moist with rugae (accordion-like folds). The cervix should be smooth and pink with a central os that may normally be scarred from childbirth.	■ A bluish color to the cervix and vaginal fornices may be a sign of pregnancy. ■ A pale cervix may be seen if the woman is anemic. ■ A cervix to the right or left of the midline may indicate a pelvic mass, uterine adhesions, or uterine mass. ■ Transverse or star-shaped cervical scars may reflect trauma that caused tearing of the cervix. ■ An enlarged cervix is associated with parity or infection. ■ **Nabothian cysts** (small, white or yellowish, raised, round cystic areas on the cervical surface) are benign but may become infected. ■ Polyps seen at the cervical os may be cervical or endometrial in origin.	■ The majority of prepubertal and adolescent girls do not require internal examination of the vagina and cervix. ■ Prior to pregnancy and in newly pregnant women, the cervix should be closed, thick, and rigid. ■ In the final weeks of pregnancy, the cervix should shorten and soften, and the opening should widen to allow passage of the fetus. ■ In older women, the vagina narrows, and the mucosa loses rugae and becomes pale and dry because of decreased estrogen. This leads to increased risk of vaginal infection.
Insert the fingers of the gloved dominant hand into the vagina. Palpate and move the cervix. Palpate the uterus and adnexa bimanually with the fingers of one hand at the cervix and the other hand on the lower abdomen.	In nonpregnant women, the cervix should be firm like the nose; in pregnant women, it should be softer like the lips. There is normally drainage from the cervical os that changes in consistency throughout the menstrual cycle. The uterus should be mobile and may be anteverted (tilted to the front), anteflexed (flexed to the front), retroverted (tilted to the back), retroflexed (flexed to the back), or midline. Uterine size varies with age and parity. If palpable, the ovaries should be the size of an almond, firm, mobile, smooth, and slightly tender.	■ Pain on movement of the cervix suggest cervicitis or pelvic inflammatory disease (PID). ■ Firm, irregular nodules on the uterine surface are likely to be myomas (fibroids). ■ Unilateral or bilateral smooth, compressible adnexal masses are usually cysts. ■ Tumors of the ovary are firm or nodular. ■ Palpable ovaries in an older, postmenopausal woman are abnormal and warrant further investigation.	■ Ovarian cysts are common in women of reproductive age and less common in postmenopausal women. ■ Postmenopausal women with ovarian cysts are at elevated risk for ovarian cancer. ■ Uterine fibroids become more common during a woman's 30s and 40s but usually shrink during menopause. ■ The uterus, fallopian tubes, and ovaries are smaller in older women. ■ Cancer of the ovary occurs most often in women over age 50. ■ The average age at diagnosis for uterine cancer is around 60.

Sources: Data from American Pregnancy Association. (2015a). *Breast changes during pregnancy.* Retrieved from http://americanpregnancy.org/pregnancy-health/breast-changes-during-pregnancy; Bickley, L., & Szilagyi, P. (2013). *Bates' guide to physical examination and history taking* (11th ed.). Philadelphia, PA: Wolters Kluwer/Lippincott Williams & Wilkins; Braverman, P. K., Breech, L., & American Academy of Pediatrics Committee on Adolescence. (2010). Gynecologic examination for adolescents in the pediatric office setting. *Pediatrics, 126*(3), 583–590; Brzyski, R. G., & Knudtson, K. (n.d.). *Effects of aging on the female reproductive system.* Retrieved from http://www.merckmanuals.com/home/women's-health-issues/biology-of-the-female-reproductive-system/effects-of-aging-on-the-female-reproductive-system; Hain, D. (2013). Assessing older women's health. In E. Youngkin, M. Davis, D. Schadewald, & C. Juve (Eds.), *Women's health: A primary care clinical guide* (4th ed., pp. 119–149). Boston, MA: Pearson; National Cancer Institute. (2015b). *Understanding breast changes: A health guide for women.* Retrieved from http://www.cancer.gov/types/breast/understanding-breast-changes; U.S. National Library of Medicine. (2014a). *Urethritis.* Retrieved from https://www.nlm.nih.gov/medlineplus/ency/article/000439.htm

Independent Interventions

Sexual health is important for physical and mental well-being. When patients are affected by sexual distress or dysfunction, they may experience anxiety, embarrassment, or physical discomfort as a result. Some issues, such as STIs, even present a physical danger to the patient. Before providing care related to sexuality, nurses must examine their own feelings about sex and sexuality to ensure they can establish a therapeutic relationship and maintain a nonjudgmental attitude while providing care.

Caring for patients with alterations related to sexuality may include any number of independent interventions. Some of the most common include:

- Teaching patients about age- and development-related changes in sexual structure and function (e.g., puberty, pregnancy, menopause)
- Educating patients about stages in the human sexual response
- Providing patients with information about different methods of birth control
- Educating patients about safer sex practices
- Instructing patients about STIs and how to prevent their transmission
- Teaching patients to perform breast or testicular self-examination
- Providing patients with information about resuming sexual activity after illness or another health-related event (e.g., heart attack, surgery, childbirth)
- Counseling patients about ways that particular conditions and/or medications may affect sexual function
- Teaching patients about diagnostic, medical, and surgical procedures
- Educating patients with physical impairment about adaptations that will allow them to resume or continue sexual activity
- Referring patients to appropriate community resources as necessary (e.g., psychologists, support groups, sex therapists)

When providing education about sexuality and sexual health, the nurse should include the patient's partner whenever possible and appropriate. By teaching both parties about the patient's condition, the nurse can help ease feelings of shame, blame, and discomfort, as well as facilitate better communication between the partners with regard to the problem for which the patient is receiving care. The nurse can also provide more effective instruction on various adaptations, devices, and methods that may assist the partners in continuing or resuming a mutually satisfying sexual relationship.

Dealing with Inappropriate Sexual Behavior

While on the job, nurses of both genders may encounter a variety of sexually inappropriate behaviors. These behaviors may be aggressive or nonaggressive. For example, patients may act out sexually by exposing themselves; asking the nurse to provide intimate physical care when they are capable of doing it themselves; touching the nurse inappropriately; making blatant sexual statements to the nurse; whistling or making comments about the nurse's attractiveness or desirability; or commenting to others about their sexual feelings about the nurse.

Patients engage in this type of behavior for many reasons, including fear or anxiety over their future ability to function sexually; unmet needs for intimacy and sexual closeness; misinterpretation of the nurse's behavior as sexual or provocative; the need for reassurance that they are still sexual beings and still sexually attractive; the need for attention or power; confusion (neurologic impairment or trauma can lead patients to use inappropriate sexual language, gestures, or behaviors); or the need for control (patients may be experiencing loss of control over their lives because of hospitalization, injury, or illness).

Before implementing nursing interventions with patients who engage in inappropriate sexual behavior, the nurse should determine whether the behavior is actually an attempt to communicate a physical need. For example, patients may expose themselves if they are febrile, pull at their penis if a catheter is uncomfortable or irritating, or reach for the nurse if they are unable to communicate verbally. If patients truly are engaging in inappropriate sexual behavior, the nurse should consider adopting one or more strategies listed in **Box 19–1** ».

Many times, nurses choose to ignore patients' inappropriate sexual behavior or simply "laugh it off." This can lead

---

Box 19–1
Nursing Strategies for Inappropriate Sexual Behavior

- Communicate that the patient's behavior is not acceptable by saying something like, "I really do not like the things you are saying" or "I see you are not dressed. I will be back in 10 minutes and will help you with breakfast when you get your clothes on."
- Tell the patient how the behavior makes you feel: "When you act like that toward me, I am uncomfortable. It embarrasses me and makes it hard for me to give you the care you need."
- Identify the behavior you expect: "Please call me by my name, not 'honey'" or "I expect you to keep yourself covered when I am in the room."
- Set firm limits: Take the patient's hand and move it away, use direct eye contact, and say, "Don't do that!"
- Try to refocus the patient from the inappropriate behavior to the patient's real concerns and fears, and offer to discuss sexuality concerns: "All morning you have been making very personal sexual comments about yourself. Sometimes individuals talk like that when they are concerned about the sexual part of their life and how their illness will affect them. Are there things that you have questions about or would like to talk about?"
- Report the incident to your nursing instructor, charge nurse, or clinical nurse specialist. Discuss the incident, your feelings, and possible interventions.
- Clarify the consequences of continued inappropriate behavior (e.g., avoidance, withdrawal of services, no chance to help resolve the patient's underlying concerns).

some patients to interpret the nurses' response (or lack thereof) as a sign of indifference toward or perhaps even approval of this behavior. Ignoring the behavior increases the likelihood that patients will continue to engage in such behaviors during future nursing encounters. Thus, nurses have a duty to try to stop this behavior before it is harmful to others.

Recognizing Sexual Abuse

Nurses also play a key role in recognizing signs of sexual abuse in patients of all ages, from children through older adults. Research suggests that approximately 10% of American children will be sexually abused before they turn 18; this includes approximately 1 out of 7 girls and 1 out of 25 boys. These figures are only estimates because up to 60% of victims of child sexual abuse never tell anyone what happened to them (Darkness to Light, 2015).

As mandatory reporters, nurses are required by law to report all instances of suspected child maltreatment—including child sex abuse—to the authorities. In some cases, nurses will see direct physical signs of sex abuse upon examination of pediatric patients. More often, nurses will come to suspect sex abuse based on emotional and behavioral signals. In children, these include avoidance or fear of physical contact; symptoms of depression or posttraumatic stress disorder; self-harm and/or suicidal behavior; difficulties at school; running away from home or school; changes in hygiene; regressive behaviors; and inappropriate knowledge of sexual topics and behaviors (Rape, Abuse, and Incest National Network, n.d.).

In the course of their practice, nurses may also encounter adult patients whom they suspect are victims of sexual abuse. Many signs of sexual abuse in adults are similar to those in children, including depression, anxiety, self-harm, suicidal behavior, posttraumatic stress disorder, and fear of contact. In addition to these signs, adult victims may experience disruptions in personal relationships and strong aversion to consensual sexual activity (U.S. Department of Justice, n.d.). Mandatory reporting requirements for adult patients vary by state and by patient. All nurses should be aware of their state's reporting requirements, and they should also familiarize themselves with local resources outside of law enforcement to whom suspected victims may be referred. (For additional information on working with patients who may be victims of abuse, refer to module on Trauma.)

Collaborative Therapies

As previously described, nurses assist healthcare providers with a number of tests and examinations related to sexual function, such as pelvic exams and Pap tests. Other collaborative measures in which the nurse may play a role include surgery, pharmacologic therapy, and various nonpharmacologic therapies. These measures are discussed in the sections that follow.

Surgery

Many types of surgery can affect a patient's sexuality. Some procedures directly involve the reproductive organs. For example, surgery to address prostate cancer may result in ED, and surgery to address ovarian cancer may result in early menopause. Other procedures may not involve the reproductive organs but nonetheless cause physical and/or psychologic changes that impede sexual function. For instance, spinal surgery may hinder a patient's mobility and complicate resumption of sexual activity, and bowel surgery may contribute to alterations in body image that decrease a patient's desire for sex.

Despite the pervasive link between surgery and sexuality, there are few surgical procedures specifically aimed at addressing sexual dysfunction. For men, those options that do exist are limited to the treatment of ED. They include implantation of prosthetic devices such as rods or inflatable balloons within the penis, reconstructing penile arteries to help blood flow, and blocking veins that drain the blood from the penis so that an erection is sustained (Hellstrom et al., 2010; Molodysky et al., 2013). For women, surgical treatments that improve or restore sexual function generally do so by addressing a related underlying condition. For example, surgery to remove tissue around the vaginal opening may be useful for women with sexual pain disorders, while surgical reconstruction of the vagina and/or pelvic floor can benefit women with congenital structural abnormalities or damage from childbirth. These procedures are not the same as the cosmetic "vaginal rejuvenation" or "designer vaginoplasty" surgeries offered by some practitioners, which the American College of Obstetricians and Gynecologists describes as medically unnecessary and potentially dangerous (American College of Obstetricians and Gynecologists, 2007/2014). Some transgender individuals may pursue sex reassignment surgery, in which their genitals and accessory structures are reshaped to match those typical of the gender with which they identify. This process requires multiple procedures and can be difficult to obtain because of its high cost and a lack of experienced providers.

Pharmacologic Therapy

Several types of medications may be used to help patients maintain sexual health and ability. Hormonal contraceptives and female infertility medications affect the woman's reproductive system in decidedly different ways. Both classes of drugs are discussed in greater detail in Exemplar 19.A on Family Planning, although hormonal contraceptives are also described in this section's Medications feature because they can be used to produce benefits unrelated to family planning. Both male and female hormone replacement therapies help maintain hormone levels and are sometimes used in the treatment of cancer. For more information on these drugs, refer to the Medications feature. Finally, for details regarding drugs used in the treatment of menopause, menstrual dysfunction, male and female sexual dysfunction, and STIs, refer to their respective exemplars in this module.

Nonpharmacologic Therapy

As mentioned previously, nonpharmacologic therapies may be appropriate for patients who are experiencing alterations in sexuality or sexual function. In some cases, nonpharmacologic therapy could be as simple as use of a mechanical or assistive device. For example, a man with ED might use a vacuum pump device to help attain an erection; a woman with orgasmic disorder might use a vibrator to increase sensations of pleasure during sexual activity; and a patient with spinal cord injury might use a harness, wedge, or other positioning device

Medications
Sexuality and Reproduction

CLASSIFICATION AND DRUG EXAMPLES	MECHANISMS OF ACTION	NURSING CONSIDERATIONS
Hormonal Contraceptives *Drug examples:* Estrogen–progestin combinations: Ortho-Novum (oral) Ortho Tri-Cyclen (oral) Triphasil (oral) Alesse (oral) NuvaRing (vaginal ring) Ortho Evra (transdermal patch)	■ These drugs prevent ovulation by inhibiting release of follicle-stimulating hormone (FSH) and luteinizing hormone (LH). ■ They cause thickening of the cervical mucus and thinning of the endometrium. ■ Benefits include decreased acne, menstrual bleeding, and menstrual pain.	■ Teach the patient how to use pills, patches, or vaginal rings. ■ Provide medication teaching, emphasizing the importance of daily dosage and what to do if a dose is missed. ■ Note that effectiveness declines with some antiseizure agents and antibiotics. The patient may need a backup contraceptive method if using these drugs. ■ Avoid use in women over age 35 or those who smoke because of increased risk of thromboembolic disorders. ■ Screen for pregnancy prior to use. ■ Monitor for hypertension. ■ Consider increased risk for gallbladder disease, depression, and rare liver problems.
Progestin-only drugs: Micronor (oral) Ovrette (oral) Depo-Provera (intramuscular or subcutaneous injection) Mirena (intrauterine system) Implanon (subcutaneous rod)	■ These drugs inhibit ovulation in variable cycles. ■ They cause thickening of the cervical mucus to prevent sperm penetration.	■ Teach the patient about drug action, how to use, and potential side effects. ■ For the patient using pills, stress the importance of taking them every day at the same time. ■ These drugs may be used in patients with a history of hypertension and deep venous thrombosis. ■ Irregular bleeding or amenorrhea is common.
Female Hormone Replacement *Drug examples:* Conjugated estrogens (oral, intramuscular, intravenous, intravaginal, transdermal): Premarin Cenestin Enjuvia Ogen	■ These drugs replace estrogen that declines in perimenopause and menopause. ■ They may be used to treat hormone-dependent cancers.	■ These drugs are contraindicated if the patient has had breast cancer, any estrogen-dependent cancer, or thromboembolic episodes. ■ They are contraindicated in pregnancy. Long-term use is contraindicated because of the increased risk of cancer, myocardial infarction, and thromboembolic disorders. ■ Teach the patient the importance of regular screening because of the increased risk for cancer. ■ If used in male patients, teach about potential feminizing changes. ■ Instruct the patient to immediately report calf tenderness, chest pain, or dyspnea. ■ These drugs should not be used without progestin in patients who still have a uterus because of the increased cancer risk.
Progestin (oral, intravaginal, transdermal): Provera Prometrium	■ These drugs decrease the action of estrogen on the endometrial lining. ■ They are typically administered in conjunction with estrogen to counteract some of estrogen's adverse effects on the uterus.	■ Explain that combination estrogen–progestin therapy is appropriate if the patient has not had a hysterectomy. ■ Teach the patient that combining progestin and estrogen increases the risk for myocardial infarction, stroke, breast cancer, dementia, and thromboembolic episodes. ■ Side effects include depression, weight gain, and fluid retention.
Selective estrogen receptor modifiers (SERMs) (oral): Duavee (combination estrogen and SERM) Osphema	■ The drugs work by mimicking the action of estrogens in some parts of the body. ■ They produce effects similar to those of estrogen–progestin combinations but with lower risk of uterine cancer. ■ They may be used in the treatment of breast cancer.	■ Teach the patient that SERMs increase the risk for endometrial cancer and deep vein thrombosis. ■ Use is contraindicated in women with a history of thromboembolic episodes.

Medications *(continued)*

CLASSIFICATION AND DRUG EXAMPLES	MECHANISMS OF ACTION	NURSING CONSIDERATIONS

Male Hormone Replacement
 	
Drug examples:
Androgens
  Danazol (oral)
  Fluoxymesterone (oral)
  Nandrolone (intramuscular)
  Striant (buccal)
  Androderm (transdermal)
  Androgel (topical)
	■ These drugs are used to treat hypogonadism resulting in insufficient testosterone. They are also used to increase sperm count when low testosterone is the cause.
	■ They are used as androgen replacement in aging men and to treat advanced prostate cancer.
	■ These drugs are used in women with endometriosis to suppress LH and FSH, thereby causing anovulation and amenorrhea.
	■ They are used to treat estrogen-dependent breast cancer.
		■ These drugs have virilizing effects (e.g., deepening voice, hirsutism) that may persist in women after therapy is stopped.
		■ Side effects include acne, weight gain, hyperglycemia, increased sperm count, priapism, renal stones, and jaundice.
		■ Monitor liver enzymes and serum electrolytes.

Leuprolide acetate: Lupron (implant, injection)	■ This drug inhibits gonadotropin release, thereby suppressing ovulation or spermatogenesis. ■ It has antitumor and contraceptive effects.	■ Warn the patient of pain at the injection site. ■ Teach the patient to report hematuria or decreased urine output immediately. ■ Teach the patient to expect hot flashes.

Source: Data from Adams, M. P., Holland, L. N., & Urban, C. (2017). *Pharmacology for nurses: A pathophysiologic approach* (5th ed.). Hoboken, NJ: Pearson Education.

to help facilitate genital-to-genital contact. A wide range of assistive devices are available; some (e.g., vacuum pumps, vaginal dilators) are best obtained from healthcare providers, while others (e.g., vibrators, lubricants) can be purchased from retailers. The nurse should assure patients that there is nothing shameful or wrong about purchasing or using these aids. The nurse may also find it useful to inform patients that such products can be purchased via catalog or the internet and shipped discreetly to their home.

Beyond assistive devices, nonpharmacologic therapies frequently involve an element of psychologic and/or relationship counseling. Some patients may benefit from one-on-one or couples counseling, during which the patient(s) and therapist discuss such things as possible psychologic or situational barriers to sexual activity, methods for enhancing communication and intimacy between partners, and ways to heighten the body's sexual response. Counseling may be provided by a general counselor or a dedicated sex therapist. Whereas general counselors often explore the deeper psychologic factors underlying sexual dysfunction, sex therapists focus specifically on the patient's symptoms. Sex therapists can provide accurate information about male and female sexual responses, encourage patients to use sensate focus exercises to boost desire and ease anxiety, and provide other suggestions to assist couples in achieving a fulfilling sexual relationship. Depending on the patient's problem, the therapist might do such things as help the patient explore and overcome negative attitudes about sex, recognize and verbalize desires, change the way he or she interacts with sexual partners, or engage in mindfulness techniques (American Psychological Association, 2015; Balon & Segraves, 2014; Faubion & Rullo, 2015; Mayo Clinic, 2013b).

One mindfulness technique commonly employed in sex therapy is **sensate focus**. Developed by Masters and Johnson in the 1960s, sensate focus involves several stages of guided touching in which patients and their partners are encouraged to explore each other's bodies, beginning with areas other than the breasts and genitals, then gradually incorporating these areas as they progress to full intercourse. During each stage, patients are instructed to focus on the pleasurable sensations they feel at that moment, rather than concentrating on achieving orgasm. A similar method called directed masturbation can be used by patients who do not wish to have a partner participate in the therapeutic process. Sensate focus and directed masturbation ideally help patients reduce their anxiety about sexual encounters and experience greater pleasure throughout the entire sexual experience (Weiner & Avery-Clark, 2014).

For many patients, the most successful treatment approach is a blend of pharmacologic and nonpharmacologic techniques. Known as integrated sex therapy, this approach involves whatever combination of medical, behavioral, and cognitive techniques the provider(s) determine will be most beneficial to the patient's particular problem.

Lifespan Considerations

The following sections take a closer look at some sexuality-related issues the nurse is likely to encounter when working with children, adolescents, young adults, pregnant patients, middle-age adults, and older adults. Additional information on lifespan-specific issues can also be found in the Nursing Assessment section.

Sexuality Considerations in Infants and Children

Development of a child's sense of sexuality begins at birth, when the infant is assigned a gender. For the first 12–18 months of life, the child does not yet understand the difference between male and female gender, or even between others and self. Rather, the assignment of gender primarily influences the way others interact with the infant. Over time, as the child comes to differentiate between self and others and develop an identity as male or female, external beliefs, expectations, and attitudes will shape the child's self-image, as well as the way he or she interacts with the world.

As infants begin to comprehend themselves as independent, gendered beings, they are likewise learning more about their physical bodies. Self-manipulation of the genitals is normal as infants begin to explore their bodies, and it is not done for sexual gratification, even though the child's external genitals are sensitive to touch. Later, between the ages of 1 and 3, most toddlers begin to engage in more purposeful body exploration and fondling of their own genitals, and they start to use names for their visible reproductive parts. Around the same age, children also become able to identify their own gender, and many have early awareness of the anatomical differences between males and females.

Between the ages of 4 and 5, preschoolers develop a fuller sense of self. Most continue to explore their own bodies, and it is not unusual for them to be curious about and/or explore playmates' body parts as well. Often, they refer to these parts using the correct names. During this stage of development, parents should answer children's questions about reproduction honestly yet simply. Parents should also be aware that overreaction to their child's genital exploration and/or masturbation can foster negative feelings about sex that persist well into the child's adult years.

As time progresses, gender roles are internalized as part of a child's total self-concept. Children also become more aware of their bodies, with increased modesty and desire for privacy. Self-stimulating behavior continues. Starting around age 8 or 9, most children become concerned about specific sex behaviors, and many approach their parents with explicit concerns about sexuality and reproduction. Here, it is important that the nurse provide parents and children with opportunities to express their concerns and ask questions regarding sex. The nurse should answer all questions with factual data and encourage parents to discuss basic information about sexual intercourse, menstruation, and reproduction with their children, beginning at 10 years of age or earlier. Many parents find it useful to give their children reading material on these topics and discuss it with them several days or weeks later.

As alluded to throughout this module, the family plays a crucial role in shaping an individual's view of sex and sexuality, beginning at birth and continuing into adolescence and beyond. Individuals develop their gender identity, body image, sexual self-concept, and capacity for intimacy within the context of family. Through family interactions, children learn about relationships, gender roles, and the expectations of others and themselves.

Sexuality Considerations in Adolescents

Between roughly age 12 and age 18, children undergo a period of rapid and dramatic change in relation to sex and sexuality. In terms of physical development, this is the time when primary and secondary sex characteristics appear, **spermarche** (onset of sperm production) or menarche occurs, and fertility begins. In terms of psychosocial development, this is often the period when individuals start to develop romantic relationships with interested partners. Parents continue to influence their children's beliefs regarding social and sexual behavior, but peer groups are increasingly important, particularly in the formation of gender roles. Masturbation is common, although many teens participate in various forms of sexual activity. Adolescence is also the time when some people begin to experiment with homosexual relationships.

The nurse's approach to the adolescent patient should be guided by consideration of the teen's cognitive and social development, especially when making decisions about issues such as parental involvement during the interview and physical examination. As with adult patients, a nonjudgmental attitude is crucial. The nurse should show a genuine interest in the teen and sustain that interest throughout the encounter. The nurse should try to focus on the adolescent, not the problem.

Many adolescents are hesitant to discuss health concerns in front of their parents, especially if those concerns are sexual in nature. It is good practice to ask parents to leave the room for a portion of the history, beginning when patients are around ages 10–11 (Szilagyi, 2013). Teenage patients should also be assured that everything they discuss with the nurse is confidential, unless it affects their safety. Even with their parents out of the room, many adolescents remain too shy, embarrassed, or scared to ask questions about sex or sexual organs. The nurse may have to start the conversation (Satterwhite, 2013). When discussing sexual topics, the nurse should use specific language and choose words that the adolescent understands. The nurse should end the interview portion of the assessment by asking the teen what other questions he or she may have about sex.

Examination of adolescent patients is much the same as for adult patients, except the nurse must assign a sex maturity rating based on Tanner staging. Pelvic examination of teen girls is done only when necessary because of a problem. The technique of speculum examination is the same as for an adult; however, the nurse should show the teen the speculum, let her handle it, and explain the procedure before proceeding. A gentle, unhurried approach is necessary, and a chaperone should be present.

For adolescent boys, an increase in the size of the testes is the first sign of puberty, and it is usually seen between ages 9 and 13 (Szilagyi, 2013). Increasing amounts of pubic hair and progressive penile growth should occur thereafter, with the genitals reaching adult size when the teen is around age 16 or 17. As with teen girls, the nurse should have a chaperone present during the examination of adolescent boys.

Education for the teenage patient is important and wide-ranging. At minimum, adolescents require information about the body changes they are currently experiencing, as well as those they can expect in the months ahead. Because many adolescents are already sexually active or may be in the near future, the nurse should provide teaching about contraceptives and precautions to take with regard to STIs.

The education portion of the patient encounter is also a good time for the nurse to discuss the importance of healthy dating relationships in which both partners feel safe and respected. This is critical because according to a 2013 survey conducted by the CDC (2013a), nearly 10% of high school students reported being the victim of physical or sexual dating violence during the prior 12 months. Much of the nursing focus on dating violence is aimed toward victims, and appropriately so. However, nurses should also be able to screen for signs that indicate a teen or young adult man is at risk of perpetrating dating or interpersonal (domestic) violence. Early warning signs include a belief that men should be in control and women should be submissive; jealous and possessive behaviors, such as checking up on the girlfriend and separating her from friends and family; threatening behaviors toward the girlfriend; use or ownership of weapons; a history of aggressive or violent behavior; blaming the girlfriend when he is violent, saying she provoked him; and a history of abusive relationships (CDC, 2015b, 2016). For more information on nursing care of individuals experiencing dating violence, see the exemplar on Rape and Rape Trauma Syndrome in the module on Trauma.

Sexuality Considerations in Young Adults

Young adulthood, or the period from about 18 to 40 years of age, is the time when most individuals fully establish their own lifestyle and values—including those related to sex. By their mid-20s, most individuals' heterosexual or homosexual identity is fully established. The majority of people in this age group engage in regular sexual activity, frequently in the context of a long-term relationship. Regular communication between partners is essential to understand each other's sexual and emotional needs, as well as to work through life problems and stresses.

When working with young adult patients, the most common sexuality-related issues nurses encounter relate to reproductive health. Young adults often need information about measures to prevent unwanted pregnancies. Education about prevention and treatment of STIs may also be necessary. On occasion, the nurse may encounter patients who demonstrate sexually compulsive behaviors, such as excessive reliance on pornography, use of prostitutes, or frequent contact with many sexual partners. Patients who are affected by sexually compulsive behavior should be referred for further medical and psychologic care (Karila et al., 2014).

Sexuality Considerations in Pregnant Women

For most women, pregnancy brings a range of physical and psychologic changes—some of which relate to sex and sexuality. Pregnant patients may ask the nurse whether it is safe to engage in sexual activity. In general, the answer is yes. Sex typically does not present a risk to either the woman or the fetus, but there are exceptions. In particular, the nurse should explain that vaginal sex may *not* be safe if the patient is experiencing vaginal bleeding or amniotic fluid leakage; has an incompetent or dilated cervix; has partial or total placenta previa; has a history of miscarriage, preterm labor, or premature birth; or is carrying multiples.

In these situations, the patient should consult with her healthcare provider before engaging in vaginal penetration of any sort. Furthermore, all pregnant patients should be advised to use a condom during sex if either they or their partner are not monogamous or if they opt to have sex with a new partner during the course of their pregnancy (March of Dimes, 2015; Mayo Clinic, 2015c).

Although sex is usually permitted during pregnancy, patients may report low desire while expecting, or they may find sex uncomfortable or physically taxing. These are normal consequences of fatigue, hormonal fluctuations, fetal growth, and physical changes in the woman's body. The nurse may recommend that the patient and her partner experiment with different sexual positions that put less pressure on the patient's pelvis, abdomen, and large blood vessels, such as side-lying and woman-on-top. The nurse may also suggest that the patient and her partner try alternative activities that enhance intimacy, including cuddling, kissing, mutual masturbation, and massage. In addition, the nurse should instruct the patient to seek immediate medical attention should she experience moderate to heavy bleeding, amniotic fluid leakage, contractions, or strong cramping during or after sexual activity (American Pregnancy Association, 2015b; March of Dimes, 2015; University of California San Francisco Medical Center, 2016).

After giving birth, patients should avoid vaginal sex for at least 6 weeks, potentially longer if the woman had tearing or required a cesarean section. Advise postpartum patients that they may become fertile before they resume menstruation, so contraceptive measures are necessary once they return to sexual activity. Because physical and hormonal changes can make sex uncomfortable after childbirth, the nurse should educate the patient about ways to enhance the sexual experience, such as by "going slowly" and using lubricants. All women who recently gave birth should be screened for postpartum depression.

Sexuality Considerations in Middle-Age Patients

Between the ages of 40 and 65, many men and women continue to enjoy sexual activity. However, age-related declines in hormone production trigger the onset of the climacteric and commonly contribute to alterations in sexual function.

As previously mentioned, the female climacteric involves reductions in estrogen and progesterone that eventually culminate in menopause. Menopause typically occurs when a woman is between 45 and 55 years old. As women enter into menopause, they often experience sexual problems related to lowered hormone levels; for example, they may report irregular lowered desire and increased vaginal dryness. The nurse should advise middle-age female patients that these changes are not their fault, but rather are the result of normal body changes. The nurse can also suggest various strategies to help patients resume a more satisfying sex life, such as increased foreplay and use of personal lubricants. Referral to a healthcare provider may also be appropriate. (For more information, see Exemplar 19.B on Menopause.)

In men, the climacteric occurs more gradually and less dramatically. Although androgen production and spermatogenesis are decreased, men retain their fertility for the remainder of their lives. Still, reduced testosterone levels and a host of other medical conditions that frequently occur in middle age (e.g., heart disease, onset of type II diabetes) mean that many patients in this age group experience ED. See Exemplar 19.D on Sexual Dysfunction for more information on ED.

Beyond the physical changes associated with the climacteric, a number of psychosocial changes can affect sexual function in middle age. As both men and women approach the end of their careers and watch their children leave home, they may find it difficult to adjust to their new roles. In some cases, these difficulties may contribute to disruptions in sexual function. Assess patients' needs, concerns, signs, and symptoms. Refer patients to counseling as appropriate.

Sexuality Considerations in Older Adults

Contrary to popular belief, interest in sexual activity often continues well into old age. Older adults may define sexuality far more broadly than younger patients, including in their definition activities and ideals such as touching, hugging, romantic gestures (e.g., giving or receiving roses), comfort, warmth, dressing up, joy, spirituality, and beauty.

Despite continued interest in sex, many older adults have alterations in sexual function related to the aging process in general or to specific disease processes. With increased age, it is normal for a woman's vaginal secretions to diminish, vaginal walls to thin, and breasts to atrophy. These changes may contribute to dyspareunia, or painful intercourse. Penetration may also be difficult because the vaginal opening may be partially obscured by the labia, tightened by atrophy, and/or lacking the lubrication needed for smooth entrance of the penis. In these cases, the nurse might advise the patient to use a vaginal lubricant as part of sexual activity and to use her hand to guide her partner's penis into the vagina.

As men enter old age, most produce fewer sperm and need more time to achieve an erection and to ejaculate. The nurse should advise patients that this is normal and suggest possible nonpharmacologic techniques for enhancing the sexual experience. Referral to a healthcare provider may also be appropriate.

In addition to aging, chronic pain and osteoarthritis are two common problems that have deleterious effects on sexual activity in older adults. Arthritis in the hip joint presents the greatest challenge to satisfying sexual activity (DeLemater, 2012), but it can be ameliorated by changes in coital position, application of heat, and timing sexual activity during the day, when joints are less painful. Warm baths can also help relieve pain and even be incorporated as foreplay.

Cardiovascular disease is another condition that affects many older adults, often causing them to question whether it is safe to engage in sexual activity. In general, if an older adult can climb two flights of stairs or walk at a rate of 2 miles per hour without chest pain or shortness of breath, then he or she should have no cardiac problems during sexual intercourse. Consideration should be given to the partner with the less stable vital signs (particularly blood pressure), and that partner should not be positioned on top. Also, older adults with heart failure who develop fatigue or shortness of breath will be more comfortable in a semireclining position or lying under their partner during sex (Levine et al., 2012).

Like cardiovascular disease, diabetes mellitus can have negative effects on the sexual expression of older adults. Diabetes is correlated with low libido in men and women, ED in men, and reductions in vaginal lubrication in women (Neithercott, 2012). Both vascular and nerve damage related to diabetes may affect sexual arousal and orgasm. When patients report these problems, the nurse should consider encouraging alternative expressions of sexuality, such as body caressing, manipulation of the partner's genitals with the hand, or mutual masturbation.

Older adults often benefit from teaching related to sexuality; however, they may be hesitant to bring up sexual topics with the nurse. To help facilitate such discussion, the nurse can first validate the older adult's desire for sexual activity. For example, the nurse may start the conversation with a neutral phrase, such as, "Many people think older adults aren't interested in sex, but that's not true. I wonder if you have any questions that I might answer for you." Additional strategies include offering specific factual information; discussing strategies such as timing of pain medication or alternating coital positions; and providing referrals to an advanced practice nurse or other expert as appropriate.

Case Study >> Part 3

Eileen Jarvis, age 65, has lived with her son Ralph and his wife Betty for the past 2 years. She has become much more active in the past 6 months as she has recovered from the shock and grief of losing her husband of 44 years. Ms. Jarvis regularly volunteers at the hospital with Betty Jarvis and goes to the Senior Center to walk and to socialize with friends. At the Senior Center, she met a man named Tom Lane, and they have been going out together. A couple of days ago, Mr. Lane asked Ms. Jarvis to marry him. She decided to say yes.

Ms. Jarvis has come to Ms. Walker, the family's nurse practitioner, for her annual checkup. After her examination, Ms. Jarvis tells Ms. Walker of her marriage plans and asks about sex. Ms. Walker congratulates Ms. Jarvis and asks her about her relationship with Mr. Lane. Ms. Walker asks, "Have you and Tom talked about sex?" and "Do you both know each other's sexual history?"

Clinical Reasoning Questions Level I

1. Communication about sexual needs and expectations promotes successful intimate relationships. Do you think Ms. Walker has helped Ms. Jarvis to plan better communication with Mr. Lane?
2. Why do you think it is important for a couple planning a sexual relationship to know about each other's sexual history before having intercourse?
3. Menopause and decreased estrogen levels can cause physical changes that make sexual intercourse uncomfortable. What are these changes?

Clinical Reasoning Questions Level II

4. *Refer to Exemplar 19.B on Menopause:* If Ms. Jarvis has dyspareunia related to sexual intercourse, one cause may be atrophic vaginitis. What are some interventions that may relieve this problem?
5. *Refer to Exemplar 19.E on STIs:* Ms. Walker knows that the incidence of STIs is increasing among older adults, but at the same time, she does not want to cause undue anxiety or problems in the relationship between Ms. Jarvis and Mr. Lane. Now that Ms. Jarvis has initiated the conversation about sex, what would you suggest Ms. Walker teach Ms. Jarvis about discussing this very private issue with her fiancé?

REVIEW The Concept of Sexuality

RELATE Link the Concepts

Linking the concept of sexuality with the concept of mood and affect:

1. Explain how psychologic factors may affect sexuality and how problems with sexuality may affect psychologic well-being.

2. What are appropriate referral resources for individuals with mood disorders who are experiencing sexual dysfunction?

Linking the concept of sexuality with the concept of elimination:

3. Explain how the proximity of the sexual organs and the organs of elimination may put patients at risk for problems with elimination.

4. What are appropriate nursing interventions for patients with elimination problems related to sexuality?

Linking the concept of sexuality with the concept of perfusion:

5. Explain how poor perfusion may affect sexuality for both men and women.

6. What nursing interventions are indicated for men and women who are experiencing sexual difficulty related to poor perfusion?

READY Go to Volume 3: Clinical Nursing Skills

- SKILL 1.10   Abdomen: Assessing
- SKILL 1.11   Anus: Assessing
- SKILL 1.12   Breasts and Axillae: Assessing
- SKILL 1.15   Genitals and Inguinal Area: Assessing
- SKILL 1.18   Mouth and Oropharynx: Assessing
- SKILL 1.25   Skin: Assessing
- SKILL 2.8   Perineal-Genital Area: Caring for
- SKILL 3.1   Pain in Newborn, Infant, Child, or Adult: Assessing
- SKILL 3.3   Pain Relief: Complementary Health Approaches
- SKILL 3.6   Sleep Promotion: Assisting
- SKILL 3.9   Dry Heat: Applying

- SKILL 4.3   Urine Specimen, Clean-Catch, Closed Drainage System for Culture and Sensitivity: Obtaining
- SKILL 14.17   Postpartum, Maternal: Assessing
- SKILL 14.18   Postpartum, Perineum: Assessing
- SKILL 15.1   Abuse: Newborn, Infant, Child, Older Adult, Assessing for

REFER Go to Pearson MyLab Nursing and eText

- Additional review materials

REFLECT Apply Your Knowledge

Qualyndria Gunderson, age 14, comes to the physician's office with her mother and requests to be seen alone while her mother sits in the waiting area. The nurse escorts Qualyndria back to the examination room. Qualyndria says she has become sexually active and would like a prescription for birth control pills but does not want her mother to know about it. She says her mother thinks she is here to discuss menstrual pain.

When the nurse goes out to the waiting room to escort another patient into the examination area, Ms. Gunderson asks to speak to the nurse. After escorting Ms. Gunderson to an area where they can talk privately, the nurse learns that Ms. Gunderson has been dodging questions from her daughter about sexuality. Ms. Gunderson says she does not want her daughter to know about such matters until she is at least 18 years old. Ms. Gunderson says she is warning the nurse because she thinks her daughter may ask these questions of the healthcare team. She also asks the nurse to avoid answering the questions or supplying her daughter with information about sex, explaining that she believes this information should come from her and that she will provide it when she feels her daughter is old enough to understand.

1. How would you respond to Ms. Gunderson?

2. How would Ms. Gunderson's request affect what you teach Qualyndria about responsible sexual behavior?

3. What would you tell Ms. Gunderson about her daughter's sexual activity?

›› Exemplar 19.A
Family Planning

Exemplar Learning Outcomes

19.A Analyze family planning as it relates to sexuality.

- Contrast family planning options.
- Describe the role of genetics in family planning.
- Outline types of contraception used in family planning.
- Summarize diagnostic tests and therapies used by interprofessional teams in the collaborative care of individuals in need of family planning.
- Differentiate considerations for care of patients with regard to family planning across the lifespan.
- Apply the nursing process in providing culturally competent care to an individual who needs family planning.

Exemplar Key Terms

Autosomes, *1476*
Carrier, *1478*
Cervical cap, *1483*
Coitus interruptus, *1481*
Combined oral contraceptives (COCs), *1485*
Condom, *1481*
Depo-Provera, *1486*
Diaphragm, *1482*
Emergency contraception (EC), *1487*
Estrogen, *1480*
Fertility awareness–based methods, *1480*
Genotype, *1478*
In vitro fertilization (IVF), *1490*
Infertility, *1475*
Intrauterine contraception (IUC), *1484*
Mendelian (single-gene) inheritance, *1478*
Monosomic, *1476*
Monosomies, *1477*
Mosaicism, *1476*
Non-Mendelian (multifactorial) inheritance, *1478*

Overview

Some of the most serious decisions couples must make relate to family planning and reproduction: whether and when to have children and how many children they want. Information provided by nurses and other health professionals can help patients make informed decisions about contraception and childbearing. Some couples are unable to fulfill their dream of having a baby because of infertility or genetic problems, but developments in medicine have helped growing numbers of couples overcome such issues. Preconception planning can help couples prepare for pregnancy and the delivery of their newborn.

Contraception

The decision to use a method of contraception may be made individually by a woman or man or jointly by a couple. The decision may be motivated by a desire to avoid pregnancy, to gain control over the number of children conceived, or to determine the spacing of future children. In choosing a specific method, consistency of use outweighs the absolute reliability of the method.

Decisions about contraception should be made voluntarily, with full knowledge of advantages, disadvantages, effectiveness, side effects, contraindications, and long-term effects. Many outside factors influence this choice, including cultural practices, religious beliefs, attitudes and personal preferences, cost, effectiveness, misinformation, practicality of method, and self-esteem. Different methods of contraception may be appropriate at different times for individuals and couples.

Preconception Counseling

Making the decision to have children is the first step a couple makes in the process of conception. For some couples, this decision is part of discussions during the dating process. Other couples do not make the choice to have children until later in their relationship. This decision involves consideration of each individual's goals, relationship expectations, and desire to be a parent. Sometimes one individual wishes to have a child but the other does not. In these situations, open discussion is essential for reaching a mutually acceptable decision.

Couples who wish to have children face a decision about the timing of pregnancy. At what point in their lives do they believe it is best to become parents? Pregnancy is a life-changing event and never proceeds just as the couple anticipates, even when the pregnancy is planned and the timing is convenient.

For couples who have religious beliefs that do not support contraception or who feel that fertility planning is unnatural, planning the timing of the pregnancy is unacceptable and irrelevant. These couples can still take steps to ensure that they are in the best possible physical and mental health if and when pregnancy occurs.

Preconception Health Measures

Most preconception recommendations focus on helping the couple attain their best possible health state so they do not enter pregnancy with unnecessary risks. The nurse begins by teaching the couple about known or suspected health risks, including the risks of smoking, secondhand smoke, caffeine, alcohol, and other drugs can pose to both mother and baby. The nurse also provides information about any prescription or over-the-counter medications the woman is taking and encourages her to discuss them with her healthcare provider.

Women with chronic health problems, such as thyroid disorders, seizures, hypertension, and diabetes, should have a preconception visit with the appropriate specialist to determine whether pregnancy is advised. Changes in medication and/or treatment plans may be warranted. Because of the possible teratogenic effects of environmental hazards, the nurse should also urge the couple contemplating pregnancy to determine possible exposure to any environmental hazards, such as radiation or chemical exposure, at work or in their community.

Physical Examination

Both partners should have a physical examination to identify any health problems so that these can be corrected if possible. These problems might include medical conditions, such as high blood pressure, diabetes, or obesity; problems that pose a threat to fertility, such as certain STIs; or conditions that keep the individual from achieving optimal health, such as anemia or colitis. If the family history indicates previous genetic disorders or if the woman is over age 35, the nurse may suggest that the couple seek genetic counseling. In addition to the history and physical exam, the woman may have a variety of laboratory tests. Before conception, the woman is also advised to have a dental examination and any necessary dental work to avoid exposure to x-rays, local anesthetics, and risk of infection while pregnant.

Nutrition

Before conception, it is recommended that the woman be at an average weight for her build and height. Women who are underweight should try to gain weight, as prepregnancy underweight increases the risk for preterm birth (Girsen et al., 2016); women who are overweight should try to get their weight down, because maternal obesity is a risk factor for pregnancy complications. The woman should be advised to follow a nutritious diet that contains ample quantities of all essential nutrients. Some nutritionists emphasize intake of calcium, protein, iron, B complex vitamins, vitamin C, and magnesium. Folic acid supplementation before conception is recommended, as folic acid decreases the risk of neural tube defects. Intake of vitamins that exceeds the recommended dietary allowance (RDA) should be avoided, because it can cause severe fetal problems. Cultural norms that affect nutritional intake should be assessed.

Exercise

A woman is advised to continue her present pattern of exercise or to establish a regular exercise plan beginning at least 3 months before she attempts to become pregnant. An exercise routine that the woman enjoys and maintains will provide the best results. Exercise that includes some aerobic conditioning and some general muscle toning will improve the woman's circulation and general health. Once an exercise program is well established, the woman is generally encouraged to continue it during pregnancy. During pregnancy, at least 150 minutes of moderate exercise per week is recommended (CDC, 2015c).

Immunizations

All women of reproductive age need to be up to date with immunizations prior to pregnancy. When a pregnancy is planned, the woman should receive immunizations for diphtheria, tetanus, pertussis, measles, mumps, rubella, and varicella. If any immunizations or boosters need to be administered, they should be finished 3 months prior to conception (Blackburn, 2013). Pregnant woman should be immunized against influenza, especially if she will be pregnant during flu season (CDC, 2014c). The flu vaccine can be given during pregnancy if needed.

Infertility Counseling

Infertility, or a lack of conception despite unprotected sexual intercourse for at least 12 months (WHO, 2015a), has profound emotional, psychologic, and economic impacts on affected couples and society. The term *sterility* is applied when there is an absolute factor preventing reproduction. **Subfertility** is used to describe a couple who has difficulty conceiving because both partners have reduced fertility. The term **secondary infertility** is applied to couples who have been unable to conceive after one or more successful pregnancies or who cannot sustain a pregnancy.

Fertility may be at risk in men who abuse alcohol, use tobacco or drugs, are exposed to environmental toxins, take certain prescription drugs for health problems, or have had treatment for cancer. Age is also a risk factor for men, but age is a much greater risk for women. Other risk factors for female infertility include excess alcohol consumption, tobacco use, stress, poor diet, being overweight or underweight, athletic training, health problems that affect hormones, or being infected with an STI (Eisenberg & Brumbaugh, 2012).

Approximately 9–14% of U.S. couples in their reproductive years are infertile (Louis et al., 2013). Public perception is that the incidence of infertility is increasing, but there has actually been no significant change in the proportion of infertile couples in the United States. Understanding the components necessary for normal fertility can help the nurse identify the many factors that may cause infertility. For example, fertility in women is supported by a healthy reproductive system with adequate hormones that is free of any obstruction between the ovaries and the uterus. Likewise, fertility in men is supported by a genital tract with normal secretions that is free of obstructions.

Normal findings are correlated with the possible causes of deviation outlined in **Table 19–2 »**. Approximately one third of the remaining couples are infertile because of a male factor, one third are infertile due to a female factor, and one

TABLE 19–2 Possible Causes of Infertility

Necessary Norms	Deviations from Normal
Female	
Favorable cervical mucus	Cervicitis, cervical stenosis, use of personal lubricants, antisperm antibodies (immunologic response)
Clear passage between cervix and tubes	Myomas, adhesions, adenomyosis, polyps, endometritis, cervical stenosis, endometriosis, congenital anomalies
Patent tubes with normal motility	Pelvic inflammatory disease (PID), peritubal adhesions, endometriosis, intrauterine contraception (IUC), salpingitis (e.g., related to chlamydia or other STIs), neoplasm, ectopic pregnancy, tubal ligation
Ovulation and release of ova	Primary ovarian failure, polycystic ovary syndrome (PCOS), hypothyroidism, pituitary tumor, lactation, periovarian adhesions, endometriosis, premature ovarian failure, hyperprolactinemia, Turner syndrome
No obstruction between ovary and tubes	Adhesions, endometriosis, PID
Endometrial preparation	Anovulation, luteal phase defect, malformation, uterine infection, Asherman syndrome
Male	
Normal semen analysis	Abnormalities of sperm or semen, polyspermia, congenital defect in testicular development, mumps after adolescence, cryptorchidism, infection, gonadal exposure to x-rays, chemotherapy, smoking, alcohol abuse, malnutrition, chronic or acute metabolic disease, medications (e.g., morphine, aspirin, ibuprofen), cocaine use, marijuana use, constrictive underclothing, heat
Unobstructed genital tract	Infections, tumors, congenital anomalies, vasectomy, strictures, trauma, varicocele
Normal genital tract secretions	Infections, autoimmunity to semen, tumors
Ejaculate deposited at the cervix	Premature ejaculation, impotence, hypospadias, retrograde ejaculation (e.g., as can happen with diabetes), spinal cord lesions, obesity (inhibiting adequate penetration)

Sources: Data from American Pregnancy Association. (2015c). *Female infertility.* Retrieved from http://americanpregnancy.org/infertility/female-infertility; American Pregnancy Association. (2015d). *Male infertility.* Retrieved from http://americanpregnancy.org/infertility/male-infertility; Centers for Disease Control and Prevention (CDC). (2015e). *What is infertility?* Retrieved from http://www.cdc.gov/reproductivehealth/infertility/; Mayo Clinic. (2014e). *Infertility: Symptoms and causes.* Retrieved from http://www.mayoclinic.org/diseases-conditions/infertility/basics/causes/con-20034770; Valentine, M., & Gardella, J. (2013). Infertility. In E. Youngkin, M. Davis, D. Schadewald, & C. Juve (Eds.), *Women's health: A primary care clinical guide* (4th ed., pp. 273–305). Boston, MA: Pearson.

third are infertile because of either an unknown cause (unexplained infertility) or a problem with both partners (Mayo Clinic, 2014d). Professional intervention can help infertile couples achieve pregnancy. The CDC reports that about 1.5% of infants born in the United States each year are conceived via assisted reproductive technology (CDC, 2015d).

Young couples with no history of reproductive disorders should be referred for infertility evaluation if they have been unable to conceive after at least 1 year of attempting to achieve pregnancy. An earlier workup is indicated in couples with a positive history for fertility-lowering disease or advancing maternal age (Eisenberg & Brumbaugh, 2012). If the woman is over age 35, she is less likely to become pregnant because her ovaries contain a smaller number of eggs and the eggs that are left may not be as healthy, and she is more prone to miscarriage.

Genetics

Once conception has occurred, families may have special reproductive concerns. The desired and expected outcome of any pregnancy is the birth of a healthy, "perfect" baby. Parents experience grief, fear, and anger when they discover that their baby has been born with a defect or genetic disease. Such an abnormality may be evident at birth or may not appear for some time. The baby may have inherited a disorder from one parent or both, which may create guilt and strife within the family.

Regardless of the type or scope of the problem, parents will have many questions: "What did I do?" "What caused the disorder?" "How do I cope with the disorder?" "Will this happen with future pregnancies?" The nurse must anticipate the couple's concerns and guide, direct, and support the family. To do so, the nurse must have a basic knowledge of genetics and genetic counseling.

Genetic Disorders

All hereditary material is carried on tightly coiled strands of deoxyribonucleic acid (DNA) found in genes that are housed in chromosomes within a cell's nucleus. Genes are the basic physical unit of inheritance (National Institutes of Health [NIH], n.d.). Completion of the Human Genome Project in 2003 has facilitated remarkable advances in genetic disease research and led to the discovery of more than 1800 disease genes (NIH, 2013).

All somatic (body) cells contain 46 chromosomes, which is the *diploid* number; the sperm and egg contain half as many (23) chromosomes, or the *haploid* number. There are 23 pairs of homologous chromosomes (matched pairs of chromosomes with one chromosome in each pair inherited from each parent). Twenty-two of the pairs are **autosomes** (non-sex chromosomes), and one pair is made up of the sex chromosomes, X and Y. A normal woman has a 46,XX chromosome constitution; a normal man has a 46,XY chromosome constitution.

Chromosome abnormalities can occur in either the autosomes or the sex chromosomes and can be divided into two categories: abnormalities of number and abnormalities of structure. Even small alterations in chromosomes can cause problems, especially in the area of growth and development. Some abnormalities can be also passed on to other offspring.

Thus, in some cases, chromosomal analysis is appropriate even if the clinical manifestations of a disorder are mild.

Abnormalities of Chromosomal Number

Abnormalities of chromosomal number are most often caused by *nondisjunction*, a failure of paired chromosomes to separate properly during cell division. If nondisjunction occurs in either the sperm or the egg before fertilization, the resulting zygote (fertilized egg) will have an abnormal chromosome makeup in all its cells. In other words, each cell that develops from the zygote will be **monosomic** (having only one copy of a particular chromosome) or **trisomic** (having three copies of a particular chromosome). If nondisjunction occurs after fertilization, the developing zygote will have cells with two or more different chromosomal makeups, evolving into two or more different cell lines (**mosaicism**). Chromosome mosaics have trisomy occurring in some but not all cells in the body, in which case the manifestations are not as severe (CDC, 2014d).

Trisomies result when a normal gamete (egg or sperm) unites with a gamete that contains an extra chromosome. When this happens, the resulting zygote has 47 chromosomes and is trisomic for the extra chromosome. Most trisomies are fatal, but several are compatible with human life (see **Table 19–3 ≫**). For example, Down syndrome is the most common trisomy observed in children (see **Figure 19–11 ≫**). With this condition, the presence of an extra copy of chromosome 21 produces distinctive clinical features (see **Figure 19–12 ≫**).

The risk of having a child with Down syndrome increases when the mother is age 35 or older because the ovum has been in a suspended state for a long time. This time span increases the likelihood that the chromosomes will divide incorrectly (American Pregnancy Association, 2015e).

Two other trisomies are trisomy 18 (Edwards syndrome) and trisomy 13 (Patau syndrome) (refer to Table 19–3). The prognosis for both trisomies 13 and 18 is extremely poor. Most children with these trisomies die within the first 3 months of life from complications related to respiratory and cardiac abnormalities. However, 5–10% survive the

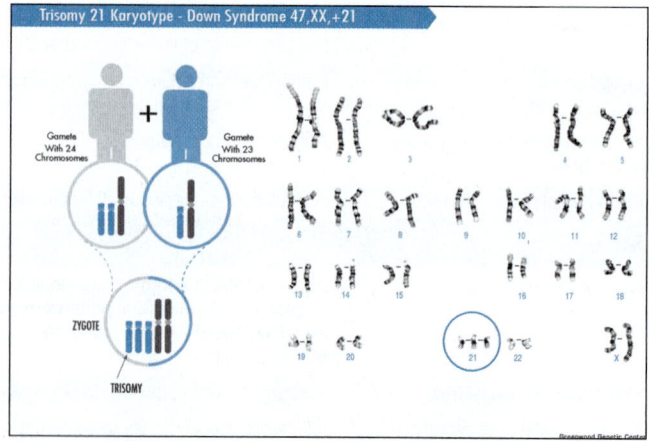

Source: From Greenwood Genetics Center. (2007). *Genetic counseling aids* (5th ed.). Greenwood, SC: Author.

Figure 19–11 ≫ Karyotype of a woman who has trisomy 21, Down syndrome. Note the extra chromosome 21.

TABLE 19–3 Chromosomal Syndromes

Altered Chromosome	Genetic Defect and Incidence	Characteristics
5P	*Genetic defect:* Deletion of short arm of chromosome 5 (cri du chat, or cat-cry, syndrome) *Incidence:* 1 in 20,000 live births	*CNS:* Severe mental retardation; a catlike cry in infancy *Head:* Microcephaly; hypertelorism (widely spaced eyes); epicanthal folds; low-set ears *Other:* Failure to thrive; various organ malformations
13	*Genetic defect:* Trisomy 13 (Patau syndrome) *Incidence:* 1 in 16,000 live births	*CNS:* Mental retardation; severe hypotonia; seizures *Head:* Microcephaly; microphthalmia and/or coloboma (keyhole-shaped pupil); malformed ears; aplasia of external auditory canal; micrognathia (abnormally small lower jaw); cleft lip and palate *Hands:* Polydactyly (extra digits); abnormal posturing of fingers; abnormal fingerprints *Other:* Congenital heart defects; hemangiomas; gastrointestinal tract defects; various malformations of other organs
18	*Genetic defect:* Trisomy 18 (Edwards syndrome) *Incidence:* 1 in 5000 live births	*CNS:* Mental retardation; severe hypotonia *Head:* Prominent occiput; low-set ears; corneal opacities; ptosis (drooping eyelids) *Hands:* Third and fourth fingers overlapped by second and fifth fingers; abnormal fingerprints; syndactyly (webbing of fingers) *Other:* Congenital heart defects; renal abnormalities; single umbilical artery; gastrointestinal tract abnormalities; rocker-bottom feet; cryptorchidism; various malformations of other organs
21	*Genetic defect:* Trisomy 21 (Down syndrome) (secondary nondisjunction or 14/21 unbalanced translocation) *Incidence:* average 1 in 700 live births; incidence variable with age of woman	*CNS:* Mental retardation; hypotonia at birth *Head:* Flattened occiput; depressed nasal bridge; epicanthal folds; white specking of the iris (Brushfield spots); protrusion of the tongue; high, arched palate; low-set ears *Hands:* Broad, short fingers; abnormalities of finger and foot; abnormal fingerprints; transverse palmar crease *Other:* Congenital heart disease
XO (sex chromosome)	*Genetic defect:* Only one X chromosome or partially missing second X chromosome in female (Turner syndrome) *Incidence:* 1 in 2500 live female births	*CNS:* No intellectual impairment; some perceptual difficulties *Head:* Low hairline; webbed neck *Trunk:* Short stature; cubitus valgus (increased carrying angle of arm); excessive nevi (congenital discoloration of skin because of pigmentation); broad, shieldlike chest with widely spaced nipples; puffy feet; no toenails *Other:* Fibrous streaks in ovaries; underdeveloped secondary sex characteristics; primary amenorrhea; usually infertile; renal anomalies; coarctation of the aorta
XXY (sex chromosome)	*Genetic defect:* Extra X chromosome in male (Klinefelter syndrome) *Incidence:* 1 in 1000 live male births, approximately 1–2% of men in institutions	*CNS:* Mild mental retardation *Trunk:* Occasional gynecomastia; eunuchoid body proportions (lack of male muscular and sexual development) *Other:* Small, soft testes; underdeveloped secondary sex characteristics; usually sterile

Sources: Data from Genetic Science Learning Center. (2015a). *Genetic disorders.* Retrieved from http://learn.genetics.utah.edu/content/disorders; Littleton-Gibbs, L. Y., & Engebretson, J. C. (2013). *Maternity nursing care* (2nd ed.). Clifton Park, NY: Delmar; U.S. National Library of Medicine. (2012). Turner syndrome. *Genetics Home Reference.* Retrieved from http://ghr.nlm.nih.gov/condition/turner-syndrome#definition; U.S. National Library of Medicine. (2016a). Trisomy 13. *Genetics Home Reference.* Retrieved from http://ghr.nlm.nih.gov/condition/trisomy-13; U.S. National Library of Medicine. (2016b). Cri-du-chat syndrome. *Genetics Home Reference.* Retrieved from https://ghr.nlm.nih.gov/condition/cri-du-chat-syndrome

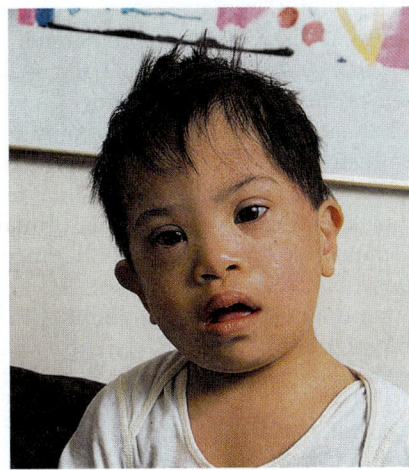

Source: Joni Hofmann/Fotolia.

Figure 19–12 ❯❯ A boy with Down syndrome.

first year of life; therefore, the family needs to plan for the possibility of long-term care of a child with severe disabilities and for family support (U.S. National Library of Medicine, 2016a, 2016c).

Monosomies occur when a normal gamete unites with a gamete that is missing a chromosome. Turner syndrome (also called XO or 45X) is a monosomy caused by the loss of the paternal X chromosome. It occurs in roughly 1 in 2500 live female births worldwide, though it is believed to be much more common among pregnancies that end in miscarriage or stillbirth (U.S. National Library of Medicine, 2012). Infants who survive with this condition are chromosome mosaics and may be sterile (see Table 19–3).

Abnormalities of Chromosome Structure

Abnormalities of chromosome structure involve only parts of a chromosome and occur in two forms: translocation and deletions or additions. Some children born with Down syndrome have an abnormal rearrangement of chromosomal material known as a *translocation*. The two types of Down syndrome are clinically indistinguishable; the only way to distinguish them is to do a chromosome analysis.

Structure abnormality is also caused by additions or deletions of chromosomal material. Any portion of a chromosome may be lost or added, generally leading to some adverse effect. Depending on how much chromosomal material is involved, the clinical effects may be mild or severe. Many types of additions and deletions have been described, such as the deletion of the short arm of chromosome 5 (cri du chat, or cat-cry, syndrome) or the deletion of the long arm of chromosome 18 (Edwards syndrome). Table 19–3 lists other chromosomal syndromes.

Sex Chromosome Abnormalities

The most common sex chromosome abnormalities are Turner syndrome in girls (45,XO with no Barr bodies present) and Klinefelter syndrome in boys (47,XXY with one Barr body present). See Table 19–3 for clinical descriptions of these abnormalities. Klinefelter syndrome is usually the result of nondisjunction of the X chromosome in the ovum. Maternal age over 35 years slightly increases the risk for this abnormality (Mayo Clinic, 2013c).

Modes of Inheritance

Many inherited diseases are produced by abnormality in a single gene or pair of genes. In such instances, the chromosomes are normal on the gross level. The defect is at the gene level. Some of these gene defects can be detected by technologies such as DNA analysis and other biochemical assays.

The two major categories of inheritance are **Mendelian (single-gene) inheritance** and **non-Mendelian (multifactorial) inheritance**. Each single-gene trait is determined by a pair of genes working together. These genes are responsible for the observable expression of the traits (e.g., brown eyes, dark skin), referred to as the **phenotype**. The total genetic makeup of an individual is referred to as the **genotype** (pattern of the genes on the chromosomes).

One of the genes for a trait is inherited from an individual's mother, the other from the father. An individual who has two identical genes at a given locus is considered to be *homozygous* for that trait. Individuals are considered to be *heterozygous* for a particular trait when they have two different alleles (alternative forms of the same gene) at a given locus on a pair of homologous chromosomes. A parent may be a **carrier** for a single-gene disorder without having any of the manifestations; that is, he or she is phenotypically normal (Genetic Science Learning Center, 2015b).

The best known modes of single-gene inheritance are autosomal dominant, autosomal recessive, and X-linked (sex-linked) recessive. There is also an X-linked dominant mode of inheritance and fragile X syndrome, both of which are uncommon.

Autosomal Dominant Inheritance

An individual is said to have an autosomal dominant inherited disorder if the disease trait is heterozygous; that is, if the abnormal gene overshadows the normal gene of the pair to produce the trait. In autosomal dominant inheritance, an affected individual generally has an affected parent, which usually results in multiple generations having the disorder.

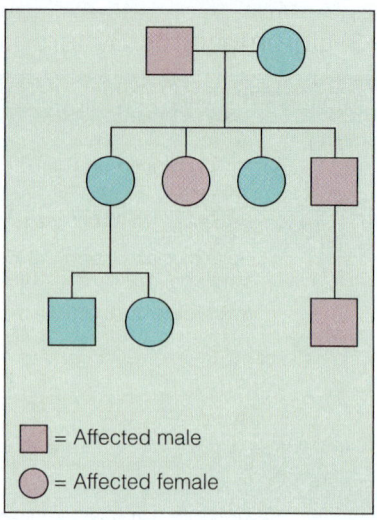

= Affected male

= Affected female

Figure 19–13 ⟫ Autosomal dominant pedigree. One parent is affected. Statistically, 50% of offspring will be affected regardless of gender.

Affected individuals have a 50% chance of passing the abnormal gene to each of their children (see **Figure 19–13 ⟫**). Men and women are equally affected, and a father can pass the abnormal gene on to his son. This is an important principle when distinguishing autosomal dominant disorders from X-linked disorders.

Autosomal dominant inherited disorders have varying degrees of presentation. This is an important factor in counseling families concerning autosomal dominant disorders. Although a parent may have a mild form of the disease, the child may have a more severe form.

Common autosomal dominant inherited disorders are Huntington disease, polycystic kidney disease, neurofibromatosis, and achondroplastic dwarfism.

Autosomal Recessive Inheritance

In an autosomal recessive inherited disorder, the individual must have two abnormal genes (one from the mother and one from the father) to be affected. In autosomal recessive inheritance, an affected individual may have clinically normal parents, but both parents are carriers of the abnormal gene (see **Figure 19–14 ⟫**). When both parents are carriers, there is a 25% chance that the abnormal gene will be passed to any of their offspring. Each pregnancy has a 25% chance of resulting in an affected child. If a child of two carrier parents is clinically normal, there is a 50% chance that the child is a carrier of the gene. Note that in autosomal recessive disorders, both male and female offspring are equally affected and there is an increased history of consanguineous matings (mating of close relatives).

Some common autosomal recessive inherited disorders are cystic fibrosis, phenylketonuria, galactosemia, sickle cell disease, Tay–Sachs disease, and most metabolic disorders.

X-linked Recessive Inheritance

X-linked, or sex-linked, disorders are those in which the abnormal gene is carried on the X chromosome. Thus, an X-linked disorder is manifested in a son who carries the abnormal gene on his X chromosome. His mother is

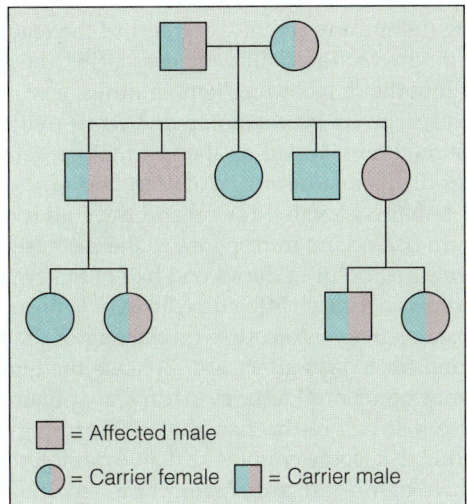

Figure 19–14 》 Autosomal recessive pedigree. Both parents are carriers. Statistically, 25% of offspring are affected regardless of gender.

considered to be a carrier when the normal gene on one X chromosome overshadows the abnormal gene on the other X chromosome. In X-linked recessive inheritance, there is no male-to-male transmission. Affected male offspring obtain the abnormal gene through the female line (see **Figure 19–15 》**). There is a 50% chance that a carrier mother will pass the normal gene to each of her sons, who will thus be unaffected. There is a 50% chance that a carrier mother will pass the abnormal gene to each of her daughters, who will become carriers. Fathers affected with an X-linked disorder cannot pass the disorder to their sons, but all their daughters become carriers of the disorder. Common X-linked recessive disorders include hemophilia, Duchenne muscular dystrophy, and color blindness.

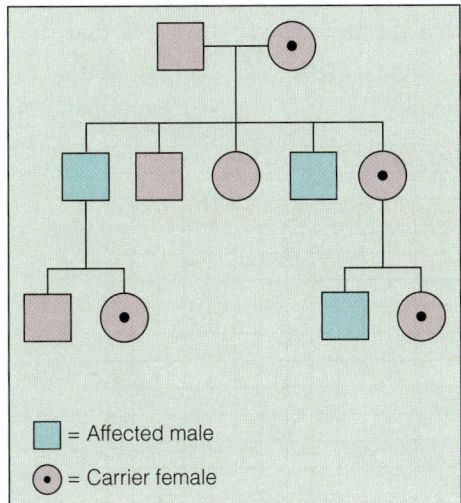

Figure 19–15 》 X-linked recessive pedigree. The mother is the carrier. Statistically, 50% of male offspring are affected, and 50% of female offspring are carriers.

X-linked Dominant Inheritance

The X-linked dominant disorders are rare, with the most common being vitamin D–resistant rickets and fragile X syndrome. When X-linked dominance does occur, the pattern is similar to that of X-linked recessive inheritance except that heterozygous female offspring are affected. It is essential to remember that in X-linked dominant inheritance, there is no male-to-male transmission. Affected fathers will have affected daughters; however, because fathers pass only the Y chromosome to male offspring, their sons will not be affected.

Fragile X syndrome is an inherited form of mental retardation; it is second only to Down syndrome among all causes of moderate mental retardation in male offspring. Fragile X syndrome is a CNS disorder linked to a "fragile" site on the X chromosome. It is characterized by moderate mental retardation, large protuberant ears, and large testes after puberty. Carrier female offspring do not have the abnormal features, but about one third have mild mental retardation.

Multifactorial Inheritance

Many common congenital malformations such as cleft palate, heart defects, spina bifida, dislocated hips, clubfoot, and pyloric stenosis are caused by the interaction of multiple genetic and environmental factors. Therefore, these conditions are multifactorial in origin. In multifactorial inheritance, the following occurs:

- Malformations may vary from mild to severe. For example, spina bifida may range in severity from mild (spina bifida occulta) to more severe (myelomeningocele). It is believed that the more severe the defect, the greater the number of genes present for that defect.

- There is often a sex bias. For example, pyloric stenosis is more common in male offspring, whereas cleft palate is more common in female offspring. When a member of the less commonly affected sex shows the condition, a greater number of genes must usually be present to cause the defect.

- In the presence of environmental influences (e.g., seasonal changes, altitude, radiation exposure, chemicals in the environment, exposure to toxic substances), fewer genes are needed to manifest the disease in the offspring.

- In contrast to single-gene disorders, multifactorial inheritance has an additive effect. The more family members who have the defect, the greater the risk that the next pregnancy will also be affected (Powell et al., 2013).

Although most congenital malformations are multifactorial, a careful family history should always be taken, because cleft lip and palate, certain congenital heart defects, and other malformations can occasionally be inherited as autosomal dominant or recessive traits. Other disorders thought to be within the multifactorial inheritance group are diabetes, hypertension, some heart diseases, and mental illness.

Contraception

Many couples use contraception to plan pregnancy and/or avoid conception. The nurse should understand the patient's cultural and religious beliefs regarding the use of contraception in order to provide information on the best contraceptive choices for the patient or couple.

Fertility Awareness Methods

Fertility awareness–based methods (FAB), also known as *natural family planning*, are based on an understanding of the changes that occur throughout a woman's ovulatory cycle. The fertility window for women occurs between days 8 and 19 of 26- to 32-day cycles (Zieman et al., 2016). All FAB methods require periods of abstinence and recording of certain events throughout the cycle; therefore, cooperation of the woman's partner is important.

FAB methods are free, safe, and acceptable to many individuals whose religious beliefs prohibit other methods. They provide increased awareness of the body, involve no artificial substances or devices, encourage a couple to communicate about sexual activity and family planning, and are useful in helping a couple plan a pregnancy. However, these methods require extensive initial counseling to be used effectively. They also require careful maintenance of records for several cycles before beginning to use them; they may be difficult or impossible for women with irregular cycles to use; and although theoretically reliable, in practice they may not be as reliable in preventing pregnancy as other methods.

The *calendar rhythm method*, also called the *standard days method*, requires the woman to record her menstrual cycles for 6 months to identify the shortest and longest cycles. The first day of menstruation is the first day of the cycle. The fertile phase is calculated from 18 days before the end of the shortest recorded cycle through 11 days from the end of the longest recorded cycle. For example, if a woman's shortest cycle is 24 days and her longest cycle is 28 days, the fertile phase would be calculated as day 6 through day 17 (United States Agency for International Development [USAID], 2012). Once this information has been obtained, the woman can identify the fertile and infertile phases of her cycle. To use this method effectively for contraception, she must abstain from intercourse during the fertile phase. The calendar method is the least reliable of the FAB methods and has largely been replaced by other, more scientific approaches.

The *basal body temperature (BBT) method* to detect ovulation requires that a woman take her BBT every morning upon awakening (before any activity) and record the readings on a temperature graph. To do this, she uses a BBT thermometer. After 3–4 months of recording temperatures, a woman with regular cycles should be able to predict when ovulation will occur. The method is based on the fact that the temperature sometimes drops just before ovulation and almost always rises and remains elevated for several days afterward. The temperature rise occurs in response to the increased progesterone levels that occur in the second half of the cycle. **Figure 19–16 》** shows a sample BBT chart. To avoid conception, the couple abstains from intercourse on the day of the temperature rise and for 3 days afterward. Because the temperature rise does not occur until after ovulation, a woman who had intercourse just before the rise is at risk of pregnancy. To decrease this risk, some couples abstain from intercourse for several days before the anticipated time of ovulation and then for 3 days afterward.

The *Billings ovulation method*, sometimes called the *cervical mucus method*, involves assessment of cervical mucus changes that occur during the menstrual cycle. The amount and character of cervical mucus change because of the influence of **estrogen** and **progesterone** (hormones responsible for female sex characteristics and fetal development). At the time of ovulation, the mucus (estrogen-dominant mucus) is clearer, more stretchable (a quality called *spinnbarkeit*), more permeable to sperm, and can prolong sperm life (Walcker & Pederson, 2013). It also shows a characteristic fern pattern when placed on a glass slide and allowed to dry. During the luteal phase, cervical mucus is thick and sticky (progesterone-dominant mucus) and forms a network that traps sperm, making their passage more difficult.

To use the cervical mucus method, the woman abstains from intercourse for the first menstrual cycle. Each day she assesses her cervical mucus for amount, feeling of slipperiness or wetness, color, clearness, and spinnbarkeit, with the goal of becoming familiar with varying characteristics. The peak day of wetness and clear, stretchable mucus is assumed to be the time of ovulation. To use this method correctly, the woman should abstain from intercourse from the time she *first* notices that the mucus is

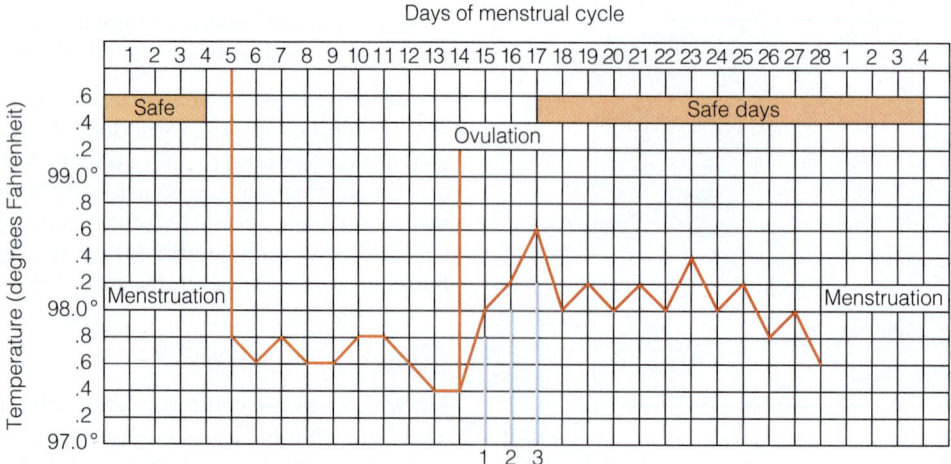

Figure 19–16 》 Sample basal body temperature chart.

becoming clear, more elastic, and slippery until 4 days *after* the last wet mucus (ovulation) day. Because this method evaluates the effects of hormonal changes, it can be used by women with irregular cycles.

The *symptothermal method* consists of various assessments made and recorded by the couple. These include information regarding cycle days, coitus, cervical mucus changes, and secondary signs such as increased libido, abdominal bloating, *mittelschmerz* (midcycle abdominal pain), and BBT. Through the various assessments, the couple learns to recognize signs that indicate ovulation. This combined approach tends to improve the effectiveness of fertility awareness as a method of birth control.

Situational Contraceptives

Abstinence can be considered a method of contraception. Like any method of contraception, its use is based on personal preference.

Coitus interruptus, or withdrawal, is one of the oldest and least reliable methods of contraception. This method requires that the man withdraw from the woman's vagina when he feels that ejaculation is impending. He then ejaculates away from the woman's external genitalia. Failure tends to occur for two reasons: (1) This method demands great self-control on the part of the man, who must withdraw just as he feels the urge for deeper penetration with impending orgasm, and (2) some preejaculatory fluid, which can contain sperm, may be released from the penis during the excitement phase before ejaculation. The fact that the quantity of sperm in a man's preejaculatory fluid is increased after a recent ejaculation is especially significant for couples who engage in repeated episodes of intercourse within a short period. Couples who use this method should be aware of postcoital contraceptive options in case the man fails to withdraw in time.

Douching after intercourse is an ineffective method of contraception and is not recommended. It may actually facilitate conception by pushing sperm farther up the birth canal.

Spermicides

The **spermicide** nonoxynol-9 (N-9), which is approved for use in the United States, is available as a cream, jelly, foam, vaginal film, and suppository. A spermicide is inserted into the vagina before intercourse. It destroys sperm by disrupting their cell membrane. A spermicide that effervesces in a moist environment offers rapid protection, and coitus may take place immediately after it is inserted. A suppository may require up to 30 minutes to dissolve and will not offer protection until it has done so. The nurse should instruct the woman to insert any of these spermicide preparations high in the vagina and to maintain a supine position.

N-9 is minimally effective when used alone. Its effectiveness increases in conjunction with a diaphragm, sponge, or condom. The major advantages of spermicides are their wide availability and low toxicity. Skin irritation and allergic reactions to spermicides are the primary disadvantages. N-9 does not offer protection against infection from the human immunodeficiency virus, which causes HIV/AIDS, or against any other STI. Moreover, N-9 may actually increase a woman's risk of HIV infection because it irritates

vaginal tissue, making it more susceptible to invasion by organisms such as HIV (U.S. Food and Drug Administration [FDA], 2015a).

Barrier Methods of Contraception

Barrier methods of contraception prevent the transport of sperm to the ovum, immobilize sperm, or are lethal against sperm.

Male and Female Condoms

The male **condom** (a sheath of synthetic material that covers the penis) offers a viable means of contraception when used consistently and properly (see **Figure 19–17 ⟫**). Acceptance of condom use has been increasing as a growing number of men assume responsibility for regulation of fertility. The condom is applied to the erect penis, rolled from the tip to the end of the shaft before vulvar or vaginal contact. A small space must be left at the end of the condom to allow for collection of ejaculate so that the condom will not break at the time of ejaculation. If the condom or vagina is dry, water-soluble lubricants such as K-Y jelly should be used to prevent irritation and possible condom breakage.

Care must be taken when removing the condom after intercourse. For optimal effectiveness, the man should withdraw his penis from the vagina while it is still erect and hold the condom rim to prevent spillage. If after ejaculation the penis becomes flaccid while still in the vagina, the man should hold onto the edge of the condom while withdrawing to avoid spilling the semen and to prevent the condom from slipping off.

The effectiveness of male condoms is largely determined by their use. Small, disposable, and inexpensive, most condoms are made of latex, although polyurethane and silicone rubber condoms are available for individuals who are allergic to latex. All condoms except natural

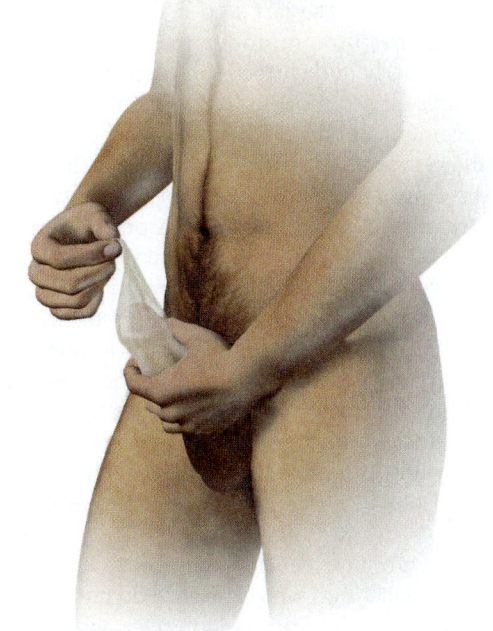

Figure 19–17 ⟫ Correct use of a condom.

"skin" condoms, made from lamb's intestines, offer protection against both pregnancy and STIs. Breakage, displacement, perineal or vaginal irritation, and dulled sensation are possible disadvantages. Condoms should not be stored in hot conditions because heat accelerates their deterioration, making them more susceptible to breaking. Thus, men should avoid placing them in a car glove box or in a wallet in their pants pocket.

The *female condom* (see **Figure 19–18** ⟩⟩) is a thin polyurethane sheath with a flexible ring at each end. The inner ring, at the closed end of the condom, serves as the means of insertion and fits over the cervix like a diaphragm. The second ring remains outside the vagina and covers a portion of the woman's perineum. It also covers the base of the man's penis during intercourse. Available over the counter and designed for one-time use, the condom may be inserted up to 8 hours before intercourse. The inner sheath is prelubricated but does not contain spermicide and is not designed to be used with a male condom. Because it also covers a portion of the vulva, it probably provides better protection than other contraceptive methods against some pathogens. High cost, noisiness during intercourse, and the cumbersome feel of the device make acceptability a problem for some couples.

Diaphragm and Cervical Cap

A **diaphragm** (see **Figure 19–19** ⟩⟩) is used with spermicidal cream or jelly and offers a good level of protection against conception. The woman must be fitted with a diaphragm and instructed in its use by trained personnel. The diaphragm should be rechecked for correct size after each childbirth and whenever a woman has gained or lost 10–15 pounds or more.

The diaphragm must be inserted before intercourse, with approximately 1 tsp (or 1.5 in. as squeezed from the tube) of spermicidal jelly placed around its rim and in the cup. This chemical barrier supplements the mechanical barrier of the diaphragm. The diaphragm is inserted through the vagina and covers the cervix. The last step in insertion is to push the edge of the diaphragm under the symphysis pubis. When fitted properly and correctly in place, the diaphragm should not cause discomfort to the woman or her partner. Correct placement of the diaphragm can be checked by touching the cervix with a fingertip through the cup. The center of the diaphragm should be over the cervix. If more than 6 hours elapse between insertion of the diaphragm and intercourse, additional spermicidal cream should be used. It is necessary to leave the diaphragm in place for at least 6 hours after coitus. If intercourse is desired again within the 6 hours, another type of contraception must be used or additional spermicidal jelly must be placed in the vagina with an applicator, taking care not to disturb the placement of the diaphragm. The diaphragm should not remain in the vagina for more than 24 hours. The diaphragm should periodically be held up to the light and inspected for tears or holes.

Diaphragms are an excellent contraceptive method for women who are lactating, who cannot or do not wish to use oral contraceptives, who are smokers over age 35, or who have infrequent sexual intercourse. A silicone diaphragm is available for women with latex allergy.

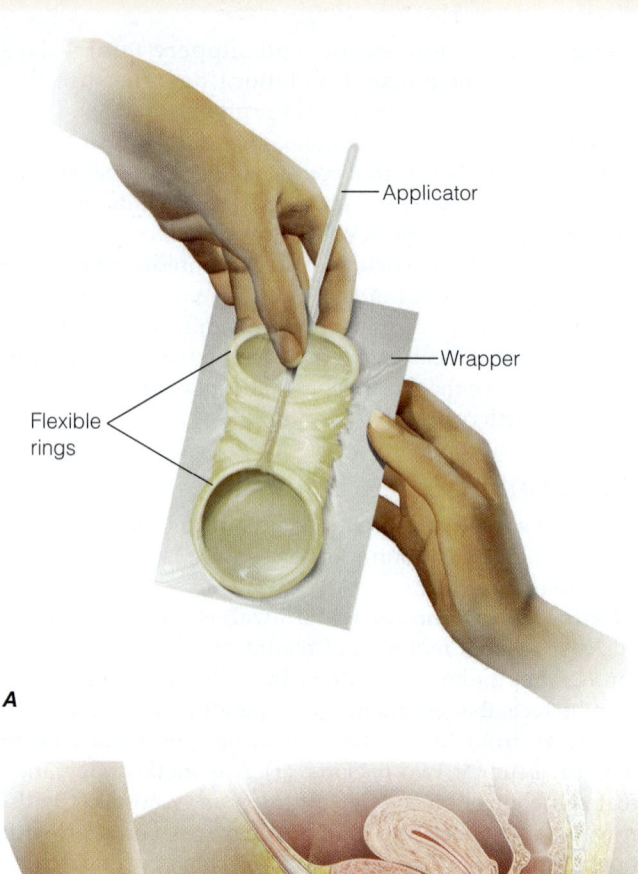

A

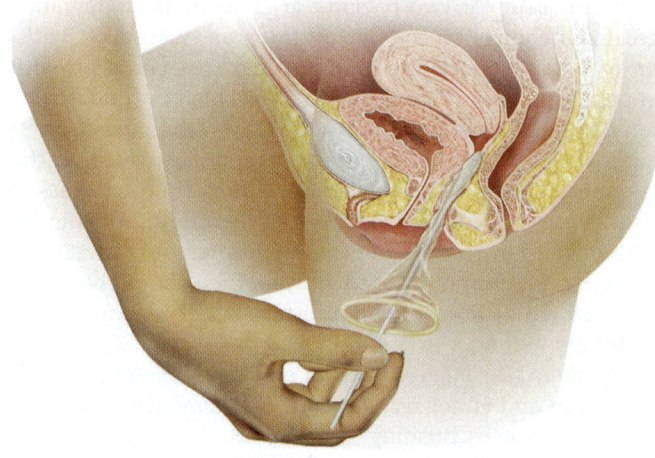

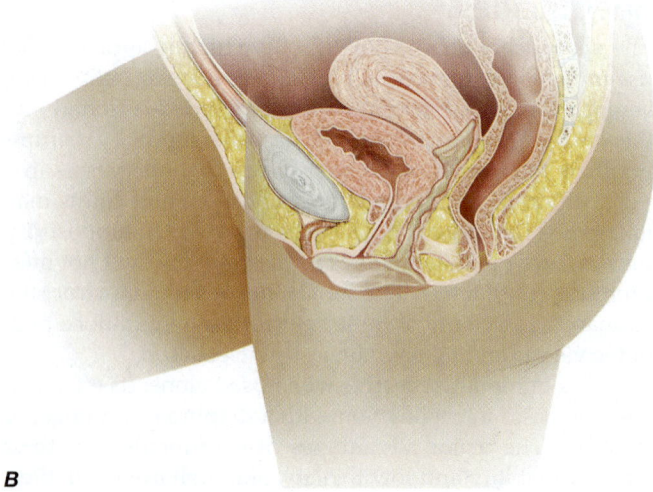

B

Figure 19–18 ⟩⟩ *A,* The female condom. *B,* When properly inserted, the outer ring should rest on the folds of the skin around the vaginal opening, and the inner ring (closed end) should fit loosely against the cervix.

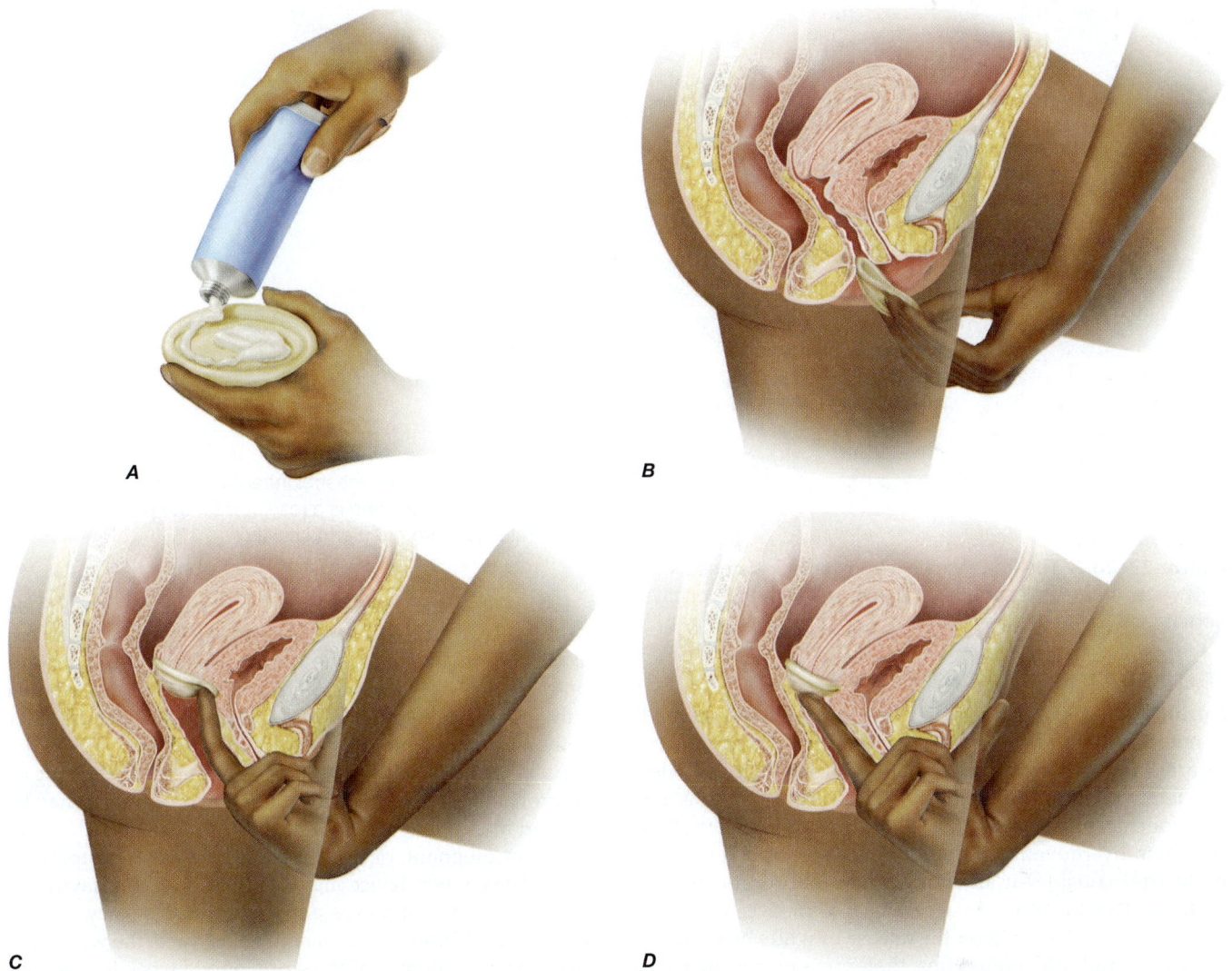

Figure 19–19 ▶ Inserting the diaphragm: **A,** Apply jelly to the rim and center of the diaphragm. **B,** Insert the diaphragm. **C,** Push the rim of the diaphragm under the pubic symphysis. **D,** Check placement of the diaphragm. The cervix should be felt through the diaphragm.

Women who object to touching their genitals to insert the diaphragm, check its placement, and remove it may find this method unsatisfactory. Women who are very obese or who have short fingers may find the diaphragm difficult to insert. The diaphragm is not recommended for women with a history of UTI, because pressure from the diaphragm on the urethra may interfere with complete bladder emptying and lead to recurrent UTIs. Women with a history of toxic shock syndrome should not use diaphragms or any of the barrier methods because they are left in place for prolonged periods. For the same reason, the diaphragm should not be used during a menstrual period or if a woman has abnormal vaginal discharge.

The only **cervical cap** available in the United States is the FemCap (Walcker & Pederson, 2013). The FemCap is made of silicone, looks like a small sailor's cap, and has a strap placed over the dome that allows for easy removal. The FemCap does not have to fit on the cervix because it is held in place by vaginal wall muscles. Spermicide is placed in the dome and in the brim of the cap so that sperm are exposed to spermicide without getting under the cap (Walcker & Pederson, 2013).

Vaginal Sponge

The *Today vaginal sponge,* available without a prescription, is a pillow-shaped, soft, absorbent synthetic sponge containing spermicide. It is made with a concave or cupped area on one side that fits over the cervix and has a loop for easy removal. The sponge is moistened thoroughly with water before insertion to activate the spermicide and then inserted into the vagina with the cupped side against the cervix (see **Figure 19–20 ▶**). It should be left in place for 6 hours following intercourse and may be worn for up to 24 hours, then removed and discarded.

The sponge has several advantages: Professional fitting is not required, it may be used for multiple acts of coitus for up to 24 hours, one size fits all, and it acts as both a barrier and a spermicide. Problems associated with the sponge include difficulty removing it and irritation or allergic reactions. Some women report vaginal dryness because the sponge absorbs vaginal secretions. For women without children, the failure rate is comparable to that of the diaphragm and cervical cap. The failure rate is higher for women who have borne children, possibly because of changes in the shape of the cervix.

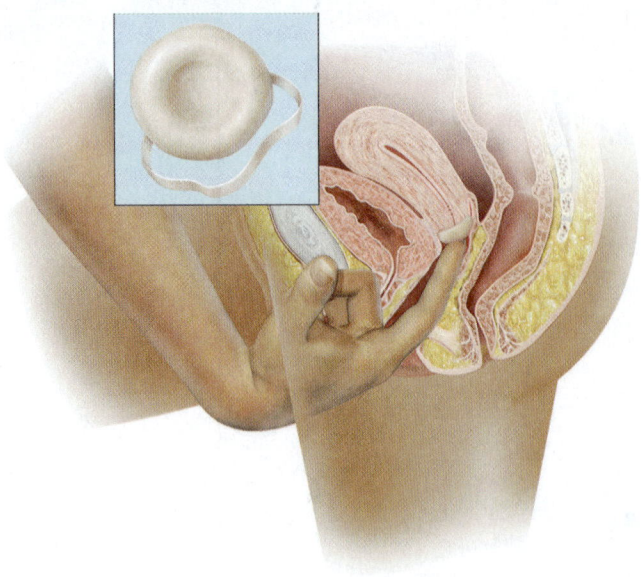

Figure 19–20 》》 The contraceptive sponge is moistened well with water and then inserted into the vagina with the concave portion positioned over the cervix.

Intrauterine Contraception

Intrauterine contraception (IUC) is a safe, effective method of reversible contraception. An IUC device is designed to be inserted into the uterus by a qualified healthcare provider and left in place for an extended period, providing continuous contraceptive protection. Some patients believe that IUC acts by preventing the implantation of a fertilized ovum and consider it an abortifacient (abortion-causing) method. This belief is not accurate. IUC devices truly are contraceptives; they trigger the release of white blood cells, enzymes, and prostaglandins that prevent sperm from reaching the ovum (Walcker & Pederson, 2013). IUC is also known to change the cervical mucus, endometrial lining, and tubal motility.

Advantages of IUC include its high rate of effectiveness, continuous contraceptive protection, and relative inexpensiveness over time, and it does not require any coitus-related activity. Possible adverse reactions to an IUC device include discomfort at insertion, increased bleeding during menses, increased risk of pelvic infection for about 3 weeks following insertion, perforation of the uterus during insertion, intermenstrual bleeding, dysmenorrhea, and expulsion of the device.

Two forms of IUC devices are currently available in the United States. The Copper T380A (ParaGard) is nonhormonal, is highly effective, and can be left in place for up to 10 years. Mirena, Skyla, and Liletta are levonorgestrel-releasing intrauterine systems (LNG-IUS), or small T-shaped frames with reservoirs that release LNG gradually (see **Figure 19–21 》》**). They are comparable in effectiveness to the Copper T380A and may be left in place for up to 5 years (Mirena) or 3 years (Skyla and Liletta). After 3 months of LNG-IUS use, the amount of bleeding and the length of menstrual cycles are reduced, and some women experience amenorrhea. Most women welcome this once they know that the absence of menses is safe and not an indication of pregnancy.

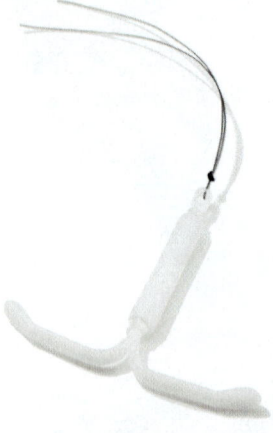

Figure 19–21 》》 Levonorgestrel intrauterine system (LNG-IUS). The section near the string is a reservoir for the progestin that is slowly released into the uterine cavity.

IUC is effective against ectopic pregnancy because of its overall effectiveness in preventing any pregnancy and a good choice for women who cannot use hormonal forms of contraception (Walcker & Pederson, 2013). Note that women with IUC devices should be encouraged to also use a barrier method of contraception to protect against STIs.

An IUC device is inserted into the uterus with its string or tail protruding through the cervix into the vagina. It may be inserted at any time during a woman's cycle, provided that she is not pregnant, or during the 4- to 6-week postpartum check. The copper device may be inserted up to 5 days after unprotected intercourse as a method of emergency contraception. After insertion, the clinician instructs the woman to check for the presence of the string once a week for the first month and then after each menses. Patient teaching includes explaining that the woman may have some cramping or bleeding intermittently for 2–6 weeks and that her first few menses may be irregular. Follow-up examination is suggested 4–8 weeks after insertion.

Women using IUC should contact their healthcare providers if they are exposed to an STI or if they develop the following warning signs: late period, abnormal spotting or bleeding, pain with intercourse, abdominal pain, abnormal discharge, signs of infection (fever, chills, and malaise), or missing string. If the woman becomes pregnant with an IUC device in place, the device should be removed as soon as possible to prevent spontaneous miscarriage (Walcker & Pederson, 2013).

Hormonal Contraceptives

Hormonal contraceptives are available in a variety of forms. The hormones used are progestin, a synthetic progesterone, and estrogen, usually ethinyl estradiol. Progestins may be used alone or in combination with estrogen.

Combined Estrogen–Progestin Approaches

Combined hormonal approaches work by inhibiting the release of an ovum, by creating an atrophic endometrium, and by maintaining a thick cervical mucus that slows sperm transport and inhibits the process that allows sperm to penetrate the ovum.

Box 19–2
Quick Start

Healthcare providers should consider suggesting the Quick Start method to patients, which allows them to start the hormonal contraceptive method on any day during the menstrual cycle. This provides patients with protection faster and more reliably, rather than waiting for days or weeks after receiving the prescription to start contraceptive use.

To use Quick Start:

■ If the last menstrual period was within the past 5 days, start the pills immediately.

■ If the last menstrual period was more than 5 days ago and a pregnancy test is negative, assess the last episode of unprotected sex to determine whether emergency contraception is needed before starting the pills.

■ If the woman had unprotected sex within the past 2 weeks, start the pills and advise the patient to return for a pregnancy test in 3 weeks.

■ Instruct the patient whose last menstrual period was more than 5 days ago to use backup contraception for 7 days.

Sources: Data from Association of Reproductive Health Professionals. (2014a). *Choosing a birth control method: Initiation of hormonal contraceptives.* Retrieved from http://www.arhp.org/Publications-and-Resources/Quick-Reference-Guide-for-Clinicians/choosing/Initiation-Hormonal-Contraceptives; Options for Sexual Health. (2013). *Using the pill.* Retrieved from https://www.optionsforsexualhealth.org/birth-control-pregnancy/birth-control-options/hormonal-methods/combined-hormonal-contraceptives/using-pill; Zieman, M., Hatcher, R. A., Allen, A. Z., Lathrop, E., & Haddad, L. (2016). *Managing contraception.* Atlanta, GA: Bridging the Gap Communications.

Combined Oral Contraceptives

Combined oral contraceptives (COCs), also called *birth control pills*, are a combination of estrogen and progestin. COCs are safe, highly effective, and rapidly reversible. COCs are generally taken daily for 21 days, typically beginning on the Sunday after the first day of the menstrual cycle. The woman can also start on day 1 of her menstrual cycle or use the Quick Start method (see **Box 19–2** »). In most cases, menses occurs 1–4 days after the last pill is taken. Seven days after taking her last pill, the woman restarts the pill. Thus, the woman always begins the pill on the same day. Some companies offer a 28-day pack with seven "blank" pills so that the woman never stops taking a pill. The pill should be taken at approximately the same time each day—usually on waking or before retiring in the evening.

Research has demonstrated that with today's low-dose COCs, the 7 hormone-free days may result in failure to completely suppress ovarian function, resulting in the development of an ovarian follicle and possible ovulation (Weisberg, 2012). As a consequence, some brands of low-dose COCs now have shortened or modified intervals. For instance, Loestrin 24 Fe has 24 active pills and only 4 placebo pills that contain iron. Extended-regimen COCs are available for women who would rather not have a monthly period. Seasonale and Seasonique are the first FDA-approved extended-regimen COCs. They both are 91-day regimens in which a woman takes an active pill daily for 84 consecutive days followed by 7 days of inactive tablets, during which the woman has a period. Thus, a woman has only four periods a year. Extended use reduces the side effects of COCs, such as bloating, headache, breast tenderness, and cramping (Options for Sexual Health, 2012). Another COC, Lybrel, has been approved by the FDA for continuous 365-day use with no scheduled hormone-free periods.

SAFETY ALERT Effectiveness of low-dose COCs may be reduced in women who take medication to control epileptic seizures. Epilepsy medications may contain liver enzyme-inducing ingredients that increase breakdown of contraceptive hormones in the body. COCs with higher doses of estrogen may reduce the risk of unexpected pregnancy, although patients may still wish to pair these medications with a barrier method to improve their effectiveness (Epilepsy Foundation of Eastern Pennsylvania, 2015).

Although they are highly effective when taken correctly, COCs may produce a variety of side effects related to either progesterone or estrogen (see **Table 19–4** »). Use of low-dose (35 mcg or less estrogen) preparations has reduced

TABLE 19–4 Side Effects Associated with Oral Contraceptives

Estrogen-Related Effects	Progestin-Related Effects
Alterations in lipid metabolism	Acne, oily skin
Breast tenderness, engorgement, increased breast size	Breast tenderness, increased breast size
Cerebrovascular accident	Decreased high-density lipoprotein (HDL) cholesterol levels
Changes in carbohydrate metabolism	Decreased libido
Chloasma	Depression
Fluid retention, cyclic weight gain	Fatigue
Headache	Hirsutism
Hepatic adenomas	Increased appetite, weight gain
Hypertension	Increased low-density lipoprotein (LDL) cholesterol levels
Leukorrhea, cervical erosion, ectopia	Oligomenorrhea, amenorrhea
Nausea	Pruritus
Nervousness, irritability	Sebaceous cysts
Telangiectasia	
Thromboembolic complications: thrombophlebitis, pulmonary embolism	

Sources: Data from Adams, M. P., Holland, L. N., & Urban, C. (2017). *Pharmacology for nurses: A pathophysiologic approach* (5th ed.). Hoboken, NJ: Pearson Education; Kee, J. L., Hayes, E. R., & McCuistion, L. E. (2015). *Pharmacology: A patient-centered nursing process approach* (8th ed., p. 847). St. Louis, MO: Elsevier Saunders; Lowdermilk, D. L., Perry, S. E., Cashion, K., & Alden, K. R. (2016). *Maternity and women's health care* (11th ed., pp. 184–185). St. Louis, MO: Elsevier; Sech, L., Segall-Gutierrez, P., Silverstein, E., & Mishell, D. (2015). *Oral contraceptives.* Retrieved from http://www.merckmanuals.com/professional/gynecology-and-obstetrics/family-planning/oral-contraceptives

the incidence of many of these side effects. The newer 20- or 25-mcg pills have even fewer side effects, but they may result in lower contraceptive effectiveness and weaker cycle control. The Evidence-Based Practice feature addresses the issue of weight gain that some women associate with use of hormonal contraceptives.

The following side effects, remembered by the mnemonic **ACHES**, are less common but more serious:

Abdominal pain

Chest pain

Headache (severe)

Eye problems (blurred vision)

Swelling or aching in the legs and thighs

Absolute contraindications to the use of oral contraceptives include pregnancy, previous history of thrombophlebitis or thromboembolic disease, acute or chronic liver disease of cholestatic type with abnormal function, presence of estrogen-dependent carcinomas, undiagnosed uterine bleeding, heavy smoking, gallbladder disease, hypertension, diabetes, and hyperlipidemia. In addition, women with the following relative contraindications need to be monitored frequently: migraine headaches, epilepsy, depression, oligomenorrhea, and amenorrhea. Women who choose this method of contraception should be fully advised of its potential side effects.

COCs also have some important noncontraceptive benefits. Many women experience relief of uncomfortable menstrual symptoms. Cramps are lessened, flow is decreased, and cycle regularity is increased. Mittelschmerz is eliminated, and incidence of functional ovarian cysts is decreased. There is also a substantial reduction in the incidence of ectopic pregnancy, ovarian cancer, endometrial cancer, iron deficiency anemia, and benign breast disease. COCs are considered a good solution to the physiologic problems some women experience during perimenopause. However, because of the increased risk of myocardial infarction, women over age 35 who smoke should not take COCs. Woman who use oral contraceptives should contact their healthcare provider if they become depressed, become jaundiced, develop a breast lump, or experience any of the following warning signs: severe abdominal pain, severe chest pain or shortness of breath, severe headaches, dizziness, vision loss or blurring, speech problems, or severe leg pain.

Another oral contraceptive is the progestin-only pill, also called the *minipill*. It is used primarily by nursing mothers because it does not interfere with breast milk production. It is also used by women who have a contraindication to the estrogen component of the combination preparation (e.g., history of thrombophlebitis) but are strongly motivated to use oral contraceptives. The major problems with this preparation are amenorrhea or irregular spotting and bleeding patterns.

Other Combined Hormonal Methods

Hormonal contraceptives may be administered transdermally via a polyester *contraceptive skin patch*. The woman applies the patch weekly for 3 weeks to one of four sites: her abdomen, buttocks, upper outer arm, or trunk (excluding the breasts). During the fourth week, no patch is worn and

menses occurs. The patch causes a more sustained serum level of hormone and contraceptive serum levels persist for at least 9 days (Association of Reproductive Health Professionals, 2014b). The patch is highly effective in women who weigh less than 198 pounds. The patch has a better rate of compliance than COCs and is generally considered as safe and reliable as COCs with similar concerns about the possibility of thrombophlebitis and pulmonary embolism (see Table 19–4).

The *vaginal contraceptive ring* is another form of low-dose, sustained-release hormonal contraceptive. It is a flexible, soft ring that the woman inserts into her vagina. The ring is left in place for 3 weeks and then removed for 1 week to allow for withdrawal bleeding. If the woman forgets to change the ring, blood levels remain therapeutic for up to 1 week (Association of Reproductive Health Professionals, 2014c). One size fits virtually all women. The ring is highly effective and has minimal side effects. The ring can be worn during intercourse and is comfortable for both the woman and her partner. Replacement rings that need to be stored for more than 4 months should be kept in the refrigerator to maintain hormone levels.

Long-acting Progestin Contraceptives

Subdermal implants prevent ovulation in most women. They also stimulate the production of thick cervical mucus, which inhibits sperm penetration. *Nexplanon*, a single 2-inch-long permeable rod implant, is inserted under the skin of the inner upper arm. It is effective for up to 3 years. It is impregnated with etonogestrel, a progestin. Nexplanon provides effective continuous contraception removed from the act of coitus. Possible side effects include spotting, irregular bleeding or amenorrhea, an increased incidence of ovarian cysts, weight gain, headaches, mood changes, and vaginal dryness (Mayo Clinic, 2015d).

Depot medroxyprogesterone acetate (DMPA) (**Depo-Provera**), another long-acting progesterone, provides highly effective birth control for 3 months when given as a single injection of 150 mg. DMPA, which acts primarily by suppressing ovulation, is safe, convenient, private, and relatively inexpensive. It also separates birth control from the act of coitus. It can safely be given to nursing mothers because it contains no estrogen. DMPA works in the same way progestin-only pills do in preventing conception. Side effects include menstrual irregularities, headache, weight gain, breast tenderness, and depression.

In a comparison of four different birth control methods, Vickery and colleagues (2013) found that average weight gain in 12 months of Depo-Provera use was about 2 pounds. Therefore, each woman choosing Depo-Provera for long-acting birth control needs counseling on typical weight gain, nutrition, and exercise. Return of fertility may be delayed for an average of 10 months (Association of Reproductive Health Professionals, 2014d).

Depo-Provera is not recommended for use for longer than 2 years without specific informed consent by the woman. It has been associated with calcium loss from the bones that may not resolve after discontinuing use. Women who remain on DMPA longer than 2 years must be educated about this serious side effect and need to exercise and take 1200 mg of calcium daily.

Evidence-Based Practice
Issues of Weight Gain Associated with Contraception

Problem

In the United States, approximately half of all pregnancies are unintended, and many end in therapeutic abortion. Many women who could use hormonal contraceptives do not initiate contraception or stop contraception prematurely because of their perception that hormonal contraceptive methods cause weight gain. Healthcare providers can provide better information and contraceptive care with a good understanding of the research evidence available about weight gain associated with hormonal contraceptive use.

Evidence

Vickery and colleagues (2013) conducted a study of the various progestin-only contraceptives and their effects on weight gain. The study compared weight gain in users of subdermal implants, LNG-IUCs, and DMPA injections to that of users of the nonhormonal copper IUC over a 12-month period. Overall, the progestin-only groups saw greater weight gain than the copper IUC group. Implant users gained an average of 2.1 pounds, LNG-IUC users gained an average of 1.0 pounds, and DMPA users gained an average of 2.2 pounds, compared with an average of 0.2 pounds for copper IUC users.

In a prospective study of 76 women new to IUC use, the women were divided into two groups, one using an LNG-IUC (Mirena) and one using the Copper T380A. The women were paired by age and body mass index and were evaluated at the time of IUC insertion and again at 1 year of use. The women in the LNG group gained an average of 6 pounds 6 ounces with an increase in fat mass in 1 year. In that same year, women in the Copper T380A group gained an average of 3 pounds 1 ounce with an increase in lean body mass. This study was limited, owing to the small number of participants and no monitoring of daily caloric intake or physical activity (Dal'Ava et al., 2012).

In a review of 49 research reports, Gallo and colleagues (2014) found few studies that compared COC methods with placebo or no hormonal method use. In the four studies reviewed, no appreciable weight gain differences were seen in the two groups. The reviewers concluded that the available evidence was insufficient to draw a conclusion about the effect of COCs on weight. They did state, however, that no large effect was evident in the available literature.

Implications

All the researchers agree that it is important for healthcare providers to give appropriate counseling about typical weight gain over time so that women are less likely to stop using hormonal contraceptive methods because of perceptions of weight gain. In addition, early counseling may help women to choose lifestyles that prevent weight gain. If a woman using a hormonal contraceptive experiences excessive weight gain that cannot be controlled with diet and exercise, then another birth control method should be chosen.

Critical Thinking Application

Consider the learning needs of women choosing hormonal contraceptive methods. Formulate a teaching plan for a woman who is going to use Depo-Provera for birth control. If a woman who is about to use a low-dose COC asks about weight gain associated with its use, how will the nurse reply using the evidence presented by these studies?

Depo-Provera 104 mg subcutaneously is an alternative to Depo-Provera 150 mg. Originally approved by the FDA for the treatment of endometriosis, it subsequently was approved as a contraceptive. Because there is 30% less drug available compared with the 150 mg preparation, it may result in less bone density loss for long-term users. It is administered subcutaneously every 10–13 weeks.

Emergency Contraception

Emergency contraception (EC) (contraception that is used after sexual activity) is indicated when a woman is worried about pregnancy because of unprotected intercourse, rape, or possible contraceptive failure (e.g., broken condom, slipped diaphragm, missed COCs, too long a time between DMPA injections). Oral progestin-only (LNG) EC is currently available without a prescription in the United States; this may be referred to by the brand name Plan B, although it is available under several other names. Ulipristal acetate (Ella), a progesterone receptor modulator, is a newer type of EC pill that requires a prescription. Insertion of the Copper T380A IUC device can also be used for EC (Office of Population Research at Princeton University & Association of Reproductive Health Professionals [ARHP], 2015).

The phrase "morning-after pill" is misleading. The woman actually takes a dose of Plan B or Ella as soon after intercourse as possible (but not longer than 120 hours postcoitus). EC taken within 120 hours can reduce the risk of pregnancy after a single act of intercourse by 75 to 95% (Office of Population Research at Princeton University & ARHP, 2015). Plan B works by stopping or delaying ovulation, causing changes in the endometrium to make it less receptive to implantation, thickening the cervical mucus, and slowing the transport of the sperm and ovum, a direct prevention of fertilization (Walcker & Pederson, 2013). It is available in two formulations: Plan B and Plan B One Step. The first involves two pills taken 12 hours apart; the second involves a single pill. Plan B One Step is gradually replacing Plan B.

Ella is a form of EC that is given as a single oral dose of 30 mg. It prevents or delays ovulation and decreases the thickness of the endometrium by binding to the progesterone receptors and producing an antiprogesterone effect. Progesterone is necessary for pregnancy to occur (Jadav & Pamar, 2012). This drug is available via prescription only.

Placement of the Copper T380A IUC device within 5 days of unprotected intercourse may reduce pregnancy risk. The IUC device produces an inflammatory response that interferes with fertilization and makes the endometrium change so that implantation does not occur (Walcker & Pederson, 2013). The Mirena IUS is not recommended for postcoital use.

Use of EC is controversial, and some women with strong beliefs about the right to life may decline them. If ovulation occurs and the sperm reaches the ovum, there is a remote chance when ECs have been used that a fertilized ovum will reach the endometrium and attempt to implant. Some individuals view this as similar to abortion and prefer not to take the medication.

Operative Sterilization

Operative sterilization is an inclusive term that refers to surgical procedures that permanently prevent pregnancy. Before sterilization is performed on either partner, the physician provides a thorough explanation of the procedure to both. Each needs to understand that sterilization is not a decision to be taken lightly or entered into when psychologic stresses, such as separation or divorce, exist. Even though procedures for both men and women are theoretically reversible, the permanence of the procedure should be stressed and understood.

The decision to have a sterilization procedure is the patient's. The nurse's responsibility is to provide patient teaching about the procedure, its permanence, and side effects (if any). The nurse should not impose his or her beliefs about sterilization on the patient and should accept the patient's decision. In addition, the nurse should not provide information in a way that makes the procedure sound intimidating or conveys any implication about the morality of the procedure. The nurse must support the patient in his or her decision, regardless of the nurse's personal beliefs about the procedure.

Male sterilization is achieved through a relatively minor procedure called a **vasectomy**. This procedure involves surgically severing the vas deferens in both sides of the scrotum. It takes about 20 ejaculations to clear the remaining sperm from the vas deferens. This can take 8 weeks or longer. During that period, the couple is advised to use another method of birth control and to bring in two or three semen samples for a sperm count. Possible side effects of a vasectomy include pain, injury to other organs, and swelling. Infection and hematoma may occur but are rare (Urology Care Foundation, 2015b). Vasectomies can sometimes be reversed by using expensive, highly specialized microsurgery techniques. Restored fertility, as measured by subsequent pregnancy, ranges from 30 to 70% (University of Iowa Hospitals and Clinics, 2015).

Female sterilization is most frequently accomplished by **tubal ligation**, in which the tubes are located through a small subumbilical incision or by minilaparotomy techniques and are clipped, ligated, electrocoagulated, banded, or plugged. Tubal ligation may be done at any time; however, the postpartum period is an ideal time to perform the procedure because the tubes are somewhat enlarged and easily located.

Complications of sterilization procedures for women are uncommon but may include coagulation burns on the bowel, perforation of the bowel, pain, infection, hemorrhage, and adverse anesthesia effects. Reversal of a tubal ligation depends on the type of procedure performed. All reversals are expensive and require major surgery and a skilled surgeon.

The *Essure* method of permanent sterilization requires no surgical incision. Insertion requires about 35 minutes in an outpatient setting. Under hysteroscopy, stainless steel microinserts are placed in the tubes, stimulating the growth of local tissue and resulting in occlusion of the fallopian tubes in 3–6 months (Association of Reproductive Health Professionals, 2014e). Essure eliminates the need for transabdominal surgery, but it does require specialized training and a hysterosalpingogram (HSG) 3 months following the procedure to confirm that the tubes are occluded. The woman should use a backup contraceptive method until the HSG confirms that her tubes are occluded.

Male Contraception

The vasectomy and the condom, discussed previously, are currently the only forms of male contraception available in the United States. Hormonal contraception for men has yet to be developed, although studies are under way. Developing safe, effective, and reversible male contraceptives is challenging: It is easier to interrupt a woman's cyclic process than to interrupt a man's continuous fertility.

Discontinuing Contraception

A woman who uses hormonal contraception—such as COCs, mini-pills, the vaginal ring, the patch, or Depo-Provera—is advised to complete the current cycle before discontinuing contraception and attempting to get pregnant. Some healthcare providers advise women to have anywhere from one to three normal menstrual periods before attempting to conceive. A woman using an IUD is advised to have it removed and wait 1 month before attempting to conceive. During the waiting period she can use barrier methods of contraception (condoms, diaphragm, or cervical cap with spermicides). Women who have used Depo-Provera should be advised that it could take up to 18 months to conceive after discontinuation.

» **Stay Current:** Nurses must be able to explain the basics of contraception to patients. They must also be able to direct patients to information about the benefits and drawbacks of various contraceptive methods. The National Campaign to Prevent Teen and Unplanned Pregnancy's Bedsider website at http://bedsider.org/ provides timely, easy-to-understand information and real-life stories about contraceptive use.

Collaboration

Care of the patient or couple seeking family planning or infertility, genetic, or contraceptive care often involves several members of the healthcare team. In addition to nurses, geneticists, psychologists, gynecologists, urologists, and infertility experts may be included in the patient's healthcare team. The care given by these providers may be supplemented by community resources such as support groups and family planning clinics. Open communication among all members of the healthcare team ensures that the patient or couple will receive the best, most sensitive care. When working with patients experiencing infertility, nurses should keep in mind that attitudes toward infertility and its treatment are culturally determined. The Focus on Diversity and Culture feature discusses some religious beliefs related to fertility and acceptable fertility treatments.

Diagnostic Tests

Diagnostic testing that may be used in the care of a patient with infertility includes the following:

- BBT recording
- Cervical mucus
- Hormonal assessments of ovulatory function (FSH, LH, estrogen, progesterone levels)

- Pregnancy tests—urine and blood for human chorionic gonadotropin (hCG)
- Sperm analysis
- Antisperm antibody test
- Postcoital test to determine sperm motility in cervical mucus
- Commercial urine test for ovulation (measures LH level)
- Endometrial biopsy
- Transvaginal and pelvic ultrasound
- Hysterosalpingography
- Hysteroscopy
- Laparoscopy.

Diagnostic tests that may be used for potential genetic issues include the following: genetic screening; genetic amniocentesis; genetic ultrasound, including nuchal translucency; percutaneous umbilical cord sampling and chorionic villus sampling (CVS); alpha-fetoprotein, hCG, inhibin, estradiol screening (quad testing); and preimplantation genetic testing.

Fertility Medications

Pharmacologic agents are commonly used for ovarian stimulation in the follicular phase, control of midcycle release, and support of the luteal phase. The pharmacologic treatment chosen depends on the specific cause of infertility. **Table 19–5 »** lists some of the drugs commonly used and their indications for use.

TABLE 19–5 Drugs Commonly Used to Treat Infertility and Indications for Use

Drugs	Indications for Use in Women	Indications for Use in Men
Clomiphene citrate (Clomid, Serophene)	■ PCOS ■ Hyperandrogenemia ■ Premature follicle rupture	■ Low levels of gonadotropins ■ Hypothalamic hypogonadism
Human menopausal gonadotropin (hMG) (Repronex, Bravelle)	■ Hypothalamic ovulatory dysfunction (after failure of clomiphene) ■ Hypopituitarism ■ PCOS (rarely) ■ Luteinized unruptured follicle syndrome (after failure of hCG alone) ■ Inadequate cervical mucus ■ In vitro fertilization (IVF), gamete intrafallopian transfer (GIFT), zygote intrafallopian transfer (ZIFT) ■ Controlled superovulation ■ Hypothalamic pituitary failure due to Kallmann syndrome or delayed puberty ■ Hypogonadotropic hypogonadism (deficiency of FSH and LH)	
Recombinant follicle-stimulating hormone (rFSH) (Follistim, Gonal-F)	■ PCOS ■ Cycles that are too long ■ IVF, GIFT, ZIFT	
Human chorionic gonadotropin (hCG) (Pregnyl, Novarel, Ovidrel)	■ Induces dominant follicle to release egg ■ Luteinized unruptured follicle syndrome	
Bromocriptine (Parlodel)	■ Pituitary adenoma	■ Hyperprolactinemia (functional or pituitary adenoma)
Cabergoline (Dostinex)	■ Hyperpituitarism	
Gonadotropin-releasing hormone (GnRH) (Factral, Lutre-pulse)	■ Hypothalamic ovulatory dysfunction—to ensure a pulsatile release of GnRH by a small pump	■ Hypothalamic pituitary failure due to Kallmann syndrome or delayed puberty (pulsed infusion)
GnRH analogs ■ Leuprolide acetate (Lupron, Eligard, Vaidur) ■ Nafarelin acetate (Synarel) ■ Goserelin acetate (Zoladex)	■ Premature follicular rupture ■ IVF, GIFT, ZIFT ■ Endometriosis	■ Hypogonadotropic hypogonadism
GnRH antagonists ■ Ganirelix acetate (Antagon) ■ Progesterone (Crinone, Prometrium, progesterone in oil)	■ Same as GnRH analogs ■ Luteal phase dysfunction ■ Luteal phase support	
Antidiabetic (metformin [Glucophage])	■ PCOS	

Sources: Data from Adams, M. P., Holland, L. N., & Urban, C. Q. (2017). *Pharmacology for nurses: A pathophysiologic approach* (5th ed.). Hoboken, NJ: Pearson Education; Valentine, M., & Gardella, J. (2013). Infertility. In E. Youngkin, M. Davis, D. Schadewald, & C. Juve (Eds.), *Women's health: A primary care clinical guide* (4th ed., pp. 273–305). Boston, MA: Pearson; Wilson, B., Shannon, M., & Shields, K. (2013). *Pearson nurse's drug guide 2013.* Upper Saddle River, NJ: Pearson.

Clinical Interruption of Pregnancy

Although abortion was legalized in the United States in 1973, the associated controversy over moral and legal issues continues. This controversy is as readily apparent in the medical and nursing professions as in other groups.

Some individuals are strongly opposed to abortion for religious, ethical, or personal reasons. Some individuals believe that access to a safe, legal abortion is every woman's right and is another aspect of self-determination. A number of physical and psychosocial factors influence a woman's decision to seek an abortion. The presence of a disease or health state that jeopardizes the mother's life and serious, life-threatening fetal problems are frequently suggested as indications for abortion. In other instances, the timing or circumstance of the pregnancy creates an inordinate stress on the woman, and she chooses an abortion. Some of these situations may involve contraceptive failure, financial considerations, interpersonal violence, sexual assault, or incest.

Medical abortion provides an effective alternative to surgical abortion for many women with unintended pregnancy. *Mifepristone* (Mifeprex), originally called RU-486, may be used to induce abortion medically during the first 7 weeks of pregnancy (up to 49 days following conception) followed by a dose of the prostaglandin misoprostol. The American College of Obstetricians and Gynecologists (2014) has endorsed an evidence-based protocol for the administration of mifepristone/misoprostol that can be used up to 63 days' gestation.

Mifepristone blocks the action of progesterone, thereby altering the endometrium. After the length of the woman's gestation is confirmed, she takes a dose of mifepristone. Between 1 and 3 days later (depending on length of gestation), she takes a dose of the prostaglandin misoprostol, which induces contractions that expel the embryo/fetus. About 14 days after taking the misoprostol, the woman is seen again to confirm that the abortion was successful.

Since being approved for use by the FDA, several deaths have been reported following the use of mifepristone and misoprostol. The majority of these deaths were related to an infection caused by a rare organism, *Clostridium sordelli* (FDA, 2015b). The FDA has determined that this is a rare occurrence (1 in 100,000 women who use mifepristone and misoprostol). However, *any* woman who has taken the oral mifepristone/oral misoprostol regimen within the past 24 hours who develops stomach pain, weakness, nausea, vomiting, or diarrhea, with or without fever, should contact her healthcare provider immediately. Mifepristone is considered safe, and use of routine prophylactic antibiotics is not recommended.

In the first trimester, surgical abortion may be performed by dilation and curettage (D&C), minisuction, or vacuum curettage. The major risks include perforation of the uterus, laceration of the cervix, systemic reaction to the anesthetic agent, hemorrhage, and infection. Second-trimester abortion may be done using dilation and extraction (D&E), hypertonic saline, systemic prostaglandins, and intrauterine prostaglandins. Surgical abortion in the first trimester is technically easier and safer than abortion in the second trimester.

Important aspects of nursing care for a woman who chooses to have an abortion include providing information about the methods of abortion and associated risks; counseling regarding available alternatives to abortion and their implications; encouraging verbalization by the woman; providing support before, during, and after the procedure; monitoring vital signs, intake, and output; providing for physical comfort and privacy throughout the procedure; and health teaching about self-care, the importance of the post-abortion checkup, and contraception review. The ANA Code of Ethics allows nurses to refuse to participate in a procedure, such as abortion, on moral grounds. However, the nurse is obliged to provide for the patient's safety, to avoid patient abandonment, and to withdraw only when assured that alternative sources of nursing care are available to the patient (ANA, 2015).

Therapeutic Insemination

Therapeutic insemination (previously known as *artificial insemination*) involves the depositing of semen at the cervical os or in the uterus by mechanical means. *Therapeutic donor insemination (TDI)* is the current term for use of donor semen, and *therapeutic husband insemination (THI)* is the current term for use of the husband's semen.

THI is generally indicated for seminal deficiencies such as oligospermia (low sperm count), asthenospermia (decreased motility), and teratospermia (low percentage, abnormal morphology); for anatomical defects accompanied by inadequate deposition of semen such as hypospadias (a congenital abnormal male urethral opening on the underside of the penis); and for ejaculatory dysfunction (e.g., retrograde ejaculation). THI is also indicated in cases of unexplained infertility and some cases of female factor infertility, such as scant or inhospitable mucus, persistent cervicitis, or cervical stenosis. In some cases, intrauterine insemination (IUI) would be indicated to bypass the cervical factor. TDI is also considered in cases of inherited male sex-linked disorders and autosomal dominant disorders.

TDI has become more complicated and expensive in the past decade because of the need for strict screening and processing procedures to prevent transmission of a genetic defect or STI to the offspring or recipient. Guidelines have been established that include mandatory medical (genetic) and infectious disease screening of both donor and recipient, the need for informed consent from all parties, the need to limit the number of pregnancies per donor, and the need for accurate means of record keeping. Finally, because of the risk of transmitting infectious diseases, donated sperm must be frozen and quarantined for 6 months from the time of acquisition, and the donor must be retested before sperm can be released for use.

SAFETY ALERT Increases in scrotal temperature adversely affect spermatogenesis. Research suggests that constrictive clothing such as tight-fitting underwear and "skinny" jeans may significantly increase scrotal temperature and lead to decreased sperm count and quality (Sharma et al., 2014).

In Vitro Fertilization

In vitro fertilization (IVF) is selectively used in cases when infertility has resulted from tubal factors, mucus abnormalities, male infertility, unexplained infertility, male and female immunologic infertility, and cervical factors. In IVF, a woman's eggs are collected from her ovaries and fertilized in the

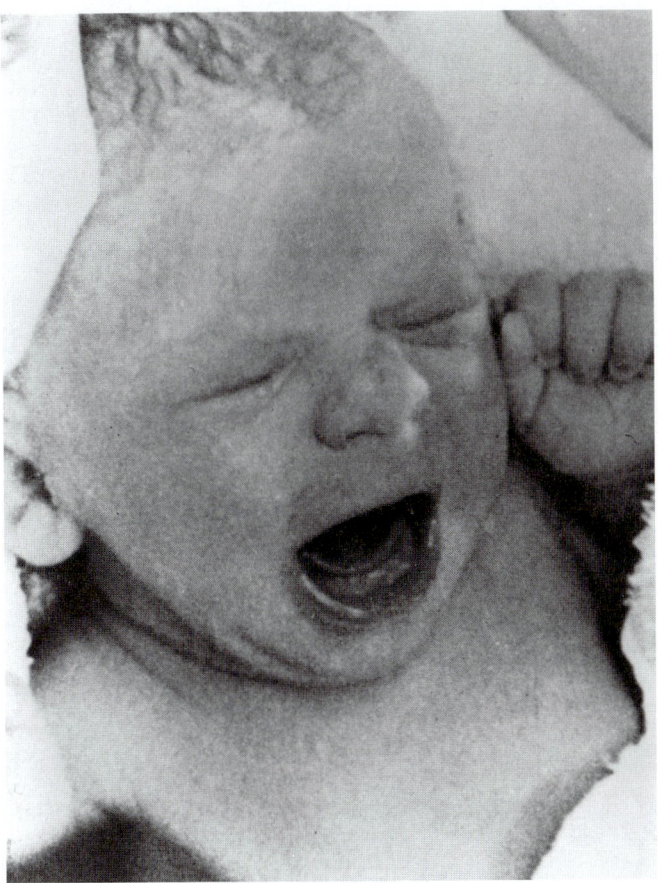

Source: Keystone/Getty Images.

Figure 19–22 》 Louise Joy Brown, the world's first "test tube baby," shown shortly after her birth by cesarean section on July 25, 1978. IVF was pioneered by Drs. Bob Edwards and Patrick Steptoe.

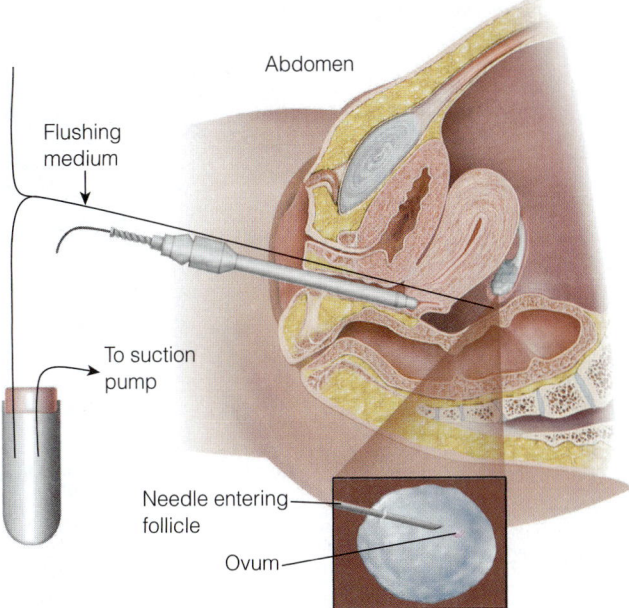

Source: Courtesy of Serono, Inc., Rockland, MA.

Figure 19–23 》 Transvaginal ultrasound-guided oocyte retrieval.

laboratory, and one or more embryos are placed into her uterus after normal development has begun. If the procedure is successful, the embryo continues to develop in the uterus, and pregnancy proceeds naturally (see **Figure 19–22** 》).

The potential for a successful pregnancy with IVF is maximized when three to four embryos (rather than one) are placed into the uterus. For this reason, fertility drugs are used to induce ovulation before the process. Follicular development and oocyte maturity are monitored frequently with ultrasound and hormonal assays. Monitoring usually begins around cycle day 5, and medications are titrated according to individual response. When follicles appear mature, hCG is given to stimulate final egg maturation and control the induction of ovulation. Egg retrieval is performed approximately 35 hours later, before ovulation occurs.

In the majority of cases, egg retrieval is performed by a transvaginal approach under ultrasound guidance (see **Figure 19–23** 》). This outpatient procedure is performed with intravenous sedation and a cervical block for anesthesia. Many follicles can be aspirated with only one puncture, and the procedure generally lasts no more than 30 minutes. Once the eggs have been fertilized and progressed to the embryo stage, the embryos are placed in the uterus. This occurs 1–2 days after conception. After the procedure, the

woman is advised to engage in only minimal activity for 12–24 hours, and progesterone supplementation is prescribed. The progesterone supplementation is given to promote implantation and support the early pregnancy; therefore, the woman will not have a period even if she is not pregnant. The pregnancy is usually determined by transvaginal ultrasound.

Sperm used to fertilize the eggs in vitro can be obtained naturally or via microsurgical epididymal sperm aspiration (MESA) or testicular sperm aspiration (TESA). These are procedures that address severe male factor infertility. MESA and TESA involve the retrieval of sperm from the gonadal tissue of men who have azoospermia or an ejaculatory disorder (see **Figure 19–24** 》). Percutaneous epididymal sperm aspiration (PESA) and TESA are replacing MESA as the preferred techniques for retrieval of sperm because they are not surgical procedures. Intracytoplasmic sperm injection (ICSI) is a microscopic procedure to inject a single sperm into the outer layer of an ovum so that fertilization will occur (Eisenberg & Brumbaugh, 2012).

Success with IVF depends on many factors, especially the woman's age and the specific indication of infertility. Women have a good chance of achieving pregnancy with an average of three cycles of IVF. Many couples find the emotional, physical, and financial costs of going beyond three cycles too great. Costs vary by treatment and by region of the country; one cycle of assisted reproductive technology (ART) averages $12,400 (American Society of Reproductive Medicine, 2015). A total of 146,244 ART procedures were reported to the CDC in 2009 (the most recent year for which data are available). Of these procedures, 60,190 resulted in live births (Sunderam et al., 2012). This means that only about 41% of ART cycles result in a live birth. Increased use of single-embryo transfer has led to lower rates of multiple fetuses, particularly in younger couples.

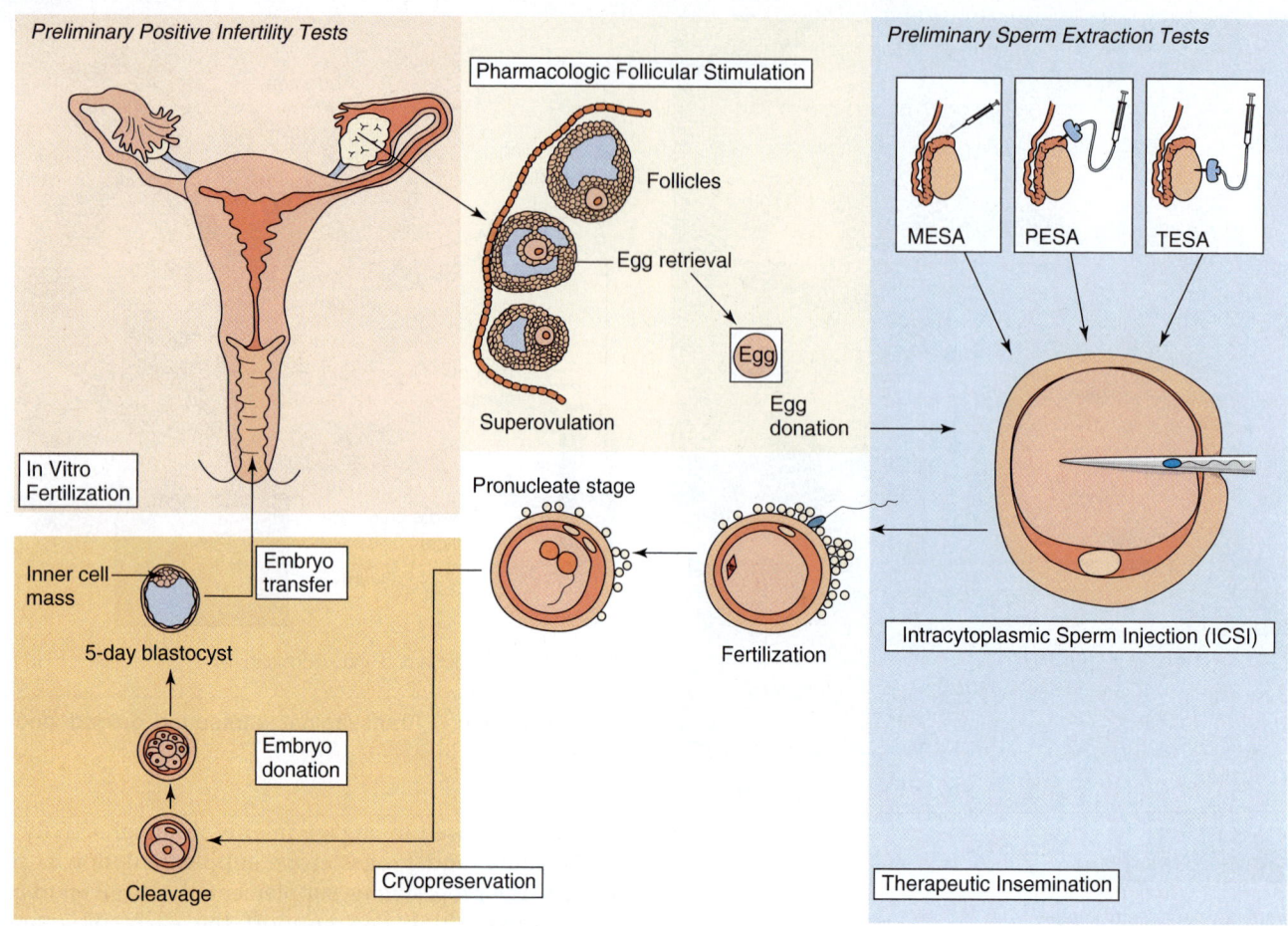

Preliminary Positive Infertility Tests

In Vitro Fertilization

Pharmacologic Follicular Stimulation

Follicles

Egg retrieval

Egg

Superovulation

Egg donation

Pronucleate stage

Inner cell mass

5-day blastocyst

Embryo transfer

Embryo donation

Cleavage

Cryopreservation

Fertilization

Preliminary Sperm Extraction Tests

MESA   PESA   TESA

Intracytoplasmic Sperm Injection (ICSI)

Therapeutic Insemination

Figure 19–24 》 Assisted reproductive techniques.

Other Assisted Reproduction Techniques

Other assisted reproductive techniques include procedures for transfer of gametes, zygotes, or embryos; cryopreservation of embryos; IVF using donor oocytes; micromanipulation techniques; and surrogacy and use of a gestational carrier.

Preimplantation Genetic Diagnosis

Recent advances in micromanipulation allow a single cell to be removed from the embryo for genetic study prior to couples deciding to use IVF. Couples at risk for having a detectable single gene or chromosomal anomaly may wish to undergo preimplantation genetic testing, called

Focus on Diversity and Culture
Belief Systems and Infertility Treatments

The acceptance of infertility treatments varies widely around the world. Some belief systems do not allow various treatments, because using a treatment is considered interfering with God's design or because the treatment itself is seen as tainted or sinful. For example, fertility practices in some cultures are influenced by traditional Muslim values that support beliefs that God decides family sizes.

In some Islamic cultures, procreation is the purpose of marriage. If a couple is infertile, it is traditionally considered the woman's problem regardless of the cause, although both infertile women and infertile men may be stigmatized. Maintaining family lineage is very important, as is conceiving in a religiously accepted manner; donor gametes and surrogacy confuse the lineage of the child and may violate religious law (Connor, Sauer, & Doll, 2012). For Sunni Muslims and the majority of Shia Muslims, the approved methods for treating infertility are limited to use of therapeutic insemination using

the husband's sperm and IVF involving the fertilization of the wife's ovum by the husband's sperm (Inhorn & Gürtin, 2012).

In Jewish cultures, infertile couples are permitted to try all possible means to have children, including egg and sperm donation. Jews believe that the ideal production of human life comes from the sex act between a husband and wife, but they accept both therapeutic insemination and IVF when fertility issues exist (Lindheim et al., 2014). The methods used to collect specimens and perform tests during the ART process may vary depending upon whether couples follow Orthodox, Reform, or Conservative teachings, particularly with regard to the collection of male ejaculate (PUAH Institute, 2015).

The Roman Catholic church opposes the use of therapeutic insemination and IVF on the grounds that these procedures separate procreation from the conjugal act between husband and wife and that they violate a child's right to be born through the holy act of intercourse within marriage (Lindheim et al., 2014).

blastomere analysis or, more recently, *preimplantation genetic diagnosis (PGD).* Results of genetic testing on the preimplantation embryos are available in 4–24 hours, so unaffected embryos may still be transferred via IVF during the required biological window of time without the need for cryopreservation.

The diagnosis of genetic disorders before implantation provides couples with the option of forgoing the attempt to establish a pregnancy and thereby avoiding a difficult decision about terminating an affected pregnancy (American Pregnancy Association, 2015f). This technology also raises several ethical issues, including the following:

- **Identification of couples at risk.** Criteria are needed to identify couples at risk for conditions that may present a significant hardship to the couple.

- **Analysis of blastomeres for sex chromosome testing when a genetic disorder carried on the sex chromosomes is suspected.** In X-linked diseases, the only way to prevent the disorder is to select only female offspring.

- **Identification of late-onset diseases.** The Human Genome Project has aided in the identification of genetic markers for late-onset diseases. Couples may wish to choose to implant blastomeres that do not carry these markers.

- **Effect on the offspring as a result of removing cells from the embryo.**

- **Selection for nonmedical reasons and potential concern of eugenics ("designer babies").**

A micromanipulation procedure called *assisted embryo hatching* has proved to be an effective adjunct therapy in IVF. IVF using a *gestational carrier* allows infertile women who are genetically sound but unable to carry a pregnancy to exercise the option of having their own biological child. Other technologies involve oocyte donation and cryopreservation of the embryo.

Genetic Counseling Referral

Genetic counseling is a communication process in which a genetic counselor, physician, or specially trained and certified nurse provides a family with the most complete and accurate current information about the occurrence or the risk of recurrence of a genetic disease in that family. Genetic counseling is an appropriate course of action for any family wondering, "Will it happen again?"

A genetic counseling referral is advised for any couple who has a child or a relative with a congenital malformation or known inheritable disorder; for any couple at risk of having a child with a metabolic disorder or biochemical defect; and any couple who has a child with a chromosomal abnormality. These criteria increase the couple's risk for having an affected child.

Couples referred to the genetics clinic are sent a form requesting information on the health status of various family members. This information assists the genetic counselor in creating the family's pedigree (see the module on Family for an overview of family pedigrees). Together, the pedigree and history facilitate identification of other family members who might also be at risk for the same disorder (see **Figure 19–25** 〉〉). The family being counseled may

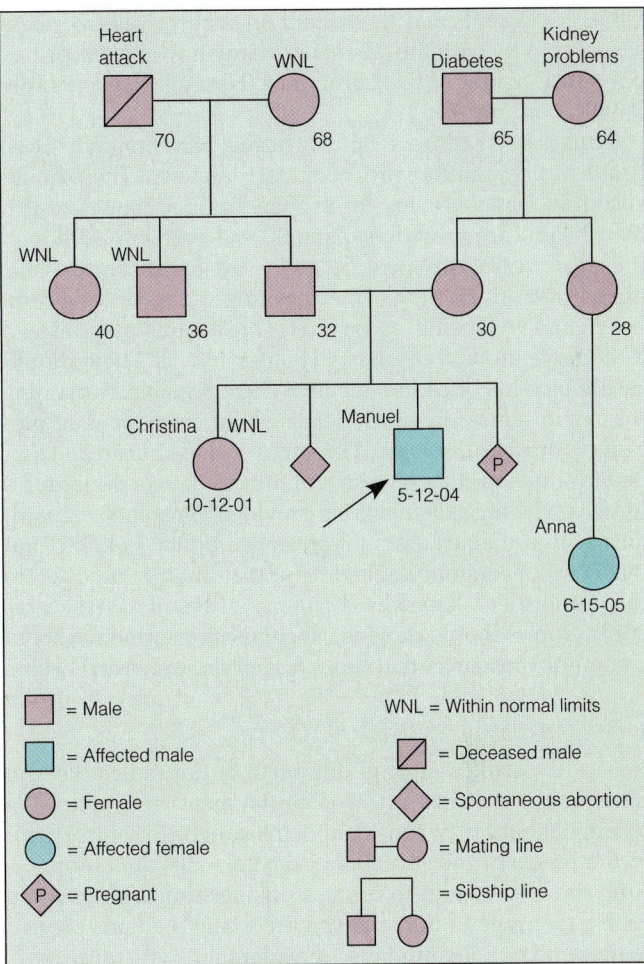

Figure 19–25 〉〉 Screening pedigree. Arrow indicates the nearest family member affected with the disorder being investigated. Basic data have been recorded. Numbers refer to the ages of the family members.

wish to notify relatives at risk so that they, too, can begin genetic counseling. When done correctly, the family history and pedigree can be powerful tools for determining a family's risk.

Lifespan Considerations

The majority of patients seeking assistance with family planning are likely to be in their 20s and 30s; however, patients outside of this age group have important needs that must be addressed. Education is a primary focus for nurses working with these individuals.

Adolescent Considerations

Education is essential for teaching adolescents about the risks inherent in unprotected sex and for helping them develop attitudes and behaviors that support sexual health. Approximately 75% of students report learning about contraception and safer sex methods in school; roughly a quarter of adolescents do not receive formal education on these topics. In addition, access to contraception and reproductive health services may be limited for adolescents because of a lack of insurance or lack of free or low-cost public health options.

Other adolescents may be hesitant or embarrassed to discuss sexual activity with the parent or guardian who is the principal policy holder of their insurance (Henry J. Kaiser Family Foundation, 2014).

Nurses must address topics of sexual behavior and sexual health in a straightforward, nonjudgmental way. They should encourage patients to engage in open dialogue about sex with their healthcare providers, parents, and partners. Although these conversations may be awkward or uncomfortable, nurses should stress that they are important for long-term health and well-being, as some STIs are incurable or can lead to complications like infertility later in life. They should assure patients of confidentiality where possible, explaining the circumstances in which details about discussions or procedures must be disclosed. These may include but are not limited to situations that represent imminent danger, procedures for which billing statements are provided to parents or guardians who are guarantors or insurance policy holders, and diagnosis of communicable disease that must be reported to the authorities (American Academy of Family Physicians, 2013). Nurses should provide patients with information about community resources that support safer sex and sexual health.

Pregnancy Considerations

Return to fertility after giving birth is unpredictable and may occur prior to the onset of regular menstrual cycles; as a result, patients must consider postpartum birth control prior to the return of menstruation. Prenatal visits are an opportune time for nurses to discuss postpartum contraception with patients and outline the issues certain methods present to new and nursing mothers. Considerations regarding postpartum contraception include:

- COCs and other forms of hormonal contraceptives can have an impact on the quantity and quality of breastmilk and increase the risk for deep vein thrombosis if used in the first month postpartum (Association of Reproductive Health Professionals, 2013).

- Changes in vaginal tone due to childbirth alter the size of the cervix and vagina and may result in improper fit of diaphragms that were used antenatally. Patients can be refitted for new devices, but refitting should take place no earlier than 6 weeks after giving birth to ensure that maximum healing has occurred. Contraceptive sponges should also be avoided until 6 weeks postpartum due to the risk of TSS.

- Patients who are breastfeeding exclusively may choose the lactational amenorrhea method (LAM). However, the effectiveness of LAM varies greatly and is affected by frequency of nursing (Association of Reproductive Health Professionals, 2013). Women who rely on LAM should be encouraged to consider a secondary method of contraception.

- Condoms and spermicides may be used for contraception in the immediate postpartum period.

- IUCs may also be used immediately postpartum, although there is a slightly elevated risk of expulsion associated with immediate insertion. As a result, some healthcare providers prefer to wait until 6 weeks postpartum to insert IUCs.

- For women who do not wish to have any more children, sterilization via tubal ligation can take place immediately postpartum.

Nurses should present pregnant women with their options for postpartum contraception several months prior to childbirth. This gives patients time to make informed, thoughtful decisions that are appropriate for their families. It also eliminates the need for patients to make important family planning decisions during the first weeks postpartum, when they are recovering from childbirth.

Considerations for Adults Over 35

In general, it takes longer for women over 35 to become pregnant due to a decrease in the quantity and quality of eggs. However, women in this age group also have a higher likelihood of giving birth to twins; this is especially true if ART methods such as IVF are used. Babies born to women over 35 are also at increased risk for chromosome abnormalities, including Down syndrome. In some cases, these abnormalities can lead to stillbirth or miscarriage, as can preexisting medical conditions. In fact, the risk of pregnancy loss increases with maternal age (Mayo Clinic, 2014f).

Women over 35 are also at increased risk for pregnancy complications, including gestational diabetes and high blood pressure. Certain complications, such as placenta previa, necessitate delivery via cesarean section, so mothers in this age group are at increased risk for cesarean delivery. Prematurity and low birth weight are also more likely (Mayo Clinic, 2014f).

Paternal age can also affect the ability to conceive and have an impact on fetal development and child health. Research suggests that partners of men over 40 may be at an increased risk of miscarriage. In addition, babies born to fathers over 40 may be more likely to have certain rare birth defects, including achondroplasia. Autism and schizophrenia are also believed to occur more frequently as paternal age increases (Mayo Clinic, 2015e).

When working with couples over age 35, the nurse should provide education about risks and encourage both partners to make healthy lifestyle choices in preparation for conception. The nurse may want to direct patients to a genetic counselor if they are concerned about their risks. The nurse should remind pregnant women in this age group about the importance of good prenatal care, healthy diet, and regular physical activity.

NURSING PROCESS

The priority of nursing care for patients with family planning considerations is to identify specific needs, provide emotional support, and teach patients about their options so they can make informed decisions.

Assessment

When assessing men and women for reproductive issues, the nurse must use a nonjudgmental attitude and open communication. Many patients are uncomfortable discussing sexuality and sexual activity. The nurse must approach the topic in a matter-of-fact manner, with reassurance of confidentiality within the law. Some assessment questions are the same for both genders. See the Nursing Assessment section in The Concept of Sexuality.

Diagnosis

Possible nursing diagnoses that may be appropriate for patients with family planning needs include the following:

- *Disturbed Body Image*
- *Sexual Dysfunction*
- *Deficient Knowledge* related to family planning, infertility, contraception, or genetics.

    (NANDA-I © 2014)

Planning

Goals of nursing care for the patient with family planning considerations include the following:

- The patient will describe options available for treatment and choose the option that best fits his or her needs, beliefs, and values.
- The patient will acknowledge the impact of the situation on existing personal relationships and lifestyle.
- The patient will describe actual changes in body function.
- The patient will maintain close social interactions and personal relationships.

Implementation

Family planning considerations can cause a great deal of stress for the couple or patient. By providing a nonjudgmental, accepting atmosphere and thorough patient teaching, the nurse can help patients resolve difficult decisions in a way that suits them best. This facilitates both the nurse–patient relationship and the patient's ability to learn and act on information.

Promote Healthy Body Image

Issues associated with family planning and infertility can create emotional stress that negatively affects body image. Individuals who are facing infertility may feel anger about what they perceive as their bodies' failings, and their sense of masculinity or femininity may be challenged. Fertility treatments may also result in patients feeling powerless or a loss of control over their own bodies (Bradley University, 2015). When working with these patients, the nurse should encourage verbalization of feelings; provide resources (pamphlets, books, tapes, referrals to support groups and counselors) as appropriate; and teach the patient (and significant other if appropriate) about reproductive physiology as it applies to use of contraceptives, infertility issues, or genetics issues.

Promote Healthy Sexual Function

Problems with sexual function can interfere with pleasure and intimacy associated with intercourse, as well as create issues in patients' relationships with their partners. These issues can compound problems with sexual function, as can misunderstandings about the causes and treatment of functional issues. Strategies to help promote healthy sexual function include:

- Encourage discussion of sexual function among the patient, partner, and healthcare provider.

Patient Teaching

Infertility Medications for Women

Infertility treatments for female patients typically involve medications that stimulate ovulation and increase the probability that healthy eggs will be released from the ovaries (Bart & Fauser, 2015). These medications may also be prescribed for women preparing to undergo IVF. Three types of medication are commonly prescribed, and patients should be educated about their method of action, dosing and delivery, and side effects.

Clomiphene or clomiphene citrate

- Clomiphene works by increasing the amount of LH in the body (Adams, Holland, & Urban, 2017; American Pregnancy Association, 2015g). It is typically used to stimulate ovulation in women with absent periods, infrequent periods, or long cycles.
- Medication is taken orally on days 3–5 of the menstrual cycle, and dosage typically starts at 50 mg per day. Dosage may be increased if ovulation does not occur. Most patients take clomiphene for 3–6 menstrual cycles.
- Side effects include hot flashes, nausea, headaches, blurred vision, breast tenderness, and mood swings. Clomiphene may also increase incidence of multiple birth or miscarriage.

Gonadotropins and hCG

- Gonadotropins work by stimulating egg growth in the ovaries (Adams et al., 2017; American Pregnancy Association, 2015g). They are typically prescribed for patients who do not respond to clomiphene or other medications that stimulate ovulation.

hCG may be used to trigger release of the egg after the follicles have developed.

- Medication is injected starting on day 2 or 3 of the menstrual cycle and continues for 7–12 days. Blood draws and transvaginal ultrasound are common during this time to monitor estrogen production and egg size.
- Side effects include abdominal discomfort, nausea, and vomiting. Gonadotropins may also increase the incidence of multiple births.

Bromocriptine or cabergoline

- Bromocriptine and cabergoline work by decreasing the amount of the hormone prolactin released by the pituitary gland (Adams et al., 2017; American Pregnancy Association, 2015g). They are typically prescribed to patients with kidney or thyroid disease or those taking medications that increase prolactin levels. High levels of prolactin can stop ovulation.
- Bromocriptine is taken orally. Dosage typically begins around 1.25 mg once per day and is gradually increased to 2.5 mg twice per day over the course of several weeks. Cabergoline is also taken orally, usually once or twice per week. Both drugs are taken for at least 1 year.
- Side effects of bromocriptine and cabergoline include nausea, vomiting, headache, dizziness, decreased blood pressure, and fainting.

- Provide information given by the healthcare provider regarding treatment options.
- Encourage the patient to discuss concerns about sexuality with a therapist or counselor.

Promote Knowledge of Sexual and Reproductive Health

Maintaining sexual and reproductive health has important implications for all patients. The most appropriate family planning options for patients depend upon their sexual behaviors, their health status, and the health status of their partners. Cultural and religious practices may inform family planning decisions. The nurse plays an essential role in helping patients understand their options and the associated risks. Strategies to facilitate informed patient decision making include:

- Teach the patient about risk factors for reproductive dysfunction. For example, STIs increase the risk of infertility.
- Teach the patient about disease prevention. For example, teach about the application of condoms.

- Teach the patient (and significant others if appropriate) about his or her specific disease and prescribed treatment. See the Patient Teaching feature for more information about treatments.

Evaluation

Patients may be evaluated according to the following expected outcomes:

- The patient makes informed decisions about treatment based on his or her disorder and individual choice.
- The patient verbalizes understanding of the information presented.
- The patient expresses his or her feelings openly.

If patient outcomes are not met, referral to a specialist in the area of treatment may be necessary. It may also be appropriate for patients to meet with a counselor or psychologist who specializes in issues associated with sexual health or infertility. Support groups may also offer social and emotional support and education about patient concerns or issues.

Nursing Care Plan
A Patient Requesting Preconception Counseling

Donner Everson and her significant other, Mola Langerson, had a child born with Tay–Sachs disease who died at 3 years of age 2 years ago. They would love to have another child but fear having another baby with this genetic disorder. They have considered adoption but would like to know whether there is any chance of having a healthy child. They report that they have attempted to conceive a few times throughout the past year, but when it did not happen immediately, they decided to return to use of contraceptives. Mr. Langerson says he is willing to "throw the dice," but Ms. Everson says she would rather be childless than deliver another child with Tay–Sachs disease. Neither of them wants to risk having to make a decision about aborting a child with Tay–Sachs. They want to make sure that if a pregnancy occurs, the child is healthy. They have come to talk with their healthcare provider to learn about their options.

ASSESSMENT

Both Ms. Everson and Mr. Langerson are healthy with no significant current, chronic, or past medical or surgical history. Vital signs are within normal limits, their weights are appropriate for their heights, and they are both physically active. Neither patient has a substance abuse issue or history, and they report an occasional glass of wine, perhaps twice a week. They are both orthodox Jews whose grandparents lived in Germany prior to World War II.

Ms. Everson's family history includes two children born with Tay–Sachs disease, one born to her maternal aunt and one to her paternal aunt. She has no siblings. Mr. Langerson had a brother who was born with Tay–Sachs disease, but there is no other family history of congenital or genetic anomalies.

Their family provider collects blood for genetic testing and refers them to a genetic counselor.

DIAGNOSES

- *Anxiety*
- *Childbearing Process, Readiness for Enhanced*
- *Decisional Conflict*
- *Deficient Knowledge* related to options for having a child without a genetic disorder

(NANDA-I © 2014)

PLANNING

- The patients will determine their chance of having a child born without Tay–Sachs disease.
- The patients will develop coping strategies for reducing anxiety.
- The patients will make an informed decision related to pregnancy, considering their risks related to genetic disorders.
- The patients will understand their options as related to conception and delivery of a healthy child.

IMPLEMENTATION

The nurse's role in caring for these patients is largely supportive. The nurse may provide the necessary teaching to help them understand what they are told and learn about any options that they are provided.

- Encourage the patients to verbalize their feelings.
- Suggest coping strategies to reduce anxiety.

- Recommend that the patients delay making a decision regarding pregnancy until they have time to gather facts and determine the options available to them.
- Describe the role of the genetic counselor and the type of information the geneticist can provide based on the blood tests collected.

Nursing Care Plan (continued)

EVALUATION

Ms. Everson and Mr. Langerson spoke with the genetic counselor and learned that there was a 50% chance that a baby conceived naturally would be born with Tay–Sachs disease. The genetic counselor told them IVF could be performed, allowing the physician to choose only sperm and ova that were free of the genetic mutation. Once conception took place, the blastocyst could be implanted into

Ms. Everson's uterus, allowing the couple 100% likelihood of conceiving a child without Tay–Sachs disease. However, the genetic counselor cautioned that this method would not eliminate risks related to other congenital or pregnancy-induced disorders. They opted to try this procedure, and Ms. Everson became pregnant and delivered a healthy baby girl.

CRITICAL THINKING

1. One of the implementations for this couple is to encourage them to delay conception until they receive information related to their options. Is this an appropriate nursing implementation? Explain your answer.

2. Define the role of the genetic counselor and explain what information genetic counseling can provide this couple.

3. Describe the in vitro process and explain how this process can reduce the risk of having a child born with Tay–Sachs disease.

REVIEW   Family Planning

RELATE Link the Concepts and Exemplars

Linking the exemplar of family planning with the concept of addiction:

1. You are working with a young couple who are planning to have a baby. The potential father smokes cigarettes. What teaching regarding the effects of paternal smoking on planned children will you provide?

2. What information about risks associated with alcohol consumption would you provide the woman who plans to become pregnant and drinks an average of four alcoholic drinks a week?

Linking the exemplar of family planning with the concept of immunity:

3. What patient teaching will you provide to a patient diagnosed with systemic lupus erythematosus who plans to become pregnant?

4. What is your priority of care for the woman diagnosed with rheumatoid arthritis who is anticipating pregnancy?

READY Go to Volume 3: Clinical Nursing Skills

REFER Go to Pearson MyLab Nursing and eText

- Additional review materials

REFLECT Apply Your Knowledge

Lisa Daniels is a 19-year-old woman recently married to her high school sweetheart, Willis. Ms. Daniels is planning to begin college in the fall to study interior decorating. Mr. Daniels is 21 and is working as the manager of a local fast-food restaurant. Ms. Daniels's family lives a few towns away and is thrilled with her marriage to Willis. Her younger brother, Tom, enjoys playing basketball with him. Mr. Daniels's family lives across the country but are very fond of Lisa and excited about the marriage.

Mr. and Ms. Daniels have come to the OB/GYN clinic to talk about planning for a family. Neither of the two has any health issues that would put them or a child at risk. Ms. Daniels feels that she can handle going to school part time and also care for a baby. Both Mr. and Ms. Daniels are very excited about the prospect of starting their family. They have just bought a house and have furnished it with hand-me-downs from family and friends. They both laugh when they talk about living paycheck to paycheck.

1. What topics will you raise with Mr. and Ms. Daniels as they consider starting a family?

2. What preconception counseling will you provide Ms. Daniels to help her optimize her status before becoming pregnant?

3. If Mr. and Ms. Daniels decide to begin attempting to conceive, what teaching will you provide this couple?

≫ Exemplar 19.B
Menopause

Exemplar Learning Outcomes

19.B Analyze menopause as it relates to sexuality.

- Describe the physiology of menopause.
- Identify the clinical manifestations of menopause.
- Summarize diagnostic tests and therapies used by interprofessional teams in the collaborative care of a woman experiencing menopause.
- Differentiate considerations for care of patients with menopause across the lifespan.
- Apply the nursing process for providing culturally competent care to a woman experiencing menopause.

Exemplar Key Terms

Hormone replacement therapy (HRT), *1499*
Menopause, *1498*

Overview

Menopause is the permanent cessation of menses and is a normal physiologic process. It is included here because it increases the risk of physical disorders and affects various aspects of women's health. The *climacteric* or *perimenopausal* period denotes the time during which reproductive function gradually ceases. For most women, the perimenopausal period lasts several years. It begins with a decline in the production of estrogen, includes permanent cessation of menstruation due to loss of ovarian function, and extends for 1 year after the final menstrual period, at which time a woman is said to be *postmenopausal*. The average woman will live one third of her life after menopause.

In the United States, the average age at which menstruation ceases is 51, although it may happen as early as a woman's 40s. Earlier menopause is associated with genetics, smoking, high altitude, and undernutrition (Gass, 2013). Certain health risks increase after menopause, including risk of heart disease, osteoporosis, macular degeneration, cognitive changes, and breast cancer.

Physiology

The menopausal period marks the natural biological end of reproductive ability. *Surgical menopause* occurs when the ovaries are removed in premenopausal women, dramatically reducing the production of estrogen and progestins. *Medical menopause* often occurs during cancer chemotherapy, when cytotoxic drugs arrest ovarian function.

As the ovaries age, they become less responsive to FSH and LH; this results in a shorter follicular phase and a shorter, less regular menstrual cycle. Over time, the number of viable follicles decreases, and the follicles that remain may not respond to hormonal stimulation (Gass, 2013). Ovarian production of estradiol (E_2) decreases, and estradiol is replaced by estrone (E_1) as the major ovarian estrogen. Estradiol is the most biologically active estrogen; estrone has only about one tenth the biological activity of estradiol and is produced in small amounts. With decreased ovarian function, progesterone production is also markedly reduced.

Levels of the hormone androstenedione also decrease during menopause. Androstenedione has few effects itself but is used in the production of estrogen (Gass, 2013). FSH and LH levels, on the other hand, increase. Estradiol controls the amount of FSH and LH released by the pituitary gland via a negative feedback system; when estradiol production decreases, this feedback system ceases to function (Elder & Thacker, 2013).

>> **Stay Current:** Menopause represents a major life transition for patients, and they may have questions about what this transition means for their health. The North American Menopause Society's website at http://www.menopause.org/ provides information for professionals and patients about all aspects of menopause.

Clinical Manifestations

Although menopause is an age-related process, not a pathologic one, some women have troublesome health experiences after the cessation of menses. As estrogen decreases, various tissues are affected. Breast tissue, body hair, skin elasticity, and subcutaneous fat decrease. The ovaries and uterus become smaller, and the cervix and vagina decrease in size and become pale in color. These changes may result in vaginal dryness, dyspareunia, urinary stress incontinence, UTIs, and vaginitis. Atrophic vaginitis may lead to urogenital infection, ulceration, and uncomfortable sexual intercourse. Vasomotor instability often results in hot flashes, palpitations, dizziness, and headaches. Other problems resulting from vasomotor instability include insomnia, frequent awakening, and perspiration (night sweats) (Coney, 2015). Hormone changes may also cause some women to experience irritability, anxiety, and depression. Long-term estrogen deprivation results in an imbalance in bone remodeling and osteoporosis, leading to fractures and kyphosis. The risk for cardiovascular diseases also increases in response to an increase in atherosclerosis (from an increase in the LDL-to-HDL cholesterol ratio).

Menopause is an individual experience that involves biocultural variation. Each woman experiencing menopause has lived through decades of physiologic responses to her environment. Nutrition, smoking, body mass index, and reproductive history all affect how a woman will respond to this physiologic transition (Davis et al., 2015). Some women may celebrate menopause; others may experience negative feelings about themselves and their body; and still others may attach no significance to it.

Manifestations of the perimenopausal period vary widely. Women can experience severe symptoms, moderate symptoms, or few or no symptoms. During perimenopause (Coney, 2015; Davis et al., 2015; Juve, 2013):

- Menstrual cycles become erratic. Menstrual flow varies widely in amount and duration and eventually ceases.
- Vaginal, vulvar, and urethral tissues begin to atrophy.
- Vaginal pH rises, predisposing the woman to bacterial infections.
- Vaginal lubrication decreases, and vaginal rugae decrease in number. This may result in dyspareunia, injury, and fungal infections.
- Vasomotor instability due to a decrease in estrogen may result in hot flashes and night sweats. A hot flash starts in the chest and moves upward toward the face and may last from seconds to several minutes.
- Psychologic symptoms may include moodiness, nervousness, insomnia, headaches, irritability, anxiety, inability to concentrate, and depression.

Collaboration

Care of the woman experiencing menopausal symptoms focuses on relieving symptoms and minimizing postmenopausal health risks. Physicians, gynecologists, nurse practitioners, nurses, and community support groups may all be involved in the provision of care. Most women entering this transitional period need reassurance, education, and support from the healthcare team.

Diagnostic Tests

As estrogen secretion diminishes, levels of FSH and LH rise and remain elevated. A woman who has not menstruated for one full year, who has a decreased estradiol level, or who

Clinical Manifestations and Therapies

Menopause

ETIOLOGY	CLINICAL MANIFESTATIONS	CLINICAL THERAPIES
Increase in vaginal pH	■ Risk of UTI; symptoms include burning, frequency, hesitancy, and urgency to urinate ■ Vaginal infection; symptoms include vaginitis and vaginal drainage	■ Medications (antibiotics or antifungals) may be prescribed. ■ Encourage adequate fluid intake. ■ Emphasize the importance of wiping from front to back. ■ Teach patients to report symptoms of UTI and vaginal infection.
Reduced vaginal lubrication	■ Dyspareunia ■ Injury ■ Fungal infections	■ Teach use of artificial water-based lubricants to reduce symptoms. ■ Treat fungal infections.
Vasomotor instability	■ Hot flashes ■ Diaphoresis ■ Trouble sleeping ■ Increased risk of heart disease	■ Teach women to dress in layers, wear cotton underwear, and drink cool liquids. ■ If instability is severe, hormone supplements may be prescribed.
Osteoporosis	■ Fractures, increased bone fragility ■ Kyphosis	■ Teach the importance of calcium, vitamin D, and phosphorus intake. ■ Suggest weight-bearing exercises.
Fluctuating estrogen levels	■ Mood swings ■ Irritability ■ Depression	■ Encourage adequate sleep and regular physical activity. ■ Teach stress-management techniques. ■ Refer the patient to a therapist, counselor, and/or support group. ■ If severe, hormone supplements and/or antidepressants may be prescribed.

has an increased FSH blood level is considered menopausal (Mayo Clinic, 2015f). Estradiol and FSH levels are not routinely measured but may be used if a woman's diagnosis is in question.

Pharmacologic Therapy

Before 2002, **hormone replacement therapy (HRT)** was a common medical choice for relieving the symptoms of menopause. Treatment options included estrogen/progestin combinations (EPT) for women who still had a uterus and estrogen only (ET) for women who had undergone hysterectomy. Research evidence had proven that the addition of progestin protects the endometrium from estrogen-induced hyperplasia and cancer.

This routine medication regimen for women experiencing menopausal symptoms changed when a landmark study from the Women's Health Initiative (WHI) concerning women using EPT was halted 3 years early (WHI, n.d.). The early data revealed that these women were at greater risk for congestive heart failure, breast cancer, pulmonary embolism, and stroke than women taking placebos. The ET arm of the study continued but was halted 1 year early because of increased incidence of stroke and breast cancer among women taking ET compared to women taking placebos (Juve, 2013). This abrupt stop to a large government-sponsored study led many women to stop HRT. It also led to a marked decrease in the number of HRT prescriptions physicians were willing to write.

In the years since the report of the WHI, experts have debated the safety and efficacy of HRT for menopausal symptoms. In 2012, the Kronos Early Estrogen Prevention Study (KEEPS) results were made available. This 4-year study included 727 participants. It demonstrated that lower dose estrogen/progestin started soon after menopause appears to be safe, relieves hot flashes and vaginal dryness, improves mood and bone density, and decreases the risk for cardiovascular disease (North American Menopause Society, 2012a). The KEEPS results, other research findings, and expert opinion about HRT use prompted the North American Menopause Society to issue a position statement on HRT. The U.S. Preventive Services Task Force also issued a recommendation statement (Moyer, 2012; North American Menopause Society, 2012b, 2013). The two documents are consistent in their recommendations, which include the following:

■ Most healthy, recently menopausal women (up to age 59 or within 10 years of menopause) can use HRT for relief of hot flashes and vaginal dryness. Treatment should be individualized.

■ HRT is the most effective treatment of menopausal hot flashes and vaginal dryness.

■ If vaginal dryness or dyspareunia are the only symptoms, then low-dose vaginal estrogen is preferred.

■ Risks for blood clots in the legs and lungs are increased with HRT, but occurrence is rare in women ages 50–59.

The risk is further lowered by using low-dose estrogen pills or transdermal patches, gels, or sprays.

- There is an increased risk of breast cancer when continuous EPT is used for 5 or more years or when ET is used for 7 or more years, but the risk ceases when the hormone is stopped.

Two new drugs for the treatment of menopause symptoms were approved by the FDA in 2013. These drugs are known as selective estrogen receptor modifiers (SERMs). They represent a new form of HRT intended to lower the risk of adverse side effects, though both carry warnings about increased risk of endometrial cancer and deep vein thrombosis. One of these drugs, Duavee, combines a SERM with conjugated estrogen to treat hot flashes and reduce risk of bone fractures. Another drug, Osphema, is used to treat dyspareunia in postmenopausal women (Adams et al., 2017). Recent research also suggests that SSRI and SNRI (serotonin-norepinephrine reuptake inhibitor) antidepressants are nearly as effective as HRT in relieving hot flashes and night sweats (Joffe et al., 2014; Shams et al., 2014).

SAFETY ALERT Use of oral HRT increases the risk of breast cancer and may also increase the risk of breast cancer recurrence. As a result, it is typically prescribed in low doses for short durations. It is also rarely prescribed for breast cancer survivors.

Nonpharmacologic Therapy

Because of the controversy surrounding the use of HRT, nontraditional or alternative therapies have become popular. Complementary health approaches, some of which are more effective than others, are used by women to reduce menopause-associated discomforts. Some of these approaches include the following:

- *Massage.* Both massage and aromatherapy massage are effective in decreasing menopause symptoms (Darsareh et al., 2012).
- *Meditation.* Randomized clinical trial evidence suggests that mindful meditation relieves vasomotor symptoms of menopause (National Center for Complementary and Integrative Health, 2016).
- *Soy.* Researchers in China evaluated the efficacy of soy in relieving menopausal hot flashes (Ye et al., 2012). The researchers found that all the women using soy had a reduction in vasomotor symptoms after 12 and 24 weeks and experienced many fewer hot flashes than the women in the placebo group. The researchers concluded that soy germ is beneficial in reducing hot flashes during menopause but more evidence is needed before soy may be recommended as an alternative to hormonal replacement.
- *Ginseng.* This botanical has many good qualities; however, it has been given an evidence grade of C for menopausal symptom control (Kim et al., 2013). This means that there is unclear or conflicting scientific evidence from multiple randomized trials that ginseng alleviates hot flashes in menopausal women.

Note that evidence supporting the use of either yoga or acupuncture in relieving symptoms of menopause is inconclusive (North American Menopause Society, 2015). Bioidentical hormones have not been proven safe or effective (Stuenkel et al., 2012). Although black cohosh has been a popular alternative to HRT for years, a Cochrane Database review (Leach & Moore, 2012) examined 16 studies for a total of 2027 participants and found that, compared to placebo, black cohosh did not decrease hot flashes and other symptoms. The authors concluded that evidence for use of black cohosh is lacking and further research is needed.

Lifespan Considerations

The average age at which women undergo menopause is 51 years, though any time during a woman's 40s or 50s is considered normal. It is possible for women under the age of 40 to enter menopause. This is known as *premature ovarian failure (POF)* or *premature menopause,* and it affects 1 in every 1000 women ages 15–29 and 1 in every 100 women ages 30–39. The average age of occurrence for POF is 27 years (American Pregnancy Association, 2015h).

Women with POF do not ovulate each month because of a low number of follicles or ovarian dysfunction. These women may still have a period, although their periods are usually irregular. They may experience typical symptoms of menopause, including hot flashes and night sweats, decrease in sex drive, dyspareunia, and vaginal dryness. FSH levels are also elevated in patients with POF. Some women may be asymptomatic; in such cases, the only indicator of POF is high FSH values (American Pregnancy Association, 2015h).

Women of any age can also undergo medical menopause or surgical menopause. Medical menopause usually results from cancer treatment or chemotherapy that damages the ovaries. Symptoms of medical menopause tend to come on gradually and typically include cessation of menstruation and vasomotor symptoms. Medical menopause may be permanent or temporary; permanence of medical menopause is linked to the age of the patient. Up to 40% of women under the age of 40 and between 70 and 90% of women over the age of 40 experience permanent medical menopause (Breastcancer.org, 2015).

Surgical menopause is caused by removal of the ovaries, known as oophorectomy. Oophorectomy may be done alone or may be combined with surgery to remove the uterus (hysterectomy) and the fallopian tubes (salpingectomy). A patient may undergo oophorectomy to treat ovarian cancer; it may also be done to treat conditions like noncancerous ovarian tumors, ovarian abscess, or endometriosis (Mayo Clinic, 2014g). Unlike medical menopause, onset of surgical menopause is abrupt. Symptoms may be severe and may be treated with HRT. Patients who are interested in having children should discuss their fertility and ART options with their doctor prior to surgery. If oophorectomy involves one ovary, patients may still be able to conceive naturally; natural conception is not an option if oophorectomy involves both ovaries.

NURSING PROCESS

Nursing care during and after the menopausal period focuses on minimizing the symptoms associated with hormonal changes; reducing the risk of cardiovascular disease, cancer, and osteoporosis; and educating the patient about lifestyle changes important to health and well-being.

Assessment

The nurse collects pertinent data through the health history and physical examination. When assessing the older woman, the nurse should be aware of normal changes associated with aging. Also, the nurse should be sensitive to the fact that patients may feel awkward discussing physical and sexual changes related to menopause. The nurse should review cancer screening history and encourage regularly scheduled Pap smears, clinical breast exams, and mammography based on current clinical guidelines and patient history (American Cancer Society, 2015a).

- *Observation and patient interview.* Review the patient's sexual history and note the occurrence of dyspareunia or changes in sexual arousal. Assess menstrual history, including changes in bleeding patterns, cycle length, and menstrual regularity. Record information related to past pregnancies, childbirth, and gynecologic surgeries. Ask about urinary problems, including frequency, urgency, or incontinence. Evaluate sleep patterns and vasomotor symptoms, including hot flashes and night sweats. Discuss changes in emotional responses. Assess alcohol, nicotine, and drug use. Evaluate diet, exercise, and vitamin or supplement use.

- *Physical examination.* Assess the patient's vital signs, height, weight, and posture. Examine the breasts for irregularities or changes in shape, skin appearance, or nipple appearance, and note the presence of masses in breast tissue or swelling in the lymph nodes. Percuss the abdomen to determine size of pelvic structures and assess for fluid collection. Palpate for tenderness, organ enlargement, and masses; be mindful of guarding and rebound tenderness. Conduct a pelvic exam, paying attention to appearance of the external genitalia, vagina, and cervix and collecting any necessary samples.

Diagnosis

Some nursing diagnoses that may apply to patients who are experiencing menopause include:

- *Deficient Knowledge*
- *Sexuality Pattern, Ineffective*
- *Self-Esteem, Situational, Low*
- *Body Image, Disturbed.*

(NANDA-I © 2014)

Planning

Goals of patient care may include the following:

- The patient will understand the process of menopause.
- The patient will learn strategies to reduce and cope with symptoms.
- The patient will undertake a program of weight-bearing exercise.

Implementation

Different women view menopause differently. It is important for the nurse to determine what menopause means to each patient before beginning implementation. Although some women may view menopause as a relief, others may see it as the end of their youth and the beginning of old age. Interventions should be aimed at helping the woman understand the process of menopause, cope with symptoms as they arise, and make healthy lifestyle choices.

Discuss Knowledge of Menopause

Because manifestations of menopause vary widely, it is difficult to predict their effect on an individual woman. However, the well-informed woman is better prepared to deal with whatever symptoms she experiences. To prepare the patient, the nurse should do the following:

- Discuss physiologic manifestations, such as hot flashes and night sweats. The underlying cause of hot flashes is unknown, but changes in estrogen levels and changes to the hypothalamus are the most likely contributors (Mayo Clinic, 2015g). Many physiologic effects of menopause are amenable to either HRT or nonpharmacologic methods of relief, such as lifestyle changes.

- Provide information about dietary recommendations. The recommended daily calcium intake for women over age 50 is 1200 mg to help prevent osteoporosis. Some women need to use calcium supplements or calcium-containing antacid tablets to meet this requirement.

- Emphasize the importance of weight-bearing exercise. Weight-bearing exercise reduces the rate of bone loss, helps maintain optimum weight, and reduces cardiovascular risk.

- Provide information about HRT. Not every woman will need or want HRT, but every woman needs to understand both the risks and the benefits of this form of therapy.

Promote Effective Sexuality Patterns

Vaginal dryness and atrophy, together with the emotional effects of menopause, can interfere with sexual expression and satisfaction. Suggesting measures to help the woman and her partner cope with these changes can enable them to continue or resume a mutually satisfying sexual relationship. Appropriate nursing actions may include the following:

- Encourage the expression of feelings and concerns about how menopause is changing the patient's sex life. Midlife and older women may not be comfortable discussing sexual behavior.

- Suggest ways to increase vaginal lubrication, such as spending more time in foreplay and/or using water-soluble gels (e.g., Replens) for vaginal lubrication. A more leisurely approach to sexual activity can be mutually gratifying for the woman and her partner. Use of water-soluble gels can prevent vaginal pain and irritation and improve the quality of the sexual experience. Plant estrogens, found in food such as brown rice, sweet potatoes, carrots, apples, corn, green beans, and tofu, are mildly estrogenic and may improve vaginal dryness.

- Explain that as women age, it may take longer for vaginal lubrication and orgasm to occur. This information is important to prevent the woman from believing something is wrong with her and to prevent her partner from believing he or she is no longer sexually exciting.

Promote Healthy Body Image and Self-Esteem

As a woman progresses through the perimenopausal period, changes in appearance and the loss of childbearing ability may combine to make her feel "old," "ugly," and "useless." Although this is far from the truth, it nevertheless is the perception of women as well as society. The physical changes women often experience include growth of facial hair, excessive perspiration and flushing of the face, and weight gain. The nurse can help the patient deal with physical changes of menopause by doing the following:

- Encourage the woman to describe her perceptions of her own body. This information is necessary to obtain data and establish an individualized plan of care.

- Encourage verbalization of feelings of concern, anger, anxiety, loss, and fear over body changes. Expressing these emotions can facilitate the grieving process and acceptance of change.

- Stress that certain physical characteristics of an individual cannot be changed; emphasize the importance of learning to recognize and appreciate one's own special strengths. This can help the woman gain acceptance and a realistic appraisal of self.

- As appropriate, offer referrals for dietary management, exercise, stress management, and cosmetic assistance (e.g., for aggravating facial hair). These actions increase wellness and a positive sense of self.

Evaluation

Expected outcomes to evaluate the patient's progress toward goals may include the following:

- The patient demonstrates a positive sense of self as evidenced by stable weight, participation in a regular exercise program, and ability to manage stress.

- The patient verbalizes feelings related to changes that have occurred.

- The patient describes strategies for maintaining health.

If patient outcomes are not met, additional patient education about health maintenance may be indicated. Emphasize the importance of peer support and encourage the patient to consider exercising with a friend who is also experiencing menopause. Referral to a counselor who specializes in issues associated with aging and the needs of menopausal women may be appropriate.

REVIEW Menopause

RELATE Link the Concepts and Exemplars

Linking the exemplar of menopause with the concept of self:

1. What interventions will you initiate for the woman entering menopause who feels that she is no longer attractive and has lost her femininity?

2. What is your priority of care for the woman experiencing menopause who has low self-esteem?

Linking the exemplar of menopause with the concept of health, wellness, and illness:

3. What health promotion interventions will be a priority for the patient entering menopause?

4. What nutritional and exercise behaviors would you promote for the woman in menopause? Explain your answer.

READY Go to Volume 3: Clinical Nursing Skills

REFER Go to Pearson MyLab Nursing and eText

- Additional review materials

REFLECT Apply Your Knowledge

Marly Cutler is a 51-year-old woman who is married to Fred. They live in a small rural community and own a farm. Mr. and Ms. Cutler have two adult children who live in the city. Mr. Cutler has hypertension that is being treated with lisinopril 10 mg/day and high cholesterol, for which he takes simvastatin 20 mg/day. Ms. Cutler has no real health issues and has yearly screening examinations. Last year, her physician told her to take calcium 1200 mg/day to reduce the risk of osteoporosis.

Ms. Cutler has come to the OB/GYN clinic today because she has missed some periods, is having night sweats, and is experiencing mood swings that are affecting her relationship with her husband. She wonders whether she has caught the flu.

1. What patient teaching will you provide for Ms. Cutler?

2. What strategies might you suggest to reduce the severity of the symptoms she reports?

3. How will you assess Ms. Cutler's mental status?

» Exemplar 19.C Menstrual Dysfunction

Exemplar Learning Outcomes

19.C Analyze menstrual dysfunction as it relates to sexuality.

- Describe the pathophysiology of menstrual dysfunction.
- Describe the etiology of menstrual dysfunction.

- Summarize risk factors and prevention of menstrual dysfunction.
- Identify the clinical manifestations of menstrual dysfunction.
- Summarize diagnostic tests and therapies used by interprofessional teams in the collaborative care of an individual with menstrual dysfunction.

- Differentiate considerations for care of patients with menstrual dysfunction across the lifespan.
- Apply the nursing process for providing culturally competent care to an individual with menstrual dysfunction.

Exemplar Key Terms

Overview

Except in rare instances, every woman will have monthly menstrual periods. Many women experience minor discomforts associated with the menstrual cycle, such as breast tenderness, uterine cramping, low back pain, and mood swings. Other women experience more serious changes that lead to visits with healthcare providers. In general, menstrual dysfunction may manifest as pain, bleeding, or both. In this exemplar, common menstrual dysfunctions and their treatment will be described.

Pathophysiology and Etiology

Menstrual dysfunction can be broadly divided into two categories: dysmenorrhea and dysfunctional uterine bleeding. **Dysmenorrhea**, or pain associated with menses, is one of the most common menstrual dysfunctions. **Dysfunctional uterine bleeding**—or **DUB**—is heavy uterine bleeding that is irregular and painless. Both types of dysfunction can negatively affect patients' lives and disrupt normal daily routines.

Pathophysiology

Dysmenorrhea may be either primary or secondary. Primary dysmenorrhea is common in young women with normal menstrual function and is hormonal in nature. The main symptom of primary dysmenorrhea is pelvic pain that radiates to the groin. Women also complain of low backache, abdominal pain lasting 12–48 hours, pain radiating to the lower back and thighs, diarrhea, headache, nausea, vomiting, anorexia, and breast tenderness. Pain may begin on the first day of menses or 1–3 days prior to the onset of menses. Pain typically peaks 24 hours after menses begins and decreases after 2 or 3 days (Pinkerton, 2015a).

Secondary dysmenorrhea is related to pathology or diseases that affect the uterus and pelvic area. These disorders are more likely to occur among women ages 30–50, and pain may occur at any time in the menstrual cycle. The pain and discomfort associated with these disorders can be very severe. Often it is described as a dull lower abdominal pain that radiates to the back and down the thighs. The pain may begin earlier in the menstrual cycle and last longer than pain experienced in primary dysmenorrhea (Cleveland Clinic, 2014b). If primary dysmenorrhea fails to respond to treatment, the patient should be re-evaluated for secondary dysmenorrhea.

Endometriosis is the most common cause of secondary dysmenorrhea and is one of the most painful gynecologic disorders. In endometriosis, cells from the endometrial tissue implant and grow outside the uterus. These tissue implants respond to estrogen and progesterone just as the endometrial lining does. Each month the implants mature, open, and bleed into the pelvic cavity, causing pain, fibrosis, and adhesions (Laubach, Lorntson, & Forrest, 2013). Endometriosis may occur anywhere in the body, but it is most likely to be seen on the organs in the lower parts of the pelvis, such as the uterus, ovaries, fallopian tubes, uterine ligaments, pelvic peritoneum, bladder, rectum, and rectovaginal septum (Office on Women's Health, 2014b). Estimates of prevalence vary widely in the medical literature, with a range of estimates from 30 to 80% of women examined because of pelvic pain being diagnosed with endometriosis. The literature also suggests that infertile women are 6–8 times more likely to have endometriosis (Practice Committee of the American Society for Reproductive Medicine, 2012).

Unlike endometriosis and other causes of dysmenorrhea, DUB involves little or no pain. DUB is characterized by profuse, painless bleeding preceded by long stretches of amenorrhea (Alswager & Durler, 2013). It is most often associated with anovulatory cycles. Over time, these cycles produce a thickened endometrial lining that begins irregular sloughing and prolonged heavy bleeding.

Etiology

Primary dysmenorrhea is caused by the release of prostaglandins that prompt the contractions of the uterus needed to expel menstrual fluid and tissue. Other inflammatory mediators produced in the endometrium may prolong these contractions and decrease blood flow. Pain may also be caused by the passage of menstrual tissue, lack of exercise, or anxiety about menses. In some cases, it may be associated with the shape and position of the reproductive organs, such as a narrowed cervix or a tilted uterus (Pinkerton, 2015a).

Although primary dysmenorrhea is the result of normal hormonal processes, secondary dysmenorrhea is the result of abnormalities or diseases of the pelvic area. Secondary dysmenorrhea may be caused by congenital malformations, though it is more commonly caused by tumors, cysts, pelvic adhesions, PID, infections, cervical stenosis, uterine leimyomas, adenomyosis, or endometriosis (Alswanger & Durler, 2013). Endometriosis is believed to have a genetic component and seems to be more common among women with relatives who have the disease (Mayo Clinic, 2013d). The cause of endometriosis is unknown, but it is thought to be due to impaired cellular and humoral immunity or an autoimmune disorder.

Like primary dysmenorrhea, DUB is linked to hormones. More specifically, it is the result of disordered hormonal processes that prevent maturation of ovarian follicles. Without ovulation, there is no corpus luteum and, therefore, a lack of progesterone. This causes changes in the endometrial lining and a loss of regular, complete shedding.

DUB presents with symptoms similar to abnormal uterine bleeding. While DUB is hormonal, abnormal uterine bleeding is caused by uterine tumors, endometrial or cervical cancer, polyps, ovarian cysts, bleeding disorders, and complications of pregnancy. Causes of abnormal uterine bleeding must be eliminated before a diagnosis of DUB can be made (Pinkerton, 2015b).

Risk Factors

Risk factors for dysmenorrhea include early age at menarche, long or heavy menstrual periods, smoking, and family history of dysmenorrhea. Endometriosis also predisposes women to secondary dysmenorrhea; risk factors for endometriosis include menarche before age 11, cycle length less than 27 days, heavy or prolonged menses, sedentary lifestyle, increased dietary fat, and having a first-degree relative with the disorder. Onset of primary dysmenorrhea typically occurs during adolescence, while secondary dysmenorrhea typically begins in adulthood unless it is the result of a congenital malformation (Pinkerton, 2015a).

A number of factors may predispose a woman to DUB. Age is a major risk factor; women in their teens and early 20s and women who are approaching menopause are more likely to experience DUB. Stress, extreme weight changes, obesity, thyroid disease, and metabolic disorders are also risk factors. Certain medications, including HRT and some types of hormonal birth control, increase the likelihood of developing DUB, as does IUC use (Behara & Price, 2015).

Prevention

Dysmenorrhea and DUB are strongly influenced by hormones, and there are no true preventive measures for these dysfunctions. However, lifestyle changes may benefit patients at risk for these conditions. Recommended changes include eating a balanced diet and avoiding sugary and salty foods, caffeine, alcohol, and cigarettes. Regular exercise and stress-relieving activities may be helpful. For patients who are overweight, a regimen of healthy, gradual weight loss may also prove beneficial. Once a diagnosis of menstrual dysfunction has been made, prevention of future episodes depends on long-term maintenance of the prescribed treatment regimen, even in the absence of symptoms (Behara & Price, 2015).

Clinical Manifestations

Clinical manifestations of primary dysmenorrhea typically begin within 6 months of menarche and include cramping and steady lower abdominal pain that radiates to the back or down to the thighs. Pain typically lasts for 2–3 days and begins around the start of menstruation. Fatigue, nausea, vomiting, and diarrhea may occur. Headache and dizziness may also accompany primary dysmenorrhea (Calis et al., 2015).

Although secondary dysmenorrhea also manifests with pain, the pain tends to take on a different pattern and be of a different nature than that of primary dysmenorrhea. Secondary dysmenorrhea typically begins in a woman's 20s or 30s following a history of painless menstruation; pain that begins immediately following menarche may indicate a congenital malformation. Pain tends to increase prior to the onset of menstruation and peaks when menstruation begins. Bloating, a heavy feeling in the pelvis, and back pain are

common, as are vaginal discharge and dyspareunia. In some cases, heavy or irregular menstrual flow may occur (Calis et al., 2015).

When secondary dysmenorrhea is a result of endometriosis, the pain may worsen each month, and, depending on where the implants are located, dyspareunia, menorrhagia, postcoital bleeding, urinary complaints, and rectal pain may occur. The pain is usually described as beginning a few days before onset of menses and becoming much worse as the period begins to decrease and stop. If the problem is long standing or there are complications such as adhesions, the pain may be constant (Kapoor et al., 2015).

DUB typically presents without pain and occurs as one of several patterns of bleeding. These patterns include amenorrhea, oligomenorrhea, menorrhagia, metrorrhagia, menometrorrhagia, and postmenopausal vaginal bleeding. These bleeding patterns may also occur in abnormal uterine bleeding, mentioned earlier.

- **Amenorrhea** is the absence of menses. Like dysmenorrhea, it may be primary or secondary. Primary amenorrhea is the absence of menstruation by age 14 without having undergone other changes associated with puberty or age 15 with having undergone normal physical changes of puberty (U.S. National Library of Medicine, 2014b). A number of conditions can give rise to amenorrhea, including incomplete formation of genital or pelvic organs, changes to the hypothalamus or pituitary gland, genetic disorders, and congenital abnormalities such as the absence of the vagina or uterus. Improper ovarian function, chronic illness, infections, tumors, and poor nutrition can also cause primary amenorrhea.

- Secondary amenorrhea occurs when a previously menstruating woman does not spot or bleed for a period of time that is three times that of her normal cycle length. Secondary amenorrhea may be pathologic or physiologic. It may be due to severe weight loss related to excessive exercise or poor diet; thyroid disorders; PCOS; or as the result of hormonal changes during early adolescence, pregnancy, or the perimenopausal period. The most common causes of secondary amenorrhea are pregnancy, breastfeeding, menopause, and contraceptive use (U.S. National Library of Medicine, 2014c).

- **Oligomenorrhea** is light or infrequent menstruation and occurs when cycles are longer than 6–7 weeks. It is usually related to hormonal imbalances such as those seen in PCOS.

- **Menorrhagia** is excessive or prolonged menstruation that occurs at regular intervals. Imbalances of estrogen and progesterone, ovarian dysfunction, uterine fibroids, and cancer may all give rise to menorrhagia. IUCs and certain medications can also cause menorrhagia. In some cases, it may be accompanied by tiredness, fatigue, and shortness of breath (Mayo Clinic, 2014h).

- **Metrorrhagia** is bleeding of variable amount between menstrual periods. It may occur as mild spotting at ovulation or breakthrough bleeding due to combination oral contraception. It may also be severe and cause heavy bleeding. Metrorrhagia may be caused by hormone imbalance, polyps, fibroids, endometriosis, or adhesions.

Clinical Manifestations and Therapies
Menstrual Dysfunction

ETIOLOGY	CLINICAL MANIFESTATIONS	CLINICAL THERAPIES
Shock due to uterine bleeding	■ Hypotension ■ Delayed capillary refill ■ Cyanosis, hypoxia, dizziness, change in level of consciousness ■ Low urine output ■ Diminished bowel motility ■ Pale skin ■ Activity intolerance ■ Tachycardia, tachypnea	■ Provide blood transfusions. ■ Administer intravenous fluids. ■ Administer intravenous estrogen. ■ Monitor ABCs. ■ Administer oxygen. ■ Measure intake and output. ■ Increase fluid intake as tolerated.
Anemia	■ Pale skin ■ Activity intolerance, fatigue	■ Blood transfusions may be needed. ■ Administer iron supplements. ■ Promote diet high in iron. ■ Encourage fluid intake.
Dysmenorrhea	■ Grimacing ■ Lying still with legs drawn up ■ On pain scale of 0 to 10, may range from 4 to 10	■ Administer analgesics as appropriate. ■ Place heating pad on lower abdomen. ■ Increase fluids.

- **Menometrorrhagia** is irregular, excessive, prolonged menstruation. It is essentially a combination of the heavy bleeding of menorrhagia and the irregularity of metrorrhagia. Bleeding is typically the result of conditions such as endometriosis, uterine fibroids, or cancers.

- **Postmenopausal bleeding** may be caused by endometrial polyps, endometrial hyperplasia, or uterine cancer. The possibility of cancer makes early evaluation and treatment essential.

Menorrhagia, severe metrorrhagia, and menometrorrhagia all involve heavy bleeding, so patients with these conditions are at increased risk of anemia. Patients reporting symptoms of these conditions and exhibiting fatigue, weakness, pale skin, and dizziness or cognitive problems should be assessed for anemia. In some cases, loss of blood may be severe enough to lead to hypovolemic shock. Confusion, decreased urine output, rapid breathing, sweating, and unconsciousness are all signs of hypovolemic shock. More information about anemia and shock related to DUB can be found in the Clinical Manifestations and Therapies feature.

>> **Stay Current:** Menstrual dysfunction can be upsetting to patients. It often prompts feelings of anxiety and gives rise to many questions. The American College of Obstetricians and Gynecologists patient portal at http://www.acog.org/Patients is an excellent source of reliable, accessible information.

Collaboration

Care of the woman with dysmenorrhea focuses on identifying the underlying cause of pain, reestablishing functional capacity, and managing pain. A careful history and physical assessment are performed to rule out any underlying organic cause of dysmenorrhea. If no organic cause is found, the diagnosis is primary dysmenorrhea. In addition, attitudes and expectations about menstruation and lifestyle disruption are identified and explored.

Care of the woman with DUB focuses on identifying and treating the underlying hormonal disorder. A careful history and physical examination are performed. Abdominal and pelvic examinations are performed to rule out abdominal masses. All women with DUB should keep a diary of menstrual patterns to help in diagnosing the cause of bleeding.

Diagnostic Tests

Various diagnostic tests are performed to identify structural abnormalities, hormonal imbalances, and pathologic conditions that could cause dysmenorrhea or DUB.

Diagnosis is made on the basis of findings from a pelvic examination and diagnostic procedures, including a Pap test for cervical dysplasia or cancer; cervical and vaginal cultures to screen for STIs or other infections; and abdominal and transvaginal ultrasound for depth of the endometrium, intrauterine or ectopic pregnancy, ovarian cysts, adnexal masses, leiomyomas, or cancer. Hysteroscopy may be used, in which a scope is placed into the uterine cavity to inspect the endometrial lining. Another procedure is saline infusion sonohysterography, in which saline is injected into the endometrial cavity via a catheter and transvaginal ultrasound is used to assess for polyps or myomas. Colposcopy is a procedure in which a large electronic microscope is used to inspect the cervix under magnification and identify areas for biopsy. Endometrial biopsy may be done to obtain tissue from the endometrium for pathologic examination. Endocervical

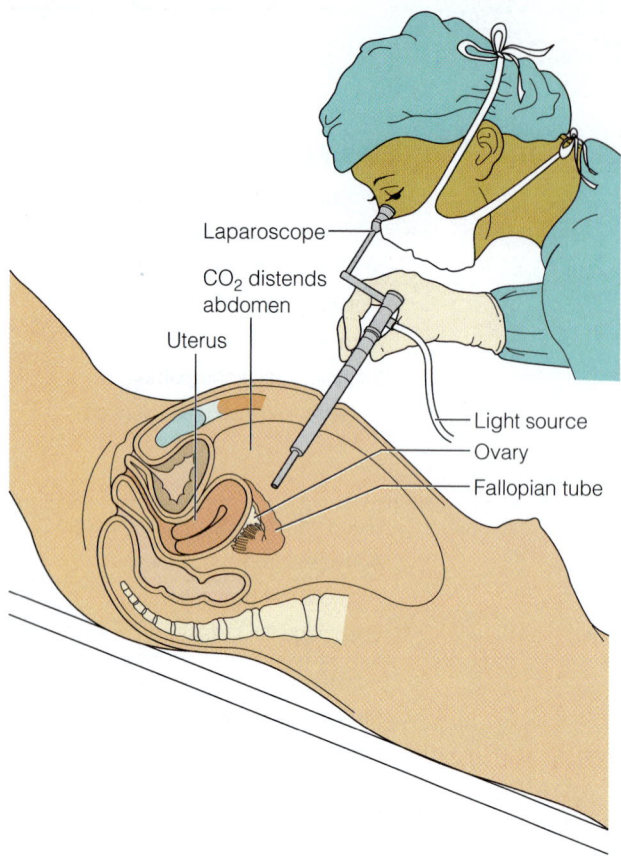

Figure 19–26 》 Laparoscopy. In this surgical procedure, a flexible, lighted instrument (laparoscope) is inserted through a periumbilical incision. Laparoscopy allows visualization of the pelvic cavity.

curettage and biopsy may be done to remove tissue from inside the cervical canal to look for evidence of dysplasia or cancer. CT scan or MRI may also be used to detect structural abnormalities, benign myomas, adenomyomas, malignancy, or infections.

Laparoscopy is used to diagnose structural defects and blockages caused by scarring, endometriosis, tumors, and cysts (see **Figure 19–26** 》).

Laboratory tests used to assess possible causes of dysmenorrhea and DUB are as follows:

- A pregnancy test determines whether pain or bleeding is a complication of pregnancy.

- FSH and LH levels are measured to assess the function of the pituitary gland. The results are correlated with the follicular phase or the luteal phase of the menstrual cycle.

- Progesterone and estradiol levels are measured to assess ovarian function.

- The thyroid-stimulating hormone test screens for thyroid dysfunction. If positive, then further testing of the thyroid is needed.

- A CBC with differential can provide evidence of anemia or infection.

- Coagulation studies reveal possible von Willebrand disease or other coagulation abnormalities (Behara & Price, 2015).

SAFETY ALERT If patients with DUB have experienced menorrhagia since menarche, have a family history of bleeding disorders, or have a personal history of bruising and bleeding of the mouth or gastrointestinal tract without obvious injury, an underlying bleeding disorder should be considered.

Surgery

For patients with menstrual dysfunction, medical treatment is preferred to surgical treatment. Primary dysmenorrhea responds well to medical treatments, while surgical interventions may be necessary to treat the underlying causes of secondary dysmenorrhea. The type of surgery required depends on the pathology or disease involved.

Most cases of DUB can be treated medically; however, surgery may be necessary in circumstances where medical treatment fails, is not tolerated, or is contraindicated. Surgical intervention emphasizes the least invasive method that provides effective relief, beginning with a therapeutic D&C, then endometrial ablation, and, finally, hysterectomy.

Therapeutic Dilation and Curettage

In a therapeutic D&C, the cervical canal is dilated and the uterine wall is scraped. Therapeutic D&C may be used to diagnose and treat DUB and other disorders of the female reproductive system. It is contraindicated in any woman who has been taking anticoagulant drugs or whose condition precludes the use of regional or general anesthesia. It may offer only temporary relief of DUB symptoms, and heavy bleeding may return during cycles following the procedure (American College of Obstetricians and Gynecologists, 2013a). The procedure can also lead to endometrial scarring (Pinkerton, 2015b).

Endometrial Ablation

Endometrial ablation destroys the uterine lining and may be done in the office setting or in surgery under general anesthesia. This procedure stops bleeding completely in most cases. Ablation may be done using extreme cold, heated fluids, microwave energy, or high-energy radio-frequency waves that vaporize the endometrial lining within 80–90 seconds (Mayo Clinic, 2012). Ablation is not recommended for women who want to become pregnant, who were recently pregnant, or who are postmenopausal. In 2013, the American College of Obstetricians and Gynecologists recommended that endometrial ablation be avoided as a primary therapy for DUB because it affects the ability to detect and diagnose endometrial cancer in the future. Patients who choose endometrial ablation should be counseled about this risk and must provide informed consent for the procedure (American College of Obstetricians and Gynecologists, 2013b).

Hysterectomy

Hysterectomy, or removal of the uterus, may be performed when medical management of DUB is unsuccessful or malignancy is present, particularly if the woman no longer wishes to bear children. In premenopausal women, the ovaries are usually left in place; in postmenopausal women, a total hysterectomy, or panhysterectomy, may be performed. A panhysterectomy involves removal of the uterus, fallopian tubes, and ovaries.

Hysterectomy may involve either an abdominal or a vaginal approach. The choice depends on the underlying disorder, the need to explore the abdominal cavity, and the preference of the surgeon and the patient.

Abdominal hysterectomy is performed when a preexisting abdominal scar is present, when adhesions are thought to be present, or when a large operating field is necessary. For example, the woman with endometriosis is more likely to have an abdominal hysterectomy because endometrial tissue implants that may be present on other abdominal organs need to be removed. The surgical incision may be longitudinal, made in the midline from umbilicus to pubis, or a Pfannenstiel incision, also known as the bikini cut.

Vaginal hysterectomy, removal of the uterus through the vagina, is desirable when the uterus has descended into the vagina or if the urinary bladder or rectum has prolapsed into the vagina. Laparoscopy-assisted vaginal hysterectomy (LAVH) is most often performed.

Pharmacologic Therapy

Medical management of dysmenorrhea relies heavily on hormonal therapies. For severe or incapacitating symptoms of dysmenorrhea, ovulation may be suppressed using COCs, Depo-Provera, danazol, or GnRH agonists. COCs and progesterone injections may also be used to relieve cramping, as may nonsteroidal anti-inflammatory drugs (NSAIDs). Other pharmacologic therapies used to treat dysmenorrhea include SSRIs such as fluoxetine (Prozac), sertraline (Zoloft), and paroxetine (Paxil, Brisdelle) to manage mood or to help patients cope with chronic pelvic pain. In addition, diuretics may be prescribed to relieve bloating.

Hormonal agents are also frequently used to correct menstrual irregularities associated with DUB. For anovulatory DUB, COCs may be prescribed for 3–6 months. As an alternative to COCs, oral medroxyprogesterone (Depo-Provera) may be prescribed for the first 12 days of each monthly cycle to regulate uterine bleeding. Hormonal IUCs such as Mirena are also effective for controlling irregular bleeding. In cases of heavy bleeding, conjugated estrogens may be administered during days 1–28 of the monthly cycle, with medroxy-progesterone added during days 15–28 (Adams et al., 2017). Other pharmacologic therapies used for DUB include NSAIDS, which may help decrease the amount of bleeding that occurs. Oral iron supplements are also commonly prescribed to replace iron lost through menstrual bleeding.

Some women may choose integrative health approaches to help manage symptoms of dysmenorrhea. See the Focus on Integrative Health feature.

Lifespan Considerations

Menstrual dysfunction affects patients differently at different stages in life. This is due in large part to hormone fluctuations associated with adolescence, pregnancy, and older adulthood.

DUB in Adolescents

Primary dysmenorrhea begins within the first three or four menstrual periods after menarche and occurs with each ovulatory cycle during a woman's teens and 20s. The pain associated with primary dysmenorrhea decreases over time and

Focus on Integrative Health
Use of Botanicals for Dysmenorrhea

Integrative therapies that may prove helpful to patients with dysmenorrhea focus on diet, exercise, relaxation, and stress management. Some of these therapies are as follows:

- Vitamin E and thiamine have been shown to be more effective than placebo in treating dysmenorrhea (Latthe, Champaneria, & Khan, 2012).
- Fish oil with B_{12} is thought to relieve dysmenorrhea by affecting the metabolism of prostaglandins, although its effectiveness has not been conclusively proven (Latthe et al., 2012).
- Exercise, adequate rest, stress management, and good nutrition are also beneficial.

is often much less after childbirth. Studies suggest that roughly 60% of adolescent girls have experienced primary dysmenorrhea, and many have missed school or work because of it (Calis et al., 2015).

Secondary dysmenorrhea is less common in adolescents than primary dysmenorrhea. If pain begins at menarche and steadily worsens, it may be the result of a congenital malformation. Pain that begins later or is resistant to hormonal treatments may be caused by endometriosis or pelvic infection (Gray, 2013).

DUB can also occur in adolescence, although it is more difficult to diagnose than dysmenorrhea. Because adolescents can experience variation in their cycles, patients and healthcare providers may have a difficult time defining what is normal for a particular patient. In general, a period lasting more than 8 days and a cycle that is less than 21 days or greater than 45 days is considered abnormal for an adolescent. Patient understanding of what constitutes excessive or heavy bleeding can also be difficult to gauge; a CBC may be especially useful in diagnosing DUB in adolescent patients (Gray, 2013).

Adolescent patients with heavy menstrual flow should also be assessed for bleeding disorders, particularly if flow has been heavy since menarche. Symptoms of anemia, large blood clots in menstrual flow, and frequent (hourly) changes of tampons or menstrual pads may all be indicative of an undiagnosed bleeding disorder (Mayo Clinic, 2014h).

DUB in Pregnant Women

Bleeding during pregnancy may manifest with symptoms similar to DUB. It is relatively common for women to bleed during the first trimester, and this does not necessarily signal complications of pregnancy; implantation bleeding and postcoital bleeding are common, nonthreatening examples. Bleeding in early pregnancy may also be caused by miscarriage, ectopic pregnancy, or molar pregnancy. When these conditions occur, bleeding may be heavy; miscarriage and ectopic pregnancy may also be accompanied by cramping and abdominal pain (American Pregnancy Association, 2015b, 2015i). Bleeding in late pregnancy may be caused by placental abruption, placenta previa, or preterm labor. These conditions pose a threat to both mother and child and require medical attention.

DUB in Older Adults

As patients enter perimenopause—the transitional stage between the childbearing years and menopause—cyclical changes in estrogen and progesterone levels become irregular. This irregularity can lead to primary dysmenorrhea as high levels of estrogen prompt the release of additional prostaglandins. These prostaglandins stimulate strong uterine contractions that can lead to pain (Centre for Menstrual Cycle and Ovulation Research, n.d.). For some patients, symptoms of primary dysmenorrhea that decreased or stopped following childbirth recur during perimenopause.

Changes in estrogen and progesterone levels can also lead to changes in perimenopausal menstrual bleeding. Irregularity and spotting become more common. Patients may experience heavy bleeding, menstruation that lasts longer than is typical, and menstruation that occurs more than once every 3 weeks (American College of Obstetricians and Gynecologists, 2011).

When patients enter menopause, pain associated with dysmenorrhea stops. DUB also stops, although a number of conditions can cause bleeding similar to that of DUB. This bleeding may be the result of natural endometrial or vaginal atrophy; prescription medications such as HRT or tamoxifen; uterine fibroids or polyps; or cancer of the uterus, cervix, or vagina. Patients should seek medical attention for any postmenopausal bleeding (Laughlin-Tommaso, 2015).

NURSING PROCESS

Nursing care for the woman with primary dysmenorrhea focuses on controlling manifestations and providing education about the normal physiology of the menstrual cycle and self-care measures. Care of the woman with secondary dysmenorrhea varies according to the cause.

Care of a patient with DUB involves symptom control as well as addressing any anxiety the woman may feel about the disorder. The patient's self-image, sexuality, or reproductive capacity may be threatened, and she may fear the possibility of cancer. She may also be embarrassed to discuss her menstrual history and hygiene practices.

Assessment

Assess the patient's menstrual patterns at each healthcare interaction. Determine the last menstrual period, normal length of menstruation and time between periods, and any symptoms associated with menstruation. Cultural influences often play a role in how a woman views and responds to menstruation and should also be assessed.

Many women view menstruation and issues surrounding it as very personal and are hesitant to discuss it, even with their healthcare providers. In addition, women may not realize that their experiences of pain or heavy menstrual bleeding are unusual, particularly if they have experienced these manifestations for several years. It is therefore essential to build rapport with patients by opening the discussion about menstruation and possible menstrual dysfunction. Asking the patient about her cycle is a simple way to start this conversation, and enquiring about menstrual regularity, bleeding, and any pain she experiences will help you gather important information. Routine health screenings offer a good opportunity for doing this, as patients may not make appointments for menstrual dysfunction out of embarrassment or failure to realize pain or discomfort are reasons to seek treatment (Fredericks, 2014).

- **Observation and patient interview.** Record information related to date of last menstrual period, typical length of cycle, and date of last OB-GYN exam. Assess menstrual history, including age at which menses began. Assess obstetric history, including past pregnancies, childbirth, and gynecologic surgeries. Ask the patient about typical sexual practices and the date of the last sexual encounter. Evaluate types of birth control used, current medications, and any preexisting conditions.
- **Physical examination.** Assess vital signs. Percuss the abdomen to determine size of pelvic structures. Palpate for tenderness, organ enlargement, and masses. Examine genitalia for any irregularities, and collect samples for a Pap test. Draw blood for hemoglobin and hematocrit testing.

Diagnosis

Nursing diagnoses appropriate for a patient with dysmenorrhea include the following:

- *Pain, Acute*
- *Coping, Ineffective.*

  (NANDA-I © 2014)

Nursing diagnoses that may be appropriate for the patient with DUB include the following:

- *Anxiety*
- *Fatigue* related to blood loss
- *Sexual Dysfunction.*

  (NANDA-I © 2014)

Planning

Goals of nursing care include the following:

- The patient's pain and discomfort will be reduced to an acceptable level.
- The patient will experience physical comfort and energy-saving rest.
- The patient will increase intake of fluids and iron-rich foods.
- The patient will become more comfortable discussing menstruation and sexual dysfunction.
- The patient will identify coping strategies to reduce anxiety.
- The patient will maintain a journal of symptoms.

Implementation

Nursing interventions for the woman with dysmenorrhea focus on relieving symptoms and providing patient teaching to decrease anxiety and increase coping skills. Assisting the patient to identify lifestyle choices that may be contributing

Patient Teaching

Dysfunctional Uterine Bleeding

The nurse should provide support, appropriate reassurance, and information to help the woman and her family better understand her disorder and the therapeutic interventions indicated. Teaching also includes self-care measures that minimize the effects of DUB on the daily functioning of the woman. The following topics should be included:

- Administration and side effects of prescribed medications, including iron
- The need to maintain a balanced diet, increasing iron-rich foods such as eggs, beans, liver, beef, and shrimp (Inform the woman that although orange juice may improve the absorption of iron, foods high in calcium and oxalic acid, such as spinach, may reduce its absorption.)
- The importance of maintaining a fluid intake of 2000–3000 mL/day
- The need to immediately report recurring episodes of abnormal uterine bleeding, particularly in postmenopausal women, to the healthcare provider.

to menstrual disorders such as heavy lifting, inadequate nutrition, and substance abuse can help the nurse implement the most effective plan of care.

Whatever the etiology and treatment of any dysmenorrhea, the nurse's teaching role is important. The Patient Teaching feature lists some of the ways in which the nurse can help the patient cope with DUB.

Relieve Acute Pain

The woman with dysmenorrhea may experience pain from headache (including migraine), lower abdominal cramps, excessive fluid retention, and backache. The nurse should teach the patient about effective pharmacologic and non-pharmacologic self-care measures to her cope with pain, including the application of heat to relieve muscle spasms and dilate blood vessels, increasing blood supply to the pelvis and uterine muscles. Relaxation techniques–such as breathing exercises, imagery techniques, or meditation—and exercise aid the release of naturally produced pain relievers called endorphins.

Relieve Anxiety

The anxiety associated with dysmenorrhea and DUB can be intense. With DUB in particular, the woman may fear cancer or other life-threatening conditions until the cause of bleeding is identified and addressed. The following nursing interventions can help the woman cope with anxiety:

- Discuss the results of tests and examinations with the woman. This allows for open exchange of information.
- Provide information about the causes, treatments, risks, long-term effects of treatments, and prognosis. This allows the woman to assume responsibility for her own health and become involved in her own treatment plan.
- Evaluate coping strategies and psychosocial support systems. Teach coping strategies if indicated. The possibility

of surgery or cancer represents a crisis for the woman and her support system. Support groups can provide assistance for the woman through crisis intervention.

- Review how fatigue may be affecting the woman's activities of daily living and suggest ways to balance rest and activity. Encourage her to ask her family to help with daily chores.

Promote Sexual Function

The woman with DUB may be unwilling to express herself sexually, particularly if bleeding is frequent or heavy. Also, fatigue may prevent her from participating in sexual activity. Some nursing interventions that address sexual dysfunction related to DUB include the following:

- Offer information about engaging in sexual activity during menstruation. Explain that conception is possible during this time if she has a 21-day menstrual cycle. Some women mistakenly believe that birth control measures are unnecessary during menstruation. Explain that orgasm may help relieve symptoms. Orgasm causes a release of tension and vascular congestion and frequently provides at least temporary relief of symptoms.
- Provide an opportunity for the patient to express concerns related to alterations in lifestyle and sexual functioning. Some women have had a prolonged period of sexual abstinence related to DUB. Allowing women to verbalize concerns can assist them in working collaboratively with the healthcare provider to minimize the impact of illness and optimize function.
- Encourage frequent rest periods. This conserves energy and may allow sexual activities to resume.
- Provide information about alternative methods of sexual expression. Methods of sexual expression other than vaginal intercourse may satisfy the needs of both partners.

Evaluation

Patient progress toward goals is evaluated on the basis of appropriate learning outcomes, which may include the following:

- The patient experiences less pain, allowing her to perform activities of daily living.
- The patient experiences less fatigue.
- The patient reports reduced anxiety.
- The patient reports return to baseline menstruation.
- The patient is able to participate in sexual activity without symptoms.

If patient outcomes are not met, additional patient teaching about lifestyle changes and other nonpharmacologic treatments for reducing pain may be appropriate. Emphasize the importance of rest and support for fatigue and anxiety, and encourage the patient to reach out to friends and loved one for assistance. If pain or heavy bleeding persist, referral to a healthcare provider who specializes in menstrual dysfunction may be appropriate.

Nursing Care Plan
A Patient with Menstrual Dysfunction

Angela Hall is a 31-year-old married accountant who relates a history of severe dysmenorrhea and menorrhagia, a feeling of pelvic heaviness, and pain that radiates down her thighs. Because of her discomfort, her husband has complained about the quality of their sex life and has expressed concerns about their plans for having children. Ms. Hall reports being so tired she does not care whether she has sex; in fact, she would really prefer not to have sex at all because of the pain it causes. Her healthcare provider suspects endometriosis, and a diagnostic laparoscopy has been scheduled.

ASSESSMENT

You interview Ms. Hall and make the following assessments: T_O 36.7°C (98.2°F); P 68 bpm; R 18/min; BP 110/70 mmHg. Ms. Hall's weight is 59 kg (130 lb) and within normal limits for her height. Review of laboratory findings indicates a hemoglobin level of 9.8 g/dL (normal range: 12–15 g/dL) and a hematocrit of 33.1% (normal range: 36–46%). Physical examination reveals pelvic tenderness on manipulation of the cervix and small masses that are palpable on abdominal/pelvic examination.

DIAGNOSES

- *Pain, Chronic,* related to endometrial pelvic implants
- *Anxiety* related to effect of endometriosis on fertility
- *Deficient Knowledge* related to diagnosis and treatment options
- *Sexuality Pattern, Inefficient,* related to the manifestations of endometriosis

(NANDA-I © 2014)

PLANNING

- The patient will use effective self-care measures to deal with the pain and discomfort.
- The patient will verbalize decreased anxiety.
- The patient will demonstrate understanding of the disease and treatment options.
- The patient will articulate an improvement in sexual functioning and a decrease in interpersonal stress between herself and her husband.

IMPLEMENTATION

- Identify the location, type, duration, and history of the pain.
- Recommend analgesics and heat therapy.
- Provide information on biofeedback, relaxation, and guided imagery to lessen pain.
- Discuss with Mr. and Ms. Hall the causes of endometriosis and its manifestations.
- Encourage the Halls to discuss their feelings about the effect of the disease on their sex life, lifestyle, and fertility.
- Refer the couple to the local mental health center if appropriate.

EVALUATION

Two years after the initiation of treatment, Mr. and Ms. Hall have become parents of a baby girl. Ms. Hall states that the discomfort and other manifestations of endometriosis have eased. Relaxation and guided imagery have effectively minimized her pain and brought about improvement in her function as wife, mother, and sexual partner. Counseling has improved the interpersonal and sexual relations between the Halls. Dietary management has improved Ms. Hall's anemia, although the menorrhagia persists. The Halls are trying to have a second child, understanding the advantages of rapid succession of pregnancies. They will be followed in the nursing clinic and referred to an infertility clinic if conception does not occur within 1 year.

CRITICAL THINKING

1. Explain the pathophysiologic basis for Ms. Hall's anemia.
2. How would you handle the situation if Mr. and Ms. Hall were extremely uncomfortable and embarrassed about discussing their sexual problems?
3. Develop a plan of care for Ms. Hall for the nursing diagnosis Situational Low Self-Esteem related to the manifestations of endometriosis.

REVIEW Menstrual Dysfunction

RELATE Link the Concepts and Exemplars

Linking the exemplar of menstrual dysfunction with the concept of elimination:

1. What teaching will you initiate for the patient with menstrual dysfunction regarding urinary health?
2. What nutritional counseling will you offer the patient with menstrual dysfunction to prevent constipation?

Linking the exemplar of menstrual dysfunction with the concept of stress and coping:

3. What assessment data would alert you that the patient with DUB is experiencing anxiety?
4. What priority interventions will you implement to help the woman with DUB cope with fears?

READY Go to Volume 3: Clinical Nursing Skills

REFER Go to Pearson MyLab Nursing and eText

- Additional review materials

REFLECT Apply Your Knowledge

Angie Able is a 35-year-old woman married to Joe. The Ables have four children: Ted, age 12; Adam, age 10; Lila, age 8; and Eva, age 4. Mr. Able is a chef who owns a very successful restaurant in town. Ms. Able is an administrative assistant to the CEO of the largest bank in the area. She is a well-organized, detail-oriented individual with high energy. She manages the children, her home, her husband, and her job with aplomb. She has enjoyed good health with only mild seasonal colds.

Ms. Able has been having heavier than usual menstrual periods during the past 6 months, and this is beginning to interfere with her work. She has needed to leave work to change clothes several times and has begun carrying extra clothing with her during her period. Besides being very embarrassed, Ms. Able is afraid that there is something seriously wrong with her. She feels tired all the time and is always thirsty. Ms. Able decides to visit her gynecologist before her next menstrual period begins.

1. What could explain Ms. Able's symptoms of fatigue and thirst?
2. What diagnostic tests do you anticipate will be ordered?
3. What teaching will you provide Ms. Able to reduce her current symptoms?

» Exemplar 19.D
Sexual Dysfunctions

Exemplar Learning Outcomes

19.D Analyze sexual dysfunctions as they relate to sexuality.

- Summarize sexual dysfunctions experienced by men.
- Summarize sexual dysfunctions experienced by women.
- Summarize diagnostic tests and therapies used by interprofessional teams in the collaborative care of an individual with sexual dysfunction.
- Differentiate considerations for care of patients with sexual dysfunction across the lifespan.
- Apply the nursing process for providing culturally competent care to an individual with sexual dysfunction.

Exemplar Key Terms

Delayed ejaculation, *1513*
Erectile disorder, *1512*
Erectile dysfunction (ED), *1512*
Female orgasmic disorder, *1514*
Female sexual interest/arousal disorder, *1514*
Genito-pelvic pain/penetration disorder, *1515*
Impotence, *1512*
Libido, *1512*
Male hypoactive sexual desire disorder, *1512*
Male orgasmic disorder, *1514*
Premature ejaculation, *1513*
Preorgasmic, *1514*
Retrograde ejaculation, *1514*
Sexual dysfunction, *1511*
Vaginismus, *1515*

Overview

Sexual dysfunction is a blanket term referring to any persistent disturbance in an individual's sexual response. Such disturbances can occur during any portion of the sexual response cycle, and they make it difficult, if not impossible, for affected individuals and their partners to experience satisfying sexual encounters (Cleveland Clinic, 2015b).

Sexual dysfunction may be linked to physical causes, psychologic causes, or a combination of both. It may be lifelong or acquired, generalized or situational. Adults of all ages and both genders may be affected; however, some dysfunctions are specific to men, and others are specific to women.

On the whole, sexual dysfunction is relatively common. Various studies put the overall prevalence rate somewhere between 30 and 45%, with men affected less frequently than women (Bhugra & Colombini, 2013). Still, some types of dysfunction are observed far more often than others. This reflects the fact that some causes of sexual dysfunction are normal consequences of aging, while others are rare or unique to affected individuals.

With the possible exception of ED, risk factors and potential causes of sexual dysfunction can vary widely from one individual to the next or may be varied or unclear; thus, prevention strategies are nonspecific. The best approach includes healthy lifestyle choices and treatment of any underlying physical or psychologic problems.

The following sections take a closer look at the causes, mechanisms, and characteristics of different types of sexual dysfunction, beginning with male disorders and moving on to female disorders.

Male Sexual Dysfunction

Within the United States, the overall prevalence rate for male sexual dysfunction is about 30% (Bhugra & Colombini, 2013; Faught, 2015). This rate accounts for all four male sexual disorders included in the DSM-5: male hypoactive sexual desire disorder, ED, premature ejaculation, and delayed ejaculation. Of these disorders, ED is the most common (and therefore receives the greatest level of coverage in this text), followed by the ejaculatory disorders and hypoactive desire disorder. Although these conditions have different causes and manifestations, they all have dramatic negative effects on a man's ability to enjoy mutually satisfying sexual experiences with a partner.

Male Hypoactive Sexual Desire Disorder

For most men, sexual desire varies from day to day, as well as over time. However, some men report a deficiency in or absence of sexual fantasies and persistently low interest or a total lack of interest in sexual activity. These individuals are said to have **male hypoactive sexual desire disorder**.

According to the DSM-5, in order for a patient to be diagnosed with male hypoactive sexual desire disorder, he must experience deficient or absent sexual thoughts or desires at least 75% of the time for a period of at least 6 months. This lack of sexual interest must not be related to another medical or psychologic disorder or to substance use or abuse. The lack of desire must also be a source of significant distress to the patient (American Psychiatric Association, 2013a). This final criterion is important, because some patients may lack sexual desire but not be troubled by this symptom. If the condition does not cause distress to the individual, no disorder is said to exist. Note that a desire discrepancy, in which a man's interest in sex is lower than his partner's, is by itself insufficient for a diagnosis of male hypoactive sexual desire disorder (Dziegielewski, 2015).

Hypoactive sexual desire is the least common male sexual dysfunction. However, many men experience problems with desire that fail to satisfy the 6-month requirement. The prevalence of these milder desire problems increases with age, affecting only 6% of men between the ages of 18 and 24 but 41% of men between the ages of 66 and 74 (American Psychiatric Association, 2013a).

Erectile Dysfunction

Erectile dysfunction (ED) is the most common male sexual problem. In basic terms, ED is the inability to attain or maintain an erection sufficient to permit mutually satisfactory sexual intercourse with a partner. ED may involve a total inability to achieve erection, an inconsistent ability to achieve erection, or the ability to sustain only brief erections. In some cases, the penis may become semi-erect but lack rigidity sufficient for intercourse. Although categorized as a disorder of arousal, ED is sometimes also associated with a loss of **libido**, or sexual desire. ED is alternatively known as **impotence** (now an outdated term) or **erectile disorder** (term preferred by the American Psychiatric Association to describe ED unrelated to physical causes).

ED occurs in men of all ages and can be chronic, intermittent, or episodic. Some men experience primary ED, meaning they have had trouble achieving erection throughout their entire life. Others experience secondary ED, meaning their problems began after a period of normal erectile function. Still other men experience situational ED, in that they have erectile difficulties only in specific circumstances.

The incidence of ED is difficult to estimate because affected men may not report the disorder and also because there are differing views on how long a man must be affected before a diagnosis can be made. A medical diagnosis of ED requires that the problem be present for at least 3 months, whereas a psychiatric diagnosis requires that the problem persist for 6 months or longer (American Psychiatric Association, 2013a; Lakin & Wood, 2012). Overall, about 52% of men report at least occasional erectile difficulties. Older men are affected at higher rates. Whereas about 40% of men experience occasional ED at age 40, roughly 70% of men are affected by age 70. Rates for chronic or complete ED are lower than those for occasional ED, but they too increase with age, going from about 5% at age 40 to about 15% at age 70 (Lakin & Wood, 2012).

ED involves a disruption in the normal process by which an erection occurs. An erection is a neurovascular event that requires functional autonomic and somatic nerves, smooth and striated muscles in the penile shaft and pelvic floor, and adequate arterial blood flow. The erectile reflex to sexual stimulation occurs when the chambers in the erectile tissue of the penis become filled with blood via arterioles that dilate in response to nitrous oxide. At the same time, pelvic muscle contractions help increase penile rigidity, and the veins of the penis constrict, blocking blood outflow until orgasm or removal of the sexual stimulus occurs (Levin, 2015).

A range of factors may disrupt any of the mechanisms in the erectile process, resulting in ED. These factors are broadly classified as either psychologic or physical; physical causes of ED can then be further described as vascular, neurologic, urologic, endocrine, respiratory, iatrogenic, or lifestyle related. The most common psychologic and physical causes of ED are described in **Table 19–6 ⟩⟩**. All of the causes listed in the table can also be considered risk factors for the development of ED.

In addition to the factors listed in Table 19–6, the aging process itself increases the risk for ED. As a man ages, the collagen in his penis becomes less elastic, leading to decreased distensibility. This interferes with the veno-occlusive mechanism, which prevents blood from prematurely "leaking" out of the penis and into the general vasculature. Problems with this mechanism result in incomplete erections. The skin's ability to sense vibrotactile stimulation also declines with age, which may in part explain why some older men require longer stimulation to achieve an erection. In addition, many older men are affected by hypogonadism, which results in decreased testosterone and may contribute to erectile problems. Finally, age increases a man's likelihood of having chronic conditions such as diabetes, kidney disease, alcoholism, atherosclerosis, and vascular disease, all of which are linked to ED—either because of the changes they cause in the body or the therapeutic interventions they require.

Prevention of ED is aimed at mitigation of risk factors. Regular exercise, eating a balanced diet, maintaining a healthy body weight, and abstaining from alcohol and tobacco are steps that can reduce any man's likelihood of ED. Other prevention strategies are specific to the physical or psychologic risk factors experienced by particular patients. For example, men with diabetes can reduce their chances of erectile difficulties by maintaining appropriate blood glucose levels, and men with depression or relationship problems can reduce their risk of ED by seeking counseling. Note, however, that many medications used in the treatment of various conditions linked to ED (e.g., heart

TABLE 19–6 Common Causes of Erectile Dysfunction

Cause	Examples
Vascular	Atherosclerosis
	Heart disease
	Hyperlipidemia
	Hypertension
	Metabolic syndrome
	Stroke
Neurologic	Multiple sclerosis
	Nerve disease
	Parkinson disease
	Spinal cord injury
Urologic	Direct injury to the penis that affects the nerves or vascular supply
	Hypospadias and epispadias
	Kidney failure
	Peyronie disease
Endocrine	Abnormal prolactin levels
	Diabetes mellitus
	Hypogonadism
	Low testosterone levels
	Thyroid disease
Respiratory	Chronic obstructive pulmonary disease
	Obstructive sleep apnea
Iatrogenic	*Medications including:*
	Antidepressants
	Antihistamines
	Antihypertensives
	Appetite suppressants
	Cimetidine
	Tranquilizers
	Procedures including:
	Bladder surgery
	Colon surgery
	Pelvic radiation or surgery
	Radical prostatectomy
	Spinal cord surgery
Lifestyle related	Alcohol use
	Excessive caffeine use
	Illicit drug use
	Lack of physical activity
	Obesity/overweight
	Tobacco use
Psychologic	Anxiety
	Depression
	Fatigue
	Fear of sexual failure
	Guilt
	Low self-esteem
	Relationship problems
	Stress

Sources: Data from American Psychiatric Association. (2013a). *Diagnostic and statistical manual of mental disorders* (5th ed.). Arlington, VA: Author; Gerber, D. (2014). Sexual problems. In B. A. Magowan, P. Owen, & A. Thomson (Eds.), *Clinical obstetrics and gynaecology* (3rd ed., pp. 191–202). Philadelphia, PA: Elsevier Health; Mayo Clinic. (2015h). *Erectile dysfunction: Causes.* Retrieved from http://www.mayoclinic.org/diseases-conditions/erectile-dysfunction/basics/causes/con-20034244

disease, depression) can themselves produce erectile problems as a side effect, as noted in Table 19–6 and discussed in the Collaboration section.

Premature Ejaculation

Two other male sexual dysfunctions involve the orgasm phase of the sexual response cycle. The first disorder, **premature ejaculation**, occurs when a man consistently ejaculates prior to or shortly after penetration—in other words, before he and his partner can achieve mutual satisfaction. In some ways, the problem is self-defined, because the man is the ultimate judge of whether he is ejaculating too soon. However, most practitioners are hesitant to assign a diagnosis of premature ejaculation unless symptoms continue for 6 months or more and the man experiences significant distress as a result (American Psychiatric Association, 2013a; Mayo Clinic, 2015i).

Premature ejaculation as an isolated event is common; between 20 and 30% of men report experiencing occasional instances in which they ejaculate earlier than they would like. However, only 1–3% of men meet all the criteria necessary for their premature ejaculation to be classified as a chronic sexual dysfunction. Some men experience premature ejaculation in all sexual situations, whereas others have a form of the disorder that occurs only with certain partners, surroundings, or types of activity. Generally speaking, younger men are more likely to experience occasional premature ejaculation (often because they have not yet learned to exert good ejaculatory control), while older men are more likely to experience premature ejaculation as a lasting sexual disorder (American Psychiatric Association, 2013a; Mayo Clinic, 2015i).

Although its physiology remains unclear, premature ejaculation is linked to a number of biological and psychologic causes. Primary premature ejaculation is frequently related to psychologic issues or events that occurred during childhood or adolescence. Men who have depression or anxiety disorders are also more likely to be affected. In addition, as mentioned previously, primary premature ejaculation may be connected to physical causes, including genetic and neurologic factors (American Psychiatric Association, 2013a; Mayo Clinic, 2015i).

As compared to the lifelong form of the disorder, secondary premature ejaculation is more likely linked to biological contributors. Risk factors include thyroid dysfunction, prostate disease, urethral infection, opioid use, abnormal hormone levels, neurotransmitter imbalances, ED, and nerve damage. Psychologic factors are also believed to play a role in many cases of secondary premature ejaculation. Again, prior experiences and high anxiety may contribute to dysfunction—especially anxiety about failure to perform sexually. Relationship difficulties between a man and his partner may also be a risk factor (American Psychiatric Association, 2013a; Mayo Clinic, 2015i).

Delayed Ejaculation

Delayed ejaculation, once called **male orgasmic disorder**, involves extreme difficulty ejaculating, despite the ability to maintain an erection for long periods (in some cases, an hour or more). Delayed ejaculation is rare; most studies report a prevalence somewhere between 1 and 4%. Although it can arise at any point after puberty, few men report delayed ejaculation until their 50s (Balon, 2015; Potts, 2012; Wincze & Weisberg, 2015).

According to the DSM-5 (American Psychiatric Association, 2013a), a diagnosis of delayed ejaculation is appropriate when a man reports marked delay, infrequency, or absence of ejaculation during all or almost all partnered sexual encounters for a period of 6 months or longer. There is no exact length of time that qualifies as a "delay"; rather, a delay is any length of time that causes distress to the man and/or his partner. Delayed ejaculation is a distinct disorder from **retrograde ejaculation**, in which ejaculation occurs but the fluid travels into the bladder instead of out through the urethra. Retrograde ejaculation nearly always occurs because of muscle and nerve damage from surgery or as a side effect of medication and thus is usually not classified as a disorder (Potts, 2012).

Researchers are not completely sure what causes delayed ejaculation. Primary delayed ejaculation seems most often related to psychologic factors. In contrast, secondary delayed ejaculation is more commonly linked to physical causes, including use of certain medications (e.g., opioids, antihypertensives, antidepressants) and various diseases, injuries, and procedures that affect nerve function in the pelvic region. Psychologic factors may also come into play, especially stress, anxiety, and relationship problems (Balon, 2015; Balon & Segraves, 2014; Wincze & Weisberg, 2015).

Female Sexual Dysfunction

On the whole, female sexual dysfunctions are more common than male sexual dysfunctions, with roughly 43% of women reporting one or more problems (Faught, 2015; Shifren et al., 2008). This rate includes all three female sexual dysfunctions described in the DSM-5—female sexual interest/arousal disorder, female orgasmic disorder, and genito-pelvic pain/penetration disorder—which collectively affect about 12% of women in the United States. It also includes related problems that fail to meet the strict DSM diagnostic criteria yet cause concern to affected individuals and their partners (Faubion & Rullo, 2015). The following sections take a closer look at the various causes and manifestations of female sexual dysfunction.

Female Sexual Interest/Arousal Disorder

Low or absent desire is by far the most common sexual complaint among women, followed by difficulties attaining adequate levels of arousal. Although many women report occasional desire and arousal issues, a smaller number are affected so severely that that they are said to have **female sexual interest/arousal disorder**. A diagnosis of female sexual interest/arousal disorder may be appropriate when a woman experiences decreased or absent sexual thoughts, interest in sexual activity, mental or physical feelings of arousal, and/or pleasurable sensation during sexual activity at least 75% of the time for a period of 6 months or more. Furthermore, the lack of desire and/or arousal must be a source of significant distress to the patient, and it must reflect more than a simple discrepancy in desire between the

woman and her partner (American Psychiatric Association, 2013a; Balon & Segraves, 2014).

Studies suggest that female sexual interest/arousal disorder has an overall prevalence rate of about 8%, making it the most common female sexual dysfunction listed in the DSM-5. Women of all ages may be affected, although middle-age women are most likely to report decreased desire accompanied by personal distress. It is likely that older women actually have lower levels of desire but are either less troubled by it or less likely to report it (Kingsberg & Woodard, 2015).

The exact pathophysiology of female sexual interest/arousal disorder is unknown, but it seems to involve a blend of physical and psychologic causes. Normal changes associated with aging, such as declines in estrogen leading to decreased vaginal lubrication and thinning of the labia, clitoris, and vaginal walls, may play a role. Beyond these physical changes, aging brings psychosocial effects that can limit a woman's desire for sex. Women may feel their aging bodies make them less attractive. Although some declines in desire and arousal are normal with age, a total or near-total lack of interest in sex is not typical and is likely indicative of a larger problem (Balon, 2015; Kingsberg & Woodard, 2015).

Numerous medical conditions may result in decreased desire. Gynecologic contributors include endometriosis, cancer, uterine fibroids, and PID. A variety of medications used in the treatment of these and other conditions can also contribute to decreased desire. Examples include antihypertensives, antidepressants, anxiolytics, antiseizure medications, and antipsychotics (Elder & Braver, 2010; Faught, 2015; Kingsberg & Woodard, 2015).

Decreased sexual interest and arousal has also been linked to a range of psychologic factors. Possible contributors include depression, anxiety disorders, schizophrenia, and posttraumatic stress disorder. Sexual abuse, childhood trauma, alterations in body image, and other factors may play a role. Cultural and religious attitudes toward sex sometimes also lead to deficiencies in desire and arousal (Balon, 2015; Gerber, 2014; Kingsberg & Woodard, 2015).

Female Orgasmic Disorder

Female orgasmic disorder is the persistent delay or absence of orgasm following a phase of normal sexual excitement. Although many women experience occasional problems achieving orgasm, the diagnostic criteria for female orgasmic disorder require that a woman have difficulties at least 75% of the time for a period of 6 months or more and experience significant distress as a result. This condition may also be diagnosed when a woman experiences orgasms but they are persistently of very low intensity (American Psychiatric Association, 2013a).

Female orgasmic disorder is the second most common female sexual dysfunction, although estimates of its prevalence vary, with some estimates as high as 40%. Up to 10% of women are **preorgasmic**, or have never experienced orgasm (American Psychiatric Association, 2013a). Most likely, the actual proportion of women with some level of orgasmic dysfunction is between 16 and 28% (Laan, Rellini, & Barnes, 2013), with approximately 6% of all women also experiencing distress related to the dysfunction and qualifying for a diagnosis of a full-fledged female orgasmic disorder (Halter, 2014).

Determining whether female orgasmic disorder is lifelong or acquired and whether it is generalized or situational can assist in identifying possible causes. Many lifelong cases can be traced to a lack of sexual experimentation, self-exploration, and/or education. Physical factors also appear to contribute to this condition. Genetic influences may account for 30–50% of a woman's variability in orgasmic frequency (Balon & Segraves, 2014; Rellini & Clifton, 2011), and research suggests that the disorder may involve disruptions in sympathetic and parasympathetic nervous function. A variety of diseases or health conditions may impair orgasmic function or make sexual activity difficult or painful, reducing the likelihood of a woman reaching orgasm. Certain gynecologic surgeries—especially hysterectomy and oophorectomy—can cause physical and psychologic changes that make orgasm difficult. Alcohol, recreational drugs, and a variety of medications are linked to female orgasmic disorder (Balon & Segraves, 2014; Rellini & Clifton, 2011).

Psychologic contributors to female orgasmic disorder are similar to those for other sexual dysfunctions and include depression, psychosis, and anxiety disorders. Sexual abuse, trauma, stress, negative body image, low self-esteem, insufficient sex education, and fear of rejection or loss of control may play a role. Relationship problems and cultural and religious influences are also frequently implicated. In addition, women who have deficiencies in arousal and/or desire are at increased risk for orgasmic disorder (Balon, 2015; Halter, 2014).

Genito-pelvic Pain/Penetration Disorder

Genito-pelvic pain/penetration disorder is persistent or recurrent dyspareunia (pain) or fear of pain before or during vaginal penetration. This disorder may also involve **vaginismus**, or involuntary tightening of the pelvic muscles that prevents penetration from occurring. Criteria for diagnosis include that these symptoms must be present at least 75% of the time for a period of 6 months or longer and that they must cause significant distress to the affected woman (American Psychiatric Association, 2013a). For some women, the condition involves the entire vulva, while for others only a portion of the vulva is affected. Likewise, some women experience pain and/or muscle tightening in all situations involving penetration or the possibility thereof, while others experience these symptoms only in specific scenarios (e.g., with sexual intercourse but not gynecologic examination, or vice versa) (Bond, Mpofu, & Millington, 2015).

Prevalence rates for this disorder are unclear. Newer studies indicate that approximately 14–34% of younger women and 6.5–45% of older women are affected (Wincze & Weisberg, 2015). Most likely, 12–21% of women in North America experience ongoing pain during sex (Biggs & Chaganaboyana, 2015). Estimated rates of vaginismus also vary, but to a lesser degree, with studies suggesting an overall prevalence somewhere between 0.4 and 6.0% (Wincze & Weisberg, 2015).

In most cases, dyspareunia is an acquired condition that arises as a result of inadequate lubrication and/or inflammation or other abnormality of the vulva and reproductive tract. Declines in estrogen are another contributor, and some contraceptive foams, creams, sponges, or latex products can irritate the vulva or vagina. Deep dyspareunia is more often linked to pelvic disease or abnormality, such as endometriosis, fibroids, PID, gynecologic cancers, scar tissue, or uterine prolapse. Women who have bowel irregularity or dysmenorrhea are also at increased risk of deep pain during sex. As opposed to dyspareunia, vaginismus tends to be primary rather than secondary. Potential physical causes of primary vaginismus include malformations of the genital tract, as well as hypertonicity and/or poor control of the muscles in the pelvic floor (Balon & Segraves, 2014; Gerber, 2014; Wincze & Weisberg, 2015).

Genito-pelvic pain/penetration disorder may be linked to sexual trauma or abuse, relationship difficulties, painful or traumatic childbirth, presence of other sexual dysfunctions, and/or high levels of anxiety or fear. Fear and sexual pain frequently have a cyclical relationship. For example, a woman may be apprehensive about engaging in sex because of a prior painful experience; this in turn may cause high levels of anxiety and physical tension that make future sexual encounters painful, thus intensifying both the woman's fear of sex and her sensation of pain during intercourse. Women who grew up in sexually repressive environments are at increased risk for genito-pelvic pain/penetration disorder, and the condition is more common in societies where women have few sexual rights and are subject to practices such as forced matrimony, child marriage, and polygamy. For many women, the disorder is the result of multiple physical and psychologic contributors (Balon & Segraves, 2014; Biggs & Chaganaboyana, 2015; Gerber, 2014; Wincze & Weisberg, 2015).

Collaboration

Patients who are affected by sexual dysfunction may be candidates for a variety of collaborative care measures. The following sections explore some of the most common collaborative procedures, beginning with those used in the treatment of male sexual dysfunction, then turning to those used in the treatment of female dysfunction.

Male Sexual Dysfunction

Treatment for men with sexual dysfunction usually starts with the least invasive methods: lifestyle changes such as quitting smoking, reducing alcohol intake, losing weight, and getting more exercise. The medical team may check for related health problems using various diagnostic measures. Medication assessment is also important: If one or more medications are thought to be contributing to sexual dysfunction, the healthcare team can determine whether these drugs can safely be decreased or replaced. If these interventions are not successful, then additional medications, surgery, assistive devices, and/or psychologic counseling may be recommended.

Diagnostic Tests

Medical management of male sexual dysfunction begins with a medical and sexual history. After that, a thorough physical examination can provide clues about systemic

Clinical Manifestations and Therapies
Sexual Dysfunction

ETIOLOGY	MANIFESTATIONS	CLINICAL THERAPIES
Sexual desire disorders (male hypoactive sexual desire disorder; female sexual interest/arousal disorder)	■ Deficient or absent sexual fantasies ■ Deficient or absent desire for sexual activity ■ In some cases, aversion to and avoidance of genital sexual contact	■ Assessment for possible physical cause ■ Hormone therapy ■ Medication (e.g., flibanserin [Addyi] for women) ■ Counseling and behavioral therapy ■ Sex therapy ■ Couples therapy
Sexual arousal disorders (erectile disorder; female sexual interest/arousal disorder)	■ Absent or inadequate vaginal lubrication in response to stimulation ■ Inadequate blood flow to the nipples and genitals in response to stimulation ■ Inability to attain or maintain an erection	■ Assessment for possible physical cause ■ Hormone therapy ■ Medication (e.g., sildenafil citrate [Viagra] or tadalafil [Cialis] for men; flibanserin [Addyi] for women) ■ Use of vaginal lubricants ■ Surgery (e.g., penile revascularization or implants for men) ■ Mechanical aids (e.g., vacuum devices for men; vibrators for women) ■ Counseling and behavioral therapy ■ Sex therapy ■ Couples therapy
Orgasmic disorders (premature ejaculation, delayed ejaculation, female orgasmic disorder)	■ Inability to attain orgasm ■ Ejaculation prior to or shortly after penetration ■ Delayed or absent ejaculation	■ Assessment for possible physical cause ■ Hormone therapy ■ Medication (e.g., addition of bupropion [Wellbutrin] to current course of antidepressant therapy) ■ Pelvic floor exercises (for women) ■ Mechanical aids (e.g., vibrators for women) ■ Counseling and behavioral therapy ■ Sex therapy ■ Couples therapy
Sexual pain disorders (genito-pelvic pain/penetration disorder)	■ Pain at entry of penis to vagina ■ Pain at deep thrusting ■ Vulvar pain that persists after sexual intercourse ■ Vaginismus	■ Assessment for possible physical cause (including vaginal infection or STI) ■ Topical anesthetics (e.g., lidocaine) ■ Hormone therapy ■ Pelvic floor exercises ■ Use of dilators to gradually increase vaginal size ■ Surgery to widen the vaginal opening or correct an anatomic abnormality ■ Medication (e.g., ospemifene [Osphena]) ■ Counseling and behavioral therapy ■ Sex therapy ■ Couples therapy

problems or structural issues within the reproductive system. A range of diagnostic tests may be ordered as part of or follow-up to the physical exam, including blood chemistry, CBC, urinalysis, lipid profile, and kidney and liver function testing. Measurement of the patient's testosterone, prolactin, thyroxine, and PSA levels can help identify metabolic and endocrine problems that may be contributing to dysfunction.

For patients with ED, nocturnal penile tumescence and rigidity monitoring can help differentiate between physical and psychogenic causes. Physically healthy men have involuntary erections during REM sleep, so declines in the number and quality of such erections suggest that a patient's ED is physically rooted, and a normal number and quality of nocturnal erections indicate that ED may be psychologically rooted. Nocturnal monitoring can be performed in a sleep laboratory or in the patient's home using portable devices. Depending on the results, further diagnostic procedures may be appropriate (Kimmel, Milrod, & Kennedy, 2014; Wespes, 2015).

Pharmacologic Therapy

A variety of medications are used in the treatment of male sexual dysfunction. For example, hormone replacement may be appropriate for men with low desire or erectile problems related to insufficient testosterone. Hormone replacements may be administered via injection, transdermal patch, or topical gel. Although such therapy can boost a man's libido and sperm count, it comes with potential side effects, including acne, weight gain, hyperglycemia, priapism, renal stones, and jaundice. Thus, men who receive hormone therapy require regular monitoring of their liver enzymes, blood glucose, and serum electrolytes. Men who use topical hormone applications must also take precautions to ensure that women and children do not come in contact with testosterone-containing gels or creams, as this can be harmful to their health (Stahlman et al., 2012).

SAFETY ALERT The U.S. Food and Drug Administration has approved prescription testosterone products only for the treatment of hormone deficiencies caused by hypogonadism secondary to disorders of the testicles, pituitary gland, or brain. Men who are taking or who wish to take these products to counter age-related declines in testosterone should be warned that such use may lead to increased risk of heart attack and stroke. Furthermore, hormone replacement has not been proven beneficial in this context (FDA, 2015c).

Other pharmacologic therapies are directed toward specific problems. ED, for example, can be treated with medications taken orally, injected into the penis, or inserted into the urethra. Oral medications include sildenafil citrate (Viagra), vardenafil hydrochloride (Levitra), tadalafil (Cialis), and avanafil (Stendra). All four drugs enhance erections only in the presence of sexual stimulation; they act by facilitating relaxation of smooth muscle in the penis, thus allowing increased blood flow. These drugs should be taken no more than once per day and should not be used by men who are taking nitrate-based drugs or alpha-adrenergic blockers (Karch, 2015).

ED can also be treated using drugs that are injected or inserted into the penis. The primary medication administered via these routes is alprostodil. Because these drugs are difficult to administer, they are rarely used today, except in patients who cannot take oral drugs like Viagra (Mayo Clinic, 2015j, 2015k).

Patients whose symptoms cannot be remedied with hormone therapy or ED medications have limited options in terms of pharmacologic treatment. There are no reliable medications aimed specifically at treatment of premature or delayed ejaculation, although some drugs that are aimed at addressing other conditions may be useful. Examples include antidepressants and topical anesthetics (Mayo Clinic, 2015l; Mirone & Fusco, 2015; Nelson, Brock, & Dean, 2014).

Nonpharmacologic Therapy

Nonpharmacologic therapy for male sexual dysfunction may include surgery, assistive devices, and counseling or other behavioral therapies.

Surgery is limited to the treatment of ED, and it is usually reserved for cases in which all other therapeutic interventions fail. Surgery may involve revascularization procedures or implantation of prosthetic devices. Venous or arterial procedures are generally not successful; often, the result is only temporary, because the underlying cause of the vascular insufficiency is not corrected. Thus, implantation of penile prostheses is usually the preferred option. A penile prosthesis may consist of either malleable rods placed inside the two corpora cavernosa or inflatable implants that can be filled with water from a reservoir in the pelvis via a pump placed in the penis or scrotum. Men are generally satisfied with their prostheses, although potential problems include increased risk of infection and difficulty adapting to the implant (Hinkle & Cheever, 2014; Townsend, 2015).

Several types of devices may be used in the treatment of male sexual dysfunction. For example, men with erectile difficulty may be prescribed a vacuum constriction device (VCD) that draws blood into the penis with a vacuum and traps it there with a constricting band at the base of the penis. Use of VCDs is beneficial for many patients, although some men cite bruising, a cold sensation at the tip of the penis, and decreased spontaneity of sexual encounters as potential drawbacks (Hirsch, 2015a).

Other devices work by either increasing or decreasing penile sensation. For instance, men who experience delayed ejaculation may benefit from penile vibratory stimulation, while men who have premature ejaculation might try using condoms to reduce genital sensation and prolong the sexual experience (Hirsch, 2015b; Nelson et al., 2014).

Female Sexual Dysfunction

Fewer diagnostic and treatment options are available for female sexual dysfunction than for male sexual dysfunction. Pharmacologic and surgical treatments are especially limited because the physiologic mechanisms of female dysfunction have yet to be determined. Diagnostic measures currently focus on identifying other disease processes that may be contributing to dysfunction; pharmacologic therapies revolve around hormone replacement; and nonpharmacologic therapies are generally limited to counseling and/or use of assistive devices.

Diagnostic Tests

Medical management of female sexual dysfunction begins with a patient history to determine the degree of the problem and reveal diseases, lifestyle habits, prior events, or medications that may be contributing to the problem. After that, a physical examination can provide clues about systemic problems or structural issues within the reproductive system. The woman's external genitalia should be inspected for atrophy and skin color, elasticity, and thickness. A focused pelvic exam is also important. During this exam, the practitioner should look for signs of infection, atrophy, prolapse, poor pelvic floor muscle tone, scars and strictures, masses, and skin diseases that may be contributing to the problem. Note that some women with vaginismus and/or dyspareunia may not tolerate use of a speculum or more than one finger during the pelvic examination (Elder & Braver, 2010; Latif & Diamond, 2013).

Laboratory tests are rarely useful in diagnosing female sexual dysfunction, but they can help confirm or rule out other conditions that could be causing a woman's symptoms. Appropriate tests may include blood chemistry; CBC; urinalysis; stool guaiac; Pap smear; and kidney, liver, and thyroid function testing. Measurement of the patient's blood glucose, estrogen, FSH, prolactin, LH, and testosterone levels might also be warranted (Bhugra & Colombini, 2013; Elder & Braver, 2010; Kingsberg & Woodard, 2015).

Pharmacologic Therapy

Pharmacologic treatments for female sexual dysfunction are severely limited. HRT is the most common choice, and it can be useful for patients with low desire, low arousal, and sexual pain. In particular, estrogen replacement can help increase genital sensitivity and lubrication, reverse vulvar and vaginal atrophy, and relieve dyspareunia. In women with a uterus, estrogen must be administered with progesterone to reduce the risk for heart attack, stroke, breast cancer, dementia, and thromboembolic episodes. Short-term use is recommended to further mitigate these risks, as is vaginal administration. A related option is use of SERMs. These medications mimic the action of estrogen in some parts of the body, and they offer benefits similar to estrogen–progestin combinations but with lower risk of cancer. Several SERMs are approved for use in the United States, the most common of which is ospemifene (Osphena) (Elder & Braver, 2010; Faubion & Rullo, 2015; Kingsberg & Woodard, 2015).

The other major form of HRT involves administration of testosterone. Although not FDA-approved for female use, testosterone is often prescribed off-label to address low desire, reduced arousal, and orgasmic difficulties in postmenopausal women. Many women report improvement after beginning testosterone treatment. However, potential risks and side effects make testosterone an inappropriate choice for many women, and they also explain why testosterone therapy has yet to gain FDA approval (Elder & Braver, 2010; Faubion & Rullo, 2015; Kingsberg & Woodard, 2015).

Outside of hormones and SERMs, pharmacologic therapy for female sexual dysfunction consists of either bupropion (Wellbutrin) or flibanserin (Addyi). Bupropion is a dopamine and norepinephrine reuptake inhibitor that is typically used as an antidepressant. Unlike most antidepressants, it can exert desire-increasing effects. For this reason, bupropion may be prescribed to premenopausal women to counter the sexual side effects of other antidepressants. Studies also suggest it may increase desire in premenopausal women who are not taking other antidepressant medications (Kingsberg & Woodard, 2015). Flibanserin is the only FDA-approved medication specifically aimed at the treatment of low desire in women. Introduced in 2015, it produces moderate improvements in desire in some women, although its mechanism of action is unknown. Flibanserin is not frequently prescribed, probably because of a combination of high cost, low effectiveness, potentially dangerous interactions with alcohol, and the small number of physicians who are certified to prescribe the drug (Edney & Colby, 2015; Puppo & Puppo, 2016).

Nonpharmacologic Therapy

Nonpharmacologic therapy for female sexual dysfunction may involve use of assistive devices and/or counseling and other behavioral therapies. Surgery is generally not appropriate unless the woman's condition is related to malformations of the genitalia (e.g., imperforate hymen) or damage from childbirth or trauma.

Several types of devices may be useful in addressing female sexual dysfunction. Women with low desire, inadequate arousal, and/or orgasmic difficulties frequently benefit from use of vibrators or clitoral vacuum devices. Lubricants and vaginal moisturizers can also enhance the sexual experience for women with these conditions or with sexual pain (Balon & Segraves, 2014; Laan et al., 2013). Although some of these products can be obtained from healthcare providers, others can be purchased from retail stores, either in person or via catalog or internet.

Vaginal dilators are another device used in the treatment of genito-pelvic pain/penetration disorder. The patient inserts a small dilator in the vagina for 5–15 minutes once or twice a day. After about 3 weeks, the woman moves to the next largest dilator, continuing until she is comfortable inserting a dilator roughly the size of an erect penis. Dilators can be purchased from a range of retailers, but patients are often advised to obtain them from a healthcare provider or medical supply company (Spadt et al., 2012).

Lifespan Considerations

Sexual dysfunction can affect adults of any age. However, certain life stages and events—namely, pregnancy, childbirth, and older adulthood—deserve special mention because they are frequently accompanied by onset of sexual difficulties.

Sexual Dysfunction in Pregnant and Postpartum Women

For many women, the changes of pregnancy and childbirth result in some level of sexual dysfunction. Studies suggest that 60–70% of women experience sexual dysfunction at some point during pregnancy and that up to 84% of couples report sexual difficulties 4 months after the birth of a child (Ahmed, Madny, & Sayed Ahmed, 2014; Brandon, 2014).

Sexual problems during pregnancy often fluctuate by trimester. The third trimester is the time when sexual difficulties are most common. At this point, most women have experienced significant changes in body size and mechanics that make certain sexual positions uncomfortable. Together with decreased androgen levels, these changes contribute to reduced likelihood and intensity of orgasm and increased likelihood of vaginal pain. Pregnancy weight gain can also disrupt a woman's body image and self-esteem, thereby decreasing her desire for sex. In addition, some women fear that penetration will harm the fetus, even though this is rarely the case. The net result is that most women report fewer sexual encounters in the third trimester, and some report total abstinence (Brandon, 2014; Lowenstein, Mustafa, & Burke, 2013; Shindel & Goldstein, 2015; Sudtelgte, 2012).

Sexual dysfunction frequently continues after childbirth and may worsen in the postpartum period. Decreased androgen and estrogen levels and increased prolactin levels (especially in breastfeeding women) cause reductions in desire and vaginal lubrication, leading to dyspareunia.

Delivery-related damage to the vulva, perineum, and pelvic floor also make sex painful for many new mothers. Fatigue and anxiety related to parenting duties can contribute to low desire and difficulty reaching orgasm, especially in women with postpartum mood disorders. Although 90% of women resume sexual intercourse by 3 months postpartum, most report some type of problem, with pain being the most common. Sexual pain usually resolves within several months (Brandon, 2014; Lowenstein et al., 2013; Shindel & Goldstein, 2015).

Despite high rates of sexual dysfunction during pregnancy and the postpartum period, there is little research regarding treatment. Nurses may recommend experimenting with different sexual positions, engaging in alternative activities that enhance intimacy, and using lubricants and assistive devices. They should advise patients that decreased desire and increased pain are common following birth and typically resolve with time. Nurses can also recommend that patients progress slowly and gently once they opt to resume sexual activity.

Sexual Dysfunction in Older Adults

Both men and women are more likely to experience sexual dysfunction as they move out of their reproductive years and into older age. For women, increasing sexual dysfunction coincides with perimenopause and menopause; for men, it coincides with a period of reduced hormone production known as the male climacteric. However, hormones are not solely responsible for age-related increases in dysfunction. Rather, sexual dysfunction in older adulthood is often linked to a number of psychologic and physical causes, including chronic disease, medication use, role changes, grief, and fear of death and/or physical decline.

In recent years, patients of both genders have become more likely to approach healthcare providers with concerns about age-related alterations in sexual function. Nonetheless, many men and women remain hesitant to discuss these issues, often because they feel it is inappropriate for older people to be interested in sex. For this reason, the nurse should assure the older adult that interest in sex is normal and encourage further conversation about sexual issues and possible treatment of sexual dysfunction.

NURSING PROCESS

The nurse may encounter patients with sexual dysfunction in any setting, either through routine examinations or careful assessment of conditions and treatments that may cause sexual dysfunction. For example, nurses who work in urology or gynecology may regularly work with patients whose primary complaint involves sexual dysfunction, whereas nurses who work in cardiology or endocrinology may encounter patients who experience dysfunction related to another disease process. Patients may report symptoms of sexual dysfunction during a regular checkup, during a period of hospitalization, or while living in a long-term care facility.

The nurse is often the first member of the healthcare team to discover that a patient is experiencing sexual difficulties. Once aware of the problem, the nurse plays a critical role in communicating information, providing emotional support, and referring the patient to other care providers.

Assessment

Whether a patient seeks care because of sexual dysfunction or dysfunction is discovered during the initial interview, the nurse must find out as much as possible about the patient's problem. This includes performing a complete physical examination that considers a range of contributing factors, such as cardiovascular disease, endocrine abnormalities, nerve disease, and problems with bowel and bladder function. In some cases, further diagnostic testing may be appropriate.

Throughout the assessment, the nurse should also ask the patient about contributing factors that may not be apparent during the physical exam. This includes questions about medications, social habits, surgical history, activity level, reproductive history, relationship status, cultural background, and overall psychologic health. When asking these questions, the nurse must seek to remain as compassionate and nonjudgmental as possible.

Diagnosis

Appropriate diagnoses for patients with sexual dysfunction vary depending on the nature of the dysfunction. However, some diagnoses are more common than others. Examples include:

- *Deficient Knowledge*
- *Sexuality Pattern, Ineffective*
- *Communication, Readiness for Enhanced*
- *Relationship, Readiness for Enhanced*
- *Sexual Dysfunction*
- *Self-Esteem, Situational Low.*

(NANDA-I © 2014)

Planning

Planning for the patient with sexual dysfunction will vary depending on the patient's diagnosis. Common goals may include:

- The patient will discuss concerns about sexual dysfunction without embarrassment or anxiety.
- The patient will articulate understanding of the diagnosis and any related teaching about any medications or other factors that may be contributing to dysfunction.
- The patient will verbalize treatment options and make an informed decision.
- The patient will communicate more effectively with his or her partner with regard to each other's thoughts, desires, and limitations.

Implementation

Although appropriate interventions vary based on the patient's needs, the nurse will typically be responsible for uncovering areas of concern, acquiring details about the patient's dysfunction, and communicating information to the primary healthcare provider as appropriate. In some cases, the nurse may provide ongoing assessment and teaching regarding the nature of the patient's sexual dysfunction as well as related treatments. The nurse should maintain a professional affect when discussing sexual dysfunction, because the patient may find it difficult to discuss sexual performance with a nurse of either sex, especially if the nurse is younger than the patient. The nurse should also be aware that many patients experience decreased self-esteem as a result of their condition, so measures to promote heightened self-esteem are often a critical component of care.

Evaluation

The nurse must evaluate the patient's progress toward the previously identified goals. This requires the nurse to determine whether certain outcomes have been achieved. Example

outcomes that may be appropriate for patients with sexual dysfunction include the following:

- The patient verbalizes an understanding of his or her diagnosis as well as contributing factors.
- The patient makes informed decisions regarding treatment options.
- The patient verbalizes that the problem is not related to or a reflection on his or her masculinity, femininity, or self-worth.
- The patient and his or her partner are able to discuss the diagnosis as well as ways they might adjust their sexual relationship in an attempt to address this problem.

REVIEW Sexual Dysfunctions

RELATE Link the Concepts and Exemplars

Linking the exemplar of sexual dysfunction with the concept of self:

1. Why might a patient's self-concept be negatively affected by sexual dysfunction?

2. What can the nurse do to help reduce this negative impact?

Linking the exemplar of sexual dysfunction with the concept of perfusion:

3. What effect might arteriosclerosis have on a man's ability to attain an erection or a woman's ability to experience desire and arousal?

4. What preventive teaching can the nurse provide to younger men and women to prevent sexual dysfunction as the result of altered perfusion?

READY Go to Volume 3: Clinical Nursing Skills

REFER Go to Pearson MyLab Nursing and eText

- Additional review materials

REFLECT Apply Your Knowledge

Steve Young is a 41-year-old man in excellent health. He has been married to his wife, Angie, for 8 years. They have two children, Kelsey and Marcus. The Youngs met in college and were married shortly after

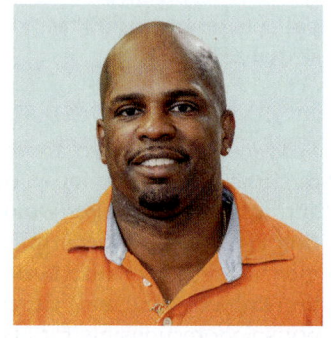

Steve graduated with a degree in accounting. Following graduation, he took the CPA exam, and he has worked for a large corporate accounting firm ever since. He has been extremely successful in his firm and has an income that easily supports his family. He is pleased that his wife is able to be a stay-at-home mother, but his success requires long working hours. Mr. Young has few outside interests and rarely exercises. His world revolves around work and home. He recognizes that his inactivity has led to weight gain during the past few years, but he is not concerned about it.

Mr. Young began smoking at age 17 and smokes about a pack per day. He knows he should quit, but he figures he can probably get away with it for a while longer without complications. Because he knows it is a source of irritation for his wife, he plans to quit smoking eventually.

1. What risk factors does Mr. Young have for developing ED?

2. What patient teaching can you provide to reduce Mr. Young's risk for ED?

3. How might you approach Mr. Young to discuss any sexual function issues he may have already experienced?

≫ Exemplar 19.E
Sexually Transmitted Infections

Exemplar Learning Outcomes

19.E Analyze sexually transmitted infections (STIs) as they relate to sexuality.

- Describe the epidemiology of STIs.
- Outline clinical manifestations and therapies of selected STIs.
- Differentiate considerations for care of patients with STIs across the lifespan.
- Apply the nursing process for providing culturally competent care to an individual with an STI.

Exemplar Key Terms

Chancres, *1524*
Chlamydia, *1523*
Genital herpes (HSV), *1522*
Genital warts, *1522*
Gonorrhea, *1523*
Sexually transmitted diseases (STDs), *1521*
Sexually transmitted infections (STIs), *1521*
Syphilis, *1524*

Overview

Sexually transmitted infections (STIs) are disorders that are transmitted by vaginal, oral, and anal intimate contact and intercourse. They can be treated and cured. **Sexually transmitted diseases (STDs)** are typically viruses that cannot be cured, such as HPV, herpes simplex virus (HSV), and HIV. Both STI and STD are general terms used to describe many different infections, and the two terms are often used interchangeably. This exemplar will use the term *STI* to refer to both infections and systemic diseases that can be transmitted sexually. This exemplar will discuss five STIs: genital herpes, HPV, chlamydia, gonorrhea, and syphilis. The initial section will include information about the incidence, prevalence, prevention, and control of these STIs in general. The subsequent sections will explore the distinct pathophysiology, etiology, risk factors, and clinical manifestations of each infection in turn.

STIs may be caused by bacteria, viruses, fungi, protozoa, and parasites. Portals of entry for these infectious agents include the mouth, genitalia, urinary meatus, anus, rectum, and skin. Although STIs are caused by various organisms, they have several characteristics in common, including that most can be prevented by using latex condoms; they can be transmitted during heterosexual and homosexual activities; and for treatment to be effective, sexual partners of the infected individual must also be treated. It is also possible for an individual to have more than one STI at the same time.

Bacterial STIs can be cured through early treatment with antibiotics. Viruses, such as genital herpes, are chronic conditions that can be managed but not cured. The most serious STI is AIDS, which is incurable; it is described in detail in the exemplar on AIDS in the module on Immunity. Treatment guidelines for STIs are updated regularly and available from the CDC.

STIs have many consequences, and the nurse has the responsibility of teaching sexually active patients how to prevent STIs, regardless of gender, age, or sexual orientation. The nurse also plays a critical role in the treatment of STIs and their associated complications.

》 Stay Current: The CDC publishes treatment guidelines for STIs on its website. These guidelines emphasize treatment but also explore prevention strategies. They can be found at http://www.cdc.gov/std/tg2015/default.htm.

Epidemiology

Incidence and Prevalence

The incidence of STIs has reached epidemic proportions worldwide. The WHO (2015b) estimates that 357 million new infections of curable STIs occur worldwide each year. In the United States, an estimated 20 million new cases of STI occur each year. STIs affect men and women of all ages, backgrounds, and socioeconomic levels. Of these 20 million annual new cases, half occur among individuals ages 15–24 (CDC, 2015f). Women have higher rates of gonorrhea, and men have higher rates of chlamydia and syphilis (CDC, 2015g). STIs can lead to infertility and other reproductive complications, and they increase the risk for acquiring and transmitting HIV (CDC, 2015f). Risk factors for contracting an STI include the following (CDC, 2013b):

- Multiple sexual partners or a new sexual partner
- Sex with someone who has sex with one or more others

- Exchange of sex for money or drugs
- Poverty, unemployment, and low education
- Young women under 25 years of age
- Drug or alcohol use that lowers inhibitions

The presence of another STI such as syphilis or HSV facilitates the transmission of HIV/AIDS, and the immune suppression caused by HIV potentiates the infectious processes of other STIs. In fact, individuals infected with STIs are at greater risk of being infected with HIV if they are exposed to the virus. This is due to several factors: Genital ulcers create a portal of entry for HIV, non-ulcerative STIs increase the concentration of cells in genital secretions that can be targets for HIV, and infection with both an STI and HIV results in increased likelihood of having HIV in genital secretions and semen.

Prevention and Control

The prevention and control of STIs are based on the principles of education, detection, effective diagnosis, and treatment of infected individuals, along with evaluation, treatment, and counseling of sex partners of infected individuals. The ability of healthcare providers to obtain an accurate sexual history is essential to prevention and control efforts. One approach to collecting accurate sexual histories is available from the CDC (2011). This approach includes the Five Ps: partners, practices, protection from STIs, past history of STIs, and prevention of pregnancy.

》 Stay Current: Opening discussion about sexual history can be awkward for both the nurse and the patient, yet these discussions are essential for providing quality care. Suggestions for starting the discussion and the types of questions to use when obtaining a sexual history can be found in the CDC's online *Guide to Taking a Sexual History* at http://www.cdc.gov/std/treatment/SexualHistory.pdf.

The most effective way to prevent transmission of STIs is to avoid sexual intercourse with an infected partner. Both partners should be tested for STIs, including HIV, before having sexual intercourse. If an individual chooses to have sex with an infected partner or one whose infection status is unknown, a new condom should be used for each act of intercourse.

SAFETY ALERT Eliminating further transmission and reinfection of STIs is critical to control. For treatable STIs, this means that referral of sex partners for diagnosis, treatment, and counseling is essential. STIs are reportable diseases in every state. When a healthcare professional refers infected patients to a local or state department of health, every effort is made to identify and contact sex partners. Reports of STI and HIV infections are maintained in strictest confidence and are protected by law from subpoena.

Selected Sexually Transmitted Infections

Human Papillomavirus

HPV is the most common STI in the United States. An estimated 79 million Americans are infected, and up to 14 million new cases are diagnosed annually (CDC, 2014e). There

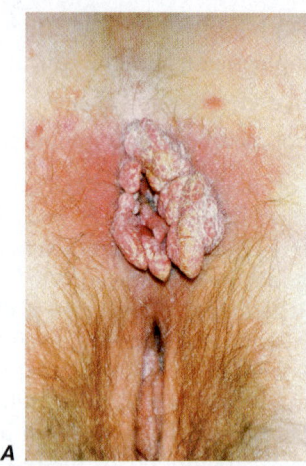

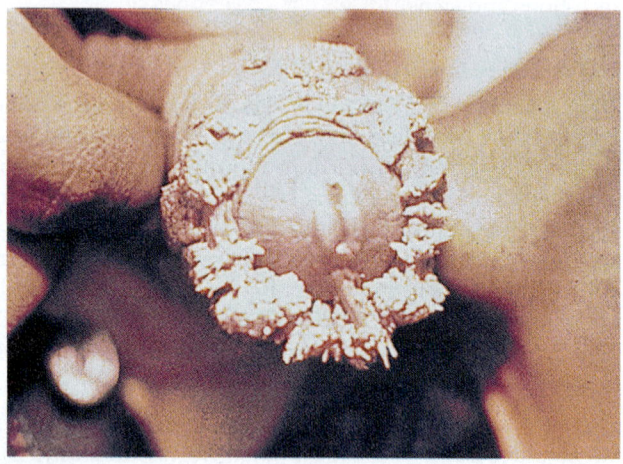

Source: *A*, BSIP SA/Alamy Stock Photo. *B*, Library of Congress.

Figure 19–27 》 Genital warts (condyloma acuminatum) on the *A*, vulva and *B*, penis.

are about 40 types of HPV that can infect the genitals of men and women (CDC, 2015h). One form of HPV infection is **genital warts**, which are painless, soft, raised or flat, large or small, flesh-colored bumps on the vulvovaginal area, perineum, penis, urethra, anus, groin, or thigh (see **Figure 19–27 》**). More important, HPV has been identified as the causative agent in many genital cancers. More than 11,000 women develop cervical cancer each year. Other HPV-caused cancers include vulvar, vaginal, penile, anal, and oropharyngeal cancer (CDC, 2014e).

HPV is so common that nearly all sexually active individuals will get at least one type of HPV at some time in their lives. Most individuals with a genital HPV infection do not know they are infected; most infections in women are diagnosed by abnormal Pap tests. Women are at greater risk for HPV genital infections because they have a larger mucosal surface area exposed in the genital area. In 90% of cases, HPV clears with no intervention within 2 years (CDC, 2013c). When HPV persists, genital warts, cervical cancer, and, less often, vulvar, penile, anal, and oropharyngeal cancers may occur.

HPV is transmitted by vaginal, anal, or oral–genital contact. This virus can be transmitted even when the infected individual has no symptoms. The incubation period is 3

weeks to 3 months (CDC, 2013c). Although some individuals with HPV may not have manifestations, others exhibit genital warts. Diagnosis of genital warts can be made on the basis of the clinical appearance on physical examination. Regular screening using Pap tests will identify precancerous lesions on the cervix early, and treatment in this early stage will prevent cancer.

No drug is available that can cure HPV itself, but genital warts can be removed with treatments applied by a healthcare provider or by the patients. Healthcare providers may use cryoprobes to freeze the warts or a chemical burn with trichloroacetic acid or bichloroacetic acid in the office setting. Patients may use imiquimod, podofilox, or sinecatechins at home to remove the warts. Extensive warts may require CO_2 laser removal (CDC, 2015i).

Genital Herpes

Genital herpes (HSV) are caused by the herpes simplex viruses HSV-1 and HSV-2. HSV-1 is associated with cold sores but may be transmitted to the genital area by oral intercourse or by self-inoculation through poor hand hygiene practices. HSV-2 is transmitted by sexual activity or during childbirth from an infected woman. HSV-2 causes most cases of genital herpes.

Like most STIs, genital herpes are most commonly found in young, sexually active adults and are associated with early onset of sexual activity and multiple sexual partners. According to the CDC, about 776,000 individuals in the United States will contract a new HSV infection this year. This accounts for 1 in 6 individuals 14–49 years of age (CDC, 2015j). There is no cure; the antivirals used to treat HSV simply lessen the severity of an outbreak and shorten its duration.

Within 2–12 days after exposure to the herpes virus, painful small vesicles appear in the genital area. In men, the lesions generally occur on the glans or shaft of the penis. In women, the lesions commonly occur on the labia, perineum, vagina, and cervix (see **Figure 19–28 》**). Anal intercourse or oral–anal sexual contact may result in lesions in and around the anus. The blisters break, shedding the highly infectious

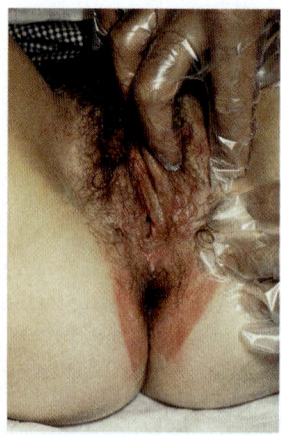

Source: Biophoto Associates/Science Source.

Figure 19–28 》 Genital herpes blisters as they appear on the labia.

virus and creating patches of painful ulcers that last 2–4 weeks. Touching these blisters and then rubbing or scratching in another place can spread the infection to other areas of the body (*autoinoculation*). Other manifestations can include flulike symptoms; regional lymphadenopathy; dysuria; urinary retention; vaginal discharge; and urinary discharge in men (CDC, 2014f).

Subsequent occurrences are usually less severe and shorter in duration than the initial outbreak. The number of outbreaks also tends to decrease over time. During the period between outbreaks, viral shedding can occur (CDC, 2015j). Prodromal symptoms of recurrent outbreaks of genital herpes can include burning, itching, tingling, or throbbing at the sites where lesions commonly appear. These sensations may be accompanied by pain in the legs, groin, or buttocks. Some authorities believe that prodromal symptoms signal increased levels of infectiousness, during which sexual contact should be avoided.

There is no cure for genital herpes. Treatment focuses on relieving symptoms and preventing spread of the infection. Antiviral medications such as acyclovir (Zovirax) help reduce the length and severity of outbreaks and are the treatment of choice for genital herpes. Antivirals are also used to suppress the virus, thereby decreasing the number of outbreaks (CDC, 2015i). Patient education is essential to prevent further transmission of the disease and to help patients integrate management of a chronic disease into their lifestyles.

Chlamydia

Chlamydia is caused by *Chlamydia trachomatis,* a bacterium that behaves like a virus, reproducing only within host cells. The bacterium is spread by sexual contact and to the neonate by passage through the birth canal of an infected mother. The infections caused by *C. trachomatis* include acute urethral syndrome, nongonococcal urethritis, mucopurulent cervicitis, and PID.

Chlamydia is the most commonly reported bacterial STI in the United States, affecting an estimated 2.86 million individuals each year. Roughly two thirds of new infections occur in 15- to 24-year-olds, and an estimated 1 in 20 sexually active teenage girls has chlamydia (CDC, 2015k). Risk factors for chlamydia include being sexually active, being female, being between ages 14 and 19, having a personal history of an STI or having a partner with such history, cervical ectopy, having multiple partners, having unprotected sex, and using drugs or alcohol that increases risky sexual behavior (CDC, 2015k; Office on Women's Health, 2014c).

Because chlamydia is asymptomatic in most women until the uterus and fallopian tubes have been invaded, treatment may be delayed, resulting in long-term complications. Chlamydia is a common cause of preventable infertility and ectopic pregnancy (CDC, 2015k). Infants born to mothers with untreated chlamydia are at risk for chlamydial conjunctivitis and pneumonia.

An estimated 90% of men with chlamydia are also asymptomatic. Reactive arthritis (formally Reiter syndrome) is the complication most likely to occur in men (CDC, 2015k). Chlamydia typically invades the cervix in women and the urethra in men. Manifestations include dysuria, urinary frequency, and discharge. Even if asymptomatic, an infected individual can spread the disease.

Untreated chlamydial infection in women may ascend into the upper reproductive tract, causing complications such as PID, which may be accompanied by endometritis and salpingitis. Chronic pelvic pain, scarring of the fallopian tubes, and systemic dissemination and septicemia may result. Scarring of the fallopian tubes may lead to ectopic pregnancy, another potentially life-threatening disorder in women. Complications of chlamydial infections in men include epididymitis, prostatitis, sterility, and reactive arthritis. The CDC recommends routine screening for sexually active women younger than 25 to minimize these serious complications (CDC, 2015k).

C. trachomatis is treated with antibiotics. Screening and diagnostic testing usually precede treatment; however, symptomatic individuals are often treated on a presumptive basis. Antibiotics recommended by the CDC for chlamydial infections in men and nonpregnant women include azithromycin (Zithromax) orally in a single dose, doxycycline (Adoxa, Apo-Doxy) orally twice daily for 7 days, or levofloxacin orally once daily for 7 days. Both sexual partners must be treated at the same time or prior to resuming sexual intercourse (CDC, 2015i).

Gonorrhea

Gonorrhea, also known as "GC" or "the clap," is caused by *Neisseria gonorrhoeae,* a gram-negative diplococcus. Gonorrhea is the second most common reportable communicable disease in the United States. The CDC (2015l) estimates that approximately 820,000 new cases occur annually, but less than half of new infections are reported each year.

Gonorrhea rates for African Americans are higher than rates for non-Hispanic Whites. Other risk factors include residence in large urban areas, being transient, early onset of sexual activity, multiple serial or consecutive sex partners, drug use, prostitution, and previous gonorrheal infection or concurrent STI (CDC, 2015g).

The causative organism of gonorrhea is a pyogenic (pusforming) bacteria that causes inflammation characterized by purulent exudate. Humans are the only host for the organism. Gonorrhea is transmitted by direct heterosexual and homosexual intercourse and during delivery as the neonate passes through an infected birth canal. The portal of entry can be the genitourinary tract, eyes, oropharynx, anorectum, or skin. The incubation period is 1–14 days after exposure in men and within 10 days in women (CDC, 2013d). The organism initially targets the female cervix and the male urethra. Without treatment, the disease ultimately disseminates (spreads widely) to other organs. In men, gonorrhea can cause acute, painful inflammation of the prostate, epididymis, and periurethral glands and can lead to sterility. In women, it can cause PID, endometritis, salpingitis, and pelvic peritonitis.

Manifestations of gonorrhea in men include dysuria and serous, milky, or purulent discharge from the penis. Some men also experience regional lymphadenopathy. Many men and most women with gonorrhea remain asymptomatic until the disease is advanced (CDC, 2015l). Women with symptoms experience dysuria, urinary frequency, abnormal menses (increased flow or dysmenorrhea), increased vaginal discharge, and dyspareunia.

Anorectal gonorrhea is seen most often in homosexual men. The manifestations include pruritus, mucopurulent rectal discharge, rectal bleeding and pain, and constipation. Gonococcal pharyngitis occurs primarily in homosexual or bisexual men or heterosexual women after oral sexual contact (fellatio) with an infected partner. The manifestations mimic those of strep throat and include fever, sore throat, and enlarged lymph glands.

The complications of untreated gonorrhea in both men and women may be permanent and serious and include blindness, infection of blood and joints, and increased susceptibility to and transmission of HIV. Untreated gonorrhea can also cause PID in women, which may lead to internal abscesses, chronic pain, ectopic pregnancy, and infertility. In men, it can cause epididymitis and prostatitis, resulting in infertility and dysuria.

The goals of treatment for the patient with gonorrhea include eradication of the organism and any coexisting disease and prevention of reinfection or transmission. Because of concerns about antimicrobial resistance in *N. gonorrhoeae*, the CDC recommends dual treatment for gonorrhea infections that includes a single injection of ceftriaxone and a single oral dose of azithromycin (Zithromax). These medications should be administered at the same time, if possible (CDC, 2015i). The nurse must emphasize the importance of abstaining from sexual contact until the infection is cured in both the patient and any partners. Condom use to prevent future infections is essential, particularly for pregnant women whose partners may be infected.

Syphilis

Syphilis is a complex systemic STI caused by the spirochete *Treponema pallidum,* an anaerobic bacteria. It can infect almost any body tissue or organ. It is transmitted from open lesions— or **chancres**—during any sexual contact (genital, oral–genital, or anal–genital). The incubation period ranges from 12 to 90 days, averaging 21 days (CDC, 2015n). If not treated appropriately, syphilis will progress in four stages and ultimately can lead to blindness, paralysis, mental illness, cardiovascular damage, and death. Syphilis may occur with one or more other STIs, such as HIV/AIDS or chlamydial infection.

In 2014, a total of 63,450 new cases of syphilis were reported in the United States. Men who have sex with men accounted for about 83% of primary and secondary syphilis cases reported. In addition, 458 cases of congenital syphilis were reported in 2014, with the highest rates of occurrence among Black and Hispanic families (CDC, 2015n).

Syphilis is generally characterized by four clinical stages: primary, secondary, latent, and tertiary. Each stage has characteristic manifestations. Syphilis remains highly infectious during the primary and secondary stages, even if no symptoms are present.

- **Primary Syphilis.** The primary stage of syphilis is characterized by the appearance of a chancre (see **Figure 19–29 »**) and by regional enlargement of lymph nodes; little or no pain accompanies these warning signs. The chancre appears at the site of inoculation (e.g., genitals, anus, mouth, breast, fingers) 3–4 weeks after the infectious contact. In women, a genital chancre may go unnoticed, disappearing within 3–6 weeks.

- **Secondary Syphilis.** Secondary syphilis is systemic, with the spirochete spreading to all major organ systems.

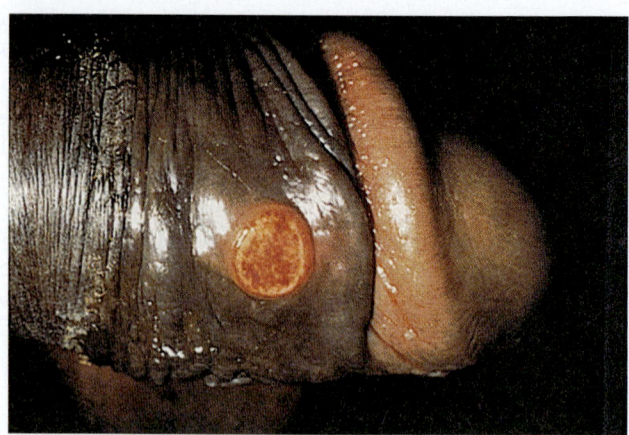

Source: Biophoto Associates/Getty Images.

Figure 19–29 » Chancre of primary syphilis on the penis.

Manifestations of secondary syphilis usually appear several weeks after the initial chancre (CDC, 2013e). These symptoms can include a rash, especially on the palms of the hands or soles of the feet; mucous patches in the oral cavity; sore throat; generalized lymphadenopathy; condyloma lata (flat, broad-based papules) on the labia, anus, or corner of the mouth; flulike symptoms; and alopecia. Manifestations generally disappear within 2–6 weeks, and an asymptomatic latency period begins.

- **Latent Syphilis.** Without treatment, the secondary lesions resolve, and a latent period occurs during which the infected individual has no symptoms. During the early part of this stage, sexual transmission is possible. The latent period may last 1 year to a lifetime (CDC, 2013e).

- **Tertiary Syphilis.** Roughly 15% of untreated individuals progress to late-stage or tertiary syphilis (CDC, 2015n). Two types of late-stage syphilis occur. Benign late syphilis has a rapid onset and is characterized by localized development of infiltrating tumors (*gummas*) in skin, bones, and liver. These tumors generally respond promptly to treatment. Cardiovascular syphilis has a more insidious onset. It is a diffuse inflammatory response involving the cardiovascular system. Though the disease can still be treated at this stage, much of the cardiovascular damage is irreversible.

Diagnosis of syphilis is complex because it mimics many other diseases. A careful history and physical examination are essential, as are laboratory evaluations of lesions and blood. Darkfield microscopy is the definitive method for diagnosing syphilis in the primary stage and involves examining a specimen from the chancre for the presence of *T. pallidum*. This method is not widely used because it requires immediate examination by a trained and experienced technician. As a result, diagnoses are most often made using blood tests (CDC, 2015n).

The goals of treatment are to inactivate the spirochete and to educate the patient about prevention of reinfection or further transmission. Treatment includes antibiotic therapy, identification and referral of partners for testing and treatment, follow-up testing, and education about condom use to prevent reinfection of self and transmission to partners. In addition, the patient should be screened for chlamydial infection and advised to have an HIV test.

Lifespan Considerations

Individuals 15–24 years of age are most commonly affected by STIs, with this age group accounting for half of all new STI infections (CDC, 2015o). As a result, it is easy to make the erroneous assumption that STIs are only an issue for young adults. In fact, STIs are a concern for patients of all ages, and these infections have important implications for patient health.

Maternal–Newborn Considerations

STIs pose particular concerns to women during pregnancy and may be contracted prior to or during gestation. Infections can have negative consequences for the woman, her child, or both.

Because women often experience few early manifestations of infection, they often do not know they are infected. All pregnant women should be tested for STIs, including HIV as part of routine medical care. STI testing typically occurs during the first prenatal visit, and treatment begins immediately upon diagnosis. Testing may be repeated during the third trimester, particularly if the patient is at high risk of infection, because complications of STIs can be more serious for mother and child if contracted during pregnancy (CDC, 2013f).

Maternal complications generally occur during pregnancy; many complications for the child occur shortly after birth, though some may not become evident for months or years (CDC, 2013f). Complications vary according to the STI involved. For example, pregnant patients with HPV may experience an increase in size and number of genital warts during pregnancy. Large, widespread warts can block the birth canal, necessitating cesarean section. Untreated chlamydia can lead to preterm labor, premature rupture of membranes, and low birth weight (CDC, 2013f). STIs fortunately can be treated during pregnancy. Antibiotics can cure bacterial infections such as chlamydia, gonorrhea, and syphilis and are safe to take during pregnancy. Viral infections such as HSV cannot be cured, but antiviral medications can reduce the risk of the infection passing from mother to child (CDC, 2013f).

STIs in Children

STI diagnosis in children under 10 years of age is suggestive of sexual abuse. In some cases, infection in young children may be the result of perinatally acquired infections that can persist for 2–3 years; however, the general rule is to consider infection evidence of abuse. STI testing should be conducted prior to initiating treatment of children exhibiting STI symptoms or signs of sexual trauma in order to obtain a reliable diagnosis (CDC, 2015i).

It is essential to examine and collect specimens from children in a manner that minimizes trauma to them. Repeat examination and testing may be indicated depending on the recency and duration of abuse. Examination and specimen collection should be conducted by a clinician with experience in the area of child sexual abuse (CDC, 2015i).

In general, presumptive treatment for STIs is not recommended because of the low incidence of infection in abused children. Infection is treated based on test results and accompanied by counseling and other psychologic care. Follow-up depends on the amount of time that has elapsed between the abuse and the initial examination; the results of testing; and the type of treatment prescribed (CDC, 2015i).

SAFETY ALERT When a prepubertal child is found to have gonorrhea or another STI, you must consider the possibility of sexual abuse. When anorectal symptoms or disease or trauma are found, suspect molestation. (See the module on Trauma for a discussion of child abuse and reporting requirements.)

STIs in Adolescents

Adolescents are at increased risk of STIs for a variety of developmental, physical, and socioeconomic reasons. Risky sexual behaviors in this group are common and stem from desire to fit in with sexually active peers; lack of education about STIs and safer sex practices; and concern or embarrassment about discussing birth control and infection prevention with parents, guardians, and healthcare providers. In addition, adolescents may have multiple sex partners at one time or move from relationship to relationship quickly. Adolescents who are sexually active at a young age and who abuse alcohol or drugs are at higher risk of acquiring an STI (CDC, 2015i).

Adolescent girls in particular are at increased risk of infection because of the presence of columnar cells in the ectocervix; in older women, these cells are located in the endocervix. This condition, known as ectopy, is normal in adolescents. It does, however, make the adolescent cervix more vulnerable to infection than that of adult women. Prevalence rates of chlamydia, gonorrhea, and HPV are highest in adolescent and young adult females (CDC, 2015i).

In spite of regulations that allow minors to consent for their own STI-related health services, adolescents may be very concerned about confidentiality and may not trust local clinics to provide confidential care. For those covered under a parent's or guardian's health insurance, issues of confidentiality are complicated by requirements to provide beneficiary information and explanations of benefits to policy holders (CDC, 2015p). In addition, sexual health is more vulnerable in those who are subject to higher rates of poverty, unemployment, low education, and income inequality. Also adolescents in detention centers, those who use injection drugs, and young men who have sex with men are at increased risk for STIs (CDC, 2015i). Many individuals in these circumstances do not have health insurance or access to healthcare.

Developmentally appropriate discussions of sexual behavior, infection risk, and safer sex practices are important preventive measures and should be discussed with all adolescents and young adults. Vaccinations for HPV and hepatitis A and B are also important, as are annual *C. trachomatis* and *N. gonorrhoeae* screenings for sexually active women. Nonjudgmental, thorough counseling and care are important for helping adolescents minimize their risk of infection (CDC, 2015i).

Focus on Diversity and Culture
STIs in Vulnerable Populations

Although any individual who engages in unprotected sex is at risk for developing an STI, those who are homeless, engage in illicit drug use, or who are sex workers carry particular risks. Commonalities among these groups that contribute to increased risk of STIs include multiple partnerships, transactional sex, lack of access to healthcare, and unstable living conditions. For those who use illicit drugs, injection drug use carries a higher risk. Lack of a stable environment and inconsistent access to healthcare increase the potential for long-term sequelae for those who abuse substances.

Patients in these groups benefit from nonjudgmental nursing care and a thorough assessment that includes assessment of personal safety. Treatment and safety planning should take into consideration available resources, such as emergency shelters, substance abuse and harm reduction programs, free healthcare clinics, supportive housing and skills training programs, and condom distribution programs.

Sources: Bryant, K. L. & Williams, S. P. (n.d.) Sexually transmitted infections among homeless persons: A literature review. Retrieved from file:///C:/Users/jamcc/Downloads/SWilliams_Poster_STI%20and%20Homelessness.pdf; CDC. (2017). Persons who use drugs (PWUD). Retrieved from: https://www.cdc.gov/pwud/Default.html; WHO. (2017). HIV/AIDS: Sex work. Retrieved from http://who.int/hiv/topics/sex_work/about/en/.

STIs in Older Adults

Older adults are living longer, healthier lives and are engaging in sex more than previous generations. Along with this increase in sexual activity comes an increase in STIs (Poynten et al., 2013). Although the number of older adults affected by STIs is not nearly as high as that of young people, older adults are faced with unique barriers to prompt recognition and treatment. Many healthcare providers do not think of their older patients as sexually active and do not assess for STIs or provide education about safe sex (Stewart & Graham, 2013). This delays diagnosis of diseases such as HIV that mimic other diseases frequently seen among older patients. In 2013, a total of 7108 new cases of HIV—or 27% of new diagnoses—occurred in individuals 50 and older. Of those cases, 1045 occurred in individuals age 65 and older (CDC, 2015m). Data from the Centers for Disease Control and Prevention (2016) also show increasing prevalence of gonorrhea, chlamydia, and other STIs in older adults.

Normal age-related changes to the body can put older adults at greater risk of infection. Postmenopausal women produce less estrogen, making the vaginal lining thinner and more prone to injury during intercourse. The resultant tears and abrasions serve as a pathway for infectious agents. Among older men, the use of drugs like sildenafil citrate (Viagra) and tadalafil (Cialis) to enhance sexual performance may prompt older men to engage in more and riskier behaviors. In addition, as the immune system ages it may be less able to fight infection and may be slower to respond to therapy (Imparato & Sanders, 2012).

Older adults may not believe themselves to be at risk of STIs (Imparato & Sanders, 2012). It is therefore essential that healthcare providers counsel older adults about using safer sex practices with new partners. As spouses die and couples divorce, older adults may begin dating for the first time in many years. From a generational standpoint, these individuals may be less aware of the risks of unprotected sex than younger individuals. Safe sex and STI education became prevalent in the 1980s; at that time, today's older adults were outside the demographic this education was intended to reach (Benjamin Rose Institute on Aging, 2015). In addition, because pregnancy is no longer a concern, older adults may not use condoms or may use them inconsistently (CDC, 2015m). Older adults may also be hesitant to discuss sexual practices with healthcare providers.

Healthcare providers should acknowledge that continuation of sexual activity is a normal part of aging and encourage patients to talk about their sexual practice. Acknowledging the personal, sensitive nature of these topics before discussing them may help put patients at ease. It is also crucial to dispel myths about the risk of infection and provide information that is relevant to the patient. This is particularly important given the current lack of STI information geared for the older adult population (Imparato & Sanders, 2012).

NURSING PROCESS

Treatment of STIs occurs most frequently in community-based clinics. No matter the setting, when providing nursing care for a patient with an STI, the nurse needs to consider both short-term and long-term implications. Although the immediate priority is symptom relief, treatment, and prevention of further transmission, the patient may need assistance coping with the diagnosis of a chronic STI and may require repeated screening for potential complications.

Although the following nursing process focuses on the patient with genital herpes, the principles addressed are applicable to patients with other STIs.

Assessment

The patient interview will guide the physical examination, and data gathered in both the interview and exam must be considered in relation to normal parameters and expectations. Therefore, the nurse must consider age, race, culture, environment, health practices, and past and concurrent problems when assessing the patient. Gender is also an essential consideration during assessment, as women and men may experience different manifestations of infection. The nurse should do the following when assessing female and male patients:

- **Observation and patient history.** Record information related to health history, preexisting conditions, and medication use. Review sexual history, including number of partners, frequency of sexual encounters, and use of condoms and other forms of birth control. Discuss symptoms of the current complaint, noting the onset, duration, and severity. Note any precipitating or relieving factors. Assess success of the patient's self-treatment of symptoms. Use follow-up questions to obtain information about the source and duration of the current complaint, as well as any measures the patient has taken to alleviate pain or other symptoms. *For women:* Assess menstrual history, noting length and frequency of cycle and unusual patterns of bleeding.

- *Physical examination—female patient.* Assess vital signs. Examine the external genitalia and perianal area for lesions, blisters, or other irregularities. Note any hemorrhoids, fissures, and infectious processes. Palpate potential sites of infection and inflammation. Conduct a pelvic examination, and collect any necessary specimens. Note the presence and color of any abnormal vaginal discharge.

- *Physical examination—male patient.* Assess vital signs. Examine genitalia and anorectal area for lesions, blisters, or irritation. Palpate testicles for tenderness or abnormal lumps. Collect specimens of any discharge, and note the color of this discharge. Collect a urethral swab if necessary.

When assessing the patient with an STI, some of the data gathered in the interview and assessment will focus on the status of the urinary system as well as the reproductive system. Because of the proximity of some of the reproductive structures to the urethra and the bladder—particularly in female patients—infection may affect both systems.

Diagnosis

Nursing diagnoses that may be appropriate for patients diagnosed with an STI may include the following:

- *Pain, Acute*
- *Sexual Dysfunction*
- *Deficient Knowledge.*

(NANDA-I © 2014)

Planning

In planning care of the patient with a diagnosed or suspected STI, the following goals may be appropriate:

- The patient will describe strategies for reducing the risk of contracting an STI.
- The patient will develop a plan for contacting anyone who may have been exposed to the diagnosed STI through sexual contact.
- The patient will abstain from sexual activity until the STI is resolved or take appropriate actions to avoid infecting others.
- The patient's pain will be reduced to a tolerable level.

Implementation

Nursing interventions for the patient with herpes primarily occur in community settings and address a number of physical and emotional issues. Pain relief is a primary concern, as is transmission prevention. Long-term symptom management and coping skills are also important given the chronic nature of herpes.

Care in the Community

In community settings such as federally funded community health centers, physicians' offices, and health department or Planned Parenthood clinics, the nurse should do the following:

- Counsel the patient about chronic disease management and strategies for preventing transmission to sexual partners.

- Discuss available antiviral therapies and differentiate between episodic and suppressive regimens.
- Stress the importance of contacting sexual partners and encouraging them to be tested.
- Arrange follow-up visits for further testing or treatment as necessary.

Herpes is not a reportable STI; however, chlamydia, gonorrhea, and syphilis are all reportable STIs. In the case of a reportable STI, the nurse may be involved with the reporting process.

Relieve Acute Pain

Herpetic lesions are very painful and can become infected. If the lesions are near the urinary meatus, dysuria and urinary retention may occur. Because the virus resides in the nerve ganglia, pain may also occur in the legs, thighs, groin, or buttocks. Although acyclovir diminishes the pain of herpes and accelerates the healing process, additional measures can relieve the discomfort further:

- Recommend oral analgesics such as acetaminophen or ibuprofen for pain relief.
- Teach the patient how to keep herpes blisters clean and dry. The area should be washed with mild soap and water daily. Lesions should be dried using a hair dryer turned to a cool setting. The patient should wear loose cotton clothing that will not trap moisture and avoid wearing panty hose and tight jeans. Keeping the lesions clean and dry reduces the possibility of secondary infection and speeds the healing process.
- For dysuria and urinary retention, suggest pouring water over the genitals to start urination and to dilute the urine. Drinking additional fluids also helps dilute the urine. Diluting the urine reduces the burning sensation.
- Suggest the use of a sitz bath (with tepid water) for 15–30 minutes several times a day. The warm water is soothing and decreases pain from ulcers and an irritated urethral meatus. It facilitates wound healing and facilitates urination.

Discuss Sexual Function

Patients who learn that they are infected with an incurable STI may believe they can no longer have a normal sex life. Many individuals fortunately have learned to live with and manage genital herpes without infecting their partners or their children. The nurse should offer factual information in a supportive, nonjudgmental environment that encourages patients to discuss feelings and ask questions. The nurse should also offer information about support groups and other resources. Information about how others cope with the disease can offset feelings of shame and hopelessness. See the Patient Teaching feature for additional information.

>> **Stay Current:** A diagnosis of herpes can leave patients feeling confused and overwhelmed. Herpes Online at http://www.herpesonline.org offers a number of useful articles and resources for individuals with herpes and other STIs.

Patient Teaching
Managing a Herpes Outbreak

Health teaching for patients with genital herpes involves helping them manage their condition with the least possible disruption in lifestyle and relationships. Understanding the disease process and the factors that affect it helps the patient regain a sense of control and see the potential for sexual intimacy without transmission of infection. The following topics should be addressed:

- Recognition of prodromal symptoms of recurrence and the factors that trigger recurrences (e.g., emotional stress)
- Abstention from sexual contact from the appearance of prodromal symptoms until 10 days following lesion healing
- Identification and culture of infected lesions and treatment of those lesions with appropriate antibiotics
- Utilization of latex condoms and careful hygiene practices (e.g., not sharing towels or other personal items) at all times in order to protect others from viral shedding
- Discussion of the herpes infection with significant others
- Maintenance of thorough hand hygiene as a means of avoiding autoinoculation of other areas.

Evaluation

Patient care may be evaluated on the basis of the following expected outcomes:

- The patient is free of the STI (for curable STIs) or free of pain and discomfort associated with the STI (for chronic STIs).
- The patient explains strategies to prevent infection of others.
- The patient abstains from sexual activity until the STI is treated.
- The patient describes barrier methods to reduce the risk of contracting an STI.

If patient outcomes are not met, additional teaching about disease management may be appropriate. Emphasize the importance of avoiding sexual contact when lesions are present, and reinforce the need for good hygiene to protect others from viral shedding and self from autoinoculation. Encourage the patient to seek help and support from resources such as the CDC National STD hotline, the National Herpes Hotline, and the American Social Health Association.

Nursing Care Plan
A Patient with Syphilis

Eddie Kratz, age 22, works as a bellman at a large hotel. For the past year, he has shared a small apartment with Maria Jones, who is 5 months pregnant with his child. Although he intends to marry Ms. Jones before the baby is born, he has continued a previous relationship with a woman named Justine Simpson. His sexual activities with Ms. Simpson have increased in frequency as Ms. Jones's pregnancy has advanced. Mr. Kratz has recently noticed a swelling in his groin and a sore on his penis.

ASSESSMENT	DIAGNOSES	PLANNING
Mr. Kratz comes to the community clinic where you work. You take a thorough medical and sexual history, including questions about drug use, allergies, difficulty with urination, urinary frequency, itching or discharge from the penis, recent sexual activities, precautions taken against infection, history of STIs, and sexual function. You determine that Mr. Kratz has been having unprotected sex with both Ms. Jones and Ms. Simpson. He believes that Ms. Jones is not having sex with anyone except him, but he is not sure. Physical assessment reveals a classic syphilitic chancre on the shaft of the penis and regional lymphadenopathy. A specimen of exudates from the chancre is sent for darkfield examination. You discuss with Mr. Kratz the likelihood that he has syphilis and the need to tell both Ms. Jones and Ms. Simpson so that they can be tested and, if necessary, treated. You also suggest that Mr. Kratz be tested for HIV, since he has been having unprotected sex with two women, at least one of whom may be sexually active with other partners. He agrees, and blood is drawn for an ELISA test. Darkfield analysis of the chancre exudate confirms the diagnosis of syphilis; the ELISA results are negative for HIV.	- *Injury, Risk for,* to the patient, his partners, and the infant, related to the disease process - *Health Maintenance, Ineffective,* related to a lack of knowledge about the disease process, its transmission, and the need for treatment - *Family Processes, Interrupted,* related to the effects of the diagnosis of syphilis on the couple's relationship - *Anxiety* related to the effects of the infection on the unborn child (NANDA-I © 2014)	- The patient will receive prompt treatment to cure syphilis. - The patient will articulate understanding of the need to abstain from sexual contact during treatment, complete all medications, return for follow-up visits, and use condoms to prevent reinfection. - The patient will verbalize an ability to cope with the effect of diagnosis and treatment on the relationship. - The patient will verbalize decreased anxiety following education and treatment.

Nursing Care Plan *(continued)*

IMPLEMENTATION

- Administer intramuscular injection of penicillin G as ordered.
- Discuss the importance of abstaining from sexual activity until Mr. Kratz and his partners are cured and of using condoms to prevent reinfection.
- Explain the need to return for follow-up testing in 3 months and again at 6 months. Provide a copy of the STI prevention checklist, and document that reminders need to be sent at 3- and 6-month intervals.

- Notify sexual partners that they need to come to the clinic for testing.
- Refer the patient to a social worker for counseling about the effect of the disease on the couple's relationship.
- Teach the couple about the importance of treatment to the health of their infant.

EVALUATION

At the 3-month follow-up visit, the chancre on Mr. Kratz's penis has healed, and he reports that he is using a condom any time he has sex. Ms. Jones has tested positive for syphilis and negative for HIV, so she, too, is given penicillin G and verbal and written follow-up instructions, including follow-up until the infant is born. The couple meets every other week with the social worker and says that their relationship is improving. Ms. Simpson has received similar test results and is given a prescription for doxycycline because she is allergic to penicillin.

CRITICAL THINKING

1. What manifestations might a patient with early syphilis experience?
2. List some appropriate questions for taking a sexual history when you suspect the presence of one or more STIs.
3. How might you counsel Mr. Kratz to help him break the news of the diagnosis to Ms. Jones?

REVIEW Sexually Transmitted Infections

RELATE Link the Concepts and Exemplars

Linking the exemplar of STIs with the concept of reproduction:

1. How will care of the pregnant patient with genital herpes differ from the care provided to a pregnant patient who does not have this infection?
2. What is your priority nursing diagnosis for the young couple contemplating pregnancy who are both diagnosed with genital warts?

Linking the exemplar of STIs with the concept of elimination:

3. Create a plan of care addressing pain management and prevention of urinary retention for the patient diagnosed with herpes.
4. What teaching will you provide a patient about using sitz baths for facilitated urination when the pain of herpes causes urinary retention?

READY Go to Volume 3: Clinical Nursing Skills

REFER Go to Pearson MyLab Nursing and eText

- Additional review materials

REFLECT Apply Your Knowledge

Maggie Lynch is a 14-year-old girl who has a 6-month-old daughter, Amy. Maggie lives with her single mother, Marcia Lynch, who has become very controlling of Maggie since she became pregnant. Ms. Lynch has forced Maggie to go back to school, which Maggie was very much against. Maggie participates very little in Amy's care. Ms. Lynch treats Amy as if she were her own child. There is a great deal of friction between Maggie and her mother.

Maggie has been skipping class occasionally to be with her 16-year-old boyfriend, Brett, who is Amy's father. Brett has no interest in Amy, but his parents make the effort to see Amy often. Maggie and Brett have resumed their physical relationship despite objections from both families.

Ms. Lynch accidentally interrupts Maggie in the bathroom and notices a foul odor. She questions Maggie and learns that Maggie has noticed a frothy yellow vaginal discharge in addition to the foul odor. Ms. Lynch arranges for Maggie to be seen by her gynecologist.

1. The nurse calls Maggie from the waiting room. Should she allow Maggie's mother to accompany them to the exam room? Explain your answer.
2. What teaching will you initiate for Maggie once diagnosis has been made and treatment ordered?
3. How will you respond to Ms. Lynch if she demands you tell her what is wrong with Maggie?

References

Adams, M. P., Holland, L. N., & Urban, C. (2017). *Pharmacology for nurses: A pathophysiologic approach* (5th ed.). Hoboken, NJ: Pearson Education.

Ahmed, M. R., Madny, E. H., & Sayed Ahmed, W. A. (2014). Prevalence of female sexual dysfunction during pregnancy among Egyptian women. *Journal of Obstetrics and Gynaecology Research, 40*(4), 1023–1029.

Alswager, K., & Durler, C. (2013). Menstruation and related problems and concerns. In E. Youngkin, M. Davis, D. Schadewald, & C. Juve (Eds.), *Women's*

health: A primary care clinical guide (4th ed., pp. 203–226). Boston, MA: Pearson.

American Academy of Family Physicians. (2013). *Adolescent health care, confidentiality*. Retrieved from http://www.aafp.org/about/policies/all/adolescent-confidentiality.html

American Academy of Pediatrics. (2015a). *Should the baby be circumcised?* Retrieved from https://www. healthychildren.org/English/ages-stages/ prenatal/decisions-to-make/Pages/Should-the-Baby-be-Circumcised.aspx

American Academy of Pediatrics. (2015b). *Physical development in boys: What to expect.* Retrieved from https://www.healthychildren.org/English/ages-stages/gradeschool/puberty/Pages/Physical-Development-Boys-What-to-Expect.aspx

American Cancer Society. (2015a). *American Cancer Society guidelines for the early detection of cancer.* Retrieved from http://www.cancer.org/healthy/findcancerearly/cancerscreeningguidelines/american-cancer-society-guidelines-for-the-early-detection-of-cancer

American Cancer Society. (2015b). *American Cancer Society recommendations for prostate cancer early detection.* Retrieved from http://www.cancer.org/cancer/prostatecancer/moreinformation/prostatecancerearlydetection/prostate-cancer-early-detection-acs-recommendations

American Cancer Society. (2015c). *What are the risk factors for testicular cancer?* Retrieved from http://www.cancer.org/cancer/testicularcancer/detailedguide/testicular-cancer-risk-factors

American Cancer Society. (2015d). *DES exposure: Questions and answers.* Retrieved from http://www.cancer.org/cancer/cancercauses/othercarcinogens/medicaltreatments/des-exposure

American Cancer Society. (2015e). *Do I have testicular cancer?* Retrieved from http://www.cancer.org/cancer/testicularcancer/moreinformation/doihavetesticularcancer/do-i-have-testicular-cancer-facts-and-risk-factors

American College of Obstetricians and Gynecologists. (2007; reaffirmed 2014). *Committee on Gynecological Practice Opinion #378: Vaginal "rejuvenation" and cosmetic vaginal procedures.* Retrieved from http://www.acog.org/Resources-And-Publications/Committee-Opinions/Committee-on-Gynecologic-Practice/Vaginal-Rejuvenation-and-Cosmetic-Vaginal-Procedures

American College of Obstetricians and Gynecologists. (2011). *Perimenopausal bleeding and bleeding after menopause.* Retrieved from http://www.acog.org/Patients/FAQs/Perimenopausal-Bleeding-and-Bleeding-After-Menopause

American College of Obstetricians and Gynecologists. (2013a). Committee opinion no. 557: Management of acute abnormal uterine bleeding in nonpregnant reproductive-aged women. *Obstetrics and Gynecology, 121*, 891–896. Retrieved from http://www.acog.org/Resources-And-Publications/Committee-Opinions/Committee-on-Gynecologic-Practice/Management-of-Acute-Abnormal-Uterine-Bleeding-in-Nonpregnant-Reproductive-Aged-Women

American College of Obstetricians and Gynecologists. (2013b). Practice bulletin no. 136: Management of abnormal uterine bleeding associated with ovulatory dysfunction. *Obstetrics and Gynecology, 122*(1), 176–185. Retrieved from https://medweb.nch.org/INTERMED/Data/ComponentFiles/1136/02_ABOG_January%202014.pdf

American College of Obstetricians and Gynecologists. (2014). Medical management of first-trimester abortion. *Practice Bulletin, 143.* Retrieved from http://www.acog.org/-/media/Practice-Bulletins/Committee-on-Practice-Bulletins—Gynecology/Public/pb143.pdf?dmc=1

American Nurses Association (ANA). (2015). *Code of ethics for nurses with interpretive statements.* Retrieved from http://nursingworld.org/

DocumentVault/Ethics-1/Code-of-Ethics-for-Nurses.html

American Pregnancy Association. (2015a). *Breast changes during pregnancy.* Retrieved from http://americanpregnancy.org/pregnancy-health/breast-changes-during-pregnancy/

American Pregnancy Association. (2015b). *Cramping during pregnancy.* Retrieved from http://americanpregnancy.org/your-pregnancy/cramping-during-pregnancy/

American Pregnancy Association. (2015c). *Female infertility.* Retrieved from http://americanpregnancy.org/infertility/female-infertility/

American Pregnancy Association. (2015d). *Male infertility.* Retrieved from http://americanpregnancy.org/infertility/male-infertility/

American Pregnancy Association. (2015e). *Down syndrome: Trisomy 21.* Retrieved from http://americanpregnancy.org/birth-defects/down-syndrome/

American Pregnancy Association. (2015f). *Preimplantation genetic diagnosis: PGD.* Retrieved from http://americanpregnancy.org/infertility/preimplantation-genetic-diagnosis/

American Pregnancy Association. (2015g). *Infertility medications.* Retrieved from http://americanpregnancy.org/infertility/infertility-medications/

American Pregnancy Association. (2015h). *Premature ovarian failure: Premature menopause.* Retrieved from http://americanpregnancy.org/womens-health/premature-ovarian-failure/

American Pregnancy Association. (2015i). *Bleeding during pregnancy.* Retrieved from http://americanpregnancy.org/pregnancy-complications/bleeding-during-pregnancy/

American Psychiatric Association. (2013a). *Diagnostic and statistical manual of mental disorders* (5th ed.). Arlington, VA: Author.

American Psychiatric Association. (2013b). *What is gender dysphoria?* Retrieved from http://www.dsm5.org/patients-families/gender-dysphoria/what-is-gender-dysphoria

American Psychological Association. (2015). *Treatment for sexual problems.* Retrieved from http://www.apa.org/topics/sex/treatment.aspx

American Society of Reproductive Medicine. (2015). *Frequently asked questions about infertility.* Retrieved from https://www.asrm.org/awards/index.aspx?id=3012

Association of Reproductive Health Professionals. (2013). *Postpartum counseling: Sexuality and contraception.* Retrieved from https://www.arhp.org/publications-and-resources/quick-reference-guide-for-clinicians/postpartum-counseling/contraception

Association of Reproductive Health Professionals. (2014a). *Choosing a birth control method: Initiation of hormonal contraceptives.* Retrieved from http://www.arhp.org/Publications-and-Resources/Quick-Reference-Guide-for-Clinicians/choosing/Initiation-Hormonal-Contraceptives

Association of Reproductive Health Professionals. (2014b). *Choosing a birth control method: Transdermal contraceptive patch.* Retrieved from https://www.arhp.org/Publications-and-Resources/Quick-Reference-Guide-for-Clinicians/choosing/Transdermal-Patch

Association of Reproductive Health Professionals. (2014c). *Choosing a birth control method: Vaginal ring.* Retrieved from https://www.arhp.org/Publications-and-Resources/Quick-Reference-Guide-for-Clinicians/choosing/Vaginal-Ring

Association of Reproductive Health Professionals. (2014d). *Choosing a birth control method: Injectable.* Retrieved from http://www.arhp.org/Publications-and-Resources/Quick-Reference-Guide-for-Clinicians/choosing/Injectable

Association of Reproductive Health Professionals. (2014e). *Choosing a birth control method: Female sterilization.* Retrieved from https://www.arhp.org/Publications-and-Resources/Quick-Reference-Guide-for-Clinicians/choosing/female-sterilization

Ball, J. W., Bindler, R. C., Cowen, K., & Shaw, M. (2017). *Principles of pediatric nursing: Caring for children* (7th ed.). Hoboken, NJ: Pearson Education.

Balon, R. (2015). Sexual dysfunctions. In L. Weiss Roberts & A. K. Louie (Eds.), *Study guide to DSM-5.* Arlington, VA: American Psychiatric Publishing.

Balon, R., & Segraves, R. T. (2014). Sexual dysfunctions. In R. E. Hales, S. C. Yudofsky, & L. Weiss Roberts (Eds.), *American Psychiatric Publishing textbook of psychiatry* (6th ed., pp. 651–678). Arlington, VA: American Psychiatric Publishing.

Bart, C., & Fauser, B. (2015). *Patient information: Infertility treatment with gonadotropins (beyond the basics).* Retrieved from http://www.uptodate.com/contents/infertility-treatment-with-gonadotropins-beyond-the-basics

Behara, M. A., & Price, T. M. (2015). *Abnormal (dysfunctional) uterine bleeding.* Retrieved from http://emedicine.medscape.com/article/257007-overview

Benjamin Rose Institute on Aging. (2015). *Sexually transmitted diseases in older adults.* Retrieved from http://www.benrose.org/Resources/article-stds-older-adults.cfm

Bhugra, D., & Colombini, G. (2013). Sexual dysfunction: Classification and treatment. *Advances in Psychiatric Treatment, 19*(1), 48–55.

Bickley, L., & Szilagyi, P. (2013). *Bates' guide to physical examination and history taking* (11th ed.). Philadelphia, PA: Wolters Kluwer/Lippincott Williams & Wilkins.

Biggs, W. S., & Chaganaboyana, S. (2015). Human sexuality. In R. E. Rakel & D. P. Rakel (Eds.), *Textbook of family medicine* (9th ed., pp. 1039–1051). Philadelphia, PA: Elsevier Saunders.

Blackburn, S. (2013). *Maternal, fetal, and neonatal physiology: A clinical perspective* (4th ed.). St. Louis, MO: Elsevier.

Bond, K. S., Mpofu, E., & Millington, M. (2015). Treating women with genito-pelvic pain/penetration disorder: Influences of patient agendas on help-seeking. *Journal of Family Medicine, 2*(4), 1033.

Bradford, J., Reisner, S., Honnold, J., & Xavier, J. (2012, November 15). Experiences of transgender-related discrimination and implications for health: Results from the Virginia Transgender Health Initiative study. *American Journal of Public Health,* e1–e10. doi:10.2105/AJPH.2012.300796

Bradley University. (2015). *The body project: Infertility and body image.* Retrieved from http://www.bradley.edu/sites/bodyproject/sexuality/infertility/

Brandon, M. (2014). Women and sexuality. In M. G. Curtis, S. T. Linares, & L. Antoniewicz (Eds.), *Glass' office gynecology* (7th ed., pp. 155–183). Philadelphia, PA: Wolters Kluwer.

Breastcancer.org. (2015). *How menopause can happen with breast cancer treatments.* Retrieved from http://www.breastcancer.org/tips/menopausal/types/treatment-induced

Brzyski, R. G., & Knudtson, K. (n.d.). *Effects of aging on the female reproductive system.* Retrieved from http://www.merckmanuals.com/home/women's-health-issues/biology-of-the-female-reproductive-system/effects-of-aging-on-the-female-reproductive-system

Burri, A., Hysi, P., Clop, A., Rahman, Q., & Spector, T. (2012). A genome-wide association study of female sexual dysfunction. *PLoS One, 7*(4), e35041. doi:10.1371/journal.pone.0035041

Calis, K. A., Erogul, M., Popat, V., Kalantaridou, S. N., & Dang, D. K. (2015). *Dysmenorrhea clinical presentation.* Retrieved from http://emedicine.medscape.com/article/253812-clinical

Carroll, J. L. (2013). *Sexuality now: Embracing diversity* (5th ed., pp. 230–237). Boston, MA: Cengage Learning.

Centers for Disease Control and Prevention (CDC). (2011). *A guide to taking a sexual history* (CDC Publication No. 99-8445). Retrieved from http://www.cdc.gov/std/treatment/SexualHistory.pdf

Centers for Disease Control and Prevention (CDC). (2013a). *National health interview survey.* Retrieved from https://www.cdc.gov/nchs/nhis/nhis_2013_data_release.htm

Centers for Disease Control and Prevention (CDC). (2013b). *Sexually transmitted disease: Fact sheets.* Retrieved from http://www.cdc.gov/std/healthcomm/fact_sheets.htm

Centers for Disease Control and Prevention (CDC). (2013c). *Ready-to-use STD curriculum: human papillomavirus (HPV).* Retrieved from http://www2a.cdc.gov/stdtraining/ready-to-use/hpv.htm

Centers for Disease Control and Prevention (CDC). (2013d). *Ready-to-use STD curriculum: Gonorrhea.* Retrieved from http://www2a.cdc.gov/stdtraining/ready-to-use/gonorrhea.htm

Centers for Disease Control and Prevention (CDC). (2013e). *Ready-to-use STD curriculum: Syphilis.* Retrieved from http://www2a.cdc.gov/stdtraining/ready-to-use/syphilis.htm

Centers for Disease Control and Prevention (CDC). (2013f). *STDs during pregnancy—CDC fact sheet.* Retrieved from http://www.cdc.gov/std/pregnancy/stdfact-pregnancy.htm

Centers for Disease Control and Prevention (CDC). (2014a). *Youth risk behavior surveillance—United States, 2013.* Retrieved from http://www.cdc.gov/mmwr/pdf/ss/ss6304.pdf?utm_source=rss&utm_medium=rss&utm_campaign=youth-risk-behavior-surveillance-united-states-2013-pdf

Centers for Disease Control and Prevention (CDC). (2014b). *Fact sheets: Excessive alcohol use and risk to men's health.* Retrieved from http://www.cdc.gov/alcohol/fact-sheets/mens-health.htm

Centers for Disease Control and Prevention (CDC). (2014c). *Preconception care and health care: Clinical care of women—Immunization.* Retrieved from http://www.cdc.gov/preconception/careforwomen/immunization.html

Centers for Disease Control and Prevention (CDC). (2014d). *Birth defects: Facts about Down syndrome.* Retrieved from http://www.cdc.gov/ncbddd/birthdefects/downsyndrome.html

Centers for Disease Control and Prevention (CDC). (2014e). *Genital HPV infection—Fact sheet.* Retrieved from http://www.cdc.gov/std/hpv/stdfact-hpv.htm

Centers for Disease Control and Prevention (CDC). (2014f). *Genital herpes—CDC fact sheet.* Retrieved from http://www.cdc.gov/std/herpes/stdfact-herpes.htm

Centers for Disease Control and Prevention (CDC). (2015a). *Sexual risk behaviors: HIV, STD, and teen pregnancy prevention.* Retrieved from http://www.cdc.gov/healthyyouth/sexualbehaviors/

Centers for Disease Control and Prevention (CDC). (2015b). *Teen dating violence.* Retrieved from http://www.cdc.gov/violenceprevention/intimatepartnerviolence/teen_dating_violence.html

Centers for Disease Control and Prevention (CDC). (2015c). *Healthy pregnant or postpartum women.* Retrieved from http://www.cdc.gov/physicalactivity/basics/pregnancy/

Centers for Disease Control and Prevention (CDC). (2015d). *Assisted reproductive technology (ART): ART success rates.* Retrieved from http://www.cdc.gov/art/reports/index.html

Centers for Disease Control and Prevention (CDC). (2015e). *What is infertility?* Retrieved from http://www.cdc.gov/reproductivehealth/infertility/

Centers for Disease Control and Prevention (CDC). (2015f). *Reported STDs in the United States: 2014 national data for chlamydia, gonorrhea, and syphilis.* Retrieved from http://www.cdc.gov/std/stats14/std-trends-508.pdf

Centers for Disease Control and Prevention (CDC). (2015g). *2014 sexually transmitted diseases surveillance.* Retrieved from http://www.cdc.gov/std/stats14/default.htm

Centers for Disease Control and Prevention (CDC). (2015h). *What is HPV?* Retrieved from http://www.cdc.gov/hpv/parents/whatishpv.html

Centers for Disease Control and Prevention (CDC). (2015i). *2015 sexually transmitted diseases treatment guidelines.* Retrieved from http://www.cdc.gov/std/tg2015/default.htm

Centers for Disease Control and Prevention (CDC). (2015j). *Genital herpes—CDC fact sheet (detailed).* Retrieved from http://www.cdc.gov/std/herpes/stdfact-herpes-detailed.htm

Centers for Disease Control and Prevention (CDC). (2015k). *Chlamydia—CDC fact sheet (detailed).* Retrieved from http://www.cdc.gov/std/chlamydia/stdfact-chlamydia-detailed.htm

Centers for Disease Control and Prevention (CDC). (2015l). *Gonorrhea—CDC fact sheet (detailed).* Retrieved from http://www.cdc.gov/std/gonorrhea/stdfact-gonorrhea-detailed.htm

Centers for Disease Control and Prevention (CDC). (2015m). *HIV among people aged 50 and older.* Retrieved from http://www.cdc.gov/hiv/group/age/olderamericans/index.html

Centers for Disease Control and Prevention (CDC). (2015n). *Syphilis—CDC fact sheet (detailed).* Retrieved from http://www.cdc.gov/std/syphilis/stdfact-syphilis-detailed.htm

Centers for Disease Control and Prevention (CDC). (2015o). *Sexually transmitted diseases: Adolescents and young adults.* Retrieved from http://www.cdc.gov/std/life-stages-populations/adolescents-youngadults.htm

Centers for Disease Control and Prevention (CDC). (2015p). *Adolescent and school health—Sexual risk behaviors: HIV, STD, & teen pregnancy prevention.* Retrieved from http://www.cdc.gov/healthyyouth/sexualbehaviors/

Centers for Disease Control and Prevention (CDC). (2016). *Intimate partner violence: Risk and protective factors.* Retrieved from http://www.cdc.gov/violenceprevention/intimatepartnerviolence/riskprotectivefactors.html

Centers for Disease Control and Prevention. (2017). *PrEP.* Retrieved from https://www.cdc.gov/hiv/basics/prep.html

Centre for Menstrual Cycle and Ovulation Research. (n.d.). *Perimenopause.* Retrieved from http://www.cemcor.ubc.ca/resources/life-phases/perimenopause

Cleveland Clinic. (2013). *Medications that affect sexual function.* Retrieved from https://my.clevelandclinic.org/health/diseases_conditions/hic_An_Overview_of_Sexual_Dysfunction/hic_Medications_that_Affect_Sexual_Function

Cleveland Clinic. (2014a). *Toxic shock syndrome.* Retrieved from http://my.clevelandclinic.org/health/diseases_conditions/hic-toxic-shock-syndrome

Cleveland Clinic. (2014b). *Diseases and conditions: Dysmenorrhea.* Retrieved from https://my.clevelandclinic.org/health/diseases_conditions/hic_Dysmenorrhea

Cleveland Clinic. (2015a). *Medications that may cause erectile dysfunction.* Retrieved from https://my.clevelandclinic.org/health/diseases_conditions/hic_Erectile_Dysfunction_Overview/hic_Medications_That_May_Cause_Erectile_Dysfunction

Cleveland Clinic. (2015b). *An overview of sexual dysfunction.* Retrieved from https://my.clevelandclinic.org/health/diseases_conditions/hic_An_Overview_of_Sexual_Dysfunction

Conaglen, H. M., & Conaglen, J. V. (2013). Drug-induced sexual dysfunction in men and women. *Australian Prescriber, 36,* 42–45.

Coney, P. (2015). *Menopause.* Retrieved from http://emedicine.medscape.com/article/264088-overview#a1

Connor, J., Sauer, C., & Doll, K. (2012). Assisted reproductive technologies and world religions: Implications for couples therapy. *Journal of Family Psychotherapy, 23,* 83–98. doi:10.1080/08975353.2012.679899

Cook, L. (2015). Where does gay America live? *U.S. News & World Report.* Retrieved from http://www.usnews.com/news/blogs/data-mine/2015/03/20/new-data-offer-picture-of-gay-america

Dahir, M. (2013). Women and sexuality. In E. Youngkin, M. Davis, D. Schadewald, & C. Juve (Eds.), *Women's health: A primary care clinical guide* (4th ed., pp. 119–149). Boston, MA: Pearson.

Dal'Ava, N., Bahamondes, L., Bahamondes, M., Santos, A., & Monteiro, I. (2012). Body weight and composition in users of levonorgestrel-releasing intrauterine system. *Contraception, 86*(2012), 350–353. doi:10.1016/j.contraception.2012.01.017

Darkness to Light. (2015). *Child sexual abuse statistics: The magnitude of the problem.* Retrieved from http://www.d2l.org/atf/cf/%7B64AF78C4-5EB8-45AA-BC28-F7EE2B581919%7D/Statistics_1_Magnitude.pdf

Darsareh, F., Taavoni, S., Joolaee, S., & Haghani, H. (2012). Effect of aromatherapy massage on menopausal symptoms: A randomized placebo-controlled clinical trial. *Menopause, 19*(9), 995–999. doi:10.1097/gme.0b013e318248ea16

Davis, S. R., Lambrinoudaki, I., Lumsden, M., Mishra, G. D., Pal, L., Rees, M., … Simoncini, T. (2015). *Nature Reviews Disease Primers: Menopause.* doi:10.1038/nrdp.2015.4

DeLemater, J. (2012). Sexual expression in later life: A review and synthesis. *Journal of Sex Research, 49*(2–3), 125–141. doi:10.1080/00224499.2011.603168

Drescher, J. (2015). Can sexual orientation be changed? *Journal of Gay and Lesbian Mental Health, 19*(1), 84–93, doi:10.1080/19359705.2014.944460

Durso, L. E., & Gates, G. J. (2012). *Serving our youth: Findings from a national survey of service providers working with lesbian, gay, bisexual, and transgender youth who are homeless or at risk of becoming homeless.* Los Angeles, CA: The Williams Institute with True Colors Fund and The Palette Fund.

Dziegielewski, S. F. (2015). *DSM-5 in action*. Hoboken, NJ: John Wiley & Sons.

Early, M. B. (2013). *Physical dysfunction practice skills for the occupational therapy assistant* (3rd ed., pp. 329–336). St. Louis, MO: Elsevier Mosby.

Edney, A., & Colby, L. (2015). *The female libido pill is no Viagra*. Retrieved from http://www.bloomberg.com/news/articles/2015-11-17/valeant-s-newest-problem-the-female-libido-pill-isn-t-selling

Eisenberg, E., & Brumbaugh, K. (Reviewers). (2012). *Infertility fact sheet*. Retrieved from http://www.womenshealth.gov/publications/our-publications/fact-sheet/infertility.html

Elder, J. A., & Braver, Y. (2010). *Female sexual dysfunction*. Retrieved from http://www.clevelandclinicmeded.com/medicalpubs/diseasemanagement/womens-health/female-sexual-dysfunction/

Elder, J. A., & Thacker, H. L. (2013). *Disease management: Menopause*. Retrieved from http://www.clevelandclinicmeded.com/medicalpubs/diseasemanagement/womens-health/menopause/

Epilepsy Foundation of Eastern Pennsylvania. (2015). *Women with epilepsy*. Retrieved from http://www.efepa.org/living-with-epilepsy/women-with-epilepsy/

Faubion, S. S., & Rullo, J. E. (2015). Sexual dysfunction in women: A practical approach. *American Family Physician, 92*(4), 281–288.

Faught, B. M. (2015, November). Female sexual dysfunction: Why is it so difficult to treat? *Women's Healthcare*, 46–48. Retrieved from http://npwomenshealthcare.com/wp-content/uploads/2015/10/WHNP_Nov15_FSH.pdf

FORGE. (2015). *Transgender rates of violence: Victim service providers' fact sheet #6*. Retrieved from http://forge-forward.org/wp-content/docs/FAQ-10-2012-rates-of-violence.pdf

Foster, V., Clark, P., Holstad, M., & Burgess, E. (2012). Factors associated with risky behaviors in older adults. *Journal of the Association of Nurses in AIDS Care, 23*(6), 487–499.

Fredericks, E. (2014). Short report: How family physicians can support discussions about menstrual issues. *Canadian Family Physician, 60*(3). Retrieved from http://www.ncbi.nlm.nih.gov/pmc/articles/PMC3952785/

Gallo, M., Lopez, L., Grimes, D., Schulz, K., & Helmerhorst, F. (2014). Combination contraceptives: Effects on weight. *Cochrane Database of Systematic Reviews* (Issue 1, Art. No. CD003987). doi:10.1002/14651858.CD003987.pub5

Gass, M., (2013). *Menopause*. Retrieved from http://www.merckmanuals.com/professional/gynecology-and-obstetrics/menopause/menopause

Genetic Science Learning Center. (2015a). *Genetic disorders*. Retrieved from http://learn.genetics.utah.edu/content/disorders/

Genetic Science Learning Center. (2015b). *Learn genetics: What are dominant and recessive?* Retrieved from http://learn.genetics.utah.edu/content/inheritance/patterns/

Gerber, D. (2014). Sexual problems. In B. A. Magowan, P. Owen, & A. Thomson (Eds.), *Clinical obstetrics and gynaecology* (3rd ed., pp. 191–202). Philadelphia, PA: Elsevier Health.

Girsen, A. I., Mayo, J. A., Carmichael, L. S., Phibbs, C. S., Shachar, B. Z., Stevenson, D. K., ... Gould, J. B. (2016). Women's prepregnancy underweight as a risk factor for preterm birth: A retrospective study. *BJOG: Journal of Obstetrics & Gynecology*, SN1471-0578. doi:10.1111/1471-0528.14027

GLAAD. (2015a). *GLAAD media reference guide: Transgender issues*. Retrieved from http://www.glaad.org/reference/transgender

GLAAD. (2015b). *Transgender FAQ*. Retrieved from http://www.glaad.org/transgender/transfaq

Gray, S .H. (2013). Menstrual disorders. *Pediatrics in Review, 34*(1). Retrieved from http://pedsinreview.aappublications.org/content/34/1/6

Greenwood Genetics Center. (2007). *Genetic counseling aids* (5th ed.). Greenwood, SC: Author.

Haas, A. P., Rodgers, P. L., & Herman, J. L. (2014). *Suicide attempts among transgender and gender non-conforming adults: Findings of the National Transgender Discrimination Survey*. Retrieved from http://williamsinstitute.law.ucla.edu/wp-content/uploads/AFSP-Williams-Suicide-Report-Final.pdf

Hain, D. (2013). Assessing older women's health. In E. Youngkin, M. Davis, D. Schadewald, & C. Juve (Eds.), *Women's health: A primary care clinical guide* (4th ed., pp. 119–149). Boston, MA: Pearson.

Halter, M. J. (2014). *Varcarolis' foundations of psychiatric health nursing* (7th ed.). St. Louis, MO: Elsevier Saunders.

Hellstrom, W. J., Montague, D. K., Moncada, I., Carson, C., Minhas, S., Faria, G., & Krishnamurti, S. (2010). Implants, mechanical devices, and vascular surgery for erectile dysfunction. *Journal of Sexual Medicine, 7*(1), 501–523.

Henry J. Kaiser Family Foundation. (2014). *Women's health policy: Sexual health of adolescents and young adults in the United States*. Retrieved from http://kff.org/womens-health-policy/fact-sheet/sexual-health-of-adolescents-and-young-adults-in-the-united-states/

Herdman, T. H. & Kamitsuru, S. (Eds.). *Nursing Diagnoses—Definitions and Classification 2015–2017*. Copyright © 2014, 1994–2014 NANDA International. Used by arrangement with John Wiley & Sons, Inc. Companion website: www.wiley.com/go/nursingdiagnoses

Hinkle, J. L., & Cheever, K. H. (2014). *Brunner and Suddarth's textbook of medical-surgical nursing*. Philadelphia, PA: Wolters Kluwer.

Hirsch, I. H. (2015a). *Erectile dysfunction*. Retrieved from http://www.merckmanuals.com/professional/genitourinary-disorders/male-sexual-dysfunction/erectile-dysfunction

Hirsch, I. H. (2015b). *Premature ejaculation*. Retrieved from https://www.merckmanuals.com/home/men's-health-issues/sexual-dysfunction-in-men/premature-ejaculation

Human Rights Campaign. (2015). *The lies and dangers of efforts to change sexual orientation or gender identity*. Retrieved from http://www.hrc.org/resources/entry/the-lies-and-dangers-of-reparative-therapy

Imparato, T., & Sanders, D. (2012). STD prevalence demands clinical awareness. *Aging Well, 5*(1), 14. Retrieved from http://www.todaysgeriatricmedicine.com/archive/012312p14.shtml

Inhorn, M. C., & Gürtin, Z. B. (2012). Infertility and assisted reproduction in the Muslim Middle East: Social, religious, and resource considerations. *Facts, Views, & Vision in ObGYN*, 24–29. Retrieved from http://www.fvvo.be/assets/265/04-Inhornetal.pdf

Jadav, S. P., & Pamar, D. M. (2012). Ulipristal acetate, a progesterone receptor modulator for emergency contraception. *Journal of Pharmacology and Pharmacotherapeutics, 3*(2), 109–111. doi:10.4103/0976-500X.95504

Joffe, H., Guthrie, K. A., LaCroix, A. Z., Reed, S. D., Ensrud, K. E., Manson, J. E., ... Cohen, L. (2014). Low-dose estradiol and the serotonin-norepinephrine reuptake inhibitor venlafaxine for vasomotor symptoms: A randomized clinical trial. *JAMA Internal Medicine, 174*(7), 1058–1066.

Juve, C. (2013). The menopausal transition. In E. Youngkin, M. Davis, D. Schadewald, & C. Juve (Eds.), *Women's health: A primary care clinical guide* (4th ed., pp. 425–459). Boston, MA: Pearson.

Kaplan, D. B., & Berkman, B. J. (2013). *Intimacy and the elderly*. Retrieved from http://www.merckmanuals.com/professional/geriatrics/social-issues-in-the-elderly/intimacy-and-the-elderly

Kapoor, D., Alderman, E., Davila, G. W., & Hiraoka, M. K. (2015). *Endometriosis clinical presentation*. Retrieved from http://emedicine.medscape.com/article/271899-clinical#b1

Karch, A. (2015). *Lippincott nursing drug guide*. Philadelphia, PA: Wolters Kluwer.

Karila, L., Wéry, A., Weinstein, A., Cottencin, O., Petit, A., Reynaud, M., & Billieux, J. (2014). Sexual addiction or hypersexual disorder: Different terms for the same problem? A review of the literature. *Current Pharmaceutical Design, 20*(25), 4012–4020.

Kee, J. L., Hayes, E. R., & McCuistion, L. E. (2015). *Pharmacology: A patient-centered nursing process approach* (8th ed., p. 847). St. Louis, MO: Elsevier Saunders.

Kim, M.-S., Lim, H.-J., Yang, H. J., Lee, M. S., Shin, B.-C., & Ernst, E. (2013). Ginseng for managing menopause symptoms: A systematic review of randomized clinical trials. *Journal of Ginseng Research, 37*(1), 30–36. http://doi.org/10.5142/jgr.2013.37.30

Kimmel, M., Milrod, C., & Kennedy, A. (2014). *Cultural encyclopedia of the penis*. London, United Kingdom: Rowman & Littlefield.

Kingsberg, S. A., & Woodard, T. (2015). Female sexual dysfunction: Focus on low desire. *Obstetrics and Gynecology, 125*(2), 477–486. Retrieved from https://medweb.nch.org/INTERMED/Data/ComponentFiles/1309/12_ABOG_May%202015.pdf

Koslov, D. S., & Andersson, K. E. (2013). Physiological and pharmacological aspects of the vas deferens—An update. *Frontiers in Pharmacology, 4*, 101.

Laan, E., Rellini, A. H., & Barnes, T. (2013). Standard operating procedures for female orgasmic disorder: Consensus of the International Society for Sexual Medicine. *Journal of Sexual Medicine, 10*(1), 74–82.

Lakin, M., & Wood, H. (2012). *Erectile dysfunction*. Retrieved from http://www.clevelandclinicmeded.com/medicalpubs/diseasemanagement/endocrinology/erectile-dysfunction/

Lamanna, M. A., Riedmann, A., & Stewart, S. D. (2014). *Marriages, families, and relationships: Making choices in a diverse society* (12th ed., pp. 102–104). Belmont, CA: Wadsworth.

Latif, E. Z., & Diamond, M. P. (2013). Arriving at the diagnosis of female sexual dysfunction. *Fertility and Sterility, 100*(4), 898–904.

Latthe, P., Champaneria, R., & Khan, K. (2012). Dysmenorrhea. *Clinical Evidence Handbook, 85*(4), 386–387. Retrieved from http://www.aafp.org/afp/2012/0215/p386.pdf

Laubach, J. M., Lorntson, R. P., & Forrest, D. E. (2013). Common gynecological pelvic disorders. In E. Youngkin, M. Davis, D. Schadewald, & C. Juve (Eds.), *Women's health: A primary care clinical guide* (4th ed., pp. 273–305). Boston, MA: Pearson.

Laughlin-Tommaso, S. K. (2015). *Bleeding after menopause: Is it normal?* Retrieved from http://www.mayoclinic.org/diseases-conditions/menopause/expert-answers/CON-20019726

Leach, M., & Moore, V. (2012). Black cohosh (Cimicifuga spp.) for menopausal symptoms. *Cochrane Database of Systematic Reviews* (Issue 9, Art. No. CD007244). doi:10.1002/14651858.CD007244.pub2

Levin, R. J. (2015). Anatomy and physiology in the male. In K. R. Wylie (Ed.), *ABC of sexual health* (3rd ed., pp. 7–11). Hoboken, NJ: John Wiley & Sons.

Levine, G., Steinke, E., Bakaeen, F., Bozkurt, B., Cheitlin, M., Conti, J., … Stewart, W. (2012). Sexual activity and cardiovascular disease: A scientific statement from the American Heart Association. *Circulation, 125,* 1058–1072. doi:10.1161/CIR.0b013e3182447787

Lindheim, S. R., Coyne, K., Avensu-Coker, L., O'Leary, K., Sinn, S., & Jaeger, A. (2014). The impact of assisted reproduction on sociocultural values and social norms. *Advances in Anthropology, 4,* 227–242. Retrieved from http://dx.doi.org/10.4236/aa.2014.44025

Lippi, G., Plebani, M., Montagnana, M., & Cervellin, G. (2012). Biochemical and genetic markers of erectile dysfunction. *Advances in Clinical Chemistry, 57,* 139–162.

Littleton-Gibbs, L. Y., & Engebretson, J. C. (2013). *Maternity nursing care* (2nd ed.). Clifton Park, NY: Delmar.

Lopushnyan, N. A., & Chitaley, K. (2012). Genetics of erectile dysfunction. *Journal of Urology, 188*(5), 1676–1683.

Louis, J. F., Thoma, M. E., Sørensen, D. N., McLain, A. C., King, R. B., Sundaram, R., … Buck Louis, G. M. (2013). The prevalence of couple infertility in the United States from a male perspective: Evidence from a nationally representative sample. *Andrology, 1*(5), 741–748. doi:10.1111/j.2047-2927.2013.00110.x

Lowdermilk, D. L., Perry, S. E., Cashion, K., & Alden, K. R. (2016). *Maternity and women's health care* (11th ed., pp. 184–185). St. Louis, MO: Elsevier.

Lowenstein, L., Mustafa, S., & Burke, Y. (2013). Pregnancy and normal sexual function: Are they compatible? *Journal of Sexual Medicine, 10,* 621–622.

Lundy, K. S., & James, S. (2016). *Community health nursing: Caring for the public's health* (3rd ed., p. 827). Burlington, MA: Jones and Bartlett.

March of Dimes. (2015). *Sex during pregnancy.* Retrieved from http://www.marchofdimes.org/pregnancy/sex-during-pregnancy.aspx

Mark, K. (2012). *What we can learn from sexual response cycles.* Retrieved from https://www.psychologytoday.com/blog/the-power-pleasure/201211/what-we-can-learn-sexual-response-cycles

Mayo Clinic. (2012). *Endometrial ablation.* Retrieved from http://www.mayoclinic.com/health/endometrial-ablation/MY01113

Mayo Clinic. (2013a). *Inguinal hernia: Causes.* Retrieved from http://www.mayoclinic.org/diseases-conditions/inguinal-hernia/basics/causes/con-20021456

Mayo Clinic. (2013b). *Sex therapy.* Retrieved from http://www.mayoclinic.org/tests-procedures/sex-therapy/basics/definition/prc-20020669

Mayo Clinic. (2013c). *Diseases and conditions: Klinefelter syndrome—Risk factors.* Retrieved from http://www.mayoclinic.org/diseases-conditions/klinefelter-syndrome/basics/risk-factors/con-20033637

Mayo Clinic. (2013d). *Diseases and conditions: Endometriosis.* Retrieved from http://www.mayoclinic.org/diseases-conditions/endometriosis/basics/definition/con-20013968

Mayo Clinic. (2014a). *Senior sex: Tips for older men.* Retrieved from http://www.mayoclinic.org/healthy-lifestyle/sexual-health/in-depth/senior-sex/art-20046465

Mayo Clinic. (2014b). *Sexual health and aging.* Retrieved from http://www.mayoclinic.org/healthy-lifestyle/sexual-health/in-depth/sexual-health/art-20046698?pg=1

Mayo Clinic. (2014c). *Enlarged breasts in men (gynecomastia).* Retrieved from http://www.mayoclinic.org/diseases-conditions/gynecomastia/basics/causes/con-20028710

Mayo Clinic. (2014d). *Disease and conditions: Infertility—Causes.* Retrieved from http://www.mayoclinic.org/diseases-conditions/infertility/basics/causes/con-20034770

Mayo Clinic. (2014e). *Infertility: Symptoms and causes.* Retrieved from http://www.mayoclinic.org/diseases-conditions/infertility/basics/causes/con-20034770

Mayo Clinic. (2014f). *Getting pregnant—Pregnancy after 35: Healthy moms, healthy babies.* Retrieved from http://www.mayoclinic.org/healthy-lifestyle/getting-pregnant/in-depth/pregnancy/art-20045756

Mayo Clinic. (2014g). *Tests and procedures: Oophorectomy (ovary removal surgery).* Retrieved from http://www.mayoclinic.org/tests-procedures/oophorectomy/basics/definition/prc-20012991

Mayo Clinic. (2014h). *Diseases and conditions: Menorrhagia (heavy menstrual bleeding).* Retrieved from http://www.mayoclinic.org/diseases-conditions/menorrhagia/basics/definition/con-20021959

Mayo Clinic. (2014i). *Diseases and conditions: Von Willebrand disease.* Retrieved from http://www.mayoclinic.org/diseases-conditions/von-willebrand-disease/basics/definition/con-20030195

Mayo Clinic. (2015a). *Painful intercourse (dyspareunia).* Retrieved from http://www.mayoclinic.org/diseases-conditions/painful-intercourse/basics/treatment/con-20033293

Mayo Clinic. (2015b). *Dense breast tissue: What it means to have dense breasts.* Retrieved from http://www.mayoclinic.org/tests-procedures/mammogram/in-depth/dense-breast-tissue/art-20123968?pg=2

Mayo Clinic. (2015c). *Healthy lifestyle: Pregnancy week by week.* Retrieved from http://www.mayoclinic.org/healthy-lifestyle/pregnancy-week-by-week/in-depth/sex-during-pregnancy/art-20045318?pg=2

Mayo Clinic. (2015d). *Test and procedures: Contraceptive implant—Risks.* Retrieved from http://www.mayoclinic.org/tests-procedures/contraceptive-implant/basics/risks/prc-20015073

Mayo Clinic. (2015e). *Getting pregnant: How does paternal age affect a baby's health?* Retrieved from http://www.mayoclinic.org/healthy-lifestyle/getting-pregnant/expert-answers/paternal-age/faq-20057873

Mayo Clinic. (2015f). *Diseases and conditions: Menopause.* Retrieved from http://www.mayoclinic.org/diseases-conditions/menopause/basics/definition/con-20019726

Mayo Clinic. (2015g). *Diseases and conditions: Hot flashes.* Retrieved from http://www.mayoclinic.org/diseases-conditions/hot-flashes/basics/definition/con-20034883

Mayo Clinic. (2015h). *Erectile dysfunction: Causes.* Retrieved from http://www.mayoclinic.org/diseases-conditions/erectile-dysfunction/basics/causes/con-20034244

Mayo Clinic. (2015i). *Premature ejaculation.* Retrieved from http://www.mayoclinic.org/diseases-conditions/premature-ejaculation/basics/definition/con-20031160

Mayo Clinic. (2015j). *Erectile dysfunction: Treatments and drugs.* Retrieved from http://www.mayoclinic.org/diseases-conditions/erectile-dysfunction/basics/treatment/con-20034244

Mayo Clinic. (2015k). *Papaverine (injection route).* Retrieved from http://www.mayoclinic.org/drugs-supplements/papaverine-injection-route/precautions/drg-20065314

Mayo Clinic. (2015l). *Premature ejaculation: Treatments and drugs.* Retrieved from http://www.mayoclinic.org/diseases-conditions/premature-ejaculation/basics/treatment/con-20031160

Mirone, V., & Fusco, F. (2015). Premature ejaculation. In V. Mirone (Ed.), *Clinical uro-andrology* (pp. 123–132). Berlin, Germany: Springer.

Molodysky, E., Liu, S.-P., Huang, S.-J., & Hsu, G.-L. (2013). Penile vascular surgery for treating erectile dysfunction: Current role and future direction. *Arab Journal of Urology, 11*(3), 254–266.

Moyer, V. (2012). Menopausal hormone therapy for the primary prevention of chronic conditions: U.S. Preventive Services Task Force recommendation statement. *Annals of Internal Medicine, 158*(1), 47–54.

National Cancer Institute. (n.d.). *Understanding prostate changes: A health guide for men.* Retrieved from http://www.cancer.gov/types/prostate/understanding-prostate-changes

National Cancer Institute. (2015a). *Human papillomavirus (HPV) vaccines.* Retrieved from http://www.cancer.gov/about-cancer/causes-prevention/risk/infectious-agents/hpv-vaccine-fact-sheet

National Cancer Institute. (2015b). *Understanding breast changes: A health guide for women.* Retrieved from http://www.cancer.gov/types/breast/understanding-breast-changes

National Center for Complementary and Integrative Health (NCCIH). (2016). *Menopausal symptoms: In depth.* Retrieved from https://nccih.nih.gov/health/menopause/menopausesymptoms

National Coalition of Anti-Violence Programs. (2014). *Lesbian, gay, bisexual, transgender, queer, and HIV-affected hate violence in 2013.* Retrieved from http://avp.org/storage/documents/2013_ncavp_hvreport_final.pdf

National Institutes of Health (NIH). (n.d.). *National Human Genome Research Institute: Talking glossary of genetic terms.* Retrieved from http://www.genome.gov/Glossary/index.cfm?id=70

National Institutes of Health (NIH). (2013). *Research Portfolio Online Reporting Tools (RePORT): Human Genome Project.* Retrieved from http://report.nih.gov/nihfactsheets/ViewFactSheet.aspx?csid=45

Neithercott, T. (2012). Sex and diabetes. *Diabetes Forecast, 65,* 48–51.

Nelson, C. J., Brock, D., & Dean, R. C. (2014). Delayed ejaculation and orgasm. In J. P. Mulhall & W. Hsiao (Eds.), *Men's sexual health and fertility* (pp. 145–158). New York, NY: Springer.

North American Menopause Society. (2012a). *KEEPS report.* Retrieved from http://www.menopause.org/annual-meetings/2012-meeting/keeps-report

North American Menopause Society. (2012b). The 2012 hormone therapy position statement of the North American Menopause Society. *Menopause, 19*(3), 257–271. doi:10.1097/gme.0b013e31824b970a

North American Menopause Society. (2013). *NAMS and USPSTF statements consistent.* Retrieved from http://www.menopause.org/publications/other-resources/nams-and-uspstf-statements-consistent

North American Menopause Society. (2015). Nonhormonal management of menopause-associated vasomotor symptoms: 2015 position statement of the North American Menopause

Society. *Menopause: The Journal of the North American Menopause Society, 22*(11). doi:10.1097/GME.0000000000000546

Office of Population Research at Princeton University & Association of Reproductive Health Professionals (ARHP). (2015). *The emergency contraception website*. Retrieved from http://ec.princeton.edu/index.html

Office on Women's Health, U.S. Department of Health and Human Services. (2014a). *Menstruation and the menstrual cycle fact sheet*. Retrieved from http://www.womenshealth.gov/publications/our-publications/fact-sheet/menstruation.html

Office on Women's Health, U.S. Department of Health and Human Services. (2014b). *Endometriosis*. Retrieved from http://www.womenshealth.gov/publications/our-publications/fact-sheet/endometriosis.html

Office on Women's Health, U.S. Department of Health and Human Services. (2014c). *Chlamydia*. Retrieved from http://www.womenshealth.gov/publications/our-publications/fact-sheet/chlamydia.html#

Options for Sexual Health. (2012). *Continuous extended use of combined hormonal contraceptives*. Retrieved from https://www.optionsforsexualhealth.org/birth-control-pregnancy/birth-control-options/hormonal-methods/combined-hormonal-contraceptives/cont

Options for Sexual Health. (2013). *Using the pill*. Retrieved from https://www.optionsforsexualhealth.org/birth-control-pregnancy/birth-control-options/hormonal-methods/combined-hormonal-contraceptives/using-pill

Pinkerton, J. V. (2015a). *Dysmenorrhea*. Retrieved from http://www.merckmanuals.com/professional/gynecology-and-obstetrics/menstrual-abnormalities/dysmenorrhea

Pinkerton, J. V. (2015b). *Dysfunctional uterine bleeding (DUB)*. Retrieved from http://www.merckmanuals.com/professional/gynecology-and-obstetrics/menstrual-abnormalities/dysfunctional-uterine-bleeding-(dub)

Planned Parenthood. (2014). *Understanding sexual pleasure*. Retrieved from https://www.plannedparenthood.org/learn/sexuality/understanding-sexual-pleasure

Planned Parenthood of the Heartland. (2015). *Transgender identity*. Retrieved from https://www.plannedparenthood.org/planned-parenthood-heartland/transgender-identity

Potts, J. M. (2012). Sexual dysfunction. In J. M. Potts (Ed.), *Essential urology: A guide to clinical practice* (2nd ed., pp. 259–276). New York, NY: Humana Press.

Powell, J. E., Henders, A. K., McRae, A. F., Kim, J., Hemani, G., Martin, N. G., …Visscher, P. M. (2013). Congruence of additive and non-additive effects on gene expression estimated from pedigree and SNP data. *PLoS Genetics, 9*(5). doi:10.1371/journal.pgen.1003502

Poynten, I., Grulich, A., & Templeton, D. (2013). Sexual transmitted infections in older populations. *Current Opinion in Infectious Disease, 26*(1), 80–85. doi:10.1097/QCO.0b013e32835c2173

Practice Committee of the American Society for Reproductive Medicine. (2012). Endometriosis and infertility: A committee opinion. *ASRM Pages, 98*(3). doi:10.1016/l.fertnstert.2012.05.031

PUAH Institute. (2015). *Collecting sperm according to halacha*. Retrieved from http://www.puahonline.org/infertility-info

Puppo, G., & Puppo, V. (2016). U.S. Food and Drug Administration approval of Addyi (flibanserin) for treatment of hypoactive sexual desire disorder. *European Urology, 69*, 376–380.

Rape, Abuse, and Incest National Network. (n.d.). *Child sexual abuse*. Retrieved from https://rainn.org/get-information/types-of-sexual-assault/child-sexual-abuse

Rellini, A. H., & Clifton, J. (2011). Female orgasmic disorder. In R. Balon (Ed.), *Sexual dysfunction: Beyond the brain-body connection*. Basel, Switzerland: Karger.

Satterwhite, C. (2013). *CDC expert commentary: Talking to adolescents and young adults about sexuality* [Podcast]. Retrieved from http://www.medscape.com/viewarticle/782515

Sech, L., Segall-Gutierrez, P., Silverstein, E., & Mishell, D. (2015). *Oral contraceptives*. Retrieved from http://www.merckmanuals.com/professional/gynecology-and-obstetrics/family-planning/oral-contraceptives

Shams, T., Firwana, B., Habib, F., Alshahrani, A., Alnouh, B., Murad, M. H., & Ferwana, M. (2014). SSRIs for hot flashes: A systematic review and meta-analysis of randomized trials. *Journal of General Internal Medicine, 29*(1), 204–213.

Sharma, R., Biedenharn, K. R., Fedor, J. M., & Agarwal, A. (2014). Lifestyle factors and reproductive health: Taking control of your fertility. *Reproductive Biology and Endocrinology, 11*, 66. doi:10.1186/1477-7827-11-66

Shifren, J. L., Monz, B. U., Russo, P. A., Segreti, A., & Johannes, C. B. (2008). Sexual problems and distress in United States women: Prevalence and correlates. *Obstetrics and Gynecology, 112*(5), 970–978.

Shindel, A. W., & Goldstein, I. (2015). Sexual function and dysfunction in the female. In A. J. Wein, L. R. Kavoussi, A. W. Partin, & C. A. Peters (Eds.), *Campbell-Walsh urology* (11th ed.). Philadelphia, PA: Elsevier.

Spadt, S. K., Iorio, J., Fariello, J. Y., & Whitmore, K. E. (2012). Vaginal dilation: When it's indicated and tips on teaching it. *OBG Management, 24*(12). Retrieved from http://www.obgmanagement.com/home/article/vaginal-dilation-when-its-indicated-and-tips-on-teaching-it/daa4d1b01f8149a4ffa0425320407e31.html

Spector, R. E. (2017). *Cultural diversity in health and illness* (9th ed.). Hoboken, NJ: Pearson Education.

Stahlman, J., Britto, M., Fitzpatrick, S., McWhirter, C., Testino, S. A., Brennan, J. J., & Zumbrunnen, T. L. (2012). Serum testosterone levels in non-dosed females after secondary exposure to 1.62% testosterone gel: Effects of clothing barrier on testosterone absorption. *Current Medical Research and Opinion, 28*(2), 291–301.

Stewart, A., & Graham, S. (2013, April). Sexual risk behavior among older adults. *Clinical Advisor, 28*, 32, 34, 38.

Stuenkel, C., Gass, M., Manson, J., Lobo, R., Pal, L., Rebar, R., & Hall, J. (2012). A decade after the Women's Health Initiative—The experts do agree. *Menopause, 19*(8), 1–2. doi:10.1097/gme.0b013e31826226f2

Sudtelgte, C. (2012). Prenatal care. In V. Berghella (Ed.), *Obstetric evidence-based guidelines* (2nd ed., pp. 12–26). London, UK: Informa Healthcare.

Sunderam, S., Kissin, D. M., Flowers, L., Anderson, J. E., Folger, S. G., Jamieson, D. J., & Barfield, W. D. (2012). Assisted reproductive technology surveillance—United States, 2009. *Surveillance Summaries, 61*(SS7), 1–23. Retrieved from http://www.cdc.gov/mmwr/preview/mmwrhtml/ss6107a1.htm

Szilagyi, P. (2013). Assessing children: Infancy through adolescence. In L. Bickley & P. Szilagyi, *Bates' guide to physical examination and history taking* (11th ed., pp. 765–875). Philadelphia, PA: Wolters Kluwer/Lippincott Williams & Wilkins.

Townsend, M. C. (2015). *Psychiatric mental health nursing* (8th ed.) Philadelphia, PA: F. A. Davis.

United States Agency for International Development (USAID). (2012). Calendar rhythm method. In *Family planning: A global handbook for providers* (Ch. 17, Sec. 7). Retrieved from https://www.fphandbook.org/calendar-rhythm-method

University of California San Francisco Medical Center. (2016). *Sex during pregnancy*. Retrieved from http://www.ucsfhealth.org/education/sex_during_pregnancy/

University of Iowa Hospitals and Clinics. (2015). *Vasectomy reversals: Frequently asked questions*. Retrieved from https://www.uihealthcare.org/vasectomy-reversals-frequently-asked-questions/

University of Rochester Medical Center. (2015). *Phimosis and paraphimosis*. Retrieved from https://www.urmc.rochester.edu/Encyclopedia/Content.aspx?ContentTypeID=90&ContentID=P03104

Urology Care Foundation. (2015). *Urologic conditions: Vasectomy*. Retrieved from http://www.urologyhealth.org/urologic-conditions/vasectomy

U.S. Department of Justice, National Sex Offender Public Website. (n.d.). *Learn the warning signs: Recognizing sexual abuse*. Retrieved from https://www.nsopw.gov/en/education/recognizingsexualabuse?AspxAutoDetectCookieSupport=1

U.S. Food and Drug Administration (FDA). (2015a). *Male condoms and sexually transmitted diseases*. Retrieved from http://www.fda.gov/forpatients/illness/hivaids/prevention/ucm126372.htm

U.S. Food and Drug Administration (FDA). (2015b). *Drugs: Mifeprex (mifepristone) information*. Retrieved from http://www.fda.gov/Drugs/DrugSafety/PostmarketDrugSafetyInformationforPatientsandProviders/ucm111323.htm

U.S. Food and Drug Administration (FDA). (2015c). *FDA drug safety communication: FDA cautions about using testosterone products for low testosterone due to aging; requires labeling change to inform of possible increased risk of heart attack and stroke with use*. Retrieved from http://www.fda.gov/Drugs/DrugSafety/ucm436259.htm

U.S. National Library of Medicine. (2014a). *Urethritis*. Retrieved from https://www.nlm.nih.gov/medlineplus/ency/article/000439.htm

U.S. National Library of Medicine. (2014b). *About menstrual periods—primary*. Retrieved from https://www.nlm.nih.gov/medlineplus/ency/article/001218.htm

U.S. National Library of Medicine. (2014c). *About menstrual periods—secondary*. Retrieved from https://www.nlm.nih.gov/medlineplus/ency/article/001219.htm

U.S. National Library of Medicine. (2016a). Trisomy 13. *Genetics Home Reference*. Retrieved from http://ghr.nlm.nih.gov/condition/trisomy-13

U.S. National Library of Medicine. (2016b). Cri-du-chat syndrome. *Genetics Home Reference*. Retrieved from https://ghr.nlm.nih.gov/condition/cri-du-chat-syndrome

U.S. National Library of Medicine. (2016c). Trisomy 18. *Genetics Home Reference*. Retrieved from http://ghr.nlm.nih.gov/condition/trisomy-18

Valentine, M., & Gardella, J. (2013). Infertility. In E. Youngkin, M. Davis, D. Schadewald, & C. Juve (Eds.), *Women's health: A primary care clinical guide* (4th ed., pp. 273–305). Boston, MA: Pearson.

Vickery, Z., Madden, T., Zhao, Q., Secura, G. M., Allsworth, J. E., & Peipert, J. F. (2013). Weight change at 12 months in users of three progestin-only contraceptive methods. *Contraception, 88*(4), 503–508. doi:10.1016/j.contraception.2013.03.004

Walcker, B., & Pederson, C. (2013). Managing contraception and family planning. In E Q. Youngkin, M. S. Davis, D. M. Schadewald, & C. Juve (Eds.), *Women's health: A primary clinical guide* (4th ed., Ch. 12). Boston, MA: Pearson.

Ward, B. W., Dahlhamer, J. M., Galinsky, A. M., & Joestl, S. S. (2014, July 15). Sexual orientation and health among U.S. adults: National Health Interview Survey, 2013. *National Health Statistics Reports, 77*. Retrieved from http://www.cdc.gov/nchs/data/nhsr/nhsr077.pdf

Weiner, L., & Avery-Clark, C. (2014). Sensate focus: Clarifying the Masters and Johnson's model. *Sexual and Relationship Therapy, 29*(3), 307–319.

Weisberg, E. (2012). A chewable low-dose oral contraceptive: A new birth control option? *Patient Preference and Adherence, 6*, 355–360. doi:10.2147/PPA.S20661

Wespes, E. (2015). Anatomy and physiology of male erectile function. In V. Mirone (Ed.), *Clinical uro-andrology* (pp. 3–14). Berlin, Germany: Springer.

Wilson, B., Shannon, M., & Shields, K. (2013). *Pearson nurse's drug guide 2013*. Upper Saddle River, NJ: Pearson.

Wincze, J. P., & Weisberg, R. B. (2015). *Sexual dysfunction* (3rd ed.). New York, NY: Guilford Press.

Women's Health Initiative. (n.d.). *The estrogen-plus-progestin study*. Retrieved from https://www.nhlbi.nih.gov/whi/estro_pro.htm

World Association of Sexual Health. (2013). *Declaration of sexual rights*. Retrieved from http://www.worldsexology.org/resources/declaration-of-sexual-rights/

World Health Organization (WHO). (2013a). *Defining sexual health*. Retrieved from http://www.who.int/reproductivehealth/topics/sexual_health/sh_definitions/en/index.html

World Health Organization (WHO). (2013b). *Gender and human rights: Sexual health*. Retrieved from http://www.who.int/reproductivehealth/topics/gender_rights/sexual_health/en/

World Health Organization (WHO). (2015a). *Sexual and reproductive health: Infertility definitions and terminology*. Retrieved from http://www.who.int/reproductivehealth/topics/infertility/definitions/en/

World Health Organization (WHO). (2015b). *Sexually transmitted infections: Fact sheet No. 110*. Retrieved from http://www.who.int/mediacentre/factsheets/fs110/en/

Ye, Y., Wang, Z., Zhuo, S., Lu, W., Liao, H., Verbruggen, M., … Su, Y. (2012). Soy germ isoflavones improve menopausal symptoms but have no effect on blood lipids in early menopausal Chinese women: A randomized placebo-controlled trial. *Menopause, 19*(7), 791–798. doi:10.1097/gam.0b013e31823dbeda

Zieman, M., Hatcher, R. A., Allen, A. Z., Lathrop, E., & Haddad, L. (2016). *Managing contraception*. Atlanta, GA: Bridging the Gap Communications.

Zunner, B. P., & Grace, P. J. (2012). The ethical nursing care of transgender patients: An exploration of bias in health care and how it affects this population. *American Journal of Nursing, 112*(12), 61–64.

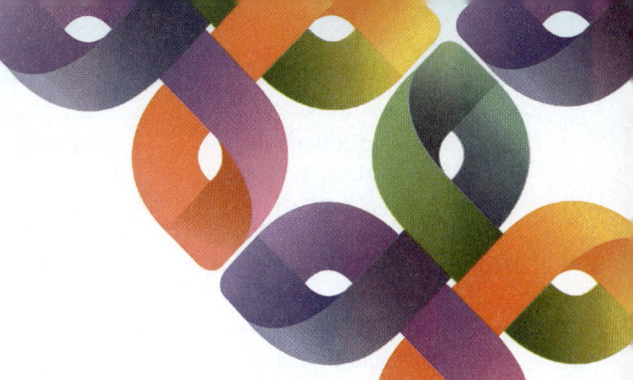

Module 20
Thermoregulation

Module Outline and Learning Outcomes

The Concept of Thermoregulation

Normal Thermoregulation

20.1 Analyze the physiology of thermoregulation.

Alterations to Thermoregulation

20.2 Differentiate among alterations in thermoregulation.

Concepts Related to Thermoregulation

20.3 Outline the relationship between thermoregulation and other concepts.

Health Promotion

20.4 Explain the promotion of thermoregulation.

Nursing Assessment

20.5 Differentiate among common assessment procedures and tests used to examine thermoregulation.

Independent Interventions

20.6 Analyze independent interventions nurses can implement for patients with alterations in thermoregulation.

Collaborative Therapies

20.7 Summarize collaborative therapies used by interprofessional teams for patients with alterations in thermoregulation.

Lifespan Considerations

20.8 Differentiate considerations related to the care of patients with alterations in thermoregulation across the lifespan.

Thermoregulation Exemplars

Exemplar 20.A Hyperthermia

20.A Analyze hyperthermia as it relates to thermoregulation.

Exemplar 20.B Hypothermia

20.B Analyze hypothermia as it relates to thermoregulation.

≫ The Concept of Thermoregulation

Concept Key Terms

Afebrile, **1538**	Chemical thermogenesis, **1538**	Febrile, **1538**	Hypothermia, **1538**	Normothermia, **1538**
Basal metabolic rate (BMR), **1538**	Conduction, **1538**	Fever, **1538**	Malignant hyperthermia, **1541**	Radiation, **1538**
Brown adipose tissue (BAT), **1547**	Convection, **1538**	Heat balance, **1537**	Neutral thermal environment (NTE), **1548**	Thermoregulation, **1537**
	Evaporation, **1538**	Heat transfer, **1538**		
		Hyperthermia, **1538**		

Thermoregulation is the body process that balances heat production and heat loss to maintain the body's temperature. It is measured in heat units called degrees. The body's surface temperature—the temperature of the skin, subcutaneous tissues, and fat—fluctuates in response to environmental factors and is therefore unreliable for monitoring a patient's health status. Nurses and other healthcare providers should monitor core body temperatures (or the deep tissues of the body) for a more reliable assessment. The body's core temperature remains relatively constant at about 37°C, or 98.6°F.

Normal Thermoregulation

The body's surface temperature rises and falls in response to the environment. However, the body's core temperature remains within a small range. The body continually produces heat as a by-product of metabolism. When the amount of heat produced by the body equals the amount of heat lost, the individual's body temperature remains within the normal range, and the individual is in **heat balance** (see **Figure 20–1 ≫**). If the body produces more heat than is lost, the

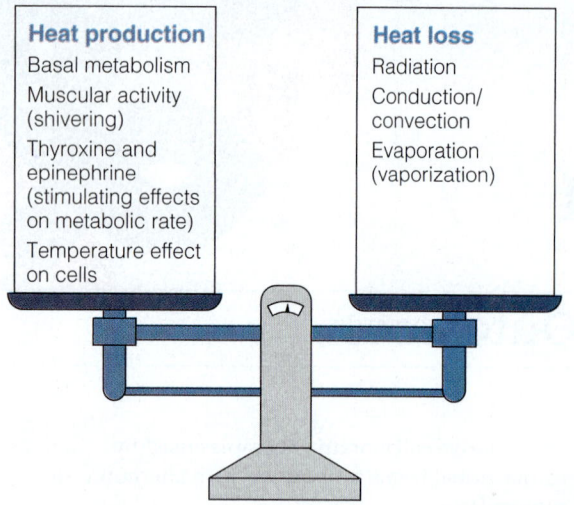

Heat production	Heat loss
Basal metabolism	Radiation
Muscular activity (shivering)	Conduction/ convection
Thyroxine and epinephrine (stimulating effects on metabolic rate)	Evaporation (vaporization)
Temperature effect on cells	

Source: From Marieb, E. N., & Hoehn, K. (2012). *Human anatomy and physiology,* (9th ed.). San Francisco, CA: Benjamin Cummings. Reprinted and Electronically reproduced by permission of Pearson Education, Inc., New York, NY.

Figure 20–1 》 As long as heat production and heat loss are properly balanced, body temperature remains constant. Factors contributing to heat production (and temperature rise) are shown on the left side of the scale; those contributing to heat loss (and temperature fall) are shown on the right side of the scale.

patient exhibits **hyperthermia**. If more heat is lost than is produced, the patient exhibits **hypothermia**.

A number of factors affect the body's heat production. The most important are these five:

1. ***Basal metabolic rate (BMR).*** The **basal metabolic rate (BMR)** is the rate of energy the body uses to maintain essential activities such as breathing. Metabolic rates decrease with age. In general, the younger the individual, the higher the BMR.
2. ***Muscle activity.*** Muscle activity, including shivering, increases the metabolic rate. All muscle activity produces heat.
3. ***Thyroxine output.*** Increased thyroxine levels cause an increase in the release of epinephrine, which, in turn, increases vasoconstriction and accelerates the cellular metabolic rate throughout the body (Huether, Rodway, & DeFriez, 2014). This effect is called **chemical thermogenesis** and is defined as the stimulation of heat production in the body through increased cellular metabolism.
4. ***Epinephrine, norepinephrine, and sympathetic stimulation/stress response.*** These hormones are neurotransmitters that mount a sympathetic nervous system response that can immediately increase the rate of cellular metabolism in many body tissues. Epinephrine and norepinephrine directly affect liver and muscle cells, thereby increasing cellular metabolism.
5. ***Fever.*** **Fever** is a protective immune response to foreign antigens within the body that causes an increase in the cellular metabolic rate that further increases the body's temperature.

To be able to predict how patients of all ages and clinical status will react to their thermal environment, the nurse should know the four ways in which **heat transfer** takes place from one place or object to another:

1. **Conduction** is the process of heat transfer through physical contact of one surface with another surface. For example, if a newborn is placed on a metal changing table, the heat from the baby would transfer to that surface, making the baby's body colder.
2. **Convection** is the process of heat transfer through the fluid motion of air or water across the skin. For example, in aquatic exercises, water flows against the moving body, and if the water is colder than the body, heat from the body is transferred to the water. To maintain body heat, the individual must keep moving.
3. **Radiation** is the process of heat transfer with no physical contact. Sunshine transfers heat to individuals enjoying the warm outdoors.
4. **Evaporation** is the process of converting water to a vapor. The evaporation of sweat, in which the heat in the sweat is transferred to the air, is a natural process to cool a heated body (Huether et al., 2014).

The system that regulates body temperature has three primary components: sensors, the hypothalamus, and an effector system that adjusts the production and loss of heat. Most sensors or sensory receptors are in the skin. The skin has more receptors for cold than warmth; therefore, skin sensors detect cold more efficiently than warmth.

When the body's skin becomes chilled, three physiologic processes occur as the body attempts to regulate its temperature: (1) Shivering increases heat production, (2) sweating is inhibited to decrease heat loss, and (3) vasoconstriction decreases heat loss.

The preoptic area of the hypothalamus is the center that controls the core temperature. When the sensors in the hypothalamus detect heat, they send out signals to reduce the body's temperature, that is, to decrease heat production and increase heat loss. In contrast, when the cold sensors are stimulated, they send out signals to increase heat production and decrease heat loss.

Alterations to Thermoregulation
Alterations and Manifestations

The usual range of core body temperature is called **normothermia**. The normal range for adults is between 36° and 38.5°C (96.8° and 101.3°F). The two primary alterations in body temperature are hyperthermia and hypothermia. Note that hyperthermia is a general term that refers to a body temperature of 38.5°C (101.3°F) and above. However, this general term applies to two categories based on clinical etiology. Fever relates to the body's controlled response to infection or other disease process that includes increasing the temperature set point of the body. The patient who has a fever is described as **febrile**; one who does not is **afebrile**. In contrast, when the term hyperthermia is used clinically, it usually refers to the body being unable to control body temperature due to exposure to excess heat as described below.

Heat-related injuries may occur with even moderate increases in temperatures (38.3–38.9°C, or 101–102°F). Heat-related illnesses or injuries include *heat exhaustion* and *heat stroke*. Heat exhaustion is defined as loss of body fluid volume caused by loss of both body fluid and salt. This low-volume state places the individual in a severe hypovolemic state beyond the body's ability to compensate for its volume deficit. As a consequence, the individual experiences low blood pressure, weakness, and in some cases, loss of consciousness.

Heat stroke occurs because of high environmental temperatures in combination with high humidity. The combination of these two environmental factors results in dysfunction of the brain's thermoregulation center. The body loses the ability to cool through sweat, and the skin becomes dry and flushed. The body's core temperature increases significantly, which may result in vascular collapse, cerebral edema, central nervous system dysfunction, organ failure, and death. Signs and symptoms of heat-related injuries include paleness, dizziness, nausea and vomiting, fatigue, low blood pressure, muscle cramps, and fainting. Late signs include irritability, confusion, stupor, and coma.

Hypothermia is a core body temperature below 35°C (95°F). Hypothermia can be classified as mild, 32–35°C (89.6–95°F); moderate, 28–32°C (82.4–89.6°F), or severe, below 28°C (less than 82.4°F). The body can tolerate temperatures as low as 33°C (91.4°F) in controlled situations such as surgery. Temperatures of 28°C (82.4°F) or lower can cause cell, tissue, and organ destruction (see **Figure 20–2 >>**). The three physiologic mechanisms of hypothermia are (1) excessive heat loss, (2) inadequate heat production to counteract heat loss, and (3) impaired hypothalamic thermoregulation.

SAFETY ALERT Extremely high temperatures of 41–43°C (105.8–109.4°F) cause cell protein coagulation, cell death, and irreversible brain damage. Uncontrolled hypothermic temperatures of 35°C (95.0°F) and below can cause vasoconstriction and lead to ischemic injuries.

Prevalence

Fever is the most common symptom among the 28 million pediatric patients seen in emergency departments annually. The most common cause of fever in children is infection. Common infections in children that produce a rise in the body temperature are colds, gastroenteritis, ear infections, croup, bronchiolitis, and urinary tract infections (Ward, 2013).

Between 2006 and 2010, approximately 3500 Americans died of heat-related injuries (Berko et al., 2014). Non-Hispanic, African American men age 75 and older had the highest heat-related mortality rate compared to women, other age groups, and other ethnicities (Berko et al., 2014).

The very young, the very old, and individuals with chronic medical conditions are the most susceptible to heat-related injuries and deaths (Centers for Disease Control and Prevention, 2013a). Heat-related injuries are preventable (Centers for Disease Control and Prevention, 2013b), yet individuals who participate in sports during the hot and humid summer months often become victims of hyperthermia. High school athletes lose an estimated 9000 days of playing time each year due to heat-related illnesses. Nonfatal high school football heat-related illnesses occur at 10–11 times the rate of all other heat-related high school sports illnesses, and lost days occur at a rate 8 times greater for high school football athletes than for eight other high school sports (Krohn, Sikka, & Olson, 2015).

In the United States, an average of 37 children die from heatstroke each year after being left in a closed vehicle. Even

Thermoregulation	Temperature	
	°C	°F
Hyperthermia	41.2	106.1
Heat stroke >41.1°C, 106°F	41.0	105.8
	40.8	105.4
	40.6	105.1
	39.2	102.6
	39.0	102.2
Heat exhaustion 38.3–38.9°C, 101–102°F	38.8	101.8
Fever >38.5°C, 101.4°F	38.6	101.5
	38.4	101.1
	38.2	100.8
	37.4	99.3
Normothermia	37.2	99.0
36–38.5°C,	37.0	98.6
96.8–101.3°F	36.8	98.2
	36.6	97.9
	36.4	97.5
	35.4	95.7
	35.2	95.4
	35.0	95.0
	34.8	94.6
	34.6	94.3
	34.4	93.9
	34.2	93.6
	34.0	93.2
Mild hypothermia	32.8	91.0
32–35°C,	32.6	90.7
89.6–95°F	32.4	90.3
	32.2	90.0
	32.0	89.6
	31.2	88.2
	31.0	87.8
	30.8	87.4
	30.6	87.1
	30.4	86.7
Moderate hypothermia	30.2	86.4
28–32°C,	30.0	86.0
82.4–89.6°F	29.8	85.6
	28.2	82.8
	28.0	82.4
	27.8	82.0
	27.6	81.7
Severe hypothermia	27.4	81.3
below 28°C, 82.4°F	27.2	81.0
	27.0	80.6

Figure 20–2 >> Terms used to describe alterations in body temperature (oral measurements) and ranges in Celsius (centigrade) and Fahrenheit scales. The 〰️ lines in the temperature columns reflect where temperatures were skipped.

mild temperatures in the 70s can cause death because the vehicle's interior temperature rises rapidly when all windows are closed (Null, 2016). Cellular dysfunction occurs at extremely high temperatures, releasing intracellular fluid into the circulation. Excess fluid causes increased blood flow to peripheral circulation as the heart works harder to pump additional fluid into circulation. Overwhelmed, the heart reaches the point when it can no longer meet the demands of the body. Cardiac output diminishes, causing collapse of the vasculature, end organ failure, and death (Kuska, 2012). See **Box 20–1 »** for more information on vehicle safety and heat-related injuries.

Between 2006 and 2010, more than 7000 deaths in the United States were attributed to cold exposure (Berko et al., 2014). Similar to heat-related deaths, most individual who died of cold weather–related deaths were non-Hispanic, African American men, age 75 and older (Berko et al., 2014). Berko and colleagues (2014) concluded that the incidence of both heat- and cold-related deaths is associated with age of greater than 75, lower income, and lack of alternatives to extreme hot or cold conditions. The individuals are often uninsured (Hughes, 2016) and tend to be socially isolated (Meiman, Anderson, & Tomasallo, 2015).

Genetic Considerations

Considerable progress has been made recently in identifying causative genes for hereditary periodic fever syndromes. These are rare clinical conditions characterized by short but repeated fevers and severe localized inflammation. Diagnosis depends on ruling out the usual childhood infections. The good news for patients is that, even without treatment, over

Box 20–1
Vehicle Safety and Heat-Related Injuries

More than 500 children died from vehicle hyperthermia between 1998 and 2012. Estimates indicate that annually hundreds of children sustain heat exhaustion, heat stroke, and thermal burns after being left in vehicles on warm days (Kuska, 2012). Leaving a child in a car with a cracked window for even a short amount of time holds the potential for lethal consequences (Duzinski et al., 2012). The National Highway Transportation Safety Administration, KidsandCars.org, and other organizations recommend several strategies to reduce the risk for heat-related illness in a vehicle, including the following (KidsandCars.org, n.d.; NHTSA, n.d.):

- Caregivers should always "Look before you lock!" Vehicles should always be locked in driveways, garages, and when not in use.
- Caregivers should place something they need (e.g., wallet, cell phone) in the back seat to ensure they check the back seat before leaving the vehicle.
- Caregivers should never leave children unattended in or around vehicles. They should store keys out of reach.
- If you see a child alone in a vehicle, call 911 immediately.

Alterations and Therapies
Thermoregulation

ALTERATION	DESCRIPTION	INTERVENTIONS AND THERAPIES
Hyperthermia	Increase in temperature as a result of more heat produced than lost	- Monitor vital signs. - Assess skin color and temperature. - Monitor EKG, white blood cell count, hematocrit value, and other pertinent laboratory reports for indication of infection or dehydration. - Reduce coverings (e.g., clothing, blankets) to allow heat loss. - Lower the room temperature. - Administer antipyretic medications. - Increase fluid intake, and provide adequate nutrition. - Measure intake and output. - Reduce physical activity to limit heat production. - Provide oral hygiene to keep mucous membranes moist. - Administer a tepid sponge bath to increase heat loss through convection. - Provide dry clothing and bed linens if the patient is perspiring. - Use a hypothermia blanket.
Hypothermia	Decrease in body temperature as a result of more heat lost than produced	- Monitor vital signs. - Assess skin color and temperature. - Apply warm blankets or warm clothing. - Provide a warm environment. - Provide dry clothing if heat loss is due to evaporation. - Keep limbs close to the body. - Cover the head with a cap or turban. - Use a hyperthermia blanket. - Administer warmed oral or intravenous (IV) fluids. - Use heat lamps, hot water bottles, or a heating pad.

time the fevers do not return. Also, patients can continue normal daily activities between episodes (Shinawi, 2013).

Malignant hyperthermia is a potentially fatal, inherited disorder that results from the body's reaction to inhalation of volatile anesthetic gases and succinylcholine, a depolarizing neuromuscular blocker. This interaction produces an increase in intercellular calcium that results in severe ongoing muscle contraction and massive oxygen and adenosine triphosphate (ATP) consumption that leads to acidosis and an increase in body temperature of approximately 1°C every 5 minutes as a result of sustained hypermetabolism (Huether et al., 2014). Cardiac dysrhythmias, hypotension, hypoxemia, hyperkalemia, central nervous system symptoms, renal injury or failure, coma and cardiac arrest follow (Huether et al., 2014). Since the introduction of dantrolene, a skeletal muscle relaxant, mortality rates associated with malignant hypertension have fallen below 5%; however, morbidity rates remain close to 35% (Kim, 2012).

There are two methods of screening for malignant hyperthermia: genetic testing and muscle biopsy also known as the caffeine halothane contracture test (CHCT). Early recognition of signs and symptoms is essential to early interventions and treatments in order to minimize potential permanent injury.

》Stay Current: Visit the website of the Malignant Hyperthermia Association of the United States at http://www.mhaus.org to learn more about the condition, testing for it, and how to manage a malignant hyperthermia crisis.

Case Study 》 Part 1

Caleb Kleinlein is a 30-year-old businessman who returned from a trip to South Africa 2 weeks ago. He has come into the physician's office today with complaints of fever and general malaise. As the intake nurse, you perform an assessment that includes taking his temperature. Mr. Kleinlein has a temperature of 38.6°C (101.5°F). He has not taken any medication for the fever today. Mr. Kleinlein tells you that he has no allergies to any medication and he prefers to take ibuprofen when he has a fever. History reveals that Mr. Kleinlein has had this fever for 3 days and has been unable to eat or drink as he normally would. The physician prescribes ibuprofen 800 mg every 6 hours, increased fluid intake, and rest.

Clinical Reasoning Questions Level I

1. What precautions should Mr. Kleinlein use to prevent side effects when taking ibuprofen?
2. If Mr. Kleinlein's fever gets higher, what should he do?

Clinical Reasoning Questions Level II

3. What education should you give to Mr. Kleinlein about management of his fever?
4. What symptoms of dehydration should you educate Mr. Kleinlein about? What advice should you give to prevent a fluid volume deficit?

Concepts Related to Thermoregulation

Infectious and inflammatory processes can cause fever, and uncontrolled hyperthermia, as seen in heat-related injuries, and can quickly result in dehydration. Both hyperthermia and hypothermia can affect patient comfort levels. The concept of thermoregulation extends to those at risk for hypo- and hyperthermia based on age and developmental factors that may increase risk for injury due to environmental extremes. Individuals diagnosed with a neurocognitive disorder such as dementia or with a severe mental illness may have a diminished ability to detect environmental changes, which may increase their risk for weather-related injuries. Individuals who are homeless or living in substandard housing are also vulnerable to injuries caused by extreme temperatures. Thermoregulation is an important public health concept for which communities, cities, municipalities, and states can develop and promote initiatives to minimize the effects of extreme temperatures on those who do not have the means to alter their environment for their own safety. The following feature links some, but not all, of the concepts related to thermoregulation. They are presented in alphabetical order.

Health Promotion

Health promotion for thermoregulation gives individuals and communities the knowledge and ability to implement and to develop initiatives that decrease the risks associated with hyperthermic and hypothermic injuries and weather-related deaths.

Hyperthermia

Awareness of the harmful combination of hot weather, high humidity, and dehydration reduces the risk of heat-related injuries: heat cramps, heat exhaustion, and heat stroke. Factors that increase the risk of heat-related injuries include age; obesity; medication; unfamiliarity with the climate; and high heat index, the combination of high temperature and high humidity. Individuals require structured health-promotion education, education reminders, reinforcements from healthcare providers, and promotional cues in mass and social media to maintain thermoregulation.

Schools, colleges, workplaces, communities, businesses, local health departments, and the government can promote thermoregulation health by providing cooling stations, shaded areas, and frequent and easy unrestricted access to fluids in high temperatures. Athletes and those who work outdoors—farmers, roofers, construction workers, lawn technicians, and others—are at increased risk for excessive heat exposure and heat-related injuries. Overexposure to heat and heat-related injuries results not only in illness but also in loss of productivity. Researchers (Singh, Hanna, & Kjellstrom, 2015) have explored the following outdoor health promotion initiatives to reduce heat-related injuries: rescheduling shifts to cooler times of the day; splitting shifts to limit heat exposure during the hottest times of the day; and promoting/providing active rehydration practices, cooling stations, lighter colored and light textured uniforms, ice vests, and frequent breaks.

Managers, teachers, parents, caregivers, coaches, athletes, and even children should be knowledgeable of the signs and symptoms of hyperthermia and appropriate actions that should be taken to promote safety in high-heat conditions. In particular, caregivers should anticipate the needs of children, older adults, and those with chronic illnesses in order to promote and provide heat-related safety measures.

》Stay Current: The Centers for Disease Control and Prevention has a wealth of information and free materials on preventing, recognizing, and treating hyperthermia at http://www.cdc.gov/disasters/extremeheat

Concepts Related to
Thermoregulation

CONCEPT	RELATIONSHIP TO THERMOREGULATION	NURSING IMPLICATIONS
Accountability	Temperature measurement and recording are delegated to medical technicians and nursing assistants; however, the nurse remains responsible for reviewing the patient's temperature.	▪ Monitor patients' temperature as frequently as necessary to prevent significant deterioration of the patients' status. ▪ Interpret changes in temperature in relation to other vital signs, level of consciousness, and glucose level. ▪ Initiate early interventions as patients' temperature begins to drift out of the normal range.
Comfort	As temperature increases or decreases significantly, comfort level and tolerance of pain decrease.	▪ Assess temperature and treat symptoms to help keep patients comfortable.
Development	Infants are more susceptible to problems caused by temperature changes both within their bodies (infections) and in the outer environment (e.g., a car with the windows closed). Children tolerate a wider range of temperature than infants. From puberty until old age, patients have fewer problems with temperature changes. After age 75, patients have an increased risk of hypothermia.	▪ Know the important role that age plays in temperature regulation; monitor patients at greater risk more often. ▪ Teach home care monitoring and basic treatment of symptoms to caregivers of infants, children, and older adults. ▪ Teach adults about vehicle safety with regard to children (see Box 20–1).
Fluids and Electrolytes	Increased temperature leads to increased sweating, which leads to fluid and electrolyte loss.	▪ Assess intake and output; act immediately to provide fluid replacement. ▪ Treat the underlying cause. ▪ Be alert for signs of dehydration or electrolyte imbalance.
Infection	Most bacteria and viruses that produce infections thrive at normal temperatures. An increase in body temperature helps the body fight the infection. Also, a fever alerts the immune system to increase production of white blood cells and antibodies.	▪ Focus on prevention and health maintenance and promotion. ▪ Assess patients' risk for infection based on concurrent conditions, comorbidities, immune system functioning, and healthcare provision, such as immunizations. ▪ Be sure to perform and teach proper hand hygiene, use standard precautions with all patients, and follow isolation techniques, when indicated.
Inflammation	In the first stage of inflammation, blood vessels constrict, then dilate. The increased blood flow (hyperemia) causes redness and heat at the injury site (localized thermic response).	▪ Do ongoing observation at the site of injury, such as monitoring to prevent IV phlebitis or to ensure wound healing. ▪ The goal is to prevent the second stage of inflammation, exudate production.

Hypothermia

Neonates and older adults are at greater risk for developing hypothermia than other age group (Mayo Clinic, 2014b). Contributing factors for hypothermia include outdoor exposure, trauma, alcohol or drug abuse, endocrine disorders, previous neurologic impairment or autonomic dysfunction, dermatologic disorders, social isolation, and socioeconomic status. Individuals may sustain frostbite and more serious hypothermic injuries without recognizing that they are in danger (Mayo Clinic, 2014c). Nurses should be mindful of patients' age, anticipate their educational needs,

and promote appropriate cold-weather safety awareness to reduce the risk of hypothermia.

Healthcare providers, public health officials, and local government officials should promote, educate, and initiate actions to prevent hypothermic injuries, including financial assistance for heating costs and shelter for the homeless, especially in extreme conditions.

>> **Stay Current:** The Centers for Disease Control and Prevention offers guidance for recognizing and treating hypothermia in the community. Visit their website at http://www.cdc.gov/disasters/winter/staysafe/hypothermia.html

Focus on Diversity and Culture
Thermoregulation in Wheelchair Tennis

Wheelchair tennis has increased in popularity around the world since its inception in 1976. Often, wheelchair tennis matches are played indoors; however, top-level matches including the Paralympics are played outdoors in temperatures greater than 30°C (86°F) and in high humidity. Players are subject to direct heat from the sun as well as radiant heat from the tennis court and from their wheelchairs. In addition, these athletes have thermoregulatory, heat sensory, and sweating impairment due to spinal cord injuries, placing them at risk for heat-related injuries (Griggs, Price, & Goosey-Tolfrey, 2015; Veltmeijer et al., 2014).

Heat acclimation over a week prior to outdoor matches, cooling vests, hats, and neck bands are possible interventions that may benefit these athletes. Although there are guidelines for breaks and cessation of play for temperatures greater than 28°C (82.4°F), specific preventive guidelines and heat-injury precautions for athletes in wheelchairs have not been established by governing tennis organizations. Acclimation, hydration, and conventional cooling are utilized at the athletes' discretion (Girard, 2015).

The patient interview includes pertinent and specific questions regarding actual and potential environmental exposure, access to hydration, and, when necessary, questions about patients' socioeconomic status.

Physical Examination

The nurse assesses thermoregulation primarily by measuring body temperature. Body temperature is measured on two scales: degrees Celsius (centigrade, abbreviated °C) and degrees Fahrenheit (abbreviated °F).

The most common sites for measuring body temperature are the mouth, rectum, armpit, tympanic membrane, and the temporal artery, which is accessed through the skin of the forehead. True core body temperature can be measured by using invasive techniques, such as placing a temperature probe in the esophagus, pulmonary artery, or bladder. Invasive core body temperature measurements are usually done only on patients who are critically ill. Each site for measuring body temperature has advantages and disadvantages (see **Table 20–1** ≫). Oral and tympanic thermometers are shown in **Figure 20–3** ≫. See also the Lifespan Considerations section.

Nursing Assessment

Although palpating the patient's skin is the most common technique for assessing a patient's thermoregulatory status, it is important to remember that patients with hyperthermia may not feel warm to the touch but may have cool, wet, and clammy skin (Mayo Clinic, 2014a). In addition to assessing the patient's skin, the nurse must assess vital signs, orientation and mental state, hydration habits and hydration status, and length of time and severity of exposure. The nurse also assesses the patient's socioeconomic status, including factors related to environmental exposure such as access to potable water and temperature-controlled shelter, and if appropriate, the patient's alcohol and drug use.

Observation and Patient Interview

The nurse observes patients' physical appearance and looks for signs of extreme temperature exposure. The nurse observes patients at risk for cold-related injuries for changes in color or texture of skin, including redness, paleness of skin, blisters, or signs of frostbite on the patients' nose, hands, and other exposed areas, and listens for cues or complaints of pain, numbness, tingling, complete loss of sensation, or itching or swelling in affected areas (Doerr, 2016a). The nurse should remember that cold weather–related injuries may occur without tissue freezing.

For patients at risk for heat-related injuries, the nurse observes for physical signs of hyperthermia, including heat rash, red bumps on the surface of the skin, significant sweating, involuntary muscle spasms, and orthostatic hypotension. The nurse listens for cues and complaints of prickly or itchy skin, dizziness, lightheadedness, headaches, nausea, or vomiting (Doerr, 2016b). In more severe cases of heat-related injuries, the nurse observes for signs of heat stroke, including weakness and confusion.

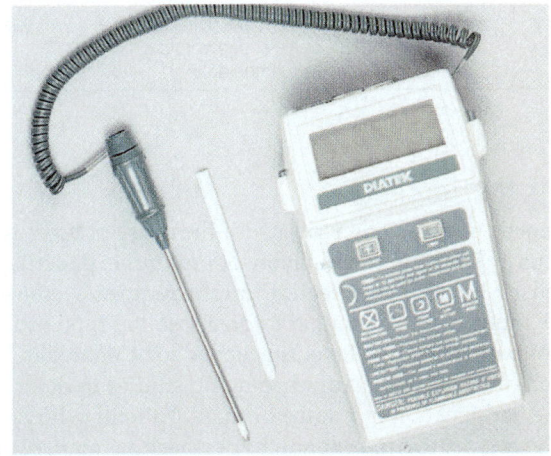

A

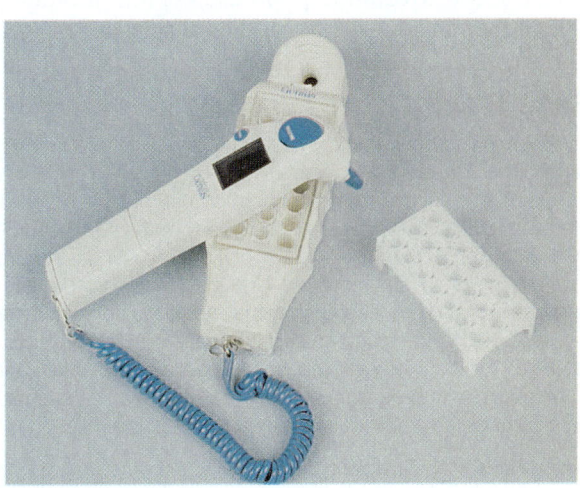

B

Figure 20–3 ≫ **A,** Oral thermometer. Note the probe and probe cover. **B,** An infrared (tympanic) thermometer used to measure the tympanic membrane temperature.

TABLE 20–1 Advantages and Disadvantages of Sites for Body Temperature Measurement

Site	Advantages	Disadvantages
Mouth (oral)	Accessible and convenient	The thermometer can break if bitten.
		This site is inaccurate if the patient has just ingested hot or cold food or fluid or has just smoked.
		This method could injure the mouth following oral surgery.
Rectum	Reliable measurement	This method is inconvenient and more unpleasant for patients; it is difficult for patients who cannot turn to the side.
		It could injure the rectum following rectal surgery.
		The presence of stool may interfere with thermometer placement. If the stool is soft, the thermometer may be embedded in stool rather than against the wall of the rectum. This method may be contraindicated in patients with cardiac problems.
Axillary	Safe and noninvasive	The thermometer must be left in place a long time to obtain an accurate measurement.
Tympanic membrane	Readily accessible; reflects the core temperature; very fast; may be less scary for small children	This method can be uncomfortable and involves risk of injuring the membrane if the probe is inserted too far.
		Repeated measurements may vary. Right and left measurements can differ.
		The presence of cerumen can affect the reading.
Temporal artery	Safe and noninvasive; very fast; less threatening for small children	This method requires electronic equipment that may be expensive or unavailable; variation in technique is needed if patients have perspiration on their foreheads.
Esophagus	Provides accurate reading of cardiac temperature if placed in the lower 25% of the esophagus; especially useful in patients who are anesthetized or intubated	It is difficult to insert the temperature probe; the probe causes irritation to nasal passages and general patient discomfort.
Pulmonary artery	Most accurate reading of core body temperature	This is the most invasive temperature monitoring technique.
Urinary bladder	Useful in patients who are catheterized; a dual-purpose catheter can both drain urine and monitor temperature	This method requires high urine flow rate to be accurate.

Diagnostic Tests

Diagnostic tests may be indicated if the cause of fever is not obvious on physical examination. For example, patients suspected of having an infection might require a complete blood count with differential to diagnose the type of infection, or patients whose fever is believed to be related to head trauma or tumor may require imaging studies to determine degree and location of trauma or mass. Patients who have a family history of malignant hyperthermia may require genetic testing to confirm the presence of this disorder, especially if they are experiencing a clinical episode.

Case Study >> Part 2

Mr. Kleinlein has been home for 24 hours since his visit to the physician's office. You are the triage nurse today and call to check on him. Mr. Kleinlein mentions that the ibuprofen has not been completely effective and that his temperature fluctuates between 37.3 and 38.9°C (99.1 and 102°F). Mr. Kleinlein mentions that he still has no appetite and is struggling to remember to drink fluids. He says that he has been lying in bed since he got home yesterday and does not remember getting up at all. As the triage nurse, you speak with the physician and determine that Mr. Kleinlein needs to be hospitalized for treatment. You tell Mr. Kleinlein to have someone bring him to the emergency department and that the physician will have orders waiting for him.

Clinical Reasoning Questions Level I

1. Why did you as the triage nurse want to speak with the physician?
2. What factors led to the decision to admit Mr. Kleinlein to the hospital?

Clinical Reasoning Questions Level II

3. What nursing diagnosis would be priority for Mr. Kleinlein?
4. What further questions could you have asked Mr. Kleinlein to determine his fluid volume status?

Independent Interventions

Interventions to Support Thermoregulation

Nurses must support patients in maintaining thermoregulation through preventive measures. Older adults and young infants may require a warmer environmental temperature than younger adults and middle-age patients. Infants and children can retain and lose more heat than adults through their disproportionately larger heads; therefore, nurses should advise caregivers that infants and children should wear hats when exposed to temperature extremes.

Nurses should advise all patients to maintain adequate hydration, especially during times of strenuous exercise and when ambient temperatures are very hot. Dehydration can present with a low-grade fever that will resolve when hydration status is corrected. Nurses should monitor the temperature of patients who are highly stressed or anxious for potential temperature elevation. In addition, when the opportunity for patient education presents itself, the nurse should teach all patients how to take and record their temperature (see the Patient Teaching feature).

Patient Teaching

Taking Temperature

- Teach the patient proper use of the thermometer and how to accurately read the temperature. Examine the thermometer the patient uses in the home for safety and for proper functioning. Encourage and facilitate the replacement of mercury-in-glass thermometers with other types.

- Observe the patient or caregiver taking and reading a temperature. Reinforce the importance of reporting the site and type of thermometer used and the value of using these consistently.

- Discuss means of keeping the thermometer clean, such as warm water and soap, and avoiding cross-contamination.

- Ensure that the patient has water-soluble lubricant when using a rectal thermometer.

- Instruct the patient or family member to notify the healthcare provider if the patient's temperature is 38.5°C (101.3°F) or higher.

- When making a home visit, take a thermometer with you in case the patient does not have a functioning thermometer.

- Check that the patient knows how to record the temperature. Provide a recording chart/table if indicated.

- Discuss environmental control modifications that should be taken during illness or extreme climate conditions (e.g., heating, air conditioning, appropriate clothing and bedding).

Interventions for Hyperthermia

The nurse carries out independent interventions to allay heat-related injuries and begin the cooling process in patients with heat exhaustion or heat stroke. The nurse supports patients with heat-related injuries both within and outside of healthcare facilities by monitoring patients' airway, breathing and ventilation, and circulation (ABCs).

Outside of the hospital, the nurse should notify emergency services immediately when heat exhaustion or heat stroke is suspected. Patients should not be left alone. If it is safe, the nurse should move patients to a shaded area, an air-conditioned vehicle, or a well-ventilated or air-conditioned room. If patients are conscious, responsive, and able to swallow, the nurse should provide cool fluids, preferably with electrolytes, to begin rehydration of both fluid and salt, but water may also be used. The nurse should remove the patients' clothing to advance the cooling process, and when possible fan or lightly mist patients with cool water to help stimulate evaporation and advance cooling. For patients with severe symptoms in which heat stroke is suspected, independent interventions include applying ice packs to the armpits and the groin and elevating lower extremities to help support blood pressure (Wedro, 2015). Cooling must begin urgently and should include fanning the face to reduce the temperature around the patients' head and brain.

For children with a history of febrile seizures, seizure precautions should be put in place once the children's temperature begins to rise (Graneto, 2016). In addition to measuring and recording temperature, pulse, respiration rate, blood pressure, and pulse oximetry, the nurse weighs pediatric patients for weight-based antipyretic, and if needed, antibiotic medication dosages.

Evidence-Based Practice

Treating Fever in the Hospitalized Patient

Problem

Fever is a common occurrence in hospitalized patients. Often, nursing staff are the first to recognize fever in patients either because of a fever spike or because of slower incremental increases in patients' temperature. Interventions and treatment modalities for patients with fever often depend on provider preference and subjective belief about the significance of a fever in light of patients' other health problems. Often, interventions are based on the provider's experience rather than on evidence-based practice (Thompson & Kagan, 2011). In fact, few evidenced-based protocols have been developed and implemented in hospitals for treating fever, and experts disagree about whether fever should even be treated in some patients (Munro, 2014).

Evidence

Rockett, Thompson, and Blissett (2015) found that nurses who used personal decision making began treating fevers earlier if (a) physicians had not provided a specific order indicating a temperature at which to begin interventions for fever, or (b) their unit or organization did not have a fever treatment protocol. In their study, Rockett and colleagues reported that nurses believed that fever, at least initially, is often not taken seriously.

Implications

Nurses recommend developing protocols to treat fevers and providing more education about fever, early interventions, and fever management to all providers (Rockett et al., 2015). Protocols based on supportive evidence for early intervention would eliminate subjectivity involved in what is the appropriate time to intervene as a patient's temperature begins to trend upward. Education should include the significance of recognizing trends in temperature measurements and less emphasis on initiating interventions when a patient's temperature reaches a certain degree. Investigating potential sources of infection from an invasive access or in blood, urine, or sputum cultures when performed earlier may decrease the severity of infection and related complications.

Critical Thinking Application

1. Have you encountered protocols for patients with fever? What independent actions would you initiate for patients who you suspect are developing a fever?

2. You are caring for a 65-year-old man who underwent coronary artery bypass surgery 2 days ago. You recognize that the hourly temperature recording shows a consistent increase in temperature. His temperature in now 37.9°C (100.2°F). What actions will you take to advocate for the patient?

3. What indications other than temperature would support that a patient may be developing an infection?

4. What independent actions would you initiate for the patient who you suspect is developing a fever?

Interventions for Hypothermia

Rewarming of patients with hypothermia must begin immediately and should proceed from core to extremities, rather than beginning with extremities. Rewarming is a slow process that usually requires collaboration of an interprofessional team, particularly for patients with hypothermia. Nurses ensure a dry environment for patients with hypothermia. Depending on the degree of severity, warm compresses or warm water bottles may be applied to the patients' core. See Exemplar 20.B on Hypothermia for more information.

Collaborative Therapies

Cooling Patients with Hyperthermia

For patients with heat-related injuries, cooling begins with independent interventions immediately upon arrival in the emergency department while the physician is notified. Collaborative measures for cooling are invasive and require diligent monitoring (Mechem, 2015). Collaborative measures for patients with heat-related injuries may include intubation and mechanical ventilation if the patients are not able to support their airway or the patients' respiratory status begins to decompensate. Patients may require invasive procedures such as placement of central lines for hemodynamic monitoring and insertion of rectal or esophageal probes for accurate core temperature readings. Patients may be given benzodiazepine medications to reduce shivering while cooling. Ice water therapy (application of cool water to the body while patients are on a porous stretcher) is used to advance cooling. Patients with severe hyperthermia may require cold peritoneal or thoracic lavage with cold water or the use of cooled oxygen. Other collaborative interventions for patients with hyperthermia include using temperature-controlled cooling blankets and administering cold IV fluid.

Collaborative care for hyperthermia can be divided into five types:

- *Prehospital care.* Singhal and colleagues (2013) found that 11% of pediatric patients with severe sepsis were transported to an emergency department by ambulance. Emergency medical service personnel pay immediate attention to the ABCs. For toxic-appearing children (children who are pale or cyanotic, and lethargic or irritable), it is important to initiate IV access. The same considerations are important for older adults.

- *Emergency department care.* For all ages, antipyretics should be administered as soon as possible after the patients enter the emergency department. If the medication brings down the fever, the lower temperature still does not signal the absence of infectious pathogen (Graneto, 2016).

- *In-patient care to pediatric, geriatric, or other designated care settings.* Newborns up to 28 days old with fevers should be admitted to the hospital (Graneto, 2016). After that age, hospitalization depends on factors in the patients' support system and medical judgment. The decision for admission or discharge with careful follow-up is often guided by protocols.

- *Admission to an intensive care unit (ICU).* Critically ill patients require admission to the ICU. The rate of fever in the ICU may be as high as 70% (McLaren & Spelman, 2015). Patients in the ICU who experience fever also have a 20% mortality rate (McLaren & Spelman, 2015).

- *Follow-up care.* If patients or caregivers have access to further communication with the primary healthcare

provider, continued monitoring can take place at home. Protocols should be in place that guide notification of positive laboratory results after discharge from the emergency department or leaving the outpatient clinic or physician's office.

Medications for lowering temperature are outlined in **Table 20–2** ⟩⟩.

Rewarming Patients with Hypothermia

The method for rewarming patients with hypothermia depends on the severity of the patients' condition. Patients with moderate to severe hypothermia and older adults with mild hypothermia require active external rewarming (AER), which entails using several rewarming methods concurrently: warm blankets, radiant heat, warm bath, forced warm air, and warm IV fluids. Zafren and Crawford Mechem (2015) advise rewarming the trunk prior to the extremities in order to prevent hypotension after extremities are warmed and vasodilatation takes effect.

Active internal rewarming (AIR) or core rewarming requires the use of warm IV fluids to rewarm the peritoneum, or the use of chest tubes to deliver warm fluid to the thorax. Endovascular rewarming, conducted via a femoral catheter placed in the femoral vein, warms circulating blood as it passes the femoral catheter tip (Zafren & Crawford Mechem, 2015).

In extreme cases of hypothermia, blood is rewarmed outside of the body via processes of extracorpeal blood rewarming, including "venovenous rewarming, hemodialysis, continuous arteriovenous rewarming (CAVR), cardiopulmonary bypass, and extracorpeal membrane oxygenation (ECMO)" (Zafren & Crawford Mechem, 2015).

Patients who fail to rewarm may have hypothyroidism. If the patients' history, medication list, or surgical scars indicate this, the patients may require an IV dose of levothyroxine. The nurse should review thyroid function test results first.

In cases of hypothermia with local injuries, patients should receive tetanus toxoid and pain medication, and the affected area should be rewarmed using a water bath. Digits should be rewarmed for no more than 30 minutes at 42°C (107.6°F) after core rewarming.

Other collaborative therapies related to treating patients with severe hypothermia include debridement or excision of damaged, dead, or infected tissue, and oral or IV pain medications, and IV antibiotics for suspected or confirmed infection.

Case Study ⟩⟩ Part 3

Mr. Kleinlein has been in the hospital now for 48 hours. He has been receiving antibiotics and ibuprofen every 6 hours since admission. He is also receiving a normal saline IV at 125 mL/hr. His output is 80 mL/hr. His appetite has increased, and he is able to eat about half of every meal.

Clinical Reasoning Questions Level I

1. Looking at the IV intake and the urine output, what would you document for intake and output?
2. What other assessments might you need to perform?

Clinical Reasoning Questions Level II

3. What is the priority nursing diagnosis for Mr. Kleinlein?
4. How would you determine whether the fluid volume deficit is resolving?

TABLE 20–2 Over-the-Counter (OTC) Antipyretics

	Acetaminophen	Ibuprofen or Naproxen	Acetylsalicylic Acid (ASA)
Brand names	Tylenol Tempra Panadol	Advil Motrin Midol Aleve Naprosyn	House brands
Category	Acetaminophen	Nonsteroidal anti-inflammatory drugs (NSAIDs)	Salicylates
Uses	Pain or fever, not inflammation	Pain, inflammation, or fever	Pain, inflammation, fever, or prevention of stroke and heart disease
Mechanism of action	Direct action at the level of the hypothalamus and dilation of peripheral blood vessels Resultant sweating dissipates heat Inhibition of production of brain prostaglandins to reduce pain	Inhibition of cyclooxygenase 1 (COX-1), necessary for production and release of brain prostaglandins and COX-2, responsible for inflammation	Inhibition of COX-1, necessary for production and release of brain prostaglandins and COX-2, responsible for inflammation
Common side effects	Generally safe with adverse effects uncommon Cause less gastric irritation than NSAIDs and do not affect blood coagulation	Stomach upset, ulcer formation, bleeding	Stomach upset, ulcer formation, bleeding
Precautions	Potential liver damage with high doses or long-term use, especially with consumption of large amounts of alcohol	Bleeding	Bleeding Chronic use: Ringing in the ears or hearing loss needs immediate attention.
Pregnancy/ lactation considerations	Relatively safe in all trimesters Detected in breast milk, but no adverse effects known, so American Academy of Pediatrics says compatible with breastfeeding	Avoid during pregnancy, since Category C prior to 30 weeks' gestation, and Category D after that No known effect on lactation	Relatively safe in intermittent doses in first and second trimesters Avoid use in third semester Detected in breast milk, so American Academy of Pediatrics urges caution on breastfeeding.
Nursing implications	Not recommended for patients who are malnourished because it can cause acute toxicity and renal failure. High doses put patients at risk for liver failure.	NSAIDs may increase the hypoglycemic effect in patients who use hypoglycemic agents or insulin. Administer with food or a full glass of water to decrease gastric irritation. Assess patients taking anticoagulants to monitor increased risk of bleeding.	Avoid use in children under age 18 because of increased risk of Reye syndrome, particularly with flu virus and varicella infections.

Source: Data from Adams, M. P., Holland, L. N., & Urban, C. (2017). *Pharmacology for nurses: A pathophysiologic approach* (5th ed.). Hoboken, NJ: Pearson Education.

Lifespan Considerations

Body temperature is affected by age. The nurse should understand the variances associated with thermoregulation across the lifespan.

Thermoregulation in Infants

Newborns have **brown adipose tissue (BAT)**, also called brown fat, that helps protect their organs from extreme temperature changes, and they have less subcutaneous fat than an adult and a thin epidermis (see **Figure 20–4 »**). Newborns are *homeothermic*; that is, they attempt to stabilize their internal (core) body temperatures within a narrow range in spite of significant temperature variations in their environment. Thermoregulation in the newborn is closely related to the rate of metabolism and oxygen consumption. Blood vessels in the newborn are closer to the skin than those of an adult. Therefore, the newborn's circulating blood is easily influenced by changes in environmental temperature, and this in turn influences the hypothalamic temperature-regulating center.

The flexed posture of the full-term newborn decreases the surface area exposed to the environment, reducing heat loss.

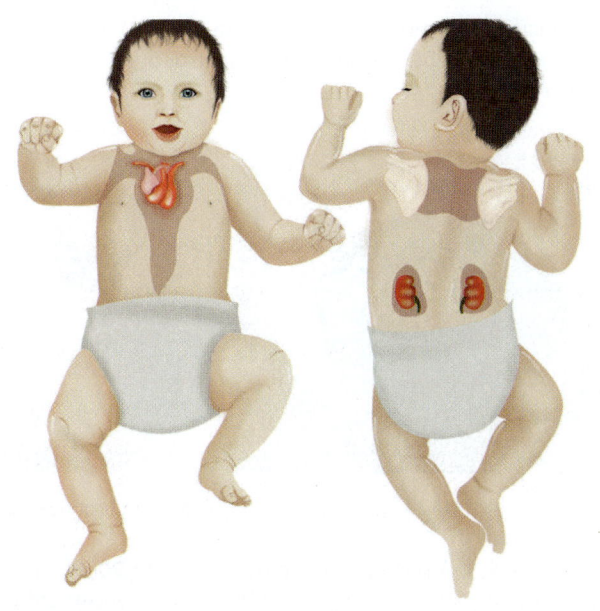

Figure 20–4 » The distribution of brown adipose tissue (brown fat) in the newborn.

Size and age may also affect the establishment of a **neutral thermal environment (NTE)**, defined as an incubator–environment temperature similar to that of a newborn's body temperature designed to minimize thermal body stress. For example, the preterm or small-for-gestational-age (SGA) newborn has less adipose tissue and is hypoflexed, requiring higher environmental temperatures to achieve an NTE. A larger, more well-insulated newborn may be able to cope with lower environmental temperatures. If the environmental temperature falls below the lower limits of the NTE, the newborn responds with increased oxygen consumption and metabolism, which results in greater heat production. Prolonged exposure to the cold may result in depleted glycogen stores and acidosis. Oxygen consumption also increases if the environmental temperature is above the NTE.

Neonates are adversely affected by heat loss through conduction, so the nurse should place padding on any surface used for diapering or examining newborns. The body temperature of newborns is extremely labile; newborns must be kept warm and dry to prevent hypothermia. Considerations for assessing temperature include:

- The tympanic route is fast and convenient. Place the infant supine and stabilize the head. Pull the pinna straight back and slightly downward. Direct the probe tip anteriorly and insert it far enough to seal the canal. The tip will not touch the tympanic membrane. Avoid this route in a child with active ear infection or tympanic membrane drainage tubes.

- If using the axillary site, the infant's arm must be held against the chest. Because the axillary area is partially exposed to the environment and because a lag time exists between changes in hypothalmic set point and axillary temperature, thermometer readings taken via this route may not be accurate (Sund-Levander & Grodzinsky, 2013).

- In using a temporal artery thermometer, it is necessary only to touch the forehead or behind the ear.

- The rectal route is least desirable in infants.

- A pacifier thermometer (see **Figure 20–5 》**) may be used in the home. The manufacturer's instructions must be followed closely.

Thermoregulation in Children and Adolescents

Until they reach puberty, children's temperatures continue to be more variable than those of adults. Children often have extremely high temperatures and tolerate them well. A healthy child can handle a temperature as high as 41°C (105.8°F) without difficulty. There are no consistent data or consensus reports to support an evidence-based practice of the most accurate method to monitor a child's temperature. Batra and Goyal (2013) found that temporal artery temperature measurements are as accurate as rectal temperature measurements in children ages 2–12 years; however, Hoffman and colleagues (2013) found the exact opposite result in their study of children younger than 36 months.

For the tympanic route, the child should be held on an adult's lap with the child's head held gently against the adult for support. The pinna is pulled straight back and upward for children over age 3 (see **Figure 20–6 》**). The tympanic route should be avoided in a child with active ear infection or tympanic membrane drainage tubes. For the axillary route, the child's arm is held against the chest (see **Figure 20–7 》**). The oral route may be used for children over age 3, but a nonbreakable electronic thermometer is recommended. For a rectal temperature, the child is placed prone across the adult's lap or in a side-lying position with the child's knees flexed. The thermometer is inserted 1 inch into the rectum.

Thermoregulation in the Pregnant Woman

The pregnant woman experiences marked changes in body temperature throughout the gestational period. The simultaneous elevation of estrogen and progesterone levels during the first trimester causes an increase in maternal body temperature. During the second and third trimesters, both estrogen and progesterone continue to increase, but estrogen outpaces progesterone, and the pregnant woman's core temperature decreases compared to the first trimester. At the same time, an increase in

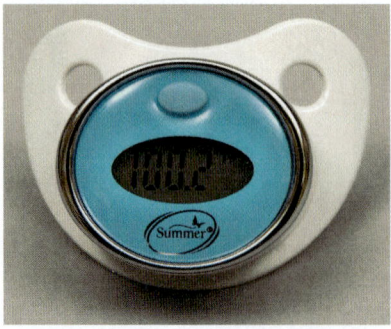

Figure 20–5 》 A pacifier thermometer can be used in the home. Parents should be cautioned to follow the manufacturer's instructions carefully for reading the temperature.

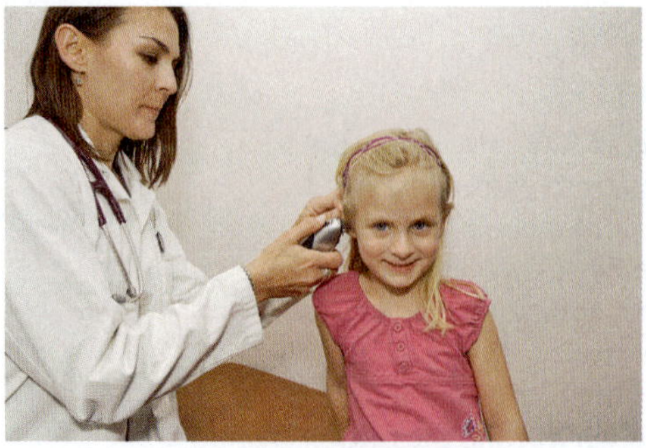

Source: Christina Kennedy/Alamy Stock Photo.

Figure 20–6 》 Pull the pinna of the ear back and up for placement of a tympanic thermometer in a child over 3 years of age; back and down for children under age 3.

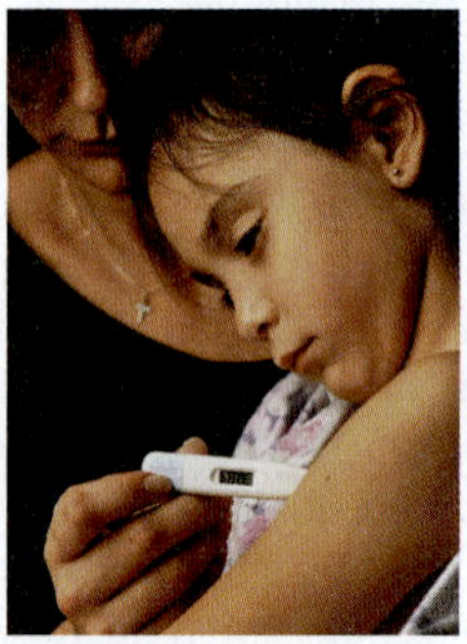

Source: Oscar Burriel/Science Source.

Figure 20–7 》 Hold the child's arm against the chest when using an axillary thermometer.

peripheral circulation occurs as core body temperature decreases; it decreases even more during exercise in the second and third trimester. These occurrences shield the fetus from hyperthermia. The woman's baseline temperature returns by the 12th week after delivery (Charkoudian & Stachenfeld, 2016).

Thermoregulation in Older Adults

Many older adults, particularly those over 75 years of age, are at risk for hypothermia (temperatures below 35°C [95°F]) for a variety of reasons, including inadequate diet, loss of subcutaneous fat, lack of activity, and reduced thermoregulatory efficiency. Older adults are particularly sensitive to extreme environmental temperatures because of decreased thermoregulatory controls. Older adults' temperature measurements tend to be lower than those of middle-

age adults. They can develop significant buildup of ear cerumen that may interfere with tympanic thermometer readings. Older adults are more likely to have hemorrhoids, so the anus should be inspected before a rectal temperature is taken.

Older adults often do not exhibit typical signs and symptoms related to illness, including infectious diseases. Providers must be aware that changes in behavior or changes in psychologic function may be the first signs of acute illness, including infection, in members of this population, and hospitalization may be required. In fact, some older adult patients may not exhibit fever as a sign of an infectious process. The three most common sources of fever in older adults are infection (30–35%); noninfectious inflammatory disorders (25–30%); and cancer (15–20%) (Kaya et al., 2013).

REVIEW The Concept of Thermoregulation

RELATE Link the Concepts

Linking the concept of thermoregulation with the concept of fluids and electrolytes:

1. What can the nurse do to provide adequate hydration to patients?
2. Why is the nurse concerned about patients' urine output?

Linking the concept of thermoregulation with the concept of safety:

3. What teaching should the nurse perform when talking with patients about hypothermia?
4. Does the teaching change when the nurse is working with adults rather than children?

Linking the concept of thermoregulation with the concept of nutrition:

5. Why is it important to maintain patients' nutritional status while they have increased temperatures?
6. If patients are unable to eat or drink, how would the nurse anticipate the patients receiving adequate nutrition?

READY Go to Volume 3: Clinical Nursing Skills

- SKILL 1.1   Appearance and Mental Status: Assessing
- SKILL 1.8   Respirations: Newborn, Infant, Child, Adult, Obtaining
- SKILL 1.9   Temperature: Newborn, Infant, Child, Adult, Obtaining
- SKILL 3.7   Cooling Blanket: Applying

- SKILL 3.8   Dry Cold: Applying
- SKILL 3.9   Dry Heat: Applying
- SKILL 3.10   Moist Pack and Tepid Sponge: Applying
- SKILL 3.11   Neonatal Incubator and Radiant Warmer: Using

REFER Go to Pearson MyLab Nursing and eText

- Additional review materials

REFLECT Apply Your Knowledge

Marilyn Sutton is 73-year-old woman who lives in an apartment complex. Her neighbor found her lying on the floor, awake but barely able to speak. Ms. Sutton did not recognize her neighbor. Her skin appeared pale and was cool to the touch. Her neighbor called 9-1-1. Upon their arrival, the paramedics noted that there was no heat in Ms. Sutton's apartment. The outside temperature was –9.5°C (15°F). Ms. Sutton was shivering, tachypneic, and unable to answer questions coherently. Her temperature was 35°C (95°F) temporal; pulse 58 bpm; respirations 10/min; and BP 88/58 mmHg. Ms. Sutton was transported to the emergency department.

1. List three nursing diagnoses appropriate for Ms. Sutton.
2. What are the priority interventions for Ms. Sutton when she arrives at the hospital?
3. What resources and support services are available in your community to assist older adults at risk for hyperthermia or hypothermia?

» Exemplar 20.A Hyperthermia

Exemplar Learning Outcomes

20.A Analyze hyperthermia as it relates to thermoregulation.

- Describe the pathophysiology of hyperthermia.
- Describe the etiology of hyperthermia.

- Compare risk factors and prevention of hyperthermia.
- Identify the clinical manifestations of hyperthermia.
- Summarize diagnostic tests and therapies used by interprofessional teams in the collaborative care of an individual with hyperthermia.

- Differentiate considerations for care of patients with hyperthermia across the lifespan.
- Apply the nursing process for providing culturally competent care to an individual with hyperthermia.

Exemplar Key Terms

Constant fever, *1550*
Endogenous pyrogens, *1550*
Febrile seizure, *1552*

Fever of unknown origin, *1550*
Fever phobia, *1555*
Fever spike, *1550*
Heat exhaustion, *1550*
Heat stroke, *1550*
Intermittent fever, *1550*
Relapsing fever, *1550*
Remittent fever, *1550*

Overview

A body temperature above 38.5°C (101.3°F) is called *hyperthermia* or, in lay terms, fever. The patient who has a fever is referred to as *febrile*; the one who does not is *afebrile*.

There are four common types of fevers: intermittent, remittent, relapsing, and constant. During an **intermittent fever**, the body temperature alternates at regular intervals between periods of fever and periods of normal or subnormal temperatures. Intermittent fever is common with some illnesses such as malaria. During a **remittent fever**, such as with a cold or influenza, a wide range of fluctuating temperatures (more than 2°C [5.3°F]), all of which are above normal, occurs over a 24-hour period. In a **relapsing fever**, short febrile periods of a few days are interspersed between periods of 1–2 days of normal temperature. During a **constant fever**, the body temperature fluctuates minimally but always remains above normal. This can occur with typhoid fever. A temperature that fluctuates from normal to fever level rapidly, and then returns to normal within a few hours, is called a **fever spike**. Bacterial blood infections often cause fever spikes.

In some conditions, an elevated temperature is not a true fever. Two such conditions are heat exhaustion and heat stroke. **Heat exhaustion** is a result of excessive heat exposure and dehydration. Signs of heat exhaustion include paleness, dizziness, nausea, vomiting, fainting, and a moderately increased temperature (38.3–38.9°C [101–102°F]). **Heat stroke**, a more serious life-threatening form of heat exhaustion, can occur when exercising or working in hot weather. Individuals with heat stroke have warm, flushed skin, and often do not sweat. They usually have a temperature of 41.1°C (106°F) or higher and may be delirious, unconscious, or have seizures.

Pathophysiology and Etiology

Pathophysiology

The clinical signs of fever vary in onset, course, and abatement stages. These signs occur as a result of changes in the set point of the temperature control mechanism regulated by the hypothalamus. Under normal conditions, whenever the core temperature rises, the rate of heat loss increases, resulting in a decrease in temperature toward the set-point level. On the contrary, when the core temperature falls, the rate of heat production increases, resulting in a rise in temperature toward the set point.

During fever, however, the set point of the hypothalamic thermostat changes suddenly from the normal level to a higher value (e.g., 39.5°C [103.1°F]). This sudden change of the hypothalamic set point may be caused by tissue destruction, pyrogenic substances, or dehydration. Although the set point changes rapidly, the core body temperature (i.e., the blood temperature) reaches this new set point after several hours. During this interval, the usual heat production responses that elevate the body temperature occur: chills, feeling cold, cold skin caused by vasoconstriction, and shivering. This is referred to as the chill phase.

When the core temperature reaches the new set point, the patient feels neither cold nor hot and no longer experiences chills (the plateau phase). Depending on the degree of temperature elevation, other signs may occur during the course of the fever. Very high temperatures of 41°C (105.8°F) and higher damage the parenchyma of cells throughout the body, particularly in the brain, where destruction of neuronal cells is irreversible. At such extreme temperatures, the body's organs, including the liver and kidneys, are at risk for significant dysfunction or failure. In some patients, this may lead to death.

In response to an infection, macrophages release **endogenous pyrogens** (interleukins, interferons, and tumor necrosis factor). These pyrogens travel through the circulatory system to the hypothalamus, the control center for body temperature regulation. In the hypothalamus, the pyrogens trigger the production of prostaglandins, which are believed to raise the body's thermoregulatory set point, causing the fever to occur. See **Figure 20–8 ≫**. Heat loss from the body is reduced, and the body temperature rises to the new temperature set point. When the temperature is elevated, the heart rate increases. One degree of temperature elevation causes an increase in respiratory rate of four breaths per minute and increases the metabolic need for oxygen by 7%. Vasodilation occurs, causing the skin to flush and become warm to the touch.

When the cause of the patient's high temperature is suddenly resolved, the hypothalamic thermostat set point reduces to a lower value, perhaps even back to the original normal level. In this instance, the hypothalamus now attempts to lower the temperature, and the usual heat loss responses that cause a reduction in body temperature occur: excessive sweating and hot, flushed skin due to sudden vasodilation. This is referred to as the flush phase.

Etiology

Hyperthermia occurs in response to viral or bacterial infections or from tissue breakdown following myocardial infarction, malignancy, surgery, or trauma. On occasion, patients will present with a **fever of unknown origin** (FUO). FUO is defined as a temperature above 38.3°C (100.9°F) that occurs on several occasions within a short time span, lasts for more than 3 weeks, and does not have a definitive cause after 1 week of clinical investigation (Chan-Tack & Bartlett, 2015). Because modern laboratory tests and imaging techniques are becoming more advanced, FUO is not seen as frequently

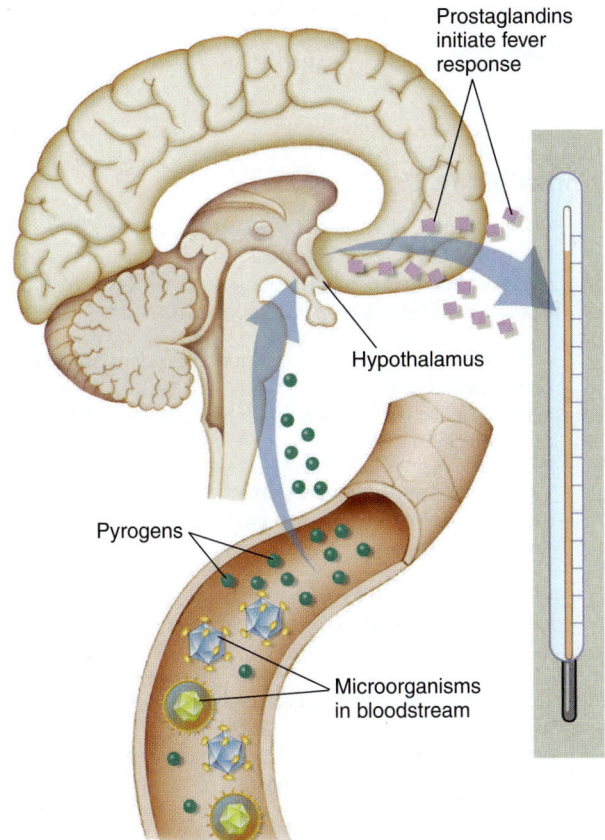

Prostaglandins initiate fever response

Hypothalamus

Pyrogens

Microorganisms in bloodstream

**Figure 20–8 ›› ** The hypothalamus functions as the body's thermostat, directing the body to conserve or dissipate heat. When microorganisms invade the body, endogenous pyrogens are released into the bloodstream. These substances travel to the hypothalamus, where they trigger the production and release of prostaglandins, which initiate the fever response. Blood is diverted from the extremities to more central vessels. This helps increase the core body temperature by decreasing heat loss. Shivering increases the metabolic action and heat production. The hypothalamus then maintains the temperature at the new set point.

today as it was in the past. After thorough investigation, FUO is usually found to be due to infections, neoplasms, autoimmune diseases, and other miscellaneous conditions (e.g., drug-induced fever). However, approximately 5–15% of cases have no known cause, even after extensive diagnostic testing. Management and treatment of FUO will depend on the underlying etiology of the fever.

Risk Factors and Prevention

Risk factors for hyperthermia include a diminished immune response, which increases the risk of infection. Risk factors for heat-related injury include age (the very young and the older adult); exertion in hot weather; sudden or prolonged exposure to hot weather; and certain chronic illnesses such as diabetes, lung disease, and heart disease.

Prevention of hyperthermia is related to methods used for preventing infection. Good hand hygiene is vital to the prevention of the spread of infection; thus, it is also useful for preventing infection. For patients in the hospital, the nurse should use interval vital sign measurement to monitor for

infections and inflammation. Interval measurements of patients' vital signs avoids the need for dramatic interventions in a crisis situation. Often, the most effective prevention activities start with graphing the vital sign data to identify a pattern or trend in the temperature rising or falling over time.

Clinical Manifestations

The clinical manifestations of fever are frequently due, at least in part, to the cause of the fever. Signs and symptoms common to all fevers include flushing, skin that is warm or hot to the touch; increased metabolic rate, producing an increased need for fluids; tachycardia; and tachypnea (see the Clinical Manifestations and Therapies feature). Fatigue, malaise, weakness, decreased responsiveness, difficulty concentrating, skin rash, poor appetite, vomiting, diarrhea, and body aches are common signs and symptoms that may accompany a fever.

Collaboration

Collaboration in treating a patient with hyperthermia will generally revolve around resolving the underlying cause of the fever. Often, the causes of fever are closely related to the age of the patient. For example, in the case of a child with history of febrile seizures, the pediatrician's office or public health clinic should work with the child's parents as well as with the child's preschool or classroom teacher. The pediatrician, the teacher, the school nurse, and the child's parents work together to ensure that all staff working with the child know what to do in the event the child has a seizure; they must also be knowledgeable about how to prevent the onset of a febrile seizure.

Treatment for fever is not always indicated. A fever can be a beneficial physiologic response that helps to slow the growth of organisms that thrive at lower body temperatures. A fever helps mobilize the immune response by increasing neutrophil production and T-cell proliferation. Fever is not inherently harmful until it reaches 41°C (105.8°F). For this reason, medical management may include postponing treatment of low-grade fevers—those under 38.9°C (102°F) in otherwise healthy children and adults—to promote the body's natural defenses against infection. The decision to treat a patient medically may be based on the patient's level of discomfort. Some individuals may also choose to treat fever using hot or cold methods, as described in the Focus on Integrative Health feature.

Acetaminophen and ibuprofen are the preferred antipyretics for children. Aspirin is no longer recommended for children because of its association with Reye syndrome, a condition that involves cerebral encephalopathy and organ injury. Antipyretics reduce fever by inhibiting prostaglandin synthesis and cause a decrease in the body's temperature set point (See the Evidence-Based Practice feature for a discussion of alternating acetaminophen and ibuprofen when treating children with fever). External cooling methods should be reserved for children who are hospitalized and critically ill.

SAFETY ALERT All prescription and over-the-counter products that contain acetaminophen carry this warning label from the U.S. Food and Drug Administration (FDA): "In rare cases, acetaminophen causes serious skin reactions." The FDA had reviewed reported reactions to acetaminophen and found evidence of a dozen fatalities and 60 hospitalizations (FDA, 2013; Kuehn, 2013).

Clinical Manifestations and Therapies
Hyperthermia

CLINICAL MANIFESTATIONS	CLINICAL THERAPIES	RATIONALES
Flushing	Correction of temperature elevation	As body temperature rises, the blood vessels vasodilate to bring more blood flow to the surface of the body. This allows the air's cooler temperature to reduce the temperature of the blood flow as heat dissipates through convection.
Warm skin	Correction of temperature elevation	As body temperature rises, the blood vessels vasodilate to bring more blood flow to the surface of the body. This causes the skin to feel warm secondary to the warmth of the blood flow.
Tachycardia	Correction of temperature elevation	With the increase in temperature, there is an increased metabolic rate that causes an increase in heart rate, pulse, and respiratory rate.
Tachypnea	Correction of temperature elevation	With the increase in temperature, the metabolic rate increases and causes an increase in heart rate, pulse, and respiratory rate.
Increased fluid requirement	Increase oral fluid intake or provide IV fluids; monitoring hydration status.	Insensible water loss increases as the result of perspiration, tachypnea, and increased metabolic rate. Dehydration can occur quickly, especially in young children and older adults if extra fluid intake is not provided.
Elevated body temperature	Treatment ranges from no treatment for a low-grade fever (less than 38.9°C [102°F] in children; less than 38.5°C [101.3°F] in adults) to the following for higher temperatures: ■ Antipyretic ■ Tepid bath ■ Reducing clothing and skin covering ■ Increasing fluid intake (at least 2000 mL/day with additional fluids in hot weather or during strenuous exercise) ■ Applying cool washcloths or ice bags to axilla, groin, forehead, and nape of neck ■ Applying a cooling blanket ■ Using a circulating fan in the patient's room	Body temperature between 36 and 38.5°C (96.8 and 101.3°F) provides an environment for normal physiologic functioning for all body systems. Core body temperatures above this range alter cellular function that, if maintained for too long, potentiates tissue and organ damage. Nursing interventions to maintain normal body temperature are aimed at aiding the body in reestablishing a core body temperature compatible with normal cellular function.

Antibiotics may be administered when the source of fever is a known or suspected infectious disease. Antibiotics have been responsible for decreasing the morbidity and mortality rates related to infections among children. However, some strains of bacteria have developed resistance to many antibiotics. Children with chronic illnesses such as cystic fibrosis, sickle cell disease, and AIDS are particularly susceptible to infection by drug-resistant pathogens.

Focus on Integrative Health
Hot and Cold Theory

Many cultures subscribe to the hot and cold theory of disease causation. "Hot" and "cold" do not refer to temperature, but to categories. Fever, a hot condition, is treated by giving the patient cold substances (foods or medicines). Cold foods include vegetables, fruits, and fish. Cold medicines include orange flower water, linden, and sage.

Lifespan Considerations
Hyperthermia in Children and Adolescents

Febrile seizures are generalized seizures that usually occur in children as the result of rapid temperature that rises above a rectal reading of 39°C (102.2°F) in association with an acute illness without evidence of intracranial infection or other defined cause. Febrile seizures usually occur in children between the ages of 6 months and 5 years, with a peak incidence in toddlers. One in every 25 children will have at least one febrile seizure. Risk factors include an immediate family member with a history of febrile seizures, first febrile seizure at less than 15 months of age, and a history of frequent fevers. More than a third of children who have a febrile seizure will have a future seizure. The older the child at the time the initial seizure occurs, the less likely that child will have additional seizures (National Institute of Neurological Disorders and Stroke, 2013).

Fever in children, including adolescents, is frequently attributed to infectious processes such as upper respiratory infections, ear infections, and urinary tract infections; however, there are instances in which fever may be attributed to a noninfectious source (Palazzi, 2016). Fever in children, especially when accompanied by other symptoms, indicates the possibility of an underlying illness. The most common causes of fever in children are infectious diseases (e.g., bacteria, viruses, fungi, mycobacteria), connective tissue diseases, and neoplasm (Palazzi, 2016); however, depending upon the child's complaint, other conditions such as appendicitis or pancreatitis may be present.

For children and adolescents with fever that does not appear to be self-limiting, it is imperative to obtain a detailed history that includes exposure to others who may have been ill, recent injuries, and social and physical activities. Even when it does not seem important, knowing children's exposure can help determine the source of fever. Consider the possibility of mononucleosis in adolescents who present with fever, pharyngitis, and lymphadenopathy (Aronson & Auwaerter, 2014).

Fever is most often a self-limiting response that can be managed at home with increased fluids and rest and with antipyretics if the child is uncomfortable. For young children, antipyretic medications should be dosed by weight.

Children should not be awakened to take medication (Ward, 2015). Although frequently used, tepid baths have not been shown to have long-term benefits in treating fever. Rubbing alcohol should not be used, and children should not be submerged in a bath as this accelerates heat loss (Ward, 2015).

When fever persists beyond 4 days, the child's condition does not improve, or the child develops a toxic appearance, the child should be evaluated by a healthcare provider (Hague, 2015).

Additional signs that indicate the child should be evaluated by a healthcare provider include pallor, not responding normally to social cues, not smiling, awakening only after prolonged stimulation, decreased activity, and swelling of a limb or joint.

Hyperthermia in Pregnancy

Hyperthermic exposure and maternal fever in the first trimester of pregnancy have been associated with congenital birth defects. Several studies indicate that in cases of maternal fever, the congenital birth defects are caused by fever and not by medication or maternal illness (Van Zutphen et al., 2012). Healthcare providers advise pregnant women to avoid hot tubs and saunas because of the known association between these types of heat exposure and neural tube defects.

Environmental exposure is of increasing concern because of ongoing climate change on the planet. In a 15-year case-control study in upstate New York, researchers examined the relationship between extremely high environmental temperatures during pregnancy and the prevalence of birth defects. The researchers found a strong association between

---

Evidence-Based Practice
Treating Fevers in Children with Alternating Ibuprofen and Acetaminophen

Problem
Should children with fever be treated with alternating doses of ibuprofen and acetaminophen?

Evidence
Clinical studies about the efficacy of alternating doses of ibuprofen and acetaminophen have historically shown mixed results; however, a recent systematic review of randomized trials involving 915 participants compared alternating antipyretic therapy versus single antipyretic therapy (Wong et al., 2013). The review concluded that while alternating therapy may shorten length of time of fever, a clinically significant difference between alternating and single medication therapy could not be established. Also, the review did not provide conclusive evidence to support alternating therapy or single therapy for improving degree of patient comfort. Furthermore, the review failed to provide consistent evidence regarding the most effective regimen of alternating therapy (Wong et al., 2013). Both the American Academy of Pediatrics and the National Institute for Health and Care Excellence oppose the use of alternating or combination therapy in treating febrile children because of the risk of dosing errors (Ward, 2015).

When fever and discomfort persist 3–4 hours after receiving acetaminophen, changing to ibuprofen may reduce fever and discomfort. Likewise, should fever and discomfort persist 3–4 hours after receiving ibuprofen, the child may benefit by changing to acetaminophen. Parents and providers should be aware that acetaminophen should not be given to children younger than 3 months of age unless an invasive bacterial infection has been ruled out. In addition, antipyretics should be given only to make the child comfortable, not simply to reduce the child's temperature to within the "normal" range, as some fever may be beneficial to fight infective organisms (MedlinePlus, 2014).

Implications
Regardless of the medication(s) chosen or pattern of administration, the nurse has a critical role in caregiver education. Because the amount of each drug contained in different preparations of the same medication may vary, the nurse must ensure that parents understand the importance of reading labels carefully, measuring doses correctly, and spacing administration with adequate intervals between doses. Liquid preparations call for particular attention to detail in order to avoid inadvertent double dosing, which may happen if over-the-counter cough and cold remedies that often include acetaminophen are given concurrently.

Critical Thinking Application
1. If a parent comes to you questioning the approach of the child's healthcare provider for fever reduction, what would be your best response?
2. What factors about the participation of children in clinical studies might have an influence on their results?
3. What is the effect of media (newspapers, TV advertisements, magazine articles) on the perception of the need to take action to reduce fevers?

high summer temperatures during weeks 4–7 of pregnancy and congenital cataracts and congenital renal defects (Van Zutphen et al., 2012).

A systematic review and meta-analysis of studies that examined fever in pregnancy found that fever in the first trimester of pregnancy is associated with a 1.5- to 3-fold increased risk of developing congenital defects, including neural tube defects, congenital cardiac defects, and cleft palate (Dreier, Andersen, & Berg-Beckhoff, 2014).

Nurses should teach pregnant women to avoid exposure to extreme temperatures, especially in the first trimester of pregnancy. High environmental temperatures, submersion in heated water, and exposure to illnesses that may cause fever increase the risk of the fetus developing congenital birth defects.

Hyperthermia in Older Adults

Thirty percent of fevers in older adults are attributed to infections such as pneumonia and urinary tract infection. Other causes of fever in older adults include giant cell arteritis (up to 19%), neoplasms, drug fever, deep venous thrombosis, and hyperthyroidism (High, 2015). As individuals age, they become more susceptible to infections. High (2015) attributes the increase in infection in the older adult population to biological (i.e., decrease in the function of the immune response; alteration in skin integrity, lungs, and other body systems; chronic diseases), societal, and cultural factors.

A significant problem in treating older adults with an infection is that early symptoms may be atypical or nonexistent, and by the time the patient seeks medical attention, the infection may be overwhelming and difficult to treat. Older adults frequently do not present with a fever that coincides with the significance of an infection. Even in cases of sepsis, it is not unusual to find that older adult patients do not perspire or complain of chills. Instead, behavioral changes and alterations in communication (e.g., delirium) are often the first observable signs that lead to suspicion of illness. High (2015) observes that while for healthy adults a temperature of 38°C (100.4°F) may not be significant, in the older adult it may reflect a serious infectious process. Temperatures below the older adult's baseline may indicate sepsis. The guidelines used to assess severity of fever in younger adults may not be applicable to adults age 65 and older.

Infection is the most common cause of fever in the older adult and may be attributed to a decrease in functional immunity. Interventions to boost and protect immunity in this population are imperative and may be accomplished by using nutritional supplements to correct deficiencies in proteins and micronutrients and ensuring that immunizations are up to date, especially for those who travel outside the United States.

NURSING PROCESS

Assessment

In caring for a patient with hyperthermia, the nurse assesses the patient's hydration status, fluid intake, vital signs, comfort level, and appetite.

- ***Observation and patient interview.*** The nurse observes the patient for seizures and a toxic appearance (lethargy, poor perfusion, hypoventilation or hyperventilation, and cyanosis), especially the pediatric patient. The patient

with a fever may be irritable and restless, sleep fitfully, and have nonspecific muscular pain. The nurse should identify the patient who may be at higher risk for a serious illness in association with a fever, including: infants and children with a toxic appearance, neonates with a temperature greater than 38°C (100.4°F), children under 4 years of age with a temperature greater than 41°C (105.8°F), patients with immunosuppression, and patients with chronic conditions. The patient with fever should be observed for other signs of infection, such as a rash, nausea and vomiting, or diarrhea, as well as generalized symptoms of poor appetite and malaise.

- ***Physical examination.*** The patient hospitalized with dehydration requires continuous assessment of mental status for subtle changes. The nurse assesses the patient's baseline mental status on admission and assesses for mental status changes during rehydration, as both fluid and electrolyte statuses shift. The nurse's initial and subsequent physical examinations must include assessment of skin turgor, mucous membranes of the oral cavity and inner eye lids, sunken eyes if present, and signs of edema to limit fluid overload with rehydration.

Diagnosis

Nursing diagnoses that may be appropriate for a patient with febrile illness include the following:

- *Hyperthermia*
- *Fluid Volume, Risk for Deficient*
- *Skin Integrity, Impaired*
- *Oral Mucous Membrane, Impaired*
- *Fluid Volume, Deficient.*

    (NANDA-I © 2014)

Planning

The nurse develops a plan for the patient with hyperthermia based on the specific needs of the patient and the cause of the temperature elevation. Goals specific to fever may include the following:

- The patient's temperature will approach normal limits within 60 minutes after administration of an antipyretic.

- The patient's temperature will remain within normal limits within 48–72 hours after beginning antibiotic therapy.

- The patient will maintain a temperature within normal range within 4 hours after application of a hypothermia blanket.

- The patient or caregiver will describe temperature elevations that should be reported to the healthcare provider immediately.

- The patient or caregiver will recognize symptoms that require consultation with the healthcare provider.

Implementation

Promote Normal Body Temperature

Body temperature between 36 and 38.5°C (96.8 and 101.3°F) provides an environment for normal physiologic functioning for all body systems. Core body temperatures above this range alter cellular function, which if maintained for too long, potentiates tissue and organ damage. Nursing interventions to maintain normal body temperature are aimed at aiding the body in reestablishing a core body temperature compatible with normal cellular function.

- Interventions to prevent and treat mild hyperthermia begin with local public health education concerning heat-related injuries, including dressing lightly to promote air circulation, remaining in rooms with ambient or comfortable temperatures to minimize heat expos ure, and informing the patient of signs and symptoms for which the patient should seek medical attention because of prolonged high heat or a combination of heat and humidity exposure.

- Additional patient education provided by the nurse should focus on those who are the most vulnerable to the effects of heat in order to minimize their risk of injury. The nurse should educate parents and caregivers about the risk of death or serious injury due to heat stroke in children left in cars on hot or even mildly warm days. The nurse should also inform the older adult patient about possible dangerous interactions between extremely hot temperatures and medications, chronic respiratory conditions, and cardiac conditions.

- The need to remain adequately hydrated and replace fluid lost through perspiration is imperative and should be reinforced at every patient–nurse interaction and opportunity.

- For the pediatric patient prone to febrile seizures, the nurse should reinforce with parents precautions and preventive measures. Adequate hydration, access to cold fluids, intermittent periods outside during hot weather, and playing in shade are reasonable measures to help prevent febrile seizures in children.

- Hospital-based nursing interventions required to promote normal body temperature center on supporting and monitoring invasive access and devices for patients in guarded and critical condition. The nurse must diligently monitor fluid intake and output to address changes in the patient's hydration state and renal function. The nurse monitors the patient's temperature every 1–2 hours or continuously if a temperature-sensing cable was placed with an indwelling Foley catheter, esophageal, or rectal probe. The nurse monitors the patient's hemodynamic status. The patient with hyperthermia requires diligent oral care, including lip lubrication since the oral cavity and cracks in the oral mucosa may serve as both a reservoir and a port of entry for infectious pathogens.

- The patient with hyperthermia requires strict monitoring of electrolytes and renal, liver, hematologic, and cardiac function. The nurse follows these physiologic functions by assessing lab work, blood gas results, and ECG results with careful attention to trends in results. Healthcare providers should be notified for both acute changes in results and suspicious trends in order to quickly intervene and minimize physiologic dysfunction.

Promote Comfort

Comfort measures are used to reduce physical discomfort, achiness, fatigue, and other physical complaints while conserving the patient's energy.

- In the community, the nurse educates the patient about drinking water to remain well hydrated or to rehydrate in mild cases of dehydration. The nurse may inform the patient about the use of over-the-counter medications such as acetaminophen or NSAIDs that may help reduce physical discomfort, but the nurse should also explain contraindications.

- The hospitalized patient may receive additional comfort measures including oral or IV medication to promote sleep, reduce anxiety or pain, and decrease nausea and vomiting. Often, these medications are ordered to be administered as needed. Nursing assessment determines the patient's need for medication alone, the need to adjust the dosage of medication, or the use of alternate interventions and therapies such as change in position or use of linen or clothing that is less irritating to the patient's skin. The nurse is able to control temperature in the patient's room and to adjust air conditioning and temperature to promote patient comfort.

Prevent Dehydration

Dehydration is the result of fluid loss that occurs as the increase in body temperature causes loss of water. This fluid loss is more pronounced with excessive perspiration and, in some cases, vomiting or diarrhea. Often, loss of fluid is accompanied by loss of electrolytes and requires both fluid and electrolyte replacement. In mild cases, fluid and electrolytes may be replaced by oral intake. Moderate or severe dehydration requires IV fluid and in some cases IV electrolyte replacement.

- The nurse can provide the patient with education to prevent and correct mild dehydration, including changing damp or wet linen as needed, avoiding or limiting time in direct sunlight, working in timed intervals when working outdoors, and knowing the signs of dehydration: dizziness, nausea, vomiting, muscle cramping. The patient should be aware of these signs as well as signs of when to seek medical attention.

- The patient should be aware of subtle signs of dehydration such as dried, cracked lips, an early indication of dehydration. Preventive and early interventions such as applying a cool towel to the neck and head and exercising in an air-conditioned room can prevent or limit dehydration.

Reduce Fear

Parents often fear a fever, believing it is a disease rather than a symptom of an illness. Their greatest fears about the harmful effects of fever typically include seizure, brain damage, and death. **Fever phobia** describes caregivers' fear about these negative results. Research on parental management of fever has shown a correlation between lower educational level and heightened concern about children's febrile condition (Monsma, Richerson, & Sloand, 2015).

- The nurse teaches parents to care for their child at home, including how and when to give antipyretics.

- The nurse should provide information and reassurance to help parents recognize the benefits of fever, proper management of fever, and when to seek medical attention (see the Patient Teaching feature for more information that is helpful to parents of children with fever).

Patient Teaching
Evaluating and Treating Fever in Children

About Fevers

- A fever is not a disease; it is the body's response to an infection. It means the child's body is using natural defenses to fight an infection.
- If the child has a fever and does not look sick, it may be better to let the body's natural defenses fight off the virus or bacteria causing the fever. Follow guidelines about when to contact the child's healthcare provider.

Treating the Fever

- Use a thermometer to check the child's temperature every 2 hours.
- Administer either acetaminophen or ibuprofen to lower a fever. Check the label to make sure the correct dosage is given—drops and syrups do not have the same concentration. Do not alternate or combine medications.
- Remove all but a light layer of the child's clothing.
- Monitor the child's behavior and response to fever medication. The fever medication will reduce the child's temperature, but the temperature may not return to normal until the child begins to recover from the illness.
- If sponging the child, give fever medication first, and then use tepid water to sponge the child. Cool water may increase shivering and discomfort.
- The child's temperature may rise again 4 hours after acetaminophen or 6 hours after ibuprofen is given. Check the temperature and give another dose of acetaminophen or ibuprofen. Follow the recommendations on the bottle for frequency of dosing and the maximum number of doses allowed per day.

Call Your Healthcare Provider *Immediately* If Any of the Following Occur

- The infant is under 2 months old and has a fever greater than 38.0°C (100.4°F).
- The child has a fever greater than 40.1°C (104.2°F) and any of the symptoms below are present:
  - The child is crying inconsolably or whimpering.
  - The child cries when moved or otherwise touched by the parent or other family members.
  - The child is difficult to awaken.
  - The child's neck is stiff.
  - Purple spots are present on the child's skin.
  - The child's breathing is difficult and does not improve after the nose is cleared.
  - The child is drooling and is unable to swallow anything.
  - The child has a convulsion or seizure.
  - The child acts or looks very sick.

Call Your Healthcare Provider Within 24 Hours If Any of the Following Occur

- The child is 2–4 months old (unless fever occurs within 48 hours of a DTaP shot and the infant has no other serious symptoms).
- The fever is higher than 40.1°C (104.2°F) (especially if the child is under 3 years old).
- The child complains of burning or pain with urination.
- The fever has been present for more than 24 hours without an obvious cause or location of infection.
- The fever went away for more than 24 hours and then returned.

Evaluation

Expected outcomes for the patient with hyperthermia include the following:

- The patient's fever is effectively managed with antipyretics.
- The patient's own defenses maintain normothermic skin and body temperature. For example, the patient sweats when hot.
- The patient maintains adequate hydration as evidenced by skin turgor, moist mucous membranes, sufficient urine output, and hematocrit within normal range.

Treating hyperthermia can be complex, especially in cases of FUO. When initial interventions to address fever do not work or when the underlying cause of the fever is not easily discernible, healthcare providers may want to consider the possibility of "drug fever." Several medications may cause fever: antimicrobial drugs, antiepileptic antihypertensive drugs, antiarrhythmic drugs, and antithyroid drugs (Bor, 2013). If there is suspicion that a patient's fever is caused by a medication, the medication should be stopped, and if necessary, replaced with a safe alternative. Other atypical causes of fever include, but are not limited to, dental abscesses, alcoholic hepatitis, adrenal insufficiency, and venous thrombosis (Bor, 2013).

REVIEW Hyperthermia

RELATE Link the Concepts and Exemplars

Linking the exemplar of hyperthermia with the concept of infection:

1. Do all infections result in fevers? Explain your answer.
2. When treating a 4-year-old patient with a viral infection and a temperature of 39.9°C (103.8°F), measured via axillary site, what independent nursing actions would you initiate? What collaborative interventions would you anticipate?

Linking the exemplar of hyperthermia with the concept of fluids and electrolytes:

3. Explain the physiology that would cause a patient to run a fever when dehydrated.
4. How does a patient's fluid requirement change when the patient has a fever? Explain the physiology behind your answer.

READY Go to Volume 3: Clinical Nursing Skills

REFER Go to Pearson MyLab Nursing and eText

- Additional review materials

REFLECT Apply Your Knowledge

Carrie Holmes is 6 weeks old, born at 38 weeks' gestation by vaginal delivery secondary to a small placental abruption attributed to her father, Casey Holmes, hitting her mother, Jessica Riley, in the abdomen. When Carrie and her mother come home from the hospital, they move into her grandmother's house with her 3-year-old brother Ryan. By 6 weeks of age, Carrie is starting to become accustomed to the daily routine. Her grandmother, Evelyn Riley, cares for her when her mother goes to work at a restaurant. Mrs. Riley feeds Carrie a bottle and lets her sit in her infant seat to watch her big brother play with his toys.

1. What factors would increase Carrie's risk of developing a fever?
2. If Ms. Riley called the pediatrician's office to report that Carrie had a fever of 38.6°C (101.5°F), taken rectally, what directions would you provide for her care? Explain the rationale for your answer.
3. If Ryan developed a fever of 38.6°C (101.5°F) taken via the axillary site, what instructions would you provide his mother and grandmother for his care?

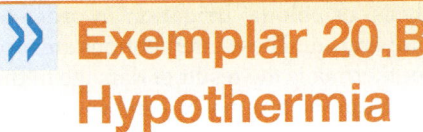

Exemplar 20.B
Hypothermia

Exemplar Learning Outcomes

20.B Analyze hypothermia as it relates to thermoregulation.

- Describe the pathophysiology of hypothermia.
- Describe the etiology of hypothermia.
- Compare risk factors and prevention of hypothermia.
- Identify the clinical manifestations of hypothermia.
- Summarize diagnostic tests and therapies used by interprofessional teams in the collaborative care of an individual with hypothermia.
- Differentiate considerations for care of patients with hypothermia across the lifespan.
- Apply the nursing process for providing culturally competent care to an individual with hypothermia.

Exemplar Key Terms

Chemical thermogenesis, *1559*
Frostbite, *1558*
Nonshivering thermogenesis, *1559*
Piloerection, *1560*

Overview

Hypothermia is a condition in which the core body temperature falls below 35°C (95°F). This occurs when the heat the body produces is less than the heat lost. Hypothermia can be a life-threatening emergency and can occur in any season and any geographic location.

Pathophysiology and Etiology

Hypothermia may be induced or accidental. Induced hypothermia is the deliberate lowering of the body temperature to decrease the metabolic rate and reduce the body's need for oxygen. Accidental hypothermia may occur as the result of immersion in cold water, exposure to cold environments, or damage to the body's thermoregulatory processes.

As the body's core temperature falls, the body tries to conserve the core temperature at the expense of the extremities. Two major routes of heat loss are from the internal core of the body to the body surface and from the external surface to the environment. The core temperature is usually higher than the skin temperature, resulting in continuous transfer or conduction of heat to the surface. The greater the difference in temperature between core and skin, the more rapidly heat transfers. The transfer is accomplished through an increase in oxygen consumption, depletion of glycogen stores, and in the newborn, brown fat metabolism.

Induced Hypothermia

Hypothermia may be induced for a variety of reasons. The most frequent reason for inducing hypothermia is to reduce metabolic rates and lower the cellular demand for oxygen in the tissues, particularly in the brain. Induced hypothermia has been used historically to reduce neurologic damage following head trauma or stroke or during cardiac surgery. Hypothermia has been shown to improve the neurologic recovery of patients resuscitated in out-of-hospital ventricular fibrillation arrest.

Other research concerning induced hypothermia has focused on its use with in-hospital cardiac arrests. Nichol and colleagues (2013) studied over 8000 patients who experienced cardiac arrest while hospitalized. The survival rate was 30% (2400). Even with considerable efforts to achieve hypothermia in about 3% (72) of the survivors, only 40% (28) of those patients' temperatures were lowered to between 32 and 34°C (89.6 and 93.2°F). Hypothermia had neither a positive nor a negative effect on survival or prevention of neurologic damage.

Accidental Hypothermia

Accidental hypothermia refers to unintentional exposure to cold temperatures that overwhelms the body, renders the individual unable to move or to shiver, and depletes the body's energy stores (Brown et al., 2012; Li, 2015). Hypothermia is described in stages based on symptoms. Patients in stage I are conscious and shiver. Patients in stage II hypothermia have impaired consciousness and have lost the ability to shiver. In stage III, patients are unconscious, unable to shiver, and have vital signs. In stage IV, patients no longer have vital signs (Brown et al., 2012). While temperatures are associated with each stage, clinical symptoms are a better indicator of the severity of hypothermia and the required medical management.

Frostbite

Frostbite is a freezing injury to the skin and its underlying tissue. If the exposure to freezing temperatures is limited, only the skin and subcutaneous tissues become involved; however, as length of exposure increases, deeper structures freeze. Skin freezes at –5°C (23°F), slightly below the freezing point of water (Fudge et al., 2015). Frostbite is most common on exposed or peripheral areas of the body, such as the nose, ears, feet, and hands.

As human tissues freeze, ice crystals form and cause an increase in the intracellular sodium content. Small blood vessels initially vasoconstrict, but then vasodilate and become more permeable, causing cells and tissues to swell. With continued exposure, vasoconstriction and increased viscosity of the blood cause infarction and necrosis of the affected tissue.

Superficial frostbite causes numbness, itching, and prickling. The skin appears cyanotic, reddened, or white. Deeper frostbite causes stiffness and paresthesias. As the skin and tissues thaw, the skin becomes white or yellow and loses its elasticity. The patient experiences burning pain. Edema, blisters, necrosis, and gangrene may appear.

Risk Factors

Common risk factors for accidental hypothermia include exposure to cold environment; immersion in cold water; lack of adequate clothing, shelter, or heat; and advanced age (Brown et al., 2012; Li, 2015; Zafren & Crawford Mechem, 2015). Hypothermia is associated with near-drowning episodes because body heat is lost more quickly in water than in air. Other causes of hypothermia include exposure to windy conditions, even in mild temperatures; trauma, especially that involving spinal cord injuries; and traumatic resuscitation. Sepsis, ingestion of alcohol that causes peripheral vasodilation and increases the rate of rapid cooling, and some medications affect sensory perception, circulation, thermoregulation, and respiratory function that may contribute to hypothermia. Skin wounds associated with burns are risk factors for hypothermia, which can contribute to increased risks in abused children and older adults (Corneli & Bolte, 2016; Zafren & Crawford Mechem, 2015). Immaturity of a newborn's temperature regulatory system and ineffective thermoregulation contribute to hypothermia.

Clinical Manifestations

Symptoms of mild hypothermia (32–35°C [89.6–95°F]) include fatigue, slurred speech, poor coordination and clumsiness, confusion and poor judgment, inappropriate behavior, shivering, tachycardia, and tachypnea. Symptoms of moderate hypothermia (28–32°C [82.4–89.6°F]) include depressed mental status, no shivering, depressed respirations, slow pulse or irregular heartbeat, hypotension, pale or cyanotic color, hallucinations, and coma. Severe hypothermia (body temperature below 28°C [82.4°F]) results in absence of respirations and pulse, ventricular fibrillation, dilated and unresponsive pupils, and coma. Zafren and Crawford Mechem (2015) warn that severity of hypothermia should not be determined based on temperature measurement, as methods of measuring temperature and degree of accuracy may differ. Clinical presentation of the patient should determine the severity of hypothermia, and all patients diagnosed with hypothermia should undergo a complete body survey.

Collaboration

After rewarming, patients with frostbite should be kept on bedrest with the affected body parts elevated. The nurse should administer pain medications and anti-inflammatory agents. Depending on the severity of frostbite, blisters may require debridement. Whirlpool therapy may be used to clean the skin and debride necrotic tissue. Recovery from frostbite is usually complete if the involved area has not become necrotic. Necrotic tissue may require amputation.

Patients with severe hypothermia may require hemodialysis, peritoneal dialysis, or colonic irrigation in order to increase core body temperature. These interventions are typically used when hypothermia is the result of damage to the hypothalamus, usually due to trauma or cerebrovascular accidents. Such damage to the hypothalamus may make return of thermoregulation physiologically impossible.

Diagnostic Tests

Diagnostic tests are recommended to thoroughly assess the effects of hypothermia, including testing for infection, acidosis, coagulopathy, and rhabdomyolysis (Zafren & Crawford Mechem, 2015). Diagnostic tests should include blood work to monitor electrolytes, renal function, and the patient's glycemic state. A complete blood count evaluates the patient's hematologic state and may indicate the onset of infection and the need to begin empirical antibiotic therapy. The patient's blood work should evaluate his or her metabolic state because patients with hypothermia are at risk for metabolic acidosis. Cardiac enzymes and electrocardiogram analyze the patient's cardiac function and assess for possible cardiac injury, including myocardial infarction. An arterial blood gas analyzes the patient's respiratory and ventilation status, and coagulation studies assess for coagulopathic injury and thrombosis. Tests for creatine kinase monitor for rhabdomyolysis, a condition in which severe muscle breakdown may lead to kidney injury or failure.

Circulatory Management

Treating the patient with hypothermia requires assessment and management of the patient's airway and support of his or her respiratory status, including intubation if warranted, and support of circulation and perfusion. In extreme cases, cardiopulmonary resuscitation (CPR) may be required for the patient who experienced cardiac arrest or the patient who has pulseless electrical activity (PEA). Hypothermia causes cardiac irritability and can lead to arrhythmias, including ventricular fibrillation, bradycardia, and asystole. Arrhythmias should be treated in accordance with American Heart Association guidelines (Zafren & Crawford Mechem, 2015).

SAFETY ALERT A pulseless, unresponsive patient with hypothermia should not be declared dead. Hypothermia reduces oxygen demands, and patients with hypothermia can survive cardiac arrest far longer than patients who experience cardiac arrest within the normal temperature range. As a result, patients in cardiac arrest who have hypothermia should be warmed and resuscitated. Only if resuscitation fails after warming should the patient be declared dead.

Clinical Manifestations and Therapies
Hypothermia

ETIOLOGY	CLINICAL MANIFESTATIONS	CLINICAL THERAPIES
Reduction in temperature results in decreased metabolic rate and reduced oxygen demands, slowing respirations and pulse rate. The body's compensatory mechanism initiates shivering to produce heat from muscle activity.	■ Decreased body temperature, pulse, and respirations ■ Severe shivering (initially) ■ Feelings of cold and chills	■ Provide a warm environment. ■ Provide dry clothing. ■ Apply warm blankets. ■ Keep limbs close to body. ■ Cover the patient's head with a cap or turban. ■ Supply warm oral or IV fluids. ■ Apply warming pads.
Hypothermia causes vasoconstriction to reduce exposure of the circulating bloodstream to the cold environment.	■ Pale, cool, waxy skin	
Vasoconstriction caused by hypothermia reduces peripheral circulation. Reduced heart rate reduces cardiac output. Blood flow to the kidneys is reduced. Blood flow to the brain is reduced secondary to slowed metabolic rate and reduced cardiac output.	■ Frostbite (nose, fingers, toes) ■ Hypotension ■ Decreased urinary output ■ Lack of muscle coordination ■ Disorientation ■ Drowsiness progressing to coma	■ Rapidly rewarm affected areas in circulating warm water, 40–40.5°C (104–104.9°F), for 20–30 minutes. ■ Do not rub or massage the areas. ■ Following rewarming, keep the patient on bedrest with the affected parts elevated. ■ Administer analgesics and anti-inflammatory agents. ■ Administer whirlpool therapy to clean skin and debride necrotic tissue. ■ Necrotic tissue may require amputation. ■ Support respiratory and cardiac function. ■ Reduce handling, because handling increases the risk of cardiac fibrillation.

Lifespan Considerations

Hypothermia in Infants

A newborn has a distinct disadvantage in maintaining a normal temperature. With a large body surface in relation to mass and a limited amount of insulating subcutaneous fat, the full-term newborn loses about 4 times more heat than an adult. Because of the risk of hypothermia and possible cold stress, minimizing heat loss in the newborn after birth is essential. Thermal conduction is a risk because of the marked difference between the newborn's core temperature and skin temperature. The newborn can respond to the air's cooler temperature with adequate peripheral vasoconstriction, but this mechanism is not entirely effective because of the minimal amount of fat insulation present, the large body surface, and ongoing thermal conduction. Minimizing the baby's heat loss and preventing hypothermia are imperative.

The newborn has several physiologic mechanisms that increase heat production, or thermogenesis. These mechanisms include increased BMR, muscular activity, and **chemical thermogenesis** (also called **nonshivering thermogenesis,** or NST) (Rozance & Rosenberg, 2012). NST is an important mechanism of heat production unique to the newborn. It occurs when skin receptors perceive a drop in the environmental temperature and, in response, transmit sensations to stimulate the sympathetic nervous system. Nonshivering

thermogenesis uses the newborn's stores of brown adipose tissue (BAT) to provide heat.

Thermoregulation in the newborn occurs without shivering (Vilinsky & Sheridan, 2014). If the newborn shivers, it means that his or her metabolic rate has already doubled. The extra muscular activity does little to produce needed heat; however, if the newborn's brown fat supply has been depleted, the metabolic response to cold is limited or lacking. An increase in basal metabolism as a result of hypothermia results in an increase in oxygen consumption. A decrease in the environmental temperature of 2°C, from 33 to 31°C (91.4 to 87.8°F), is sufficient to double the oxygen consumption of a term newborn. Keeping the term newborn warm promotes normal oxygen requirements, whereas chilling can cause signs of respiratory distress in the newborn.

Refer to the exemplar on Newborn Care in the module on Reproduction for more information on thermoregulation in newborns.

Hypothermia in Children and Adolescents

Young children are at increased risk for hypothermia because of their larger ratio of surface area to mass. In addition, young children may not be able to recognize signs of frostbite and hypothermia and may lack the knowledge of how to avoid or escape severe cold exposure. Because of their small size, children have relatively small amounts of glycogen stores and are not as readily able to support heat production compared with adults. Furthermore, children do not require extreme temperatures to develop hypothermia. Strong winds on mild days have the potential to cause hypothermia in a child. Children who are abused, neglected, or who are victims of extreme poverty and lack adequate shelter are also at risk for hypothermia (Corneli & Bolte, 2016). Guidelines for rewarming children with hypothermia are similar to rewarming adults with hypothermia.

Hypothermia in Pregnant Women

Treatment for hypothermia in the pregnant woman should follow the guidelines for adults with hypothermia with appropriate obstetric consultation and involvement for fetal monitoring. Pregnancy is a contraindication to therapeutic hypothermia (Scirica, 2013). There have been four documented cases of pregnant women who experienced cardiac arrest with successful resuscitation and who were then treated with therapeutic hypothermia. All four women survived. Three delivered healthy babies; one delivered a stillborn fetus (Oguayo et al., 2015).

Hypothermia in Older Adults

Older adults are at increased risk for hypothermia because their bodies are less able to maintain a constant internal temperature. Older adults are also more sensitive than young and middle-age adults to variations in environmental temperature. This increased sensitivity may be due to the decreased thermoregulatory control and loss of subcutaneous fat common in older adults, or it may be due to environmental factors such as lack of activity, inadequate diet, or lack of central heating. Illness or a central nervous system disorder may impair the thermostatic function of the hypothalamus. Chronic conditions (e.g., diabetes, peripheral neuropathy, hypothyroidism), medication use, reduced sensory perception, and cognitive disorders can increase the risk of hypothermia in older adults. Hypothermia in older adults is extremely dangerous, as members of this age group lack "physiologic reserve" and are often on medications that affect the body's ability to compensate for colder temperatures. Some older adults are also at risk for hypothermia because of social isolation. In older adults, hypothermia may be a sign of overwhelming sepsis (Zafren & Crawford Mechem, 2015).

Treatment of hypothermia in older adults is similar to treatment for hypothermia at any age. Once hypothermia is resolved, the nurse should assess for issues that may place the older adult patient at increased risk for recurrent hypothermia. These may include nutritional status, financial concerns that limit the patient's ability to heat his or her home, and self-care deficits.

NURSING PROCESS

Assessment

- ***Observation and patient interview.*** The nurse's ability to assess the patient with hypothermia varies with the patient's presentation and the severity of condition. The nurse may observe shivering, confusion when responding to questions, rapid breathing, and a lack of coordination.

The patient's subjective complaints may include nausea, fatigue, and dizziness. With moderate to severe hypothermia, the nurse may observe that the patient does not shiver but exhibits slurred speech and clumsy movements. The patient with moderate to severe hypothermia may be confused and drowsy and fail to exhibit concern for his or her condition (Mayo Clinic, 2014d). If the patient is able, ask the patient about precipitating factors, duration of exposure to cold temperatures, and health conditions that may increase the patient's risk of hypothermia.

- ***Physical examination.*** The nurse's physical assessment may identify defining characteristics of hypothermia, including body temperature below normal range, cool skin, cyanotic nail beds, pallor, **piloerection** (goosebumps), shivering, no shivering, slow capillary refill, weak pulse, and tachycardia.

Diagnosis

Nursing diagnoses for the patient with hypothermia may include the following:

- *Body Temperature, Risk for Imbalanced*
- *Hypothermia.*

    (NANDA-I © 2014)

Planning

Prevention is a primary nursing goal.

- The patient will demonstrate a balance between heat production, heat gain, and heat loss.
- The patient will maintain core body temperature within normal range.

Implementation

The severity of hypothermia—mild, moderate, or severe—the patient's health status, and the precipitating factors related to the hypothermic state determine the method of rewarming appropriate for the patient. See the Clinical Manifestations and Therapies feature and Collaboration section for medical interventions used to treat the patient with hypothermia.

Promote Normal Body Temperature

Nursing interventions to re-establish normal body temperature in the patient with hypothermia focus on the return of cellular and tissue function to areas of the body that have been exposed to extreme temperatures. In the patient with severe hypothermia, rewarming the body's core precedes rewarming extremities in order to avoid additional complications such as hypotension caused by vasodilation of the extremities. Even for the patient with mild hypothermia, rewarming the body to normal temperature is a slow and cautious process. The patient with hypothermia should be handled gently to avoid cardiac stimulation that could lead to cardiac arrest.

In emergency situations in the community:

- Body heat is the most efficient way to begin rewarming and requires removing clothing for skin-to-skin contact while both parties are covered with a blanket. Rewarming of the patient with hypothermia must begin immediately.

If available, warm compresses should be applied to the patient's neck, chest, and groin. A warm towel or warm water in a plastic bottle may be used instead. Do not apply compresses to extremities first as this will force cold blood toward organs and cause the core temperature to drop. Direct heat should not be applied to the body because of the potential for skin damage and dysrhythmias. The patient with hypothermia who is conscious, responsive, and able to swallow should be provided with a high-calorie warm beverage. If the patient is not breathing or does not have a pulse, CPR should be started immediately.

- The nurse should educate parents to layer their child's clothing and use hats in cold climates. The child should be taught to recognize signs of hypothermia, to decrease time of exposure to cold, and, if old enough, to treat mild hypothermia.

In the hospital:

- The nurse caring for the hospitalized patient with mild hypothermia who is able to generate his or her own heat and who does not require invasive rewarming may begin passive external rewarming (PER) and undertake similar measures for the adult patient as listed previously. The nurse should ensure that the patient's room is at least 28°C (82.4°F) and that the patient does not rewarm faster than 2°C per hour.

- For the patient with moderate to severe hypothermia, the nurse rewarms the patient's digits in a warm bath for no more the 30 minutes at 42°C (107.6°F) after core rewarming has been completed. The nurse is diligent in monitoring intake and output, including quantity and characteristic of urine output, vital signs, lab work, and ECG.

Promote Comfort

The patient who is exposed to extreme cold experiences pain during the rewarming process. The severity and length of exposure factors into the patient's level of pain; however, pain is subjective and should be addressed and treated to provide the patient with comfort.

- Advise the patient to limit use of the affected area and soak digits, hands, or feet in warm (not hot) water.

- The nurse may advise the patient to take over-the-counter ibuprofen as directed for pain and inform the patient that tingling and burning sensations can be expected as blood flow returns but that these sensations should resolve.

- For all patients at risk for environmental exposure, the nurse notifies social services to assess the patient's ability to meet heating costs, to determine if the patient is able to support a comfortable environmental temperature without financial constraints, and to assess if the patient has adequate shelter and clothing. Mandatory reporting is required if the nurse suspects the patient with hypothermia is a victim of neglect or abuse.

Evaluation

Expected outcomes for the patient with hypothermia include the following:

- The patient does not exhibit piloerection or shivering.
- The patient maintains core temperature within normal ranges.
- The patient reports thermal comfort.
- The patient describes adaptive measures to minimize fluctuations in body temperature.
- The patient reports early signs and symptoms of hypothermia (Wilkinson & Ahern, 2013).

Additional interventions include age-appropriate patient or caregiver education that focuses on eliminating and avoiding risks that may predispose an individual to hypothermia. The patient should be informed of and verbalize understanding that even mild hypothermia may have serious, lifelong effects. The patient should also express practical interventions he or she can take to avoid overexposure and cold weather–related injuries.

Nursing Care Plan
A Patient with Hypothermia

Jerry Karpinski, an 87-year-old man, is brought to the emergency department after his son finds him unresponsive. The son reports that the patient has lived alone in a single-family home in Minnesota since his wife died 3 years ago. Mr. Karpinski depends on his Social Security income as his sole means of financial support and has been trying to keep his utility bills low by setting his thermostat to 15°C (about 60°F). His son checks on him every day, and today he found Mr. Karpinski lying on the kitchen floor near the stove.

ASSESSMENT	DIAGNOSIS	PLANNING
Mr. Karpinski has a history of hypothyroidism and hypertension. He recently began taking sedatives to help him sleep at night. His vital signs are temperature 29°C (84.2°F) rectal, and BP 82/36 mmHg. His height is 183 cm (6 ft), and his weight is 72.7 kg (160 lb). Mr. Karpinski's skin is pale and cool to the touch; his nail beds are cyanotic. His breath sounds are diminished throughout, and his pulse is weak and thready. Mr. Karpinski is nonresponsive to voice or stimulation. (Deep pain response was not evaluated secondary to hypothermia.)	• *Hypothermia* as evidenced by rectal temperature of 29°C (NANDA-I © 2014)	Mr. Karpinski will demonstrate thermoregulation as evidenced by the following indicators: • Body temperature within normal limits • Skin color becoming pink and less pale • No signs of piloerection or shivering • Reported thermal comfort.

(continued on next page)

Nursing Care Plan (continued)

IMPLEMENTATION

- Gradually rewarm the patient using a heating blanket until his temperature reaches 36°C (96.8°F).
- Administer warm IV solutions.
- Utilize a continuous core temperature monitoring device.
- Monitor the patient continuously, and record his vital signs and cardiac rhythm on a cardiorespiratory monitor.

- Make a referral to social services.
- Teach the patient and family how to prevent hypothermia.
- Teach the patient and family indications of hypothermia and appropriate emergency treatment.
- Reduce manual stimulation.

EVALUATION

Mr. Karpinski's core temperature is approaching the normal range, he is increasingly more alert, and his vital signs have returned to normal ranges. Mr. Karpinski was at increased risk for hypothermia because of his age and poorly controlled hypothyroidism. Prior to discharge, Mr. Karpinski and his son were able to explain signs of early hypothermia, strategies for preventing hypothermia, and the importance of taking his thyroid hormone supplement every day. Social services contacted a local agency that can help Mr. Karpinski pay for his prescription medications, freeing him to pay his utility bills to maintain an acceptable environmental temperature.

CRITICAL THINKING

1. What factors contributed to Mr. Karpinski's development of hypothermia?
2. The care plan focuses on the acute care of Mr. Karpinski's hypothermia. Once the patient's temperature returns to normal range, what nursing care will this patient require? Why will that care be required?
3. What patient teaching (other than that mentioned in the plan of care) would the nurse initiate? Why?
4. Does this event indicate that Mr. Karpinski is no longer able to care for himself? Explain the assessments you would perform to reach a decision about his competence for self-care.

REVIEW Hypothermia

RELATE Link the Concepts and Exemplars

Linking the exemplar of hypothermia with the concept of safety:

1. When teaching a class on safety at a long-term care facility, what teaching points would the nurse discuss regarding prevention of hypothermia in the older adult patient?
2. What safety measures should the nurse teach the new mother of a baby born prematurely to avoid hypothermia?

Linking the exemplar of hypothermia with the concept of addiction:

3. Why is the patient who abuses alcohol at increased risk for hypothermia?
4. A patient is brought to the emergency department with no pulse, an elevated blood alcohol level, and a core temperature of 31.3°C (88.4°F). What is the priority nursing action? Explain the rationale for your answer.

READY Go to Volume 3: Clinical Nursing Skills

REFER Go to Pearson MyLab Nursing and eText

- Additional review materials

REFLECT Apply Your Knowledge

Baby girl Cho is born at 34 weeks' gestation to Jenny and Brian Cho. This is their first child. The parents attended Lamaze classes because they wanted to deliver the baby using natural childbirth methods, and they avoided all medications during labor. The baby has made a successful transition to extrauterine life and is breathing independently and maintaining oxygenation without assistance. After spending 30 minutes bonding with her parents, the baby is taken to the newborn nursery. The baby's axillary temperature is 34.2°C (93.6°F), and she begins to demonstrate mild substernal and intercostal retractions and nasal flaring. Her respiratory rate is 52, and her apical pulse is 148.

1. What factors may contribute to the baby's development of respiratory distress?
2. What are the priority nursing interventions for this newborn?
3. What nursing interventions would be appropriate to warm the newborn?

References

Adams, M. P., Holland, L. N., & Urban, C. (2017). *Pharmacology for nurses: A pathophysiologic approach* (5th ed.). Hoboken, NJ: Pearson Education.

Aronson, M. D., & Auwaerter, P. G. (2014). Infectious mononucleosis in adults and adolescents. In M. S. Hirsch, S. L. Kaplan & J. Mitty (Eds.), *UpToDate*.

Retrieved from http://www.uptodate.com/contents/infectious-mononucleosis-in-adults-and-adolescents

Batra, P., & Goyal, S. (2013). Comparison of rectal, axillary, tympanic, and temporal artery thermometry in the pediatric emergency room. *Pediatric Emergency Care, 29*(1), 63–66. doi:10.1097/PEC.0b013e31827b5427

Berko, J., Ingram, D. D., Saha, S., & Parker, J. D. (2014). *National Health Statistics: Death attributed to heat, cold, and other weather events in the United States, 2006–2010.* (Report No. 76.). Retrieved from U.S. Department of Health and Human Services Centers for Disease Control and Prevention website: http://www.cdc.gov/nchs/data/nhsr/nhsr076.pdf

Bor, D. H. (2013). Etiologies of fever of unknown origin in adults. In P. F. Weller & A. R. Thorner (Eds.), *UpToDate.* Retrieved from http://www.uptodate.com/contents/etiologies-of-fever-of-unknown-origin-in-adults?source=search_result&search=fever+of+unknown+origin+adult&selectedTitle=2%7E62

Brown, D. J., Brugger, H., Boyd, J., & Paal, P. (2012). Accidental hypothermia. *New England Journal of Medicine, 367*(20), 1930–1938. doi:10.1056/NEJMra1114208

Centers for Disease Control and Prevention. (2013a). *Emergency preparedness and response: Extreme heat prevention guide.* Retrieved from http://emergency.cdc.gov/disasters/extremeheat/index.asp

Centers for Disease Control and Prevention. (2013b). *CDC urges everyone: Get ready to stay cool before temperatures soar.* Retrieved from http://www.cdc.gov/media/releases/2013/p0606-extreme-heat.html

Chan-Tack, K. M., & Bartlett, J. (2015). *Fever of unknown origin.* Retrieved from http://emedicine.medscape.com/article/217675-overview

Charkoudian, N., & Stachenfeld, N. (2016). Sex hormone effects on autonomic mechanisms of thermoregulation in humans. *Autonomic Neuroscience, 196*, 75–80. doi:10.1016/j.autneu.2015.11.004

Corneli, H. M., & Bolte, R. G. (2016). Hypothermia in children: Clinical manifestations and diagnosis. In D. F. Danzi & J. F. Wiley II (Eds.), *UpToDate.* Retrieved from http://www.uptodate.com/contents/hypothermia-in-children-clinical-manifestations-and-diagnosis

Doerr, S. (2016a). Frostbite and cold weather-related injuries. In C. P. Davis (Ed.), *Medicinenet.* Retrieved from http://www.medicinenet.com/frostbite/article.htm

Doerr, S. (2016b). Heat-related illnesses. In W. C. Shiel, Jr. (Ed.), *Medicinenet.* Retrieved from http://www.medicinenet.com/hyperthermia/page4.htm

Dreier, J. W., Andersen, A. M., & Berg-Beckhoff, G. (2014). Systematic review and meta-analyses: Fever in pregnancy and health impacts in the offspring. *Pediatrics, 133*(3), e674–e688. doi:10.1542/peds.2013-3205

Duzinski, S. V., Barczyk, A. N., Wheeler, T. C., Iyer, S. S., & Lawson, K. A. (2014). Threat of paediatric hyperthermia in an enclosed vehicle: A year-round study. *Injury Prevention, 20*(4), 220–225. doi:10.1136/injuryprev-2013-040910

Fudge, J. R., Bennett, B. L., Simanis, J. P., & Roberts, W. O. (2015). Medical evaluation for exposure extremes: Cold. *Clinical Journal of Sports Medicine, 25*(1), 432–436.

Girard, O. (2015). Thermoregulation in wheelchair tennis: How to manage heat stress? *Frontiers in Physiology, 6*, 175. doi:10.3389/fphys.2015.00175

Graneto, J. W. (2016). Emergent management of pediatric patients with fever. *Medscape.* Retrieved from http://emedicine.medscape.com/article/801598-overview

Griggs, K. E., Price, M. J., & Goosey-Tolfrey, V. L. (2015). Cooling athletes with a spinal cord injury. *Sports Medicine, 45*(1), 9–21. doi:10.1007/s40279-014-0241-3

Hague, R. (2015). Managing the child with a fever. *Practitioner, 259*(1784), 17–21, 12–13.

Herdman, T. H. & Kamitsuru, S. (Eds.). *Nursing Diagnoses—Definitions and Classification 2015–2017.* Copyright © 2014, 1994–2014 NANDA International. Used by arrangement with John Wiley & Sons, Inc. Companion website: www.wiley.com/go/nursingdiagnoses

High, K. (2015). Evaluation of infection in the older adult. In K. E. Schmader & L. Park (Eds.), *UpToDate.* Retrieved from http://www.uptodate.com/contents/evaluation-of-infection-in-the-older-adult?source=search_result&search=evaluation+of+infection+in+the+older&selectedTitle=1%7E150

Hoffman, R. J., Etwaru, K., Dreisinger, N., Khokhar, A., & Husk, G. (2013). Comparison of temporal artery thermometry and rectal thermometry in febrile pediatric emergency department patients. *Pediatric Emergency Care, 29*(3), 301–304. doi:10.1097/PEC.0b013e3182850421

Huether, S., Rodway, G., & Defriez, C. (2014). Pain, temperature, regulation, sleep, and sensory function. In K. L. McCance, S. E. Huether, V. L. Brashers, & N. S. Rote (Eds.), *Pathophysiology: The biologic basis for disease in adults and children* (pp. 484–526). St. Louis, MO: Mosby.

Hughes, A. (2016). Poor, homeless, and underserved populations. In N. Coyle & B. R. Ferrell (Eds.), *Legal and ethical aspects of care* (pp. 89–116). New York, NY: Oxford University Press.

Kaya, A., Ergul, N., Kaya, S. Y., Kilic, F., Yilmaz, M. H., Besirli, K., & Ozaras, R. (2013). The management and the diagnosis of fever of unknown origin. *Expert Review of Anti-Infective Therapy, 11*(8), 805–815. doi:10.1586/14787210.2013.814436

KidsandCars.org. (n.d.). *Safety tips from KidsandCars.org.* Retrieved from http://www.kidsandcars.org/userfiles/dangers/heat-stroke/heat-stroke-safety-tips.pdf

Kim, D. C. (2012). Malignant hyperthermia. *Korean Journal of Anesthesiology, 63*(5), 391–401. doi:10.4097/kjae.2012.63.5.391

Krohn, A. R., Sikka, R., & Olson, D. E. (2015). Heat illness in football: Current concepts. *Current Sports Medicine Reports, 14*(6), 463–471. doi:10.1249/JSR.0000000000000212

Kuehn, B. M. (2013). FDA: Acetaminophen may trigger serious skin problems. *JAMA: Journal of the American Medical Association, 310*(8), 785. doi:10.1001/jama.2013.276938

Kuska, T. (2012). Hyperthermia and children left in cars. *Journal of Emergency Nursing, 38*(3), 287–288. doi:10.1016/j.jen.2012.01.006

Li, J. (2015). Hypothermia. In J. Alcock (Ed.), *Medscape.* Retrieved from http://emedicine.medscape.com/article/770542-overview

Marieb, E. N, & Hoehn, K. (2012). *Human anatomy and physiology* (9th ed.). San Francisco, CA: Benjamin Cummings. Reprinted and Electronically reproduced by permission of Pearson Education, Inc., New York, NY.

Mayo Clinic. (2014a). *Heat exhaustion.* Retrieved from http://www.mayoclinic.org/diseases-conditions/heat-exhaustion/basics/prevention/con-20033366

Mayo Clinic. (2014b). *Hypothermia risk factors.* Retrieved from http://www.mayoclinic.org/diseases-conditions/hypothermia/basics/risk-factors/con-20020453

Mayo Clinic. (2014c). *Hypothermia: Prevention: Staying warm in cold weather.* Retrieved from http://www.mayoclinic.org/diseases-conditions/hypothermia/basics/prevention/con-20020453

Mayo Clinic. (2014d). *Hypothermia: Symptoms.* Retrieved from http://www.mayoclinic.org/diseases-conditions/hypothermia/basics/symptoms/con-20020453

McLaren, G., & Spelman, D. (2015). Fever in the intensive care unit. In S. Manaker & G. Finlay (Eds.). *UpToDate.* Retrieved from http://www.uptodate.com/contents/fever-in-the-intensive-care-unit?source=search_result&search=fever+in+the+icu&selectedTitle=1%7E100

Mechem, C. C. (2015). Severe nonexertional hyperthermia (classic heat stroke) in adults. In D. F. Danzi & J. Grayzel (Eds.), *UpToDate.* Retrieved from http://www.uptodate.com/contents/severe-nonexertional-hyperthermia-classic-heat-stroke-in-adults

MedlinePlus. (2014). *Fever.* Retrieved from https://medlineplus.gov/ency/article/003090.htm

Meiman, J., Anderson, H., & Tomasallo, C. (2015). Hypothermia-related deaths—Wisconsin, 2014, and United States, 2003–2013. *MMWR Morbidity and Mortality Weekly Report, 64*(6), 141–143.

Monsma, J., Richerson, J., & Sloand, E. (2015). Empowering parents for evidence-based fever management: An integrative review. *Journal of the American Association of Nurse Practitioners, 27*(4), 222–229. doi:10.1002/2327-6924.12152

Munro, N. (2014). Fever in acute and critical care: A diagnostic approach. *AACN Advanced Critical Care, 25*(3), 237–248.

National Highway Transportation Safety Administration. (n.d.). *Prevent child heatstroke in cars.* Retrieved from http://www.safercar.gov/parents/InandAroundtheCar/heatstroke.htm

National Institute of Neurological Disorders and Stroke. (2013, April). *Febrile seizures fact sheet.* Retrieved from http://www.ninds.nih.gov/disorders/febrile_seizures/detail_febrile_seizures.htm

Nichol, G., Huszti, E., Kim, F., Fly, D., Parnia, S., Donnino, M., … Callaway, C. W. (2013). Does induction of hypothermia improve outcomes after in-hospital cardiac arrest? *Resuscitation, 84*(5), 620–625. doi:10.1016/j.resuscitation.2012.12.009

Null, J. (2016). *Heatstroke deaths of children in vehicles.* Retrieved from http://www.ggweather.com/heat

Oguayo, K. N., Oyetayo, O. O., Stewart, D., Costa, S. M., & Jones, R. O. (2015). Successful use of therapeutic hypothermia in a pregnant patient. *Texas Heart Institute Journal, 42*(4), 367–371. doi:10.14503/THIJ-14-4331

Palazzi, D. L. (2016). Fever of unknown origin in children: Etiology. In M. S. Edwards, R. Sundel, J. E. Drutz, & M. M. Torchia (Eds.), *UpToDate.* Retrieved from http://www.uptodate.com/contents/fever-of-unknown-origin-in-children-evaluation

Rockett, H., Thompson, H. J., & Blissitt, P. A. (2015). Fever management practices of neuroscience nurses: What has changed? *Journal of Neuroscience Nursing, 47*(2), 66–75. doi:10.1097/JNN.0000000000000118

Rozance, P. J., & Rosenberg, A. A. (2012). The neonate. In S. G. Gabbe, J. R. Niebyl, H. L. Galan, E. R. M. Jauniaux, M. B. Landon, J. L. Simpson, & D. A. Driscoll (Eds.), *Obstetrics: Normal and problem pregnancies* (6th ed., p. 528). Philadelphia, PA: Saunders.

Scirica, B. M. (2013). Therapeutic hypothermia after cardiac arrest. *Circulation, 127*(2), 244–250. doi:10.1161/CIRCULATIONAHA.111.076851

Shinawi, M. (2013). Hereditary periodic fever syndromes. *Medscape*. Retrieved from http://emedicine.medscape.com/article/952254-overview

Singh, S., Hanna, E. G., & Kjellstrom, T. (2015). Working in Australia's heat: Health promotion concerns for health and productivity. *Health Promotion International, 30*(2), 239–250. doi:10.1093/heapro/dat027

Singhal, S., Allen, M. W., McAnnally, J. R., Smith, K. S., Donnelly, J. P., & Wang, H. E. (2013). National estimates of emergency department visits for pediatric severe sepsis in the United States. *Peer Journal, 1*, e79. doi:10.7717/peerj.79

Sund-Levander, M., & Grodzinsky, E. (2013). Assessment of body temperature measurement options. *British Journal of Nursing, 22*(15), 880, 882–888.

Thompson, H. J., & Kagan, S. H. (2011). Clinical management of fever by nurses: Doing what works. *Journal of Advanced Nursing, 67*(2), 359–370.

U.S. Food and Drug Administration. (2013). *FDA warns of rare acetaminophen risk*. Retrieved from http://www.fda.gov/downloads/ForConsumers/ConsumerUpdates/UCM363067.pdf

Van Zutphen, A. R., Lin, S., Fletcher, B. A., & Hwang, S. A. (2012). A population-based case-control study of extreme summer temperature and birth defects. *Environmental Health Perspectives, 120*(10), 1443–1449. doi:10.1289/ehp.1104671

Veltmeijer, M. T., Pluim, B., Thijssen, D. H., Hopman, M. T., & Eijsvogels, T. M. (2014). Thermoregulatory responses in wheelchair tennis players: A pilot study. *Spinal Cord, 52*(5), 373–377. doi:10.1038/sc.2014.27

Vilinsky, A., & Sheridan, A. (2014). Hypothermia in the newborn: An exploration of its cause, effect and prevention. *British Journal of Midwifery, 22*(8), 557–562.

Ward, M. A. (2013). Patient information: Fever in children (beyond the basics). *UpToDate*. Retrieved from http://www.uptodate.com/contents/fever-in-children-beyond-the-basics

Ward, M. A. (2015). Fever in infants and children: Pathophysiology and management. In M. S. Edwards & M. M. Torchia (Eds.). *UpToDate*. Retrieved from http://www.uptodate.com/contents/fever-in-infants-and-children-pathophysiology-and-management

Wedro, B. (2015). Heat exhaustion. In M. Conrad Stoppler (Ed.), *Medicinenet*. Retrieved from http://www.medicinenet.com/heat_exhaustion/page5.htm#what_is_the_treatment_for_heat_exhaustion

Wilkinson, J. M., & Ahern, N. R. (2013). *Nursing diagnosis handbook* (10th ed.). Upper Saddle River, NJ: Prentice Hall.

Wong, T., Stang, A. S., Ganshorn, H., Hartling, L., Maconochie, I. K., Thomsen, A. M., & Johnson, D. W. (2013). Combined and alternating paracetamol and ibuprofen therapy for febrile children. *Cochrane Database Systematic Reviews, 10*, CD009572. doi:10.1002/14651858.CD009572.pub2

Zafren, K., & Crawford Mechem, C. (2015). Accidental hypothermia in adults. In D. F. Danzi & Grayzel, J. (Eds.). *UpToDate*. Retrieved from http://www.uptodate.com/contents/accidental-hypothermia-in-adults?source=search_result&search=accidental+hypothermia+in+adults&selectedTitle=1%7E150

Module 21
Tissue Integrity

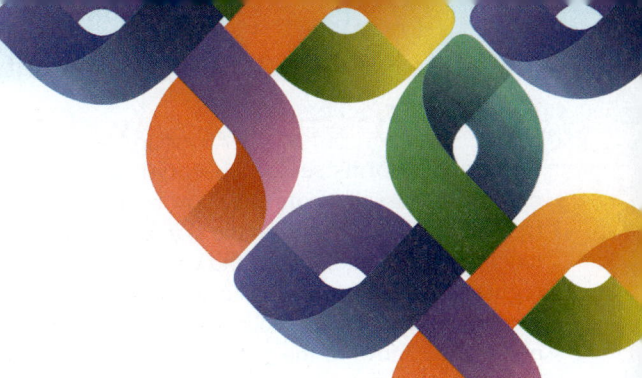

Module Outline and Learning Outcomes

The Concept of Tissue Integrity

Normal Tissue Integrity

21.1 Analyze the physiology of tissue integrity in the body.

Alterations to Tissue Integrity

21.2 Differentiate alterations in tissue integrity.

Concepts Related to Tissue Integrity

21.3 Outline the relationship between tissue integrity and other concepts.

Health Promotion

21.4 Explain the promotion of healthy tissue integrity.

Nursing Assessment

21.5 Differentiate among common assessment procedures and tests used to examine tissue integrity.

Independent Interventions

21.6 Analyze independent interventions nurses can implement for patients with alterations in tissue integrity.

Collaborative Therapies

21.7 Summarize collaborative therapies used by interprofessional teams for patients with alterations in tissue integrity.

Lifespan Considerations

21.8 Differentiate considerations related to the care of patients with alterations in tissue integrity across the lifespan.

Tissue Integrity Exemplars

Exemplar 21.A Burns

21.A Analyze burns as they relate to tissue integrity.

Exemplar 21.B Pressure Injuries

21.B Analyze pressure injuries as they relate to tissue integrity.

Exemplar 21.C Wound Healing

21.C Analyze wound healing as it relates to tissue integrity.

≫ The Concept of Tissue Integrity

Concept Key Terms

The body's **integumentary system** includes the skin, hair, and nails and the sebaceous, sweat, and mammary glands. The skin is the largest organ in the body, and it serves a variety of important functions in maintaining health and protecting the individual from injury. Important nursing functions are maintaining skin integrity and promoting wound healing. Impaired skin integrity—that is, alterations to the dermis and epidermis—is not a serious problem for most healthy individuals, but it is a threat to older adults; to patients with restricted mobility, chronic illnesses, or trauma;

and to those undergoing invasive healthcare procedures. To protect the skin and manage wounds effectively, the nurse must understand the factors that affect skin integrity, the physiology of wound healing, and specific measures that promote optimal conditions for the skin.

Tissue integrity includes integumentary, mucous membrane, corneal, or subcutaneous tissues uninterrupted by wounds. Tissue integrity is influenced by internal factors such as genetics, age, and the underlying health of the individual, as well as by external factors such as activity and injury.

Normal Tissue Integrity

The skin performs several essential functions. It protects underlying tissues from invasion by microorganisms and from trauma. The nerves in the skin enable the perception of touch, pain, pressure, heat, and cold. The skin also assists in regulating temperature. Dilation of blood vessels and the secretion of sweat by the eccrine sweat glands, which function under the control of the central nervous system, enable the body to release excess heat. The sweat glands, secreting a solution of water, electrolytes, and urea, also help rid the body of toxins. The skin supplements the body's intake of vitamin D by synthesizing this vitamin from ultraviolet (UV) light.

Newborns and infants have thinner skin than that of adults. Their skin becomes thicker and less hydrated as they grow and develop. Older adults begin to develop thinner, less elastic skin, a change that occurs as a normal part of the aging process. See the Lifespan Considerations section.

Physiology Review

The skin has three distinct layers: the epidermis, the dermis, and the subcutaneous fatty layer that separates the skin from the underlying tissue (see **Figure 21–1 》**).

Epidermis

The **epidermis**, which is the surface or outermost part of the skin, consists of epithelial cells. The epidermis has either four or five layers, depending on location: five layers over the palms of the hands and the soles of the feet, and four layers over the rest of the body.

The outermost layer of the epidermis, the stratum corneum, is also the thickest, making up about 75% of the total thickness of the epidermis. It consists of about 20–30 sheets of dead cells filled with keratin fragments arranged in "shingles" that flake off as dry skin. **Keratin** is a fibrous, water-repellent protein that gives the epidermis its tough, protective quality.

In areas of thick skin, such as the palms of the hands and the soles of the feet, the stratum lucidum lies below the stratum corneum. The stratum lucidum is made up of dead, flattened cells called keratinocytes, which produced keratin prior to their death.

The stratum granulosum is the next innermost layer and is only two to three cells thick. The cells of the stratum granulosum contain a glycolipid that slows water loss across the epidermis. Keratinization, a thickening of the cells' plasma membranes, begins in the stratum granulosum.

The next layer of the epidermis is the stratum spinosum. Several cells thick, this layer contains abundant cells that arise from the bone marrow and migrate to the epidermis. Mitosis occurs at this layer, although not as abundantly as in the deepest epidermal layer, the stratum basale.

The stratum basale contains keratinocytes and melanocytes, which are the cells that produce the pigment melanin. **Melanin** forms a shield that protects the keratinocytes and

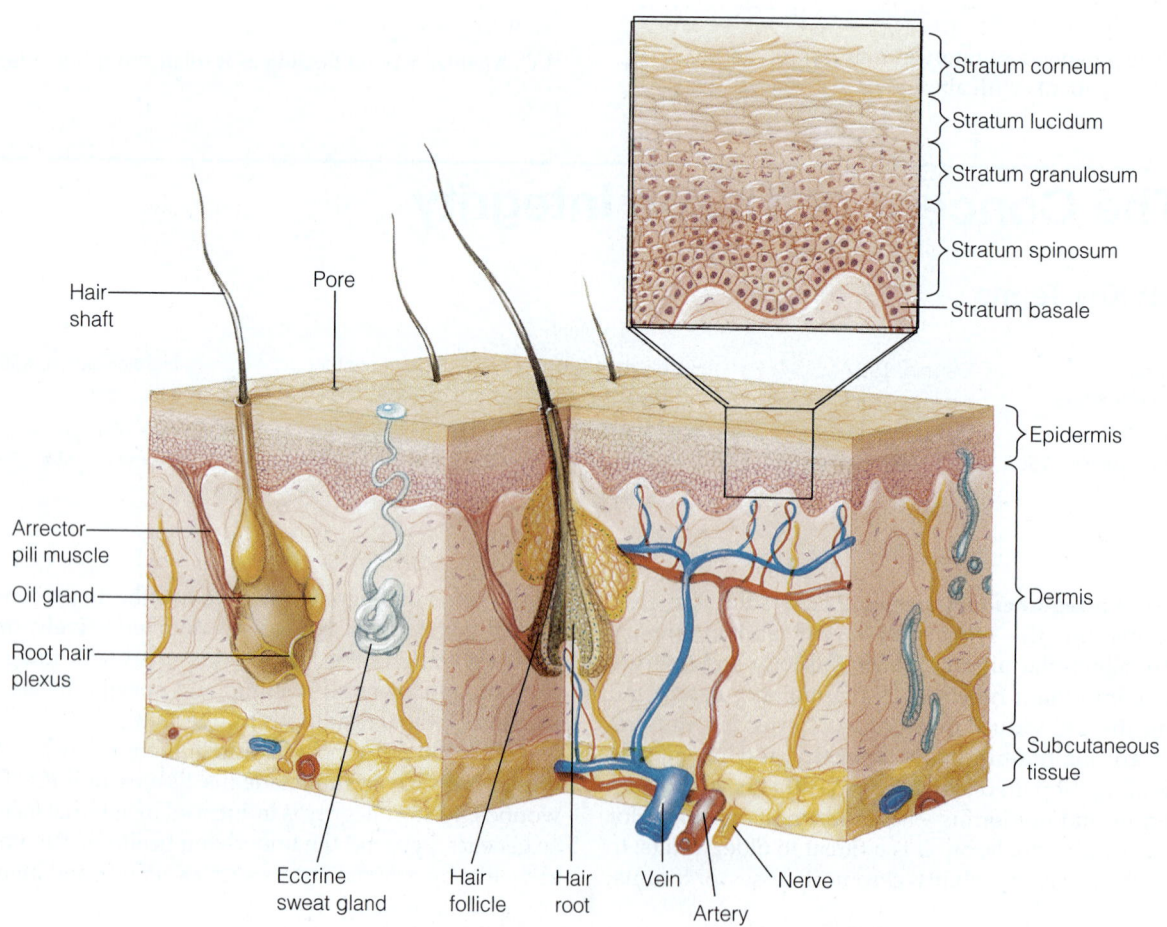

Figure 21–1 》 Three-dimensional view of the skin, subcutaneous tissue, glands, and hairs.

the nerve endings in the dermis from the damaging effects of UV light. Melanocyte activity probably accounts for the difference in skin color in humans. As keratinocytes mature, they move upward through the epidermal layers, eventually becoming dead cells at the surface of the skin. Millions of these cells are worn off by abrasion each day, but millions more are simultaneously produced in the stratum basale.

Dermis

The **dermis** is the second, deeper layer of skin. Made of a flexible connective tissue, this layer is richly supplied with blood cells, nerve fibers, and lymphatic vessels. Most of the hair follicles, sebaceous glands, and sweat glands are located in the dermis.

The dermis consists of a papillary and a reticular layer. The papillary layer contains ridges that indent the overlying epidermis. It also contains capillaries and receptors for pain and touch. The deeper reticular layer contains blood vessels, sweat and sebaceous glands, deep pressure receptors, and dense bundles of collagen fibers. The regions between these bundles form lines of cleavage in the skin. Surgical incisions parallel to these lines of cleavage heal more easily and with less scarring than do incisions or traumatic wounds across cleavage lines.

Subcutaneous Tissue

The **hypodermis**—more commonly known as the **subcutaneous tissue**—lies below the dermis. This layer consists of loose connective tissue and stores roughly half the fat cells in the body. Subcutaneous tissue serves as both an insulator and a cushion for the body. It also stores energy in the form of fat.

Cultural Considerations

Skin color is a significant biologic variation that can affect the delivery of culturally competent nursing care (Yoost & Crawford, 2015). Variations in skin color are associated with the amount of melanin in the skin. In general, individuals with light skin tones produce less melanin than individuals with dark skin tones. Melanin helps protect skin from UV damage, and the darkest skin tones are found in individuals from the hottest climates or whose ancestors lived in the hottest climates. The assessment of a patient with darker skin can be more challenging, and the procedures used are quite different from those used to assess lighter skinned patients.

Skin color can vary between ethnicities in conditions such as jaundice, pallor, and some rashes. When assessing patients with darker skin for alterations in oxygenation, it is important to examine the least pigmented areas, such as the buccal mucosa, lips, tongue, nail beds and palms of the hands, or soles of the feet (Yoost & Crawford, 2015). Pallor may present in darker skinned patients as a yellowish-brown tinge or an ashen gray color. Cyanosis may be more prevalent in the nail beds, lips, and buccal mucosa. Nurses should also take care not to confuse jaundice (a yellowish tinge) with the normal yellow pigmentation in the sclera of darker skinned patients. If jaundice is suspected, the palms of the hands and soles of the feet can also have yellow discoloration and should be assessed for this alteration. It is important for a baseline skin color to be established, and the examiner should not rely on skin tone alone.

Focus on Diversity and Culture
Color Awareness

Color awareness recognizes that skin color is relevant to an individual's health and should not be ignored. Healthcare providers who apply color awareness to health assessment practices are able to more appropriately identify manifestations of specific conditions that present differently in patients of various ethncities. Differences in the complexions and skin tones of these patients, which can vary from light to very dark, can also alter the symptom presentation. Some skin disorders are more common among specific ethnic populations. For example, a major skin disorder among the African American population is postinflammatory hyperpigmentation, in which inflammatory processes affect either the synthesis or release of melanin as a result of injury, or following treatment from certain electromagnetic devices, such as ultrasound (Schwartz, 2016a). African Americans also experience a disproportionate amount of vitiligo, a loss of skin color in blotches or sections that occurs when the cells that produce melanin die or stop functioning (Purnell, 2013).

Individual skin color should also be considered when evaluating pressure points for early signs of skin breakdown or when assessing an existing wound for color changes that could indicate healing or worsening of infection. Patients with lighter skin normally have an identifiable blanch response indicating adequate tissue perfusion, whereas patients with darker skin rarely have the same response to light skin pressure. This makes it difficult to determine when a darker skinned patient may be at risk for pressure ulcers. In patients with darker skin, pressure ulcer assessment should include the application of light pressure and observation for an area that is darker than the surrounding skin or that is taught, shiny, or indurated (Everett, Budescu, & Sommers, 2012).

Alterations to Tissue Integrity

In its role as the body's primary protective barrier, the skin is subject to a vast number of environmental agents and insults. Alterations in tissue integrity can influence the patient's level of wellness in numerous areas.

Alterations and Manifestations

The term *intact skin* refers to the presence of normal skin and skin layers uninterrupted by wounds. The appearance of the skin and skin integrity are influenced by internal factors such as genetics, age, and the underlying health of the individual, as well as by external factors such as activity. The melanocytes of darker skinned individuals have a tendency to show an exaggerated response to skin injury, causing discoloration in areas where lesions have healed (Saedi & Ganesan, 2013). In addition, patients with darker skin tones are prone to a condition called melasma, in which too much melanin is produced. This condition causes discolored patches on areas of the face that receive excessive sun exposure, including the cheeks, the upper lip, the chin, and the forehead. Patients may be sensitive or embarrassed about these areas and seek to cover them with makeup or treat them with bleaching creams. These treatments may irritate the skin or negatively interact with topical medications (Lyford, 2016).

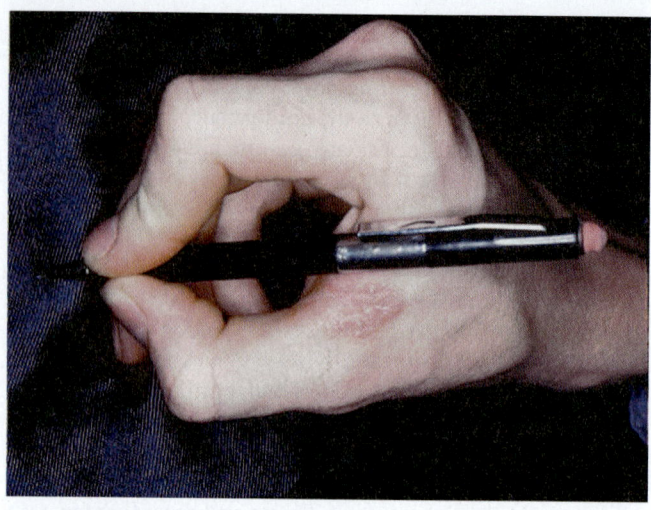

Figure 21–2 ▶▶ Contact dermatitis.

Classification of Skin Disorders

Skin disorders are diverse, and symptoms are often vague, such as itching, inflammation, and redness. As a result, skin disorders can be difficult to classify. One method is to classify these disorders as acute or chronic conditions. Another common, simple classification method groups disorders into three categories:

- *Infectious.* Caused by bacterial, fungal, viral, or parasitic agents. Examples include impetigo (bacterial), athlete's foot (fungal), chickenpox (viral), and lice (parasitic).

- *Inflammatory.* Caused by pathologies such as acne, burns, eczema, dermatitis, and psoriasis. Examples include atopic, seborrheic, and stasis dermatitis.

- *Neoplastic.* Caused by skin cancers. Examples include squamous cell carcinoma, basal cell carcinoma, and malignant melanoma. Melanoma is the most serious type of neoplasm. (For further discussion of skin cancer, see the exemplar on Skin Cancer in the module on Cellular Regulation.)

The infectious classification covers the most diverse collection of disorders. Bacterial and viral agents are the most common causes of infectious skin disease; however, fungal infections can be especially damaging to patients who are immunocompromised. In addition, certain viral skin infections, such as human papillomavirus (HPV), increase patients' likelihood of developing cancerous tumors in the genital and gastrointestinal tracts (Centers for Disease Control and Prevention [CDC], 2016a; National Institutes of Health [NIH], 2014).

Overactive glands and increased hormone production are common in inflammatory disorders, as are itching and cracking of the skin. **Contact dermatitis** is an inflammatory disorder of the skin (see **Figure 21–2 ▶▶**). There are two types: allergic and irritant. Contact dermatitis is characterized by damage to the dermis and epidermis that generally takes the form of a red, pruritic rash. This rash is usually confined to the area of skin that came into contact with the allergen or irritant. Bullae, vesicles, or wheals may also form and take on the pattern or shape of the object that caused the

irritation if it is an allergic response, as in **allergic contact dermatitis**. **Irritant contact dermatitis** is not a hypersensitivity response and results from contact with chemicals (e.g., acids), soaps, dyes, detergents, metals, and perfumes. Individuals with impaired skin barrier function and slower healing processes are at an increased risk of developing contact dermatitis. Research has suggested that older adults are more likely to develop allergic contact dermatitis than younger adults, but are less likely to develop irritant contact dermatitis. One possible explanation for this occurrence is that over time, older adults experience greater exposure and sensitization to allergens (Zhai et al., 2012a). Irritant response is enhanced in younger skin, whereas older skin has a slower, less intense reaction. The decreased effectiveness of the circulatory system and slower turnover of the stratum corneum with age may account for this decreased response (Zhai et al., 2012b).

The inflammatory classification includes conditions caused by exposure to environmental stresses and injury to skin, such as sunburn. Prolonged exposure to sunlight can also give rise to the cancerous cells found in neoplastic skin disorders.

Not all skin abnormalities indicate skin disorders; in fact, the skin often reflects disease processes elsewhere in the body. For example, dry skin accompanied by loss of body hair on the arms and legs can indicate hypothyroidism. Skin **lesions**, or observable changes from normal skin structure, may also indicate disorders in other systems and organs. Skin lesions vary in size, shape, color, and texture. Primary lesions arise from previously healthy skin and include macules, patches, papules, nodules, tumors, vesicles, pustules, bullae, and wheals. Secondary lesions result from changes in primary lesions. They include crusts, scales, **lichenification** (thickening of the skin), scars, keloids, excoriation, fissures, erosion, and ulcers. It is important for the nurse to be able to identify and describe the primary and secondary skin lesions and understand their underlying cause and treatment.

Primary and secondary skin lesions are described and illustrated in **Tables 21–1 ▶▶** and **21–2 ▶▶**. The terms from these tables are used throughout the module.

TABLE 21–1 Primary Skin Lesions

Lesion	Description and Examples	Lesion	Description and Examples
Macule, patch	Flat, nonpalpable change in skin color. Macules are smaller than 1 cm, with a circumscribed border, and patches are larger than 1 cm and may have an irregular border. *Examples:* Macules: freckles, measles, and petechiae. Patches: Mongolian spots, port-wine stains, vitiligo, and chloasma.	Vesicle, bulla	Elevated, fluid-filled, round or oval-shaped, palpable mass with thin, translucent walls and circumscribed borders. Vesicles are smaller than 0.5 cm; bullae are larger than 0.5 cm. *Examples:* Vesicles: herpes simplex, zoster, early chickenpox, poison ivy, and small burn blisters. Bullae: contact dermatitis, friction blisters, and large burn blisters.
Papule, plaque	Elevated, solid, palpable mass with circumscribed border. Papules are smaller than 0.5 cm; plaques are groups of papules that form lesions larger than 0.5 cm. *Examples:* Papules: elevated moles, warts, and lichen planus. Plaques: psoriasis, actinic keratosis, and lichen planus.	Wheal	Elevated, often reddish area with irregular border caused by diffuse fluid in tissues rather than free fluid in a cavity, as in vesicles. Size varies. *Examples:* Insect bites and hives (extensive wheals).
Nodule, tumor	Elevated, solid, hard or soft palpable mass extending deeper into the dermis than a papule. Nodules have circumscribed borders and are 0.5–2 cm; tumors may have irregular borders and are larger than 2 cm. *Examples:* Nodules: small lipoma, squamous cell carcinoma, fibroma, and intradermal nevi. Tumors: large lipoma, carcinoma, and hemangioma.	Pustule	Elevated, pus-filled vesicle or bulla with circumscribed border. Size varies. *Examples:* Acne, impetigo, and carbuncles (large boils).
Cyst	Elevated, encapsulated, fluid-filled or semi-solid mass originating in the subcutaneous tissue or dermis, usually 1 cm or larger. *Examples:* Varieties include sebaceous cysts and epidermoid cysts.		

TABLE 21–2 Secondary Skin Lesions

Lesion	Description and Examples	Lesion	Description and Examples
Atrophy	A translucent, dry, paperlike, sometimes wrinkled skin surface resulting from thinning or wasting of the skin due to loss of collagen and elastin. *Examples:* Striae and aged skin.	Ulcer	Deep, irregularly shaped area of skin loss extending into the dermis or subcutaneous tissue. Ulcers may bleed or leave a scar. *Examples:* Decubitus ulcers (pressure sores), stasis ulcers, and chancres.
Erosion	Wearing away of the superficial epidermis causing a moist, shallow depression. Because erosions do not extend into the dermis, they heal without scarring. *Examples:* Scratch marks and ruptured vesicles.	Fissure	Linear crack with sharp edges, extending into the dermis. *Examples:* Cracks at the corners of the mouth or on the hands and athlete's foot.

(continued on next page)

TABLE 21–2 Secondary Skin Lesions *(continued)*

Lesion	Description and Examples	Lesion	Description and Examples
Lichenification 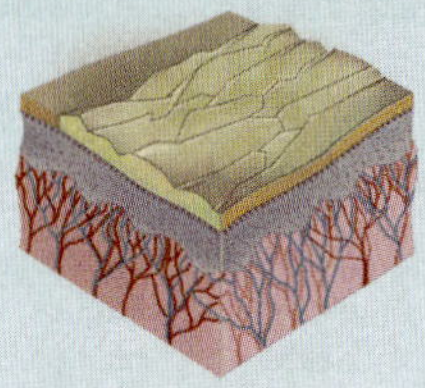	Rough, thickened, hardened area of epidermis resulting from chronic irritation such as scratching or rubbing. *Examples:* Chronic dermatitis.	Scar 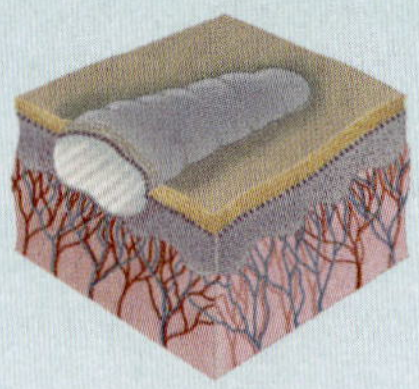	Flat, irregular area of connective tissue left after a lesion or wound has healed. New scars may be red or purple; older scars may be silvery or white. *Examples:* Healed surgical wound or injury and healed acne.
Scales 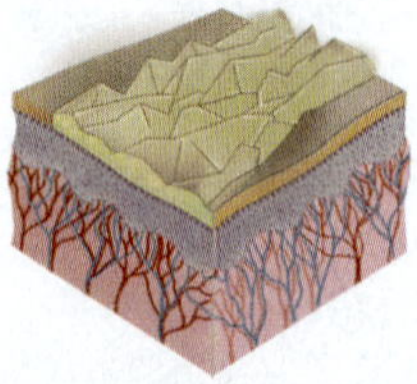	Shedding flakes of greasy, keratinized skin tissue. Color may be white, gray, or silver. Texture may vary from fine to thick. *Examples:* Dry skin, dandruff, psoriasis, and eczema.	Keloid 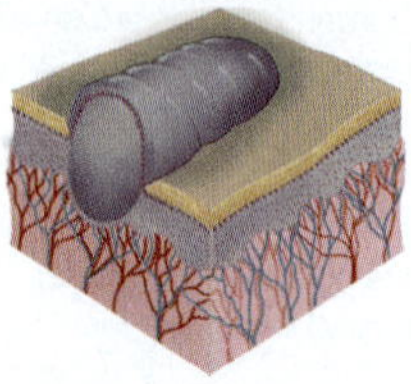	Elevated, irregular, darkened area of excess scar tissue caused by excessive collagen formation during healing. Keloids extend beyond the site of the original injury. There is a higher incidence in individuals of African descent. *Examples:* Keloid from ear piercing or surgery.
Crust 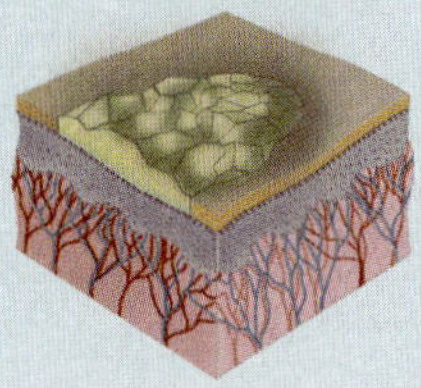	Dry blood, serum, or pus left on the skin surface when vesicles or pustules burst. Crusts can be red-brown, orange, or yellow. Large crusts that adhere to the skin surface are called scabs. *Examples:* Eczema, impetigo, herpes, or scabs following abrasion.		

Common Skin Disorders

Disorders of the skin can vary greatly in their presentation and severity of symptoms. Skin disorders, such as bacterial infections or dermatitis, can be temporary or acute in duration, whereas genetic disorders and changes in pigmentation are permanent or chronic. Acute skin disorders generally have situational causes; treatment includes reduction of inflammation and avoidance of the trigger, if applicable.

Selected common skin disorders are outlined in **Table 21–3 》》**. The chronic disorders can be present from birth or may suddenly appear later in life, and often their cause is unknown. Selected common chronic skin disorders are outlined in **Table 21–4 》》**. Effective treatments are available that provide extended periods of remission for certain chronic skin disorders; however, these treatments do not provide a cure (Brind'Amour, 2016).

TABLE 21–3 Common Acute Skin Disorders

Disorder	Description
Bacterial Skin Infections	
Methicillin-resistant **Staphylococcus aureus (MRSA)**	A common cause of cellulitis, MRSA enters the skin through a crack or cut in the skin. This infection is most common in the lower extremities and is typically unilateral. The skin over the infected area is hot, erythematous, edematous, and tender to the touch. The most common way MRSA is transmitted is through contact with infected skin or sharing personal items with someone who is infected (CDC, 2016b).
Impetigo 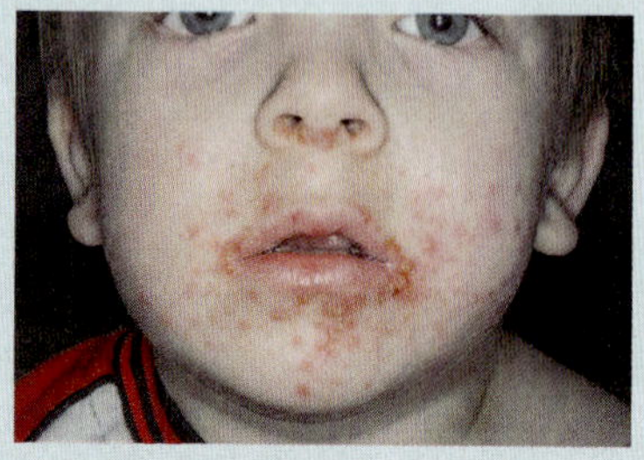	Impetigo is a superficial skin infection common in children that is caused by *Streptococci*, *Staphylococci*, or both. It presents as an itchy rash with clusters of fluid-filled vesicles that rupture easily (see **Figure 21–3 》》**). Ruptured vesicles develop a honey-colored crust over the lesions. It is most commonly seen on the face, arms, and legs. General risk factors include poor hygiene, a moist environment, or chronic nasopharyngeal infection with the causative bacteria.

Source: Scott Camazine/Alamy Stock Photo.

Figure 21–3 》》 Child with a rash from impetigo.

TABLE 21–3 Common Acute Skin Disorders *(continued)*

Disorder	Description
Folliculitis	Folliculitis is an infection of hair follicles that is usually caused by *Staphylococcus aureus* but can be caused by other organisms. It is characterized by mild pain, pruritus or irritation, and superficial pustules or nodules around the hair follicle.
Furuncles and carbuncles	Furuncles, or boils, are caused by staphylococcal bacteria and involve a hair follicle and surrounding tissue. MRSA is a common cause. Furuncles occur more frequently on the neck, breasts, face, and buttocks. Carbuncles are clusters of furuncles connected beneath the skin that cause deeper pus formation and scarring. Both types of infection can affect healthy individuals but are more common among those who are obese, are immunocompromised, have diabetes, or are older adults.
Paronchyia	This soft tissue infection around the fingernail can be acute or chronic. Acute infections are frequently caused by staphylococci, whereas chronic infections are usually caused by a fungus. This is the most common hand infection in the United States. It generally begins as cellulitis and can progress to a painful, purulent abscess. The affected area often appears erythematous and swollen. Pus may collect under the skin next to the nail bed in more advanced cases.

Fungal Skin Infections

Candidiasis

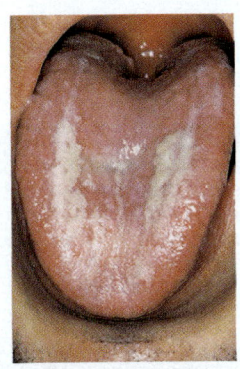

Source: Mediscan/Alamy Stock Photo.

Figure 21–4 » Candidiasis (thrush) in an adult.

Candidiasis is infection with the *Candida* species, most commonly *Candida albicans*, also referred to as thrush. These infections are most commonly seen in skinfolds or areas where skin rubs together (groin, axilla, gluteal folds, beneath the breasts), genitals, the oral mucosa, and between fingers and toes (see **Figure 21–4** »). *Candida* is a harmless yeast that is always present on the skin and mucous membranes until conditions provide an environment for it to grow. Risk factors include hot weather, poor hygiene, infrequent diaper or undergarment changes, altered flora due to antibiotic therapy, and immunosuppression. Thrush may also be seen in patients receiving chemotherapy and in organ transplant recipients. Infection presents as pruritic, well-demarcated, erythematous patches that vary in size. Papules and pustules may be present around the primary patches of infection, as is often seen with thrush in the diaper region. Infection in the oropharyngeal area or oral thrush causes white plaques on oral mucous membranes that may bleed when scraped.

Tinea   *Tinea capitis*

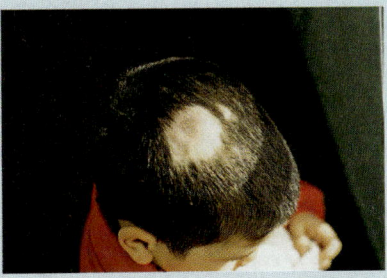

Source: PR Bouree/BSIP SA/Alamy Stock Photo.

Figure 21–5 » *Tinea capitis* (scalp ringworm).

Tinea pedis (athlete's foot)

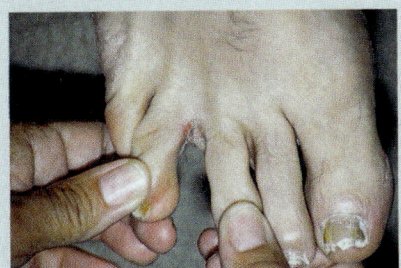

Source: Ted Foxx/Alamy Stock Photo.

Figure 21–6 » *Tinea pedis* (athlete's foot).

This group of dermatophyte infections is caused by a fungus. These types of infections are generally not serious but can be uncomfortable. They can be spread between individuals (by touching an infected person), from a damp surface such as a shower floor, or from a pet. The presentation of symptoms depends on the area of the body affected.

- Tinea capitis, also known as scalp ringworm, is a contagious infection of the scalp that mainly affects children. It causes the gradual appearance of round patches of dry scales, alopecia, or both (see **Figure 21–5** »).
- Tinea corporis, also known as body ringworm, is an infection of the face, trunk, and extremities. This infection causes pink to red ring-shaped patches and plaques with raised scaly borders and a clear center.
- Tinea cruris, or jock itch, is primarily associated with a moist environment and restrictive clothing. This infection affects male patients more frequently than female patients due to the close proximity between the scrotum and thigh; it is more common during warm weather.
- Tinea onychomycosis or tinea unguium occurs in approximately 10% of individuals and is a fungal infection of the nail bed, nail plate, or both. The toenails are more commonly infected than the fingernails.
- Tinea pedis, or athlete's foot, is the most common of the tinea infections. The infection develops because of sweating of the feet, which allows moisture to accumulate in the warm areas between the toes, facilitating fungus growth (see **Figure 21–6** »).
- Tinea versicolor is an infection caused by the yeast *Malassezia furfur*, which is a harmless yeast that lives on the skin. This infection is common, especially among young adults.

(continued on next page)

TABLE 21–3 Common Acute Skin Disorders *(continued)*

Disorder	Description
Viral Skin Disorders	
Varicella zoster (chickenpox) 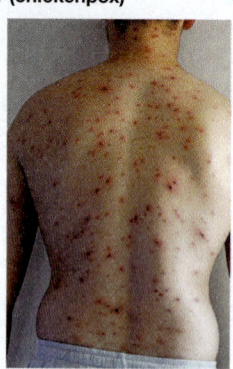 *Source:* Chris Deeney/Alamy Stock Photo. **Figure 21–7** ›› Varicella zoster (chickenpox) in an adult.	This acute systemic infection, which usually occurs during childhood, is caused by the varicella-zoster virus. This infection is extremely contagious and is spread by airborne droplets or aerosolized particles, or through direct contact with the viral skin lesions. It is most communicable from 48 hours prior to eruption of the first skin lesions until the final lesions have crusted. Individuals may experience mild headache, moderate fever, and malaise 10–21 days after exposure to the virus, which is approximately 24–36 hours before lesions appear. The initial macular rash first appears on the face and trunk, erupting in successive crops. The macules progress to papules within a few hours, then to vesicles on red bases, which are accompanied by intense pruritus (see **Figure 21–7** ››). These lesions become pustular and then crust. Crusts typically disappear within 20 days after onset. Infected individuals should not be in close contact with individuals who do not have immunity until the final lesions have crusted. A vaccine is available to provide immunity against the virus.
Dermatitis	
Contact dermatitis	Contact dermatitis is inflammation of the skin caused by direct contact with an allergen or irritant. It typically manifests as a localized red, pruritic rash or irritation in the superficial layers of the skin; edematous vesicles or bullae may be present in the case of allergic contact. The rash may not appear until several days after exposure and is usually confined to the area of skin that was in contact with the irritant or allergen. Healing may take several weeks and is slowed if the skin is continually exposed to the allergen or irritant. There are two types: allergic and irritant.
Seborrheic dermatitis	This inflammation occurs in skin regions that have a large number of sebaceous glands, such as the face, scalp, or upper trunk. The pathophysiology is unclear, but there has been a link between its development and the amount of *Malassezia* yeast present on the skin. This disorder occurs most often in infants, usually within the first 3 months of life, and in adults ages 30–70 years. The symptoms tend to develop gradually and are usually apparent only as dry or greasy diffuse scaling of the scalp. In newborns, a thick, yellow, crusted scalp lesion (cradle cap) and yellow scaling behind the ears may develop. In adults, if the disease is severe, yellow-red scaling papules may appear along the hairline, behind the ears, in the ear canals, on the eyebrows, in the axilla, on the bridge of the nose, around the nose, and over the sternum. The incidence and severity of the disease appears to be affected by climate (worse in cold weather), genetic factors, neurologic disorders (especially Parkinson disease), and emotional or physical stress.
Urticaria *Source:* Mediscan/Alamy Stock Photo. **Figure 21–8** ›› Urticaria (hives).	This disorder consists of erythematous, raised, pruritic, slightly elevated areas with clearly defined borders (see **Figure 21–8** ››). These areas typically appear and disappear randomly, leaving normal-looking skin behind. Urticaria results from the release of histamine, bradykinin, and other vasoactive substances within the superficial dermis. This can be an acute disorder, such as a response to an allergen, or a chronic disorder resulting from autoimmune disorders. Urticaria is often self-resolving, but pharmacologic measures can be used to relieve pruritus and other symptoms.
Lichen planus	This recurrent, pruritic, inflammatory eruption is thought to be caused by a T-cell–mediated autoimmune reaction. Certain medications such as nonsteroidal anti-inflammatory drugs (NSAIDs), angiotensin-converting–enzyme (ACE) inhibitors, beta blockers, and sulfonylureas can also cause the development of this disorder. It is characterized by small, individual, polygonal, flat-topped, purple-colored papules that may merge into rough scaly plaques. These lesions are usually symmetrically distributed and are most commonly seen on the inner surfaces of the wrists, legs, trunk, glans penis, and oral and vaginal mucosa. Approximately 50% of those who develop the disorder also develop it in the mouth, where it presents as a lacy, bluish-white patch that forms in lines called Wickham striae. The disorder can last for 1–2 years and usually disappears on its own. Children are not frequently affected.

TABLE 21–3 Common Acute Skin Disorders *(continued)*

Disorder	Description
Insect and Spider Bites	
Bees and wasps	Stinging insect venom can cause local toxic reactions in all individuals and allergic reactions only in those who have been previously sensitized. The severity of the reaction is related to the dose of venom and the degree of previous sensitization. Individuals who are exposed to large amounts of venom at one time (i.e., from a swarm attack) and those with highly venom-specific IgE levels are most at risk for an anaphylactic reaction. Reactions to insect bites typically present as immediate burning, transient pain, and pruritus, an erythematous area, swelling, and induration up to a few centimeters in diameter. An allergic reaction can present with urticaria, angioedema, bronchospasm, refractory hypotension, or a combination of these symptoms. Individuals with a known hypersensitivity to insect stings should carry an epinephrine autoinjector.
Ticks *Lyme disease* 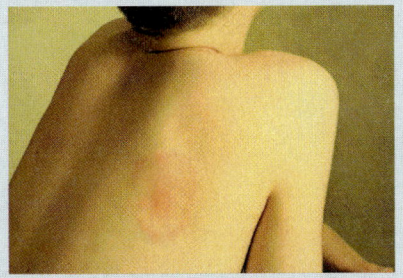 *Source:* Kevin Shields/Alamy Stock Photo. **Figure 21–9 》** Child with a classic bull's-eye rash of Lyme disease.	Tick bites are painless and often cause a red papule at the site of the bite. Disease transmission is the main concern, and the risk of transmission increases the longer the tick is attached to the body. Lyme disease is an infection transmitted by ticks and is caused by the spirochete *Borrelia burgdorferi.* Early manifestations of the disease include an erythema migrans rash, which is the hallmark and best clinical indicator of this disease (see **Figure 21–9 》**). This rash can appear 3–32 days after the tick bite and resembles a bull's-eye in appearance. The area may or may not be hot to touch or indurated. Individuals can develop cardiac, neurologic, or joint abnormalities within weeks to months after the presentation of erythema migrans.
Spiders	Almost all species of spiders are venomous; however, the fangs of most species are either too fragile or too short to penetrate the skin. The two species that most frequently cause serious systemic reactions from their bites are brown spiders (i.e., violin, fiddleback, and recluse) and widow spiders (i.e., black widow).
Brown spider bite	■ Brown spider bites are the most common in the United States. The area of the bite is initially painless, but pain, which can be severe, develops within 30–60 minutes and can involve the entire extremity. The area of the bite appears erythematous and ecchymotic; generalized pruritus may also be present. A central bleb forms at the site of the bite, and the area develops a bull's-eye–like appearance. The bleb increases in size, fills with blood, and ruptures, leaving an ulcerated area. A black eschar forms over the ulcerated area and eventually sloughs off. Individuals can also experience systemic effects, including fever, chills, nausea, vomiting, arthralgias, myalgias, generalized rash, seizures, disseminated intravascular coagulation, hemolysis, or renal failure.
Black widow bite	■ The bite of the black widow spider usually causes an immediate, sharp, stinging sensation. Localized, persistent pain; diaphoresis; erythema; and piloerection develop within 1 hour after the bite occurs. These bites are graded as mild, moderate, or severe based on the presentation of symptoms. If the bite is severe, the individual develops a systemic syndrome, which can last up to 3 days, but residual symptoms may last for weeks to months.
Infestations	
Pediculosis 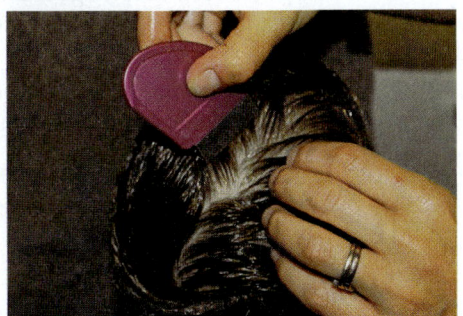 *Source:* Naomi Aylott/Alamy Stock Photo. **Figure 21–10 》** Child with nits from a lice infestation.	Pediculosis can infect the scalp, body, pubis, and eyelashes and is transmitted by contact. Manifestations differ by location. ■ Scalp infestations are most common among girls ages 5–11, but can affect almost anyone (see **Figure 21–10 》**). These infestations are rare in African Americans. Scalp infestations cause severe pruritus and scalp excoriations, and posterior cervical adenopathy can be present. ■ Body pediculosis live primarily in bedding and on clothing, not people. Their bites are identified by the presence of small red puncta that cause pruritus and associated linear scratch marks. Manifestations are most commonly seen on the shoulders, buttocks, and abdomen. ■ Pubic pediculosis most commonly infest the pubic and perianal hairs, but may spread to the thighs, trunk, and facial hair. This infestation causes pruritus, and some individuals may have excoriations and regional lymphadenopathy.

(continued on next page)

TABLE 21–3 Common Acute Skin Disorders *(continued)*

Disorder	Description
Scabies	Scabies is an infestation of the skin caused by a mite (*Sarcoptes scabiei*) that lives in burrowed tunnels in the stratum corneum. Transmission occurs through physical contact, and the primary risk factor is crowded conditions. The main symptom is intense pruritus that is classically worse at night. This infestation initially presents as erythematous papules in the finger web spaces, internal surfaces of the wrists and elbows, axillary folds, along the beltline, or on the lower buttocks. The papules can affect any area of the body. Burrows are usually seen on the wrists, hands, or feet and present as fine, wavy, slightly scaly lines. They can be up to 1 cm in length. The mite is often visible as a tiny dark papule at the end of the burrow.
Bed bugs *Source:* Kuttig–RF–Kids/Alamy Stock Photo. .... **Figure 21–11 》** Cluster of raised red bed bug bites.	Bed bugs are small oval insects that are attracted to humans by warmth and carbon dioxide and bite exposed skin, usually at night. They hide in cracks and crevices of mattresses, cushions, bedframes, and other structures. Lesions from the bites can develop in the morning up to 10 days after being bitten. They may appear as puncta only; purpuric macules; erythematous, pruritic macules, papules, or wheals, each with a central hemorrhagic punctum; or bullae (blisters). The lesions may form a linear pattern or be seen in clusters and usually resolve in approximately 1 week (see **Figure 21–11 》**).
Adolescent and Adult Skin	
Acne vulgaris	Acne vulgaris is the most common skin disease in the United States and can be classified as inflammatory or noninflammatory. Noninflammatory acne is characterized by comedones, which are sebaceous plugs impacted within follicles. Inflammatory acne occurs when papules and pustules develop within the closed comedones. The inflamed follicle can rupture into the dermis, causing an additional inflammatory reaction and papule production. Nodules and cyst formation, which can be painful, are also manifestations of inflammatory acne.

Sources: Based on Billingsley, E. M. (2016). Paronychia. *Medscape.* Retrieved from http://emedicine.medscape.com/article/1106062-overview; *Dermatologic disorders.* (n.d.). Retrieved from Merck Manual Professional Version website: http://www.merckmanuals.com/professional/dermatologic-disorders; *Infectious diseases.* (n.d.). Retrieved from Merck Manual Professional Version website: http://www.merckmanuals.com/professional/infectious-diseases; *Injuries and poisoning.* (n.d.). Retrieved from Merck Manual Professional Version website: http://www.merckmanuals.com/professional/injuries-poisoning

Wounds

Body wounds are either intentional or unintentional. Intentional trauma occurs during therapy; for example, an operation or a venipuncture. Although removing a tumor, for example, is therapeutic, cutting into tissues traumatizes them. Unintentional wounds are accidental, such as a fractured arm that occurs in a skating accident. When the tissues are traumatized without a break in the skin, the wound is closed. When the skin or mucous membrane surface is broken, the wound is open.

Wounds may be described according to how they are acquired (see **Table 21–5 》**). They also can be described according to the likelihood and degree of wound contamination.

- *Clean wounds* are uninfected wounds in which minimal inflammation is encountered and the respiratory, alimentary, genital, and urinary tracts are not entered. Clean wounds are primarily closed wounds.
- *Clean contaminated wounds* are surgical wounds in which the respiratory, alimentary, genital, or urinary tract has been entered. Such wounds show no evidence of infection.
- *Contaminated wounds* include open, fresh, accidental wounds and surgical wounds that involve a major break in sterile technique or a large amount of spillage from the gastrointestinal tract. Contaminated wounds show evidence of inflammation.
- *Dirty or infected wounds* include wounds containing dead tissue and wounds with evidence of a clinical infection, such as purulent drainage.

Wounds, excluding pressure injuries and burns, are classified by depth, that is, the tissue layers involved in the wound:

- *Partial-thickness wounds* are confined to the skin, that is, the dermis and epidermis; they heal by regeneration.
- *Full-thickness wounds* involve the dermis, epidermis, subcutaneous tissue, and possibly muscle and bone; they require connective tissue repair.

TABLE 21–4 Common Chronic Skin Disorders

Disorder	Description
Viral Skin Infections	
Herpes simplex types 1 and 2	The herpes simplex viruses (type 1 and type 2) are often the cause of recurrent infection of the skin, mouth, lips, eyes, and genitals. Transmission results from close contact with a person who is actively shedding the virus and can occur whether or not lesions are present. Out-breaks are generally preceded by a prodromal period of tingling discomfort or itching. Within 6 hours of this period, clusters of small, tense vesicles appear on an erythematous base. These lesions can be painful depending on their location. The vesicles typically last for a few days before rupturing and forming a thin, dry, yellowish crust. Lesions generally heal within 10–19 days after their initial appearance in a primary infection or within 5–10 days in recurrent infection.
Herpes zoster 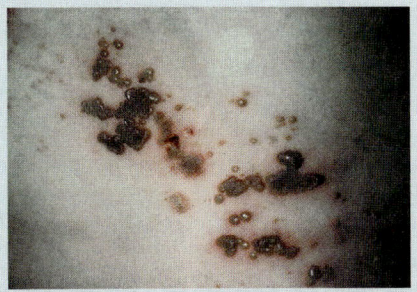 *Source:* Centers for Disease Control and Prevention (CDC). .... **Figure 21–12** ≫ Herpes zoster (shingles) is characterized by clusters of painful vesicles.	Herpes zoster infection results from the same virus that causes chickenpox. It frequently occurs in older adults and those who are immunocompromised. It is characterized by pain, tingling, or itching on a unilateral area of skin (a dermatome). In 2–3 days following the initial sensations, clusters of small vesicles on an erythematous base develop; lesions can continue to form for 3–5 days (see **Figure 21–12** ≫). The site is generally in the thoracic or lumbar region. Adults age 60 and older should receive the zoster vaccine whether they have had the virus or not, as it has been shown to decrease the incidence of zoster infection.
Warts	Warts are named by their location and appearance; they can be caused by more than 100 human papillomavirus (HPV) subtypes. Most forms are asymptomatic and spread by autoin-oculation. Common warts have edges that are sharply demarcated, rough, round or irregular, and firm; they can be light gray, yellow, brown, or gray-black in color. They can range in size from 2 to 10 mm in diameter. These warts most often appear on areas of the body subject to trauma, such as fingers, elbows, or knees, but may spread to other areas. Flat warts are smooth, flat-topped, yellow-brown, or pink or flesh-colored papules. They are most often located on the face and along scratch marks. This type of wart is more commonly seen among children and young adults. Palmar and plantar warts occur on the palms of the hands and soles of the feet. They are flattened by pressure, surrounded by cornified epithelium, and are often tender or mildly painful because of their location.
Genetic Disorders	
Eczema	Eczema is an immune-mediated inflammation of the skin that primarily affects children but can also be seen in adults. It appears to result from an interaction between genetic and environmental factors. Eczema is characterized by a rash that develops and often recurs in only one or a few areas, usually the hands, upper arms, antecubital space, or behind the knees. The rash is always pruritic, although the color, intensity, and location may vary. The intense itching often leads to uncontrollable scratching that triggers an itch-scratch-itch cycle, making the problem worse. The continuous scratching causes lichenification (thickening) of the skin.
Psoriasis 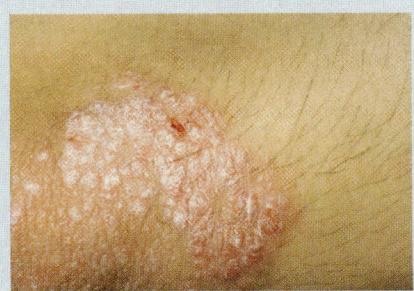 *Source:* Olavs/Shutterstock. .... **Figure 21–13** ≫ Psoriasis is characterized by raised red lesions covered with thick, silvery scales.	Psoriasis is an inflammatory disease and most commonly presents as well-circumscribed, erythematous papules and plaques covered with silvery scales (see **Figure 21–13** ≫). The lesions can be completely asymptomatic or pruritic and are most often localized on the elbows and knees, scalp, sacrum, buttocks, and genitals. In some cases, the eyebrows, axilla, nails, and umbilicus may also be affected. Multiple factors, including genetics, contribute to the development of this disease, and common triggers include trauma, infection, emotional stress, tobacco use, alcohol consumption, and certain drugs.

(continued on next page)

TABLE 21–4 Common Chronic Skin Disorders *(continued)*

Disorder	Description
Benign Neoplasms	

Note: *Malignant skin neoplasms are covered in the exemplar on Skin Cancer in the module on Cellular Regulation.*

Disorder	Description
Photodermatitis and actinic keratosis	Photodermatitis is an abnormal skin reaction to UV rays. The level of exposure and reaction varies by individual. It presents as pruritic macules, vesicles, or papules; lesions that resemble eczema; pain; erythema; swelling; chills; headache; fever; and nausea. Risk factors include diseases causing the skin to be sensitive to light, such as lupus or eczema; genetic or metabolic factors; and reactions to chemicals or medications. Those at greatest risk are individuals who have fair to light skin, red or blond hair, and green or blue eyes; individuals with lupus, porphyria, or polymorphous light eruptions; and individuals exposed to UV rays for 30 minutes to several hours per day. Actinic keratosis is precancerous changes in skin cells that occur from many years of sun exposure. These lesions are usually pink or red in color, poorly marginated, and feel rough and scaly when palpated. Those at greater risk include individuals who are continuously exposed to the sun, such as farmers, ranchers, sailors, athletes, and frequent sunbathers or tanning salon users.
Hemangiomas	Hemangiomas are the most common tumor of infancy, affecting 10–12% of infants by age 1 year. The preferred term for these lesions is *infantile hemangioma*. Lesions that are superficial have a bright red appearance, whereas deeper lesions are bluish in color. Minor trauma can cause these lesions to bleed or ulcerate, and the ulcers may be painful. Certain locations of lesions can interfere with function, such as those on the face, or may indicate underlying anomalies.
Moles and nevi	These flesh- to brown-colored macules, papules, or nodules are composed of clusters of melanocytes or nevus cells. The only significance of these lesions, aside from cosmetic, is their resemblance to melanoma. Benign lesions are typically symmetrical in appearance with round or oval borders, have even pigmentation, and are smaller than 6 cm in diameter. Most lesions typically change in consistency over the lifespan of an individual, becoming softer and boggy or firmer and less pigmented. The lifetime risk of an individual mole becoming malignant is low; however, those with large numbers of benign moles (more than 50) have an increased risk.
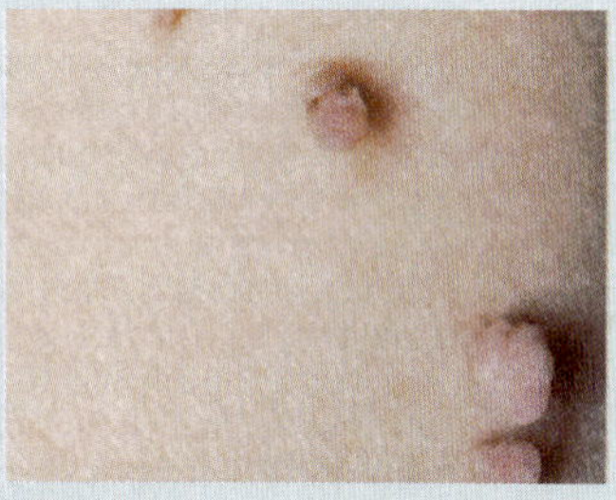 **Skin tags**	Skin tags are common soft, small, flesh-colored or hyperpigmented, pedunculated lesions and are usually multiple in number (see **Figure 21–14 »**). They are typically found on the neck, groin, and axilla. Although they are usually asymptomatic, they may be irritating and can be removed by freezing with liquid nitrogen, excision with a scalpel or scissors, or light eletrodesiccation.

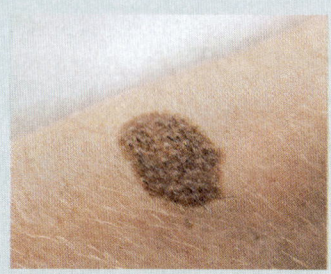

Source: Jodi Jacobson/E+/Getty Images.

Figure 21–14 » Skin tags.

Disorder	Description
Changes in Pigmentation	
Vitiligo	Vitiligo is a loss of melanocytes in the skin that causes areas of depigmentation that vary in size. The cause is unclear but may be related to genetic and autoimmune factors. This disorder is characterized by hypo- or depigmented areas on the skin that usually have sharply defined borders and are normally symmetric. These depigmented areas may be localized, involving only one or two spots, or entire body segments; rarely it may be generalized, involving most of the skin surface. It most commonly involves the face (especially around the orifices), digits, dorsal surface of the hands, inner surface of the wrists, knees, elbows, or shins; dorsal surface of the ankles, axilla, inguinal area, anogenital area, umbilicus, and nipples.
Café au lait spots	Café au lait spots are hyperpigmented freckle-like macules that can vary in color from light brown to dark brown, with borders that may be smooth or irregular (see **Figure 21–15 »**). These lesions can vary in size and number and are most commonly distributed over the trunk, pelvis, knees, and elbows. They are usually the earliest manifestation of the genetic disorder neurofibromatosis.

Source: Wakila/E+/Getty Images.

Figure 21–15 » Café au lait spots.

TABLE 21–4 Common Chronic Skin Disorders *(continued)*

Disorder	Description
Lentigo	Commonly caused by chronic sun exposure, lentigo is a flat, tan-to-brown, oval macule that occurs most frequently on the face and dorsal surface of the hands. These lesions typically first appear during middle age and increase in number as the individual ages. Although there has not been a link established between these lesions and melanoma, they are a risk factor. There are systemic disorders that may also cause these lesions to appear.
Mongolian spot	Mongolian spots are congenital, nonblanching, hyperpigmented patches most commonly seen over the lumbosacral area. Usually present at birth or during the first few weeks of life, these lesions are most commonly seen in individuals of Asian or African ethnicity but may also be seen in Hispanic individuals. They usually resolve by 1–2 years of age and rarely persist into adulthood. The lesions are generally bluish-green to black in color and can be oval or irregular in shape. Sometimes lesions are located in abnormal locations, such as the shoulders, limbs, mandibular area, or occiput, and may be confused with other melanocyte disorders or bruises secondary to child abuse, necessitating documentation at birth. Once believed to be benign, research has indicated that there is an association between these lesions and other conditions.
Acanthosis nigricans	Acanthosis nigricans is dark, thickened, velvety discoloration in body folds and creases, usually around the neck, axilla, and groin. The affected area may also be pruritic or have an odor. One of the most common causes of this disorder is hyperglycemia. This disorder has rapidly increased in prevalence since the rate of prediabetes and type 2 diabetes has increased. It may also be caused by hormonal disorders or certain medications, such as birth control pills or corticosteroids. In rare cases, this condition can be a warning sign of malignancy in the liver, colon, or stomach.
Vascular Lesions	
Spider angioma	This small, bright red vascular lesion consists of a central dilated blood vessel or punctum surrounded by a radial pattern of slender dilated capillaries that resemble legs. These asymptomatic lesions range in size from 0.5 to 10 mm in diameter and are most frequently found on exposed areas of the body, such as the face, neck, upper trunk, and arms. They are an acquired condition and can develop during pregnancy, after contraceptive use, or as a result of internal disease such as cirrhosis.
Nevus flammeus (port-wine stain)	These flat pink, red, or purplish lesions are present at birth and can appear anywhere on the body; however, most involve the head and neck. The growth of the lesion is proportionate with the child and becomes darker and more palpable with age. Lesions are usually unilateral and can be an indication of other syndromes.
Adolescent/Adult Skin	
Rosacea 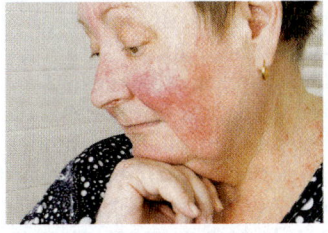 *Source:* Milan Lipowski/Alamy Stock Photo.	Rosacea is a chronic inflammatory disorder that affects the face and scalp and is most commonly seen in individuals with fair complexions who are from ages 30 to 50. It is characterized by facial flushing, erythema, telangiectasias, papules, pustules, and in severe cases, rhinophyma (red, bulbous appearance of the nose) (see **Figure 21–16 »**). This disorder generally manifests itself in four sequential phases, and treatment may cause the disorder to return to an earlier stage. Progression of the disorder to the late stage is not unavoidable.

Figure 21–16 » Woman with a red face rash characteristic of rosacea.

Sources: Based on Centers for Disease Control and Prevention (CDC). (2016c). *Psoriasis.* Retrieved from https://www.cdc.gov/psoriasis; *Dermatologic disorders.* (n.d.). Retrieved from Merck Manual Professional Version website: http://www.merckmanuals.com/professional/dermatologic-disorders; Ehrlich, S. D. (2015). *Photodermatitis.* Retrieved from University of Maryland Medical Center: http://umm.edu/health/medical/altmed/condition/photodermatitis; Gupta, D., & Thappa, D. M. (2013). Mongolian spots: How important are they? *World Journal of Clinical Cases, 1*(8), 230–232. doi:10.12998/wjcc.v1.i8.230; *Infectious diseases.* (n.d.). Retrieved from Merck Manual Professional Version website: http://www.merckmanuals.com/professional/infectious-diseases; James, W. D. (2016). Café au lait spots. *Medscape.* Retrieved from http://emedicine.medscape.com/article/911900-overview; Mayo Clinic. (2015). *Acanthosis nigricans.* Retrieved from http://www.mayoclinic.org/diseases-conditions/acanthosis-nigricans/basics/definition/con-20025600; *Neurofibromatosis.* (n.d.). Retrieved from Merck Manual Professional Version: http://www.merckmanuals.com/professional/pediatrics/neurocutaneous-syndromes; Pinney, S. S. (2016). Nevus araneus (Spider nevus). *Medscape.* Retrieved from http://emedicine.medscape.com/article/1084388-overview#a5

Untreated Wounds

Untreated wounds usually are seen shortly after an injury (e.g., at the scene of an accident, in the emergency department). The following are guidelines for treatment:

- Control severe bleeding by (a) applying direct pressure over the wound and (b) elevating the involved extremity.

- Prevent infection by (a) cleaning or flushing abrasions or lacerations with normal saline and (b) covering the wound with a clean dressing if possible (a sterile dressing is preferred). When applying a dressing, wrap the wound tightly enough to apply pressure, and approximate the wound edges if possible. If the first layer of dressing becomes saturated with blood, apply a second layer. Do so without removing the first layer of dressing, because

TABLE 21–5 Types of Wounds

Type	Cause	Description and Characteristics
Incision	Sharp instrument (e.g., knife, scalpel)	Open wound; deep or shallow
Contusion	Blow from a blunt instrument	Closed wound; skin appearing ecchymotic (bruised) because of damaged blood vessels
Abrasion	Surface scrape, either unintentional (e.g., scraped knee from a fall) or intentional (e.g., dermal abrasion to remove pockmarks)	Open wound involving the skin
Puncture	Penetration of the skin and often the underlying tissues by a sharp instrument, either intentional or unintentional	Open wound
Laceration	Tissues torn apart, often from accidents (e.g., with machinery)	Open wound; edges often jagged
Penetrating wound	Penetration of the skin and the underlying tissues, usually unintentional (e.g., from a bullet or metal fragments)	Open wound

removing it might disturb the clotting blood, resulting in more bleeding.

- Control swelling and pain by applying ice over the wound and surrounding tissues.
- If bleeding is severe or internal bleeding is suspected and if emergency equipment is available, assess the patient for signs of shock (rapid, thready pulse; cold, clammy skin; pallor; lowered blood pressure).

Treated Wounds

Treated or sutured wounds usually need to be observed for determination of the progress of healing. These wounds may be inspected when a dressing is changed. If the wound itself cannot be directly inspected, the dressing is inspected and other data regarding the wound (e.g., the presence of pain) are assessed. See Exemplar 21.C on Wound Healing for more information.

Prevalence

Skin disorders are one of the most common human illnesses. They occur in all cultures and age groups and affect 30–70% of individuals in the United States at any given time (Hay et al., 2013). Some of the most common disorders in the general population are dermatitis, inflammatory reactions to topical drugs, and infectious diseases of the skin. Acne is one of the most common skin disorders, affecting approximately 50 million Americans each year; close to 100% of adolescents have at least mild acne. Other common skin diseases include contact dermatitis (72.3 million), hair and nail disorders (70.5 million), herpes simplex or herpes zoster (165 million), warts (58.5 million), seborrheic keratosis (83.8 million), and damage from solar radiation (123.1 million). Skin disorders also include fungal infections (29.4 million), rosacea (14.7 million), psoriasis (6.7 million), and skin ulcers and wounds (4.8 million) (American Academy of Dermatology [AAD], 2016). Skin cancer is the most common form of cancer in the United States; an estimated 71,943 individuals were diagnosed with and 9394 individuals died from melanoma in 2013, the most recent year for which the Centers for Disease Control and Prevention (CDC) has statistics (CDC, 2016d).

Genetic Considerations and Risk Factors

Having one or both parents, a sibling, or another closely related family member with a particular skin disorder increases an individual's likelihood of developing that disorder. Skin conditions often occur as part of a genetically related metabolic disorder or a disease that affects multiple body systems (Uitto, 2012). Heritable skin disorders include epidermolysis bullosa (a blistering disorder), ichthyosis (a disorder in which the skin becomes thick and scaly), and albinism (a disorder in which too little melanin is produced). Ethnicity and age are also nonmodifiable risk factors for a number of skin diseases.

Differences in gender and age also play a role in individual susceptibility to some skin disorders (Firooz et al., 2012). Men are generally more affected by infectious skin disorders, whereas women more commonly experience pigmentary and autoimmune disorders (Brown, 2016; Ngoa, Steyna, & McCombeb, 2014). Although not completely understood, research has suggested a correlation between this occurrence and sex hormones. There are also indications that as the amount of sex hormones decreases with age, patients experience changes in skin thickness, surface pH, and quality of wound healing. These changes predispose older adults to a number of skin disorders (Brown, 2016).

Skin color also influences an individual's risk for certain skin disorders that include keloids, dyschromia, pseudofolliculitis, and dermatosis papulosa nigra, which are more common among patients with dark skin tones, and conditions such as vitiligo and depigmentation, which are more difficult to treat in individuals with darker skin. Other conditions such as psoriasis, atopic dermatitis, and eczema present differently in patients with dark skin tones than in patients with light skin tones (Kundu & Patterson, 2013; Lawson et al., 2015). Although darker toned skin is less susceptible to sun damage, all types and tones of skin can be damaged by exposure to UV light. Nurses, therefore, should encourage all patients to use sunscreen, cover their heads, and wear protective clothing outdoors whenever possible to prevent sunburn and the future development of skin cancer.

Alterations and Therapies
Tissue Integrity

ALTERATION	DESCRIPTION/ DEFINITION	MANIFESTATIONS	INTERVENTIONS AND TREATMENTS
Impaired skin integrity	Disruption or damage to the epidermal and/or dermal layers of skin as a result of a cut, scrape, burn, or other injury	▪ Open wound of varying severity, depth, and size (e.g., incision, severe burn, ulcer) ▪ Closed wound affecting the superficial (e.g., sunburn) or deeper (e.g., bruise) layers of skin ▪ Changes in skin color, especially after burn	▪ Cleanse wound. ▪ Close open wounds with sutures or staples if edges can be approximated. ▪ Use moist wound management. ▪ Apply a sterile bandage. ▪ Apply ointment, cream, or gel as prescribed. ▪ Promote good nutrition and fluid intake; administer enteral or parenteral nutrition or intravenous (IV) fluids as ordered. ▪ Refer to a nutritionist or dietitian if needed. ▪ Monitor for infection and other complications.
Pain	Discomfort related to impaired skin integrity	▪ Acute pain at the site of injury ▪ Pain rating of higher than 1 on a 0–10 scale ▪ Elevated blood pressure ▪ Increased heart rate ▪ Anxiety ▪ Decreased ability to perform activities of daily living (ADLs)	▪ Provide opioid or nonopioid analgesics. ▪ Use nonpharmacologic pain management techniques (e.g., relaxation, distraction).
Inflammation	Innate immune response to tissue damage or foreign organisms or particles	▪ Pain ▪ Redness ▪ Swelling ▪ Heat ▪ Impaired function	▪ Apply heat or ice. ▪ Apply compression. ▪ Use analgesics. ▪ Encourage movement and exercise. ▪ Elevate limbs.
Infection	Invasion of the wound with microorganisms such as bacteria, viruses, fungi, or parasites	▪ Inflammation ▪ Purulent drainage ▪ Foul smell ▪ Elevated body temperature ▪ Impaired oxygenation (if infection is in the lungs) ▪ Restlessness ▪ Fatigue ▪ Sweating, chills	▪ Obtain a culture of wound exudate for sensitivity testing. ▪ Treat with topical or oral antibiotics as prescribed. ▪ If infection is not bacterial, administer other anti-infective agents as needed. ▪ Debride wound. ▪ Use good wound hygiene. ▪ Administer antipyretics as ordered. ▪ Provide cool compresses or blankets as needed.

Pruritus	Itching of the skin	▪ Rash
		▪ Redness
		▪ Rough, dry skin
		▪ Scaly skin
			▪ Administer medications as ordered:
			  • Topical or oral corticosteroids
			  • Antihistamines
			  • Topical anesthetics
			▪ Apply soothing lotions or creams to the affected site.
			▪ Teach the patient to avoid scratching.

(continued on next page)

Alterations and Therapies (continued)

ALTERATION	DESCRIPTION/ DEFINITION	MANIFESTATIONS	INTERVENTIONS AND TREATMENTS
			▪ Monitor for open wounds caused by scratching. ▪ Monitor for infection. ▪ Apply mittens. ▪ Apply cool compresses or give a cool bath. ▪ Avoid substances that stimulate pruritus.
Eschar	Hard crust covering an open wound consisting of dried plasma proteins and dead cells	▪ Leathery and rigid crust over wound ▪ Circumferential constriction of the torso or extremity ▪ Gangrene (severe cases)	▪ Remove eschar by debridement. ▪ Perform escharotomy. ▪ Use hydrotherapy.
Edema	Fluid accumulation under the skin	▪ Swelling ▪ Spongy or boggy skin upon palpation ▪ Increased compartment pressure ▪ Pitting upon pressure In lungs: ▪ Atelectasis ▪ Labored breathing ▪ Stridor	▪ Elevate edematous area. ▪ Apply compression to stimulate blood flow (contraindicated if pressure will cut off blood flow). ▪ Administer diuretics (contraindicated in patients at risk for deficient fluid volume). ▪ Maintain patent airway. ▪ Ensure adequate fluid intake. ▪ Monitor fluid intake and output. ▪ Use vacuum-assisted closure (VAC).
Exudate	Fluid drainage from a wound	▪ Clear or straw-colored exudate (serous) ▪ Milky exudate full of cells and necrotic debris (purulent); color may be blue, green, or yellow ▪ Bright or dark red exudate containing red blood cells (sanguineous)	▪ Cleanse exudate from wound. ▪ Cover with sterile, absorptive bandage. ▪ Collect purulent exudate for culture. ▪ Apply antibacterial ointments as prescribed. ▪ Apply pressure to bleeding wound, or cover with pro-coagulant bandage.
Bruising	Bleeding underneath the epidermal layer of skin caused by broken blood vessels or capillaries	▪ Discoloration of skin at the site of injury ("black-and-blue," red, or purple for fresh bruises; yellow or green for older bruises) ▪ Discomfort upon movement or pressure	▪ Apply ice to bruised area. ▪ Administer analgesics if ordered. ▪ Most bruises heal on their own with no treatment.

Case Study » Part 1

Arthur Sullivan is a 52-year-old man who was scheduled for neurosurgery to remove a pituitary tumor. Mr. Sullivan is a large man, standing 6'3" tall and weighing 342 lb. After surgery, an external ventricular drainage device was inserted to prevent cerebrospinal fluid accumulation at the surgical site to promote healing. Upon the surgeon's orders, Mr. Sullivan must remain on restricted mobility in a supine position at a 20-degree angle or less for 3 days after surgery. Because of his restricted mobility, intermittent pneumatic compression pumps are placed on his legs to stimulate blood flow. However, because of Mr. Sullivan's large size, the pumps do not fit well, even though they are the largest size available in the intensive care unit (ICU).

Two days after surgery, Mr. Sullivan develops deep vein thrombosis (DVT) in his left leg. Because it is too soon after surgery to administer anticoagulant or thrombolytic drugs, the attending physician decides that the best course of treatment is insertion of an inferior vena cava filter to prevent thromboses from traveling to the lungs, heart, and brain. As the filter clogs with additional blood clots, Mr. Sullivan experiences severe edema in both legs. In spite of continued use of the compression pumps, Mr. Sullivan does not obtain relief from the edema. One week after surgery, he is placed on IV heparin (titrated to a partial thromboplastin time [PTT] of 60) to prevent further DVT. Three days after the heparin regimen has been initiated, Mr. Sullivan calls the nurse because his lower left leg has suddenly started "squirting blood." Upon inspection, the nurse finds that a varicose vein has ruptured over Mr. Sullivan's mid-tibia.

Clinical Reasoning Questions Level I

1. What assessment techniques are required to determine the source of the bleeding?
2. What are the immediate nursing priorities for Mr. Sullivan?

3. What risk factors does Mr. Sullivan have for developing edema after insertion of the inferior vena cava (IVC) filter?

Clinical Reasoning Questions Level II

4. What factors may have contributed to the rupture of a vein?
5. Once the bleeding is controlled, what responsibilities does the nurse have in caring for Mr. Sullivan's wound?
6. What additional nursing interventions should have been implemented after surgery to prevent blood clots and edema?

Concepts Related to Tissue Integrity

The immune system and the skin are intricately linked through their roles as protectors of the body. Impaired tissue integrity can lead to an immune response. Immune responses—such as allergic reactions and inflammation— conversely can lead to issues with tissue integrity. For example, when allergic reactions occur, they may result in contact dermatitis; the resulting discomfort may lead to scratching, which leads to impaired skin integrity. When inflammation occurs, scars or abscesses may form; if healing is slow or impaired, these breaks in the skin can lead to infection.

Infection is the invasion of body tissue by microorganisms that have the potential to cause illness. Microorganisms grow on intact skin and can enter the body through a number of portals. The majority of microorganisms on the skin are harmless; however, if their growth is unchecked or if they enter the body through breaks in the skin, even normally harmless microorganisms can cause disease. These problems are further compounded if the immune system is compromised.

Concepts Related to
Tissue Integrity

CONCEPT	RELATIONSHIP TO TISSUE INTEGRITY	NURSING IMPLICATIONS
Immunity	Impaired tissue integrity triggers immune responses; immune responses can also lead to impaired tissue integrity.	■ Assess for rash and inflammation. ■ Be alert to topical and latex allergies that could worsen symptoms. ■ Be alert to abscess formation. ■ *Anticipate:* Use of aspirin, antipyretics, and cold packs
Infection	Microorganisms grow on the skin, and breaks in the skin serve as portals for these microorganisms to enter the body.	■ Assess for complications of infectious disease. ■ Exercise infection control measures, and use personal protective equipment. ■ *Anticipate:* Blood cultures, antibiotics, and isolation practices
Mobility	Impaired mobility may lead to skin breakdown and the development of pressure ulcers.	■ Assess for skin breakdown at least once per shift; pay special attention to bony prominences. ■ *Anticipate:* Repositioning, wound care, comfort measures, hygiene care, and infection control measures ■ Educate patient about how to care for impaired skin.
Nutrition	Adequate nutritional intake is essential for the maintenance of tissue integrity, healing, and recovery.	■ Assess nutritional intake. ■ Identify signs of poor nutritional status (e.g., pale, dry skin; subcutaneous tissue loss). ■ *Anticipate:* Laboratory testing (CBC, transferrin, serum albumin and serum electrolyte values; protein supplements)
Perfusion	↓ Blood flow to tissues →↓ oxygen and nutrient delivery. If prolonged, damage or death may occur.	■ Assess for signs of decreased tissue perfusion (i.e., changes in skin temperature, color, characteristics or sensation; or weak or absent pulses at least once per shift). ■ Identify conditions or contributing factors, such as position, mobility level, or constrictive devices that place the patient at risk for impaired tissue perfusion. ■ *Anticipate:* Repositioning, wound care
Safety	Impaired safety may lead to alterations in tissue integrity.	■ Assess for barriers to safety. ■ Identify patients at increased risk for alterations in safety. ■ *Anticipate:* Use of mechanical devices for patient transfer, bed alarms ■ Educate the patient on ways to promote safety in the environment.
Self	Alterations in tissue integrity can affect perceptions of self in relation to body image and functional ability.	■ Perform a psychosocial assessment. ■ *Anticipate:* Cognitive–behavioral therapy; antidepressants, anxiolytics

Patients with alterations in mobility may be at an increased risk for impaired skin integrity—and subsequently infection—as a result of pressure ulcers. Pressure ulcers are areas of skin that break down as a result of pressure on that particular area. This pressure essentially reduces blood flow to that area of skin, causing the skin to die. The weight of the body pressing down on areas such as the buttocks, shoulders, and elbows of patients who are bedridden can lead to ulcerations. Bony protuberances are particularly susceptible. Repeated irritation of the skin—as from constant friction of bed linens or moisture from urinary incontinence—can lead to ulcerations as well.

Perfusion has an important role in tissue integrity. Blood is responsible for the delivery of oxygen and nutrients to the organs and tissues of the body. Delivery of these substances is impaired when blood flow is decreased or interrupted. If perfusion to organs or tissue is decreased for an extended period, damage or death may occur. Specific disease processes such as diabetes mellitus and coronary artery disease can affect tissue perfusion. All patients should be routinely assessed for adequate tissue perfusion, and those identified as having increased risk should be assessed more frequently.

Nutrition is also important in relationship to tissue integrity. Adequate nutrition is required not only for maintenance of tissue integrity, but also for proper healing and recovery. Patients who are at risk for or have actual impaired tissue integrity should have their nutritional intake monitored, especially protein, to ensure it is appropriate for their body's demands.

Alterations in tissue integrity can affect a patient's perception of self. This can be related to the patient's body image or functional ability caused by damage to an area from a wound. Patient safety can affect tissue integrity due to falls or other safety concerns. Education of the patient regarding ways to prevent injury by monitoring the safety of their environment can decrease the incidence of this problem.

The Concepts Related to Tissue Integrity feature links some, but not all, of the concepts integral to tissue integrity. They are presented in alphabetical order.

Health Promotion

Skin disorders can cause intense pain and discomfort for patients and can affect their overall health and self-concept. Many of these disorders are preventable; even individuals with genetic predispositions for certain disorders can benefit from taking simple preventive measures. Because increased melanin levels make darker toned skin less susceptible to problems associated with overexposure, some patients may mistakenly believe they are not at risk of developing skin cancer. All patients, regardless of skin tone, should understand the risks and be coached on preventive measures. Preventive measures for skin disorders include those listed in the Patient Teaching feature.

Modifiable Risk Factors

Proper skin care and maintenance are important for preventing many infectious disorders, especially for patients with compromised immune systems, diabetes, HIV/AIDS, or

Patient Teaching
How to Reduce Dry Skin and Relieve Pruritus

- Wash clothing in a mild detergent and rinse twice; do not use fabric softeners.
- Avoid using perfumes and lotions containing alcohol.
- Apply skin lubricants after a bath to help retain moisture.
- Because soaps and hot water are drying, clean the skin with tepid water and either a mild soap or cleansing creams. If soap is used, rinse it off carefully.
- It is not necessary to take a bath every day.
- If bath oils are used, add them to the bath water at the end of the bath (the moist skin is more likely to retain the oil). Bath oils make the tub surface slippery, so they may be contraindicated for use by patients with poor balance and patients who are already at risk for falls.
- Use a humidifier to humidify the air.
- Apply creams and lotions when the skin is slightly damp after bathing.
- Increase fluid intake.
- Keep nails trimmed short, wear loose clothing, and keep the environment cool.
- A brief application of pressure or cold may relieve pruritus.
- Cotton gloves may be worn at night if scratching during sleep causes skin excoriation.
- Distraction or relaxation techniques may prove helpful.

obesity. Skin should be kept clean, dry, and moisturized; when wounds occur, they should be kept clean and covered to decrease the risk of infection. Children and others who are in close contact in a community setting should be coached to avoid sharing personal items—such as combs, brushes, and hats—with others to decrease the likelihood of parasite transfer.

Risk for inflammatory disorders can be decreased through avoidance of irritants or allergens known to inflame patients' skin, such as harsh chemical cleaners, dyes, perfumes, poison plants (ivy, oak, sumac), latex, and certain metals. Skin should be kept clean, but excessive cleansing should be avoided as it can cause the skin to become overly dry. Use of moisturizers may also be helpful. Parents of children in diapers should be taught proper diaper-area care and coached to change wet or soiled diapers as soon as the parent becomes aware of them.

Many chronic illnesses and their treatments increase the risk for impaired skin integrity. Impaired peripheral arterial circulation in the lower extremities may produce skin that appears shiny, has lost its hair, and damages easily. Some medications, such as corticosteroids, cause thinning of the skin, making it much more easily injured. Many medications increase sensitivity to sunlight and can predispose the individual to severe sunburns. Some of the most common medications that cause this kind of damage are certain antibiotics, chemotherapy drugs for cancer, and some psychotherapeutic drugs. Poor nutrition alone can also interfere with the appearance and function of normal skin.

Screenings

All patients benefit from regular self-examination of the skin. The benefits of these examinations are twofold: Patients are able to identify and recognize problems as they occur, and patients develop a familiarity with their skin. This familiarity makes it easier for patients to identify changes (e.g., appearance of new wounds in patients with diabetic neuropathy). Examinations should focus on areas that receive the most exposure to sunlight and toxins: the face, neck, ears, scalp, arms, and legs. The trunk, chest, and feet should also be examined.

Next to self-examinations of the skin, professional examinations are perhaps the most common screening method for identifying skin disorders. During a professional examination, a physician—often a dermatologist—conducts a head-to-toe inspection of the skin and identifies any problem areas. Diagnostic tests—such as biopsy, cultures, and patch tests—are ordered on the basis of these findings. These and other common diagnostic tests are discussed in detail later in the module.

Nursing Assessment

General physical assessment always includes the integumentary system. Even when providing routine care, such as during a regular healthcare visit or well-child visit, or when assisting with personal hygiene, the nurse should be alert to skin abnormalities.

Observation and Patient Interview

Conduct a general observation of the patient's skin during the interview, noting the color, presence of erythema, dryness, rashes, lesions or areas of hyper- or hypopigmentation. During the review of systems as part of the history, obtain information about skin diseases, previous bruising, general skin condition, skin lesions, and usual healing of sores.

Many mainstream skin and hair care products do not adequately address the health needs of people of color. As a result, patients may rely on home remedies and alternative products that contain ingredients such as olive oil, honey, or lemon juice; some of these remedies and products are culturally significant. It is important to understand individual patients' skin care regimens and the potential impact of these regimens on medical treatments.

Skin color and skin care are emotionally charged subjects for many patients, as is exposure of skin through either removal of clothing or removal of makeup. It is imperative that the nurse be sensitive to these emotions when discussing patients' skin conditions and care regimens and when examining the skin itself.

The following are questions the nurse asks in assessing the patient's skin and tissue integrity:

- Do you have a history of skin problems? If so, what were the problems and when did they occur?
- If the problems were acute, have they ever recurred? If the problems were chronic, how are you currently managing them?
- What treatments have been effective for previous skin problems?
- Are lesions, sores, ulcers, or rashes on your skin slow to heal?

- When did you first notice your current skin problem? Where did it originate? Where and when did it spread?
- Is your skin problem accompanied by other symptoms, such as fever or chills?
- Do you notice the problems occurring after exposure to certain chemicals, toxins, items of clothing, or items of jewelry?
- Have you recently switched soap, shampoo, detergent, or moisturizer, or started taking new medications? Has your diet changed recently?
- Have you traveled or been exposed to extreme temperatures recently?
- Have you noticed any drainage from affected areas? If so, what did it look and smell like?
- How frequently is your skin exposed to direct sunlight? Do you take proper protective measures—such as sunscreens, protective clothing, and hats—during exposure?
- How does your skin react to sun exposure? Does it burn or become red easily? Have you ever developed blisters as a result of exposure?
- Do you have any tattoos, piercings, or brands? How long have you had your tattoos, piercings, or brands, and have you ever noticed any skin problems in those areas?
- Have you noticed any long-term changes in your skin over the past few years?
- Are you under a high level of stress, or have you ever experienced intermittent or prolonged anxiety?
- Do your skin problems negatively affect your personal or social relationships in any way?

Physical Examination

Inspection and palpation of the skin focus on determining skin color distribution, skin turgor, presence of **edema** (swelling caused by excess fluid trapped in body tissue; see **Figure 21–17 »**), and characteristics of any lesions that are present. Particular attention is paid to skin condition in areas that are most likely to break down: in skinfolds, such as under the breasts; in areas that are frequently moist, such as the perineum; and in areas that receive extensive pressure, such as the bony prominences. See the Integumentary Assessment feature. Antiemboli stockings, braces, or other medical or assistive devices must be removed to assess the condition of the skin underneath. Detection of variations in skin color and identification of lesions require good lighting.

Diagnostic Tests

The results of diagnostic tests of the structure and function of the integumentary system are used to support the diagnosis of a specific injury or disease. Diagnostic tests also provide information used to identify or modify the appropriate medications or treatments for the disease and help the nurse monitor the patient's response to nursing care interventions. Diagnostic tests to assess the integumentary system are summarized in the following list:

- One of the most common diagnostic tests is a skin biopsy, which is used to differentiate a benign skin lesion from a

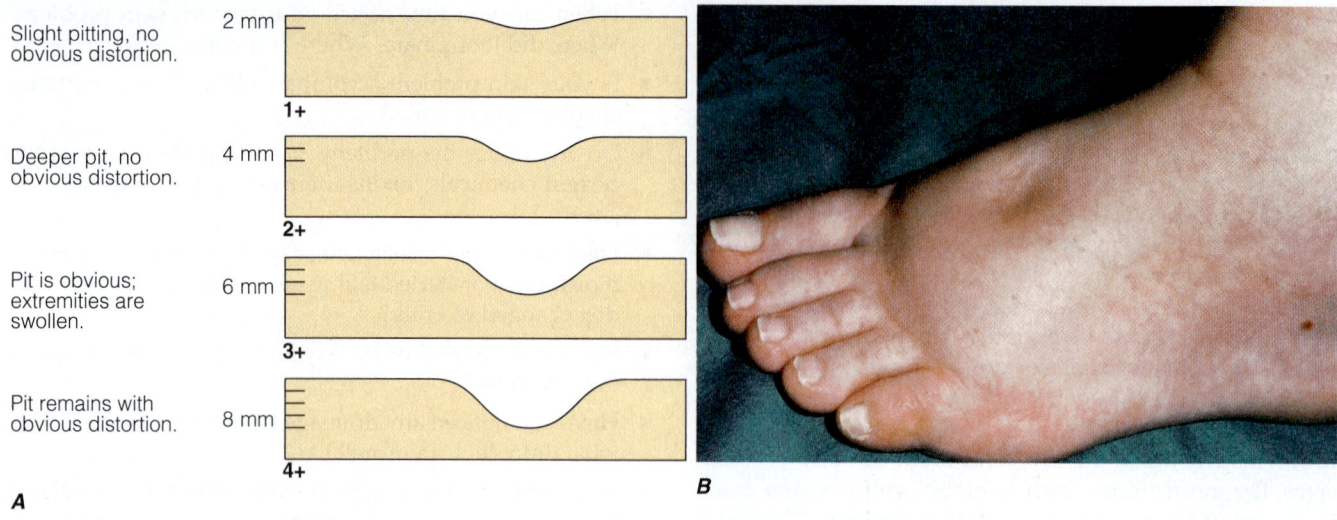

Slight pitting, no obvious distortion. 2 mm — 1+

Deeper pit, no obvious distortion. 4 mm — 2+

Pit is obvious; extremities are swollen. 6 mm — 3+

Pit remains with obvious distortion. 8 mm — 4+

A

B

Source: B, Dr. P. Marazzi/Science Source.

Figure 21–17 》 A, Degrees of pitting in edema. **B,** 4+ pitting.

skin cancer. Skin biopsies can be obtained by a punch technique, incision, excision, or shaving.

- Cultures used to identify infections may be conducted on tissue samples, on drainage and exudate (material, such as fluid and cells, that has escaped from blood vessels during the inflammatory process and is deposited in tissue or on tissue surfaces) from lesions, and (if an illness is generalized) on serum.

- Tests that are used to identify infections include immunofluorescence studies, Wood lamp, potassium hydroxide, and the Tzanck test.

- Tests used to identify allergens include scratch, intradermal, and patch testing. Scratch, or skin prick, testing is performed by applying small amounts of allergens to the skin, usually on the back, and using a needle to penetrate the skin underneath with the allergen. Intradermal testing uses needles to inject small amounts of allergen into the skin on the arm, and may be used to clarify or confirm negative or inconsistent results of a scratch test. Scratch and intradermal testing are not appropriate for all individuals, especially those who have had previous life-threatening allergic reactions. Skin prick and intradermal testing both provide an immediate reaction. Patch testing, which provides a delayed reaction, involves the placement of an adhesive patch containing common allergens on the back between the scapulae.

Some studies are conducted to identify bacterial carriers. For example, if patients have repeated bacterial skin infections or if a healthcare unit or agency experiences numerous bacterial infections of patients, nasal cultures may be performed to determine whether the patients or healthcare workers are carriers of the bacteria. Regardless of the type of diagnostic test, the nurse is responsible for explaining the procedure to the patient; explaining any special preparation needed, including fasting or avoiding allergy medications prior to testing; assessing for medication use that may affect the outcome of the tests; supporting the patient during the

examination as necessary; documenting the procedures as appropriate; and monitoring the results of the tests.

Laboratory data can also support the nurse's clinical assessment of a wound's progress in healing. A decreased leukocyte count can delay healing and increase the possibility of infection. A hemoglobin level below the normal range indicates poor oxygen delivery to the tissues. Blood coagulation studies are also significant. Prolonged coagulation times can result in excessive blood loss and prolonged clot absorption. Hypercoagulability can lead to intravascular clotting. Intra-arterial clotting can result in a deficient blood supply to the wound area. Serum protein analysis provides an indication of the body's nutritional reserves for rebuilding cells. Albumin is an important indicator of nutritional status. A value below 3.5 g/dL indicates poor nutrition and may increase the risk of poor healing and infection. Wound cultures can either confirm or rule out the presence of infection. Sensitivity studies are helpful in the selection of appropriate antibiotic therapy. The nurse obtains a wound culture whenever an infection is suspected.

Case Study 》 Part 2

Because of Mr. Sullivan's complications, his hospital stay extends to 8 weeks. His surgical site is healing well, and he is no longer on restricted mobility. Mr. Sullivan is undergoing physical therapy to regain his ability to walk after the extended bedrest and edema. Treatment to reduce edema in his legs includes elevation of his legs; compression stockings (custom-fit stockings have been ordered and fit well); furosemide 80 mg daily; and sustained ambulation of 15 minutes or more at least three times daily. Edema has steadily decreased over the weeks but is still significant. He is now on oral warfarin 4 mg daily (adjusted to maintain an international normalized ratio [INR] of 2.5) to prevent additional DVT.

Over the 6 weeks since his varicose vein ruptured, Mr. Sullivan has been diagnosed with chronic venous disease. He has experienced four episodes of hemorrhage from the site, and bleeding is difficult to stop because of the anticoagulant he is taking for DVT. The site of rupture has developed into a grade C6 (open venous ulcer) on the CEAP venous disease scale. The ulcer is 2.8 cm long, 2.3 cm wide, and 0.6 cm deep. When the ulcer is not bleeding profusely, it is exuding a dark reddish-brown serosanguineous fluid. No signs of

Integumentary Assessment

ASSESSMENT/ METHOD	NORMAL FINDINGS	ABNORMAL FINDINGS	LIFESPAN OR DEVELOPMENTAL CONSIDERATIONS
General Assessment			
Inspect the skin color, and note any odors coming from the skin.	Skin color should be even, appropriate to the age and race of the patient, and without foul odors.	■ A strong odor of perspiration may indicate poor hygiene. ■ A foul odor may indicate a disorder of the sweat glands. ■ Pallor or cyanosis is seen with exposure to cold and with decreased perfusion and oxygenation. ■ Redness, swelling, and pain are seen with various rashes, inflammations, infections, and burns. ■ First-degree burns cause areas of **erythema** (redness of the skin) and swelling; second-degree burns cause red, painful blisters; third-degree burns cause white or blackened areas. ■ Abnormal loss of melanin in patches of the face, hands, or groin may indicate the autoimmune disorder vitiligo.	■ Hormone fluctuations during pregnancy may cause skin discoloration, which is more pronounced in women with darker skin tones. In most cases, the discoloration resolves itself postpartum without treatment. Oral contraceptives causes similar discoloration in some women.
Assessment of Skin with Impaired Integrity			
Inspect skin for lesions and alterations, including calluses, scars, tattoos, and piercings. Include inspection of skin creases and folds.	Skin should be intact without abnormal lesions.	■ Primary, secondary, and vascular lesions may be present. ■ Pearly edged nodules with a central ulcer may indicate basal cell carcinoma. ■ Scaly, red, fast-growing papules may indicate squamous cell carcinoma. ■ Dark, asymmetrical, multicolored patches with irregular edges may indicate malignant melanoma. ■ Circular lesions may indicate ringworm or tinea versicolor. ■ Grouped vesicles may be seen in contact dermatitis. ■ Linear lesions may indicate poison ivy or herpes zoster. ■ In herpes zoster, vesicles appear along sensory nerve paths, turn into pustules, and crust over. ■ **Urticaria** (also known as hives) appears as patches of pale, itchy wheals in an erythematous area. ■ In psoriasis, scaly red patches appear on the scalp, knees, back, and genitals. ■ Bruises in various stages of healing may be indicators of trauma or abuse.	■ Some skin conditions, such as psoriasis, eczema, and atopic dermatitis, are more difficult to diagnose in darker skin. If undiagnosed or treated improperly, lesions can darken. These dark spots often remain for years. ■ Pseudofolliculitis barbae (razor bumps) is common in individuals who have darker skin or curly hair. In some cases, this condition results in scarring, infection, and keloid formation. ■ Note location of birthmarks.
Skin Temperature Assessment			
Palpate skin temperature.	Skin should be warm.	■ Warm, red skin indicates inflammation and elevated body temperature. ■ Decreased skin temperature indicates decreased blood flow to the skin; it may be generalized (as in shock) or localized (as in arteriosclerosis).	■ Temperature regulation in infants is inefficient, and skin may feel warm or cool in the absence of inflammation or decreased blood flow.

(continued on next page)

Integumentary Assessment *(continued)*

ASSESSMENT/ METHOD	NORMAL FINDINGS	ABNORMAL FINDINGS	LIFESPAN OR DEVELOPMENTAL CONSIDERATIONS
Skin Texture Assessment			
Palpate skin moisture.	Skin should be dry.	■ Excessively dry skin may be present in older adults and patients with hypothyroidism. ■ Oily skin may be present in adolescents and young adults; this finding may be normal or may indicate a skin disorder like acne vulgaris. ■ Excessive perspiration may be associated with shock, fever, increased activity, or anxiety.	■ In darker skin tones, an ashy appearance indicates excessive dryness.
Skin Turgor Assessment			
Palpate skin turgor. Pinch skin gently over the sternum or collarbone.	Skinfold should return rapidly to the normal positions.	■ Skin turgor is decreased in dehydration. It is increased in edema and scleroderma.	■ Tenting, in which the skin remains pinched for a few moments before resuming its normal position, is common among thin older adults.
Edema Assessment			
Assess edema by depressing the patient's skin for a minimum of 2–3 seconds (see Figure 21–17) Record findings on a 4-point scale: ■ 1+: Slight pitting, no obvious distortion. ■ 2+: Deeper pit, no obvious distortion. ■ 3+: Pit is obvious; extremities are swollen. ■ 4+: Pit remains with obvious distortion.	No edema should be present.	■ Edema commonly occurs in cardiovascular disorders, renal failure, and cirrhosis of the liver.	■ Edema is a side effect of some medications, including calcium channel blockers, NSAIDs, and estrogens. Pregnant women may also exhibit mild edema.
Assessment of Hair Distribution and Quality			
Visual assessment.	Hair should be evenly distributed for the patient's gender.	■ **Alopecia** (hair loss) may be related to changes in hormones, chemical or drug treatment, or radiation. ■ **Hirsutism** (increased growth of coarse hair on the face and trunk) is seen in Cushing syndrome, acromegaly, and ovarian dysfunction. ■ A deviation in normal hair distribution in the genital area may indicate an endocrine disorder.	■ In adult men whose hair loss follows the normal male pattern, the cause is usually genetic. ■ Excess hair is a common problem for individuals with darker skin; laser hair removal should be used cautiously, because certain types of lasers cause changes in skin pigment.

Integumentary Assessment (continued)

ASSESSMENT/ METHOD	NORMAL FINDINGS	ABNORMAL FINDINGS	LIFESPAN OR DEVELOPMENTAL CONSIDERATIONS
Hair Texture Assessment			
Palpate hair texture.	Hair should be of even texture.	■ Systemic diseases cause changes to the texture of the hair. ■ Hypothyroidism causes the hair to coarsen. ■ Hyperthyroidism causes the hair to become fine.	■ Gradual changes in hair texture normally occur across the lifespan. Infants have fine, soft hair that thickens in diameter through childhood and adolescence. During middle and old age, the diameter gradually decreases, and hair becomes finer again.
Scalp Assessment			
Inspect the scalp for lesions.	There should be no lesions on the scalp.	■ Mild dandruff is normal, but excessive or greasy flakes indicate seborrhea. ■ Hair loss, pustules, and scales appear on the scalp in tinea capitis. ■ Red, swollen pustules that appear around infected hair follicles indicate folliculitis. ■ Head lice may be seen as oval nits adhering to the base of the hair shaft. Head lice are usually accompanied by itching.	■ Head lice are common among children, but may be particularly embarrassing for those in late elementary school or middle school. Children in this age group may be subject to ridicule by their peers.
Nail Assessment			
Inspect nail curvature.	Nail surfaces should be smooth and nail folds firm, without redness.	■ Inflammation and transverse rippling of the nail are associated with chronic paronychia and/or eczema. ■ The nail plate may separate from the nail bed in trauma, psoriasis, and *Pseudomonas* and *Candida* infections. This separation is called *oncolysis*. ■ Nail grooves may be caused by inflammation, planus, or nail biting. ■ Nail pitting may be seen with psoriasis. ■ A transverse groove (Beau line) may be seen in trachoma or acute disease. ■ Thin, spoon-shaped nails are common in anemia.	■ Spoon-shaped concave nails occur normally in young children and usually resolve with age.
Inspection of Nail Color			
Visual assessment.	Nail color should be even.	■ The sudden appearance of a pigmented band may indicate melanoma in Caucasians. ■ Yellowish nails are seen in psoriasis and fungal infections. ■ Dark nails occur with trauma, *Candida* infections, and hyperbilirubinemia. ■ Blackish-green nails are apparent in injury and in *Pseudomonas* infection. ■ Red splinter longitudinal hemorrhages may be seen in injury and/or psoriasis.	■ Pigmented bands are normally found in more than 90% of African Americans. ■ Certain foods, chemicals, and nail polishes can stain the nails yellow; this condition may be particularly noticeable in individuals who wear nail polish the majority of the time.

(continued on next page)

Integumentary Assessment *(continued)*

ASSESSMENT/METHOD	NORMAL FINDINGS	ABNORMAL FINDINGS	LIFESPAN OR DEVELOPMENTAL CONSIDERATIONS
Inspection of Nail Thickness			
Visual assessment.	Nails should not be excessively thick.	■ Trauma to the nails usually causes thickening. Other causes of thick nails include psoriasis, fungal infections, and decreased peripheral vascular blood supply.	■ Thickening of the nails is common in older patients and not necessarily indicative of disease in this population.

infection are present. The surrounding skin has turned purple in an area approximately 19 cm long and 11 cm wide. However, there is no sign of additional ulceration in the area. Daily care of the wound includes cleansing the area with sterile saline and applying an alginate dressing and topical sucralfate. The wound site is then wrapped in an elastic bandage, and the compression stocking is placed over the top.

Clinical Reasoning Questions Level I

1. What nursing assessments are necessary to monitor the status of the venous ulcer?
2. Why has the skin around the venous ulcer turned purple?
3. Based on the location and dimensions of Mr. Sullivan's ulcer, which layers of skin may be affected? What implications does this have for any symptoms he may experience and how the ulcer should be treated?

Clinical Reasoning Questions Level II

4. How would Mr. Sullivan's nursing plan change if the ulcer develops an infection?
5. What other treatments are available to help heal the venous ulcer?
6. Mr. Sullivan's case is complicated because he needs both anticoagulation to prevent DVT and procoagulation to prevent hemorrhage of the ulcer. Which treatment is a higher priority for Mr. Sullivan at this point in his healing process? Why?

Independent Interventions

Clinical management of alterations in tissue integrity is based on the cause and severity of the condition. The goals of treatment are to control the severity of the disease, prevent infection, and promote healing. Palliative care may also be necessary, depending on the severity of the problem and the level of discomfort it presents for the patient. For patients in the community, the nurse should ask questions to determine whether the patient is doing anything at home to relieve discomfort that could unintentionally inhibit healing.

Where appropriate, the nurse should teach the patient about good hygiene, that is, daily bathing for most adults for the purpose of keeping skin clean and free of odors. Children and older adults may need to bathe only every other day. Because soap can cause the skin to become dry, the nurse should encourage the patient to rinse thoroughly; liquid cleansers may be appropriate rather than bar soap for individuals with very dry skin. Use of moisturizing lotions after bathing should be encouraged. The nurse should also provide information about home remedies that may provide comfort while promoting healing.

The patient with impaired skin integrity or chronic skin conditions should be taught infection prevention measures. These include proper cleaning and dressing of wounds; use of antibiotic ointments on wounds may also be appropriate. The patient should be taught proper hand hygiene technique and instructed to cleanse the hands before and after touching the wound; the patient should also learn how to properly dispose of soiled dressings. In addition, the nurse should teach the patient how to recognize a wound that has become infected or necrotic and emphasize the importance of contacting a healthcare provider if infection occurs.

The nurse should also emphasize exercise and nutrition. Exercise improves blood flow and is important for maintaining overall well-being. Patients who are bedridden and susceptible to pressure ulcers should do simple exercises appropriate to their condition that can be performed while seated or lying down. Proper nutrition is also important for wound healing. During the healing process, the body requires increased amounts of calories, proteins, and vitamins A and C (Cleveland Clinic, 2015). Eating a variety of foods—including whole grains, leafy vegetables, citrus fruits, fortified dairy products, and lean proteins—enables the patient to get these vitamins and minerals. If the patient has difficulty consuming the necessary calories and nutrients in three large meals per day, the nurse should encourage the patient to eat smaller, more frequent meals or healthy snacks between meals. Nutritional supplements and multivitamins may also be appropriate for some patients.

Collaborative Therapies

The use of interprofessional teams in the healthcare setting has been shown to improve patient outcomes. When treating skin conditions, a variety of team members may participate in and manage the care of the patient, including: nurses and UAPs providing direct patient care, wound care nurses, nurse case managers, the attending healthcare provider, dermatologists, oncologists, and surgeons. These team members enhance the quality and safety of patient care through improved communication and decreased risk of complications (Epstein, 2014).

Pharmacologic Therapy

In some cases, treatment of skin disorders requires pharmacologic therapy. Over-the-counter (OTC) medications are suitable for less serious conditions, such as lice infestation, minor sunburns, and mild to moderate acne. The majority of OTC medications are topical; the efficacy of these medications depends upon the severity of the disorder, the patient's skin type, and the patient's skin care practices. For example, there are a variety of OTC acne medications on the market with active ingredients, most of which contain either benzoyl peroxide or salicylic acid. These ingredients may effectively treat acne in some patients, but may cause excessive dryness, redness, or burning sensations in others. Of these, benzoyl peroxide is generally considered the first-line treatment for acne. Its antiseptic properties help reduce bacteria in the skin and unplug oil ducts (American Academy of Pediatrics, 2015). Salicylic acid exfoliates and reduces inflammation.

Dark skin tones differ from light skin tones in terms of certain biological characteristics, such as sebum production,

making dark skin more prone to inflammation than light skin. These differences can cause topical medications that are effective in treating certain disorders in patients with lighter toned skin to be either ineffective or too harsh in treating the same conditions in patients with darker skin. Patients with darker skin tones may be candidates for combination therapy, which uses microdermabrasion or chemical peels in addition to topical therapy (AAD, 2013).

More serious disorders, such as eczema, dermatitis, and psoriasis, often require extensive or prolonged prescription therapy. These regimens are used under a doctor's supervision and may include a combination of oral and topical preparations. The Medications feature provides information about the different classes and actions of drugs used to treat skin disorders.

Medications
Tissue Integrity

CLASSIFICATION AND DRUG EXAMPLES	MECHANISMS OF ACTION	NURSING CONSIDERATIONS
Topical Corticosteroids Alclometasone Amcinonide Betamethasone Clobetasol Clocortolone Diflorasone Desonide Desoximetasone Fluocinolone Fluocinonide Halcinonide Hydrocortisone Mometasone Triamcinolone ***Drug examples:*** Alclovate, Cyclocort, Diprolene, Clobex, Cloderm, Florone, Tridesilon, Topicort, Fluoderm, Vanos, Halog, Cetacort, Elocon, Triderm	Relieve inflammatory and pruritic manifestations of corticosteroid-responsive dermatoses ***May also be used for:*** ■ Immunosuppression	■ Encourage the patient to apply a thin layer of medication after bathing. ■ Advise the patient against self-diagnosis and treatment with OTC preparations for more than 7 days. ■ Monitor for skin thinning and atrophy, acne, hypo- and hyperpigmentation, and allergic reaction; these effects are more severe on areas of thin skin, such as the face. ■ Assess for systemic toxicity in small children; do not use in children younger than 2.
Antiacne Adapalene Tazarotene Tretinoin ***Drug examples:*** Differin Tazorac Avita	Promote cell turnover and prevent blocking of follicles; may be used in combination with antibiotics ***May also be used for:*** ■ Treatment of plaque psoriasis ■ Treatment of hypo- and hyperpigmentation	■ Advise the patient that acne may worsen during the initial weeks of treatment. ■ Encourage the patient not to use in combination with OTC preparations containing salicylic acid, benzoyl peroxide, or sulfur. ■ Advise the patient to minimize sun exposure during treatment. ■ Monitor for pruritus, erythema, inflammation, and contact dermatitis.

(continued on next page)

Medications (continued)

CLASSIFICATION AND DRUG EXAMPLES	MECHANISMS OF ACTION	NURSING CONSIDERATIONS
Antibacterials Erythromycin Methotrexate Tetracycline *Drug examples:* EryPed Trexall Tetracap	Interfere with bacterial DNA and protein synthesis, causing cell death *May also be used for:* ■ Prophylaxis for neonatal eye infection (erythromycin) ■ Treatment of rheumatoid arthritis (methotrexate) ■ Treatment of chlamydia and rickettsial infections (tetracycline)	■ Encourage the patient using oral medications to take with a full glass of water on an empty stomach; if stomach upset occurs, medications can be taken with foods that are not high in calcium. ■ Advise the patient to avoid exposure to sunlight and UV light. ■ Encourage the patient to check expiration dates on antibacterial medications and dispose of those that have expired. ■ Monitor for urticaria, pruritus, and skin eruptions.
Antibiotics Bacitracin Gentamicin Polysporin Silver sulfadiazine *Drug example:* Silvadene	Interfere with bacterial replication and synthesis; used to treat infection *May also be used for:* ■ Superficial infection of external eye ■ Prevention and treatment of sepsis in burns	■ Encourage the patient to clean the affected area prior to application and cover with a sterile bandage or gauze after application. ■ Advise the patient against applying to large areas because of risk of systemic absorption and toxicity. ■ Monitor for hypersensitivity, local allergic reaction, and photosensitivity.
Antifungals Clotrimazole Ketoconazole Miconazole Nystatin *Drug examples:* Lotrimin Nizoral Monistat Mycostatin	Alter fungal membrane structure, causing cell death; each preparation is specific to a particular organism	■ Emphasize the importance of keeping affected areas clean and dry. ■ Advise the patient against covering areas with occlusive dressings unless instructed by the physician. ■ Monitor for erythema, irritation, pruritus, contact dermatitis, and allergic reaction.
Antivirals Acyclovir Famciclovir *Drug examples:* Zovirax Famvir	Inhibit viral DNA replication *May also be used for:* ■ Prophylaxis for cytomegalovirus ■ Prophylaxis for varicella	■ Advise the patient that full therapeutic effect may take several weeks. ■ Encourage adequate fluid intake. ■ Explain that antivirals do not cure the herpes virus. ■ Teach the patient about standard precautions to prevent the spread of infection. ■ Monitor for effectiveness and viral resistance. ■ Monitor for urticaria, pruritus, burning, and irritation.
Anesthetics Lidocaine hydrochloride *Drug example:* Xylocaine	Decrease pain through reversible nerve conduction blockade *May also be used for:* ■ Treatment of postherpetic neuralgia	■ Advise the patient against applying to large areas or broken skin. ■ Advise the patient to avoid contact with eyes.
Creams *Drug examples:* *Aquacare* Curel Nutra*derm*	Moisturize the skin	■ Encourage the patient to apply after bathing while skin is slightly damp. ■ Advise the patient to rub cream in completely. ■ Monitor for redness and itching.
Ointments *Drug examples:* Aquaphor Vaseline	Lubricate the skin; retard water loss	■ Advise the patient to cleanse the affected area with warm water and soap prior to application. ■ Encourage the patient to apply in a thin layer so air can reach the wound. ■ Advise the patient to avoid the nose and mouth area. ■ Monitor for redness and itching.

Medications *(continued)*

CLASSIFICATION AND DRUG EXAMPLES	MECHANISMS OF ACTION	NURSING CONSIDERATIONS
Lotions *Drug examples:* Alpha-Keri Dermassage Lubriderm	Moisturize the skin; lubricate the skin	▪ Encourage the patient to apply after bathing while the skin is slightly damp. ▪ Advise the patient to rub lotion in completely. ▪ Monitor for redness and itching.

Nonpharmacologic Therapy

Patients with skin disorders can benefit from a variety of nonpharmacologic interventions provided by an interprofessional team. These interventions are generally associated with proper wound management, which can include multiple techniques and procedures, as well as nutritional therapies. Some therapies used are similar, and some differ depending on the type of skin disorder being treated.

Infection prevention and adequate nutrition are important for all patients. Patients with burn wounds may also require additional therapies such as daily debridement and dressing changes. Therapies used for pressure ulcer management can vary based on facility protocol, provider orders, and stage of the wound. Wounds with impaired healing may require the use of vacuum devices to assist with closure.

Complementary Health Approaches

Patients with skin conditions often seek the use of complementary health approaches as treatment. The therapies may include the use of vitamin, mineral, and herbal supplements. The use of herbal supplements such as topical aloe vera gel and chamomile and oral evening primrose oil have been noted to soothe irritation and discomfort associated with skin inflammation and eczema. These supplements have also been useful in promoting healing of superficial burns, wounds, and abrasions. Despite the growing interest in these complementary health approaches, there is insufficient evidence to either recommend or dismiss the use of these treatments. The nurse should ask patients about the use of any complementary health approaches, as some can interact with prescription medications or other integrative therapies. Anyone using complementary health approaches should be monitored for allergic reactions (National Center for Complementary and Integrative Health, 2016; National Institutes of Health, 2014).

Lifespan Considerations

The aging of the skin is an unavoidable occurrence that every individual must face. This process is affected by both intrinsic and extrinsic factors. The intrinsic process occurs over the lifespan regardless of external influences and generally begins around 20 years of age. The pace of exfoliation of the skin decreases around that time, causing dead skin cells to adhere to each other for longer periods of time. Moisture transfer from the dermis to epidermis declines as individuals reach their 30s, and fat cells in the skin begin to decrease in size; these effects cause the skin to appear dull and thin. As individuals reach their 40s, collagen production comes to an end, causing the appearance of fine aging lines and wrinkles. Next, the sebaceous glands decrease in size. This results in skin that is dry and easily bruised, damaged, or broken. During menopause, women experience a decrease in estrogen levels, which leaves the skin drier, thinner, more sensitive, and less toned.

Extrinsic aging of the skin can be controlled because it results from environmental damage. This form of aging appears as thickening of the cornified layer, precancerous changes, skin cancer development, freckle formation, and vast losses of collagen and elastin. These processes cause the skin to become rough, uneven in tone, and wrinkled. Free radicals cause chemical changes to occur in the skin, which accelerate wrinkling and result from environmental influences such as pollution, smoking, and UV radiation. Prevention of extrinsic damage plays a key role in minimizing the development of wrinkles (Leal, 2013).

Tissue Integrity in Newborns

The newborn's skin is covered by vernix caseosa in utero, a waxy substance containing sebum, shed cells, and lipids that covers and protects the fetal skin from amniotic fluid and loss of fluids and electrolytes. It has many important properties, including anti-infective, thermoregulatory, antioxidant, moisturizing, and wound-healing agents (Kaneshiro, 2015; Van Onselen, 2015).

Certain conditions may be present on the newborn's skin at birth. Milia (tiny, pearly-white, firm raised bumps) may be present on the face. These generally require no treatment and disappear on their own. Mild acne, caused by hormones from the mother, may be present but usually resolves within a few weeks. A common, harmless rash known as erythema toxicum (small pustules on a red base) can appear 1–3 days after delivery, most commonly on the face, trunk, and extremities; it also resolves by 1 week of age. Some newborns have "stork bites" (small red patches caused by stretching of blood vessels) on the forehead, eyelids, back of the neck, or upper lip. Stork bites generally resolve within 18 months after birth. Other changes that may be noted include congenital nevi, Mongolian or café au lait spots, port-wine stains, or hemangiomas (Kaneshiro, 2015). See Table 21–4 for information on common chronic skin disorders.

At birth, the newborn's skin is between 40 and 60% thinner than an adult's skin and has little underlying subcutaneous fat. As a result, the infant loses heat more rapidly, has greater difficulty regulating body temperature, and becomes chilled more quickly than an older child or an adult. The infant's thinner skin also allows increased absorption of harmful chemical substances and topical medications. It also contains more water than an adult's and has loosely attached cells. As the infant grows, the skin toughens and becomes less hydrated, so it is less susceptible to bacteria (Ball et al., 2017).

Tissue Integrity in Children

Children have a proportionately larger body surface area (BSA) than adults, placing children at greater risk for excessive loss of heat and fluids. Because of their larger BSA and thinner skin, children are also more easily and rapidly affected by toxins or other agents that are absorbed through the skin. As individuals mature, their skin progressively thickens until they reach their 40s and 50s (Amirlak, 2015). Fungal (tinea), viral (varicella, warts), and parasitic (scabies, lice) skin infections are not uncommon in this age group. See Table 21–3 for information on common acute skin disorders. In addition to these skin disorders, children may commonly be affected by viral infections such as erythema infectiosum (fifth disease), pityriasis rosea, and roseola infantum.

Erythema infectiosum is caused by the virus PV-B19, a member of the *Parvoviridae* family. This disorder is characterized by a classic slapped-cheek appearance and lacy exanthema. It is self-limiting, lasting between 4 and 21 days, and commonly occurs during the winter and early spring. Symptom management, fluids, and rest are the recommended treatment for this infection.

Pityriasis rosea is a benign scaly rash, thought to be viral in origin; however, the exact cause is not known. This self-limiting condition evolves rapidly and generally begins with a "herald patch" that appears on the chest or back. An eruption of pink or tan patches will follow within a few weeks, appearing on the neck, back, arms, and legs. The duration of this outbreak usually is 4–8 weeks, and treatment is symptomatic.

Roseola infantum is most commonly caused by human herpes virus 6 (HHV-6) and is mainly seen during the spring and fall in children younger than age 3 years. This contagious disorder is marked by a high fever and rash that develops as the fever decreases. A child with roseola is most contagious during the period of high fever, prior to the appearance of the rash. It can take 5–15 days for symptoms to develop after exposure to the virus. The most serious complication is the occurrence of febrile seizures (Children's National Health System, 2016a, 2016b; Gorman, 2016; Schwartz, 2016b; Zellman, 2016).

Tissue Integrity in Adolescents

The skin of an adolescent undergoes physiologic changes. Testosterone, one of the hormones released during puberty, is responsible for an increase in sebum production and axillary sweating. Hormonal fluctuations caused by the menstrual cycle in female adolescents also cause changes in the skin and can cause premenstrual exacerbations of preexisting skin disorders (psoriasis, eczema, lupus erythematosus). Specific skin disorders that have a tendency to appear during adolescence include: acne vulgaris, seborrheic dermatitis, psoriasis, and tinea versicolor (Wong, 2014). This age group can also have a higher incidence of warts and fungal tinea infections due to involvement with sports and use of public shower facilities (Vocal, 2014). See Table 21–3 for information on common acute skin disorders.

Tissue Integrity in Pregnant Women

Skin changes during pregnancy are not uncommon. Of these, hyperpigmentation, striae distensae (stretch marks), and pruritus gravidarum are more commonly seen and are specifically related to the hormonal increases that occur during pregnancy. Other skin changes related to exacerbation of preexisting skin conditions such as acne, eczema, psoriasis, or rosacea may also occur due to increased hormone levels. Treatment goals for specific skin conditions during pregnancy are to control pruritus and skin lesions; however, treatment depends on gestational age and disease severity (Jones, Ambros-Rudolph, & Nelson-Piercy, 2014).

Atopic eruption of pregnancy (AEP) is a common pregnancy-specific skin disorder, occurring in approximately 50% of all pregnancies. Its development is thought to be initiated by pregnancy-related immune system changes and is characterized by the appearance of eczematous skin changes, most often around the neck and flexor surfaces of the body. AEP generally develops prior to the third trimester of pregnancy, responds well to treatment, and spontaneously resolves during the postpartum period. The fetus is unaffected but is at increased risk for the development of atopic dermatitis as an infant. Women who develop AEP are more likely to experience this disorder with future pregnancies (White et al., 2014).

Tissue Integrity in Older Adults

Skin changes are a normal part of the aging process (see **Table 21–6 »**); most changes occur slowly. Disorders of the skin are very common among older adults, making it difficult to differentiate normal changes of aging from those related to a disorder. Skin disorders in older adults can be caused by multiple factors, including disease processes, nutritional deficiencies, obesity, stress, medication reactions, allergic reactions, and sun exposure (Hurd, 2014).

As individuals age, the skin's thickness and collagen content decrease, causing skin to become thinner and less elastic over time. This change gives rise to wrinkled and sagging skin on the face, neck, and upper arms; these cosmetic changes often receive more attention than the functional changes, carry a social stigma, and can negatively affect self-esteem. Environmental factors such as sun exposure, chemical exposure, and nutrition can also affect skin's function and appearance. Sebaceous glands decrease their oil production, epidermal cell turnover declines, and the subcutaneous fat layer decreases and is redistributed. These variations result in a number of functional changes, including decreased sensation, increased healing time, increased risk for injury, and decreased thermoregulation (Hurd, 2014).

The number of melanocytes in aging skin decreases, causing it to appear more pale and translucent. Older adults commonly develop large hyperpigmented lesions (age or liver spots) on areas exposed to the sun. Blood vessels of the dermis become more fragile, increasing the risk for bleeding under the skin, often termed *senile purpura* (Hurd, 2014).

The loss and redistribution of fat in the subcutaneous tissue that occurs during the aging process is especially noticeable in the face and hands, which lose fat, and in the thighs and abdomen, which gain it. These changes make older individuals more prone to problems with thermoregulation, pressure ulcers over bony areas, and medication absorption (Hurd, 2014).

TABLE 21–6 Age-Related Skin Changes

Age-Related Change	Significance
Epidermis: ↓ thickness and miotic activity	■ Skin more fragile and at greater risk for tears or injury ■ Delayed wound healing ■ Hyperkeratosis and skin cancer more evident in sun-exposed areas
Epidermis: ↑ permeability, ↓ Langerhans cells	■ Increased risk of reactions to irritants ■ Decreased inflammatory response
Epidermis: ↓ number of active melanocytes	■ Increased susceptibility to skin damage from sun exposure
Epidermis: hyperplasia of melanocytes, especially in sun-exposed areas	■ Small areas of hyperpigmentation (liver spots) and hypopigmentation (age spots), especially on the hands
Epidermis: ↓ vitamin D production	■ Increased risk of osteomalacia and osteoporosis
Epidermis: flattened dermal–epidermal junction	■ Increased risk of skin tears, purpura, and pressure ulcers
Dermis: ↓ perfusion	■ Greater susceptibility to dry skin ■ Decreased sensation (pain, touch, temperature, and peripheral vibration) ■ Increased risk of injury
Dermis: ↓ vasomotor response	■ Greater risk of hyperthermia and hypothermia
Dermis: elastic fiber degeneration	■ Decreased tone and elasticity, with wrinkle formation
Dermis: proliferation of capillaries	■ Cherry hemangiomas common
Subcutaneous skin layer: thinning	■ Greater risk of hypothermia ■ Increased risk of pressure ulcers
Subcutaneous skin layer: redistribution of adipose tissue	■ Cellulite formation ■ Bags over and under the eyes ■ Double chin formation ■ Increase in abdominal fat ■ Sagging of breasts ■ Skin slower to return to normal when pinched (tenting)
Glands: ↓ eccrine and apocrine activity	■ Dry skin common ■ Absent perspiration

Case Study » Part 3

Three years after his release from the hospital following his neurosurgery, Mr. Sullivan's venous ulcer has improved but is still not healed completely. The ulcer is now 2.5 cm long, 1.8 cm wide, and 0.4 cm deep. The purple area around the ulcer has measured at 22 cm long and 13 cm wide for the past 2 years. Mr. Sullivan has experienced no further episodes of hemorrhage since he was taken off all anticoagulants. However, because of the open wound and skin discoloration, Mr. Sullivan has developed a disturbed body image.

Mr. Sullivan has been seeing a dermatologist for treatment of his ulcer and has tried several treatments over time, all of which have failed. As a result, his dermatologist has scheduled sclerotherapy to collapse the damaged veins. After the procedure, Mr. Sullivan continues treatment with daily topical sucralfate covered by simple gauze. Compression with an elastic bandage and compression stockings also continues. Six months after sclerotherapy, the ulcer measures 1.3 cm long, 0.8 cm wide, and 0.2 cm deep. However, the purple area surrounding the wound has not decreased. Mr. Sullivan and his dermatologist hope that the ulcer will be completely healed within a year after the procedure.

Clinical Reasoning Questions Level I

1. As the dermatologist's nurse, what patient teaching will you perform prior to sclerotherapy?
2. How does ablation of damaged veins contribute to ulcer healing?
3. Once Mr. Sullivan's ulcer has healed completely, what maintenance therapy may be beneficial for continued healing of the damaged area?

Clinical Reasoning Questions Level II

4. What may be the long-term consequences of Mr. Sullivan's venous ulcer?
5. What patient teaching is necessary to help Mr. Sullivan prevent future development of venous ulcers?
6. What nursing interventions are appropriate for the nursing diagnosis *Disturbed Body Image*?

REVIEW   The Concept of Tissue Integrity

RELATE Link the Concepts

Linking the concept of tissue integrity with the concept of comfort:

1. You are caring for a 2-year-old patient with nonbullous impetigo. What actions can you take to improve the child's comfort?
2. What patient teaching would you provide the child's caretaker to improve the child's comfort?

Linking the concept of tissue integrity with the concept of development:

3. You are caring for a 12-year-old who was just diagnosed with vitiligo. How can you explain the child's condition to him in a developmentally appropriate way? What psychosocial considerations are especially important for a patient in this age group?

4. What psychologic and cognitive aspects should you consider when explaining impaired tissue integrity related to pressure ulcers to a patient in his 80s who is bedridden?

READY Go to Volume 3: Clinical Nursing Skills

- SKILL 1.16   Hair: Assessing
- SKILL 1.20   Nails: Assessing
- SKILL 1.25   Skin: Assessing
- SKILL 16.1   Wound Drainage Specimen: Obtaining
- SKILLS 16.2–16.9   Dressings and Binders
- SKILLS 16.10–16.19 Wound Care

REFER Go to Pearson MyLab Nursing and eText

- Additional review materials

REFLECT Apply Your Knowledge

Gavin Clairmont, a 15-year-old boy, has been brought to the pediatrician's office by his mother. She is concerned about the rash on his face. When questioned by the nurse about the rash, Gavin indicates that these "bumps" have gotten worse and are spreading onto his chest and back. The lesions do not itch and are not painful. He has not had a fever or other symptoms of illness. Gavin has tried washing his face with soap but has not used any medications to try to make the rash better. He is upset about these "bumps" because classmates at school are making jokes about it.

1. What additional questions about Gavin's skin rash would be important for the nurse to ask?
2. Are there any psychosocial factors that might place him at increased risk for developing a skin rash?
3. When conducting the physical assessment, what findings should the nurse note about Gavin's skin?
4. Are there any additional body systems that should be assessed as part of this complaint?

» Exemplar 21.A
Burns

Exemplar Learning Outcomes

21.A Analyze burns as they relate to tissue integrity.

- Describe the pathophysiology, etiology, risk factors, and prevention of burns.
- Identify the clinical manifestations of burns.
- Summarize diagnostic tests and therapies used by interprofessional teams in the collaborative care of an individual with burns.
- Differentiate considerations for care of patients with burns across the lifespan.
- Apply the nursing process in providing culturally competent care to an individual with burns.

Exemplar Key Terms

Allograft, *1611*
Autografting, *1609*
Burn, *1594*
Burn shock, *1601*
Compartment syndrome, *1602*
Contracture, *1598*
Curling ulcers, *1603*
Debridement, *1605*
Eschar, *1602*
Escharotomy, *1609*
Fascial excision, *1609*
Fasciectomy, *1609*
Fluid resuscitation, *1607*
Full-thickness burns, *1598*
Heterograft, *1611*
Homograft, *1611*
Hypertrophic scar, *1600*
Keloid, *1600*
Partial-thickness burns, *1597*
Superficial burns, *1597*
Surgical debridement, *1609*
Tangential excision, *1609*
Xenograft, *1611*

Overview

A **burn** is a type of injury caused by exposure to heat, certain chemicals, electricity, or radiation. When energy from one of these sources is transferred to an individual's body, it initiates a sequence of physiologic events that, in the most severe cases, lead to irreversible tissue destruction. Burns range in severity from minor losses of small segments of the epidermis to complex multisystem injuries. Thus, treatment may involve anything from simple first aid to delivery of complex, interprofessional team care in the aseptic environment of a hospital burn center.

Pathophysiology and Etiology

Burns are among the most common types of injuries, in part because they arise from many different causes. Although burns affect individuals from all walks of life, some individuals are at elevated risk because of factors such as age, occupation, and preexisting conditions.

Types of Burns

Burns may be caused by heat, chemicals, electricity, or radiation. Although all four types of burns can result in generalized tissue damage and multisystem involvement, each type exhibits unique characteristics and requires unique priority treatment measures.

Thermal Burns

As their name suggests, thermal burns result from exposure to heat, either dry (e.g., flames) or moist (e.g., steam, hot liquids). Thermal burns are the most common type of burn injury and most often affect children and older adults (see

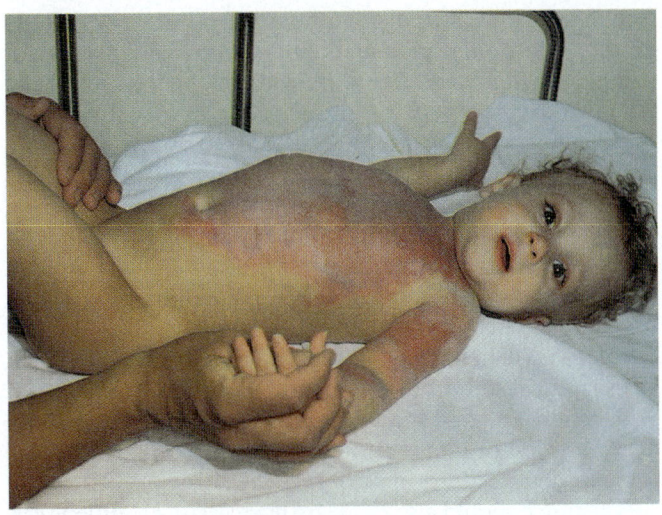

Figure 21–18 》 Thermal (scald) burns are the most common burn injury in infants. Notice the distribution of the burned skin, a wide area on the upper chest and arm where the hottest liquid fell, with a narrower area near the umbilicus, indicating that the liquid cooled as it traveled down the chest.

Figure 21–18 》). With thermal burns, direct exposure to the heat source causes cellular destruction and may result in charring of vascular, bony, muscle, and nervous tissue.

Chemical Burns

Chemical burns result from direct contact between skin and certain acids, alkaline agents, or organic compounds. The destruction that these chemicals cause in the proteins in the individual's tissues leads to necrosis.

More than 25,000 products found in the home or workplace can cause chemical burns, including those listed in **Box 21–1** 》. Of these products, acids (e.g., hydrochloric acid) produce burns through coagulative necrosis of the superficial tissue. Alkalis (e.g., lye) produce burns through liquefaction necrosis, and organic compounds (e.g., petroleum distillates) produce burns by dissolving cells' lipid membranes. Burns from alkalis are more difficult to neutralize than burns caused by acids and tend to be deeper and more severe. Organic compound burns also pose a special threat because their causative agents may trigger renal and liver failure if absorbed. For all chemical burns, the severity of an individual's injury is related to the type and concentration of chemical agent, the mechanism of action, the duration of contact, and the amount of BSA exposed (Gnaneswaran et al., 2015).

Box 21–1
Household Chemicals that May Cause Burns

- Drain cleaners
- Lye
- Ammonia
- Oven cleaners
- Toilet bowl cleaners
- Dishwasher detergents
- Bleach

Electrical Burns

Electrical burns vary in severity depending on the type and duration of current and the amount of voltage. Assessment of electrical burn injuries is difficult because electricity follows the path of least resistance. This path tends to lie along muscles, bone, blood vessels, and nerves so that the extent and depth of an individual's injury may not be evident until weeks after the initial burn event. Furthermore, the small entry and exit wounds from electricity mask widespread tissue damage underneath the outer layer of the skin. Tissue necrosis frequently results from impaired flow secondary to blood coagulation at the site of an electrical injury. If this necrosis is severe, an individual may develop gangrene that necessitates amputation (Yale Medicine, 2016).

The nurse should be aware that different types of electric current tend to produce characteristic patterns of injury. In general, alternating current (AC), like that found in most U.S. households, produces repeated electrical surges that lead to tetanic muscle contractions. These sustained contractions inhibit an individual's respiratory efforts for the duration of contact and may result in respiratory arrest. The contractions may also cause the individual to clamp down on the power source (e.g., an electrical cord) and thereby increase the duration of contact with the source. In comparison, direct current (DC), as in injury from a lightning bolt, exposes the body to very high voltage for an instant. However, few individuals experience the full energy of a lightning strike because only a small percentage of injuries are from a direct strike. Lightning injuries can range from mild to severe and have varying outcomes. Mild injury is rarely associated with superficial burns, but the individual may experience loss of consciousness, amnesia, tingling, and a variety of other non-specific symptoms. Moderate injury may cause seizures, respiratory arrest, or cardiac standstill; superficial burns are common 》. Severe or high-voltage injury usually results in cardiopulmonary arrest, and survival is rare unless resuscitative efforts are begun immediately. In some high-voltage lightning strikes, a phenomenon known as the *flashover effect* occurs. Here, the lightning bolt flashes over the individual, and the current travels over the moist surface of the skin rather than through deeper structures, often saving the individual from death. Other possible outcomes from severe lightening injury include brain injury, resulting in loss of consciousness or coma; injuries to the eyes and ears; temporary paralysis; nerve damage; and burns from metal jewelry or coins that are heated by the lightning. Many who survive have no memory of the event, but may experience ongoing symptoms, including seizures (Cooper, 2016).

Radiation Burns

Radiation burns are usually associated with sunburn or radiation treatment for cancer. These kinds of burns tend to be superficial, involving only the outermost layers of the epidermis. All functions of the skin remain intact. Symptoms are limited to mild systemic reactions, including headache, chills, local discomfort, nausea, and vomiting.

More extensive exposure to radiation or radioactive substances, as in nuclear power accidents, leads to the same degree of tissue damage and multisystem involvement associated with other types of burns.

Etiology

Researchers estimate that U.S. hospitals and emergency departments treat 500,000 individuals with burn injuries each year. Of these, approximately 40,000 require hospital admission; 30,000 receiving care in specialized burn centers (Fonseca, 2016). Each year, nearly 3500 Americans die from burns, with more than 3400 of these fatalities being caused by fires, and the remainder by other sources (American Burn Association, 2016; U.S. Department of Homeland Security, 2016). In the United States, burn injuries are listed as one of the top six leading causes of accidental death for children ages 1–14, and the eighth leading cause for adults greater than age 65 (CDC, 2016e).

Burns are especially common among children. According to the American Burn Association (2016), approximately 250,000 children under age 17 require medical attention for burn injuries each year. Burns in children under age 4 are primarily caused by contact with hot surfaces or scalding liquids; older children can receive burn injuries from varied heat sources, with flame injury being the most common cause of serious burns (Edlich, 2015). Fires kill approximately 488 children under age 14 each year, and 90% of these blazes occur in residences. Another 116,600 children are injured from a fire- or burn-related incident but do not die from their wounds (Blank Children's Hospital, 2016). Common causes of residential fires include cooking equipment, heating equipment, and smoking. Three of five residential fire deaths occur in homes that did not have smoke detectors or in which smoke detectors were not working—a sobering statistic that highlights the importance of properly installing and maintaining such equipment (Ahrens, 2016).

Risk Factors

Several factors increase an individual's likelihood of burns. The main factor among these is age, with children age 4 and younger and adults age 65 and older having the greatest risk (Ahrens, 2016; Edlich, 2015). One reason young children are so vulnerable to burns is that they simply do not understand the dangers presented by everyday objects such as hot tap water and electrical outlets. Children are also innately curious, and therefore more likely to play with items such as matches, lighters, fireworks, microwaves, and stoves if left unattended. In addition, children's lower height and ability to climb, stretch, and reach objects over their heads places them at increased risk of burns from spills or hot surfaces (Akansel et al., 2013). Finally, abuse is a factor in many childhood burn injuries; experts estimate that between 1 and 35% of children who are admitted to burn units sustained intentional burns (Hornor, 2012).

Older adults are also at increased risk for burns. Slower reaction times, impaired mobility, and sensory impairment account for much of this risk. Dementia is another age-related factor that can increase an individual's likelihood of injury. Furthermore, age-related thinning of the skin means that older adults are more susceptible to deep burns, even from sources that would cause only minor to moderate burns in a younger individual.

Other factors associated with heighted burn risk include gender, with male patients being more likely to sustain burns than female patients (American Burn Association, 2016). Individuals of lower socioeconomic status are at increased risk for burns, often because they live in unsafe homes, lack smoke detectors, and/or rely on portable heating devices. African Americans and Native Americans have a higher incidence of burn injuries, as do patients who smoke or use tobacco, drugs, or alcohol.

Individuals with physical and/or mental disabilities may not understand the risk posed by various hazards, may have decreased reaction times, and/or may be physically unable to escape fires and other dangers. Individuals who work with chemicals, gasoline, electricity, or extreme heat sources are more likely to be burned than individuals in other occupations.

The nurse should also be aware that certain conditions can increase a patient's risk of burn-related complications and morbidity. Examples include preexisting cardiac, pulmonary, or renal disorders; diabetes mellitus; and alcoholism.

Prevention

Methods for preventing burns vary by setting and causative agent. Many of these measures involve taking proper precautions in the home, especially when children are present. See **Box 21–2 »** for examples. Other methods are specific to the workplace. For instance, individuals who work with hazardous chemicals should be aware of proper handling protocols and what to do if a spill, fire, or other accident

Box 21–2
Burn Prevention in the Home

The following measures can greatly reduce burn risk in the home:

- Be sure working smoke detectors are installed in each level of the home. Test the devices monthly, and change the batteries at least once per year.
- Create an emergency escape plan, and practice it with all members of the household.
- When cooking, do not wear clothes with loose-fitting sleeves, and keep pot handles turned away from the front of the stove.
- Never leave cooking food or open flames (even in a grill or fireplace) unattended.
- Keep fire extinguishers near possible sources of ignition.
- Use caution when carrying hot foods and liquids around children.
- Install childproofing devices on electrical outlets, oven knobs, and cabinets that contain hazardous chemicals. Keep matches, lighters, and fireworks stored out of children's reach.
- Set the home's water heater temperature at 120–130°F.
- Keep electrical appliances away from water, and unplug them when they are not in use.
- Check all electrical cords for wear, and replace the cords as needed.
- Avoid overloading outlets and extension cords.
- Always test the temperature of a child's bathwater before placing the child in the tub.
- Never leave young children in the bathroom or kitchen unsupervised.

occurs. Individuals who work with electricity should be sure to use proper safety equipment at all times. Of course, all employees in all workplaces should know and be familiar with a planned escape route in case of fires or other emergencies.

Other burn prevention tips apply specifically to individuals who smoke. Smokers should always use safe, heat-resistant ashtrays, and they should be sure all ashes, butts, used matches, and related materials are completely cool before placing them in the trash. Individuals should also avoid smoking in bed, as well as during periods when they are sleepy or under the influence of alcohol or medications that can induce drowsiness. Finally, matches and lighters should be kept out of children's reach, and working smoke detectors should be installed in rooms where smoking most often occurs.

Clinical Manifestations

Regardless of their cause, all burns are classified according to the same basic system and heal by way of a similar process. Still, different burns can affect an individual's body systems in a number of different ways depending on their source, type, and severity.

Classification of Burns

Tissue damage following a burn is determined primarily by two factors: the depth of the burn (i.e., how many layers of underlying tissue are affected) and the extent of the burn (i.e., the percentage of BSA involved). Although once many

classified burn injuries by degree (first, second, third), that method of classification has been replaced by assessing the depth of the burn (Kearns, Holmes, & Cairns, 2013).

Depth of the Burn

The depth of a burn injury is determined by which elements of the skin have been damaged or destroyed. Burn depth depends on the temperature of the burning agent and the length of contact. Based on depth, burns are classified as superficial, partial thickness, or full thickness (see **Figure 21–19 》》**).

Superficial burns involve only the epidermal layer of the skin. They most often result from sunburn, UV light, minor flash injury (from a sudden ignition or explosion), or mild radiation associated with cancer treatment. Because the skin remains intact, superficial burns are not calculated into estimates of burn extent.

Skin affected by superficial burns ranges in color from pink to bright red and may be accompanied by slight edema over the burned area. If a significant portion of the body is burned, additional symptoms may include chills, headache, nausea, and vomiting. Superficial burns usually heal in 3–6 days, with dryness and peeling of the outer layer of skin and no scar formation. Treatment typically involves administration of mild analgesics and application of water-soluble lotions. However, extensive superficial burns may require IV fluid treatment, especially in older adults.

Partial-thickness burns are deeper than superficial burns, involving both the epidermis and the dermis.

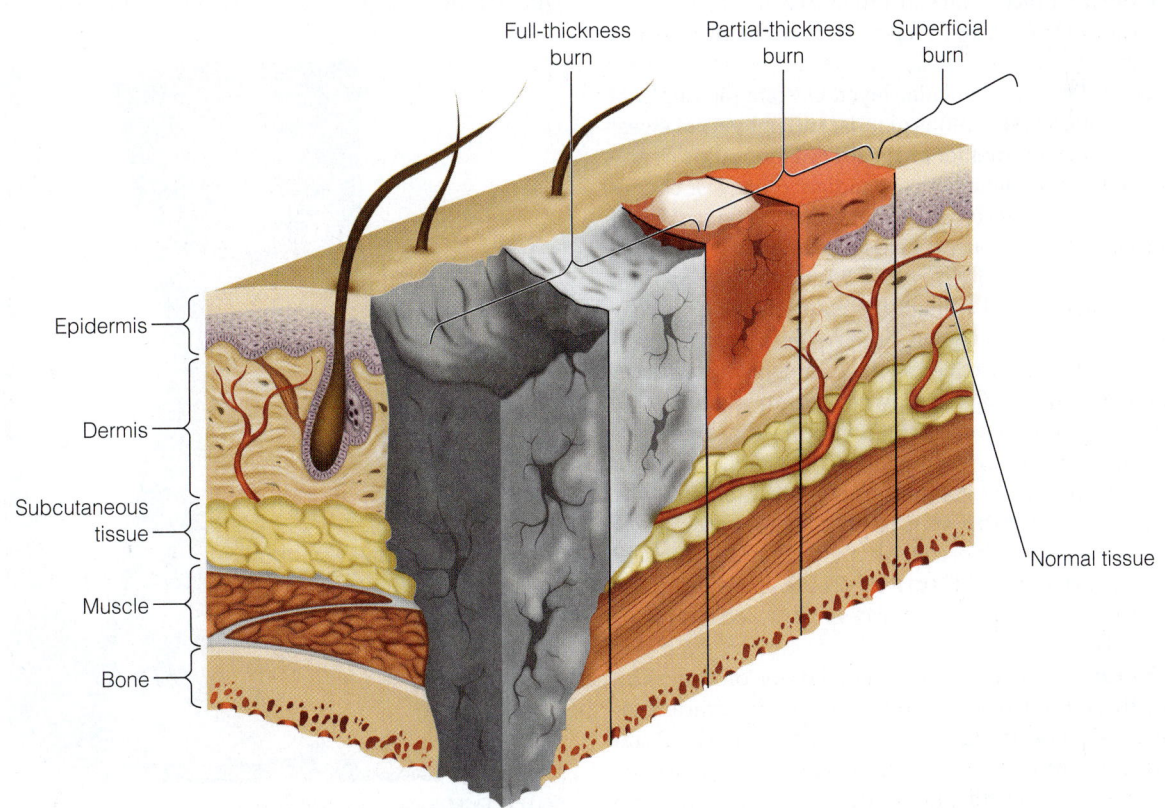

Figure 21–19 》》 Characteristics of burns by depth of injury.

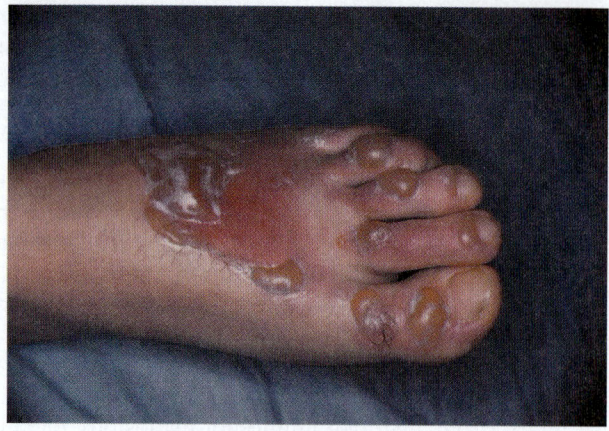

Source: Charles Stewart MD, EMDM, MPH.

Figure 21–20 》 Partial-thickness burn injury.

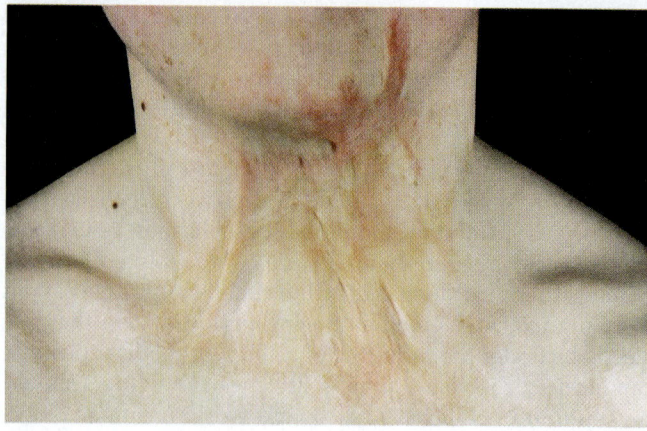

Source: Biophoto Associates/Science Source.

Figure 21–21 》 Burn contracture.

Depending on their depth, partial-thickness burns may be further categorized as either superficial or deep.

A *superficial partial-thickness burn* (see **Figure 21–20 》**) extends from the skin's surface into the papillary layer of the dermis. This type of burn may result from brief exposure to a flash flame or dilute chemical agents or contact with a hot surface. Superficial partial-thickness burns are often bright red and have a moist, glistening appearance with blister formation. The burned area blanches on pressure, and touch and pain sensation remains intact. Pain in response to temperature and air exposure is usually severe. These burns typically heal within 21 days with minimal or no scarring, but pigment changes are common. Analgesics may be administered, and if large blistered areas are disrupted, skin substitutes may be used.

A *deep partial-thickness burn* also involves the dermis but extends deeper than a superficial partial-thickness burn, past the papillae and into the reticular layer. Despite the depth of damage, hair follicles, sebaceous glands, and epidermal sweat glands remain intact (Huether et al., 2017). Hot liquids or solids, flash flame, direct flame, intense radiant energy, or chemical agents may cause this level of burn wound. The surface of a deep partial-thickness burn appears pale and waxy and may be moist or dry. Large, easily ruptured blisters may be present, or the blisters may look like flat, dry tissue paper. Capillary refill time is decreased. The wound is less painful than a superficial partial-thickness burn, because sensation is decreased at the site. However, areas of pain may be present, and sensation to deep pressure will remain intact. Deep partial-thickness burn wounds often require more than 21 days for healing and may convert to full-thickness injuries if necrosis extends the depth of the wound. **Contracture**, or permanent shortening of connective tissue, is possible, as are hypertrophic scarring and functional impairment (see **Figure 21–21 》**). Excision of the wound and skin grafting may be necessary to decrease scarring and loss of function.

Full-thickness burns involve all layers of the skin, including the epidermis, the dermis, and the epidermal appendages (see **Figure 21–22 》**). The wound may extend below the skin into subcutaneous fat, connective tissue, muscle, and bone. Full-thickness burns are caused by prolonged contact with flames, steam, chemicals, or high-voltage electric current.

Depending on the cause of injury, a full-thickness burn wound may appear pale, waxy, yellow, brown, mottled, charred, or nonblanching red. The wound's surface is dry, leathery, and firm to the touch. Thrombosed blood vessels may be visible under the surface of the wound. There is no sensation of pain or light touch at the site because pain and touch receptors have been destroyed. Full-thickness burns require skin grafting to heal.

Extent of the Burn

The extent of a burn injury is expressed as a percentage of the affected individual's total body surface area (TBSA). Several methods are used to determine this percentage. The rule of nines is a quick method of estimation used during the

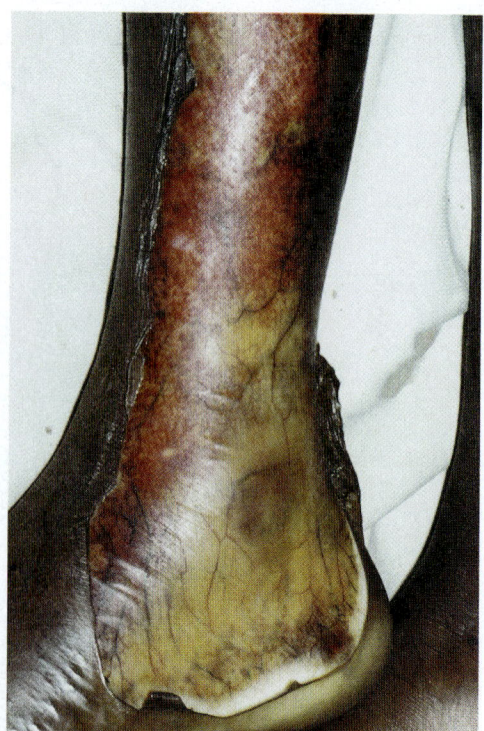

Source: Dr M.A. Ansary/Science Source.

Figure 21–22 》 Full-thickness burn injury.

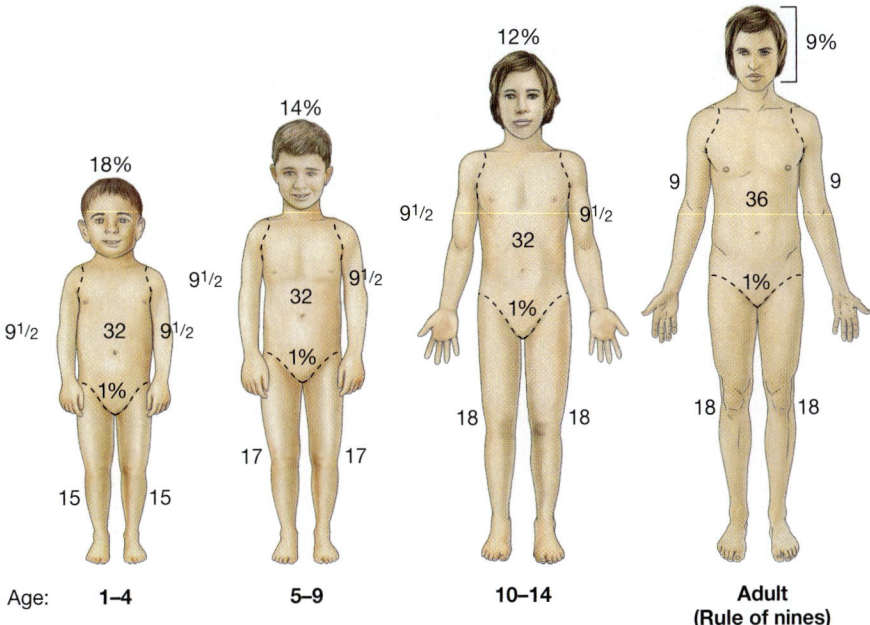

Figure 21–23 ❯❯ The rule of nines is one method for quickly estimating the percentage of TBSA affected by a burn injury. Although useful in emergency care situations, the rule of nines is not accurate for estimating TBSA for adults who are short, obese, or very thin.

prehospital and emergency care phases. In the rule of nines method, the adult body is divided into five surface areas—head, trunk, arms, legs, and perineum—and percentages that equal or total a sum of nine are assigned to each body area; different percentages are assigned for children (see **Figure 21–23** ❯❯). For example, an adult patient with burns of the face, anterior right arm, and anterior trunk would have burn injury involving 27% of TBSA. (In this example, face = 4.5%, arm = 4.5%, and trunk = 18%, for an overall total of 27%.) Again, only partial- and full-thickness burns are included in the estimation.

Later, upon the patient's admission to the hospital, critical care unit, or burn center, more accurate methods for estimating the extent of injury can be employed. For example, the Lund and Browder method (see **Figure 21–24** ❯❯) determines surface area measurements for each body part according to the age of the patient.

Another widely recognized system for describing burn injuries, developed by the American Burn Association, uses both the extent and the depth of injury to classify burns as minor, moderate, or major (see **Table 21–7** ❯❯). Also see the Clinical Manifestations and Therapies feature later in this exemplar for information on therapeutic measures appropriate for each class of burn.

Burn Wound Healing

Burns heal through the same processes as do other wounds, but the healing phases occur more slowly and last longer. There are three phases in the burn healing process: inflammation, proliferation, and remodeling (Huether et al., 2017).

Inflammation

The inflammation phase begins immediately following a burn injury, as platelets come into contact with the damaged tissue and start to aggregate. Fibrin is deposited, trapping additional platelets, and a thrombus forms. The thrombus, combined with local vasoconstriction, causes hemostasis, which walls off the wound from the systemic circulation.

TABLE 21–7 American Burn Association Classification of Burn Injury

Minor Burn Injury	Moderate Burn Injury	Major Burn Injury
Excludes electrical injury, inhalation injury, complicated injuries (e.g., multiple trauma), and all patients who are considered at high risk (e.g., older adults, those with chronic illnesses)	Excludes electrical injury, inhalation injury, complicated injuries (e.g., multiple trauma), and all patients who are considered at high risk (e.g., older adults, those with chronic illnesses)	Includes all burns of the hands, face, eyes, ears, feet, and perineum; all electrical injuries, inhalation injuries, and multiple-trauma injuries; and all patients who are considered at high risk
Includes partial-thickness burns of less than 15% of TBSA in adults	Includes partial-thickness burns of 15–25% of TBSA in adults	Includes partial-thickness burns of greater than 25% of TBSA in adults
Includes full-thickness burns of less than 2% of TBSA not involving special care areas (i.e., eyes, ears, face, hands, feet, joints, perineum)	Includes full-thickness burns of less than 10% of TBSA not involving special care areas (i.e., eyes, ears, face, hands, feet, joints, perineum)	Includes all full-thickness burns of 10% or greater of TBSA

Note: The injuries described in this table (except minor burns) should be treated in a specialized burn center. These criteria have been established by the American Burn Association.

Area	Age (years)					% 1°	% 2°	% 3°	% Total
	0–1	1–4	5–9	10–15	Adult				
Head	19	17	13	10	7				
Neck	2	2	2	2	2				
Ant. trunk	13	13	13	13	13				
Post. trunk	13	13	13	13	13				
R. buttock	2½	2½	2½	2½	2½				
L. buttock	2½	2½	2½	2½	2½				
Genitalia	1	1	1	1	1				
R.U. arm	4	4	4	4	4				
L.U. arm	4	4	4	4	4				
R.L. arm	3	3	3	3	3				
L.L. arm	3	3	3	3	3				
R. hand	2½	2½	2½	2½	2½				
L. hand	2½	2½	2½	2½	2½				
R. thigh	5½	6½	8½	8½	9½				
L. thigh	5½	6½	8½	8½	9½				
R. leg	5	5	5½	6	7				
L. leg	5	5	5½	6	7				
R. foot	3½	3½	3½	3½	3½				
L. foot	3½	3½	3½	3½	3½				
								Total	

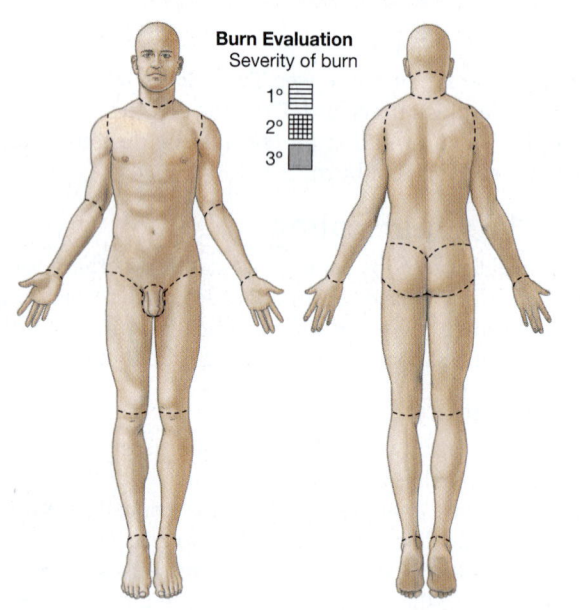

Burn Evaluation
Severity of burn

1°
2°
3°

Figure 21–24 》 The Lund and Browder burn assessment chart. This method of estimating TBSA affected by a burn injury is more accurate than the rule of nines because it accounts for changes in the body surface area across the lifespan.

Local vasodilation and an increase in capillary permeability follow hemostasis. Neutrophils infiltrate the wound and peak in about 24 hours, at which point monocytes predominate. The monocytes are converted into macrophages, which consume pathogens and dead tissue and secrete various growth factors. These growth factors stimulate the proliferation of fibroblasts and the deposit of a provisional wound matrix.

Proliferation

The proliferation phase begins about 2–3 days postburn. At this point, the wound contains primarily fibroblasts. Their number peaks about 14 days after the injury. Granulation tissue begins to form, with complete re-epithelialization occurring during this stage. Epithelial cells gradually cover the wound as each cell stretches across the wound's surface to join with other epithelial cells on the opposite side of the wound. The proliferation phase lasts until complete re-epithelialization occurs by epithelial cell migration, surgical intervention, or a combination of the two.

Remodeling

With burn wounds, the remodeling phase may last for years. Over time, collagen fibers that were laid down during the proliferative phase reorganize into more compact areas. Scars also gradually contract and fade in color. In normal healing following a minor burn injury, the newly formed skin closely resembles its neighboring tissue. However, when a burn injury extends into the dermal layer of skin, two types of excessive scar may develop. A **hypertrophic scar** is an overgrowth of dermal tissue that remains within the boundaries of the wound. A **keloid** is a scar that extends beyond the boundaries of the original wound. Patients with dark skin are at greater risk for hypertrophic scars and keloids.

Systemic Effects of Burn Injuries

The pathophysiologic changes that result from major burn injuries involve all body systems. Extensive loss of skin (the body's protective barrier) can result in massive infection, fluid and electrolyte imbalances, and hypothermia. Often, the affected individual inhales the products of combustion, thus compromising respiratory function. Cardiac dysrhythmias and circulatory failure are also common manifestations of serious burn injuries.

Meanwhile, the profound catabolic state associated with a severe burn dramatically increases an individual's caloric expenditure and nutritional deficiencies. Alterations in gastrointestinal motility predispose the patient to developing paralytic ileus, and hyperacidity can lead to gastric and duodenal ulcerations. Dehydration slows glomerular filtration rates and renal clearance of toxic wastes and may lead to acute tubular necrosis and renal failure. As a result of these effects, a significant burn injury may profoundly alter an individual's metabolism. Systemic responses to burns are shown in **Figure 21–25 》**. More specific systemic responses to burns are discussed in the following sections.

Respiratory System

Pulmonary damage sometimes results from the systemic response to a burn injury. More commonly, however, breathing in hot gases and smoke causes direct damage to an individual's pulmonary tissues. In fact, inhalation injury is a frequent and often lethal complication of burns. The injury may range from mild respiratory inflammation to massive pulmonary failure, such as acute respiratory distress syndrome (ARDS).

Exposure to heat, asphyxiants, and smoke initiates the pathophysiologic process associated with inhalation injury. Inflammation occurs at localized sites in the airway and is

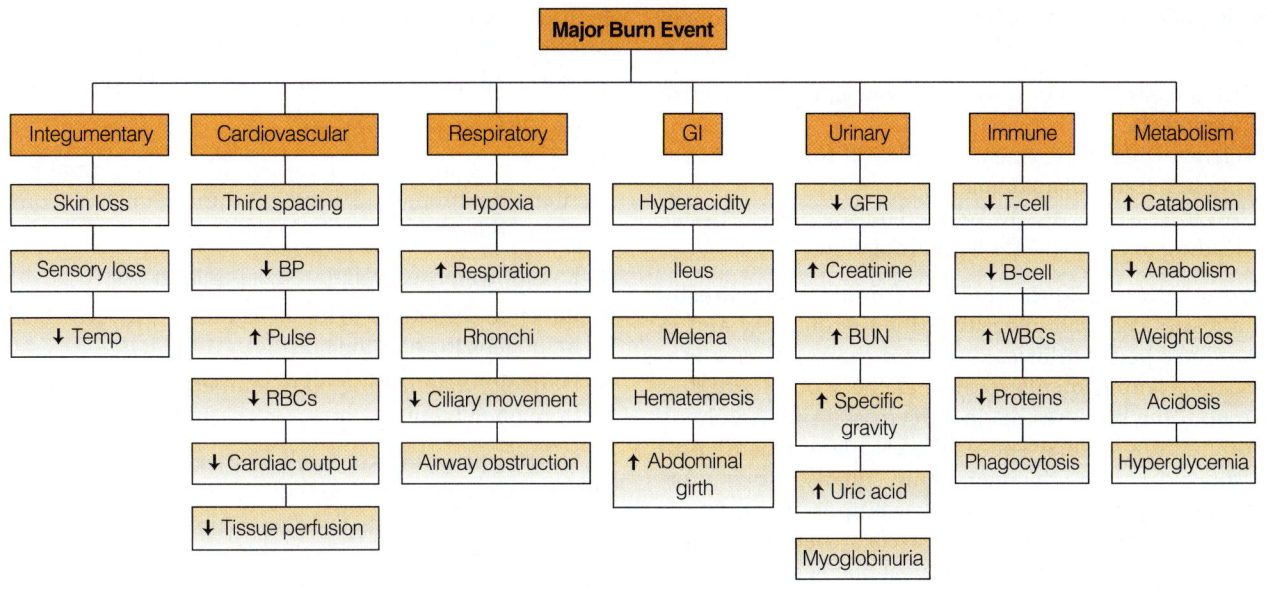

Figure 21–25 ≫ Effects of a severe burn on major body systems and metabolism.

manifested as hyperemia (increased blood supply). As a result, cells are destroyed, and the bronchial cilia are rendered inactive. Because the mucociliary transport mechanism no longer functions, the patient may develop bronchial congestion and infection. Interstitial pulmonary edema develops secondary to the escape of fluid from the pulmonary vasculature into the interstitial compartment of the lung tissue. Surfactant is inactivated, and the result is atelectasis (collapse of lung tissue) and alveolar collapse. Sloughing of the damaged and dead lung tissue occasionally produces debris that may lead to complete airway obstruction.

Upper airway thermal injury (above the level of the glottis) can also result from the inhalation of heated air or chemicals dissolved in water. This type of injury should be suspected when a patient has singed facial, scalp, or nasal hair. Physical findings include the presence of soot, charring, edema, blisters, and ulcerations along the mucosal lining of the oropharynx and larynx. The resulting edema in the airway peaks within the first 24–48 hours of injury. Ominous signs of hoarseness, labored breathing, or stridor indicate possible airway obstruction due to edema.

Lower airway thermal injury is a much less common occurrence. Because the lower airway is protected by laryngeal reflexes, thermal injury below the vocal cords is uncommon. When it does occur, it is typically associated with the inhalation of steam or explosive gases or the aspiration of hot liquids. Sputum containing soot or carbon particles is a classic manifestation of lower airway thermal injury (Bishop & Maguire, 2012).

Smoke poisoning results when toxic gases and particulate matter, the products of incomplete combustion, deposit directly on the pulmonary mucosa. The composition of the products of combustion depends on the combustible material, the rate at which the temperature increases, and the amount of ambient oxygen present. Irritant gases and particulate matter have a direct cytotoxic effect. The degree of injury is determined by the solubility in water of the irritant,

the duration of exposure, and the size of the particulate or aerosol droplet.

One product of combustion that deserves special mention is carbon monoxide, which is an extremely common asphyxiant. Carbon monoxide is a colorless, tasteless, odorless gas that has a 200 times greater affinity for hemoglobin than does oxygen. Thus, carbon monoxide easily displaces oxygen to bind with hemoglobin, forming a complex called *carboxyhemoglobin*. When this occurs, the resulting decrease in an individual's arterial oxyhemoglobin produces tissue hypoxia. Carbon monoxide impairs both oxygen delivery and cellular oxygen use. Clinical manifestations of carbon monoxide poisoning range from headache, nausea, and dizziness to coma and death.

Another notable product of combustion is cyanide gas, which is released when plastic, polyurethane, nylon, or silk is burned. Cyanide gas impedes cellular respiration. Of the various organs, the brain and heart are most vulnerable to cyanide poisoning. Manifestations of this condition include headache, dizziness, seizures, tachycardia, and lethal dysrhythmias.

Cardiovascular System

The effects of a major burn are also manifested in all components of the vascular system. These effects include hypovolemic shock (burn shock), cardiac dysrhythmias (e.g., ventricular fibrillation), cardiac arrest, and vascular compromise.

Hypovolemic Shock (Burn Shock)

Within minutes after a major burn injury, a cascade of cellular events is initiated, and a massive amount of fluid shifts from the intracellular and intravascular compartments into the interstitium. This shift is a type of hypovolemic shock called **burn shock**, which continues until capillary integrity is restored, usually within 24–36 hours after the injury.

Although the pathophysiologic mechanisms of postburn vascular changes and fluid volume shifts are not clearly understood, three processes occur early in the postburn phase in patients who have burns involving 40% or more of their TBSA:

1. An increase in microvascular permeability at the burn wound site
2. Generalized impairment of cell wall function, resulting in intracellular edema
3. An increase in osmotic pressure of the burned tissue, leading to extensive fluid accumulation.

During burn shock, the shifting of fluid results directly from a loss of cell wall integrity at the site of injury and in the capillary bed. Fluid leaking from the capillaries into interstitial compartments located at the wound site and throughout the body results in a decrease in fluid volume within the intravascular space. The escape of plasma proteins and sodium into the interstitium enhances edema formation. Blood pressure falls as cardiac output diminishes.

Vasoconstriction results as the vascular system attempts to compensate for fluid loss. Abnormal platelet aggregation and white blood cell (WBC) accumulation result in ischemia (insufficient blood supply) in the deeper tissue below the burn, leading to eventual thrombosis. Red blood cells (RBCs) and WBCs remain in the circulation, producing an elevation in erythrocyte and leukocyte counts secondary to hemoconcentration.

The leakage of fluid into the interstitium compromises the lymphatic system, resulting in intravascular hypovolemia and edema at the burn wound site. Edematous body surfaces impair peripheral circulation and result in necrosis of the underlying tissue. During burn shock, potassium ions leave the intracellular compartment, a process that puts the patient at risk for cardiac dysrhythmia due to hypokalemia. The process of burn shock continues until capillary integrity is restored, usually within 24 hours after the injury.

Burn shock reverses when fluid is reabsorbed from the interstitium into the intravascular compartment. As this happens, the patient's blood pressure rises, cardiac output increases, and urinary output improves. Diuresis continues from several days to 2 weeks postburn. During this phase, the extra cardiac workload may predispose older patients or patients with cardiovascular disease to fluid volume overload.

Cardiac Rhythm Alterations

Burns on more than 40% of an individual's TBSA cause significant myocardial dysfunction, with a decrease in myocardial contractibility and cardiac output. These changes, which occur prior to a decrease in plasma volume, are believed to be due to the release of substances and oxygen-free radicals from the burn wound and from ischemic myocardial cells. In addition, electrical burns often result in cardiac dysrhythmias or cardiopulmonary arrest caused by heat damage to the myocardium or by electrical interference with cardiac electrical activity.

Peripheral Vascular Compromise

Circumferential burns are those that result from injury that encircles an extremity. As scar tissue develops, the circumferential burn tightens, much like a rubber band, reducing or eliminating blood supply below the burn. Circulation to extremities may be further impaired by edema and by peripheral vasoconstriction that occurs during burn shock.

In addition, **compartment syndrome** may result. With this condition, tissue pressure in a muscle compartment exceeds microvascular pressure, interrupting cellular perfusion.

Integumentary System

The loss of skin in burn injuries interrupts normal integumentary functions and protective mechanisms. Common results of burn injuries include the following:

- Loss of water secondary to evaporation
- Infection secondary to loss of skin integrity, which allows pathogens to enter the body
- Difficulty maintaining body temperature due to heat loss from open wounds.

Heat transfer to skin is a complex phenomenon. If the skin's microcirculation remains intact during burning, it both cools and protects the deeper portions of the skin and cools the skin's outer surface once the heat source is removed. With extensive burn injury, however, the integrity of the microcirculation is lost, and the burning process continues even after the heat source is removed. For this reason, stopping the burning process is critical in extensive burn injuries.

Burns have a characteristic surface appearance that resembles a bull's-eye, with the most severe part of the burn located centrally and the less severe portions of the burn located along the peripheral wound edges. Depending on their intensity, burns consist of one, two, or three concentric three-dimensional zones closely corresponding on the skin surface to the depth of the burn (see **Figure 21–26** 》):

- The outer zone of hyperemia consists of unburned tissue, blanches on pressure, and heals in 2–7 days postburn.
- The medial zone of stasis is initially moist, red, and blistered, and it blanches on pressure. It may recover or become pale and necrotic between 3–7 days postburn due to decreased perfusion or infection.
- The inner zone of coagulation immediately appears leathery and coagulated. It may merge with the zone of stasis from 3–7 days postburn.

The overall thickness of the dermis and epidermis varies considerably from one area of the body to another. For example, in adults, the skin covering the medial aspect of the forearm is thinner and more easily damaged than the skin covering the back of the body. As a result, similar temperatures produce different depths of injury in different body parts. Skin dissipates heat maximally in the areas of greatest vascularization. When heat absorption exceeds the rate of dissipation, cellular temperatures rise and skin tissue is destroyed.

Burn injuries result in the formation of necrotic skin and subcutaneous tissue. During the acute stage of a burn injury, a hard crust called an **eschar** forms, covering the wound and harboring necrotic tissue. The eschar is characteristically leathery and rigid. Removal of the eschar facilitates healing.

Gastrointestinal System

Dysfunction of the gastrointestinal system is directly related to the size of a burn wound. Patients with burns involving 20% or more of their TBSA experience decreased peristalsis,

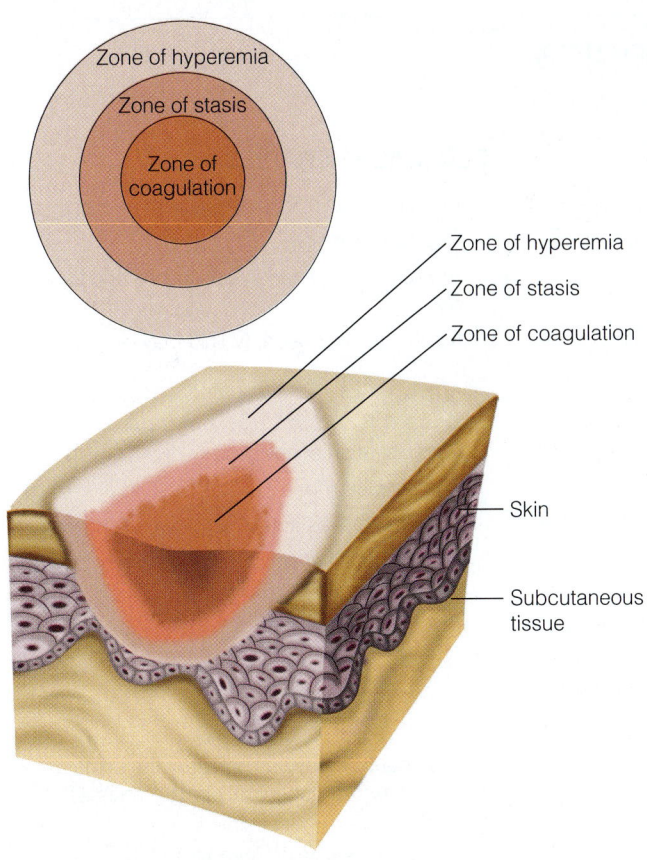

Zone of hyperemia
Zone of stasis
Zone of coagulation
Skin
Subcutaneous tissue

Figure 21–26 》 The zones of injury.

with resultant gastric distention and increased risk of aspiration. A decrease in or absence of bowel sounds is a manifestation of paralytic ileus (adynamic bowel) secondary to burn trauma. The resulting cessation of intestinal motility leads to gastric distention, nausea, vomiting, and hematemesis.

Stress ulcers (**Curling ulcers**) are acute ulcerations of the stomach or duodenum that may form after a burn injury. Abdominal pain, acidic gastric pH levels, hematemesis, and blood in the stool may all indicate a gastric ulcer.

Urinary System

During the early stages of a burn injury, renal blood flow and glomerular filtration rates are greatly reduced due to decreased intravascular blood volume and the release of antidiuretic hormone (ADH) by the posterior pituitary. Urine output decreases, and serum creatinine and blood urea nitrogen (BUN) increase.

Dark brown concentrated urine may indicate myoglobinuria or hemoglobinuria, the result of underlying muscle damage or the release of large amounts of dead or damaged erythrocytes after a major burn injury. When large amounts of these pigments are released, the liver cannot keep pace with conjugation, and the pigments pass through the glomeruli. These pigments can occlude the renal tubules and cause renal failure, especially when dehydration, acidosis, or shock is also present.

Immune System

The capillary leak that occurs in the early stages of a burn continues throughout the burn shock phase and impairs the active components of both the cell-mediated and the humoral immune systems.

The humoral immune system relies on B cells to produce antibodies or immunoglobulins. However, in the patient with burns, the serum levels of all immunoglobulins are significantly diminished. Serum protein levels remain persistently low throughout the clinical course until wound closure occurs. At the same time, a marked decrease in T-cell counts results in reduction of cytotoxic activity and suppression of the cell-mediated immune system.

Burn-related compromises in the humoral and cell-mediated immune systems cause a state of acquired immunodeficiency, which places the patient at risk for infection. The period of vulnerability is transient and may last 1–4 weeks after the onset of the burn injury. During this time, opportunistic infections may be fatal despite aggressive antimicrobial therapy.

Metabolism

Two distinct phases characterize the body's metabolic response to a burn injury. The ebb phase, which occurs during the first 3 days of the injury, is manifested by decreased oxygen consumption, fluid imbalance, shock, and inadequate circulating volume. These responses protect the body from the initial impact of the injury.

The second phase, called the flow phase, occurs when adequate burn resuscitation has been accomplished. This phase is characterized by increases in cellular activity and protein catabolism, lipolysis, and gluconeogenesis. The patient's basal metabolic rate (BMR) significantly increases, reaching twice the normal rate. Meanwhile, body weight and heat drop dramatically. Total energy expenditure may exceed 100% of the patient's normal BMR. Hypermetabolism persists until after wound closure has been accomplished, and it may reappear if complications occur.

Collaboration

A burn team is an interprofessional group of healthcare professionals who plan the care and treatment of the patient with a burn injury during the acute and rehabilitative stages. This team typically consists of the nurse, physician, physical and/or occupational therapist, dietitian, and a nurse case manager. A member of the spiritual care team or mental health professional may also be involved. The team members meet regularly to discuss patient progress and collaboratively determine the most effective regimen of care and psychosocial support.

Treatment for burns depends on the amount of BSA involved, the depth of skin damage, and the location of the burn. Burns that involve the airway require more careful monitoring than those involving extremities. Treatment often begins on scene, where it may be provided by family members, emergency services personnel, or specially trained personnel in occupational settings. Later, the patient may receive more advanced treatment in an outpatient facility, hospital, or burn center.

Minor Burns

Minor burn injuries are usually treated on an outpatient basis. The goals of therapy are to promote wound healing, eliminate discomfort, maintain mobility, and prevent infection.

Clinical Manifestations and Therapies
Burns

ETIOLOGY	CLINICAL MANIFESTATIONS	CLINICAL THERAPIES
Superficial burns	<ul><li>Only the epidermis is affected.</li><li>Skin is dry and pink to bright red.</li><li>Slight edema may be present over the burned area.</li><li>Burns may be accompanied by chills, headache, nausea, and vomiting.</li><li>Burns usually heal in 3–6 days with no scarring.</li></ul>	<ul><li>Administration of mild analgesics</li><li>Regular cleaning</li><li>Application of water-soluble lotions and topical agents</li><li>If burns are extensive, IV fluid may be required</li></ul>
Partial-thickness burns *Superficial partial-thickness burns*	<ul><li>Both the epidermis and dermis (papillary layer) are affected.</li><li>Skin is bright red and has a moist appearance.</li><li>Blister formation is common.</li><li>Burned area blanches upon pressure.</li><li>Patient may experience severe pain in response to temperature and air exposure.</li><li>Burns usually heal within 21 days with minimal to no scarring.</li></ul>	<ul><li>Administration of analgesics</li><li>Regular cleaning</li><li>Use of skin substitutes if large area is burned</li><li>Administration of antipyretics in case of fever associated with thermal burns</li></ul>
Deep partial-thickness burns	<ul><li>Both the epidermis and dermis (papillary and reticular layers) are affected.</li><li>Burn area is pale and waxy and may be moist or dry.</li><li>Blisters are present and may be large and easily ruptured or flat and dry like tissue paper.</li><li>Capillary refill is decreased.</li><li>Sensation to deep pressure remains intact, although other forms of sensation (including pain) are decreased.</li><li>Burns may require more than 21 days to heal.</li><li>Burns may convert to full-thickness injury if necrosis extends to the depth of the wound.</li><li>Contractures are possible.</li><li>Hypertrophic scarring and functional impairment may occur.</li></ul>	<ul><li>Therapeutic measures generally the same as those used for superficial partial-thickness burns</li><li>Excision and grafting possibly necessary to decrease scarring and lack of function</li></ul>
Full-thickness burns	<ul><li>Epidermis, dermis, and underlying tissues are all affected.</li><li>Burn area may appear pale, waxy, yellow, brown, mottled, charred, or nonblanching red.</li><li>Wound surface is dry and leathery, with thrombosed vessels visible.</li><li>Sensation to pain and light touch is absent at the burn site.</li><li>Skin grafting is required for the wound to heal.</li></ul>	<ul><li>Regular cleaning</li><li>Application of topical agents</li><li>Use of skin substitutes</li><li>Excision of eschar</li><li>Skin grafting</li></ul>

Sunburn is one of the most common types of minor burns. Independent nursing interventions relevant to care of the patient with a sunburn generally consist of applying mild lotions, increasing liquid intake, and maintaining warmth. Older adults and young children should be monitored for evidence of dehydration. The patient should be taught that using sunscreen properly and limiting sun exposure to the less hazardous hours of the day (before 10 a.m. and after 3 p.m.) can prevent sunburn. For all types of minor burns, patient education should also include teaching regarding the application of skin dressings and antibiotic solutions as ordered by the primary care provider. In addition, the nurse should reinforce the need to maintain adequate nutritional intake for promotion of wound healing.

Collaborative nursing interventions may include administration of mild analgesics as ordered by the primary

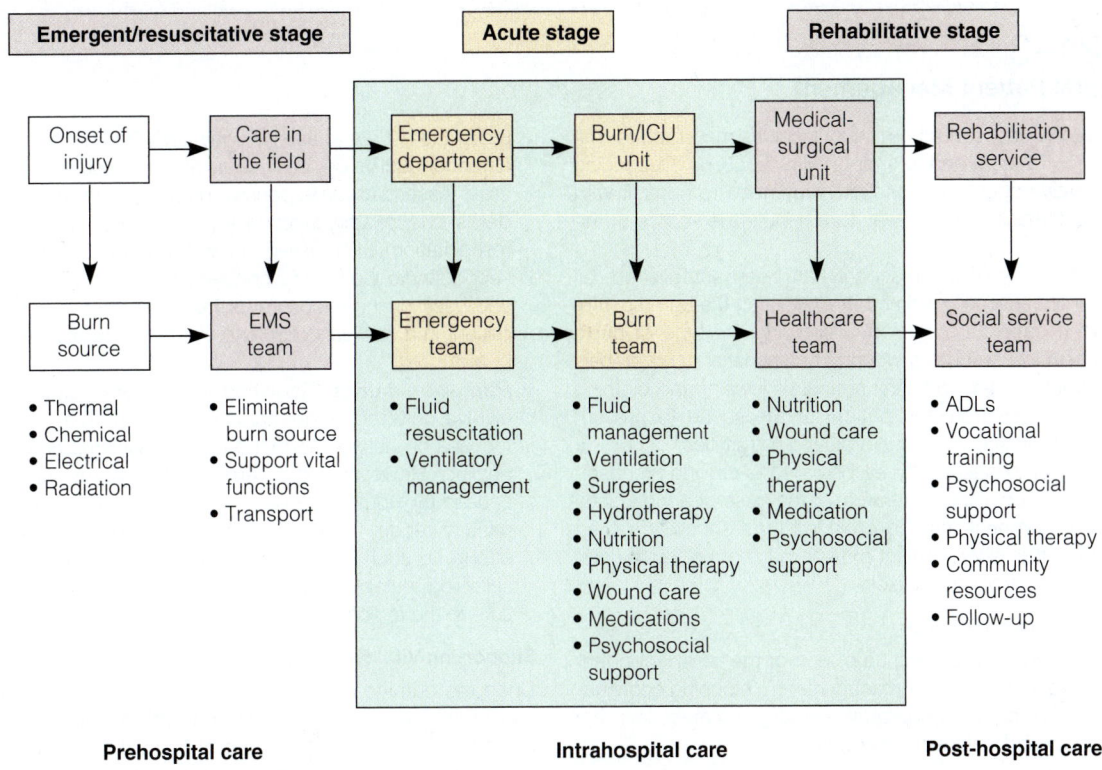

| Emergent/resuscitative stage | | Acute stage | | Rehabilitative stage |

| Onset of injury | Care in the field | Emergency department | Burn/ICU unit | Medical-surgical unit | Rehabilitation service |

| Burn source | EMS team | Emergency team | Burn team | Healthcare team | Social service team |

- Thermal
- Chemical
- Electrical
- Radiation

- Eliminate burn source
- Support vital functions
- Transport

- Fluid resuscitation
- Ventilatory management

- Fluid management
- Ventilation
- Surgeries
- Hydrotherapy
- Nutrition
- Physical therapy
- Wound care
- Medications
- Psychosocial support

- Nutrition
- Wound care
- Physical therapy
- Medication
- Psychosocial support

- ADLs
- Vocational training
- Psychosocial support
- Physical therapy
- Community resources
- Follow-up

Prehospital care   Intrahospital care   Post-hospital care

Figure 21–27 》 The patient's progression through the healthcare system during the emergent, acute, and rehabilitative stages of burn injury.

care provider. In addition, if blistering is present, the lesions may be either left intact or debrided. **Debridement** is the process of removing necrotic material (including all loose tissue, wound debris, and eschar) from the wound. Follow-up care for the minor burn injury includes twice-daily wound cleansing with application of a topical ointment, range-of-motion (ROM) exercises for affected joints, and weekly clinic appointments until the wound heals completely.

Severe Burns

The clinical course of treatment for a patient with a severe burn injury is divided into three stages: emergent/resuscitative, acute, and rehabilitative. Although these stages are useful in helping plan the patient's care, the process of burn injury is dynamic. In many cases, the clinical stage may not be clearly delineated. This is one of the many reasons ongoing assessment is necessary throughout the course of treatment. **Figure 21–27 》** shows the typical progression of a patient with a burn injury through the healthcare system. During each stage of care, different groups of nurses, physicians, and other healthcare specialists collaborate to manage the patient's recovery, as described in the following sections.

Emergent/Resuscitative Stage

The emergent/resuscitative stage lasts from the onset of a burn injury through successful fluid resuscitation. During this stage, healthcare workers estimate the extent of the burn injury, institute first-aid measures, and implement fluid resuscitation therapies. The patient is assessed for

shock and evidence of respiratory distress. If indicated, IV lines are inserted, and the patient may be prophylactically intubated. These actions frequently are performed at the scene of the injury rather than in a hospital setting. See **Box 21–3 》** for more information on prehospital patient management.

Toward the end of the emergent/resuscitative stage, healthcare workers must often determine whether the patient will be transported to a burn center for the complex intervention strategies of the professional interprofessional burn team. According to American Burn Association (2016) guidelines, adult patients who should be treated at burn centers include the following:

- Individuals older than age 50 who have second- or third-degree burns on more than 10% of their TBSA
- Individuals younger than age 50 who have second- or third-degree burns on more than 20% of their TBSA
- Adults of any age who have third-degree burns on more than 5% of their TBSA
- Individuals with electrical (including lightning), chemical, and inhalation injuries
- Individuals with circumferential burns of the extremities and/or chest
- Any burned individuals with extenuating problems, pre-existing illness, fractures, or other trauma

Acute Stage

The acute stage begins with the start of diuresis and ends with closure of the burn wound (either by natural healing or

Box 21–3
Prehospital Patient Management

Treatment at the scene of a burn injury includes measures to limit the severity of the burn and to support vital functions. Depending on the causative agent, the rescuers may need to consult with experts to determine the best way to eliminate the source of the injury.

Once the safety of the rescuers has been established, all prehospital interventions are aimed at eliminating the burn source, stabilizing the patient's condition, identifying the type of burn, preventing heat loss, reducing wound contamination, and preparing for emergency transport. Any restrictive jewelry and clothing should be removed from the patient at the scene to prevent circumferential constriction of the torso and extremities.

Emergency personnel ideally will be called to provide prehospital treatment for a patient with burns. In the case of a workplace injury, onsite treatment may be provided by a specially trained employee, and the injured patient may or may not be treated and transported by emergency services.

Stopping the Burning Process

Regardless of who is providing care, one of the most important elements of prehospital patient management is stopping continuation of the burning process. Appropriate emergency measures vary by type of injury and include the following:

- *Thermal burns.* If a thermal injury has been caused by dry heat, smother inflamed clothing or lavage with water. Help the patient to "Stop, drop, and roll" to extinguish the flame and limit the extent of burn. Once the flame has been extinguished, cover the patient's body to prevent hypothermia. If the thermal injury has been caused by moist heat, lavage the area with cool water. Ice should not be used for cooling because it causes vasoconstriction and may result in further injury.
- *Chemical burns.* For chemical burns, immediately remove the patient's clothing, and use a hose or shower to lavage the involved area thoroughly for a minimum of 20 minutes. Many chemicals come in powder form; as much dry chemical as possible needs to be removed from the skin before its surface is flushed with water. Unusual chemicals may require consultation with a Poison Control Center about appropriate treatment. The rescuer should wear protective clothing during this portion of the care process for personal protection from chemical exposure. Chemical splashes in or near the eye require immediate eye irrigation with clean, cool water or saline solution.
- *Electrical burns.* Electrical injuries pose the potential of serious harm to both the rescuer and the patient with a burn injury. Thus, before assisting the patient, ensure that the source of electrical current has been disconnected. If this is not possible,

move the patient to safety, away from the energy source, using a nonconductive device such as an unpainted nonmetal broomstick. Assess an unresponsive patient for the presence of cardiac and respiratory function. If indicated, begin cardiopulmonary resuscitation (CPR). Keep in mind a possible spinal cord injury secondary to the forceful contraction of the muscles of the neck and back during exposure to the current. If possible, place the patient in a cervical collar, and transport the patient on a spinal board.
- *Radiation burns.* Radiation injuries are usually minor and involve only the epidermal layer of skin. Treatment therefore focuses on helping normal body mechanisms promote wound healing. However, for severe radiation burns, such as those caused by industrial radiation accidents, trained personnel may need to render the area safe for entry prior to beginning rescue efforts. In such cases, appropriate interventions are aimed at shielding, establishing distance, and limiting the time of exposure to the radioactive source.

Supporting Vital Function

Once the burning process has been stopped, rescue personnel should take steps to support the patient's respiratory and circulatory function. Initial assessment of the patient's respiratory and hemodynamic status begins with an evaluation of the patient's airway, breathing, and circulation, as well as disability status and exposure to the source of the burn. These five elements (Airway, Breathing, Circulation, Disability, and Exposure) collectively are known as the **ABCDE** bundle of trauma care:

Airway
Breathing
Circulation
Disability
Exposure

Depending on the results of the ABCDE evaluation, a number of interventions may be appropriate, including lifesaving measures such as CPR. Positioning, administering humidified oxygen, and nasotracheal suctioning may be necessary to ensure airway patency. Emergency personnel will continually assess airway patency and monitor respiratory status as well as monitor for cardiac dysrhythmias or arrest, changes in level of consciousness, and changes in blood pressure.

For nonsuperficial burn wounds that involve more than 15% of the patient's TBSA, emergency personnel will initiate fluid replacement therapy. The patient will be covered to maintain body temperature and to prevent further wound contamination and tissue damage.

---

by use of skin grafts). During this stage, the following therapies are implemented:

- *Wound care.* Hydrotherapy and excision and grafting of full-thickness wounds are performed as soon as possible after injury.
- *Nutrition therapy.* Enteral and parenteral nutritional interventions are started early in the treatment plan to address caloric needs resulting from extensive energy expenditure.
- *Infection prevention.* Measures to combat infection are also implemented during this stage, including administration of topical and systemic antimicrobial agents.

- *Pain management.* Pain management constitutes a significant segment of the nursing care plan throughout the entire course of burn treatment. Administration of opioid analgesics must precede all invasive procedures to maximize patient comfort and reduce anxiety associated with wound debridement and intensive physical therapy.

Rehabilitative Stage

The rehabilitative stage begins with wound closure and ends when the patient returns to the highest level of health restoration, which may take years. During this stage, the primary focus is the biopsychosocial adjustment of the patient, which may include the following measures:

- Prevention of contractures and scars
- The patient's successful resumption of work, family, and social roles through physical, vocational, occupational, and psychosocial rehabilitation
- ROM exercises to enhance mobility and to support injured joints.

Emergency and Acute Care

Immediately upon the patient's arrival at the hospital, the nurse should assess the patient's airway and efficacy of breathing, including thorough auscultation of breath sounds and continuous pulse oximetry monitoring. Patients who sustain severe burns or who may be at risk for inhalation injury have often undergone tracheal intubation by emergency medical personnel prior to hospital arrival. Assessment of circulatory status includes obtaining and continuing to monitor the patient's blood pressure, heart rate, and electrocardiogram (ECG). The nurse should obtain a history of the injury (including any medical interventions already implemented), estimate the depth and extent of the burn, begin fluid resuscitation as per medical orders, and continue to support ventilation according to protocol. These measures generally precede diagnostic testing and any surgical or pharmacologic therapies, with the exception of administration of analgesics.

After stabilization in the emergency department, the patient is transferred to the critical care unit or a facility that specializes in the treatment of patients with burns. In both settings, continuous support and monitoring of the patient's physiologic status, administration of medications, pain control, wound management, and nutrition support therapies constitute the initial plan of care.

Airway and Ventilatory Management

Intubation is indicated for all patients with burns of the chest, face, or neck. As stated earlier, intubation may well have been done as part of prehospital management by emergency services personnel. The primary treatment plan is oriented toward preventing atelectasis and maintaining alveolar oxygen exchange. The following interventions should be initiated:

- Maintain the head of the bed at 30 degrees or greater to maximize the patient's ventilatory efforts. Turn the patient from side to side every 2 hours to prevent hypostatic pneumonia.
- To keep airway passages clear, suction the patient frequently, encourage the patient to use incentive spirometry hourly, and help the patient perform coughing and deep-breathing exercises every 2 hours.
- In the face of impending airway obstruction, the patient will require immediate intubation. Endotracheal intubation is reserved for short-term ventilatory management. For long-term ventilatory management (i.e., greater than 3 weeks), a tracheostomy should be performed.
- Humidification of either room air or oxygen helps prevent drying of tracheal secretions. The choice of ambient

air or oxygen flow is based on arterial blood gas (ABG) results. The patient may be placed on a face mask, steam collar, T-piece, mechanical ventilation with positive end-expiratory pressure, pressure support ventilation, or high-frequency jet ventilation. The goal of all therapies is to maintain adequate tissue oxygenation with the least amount of inspired oxygen flow necessary.

- Medications to dilate constricted bronchial passages may be administered intravenously and/or as inhalants to control bronchospasms and wheezing. Mucolytic agents can be used to liquefy tenacious sputum and aid in expectoration.
- An arterial line is placed in the patient with a major burn injury for continuous assessment of ABGs. Pulmonary artery pressure (PAP) catheters may be inserted to measure pulmonary vascular resistance (PVR), PAP, pulmonary artery wedge pressure (PAWP), and mixed venous oxygen saturation (SvO_2). The patient's PVR and PAP rises in the presence of hypoxia. The SvO_2 is the average percentage of hemoglobin bound with oxygen in the venous blood, and it reflects overall tissue utilization of oxygen. Pulse oximetry may also be used to monitor arterial oxygen saturation levels.
- In the presence of carbon monoxide (CO) poisoning, the patient's carboxyhemoglobin (COHgb) levels must be monitored. Pulse oximetry cannot distinguish between oxyhemoglobin and COHgb; thus, a false normal or high pulse oximetry reading is seen. High-flow 100% oxygen should be given immediately by nonrebreather mask. Patients with COHgb greater than 15% may also require hyperbaric oxygen therapy to replace the CO.

SAFETY ALERT High levels of carbon monoxide in the bloodstream can skew pulse oximetry readings, giving the appearance of adequate oxygen saturation even in patients with hypoxia. Make patient assessment your primary data source, and do not rely on monitors as a replacement for assessment.

Circulatory Support and Fluid Resuscitation

Fluid resuscitation is the administration of IV fluids to restore the circulating blood volume during the acute period of increasing capillary permeability, thus counteracting the effects of burn shock. The American Burn Association's practice guidelines recommend formal fluid replacement for any patient with nonsuperficial burn wounds that involve 15% or more of TBSA (Rice & Orgill, 2015).

During fluid resuscitation, crystalloid fluids are administered through a large-bore (14- to 16-gauge) IV catheter, preferably inserted through unburned skin. If TBSA is greater than 40%, then two large-bore IV catheters are preferred (Pukar et al., 2015). Although the ideal solution has not been determined, warmed lactated Ringer's is typically used during the first 24 hours after a burn injury because it most closely approximates the body's extracellular fluid composition (Rice & Orgill, 2015). Multiple formulas may be used to replace fluid loss, including Parkland formula and its variations, which have become the universal standard, and the modified Brooke formula. These formulas provide guidelines for the volume of fluid to be infused over the first 24 hours from the time of the burn injury. According to the Parkland formula, adult fluid requirements during the first 24 hours of treatment are 4 mL/kg, with 50% of the fluid to be infused during the first 8 hours, followed by the remaining 50% divided equally over the next 16 hours (Pukar et al., 2015; Rice & Orgill, 2015).

Pediatric patients with burn injuries require a different approach to fluid resuscitation. They require maintenance fluid in addition to the calculated fluid resuscitation volumes, and this fluid should contain dextrose because of the decreased glycogen stores compared to adults. The Parkland formula can be used to estimate fluid replacement requirements for this population; however, the Galveston formula is an alternative based on TBSA rather than body weight. Although more time-consuming to calculate, it is believed to provide a more accurate indication of the initial fluid resuscitation needs of the pediatric patient. The fluid requirements using the Galveston formula are calculated as 5000 mL/m^2 per percent TBSA and add 2000 mL/m^2 per day for maintenance requirements (Joffe, 2015; Rice & Orgill, 2015; Schraga, 2016).

Hourly urine output is considered the most effective indicator of fluid resuscitation. In adult patients with burn injuries, urine production of 0.5–1 mL/kg/hr is considered adequate. In pediatric patients with burns, the targeted hourly urine output is 1–2 mL/kg/hr for children weighing less than 30 kg and 0.5–1 mL/kg/hr for children weighing 30 kg or more (Joffe, 2015; Krishnamoorthy, Ramaiah, & Bhananker, 2012). Patients who sustain electrical burns often have injuries that are not visible, making the extent or volume of tissue damage difficult to assess. For these patients, conventional fluid resuscitation formulas, which rely upon calculation of the percentage of the patient's body that is burned, may underestimate fluid requirements. Emergency fluid resuscitation of the patient with a major electrical injury should begin at 500 mL/hr (250 mL/hr per IV site) until urinary catheterization can occur. Once urine output can be evaluated and measured, IV fluids can be titrated to maintain urine output of approximately 1 mL/kg/hr in adult patients and 1.5 mL/kg/hr in pediatric patients (Kearns et al., 2014).

Another indicator is heart rate; if fluid resuscitation is adequate, the rate should be less than 110 beats per minute or in the upper limits of normal for age. However, underlying conditions and the fear, anxiety, and pain that accompany burn injuries often increase heart rate. Blood pressure changes are less reliable because significant hypotension does not develop until volume losses exceed 30% due to the body's compensatory mechanisms. Rather, assessment for narrowed pulse pressure (a more sensitive indicator of shock) should be considered along with urine output to monitor adequacy of fluid resuscitation. Heart rate is a better indicator of circulatory status in pediatric patients than blood pressure (Joffe, 2015; Weavind, 2016).

During the fluid resuscitation stage, the patient may require invasive hemodynamic monitoring. A pulmonary artery catheter may be used to monitor cardiac output, cardiac index, and PAWPs. All measurements must be maintained within normal limits to effect adequate fluid resuscitation.

Diagnostic Tests

Upon the patient's admission to the emergency department, following assessment and management of all acute life-threatening issues, several diagnostic tests should be completed. The following tests are particularly useful in establishing a baseline and evaluating the response of a patient with burn injury to therapeutic interventions throughout the entire hospitalization period:

- *Pulse oximetry* generally allows for continuous assessment of oxygen saturation levels, except in patients with carbon monoxide poisoning. For these patients, pulse oximetry readings may be falsely elevated because of carbon monoxide that is bound to hemoglobin.

- *Carboxyhemoglobin measurement,* which may be performed using venous or arterial blood, measures the percentage of hemoglobin that is bound to carbon monoxide.

- *Serial ABGs* indicate the presence of hypoxia and acid–base disturbances and help measure patient response to changes in oxygen therapies. The patient with a burn injury may demonstrate elevated or lowered pH, decreased PCO$_2$, decreased PO$_2$, and low-normal bicarbonate levels.

- *Serial 12-lead ECGs* are necessary to monitor the development of dysrhythmias, especially those associated with hypokalemic and hyperkalemic states.

- *Serial chest x-ray studies* document changes within the first 24–48 hours after injury that may reflect the presence of atelectasis, pulmonary edema, or ARDS.

- *Urinalysis* indicates the adequacy of renal perfusion and the patient's nutritional status. In catabolic states, nitrogen is excreted in large amounts into the urine. Nitrogen loss is measured through 24-hour urine collection and testing for total nitrogen, urea nitrogen, and amino acid nitrogen. Myoglobinuria, which manifests as dark brown or wine-colored urine, signals the development of acute tubular necrosis. Loss of plasma protein and dehydration often lead to proteinuria and elevated urine specific gravity. Glycosuria is also a transient development following major burn injury, and it indicates a need to adjust the nutritional program.

- *Complete blood count (CBC)* must be monitored regularly. Hematocrit may be elevated secondary to hemoconcentration and fluid shifts from the intravascular compartment, and hemoglobin may be decreased secondary to hemolysis. WBCs are also elevated if infection is present.

- *Serum electrolytes* should also be regularly monitored. Sodium levels are generally decreased secondary to massive fluid shifts into the interstitium. Potassium levels are initially elevated during burn shock as a result of cell lysis and fluid shifts into the extracellular space. However, potassium levels decrease after burn shock resolves as fluid shifts back to the intracellular and intravascular compartments.

- *Renal function* test results are critical. In patients with burn injuries, BUN is elevated secondary to dehydration. Creatinine is also elevated in the presence of renal insufficiency.

- *Total protein, albumin, transferrin, prealbumin, retinol binding protein, α_1-acid glycoprotein, and C-reactive protein levels* indicate protein synthesis and nutritional status. However, because of the fluid shifts that occur during the early stages of a burn injury, these measurements are more useful during the rehabilitative phase of care.
- *Creatine kinase (CK)* is elevated following an electrical burn, secondary to extensive muscle damage.
- Finally, *blood glucose* is transiently elevated after any major burn injury.

Surgery

Three surgical interventions are commonly employed to manage burn wounds: escharotomy, surgical debridement, and autografting.

Escharotomy

When burn eschar forms circumferentially around the torso or extremities, it acts as a tourniquet, impairing circulation. If this eschar is left unchecked, the affected body part will become gangrenous. To prevent circumferential constriction of the torso or extremity, the healthcare provider may perform an **escharotomy**, removing the eschar with a scalpel or by electrocautery. During this procedure, a sterile surgical incision is made longitudinally along the extremity or trunk to release taut skin and allow for expansion caused by edema formation. In the first 24 hours following the procedure, the incision should be gently packed with fine-mesh gauze. After 24 hours, the site may be treated with direct application of a topical antimicrobial agent.

Surgical Debridement

Surgical debridement is the process of excising a wound to the level of fascia (**fascial excision**) or sequentially removing thin slices of the wound to the level of viable tissue (**tangential excision**). Because fascial excision, or **fasciectomy**, sacrifices potentially viable fat and lymphatic tissue, its use is reserved for patients with extensive or full-thickness burns. The most common technique is electrocautery with cutting and coagulating current capabilities. Tangential excision, by contrast, is performed with the use of a dermatome. Shallow burns and some burns of moderate depth bleed briskly after one slice. If bleeding does not occur, the procedure is repeated until a viable bed of dermis or subcutaneous fat is reached. Following surgical debridement, the patient is returned to the burn unit.

Autografting

Autografting is a procedure performed in the surgical suite in which part of the patient's healthy skin is removed and used to effect permanent skin coverage over the wound area. Early burn wound excision and skin grafting decrease the patient's hospital stay and enhance rehabilitation.

During an autografting procedure, skin is removed from healthy tissue (the donor site) of the patient with a burn injury and applied to the burn wound. After the autograft is applied, the grafted area is immobilized. The site is assessed daily for evidence of adherence. The patient resumes ROM exercises 5 days postgraft. As the wound heals, the patient may complain of itching, which can be treated with mild lotions.

Cultured epithelial autografting is a technique in which skin cells are removed from unburned sites on the patient's body, then minced and placed in a culture medium for growth. Over a 5- to 7-day period, the cells grow to 50–70 times the size of the initial biopsies. The cells are again separated out and placed in a new culture medium for continued growth. With this technique, enough skin can be grown over a period of 3–4 weeks to cover an entire human body. The cells are prepared in sheets and attached to petroleum jelly gauze backing, which is applied to the burn wound site. Although this procedure is often successful, problems with infection and lack of attachment may occur.

Pharmacologic Therapy

Patients with burns typically receive medications to control pain, prevent infection (including tetanus), and reduce the risk of peptic ulcer disease. IV fluids and other medications to support vital functions may also be indicated in individuals with severe burns.

Analgesia

Burns often cause excruciating pain. In the emergent stages of care, opioid analgesics such as morphine, oxycodone, or fentanyl are the best means of managing pain. Morphine is generally the drug of choice, and it may be given orally or intravenously. Oxycodone is an effective alternative to morphine, and it, too, may be administered either orally or intravenously. While also a fast-acting opiate, fentanyl differs from morphine and oxycodone in that it may be given intravenously, orally, or transmucosally (often via intranasal sprays or lozenges that permit absorption through the buccal mucosa). For all three drugs, the nurse should avoid oral administration until the patient has resumed hemodynamic stability and normal gastric emptying. IV and/or transmucosal preparations also offer the benefit of faster pain relief and are thus preferred during the early stages of care.

Later, during the acute stage of burn care, opioids should be administered around the clock to provide consistent plasma levels of analgesics and decrease pain that occurs at rest. Prior to undergoing any procedures, the patient typically receives a larger dose of opioid analgesic medication. Ongoing pain management may also be provided through the use of nonopioid analgesics, such as acetaminophen (which has an enhanced effect when combined with opiates) and nonsteroidal anti-inflammatory drugs (NSAIDs). In many cases, patient-controlled analgesia (PCA) enhances the patient's ability to cope with pain. Because burn treatments and the trauma associated with experiencing a major burn can produce high levels of anxiety, the scheduled administration of a benzodiazepine such as lorazepam may be beneficial in decreasing the level of pain experienced, especially when administered 1 hour before wound care (Wiechman, & Sharar, 2015).

Antimicrobials

Systemic infection is the most common cause of morbidity and mortality in patients with major burns. Microorganisms that primarily infect burn wounds are gram-positive bacteria such as methicillin-resistant *Staphylococcus aureus* (MRSA) and gram-negative bacteria such as *Pseudomonas aeruginosa* and *Klebsiella* species. Fungal pathogens, most commonly

Candida albicans, can also infect burn wounds. These infections generally develop later, after the administration of broad-spectrum antibiotics or delayed wound care. The use of routine wound cultures for infection surveillance purposes has not been shown to improve patient outcomes (Fonseca, 2016).

Depending on protocol, topical antimicrobial therapy may be used to eliminate infection on the surface of a burn wound. In general, topical antimicrobials are not applied until the patient is admitted to a burn unit. Of the many antimicrobial agents available, the most widely used are mafenide acetate (Sulfamylon) cream, silver nitrate 0.5% soaks, and silver sulfadiazine (Silvadene) cream. All three are broad-spectrum antibiotics. The choice of topical antibiotic is based on the extent of the burn wound; the presence of identified bacterial organisms; the method of treatment (i.e., whether open to the air or closed using bulky dressings); and patient response.

Despite antimicrobial therapy, patients with major burn assault have a greater risk for sepsis and septic shock. Therefore, patients with major burns are usually given prophylactic antibiotics. Systemic antimicrobial therapy is indicated in the immediate preoperative and postoperative periods associated with excision and autografting. Postoperatively, antibiotic therapy is discontinued as soon as the patient's hemodynamic status returns to normal, usually within the first 24 hours. In the long-term treatment of identified infectious processes, drug administration is limited to the least amount of time required to eradicate the infection.

Tetanus Prophylaxis

If the patient's immunization status is in doubt, tetanus toxoid should be administered intramuscularly early in the acute phase of care to prevent *Clostridium tetani* infection. If the patient's tetanus immunization is older than 5 years, a booster should be administered.

Antacids

With patients with burn injuries, hyperacidity must be controlled to prevent Curling ulcer. A nasogastric tube is placed during the emergent phase of care, and gastric aspirant is obtained hourly. The gastric pH should be assessed and maintained at levels above 5. To control gastric acid secretion during the acute phase of care, histamine H_2 blockers (e.g., famotidine [Pepcid]) or proton pump inhibitors (e.g., pantoprazole [Protonix]) can be administered intravenously, either intermittently or as continuous infusions. As soon as bowel sounds become audible, the patient is placed on an antacid regimen.

Nonpharmacologic Therapy

Patients with burn wounds can benefit from a range of nonpharmacologic interventions delivered by a multidisciplinary team of professionals. In general, these interventions revolve around proper wound management and nutritional therapies.

Wound Management

The main goal of burn wound management is to close the wound within the first 5 days after the burn (Gauglitz & Williams, 2016). To help patients with major burns achieve this goal, the healthcare team must prevent and treat infection through daily topical wound care, wound monitoring, and wound excision and closure. This treatment includes proper debridement and use of dressings, as described in the following sections.

Debridement

Burned tissue releases chemical mediators that stimulate phagocytosis in an attempt to digest debris left by decaying necrotic tissue. Necrotic tissue that remains despite phagocytic action retards healing and prolongs inflammation. To prevent this from happening, the necrotic tissue must be removed by one of three methods: mechanical, enzymatic, or surgical debridement.

As previously described, surgical debridement is the cutting away of necrotic tissue. Mechanical debridement also involves the removal of dead tissue, but in this case, the nurse does so by applying and removing gauze dressings (wet-to-dry or wet-to-moist) or by using hydrotherapy, irrigation, or scissors and tweezers (sharp debridement). Although removal of gauze dressings is perhaps the simplest method, it can cause pain and possibly damage granulation tissue. To prevent these problems, hydrotherapy is sometimes preferable. During hydrotherapy (in an immersion tank, in a shower, or on a spray table), the burn injury is gently washed with a mild, nonperfumed antimicrobial soap or wound cleanser solution to remove dead skin and to separate eschar. The solution is then rinsed off with warm saline or tap water. Within the burn, body hair (except for eyebrows) is shaved to within 2.5 cm of the wound edges. Blistered skin is then grasped with dry gauze and gently removed. Next, the edges of blisters or eschar are trimmed with blunt scissors, and the wound is covered with a topical antimicrobial agent.

Enzymatic debridement is similar but involves the use of a topical agent to dissolve and remove necrotic tissue and lift eschar. An enzyme preparation such as collagenase (Santyl), papain, papain-urea, or fibrinolysin-deoxyribonuclease (Elase) is applied in a thin layer only within the wound area and covered with one layer of fine-mesh gauze. A topical antimicrobial agent is then applied and covered with a bulky wet dressing, and the wound is immobilized with expandable mesh gauze. Enzymatic agents are discontinued once the eschar is removed and granulation tissue appears.

Dressing the Wound

Once the burn wound has been cleaned and debrided, it may be dressed by one of two methods. In the open method, the wound remains open to air, covered by only a topical antimicrobial agent. This method allows easy access to the wound. Topical agents must be reapplied frequently because they tend to rub off onto the bedding. The open method also increases the risk for hypothermia.

In the closed method, a topical antimicrobial agent is applied to the wound site, and the site is then covered with gauze or a nonadherent dressing and gently wrapped with a gauze roll bandage. With the closed method, burn wounds are usually dressed twice daily and as needed. Dressings are applied circumferentially in a distal-to-proximal manner. All fingers and toes are wrapped separately. Dressings are held in place with stockinettes rather than tape to prevent further skin injury. The closed method decreases heat loss but may impair ROM.

Applying uniform pressure can prevent or reduce hypertrophic scarring. Accordingly, tubular support bandages may be applied 5–7 days postgraft to maintain tension ranging from 10 to 20 mmHg. The patient may also wear custom-made elastic pressure garments (e.g., Jobst pressure garments) for 6 months to a year postgraft.

Using Biological and Biosynthetic Dressings

The terms *biological dressing* and *biosynthetic dressing* refer to any temporary material that rapidly adheres to the wound bed, promotes healing, and/or prepares the burn wound for permanent autograft coverage. These kinds of dressings ideally are inexpensive, nonantigenic, elastic, and easy to apply and remove. They should also reduce pain, serve as a bacterial barrier, and enhance the natural healing process. Such dressings are applied to the burn wound as soon as possible. Covering the wound eliminates the loss of water through evaporation, reduces infection, and promotes wound healing. Types of biological and biosynthetic dressings currently in use include homograft (allograft), heterograft (xenograft), amnionic membranes, and synthetic materials.

Homograft, also called **allograft**, is human skin that has been harvested from cadavers. It is stored in skin banks located throughout the nation. The development of methods to achieve prolonged storage of viable frozen skin has increased use of this dressing; however, its short supply and high expense still pose problems. Homograft is cut to match the pattern of a patient's burn and applied by the use of sterile technique. As with any transplanted tissue, rejection is always a concern. Under normal circumstances, a homograft demonstrates rejection within 14–21 days following application if it is not accepted. Still, even with rejection, the homograft acts as a covering to reduce infection and promote healing for as long as it remains in place.

Heterograft, or **xenograft**, is skin obtained from an animal, usually a pig. Although fresh porcine heterograft is available at some centers, frozen heterograft is more commonly used. Once applied, heterograft appears to undergo early softening and lysis from enzymatic action in the wound. As a result, frequent changes of the heterograft dressing are necessary. Because of high infection rates associated with this type of dressing, researchers have developed silver nitrate–treated porcine heterograft to help retard microbial growth.

The multiple problems associated with the use of biological dressings have driven the development of synthetic substitutes. One such material is Biobrane, a composite material consisting of nylon mesh bonded to silicone that has been used successfully in the temporary coverage of second- and third-degree burns. Whereas Biobrane adheres well to moderately clean wounds, it unfortunately cannot adhere to, or lower bacterial counts in, grossly contaminated wounds. Biobrane dressing is supplied in various sizes, cut to fit the wound site, and secured with tape or Steri-Strips. It spontaneously separates from the wound when the underlying tissue heals. Hydrocolloid dressings are another type of biosynthetic dressing that consists of occlusive wafers of gumlike materials that provide a water-resistant outer layer for coverage of the donor site. Hydrocolloid dressings protect healing tissue from excessive drying, liquefy necrotic tissue, and absorb wound drainage.

If dermal thickness is lost in deep partial-thickness or full-thickness burns, several products can serve as a dermal replacement. Integra is a synthetic dermal substitute, and AlloDerm is human cadaver allograft dermis that is nonimmunogenic. These products are placed in the wound, and split-thickness autografts are then placed over the dermal replacement. They provide temporary wound coverage, reduce pain, and facilitate healing.

Two more recently developed temporary skin substitutes are TransCyte and Apligraf. TransCyte is a bioengineered substance derived from human fibroblast cells grown within mesh. As the cells grow, they secrete human dermal collagen, matrix proteins, and growth factors. The product is produced, extensively tested for infectious agents, and then frozen. It is used as a temporary covering for surgically debrided full-thickness and deep partial-thickness burn wounds and is an alternative to silver sulfadiazine and cadaver skin. TransCyte forms a transparent protective barrier over the wound surface and is typically applied only once. The best results have been obtained when TransCyte was applied within 24 hours of injury. Apligraf is a bilayered skin substitute cultured from neonatal foreskin, and it is used similarly.

A more recent advancement in the treatment for burn wounds involves use of a vacuum-assisted closure (VAC) device. With this treatment method, negative pressure is applied to a special dressing positioned over the wound and draws the edges of the wound toward the center of the site. The application of negative pressure assists in removing the excess fluid that causes edema, stimulates cellular growth, increases blood flow, and promotes an increased healing response (Wake Forest Baptist Health, 2016). These devices have been found to shorten the time required to prepare burn wounds prior to skin grafting (Huang et al., 2014).

>> **Stay Current:** Recent clinical evidence supports the use of honey as a biologic wound dressing. Studies have shown that honey contains multiple bioactivities that expedite the healing process. Manuka honey, currently used in wound care products, has broad-spectrum antibacterial activity, as well as the ability to suppress inflammation and bring about rapid autolytic debridement. Read more about the use of honey in wound care management at http://www.woundsresearch.com/article/honey-biologic-wound-dressing.

Nutritional Support

The patient with a major burn is in a hypermetabolic and catabolic state. In fact, an individual's resting energy expenditure after severe burn injury can increase by as much as 100% over normal levels depending on the extent of catabolism and the patient's physical activity, size, age, and gender. This increase is believed to be due to heat loss from the burn wound, an increase in beta-adrenergic activity, pain, and infection. As a result, the patient's total caloric needs may be as great as 4000–6000 kcal/day.

Traditional dietary management based on oral intake seldom meets the kilocalorie requirements necessary to reverse negative nitrogen balance and begin the healing process. Therefore, enteral feedings with a nasointestinal feeding tube are instituted within 24–48 hours after the burn injury to offset hypermetabolism, improve nitrogen balance, decrease sepsis, and decrease length of hospital stay. A nasointestinal feeding tube is placed under fluoroscopy, with the tip extending past the pylorus to prevent reflux and aspiration.

Although enteral feeding is the preferred nutritional therapy, it is contraindicated in Curling ulcer, bowel obstruction, feeding intolerance, pancreatitis, and septic ileus. When the enteral route cannot be used, a central venous catheter is inserted via the subclavian or jugular vein for administration of total parenteral nutrition.

Lifespan Considerations

Injuries from burns are normally attributed to an extreme source of heat but may also result from electricity, radiation, or chemical exposure. The majority of burns are minor and do not require emergent medical treatment; however, burns involving large areas of the body, critical body parts, or the pediatric or geriatric population can benefit from specialized treatment in a burn center (Hockenberry & Wilson, 2014).

Burns in Infants and Children

Burns involving infants and children can be caused by hot liquids, hot objects, fires, chemicals, radiation (sunburn), and electricity. Children at different developmental stages are at risk for different types of burns, and the majority of these burns occur in the home. Children age 5 and under are most vulnerable to death and injury from a fire in the home; this population also accounts for nearly all scald deaths (Hockenberry & Wilson, 2014).

Interview of a parent about a burn injury involving an infant or child can be challenging. If the injury was preventable, the parent may be experiencing feelings of guilt. The nurse should use caution during the interview process to avoid sounding accusatory when questioning the parent about the injury.

The nurse should also be alert to signs of child abuse when the history does not match the burn injury (e.g., glove and stocking burns; burns that spare flexor surfaces; contact burns from objects such as curling irons, cigarettes, and irons; zebra burn lines from contact with a hot grate). Photographs may be taken to document these burn injuries. Child neglect may be a factor in the burn of a child who was not adequately supervised.

Infants are most often injured by thermal burns, such as burns from scalding liquids, excessively hot bathwater, and house fires. As their mobility increases, toddlers are also at higher risk for thermal burns from pulling hot liquids or grease onto themselves. Electrical burns can result from biting electrical cords, and contact burns and chemical burns can be caused by the ingestion of cleaning agents and other substances associated with exploring their environment. Preschool-age children, who have not yet fully developed thinking and reasoning skills, are most often injured by scalding or contact with hot appliances such as curling irons and ovens.

School-age children are at risk for thermal, electrical, and chemical burns. This age group is very curious and enjoys experimentation. These burns may result from playing with matches and fireworks, climbing high-voltage towers, or climbing trees and making contact with electrical wires, or from conducting combustion experiments.

Children who are recovering from burns are encouraged to participate in play therapy, even if they can only observe initially. For the child with a major burn, play therapy provides an outlet for frustration, independence, and creativity; promotes activities that challenge ROM; normalizes the child's daily routine; and encourages the child, who sees the progress that other children make day by day.

Burns in Adolescents

Adolescents also experience thermal, chemical, and electrical burns, as well as radiation burns associated with sunbathing. Although the death rate from fire and burn injury has greatly declined among children 14 years of age and under, fire and burns remain the fourth leading cause of unintentional injury for this age group. Burns involving flammable liquids are also more prevalent in children over 8 years of age, due to risk-taking behaviors associated with this group (Hockenberry & Wilson, 2014).

Families of children and adolescents with major burns are at risk for emotional stress. They should be forewarned to expect edema and changes in the child's body with the injury response. Fear usually results from lack of knowledge about the severity of the burn and the child's status, especially in the early stages of burn care and admission to the hospital's ICU. The nurse should include the family in the patient's care when possible. The family must be given information and frequent updates to promote the development of trust between the family and the healthcare team. Parents often feel guilty and responsible for the occurrence of the injury. It is important to help parents focus on recovery rather than past actions.

Burns in Pregnant Women

Severe burn injuries during pregnancy are rare. The maternal morbidity and mortality rates are significantly higher for these patients than patients with the same degree of injury who are not pregnant. There has also been a relationship noted between percentage of BSA involved and fetal–maternal survival.

Burn injuries that occur during pregnancy not only complicate treatment for the mother, but also threaten the life of the fetus. It is imperative that accurate gestational age be assessed to allow for proper selection of treatment. A fetus at or near term may be delivered in order to prevent fetal distress and risk of drug toxicity due to maternal treatment. Further research in this area is needed (Shi et al., 2015).

Burns in Older Adults

Older adults sustain fewer serious burns than other age groups each year; however, the major cause of these injuries is flame and scalding burns from hot water and grease. This population is at greater risk for burns of all degrees of severity, burns and fires being a major cause of death. Most burns received by older adults are accidental, resulting from slower reaction times, decreased mobility, visual deficits, decreased sense of smell, forgetfulness, and impaired sensation. Many older adults are burned by stoves, hot water, hot food, irons, cookware, and heating pads. Older adults with cognitive impairment or dementia may start fires by leaving foods cooking unattended. The most common burns in this age group result from clothing catching fire and from tap water that is too hot.

Age has a significant impact on an individual's response to burn injury, with older adults at greatest risk for death as a result of their wounds. In fact, studies reveal that the risk of older adults dying in a fire is 2.6 times greater than that of the general population, and the mortality rate among older adults with burn injuries is two to three times higher compared to pediatric patients (Collins, 2015; U.S. Fire Administration, 2016).

Multiple factors account for the higher rate of mortality in the older adult population. This population is more likely to sustain burns to a greater percentage of their TBSA, largely because their skin is so much thinner and therefore more delicate than that of younger individuals. The greater the amount of TBSA affected, the more likely an individual is to die from a burn. Older adults also tend to experience inhalation injury at greater rates than members of other age groups, and inhalation injury is a leading cause of burn-related mortality (Fonseca, 2016).

Care of the older adult with burns often presents unique challenges. Older adults may delay seeking treatment, thus increasing the risk of infection. These patients are also far more likely to have chronic conditions that increase their risk of complications and impair their ability to heal from burn wounds. Common examples of such conditions are diabetes, cardiovascular disease, respiratory disease, kidney disease, and arthritis (Collins, 2015). In addition, older adults may live alone and have no one to care for them during rehabilitation. Thus, even small burns have the potential to become lethal in older adults.

To help prevent burn injuries, the nurse should emphasize ways to prevent fires and burn injuries when working with older adults. The nurse should encourage individuals in this age group to have a relative or neighbor routinely check for the odor of gas and check the smoke detector battery once a month. Older adults should wear close-fitting clothing when cooking and use a cooking timer with a loud alarm to prevent fires from burned food. They should be instructed to not place any items over a heating device, as this is a common cause of residential fires, especially during the colder months. Older adults should have the temperature of the water heater set no higher than 120°F to prevent scald burns and install antiscald devices in bathroom plumbing. They should also be encouraged not to smoke in the house.

NURSING PROCESS

The patient with a major burn has complex multisystem needs. During the acute phase, life support and monitoring take priority. While beginning to heal, the patient must cope with scarring, hair loss, and powerlessness. The nurse must consider altered body image and loss of independence for a significant period of time, sometimes lifelong, when planning care.

Assessment

Nursing assessment is continuous from the initial contact with the patient with a burn injury. Once the patient arrives at the emergency department, the staff must act quickly to obtain the history of the burn injury, including the time of occurrence, causative agents, and any early treatment that

has been provided. The nurse should inquire about the patient's medical history (including medication use), age, and body weight. In most cases, the patient is awake and oriented and can relate the information during the emergent phase of care. Because changes in sensory abilities become evident within the first few hours following a major burn injury, the nurse should obtain as much information as possible immediately upon the patient's arrival. Some guidelines for information gathering are as follows:

- *Time of injury.* In many cases, the patient is admitted to the emergency department an hour or more after the injury occurred. The time of the burn injury must be documented as precisely as possible at the scene because all fluid resuscitation calculations are based on the time of the injury, *not* on the patient's time of arrival at the emergency department.

- *Cause of the injury.* Because the type of burn injury determines which nursing measures take priority, it is important to identify the specific causative agent. This information allows the nurse to establish the appropriate plan of care.

- *First-aid treatment.* Prior to the arrival of medical personnel, the patient or family may have applied home remedies to treat the burn wound. It is important for the nurse to ascertain and document the nature of all home treatment interventions, including the application of neutralizing agents, liquids, and immobilizing devices used to splint associated injuries.

- *Past medical history.* Obtaining a medical history is important because more intense observation is required for the patient with a history of respiratory, cardiac, renal, metabolic, neurologic, gastrointestinal, or skin diseases; alcohol abuse; or altered immune states. The nurse must also obtain information about known allergies.

- *Medications.* Any drugs (either prescribed or recreational) taken by the patient prior to the burn injury may further complicate the treatment regimen. Drugs that affect any of the major body systems or cause mood alterations need to be factored into the treatment plan. Thus, as part of the early assessment, the nurse must obtain and document blood levels of therapeutic pharmaceutical agents and mood-altering substances.

- *Age.* Age is an important consideration in the treatment of patients with burn injuries, as children and older adults tend to require more supportive care.

- *Body weight.* During the acute and rehabilitative phases of the burn injury, patients lose as much as 20% of their preburn weight. This fact has significant implications for all patients, especially those who are underweight at the time of injury.

Diagnosis

Each patient's condition warrants individualized nursing diagnoses based on assessment data. Nursing diagnoses that may be appropriate for inclusion in the plan of care for the patient with burns include the following:

- *Airway Clearance, Ineffective*
- *Gas Exchange, Impaired*
- *Aspiration, Risk for*
- *Cardiac Tissue Perfusion, Risk for Decreased*

- *Fluid Volume, Deficient*
- *Ineffective Renal Perfusion, Risk for*
- *Infection, Risk for*
- *Imbalanced Nutrition: Less Than Body Requirements*
- *Pain, Acute*
- *Physical Mobility, Impaired*
- *Powerlessness.*

(NANDA-I © 2014)

Planning

A major burn affects virtually every body system, as well as the patient's social, cultural, economic, psychologic, and spiritual well-being. As was discussed earlier in this exemplar, for the patient who has sustained life-threatening injuries, the three priorities of care are ensuring proper airway management, maintaining effective breathing, and promoting adequate cardiovascular circulation. The plan of care changes as the patient moves from stage to stage, and it requires frequent updating in response to the patient's changing condition. For the stable patient who has sustained a burn, goals of patient care often include the following:

- The patient will maintain a clear, unobstructed airway.
- The patient will maintain ABG values and pulse oximetry readings that are within normal limits.
- The patient will demonstrate no cardiac dysrhythmias.
- The patient will receive adequate nutrition to meet body needs.
- The patient will maintain adequate fluid volume, as evidenced by hourly urine output that meets minimum acceptable guidelines.
- The patient's blood pressure and heart rate will range within acceptable limits.
- The patient will demonstrate adequate wound healing.
- The patient will maintain adequate pain control, reporting pain as a 3 or less on a scale of 0–10.
- The patient will not develop a healthcare-associated infection.
- The patient will maintain full ROM following recovery.

Implementation

Nursing interventions related to ensuring airway patency, effective ventilation, and adequate circulation were described earlier in this exemplar. Additional elements included in the care of the patient who sustains a burn injury include fluid and nutritional considerations, pain management, wound care, and infection prevention. Continuous assessment is necessary until well into the healing process and should include assessment of the patient's and family's feelings regarding the injury and its long-term effects.

Promote Fluid Volume Balance

Fluid resuscitation rates are adjusted periodically throughout the emergent stage of care. The nurse should be particularly aware of several situations that may warrant administration of fluids at rates in excess of the calculations needed to maintain adequate urine output. These situations include initial underestimation of burn size, sequestration of fluid in lung tissue in an inhalation injury, electrical injury full-thickness burns, and inordinately delayed starts of fluid resuscitation. To most effectively promote fluid volume balance, the nurse should also do the following:

- Monitor intake and output hourly. Report decreased or inadequate urine output.
- Regularly assess narrowed pulse pressure, which is an earlier and more accurate indicator of shock than blood pressure or heart rate.
- Monitor hemodynamic status; inadequate fluid resuscitation is manifested by a drop in central venous pressure (CVP) and PAWP.
- Follow prescribed protocols for IV fluid resuscitation. Therapy for burn shock is aimed at supporting the patient through the period of hypovolemic instability.
- Weigh the patient daily. Body weight is used to calculate fluid requirements.
- Test all stools and emesis for the presence of blood. Occult blood in emesis or stool indicates gastrointestinal bleeding.
- Maintain a warm environment. Hypothermia leads to shivering and further loss of body fluid through increased energy expenditure and catabolism.
- Monitor for fluid volume overload. Older patients and patients with underlying cardiac disease may demonstrate symptoms of heart failure during the fluid resuscitation stage.

SAFETY ALERT Patients with major burns receive 10 or more liters of fluid and gain weight due to fluid shifts. When their capillary membrane integrity resumes, these patients have a high CVP and urine output that necessitates monitoring of urine electrolytes.

Provide Effective Pain Management

All partial-thickness burns, along with extensive superficial burns, can cause excruciating pain, as can wound care and physical therapy. Increased levels of anxiety about treatments and outcomes may increase a patient's perception of pain. To help manage this pain, the nurse should take the following actions:

- Measure the patient's level of pain using a consistent measurement tool. The term *pain tolerance* refers to the duration and intensity of pain that the patient is able to endure. Pain tolerance differs from one patient to the next and may vary in the same patient in different situations. A description of pain management tools can be found in the exemplar on Acute and Chronic Pain in the module on Comfort.
- Administer pain medication before painful procedures, and determine when PCA is appropriate. Remember that inability to manage pain often results in feelings of despair and frustration for the patient.
- Administer IV opioid analgesics as prescribed. Nurses' fears of precipitating addiction often make them reluctant to administer narcotics. During the acute stage of burn injury, however, invasive procedures and exposed neurosensory nerve endings dictate the need for narcotic pharmaceutical agents.

- Explain all procedures and expected levels of discomfort. Patients experience less stress when they are prepared for painful procedures and know beforehand the actual sensations they will feel.

- Use methods of nonopioid pain control in combination with medications for pain. Noninvasive pain relief measures (e.g., relaxation, massage, distraction) can enhance the therapeutic effects of pain relief medications.

- Allow the patient to verbalize the pain experience. Be aware that every individual experiences and expresses pain differently, using various sociocultural adaptation techniques.

SAFETY ALERT Narcotics should be administered intravenously (rather than orally, subcutaneously, or intramuscularly) in the emergent or acute stage of a burn because of decreased circulation and absorption of medications.

Protect Skin Integrity

A burn injury significantly impairs the patient's skin integrity, although the severity of impairment varies according to the depth and extent of the burn. General treatment measures are designed to restore normal skin function as quickly as possible. Nursing care focuses on assessing and cleaning the wound and controlling infection. In this capacity, the nurse generally does the following:

- Estimate the extent and depth of the burn wound and recalculate the extent of unhealed burns weekly. The severity of the burn injury is the basis for determining which types of interventions are appropriate. Regular reassessment is necessary to monitor the healing process.

- Provide daily wound care (including debridement, dressing, and medication administration) as prescribed to remove dead tissue, control infection, and promote re-epithelialization as soon as possible. During all wound care, take steps to avoid cross-contamination of wounds.

- Elevate burned or newly skin-grafted extremities at or above heart level to increase venous return and prevent edema formation.

- Immobilize skin graft sites for 3–5 days or as ordered to promote graft adherence and prevent loss of newly grafted skin.

SAFETY ALERT Move the patient slowly and carefully across bed sheets to prevent shearing or dislodging new skin grafts.

- Provide special skin care to sensitive body areas as follows:
  a. Clean burns involving the eyes using normal saline or sterile water to prevent corneal and conjunctival drying and adherence. If contracture of the eyelid develops, apply drops or ointment to the eye to prevent corneal abrasion.
  b. Gently wipe burns of the lips with saline-soaked pads. Apply an antibiotic ointment as prescribed. Assess the mouth frequently, and perform mouth care routinely. If an oral endotracheal tube is in place, reposition it often to prevent pressure ulcer formation.
  c. Gently debride burns of the nose and apply mafenide acetate (Sulfamylon) cream. Position nasogastric and nasotracheal tubes to prevent excessive pressure.
  d. Apply mafenide acetate (Sulfamylon) cream to burns of the ear. Gently debride and thoroughly clean the wound with a water spray. Do not cover ears with dressings. Do not use pillows; to reduce pressure to the area, use a foam doughnut instead. Burns of the ears are prone to infection, and special positioning devices are necessary to decrease pressure ulcer formation.

Prevent Infection

From the onset of a burn injury, loss of the body's natural barrier to the external environment increases the risk of infection. Appropriate nursing interventions therefore focus on controlling infectious processes and include the following:

- Monitor daily for manifestations of wound infection. Be sure to remove topical medications and wound exudate and examine the entire wound. Early manifestations of infection include swelling and inflammation of intact skin surrounding the wound; a change in the color, odor, or amount of exudate; increased pain; and loss of previously healed skin grafts.

SAFETY ALERT An increase in body temperature without other manifestations of infection does not indicate infection in patients with large burn wounds, because the hypermetabolic response resets their core temperature to a higher level.

- Monitor for positive blood cultures, which indicate bacteremia.

- Monitor for hyperemia, cough, chest pain, wheezing, rhonchi, decreased oxygen saturation, and purulent sputum, all of which are manifestations of pneumonia.

- Monitor for the presence of bacteriuria, fever, urgency, frequency, dysuria, and suprapubic pain, which are all manifestations of urinary tract infection.

SAFETY ALERT If the patient has an indwelling catheter, assess the urine for cloudiness and a foul odor, and obtain a urine culture and sensitivity at least weekly.

- Obtain daily WBC counts. Leukocyte counts are indicators of immune system function and increase in the presence of infection.

- Determine tetanus immunization status. Patients who have burn injuries are at risk for anaerobic infection caused by *Clostridium tetani*.

- Maintain a high-kilocalorie intake. Nutritional support provides the nutrients needed to maintain the body's defense mechanisms.

- Maintain an aseptic environment using standard precautions (including gloving, gowning, and sterile procedures). Strict isolation technique deters the development of healthcare-associated infections.

- Culture all wounds and body secretions per protocol. Culture and sensitivity reports identify the presence of infectious microbes and indicate appropriate antimicrobial therapies.

- Administer prescribed antimicrobial medications to decrease invasive wound infections.

Maintain Physical Mobility

As a patient's burn wound heals and new skin tissue forms, the involved area tends to shrink. Contractures often form at the site and significantly limit mobility, especially when a joint is involved. Physical therapy is therefore important, beginning in the early stages of treatment. The nurse plays an important role in physical therapy and preservation of patient mobility by way of the following interventions:

■ Perform active or passive ROM exercises to all joints every 2 hours, and assist the patient in ambulating once stable. Regular exercise prevents further loss of motion, restores movement, and improves functional status.

■ Apply splints as prescribed. Maintain antideformity positions, and reposition the patient hourly. Splinting and positioning retard the formation of contractures.

■ Maintain limbs in functional alignment to preserve joint mobility.

■ Anticipate the need for analgesia. Administering analgesics promotes the patient's comfort during exercise sessions.

SAFETY ALERT Assess all patients, especially older adults, for indications of pressure ulcer formation under splints.

Promote Balanced Nutrition

A burn injury initiates a complex series of events that have a profound effect on the body's use of nutrients and expenditure of energy. The dietitian determines a patient's daily kilocalorie requirements, and as soon as possible, enteral or parenteral feedings are initiated. Associated nursing measures focus on assessing feeding tolerance and use of nutrients and include the following:

■ Maintain nasogastric or nasointestinal tube placement. Correct tube placement ensures appropriate absorption of nutrients and prevents aspiration.

■ Maintain enteral or parenteral nutritional support as prescribed. Observe and report any evidence of feeding intolerance, such as diarrhea, vomiting, excessive gastric residual, abdominal distention, absent bowel sounds, and constipation. The dietitian, in collaboration with the physician, selects and individualizes the feeding formula according to the patient's daily energy expenditure requirements and feeding tolerance. Failure to maintain rates of infusion predisposes the patient to continued catabolism and negative nitrogen balance.

■ Weigh the patient daily. Weight indicates the adequacy of nutritional support therapies.

■ Obtain daily laboratory values for protein, iron, CBC, glucose, and albumin. Decreased serum values indicate inadequate nutritional intake.

Facilitate Empowerment

The patient with a major burn injury usually endures a lengthy hospital stay involving many treatments and care protocols that are beyond the patient's control. During the early stages, much of the care regimen involves excruciating pain. Further, the foreign environment of the burn unit makes it difficult for the patient to relate to the immediate surroundings. For example, the need to control infection in the burn unit requires hospital personnel and family members to don sterile clothing before coming to the patient's bedside. Family members and nursing personnel appear radically different when they are masked and gowned, and their odd appearance can add to the patient's sense of alienation. Furthermore, the patient's body image is often altered depending on the extent and location of the burn injury. To help address feelings of powerlessness, the nurse should take the following actions:

■ Allow the patient as much control over surroundings and daily routine as possible. For example, allow the patient to choose times of dressing changes. Powerlessness derives from the belief that one is unable to influence the outcome of a situation.

■ Keep needed items (e.g., call bell, urinal, water pitcher, tissues) within the patient's reach to reinforce the patient's feeling of control.

■ Encourage the patient to express feelings. The nurse can help the patient cope by therapeutically listening, displaying a caring presence, clarifying misconceptions, and providing positive feedback.

■ Set short-term, realistic goals for the patient (e.g., to ambulate from bedside to chair twice daily). Small incremental gains are easiest to achieve and allow for frequent positive reinforcement.

Table 21–8 » lists overall interventions for the emergent, acute, and rehabilitative stages of burn injury.

Evaluation

The patient with a severe burn must be constantly evaluated, and the plan of care changes to meet emerging or diminishing needs. It is not unusual for a patient with a severe burn to be hospitalized for extended periods of time, requiring new care plan modifications as the patient moves through the recovery process. Expected outcomes used to evaluate patient progress may include the following:

■ The patient maintains stable vital signs, as evidenced by values within normal limits.

■ The patient receives adequate pain management to allow for comfort, as evidenced by being able to rest and reporting a pain level of 3 or less.

■ The patient's nutritional needs are being met, as evidenced by stable weight, balanced intake and output, and laboratory values within normal range.

■ The patient is infection free, as evidenced by CBC within normal range and wound healing.

The prevention of complications from burn wounds requires an interprofessional team approach. Infection is the most common complication and can cause a cascade of other events to occur, such as development of sepsis and loss of grafts. Because manifestations of burn wound infections are difficult to identify, careful wound monitoring is imperative. Patients with severe burn injuries can also develop multiple organ dysfunction syndrome, a progressive disorder caused by the systemic inflammatory response, which can result in death (Gauglitz & Williams, 2016). Any of these changes in patient condition require re-evaluation and modification of goals, interventions, and treatments previously identified for the patient.

TABLE 21–8 Interventions in Various Stages of Burn Injury

Stage of Burn Injury	Onset	End Point	Interventions
Emergent/resuscitative	Occurrence of burn injury	Successful fluid resuscitation	Remove patient from heat source.
			Initiate first aid.
			Assess extent of burn injury.
			Prevent hypothermia.
			Assess for shock.
			Determine need for intubation.
			Determine need for IV therapy.
			Follow protocol for fluid resuscitation.
			Obtain history.
			Transport to tertiary care facility.
Acute	Diuresis	Wound closure	Begin hydrotherapy.
			Determine need for excision of burn wound.
			Control spread of infection.
			Institute wound care.
			Start nutrition support.
			Graft burn wound.
			Initiate physical therapy.
			Manage pain.
Rehabilitative	Wound closure	Return to highest level of health restoration	Prevent scar formation.
			Continue physical therapy.
			Address psychosocial, cultural, and spiritual needs.
			Consider occupational therapy.
			Consider vocational training.
			Assess home maintenance management.

Patient Teaching

Burn Care

Patient and family teaching is an important component of all phases of burn care. As treatment progresses, the nurse encourages family members to assume more responsibility in providing care. However, many burn centers perform dressing changes in a burn clinic because family members find it difficult to perform procedures they know will inflict pain on the patient. If family members perform dressing changes, the nurse should provide patient teaching regarding how to change the dressing(s) and how soon before the dressing change to give pain medication. Specific guidelines for dressing changes should be outlined so that family members and healthcare team members have the same focus.

From admission to discharge, the nurse teaches the patient and family to assess all findings, implement therapies, and evaluate progress. The nurse should address the following topics when preparing the patient and family for home care:

- Long-term goals of rehabilitation care (including preventing soft tissue deformity, protecting skin grafts, maintaining physiologic function, managing scars, and returning the patient to an optimal level of independence)
- Necessity of avoiding exposure to individuals with colds or infections and meticulously following aseptic technique when caring for the wound

- Need for progressive physical activity
- Procedures for applying splints, pressure support garments, and other assistive devices
- Dietary requirements with increased kilocalorie amounts
- Alternative pain control therapies such as guided imagery, relaxation techniques, and diversional activities
- Care of the graft and donor sites
- Referral for occupational therapy, social services, clergy, and/or psychiatric services as appropriate
- Referral to any of the following organizations dedicated to helping burn survivors:
  - American Burn Association (http://www.ameriburn.org)
  - International Society for Burn Injuries (http://www.world-burn.org)
  - American Academy of Facial Plastic and Reconstructive Surgery (http://www.aafprs.org)
  - The Phoenix Society for Burn Survivors (http://www.phoenix-society.org)

Nursing Care Plan
A Patient with a Severe Burn

Craig Howard, a 39-year-old truck driver, is admitted to the hospital following an accident in which the cab of his truck caught fire. Mr. Howard was freed from the truck by a passing motorist, who stayed with him until the rescue team arrived to transport him to a local emergency department. Mr. Howard's wife, Mary, and twin daughters, Jessica and Jane, age 10, have been notified of the accident.

ASSESSMENT	DIAGNOSES	PLANNING
On his admission to the emergency department, Mr. Howard is diagnosed with deep partial-thickness and full-thickness burns of the anterior chest, arms, and hands. A quick assessment based on the rule of nines estimates the extent of his burn injury at 36% of TBSA. His vital signs are as follows: T 35.6°C rectal (96.2°F), P 140 bpm, R 40/min, BP 98/60 mmHg. In the field, the paramedics inserted a large-bore central line into Mr. Howard's right subclavian vein and started the rapid infusion of lactated Ringer's solution. Mr. Howard is also receiving 40% humidified oxygen via face mask. Initial ABGs are pH 7.49, PO_2 60 mmHg, PCO_2 32 mmHg, and bicarbonate 22 mEq/L. Lung sounds indicate inspiratory and expiratory wheezing, and a persistent cough reveals sooty sputum production. A Foley catheter is inserted and initially drains a moderate amount of dark concentrated urine. A nasogastric tube is connected to low intermittent suction. Mr. Howard is alert and oriented and complains of severe pain associated with the burn injuries. The burn unit is notified, and Mr. Howard is transferred there.	■ *Risk for Ineffective Airway Clearance* related to increasing lung congestion secondary to smoke inhalation ■ *Deficient Fluid Volume* related to abnormal fluid loss secondary to burn injury ■ *Risk for Ineffective Peripheral Tissue Perfusion* related to peripheral constriction secondary to circumferential burn wounds of the arms (NANDA-I © 2014)	Goals of nursing care for Mr. Howard include the following: ■ The patient will demonstrate a patent airway as evidenced by clear breath sounds; absence of cyanosis; and vital signs, chest x-ray findings, and ABGs within normal limits. ■ The patient will demonstrate adequate fluid volume and electrolyte balance as evidenced by urine output, vital signs, mental status, and laboratory findings within normal limits. ■ The patient will demonstrate adequate tissue perfusion as evidenced by palpable pulses, warm extremities, normal capillary refill, and absence of paresthesia.

IMPLEMENTATION

■ Prepare for prophylactic nasotracheal intubation to maintain airway patency.

■ Initiate fluid resuscitation therapy using the Parkland formula to calculate IV fluid rate for the first 24 hours postburn.

■ Assist the healthcare provider in performing escharotomies of both upper extremities.

EVALUATION

The nurse anesthetist inserted a nasotracheal tube and connected Mr. Howard to a T-piece delivering 40% oxygen. Vigorous respiratory toileting has significantly improved his ABGs. Bronchodilators have been parenterally administered and mucolytic agents added to his respiratory treatments. Mr. Howard's tracheal secretions have begun to show evidence of clearing. Hourly urine outputs indicate adequate fluid resuscitation. Urine output has been maintained at 50 mL/hr, and color and concentration have improved. CVP readings have been maintained at 6 cm H_2O, and blood pressure has increased to 100/64 mmHg. Pulse rate has decreased to 100 bpm.

To improve tissue perfusion of both arms, the healthcare provider has performed bilateral escharotomies, and the wounds have been dressed using sterile procedure. The extremities consequently have demonstrated improved circulation.

CRITICAL THINKING

1. Explain the rationale for the immediate insertion of a Foley catheter and nasogastric tube.

2. An escharotomy was performed on both arms. Why was this procedure necessary in Mr. Howard's case?

3. What is the rationale supporting the IV administration of narcotics to control Mr. Howard's pain?

4. Explain the sequence of events that led to a fluid and electrolyte shift during the first 24–48 hours after Mr. Howard sustained his injury.

REVIEW Burns

RELATE Link the Concepts and Exemplars

Linking the exemplar of burns with the concept of comfort:

1. When providing care to the patient with deep full-thickness burns involving the entire right arm, will the nurse need to administer analgesics? Explain your answer.

2. A patient is brought to the emergency department with partial-thickness burns of the chest and neck. The patient is crying in pain. What nursing considerations will affect the plan for pain management for this patient?

Linking the exemplar of burns with the concept of development:

3. In the care of a 12-year-old patient admitted following a major burn, what pain scale is most appropriate for assessing pain? Explain your choice.

4. Once this patient's physical condition stabilizes, how can the nurse address the patient's developmental issues?

READY Go to Volume 3: Clinical Nursing Skills

REFER Go to Pearson MyLab Nursing and eText

- Additional review materials

REFLECT Apply Your Knowledge

David Newton, age 54, was smoking a cigarette and fell asleep, dropping the cigarette and igniting his bed linens. A neighbor saw the fire and called 9-1-1, and Mr. Newton was rescued by the fire department. He sustained full-thickness burns over the upper half of his chest and back and the posterior aspects of both upper arms. He also sustained superficial partial-thickness burns to his anterior and posterior head and neck.

Mr. Newton was initially treated in the local emergency department and then transported via life flight to a specialized burn unit located 150 miles from his home. Upon his arrival in the burn unit, 5 hours after injury, the nurse notes the presence of a Foley catheter that is draining burgundy-colored urine. Mr. Newton also has a nasogastric tube that is draining dark yellow-green liquid. He was intubated in the emergency department and is now placed on a ventilator in the burn unit. Upon admission to the burn unit, Mr. Newton's vital signs are as follows: temperature 99.9°F oral; pulse 102 bpm; respirations 24/min; and BP 98/52 mmHg. His pain level is reported as a 9 on a 0–10 scale, and he is medicated with morphine sulfate 10 mg IV by the physician's order.

1. The initial assessment in the emergency department is that Mr. Newton has sustained burns over 36% of his body. Using the rule of nines, how does the nurse analyze this total percentage?

2. Mr. Newton is in the phase of burn shock. His urinary output for the past 5 hours has been 150 mL. On the basis of his urinary output and vital signs, what is the nurse's explanation for the physiology of shock related to a major burn injury?

3. Mr. Newton's diagnosis is *Impaired Gas Exchange* related to swelling secondary to inhalation injury manifested by need for intubation and mechanical ventilation. Why was intubation necessary for Mr. Newton? What important nursing interventions are related to this choice?

4. Why was Mr. Newton's Foley catheter draining burgundy-colored urine at the time of admission to the burn unit?

5. Mr. Newton is put on enteral feeding during the recovery phase of the burn injury, and the related nursing diagnosis is *Imbalanced Nutrition: Less Than Body Requirements* related to hypermetabolic and catabolic stage secondary to a major burn. What is the rationale for this diagnosis?

» Exemplar 21.B Pressure Injuries

Exemplar Learning Outcomes

21.B Analyze pressure injuries as they relate to tissue integrity.

- Describe the pathophysiology, etiology, risk factors, and prevention of pressure injuries.
- Identify the clinical manifestations of pressure injuries.
- Summarize diagnostic tests and therapies used by interprofessional teams in the collaborative care of an individual with pressure injuries.
- Apply the nursing process in providing culturally competent care to an individual with pressure injuries.

Exemplar Key Terms

Debridement, *1624*
Eschar, *1624*
Excoriation, *1620*
Immobility, *1620*
Maceration, *1620*
Necrosis, *1619*
Pressure injury, *1619*
Shearing forces, *1620*

Overview

Pressure injuries are ischemic lesions of the skin and underlying tissue caused by external pressure that impairs the flow of blood and lymph (Huether et al., 2017). The ischemia causes tissue **necrosis** (dead tissue) and eventual ulceration. These injuries, which have previously been called *bedsores* or *decubitus ulcers*, tend to develop over a bony prominence (e.g., heels, greater trochanter, sacrum, ischia), but they may appear on the skin of any part of the body that is subjected to external pressure, friction, or shearing forces.

The incidence of pressure injuries in hospitals, long-term care facilities, and home settings is high enough to warrant concern among healthcare providers. The incidence in hospitals has been reported to be as high as 8%; the incidence in long-term care facilities is reported to range from 2.4 to 23% (Huether et al., 2017). Little research has been done to determine the extent of the problem in the home setting. However, with increasing numbers of patients (especially older adult patients) being cared for in the home, it is probable that the incidence is great enough to warrant plans of care to prevent their occurrence.

Pathophysiology and Etiology

Pathophysiology

When an individual lies or sits in one position for an extended length of time without moving, pressure on the tissue between a bony prominence and the external surface of the body distorts capillaries and interferes with normal blood flow. If the pressure is relieved, blood flow to the area increases, and a brief period of reactive hyperemia occurs without permanent damage. If the pressure continues, platelets aggregate in the endothelial cells surrounding the capillaries and form microthrombi. These microthrombi impede blood flow; the result is ischemia and hypoxia of tissues. The cells and tissues of the immediate area of pressure and of the surrounding area eventually die and become necrotic.

Alterations in the involved tissue depend on the depth of the injury. Injury to superficial layers of skin results in blister formation; damage to deeper structures causes the pressure injury area to appear dark reddish-blue. As the tissues die, the ulcer becomes an open wound that may be deep enough to expose the bone. The necrotic tissue elicits an inflammatory response, and the patient experiences increases in temperature, pain, and WBC count. Secondary bacterial invasion is common. Enzymes from bacteria and macrophages dissolve necrotic tissue; the result is a foul-smelling drainage.

Etiology

Pressure injuries develop from external pressure that compresses blood vessels or from friction and shearing forces that tear and damage vessels. Both of these elements can cause traumatic damage and initiate the process of pressure injury development.

External pressure that is greater than capillary pressure and arteriolar pressure interrupts blood flow in capillary beds. When pressure is applied to skin over a bony prominence for 2 hours, tissue ischemia and hypoxia from external pressure cause irreversible tissue damage. A given amount of pressure causes more damage when it is applied to a small area than when it is distributed over a large surface.

Shearing forces result when one tissue layer slides over another. The stretching and bending of blood vessels cause injury and thrombosis. The patient in a hospital bed is subject to shearing forces when the head of the bed is elevated and the torso slides down toward the foot of the bed. Pulling the patient up in bed also subjects the patient to shearing forces. (For this reason, the nurse should always lift the patient up in bed instead of pulling.) In both cases, friction and moisture cause the skin and superficial fascia to remain fixed to the bedsheet, while the deep fascia and bony skeleton slide in the direction of body movement.

Risk Factors

Although a pressure injury may develop in any adult who has impaired mobility, those who are most at risk are older adults with limited mobility, individuals with quadriplegia, and patients in the critical care setting (Huether et al., 2017).

Several factors contribute to the formation of pressure injuries: immobility and inactivity, inadequate nutrition, fecal and urinary incontinence, decreased mental status, diminished sensation, excessive body heat, advanced age, and the presence of certain chronic conditions.

Immobility

Immobility is a reduction in the amount and control of movement. Individuals normally move when they experience discomfort from pressure on an area of the body. Healthy individuals rarely exceed their tolerance to pressure. However, paralysis, extreme weakness, pain, or any cause of decreased activity can hinder an individual's ability to change positions independently and relieve the pressure, even if the individual can perceive the pressure.

Inadequate Nutrition

Prolonged inadequate nutrition causes weight loss, muscle atrophy, and the loss of subcutaneous tissue. These processes reduce the amount of padding between the skin and the bones, thus increasing the risk of pressure injury development. More specifically, inadequate intake of protein, carbohydrates, fluids, zinc, and vitamin C contributes to pressure ulcer formation.

Hypoproteinemia (abnormally low protein content in the blood), due to either inadequate intake or abnormal loss, predisposes the patient to dependent edema. Edema (swelling caused by excess fluid trapped in body tissue) makes skin more prone to injury by decreasing its elasticity, resilience, and vitality. Edema increases the distance between the capillaries and the cells, thereby slowing the diffusion of oxygen to the tissue cells and of metabolites away from the cells.

Fecal and Urinary Incontinence

Moisture from incontinence promotes skin **maceration** (tissues softened by prolonged wetting or soaking) and makes the epidermis more easily eroded and susceptible to injury. Digestive enzymes in feces, gastric tube drainage, and urea in urine also contribute to skin **excoriation** (the area of loss of the superficial layers of the skin, also known as a *denuded area*). Any accumulation of secretions or excretions is irritating to the skin, harbors microorganisms, and makes the skin prone to breakdown and infection.

Decreased Mental Status

Individuals with a reduced level of awareness, including those who are unconscious, are heavily sedated, or have dementia, are at risk for pressure injuries because they are less able to recognize and respond to pain associated with prolonged pressure.

Diminished Sensation

Paralysis, stroke, or other neurologic disease may cause loss of sensation in a body area. Loss of sensation reduces an individual's ability to respond to trauma, to injurious heat and cold, and to the tingling ("pins and needles") that signals loss of circulation. Sensory loss also impairs the body's ability to recognize and provide healing mechanisms for a wound. In older adults, diminished pain perception due to a reduction in the number of cutaneous end organs responsible for the sensation of pressure and light touch increases risk for impaired skin integrity.

Excessive Body Heat

Body heat is another factor in the development of pressure injuries. An elevated body temperature increases the metabolic rate, thus increasing the cells' need for oxygen. This increased need is particularly severe in the cells of an area under pressure, which are already oxygen deficient. Severe infections with accompanying elevated body temperatures may affect the body's ability to deal with the effects of tissue compression.

Advanced Age

The aging process brings about several changes in the skin and its supporting structures, making the older individual more prone to impaired skin integrity. These changes include loss of lean body mass, generalized thinning of the epidermis, decreased strength and elasticity of the skin, and diminished venous and arterial flow due to aging vascular walls. Increased dryness due to a decrease in the amount of oil produced by the sebaceous glands also increases risk for impaired skin integrity in older adults.

Chronic Medical Conditions

Certain chronic conditions, such as diabetes and cardiovascular disease, are risk factors for skin breakdown and delayed healing. These conditions compromise oxygen delivery to tissues; the result is poor and delayed healing and increased risk of pressure injuries.

Other Factors

Other factors contributing to the formation of pressure injuries are poor lifting and transferring techniques, incorrect positioning, hard support surfaces, and incorrect application of pressure-relieving devices.

Prevention

Preventing pressure ulcer development requires a multifaceted approach. Nursing interventions combine actively promoting optimal skin integrity with educating the patient, support people, and caregivers about how to prevent pressure ulcers. Key preventive measures incorporate nutrition, skin hygiene and protection, and use of supportive devices.

Providing Nutrition

Because an inadequate intake of calories, protein, vitamins, and iron is believed to be a risk factor for pressure ulcer development, nutritional supplements should be considered for patients who are nutritionally compromised. The diet should be similar to one that supports wound healing, as discussed earlier. The nurse should monitor weight regularly to help assess nutritional status. Pertinent lab work should also be monitored, including lymphocyte count, protein (especially albumin), and hemoglobin.

Maintaining Skin Hygiene

The nurse should obtain baseline data using the established tool and then reassess the skin at least daily in the hospital and weekly at home. When bathing the patient, the nurse should minimize the force and friction applied to the skin, using mild cleansing agents that minimize irritation and dryness and do not disrupt the skin's "natural barriers." Also, the nurse should avoid using hot water, which increases skin dryness and irritation. The nurse can minimize dryness by avoiding exposure of the patient's skin to cold and low humidity. Dry skin is best treated with moisturizing lotions applied while the skin is moist after bathing. The patient's skin should be kept clean and dry and free of irritation and maceration by urine, feces, sweat, or incomplete drying after a bath. The nurse applies skin protection if indicated. Dimethicone-based creams or alcohol-free barrier films, which are available in liquid, spray, and moist-wipe preparations, are very effective in preventing moisture or drainage from collecting on the skin. In most cases, the nurse can apply these without a primary care provider's order. Use of petroleum-based creams and ointments is not advised because of their poor overall skin protection and interference with diaper or incontinence product absorption.

Avoiding Skin Trauma

Providing the patient with a smooth, firm, and wrinkle-free foundation on which to sit or lie helps prevent skin trauma. To prevent injury due to friction and shearing forces, the patient must be positioned, transferred, and turned correctly. For a patient who is bedridden, shearing force can be reduced by elevation of the head of the bed to no more than 30 degrees if this position is not contraindicated by the patient's condition (e.g., a patient with respiratory disorders may find it easier to breathe in Fowler position). When the head of the bed is raised, the skin and superficial fascia may stick to the bed linen, while the deep fascia and skeleton slide down toward the bottom of the bed. As a result, blood vessels in the sacral area become twisted, and the tissues in the area can become ischemic and necrotic. Baby powder and cornstarch are never used for friction or moisture prevention. These powders create harmful abrasive grit that is damaging to tissues, and they are considered a respiratory hazard when airborne. Instead, moisturizing creams and protective films, such as transparent dressings and alcohol-free barrier films, are used.

Frequent shifts in position, even if only slight, effectively change pressure points. The patient who is able should shift weight 10–15 degrees every 15–30 minutes and, whenever possible, exercise or ambulate to stimulate blood circulation.

When lifting a patient to change position, the nurse should use a lifting device such as a trapeze rather than dragging the patient across or up in bed. The friction that results from dragging the skin against a sheet can cause blisters and abrasions, which may contribute to more extensive tissue damage. Therefore, using a device that lifts the patient's weight off the bed surface is the method of choice. To deter shearing forces, the nurse should place a draw sheet that covers the bed from an individual's chest to buttocks and is folded to be wide enough to tuck under the mattress on either side when not in use.

Any at-risk patient who is confined to bed—even when a special support mattress is used—should be repositioned at least every 2 hours, depending on the patient's need, to

TABLE 21–9 Mechanical Devices for Reducing Pressure on Body Parts

Device	Description/Comments
Gel flotation pads	Polyvinyl, silicone, or Silastic pads are filled with a gelatinous substance similar to fat.
Pillows and wedges (foam, gel, air, fluid)	Pillows and wedges support positioning and offload bone-on-bone contact.
Heel protectors (sheepskin boots, padded splints, off-loading inflatable boots, foam blocks)	Heel protectors can raise or "float" a body part (e.g., heels) off the surface; they prevent shearing and limit pressure on the heel area.
Memory foam mattresses or chair pads	These devices distribute weight over bony areas evenly; they mold to the body.
Alternating pressure mattresses	Alternating pressure mattresses are composed of a number of cells in which the pressure alternately increases and decreases; they use a pump.
Waterbeds	The support surface of waterbeds is filled with water; the water temperature is controllable.
Static low-air-loss (LAL) beds	Static LAL beds consist of many air-filled cushions divided into four or five sections. (Separate controls permit each section to be inflated to a different level of firmness; thus, pressure can be reduced on bony prominences but increased under other body areas for support.)
Active or second-generation LAL beds	These beds are like static LAL beds but also gently pulsate or rotate from side to side, thus stimulating capillary blood flow and facilitating movement of pulmonary secretions.
Air-fluidized (AF) beds (static high-air-loss beds)	AF beds consist of millions of tiny silicone-coated beads, around which forced temperature-controlled air circulates, producing a fluidlike movement. They provide uniform support to body contours and decrease skin maceration by their drying effect. (Moisture from the patient penetrates the linens and soaks the beads. Air flow forces the beads away from the patient and rapidly dries the sheets. A major disadvantage is that the head of the bed cannot be elevated. Some beds are a unique combination of AF therapy and LAL therapy on an articulating frame. These are used with patients who require head elevation.)

allow another body surface to bear the weight. Six body positions can usually be used: prone, supine, right and left lateral (side-lying), and right and left Sims positions. When a lateral position is used, the nurse should avoid positioning the patient directly on the trochanter and should instead position the patient at a 30-degree angle. A written schedule should be established for turning and repositioning.

Providing Supportive Devices

For circulation to remain uncompromised and development of pressure injuries avoided, external pressure on the bony prominences should remain below capillary pressure for as much time as possible through a combination of turning, positioning, and use of pressure-relieving surfaces. External pressure greater than the arterial capillary pressure (32 mmHg) for an extended period can impair blood flow to soft tissue (Kirman, 2016). Some research has evaluated the effectiveness of pressure-reducing support surfaces in preventing pressure injuries in patients at low, intermediate, or high risk; however, the results have been inconclusive (McInnes et al., 2015). The nurse should review the manufacturer's product descriptions that report the amount of time that the pressure between the surface and the bony prominence is above or below specified levels and determine whether this amount of time is adequate to protect a particular patient.

For patients who are confined to bed, three types of support surfaces can be used to relieve pressure:

1. An overlay mattress is applied on top of the standard bed mattress. Most overlay mattresses are made of foam and gel combinations.
2. Specialty beds replace hospital beds. They provide pressure relief, eliminate shearing and friction, and reduce moisture. Examples are high-air-loss beds, low-air-loss beds, and beds that provide kinetic therapy.
3. Kinetic beds provide continuous passive motion or oscillation therapy, both of which are intended to counteract the effects of a patient's immobility.

When a patient is confined to bed or to a chair, pressure-reducing devices, such as pillows made of foam, gel, air, or a combination of these, can be used. When the patient is sitting, weight should be distributed over the entire seating surface so that pressure does not center on just one area. To protect a patient's heels in bed, supports such as wedges or pillows can be used to raise the heels completely off the bed. Doughnut-type devices should not be used, because they limit blood flow and can cause tissue damage to the areas in direct contact with the device. **Table 21–9 》** lists mechanical devices for reducing pressure on body parts.

Clinical Manifestations

Pressure injuries can manifest in different ways depending upon their severity. This variation is attributed to the soft tissue, muscle, and skin resisting pressure to differing degrees. Muscle is generally the least resistant to pressure and will become necrotic prior to skin breaking down. In addition, pressure is not distributed equally from a bony prominence, where it is greatest, to the overlying skin. Pressure decreases gradually from the bony area toward the periphery, and a small area of skin breakdown may not be representative of what lies underneath (Kirman, 2016).

Pressure injuries range from discoloration to blisters or areas of denuded superficial skin to deep tissue damage with necrosis. As a result, pressure injuries are graded or staged to classify the degree of tissue damage. The stages are listed in **Table 21–10 》**, and clinical manifestations and therapies are listed in the feature box.

TABLE 21–10 Pressure Injury Staging

Stage	Description
Stage 1	

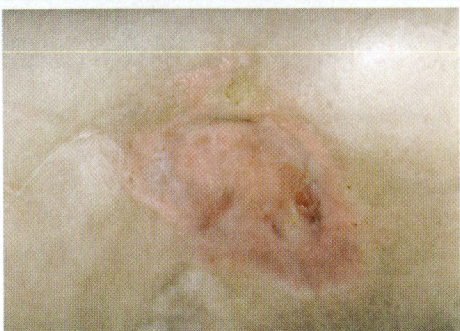

Source: Mediscan/Alamy Stock Photo.

The patient experiences nonblanchable erythema of intact skin, the heralding lesion of skin ulceration. Stage 1 pressure injuries usually occur in a localized area over a bony prominence. Identification may be difficult in patients with darkly pigmented skin.

Note: Affected areas may be painful and have a different temperature and consistency than surrounding skin.

Stage 2

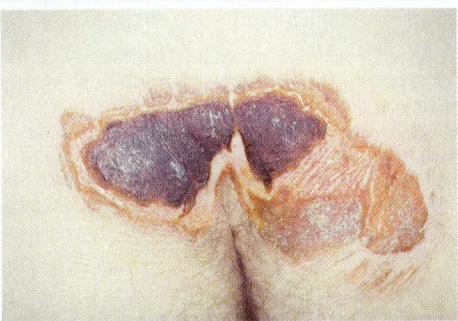

Source: Mediscan/Alamy Stock Photo.

The patient experiences partial-thickness skin loss involving the dermis. Stage 2 pressure injuries present as shallow, open ulcers with a viable pink or red moist wound bed. Granulation tissue, slough, and eschar are not present. These injuries may also present as intact or open serum-filled blisters.

Note: Skin tears, tape burns, incontinence-associated dermatitis, maceration, and excoriation are not included in this classification.

Stage 3

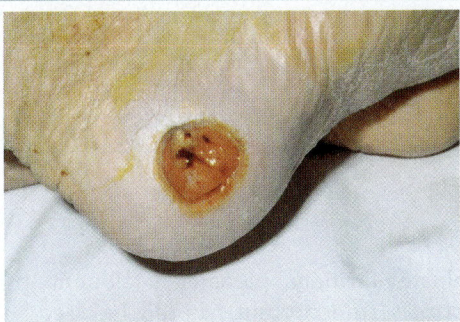

Source: Mediscan/Alamy Stock Photo.

The patient experiences full-thickness skin loss involving damage or necrosis of subcutaneous tissue; adipose tissue is visible within the ulcer. Granulation and rolled wound edges are often present. Bone, tendon, and muscle are not exposed. The ulcer presents clinically as a deep crater with or without undermining and tunneling of adjacent tissue. Slough and/or eschar may be present.

Note: Depth of stage 3 pressure injuries varies by anatomic location; in areas without adipose tissue, ulcers may be very shallow. The presence of slough or eschar that obscures the extent of tissue loss deems the injuries unstageable.

Stage 4

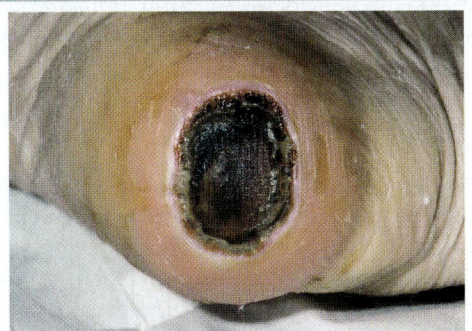

Source: Dr P. Marazzi/Science Source.

The patient experiences full-thickness skin loss with extensive tissue damage and necrosis. Fascia, muscle, ligament, cartilage, tendon, and/or bone are exposed and directly palpable; slough or eschar may be present. Undermining and tunneling, and rolled wound edges are usually present.

Note: Depth can vary by anatomic location, and injuries can extend into muscle and supporting structures (including fascia, tendons, or joint capsules), increasing the likelihood of osteomyelitis. The presence of slough or eschar that obscures the extent of tissue loss deems the injuries unstageable.

(continued on next page)

TABLE 21–10 Pressure Injury Staging *(continued)*

Stage	Description
Unstageable	
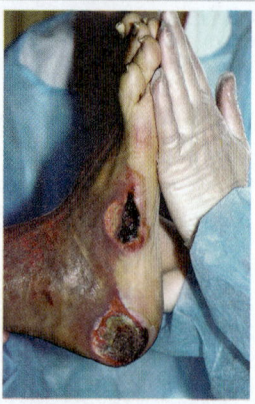 Source: BSIP/UIG/Getty Images.	The patient experiences full-thickness tissue loss with depth completely obscured by slough or eschar in the wound bed. Depth of the wound cannot be determined until slough or eschar is removed; once it is removed, the injury will be classified as stage 3 or 4. *Note:* Stable eschar on the heels serves as a natural biological cover and should not be removed.
Suspected Deep Tissue Injury	
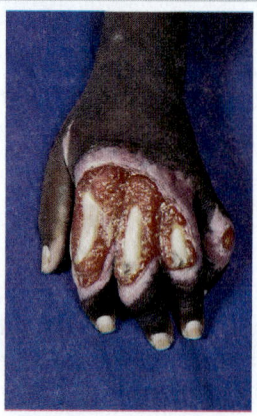 Source: Dr M.A. Ansary/Science Source.	The patient experiences intact or nonintact skin with localized, nonblanchable maroon, deep red, or purple discoloration or blood-filled blister. These injuries indicate damage of underlying soft tissue from pressure or shear. They may rapidly evolve into thin blisters over dark wound beds or develop thin eschar. They may be difficult to detect in patients with darkly pigmented skin. *Note:* Discoloration or blister may be preceded by painful tissue that is a different temperature and consistency from surrounding skin.

Source: Based on National Pressure Ulcer Advisory Panel (NPUAP). (2016). *NPUAP pressure injury stages*. Retrieved from http://www.npuap.org/resources/educational-and-clinical-resources/npuap-pressure-injury-stages

Collaboration

The primary objective for the patient at risk for developing pressure injury is prevention. Members of the healthcare team should assess patients for ulcer development regularly and reposition them following an established schedule. In repositioning, proper technique is essential to prevent injuries related to shear. When ulcers develop, they should be regularly assessed to ensure that they do not advance to a more severe stage. The patient and family members should be taught how to protect and treat ulcers and assess for stage changes.

Diagnostic Tests

Diagnostic tests are conducted to determine the presence of a secondary infection and to differentiate the cause of the pressure injury. WBC counts can be used to indicate the degree of inflammation or invasive infection. Evaluation of the erythrocyte sedimentation rate (ESR) is useful in determining the presence of osteomyelitis. Laboratory studies that evaluate nutritional parameters (albumin, prealbumin, transferrin, serum protein) should be used to assess a patient's nutritional status, as adequate nutrition is needed for wound healing. Other laboratory studies such as urine, stool, or blood cultures may be required if indicated by specific patient situations (Kirman, 2016). If the pressure injury is deep or appears infected, drainage or biopsied tissue is cultured to determine the causative organism.

Surgery

Nonviable tissue must be removed from a wound before the wound can be staged or heal. Surgical **debridement** (removal of necrotic material) may be necessary if the pressure ulcer is deep, if subcutaneous tissues are involved, or if **eschar** (a scab or dry crust consisting of dried plasma proteins and dead cells that forms over skin damaged by burns, infections, or excoriations) has formed over the ulcer, preventing healing by granulation.

Clinical Manifestations and Therapies
Pressure Injuries

ETIOLOGY	CLINICAL MANIFESTATIONS	CLINICAL THERAPIES
Pressure injuries with nonblanchable erythema (stage 1)	■ Intact skin with localized redness that does not blanch (lose redness) when pressed	■ Cleansing of ulcer and surrounding area ■ Application of barrier cream ■ Application of protective dressing ■ Introduction of appropriate support surfaces and other measures to redistribute pressure ■ Frequent repositioning
Pressure injuries with partial-thickness loss of dermis (stage 2)	■ Shallow open wound or blister without slough	■ Cleansing of ulcer and surrounding area ■ Application of moisture-retaining protective dressing ■ Assessment for necrosis and infection ■ Frequent repositioning ■ Comfort measures
Pressure injuries with full-thickness tissue loss (stages 3 and 4; unstageable)	■ Deep, open wound bed; necrosis of subcutaneous tissue and possible exposure of underlying bone, muscle, and support structure ■ Slough or eschar present	■ Cleansing of ulcer and surrounding area ■ Debridement of wound bed and edges ■ Surgical removal of necrotic tissue ■ Application of medicated moisture-retaining dressing that maintains contact with skin ■ Assessment for and treatment of infection ■ Pain management
Suspected deep tissue injury	■ Intact skin with localized purple discoloration ■ Possibly quick development of a thin blister or eschar	■ Cleansing of injury and surrounding area ■ Application of moisturizers or barrier creams ■ Application of nonadhesive protective dressing ■ Introduction of appropriate support surfaces and other measures to remove all pressure ■ Elevation of affected area (if possible) ■ Monitoring for pressure injury development

In addition to the surgical, mechanical, and enzymatic methods of debridement discussed in Exemplar 21.A on Burns, autolytic debridement may be used to treat pressure ulcers. In autolytic debridement, dressings that contain wound moisture, such as hydrocolloid and clear absorbent acrylic dressings, trap the wound drainage against the eschar. The body's own enzymes in the drainage break down the necrotic tissue. Although this method takes longer than the other three, it is the most selective and therefore causes the least damage to healthy surrounding and healing tissues.

Over the past decade, the use of fly larvae (maggots, *Phaenicia sericata*) has received increased attention, especially in the areas of antimicrobial and growth-promoting activity. In the past, larval therapy was known to be extremely effective in debriding chronic wounds because the maggots secrete and excrete digestive enzymes that break down necrotic tissue while leaving healthy tissue untouched. Research has shown that these larvae also secrete and excrete potent antimicrobial compounds, which reduce bacterial growth, and just their presence contributes to the healing process (Sherman, 2014). Large wounds may require skin grafting for complete closure.

Pharmacologic Therapy

Topical and systemic antibiotics specific to the infectious organism eradicate any infection present. In addition, a variety of topical products promote healing. For pressure injuries that are clean and granulating, dressings that maintain moisture are typically used, such as hydrocolloid and transparent film dressings. In addition to maintaining moisture, these dressings protect the wound from friction and bacterial colonization. Dressings may be impregnated with substances that offer microbial benefits, such as silver sulfadiazine and medical-grade honey. For deep, exudative wounds, alginate, foam, and iodine dressings may be preferable. The type of dressing used changes over time as the wound either heals or worsens (NPUAP, European Pressure Ulcer Advisory Panel [EPUAP], & PAN Pacific Pressure Injury Alliance [PPPPIA], 2014). Some examples of common dressings and the stages at which they are used are listed in **Table 21–11 》**.

TABLE 21–11 Products Used to Treat Pressure Injuries

Product	Purpose
Stage 1	
Skin prep Granulex	Toughens intact skin and preserves skin integrity; prevents skin breakdown, increases blood supply, adds moisture, contains trypsin to aid in removal of necrotic tissue
Hydrocolloid dressing (e.g., DuoDERM)	Prevents skin breakdown and promotes healing without the formation of a crust over the ulcer; is permeable to air and water vapor; prevents the growth of anaerobic organisms
Transparent dressing (e.g., Tegaderm)	Prevents skin breakdown; prevents entrance of moisture and bacteria but allows oxygen and moisture vapor permeability
Stage 2	
Transparent dressing	Enhances healing (see transparent dressing for stage 1)
Hydrocolloid dressing	Enhances healing (see hydrocolloid dressing for stage 1) *Note:* If infection is present, these types of dressings are contraindicated. A sterile dressing should be applied instead.
Wet-to-dry gauze dressing with sterile normal saline	Allows necrotic material to soften and adhere to the gauze so that the wound is debrided
Hydrocolloid dressing	Enhances healing (see above)
Proteolytic enzymes (e.g., Elase)	Serve as debriding agents in inflamed and infected lesions
Wet-to-dry gauze dressing with sterile normal saline	Enhances healing (see above) *Note:* Transparent or hydrocolloid dressings or skin barriers are contraindicated.
Vacuum-assisted closure (VAC)	Creates a negative pressure to help reduce edema, increase blood supply and oxygenation, and decrease bacterial colonization; helps promote moist wound healing and the formation of granulation tissue

Nonpharmacologic Therapy

Pressure injuries are a challenge for nurses because of the number of variables involved (e.g., risk factors, types of ulcers, degrees of impairment) and the numerous treatment measures advocated. Infection is the most serious complication of pressure injury. When treating pressure injuries, the nurse should follow the agency protocols and the primary care provider's orders. Prompt treatment can prevent further tissue damage and pain and can facilitate wound healing.

Following are the nursing care activities in treating pressure injuries:

- Minimize direct pressure on the ulcer. Reposition the patient at least every 2 hours. Make a schedule, and record position changes on the patient's chart. Provide devices to minimize or float pressure areas.
- Clean the pressure injury with every dressing change. The method of cleaning depends on the stage of the ulcer, the products available, and agency protocol.
- Clean and dress the ulcer using surgical asepsis. Never use alcohol or hydrogen peroxide, as they are cytotoxic to tissue beds.
- If the pressure injury is infected, obtain a sample of the drainage to culture and test for sensitivity to antibiotic agents.
- Teach the patient how to move to alleviate pressure. Even slight movements can be beneficial; provide assistive devices such as trapeze bars to facilitate movement.
- Provide ROM exercises and mobility out of bed as the patient's condition permits.

Nurses may find themselves collaborating with a number of individuals when providing care for a patient who has or is at risk for pressure injuries. Nurses frequently collaborate with physical therapists, especially in hospitals, rehabilitation centers, and nursing homes. When caring for a patient who is living at home, the nurse often collaborates with the individual's primary caregiver, be that a family member or a hired professional. Because many patients with pressure injuries are older or have other serious illnesses, a caregiver may require teaching in the following areas:

- General information about pressure injuries
- Risk factors for the development of pressure injuries
- Skin care and ways to avoid development of pressure injuries
- Diet and nutrition.

Depending on the stage of the pressure injury, the nurse teaches the patient or caregiver how to care for ulcers that are already present: how to change dressings, apply skin barriers, and avoid injury and infection. Referrals to a home health agency or community health department can help the family through the lengthy healing process.

NURSING PROCESS

Prevention is the goal for the patient at risk for pressure injuries. The patient with one or more pressure injuries not only has impaired skin integrity but also is at increased risk for infection, pain, and decreased mobility. Pressure injuries prolong treatment for other health problems, increase healthcare costs, and diminish the patient's quality of life.

Assessment

It is important to ensure that the lighting is good; natural or fluorescent lighting is preferable, because incandescent lights can create a transilluminating effect. The room should be neither too hot nor too cold. Heat can cause the skin to flush; cold can cause the skin to blanch or become cyanotic.

The nurse inspects pressure areas for discoloration (see **Figure 21–28** »), which can result from impaired blood

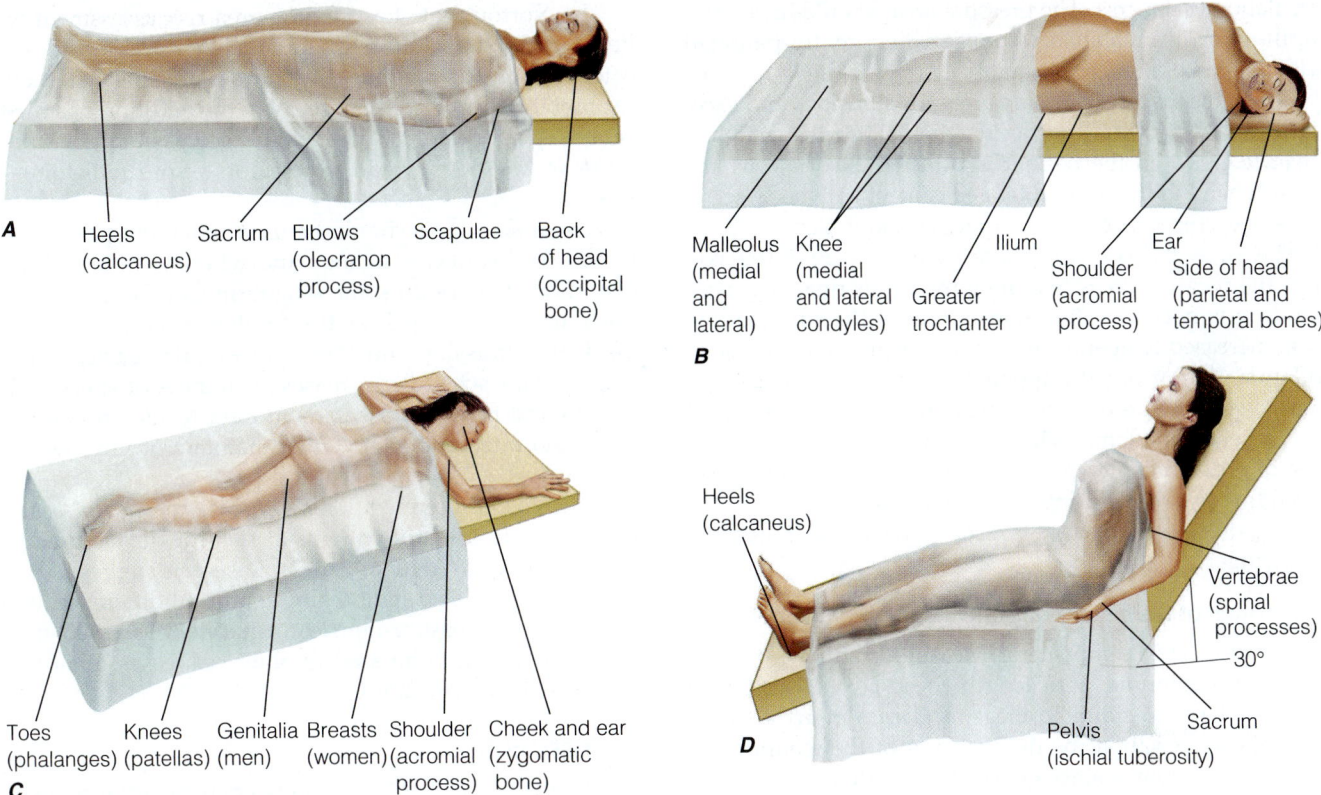

A

Heels (calcaneus) Sacrum Elbows (olecranon process) Scapulae Back of head (occipital bone)

B

Malleolus (medial and lateral) Knee (medial and lateral condyles) Greater trochanter Ilium Shoulder (acromial process) Ear Side of head (parietal and temporal bones)

C

Toes (phalanges) Knees (patellas) Genitalia (men) Breasts (women) Shoulder (acromial process) Cheek and ear (zygomatic bone)

D

Heels (calcaneus) Vertebrae (spinal processes) 30° Pelvis (ischial tuberosity) Sacrum

Figure 21–28 》 Body pressure areas in **A,** supine position; **B,** lateral position; **C,** prone position; **D,** Fowler position.

Pressure Injury Assessment

ASSESSMENT/ METHOD	NORMAL FINDINGS	ABNORMAL FINDINGS	LIFESPAN OR DEVELOPMENTAL CONSIDERATIONS
Pressure Area Assessment			
Inspect pressure areas for discoloration, abrasion, and excoriation.	Pressure areas should have brisk capillary refill or blanch response when gently palpated with the end of a finger or thumb. Skin over pressure areas should be intact.	▪ Nonblanching redness ▪ Abrasions in areas where skin rubs on linens or bedding ▪ Excoriations in areas exposed to body secretions or excretions and in skinfolds	▪ Older patients—even those in generally good health—may have mobility limitations. Do not discount early signs of pressure injuries in patients who are not bedridden.
Skin Temperature Assessment			
Palpate the surface temperature of the skin over the pressure area.	Temperature of pressure areas is the same as that of surrounding skin.	▪ Increased temperature indicates inflammation or trapping of blood in the pressure area. ▪ Decreased temperature indicates lack of blood flow.	▪ Because of decreased subcutaneous tissue in the extremities, older patients may have trouble regulating body temperature and have skin that is cool to the touch. Cool skin on its own does not necessarily indicate a problem; always compare the temperature of the pressure area to that of the surrounding skin.
Inspection of Bony Prominences			
Palpate the skin over bony prominences.	Tissue should be firm but not hard and have the same consistency as the surrounding area.	▪ Spongy or boggy tissue or skin is indicative of edema.	▪ Regardless of age, patients with spinal cord injuries who rely on wheelchairs are prone to pressure injuries over the bony prominences of the pelvic bones.

circulation to the area. The pressure areas should have brisk capillary refill or blanch response when gently palpated with the end of a finger or thumb.

The nurse inspects pressure areas for abrasions and excoriations. An abrasion can occur when skin rubs against a sheet (e.g., when the patient is pulled). Excoriations can occur when the skin has prolonged contact with body secretions or excretions or with dampness in skinfolds.

The nurse palpates the surface temperature of the skin over the pressure areas (warming the hands first). The temperature is normally the same as that of the surrounding skin. Increased temperature is abnormal and may be due to inflammation or blood trapped in the area. The nurse palpates over bony prominences and dependent body areas for the presence of edema, which feels spongy or boggy. If an area of pressure injury is open or visibly infected, the nurse should wear gloves during the examination.

If a pressure injury is present, the nurse notes the following:

- Location of the injury related to a bony prominence
- Size of ulcer in centimeters. (Measure length, width, and depth, beginning with length [head to toe] and then width [side to side]. To measure depth, insert a sterile applicator swab at the deepest part of the wound, and then measure it against a measuring guide.)
- Presence of undermining or sinus tracts, assessed as face on a clock, where 12 o'clock is the patient's head
- Stage of the injury (see Table 21–10)
- Color of the wound bed and location of necrosis or eschar
- Condition of the wound margins
- Integrity of surrounding skin
- Clinical signs of infection, such as redness, warmth, swelling, pain, odor, and exudate (note color of exudate)
- Patient complaints of pain or discomfort at the wound site
- Signs of infection, such as fever, chills, or elevated WBC count.

The nurse documents the status of the patient's skin and wounds on the standard agency form. It is important to be able to determine how these change over time.

Several available risk assessment tools provide the nurse with systematic means of identifying patients at high risk for pressure injury development. The National Pressure Ulcer Advisory Panel (NPUAP, EPUAP, & PPPIA, 2014) recommends that these tools consider mental status; exposure to moisture; incontinence; device-related pressure, friction, and shear; immobility; inactivity; and nutritional deficits.

The most commonly used assessment tool in the United States is the Braden Scale for Predicting Pressure Sore Risk. The scale was developed in 1987 by Bergstrom, Braden, Laguzza, and Holman, and consists of six subscales: sensory perception, moisture, activity, mobility, nutrition, and friction and shear (see **Figure 21–29 »**). A total of 23 points is possible. An adult who scores below 18 points is considered at risk (Agency for Healthcare Research and Quality [AHCRQ], 2012). For best results, the nurse should be trained in proper use of the scale.

The Norton Scale for pressure area risk assessment was developed in the United Kingdom in 1962 and includes the categories of general physical condition, mental state, activity, mobility, and incontinence. With the addition of a medications category in 1987, the possible score is 24. Scores of 15 or 16 should be viewed as indicators—not predictors—of risk.

Assessment tools should be used when the patient first enters the healthcare agency and whenever the patient's condition changes. In some long-term care facilities, a risk assessment scale, such as the Braden or Norton scale, is used on admission and then on a regular basis, usually weekly. This schedule increases awareness of specific risk factors and provides assessment data to use in planning goals and interventions to either maintain or improve skin integrity.

Professional organizations advocate the use of assessment tools to identify patients at risk for development of pressure injury (AHCRQ, 2012). Research suggests, however, that there is no statistically significant difference in the incidence of pressure injuries in patients assessed using the Braden scale compared to other risk assessment tools (Moore & Cowman, 2014).

Diagnosis

The following NANDA-I diagnoses may be appropriate for the patient with a pressure ulcer:

- *Impaired Skin Integrity, Risk for*
- *Skin Integrity, Impaired*
- *Infection, Risk for*
- *Imbalanced Nutrition: Less Than Body Requirements*
- *Compromised Human Dignity, Risk for*
- *Situational Low Self-Esteem.*

(NANDA-I © 2014)

Planning

Outcomes to be developed in collaboration with the patient and caregivers include the following:

- The patient who is immobile or on bedrest will be repositioned every 2 hours. Appropriate positioning devices may be used.
- The patient who is mobile will maintain or improve activity levels.
- The patient will report any alterations, such as changes in pain level, redness, numbness, tingling, or increased drainage.
- The patient will articulate the importance of maintaining adequate nutrition and hydration.
- The patient will describe measures to protect and heal tissue.

Implementation

Nursing implementations depend on the patient's mobility, risk factors for developing pressure ulcers, and staging of existing ulcers. Nursing care focuses on ulcer and infection prevention.

BRADEN SCALE FOR PREDICTING PRESSURE SORE RISK

Patient's Name _____ Evaluator's Name _____ Date of Assessment _____

SENSORY PERCEPTION
Ability to respond meaningfully to pressure-related discomfort

1. **Completely Limited:** Unresponsive (does not moan, flinch, or grasp) to painful stimuli, due to diminished level of consciousness or sedation, OR limited ability to feel pain over most of body surface.

2. **Very Limited:** Responds only to painful stimuli. Cannot communicate discomfort except by moaning or restlessness, OR has a sensory impairment which limits the ability to feel pain or discomfort over 1/2 of body.

3. **Slightly Limited:** Responds to verbal commands but cannot always communicate discomfort or need to be turned, OR has some sensory impairment which limits ability to feel pain or discomfort in 1 or 2 extremities.

4. **No Impairment:** Responds to verbal commands. Has no sensory deficit which would limit ability to feel or voice pain or discomfort.

MOISTURE
Degree to which skin is exposed to moisture

1. **Constantly Moist:** Skin is kept moist almost constantly by perspiration, urine, etc. Dampness is detected every time patient is moved or turned.

2. **Moist:** Skin is often but not always moist. Linen must be changed at least once a shift.

3. **Occasionally Moist:** Skin is occasionally moist, requiring an extra linen change approximately once a day.

4. **Rarely Moist:** Skin is usually dry; linen requires changing only at routine intervals.

ACTIVITY
Degree of physical activity

1. **Bedfast:** Confined to bed.

2. **Chairfast:** Ability to walk severely limited or nonexistent. Cannot bear own weight and/or must be assisted into chair or wheelchair.

3. **Walks Occasionally:** Walks occasionally during day but for very short distances, with or without assistance. Spends majority of each shift in bed or chair.

4. **Walks Frequently:** Walks outside the room at least twice a day and inside room at least once every 2 hours during waking hours.

MOBILITY
Ability to change and control body position

1. **Completely Immobile:** Does not make even slight changes in body or extremity position without assistance.

2. **Very Limited:** Makes occasional slight changes in body or extremity position but unable to make frequent or significant changes independently.

3. **Slightly Limited:** Makes frequent though slight changes in body or extremity position independently.

4. **No Limitations:** Makes major and frequent changes in position without assistance.

NUTRITION
Usual food intake pattern

1. **Very Poor:** Never eats a complete meal. Rarely eats more than 1/3 of any food offered. Eats 2 servings or less of protein (meat or dairy products) per day. Takes fluids poorly. Does not take a liquid dietary supplement, OR is NPO and/or maintained on clear liquids or IV's for more than 5 days.

2. **Probably Inadequate:** Rarely eats a complete meal and generally eats only about 1/2 of any food offered. Protein intake includes only 3 servings of meat or dairy products per day. Occasionally will take a dietary supplement, OR receives less than optimum amount of liquid diet or tube feeding.

3. **Adequate:** Eats over half of most meals. Eats a total of 4 servings of protein (meat, dairy products) each day. Occasionally will refuse a meal, but will usually take a supplement if offered, OR is on a tube feeding or TPN regimen, which probably meets most of nutritional needs.

4. **Excellent:** Eats most of every meal. Never refuses a meal. Usually eats a total of 4 or more servings of meat and dairy products. Occasionally eats between meals. Does not require supplementation.

FRICTION AND SHEAR

1. **Problem:** Requires moderate to maximum assistance in moving. Complete lifting without sliding against sheets is impossible. Frequently slides down in bed or chair, requiring frequent repositioning with maximum assistance. Spasticity, contractures, or agitation leads to almost constant friction.

2. **Potential Problem:** Moves feebly or requires minimum assistance. During a move skin probably slides to some extent against sheets, chair, restraints, or other devices. Maintains relatively good position in chair or bed most of the time but occasionally slides down.

3. **No Apparent Problem:** Moves in bed and in chair independently and has sufficient muscle strength to lift up completely during move. Maintains good position in bed or chair at all times.

Total Score _____

Figure 21–29 ≫ Braden Scale for Predicting Pressure Sore Risk.

Maintain Skin Integrity

Interventions for patients with or at risk for impaired skin integrity include the following:

- Conduct a systematic skin inspection at least once a day, paying particular attention to the bony prominences. Systematic, comprehensive, and routine skin care may decrease pressure ulcer incidence (although the exact role is unknown). Skin inspection provides data the nurse uses in designing interventions to reduce risk and in evaluating outcomes of those interventions.

- Clean the skin at the time of soiling and at routine intervals, as frequently as the patient's need or preference dictates. Avoid hot water, use a mild cleansing agent, and clean the skin gently, applying as little force and friction as possible. Metabolic wastes and environmental contaminants accumulate on the skin; these potentially irritating substances should be removed frequently. Feces and urine cause chemical irritation and should be removed as soon as possible.

- Minimize environmental factors leading to skin drying, such as low humidity and exposure to cold. Treat dry skin with moisturizers. Well-hydrated skin resists mechanical trauma. Hydration decreases as the ambient air temperature decreases, especially when the air humidity is low. Poorly hydrated skin is less pliable, and severe dryness is associated with fissuring and cracking of the stratum corneum.

- Avoid massaging over bony prominences. Although massage has been practiced for years, evidence now suggests that massage over bony prominences may lead to deep tissue trauma in patients at risk for, or with beginning, skin manifestations of a pressure injury.

- Minimize skin exposure to moisture due to incontinence, perspiration, or wound drainage. When these sources of moisture cannot be controlled, use underpads or briefs made of materials that absorb moisture and present a quick-drying surface to the skin. Change underpads and briefs frequently. Do not place plastic directly against the skin. Moisture from incontinence, perspiration, or wound drainage may contain factors that irritate the skin; moisture alone can increase the susceptibility of the skin to injury.

- To minimize skin injury due to friction and shearing forces, use proper positioning, transferring, and turning techniques. Shear injury occurs when skin remains stationary and the underlying tissue shifts. This shift diminishes the blood supply to the skin; the result is ischemia and tissue damage. Proper positioning, however, can eliminate most shear injuries. Friction injuries occur when the skin moves across a coarse surface, such as bed linens. Most friction injuries can be prevented by the use of appropriate techniques to move the patient so that the skin is never dragged across the linens. Any agent that eliminates contact or decreases the friction between the skin and the linens reduces the potential for injury.

- For the patient who is immobile or on bedrest, provide interventions against the adverse effects of external mechanical forces of pressure, friction, and shear:
  a. Reposition the at-risk patient at least every 2 hours, using a written schedule for systematic turning and repositioning. Immobility increases the risk for pressure injury development, and position changes optimize circulation to all tissues and relieve pressure.
  b. For the patient on bedrest, use positioning devices, such as pillows or foam wedges, to protect bony prominences.

- For the patient who is completely immobile, use devices to relieve pressure on the heels (the most common method is to raise the heels off the bed). Do not use doughnut-type devices. Patients who spend an increased amount of time on one surface need a pressure reduction or pressure relief device to reduce the risk of pressure injury. Doughnut-type devices can create areas of increased pressure that may damage tissue.

- Avoid placing the patient in the side-lying position directly on the trochanter. This bony prominence area places the patient at greater risk for pressure injury resulting from tissue ischemia from compression against a hard surface.

- Maintain the head of the bed at the lowest degree of elevation consistent with the patient's medical condition and other restrictions. Limit the amount of time the head of the bed is elevated. This decreases the risk for pressure injury to bony prominence areas such as the sacrum.

- Use assistive devices, such as a trapeze or bed linen, to move the patient in bed who cannot assist during transfers and position changes. The use of these devices helps reduce the risk of sheer or friction injury.

- For the patient who is chair-bound, use pressure-reducing devices. Consider postural alignment, distribution of weight, balance and stability, and pressure relief when positioning the patient. Avoid uninterrupted sitting in a chair or wheelchair. Reposition the patient every hour. Teach patients who can do so to shift their weight every 15 minutes. Use a written plan for positioning, movement, and the use of positioning devices.

Prevent Infection of Pressure Injuries

Untreated pressure injuries can become infected quickly. The nurse working with a patient who is at risk for pressure injuries should teach the patient to guard against infection by doing the following:

- Maintaining skin hygiene. Keeping the skin clean, dry, and moisturized is important to prevent the development of pressure injury.

- Maintaining appropriate nutrition and hydration. Adequate nutrition, especially protein and carbohydrate intake, as well as hydration status are important in maintenance of skin integrity and promotion of wound healing.

- Recognizing the early stages of a pressure injury. This allows for early intervention and prevention of additional injury.

- Contacting the healthcare provider at the earliest appearance of a pressure injury or change in skin integrity. This allows for immediate assessment and intervention to prevent development of further tissue injury.

- Maintaining or improving current activity levels. This increases patient independence, improves self-esteem, and reduces the potential for the development of immobility and pressure injury.

Prevent Nutritional Imbalance

Although the role nutrition plays in the development of (and to a lesser degree, the healing of) pressure injuries is not well understood, poor dietary intake of kilocalories, protein, and iron has been associated with the development of pressure injuries. The nurse should assess factors related to dietary intake, offer nutritional supplements, and provide support as necessary during mealtimes to ensure adequate dietary intake. If barriers to adequate nutrition are found on assessment, the nurse works with the patient to find solutions to reduce or eliminate these barriers. If, after interventions and support, the patient's dietary intake remains inadequate, the nurse consults with a dietitian for strategies to improve the patient's nutritional status.

Prevent Compromised Human Dignity and Situational Low Self-Esteem

The patient who is immobile or nearly immobile is at the mercy of the individuals who are responsible for caregiving. If family members or caregivers do not implement interventions necessary to inhibit the growth of pressure injuries and maintain patient hygiene, the patient is at risk for compromised human dignity, which can affect a patient's moods and perception of self, in turn putting the patient at risk for situational

low self-esteem. Depression can follow quickly. The nurse can assist the patient in these areas by doing the following:

- Assessing the patient for indicators of abuse or neglect at each healthcare interaction
- Developing a trusting, caring relationship to promote the patient's comfort with discussing issues related to dignity and self-esteem
- Providing essential patient and family teaching to reduce the risk of pressure injury development and promote the dignity of the patient
- Assisting patients and family members with obtaining supportive devices to help the patient maintain appropriate positioning.

Evaluation

For the patient who is immobile or on bedrest, the treatment plan may need to be evaluated and modified as often as daily, depending on the assessment of the patient's skin integrity, patient comfort and pain level, and whether or not the written repositioning plan has been followed. Patients who are in bed for long periods of time can experience a diminished appetite. For a patient who is not maintaining adequate dietary intake, even with changes to the nutrition plan, the nurse may need to consult with a nutritionist or dietitian. The nurse should inform patients who are mobile when to call the office if they discover another potential pressure ulcer or change in skin integrity.

Nursing Care Plan
A Patient with a Pressure Injury

Agnes Pimm, age 74, recently underwent knee replacement surgery. She was hospitalized for a week following her surgery, after which she spent 4 weeks at a rehabilitation facility. She returned to her home earlier this week and has arranged for a home health agency nurse to visit her daily. Her surgical incision and the bone are healing nicely; during her time at the rehabilitation facility, how-

ever, she developed a stage 3 pressure injury on the leg where her supportive knee brace rubs against her skin. She does not want to take the brace off because she does not want to leave her knee unsupported; however, the ulcer is causing her a great deal of pain, especially since she has been weaned off the prescription pain medication she was taking postoperatively.

ASSESSMENT	DIAGNOSES	PLANNING
Jessi Fletcher, RN, is the agency nurse assigned to Ms. Pimm. During her visit to Ms. Pimm's home, she obtains a history and does a physical examination. Nurse Fletcher notes that Ms. Pimm's husband died 6 months ago after a lengthy battle with prostate cancer; since her husband's death, Ms. Pimm has not "felt much like eating" and states that what she does eat is canned or frozen. As a result, Ms. Pimm's diet is high in sodium and low in protein. The sodium is of particular concern in light of Ms. Pimm's history of hypertension. Ms. Pimm also indicates that she is a smoker; she has smoked on and off for 50 years, having quit for several years at a time during that span. She indicates that she always returned to smoking during particularly stressful times; her most recent return to cigarettes came during her husband's illness. Ms. Pimm is very proud that her husband remained at home for the duration of his illness, and she wants to be as independent as possible during her own recovery; therefore, she has turned down an offer from her son to stay with him until she recovers. She also does not want to return to the rehabilitation facility because it made her feel "very cramped and claustrophobic."	■ *Risk for Infection* related to pressure injury ■ *Impaired Tissue Integrity* related to prolonged pressure, inadequate nutrition, and decreased vascular perfusion associated with smoking ■ *Acute Pain* related to stage 3 injury and postoperative recovery ■ *Imbalanced Nutrition: Less Than Body Requirements* related to loss of appetite and grieving ■ *Grieving* related to loss of spouse (NANDA-I © 2014)	Goals for Ms. Pimm's care include the following: ■ The patient will describe measures to protect and heal the tissue. ■ The patient will demonstrate no signs or symptoms of infection. ■ The patient will report any additional symptoms or changes immediately. ■ The patient will demonstrate an understanding of nutrition that supports wound healing.

(continued on next page)

Nursing Care Plan (continued)

ASSESSMENT	DIAGNOSES	PLANNING
Ms. Pimm is clean and well-groomed, and her home is tidy. She is thin but is very strong and shows no signs of frailty. She is capable of performing most ADLs but mentions that the surgery and the pain from the ulcer have slowed her down and that she "sometimes takes all day" to get washed and dressed and the house picked up. Ms. Pimm's vital signs include temperature 98.3°F oral; pulse 75 bpm; respirations 20/min; and BP 141/84 mmHg. Upon inspection of the pressure injury, Nurse Fletcher notes that it is a roughly 4-cm × 4-cm stage 3 ulcer that involves full-thickness skin loss with damage to the subcutaneous tissue. No necrotic tissue is present, and the underlying bone, tendon, and muscle are not exposed. Undermining and tunneling are not present, and there are no signs of inflammation or infection. She cleanses the wound and applies a hydrocolloid dressing, which should be changed every third day. Nurse Fletcher then contacts Ms. Pimm's surgeon, who indicates that she no longer needs to wear the immobilizer brace she has been wearing. He states that if Ms. Pimm feels more comfortable with some kind of support on the area, she can wear a soft elastic sleeve-type brace and should wear it only when sleeping or walking. He also indicates that OTC ibuprofen is appropriate for both postoperative and ulcer pain if needed, and that it should be taken according to the directions on the package.		■ The patient will decrease her per-day consumption of cigarettes. ■ The patient will remain in her home and maintain independence.

IMPLEMENTATION

- Administer antibiotics as ordered.
- Teach about wound care and infection prevention, and demonstrate the proper method for cleaning and dressing the pressure ulcer.
- Describe changes to the wound that indicate the development of infection or a deterioration of the wound site.

- Demonstrate how to use a soft elastic brace, and review when and how it should be used.
- Teach about nutrition that promotes wound healing.
- Provide information about smoking cessation and support groups.

EVALUATION

Nurse Fletcher initially changes Ms. Pimm's dressing and cleanses her wound every third day. Over time, Ms. Pimm takes over this responsibility and is very serious about wound care and infection prevention. Nurse Fletcher is able to decrease the frequency of her visits to Ms. Pimm's home from every day to three times per week. The wound remains infection free and, after a month with the hydrocolloid dressings, is restaged as a stage 2 injury. At this point, treatment continues with hydrocolloid dressings that require changing every fifth day, rather than every third day.

Nurse Fletcher also refers Ms. Pimm to a dietitian, who outlines a meal plan that promotes wound healing, appeals to Ms. Pimm's tastes, is appropriate for someone with hypertension, and is easy to prepare. Ms. Pimm struggles with her diet a bit, because it is difficult for her to visit the store and purchase fresh foods and because she continues to struggle with a lack of appetite. However, she verbalizes an understanding of the need to eat a healthier diet and makes an effort to follow the dietitian's meal plan as best she can.

Finally, Ms. Pimm continues to struggle with smoking cessation. She has tried several methods to decrease her cigarette consumption but states that continued stress about her husband's death and her current condition prevents her from making much progress. Nurse Fletcher refers Ms. Pimm to several community resources for smoking cessation.

CRITICAL THINKING

1. How would you adapt Ms. Pimm's care plan if the surgeon indicated that she was required to wear the brace that caused the ulcer?
2. Suppose that Ms. Pimm's ulcer had progressed to stage 4 after a month of treatment rather than improving to stage 2. How would her treatment regimen change? Would the goals and implementation for her care change as well?
3. Develop a care plan for the nursing diagnosis *Impaired Tissue Integrity* related to physical immobilization.

REVIEW Pressure Injuries

RELATE Link the Concepts and Exemplars

Linking the exemplar of pressure ulcers with the concept of infection:

1. What assessment findings would cause you to believe a pressure injury is infected?

2. What nursing interventions can be implemented to reduce the risk of infection of a pressure injury?

Linking the exemplar of pressure ulcers with the concept of mobility:

3. Contrast appropriate nursing interventions to prevent pressure injuries in patients age 6, 30, and 80 with limited mobility.

4. You are caring for a child who was involved in a bicycle accident resulting in below-the-waist paraplegia. How will you teach the parents to reduce the risk of pressure injuries?

READY Go to Volume 3: Clinical Nursing Skills

REFER Go to Pearson MyLab Nursing and eText

- Additional review materials

REFLECT Apply Your Knowledge

Lydia Ocampo is a 69-year-old widow who has recently been moved from a rehabilitation center to the skilled nursing wing of a nursing facility. She is still receiving care related to surgery on a broken hip a couple of months before. Before that, she had lived in the home that she shared with her husband of 50 years. Her husband died a few weeks ago. Ms. Ocampo has Alzheimer disease. At the nursing home, she exhibits intermittent confusion and is alternately passive and uncooperative with the staff. Over the course of the next month, her condition deteriorates. She eats very little and is fairly unresponsive to caregivers. She sleeps often.

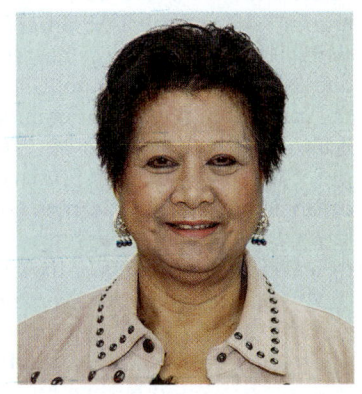

1. What data suggest that Ms. Ocampo is particularly vulnerable to pressure injury development?

2. What additional information do you need in order to use the Braden scale to determine Ms. Ocampo's potential for pressure ulcer development?

3. What independent measures can you take to protect Ms. Ocampo's skin from further breakdown?

4. Considering that Ms. Ocampo does not have any areas of skin breakdown, why is it important to institute treatment for pressure injuries at this time?

» Exemplar 21.C
Wound Healing

Exemplar Learning Outcomes

21.C Analyze wound healing as it relates to tissue integrity.

- Describe the phases of wound healing, risk factors for complications, and health promotion for good wound healing.
- Identify the clinical manifestations of wounds.
- Summarize diagnostic tests and therapies used by interprofessional teams in the collaborative care of an individual with a wound.
- Differentiate considerations for care of patients with wounds across the lifespan.
- Apply the nursing process in providing culturally competent care to an individual with a wound.

Exemplar Key Terms

Approximated, *1634*
Collagen, *1635*
Dehiscence, *1635*
Evisceration, *1635*
Exudate, *1636*
Fibrin, *1634*
Granulation tissue, *1635*
Hematoma, *1635*
Hemorrhage, *1635*
Hemostasis, *1634*
Keloid, *1635*
Macrophages, *1634*
Phagocytosis, *1635*
Primary intention healing, *1634*
Purulent exudate, *1636*
Pus, *1636*
Pyogenic bacteria, *1636*
Regeneration, *1633*
Sanguineous (hemorrhagic) exudate, *1636*
Secondary intention healing, *1634*
Serosanguineous exudate, *1636*
Serous exudate, *1636*
Suppuration, *1636*
Tertiary intention healing, *1634*

Overview

Healing is a quality of living tissue; it is also referred to as **regeneration** (renewal) of tissues. Healing can be considered in terms of *types of healing,* having to do with the caregiver's decision about whether to allow the wound to seal itself or to purposefully close the wound, and *phases of healing,* which refer to the steps in the body's natural processes of tissue repair. The phases are the same for all wounds, but the rate of healing depends on factors such as the type of healing, the location and size of the wound, and the patient's health.

Physiology

There are two types of healing, each influenced by the amount of tissue loss. **Primary intention healing** occurs where the tissue surfaces have been **approximated** (closed) and there is minimal or no tissue loss; it is characterized by the formation of minimal granulation tissue and scarring. It is also called *primary union* or *first intention healing*. An example of wound healing by primary intention is a closed surgical incision. Other examples would be the use of staples, tapes (Steri-Strips), or tissue adhesive, a liquid "glue," used to seal clean lacerations or incisions (Olin, 2012).

A wound that is extensive and involves considerable tissue loss and in which the edges cannot or should not be approximated heals by **secondary intention healing**. An example of wound healing by secondary intention is a pressure ulcer. Secondary intention healing differs from primary intention healing in three ways: The repair time is longer, the scarring is greater, and the susceptibility to infection is greater.

Those wounds that are left open for 3–5 days to allow edema or infection to resolve or to permit exudate to drain and then are closed with sutures, staples, or adhesive skin closures, undergo **tertiary intention healing**. This is also called *delayed primary intention healing*.

Phases of Wound Healing

Wound healing can be broken down into three phases: inflammatory, proliferative, and maturation or remodeling (see **Figure 21–30 »**).

Inflammatory Phase

The inflammatory phase is initiated immediately after injury and lasts 3–6 days. Two major processes occur during this phase: hemostasis and phagocytosis.

Hemostasis (the cessation of bleeding) results from vasoconstriction of the larger blood vessels in the affected area, the retraction (drawing back) of injured blood vessels, the deposition of **fibrin** (connective tissue), and the formation of blood clots in the area. The blood clots, formed from blood platelets, provide a matrix of fibrin that becomes the framework for cell repair. A scab also forms on the surface of the wound. Consisting of clots and dead and dying tissue, the scab aids hemostasis and inhibits contamination of the wound by microorganisms. Below the scab, epithelial cells migrate into the wound from the edges. The epithelial cells serve as a barrier between the body and the environment, preventing the entry of microorganisms.

The inflammatory phase also involves vascular and cellular responses intended to remove any foreign substances as well as dead and dying tissues. The blood supply to the wound increases, bringing with it oxygen and nutrients needed in the healing process. As a result, the area appears reddened and edematous. Exudate of fluid and cell debris is a normal accumulation and helps cleanse the wound. Overproduction of this exudate and other factors can impair wound healing, especially of chronic wounds (Bianchi, 2012).

During cell migration, leukocytes (specifically, neutrophils) move into the interstitial space. These are replaced about 24 hours after injury by **macrophages** (large cells of

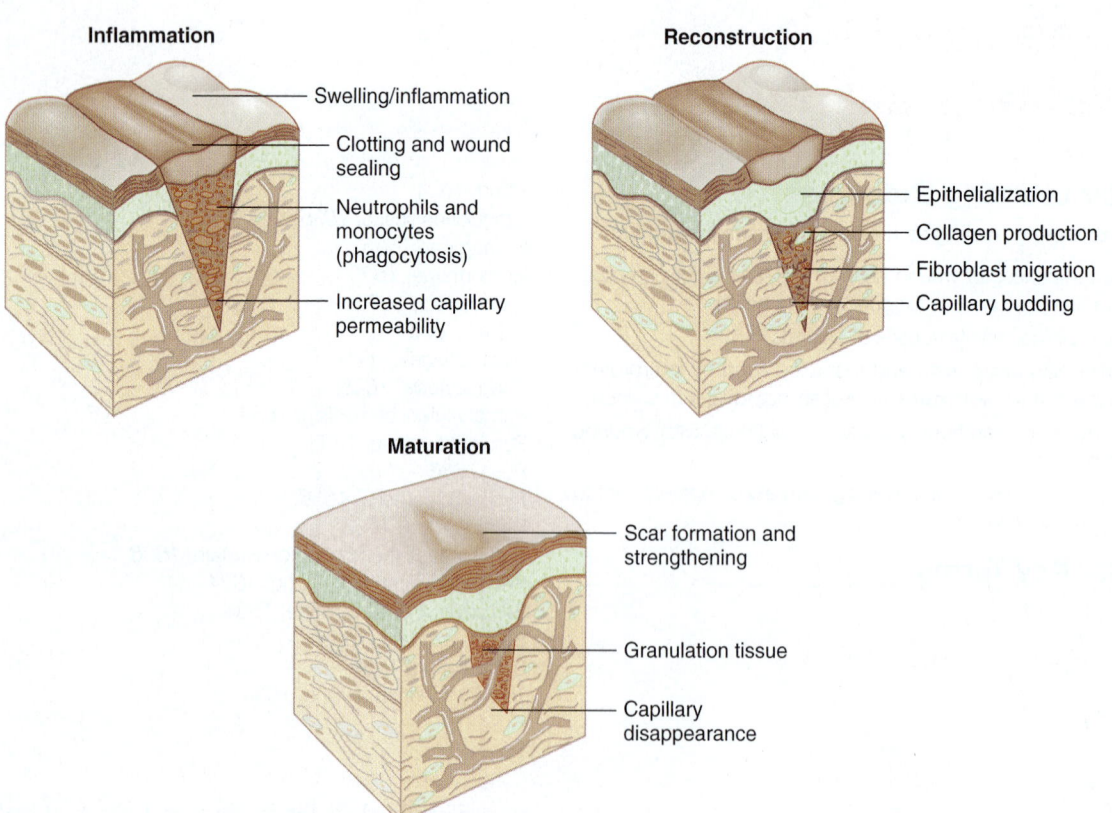

Inflammation
- Swelling/inflammation
- Clotting and wound sealing
- Neutrophils and monocytes (phagocytosis)
- Increased capillary permeability

Reconstruction
- Epithelialization
- Collagen production
- Fibroblast migration
- Capillary budding

Maturation
- Scar formation and strengthening
- Granulation tissue
- Capillary disappearance

Source: Data from Nicol, N. H., Heuther, S. E., & Weber, R. (2006). Structure, function, and disorders of the integument. In K. L. McCance & S. E. Huether (Eds.), *Pathophysiology: The biologic basis for disease in adults and children* (5th ed., pp. 1573–1607). St. Louis, MO: Elsevier Mosby.

Figure 21–30 » Wound healing occurs in three overlapping phases.

the immune system that remove waste and harmful micro-organisms), which arise from the blood monocytes. These macrophages engulf microorganisms and cellular debris by a process known as **phagocytosis**. The macrophages also secrete an angiogenesis factor, which stimulates the formation of epithelial buds at the end of injured blood vessels. The microcirculatory network that results sustains the healing process and the wound during its life. This inflammatory response is essential to healing. Measures that impair inflammation, such as steroid medications, can place the healing process at risk.

Proliferative Phase

The proliferative phase, the second phase in healing, extends from day 3 or 4 to about day 21 postinjury. Fibroblasts (connective tissue cells), which migrate into the wound starting about 24 hours after injury, begin to synthesize collagen. **Collagen** is a whitish protein substance that adds tensile strength to the wound. As the amount of collagen increases, so does the strength of the wound; therefore, the chance that the wound will remain closed increases progressively. If the wound is sutured, a raised "healing ridge" appears under the intact suture line. In a wound that is not sutured, the new collagen is often visible.

Capillaries grow across the wound, increasing the blood supply. Fibroblasts move from the bloodstream into the wound, depositing fibrin. As the capillary network develops, the tissue becomes a translucent red. This tissue, called **granulation tissue**, is fragile and bleeds easily.

When the skin edges of a wound are not sutured, the area must be filled in with granulation tissue. When the granulation tissue matures, marginal epithelial cells migrate to it, proliferating over this connective tissue base to fill the wound. If the wound does not close by epithelialization, the area becomes covered by a scab or dry crust, called eschar, formed by dried plasma proteins and dead cells. Wounds healing by secondary intention initially seep blood-tinged (serosanguineous) drainage. Later, if the wounds are not covered by epithelial cells, they become covered with thick, gray, fibrinous tissue that is eventually converted into dense scar tissue.

Maturation Phase

The maturation phase begins about day 21 and can extend 1–2 years after the injury. Fibroblasts continue to synthesize collagen. The collagen fibers themselves, which were initially laid haphazardly, reorganize into a more orderly structure. During maturation, the wound site is remodeled and contracted. The scar becomes stronger, but the repaired area is never as strong as the original tissue. In some individuals, particularly those with dark skin, an abnormal amount of collagen appears. The result can be a hypertrophic scar or **keloid**.

Risk Factors for Complications

Several untoward events can interfere with the healing of a wound: hemorrhage, infection, dehiscence, and evisceration.

Hemorrhage

Some escape of blood from a wound is normal. **Hemorrhage** (massive bleeding), however, is abnormal. A dislodged clot, a slipped stitch, or an erosion of a blood vessel may cause severe bleeding.

Internal hemorrhage may be indicated by swelling or distention in the area of the wound and, possibly, by sanguineous drainage from a surgical drain. Some patients have a **hematoma**, a localized collection of blood underneath the skin that may appear as a reddish blue swelling (bruise). A large hematoma may be dangerous because it can place pressure on blood vessels, thereby obstructing blood flow.

The risk of hemorrhage is greatest during the first 48 hours after surgery. Hemorrhage is an emergency; the nurse applies pressure dressings to the area and monitors the patient's vital signs. In many instances, the patient must be taken to the operating room for surgical intervention.

Infection

Contamination of a wound surface with microorganisms (colonization) is inevitable. Because the colonizing organisms compete with new cells for oxygen and nutrition and because their by-products can interfere with a healthy surface condition, the presence of contamination can impair wound healing and lead to infection. When the microorganisms colonizing the wound multiply excessively or invade tissues, infection occurs. Infection is suggested by a change in wound color, pain, or drainage and is confirmed by a culture of the wound. Severe infection causes fever and elevated WBC count. Patients who are immunosuppressed, such as those with HIV infection or those receiving myelosuppressive treatment for cancer, are especially susceptible to wound infections.

A wound can be infected with microorganisms at the time of injury, during surgery, or postoperatively. Wounds that occur as a result of injury (e.g., bullet and knife wounds) are most likely to be contaminated at the time of injury. Surgery involving the intestines can also result in infection from microorganisms inside the intestine. Surgical infection becomes apparent 2–11 days postoperatively.

Dehiscence with Possible Evisceration

Dehiscence is the partial or total rupture of a sutured wound. Dehiscence usually involves an abdominal wound in which the layers below the skin also separate. **Evisceration** is the protrusion of the internal viscera through an incision. A number of factors, including obesity, poor nutrition, multiple trauma, failure of suturing, excessive coughing, vomiting, and dehydration heighten a patient's risk of wound dehiscence. Comorbidities such as diabetes place patients at additional risk. Wound dehiscence is most likely to occur 4–5 days postoperatively, before extensive collagen has been deposited in the wound.

Sudden straining, such as coughing or sneezing, may precede dehiscence. It is not unusual for a patient to feel that "something has given way." When dehiscence or evisceration occurs, the wound should be supported quickly by large sterile dressings soaked in sterile normal saline. The nurse should place the patient in bed with knees bent to decrease pull on the incision. The surgeon must be notified because immediate surgical repair of the area may be necessary.

Health Promotion

Characteristics of the individual, such as age, nutritional status, lifestyle, and medications influence the speed of wound healing. The modifiable factors among this group affect the overall health of an individual. In general, habits that promote overall good health—such as eating a balanced diet and exercising—promote wound healing; conversely, habits that do not promote good health can lead to impaired healing.

Nutrition

Wound healing places additional demands on the body. The patient requires a diet rich in protein; carbohydrates; lipids; vitamins A and C; and minerals such as iron, zinc, and copper. Patients who are malnourished may require time to improve their nutritional status—before surgery, if possible. Patients who are obese are at increased risk of wound infection and slower healing because adipose tissue usually has a minimal blood supply.

Lifestyle

Patients who exercise regularly tend to have good circulation and are more likely to heal quickly because blood brings oxygen and nourishment to the wound. Smoking constricts arterioles and reduces the amount of functional hemoglobin in the blood, thus limiting the oxygen-carrying capacity of the blood. As a result, smokers are at risk for delayed healing.

Medications

Anti-inflammatory drugs (e.g., steroids, aspirin) and antineoplastic agents interfere with healing. Prolonged use of antibiotics may make an individual susceptible to wound infection by resistant organisms.

Clinical Manifestations

Exudate is material, such as fluid and dead phagocytic cells, that has escaped from blood vessels during the inflammatory process and is deposited in tissue or on tissue surfaces. The nature and amount of exudate vary according to the tissue involved, the intensity and duration of the inflammation, and the presence of microorganisms.

There are three major types of exudate: serous, purulent, and sanguineous (hemorrhagic). A **serous exudate** typically accompanies mild inflammation and presents as clear or straw colored. It is thin and watery and has few cells. An example is the fluid in a blister from a burn.

A **purulent exudate** is thicker than serous exudate and consists of a large quantity of cells and necrotic debris; it is usually opaque or milky in appearance. The formation of purulent exudate, commonly known as **pus**, is referred to as **suppuration**, and the bacteria that produce pus are called **pyogenic bacteria**. Not all microorganisms are pyogenic. Purulent exudates can vary in color, sometimes acquiring tinges of blue, green, or yellow. The color may depend on the causative organism.

A **sanguineous (hemorrhagic) exudate** consists of large amounts of RBCs, indicating damage to capillaries that is severe enough to allow the escape of RBCs from plasma. Bright sanguineous exudate indicates fresh bleeding, while dark sanguineous exudate denotes older bleeding. This type of exudate is frequently seen in open wounds.

Mixed types of exudates are often observed. A **serosanguineous exudate** (consisting of clear and blood-tinged drainage) is commonly seen in surgical incisions. A purosanguineous discharge (consisting of pus and blood) is often seen in a new wound that is infected.

Collaboration

Under normal circumstances, collaborative efforts related to wound healing are wellness oriented. Efforts should focus on promoting healing and preventing infection. The patient should be taught how to recognize signs of infection and other complications of impaired healing and be coached to contact the healthcare provider immediately if symptoms develop. When healing is impaired, the first priority is addressing any life-threatening complications, such as hemorrhage or evisceration. The focus then shifts back to promotion of healing and prevention of infection. Impaired healing

Clinical Manifestations and Therapies
Impaired Wound Healing

ETIOLOGY	CLINICAL MANIFESTATIONS	CLINICAL THERAPIES
Massive bleeding (hemorrhage)	■ Swelling, wound distention, sanguineous drainage, and hematoma indicate internal hemorrhage. ■ Rapid loss of blood and the onset of shock indicate external hemorrhage.	■ Pressure dressings ■ Emergency surgery
Infection by colonized microorganisms	■ Wound color changes, and pain or drainage increases. ■ Edema may develop, and skin may become red and warm to the touch.	■ Antibiotics ■ Debridement ■ Protective dressings ■ Infection prevention measures
Rupture of a sutured wound (dehiscence)	■ Wound opens spontaneously with possible bleeding, pain, or inflammation. ■ Protrusion of underlying tissue or organs indicates evisceration.	■ Supportive dressings ■ Positioning to decrease pressure ■ Antibiotics ■ Debridement ■ Emergency surgery

may also result in significant discomfort for the patient, so pain management strategies may also be appropriate.

Diagnostic Tests

If infection is suspected, a culture and sensitivity test may be performed. The culture identifies the causative organism, and the sensitivity test determines which medication is most appropriate for treating the infection. For a culture, drainage or tissue is collected from the wound and placed in a medium that promotes bacterial growth. In most cases, the sensitivity test indicates an antibiotic.

Surgery

In the event of life-threatening complications, surgery may be performed to repair damaged tissues or vessels and to reclose the wound. In nonemergency situations, surgery may also be indicated if healing is ineffective. The presence of slough, eschar, or necrotic tissue indicates ineffective healing.

Surgical debridement is appropriate for wounds with large amounts of infected and necrotic tissue. It may also be used to treat wounds that abscess. During this procedure, the wound is flushed with saline solution, and topical anesthetic is applied. Forceps are used to grip the necrotic tissue, which is then cut away with a scalpel. Depending upon the extent of the necrosis and the amount of living tissue affected, debridement may take place in multiple sessions. In some cases, a laser rather than a scalpel is used to cut away the dead tissue.

Escharotomy is performed to treat full-thickness wounds that encircle or nearly encircle a body part and have formed eschar; these wounds are often caused by burns. The inelasticity of the eschar restricts the flow of blood and extracellular fluids and can lead to fluid accumulation and increased pressure inferior to the wound. If left untreated, this pressure can cause compartmental tissue damage. Escharotomy is the surgical removal of the eschar. During the procedure, incisions are made along the damaged area to release pressure; the swelling of the tissue causes the incisions to spread and exposes the underlying tissue and structures. The patient is usually sedated during the procedure, and the wound is covered with a moist dressing after the procedure.

Pharmacologic Therapy

Pharmacologic therapy of wounds depends upon whether wound healing is normal or impaired. For normal wound healing, therapies may include antibacterial ointments, prophylactic antibiotics, and analgesics for pain. Alternative therapies such as products containing aloe vera may also be used (see the Evidence-Based Practice feature).

Treatment for wounds with impaired healing depends upon the particular complication. Infected wounds are treated with antibiotics specific to the causative organism. In some cases, growth factors may be prescribed to promote healing; these factors simulate the body's own growth factor production and stimulate collagen and keratinocyte production and migration to wound sites. Growth factors for wound therapy often come in the form of topical gels that are applied directly to the wound, though some may be administered via injection. Other forms can be incorporated into wound dress-

ing or commercial skin graft products (Wound Care Centers, 2012). Opioids and NSAIDs may also be appropriate for management of pain associated with the wound.

Nonpharmacologic Therapy

Nonpharmacologic therapies for wound healing are diverse and include a number of techniques and procedures. For wounds with normal healing, these may include infection prevention measures; compression bandages or hosiery; and diets high in protein, carbohydrates, and vitamins to promote healing.

For wounds with impaired healing, VAC may be used. Vacuum-assisted wound closure is generally used only after traditional therapies have failed or if the wound is large; the FDA has approved this process for the management of poorly healing wounds. This noninvasive procedure involves the use of an open-pore foam placed in the wound cavity, a semi-occlusive dressing, suction tubing, and a suction device. Negative pressure is applied to remove excess fluid from the wound, thus improving oxygenation and blood flow to the area and promoting formation of granulation tissue. Vacuum-assisted closure has been indicated for use with a variety of wound types, including: chronic, acute, traumatic, and dehisced wounds; partial-thickness burns; and ulcers (diabetic, pressure venous insufficiency), flaps, and grafts. These devices should not be used on wounds with eschar, necrotic tissue, or malignancy present; untreated osteomyelitis; or wounds with exposed vessels, nerves, anastomotic sites, or organs (Huang et al., 2014).

The effects of VAC therapy have been found to be both location and disease specific. Patients who have wounds related to chronic disease process (e.g., diabetes, peripheral vascular disease) should also receive treatment for the comorbidity in conjunction with VAC therapy. VAC can be used postoperatively for closure of large wounds and is commonly used in preparation of skin graft sites (Huang et al., 2014). There is currently limited research related to the effectiveness of VAC therapy on surgical wounds that are healing by secondary intention (Dumville et al., 2015).

Other regenerative therapies include cellular therapies that introduce rapidly regenerating new cells—such as stem cells—into wounds to promote healing. This is especially promising in the older population (Duscher et al., 2016). Skin or tissue grafts—either of the patient's own skin or of donor skin—may also be appropriate in some cases.

Biosurgery may be used in nonhealing wounds with necrotic tissue or slough; in this procedure, sterile maggots are placed on the wound and digest the damaged tissue. The damage to surrounding healthy tissue is minimal. In some cases, biosurgery is preferable to surgical debridement of necrotic wounds.

For many patients, a combination of therapies is used. As a result, patients with wounds may receive care from a number of healthcare providers. Surgeons, nurses, scrub persons, anesthetists, phlebotomists, x-ray technicians, registration clerks, and emergency transporters are often involved in securing the safety and health of patients. Case managers and social workers are available based on patients' postdischarge needs. This interprofessional approach focuses on placing the patient in the best possible health status to achieve successful wound healing.

Evidence-Based Practice
Aloe Vera and Wound Healing

Problem

Many alternative health approaches are available for promotion of wound healing, including honey, iodine, aloe vera, phenytoin, and electrical stimulation. However, the research that supports the use of these practices is variable, and solid scientific evidence for their use is often lacking. It is the nurse's responsibility to understand the benefits and risks of using alternative therapies for wound healing.

Evidence

One of the most widely accepted, frequently used alternative therapies for wound healing is application of aloe vera. It is used for burns, sunburns, frostbite, psoriasis, cold sores, surgical wounds, pressure ulcers, inflammatory skin disorders, and other minor wounds (Pereira & Bártolo, 2016; World Health Organization [WHO], 2013). Aloe vera (*Aloe barbadensis miller*) is a cactuslike plant that produces a clear gel and yellow latex. The gel has proven to be most valuable in treatment of skin lesions; many Food and Drug Administration (FDA)–approved wound dressings and OTC topical gels contain aloe vera. Active components of aloe vera include vitamins A, B, C, and E; enzymes; minerals; sugars; anthraquinones; fatty acids; hormones; amino acids; lignin; and saponins, among others. These components give aloe vera its healing properties: reducing inflammation, neutralizing free radicals, preventing infection, reducing pain, stimulating fibroblast proliferation and activity, promoting wound closure, and binding moisture into the skin. Multiple studies have investigated the usefulness of aloe vera for treating a variety of acute and chronic wounds. One study examined the effectiveness of aloe vera gel in the wound-healing process of surgical wounds. This study showed a significant increase in stimulation of biologic activity and wound closure (Pereira & Bártolo, 2016). The effects are thought to be due to the improved infiltration of aloe vera into the skin tissue compared to other products. Another study of 30 patients conducted by Khorasani and colleagues in 2009, showed a beneficial effect of aloe vera cream (0.5% of aloe vera gel powder) compared to silver sulfadiazine for patients with second-degree burns. Patients in this study who were treated with aloe vera demonstrated a significantly faster re-epithelialization rate and faster wound-healing times (Pereira & Bártolo, 2016). Other studies have shown no difference in the results between the two treatments. A benefit of aloe vera application was also seen when it was applied to hemorrhoidectomy incisions but not when used to treat skin biopsy wounds or pressure ulcers (Dat et al., 2012).

Implications

Although generally safe when applied topically to minor wounds and burns, aloe vera is not clinically supported for all wounds. Before applying aloe, the nurse should fully research its known effects for the patient's specific type of wound. Because many products that contain aloe are available OTC and do not require a prescription, the nurse must use best judgment based on clinical research and personal experience before providing this treatment to patients. In addition, adverse reactions to aloe vera have been reported, including contact dermatitis, burning sensations, and allergic reaction. These reactions appear to be associated with anthraquinones found in the aloe latex. Aloe should not be used in patients with a known allergy to plants in the Liliaceae family (WHO, 2013). Before applying a lotion, cream, gel, or wound dressing containing aloe, the nurse should ask the patient about any known allergies or previous adverse reactions to aloe.

Critical Thinking Application

1. What are the advantages and disadvantages of using aloe vera to treat open wounds (e.g., cuts, surgical wounds) versus closed wounds (e.g., sunburns, psoriasis)?

2. What nursing interventions would you implement for a patient who develops contact dermatitis after being treated with a wound dressing containing aloe vera?

3. Develop a strategy for teaching patients about three alternative wound-healing treatments using clinical evidence that supports or opposes each treatment.

>> **Stay Current:** Advances have been made in the area of skin grafts. The American Podiatric Medical Association (APMA) has approved the use of placental allografts. These grafts are derived from dehydrated human placenta tissue and can be used in the treatment of chronic nonhealing wounds such as diabetic foot ulcers, venous leg ulcers, and pressure injuries. Read more about these grafts at http://www.woundsresearch.com/news/seal-approval-granted-2-allografts.

Lifespan Considerations

Healthy children and adults often heal more quickly than do older adults, who are more likely to have chronic diseases that hinder healing. For example, reduced liver function can impair the synthesis of blood clotting factors. Older adults are also at an increased risk of developing nutritional deficiencies. These deficiencies may reduce the numbers of RBCs and leukocytes, thus impeding the delivery of oxygen and the inflammatory response essential for wound healing. Diabetes, chronic lung disease, and cardiovascular disease also impair oxygen delivery to body tissues. In addition, vascular changes—such as atherosclerosis and atrophy of capillaries in the skin—impair blood flow to wounds.

Older adults who do not have chronic diseases may still experience slowed healing as a result of normal cellular and molecular changes. Chief among these changes is a delayed inflammatory response with fewer macrophages and decreased phagocytic activity. Cell renewal and collagen synthesis also slow with age. Vascularity is reduced, and collagen tissue is less flexible. These alterations in aging skin not only have an impact on the healing process, but they also make the skin more susceptible to damage from pressure, friction, and shearing. Scar maturation appears to be improved in comparison to younger individuals (Sgonc & Gruber, 2013).

Wound Healing in Newborns, Infants, and Children

The skin of newborns and infants is more fragile than that of older children and adults and is more susceptible to infection, shearing from friction, and burns. Newborns and infants in neonatal intensive care units (NICUs) may commonly experience contact irritation, surgical wounds, pressure injuries, or shear or IV infiltration injuries. Newborns who are extremely premature are at greater risk for abrasions and skin tears. This population is also at greater risk for bacterial and fungal infections due to decreased immunity levels, use of foreign devices, prolonged use of antibiotics, and environmental exposure (Amaya, 2013).

The two major infectious agents affecting the skin of children are *Staphylococcus* and fungi. Abrasions or small lacerations, commonly experienced by children, provide an entry in the skin for these organisms. Minor wounds should be cleaned with warm, soapy water, and covered with a sterile bandage; the nurse should instruct children not to touch the wound. Children with more serious skin lesions should be reminded not to touch the wound, drains, or dressing. These wounds should be covered with an appropriate bandage that will remain intact during the child's usual activities. If the wound is visually disturbing to the child, the transparent dressing can be covered with opaque material. In the case of younger children, wound care can be demonstrated on a doll. The nurse should reassure the child that the wound will not be permanent and that nothing will fall out of the child's body. Children should be restrained only when all alternatives to prevent bandage removal have been tried and when absolutely necessary.

Wound Healing in Older Adults

The older adult's skin is more fragile and can easily tear with removal of tape (especially adhesive tape). Paper tape and tape remover should be used as indicated, keeping tape use to the minimum required; extreme caution should be used during tape removal. Wrinkled skin should be held taut during application of a transparent dressing, and assistance should be obtained if needed. Older adults in long-term care facilities are often subject to factors such as immobility, malnutrition, and incontinence, all of which increase the risk for development of skin breakdown. Skin breakdown in this population can occur as quickly as within 2 hours, so skin assessments should be done with each repositioning of the patient. In addition, a thorough assessment of a patient's heels should be performed every shift; this area is at risk for breakdown because of friction and pressure on the bed.

NURSING PROCESS

Nursing care related to wounds is primarily directed toward promotion of healing and prevention of infection and other complications. This goal involves not only care and aseptic procedures when the patient is in the healthcare setting, but also patient teaching focused on ongoing care of the wound at home. The patient should understand not only how to clean, dress, and promote healing of wounds, but also how to identify signs of complications in the healing process.

Assessment

Nurses commonly assess both untreated and treated wounds. Untreated wounds usually are seen shortly after an injury (e.g., at the scene of an accident, in an emergency department). Assessment for these wounds is as follows:

- Assess the location and extent of tissue damage (e.g., partial thickness, full thickness). Measure the length, width, and depth of the wound.

- Inspect the wound for bleeding. The amount of bleeding varies with the type of wound and its location. Penetrating wounds may cause internal bleeding.

- Inspect the wound for foreign bodies (soil, broken glass, shreds of cloth, or other foreign substances).

- Assess associated injuries such as fractures, internal bleeding, spinal cord injuries, or head trauma.

- If the wound is contaminated with foreign material, determine when the patient last had a tetanus toxoid injection. A tetanus immunization or booster may be necessary.

Assessment of a treated (sutured) wound involves observation of its appearance, size, and drainage; the presence of swelling and pain; and the status of drains or tubes. In some long-term facilities, home care situations, and outpatient clinics, photographs are taken weekly for a visual record of the progress of pressure ulcers and wounds. Other assessments are documented and dated along with the photograph.

Estimating the amount of wound drainage can be difficult. One recommendation is to describe the degree to which the dressing is saturated. Wound tissues that are moist, with no measurable exudate, are said to have scant drainage. Small or minimal drainage covers less than 25% of the dressing; moderate drainage involves 25–75% of the dressing without leakage prior to scheduled dressing changes; and large or copious drainage involves more than 75% of the dressing and may completely saturate the dressing prior to scheduled changes (Morgan, 2015). These terms, plus the description of the drainage and the amount and type of dressing material used, should be well understood by all care providers.

Sometimes the wound reaches under the skin surface (called *undermining*). The edges of the wound around an open center may be raw or appear healed, but the undermining can result in a sinus tract or tunnel that extends the wound many centimeters beyond the main wound surface. To assess the size of the wound, gently explore the undermined area with a thin, flexible probe. Do not use a cotton-tipped swab, since it can leave fibers in the wound. Once the end of the tract is reached, gently raise the probe so that the bulge created by the end can be seen and its length can be measured on the skin surface. Sinus tracts are often caused by infection and have significant drainage. They may be treated with antibiotics, irrigation, surgical incision to open and drain the tract, or vacuum therapy for large tracts.

Diagnosis

The following nursing diagnoses relate to patients who have skin wounds or who are at risk for skin breakdown:

- *Infection, Risk for*
- *Impaired Skin Integrity, Risk for*
- *Skin Integrity, Impaired*
- *Tissue Integrity, Impaired*
- *Pain, Acute.*

(NANDA-I © 2014)

If the skin impairment is severe, the patient is immunosuppressed, or the wound is caused by trauma, the potential for infection is even greater.

Impaired Skin Integrity commonly applies to pressure ulcers and wounds that extend through the epidermis but not through the dermis. *Impaired Tissue Integrity* applies to pressure ulcers and wounds that extend into subcutaneous tissue, muscle, or bone. Pain is also a concern, particularly related to nerve involvement within the tissue impairment or as a consequence of procedures used to treat the wound.

Planning

The major goals for the patient at *Risk for Impaired Skin Integrity* are to maintain skin integrity and avoid potential associated risks. The outcomes associated with these goals may be as follows:

- The patient will demonstrate progressive wound healing and regain intact skin within a specified time.
- The patient will describe measures to protect and heal tissue and prevent further injury within a specified time.

Implementation

The four major areas in which the nurse can help the patient develop optimal conditions for wound healing are maintaining moist wound healing, providing sufficient nutrition and hydration, preventing wound infections, and using proper positioning. Interventions addressing these four areas differ depending upon the age and condition of the patient. Patient education for home care management focuses on maintaining skin integrity.

Facilitate Wound Healing

The dressing and frequency of change should support moist wound bed conditions. Wound beds that are too dry or disturbed too often fail to heal. See the Evidence-Based Practice feature in the exemplar on Cellulitis in the module on Infection for more information about moist wound management.

Promote Optimal Nutrition and Hydration

The patient should be assisted to take in at least 2500 mL of fluids a day, unless other health conditions contraindicate this amount. Although there is no evidence that excessive doses of vitamins or minerals enhance wound healing, adequate amounts are extremely important. The nurse should ensure that the patient receives sufficient protein; vitamins C, A, B, and B_5; and zinc. A consultation with a registered dietitian helps to ensure that correct supplementation needs are met. The nurse and those planning the patient's meals should take into account the patient's personal and religious food preferences.

Prevent Infection

There are two main aspects to controlling wound infection: preventing microorganisms from entering the wound and preventing the transmission of bloodborne pathogens between the patient and others.

Position to Minimize Pressure on the Wound

To promote wound healing, position the patient to keep pressure off the wound (sometimes referred to as off-loading). Changes of position and transfers can be accomplished without shear or friction damage. In addition to proper positioning, the nurse should assist the patient to be as mobile as possible, because activity enhances circulation. If the patient cannot move independently, ROM exercises and a turning schedule are implemented (see the Nursing Care Plan).

Plan for Discharge

In planning home care for the patient with a wound, the nurse needs to assess the following factors. This assessment will guide individualization of interventions to aid in prevention of serious complications.

- Patient's current level of knowledge: understanding of the cause of the wound or risk for developing a pressure ulcer; prevention or treatment strategies
- Patient's self-care abilities for mobility: physical ability to change position, ambulate, and transfer, including the use of assistive devices
- Patient's self-care abilities for wound care: manual dexterity and visual acuity necessary to perform skin assessments and wound treatments
- Facilities: bathroom with running water and garbage container needed to perform wound care and contain potentially infectious materials
- Patient's current level of nutrition: eating habits and preferences, laboratory values indicating need for teaching or other intervention
- Caregiver availability, skills, and responses: understanding of the cause of the wound or risk for developing a pressure ulcer, prevention or treatment strategies, willingness to assist with wound care, and actions to prevent pressure ulcers
- Family role changes and coping: effect on financial status, parenting and spousal roles, sexuality, and social roles
- Alternative potential primary or respite caregivers: for example, other family members, volunteers, church members, paid caregivers, or housekeeping services; available community respite care (e.g., adult day care, senior centers)
- Resources: availability and familiarity with possible sources of assistance, such as equipment and supply companies, organizations that offer medical supplies or financial assistance, home health agencies, and transportation to and from medical appointments, if needed.

Evaluation

Regular evaluation during the wound-healing process is important for a patient with a wound. Expected outcomes of nursing care include the following:

- The patient's skin and tissue integrity is maintained.
- The wound has decreased in size.
- The patient demonstrates an understanding of preventive care measures.

Patients with wounds may develop complications during hospitalization or after discharge that require additional intervention by the healthcare team. Infection is one of the most common complications. Infection development after discharge is most often related to self-care or care-giver abilities. Depending on the type of wound involved, infection can lead to further, more serious complications. The occurrence of any changes in patient condition related to wound healing require re-evaluation and modification of goals, interventions, and treatments previously identified for the patient.

Nursing Care Plan
A Patient with a Postoperative Wound

Tara Overbeck, 44 years old, underwent bariatric surgery 4 days ago. She says she knew it was time to do something dramatic when her doctor diagnosed both hypertension and type 2 diabetes mellitus on the same day.

ASSESSMENT

She has an 8 in. midline abdominal incision that appeared slightly red and began to ooze purulent drainage yesterday. The incision is stapled and has dissolvable sutures internally. Ms. Overbeck is NPO because of absent bowel sounds, with an IV solution of dextrose and water infusing at 100 mL/h per infusion pump. The antibiotic ciprofloxacin hydrochloride (Cipro) is to be administered every 6 hours IV. Other medications include Humulin 70/30 insulin administered on a sliding scale based on finger-stick glucose levels, clevidipine butyrate (Cleviprex) administered prn for hypertension, acetaminophen suppository prn for fever greater than 100°F, and morphine sulfate prn for pain.

Assessment findings include:

- Ms. Overbeck is drowsy but arousable and oriented.
- Skin is pale and slightly cool.
- Ms. Overbeck states that she is cold and requests additional covers.
- Ms. Overbeck states that she is in no pain and would like to sleep.
- Her respirations are unlabored.
- Vital signs: temperature 101.2°F oral; pulse 96 bpm; respirations 18/min; and BP 122/86 mmHg.
- She has a large abdominal dressing over a midline abdominal incision with purulent drainage the size of a silver dollar and a Jackson Pratt suction device connected to a drain with 10 mL dark red serosanguineous drainage coming from the distal part of the wound.
- An indwelling catheter is in place with 210 mL clear amber urine.
- This morning's lab results include: fasting blood sugar 110 mg/dL, hemoglobin within normal limits, WBC 12,400 mm^3, serum albumin 2.6 g/dL.

DIAGNOSES

- *Ineffective Thermoregulation* related to surgical procedure
- *Risk for Fluid Volume Deficit* related to altered postoperative intake
- *Impaired Skin Integrity* related to surgical incision
- *Delayed Surgical Recovery* related to postoperative surgical site infection

(NANDA-I © 2014)

PLANNING

Goals for Ms. Overbeck's plan of care include:

- The patient will engage in activities that promote wound healing.
- The patient will maintain adequate hydration.
- The patient's temperature will be controlled within acceptable limits until fever subsides.
- The patient's risk for complications secondary to wound infection will be reduced.

IMPLEMENTATION

- Use aseptic technique while changing the patient's dressing.
- Monitor the patient's temperature every 4 hours, with repeat measurement in 1 hour following administration of antipyretic if elevated higher than 100°F.
- Assess the wound every 4 hours for purulent drainage and odor; assess the edges of the wound for approximation, edema, redness, and inflammation.
- Teach the patient how to use aseptic technique when caring for her wound.
- Promote comfort through appropriate pain management, both pharmacologic and nonpharmacologic.
- Monitor intake and output, daily weight, and hydration status.
- Assess blood glucose four times per day, and administer insulin on a sliding scale as ordered.
- Empty the Jackson Pratt wound drain every 4 hours, and notify the primary care provider if drainage increases beyond acceptable limits based on baseline drainage to date.
- Assist the patient to change positions at least every 2 hours.
- Teach the patient proper nutrition to promote wound healing in keeping with postop bariatric surgical requirements.

EVALUATION

Expected outcomes for Ms. Overbeck include the following:

- The patient attains skin integrity of the abdominal incision.
- The patient demonstrates proper aseptic technique while performing dressing changes.
- The patient reports control of pain at incision site.
- The patient's temperature returns to acceptable limits within 1 hour of receiving antipyretic.

CRITICAL THINKING

1. In addition to the nursing diagnoses identified in this plan of care, what other nursing diagnoses would be appropriate for Ms. Overbeck's care?

2. Assess Ms. Overbeck's nutritional status based on the data provided. Is it adequate to promote wound healing? Explain your answer, and devise interventions as needed based on your response.

3. What impact will Ms. Overbeck's preexisting conditions of hypertension and type 2 diabetes mellitus have on her wound healing?

4. Other than the implementations listed in the plan of care, what else could you do to promote wound healing?

5. What discharge teaching will you provide Ms. Overbeck to promote wound healing?

REVIEW Wound Healing

RELATE Link the Concepts and Exemplars

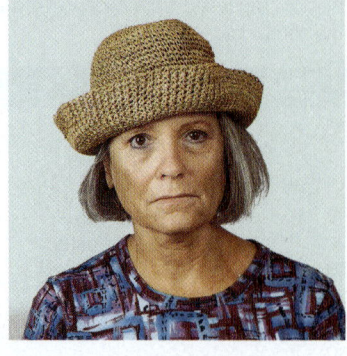

Norma James, a 65-year-old widow who lives alone, presents at the geriatric nursing clinic at the local senior center with a wound on her ankle about the size of a quarter. The wound is sore, with yellowish drainage. The skin around the wound is red and inflamed. Ms. James says that she has had the sore about 3 weeks and that she treated it with butter for a while, but the butter seemed to make it worse. Ms. James says that her foot hurts when she walks on it. The nurse at the clinic smells cigarette smoke on Ms. James clothing. When asked, Ms. James reports that she smokes about a pack a day. In response to a question from the nurse, Ms. James says that she has diabetes and high blood pressure. Ms. James is not able to say what medicines she takes but estimates that she takes "about four different ones."

Linking the exemplar of wound healing with the concept of metabolism:

1. What metabolic factors will increase the risk of delayed wound healing?

2. What teaching can the nurse provide Ms. James to promote wound healing in relation to metabolic concerns?

Linking the exemplar of wound healing with the concept of perfusion:

3. What factors related to perfusion will increase the risk of delayed wound healing for Ms. James?

4. What teaching will you provide Ms. James to reduce these risks related to perfusion?

READY Go to Volume 3: Clinical Nursing Skills

REFER Go to Pearson MyLab Nursing and eText

- Additional review materials

REFLECT Apply Your Knowledge

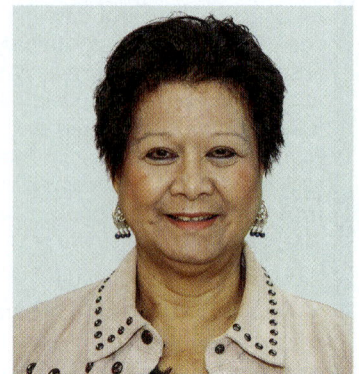

Lydia Ocampo, 69, wakes during the night to urinate but falls on the way to the bathroom. An ambulance takes her to the emergency department, where she is diagnosed with a left hip fracture. She is sent to the operating room for an open reduction internal fixation of the left hip. She is admitted to the medical-surgical floor following surgery.

Ms. Ocampo remains at the hospital because she has developed an infection in her incision and needs IV antibiotics and dressing changes. Her oral intake has been inadequate, but she has been well hydrated by IV fluids. She has been incontinent ever since the Foley catheter was removed. Attempts at physical therapy have been unproductive. The physical therapists are successful at transferring her from the bed to a chair, but this maneuver requires nearly full assistance.

1. Identify priority nursing diagnoses for Ms. Ocampo.

2. List factors that put Ms. Ocampo at risk for *Impaired Tissue Integrity*.

References

Agency for Healthcare Research and Quality (AHCRQ). (2012). Pressure ulcer risk assessment and prevention: A comparative effectiveness review. *Evidence-Based Practice Center Systematic Review Protocol*. Retrieved from http://effectivehealthcare.ahrq.gov/index.cfm/search-for-guides-reviews-and-reports/?pageaction=displayproduct&productid=926

Ahrens, M. (2016). *Report: National Fire Protection Association's "Home structure fires."* Retrieved from http://www.nfpa.org/news-and-research/fire-statistics-and-reports/fire-statistics/fires-by-property-type/residential/home-structure-fires

Akansel, N., Yilmaz, S., Aydin, N., & Kahveci, R. (2013). Etiology of burn injuries among 0–6 aged children in one university. *International Journal of Caring Sciences, 6*(2). Retrieved from http://www.internationaljournalofcaringsciences.org/docs/10.%20AKansel%20Burn%20Injuries.pdf

Amaya, R. (2013). *Neonatal wound management. Pediatric Wound Care Center of Houston.* Retrieved from https://www.utmb.edu/kaleidoscope/Neonatal%20Wound%20Care.pdf

American Academy of Dermatology. (2013). *Variety of options available to treat pigmentation problems.* Retrieved from https://www.aad.org/media/news-releases/variety-of-options-available-to-treat-pigmentation-problems

American Academy of Dermatology. (2016). *Acne.* Retrieved from https://www.aad.org/media/stats/conditions

American Academy of Pediatrics. (2015). *Teens and acne treatment.* Retrieved from https://www.healthychildren.org/English/ages-stages/teen/Pages/Teens-and-Acne.aspx

American Burn Association. (2016). *Burn incidence and treatment in the United States: 2016 fact sheet.* Retrieved from http://www.ameriburn.org/resources_factsheet.php

Amirlak, B. (2015). Skin anatomy. *Medscape.* Retrieved from http://emedicine.medscape.com/article/1294744-overview#

Ball, J. W., Bindler, R. C., Cowen, K., & Shaw, M. (2017). *Principles of pediatric nursing: Caring for children* (7th ed.). Hoboken, NJ: Pearson Education.

Behrman, A. J. (2016). Latex allergy. *Medscape.* Retrieved from http://emedicine.medscape.com/article/756632-overview#a6

Bianchi, J. (2012). The effective management of exudate in chronic wounds. *Wounds International, 3*(4). Retrieved from http://www.woundsinternational.com/practice-development/the-effective-management-of-exudate-in-chronic-wounds

Billingsley, E. M. (2016). Paronychia. *Medscape.* Retrieved from http://emedicine.medscape.com/article/1106062-overview

Bishop, S., & Maguire, S. (2012). Anaesthesia and intensive care for major burns. *Continuing Education in Anaesthesia, Critical Care, and Pain, 12*(3), 118–122.

Blank Children's Hospital, Unity Point Health. (2016). *Fire safety statistics.* Retrieved from https://www.unitypoint.org/blankchildrens/fire-statistics.aspx

Brind'Amour, K. (2016). *Common skin disorders.* Retrieved from http://www.healthline.com/health/skin-disorders#7

Brown, L. L. (2016). Infectious diseases are more closely linked to sex and gender than we think.

Huffington Post. Retrieved from http://www.huffingtonpost.com/society-for-womens-health-research/infectious-diseases-are-more-closely-linked-to-sex-and-gender-than-we-think_b_8490626.html

Centers for Disease Control and Prevention (CDC). (2016a). *Human papillomavirus: Genital HPV infection fact sheet.* Retrieved from http://www.cdc.gov/std/hpv/stdfact-hpv.htm

Centers for Disease Control and Prevention (CDC). (2016b). *General information about MRSA in the community.* Retrieved from https://www.cdc.gov/mrsa/community

Centers for Disease Control and Prevention (CDC). (2016c). *Psoriasis.* Retrieved from https://www.cdc.gov/psoriasis

Centers for Disease Control and Prevention (CDC). (2016d). *Skin cancer statistics.* Retrieved from https://www.cdc.gov/cancer/skin/statistics

Centers for Disease Control and Prevention (CDC). (2016e). *Injury prevention & control: Data & statistics (WISQRATM) ten leading causes of death and injury.* Retrieved from https://www.cdc.gov/injury/wisqars/pdf/leading_causes_of_injury_deaths_highlighting_unintentional_injury_2014-a.pdf

Children's National Health System. (2016a). *Pediatric common skin disorders.* Retrieved from http://childrensnational.org/choose-childrens/conditions-and-treatments/skin-disorders/common-skin-disorders

Children's National Health System. (2016b). *Pediatric non-infectious skin conditions.* Retrieved from https://childrensnational.org/choose-childrens/conditions-and-treatments/skin-disorders/noninfectious-skin-conditions

Cleveland Clinic. (2015). *Nutrition guidelines to improve wound healing.* Retrieved from http://my.clevelandclinic.org/healthy_living/nutrition/hic_nutrition_guidelines_to_improve_wound_healing.aspx

Collins, J. (2015). Preventing burn trauma. *Today's Geriatric Medicine, 8*(5), 28. Retrieved from http://www.todaysgeriatricmedicine.com/archive/0915p28.shtml

Cooper, M. A. (2016). *Lightning injuries.* Retrieved from http://emedicine.medscape.com/article/770642-overview#a4

Dat, A. D., Poon, F., Pham, K. B., & Doust, J. (2012). Aloe vera for treating acute and chronic wounds. *Cochrane Database of Systematic Reviews, 2,* CD008762. doi:10.1002/14651858.CD008762.pub2

Dermatologic disorders. (n.d.). Retrieved from Merck Manual Professional Version website: http://www.merckmanuals.com/professional/dermatologic-disorders

Dumville, J. C., Owens, G. L., Crosbie, E. J., Peinemann, F., & Liu, Z. (2015). *Negative pressure wound therapy for treating surgical wounds healing by secondary intention (open surgical wounds).* Retrieved from http://www.cochrane.org/CD011278/WOUNDS_negative-pressure-wound-therapy-for-treating-surgical-wounds-healing-by-secondary-intention-open-surgical-wounds

Duscher, D., Barrera, J., Wong, V. W., Maan, Z. N., Whittam, A. J., Januszyk, M., & Gurtner, G. C. (2016). Stem cells in wound healing: The future of regenerative medicine? A mini-review. *Gerontology, 62*(2), 216–225. doi:10.1159/000381877

Edlich, R. F. (2015). Thermal burns. *Medscape.* Retrieved from http://emedicine.medscape.com/article/1278244-overview#a1

Ehrlich, S. D. (2015). *Photodermatitis.* Retrieved from University of Maryland Medical Center: http://umm.edu/health/medical/altmed/condition/photodermatitis

Epstein, N. E. (2014). Multidisciplinary in-hospital teams improve patient outcomes: A review. *Surgical Neurology International, 5*(Suppl. 7), S295–S303. doi:10.4103/2152-7806.139612

Everett, J. S., Budescu, M., & Sommers, M. S. (2012). Making sense of skin color in clinical care. *Clinical Nurse Research, 21*(4), 495–516. doi:10.1177/1054773812446510

Firooz, A., Sadr, B., Babakoohi, S., Sarraf-Yazdy, M., Fanian, F., Kazerouni-Timsar, A., … Dowlati, Y. (2012). Variation of biophysical parameters of the skin with age, gender and body region. *Scientific World Journal.* doi:http://dx.doi.org/10.1100/2012/386936

Fonseca, J. A. (2016). Burn wound infections. *Medscape.* Retrieved from http://emedicine.medscape.com/article/213595-overview#a4

Gauglitz, G. G., & Williams, F. N. (2016). *Complications and long-term outcomes of a severe burn.* Retrieved from https://www.uptodate.com/contents/complications-and-long-term-outcomes-of-a-severe-burn

Gnaneswaran, N., Perera, E., Perera, M., & Sawhney, R. (2015). Cutaneous chemical burns: Assessment and early management. *Australian Family Physician, 44*(3), 135–139. Retrieved from http://search.proquest.com.proxy092.nclive.org/docview/1662641601/fulltextPDF/380128E495EA42B2PQ/1?accountid=14003

Gorman, C. R. (2016). Roseola infantum. *Medscape.* Retrieved from http://emedicine.medscape.com/article/1133023-overview#a4

Gupta, D., & Thappa, D. M. (2013). Mongolian spots: How important are they? *World Journal of Clinical Cases, 1*(8), 230–232. doi:10.12998/wjcc.v1.i8.230

Hay, R. J., Johns, N. E., Williams, H. C., Bolliger, I. W., Dellavalle, R. P., Margolis, D. J., … Naghavi, M. (2013). *The global burden of skin disease in 2010: An analysis of the prevalence and impact of skin conditions.* doi:http://dx.doi.org/10.1038/jid.2013.446

Herdman, T. H. & Kamitsuru, S. (Eds.). *Nursing Diagnoses—Definitions and Classification 2015–2017.* Copyright © 2014, 1994–2014 NANDA International. Used by arrangement with John Wiley & Sons, Inc. Companion website: www.wiley.com/go/nursingdiagnoses

Hockenberry, M. J., & Wilson, D. (2014). *Wong's nursing care of infants and children* (10th ed.). St. Louis, MO: Mosby.

Hornor, G. (2012). Medical evaluation for child physical abuse: What the PNP needs to know. *Journal of Pediatric Health Care, 26*(3), 163–170.

Huang, C., Leavitt, T., Bayer, L. R., & Orgill, D. P. (2014). Effect of negative pressure wound therapy on wound healing. *Current Problems in Surgery, 51*(7), 301–331. doi:http://dx.doi.org/10.1067/j.cpsurg.2014.04.001

Huether, S. E., McCance, K. L., Brashers, V. L., & Rote, N. S. (2017). *Understanding pathophysiology* (6th ed.). St. Louis, MO: Elsevier.

Hurd, R. (2014). Aging changes in skin. *MedlinePlus.* Retrieved from https://medlineplus.gov/ency/article/004014.htm

Infectious diseases. (n.d.). Retrieved from Merck Manual Professional Version website: http://www.merckmanuals.com/professional/infectious-diseases

Injuries and poisoning. (n.d.). Retrieved from Merck Manual Professional Version website: http://www.merckmanuals.com/professional/injuries-poisoning

James, W. D. (2016). Café au lait spots. *Medscape.* Retrieved from http://emedicine.medscape.com/article/911900-overview

Joffe, M. D. (2015). *Emergency care of moderate and severe thermal burns in children.* Retrieved from https://www.uptodate.com/contents/emergency-care-of-moderate-and-severe-thermal-burns-in-children

Jones, S. V., Ambros-Rudolph, C., & Nelson-Piercy, C. (2014). Skin disease in pregnancy. *BMJ.* doi:http://dx.doi.org/10.1136/bmj.g3489

Kaneshiro, N. K. (2015). Skin findings in newborns. *Medline Plus.* Retrieved from https://medlineplus.gov/ency/article/002301.htm

Kearns, R. D., Holmes, J. H., & Cairns, B. A. (2013). Burns injury: What's in a name? Labels used for burn injury classification: A review of the data from 2000–2012. *Annals of Burns and Fire Disasters, 26*(3), 115–120.

Kearns, R. D., Rich, P. B., Cairns, C. B., Holmes, J. H., & Cairns, B. A. (2014). *Electrical injury and burn care: A review of best practices.* Retrieved from http://www.emsworld.com/article/11621404/electrical-injury-electrocution-and-burn-care

Khorasani, G., Hosseinimehr, S. J., Azadbakht, M., Zamani, A., & Mahdavi, M. R. (2009). Aloe versus silver sulfadiazine creams for second-degree burns: A randomized controlled study. *Surgery Today, 39*(7), 587–591. doi:10.1007/s00595-008-3944-y

Kirman, C. N. (2016). Pressure injuries (pressure ulcers) and wound care. *Medscape.* Retrieved from http://emedicine.medscape.com/article/190115-overview#a4

Krishnamoorthy, V., Ramaiah, R., & Bhananker, S. M. (2012). Pediatric burn injuries. *International Journal of Critical Illness & Injury Science, 2*(3), 128–134. doi:10.4103/2229-5151.100889

Kundu, R. V., & Patterson, S. (2013). Dermatologic conditions in skin of color: Part II. Disorders occurring predominantly in skin of color. *American Family Physician, 87*(12), 859–865. Retrieved from http://www.aafp.org/afp/2013/0615/p859.html

Lawson, C. N., Hollinger, J., Sethi, S., Rodney, I., Sarkar, R., Dlova, N., & Callender, V. D. (2015). Updates in the understanding and treatments of skin and hair disorders in women of color. *International Journal of Women's Dermatology,* 59–75. doi:http://dx.doi.org/10.1016/j.ijwd.2015.04.002

Leal, A. C. (2013). Why does your skin age? *Dartmouth Undergraduate Journal of Science.* Retrieved from http://dujs.dartmouth.edu/2013/01/why-does-your-skin-age/#.WFgv3fkrK00

Lyford, W. H. (2016). Melasma. *Medscape.* Retrieved from http://emedicine.medscape.com/article/1068640-overview#a4

Mayo Clinic. (2015). *Acanthosis nigricans.* Retrieved from http://www.mayoclinic.org/diseases-conditions/acanthosis-nigricans/basics/definition/con-20025600

McInnes, E., Jammali-Blasi, A., Bell-Syer, S. E. M., Dumville, J. C., Middleton, V., & Cullum, N. (2015). Support surfaces for pressure ulcer prevention. *Cochrane Database of Systematic Reviews, 5.* doi:10.1002/14651858.CD001735.pub5

Moore, Z. E., & Cowman, S. (2014). Risk assessment tools for the prevention of pressure ulcers. *Cochrane Database System Review, 5*(2). doi:0.1002/14651858.CD006471.pub3.

Morgan, N. (2015). How to assess wound exudate. *Wound Care Advisor, 4*(5). Retrieved from https://woundcareadvisor.com/how-to-assess-wound-exudate-vol3-no2

National Center for Complementary and Integrative Health. (2016). *Aloe vera.* Retrieved from https://nccih.nih.gov/health/aloevera

National Institutes of Health. (2014). Skin infections. *Medline Plus.* Retrieved from https://medlineplus.gov/skininfections.html#summary

National Pressure Ulcer Advisory Panel (NPUAP). (2016). *NPUAP pressure injury stages.* Retrieved from http://www.npuap.org/resources/educational-and-clinical-resources/npuap-pressure-injury-stages

National Pressure Ulcer Advisory Panel (NPUAP), European Pressure Ulcer Advisory Panel (EPUPA), & PAN Pacific Pressure Injury Alliance (PPPIA). (2014). *Prevention and treatment of pressure ulcers: Quick reference guide.* Retrieved from http://www.npuap.org/wp-content/uploads/2014/08/Quick-Reference-Guide-DIGITAL-NPUAP-EPUAP-PPPIA-Jan2016.pdf

Neurofibromatosis. (n.d.). Retrieved from Merck Manual Professional Version: http://www.merckmanuals.com/professional/pediatrics/neurocutaneous-syndromes

Ngoa, S. T., Steyna, F. J., & McCombeb, P. A. (2014). Gender differences in autoimmune disease. *Frontiers in Neuroendocrinology, 35*(3), 347–369. doi:http://dx.doi.org/10.1016/j.yfrne.2014.04.004

Olin, J. (2012). *Wound healing: A process almost all RNs encounter.* Retrieved from http://www.rncentral.com/blog/2012/wound-healing-a-process-almost-all-rns-encounter

Pereira, R. F., & Bártolo, P. J. (2016). Traditional therapies for skin wound healing. *Advances in Wound Care, 5*(5), 208–229. doi:10.1089/wound.2013.0506

Pinney, S. S. (2016). Nevus araneus (spider nevus). *Medscape.* Retrieved from http://emedicine.medscape.com/article/1084388-overview#a5

Pukar, M., Rajshakha, A., Mewada, S., & Lakhani, D. (2015). Outcome of heliotherapy and modified Parkland's formula for fluid resuscitation in management of moderate degree of burns: A single centre observational study. *IJSS Journal of Surgery, 1*(3). doi:10.17354/SUR/2015/17

Purnell, L. D. (2013). People of African American heritage. In *Transcultural health care: A culturally competent approach* (4th ed., pp. 97, 98, 238). Philadelphia, PA: F. A. Davis.

Rice, P. L., & Orgill, D. P. (2015). *Emergency care of moderate and severe thermal burns in adults.* Retrieved from http://www.uptodate.com/contents/emergency-care-of-moderate-and-severe-thermal-burns-in-adults

Saedi, N., & Ganesan, A. K. (2013). Treating hyperpigmentation in darker-skinned patients. *Journal of Dermatology, 12*(5), 563. Retrieved from http://jddonline.com/articles/dermatology/S1545961613P0563X/1

Schraga, E. D. (2016). Emergent management of thermal burns. *Medscape.* Retrieved from http://emedicine.medscape.com/article/769193-overview

Schwartz, R. A. (2016a). *Postinflammatory hyperpigmentation.* Retrieved from http://emedicine.medscape.com/article/1069191-overview#a4

Schwartz, R. A. (2016b). Pityriasis rosea. *Medscape.* Retrieved from http://emedicine.medscape.com/article/1107532-overview

Sgonc, R., & Gruber, J. (2013). Age-relate aspects of cutaneous wound healing: A mini review. *Gerontology, 59*(2), 159–164. doi:10.1159/000342344

Sherman, R. A. (2014). Mechanisms of maggot-induced wound healing: What do we know, and where do we go from here? *Evidence Based Complementary Alternative Medicine.* doi:10.1155/2014/592419

Shi, Y., Zhang, X., Huang, B., Wang, W., & Liu, Y. (2015). Severe burn injury in late pregnancy: A case report and literature review. *Burns and Trauma, 3*(2). Retrieved from https://burnstrauma.biomedcentral.com/articles/10.1186/s41038-015-0002-z

Uitto, J. (2012). Milestones in genetics of structural skin disorders. *Journal of Investigative Dermatology, 132,* E1. doi:10.1038/skinbio.2012

U.S. Department of Homeland Security. (2016). Fire risk in 2014. *U.S. Fire Administration National Fire Data Center Topical Fire Report Series, 17*(7). Retrieved from https://www.usfa.fema.gov/downloads/pdf/statistics/v17i7.pdf

U.S. Fire Administration. (2016). *Fire death rates.* Retrieved from https://www.usfa.fema.gov/data/statistics/fire_death_rates.html

Van Onselen, J. (2015). Infant skin care: Best practice and parental advice. *Nursing in Practice Health Visitor Supplement.* Retrieved from http://www.nursinginpractice.com/article/infant-skin-care-best-practice-and-parental-advice

Vocal, A. (2014). *Common skin disease during adolescence.* Retrieved from http://www.slideshare.net/AllynVocal/common-skin-diseases-during-adolescence?qid=a36c8687-44d0-412f-90b7-4bd24b66a336&v=&b=&from_search=1

Wake Forest Baptist Health. (2016). *Vacuum-assisted closure.* Retrieved from http://www.wakehealth.edu/Plastic-Surgery/Wound-Care/Vacuum-Assisted-Closure.htm

Weavind, L. (2016). Burn shock: Resuscitation of burn shock. *Journal of Family Practice.* Retrieved from http://www.mdedge.com/node/5334/path_term/30

White, S., Philips, R., Neill, M. M., & Kelly, E. (2014). Pregnancy-specific skin disorders. *Skin Therapy Letter, 19*(5). Retrieved from http://www.medscape.com/viewarticle/832816_2

Wiechman, S., & Sharar, S. R. (2015). Burn pain: Principles of pharmacologic and nonpharmacologic management. Retrieved from https://www.uptodate.com/contents/burn-pain-principles-of-pharmacologic-and-nonpharmacologic-management

Wong, D. (2014). *Skin changes at puberty.* Retrieved from the New Zealand Dermatological Society website: http://www.dermnetnz.org/topics/skin-changes-at-puberty

World Health Organization (WHO). (2013). *Aloe vera gel.* Retrieved from http://apps.who.int/medicinedocs/en/d/Js2200e/6.html#Js2200e.6

Wound Care Centers. (2012). *Growth factor therapy.* Retrieved from http://www.woundcarecenters.org/article/wound-therapies/growth-factor-therapy

Yale Medicine. (2016). *Gangrene.* Retrieved from https://www.yalemedicine.org/conditions/gangrene

Yoost, B. L., & Crawford, L. R. (2015). *Fundamentals of nursing: Active learning for collaborative practice.* St. Louis: MO: Elsevier.

Zellman, G. L. (2016). Erythema infectiosum. *Medscape.* Retrieved from http://emedicine.medscape.com/article/1132078-overview#a1

Zhai, H., Meier-Davis, S. R., Cayme, B., Shudo, J., & Maibach, H. (2012a). Allergic contact dermatitis: Effect of age. *Cutaneous and Ocular Toxicology, 31*(1), 20–25. doi:10.3109/15569527.2011.595749

Zhai, H., Meier-Davis, S. R., Cayme, B., Shudo, J., & Maibach, H. (2012b). Irritant contact dermatitis: Effect of age. *Cutaneous and Ocular Toxicology, 31*(2), 138–143. doi:10.3109/15569527.2011.618472

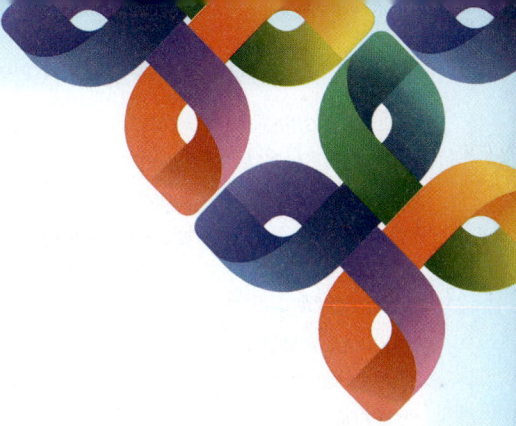

Appendix A
NANDA-Approved Nursing Diagnoses 2015–2017

Activity, Deficient Diversional

Activity Intolerance

Activity Intolerance, Risk for

Activity Planning, Ineffective

Activity Planning, Risk for Ineffective

Adaptive Capacity: Intracranial, Decreased

Adverse Reaction to Iodinated Contrast Media, Risk for

Airway Clearance, Ineffective

Allergy Response, Risk for

Allergy Response, Latex

Allergy Response, Latex, Risk for

Anxiety

Anxiety, Death

Aspiration, Risk for

Attachment, Risk for Impaired

Bleeding, Risk for

Blood Glucose Level, Risk for Unstable

Body Image, Disturbed

Body Temperature: Imbalanced, Risk for

Bowel Incontinence

Breast Milk, Insufficient

Breastfeeding, Ineffective

Breastfeeding, Interrupted

Breastfeeding, Readiness for Enhanced

Breathing Pattern, Ineffective

Cardiac Output, Decreased

Cardiac Output, Decreased, Risk for

Cardiovascular Function, Impaired, Risk for

Caregiver Role Strain

Caregiver Role Strain, Risk for

Childbearing Process, Ineffective

Childbearing Process, Readiness for Enhanced

Childbearing Process, Risk for Ineffective

Chronic Pain Syndrome

Comfort, Impaired

Comfort, Readiness for Enhanced

Communication, Readiness for Enhanced

Communication: Verbal, Impaired

Confusion, Acute

Confusion, Chronic

Confusion, Risk for Acute

Constipation

Constipation, Perceived

Constipation, Risk for

Contamination

Contamination, Risk for

Coping: Community, Ineffective

Coping: Community, Readiness for Enhanced

Coping, Defensive

Coping: Family, Compromised

Coping: Family, Disabled

Coping: Family, Readiness for Enhanced

Coping: Readiness for Enhanced

Coping, Ineffective

Corneal Injury, Risk for

Decision Making, Readiness for Enhanced

Decisional Conflict (Specify)

Denial, Ineffective

Dentition, Impaired

Development: Delayed, Risk for

Diarrhea

Disuse Syndrome, Risk for

Dry Eye, Risk for

Dysreflexia, Autonomic

Dysreflexia, Autonomic, Risk for

Electrolyte Imbalance, Risk for

Emancipated Decision-Making, Impaired

Emancipated Decision-Making, Impaired, Risk for

Emancipated Decision-Making, Readiness for Enhanced

Emotional Control, Labile

Falls, Risk for

Family Processes, Dysfunctional

Family Processes, Interrupted

Family Processes, Readiness for Enhanced

Fatigue

Fear

Fluid Balance, Readiness for Enhanced

Fluid Volume: Deficient

Fluid Volume: Deficient, Risk for

Fluid Volume: Excess

Fluid Volume: Imbalanced, Risk for

Frail Elderly Syndrome

Frail Elderly Syndrome, Risk for

Functional Constipation, Chronic

Gas Exchange, Impaired

Gastrointestinal Motility, Risk for Dysfunctional

Gastrointestinal Motility, Dysfunctional

Grieving

Grieving, Complicated

Grieving, Risk for Complicated

Growth: Disproportionate, Risk for

Health: Community, Deficient

Health Behavior, Risk-Prone

Health Maintenance, Ineffective

Health Management, Family, Ineffective

Health Management, Ineffective

Health Management, Readiness for Enhanced

Home Maintenance, Impaired

Hope, Readiness for Enhanced

Hopelessness

Human Dignity, Risk for Compromised

Hyperthermia

Hypothermia

Hypothermia, Risk for

Impulse Control, Ineffective

Infant Behavior: Disorganized

Infant Behavior: Disorganized, Risk for

Infant Behavior: Organized, Readiness for Enhanced

Infant Feeding Pattern, Ineffective

Infection, Risk for

Injury, Risk for

Insomnia

Jaundice, Neonatal

Jaundice, Neonatal, Risk for

Knowledge, Deficient

Knowledge, Readiness for Enhanced

Labor Pain

Lifestyle, Sedentary

Liver Function, Risk for Impaired

Loneliness, Risk for

Maternal/Fetal Dyad, Risk for Disturbed

Memory, Impaired

Mobility: Bed, Impaired

Mobility: Physical, Impaired

Mobility: Wheelchair, Impaired

Mood Regulation, Impaired

Moral Distress

Nausea

Neglect, Unilateral

Neurovascular Dysfunction: Peripheral, Risk for

Noncompliance

Nutrition, Imbalanced: Less than Body Requirements

Nutrition, Readiness for Enhanced

Mucous Membrane: Oral, Impaired

Mucus Membrane: Oral, Impaired, Risk for

Obesity

Overweight

Overweight, Risk for

Pain, Acute

Pain, Chronic

Parenting, Impaired

Parenting, Readiness for Enhanced

Parenting, Risk for Impaired

Perfusion: Gastrointestinal, Risk for Ineffective

Perfusion: Renal, Risk for Ineffective

Perioperative Hypothermia, Risk for

Perioperative Positioning Injury, Risk for

Personal Identity: Disturbed

Personal Identity: Disturbed, Risk for

Poisoning, Risk for

Post-Trauma Syndrome

Post-Trauma Syndrome, Risk for

Power, Readiness for Enhanced

Powerlessness

Powerlessness, Risk for

Pressure Ulcer, Risk for

Protection, Ineffective

Rape-Trauma Syndrome

Relationship, Ineffective

Relationship, Risk for Ineffective

Relationship, Readiness for Enhanced

Religiosity, Impaired

Religiosity, Readiness for Enhanced

Religiosity, Risk for Impaired

Relocation Stress Syndrome

Relocation Stress Syndrome, Risk for

Resilience, Impaired

Resilience, Readiness for Enhanced

Resilience, Risk for Impaired

Role Conflict, Parental

Role Performance, Ineffective

Self-care, Readiness for Enhanced

Self-care Deficit: Bathing

Self-care Deficit: Dressing

Self-care Deficit: Feeding

Self-care Deficit: Toileting

Self-Concept, Readiness for Enhanced

Self-Esteem, Chronic Low

Self-Esteem, Chronic Low, Risk for

Self-Esteem, Situational Low

Self-Esteem, Situational Low, Risk for

Self-Mutilation

Self-Mutilation, Risk for

Self Neglect

Sexual Dysfunction

Sexuality Pattern, Ineffective

Shock, Risk for

Sitting, Impaired

Skin Integrity, Impaired

Skin Integrity, Risk for Impaired

Sleep Deprivation

Sleep Pattern, Disturbed

Sleep, Readiness for Enhanced

Social Interaction, Impaired

Social Isolation

Sorrow, Chronic

Spiritual Distress

Spiritual Distress, Risk for

Spiritual Well-Being, Readiness for Enhanced

Standing, Impaired

Sudden Infant Death Syndrome, Risk for

Stress Overload

Suffocation, Risk for

Suicide, Risk for

Surgical Recovery, Delayed

Surgical Recovery, Delayed, Risk for

Swallowing, Impaired

Thermal Injury, Risk for

Thermoregulation, Ineffective

Tissue Integrity, Impaired

Tissue Integrity, Impaired, Risk for

Tissue Perfusion: Cardiac, Risk for Decreased

Tissue Perfusion: Cerebral, Risk for Ineffective

Tissue Perfusion: Peripheral, Ineffective

Tissue Perfusion: Peripheral, Risk for Ineffective

Transfer Ability, Impaired

Trauma, Risk for

Trauma: Vascular, Risk for

Urinary Elimination, Impaired

Urinary Elimination, Readiness for Enhanced

Urinary Incontinence, Functional

Urinary Incontinence, Overflow

Urinary Incontinence, Reflex

Urinary Incontinence, Stress

Urinary Incontinence, Urge

Urinary Incontinence, Urge, Risk for

Urinary Retention

Urinary Tract Injury, Risk for

Ventilation: Spontaneous, Impaired

Ventilatory Weaning Response, Dysfunctional

Violence: Other-Directed, Risk for

Violence: Self-Directed, Risk for

Walking, Impaired

Wandering

Glossary

ABC The essential functions of airway, breathing, and circulation.

ABCD An enhancement of the **ABC** mnemonic, with the **D** representing one of four indicators depending on agency use: defibrillation, deficiency, deadly bleeding, or disability.

Abortion Loss of pregnancy before the fetus is viable outside the uterus. Also called *miscarriage*.

Absence seizures Also called petit mal seizures, absence seizures involve both hemispheres of the brain as well as deeper structures such as thalamus, basal ganglia, and upper brainstem. They are considered a type of generalized seizure.

Absorption The process of moving nutrients and fluid from the external environment of the gastrointestinal tract to the internal environment. May also refer to the intake of any specific nutrient.

Abstinence Voluntarily going without alcohol, drugs, or other pleasurable substances or activities.

Abuse of power An attempt by an individual to use his or her position or authority in a manner that shames, controls, demeans, humiliates, or denigrates another individual to gain emotional, psychologic, or physical advantage over that individual.

Accelerations A transient increase in the fetal heart rate normally caused by fetal movement.

Accommodation 1. The ability of the eye to adjust to variations in distance. 2. The process of a change whereby cognitive processes mature sufficiently to allow an individual to solve problems that were unsolvable before.

Accountability The ability and willingness of an individual to assume responsibility for his or her actions and to accept the consequences of his or her behavior.

Accreditation A peer review process that evaluates and certifies the quality of an organization.

Acculturation The process of adapting to the majority culture and accepting it as one's own.

Acid indigestion A condition in which an individual can taste the stomach acid when it flows back into the esophagus.

Acidosis The condition that results when hydrogen ion concentration increases above normal, causing the pH to drop below 7.35.

Acids Substances that release hydrogen ions in solution.

Acquaintance phase The first few days after a child's birth, when the new mother applies herself to the task of getting to know her baby.

Acquaintance rape A broad term used to describe a rape committed by an acquaintance or other familiar individual.

Acquired immunity Immunity developed after exposure to a pathogen.

Acquired immunodeficiency syndrome (AIDS) An immune system deficit induced by infection with the human immunodeficiency virus (HIV). AIDS is characterized by opportunistic infections.

Acrocyanosis A bluish discoloration of the hands and feet.

Acromegaly Excessive growth of bone from growth hormone hypersecretion.

Actinic keratosis An epidermal skin lesion directly related to chronic sun exposure and photodamage. Also called *senile keratosis* or *solar keratosis*.

Action potential The electrical activity produced by movement of ions across cell membranes that stimulates muscle contraction.

Active acquired immunity Antibodies formed in response to an illness or an immunization while a woman is pregnant.

Active euthanasia Actions to bring about a patient's death directly, with or without patient consent.

Active immunity Production of antibodies or development of immune lymphocytes against specific antigens.

Active listening Fully concentrating on both the content and emotion of a person's message, rather than just passively hearing the words a person says.

Active transport A method that requires additional energy (in the form of adenosine triphosphate) to move substances against the concentration gradient (from low concentration to high concentration).

Activities of daily living (ADLs) Activities used routinely in daily life, such as grooming, eating, bathing, and dressing.

Activity-exercise pattern An individual's routine of exercise, activity, leisure, and recreation, including activities of daily living that require energy expenditure.

Activity tolerance The type and amount of exercise or daily living activities that an individual is able to perform without experiencing adverse effects.

Actual loss A change in or unavailability of something or someone of value that can be recognized by others.

Acute coronary syndrome (ACS) Any condition that develops due to sudden, reduced blood flow to the heart.

Acute fatigue A sudden onset of physical and mental exhaustion or weariness, particularly after a period of mental or physical stress.

Acute illness An alteration in health or functioning characterized by severe symptoms of relatively short duration.

Acute infection An infection that appears suddenly and lasts for a short time.

Acute kidney injury (AKI) Proposed as a more accurate term for *acute renal failure*, AKI is defined as a sudden decline in kidney function that causes disturbances in fluid, electrolyte, and acid–base balances.

Acute lymphocytic leukemia (ALL) The most common type of leukemia in children and adolescents, marked by the proliferation of malignant cells that resemble immature lymphocytes.

Acute myeloid leukemia (AML) A disorder characterized by uncontrolled proliferation of myeloblasts and hyperplasia of the bone marrow and spleen.

Acute myocardial infarction (AMI) A life-threatening condition that occurs when blood flow to a portion of the cardiac muscle is blocked. If circulation to the affected myocardium is not promptly restored, loss of functional myocardium affects the heart's ability to maintain an effective cardiac output, ultimately leading to cardiogenic shock and death.

Acute pain Temporary, localized, and sudden pain that lasts for less than 6 months and has an identifiable cause, such as trauma, surgery, or inflammation.

Acute pancreatitis An inflammatory disorder that involves self-destruction of the pancreas by its own enzymes through autodigestion.

Acute postinfectious glomerulonephritis (APIGN) Inflammation of the glomerular capillary membrane that is most often seen in children as a response to a group A beta-hemolytic streptococcal infection of the skin or pharynx or as a result of infection by *Staphylococcus, Pneumococcus,* or Coxsackie virus.

Acute renal failure (ARF) A rapid decline in renal function with azotemia, fluid, and electrolyte imbalances. ARF may be reversed with prompt intervention.

Acute respiratory distress syndrome (ARDS) A disorder with rapid onset characterized by noncardiac pulmonary edema and progressive refractory hypoxemia. ARDS is a life-threatening emergency.

Acute retroviral syndrome (ARS) Primary human immunodeficiency virus infection.

Acute stress disorder A condition that may occur following an individual experiencing, learning of, or witnessing an extremely stressful event that involves the threat of death, actual or threatened serious injury, or actual or threatened physical or sexual violation.

Acute tubular necrosis (ATN) The destruction of tubular epithelial cells, which causes an abrupt and progressive decline of renal function.

Adaptation 1. The ability to handle the demands made by the environment. Also called *coping behavior*. 2. The return to normal functioning, even when homeostasis cannot be regained.

Adaptation phase The phase during a crisis in which the individual meets the challenges presented and uses his or her resources to successfully resolve the crisis.

Adaptive behavior Everyday skills, including conceptual skills, social skills, and practical skills.

Adaptive functioning The ability of an individual to meet the standards expected for his or her cultural group.

Adaptive mechanisms Methods the ego uses to fulfill the needs of the id in a socially acceptable manner. Also called *defense mechanisms*.

Addiction A psychologic or physical need for a substance (such as alcohol) or process (such as gambling) to the extent that the individual will risk negative consequences in an attempt to meet the need.

Addictive behaviors Compulsive, problematic patterns of action resulting in psychologic and/or physiologic dependence.

Addison disease A disorder that results from adrenal insufficiency, particularly a cortisol deficiency.

Adherence Commitment or attachment to a regimen. Also called *compliance*.

Adhesions Fibrous bands of scar tissue.

Adjustment disorder with depressed mood A maladaptive reaction to an identifiable psychosocial stressor or stressors that occurs within 3 months after the onset of the stressor and has persisted for no longer than 6 months. Also called *adjustment disorder* or *situational depression*.

Adjustment phase Initial phase experienced in response to crisis, characterized by disorganization and unsuccessful attempts to meet the crisis.

Adjustment reaction to depressed mood See Postpartum blues.

Administrative laws Responsibilities that may be interpreted and enforced by an agency that has been delegated the power of oversight by the governing legislation.

Adolescent family A family in which one or more parents are adolescents.

Advance healthcare directives Legal documents that allow an individual to plan for healthcare and/or financial affairs in the event of incapacity. Also called *advance directives* or *healthcare advance directives*.

Advocacy Protecting an individual by expressing and defending the individual's cause on his or her behalf.

Advocate An individual who expresses and defends the cause of another.

Aerobic exercise An activity during which the amount of oxygen taken into the body is greater than that used to perform the activity.

Aesthetic knowing The subjective elements and personal style a nurse uses when delivering care, including empathy, holistic thinking, compassion, and sensitivity.

Afebrile Without fever.

Affect The immediate and observable emotional expression of mood, which people communicate verbally and nonverbally; the outward manifestation of what the individual is feeling.

Affective commitment An attachment to a profession that includes identification with and involvement in the profession.

Affective domain The learning domain encompassing an individual's emotional response to tasks, including feelings, emotions, interests, attitudes, and appreciation. Also called the *feeling domain*.

Afterload The force that ventricles must overcome to eject their blood volume.

Afterpains Cramplike pains caused by intermittent contractions of the uterus that occur after childbirth.

Age-related macular degeneration (AMD) A gradual degeneration in the macular area of the retina that is the leading cause of blindness in people over age 65.

Ageism A deep and profound prejudice in American society against older adults.

Aggravated assault An unlawful attack by one individual on another for the purpose of inflicting severe or aggravated bodily injury. This type of assault usually is accompanied by the use of a weapon or by means likely to produce death or great bodily harm.

Aggression Any form of behavior directed toward the goal of harming or injuring another living being.

Aggressive behavior Behavior directed toward getting what one wants without considering the feelings of others.

Aggressive communicators Individuals who tend to focus on their own needs and become impatient when these needs are not met.

Agnosia The inability to recognize one or more objects that previously were familiar.

Agoraphobia A condition that is characterized by anxiety associated with two or more of the following situations: being in enclosed spaces, being in open spaces, using public transportation, being in a crowd or standing in a line of people, or being alone outside the home environment.

Agraphia The inability to write properly.

AIDS dementia complex The most common cause of mental status changes for patients with HIV infection. This dementia results from a direct effect of the virus on the brain and affects cognitive, motor, and behavioral functioning. Fluctuating memory loss, confusion, difficulty concentrating, lethargy, and diminished motor speed are typical manifestations.

Air trapping Decreased airflow with exhalation caused by edema of the air passages.

Airborne precautions Used for patients who are known to have or suspected of having serious illnesses transmitted by airborne droplet nuclei smaller than 5 microns, such as tuberculosis.

Airway clearance techniques Nonpharmacologic strategies for clearing the airway. Examples include coughing, huffing, and **chest physical therapy**.

Airway remodeling Structural changes of the airway caused by a disease, such as asthma, resulting in progressive or permanent loss of lung function.

Airway resistance The effort or force needed to move oxygen through the trachea to the lungs.

Akathisia Restlessness.

Alcohol dependence A primary, chronic disease characterized by use or abuse of alcohol; genetic, psychosocial, and environmental factors influence its development and manifestations. Also called *alcoholism*.

Alcohol poisoning A toxic condition that results from excessive consumption of large amounts of alcohol in a very short period of time.

Alcohol withdrawal delirium A medical emergency usually occurring 3–5 days following alcohol withdrawal and lasting 2–3 days. Characterized by paranoia, disorientation, delusions, visual hallucinations, elevated vital signs, vomiting, diarrhea, and diaphoresis. Also known as *delirium tremens (DTs)*.

Alcohol withdrawal syndrome Condition that typically begins about 6–8 hours after an individual with alcoholism takes his or her last drink. Early symptoms include irritability, anxiety, insomnia, tremors, sweating, and a mild tachycardia.

Alcoholic cirrhosis A progressive, irreversible liver disorder resulting from excessive consumption of alcohol. Also called *Laënnec cirrhosis*.

Alcoholism A primary, chronic disease characterized by use or abuse of alcohol; genetic, psychosocial, and environmental factors influence its development and manifestations. Also called *alcohol dependence*.

Alkalosis The condition that results when hydrogen ion concentration falls below normal and the pH level rises above 7.45.

Allen test A measurement of radial or ulnar artery patency; either the radial or ulnar artery is digitally compressed by the examiner after blood has been forced out of the hand by clenching it into a fist.

Allergen An environmental or exogenous antigen that provokes a hypersensitivity response.

Allergic contact dermatitis A cell-mediated or delayed hypersensitivity to a wide variety of allergens.

Allergy A hypersensitivity response to environmental or exogenous antigens.

Allogeneic blood transfusion A transfusion using blood that has been donated by the community.

Allogeneic bone marrow transplant A transplant using bone marrow from a matched donor.

Allografts Grafts between members of the same species who have different genotypes and HLA antigens. Human skin that has been harvested from cadavers is usually used. Also called *homograft*.

Alloimmunization The reaction of the immune system to donated tissue.

Allostasis Necessary changes that must occur to achieve the characteristic stability of homeostasis.

Allostatic load The physical cost of adaptation to physiologic or psychosocial stressors.

Alogia Limited or impoverished speech.

Alopecia Hair loss.

Alternative therapies (also referred to as *alternative medicine*) A term used to describe use of these diverse therapies *instead of* conventional therapies, including acupuncture; cultural practices related to food preparation or practices at specific times of the day or during the week.

Altruism A concern for the welfare and well-being of others.

Alveoli Terminal structures of the respiratory system where gas exchange occurs.

Alzheimer disease (AD) The most common kind of dementia, Alzheimer disease involves progressive dementia, memory loss, and the inability to care for one's self.

Ambulation The ability to walk from place to place independently with or without an assistive device.

Amblyopia Lazy eye; one eye has reduced vision even with no identifiable cause, and the reduced vision is not correctable by corrective lenses.

Amenorrhea The absence of menstruation.

Amniocentesis A procedure used to obtain amniotic fluid for genetic testing to determine fetal abnormalities or fetal lung maturity in the third trimester of pregnancy.

Amnion A thin protective membrane that contains amniotic fluid.

Amniotic fluid The liquid surrounding the fetus in utero. It absorbs shocks, permits fetal movement, and prevents heat loss.

Amphetamine A powerful stimulant that, when used improperly or abused, poses a severe health risk due to its devastating physical and neurologic consequences, including amphetamine-induced mental disorders.

Ampulla The outer third of the fallopian tube, where fertilization usually occurs.

Amyloid plaques Seen in Alzheimer disease and formed when groups of nerve cells degenerate and clump around the amyloid core in the spaces between the neurons in the brain. Amyloid plaques consist primarily of insoluble deposits of beta-amyloid, a protein fragment from a larger protein called amyloid precursor protein, mixed with other neurons and nonnerve cells.

Anaerobic exercise Activity in which the muscles cannot draw out enough oxygen from the bloodstream, and anaerobic pathways are used to provide additional energy for storing for a short time.

Anal stimulation The stimulation of the anus with the fingers, mouth, or sex toys for sexual pleasure.

Anaphylactic shock Shock resulting from a widespread hypersensitivity reaction. Also called *anaphylaxis*.

Anaphylaxis An acute systemic type I hypersensitivity (allergic) response that may result in shock and death. It occurs in highly sensitive persons following exposure to a specific antigen, usually through injection or ingestion.

Anaplasia The regression of a cell to an immature or undifferentiated cell type.

Anasarca Severe, generalized edema.

Andragogy The art and science of teaching adults.

Androgen A hormone that stimulates the development and maintenance of male sex characteristics.

Androgyny Flexibility in gender roles.

Anemia An abnormally low number of circulating red blood cells, low hemoglobin concentration, or both.

Anergic Unable to react to common antigens.

Anergy Fatigue and decreased energy associated with a depressive disorder. Also called *anergia*.

Anger A subjective sense of intense displeasure, irritation, or animosity.

Angina pectoris Chest pain resulting from reduced coronary blood flow caused by a temporary imbalance between myocardial blood supply and demand. Also called *angina*.

Angle-closure glaucoma A type of glaucoma that results from a narrowing of the anterior chamber angle due to corneal flattening or bulging of the iris into the anterior chamber. Also called *narrow-angle* or *closed-angle glaucoma*.

Anhedonia The inability to feel pleasure.

Animism Giving lifelike qualities to nonliving things.

Anion Ion that carries a negative charge.

Anomia Difficulty naming people and things.

Anorexia Loss of appetite.

Anorexia nervosa (AN) A potentially life-threatening disorder characterized by extreme perfectionism, weight fear, significant weight loss, body image disturbances, strenuous exercising, peculiar food-handling patterns, and reductions in heart rate, blood pressure, metabolic rate, and the production of estrogen or testosterone.

Anorgasmia Absence of orgasm.

Antagonism One of the six trait domains associated with personality disorders that is composed of manipulativeness, deceitfulness, callousness, hostility, grandiosity, and attention seeking.

Antepartum Time between conception and the onset of labor; usually used to describe the period during which a woman is pregnant.

Anthropometric measurements Measurements that can help identify individuals who are at risk for undernutrition or overnutrition. Specific measurements include height, length (in babies), weight, body mass index, waist-to-hip circumference, and skinfold thickness.

Antibodies Proteins that work against antigens.

Antibody-mediated (humoral) immune response Activation of B cells to produce antibodies to respond to antigens such as bacteria, bacterial toxins, and free viruses.

Anticipatory grief Grief experienced in advance of a loss, such as the wife who grieves before her ailing husband dies.

Anticipatory guidance Information about developmental changes that can be expected in the future. Including the recognition of the potential for a crisis and assistance with identifying potential methods for averting the crisis.

Anticipatory learning Learning necessary to effectively reach a desired outcome or in anticipation of a need for information that has not yet occurred.

Anticipatory loss A loss that is experienced before the loss actually occurs. For example, the gradual decline and eventual death of a family member who has Alzheimer disease.

Anticipatory problem solving Initial information is presented to a learner, who is then asked a question or presented with a situation related to the information. The learner applies the new information to the situation and decides what to do.

Antigen Foreign substance that triggers the immune response.

Antigen-antibody complex The complex formed by the binding of an antibody to an antigen.

Antigenic drift Describes small changes that occur continuously as a virus makes copies of itself.

Antigenic shift When two different strains of a virus infect the same cell and exchange genetic material to create a new subtype of the virus.

Antiretroviral therapies Pharmacologic therapies that stop or suppress the activity of a retrovirus, preventing further weakening of the immune system and thereby minimizing opportunistic infections.

Antiseptics Agents that inhibit the growth of some microorganisms.

Antisocial personality disorder (ASPD) One of several types of personality disorders defined by the DSM-5, it is characterized by a pattern of disregard for and violation of the rights of others.

Anuria The failure of the kidneys to produce urine, resulting in a total lack of urination or output of less than 100 mL/day in an adult.

Anxiety A stress response characterized by feelings of apprehension, dread, mental uneasiness, and a sense of helplessness in response to an actual or perceived threat to the well-being of oneself or others.

Anxious distress A combination of symptoms often associated with anxiety, including restlessness, impaired concentration due to worry, fear of something awful happening, and fear of losing control. Anxious distress often manifests in patients with depression and bipolar disorders and is associated with an increased risk for suicide.

Aortic stenosis Narrowing of the aortic valve that obstructs blood flow to systemic circulation.

Apathy A lack of interest or enthusiasm.

Apgar score A physical assessment of a newborn at 1 minute and 5 minutes after birth on a scale from 1 to 10 that includes heart rate, respiratory effort, muscle tone, reflex irritability, and skin color.

Aphakia Absence of the lens of the eye (e.g., after surgical removal of a cataract).

Aphasia Defective or absent language function.

Apical-radial pulse A comparison of the apical and radial pulses, which are normally identical. A pulse deficit can indicate certain cardiovascular disorders.

Aplastic anemia A disorder that results when the bone marrow fails to produce all three types of blood cells.

Apnea Absence of breathing.

Apnea of prematurity Absence of breathing for 20 seconds or longer, or for less than 20 seconds when associated with cyanosis, pallor, and bradycardia. A common problem in a preterm infant of less than 36 weeks' gestation, usually presenting between day 2 and day 7 of life.

Appendectomy Surgical removal of the appendix.

Appendicitis Inflammation of the vermiform appendix.

Appendicular skeleton Pectoral girdles, upper limbs, pelvic girdle, and lower limbs.

Approach-coping The use of confrontation to change the stressor by taking direct action.

Approximated Term describing successful closure of a wound with little or no tissue loss.

Apraxia The inability to perform purposeful movements and use objects correctly.

Areflexia The loss of reflex function.

Areola Pigmented ring surrounding the nipple of the breast.

Arousal In the brain, arousal, or alertness, is regulated by the **reticular activation system**.

Arrhythmogenic tissue Tissue that affects the generation and conduction of electrical impulses in the heart.

Arrogance Excessive pride and a feeling of superiority.

Arrhythmogenic right ventricular dysplasia (ARVD) A condition that results when the body progressively replaces the muscle of the right ventricle with fatty and fibrous tissue.

Arterial blood gas (ABG) A laboratory test used to evaluate oxygen and carbon dioxide exchange and the acid–base balance within the blood.

Arterial blood pressure A measure of the pressure exerted by the blood as it flows through the arteries.

Arteriosclerosis An arterial disorder characterized by thickening, loss of elasticity, and calcification of arterial walls.

Arteriovenous (AV) fistula An artificial connection between a vein and an artery created for long-term vascular access.

Arthrodesis A procedure that permanently fuses two or more bones together at a joint using pins, plates, screws, and rods. Also called *joint fusion*.

Arthroplasty Total joint replacement.

Arthroscopy A surgical procedure in which a thin, lighted tube with a camera in one end is inserted into a joint in order to allow a surgeon to visualize joint structure more easily.

Artificial disc surgery Surgery to replace a herniated disc with an artificial disc in order to maintain flexibility of the spinal joint.

Artificial rupture of membranes A process of rupturing of the membranes by the certified nurse-midwife or physician using an instrument called an amniohook. Completed if spontaneous rupture of membranes does not occur.

ASA Physical Classification Scale A physical risk classification category that determines the type and dosage of sedation a patient can receive.

Ascites Excess fluid in the peritoneal cavity.

Asepsis The absence of disease-causing organisms.

Assault The action of creating an apprehension of offensive, insulting, or physically injurious touching.

Assertive behavior Behavior that consists of expressing one's wishes and opinions, or taking care of oneself, but not at the expense of others.

Assertive communicators Individuals who tend to declare and affirm their opinions. In doing this, however, they respect the rights of others to communicate in the same fashion.

Assertive community treatment (ACT) A therapeutic regimen for individuals with moderate to severe mental illness that provides patients with individually tailored services within their communities.

Assessment The systematic and continuous collection of data about a patient for the purpose of determining the patient's current and ongoing health status, predicting the patient's health risks, and identifying appropriate health-promoting activities.

Assignment The transfer of responsibility to accomplish a task, without the transfer of authority.

Assimilation 1. The process of adapting to and integrating characteristics of the dominant culture as one's own. 2. The process by which humans encounter and react to new situations by using the mechanisms they already possess.

Assisted suicide Self-administration of a lethal dose of medication provided by a physician or healthcare provider in order to intentionally end a patient's life with the goal of relieving pain and suffering.

Associative play A stage of play in which children play together or share tasks during play.

Astereognosis The inability to identify objects by touch.

Asthma A chronic inflammatory disease of the lungs characterized by recurrent episodes of wheezing, breathlessness, chest tightness, and coughing.

Asynclitism A condition that occurs when the sagittal suture is directed toward either the symphysis pubis or the sacral promontory and is felt to be misaligned.

Asystole Cardiac standstill.

Ataxia Lack of muscle coordination.

Atelectasis Collapse of lung tissue following obstruction of the bronchus or bronchioles.

Atherectomy A procedure to remove plaque from a lesion, specifically an **atheroma**.

Atheroma Complex lesion consisting of lipids, fibrous tissue, collagen, calcium, cellular debris, and capillaries. The formation of atheromas is the final stage of **atherosclerosis**.

Atherosclerosis A form of arteriosclerosis in which deposits of fat and fibrin obstruct and harden the arteries.

Atrial gallop (S₄) A heart sound produced by atrial contraction and ejection of blood into the ventricle during late diastole. Also called the *fourth heart sound*.

Atrial kick An extra bolus of blood delivered to the ventricles before they contract.

Atrial natriuretic factor (ANF) A peptide hormone released from cells in the atrium of the heart in response to excess blood volume and stretching of the atrial walls.

Atrial septal defect (ASD) An opening in the atrial septum that permits left-to-right shunting of blood.

Atrioventricular (AV) canal defect A combination of defects in the atrial and ventricular septa and portions of tricuspid and mitral valves. A complete AV canal defect allows blood to travel freely among all four chambers of the heart. Also called *endocardial cushion defect*.

Atrophy The wasting away or decrease in size of an organ, muscle, or tissue.

Attention deficit disorder (ADD) A variation in central nervous system processing characterized by developmentally inappropriate behaviors involving inattention.

Attention-deficit/hyperactivity disorder (ADHD) A variation in central nervous system processing characterized by developmentally inappropriate behaviors involving inattention, hyperactivity, and impulsivity.

Attention impairment A condition marked by an inability to process information and respond to such information appropriately; a patient with attention impairment will have poor concentration and be easily distracted.

Attentive listening The process of listening actively, using all the senses. Also called *mindful listening*.

Attributes of safety The quality or properties of remaining safe.

Audiologist A healthcare professional specializing in identifying, diagnosing, treating, and monitoring disorders of the auditory and vestibular portions of the ear.

Audit An examination of records to verify accuracy and proper use.

Auditory Of or relating to hearing.

Aura An olfactory or visual sensory sensation that may provide an early warning sign of a seizure.

Auscultation Listening to the sounds produced within the body. Auscultation can be direct using the unaided ear or indirect using a stethoscope or other listening device.

Authority 1. The power to command other individuals and direct their activities. 2. The right to act or to accomplish the task.

Autism spectrum disorders (ASDs) A developmental disorder in which individuals have persistent deficits in social communication and social interaction, and restricted, repetitive patterns of behavior, interest, or activities.

Autoantibodies Antibodies that react to the individual's own tissues.

Autocratic (authoritarian) leader A leader who makes decisions for the group based on the belief that individuals are externally motivated and are incapable of independent decision making.

Autografting A procedure performed in the surgical suite in which part of a patient's healthy skin is removed and used to effect permanent skin coverage over a wound area.

Autoimmune disorder/disease Failure of immune system to recognize itself, resulting in normal host tissue being targeted by immune defenses.

Autologous blood transfusion A blood transfusion using a patient's own blood.

Autologous bone marrow transplant Bone marrow transplant using a patient's own bone marrow.

Automatism A repetitive reaction that occurs automatically, without conscious thought. Examples include lip smacking, eyelid fluttering, aimless walking, picking at clothing, and swallowing.

Autonomic dysreflexia An abrupt onset of excessively high blood pressure as the result of an overactive autonomic nervous system. An exaggerated sympathetic response that occurs in patients with spinal cord injuries at or above the T6 level. Also called *autonomic hyperreflexia*.

Autonomy 1. The state of being independent and self-directed without outside control. 2. The right to make one's own decisions.

Autosomal chromosomes Genetic material found in a cell nucleus that determines physical characteristics (excluding gender) of the individual.

Autosome A single chromosome from any one of the 22 pairs of chromosomes not involved in sex determination (X or Y); humans have 22 pairs of autosomes.

Avascular necrosis The death of bone tissue due to lack of blood supply. Also called *osteonecrosis*.

Avian influenza Also known as "bird flu," it is a form of influenza that commonly infects birds. This virus has not yet demonstrated the ability to spread among humans; however, concerns are that it will mutate to allow person-to-person spread. This viral strain has a mortality rate of greater than 50% in people who have been infected due to close association with infected birds.

Avoidance-coping The use of both behaviors and cognitive processes to avoid a stressor.

Avoidant personality disorder (APD) One of several types of personality disorders recognized by the DSM-5, APD is characterized by a pattern of social withdrawal along with a sense of inadequacy, fear, and hypersensitivity to potential rejection or shame.

Avolition The inability to persist in goal-directed activities.

Awareness The ability to perceive environmental stimuli and body reactions and to respond appropriately through thought and action.

Axial loading The application of vertical force to the spinal column.

Axial skeleton Ribs, sternum, vertebral column, and skull.

Axon A nerve fiber.

Azotemia Increased levels of nitrogenous wastes in the blood.

B lymphocytes (B cells) Integral to specific immune response, they are activated and mature into either plasma cells, which secrete antibodies, or memory cells.

Babinski reflex The fanning and extension of the toes or flexion of the toes due to gentle stroking on the sole of the foot. Also called the *Babinski response.*

Bacilli Rod-shaped bacteria.

Background questions General questions asked of a patient that seek more information about a topic, such as diseases and medications.

Bacteremia The presence of bacteria in the blood.

Bacteria The most common category of infection-causing microorganisms.

Bactericidal agent Destroys bacteria.

Bacteriostatic agent Prevents the growth and reproduction of some bacteria.

Balanitis Inflammation of the glans.

Balloon tamponade The inflation of the balloon tip of a multiple-lumen nasogastric tube to control bleeding.

Barlow maneuver A procedure used to evaluate an infant for hip dislocation or instability in which the healthcare provider grasps and adducts the infant's thigh and then applies gentle downward pressure.

Barotrauma Lung injury caused by alveolar overdistention. Also called *volutrauma.*

Barrel chest An increase in the anteroposterior chest diameter resulting from air trapping and hyperinflation.

Basal cell carcinoma An epithelial tumor believed to originate either from the basal layer of the epidermis or from cells in the surrounding dermal structures. Also called *basal cell cancer.*

Basal metabolic rate (BMR) The amount of energy expended by the body at rest.

Base excess (BE) A calculated value also known as *buffer base capacity.* The BE measures substances that can accept or combine with hydrogen ions. It reflects the degree of acid–base imbalance by indicating the status of the body's total buffering capacity.

Baseline fetal heart rate The average fetal heart rate (FHR) rounded to increments of 5 bpm observed during a 10-minute period of monitoring. This excludes periodic or episodic changes, periods of marked variability, and segments of the baseline that differ by more than 25 bpm.

Baseline fetal heart rate variability Fluctuation in the FHR baseline of 2 cycles per minute or greater, with irregular amplitude and inconstant frequency.

Bases Substances that accept hydrogen ions in solution. Also called *alkalis.*

Basic needs The physical needs of an individual, such as eating, sleeping, resting, self-care, and physical stability.

Battery The willful touching of another individual, an individual's clothes, or even something the individual is carrying that is unwanted, embarrassing, or unwarranted.

Behavioral therapy A form of therapy in which patients learn techniques to modify or change maladaptive behaviors.

Behaviorist theory A theory that suggests that learning takes place when an individual's reaction to a stimulus is either positively or negatively reinforced.

Belief An interpretation or conclusion that one accepts as true.

Belief system The way in which a culture explains the mysteries of the universe and life.

Belt restraint Restraint used to ensure the safety of patients who are transported by wheelchair or gurney, or to protect patients confined to a bed or a chair. Also called *safety strap body restraint.*

Benchmarking A method used to compare the performance of an individual or organization to industry standards.

Beneficence The act of doing good or beneficial actions.

Benign Referring to a growth or tumor that does not endanger life or health and tends to not recur after treatment.

Benign prostatic hyperplasia (BPH) Nonmalignant enlargement of the prostate gland commonly seen in the aging man.

Bereavement The subjective response experienced by the surviving loved ones after the death of an individual with whom they have shared a significant relationship.

Bias The favoring of a group or individual over another.

Bidirectional influence Influences exerted between an individual and his or her family that may negatively affect the emotional health of the individual, the family, or both.

Bilevel ventilator (BiPAP) Mechanical ventilation that provides inspiratory positive airway pressure as well as airway support during expiration.

Biliary colic A severe, steady pain in the epigastric region or right upper quadrant of the abdomen.

Binge drinking The consumption of five or more drinks containing alcohol in a single session.

Binge eating The ingestion of huge amounts of food (about 3,500 kcal) within a short time (about 1 hour).

Binge eating disorder (BED) An eating disorder characterized by recurring episodes of binge eating, a sense of lack of control, and negative feelings about oneself, but without intervening periods of behavior such as self-induced vomiting, purging by laxatives, fasting, or prolonged exercise.

Binuclear family A postdivorce family in which the biologic children are members of two nuclear households—that of the father and that of the mother—and the children alternate between the two homes.

Bioethics The application of ethics to issues of human life or health (e.g., to decisions about abortion or euthanasia).

Bioethical dilemmas Ethical dilemmas of human life or health that arise in the care of patients and families; they often emerge from a combination of causative factors.

Biologic rhythm A cyclical event or function that consists of repeated occurrences and repeated, regular intervals between occurrences. Biologic rhythms can refer to both physical and psychologic patterns.

Biomedical informatics The interprofessional science that deals with biomedical information's structure, acquisition, and use.

Bioterrorism The deliberate release of viruses, bacteria, or other microbes as weapons.

Bipolar disorder A mood disorder characterized by alternating depression and elation, with periods of normal mood in between. Formerly called *manic–depressive disorder.*

Birthing room A single room in a hospital where a pregnant woman and her partner or other family members will stay for the labor, birth, recovery, and possibly the postpartum period.

Bisexual An individual who is attracted to members of both sexes.

Bisphosphonates Drugs used to treat osteoporosis that inhibit bone reabsorption by suppressing osteoclast activity.

Blackouts A form of amnesia about events that occurred during a drinking period. This is often seen in the early stages of alcoholism.

Bladder training Gradually increases the bladder capacity by increasing the intervals between voidings and resisting the urge to void.

Blame-free environment An environment in which healthcare providers can report errors or near misses without the fear of punishment.

Blended family A family formed after the death or divorce of a parent; may include stepparents on both sides, stepchildren, half-siblings.

Blepharism Spasms that cause the eye to blink continuously.

Blighted ovum One of the most common causes of miscarriage, it occurs when the egg has been fertilized and both the membrane and placenta have formed, but the embryo has not formed.

Blood flow The volume of blood transported in a vessel, in an organ, or throughout the entire circulation over a given period of time.

Blood pressure The force that blood exerts against the walls of the arteries as it is pumped from the heart.

Blood urea nitrogen (BUN) A measure of blood level of urea, the end product of protein metabolism.

Bloodborne pathogens Microorganisms carried in blood and body fluids that are capable of infecting other individuals with serious and difficult-to-treat viral infections.

Bloody show The pink-tinged secretions resulting from a small amount of blood loss from the exposed cervical capillaries during pregnancy.

Blunt trauma Trauma that occurs without any communication between the damaged tissues and the outside environment.

Body fluid Any fluid that is essential to homeostasis; water is the primary body fluid.

Body image The mental image of the physical self.

Body mass index (BMI) A method of comparing weight to height as an indirect measure of body fat.

Body substance isolation (BSI) System that employs generic infection control precautions for all patients, except those with the few airborne diseases.

Body surface area (BSA) The relationship between height and weight measured in square meters.

Body temperature The core or surface measurement of a patient's internal heat production and loss.

Bone marrow transplant The treatment of disease by infusing a patient with his or her own bone marrow or that of a healthy donor.

Borborygmus Hyperactive, high-pitched, tinkling, rushing, or growling bowel sounds heard in diarrhea or at the onset of bowel obstruction.

Borderline personality disorder (BPD) One of several personality disorders defined in the DSM-5, BPD is marked by unstable interpersonal relationships, self-image, affect, and impulsiveness.

Bouchard nodes Bony lumps in the middle joint of the digit.

Boundaries The invisible lines that define the amount and kind of contact allowable among members of a family and between the family and outside systems.

Boutonnière deformity A flexion deformity of the PIP joints with extension of the DIP joint.

Bowel incontinence The inability to voluntarily control the passage of fecal contents and intestinal gas through the anal sphincter. Also called *fecal incontinence.*

Brachytherapy Radiation treatment given by placing radioactive material directly in or near the target, which is often a tumor.

Bradycardia A heart rate in an adult of less than 60 bpm.

Bradydysrhythmia Abnormally slow rhythms.

Bradykinesia Slowed movements due to muscle rigidity.

Bradyphrenia Slowed thinking and a decreased ability to form thoughts, to plan, or to make decisions.

Bradypnea A respiratory rate of less than 10 breaths per minute in adults.

Brain death The cessation and irreversibility of all brain functions, including those of the brainstem.

Brainstem Contains the midbrain, pons, and medulla oblongata. Located between the cerebrum and spinal cord, the brainstem connects pathways between the higher and lower structures. Ten of the 12 pairs of cranial nerves originate in the brainstem.

Brainstorming A decision-making method in which group members meet and generate diverse ideas about the nature, cause, definition, or solution to a problem.

Braxton Hicks contractions Intermittent painless uterine contractions that may occur every 10–20 minutes and occur more frequently near the end of pregnancy.

Brazelton neonatal behavioral assessment scale A scale developed to assess a newborn's state changes, temperament, and individual behavioral patterns.

Breach of care See Breach of duty.

Breach of duty A deviation from the standard of care owed a patient. Also called *breach of care.*

Breakthrough pain A sudden flare or increase in pain despite comfort with or without baseline analgesia.

Breast Mammary gland.

Breast cancer The unregulated growth of abnormal cells in breast tissue.

Breathing exercises Techniques used to slow the breathing rate by focusing on taking regular and deep breaths from the diaphragm.

Brief psychotic disorder Rapid onset of at least one of the following psychotic symptoms: delusions, hallucinations, disorganized speech, or disorganized behavior. The episode lasts at least 1 day but less than 1 month, after which the person returns to the premorbid level of functioning.

Bronchial sounds Loud, high-pitched sounds heard over the trachea that are longer on exhalation than inhalation.

Bronchiectasis Chronic dilation of the bronchi and bronchioles.

Bronchiolitis A lower respiratory tract illness that occurs when an infecting agent (virus or bacterium) causes inflammation and obstruction of the small airways.

Bronchitis Inflammation of the mucous membranes of the bronchial tubes.

Bronchogenic carcinomas Tumors of the airway epithelium.

Bronchoscopy A procedure that allows direct visualization of the lungs by inserting a bronchoscope orally into the trachea and advancing it to the bronchi bifurcation.

Bronchovesicular sound The sound created as air moves within the bronchial tree.

Brown adipose tissue (BAT) A specific store of fat in newborn infants that appears dark brown due to enriched blood supply, dense cellular content, and abundant nerve endings.

Bruits Blowing sound sometimes heard due to restriction of blood flow through the vessels.

Buffers Substances that prevent major changes in pH by releasing hydrogen ions.

Bulimia nervosa (BN) A type of eating disorder characterized by an obsessive focus on weight and body size and cycles of binge eating followed by purging.

Bullying Any unwanted aggressive behavior committed against another who is not a sibling or dating partner.

Bureaucratic leader A leader who relies on the organization's rules, policies, and procedures to direct the group's work efforts.

Burn An injury resulting from exposure to heat, chemicals, radiation, or electric current.

Burn shock Hypovolemic shock resulting from the shift of a massive amount of fluid from the intracellular and intravascular compartments into the interstitium following burn injury. Also called *hypovolemic shock.*

Burnout A complex syndrome resulting from unmanaged stress that manifests as physical and emotional depletion, a negative attitude and self-concept, and feelings of helplessness and hopelessness.

Cachexia Physical wasting from weight loss and loss of muscle mass due to the rapid growth and reproduction of cancer cells and their need for increased nutrients.

Caffeine A stimulant that increases the heart rate and acts as a diuretic.

Calcium oxalate A chemical compound from which kidney stones may form.

Calcium phosphate A chemical compound from which kidney stones may form.

Calculi Renal stones.

Cancellous bone The spongy tissue of bone.

Cancer A family of complex diseases with manifestations that vary according to body system and type of tumor cells.

Cancer pain Pain that may result from the direct effects of the cancerous disease and its treatment, or it may be unrelated to the disease and its treatment in individuals with cancer.

Candidiasis A common, opportunistic fungal infection in patients with AIDS.

Cannabis sativa The plant source of marijuana.

Caput succedaneum A localized, easily identifiable, soft area of the scalp, generally resulting from a long and difficult labor or vacuum extraction.

Carbohydrate One of the three major macronutrients primarily derived from plant foods. These foods contain simple and complex sugars, and starches.

Carcinogen A substance that causes cancer.

Carcinogenesis The production or origin of cancer.

Cardiac arrest The cessation of heart function that precedes biologic death.

Cardiac cycle One contraction and relaxation of the heart; a single heartbeat.

Cardiac index The cardiac output adjusted for the patient's body size or body surface area (BSA).

Cardiac markers Proteins released from necrotic heart muscle.

Cardiac output (CO) The amount of blood pumped by the ventricles into the pulmonary and systemic circulations in 1 minute.

Cardiac rehabilitation A medically supervised program designed to aid people with their recovery from heart attacks, heart surgeries, and percutaneous coronary interventions.

Cardiac reserve The heart's ability to respond to the body's changing need for cardiac output.

Cardiac tamponade Compression of the heart caused by collected blood or fluid in the pericardium.

Cardinal ligament Major ligament of the uterus containing the uterine artery and vein.

Cardinal movements A series of changes in position that allow the fetus to move through the birth canal. Also called *mechanisms of labor*.

Cardiogenic shock Shock that occurs when the heart's pumping ability is compromised to the point that it cannot maintain cardiac output and adequate tissue perfusion.

Cardiomyopathy Disease that affects the heart muscle's ability to pump effectively. Primary abnormality of the heart muscle that affects its structural or functional characteristics.

Cardiopulmonary resuscitation (CPR) A mechanical attempt to maintain tissue perfusion and oxygenation using oral resuscitation and external cardiac compressions.

Care coordination The means by which a multidisciplinary team works with a patient to ensure that the care received across the healthcare continuum meets the patient's needs.

Care management model Planning, assessment, and coordination of health services to provide an integrated continuum of clinical services, including medical care, health promotion, disease prevention, costs, and use of resources.

Care map Expected outcomes and care strategies developed through collaboration by the healthcare team. Also called a *critical pathway*.

Caring To feel interest, concern, and respect for a patient while demonstrating sensitivity, sincerity, honesty, and patience.

Caring for the dying The act of helping patients live as comfortably as possible until death and helping the patient's support individuals cope with death.

Carpal spasm Involuntary contraction of the hand and fingers due to decreased calcium levels.

Carphologia Involuntary, repeated lint picking.

Carrier Human or animal reservoir of a specific infectious agent that usually does not manifest any clinical signs of the disease.

Cartilage A type of flexible connective tissue found throughout the body.

Case management (CM) The coordination of patient care over time using the combination of health and social services necessary to meet the individual patient's needs.

Case managers Individuals who help manage the care of certain patient populations, including patients with chronic medical conditions, such as diabetes; patients recovering from acute conditions, such as those receiving joint replacement; and patients managing psychiatric disorders.

Case method A patient-centered method of managing care in which one nurse is assigned to, and is responsible for, the comprehensive care of a group of patients during an 8- or 12-hour shift.

Caseation necrosis A process in which tissue infected with *Mycobacterium tuberculosis* dies and forms a cheeselike center in the infectious bacilli.

Cast A rigid device applied to immobilize injured bones and promote healing.

Catabolism The breakdown of body proteins.

Cataract An opacification (clouding) of lens of the eye due to a breakdown of proteins within the lens.

Catatonia Unresponsiveness to the environment or others.

Catatonic excitement Includes hyperactivity and bizarre behavior and is a positive symptom of schizophrenia.

Catatonic inhibition Involves decreased activity level; limited speech; minimal self-care; and, at times, a trancelike state. Catatonic inhibition is a negative symptom of schizophrenia.

Cation Ion that carries a positive charge.

Cauda equina syndrome (CES) A condition that occurs when the nerve roots of the cauda equine are compressed. It may result in permanent neurologic impairment, including urinary incontinence and paralysis.

Causation To make a successful claim for malpractice, an injury must have occurred as a direct consequence of a nurse's or other healthcare professional's breach of duty.

Cavitation Formation of a cavity or bubble.

Celiac disease A chronic immune-mediated disorder of the small intestine in which the absorption of nutrients, particularly fats, is impaired. Also known as celiac sprue or nontropical sprue.

Cell cycle The four phases of cell growth and development.

Cell-mediated (cellular) immune response Direct or indirect inactivation of antigen by lymphocytes.

Cellulitis An acute bacterial infection of the dermis and underlying connective tissue. Cellulitis is characterized by red or lilac, tender, warm, edematous skin that may have an ill-defined, nonelevated border.

Central nervous system (CNS) One of two principal parts of the neurologic system, the central nervous system consists of the brain and the spinal cord.

Central nervous system (CNS) depressants A type of drug that acts to slow brain function, decreasing levels of alertness and awareness. CNS depressants include barbiturates, benzodiazepines, paraldehyde, meprobamate, and chloral hydrate.

Central pain 1. A type of pain related to a lesion in the brain that may spontaneously produce high-frequency bursts of impulses that are perceived as pain. 2. A type of pain caused by damage to the central nervous system that may manifest in constant pain, pain paroxysms, evoked pain, or allodynia. Patients may describe their pain as "pins and needles," aching, or lacerating.

Centration Focusing only on one particular aspect of a situation or the ability to concentrate.

Cephalocaudal development Growth that proceeds in the direction from head to toe.

Cephalohematoma A collection of blood resulting from ruptured blood vessels between the surface of a cranial bone and the periosteal membrane. Also called an *entrapped hemorrhage*.

Cerebellum Located below the cerebrum and behind the brainstem, it coordinates stimuli from the cerebral cortex to provide precise timing for skeletal muscle coordination and smooth movements.

Cerebral palsy (CP) A group of chronic conditions affecting body movement, coordination, and posture that results from a nonprogressive abnormality of the immature brain.

Cerebral perfusion pressure (CPP) The pressure it takes for the heart to provide the brain with blood. It is calculated by finding the difference between arterial pressure and intracranial pressure. Normal CPP is 0–95 mmHg.

Cerebrum The largest portion of the brain, it is composed of gray matter and has two hemispheres divided into four regions or lobes.

Certification The credentialing process by which a nongovernmental agency or association recognizes the professional competence of an individual who has met the predetermined qualifications specified by the agency or association.

Cerumen Earwax.

Cervical cap A latex cup-shaped contraceptive device, used with spermicidal cream or jelly, that fits snugly over the cervix and is held in place by suction.

Cervical collar A device that stabilizes and maintains neutral alignment of the cervical spine; it is used with patients with potential or suspected cervical spine injury. Also called *C-collar*.

Cervical ripening The softening and effacing of the cervix.

Cervix The narrow neck of the uterus.

Cesarean birth The birth of an infant through an abdominal and uterine incision.

CFTR modulators A treatment for **cystic fibrosis** that attacks the cause of the problem—issues with the CFTR protein—rather than just CF's clinical manifestations.

Chain of command The hierarchy of authority and responsibility within an organization.

Chancre A painless ulceration formed during the first stage of syphilis.

Change-of-shift report A type of handoff communication given to all nurses on the next shift.

Channel A medium used to convey messages.

Charcot-Marie-Tooth disease The most common inherited form of **peripheral neuropathy,** it is characterized by a slowly progressive degeneration of the muscles of the foot, lower leg, hand, and forearm. Symptoms usually present between adolescence and young adulthood.

Charismatic leader A rare type of leader who is characterized by a strong, emotional relationship between the leader and the group members.

Chart A formal, legal document that provides evidence of a patient's care. Also called a *patient record* or a *clinical record*.

Charting The process of making an entry on a patient record. Also called *recording* or *documenting*.

Charting by exception (CBE) A documentation system in which only abnormal or significant findings or exceptions to norms are recorded.

CHCT A biopsy of thigh skeletal muscle tissue to determine sensitivity to caffeine and halothane.

Cheilosis Cracking of lips.

Chemical conjunctivitis An irritation of the conjunctiva by chemicals used to treat the eyes.

Chemical restraints Pharmacologic agents administered for the purpose of controlling hyperactive behavior in agitated patients.

Chemical thermogenesis The stimulation of heat production in the body through increased cellular metabolism. Also called *nonshivering thermogenesis* or *NST*.

Chemotaxis The movement of cells in response to a chemical stimulus.

Chemotherapy Cancer treatment involving the use of cytotoxic medications to decrease tumor size, adjunctive to surgery or radiation therapy; or to prevent or treat suspected metastases.

Chest physical therapy An **airway clearance technique** that involves clapping and **percussion**.

Chest x-ray Allows for two-dimensional visualization of the contents of the thoracic cavity.

Child abuse Any act or failure to act on the part of a parent or caretaker which results in the death, serious physical or emotional harm, sexual abuse, or exploitation of a child.

Child Health Insurance Program (CHIP) State and federal funded healthcare coverage for children under the age of 19 whose families earn more than the Medicaid limits but cannot afford to purchase private healthcare coverage.

Childhood traumatic grief A grief reaction that occurs when an important person in a child's life dies as the result of a traumatic event or circumstances the child views as traumatic.

Childfree family A family without children.

Chlamydia A group of sexually transmitted infections caused by *Chlamydia trachomatis*.

Chloasma Brownish pigmentation over the bridge of the nose and the cheeks during pregnancy and in some women who are taking oral contraceptives. Also called *melasma gravidarum* or *mask of pregnancy*.

Cholangitis Duct inflammation.

Cholecystitis Inflammation of the gallbladder.

Cholelithiasis The formation of stones (*calculi* or *gallstones*) in the gallbladder or biliary duct system.

Chromosomes Tightly coiled strands of DNA within the nucleus that contain genetic information.

Chronic bronchitis A disorder of excessive bronchial mucous secretion.

Chronic fatigue Profound fatigue of long duration that is not improved by rest.

Chronic fatigue syndrome A complex disorder in which the patient experiences unrelenting fatigue and associated symptoms that are not alleviated by substantial rest and that cannot be otherwise explained for a period of 6 months or longer. Also called *myalgic encephalomyelitis*.

Chronic illness An alteration in health or function that lasts for an extended period of time, usually 6 months or longer, and often for the duration of the individual's life.

Chronic infection An infection that develops slowly and persists for months or sometimes years.

Chronic intermittent colitis A recurrent form of ulcerative colitis characterized by insidious onset, few systemic manifestations, and attacks lasting 1–3 months that occur at intervals of months to years.

Chronic kidney disease A type of renal failure that progresses slowly with few symptoms until the kidneys are severely damaged and unable to meet the excretory needs of the body. Also called *chronic renal failure.*

Chronic lymphocytic leukemia (CLL) A disorder characterized by the proliferation and accumulation of small, abnormal, mature lymphocytes in the bone marrow, peripheral blood, and body tissues.

Chronic myeloid leukemia (CML) A disorder characterized by abnormal proliferation of all bone marrow elements.

Chronic obstructive pulmonary disease (COPD) A specific progressive disorder that slowly alters the structures of the respiratory system over time, irreversibly affecting lung function.

Chronic pain Prolonged pain, usually lasting longer than 6 months. It is not always associated with an identifiable cause and is often unresponsive to conventional medical treatment.

Chronic pancreatitis An irreversible process characterized by chronic inflammation, fibrosis, and gradual destruction of functional pancreatic tissue.

Chronic traumatic encephalopathy (CTE) A form of dementia associated with a history of multiple concussions.

Chronic renal failure See Chronic kidney disease.

Chronic venous insufficiency (CVI) A disorder of inadequate venous return over a prolonged period of time.

Chvostek sign Facial grimacing caused by repeated contractions of the facial muscle. A test used to check for hypocalcemia.

Circadian rhythms Regular fluctuations in the body's physiologic processes occurring in a 24-hour cycle.

Circumcision A surgical procedure in which the prepuce, an epithelial layer covering the penis, is separated from the glans penis and excised. This procedure permits exposure of the glans for easier cleaning.

Cirrhosis The end stage of chronic liver disease. It is a progressive, irreversible disorder, eventually leading to liver failure.

Civil law The area of law that deals with the rights and duties of private persons or citizens and is most often enforced through the awarding of damages or compensation.

CK-MB A subset of CK enzyme specific to cardiac muscle. Elevated CK-MB is an indicator of myocardial infarction. Also called *MB-bands.*

Clang Repetition of rhyming words without apparent meaning.

Classism The oppression of groups of people based on their socioeconomic status.

Clean A state of medical asepsis in which almost all microorganisms are absent.

Client An individual who engages the advice or services of another person who is qualified to provide this service.

Clinical database The full extent of information about a patient, including the nursing health history, physical assessment, primary care provider's history and physical examination, results of laboratory and diagnostic tests, and material contributed by other health personnel.

Clinical decision support system A system that analyzes data and provides information about evidence-based practices. These systems can help improve patient safety and quality of care when used with sound nursing and medical judgment.

Clinical information system A software-based system that allows multiple disciplines to simultaneously access the patient's chart and record data that can be viewed and analyzed by a number of healthcare providers in real time. These systems are designed to provide the most accurate and current information about the patient so that the best decisions concerning the care of that patient can be made.

Clinical pathway A standardized, evidence-based, multidisciplinary plan that outlines the expected care required for patients with common, predictable—usually medical—conditions.

Clonic phase Typically the second phase in a generalized or tonic–clonic seizure, characterized by alternating muscular contraction and relaxation.

Closed fracture A bone fracture in which the skin remains intact. Also called a *simple fracture.*

Closed questions Restrictive questions in an interview that require only a "yes" or "no" or short, specific answer.

Clotting Also known as **coagulation,** the process by which blood changes from liquid into a gel-like substance in order to stop bleeding from a damaged vessel.

Club drugs Substances popular among adolescents and young adults who frequent dance clubs and "raves." The most common is MDMA (methylenedioxymethamphetamine), better known as Ecstasy.

Coaching The process that encourages the development of individuals through personal interaction within an organization.

Coagulation Also known as **clotting,** the process by which blood changes from liquid into a gel-like substance for the purpose of forming a clot to stop bleeding from a damaged vessel.

Coagulation cascade A process that activates clotting factors, plasma proteins used in the formation of blood clots.

Coanalgesics Drugs that have analgesic properties, potentiate the effects of pain medications, relieve other discomforts, or reduce the side effects of analgesic drugs. Coanalgesics are especially effective at reducing neuropathic pain.

Coarctation of the aorta Narrowing or constriction in the descending aorta, often near the ductus arteriosus or left subclavian artery, which obstructs the systemic blood outflow.

Cobb angle A technique to estimate the degree of curvature of the spine using lines drawn from the vertebrae at the upper and lower limits of the curve that tilt most dramatically toward the apex of the curve.

Cocaine A powerful stimulant of natural origin that acts at the nerve terminals to prevent the reuptake of dopamine and norepinephrine, which in turn results in vasoconstriction, tachycardia, and hypertension.

Code of ethics A general guide for a profession's membership and a social contract with the public that it serves.

Codependence A cluster of maladaptive behaviors exhibited by significant others of a substance-abusing individual that serves to enable and protect the abuse at the expense of living a full and satisfying life.

Cognition The complex set of mental activities through which individuals acquire, process, store, retrieve, and apply information.

Cognitive appraisal The process of appraising, sorting, assessing, categorizing, evaluating, and framing the significance of an event or stressor with respect to an individual's own well-being.

Cognitive–behavioral therapy (CBT) The use of cognitive techniques and behavior modification to change detrimental beliefs and thought patterns.

Cognitive development The manner in which people learn to think, reason, and use language.

Cognitive domain The learning domain that includes the six intellectual abilities and thinking processes: knowing, comprehending, applying, analysis, synthesis, and evaluation. Also called the *thinking domain.*

Cognitive skills Intellectual skills or thought processes that include problem solving, decision making, critical thinking, and creativity.

Cognitive symptoms Cognitive symptoms of schizophrenia include deficits in memory, attention, language, visual-spatial awareness, social and emotional perception, and intellectual and executive function.

Cognitive theory A learning theory that recognizes the developmental level of learners and acknowledges the learner's motivation and environment. Also called *cognitivism.*

Coitus interruptus A method of contraception in which the man withdraws from the woman's vagina when he feels that ejaculation is impending.

Cold zone When a disaster occurs, this zone, located outside the warm zone, is where decontaminated victims are triaged and treated. Also called the *green zone* or the *support zone.*

Colectomy Surgical resection and removal of the colon.

Collaboration Two or more people working toward a common goal.

Collaborative intervention The actions a nurse carries out in collaboration with other healthcare team members, such as physical therapists, social workers, dietitians, and physicians.

Collagen A whitish protein substance that adds tensile strength to a wound.

Collateral channels Small blood vessels that develop to connect small arteries. Also called *collateral circulation.*

Colloid osmotic pressure A pulling force exerted by colloids that helps maintain the water content of blood by pulling water from the interstitial space into the vascular compartment. Also called *oncotic pressure.*

Colloids Substances such as large protein molecules that do not readily dissolve into true solutions.

Colon cancer Cancer of the third segment of the large bowel that may or may not include the anus.

Colonization The process by which strains of microorganisms become resident flora, capable of growing and multiplying.

Colorectal cancer Cancer of both the colon and rectum.

Colostomy A surgical opening into the colon.

Colostrum The initial milk that begins to be secreted during midpregnancy and that is immediately available to the baby at birth.

Column plan A nursing care plan that uses columns to categorize data for each phase of the nursing process. This type of care plan may include four columns: (1) nursing diagnoses, (2) goals/desired outcomes, (3) nursing interventions, and (4) evaluation. Some include only three columns.

Combined oral contraceptives (COCs) A safe, highly effective contraceptive pill combining estrogen and progestin. Also called *birth control pills.*

Comfort To ease the grief or trouble of others; to give hope.

Commitment The state or an instance of being obligated or emotionally impelled.

Communicable disease An illness that is transmitted directly from one person or animal to another by contact with body fluids, or that is indirectly transmitted by contact with contaminated objects or vectors.

Communication The exchange of information, feelings, thoughts, and ideals through verbal or other techniques.

Communication deviance Communication patterns that are distracting and confusing to listeners who are trying to share a common focus or meaning with a speaker. Communication deviance has been identified as a social-environmental trigger for schizophrenia symptoms.

Communicator style The manner in which an individual communicates; includes the way the individual interacts with others.

Community-based care Care that focuses on the political, social, institutional, and physical environments of the patient.

Community Emergency Response Team (CERT) program A Federal Emergency Management Agency–organized program that prepares participants to safely assist themselves, their families, and their neighbors in case of a disaster.

Comorbidity The presence of two or more disease processes.

Compartment syndrome A condition in which the tissue pressure in a muscle compartment exceeds the microvascular pressure, interrupting cellular perfusion.

Compassion An awareness of and concern for other individuals' suffering.

Competence Possessing the knowledge and skills necessary to perform one's job appropriately and safely.

Complementary health approaches (also referred to as alternative therapies) Any of the diverse array of practices, therapies, and supplements that are not considered part of conventional or traditional medicine that are used in addition to conventional treatments.

Complete spinal cord injury An injury that involves a total loss of all sensory and motor function below the level of the injury; usually the damage is irreversible.

Compliance 1. The relationship between the volume of the intracranial components and intracranial pressure. 2. The amount of distention or expansion the ventricles can achieve to increase stroke volume. 3. The extent to which an individual's behavior coincides with medical or health advice.

Complicated grief A form of grief in which the individual's strategies to cope with a loss are maladaptive. Also called *prolonged grief disorder (PGD).*

Compression A condition that occurs when a vertical force is applied to the spinal column, such as occurs by falling and landing on the feet or buttocks or diving into shallow water.

Compromised host An individual who is at increased risk of infection.

Compulsion A repetitive behavior or mental activity used in response to obsessive thoughts that helps the individual lower his or her anxiety level.

Compulsivity One of the six trait domains associated with personality disorders that is distinguished by extreme inflexibility in a quest for perfection, in relation to both the individual's own actions and others' behaviors.

Computer vision syndrome The most common sequela of computer use. Symptoms include eye fatigue, headaches, blurred vision, dry eyes, and changes in color perception. Also called *eye strain.*

Concept map A visual representation of a nursing plan of care in a patterned diagram with data and ideas. Various shapes and colors are used to show relationships and connections in combination with lines or arrows.

Concrete thinking A type of thinking characterized by a focus on facts and details coupled with an inability to generalize or think abstractly.

Concurrent audit An evaluation of the adequacy of the nursing care a patient is receiving and a determination of whether desired outcomes are being met while the individual is still undergoing care at the healthcare facility.

Concussion Mild **traumatic brain injury**.

Condom A sheath of synthetic material that covers the penis to prevent conception or disease.

Conduction The process of heat transfer through physical contact of one surface with another surface.

Confabulation Making up information to fill memory gaps; used as a defensive mechanism to protect the person's attempt to protect self-esteem when confronted with memory loss.

Confidentiality The assurance the patient has that private information will not be disclosed without the patient's consent.

Conflict A situation that occurs when an agreement cannot be reached with regard to significant issues and concerns or when emotional opposition creates discord within an individual or among individuals, groups, or organizations.

Conflict competence Purposeful development of cognitive, behavioral, and emotional skills that assist individuals in preventing and reducing conflict.

Confusion An alteration in cognition that makes it difficult to think clearly, focus attention, or make decisions.

Confusion assessment method (CAM) A two-part test that differentiates between delirium and dementia. It is specifically designed to account for and control ageism.

Congenital cataracts A type of cataract that may appear in a child at birth or in childhood, usually in both eyes.

Congenital glaucoma A primary form of **glaucoma** caused by an abnormal development in the ocular drainage system that is sometimes diagnosed at birth but is usually diagnosed within the first year.

When diagnosed within the first year, it is often referred to as **infantile glaucoma**. When diagnosed after age 3, it may be referred to as **juvenile glaucoma**.

Congenital heart defect   A defect of the heart or great vessels that is present at birth.

Congruent communication   Communication in which the verbal and nonverbal aspects of the message match.

Conjugate vera   The true conjugate, which extends from the middle of the sacral promontory to the middle of the pubic crest.

Conjunctiva   The thin, transparent membrane that covers the anterior surface of the eye and lines the inner surfaces of the eyelids.

Conjunctivitis   Inflammation of the conjunctiva. The most common eye disease, conjunctivitis is usually caused by a bacterial or viral infection.

Connective tissue   Tissue made of fiber that forms the framework for support of the body's tissue and organs.

Consciousness   A condition in which the individual is aware of self and environment and is able to respond appropriately to stimuli. Full consciousness requires both normal arousal and full cognition.

Consequence-based (teleologic) theories   Theories that look to the outcomes (consequences) of an action in judging whether that action is right or wrong.

Conservation   The concept that matter is not changed when its form is altered.

Consolidation   Solidification of damaged cells and tissue during immune response to inflammation, specifically in the lungs.

Constant fever   A condition that occurs when the body temperature fluctuates minimally but always remains above normal.

Constipation   Fewer than three bowel movements per week or the difficult passage of stools.

Constructivism   A collection of theories with the common thread of individuals actively constructing knowledge in order to solve realistic problems, often in collaboration with others.

Consumer   An individual, a group of people, or a community that uses a service or commodity.

Consumer-driven healthcare plan (CDHP)   A type of employer-sponsored coverage that combines a private insurance plan with a Health Savings Account (HSA) or Health Reimbursement Account (HRA).

Contact dermatitis   An inflammation of the skin that occurs in response to direct contact with an allergen or irritant.

Contact precautions   Used for patients who are known to have or suspected of having serious illnesses that are easily transmitted by direct contact with the patient or by contact with items in the environment, such as *Shigella*.

Contingency contracts   A reinforcement process. Contingency contracts operate by "if–then" rules. If the patient performs a targeted response, such as abstinence from the addictive behavior (gambling, drug use, cutting, and so on), then the patient receives desired reinforcers.

Contingency planning   The process of identifying and managing unplanned and unexpected events that interfere with getting work done efficiently, effectively, and in a timely manner.

Continuance commitment   The awareness of costs associated with leaving a profession that inhibit an individual from leaving that profession. Considered the weakest type of commitment to a profession.

Continuous bladder irrigation (CBI)   A method used to prevent the formation of blood clots.

Continuous positive airway pressure (CPAP)   Mechanical ventilation that applies positive pressure to the airways of a patient who is breathing spontaneously. Breathing is patient triggered and pressure controlled. CPAP is used to help maintain open airways and alveoli, decreasing the work of breathing.

Continuous quality improvement (CQI)   A structured organizational process for involving personnel in planning and executing a continuous flow of improvements to provide quality healthcare that meets or exceeds expectations.

Continuous renal replacement therapy (CRRT)   A form of dialysis in which blood is continuously circulated through a highly porous hemofilter from artery to vein or vein to vein.

Contractility   The inherent capability of the cardiac muscle fibers to shorten.

Contraction stress test (CST)   A method of evaluating the respiratory function (oxygen and carbon dioxide exchange) of a placenta.

Contracture   Permanent shortening of connective tissue.

Contralateral deficit   Loss or impairment of sensorimotor functions on the side of the body opposite the side of the brain that is damaged by stroke.

Contrecoup injury   This injury occurs when the brain strikes the side of the skull opposite to the side of impact.

Controlled Substance Act (CSA)   A federal law that requires drugs to be classified based on the substance's medical use, potential for abuse, and safety risks.

Controlling   The managerial process of comparing actual results with projected results, similar to the evaluation step in the nursing process. Controlling includes establishing performance standards, determining how to measure performance and creating the tools that will permit consistent measurement, evaluating performance, and providing feedback.

Convection   The process of heat transfer through the fluid motion of air or water across the skin.

Convergence   The medial rotation of the eyeballs so that each is directed toward the viewed object.

Co-occurring disorders   Concurrent diagnosis of a substance use disorder and a psychiatric disorder. One disorder can precede and cause the other, such as the theorized relationship between alcoholism and depression.

Cooperative play   The stage of play in which children work together to contribute to a unified whole, such as forming a sports team or dancing in an ensemble.

Copayment   The set payment owed by an insured individual at the time a covered service is rendered.

Coping   A dynamic process through which an individual applies cognitive and behavioral measures to handle internal and external demands that are perceived by the individual as exceeding available resources.

Cor pulmonale   Right-sided heart failure.

Corneal abrasion   Disruption of the superficial epithelium of the cornea.

Corneal reflex   Closure of eyelids (blinking) due to corneal irritation.

Cornu   The elongated portion of the uterus where the fallopian tubes enter.

Coronary artery bypass grafting (CABG)   A procedure in which a section of a vein or artery is used to create a connection, or bypass, between the aorta and the blocked coronary artery beyond the obstruction.

Coronary artery disease (CAD)   The most common type of heart disease, CAD is caused by impaired blood flow to the myocardium.

Coronary circulation   A network of vessels that supply the heart muscle.

Corpus   The upper triangular portion of the uterus. Also called the *uterine body*.

Corpus luteum   A small yellow body that develops within a ruptured ovarian follicle.

Corrective action   The steps taken to overcome a job performance problem.

Coryza   Inflammation of the mucous membranes lining the nose, usually associated with nasal discharge.

Countershock phase The second part of an alarm reaction during which the sympathetic nervous system stimulation triggers the body's defenses.

Coup injury An injury that occurs when the brain strikes the same side of the skull as the side of impact.

Coup-contrecoup injury In this type of injury, the brain strikes the coup side, then bounces back and strikes the contrecoup side, resulting in contusions on both sides of the brain.

Couplet Two premature ventricular contractions in a row.

Couvade In some cultures, the man's observance of certain rituals and taboos to signify the transition to fatherhood.

Covert conflict Conflict that is avoided, ignored, or not discussed openly.

Crack A form of freebase cocaine that is made of baking soda, water, and cocaine mixed into a paste and microwaved to form a rock.

Crackles High-pitched popping sounds heard on inspiration due to fluid associated with or resulting from inflammation, or exudates, within the lung fields, or localized atelectasis.

Creatinine clearance A test that uses 24-hour urine and serum creatinine levels to determine the glomerular filtration rate; a sensitive indicator of renal function.

Creatine kinase (CK) An enzyme important for cellular function that is found principally in cardiac and skeletal muscle and the brain.

Creativity The ability to find or create a unique solution to a unique problem when traditional interventions are not effective.

Creativity techniques Strategies, such as brainstorming sessions, that use the creative potential of the group to generate a large number of possible options quickly.

Credentialing The formal identification of professionals who meet predetermined standards of professional skill or competence.

Credibility The quality of being truthful, trustworthy, and reliable.

Crepitation A grating or cracking sound.

Crime An act prohibited by statute or by common law principles.

Criminal law The area of law that deals with conduct that is harmful to another individual or to society as a whole and that may be punishable by fines or imprisonment.

Crisis An event or circumstance that overwhelms an individual's inherent ability to resolve, manage, or process the event or circumstance.

Crisis counseling A meeting that focuses on brief solutions, focused interventions, and supportive care during or after a crisis. It also considers the individual's physical vulnerability and degree of emotional stability.

Crisis intervention An emergent approach to care that is intended to assist patients with recognizing a crisis situation, and identifying and implementing an immediate, short-term solution.

Crisis intervention centers Organizations that provide telephone counseling for patients in crisis. Some organizations also provide consultation through email and online chatting.

Critical pathway Expected outcomes and care strategies developed through collaboration by the healthcare team. Also called a *case map*.

Critical thinking All or part of the process of questioning, analysis, synthesis, interpretation, inference, inductive and deductive reasoning, intuition, application, and creativity.

Crohn disease A chronic, relapsing inflammatory bowel disorder affecting the gastrointestinal tract. Also known as *regional enteritis*.

Cross-dressing Occurs when an individual of one gender (typically male) dresses in clothing specific to the opposite gender.

Crowning During birth, the appearance of the newborn's head or presenting fetal part at the vaginal orifice.

Crystalloids Salts that dissolve readily into true solutions.

Cultural deprivation A lack of culturally assistive, supportive, or facilitative acts.

Cultural groups Racial, ethnic, religious, or social groups with specific group behaviors and characteristics that are learned and shared, including language, customs, beliefs, and values.

Cultural humility The recognition that a healthcare provider's personal cultural values are not superior to the cultural values of others, thus preventing an abuse of power.

Cultural values Preferred ways of behaving or thinking that are sustained over time and used to govern a cultural group's actions and decisions.

Culture The patterns of behavior and thinking that people living in social groups learn, develop, and share.

Cultures Laboratory cultivations used to identify probable microorganisms by their characteristics, such as shape, growth patterns, and Gram-staining qualities.

Curling ulcers Acute ulcerations of the stomach or duodenum that form following a burn injury.

Cushing syndrome A disorder resulting from too much cortisol in the body. It can develop in individuals who take too much exogenous glucocorticosteroid for asthma or other disorders, or it can develop as a result of the overproduction of endogenous cortisol due to a pituitary or adrenal tumor.

Cyanosis Gray to blue or purple skin color caused by deoxygenated hemoglobin.

Cyber-bullying Aggression or bullying that occurs through the use of technology (e.g., social media, texting, or email).

Cycle of violence Violence that occurs with a patterned frequency, usually in three phases: initial tension due to communication failures, an abusive incident, and a honeymoon stage in which the aggressor may show love and affection. Cycle of violence may also refer to violence that spans multiple generations in a family.

Cyclothymic disorder A type of bipolar disorder characterized by chronic, fluctuating mood disturbances involving numerous periods of hypomanic symptoms and numerous periods of depressive symptoms.

Cystic fibrosis (CF) An inherited disorder that affects the secretory glands, particularly the glands that are responsible for secreting mucus, digestive enzymes, and sweat.

Cystic fibrosis transmembrane conductance regulator (CFTR) protein. A protein that is central to the movement of chloride into and out of the body cells.

Cystitis Inflammation of the urinary bladder.

Cystoscopy Endoscopy of the urinary tract. Also called *catheterization*.

Cytokines Proteins that carry messages for immune system function.

Damages Compensation sufficient to restore the plaintiff to his or her original position, so far as is financially possible.

Dashboard An interface that gathers, organizes, and displays a healthcare facility's key performance indicators in an easy-to-read format, often with charts or graphs.

Dashboard knee Tearing of the posterior cruciate ligament or any knee injury resulting from an individual's knee slamming into the dashboard or back of a seat during a motor vehicle collision.

Database A compilation of all information about a patient, including the nursing health history, physical assessment, primary care provider's history, physical examination, and test results.

Date rape A term used when dating violence takes the form of rape.

Dating violence A type of intimate partner abuse; this type occurs most often in relationships among youth.

Dawn phenomenon A rise in blood glucose between 4 a.m. and 8 a.m. that is not a response to hypoglycemia.

Dead space Areas of the lung that are ventilated but not perfused.

Death anxiety Worry or fear related to death or dying.

Debridement The process of removing painful or necrotic material, including all loose tissue, wound debris, and dead tissue, from a wound.

Decelerations The periodic decreases in fetal heart rate from the normal baseline.

Decerebrate posturing An abnormal posture adopted by an unconscious individual that indicates deteriorating brain function. It is characterized by an extended neck; clenched jaw; arms pronated, extended, and close to the sides; legs extended and feet plantar flexed.

Decibels (dB) Units of loudness.

Decision tree A graphic model that visually represents the choices, outcomes, and risks to be anticipated.

Declarative memory Memory that is related to people and facts, is consciously accessible, and can be verbally expressed.

Decode The process of relating the message perceived to the receiver's storehouse of knowledge and experience and sorting out the meaning of the message.

Decompensation Loss of effective compensation.

Decorticate posturing An abnormal posture adopted by an unconscious individual that indicates deteriorating brain function. It is characterized by the upper arms kept close to the sides; the elbows, wrists, and fingers flexed; the legs extended and internally rotated; and the feet plantar flexed.

Deductible A set annual cost for healthcare paid by an individual or family participating in a health insurance plan.

Deductive reasoning A "top-down" method of logical thinking that starts with a conclusion and analyzes the situation for valid, significant cues. One of two methods of logical thinking that are used to determine if decisions are reasonable.

Deep brain stimulation (DBS) A procedure in which a neurostimulator is implanted into the individual to send electrical signals to one of three brain regions—the subthalamic nucleus, the globus pallidus, or the thalamus—in order to reduce symptoms of Parkinson disease.

Deep venous thrombosis (DVT) A blood clot that forms along the intimal lining of a large vein, usually in a leg.

Defecation The expulsion of feces from the anus and rectum.

Defense mechanism See Adaptive mechanisms.

Defibrillation An emergency procedure that delivers an electrical shock to stop ventricular fibrillation and return to a rhythm that promotes cardiac output sufficient to sustain life.

Deficiency A term used to describe when intake of a nutrient is less than recommended.

Defining characteristics The cluster of signs and symptoms that indicate the presence of a particular diagnostic label.

Deformation The alteration of the spinal cord and soft tissues caused by abnormal movement.

Dehiscence An unintended separation of wound margins due to incomplete healing.

Dehydration A condition that occurs when a body does not take in as much water as it loses or lacks sufficient reserves to maintain proper function.

Delayed ejaculation Once called **male orgasmic disorder**, involves extreme difficulty ejaculating, despite the ability to maintain an erection for long periods (in some cases, an hour or more).

Delayed union The delayed healing of bones beyond the expected time period.

Delegate An individual who assumes responsibility for the actual performance of an assigned task or procedure.

Delegation The transfer of responsibility and authority for completing an activity to a qualified individual.

Delegator An individual who assigns a task to another individual to perform, but retains accountability for the outcome.

Delirium An acute cognitive disorder that affects functional independence.

Delirium tremens (DTs) A medical emergency usually occurring 3–5 days following alcohol withdrawal and lasting 2–3 days. Characterized by paranoia, disorientation, delusions, visual hallucinations, elevated vital signs, vomiting, diarrhea, and diaphoresis. Also known as *alcohol withdrawal delirium.*

Delusions False ideas or beliefs not based in reality.

Dementia The progressive, irreversible loss of cognitive function.

Democratic leader A leader who assumes that individuals are internally motivated, are capable of making decisions, and value independence. Democratic leaders typically provide constructive feedback, offer information, make suggestions, and ask questions to gain information or to help group members grow in their ability to make decisions.

Demography The study of population, including statistics about distribution by age and place of residence, mortality, and morbidity.

Demyelination A condition in which cells of the immune system, such as lymphocytes and macrophages, cross the blood–brain barrier and attack and destroy the myelin sheath.

Denominations Groups of members that adhere to the same practices and beliefs.

Dental caries Cavities.

Deoxyribonucleic acid (DNA) One of two types of nucleic acid made by cells, DNA contains the genetic instructions for the development and functioning of human beings.

Dependence A physiologic need for a substance that the patient cannot control, and which results in withdrawal symptoms if the substance is withheld.

Dependent intervention Activities carried out under a physician's orders or supervision, or according to specified routines or protocols.

Dependent personality disorder (DPD) One of several personality disorders defined in the DSM-5, it is marked by a pervasive, excessive, and unrealistic need to be cared for; fear of separation; lack of self-confidence; an inability to make decisions; and an inability to function independently.

Depersonalization A feeling of strangeness or unreality about the physical self.

Depolarization 1. The rapid inflow of sodium ions, causing an electrical change in which the inside of a cell becomes positive in relation to the outside. 2. The phase in which the heart contracts as a result of ion channel functions.

Depo-Provera A long-acting progesterone that provides highly effective birth control for 3 months when given as a single injection.

Depression A disorder characterized by a sad or despondent mood or loss of interest in usual activities.

Depressive disorder with peripartum onset See Postpartum depression.

Derealization A feeling of disconnection from an individual's own body or the environment.

Dermatome An area of skin innervated by the cutaneous branch of one spinal nerve.

Dermis The second layer of skin, which is made of a flexible connective tissue. It is richly supplied with blood cells, nerve fibers, and lymphatic vessels, as well as most of the hair follicles, sebaceous glands, and sweat glands.

Desaturated blood Blood that is low in oxygen as a result of oxygenated and deoxygenated blood mixing due to a congenital heart defect.

Desire phase The first phase of the sexual response cycle is the arousal of sexual interest by means of real or symbolic stimuli.

Detachment One of the six trait domains associated with personality disorders that is broken down into withdrawal, intimacy avoidance, anhedonia, and restricted affectivity.

Detrusor muscle The smooth muscle layers of the bladder wall, the detrusor muscle allows the bladder to expand as it fills with urine and contract as it releases urine during voiding.

Development An increase in the complexity and function of skill progression, the individual's capacity and skill to adapt to the environment. Related to growth.

Developmental disability Any of a variety of chronic conditions characterized by mental and/or physical impairment.

Developmental stage A level of achievement for a particular segment of an individual's life.

Developmental task A skill or behavior pattern learned during stages of development.

Device integration Real-time, accurate data is recorded in the patient's chart directly from a device (e.g., blood pressure monitor). Device integration allows the nurse to more quickly analyze and interpret that data and make adjustments to the plan of care based on the most current information.

Diabetes mellitus Group of chronic disorders of the endocrine pancreas, all categorized under a broad diagnostic label. The condition is characterized by inappropriate hyperglycemia caused by a relative or absolute deficiency of insulin or by a cellular resistance to the action of insulin. Also called *diabetes*.

Diabetic ketoacidosis (DKA) A form of metabolic acidosis that develops when there is an absolute deficiency of insulin and an increase in the insulin counterregulatory hormones. It may also be induced by stress in an individual with type 1 diabetes.

Diabetic nephropathy Disease of the kidneys in patients with diabetes that is characterized by the presence of albumin in the urine, hypertension, edema, and progressive renal insufficiency.

Diabetic neuropathy A disorder of the peripheral nerves and the autonomic nervous system in patients with diabetes, which manifests in one or more of the following: sensory and motor impairment, muscle weakness and pain, cranial nerve disorders, impaired vasomotor function, impaired gastrointestinal function, and impaired genitourinary function.

Diabetic retinopathy The collective name for the changes in the retina that occur in the person with diabetes. The retinal capillary structure undergoes alterations in blood flow, leading to retinal ischemia and a breakdown in the blood–retinal barrier.

Diagnosis-related groups (DRGs) A system of price control regulation that classifies patient illnesses based on diagnoses and pays hospitals a predetermined sum for each specific diagnosis regardless of the actual cost of services, the length of stay, or the acuity or complexity of the patient's illness.

Diagnostic label Standardized NANDA names for nursing diagnoses.

Diagonal conjugate Distance from the lower posterior border of the symphysis pubis to the sacral promontory.

Dialysate Dialysis solution.

Dialysis A process by which fluids and molecules pass through a semipermeable membrane from an area of higher solute concentration to one of lower solute concentration according to the rules of osmosis. Dialysis is used to remove excess fluid and metabolic waste products in renal failure.

Diaphragm A flexible disc that covers the cervix to prevent conception.

Diaphysis The shaft of a bone.

Diarrhea The passage of liquid feces and an increased frequency of defecation.

Diastasis recti abdominis A separation of the abdominal muscle.

Diastole The phase of ventricular relaxation between heartbeats.

Diastolic blood pressure The minimum pressure within the arteries during diastole.

Diathermy Treatment with heat generated by high-frequency electrical currents.

Diencephalon Area of the brain consisting of the thalamus (sometimes called the dorsal thalamus), hypothalamus, epithalamus, and subthalamus.

Diet recall Patient history of intake over a specified period of time.

Dietary Reference Intakes (DRIs) A standardized, recommended nutrient intake to support a healthy diet often provided by health organizations.

Differentiated practice A system in which each nurse's educational preparation and skill sets are evaluated and used to determine how he or she will be best used.

Differentiation A process occurring over many cell cycles that allows cells to specialize in certain tasks.

Diffuse axonal injury An injury that occurs because of a rotational deceleration that is dramatic enough to cause damage to the brain's white matter in the form of widespread disruption of axon fibers and myelin sheaths.

Diffusion The continual intermingling of molecules in liquids, gases, or solids brought about by the random movement of the molecules.

Digestion The conversion of food by means of its mechanical and chemical breakdown into absorbable substances in the gastrointestinal tract.

Digital rectal examination (DRE) An examination to detect for abnormalities in the rectum that can be detected through palpation.

Dihydrotestosterone (DHT) The androgen that mediates prostatic growth at all ages; formed in the prostate from testosterone.

Dilated cardiomyopathy The most common form of cardiomyopathy, it is characterized by the dilation of the heart chambers and impaired ventricular contraction.

Directing The managerial process of effectively motivating, communicating, and delegating tasks in order to complete an organization's work.

Directive interview A highly structured interview that elicits specific health information.

Dirty In medical asepsis, a term used to indicate that microorganisms are likely to be present.

Disaster An event that occurs with little or no warning in which available personnel and emergency services are initially overwhelmed and a serious threat to life, public health, and the environment is posed.

Discharge planning A plan of care that prepares the patient for discharge, including training in any necessary health skills.

Discipline A method of teaching children the rules for how to behave in society and what is expected in different circumstances.

Discoid lesions Raised, scaly, circular lesions with an erythematous rim.

Discovery The legal process of obtaining information before a trial.

Discrimination The differential treatment of individuals or groups, based on categories such as race, age, weight, gender, or social class, that occurs when an individual acts on prejudice and denies other people one or more of their fundamental rights.

Discussion An informal oral consideration of a subject by two or more healthcare personnel to identify a problem or establish strategies to resolve a problem.

Disease A detectable alteration in body function resulting from infection by microorganisms that causes a reduction of capacities or a shortening of the normal lifespan. Also called *pathogenesis*.

Disease surveillance Monitoring patterns of disease occurrence from cases of infections and communicable diseases reported by healthcare workers to state officials.

Diseases of adaptation Stress-related illnesses, such as peptic ulcers and hypertension.

Disenfranchised grief Grief that occurs when an individual is unable to acknowledge a loss to other persons. Also called *ambiguous loss*.

Disinfectants Agents that destroy pathogens other than spores.

Disinhibition One of the six trait domains associated with personality disorders that is noted for the presence of irresponsibility, impulsivity, and risk taking.

Disc Fluid-filled "shock absorber" that holds together and insulates the vertebrae. Also called *spinal disc*.

Discectomy The removal of all or part of the nucleus pulposus of an intervertebral disc.

Dismissal Termination of employment.

Disorganized behavior The inability to start or finish goal-oriented activities to a degree that it interferes with an individual's ability to lead a normal life.

Disorganized thinking Difficulty logically connecting thoughts, leading to garbled speech.

Dissatisfaction problems Issues that arise from unmet sexual needs and expectations.

Disseminated intravascular coagulation (DIC) A disruption of hemostasis characterized by widespread intravascular clotting and bleeding. It may be acute and life threatening, or it may be relatively mild.

Distracted driving The act of driving a motor vehicle while doing any activity that takes attention away from the road. Activities include texting, talking on the phone, eating, drinking, reading a map, talking to passengers, looking at a GPS, and adjusting the radio.

Distress A stress that is associated with inadequacy, insecurity, and loss.

Distributive shock Shock that results from widespread vasodilation and decreased peripheral resistance. Also called *vasogenic shock*.

Diuresis The production and excretion of abnormally large amounts of urine. Also called *polyuria*.

Diuretics Pharmacologic agents that increase urine formation and secretion.

Diversity The unique variations among and between individuals, variations that are informed by genetics and cultural background, but that are refined by experience and personal choice.

Diverticula Saclike projections of mucosa through the muscular layer of the wall of a canal or organ, e.g., the bladder wall, colon, or large intestine.

Documenting The process of making an entry on a patient record. Also called *recording* or *charting*.

Doll's eye reflex An oculomotor response in which the eyes move in opposite direction as head turns to the side. Also called the **oculocephalic reflex**.

Domestic partner An unmarried partner of the same or opposite sex.

Do-not-intubate (DNI) order Usually written by the physician for the patient who has a terminal illness or is near death, this order is usually based on the wishes of the patient and family that no lifesaving measures be provided once the patient stops breathing.

Do-not-resuscitate (DNR) order Usually written by the physician for the patient who has a terminal illness or is near death, this order is usually based on the wishes of the patient and family that no cardiopulmonary resuscitation be performed for respiratory or cardiac arrest. Also called a *no-code order*.

Dopamine A brain neurotransmitter that regulates voluntary movement, reward-seeking behavior, memory and learning, attention, sleep, affect, and many other functions.

Dormant Temporarily inactive but not dead.

Double-bind theory The theory that schizophrenia symptoms are partially an expression of contradictory family interactions.

Double depression A term used to describe a situation in which an individual experiences dysthymic disorder in combination with major depressive disorder.

Doula A paid caregiver who has typically received special training and may even be certified in caring for laboring women.

Down syndrome A developmental disorder that occurs when an individual is born with an extra full or partial chromosome. Down syndrome is associated with intellectual disability and a wide variety of physical impairments that can range from mild to severe.

Dramatic play The stage of play in which individuals use props to act out the drama of human life.

Dressler syndrome A symptom complex characterized by fever and chest pain that may develop days to weeks after an AMI. It is thought to be a hypersensitivity response to necrotic tissue or an autoimmune disorder.

Droplet nuclei Residue of evaporated droplets emitted by an infected host; can remain in the air for long periods of time.

Droplet precautions Used for patients who are known to have or suspected of having serious illnesses transmitted by particle droplets larger than 5 microns, such as pertussis or pneumonia.

Dual diagnosis Term used to refer to concurrent diagnoses of a psychiatric disorder and a substance use disorder.

Dubowitz tool A tool for assessing newborns that includes neuromuscular tone assessments, such as head lag, ventral suspension, and leg recoil.

Dullness A thudlike sound produced by dense tissue such as the liver, spleen, or heart.

Duodenal ulcer A peptic ulcer occurring in the duodenum.

Durable power of attorney A legal document that can delegate the authority to make health, financial, and/or legal decisions on an individual's behalf.

Durable power of attorney for healthcare A legal designation of another individual, usually a family member, significant other, or close personal friend, to make healthcare decisions on an individual's behalf.

Duration 1. The length of a sound. 2. The length of time from the beginning of a contraction to the completion of that same contraction.

Duty A legally enforceable obligation to conform to a particular standard of conduct that is owed to the patient.

Dwarfism Excessively short stature caused by insufficient growth hormone, typically resulting from a genetic abnormality.

Dysfunctional uterine bleeding (DUB) Vaginal bleeding that is usually painless but abnormal in amount, duration, or time of occurrence. Also called *abnormal uterine bleeding*.

Dysmenorrhea Painful menstruation.

Dyspareunia Painful intercourse.

Dysphagia Difficulty swallowing.

Dysplasia A loss of DNA control over differentiation occurring in response to adverse conditions.

Dyspnea Shortness of breath or difficulty breathing that is uncomfortable or painful; or when breathing is insufficient to meet oxygen demand.

Dysrhythmia Abnormal heart rate or rhythm. Also called *arrhythmia*.

Dysthymia A chronic depressive disorder with symptoms that are less severe than those of major depressive disorder. Also called *persistent depressive disorder* or *dysthymic disorder*.

Dystonia Severe muscle spasms, particularly of the back, neck, tongue, and face.

Dysuria Difficult or painful urination.

Early deceleration During birth, a condition that occurs when the fetal head is compressed and cerebral blood flow decreases, causing central vagal stimulation. Usually associated with the onset of uterine contractions.

Early (primary) postpartum hemorrhage Hemorrhage that occurs in the first 24 hours after childbirth.

Eating disorder A set of maladaptive responses to stress or anxiety characterized by obsessions with food and weight, often to the extent that daily functioning is impaired and physical and psychologic health are threatened.

Echolalia The compulsive parroting of a word or phrase just spoken by another.

Echopraxia The compulsive imitation of the movements of another.

Eclampsia A major complication of pregnancy characterized by hypertension, albuminuria, oliguria, tonic and clonic convulsions, and coma.

Ecologic theory A theory of development that emphasizes the presence of mutual interactions between the individual and all of life's settings.

Ecomap Visual representation of how the family unit interacts with the external community environment, including schools, religious institutions, occupational duties, and recreational pursuits.

Ectopic beats Impulses originating outside normal conduction pathways of the heart that interrupt the normal conduction sequence and may not initiate a normal muscle contraction.

Edema Swelling caused by excess fluid trapped in body tissue.

Effacement The drawing up of the internal os and the cervical canal into the uterine side walls.

Effectiveness In healthcare, effectiveness is providing services based on scientific knowledge to all who could benefit and refraining from providing services to those not likely to benefit.

Efficiency In healthcare, efficiency is avoiding waste of equipment, supplies, ideas, and energy.

Ego defense mechanisms Unconscious psychologic processes developed for the purpose of defending the personality. Also called *defense mechanisms.*

Egocentrism Ability to see things only from one's own point of view.

Ego-syntonic The perception that one's behaviors and beliefs are normal and any difficulties with other people are external to oneself.

E-health Electronic information that can be retrieved and transferred online or through a mobile device to improve a person's health or healthcare.

Ejection fraction The fraction or percentage of the diastolic volume that is ejected from the heart during systole.

Elasticity of the arterial wall An indicator of the health of an artery. A healthy, normal artery feels straight, smooth, soft, and pliable. Older adults often have inelastic arteries that feel twisted (tortuous) and irregular upon palpation.

Elder abuse The intentional physical, emotional, or sexual mistreatment or neglect of an individual 65 years of age or older.

Elderspeak A speech style similar to baby talk that communicates a message of dependence and incompetence to older adults.

Elective surgery Performed when surgical intervention is the preferred treatment for a condition that is not imminently life threatening (but may ultimately threaten life or well-being) or to improve the patient's life.

Electrocardiogram (ECG) A graphic record of the heart's activity.

Electrocardiography A diagnostic test of cardiac function.

Electroconvulsive therapy (ECT) A treatment procedure during which an electric current is passed through the brain. It is useful to patients with severe depression, acute mania, some psychotic conditions, and those who are acutely suicidal.

Electroencephalogram (EEG) Measures and records the brain's electrical activity.

Electrolyte A charged ion capable of conducting electricity.

Electromyogram A diagnostic technique that measures the electrical activity of the muscles at rest and during contraction.

Electronic communication Transmitting information though email, social networking, text messaging, and other electronic means.

Electronic fetal monitoring (EFM) The measurement and tracing of the fetal heart rate (FHR), which allows many characteristics of the FHR to be visually assessed.

Electronic health record (EHR) A health record system that is designed so that multiple clinicians from multiple disciplines (e.g., family practice, nursing, pharmacy, specialists) can all have simultaneous access to the patient's health information.

Electronic medical record (EMR) A system focused on diagnosis and treatment. EMRs track information over time (weight, blood pressure, cholesterol readings) and identify when patients are due for routine preventive health maintenance such as vaccines and mammograms.

Elimination The secretion and excretion of body wastes from the kidneys and intestines.

Embolus A particle or aggregate of blood, fat, or pathogens or a bubble of air that obstructs a blood vessel.

Embryo The early stage of development of the young of any organism. In humans the embryonic period is from about 2 to 8 weeks' gestation and is characterized by cellular differentiation and predominantly hyperplastic growth.

Embryonic membranes The amnion and chorion.

Emergency A sudden, often unforeseen event that threatens health or safety.

Emergency preparedness The act of making plans to prevent, respond to, and recover from emergencies.

Emergency response The implementation of emergency preparedness plans.

Emergency surgery Surgery that is performed immediately to preserve function or the life of the patient.

Emesis The act of vomiting; occurs when inspiratory muscles of the thorax (including the diaphragm) and abdomen contract, increasing intrathoracic and intra-abdominal pressures.

Emigration The movement of leukocytes through the blood vessel wall into affected tissue spaces in response to illness or injury.

Emotion-focused coping The regulation of emotional responses to distress when the stressor is perceived to be beyond the individual's control.

Emotional availability The quality of parent–child interactions, including parental sensitivity, structuring, and degree of intrusiveness and hostility.

Emotions Feeling responses to a wide variety of emotional stimuli.

Emphysema A progressive pulmonary disease characterized by destruction of the walls of the alveoli, with resulting enlargement of abnormal air spaces.

Empirical knowing The twofold understanding of facts and observations relevant to nursing, and of the analyses and theories that attempt to explain them. Also called the *science of nursing.*

Empyema Accumulation of purulent (infected) exudate in a space, for example, the pleural cavity or the gallbladder.

Enabling behavior Any action by an individual that consciously or unconsciously facilitates substance dependence.

Enamel A hard substance that encapsulates the crown, the uppermost part of the tooth.

Encapsulated Enclosed.

Encoding The selection of specific signs or symbols to transmit a message, such as which language and words to use, how to arrange the words, and what tone of voice and gestures to use.

Encopresis Abnormal elimination pattern characterized by recurrent soiling or passage of stool at inappropriate times.

Enculturation The process by which children learn culture from adults. Also called *cultural transmission.*

End-of-dose medication failure Pain experienced at the end of one dose of medication before the next dose is scheduled.

End of life The final weeks of life when death is imminent.

End-of-life care The nursing care provided to a patient who is dying or who is near death.

End-stage renal disease (ESRD) The final stage of chronic kidney disease, when the kidneys are unable to excrete metabolic wastes and regulate fluid and electrolyte balance adequately.

Endocardial cushion defect A combination of defects in the atrial and ventricular septa and portions of the tricuspid and mitral valves. A complete AV canal defect allows blood to travel freely among all four chambers of the heart. Also called *atrioventricular (AV) canal defect.*

Endocardial cushions Fetal growth centers for mitral and tricuspid valves and AV septum.

Endogenous Developing from within.

Endogenous insulin Insulin that is produced by an individual's own body.

Endogenous pyrogens Interleukins, interferons, and tumor necrosis factor released by macrophages in response to an infection.

Endometriosis A condition that occurs when endometrial tissue implants on organs outside the uterus, causing pain, fibrosis, and adhesions.

Endometrium The innermost mucosal layer of the uterus.

Endotoxins Found in the cell wall of gram-negative bacteria, endotoxins are released only when the cell is disrupted. They act as activators of many human regulatory systems, producing fever, inflammation, and potentially clotting, bleeding, or hypotension when released in large quantities.

Engagement The passing of the fetus into the pelvic inlet in preparation for birth.

Engrossment The characteristic sense of absorption, preoccupation, and interest in an infant demonstrated by fathers during early contact.

Enophthalmos Sunken appearance of the eyes.

Enteral nutrition Tube feeding used to meet calorie and protein requirements in patients who are unable to consume enough food on their own.

Entropion Inversion of the eyelid.

Enuresis Involuntary passing of urine in children after bladder control is achieved.

Environmental health hazards Factors that impede individual and community health and include natural or human-made substances, states, or events which affect the natural environment, produce negative effects on the human ecosphere, and adversely affect health.

Environmental quality One of the 12 leading health indicators identified by *Healthy People 2020,* environmental quality refers to the ability of the environment to promote and sustain individual and community health.

Enzymes Chemicals that induce a chemical reaction in order to assist in the breakdown of nutrients.

Eosinophil A type of leukocyte found in large numbers in the respiratory and gastrointestinal tracts. Eosinophils are thought to be responsible for protecting the body from parasitic worms. They also play a role in the hypersensitivity response by inactivating some of the inflammatory chemicals released during the inflammatory response.

Epidemic Widespread outbreak of infectious disease with many infected people.

Epidermis The surface or outermost part of the skin consisting of four to five layers of epithelial cells.

Epigenetic External influences or effects on gene expression.

Epilepsy A chronic disorder characterized by recurrent, unprovoked seizures secondary to a central nervous system disorder.

Epiphyseal plate Cartilage between the epiphysis and diaphysis found in the long bones of children.

Episiotomy A surgical incision of the perineal body to enlarge the outlet.

Epispadias Congenital abnormality in which the meatus is located on the upper side of the glans.

Epstein's pearls Small, glistening, white specks that feel hard to the touch on the hard palate and gum margins.

Erb-Duchenne paralysis Damage affecting the upper arm between the fifth and sixth cervical nerves, causing paralysis. Also called *Erb palsy.*

Erectile disorder Term used to describe **erectile dysfunction** when the cause of the disorder is unrelated to physical causes (for example, it results as a side effect of a substance or medication).

Erectile dysfunction (ED) The inability of a man to attain and maintain an erection sufficient to permit satisfactory sexual intercourse.

Ergonomics The science of fitting workplace conditions and job demands to the capabilities of the working population.

Erik Erikson A German-born psychologist and psychoanalyst who created a theory of development comprising eight stages or age-related tasks faced by an individual throughout the lifespan.

Erythema A reddening of the skin.

Erythema toxicum An eruption of lesions in the area surrounding a hair follicle that are firm, vary in size from 1 to 3 mm, and consist of a white or pale yellow papule or pustule with an erythematous base. Also called *newborn rash* or *flea bite dermatitis.*

Eschar Hard, leathery crust that covers a burn wound and harbors necrotic tissue.

Escharotomy Surgical removal of eschar from the torso or extremity to prevent circumferential constriction.

Essential nutrients The macro- and micronutrients needed for the body's survival.

Essential tremors Tremors that are not associated with another condition and may be genetic in origin.

Estimated date of birth (EDB) The approximated date of childbirth. Also called estimated date of delivery.

Estrogen The primary hormone responsible for female sex characteristics.

Ethical knowing Understanding and applying the ethical codes by which nurses are expected to abide, as well as upholding the various philosophical, cultural, and moral frameworks of the institution and of the patient. Also called the *moral component.*

Ethics The rules or principles that govern right or moral conduct.

Ethnic group Group of individuals who have common racial characteristics and share a cultural heritage.

Etiology A causal relationship between a problem and its related or risk factors.

Eupnea Breathing within the expected respiratory rates.

Eustachian tube Connects the middle ear with the nasopharynx to help equalize the pressure in the middle ear with the atmospheric pressure.

Eustress Good stress that is associated with accomplishment and victory.

Euthanasia From the Greek for *painless, easy, gentle,* or *good death,* now commonly used to signify a killing prompted by a humanitarian motive.

Euthymia Stable or normal mood.

Euthyroid A normal thyroid state.

Evaluation Reassessment of a patient following nursing or medical intervention or therapy.

Evaluation statement A written comment on the care plan or in the nurse's notes about progress following an evaluation. An evaluation statement must contain the date and time evaluation was done; a conclusion statement determining goal met, partially met, or not met; and a supporting statement giving the results of how the patient did or did not achieve the goal.

Evaporation The process of converting water to a vapor.

Evidence Clinical knowledge, expert opinion, or information resulting from research.

Evidence-based nursing An integration of the best evidence available, nursing expertise, and the values and preferences of the individuals, families, and communities who are served.

Evidence-based practice The application of research in areas that are of interest to nursing and in the actual practice of nursing.

Evisceration Protrusion of internal viscera through a surgical wound.

Exacerbation A reappearance of symptoms of a chronic illness. Also called a *flare*.

Excess More than is needed in order for the body to survive and remain productive.

Excitement phase This second phase of the sexual response cycle is marked by an increase in blood flow to various body parts, resulting in erection of the penis and clitoris and swelling of the labia, testes, and breasts.

Excoriation Area of loss of the superficial layers of the skin. Also called *denuded area*.

Executive function The mental skills involved in planning and executing complex tasks.

Exercise Physical activity that is planned, structured, and involves repetitive body movements; the goal is to improve or maintain one or more components of physical fitness.

Exercise addiction Excessive pattern of exercising regardless of physical injury, personal inconvenience, or disruption to other areas of life, including marital strain, interference with work, and lack of time for other activities.

Exercise intolerance Decreased ability to participate in activities using large skeletal muscles because of fatigue or dyspnea.

Exogenous Developing from outside sources.

Exogenous insulin Insulin from a source outside the body.

Exophthalmos Protruding eyes.

Exotoxins Soluble proteins that microorganisms secrete into surrounding tissue. Exotoxins are highly poisonous, causing cell death or dysfunction.

Expectorate To expel or spit out.

Expiration The act of exhaling air in respiration.

Expressed consent An oral or written agreement.

Expressive jargon Using unintelligible words with normal speech intonations as if truly communicating in words.

Expressive speech The ability to speak and be understood by others.

Extended family The relatives of nuclear families, such as grandparents, aunts, and uncles.

Extended kin network family A form of extended family in which two nuclear families of primary or unmarried kin live in proximity to each other and share a social support network, goods, and services.

External patients The individuals who seek healthcare as well as their family members and significant others; and other individuals and entities with whom internal patients interact, such as insurance companies, managed care organizations, equipment or material suppliers, social service agencies, and law enforcement officials.

External environmental stressors Triggers outside of an individual that demand change or disrupt homeostasis.

External locus of control The belief that an individual's health is controlled by forces outside of his or her control such as chance or fate.

Extracapsular extraction A surgical treatment for cataracts in which the anterior capsule, nucleus, and cortex of the lens are removed, leaving the posterior capsule intact.

Extracapsular hip fracture A hip fracture involving the trochanteric region between the neck and diaphysis of the femur.

Extracellular fluid (ECF) Fluid found outside the cells. It accounts for about one third of total body fluid and is subdivided into compartments. The two main compartments of ECF are intravascular and interstitial.

Extracorporeal shock wave lithotripsy (ESWL) A noninvasive technique for fragmenting kidney stones using shock waves generated outside the body.

Extrapulmonary tuberculosis Results when tuberculosis spreads through the blood and lymph system to other organs.

Extrapyramidal side effects (EPS) A particularly serious set of adverse reactions to antipsychotic drugs. EPS includes acute dystonia, akathisia, parkinsonism, and tardive dyskinesia.

Extubation The process of withdrawing a breathing tube on completion of anesthesia and the surgical case.

Exudate Material, such as fluid and cells, that has escaped from blood vessels during the inflammatory process and is deposited in tissue or on tissue surfaces.

Exudative macular degeneration A form of macular degeneration characterized by the formation of new, weak blood vessels in the potential space between the choroid and the retina. Also referred to as the wet form of macular degeneration.

Eye movement desensitization and reprocessing (EMDR) A form of psychotherapy that contains elements of a number of types of therapy, including cognitive–behavioral therapy and body-centered therapy.

Failure to thrive (FTT) 1. Inability to meet or maintain developmental milestones related to physical growth due to undernutrition. 2. A syndrome in which an infant falls below the fifth percentile for weight and height on a standard growth chart or is falling in percentiles on a growth chart.

Faith To believe in or be committed to something or someone.

Fallopian tubes Tubes that extend from the lateral angle of the uterus and terminate near the ovary. Also called *oviducts* and *uterine tubes*.

False imprisonment The unjustifiable detention of an individual without legal warrant to confine the person.

False pelvis The portion of the pelvis above the linea terminalis that supports the enlarged pregnant uterus.

Familial AD (FAD) One of the two basic types of Alzheimer disease, it has a strong inherited component and usually manifests before the age of 65. Also called *early-onset Alzheimer disease*.

Family Individuals who are joined together by marriage, blood, adoption, or residence in the same household.

Family burden The overall level of distress experienced by a family as a result of a family member's illness.

Family-centered care A model of healthcare service that is provided in partnership with the patient and family.

Family-centered nursing Nursing that considers the health of the family as a unit in addition to the health of individual family members.

Family cohesion The emotional bonding between family members.

Family communication Includes listening, speaking, self-disclosure, and tracking abilities of the family as a group.

Family coping mechanisms The behaviors families use to deal with stress or changes imposed from either within or without the family.

Family development The dynamics or changes a family experiences over time, including changes in relationships, communication patterns, roles, and interactions.

Family flexibility The amount of change in a family's leadership, role relationships, relationship rules, and ability to respond to stress.

Family recovery Family response to a member's mental illness.

Family support Support from family members as they care for other family members; for example, one sister relieves another to care for their aging mother over the weekend.

Family therapy A form of therapy in which the family system is treated as a unit and the focus is on family dynamics.

Fascial excision Excising a wound to the level of fascia. Also called *fasciectomy*.

Fasciculation An irregular movement or a twitch.

Fasciectomy Excising a wound to the level of fascia. Also called *fascial excision*.

Fat embolism syndrome (FES) Occurs when fat globules lodge in the pulmonary vascular bed or peripheral circulation.

Fatigue A condition characterized by a lack of energy and motivation that may or may not be accompanied by drowsiness.

Fear A sense of apprehension triggered by a perceived threat to safety or well-being, including a painful stimuli or dangerous event.

Febrile Having a fever.

Febrile seizures Generalized seizures that usually occur in children as the result of rapid temperature rise above 39°C (102°F), usually in association with an acute illness. No evidence of intracranial infection or other defined cause is found in relation.

Fecal impaction A mass or collection of hardened feces in the folds of the rectum.

Fecal incontinence The loss of voluntary ability to control fecal and gaseous discharges through the anal sphincter. Also called *bowel incontinence*.

Fecalith A hard mass of feces.

Feces Body wastes and undigested food eliminated from the bowel. Also called *stool*.

Feedback 1. The mechanisms by which some of the output of a system is returned to the system as input. 2. The response a receiver of a message gives to the message's sender.

Female orgasmic disorder The persistent delay or absence of orgasm following a phase of normal sexual excitement.

Female reproductive cycle (FRC) The monthly rhythmic changes in sexually mature women; composed of the ovarian cycle, during which ovulation occurs, and the uterine cycle, during which menstruation occurs.

Female sexual interest/arousal disorder Persistent decreased or absent sexual thoughts, interest in sexual activity, mental or physical feelings of arousal, and/or pleasurable sensation during sexual activity.

Fertility awareness-based methods Contraception based on an understanding of the changes that occur throughout a woman's ovulatory cycle. Also called *natural family planning*.

Fertilization The process by which a sperm fuses with an ovum to form a new diploid cell, or zygote.

Festination Rapid, small steps, as if an individual is trying to run.

Fetal alcohol spectrum disorder See Fetal alcohol syndrome (FAS).

Fetal alcohol syndrome (FAS) A developmental disorder that occurs when a developing fetus is exposed to ethyl alcohol. Fetal alcohol syndrome is associated with physical, intellectual, behavioral, and/or learning disabilities. Also called *fetal alcohol spectrum disorder*.

Fetal attitude The flexion or extension of the fetal body and extremities.

Fetal bradycardia A fetal heart rate of less than 110 bpm during a 10-minute period or longer.

Fetal demise Death of a fetus that occurs after 20 weeks' gestation. Also called a *stillbirth* or *intrauterine fetal death (IUFD)*.

Fetal heart rate (FHR) The number of times the fetal heart beats per minute; normal range is 120–160.

Fetal lie The relationship of the cephalocaudal axis, or spinal column, of the fetus to the cephalocaudal axis, or spinal column, of the woman. The fetus may be in a longitudinal or transverse lie.

Fetal movement record A noninvasive technique that enables the pregnant woman to monitor and record movements easily and without expense.

Fetal position The relationship of the landmark on the presenting fetal part to the front, sides, or back of the maternal pelvis.

Fetal presentation The body part of the fetus entering the pelvis in a single or multiple pregnancy.

Fetal tachycardia A fetal heart rate of 161 bpm or more during a 10-minute period of continuous monitoring.

Fetoscope An adaptation of a stethoscope that facilitates auscultation of the fetal heart rate.

Fetoscopy A technique for directly observing the fetus and obtaining a sample of fetal blood or skin.

Fetus The child in utero from about the seventh to ninth week of gestation until birth.

Fever A protective immune response to foreign antigens within the body that increases the cellular metabolic rate, thus increasing the body's temperature.

Fever of unknown origin A temperature above 100.9°F (38.3°C) that occurs on several occasions within a short time span, lasts for more than 3 weeks, and does not have a definitive cause after 1 week of clinical investigation.

Fever phobia Fear felt by caregivers about the harmful effects of a fever on a child, such as seizure, brain damage, and death.

Fever spike A temperature that rises to fever level rapidly, following a normal temperature, and then returns to normal within a few hours.

Fiber A polysaccharide that contributes to disease prevention, especially in the gastrointestinal tract and the cardiovascular system.

Fibrin Connective tissue.

Fibrin degradation products Potent anticoagulants.

Fibromyalgia A chronic disorder characterized by widespread musculoskeletal pain, fatigue, and multiple tender points.

Fidelity A moral principle that obligates an individual to be faithful to agreements and responsibilities one has undertaken.

Filtration A process whereby fluid and solutes move together across a membrane from a compartment with higher pressure to a compartment with lower pressure.

Filtration pressure The pressure in the compartment that results in the movement of the fluid and substances dissolved in fluid out of the compartment.

Fimbria A funnel-like enlargement of the fallopian tube with many fingerlike projections (fimbriae) reaching out to the ovary.

First heart sound (S$_1$) The heart sound produced by the closure of the AV valve; characterized by the syllable "lub."

Five P's neurovascular assessment An assessment checklist for pain, pulse, pallor, paralysis/paresis, and paresthesia.

Fixation The immobilization or inability of an individual to proceed to the next developmental stage because of anxiety.

Flaccidity Absence of muscle tone. Also called *hypotonia*.

Flashbacks The recurrence of images, sounds, smells, or feelings from a traumatic event; often triggered by daily events, such as a car backfiring on the street or the smell of a perpetrator's cologne.

Flat affect Minimal facial expression and movement, sometimes monotone speech patterns.

Flatness An extremely dull sound produced by very dense tissue, such as muscle or bone.

Flatulence The presence of excessive amounts of gas in the stomach or intestines.

Flatus Gas or air normally present in the stomach or intestines.

Flight of ideas Rapidly changing, fragmentary thoughts.

Flow sheet A specific assessment criteria in a particular format, such as human needs or functional health patterns.

Fluid resuscitation The administration of intravenous (IV) fluids to restore circulating blood volume during an acute period of increasing capillary permeability.

Fluid volume deficit (FVD) Substantial loss of both water and electrolytes in similar proportions from the extracellular fluid. Also called *hypovolemia*.

Fluid volume excess (FVE) Excessive fluid retained by the body. The retention of both water and sodium in similar proportions to normal extracellular fluid (ECF). Also called *hypervolemia*.

Fluoroscope A scope used to project visual examination images on a fluorescent screen.

Focal seizures Seizures that are caused by abnormal electrical activity in one hemisphere or in a specific area of the cerebral cortex, most often the temporal, frontal, or parietal lobes. The seizure may spread regionally, and the symptoms are related to the region of the cortex that is affected. Also known as *partial seizures*.

Focus charting Date and time, focus, and progress notes are recorded for a specific condition, nursing diagnosis, and behavior to make the patient and the patient's concerns and strengths the focus of care.

Folic acid A vitamin that is required for normal growth, reproduction, and lactation and that prevents the macrocytic, megaloblastic anemia of pregnancy.

Follicle-stimulating hormone (FSH) Hormone produced by the anterior pituitary during the first half of the menstrual cycle, stimulating development of the graafian follicle.

Fontanels The intersections of membranous spaces between the cranial bones of a fetus.

Food choice An individual's decision of what and how much to eat of a specific food. This decision can be influenced by a number of conscious and unconscious factors such as taste, preparation, smell, habits, convenience, availability, and cost.

Food insecurity Results when one or more members of a household must reduce their eating patterns due to a lack of money or lack of resources to access appropriate amounts and varieties of food.

Food security Results when all members of a household have sufficient resources to access appropriate amounts and varieties of food.

Foramen ovale An opening between the atria of the fetal heart.

Foraminotomy An enlargement of the opening between the disc and the facet joint to remove bony overgrowth.

Forced expiratory volume in 1 second (FEV$_1$) The amount of air that can be exhaled in 1 second as measured by a spirometer.

Forceps-assisted birth The use of forceps to assist the birth of a fetus by providing traction or by providing the means to rotate the fetal head to an occiput-anterior position. Also called an *instrumental delivery*, *operative delivery*, or *operative vaginal delivery*.

Forceps marks Reddened areas over the cheeks and jaws on an infant caused by a difficult forceps birth.

Foreground question Questions that are narrow in focus about a specific clinical issue.

Foreseeability The ability to foresee events that reasonably may be expected to cause specific results.

Formal group A group with formalized goals, designated management, and only partly voluntary membership.

Formal leader A leader who is selected by an organization and given official authority to make decisions and act.

Formation The process that facilitates the transformation of an individual from a layperson to a professional nurse.

Foster family A family consisting of one or more adults caring for one or more children from other families when the children can no longer live with their birth parents.

Fourth heart sound (S$_4$) A heart sound produced by atrial contraction and ejection of blood into the ventricle during late diastole. Also called *atrial gallop*.

Fracture A break in the continuity of a bone.

Fragile X syndrome A developmental disorder caused by a single recessive gene abnormality on the X chromosome. Fragile X syndrome is associated most notably with intellectual disability, often accompanied by ADHD and other behavioral problems.

Frank–Starling mechanism An increase in venous return increases ventricular filling and myocardial stretch, which increases the force of contraction.

Free-floating anxiety Excessive worry about everyday events; worry that is hard to control and the focus of which may shift from moment to moment.

Freezing A condition in which an individual feels like his or her feet are stuck to the floor.

Frequency The time between the beginning of one contraction and the beginning of the next contraction.

Friend support Support or assistance from nonfamily members, such as friends or coworkers, for a family during a time of illness or stress.

Frostbite An injury of the skin resulting from freezing.

Frustration An emotion that occurs when an individual is prevented from reaching a desired goal. Intense frustration may trigger violent aggressive tendencies resulting in assault or homicide.

Fulguration A procedure that destroys tissue with electrical current.

Full-thickness burn A burn that involves all layers of the skin, including the epidermis, the dermis, and the epidermal appendages.

Fulminant colitis An acute form of ulcerative colitis that involves the entire colon; manifestations include severe bloody diarrhea, acute abdominal pain, and fever.

Functional assessments Typically a combination of assessments that includes observations of child behavior, responses, and abilities. It is used to assess how a child functions on a daily basis in his or her environment and to determine if the child has any developmental delays or special needs.

Functional method A method of coordinating care that focuses on the jobs to be completed as part of patient care (e.g., bed making and temperature measurement). In this task-oriented approach, personnel with less educational preparation than the professional nurse (e.g., unlicensed assistive personnel) perform aspects of care with less complex requirements.

Functional nursing A task-oriented approach to care delivery used in situations of inadequate staffing or nursing shortages.

Functional strength The body's ability to perform work.

Fundus The rounded, uppermost portion of the uterus.

Fungi A type of microorganism capable of producing infection. Yeasts and molds are common types of fungi.

Galanin A neuropeptide that is released by neurons as they are injured or die. Often associated with Alzheimer disease, although the exact role galanin plays in the disease is unknown.

Gallstone ileus A large gallstone.

Gambling disorder An **addiction** to gambling characterized by gambling despite the risk of losing something of value (e.g., a home) and an inability to stop gambling.

Gamete Female or male germ cell; contains a haploid number of chromosomes.

Gametogenesis The process by which germ cells are produced.

Gastric lavage Irrigation of the stomach with large quantities of normal saline.

Gastric outlet obstruction Obstruction of the pyloric region of the stomach and duodenum that impairs gastric outflow; a potential complication of peptic ulcer disease.

Gastric ulcer A peptic ulcer that occurs in the stomach.

Gastrocolic reflex The increased peristalsis of the colon after food has entered the stomach.

Gastroesophageal reflux disease (GERD) A disease in which stomach contents flow back up into the esophagus.

Gate control theory Melzack and Wall's 1965 theory stating that the perception of pain is controlled by the overall activity of small-diameter (pain) fibers vs. large-diameter (heat, cold, mechanical) fibers.

Gender identity One's self-image as a female or male.

Gender-role behavior The outward expression of an individual's sense of maleness or femaleness as well as the expression of what is perceived as gender-appropriate behavior.

General adaptation syndrome (GAS) A three-stage chain of events in an individual's stress response.

Generalized anxiety disorder (GAD) A condition that occurs when an individual experiences intense tension and worry, even if no external stressors are present.

Generalized seizures The result of diffuse electrical activity that often begins in both hemispheres of the brain simultaneously, then spreads throughout the cortex into the brainstem. As a result, movements and spasms displayed by the patient are bilateral and symmetric.

Generational cohort Individuals born in the same general time span who share key life experiences, including historical events, public heroes, pastimes, and early work experiences.

Genital herpes A sexually transmitted infection caused by the herpes simplex virus.

Genital intercourse Penetration of the vagina by the penis. Also called *coitus*.

Genital warts A sexually transmitted infection caused by the human papillomavirus (HPV).

Genito-pelvic pain/penetration disorder Persistent or recurrent dyspareunia (pain) or fear of pain before or during vaginal penetration.

Genogram Visual representation of gender showing lines of birth descent through the generations.

Genotype The pattern of genes on chromosomes.

Geographic information system (GIS) A system that relies on satellite imaging and global positioning systems to capture, manage, and analyze geographical data.

Geragogy The process of stimulating and helping older adults to learn.

Geriatric failure to thrive (GFTT) A condition in which older patients experience a multidimensional decline in physical functioning that is characterized by weight loss of more than 5% of baseline body weight, decreased appetite, undernutrition, dehydration, depression, and cognitive and immune impairment.

Gestation Period of intrauterine development from conception through birth; pregnancy.

Gestational age assessment tools Methods to determine an infant's age at birth assessing external physical characteristics and neurologic or neuromuscular development.

Gestational diabetes mellitus (GDM) A carbohydrate intolerance of variable severity with onset or first recognition during pregnancy.

Gingiva The gum.

Gingivitis Red, swollen gingiva.

Glaucoma A condition characterized by optic neuropathy with gradual loss of peripheral vision and, usually, increased intraocular pressure of the eye.

Global evaluative dimension of the self The degree to which an individual likes him- or herself overall, as a whole being. Also called *global self-esteem*.

Global self The collective beliefs and images an individual holds about him- or herself.

Global self-esteem See Global evaluative dimension of the self.

Glomerular filtration rate (GFR) The rate at which fluid is filtered through the kidneys.

Glomerulonephritis Inflammation of the glomerular capillary membrane.

Glomerulus Found in the nephrons of the kidneys, a tuft of capillaries surrounded by the Bowman capsule.

Glucagon Produced by alpha cells, glucagon is a hormone that decreases glucose oxidation and promotes an increase in the blood glucose level by signaling the liver to release glucose from glycogen stores. In addition to stimulating the breakdown of glycogen in the liver, glucagon stimulates the formation of carbohydrates in the liver and the breakdown of lipids in both the liver and adipose tissue.

Gluconeogenesis The formation of glucose from fats and proteins.

Glucosuria The excretion of glucose in the urine.

Glycogenolysis The breakdown of liver glycogen.

Glycosuria The excretion of carbohydrates into the urine.

Goiter An enlarged thyroid gland

Gonadotropin-releasing hormone (GnRH) A hormone secreted by the hypothalamus that stimulates the anterior pituitary to secrete follicle-stimulating hormone and luteinizing hormone.

Gonorrhea A sexually transmitted infection caused by *Neisseria gonorrhoeae*.

Good-faith immunity Law or laws that protect healthcare workers from civil or criminal liabilities when they report suspected child abuse in good faith, even if the subsequent investigation does not make a determination of abuse.

Good Samaritan laws Specific laws designed to protect healthcare workers from potential liability when volunteering their skills outside of an employment contract.

Goodpasture syndrome A rare autoimmune disorder of unknown etiology that is characterized by formation of antibodies to the glomerular basement membrane.

Governance The establishment and maintenance of social, political, and economic arrangements by which professionals control their practice, their self-discipline, their working conditions, and their professional affairs.

Graafian follicle The ovarian cyst containing the ripe ovum, which secretes estrogens.

Grading A standardized method of judging a tumor's aggressiveness based on the level of differentiation and mitotic rate; where the least malignant cells are classified grade 1 and the most aggressive malignant cells are classified grade 4.

Graft-versus-host disease (GVHD) A series of immunologic reactions in response to transplanted cells.

Gram stain A diagnostic test conducted to identify infecting organisms in urine by shape and characteristic.

Granulation tissue Young connective tissue with new capillaries formed in the healing process.

Grasping reflex The closing and grasping of an infant's fingers in response to a finger placed in the palm of the infant's hand.

Graves disease An autoimmune disorder marked by an enlarged thyroid and signs of hyperthyroidism.

Grief The total psychologic, biological, and behavioral response to the emotional experience related to loss.

Group Three or more individuals who have a common purpose, interact with each other, influence each other, and are interdependent.

Group therapy A form of therapy that allows group members to help each other with psychologic, cognitive, behavioral, and spiritual dysfunctions through a process of change, aided by a professional group therapist.

Groupthink A type of decision making characterized by a group's failure to critically examine their own processes and practices or to recognize and respond to change.

Growth Physical change and increase in size.

Guillain-Barré syndrome (GBS) An acute inflammatory demyelinating disorder of the peripheral nervous system characterized by an acute onset of motor paralysis (usually ascending).

Gustatory Of or relating to taste.

Gynecomastia Abnormal enlargement of the breast(s) in men.

H₁ receptors Cellular histamine receptors that are present in the smooth muscle of the vascular system, the bronchial tree, and the digestive tract. Stimulation of these receptors results in itching, pain, edema, bronchoconstriction, and other characteristic symptoms of inflammation and allergy.

H1N1 influenza A form of the influenza virus that consists of avian genes, human genes, and genes from flu viruses typically found in pigs from Asia and Europe. Once mistakenly called *swine flu*, it can be spread through human-to-human transmission.

H₂ receptors Cellular histamine receptors present primarily in the stomach; their stimulation results in the secretion of large amounts of hydrochloric acid.

Habit training Attempts to keep patients dry by having them void at regular intervals.

Habituation The newborn's ability to process and respond to complex stimulations.

Hallucination The perception of seeing, hearing, or feeling something that is not present in reality.

Hallucinogen A type of drug that induces the same types of thoughts, perceptions, and feelings that occur in dreams. Hallucinogens include PCP, 3,4-MDMA, ᴅ-lysergic acid diethylamide (LSD), mescaline, dimethyltryptamine (DMT), and psilocin.

Hand restraints A device used to protect confused patients from scratching or injuring their skin, or dislodging intravenous access devices. Also called *mitt restraints.*

Handoff The transfer of information along with authority and responsibility during transitions in care across the continuum.

Handoff communication A verbal or written exchange of information. It encompasses the nursing team and all other members of the healthcare team who care for a patient at any given time.

Hardware The physical component of technology, including computers, keyboards, and display screens.

Harlequin sign A reddening of the skin on one side of an infant's body while the other side remains pale. Also called *clown color change.*

Hashimoto thyroiditis An autoimmune disorder in which antibodies destroy thyroid tissue.

Hassles Day-to-day tension/stressors.

Health A state of complete physical, mental, and social well-being.

Health beliefs Concepts about health that an individual believes are true, regardless of whether or not they are founded in fact.

Health Insurance Portability and Accountability Act (HIPAA) Legislation enacted by Congress to minimize the exclusion of preexisting conditions as a barrier to healthcare insurance, designate special rights for those who lose other health coverage, and eliminate medical underwriting in group plans. The act includes the Privacy Rule, which creates a national standard for of the disclosure of private health information.

Health Level Seven (HL7) A framework designed for the exchange, integration, sharing, and retrieval of electronic health information that supports clinical practice and the management, delivery, and evaluation of health services.

Health literacy The ability to read, understand, and act on health information, including such tasks as comprehending prescription labels, interpreting appointment slips, completing health insurance forms, and following instructions for diagnostic tests.

Health maintenance organization (HMO) The most restrictive type of private health insurance plan. HMO participants must select a primary care provider who provides basic medical services and, as the gatekeeper to care, refers the patient to in-network hospitals and specialists when additional care is needed.

Health policy The actions and decisions by government bodies and professional organizations that affect whether or not healthcare organizations and individuals working within the healthcare system can achieve their healthcare goals.

Health promotion A way of thinking and acting in order to increase individuals' overall health and well-being regardless of their health and illness status or age.

Health restoration Care focusing on the ill patient that extends from early detection of disease through helping the patient during the recovery period.

Healthcare advance directive Legal document that allows an individual to plan for healthcare and/or financial affairs in the event of incapacity. Also called *advance directive* or *advance healthcare directive.*

Healthcare-associated infection (HAI) Infections associated with the delivery of healthcare services in a facility such as a hospital or nursing home. Also called a *nosocomial infection.*

Healthcare disparity A difference in a measurement of access to or quality of healthcare services between an individual or group possessing a defined characteristic when other variables have been controlled, such as individual health choices, disease courses, and other variations from the normative measure.

Healthcare proxy An individual selected to speak to physicians and other healthcare providers on behalf of a patient to determine the best course of treatment.

Healthcare surrogate An individual selected to make medical decisions when someone is no longer able to make them for him- or herself.

Heart block A block in the normal electrical conduction of the heart.

Heart failure The inability of the heart to pump adequate blood to meet the metabolic demands of the body.

Heart murmur Harsh, blowing sounds caused by disruption of blood flow into the heart, between the chambers of the heart, or from the heart into the pulmonary or aortic systems.

Heartburn A burning sensation in the chest or throat. Also called *pyrosis.*

Heat balance When the amount of heat produced by the body equals the amount of heat lost.

Heat exhaustion Excessive heat exposure and dehydration that causes paleness, dizziness, nausea, vomiting, fainting, and a moderately increased temperature (38.3°–38.9°C [101°–102°F]).

Heat stroke A serious form of heat exhaustion that can be life threatening, generally caused by exercising in hot weather. Patients will have warm, flushed skin, often do not sweat, and have a temperature of 41°C (106°F) or higher. A patient may be also delirious, unconscious, or having seizures.

Heat transfer The four ways heat moves from one place or object to another place or object.

Heaving Lifting of the chest wall during contraction.

Heberden nodes Bony lumps on the end joint of a digit.

Helper T cells Play a vital role in normal immune system function, recognizing foreign antigens and infected cells and activating antibody-producing B cells. They are the primary cells infected by the human immunodeficiency virus.

HELPP syndrome A cluster of changes, including hemolysis, elevated liver enzymes, and low platelet count, sometimes associated with preeclampsia.

Hematochezia Bright blood in the stool.

Hematocrit The proportion of cells and plasma in blood. Also refers to the laboratory test that measures the hematocrit. This test can also be used to detect severe dehydration or overhydration.

Hematogenous spread Describes the spread of infection or disease through the blood.

Hematoma A localized collection of blood underneath the skin that may appear as a bruise.

Hematopoiesis Blood cell formation.

Hematuria The presence of blood in the urine.

Hemianopia The loss of half of the visual field of one or both eyes.

Hemiarthroplasty Hip replacement that involves replacement of the ball, the head, or the femur.

Hemiarthroscopy The surgical replacement of the femoral head with a smooth metal sphere.

Hemiparesis Weakness of the left or right half of the body.

Hemiplegia Paralysis of the left or right half of the body.

Hemispheres The two halves created by the division of the cerebrum by the deep fold.

Hemodialysis A process by which a patient's blood flows through vascular catheters, passes by the dialysate in an external machine, and then returns to the patient.

Hemodynamics The study of forces involved in blood circulation.

Hemoglobin The oxygen-carrying molecule within red blood cells; a laboratory test to measure the amount of hemoglobin.

Hemoglobinopathy A disorder of hemoglobin.

Hemolysis The destruction of red blood cells; releases hemoglobin into the circulation.

Hemolytic anemia A disorder that results from the premature destruction of red blood cells.

Hemoptysis Bloody sputum.

Hemorrhage Rapid or excessive bleeding.

Hemosiderosis The storage of excessive iron in tissues and organs.

Hemostasis The cessation of bleeding.

Hemotympanum Bleeding into or behind the tympanic membrane.

Hepatitis The inflammation of the liver triggered by a virus, alcohol, medications, toxins, autoimmune disorder, or other pathogens.

Here-and-now concept A concept used in group therapy that recognizes that only in the present moment of a group's experience can change be made.

Hernia A protrusion in the intestine through the inguinal wall or canal.

Herniated intervertebral disc A rupture of the cartilage surrounding the intervertebral disc with protrusion of the nucleus pulposus. Also called a *ruptured disc*, *slipped disc*, or *herniated nucleus pulposus*.

Heroin An illicit, central nervous system depressant narcotic that alters perception and produces euphoria.

Heterograft Skin used for transplantation that was obtained from an animal, usually a pig. Also called a *xenograft*.

Heterosexism The view that heterosexuality is the only correct sexual orientation.

Heterosexual An individual who is attracted to members of the opposite sex.

Highly active antiretroviral therapy (HAART) Effective treatment of AIDS that combines at least three medications to inhibit HIV replication.

Hip fracture A fracture of the femur at the head, neck, or trochanteric regions.

Hippocampus A small, curved body in the brain. Part of the limbic system, it plays a major role in memory formation.

Hirsutism An increased growth of coarse hair on the face and trunk.

Histamine A key chemical mediator of inflammation.

Histrionic personality disorder (HPD) One of several personality disorders defined in the DSM-5, it is characterized by a lifelong tendency for dramatic, egocentric, attention-seeking response patterns.

Hoarding compulsion An excessive collection and accumulation of objects, extreme cluttering of the living environment, accompanied by a lack of regard for the embarrassment of family member or others whose living is impacted.

Holistic health A clinical mindset that considers more than the physiologic health status of an individual.

Holosystolic Term used to describe the sounds heard during the entire phase of systole.

Holy day A day set aside for special religious observance.

Homan sign Pain in the calf when the foot is dorsiflexed.

Homeostasis The body's ability to maintain a state of physiologic balance in the presence of constantly changing conditions.

Homicide The killing of one individual by another; for legal purposes, this act is further specified by whether the act was intentional or due to negligence.

Homocysteine An amino acid that is a homologue of cysteine.

Homograft Grafts between members of the same species who have different genotypes and HLA antigens. Usually human skin that has been harvested from cadavers. Also called an *allograft*.

Homologous chromosomes The two paired chromosomes that are inherited, one from each parent.

Homophobia The fear, hatred, or mistrust of gays and lesbians often expressed in overt displays of discrimination.

Homosexual An individual who is attracted to members of the same sex.

Hope To expect or desire with confidence.

Horizontal violence (HV) Aggressive acts committed against a nurse by one or more nursing colleagues.

Hormone replacement therapy (HRT) Administration of hormones, usually estrogen and a progestin, to alleviate the symptoms of menopause.

Hormones Chemical messengers secreted by various glands that exert controlling effects on the cells of the body.

Hospice An organization that provides end-of-life care for patients either in their homes or in a hospital setting.

Hospice care The support and care for persons in the last phase of an incurable disease so that they may live as fully and comfortably as possible until their death.

Hot zone When a disaster occurs, the hot zone is the most dangerous zone because it is located immediately adjacent to the site of the disaster. All responders who enter the area must be protected by personal protective equipment.

Human chorionic gonadotropin (HCG) A hormone produced by the chorionic villi that is found in the urine of pregnant women. Also called *prolan*.

Human dignity The inherent worth and uniqueness of individuals and populations.

Human immunodeficiency virus (HIV) A primary immunodeficiency disorder that is spread primarily through sexual contact with an infected person. HIV is the virus that causes acquired immunodeficiency syndrome (AIDS).

Human leukocyte antigen (HLA) The major histocompatibility complex gene.

Humanistic learning theory A learning theory that focuses on the unique cognitive and affective qualities of a learner.

Humoral immune response Hyperreactive response of B cells characteristic of systemic lupus erythematosus (SLE).

Hunger The feeling that makes individuals think of food and encourages them to satisfy this feeling by eating.

Hyaluronic acid (HA) A lubricating substance in cartilage and joint synovial fluid.

Hydrocephalus A condition characterized by enlargement of the head caused by inadequate drainage of cerebrospinal fluid.

Hydronephrosis An accumulation of urine in the renal pelvis as a result of obstructed outflow.

Hydrostatic pressure The pressure a fluid exerts within a closed system on the walls of its container. The hydrostatic pressure of blood is the force blood exerts against the vascular walls (e.g., the artery walls). The principle involved in hydrostatic pressure is that fluids move from an area of greater pressure to an area of lesser pressure.

Hydroureter Distention of the ureter with urine.

Hyperalgesia Increased response to a pain stimulus because of peripheral sensitization.

Hypercalcemia Elevated blood levels of calcium.

Hypercapnia A condition marked by a $PaCO_2$ level above 45 mmHg. Also known as **hypercarbia**.

Hypercarbia See Hypercapnia.

Hyperchloremia Elevated chloride levels in the blood.

Hypercyanotic episode A potentially life-threatening episode of hypoxia. Also called a *tet episode*.

Hyperemia Increased blood flow to an area.

Hyperextension Forcible backward bending.

Hyperflexion Forcible forward bending.

Hyperglycemia Elevated glucose levels.

Hyperkalemia Elevated potassium levels in the blood.

Hypermagnesemia Elevated magnesium levels in the blood.

Hypernatremia Elevated sodium levels in the blood.

Hyperopia Farsightedness.

Hyperosmolar hyperglycemic state (HHS) A disorder characterized by a plasma osmolarity of 340 mOsm/L or greater, greatly elevated blood glucose levels, and altered levels of consciousness. It occurs in individuals who have type 2 diabetes mellitus.

Hyperphosphatemia Increased blood levels of phosphate.

Hyperplasia An increase in the number or density of normal cells.

Hyperresonance An abnormal, booming sound that can be heard over an emphysematous lung.

Hyperresponsiveness An exaggerated response, as with bronchoconstriction in asthma.

Hypersensitivity An overreaction of the immune system to an antigen or antigens.

Hypersomnia The inability to stay awake during the day, despite obtaining sufficient sleep at night.

Hypertension Excess pressure in the arterial portion of the circulatory system, specifically a systolic blood pressure of 140 mmHg or higher or a diastolic blood pressure of 90 mmHg or higher.

Hypertensive crisis A systolic blood pressure greater than 180 mmHg and diastolic blood pressure higher than 120 mmHg. Also called *malignant hypertension*.

Hypertensive encephalopathy A syndrome characterized by extremely high blood pressure, altered level of consciousness, increased intracranial pressure, papilledema, and seizures.

Hyperthermia A condition that occurs when a body produces more heat than is lost.

Hyperthermia blanket An electronically controlled blanket that provides a specified temperature

Hyperthermic A body temperature above 37.8°C (100°F).

Hyperthyroidism A disorder caused by excessive delivery of thyroid hormone to the peripheral tissues. Also called *thyrotoxicosis*.

Hypertonic Refers to solutions that have a higher osmolality than body fluids; 3% sodium chloride is a hypertonic solution.

Hypertonic dehydration Occurs when sodium loss is proportionately less than water loss. Also called *hypernatremic dehydration*.

Hypertrophic cardiomyopathy A disorder characterized by decreased compliance of the left ventricle and hypertrophy of the ventricular muscle mass.

Hypertrophic scar An overgrowth of dermal tissue that remains within the boundaries of the wound.

Hypertrophy An enlargement of glandular cells or muscles.

Hyperventilation Unusually fast respirations, or overbreathing causing an imbalance of oxygen and carbon dioxide.

Hypervolemia The excessive retention of both water and sodium in similar proportions to normal extracellular fluid (ECF). Also called *fluid volume excess*.

Hyphema Bleeding into the anterior chamber of the eye.

Hypoactive sexual desire disorder A deficiency in or absence of sexual fantasies and persistently low interest or a total lack of interest in sexual activity.

Hypocalcemia Decreased blood levels of calcium.

Hypocapnia A condition that results when $PaCO_2$ falls below 35 mmHg. Also called **hypocarbia**.

Hypocarbia See Hypocapnia.

Hypochloremia Decreased blood levels of chloride.

Hypodermis The layer of loose connective tissue and fat cells that lies below the dermis. Also called *subcutaneous tissue*.

Hypodermoclysis Fluid administered subcutaneously.

Hypoglycemia Diminished glucose levels.

Hypokalemia Decreased blood levels of potassium.

Hypomagnesemia Decreased blood levels of magnesium.

Hypomania A less extreme form of mania that is not severe enough to markedly impair functioning or require hospitalization.

Hyponatremia Decreased blood levels of sodium.

Hypoperfusion Decreased blood flow.

Hypophonia A lowered voice volume.

Hypophosphatemia Decreased blood levels of phosphate.

Hypoplastic left heart syndrome (HLHS) One of the most severe congenital heart defects, characterized by absence or stenosis of mitral and aortic valves, an abnormally small left ventricle, a small aorta, and aortic or mitral stenosis or atresia.

Hypotension A below-normal blood pressure reading between 85 and 110 mmHg.

Hypothalamic-pituitary axis In the brain, the HPA is responsible for the regulation of endocrine glands, and consequently, hormones.

Hypothermia A condition that occurs when a body loses more heat than it produces.

Hypothermic A body temperature below 36°C (97°F).

Hypothyroidism A disorder resulting when the thyroid gland produces an insufficient amount of thyroid hormone.

Hypotonic Refers to solutions that have a lower osmolality than body fluids, such as one half normal saline.

Hypotonic dehydration Occurs when fluid loss is characterized by a proportionately greater loss of sodium than water. Also called *hyponatremic dehydration*.

Hypoventilation An abnormally slow respiratory rate leads to inadequate oxygen delivery to the lungs as well as an increase in retention of carbon dioxide.

Hypovolemia Loss of both water and electrolytes in similar proportions from extracellular fluid. Also called *fluid volume deficit*.

Hypovolemic shock Shock caused by a decrease in intravascular volume of 15% or more.

Hypoxemia Decreased oxygen levels in the blood that result when PaO_2 falls below 80 mmHg.

Hypoxia Decreased delivery of oxygen to the tissues.

Iatrogenic Refers to a condition induced by the effects of treatment.

Iatrogenic infection A type of infection that results directly from diagnostic or therapeutic procedures.

Ideal body image A mental representation of what an individual believes his or her body should look like.

Ideal self How the individual thinks he or she should be or would prefer to be.

Idiopathic pain A type of pain that occurs unpredictably and is not associated with any known cause, making it difficult to treat.

Ileostomy A surgical opening made in the ileum of the small intestine.

Ileus A condition that causes a temporary cessation of the passage of material through the intestines, usually lasting 24–48 hours.

Illness A state in which an individual's physical, emotional, intellectual, social, developmental, or spiritual functioning is diminished.

Illness behavior A coping mechanism that includes the ways in which an individual describes, monitors, and interprets symptoms, and the individual's ability to take remedial action and use the healthcare system.

Illness prevention Healthcare focusing on maintaining optimal health by preventing disease through programs on immunizations, prenatal and infant care, and prevention of sexually transmitted infections.

Illusion A distorted perception of actual sensory stimuli.

Imagery A relaxation technique in which the patient focuses on pleasant images such as a beach or a garden to replace negative images such as pain and darkness. Also called *guided imagery*.

Imitation The process by which individuals copy or reproduce what they have observed.

Immobility A reduction in the amount and control of one's movement.

Immunity The body's natural or induced response to infection and the conditions associated with its response.

Immunization Introduces an antigen into the body, allowing immunity against a disease to develop naturally.

Immunocompetent Term used to describe patients who have an immune system that identifies antigens and effectively destroys or removes them.

Immunodeficiency A condition that develops when the immune system is incompetent or unable to respond effectively.

Immunoglobulin (Ig) A protein that functions as an antibody.

Immunosuppression Inability of the immune system to respond to an antigen. Occurs in response to disease or medications; may be intentional to prevent rejection of transplants or a side effect of some medications.

Implied consent Nonverbal consent indicated by a patient's cooperative actions.

Impotence Inability to achieve or maintain an erection.

Impulse conduction The transmission of an impulse along the nerve pathways to the spinal cord and directly to the brain.

Impulsiveness Acting without considering the consequences of one's behavior. Also called *impulsivity*.

In vitro fertilization A process in which a woman's eggs are collected from her ovaries, fertilized in the laboratory, and then placed into her uterus after normal embryo development has begun.

Incentive spirometry A breathing exercise using an incentive spirometer that helps patients breathe deeply to expand the lungs. This process can help patients clear mucus secretions and increase the amount of oxygen delivered to the bronchi and alveoli.

Incident pain A type of breakthrough pain that is predictable because it is precipitated by an event or activity such as coughing or changing position.

Incident report An agency record of an accident or incident occurring within the agency. This record is designed to collect adequate information to assist personnel in preventing future incidents or occurrences. Also called *variance reports* or *unusual occurrence reports*.

Incomplete spinal cord injury An injury that involves only a partial loss of sensory and motor function below the level of the injury.

Increased intracranial pressure (IICP) Sustained, elevated pressure (15 mmHg or higher in adults) in the cranial cavity.

Indemnity plan A type of health insurance program that allows the insured to self-select healthcare providers and has no predefined network.

Independent intervention The activities that nurses are licensed to do within their scope of practice; in other words, areas of healthcare that are unique to nursing and separate and distinct from medical management.

Indicator A statistic that reflects the organization's performance in a specific area.

Inductive reasoning A "bottom-up" method of logical thinking that starts with putting significant cues together in order to reach a conclusion. It is a method of logical thinking that is used to determine if decisions are reasonable.

Infantile glaucoma **Congenital glaucoma** diagnosed within the first year of life.

Infection An invasion of the body tissue by microorganisms with the potential to cause illness or disease.

Infectious disease Any communicable disease that is caused by microorganisms that are commonly transmitted from one person to another or from an animal to an individual.

Infertility A lack of conception despite unprotected sexual intercourse for at least 12 months.

Inflammation An adaptive response to what the body sees as harmful, such as an allergen, illness, or injury. Inflammation typically is characterized by pain, heat, redness, and swelling. Also called *inflammatory response*.

Inflammatory bowel disease (IBD) Chronic inflammation of the bowel common to a group of conditions that includes Crohn disease and ulcerative colitis.

Influenza A highly contagious viral respiratory disease characterized by coryza (inflammation of the mucous membranes lining the nose usually associated with nasal discharge), fever, cough, and systemic symptoms such as headache and malaise (vague feeling of physical discomfort).

Informal groups A type of group that functions with much less structure than a formal or semiformal group. Characteristics of informal groups include easily recognized, basic objectives; rotational leadership; and no set of written rules or regulations.

Informal leader A leader who is not officially appointed to direct the activities of others but, because of seniority, age, or special abilities, is recognized by the group as a leader and plays an important role in influencing colleagues, coworkers, or other group members to achieve the group's goals.

Informed consent 1. A patient's legal and ethical rights to be informed of and give permission for any healthcare procedure or treatment. 2. A study volunteer's legal right to be informed with full disclosure of the study's purpose, required procedures, length of the study, expectations, risks, and possible benefits before consenting to participate. Informed consent also includes the right to withdraw from the study at any time.

Infundibulopelvic ligament A ligament that suspends and supports the ovaries.

Inhalant A substance inhaled to produce euphoria. Categorized into three types: anesthetics, volatile nitrites, and organic solvents.

Injury An act or event that causes damage, harm, or loss to a body's functioning.

Input Information, material, or energy that enters a system.

Inquiry A search for knowledge or facts in order to gain clarification and find solutions to problems.

Insensible fluid loss Fluid loss that is not perceptible to the individual and cannot be measured.

Insomnia The inability to fall asleep or remain asleep.

Inspection A visual, auditory, and olfactory examination or assessment of a patient to note health condition.

Inspiration The act of inhaling air in respiration.

Instrumental aggression Aggression executed in the absence of emotional arousal.

Insubordination Defiance of authority, such as the refusal to complete a task as assigned.

Insulin A hormone that facilitates the uptake and use of glucose by cells and prevents an excessive breakdown of glycogen in the liver and muscle. In doing so, insulin acts to decrease blood glucose levels.

Insulin reaction Low blood glucose levels, or hypoglycemia. Also called *insulin shock.*

Integrative health The process of incorporating **complementary health approaches** into mainstream Western healthcare.

Integrity Adherence to a strict moral or ethical code.

Integumentary system The body's system that includes skin, hair, and nails and the sebaceous, sweat, and mammary glands.

Intellect The ability to learn and understand knowledge; the capacity for thinking and reasoning intelligently.

Intellectual disability Significant limitations in intellectual functioning and adaptive behavior prior to the age of 18. Previously called *mental retardation.*

Intellectual functioning General intelligence or mental capacity, including an individual's abilities to learn, use logic, and solve problems.

Intensity 1. The amplitude of a sound produced. 2. The strength of the contraction during acme, the peak of a uterine contraction during the birth process.

Interdisciplinary assessment An assessment that involves more than one discipline such as nursing and physical therapy. Also called *interprofessional assessment.*

Interdisciplinary team A team that seeks to achieve a common goal, though the team members are professionals with varied backgrounds. Also called *interprofessional team.*

Intergroup conflict Conflict that occurs between teams that are in competition or opposition to one another.

Intermittent claudication A cramping or aching pain in the calves of the legs, the thighs, and the buttocks that occurs with a predictable level of activity

Intermittent fever Occurs when body temperature alternates at regular intervals between periods of fever and periods of normal or subnormal temperatures.

Internal environment The physical, spiritual, cognitive, emotional, and psychologic well-being of an individual that depends on the satisfaction of these basic human needs.

Internal locus of control A belief that an individual can impact her or his own health and well-being.

Internet gaming disorder The persistent use of the internet to engage in games, often with other players, leading to clinically significant impairment or distress. May also be referred to as *internet gaming addiction.*

Interdisciplinary Referring to professionals or paraprofessionals from various disciplines.

Interorganizational conflict Usually conflict that occurs between two organizations that exist within one market.

Interpersonal conflict Conflict that occurs between two or more individuals due to differences, competition, or concern about territory, control, or loss.

Interpersonal violence Violence that occurs within relationships, between family members, intimate partners, acquaintances, or strangers that does not aim to further the goals of a formal group or cause.

Interprofessional Referring to professionals from multiple or various disciplines.

Interprofessional team A team that seeks to achieve a common goal, though the team members are professionals with varied backgrounds. Also called *interdisciplinary team.*

Intersex A general term used to describe a variety of conditions in which reproductive or sexual anatomy does not fit the typical definitions of male or female.

Interstitial fluid Accounts for approximately 75% of extracellular fluid; interstitial fluid surrounds the cells.

Intervention Activities conducted or attempts made by the nurse to influence a positive change in a patient's health status or behavior; a personalized confrontation that prevents an addict from denying the addiction problem and forces them to face the negative aspects of their behavior and enroll in treatment.

Intimacy A relationship that entails commitment, companionship, affective intimacy, social support, physical closeness, and mutuality.

Intimate distance Communication that is characterized by body contact, heightened sensations of body heat and smell, and vocalizations that are low.

Intimate partner violence (IPV) The act of inflicting sexual, emotional, or physical harm on a current or previous partner or spouse.

Intra-aortic balloon pump (IABP) Also called intra-aortic balloon counterpulsation, the IABP is a mechanical circulatory support device that may be used after cardiac surgery or to treat cardiogenic shock following AMI. The IABP temporarily supports cardiac function, allowing the heart to recover gradually by decreasing myocardial workload and oxygen demand and increasing perfusion of the coronary arteries.

Intracapsular hip fracture A hip fracture involving the head or neck of the femur.

Intracellular fluid (ICF) Fluid found within the body cells that contains solute vital to the metabolic processes of the cells. Also called *cellular fluid.*

Intracranial hypertension A sustained state of increased intracranial pressure that is potentially life threatening.

Intracranial regulation The processes that affect intracranial compensation and adaptive neurologic function.

Intractable seizures Seizures that continue to occur even with optimal medical management.

Intradiscal electrothermal therapy (IDET) The use of thermal energy to treat pain from a bulging spinal disc.

Intradisciplinary assessment An evaluation that occurs within a group of individuals with a similar position in the healthcare system, such as a group of nurses or a group of surgeons, to identify areas of improvement at each level of care.

Intradisciplinary team A team that seeks to achieve a common goal with team members from the same background.

Intergenerational family A family in which more than two generations live together.

Internal patients Employees of a healthcare organization, such as nurses, physicians, therapists, medical record staff, billing specialists, and other employees.

Intraocular pressure A force within the eye that causes tissue damage.

Intraoperative The phase of an operative process in which the surgical procedure actually takes place.

Intrapartum The time from the onset of true labor until the birth of the infant and expulsion of the placenta.

Intrapersonal conflict Conflict that occurs within an individual, arising from stress or tension that results from real or perceived pressure generated by incompatible expectations or goals.

Intrauterine contraception (IUC) A safe, effective method of reversible contraception that is designed to be inserted into the uterus by a qualified healthcare provider and left in place for an extended period, providing continuous contraceptive protection.

Intrauterine device (IUD) A small plastic or metal form that is placed in the uterus to prevent implantation of a fertilized ovum.

Intrauterine fetal death (IUFD) Death of a fetus that occurs after 20 weeks' gestation. Often referred to as *stillbirth* or *fetal demise.*

Intrauterine pressure catheter (IUPC) A device that measures the pressure in the uterine cavity.

Intravascular fluid Accounts for approximately 20% of the extracellular fluid and is found within the vascular system. Also called *plasma*.

Intravenous pyelography (IVP) A diagnostic test used to evaluate the structure and excretory function of the kidneys, ureters, and bladder.

Introspection The personal exploration and evaluation of one's own thoughts, emotions, behaviors, and values incorporating both verbal and nonverbal feedback from others.

Intubation The process of inserting a breathing tube.

Intuition The use of nursing knowledge, experience, and expertise for understanding without the conscious use of reasoning.

Invasion Occurs when cancerous cells overtake adjacent tissues.

Involuntary admission The detention of a patient in a psychiatric or medical facility against the patient's will, normally reserved for cases in which the patient is a danger to himself or others.

Involution The rapid reduction in size of the uterus and the return of the uterus to a nonpregnant state.

Ions Electrically charged particles.

Iron deficiency anemia A disorder that results when the supply of iron in the body is insufficient for the formation of red blood cells.

Irritant contact dermatitis An inflammation of the skin from irritants; it is not a hypersensitivity response.

Ischemia Insufficient blood supply.

Ischemic Deprived of oxygen.

Ischial spines Prominences that arise near the junction of the ilium and ischium and jut into the pelvic cavity.

Isoelectric line A straight line on an electrocardiograph that indicates the absence of electrical activity.

Isokinetic exercises Resistive exercises that involve muscle contraction or tension against resistance; can be either isotonic or isometric.

Isolation Measures designed to prevent the spread of infection to health personnel, patients, and visitors.

Isometric exercises Static or sitting exercises in which muscles contract without moving the joint.

Isotonic A solution that has the same osmolality as body fluids. Normal saline, 0.9% sodium chloride, is an isotonic solution.

Isotonic dehydration A type of fluid imbalance that occurs when fluid loss is not balanced by intake and the losses of water and sodium are in proportion. Also called *isonatremic dehydration*.

Isotonic exercises Dynamic exercises in which the muscle shortens to produce muscle contractions and active movement.

Isotonic fluid volume deficit A type of fluid imbalance that occurs when electrolytes are lost along with fluid.

Isotonic imbalance A fluid imbalance that occurs when water and electrolytes are lost or gained in equal proportions, so that the osmolality of body fluids remains constant.

Isthmus That portion of the uterus between the internal cervical os and the endometrial cavity.

Jaundice A yellow pigmentation of body tissues caused by the presence of bile pigments.

Joint arthroplasty The reconstruction or replacement of a joint.

Joint custody Occurs when two parents who are not married have equal responsibility and legal rights for their shared children.

Joint fusion A procedure that permanently fuses two or more bones together at a joint using pins, plates, screws, and rods. Also called *arthrodesis*.

Joint irrigation A fluid injected into the joint to allow the surgeon to visualize joint structures more easily and to help remove debris and infection in the joint.

Joint resurfacing A procedure in which a little bone is removed at the articulating surface of the joint and a metal replacement is fitted over the end of the bone.

Just culture An attempt to balance the blame-free environment with appropriate accountability by focusing on correcting problems that lead individuals to engage in unsafe behavior while maintaining individual accountability by establishing zero tolerance for reckless behavior.

Justice Fairness.

Juvenile glaucoma Congenital glaucoma diagnosed after age 3.

Juvenile idiopathic arthritis (JIA) See Juvenile rheumatoid arthritis (JRA).

Juvenile macular degeneration A pediatric form of **age-related macular degeneration** that is inherited rather than acquired.

Juvenile rheumatoid arthritis (JRA) A chronic inflammatory autoimmune disease diagnosed in children that is characterized by joint inflammation resulting in decreased mobility, swelling, and pain.

Kaposi sarcoma (KS) Often the presenting symptom of AIDS, it remains the most common cancer associated with the disease. Kaposi sarcoma is caused by a virus called the Kaposi sarcoma–associated herpes virus, also known as human herpes virus 8.

Kardex A widely used, concise method of organizing and recording data about a patient, making information quickly accessible to all healthcare professionals.

Karyotype A pictorial analysis of chromosomes.

Kcalorie See Kilocalories.

Kegel exercises The act of tightening the perineal muscle in order to strengthen the pubococcygeus muscle and increase its elasticity.

Keloid A scar that extends beyond the boundaries of the original wound.

Keratin A fibrous, water-repellent protein that gives the epidermis its tough, protective quality.

Keratotic basal cell carcinoma A type of skin cancer.

Ketonuria The presence of ketones in the urine.

Ketosis An accumulation of ketone bodies produced during oxidation of fatty acids.

Kilocalories A term used to identify the energy-producing ability of nutrients. Also called *Kcalories* or *kcal*.

Kindling Long-term changes in brain neurotransmission that occur after repeated detoxifications.

Kinesthesia The ability to perceive movement and sense of position.

Kinesthetic A term referring to awareness of the position and movement of body parts.

Korotkoff sounds The series of sounds identified while taking a blood pressure using a stethoscope.

Korsakoff psychosis A condition typically seen in alcoholics that is characterized by intact intellectual functioning but an inability to retrieve long-term memory events or retain new information.

Kosher Acceptable to or prepared according to Jewish law.

Kussmaul respirations Deep, rapid respirations associated with compensatory mechanisms.

Kyphosis A convex curvature of the spine that may decrease mobility.

Labor induction The stimulation of uterine contractions before the spontaneous onset of labor, with or without ruptured fetal membranes, for the purpose of accomplishing birth.

Labyrinthitis Inflammation of the inner ear. Also called *otitis interna*.

Laceration Disruption of the brain tissue caused by the entrance of a foreign object such as a bullet, knife, or skull fragment.

Lactase deficiency An individual's inability to digest lactose because of a deficiency of lactase, the enzyme that breaks down lactose into monosaccharides. Also called *lactose intolerance*.

Lactation consultant A specially trained individual who provides breastfeeding support and care to mothers, infants, children, families, and communities.

Lacto-ovovegetarians Vegetarians who include milk, dairy products, and eggs in their diets.

Lactase deficiency Occurs when the body lacks that substance that triggers the chemical breakdown to metabolize lactose.

Lactose intolerance An individual's inability to digest lactose because of a deficiency of lactase, the enzyme that breaks down lactose into monosaccharides. Also called *lactose deficiency*.

Lactovegetarians Vegetarians who include dairy products but no eggs in their diets.

Laënnec cirrhosis A progressive, irreversible liver disorder resulting from excessive alcohol consumption. Also called *alcoholic cirrhosis*.

Laissez-faire leader A leader who recognizes a group's need for autonomy and self-regulation. The leader assumes a "hands-off" approach, being less directive and more permissive than other types of leaders.

Lamellar A type of bone that is stronger and more compact with better blood circulation compared to woven bone.

Laminectomy The surgical removal of the vertebral lamina.

Laminotomy The surgical removal of part of the vertebral lamina.

Lanugo A large quantity of fine hair found on some newborns.

Laparoscopic cholecystectomy Removal of the gallbladder using an endoscope.

Late deceleration A condition caused by uteroplacental insufficiency resulting from decreased blood flow and oxygen transfer to the fetus through the intervillous spaces during uterine contractions.

Late (secondary) postpartum hemorrhage Postpartum hemorrhage that occurs from 24 hours to 6 weeks after birth.

Law The sum total of the rules and regulations by which a society is governed.

Laxatives Medications that stimulate bowel activity and assist in fecal elimination.

Lead An insulated wire that connects an electrocardiograph to the electrodes attached to a patient.

Leader An individual with the ability to rule, guide, or inspire others to think or act as that individual recommends.

Leading question A closed question that gives the patient an opportunity to decide whether the answer is true or not.

Lean Six Sigma A methodology used to reduce waste and provide consistency in the quality of care.

Learned helplessness A sense of helplessness that nothing the individual does can change an aspect of a situation or stressor; often reinforced by repeated failures, learned helplessness is common in individuals with major depressive disorder.

Learning A change in human disposition or capability that persists and that cannot be solely accounted for by growth.

Learning disabilities Disorders that impair an individual's ability to receive and process information, causing reduced functioning in verbal, linguistic, reasoning, and academic skills; neurologic conditions in which the brain cannot receive or process information normally.

Learning need A desire or a requirement to know something that is presently unknown to the learner.

Lecithin/sphingomyelin (L/S) ratio The measurement of lecithin and sphingomyelin in order to determine the lung maturity of a fetus.

Leopold maneuvers A systematic way to evaluate the maternal abdomen.

Lesbian A woman who prefers relationships with other women.

Lesion An observable change in skin structure that may indicate disorders in other systems and organs.

Leukemia A group of chronic malignant disorders of white blood cells (WBCs) and WBC precursors.

Leukocytes The primary cells involved in both nonspecific and specific immune system responses. Also known as *white blood cells (WBCs)*.

Leukocytosis An increase in the number of leukocytes in the blood (above $10,000/mm^3$), in response to infection or inflammation.

Leukopenia A decrease in the number of circulating leukocytes.

Level of injury The vertical location of an injury along the spinal column.

Lewy bodies Abnormal aggregates of proteins, including alpha-synuclein.

Liability The state of being legally obliged and responsible.

Libido Sexual desire.

Licensed practical nurses (LPNs) Members of a nursing team who provide direct patient care under the direction of an RN, physician, or other licensed practitioner.

Lichenification The thickening of the skin.

Lifestyle An individual's general way of living, including living conditions and individual patterns of behavior that are influenced by sociocultural factors and personal characteristics.

Ligaments Connective tissue between bones to create joints.

Lightening The effects that occur when the fetus begins to settle into the pelvic inlet.

Limb restraints A device typically made of cloth that may be used when limb immobilization is needed for therapeutic purposes, for example, to prevent dislodgement of an intravenous infusion device.

Limbic system A set of structures located deep inside the brain; includes the hippocampus.

Limit setting Establishing clear and consistent rules or guidelines for child or patient behavior.

Line authority The power to direct the activities of subordinates within an organization.

Lipids The macronutrient that provides most of the body's energy at 9 kcal/g. There are three categories of lipids: triglycerides, phospholipids, and sterols. Also called *fats*.

Lipoatrophy Atrophy of subcutaneous tissues.

Lipodystrophy Excessive growth of subcutaneous tissue.

Lithiasis Stone formation.

Lithotripsy The preferred treatment for urinary calculi; uses sound or shock waves to crush a stone.

Living will A document that provides written directions about life-prolonging procedures to provide instructions when an individual can no longer communicate in a life-threatening situation.

Lobes Specialized cognitive regions in the hemispheres of the brain.

Local adaptation syndrome (LAS) A stress response that affects only one organ or body system.

Local emergency management agency (LEMA) A governmental agency with expertise in public safety, emergency medical services, and management.

Local infection Invasion by a microorganism that is limited to the specific part of the body where the microorganism remains.

Localized responses Common manifestations of type I hypersensitivity, they are typically atopic responses; that is, they have a strong genetic predisposition. Atopic reactions are the result of localized, rather than systemic, IgE-mediated responses to an allergen. They are prompted by contact of the allergen with IgE in the bronchial tree, nasal mucosa, and conjunctival tissues.

Lochia The discharge through which the uterus rids itself of the debris remaining after birth. The discharge should change appearance and contents as healing commences.

Lochia alba The final discharge as the uterus completes healing; composed primarily of leukocytes, decidual cells, epithelial cells, fat, cervical mucus, cholesterol crystals, and bacteria.

Lochia rubra The dark red initial discharge as the uterus eliminates epithelial cells, erythrocytes, leukocytes, shreds of decidua, and occasionally fetal meconium, lanugo, and vernix in the first 1–2 days following birth.

Lochia serosa A light pink discharge of serous exudate, shreds of degenerating decidua, erythrocytes, leukocytes, cervical mucus, and numerous microorganisms from the uterus 3–10 days following birth.

Locked-in syndrome A state of consciousness in which the patient is alert and fully aware of the environment and has intact cognitive abilities but is unable to communicate through speech or movement because of blocked efferent pathways from the brain. Motor paralysis affects all voluntary muscles, although the upper cranial nerves (I through IV) may remain intact, allowing the patient to communicate through eye movements and blinking.

Locus of control (LOC) The extent to which patients believes their health status is under their own or others' control.

Long-term memory The final process or destination for information to be stored indefinitely.

Longboard spinal immobilization A device that provides support and immobilization of the entire spine below the level of the neck, instituted for patients with a potential or suspected spinal cord injury from a motor vehicle collision.

Loose association An indication of disordered thinking characterized by the shifting of verbal ideas from one topic to another, with no apparent relationship between thoughts, and the person speaking being unaware that the topics are unconnected. Commonly seen in schizophrenia.

Lordosis A concave curvature of the spine that may decrease mobility.

Loss A situation in which someone or something that is valued becomes altered or no longer available.

Lower body obesity Identified by a waist-to-hip ratio of less than 0.8; more commonly seen in women. Also called *peripheral obesity*.

Lumpectomy Removal of a tumor and the surrounding margin of breast tissue followed by radiation therapy. Also called *segmental mastectomy* or *breast conservation surgery*.

Lung abscess A local area of necrosis and pus formation within the lung.

Lupus nephritis Inflammation of the kidneys resulting from systemic lupus erythematosus (SLE).

Luteinizing hormone (LH) Anterior pituitary hormone responsible for stimulating ovulation and for development of the corpus luteum.

Lymphadenopathy The enlargement of lymph nodes with or without tenderness. It may be caused by inflammation, infection, or malignancy of the nodes or the regions drained by the nodes.

Lymphangitis Inflammation of a lymph vessel.

Lymphedema Accumulation of fluid in the soft tissues of the arm caused by removal of lymph channels.

Lymphocytes The principal effector and regulator cells of specific immune responses to protect the body from microorganisms, foreign tissue, and cell mutations or alterations.

Lyse Disintegrate.

Maceration Tissues softened by prolonged wetting or soaking.

Macronutrients Essential nutrients needed by the body in large amounts to survive: carbohydrates, proteins, and fats.

Macrophages Large phagocytes that are important in the body's defense against chronic infections.

Macular degeneration A progressive disorder involving loss of central vision due to damage to the retina.

Magical thinking Believing that events occur because of one's thoughts or actions.

Major depressive disorder (MDD) A mood disorder characterized by loss of interest in life and unresponsiveness, moving from mild to severe, with severe symptoms lasting at least 2 weeks. Also called *unipolar depression*.

Major depressive episode Characterized by a change in several aspects of an individual's emotional state and functioning consistently over a period of 14 days or longer.

Major trauma A serious single-system injury (such as the amputation of a leg) or multiple-system injuries (simultaneous injuries such as a punctured lung, traumatic brain injury, and crushed bones in the arms and legs). Also called *multisystem trauma*.

Malabsorption A condition in which the intestinal mucosa is unable to absorb nutrients, resulting in nutrients being excreted in the stool.

Malaise Vague feeling of physical discomfort.

Maldigestion A condition in which there is inadequate preparation of chyme for absorption of nutrients; also can result in malabsorption.

Male hypoactive sexual desire disorder A deficiency in or absence of sexual fantasies and persistently low interest or a total lack of interest in sexual activity.

Male orgasmic disorder A condition that occurs when a man can maintain an erection for long periods, but has difficulty ejaculating.

Malignant Term used to refer to a cell or growth that, if not treated, will recur, continue to grow, and spread to other sites in the body, ending in death.

Malignant hyperthermia A musculoskeletal disorder resulting from an inherited cellular deficit that places the patient in a hypermetabolic state.

Malnutrition Health effects due to insufficient nutrient intake or stores. Also called *undernutrition*.

Malpractice Conduct deviating from the standard of practice dictated by a profession.

Malpresentation A condition that occurs when a fetus passes into the pelvic inlet with a breech or shoulder presentation. These presentations are associated with difficulties during labor.

Malunion The healing of bones in an anatomically incorrect position. Surgical correction may be needed.

Managed care A healthcare delivery system designed to provide cost-effective, high-quality care for groups of patients from the time of their initial contact with the health system through the conclusion of their health problem.

Manager An individual employed by an organization and granted the required authority, responsibility, accountability, and power to accomplish the organization's goals.

Mandatory health insurance Health insurance is provided by large, nonprofit health organizations centered around large employers or work-based associations or else is provided by government-sponsored programs. Everyone belongs to one of these two types of insurance plans, thus ensuring universal coverage.

Mandatory reporting A legal requirement to report an act, event, or situation that is designated by state or local law as a reportable event.

Mania An abnormal and persistently elevated, expansive, or irritable mood lasting at least 1 week, significantly impairing social or occupational functioning and generally requiring hospitalization.

Manipulation Controlling behavior used to exploit others for personal gain.

Margination The accumulation of leukocytes along the inner surface of blood vessels. Occurs as part of the inflammatory process.

Marital rape Rape that occurs when one spouse forces the other to have sex against his or her will.

Maslow's hierarchy of needs A concept proposed by Abraham Maslow in which he proposed the existence of levels of human needs that could be organized into five categories: physiologic, safety, love and belonging, esteem, and self-actualization.

Massage therapy The scientific manipulation of the soft tissues of the body for the purposes of promoting healing and wellness.

Massive transfusion A series of blood parcels, including packed red blood cells, fresh frozen plasma, cryo units, and platelet pheresis administered to a patient who has lost a substantial amount of blood.

Mast cells Leukocytes that detect foreign agents or injury and respond by releasing histamine, thereby activating the inflammatory process.

Masturbation The self-stimulation of one's genitals for sexual pleasure.

Maternal role attainment (MRA) The process by which a woman learns mothering behaviors and becomes comfortable with her identity as a mother.

Maturational crisis A crisis that occurs normally as an individual progresses through the life cycle.

Mature milk A white or slightly blue-tinged color milk that presents by 2 weeks postpartum and continues thereafter until lactation ceases.

McDonald sign A probable sign of pregnancy characterized by an ease in flexing the body of the uterus against the cervix.

Mean arterial pressure (MAP) The average pressure in the arterial circulation throughout the cardiac cycle.

Meaning-focused coping The use of revaluation to reduce the appraisal of a threat.

Meatus A body passage or opening.

Meconium The first fecal material passed by a newborn, normally within 8–24 hours after birth.

Medicaid A state-administered health insurance program available to certain lower-income individuals and families, older adults, and people with disabilities.

Medical asepsis All practices intended to confine a specific microorganism to a specific area, thus limiting the number, growth, and transmission of the microorganism.

Medicare A federally funded health insurance program available to people ages 65 or older, younger people with disabilities, and people with end-stage renal disease.

Medigap policy A private health insurance plan designed to supplement Medicare coverage. It may pay copayments, coinsurance, deductibles, and "gaps" in Medicare coverage (i.e., noncovered healthcare costs). Also called *Medicare supplemental insurance.*

Meditation The act of focusing one's thoughts or engaging in self-reflection or contemplation.

Meiosis A reductive division of sex cells, producing ova or sperm with a half set (haploid) of chromosomes.

Melanin A shield that protects the keratinocytes and the nerve endings in the dermis from the damaging effects of ultraviolet light.

Melanoma A type of malignant skin cancer.

Melasma gravidarum See Chloasma.

Mendelian inheritance Traits that are passed on by a single gene. Also called *single-gene inheritance.*

Meninges Three connective tissue membranes that cover, protect, and nourish the central nervous system.

Menometrorrhagia Irregular, excessive, prolonged menstruation.

Menopause The permanent cessation of menses.

Menorrhagia Excessive or prolonged menstruation that occurs at regular intervals.

Menstrual cycle The cyclic phases of menstruation that normally occur about every 28 days.

Menstruation The periodic shedding of the uterine lining in a woman of childbearing age who is not pregnant.

Mental health A state of well-being in which an individual is able to work productively, cope with change and adversity, engage in meaningful relationships, and realize his own potential.

Mental illness A condition that affects emotions, thinking, behavior, or any combination of the three; mental illness is characterized by symptoms that are severe enough to impair functioning.

Mental retardation See Intellectual disability.

Mentor A competent, experienced professional who develops a relationship with a novice for the purpose of providing advice, support, information, and feedback in order to encourage development of the individual.

Message Content that is actually said or written, the body language that accompanies the words, and how the words are transmitted.

Metabolic acidosis This bicarbonate deficit is characterized by a low pH (<7.35), low bicarbonate (<24 mEq/L), and $PaCO_2$ less than 38 mmHg. It may be caused by excess acid in the body or loss of bicarbonate from the body.

Metabolic alkalosis This bicarbonate excess is characterized by a high pH (>7.45), a high bicarbonate (>28 mEq/L), and $PaCO_2$ higher than 45 mmHg. It may be caused by loss of acid or excess bicarbonate in the body.

Metabolic syndrome A disorder characterized by the presence of three or more of the following: increased waist circumference, hypertension, elevated blood triglycerides and fasting blood glucose, and low HDL cholesterol.

Metabolism The complex process of biochemical reactions occurring in the body's cells necessary to produce energy, repair cells, and sustain life.

Metacognition The human ability to think about thinking.

Metaphysis The portion of the bone between the diaphysis and the epiphysis.

Metaplasia A change in the normal pattern of differentiation such that dividing cells differentiate into cell types not normally found at that location in the body.

Metastasis The process by which spreading of malignant neoplasms occurs; the transfer of disease from one organ or part to another.

Metrorrhagia Bleeding between menstrual periods.

Microalbuminuria An abnormally low level of albumin in the urine.

Micronutrients Essential nutrients needed by the body in small quantities, such as vitamins and minerals.

Microstaging The assessment of the level of invasion of a malignant melanoma and the maximum tumor thickness.

Micturition Releasing urine from the urinary bladder. Also called *voiding* or *urination.*

Middle ear effusion Results when negative pressure in the middle ear causes sterile serous fluid to move from the capillaries into the space.

Milia Exposed sebaceous glands that appear as raised white spots on the face, especially across the nose on infants within the first month after birth.

Miliary tuberculosis Results from hematogenous spread (through the blood) of the tuberculosis bacilli throughout the body.

Milieu therapy A therapeutic recovery environment that supports behavior changes, teaches new coping skills, and helps the patient move from addiction to sobriety.

Milliequivalent The chemical combining power of the ion, or the capacity of cations to combine with anions to form molecules.

Minerals Salts dissolved in water that carry electrical charge and work with other nutrients to maintain fluid balance throughout the body. Also called *electrolytes.*

Minimal enteral nutrition Small-volume feedings of formula or human milk (usually <24 mL · kg^{-1} · day^{-1}) designed to "prime" the premature infant's intestinal tract and stimulate many of its hormonal and enzymatic functions.

Minor trauma Trauma that affects a single part or system of the body and is usually treated in a physician's office or in a hospital's emergency department.

Miscarriage The loss of a fetus prior to 20 weeks' gestation. Also called a *spontaneous abortion.*

Mitigation A phase that takes place before and after an emergency that consists of identifying potential hazards, minimizing effects, and reducing the likelihood of their occurrence.

Mitosis The process of cell division.

Mitt restraints A device used to protect confused patients from scratching or injuring their skin or dislodging intravenous access devices. Also called *hand restraints.*

Modeling Observing the behavior of people who have successfully achieved a goal that they have set for themselves and, through observing, acquiring ideas for behavior and coping strategies.

Modified radical mastectomy The removal of the breast tissue and lymph nodes under the arm, leaving the chest wall muscles intact.

Molding The asymmetrical appearance of an infant's head caused by overlapping of the cranial bones during labor and birth.

Mongolian spots Macular areas of bluish-black or gray-blue pigmentation on the dorsal area and the buttocks; common in newborns of Asian, Hispanic, and African descent and in newborns of other dark-skinned races.

Monoamine oxidase inhibitor (MAOI) A drug that inhibits monoamine oxidase, an enzyme that terminates the actions of neurotransmitters such as dopamine, norepinephrine, epinephrine, and serotonin. These drugs are used to treat individuals who have not responded to typical treatments for depression.

Mononeuropathies Isolated peripheral neuropathies that affect a single nerve.

Monophasic A term used to describe rheumatoid arthritis when it occurs for a limited time and then improves.

Monopolizing The domination of a discussion by one member of a group.

Monosomy Absence of a chromosome.

Monro-Kellie hypothesis A hypothesis that states if the volume of any of the three intracranial components (the brain, cerebrospinal fluid, and blood) increases, the volume of the others must decrease to maintain normal pressures in the cranial cavity.

Mood An individual's internal, subjective, sustained emotional state.

Mood stabilizers Drugs used for treatment of bipolar disorder because they moderate extreme shifts in emotions between mania and depression.

Moral behavior The way in which an individual perceives and responds to society's requirements.

Moral development 1. The process of learning to tell the difference between right and wrong and of learning what ought and ought not to be done. 2. The pattern of change in moral behavior that occurs with age.

Moral principles Statements about broad, general, philosophical concepts such as autonomy and justice.

Moral rules Specific prescriptions for actions.

Morality Private, personal standards of what is right and wrong in conduct, character, and attitude; the requirements necessary for people to live together in society.

Morbid obesity A condition in which an individual weighs more than 200% of his or her ideal body weight or has a BMI >40 kg/m^2.

Morning sickness A term that refers to the nausea and vomiting that a woman may experience in early pregnancy. This lay term is sometimes used because these symptoms frequently occur in the early part of the day and disappear within a few hours.

Moro reflex In response to being lifted, then suddenly lowered or surprised by a loud noise, a newborn will straighten the arms and hands outward while the knees flex. Slowly, the arms return to the chest, as in an embrace. The fingers spread, forming a "C," and the newborn may cry.

Morpheaform basal cell carcinoma A type of skin cancer.

Morula Developmental stage of the fertilized ovum in which there is a solid mass of cells.

Mosaicism The expression of two cell lines, each with a different chromosomal number, in an individual.

Motility The process of moving food and fluid through the gastrointestinal tract from the mouth to the anus.

Motivation to learn The individual's personal desire and need to learn that affects how much and how fast the individual will learn.

Motor vehicle crash (MVC) The unintentional collision of one or more motor vehicles with another vehicle or object.

Mottling A lacy pattern of dilated blood vessels under the skin.

Mourning The behavioral process through which grief is eventually resolved or altered; it is often influenced by culture, spiritual beliefs, and custom.

Movement disorder A disorder associated with schizophrenia. There are two general forms: The first involves increased body movements that may appear agitated, repetitious, or purposeless. The second form involves catatonia, or unresponsiveness to the environment or others.

Movement technique A relaxation technique, such as yoga or tai chi, designed to improve strength, balance, and mental calmness.

Mucolytics Medications that help break up thick mucus secretions in the airways.

Multi-payer system Healthcare insurance coverage or payment system in which funds come from multiple sources.

Multiculturalism Characterized by many subcultures coexisting within a given society in which no one culture dominates.

Multidisciplinary team approach An approach to healthcare in which team members work together to deliver patient care, but a single team member—usually a physician—makes the treatment decisions.

Multifocal A term used to describe premature ventricular contractions (PVCs) that arise from different ectopic sites and appear distinct on the ECG.

Multigravida Term used to describe a woman who has been pregnant more than once.

Multipara Term used to describe a woman who has had more than one pregnancy in which the fetus was viable.

Multiple pregnancy More than one fetus in the uterus at the same time.

Multiple sclerosis (MS) A chronic demyelinating neurologic disease of the central nervous system associated with an abnormal immune response to an environmental factor.

Multiple trauma Trauma that involves serious single-system injury or multiple-system injuries. Also called *major trauma.*

Mural thrombi Blood clots in the heart wall.

Muscle relaxation A relaxation technique that involves consciously tightening and then relaxing each muscle progressively from either head to toe or toe to head.

Mutual recognition model A licensing system that allows a nurse to have a single license that confers the privilege to practice in other states that are part of the Nurse Licensure Compact.

Mutual respect A state in which two or more individuals show or feel honor or esteem toward one another.

Mycobacterium tuberculosis The bacteria that causes tuberculosis.

Mydriasis Abnormal or excessive dilation of the pupil of the eye, usually caused by a disease or drug.

Myelin The fatty, segmented wrappings that normally protect and insulate nerves. Also called *myelin sheath.*

Myelogram A diagnostic technique in which dye is injected into the spinal fluid and visualized by x-ray in order to identify areas of pressure on the spinal cord or nerves due to herniated discs.

Myocardial hypertrophy An increase in the size of muscle cells of the myocardium.

Myometrium The middle muscular layer of the uterus.

Myopia Nearsightedness.

MyPlate A nutrient intake guide from the U.S. Department of Agriculture that outlines suggested food intake by food groups.

Myringotomy A surgical incision of the tympanic membrane.

Myxedema The hypothyroid state with characteristic accumulation of nonpitting edema in the connective tissues throughout the body.

Myxedema coma A life-threatening complication of long-standing, untreated hypothyroidism, usually triggered by an acute illness or trauma.

Nägele rule A common method of determining the estimated date of birth using the first day of the last menstrual period, subtracting 3 months, and adding 7 days.

NANDA The acronym for North American Nursing Diagnosis Association.

Narcissism Self-centered behavior in which the individual feels entitled to special favors due to a mistaken perception that they are superior to others.

Narcissistic personality disorder (NPD) One of several personality disorders defined in the DSM-5, it is marked by in a pattern of grandiosity, difficulty regulating self-esteem, and the need for admiration and attention from others.

Narcolepsy A disorder characterized by daytime sleep attacks or excessive daytime sleepiness.

Narcotics See Opioids.

Narrative charting A traditional part of the source-oriented record. It consists of written notes that include routine care, normal findings, and patient problems.

National Institute for Occupational Safety and Health (NIOSH) An organization that focuses on generating new knowledge in the field of occupational safety and health and transferring that knowledge into practice for the betterment of workers.

National Patient Safety Goals (NPSGs) Formulated goals to assist accredited organizations with specific topics about patient safety.

Natural killer (NK) cells Large, granular cells found in the spleen, lymph nodes, bone marrow, and blood. NK cells provide immune surveillance and resistance to infection, and they play an important role in the destruction of early malignant cells.

Nature The genetic or hereditary capability of the individual.

Nausea A vague, but unpleasant, subjective sensation of sickness or queasiness.

Necrosis Dead tissue.

Negative affectivity One of the six trait domains associated with personality disorders that is distinguished by anxiousness, emotional lability, separation insecurity, depressive tendencies, perseveration, and suspicion.

Negative airflow room A room where airflow is controlled to prevent the air from circulating into the hallway or other rooms. Multiple fresh-air exchanges dilute the concentration of droplet nuclei in a negative airflow room. Also called *negative flow room.*

Negative feedback Output of a system that returns to the system as input and which inhibits system change.

Negative pressure ventilators A device that creates negative pressure externally to draw the chest outward and air into the lungs, mimicking spontaneous breathing.

Negative punishment The removal of a positive reward if an undesirable behavior occurs.

Negative symptom Loss or absence of a normal function seen in mentally healthy adults, such as the ability to care for one's self; commonly seen in schizophrenia.

Neglect syndrome A disorder of attention that can result from stroke, which is characterized by the inability to integrate and use perceptions from the affected side. Also called *unilateral neglect.*

Negligence Any conduct that deviates from what a reasonable person would do in a particular circumstance.

Neologisms Use of meaningless words that only have meaning to the individual using them.

Neonatal abstinence syndrome (NAS) A combination of neonatal signs and symptoms caused by withdrawal of gestational opioid exposure.

Neonatal anemia A disorder caused by blood loss, hemolysis, and impaired red blood cell production related to birth.

Neonatal mortality risk An infant's chance of death within the first 28 days of life.

Neonatal transition The first few hours after birth, in which a newborn's body systems adapt to extrauterine life.

Neonatology The field of medicine providing care for sick and premature infants.

Neoplasm A mass of new tissue that grows independently of its surrounding structures and has no physiologic purpose.

Nephrectomy Removal of a kidney.

Nephritis Inflammation of the kidneys.

Nephrolithiasis The formation of stones in the kidney.

Nephrolithotomy A procedure for removal of a staghorn calculus that invades the calyces and renal parenchyma.

Nephrotoxins Substances that damage nerves or nerve tissue.

Nerve block A chemical interruption of a nerve pathway, effected by injecting a local anesthetic into the nerve.

Networking The act of developing and maintaining relationships with others within and outside of the nursing profession and affiliated organizations to improve nursing practice, advance career goals, offer support, share information, and provide advice.

Neurofibrillary tangles Seen in patients with Alzheimer disease, they are thick, insoluble clots of protein inside the damaged brain cells or neurons.

Neurogenic bladder Interference with the normal mechanisms of urine elimination in which the patient does not perceive bladder fullness and is unable to control the urinary sphincters; usually the result of impaired neurologic function.

Neurogenic shock The result of an imbalance between parasympathetic and sympathetic stimulation of vascular smooth muscle.

Neuroleptic malignant syndrome (NMS) A potentially fatal condition caused by antipsychotic medications that block dopamine receptors. It is characterized by fever, rigidity, and increased prolactin levels.

Neuron The basic or specialized cell of the nervous system that carries electrical impulses throughout the body.

Neuropathic pain A type of pain experienced by people who have damaged or malfunctioning nerves.

Neurotransmitters Chemical messengers that carry information between neurons.

Neutral question An open-ended question the patient can answer without direction or pressure.

Neutral thermal environment (NTE) A specific environmental temperature range in which the rates of oxygen consumption and metabolism are minimal and the internal body temperature is maintained because of thermal balance.

Never events Preventable hazards that can result in injury or death, and that should never happen to patients.

Nevi Moles.

Nevus flammeus A capillary angioma directly below the epidermis. It is a nonelevated, sharply demarcated, red-to-purple area of dense capillaries. In infants of African descent, it may appear as a purple-black stain. Also called *port-wine stain.*

Nevus vasculosus A capillary hemangioma consisting of newly formed and enlarged capillaries in the dermal and subdermal layers. It is a raised, clearly delineated, dark red, rough-surfaced birthmark commonly found in the head region. Also called a *strawberry mark.*

New Ballard score Specific criteria designed for accurate assessment of the gestational age of newborns between 20 and 28 weeks of gestation and weighing less than 1500 g.

Newborn Infant from birth through the first 28 days of life.

Nicotine A highly addictive chemical that is found in tobacco and enters the body via the lungs (cigarettes, pipes, and cigars) and oral mucous membranes (chewing tobacco as well as smoking).

Nicotine replacement therapy (NRT) A pharmacologic therapy designed to relieve some of the physiologic effects of withdrawal, including cravings, for patients trying to quit smoking or using tobacco. NRT transdermal patches and gums are available over the counter; nicotine inhalers and nasal sprays are available by prescription only.

Nicotinic receptors Found in the hippocampus and involved with new sensory information and memory formation, they are thought to be impaired in patients with schizophrenia.

Nidation The cyclical preparation of the uterine lining by steroid hormones for implantation of the embryo.

Nociceptive pain A type of pain resulting from external stimuli on an uninjured, fully functional nervous system.

Nociceptors The nerve receptors for pain.

Nocturia Voiding two or more times at night.

Nocturnal emissions Orgasm and emission of semen during sleep. Also called *wet dreams.*

Nocturnal enuresis Involuntary urination at night after bladder control has been achieved. Also called *bed wetting.*

Nocturnal frequency The need for older adults to arise during the night to urinate.

Nodular basal cell carcinoma A type of skin cancer.

Noise-induced hearing loss (NIHL) A condition associated with prolonged exposure to sound of greater than or equal to 85 dB.

Nolo contendere A term used when an individual neither admits to nor denies committing a crime but agrees to a punishment as if guilty.

Nominal group technique (NGT) A process that alternates between individual work and group work. Individuals meet as a group, but they write their responses without any discussion.

Nondirective interview An unstructured interview in which the nurse allows the patient to control the purpose, subject matter, and pacing.

Nonexudative macular degeneration The most common form of macular degeneration, it is characterized by the accumulation of deposits beneath the pigment epithelium of the retina, causing the pigment epithelium to detach and interfere with the sensory function of the macula. Also referred to as the dry form of macular degeneration.

Noninvasive ventilation (NIV) Ventilator support using a tight-fitting face mask, thus avoiding intubation.

Nonmaleficence The duty to do no harm.

Non-Mendelian inheritance Traits that are passed on by the influence of multiple genes. Also called *multifactorial inheritance.*

Nonpenetrating injury Also called a close injury, this type of injury is associated with blunt-force injuries that do not result in the entrance of a foreign object into the body.

Nonshivering thermogenesis (NST) The stimulation of heat production in the body through increased cellular metabolism. Also called *chemical thermogenesis.*

Non-small-cell carcinoma Lung cancers other than small-cell carcinoma.

Nonstress test (NST) A widely used method of evaluating fetal status; may be used alone or as part of a more comprehensive diagnostic assessment called a biophysical profile.

Non-suicidal self-injury behaviors (NSSI) Intentional self-inflicted acts of harm to body tissue without the intent of suicide.

Nonunion Failure of the ends of a fracture to heal together after at least 3 months.

Nonverbal communication Transmitting information through gestures, facial expressions, or touch.

Normal sinus rhythm (NSR) The normal heart rhythm, in which impulses originate in the sinus node and travel through all normal conduction pathways without delay.

Normative commitment A feeling of obligation to continue in the profession due to benefits or positive experiences derived from the profession.

Normothermia Normal body temperature.

Nosocomial infections Infections that are associated with the delivery of healthcare services in a facility such as a hospital or nursing home. Also called *healthcare-associated infections (HAIs).*

NREM Sleep Non-rapid-eye-movement sleep occurs when activity in the *reticular activating system* is inhibited.

Nuclear family A family structure consisting of a husband and wife and their biological children.

Nucleation The formation of a crystal from a liquid.

Nucleotomy The surgical removal of a herniated disc.

Nulligravida Term used to describe a woman who has never been pregnant.

Nullipara Term used to describe a woman who has not given birth to a viable fetus.

Nurse practice act (NPA) State-level statutes that define and regulate nursing practices.

Nursing clinical research Research that seeks to answer questions that ultimately will improve patient care.

Nursing diagnosis A clinical judgment about individual, family, or community responses to actual and potential health problems/life processes.

Nursing ethics Ethical issues that occur in nursing practice.

Nursing informatics (NI) A specialty that integrates nursing science, computer science, and information science to manage and communicate data, information, knowledge, and wisdom in nursing practice.

Nursing plan of care A written or electronic guideline that organizes information about an individual patient's or family's care.

Nursing process The process used to identify a patient's health status and actual or potential healthcare problems or needs, to establish plans to meet the identified needs, to deliver specific nursing interventions to meet those needs, and to evaluate the success of those interventions.

Nursing research A systematic and strict scientific process that tests hypotheses about health-related illness and conditions and processes of nursing care practices.

Nursing transactional model The relationship among the nurse, the patient, and the environment in which they interact.

Nurture The effects of the environment on an individual's performance.

Nutrient density The ratio of good nutrients to calories a food contains.

Nutrients Substances found in food used by the body to promote growth, maintenance, and repair.

Nutrition The process by which the body ingests, absorbs, transports, uses, and eliminates nutrients in food.

Nutritional health The physical result of the balance between nutrient intake and nutritional requirements.

Nystagmus Involuntary rapid eye movement.

Obesity An excess of adipose tissue.

Object permanence The ability to understand that when something is out of sight it still exists.

Objective data Information that is detectable by an observer or can be measured or tested against an accepted standard. Also called *overt data* or *signs.*

Objective family burden Actual, identifiable family problems associated with the mental illness of a family member.

Obligatory losses Essential fluid losses required to maintain body functioning.

Observational learning The acquisition of new skills or the alteration of old behaviors simply by watching other children and adults.

Obsession A recurrent, unwanted, and often distressing thought or image that leads to feelings of fear and anxiety.

Obsessive-compulsive disorder (OCD) A disabling disorder characterized by obsessive thoughts and compulsive, repetitive behaviors that dominate an individual's life.

Obsessive–compulsive personality disorder (OCPD) One of several personality disorders defined in the DSM-5, it is marked by fear and anxiety concerning loss of control over situations, objects, or people.

Obstetric conjugate The distance from the middle of the sacral promontory to an area approximately 1 cm below the pubic crest.

Obstructive shock Shock caused by an obstruction in the heart or great vessels that either impedes venous return or prevents effective cardiac pumping action.

Occult blood Blood in stool that cannot be seen with the naked eye.

Occupational exposure Skin, eye, mucous membrane, or parenteral contact with blood or other potentially infectious materials that may result from the performance of an employee's duties.

Occupational Safety and Health Administration (OSHA) An organization that enforces the guidelines presented in the OSHA Act of 1970, requiring its covered employees to report specific incidents and illnesses in a timely manner.

Oculocephalic reflex An oculomotor response in which the eyes move in opposite direction as head turns to the side. Also called **doll's eye reflex**.

Olfactory Of or relating to smell.

Oligodendrocytes Cells that produce myelin.

Oligomenorrhea Light or infrequent menstruation and occurs when cycles are longer than 6–7 weeks. Usually related to hormonal imbalances such as those seen in polycystic ovary syndrome.

Oliguria The production of abnormally small amounts of urine by the kidney.

On–off effect A sudden lack of symptom control and unexpected dyskinesias appearing as drug effectiveness diminishes.

Oncogenes Genes that promote cell proliferation and are capable of triggering cancerous characteristics.

Oncology The study of cancer.

Oncotic pressure A pulling force exerted by colloids that helps maintain the water content of blood by pulling water from the interstitial space into the vascular compartment. Also called *colloid osmotic pressure*.

Online shopping addiction Excessive online shopping, often associated with overspending and aided by the internet, and characterized by compulsive and addictive forms of consumption and buying behavior.

Oogenesis The process that produces the female gamete, called an ovum (egg).

Open-angle glaucoma The most common form of glaucoma, it is a chronic, gradually progressive disease that typically affects both eyes.

Open-ended question A question that allows patients to discover, explore, elaborate, clarify, or illustrate their thoughts or feelings.

Open fracture A fracture in which the skin integrity is disrupted. Also called a *compound fracture*.

Open reduction and internal fixation (ORIF) The surgical insertion of nails, screws, plates, or pins to hold fractured bones in place.

Opiates A type of drug derived from natural or synthetic opiates that is used as a pain reliever. Opiates include morphine, meperidine, codeine, hydrocodone, and oxycodone.

Opioids Drugs that act on one or more of three opioid receptors: mu, delta, and kappa. They are controlled substances due to their potential for abuse. Also called *narcotics*.

Opportunistic infection An invasion of the body tissue by microorganisms appearing in an individual with immunodeficiency that would normally not affect an individual with an intact immune system.

Opportunistic pathogen A microorganism that causes disease only in susceptible individuals.

Optimism A feeling that things will turn out for the best.

Oral–genital sex Kissing, licking, or sucking of the genitals for sexual pleasure.

Orchiectomy Surgical removal of the testes.

Organizational chart A chart that depicts the formal hierarchical structure and related responsibilities within a traditional organization.

Organizational commitment The relative strength of an individual's relationship and sense of belonging to an organization.

Organizing The process of coordinating the work to be done. Formally, it involves identifying the work of the organization, dividing the labor, developing the chain of command, and assigning authority.

Orgasmic phase The phase of the sexual response cycle that is marked by the involuntary release of sexual tension accompanied by physiologic and psychologic release.

Orientation 1. A structured program of activities to help new employees adapt to their new workplace; it is geared toward helping newly employed nurses to be successful. 2. A newborn's ability to be alert to, follow, and fixate on appealing and attractive, complex visual stimuli. 3. A component of normal perception that includes four basic elements: person, place, time, and situation.

Orthopnea Difficulty breathing when supine.

Orthopneic position A body position with the head and arms supported on the overbed table to facilitate breathing.

Orthotic devices Orthopedic devices that may include splints or braces applied to reduce strain on a joint.

Ortolani maneuver A procedure used to evaluate an infant for developmental dysplastic hip.

Osmolality A measure of the concentration of solutes in body fluids. Osmolality is determined by the total solute concentration within a fluid compartment and is measured as parts of solute per kilogram of water.

Osmolar imbalance A fluid imbalance that involves the loss or gain of only water, so that the osmolality of the serum is altered.

Osmosis The movement of water across cell membranes, from a less concentrated solution to a more concentrated solution.

Osmotic pressure The power of a solution to draw water across a semipermeable membrane.

Ossification The development of bone.

Osteoarthritis (OA) The most common form of arthritis in older adults. It is caused by chronic degenerative changes in the cartilage and synovial membranes of the joints.

Osteoblasts Cells that form bone.

Osteoclasts Cells that resorb bone.

Osteocytes Cells that maintain bone matrix.

Osteodystrophy A complex bone disease process of chronic kidney disease in which chronic hyperparathyroidism causes increased resorption of bone.

Osteomyelitis Infection of the bone in a compound fracture.

Osteophytes Bony spurs that form as cartilage deteriorates.

Osteoporosis A metabolic bone disorder characterized by loss of bone mass, increased bone fragility, and increased risk of fractures.

Osteotomy 1. Surgical removal of a wedge of bones above or below a joint to realign the joint and shift weight away from the damaged potion of a joint. 2. An incision into or transection of the bone.

Otitis externa Inflammation of the ear canal. It is often called *swimmer's ear* because it is most frequently found in people who spend significant time in the water.

Otitis interna An inflammation of the inner ear. Also called *labyrinthitis*.

Otitis media Inflammation of the middle ear.

Otoscope A handheld instrument with a light and a cone-shaped attachment; known as an *ear speculum*.

Outcome The specific, observable criteria used to evaluate whether goals have been met and the effectiveness of nursing actions.

Outcome standards Standards that focus on the performance of a process, such as the number of bedridden patients who develop a pressure injury.

Outcomes management Management process that uses patient experiences to guide improvement in all areas of healthcare by providing a link between medical interventions and health outcomes and between health outcomes and the cost of care.

Output Energy, material, or information that a system gives out as a result of its processes.

Ovarian cycle The three cyclical phases of oogenesis that occur about every 28 days.

Ovarian ligaments Ligaments that anchor the lower pole of the ovary to the uterus.

Ovaries Female sex glands in which the ova are formed and in which estrogen and progesterone are produced. Normally, a woman has two ovaries.

Overdelegation A situation that occurs when a delegator loses control over a situation by providing a delegate with too much authority or too much responsibility. This places the delegator in a risky position, increasing the potential for liability.

Overnutrition Health effects caused by excessive or accelerated nutrient intake or stores, such as obesity, hypertension, hypercholesterolemia, or toxic levels of stored vitamins or minerals.

Overt conflict Conflict that is addressed openly and is generally obvious to the individuals involved.

Ovulation Normal process of discharging a mature ovum from an ovary approximately 14 days before the onset of menses.

Oxygenation The mechanism that facilitates or impairs the body's ability to supply oxygen to all cells of the body.

Pacemaker An external or implanted pulse generator used to provide an electrical stimulus to the heart when the heart fails to generate or conduct its own stimulus at a rate that maintains the cardiac output.

PaCO₂ A measure of the pressure exerted by dissolved carbon dioxide in the blood; it reflects the respiratory component of acid–base regulation and balance because it is regulated by the lungs.

Pain An unpleasant sensory and emotional experience associated with actual or potential tissue damage.

Pain threshold The point at which pain is initially perceived.

Pain tolerance The duration of time or intensity of pain an individual will endure before demonstrating pain responses.

Palliation Measures taken not to cure a disease, but to relieve disease-related symptoms and enhance the patient's quality of life. See also Palliative care.

Palliative care Nursing care that improves the quality of life of patients and their families facing life-threatening illness by preventing, assessing, and treating pain and other physical, psychosocial, and spiritual problems.

Palliative procedure A surgical or interventional cardiac catheterization procedure that does not create normal anatomic or hemodynamic results but allows adequate blood flow to oxygenate the tissues.

Pallidotomy A surgical technique for Parkinson disease in which the neurosurgeon locates the affected areas of the globus pallidus and destroys the involved tissue in order to improve tremors and mobility.

Palpation A method of assessment that involves touching the areas related to the body system to determine symmetry, equality of the size, shape, or condition of opposite sides of the body.

Pancreatitis Inflammation of the pancreas that occurs when pancreatic enzymes are released into the pancreas itself, causing autodigestion of pancreatic tissues.

Pandemic Widespread global outbreak of an infectious disease.

Panic disorder A sudden attack of terror, sometimes accompanied by a pounding heart, sweating, fainting, or dizziness.

Pannus An abnormal tissue layer that includes newly formed blood vessels. Pannus leads to scar tissue formation that immobilizes joints.

PaO₂ A measure of the pressure exerted by oxygen that is dissolved in the plasma.

Para Term used to describe a woman who has borne offspring who reached the age of viability.

Paracentesis Aspiration of fluid from the peritoneal cavity.

Parallel play A stage of play in which toddlers play side by side with similar objects, but do not play together.

Paranoia An extreme suspicion that others are "out to get you" and delusions that one is being followed and that others are trying to harm oneself; experienced by some individuals with psychosis.

Paranoid personality disorder (PPD) One of several personality disorders defined in the DSM-5, it is characterized by the inability to trust others, hypervigilance, pathologic jealousy, and prejudicial and judgmental tendencies.

Paraplegia Paralysis of all or part of the lower portion of the body.

Paraphimosis Condition in which the retracted foreskin becomes trapped over the glans and tightens on the penis, causing painful swelling.

Parasite One of the four categories of microorganisms, parasites live on other organisms.

Parasomnias Abnormal behaviors that may interfere with sleep and may occur during sleep.

Parenteral nutrition (PN) The intravenous administration of amino acids, often with added carbohydrates, fats, electrolytes, vitamins, and minerals.

Parenting The ongoing act of guiding children to learn acceptable behaviors, morals, and rituals of the family and of teaching them to become socially responsible, contributing members of society.

Paresis Weakness.

Paresthesia Sensation of prickling, tingling, or numbing.

Parkinson disease (PD) A degenerative disorder of the central nervous system resulting from the death of neurons that produce the brain neurotransmitter dopamine.

Parkinsonian gait Altered gait characterized by small, shuffling steps, as well as bradykinesia or festination.

Parkinsonism The motor symptoms of Parkinson disease: tremors, muscle rigidity, postural instability, and bradykinesia.

Paroxysmal Occurring in bursts with an abrupt onset and termination.

Paroxysmal nocturnal dyspnea A sudden episode of shortness of breath occurring at night during sleep.

Partial-thickness burns Burns that involve the entire dermis and the papillae of the dermis (superficial partial-thickness burns) or extend into the hair follicles (deep partial-thickness burns).

Passive acquired immunity A condition that occurs when a pregnant woman passes IgG antibodies to a fetus in utero.

Passive behavior Behavior that seeks to avoid conflict at any cost, even at the expense of one's own happiness.

Passive communicators Individuals who focus on the needs of others. They often deny themselves any sort of power, which causes them to become frustrated.

Passive immunity Temporary protection—provided by antibodies produced by other people or animals—against disease-producing antigens. Protection is gradually lost when these acquired antibodies are used up either by natural degradation or by combining with the antigen.

Patch testing A test used to identify allergens causing dermatitis. An adhesive patch with common allergens is placed on the back between the scapulae. The patch is generally removed after several days; if there is no reaction to a particular allergen, that allergen is eliminated as a possible cause of dermatitis.

Patent airway An airway that is open and free of obstruction.

Patent ductus arteriosus (PDA) A congenital connection between the great vessels that normally closes after birth, allowing blood from the right and left side of the heart to mix.

Pathogen A microorganism that causes disease.

Pathogenicity The ability to produce disease.

Pathologic fracture A fracture that results from disease that has weakened the bone.

Patient An individual who is waiting for or undergoing medical treatment and care.

Patient advocacy Process or strategy for acting on behalf of others, including patients, families, groups, or communities, to help them obtain services and rights that they might not otherwise receive but that they need to advance their well-being.

Patient-centered medical home A model of care in which a patient's primary care provider works with the patient and family to develop a personalized plan that addresses the patient's physical and mental health needs across the lifespan.

Patient-controlled analgesia (PCA) A pump with a control mechanism that allows the patient to self-manage pain.

Patient-focused care A delivery model that organizes healthcare around the expressed physical and emotional needs of the patient.

Patient Protection and Affordable Care Act (PPACA or ACA) A law enacted during the presidency of Barak Obama designed to increase access to and affordability of healthcare. Also called *Obamacare*.

Patient record A formal, legal document that provides evidence of a patient's care. Also called a *chart* or a *clinical record*.

Patient Self-Determination Act (PSDA) A federal law that requires every competent adult to be informed in writing on admission to a healthcare institution about his or her rights to accept or refuse medical care and to use advance directives.

Pauciarticular arthritis A form of juvenile rheumatoid arthritis that primarily affects the knees, ankles, and elbows; it occurs more frequently in females.

Peak expiratory flow rate (PEFR) A measurement used to monitor the ability of an individual to exhale a specific volume of air related to the individual's age, gender, height, and weight.

Pedagogy The study or science of teaching, specifically referring to children and adolescents.

Pedigree The graphic representation of a family tree, usually to trace genetic abnormalities.

Peer review A method to professionally critique a colleague's work based on predetermined standards.

Pelvic cavity Bony portion of the birth passage; a curved canal with a longer posterior than anterior wall.

Pelvic diaphragm Part of the pelvic floor, composed of deep fascia and the levator ani and the coccygeal muscles.

Pelvic floor exercises Isometric exercises to strengthen the pelvic floor muscles for increased support of the neighboring organs.

Pelvic inlet Upper border of the true pelvis.

Pelvic outlet Lower border of the true pelvis.

Pelvic tilt An exercise that helps prevent or reduce back strain as it strengthens abdominal muscles. Also called *pelvic rocking*.

Penetrating injury Also called an open injury, a penetrating injury causes an open wound with focal damage around the site of the injury. When referring to eye injuries specifically, in a penetrating injury, the layers of the eye spontaneously reapproximate after entry of a sharp-pointed object or small missile (e.g., a BB) into the globe.

Penetrating trauma Trauma that occurs when a foreign object enters the body, causing damage to body structures.

Penta screen Maternal screening that measures five indicators whose presence may suggest fetal complications: AFP, beta hCG, unconjugated estriol, inhibin A, and invasive trophoblast antigen.

Penumbra A band of minimally perfused cells that surrounds a central core of dead or dying cells.

Peplau, Hildegard A nursing theorist who is widely considered the mother of psychiatric nursing; she presented nursing as a therapeutic interpersonal process, rather than as a task-oriented process.

Peptic ulcer A break in the mucosal lining of the GI tract exposed to acid-pepsin secretions, including the esophagus, stomach, and duodenum.

Peptic ulcer disease (PUD) A break in the mucous lining of the GI tract where it comes in contact with gastric juice.

Perceived loss A loss that is experienced by one person but cannot be verified by others.

Perception Awareness and interpretation of stimuli; the ability of the individual to interpret the environment.

Percussion A method of tapping the chest or back to assess underlying structures. More forceful striking of the skin with cupped hands is sometimes called *clapping*.

Percutaneous coronary revascularization (PCR) Procedures are used to restore blood flow to the ischemic myocardium in patients with CAD.

Percutaneous transluminal coronary angioplasty (PTCA) A type of PCR (see above entry) in which a balloon-tipped catheter is threaded over the guidewire, with the balloon positioned across the area of narrowing.

Perforating injury A type of eye injury in which the layers of the eye do not spontaneously reapproximate after the entry of a sharp-pointed object or small missile (e.g., a BB) into the globe, which results in rupture of the globe and potential loss of ocular contents.

Perforation Rupture, as in the penetration of ulcer through mucosal wall.

Performance improvement Quality of care improvement is directly linked to the performance of an individual, team, unit, or organization.

Pericarditis Inflammation of the pericardial tissue surrounding the heart.

Pericardium A double layer of fibroserous membrane that encases and anchors the heart.

Perimenopause A period of hormonal change during which the body gradually transitions toward permanent infertility.

Perimetrium The outermost layer of the uterus.

Perinatal loss Death of a fetus or infant that occurs between the time of conception and the end of the newborn period 28 days after birth.

Perineal body The wedge-shaped mass of fibromuscular tissue between the lower part of the vagina and the anus.

Periodic breathing A breathing pattern characterized by pauses lasting 5–15 seconds.

Periodontal disease Gum disease.

Perioperative The three phases of a surgical procedure: the preoperative phase, intraoperative phase, and postoperative phase.

Perioperative nursing care Nursing care provided during any or all of the three phases of surgery: preoperative, intraoperative, and postoperative.

Peripartum cardiomyopathy A rare but serious dysfunction of the left ventricle that occurs in the last month of pregnancy or the first 5 months postpartum in a woman with no previous history of heart disease.

Peripheral nervous system (PNS) One of two principal parts of the neurologic system, the peripheral nervous system consists of the cranial nerves and the spinal nerves.

Peripheral neuropathy A condition that results when trauma or a disease process interferes with innervation of peripheral nerves.

Peripheral pulse A pulse located away from the heart, in the foot or the wrist.

Peripheral vascular disease (PVD) A disorder in which arteriosclerosis and atherosclerosis affect circulation to peripheral tissues, particularly the lower extremities.

Peripheral vascular resistance The opposing forces or impedance to blood flow as the arterial channels become more and more distant from the heart.

Peristalsis The process of wavelike muscular contractions that propels food and digestive products through the digestive tract.

Peritoneal dialysis The process by which dialysate is instilled into the abdominal cavity through a catheter, allowed to rest there while fluids and molecules exchange, and then removed through the catheter.

Peritonitis Inflammation and bacterial infection of the abdominal area.

Pernicious anemia A disorder that results from a failure to absorb dietary vitamin B_{12}.

Perseveration Use of the same words or phrases repetitively.

Persistent A term used to describe a disease or disorder (such as rheumatoid arthritis) that lasts for a period of 3–6 months or longer.

Persistent bacteriuria The reappearance of bacteria in urine due to a persistent source of infection causing repeated infection after the initial cure.

Persistent depressive disorder Chronic depression that affects an individual for the majority of most days for at least 2 years (1 year for children and adolescents). May be interrupted by periods of normal mood that do not exceed 2 months over the course of the 2 years. Also called *dysthymic disorder*.

Persistent vegetative state A permanent condition of complete unawareness of self and the environment and loss of all cognitive functions. Also called *irreversible coma*.

Personal distance Communication characterized by moderate voice tones, less noticeable body heat and smell. Physical contact such as a handshake or touching a shoulder is possible.

Personal identity The conscious sense of individuality and uniqueness that is continually evolving throughout life.

Personal knowing A nurse's commitment to ongoing, individual self-exploration and self-actualization.

Personal space The distance people prefer in interactions with others.

Personality The individual qualities, including habitual behavior patterns, that make an individual unique; the outward expression of the inner self.

Personality disorder (PD) Rigid, stereotyped behavioral patterns that deviate markedly from the norm of an individual's culture and persist throughout the person's life. Personality disorders are characterized by a lifelong maladaptive pattern of perceiving, thinking, and relating that impairs social or occupational functioning.

Personality traits The elements and patterns that make up an individual's personality.

Pessimism A feeling that a situation is always bad and may become worse.

pH A measurement of the hydrogen ion concentration of a solution.

Phagocytosis A process by which a foreign agent or target cell is engulfed, destroyed, and digested. Neutrophils and macrophages, known as phagocytes, are the primary cells involved in phagocytosis.

Phantom pain A confusing pain syndrome that occurs following surgical or traumatic amputation of a limb. The patient experiences pain in the missing body part even though there is complete mental awareness that the limb is gone. Also called *phantom limb syndrome*.

Phase of mutual regulation Time period during which a mother and her infant seek to determine the degree of control each partner in their relationship will exert. In this phase of adjustment, a balance is sought between the needs of the mother and the needs of the infant.

Phenotype The observable expression of genetic traits.

Philadelphia chromosome The balanced translocation of chromosome 22 to chromosome 9; associated with chronic myeloid leukemia.

Phimosis Tightness of the prepuce that prevents retraction of the foreskin.

Phobia An intense, persistent, irrational fear of a simple thing or social situation that compels the individual to avoid the stressor that elicits the fear.

Photophobia Sensitivity to light.

Physical activity Body movement produced by skeletal muscle contraction that increases energy expenditure.

Physical fitness The ability to carry out tasks with vigor and alertness and without fatigue, while still maintaining enough energy for other tasks.

Physical attending The conveyed act of being with another individual through physical posturing.

Physical restraint Any manual method, material, device, or equipment that is attached to the patient's body with the intention of limiting or restricting free movement of the patient's head, arms, legs, or body.

Physiologic anemia of infancy A type of anemia that occurs as a result of the normal, gradual drop in hemoglobin for the first 6–12 weeks of life.

Physiologic anemia of pregnancy Apparent anemia that results because during pregnancy the plasma volume increases more than the erythrocytes increase. Also called *pseudoanemia*.

Physiologic jaundice A yellow discoloration of the skin caused by accelerated destruction of fetal red blood cells, impaired conjugation of bilirubin, and increased bilirubin reabsorption from the intestinal tract.

Physiologic pain Experienced when an intact, properly functioning nervous system sends signals that tissues are damaged, requiring attention and proper care.

Physiologic tremors Tremors that occur normally as a result of physiologic exhaustion or emotional stress.

Pica The craving for and persistent eating of nonnutritive substances not ordinarily considered to be edible or nutritionally valuable, such as soil, clay, and soap.

PICOT A mnemonic method used by clinicians to define and formulate a clinical question driving the search for evidence-based practice. PICOT stands for Population of a group, Intervention or activity focus, Comparison group, Outcome(s) or desired effects, and Time frame.

Pigmented basal cell carcinoma A type of skin cancer.

Pill-rolling Rubbing of the thumb and fingers together accompanying other tremors.

Piloerection Goosebumps.

Pilot projects Limited trials to determine problems with problem-solving alternatives. Pilot project strategies may resemble research projects and may be linked to quality improvement initiatives.

Pitch The frequency of vibrations in a sound.

Pitfall A hidden trap that catches people unaware and undermines their plans.

Pitting edema Edema that retains indentation caused by pressure.

Placenta A flat, disc-shaped organ that is highly vascular and normally forms in the upper segment of the endometrium of the uterus; exchanges nutrients and gases between the fetus and the mother.

Placenta previa Occurs when the placenta partially or totally covers the mother's cervix; can result in severe bleeding before or during delivery.

Placental abruption A condition that occurs when the placenta detaches from the uterine wall before delivery. May or may not result in fetal demise, but a fetus's survival depends on the stage of development and prompt medical treatment.

Plan–do–study–act (PDSA) A system of quality improvement most often associated with total quality management.

Planning The four-stage managerial process that establishes objectives, evaluates the present situation in order to predict future trends and events, formulates a planning statement, and converts the plan into an action statement.

Plaque 1. An invisible soft film that adheres to the enamel surface of teeth. Consists of bacteria, saliva molecules, and remnants of epithelial cells and leukocytes. 2. Scar tissue on myelin sheath due to repeated attacks by the immune system.

Plateau phase A phase of the **sexual response cycle** during which individuals experience strong, prolonged sexual arousal. The plateau phase is typically maintained by physical stimulation.

Plasmapheresis Removal of a harmful component from plasma. Also called *plasma exchange therapy*.

Play therapist A therapist who designs and provides recreational activities to promote emotional and/or physical healing and wellness.

Pleural effusion Accumulation of excess fluid in the pleural cavity.

Pleural friction rub Associated with pleural inflammation, it occurs when inflamed pleural surfaces slide across one another. This low-pitched, crackling sound typically is present during both inspiration and expiration.

Pleural space The region between the visceral and parietal pleura.

Pleuritic pain Sharp localized chest pain that increases with breathing and coughing.

Pleuritis Local extension of an infection to involve the pleura.

Pleximeter The middle finger of the nondominant hand. Often used in indirect percussion techniques.

Plexor The middle finger of the dominant hand. Often used in indirect percussion techniques.

Pneumatic retinopexy A surgical procedure to correct retinal detachment in which air is injected into the vitreous cavity and the patient is positioned so that the air bubble pushes the detached portion of the retina into contact with the choroid.

Pneumocystis jirovecii **pneumonia** An opportunistic infection that is not pathogenic in those with intact immune systems.

Pneumomediastinum The presence of air in the mediastinum.

Pneumonia Inflammation of the lung parenchyma (the respiratory bronchioles and alveoli).

Pneumopericardium Air in the pericardial sac.

Pneumothorax A partial lung collapse due to air or gas collecting in the lung or in the pleural space that surrounds the lungs.

Point of care Interventions or testing that provides on-the-spot information about the patient rather than having to send blood or urine samples down to the laboratory and wait for results to be returned.

Point of maximal impulse (PMI) A pulse located at the apex of the heart. Also called the *apical pulse*.

Point-of-service (POS) plan An insurance plan that allows the insured to choose between a health maintenance organization or a preferred provider organization each time they seek healthcare.

Polyarticular arthritis A form of juvenile rheumatoid arthritis that involves many joints (five or more), particularly the small joints of the hands and fingers. It may also affect the hips, knees, feet, ankles, and neck.

Polycyclic Describes a periodically recurring course of rheumatoid arthritis.

Polycythemia An increase in the production of red blood cells.

Polydipsia Excessive thirst.

Polyneuropathies Bilateral sensory disorders; they are the most common types of neuropathy associated with diabetes.

Polyp A small vascular growth on the surface of any mucous membrane.

Polyphagia Excessive hunger.

Polysomnography (PSG) A recording of the biophysical changes that a patient experiences during sleep.

Polysubstance abuse The simultaneous use of many substances.

Polyuria The production of abnormally large amounts of urine. Also called *diuresis*.

Pop-ups Unexpected things or events occurring during the day that require time and attention in addition to the regular plan for the day.

Positive end-expiratory pressure (PEEP) Mechanical ventilation in which a positive pressure is maintained in the airways during exhalation and between breaths to help keep alveoli open.

Positive feedback Output of a system that returns to the system as input and which promotes system change.

Positive pressure ventilator A mechanical device that pushes air into the lungs through an invasive device such as an endotracheal tube or tracheostomy tube, rather than drawing air in by negative pressure.

Positive punishment The addition of a negative consequence if undesirable behavior occurs.

Positive reinforcement Giving rewards such as praise or encouragement for a learner's achievements.

Positive symptoms Excessive or added behaviors that are not normally seen in healthy adults, such as delusions; commonly seen in schizophrenia.

Postanesthesia care unit (PACU) Designated unit for postoperative recovery of patients who do not require intensive care following a surgical procedure with anesthesia.

Postcoital contraception A drug taken after intercourse to avoid pregnancy. Also called *Plan B* or the *morning after pill*.

Postconception age periods Period of time in embryonic/fetal development calculated from the time of fertilization of the ovum.

Postconcussion syndrome A series of concussion-like symptoms that occur 7–10 days after a concussion. Manifestations include nausea, headache, dizziness, fatigue, memory problems, difficulty concentrating, insomnia, light and noise sensitivity, and/or personality changes.

Postictal period A period immediately following seizure activity in which level of consciousness is decreased. The length of the postictal period varies.

Postmenopausal bleeding Bleeding that occurs after menopause has occurred; may be caused by endometrial polyps, endometrial hyperplasia, or uterine cancer.

Postoperative The third phase of an operative process in which recovery occurs.

Postpartal hemorrhage A loss of blood of greater than 500 mL following birth. The hemorrhage is classified as *early* if it occurs within the first 24 hours and *late* if it occurs after the first 24 hours.

Postpartum After childbirth.

Postpartum blues A maternal adjustment reaction occurring in the first few postpartum days, characterized by mild depression, tearfulness, anxiety, headache, and irritability. Also called *adjustment reaction to depressed mood*.

Postpartum depression A severe form of depression that affects new mothers, often beginning within 3 months of delivery but which may strike at any time during the first year after having a child. Also called *depressive disorder with peripartum onset*.

Postpartum endometritis (metritis) An inflammation of the endometrium portion of the uterine lining occurring anytime up to 6 weeks postpartum.

Postpartum psychosis Severe psychosis occurring within the first 3 months after birth that usually requires hospitalization.

Postterm labor Labor that occurs after 42 weeks' gestation.

Postterm newborn Any infant born after 42 weeks' gestation.

Postterm pregnancy Pregnancy that lasts beyond 42 weeks' gestation.

Posttraumatic stress disorder (PTSD) A trauma- and stressor-related disorder that can evolve after exposure to a traumatic or overwhelming event in which an individual's physical health was endangered.

Postural drainage The drainage by gravity of secretions from various lung segments.

PPD Tuberculin skin test. See Purified protein derivative.

Prader–Willi syndrome (PWS) A congenital disorder of the 15th chromosome that causes an unrelenting feeling of hunger, but also low muscle tone, short stature, incomplete sexual development, mild to severe mental retardation, and behavioral problems.

Prayer Human communication with divine and spiritual entities.

Preceptor An experienced nurse who provides knowledge and emotional support, as well as a clarification of role expectations, on a one-to-one basis.

Precipitating factor A practice, behavior, or environmental factor that gives rise to a specific incident of violence.

Predisposing factor A practice, behavior, or environmental factor that increases the potential of an individual's risk of violent victimization or perpetration of violence.

Preeclampsia An increase in blood pressure after 20 weeks of gestation accompanied by proteinuria. May also be accompanied by albuminuria and edema. Also called *toxemia of pregnancy*.

Preferred provider organization (PPO) A type of health insurance program that does not require its insureds to select a primary care provider. PPOs usually have larger networks of providers than health maintenance organizations (HMOs) and provide financial incentives that encourage insureds to seek care from in-network providers. They are less restrictive than HMOs but typically have higher copayments.

Prejudice A negative belief or preference that is generalized about a group that leads to prejudgment.

Preload The amount of cardiac muscle fiber tension, or stretch, that exists at the end of diastole.

Premature ejaculation Ejaculation that occurs consistently before or shortly after penetration; i.e., before both partners are able to achieve satisfaction.

Premature junctional contractions Heartbeats that occur before the next expected beat of the underlying rhythm.

Premature rupture of membranes (PROM) Spontaneous rupture of membranes and leakage of amniotic fluid before the onset of labor at any gestational age.

Premenstrual syndrome (PMS) A complex of manifestations (e.g., mood swings, breast tenderness, fatigue, irritability, food cravings, and depression) that occurs 3–14 days before menstruation and is relieved by the onset of menses.

Prenatal education Programs offered to expectant families, adolescents, women, or partners to provide education regarding the pregnancy, labor, and birth experience.

Preoperative The first phase of an operative process in which the patient is identified as a candidate for surgical intervention, assessed, and prepared for surgery.

Preorgasmic Never having had an orgasm.

Preparedness The phase that takes place before an emergency occurs during which risks are assessed and plans are developed to address them.

Preprocedure verification process A standardized process used to verify that the correct procedure is being implemented on the correct patient at the correct site, and that all items necessary for the procedure are available.

Presbycusis Age-related loss of the ability to hear high-frequency sounds; may occur because of cochlear hair cell degeneration or loss of auditory neurons in the organ of Corti.

Presbyopia Impaired near vision resulting from a loss of elasticity of the lens related to aging.

Presencing Being present with a patient and being open, receptive, and available at all levels without judging or labeling.

Presenting part The first part of the fetus to enter and settle in the pelvic inlet during fetal presentation.

Pressure injury Ischemic lesions of the skin and underlying tissue caused by external pressure that impairs the flow of blood and lymph.

Preterm infant An infant born at less than 37 completed weeks of gestation.

Preterm premature rupture of the membranes (PPROM) A condition that occurs when membranes rupture and amniotic fluid leaks from the vagina before 37 weeks of gestation.

Pretibial myxedema The bilateral formation of edematous, erythematous, and sometimes hyperpigmented plaques and nodules over the shins and dorsal surface of the feet. A characteristic sign of Graves disease.

Priapism Persistent, painful erection of the penis.

Primary appraisal The evaluation of an event or circumstance in terms of its potential to harm, benefit, threaten, or challenge the individual.

Primary care provider (PCP) A healthcare provider who provides basic medical service and acts as a gatekeeper to more specialized care, referring patients to in-network hospitals and specialists.

Primary group A small, intimate group in which the relationships among members are personal, spontaneous, sentimental, cooperative, and inclusive.

Primary hypertension A persistently elevated systemic blood pressure. Also called *essential hypertension*.

Primary immune response When an individual is exposed to an antigen, the B-lymphocyte system produces antibodies that react specifically with that antigen over the first 3 days.

Primary intention healing Healing that occurs where the tissue surfaces have been closed and there is minimal or no tissue loss. It is characterized by the formation of minimal granulation tissue and scarring. Also called *primary union* or *first intention healing*.

Primary nursing A model in which one nurse has 24/7 authority and responsibility for the care of an assigned group of patients.

Primary prevention Methods designed to focus on health promotion and illness prevention.

Primary sex characteristics The reproductive organs.

Primigravida A woman who is pregnant for the first time.

Primipara Term used to describe a woman who has given birth to her first child (past the point of viability), whether or not that child is living or was alive at birth.

Principles-based (deontologic) theories Theories that involve logical and formal processes and emphasize individual rights, duties, and obligations.

Prioritizing care A process that helps nurses manage time and establish an order for completing responsibilities and care interventions for a single patient or for a group of patients.

Priority Something given or meriting attention before competing alternatives.

Privacy The right of individuals to keep their personal information from being disclosed.

Private insurance Health insurance provided by private or publicly owned companies such as Blue Cross Blue Shield, Kaiser, or Aetna.

Probiotics Microorganisms that aid in digestion and help to protect the body from harmful bacteria.

Problem-focused coping Managing or altering a stressor, event, or circumstance in response to distress.

Problem, intervention, evaluation (PIE) An assessment system consisting of patient care flow sheets and progress notes.

Problem-oriented medical record (POMR) A recording system in which data are arranged according to the problems the patient has rather than the source of the information. Also called *problem-oriented record (POR)*.

Problem-oriented record (POR) See Problem-oriented medical record (POMR).

Procedural memory Recall of information that does not require conscious awareness and involves the memory of motor skills and procedures.

Process addictions Compulsive behaviors that serve to reduce anxiety such as workaholism, gambling, shopping, cutting, pornography, spending and indebtedness, internet surfing or gaming, eating disorders, and sexual addictions.

Process standards Standards that focus on the steps used to lead to a particular outcome. It is used to determine if a set of steps exists and if those steps are being followed.

Productivity The performance measure of both the effectiveness and efficiency of nursing care.

Profession An occupation that requires extensive education or a calling that requires special knowledge, skill, and preparation.

Professional behaviors Effective nursing actions based on ethical principles, clinical reasoning, and technical knowledge and expertise that form helping relationships.

Professional development Continued staff education, planned activities to enhance role performance, and defined goals to improve patient outcomes. Also called *staff development*.

Professional support Assistance provided by professionals in the community who exhibit a nonblaming and respectful attitude toward families and patients and who provide information and help locating community resources.

Professionalism Acting with the knowledge, skill, and preparation of a professional.

Professionalization The process of establishing qualifications, ethical guidelines, and a standardized knowledge base by which an occupation transforms itself into a profession.

Progesterone Hormone produced by the corpus luteum, adrenal cortex, and placenta whose function is to stimulate proliferation of the endometrium to facilitate growth of the embryo.

Projectile vomiting Vomiting in which emesis may be spewed up to 2–3 feet out of a baby's mouth. A major symptom of pyloric stenosis.

Prone Face-down.

Proprioception The body's sense of its position.

Proptosis Forward displacement of the eye.

Prospective payment system (PPS) A system in which hospitals determine the amount to be billed to the insurance company before the patient is ever admitted to the hospital.

Prostaglandins (PGs) Complex lipid compounds synthesized by many cells of the body.

Prostate specific antigen (PSA) A protein produced in the cells of the prostate gland.

Prostatectomy Surgical removal of part or all of the prostate gland.

Prostatitis An inflammation of the prostate gland.

Prostatodynia A condition in which the patient experiences the symptoms of prostatitis, but shows no evidence of inflammation or infection.

Protected health information Personal information or healthcare data that could identify an individual. This information is protected and defined by HIPAA's Privacy Rule.

Protective factor 1. A practice, behavior, or environmental factor that provides strength and assistance to children and families in dealing with crises and risk factors. 2. A practice, behavior, or environmental factor that decreases the potential of an individual to perpetuate violence or victimization.

Protein A macronutrient that contains nitrogen and is a critical component of all tissues in the human body, including muscle, bone, and blood.

Protein-calorie malnutrition Problem of patients with long-term deficiencies in caloric intake; characteristics include depressed visceral proteins (e.g., albumin), weight loss, and visible muscle and fat wasting.

Proteinuria Excess protein in urine.

Proxemics The study of distance between people in their interactions.

Proximodistal Growth that proceeds from the center of the body outward.

Proximodistal development Development that proceeds from the center of the body outward.

Pruritus Itching of the skin.

Pseudoaddiction A term applied to patients who display drug-seeking behaviors but differ from addicts in that they have true underlying pain for which they are seeking relief. These behaviors will generally stop when adequate pain control is achieved.

Pseudoexacerbation A temporary aggravation of symptoms that is directly related to a trigger and subsides as soon as the trigger is removed.

Pseudomenstruation Blood or whitish discharge may occasionally be observed on the diapers of female newborns caused by the withdrawal of maternal hormones.

Purified protein derivative (PPD) Used to screen for tuberculosis in a tuberculin test. A small amount of the PPD is injected and the body's response interpreted.

Purulent exudate A large quantity of cells and necrotic debris that form an opaque or milky discharge that is thicker than serous exudate. Also called *pus* or *suppuration*.

Pus The common name for *purulent exudate*.

Psychoanalytic theory A framework for personality development that emphasizes the presence of unconscious impulses and their influence on behaviors and the formation of self; developed by Sigmund Freud (1856–1939).

Psychogenic pain Pain that is experienced in the absence of any diagnosed physiologic cause or event.

Psychomotor domain The learning domain that includes fine motor skills. Also called the *skill domain*.

Psychomotor retardation A state in which thinking and body movements are noticeably slower than normal and speech is slowed or absent.

Psychosis A mental health condition characterized by delusions, hallucinations, illusions, disorganized behavior, and a difficulty relating to others. Also called *psychotic disorder*.

Psychosocial skills Skills that enable an individual in crisis to maintain relationships with family and friends throughout and after the crisis period.

Psychostimulants Stimulants that have a high potential for abuse. Psychostimulants include cocaine and amphetamines.

Psychoticism One of the six trait domains associated with personality disorders that is composed of eccentricity, cognitive and perceptual dysregulation, and unusual beliefs and experiences.

Ptosis Drooping of the eyelid.

Ptyalism Excessive, often bitter salivation.

Puberty The stage during which an individual reaches sexual maturity.

Pubis Pertaining to the pubes or pubic area.

Public distance Communication that requires loud, clear vocalizations with careful enunciation.

Public insurance Health insurance financed by the government.

Public self How the individual wishes to be perceived by others.

Puerperium That time immediately following childbirth during which physiologic changes that occurred during pregnancy begin to return to normal. Also called *postpartum period*.

Pulmonary atresia The absence of communication between the right ventricle and the pulmonary artery.

Pulmonary circulation Circulation through the right side of the heart, the pulmonary artery, the pulmonary capillaries, and the pulmonary vein.

Pulmonary edema An abnormal accumulation of fluid in the interstitial tissue and alveoli of the lung.

Pulmonary embolism (PE) The obstruction of blood flow in part of the pulmonary vascular system by an embolus. Also called *pulmonary thromboembolism*.

Pulmonary function test (PFT) A test designed to provide information about ventilation airflow, lung volume, and the capacity and diffusion of gas.

Pulmonary vascular resistance The force or resistance of the blood in the pulmonary circulation.

Pulse A wave of blood created by the contraction of the left ventricle of the heart.

Pulse oximetry A noninvasive method of assessing arterial blood oxygenation.

Pulse pressure The difference between the systolic and diastolic pressure.

Pulse rhythm The pattern of the beats and the intervals between the beats.

Punctual On time.

Punishment 1. Action taken to enforce rules when a child misbehaves. 2. Consequences that lead to a decrease in undesirable behavior.

Pupillary light reflex Reflex in which the pupil contracts in response to a bright light.

Purging Self-induced vomiting or misuse of laxatives, diuretics, or enemas.

Pursed-lipped breathing Exhaling through a narrow opening between the lips to prolong the expiratory phase in an effort to promote more alveolar emptying while maintaining open alveoli.

Pyelolithotomy An incision into and removal of a stone from the kidney pelvis.

Pyelonephritis Inflammation of the renal pelvis and parenchyma, the functional kidney tissue.

Pyloric stenosis A thickening of the pyloric muscle resulting in a narrowing of the pyloric sphincter between the stomach and small intestine.

Pyogenic bacteria Bacteria that produces purulent exudate or pus.

Pyorrhea Advanced periodontal disease.

Pyuria Cloudy or pus-filled urine.

Quadriplegia Complete loss of function of the upper and lower body, including the arms, trunk, legs, and pelvic organs. Also called *tetraplegia*.

Quadruple screen The most widely used test to screen for Down syndrome (trisomy 21), trisomy 18, and neural tube defects.

Qualifiers Words that have been added to some NANDA nursing diagnosis labels to give additional meaning to the diagnostic statement.

Qualitative research Investigates a question through narrative data from interviews, storytelling, and description of observation to provide a better understanding of the patient's perspective.

Quality 1. A subjective description of a sound, for example: whistling, gurgling, or snapping. 2. The degree to which health services for individuals and populations increase the likelihood of desired health outcomes and are consistent with current professional knowledge.

Quality and Safety Education for Nurses (QSEN) A program designed to identify and standardize the six core competencies or nursing: patient-centered care, teamwork and collaboration, evidence-based practice, quality improvement, safety, and informatics.

Quality assurance The process of collecting data related to a problem and then analyzing the data based on benchmark standards to determine if standards are being met.

Quality improvement The process of using systematic and continuous actions that lead to measurable improvement in healthcare services and the health status of targeted patient groups.

Quality management The evaluation of medical and nursing processes for quality and effectiveness compared to accepted standards in order to correct problems before they harm patients and to prevent errors in treatment.

Quantitative research Uses precise measurements for data collection and employs statistical analysis to provide specific and objective data about a topic.

Quickening The mother's perception of fetal movement.

Race A term used to describe socially defined populations that share genetically transmitted physical characteristics, such as skin color and bone structure.

Racism The oppression of a group of people based on their perceived race.

Radiation The process of heat transfer with no physical contact.

Radiation cataracts A type of cataract that may result from long-term exposure to radiation.

Radical mastectomy The removal of an entire affected breast, its underlying chest muscles, and the lymph nodes under the arms. Compare with Simple mastectomy.

Range of motion (ROM) The degree to which a joint can be moved; a measurement of flexion and extension.

Range-of-motion (ROM) exercises Exercises designed to take each joint through all possible movements to maintain flexibility and movement in the joint.

Rape Any penetration, no matter how slight, of the vagina or anus with any body part or object, or oral penetration by a sex organ of another person, without the consent of the victim.

Rape-trauma syndrome (RTS) A series of psychologic sequelae that many victims experience following rape in addition to physiologic sequelae.

Rapport An understanding between two or more people.

Readiness to learn The demonstration of behaviors or cues that reflect a learner's motivation to learn at a specific time.

Real self The perceived true self.

Reappraisal An individual's ongoing evaluation and reinterpretation of an event or circumstance, as well as continued evaluation of the efficacy of the coping strategies.

Receiver This is the third component of the communication process. The receiver is the listener, who listens, observes, and attends.

Receptive speech The ability to understand the spoken word.

Receptor A nerve cell that converts a stimulus to a nerve impulse. Most receptors are specific, that is, sensitive to only one type of stimulus.

Record A formal, legal document that provides evidence of a patient's care. Also called a *patient record* or a *clinical chart*.

Recording The process of making an entry on a patient record. Also called *charting* or *documenting*.

Recovery 1. Return to (or exceed) preillness levels of functioning. 2. A continued state of voluntary sobriety in which an individual maintains personal health and functions normally. 3. A phase of mental illness in which symptoms of the disorder are present but under control.

Recurrence A later recurrence of a disorder after recovery.

Red blood cells (RBCs) Blood cells shaped like biconcave discs that contain the hemoglobin required for oxygen transport to body tissues; the most common type of blood cell. Also called *erythrocytes*.

Reduction Surgical placement of a broken bone in the correct alignment.

Referred pain Pain that is perceived in an area distant from the site of the stimuli.

Reflection The action of making sense of occurrences, situations, or decisions by carefully considering the totality of the experience: what worked or did not work, what could have been done differently to achieve better outcomes, what was done well, what necessary resources were available, and so on.

Reflexes The rapid, involuntary, predictable motor responses to a stimulus.

Reflux A backward flow of acidic secretions into the lower esophagus.

Refraction The bending of light rays as they pass from one medium to another medium of different optical density.

Refractory hypoxemia The decrease of particle arterial oxygen despite administration of oxygen at high flow rates.

Refractory period A phase during which myocardial cells resist stimulation.

Refractory septic shock A persistently low mean arterial blood pressure despite vasopressor therapy and adequate fluid resuscitation.

Regeneration The replacement or renewal of destroyed tissue cells by cells that are identical or similar in structure and function.

Registered nurses (RNs) The members of a nursing team who are specially licensed and trained to deliver direct patient care, including patient assessment, identification of health problems, and development and coordination of care.

Regurgitation The backflow of blood into the atria during systole.

Rehabilitation A level of wellness in which symptoms of the condition are under control to the extent that the affected individual can engage in goal-directed activities.

Reinfection The development of a new infection with a different pathogen following successful treatment.

Reinforcement Consequences that lead to an increase in a particular behavior.

Relapse Return of an acute phase of illness after recovery.

Relapsing fever Short febrile periods of a few days are interspersed with periods of 1–2 days of normal temperature.

Relationship-based (caring) theories Theories that stress courage, generosity, commitment, and the need to nurture and maintain relationships.

Relaxation response A healthful physiologic state that can be elicited through deep relaxation breathing with emphasis on a prolonged exhalation phase.

Religion A set of doctrines accepted by a group of people who gather together regularly to worship that offers a means to relate to God or a higher power; an organized system of beliefs and practices.

REM sleep Rapid-eye-movement sleep that occurs during sleep about every 90 minutes and lasts 5–30 minutes. The brain is highly active in this phase, and most dreams will take place during REM sleep.

Remission 1. A period during a chronic illness in which the symptoms of the illness disappear. 2. A sustained recovery lasting 8 weeks or more.

Remittent fever A wide range of fluctuating temperatures (more than 2°C [3.6°F]), all of which are above normal and occur over a 24-hour period.

Remyelination Repair of the damaged myelin sheath by oligodendrocytes.

Renal colic Acute, severe flank pain on an affected side that develops when a stone obstructs the ureter, causing ureteral spasm.

Renal failure A condition in which the kidneys are unable to remove accumulated metabolites from the blood or produce urine, resulting in altered fluid, electrolyte, and acid–base balance.

Renal insufficiency Decrease in the kidneys' ability to conserve sodium and concentrate the urine.

Renin–angiotensin–aldosterone system System initiated by specialized receptors in the juxtaglomerular cells of the kidney nephrons that respond to changes in renal perfusion.

Repetitive strain injury A nerve, tendon, or muscle condition that occurs when the limbs are subjected to repetitive use, awkward positions, or forced positions. Also called *repetitive motion disorder.*

Repolarization The process that returns the cell to its resting, polarized state.

Report An oral, written, or electronic communication intended to convey information to others.

Research participants Volunteers for a specific study project that meet all the inclusion criteria, have been informed of all aspects of the study, and have signed informed consent.

Reservoir A source of microorganisms.

Residual urine Urine that remains in the bladder after voiding.

Resilience/resiliency The ability to function with healthy responses, even when experiencing significant stress or adversity; the personal patterns, behaviors, or processes that promote an individual's recovery from or adaptation to adversity.

Resolution phase The fourth and final phase of the sexual response cycle is marked by a return to an unaroused state.

Resonance A hollow sound, such as the sound produced by lungs filled with air.

Resource An asset that helps nurses meet patient needs.

Resource allocation The distribution of resources among competing groups of people or programs.

Respiration The act of inhaling (inspiration) and exhaling (expiration) air to transport oxygen to the alveoli so that oxygen may be exchanged for carbon dioxide, and the carbon dioxide expelled from the body.

Respiratory acidosis A condition that is caused by an excess of dissolved carbon dioxide, or carbonic acid. It is characterized by a pH of less than 7.35 and a $PaCO_2$ greater than 45 mmHg. It may be caused by hypoventilation.

Respiratory alkalosis A condition that results when pH rises above 7.45 and $PaCO_2$ falls below 35 mmHg. It is caused by hyperventilation (unusually fast respiration, or overbreathing), leading to a carbon dioxide deficit.

Respiratory depression A decrease in the depth and rate of breathing.

Respiratory syncytial virus (RSV) A highly contagious respiratory infection that affects almost all children before 2 years of age.

Response This is the fourth component of the communication process; it is the message that the receiver returns to the sender. Also called *feedback.*

Responsibility The specific accountability or liability associated with the performance of duties of a particular role.

Rest pain Cramping or aching pain in the calves of the legs, the thighs, and the buttocks that occurs while at rest.

Restless leg syndrome A neurologic sensorimotor disorder that is characterized by an overwhelming urge to move the legs when at rest.

Restraints Any devices or medications intended to protect the patient from injuring self or others through partially or fully limiting the patient's mobility.

Restrictive cardiomyopathy A disorder characterized by rigid ventricular walls that impair diastolic filling.

Reticular activating system Modulation of sleep–wake transitions that occurs when the reticular formation, a network of ascending nerves, relays information about alertness and arousal to the cerebral cortex and directs the brain's attention to sensory events.

Retinal detachment Separation of the retina or sensory portion of the eye from the choroid.

Retractions Visible sinking of the chest wall, or sunken areas seen between the ribs during inspiration.

Retrograde conduction Cardiac conduction against the normal flow or pattern.

Retrograde ejaculation Ejaculation that occurs with fluid traveling into the bladder instead of out through the urethra.

Retropulsion The tendency to topple backward when bumped or when rising, standing, or turning.

Retrospective audit An evaluation performed after a patient's discharge comparing the care provided to the patient with care provided to patients with similar conditions.

Reverse delegation A situation that occurs when someone with a lower rank delegates to someone with more authority.

Reverse triage A method in which the most severely injured or ill victims who require the greatest resources are treated last to allow the greatest number of victims to receive medical attention.

Revision surgery The replacement of an artificial joint after 10 years or more.

Reward deficiency syndrome The decreased ability to experience pleasure. Reward deficiency syndrome drives the person to seek external forms of gratification through the use of substances, pathologic gambling, or other high-risk behaviors.

Rh disease A rare condition where the mother is Rh negative while the child is Rh positive. If this condition arises, the mother's body will see the Rh-positive cells in the fetus as foreign, and will then produce antibodies to fight off the Rh-positive cells. May result in fetal demise in extreme cases.

Rheumatoid arthritis (RA) A chronic systemic autoimmune disease that causes inflammation of connective tissue, primarily in the joints.

Rhinorrhea Drainage of mucus from the nose. Commonly known as a runny nose.

Rhonchi A long, low-pitched sound that continues throughout inspiration suggesting a blockage of large airway passages.

Ribonucleic acid (RNA) One of two types of nucleic acid made by cells. Ribonucleic acid is made up of ribose rather than deoxyribose and contains information that has been copied from DNA (the other type of nucleic acid).

Rigidity Resistance to movement because of the involuntary contraction of all skeletal muscles.

Risk diagnosis A clinical judgment that a problem does not exist, but the presence of risk factors indicates a problem is likely to develop unless the nurse intervenes.

Risk factor A practice, behavior, or environmental factor that increases the potential of negative effects on an individual's health.

Risk management Preventive policies and processes that focus on limiting a healthcare agency's financial and legal risk associated with the delivery of care, particularly in terms of lawsuits.

Role A set of expectations about how an individual occupying one position behaves.

Role ambiguity Occurs when expectations are unclear and when people do not know how to perform their roles and/or are unable to predict the reactions of others to their behavior.

Role conflict Emotional conflict arising when competing demands are made on an individual in the fulfillment of his or her multiple social roles.

Role development Teaching and modeling the behaviors needed to successfully assume a particular role.

Role mastery Occurs when an individual's behaviors meet or exceed social expectations.

Role performance The demonstration of behaviors or actions associated with a given role.

Role strain The stress or strain experienced by an individual when incompatible behavior, expectations, or obligations are associated with a single social role.

Root cause analysis An evaluation required by the Joint Commission that is focused on identifying areas of improvement that would decrease the likelihood of future adverse events and to develop an action plan for improvement.

Rooting reflex In response to a light touch of a finger on an infant's cheek close to the mouth, the infant's head will rotate toward the stimulation and attempt to suck the finger.

Rotational injury An injury caused by lateral flexion or twisting of the head and neck.

Round ligaments The ligaments that hold the ovaries in place.

Rupture of membranes The rupturing of amniotic membranes before the onset of labor.

Sacral promontory A projection into the pelvic cavity on the anterior upper portion of the sacrum, which serves as a landmark for pelvic measurements.

Sarcopenia The process of atrophy due to age.

Safety Decreasing risks of dangers or hazards to prevent accidents, injuries, mistakes, and harm.

Safety culture A general feeling of shared attitudes, values, practices, and beliefs which result in behaviors and feelings of responsibility for safety in all daily routines.

Safety strap body restraint Restraints used to ensure the safety of patients who are transported by wheelchair or gurney, or to protect patients confined to a bed or a chair. Also called *belt restraint.*

Salient cue The leading, most noticeable, or most important information about a patient's health status.

Saline An isotonic solution of 0.9% sodium chloride.

Sanguineous exudate A large amount of red blood cells that form a bright or dark red discharge indicating new or old damage to capillaries. Also called *hemorrhagic exudate.*

Satiety The sensation of fullness and satisfaction that should inhibit eating until the next meal.

Saturated fat A triglyceride fat that contains all of the hydrogen ions it is capable of holding.

SBAR A method of reporting information about a patient in the following order: situation, background, assessment, and recommendation.

Scaling The rating of the severity of symptoms or problems.

Scapegoat An individual who has been selected to take the blame for another individual or for a group.

Scenario planning A group process strategy that encourages members of a group to create hypothetical or "possible future" situations.

Scheduled toileting Toileting at regular intervals.

Schemes Adaptive cognitive structures formed in response to environmental stimuli according to Jean Piaget's theory of cognitive development.

Schistocytes Fragmented red blood cells.

Schizoaffective disorder A psychotic disorder with features of both schizophrenia and mood disorders.

Schizoid personality disorder (SPD) One of several personality disorders defined in the DSM-5, it is characterized by a lifelong pattern of indifference to others, absence of humor, and social isolation.

Schizophrenia The most common psychotic disorder, schizophrenia is a combination of disordered thinking, perceptual disturbances, behavioral abnormalities, affective disruptions, and impaired social competency.

Schizophreniform disorder A disorder with rapid onset of psychotic symptoms, very similar to schizophrenia, lasting less than 6 months.

Schizotypal personality disorder One of several personality disorders defined in the DSM-5, it is characterized by a pattern of disturbed interpersonal relationships, thought patterns, appearance, and behavior.

Sciatica Lumbar back pain that radiates down the posterior leg to the ankle due to irritation or compression of all or part of the sciatic nerve.

Scleral buckling A surgical procedure to correct retinal detachment.

Scoliometer A diagnostic test used to measure a patient's rib hump when in the Adam position.

Scoliosis A lateral, or sideways, curvature of the spine.

Scoop method A safe method of recapping sharps in which the cap is placed on a needle or a hard surface and the needle is guided into the cap.

Seasonal affective disorder (SAD) A mood disorder typically characterized by depression during fall and winter and normal mood or hypomania during spring and summer.

Second heart sound (S_2) The heart sound produced by closure of the semilunar valves; characterized by the syllable "dub."

Second impact syndrome (SIS) A constellation of clinical manifestations that can occur when an individual receives a second concussion before the initial concussion is completely healed.

Secondary appraisal Evaluation of an individual's available coping resources and potential options for responding to an event or circumstance.

Secondary cataracts A type of cataract that may form after surgery to treat another eye disorder, such as glaucoma, or as an effect of medication or another primary disorder.

Secondary group A group that is larger, more impersonal, and less sentimental than a primary group.

Secondary hypertension Elevated blood pressure resulting from an identifiable underlying process.

Secondary immune response Subsequent encounters with an antigen following the primary immune response that result in triggering memory cells.

Secondary infertility The inability to conceive after one or more successful pregnancies, or the inability to sustain a pregnancy.

Secondary intention healing Healing that occurs when a wound's edges cannot or should not close. Repair time is typically longer, scarring is greater, and susceptibility to infection is greater.

Secondary prevention Methods that focus on the diagnosis and treatment of disease.

Secondary sex characteristics Bodily traits that develop over time and are influenced by a person's sex but not directly involved in reproduction.

Segmental mastectomy See *Lumpectomy*.

Seizures Periods of abnormal electrical discharges in the brain that cause involuntary movement, as well as behavior and sensory alterations.

Selective perception The process of filtering out unnecessary and distracting information in order to focus on what is important at any given moment.

Selective serotonin reuptake inhibitor (SSRI) A drug that selectively inhibits the reuptake of serotonin into nerve terminals; used mostly for depression.

Selectively permeable Refers to membranes separating body fluid compartments across which solutes can move with relative ease.

Self The entirety of an individual's being, including body, sensations, emotions, and thoughts, as well as a conscious awareness of one's own being.

Self-awareness The relationship between an individual's perception of himself or herself and others' perceptions of him or her.

Self-concept The personal perception of the self formed in response to interactions with others and the environment throughout the course of an individual's lifetime.

Self-efficacy The expectation that someone can produce a desired outcome.

Self-esteem One's judgment of one's own worth.

Self-help group A group of individuals who come together to face a common problem or difficulty.

Self-quieting ability The ability of newborns to use their own resources to quiet and comfort themselves.

Semen Sperm mixed with seminal fluid, ejaculated during sexual activity.

Semiformal group A group with formalized structure, delineated hierarchy, and voluntary, but selective, membership.

Sender An individual or group who wishes to convey a message to another; can be considered the *source-encoder*.

Sensate focus A mindfulness technique commonly employed as part of sex therapy.

Sensitization An increased reaction to pain over time, or a reduced threshold for reaction to painful stimuli.

Sensory memory The earliest stage of memory in which visual input and auditory information are retained for less than a few seconds.

Sensory perception The conscious organization and translation of external data or stimuli into meaningful information.

Sensory reception The process of receiving external stimuli or data. External stimuli are visual (sight), auditory (hearing), olfactory (smell), tactile (touch), and gustatory (taste).

Sentinel event An unexpected occurrence involving death or serious physical or psychologic injury, or the risk thereof.

Sepsis 1. A whole-body inflammatory process resulting in acute illness. 2. A state of infection.

Septal defect A congenital heart defect that connects the right and left side of the heart.

Septic shock Altered perfusion resulting from a systemic infection that manifests with hypotension, delayed capillary refill, and inadequate perfusion and oxygenation of vital body tissues. Also called *septicemia*.

Septicemia See Septic shock.

Serious mental illness Mental illness that is severe enough to impair daily functioning and the ability to achieve life goals.

Seroconversion Antibody response to a disease or vaccine.

Serosanguineous exudate A clear or blood-tinged discharge commonly seen in surgical incisions.

Serotonin syndrome A condition that may occur in individuals taking two or more medications that increase serotonin levels. Symptoms include hypertension or hypotension, agitation, shivering, changes in mental status, symptoms of gastrointestinal distress, restlessness, tremor, muscle rigidity, unreactive pupils, and tachypnea.

Serous exudate A watery, clear or straw-colored discharge that accompanies mild inflammation.

Serum bicarbonate (HCO_3) A value that reflects the renal regulation of acid–base balance. The normal HCO_3 value is 24–28 mEq/L.

Serum sickness A systemic type III hypersensitivity response, usually in response to a drug such as penicillin or a sulfonamide.

Servant leadership A theory of leadership rooted in the belief that the most effective leaders are those who are motivated primarily by a desire to serve, rather than a desire to lead.

Severe sepsis Sepsis associated with acute organ failure.

Seven rights of medication administration Right person, right assessment, right drug, right dose, right route, right time, right documentation.

Sex addiction Persistent, excessive sexual behaviors.

Sex chromosomes The 23rd pair of chromosomes found in a cell's nucleus; it determines an individual's gender.

Sexism When male values, beliefs, or activities are preferred over female ones.

Sexual abuse Any sexual act that is perpetrated against someone's will including rape, attempted sexual acts, unwanted sexual contact, voyeurism, and sexual harassment. Also called *sexual violence*.

Sexual aversion disorder A disorder characterized by severe distaste for sexual activity or the thought of sexual activity.

Sexual dysfunction Any persistent disturbance in an individual's sexual response.

Sexual health A state of physical, emotional, mental, and social well-being in relation to sexuality, not merely the absence of disease, dysfunction, or infirmity. Sexual health requires a positive and respectful approach to sexuality and sexual relationships.

Sexual orientation The sexual attraction of an individual to the same sex, the opposite sex, or both sexes.

Sexual self-concept How one values oneself as a sexual being.

Sexually transmitted infections (STIs) Infections transmitted by vaginal, oral, and anal intimate contact and intercourse.

SHARE A method of handoff reporting: Standardize critical content; hardwire within your system; allow opportunity to ask questions; reinforce quality and measurement; educate and coach.

Shared governance A method that aims to distribute decision making among a group of people.

Shared leadership The concept that a professional workplace is made up of many leaders.

Shared psychotic disorder A condition that results when an individual who is in a close relationship with another person who is delusional comes to share the delusional beliefs.

Shearing force A condition that results when one tissue layer slides over another.

Shock A clinical syndrome characterized by a systemic imbalance between oxygen supply and demand.

Shock phase The initial part of an alarm reaction during which the sympathetic nervous system is suppressed and an individual may experience manifestations such as hypotension, decreased body temperature, and decreased muscle tone.

Short bowel syndrome A condition in which the transit time of ingested foods and fluids is reduced and digestive processes are impaired because of a resection of significant portions of the small intestine.

Short-term memory Information held in the brain for immediate use; what an individual has in mind at a given moment.

Shunt A natural or artificially created tunnel or passage that allows blood to flow through an area.

Sickle cell anemia An inherited chronic hemolytic anemia, sickle cell anemia is the most common form of sickle cell disease.

Sickle cell crisis Severe episodes of fever and intense pain that are the hallmark of sickle cell disease. Also called *vaso-occlusive crisis.*

Sickle cell disease A hereditary hemoglobinopathy characterized by replacement of normal hemoglobin with abnormal hemoglobin S (Hgb S) in RBCs.

Sickle cell trait Carrying one copy of the defective sickle cell gene, which can be passed on to children but does not usually cause the illness.

Sickling A process in which red blood cells take on the characteristic sickle shape following deoxygenation in patients who have sickle cell disease.

Sick-role behavior A combination of illness behaviors, such as engaging in self-care and using the healthcare system, combined with dependent behaviors, such as avoiding usual responsibilities.

Signs See Objective data.

Simple assault An unlawful physical attack by one person upon another in which neither the offender displays a weapon, nor the victim suffers any obvious severe or aggravated bodily injury involving apparent broken bones, loss of teeth, possible internal injury, severe laceration, or loss of consciousness.

Simple mastectomy The removal of a complete breast only. Compare with Radical mastectomy.

Single-parent family A family in which only one parent resides in the home and is the primary caretaker and provider for the family.

Single-payer system Healthcare coverage arising from a single source, usually the government.

Situational crisis A crisis that involves an unexpected stressor or circumstance that occurs in the course of daily living.

Situational depression A maladaptive reaction to an identifiable psychosocial stressor or stressors that occurs within 3 months after the onset of the stressor and has persisted for no longer than 6 months. Also called *adjustment disorder with depressed mood.*

Situational leader A leader who is flexible in task and relationship behaviors, considers the staff members' abilities, knows the nature of the task to be done, and is sensitive to the context or environment in which the task takes place.

Six Sigma A quality improvement program originally implemented by Motorola and General Electric that focuses on reducing variation within a process to produce a near-perfect product.

Skin turgor The elasticity of skin.

Sleep An altered state of consciousness in which an individual's perception and reaction to the environment are decreased.

Sleep apnea A disorder characterized by frequent short breathing pauses during sleep.

Sleep architecture The basic organization of normal sleep.

Sleep hygiene Interventions used to promote quality sleep at night.

Sleep loss A duration of sleep shorter than the recommended 7–8 hours a night for an adult.

Small cell carcinoma A highly malignant cancer usually associated with the lung.

SMART An acronym to provide assistance in writing a patient-centered goal statement. SMART is Single action (choose a specific, single action to focus on), Measurable result (observable or measurable result), Attainable (level appropriate), Relevant (customized specifically for patient's needs), and Time-limited (specific time frame for goal to be completed).

SOAP An acronym for collective data in a progress note; it stands for subjective data, objective data, assessment, and planning.

SOAPIER Short for subjective data, objective data, assessment, plan of care, intervention, evaluation, and revision.

Sobriety A state of habitually refraining from using alcohol or drugs.

Social cognition The ability to process and apply social information accurately and effectively.

Social distance Communication characterized by a clear visual perception of the whole person. Body heat and odor are imperceptible, eye contact is increased, and vocalizations are loud enough to be overheard by others.

Social justice A framework in which to explore the complexities surrounding the variety of factors that impact diverse and vulnerable populations.

Social microcosm The concept that group members eventually behave in a therapy group the same way they behave with family and friends.

Social phobia A condition that is characterized by a pervasive, extreme fear of one or more social situations that may lead to scrutiny by others. Also called *social anxiety disorder.*

Socialization The process by which individuals learn to become members of groups and society and learn the social rules defining relationships into which they will enter.

Socialized insurance A system in which all medically necessary services are covered, including physician care, hospital services, and to some extent, prescription drugs.

Socialized medicine State government-owned and controlled healthcare services.

Solitary play A stage of play in which an infant still plays primarily alone, but enjoys the presence of others.

Solute Substance that dissolves in liquid.

Solvent The component of a solution that can dissolve a solute.

Somatic cells Cells that make up the tissue of the body, with a full complement (diploid) of chromosomes, as opposed to sex cells.

Somatic pain Pain arising from nerve receptors originating in the skin or close to the surface of the body.

Somatization The process by which psychologic distress is experienced and communicated in the form of somatic symptoms.

Somatostatin A substance, believed to be a neurotransmitter, that inhibits the production of both glucagon and insulin.

Somnology The study of sleep.

Somogyi phenomenon A combination of hypoglycemia during the night with a rebound, morning rise in blood glucose to hyperglycemic levels.

Source-oriented record Patient record in which each healthcare provider or department member makes notations in a separate section or sections of the patient's chart.

Spasticity Increased muscle tone, usually with some degree of weakness.

Specific defenses Immune system responses directed against identifiable bacteria, viruses, fungi, or other infectious agents.

Specific gravity An indicator of urine concentration that can be performed quickly and easily by nursing personnel.

Specific phobia An intense or extreme fear with regard to a particular object or situation.

Specific self-esteem How much one approves of a certain parts of oneself.

Spermatogenesis The process by which mature spermatozoa are formed.

Spermicide A cream, jelly, foam, vaginal film, or suppository that is inserted into the vagina before intercourse to destroy sperm and prevent conception.

Spinal cord A continuation of the medulla oblongata, it has the ability to transmit impulses to and from the brain via the ascending and descending pathways.

Spinal cord injury (SCI) Trauma to the spinal cord that results from excessive force to the spinal column.

Spinal cord stimulation (SCS) A form of therapy used with persistent pain that has not been controlled with less invasive therapies. SCS involves the insertion of an electrode (a single channel or multichannel device) adjacent to the spinal cord in the epidural space. The electrode(s) is attached to an impulse-generator (external or implanted) that sends electric impulses to the spinal cord to control pain.

Spinal fusion The insertion of a wedge-shaped piece of bone or bone chips between the vertebrae to stabilize them and reduce pain.

Spinal shock A condition that is characterized by spinal cord swelling, decreased blood flow and blood pressure, and complete loss of motor function, spinal reflexes, and autonomic function below the level of injury.

Spiritual distress A challenge to the spiritual well-being or to the belief system that provides strength, hope, and meaning to life; a feeling of being separated from interconnectedness with others or with a higher power.

Spiritual health The overall feeling of strength, hope, and fulfillment that encourages people to find life-sustaining and enriching opportunities.

Spiritual skills Skills that help an individual find meaning in and understand the personal significance of an unexpected event.

Spiritual support Assistance to patients and families in providing meaning and sustaining courage during difficult times.

Spiritual well-being A feeling of inner peace and of being generally alive, purposeful, and fulfilled; the feeling is rooted in spiritual values and/or specific religious beliefs.

Spirituality The part of being human that seeks meaningfulness through personal connection, which may include belief in or relationship with some higher power, creative force, driving being, or infinite source of energy.

Spirometry A means of measuring inhalation and exhalation, although the key measurements are forced expiratory volume over 1 second (FEV_1) and the ratio of FEV_1 to forced vital capacity (FEV_1/FVC). In other words, how much and how quickly an individual exhales air as measured by spirometry is an indicator of the degree of pulmonary function deficit.

Splint An easily adjustable device that stabilizes injuries, usually before swelling has subsided or after the reparative phase of healing.

Splitting 1. The inability to integrate contradictory experiences. 2. The inclination to perceive people or situations as one extreme or the other.

Spontaneous abortion The loss of a fetus prior to 20 weeks of gestation. Also called *miscarriage*.

Spontaneous rupture of membranes (SROM) The rupturing of membranes during the height of an intense contraction with a gush of fluid out of the vagina.

Sporadic AD One of the two basic types of Alzheimer disease, it shows no clear pattern of inheritance, although genetic factors may contribute to the disorder. Sporadic AD typically does not develop until after the age of 65. Also called *late-onset Alzheimer disease*.

Sprain A stretching or tearing of ligaments.

Sputum Mucus or mucopurulent matter expectorated from the lungs.

Squamous cell carcinoma A malignant tumor of the squamous epithelium of the skin or mucous membranes.

Staff authority The power to provide advice and support to employees or departments but not to assign tasks.

Staff development Continued staff education, planned activities to enhance role performance, and defined goals to improve patient outcomes. Also called *professional development*.

Stage of exhaustion Stage in which the body ceases to maintain its adaptation to a stressor; the stressor overwhelms the individual's ability to cope or mount a continued defense, resulting in the depletion of energy and resources.

Stage of resistance Stage in which the body attempts to move toward restoration of homeostasis while continuing to respond to the stressor.

Staghorn calculi A type of calculi associated with a urinary tract infection caused by urease-producing bacteria such as *Proteus*. These stones can grow to become very large, filling the renal pelvis and calyces. Also called *struvite calculi*.

Staging A system of classifying cancer according to the size of the tumor, involvement of lymph nodes, and metastasis to distant sites.

Standard precautions Safety guidelines, such as proper hand hygiene, use of proper protective equipment, safe injection practices, and effective management of potentially contaminated surfaces or equipment, that are designed to decrease the risk of transmitting unidentified pathogens. Also called *universal precautions* and *body substance isolation (BSI)*.

Standardized plan A nursing care plan that specifies the nursing care for groups of patients with common needs (e.g., all patients with myocardial infarction).

Standards Models of high-quality performance that may reflect the performance of industry leaders, scientific or clinical research, or recommendations of professional organizations such as the ANA.

Standards of care Guidelines used to determine what a nurse should or should not do, and may be defined as a benchmark of achievement based on a desired level of excellence.

Standards of practice A standardized description of the responsibilities for which nurses are responsible.

Standards of professional performance The behaviors expected in the professional nursing role by the American Nurses Association.

Station The location of the fetal presenting part in the maternal pelvis in relation to the ischial spine.

Status asthmaticus A severe, prolonged form of asthma that is difficult to treat.

Status epilepticus A continuous seizure that lasts for more than 30 minutes or a series of seizures during which time consciousness is not regained.

Statute of limitations The limit to the amount of time that can pass between recognition of harm and bringing a suit.

Statutory laws Laws made by any legislative branch of the government, including the U.S. Congress, state legislatures, and city and county governments.

Steatorrhea Fatty, frothy, foul-smelling stools caused by a decrease in pancreatic enzyme secretion.

Stem cell transplant The infusion of immature stem cells to replenish a patient's blood cell lines; used as an alternative to bone marrow transplantation.

Stenosis Narrowing of the valve, valve area, or great artery above the valve.

Stent A short, narrow tube inserted into the lumen of a vessel (e.g., artery) to relieve blockage.

Step-down therapy A gradual reduction in the dosage and number of drugs used in a therapeutic regimen.

Stepfamily Consists of a biological parent with children and a new spouse who may or may not have children.

Stereognosis The ability to perceive and understand an object through touch.

Stereotaxic thalamotomy An x-ray taken during neurosurgery to guide the insertion of a needle into a specific area of the brain.

Stereotyping The act of generalizing that all people in a group are the same.

Stereotypy Rigid and obsessive behavior.

Sterile field An area free of microorganisms.

Sterile technique Practices that keep an area or object free of all microorganisms. Also known as *surgical asepsis*.

Sterilization 1. A process that destroys all microorganisms, including spores and viruses. 2. An inclusive term that refers to surgical procedures that permanently prevent pregnancy.

Stigma A collection of negative attitudes and beliefs that lead people to fear, reject, avoid, and discriminate against people with mental illness.

Stillbirth Death of a fetus that occurs after 20 weeks of gestation. Also called *fetal demise* or *intrauterine fetal death (IUFD)*.

Stimulus The agent or act that stimulates a nerve receptor.

Stimulus-based stress model A model that defines stress as being a life event that requires change or adaptation on the part of the individual who is experiencing the life event.

Stoma An artificial opening in the abdominal wall; it may be permanent or temporary.

Stool Body wastes and undigested food eliminated from the bowel. Also called *feces*.

Strabismus Misalignment of the eyes.

Strain A stretching or tearing of a muscle or tendon.

Strategic planning The process of continual assessment, planning, and evaluation to guide future decisions and developments.

Stress The body's general, nonspecific response to the demands placed on it by a stressor.

Stress fracture A fracture that results from disease that has weakened the bone.

Stress mediators Hormonal triggers that are intended to promote adaptation through mechanisms such as triggering a necessary increase in heart rate and blood pressure when faced with physical danger.

Stress response Physiologic changes triggered by stress; includes activation of the neural, neuroendocrine, and endocrine systems, as well as activation of target organs.

Stressor An external influence that threatens to disrupt the equilibrium that is needed to maintain homeostasis.

Striae Whitish-silver stretch marks seen in obesity and during or after pregnancy.

Stridor A high-pitched sound within the trachea and larynx that suggests narrowing of the tracheal passage.

Stroke A condition in which neurologic deficits result from a sudden decrease in blood flow to a localized area of the brain. Also called *cerebrovascular accident* or *brain attack*.

Stroke volume (SV) The amount of blood pumped into the aorta with each contraction of the left ventricle that is measured by the difference between the end-diastolic volume and the end-systolic volume.

Structural-functional theory Focuses on family structure and function, examining family relationships and how they affect the functions of the family and relationships with other systems.

Structure standards Standards related to material resources, human resources, and general organizational structure.

Struvite calculi A type of calculi associated with a urinary tract infection caused by urease-producing bacteria such as *Proteus*. These stones can grow to become very large, filling the renal pelvis and calyces. Also called *staghorn stones*.

Subconjunctival hemorrhage Temporary, nonpathogenic hemorrhages that are caused by the changes in vascular tension or ocular pressure during birth.

Subculture groups Minority groups characterized by specific norms, beliefs, and values that coexist with a dominant culture.

Subcutaneous tissue The layer of loose connective tissue and fat cells that lies below the dermis. Also called *hypodermis*.

Subdermal implant Capsules implanted within the skin that slowly release medication, such as for contraception.

Subfertility Occurs when both partners of a couple have reduced fertility.

Subinvolution A slowing of the descent of the uterus during the post-pregnancy healing process.

Subjective data Information that is apparent to only the patient affected and can be described or verified by only that patient. Also called *symptoms* or *covert data*.

Subjective family burden The psychologic distress of family members in relation to the objective family burden of having a family member with a mental illness.

Substance abuse The use of any chemical in a fashion inconsistent with medical or culturally defined social norms despite physical, psychologic, or social adverse effects.

Substance dependence A condition in which the patient can no longer control use of the substance, continues to use it despite adverse effects, and experiences withdrawal symptoms without continued use of the substance.

Subsystem A component of a larger system.

Sucking reflex Occurs in response to a finger or nipple inserted into an infant's mouth; the infant responds by beginning to rhythmically suck on the finger.

Suctioning Aspirating secretions through a catheter connected to a suction machine or wall suction outlet.

Sudden cardiac death (SCD) Unexpected death occurring within 1 hour of the onset of cardiovascular symptoms.

Sudden infant death syndrome (SIDS) The sudden death of an apparently healthy infant that remains unexplained after other possible causes have been ruled out through autopsy, death scene investigation, and review of the medical history.

Sudden unexpected death in epilepsy (SUDEP) Sudden and unexpected death in an individual diagnosed with epilepsy.

Suicidal ideation A case of an individual constantly considering, planning, or thinking about suicide.

Suicide An act of an individual inflicting self-harm resulting in death.

Suicide attempt An act of an individual inflicting self-harm with the intent to cause death that is not successful.

Sundowning A behavioral change commonly seen in patients with dementia, characterized by increased agitation, time disorientation, and wandering behaviors during afternoon and evening hours; it is accelerated on overcast days.

Superficial basal cell carcinoma A type of skin cancer.

Superficial burn A burn that involves only the epidermal layer of the skin.

Superficial thrombophlebitis A blood clot blocking one or more veins near the skin's surface.

Superimposed preeclampsia Occurs when a woman previously diagnosed with chronic hypertension develops hypertension-related end-organ dysfunction in pregnancy or worsening hypertension that is resistant to treatment.

Supersaturated urine A condition that results when the concentration of salt in the urine is very high.

Supine On the back.

Suppuration A large quantity of cells and necrotic debris that form an opaque or milky discharge that is thicker than serous exudate. Also called *pus* or *purulent exudate*.

Suprasystem An overarching system to which smaller systems or subsystems belong. For example, the family is the suprasystem of the individual.

Surface temperature Body temperature taken at the skin's surface that may rise or fall in response to the environment.

Surfactant Specialized cells that control surface tension and keep alveoli from collapsing and sticking to themselves.

Surge capacity A community's ability to rapidly meet the increased demand for qualified personnel and resources, including healthcare resources, in the event of a disaster.

Surgical asepsis Practices that keep an area or object free of all microorganisms. Also called *sterile technique*.

Surgical debridement The process of excising a wound to the level of fascia or sequentially removing thin slices of a burn wound to the level of viable tissue.

Sutures The membranous spaces between the cranial bones of a fetus.

Swan-neck deformity Caused by rheumatoid arthritis, it is characterized by hyperextension of the proximal interphalangeal joints with compensatory flexion of the distal interphalangeal joints.

Sweat test Typically administered twice, it measures the amount of salt in the baby's sweat and is most effective for a CF diagnosis; a high level of salt confirms the diagnosis.

Switching A term used in disorders of mood and affect to describe a new illness phase (manic or depressed) without recovery.

Symmetry Equality of the size, shape, or condition of opposite sides of the body.

Sympathetic tone A state of partial smooth muscle contraction around arteries and veins.

Symphysis pubis Fibrocartilaginous joint between the pelvic bones in the midline.

Symptom See Subjective data.

Synchronized cardioversion Delivery of direct electrical current synchronized with the patient's heart rhythm.

Synclitism A condition that occurs when the sagittal suture is midway between the symphysis pubis and the sacral promontory and is felt to be aligned.

Syncope Transient loss of consciousness and muscle tone after exercise or activity.

Syndrome diagnosis A cluster of nursing diagnoses that occur together and may result in best patient outcomes if addressed at the same time.

Synovectomy Excision of synovial membrane; this procedure is used as a treatment for rheumatoid arthritis.

Synovitis Inflammation of the synovial membrane lining the articular capsule of a joint.

Syphilis A complex systemic sexually transmitted infection caused by the spirochete *Treponema pallidum*.

System A set of interacting identifiable parts or components.

Systematized delusions A manifestation of schizophrenia characterized by an extensively developed central delusional theme from which conclusions are deduced.

Systemic arthritis A form of juvenile rheumatoid arthritis that characteristically is manifested by high fever, polyarthritis, and rheumatoid rash. Systemic arthritis also affects internal organs and joints.

Systemic circulation Circulation through the left side of the heart, the aorta and its branches, the capillaries that supply the brain and peripheral tissues, the systemic venous system, and the vena cava.

Systemic infection Occurs when an invading microorganism spreads and damages different parts of the body.

Systemic inflammatory response syndrome (SIRS) Describes the body's response to a critical illness that can result from an infectious or noninfectious cause precipitating a whole-body inflammatory process.

Systemic lupus erythematosus (SLE) A chronic, inflammatory connective tissue disease.

Systemic response Results because of a widespread antibody-antigen reaction. Systemic responses include anaphylaxis, urticaria, or angioedema.

Systemic vascular resistance The force or resistance of the blood in the body's blood vessels that helps return blood to the heart.

Systems theory The study of how a system operates, including how it interacts with other systems and how its components interact with each other within the system itself.

Systole The phase of ventricular contraction.

Systolic blood pressure The maximum pressure exerted within the arteries when the heart compresses.

T lymphocyte (T cells) A type of leukocyte that matures in the thymus gland and is integral to the specific immune response.

Tachycardia An excessively fast heart rate greater than 100 bpm in an adult.

Tachypnea A respiratory rate greater than 20 bpm in adults.

Tactile Of or relating to touch.

Tangential excision The sequential removal of thin slices of a burn wound to the level of viable tissue.

Tanner stages Stages of physical growth of the breasts and pubic hair in girls and the genitalia and pubic hair in boys.

Tardive dyskinesia A condition characterized by repetitive, involuntary body movement of varying severity that may not cease after medication cessation; includes unusual tongue and face movements such as lip smacking and wormlike motions of the tongue.

Tartar A visible, hard deposit of plaque and dead bacteria that forms at the gumlines. Also called *dental calculus*.

Tau A protein found in the neurons.

Teach-back method A patient teaching strategy in which the nurse provides information to a patient and asks the patient to restate the information to ensure that the patient understands it correctly.

Teaching A system of activities intended to produce learning.

Team Two or more individuals who agree to work in tandem to accomplish a common goal.

Team nursing The delivery of individualized nursing care to a group of patients by a team led by a professional nurse.

Telangiectatic nevi Pale pink or red spots frequently found on the eyelids, nose, lower occipital bone, and nape of the neck of young children. These areas have no clinical significance and usually fade by the second birthday. Also called *stork bites*.

Telecommunication The transmission of information from one site to another, using equipment to send information in the form of signs, signals, words, or pictures by cable, radio, or other systems.

Telehealth A system that employs the use of telecommunications technologies (e.g., videoconferencing, streaming media, real-time forwarding imaging, and land-based and wireless communications) to allow patients access to care that they might not otherwise be able to obtain. Also called *telemedicine* or *remote patient monitoring*.

Telenursing The provision of nursing care via **telecommunication**.

Temperament The combination of biological and physical characteristics that influence personality and behavior specific to each individual.

Tender points Tenderness that occurs in precise, localized areas, particularly in the neck, spine, shoulders, and hips.

Tendon Tissue that connects bones to muscles and carries the contractile forces from the muscle to the bone to cause movement.

Tendonitis Inflammation of a tendon.

Teratogen Any substance that adversely affects the normal growth and development of the fetus.

Terminal weaning The gradual withdrawal of mechanical ventilation when survival without assisted ventilation is not expected.

Territoriality A concept of the space and things that an individual considers as belonging to the self.

Tertiary intention healing Healing that occurs after closing a wound that has been left open for 3–5 days to allow edema or infection to resolve. Also called *delayed primary intention*.

Tertiary prevention Methods that focus on the restoration of health following an illness or accident and include rehabilitation and palliative services.

Testosterone The primary male sex hormone produced by the testes.

Tetany Tonic muscle spasms.

Tetralogy of Fallot A rare disease that consists of four defects: pulmonic stenosis, right ventricular hypertrophy, ventricular-septal defect, and an overriding aorta.

Tetraplegia Complete loss of function of the upper and lower body, including the arms, trunk, legs, and pelvic organs. Also called *quadriplegia*.

Thalassemia Inherited disorder of hemoglobin synthesis in which either the alpha or beta chains of the hemoglobin molecule are missing or defective.

Thelarche The beginning of breast development in females.

Therapeutic communication An interactive process between the nurse and the patient that helps the patient to overcome temporary stress, to get along with other people, to adjust to situations that cannot be altered, and to overcome any psychologic blocks that may stand in the way of self-realizations.

Therapeutic insemination The process of depositing semen at the cervical os or in the uterus by mechanical means.

Therapeutic relationship Nurse–patient relationship that is focused on helping patients manage problems and become better at helping themselves.

Thermoregulation The body process that balances heat production and heat loss to maintain the body's temperature.

Third heart sound (S₃) Heart sound that is sometimes heard after the second heart sound in children, young adults, and pregnant women during the third trimester. Also called a *ventricular gallop*.

Third spacing A shift of fluid from the vascular space into an area where it is not available to support normal physiologic processes.

Thoracentesis Needle insertion into the pleural space to remove fluid accumulation.

Thoracolumbar sacral orthosis (TLSO) A brace contoured to conform to the body and support the spine. Also called an *underarm brace* or *Boston brace*.

Thought blocking Speech stopped in midsentence as if the thought disappeared from the individual's head.

Thought disorders Disorders associated with schizophrenia that involve an abnormal way of thinking, such as disorganized thinking, sensory overload, thought blocking, neologisms, loose association, clang, and perseveration.

Threshold potential The point at which an action potential is capable of being generated.

Thrill A palpable vibration over the precordium or an artery.

Thromboemboli Emboli created by a blood clot.

Thrombophlebitis Sometimes called phlebitis, condition in which a blood clot forms and blocks one or more veins. Clots typically form in the legs but can form in the arms and neck in rare instances.

Throughput The process by which information, energy, or material that enters a system (input) is used by the system.

Thrush White patches that look like milk curds that adhere to the mucous membranes usually caused by an infected vaginal tract during birth, antibiotic use, or poor hand hygiene. Bleeding may occur if patches are removed.

Thyroid crisis See Thyroid storm.

Thyroid storm An extreme state of hyperthyroidism. Now extremely rare due to improved diagnosis and treatment methods. Also called *thyroid crisis*.

Thyroidectomy Surgical removal of all or part of the thyroid gland.

Thyroiditis Inflammation of the thyroid gland.

Thyrotoxicosis A disorder caused by excessive delivery of thyroid hormone to the peripheral tissues. Also called *hyperthyroidism*.

Tics Semi-involuntary movements that are sudden, repetitive, and non-rhythmic. They may involve muscle groups or vocalizations (motor or phonic).

Time constraints Deadlines for completion.

Time-out A preprocedure verification to ensure the correct procedure is being performed at the right site on the right patient.

Time priority A time constraint to complete an action.

Tine test Test in which a multiple-puncture device is used to introduce tuberculin into the skin.

Tinea pedis Fungal infection of the feet. Also called *athlete's foot*.

Tinnitus The perception of sound or noise in the ears without stimulus from the environment.

Token economies Formalized programs of contingency contracts.

Tolerance State in which a particular dose elicits a smaller response than it formerly did. With increased tolerance, the individual needs higher and higher doses to obtain the desired response.

Tone 1. The amount of tension or resistance to movement in a muscle. 2. The ability of vessels to constrict or dilate to maintain normal pressure.

Tonic–clonic seizures Alternating contraction (tonic phase) and relaxation (clonic phase) of muscles during seizure activity.

Tonic neck reflex In response to an infant's head being turned to one side while the infant lies on the back, the infant will extend the arm and leg on the side the infant faces while the opposite arm and leg will be flexed.

Tonic phase Initial phase of a generalized seizure, manifested by unconsciousness and continuous muscular contraction.

Tonicity The osmolality of a solution. Solutions may be termed *isotonic*, *hypertonic*, or *hypotonic*.

Torsades de pointes A type of ventricular tachycardia associated with a prolongation of the QT interval.

Tort A civil wrong committed against an individual or an individual's property.

Total anomalous pulmonary venous return The pulmonary veins empty into the right atrium or into veins leading to the right atrium, rather than into the left atrium.

Total lymphoid irradiation A procedure sometimes used in the treatment of rheumatoid arthritis; it decreases total lymphocyte levels.

Total quality management (TQM) A comprehensive management philosophy that improves quality and productivity by using data and statistics to improve system processes.

Toxic multinodular goiter A tumor characterized by small, discrete, independently functioning nodules in the thyroid gland tissue that secrete excessive amounts of thyroid hormone.

Toxoplasmosis Space-occupying lesions common in patients with AIDS that may cause headache, altered mental status, and neurologic deficits.

Trachoma A chronic conjunctivitis caused by *Chlamydia trachomatis*. It is a significant preventable cause of blindness worldwide.

Traction The application of a straightening or pulling force to return or maintain fractured bones in their normal anatomic position.

Traditional family An autonomous unit in which both parents reside in the home with their children, the mother assuming the nurturing role and the father providing the necessary economic resources.

Transactional leader A leader who has a relationship with followers based on an exchange of some resource valued by the follower.

Transcellular fluid One of the compartments where extracellular fluid is found. Examples of transcellular fluid are cerebrospinal, pericardial, pancreatic, pleural, intraocular, biliary, peritoneal, and synovial fluids.

Transcendence A person's recognition that there is something other or greater than the self and a seeking and valuing of that greater other, whether it is an ultimate being, force, or value.

Transcranial magnetic stimulation (TMS) A promising alternative therapy for individuals with schizophrenia that uses electromagnetic stimulus to affect brain activity in the cerebral cortex.

Transductive reasoning Connecting two events in a cause-and-effect relationship simply because they occur together in time.

Transection An injury that occurs when an individual is injured by a gunshot, stabbing, or similar force, which may partially or completely sever the spinal cord.

Transference The transfer of feelings that were originally evoked by one's parents or significant others to people in the present setting.

Transformational leader A leader who fosters creativity, risk taking, commitment, and collaboration by empowering a group to share in an organization's vision. The leader inspires others with a clear, attractive, and attainable goal and enlists them to participate in attaining the goal.

Transfusion reaction A type II or cytotoxic hypersensitivity reaction to blood of an incompatible type.

Transgender Gradations of human characteristics running from female to male; more commonly, an individual who expresses a gender identity different from that with which he or she was born.

Transient ischemic attack (TIA) A brief period of localized cerebral ischemia that causes neurologic deficits lasting for less than 24 hours. Also called a *mini-stroke*.

Transitional milk A light yellow milk that is more copious than colostrum and contains more fat, lactose, water-soluble vitamins, and calories; it usually presents between the second and fifth day following birth.

Transjugular intrahepatic portosystemic shunt (TIPS) An expandable metal stent inserted through a transcutaneous needle to channel blood from the portal vein into the hepatic vein, bypassing the cirrhotic liver.

Translational research A systematic approach of converting research knowledge into applications of healthcare for improved patient outcomes.

Transplacental immunity Passive immunity transferred from mother to infant.

Transposition of the great arteries (TGA) A congenital heart defect in which the pulmonary artery, the outflow tract for the left ventricle, and the aorta, the outflow tract for the right ventricle, are transposed.

Transsexual An individual who feels his or her sexual anatomy is not consistent with his or her gender identity.

Transurethral incision of the prostate (TUIP) Small incisions are made in the smooth muscle where the prostate is attached to the bladder in order to reduce pressure on the urethra.

Transurethral needle ablation (TUNA) A procedure that uses low-level radio-frequency through twin needles to burn away a region of the enlarged prostate in order to improve the flow of urine.

Transurethral resection of the prostate (TURP) A procedure that removes obstructing prostate tissue using the wire loop of a resectoscope and electrocautery inserted through the urethra.

Transverse diameter The largest diameter of the pelvic inlet; helps determine the shape of the inlet.

Trauma An injury to human tissues and organs resulting from the transfer of energy from an external environmental source, such as a motor vehicle, a fire, or a sharp object.

Traumatic brain injury (TBI) An injury resulting from an external physical force, such as a blow or jolt to the head, that causes displacement of the brain within the skull and disruption of normal brain function.

Traumatic cataracts A type of cataract that may result from an injury to the eye.

Tremors Rhythmic, involuntary movements or twitching of the extremities.

Triage The process of identifying priorities for implementing care.

Trial and error A group decision strategy in which the most viable solution is attempted.

Tricuspid atresia The absence of the tricuspid valve.

Tricyclic antidepressant (TCA) A class of drugs that inhibit the reuptake of both norepinephrine and serotonin into presynaptic nerve terminals. TCAs are primarily used in the pharmacotherapy of depression.

Triglycerides Substances converted from dietary fats and carbohydrates to store energy in fat cells.

Triplet Three premature ventricular contractions in a row.

Tripod position A position of sitting and leaning forward; often used by patients who are having difficulty breathing.

Trisomy An extra chromosome.

Trisomy 21 A condition that occurs when an individual born with Down syndrome has an additional full chromosome present.

Troponins Proteins released during a myocardial infarction that are sensitive indicators of myocardial damage.

Trousseau sign Spasmodic contraction of the hand and fingers in response to occlusion of the blood supply by a blood pressure cuff; caused by decreased blood calcium levels. A test used to check for hypocalcemia.

True pelvis The portion that lies below the linea terminalis; made up of the inlet, cavity, and outlet.

Truncus arteriosus A heart defect in which a single large vessel empties both ventricles and provides circulation for the pulmonary, systemic, and coronary circulations.

Trunk incurvation In response to stroking an infant's spine, the infant's pelvis will turn toward the stimulated side. Also called *Galant reflex*.

Tubal ligation A surgical procedure to clip, tie off, band, or plug the fallopian tubes to sterilize a female patient.

Tubercle A granulomatous lesion (a sealed-off colony of bacilli) formed from *Mycobacterium tuberculosis*.

Tuberculosis (TB) A chronic, recurrent infectious disease caused by *Mycobacterium tuberculosis.* TB usually affects the lungs, but any organ can be affected.

Tubular sound The sound air makes moving through a clear and functioning trachea.

Tumor lysis syndrome (TLS) A condition that occurs when tumor cells dissolve and release intracellular contents into circulation, causing hyperkalemia, hyperuricemia, and hyperphosphatemia.

Tumor marker A protein molecule detectable in serum or other body fluids that is used to highlight suspicious regions for follow-up.

TURP syndrome A condition that is characterized by hyponatremia, decreased hematocrit, hypertension, bradycardia, nausea, and confusion.

Two-career family A family in which both partners are employed by choice or necessity. A two-career family may or may not have children.

Tympanic membrane A thin, tense membrane that separates the middle ear from the external auditory canal, protecting the middle ear from the external environment.

Tympanocentesis A surgical incision of the tympanic membrane. Also called *myringotomy.*

Tympanogram A test that provides a graph of the middle ear's ability to transmit sound.

Tympanostomy tubes Pressuring-equalizing tubes inserted to provide the middle ear with ventilation and drainage during healing.

Tympany A musical or drumlike sound produced from an air-filled stomach.

Type 1 diabetes mellitus An absolute deficiency of insulin related to pancreatic beta cell destruction that results in severe hyperglycemia and diabetic ketoacidosis, among other symptoms.

Type 2 diabetes mellitus A relative deficiency of insulin, which may be related to insulin resistance and inadequate secretion of insulin to meet body needs. Both of these components are usually present at time of diagnosis.

Ulcer A break in the GI mucosa that develops when the mucosal barrier is unable to protect the mucosa from damage by hydrochloric acid and pepsin, the gastric digestive juices.

Ulcerative colitis A chronic inflammatory bowel disorder that affects the mucosa and submucosa of the colon and rectum.

Ultrafiltration Removal of excess body water using a hydrostatic pressure gradient.

Ultrasound A test using intermittent ultrasonic waves transmitted by an alternating current to a transducer and applied to the abdomen.

Unconscious mind The part of an individual's mental life of which he or she is unaware.

Underinsured Individuals whose healthcare coverage is insufficient to meet their needs.

Undernutrition Health effects due to insufficient or diminished nutrient intake or stores. Also known as *malnutrition.*

Unifocal When a ventricular impulse arises from one ectopic site.

Unilateral lobar pneumonia A pattern of pneumonia in which bacteria tend to be distributed evenly throughout one or more lobes of a single lung.

Uninsured Individuals who are without any type of healthcare coverage.

Unipolar depression A mood disorder characterized by loss of interest in life and unresponsiveness, moving from mild to severe, with severe symptoms lasting at least 2 weeks. Also called *major depressive disorder (MDD).*

Universal precautions (UP) Safety guidelines, such as proper hand hygiene, use of proper protective equipment, safe injection practices, and effective management of potentially contaminated surfaces or equipment, that are designed to decrease the risk of transmitting

unidentified pathogens. Also called *standard precautions* and *body substance isolation (BSI).*

Universal protocol Established guidelines for healthcare professionals to prevent errors during surgical procedures, including wrong-site surgery.

Unlicensed assistive personnel (UAP) Members of a nursing team who assume delegated aspects of basic patient care such as bathing, assisting with feeding, and collecting specimens. UAPs include certified nurse assistants, hospital attendants, nurse technicians, and orderlies.

Unresolved bacteriuria The presence of bacteria in urine that fails to resolve with treatment.

Unsaturated fat A triglyceride fat that does not contain all of the hydrogen ions it is capable of holding.

Upper body obesity Identified by a waist-to-hip ratio of greater than 1 in men or 0.8 in women. Also called *central obesity.*

Uremia Excessive amounts of urea in the blood.

Uremic fetor A urine-like breath odor often associated with a metallic taste in the mouth.

Uremic frost Crystallized deposits of urea on the skin.

Ureteral stent A thin catheter inserted into the ureter to provide for urine flow and ureteral support.

Ureterolithotomy An incision in the affected ureter to remove a calculus.

Ureteroplasty The surgical repair of a ureter.

Urgency The sudden, strong desire to void.

Urgency factor A way to illustrate how much time can safely lapse before doing interventions without compromising patient outcomes.

Uric acid stones Develop when the urine concentration of uric acid is high.

Urinary calculi Stones in the urinary tract.

Urinary drainage system Those organs required to drain urine from the kidneys, including the ureters, urinary bladder, and urethra.

Urinary frequency The need to urinate often, specifically more than four to six times a day.

Urinary hesitancy A delay and difficulty in initiating voiding; often associated with dysuria.

Urinary incontinence Involuntary urination due to the temporary or permanent inability of the external sphincter muscles to control the flow of urine from the bladder. Also called *involuntary urination.*

Urinary reflux Backward flow of urine.

Urinary retention The accumulation of urine in the bladder and inability of the bladder to empty itself, resulting in overdistention of the bladder.

Urinary stasis Stagnation of urinary flow.

Urination Releasing urine from the urinary bladder. Also called *voiding* or *micturition.*

Uroflowmetry A method of measuring urine flow rate.

Urolithiasis The formation of stones in the urinary tract.

Urticaria Patches of pale, itchy wheals in an erythematous area. Also known as *hives.*

Uterine atony The relaxation of uterine muscle tone.

Uterosacral ligaments Ligaments that provide support for the uterus and cervix at the level of the ischial spines.

Uterus The hollow muscular organ in which the fertilized ovum is implanted and in which the developing fetus is nourished until birth.

Utilitarianism A form of consequentialist theory that views a good act as one that brings the most good and the least harm for the greatest number of people. This is called the principle of utility.

Utility See Utilitarianism.

Utilization review An evaluation of the use of resources to identify areas of overuse, misuse, and underuse.

Uveitis Inflammation of the middle layer of the eye called the uvea.

Vaccine Suspensions of whole or fractionated bacteria or viruses that have been treated to make them nonpathogenic; introduced by immunization to provoke active immunity.

Vacuum extraction An obstetric procedure used by physicians and CNMs to assist the birth of a fetus by applying suction to the fetal head.

Vagina The muscular and membranous tube that connects the external genitals with the uterus.

Vaginal birth after cesarean (VBAC) An option for a mother to choose a trial of labor and vaginal birth after having a cesarean for a previous child, provided the previous cesarean was required due to a nonrecurring indication and the mother meets the guidelines established by the American College of Obstetricians and Gynecologists.

Vaginismus The involuntary spasm of the outer one third of the vaginal muscles, making penetration of the vagina painful and sometimes impossible.

Validation The act of verifying the accuracy and factuality of data.

Valsalva maneuver Forced exhalation against a closed glottis.

Values Personal beliefs about truth and the worth of behaviors or objects; standards that influence behavior.

Values clarification A process of consciously identifying, examining, and developing individual values that helps nurses gain the ability to choose actions on the basis of deliberately adopted values.

Variable decelerations A condition that occurs if the umbilical cord becomes compressed, reducing blood flow between the placenta and fetus. Fetal hypertension stimulates the baroreceptors in the aortic arch and carotid sinuses, slowing the fetal heart rate.

Variance 1. An unmet goal. 2. An incident or accident that affects a patient or a visitor in a healthcare facility.

Vasectomy A procedure to surgically sever the vas deferens on both sides of the scrotum to sterilize a male patient.

Vasogenic shock Shock that results from widespread vasodilation and decreased peripheral resistance. Also called *distributive shock.*

Vaso-occlusive crisis See Sickle cell crisis.

Vegan A type of vegetarian diet that excludes all animal and fish products, including dairy, meat, eggs, and honey.

Venous stasis The collection and stagnation of blood in the lower extremities.

Venous thrombectomy Surgical removal of a blood clot from the femoral vein to prevent pulmonary embolism or gangrene.

Venous thrombosis A condition in which a blood clot (thrombus) forms on the wall of a vein, accompanied by inflammation of the vein wall and some degree of obstructed venous blood flow. Also called *thrombophlebitis.*

Ventilation The exchange of oxygen and carbon dioxide.

Ventilation-perfusion (V-Q) The movement of oxygen across the alveolar–capillary membrane into a well-perfusing capillary.

Ventricular aneurysm An outpouching of the ventricular wall that does not contract during systole, causing stroke volume to decrease.

Ventricular bigeminy A premature ventricular contraction following each normal beat.

Ventricular gallop (S_3) Heart sound sometimes heard after the second heart sound in children, young adults, and pregnant women during the third trimester. Also called the *third heart sound.*

Ventricular septal defect (VSD) An opening in the ventricular septum that causes increased pulmonary blood flow.

Ventricular trigeminy A premature ventricular contraction every third beat.

Veracity A moral principle that holds that an individual should tell the truth and not lie.

Verbal abuse The use of berating, humiliating, ridiculing, blaming, or threatening language toward an individual.

Verbal communication Transmitting information through the spoken or written word.

Vernix caseosa A whitish, cheeselike substance that covers a fetus while in utero.

Vertical rotation The degree of rotation of the vertebrae.

Vertical transmission Perinatal transmission of an infection, such as the human immunodeficiency virus, from mother to infant.

Vertigo A sensation of whirling or rotation.

Very-low-calorie diets A program providing a protein-sparing modified fast (400–800 kcal/day or less) under close medical supervision.

Vesicoureteral reflux A condition in which urine moves from the bladder back toward the kidney. A common risk factor in children who develop pyelonephritis that may also be seen in adults whose bladder outflow is obstructed.

Vesicular sounds The soft and breezy sounds of air moving in and out of the lobes at the alveolar level.

Vestibulitis Pain of the outer portion of the vagina upon touch or attempted penetration.

Vibration A series of vigorous quiverings produced by hands that are placed flat against the patient's chest wall.

Violence The use of excessive force against other individuals or oneself, often resulting in physical or psychologic injuries or death.

Virchow triad Three factors associated with thrombophlebitis: stasis of blood, vessel damage, and increased blood coagulability.

Virions Virus particles unable to grow and reproduce outside a host.

Virulence The ability of a microorganism to produce disease.

Virus A type of microorganism that must enter living cells in order to reproduce.

Visceral Of or relating to any large organ in the body.

Visceral pain Pain arising from body organs. It is dull and poorly localized because of the low number of nociceptors.

Viscosupplementation A treatment for osteoarthritis of the knee that involves injecting lubricating substances directly into the knee.

Visual Of or relating to sight.

Vitamins Micronutrient compounds that are involved in regulating body functioning. Most vitamins, with the exceptions of vitamins D and K, cannot be manufactured within the body and must be consumed through dietary intake.

Vitiligo An autoimmune disorder that results in loss of melanin in patches of the face, hands, or groin.

Voiding Releasing urine from the urinary bladder. Also called *urination* or *micturition.*

Voiding cystourethrography Use of a contrast medium and x-rays to assess the bladder and urethra when filled and during voiding.

Volatile acid Acids eliminated from the body as a gas.

Volkmann contracture Impaired mobility of the arm and inability to extend the arm completely, which is a common complication of elbow fractures.

Voluntary admission The detention of a patient in a psychiatric or medical facility at the patient's request.

Voluntary insurance Healthcare insurance that provides no guarantee of universality because coverage may be expensive and difficult to purchase.

Vomiting The forceful expulsion of the contents of the upper gastrointestinal tract resulting from contraction of muscles in the gut and abdominal wall.

Vulnerability An individual's susceptibility to react to a specific stressor.

Vulnerability factors A practice, behavior, or environmental factor that increases the potential of an individual becoming a victim of violence.

Vulnerable populations Social groups with inadequate access to healthcare because they lack resources and are exposed to more risk factors.

Vulva The external female genitals.

Vulvodynia Constant, unremitting burning that is localized to the vulva with an acute onset.

Warm zone When a disaster occurs, this zone, located at least 300 feet from the outer edge of a hot zone, is where decontamination occurs and rapid triage and emergency treatment are given to stabilize victims. Also called the *yellow zone*, *contamination zone*, or *contamination reduction zone*.

Water An essential nutrient for the body's survival, it contributes to fluid balance and plays an important role in nerve and muscle functioning and in the transport of nutrients to all body systems.

Weaning 1. The process of removing ventilator support and reestablishing spontaneous, independent respirations. 2. The process of discontinuing breastfeeding and transitioning an infant to another feeding method.

Well-being A subjective perception of feeling well that can be described objectively and measured.

Wellness A state of well-being that encompasses self-responsibility, dynamic growth, nutrition, physical fitness, emotional health, preventive healthcare, and the whole being of the individual.

Wellness diagnosis A term that describes human responses to levels of wellness in an individual, family, or community that have a readiness for enhancement. For example, *Readiness for Enhanced Coping*.

Wernicke encephalopathy A condition typically seen in people with alcoholism that is characterized by ataxia (lack of coordination), abnormal eye movements, and confusion.

Wheezing A high-pitched whistling sound most often heard on expiration and caused by the narrowing of bronchi; wheezes can also be heard on inspiration.

Whiplash An injury that results from sudden impact to a motor vehicle that causes an individual's head and neck to be forcibly contorted, resulting in injury to the spine.

Whistleblower A nurse or other individual who goes outside of an organization for the public's best interest when the organization fails to follow procedures regarding safety and patient care.

Whistleblowing The act of going outside of an organization for the public's best interest when an organization fails to follow procedures regarding safety and patient care.

White blood cells (WBCs) See Leukocytes.

Withdrawing or withholding life-sustaining therapy (WWLST) The withdrawal of extraordinary means of life support, such as removing a ventilator or withholding special attempts to revive a patient, and allowing the patient to die of the underlying medical condition.

Work ethic A belief in the importance and moral worth of work.

Workplace bullying Malicious, repeated, harmful mistreatment of an individual with whom one works, regardless of whether that individual is an equal, a superior, or a subordinate.

Workplace violence Any physical assault, threatening behavior, or verbal abuse occurring in the workplace.

Worldview The way in which people in a culture perceive ideas and attitudes about the world, other people, and life in general.

Worst-case scenario Technique designed to help groups make decisions that involve risk. The worst-case outcome is outlined for each alternative, and then the scenario with the comparatively best outcome is selected as the preferred outcome. This technique helps ensure that the "least of all evils" is selected.

Wrong-site surgery (WSS) A surgical operation that is performed at the wrong location on a patient's body due to error.

Xenograft Skin used for transplantation that was obtained from an animal, usually a pig. Also called *heterograft*.

Xenophobia The fear or dislike of people different from one's self.

Xerostomia Dry mouth that occurs when an individual's supply of saliva is reduced.

Zollinger-Ellison syndrome A form of peptic ulcer disease caused by a gastrinoma, or gastrin-secreting tumor of the pancreas, stomach, or intestines.

Zygote A fertilized egg.

Index

Special Features

CONCEPTS RELATED TO

EVIDENCE-BASED PRACTICE

FOCUS ON DIVERSITY AND CULTURE

FOCUS ON INTEGRATIVE HEALTH

MEDICATIONS